HAROLD R. YEARY LIBRARY

# PDR® 2011 EDITION NURSE'S DRUG HANDBOOK



THE INFORMATION STANDARD FOR PRESCRIPTION DRUGS AND NURSING CONSIDERATIONS

# PDR® NURSE'S DRUG HANDBOOK

2011 EDITION

*Senior Director, Editorial & Publishing:* Bette Kennedy
*Director, Clinical Services:* Sylvia Nashed, PharmD
*Manager, Clinical Services:* Nermin Shenouda, PharmD
*Drug Information Specialists:* Peter Leighton, PharmD; Kristine Mecca, PharmD; Anila Patel, PharmD; Christine Sunwoo, PharmD
*Contributing Clinical Editor:* Majid Kerolous, PharmD
*Manager, Editorial Services:* Lori Murray
*Associate Editor:* Jennifer Reed
*Project Manager:* Gary Lew
*Director, Marketing:* Kim Marich
*Manager, Production Purchasing:* Thomas Westburgh
*Manager, Art Department:* Livio Udina
*Electronic Publishing Designer:* Carrie Spinelli Faeth





ISBN: 978-1-56363-782-7

Printed in Canada

# Contents

# Foreword

Nursing professionals are at the forefront when it comes to safe medication use and patient education, and they play an especially crucial role in the new era of healthcare reform. Nurses must decipher the constantly changing information regarding medications, new therapies, and interactions, and rapidly assess patient responses to multiple variables important to medication administration. A reference that provides accurate and easily accessible drug information is vital. The *PDR® Nurse's Drug Handbook, 2011 Edition* fulfills this need.

*Physicians' Desk Reference®* is a well-known and trusted resource for medication information—and *PDR Nurse's Drug Handbook* follows this tradition. This important reference is specifically designed for nurses, with each entry providing the following when applicable: therapeutic class, indications, dosage, how the medication is supplied, relevant warnings and precautions, key adverse reactions, interactions, pregnancy category, mechanism of action, pharmacokinetics, and nursing considerations—a special section that includes content specific to assessing, monitoring, and counseling patients and administering medications.

The *PDR Nurse's Drug Handbook* is organized to foster quick identification of key drug information. Medications can be identified by generic and brand names as well as therapeutic class. Special sections provide important considerations when caring for women who are pregnant or breastfeeding, children, and older adults. Other useful resources include more than 100 charts and tables about medications for specific chronic problems such as hypertension, headache, HIV, hepatitis, and diabetes; immunizations; poison antidotes; lactose-, galactose-, and sugar-free products; cytochrome P450 enzyme inhibitors, substrates, and inducers; and a full-color visual identification guide. New for this year are tables providing detailed information about treatments for prostate cancer and erectile dysfunction.

The *PDR® Nurse's Drug Handbook, 2011 Edition* is an essential reference for enhancing nursing practice and patient education efforts. Its convenient size and clear layout provide fast access to concise, authoritative drug information, making this book a trusted resource among nurses.

**Ivy M. Alexander, PhD, APRN, ANP-BC, FAAN**
Professor
Director–Adult, Family, Gerontological, and
Women's Health Primary Care Specialty
Yale University School of Nursing

# How to Use This Book

The *PDR® Nurse's Drug Handbook, 2011 Edition* allows you to quickly locate important drug information so you can care for patients with confidence. The guide includes over 1,100 monographs providing current, organized information for more than 1,500 of the most commonly used drugs. This handy reference is the perfect companion for practicing nurses, nursing students, and other healthcare professionals.

This compact guide is divided into four discrete sections. The **first section** consists of **concise drug monographs** based on FDA-approved prescribing information. These monographs are organized alphabetically by brand name. When a brand is no longer available, the generic name is used. Monographs may include:

- Brand Name
- Generic Name
- Manufacturer
- FDA/DEA Schedule
- Black Box Warnings
- Therapeutic Class
- Indications
- Dosage (adults, pediatrics, special populations)
- How Supplied (dosage form/strength)
- Contraindications
- Warnings/Precautions
- Adverse Reactions
- Interactions
- Pregnancy Category/Breastfeeding Precautions
- Mechanism of Action
- Pharmacokinetics
- Nursing Considerations
    - —Assessment
    - —Monitoring
    - —Patient Counseling
    - —Administration and Storage

The **second section** comprises an extensive collection of **tables and key references** to help nurses assess drug therapy and patient safety. Tables provided include Rx and OTC drug comparisons; the most common abbreviations, acronyms, and symbols used by healthcare professionals; and professional associations for nurses. Within the drug comparison tables, drugs are organized alphabetically and by class for easy access. These tables and references may include, but are not limited to:

- Brand/Generic Name
- How Supplied (dosage form/strength)
- Indications
- Initial and Max Dosages
- Usual Dosage Range
- Most Common Side Effects

The **third section** contains two **indices**—one with drugs indexed by brand and generic name and the other organized by therapeutic class.

The **final section** contains a **Visual Identification Guide** featuring product images listed by brand name. This section helps you quickly verify the identity of a capsule, tablet, or other solid oral medication. Each product image contains both the generic and brand name, strength, and the name of its supplier. Other strengths and dosage forms may be available; please check FDA-approved prescribing information for a complete listing of all strengths and dosage forms.

**Important Information About Product Labeling**

Entries in the *PDR® Nurse's Drug Handbook, 2011 Edition* are drawn from FDA-approved product labeling as published in *Physicians' Desk Reference®* or supplied by the manufacturer. The entries are compiled and updated on a regular basis by a staff of experienced pharmacists. While diligent efforts have been made to ensure the accuracy of each entry, it is essential to bear in mind that the information presented here is merely a synopsis of key points in the official labeling, and that the complete labeling contains additional precautionary information that may be of significance in specific cases. Similarly, please remember that only common and dangerous adverse reactions and interactions are included here, and that numerous less-prevalent adverse effects may be reported in the complete labeling. If an entry leaves any question unanswered, be sure to consult *Physicians' Desk Reference* or the manufacturer for additional information.

The function of the Publisher is the compilation, organization, and distribution of this information. In organizing and presenting the material in the *PDR® Nurse's Drug Handbook, 2011 Edition*, the Publisher does not warrant or guarantee any of the products described, or perform any independent analysis in connection with any of the product information contained herein.

The Publisher assumes no obligation to obtain and include any information in these entries other than that provided by the manufacturer. The Publisher does not warrant, guarantee, or advocate the use of any product described herein. The Publisher and editors do not assume, and expressly disclaim, any liability for errors, omissions, or typographical errors in the information contained herein or for misuse of any of the products listed.

# Drug Monograph Key[1, 2]

**Brand Name** FDA/DEA Class*

generic (Manufacturer)

**Boxed Warning: A brief description of the black box warning(s) that appear in the beginning of the official FDA-approved labeling for the drug.**

**OTHER BRAND NAMES:** Brand name drugs that have the same generic components as the monograph drug.

**THERAPEUTIC CLASS:** Based on the active ingredients and their mechanism of action.

**INDICATIONS:** Only includes FDA-approved indications.

**DOSAGE:** Dosages for adults, pediatrics, and/or special populations as indicated in the official FDA-approved labeling.

**HOW SUPPLIED:** Product description including strength, formulation, [package size], and scored tablet information.

**CONTRAINDICATIONS:** Details harmful conditions related to the use of the drug and disease states or patient populations in which use of the monograph drug should be avoided.

**WARNINGS/PRECAUTIONS:** Details harmful conditions related to the use of the drug and disease states or patient populations where caution is dictated.

**ADVERSE REACTIONS:** Denotes side effects and adverse reactions listed in the official FDA-approved labeling as occurring with greater frequency (generally at a rate of ≥3%) or deemed significant based on the clinical judgment of the editors. Other side effects may be included if deemed serious or life-threatening. For a complete list of adverse reactions, please refer to the official FDA-approved labeling.

**INTERACTIONS:** Includes the effects and implications of other drugs and food on the monograph drug based on official FDA-approved labeling.

**PREGNANCY:** Indicated pregnancy and breastfeeding precautions and, when available, the FDA pregnancy rating system category.†

**MECHANISM OF ACTION:** Includes pharmacologic drug class and a brief description, or proposed mechanism, of how the drug produces its therapeutic effect.

**PHARMACOKINETICS:** Brief description of the important parameters described in the FDA-approved labeling related to the absorption, distribution, metabolism, and elimination of the drug. The majority of parameters included are an average or the approximate values provided in the FDA-approved labeling. Only a select group of parameters are included. Refer to the full prescribing information for more detailed pharmacokinetics information.

- **Absorption:** The process by which the drug enters the bloodstream and becomes bioavailable. Absorption parameters may include time to peak plasma concentration ($T_{max}$), area under the curve (AUC), peak plasma concentration ($C_{max}$), and absolute bioavailability.
- **Distribution:** Parameters related to the dispersion and dissemination of the monograph drug through bodily fluids and tissues. Distribution parameters may include plasma protein binding and volume of distribution ($V_d$).
- **Metabolism:** Summary of the biotransformation or detoxification of the parent compound into metabolites. Associated enzymes and active metabolites are included if applicable.
- **Elimination:** The parameters associated with the removal of the drug from the body. Elimination parameters may include elimination/terminal half-life ($T_{1/2}$) and percentage eliminated through urine or feces.

## NURSING CONSIDERATIONS

**Assessment:** Contains specific parameters and laboratory tests that the patient must be assessed for or undergo prior to starting treatment with the drug.

**Monitoring:** Information used for monitoring patients currently treated with the drug. Monitoring points may include specific lab tests and drug-related or condition-specific information.

**Patient Counseling:** A compilation of important treatment information to discuss with the patient.

**Administration:** Guidelines for preparing the monograph drug for administration, rate of administration, proper administration technique, and/or compatibility. Please see the Dosage section. For more details on the step-by-step administration process, refer to the full prescribing information for the drug. **Storage:** Instructions for safe storage and disposal of the monograph drug.

[1] Drug monographs contain concise information. Not all fields described in the Drug Monograph Key are included in every monograph. For more detailed information, please see the full FDA-approved labeling information for the drug.

[2] To identify abbreviated terms used within monographs, refer to the Abbreviations, Acronyms, and Symbols table in the appendix on page A1.

### *FDA/DEA CLASS

| | |
|---|---|
| **OTC:** | Available over-the-counter. |
| **RX:** | Requires a prescription. |
| **CII:** | Controlled substance; high potential for abuse. |
| **CIII:** | Controlled substance; some potential for abuse. |
| **CIV:** | Controlled substance; low potential for abuse. |
| **CV:** | Controlled substance; subject to state and local regulation. |

### †FDA USE-IN-PREGNANCY RATINGS

The FDA use-in-pregnancy rating system weighs the degree to which available information has ruled out risk to the fetus against the drug's potential benefit to the patient. The ratings, and the interpretation, are as follows:

| CATEGORY | INTERPRETATION |
|---|---|
| A | **CONTROLLED STUDIES SHOW NO RISK.** Adequate, well-controlled studies in pregnant women have failed to demonstrate a risk to the fetus in any trimester of pregnancy. |
| B | **NO EVIDENCE OF RISK IN HUMANS.** Adequate, well-controlled studies in pregnant women have not shown increased risk of fetal abnormalities despite adverse findings in animals, or, in the absence of adequate human studies, animal studies show no fetal risk. The chance of fetal harm is remote, but remains a possibility. |
| C | **RISK CANNOT BE RULED OUT.** Adequate, well-controlled human studies are lacking, and animal studies have shown a risk to the fetus or are lacking as well. There is a chance of fetal harm if the drug is administered during pregnancy; but the potential benefits may outweigh the potential risk. |
| D | **POSITIVE EVIDENCE OF RISK.** Studies in humans, or investigational or post-marketing data, have demonstrated fetal risk. Nevertheless, potential benefits from the use of the drug may outweigh the potential risk. For example, the drug may be acceptable if needed in a life-threatening situation or serious disease for which safer drugs cannot be used or are ineffective. |
| X | **CONTRAINDICATED IN PREGNANCY.** Studies in animals or humans, or investigational or post-marketing reports, have demonstrated positive evidence of fetal abnormalities or risk which clearly outweighs any possible benefit to the patient. |

# Concise Drug Monographs

# ABBOKINASE RX

urokinase (Abbott)

**THERAPEUTIC CLASS:** Thrombolytic agent

**INDICATIONS:** Lysis of acute massive pulmonary emboli (PE) and PE accompanied by unstable hemodynamics.

**DOSAGE:** *Adults:* LD: 4400 IU/kg IV at 90mL/hr over 10 min. Maint: 4400 IU/kg/hr IV at 15mL/hr for 12 hrs. Flush line after each cycle. For IV use only.

**HOW SUPPLIED:** Inj: 250,000 IU

**CONTRAINDICATIONS:** Active internal bleeding, intracranial neoplasm, arteriovenous malformation, aneurysm, bleeding diathesis, severe uncontrolled arterial HTN. Recent (within 2 months) CVA, intracranial or intraspinal surgery, trauma including resuscitation.

**WARNINGS/PRECAUTIONS:** Prior to use obtain Hct, platelet count, and activated partial thromboplastin time (aPTT). Increased risk of bleeding; fatalities due to hemorrhage, including intracranial and retroperitoneal, reported. Avoid IM injections, nonessential patient handling, frequent venipunctures. Use upper extremity vessels when performing arterial punctures. Increased risk of bleeding with recent (within 10 days) major surgery, obstetrical delivery, organ biopsy, previous puncture of noncompressible vessels, serious GI bleeding, high likelihood of left heart thrombus, subacute bacterial endocarditis, hemostatic defects including those secondary to severe hepatic or renal disease, pregnancy, cerebrovascular disease, diabetic hemorrhagic retinopathy, and any other condition in which bleeding may be a significant hazard or difficult to manage. May carry risk of transmitting infectious agents.

**ADVERSE REACTIONS:** Bleeding, fatal hemorrhage, anaphylaxis, allergic-type or infusion reactions.

**INTERACTIONS:** Increased risk of serious bleeding with other thrombolytic agents, anticoagulants, or agents inhibiting platelet function (eg, ASA, other NSAIDs, dipyridamole, GP IIb/IIIa inhibitors).

**PREGNANCY:** Category B, caution in nursing.

**MECHANISM OF ACTION:** Thrombolytic agent; acts on the endogenous fibrinolytic system. Converts plasminogen to the enzyme plasmin. Plasmin degrades fibrin clots, fibrinogen, and some plasma proteins.

**PHARMACOKINETICS: Distribution:** $V_d$=11.5L. **Metabolism:** Liver. **Elimination:** Bile, urine; $T_{1/2}$=12.6 min.

## NURSING CONSIDERATIONS

**Assessment:** Assess for active internal bleeding, recent (within 2 months) cerebrovascular accident or intracranial or intraspinal surgery; recent trauma (eg, cardiopulmonary resuscitation), intracranial neoplasm, arteriovenous malfunction, aneurysms, bleeding diathesis, and severe uncontrolled arterial HTN. Assess use in patients who had recent (within 10 days) major surgery, obstetrical delivery, organ biopsy, or previous puncture of non-compressing vessels. Assess use in patients with recent (eg, within 10 days) GI bleeding, patients at risk for left heart thrombus, presence of subacute bacterial endocarditis, hemostatic defects (eg, secondary to severe hepatic or renal disease), pregnancy, cerebrovascular disease, diabetic hemorrhagic retinopathy, and any condition in which bleeding might constitute a significant hazard. Assess for drug interactions. Obtain baseline Hct, platelet count, and an aPTT.

**Monitoring:** Monitor for signs/symptoms of bleeding (eg, intracranial hemorrhage, retroperitoneal bleeding), anaphylaxis, and other infusion reactions (eg, fever, hypoxia, cyanosis, dyspnea, hypotension), cholesterol embolization (eg, livedo reticularis, "purple toe" syndrome, acute renal failure, cerebral infarction), and transmission of infectious disease. Monitor for clinical response, vital signs (BP), Hct, platelet count, and aPTT.

**Patient Counseling:** Instruct to contact physician immediately if allergic reactions (eg, anaphylaxis, bronchospasm, orolingual edema, urticaria, skin rash, and pruritus) or bleeding occur. Counsel about the risk of viral transmission from medication.

**Administration:** IV route. Do not reconstitute until immediately before use. Discard any unused portion. 1) Reconstitute. Aseptically add 5 mL of SWFI, without preservatives to vial. Do not use bacteriostatic water. 2) After reconstituting, visually inspect vial for discoloration or presence of particulate matter. Solution should be pale and straw-colored. 3) Further dilute using 0.9% NS or D5W, USP. **Storage:** Refrigerate at 2-8°C (36-46°F).

## ABELCET RX

amphotericin B lipid complex (Enzon)

**THERAPEUTIC CLASS:** Polyene antifungal

**INDICATIONS:** Treatment of invasive fungal infections in patients refractory to or intolerant of conventional amphotericin B therapy.

**DOSAGE:** *Adults:* 5mg/kg IV at 2.5mg/kg/hr.
*Pediatrics:* ≥16 yrs: 5mg/kg IV at 2.5mg/kg/hr.

**HOW SUPPLIED:** Inj: 5mg/mL

**WARNINGS/PRECAUTIONS:** Anaphylaxis reported. D/C if respiratory distress occurs. Monitor SrCr, LFTs, serum electrolytes, CBC during therapy.

**ADVERSE REACTIONS:** Chills, fever, increased SrCr, multi-organ failure, N/V, hypotension, respiratory failure, dyspnea, sepsis, diarrhea, headache, heart arrest, HTN, hypokalemia, infection, kidney failure, pain, thrombocytopenia.

**INTERACTIONS:** Antineoplastics may potentiate renal toxicity, bronchospasm, hypotension. Corticosteroids and corticotropin may potentiate hypokalemia, predisposing patients to cardiac dysfunction. May potentiate digitalis toxicity. Increased risk of flucytosine toxicity. Acute pulmonary toxicity reported with leukocyte transfusions. Nephrotoxic drugs (eg, aminoglycosides, pentamidine) enhance potential for renal toxicity. Cyclosporine within several days of bone marrow ablation associated with nephrotoxicity. Hypokalemia effect may enhance curariform effect of skeletal muscle relaxants. May cause increased myelotoxicity and nephrotoxicity with concomitant zidovudine.

**PREGNANCY:** Category B, not for use in nursing.

**MECHANISM OF ACTION:** Acts by binding to sterols in cell membrane of susceptible fungi, with resultant change in membrane permeability.

**PHARMACOKINETICS: Absorption:** $C_{max}$=1.7mcg/mL, AUC=14mcg•h/mL. **Distribution:** $V_d$=131L/kg. **Elimination:** $T_{1/2}$=173.4 hrs.

### NURSING CONSIDERATIONS

**Assessment:** Assess for hepatic/renal impairment and possible drug interactions.

**Monitoring:** Monitor for anaphylatic reaction, hypotension, bronchospasm or respiratory distress, arrhythmias, shock, chills, and fever. Frequently monitor creatinine, LFTs, serum electrolytes (Mg, K+) and CBC.

**Patient Counseling:** Inform about risks/benefits.

**Administration:** IV infusion. Do not dilute with saline solution or mix with other drugs or electrolytes. **Storage:** 2-8°C (36-46°F); admixture stable for 48 hrs at 2-8°C (36-46°F) and additional 6 hrs at room temperature. Avoid light exposure and freezing.

## ABILIFY RX

aripiprazole (Bristol-Myers Squibb/Otsuka America)

**Elderly patients with dementia-related psychosis treated with atypical antipsychotic drugs are at an increased risk of death; most appeared to be cardiovascular (eg, heart failure, sudden death) or infectious (eg, pneumonia) in nature. Not approved for the treatment of patients with dementia-related psychosis. Children, adolescents, and young adults taking antidepressants for major depressive disorder and other psychiatric disorders are at increased risk of suicidal thinking and behavior.**

**OTHER BRAND NAMES:** Abilify Discmelt (Bristol-Myers Squibb/Otsuka America)

**THERAPEUTIC CLASS:** Partial $D_2/5HT_{1A}$ agonist/$5HT_{2A}$ antagonist

**INDICATIONS:** (PO) Acute and maintenance treatment of schizophrenia in adults and adolescents (13-17 yrs). Monotherapy for acute and maintenance treatment of manic and mixed episodes associated with bipolar I disorder and as adjunct therapy to lithium or valproate for acute treatment of manic and mixed episodes in adults and pediatrics (10-17 yrs). Adjunctive therapy to antidepressants for acute treatment of major depressive disorder (MDD) in adults. Treatment of irritability associated with autistic disorder in pediatric patients (6-17 yrs). (Inj) Acute treatment of agitation associated with schizophrenia or bipolar disorder, manic or mixed, in adults.

**DOSAGE:** *Adults:* (PO) Schizophrenia: Initial/Target: 10-15mg qd. Titrate: Should not increase before 2 weeks. Usual: 15-30mg/day. Bipolar Disorder (Monotherapy or Adjunct to lithium or valproate): Initial/Target: 15mg/day. Titrate: May increase to 30mg/day based on clinical response. Max: 30mg/day. MDD: Initial: 2-5mg/day. Titrate: May adjust dose at increments up to 5mg/day at intervals ≥1 week. Usual: 2-15mg/day. Periodically reassess need for maintenance therapy. Oral sol can be given on mg-per-mg basis up to 25mg. Patients receiving 30mg tabs should receive 25mg of oral sol. (Inj) Schizophrenia or Bipolar Mania: 9.75mg IM. Usual: 5.25-15mg IM. Max: 30mg/day. Do not give additional doses more frequently than every 2 hrs. Concomitant Strong CYP3A4 Inhibitors (eg, ketoconazole, clarithromycin): Reduce usual dose by 50%. Concomitant CYP2D6 Inhibitors (eg, quinidine, fluoxetine, paroxetine): Reduce usual dose by 50%. Concomitant CYP3A4 Inducers (eg, carbamazepine): Double the dose.
*Pediatrics:* Schizophrenia (13-17 yrs)/Bipolar Disorder (Monotherapy or Adjunct) (10-17 yrs): Initial: 2mg/day. Titrate: May increase by 5mg/day every 2 days to a target dose of 10mg/day. Usual: 10-30mg/day. Irritability Associated with Autistic Disorder (6-17 yrs): Individualize dosing according to tolerability and response. Initial: 2mg/day. Titrate: Increase to 5mg/day gradually at intervals ≥1 week. May increase to 10-15mg/day if necessary. Usual: 5mg-15mg/day. Max: 15mg/day. Periodically reassess need for maintenance therapy. Oral sol can be given on mg-per-mg basis up to 25mg. Patients receiving 30mg tabs should receive 25mg of oral sol. Concomitant Strong CYP3A4 Inhibitors (eg, ketoconazole, clarithromycin): Reduce usual dose by 50%. Concomitant CYP2D6 Inhibitors (eg, quinidine, fluoxetine, paroxetine): Reduce usual dose by 50%. Concomitant CYP3A4 Inducers (eg, carbamazepine): Double the dose.

**HOW SUPPLIED:** Tab, Orally Disintegrating: (Discmelt) 10mg, 15mg; Tab: 2mg, 5mg, 10mg, 15mg, 20mg, 30mg; Sol: 1mg/mL; Inj: 7.5mg/mL

**WARNINGS/PRECAUTIONS:** May develop tardive dyskinesia (TD) or neuroleptic malignant syndrome (NMS). Monitor for hyperglycemia, worsening of glucose control with diabetes mellitus (DM), and fasting blood glucose (FBG) levels with diabetes risk. Increased incidence of cerebrovascular adverse events (eg, stroke, and transient ischemic attack) in elderly dementia patients. Orthostatic hypotension reported, caution with cardiovascular disease, conditions that predispose to hypotension (eg, dehydration, hypovolemia). May lower seizure threshold. May impair physical/mental abilities. May disrupt body's temperature regulation. Possible esophageal dysmotility and aspiration; caution in patients at risk for aspiration pneumonia. Exercise vigilance when treating psychosis associated with Alzheimer's; monitor for emergence of difficulty swallowing or excessive somnolence. Leukopenia/neutropenia and agranulocytosis reported; d/c if severe neutropenia (absolute neutrophil count is <1000/$mm^3$) occurs. Monitor carefully for fever or other signs/symptoms of infection.

**ADVERSE REACTIONS:** Headache, blurred vision, cough, tremor, anxiety, insomnia, N/V, somnolence, constipation, akathisia, extrapyramidal disorder, nasopharyngitis, dizziness, restlessness.

**INTERACTIONS:** May potentiate effect of antihypertensives. Caution with anticholinergic agents, other centrally acting drugs. Avoid alcohol. CYP3A4 inducers (eg, carbamazepine) may lower blood levels. CYP3A4 inhibitors (eg, ketoconazole, itraconazole) or 2D6 inhibitors (eg, quinidine, fluoxetine, paroxetine) may increase blood levels.

**PREGNANCY:** Category C, not for use in nursing.

**MECHANISM OF ACTION:** Partial $D_2$/$5HT_{1A}$ agonist/$5HT_{2A}$ antagonist; mechanism not established.

**PHARMACOKINETICS: Absorption:** Absolute bioavailability 87% (PO), 100% (IM); $T_{max}$=3-5 hrs (PO), 1-3 hrs (IM). **Distribution:** $V_d$=404L or 4.9L/kg (IV); plasma protein binding 99% (IV). **Metabolism:** Hepatic via dehydrogenation, hydroxylation, and N-dealkylation. Dehydro-aripiprazole (active metabolite) CYP3A4 and 2D6 enzymes (PO). Not systemically evaluated (IM). **Elimination:** Urine (25%), feces (55%); $T_{1/2}$=75 hrs.

## NURSING CONSIDERATIONS

**Assessment:** Assess for dementia-related psychosis, risk of suicidal behavior in children or adolescents/young adults, clinical diagnosis of bipolar disorder, use of drug in patients who have a history of cardiovascular or cerebrovascular disease or history of seizures, risk of aspiration pneumonia, autistic disorder, pregnancy/nursing status, and possible drug interactions. Assess baseline FBG levels in patients at risk for hyperglycemia.

**Monitoring:** If patient remains on therapy for longer than 6 weeks, perform periodic clinical evaluations to determine treatment responsiveness. Monitor for unusual changes in behavior, signs of worsening depression, risk of suicidality, signs/symptoms of NMS, TD, hyperglycemia, hypotension, dysphagia, dystonia, and extrapyramidal symptoms while on therapy. Measure FBG levels if symptoms develop. Periodically evaluate serum glucose levels in patients at risk for DM.

**Patient Counseling:** Counsel caregivers to be alert to signs of agitation, anxiety, panic attacks, insomia, hostility, aggressiveness, impulsivity, akathisia, hypomania, mania, irritability, worsening of depression, changes in behavior, or suicidal ideation; d/c and notify physician. Counsel about cognitive/motor impairment; use caution when operating machinery/driving. Avoid alcohol consumption. Medication may affect body's ability to lower body temperature; instruct to take appropriate measures (eg, adequate hydration when performing strenuous activities or exposed to extreme heat, on concomitant medications with anticholinergic activity). Explain the need to monitor CBC frequently during the first few months of therapy and discontinuation.

**Administration:** Oral/IM route. **Storage:** 25°C (77°F); excursions permitted to 15-30°C (59-86°F). Opened bottles of oral solution may be used for up to 6 months after opening, not beyond expiration date. Store injections in original container, protect from light.

# ABRAXANE RX

paclitaxel protein-bound particles (Abraxis)

**Should not be administered to patients with metastatic breast cancer who have baseline neutrophil counts of <1,500 cells/mm³. Recommended that frequent peripheral blood cell counts should be performed on all patients to monitor for the occurrence of bone marrow suppression, primarily neutropenia. Should be administered under the supervision of a physician experienced in the use of cancer chemotherapeutic agents. Do not substitute for or with other paclitaxel formulations.**

**THERAPEUTIC CLASS:** Antimicrotubule agent

**INDICATIONS:** Treatment of breast cancer after failure of combination chemotherapy for metastatic disease or relapse within 6 months of adjuvant chemotherapy. Prior therapy should have included an anthracycline unless clinically contraindicated.

**DOSAGE:** *Adults:* 260mg/m² IV over 30 min every 3 weeks. Severe Neutropenia (neutrophil <500 cells/mm³ for week or longer) or Severe Sensory Neuropathy During Therapy: Reduce dose to 220mg/m² for subsequent courses. For recurrence of severe neutropenia or severe sensory neuropathy, additional dose reduction should be made to 180mg/m². For grade 3 sensory neuropathy, hold treatment until resolution to grade 1 or 2, followed by a dose reduction for all subsequent courses. Moderate Hepatic Impairment (AST<10xULN, Bilirubin 1.26-2.0xULN): 200mg/m$^2$. Severe Hepatic Impairment (AST<10xULN, Bilirubin 2.01-5.0xULN): 130mg/m$^2$. Do not give if AST>10xULN or Bilirubin>5.0xULN.

**HOW SUPPLIED:** Inj: 100mg

**CONTRAINDICATIONS:** Patients with baseline neutrophil counts of <1,500 cells/mm$^3$.

**WARNINGS/PRECAUTIONS:** Bone marrow suppression is dose dependent and a dose-limiting toxicity; do not retreat until neutrophils recover to >1,500 cells/mm$^3$ and platelets recover to >100,000 cells/mm$^3$. Use has not been studied in patients with renal dysfunction. May cause fetal harm. Men should be advised not to father a child while receiving treatment. Remote risk for transmission of viral diseases; theoretical risk for transmission of Creutzfeldt-Jakob disease (CJD). Sensory neuropathy occurs frequently. Injection-site reactions reported. Caution with hepatic impairment. May affect ability to drive and use machines.

**ADVERSE REACTIONS:** Neutropenia, infections, anemia, ECG abnormalities, dyspnea, fluid retention/edema, sensory neuropathy, ocular/visual disturbances, arthralgia/myalgia, N/V, asthenia, diarrhea, alopecia, alkaline phosphatase elevations, AST elevations.

**INTERACTIONS:** Caution with concomitant use of medications known to inhibit (eg, ketoconazole and other imidazole antifungals, erythromycin, fluoxetine, gemfibrozil, cimetidine, ritonavir, saquinavir, indinavir, nelfinavir) or induce (eg, rifampicin, carbamazepine, phenytoin, efavirenz, nevirapine) either CYP2C8 or CYP3A4; pharmacokinetics of drug may be altered by interactions with substrates, inducers or inhibitors of CYP2C8 and/or CYP3A4. Concomitant or previous use with neurotoxic agents may influence the frequency or severity of neurological manifestations.

**PREGNANCY:** Category D, not for use in nursing.

**MECHANISM OF ACTION:** Antimicrotubule agent; promotes assembly of microtubules from tubulin dimers and stabilizes microtubules by preventing depolymerization. This stability results in inhibition of the normal dynamic reorganization of the microtubule network that is essential for vital interphase and mitotic cellular functions.

**PHARMACOKINETICS: Absorption:** $C_{max}$=18,741ng/mL. **Distribution:** $V_d$=632L/m$^2$, plasma protein binding (89-98%). **Metabolism:** Liver, via CYP2C8 (6α-hydroxypaclitaxel, major metabolite) and CYP3A4 (3'-*p*-hydroxypaclitaxel and 6α, 3'-*p*-dihydroxypaclitaxel, minor metabolites). **Elimination:** Urine (4% unchanged, <1% metabolite), feces (approximately 20%), $T_{1/2}$=27 hrs.

## NURSING CONSIDERATIONS

**Assessment:** Assess for history of heart disease, hepatic/renal impairment, pregnancy/nursing status, and for possible drug interactions. Assess that baseline neutrophil count is ≥1,500 cells/mm$^3$.

**Monitoring:** Monitor for signs/symptoms of bone marrow suppression, viral infections, sensory neuropathy, and injection-site rections. Perform frequent peripheral blood cell counts.

**Patient Counseling:** Inform of risks and benefits of therapy. Advise women of childbearing potential to avoid becoming pregnant and men not to father a child while on therapy. Counsel to immediately report any signs of fever or other signs of infection. Instruct to avoid contact with skin; if contact occurs wash skin immediately and thoroughly with soap and water. Inform that may affect ability to drive or use machines.

**Administration:** IV route. See PI for reconstitution instructions. **Storage:** Store vials in original cartons at 20-25°C (68-77°F). Retain in original package to protect from light.

## ACANYA RX

clindamycin phosphate - benzoyl peroxide (Valeant)

**THERAPEUTIC CLASS:** Antibacterial/keratolytic

**INDICATIONS:** Topical treatment of acne vulgaris in patients ≥12 yrs.

**DOSAGE:** *Adults:* Apply pea-sized amount to face qd. Not for oral, ophthalmic, or intravaginal use.
*Pediatrics:* ≥12 yrs: Apply pea-sized amount to face qd. Not for oral, ophthalmic, or intravaginal use.

**HOW SUPPLIED:** Gel: (Clindamycin-Benzoyl Peroxide) 1.2%-2.5% [50g]

**CONTRAINDICATIONS:** History of regional enteritis, ulcerative colitis, or antibiotic-associated colitis.

**WARNINGS/PRECAUTIONS:** Diarrhea, bloody diarrhea, and colitis (eg, pseudomembranous colitis) reported; d/c if significant diarrhea occurs. Antiperistaltic agents (eg, opiates, diphenoxylate with atropine) may prolong and/or worsen severe colitis, and may result in death. Minimize exposure to natural and artificial sunlight after application.

**ADVERSE REACTIONS:** Erythema, scaling, itching, burning, and stinging.

**INTERACTIONS:** Avoid with topical or oral erythromycin. Caution with concomitant topical acne therapy (eg, peeling, desquamating, or abrasive agents). May potentiate neuromuscular blockers.

**PREGNANCY:** Category C, not for use in nursing.

**MECHANISM OF ACTION:** Clindamycin: Binds to 50S ribosomal subunits of susceptible bacteria and prevents elongation of peptide chains, thereby suppressing bacterial protein synthesis. Benzoyl peroxide: Oxidizing agent with bacteriocidal and keratolytic effects.

### NURSING CONSIDERATIONS

**Assessment:** Assess for history of regional enteritis, ulcerative colitis, or antibiotic-associated colitis, diarrhea, bloody diarrhea, and active colitis, possible drug interactions, and pregnancy/nursing status.

**Monitoring:** Monitor for erythema, scaling, itching, burning, and stinging.

**Patient Counseling:** Instruct to apply medication as directed and avoid direct contact with mouth, eyes, vagina, or lips. Avoid applying on cuts or open wounds and washing of face more than 3 times a day. Instruct to wash hands with soap and water after application. Advise not use more than the recommended amount and not to apply more often than once daily. Instruct to notify physician if any signs or symptoms of local skin irritation, pregnant or intend to be pregnant. Advise to minimize exposure to natural and avoid artificial sunlight; to minimize exposure to sunlight wear a wide-brimmed hat or other protective clothing and use a sunscreen with SPF 15 rating or higher during treatment.

**Administration:** Topical route. See PI for admixing instructions. **Storage:** Store at room temperature up to 25°C (77°F). Do not freeze. Keep jar tightly closed.

## ACCOLATE RX

zafirlukast (AstraZeneca)

**THERAPEUTIC CLASS:** Leukotriene receptor antagonist

**INDICATIONS:** Prophylaxis and chronic treatment of asthma.

**DOSAGE:** *Adults:* 20mg bid. Administer 1 hr ac or 2 hrs pc.
*Pediatrics:* ≥12 yrs: 20mg bid. 5-11 yrs: 10mg bid. Administer 1 hr ac or 2 hrs pc.

**HOW SUPPLIED:** Tab: 10mg, 20mg

**WARNINGS/PRECAUTIONS:** Cases of life-threatening hepatic failure reported; if suspected, d/c therapy. Not for reversal of bronchospasm in acute asthma attacks. Systemic eosinophilia, eosinophilic pneumonia, and vasculitis consistent with Churg-Strauss syndrome have been reported rarely. Neuropsychiatric events (eg, insomnia and depression) reported.

**ADVERSE REACTIONS:** Headache, infection, nausea.

**INTERACTIONS:** Coadministration with warfarin increases PT time; monitor closely. Caution with drugs metabolized by CYP2C9 (eg, tolbutamide, phenytoin, carbamazepine) or CYP3A4 (eg, dihydropyridine CCBs, cyclosporine, cisapride, astemizole). Increased levels with ASA. Decreased levels with erythromycin, theophylline. May increase theophylline levels.

**PREGNANCY:** Category B, not for use in nursing.

**MECHANISM OF ACTION:** Leukotriene receptor antagonist; selective and competitive receptor antagonist of leukotriene $D_4$ and $E_4$ ($LTD_4$ and $LTE_4$), components of slow-reacting substance of anaphylaxis (SRSA); inhibits bronchoconstriction.

**PHARMACOKINETICS: Absorption:** Rapid. (Adult) $C_{max}$=326ng/mL; $T_{max}$=2 hrs; AUC=1137ng•h/mL. (7-11 yrs) $C_{max}$=601ng/mL; $T_{max}$=2.5 hrs; AUC=2027ng•h/mL. (5-6 yrs) $C_{max}$=756ng/mL; $T_{max}$=2.1 hrs; AUC=2458ng•h/mL. **Distribution:** $V_d$=approximately 70L; plasma protein binding (>99%). **Metabolism:** Liver, hydroxylation via CYP2C9. **Elimination:** $T_{1/2}$=10 hrs.

## NURSING CONSIDERATIONS

**Assessment:** Assess for hepatic dysfunction, bronchospasm (status asthmaticus), nursing status, and possible drug interactions. Obtain baseline LFTs.

**Monitoring:** Monitor LFTs and PT, signs/symptoms of hepatotoxicity, eosinophilia, vasculitic rash, worsening pulmonary symptoms, cardiac complications, neuropathy, neuropsychiatric events (eg, insomnia, depression), and hypersensitivity reactions (eg, urticaria, angioedema, rash).

**Patient Counseling:** Counsel to take drug at least 1 hr before or 2 hrs after meals. Do not decrease dose or stop taking other anti-asthma medications unless instructed by physician. Instruct to seek medical attention if symptoms of liver dysfunction (eg, right upper quadrant abdominal pain, nausea, fatigue, lethargy, pruritus, jaundice, flu-like symptoms, anorexia), eosinophilia, vasculitic rash, worsening pulmonary symptoms, cardiac complications, neuropathy, neuropsychiatric events, and hypersensitivity reactions (eg, urticaria, angioedema, rash) occur. Advise against use if nursing.

**Administration:** Oral route. **Storage:** 20-25°C (68-77°F). Protect from light and moisture. Dispense in original air-tight container.

# AccuNeb RX

albuterol sulfate (Dey)

**THERAPEUTIC CLASS:** $Beta_2$-agonist

**INDICATIONS:** Relief of bronchospasm with asthma.

**DOSAGE:** *Pediatrics:* 2-12 yrs: Initial: 0.63mg or 1.25mg tid-qid via nebulizer. 6-12 yrs with severe asthma, >40kg or 11-12 yrs: Initial: 1.25mg tid-qid.

**HOW SUPPLIED:** Sol, Inhalation: 1.25mg/3mL, 0.63mg/3mL [3mL, $25^s$]

**WARNINGS/PRECAUTIONS:** Hypersensitivity reactions reported. Fatalities reported with excessive use. Caution with cardiovascular disorders, especially coronary insufficiency, arrhythmias and HTN. May need concomitant anti-inflammatory agents. Can produce paradoxical bronchospasm. Caution with DM. May cause hypokalemia.

**ADVERSE REACTIONS:** Asthma exacerbation, otitis media, allergic reaction, gastroenteritis, cold symptoms.

**INTERACTIONS:** Avoid other short-acting sympathomimetic bronchodilators and epinephrine. Extreme caution within 2 weeks of MAOI or TCA use. Monitor digoxin. ECG changes and/or hypokalemia with non-$K^+$-sparing diuretics may worsen. May be antagonized by β-blockers.

**PREGNANCY:** Category C, not for use in nursing.

**MECHANISM OF ACTION:** $\beta_2$ adrenergic agonist; stimulates adenyl cyclase, enzyme that catalyzes formation of ATP.

**PHARMACOKINETICS: Absorption:** (3mg): $C_{max}$=2.1ng/mL, $T_{max}$=0.5 hrs. **Elimination:** (4 mg): $T_{1/2}$=5-6 hrs.

## NURSING CONSIDERATIONS

**Assessment:** Assess for CVD (coronary insufficiency, cardiac arrhythmias, HTN), hyperthyroidism, DM, and possible drug interactions.

**Monitoring:** Monitor for signs/symptoms of cardiovascular effects (eg, increased BP, palpitations), worsening of symptoms, paradoxical bronchospasm, destabilization of asthma, and hypersensitivity reactions (eg, anaphylactic, urticaria, angioedema, rash, bronchospasm, oropharyngeal edema).

**Patient Counseling:** Instruct not for relief of acute respiratory symptoms. Seek medical attention if symptoms worsen, therapy becomes less effective, need more inhalation from short-acting $\beta_2$-agonist than usual, or if experience destabilization of asthma, paradoxical bronchospams, and hypersensitivity (eg, anaphylactic, urticaria, angioedema, rash, bronchospasm, oropharyngeal edema).

**Administration:** Inhalation route. **Storage:** Between 2-25°C (36-77°F). Protect from light and excessive heat. Store vials in protective foil pouch at all times. Once removed, use within 1 week. Discard if solution not colorless.

# ACCUPRIL — RX

quinapril HCl (Parke-Davis)

**ACE inhibitors can cause death/injury to the fetus during 2nd and 3rd trimesters. D/C if pregnancy is detected.**

**THERAPEUTIC CLASS:** ACE inhibitor

**INDICATIONS:** Treatment of hypertension alone or in combination with thiazide diuretics. Management of heart failure with diuretics and/or digitalis as adjunct therapy.

**DOSAGE:** *Adults:* HTN: If possible, d/c diuretic 2-3 days prior to therapy. Initial: 10mg or 20mg qd; 5mg qd with concomitant diuretic. Titrate: May adjust dosage based on BP response at intervals of at least 2 weeks. Usual: 20-80mg/day given qd-bid. CrCl >60mL/min: Initial: 10mg/day. CrCl 30-60mL/min: Initial: 5mg/day. CrCl 10-30mL/min: Initial: 2.5mg/day. Elderly: Initial: 10mg qd. Titrate: Increase to the optimal response. Heart Failure: Initial: 5mg bid. Titrate: May adjust dosage at weekly intervals. Usual: 20-40mg given bid. CrCl >30mL/min: Initial: 5mg/day. CrCl 10-30mL/min: Initial: 2.5mg/day. If inital dose is well tolerated, succeeding days may be given bid. Titrate dose at weekly intervals based on clinical and hemodynamic response. Elderly: Start at low end of dosing range.

**HOW SUPPLIED:** Tab: 5mg*, 10mg, 20mg, 40mg *scored

**CONTRAINDICATIONS:** History of ACE inhibitor-associated angioedema.

**WARNINGS/PRECAUTIONS:** D/C if angioedema, jaundice, or marked LFT elevation occurs. Risk of hyperkalemia with DM, renal dysfunction. Persistent nonproductive cough reported. Monitor WBCs in renal or collagen vascular disease. Anaphylactoid reactions reported. Monitor for hypotension in high-risk patients (heart failure, surgery/anesthesia, hyponatremia, high-dose diuretic therapy, recent intensive diuresis, dialysis, or severe volume and/or salt depletion). Caution with CHF, renal dysfunction, and renal artery stenosis. Less effective on BP in blacks and higher rates of angioedema than nonblacks. Caution in elderly.

**ADVERSE REACTIONS:** Headache, dizziness, cough.

**INTERACTIONS:** Decreases tetracycline absorption (possibly due to magnesium content in quinapril); consider interaction with drugs that interact with magnesium. May increase lithium levels and risk of toxicity. Hypotension risk with diuretics. Increased risk of hyperkalemia with $K^+$-sparing diuretics, $K^+$ supplements, or $K^+$-containing salt substitutes. May attenuate $K^+$ loss with thiazide diuretics. Nitritoid reactions reported (eg, facial flushing, N/V, hypotension) rarely with injectable gold (eg, sodium aurothiomalate).

**PREGNANCY:** Category C (1st trimester) and D (2nd and 3rd trimesters), caution in nursing.

**MECHANISM OF ACTION:** Angiotensin-converting enzyme inhibitor; inhibits ACE activity, reducing angiotensin II formation.

**PHARMACOKINETICS: Absorption:** $T_{max}$=1hr. (Quinaprilat) $T_{max}$=2 hrs. **Distribution:** Plasma protein binding (97%); found in breast milk. **Metabolism:** De-esterification. Quinaprilat (active metabolite). **Elimination:** (Quinaprilat) Renal; $T_{1/2}$=2hrs.

## NURSING CONSIDERATIONS

**Assessment:** Assess for volume/salt depletion, collagen vascular disease (systemic lupus erythematosus [SLE], scleroderma), CHF, DM, possible drug interactions, ischemic heart disease, cerebrovascular disease, renal impairment, pregnancy/nursing status, and possible drug interactions.

**Monitoring:** Monitor renal function for 1st few weeks, WBC periodically in patients with collagen vascular disease. Monitor for signs/symptoms of hypotension, anaphylactoid or hypersensitivity reactions, head/neck and intestinal angioedema, agranulocytosis, hyperkalemia, and renal dysfunction.

**Patient Counseling:** Inform of pregnancy risks; d/c therapy if pregnancy detected. Instruct that inadequate fluid intake or fluid loss may lead to drop in BP resulting in lightheadedness or syncope; avoid $K^+$ supplements or salt substitutes. Advise to seek medical attention if symptoms of hypotension (syncope), anaphylactoid or hypersensitivity reactions, angioedema (head/neck; abdominal pain with/without N/V), infection (sore throat, fever), or hyperkalemia occur.

**Administration:** Oral route. **Storage:** 15-30°C (59-86°F). Protect from light.

# ACCURETIC RX

quinapril HCl - hydrochlorothiazide (Parke-Davis)

**ACE inhibitors can cause death/injury to developing fetus during 2nd and 3rd trimesters. D/C therapy if pregnancy detected.**

**THERAPEUTIC CLASS:** ACE inhibitor/thiazide diuretic

**INDICATIONS:** Treatment of hypertension.

**DOSAGE:** *Adults:* Initial (if not controlled on quinapril monotherapy): 10mg-12.5mg or 20mg-12.5mg tab qd. Titrate: May increase after 2-3 weeks based on clinical response. Initial (if controlled on HCTZ 25mg/day but significant $K^+$ loss): 10mg-12.5mg or 20mg-12.5mg tab qd. If previously treated with 20mg quinapril and 25mg HCTZ, may switch to 20mg-25mg tab qd. Elderly: Start at low end of dosing range.

**HOW SUPPLIED:** Tab: (Quinapril-HCTZ) 10mg-12.5mg*, 20mg-12.5mg*, 20mg-25mg *scored

**CONTRAINDICATIONS:** History of ACE inhibitor-associated angioedema, anuria, sulfonamide hypersensitivity.

**WARNINGS/PRECAUTIONS:** D/C if angioedema, jaundice, or marked LFT elevation occurs. Risk of hyperkalemia with DM, renal dysfunction. Persistent nonproductive cough reported. Monitor WBCs in renal or collagen vascular disease. Anaphylactoid reactions reported. Monitor for hypotension in high-risk patients (eg, heart failure, surgery/anesthesia, hyponatremia, severe volume/salt depletion, etc). Caution with CHF, renal or hepatic dysfunction, and renal artery stenosis. Less effective on BP in blacks and more reports of angioedema than nonblacks. May exacerbate or activate systemic lupus erythematosus (SLE). Monitor serum electrolytes. Avoid if CrCl ≤30mL/min/1.73m². May increase cholesterol, TG, magnesium, calcium, and uric acid levels. May decrease glucose tolerance, serum protein-bound iodine levels without signs of thyroid disturbance. D/C for a few days before parathyroid function tests. Not for initial therapy. Caution in elderly.

**ADVERSE REACTIONS:** Dizziness, headache, cough, increases in serum creatinine and BUN levels.

**INTERACTIONS:** Quinapril: Decreases tetracycline absorption (possibly due to magnesium content in quinapril); consider interaction with drugs that interact with magnesium. Increased risk of hyperkalemia with $K^+$-sparing diuretics, $K^+$ supplements, or $K^+$-containing salt substitutes. May increase lithium levels and risk of toxicity. Nitritoid reactions reported (eg, facial flushing, N/V, hypotension) rarely with injectable gold (eg, sodium aurothiomalate). HCTZ: Potentiates orthostatic hypotension with alcohol, barbiturates, and narcotics. Adjust antidiabetic drugs (eg, insulin, oral hypoglycemic agents). Impaired absorption with cholestyramine, colestipol. Corticosteroids and ACTH deplete electrolytes. May decrease response to pressor amines. Potentiates other antihypertensives. May increase responsiveness to non-depolarizing skeletal muscle relaxants. Risk of lithium toxicity. NSAIDs decrease diuretic, natriuretic, and antihypertensive effects.

**PREGNANCY:** Category C (1st trimester) and D (2nd and 3rd trimesters), not for use in nursing.

**MECHANISM OF ACTION:** Quinapril: Angiotensin-converting enzyme inhibitor; inhibits ACE activity, reducing angiotensin II formation. HCTZ: Thiazide diuretic; affects renal tubular mechanism of electrolyte reabsorption directly increasing excretion of $Na^+$ and $Cl^-$, and indirectly reducing plasma volume.

**PHARMACOKINETICS: Absorption:** Quinapril: $T_{max}$=1 hr. (Quinaprilat) $T_{max}$=2 hrs. **Distribution:** Quinapril: Plasma protein binding (97%). HCTZ: $V_d$=3.6-7.8L/kg; plasma protein binding (67.9%); crosses placenta; found in breast milk. **Metabolism:** Quinapril: De-esterification. Quinaprilat (metabolite). **Elimination:** Quinaprilat: Renal; $T_{1/2}$=2 hrs. HCTZ: Kidney (61%, unchanged); $T_{1/2}$=4-15 hrs.

## NURSING CONSIDERATIONS

**Assessment:** Assess for volume/salt depletion, collagen vascular disease (SLE, scleroderma), CHF, DM, ischemic heart disease, cerebrovascular disease, anuria, sulfonamide hypersensitivity, renal/hepatic impairment, pregnancy/nursing status, and possible drug interactions.

**Monitoring:** Monitor renal function for 1st few weeks; WBC periodically in patients with collagen vascular disease. Monitor cholesterol, TG, magnesium, calcium and uric acid levels. Monitor for signs/symptoms of hypotension, anaphylactoid or hypersensitivity reactions, head/neck and intestinal angioedema, agranulocytosis, hyperkalemia, electrolyte imbalance, exacerbation or activation of SLE, precipitation of gout, hyperglycemia, renal/hepatic dysfunction.

**Patient Counseling:** Inform of pregnancy risks. Advise that inadequate fluid intake or loss of fluids may lead to drop in BP resulting in lightheadedness or syncope. Advise to seek medical attention if symptoms of angioedema (head/neck; abdominal pain with/without N/V), infection (sore throat, fever), hypotension (syncope), hypersensitivity reactions, hyperkalemia, or electrolyte imbalance (dry mouth, thirst, weakness) occurs.

**Administration:** Oral route. **Storage:** 20-25°C (68-77°F).

# ACEON RX

perindopril erbumine (Solvay)

> **ACE inhibitors can cause death/injury to developing fetus during the 2nd and 3d trimester. D/C therapy if pregnancy detected.**

**THERAPEUTIC CLASS:** ACE inhibitor

**INDICATIONS:** Treatment of hypertension (HTN); may be used alone or with other classes of antihypertensives, especially thiazide diuretics. To reduce the risk of cardiovascular mortality or nonfatal myocardial infarction (MI) in patients with stable coronary artery disease (CAD); may be used with conventional treatment for management of CAD (eg, antiplatelet, antihypertensive, or lipid lowering therapy).

**DOSAGE:** *Adults:* CAD: Initial: 4mg qd for 2 weeks. Maint: 8mg qd. Elderly (>70 yrs): Initial: 2mg qd for 1 week. Titrate: 4mg qd for Week 2. Maint: 8mg qd. HTN: If possible, d/c diuretic 2-3 days prior to therapy. Initial: 4mg qd; 2-4mg/day given qd-bid with concomitant diuretic. Maint: 4-8mg/day given qd-bid. Resume diuretic if BP not controlled. Max: 16mg/day. Elderly (>65 yrs): Initial: 4mg/day given qd-bid. Max (usual): 8mg/day. Renal Impairment: CrCl >30mL/min: Initial: 2mg/day. Max: 8mg/day.

**HOW SUPPLIED:** Tab: 2mg*, 4mg*, 8mg* *scored

**CONTRAINDICATIONS:** History of ACE inhibitor-associated angioedema.

**WARNINGS/PRECAUTIONS:** Head, neck, and intestinal angioedema reported; d/c if angioedema occurs. Anaphylactoid reactions during desensitization and during membrane exposure reported. Monitor for hypotension in high-risk patients (eg, heart failure, surgery/anesthesia, ischemic heart disease or cerebrovascular disease, volume and/or salt depletion). May cause agranulocytosis. Fetal/neonatal morbidity and death reported. Rarely associated with cholestatic jaundice that progresses to fulminant hepatic necrosis and sometimes death; d/c if jaundice or marked elevations of hepatic enzymes occur. May cause changes in renal function; caution in patients with severe CHF, renal artery stenosis, or pre-existing renal impairment. May cause hyperkalemia; caution in patients with risk factors for hyperkalemia (eg, diabetes mellitus [DM]), renal dysfunction). Persistent nonproductive cough reported. Less effective on BP in blacks and more reports of angioedema than nonblacks. Avoid if CrCl <30mL/min. Caution in elderly.

**ADVERSE REACTIONS:** Cough, back pain, sinusitis, viral infection, dizziness, headache, URI, asthenia, rhinitis, low extremity pain, diarrhea, edema, pharyngitis.

**INTERACTIONS:** May increase lithium levels. Hypotension risk with diuretics, anesthetics. Increased risk of hyperkalemia with $K^+$-sparing diuretics (eg, spironolactone, amiloride, triamterene), drugs that increase serum $K^+$, or $K^+$ supplements. Caution with gentamicin. Nitritoid reactions (eg, facial flushing, N/V, hypotension) reported rarely with injectable gold.

**PREGNANCY:** Category D, caution in nursing.

**MECHANISM OF ACTION:** Angiotensin-converting enzyme inhibitor; inhibits ACE activity resulting in decreased plasma angiotensin II, leading to decreased vasoconstriction, increased plasma renin activity, and decreased aldosterone secretion.

**PHARMACOKINETICS: Absorption:** Rapid; absolute bioavailability (75%); $T_{max}$=1 hr. Perindoprilat: Absolute bioavailability (25%); $T_{max}$=3-7 hrs. **Distribution:** Plasma protein binding (60%); crosses the placenta. Perindoprilat: Plasma protein binding (10-20%). **Metabolism:** Hepatic esterases (hydrolysis), glucuronidation, cyclization. Perindoprilat (active metabolite). **Elimination:** Urine (4-12%); $T_{1/2}$=0.8-1 hr. Perindoprilat: $T_{1/2}$=3-10 hrs.

## NURSING CONSIDERATIONS

**Assessment:** Assess for volume and/or salt depletion, CHF, renal artery stenosis, ischemic heart disease, cerebrovascular disease, pregnancy/nursing status, hepatic/renal impairment, hypersensitivity, and for possible drug interactions. Assess for risk factors for developing hyperkalemia (eg, DM).

**Monitoring:** Monitor for signs/symptoms of anaphylactoid reactions, head/neck and intestinal angioedema, hypotension, agranulocytosis, hepatic failure, hyperkalemia, persistent nonproductive cough, and hypersensitivity reactions. Monitor hepatic/renal function.

**Patient Counseling:** Inform that angioedema, including laryngeal edema may occur during therapy; instruct to immediately report to physician any signs/symptoms of angioedema (eg, swelling of the face, extremities, eyes, lips, tongue, difficulty swallowing or breathing) and to not take any more drug until physician is contacted. Instruct to contact physician if lightheadedness occurs and d/c therapy if fainting occurs. Advise to avoid potassium supplements or salt substitutes unless physician has been notified. Counsel to report any signs of infection (eg, sore throat, fever). Inform of potential risks if used during pregnancy.

**Administration:** Oral route. **Storage:** 20-25°C (68-77°F). Protect from moisture.

## ACETYLCYSTEINE RX
acetylcysteine (Various)

**THERAPEUTIC CLASS:** Acetaminophen antidote/Mucolytic

**INDICATIONS:** Adjunctive mucolytic therapy in acute and chronic bronchopulmonary disease; pulmonary complications of cystic fibrosis and surgery; tracheostomy care; during anesthesia; post-traumatic chest conditions; atelectasis; diagnostic bronchial studies. Antidote for acute acetaminophen (APAP) toxicity.

**DOSAGE:** *Adults:* Antidote: Empty stomach by lavage or emesis before administration. Administer immediately, regardless of quantity, if APAP ingestion ≤24hrs. LD: 140mg/kg PO then 70mg/kg PO q4h for 17 doses starting 4 hrs after LD. D/C if predetoxification APAP level is in nontoxic range and overdose occurred at least 4 hrs before assay. Obtain 2nd plasma level if range is nontoxic and time of ingestion is unknown or <4 hrs. Mucolytic: Nebulization (face mask, mouth piece, tracheostomy): 1-10mL of 20% or 2-10mL of 10% q2-6h. Usual: 3-5mL of 20% or 6-10mL of 10% 3-4 times/day. Closed Tent or Croupette: Up to 300mL of 10% or 20%. Direct Instillation: 1-2 mL of 10% or 20% q1-4h. Percutaneous Intratracheal Catheter: 1-2mL of 20% or 2-4mL of 10% q1-4h. Diagnostic Bronchograms: Give before procedure. 2-3 doses of 1-2mL of 20% or 2-4mL of 10%.
*Pediatrics:* Antidote: Empty stomach by lavage or emesis before administration. Administer immediately, regardless of quantity, if APAP ingestion ≤24hrs. LD: 140mg/kg PO then 70mg/kg PO q4h for 17 doses starting 4 hours after LD. D/C if predetoxification APAP level is in nontoxic range and overdose occurred at least 4 hrs before assay. Obtain 2nd plasma level if range is nontoxic and time of ingestion is unknown or <4 hrs. Mucolytic: Nebulization (face mask, mouth piece, tracheostomy): 1-10mL of 20% or 2-10mL of 10% q2-6h. Usual: 3-5mL of 20% or 6-10mL of 10% 3-4 times/day. Closed Tent or Croupette: Up to 300mL of 10% or 20%. Direct Instillation: 1-2 mL of 10% or 20% q1-4h. Percutaneous Intratracheal Catheter: 1-2mL of 20% or 2-4mL of 10% q1-4h. Diagnostic Procedures: Give before procedure. 2-3 doses of 1-2mL of 20% or 2-4mL of 10%.

**HOW SUPPLIED:** Sol: 10%, 20%

**WARNINGS/PRECAUTIONS:** (Oral) D/C if generalized urticaria or encephalopathy due to hepatic failure develops. May aggravate vomiting; evaluate with risk of gastric hemorrhage. (Inhalation) Monitor asthmatics. D/C if bronchospasm progresses.

**ADVERSE REACTIONS:** (Oral) N/V, other GI symptoms. (Inhalation) Stomatitis, N/V, fever, rhinorrhea, drowsiness, clamminess, chest tightness, bronchoconstriction.

**PREGNANCY:** Category B, caution in nursing.

**MECHANISM OF ACTION:** N-acetyl derivative. Mucolytic: Opens disulfide linkages in mucus, thereby lowering viscosity. Antidote: Protects liver by maintaining or restoring glutathione levels, or by acting as alternate substrate for conjugation with, and thus detoxification of reactive metabolites, reducing extent of liver injury.

**PHARMACOKINETICS: Metabolism:** Deacetylation, oxidation.

### NURSING CONSIDERATIONS

**Assessment:** Assess for possible drug interactions, asthma, esophageal varices, and peptic ulcers.

**Monitoring:** Monitor for signs/symptoms of bronchospasm, encephalopathy, gastric hemorrhage, and hypersensitivity reactions.

**Patient Counseling:** Advise to seek medical attention if symptoms of bronchospasm, encephalopathy, gastric hemorrhage, or hypersensitivity reactions (urticaria) occur.

**Administration:** Mucolytic: Inhalation route. Antidote: Oral route. Dilute 20% solution with NS for injection or sterile water for inhalation. Refer to full PI for administration techniques. **Storage:** 20-25°C (68-77°F), or 2-8°C (36-46°F) after opening; stable for 96 hrs.

## ACIPHEX RX

rabeprazole sodium (Eisai/PRICARA)

**THERAPEUTIC CLASS:** Proton pump inhibitor

**INDICATIONS:** Short-term treatment in the healing and symptomatic relief of erosive or ulcerative gastroesophageal reflux disease (GERD). Maintenance of healing and reduction in relapse rates of heartburn symptoms in patients with erosive or ulcerative GERD. Treatment of daytime and nighttime heartburn and other symptoms associated with GERD. Short-term treatment in the healing and symptomatic relief of duodenal ulcers (DU). In combination with amoxicillin and clarithromycin as a 3-drug regimen for the treatment of patients with *H.pylori* infection and DU disease (active or history within the past 5 yrs) to eradicate *H.pylori* and reduce the risk of DU recurrence. Long-term treatment of pathological hypersecretory conditions, including Zollinger-Ellison syndrome.

**DOSAGE:** *Adults:* Erosive/Ulcerative GERD: Healing: 20mg qd for 4-8 weeks. May repeat for 8 weeks if needed. Maint: 20mg qd. Symptomatic GERD: 20mg qd for 4 weeks. May repeat for 4 weeks if needed. DU: 20mg qd after morning meal for up to 4 weeks. May need additional therapy. *H.pylori* Triple Therapy: 20mg + clarithromycin 500mg + amoxicillin 1g, all bid (qam and qpm) with food for 7 days. Pathological Hypersecretory Conditions: Initial: 60mg qd. Titrate: Adjust according to need. Maint: Up to 100mg qd or 60mg bid. May treat up to 1 yr. Swallow tabs whole; do not chew, crush, or split.
*Pediatrics:* ≥12 yrs: Symptomatic GERD: 20mg qd for up to 8 weeks.

**HOW SUPPLIED:** Tab, Delayed-Release: 20mg

**WARNINGS/PRECAUTIONS:** Symptomatic response does not preclude the presence of gastric malignancy. Caution with severe hepatic impairment.

**ADVERSE REACTIONS:** Headache, diarrhea, N/V, abdominal pain, and taste perversion with triple therapy.

**INTERACTIONS:** May alter absorption of pH-dependent drugs (eg, ketoconazole, digoxin). May inhibit cyclosporine metabolism. May increase digoxin plasma levels and decrease ketoconazole levels. Concomitant use with warfarin increases the INR and PT time; monitor PT/INR. Increased rabeprazole and clarithromycin levels with triple therapy.

**PREGNANCY:** Category B, not for use in nursing.

**MECHANISM OF ACTION:** Proton pump inhibitor; suppresses gastric acid secretion by inhibiting the gastric ($H^+$, $K^+$)-ATPase enzyme at the secretory surface of the gastric parietal cell. Blocks the final step of gastric acid secretion.

**PHARMACOKINETICS: Absorption:** $T_{max}$=2-5 hrs; absolute bioavailability (52%). **Distribution:** Plasma protein binding (96.3%). **Metabolism:** Extensive. Liver via CYP3A4 to sulphone (primary metabolite) and CYP2C19 to desmethyl rabeprazole (primary metabolite). **Elimination:** Urine (90%), feces; $T_{1/2}$=1-2 hrs.

## NURSING CONSIDERATIONS

**Assessment:** Assess for hypersensitivity to other proton pump inhibitors, presence of gastric malignancy, severe hepatic impairment, pregnancy/nursing status, and possible drug interactions.

**Monitoring:** Monitor for allergic reactions, clinical improvement, and pathological changes in gastric mucosa. If on concomitant therapy with antibacterial agents, monitor for signs/symptoms of *C. difficile*.

**Patient Counseling:** Instruct to swallow tablet whole with water; do not chew, crush, or split tablet. May take with/without food. Inform if dose is missed, take drug as soon as possible. If almost time for the next dose, skip missed dose and go back to normal schedule; do not take 2 doses at same time.

Instruct to contact physician if signs of hypersensitivity reaction (hives, swelling of face, eyelids, lips, tongue, or throat) occur.

**Administration:** Oral route. **Storage:** 15-30°C (59-86°F); store in dry place, out of reach of children.

## ACLOVATE RX

alclometasone dipropionate (GlaxoSmithKline)

**THERAPEUTIC CLASS:** Corticosteroid

**INDICATIONS:** Relief of the inflammatory and pruritic manifestations of corticosteroid-responsive dermatoses.

**DOSAGE:** *Adults:* Apply bid-tid. Reassess if no improvement after 2 weeks. *Pediatrics:* ≥1 yr: Apply bid-tid. Reassess if no improvement after 2 weeks.

**HOW SUPPLIED:** Cre, Oint: 0.05% [15g, 45g, 60g]

**WARNINGS/PRECAUTIONS:** May produce reversible HPA axis suppression, manifestations of Cushing's syndrome, hyperglycemia, and glucosuria. Use appropriate antifungal or antibacterial agent with dermatological infections. Peds may be more susceptible to systemic toxicity. Avoid occlusive dressings. Avoid diaper area. Not for use in diaper dermatitis. D/C if irritation occurs. Caution in peds.

**ADVERSE REACTIONS:** Itching, burning, erythema, dryness, irritation, papular rash, folliculitis, acneiform eruptions, hypopigmentation, perioral dermatitis, allergic contact dermatitis, secondary infection, skin atrophy, striae.

**PREGNANCY:** Category C, caution in nursing.

**MECHANISM OF ACTION:** Corticosteroid; has anti-inflammatory, antipruritic, and vasoconstrictive properties. Anti-inflammatory mechanism not established. Suspected to act by the induction of phospholipase $A_2$ inhibitory proteins (lipocortins), which may control the biosynthesis of potent mediators of inflammation (eg, prostaglandins, leukotrienes) by inhibiting the release of their common precursor, arachidonic acid. Arachidonic acid is released from membrane phospholipids by phospholipase $A_2$.

**PHARMACOKINETICS: Distribution:** Systemically administered corticosteroids are found in breast milk.

### NURSING CONSIDERATIONS

**Assessment:** Assess use in pregnant/nursing females.

**Monitoring:** Monitor for occurrence of HPA axis suppression through periodic monitoring of ACTH stimulation, a.m. plasma cortisol, and urinary-free cortisol tests. Monitor for manifestations of Cushing's syndrome, hyperglycemia, and glucosuria while on therapy. Monitor for development of skin irritation. If present, d/c medication. Monitor for signs of allergic contact dermatitis (eg, failure to heal) and signs of concomitant skin infections. In pediatric patients, monitor for HPA axis suppression, Cushing's syndrome, linear growth retardation, delayed weight gain, and intracranial HTN.

**Patient Counseling:** Instruct to use externally and as directed. Counsel to avoid contact with eyes and that treated skin area should not be bandaged. Instruct not to use medication on face, underarms, or groin areas unless directed by a physician. Counsel to notify physician if any signs of improvement do not occur within 2 weeks of starting medication.

**Administration:** Apply topically. **Storage**: 2-30°C (36-86°F).

## ACTEMRA RX

tocilizumab (Genentech)

**Increased risk for developing serious infections that may lead to hospitalization or death. If serious infections develop, interrupt treatment until infection is controlled. Reported infections include active tuberculosis (TB), invasive fungal infections (eg, candidiasis, aspergillosis, and pneumocystis), bacterial, viral and other infections due to opportunistic pathogens. Perform test for latent TB and treat prior to initiation of therapy. Risks and benefits should be considered prior to treatment. Closely monitor for development of signs and symptoms of infection during and after treatment.**

**THERAPEUTIC CLASS:** Interleukin-6 receptor antagonist

**INDICATIONS:** Treatment of moderate to severe active rheumatoid arthritis in adult patients who have had inadequate response to one or more tumor necrosis factor (TNF) antagonist therapies.

**DOSAGE:** *Adults:* Monotherapy/Combination Therapy with MTX or other Disease-Modifying Antirheumatic Drugs: Initial: 4mg/kg q4 weeks as 60-min IV drip infusion. Titrate: Increase to 8mg/kg based on clinical response. Max: 800mg per infusion. Refer to PI for dose modifications based on liver enzyme abnormalities, absolute neutrophil count (ANC), and platelet count. Do not initiate treatment if ANC <2,000 cells/mm$^3$, platelets <100,000 cells/mm$^3$, or ALT/AST >1.5x ULN. D/C if liver enzymes >5x ULN, ANC <500 cells/mm$^3$, or platelets <50,000 cells/mm$^3$.

**HOW SUPPLIED:** Inj: 20mg/mL [80mg/4mL, 200mg/10mL, 400mg/20mL]

**WARNINGS/PRECAUTIONS:** Avoid with active infection, including localized infections. D/C if serious infection, opportunistic infection, or sepsis develop. Weigh risks and benefits of treatment in patients with chronic or recurrent infections, history of serious or an opportunistic infections, with exposure to TB, or who travel in areas where TB/mycoses are endemic. Viral reactivation reported with immunosuppressive biologic therapies and herpes zoster exacerbation observed. GI perforation reported; caution in patients at risk for GI perforation. Neutropenia, thrombocytopenia, elevation of liver enzymes, and increase in lipid parameters reported; monitor with appropriate tests every 4 to 8 weeks. Severe hypersensitivity reactions (eg, anaphylaxis) may occur. May result in an increased risk of malignancies. Multiple sclerosis (MS) and chronic inflammatory demyelinating polyneuropathy reported rarely; caution with pre-existing or recent onset demyelinating disorders. Avoid with active hepatic disease or hepatic impairment. Caution in elderly.

**ADVERSE REACTIONS:** Upper respiratory tract infections, nasopharyngitis, headache, HTN, increased ALT, dizziness, bronchitis.

**INTERACTIONS:** Avoid with live vaccines. Caution when coadministered with CYP3A4 substrates (eg, oral contraceptives, lovastatin, atorvastatin, simvastatin, omeprazole); may decrease effectiveness. May decrease dextromethorphan levels. Monitor therapeutic effect of warfarin, and concentration of cyclosporine and theophylline if coadministered; dose adjustments may be necessary. Avoid combination therapy with biological DMARDs such as TNF antagonists, IL-1R antagonists, anti-CD20 monoclonal antibodies, and selective costimulation modulators.

**PREGNANCY:** Category C, not for use in nursing.

**MECHANISM OF ACTION:** Interleukin-6 (IL-6) receptor monoclonal antibody; toclizumab binds specifically to both soluble and membrane-bound IL-6 receptors (sIL-6R and mIL-6R) and has been shown to inhibit IL-6 mediated signaling through these receptors.

**PHARMACOKINETICS: Absorption:** (4mg/kg) $C_{max}$=88.3mcg/mL; AUC=13000mcg•h/mL, (8mg/kg) $C_{max}$=183mcg/mL; AUC=35000mcg•h/mL. **Distribution:** $V_d$=6.4L. **Elimination:** (4mg/kg) $T_{1/2}$=11 days, (8mg/kg) $T_{1/2}$=14 days.

### NURSING CONSIDERATIONS

**Assessment:** Assess for infections (eg, bacteria, fungi, or viruses), including TB infections. Assess for hypersensitivity reactions, MS and chronic inflammatory demyelinating polyneuropathy, GI disorders. Check lipid levels, platelet and neutrophil count, pregnancy status and possible drug interactions.

**Monitoring:** Monitor for signs and symptoms of TB, bacterial, viral, fungal infections. Monitor for hypersensitivity reactions, GI disorders, and other side effects. Check CBC, platelet, LFTs, lipid levels every 4 to 8 weeks.

**Patient Counseling:** Advise of the potential risks/benefits of therapy. Inform that therapy may lower resistance to infections and some patients treated have had serious GI side effects; contact physician if symptoms of infection or severe, persistent abdominal pain appear. Advise to inform physician of travel history, especially in places that are endemic for TB/mycoses.

**Administration:** IV route. See PI for proper administration technique. Do not administer as an IV bolus or push. **Storage:** Refrigerate at 2-8°C (36-46°F). Do not freeze. Protect vials from light; keep in original package until time of use. Fully diluted solutions may be stored at room temperature for up to 24 hrs.

## ACTIGALL RX

ursodiol (Watson)

**THERAPEUTIC CLASS:** Bile acid

**INDICATIONS:** Treatment of radiolucent, noncalcified gallbladder stones <20mm in diameter in patients unable to undergo cholecystectomy. Prevention of gallstone formation in obese patients experiencing rapid weight loss.

**DOSAGE:** *Adults:* Treatment: 8-10mg/kg/day given bid-tid. Obtain ultrasound at 6 month intervals for 1 yr. Continue therapy after stones have dissolved and confirm with repeat ultrasound within 1-3 months. Prevention: 300mg bid.

**HOW SUPPLIED:** Cap: 300mg

**CONTRAINDICATIONS:** Calcified cholesterol stones, radiopaque stones, radiolucent bile pigment stones, unremitting acute cholecystitis, cholangitis, biliary obstruction, gallstone pancreatitis, biliary-gastrointestinal fistula, bile-acid hypersensitivity.

**WARNINGS/PRECAUTIONS:** Therapy is not associated with liver damage. Monitor SGOT (AST) and SGPT (ALT) at the initiation of therapy and periodically thereafter. Caution in elderly.

**ADVERSE REACTIONS:** Abdominal pain, constipation, diarrhea, dyspepsia, flatulence, N/V, arthralgia, coughing, viral infection, bronchitis, pharyngitis, back pain, myalgia, headache, sinusitis.

**INTERACTIONS:** Decreased absorption with bile acid sequestrants and aluminum-based antacids. May increase hepatic cholesterol secretion, and encourage gallstone formation with estrogens, oral contraceptives, and clofibrate.

**PREGNANCY:** Category B, caution in nursing.

**MECHANISM OF ACTION:** Bile acid; suppresses hepatic synthesis, cholesterol secretion, and inhibits intestinal cholesterol absorption; actions combine to change bile from cholesterol-precipitating to solubilizing, resulting in bile conducive to cholesterol stone dissolution.

**PHARMACOKINETICS: Absorption:** Small bowel (90%). **Metabolism:** Liver (1st pass, conjugation). **Elimination:** Feces.

### NURSING CONSIDERATIONS

**Assessment:** Assess for type of bile pigment stones (calcified cholesterol, radiopaque, radiolucent), unremitting acute cholecystitis, cholangitis, biliary obstruction, gallstone pancreatitis, biliary GI fistula, nursing status, and possible drug interactions. Obtain baseline SGOT (AST) and SGPT (ALT).

**Monitoring:** Ultrasound should be taken in 6-month intervals for first year. If appear dissolved, continue therapy and confirm on repeat ultrasound within 1-3 months. If partial dissolution not seen by 12 months, success is greatly reduced. Monitor SGOT (AST) and SGPT (ALT) periodically. Signs/symptoms of hypersensitivity reactions.

**Patient Counseling:** Seek medical attention if symptoms of hypersensitivity or allergic reactions occur. Advise patient that gallbladder stone dissolution requires months of therapy.

**Administration:** Oral route. **Storage:** 25°C (77°F); excursions permitted to 15-30°C (59-86°F). Dispense in tight container.

## ACTIQ CII

fentanyl citrate (Cephalon)

**May cause life-threatening respiratory depression, even death, in opioid non-tolerant patients. Contains fentanyl, with abuse liability similar to other opioid analgesics. Substitution for any other fentanyl product may result in fatal overdose. Use only in the care of cancer patients and only by oncologists and pain specialists who are skilled/knowledgeable in the use of Schedule II opioids to treat cancer patients. Only for breakthrough cancer pain in opioid-tolerant patients with malignancies who are already receiving and who are tolerant to around-the-clock opioid therapy for their underlying persistent cancer pain. Keep out of reach of children and discard properly. Concomitant use with moderate and strong CYP3A4 inhibitors may cause fatal respiratory depression.**

**THERAPEUTIC CLASS:** Opioid analgesic

**INDICATIONS:** Management of breakthrough cancer pain in patients ≥16 yrs old with malignancies who are already receiving and are tolerant to around-the-clock opioid therapy.

**DOSAGE:** *Adults:* Initial: 200mcg (consume over 15 min). Titrate: Redose 15 min after previous dose is completed if breakthrough pain episode not relieved; take only 1 additional dose of the same strength. No more than 2 units per breakthrough pain episode. Wait at least 4 hrs before treating another episode of breakthrough pain. May increase to next highest available strength if several breakthrough episodes require more than 1 unit per pain episode. Repeat titration for each new dose. Prescribe an initial titration supply of six 200mcg units. Maint: Once titrated to an effective dose, use only 1 unit of the appropriate strength per breakthrough pain episode. If experience >4 breakthrough pain episodes per day, re-evaluate maint dose. Upon d/c, gradually titrate dose downward.

*Pediatrics:* ≥16 yrs: Initial: 200mcg (consume over 15 min). Titrate: Redose 15 min after previous dose is completed if breakthrough pain episode not relieved; take only 1 additional dose of the same strength. No more than 2 units per breakthrough pain episode. Wait at least 4 hrs before treating another episode of breakthrough pain. May increase to next highest available strength if several breakthrough episodes require more than 1 unit per pain episode. Repeat titration for each new dose. Prescribe an initial titration supply of six 200mcg units. Maint: Once titrated to an effective dose, use only 1 unit of the appropriate strength per breakthrough pain episode. If experience >4 breakthrough pain episodes per day, re-evaluate maint dose. Upon d/c, gradually titrate dose downward.

**HOW SUPPLIED:** Loz: 200mcg, 400mcg, 600mcg, 800mcg, 1200mcg, 1600mcg

**CONTRAINDICATIONS:** Opioid non-tolerant patients and management of acute or postoperative pain, including headache/migraine.

**WARNINGS/PRECAUTIONS:** There are no safe conversion directions available for patients on any other fentanyl products, including oral, transdermal or parenteral formulations. Caution with chronic obstructive pulmonary disease (COPD), pre-existing medical conditions predisposing to respiratory depression, hepatic or renal dysfunction and the elderly. Risk of clinically significant respiratory depression. Extreme caution with evidence of increased intracranial pressure (ICP) or impaired consciousness. May obscure clinical course of head injuries. Dental decay of varying severity may occur (eg, dental caries, tooth loss, gum line erosion). Caution with bradyarrhythmias. May impair mental and/or physical status. Anaphylaxis and hypersensitivity reported. Maybe fatal to children.

**ADVERSE REACTIONS:** Respiratory depression, circulatory depression, headache, hypotension, shock, N/V, constipation, dizziness, dyspnea, anxiety, somnolence, asthenia, confusion, depression, rash.

**INTERACTIONS:** See Black Box Warning. Respiratory depression may occur more readily when given with other agents that depress respiration. Concomitant use with other CNS depressants, including opioids, sedatives, hypnotics, general anesthetics, phenothiazines, tranquilizers, skeletal muscle relaxants, sedating antihistamines, strong inhibitors of CYP3A4 (eg, ketoconazole, itraconazole, ritonavir, troleandomycin, clarithromycin, nelfinavir and nefazodone) or moderate inhibitors (eg, amprenavir, aprepitant, diltiazem, erythromycin, fluconazole, fosamprenavir, and verapamil) and alcohol may result in increased plasma concentrations of fentanyl resulting in increased depressant effect; adjust dose if warranted. Avoid grapefruit and grapefruit juice. Opposite effect with CYP3A4 inducers. Not recommended with or within 14 days of d/c of MAOIs.

**PREGNANCY:** Category C, not for use in nursing.

**MECHANISM OF ACTION:** Opioid analgesic: μ-opioid receptor agonist. Principal therapeutic effect is analgesia; exact mechanism not established. Specific CNS opioid receptors for endogenous compounds have been identified throughout brain and spinal cord and play a role in analgesic effects.

**PHARMACOKINETICS: Absorption:** Rapidly absorbed from buccal mucosa; slow absorption of swallowed fentanyl from GI tract. Absolute bioavailability (50%); (200mcg) $C_{max}$= 0.39ng/mL, AUC= 102ng/mL•min, $T_{max}$= 40 min; (400mcg) $C_{max}$= 0.75ng/mL, AUC= 243ng/mL•min, $T_{max}$=25 min; (800mcg) $C_{max}$=1.55ng/mL, AUC= 573ng/mL•min, $T_{max}$=25 min; (1600mcg) $C_{max}$= 2.51ng/mL, AUC= 1026ng/mL•min, $T_{max}$=20 min. **Distribution:** $V_d$=4L/kg; plasma protein binding (80-85%). Readily crosses placenta; found in breast milk. **Metabolism:** Liver and intestinal mucosa via CYP3A4; norfentanyl (metabolite). **Elimination**: Urine (<7%, unchanged) (major), feces (1%, unchanged); $T_{1/2}$= 193 min (200mcg), 386 min (400mcg), 381 min (800mcg), 358 min (1600mcg).

## NURSING CONSIDERATIONS

**Assessment:** Assess for risk of drug misuse, abuse, or diversion, acute/chronic post-op pain, opioid intolerance, COPD, pre-existing medical conditions predisposing to respiratory depression, increased ICP, impaired consciousness, hepatic/renal function, bradyarrhythmias, pregnancy/nursing status and drug interactions.

**Monitoring:** Monitor for signs/symptoms of respiratory and CNS depression, bradycardia, circulatory depression, hypotension, shock, impairment of mental/physical abilities, abuse/addiction, dental decay, and hypersensitivity reactions. Monitor glucose levels with DM.

**Patient Counseling:** Inform that medication must be kept out of reach of children; may be fatal to child. Seek immediate help if child accidentally consumes medication. Instruct to properly discard partially used units. Inform that use may impair mental/physical abilities and to use caution if performing hazardous tasks (eg, operating machinery/driving). Notify physician of all concurrently used medications or before taking any other medications. Avoid consumption of grapefruit juice and alcohol. Instruct to maintain proper dental hygiene during therapy and consult dentist to ensure proper dental care. Advise diabetics that medication contains approximately 2g sugar/unit. Advise to contact physician for any signs of respiratory depression (eg, difficulty breathing, extreme drowsiness with slowed breathing, slow shallow breathing, faintness, dizziness, confusion). Instruct to avoid abrupt withdrawal. Patient may drink water prior to use, but should not eat or drink anything during use. Advise that if dizziness, nausea, or sleepiness develops before medication is completely dissolved, to remove medication from mouth. Notify physician if have 4 episodes of breakthrough pain.

**Administration:** Oral route. The lozenge should be sucked, not chewed, and consumed over 15 min. Refer to PI for proper administration. **Storage:** 20-25°C (68-77°F); excursions permitted between 15-30°C (59-86°F). Protect from freezing and moisture. Do not use if blister package has been opened.

## ACTIVASE RX

alteplase (Genentech)

**THERAPEUTIC CLASS:** Thrombolytic agent

**INDICATIONS:** Management of acute myocardial infarction (AMI) for the improvement of ventricular function following AMI, the reduction of incidence of congestive heart failure (CHF) and reduction of mortality with AMI. Management of acute ischemic stroke and acute massive pulmonary embolism (PE).

**DOSAGE:** *Adults:* AMI: Accelerated Infusion: >67kg: 15mg IV bolus, then 50mg over next 30 min, and then 35mg over next 60 min. ≤67kg: 15mg IV bolus, then 0.75mg/kg (max 50mg) over next 30 min, then 0.50mg/kg (max 35mg) over next 60 min. Max: 100mg total dose. 3-Hr Infusion: ≥65kg: 60mg in 1st hr (give 6-10mg as IV bolus), then 20mg over 2nd hr, and 20mg over 3rd hr. <65kg: 1.25mg/kg over 3 hrs as described above. Acute Ischemic Stroke: 0.9mg/kg IV over 1 hr (max 90mg total dose). Administer 10% of total dose as IV bolus over 1 min. PE: 100mg IV over 2 hrs. Start heparin at end or immediately after infusion when PTT or PT ≤2x normal.

**HOW SUPPLIED:** Inj: 50mg, 100mg

**CONTRAINDICATIONS:** (AMI, PE) Active internal bleeding, history of cerebrovascular accident (CVA), recent intracranial/intraspinal surgery or trauma, intracranial neoplasm, arteriovenous (AV) malformation, aneurysm, bleeding diathesis, severe uncontrolled HTN. (Acute Ischemic Stroke) Active internal bleeding, AV malformation, intracranial neoplasm, history or evidence of intracranial hemorrhage, aneurysm, bleeding diathesis, uncontrolled HTN, subarachnoid hemorrhage, seizure at stroke onset. Recent (within 3 months) intracranial or intraspinal surgery, serious head trauma, previous stroke.

**WARNINGS/PRECAUTIONS:** Weigh benefits/risks with recent major surgery, cerebrovascular disease, recent GI or genitourinary (GU) bleeding, recent trauma, HTN (systolic BP ≥175mmHg and/or diastolic BP >110mmHg), left heart thrombus, acute pericarditis, subacute bacterial endocarditis, hemostatic defects, severe hepatic dysfunction, pregnancy, diabetic hemorrhagic retinopathy or other hemorrhagic ophthalmic conditions, septic thrombophlebitis or occluded AV cannula at a seriously infected site, advanced age or elderly, any other bleeding condition that is difficult to manage. For stroke, also weigh benefits/risks with severe neurological deficit or major early infarct signs on CT. Cholesterol embolism and internal/superficial bleeding reported. Arrhythmias may occur with reperfusion. Avoid IM injection, noncompressible arterial puncture, and internal jugular or subclavian venous puncture. Caution with readministration. D/C therapy if anaphylactoid reaction occurs.

**ADVERSE REACTIONS:** Bleeding, orolingual angioedema.

**INTERACTIONS:** Increased risk of bleeding with warfarin, heparin, vitamin K antagonists, drugs that alter platelets (eg, ASA, dipyridamole, abciximab) given before, during, or after alteplase therapy. Orolingual angioedema with ACE inhibitors.

**PREGNANCY:** Category C, caution in nursing.

**MECHANISM OF ACTION:** Tissue plasminogen activator (t-PA); serine protease enzyme that has property of fibrin-enhanced conversion of plasminogen to plasmin. Produces limited conversion of plasminogen in absence of fibrin. Binds to fibrin in thrombus and converts entrapped plasminogen to plasmin. Initiates local fibrinolysis with limited systemic proteolysis.

**PHARMACOKINETICS: Metabolism**: Liver. **Elimination:** $T_{1/2}$=<5 min (initial).

### NURSING CONSIDERATIONS

**Assessment:** In patients with acute MI or PE, assess for presence of active internal bleeding, history of cerebrovascular accident, trauma, aneurysm, known bleeding diathesis, and severe uncontrolled HTN. In patients with acute ischemic stroke, assess for presence or history of hemorrhage, surgery, serious head trauma, previous stroke, uncontrolled HTN, and possible drug interactions.

**Monitoring:** Monitor for signs/symptoms of bleeding (eg, internal, superficial, surface bleeding), cholesterol embolism (eg, livedo reticularis, "purple toe" syndrome, acute renal failure, gangrenous digits), and for allergic reactions (eg, anaphylactoid reaction, laryngeal edema, orolingual angioedema, rash, urticaria). Monitor BP frequently and arrhythmias with acute MI.

**Patient Counseling:** Inform about risk of bleeding with medication. Instruct to notify physician if any type of allergic reaction develops during therapy.

**Administration:** IV route. Reconstitute using appropriate volume of SWFI (without preservatives) to vial. Do not use Bacteriostatic Water for Inj, USP. Reconstitute to a final concentration of 1mg/mL. Reconstitute just prior to use. May further dilute using an equal volume of 0.9% NS or D5W to yield concentration of 0.5mg/mL. Do not add any other medication to infusion solutions containing drug. Discard any unused infusion solution. Do not use if vacuum is not present in 50mg vials. **Storage:** Lyophilized: Controlled room temperature not to exceed 30°C (86°F), or under refrigeration 2-8°C (36-46°F). Protect from excessive exposure to light. Reconstituted: 2-30°C (36-86°F); use within 8 hrs.

## ACTIVELLA — RX

norethindrone - estradiol (Novo Nordisk)

**Estrogens and progestins should not be used for the prevention of cardiovascular disease or dementia. Increased risk of MI, stroke, invasive breast cancer, PE, and DVT in postmenopausal women (50-79 yrs of age) reported. Increased risk of developing probable dementia in postmenopausal women ≥65 yrs of age reported.**

**THERAPEUTIC CLASS:** Estrogen/progestogen combination

**INDICATIONS:** For women with intact uterus, treatment of moderate to severe vasomotor symptoms associated with menopause, vulvar/vaginal atrophy and prevention of postmenopausal osteoporosis.

**DOSAGE:** *Adults:* 1 tab qd.

**HOW SUPPLIED:** Tab: (Estradiol-Norethindrone) 1mg-0.5mg, 0.5mg-1mg

**CONTRAINDICATIONS:** Pregnancy, breast cancer, abnormal genital bleeding, estrogen-dependent neoplasia, DVT, thromboembolic disorders, stroke, liver dysfunction or disease.

**WARNINGS/PRECAUTIONS:** Risk of gallbladder disease, endometrial and breast cancer, fetal congenital reproductive tract disorder, elevated BP, and hypercalcemia with breast cancer or bone metastases. Possible risk of cardiovascular disease. Increased risk of DVT, stroke, and PE; increased risk of endometrial, breast, and ovarian cancer with prolonged use. Risk of probable dementia-unknown risk in postmenopausal women under 65 years of age. Monitor for fluid retention with asthma, epilepsy, migraine, and cardiac/renal dysfunction. Avoid in post-menopausal women without a uterus. D/C if vision disturbances or thrombotic disorders occur. Caution with depression, DM, severe hypocalcemia. Acceleration of PT, PTT. Hypercoagulability effects. Impaired glucose tolerance. Increased triglycerides, fibrin/fibrinogen, and plasmin/plasminogen activity.

**ADVERSE REACTIONS:** Back pain, headache, nasopharyngitis, sinusitis, insomnia, upper respiratory tract infection, breast pain, postmenopausal bleeding/vaginal hemorrhage, endometrial thickening, uterine fibroid, pain in extremities, nausea, and diarrhea.

**INTERACTIONS:** CYP3A4 inducers (eg, St. John's wort, phenobarbital, carbamazepine, rifampin) may reduce estrogen levels. CYP3A4 inhibitors (eg, erythromycin, clarithromycin, ketoconazole, itraconazole, ritonavir, grapefruit juice) may increase estrogen levels.

**PREGNANCY:** Category X, caution in nursing.

**MECHANISM OF ACTION:** Estrogen/progestogen combination. Estradiol: Binds to nuclear receptors in estrogen-responsive tissues and modulating pituitary secretion of gonadotropins, luteinizing hormone (LH) and follicle-stimulating hormone (FSH), through negative-feedback mechanism.

Norethindrone: Exerts effect in target cells by binding to specific progesterone receptors that interact with progesterone-response elements in target genes. Enhances cellular differentiation and opposing actions of estrogens by decreasing estrogen receptor levels, increasing local metabolism of estrogens to less active metabolites, and inducing gene products that blunt cellular responses to estrogen.

**PHARMACOKINETICS: Absorption:** Estradiol ($E_2$): Well-absorbed, $T_{max}$=5-8 hrs. Norethindrone (NET): Rapid. **Distribution:** Estrogens found in breast milk. $E_2$: Sex-hormone-binding globulin (37%); albumin (61%); unbound (1-2%). NET: Sex-hormone-binding globulin (36%); albumin (61%). **Metabolism:** $E_2$: Liver to estrone, $E_1$ (metabolite); estriol (major urinary metabolite); enterohepatic recirculation via sulfate and glucuronide conjugation; biliary secretion of conjugates into the intestine, and hydrolysis in intestine; CYP3A4 (partial). NET: 5α-dihydro-norethindrone and tetrahydro-norethindrone (metabolites). **Elimination:** $E_2$: Urine; $T_{1/2}$=12-14 hrs. $E_1$: Urine; $T_{1/2}$=12-14 hrs. NET: $T_{1/2}$=8-11 hrs.

## NURSING CONSIDERATIONS

**Assessment:** Assess for abnormal genital bleeding, presence or history of breast cancer, estrogen-dependent neoplasias, DVT, PE, active or recent (within past yr) arterial thromboembolic disease (eg, stroke, MI), liver dysfunction/disease, and known/suspected pregnancy. Assess use in patients undergoing surgery associated with increased risk of thromboembolism, under prolonged immobilization, and with history of hypertriglyceridemia, hypothyroidism, renal dysfunction, or presence of severe hypocalcemia. Assess use in women ≥65 yrs old, nursing patients, and those with DM, asthma, epilepsy, migraines or porphyria, SLE, and hepatic hemangiomas. Assess for possible drug and lab test interactions.

**Monitoring:** Monitor for signs/symptoms of cardiovascular disorders (eg, MI, stroke, venous thrombosis, PE), malignant neoplasms (eg, breast, endometrial, ovarian cancer), dementia, gallbladder disease, hypercalcemia, visual abnormalities (eg, retinal vascular thrombosis), increased BP, hypertriglyceridemia, hypothyroidism, fluid retention, cholestatic jaundice, exacerbation of endometriosis and other conditions (eg, asthma, DM, epilepsy, migraine, porphyria, SLE, and hepatic hemangiomas). Perform annual mammography and periodic monitoring of BP. Monitor thyroid function if patient on thyroid hormone replacement therapy. In cases of undiagnosed, persistent, or recurrent vaginal bleeding in women with uterus, perform adequate diagnostic measures (eg, endometrial sampling) to rule out malignancies.

**Patient Counseling:** Inform that estrogens may increase risk for uterine and breast cancer, heart attack, stroke, blood clots, and dementia. Report any unusual vaginal bleeding, breast lumps, dizziness or faintness, changes in speech, severe headaches, chest pain, SOB, leg pain, changes in vision, or vomiting. Advise to perform monthly self breast exam, and have annual gynecologic exam (breast exam, mammography).

**Administration:** Oral route. **Storage:** Store in dry place; protect from light. Store at room temperature, 25°C (77°F), excursions permitted to 15-30°C (59-86°F).

# ACTONEL RX

risedronate sodium (Procter & Gamble)

**THERAPEUTIC CLASS:** Bisphosphonate

**INDICATIONS:** Treatment and prevention of osteoporosis in postmenopausal women and glucocorticoid-induced osteoporosis in men and women who are either initiating or continuing systemic glucocorticosteroids. Increase bone mass in men with osteoporosis. Treatment of Paget's Disease of bone in men and women.

**DOSAGE:** *Adults:* Postmenopausal Osteoporosis Prevention/Treatment: 5mg qd or 35mg once weekly or 75mg on 2 consecutive days each month or 150mg once a month. Glucocorticoid-Induced Osteoporosis: 5mg qd. Increase Bone Mass in Men with Osteoporosis: 35mg once weekly. Paget's Disease:

30mg qd for 2 months. May retreat after 2 months. Take at least 30 min before 1st food or drink of day other than water. Swallow tab in upright position with 6-8 oz plain water. Do not lie down for 30 min after dose.

**HOW SUPPLIED:** Tab: 5mg, 30mg, 35mg, 150mg

**CONTRAINDICATIONS:** Hypocalcemia, inability to stand or sit upright for at least 30 min and abnormalities of the esophagus that delay esophageal emptying (eg, stricture or achalasia).

**WARNINGS/PRECAUTIONS:** May cause upper GI disorders (eg, dysphagia, esophagitis, esophageal or gastric ulcer); d/c if new or worsening symptoms occur. Treat hypocalcemia and other disturbances of bone and mineral metabolism before therapy. Give supplemental calcium and vitamin D if dietary intake is inadequate. Osteonecrosis of the jaw (ONJ) associated with tooth extraction and/local infection with delayed healing has been reported. Caution if with risk facts for ONJ including invasive dental procedures, cancer diagnosis and comorbid disorders (eg, anemia, coagulopathy, periodontal and/or preexisting dental disease, infection, ill-fitting dentures). Postmarketing reports of severe and occasionally incapacitating bone, joint, and/or muscle pain. Before initiating therapy for the treatment and prevention of glucocorticoid-induced osteoporosis, ascertain sex steroid hormonal status of both men and women and consider appropriate replacement. May interfere with the use of bone-imaging agents. Avoid with severe renal impairment (CrCl <30mL/min). Not for use in pediatrics.

**ADVERSE REACTIONS:** Diarrhea, abdominal pain, nausea, constipation, arthralgia, headache, infection, back pain, pain, flu syndrome, hypertension, dyspepsia, rash, bronchitis, UTI.

**INTERACTIONS:** Calcium supplements, antacids, or oral medications containing divalent cations (aluminum, magnesium) interfere with absorption of bisphosphonates; such supplements should be taken at a different time of the day. Risk of ONJ with concomitant therapies (eg, corticosteroids, chemotherapy).

**PREGNANCY:** Category C, not for use in nursing.

**MECHANISM OF ACTION:** Bisphosphonate; has an affinity for hydroxyapatite crystals in bone and acts as an antiresorptive agent. Inhibits osteoclast-mediated bone resorption and modulates bone metabolism.

**PHARMACOKINETICS: Absorption**: $T_{max}$=1 hr; (30mg) absolute bioavailability (0.63%). **Distribution**: $V_d$=13.8L/kg; plasma protein binding (24%). **Elimination**: Urine, feces (unabsorbed dose); $T_{1/2}$=561 hrs.

## NURSING CONSIDERATIONS

**Assessment:** Assess for hypocalcemia and other bone disturbances or problems with mineral metabolism; treat appropriately. Assess for ability to stand or sit upright for 30 min, esophageal abnormalities (eg, strictures, achalasia), severe renal impairment (CrCl <30mL/min), risk factors for developing ONJ, pregnancy/nursing status and possible drug interactions. Assess hormonal status if treatment is for glucocorticoid-induced osteoporosis; consider appropriate replacement therapy.

**Monitoring:** Monitor for signs/symptoms of upper GI disorders (eg, dysphagia, esophagitis, esophageal or gastric ulcers), ONJ and musculoskeletal pain.

**Patient Counseling:** Instruct to take at least 30 min before first food or drink of the day other than water. Advise to take in an upright position (while sitting or standing) with a full glass of plain water (6 to 8 oz). Inform that should not lie down for 30 min after taking medication. Advise to avoid chewing or sucking tablet. Instruct to contact physician if develop symptoms of esophageal disease (eg, difficulty or pain with swallowing, retrosternal pain, worsening heartburn) before continuing medication. Advise to take supplemental calcium and vitamin D if dietary intake is inadequate; take supplement at a different time of the day than risedronate. Advise to consider weight-bearing exercises as well as modification of behavioral factors (eg, excessive cigarette smoking, alcohol consumption). Instruct patients to read the PI before starting therapy and to re-read each time the prescription is renewed. Refer to PI for instructions on missed doses. Inform not to take two 35mg-tabs on the same day, or >two 75mg-tabs within 7 days, or >one 150mg-tab within 7 days.

**Administration:** Oral route. **Storage**: 20-25°C (68-77°F).

## ACTONEL WITH CALCIUM RX

risedronate sodium - calcium carbonate (Procter & Gamble)

**THERAPEUTIC CLASS:** Bisphosphonate

**INDICATIONS:** Treatment and prevention of postmenopausal osteoporosis.

**DOSAGE:** *Adults:* Risedronate: 35mg once weekly (Day 1 of 7-day treatment cycle). Take at least 30 min before 1st food or drink of day other than water. Swallow tab in upright position with 6-8oz of plain water. Do not lie down for 30 min after dose. Calcium: 1250mg qd with food on each of remaining 6 days (Days 2-7 of the 7-day treatment cycle).

**HOW SUPPLIED:** Tab: (Risedronate Sodium) 35mg; Tab: (Calcium Carbonate) 1250mg

**CONTRAINDICATIONS:** (Risedronate) Hypocalcemia; inability to stand or sit upright for at least 30 min. (Calcium) Hypercalcemia from any cause (eg, hyperparathyroidism, hypercalcemia of malignancy, sarcoidosis).

**WARNINGS/PRECAUTIONS:** (Risedronate) May cause upper GI disorders (eg, dysphagia, esophagitis, esophageal or gastric ulcer). Treat hypocalcemia and other disturbances of bone and mineral metabolism before therapy. May cause osteonecrosis, primarily in jaw. Avoid with severe renal impairment (CrCl <30mL/min). (Calcium) Should not be used to treat hypocalcemia. Daily intake above 2000mg has been associated with increased risk of adverse effects, including hypercalcemia and kidney stones. Patients with achlorhydria may have decreased absorption of calcium. Severe and occasionally incapacitating bone, joint, and/or muscle pain in patient taking bisphosphonates reported.

**ADVERSE REACTIONS:** Risedronate: Infection, pain, flu syndrome, abdominal pain, headache, asthenia, HTN, constipation, dyspepsia, arthralgia, nausea, diarrhea, dizziness, myalgia. Calcium: Constipation, flatulence, nausea, abdominal pain, and bloating.

**INTERACTIONS:** Risedronate: Calcium supplements, and calcium-, aluminum-, and magnesium-containing agents may interfere with absorption; space doses. Calcium: May reduce absorption of levothyroxine, fluoroquinolones, tetracycline. Calcium absorption reduced when taken with systemic glucocorticoids. Reduced urinary excretion of calcium with use of thiazide diuretics. Absorption of calcium increased with use of vitamin D and analogues. May interfere with absorption of iron. Take iron and calcium at different times of the day.

**PREGNANCY:** Category C, not for use in nursing.

**MECHANISM OF ACTION:** Risedronate: Bisphosphonate; inhibits osteoclast-mediated bone resorption and modulates bone metabolism. Calcium: Major substrate for mineralization; has antiresorptive effect on bone. Suppresses PTH secretion and decreases bone turnover.

**PHARMACOKINETICS: Absorption**: Risedronate: Relatively rapid. $T_{max}$=1 hr; absolute bioavailability (30mg): (0.63%). **Distribution**: Risedronate: $V_d$=6.3L/kg, plasma protein binding (24%). Calcium: Plasma protein binding (40%). **Elimination**: Risedronate: Urine, feces (unabsorbed dose); $T_{1/2}$=480 hrs. Calcium: Renal, feces (unabsorbed dose).

### NURSING CONSIDERATIONS

**Assessment:** Assess for hypocalcemia and other bone disturbances; treat appropriately prior to therapy. Assess for hypercalcemia from any cause (eg, hyperparathyroidism, hypercalcemia of malignancy, sarcoidosis), inability to stand or sit upright for 30 min, severe renal impairment (CrCl <30mL/min), risk of osteonecrosis, history of kidney stones or hypercalciuria, achlorhydria, pregnancy/nursing status, and possible drug interactions.

**Monitoring:** Monitor for signs/symptoms of GI disorders (eg, dysphagia, esophagitis, esophageal or gastric ulcers), osteonecrosis, musculoskeletal pain, and kidney stone formation. Perform periodic monitoring of urinary calcium excretion in patients with kidney stones.

**Patient Counseling:** Actonel: Advise to take as directed. Take at least 30 min before first food or drink of day other than water. Take in an upright position (eg, sitting or standing) with a full glass of plain water and avoid lying down for 30 min after administration. Avoid chewing or sucking medication. Contact physician if develop symptoms of esophageal disease (eg, difficulty or pain swallowing, worsening heartburn). If patient misses one 35mg dose taken once weekly, instruct to take 1 tablet the morning after remembering and return to taking 1 tab once a week on originally scheduled day; avoid taking 2 tabs in one day. Advise to take supplemental calcium and vitamin D if dietary intake is inadequate. Counsel to consider weight-bearing exercises and modification of certain behavioral factors (eg, excessive cigarette smoking, alcohol consumption). Calcium: Instruct to take with food.

**Administration:** Oral route. **Storage**: 20-25°C (68-77°F); excursions permitted to 15-30°C (59-86°F).

## ACTOPLUS MET — RX

pioglitazone HCl - metformin HCl (Takeda)

**Thiazolidinediones may cause or exacerbate CHF in some patients. After initiation and dose increases, observe patients for signs/symptoms of HF; if they develop, heart failure should be managed according to current standards of care and d/c or dose reduction of drug must be considered. Not recommended in patients with symptomatic HF.**

**THERAPEUTIC CLASS:** Thiazolidinedione/biguanide

**INDICATIONS:** Adjunct to diet and exercise to improve glycemic control in adults with type 2 diabetes mellitus who are already treated with a thiazolidinedione and metformin or who have inadequate glycemic control on a thiazolidinedione alone or metformin alone.

**DOSAGE:** *Adults:* Individualize dose. Prior Pioglitazone/Metformin: Base on current regimen. Prior Pioglitazone Monotherapy or Metformin Monotherapy: (Actoplus Met) Initial: 15mg-500mg or 15mg-850mg qd-bid with food. Titrate: Gradually increase after assessing adequacy of therapeutic response. Max: 45mg-2550mg. Elderly/Debilitated/Malnourished: Conservative dosing; do not titrate to max dose.

**HOW SUPPLIED:** Tab: (Pioglitazone-Metformin) 15mg-500mg, 15mg-850mg

**CONTRAINDICATIONS:** Established NYHA Class III or IV HF, renal disease or dysfunction (eg, SrCr ≥1.5mg/dL [males], ≥1.4mg/dL [females], or abnormal CrCl), and acute or chronic metabolic acidosis, including diabetic ketoacidosis. Temporarily d/c in patients undergoing radiologic studies involving intravascular iodinated contrast materials.

**WARNINGS/PRECAUTIONS:** (Metformin) Lactic acidosis may occur due to metformin accumulation; d/c product if acidosis is suspected. Increased risk with renal dysfunction, increased age, DM, CHF, and other conditions with risk of hypoperfusion and hypoxemia. Avoid in patients ≥80 yrs unless renal function is normal. Monitor renal function and for ketoacidosis and metabolic acidosis. Avoid in renal/hepatic impairment. D/C in hypoxic states (eg, CHF, shock, acute MI), loss of blood glucose control due to stress (give insulin), acidosis, dehydration, sepsis. Temporarily d/c prior to surgery (due to restricted food intake) and procedures requiring IV iodinated contrast materials. May decrease serum $B_{12}$ levels. Increased risk of hypoglycemia in elderly, in debilitated/malnourished, with adrenal or pituitary insufficiency, or with alcohol intoxication. Alcohol known to potentiate effect of metformin on lactate metabolism. (Pioglitazone) May cause fluid retention and exacerbation/initiation of heart failure; d/c if cardiac status deteriorates. Use lowest approved dose if systolic HF (NYHA Class II). Not for use in type 1 diabetes or for diabetic ketoacidosis treatment. Caution with edema. Dose-related wt gain reported. Ovulation in premenopausal anovulatory patients may occur; risk of pregnancy with inadequate contraception. May decrease Hgb and Hct. Avoid with active liver disease, if ALT levels >2.5x ULN. D/C if jaundice occurs or ALT

>3x ULN on therapy. Macular edema reported. Increased risk of fractures in female patients.

**ADVERSE REACTIONS:** Upper respiratory tract infection, diarrhea, nausea, headache, UTI, sinusitis, dizziness.

**INTERACTIONS:** (Pioglitazone) Possible loss of contraception with ethinyl estradiol and norethindrone; caution when coadministering. Ketoconazole may inhibit pioglitazone metabolism; evaluate for glycemic control more frequently. Risk of hypoglycemia with insulin or oral hypoglycemic agents. May cause reduction of midazolam levels. CYP2C8 inhibitors (eg, gemfibrozil) may significantly increase AUC of pioglitazone. CYP2C8 inducers (eg, rifampin) may significantly decrease AUC of pioglitazone. (Metformin) Furosemide, nifedipine, cimetidine, cationic drugs (eg, digoxin, amiloride, procainamide, quinidine, quinine, ranitidine, trimethoprim, vancomycin, triamterene, morphine) may increase metformin levels. Thiazides, other diuretics, corticosteroids, phenothiazines, thyroid products, estrogens, oral contraceptives, phenytoin, nicotinic acid, sympathomimetics, CCBs, or isoniazid may cause hyperglycemia. Risk of hypoglycemia with alcohol; excess alcohol may increase potential for lactic acidosis. May decrease furosemide levels.

**PREGNANCY:** Category C, not for use in nursing.

**MECHANISM OF ACTION:** Pioglitazone: Thiazolidinedione; insulin sensitizing agent, enhances peripheral glucose utilization, decreases insulin resistance in periphery and liver resulting in increased insulin-dependent glucose disposal and decreased hepatic glucose output. Metformin: Biguanide; decreases endogenous hepatic glucose production, also decreases intestinal absorption of glucose and improves insulin sensitivity, improves glucose tolerance in patients with type 2 DM.

**PHARMACOKINETICS: Absorption:** Variable doses resulted in different pharmacokinetic parameters. Refer to PI. **Distribution:** Pioglitazone: $V_d$ =0.63L/kg, plasma protein binding (>99%). Metformin: $V_d$ =654L. **Metabolism:** Pioglitazone: Hydroxylation and oxidation (extensive). Via CYP450 (2C8, 3A4, 1A1). (Active metabolites) M-II [hydroxy derivative], M-III [keto derivative], M-IV [hydroxy derivative]. Metformin: No hepatic metabolism. **Elimination:** Refer to PI for $T_{1/2}$ values. Pioglitazone: Urine (15%-30%), bile/feces. Metformin: Urine (unchanged)

## NURSING CONSIDERATIONS

**Assessment:** Obtain baseline LFTs, renal function tests, CBC. Assess for lactic acidosis, metabolic acidosis, CHF, macular edema, type 1 DM, diabetic ketoacidosis, hypersensitivity, and possible drug interactions. Assess for history of hepatic insufficiency, and renal impairment (eg, abnormal CrCl). Assess pregnancy/nursing status.

**Monitoring:** Monitor FPG and $HbA_{1c}$ periodically for glycemic control and therapeutic response. Perform LFTs, hematologic parameters, renal function, and eye exams periodically. Monitor for signs/symptoms of heart failure, edema, lactic acidosis, diabetic ketoacidosis, fractures.

**Patient Counseling:** Inform to d/c with unexplained hyperventilation, myalgia, malaise, unusual somnolence symptoms. Counsel to report unexplained GI symptoms, rapid increase in weight or edema, SOB, N/V, abdominal pain, fatigue, anorexia, or dark urine. Inform to avoid excessive alcohol intake. Counsel females about use of reliable contraception. Advise on importance of regular follow-up visits.

**Administration:** Oral route. **Storage:** 25°C (77°F); excursions permitted to 15-30°C (59-86°F). Keep container tightly closed. Protect from moisture and humidity.

# ACTOS

RX

pioglitazone HCl (Takeda)

**Thiazolidinediones may cause or exacerbate CHF in some patients. Pioglitazone is not recommended in patients with symptomatic heart failure.**

**THERAPEUTIC CLASS:** Thiazolidinedione

**INDICATIONS:** Adjunct to diet and exercise, to improve glycemic control in type 2 diabetes mellitus.

**DOSAGE:** *Adults:* Monotherapy: Initial: 15-30mg qd. Max: 45mg/day. Combination Therapy: Initial: 15-30mg qd. Max: 30mg/day. Decrease insulin dose by 10-25% if hypoglycemia occurs or if plasma glucose is <100mg/dL. Decrease sulfonylurea dose with hypoglycemia also.

**HOW SUPPLIED:** Tab: 15mg, 30mg, 45mg

**CONTRAINDICATIONS:** Established NYHA Class III or IV heart failure.

**WARNINGS/PRECAUTIONS:** May cause fluid retention and exacerbation/initiation of heart failure; d/c if cardiac status deteriorates. Avoid if NYHA Class III or IV cardiac status. Use lowest approved dose if systolic heart failure (NYHA Class II). Not for use in type 1 diabetes or for diabetic ketoacidosis treatment. Caution with edema. Dose-related wt gain reported. Ovulation in premenopausal anovulatory patients may occur; risk of pregnancy with inadequate contraception. May decrease Hgb and Hct. Avoid with active liver disease, if ALT levels >2.5x ULN. Check LFTs before therapy, every 2 months for 1 yr, and periodically thereafter, or if hepatic dysfunction symptoms occur. D/C if jaundice occurs or ALT >3x ULN on therapy. Macular edema reported. Increased incidence of bone fracture was noted in female patients.

**ADVERSE REACTIONS:** Upper respiratory tract infection, myalgia, tooth disorder, headache, sinusitis, pharyngitis, transient CPK level elevations, CHF, weight gain, aggravated DM, edema, dyspnea, new onset or worsening of diabetic macular edema.

**INTERACTIONS:** Possible loss of contraception with ethinyl estradiol and norethindrone; caution when co-administering. Ketoconazole may inhibit pioglitazone metabolism; evaluate glycemic control more frequently. Risk for hypoglycemia with insulin or oral hypoglycemic agents. May cause reduction of midazolam levels. An enzyme inhibitor of CYP2C8 (such as gemfibrozil) may significantly increase the AUC of pioglitazone and an enzyme inducer of CYP2C8 (such as rifampin) may significantly decrease the AUC of pioglitazone.

**PREGNANCY:** Category C, not for use in nursing.

**MECHANISM OF ACTION:** Thiazolidinedione; decreases insulin resistance in the periphery and liver resulting in increased insulin-dependent glucose disposal and decreased hepatic glucose output.

**PHARMACOKINETICS: Absorption:** $T_{max}$=within 2 hrs (fasting), 3-4 hrs (with food). **Distribution:** $V_d$=0.63±0.41 L/kg; plasma protein binding (>99%). **Metabolism:** Hydroxylation and oxidation; active metabolites: M-II and M-IV (hydroxy derivatives), M-III (keto derivative); CYP450 enzymes: 2C8, 3A4. **Elimination:** Urine (15-30%), bile (unchanged), feces (metabolites); $T_{1/2}$=3-7 hrs (pioglitazone), 16-24 hrs (total pioglitazone).

## NURSING CONSIDERATIONS

**Assessment:** Assess for history of insulin-induced hypoglycemia, serum ALT, $HbA_{1c}$, active liver disease, class III or IV symptomatic heart failure, and other drug interactions. After initiation and dose increases, observe carefully for signs/symptoms of heart failure, including excessive and rapid weight gain, dyspnea, and/or edema.

**Monitoring:** Perform FPG and $HbA_{1c}$ measurements periodically to monitor glycemic control and therapeutic response. Monitor for signs/symptoms of heart failure, liver function tests (serum ALT), and hematological parameters (Hgb/Hct). Monitor adverse events related to fluid retention after initiation and with dose increases.

**Patient Counseling:** Advise to adhere to dietary instructions and to regularly test blood glucose and glycosylated hemoglobin. Drug can be taken with/without meals once daily; if dose is missed, do not double dose the following day. Instruct to immediately report SOB, rapid increase in weight or edema, unexplained N/V, anorexia, fatigue, and dark urine.

**Administration:** Oral route. **Storage:** 25°C (77°F); excursions permitted to 15-30°C (59-86°F). Keep container tightly closed. Protect from moisture and humidity.

## Acular RX

ketorolac tromethamine (Allergan)

**THERAPEUTIC CLASS:** NSAID

**INDICATIONS:** Ocular itching due to seasonal allergic conjunctivitis. Postoperative inflammation in cataract extraction.

**DOSAGE:** *Adults:* 1 drop qid. Post-op Inflammation: Begin 24 hrs post-op and continue for 2 weeks.
*Pediatrics:* ≥3 yrs: 1 drop qid. Post-op Inflammation: Begin 24 hrs post-op and continue for 2 weeks.

**HOW SUPPLIED:** Sol: 0.5% [3mL, 5mL, 10mL]

**WARNINGS/PRECAUTIONS:** May increase ocular tissue bleeding in conjunction with ocular surgery. Avoid use with contact lenses. D/C if corneal epithelium breakdown occurs. Caution in known bleeding tendencies, complicated ocular surgeries, corneal denervation, corneal epithelial defects, diabetes mellitus (DM), ocular surface diseases (eg, dry eye syndrome), rheumatoid arthritis, or repeat ocular surgeries within a short period of time. Caution if used >24 hrs prior to surgery and use beyond 14 days post-surgery.

**ADVERSE REACTIONS:** Transient stinging/burning, superficial keratitis or infections, allergic reactions, ocular inflammation, corneal edema, iritis.

**INTERACTIONS:** Potential for cross-sensitivity to acetylsalicylic acid, phenylacetic acid derivatives, and other NSAIDs. Caution with agents that may prolong bleeding time. Increased potential for healing problems with topical steroids.

**PREGNANCY:** Category C, caution in nursing.

**MECHANISM OF ACTION:** NSAID; inhibits prostaglandin biosynthesis.

**PHARMACOKINETICS: Absorption:** $C_{max}$=95ng/mL; $T_{max}$=12hrs.

### NURSING CONSIDERATIONS

**Assessment:** Assess for drug hypersensitivity, cross-sensitivity reactions, bleeding tendencies, complicated ocular surgeries, corneal denervation, corneal epithelial defects, DM, ocular surface disease (dry eye syndrome), rheumatoid arthritis, possible drug interactions.

**Monitoring:** Monitor for bleeding of ocular tissues (hyphema), healing problems, keratitis, epithelial breakdown, corneal thinning/erosion/ulceration/perforation.

**Patient Counseling:** Advise not to use while wearing contact lenses. Caution during nursing/late pregnancy.

**Administration:** Intraocular route. **Storage:** 15-25°C (59-77°F), protect from light.

## Adalat CC RX

nifedipine (Schering)

**OTHER BRAND NAMES:** Afeditab CR (Watson)

**THERAPEUTIC CLASS:** Calcium channel blocker (dihydropyridine)

**INDICATIONS:** Treatment of hypertension alone or in combination with other antihypertensive agents.

**DOSAGE:** *Adults:* Initial: 30mg qd. Titrate over 7-14 days. Usual: 30-60mg qd. Max: 90mg/day. Elderly: Start at low end of dosing range. Take on empty stomach. Swallow tab whole; do not bite or divide.

**HOW SUPPLIED:** Tab, Extended-Release: (Adalat CC, Afeditab CR) 30mg, 60mg, (Adalat CC) 90mg

**WARNINGS/PRECAUTIONS:** May cause hypotension; monitor BP initially or with titration. May exacerbate angina from β-blocker withdrawal. CHF risk, especially with aortic stenosis or β-blockers. Peripheral edema reported. May increase angina or MI with severe obstructive CAD. Caution in elderly.

**ADVERSE REACTIONS:** Headache, flushing, heat sensation, dizziness, peripheral edema, fatigue, asthenia.

**INTERACTIONS:** β-blockers may increase risk of CHF, severe hypotension, or angina exacerbation. Possible hypotension with fentanyl. Monitor digoxin, quinidine, and coumarin levels. Caution with diltiazem. Enhanced hypotensive effect with benazepril, timolol. CYP3A4 inhibitors (eg, verapamil, ketoconazole, itraconazole, fluconazole, erythromycin, protease inhibitors) may increase levels. Avoid with grapefruit juice. Cimetidine may increase levels. CYP3A4 inducers (eg, carbamazepine, phenytoin, phenobarbitone, rifampin, rifapentine, St. John's wort) may decrease levels. Hyperglycemia and loss of glucose control may occur; monitor blood glucose level and consider dose adjustment when co-administering with acarbose.

**PREGNANCY:** Category C, not for use in nursing.

**MECHANISM OF ACTION:** Calcium channel blocker; involved in peripheral arterial vasodilation and consequently reduction in peripheral vascular resistance.

**PHARMACOKINETICS: Absorption:** Complete; absolute bioavailability (84-89%); $C_{max}$=115ng/mL; $T_{max}$=2.5-5 hrs. **Distribution:** Plasma protein binding (92-98%); found in breast milk. **Metabolism:** Liver (extensive). **Elimination:** Urine (60-80% as metabolite/unchanged), feces (metabolite); $T_{1/2}$=7 hrs.

## NURSING CONSIDERATIONS

**Assessment:** Assess for hypotension, CHD, aortic stenosis, hepatic/renal impairment, pregnancy/nursing status, and possible drug interactions.

**Monitoring:** Carefully monitor BP and HR during initial administration and titration. Monitor for signs/symptoms of CHF, hypotension, cholestasis with/without jaundice, peripheral edema, angina, MI, lab tests (eg, elevations in alkaline phosphatase, CPK, LDH, SGOT, and SGPT), decrease in platelet aggregation, increased bleeding time, positive direct Coombs' test with/without hemolytic anemia, and reversible elevation in BUN and serum creatinine.

**Patient Counseling:** Instruct to swallow whole; do not bite or divide. Take on empty stomach. Do not take with grapefruit juice. Inform about potential benefits/risks and to report any adverse reactions to physician. Notify if pregnant/nursing.

**Administration:** Oral route. **Storage:** Below 30°C (86°F); in tight, light-resistant container. Protect from light and moisture.

# ADDERALL

CII

amphetamine salt combo (Shire)

**High potential for abuse; avoid prolonged use. Misuse of amphetamine may cause sudden death and serious cardiovascular adverse events.**

**THERAPEUTIC CLASS:** Sympathomimetic amine

**INDICATIONS:** Treatment of attention deficit disorder with hyperactivity (ADHD) and narcolepsy.

**DOSAGE:** *Adults:* Narcolepsy: Initial: 10mg/day. Titrate: May increase by 10mg/day every week. Usual: 5-60mg/day. Give 1st dose upon awakening, and additional doses q4-6h.

*Pediatrics:* ADHD: 3-5 yrs: Initial: 2.5mg qd. Titrate: May increase by 2.5mg weekly. ≥6 yrs: 5mg qd-bid. May increase by 5mg weekly. Max (usual): 40mg/day. Narcolepsy: 6-12 yrs: Initial: 5mg/day. May increase by 5mg weekly. ≥12 yrs: Initial: 10mg/day. Titrate: May increase by 10mg/day every week. Usual: 5-60mg/day. Give 1st dose upon awakening, and additional doses q4-6h.

**HOW SUPPLIED:** Tab: 5mg*, 7.5mg*, 10mg*, 12.5mg*, 15mg*, 20mg*, 30mg* *scored

**CONTRAINDICATIONS:** Advanced arteriosclerosis, symptomatic cardiovascular disease, moderate to severe HTN, hyperthyroidism, glaucoma, agitated states, history of drug abuse, during or within 14 days of MAOI use.

**WARNINGS/PRECAUTIONS:** May exacerbate symptoms of behavior disturbance and thought disorder in psychotic patients. Caution when using stimulants to treat patients with comorbid bipolar disorder because of concern for possible induction of mixed/manic episode in such patients. Stimulants at usual doses can cause treatment emergent psychotic or manic symptoms (eg, hallucinations, delusional thinking, mania) in children and adolescents without prior history of psychotic illness. Aggressive behavior or hostility reported in clinical trials and the postmarketing experience of some medications indicated for the treatment of ADHD. Monitor growth in children. May lower convulsive threshold; d/c in presence of seizures. Visual disturbances reported with stimulant treatment. May exacerbate Tourette's syndrome and phonic or motor tics. Caution with HTN and monitor BP. Interrupt occasionally to determine if patient requires continued therapy. Sudden death reported in children with structural cardiac abnormalities; avoid with known structural cardiac abnormalities or other serious cardiac problems.

**ADVERSE REACTIONS:** HTN, tachycardia, palpitations, CNS overstimulation, dry mouth, GI disorders, anorexia, impotence, urticaria, rash, angioedema, anaphylaxis, Stevens-Johnson syndrome.

**INTERACTIONS:** GI acidifying agents (eg, guanethidine, reserpine, glutamic acid, etc.) and urinary acidifying agents (eg, ammonium chloride, etc.) decrease efficacy. MAOIs may cause hypertensive crisis. Potentiated by GI and urinary alkalinizers, propoxyphene overdose. Potentiated effects of both agents with TCAs. May delay absorption of phenytoin, ethosuximide, phenobarbital. Potentiates meperidine, norepinephrine, phenobarbital, phenytoin. Antagonized by haloperidol, chlorpromazine, lithium. Antagonizes adrenergic blockers, antihistamines, antihypertensives, veratrum alkaloids (antihypertensive). Avoid coadministration with alkalinizing agents (eg, antacids).

**PREGNANCY:** Category C, not for use in nursing.

**MECHANISM OF ACTION:** CNS stimulant; thought to block reuptake of norepinephrine and dopamine into presynaptic neuron and increase release of these monoamines into extraneuronal space.

**PHARMACOKINETICS: Absorption**: $T_{max}$=approximately 3 hrs (fasted). **Metabolism**: CYP2D6 (oxidation): 4-hydroxy-amphetamine and norephedrine. **Elimination**: Urine, $T_{1/2}$=9.77-11 hrs (d-amphetamine), 11.5-13.8 hrs (l-amphetamine).

## NURSING CONSIDERATIONS

**Assessment:** Assess for agitation, glaucoma, tics, family history of Tourette's syndrome, cardiovascular conditions (eg, severe HTN, angina pectoris, cardiac abnormalities, arrhythmias, heart failure, recent MI), hyperthyroidism or thyrotoxicosis, bipolar illness, history of drug dependence or alcoholism.

**Monitoring:** Monitor for cardiac abnormalities, exacerbations of behavior disturbances and thought disorder, bipolar illness, aggression, seizures, and visual disturbances. Periodic monitoring of CBC, differential and platelet count, LFTs. Monitor height and weight in children.

**Patient Counseling:** Inform about risks of treatment, appropriate use, drug abuse/dependence. Caution while operating machinery/driving.

**Administration:** Oral route. **Storage**: 20-25°C (68-77°F).

# ADDERALL XR

CII

amphetamine salt combo (Shire)

**High potential for abuse; avoid prolonged use. Misuse of amphetamine may cause sudden death and serious cardiovascular adverse events.**

## ADDERALL XR

**THERAPEUTIC CLASS:** Sympathomimetic amine

**INDICATIONS:** Treatment of attention deficit hyperactivity disorder (ADHD).

**DOSAGE:** *Adults:* Initial: 20mg qam. Currently Using Adderall: Switch to Adderall XR at the same total daily dose, taken once daily. Titrate at weekly intervals as needed. Swallow cap whole or open cap and sprinkle contents on applesauce; do not chew beads.
*Pediatrics:* ≥6 yrs: Initial: 10mg qam. Titrate: May increase weekly by 5-10mg/day. Max: 30mg/day. 13 to 17 yrs: Initial: 10mg/day. Titrate: May increase to 20mg/day after one week. Currently Using Adderall: Switch to Adderall XR at the same total daily dose, taken once daily. Titrate at weekly intervals as needed. Swallow cap whole or open cap and sprinkle contents on applesauce; do not chew beads.

**HOW SUPPLIED:** Cap, Extended-Release: 5mg, 10mg, 15mg, 20mg, 25mg, 30mg

**CONTRAINDICATIONS:** Advanced arteriosclerosis, symptomatic cardiovascular disease, moderate to severe HTN, hyperthyroidism, glaucoma, agitated states, history of drug abuse, during or within 14 days of MAOI use.

**WARNINGS/PRECAUTIONS:** May exacerbate symptoms of behavior disturbance and thought disorder in psychotic patients. Caution when using stimulants to treat patients with comorbid bipolar disorder because of concern for possible induction of mixed/manic episode in such patients. Stimulants at usual doses can cause treatment emergent psychotic or manic symptoms (eg, hallucinations, delusional thinking, mania) in children and adolescents without prior history of psychotic illness. Aggressive behavior or hostility reported in clinical trials and postmarketing experience of some medications indicated for the treatment of ADHD. Monitor growth in children. May lower convulsive threshold; d/c in presence of seizures. Visual disturbances reported with stimulant treatment. May exacerbate Tourette's syndrome and phonic or motor tics. Caution with HTN and monitor BP. Interrupt occasionally to determine if patient requires continued therapy. Sudden death reported in children with structural cardiac abnormalities; avoid with known structural cardiac abnormalities or other serious cardiac problems. May decrease appetite.

**ADVERSE REACTIONS:** Abdominal pain, asthenia, fever, infection, viral infection, loss of appetite, diarrhea, N/V, emotional lability, insomnia, nervousness, weight loss, dry mouth, headache, urticaria, anaphylaxis.

**INTERACTIONS:** GI acidifying agents (guanethidine, reserpine, glutamic acid, etc) and urinary acidifying agents (ammonium chloride, etc) decrease efficacy. MAOIs may cause hypertensive crisis. Potentiated by GI and urinary alkalinizers, propoxyphene overdose. Potentiated effects of both agents with TCAs. May delay absorption of phenytoin, ethosuximide, phenobarbital. Potentiates meperidine, norepinephrine, phenobarbital, phenytoin. Antagonized by haloperidol, chlorpromazine, lithium. Antagonizes adrenergic blockers, antihistamines, antihypertensives, veratrum alkaloids (antihypertensive). Avoid coadministration of alkalinizing agents (eg, antacid).

**PREGNANCY:** Category C, not for use in nursing.

**MECHANISM OF ACTION:** CNS stimulant; thought to block reuptake of norepinephrine and dopamine into presynaptic neuron and increase release of these monoamines into extraneuronal space.

**PHARMACOKINETICS: Absorption**: $T_{max}$=7 hrs. **Metabolism**: CYP2D6 (oxidation): 4-hydroxy-amphetamine and norepinephrine (metabolites). **Elimination**: Urine (30-40%). D-amphetamine: $T_{1/2}$=10 hrs (adults), 11 hrs (adolescents aged 13-17 years), 9 hrs (6-12 years). l-amphetamine: $T_{1/2}$=13 hrs (adults), 13-14 hrs (adolescents aged 13-17), 11 hrs (6-12 yrs).

### NURSING CONSIDERATIONS

**Assessment:** Assess for agitation, glaucoma, tics, family history of Tourette's syndrome, cardiovascular conditions (eg, severe HTN, angina pectoris, cardiac abnormalities, arrhythmias, heart failure, recent MI), hyperthyroidism or thyrotoxicosis, bipolar illness, history of drug dependence or alcoholism.

**Monitoring:** Monitor for cardiac abnormalities, exacerbations of behavior disturbances and thought disorder, bipolar illness, aggression, seizures, and visual disturbances. Periodic monitoring of CBC, differential and platelet count, LFTs. Monitor height and weight in children.

**Patient Counseling:** Inform about risk of treatment, appropriate use, and drug abuse/dependence. Caution while operating machinery/driving.

**Administration:** Oral route. **Storage**: 15-30°C (59-86°F).

## ADRENACLICK RX

epinephrine (Sciele)

**THERAPEUTIC CLASS:** Sympathomimetic catecholamine

**INDICATIONS:** Emergency treatment of severe allergic reactions (Type 1) including anaphylaxis to stinging insects (eg, Order Hymenoptera, which includes bees, wasps, hornets, yellow jackets and fire ants), and biting insects (eg, triatoma, mosquitoes), allergen immunotherapy, foods, drugs, diagnostic testing substances (eg, radiocontrast media), and other allergens, as well as anaphylaxis to unknown substances (idiopathic anaphylaxis) or exercise-induced anaphylaxis. For immediate administration with history of anaphylactic reactions.

**DOSAGE:** *Adults:* 15-30kg: Inject 0.15mg IM/SQ into the anterolateral aspect of the thigh. ≥30kg: Inject 0.30mg IM/SQ into the anterolateral aspect of the thigh.
*Pediatrics:* IM/SQ: 15-30kg: Inject 0.15mg IM/SQ into the anterolateral aspect of the thigh. ≥30kg: Inject 0.30mg IM/SQ into the anterolateral aspect of the thigh.

**HOW SUPPLIED:** Inj: 1mg/ml [0.15mg, 0.3mg]

**WARNINGS/PRECAUTIONS:** Avoid injecting into the hands, feet, or buttock; may result in loss of blood flow if accidentally injected into these areas. Avoid IV use or possible inadvertent intravascular administration; may result in cerebral hemorrhage due to sharp rise in BP if accidentally injected. Caution with cardiac arrhythmias, coronary artery or heart disease, or HTN. May precipitate/aggravate angina pectoris and produce ventricular arrhythmias in patients with coronary insufficiency or ischemic heart disease. High risk of developing adverse reactions with hyperthyroidism, cardiovascular disease, HTN, DM, elderly, and pregnant women.

**ADVERSE REACTIONS:** Anxiety, apprehensiveness, restlessness, tremor, weakness, dizziness, sweating, palpitations, pallor, N/V, headache, respiratory difficulties.

**INTERACTIONS:** Monitor for cardiac arrhythmias with cardiac glycosides and diuretics. Effects may be potentiated by tricyclic antidepressants, MAOIs, sodium levothyroxine, and certain antihistamines (eg, chlorpheniramine, tripelennamine, diphenhydramine). Cardiostimulating and bronchodilating effects antagonized by β-adrenergic blockers (eg, propranolol). Vasoconstricting and hypertensive effects antagonized by α-adrenergic blockers (eg, phentolamine). Ergot alkaloids and phenothiazines may reverse pressor effects.

**PREGNANCY:** Category C, safety not known in nursing.

**MECHANISM OF ACTION:** Sympathomimetic catecholamine; acts on α-adrenergic receptors by lessening the vasodilation and increasing permeability that occurs during anaphylactic reaction, leading to loss of intravascular fluid volume and hypotension. Acts on β-adrenergic receptors causing bronchial smooth muscle relaxation that helps alleviate bronchospasm, wheezing, and dyspnea that may occur during anaphylaxis. Helps alleviate pruritus, urticaria, and angioedema, and may be effective in relieving GI and genitourinary symptoms of anaphylaxis because of its relaxer effects on the smooth muscle of the stomach, intestine, uterus, and urinary bladder.

### NURSING CONSIDERATIONS

**Assessment:** Assess for arrhythmias, coronary artery or organic heart disease, HTN, hyperthyroidism, cardiovascular disease, DM, Parkinson's disease, pregnancy status, and possible drug interactions.

**Monitoring:** Monitor BP, HR, blood glucose, signs of cerebral hemorrhage, ventricular arrhythmia, HTN, anginal pain, and other adverse reactions.

**Patient Counseling:** Inform about side effects of therapy (eg, increased pulse rate, sensation of a more forceful heartbeat, palpitations, throbbing headache, pallor, feelings of overstimulation, anxiety, weakness, shakiness, dizziness, or nausea). Side effects may subside rapidly, especially with rest, quiet, and recumbency. Advise to avoid injecting into the hands, feet, or buttocks and to avoid IV route. Advise to inform physician if accidental injection occurs into these areas. Instruct to inspect the solution for particulate matter and discoloration.

**Administration:** SQ or IM route. Inject only at the anterolateral aspect of the thigh. **Storage:** 20-25°C (68-77°F); excursions permitted to 15-30°C (59-86°F). Light sensitive; store in the carrying case provided. Protect from light and freezing. Do not refrigerate. Discard if discolored.

## ADVAIR RX

salmeterol xinafoate - fluticasone propionate (GlaxoSmithKline)

**Long-acting $\beta_2$-adrenergic agonists, such as salmeterol, may increase risk of asthma-related deaths. Use of diskus should be reserved for patients not adequately controlled on other medications or whose disease severity warrants initiation with two maintenance therapies.**

**THERAPEUTIC CLASS:** Corticosteroid/beta$_2$ agonist

**INDICATIONS:** Long-term, maintenance treatment of asthma in patients ≥4 yrs. 250/50: Maintenance treatment of airflow obstruction in patients with COPD, including chronic bronchitis and/or emphysema; to reduce exacerbations of COPD in patients with history of exacerbations.

**DOSAGE:** *Adults:* Asthma: 1 inh q12h (am/pm). Without Prior Inhaled Corticosteroid (CS) Therapy/Inadequate Control on Current Inhaled CS: Initial: 100/50 or 250/50 bid. Max: 500/50 bid. If no response after 2 weeks, may increase to higher strength. Titrate to lowest effective strength after adequate asthma stability is achieved. COPD: (250/50 only): 1 inh q12h (am/pm). If SOB occurs in the period between doses, an inhaled, short-acting beta$_2$-agonist should be taken for immediate relief.
*Pediatrics:* ≥12 yrs*:* Asthma: 1 inh q12h (am/pm). Without Prior Inhaled Corticosteroid (CS) Therapy/Inadequate Control on Current Inhaled CS: Initial: 100/50 or 250/50 bid. Max: 500/50 bid. If no response after 2 weeks, may increase to higher strength. Titrate to lowest effective strength after adequate asthma stability is achieved. (100/50 only): 4-11 yrs: Symptomatic on Inhaled CS: 1 inh of 100/50 q12h (am/pm).

**HOW SUPPLIED:** Disk (Inhalation): (Fluticasone-Salmeterol) (100/50) 0.1mg-0.05mg/inh, (250/50) 0.25mg-0.05mg/inh, (500/50) 0.5mg-0.05mg/inh [14 blisters, 60 blisters]

**CONTRAINDICATIONS:** Primary treatment of status asthmaticus or other acute episodes of asthma or COPD episodes where intensive measures are required; hypersensitivity to milk proteins.

**WARNINGS/PRECAUTIONS:** Should not be initiated during rapidly deteriorating or potentially life-threatening episodes of asthma or COPD. Increased use of inhaled, short-acting $\beta_2$-agonist is marker of deteriorating asthma; reevaluate and reassess treatment regimen. Should not use more often than recommended or at higher dose as recommended; cardiovascular (CV) effects and fatalities reported. Should not be used for the relief of acute symptoms; use short-acting $\beta_2$-agonist to relieve acute symptoms. At treatment initiation, regular use of oral or inhaled, short-acting beta$_2$-agonists should be d/c. Localized infections of the mouth and pharynx with *Candida albicans* reported; if develops, treat accordingly. Lower respiratory tract infections including pneumonia reported in patients with COPD. More susceptible to infections. Caution with active or quiescent TB infections of the respiratory tract, untreated systemic fungal, bacterial, viral, or parasitic infections, or ocular herpes simplex. Deaths due to adrenal insufficiency have occurred with transfer from systemic corticosteroids to inhaled corticosteroids. Resume oral corticosteroids during period of stress or a severe asthma attack. Monitor for systemic corticosteroid effects such as hypercorticism and adrenal suppression; if effects occur reduce dose slowly. May produce paradoxical bronchospasm; d/c immediately, treat, and institute alternative therapy. Immediate hypersensitivity reactions (eg, urticaria, angioedema, rash, bronchospasm) may occur. Upper airway symptoms (eg, laryngeal spasm, irritation, swelling, stridor, choking) reported. CV effects may occur; caution in patients with CV disorders especially coronary insufficiency, cardiac arrhythmias, and HTN. Prolonged use may result to loss of bone mineral density, glaucoma, increased IOP, and cataracts. May cause reduction in growth velocity in pediatric patients. In rare cases, eosinophilic conditions may occur. Caution in patient with convulsive disorder, thyrotoxicosis, elderly, and in those who are unusually responsive to sympathomimetic amines. Changes in blood glucose and/or serum potassium reported.

**ADVERSE REACTIONS:** Asthma: Upper respiratory tract infection/inflammation, pharyngitis, dysphonia, oral candidiasis, bronchitis, cough, headache, N/V. COPD: Pneumonia, oral candidiasis, throat irritation, dysphonia, viral respiratory infection, headache, musculoskeletal pain.

**INTERACTIONS:** Extreme caution with TCAs or MAOIs during or within 2 weeks of d/c such products. Antagonized by β-blockers. Caution with non-$K^+$-sparing diuretics (eg, loop or thiazide diuretics); ECG changes, hypokalemia may develop. Concomitant use with strong CYP3A4 inhibitors (eg, ritonavir, atazanavir, clarithromycin, indinavir, itraconazole, nefazodone, nelfinavir, saquinavir, ketoconazole, telithromycin) is not recommended. Avoid use with other medications containing long-acting $beta_2$-agonists.

**PREGNANCY:** Category C, caution in nursing.

**MECHANISM OF ACTION:** Fluticasone: Corticosteroid with anti-inflammatory activity; inhibits multiple cell types (eg, mast cells, eosinophils, neutrophils, macrophages, lymphocytes) and mediators (eg, histamine, eicosanoids, leukotrienes, cytokines) involved in inflammation and asthmatic response. Salmeterol: Long-acting $\beta_2$-adrenergic agonist; stimulates intracellular adenyl cyclase, which catalyzes conversion of ATP to cAMP, producing relaxation of bronchial smooth muscle and inhibition of release of immediate hypersensitivity mediators from cells (eg, mast cells).

**PHARMACOKINETICS: Absorption:** Fluticasone: (Asthma, 500 bid) $C_{max}$=110pg/mL, (COPD, 250 bid) 53pg/mL. Salmeterol: $C_{max}$=167pg/mL, $T_{max}$=20 min. **Distribution:** Fluticasone: $V_d$=4.2L/kg; plasma protein binding (91%). Salmeterol: Plasma protein binding (96%); Xinafoate Moiety: Plasma protein binding (>99%). **Metabolism:** Fluticasone: Liver via CYP3A4. Salmeterol: Liver, via CYP3A4 to α-hydroxysalmeterol (metabolite). **Elimination:** Urine, feces; Fluticasone: $T_{1/2}$=7.8 hrs. Salmeterol: $T_{1/2}$=5.5 hrs; Xinafoate Moiety: $T_{1/2}$=11 days.

## NURSING CONSIDERATIONS

**Assessment:** Assess if asthma is controlled by inhaled corticosteroids and occasional use of short-acting $\beta_2$-agonists. Assess for hypersensitivity to milk proteins, acute bronchospasm; rapidly deteriorating asthma or COPD, risk factors for decreased bone mineral content (eg, tobacco use, advanced age, prolonged immobilization, poor nutrition, family history of osteoporosis, drugs that decrease bone mass); CVD (eg, coronary insufficiency, cardiac arrhythmia, HTN); convulsive disorder; thyrotoxicosis; DM; history of increased IOP; glaucoma; cataracts; active or quiescent pulmonary TB; ocular herpes simplex; untreated systemic fungal, bacterial, parasitic or viral infections; pregnancy/nursing status; and for possible drug interactions. Obtain baseline bone mineral density, eye exam, and lung function prior to therapy.

**Monitoring:** Monitor for localized oral infections with *Candida albicans*, decreased bone mass, upper airway symptoms (eg, laryngeal spasm, irritation, swelling), worsening or acutely deteriorating asthma (eg, increased use of inhaled $\beta_2$-agonist, decreased lung function), development of glaucoma, increased IOP, cardiovascular effects, CNS effects, cataracts, hypercorticism, adrenal suppression, paradoxical bronchospasm, eosinophilic conditions, hypokalemia, hyperglycemia, and for hypersensitivity reactions. Monitor bone mineral density and lung function periodically. Perform periodic eye exams.

Monitor growth in pediatric patients. Monitor for lower respiratory tract infections (eg, pneumonia) in patients with COPD.

**Patient Counseling:** Inform that salemeterol, a component of Advair, may increase the risk of asthma-related death. Advise that medication is not for the relief of acute asthma symptoms or exacerbations of COPD and extra doses should not be used for this purpose. Inform not to d/c therapy unless directed by physician. Instruct to never exhale into diskus or to take diskus apart. Inform to use in horizontal position, never wash mouthpiece or any part of the diskus, and to keep diskus in a dry place. Advise to rinse mouth after inhalation and to spit water out, do not swallow water. Inform may cause reduction in growth velocity (pediatric) and may also unmask conditions (eg, rhinitis, conjunctivitis, eczema). Instruct to avoid exposure to chickenpox or measles. Instruct to seek medical attention if exposed to chickenpox or measles, if existing TB infections or ocular herpes simplex symptoms that do not improve or worsen, during periods of stress or severe asthmatic attack, or if adrenal insufficiency, paradoxical bronchospasm or hypersensitivity reactions occur.

**Administration:** Oral inhalation. More frequent administration or higher number of inhalations (> 1 inhalation bid) is not recommended. After inhalation, rinse mouth with water without swallowing. Refer to PI for further instructions regarding administration. **Storage:** 20-25°C (68-77°F). Store in a dry place, away from direct heat or sunlight. Discard 1 month after removal from pouch or when indicator reads "0", whichever comes first.

## ADVAIR HFA — RX

salmeterol xinafoate - fluticasone propionate (GlaxoSmithKline)

**Long-acting $\beta_2$-adrenergic agonists, such as salmeterol, may increase risk of asthma-related deaths; prescribe only in patients not adequately controlled on other asthma-controller medications or whose disease severity clearly warrants initiation of treatment with 2 maintenance therapies.**

**THERAPEUTIC CLASS:** Corticosteroid/beta$_2$ agonist

**INDICATIONS:** For long-term, maintenance treatment of asthma in patients ≥12 yrs.

**DOSAGE:** *Adults:* Asthma: 2 inh q12h. Without Prior Inhaled Corticosteroid (CS): Initial: 2 inh bid of 45/21 or 115/21. Max: 2 inh of 230/21 bid. Current Inhaled CS: Beclomethasone: ≤160mcg/day use 2 inh of 45/21 bid, 320mcg/day use 2 inh of 115/21 bid, 640mcg/day use 2 inh of 230/21 bid. Budesonide: ≤400mcg/day use 2 inh of 45/21 bid, 800-1200mcg/day use 2 inh of 115/21 bid, 1600mcg/day use 2 inh of 230/21 bid. Flunisolide: ≤1000mcg/day use 2 inh of 45/21 bid, 1250-2000mcg/day use 2 inh of 115/21 bid. Flunisolide HFA: ≤320mcg/day use 2 inh of 45/21 bid, 640mcg/day use 2 inh of 115/21 bid. Fluticasone Aerosol: ≤176mcg/day use 2 inh of 45/21 bid, 440mcg/day use 2 inh of 115/21 bid, 660-880mcg/day use 2 inh of 230/21 bid. Fluticasone Powder: ≤200mcg/day use 2 inh of 45/21 bid, 500mcg/day use 2 inh of 115/21 bid, 1000mcg/day use 2 inh of 230/21 bid. Mometasone Powder: 220mcg/day use 2 inh of 45/21 bid, 440mcg/day use 2 inh of 115/21 bid, 880mcg/day use 2 inh of 230/21 bid. Triamcinolone: ≤1000mcg/day use 2 inh of 45/21 bid, 1100-1600mcg/day use 2 inh of 115/21 bid. If no response within 2 weeks, increase to higher strength.

*Pediatrics:* ≥12 yrs: Asthma: 2 inh q12h. Without Prior Inhaled Corticosteroid (CS): Initial: 2 inh bid of 45/21 or 115/21. Max: 2 inh of 230-21 bid. Current Inhaled CS: Beclomethasone: ≤160mcg/day use 2 inh of 45/21 bid, 320mcg/day use 2 inh of 115/21 bid, 640mcg/day use 2 inh of 230/21 bid. Budesonide: ≤400mcg/day use 2 inh of 45/21 bid, 800-1200mcg/day use 2 inh of 115/21 bid, 1600mcg/day use 2 inh of 230/21 bid. Flunisolide: ≤1000mcg/day use 2 inh of 45/21 bid, 1250-2000mcg/day use 2 inh of 115/21 bid. Flunisolide HFA: ≤320mcg/day use 2 inh of 45/21 bid, 640mcg/day use 2 inh of 115/21 bid. Fluticasone Aerosol: ≤176mcg/day use 2 inh of 45/21 bid, 440mcg/day use 2 inh of 115/21 bid, 660-880mcg/day use 2 inh of 230/21 bid. Fluticasone Powder: ≤200mcg/day use 2 inh of 45/21 bid, 500mcg/day use 2 inh of 115/21 bid, 1000mcg/day use 2 inh of 230/21 bid. Mometasone powder:

220mcg/day use 2 inh of 45/21 bid, 440mcg/day use 2 inh of 115/21 bid, 880mcg/day use 2 inh of 230/21 bid. Triamcinolone: ≤1000mcg/day use 2 inh of 45/21 bid, 1100-1600mcg/day use 2 inh of 115/21 bid. If no response within 2 weeks, increase to higher strength.

**HOW SUPPLIED:** MDI: (Fluticasone-Salmeterol) (45/21) 45mcg-21mcg/inh, (115/21) 115mcg-21mcg/inh, (230/21) 230mcg-21mcg/inh [60 inhalations,120 inhalations]

**CONTRAINDICATIONS:** Primary treatment of status asthmaticus or other acute episodes of asthma where intensive measures are required.

**WARNINGS/PRECAUTIONS:** Should not be initiated in patients during rapidly deteriorating or potentially life-threatening episodes of asthma. Should not be used to treat acute symptoms of shortness of breath; an inhaled, short-acting beta$_2$-agonist (eg, albuterol) should be used for treatment of shortness of breath. Should not use more than 2 inhalations twice daily or exceed recommended dose; prolongation of QTc interval, which may lead to ventricular arrhythmias, reported. Should not be used for transferring patients from systemic corticosteroids to inhaled corticosteroids; deaths from adrenal insufficiency reported. During stress or severe asthma attacks, resume oral corticosteroids. May cause life-threatening paradoxical bronchospasm; treat immediately with an inhaled, short-acting bronchodilator and d/c Advair HFA immediately. Immediate hypersensitivity reactions (eg, urticaria, angioedema, rash, bronchospasm) may occur. Upper airway symptoms (eg, laryngeal spasm, irritation, or swelling, stridor and choking) reported. Avoid exposure to chickenpox or measles; more serious or even fatal course may occur. Caution in CVD, convulsive disorders, thyrotoxicosis, patients unusually responsive to sympathomimetic amines, active or quiescent TB, untreated systemic fungal, bacterial, viral, or parasitic infection, and ocular herpes simplex. Changes in blood glucose and/or serum potassium reported. Monitor for systemic corticosteroid effects such as hypercorticism and adrenal suppression; if effects occur reduce dose slowly. Long-term use may result in loss of bone mineral density; glaucoma, increased IOP, and cataracts. Lower respiratory tract infections (eg, pneumonia) and localized infections of the pharynx with *Candida albicans* reported; treat with appropriate local or systemic therapy. In rare cases, eosinophilic conditions may occur.

**ADVERSE REACTIONS:** Upper respiratory tract infection, throat irritation, upper respiratory tract inflammation, headaches, dysphonia, N/V, musculoskeletal pain, menstruation symptoms, dizziness, gastrointestinal signs/symptoms, intoxication.

**INTERACTIONS:** Extreme caution with TCAs or MAOIs during or within 14 days of use. Should not be used in conjunction with inhaled, long-acting $\beta_2$-agonists. β-blockers blocks the pulmonary effects of β-agonists. Caution with non-potassium sparing diuretics; ECG changes, hypokalemia may develop. Potentiated by ketoconazole, ritonavir, erythromycin, and other CYP3A4 inhibitors; avoid concomitant use with strong CYP3A4 inhibitors.

**PREGNANCY:** Category C, caution in nursing.

**MECHANISM OF ACTION:** Fluticasone: Corticosteroid with anti-inflammatory activity; inhibits multiple cell types (eg, mast cells, eosinophils, neutrophils, macrophages, lymphocytes) and mediators (eg, histamine, eicosanoids, leukotrienes and cytokines) Involved in inflammation and asthmatic response. Salmeterol: $\beta_2$-adrenergic agonist; stimulates intracellular adenyl cyclase, which catalyzes conversion of ATP to cAMP, producing relaxation of bronchial smooth muscle and inhibition of release of immediate hypersensitivity mediators from cells (eg, mast cells).

**PHARMACOKINETICS: Absorption:** Fluticasone: Absolute Bioavailability (5.3%); Salmeterol: $C_{max}$=150pg/mL; $T_{max}$=5-10 mins. **Distribution:** Fluticasone: $V_d$=4.2L/kg; plasma protein binding (99%). Salmeterol: Plasma protein binding (96%). **Metabolism:** Fluticasone: Liver, via CYP3A4. Salmeterol: Extensive by hydroxylation. **Elimination:** Fluticasone: Feces (major), urine (<5%); $T_{1/2}$=7.8 hrs. Salmeterol: Feces (60%), urine (25%); $T_{1/2}$=5.5 hrs.

## NURSING CONSIDERATIONS

**Assessment:** Assess if asthma is controlled by inhaled corticosteroids and occassional use of short-acting $\beta_2$-agonists. Assess for risk factors for decreased bone mineral content (eg, tobacco use, sedentary lifestyle, family history of osteoporosis, drugs that decrease bone mass), CVD (eg, coronary insufficiency, cardiac arrhythmia, HTN), convulsive disorder, thyrotoxicosis, DM, history of increased IOP, glaucoma, cataracts, concomitant diseases like status asthmaticus, active or quiescent pulmonary TB, ocular herpes simplex, untreated systemic fungal, bacterial, parasitic or viral infections, and possible drug interactions, and pregnancy/nursing status. Obtain baseline bone mineral density, eye exam, and lung function prior to therapy.

**Monitoring:** Monitor asthma severity, response to short-acting β-agonist, signs and symptoms of paradoxical bronchospasm, hypersensitivity reactions, cardiovascular effects (eg, ECG changes), infections (eg, pneumonia, *Candida albicans*), changes in blood glucose and serum potassium, and systemic corticosteroid effects (eg, hypercorticism, adrenal suppression). Monitor for eosinophilic conditions presenting as eosinophilia, vasculitic rash, worsening pulmonary symptoms, cardiac complications, and/or neuropathy. For long-term use, monitor bone mineral density, intraocular pressure and signs and symptoms of cataract development. Perform periodic eye exam. After withdrawal, monitor for signs and symptoms of adrenal insufficiency.

**Patient Counseling:** Inform that therapy is not to relieve acute asthma symptoms and extra dose should not be used for that purpose. Instruct to use at regular intervals as directed. Instruct not use more than the prescribed dosage and contact physician if symptoms do not improve or if condition worsens. Inform not to d/c therapy unless directed by physician. Counsel about $\beta_2$-agonists common adverse reactions (eg, palpitations, chest pain, rapid HR, tremor, or nervousness) during therapy. Instruct to get regular eye examinations. Instruct not to use other medications for asthma unless instructed by a physician. Advise to avoid exposure to chickenpox or measles and if exposed, instruct to immediately consult physician. Counsel on appropriate use including priming inhaler before use, rinsing mouth after inhalation, and cleaning inhaler once a week.

**Administration:** Oral inhalation. Prime inhaler before use for first time by releasing 4 test sprays into air, away from face, shaking well for 5 seconds before each spray. If not used for 4 weeks or dropped, reprime by releasing 2 test sprays into air, shaking well before each spray. **Storage:** 25°C (77°F); excursions permitted to 15-30°C (59-86°F). Store with mouthpiece down. Do not puncture. Do not use or store near heat or open flame.

# ADVICOR — RX

lovastatin - niacin (Abbott)

**THERAPEUTIC CLASS:** B-complex vitamin/HMG-CoA reductase inhibitor

**INDICATIONS:** As an adjunct to diet, for the treatment of hypercholesterolemia when use of both Niaspan (niacin ER) and lovastatin is appropriate. (Niacin ER) As adjunct to diet for the treatment of primary hypercholesterolemia and mixed dyslipidemia, as an adjunct for the treatment of hypertriglyceridemia, and for the secondary prevention of cardiovascular events. (Lovastatin) Adjunct to diet for the treatment of primary hypercholesterolemia, and for primary and secondary prevention of cardiovascular events. See individual labeling for further details.

**DOSAGE:** *Adults:* ≥18 yrs: Initial: 500mg-20mg qhs. Titrate: Increase by no more than 500mg of niacin every 4 weeks. Max: 2000mg-40mg qd. Concomitant Cyclosporine/Danazol: Initial: 10mg/day of lovastatin. Max Lovastatin: 20mg/day. Concomitant Amiodarone/Verapamil: Max Lovastatin: 40mg/day. Swallow tab whole. Take with low-fat snack. May pretreat 30 min prior with ASA or other NSAID to reduce flushing. If d/c for an extended period of time (>7 days), reinstitute at the lowest dose.

**HOW SUPPLIED:** Tab: (Extended-Release Niacin- Immediate-Release Lovastatin) 500mg-20mg, 750mg-20mg, 1000mg-20mg, 1000mg-40mg

**CONTRAINDICATIONS:** Active liver disease or unexplained persistent elevations in serum transaminases, active peptic ulcer disease (PUD), arterial bleeding, pregnancy, nursing mothers.

**WARNINGS/PRECAUTIONS:** Do not substitute for equivalent dose of immediate-release niacin. Myopathy, rhabdomyolysis, severe hepatotoxicity reported. Caution with history of liver disease or jaundice, heavy alcohol use, hepatobiliary disease, history of peptic ulcer, diabetes, unstable angina, acute phase of MI, gout, renal dysfunction. Monitor LFTs prior to therapy, every 6-12 weeks for first 6 months, and periodically thereafter. May elevate PT, uric acid levels. Lovastatin may elevate CPK and transaminase levels and produce optic nerve degeneration. D/C if AST or ALT ≥3x ULN persists, if myopathy diagnosed or suspected, and a few days before surgery. May reduce phosphorous levels. May cause endocrine dysfunction. May cause CNS toxicity. Niacin may produce false elevations in some fluorometric determinations of plasma or urinary catecholamines and may give false positive reactions with cupric sulfate solution in urinary glucose tests. May disrupt therapy during a course of treatment with systemic antifungal azole, a macrolide antibiotic or ketolide antibiotic.

**ADVERSE REACTIONS:** Flushing, asthenia, flu syndrome, headache, infection, pain, back pain, diarrhea, nausea, hyperglycemia, myalgia, pruritus, rash.

**INTERACTIONS:** May potentiate ganglionic blockers, vasoactive drugs. Decreased niacin clearance with ASA. Separate bile acid sequestrants by 4-6 hrs. Avoid concomitant alcohol and hot drinks; may increase flushing and pruritus. Antidiabetic agents may need adjustment. Caution with niacin-containing nutritional supplements. Increased risk of skeletal muscle disorders with CYP3A4 inhibitors (eg, cyclosporine, itraconazole, ketoconazole, erythromycin, clarithromycin, telithromycin, danazol, HIV protease inhibitors, nefazodone, >1 quart/day of grapefruit juice), verapamil, fibrates (eg, gemfibrozil). Caution with drugs that diminish levels or activity of steroid hormones (eg, ketoconazole, spironolactone, cimetidine). Caution with acute MI and vasoactive drugs (eg, nitrates, CCBs, adrenergic blockers). Monitor PT before initiating therapy and during early treatment in patients on anticoagulants (eg, warfarin).

**PREGNANCY:** Category X, not for use in nursing.

**MECHANISM OF ACTION:** Niacin: Vitamin B complex; not completely understood and may include various actions, including partial inhibition of free fatty acids from adipose tissue and increased lipoprotein lipase activity. Decreases hepatic synthesis rate of VLDL-C and LDL-C. Lovastatin: Inhibits HMG-CoA reductase enzyme, which is needed for conversion of HMG-CoA to mevalonate. Has LDL-lowering effect by involving both reduction of VLDL-C concentration and induction of the LDL receptor, leading to reduction of production and/or increased catabolism of LDL-C.

**PHARMACOKINETICS: Absorption:** Niacin: $C_{max}$=18mcg/mL, $T_{max}$=5 hrs. Lovastatin: Incomplete, $C_{max}$=11ng/mL, $T_{max}$=2 hrs. **Distribution:** Niacin: Serum protein binding (<20%), found in breast milk. Lovastatin: Plasma protein binding (>95%), crosses blood-brain/placental barrier. **Metabolism:** Niacin: Rapid and extensive. Liver to nicotinamide adenine dinucleotide (NAD) metabolite and other metabolites; conjugation to nicotinuric acid (NUA) (metabolite). Lovastatin: Liver (extensive) via CYP3A4. Lovastatin acid, 6'-hydroxy (active metabolites). **Elimination:** Niacin: Urine (60%); $T_{1/2}$=20-48 min. Lovastatin: Urine (10%), feces (83%), bile; $T_{1/2}$=4.5 hrs.

## NURSING CONSIDERATIONS

**Assessment:** Assess for presence or history of liver disease, unexplained persistent serum transaminase elevations, active peptic ulcer disease or arterial bleeding, pregnancy/nursing status, alcohol intake, DM, upcoming surgery, unstable angina, acute phase of MI, gout, renal impairment, and for possible drug interactions. Perform LFTs prior to therapy. Attempt to control dyslipidemia with appropriate diet, exercise, and weight reduction in obese patients and treat other underlying medical problems before instituting therapy.

**Monitoring:** Monitor for signs and symptoms of hepatotoxicity, myopathy (muscle pain, tenderness, weakness), rhabdomyolysis with or without acute renal failure, endocrine dysfunction, CNS toxicity, and for laboratory test interactions. Perform periodic determinations of CK levels, phosphorus levels, glucose levels, uric acid levels, platelet count, and PT. Monitor LFTs every 6-12 weeks during the first 6 months of therapy and periodically thereafter.

**Patient Counseling:** Instruct to take as prescribed. Inform about risks/benefits of therapy and instruct to report promptly any signs of unexplained muscle pain, tenderness, or weakness. Advise to avoid alcohol and hot drinks around time of drug administration. Counsel to avoid administration with grapefruit juice. Instruct to notify physician if pregnant/nursing or if dizziness occurs. Inform that flushing is a common side effect of drug and inform that taking aspirin or another NSAID (eg, ibuprofen) 30 min before administration may minimize it.

**Administration:** Oral route. Take drug whole at bedtime; do not crush or chew. Do not take on empty stomach or with grapefruit juice. **Storage:** 20-25°C (68-77°F).

## AEROBID RX

flunisolide (Forest)

**OTHER BRAND NAMES:** Aerobid-M (with menthol) (Forest)

**THERAPEUTIC CLASS:** Corticosteroid

**INDICATIONS:** Maintenance treatment of asthma as prophylactic therapy in patients ≥6 years and to reduce or eliminate the need for oral systemic corticosteroidal therapy.

**DOSAGE:** *Adults:* Initial: 2 inh bid. Max: 4 inh bid. Rinse mouth after use. *Pediatrics:* 6-15 yrs: 2 inh bid. Rinse mouth after use.

**HOW SUPPLIED:** MDI: 0.25mg/inh [7g]

**CONTRAINDICATIONS:** Primary treatment of status asthmaticus or other acute asthma attacks.

**WARNINGS/PRECAUTIONS:** Deaths due to adrenal insufficiency have occurred with transfer from systemic corticosteroids to inhaled corticosteroids. Resume oral corticosteroids during stress or severe asthma attack. Observe for adrenal insufficiency, systemic corticosteroid withdrawal effects, and growth suppression (children). More susceptible to infections. Not for acute bronchospasm. D/C if bronchospasm occurs after dosing. Caution with tuberculosis of the respiratory tract; untreated systemic fungal, bacterial, viral, or parasitic infections; or ocular herpes simplex. *Candida* infection of the mouth and pharynx reported.

**ADVERSE REACTIONS:** Upper respiratory infection, diarrhea, stomach upset, cold symptoms, nasal congestion, headache, N/V, sore throat, unpleasant taste.

**PREGNANCY:** Category C, caution with nursing.

**MECHANISM OF ACTION:** Corticosteroid; demonstrated marked anti-inflammatory and anti-allergic activity in test systems.

**PHARMACOKINETICS: Metabolism:** Liver (1st pass). Metabolite (6β-OH). **Elimination:** $T_{1/2}$=1.8 hrs.

### NURSING CONSIDERATIONS

**Assessment:** Assess for concomitant diseases such as status asthmaticus, active or quiescent pulmonary TB, untreated systemic fungal, bacterial or parasitic or viral infections, and possible drug interactions.

**Monitoring:** Monitor for localized oral infections with *Candida albicans*, body height in children, adrenal insufficiency, paradoxical bronchospasm, pulmonary infiltrates with eosinophilia, and hypersensitivity reactions.

**Patient Counseling:** Inform that medication is not for relief of acute bronchospasm. Inform that therapy may unmask allergies (eg, rhinitis, conjunctivitis, eczema). Warn to avoid exposure to chickenpox or measles. Advise to seek medical attention if exposed to chickenpox or measles, symptoms worsen or do not improve, during periods of stress or severe asthmatic attack, adrenal insufficiency, paradoxical bronchospasm or hypersensitivity reactions occur.

**Administration:** Oral inhalation. **Storage:** Do not puncture. Do not use or store near heat or open flame. Exposure to temperatures above 49°C (120°F) may cause container to explode. Never throw container into fire or incinerator. Keep out of reach of children.

## AFLURIA RX

influenza virus vaccine (CSL Biotherapies)

**THERAPEUTIC CLASS:** Vaccine

**INDICATIONS:** Active immunization of individuals ≥6 months against influenza disease caused by influenza virus subtypes A and type B present in the vaccine.

**DOSAGE:** *Adults*: ≥18 yrs: 0.5mL IM in deltoid muscle of upper arm. *Pediatrics:* ≥9 yrs: 0.5mL IM. ≥36 months-8 yrs: Unvaccinated/Previously vaccinated once with 1 dose last season: Give 2 doses of 0.5mL, 1 on day 1 followed by another 4 weeks later. Previously vaccinated with 2 doses last season or 1 dose ≥2 yrs ago: Give 1 dose of 0.5mL. ≥6 months-35 months: Unvaccinated/Previously vaccinated once with 1 dose last season: Give 2 doses of 0.25mL IM, 1 on day 1 followed by another 4 weeks later. Previously vaccinated with 2 doses last season or 1 dose ≥2 yrs ago: Give 1 dose of 0.25mL IM. Preferred sites for IM are the anterolateral aspect of the thigh in infants or deltoid muscle of the upper arm in toddlers and young children.

**HOW SUPPLIED:** Inj: 0.25mL [10 syringes], 0.5mL [10 syringes], MDV: 5mL [10 doses]

**CONTRAINDICATIONS:** Hypersensitivity to eggs, neomycin, or polymyxin, or life-threatening reaction to previous influenza vaccination.

**WARNINGS/PRECAUTIONS:** Caution if Guillain-Barre syndrome (GBS) has occurred within 6 weeks of previous influenza vaccination. Caution in immunocompromised and those receiving immunosuppressive therapy. Medical treatment and supervision must be available to manage possible anaphylactic reaction. Influenza virus vaccine may not protect all individuals.

**ADVERSE REACTIONS:** Local site reactions (tenderness, pain, redness, swelling, bruising), headache, malaise, muscle aches, nausea, chills/shivering, fever, cough, loss of appetite, vomiting/diarrhea, irritability, rhinitis, sore throat.

**INTERACTIONS:** Do not mix with any other vaccine in the same syringe or vial. Administer at different injection sites if given at the same time as another injectable vaccine. May diminish immune response with corticosteroid and immunosuppressive therapies.

**PREGNANCY:** Category C, caution in nursing.

**MECHANISM OF ACTION:** Vaccine; stimulates the immune system to elicit an immune response that produces antibodies that may protect against influenza disease.

### NURSING CONSIDERATIONS

**Assessment:** Assess for allergies, immunosuppression, pregnancy/nursing status, possible drug interactions and local injection-site reactions (eg, tenderness, pain, redness, swelling). Assess potential benefits/risks if GBS occurred with previous influenza vaccination.

**Monitoring:** Monitor for hypersensitivity reactions, injection-site reactions, fever, headache, myalgia, irritability, insomnia, neurological complications (GBS) and anaphylactic shock.

**Patient Counseling:** Inform that effect is achieved approximately 3 weeks after vaccination; annual revaccination is recommended. Instruct to report any severe or unusual adverse reactions.

**Administration:** Inspect visually for particulate matter and discoloration; do not use if present. 1) Administered as a single 0.5mL IM injection, preferably in deltoid muscle of upper arm. 2) When using preservative-free, single-dose syringe, shake syringe and administer dose immediately. 3) When using multi-dose vial, shake vial before withdrawing each dose and administer dose immediately. See PI for full administration instructions. **Storage:** 2-8°C (36-46°C). Do not freeze. Protect from light. Pierced vial must be discarded within 28 days.

## AGGRASTAT RX

tirofiban HCl (Medicure)

**THERAPEUTIC CLASS:** Glycoprotein IIb/IIIa inhibitor

**INDICATIONS:** In combination with heparin, for treatment of acute coronary syndrome, in patients being medically managed or undergoing PTCA or atherectomy.

**DOSAGE:** *Adults:* Initial: 0.4mcg/kg/min IV for 30 min. Maint: 0.1mcg/kg/min IV. Continue through angiography and for 12-24 hrs after angioplasty or atherectomy. CrCl <30mL/min: Administer at half of usual rate of infusion.

**HOW SUPPLIED:** Inj: 0.05mg/mL, 0.25mg/mL

**CONTRAINDICATIONS:** Active internal bleeding, acute pericarditis, severe HTN, concomitant parenteral GP IIb/IIIa inhibitor, hemorrhagic stroke, aortic dissection, thrombocytopenia with prior exposure. Bleeding diathesis, stroke, major surgical procedure, or severe physical trauma within past 30 days. History of intracranial hemorrhage or neoplasm, arteriovenous malformation, aneurysm.

**WARNINGS/PRECAUTIONS:** Bleeding reported. Monitor platelets, Hgb, Hct before treatment, within 6 hrs after loading infusion, and daily during therapy. Monitor platelets earlier if previous GP IIb/IIIa inhibitor use. Determine aPTT before and during therapy with heparin. Caution with platelets <150,000/$mm^3$, hemorrhagic retinopathy, chronic hemodialysis patients, femoral access site in percutaneous coronary intervention. Minimize vascular and other trauma. D/C if thrombocytopenia confirmed or if bleeding cannot be controlled by pressure.

**ADVERSE REACTIONS:** Bleeding, nausea, fever, headache, edema, anaphylaxis.

**INTERACTIONS:** Avoid other parenteral GP IIb/IIIa inhibitors. Increased bleeding with heparin and ASA. Caution with other drugs that affect hemostasis (eg, warfarin). Increased clearance with levothyroxine, omeprazole.

**PREGNANCY:** Category B, not for use in nursing.

**MECHANISM OF ACTION:** Glycoprotein IIb/IIIa inhibitor; reversible antagonist of fibrinogen binding to the GP IIb/IIIa receptor, the major platelet surface receptor involved in platelet aggregation. Inhibits platelet aggregation.

**PHARMACOKINETICS: Absorption:** $C_{max}$=0.01-25mcg/mL. **Distribution**: $V_d$=22-43L; plasma protein binding (35%). **Metabolism:** Limited. **Elimination**: Urine (65%), feces (25%); $T_{1/2}$=2 hrs.

### NURSING CONSIDERATIONS

**Assessment:** Assess for presence or history (within previous 30 days) of internal bleeding; history of intracranial hemorrhage, intracranial neoplasm, arteriovenous malformation, or aneurysm; history of thrombocytopenia following previous exposure to the medication; history of any stroke; major recent surgical procedure or severe trauma; history, symptoms, or findings of aortic dissection; severe HTN; concomitant use of another parenteral GP IIb/IIIa inhibitor; and acute pericarditis. Assess use in patients with platelet counts <150,000/$mm^3$, presence of hemorrhagic retinopathy, and those on chronic hemodialysis. Assess for drug interactions. Obtain baseline platelet counts, Hgb, and Hct.

**Monitoring:** Monitor for signs/symptoms of bleeding, allergic reactions (eg, anaphylaxis), and thrombocytopenia. Monitor platelet counts, Hgb, and Hct within 6 hours of loading infusion, and at least daily thereafter.

**Patient Counseling:** Counsel to notify physician if allergic reaction (eg, anaphylaxis) or bleeding occurs.

**Administration:** IV route. Dilute. 1) If using 500mL of 0.9% NS or D5W, withdraw and discard 100mL from bag and replace this volume with 100mL of drug injection from two 50mL vials. 2) If using 250mL of 0.9% NS or D5W, withdraw and discard 50mL from bag and replace this volume with 50mL of drug injection from one 50mL vial. Mix well prior to administration. **Storage:** 25°C (77°F) with excursions permitted between 15-30°C (59-86°F). Protect from light. Do not freeze.

## AGGRENOX RX

dipyridamole - aspirin (Boehringer Ingelheim)

**THERAPEUTIC CLASS:** Platelet aggregation inhibitor

**INDICATIONS:** Reduce risk of stroke in patients with transient brain ischemia or complete ischemic stroke due to thrombosis.

**DOSAGE:** *Adults:* 1 cap bid (am and pm).

**HOW SUPPLIED:** Cap: (Dipyridamole Extended-Release/ASA) 200mg-25mg

**CONTRAINDICATIONS:** NSAID allergy, children or teenagers with viral infections, syndrome of asthma, rhinitis, nasal polyps.

**WARNINGS/PRECAUTIONS:** Increased risk of bleeding with chronic, heavy alcohol use. Caution with inherited or acquired bleeding disorders, severe CAD, and hypotension. Monitor for signs of GI ulcers and bleeding. Avoid with history of peptic ulcer disease, severe renal failure (CrCl <10mL/min). Risk of hepatic dysfunction. Not interchangeable with individual components of ASA and Persantine tabs. Avoid in 3rd trimester of pregnancy.

**ADVERSE REACTIONS:** Headache, dyspepsia, abdominal pain, N/V, diarrhea, fatigue, arthralgia, pain, hemorrhage.

**INTERACTIONS:** May decrease effects of ACE inhibitors, cholinesterase inhibitors, phenytoin, β-blockers. Potentiates adenosine, acetazolamide, methotrexate, oral hypoglycemics, valproic acid. Anticoagulants increase risk of bleeding. Decreased effects of diuretics in renal or cardiovascular disease. NSAIDs may increase risk of bleeding and decrease renal function. May antagonize uricosuric agents.

**PREGNANCY:** Category D, caution in nursing.

**MECHANISM OF ACTION:** Dipyridamole: Platelet aggregation inhibitor. Inhibits uptake of adenosine into platelets, endothelial cells, and erythrocytes. Leads to increase in adenosine, which acts on platelet $A_2$-receptor to stimulate platelet adenylate cyclase and increase platelet cyclic-3',5'-adenosine monophosphate (cAMP) levels. Platelet aggregation is then inhibited in response to stimuli such as platelet activation factor (PAF), collagen, and adenosine diphosphate (ADP). Also responsible for inhibiting phosphodiesterase (PDE). Weakly inhibits cAMP-PDE. Therapeutic levels of dipyridamole inhibit cyclic-3',5'-guanosine monophosphate-PDE (cGMP-PDE), which helps to augment the increases in cGMP that are produced by endothelium-derived relaxing factor (EDRF). ASA: Platelet aggregation inhibitor. Irreversibly inhibits platelet cyclooxygenase. Leads to inhibition in the generation of thromboxane $A_2$, a powerful inducer of platelet aggregation and vasoconstriction.

**PHARMACOKINETICS: Absorption:** Dipyridamole: $C_{max}$=1.98mcg/mL; $T_{max}$=2 hrs. ASA: $C_{max}$=319ng/mL; $T_{max}$=0.63 hrs. **Distribution:** Dipyridamole/ASA found in breast milk. Dipyridamole: $V_d$=92L; plasma protein binding (99%). ASA: $V_d$=10 L; plasma protein binding (poor); salicylic acid (ASA metabolite): highly protein bound (concentration dependent). **Metabolism:** Dipyridamole: Liver (conjugation); monoglucuronide (metabolite) (low activity). ASA: Liver (conjugation); salicylic acid (metabolite). **Elimination:** Dipyridamole: Feces (95%), urine (low); $T_{1/2}$=15.5 hrs. ASA: Urine; $T_{1/2}$=0.33 hrs, $T_{1/2}$=1.71 hrs (metabolite).

## NURSING CONSIDERATIONS

**Assessment:** Assess for hypersensitivity to NSAIDs, asthma, rhinitis, nasal polyps, severe renal failure, and severe hepatic dysfunction. Assess use in presence of inherited or acquired bleeding disorders (eg, liver disease, vitamin K deficiency), pregnancy/nursing, history of active peptic ulcer disease, presence of severe coronary artery disease (eg, unstable angina or recently sustained MI), and hypotension. Assess for drug interactions.

**Monitoring:** Monitor for signs/symptoms of allergic reactions (eg, urticaria, angioedema, bronchospasm), coagulation abnormalities (including bleeding time), GI effects (eg, stomach pain, heartburn, N/V), elevated hepatic enzymes (hepatic failure), bleeding (eg, GI, intracranial hemorrhage), increased BUN, increased serum creatinine, hyperkalemia, and proteinuria. If used in pediatrics, monitor for Reye's syndrome.

**Patient Counseling:** Inform patients who consume ≥3 alcoholic drinks every day are at increased risk for bleeding. Advise to contact physician if any signs of abnormal bleeding or allergic reactions occur. Instruct to swallow medication whole, with/without food. If intolerable headaches occur during initial treatment, advise to switch to 1 capsule at bedtime and low-dose aspirin in the morning. Advise to return to normal treatment regimen as soon as possible, usually within 1 week.

# AGRIFLU RX

influenza virus vaccine (Novartis)

**THERAPEUTIC CLASS:** Vaccine

**INDICATIONS:** Active immunization of persons ≥18 yrs for prevention of disease caused by influenza virus subtypes A and type B contained in the vaccine.

**DOSAGE:** *Adults:* 0.5mL IM as a single dose, preferably in the deltoid muscle of the upper arm.

**HOW SUPPLIED:** Inj: 0.5mL

**CONTRAINDICATIONS:** Hypersensitivity reactions to egg proteins, kanamycin and neomycin or life-threatening reaction to previous administration of any influenza vaccine.

**WARNINGS/PRECAUTIONS:** Do not inject in gluteal area or areas with major nerve trunk. Caution if Guillain-Barre syndrome has occured within 6 weeks of receipt of prior influenza vaccine. May not obtain expected immune response in immunocompromised persons. Have appropriate medical treatment available to manage possible anaphylactic reactions. May not protect all recipients.

**ADVERSE REACTIONS:** Local reaction (pain, induration, swelling, erythema), headache, myalgia, malaise, anaphylactic shock.

**INTERACTIONS:** Immunosuppressive therapies may reduce effectiveness.

**PREGNANCY:** Category B, caution in nursing.

**MECHANISM OF ACTION:** Vaccine; elicits the formation of antibodies that may protect against influenza virus subtypes A and B.

## NURSING CONSIDERATIONS

**Assessment:** Assess immunity and current health status, known hypersensitivity to egg proteins, immunization history, pregnancy/nursing status, and possible drug interactions. Assess potential benefits and risks if Guillain-Barre syndrome occurred with previous influenza vaccination.

**Monitoring:** Monitor hypersensitivity reactions, local injection-site reactions (eg, pain, induration, swelling, erythema), systemic adverse events (eg, headache, myalgia, malaise) and serious allergic reactions (eg, anaphylactic shock).

**Patient Counseling:** Inform of potential benefits and risks of immunization. Explain that contains noninfectious particles and cannot cause influenza and is intended to provide protection against illness due to influenza viruses only; cannot protect against other respiratory illnesses. Instruct to report any adverse reaction to healthcare provider. Instruct that annual vaccination is recommended.

**Administration:** IM route; inject into deltoid muscle of upper arm. **Storage:** 2-+8°C (35-46°F). Do not freeze. Protect from light.

## AGRYLIN RX

anagrelide HCl (Shire)

**THERAPEUTIC CLASS:** Platelet-reducing agent

**INDICATIONS:** Treatment of thrombocythemia, secondary to myeloproliferative disorders, to reduce the elevated platelet count and the risk of thrombosis and to ameliorate associated symptoms (eg, thrombo-hemorrhagic events).

**DOSAGE:** *Adults:* Initial: 0.5mg qid or 1mg bid (2 caps of 0.5mg bid) for at least 1 week. Moderate Hepatic Impairment: Initial: 0.5mg qd for at least 1 week. Titrate: Increase by no more than 0.5mg/day per week. Max: 10mg/day or 2.5mg/dose. Adjust to lowest effective dose to reduce and maintain platelets <600,000/μL. Monitor platelet counts every 2 days during first week, then weekly thereafter until maintenance dosage reached.
*Pediatrics:* Initial: 0.5mg qd. Titrate: Increase by no more than 0.5mg/day per week. Max: 10mg/day or 2.5mg/dose. Adjust to lowest effective dose to reduce and maintain platelets <600,000/μL. Monitor platelet counts every 2 days during first week, then weekly thereafter until maintenance dosage reached.

**HOW SUPPLIED:** Cap: (Agrylin) 0.5mg, (Generic) 0.5mg, 1mg

**CONTRAINDICATIONS:** Severe hepatic impairment.

**WARNINGS/PRECAUTIONS:** Caution with heart disease, renal or hepatic dysfunction. Perform pre-treatment cardiovascular exam and monitor during treatment; may cause cardiovascular effects (eg, vasodilation, tachycardia, palpitations, congestive heart failure). Reduce dose in moderate hepatic impairment. Interstitial lung diseases (eg, allergic alveolitis, eosinophilic pneumonia, interstitial pneumonitis) reported. Monitor blood counts (Hgb, WBC), liver function (AST, ALT), and renal function (SrCr, BUN) while platelet count is being lowered. Interruption of treatment is followed by an increase in platelet count.

**ADVERSE REACTIONS:** Headache, palpitations, diarrhea, asthenia, edema, N/V, abdominal pain, dizziness, pain, dyspnea, flatulence, fever, peripheral edema, rash (including urticaria), chest pain.

**INTERACTIONS:** Sucralfate may interfere with absorption. Exacerbated effects of products that inhibit cyclic AMP PDE III (inotropes: milrinone, enoximone, amrinone, olprinone, cilostazol). Concomitant use with CYP1A2 inhibitors (eg, fluvoxamine) may adversely affect the clearance of anagrelide. Caution with concomitant use with other CYP1A2 substrates (eg, theophylline). Assess prior to coadministration, the potential risks and benefits of concomitant use of anagrelide with aspirin, particularly in patients with a high risk profile for hemorrhage.

**PREGNANCY:** Category C, not for use in nursing.

**MECHANISM OF ACTION:** Platelet-reducing agent; not established. Suspected to reduce platelet production resulting from a decrease in megakaryocyte hypermaturation. Inhibits cyclic AMP phosphodiesterase III (PDEIII). PDEIII inhibitors can also inhibit platelet aggregation.

**PHARMACOKINETICS: Metabolism:** Liver, CYP1A2 (partial). RL603 and 3-hydroxy anagrelide (major metabolites). **Elimination**: Urine (70%); $T_{1/2}$=1.3 hrs.

### NURSING CONSIDERATIONS

**Assessment:** Assess for severe hepatic impairment, pregnancy/nursing status, and for possible drug interactions. Assess use in presence of known or suspected heart disease, presence of moderate hepatic impairment, and in the presence of renal insufficiency. Perform pretreatment cardiovascular exam.

**Monitoring:** Monitor for signs/symptoms of cardiovascular effects (eg, palpitations, vasodilation, tachycardia, congestive heart failure), thrombocytopenia, and for interstitial lung diseases (eg, allergic alveolitis, eosinophilic pneumonia, interstitial pneumonitis). Monitor platelet counts every 2 days during first week of treatment and at least weekly thereafter until maintenance dose is reached. Perform periodic monitoring of blood counts (Hgb, WBC), liver function (AST, ALT), and renal function (SrCr, BUN).

**Patient Counseling:** Instruct to notify physician if any cardiovascular effects (eg, palpitations) develop. Advise that periodic laboratory tests will need to be performed while on therapy. Inform that platelet counts begin to respond within 7-14 days of therapy at the proper dosage.

**Administration:** Oral route. **Storage:** 25°C (77°F); excursions permitted to 15-30°C (59-86°F). Store in light-resistant container.

## ALAMAST RX
pemirolast potassium (Vistakon)

**THERAPEUTIC CLASS:** Mast cell stabilizer

**INDICATIONS:** Prevention of ocular itching due to allergic conjunctivitis.

**DOSAGE:** *Adults:* 1-2 drops in affected eye qid.
*Pediatrics:* ≥3 yrs: 1-2 drops in affected eye qid.

**HOW SUPPLIED:** Sol: 0.1% [10mL]

**WARNINGS/PRECAUTIONS:** May reinsert soft contact lens after 10 min, if eyes are not red. Contains lauralkonium chloride; may be absorbed by soft contact lens.

**ADVERSE REACTIONS:** Headache, rhinitis, cold/flu symptoms, ocular burning/discomfort, dry eye, foreign body sensation.

**PREGNANCY:** Category C, caution in nursing.

**MECHANISM OF ACTION:** Mast cell stabilizer; inhibits type I immediate hypersensitivity reaction, antigen-induced release of inflammatory mediators (eg, histamine, leukotriene $C_4$, $D_4$, $E_4$) from human mast cell; also inhibits the chemotaxis of eosinophils into ocular tissue, blocks the release of mediators from human eosinophils, and prevents calcium influx into mast cells upon antigen stimulation (not established).

**PHARMACOKINETICS: Absorption:** $C_{max}$=4.7ng/mL, $T_{max}$=0.42 hrs. **Elimination:** Urine (10-15% unchanged); $T_{1/2}$=4.5 hrs.

### NURSING CONSIDERATIONS

**Assessment:** Assess for known drug hypersensitivity.

**Monitoring:** Monitor for anaphylaxis and adverse reactions.

**Patient Counseling:** Counsel not to touch dropper tip to eyelid or surrounding areas and not to wear contact lenses if eye is red.

**Administration:** Intraocular route. **Storage:** 15-25°C (59-77°F).

## ALBUTEROL RX
albuterol sulfate (Various)

**THERAPEUTIC CLASS:** $Beta_2$-agonist

**INDICATIONS:** (Aerosol) Prevention and treatment of bronchospasm with reversible obstructive airway disease. Prevention of Exercise-Induced Bronchospasm (EIB). (Sol) Relief of bronchospasm with reversible obstructive airway disease and acute attacks of bronchospasm in patients ≥12 yrs. (Tab; Tab, Extended-Release) Relief of bronchospasm with reversible obstructive airway disease in patients ≥6 yrs. (Syrup) Relief of bronchospasm in patients ≥2 yrs with reversible obstructive airway disease.

**DOSAGE:** *Adults:* Bronchospasm: (Aerosol) 2 inh q4-6h or 1 inh q4h. (Repetabs) Initial: 4-8mg q12h. Max: 32mg/day. (Sol) 2.5mg tid-qid by nebulizer. (Syrup, Tabs) 2-4mg tid-qid. Max: 32mg/day (8mg qid). Elderly/β-Adrenergic Sensitivity: (Syrup, Tabs) Initial: 2mg tid-qid. Max: (Tabs) 8mg tid-qid. EIB: (Aerosol) 2 inh 15 min before activity.

*Pediatrics:* Bronchospasm: >14 yrs: (Syrup) Initial: 2-4mg tid-qid. Max: 8mg qid. ≥12 yrs: (Aerosol) 2 inh q4-6h or 1 inh q4h. (Sol) 2.5mg tid-qid by nebulizer. (Tabs) Initial: 2-4mg tid-qid. Max: 8mg qid. >12 yrs: (Repetabs) Initial: 4-8mg q12h. Max: 32mg/day. 6-14 yrs: (Syrup) Initial: 2mg tid-qid. Max: 24mg/day. 6-12 yrs: (Repetabs) Initial: 4mg q12h. Max: 24mg/day. (Tabs) Initial: 2mg tid-qid. Max: 24mg/day. 2-6 yrs: (Syrup) Initial: 0.1mg/kg tid (not to exceed 2mg tid). Titrate: May increase to 0.2mg/kg/day. Max: 4mg tid. EIB: ≥12 yrs: (Aerosol) 2 inh 15 min before activity.

**HOW SUPPLIED:** MDI: 0.09mg/inh [17g]; Sol (neb): 0.083% [3mL, 25[s]], 0.5% [20mL]; Syrup: 2mg/5mL; Tab: 2mg*, 4mg*; Tab, Extended-Release (Repetabs): 4mg *scored

**WARNINGS/PRECAUTIONS:** Hypersensitivity reactions reported. Monitor for worsening asthma. Fatalities reported with excessive use. Caution with cardiovascular disorders, especially coronary insufficiency, arrhythmias and HTN. May need concomitant corticosteroids. Can produce paradoxical bronchospasm. Caution with DM, hyperthyroidism, seizures. May cause transient hypokalemia.

**ADVERSE REACTIONS:** Tachycardia, increased BP, tremor, nervousness, dizziness, N/V, palpitations, paradoxical bronchospasm, heartburn, rhinitis, respiratory tract infection.

**INTERACTIONS:** Avoid other sympathomimetic agents. Extreme caution with MAOIs and TCAs. Monitor digoxin. May worsen ECG changes and/or hypokalemia with non-$K^+$-sparing diuretics. Antagonized by β-blockers.

**PREGNANCY:** Category C, not for use in nursing.

**MECHANISM OF ACTION:** $\beta_2$-adrenergic agonist; stimulates intracellular adenyl cyclase, which catalyzes conversion of ATP to cAMP to produce relaxation of bronchial smooth muscle and inhibition of release of mediators of immediate hypersensitivity from cells (mast cells).

**PHARMACOKINETICS: Absorption:** (Aerosol) $T_{max}$=2-4 hrs. (Syrup, Tab) Rapid. $C_{max}$=18ng/mL; $T_{max}$=2 hrs. **Elimination:** (Aerosol) Urine (28%); $T_{1/2}$=3.8 hrs. (Syrup, Tab) $T_{1/2}$=5 hrs.

## NURSING CONSIDERATIONS

**Assessment:** Assess for CVD (coronary insufficiency, cardiac arrhythmias, HTN), convulsive disorder, hyperthyroidism, DM, and possible drug interactions.

**Monitoring:** Monitor for signs/symptoms of CV effects (increased BP, palpitations), worsening of symptoms, destabilization of asthma, paradoxical bronchospasm, and hypersensitivity reactions (anaphylactic, urticaria, angioedema, rash, bronchospasm).

**Patient Counseling:** Seek medical attention if worsening of symptoms, therapy becomes less effective, need more inhalation from short-acting $\beta_2$-agonist than usual, paradoxical bronchospams, and hypersensitivity (anaphylactic, urticaria, angioedema, rash, bronchospasm) occur.

**Administration:** Oral inhalation, oral route. (Aerosol) 1) Shake well. 2) Breathe out fully through mouth. 3) While breathing in deeply and slowly through mouth, depress the top of metal canister. 4) Hold breath as long as possible. 5) Cleanse inhaler thoroughly and frequently. 6) Recommend "test spray" into air before using for first time. **Storage:** (Inhalation) 2-25°C (36-77°F). Protect from light. Store in pouch until time of use. (Aerosol) 15-30°C (59-86°F). Shake well before using. (Tab) 20-25°C (36-77°F). Protect from light. Dispense in tight, light-resistant container. (Syrup) 15-30°C (59-86°F). Dispense in tight, light-resistant container.

# ALCORTIN RX

iodoquinol - hydrocortisone (Primus)

**THERAPEUTIC CLASS:** Corticosteroid/Anti-infective

**INDICATIONS:** "Possibly" Effective: Contact or atopic dermatitis, impetiginized eczema, nummular eczema, endogenous chronic infectious dermatitis, stasis dermatitis, pyoderma, nuchal eczema and chronic eczematoid otitis externa, acne urticata, localized or disseminated neurodermatitis, lichen simplex chronicus, anogenital pruritus (vulvae, scroti, ani), folliculitis, bacterial dermatoses, mycotic dermatoses such as tinea (capitis, cruris, corporis, pedis), monliasis, intertrigo.

**DOSAGE:** *Adults:* Apply to affected area(s) tid-qid.
*Pediatrics:* ≥12 yrs: Apply to affected area(s) tid-qid.

**HOW SUPPLIED:** Gel: (Hydrocortisone-Iodoquinol) 2%-1% [2g]

**WARNINGS/PRECAUTIONS:** For external use only. Avoid eyes. D/C if irritation develops. May stain skin, hair, or fabrics. Risk of systemic absorption with treatment of extensive areas or use of occlusive dressings. Increased risk of systemic absorption in children. Iodoquinol may interfere with thyroid tests. False-positive phenylketonuria test reported. Prolonged use may result in overgrowth of nonsusceptible organisms.

**ADVERSE REACTIONS:** Burning, itching, irritation, dryness, folliculitis, hypertrichosis, acneiform eruptions, hypopigmentation, perioral dermatitis, allergic dermatitis, skin maceration, secondary infection, skin atrophy, striae, miliaria.

**PREGNANCY:** Category C, caution in nursing.

**MECHANISM OF ACTION:** Corticosteroid/Anti-infective. Hydrocortisone: Corticosteroid; possesses anti-inflammatory, antipruritic, and vasoconstrictive properties. Anti-inflammatory effect unclear; however, there is a recognizable correlation between vasoconstrictor potency and therapeutic efficacy. Iodoquinol: Anti-infective; possesses both antifungal and antibacterial properties.

**PHARMACOKINETICS: Absorption:** Hydrocortisone: Absorbed from normal intact skin. Inflammation of skin increases absorption. **Metabolism:** Hydrocortisone: Liver and most body tissues. Tetrahydrocortisone and tetrahydrocortisol (metabolites). **Elimination:** Hydrocortisone: Urine (unchanged and glucuronides). Iodoquinol: Urine (3-5% glucuronide).

## NURSING CONSIDERATIONS

**Assessment:** Assess for known hypersensitivity to aloe vera, glycine, histidine, lysine, or palmitic acid. Assess use in pregnant/nursing females.

**Monitoring:** Monitor for development of systemic toxicity in children if large areas of body are treated or if occlusive dressings used (eg, diapers, plastic pants) on treated areas. With prolonged therapy, monitor for occurrence of overgrowth of non-susceptible bacteria. Monitor for lab test interactions (eg, thyroid function tests, ferric chloride tests for phenylketonuria [PKU]). If necessary, perform thyroid function tests 1 month after therapy end.

**Patient Counseling:** Instruct parents of pediatric patients not to use tight-fitting diapers or plastic pants on child being treated in diaper area. Counsel to keep medication away from eyes. If contact occurs and irritation develops, counsel to d/c medication and apply appropriate therapy. Inform that medication may cause staining of skin, hair, or fabrics and burning, itching, irritation, or dryness.

**Administration:** Topical route; external use only. **Storage:** Store at room temperature, 15-30°C (59-86°F). Keep out of reach of children. Keep tightly closed.

## ALDACTAZIDE RX

hydrochlorothiazide - spironolactone (Pharmacia & Upjohn)

**Tumorigenic in chronic toxicity animal studies; avoid unnecessary use. Not for initial therapy.**

**THERAPEUTIC CLASS:** $K^+$-sparing diuretic/thiazide diuretic

**INDICATIONS:** Management of edematous conditions (CHF, hepatic cirrhosis with edema/ascites, nephrotic syndrome) and hypertension.

**DOSAGE:** *Adults:* Edema: 100mg/day per component qd or in divided doses. Maint: 25-200mg/day per component. HTN: 50-100mg/day per component qd or in divided doses.

**HOW SUPPLIED:** Tab: (Spironolactone-HCTZ) 25mg-25mg, 50mg-50mg* *scored

**CONTRAINDICATIONS:** Acute renal impairment, significantly impaired renal excretory function, hyperkalemia, acute or severe hepatic dysfunction, anuria, sulfonamide hypersensitivity.

**WARNINGS/PRECAUTIONS:** Monitor for fluid/electrolyte imbalance. Caution with renal and hepatic dysfunction. Hyperchloremic metabolic acidosis reported with decompensated hepatic cirrhosis. Mild acidosis, gynecomastia, transient BUN elevation, hypercalcemia, hyperglycemia, hyperuricemia, hypomagnesemia, and sensitivity reactions may occur. D/C if hyperkalemia occurs. Risk of dilutional hyponatremia. Enhanced effects in post-sympathetectomy patient. May increase cholesterol and TG levels. May manifest latent DM.

**ADVERSE REACTIONS:** Gastric bleeding, ulceration, gynecomastia, impotence, agranulocytosis, fever, urticaria, confusion, ataxia, renal dysfunction, blood dyscrasias, electrolyte disturbances, weakness, irregular menses, amenorrhea.

**INTERACTIONS:** Risk of hyperkalemia with $K^+$-sparing diuretics, $K^+$ supplements, NSAIDs, ACE inhibitors. Alcohol, barbiturates, or narcotics potentiate orthostatic hypotension. Corticosteroids, ACTH may intensify electrolyte depletion. Reduced vascular response to norepinephrine. Increased response to nondepolarizing skeletal muscle relaxants. Risk of digoxin, lithium toxicity. NSAIDs may reduce effects. Antidiabetic agents may need adjustment.

**PREGNANCY:** Category C, not for use in nursing.

**MECHANISM OF ACTION:** Spironolactone: Aldosterone antagonist; competitively binds to receptors at aldosterone-dependent sodium-potassium exchange site. HCTZ: Thiazide diuretic; promotes excretion of sodium and water by inhibiting reabsorption.

**PHARMACOKINETICS: Absorption:** Spironolactone: $C_{max}$=80ng/mL; $T_{max}$=2.6 hrs. HCTZ: Rapid; $T_{max}$=1-2 hrs. **Distribution:** Spironolactone: Plasma protein binding (90%). **Elimination:** Spironolactone: Urine (major), bile (minor). HCTZ: Urine.

## NURSING CONSIDERATIONS

**Assessment:** Assess for renal impairment (insufficiency, anuria, impairment of excretion), hepatic impairment (failure), hyperkalemia, pregnancy status, possible drug interactions, SLE, DM, sulfonamide hypersensitivity, history of allergy or bronchial asthma.

**Monitoring:** Monitor serum electrolytes, serum $K^+$, and renal function periodically. Monitor for signs/symptoms of electrolyte imbalance, hyperkalemia, gynecomastia, hyperglycemia, exacerbation or activation of SLE, hyperuricemia or precipitation of gout, hypersensitivity reactions, hepatic/renal impairment.

**Patient Counseling:** Instruct to avoid $K^+$ supplements and foods containing high levels of $K^+$. Inform of pregnancy risks. Advise to seek medical attention if symptoms of electrolyte imbalance (dry mouth, thirst, weakness), hyperkalemia (paresthesia, fatigue, muscle weakness), or hypersensitivity reactions occur.

**Administration:** Oral route. **Storage:** Below 25°C (77°F).

# ALDACTONE RX

spironolactone (G.D. Searle)

**Tumorigenic in chronic toxicity animal studies; avoid unnecessary use.**

**THERAPEUTIC CLASS:** $K^+$-sparing diuretic

**INDICATIONS:** Management of primary hyperaldosteronism (diagnosis, short-term preoperative and long-term maintenance treatment), edematous conditions (CHF, hepatic cirrhosis with edema/ascites, nephrotic syndrome, pathological causes of edema in pregnancy), essential hypertension. Treatment and prophylaxis of hypokalemia. In addition to standard therapy in severe heart failure (NYHA Class III-IV).

**DOSAGE:** *Adults:* Primary Hyperaldosteronism: (Diagnostic) 400mg/day for 3-4 weeks or 400mg/day for 4 days. (Preoperative) 100-400mg/day. (Unsuitable for Surgery) Maint: Lowest effective dose. Edema: Initial: 100mg/day given qd or in divided doses for at least 5 days. Maint: 25-200mg/day given qd-bid. HTN: Initial: 50-100mg/day given qd or in divided doses. Titrate: Adjust at 2-week intervals. Diuretic-Induced Hypokalemia: 25-100mg/day. Severe Heart Failure (Sr$K^+$ ≤5.0mEq/L, SrCr ≤2.5mg/dL): Initial: 25mg qd. May increase to 50mg qd if tolerated or reduce to 25mg every other day if not tolerated.

**HOW SUPPLIED:** Tab: 25mg, 50mg*, 100mg* *scored

**CONTRAINDICATIONS:** Anuria, acute renal insufficiency, significantly impaired renal excretory function, hyperkalemia.

**WARNINGS/PRECAUTIONS:** Monitor for fluid/electrolyte imbalance. Caution with renal and hepatic dysfunction. Hyperchloremic metabolic acidosis reported with decompensated hepatic cirrhosis. Mild acidosis, gynecomastia, transient BUN elevation may occur. D/C and monitor ECG and $K^+$ levels if hyperkalemia occurs. May cause/aggravate dilutional hyponatremia.

**ADVERSE REACTIONS:** Gastric bleeding, ulceration, gynecomastia, agranulocytosis, fever, urticaria, confusion, ataxia, renal dysfunction, irregular menses, postmenopausal bleeding.

**INTERACTIONS:** Risk of hyperkalemia with $K^+$-sparing diuretics, $K^+$ supplements, NSAIDs (eg, indomethacin) , ACE inhibitors. Alcohol, barbiturates, or narcotics potentiate orthostatic hypotension. Corticosteroids, ACTH may intensify electrolyte depletion, particularly hypokalemia. Reduced vascular response to norepinephrine; caution in patients subjected to regional or general anesthesia. Increased response to nondepolarizing skeletal muscle relaxants (eg, tubocurarine). Risk of digoxin, lithium toxicity. NSAIDs may reduce effects.

**PREGNANCY:** Category C, not for use in nursing.

**MECHANISM OF ACTION:** Aldosterone antagonist; competitively binds to receptors at aldosterone-dependent $Na^+$-$K^+$ exchange site in distal convoluted renal tubule, causing increased $Na^+$ and water excretion and $K^+$ retention.

**PHARMACOKINETICS: Absorption:** $C_{max}$=80ng/mL; $T_{max}$=2.6 hrs. **Distribution:** Plasma protein binding (>90%). **Elimination:** Urine (major), bile (minor).

## NURSING CONSIDERATIONS

**Assessment:** Assess for renal impairment (insufficiency, anuria, impairment of excretion), hepatic impairment, hyperkalemia, pregnancy/nursing status and possible drug interactions.

**Monitoring:** Monitor serum $K^+$, electrolytes, ECG and renal function (eg, BUN, creatinine) periodically. Monitor for signs/symptoms of fluid/electrolyte imbalance, dilutional hyponatremia, hyperkalemia, acidosis, gynecomastia, hypersensitivity reactions, renal/hepatic dysfunction.

**Patient Counseling:** Instruct to avoid $K^+$ supplements and foods containing high levels of $K^+$, including salt substitutes. Advise to seek medical attention if symptoms of electrolyte imbalance (dry mouth, thirst, weakness), hyperkalemia (paresthesia, fatigue, muscle weakness) or hypersensitivity reactions occur.

**Administration:** Oral route. **Storage:** <25°C (77°F).

## ALDARA
imiquimod (Graceway)

**RX**

**THERAPEUTIC CLASS:** Immune response modifier

**INDICATIONS:** Actinic keratoses on face or scalp in immunocompetent adults. External genital and perianal warts/condyloma acuminata. Biopsy-confirmed, primary superficial basal cell carcinoma (sBCC) in immunocompetent adults, with a maximum tumor diameter of 2cm, located on trunk (excluding anogenital skin), neck, or extremities (excluding hands and feet), only when surgical methods are medically less appropriate and follow-up can be assured.

**DOSAGE:** *Adults:* Use before bedtime. Actinic Keratosis: Usual: Apply 2x/week to defined area on face or scalp (but not both concurrently). Wash off after 8 hrs with soap and water. Max: 36 packets for 16 weeks. External Genital and Perianal Warts/Condyloma: Usual: Apply 3x/week. Wash off after 6-10 hrs with soap and water. Use until warts are totally cleared. Max: 16 weeks. May suspend use for several days to manage local reactions. Do not occlude treatment area. sBCC: Apply 5x/week for 6 weeks. If tumor diameter is 0.5 to <1cm, use 4mm (10mg) of cream. If tumor is ≥1 to <1.5cm, use 5mm (25mg) of cream. If tumor is ≥1.5 to 2cm, use 7mm (40mg) of cream. Max diameter of tumor: ≤2cm. Treatment area should include a 1cm margin of skin around the tumor. Wash off after 8 hrs with soap and water. Max: 36 packets for 16 weeks. *Pediatrics:* ≥12 yrs: External Genital and Perianal Warts/Condyloma: Usual: Apply 3x/week before bedtime. Wash off after 6-10 hrs with soap and water. Use until warts are totally cleared. Max: 16 weeks. May suspend use for several days to manage local reactions. Do not occlude treatment area.

**HOW SUPPLIED:** Cre: 5% [250mg, 24[s]]

**WARNINGS/PRECAUTIONS:** Not for urethral, intra-vaginal, cervical, rectal, or intra-anal human papilloma viral disease. Not for repeated use in treatment of actinic keratosis in same area; not for treatment of actinic keratosis on areas of skin >25cm². Avoid sexual contact while cream is on skin. May weaken condoms and diaphragms; avoid concurrent use. Avoid or minimize exposure to sunlight. Avoid contact with eyes, lips, nostrils. Avoid after surgery or with sunburn until tissue is healed. May exacerbate inflammatory skin conditions; interruption of dosing should be considered, if systemic reactions (eg, flu-like signs/symptoms) occur. Not recommended for treatment of basal cell carcinoma subtypes, other than sBCC.

**ADVERSE REACTIONS:** Application-site reactions, upper respiratory tract infection, sinusitis, headache, squamous cell carcinoma, diarrhea, back pain, rhinitis, lymphadenopathy, flu-like symptoms.

**PREGNANCY:** Category C, caution in nursing.

**MECHANISM OF ACTION:** Immune response modifier; not established. In basal cell carcinoma, suspected to increase infiltration of lymphocytes, dendritic cells, and macrophages in the tumor lesion. In external genital warts, suspected to induce mRNA encoding cytokines, including interferon-α at the treatment site.

**PHARMACOKINETICS: Absorption:** $C_{max}$=0.1ng/mL (12.5mg, face), 0.2ng/mL (25mg, scalp), 3.5ng/mL (75mg, hands/arms). **Elimination:** Urine: Male (0.11%), female (2.41%).

### NURSING CONSIDERATIONS

**Assessment:** Assess use with pre-existing autoimmune conditions, immunosuppression, basal cell nevus syndrome or xeroderma pigmentosum. For treatment of superficial basal cell carcinoma, assess proper diagnosis (eg, biopsy). Assess use in inherent sensitivity to sunlight, current sunburn, and in pregnancy/nursing. Assess for possible drug interactions.

**Monitoring:** Monitor for signs/symptoms of local inflammatory reactions (eg, weeping or erosion) and for systemic reactions (eg, flu-like symptoms: malaise, fever, nausea, myalgias). Monitor for clinical signs of improvement.

**Patient Counseling:** Inform to wash hands before and after applying cream. Before applying, wash treatment area with mild soap and water and allow area to dry thoroughly (at least 10 min). Avoid contact with eyes, lips, and nostrils. Warn to avoid exposure to sunlight (including sunlamps) and to use protective clothing (eg, hat) or sunscreen when using medication. Advise patients with sunburns not to use the cream until fully recovered. Advise female patients to take special care when applying the cream at the vaginal opening because of local skin reactions on the delicate moist surfaces, which may result in pain or swelling and may cause difficulty in passing urine. When using for the treatment of actinic keratosis or superficial basal cell carcinoma, wash the treatment area with mild soap and water 8 hrs following application of the cream. When using for the treatment of external genital warts, wash treatment area with mild soap and water 6-10 hrs following application of cream.

**Administration:** Topical application. **Storage:** Store at 4-25°C (39-77°F). Do not freeze.

## ALESSE — RX

ethinyl estradiol - levonorgestrel (Wyeth)

**OTHER BRAND NAMES:** Aviane (Duramed) - Lessina (Barr)

**THERAPEUTIC CLASS:** Estrogen/progestogen combination

**INDICATIONS:** Prevention of pregnancy.

**DOSAGE:** *Adults:* 1 tab qd for 28 days, then repeat. Start 1st Sunday after menses begin or 1st day of menses.

**HOW SUPPLIED:** Tab: (Ethinyl Estradiol-Levonorgestrel) 0.02mg-0.1mg

**CONTRAINDICATIONS:** Thrombophlebitis, DVT or thromboembolic disorders, pregnancy, cerebrovascular or coronary artery disease, undiagnosed abnormal genital bleeding, cholestatic jaundice of pregnancy or jaundice with prior pill use, hepatic adenomas or carcinomas, active liver disease (as long as liver function has not returned to normal), breast cancer or other estrogen-dependent neoplasia, thrombogenic valvulopathies, thrombogenic rhythm disorders, diabetes with vascular involvement, uncontrolled HTN.

**WARNINGS/PRECAUTIONS:** Cigarette smoking increases risk of serious cardiovascular side effects; risk increases with age (especially >35 yrs) and heavy smoking. Increased risk of MI, vascular disease, thromboembolism, stroke and gallbladder disease. Retinal thrombosis, hepatic neoplasia, carcinoma of breast and reproductive organs reported. May cause glucose intolerance. May increase BP, elevate LDL levels or cause other lipid changes, fluid retention, breakthrough bleeding, and spotting. May cause or exacerbate migraine. May develop visual changes with contact lens. Diarrhea and/or vomiting may reduce absorption. Increased risk of MI with HTN, hyperlipidemia, obesity, and diabetes. D/C if jaundice, significant depression or ophthalmic irregularities develop. Perform annual physical exam. Use before menarche is not indicated. May affect certain endocrine, LFTs and blood components.

**ADVERSE REACTIONS:** N/V, breakthrough bleeding, spotting, amenorrhea, migraine, depression, vaginal candidiasis, edema, weight changes.

**INTERACTIONS:** Reduced effects, increased breakthrough bleeding, and menstrual irregularities with rifampin, barbiturates, phenylbutazone, phenytoin, griseofulvin, topiramate, some protease inhibitors, modafinil, ampicillin, tetracyclines, and possibly with St. John's wort. Troleandomycin may increase risk of intrahepatic cholestasis. Ascorbic acid, APAP, CYP3A4 inhibitors (eg, indinavir, fluconazole, troleandomycin), atorvastatin may increase plasma levels. Increased plasma levels of cyclosporine, theophylline, and corticosteroids.

**PREGNANCY:** Category X, not for use in nursing.

**MECHANISM OF ACTION:** Oral contraceptive: Inhibits ovulation by suppression of gonadotropins. Causes changes in cervical mucus (increases difficulty of sperm entry into uterus) and in endometrium (reduces likelihood of implantation).

**PHARMACOKINETICS: Absorption:** Levonorgestrel: Rapid and complete, bioavailability (100%), $C_{max}$=2.8ng/mL (single dose), 6.0ng/mL (multiple doses), $T_{max}$=1.6 hrs (single dose), 1.5 hrs (multiple doses); Ethinyl Estradiol: Rapid, bioavailability; (38-48%); $C_{max}$=62pg/mL (single dose), 77pg/mL (multiple doses), $T_{max}$=1.5 hrs (single dose), 1.3 hrs (multiple doses). **Distribution:** Levonorgestrel: Primarily bound to SHBG. Ethinyl estradiol: Plasma protein binding (97%). **Metabolism:** Levonorgestrel: Reduction, hydroxylation, and conjugation. Ethinyl Estradiol: Hepatic, via CYP3A4 (hydroxylation), methylation, and glucuronidation. **Elimination:** Levonorgestrel: Urine (40-68%), feces (16-48%); $T_{1/2}$=36 hrs. Ethinyl Estradiol: $T_{1/2}$=18 hrs.

## NURSING CONSIDERATIONS

**Assessment:** Assess for thromboembophlebitis or thromboembolic disorder, past history of DVT, CVD, CAD, uncontrolled HTN, thrombogenic valvulopathies, thrombogenic rhythm disorders, major surgery with prolonged immobilization, DM, headache with focal neurological symptoms, known/suspected or history of carcinoma (of breast, endometrium) or known/suspected estrogen-dependent neoplasia, undiagnosed abnormal genital bleeding, cholestatic jaundice of pregnancy or jaundice with prior pill use, hepatic adenomas or carcinomas, active liver disease, and known/suspected pregnancy. Assess use in patients who are >35 years and heavy smokers (≥15 cigarettes/day). Assess use with HTN, hyperlipidemias, obesity, DM, or in patients at increased risk for thrombosis. Assess for possible drug interactions.

**Monitoring:** Monitor for venous and arterial thrombotic and thromboembolic events (eg, MI, thromboembolism, and stroke), hepatic neoplasia, gallbladder disease, ocular lesions, HTN, bleeding irregularities, onset or exacerbation of headaches or migraines, and ectopic pregnancy. Monitor fasting blood glucose levels in DM and prediabetic patients, BP with history of HTN, lipid levels with a history of hyperlipidemia. Monitor for signs of liver dysfunction (eg, jaundice) and signs of depression with previous history. Refer patients with contact lenses to an ophthalmologist if visual changes occur. Perform annual history and physical exam.

**Patient Counseling:** Inform that drug does not protect against HIV infection and other STDs. Instruct women who are initiating therapy to use additional method of protection during first 7 days of use. Take exactly as directed and at intervals not exceeding 24 hrs. Advise that if pill missed, take as soon as remembered; take next dose at regularly scheduled time. Inform may experience spotting, light bleeding, or stomach upset during first 1-3 packs of pills. Instruct to continue using therapy and to contact physician if symptoms persist. Counsel to avoid smoking while on medication.

**Administration:** Oral route. **Storage:** Store at controlled room temperature 20-25°C (68-77°F).

## ALIMTA — RX

pemetrexed disodium (Lilly)

**THERAPEUTIC CLASS:** Antifolate

**INDICATIONS:** In combination with cisplatin for the initial treatment of locally advanced or metastatic nonsquamous non-small cell lung cancer (NSCLC). Maintenance treatment in patients with locally advanced or metastatic nonsquamous NSCLC whose disease has not progressed after 4 cycles of platinum-based first-line chemotherapy. Single agent for the treatment of patients with locally advanced or metastatic nonsquamous NSCLC after prior chemotherapy. In combination with cisplatin for the treatment of patients with malignant pleural mesothelioma whose disease is unresectable or who are otherwise not candidates for curative surgery.

**DOSAGE:** *Adults:* Premedication: Dexamethasone (or equivalent): 4mg PO bid day before, day of, and day after administration. Folic Acid: At least 5 daily doses (350-1000mcg) during 7 days prior to first dose. Continue throughout therapy and for 21 days after last dose. Vitamin $B_{12}$: 1000mcg IM once during week preceding first dose and every 3 cycles thereafter. Combination with Cisplatin: Nonsquamous NSCLC/ Mesothelioma: 500mg/m² IV over 10 min on Day 1 of each 21-day cycle; Cisplatin 75mg/m² infused over 2 hrs beginning

30 min after pemetrexed. Patient should receive appropriate hydration prior to and/or after receiving cisplatin. Single Agent: Nonsquamous NSLC: 500mg/m² IV over 10 minutes on Day 1 of each 21-day cycle. Refer to PI for dose adjustments for hematologic, nonhematologic, and neurotoxicities.

**HOW SUPPLIED:** Inj: 100mg, 500mg

**WARNINGS/PRECAUTIONS:** Premedicate with folic acid and vitamin $B_{12}$ to reduce hematologic and GI toxicity and with dexamethasone or its equivalent to reduce the incidence and severity of cutaneous reactions. Bone marrow suppression may occur; myelosuppression is usually the dose-limiting toxicity. Caution with renal/hepatic dysfunction and the elderly. Avoid in patients with CrCl <45mL/min. D/C if with ≥Grade 3 nonhematologic toxicities (including neurotoxicity). Do not start new cycle unless CrCl ≥45mL/min, ANC ≥1500 cells/mm³, platelet count ≥100,000 cells/mm³. May cause fetal harm; use effective contraception to prevent pregnancy. In patients with clinically significant third space fluid, consider draining the effusion prior to therapy.

**ADVERSE REACTIONS:** Anemia, anorexia, fatigue, increased ALT/AST, leukopenia, N/V, stomatitis, neutropenia, rash/desquamation, thrombocytopenia, constipation, pharyngitis, diarrhea.

**INTERACTIONS:** Delayed clearance with nephrotoxic or tubularly secreted drugs (eg, probenecid). Reduced clearance with ibuprofen; caution with concomitant use of ibuprofen in patients with mild-moderate renal insufficiency (CrCl from 45-79 mL/min). In mild-moderate renal insufficiency, avoid NSAIDs with short elimination half-lives for a period of 2 days before, the day of, and 2 days following therapy. Interrupt dosing of NSAIDs with longer half-lives for at least 5 days before, the day of, and 2 days following therapy.

**PREGNANCY:** Category D, not for use in nursing.

**MECHANISM OF ACTION:** Antifolate; disrupts folate-dependent metabolic processes essential for cell replication. Inhibits thymidylate synthase, dihydrofolate reductase and glycinamide ribonucleotide formyltransferase.

**PHARMACOKINETICS: Distribution:** $V_d$=16.1L. Plasma protein binding (81%). **Elimination:** Urine (70-90%; unchanged); $T_{1/2}$=3.5 hrs.

## NURSING CONSIDERATIONS

**Assessment:** Assess for renal/hepatic impairment, pregnancy/nursing status, hypersensitivity reaction to the drug, significant third space fluid (eg, ascites, pleural effusion) and possible drug interactions. Obtain baseline ANC, CBC with platelet and CrCl.

**Monitoring:** Monitor for signs and symptoms of bone marrow suppression (eg, neutropenia, thrombocytopenia, anemia), GI toxicity (eg, diarrhea), neurotoxicity, cutaneous reaction (eg, rash) and hypersensitivity reactions. Monitor CBC including platelet count, renal function (CrCl), and hepatic function.

**Patient Counseling:** Instruct to take folic acid and vitamin $B_{12}$ as prophylactic measures to reduce treatment-related hematological and GI toxicities. Inform about risks of low blood counts. Instruct to contact physician if any sign of infection (eg, fever), bleeding, anemia, vomiting, diarrhea, or dehydration occur. Advise women of childbearing potential to avoid becoming pregnant and to use effective contraceptive measures to prevent pregnancy during treatment.

**Administration:** IV route. Refer to PI for further details on preparation and administration. Reconstitution and further dilution is only recommended with 0.9% NaCl injection (preservative free). Physically incompatible with calcium-containing diluents (eg, Lactated Ringer). **Storage:** 25°C (77°F); excursions permitted to 15-30°C (59-86°F). Reconstituted and infusion solution can be used up to 24 hrs following initial reconstitution, when stored refrigerated, 2-8°C (36-46°F) or at 25°C (77°F); excursions permitted to 15-30°C (59-86°F). Discard unused portion.

# ALINIA — RX

nitazoxanide (Romark)

**THERAPEUTIC CLASS:** Antiprotozoal agent

**INDICATIONS:** Treatment of diarrhea caused by *Cryptosporidium parvum* and *Giardia lamblia.*

**DOSAGE:** *Adults:* ≥12 yrs: *G.lamblia* Diarrhea: 500mg q12h for 3 days. Take with food.
*Pediatrics: C.parvum/G.lamblia* Diarrhea: 1-3 yrs: 100mg (5mL) q12h for 3 days. 4-11yrs: 200mg (10mL) q12h for 3 days. *G.lamblia* Diarrhea: ≥12 yrs: 500mg (1 tab or 25mL) q12h for 3 days. Take with food.

**HOW SUPPLIED:** Sus: 100mg/5mL [60mL]; Tab: 500mg [60[s], 3-Day Therapy Packs, 6[s]]

**WARNINGS/PRECAUTIONS:** Caution with hepatic and biliary disease, renal disease. Contains 1.48g sucrose/5mL. Safety and effectiveness have not been established in HIV positive or immunodeficient patients.

**ADVERSE REACTIONS:** Abdominal pain, diarrhea, headache, nausea.

**INTERACTIONS:** Highly protein bound; caution with other highly plasma protein-bound drugs with narrow therapeutic indices.

**PREGNANCY:** Category B; caution in nursing.

**MECHANISM OF ACTION:** Antiprotozoal agent; interferes with the pyruvate, ferredoxin oxidoreductase enzyme-dependent electron transfer reaction, which is essential to anaerobic energy metabolism.

**PHARMACOKINETICS: Absorption**: Tizoxanide: (Tab, 500mg) 12-17 yrs: $C_{max}$=9.1mcg/mL, $T_{max}$=4 hrs, AUC=39.5mcg•hr/mL; ≥18 yrs: $C_{max}$=10.6mcg/mL, $T_{max}$=3 hrs, AUC=41.9mcg•hr/mL. (Sus, 100mg) 1-3 yrs: $C_{max}$=3.11mcg/mL, $T_{max}$=3.5 hrs, AUC=11.7mcg•hr/mL; 4-11 yrs: $C_{max}$=3mcg/mL, $T_{max}$=2 hrs, AUC=13.5mcg•hr/mL. **Distribution**: Tizoxanide: Plasma protein binding (>99%). **Metabolism**: Hydrolysis, glucuronidation: Tizoxanide and tizoxanide glucuronide (active). **Elimination**: Urine (33%), bile and feces (66%). Refer to PI for complete kinetics information.

## NURSING CONSIDERATIONS

**Assessment:** Assess for hepatic, renal/biliary impairment, HIV infection, DM, possible drug interactions.

**Monitoring:** Monitor for abdominal pain, diarrhea, nausea, LFTs, and CBC.

**Patient Counseling:** Counsel to take exactly as directed. Shake well prior to administration. Report lack of response or adverse effects.

**Administration:** Oral route, should be taken with food. Reconstitute with 48mL of water and keep tightly closed. Sus may be stored for 7 days. **Storage**: 25°C (77°F); excursions permitted to 15-30°C (59-86°F).

# ALLEGRA RX

fexofenadine HCl (Sanofi-Aventis)

**THERAPEUTIC CLASS:** $H_1$-antagonist

**INDICATIONS:** Relief of symptoms associated with seasonal allergic rhinitis in adults and children ≥2 years of age. Treatment of uncomplicated skin manifestations of chronic idiopathic urticaria in adults and children ≥6 months of age.

**DOSAGE:** *Adults:* Tab: Rhinitis/Urticaria: 60mg bid or 180mg qd. Renal Dysfunction: Initial: 60mg qd.
*Pediatrics:* Tab: ≥12 yrs: Rhinitis/Urticaria: 60mg bid or 180mg qd. Renal Dysfunction: Initial: 60mg qd. 6-11 yrs: Rhinitis/Urticaria: 30mg bid. Renal Dysfunction: Initial: 30mg qd. ODT: Rhinitis/Urticaria: 6-11 yrs: 30mg bid. Renal Dysfunction: 30mg qd. Sus: Rhinitis: 2-11 yrs: 30mg (5mL) bid. Renal Dysfunction: 30mg (5mL) qd. Urticaria: 2-11 yrs: 30mg (5mL) bid. Renal Dysfunction: 30mg (5mL) qd. 6 months to <2 yrs: 15mg (2.5mL) bid. Renal Dysfunction: 15mg (2.5mL) qd.

**HOW SUPPLIED:** Tab: 30mg, 60mg, 180mg; Tab, Orally Disintegrating: 30mg; Sus: 30mg/5mL

**WARNINGS/PRECAUTIONS:** Oral disintegrating tablet contains phenylalanine, a component of aspartame. Hypersensitivity reactions reported. Caution in elderly.

**ADVERSE REACTIONS:** Vomiting, headache, cough, diarrhea

**INTERACTIONS:** Increased plasma levels with erythromycin or ketoconazole. Avoid concomitant aluminum- and magnesium-containing antacids. Fruit juices (eg, grapefruit, orange, and apple) may decrease levels.

**PREGNANCY:** Category C, caution in nursing.

**MECHANISM OF ACTION:** Antihistamine with selective peripheral $H_1$-receptor antagonist activity; prevents antigen-induced bronchospasm and histamine release from peritoneal mast cells.

**PHARMACOKINETICS: Absorption:** Rapid; (Cap, 120mg) $T_{max}$=2.6 hrs; (Cap, 60mg) $C_{max}$=131ng/mL; (Tab, 60mg) $C_{max}$=142ng/mL; (Tab, 180mg) $C_{max}$=494ng/mL; (Sus, 30mg) $C_{max}$=118.0ng/mL, $T_{max}$=1.0 hrs. **Distribution:** Plasma protein binding (60%). **Metabolism:** Liver (5%). **Elimination:** Urine (80%), feces (11%); $T_{1/2}$=14.4 hrs.

## NURSING CONSIDERATIONS

**Assessment:** Assess for hepatic/renal impairment, pregnancy/nursing status, and possible drug interactions.

**Monitoring:** Monitor for side effects and treatment efficacy.

**Patient Counseling:** Advise to take as prescribed and not to exceed recommended dose. D/C and consult physician if adverse effects occur. Advise not to take with fruit juices.

**Administration:** Oral route. Take with water. Oral disintegrating tablet can be taken with or without water and on an empty stomach. Shake suspension bottle before use. **Storage:** 20-25°C (68-77°F).

# ALLEGRA-D **RX**

fexofenadine HCl - pseudoephedrine HCl (Sanofi-Aventis)

**THERAPEUTIC CLASS:** $H_1$-antagonist/sympathomimetic amine

**INDICATIONS:** Relief of symptoms of seasonal allergic rhinitis.

**DOSAGE:** *Adults:* 60mg-120mg tab bid or 180mg-240mg tab qd without food. Renal Dysfunction: Initial: 60mg-120mg tab qd; avoid 180mg-240mg tab. Do not crush or chew.
*Pediatrics:* ≥12 yrs: 60mg-120mg tab bid or 180mg-240mg tab qd without food. Renal Dysfunction: Initial: 60mg-120mg tab qd; avoid 180mg-240mg tab. Do not crush or chew.

**HOW SUPPLIED:** Tab, Extended-Release: (Fexofenadine-Pseudoephedrine) (12-Hour) 60mg-120mg, (24-Hour) 180mg-240mg

**CONTRAINDICATIONS:** Narrow-angle glaucoma, urinary retention, severe HTN, severe CAD, within 14 days of MAOI therapy.

**WARNINGS/PRECAUTIONS:** Caution with HTN, DM, ischemic heart disease, increased IOP, hyperthyroidism, renal impairment, or prostatic hypertrophy. May produce CNS stimulation with convulsions or cardiovascular collapse with hypotension.

**ADVERSE REACTIONS:** Headache, insomnia, nausea, dry mouth, dyspepsia, throat irritation.

**INTERACTIONS:** Increased plasma levels with erythromycin or ketoconazole. Avoid MAOIs. Increased ectopic pacemaker activity can occur with digitalis. Caution with other sympathomimetic amines. Reduced effects of antihypertensive drugs which interfere with sympathetic activity (eg, methyldopa, mecamylamine, reserpine).

**PREGNANCY:** Category C, caution with nursing.

**MECHANISM OF ACTION:** $H_1$-receptor antagonist/sympathomimetic amine. Fexofenadine: Selective peripheral $H_1$-receptor antagonist; inhibits antigen-induced bronchospasm and histamine release from peritoneal mast cells. Pseudoephedrine: Exerts a decongestant action on the nasal mucosa.

**PHARMACOKINETICS: Absorption:** Fexofenadine: Rapidly absorbed; $C_{max}$=634ng/mL (single dose), 674ng/mL (multiple doses); $T_{max}$=1.8-2 hrs.

Pseudoephedrine: $C_{max}$=394ng/mL (single dose), 495ng/mL (multiple doses); $T_{max}$=12 hrs. **Distribution:** Fexofenadine: Plasma protein binding (60-70%). Pseudoephedrine: $V_d$=2.6-3.5L/kg. **Metabolism:** Fexofenadine and pseudoephedrine: Hepatic (5% of fexofenadine; <1% of pseudoephedrine). **Elimination:** Fexofenadine: Feces (80%), urine (11%); $T_{1/2}$=14.6 hrs. Pseudoephedrine: $T_{1/2}$=7 hrs.

## NURSING CONSIDERATIONS

**Assessment:** Assess for narrow-angle glaucoma, urinary retention, MAOI therapy presently or within past 14 days, severe HTN, and severe CAD. Assess for idiosyncrasies to adrenergic agents or other drugs of similiar chemical structure. Assess use in patients with HTN, DM, ischemic heart disease, increased IOP, hyperthyroidism, renal impairment, prostatic hypertrophy, and in pregnant/nursing females. Assess for drug interactions.

**Monitoring:** Monitor for signs/symptoms of CNS stimulation with convulsions and for cardiovascular collapse with accompanying hypotension.

**Patient Counseling:** Instruct to take on empty stomach with water; swallow tab whole, do not break or chew. Instruct not to exceed recommended dose. Counsel to d/c and contact physician if nervousness, dizziness, or sleeplessness occur. Avoid concurrent use with OTC antihistamines and decongestants.

**Administration:** Oral route. **Storage:** 20-25°C (68-77°F). Store in tightly-closed container in a cool, dry place, away from children.

# ALOPRIM RX

allopurinol sodium (Bioniche)

**THERAPEUTIC CLASS:** Xanthine oxidase inhibitor

**INDICATIONS:** Management of elevated serum and urinary uric acid levels in patients with leukemia, lymphoma, and solid tumor malignancies receiving cancer therapy when oral therapy is not tolerated.

**DOSAGE:** *Adults:* Usual: 200-400mg/m²/day IV infusion qd or in equally divided infusions every 6, 8, or 12 hrs. Max: 600mg/day. CrCl 10-20mL/min: 200mg/day. CrCl 3-10mL/min: 100mg/day. CrCl <3mL/min: 100mg/day at extended intervals. Elderly: Start at lower end of dosing range.
*Pediatrics:* Usual: 200mg/m²/day IV qd or in divided doses every 6, 8, or 12 hrs.

**HOW SUPPLIED:** Inj: 500mg

**WARNINGS/PRECAUTIONS:** D/C at first appearance of hypersensitivity (skin rash or other signs which indicate an allergic reaction); increased risk in patients with decreased renal function. Caution with renal/hepatic impairment or concurrent illnesses affecting renal function such as HTN and diabetes mellitus (DM). Hepatotoxicity may occur; monitor LFTs during early stages of therapy if with pre-existing liver disease. Monitor renal function and uric acid levels; adjust dose if needed. Maintain sufficient fluid intake to yield a daily urinary output ≥2L and maintain neutral/slightly alkaline urine. May impair mental/physical abilities. Drowsiness and bone marrow suppression reported. Caution in elderly.

**ADVERSE REACTIONS:** Skin rash, eosinophilia, local injection-site reaction, N/V, diarrhea, renal failure/insufficiency.

**INTERACTIONS:** Inhibits oxidation of mercaptopurine and azathioprine; reduce mercaptopurine and azathioprine dose to 1/3-1/4 of usual dose. Increased frequency of skin rash with ampicillin and amoxicillin. Increased allopurinol toxicity and risk of hypersensitivity in patients with renal dysfunction with concomitant thiazide diuretics; monitor renal function. Increased risk of hypoglycemia in the presence of renal insufficiency with concomitant chlorpropamide. Enhanced bone marrow suppression when used with cyclophosphamide and other cytotoxic agents among patients with neoplastic disease, except leukemia. May increase cyclosporine levels; monitor cyclosporine levels and possible adjustment of cyclosporine dose may be needed when coadministered. Decreased inhibition of xanthine oxidase by oxypurinol and increased urinary excretion of uric acid with uricosuric agents. Prolongs half-life of dicumarol; monitor PT with concomitant use.

**PREGNANCY:** Category C, caution in nursing.

**MECHANISM OF ACTION:** Xanthine oxidase inhibitor; reduces production of uric acid by inhibiting the biochemical reactions immediately preceding its formation.

**PHARMACOKINETICS: Absorption:** Absolute bioavailability (100%); $C_{max}$=1.58µg/mL (100mg), 5.12µg/mL (300mg); $T_{max}$=0.5 hrs; AUC=1.99 hr•µg/mL (100mg), 7.1 hr•µg/mL (300mg). **Distribution:** $V_d$=0.84L/kg (100mg), 0.87L/kg (300mg); found in breast milk. **Metabolism:** Oxidative; oxypurinol (active metabolite). **Elimination:** Urine (12% unchanged, 76% as oxypurinol); $T_{1/2}$=(100mg) 1 hr (parent), 24.1 hrs (oxypurinol), (300mg) 1.21 hrs (parent), 23.5 hrs (oxypurinol).

## NURSING CONSIDERATIONS

**Assessment:** Assess for renal/hepatic impairment, concurrent illnesses affecting renal function (eg, HTN, DM), hypersensitivity reactions (eg, skin rash, Stevens-Johnson syndrome), pregnancy/nursing status and possible drug interactions. Obtain serum uric acid to provide correct dosage and schedule.

**Monitoring:** Monitor for allergic reactions, severe hypersensitivity reactions (eg, exfoliative, urticarial, purpuric lesions, Stevens-Johnson syndrome), generalized vasculitis, hepatotoxicity, drowsiness, bone marrow suppression and fluid intake. Monitor LFTs, serum uric acid, BUN and SrCr.

**Patient Counseling:** Inform about benefits/risks of therapy. Inform may impair mental/physical abilities. Advise to take sufficient fluid to yield a daily urinary output of at least 2L in adults and the need to maintain a neutral or preferably slightly alkaline urine. Advise to report any adverse events to physician.

**Administration:** IV infusion. Refer to PI for reconstitution and dilution. Rate of infusion depends on the volume of infusate. Whenever possible, initiate therapy 24-48 hrs before the start of chemotherapy known to cause tumor cell lysis (including adrenocorticosteroids). Do not mix or administer through the same IV port with agents which are incompatible in solution (refer to PI). Begin administration within 10 hrs after reconstitution. **Storage:** 25°C (77°F); excursions permitted to 15-30°C (59-86°F). After dilution, store solution at 20-25°C (68-77°F). Do not refrigerate the reconstituted and/or diluted product.

# ALOXI RX

palonosetron HCl (MGI Pharma)

**THERAPEUTIC CLASS:** 5-$HT_3$ receptor antagonist

**INDICATIONS:** Prevention of acute and delayed N/V associated with initial and repeat courses of moderately emetogenic cancer chemotherapy and prevention of acute N/V associated with initial and repeat courses of highly emetogenic cancer chemotherapy. Prevention of postoperative nausea and vomiting (PONV) for up to 24 hrs following surgery.

**DOSAGE:** Chemotherapy-Induced N/V: 0.25mg IV single dose over 30 sec. Dosing should occur approximately 30 min before the start of chemotherapy.

**HOW SUPPLIED:** Inj: 0.25mg/5mL

**WARNINGS/PRECAUTIONS:** Hypersensitivity reactions may occur in patients who have exhibited hypersensitivity to other 5-$HT_3$ receptor antagonists. Routine prophylaxis is not recommended in patients in whom there is little expectation that nausea and/or vomiting will occur postoperatively.

**ADVERSE REACTIONS:** Headache, constipation, QT prolongation, bradycardia.

**PREGNANCY:** Category B, not for use in nursing.

**MECHANISM OF ACTION:** 5-$HT_3$ receptor antagonist with antiemetic and antinauseant properties.

**PHARMACOKINETICS: Absorption:** (IV, 3mcg/kg) $C_{max}$=5.6ng/mL, AUC=35.8ng•hr/mL. **Distribution:** $V_d$=8.3L/kg; plasma protein binding

(62%). **Metabolism:** 50% metabolized via CYP2D6, CYP3A4, CYP1A2; N-oxide-palonosetron and 6-S-hydroxy-palonosetron (primary metabolites). **Elimination:** Urine (40%); $T_{1/2}$=40 hrs.

## NURSING CONSIDERATIONS

**Assessment:** Assess for previous hypersensitivity to other 5-$HT_3$ receptor antagonists and for pregnancy/nursing status.

**Monitoring:** Monitor ECG for QT interval prolongation. Monitor for hypersensitivity reactions.

**Patient Counseling:** Advise to report to physician of all medical conditions, any pain, redness, or swelling around infusion site. Instruct to read patient insert.

**Administration:** IV route. **Storage:** 20-25°C (68-77°F); excursions permitted to 15-30°C (59-86°F). Protect from light and freezing.

# ALPHAGAN P — RX

brimonidine tartrate (Allergan)

**THERAPEUTIC CLASS:** Selective $alpha_2$ agonist

**INDICATIONS:** Treatment of open-angle glaucoma and ocular hypertension.

**DOSAGE:** *Adults:* 1 drop in the affected eye(s) q8h. Space dosing of other topical products that lower IOP by 5 min.
*Pediatrics:* ≥2 yrs: 1 drop in the affected eye(s) q8h. Space dosing of other topical products that lower IOP by 5 min.

**HOW SUPPLIED:** Sol: 0.1% [5mL, 10mL, 15mL], 0.15% [5mL, 10mL, 15mL]

**CONTRAINDICATIONS:** Concomitant MAOI therapy.

**WARNINGS/PRECAUTIONS:** Caution with severe CV disease, hepatic or renal dysfunction, depression, cerebral or coronary insufficiency, Raynaud's phenomenon, orthostatic hypotension, thromboangiitis obliterans.

**ADVERSE REACTIONS:** Oral dryness, ocular hyperemia, ocular pruritus, burning, stinging, ocular allergic reaction, blurred vision, foreign-body sensation, fatigue, drowsiness, headache, conjunctival follicles.

**INTERACTIONS:** See Contraindications. May potentiate CNS depressants. May reduce BP; caution with β-blockers, antihypertensives, cardiac glycosides, TCAs. May be given with other topical products that lower IOP.

**PREGNANCY:** Category B, not for use in nursing.

**MECHANISM OF ACTION:** Selective $\alpha_2$ agonist; reduces aqueous humor production and increases uveoscleral outflow.

**PHARMACOKINETICS: Absorption:** $T_{max}$=0.5-2.5 hrs. **Metabolism:** Liver (extensive). **Elimination:** $T_{1/2}$=2 hrs.

## NURSING CONSIDERATIONS

**Assessment:** Assess for depression, cerebral or coronary insufficiency, Raynaud's phenomenon, orthostatic hypotension, or thromboangiitis obliterans. Assess renal/hepatic function prior to therapy, for MAOI therapy, other drug interactions, and pregnancy/nursing status.

**Monitoring:** Perform routine monitoring of IOP while on therapy. Monitor for signs of decreased pulse rate and BP levels while on medication.

**Patient Counseling:** Advise drug may cause fatigue and/or drowsiness; use caution during hazardous activities that require mental alertness. Advise that concomitant ophthalmic products should be seperated by at least 5 min.

**Administration:** Ocular route. **Storage:** 15-25°C (59-77°F).

## ALREX RX
loteprednol etabonate (Bausch & Lomb)

**THERAPEUTIC CLASS:** Corticosteroid

**INDICATIONS:** Relief of signs and symptoms of seasonal allergic conjunctivitis.

**DOSAGE:** *Adults:* 1 drop qid.

**HOW SUPPLIED:** Sus: 0.2% [5mL, 10mL]

**CONTRAINDICATIONS:** Viral diseases of the cornea and conjunctiva, including epithelial herpes simplex keratitis, vaccinia, and varicella. Mycobacterial infection and fungal diseases of the eye.

**WARNINGS/PRECAUTIONS:** Caution with glaucoma, herpes simplex, diseases causing thinning of cornea/sclera and other ocular viral infections. Prolonged use can cause glaucoma or secondary ocular infections (eg, fungal). Monitor IOP beyond 10 days of therapy. Wait 10 min after instillation before inserting soft contact lenses. Re-evaluate if no response after 2 days.

**ADVERSE REACTIONS:** Elevated IOP, foreign body sensation, itching, chemosis, epiphora, blurred vision, burning on instillation, discharge, dry eyes, photophobia.

**PREGNANCY:** Category C, caution in nursing.

**MECHANISM OF ACTION:** Corticosteroid; anti-inflammatory agent, not established. Inhibits edema, fibrin deposition, capillary dilation, leukocyte migration, fibroblast proliferation, deposition of collagen, and scar formation associated with inflammation by induction of phospholipase $A_2$ inhibitory protein lipocortin.

**PHARMACOKINETICS: Absorption:** $C_{max}$<1ng/mL.

### NURSING CONSIDERATIONS

**Assessment:** Assess for viral diseases of the cornea and conjunctiva (eg, epithelial herpes simplex, keratitis (dendritic keratitis), vaccinia and varicella, mycobacterial infection of the eye and fungal diseases of ocular structure, known hypersensitivity to drug components, glaucoma, and possible drug interactions.

**Monitoring:** Monitor for secondary ocular infections, fungal infections, masking or enhancement of existing infections, thinning of the cornea or sclera, perforation, glaucoma, damage to optic nerve, defects in visual acuity, and posterior subcapsular cataract formation.

**Patient Counseling:** Avoid touching dropper tip to eyes, fingers, or any surface. Notify physician if symptoms persist or worsen. Do not wear contact lenses if eyes are red or irritated.

**Administration:** Intraocular route. **Storage:** 15-25°C (59-77°F). Do not freeze.

## ALTABAX RX
retapamulin (GlaxoSmithKline)

**THERAPEUTIC CLASS:** Pleuromutilin antibacterial

**INDICATIONS:** Topical treatment of impetigo caused by susceptible strains of microorganisms, in patients ≥9 months.

**DOSAGE:** *Adults*: Apply thin layer (up to 100 cm² in total area) bid for 5 days. May cover with sterile bandage or gauze.
*Pediatrics:* 9 mos-17yrs: Apply thin layer (up to 2% total BSA) bid for 5 days. May cover with sterile bandage or gauze.

**HOW SUPPLIED:** Oint: 1% [5g, 10g, 15g, 30g]

**WARNINGS/PRECAUTIONS:** D/C if sensitization or irritation occurs. Not intended for oral, intranasal, ophthalmic or intravaginal use. May cause superinfection during therapy.

**ADVERSE REACTIONS:** Application-site reactions.

**INTERACTIONS:** Coadministration with ketoconazole may increase levels.

**PREGNANCY:** Category B, caution in nursing.

**MECHANISM OF ACTION:** Pleuromutilin antibacterial; selectively inhibits bacterial protein synthesis by interacting at a site on the 50S subunit of the bacterial ribosome. The binding site involves ribosomal protein L3 and is in the region of the ribosomal P site and peptidyl transferase center. By binding to this site, peptidyl transfer is inhibited, P-site interactions are blocked, and the formation of normal active 50S ribosomal subunits is prevented.

**PHARMACOKINETICS: Absorption:** Low systemic exposure. Following application to 800cm$^2$ of intact skin: $C_{max}$=3.5ng/mL (multiple doses). Following application to 200cm$^2$ of abraded skin: $C_{max}$=11.7ng/mL (single dose), 9.0ng/mL (multiple doses). **Distribution:** Plasma protein binding (94%). **Metabolism:** Liver via CYP3A4 (mono-oxygenation, N-demethylation).

## NURSING CONSIDERATIONS

**Assessment:** Assess for proper diagnosis of bacterial organisms, use in nursing females, and possible drug interactions.

**Monitoring:** Monitor for signs/symptoms of sensitization reactions or severe local irritation, and for the development of overgrowth of nonsusceptible organisms (superinfection).

**Patient Counseling:** Counsel drug is for external use only; avoid contact with eyes, mouth, inside of nose, or inside of female genital area. May use sterile bandage or gauze dressing after applying ointment. Wash hands following application (if hands are not the treatment area). Take the medication for full recommended time; notify physician if symptoms do not improve within 3-4 days after starting treatment or if irritation, redness, itching, burning, blistering, oozing at treatment site develops.

**Administration:** Topical route. Do not use in eyes, mouth, lips, or inside the nose. **Storage**: Store at 25°C (77°F); excursions permitted to 15-30°C (59-86°F).

# ALTACE — RX

ramipril (Monarch Pharmaceuticals Inc.)

**ACE inhibitors can cause death/injury to developing fetus during 2nd and 3rd trimesters. Stop therapy if pregnancy detected.**

**THERAPEUTIC CLASS:** ACE inhibitor

**INDICATIONS:** Hypertension, alone or with thiazide diuretics. To decrease hospitalization and mortality in stable post-MI patients who show signs of congestive heart failure (CHF). To reduce risk of MI, stroke, and cardiovascular (CV) death in patients ≥55 yrs who are at risk due to history of coronary artery disease, stroke, peripheral vascular disease, or diabetes with at least one other CV risk factor.

**DOSAGE:** *Adults:* HTN: Initial: 2.5mg qd. Maint: 2.5-20mg/day given qd or bid. Add diuretic if BP not controlled. CrCl <40mL/min: Initial: 1.25mg qd. Titrate/Max: 5mg/day. CHF Post-MI: Initial: 2.5mg bid, 1.25mg bid if hypotensive. Titrate: Increase to 5mg bid at 3 weeks interval. CrCl <40mL/min: Initial: 1.25mg qd. Titrate: May increase to 1.25mg bid. Max: 2.5mg bid. Risk Reduction of MI, Stroke, Death ( ≥55 yrs): Initial: 2.5mg qd for 1 week. Increase to 5mg qd for next 3 weeks. Maint: 10mg qd. Reduce or d/c diuretic if possible. With Volume Depletion/Renal Artery Stenosis: Initial: 1.25mg qd.

**HOW SUPPLIED:** Cap: 1.25mg, 2.5mg, 5mg, 10mg. Tab: 1.25mg, 2.5mg, 5mg, 10mg

**CONTRAINDICATIONS:** History of ACE inhibitor-associated angioedema.

**WARNINGS/PRECAUTIONS:** D/C if angioedema, jaundice/hepatic necrosis, or if marked LFT elevation occurs. Risk of hyperkalemia with diabetes mellitus (DM), renal dysfunction. Persistent nonproductive cough and anaphylactoid reactions reported. Monitor WBCs in renal and collagen vascular disease. Fetal/neonatal injury including hypotension, neonatal skull hypoplasia, anuria, renal failure, and death reported. Monitor for hypotension in high-risk patients (heart failure, surgery/anesthesia, hyponatremia, high-dose diuretic therapy, recent intensive diuresis, dialysis, or severe volume and/or salt depletion, etc). Caution with CHF, renal dysfunction, severe liver cirrhosis and/or ascites, and renal artery stenosis. Less effective on BP in blacks and more reports of angioedema than nonblacks. May reduce RBCs, Hgb, WBCs, or platelets. May cause agranulocytosis, pancytopenia, and bone marrow depression.

**ADVERSE REACTIONS:** Hypotension, cough, dizziness, fatigue, angina, headache.

**INTERACTIONS:** May increase lithium levels; if coadministered monitor levels and symptoms of lithium toxicity. Hypotension risk with diuretics. Increased risk of hyperkalemia with $K^+$-sparing diuretics, $K^+$ supplements, or $K^+$-containing salt substitutes. NSAIDs may worsen renal failure and increase serum potassium. Nitritoid reactions (eg, facial flushing, N/V, hypotension) reported rarely with injectable gold. Concomitant with telmisartan is not recommended. Hypotension reported with anesthesia agents.

**PREGNANCY:** Category C (1st trimester) and D (2nd and 3rd trimesters), not for use in nursing.

## NURSING CONSIDERATIONS

**Assessment:** Assess for pregnancy status, possible drug interactions, hypersensitivity, volume/salt depletion, DM, collagen vascular disease, CHF, hepatic/renal impairment. Obtain baseline BP, renal function and WBC with differential (impaired renal function).

**Monitoring:** Monitor renal function periodically; BP in first 2 weeks and at dosage change. If impaired renal function, monitor WBC with differential before therapy, at 2-week intervals for 3 months, and then periodically during therapy. Monitor for signs/symptoms of hypotension, anaphylactoid or hypersensitivity reactions, head/neck and intestinal angioedema, infection, and neutropenia/agranulocytosis.

**Patient Counseling:** Inform of pregnancy risks. Instruct that inadequate fluid intake or loss of fluids may lead to drop in BP resulting in lightheadedness or syncope; avoid $K^+$ or salt substitutes. Advise to seek medical attention if symptoms of angioedema (head/neck, intestinal), infection (sore throat, fever), syncope, or hypersensitivity reactions occur.

**Administration:** Oral route. **Storage:** (Cap) 59°-86°F, (Tab) 20°-25°C (68°-77°F); excursion permitted between 15°-30°C (59°-86°F).

# ALTOPREV RX

lovastatin (Sciele)

**THERAPEUTIC CLASS:** HMG-CoA reductase inhibitor

**INDICATIONS:** Adjunct to diet, to slow progression of coronary atherosclerosis in coronary heart disease. Adjunct to diet, for reduction of elevated total cholesterol (total-C), LDL-C, Apo B, and TG, and to increase HDL-C in patients with primary hypercholesterolemia (heterozygous familial and non-familial) and mixed dyslipidemia (Fredrickson types IIa and IIb). To reduce risk of MI, unstable angina, and coronary revascularization procedures in patients without symptomatic cardiovascular disease, average to moderately elevated Total-C and LDL-C, and below average HDL-C.

**DOSAGE:** *Adults:* Individualize dosing. Initial: 20, 40, or 60mg qhs. Range: 20-60mg/day. Consider immediate-release lovastatin in patients requiring smaller reductions. May adjust at intervals of ≥4 weeks. Elderly (>65 yrs)/Renal Insufficiency/Diabetes Mellitus: Initial: 20mg qhs. Severe Renal Insufficiency (CrCl <30mL/min): Consider dose increase of >20mg/day carefully and implement cautiously. Concomitant Fibrates/Niacin ( ≥1g/day): Try to avoid. Max: 20mg/day. Concomitant Amiodarone/Verapamil: Max: 20mg/day. Swallow whole; do not chew, crush or cut.

**HOW SUPPLIED:** Tab: Extended-Release: 20mg, 40mg, 60mg

**CONTRAINDICATIONS:** Active liver disease, unexplained persistent elevations of serum transaminases, pregnancy, nursing mothers.

**WARNINGS/PRECAUTIONS:** Myopathy and rhabdomyolysis with or without acute renal failure secondary to myoglobinuria reported. May increase serum transaminases and CPK levels; consider in differential diagnosis of chest pain. D/C if AST or ALT ≥3x ULN persists, if myopathy diagnosed or suspected, and a few days before major surgery. Monitor LFTs prior to therapy, at 6 weeks and 12 weeks after initiation of therapy or elevation of dose, and then periodically thereafter. Caution with heavy alcohol use and/or history of hepatic disease. Caution with dose escalation in renal insufficiency. May cause endocrine dysfunction and CNS toxicity. Lovastatin immediate-release found to be less effective with homozygous familial hypercholesterolemia.

**ADVERSE REACTIONS:** Nausea, abdominal pain, insomnia, dyspepsia, headache, asthenia, myalgia, diarrhea, back pain, flu syndrome, infection, arthralgia, sinusitis.

**INTERACTIONS:** Due to increased risk of myopathy, suspend lovastatin if itraconazole, ketoconazole, erythromycin, or clarithromycin must be used. Avoid other CYP3A4 inhibitors unless benefits outweigh the risk (eg, HIV protease inhibitors, nefazodone, >1 quart/day grapefruit juice). Avoid use with cyclosporine. Avoid use with gemfibrozil, other fibrates, or lipid lowering doses of (>1g/day) of niacin; if necessary, lovastatin dose should not exceed 20mg/day. Avoid lovastatin doses >20 mg/day if used with amiodarone or verapamil. Monitor PT in patients taking anticoagulants (eg, warfarin) before starting lovastatin and following initiation of therapy. Caution with drugs that may decrease the levels or activity of endogenous steroid hormones (eg, ketoconazole, spironolactone, cimetidine).

**PREGNANCY:** Category X, not for use in nursing.

**MECHANISM OF ACTION:** HMG-CoA reductase inhibitor; inhibits the conversion of HMG-CoA to mevalonate which is an early step in the biosynthetic pathway for cholesterol. Reduces LDL-C and total-C.

**PHARMACOKINETICS: Absorption:** Lovastatin: $C_{max}$=5.5ng/mL, $T_{max}$=14.2 hrs, AUC=77ng•hr/mL. Lovastatin acid: $C_{max}$=5.8ng/mL, $T_{max}$=11.8 hr, AUC=87ng•hr/mL. **Distribution:** Plasma protein binding (>95%). Crosses blood brain/placental barriers. **Metabolism:** Liver (extensive), β-hydroxy acid, 6'-hydroxy derivative, and two additional metabolites (major active metabolites). **Elimination:** Urine, bile.

## NURSING CONSIDERATIONS

**Assessment:** Assess for active liver disease or unexplained persistent elevations in serum transaminases, pregnancy/nursing status, renal insufficiency, homozygous familial hypercholesterolemia, and for possible drug interactions. Assess use in patients who consume substantial quantities of alcohol and/or have a past history of liver disease. Assess LFTs prior to therapy.

**Monitoring:** Monitor for signs/symptoms of myopathy/rhabdomyolysis (eg, pain, tenderness, or weakness), increases in serum transaminases, CNS toxicity, and endocrine dysfunction. Monitor creatine kinase levels. Monitor LFTs at 6 and 12 weeks after initiation of therapy or dose elevations, and periodically thereafter.

**Patient Counseling:** Inform about risks/benefits of therapy. Instruct to promptly report unexplained muscle pain, tenderness, or weakness. Advise to avoid grapefruit juice. Instruct to swallow tablet whole and to not chew, crush, or cut tablet. Counsel to inform physician of all medical conditions and medicines being taken.

**Administration:** Oral route. Take drug whole; do not crush, chew or cut. **Storage:** 20-25°C (68-77°F); excursions permitted to 15-30°C (59-86°F). Avoid excessive heat and humidity.

# ALVESCO RX

ciclesonide (Sepracor)

**THERAPEUTIC CLASS:** Non-halogenated glucocorticoid

**INDICATIONS:** Maintenance treatment of asthma as prophylactic therapy in adults and adolescents ≥12 yrs.

**DOSAGE:** *Adults:* Previous Bronchodilator Alone: Initial: 80mcg bid. Max: 160mcg bid. Previous Inhaled Corticosteroid Therapy: Initial: 80mcg bid. Max: 320mcg bid. Previous Oral Corticosteroid Therapy: Initial: 320mcg bid. Max: 320mcg bid.

*Pediatrics:* ≥12 yrs: Previous Bronchodilator Alone: Initial: 80mcg bid. Max: 160mcg bid. Previous Inhaled Corticosteroid Therapy: Initial: 80mcg bid. Max: 320mcg bid. Previous Oral Corticosteroid Therapy: Initial: 320mcg bid. Max: 320mcg bid.

**HOW SUPPLIED:** MDI: 80mcg/actuation [60 actuations], 160mcg/actuation [60 or 120 actuations]

**CONTRAINDICATIONS:** Status asthmaticus or other acute episodes of asthma.

**WARNINGS/PRECAUTIONS:** *Candida albicans* infections of mouth and pharynx may occur; examine periodically and treat accordingly. Advise to rinse mouth after inhalation. Caution with active or quiescent TB infections, untreated local/systemic bacterial/fungal infections, systemic viral or parasitic infections, or ocular herpes simplex. Risk for more severe/fatal course of infections (eg, chickenpox, measles); avoid exposure in patients who have not had the disease or been properly immunized. Risk of adrenal insufficiency and withdrawal symptoms when replacing oral corticosteroids with inhaled corticosteroids; monitor closely. Taper dose if symptoms of hypercorticism and adrenal suppression occur. May cause reduced growth velocity in pediatrics. May decrease bone mineral density (BMD) with prolonged treatment; monitor and treat accordingly. Caution with history of glaucoma, increased IOP, and cataracts; monitor closely. Acute asthma episodes or bronchospasm may occur; d/c use and institute alternative treatment if occur.

**ADVERSE REACTIONS:** Headache, nasopharyngitis, sinusitis, pharyngolaryngeal pain, upper respiratory infection, arthralgia, nasal congestion, pain in extremity, back pain.

**INTERACTIONS:** Ketoconazole may increase levels of the pharmacologically active metabolite des-ciclesonide; coadminister with caution.

**PREGNANCY:** Category C, caution in nursing.

**MECHANISM OF ACTION:** Corticosteroid: exerts anti-inflammatory actions with affinity to glucocorticoid receptor that inhibits activities of multiple cell types (mast cells, eosinophils, basophils, lymphocytes, macrophages, and neutrophils) and mediators (histamine, eicosanoids, leukotrienes, and cytokines) involved in asthmatic response.

**PHARMACOKINETICS: Absorption:** Ciclesonide: Absolute bioavailability: 22%. Des-ciclesonide (active metabolite): 63%; $C_{max}$=1.02ng/mL in asthmatic patient. **Distribution:** Ciclesonide: $V_d$=2.9L/kg. Des-ciclesonide: $V_d$=12.1L/kg. **Metabolism:** Liver, via CYP3A4, CYP2D6 (hydrolysis); des-ciclesonide (active metabolite). **Elimination:** Feces (60%), urine (≤20%), and bile. $T_{1/2}$=ciclesonide (0.71 hrs), des-ciclesonide (6-7 hrs).

## NURSING CONSIDERATIONS

**Assessment:** Assess for risk of impaired adrenal function, presence of status asthmaticus or other acute episodes of asthma and potential worsening of current infection (TB, ocular herpes simplex), history of increased IOP, glaucoma, and/or cataracts, under systemic corticosteroid therapy, and hypersensitivity to drug.

**Monitoring:** Monitor for signs of adverse effects in oral cavity, change of vision, growth velocity measurement (stadiometry) especially for pediatrics, BMD, corticosteroid effects of hypercorticism and adrenal suppression, and urinary cortisol level.

**Patient Counseling:** Advise that drug is not a bronchodilator and not intended to provide rapid relief of breathing difficulties during asthmatic attack. Instruct that medication must be taken at regular intervals as recommended, and not as emergency measure. Caution to not inhale more often than what is advised. Instruct that it may take 4 weeks or longer to feel full benefit. Instruct to report if symptoms do not improve in that time frame or if condition worsens at any point during treatment. Instruct to not stop treatment even if feeling better unless told to do so. Inform that if dose is missed, wait and take regularly scheduled next dose. Advise to test spray inhaler on 1st use or if it has not been used for more than 10 days.

**Administration:** Inhalation route. Inhaler is fitted with dose indicator which shows how much medication is left during use. Dose indicator display will move every 10th time puff is taken. Dose indicator display window will turn red when there are only 20 puffs remaining; this means that inhaler must be replaced soon. Inhalation Steps: 1) Close lips around mouthpiece, keeping tongue below it. 2) While breathing in deeply and slowly, press down on center of dose. Fully depress canister until it stops moving in adapter while delivering dose. When finished breathing in, hold breath for about 10 sec, or for as long as is comfortable. Breathe out gently. 3) After taking dose, rinse mouth with water and spit out; do not swallow. Do not wash inhaler in water.
**Storage:** Store at room temperature. Keep out of reach of children. Contents under pressure. Do not puncture. Temperature above 120°F (49°C) may cause bursting. Never throw into fire.

## AMARYL RX

glimepiride (Sanofi-Aventis)

**THERAPEUTIC CLASS:** Sulfonylurea (2nd generation)

**INDICATIONS:** Adjunct to diet and exercise, to improve glycemic control in type 2 diabetes mellitus. May use in combination with metformin or insulin.

**DOSAGE:** *Adults:* Initial: 1-2mg qd with breakfast or 1st main meal. Titrate: After 2mg, may increase by up to 2mg every 1-2 weeks. Maint: 1-4mg qd. Max: 8mg qd. Amaryl/Metformin: Add Metformin to 8mg qd for better glucose control. Amaryl/Insulin Therapy: If FBG >150mg/dL on 8mg qd, add low-dose insulin; increase insulin weekly as needed. Renal Insufficiency: Initial: 1mg qd. Elderly/Debilitated/Malnourished/Hepatic Insufficiency: Dose conservatively to avoid hypoglycemia.

**HOW SUPPLIED:** Tab: 1mg, 2mg, 4mg

**CONTRAINDICATIONS:** Diabetic ketoacidosis with or without coma.

**WARNINGS/PRECAUTIONS:** Increased CV mortality. Hypoglycemia risk if debilitated, malnourished, or with adrenal, pituitary, renal or hepatic insufficiency. Hypoglycemia may be masked in elderly and patients with autonomic neuropathy. May lose blood glucose control with stress (eg, fever, trauma, infection, or surgery). Secondary failure may occur. Risk of hemolytic anemia reported with G6PD deficiency; use with caution and consider alternative therapy. Allergic reaction may develop if allergic to other sulfonamide derivatives.

**ADVERSE REACTIONS:** Dizziness, nausea, asthenia, headache, hypoglycemia.

**INTERACTIONS:** Potentiates hypoglycemia with alcohol, NSAIDs, insulin, metformin, highly protein-bound drugs, such as salicylates, sulfonamides, chloramphenicol, coumarin, probenecid, MAOIs, miconazole, β-blockers, disopyramide, fluoxetine, quinolones, and clarithromycin. Risk of hyperglycemia with diuretics, corticosteroids, phenothiazines, thyroid products, estrogens, oral contraceptives, phenytoin, nicotinic acid, sympathomimetics, and isoniazid. Monitor for hypoglycemia when switching from long-acting sulfonylurea, and with combination therapy with insulin and metformin. Hypoglycemia may be masked with β-blockers or other sympatholytic agents.

**PREGNANCY:** Category C, not for use in nursing.

**MECHANISM OF ACTION:** Sulfonylurea; lowers blood glucose by stimulating insulin release from functioning pancreatic β cells.

**PHARMACOKINETICS: Absorption:** Administration of variable doses resulted in different parameters. Complete (GI tract, 100%); $T_{max}$=2-3 hrs; **Distribution:** (IV) $V_d$=8.8L; plasma protein binding (99.5%). **Metabolism:** Complete (liver); CYP2C9; major metabolites: M1 & M2. **Elimination:** Urine (60%), feces (40%).

## NURSING CONSIDERATIONS

**Assessment:** Assess for signs/symptoms of hypoglycemia, loss of glucose control (fever, trauma, infection), risk of CV mortality, hepatic porphyria, hyponatremia, allergic reactions, thrombocytopenia, leukopenia, agranulocytosis, and hepatitis (eg, cholestasis, jaundice), G6PD deficiency, pregnancy/nursing status, and potential drug interactions.

**Monitoring:** Monitor fasting blood glucose and glycosylated hemoglobin (every 3-6 months) to determine response to therapy and glycemic control.

**Patient Counseling:** Instruct to have a proper diet and exercise and regularly test blood glucose. Inform about risks of hypoglycemia (symptoms, treatment) and conditions that predispose to development. Inform risks, advantages, and alternative modes of therapy.

**Administration:** Oral route. **Storage:** 15-30°C (59-86°F). Dispense in tightly closed container.

# AMBIEN

**CIV**

zolpidem tartrate (Sanofi-Aventis)

**THERAPEUTIC CLASS:** Imidazopyridine hypnotic

**INDICATIONS:** Short-term treatment of insomnia characterized by difficulties with sleep initiation.

**DOSAGE:** *Adults:* Tab: Usual: 10mg qhs. Elderly/Debilitated/Hepatic Insufficiency: Initial: 5mg. Decrease dose with other CNS depressants. Max: 10mg qd. Re-evaluate if insomnia persists after 7-10 days.

**HOW SUPPLIED:** Tab: 5mg, 10mg

**WARNINGS/PRECAUTIONS:** Severe anaphylactic/anaphylactoid reactions reported. Abnormal thinking, behavior changes and complex behaviors (eg, sleep driving) reported. Worsening of depression or suicidal thinking may occur; use lowest feasible amount to avoid intentional overdose. Withdrawal symptoms may occur with rapid dose reduction or d/c. Potential impairment of activities requiring complete mental alertness (eg, operating machinery) after ingestion and following day. Monitor elderly and debilitated patients for impaired motor performance. Caution with hepatic impairment, mild to moderate COPD or sleep apnea, impaired drug metabolism or hemodynamic responses. Avoid if a full night's sleep not possible.

**ADVERSE REACTIONS:** Drowsiness, dizziness, headache, nausea, diarrhea, drugged feeling, dyspepsia, myalgia, lethargy, memory loss, anxiety, abnormal thoughts and behavior, tongue or throat swelling.

**INTERACTIONS:** Decreased alertness with imipramine. Impaired alertness and psychomotor performance with chlorpromazine. Additive psychomotor impairment with alcohol and other CNS depressants. Rifampin may decrease effects. Flumazenil may reverse effect.

**PREGNANCY:** Category B, not for use in nursing.

**MECHANISM OF ACTION:** Imidazopyridine, a non-benzodiazepine hypnotic; binds to $GABA_A$ receptor complex at the α-subunit/benzodiazepine receptor, the major modulatory site. GABA receptor complex modulation is hypothesized to be responsible for the sedative, anticonvulsant, anxiolytic, myorelaxant properties.

**PHARMACOKINETICS: Absorption:** Rapid. $C_{max}$=59ng/mL (5mg), 121ng/mL (10mg). $T_{max}$=1.6 (5mg, 10mg). **Distribution:** Plasma protein binding (92.5%). **Metabolism**: CYP450. **Elimination**: Renal; $T_{1/2}$=2.6 hrs (5mg), 2.5 hrs (10mg).

## NURSING CONSIDERATIONS

**Assessment:** Carefully assess for primary psychiatric and/or medical illness or depression prior to initiation. Assess for presence of pre-existing respiratory impairment (eg, myasthenia gravis, sleep apnea syndrome, COPD), hepatic/renal impairment, possible drug interaction, and history of addiction or abuse of drugs or alcohol.

**Monitoring:** Monitor for anaphylactic/anaphylactoid reactions, insomnia, abnormal thinking, behavioral changes, complex behaviors (eg, sleep driving, suicidal thinking), visual and auditory hallucinations. Monitor patients with hepatic/renal impairment, and for drug abuse/dependence with long-term treatment.

**Patient Counseling:** Counsel to take immediately before bedtime and not with or right after meals. Inform about benefits/risks with long-term use. Caution needed when performing hazardous tasks (eg, operating machinery/driving). Counsel on tolerance, dependence, and withdrawal signs/symptoms. Do not take with alcohol.

**Administration:** Oral route. **Storage:** 20-25°C (68-77°F).

# AMBIEN CR

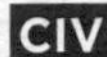


zolpidem tartrate (Sanofi-Aventis)

**THERAPEUTIC CLASS:** Imidazopyridine hypnotic

**INDICATIONS:** Treatment of insomnia, characterized by difficulties with sleep onset and/or sleep maintenance.

**DOSAGE:** *Adults:* 12.5mg qhs. Elderly/Debilitated/Hepatic Insufficiency: 6.25mg qhs. Swallow whole; do not divide, crush, or chew.

**HOW SUPPLIED:** Tab, Extended-Release: 6.25mg, 12.5mg

**WARNINGS/PRECAUTIONS:** Use smallest possible effective dose, especially in elderly. Abnormal thinking and behavior changes reported with use of sedative/hypnotics. Caution with depression and conditions that could affect metabolism or hemodynamic responses. Signs and symptoms of withdrawal reported with abrupt d/c of sedative/hypnotics. Monitor elderly and debilitated patients for impaired motor and/or cognitive performance.

**ADVERSE REACTIONS:** Headache, somnolence, dizziness, nausea, hallucinations, back pain, myalgia, fatigue.

**INTERACTIONS:** Increased effect with alcohol and other CNS depressants. Rifampin may decrease effects. Flumazenil reverses effect.

**PREGNANCY:** Category C, not for use in nursing.

**MECHANISM OF ACTION:** Imidazopyridine, non-benzodiazepine hypnotic; binds to $GABA_A$ receptor complex at the α-subunit/benzodiazepine receptor, the major modulatory site. GABA receptor complex modulation is hypothesized to be responsible for the sedative, anticonvulsant, anxiolytic, myorelaxant properties.

**PHARMACOKINETICS: Absorption:** Rapid; 12mg: $C_{max}$=134ng/mL, $T_{max}$=1.5 hrs, AUC=740ng•hr/mL. **Distribution:** Plasma protein binding (92.5%). **Metabolism**: CYP450. **Elimination:** Urine; $T_{1/2}$=2.8 hrs.

## NURSING CONSIDERATIONS

**Assessment:** Assess for primary psychiatric illness or depression, pre-existing respiratory impairment (eg, COPD, sleep apnea syndrome), hypersensitivity reactions, hepatic/renal impairment, possible drug interactions, and history of alcohol abuse.

**Monitoring:** Monitor for anaphylactic/anaphylactoid reactions, abnormal thinking, behavioral changes, complex behavior (eg, sleep driving, hallucinations). Monitor patients with hepatic/renal impairment, and those on long-term treatment for drug abuse/dependence.

**Patient Counseling:** Counsel to take just before bedtime without food; do not crush, divide, or chew, and do not take when drinking alcohol. Caution against hazardous tasks (eg, driving/operating machines). Inform about risks/benefits of use.

**Administration:** Oral route. **Storage:** 15-25°C (59-77°F).

## AmBisome RX

amphotericin B liposome (Astellas)

**THERAPEUTIC CLASS:** Polyene antifungal

**INDICATIONS:** Empirical therapy for presumed fungal infection in febrile, neutropenic patients. Treatment of *Aspergillus, Candida,* or *Cryptococcus* infections refractory to amphotericin B deoxycholate or where renal impairment or unacceptable toxicity precludes its use. Treatment of cryptococcal meningitis in HIV-infected patients. Treatment of visceral leishmaniasis.

**DOSAGE:** *Adults:* Empiric Therapy: 3mg/kg/day IV. Systemic Infections (*Aspergillus, Candida, Cryptococcus*): 3-5mg/kg/day IV. Cryptococcal Meningitis in HIV: 6mg/kg/day IV. Visceral Leishmaniasis: Immunocompetent: 3mg/kg/day IV on Days 1-5, 14, 21. May repeat course if needed. Immunocompromised: 4mg/kg/day IV on Days 1-5, 10, 17, 24, 31, 38. *Pediatrics:* 1 month-16 yrs: Empirical Therapy: 3mg/kg/day IV. Systemic Infections (*Aspergillus, Candida, Cryptococcus*): 3-5mg/kg/day IV. Cryptococcal Meningitis in HIV: 6mg/kg/day IV. Visceral Leishmaniasis: Immunocompetent: 3mg/kg/day IV on Days 1-5, 14, 21. May repeat course if needed. Immunocompromised: 4mg/kg/day IV on Days 1-5, 10, 17, 24, 31, 38.

**HOW SUPPLIED:** Inj: 50mg

**WARNINGS/PRECAUTIONS:** If anaphylaxis occurs, d/c all further infusions. Significantly less toxic than amphotericin B deoxycholate. Monitor renal, hepatic, hematopoietic function and electrolytes (especially $K^+$, $Mg^{++}$).

**ADVERSE REACTIONS:** Chills, asthenia, back pain, pain, infection, chest pain, HTN, hypotension, tachycardia, GI hemorrhage, diarrhea, N/V, hyperglycemia, hypokalemia, dyspnea.

**INTERACTIONS:** Concurrent use of antineoplastic agents may potentiate renal toxicity, bronchospasm, hypotension. Corticosteroids and corticotropin may potentiate hypokalemia. May potentiate digitalis toxicity. May increase flucytosine toxicity. Acute pulmonary toxicity with leukocyte transfusions reported. Nephrotoxic drugs enhance potential for renal toxicity. May enhance curariform effect of skeletal muscle relaxants due to hypokalemia. Imidazoles (eg, ketoconazole, miconazole, clotrimazole, fluconazole) may induce fungal resistance; caution with combination therapy, especially in immunocompromised patients.

**PREGNANCY:** Category B, not for use in nursing.

**MECHANISM OF ACTION:** Antifungal agent; acts by binding to the sterol component of the cell membrane, which leads to changes in cell permeability and cell death in susceptible fungi. Also binds to the cholesterol component of the mammalian cell, leading to cytotoxicity.

**PHARMACOKINETICS: Absorption:** IV administration of variable doses resulted from different parameters. **Metabolism:** Not known.

### NURSING CONSIDERATIONS

**Assessment:** Assess cultures, renal function, and possible drug interactions.

**Monitoring:** Monitor for acute infusion reactions (eg, chills, hypotension, hypoxia, rash), renal, hepatic and hematopoietic function, and serum electrolytes (particularly $Mg^+$ and $K^+$).

**Patient Counseling:** Seek medical attention if symptoms of acute reaction occur (eg, fevers, chills, respiratory symptoms). May receive pretreatment medication to help prevent acute infusion reactions. Infusion time may be reduced to approximately 60 min if treatment is well tolerated.

**Administration:** IV infusion. Reconstitute. 1) Add 12mL of Sterile Water For Inj, USP to vial. 2) Shake vial until all solids are completely dispersed. 3) Further dilute using 5% Dextrose. Must be diluted to a final concentration of

1.0-2.0 mg/mL in adults, (0.2-0.5mg/mL may be appropriate for infants and children). Discard partially used vials. Infuse over a period of 120 min. If using an existing IV line, must flush with 5% Dextrose prior to infusion. Otherwise, another IV line must be used. **Storage:** Unopened vials: 25°C (77°F). Reconstituted: 2-8°C (36-46°F) stored for 24 hrs. Diluted Product: Injection should commence within 6 hrs of dilution with 5% Dextrose Injection.

## AMERGE RX

naratriptan HCl (GlaxoSmithKline)

**THERAPEUTIC CLASS:** 5-$HT_{1B/1D}$ agonist

**INDICATIONS:** Acute treatment of migraine with or without aura.

**DOSAGE:** *Adults:* ≥18 yrs: 1mg or 2.5mg taken with fluids; may repeat dose once after 4 hrs. Max: 5mg/24 hrs. Mild-Moderate Renal/Hepatic Impairment: Initial: Lower dose. Max: 2.5mg/24 hrs. Safety of treating >4 headaches/30 days not known.

**HOW SUPPLIED:** Tab: 1mg, 2.5mg

**CONTRAINDICATIONS:** Uncontrolled HTN, ischemic cardiac disease, cerebrovascular or peripheral vascular syndromes, other significant CVD, severe renal or hepatic impairment, basilar or hemiplegic migraine, within 24 hrs of another 5-$HT_1$ agonist, ergotamine-containing or ergot-type drugs (eg, dihydroergotamine, methysergide).

**WARNINGS/PRECAUTIONS:** Confirm diagnosis. Supervise 1st dose and monitor cardiac function in those at risk of CAD (eg, HTN, hypercholesterolemia, smoker, obesity, diabetes, CAD family history, postmenopausal women, males >40 yrs). Monitor cardiovascular function with long-term intermittent use. May cause vasospastic reactions or cerebrovascular events. Serotonin syndrome may occur; symptoms may include mental status changes, autonomic instability, neuromuscular aberrations, and GIT symptoms. Caution with renal or hepatic dysfunction. Avoid in elderly.

**ADVERSE REACTIONS:** Paresthesias, dizziness, drowsiness, malaise/fatigue, throat and neck symptoms (eg, pain/pressure sensation).

**INTERACTIONS:** Ergotamine-containing and ergot-type drugs (eg, dihydroergotamine, methysergide) drugs may cause prolonged vasospastic reactions. Avoid other 5-$HT_1$ agonist drugs within 24-hr period due to additive effects. Serotonin syndrome reported with combined use of an SSRI or SNRI.

**PREGNANCY:** Category C, caution in nursing.

**MECHANISM OF ACTION:** Selective 5-$HT_1$ receptor agonist; binds with high affinity to 5-$HT_{1D/1B}$ receptors; two theories explain its efficacy in migraine. One theory suggests that activation of 5-$HT_{1D/1B}$ receptors located on intracranial blood vessels, including those on arteriovenous anastomoses, leads to vasoconstriction that correlates with relief of migraine. Another suggests that activation of 5-$HT_{1D/1B}$ receptors in the trigeminal system results in inhibition of pro-inflammatory neuropeptide release.

**PHARMACOKINETICS: Absorption:** Well-absorbed; bioavailability (70%); $T_{max}$=2-3 hrs. **Metabolism:** Via CYP450 isoenzymes. **Distribution:** $V_d$=170L, plasma protein binding (28-31%); found in breast milk. **Elimination:** Urine (50% unchanged, 30% metabolites); $T_{1/2}$=6 hrs.

### NURSING CONSIDERATIONS

**Assessment:** Confirm diagnosis of migraine before therapy. Assess for IHD (eg, angina pectoris, Prinzmetal's variant angina, MI or documented silent MI), HTN, hemiplegic/basilar migraine, presence of risk factors (eg, hypercholesterolemia, smoking, obesity, DM, strong family history of CAD, female with surgical/physiological menopause, or male >49 yrs), ECG changes, hepatic/renal impairment, pregnancy/nursing status, and possible drug interactions.

**Monitoring:** Administration of 1st dose should be in physician's office or medically staffed and equipped facility as cardiac ischemia may occur in absence of clinical symptoms; ECG should be obtained immediately during interval in those with risk factors. Monitor for signs/symptoms of cardiac events (eg, coronary vasospasm, acute MI, arrhythmia, ECG changes, follow-up coronary angiography), cerebrovascular events (eg, hemorrhage, stroke, TIAs), peripheral vascular ischemia, colonic ischemia with bloody diarrhea and abdominal pain, serotonin syndrome (eg, mental status changes, autonomic instability, neuromuscular aberrations and/or GI symptoms), ophthalmic effects, increased BP, and anaphylaxis/anaphylactoid reactions.

**Patient Counseling:** Inform about potential risks of therapy (eg, symptoms of serotonin syndrome such as confusion, hallucinations, fast heartbeat, fever, sweating, muscle spasms, and diarrhea), especially if taken with SSRIs or SNRIs. Instruct to report adverse reactions to physician. Advise to take exactly as directed. Instruct to notify if pregnant/nursing or planning to become pregnant.

**Administration:** Oral route. **Storage:** 20-25°C (68-77°F).

## AMEVIVE RX

alefacept (Astellas)

**THERAPEUTIC CLASS:** Immunosuppressive agent

**INDICATIONS:** Treatment of moderate to severe chronic plaque psoriasis for candidates of systemic therapy or phototherapy.

**DOSAGE:** *Adults:* 15mg IM once weekly for 12 weeks. May initiate retreatment with an additional 12-week course if CD4+ T-lymphocyte counts are within normal range and a 12-week minimum interval has passed since the previous course of treatment. If CD4+ T-Lymphocyte Counts <250 cells/µL, withhold dose. D/C if counts remain below 250 cells/µL for 1 month.

**HOW SUPPLIED:** Inj: 15mg

**CONTRAINDICATIONS:** HIV.

**WARNINGS/PRECAUTIONS:** Dose-dependent reductions in circulating CD4+ and CD8+ T-lymphocyte counts reported. Do not initiate with CD4+ T-lymphocyte counts below normal; monitor every 2 weeks. May increase risk of malignancies; do not administer to patients with history of systemic malignancy. May increase risk of infection or reactivate latent, chronic infections; avoid with clinically important infections, caution with chronic infection or history of recurrent infections; d/c if serious infection develops. D/C if serious hypersensitivity reactions occur. Liver injury (fatty infiltration, hepatitis) reported; d/c if significant clinical signs of liver injury develop. Caution in elderly. Avoid concurrent phototherapy.

**ADVERSE REACTIONS:** Lymphopenia, malignancies, serious infections, hypersensitivity reactions, pharyngitis, dizziness, increased cough, nausea, pruritus, myalgia, chills, injection-site pain/inflammation.

**INTERACTIONS:** Avoid with other immunosuppressive agents.

**PREGNANCY:** Category B, not for use in nursing.

**MECHANISM OF ACTION:** Immunosuppressive agent; interferes with lymphocyte activation by specifically binding to the lymphocyte antigen CD2, and inhibiting LFA-2/CD2 interaction. Reduces subsets of CD2+ T lymphocytes (primarily CD45RO+), presumably by bridging between CD2 on target lymphocytes and immunoglobulin Fc receptors on cytotoxic cells, such as natural killer cells, which results in reduction of circulating total CD4+ and CD8+ T-lymphocyte counts.

**PHARMACOKINETICS: Absorption:** Bioavailability (63%). **Distribution:** $V_d$=94mL/kg. **Elimination:** $T_{1/2}$=270 hrs.

### NURSING CONSIDERATIONS

**Assessment:** Assess for HIV infection, history of systemic malignancy or risk of malignancy, chronic infections or history of recurrent infection, immunosuppressants or phototherapy, immunization status, hepatic impairment, pregnancy/nursing status, and possible drug interactions. Prior to initiation or subsequent course of therapy, patient should have normal CD4+ T lymphocytes.

**Monitoring:** Requires monitoring of CD4+ T lymphocyte counts every 2 weeks throughout the course of the 12-week dosing regimen. Monitor for signs/symptoms of infection during or after a course of therapy. Monitor for new infections, malignancies, hypersensitivity reactions (urticaria, angioedema, anaphylactic reactions, or serious allergic reaction), signs/symptoms of hepatic injury, and WBCs.

**Patient Counseling:** Inform about potential risks/benefits of therapy and to report any signs/symptoms of infections, malignancy, or liver injury (eg, N/V, fatigue, jaundice, dark urine) to physician. Notify physician if pregnant/nursing or planning to become pregnant.

**Administration:** IM route. Use only under supervision of a physician. **Storage:** 2-8°C (36-46°F). Protect from light, retain in carton or drug/diluent pack until time of use.

## AMICAR — RX

aminocaproic acid (Xanodyne)

**THERAPEUTIC CLASS:** Monoamino carboxylic acid anti-fibrinolytic

**INDICATIONS:** To enhance hemostasis when fibrinolysis contributes to bleeding.

**DOSAGE:** *Adults:* IV: 16-20mL (4-5g) in 250mL diluent during 1st hr, then 4mL/hr (1g) in 50mL of diluent. PO: 5g during 1st hr, then 5mL (syr) or 1g (tabs) per hr. Continue therapy for 8 hrs or until bleeding is controlled.

**HOW SUPPLIED:** Inj: 250mg/mL [20mL]; Syrup: 1.25g/5mL; Tab: 500mg*, 1000mg* *scored

**CONTRAINDICATIONS:** Active intravascular clotting process, disseminated intravascular coagulation without concomitant heparin.

**WARNINGS/PRECAUTIONS:** Avoid in hematuria of upper urinary tract origin due to risk of intrarenal obstruction from glomerular capillary thrombosis or clots in renal pelvis and ureters. Skeletal muscle weakness with necrosis of muscle fibers reported after prolonged therapy. Consider cardiac muscle damage with skeletal myopathy. Avoid rapid IV infusion. Thrombophlebitis may occur. Contains benzyl alcohol; do not administer to neonates due to risk of fatal "gasping syndrome." Do not administer without a definite diagnosis of hyperfibrinolysis.

**ADVERSE REACTIONS:** Edema, headache, anaphylactoid reactions, injection-site reactions, pain, bradycardia, hypotension, abdominal pain, diarrhea, N/V, agranulocytosis, increased CPK, confusion, dyspnea, pruritus, tinnitus.

**INTERACTIONS:** Increased risk of thrombosis with Factor IX complex concentrates, anti-inhibitor coagulant concentrates.

**PREGNANCY:** Category C, caution in nursing.

**MECHANISM OF ACTION:** Monoamino carboxylic acid anti-fibrinolytic; fibrinolysis inhibitory effects are exerted principally by inhibition of plasminogen activators and, to a lesser extent, through antiplasmin activity.

**PHARMACOKINETICS: Absorption:** (PO) $C_{max}$=164mcg/mL; $T_{max}$=1.2 hrs. **Distribution:** (PO) $V_d$=23.1L; (IV) $V_d$=30L. **Metabolism:** Adipic acid (metabolite). **Elimination:** Renal: Urine (65% unchanged), (11% metabolite); $T_{1/2}$=2 hrs.

### NURSING CONSIDERATIONS

**Assessment:** Assess for evidence of active intravascular clotting, proper diagnosis of hyperfibrinolysis (hyperplasminemia), pregnancy/nursing status, and possible drug interactions. Assess use in presence of hematuria of the upper urinary tract origin.

**Monitoring:** Monitor for signs/symptoms of subendocardial hemorrhages, fatty degeneration of the myocardium, skeletal muscle weakness with necrosis of muscle fibers (rhabdomyolysis, myoglobinuria, acute renal failure), cardiac muscle damage, thrombophlebitis, and neurological deficits (eg, hydrocephalus, cerebral ischemia, cerebral vasospasm). In patients with upper urinary tract bleeding, monitor for signs/symptoms of intrarenal obstruction (eg, glomerular capillary thrombosis, clots in renal pelvis and ureters). If used in pediatrics, monitor for "gasping syndrome" in neonates. Monitor CPK levels in patients on long-term therapy. Perform periodic monitoring to determine amount of fibrinolysis present.

**Patient Counseling:** Advise not to administer without definite diagnosis (laboratory finding indicative of hyperfibrinolysis). Instruct to contact physician if unusual muscle weakness or pain develops.

**Administration:** IV or Oral routes. IV: Use compatible intravenous vehicles (eg, Sterile Water for Injection, Sodium Chloride for Injection, 5% Dextrose or Ringer's Injection). Rapid IV administration may induce hypotension, bradycardia, and/or arrhythmias. **Storage:** 15-30°C (59-86°F).

## AMIKACIN — RX

amikacin sulfate (Various)

**Potential for ototoxicity and nephrotoxicity. Neuromuscular blockade, respiratory blockade reported. Avoid potent diuretics and other neurotoxic, nephrotoxic, and ototoxic drugs.**

**THERAPEUTIC CLASS:** Aminoglycoside

**INDICATIONS:** Short-term treatment of serious infections due to susceptible strains of gram-negative bacteria. Shown to be effective in bacterial septicemia; respiratory tract, bone/joint, CNS (including meningitis), skin and soft tissue, and intra-abdominal infections; burns and postoperative infections; complicated and recurrent urinary tract infections (UTI) due to susceptible strains of microorganisms.

**DOSAGE:** *Adults:* IM/IV: 15mg/kg/day given q8h or q12h. Max: 15mg/kg/day. Heavier Wt Patients: Max: 1.5g/day. Recurrent Uncomplicated UTI: 250mg bid. Usual Duration: 7-10 days. D/C therapy if no response after 3-5 days. D/C if azotemia increases or if progressive decrease in urinary output occurs. Renal Impairment: Reduce dose.
*Pediatrics:* 15mg/kg/day given q8h or q12h. Newborns: LD: 10mg/kg. Maint: 7.5mg/kg q12h. Usual Duration: 7-10 days. D/C therapy if no response after 3-5 days. D/C if azotemia increases or if progressive decrease in urinary output occurs. Renal Impairment: Reduce dose.

**HOW SUPPLIED:** Inj: 50mg/mL, 250mg/mL

**CONTRAINDICATIONS:** History of serious toxic reactions to aminoglycosides.

**WARNINGS/PRECAUTIONS:** May aggravate muscle weakness; caution with muscular disorders (eg, myasthenia gravis, parkinsonism). May cause fetal harm in pregnancy. Contains sodium metabisulfite, allergic reactions may occur especially in asthmatics. Maintain adequate hydration. Assess kidney function before therapy, then daily.

**ADVERSE REACTIONS:** Ototoxicity, neuromuscular blockage, nephrotoxicity, skin rash, drug fever, headache, paresthesia, tremor, nausea, arthralgia, anemia, hypotension.

**INTERACTIONS:** Increased nephrotoxicity with cephalosporins. Significant mutual inactivation may occur with β-lactams (eg, penicillin, cephalosporins). Cross-allergenicity between aminoglycosides. Avoid potent diuretics (eg, ethacrynic acid, furosemide), bacitracin, cisplatin, amphotericin B, paromomycin, polymyxin B, colistin, vancomycin, other aminoglycosides, and other neurotoxic, nephrotoxic and ototoxic drugs. Increased risk of neuromuscular blockade and respiratory paralysis with anesthetics, neuromuscular blockers, or massive transfusions of citrate-anticoagulated blood.

**PREGNANCY:** Category D, not for use in nursing.

**MECHANISM OF ACTION:** Semi-synthetic aminoglycoside antibiotic derived from kanamycin.

**PHARMACOKINETICS: Absorption**: Rapidly absorbed after IM administration. (IV) $C_{max}$=38mcg/mL. **Distribution**: $V_d$=24L; plasma protein binding (0-11%); crosses placenta. **Elimination**: Urine; $T_{1/2}$ ≥2 hr; (IM) 91.9% at 8 hrs, 98.2% at 24 hrs; (IV) 84% at 9 hrs, 94% at 24 hrs.

## NURSING CONSIDERATIONS

**Assessment:** Assess for pregnancy/nursing status, renal impairment, muscular disorders (eg, myasthenia gravis, parkinsonism) and for possible drug interactions. Assess renal function tests prior to and throughout therapy.

**Monitoring:** Periodic monitoring of urea, creatinine, CrCl, audiometric testing changes, 8th nerve function, serum concentrations of the drug and urine (specific gravity, proteins, presence of cells/casts). Monitor for signs/symptoms of nephrotoxicity, neurotoxicity (vestibular and permanent bilateral auditory ototoxicity, vertigo, numbness, skin tingling, muscle twitches, and convulsions), cochlear damage, neuromuscular blockade, respiratory paralysis, and CDAD.

**Patient Counseling:** Inform about potential risks/benefits of therapy and to report signs of ototoxicity (eg, dizziness, vertigo, tinnitus, roaring in the ears, and hearing loss). Notify physician if pregnant/nursing or planning to become pregnant. Inform that drug treats bacterial infections only. Take as prescribed.

**Administration:** IV, IM route. Obtain pretreatment body weight to calculate correct dosage. **Storage**: 20-25°C (68-77°F).

# AMILORIDE/HCTZ RX

amiloride HCl - hydrochlorothiazide (Various)

**THERAPEUTIC CLASS:** $K^+$-sparing diuretic/thiazide diuretic

**INDICATIONS:** Treatment of hypertension or congestive heart failure if hypokalemia occurs on thiazides or kaliuretic diuretics alone, or if maintenance of normal serum $K^+$ levels is clinically important.

**DOSAGE:** *Adults:* Initial: 1 tab qd. Titrate: May increase to 2 tabs qd or in divided doses. Max: 2 tabs/day. May give intermittently once diuresis is achieved. Take with food.

**HOW SUPPLIED:** Tab: (Amiloride-HCTZ) 5mg-50mg* *scored

**CONTRAINDICATIONS:** Hyperkalemia, anuria, sulfonamide hypersensitivity, acute or chronic renal insufficiency, diabetic neuropathy. Concomitant $K^+$-sparing agents (eg, spironolactone, triamterene), $K^+$ supplements, salt substitutes, $K^+$-rich diet (except with severe hypokalemia).

**WARNINGS/PRECAUTIONS:** Risk of hyperkalemia ( ≥5.5mEq/L), especially with renal impairment or DM; d/c if hyperkalemia occurs. Monitor for fluid/electrolyte imbalance; hyponatremia and hypochloremia may occur. Caution in severely ill (risk of respiratory or metabolic acidosis). Increases BUN, cholesterol, and TG levels. D/C at least 3 days before glucose tolerance test. May precipitate gout or exacerbate SLE. May precipitate azotemia with renal disease.

**ADVERSE REACTIONS:** Nausea, anorexia, rash, headache, weakness, hyperkalemia, dizziness.

**INTERACTIONS:** May potentiate other antihypertensives. Risk of lithium toxicity. Increased risk of hyperkalemia with ACE inhibitors, angiotensin II receptor antagonists, indomethacin, cyclosporine, tacrolimus. May increase responsiveness to nondepolarizing muscle relaxants. May decrease response to norepinephrine. Antidiabetic agents may need adjustment. Alcohol, barbiturates, or narcotics may potentiate orthostatic hypotension. NSAIDs may decrease effects. Cholestyramine, colestipol impair absorption. ACTH, corticosteroids intensify electrolyte depletion.

**PREGNANCY:** Category B, not for use in nursing.

**MECHANISM OF ACTION:** Amiloride: Antikaliuretic-diuretic; inhibits $Na^+$ reabsorption at tubules and collecting duct, decreasing potential of tubular lumen, reducing $K^+$ and $H^+$ secretion and excretion. HCTZ: Thiazide diuretic; affects distal renal tubular mechanism of electrolyte reabsorption, increasing $Na^+$ and $Cl^-$ excretion.

**PHARMACOKINETICS: Absorption:** Amiloride: $T_{max}$=3-4 hrs. **Distribution:** HCTZ: Crosses placenta; excreted in breast milk. **Elimination:** Amiloride: Urine (50%), feces (40%); $T_{1/2}$=6-9 hrs. HCTZ: Kidney (61%); $T_{1/2}$=5.6-14.8 hrs.

## NURSING CONSIDERATIONS

**Assessment:** Assess for hyperkalemia, anuria, renal impairment, DM, systemic lupus erythematosus (SLE), sulfonamide hypersensitivity, possible drug interactions, metabolic or respiratory acidosis, and history of allergy or bronchial asthma. Obtain baseline serum $K^+$ levels.

**Monitoring:** Monitor serum electrolytes, renal function, acid-base balance, and serum $K^+$ levels periodically. Monitor for signs/symptoms of electrolyte imbalance, hyper/hypokalemia, hypersensitivity reactions, renal dysfunction, hypo/hyperglycemia, hyperuricemia or precipitation of gout, and exacerbation or activation of SLE.

**Patient Counseling:** Instruct to take with food; avoid use of $K^+$ supplements or salt substitutes. Seek medical attention if symptoms of hyperkalemia (paresthesias, muscle weakness, fatigue), electrolyte imbalance, or hypersensitivity reactions occur.

**Administration:** Oral route. **Storage:** 15-30°C (59-86°). Protect from light.

# AMIODARONE IV — RX

amiodarone HCl (Various)

**THERAPEUTIC CLASS:** Class III antiarrhythmic

**INDICATIONS:** Initiation of treatment and prophylaxis of frequently recurring ventricular fibrillation and hemodynamically unstable ventricular tachycardia refractory to other therapies.

**DOSAGE:** *Adults:* LD: 150mg over 1st 10 min (15mg/min), then 360mg over next 6 hrs (1mg/min), then 540mg over remaining 18 hrs (0.5mg/min). Maint: 0.5mg/min for 2-3 weeks. Breakthrough Ventricular Tachycardia/Ventricular Fibrillation: 150mg supplement IV over 10 min. Increase rate to achieve suppression. Elderly: Start at low end of dosing range. Administer infusions >2 hrs in a glass or polyolefin bottle containing $D_5W$. Amiodarone leaches out plasticizers (eg, DEHP from IV tubing) especially at higher infusion concentrations, and lower flow rates.

**HOW SUPPLIED:** Inj: 50mg/mL [3mL]

**CONTRAINDICATIONS:** Cardiogenic shock, marked sinus bradycardia, 2nd- or 3rd-degree AV block (unless a functioning pacemaker is available). Hypersensitivity to iodine.

**WARNINGS/PRECAUTIONS:** Bradycardia and AV block reported. Hypotension reported; do not exceed initial rate of infusion. Correct hypokalemia or hypomagnesemia before therapy to prevent exaggeration of $QT_c$ prolongation. Congenital goiter/hypothyroidism, hyperthyroidism, postoperative ARDS reported with oral therapy. Hyperthyroidism may result in thyrotoxicosis and/or the possibility of arrhythmia breakthrough or aggravation. Elevations of hepatic enzymes reported. May worsen or precipitate a new arrhythmia; monitor for $QT_c$ prolongation. Adult respiratory distress syndrome (ARDS) reported. Pulmonary toxicity reported. Contains benzyl alcohol. Caution in elderly.

**ADVERSE REACTIONS:** Hypotension, fever, bradycardia, CHF, heart arrest, ventricular tachycardia, abnormal LFTs, nausea.

**INTERACTIONS:** Risk of interactions may persist after discontinuation due to long half-life. May increase PT with warfarin. May elevate plasma levels of cyclosporine, digoxin, quinidine, procainamide, phenytoin, disopyramide, HMG-CoA reductase inhibitors. May increase QT prolongation with disopyramide. Reduce flecainide dose to maintain therapeutic plasma levels. Cholestyramine may decrease levels and half-life. Decreased levels with phenytoin. Risk of bradycardia, hypotension with β-blockers, fentanyl. Increased risk of AV block with verapamil or diltiazem and hypotension with CCBs. May increase sensitivity to myocardial depressant and conduction defects of halogenated inhalational anesthetics. CYP3A4 inhibitors (eg, protease inhibitors, cimetidine, grapefruite juice) may increase levels. QT prolongation and torsades de pointes with $H_1$ antagonists (eg, loratadine) and antidepressants (eg, trazodone) reported. Concomitant use with clopidogrel may result in ineffective inhibition of platelet aggregation. CYP3A4 inducers (eg, rifampin, St. John's wort) may decrease levels. Concomitant use with fentanyl may cause hypotension, bradycardia, and decreased cardiac output. $QT_c$ prolongation reported with fluoroquinolones, macrolides, and azoles. Concomitant administration with propranolol, diltiazem, and verapamil may result in hemodynamic and electrophysiologic interactions.

**PREGNANCY:** Category D, not for use in nursing.

**MECHANISM OF ACTION:** Class III antiarrhythmic; blocks sodium, calcium, and potassium channels; exerts noncompetitive antisympathetic action, and negative chronotropic and dromotropic effects; lengthens cardiac action potential, decreases cardiac workload and myocardial oxygen consumption.

**PHARMACOKINETICS: Absorption:** $C_{max}$=5-41mg/L. **Distribution:** Plasma protein binding (>96%). **Metabolism:** CYP3A4, 2C8; N-desethylamiodarone (major active metabolite). **Elimination:** Urine, bile; $T_{1/2}$=20-47 days.

## NURSING CONSIDERATIONS

**Assessment:** Assess for cardiogenic shock, marked sinus bradycardia, 2nd- or 3rd-degree AV block, functioning pacemaker, thyroid dysfunction, pulmonary disorders, pregnancy/nursing status, and possible drug interaction. Prior to initiation, hypokalemia and hypomagnesemia should be corrected with special attention to electrolyte and acid-base balance in patients experiencing severe/prolonged diarrhea or concomitantly receiving diuretics.

**Monitoring:** Monitor for hypotension, bradycardia, AV block, acute/centrolobular confluent hepatocelluar necrosis, hepatic coma, acute renal failure, worsening of existing or precipitation of new arrhythmia, ARDS, pulmonary fibrosis, optic neuropathy/neuritis, visual impairment, thyrotoxicosis, and congenital goiter/hypothyroidism in infants. Monitor LFTs and thyroid function. Perioperative monitoring for myocardial depression recommended.

**Patient Counseling:** Advise that corneal refractive laser surgery is contraindicated with concurrent use. Inform about benefits/risks and report any adverse reactions promptly.

**Administration:** IV route. **Storage:** 15-25°C (59-77°F). Protect from light.

# AMITIZA — RX

lubiprostone (Sucampo/Takeda)

**THERAPEUTIC CLASS:** Chloride channel activator

**INDICATIONS:** Treatment of chronic idiopathic constipation in adults. Treatment of the irritable bowel syndrome with constipation (IBS-C) in women ≥18 yrs.

**DOSAGE:** *Adults:* Chronic Idiopathic Constipation: 24mcg bid with food. IBS-C: 8mcg bid with food.

**HOW SUPPLIED:** Cap: 8mcg, 24mcg

**CONTRAINDICATIONS:** History of mechanical gastrointestinal obstruction.

**WARNINGS/PRECAUTIONS:** Potential to cause fetal loss; women who could become pregnant should have a negative pregnancy test prior to initiation of therapy and comply with effective contraceptive measures. May cause nausea. Do not prescribe to patients with severe diarrhea. Dyspnea reported. Confirm absence of mechanical GI obstruction prior to initiating therapy.

**ADVERSE REACTIONS:** Nausea, diarrhea, abdominal distention/pain/discomfort, flatulence, vomiting, loose stools, sinusitis, urinary/upper respiratory tract infections, headache, dizziness, peripheral edema, arthralgia.

**PREGNANCY:** Category C, not for use in nursing.

**MECHANISM OF ACTION:** Chloride channel activator; enhances chloride-rich intestinal fluid secretion, increasing motility in the intestine, thereby facilitating the passage of stool.

**PHARMACOKINETICS: Absorption:** (M3) $C_{max}$=41.5pg/mL, $T_{max}$=1.1 hrs, AUC=57.1pg•hr/mL. **Distribution:** Plasma protein binding (94%). **Metabolism:**

Stomach, jejunum (biotransformation via carbonyl reductase). (Metabolite) M3. **Elimination:** (M3) $T_{1/2}$=0.9-1.4hrs.

## NURSING CONSIDERATIONS

**Assessment:** Assess for known mechanical GI obstruction, severe diarrhea, and pregnancy status. Perform pregnancy test and thorough evaluation to confirm absence of obstruction (if symptoms suggestive of mechanical obstruction) prior to therapy.

**Monitoring:** Monitor for symptoms of hypersensitivity reactions and severe diarrhea.

**Patient Counseling:** Advise to take with food to reduce symptoms of nausea. Report severe nausea or diarrhea to physician.

**Administration**: Oral route. **Storage:** 25°C (77°F); excursions permitted to 15-30°C (59-86°F). Protect from extreme temperatures.

# AMITRIPTYLINE RX

amitriptyline HCl (Mylan)

**Antidepressants increased the risk of suicidal thinking and behavior (suicidality) in short-term studies in children, adolescents, and young adults with major depressive disorder (MDD) and other psychiatric disorders. Monitor for clinical worsening, suicidality, or unusual changes in behavior. Not approved for pediatric patients.**

**THERAPEUTIC CLASS:** Tricyclic antidepressant

**INDICATIONS:** Relief of symptoms of depression, especially endogenous depression.

**DOSAGE:** *Adults:* PO: Initial: (Outpatient) 75mg/day in divided doses or 50-100mg qhs. (Inpatient) 100mg/day. Titrate: (Outpatient) Increase by 25-50mg qhs. (Inpatient) Increase to 200mg/day. Increases are made preferably in the late afternoon and/or bedtime doses. Maint: 50-100mg qhs. Max: (Outpatient) 150mg/day. (Inpatient) 300mg/day. Elderly: 10mg tid and 20mg qhs. *Pediatrics:* >12 yrs: Adolescents: 10mg tid and 20mg qhs.

**HOW SUPPLIED:** Tab: 10mg, 25mg, 50mg, 75mg, 100mg, 150mg

**CONTRAINDICATIONS:** MAOI use or within 14 days; acute recovery period following MI; concurrent cisapride.

**WARNINGS/PRECAUTIONS:** Screen for risk for bipolar disorder. Caution with history of seizures, urinary retention, angle-closure glaucoma, increased IOP, hyperthyroidism, cardiovascular disorders, liver dysfunction. Increases symptoms with schizophrenia and bipolar disorder. D/C several weeks before elective surgery. May alter blood glucose levels. May impair physical/mental abilities. Caution in elderly.

**ADVERSE REACTIONS:** MI, stroke, seizure, paralytic ileus, urinary retention, constipation, blurred vision, dry mouth, hyperpyrexia, rash, bone marrow depression, testicular swelling, gynecomastia (male), breast enlargement (female), alopecia, edema.

**INTERACTIONS:** See Contraindications. May block antihypertensive effects of guanethidine. Potentiates other CNS depressants, alcohol, barbiturates. Increased levels with CYP2D6 inhibitors (eg, quinidine, cimetidine, SSRIs). Avoid within 5 weeks of fluoxetine use. Caution with thyroid drugs. Delirium reported with disulfiram and ethchlorvynol. Paralytic ileus and hyperpyrexia with anticholinergics. Monitor with sympathomimetics and neuroleptics. Increased plasma levels with cimetidine. Very rare cases of serotonin syndrome (SS) have been reported with other drugs that have a recognized association with SS.

**PREGNANCY:** Category C, not for use in nursing.

**MECHANISM OF ACTION:** Dibenzocycloheptadiene derivative; suspected to inhibit the membrane pump mechanism responsible for uptake of norepinephrine and serotonin in adrenergic and serotonergic neurons.

**PHARMACOKINETICS: Absorption:** Rapid. **Distribution:** Excreted in breast milk; crosses the placenta. **Metabolism:** N-demethylation and hydroxylation.

## NURSING CONSIDERATIONS

**Assessment:** Assess if acute recovery period after MI, for bipolar disorder risk, history of mania, paranoia, seizures, unrecognized/history of schizophrenia, CVD, hyperthyroidism, IOP, narrow-angle glaucoma, urinary retention, hepatic impairment, hypersensitivity, pregnancy/nursing status, and possible drug interactions.

**Monitoring:** Periodically monitor LFTs, thyroid function tests, blood glucose, and CBC. Monitor for signs/symptoms of clinical worsening (suicidality, unusual changes in behavior), mania, cardiovascular events, increasing psychosis or paranoia, mydriasis, hypo/hyperglycemia, seizures, hepatic dysfunction, cognitive/motor impairment, and hypersensitivity reactions.

**Patient Counseling:** Advise to avoid alcohol. Seek medical attention for symptoms of mania, clinical worsening (suicidal ideation, unusual changes in behavior), cardiovascular events, increasing psychosis or paranoia, mydriasis, hypo/hyperglycemia, seizures, and discontinuation symptoms (irritability, agitation, dizziness, anxiety, headache, insomnia). Caution in engaging hazardous tasks (eg, driving automobile).

**Administration:** Oral route. **Storage:** 20-25°C (68-77°F). Dispense in tight, light-resistant container. Keep out the reach of children

# AMOXIL RX

amoxicillin (GlaxoSmithKline)

**THERAPEUTIC CLASS:** Semisynthetic ampicillin derivative

**INDICATIONS:** Treatment of infections of the ear, nose, throat, genitourinary tract (GU), skin and skin structure (SSSI), lower respiratory tract (LRTI); acute, uncomplicated gonorrhea due to susceptible (β-lactamase negative) strains of microorganisms. Combination therapy for *H.pylori* eradication to reduce the risk of duodenal ulcer recurrence.

**DOSAGE:** *Adults:* Ear/Nose/Throat/SSSI/GU: (Mild/Moderate) 500mg q12h or 250mg q8h. (Severe) 875mg q12h or 500mg q8h. LRTI: 875mg q12h or 500mg q8h. Gonorrhea: 3g as single dose. *H.pylori:* (Dual Therapy) 1g + 30mg lansoprazole, both tid x 14 days. (Triple Therapy) 1g + 30mg lansoprazole + 500mg clarithromycin, all q12h x 14 days. (Amoxicillin) GFR 10-30mL/min: 250-500mg q12h. GFR<10mL/min: 250-500mg q24h. Hemodialysis: 250-500mg q24h, additional dose during and at end of dialysis.
*Pediatrics:* Neonates: ≤12 weeks: Max: 30mg/kg/day divided q12h. >3 months: Ear/Nose/Throat/SSSI/GU: (Mild/Moderate) 25mg/kg/day given q12h or 20mg/kg/day given q8h. (Severe): 45mg/kg/day given q12h or 40mg/kg/day given q8h. LRTI: 45mg/kg/day given q12h or 40mg/kg/day given q8h. Gonorrhea: (Prepubertal) 50mg/kg with 25mg/kg probenecid as single dose. (Not for <2yrs). >40kg: Dose as adult.

**HOW SUPPLIED:** (Amoxil) Cap: 500mg; Sus: 50mg/mL [30mL], 250mg/5mL [100mL, 150mL], 400mg/5mL [100mL]. (Generic) Cap: 250mg, 500mg; Sus: 125mg/5mL [80mL, 100mL, 150mL], 200mg/5mL [50mL, 75mL, 100mL], 250mg/5mL [80mL, 100mL, 150mL], 400mg/5mL [50mL, 75mL, 100mL]; Tab: 500mg, 875mg; Tab, Chewable: 125mg, 200mg, 250mg, 400mg

**WARNINGS/PRECAUTIONS:** Serious, sometimes fatal, hypersensitivity reactions reported with PCN therapy. *Clostridium difficile*-associated diarrhea (CDAD) has been reported. May develop superinfection with mycotic or bacterial pathogens; d/c if superinfection occurs. Erythematosus rash may develop in patients with mononucleosis; avoid use in patients with mononucleosis. Prescribing in absence of a proven or strongly suspected bacterial infection or a prophylactic indication is unlikely to provide benefit and increases risk of developing drug-resistant bacteria. Perform periodic assessment of renal, hepatic, and hematopoietic function with prolonged use. The 200mg and 400mg chewable tabs contain phenylalanine. All patients with gonorrhea should have a serologic test for syphilis at the time of diagnosis; patients treated with amoxicillin should have a follow-up serologic test for syphilis after 3 months. In pregnant women, may cause a transient decrease in plasma concentrations of total conjugated estriol, estriol-glucuronide, conjugated estrone, and estradiol. False (+) for urine glucose with Clinitest, Benedict's or Fehling's solution.

**ADVERSE REACTIONS:** N/V, diarrhea, black hairy tongue, pseudomembranous colitis, hypersensitivity reactions, blood dyscrasias, hepatic dysfunction, tooth discoloration.

**INTERACTIONS:** Increased and prolonged levels with probenecid. Abnormal prolongation of PT may occur when used concomitantly with oral anticoagulants; monitor PT and adjust dose appropriately. May reduce efficacy of combined oral estrogen/progesterone contraceptives. Chloramphenicol, macrolides, sulfonamides, tetracyclines may interfere with bactericidal effects.

**PREGNANCY:** Category B, caution in nursing.

**MECHANISM OF ACTION:** Ampicillin analog; has broad-spectrum bactericidal activity against susceptible organisms during active multiplication; acts through inhibition of biosynthesis of cell-wall mucopeptide.

**PHARMACOKINETICS: Absorption:** Rapid. Cap (250mg): $T_{max}$=1-2 hrs. $C_{max}$=3.5-5mcg/mL. Cap (500mg): $T_{max}$=1-2 hrs. $C_{max}$=5.5-7.5mcg/mL. Tab (875mg): $C_{max}$=13.8mcg/mL, AUC=35.4mcg•hr/mL. Oral suspension (400mg): $C_{max}$=5.92mcg/mL, AUC=17.1mcg•hr/mL. Chewable tab (400mg): $C_{max}$=5.18mcg/mL, AUC=17.9mcg•hr/mL. Oral suspension (125mg): $T_{max}$=1-2 hrs, $C_{max}$=1.5-3mcg/mL. Oral Suspension (250mg) $T_{max}$=1-2 hrs, $C_{max}$=3.5-5mcg/mL. **Distribution:** Plasma protein binding, (20%). Found in breast milk. Diffuses to spinal fluid and brain only if meninges inflamed. **Elimination:** Urine (unchanged); $T_{1/2}$=61.3 min.

## NURSING CONSIDERATIONS

**Assessment:** Assess for history of allergic reaction to PCNs, cephalosporins, or other allergens, infectious mononucleosis, phenylketonurics, pregnancy/nursing status, and for possible drug interactions.

**Monitoring:** Monitor for serious anaphylactic reactions, erythematous skin rash, development of drug resistance or superinfection with mycotic or bacterial pathogen, signs/symptoms of CDAD (may range from mild diarrhea to fatal colitis). Monitor for false (+) reactions for urinary glucose test if Clinitest, Benedict's/Fehling's solutions are used, and transient decrease in plasma concentration of total conjugated estriol, estriol-glucuronide, conjugated estrone and estradiol if given to pregnant women. In patients on prolonged therapy, periodically monitor renal, hepatic, and hematopoietic function. Perform serologic test for syphilis at diagnosis of gonorrhea and after 3 months of treatment with amoxicillin.

**Patient Counseling:** Inform drug treats bacterial, not viral, infections. Instruct to take exactly as directed; skipping doses or not completing full course may decrease effectiveness and increase resistance. Inform about potential benefits/risks; notify physician if watery/bloody diarrhea (with/without stomach cramps and fever) develop (may occur as late as 2 months after treatment). Notify if pregnant/nursing.

**Administration:** Oral route. **Storage:** ≤20°C (68°F) for caps and (250mg) unreconstituted powder; ≤25°C (77°F) for unreconstituted powder (200-400mg), chewable tabs, and tabs. Store in tight container.

# AMPHOTEC RX

amphotericin B cholesteryl sulfate (Three Rivers)

**THERAPEUTIC CLASS:** Polyene antifungal

**INDICATIONS:** Treatment of invasive aspergillosis in patients with renal impairment, unacceptable toxicity, or previous failure to amphotericin deoxycholate.

**DOSAGE:** *Adults:* Test Dose: Infuse small amount over 15-30 min. Treatment: 3-4mg/kg/day IV at 1mg/kg/hr.
*Pediatrics:* Test Dose: Infuse small amount over 15-30 min. Treatment: 3-4mg/kg/day IV at 1mg/kg/hr.

**HOW SUPPLIED:** Inj: 50mg, 100mg

**WARNINGS/PRECAUTIONS:** Anaphylaxis may occur. D/C if severe respiratory distress occurs. Acute reactions (eg, fever, shaking chills, hypotension, nausea, tachypnea) 1-3 hrs after starting infusion. Monitor renal/hepatic function, electrolytes, CBC, PT during therapy.

**ADVERSE REACTIONS:** Chills, fever, headache, hypotension, tachycardia, HTN, N/V, thrombocytopenia, increased creatinine, hypokalemia, dyspnea, hypoxia.

**INTERACTIONS:** Antineoplastics may potentiate renal toxicity, bronchospasm, hypotension. Corticosteroids and corticotropin may potentiate hypokalemia. May increase flucytosine toxicity. Caution with imidazoles (eg, ketoconazole, clotrimazole, miconazole, fluconazole). Increased risk of renal toxicity with nephrotoxic drugs (eg, aminoglycosides, cyclosporine, pentamidine). May enhance curariform effect of skeletal muscle relaxants (eg, tubocurarine) or digitalis toxicity with hypokalemia.

**PREGNANCY:** Category B, not for use in nursing.

**MECHANISM OF ACTION:** Polyene antibiotic; binds to sterols (primarily ergosterol) in cell membranes of sensitive fungi, with subsequent leakage of intracellular contents and cell death. Also binds to cholesterol in mammalian cell membranes, which may account for human toxicity.

**PHARMACOKINETICS: Administration:** Variable doses resulted in altered parameters. **Absorption:** 3mg/kg/day: AUC=29µg/mL•hr, $C_{max}$=2.6µg/mL. 4mg/kg/day: AUC=36µg/mL•hr, $C_{max}$=2.9µg/mL. **Distribution:** 3mg/kg/day: $V_d$=3.8L/kg. 4mg/kg/day: $V_d$=4.1L/kg. **Metabolism:** Unknown. **Elimination:** 3mg/kg/day: $T_{1/2}$=27.5 hrs. 4mg/kg/day: $T_{1/2}$=28.2 hrs.

## NURSING CONSIDERATIONS

**Assessment:** Assess cultures, renal function, and possible drug interactions.

**Monitoring:** Monitor for acute infusion reactions (fevers, chills, hypoxia, hypotension), hepatic function, serum electrolytes, CBC, PT, and possible drug interactions.

**Patient Counseling:** Seek medical attention if symptoms of acute reaction occur (fever, chills, respiratory symptoms).

**Administration:** IV route. Infusion time may be shortened to 2 hrs for patients who show no evidence of intolerance or infusion-related reactions. If reaction occurs or if infusion is not tolerated, infusion time may be extended. Do not reconstitute lyophilized powder with saline or dextrose solutions, or admix the reconstituted liquid with saline or electrolytes. Do not mix infusion admixture with other drugs. If using an existing IV line, flush with 5% Dextrose prior and following infusion, or administer via a separate line. 1) Reconstitute: Add Sterile Water for Inj, USP to vial. If using 50mg/vial, add 10mL of Sterile Water. If using 100mg/vial, add 20mL of Sterile Water. 2) Shake vial until all solids have dissolved. 3) Further dilute using 5% Dextrose Inj, USP. **Storage:** Unopened vial: 15-30°C (59-86°F). Store in unopened carton. Reconstituted: Refrigerate 2-8°C (36-46°F). Use within 24 hrs, do not freeze. Further diluted with 5% Dextrose: Refrigerate 2-8°C. Use within 24 hrs.

# AMPHOTERICIN B — RX

amphotericin B (Various)

**Treatment primarily for progressive and potentially life-threatening fungal infections. Not for noninvasive fungal disease (eg, oral thrush, vaginal and esophageal candidiasis) in patients with normal neutrophil counts. Exercise caution to prevent inadvertent overdosage; verify product name and dose especially if dose >1.5mg/kg.**

**OTHER BRAND NAMES:** Fungizone (Geneva)

**THERAPEUTIC CLASS:** Polyene antifungal

**INDICATIONS:** Treatment of progressive, potentially life-threatening fungal infections including aspergillosis, cryptococcosis, North American blastomycosis, systemic candidiasis, coccidioido-mycosis, histoplasmosis, zygomycosis including mucormycosis due to susceptible species of the genera (*Absidia,*

*Mucor* and *Rhizopus*), sporotrichosis, and infections due to susceptible species of *Conidiobolus* and *Basidiobolus*. May be useful for treatment of American mucocutaneous leishmaniasis.

**DOSAGE:** *Adults:* Administer by slow IV infusion. Test dose: 1mg in 20mL of D5W over 20-30 min. Treatment: Initial: 0.25mg/kg. Severe or rapidly progressive Infection: Initial: 0.3mg/kg. Give smaller initial dose if impaired cardio-renal function or severe reaction to test dose. Titrate: May increase by 5-10mg/day, depending on cardio-renal status, up to 0.5-0.7mg/kg/day. Max: 1mg/kg/day or 1.5mg/kg/day when given on alternate days. Sporotrichosis: Therapy has ranged up to 9 months with total dose up to 2.5g. Aspergillosis: Total dose up to 3.6g for 11 months. Rhinocerebral Phycomycosis: Cumulative dose of at least 3g is recommended. Whenever therapy is interrupted for >7 days, resume with lowest dose.

**HOW SUPPLIED:** Inj: 50mg

**WARNINGS/PRECAUTIONS:** Acute reactions (eg, fever, shaking chills, hypotension, anorexia, N/V, headache, tachypnea) 1-3 hrs after starting infusion may occur. Avoid rapid IV infusion; may cause hypotension, hypokalemia, arrhythmias and shock. Caution with renal impairment. Reduced risk of nephrotoxicity with hydration and sodium repletion before drug administration. Leukoencephalopathy reported.

**ADVERSE REACTIONS:** Fever, malaise, weight loss, hypotension, tachypnea, anorexia, N/V, diarrhea, dyspepsia, normochromic normocytic anemia, injection site pain, renal dysfunction, phlebitis, headache, azotemia.

**INTERACTIONS:** Antineoplastics (eg, nitrogen mustard) may potentiate renal toxicity, bronchospasm, hypotension; caution when coadministering. Corticosteroids and corticotropin may potentiate hypokalemia; monitor serum electrolytes and cardiac function during co-administration. May increase flucytosine toxicity. Caution with imidazoles (eg, ketoconazole, clotrimazole, miconazole, fluconazole), especially in immunocompromised patients. Increased risk of renal toxicity with nephrotoxic drugs (eg, aminoglycosides, cyclosporine, pentamidine). May enhance curariform effect of skeletal muscle relaxants (eg, tubocurarine) or digitalis toxicity with amphotericin B-induced hypokalemia. Acute pulmonary reactions reported with leukocyte transfusions; separate infusions and monitor pulmonary function.

**PREGNANCY:** Category B, not for use in nursing.

**MECHANISM OF ACTION:** Fungistatic or fungicidal; binds to sterols in cell membranes of susceptible fungi, resulting in change in membrane permeability, allowing leakage of intracellular components.

**PHARMACOKINETICS: Absorption:** $C_{max}$= approximately 0.5-2mcg/mL. **Distribution:** Plasma protein binding (>90%). **Elimination:** Renal excretion. Urine (approximately 40%, urinary output over 7-day period); $T_{1/2}$= approximately 15 days.

## NURSING CONSIDERATIONS

**Assessment:** Assess cultures, renal function, hematological effects (normocytic anemia), hepatic function, nursing status and possible drug interactions.

**Monitoring:** Monitor for signs/symptoms of acute reaction (fever, shaking, chills, hypotension, tachypnea), serum electrolytes (Mg, K+), liver function, frequent renal function tests, Hgb, CBC, pulmonary function. Monitor temperature, pulse, respiration, and BP every 30 min for 2-4 hrs after initial (test) dose.

**Patient Counseling:** Advise to seek medical attention if symptoms of acute reactions (fever, shaking, chills, respiratory symptoms) occur. Maintain adequate hydration.

**Administration:** IV route. Observe aseptic technique strictly in all handling. 1) Reconstitute (add 10mL of Sterile Water for Inj, USP into vial). 2) Shake vial until sol is clear. 3) Dilute using 5% Dextrose Inj, USP. **Storage:** Refrigerate; protect against exposure to light. The concentrate may be stored in dark, at room temperature for 24 hrs or refrigerator for 1 week with minimal loss of potency and clarity. Discard unused material. Protect from light during administration.

# AMPICILLIN INJECTION RX

ampicillin sodium (Various)

**THERAPEUTIC CLASS:** Semisynthetic penicillin derivative

**INDICATIONS:** Treatment of respiratory tract, urinary tract, and GI infections, bacterial meningitis, septicemia, and endocarditis caused by susceptible strains of microorganisms.

**DOSAGE:** *Adults:* IM/IV: Respiratory Tract/Soft Tissues: ≥40kg: 250-500mg q6h. <40kg: 25-50mg/kg/day given q6-8h. GI/GU Tract Infections: ≥40kg: 500mg q6h. <40kg: 50mg/kg/day given q6-8h. Urethritis (Caused by *N.gonorrhoeae* in Males): 500mg q8-12h for 2 doses; may retreat if needed. Bacterial Meningitis: 150-200mg/kg/day given q3-4h. Septicemia: 150-200mg/kg/day IV for 3 days, continue with IM q3-4h. Treatment of all infections should be continued for a minimum of 48-72 hrs after becoming asymptomatic or evidence of bacterial eradication has been obtained. Minimum of 10 days treatment recommended for Group A β-hemolytic streptococci. *Pediatrics:* Bacterial Meningitis: 150-200mg/kg/day given q3-4h. Septicemia: 150-200mg/kg/day IV for 3 days, continue with IM q3-4h. Treatment of all infections should be continued for a minimum of 48-72 hrs after becoming asymptomatic or evidence of bacterial eradication has been obtained. Minimum of 10 days treatment recommended for Group A β-hemolytic streptococci.

**HOW SUPPLIED:** Inj: 125mg, 250mg, 500mg, 1g, 2g, 10g

**WARNINGS/PRECAUTIONS:** Serious, sometimes fatal, hypersensitivity reactions reported; d/c if occurs. Prior to therapy, assess for previous hypesensitivity reactions to penicillins, cephalosporins, and other allergens. *Clostridium difficile*-associated diarrhea (CDAD) reported and may range from mild diarrhea to fatal colitis. D/C if superinfection develops. Avoid in infectious mononucleosis; skin rash reported. May increase risk of development of drug-resistant bacteria in the absence of proven or strongly suspected bacterial infection or a prophylactic indication. False-positive glucose reactions reported with Clinitest, Benedict's Solution, or Fehling's solution. Perform periodic assessment of renal, hepatic, and hematopoietic function during prolonged therapy. Rapid direct IV administration may result in convulsive seizures.

**ADVERSE REACTIONS:** Skin rashes, urticaria, glossitis, N/V, diarrhea, stomatitis, enterocolitis, anemia, thrombocytopenia, eosinophilia, leukopenia, agranulocytosis.

**INTERACTIONS:** May delay excretion with probenecid. Increased incidence of skin rash with allopurinol.

**PREGNANCY:** Category B, caution in nursing.

**MECHANISM OF ACTION:** Penicillin derivative; bactericidal against penicillin-susceptible gram-positive organisms and many common gram-negative pathogens.

**PHARMACOKINETICS: Distribution:** Plasma protein binding (20%), found in breast milk. Penetrates to CSF and brain only if meninges are inflamed. **Elimination:** Urine (unchanged).

## NURSING CONSIDERATIONS

**Assessment:** Assess for proper diagnosis, hypersensitivity to penicillins/cephalosporins or other allergens, infectious mononucleosis, pregnancy/nursing status, and for possible drug interactions.

**Monitoring:** Monitor for signs/symptoms of hypersensitivity reactions, CDAD, superinfection, and for skin rash. Perform periodic monitoring of renal, hepatic and hematopoietic function.

**Patient Counseling:** Inform that drug treats bacterial, not viral, infections. Instruct to take exactly as directed to prevent drug resistance. Instruct to notify physician if pregnant/nursing. Advise to contact physician if watery and bloody stools developed even after 2 or more months after therapy.

**Administration:** IM/IV routes. Administer within 1 hr after preparation. Administer IV slowly, over at least 10-15 min to avoid convulsive seizures. Refer to PI for information regarding dilution and storage instructions.

## AMPICILLIN ORAL RX
ampicillin (Various)

**THERAPEUTIC CLASS:** Semisynthetic penicillin derivative

**INDICATIONS:** Genitourinary tract (GU) infections, including gonorrhea, respiratory and GI tract infections, and meningitis.

**DOSAGE:** *Adults:* GI/GU: 500mg qid. Use larger doses in chronic or severe infections. Gonorrhea: 3.5g single dose with 1g probenecid. Respiratory: 250mg qid. Treat minimum 48-72 hrs after eradication. Treat minimum 10 days for hemolytic strains of strep.
*Pediatrics:* >20kg: GI/GU: 500mg qid. Respiratory: 250mg qid. ≤20kg: GI/GU: 25mg/kg qid. Respiratory: 50mg/kg/day given tid-qid. Do not exceed adult doses. Use larger doses in chronic or severe infections. Treat minimum 48-72 hrs after eradication. Treat minimum 10 days for hemolytic strains of strep.

**HOW SUPPLIED:** Cap: 250mg, 500mg; Sus: 125mg/5mL, 250mg/5mL [100mL, 200mL]

**CONTRAINDICATIONS:** Infections caused by penicillinase-producing organisms.

**WARNINGS/PRECAUTIONS:** Possible cross-sensitivity with cephalosporins. Pseudomembranous colitis and anaphylatic reactions may occur.

**ADVERSE REACTIONS:** Stomatitis, N/V, diarrhea, rash, SGOT elevation, blood dyscrasias, eosinophilia, thrombocytopenic purpura, hypersensitivity reactions, superinfection (prolonged use).

**INTERACTIONS:** Increased risk of rash with allopurinol. Bacteriostatic antibiotics (eg, chloramphenicol, erythromycins, sulfonamides or tetracyclines) may interfere with bactericidal activity. May decrease the effectiveness of oral contraceptives. Increased blood levels with probenecid.

**PREGNANCY:** Category B, not for use in nursing.

**MECHANISM OF ACTION:** Penicillin derivative; bactericidal against gram-positive and gram-negative organisms.

**PHARMACOKINETICS: Absorption:** Well-absorbed; (500mg Cap) $C_{max}$=3mcg/mL; (250mg Sus) $C_{max}$=2.3mcg/mL. **Distribution:** Plasma protein binding (20%). **Elimination:** Urine (unchanged).

### NURSING CONSIDERATIONS

**Assessment:** Assess for previous hypersensitivity reactions to PCNs and possible drug interactions. Conduct susceptibility testing as guide to therapy.

**Monitoring:** Monitor for hypersensitivity reactions, pseudomembranous colitis, overgrowth of nonsusceptible organisms with prolonged use, and renal/hepatic/hematopoietic systems periodically with prolonged therapy. Upon completion, obtain cultures to determine organism eradication.

**Patient Counseling:** Instruct to notify physician of history of hypersensitivity to PCNs/cephalosporins. Inform diabetics to consult with physician prior to changing diet or dosage of diabetic medication. Instruct to take with full glass of water, 1/2 hr before or 2 hrs after meals. Take exactly as directed; skipping doses or not completing full course decreases effectiveness and increases resistance. D/C and notify physician if side effects occur. Inform that therapy only treats bacterial, not viral, infections.

**Administration:** Oral route. **Storage:** 20-25°C (68-77°F). Dispense in a tight container.

## AMPYRA RX
dalfampridine (Acorda)

**THERAPEUTIC CLASS:** Potassium channel blocker

**INDICATIONS:** Treatment to improve walking in patients with multiple sclerosis (MS).

**DOSAGE:** *Adults:* 10mg bid (approximately 12 hrs apart). Max recommended dose of 10mg bid should not be exceeded. Do not double dose or take extra if a dose is missed. Take whole; do not divide, crush, chew, or dissolve.

**HOW SUPPLIED:** Tab, Extended Release: 10mg

**CONTRAINDICATIONS:** History of seizure, and moderate or severe renal impairment.

**WARNINGS/PRECAUTIONS:** Increased incidence of seizure has been observed. D/C and do not restart if experience seizure while on treatment. The risk for seizures with mild renal impairment (CrCl 51-80mL/min) is unknown but dalfampridine plasma levels in these patients may approach those seen with 15mg bid, a dose that may increase the risk of seizures. CrCl should be estimated prior to initiating treatment.

**ADVERSE REACTIONS:** Seizure, urinary tract infection, insomnia, dizziness, headache, nausea, asthenia, multiple sclerosis relapse, paresthesia.

**INTERACTIONS:** Avoid use with other forms of 4-aminopyridine.

**PREGNANCY:** Category C, not use for nursing

**MECHANISM OF ACTION:** Broad spectrum potassium channel blocker; therapeutic effect has not been fully elucidated. In animal studies it has been shown to increase conduction of action potentials in demyelinated axons through inhibition of potassium channels.

**PHARMACOKINETICS: Absorption:** Rapid and complete; relative bioavailability (96%); (Tab) $C_{max}$=17.3-21.6ng/mL (fasted) $T_{max}$=3-4 hrs (fasted). **Distribution:** $V_d$=2.6L/kg. **Metabolism:** CYP2E1 (major). **Elimination:** Urine (95.9%); feces (0.5%); $T_{1/2}$=5.2-6.5 hrs.

## NURSING CONSIDERATIONS

**Assessment:** Assess for history of seizure, moderate or severe renal impairment, concomitant use of 4-aminopyridine, pregnancy/nursing status, and possible drug interactions. Obtain baseline CrCl.

**Monitoring:** Monitor for seizure, urinary tract infection, headache, dizziness and relapse of multiple sclerosis.

**Patient Counseling:** Inform patients that medication may cause seizures in a dose-dependent fashion, and that they must d/c use if experience a seizure. Instruct patients to take medication exactly as prescribed. Instruct to take tablet whole, do not crush, chew, or dissolve. Instruct not to take more than 2 tablets in a 24-hour period and to make sure that there is a 12-hour interval between doses.

**Administration:** Oral route. **Storage:** 25°C (77°F). Excursions permitted 15-30°C (59-86°F).

# AMRIX — RX

cyclobenzaprine HCl (Cephalon)

**THERAPEUTIC CLASS:** Skeletal muscle relaxant (central-acting)

**INDICATIONS:** Adjunct to rest and physical therapy to relieve muscle spasm associated with acute, painful musculoskeletal conditions. Use for only short periods of time (up to 2-3 weeks).

**DOSAGE:** *Adults:* Usual: 15mg qd. Titrate: May increase to 30mg qd if needed. Use for longer than 2-3 weeks not recommended.

**HOW SUPPLIED:** Cap, Extended-Release: 15mg, 30mg

**CONTRAINDICATIONS:** MAOI use during or within 14 days. Hyperpyretic crisis seizures and deaths associated with concomitant use of cyclobenzaprine (or drugs structurally similar to TCAs) and MAOIs reported. Acute recovery phase of MI, arrhythmias, heart block conduction disturbances, CHF, hyperthyroidism.

**WARNINGS/PRECAUTIONS:** Avoid in hepatic impairment and elderly patients. Caution with history of urinary retention, angle-closure glaucoma, increased IOP, and use of anticholinergic medication. May impair mental and/or physical performance.

**ADVERSE REACTIONS:** Drowsiness, dry mouth, dizziness, somnolence, headache.

**INTERACTIONS:** Contraindicated with MAOIs. Enhances effects of alcohol, barbiturates and other CNS depressants. TCAs may block antihypertensive action of guanethidine and similar compounds and may enhance seizure risk with tramadol.

**PREGNANCY:** Category B, caution in nursing.

**MECHANISM OF ACTION:** Skeletal muscle relaxant; acts primarily within the CNS at brain stem as opposed to spinal cord level, although overlapping action on the latter may contribute to its overall skeletal muscle relaxant activity; suggested to reduce tonic somatic motor activity influencing both gamma and α motor systems.

**PHARMACOKINETICS: Absorption:** $C_{max}$=8.3ng/mL, $T_{max}$=8.1 hrs, AUC=354.1ng•h/mL; see Full PI for more detailed information. **Metabolism:** Extensive; via CYP3A4, 1A2, and 2D6 through N-demethylation pathway. **Elimination:** Urine (glucuronides); $T_{1/2}$=33.4 hrs.

## NURSING CONSIDERATIONS

**Assessment:** Assess for hepatic impairment, seizures, hyperthyroidism, urinary retention, angle-closure glaucoma, IOP, recent MI, arrhythmias, heart block, CHF, alcohol intake, pregnancy/nursing status, and possible drug interactions (eg, MAOIs if concomitant use or within 14 days after d/c, and anticholinergic medications).

**Monitoring:** Monitor for cardiac arrhythmias, sinus tachycardia, MI, stroke, IOP, CBC, and LFTs.

**Patient Counseling:** Caution against performing hazardous tasks (eg, operating machinery/driving); avoid alcohol and other CNS depressants. Notify if pregnant/nursing.

**Administration:** Oral route; take at same time each day. **Storage:** 25°C (77°F); excursions permitted to 15-30°C (59-86°F); in tight, light-resistant container. Keep out of reach of children.

# ANAPROX DS — RX

naproxen sodium (Roche Labs)

**NSAIDs may cause an increased risk of serious cardiovascular thrombotic events, MI, stroke, and serious GI adverse events including bleeding, ulceration, and perforation of the stomach or intestines. Contraindicated for the treatment of perioperative pain in the setting of coronary artery bypass graft (CABG) surgery.**

**OTHER BRAND NAMES:** Anaprox (Roche Labs)

**THERAPEUTIC CLASS:** NSAID

**INDICATIONS:** Relieves signs and symptoms of rheumatoid arthritis (RA), osteoarthritis (OA), ankylosing spondylitis (AS), juvenile arthritis (JA), tendinitis, bursitis, and acute gout. Management of pain and primary dysmenorrhea.

**DOSAGE:** *Adults:* RA/OA/AS: 275mg bid or 550mg bid. Acute Gout: 825mg followed by 275mg q8h. Pain/Dysmenorrhea/Tendinitis/Bursitis: 550mg followed by 550mg q12h or 275mg q6-8h prn. Max: 1375mg on Day 1, then 1100mg/day.

**HOW SUPPLIED:** (Anaprox) Tab: 275mg; (Anaprox DS) Tab: 550mg* *scored

**CONTRAINDICATIONS:** Asthma, urticaria, or other allergic-type reactions with aspirin (ASA) or other NSAIDs. Treatment of perioperative pain in the setting of CABG surgery.

**WARNINGS/PRECAUTIONS:** May lead to onset of new HTN or worsening of pre-existing HTN; monitor BP closely. Fluid retention, edema, and peripheral edema reported; caution with fluid retention, HTN, or heart failure. Renal papillary necrosis and other renal injury reported after long-term use. Not recommended for use with advanced renal disease; if therapy must be initiated, monitor renal function closely. Anaphylactoid reactions may occur. May cause serious skin adverse events (eg, exfoliative dermatitis, Stevens-Johnson syndrome, toxic epidermal necrolysis). Avoid in late pregnancy; may cause premature closure of ductus arteriosus. Not a substitute for corticosteroid or to treat corticosteroid insufficiency. Monitor for visual changes or disturbances. May cause elevations of LFTs; d/c if liver disease develops or systemic manifestations occur. Caution with high doses in chronic alcoholic liver disease and elderly. Anemia may occur with long-term use; monitor Hgb/Hct if signs or symptoms of anemia develop or if initial Hgb ≤10g. May inhibit platelet aggregation and prolong bleeding time; monitor with coagulation disorders. Caution with asthma and avoid with ASA-sensitive asthma.

**ADVERSE REACTIONS:** Edema, drowsiness, dizziness, constipation, heartburn, abdominal pain, nausea, headache, tinnitus, dyspnea, pruritus, skin eruptions, ecchymoses.

**INTERACTIONS:** Avoid other products containing naproxen. Potential for increased adverse effects with ASA. May reduce tubular secretion of methotrexate; monitor for toxicity. May diminish antihypertensive effect and potentiate renal disease with ACE inhibitors. May reduce natriuretic effect of furosemide and thiazides. May increase lithium levels; monitor for toxicity. Increase risk of GI bleeding with SSRIs, oral corticosteroids, and anticoagulants. Synergistic effects on GI bleeding with warfarin. Observe for dose adjustment with hydantoins, sulfonamides, or sulfonylureas. May reduce antihypertensive effects of propranolol and other β-blockers. Probenecid increases half-life significantly. Antacids (magnesium oxide or aluminum hydroxide) and sucralfate may delay absorption. May impair response of thiazides or loop diuretics.

**PREGNANCY:** Category C, not for use in nursing.

**MECHANISM OF ACTION:** NSAID; unknown, related to prostaglandin synthetase inhibition.

**PHARMACOKINETICS: Absorption:** Rapid and complete. Bioavailability (95%). $T_{max}$=1-2 hrs. **Distribution:** $V_d$=0.16 L/kg; plasma protein binding (>99%). **Metabolism:** Hepatic, metabolite (6-O-desmethyl naproxen). **Elimination:** Urine (95%), feces (≤3%), $T_{1/2}$=12-17 hrs.

## NURSING CONSIDERATIONS

**Assessment:** Assess for history of asthma, CV disease (pre-existing HTN, CHF) or risk factors for disease, fluid retention, edema, CV thrombotic events, MI, stroke, CABG surgery, pregnancy status, risk factors for GI events (bleeding, ulceration, perforation), possible drug interactions, renal/hepatic dysfunction.

**Monitoring:** Monitor BP, CBC, LFTs, renal function, and chemistries periodically. Monitor for signs/symptoms of GI events (bleeding, ulceration, perforation), CV thrombotic events, CHF, HTN, anemia, salt depletion, renal/liver dysfunction.

**Patient Counseling:** Seek medical attention if symptoms of hepatotoxicity (eg, nausea, fatigue, pruritus), anaphylactic reaction (eg, difficulty breathing, swelling of face/throat), hypersensitivity reaction (eg, rash), CV events (eg, chest pain, SOB, weakness, slurring of speech), GI ulceration and bleeding (eg, epigastric pain, dyspepsia, melena, hematemesis), weight gain, or edema occur. Inform of pregnancy risks. Caution if drowsiness, dizziness, vertigo, or depression is experienced during therapy.

**Administration:** Oral route. **Storage:** 15-30°C (59-86°F) in well-closed containers.

# ANDRODERM CIII

testosterone (Physicians Total Care, Inc)

**THERAPEUTIC CLASS:** Androgen

**INDICATIONS:** Testosterone replacement therapy in men for conditions associated with a deficiency or absence of endogenous testosterone (eg, primary or secondary hypogonadism).

**DOSAGE:** *Adults:* Initial: 5mg/day. Maint: 2.5mg-7.5mg/day. Apply patch nightly to intact skin of back, abdomen, upper arm, or thigh. Rotate sites; avoid same site for 7 days. Do not apply to scrotum or oily, damaged, irritated areas. May apply 2 patches at same time.
*Pediatrics:* ≥15 yrs: Initial: 5mg/day. Maint: 2.5mg-7.5mg/day. Apply patch nightly to intact skin of back, abdomen, upper arm, or thigh. Rotate sites; avoid same site for 7 days. Do not apply to scrotum or oily, damaged, irritated areas. May apply 2 patches at same time.

**HOW SUPPLIED:** Patch: 2.5mg/24 hrs [60[s]], 5mg/24 hrs [30[s]]

**CONTRAINDICATIONS:** Breast or known or suspected prostate cancer in men. Women.

**WARNINGS/PRECAUTIONS:** Prolonged use is associated with serious hepatic effects (eg, peliosis hepatis, cholestatic jaundice, hepatic neoplasms). Increased risk for prostatic hyperplasia/carcinoma in elderly. Risk of edema with pre-existing cardiac, renal, or hepatic disease; d/c if edema occurs. Gynecomastia may develop. Risk of virilization of female sex partner. Monitor LFTs, Hgb, Hct, prostate specific antigen (PSA), cholesterol, lipids. May decrease thyroxine-binding globulin leading to changes in $T_3$ and $T_4$ levels; free thyroid hormone unchanged.

**ADVERSE REACTIONS:** Gynecomastia, pruritus/erythema/vesicles/blister/burning/induration at application site, prostate abnormalities, headache, depression.

**INTERACTIONS:** May potentiate effects of anticoagulants, oxyphenbutazone. May decrease blood glucose and insulin requirements in diabetics. Pretreatment with ointments may reduce testosterone absorption.

**PREGNANCY:** Category X, not for use in nursing.

**MECHANISM OF ACTION:** Endogenous androgen; responsible for normal growth and development of male sex organs and for maintenance of secondary sex characteristics.

**PHARMACOKINETICS: Absorption:** $C_{max}$=753ng/dL; $T_{max}$=7.9 hrs. **Distribution:** Sex hormone-binding globulin and albumin binding. **Metabolism:** Liver; estradiol and dihydrotestosterone (major metabolites). **Elimination:** (IM) Urine (90% glucuronide and sulfate conjugates), feces (6% unconjugated); $T_{1/2}$=71 min.

## NURSING CONSIDERATIONS

**Assessment:** Assess for breast or prostate carcinoma, cardiac or renal/hepatic disease, hypersensitivity to components, pregnancy/nursing status of female partner, and possible drug interactions.

**Monitoring:** Periodically monitor Hgb, Hct, LFTs, PSA, cholesterol and HDL, and serum testosterone levels after initiation of therapy. Monitor for signs/symptoms of hypersensitivity reactions, edema with/without CHF, gynecomastia, prostatic hyperplasia/carcinoma in geriatrics.

**Patient Counseling:** Advise not to apply to the scrotum or over a bony prominence or any part of the body that could be subject to prolonged pressure during sleep or sitting. Instruct to contact physician if changes in body hair distribution, increase in acne, virilization of female partner, too frequent or persistent erections, changes in skin color, ankle swelling, unexplained N/V, or hypersensitivity reactions occur.

**Administration:** Transdermal patch system. Apply adhesive side of the system to a clean, dry area of the skin on the back, abdomen, upper arms, or thighs. Rotate application site with an interval of 7 days between applications to the same site. **Storage:** 25° (77°F); excursions permitted to 15-30°C (59-86°F). Do not store outside pouch provided.

# ANDROGEL

testosterone (Solvay)

CIII

**Virilization reported in children secondarily exposed to testosterone gel. Children should avoid contact with unwashed or unclothed application sites in men using testosterone gel. Healthcare providers should advise patients to strictly adhere to recommended use instructions.**

**THERAPEUTIC CLASS:** Androgen

**INDICATIONS:** Testosterone replacement in males with congenital or acquired primary hypogonadism or hypogonadotropic hypogonadism.

**DOSAGE:** *Adults:* Initial: Apply 5g qd, preferably in the am, to clean, dry, intact skin of shoulders and upper arms and/or abdomen limited to area covered by short sleeved shirt. Allow to dry prior to dressing. Titrate: May increase to 7.5g qd, then 10g qd if response not achieved or serum concentration is below normal range. If serum concentration consistently exceeds the normal range at a daily dose of 5g, d/c therapy. Do not apply to scrotum/genitals; wash hands after application. Pump: 4 actuations (5g), 6 actuations (7.5g), 8 actuations (10g).

**HOW SUPPLIED:** Gel: 1% [2.5g, 5g pkts; 75g pump]

**CONTRAINDICATIONS:** Breast or prostate carcinoma in men, women who are or may become pregnant or who are nursing. Hypersensitivity to alcohol or soy products.

**WARNINGS/PRECAUTIONS:** Patients with BPH may be at increased risk for worsening of signs/symptoms of BPH. May be at increased risk for prostate cancer; evaluate for prostate cancer prior to therapy and during therapy. May increase PSA levels. Risk of virilization in children (eg, enlarged penis/clitoris, pubic hair, increased erection/libido, aggressive behavior, advanced bone age) and women (eg, changes in body hair distribution, significant increase in acne) due to secondary skin exposure from contact with men using testosterone-containing gel products. Women/children should avoid contact with unwashed or unclothed application site. Should only be applied to shoulders, upper arms, and/or abdomen (application should be limited to area that will be covered by short sleeve t-shirt). Wash hands immediately with soap and water following application. Cover application site after gel has dried. Prior to situation where skin to skin contact is anticipated, wash application site throughly to remove any testosterone residue. If skin of another person comes in direct contact with unwashed or unclothed drug application site, wash contact area of other person with soap and water as soon as possible. Not indicated for use in women. Suppressed spermatogenesis may occur. Risk of edema with pre-existing cardiac, renal, or hepatic disease. Risk of gynecomastia. May potentiate sleep apnea especially with obesity or chronic lung diseases. Increases in Hct, red blood cell mass, and changes in serum lipid profile reported; adjust dose. Prolonged use may cause serious hepatic effects (eg, peliosis hepatis, hepatic neoplasms, cholestatic hepatitis, jaundice). Gel is flammable; avoid fire, flame, or smoking during use. Caution in cancer patients at risk of hypercalcemia.

**ADVERSE REACTIONS:** Acne, application-site reaction, headache, emotional lability, gynecomastia, HTN, nervousness, breast pain, abnormal lab tests, prostate disorders, asthenia, decreased libido, urinary symptoms.

**INTERACTIONS:** May decrease blood glucose and insulin requirements. Concurrent use with ACTH or corticosteroids may increase fluid retention. Changes in anticoagulant activity may be seen with androgens; increase frequency of monitoring INR and PT.

**PREGNANCY:** Category X, not for use in nursing.

**MECHANISM OF ACTION:** Androgen; responsible for normal growth and development of male sex organs and for maintenance of secondary sex characteristics.

**PHARMACOKINETICS: Absorption:** 10% absorbed systemically. **Distribution:** Sex hormone-binding globulin (SHBG) binding (40%), albumin- and plasma protein-binding (58%), unbound (2%). **Metabolism:** Estradiol and DHT (active metabolites). **Elimination:** Urine (90% glucuronic and sulfuric acid conjugates), feces (6% unconjugated); $T_{1/2}$=10-100 min.

## NURSING CONSIDERATIONS

**Assessment:** Assess for hypersensitivity to alcohol and soy, breast or prostate carcinoma, BPH, cardiac or renal/hepatic disease, obesity, chronic lung disease, pregnancy/nursing status of female partner, and for possible drug interactions. Assess use in cancer patients at risk of hypercalcemia.

**Monitoring:** Monitor for signs/symptoms of hypersensitivity reactions, prostate carcinoma, inhibition of spermatogenesis, hepatic toxicity, edema with or without CHF, gynecomastia, and potentiation of sleep apnea. In patients with BPH, monitor for signs/symptoms of worsening of BPH. Perform periodic monitoring of Hgb, Hct, PSA, serum lipid profile, LFTs, PSA, and serum testosterone levels. In cancer patients at risk for hypercalcemia, perform regular monitoring of serum calcium levels.

**Patient Counseling:** Inform of pregnancy risks; avoid contact with application sites in children and women; instruct to wash area immediately with soap and water if contact occurs. Advise to cover application site with clothing after gel dries. Instruct to wash application site with soap and water prior to direct skin-to-skin contact with others. Inform that drug is flammable until dry. Inform to contact physician if experience changes in body hair distribution, increase in acne, virilization of female partner or child, too frequent or persistent erections, changes in skin color, ankle swelling, unexplained N/V, breathing disturbances, or hypersensitivity reactions. Advise of the importance of adhering to all recommended monitoring. Advise to read Medication Guide before therapy and reread each time the prescription is renewed.

**Administration:** Topical route. Multi-Dose Pump: Prime the pump before using it for the first time by depressing pump 3 times and discarding the portion to ensure precise dose delivery. Refer to Full Prescribing Information for administration details. **Storage:** 25°C (77°F); excursions permitted to 15-30°C (59-86°F). Keep out of reach of children.

# ANGELIQ — RX

drospirenone - estradiol (Bayer Healthcare)

**Estrogens and progestins should not be used for prevention of cardiovascular disease or dementia. Increased risk of MI, stroke, invasive breast cancer, PE, and DVT in postmenopausal women (50-79 yrs of age) reported. Increased risk of developing probable dementia in postmenopausal women ≥65 yrs of age reported.**

**THERAPEUTIC CLASS:** Estrogen/progestogen combination

**INDICATIONS:** Treatment of moderate to severe vasomotor symptoms and/or vulvar/vaginal atrophy associated with menopause.

**DOSAGE:** *Adults:* 1 tab qd. Re-evaluate after 3-6 months.

**HOW SUPPLIED:** Tab: (Drospirenone-Estradiol) 0.5mg-1mg

**CONTRAINDICATIONS:** Pregnancy, undiagnosed abnormal genital bleeding, breast cancer, estrogen-dependent neoplasia, DVT/PE, active or recent (eg, within past year) arterial thromboembolic disease (eg, stroke, MI), liver dysfunction or disease, renal insufficiency, adrenal insufficiency.

**WARNINGS/PRECAUTIONS:** Not for use in renal insufficiency, hepatic dysfunction, and adrenal insufficiency due to increased risk of hyperkalemia. May increase risk of cardiovascular events (eg, MI, stroke), venous thrombosis, and PE; d/c immediately if any of these events occur or are suspected. May increase risk of breast/endometrial cancer, and gallbladder disease. May lead to severe hypercalcemia with breast cancer and bone metastases; monitor and d/c if hypercalcemia occurs. Retinal vascular thrombosis reported; monitor and d/c if papilledema or retinal vascular lesions occur. May elevate BP; monitor at regular intervals. May cause elevations of plasma triglycerides with pre-existing hypertriglyceridemia. Caution with history of cholestatic jaundice associated with past estrogen use or with pregnancy; d/c with recurrence. May lead to increased thyroid-binding globulin levels; monitor thyroid function. May cause fluid retention; caution with cardiac/renal dysfunction. Caution with severe hypocalcemia. May increase risk of ovarian cancer. May exacerbate endometriosis, asthma, DM, epilepsy, migraine, porphyria, SLE, and hepatic hemangiomas; use with caution.

**ADVERSE REACTIONS:** Abdominal pain, pain in extremity, back pain, flu syndrome, enlarged abdomen, headache, upper respiratory infection, sinusitis, breast pain, vaginal hemorrhage.

**INTERACTIONS:** CYP3A4 inducers (eg, St. John's wort, phenobarbital, carbamazepine, rifampin) may decrease levels which may decrease therapeutic effects and/or change uterine bleeding profile. CYP3A4 inhibitors (eg, erythromycin, clarithromycin, ketoconazole, itraconazole, ritonavir, grapefruit juice) may increase levels which may result in side effects. Increased risk of hyperkalemia with ACE inhibitors, angiotensin receptor blockers, NSAIDs, potassium-sparing diuretics, potassium supplements, and heparin.

**PREGNANCY:** Contraindicated in pregnancy, caution in nursing.

**MECHANISM OF ACTION:** Estrogen/progestogen combination. Estradiol: Binds to nuclear receptors in estrogen-responsive tissues. Modulates pituitary secretion of gonadotropins, leuteinizing hormone (LH) and follicle stimulating hormone (FSH), through negative feedback mechanism. Drospirenone (DRSP): Synthetic progestin and spironolactone analog with antimineralocorticoid activity. Possesses anti-androgenic activity. Counters estrogenic effects by decreasing number of nuclear estradiol receptors and suppressing epithelial DNA synthesis in endometrial tissue.

**PHARMACOKINETICS: Absorption:** DRSP: $C_{max}$=18.3ng/mL; $T_{max}$=1.0 hr; $AUC_{0-24hr}$=208ng•hr/mL. Absolute bioavailability (76-85%) Estradiol; $C_{max}$=43.8pg/mL; $T_{max}$=2.5 hrs; $AUC_{0-24\,hr}$=665pg•hr/mL. Estrone (metabolite): $C_{max}$=245pg/mL; $T_{max}$=4 hrs; $AUC_{0-24\,hr}$=3814pg•hr/mL. **Distribution:** Estrogens and DRSP found in breast milk. DRSP: $V_d$=4.2L/kg, serum protein binding (97%). Estradiol: Sex hormone binding globulin (SHBG) (37%); albumin binding (61%). **Metabolism:** DRSP: Extensive; CYP3A4 (minor). Estradiol: Liver to estrone (metabolite); estriol (major urinary metabolite); enterohepatic recirculation via sulfate and glucuronide conjugation in the liver; biliary secretion of conjugates in the intestine; hydrolysis in the gut; reabsorption. **Elimination:** DRSP: Urine (38-47%, glucuronide and sulfate conjugates), feces (17-20%, glucuronide and sulfate conjugates); $T_{1/2}$=36-42 hrs. Estradiol: Urine. Estrone: Urine; $T_{1/2}$=23 hrs.

## NURSING CONSIDERATIONS

**Assessment:** Assess for abnormal genital bleeding, known or history of breast cancer, estrogen-dependent neoplasias, DVT or PE, present or recent (within past yr) arterial thromboembolic disease (eg, stroke, MI), renal insufficiencies, liver dysfunction/disease, adrenal insufficiencies, and known/suspected pregnancy. Assess use in patients undergoing surgeries associated with risk of thromboembolism, with prolonged immobilization, ≥65 yrs old, presence of hypothyroidism or hypocalcemia, and in nursing females. Assess for drug or lab interactions.

**Monitoring:** Monitor for signs/symptoms of cardiovascular disorders (eg, MI, stroke, venous thrombosis, PE), malignant neoplasms (eg, endometrial, breast, or ovarian cancer), dementia, gallbladder disease, cholestatic jaundice, hypercalcemia, visual abnormalities (eg, retinal vascular thrombosis), increased BP levels, fluid retention, hyponatremia, hypertriglyceridemia, hypothyroidism, exacerbation of endometriosis, and exacerbation of other conditions (eg, asthma, DM, epilepsy, migraines, porphyria, SLE, and hepatic hemangiomas). Periodically monitor BP levels, thyroid function in patients on thyroid hormone replacement therapy, serum potassium levels during first cycle of therapy in patients at risk for hyperkalemia. Perform proper diagnostic testing (eg, endometrial sampling) in patients with undiagnosed, persistent, or recurring vaginal bleeding. Perform annual breast exam (eg, mammography). Monitor use of therapy every 3-6 months.

**Patient Counseling:** Inform drug may increase risk for heart attack, stroke, breast cancer, blood clots, and dementia. Report any breast lumps, unusual vaginal bleeding, dizziness and faintness, changes in speech, severe headaches, chest pain, SOB, leg pains, changes in vision, or vomiting. Instruct to perform monthly breast exam.

**Administration:** Oral route. **Storage:** 25°C (77°F); excursions permitted to 15-30°C (59-86°F). Do not store above 30°C (86°F).

## ANGIOMAX RX

bivalirudin (The Medicines Company)

**THERAPEUTIC CLASS:** Thrombin inhibitor

**INDICATIONS:** Adjunct to aspirin for anticoagulation in patients with unstable angina undergoing percutaneous transluminal coronary angioplasty (PTCA) or percutaneous coronary intervention (PCI). Patients with, or at risk of, HIT/HITTS undergoing PCI.

**DOSAGE:** *Adults:* Initial: 0.75mg/kg IV bolus, then 1.75mg/kg/hr for duration of PCI procedure. Additional bolus of 0.3mg/kg can be given if needed based on ACT. Continuation of infusion for up to 4 hrs post-procedure is optional. After 4 hrs, if needed, an additional 0.2mg/kg/hr IV for up to 20 hrs may be initiated. Renal Impairment: CrCl <30mL/min: 1mg/kg/hr infusion. Hemodialysis: 0.25mg/kg/hr infusion. Reduction in bolus dose not necessary; monitor anticoagulation.

**HOW SUPPLIED:** Inj: 250mg

**CONTRAINDICATIONS:** Active major bleeding.

**WARNINGS/PRECAUTIONS:** Not for IM administration. Hemorrhage can occur at any site. D/C with unexplained symptoms, fall in BP or Hct. There is no known antidote to treatment, but can be hemodialyzable. Caution when used during brachytherapy procedures.

**ADVERSE REACTIONS:** Bleeding, back pain, pain, N/V, headache, hypotension, HTN, bradycardia, dyspepsia, urinary retention, insomnia, anxiety, abdominal pain, fever, nervousness.

**INTERACTIONS:** Increased risk of major bleed with heparin, warfarin, thrombolytics, glycoprotein IIb/IIIa inhibitors.

**PREGNANCY:** Category B, caution in nursing.

**MECHANISM OF ACTION:** Reversible direct thrombin inhibitor; inhibits thrombin by specifically binding to catalytic site and to anion-binding exosite of circulating and clot-bound thrombin.

**PHARMACOKINETICS: Metabolism:** Renal mechanisms and proteolytic cleavage. **Elimination:** Urine; $T_{1/2}$=25 min.

### NURSING CONSIDERATIONS

**Assessment:** Assess for active major bleeding, renal impairment, and drug interactions. Assess use in patients with disease states associated with increased risk of bleeding.

**Monitoring:** Monitor for signs/symptoms of hemorrhage (eg, decreases in BP or Hct), and thrombus formation. For patients with renal impairment, monitor anticoagulant status.

**Patient Counseling:** Advise about increased risk of bleeding events and instruct to contact physician if any occur.

**Administration:** IV route. Not for IM administration. Reconstitute: 1) To each 250mg vial, add 5mL of sterile water for injection. 2) Gently swirl until all material is dissolved. Further dilute: 3) Use 500mL D5W or 0.9% NaCl for injection to yield a final concentration of 0.5mg/mL. 4) Infusion rate to be administered is adjusted according to patient's weight. During brachytherapy, maintain meticulous catheter technique (eg, frequent aspiration and flushing). **Storage:** 20-25°C (68-77°F); excursion permitted to 15-30°C. Do not freeze. Reconstituted: May be stored at 2-8°C for up to 24 hrs. Diluted preparation is stable at room temperature for up to 24 hrs.

# ANSAID RX

flurbiprofen (Pharmacia & Upjohn)

**NSAIDs may cause an increased risk of serious cardiovascular thrombotic events, MI, stroke, and serious GI adverse events including bleeding, ulceration, and perforation of the stomach or intestines. Contraindicated for the treatment of perioperative pain in the setting of coronary artery bypass graft (CABG) surgery.**

**THERAPEUTIC CLASS:** NSAID

**INDICATIONS:** Relief of the signs and symptoms of rheumatoid arthritis or osteoarthritis.

**DOSAGE:** *Adults:* Initial: 200-300mg/day given bid, tid or qid. Max: 300mg/day or 100mg/dose.

**HOW SUPPLIED:** Tab: 50mg, 100mg

**CONTRAINDICATIONS:** ASA, with ASA triad, or other NSAID allergy that precipitates acute asthmatic attack, urticaria, or rhinitis. Treatment of perioperative pain in the setting of CABG surgery.

**WARNINGS/PRECAUTIONS:** May lead to onset of new HTN or worsening of pre-existing HTN; monitor BP closely. Fluid retention and edema reported; caution with fluid retention or heart failure. Renal papillary necrosis and other renal injury reported after long-term use. Not recommended for use with advanced renal disease; if therapy must be initiated, monitor renal function. Anaphylactoid reactions may occur. Avoid in late pregnancy; may cause premature closure of ductus arteriosus. May cause elevations of LFTs; d/c if liver disease develops or systemic manifestations occur. Caution in elderly. Anemia may occur; monitor Hgb/Hct with long-term use. May inhibit platelet aggregation and prolong bleeding time; monitor with coagulation disorders. Caution with asthma and avoid with ASA-sensitive asthma. Monitor for visual changes or disturbances. Risk of GI ulceration, bleeding, and perforation. May cause serious skin adverse events (eg, exfoliative dermatitis, Stevens-Johnson syndrome, toxic epidermal necrolysis).

**ADVERSE REACTIONS:** Dyspepsia, diarrhea, abdominal pain, constipation, headache, nausea, edema.

**INTERACTIONS:** Caution with anticoagulants; serious bleeding reported. Concomitant ASA is not recommended. May decrease hypotensive effects of β-blockers, decrease diuretic effects and diminish the antihypertensive effects of ACE inhibitors. May elevate plasma lithium levels and could enhance the toxicity of methotrexate.

**PREGNANCY:** Category C, not for use in nursing.

**MECHANISM OF ACTION:** NSAID; suspected to inhibit prostaglandin synthetase and exerts anti-inflammatory, analgesic, and antipyretic actions.

**PHARMACOKINETICS: Absorption:** Rapid; bioavailability 96%; $T_{max}$=2 hrs. **Distribution:** $V_d$=0.12L/kg; plasma protein binding (99%); found in breast milk. **Metabolism:** CYP2C9. 4'-hydroxy-flurbiprofen (major metabolite). **Elimination:** Urine (≤3% unchanged) (70% parent drug and metabolites); $T_{1/2}$=4.7 hrs (R-flurbiprofen), 5.7 hrs (S-flurbiprofen).

## NURSING CONSIDERATIONS

**Assessment:** Assess LFTs, renal function, CBC, and coagulation profile. Assess for history of CABG surgery, asthma and allergic reactions to aspirin or other NSAIDs, active ulceration or chronic inflammation of GI tract, CVD, asthma, pregnancy status. Note other diseases/conditions and drug therapies.

**Monitoring:** Monitor for hypersensitivity reactions, cardiac complications, stroke, GI bleeding, asthma, skin side effects, BP, LFTs, renal function, CBC with differential and platelet count, coagulation profile, ophthalmic exams.

**Patient Counseling:** Counsel about side effects; seek medical attention if any develop. Avoid alcohol and smoking during treatment. Instruct to take exactly as prescribed. Caution women against using medication late in pregnancy.

**Administration:** Oral route. **Storage:** 20-25°C (68-77°F).

# ANTARA

## fenofibrate (Oscient)

RX

**THERAPEUTIC CLASS:** Fibric acid derivative

**INDICATIONS:** Adjunct to diet, to reduce elevated LDL-C, Total-C, TG, Apo B, and to increase HDL-C in adult patients with primary hypercholesterolemia or mixed dyslipidemia (Fredrickson Types IIa and IIb). Adjunct to diet, for treatment of hypertriglyceridemia (Fredrickson Types IV and V hyperlipidemia) in adult patients.

**DOSAGE:** *Adults:* Hypercholesterolemia/Mixed Hyperlipidemia: Initial: 130mg qd. Hypertriglyceridemia: Initial: 43-130mg/day. Titrate: Adjust if needed after repeat lipid levels at 4-8 week intervals. Max: 130mg/day. Renal Dysfunction/ Elderly: Initial: 43mg/day. Take without regard to meals.

**HOW SUPPLIED:** Cap: 43mg, 130mg

**CONTRAINDICATIONS:** Hepatic or severe renal dysfunction (including primary biliary cirrhosis), unexplained persistent hepatic function abnormality, pre-existing gallbladder disease.

**WARNINGS/PRECAUTIONS:** Hepatocellular, chronic active, and cholestatic hepatitis and cirrhosis (rare) reported. Increases in serum transaminases reported; monitor LFTs regularly; d/c if >3x ULN. May cause cholelithiasis; d/c if gallstones found. May cause myositis, myopathy, or rhabdomyolysis; d/c if myopathy/myositis is suspected or diagnosed or if markedly elevated CPK levels occur. Acute hypersensitivity reactions (rare) and pancreatitis reported. Pulmonary embolus (PE) and deep vein thrombosis (DVT) were observed. Decreased Hgb, Hct, WBCs, thrombocytopenia, and agranulocytosis reported; monitor CBC during first 12 months of therapy. Minimize dose in severe renal impairment. Caution in elderly. Prior to therapy, attempt to control lipid levels with appropriate diet, exercise, and weight loss in obese patients and attempt to control any medical problems (eg, diabetes mellitus [DM]), hypothyroidism) that are contributing to lipid abnormalities. Measure lipid levels prior to therapy and during initial treatment; d/c use if inadequate response after 2 months on maximum recommended dose of 130mg/day.

**ADVERSE REACTIONS:** Abdominal pain, back pain, headache, abnormal LFTs, respiratory disorder, increased creatinine phosphokinase, increased AST, increased ALT.

**INTERACTIONS:** Caution with anticoagulants because may potentiate coumarin anticoagulants; reduce anticoagulant dose to maintain desirable INR and PT. Avoid HMG-CoA reductase inhibitors unless benefits outweigh risks. Bile acid sequestrants may impede absorption; take at least 1 hr before or 4-6 hrs after bile acid binding resin. Evaluate benefits/risks with immunosuppressants (eg, cyclosporine) and other nephrotoxic agents. Prior to therapy, d/c or change if possible, medications known to exacerbate hypertriglyceridemia (eg, beta-blockers, thiazides, estrogens). Caution with drugs that are substrates of CYP2C19, CYP2A6, or CYP2C9.

**PREGNANCY:** Category C, not for use in nursing.

**MECHANISM OF ACTION:** Fibric acid derivative; activates peroxisome proliferator activated receptor α (PPARα), increasing lipolysis and elimination of triglyceride-rich particles from plasma by activating lipoprotein lipase and reducing production of apoprotein C-III. Decreased triglycerides produces an alteration in the size and composition of LDL particles. LDL particles then have a greater affinity for cholesterol receptors and are catabolized rapidly. Activation of PPARα also induces an increase in the synthesis of apoproteins A-I, A-II, and HDL cholesterol. Also reduces serum acid uric levels in hyperuricemic and normal individuals by increasing the urinary excretion of uric acid.

**PHARMACOKINETICS: Absorption:** Well absorbed; $T_{max}$=4-8 hrs. **Distribution:** Plasma protein binding (99%). **Metabolism:** Rapid, via hydrolysis by esterases to fenofibric acid (active metabolite), conjugation. **Elimination:** Urine (60%), feces (25%); $T_{1/2}$=23 hrs.

## NURSING CONSIDERATIONS

**Assessment:** Assess for renal impairment, hepatic impairment or primary biliary cirrhosis, pre-existing gallbladder disease, pregnancy/nursing status, and for possible drug interactions. Prior to therapy, attempt to control serum lipids with appropriate diet, exercise, and weight loss in obese patients and attempt to control medical problems (eg, DM, hypothyroidism) that are contributing to lipid abnormalities. Measure lipid levels and LFTs prior to therapy.

**Monitoring:** Monitor for signs/symptoms of myositis, myopathy, and rhabdomyolysis; measure CPK levels if myopathy is suspected. Monitor for signs/symptoms of increases in serum transaminase levels, hepatocellular, chronic active and cholestatic hepatitis; perform periodic monitoring of LFTs. Monitor for signs/symptoms of venothromboembolic disease (eg, PE, DVT), pancreatitis, and for hypersensitivity reactions (eg, severe skin rashes). Monitor for hematological changes (eg, thrombocytopenia, agranulocytosis); perform periodic monitoring of blood counts. Monitor for signs/symptoms of cholelithiasis; perform gallbladder studies if cholelithiasis is suspected. Perform periodic monitoring of lipid levels.

**Patient Counseling:** Inform about risks/benefits of therapy. Counsel need to be on a lipid-lowering diet while on therapy. Inform that may be taken without regard to meals. Instruct to promptly report to physician any signs of myopathy (eg, unexplained muscle pain, weakness, or tenderness) particularly if accompanied by malaise and fever. Inform to notify physician if pregnant or nursing.

**Administration:** Oral route. **Storage:** 25°C (77°F); excursions permitted to 15-30°C (59-86°F).

# ANTIVERT RX

meclizine HCl (Pfizer)

**THERAPEUTIC CLASS:** Antihistamine

**INDICATIONS:** Management of nausea, vomiting and dizziness associated with motion sickness. Management of vertigo associated with diseases affecting the vestibular system.

**DOSAGE:** *Adults:* Motion Sickness: 25-50mg 1 hr prior to trip/departure, repeat q24h prn. Vertigo: 25-100mg/day in divided doses.
*Pediatrics:* ≥12 yrs: Motion Sickness: 25-50mg 1 hr prior to trip/departure, repeat q24h prn. Vertigo: 25-100mg/day in divided doses.

**HOW SUPPLIED:** Tab: 12.5mg, 25mg, 50mg* *scored

**WARNINGS/PRECAUTIONS:** Caution with asthma, glaucoma, prostatic hypertrophy.

**ADVERSE REACTIONS:** Drowsiness, dry mouth, blurred vision (rare).

**INTERACTIONS:** Avoid alcoholic beverages.

**PREGNANCY:** Category B, safety in nursing is not known.

**MECHANISM OF ACTION:** Antihistaminic agent; blocks vasodepressor response to histamine; slight blocking against acetylcholine.

## NURSING CONSIDERATIONS

**Assessment:** Assess for asthma, glaucoma, prostate enlargement, alcohol intake, and possible drug interactions.

**Monitoring:** Monitor for drowsiness.

**Patient Counseling:** Caution against performing hazardous tasks (eg, operating machinery/driving).

**Administration:** Oral route.

# ANZEMET RX

dolasetron mesylate (Sanofi-Aventis)

**THERAPEUTIC CLASS:** $5\text{-}HT_3$ receptor antagonist

**INDICATIONS:** (Inj) Prevention of N/V associated with initial and repeat courses of emetogenic cancer chemotherapy, including high-dose cisplatin. Prevention and treatment of postoperative nausea and vomiting (PONV). (Tab) Prevention of N/V associated with moderately emetogenic cancer chemotherapy, including initial and repeat courses. Prevention of PONV.

**DOSAGE:** *Adults:* Prevention of Chemotherapy-Induced N/V: (Inj) 1.8mg/kg IV single dose or 100mg IV fixed dose over 30 seconds, approximately 30 min before chemotherapy. (Tab) 100mg PO within 1 hr before chemotherapy. Prevention/Treatment of PONV: (Inj) 12.5mg IV single dose 15 min before cessation of anesthesia or as soon as N/V presents. (Tab) 100mg PO within 2 hrs before surgery.
*Pediatrics:* 2-16 yrs: (Inj) Prevention of Chemotherapy-Induced N/V: 1.8mg/kg IV single dose, approximately 30 min before chemotherapy. May mix 1.8mg/kg inj in apple or grape juice and administer orally within 1 hr before chemotherapy. Max: 100mg. (Tab) 1.8mg/kg PO within 1 hr before chemotherapy. Max: 100mg. Prevention/Treatment of PONV: (Inj) 0.35mg/kg IV single dose 15 min before cessation of anesthesia or as soon as N/V presents. Max: 12.5mg single dose. May mix 1.2mg/kg inj in apple or grape juice and administer orally within 2 hrs before surgery. Max: 100mg/dose. (Tab) 1.2mg/kg PO within 2 hrs before surgery. Max: 100mg.

**HOW SUPPLIED:** Inj: 20mg/mL [0.625mL, 5mL, 25mL]; Tab: 50mg, 100mg

**WARNINGS/PRECAUTIONS:** Can cause ECG interval changes (PR, $QT_c$, JT prolongation, and QRS widening); CV consequences, including heart block or cardiac arrhythmias, rarely reported. Caution in patients who have or may develop prolongation of cardiac conduction intervals, particularly $QT_c$, including patients with congenital QT syndrome, hypokalemia, and hypomagnesemia. Rare cases of supraventricular and ventricular arrhythmias, cardiac arrest leading to death, and MI reported in children and adolescents. Cross hypersensitivity reported in patients who received other selective $5\text{-}HT_3$ antagonists.

**ADVERSE REACTIONS:** (Inj, Tab) Headache, diarrhea, fever, fatigue, dizziness, hypotension, bradycardia, dyspepsia, HTN. (Inj) Abnormal hepatic function, abdominal pain. (Tab) Tachycardia, pruritus.

**INTERACTIONS:** Increased risk of prolongation of cardiac conduction intervals with diuretics, antiarrhythmics or other drugs which lead to QT prolongation, and cumulative high-dose anthracycline therapy. Increased levels with cimetidine. Decreased levels with rifampin. Decreased clearance with IV atenolol. Cardiac abnormality may be observed when concomitantly administered with verapamil.

**PREGNANCY:** Category B, caution in nursing.

**MECHANISM OF ACTION:** $5\text{-}HT_3$ receptor antagonist; antinauseant and antiemetic.

**PHARMACOKINETICS: Absorption:** (Inj) $T_{max}$=0.6 hr (metabolite). (Tab) Absolute bioavailability (75%); $T_{max}$=1 hr (metabolite). **Distribution:** $V_d$=5.8L/kg (metabolite); plasma protein binding (69-77%) (metabolite). **Metabolism:** Complete. Reduction via carbonyl reductase to hydrodolasetron (major metabolite); CYP2D6 (hydroxylation); N-oxidation of hydrodolasetron via CYP3A and flavin monooxygenase. **Elimination:** (Inj) Rapid; Urine (53%, unchanged hydrodolasetron), feces; $T_{1/2}$=<10 min, 7.3 hrs (metabolite). (Tab) Urine (61%, unchanged hydrodolasetron), feces; $T_{1/2}$=8.1 hrs (metabolite). Refer to PI for the Pharmacokinetic Values.

## NURSING CONSIDERATIONS

**Assessment:** Assess for possibility of cardiac prolongation of conduction interval (particularly $QT_c$), hypokalemia, hypomagnesemia, congenital QT syndrome, pregnancy/nursing status, and for possible drug interactions.

**Monitoring:** Monitor for ECG interval changes (PR, $QT_c$, JT prolongation and QRS widening), heart block, cardiac arrhythmias, supraventricular arrhythmias, ventricular arrhythmias, cardiac arrest and MI.

**Patient Counseling:** Inform about potential risks/benefits of therapy. Advise to contact physician if any adverse reactions develop or if pregnant/nursing. Instruct to not exceed the recommended dose.

**Administration:** IV and Oral route.(Inj) Dilute in a compatible IV solution to 50mL and infused over 15 min. Flush the infusion line before and after administration. **Storage:** 20-25°C (68-77°F); protect from light. (Inj) Excursions permitted to 15-30°C (59-86°F). Diluted product may be kept up to 24 hrs at room temperature or under refrigeration for up to 48 hrs. Mixed with apple or apple-grape juice, may be kept up to 2 hrs at room temperature before use.

## APIDRA — RX

insulin glulisine, rdna (Sanofi-Aventis)

**OTHER BRAND NAMES:** Apidra Solostar (Sanofi-Aventis)

**THERAPEUTIC CLASS:** Insulin

**INDICATIONS:** Indicated to improve glycemic control in adults and children with diabetes mellitus (DM).

**DOSAGE:** *Adults:* Individualize dose. Usual requirement: 0.5-1 unit/kg/day. Inject SQ within 15 min before a meal or within 20 min after starting a meal. Rotate inj site (abdomen, thigh, or deltoid). May be administered IV under medical supervision. Use concentration of 0.05-1 U/mL in infusion systems using polyvinyl chloride (PVC) bags.
*Pediatrics:* ≥4 yrs: Individualize dose. Usual requirement: 0.5-1 unit/kg/day Inject SQ within 15 min before a meal or within 20 min after starting a meal. Rotate inj site (abdomen, thigh, or deltoid). May be administered IV under medical supervision. Use concentration of 0.05-1 U/mL in infusion systems using polyvinyl chloride (PVC) bags.

**HOW SUPPLIED:** Inj: (Apidra) 100 U/mL [10mL vial, 3mL cartridge]; Pre-filled: (Apidra-Solostar) 100 U/mL [3mL pen]

**CONTRAINDICATIONS:** Episodes of hypoglycemia.

**WARNINGS/PRECAUTIONS:** Hypoglycemia and hypokalemia may occur; monitor glucose and potassium levels frequently. Rapid onset and short duration of action; follow dosage directions. Adjust dose if change in physical activity or usual meal plan. Whether using an external pump for SQ infusion or administering intravenously, do not dilute or mix with any other insulin. Caution when changing insulin strength, manufacturer, type, or species. Concomitant antidiabetic therapy may need adjustment. Severe, generalized allergy including anaphylaxis may occur.

**ADVERSE REACTIONS:** Allergic reactions, injection-site reactions, lipodystrophy, pruritus, rash, hypoglycemia, influenza, nasopharyngitis, urinary tract infection, arthralgia, HTN, headache, peripheral edema.

**INTERACTIONS:** Decreased effect with corticosteroids, danazol, niacin, diuretics, sympathomimetic agents (eg, epinephrine, albuterol, terbutaline), glucagon, isoniazid, phenothiazine derivatives, somatropin, thyroid hormones, estrogens, progestogens (eg, in oral contraceptives), protease inhibitors, and atypical antipsychotic medications (eg, olanzapine and clozapine). Increased effect with ACEIs, MAOIs, oral antidiabetics, disopyramide, fibrates, fluoxetine, pentoxifylline, propoxyphene, salicylates, sulfonamide antibiotics, somastatin analogs and pramlintide. Decreased or increased effect with β-blockers, clonidine, lithium salts, and alcohol. Pentamidine may cause hypoglycemia followed by hyperglycemia. β-blockers, clonidine, guanethidine, and reserpine may reduce or mask signs of hypoglycemia.

**PREGNANCY:** Category C, caution in nursing.

**MECHANISM OF ACTION:** Insulin glulisine (rDNA origin); lowers blood glucose by stimulating peripheral glucose uptake by skeletal muscle and fat and by inhibiting hepatic glucose production.

**PHARMACOKINETICS: Absorption:** $C_{max}$=83, 84μU/mL (0.15, 0.2 IU/kg); $T_{max}$=60, 100 min (0.15, 0.2 IU/kg); Absolute bioavailability, 70% (SQ). **Distribution:** $V_d$=13L. **Elimination:** Rapidly eliminated; $T_{1/2}$=42 min.

## NURSING CONSIDERATIONS

**Assessment:** Assess FPG, $HbA_{1c}$, renal function, LFTs, episodes of hyperglycemia, infections, alcohol consumption, exercise routines, pregnancy/nursing status, and possible drug interactions.

**Monitoring:** Monitor glucose and potassium levels, FPG, $HbA_{1c}$, hypokalemia, renal function, diabetic ketoacidosis, vision changes, lipodystrophy, allergic reactions. Monitor for signs of hypoglycemia (sweating, palpitations, seizures, disorientation, tremors).

**Patient Counseling:** Use only if the solution is clear and colorless with no visible particles. Do not dilute or mix with other insulins or solutions. Counsel about signs/symptoms of hypoglycemia, hyperglycemia, diabetic ketoacidosis, the importance of frequent monitoring of blood glucose levels, and the need for eating a balanced diet and exercising regularly. Advise to avoid excessive alcohol use. During periods of stress (eg, trauma, infection, surgery), insulin requirements may be changed; advise patients to seek prompt medical advice. Counsel on proper administration techniques.

**Administration:** SQ/ IV route. Refer to Full Prescribing Information for administration techniques. **Storage:** Unopened vial/cartridge/prefilled pen: 2-8°C (36-46°F). Open (in-use): 25°C (77°F). Discard after 28 days. Protect from light. Insulin exposed to temperatures >37°C (98°F) should be discarded.

# APLENZIN — RX

## bupropion hydrobromide (Sanofi-Aventis)

**Antidepressants increased the risk of suicidal thinking and behavior (suicidality) in short-term studies in children, adolescents, and young adults with major depressive disorder (MDD) and other psychiatric disorders. Bupropion is not approved for use in pediatric patients.**

**THERAPEUTIC CLASS:** Aminoketone

**INDICATIONS:** Treatment of major depressive disorder (MDD).

**DOSAGE:** *Adults:* ≥18 yrs: Initial: 174mg qam. Titrate: May increase to 348mg qd on Day 4 if tolerated. Max: 522mg/day given as single dose if no clinical improvement after several weeks. Switching from Wellbutrin, Wellbutrin SR, or Wellbutrin XL: Give equivalent dose. 522mg bupropion HBr = 450mg bupropion HCl, 348mg bupropion HBr = 300mg bupropion HCl, 174mg bupropion HBr = 150mg bupropion HCl. Mild-Moderate Hepatic Cirrhosis/Renal Impairment: Reduce frequency and/or dose. Severe Hepatic Cirrhosis: Max: 174mg every other day.

**HOW SUPPLIED:** Tab, Extended-Release: 174mg, 348mg, 522mg

**CONTRAINDICATIONS:** Seizure disorder, bulimia or anorexia nervosa, within 14 days of MAOIs, other forms of bupropion, abrupt d/c of alcohol or sedatives (including benzodiazepines).

**WARNINGS/PRECAUTIONS:** May worsen depression and/or emergence of suicidal ideation and behavior; monitor closely. May precipitate manic episodes in bipolar disorder. Dose-related risk of seizures; d/c and do not restart if seizures occur. Extreme caution with history of seizures, cranial trauma, severe hepatic cirrhosis, concomitant medications that lower seizure threshold. Agitation, insomnia, psychosis, confusion and other neuropsychiatric signs reported. Caution with hepatic impairment (including mild to moderate hepatic cirrhosis). Anorexia/weight loss may occur. HTN reported; caution with recent history of MI or unstable heart disease. Anaphylactoid/anaphylactic reactions reported; d/c if any occur.

**ADVERSE REACTIONS:** Dry mouth, nausea, insomnia, dizziness, pharyngitis, abdominal pain, agitation, anxiety, tremor, palpitation, tremor, sweating, tinnitus, myalgia.

**INTERACTIONS:** See Contraindications. Extreme caution with drugs that lower seizure threshold (eg, antidepressants, antipsychotics, theophylline, systemic steroids). Increased seizure risk with opioids, cocaine, or stimulant addiction, OTC stimulants or anorectics, oral hypoglycemics, insulin, excessive use or abrupt d/c of alcohol or sedatives. Caution with levodopa, amantadine, and drugs that are metabolized by CYP2D6 (eg, SSRIs, TCAs, antipsychotics, β-blockers, Class 1C antiarrhythmics); use low initial dose and gradually titrate. Monitor HTN with transdermal nicotine. Caution with CYP2B6 substrates or inhibitors (eg, orphenadrine, cyclophosphamide, thiotepa). Carbamazepine, phenytoin, cimetidine, and phenobarbital may induce metabolism of bupropion. Infrequently associated with hemorrhagic or thrombotic complications when used with warfarin. Minimize or avoid alcohol.

**PREGNANCY:** Category C, not for use in nursing.

**MECHANISM OF ACTION:** Aminoketone antidepressant; MOA not established, presumed that action is mediated by noradrenergic and/or dopaminergic mechanisms.

**PHARMACOKINETICS: Absorption**: $T_{max}$=5 hrs. **Distribution**: Plasma protein binding (84%). **Metabolism**: Extensive to hydroxybupropion (CYP2B6) via hydroxylation; threohydrobupropion, erythrohydrobupropion via reduction of carbonyl group. **Elimination**: Urine (87%), feces (10%), (0.5% unchanged). $T_{1/2}$= 21 hrs, 24 hrs, 31 hrs, 50 hrs (bupropion, hydroxybupropion, erythrohydrobupropion, threohydrobupropion respectively).

## NURSING CONSIDERATIONS

**Assessment:** Assess for history of seizures, bulimia/anorexia nervosa, LFTs, renal function tests, DM, head trauma, use of alcohol, opiate sedatives, history of MI or unstable heart disease, psychosis, mixed/manic eposodes. Note other diseases/conditions and drug therapies especially other bupropion products.

**Monitoring:** Monitor for clinical worsening, suicidality, or unusual changes in behavior, seizures, increased restlessness, agitation, anxiety, insomnia, neuropsychiatric signs/symptoms (eg, delusions, hallucinations, psychosis, concentration disturbances, paranoia, and confusion), weight loss, loss of appetite, arthralgia, myalgia, HTN, and fever with rash.

**Patient Counseling:** Advise families and caregivers of need for close observation of clinical worsening and suicidal risks. Avoid alcohol, sedatives, and OTC drugs. Exercise caution while driving or operating machinery. Advise not to use in combination with other medications that contains the same active ingredient. Advise that something that looks like a tablet may appear in the stool; this is the non-absorbable empty shell that is eliminated from the body. D/C and do not restart if seizures are experienced while on treatment.

**Administration:** Oral route. Swallow whole; do not chew, divide or crush tablets. **Storage**: 25°C (77°F); excursions permitted to 15-30°C (59-86°F).

# APRISO — RX

mesalamine (Salix)

**THERAPEUTIC CLASS:** Anti-inflammatory Agent

**INDICATIONS:** Maintenance of remission of ulcerative colitis in patients ≥18 yrs.

**DOSAGE:** *Adults:* 1.5g (4 caps) qam. Take with or without food.

**HOW SUPPLIED:** Cap, Extended Release: 0.375g

**WARNINGS/PRECAUTIONS:** Renal impairment, including minimal change nephropathy, acute and chronic interstitial nephritis, renal failure (rare), reported. Evaluate renal function prior to initiation of therapy and periodically while on therapy. Caution in patients with known renal dysfunction or a history of renal disease. D/C if acute intolerance syndrome occurs (eg, acute abdominal pain, cramping, bloody diarrhea). Re-evaluate periodically. Caution with sulfasalazine hypersensitivity. Caution in patients with liver disease and elderly.

**ADVERSE REACTIONS:** Headache, diarrhea, upper abdominal pain, nausea, nasopharyngitis, influenza or influenza-like illness, and sinusitis.

**INTERACTIONS:** Avoid coadministration with antacids.

**PREGNANCY:** Category B, caution in nursing.

**MECHANISM OF ACTION:** Anti-inflammatory agent; not established; possible that 5-ASA diminishes inflammation by blocking production of arachidonic acid metabolites.

**PHARMACOKINETICS: Absorption:** $T_{max}$=4 hrs, $C_{max}$=2.1µg/mL, $AUC_{0-24}$=11µg*h/mL. $AUC_{0-inf}$= 14 µg*h/mL. **Distribution:** Plasma protein binding (43%). **Metabolism:** Liver and intestinal mucosa via N-acetyltransferase activity; N-acetyl-5-aminosalicylic acid (major metabolite). **Elimination:** $T_{1/2}$=9 hrs. Urine (2%, unchanged).

## NURSING CONSIDERATIONS

**Assessment:** Assess for pre-existing renal/liver disease, hepatic/renal impairment, obtain baseline LFTs, BUN, creatinine, and urinalysis (protein).

**Monitoring:** Monitor LFTs, BUN, creatinine, and urinalysis (protein) periodically. Monitor acute intolerance syndrome, hypersensitivity, and allergic reactions.

**Patient Counseling:** Instruct not to take with antacids. Seek medical consultation if ulcerative colitis symptoms worsen.

**Administration:** Oral route. **Storage:** Store at 20-25°C (68-77°F); excursions permitted between 15-30°C (59-86°F).

# APTIVUS — RX

tipranavir (Boehringer Ingelheim)

**Both fatal and nonfatal intracranial hemorrhage reported. Clinical hepatitis and hepatic decompensation, including some fatalities, have been reported. Extra vigilance needed in patients with chronic hepatitis B or hepatitis C coinfection due to increased risk of hepatotoxicity.**

**THERAPEUTIC CLASS:** Protease inhibitor

**INDICATIONS:** Coadministered with ritonavir for combination antiretroviral treatment of HIV-1-infected patients who are treatment-experienced and have HIV-1 strains resistant to more than one protease inhibitor (PI).

**DOSAGE:** *Adults:* 500mg (two 250mg or 5mL) with 200mg ritonavir bid with or without food.
*Pediatrics:* 2-18 yrs: 14mg/kg with 6mg/kg ritonavir (or 375mg/m² with ritonavir 150mg/m²) bid. Max: 500mg with 200mg ritonavir bid. Intolerance or Toxicity: Decrease dose to 12mg/kg with 5mg/kg ritonavir (or 290mg/m² with ritonavir 115mg/m²) bid. If unable to swallow caps; may switch to oral sol.

**HOW SUPPLIED:** Cap: 250mg; Sol: 100mg/mL

**CONTRAINDICATIONS:** Moderate to severe (Child-Pugh Class B and C) hepatic impairment. Concomitant administration with amiodarone, bepridil, flecainide, propafenone, quinidine, rifampin, dihydroergotamine, ergonovine, ergotamine, methylergonovine, cisapride, St. John's wort, lovastatin, simvastatin, pimozide, oral midazolam and triazolam.

**WARNINGS/PRECAUTIONS:** Must be coadministered with ritonavir. Not recommended for use in treatment-naive patients. Caution with mild hepatic impairment (Child-Pugh Class A) and/or with chronic hepatitis B or C coinfection; monitor LFTs prior to therapy and during therapy. D/C if signs and symptoms of clinical hepatitis develop. D/C if asymptomatic elevations in AST or ALT >10X the ULN or if asymptomatic elevations in AST or ALT between 5-10X the ULN and increases in total bilirubin >2.5X the ULN occur. Caution in patients at risk of increased bleeding from trauma, surgery or other medical conditions. Reports of new-onset DM, exacerbation of pre-existing DM, diabetic ketoacidosis, hyperglycemia and increased bleeding with hemophilia types A and B. Spontaneous bleeding may occur, and additional factor VIII may be required. Rash (eg, urticarial/maculopapular) and possible photosensitivity and rash accompanied with joint pain/stiffness, throat tightness, generalized pruritus reported; d/c with severe rash. Increased total cholesterol and TG reported; assess lipid levels prior to and during therapy. Caution with known sulfonamide allergy. Possible redistribution/accumulation of body fat. Immune reconstitution syndrome reported with combination therapy. Caution in elderly.

**ADVERSE REACTIONS:** Diarrhea, N/V, abdominal pain, pyrexia, fatigue, asthenia, bronchitis, headache, cough, rash, anemia, weight decrease, hypertriglyceridemia, intracranial hemorrhage, hepatitis.

**INTERACTIONS:** See Contraindications. Combination therapy with other PIs not recommended. Decreased levels of abacavir, atazanavir, didanosine, zidovudine, amprenavir, lopinavir, saquinavir, valproic acid, methadone, meperidine and omeprazole. Increased levels of fluoxetine, paroxetine, sertraline, atorvastatin, rosuvastatin, tadalafil, trazodone and desipramine. Weigh risks/benefits with fluticasone; coadministration not recommended. Decreased levels with buprenorphine, naloxone, carbamazepine, phenobarbital and phenytoin. Increased levels with fluconazole and enfuvirtide. Caution with itraconazole, ketoconazole, voriconazole, diltiazem, felodipine, nicardipine, nisoldipine, verapamil, disulfiram/metronidazole, fluticasone, cyclosporine, sirolimus and tacrolimus. Starting dose of sildenafil should not exceed 25mg within 48 hours, tadalafil 10mg every 72 hours, and vardenafil 2.5mg every 72 hours. Decreased levels of ethinyl estradiol; use alternative forms of birth control. Dosage reduction needed for clarithromycin by 50% if CrCl 30-60mL/min and 75% if <30mL/min; concomitant rifabutin by 75%. Dose reduction and concentration monitoring for desipramine. Monitor glucose with glimepiride, glipizide, glyburide, pioglitazone, repaglinide or tolbutamine. Caution with antiplatelet and anticoagulants; may increase risk of bleeding. Monitor INR with warfarin. Caution with parenteral midazolam; monitor for respiratory depression/prolonged sedation and consider dose adjustments. See Prescribing information for complete information.

**PREGNANCY:** Category C, not for use in nursing.

**MECHANISM OF ACTION:** HIV-1 protease inhibitor; inhibits processing of Gag and Gag-Pol polyproteins, preventing formation of mature virions.

**PHARMACOKINETICS: Absorption:** Tipranavir/Ritonavir: (female) $C_{max}$=94.8µM, $T_{max}$=2.9 hrs, AUC=851µM•h. (male) $C_{max}$=77.6µM, $T_{max}$=3.0 hrs, AUC=710µM•h. **Distribution:** Plasma protein binding (>99.9%). **Metabolism:** Liver via CYP3A4. **Elimination:** Feces (82.3%), urine (4.4%). Tipranavir/Ritonavir: (healthy) $T_{1/2}$=4.8 hrs. (HIV-infected) $T_{1/2}$=6.0 hrs.

## NURSING CONSIDERATIONS

**Assessment:** Assess for HBV or HCV infection, hepatic impairment, hemophilia, sulfonamide allergy, DM, pregnancy and possible drug interactions. Determine baseline LFTs and lipid levels.

**Monitoring:** Monitor for signs and symptoms of clinical hepatitis, severe skin reaction, DM and bleeding. LFTs and lipid levels should be monitored periodically during treatment. May enroll patients in the Antiretroviral Pregnancy Registry if they become pregnant while on treatment.

**Patient Counseling:** Inform that therapy is not cure for HIV, does not reduce risk of transmission of HIV and that opportunistic infections may develop. Advise to seek medical attention for symptoms of hepatitis (eg, fatigue, malaise, anorexia, nausea), bleeding, severe skin reaction, infections and hyperglycemia. Advise to inform healthcare provider about all medications, including prescription or nonprescription medications (eg, St. John's wort) before initiating therapy. Report any history of sulfonamide allergy. Avoid vitamin E supplements. Instruct to use additional or alternative contraceptive measures for patients taking estrogen-based hormonal contraceptives. Do not alter or d/c therapy without consulting physician. Inform that if a dose is missed, take dose as soon as possible and then return to normal schedule. Instruct not to double the next dose.

**Administration:** Oral route. **Storage:** Must be used within 60 days of opening. (Cap) Refrigerate at 2-8°C (36-46°F) prior to opening the bottle. After open store at 25°C (77°F); excursions permitted to 15-30°C (59-86°F). (Sol) Store at 25°C (77°F); excursions permitted to 15-30°C (59-86°F); do not refrigerate or freeze.

## ARANESP RX

darbepoetin alfa (Amgen)

**Increase mortality, serious CV events and stroke in CRF patient when administered to target Hgb levels of ≥13g/dL. Individualize dosing to achieve and maintain Hgb levels within range of 10-12g/dL. Shortened overall survival and/or increased risk of tumor progression or recurrence in patients with breast, non-small cell lung, head and neck, lymphoid, and cervical cancers. To decrease these risks, as well as risk of serious cardio- and thrombovascular events, use lowest dose needed to avoid RBC transfusions. Because of these risks, prescribers and hospitals must enroll in and comply with the ESA APPRISE Oncology Program to prescribe and/or dispense to patients with cancer. Use only for treatment of anemia due to concomitant myelosuppressive chemotherapy. Not indicated for patients receiving myelosuppressive therapy when anticipated outcome is cure. D/C following completion of chemotherapy course.**

**THERAPEUTIC CLASS:** Erythropoiesis stimulator

**INDICATIONS:** Treatment of anemia associated with chronic renal failure (CRF), and anemia in patients due to chemotherapy with metastatic, non-myeloid malignancies due to chemotherapy.

**DOSAGE:** *Adults:* CRF: Initial: 0.45mcg/kg IV/SQ weekly or 0.75mcg/kg SQ once q2 weeks for patient not in dialysis. Titrate: Adjust to target Hgb 10-12g/dL. If Hgb increases >1g/dL in a 2-week period or is approaching 12g/dL, reduce dose by 25%. If Hgb continues to increase, hold dose until Hgb begins to decrease, and reinitiate at 25% below previous dose. Do not increase more than once monthly. If Hgb increases <1g/dL over 4 weeks, with adequate iron stores, increase dose by 25% of the previous dose. If Hgb of 10-12g/dL is not attained in 12 weeks, do not give higher dose and use the lowest dose to maintain Hgb at levels sufficient to avoid transfusion. Evaluate for other causes of anemia. Conversion from Epoetin Alfa: Base dose on weekly epoetin dose. Administered less frequently than Epoetin alfa. (See PI for details). Malignancy: Initial: 2.25mcg/kg SQ weekly or 500mcg once q3 weeks. Do not initiate therapy if Hgb ≥10g/dL. Titrate: If Hgb increases by >1g/dL in a 2-week period or if Hgb >12g/dL, decrease dose by 40%. If Hgb >12g/dL, hold dose until Hgb approaches a level where transfusions may be required. Reinitiate at 40% below previous dose. If given weekly and <1g/dL Hgb increase after 6 weeks, may increase up to 4.5 mcg/kg. D/C after 8 weeks if no response or transfusions are still required.
*Pediatrics:* ≥1 year: CRF: Conversion from Epoetin Alfa: Base dose on weekly epoetin dose. Administered less frequently than Epoetin alfa.(See Full PI for details).

**HOW SUPPLIED:** Inj: Autoinjector/Prefilled Syringe: 0.025mg/0.42mL, 0.04mg/0.4mL, 0.06mg/0.3mL, 0.1mg/0.5mL, 0.15mg/0.3mL, 0.2mg/0.4mL, 0.3mg/0.6mL, 0.5mg/mL; SDV: 0.025mg/mL, 0.04mg/mL, 0.06mg/mL, 0.1mg/mL, 0.15mg/0.75mL, 0.2mg/mL, 0.3mg/mL, 0.5mg/mL.

**CONTRAINDICATIONS:** Uncontrolled HTN.

**WARNINGS/PRECAUTIONS:** Pure red cell aplasia and severe anemia (with or without other cytopenias) may occur. Evaluate etiology if lack/loss of response occurs; test for presence of antibodies to erythropoietin; if present d/c permanently. Seizures reported. Rare reports of allergic reactions; permanently d/c if serious allergic reaction occurs. Formulation with albumin may carry risk for transmission of viral diseases. May increase BP; monitor and control BP during therapy. Avoid in patients with underlying hematologic disease (eg. hemolytic anemia, sickle cell anemia, thalassemia, porphyria). May cause allergic reaction in latex sensitive individuals. May need interval of 2-6 weeks between dose adjustment and response. Monitor Hgb and BP especially in CRF patient not on dialysis and patients transitioning to dialysis. May reduce dialysis efficiency; may require adjustment in dialysis prescription. Monitor Hgb weekly until stabilized and maintenance dose established, and for at least 4 weeks after dose adjustment. Supplemental iron is recommended if ferritin is <100mcg/L or serum transferrin is <20%.

**ADVERSE REACTIONS:** Thrombotic events, infection, myalgia, HTN, hypotension, headache, diarrhea, fatigue, edema, N/V, fever, dyspnea.

**PREGNANCY:** Category C, caution in nursing.

**MECHANISM OF ACTION:** Erythropoiesis stimulating protein; stimulates erythropoiesis (same mechanism as endogenous erythropoietin) in response to hypoxia. Erythropoietin interacts with progenitor stem cells to increase RBC production.

**PHARMACOKINETICS: Absorption: Adults:** (SQ) Slow. $T_{max}$=48 hrs. Bioavailability (37%). (6.75mcg/kg) $T_{max}$=71 hrs; (2.25mcg/kg) $T_{max}$=90 hrs. **Pediatrics:** Bioavailability (54%). Elimination: (IV) $T_{1/2}$=21 hrs. (SQ): $T_{1/2}$=74 hrs.

## NURSING CONSIDERATIONS

**Assessment:** Assess for cause of anemia. Assess for uncontrolled HTN, latex allergy, underlying hematologic disease (hemolytic anemia, sickle cell anemia, thalassemia, porphyria), and hypersensitivity to active substance or any of the excipients. Obtain baseline iron status, Hgb, BP, renal function, and electrolytes.

**Monitoring:** Monitor for signs/symptoms of allergic reactions especially in latex-sensitive patients, pure red cell aplasia, severe anemia, HTN, CV events, thromboembolic events, stroke, iron status and seizures. In cancer patient, monitor for progression and recurrence of tumor. If lack/loss of response, check for presence of antibodies. Monitor Hgb , BP, renal function and electrolyte balance periodically especially in CRF patient not on dialysis and patient transitioning to dialysis. In patient on dialysis, monitor for dialysis efficiency.

**Patient Counseling:** Counsel on importance of compliance with treatment, dietary and dialysis prescription; stress importance of judicious monitoring of BP and Hgb concentrations. Advise to seek medical attention if symptoms of anaphylactic reactions, lack/loss of response, pure red cell aplasia, viral diseases, HTN, CV events, thrombosis, or seizures occur. Inform of increased risks of mortality, serious cardiovascular events, thromboembolic events and increased risk of tumor progression/recurrence.

**Administration:** Syringe/SDV: IV route. Prefilled Autoinjector: SQ route. In patients on hemodialysis IV route is recommended. Autoinjectors are designed to administer full content and should be used only for patients who need full dose. **Storage:** 2-8°C (36-46°F). Do not freeze or shake. Do not use if it has been frozen. Protect from light.

# ARAVA — RX

leflunomide (Sanofi-Aventis)

**Avoid pregnancy during treatment or before completion of drug elimination procedure after treatment.**

**THERAPEUTIC CLASS:** Pyrimidine synthesis inhibitor

**INDICATIONS:** Treatment of active rheumatoid arthritis to reduce signs/symptoms, inhibit structural damage, or improve physical function in adults.

**DOSAGE:** *Adults:* LD: 100mg qd for 3 days. Maint: 20mg qd. If not tolerated and/or ALT elevations >2 but ≤3x ULN: Reduce to 10mg qd. If elevations persist or >3x ULN, d/c and give cholestyramine or charcoal. Max: 20mg/day.

**HOW SUPPLIED:** Tab: 10mg, 20mg, 100mg

**CONTRAINDICATIONS:** Pregnancy.

**WARNINGS/PRECAUTIONS:** May cause immunosuppression. Avoid with severe immunodeficiency, bone marrow dysplasia, severe, uncontrolled infections, significant hepatic impairment, or evidence of hepatitis B or C. May cause patients to be more susceptible to infections esp. *Pneumocystis jirovecii* pneumonia (PCP), tuberculosis, aspergillosis. Rare reports of sepsis, pancytopenia, agranulocytosis, thrombocytopenia, Stevens-Johnson syndrome (SJS), toxic epidermal necrolysis (TEN), and potentially fatal severe liver injury. Monitor WBCs, platelets, Hgb, Hct, LFTs (esp ALT) at baseline then monthly for 6 months, and every 6-8 weeks thereafter; monitor monthly with concomitant MTX and/or other immunosuppressive agents. D/C with evidence of bone marrow suppression. Women of childbearing potential must have negative pregnancy test. Interstitial lung disease reported. Caution with renal impairment. Screen for latent tuberculosis infection with a tuberculin skin test prior to initiating therapy. Monitor for BP before start of therapy and periodically thereafter.

**ADVERSE REACTIONS:** Diarrhea, respiratory infections, HTN, alopecia, rash, nausea, bronchitis, abdominal/back pain, abnormal liver enzymes, urinary tract infections, dyspepsia.

**INTERACTIONS:** Decreased levels with cholestyramine or activated charcoal. Increased side effects with hepatotoxic substances. Increased levels with rifampin; caution with concomitant use. May increase levels of diclofenac, ibuprofen, or tolbutamide. Avoid vaccination with live vaccines. Increased INR when coadministered with warfarin (rare).

**PREGNANCY:** Category X, not for use in nursing.

**MECHANISM OF ACTION:** Pyrimidine synthesis inhibitor; immunomodulatory agent. Inhibits dihydroorotate dehydrogenase. Produces antiproliferative activity.

**PHARMACOKINETICS: Absorption**: A77 1726 (M1) (major active metabolite): $T_{max}$=6-12 hrs. Oral administration of various doses led to different parameters. **Distribution**: (M1) $V_d$=0.13L/kg; plasma protein binding (>99.3%). **Metabolism**: M1 and many minor metabolites. **Elimination**: Urine (43%), feces (48%).

## NURSING CONSIDERATIONS

**Assessment:** Assess for severe immunodeficiency, bone marrow dysplasia, severe infections, hepatic dysfunction or evidence of hepatitis B or C, renal insufficiencies, pregnancy/nursing status, and possible drug interactions. Obtain baseline platelet, WBC count, Hgb, Hct, and ALT levels.

**Monitoring:** Monitor for signs/symptoms of immunosuppression and opportunistic infections (eg, PCP, TB, aspergillosis), sepsis, bone marrow suppression, pancytopenia, agranulocytosis, thrombocytopenia, severe liver injury, skin reactions (eg, SJS, TEN), interstitial lung disease. Monitor platelets, WBC count, Hgb/Hct, and ALT levels monthly for 6 months and every 6-8 weeks thereafter.

**Patient Counseling:** Advise women of increased risks of having a child with birth defects if taking medication while pregnant or if become pregnant when medication has not been completely eliminated from body. Instruct women of childbearing potential to use reliable form of contraception while on therapy. Advise to promptly inform physician if there is any possibility of pregnancy. Advise to contact physician if develop any type of skin rash or mucous membrane lesions, hepatotoxicity (eg, tiredness, abdominal pain or jaundice), pancytopenia (eg, easy bruising, bleeding, recurrent infections), and interstitial lung disease. Inform that will need periodic lab monitoring of liver enzymes and hematological parameters while on therapy.

**Administration:** Oral route. **Storage**: 25°C (77°F); excursions permitted to 15-30°C (59-86°F). Protect from light.

# AREDIA — RX

pamidronate disodium (Novartis)

**THERAPEUTIC CLASS:** Bisphosphonate

**INDICATIONS:** Treatment of moderate to severe hypercalcemia of malignancy, with or without bone metastasis. Treatment of moderate to severe Paget's disease of the bone. Adjunct to standard antineoplastic therapy for treatment of osteolytic bone metastases of breast cancer and osteolytic lesions of multiple myeloma.

**DOSAGE:** *Adults:* Moderate Hypercalcemia: 60-90mg IV single dose over 2-24 hrs. Severe Hypercalcemia: 90mg IV single dose over 2-24 hrs. Retreatment: Minimum of 7 days should elapse before retreatment to allow for full response to initial dose. Paget's Disease: 30mg IV over 4 hrs for 3 consecutive days.

Retreatment: When indicated, retreat at the dose of initial therapy. Osteolytic Bone Lesions of Multiple Myeloma: 90mg IV over 4 hrs once a month. Osteolytic Bone Metastases of Breast Cancer: 90mg IV over 2 hrs every 3-4 weeks. Max: 90mg/single dose for all indications. Give oral calcium and vitamin D supplementation to minimize hypocalcemia. Renal Dysfunction With Bone Metastases: Withhold dose if SrCr increases by 0.5mg/dL (normal baseline) or by 1mg/dL (abnormal baseline). Resume when SrCr returns to within 10% of baseline. Elderly: Start at low end of dosing range.

**HOW SUPPLIED:** Inj: 30mg, 90mg

**WARNINGS/PRECAUTIONS:** Associated with renal toxicity; assess SrCr prior to each treatment. Focal segmental glomerulosclerosis with or without nephrotic syndrome reported. Do not use during pregnancy; may cause fetal harm. Asymptomatic cases of hypophosphatemia, hypokalemia, hypomagnesemia, and hypocalcemia reported. Rare cases of symptomatic hypocalcemia (including tetany) reported. Increase risk of hypocalcemia in patients with previous thyroid surgery and hypoparathyroidism. Monitor serum calcium, electrolytes, phosphate, magnesium, CBC with differential, Hct/Hgb closely. Monitor for 2 weeks post-treatment if pre-existing anemia, leukopenia, or thrombocytopenia exists. Increased risk of renal adverse reactions with renal impairment. Avoid treatment of bone metastases in severe renal impairment. Osteonecrosis of the jaw (ONJ) reported in cancer patients; avoid invasive dental procedures. Severe and occasionally incapacitating bone, joint/and or muscle pain is reported. Do not mix with calcium-containing infusion solutions (eg, Ringer's solution); should be given in a single IV solution in line separate from all other drugs. Caution in elderly.

**ADVERSE REACTIONS:** Fever, infusion-site reaction, anorexia, constipation, dyspepsia, N/V, upper respiratory tract infection, leukopenia, uremia, hypocalcemia, hypokalemia, hypomagnesemia, hypophosphatemia, rhinitis, atrial fibrillation.

**INTERACTIONS:** Concurrent use with thalidomide increases risk of renal dysfunction in multiple myeloma. Caution with other potential nephrotoxic drugs.

**PREGNANCY:** Category D, caution in nursing.

**MECHANISM OF ACTION:** Bone resorption inhibitor; mechanism of antiresorptive action not established. Adsorbs to calcium phosphate crystals in bone and may directly block dissolution of this mineral component of bone. Inhibition of osteoclast activity contributes to inhibition of bone resorption.

**PHARMACOKINETICS: Elimination**: Urine (46% unchanged); $T_{1/2}$=28 hrs.

## NURSING CONSIDERATIONS

**Assessment:** Assess for renal impairment, history of thyroid surgery, pregnancy/nursing status, and for possible drug interactions. Assess SrCr prior to each treatment. In cancer patients, obtain dental exam with preventive dentistry prior to treatment.

**Monitoring:** Monitor for signs/symptoms of hypocalcemia, hypophosphatemia, hypokalemia, hypomagnesemia, renal toxicity, osteonecrosis of the jaw, and for musculoskeletal pain. Monitor serum calcium, electrolytes, phosphate, magnesium, and CBC, differential, and Hct/Hgb.

**Patient Counseling:** Instruct women of child bearing potential, to avoid pregnancy during therapy. Inform cancer patients to maintain good oral hygiene and avoid invasive dental procedures during therapy. Inform that periodic laboratory monitoring is required during treatment.

**Administration:** IV route. Reconstitute. 1) Add 10mL of Sterile Water for Injection to each vial resulting in a solution of 30mg/10mL or 90mg/10mL. Do not mix with calcium-containing infusion solutions (eg, Ringer's solution); administer in single IV sol and line separate from all other drugs. **Storage**: Vial: Do not store above 30°C (86°F). Reconstituted: Refrigerate at 2-8°C (36-46°F) for up to 24 hrs.

## ARGATROBAN RX

argatroban (GlaxoSmithKline)

**THERAPEUTIC CLASS:** Direct thrombin inhibitor

**INDICATIONS:** Prophylaxis or treatment of thrombosis in heparin-induced thrombocytopenia (HIT). As an anticoagulant in patients with or at risk for HIT undergoing percutaneous coronary intervention (PCI).

**DOSAGE:** *Adults:* Thrombosis: D/C heparin and obtain baseline aPTT. Initial: 2mcg/kg/min IV. Check aPTT after 2 hrs. Titrate: Increase dose until aPTT is 1.5-3x initial baseline. Max: 10mcg/kg/min. Moderate Hepatic Impairment: Initial: 0.5mcg/kg/min. PCI: Initial: 350mcg/kg bolus with 25mcg/kg/min IV. Check activated clotting time (ACT) 5-10 min after bolus. Proceed with PCI if ACT >300 sec. If ACT <300 sec, give additional 150mcg/kg bolus and increase infusion to 30mcg/kg/min. Check ACT 5-10 min later. If ACT >450 sec, decrease to 15mcg/kg/min and check ACT 5-10 min later. Continue infusion dose at therapeutic ACT (300-450 sec) during procedure. May give additional 150mcg/kg bolus and increase infusion to 40mcg/kg/min if dissection, impending abrupt closure, thrombus formation, or inability to achieve/maintain ACT >300 sec. After PCI, may use lower infusion rate if anticoagulation is needed.

**HOW SUPPLIED:** Inj: 100mg/mL

**CONTRAINDICATIONS:** Overt major bleeding.

**WARNINGS/PRECAUTIONS:** D/C all parenteral anticoagulants before administering. Extreme caution in conditions associated with an increased danger of hemorrhage (eg, severe HTN, immediately following lumbar puncture, bleeding disorder, GI lesions, spinal anesthesia, major surgery, etc). Caution in hepatic impairment. Avoid high doses in PCI patients with significant hepatic disease or AST/ALT ≥3x ULN. Monitor aPTT. For PCI, obtain ACT before dose, 5-10 min after bolus and infusion rate change, at the end of PCI, and every 20-30 min during prolonged procedures.

**ADVERSE REACTIONS:** GI bleed, GU bleed, Hct/Hgb decrease, hypotension, fever, diarrhea, sepsis, cardiac arrest, N/V, ventricular tachycardia, allergic reactions, chest pain (in PCI).

**INTERACTIONS:** Initiate after cessation of heparin therapy; allow time for heparin's effect on the aPTT to decrease. Prolongation of PT/INR with warfarin. Antiplatelets, thrombolytics, and other anticoagulants may increase risk of bleeding. Discontinue all anticoagulants before argatroban administration.

**PREGNANCY:** Category B, not for use in nursing.

**MECHANISM OF ACTION:** Direct thrombin inhibitor; reversibly binds to thrombin active site. Exerts anticoagulant effects by inhibiting thrombin-catalyzed or thrombin-induced reactions, including fibrin formation; activation of coagulation factors V, VIII, XIII; activation of protein C; and platelet aggregation. Capable of inhibiting both free and clot-associated thrombin.

**PHARMACOKINETICS: Distribution:** $V_d$=174mL/Kg; plasma protein binding (54%). **Metabolism:** Liver, via hydroxylation and aromatization; CYP3A4/5; M1 (primary metabolite). **Elimination:** Feces (primary), urine; $T_{1/2}$=39-51 min.

### NURSING CONSIDERATIONS

**Assessment:** Assess for hepatic impairment, overt major bleeding, and for drug interactions. Assess use in patients with disease states at risk for a hemorrhagic event (eg, severe HTN). Obtain baseline aPTT and activated clotting time (ACT).

**Monitoring:** Monitor for signs/symptoms of hemorrhagic events (eg, unexplained fall in Hct, decrease in BP) and for allergic reactions. Monitor aPTT 2 hrs after initiation of therapy to confirm desired therapeutic range. Monitor ACT 5-10 min after bolus dosing, after changes in infusion rate, and at end of PCI procedure.

**Patient Counseling:** Inform about risk of hemorrhagic events. Instruct to contact physician if unusual bleeding or allergic reactions occur.

**Administration:** IV route. Do not mix with other drugs prior to dilution. 2.5 mL vial: 1) Dilute (0.9% NS, D5W, or LR) to a final concentration of 1 mg/mL. Each 2.5mL vial should be diluted 100-fold by mixing with 250mL of diluent. 2) Mix repeatedly by inversion for 1 min. **Storage:** Vial: 25°C (77°F); excursions permitted to 15-30°C. Retain in original carton to protect from light. Prepared Solution: 25°C (77°F); excursions permitted to 15-30° (59-86°F) in ambient indoor light for 24 hrs. Stable for 96 hrs when protected from light and stored at controlled room temperature, 20-25°C (68-77°F) or refrigerated, 5°C ± 3°C (41°F ± 5°F).

## ARICEPT RX

donepezil HCl (Eisai/Pfizer)

**OTHER BRAND NAMES:** Aricept ODT (Eisai/Pfizer)

**THERAPEUTIC CLASS:** Acetylcholinesterase inhibitor

**INDICATIONS:** Treatment of dementia of the Alzheimer's type.

**DOSAGE:** *Adults:* Take hs. Mild to Moderate Alzheimer's Disease: Usual: 5mg to 10mg qd. Initial: 5mg qd. Titrate: May increase to 10mg after 4-6 weeks. Severe Alzheimer's Disease: Usual: 10mg qd. Initial: 5mg qd. Titrate: May increase to 10mg after 4-6 weeks. Swallow tab whole with water or dissolve ODT tab on tongue and follow with water.

**HOW SUPPLIED:** Tab: 5mg, 10mg; Tab, Disintegrating: (ODT) 5mg, 10mg

**CONTRAINDICATIONS:** Hypersensitivity to piperidine derivatives.

**WARNINGS/PRECAUTIONS:** May exaggerate succinylcholine-type muscle relaxation during anesthesia. May have vagotonic effects on sinoatrial and atrioventricular node; may cause bradycardia or heart block. May increase gastric acid secretion; monitor for GI bleeding. May cause bladder outflow obstruction. May increase risk for seizures. Caution with asthma or COPD.

**ADVERSE REACTIONS:** Nausea, diarrhea, insomnia, vomiting, muscle cramps, fatigue, anorexia, dizziness, depression, weight decrease, infection, HTN, back pain, abnormal dreams, ecchymosis.

**INTERACTIONS:** Synergistic effect with neuromuscular blocking agents (eg, succinylcholine) and cholinergic agonists (eg, bethanechol). May interfere with anticholinergic medications. CYP2D6 and CYP3A4 inducers (eg, phenytoin, carbamazepine, dexamethasone, rifampin, phenobarbital) may increase elimination rate. Ketoconazole and quinidine inhibitors of CYP450, 3A4, and 2D6, respectively, inhibit donepezil metabolism.

**PREGNANCY:** Category C, not for use in nursing.

**MECHANISM OF ACTION:** Acetylcholinesterase inhibitor; postulated to exert effect by increasing acetylcholine concentrations through inhibition of its hydrolysis by AChE.

**PHARMACOKINETICS: Absorption**: Absolute bioavailability (complete); $T_{max}$=3-4 hrs. **Distribution:** Plasma protein binding (96%). **Metabolism:** Hepatic (glucoronidation) via CYP2D6 and CYP3A4. **Elimination:** Urine (57%), feces (15%); $T_{1/2}$=70 hrs.

### NURSING CONSIDERATIONS

**Assessment:** Assess for history of CV conditions, ulcer disease, NSAID usage, GI bleed, asthma, COPD, possible drug interactions, renal/hepatic function.

**Monitoring:** Monitor renal/hepatic function, signs/symptoms of GI bleeding.

**Patient Counseling:** Can be taken without regard to meals. Seek medical attention if symptoms of GI bleeding occur. Caution with use of NSAIDs.

**Administration:** Oral route. **Storage:** 15-30°C (59-86°F).

## ARIMIDEX RX

anastrozole (AstraZeneca)

**THERAPEUTIC CLASS:** Nonsteroidal aromatase inhibitor

**INDICATIONS:** Adjuvant treatment of postmenopausal women with hormone receptor-positive early breast cancer. First-line treatment of postmenopausal women with hormone receptor positive or hormone receptor-unknown locally advanced or metastatic breast cancer. Treatment of advanced breast cancer in postmenopausal women with disease progression following tamoxifen therapy. Patients with ER-negative disease and patients who did not respond to previous tamoxifen therapy rarely respond.

**DOSAGE:** *Adults:* 1mg qd. Continue until tumor progression with advanced breast cancer.

**HOW SUPPLIED:** Tab: 1mg

**CONTRAINDICATIONS:** Pregnancy and premenopausal women.

**WARNINGS/PRECAUTIONS:** Increased incidence of ischemic cardiovascular events in patients with pre-existing ischemic heart disease reported. May cause reduction in bone mineral density. May elevate serum cholesterol.

**ADVERSE REACTIONS:** Hot flashes, asthenia, arthritis, pain, arthralgia, pharyngitis, HTN, depression, N/V, rash, osteoporosis, fractures, back pain, insomnia, headache, bone pain, peripheral edema, increased cough, dyspnea, pharyngitis, and lymphedema.

**INTERACTIONS:** Concurrent use with tamoxifen decreases plasma levels. Avoid with estrogen-containing therapies.

**PREGNANCY:** Category X, not for use in nursing.

**MECHANISM OF ACTION:** Nonsteroidal aromatase inhibitor; lowers estradiol concentrations and has no detectable effect on formation of adrenal corticosteroids or aldosterone.

**PHARMACOKINETICS: Distribution:** Plasma protein binding (40%). **Metabolism:** Liver via N-dealkylation, hydroxylation, and glucuronidation. **Elimination**: Hepatic (major), renal (minor); urine (10%); $T_{1/2}$=50 hrs.

### NURSING CONSIDERATIONS

**Assessment:** Assess for pre-existing ischemic cardiac disease, pregnancy/nursing status, menopausal status, and hepatic/renal impairment.

**Monitoring:** Monitor bone mineral density and LFTs.

**Patient Counseling:** Instruct to notify physician if pregnant/nursing or intend to become pregnant.

**Administration:** Oral route. **Storage:** 20-25°C (68-77°F).

## ARIXTRA RX

fondaparinux sodium (GlaxoSmithKline)

**Epidural or spinal hematomas resulting in long-term or permanent paralysis may occur in patients anticoagulated with low molecular weight heparins, heparinoids, or fondaparinux sodium and who are receiving neuraxial anesthesia or undergoing spinal puncture. Increased risk with indwelling epidural catheters, concomitant use of other drugs that affect hemostasis (eg, NSAIDs, platelet inhibitors, other anticoagulants), history of traumatic or repeated epidural or spinal puncture, or a history of spinal deformity or spinal surgery. Monitor frequently for signs/symptoms of neurologic impairment; if neurologic compromise noted, urgent treatment is necessary. Consider benefit and risks before neuraxial intervention in patients anticoagulated or to be anticoagulated for thromboprophylaxis.**

**THERAPEUTIC CLASS:** Specific factor Xa inhibitor

**INDICATIONS:** Prophylaxis of deep vein thrombosis (DVT) in patients undergoing hip fracture surgery, including extended prophylaxis; hip replacement surgery; knee replacement surgery; abdominal surgery who are at risk of thromboembolic complications. Treatment of acute DVT when administered in conjunction with warfarin sodium. Treatment of acute pulmonary embolism (PE) when administered in conjunction with warfarin sodium when initial therapy is administered in the hospital.

**DOSAGE:** *Adults:* DVT Prophylaxis: 2.5mg SQ qd, starting 6-8 hrs post-op for 5-9 days. Hip Fracture Surgery Prophylaxis: Extended prophylaxis up to 24 additional days is recommended. DVT/PE Treatment: <50kg: 5mg SQ qd. 50-100kg: 7.5mg SQ qd. >100kg: 10mg SQ qd. Initiate concomitant warfarin as soon as possible, usually within 72 hrs. Continue treatment with fondaparinux for at least 5 days and until therapeutic anticoagulant effect is established (INR=2-3).

**HOW SUPPLIED:** Inj: 2.5mg/0.5mL, 5mg/0.4mL, 7.5mg/0.6mL, 10mg/0.8mL

**CONTRAINDICATIONS:** Severe renal impairment (CrCl <30mL/min), active major bleeding, bacterial endocarditis, thrombocytopenia associated with a positive *in vitro* test for antiplatelet antibody in the presence of fondaparinux sodium, body weight <50kg (for venous thromboembolism [VTE] prophylaxis only).

**WARNINGS/PRECAUTIONS:** Not for IM injection. Cannot be compared with activities of heparin or low molecular weight heparins. Extreme caution in conditions with an increased risk of hemorrhage (eg, congenital or acquired bleeding disorders, active ulcerative and angiodysplastic GI disease; hemorrhagic stroke, uncontrolled arterial HTN, diabetic retinopathy, shortly after brain, spinal, or ophthalmological surgery). Administration earlier than 6 hrs after surgery increases risk of major bleeding. Risk of bleeding increases with renal impairment; monitor renal function periodically. Caution if CrCl 30-50mL/min. Increased risk of bleeding in patients <50kg. Thrombocytopenia reported; d/c if platelets <100,000/mm$^3$. D/C if unexpected changes in coagulation parameters or major bleeding occurs during therapy. Perform routine CBC (including platelet count), SrCr, and stool occult blood tests during treatment. May cause allergic reaction in latex-sensitive individuals. Caution with hepatic impairment and in the elderly.

**ADVERSE REACTIONS:** Bleeding complications, thrombocytopenia, local reactions (eg, rash, pruritus), anemia, insomnia, hypokalemia, purpura, hypotension, dizziness, increased wound drainage, confusion, bullous eruption, hematomas.

**INTERACTIONS:** See BlackBox Warning. Agents that may enhance the risk of hemorrhage should be d/c prior to initiation of therapy unless these agents are essential; if coadministration is necessary, monitor closely for hemorrhage.

**PREGNANCY:** Category B, caution in nursing.

**MECHANISM OF ACTION:** Specific factor Xa inhibitor; selectively binds to antithrombin III (ATIII). Potentiates the innate neutralization of Factor Xa by ATIII thereby interrupting the blood coagulation cascade and inhibiting thrombin formation and thrombus development.

**PHARMACOKINETICS: Absorption:** Rapid, complete; absolute bioavailability (100%); $C_{max}$=0.39-0.5mg/L (2.5mg QD); 1.2-1.26mg/L (5mg, 7.5mg, 10mg QD); $T_{max}$=3 hrs (2.5mg QD). **Distribution:** $V_d$=7-11L; bound to ATIII (94%). **Elimination:** Urine (77%, unchanged); $T_{1/2}$=17-21 hrs.

## NURSING CONSIDERATIONS

**Assessment:** Assess for renal/hepatic impairment, presence of active major bleeding, bacterial endocarditis, thrombocytopenia, weight of patient, conditions that increase the risk of hemorrhage (eg, congenital or acquired bleeding disorders, active ulcerative and angiodysplastic GI disease, hemorrhagic stroke, uncontrolled arterial HTN, diabetic retinopathy), latex sensitivity, nursing/pregnancy status, and for possible drug interactions.

**Monitoring:** Monitor for signs/symptoms of bleeding and thrombocytopenia. In patients undergoing neuraxial anesthesia or spinal puncture, monitor for epidural or spinal hematomas and neurologic impairment. Perform periodic monitoring of CBC (including platelet count), SrCr, and stool occult blood tests.

**Patient Counseling:** Instruct on the proper technique of administration: do not inject IM; do not mix with other injections or infusions; do not expel air bubble from prefilled syringe; administer in fatty tissue, alternating injection sites. Counsel on signs and symptoms of possible bleeding. Inform that it may take longer than usual to stop bleeding and may bruise and/or bleed more easily while on therapy. Instruct to report any unusual bleeding, bruising, or signs of thrombocytopenia (eg, rash of dark red spots under the skin). Advise to notify physician or dentist of all prescription and nonprescription medications currently taking. Instruct to watch for signs and symptoms of spinal or epidural hematomas such as tingling, numbness and muscular weakness; contact physician immediately if symptoms occur.

**Administration:** SQ route. Refer for PI on Instructions for Use. Do not inject IM. Do not mix with other injections or infusions. Do not expel air bubble from prefilled syringe. Administer in fatty tissue, alternating injection sites. **Storage:** 25°C (77°F); excursions permitted to 15-30°C (59-86°F).

## ARMOUR THYROID — RX

thyroid (Forest)

**THERAPEUTIC CLASS:** Thyroid replacement hormone

**INDICATIONS:** Treatment of hypothyroidism. As a pituitary TSH suppressant in the treatment or prevention of various types of euthyroid goiters. Diagnostic agent in suppression tests to differentiate suspected mild hyperthyroidism or thyroid gland autonomy. Management of thyroid cancer.

**DOSAGE:** *Adults:* Hypothyroidism: Initial: 30mg qd. Titrate: Increase by 15mg q2-3 weeks. Myxedema with Cardiovascular Disorder: 15mg qd. Maint: 60-120mg/day. Thyroid Cancer: Higher doses than replacement therapy are required. Myxedema Coma: Levothyroxine Sodium: Initial: 400mcg IV then 100-200mcg/day IV. Continue with oral therapy when stabilized. Thyroid Suppression: 1.56mg/kg/day for 7-10 days. Elderly: Initial: Use lower dose (eg, 15-30mg qd).

*Pediatrics:* Hypothyroidism: 0-6 months: 4.8-6mg/kg/day; 6-12 months: 3.6-4.8mg/kg/day; 1-5 yrs: 3-3.6mg/kg/day; 6-12 yrs: 2.4-3mg/kg/day; >12 yrs: 1.2-1.8mg/kg/day.

**HOW SUPPLIED:** Tab: 15mg, 30mg, 60mg, 90mg, 120mg, 180mg*, 240mg, 300mg* *scored

**CONTRAINDICATIONS:** Untreated thyrotoxicosis; uncorrected adrenal cortical insufficiency.

**WARNINGS/PRECAUTIONS:** Do not use in the treatment of obesity; larger doses in euthyroid patients can cause serious or even life-threatening toxicity. Caution with cardiovascular disease, DM, diabetes insipidus, elderly, and adrenal cortical insufficiency.

**INTERACTIONS:** May increase insulin or oral hypoglycemic requirements. Reduced absorption with cholestyramine and colestipol; space dosing by 4-5 hrs. Altered effect of oral anticoagulants; monitor PT/INR. Estrogens increase thyroxine-binding globulin; increase in thyroid dose may be needed. Serious or life-threatening side effects can occur with sympathomimetic amines. Androgens, corticosteroids, estrogens, iodine-containing preparations, and salicylates may interfere with thyroid lab tests.

**PREGNANCY:** Category A, caution in nursing.

**MECHANISM OF ACTION:** Thyroid hormone; not established, suspected to enhance oxygen consumption by most body tissues, increase the basal metabolic rate and metabolism of carbohydrates, lipids, and proteins.

**PHARMACOKINETICS: Abosrption:** ($T_3$) Completely absorbed; $T_{max}$=4 hrs; ($T_4$) partially absorbed. **Distribution:** Plasma protein binding (>99%), found in breast milk. **Metabolism:** Deiodination in liver, kidneys, other tissues.

### NURSING CONSIDERATIONS

**Assessment:** Assess for diagnosed but uncorrected adrenal cortical insufficiency, untreated thyrotoxicosis, hypersensitivity to any of its active or extraneous constituents, cardiovascular system, angina, DM, myxedema coma, and possible drug and test interactions.

**Monitoring:** Monitor urinary glucose levels in patients with DM, PT in patients receiving anticoagulants, and periodic assessment of thyroid status (TSH suppression test, serum $T_4$ levels, free $T_4$; if TSH is normal, total $T_4$ is low), free $T_3$, $T_4$, signs/symptoms of thyroid hormone toxicity (chest pain, increased pulse rate, palpitations, excessive sweating, heat intolerance, and nervousness), partial hair loss in children.

**Patient Counseling:** Inform that replacement therapy is to be taken essentially for life, with the exception of cases of transient hypothyroidism, which associated with thyroiditis, and those patients receiving a therapeutical trial of the drug. Report immediately any signs/symptoms of thyroid toxicity.

**Administration:** Oral route. **Storage**: Store at 15-30°C (59-86°F).

## AROMASIN RX

exemestane (Pharmacia & Upjohn)

**THERAPEUTIC CLASS:** Aromatase inactivator

**INDICATIONS:** In postmenopausal women, treatment of advanced breast cancer that has progressed after tamoxifen therapy. Adjuvant treatment of postmenopausal women with estrogen-receptor positive early breast cancer who have received 2-3 yrs of tamoxifen and are switched to exemestane for a total completion of 5 consecutive yrs to adjuvant hormonal therapy.

**DOSAGE:** *Adults:* Early/Advanced: 25mg qd after a meal. Continue in the absence of recurrence of contralateral breast cancer until completion of 5 yrs of adjuvant endocrine therapy in postmenopausal women with early breast cancer treated with 2-3 yrs of tamoxifen. Continue until tumor progression is evident. Concomitant Potent CYP3A4 Inducers (eg, rifampicin, phenytoin): 50mg qd after a meal.

**HOW SUPPLIED:** Tab: 25mg

**WARNINGS/PRECAUTIONS:** Fetal harm in pregnancy. Avoid in premenopausal women.

**ADVERSE REACTIONS:** Fatigue, N/V, hot flashes, pain, depression, insomnia, anxiety, dyspnea, dizziness, headache, increased sweating, edema, HTN, anorexia.

**INTERACTIONS:** Avoid coadministration with estrogen-containing agents. Potent CYP3A4 inducers (eg, rifampin, phenytoin, carbamazepine, phenobarbital, St. John's wort) may decrease plasma levels.

**PREGNANCY:** Category D, caution in nursing.

**MECHANISM OF ACTION:** Irreversible steroidal aromatase inactivator; acts as. false substrate for aromatase enzyme; processed to intermediate that binds irreversibly to active site of enzyme, causing inactivation.

**PHARMACOKINETICS: Absorption:** Rapid. (Healthy) $T_{max}$=2.9 hrs; AUC=41.4ng•h/mL. (Breast cancer) $T_{max}$=1.2 hrs; AUC=75.4ng•h/mL. **Distribution:** Plasma protein binding (90%). **Metabolism:** Oxidation via CYP3A4; reduction. **Elimination:** Urine (<1%), $T_{1/2}$=24 hrs.

### NURSING CONSIDERATIONS

**Assessment:** Assess for possible drug interactions, renal/hepatic functions.

**Monitoring:** Monitor for hematological abnormalities, LFTs, creatinine, and bone mineral density.

**Patient Counseling:** Inform of pregnancy risks. Advise to take after meal.

**Administration:** Oral route. **Storage:** 25°C (77°F); excursions permitted to 15-30°C (59-86°F).

## ARTHROTEC RX

diclofenac sodium - misoprostol (G.D. Searle)

**Contraindicated in pregnancy; misoprostol may cause abortion, premature birth or birth defects. Uterine rupture reported when used to induce labor and abortion beyond 8 weeks of pregnancy. Use only in women of child-bearing age if at high risk for developing NSAID-associated gastric or duodenal ulcers and its complications. Such patients should have a negative pregnancy test within 2 weeks prior to beginning therapy, received both oral and written warnings on the hazards of misoprostol, be capable of effective contraceptive means, and will begin Arthrotec only on the 2nd or 3rd day of the next normal menstrual period. NSAIDs may cause an increased risk of serious cardiovascular thrombotic events, MI, stroke, and serious GI adverse events including bleeding, ulceration, and perforation of the stomach or intestines. Contraindicated for the treatment of perioperative pain in the setting of coronary artery bypass graft (CABG) surgery.**

**THERAPEUTIC CLASS:** NSAID/prostaglandin $E_1$ analogue

**INDICATIONS:** Treatment of the signs and symptoms of osteoarthritis (OA) or rheumatoid arthritis (RA) in patients at high risk of developing NSAID-induced gastric and duodenal ulcers and their complications.

**DOSAGE:** *Adults:* OA: 50mg tid. Max: (Diclofenac)150mg/day. RA: 50mg tid-qid. Max: (Diclofenac) 225mg/day. OA/RA: If not tolerable, give 50-75mg bid (less effective in preventing ulcers). Swallow whole; tab should not be crushed, chewed, or dissolved. Misoprostol dose should not exceed 0.8mg/day.

**HOW SUPPLIED:** Tab: (Diclofenac-Misoprostol) 50mg-0.2mg, 75mg-0.2mg

**CONTRAINDICATIONS:** See Black Box Warning. Pregnancy, patients who experienced asthma, urticaria or other allergic type reactions to ASA or other NSAIDs.

**WARNINGS/PRECAUTIONS:** May lead to onset of new HTN or worsening of pre-existing HTN. Caution in patients with HTN; monitor BP closely. Fluid retention and edema reported; caution in patients with fluid retention or heart failure. Caution with history of ulcer disease or GI bleeding. Renal papillary necrosis and other renal injury reported after long-term use. Renal toxicity also reported in patients in whom renal prostaglandins have a compensatory role in the maintenance of renal perfusion; caution with impaired renal function, heart failure, liver dysfunction, and the elderly. Not recommended for use with advanced renal disease; if therapy must be initiated, monitor renal function. May cause elevations of LFTs; d/c if abnormal LFTs persist/worsen, liver disease develops, or if systemic manifestations occur. Anaphylactic reactions may occur. May cause serious skin adverse events (eg, exfoliative dermatitis, Stevens-Johnson syndrome, toxic epidermal necrolysis). Use late in pregnancy may cause premature closure of the ductus arteriosis. Not a substitute for corticosteroids or for the treatment of corticosteroid insufficiency. Anemia may occur; with long-term use, monitor Hgb/Hct if signs or symptoms of anemia develop. May inhibit platelet aggregation and prolong bleeding time; monitor with coagulation disorders. Caution with asthma and avoid with ASA-sensitive asthma. Aseptic meningitis with fever and coma reported. Avoid with hepatic porphyria.

**ADVERSE REACTIONS:** Abdominal pain, diarrhea, dyspepsia, nausea, flatulence, GI disorders.

**INTERACTIONS:** Concomitant use with ACE inhibitors may diminish the antihypertensive effect of ACE inhibitors and increase the risk of renal toxicity. Concomitant use with antacids may reduce the bioavailability of misoprostol acid and delay the absorption of diclofenac sodium. Avoid coadministration with magnesium-containing antacids; misoprostol-associated diarrhea may be exacerbated when used concomitantly. Concomitant use with diuretics may increase the risk of renal toxicity; may reduce the natriuretic effect of furosemide and thiazides. Increased serum potassium with $K^+$-sparing diuretics. Synergistic GI bleeding effects when used concomitantly with warfarin. May increase risk of serious GI bleeding when used concomitantly with oral corticosteroids, anticoagulants, or alcohol. May alter response to insulin or oral hypoglycemics. Monitor for digoxin, methotrexate, cyclosporine, phenobarbital, and lithium toxicities. Caution with concomitant use of drugs that are known to be potentially hepatotoxic (eg, antibiotics, anti-epileptics). Avoid with ASA.

**PREGNANCY:** Category X, caution in nursing.

**MECHANISM OF ACTION:** Diclofenac: NSAID; not established. May be related to prostaglandin synthetase inhibition. Possesses anti-inflammatory, analgesic, and antipyretic properties. Misoprostol: Prostaglandin $E_1$ analog with gastric antisecretory and mucosal protective properties.

**PHARMACOKINETICS: Absorption**: Oral administration of a single dose or multiple doses of medication are similar to pharmacokinetics of two individual components. Refer to PI for further information. **Distribution:** Diclofenac: $V_d$=550mL/kg; albumin binding (>99%); found in breast milk. Misoprostol: Plasma protein binding (<90%); found in breast milk. **Metabolism:** Diclofenac: Glucuronide and sulfate conjugation. Misoprostol: Rapidly, to misoprostol acid (active metabolite). **Elimination:** Diclofenac: Urine (65%), bile (35%); $T_{1/2}$=2 hrs. Misoprostol: Urine (70%); $T_{1/2}$=30 min.

## NURSING CONSIDERATIONS

**Assessment:** Assess for history of hypersensitivity reaction to aspirin or other NSAIDs, CVD (eg, pre-existing HTN, CHF) or risk factors for CVD, fluid retention, risk factors for a GI event (eg, prior history of ulcer disease or GI bleeding, smoking), renal/hepatic dysfunction, coagulation disorders, asthma, hepatic porphyria, SLE, connective tissue diseases, nursing status, and for possible drug interactions. Assess pregnancy status (negative pregnancy test within 2 weeks prior to therapy) and assess ability to maintain effective contraceptive measures.

**Monitoring:** Monitor for signs/symptoms of CV thrombotic events, new onset or worsening of pre-existing HTN, fluid retention and edema, GI effects (eg, bleeding, ulceration, perforation of stomach, small intestine, or large intestine), renal effects (eg, renal papillary necrosis), hepatic effects (eg, elevations in LFTs, liver necrosis, jaundice), anaphylactic reactions, skin reactions (eg, exfoliative dermatitis, Stevens-Johnson syndrome, toxic epidermal necrolysis), hematological effects (eg, anemia, prolongation of bleeding time), bronchospasm, aseptic meningitis, and porphyria. Monitor BP at initiation of and during therapy. If anemia is suspected, monitor Hgb/Hct. Monitor renal function if renal disease present. If on long-term therapy, monitor transaminases 4-8 weeks after initiating therapy and periodically monitor CBC and chemistry profile.

**Patient Counseling:** Inform women of childbearing potential, they must not be pregnant when therapy is initiated and must remain on an effective form of contraception during treatment. Advise of pregnancy/fetal risks. Instruct to not give medication to other individuals. Instruct to contact physician if signs/symptoms of CV effects (eg, chest pain, SOB, slurring of speech), GI effects (eg, epigastric pain, dyspepsia, melena, hematemesis), or unexplained weight gain and edema occur. Contact physician and d/c treatment if signs of skin reactions or hepatotoxicity (eg, nausea, fatigue, jaundice, RUQ tenderness) occur. Instruct to seek immediate emergency attention if signs of an anaphylactic reaction occur (eg, breathing difficulty, facial or throat swelling).

**Administration:** Oral route. **Storage:** At or below 25°C (77°F), in a dry area.

# ASACOL — RX

mesalamine (Procter & Gamble)

**OTHER BRAND NAMES:** Asacol HD (Procter & Gamble)

**THERAPEUTIC CLASS:** Anti-inflammatory Agent

**INDICATIONS:** (Asacol): Treatment of mildly to moderately active ulcerative colitis and for the maintenance of remission of ulcerative colitis. (Asacol HD): Treatment of moderately active ulcerative colitis.

**DOSAGE:** *Adults:* (Asacol): Mild-Moderately Active Ulcerative Colitis: Usual: 2 tabs of 400mg tid for 6 weeks. Maintenance of Remission of Ulcerative Colitis: 1.6g/day in divided doses. (Asacol HD): Moderately Active Ulcerative

Colitis: Usual: 2 tabs of 800mg tid for 6 weeks. One Asacol HD 800mg tab has not been shown to be bioequivalent to two Asacol 400mg tabs.

**HOW SUPPLIED:** Tab, Delayed-Release: 400mg (Asacol), 800mg (Asacol HD).

**CONTRAINDICATIONS:** Hypersensitivity to salicylates.

**WARNINGS/PRECAUTIONS:** Caution in patients with pyloric stenosis, may prolong gastric retention which could delay mesalamine release in the colon. Exacerbation of symptoms of colitis reported; symptoms abate with discontinuation. Caution with sulfasalazine hypersensitivity. Renal impairment, including minimal change nephropathy, acute and chronic interstitial nephritis, and rarely renal failure reported; caution with renal dysfunction or history of renal disease. Monitor renal function prior to therapy and periodically thereafter. Caution in elderly. Reports of hepatic failure in patients with pre-existing liver disease; caution in patients with liver disease.

**ADVERSE REACTIONS:** (Asacol): Headache, abdominal pain, eructation, pain, nausea, pharyngitis, dizziness, asthenia, diarrhea, back pain, fever, rash, dyspepsia. (Asacol HD): Headache, nausea, nasopharyngitis, abdominal pain, exacerbation of ulcerative colitis, diarrhea.

**PREGNANCY:** Category B, caution in nursing.

**MECHANISM OF ACTION:** Anti-inflammatory agent; unknown. Possibly diminishes inflammation by blocking cyclooxygenase and inhibiting prostaglandin production in the colon.

**PHARMACOKINETICS: Absorption:** (400 mg) $T_{max}$=4-12 hrs. (800mg): $C_{max}$ =5mcg/mL, ($AUC_{tau}$=20mcg• h/mL). **Distribution:** (400mg, 800mg): Found in breast milk. (800mg): Crosses placental barrier. **Metabolism:** Gut mucosal wall and liver via rapid acetylation. Metabolite (N-acetyl-5-aminosalicylic acid). **Elimination:** Renally excreted as metabolite. (400mg): $T_{1/2}$=2-15 hrs. (800mg) $T_{1/2}$=12.6 hrs.

## NURSING CONSIDERATIONS

**Assessment:** Assess for renal dysfunction or history of renal disease, liver disease, pyloric stenosis, and pregnancy/nursing status. Obtain baseline renal function, LFTs, CBC, and cardiac function.

**Monitoring:** Monitor for signs and symptoms of renal impairment including nephropathy, acute and chronic interstitial nephritis, and renal failure. Monitor for signs and symptoms of a colitis exacerbation (eg, cramping, abdominal pain, bloody diarrhea) and for hypersensitivity reactions. If pyloric stenosis exists, monitor for prolonged gastric retention. If pre-existing liver disease exists, monitor for signs and symptoms of hepatic failure. Perform periodic monitoring of renal function, LFTs, and CBC.

**Patient Counseling:** Instruct to swallow whole; do not break, cut, or chew tabs. Advise to report if intact or partially intact tablet is seen in stool. Inform that ulcerative colitis rarely remits completely, and the risk of relapse can be substantially reduced by continued administration of medication. Instruct to seek medical attention if an exacerbation of colitis (cramping, abdominal pain, bloody diarrhea) occurs or if a hypersensitivity reaction develops. Inform that Asacol cannot be substituted with Asacol HD.

**Administration:** Oral route. **Storage:** 20-25°C (68-77°F).

# ASMANEX — RX

mometasone furoate (Schering)

**THERAPEUTIC CLASS:** Corticosteroid

**INDICATIONS:** Maintenance treatment of asthma as prophylactic therapy in patients ≥4 yrs.

**DOSAGE:** *Adults:* Previous Therapy with Bronchodilators Alone or Inhaled Corticosteroids: Initial: 220mcg qpm. Max: 440mcg qpm or 220mcg bid. Previous Therapy with Oral Corticosteroids: Initial: 440mcg bid. Max: 880mcg/day. Titrate to lowest effective dose once asthma stability achieved.

*Pediatrics:* ≥12 yrs: Previous Therapy with Bronchodilators Alone or Inhaled Corticosteroids (CS): Initial: 220mcg qpm. Max: 440mcg qpm or 220mcg bid. Previous Therapy with Oral CS: Initial: 440mcg bid. Max: 880mcg/day. 4-11 yrs: 110mcg qpm regardless of prior therapy. Titrate to lowest effective dose once asthma stability achieved.

**HOW SUPPLIED:** Twisthaler: 110mcg/inh, 220mcg/inh

**CONTRAINDICATIONS:** Primary treatment of status asthmaticus or other acute episodes of asthma where intensive measures are required.

**WARNINGS/PRECAUTIONS:** Deaths due to adrenal insufficiency have occurred with transfer from systemic corticosteroids to inhaled corticosteroids. Wean slowly from systemic corticosteroid therapy. Resume oral corticosteroids during stress or severe asthma attack. May unmask allergic conditions previously suppressed by systemic corticosteroid therapy. May increase susceptibility to infections. Not for rapid relief of bronchospasm or other acute episodes of asthma. D/C if bronchospasm occurs after dosing. Observe for systemic corticosteroid withdrawal effects, hypercorticism, reduced bone mineral density, and adrenal suppression; reduce dose slowly if needed. Decreased growth velocity may occur in pediatrics. *Candida* infections in the mouth and pharynx reported. Caution with active or quiescent TB infection of respiratory tract; untreated systemic fungal, bacterial, viral, or parasitic infections; or ocular herpes simplex. Glaucoma, increased IOP, and cataracts reported.

**ADVERSE REACTIONS:** Headache, allergic rhinitis, pharyngitis, upper respiratory tract infection, sinusitis, oral candidiasis, dysmenorrhea, musculoskeletal pain, back pain, dyspepsia, myalgia, abdominal pain, nausea.

**INTERACTIONS:** Ketoconazole may increase plasma levels.

**PREGNANCY:** Category C, caution in nursing.

**MECHANISM OF ACTION:** Corticosteroid; shown to have inhibitory effects on multiple cell types (mast cells, eosinophils, neutrophils, macrophages, and lymphocytes) and mediators (histamine, eicosanoids, leukotrienes and cytokines), involved in inflammatory and asthmatic response.

**PHARMACOKINETICS: Absorption:** Absolute bioavailability (≤1%); $C_{max}$=94-114pcg/mL; $T_{max}$=1.0-2.5 hrs. **Distribution:** $V_d$=152L; plasma protein binding (98-99%). **Metabolism:** Liver, via CYP3A4. **Elimination:** $T_{1/2}$=5 hrs.

## NURSING CONSIDERATIONS

**Assessment:** Assess for risk factors for decreased bone mineral content (eg, prolonged immobilization, family history of osteoporosis, drugs that decrease bone mass), history of increased IOP, glaucoma, cataracts, concomitant diseases such as status asthmaticus, active or quiescent pulmonary TB, ocular herpes simplex, untreated systemic fungal, bacterial, parasitic or viral infections, and possible drug interactions.

**Monitoring:** Monitor for localized oral infections with *Candida albicans*, decreased bone mass, asthma instability (serial objective measures of airflow), body height in children, development of glaucoma, increased IOP, posterior subcapsular cataracts, adrenal insufficiency (eg, fatigue, weakness, N/V, hypotension), paradoxical bronchospasm, and hypersensitivity reactions.

**Patient Counseling:** Instruct to discard inhaler 45 days after opening foil pouch or when dose counter reads "00" and final dose inhaled, whichever comes first. If dose counter not working correctly, do not use and bring to physician or pharmacist. Inform that medication is not a bronchodilator and should not be used for sudden symptoms of SOB or acute bronchospasm. Advise to rinse mouth after inhalation. Inform drug may cause reduction in growth rate (pediatrics) and may also unmask allergies (eg, rhinitis, conjunctivitis, eczema). Avoid exposure to chickenpox or measles; seek medical attention if exposed to chickenpox or measles, worsening of existing TB, infections, or ocular herpes simplex, symptoms do not improve or worsen, during periods of stress or severe asthmatic attack, adrenal insufficiency (eg, fatigue, weakness, N/V and hypotension), paradoxical bronchospasm or hypersensitivity reactions occur.

**Administration:** Oral inhalation. Inhale rapidly and deeply. **Storage:** Dry place at 25°C (77°F); excursions permitted to 15-30°C (59-86°F). Discard inhaler 45 days after opening foil pouch or when dose counter reads "00" and final dose has been inhaled, whichever comes first.

## ASTELIN RX
azelastine HCl (Meda)

**THERAPEUTIC CLASS:** Antihistamine

**INDICATIONS:** Treatment of the symptoms of seasonal allergic rhinitis and vasomotor rhinitis.

**DOSAGE:** *Adults:* 2 sprays per nostril bid.
*Pediatrics:* Seasonal Allergic/Vasomotor Rhinitis: ≥12 yrs: 2 sprays per nostril bid. Seasonal Allergic Rhinitis: 5-11 yrs: 1 spray per nostril bid.

**HOW SUPPLIED:** Spray: 137mcg/spray [30mL]

**ADVERSE REACTIONS:** Bitter taste, somnolence, weight increase, headache, nasal burning, pharyngitis, paroxysmal sneezing, dry mouth, nausea, atrial fibrillation, palpitations.

**INTERACTIONS:** Avoid alcohol or other CNS depressants; additive CNS impairment may occur. Increased azelastine levels with cimetidine.

**PREGNANCY:** Category C, caution in nursing.

**MECHANISM OF ACTION:** Phthalazinone derivative; inhibits histamine $H_1$ receptor activity.

**PHARMACOKINETICS: Absorption:** $T_{max}$=2-3 hrs. **Distribution:** Azelastine: plasma protein binding (88%). Desmethylazelastine: $V_d$=14.5L/kg; plasma protein binding (97%).

### NURSING CONSIDERATIONS

**Assessment:** Assess for liver/renal functions, alcohol intake, and possible drug interactions.

**Monitoring:** Monitor for somnolence.

**Patient Counseling:** Caution against hazardous activities (eg, operating machinery/driving). Avoid concomitant use of drugs (eg, other antihistamines, CNS depressants) or alcohol. Avoid spraying in eyes. Consult physician if pregnant/nursing or planning to become pregnant.

**Administration:** Intranasal route. **Storage:** 20-25°C (68-77F°). Protect from freezing. Store bottle upright with pump tightly closed.

## ASTEPRO RX
azelastine HCl (Meda)

**THERAPEUTIC CLASS:** $H_1$-antagonist

**INDICATIONS:** Relief of symptoms of seasonal and perennial allergic rhinitis in patients ≥12 yrs.

**DOSAGE:** *Adults:* Seasonal allergic rhinitis: (0.1%, 0.15%): 1 or 2 sprays per nostril bid. (0.15%): May be administered as 2 sprays per nostril qd. Perennial allergic rhinitis: (0.15%): 2 sprays per nostril bid. Elderly: Start at the low end of dosing range.
*Pediatrics:* ≥12 yrs: Seasonal allergic rhinitis: (0.1%, 0.15%): 1 or 2 sprays per nostril bid. (0.15%): May be administered as 2 sprays per nostrils qd. Perennial allergic rhinitis: (0.15%): 2 sprays per nostril bid.

**HOW SUPPLIED:** Spray: (0.1%) 137mcg; (0.15%) 205.5mcg

**WARNINGS/PRECAUTIONS:** Somnolence reported. May impair physical/mental abilities. Administer by intranasal route only. Caution in elderly.

**ADVERSE REACTIONS:** Bitter taste, somnolence, epistaxis, headache, nasal discomfort, fatigue, sneezing.

**INTERACTIONS:** Avoid concurrent use with alcohol or other CNS depressants; additional reductions in alertness and impairment of CNS performance may occur. Increased levels with cimetidine.

**PREGNANCY:** Category C, caution in nursing.

**MECHANISM OF ACTION:** $H_1$-receptor antagonist; phthalazinone derivative which exhibits histamine $H_1$-receptor activity in isolated tissues, animal models, and humans; desmethylazelastine (major metabolite) also possesses $H_1$-receptor antagonist activity.

**PHARMACOKINETICS: Absorption:** Bioavailability (40%); (0.1%) $C_{max}$=200pg/mL; $T_{max}$=3 hrs; AUC =5122 pg•hr/mL. (0.15%) $C_{max}$=409pg/mL; $T_{max}$=4 hrs; AUC=9312pg•hr/mL. Desmethylazelastine: (0.1%) $C_{max}$=23pg/mL; $T_{max}$=24 hrs; AUC =2131 pg•hr/mL. (0.15%) $C_{max}$=38pg/mL; $T_{max}$=24 hrs; AUC=3824pg•hr/mL. **Distribution:** Plasma protein binding (azelastine, desmethylazelastine [major metabolite]): (88%, 97% respectively). $V_d$=14.5L/kg. **Metabolism:** Oxidation via CYP450 enzyme system. Desmethylazelastine (major metabolite). **Elimination:** Azelastine: Feces (75%, <10% unchanged); $T_{1/2}$=22-25 hrs. Desmethylazelastine: $T_{1/2}$=52-57 hrs.

## NURSING CONSIDERATIONS

**Assessment:** Assess for hepatic/renal functions, alcohol intake, and possible drug interactions. Assess pregnancy/nursing status.

**Monitoring:** Monitor for somnolence, bitter taste, epistaxis, headache, nasal discomfort, fatigue, and sneezing.

**Patient Counseling:** Instruct to use exactly as prescribed. Instruct to use caution while engaging in hazardous activities (eg, operating machinery/driving) that require complete mental alertness and motor coordination. Advise to avoid alcohol or other CNS depressants. Must notify physician if pregnant/nursing or planning to become pregnant. Advise to prime medication before intial spray by releasing 6 sprays or until a fine mist appears. When medication has not been used for ≥3 days, counsel to reprime with 2 sprays or until a fine mist appears. Avoid spraying into eyes. Keep out of the reach of children.

**Administration:** Intranasal route. **Storage:** 20°-25°C (68°-77°F). Protect from freezing.

# ASTRAMORPH PF — CII

morphine sulfate (Abraxis)

**THERAPEUTIC CLASS:** Opioid analgesic

**INDICATIONS:** Management of pain unresponsive to non-narcotic analgesics.

**DOSAGE:** *Adults:* IV: Initial: 2-10mg/70kg. Epidural Injection: Initial: 5mg in lumbar region. Titrate: If inadequate pain relief within 1 hr, increase by 1-2mg. Max: 10mg/24hrs. Continuous Epidural: Initial: 2-4mg/24hrs. Give additional 1-2mg if needed. Intrathecal: 0.2-1mg single dose, do not repeat; may follow with 0.6mg/hr naloxone infusion to reduce incidence of side effects. Elderly/Debilitated: Epidural: <5mg/24hrs. Intrathecal: Lower dose.

**HOW SUPPLIED:** Inj: 0.5mg/mL, 1mg/mL

**CONTRAINDICATIONS:** Allergy to opiates, acute bronchial asthma, upper airway obstruction. Epidural/intrathecal routes with injection site infection, anticoagulants, bleeding diathesis, within 2 weeks of IV corticosteroids.

**WARNINGS/PRECAUTIONS:** Have resuscitation equipment, trained personnel and narcotic antagonists available; severe respiratory depression may occur. Avoid rapid administration. May be habit-forming. Caution with head injury, increased intracranial/intraocular pressure, decreased respiratory reserve, hepatic/renal dysfunction, elderly, debilitated. High doses may cause seizures. Smooth muscle hypertonicity may cause biliary colic, urinary difficulty or retention. Orthostatic hypotension may occur with hypovolemia or myocardial dysfunction. Acute respiratory failure reported with COPD or acute asthmatic attack. Limit epidural/intrathecal route to lumbar area.

**ADVERSE REACTIONS:** Respiratory depression, hypotension, pruritus, urinary retention, NV, constipation, anxiety, cough reflex depression, oliguria.

**INTERACTIONS:** CNS depressants (eg, alcohol, sedatives, antihistamines) and psychotropics (eg, MAOIs, phenothiazines, TCAs) potentiate CNS depression. Neuroleptics may increase respiratory depression.

**PREGNANCY:** Category C, safety in nursing not known.

**MECHANISM OF ACTION:** Opioid analgesic. Analgesic effect involves 3 areas of CNS; periaqueductal periventricular gray matter, ventromedial medulla, and spinal cord. Interacts predominantly with the μ-receptor to produce analgesic effects; μ-binding sites are found in the brain, spinal cord, and in the trigeminal nerve.

**PHARMACOKINETICS: Absorption:** (Epidural) $C_{max}$=33-40ng/mL; (intrathecal) $C_{max}$≤1-7.8ng/mL; (epidural, intrathecal) $T_{max}$=5-10 min. **Distribution:** (IV) $V_d$= 1-4.7L/kg; (intrathecal) $V_d$=22 mL. Plasma protein binding (36%), muscle tissue binding (54%). **Metabolism:** Hepatic glucuronidation. Found in breast milk. **Elimination:** Urine (major), feces (10%). (IV) $T_{1/2}$=1.5-2 hrs; (Epidural) $T_{1/2}$=39-249 min.

## NURSING CONSIDERATIONS

**Assessment:** Assess for hypersensitivity to other opioids, acute bronchial asthma or COPD, infection at the injection site, bleeding diathesis, hypotension, seizure disorder, head injury or increased intracranial pressure, age of patient, renal/hepatic function, biliary tract disorders, nursing/pregnancy status, and drug interactions.

**Monitoring:** Monitor for signs/symptoms of respiratory depression, hypotension, myoclonic-like spasms, seizures, urinary retention, and drug dependence. If administered via epidural intrathecally, monitor patients for 24 hrs for signs of respiratory depression.

**Patient Counseling:** Instruct to report if any signs/symptoms of respiratory depression (eg, difficulty breathing) occur. Inform physician of all medications currently taking. Advise to avoid consumption of alcohol or other CNS depressants. Inform drug may be habit forming. Avoid abrupt withdrawal.

**Administration:** IV, epidural, or intrathecal route. Administer in a setting where proper monitoring and resuscitative equipment are available. For epidural administration, proper placement of the needle or catheter in the epidural space should be verified before medication is injected. **Storage:** Store in a carton 20-25°C (68-77°F); excursions permitted to 15-30°C (59-86°F). Do not freeze. Discard any unused portion. Do not heat-sterilize.

# ATACAND RX

candesartan cilexetil (AstraZeneca)

**Can cause injury/death to developing fetus during 2nd and 3rd trimesters. D/C therapy if pregnancy is detected.**

**THERAPEUTIC CLASS:** Angiotensin II receptor antagonist

**INDICATIONS:** Treatment of hypertension, alone or with other antihypertensives. Treatment of heart failure (NYHA class II-IV, ejection fraction ≤40%) to reduce risk of death and hospitalizations.

**DOSAGE:** *Adults:* Individualize dosing. HTN: Monotherapy Without Volume Depletion: Initial: 16mg qd. Usual: 8-32mg/day given qd-bid. May add diuretic if BP not controlled. Intravascular Volume Depletion/Moderate Hepatic Impairment: Lower initial dose. Heart Failure: Initial: 4mg qd. Usual: 32mg qd. Titrate: Double dose every 2 weeks, as tolerated.

**HOW SUPPLIED:** Tab: 4mg*, 8mg*, 16mg*, 32mg* *scored

**WARNINGS/PRECAUTIONS:** Can cause fetal injury/death. Correct volume or salt depletion before therapy or monitor closely. Changes in renal function may occur; caution with renal artery stenosis, CHF. Consider low initial dose in patients with moderate hepatic impairment. Risk of hypotension; caution in major surgery and anesthesia, or when initiating therapy in heart failure. May cause hyperkalemia in heart failure patients; monitor serum potassium.

**ADVERSE REACTIONS:** Back pain, dizziness, upper respiratory tract infection.

**INTERACTIONS:** May increase lithium levels when coadministered; monitor serum lithium levels carefully.

**PREGNANCY:** Category C (1st trimester) and D (2nd and 3rd trimesters), not for use in nursing.

**MECHANISM OF ACTION:** Angiotensin II receptor antagonist; blocks the vasoconstrictor and aldosterone-secreting effects of angiotensin II by selectively blocking the binding of angiotensin II to the $AT_1$ receptor in many tissues, such as vascular smooth muscle and adrenal gland.

**PHARMACOKINETICS: Absorption:** Rapid, complete; absolute bioavailability (15%); $T_{max}$=3-4 hrs. **Distribution:** $V_d$=0.13L/kg; plasma protein binding (>99%). **Metabolism:** GIT via ester hydrolysis, liver via O-deethylation (minor); candesartan (metabolite). **Elimination**: Biliary, feces (unchanged), urine (26%, unchanged); $T_{1/2}$=9 hrs.

## NURSING CONSIDERATIONS

**Assessment:** Assess for hepatic impairment, CHF, cardiovascular disease, renal artery stenosis, volume changes, salt-depletion status, hypersensitivity, pregnancy/nursing status, and possible drug interactions.

**Monitoring:** In renal impairment, monitor serum $K^+$, serum creatinine, BUN, and BP periodically. Monitor for signs/symptoms of hypotension, CV events, hypersensitivity reactions, liver/renal dysfunction.

**Patient Counseling:** Inform patient of pregnancy/nursing risks. Advise to seek medical attention if symptoms of hypotension, CV events, or hypersensitivity reactions occur. Take without regard to food.

**Administration:** Oral route. **Storage:** 25°C (77°F); excursions permitted to 15-30°C (59-86°F).

# ATACAND HCT — RX

candesartan cilexetil - hydrochlorothiazide (AstraZeneca)

> **Can cause injury/death to developing fetus during 2nd and 3rd trimesters. D/C therapy if pregnancy detected.**

**THERAPEUTIC CLASS:** Angiotensin II receptor antagonist/thiazide diuretic

**INDICATIONS:** Treatment of hypertension.

**DOSAGE:** *Adults:* Initial: If BP Not Controlled on HCTZ 25mg/day or Controlled But Serum $K^+$ Decreased: 16mg-12.5mg tab qd. If BP not controlled on 32mg candesartan/day, give 32mg-12.5mg qd; may increase to 32mg-25mg qd. Replacement Therapy: Combination may be substituted for titrated components.

**HOW SUPPLIED:** Tab: (Candesartan-HCTZ) 16mg-12.5mg*, 32mg-12.5mg*, 32mg-25mg* *scored

**CONTRAINDICATIONS:** Anuria, history of sulfonamide hypersensitivity.

**WARNINGS/PRECAUTIONS:** Can cause fetal injury/death. Correct volume or salt depletion before therapy. Caution with hepatic or renal dysfunction, renal artery stenosis, severe CHF, and history of allergies and asthma. May exacerbate or activate systemic lupus erythematosus (SLE). Avoid if CrCl ≤30mL/min. Hyperuricemia, hyperglycemia, hypokalemia, hypomagnesemia, hyponatremia, hypercalcemia may occur. Enhanced effects in post-sympathectomy patient. May increase cholesterol and triglyceride levels. Risk of hypotension; caution in major surgery or anesthesia. Not for initial therapy. Start a low dose in patients with moderate hepatic impairment.

**ADVERSE REACTIONS:** Upper respiratory tract infection and back pain.

**INTERACTIONS:** Candesartan: Increases lithium levels. HCTZ: Potentiates orthostatic hypotension with alcohol, barbiturates, and narcotics. Adjust dosage of insulin and antidiabetic drugs. Impaired absorption with cholestyramine, colestipol. Corticosteroids and ACTH deplete electrolytes. May decrease response to pressor amines. Potentiates other antihypertensives. May increase responsiveness to skeletal muscle relaxants. Risk of lithium toxicity; monitor lithium levels during concomitant use. NSAIDs decrease diuretic effects.

**PREGNANCY:** Category C (1st trimester) and D (2nd and 3rd trimesters), not for use in nursing.

**MECHANISM OF ACTION:** Candesartan: Angiotensin II receptor antagonist; blocks vasoconstrictor and aldosterone-secreting effects of angiotensin II by blocking binding of angiotensin II to $AT_1$ receptors. HCTZ: Thiazide diuretic; mechanism not established. Affects renal tubular mechanism of electrolyte reabsorption, directly increasing excretion of $Na^+$ and $Cl^-$, and indirectly reducing plasma volume.

**PHARMACOKINETICS: Absorption:** Candesartan: Rapid and complete; absolute bioavailability (15%); $T_{max}$=3-4 hrs. **Distribution:** Candesartan: Plasma protein binding (>99%); $V_d$=0.13L/kg. HCTZ: Crosses placenta; excreted in breast milk. **Metabolism:** Candesartan: GIT via ester hydrolysis, liver via O-deethylation (minor); candesartan (metabolite). **Elimination:** Candesartan: Biliary, feces (unchanged), urine (26%, unchanged); $T_{1/2}$=9 hrs. HCTZ: Urine (61%); $T_{1/2}$=5.6-14.8 hrs.

## NURSING CONSIDERATIONS

**Assessment:** Assess for pregnancy/nursing status, possible drug interactions, volume/salt depletion, SLE, DM, anuria, hypersensitivity to sulfonamide, history of allergies or bronchial asthma, hepatic/renal impairment.

**Monitoring:** Monitor serum electrolytes periodically. Monitor for signs/symptoms of electrolyte imbalance, exacerbation or activation of SLE, hypotension, hyperglycemia, hyperuricemia or precipitation of gout, hypersensitivity reactions, renal/hepatic dysfunction.

**Patient Counseling:** Instruct not to use $K^+$ supplements or salt substitutes. Inform of pregnancy risks. Advise that inadequate fluid intake, excessive perspiration, diarrhea, or vomiting may result in drop of BP leading to lightheadedness or syncope. Advise to seek medical attention if syncope, symptoms of electrolyte imbalance (dry mouth, thirst, weakness, lethargy), or hypersensitivity reactions occur. Take without regard to food.

**Administration:** Oral route. **Storage:** 25°C (77°F); excursions permitted to 15-30°C (59-86°F).

# ATIVAN

lorazepam (Biovail) **CIV**

**THERAPEUTIC CLASS:** Benzodiazepine

**INDICATIONS:** Management of anxiety disorders or for short-term relief of the symptoms of anxiety or anxiety associated with depressive symptoms.

**DOSAGE:** *Adults:* Initial: 2-3mg/day given bid-tid. Usual: 2-6mg/day in divided doses. Insomnia: 2-4mg qhs. Elderly/Debilitated: 1-2mg/day in divided doses. *Pediatrics:* >12 yrs: Initial: 2-3mg/day given bid-tid. Usual: 2-6mg/day in divided doses. Insomnia: 2-4mg qhs.

**HOW SUPPLIED:** Tab: 0.5mg, 1mg*, 2mg* *scored

**CONTRAINDICATIONS:** Acute narrow-angle glaucoma.

**WARNINGS/PRECAUTIONS:** Avoid with primary depression or psychosis. Withdrawal symptoms with abrupt d/c. Careful supervision if addiction-prone. Caution in patients with compromised respiratory function. Caution with elderly, and renal or hepatic dysfunction. Monitor for GI disease with prolonged therapy. Periodic blood counts and LFTs with long-term therapy.

**ADVERSE REACTIONS:** Sedation, dizziness, weakness, unsteadiness, transient amnesia, memory impairment, visual disturbance, depression, respiratory depression, constipation, vertigo, change in appetite, headache.

**INTERACTIONS:** CNS-depressant effects with barbiturates, alcohol. Diminished tolerance to alcohol and other CNS depressants. Increased plasma levels with valproate and probenecid, decrease dose by 50%.

**PREGNANCY:** Not for use in pregnancy or nursing.

**MECHANISM OF ACTION:** Benzodiazepine; antianxiety agent, interacts with GABA-benzodiazepine receptor complex.

**PHARMACOKINETICS: Absorption:** Absolute bioavailability (90%); $C_{max}$=20ng/mL (2mg PO); $T_{max}$=2 hrs. **Distribution:** Plasma protein binding (85%). **Metabolism:** Glucuronidation. **Elimination:** Urine; $T_{1/2}$=12 hrs.

## NURSING CONSIDERATIONS

**Assessment:** Assess for acute narrow-angle glaucoma, pre-existing depression and/or psychosis, compromised respiratory function (eg, COPD, sleep apnea syndrome), impaired renal/hepatic function, and possible drug interactions. Assess addiction-prone individuals (eg, drug addicts, alcoholics).

**Monitoring:** Monitor worsening of depression and/or suicidal thinking, physical/psychological dependence, paradoxical reactions, CNS depression, lab tests (CBC, LFTs, LDH).

**Patient Counseling:** Inform that psychological/physical dependence may result; consult physician before increasing dose or abruptly d/c drug. Caution with hazardous tasks (eg, operating machinery/driving); do not drink alcohol or take other CNS depressants concomitantly.

**Administration:** Oral route. **Storage:** 20-25°C (68-77°F). Keep tightly closed.

# Ativan Injection CIV

lorazepam (Baxter)

**THERAPEUTIC CLASS:** Benzodiazepine

**INDICATIONS:** Treatment of status epilepticus and preanesthetic medication in adults.

**DOSAGE:** *Adults:* ≥18 yrs: Status Epilepticus: 4mg IV (given slowly at 2mg/min); may repeat 1 dose after 10-15 min if seizures recur or fail to cease. Preanesthetic Sedation: Usual: (IM) 0.05mg/kg given at least 2 hrs prior to operation; (IV) 2mg or 0.044mg/kg IV (whichever is smaller) 15-20 min prior to procedure. Max: 4mg IM/IV. Elderly: Start at the low end of the dosing range.

**HOW SUPPLIED:** Inj: 2mg/mL, 4mg/mL [1mL, 10mL]

**CONTRAINDICATIONS:** Acute narrow-angle glaucoma, sleep apnea syndrome, severe respiratory insufficiency. Not for intra-arterial injection.

**WARNINGS/PRECAUTIONS:** May produce heavy sedation; airway obstruction and respiratory depression may occur; ensure airway patency and monitor respiration. May impair mental/physical abilities. Avoid intra-arterial administration. Avoid in patients with hepatic and/or renal failure; caution in patients with hepatic and/or renal impairment. May cause fetal damage during pregnancy. When used for peroral endoscopic procedures; adequate topical/regional anesthesia is recommended to minimize reflex activity. Extreme caution when administering injections to elderly, very ill, or to patients with limited pulmonary reserve as hypoventilation and/or hypoxic cardiac arrest may occur. Paradoxical reaction, propylene glycol toxicity (eg, lactic acidosis, hyperosmolality, hypotension) and polyethylene glycol toxicity (eg, acute tubular necrosis) reported; premature and low birth weight infants as well pediatric patients receiving high-doses may be at higher risk. Pediatric patients may exhibit sensitivity to benzyl alcohol; "gasping syndrome" associated with administration of IV solutions containing benzyl alcohol in neonates. Repeated doses over a prolonged period of time may result in physical and psychological dependence and withdrawal symptoms following abrupt d/c.

**ADVERSE REACTIONS:** Respiratory depression/failure, hypotension, somnolence, headache, hypoventilation, injection-site reactions (eg, pain, burning, redness), paradoxical excitement.

**INTERACTIONS:** Additive CNS depression with other CNS depressants (eg, ethyl alcohol, phenothiazines, barbiturates, MAOIs, antidepressants). Increased sedation, hallucinations and irrational behavior with scopolamine. Reduce dose by 50% when given in combination with valproate or probenecid due to decreased clearance. Increased clearance with oral contraceptives. Severe adverse effects with clozapine, loxapine, and haloperidol reported. Prolonged and profound effect with concomitant sedatives, tranquilizers, narcotic analgesics.

**PREGNANCY:** Category D, not for use in nursing.

**MECHANISM OF ACTION:** Benzodiazepine; antianxiety, sedative and anticonvulsant effects. Interacts with GABA-benzodiazepine receptor complex in human brain. Exhibits relatively high and specific affinity for its recognition site but does not displace GABA. Attachment to the specific binding site enhances the affinity of GABA for its receptor site on the same receptor complex.

**PHARMACOKINETICS: Absorption:** Complete, rapid; (IM) $C_{max}$=48ng/mL, $T_{max}$=within 3 hrs. **Distribution:** $V_d$=1.3L/kg, plasma protein binding (91%), crosses blood brain barrier. **Metabolism:** Liver. **Elimination:** Urine (88%), feces (7%), (0.3% unchanged); $T_{1/2}$=14 hrs.

## NURSING CONSIDERATIONS

**Assessment:** Comprehensive review of benefits/risks in status epilepticus. Assess for hypersensitivity to benzodiazepine or its vehicle, acute-angle glaucoma, pre-existing respiratory impairment, hepatic/renal impairment, pregnancy/nursing status, and possible drug interactions.

**Monitoring:** "Gasping syndrome" in very low body weight neonates, which manifests by CNS depression, metabolic acidosis, gasping respiration. Monitor for respiratory depression, airway obstruction, heavy sedation, drowsiness, excessive sleepiness, hypoglycemia and hyponatremia in status epilepticus, seizures, myoclonus, somnolence, injection-site reactions (eg, pain, burning sensation, and redness), and paradoxical reactions (eg, mania, agitation, psychosis). Signs of toxicity to the vehicle's components (eg, lactic acidosis, hyperosmolarity, hypotension, and acute tubular necrosis). Monitor for hypersensitivity reactions.

**Patient Counseling:** Inform of risks/benefits. Caution with hazardous tasks (eg, operating machinery/driving). Do not get out of bed unassisted. Avoid alcoholic beverages for at least 24-48 hrs after receiving drug. Advise about potential for physical/psychological dependence and withdrawal symptoms.

**Administration:** IM/IV route. **Storage:** Refrigerate; protect from light.

# ATRIPLA — RX

tenofovir disoproxil fumarate - emtricitabine - efavirenz (Bristol-Myers Squibb/Gilead Sciences)

**Lactic acidosis and severe hepatomegaly with steatosis, including fatal cases, have been reported with the use of nucleoside analogs, including tenofovir disproxil fumarate, in combination with other antiretrovirals. Not approved for the treatment of chronic hepatitis B virus (HBV) infection. Severe acute exacerbations of hepatitis B have been reported in patients who have discontinued Emtriva or Viread. Hepatic function should be monitored closely for at least several months in patients coinfected with HIV-1 and HBV and discontinue therapy. Initiation of anti-hepatitis B therapy may be warranted.**

**THERAPEUTIC CLASS:** Non-nucleoside reverse transcriptase inhibitor/nucleoside analog combination

**INDICATIONS:** For use alone as a complete regimen or in combination with other antiretroviral agents for the treatment of HIV-1 infection in adults.

**DOSAGE:** *Adults:* ≥18 yrs: 1 tab qd on empty stomach. Bedtime dosing may improve tolerability of nervous system symptoms.

**HOW SUPPLIED:** Tab: (Efavirenz-Emtricitabine-Tenofovir DF) 600mg-200mg-300mg

**CONTRAINDICATIONS:** Concomitant use with voriconazole, dihydroergotamine, ergonovine, ergotamine, methylergonovine, midazolam, triazolam, bepridil, cisapride, pimozide, St. John's wort.

**WARNINGS/PRECAUTIONS:** Caution in patients with risk factors for liver disease; monitor LFTs before and during treatment in patients with underlying hepatic disease; suspend treatment if clinical or laboratory findings suggestive of lactic acidosis or pronounced hepatotoxicity. Test for presence of chronic HBV prior to initiation; post-treatment exacerbations reported. Serious psychiatric (eg, depression, suicidal ideation) reported. CNS symptoms (eg, dizziness, insomnia) reported; may impair mental/physical abilities. May cause renal impairment; avoid with moderate or severe renal impairment (CrCl <50mL/min); assess CrCl prior to therapy; monitor CrCl and phosphorous with risk or history of renal dysfunction. Avoid pregnancy during therapy; use of adequate contraceptive measures for 12 weeks after d/c is recommended and perform pregnancy testing prior to therapy. Skin rash reported; d/c if severe rash associated with blistering, desquamation, mucosal involvement, or fever develop. Monitor BMD in patients with history of pathological fractures or if at risk for osteopenia. Caution in patients with history of seizures; convulsions reported. May cause redistribution/accumulation of body fat. Immune reconstitution syndrome reported.

**ADVERSE REACTIONS:** Diarrhea, nausea, fatigue, depression, sinusitis, upper respiratory tract infections, dizziness, rash, headache, anxiety, insomnia, nasopharyngitis, abnormal dreams, laboratory abnormalities, lactic acidosis, severe hepatomegaly with steatosis.

**INTERACTIONS:** See Contraindications. Avoid with concurrent or recent use of a nephrotoxic agent. Avoid concomitant use with drugs with the same active components. Should not be coadministered with drugs containing lamivudine. May cause additive CNS effects when used with alcohol or psychoactive drugs. Coadministration with atazanavir is not recommended. Additional 100mg/day of ritonavir needed when concomitantly used with fosamprenavir/ritonavir once daily. Monitor LFTs when coadministered with ritonavir. Coadministration with didanosine may increase didanosine concentrations; monitor for didanosine-associated adverse effects and reduce didanosine dose to 250mg in adults weighing >60kg. May decrease plasma concentrations of rifabutin; increase rifabutin daily dose by 50%. May decrease the levels of the active metabolites of norgestimate and etonogestrel; use reliable method of barrier contraception. Lactic acidosis and severe hepatomegaly reported with tenofovir disoproxil fumarate in combination with other antiretrovirals. Efavirenz: May decrease plasma concentrations of CYP3A substrates. May alter plasma concentrations of drugs metabolized by 2C9, 2C19, and 3A4. Drugs that induce CYP3A activity (eg, phenobarbital, rifampin, rifabutin) may increase clearance resulting in lowered plasma concentrations. May decrease levels of indinavir, lopinavir, and saquinavir. May decrease the plasma levels of the anticonvulsants phenytoin, carbamazepine, and phenobarbital; monitor plasma levels. May decrease the levels of sertraline, ketoconazole, itraconazole, clarithromycin, calcium channel blockers that are CYP3A substrates (eg, diltiazem, felodipine, nicardipine, nifedipine, verapamil), and the HMG-CoA reductase inhibitors atorvastatin, pravastatin, and simvastatin. May decrease methadone concentrations; monitor for signs of withdrawal. Concomitant use with rifampin may decrease efavirenz concentrations. May increase or decrease warfarin concentrations. Emtricitabine (FTC) and Tenofovir DF (TDF): Coadministration with drugs that reduce renal function or compete for active tubular secretion (eg, acyclovir, adefovir dipivoxil, cidofovir, ganciclovir, valacyclovir, valganciclovir) may increase concentrations of FTC, TDF, and/or the coadministered drug. Concomitant use with lopinavir/ritonavir may increase TDF concentrations and may potentiate TDF-associated adverse events. May increase the levels of cyclosporine, tacrolimus, sirolimus, and other immunosuppressants metabolized by CYP3A; dosage adjustment of the immunosuppressant may be required and close monitoring of immunosuppressant concentrations for at least 2 weeks should occur when starting or stopping Atripla. See PI for complete information.

**PREGNANCY:** Category D, not for use in nursing.

**MECHANISM OF ACTION:** Efavirenz: Non-nucleoside reverse transcriptase inhibitor; noncompetitive inhibition of HIV-1 reverse transcriptase (RT). Emtricitabine: Nucleoside analog of cytidine; inhibits activity of HIV-1 RT by competing with natural substrate deoxycytidine 5'-triphosphate and incorporating into nascent viral DNA, resulting in chain termination. Tenofovir DF: Acyclic nucleoside phosphonate diester analog of adenosine monophosphate; inhibits activity of HIV-1 RT by competing with the natural substrate deoxyadenosine 5'-triphosphate and, after incorporation into the DNA, by DNA chain termination.

**PHARMACOKINETICS: Absorption:** Efavirenz: $C_{max}$=12.9µM, $T_{max}$=3-5 hrs, AUC=184µM•hr. Emtricitabine: Rapid; absolute bioavailability (93%), $C_{max}$=1.8mcg/mL, $T_{max}$=1-2 hrs, AUC=10µg•hr/mL. Tenofovir DF: $C_{max}$=296mcg/mL, $T_{max}$=1hr, AUC=2287ng•hr/mL. **Distribution:** Efavirenz: Plasma protein binding (99.5-99.75%). Emtricitabine: Plasma protein binding (<4%). Tenofovir DF: Plasma protein binding (<0.7%). **Metabolism:** Efavirenz: Hepatic via CYP3A and CYP2B6. **Elimination:** Efavirenz: Urine (14-34%), feces (16-61%); $T_{1/2}$=52-76 hrs (single dose), 40-55 hrs (multiple doses). Emtricitabine: Urine (86%); $T_{1/2}$=10 hrs. Tenofovir DF: Urine (70-80%); $T_{1/2}$=17 hrs.

## NURSING CONSIDERATIONS

**Assessment:** Assess for liver dysfunction or risk factors for liver disease, renal impairment, HBV or HCV infection, psychiatric history, history of injection drug use, pregnancy/nursing status, history of seizures, and for possible drug interactions. Obtain baseline LFTs, CrCl, and serum phosphorus levels. Obtain pregnancy test in women of child bearing potential. Assess bone mineral density (BMD) in patients with a history of pathological bone fracture or those at risk for osteopenia.

**Monitoring:** Monitor for signs/symptoms of lactic acidosis, severe hepatomegaly with steatosis, acute exacerbation of hepatitis B, psychiatric symptoms (eg, severe depression, suicidal ideations, aggressive behavior) nervous system symptoms (eg, dizziness, insomnia, impaired concentration), new onset or worsening renal impairment, skin rash, decreases in BMD, convulsions, immune reconstitution syndrome, and for fat redistribution. Monitor $CD4^+$ cell count, HIV-1 RNA levels, LFTs, CrCl, serum phosphorus, and LFTs. Monitor BMD in patients with a history of pathologic bone fracture or those at risk for osteopenia.

**Patient Counseling:** Inform that therapy is not a cure for HIV-1 infection and may continue to experience illnesses associated with HIV-1 and may still transmit the infection to others through sexual contact or blood contamination. Instruct to take on an empty stomach, to take on a regular dosing schedule, and to avoid missing doses. Instruct to contact physician if develop symptoms of lactic acidosis or severe hepatomegaly with steatosis (eg, nausea, vomiting, unusual stomach discomfort, weakness), new onset or worsening renal impairment, psychiatric symptoms (eg, aggressive behavior, depression, suicide attempts, delusions, paranoia), CNS symptoms (eg, dizziness, insomnia, somnolence, abnormal dreams), or if a skin rash develops. Advise that fat redistribution or accumulation may occur. Counsel to avoid pregnancy while on therapy; instruct that a barrier contraception must always be used in combination with other methods of contraception. Advise to avoid potentially hazardous tasks (eg, driving, operating machinery) if experience CNS symptoms such as dizziness, impaired concentration, and/or drowsiness. Advise that severe acute exacerbation of hepatitis B may occur if co-infected with HBV and HIV-1.

**Administration:** Oral route. Take on an empty stomach. **Storage:** 25°C (77°F); excursions permitted to 15-30°C (59-86°F). Keep in original container, tightly closed.

## ATROVENT HFA RX

ipratropium bromide (Boehringer Ingelheim)

**THERAPEUTIC CLASS:** Anticholinergic bronchodilator

**INDICATIONS:** Maintenance treatment of bronchospasm associated with COPD, including chronic bronchitis and emphysema.

**DOSAGE:** *Adults:* Initial: 2 inh qid. Max: 12 inh/24hrs.

**HOW SUPPLIED:** MDI: 0.017mg/inh [12.9g]

**CONTRAINDICATIONS:** Hypersensitivity to atropine or its derivatives.

**WARNINGS/PRECAUTIONS:** Not for acute episodes. Immediate hypersensitivity reaction reported. Caution with narrow-angle glaucoma, prostatic hypertrophy or bladder-neck obstruction.

**ADVERSE REACTIONS:** Back pain, bronchitis, dyspnea, dizziness, headache, nausea, blurred vision, dry mouth, exacerbation of symptoms.

**INTERACTIONS:** Caution with anticholinergic-containing drugs.

**PREGNANCY:** Category B, caution in nursing.

**MECHANISM OF ACTION:** Anticholinergic; inhibits vagally-mediated refluxes by antagonizing the action of acetylcholine; prevents increase in intracellular concentration of cGMP caused by interaction of acetylcholine with muscarinic receptors on bronchial smooth muscle (animal studies).

**PHARMACOKINETICS: Absorption:** $C_{max}$=59pg/mL. **Distribution:** Plasma protein binding (0-9%). **Metabolism:** Partial. **Elimination:** $T_{1/2}$=2 hrs.

### NURSING CONSIDERATIONS

**Assessment:** Assess for hypersensitivity to atropine or derivative, narrow-angle glaucoma, prostatic hyperplasia, bladder-neck obstruction, and possible drug interactions.

**Monitoring:** Monitor for urinary retention, mydriasis, GI distress (diarrhea, NV), paradoxical bronchospasm and allergic type-reaction (pruritus, angioedema of tongue, lips and face, urticaria, laryngospasm, anaphylaxis).

**Patient Counseling:** Advise not to increase dose or frequency. Not for acute periods of bronchospasm. Avoid spraying in the eyes. Seek medical attention if symptoms of precipitation or worsening of narrow-angle glaucoma, mydriasis, increased IOP, acute eye pain/discomfort, blurring of vision, visual halos or colored images with red eyes from conjunctival and corneal congestion, or allergic/hypersensitivity reactions occur.

**Administration:** Oral inhalation. Prime pump: Before first use, prime with 2 sprays. If not used for >3 days, reprime with 2 sprays. **Storage:** 25°C (77°F); excursions permitted to 15-30°C (59-86°F). Do not puncture, use or store near heat or open flame.

## ATROVENT NASAL RX

ipratropium bromide (Boehringer Ingelheim)

**OTHER BRAND NAMES:** Ipratropium Bromide (Various)

**THERAPEUTIC CLASS:** Anticholinergic

**INDICATIONS:** (0.03%) Symptomatic relief of rhinorrhea associated with allergic and nonallergic perennial rhinitis in adults and children ≥6 yrs. (0.06%) Symptomatic relief of rhinorrhea associated with the common cold or seasonal allergic rhinitis in adults and children ≥5 yrs.

**DOSAGE:** *Adults:* Rhinorrhea with Allergic/Nonallergic Perennial Rhinitis: (0.03%) 2 sprays per nostril bid-tid. Rhinorrhea w/Common Cold: (0.06%) 2 sprays per nostril tid-qid. Rhinorrhea w/Seasonal Allergic Rhinitis: (0.06%) 2 sprays per nostril qid.
*Pediatrics:* ≥6 yrs: Rhinorrhea with Allergic/Nonallergic Perennial Rhinitis: (0.03%) 2 sprays per nostril bid-tid. Rhinorrhea w/Common Cold: ≥12 yrs: (0.06%) 2 sprays per nostril tid-qid. 5-11 yrs: (0.06%) 2 sprays per nostril tid.

≥5 yrs: Rhinorrhea w/Seasonal Allergic Rhinitis: (0.06%) 2 sprays per nostril qid.

**HOW SUPPLIED:** Spray: (0.03%) 21mcg/spray [31.1g], (0.06%) 42mcg/spray [16.6g]

**CONTRAINDICATIONS:** Hypersensitivity to atropine or its derivatives.

**WARNINGS/PRECAUTIONS:** Immediate hypersensitivity reactions reported. Caution with narrow-angle glaucoma, prostatic hypertrophy, or bladder-neck obstruction. Caution in patients with hepatic or renal insufficiency.

**ADVERSE REACTIONS:** Headache, epistaxis, pharyngitis, nasal dryness, upper respiratory tract infection, dry mouth/throat.

**INTERACTIONS:** May produce additive effects with other anticholinergic agents.

**PREGNANCY:** Category B, caution in nursing.

**MECHANISM OF ACTION:** Anticholinergic; inhibits vagally-mediated reflexes by antagonizing action of acetylcholine at the cholinergic receptor. Inhibits secretions from serous and seromucous glands lining the nasal mucosa.

**PHARMACOKINETICS: Absorption:** Poorly absorbed into systemic circulation. **Distribution:** Plasma protein binding (0-9%). **Metabolism:** Partial; ester hydrolysis. **Elimination:** 6-18 yrs old: Urine (8.6-11.1%, unchanged). **Adults:** Urine (3.7-5.6%, unchanged). (IV) $T_{1/2}$=1.6 hrs.

## NURSING CONSIDERATIONS

**Assessment:** Assess for hypersensitivity to atropine or its derivatives, narrow-angle glaucoma, prostatic hypertrophy, bladder-neck obstruction, hepatic/renal insufficiency, pregnancy/nursing status, and for possible drug interactions.

**Monitoring:** Monitor for signs and symptoms of hypersensitivity reactions, nasal bleeding, and for nasal dryness. If contact with the eyes occur, monitor for blurring of vision, precipitation or worsening of narrow-angle glaucoma, mydriasis, increased IOP, acute eye pain or discomfort, and for visual halos or colored images in association with red eyes from conjunctival and corneal congestion.

**Patient Counseling:** Advise not to alter size of nasal spray opening. Instruct to avoid spraying medication into the eyes. Inform that temporary blurring of vision, precipitation or worsening of narrow angle glaucoma, mydriasis, increased IOP, acute eye pain or discomfort, visual halos or colored images in association with red eyes from conjunctival and corneal congestion may occur if medication comes into direct contact with the eyes. Instruct to contact physician if eye pain, blurred vision, excessive nasal dryness, or episodes of nasal bleeding occur.

**Administration:** Intranasal. Prime the nasal spray pump and blow nose to clear nostrils before first use. Refer to PI for proper administration. **Storage:** 25°C (77°F); excursions permitted to 15-30°C (59-86°F) . Avoid freezing.

# AUGMENTIN RX

clavulanate potassium - amoxicillin (GlaxoSmithKline)

**THERAPEUTIC CLASS:** Aminopenicillin/beta lactamase inhibitor

**INDICATIONS:** Treatment of lower respiratory tract (LRTI), skin and skin structure (SSSI), and urinary tract infections (UTI), otitis media (OM), sinusitis caused by susceptible strains of microorganisms.

**DOSAGE:** *Adults:* (Dose based on amoxicillin) 500mg q12h or 250mg q8h. Severe Infections/RTI: 875mg q12h or 500mg q8h. May use 125mg/5mL or 250mg/5mL sus in place of 500mg tab and 200mg/5mL sus or 400mg/5mL sus in place of 875mg tab. CrCl <30mL/min: Do not give 875mg tab. CrCl 10-30mL/min: 250-500mg q12h. CrCl <10mL/min: 250-500mg q24h. Hemodialysis: 250-500mg q24h, give additional dose during and at end of dialysis.

*Pediatrics:* (Dose based on amoxicillin) ≥40kg: Use adult dose. ≥12 weeks: Sinusitis/Otitis Media/LRTI/Severe Infections: (Sus/Tab, Chewable)

45mg/kg/day given q12h or 40mg/kg/day given q8h. Treat otitis media for 10 days. Less Severe Infections: 25mg/kg/day given q12h or 20mg/kg/day given q8h. <12 weeks: 15mg/kg q12h (use 125mg/5mL sus).

**HOW SUPPLIED:** (Amoxicillin-Clavulanate) Sus: 125-31.25mg/5mL [75mL, 100mL, 150mL], 200-28.5mg/5mL [50mL, 75mL, 100mL], 250-62.5mg/5mL [75mL, 100mL, 150mL], 400-57mg/5mL [50mL, 75mL, 100mL]; Tab: 250-125mg, 500-125mg, 875-125mg*; Tab, Chewable: 125-31.25mg, 200-28.5mg, 250-62.5mg, 400-57mg *scored

**CONTRAINDICATIONS:** History of PCN allergy or amoxicillin clavulanate-associated cholestatic jaundice/hepatic dysfunction.

**WARNINGS/PRECAUTIONS:** Serious, sometimes fatal, hypersensitivity reactions reported with PCN therapy. *Clostridium difficile*-associated diarrhea (CDAD) reported. Possibility of superinfection. Caution with hepatic dysfunction. Monitor renal, hepatic, and hematopoietic functions with prolonged use. Avoid with mononucleosis. Take with food to reduce GI upset. The 200mg and 400mg chewable tabs and 200mg/5mL and 400mg/5mL sus contain phenylalanine. The 250mg tab and chewable tab are not interchangeable due to unequal clavulanic acid amounts. Only use 250mg tab in pediatrics ≥40kg. False (+) for urine glucose with Clinitest and Benedict's or Fehling's solution.

**ADVERSE REACTIONS:** Diarrhea/loose stools, nausea, skin rashes, urticaria, pruritus, angioedema, hepatitis, cholestatic jaundice, serum sickness-like reactions, erythema multiforme, acute generalized exanthematous pustulosis, hypersensitivity vasculitis, exfoliative dermatitis, and hepatitis.

**INTERACTIONS:** Increased and prolonged plasma levels with probenecid. May reduce effects of oral contraceptives. Allopurinol may increase incidence of rash. May increase PT with anticoagulant therapy.

**PREGNANCY:** Category B, caution in nursing.

**MECHANISM OF ACTION:** Amoxicillin: Semisynthetic antibiotic with broad-spectrum of bactericidal activity against gram-positive and gram-negative organisms. Clavulanate: β-lactamase inhibitor; possesses ability to inactivate a wide range of β-lactamase enzymes commonly found in microorganisms resistant to PCN and cephalosporins.

**PHARMACOKINETICS: Absorption:** Well absorbed from GI tract. $C_{max}$ and AUC varied according to dose and regimen; see Full PI for more information. (Tab, Sol) $T_{max}$=1.5 hrs, 1 hr. **Distribution:** Found in breast milk. Amoxicillin: Diffuses readily in body tissues and fluids. Clavulanic acid: Well distributed in body tissues. Plasma protein binding: Amoxicillin (18%), clavulanic acid (25%). **Elimination:** Urine, (amoxicillin) (50-70% unchanged), (clavulanic acid) (25-40% unchanged); $T_{1/2}$=1.3 hrs (amoxicillin), 1 hr (clavulanic acid).

## NURSING CONSIDERATIONS

**Assessment:** Assess for history of allergic reactions to penicillins or cephalosporins or other allergens, hepatic or renal or hematopoietic function, pregnancy/nursing status, and possible drug interactions.

**Monitoring:** Periodically monitor renal, hepatic, and hematopoietic functions. Monitor for anaphylactic reactions, hepatic toxicity, cholestatic jaundice, superinfection with mycotic or bacterial pathogen, drug resistance, and pseudomembranous colitis/CDAD.

**Patient Counseling:** Inform drug only treats bacterial, not viral, infections. Instruct to take as directed; skipping doses or not completing full course may decrease effectiveness and increase resistance. Inform about potential benefits/risks of therapy. Advise to d/c therapy and consult physician if allergic reactions or watery/bloody diarrhea (with/without stomach cramps) occur (may occur up to 2 months after therapy). Advise to notify physician if pregnant/nursing.

**Administration:** Oral route. Take at start of meals or snacks. **Storage:** Tabs/Dry Powder at or below 25°C (77°F); store in original containers. Refrigerate reconstituted sus; shake well before using; discard after 10 days.

# AUGMENTIN ES-600 RX

clavulanate potassium - amoxicillin (GlaxoSmithKline)

**THERAPEUTIC CLASS:** Aminopenicillin/beta lactamase inhibitor

**INDICATIONS:** Treatment of pediatric patients with recurrent or persistent acute otitis media due to susceptible strains of microorganisms.

**DOSAGE:** *Pediatrics:* ≥3 months: <40kg: (Dose based on amoxicillin content) 45mg/kg q12h for 10 days.

**HOW SUPPLIED:** Sus: (Amoxicillin-Clavulanate) 600mg-42.9mg/5mL [75mL, 125mL, 200mL]

**CONTRAINDICATIONS:** History of PCN allergy or amoxicillin-clavulanate associated cholestatic jaundice/hepatic dysfunction.

**WARNINGS/PRECAUTIONS:** Serious, sometimes fatal, hypersensitivity reactions reported with PCN therapy. *Clostridium difficile*-associated diarrhea (CDAD) reported. Possibility of superinfection with mycotic or bacterial pathogens. Caution with hepatic dysfunction. Avoid with mononucleosis.

**ADVERSE REACTIONS:** Diaper rash, coughing, vomiting, fever, upper respiratory infection, skin rashes, pruritus, urticaria, angioedema, serum sickness-lke reactions, erythema multiforme, hypersensitivity vasculitis, exfoliative dermatitis. Hepatitis and cholestatic jaundice reported.

**INTERACTIONS:** Increased and prolonged plasma levels with probenecid. Avoid with probenecid. May reduce effects of oral contraceptives. May increase PT with anticoagulant agents.

**PREGNANCY:** Category B, caution in nursing.

**MECHANISM OF ACTION:** Amoxicillin: Semisynthetic antibiotic with broad spectrum of bactericidal activity against gram-positive and gram-negative organisms. Clavulanate: β-lactamase inhibitor. Possesses ability to inactivate a wide range of β-lactamase enzymes commonly found in microorganisms resistant to PCN and cephalosporins.

**PHARMACOKINETICS: Absorption:** Amoxicillin: $C_{max}$=15.7mcg/mL; $T_{max}$=2.0 hr; AUC=59.8mcg•hr/mL. Clavulanic acid: $C_{max}$=1.7mcg/mL; $T_{max}$=1.1 hr; AUC=4.0mcg•hr/mL. **Distribution:** Plasma protein binding 18% (amoxicillin), 25% (clavulanic acid). Well distributed in bodily tissues except brain and spinal fluid. **Elimination:** Urine (unchanged) amoxicillin (50-70%); clavulanic acid (25-40%).

## NURSING CONSIDERATIONS

**Assessment:** Assess for history of allergic reactions to PCNs, cephalosporins or other allergens, cholestatic jaundice, hepatic dysfunction, infectious mononucleosis, phenylketonuria, pregnancy/nursing status, and possible drug interactions.

**Monitoring:** Periodically monitor renal, hepatic and hematopoietic organ functions. Monitor for anaphylactic reactions, hepatic toxicity, cholestatic jaundice, development of superinfection with mycotic or bacterial pathogen, development of drug resistance, skin rash, diarrhea, pseudomembranous colitis/CDAD, false-positive reaction of urinary glucose if Benedict's or Fehling's solution or Clinitest are used, and for transient decrease in plasma concentration of total conjugated estriol, estriol-glucuronide, conjugated estrone and estradiol if given to pregnant women.

**Patient Counseling:** Inform drug only treats bacterial, not viral, infections. Instruct to take as directed; skipping doses or not completing full course may decrease effectiveness and increase resistance. Inform about potential benefits/risks of therapy. Advise to d/c therapy and consult physician if allergic reactions or watery/bloody diarrhea (with or without stomach cramps) occur (may occur up to 2 months or more after treatment). Advise to notify physician if pregnant/nursing.

**Administration:** Oral route. Take at start of meals or snacks to prevent gastric upset. Shake well before using. **Storage:** Store dry powder at or below 25°C (77°F); original container. Refrigerate reconstituted sus; discard after 10 days.

# AUGMENTIN XR RX

clavulanate potassium - amoxicillin (GlaxoSmithKline)

**THERAPEUTIC CLASS:** Aminopenicillin/beta lactamase inhibitor

**INDICATIONS:** Treatment of community-acquired pneumonia (CAP) or acute bacterial sinusitis due to confirmed or suspected β-lactamase producing pathogens and *S.pneumoniae* with reduced susceptibility to PCN.

**DOSAGE:** *Adults:* Sinusitis: 2 tabs q12h for 10 days. CAP: 2 tabs q12h for 7-10 days. Take at start of a meal.
*Pediatrics:* ≥16 yrs: Sinusitis: 2 tabs q12h for 10 days. CAP: 2 tabs q12h for 7-10 days. Take at the start of a meal.

**HOW SUPPLIED:** Tab, Extended-Release: (Amoxicillin-Clavulanate) 1000mg-62.5mg

**CONTRAINDICATIONS:** History of PCN allergy or amoxicillin clavulanate-associated cholestatic jaundice/hepatic dysfunction, severe renal impairment (CrCl <30mL/min), hemodialysis.

**WARNINGS/PRECAUTIONS:** Serious, sometimes fatal, hypersensitivity reactions reported with PCN therapy. *Clostridium difficile*-associated diarrhea (CDAD) reported. Possibility of superinfection. Caution with hepatic dysfunction. Monitor renal, hepatic, and hematopoietic functions with prolonged use. Avoid with mononucleosis. False (+) for urine glucose with Clinitest and Benedict's or Fehling's solution.

**ADVERSE REACTIONS:** Diarrhea, nausea, genital moniliasis, abdominal pain, vaginal mycosis, skin rashes, pruritus, urticaria, angioedema, hepatitis, cholestatic jaundice, serum sickness-like reactions, erythema multiforme, acute generalized exanthematous pustulosis, hypersensitivity vasculitis, exfoliative dermatitis.

**INTERACTIONS:** Increased and prolonged plasma levels with probenecid. May reduce effects of oral contraceptives. Allopurinol may increase incidence of rash. May increase PT with anticoagulant therapy.

**PREGNANCY:** Category B, caution in nursing.

**MECHANISM OF ACTION:** Amoxicillin: Semisynthetic antibiotic with broad spectrum of bactericidal activity against gram-positive and gram-negative organisms. Clavulanate: β-lactamase inhibitor; possesses ability to inactivate a wide range of β-lactamase enzymes commonly found in microorganisms resistant to PCN and cephalosporins.

**PHARMACOKINETICS: Absorption:** Well-absorbed. Amoxicillin: $C_{max}$=17 mcg/mL, $T_{max}$=1.5 hrs, AUC=71.6mcg•hr/mL. Clavulanate potassium: $C_{max}$=2.05mcg/mL, $T_{max}$=1.03 hrs, AUC=5.29mcg•hr/mL. **Distribution:** Plasma protein binding: Amoxicillin (18%); Clavulanate potassium (25%). Found in breast milk. Well distributed to body tissues except brain and spinal fluid. **Elimination:** Urine: Amoxicillin (60-80% unchanged); $T_{1/2}$=1.27 hrs. Clavulanate potassium: (30-50% unchanged); $T_{1/2}$=1.03 hrs.

## NURSING CONSIDERATIONS

**Assessment:** Assess for history of allergic reactions to PCNs, cephalosporins or other allergens, cholestatic jaundice, hepatic/renal impairment or hemodialysis patients, infectious mononucleosis, pregnancy/nursing status, and possible drug interactions.

**Monitoring:** Periodically monitor renal, hepatic and hematopoietic organ functions. Monitor for anaphylactic reactions, hepatic toxicity, cholestatic jaundice, development of superinfection with mycotic or bacterial pathogen, development of drug resistance, skin rash, diarrhea, pseudomembranous colitis/CDAD, false-positive reaction of urinary glucose if Benedict's, Fehling's solution or Clinitest are used. Monitor for transient decrease in plasma concentration of total conjugated estriol, estriol-glucuronide, conjugated estrone and estradiol if given to pregnant women.

**Patient Counseling:** Inform drug only treats bacterial, not viral, infections. Instruct to take as directed; skipping doses or not completing full course may decrease effectiveness and increase resistance. Inform about potential benefits/risks of therapy. Advise to d/c and consult physician if allergic reactions or watery/bloody diarrhea (with/without stomach cramps) occur (may occur up to 2 months or more after treatment). Advise to notify physician if pregnant/nursing.

**Administration:** Oral route. Take at start of meals or snacks to reduce possible GI upset. **Storage:** At or below 25°C (77°F); store in original container; discard unused medicine.

## AVALIDE — RX

irbesartan - hydrochlorothiazide (Bristol-Myers Squibb/Sanofi-Aventis)

**Can cause death/injury to developing fetus during 2nd and 3rd trimesters. Stop therapy if pregnancy detected.**

**THERAPEUTIC CLASS:** Angiotensin II receptor antagonist/thiazide diuretic

**INDICATIONS:** Treatment of hypertension. May be used in patients not adequately controlled with monotherapy. May be used as initial therapy in patients likely to need multiple drugs to achieve BP goals.

**DOSAGE:** *Adults:* Not controlled on Monotherapy: 150mg/12.5mg qd. Titrate: May increase to 300mg/12.5mg qd, then 300mg/25mg qd if needed. Initial Therapy: Initiate with 150mg/12.5mg qd for 1 to 2 weeks. Titrate: As needed to maximum 300mg/25mg qd. Replacement Therapy: May substitute for titrated components. Avoid with CrCl <30mL/min.

**HOW SUPPLIED:** Tab: (Irbesartan-HCTZ) 150mg-12.5mg, 300mg-12.5mg, 300mg-25mg

**CONTRAINDICATIONS:** Anuria, sulfonamide hypersensitivity.

**WARNINGS/PRECAUTIONS:** Can cause fetal injury/death when administered to a pregnant women. Correct volume or salt depletion before therapy; risk of hypotension exists. Caution in elderly. Caution with impaired hepatic function or progressive liver disease; may precipitate hepatic coma. Avoid if CrCl<30mL/min. May cause changes in renal function; if progressive renal impairment becomes evident, consider d/c or withholding diuretic therapy. Caution in patients with renal disease, may precipitate azotemia. In patients whose renal function is dependent on the activity of the renin angiotensin aldosterone system (eg, severe CHF), may cause oliguria and/or progressive azotemia, renal failure, and possibly death. If unilateral or bilateral renal artery stenosis is present, may increase SrCr and BUN. Hypersensitivity reactions may occur; caution with history of allergy or bronchial asthma. May exacerbate or activate systemic lupus erythematosus (SLE). Monitor serum electrolytes. Hyponatremia (including dilutional hyponatremia in edematous patients in hot weather), hypochloremic alkalosis, hyperuricemia (or frank gout), hyperglycemia, hypomagnesemia, and hypercalcemia may occur. Hypokalemia may occur and may cause cardiac arrhythmias and may sensitize or exaggerate the response of the heart to the toxic effects of digitalis (eg, increased ventricular irritability). Enhanced effects may occur in the post-sympathectomy patient. May increase cholesterol and triglyceride levels.

**ADVERSE REACTIONS:** Dizziness, fatigue, musculoskeletal pain, influenza, edema, N/V.

**INTERACTIONS:** Potentiation of orthostatic hypotension may occur with alcohol, barbiturates, and narcotics. Dosage adjustment of insulin or oral hypoglycemic agents may be required. Impaired absorption with cholestyramine, colestipol resins. Corticosteroids and ACTH deplete electrolytes, particularly potassium. May decrease response to pressor amines (eg, norepinephrine). Potentiation/additive effect with other antihypertensives. May increase responsiveness to nondepolarizing skeletal muscle relaxants (eg, tubocurarine). Increased risk of lithium toxicity; avoid concomitant use. NSAIDs may reduce diuretic effects.

**PREGNANCY:** Category D, not for use in nursing.

**MECHANISM OF ACTION:** Irbesartan: Angiotensin II receptor antagonist; blocks the vasoconstrictor and aldosterone-secreting effects of angiotensin II by selectively blocking binding to the $AT_1$ angiotensin II receptor. HCTZ:

Thiazide diuretic; antihypertensive effect not fully understood; believed to affect renal tubular mechanisms of electrolyte reabsorption, directly increasing $Na^+$ and $Cl^-$ excretion in approximately equivalent amounts, and indirectly reducing plasma volume.

**PHARMACOKINETICS: Absorption:** Irbesartan: Rapid, complete; absolute bioavailability (60-80%); $T_{max}$=1.5-2 hrs. **Distribution:** Irbesartan: $V_d$=53-93L; plasma protein binding (90%); crosses placenta and blood brain barrier; excreted in breast milk. HCTZ: Crosses placenta, excreted in breast milk. **Metabolism:** Irbesartan: CYP2C9 (oxidation), glucuronide conjugation. **Elimination:** Irbesartan: Kidney, biliary. Urine (20%), feces (remainder). $T_{1/2}$=11-15 hrs. HCTZ: Kidney (61%); $T_{1/2}$=5.6-14.8 hrs.

## NURSING CONSIDERATIONS

**Assessment:** Assess for anuria, sulfonamide hypersensitivity, pregnancy/nursing status, volume/salt depletion, history of allergy or bronchial asthma, hepatic impairment or progressive liver disease, SLE, renal impairment, and for possible drug interactions.

**Monitoring:** Monitor serum electrolytes periodically. Monitor for signs/symptoms of electrolyte imbalance, exacerbation or activation of SLE, hypotension, hyperglycemia, hyperuricemia or precipitation of gout, hypersensitivity reactions, hepatic/renal dysfunction.

**Patient Counseling:** Inform of pregnancy risks; instruct to notify physician if become pregnant during therapy. Inform patients that they may feel lightheaded during first days of use; d/c use if fainting occurs and notify health care provider. Inform that becoming dehydrated while on therapy can lower BP too much and lead to lightheadedness and possibly fainting. Inform that dehydration may occur with excessive sweating, diarrhea, vomiting, and with not drinking enough liquids.

**Administration:** Oral route. **Storage:** 25°C (77°F); excursions permitted 15-30°C (59-86°F).

# AVANDAMET RX

metformin HCl - rosiglitazone maleate (GlaxoSmithKline)

**Thiazolidinediones may cause or exacerbate CHF in some patients. Avandamet is not recommended in patients with symptomatic heart failure. Meta-analysis of studies has shown rosiglitazone to be associated with an increased risk of myocardial ischemic events. Lactic acidosis may occur due to metformin accumulation.**

**THERAPEUTIC CLASS:** Thiazolidinedione/biguanide

**INDICATIONS:** Adjunct to diet and exercise, to improve glycemic control in type 2 diabetes mellitus (DM) when treatment with dual rosiglitazone and metformin therapy is appropriate.

**DOSAGE:** *Adults:* Prior Metformin Therapy of 1000mg/day: Initial: 2mg-500mg tab bid. Prior Metformin Therapy of 2000mg/day: Initial: 2mg-1000mg tab bid. Prior Rosiglitazone Therapy of 4mg/day: Initial: 2mg-500mg tab bid. Prior Rosiglitazone Therapy of 8mg/day: 4mg-500mg tab bid. Titrate: May increase by increments of 4mg rosiglitazone and/or 500mg metformin. Max: 8mg-2000mg/day. Drug-Naive Patients: Initial: 2mg-500mg qd-bid. If $HbA_{1c}$ >11% and FPG >270mg/dL: Initial: 2mg-500mg bid. Titrate: After 4 weeks, may increase by increments of 2mg-500mg per day. Max: 8mg-2000mg per day. Elderly/Debilitated/Malnourished: Conservative dosing; do not titrate to max dose. Take with meals.

**HOW SUPPLIED:** Tab: (Rosiglitazone-Metformin) 2mg-500mg, 4mg-500mg, 2mg-1000mg, 4mg-1000mg

**CONTRAINDICATIONS:** Established NYHA Class III or IV heart failure, renal disease/dysfunction (SrCr ≥1.5mg/dL [males], ≥1.4mg/dL [females], or abnormal CrCl), metabolic acidosis, including diabetic ketoacidosis. D/C temporarily (48 hrs) for radiologic studies with intravascular iodinated contrast materials.

**WARNINGS/PRECAUTIONS:** Lactic acidosis reported; increased risk with renal dysfunction, increased age, DM, CHF, and other conditions with risk of hypoperfusion and hypoxemia. Avoid use in patients ≥80 yrs unless renal function is normal. Monitor renal function and for ketoacidosis and metabolic acidosis. D/C in hypoxic states (eg, CHF, shock, acute MI), loss of blood glucose control due to stress, acidosis, and prior to surgical procedures (due to restricted food intake). May decrease serum vitamin $B_{12}$ levels. Increased risk of hypoglycemia with concomitant use with other hypoglycemic agents, elderly, debilitated/malnourished, adrenal or pituitary insufficiency, or alcohol intoxication. May cause fluid retention and exacerbation/initiation of heart failure; d/c if cardiac status deteriorates. Initiation not recommended in patients experiencing an acute coronary event. Avoid with NYHA Class III or IV cardiac status. Not for use in type 1 diabetes or for diabetic ketoacidosis treatment. Caution with edema. Dose-related weight gain reported. Ovulation in premenopausal anovulatory patients may occur; risk of pregnancy with inadequate contraception. May decrease Hgb and Hct. Avoid with active liver disease, if ALT levels >2.5x ULN, or if jaundice occurred with troglitazone. Check LFTs before therapy, every 2 months for 1 yr, and periodically thereafter, or if hepatic dysfunction symptoms occur. D/C if ALT >3x ULN on therapy. Increased incidence of bone fracture was noted in female patients.

**ADVERSE REACTIONS:** Upper respiratory tract infection, headache, back pain, hypoglycemia, fatigue, sinusitis, diarrhea, viral infection, arthralgia, anemia, dyspepsia, dizziness, abdominal pain, N/V.

**INTERACTIONS:** Furosemide, nifedipine, cimetidine, and cationic drugs (eg, digoxin, amiloride, procainamide, quinidine, quinine, ranitidine, trimethoprim, vancomycin, triamterene, morphine) may increase metformin levels. Thiazides and other diuretics, corticosteroids, phenothiazines, thyroid products, estrogens, oral contraceptives, phenytoin, nicotinic acid, sympathomimetics, CCBs, and isoniazid may cause hyperglycemia. Risk of hypoglycemia with alcohol. Excess alcohol may increase potential for lactic acidosis. May decrease furosemide levels. Inhibitors of CYP2C8 (eg, gemfibrozil) may increase rosiglitazone AUC. Inducers of CYP2C8 (eg, rifampin) may decrease rosiglitazone AUC. Coadministration with insulin or nitrates is not recommended.

**PREGNANCY:** Category C, not for use in nursing.

**MECHANISM OF ACTION:** Rosiglitazone: Thiazolidinedione; insulin sensitizing agent that acts by enhancing peripheral glucose utilization. Metformin: Biguanide; decreases hepatic glucose production, decreases intestinal absorption of glucose, and increases peripheral glucose uptake and utilization.

**PHARMACOKINETICS: Absorption:** Rosiglitazone: Absolute bioavailability (99%). (4mg) $C_{max}$=242ng/mL. $T_{max}$=1 hr. Metformin: Absolute bioavailability (50-60%). (500mg) $C_{max}$=1106ng/mL; $T_{max}$=3 hrs. **Distribution:** Rosiglitazone: $V_d$=17.6L; plasma protein binding (99.8%). Metformin: $V_d$=654L. **Metabolism:** Rosiglitazone: Liver (extensive); CYP2C8 (major), 2C9 (minor). Metformin: No hepatic metabolism. **Elimination:** Rosiglitazone: Urine (64%), feces (23%); $T_{1/2}$=3-4 hrs. Metformin: Urine (unchanged); $T_{1/2}$=6.2 hrs (plasma).

## NURSING CONSIDERATIONS

**Assessment:** After initiation or dose increases, observe carefully for signs/symptoms of heart failure (including excessive and rapid weight gain, dyspnea, edema). Prior to initiation or escalation, investigate and treat secondary causes of poor glycemic control (eg, infection). Before initiation and at least annually thereafter, assess renal function and liver enzymes and verify as normal.

**Monitoring:** Measure fasting blood glucose and glycosylated hemoglobin to monitor therapeutic response. Monitor liver enzymes, hematologic parameters (Hct/Hgb), and renal function periodically. Monitor for signs/symptoms of lactic acidosis.

**Patient Counseling:** Inform of importance of diet and regular exercise, regular testing of blood glucose, $HbA_{1c}$, renal function, and hematologic parameters. Advise to d/c and notify physician if unexplained hyperventilation, myalgia, malaise, unusual somnolence, or nonspecific symptoms occur. Warn against excessive alcohol intake.

**Administration:** Oral route. **Storage:** Store at 25°C (77°F); excursions permitted to 15-30°C (59-86°F). Keep out of reach of children.

# AVANDARYL RX

rosiglitazone maleate - glimepiride (GlaxoSmithKline)

**Thiazolidinediones may cause or exacerbate CHF in some patients. Avandaryl is not recommended in patients with symptomatic heart failure. Meta-analysis has shown rosiglitazone to be associated with an increased risk of myocardial ischemic events.**

**THERAPEUTIC CLASS:** Thiazolidinedione/sulfonylurea

**INDICATIONS:** Adjunct to diet and exercise to improve glycemic control in type 2 DM when treatment with both rosiglitazone and glimepiride therapy is appropriate.

**DOSAGE:** *Adults:* Individualize dose. Initial: 1mg-4mg qd with 1st meal of day. Already Treated with Sulfonylurea or Thiazolidinedione: Initial: 2mg-4mg qd. Switching From Prior Combination Therapy: Start with dose of each component already being taken. Previously treated with Thiazolidinedione Monotherapy and Switched to Avandaryl: If inadequate control after 1-2 weeks, titrate glimepiride component to no more than 2mg increments at 1-2 week intervals. Previously treated with Sulfonylurea Monotherapy and Switched to Avandaryl: If inadequate control after 8-12 weeks, titrate rosiglitazone component at intervals of 2-3 months. Max: (Glimeperide-Rosiglitazone) 4mg-8mg qd. Elderly/Debilitated/Malnourished/Renal, Hepatic, or Adrenal Insufficiency: Initial: 1mg-4mg qd. Titrate carefully.

**HOW SUPPLIED:** Tab: (Glimepiride-Rosiglitazone) 1mg-4mg, 2mg-4mg, 4mg-4mg, 2mg-8mg, 4mg-8mg

**CONTRAINDICATIONS:** Established NYHA Class III or IV heart failure.

**WARNINGS/PRECAUTIONS:** Should not be used in patients with type 1 diabetes or for the treatment of diabetic ketoacidosis. Avoid with active liver disease, if ALT levels >2.5x ULN. Check LFTs before therapy, and periodically thereafter, or if hepatic dysfunction symptoms occur. D/C if ALT >3x ULN on therapy. May lose blood glucose control with stress; perform fasting glucose and HbA1C measurements to monitor therapeutic response. (Glimepiride) Increased cardiovascular mortality. Hypoglycemia risk if debilitated, malnourished, or with adrenal, pituitary, renal or hepatic insufficiency. May elevate liver enzyme levels in rare cases. Hemolytic anemia reported. Caution with G6PD deficiency. Hypoglycemia may be masked in elderly. (Rosiglitazone) D/C if cardiac status deteriorates. Increased risk of CV events with NYHA Class I and II heart failure. Initiation not recommended for patients experiencing an acute coronary event and d/c during this acute phase. Caution with edema. May cause macular edema. Dose-related wt gain reported. Ovulation in premenopausal anovulatory women may occur; risk of pregnancy with inadequate contraception. May decrease Hgb and Hct. Increased incidence of bone fracture was noted in female patients. Increase in serum lipids observed.

**ADVERSE REACTIONS:** Headache, hypoglycemia, anemia, edema, nasopharyngitis, HTN.

**INTERACTIONS:** Risk of severe hypoglycemia with oral miconazole. Use with insulin or nitrates is not recommended. Glimepiride: Risk of hyperglycemia with thiazides, corticosteroids, phenothiazines, thyroid products, estrogens, oral contraceptives, phenytoin, nicotinic acid, sympathomimetics, and isoniazid. Hypoglycemic action may be potentiated by certain drugs including NSAIDs, and other drugs that are highly protein bound, such as salicylates, sulfonamides, chloramphenicol, coumarins, probenecid, MAO inhibitors, and beta-blockers. Rosiglitazone: CYP2C8 inhibitors (eg, gemfibrozil) may increase the AUC. CYP2C8 inducers (eg, rifampin) may decrease the AUC.

**PREGNANCY:** Category C, not for use in nursing.

**MECHANISM OF ACTION:** Glimepiride: Sulfonylurea; stimulates insulin release from functional pancreatic β cells. Rosiglitazone: Thiazolidinedione; insulin sensitizing agent that acts by enhancing peripheral glucose utilization.

**PHARMACOKINETICS: Absorption:** Glimepiride: Complete; $T_{max}$=2-3 hrs; (4mg) $C_{max}$=151ng/mL. Rosiglitazone: Absolute bioavailability (99%); $T_{max}$=1 hr; (4mg) $C_{max}$=257ng/mL. **Distribution:** Glimepiride: (IV) $V_d$=8.8L; protein binding (>99.5%). Rosiglitazone: $V_d$=17.6L; plasma protein binding (99.8%).

**Metabolism:** Glimepiride: Liver (complete); major metabolites M1 & M2; CYP2C9. Rosiglitazone: N-demethylation & hydroxylation followed by conjugation; CYP2C8 (major), 2C9 (minor). **Elimination:** Glimepiride: Urine (60%), feces (40%). Rosiglitazone: Urine (64%), feces (23%); $T_{1/2}$=3-4 hrs.

## NURSING CONSIDERATIONS

**Assessment:** Assess for signs/symptoms of heart failure (excessive and rapid weight gain, dyspnea, and edema), liver failure (N/V, loss of appetite, dark urine, unusual fatigue, and jaundice). Check liver enzymes prior to therapy.

**Monitoring:** Monitor fasting blood glucose, glycosylated hemoglobin to check therapeutic response, and liver enzymes periodically.

**Patient Counseling:** Inform of importance of adherence to dietary instructions, weight loss, and exercise program. Instruct regarding regular blood glucose testing and $HbA_{1c}$. Inform to report unexplained N/V, anorexia, abdominal pain, or dark urine. Instruct to also report any edema, SOB, or other symptoms of heart failure. Inform that there are multiple medications available to treat type 2 diabetes but the benefits and risks should be taken into account when choosing a particular medication. Inform that diet control is included in management of diabetes. Explain to patients and their family members the risks, symptoms, treatment and conditions that predispose to the development of hypoglycemia. Adequate contraception in premenopausal women is recommended.

**Administration:** Oral route. **Storage:** Store at 25°C (77°F); excursions permitted to 15-30°C (59-86°F). Dispense in a tight, light-resistant container.

# AVANDIA RX

rosiglitazone maleate (GlaxoSmithKline)

**Thiazolidinediones may cause or exacerbate CHF in some patients. Rosiglitazone is not recommended in patients with symptomatic heart failure. Studies have shown rosiglitazone to be associated with an increased risk of myocardial ischemic events, such as angina or MI.**

**THERAPEUTIC CLASS:** Thiazolidinedione

**INDICATIONS:** Adjunct to diet and exercise to improve glycemic control in type 2 diabetes mellitus.

**DOSAGE:** *Adults:* ≥18 yrs: Initial: 2mg bid or 4mg qd. Titrate: May increase after 8-12 weeks to 8mg daily as monotherapy or in combination with metformin, sulfonylurea, or sulfonylurea plus metformin. Max: 8mg/day.

**HOW SUPPLIED:** Tab: 2mg, 4mg, 8mg

**CONTRAINDICATIONS:** Established NYHA Class III or IV heart failure.

**WARNINGS/PRECAUTIONS:** May cause fluid retention and exacerbation/initiation of heart failure; d/c if cardiac status deteriorates. Increased risk of CV events with NYHA Class I or II cardiac status; avoid with NYHA Class III or IV cardiac status. An increased risk of myocardial ischemic events has been observed. CHF and MI during coadministration with insulin. Coadministration with insulin or nitrates is not recommended. Not for use in type 1 diabetes or diabetic ketoacidosis treatment. Caution with edema. Macular edema reported. Dose-related weight gain and anemia reported. Avoid with active liver disease, if ALT levels >2.5x ULN, or if jaundice occurred with troglitazone. Check LFTs before therapy, every 2 months for 1 year, and periodically thereafter, or if hepatic dysfunction symptoms occur. D/C if ALT >3x ULN on therapy. Increased incidence of bone fracture in female patients. May decrease Hgb and Hct. Risk for hypoglycemia. Monitor blood glucose and $HbA_{1c}$ measurements. Ovulation in premenopausal anovulatory patients may occur; risk of pregnancy with inadequate contraception.

**ADVERSE REACTIONS:** Upper respiratory tract infection, injury, headache, back pain, hyperglycemia, fatigue, sinusitis, anemia, edema.

**INTERACTIONS:** Risk of hypoglycemia when used in combination with other hypoglycemic agents. CYP2C8 inhibitors (eg, gemfibrozil) may increase

AUC of rosiglitazone. CYP2C8 inducers (eg, rifampin) may decrease AUC of rosiglitazone. Use with insulin or nitrates is not recommended.

**PREGNANCY:** Category C, not for use in pregnancy or nursing.

**MECHANISM OF ACTION:** Thiazolidinedione; acts by improving insulin sensitivity.

**PHARMACOKINETICS: Absorption:** Absolute bioavailability (99%); $T_{max}$=1 hr. **Distribution:** $V_d$=17.6L; plasma protein binding (99.8%). **Metabolism:** CYP450, 2C8 (major) & 2C9 (minor); N-demethylation & hydroxylation then conjugation. **Elimination**: Urine (64%), feces (23%); $T_{1/2}$=3-4 hrs.

## NURSING CONSIDERATIONS

**Assessment:** Check liver enzymes prior to initiation and periodically after initiation; assess for elevated liver enzymes prior to therapy. Assess for risk of hypoglycemia, its symptoms and predisposing conditions.

**Monitoring:** Regularly monitor fasting blood glucose and glycosylated hemoglobin levels to measure therapeutic response. Monitor liver function tests periodically. Monitor for signs/symptoms of heart failure (eg, excessive rapid weight gain, dyspnea, edema).

**Patient Counseling:** Instruct to report any rapid increase in weight or edema, SOB, or other symptoms of heart failure. Instruct to report anorexia, N/V, dark urine, abdominal pain. Inform of importance of caloric restriction, weight loss, and exercise for glycemic control. Educate on importance of testing blood glucose and glycosylated hemoglobin regularly.

**Administration:** Oral route. **Storage**: 25°C (77°F). Dispense in tight, light-resistant container.

# AVAPRO RX

irbesartan (Bristol-Myers Squibb/Sanofi-Aventis)

**May cause death/injury to developing fetus during 2nd and 3rd trimesters. D/C if pregnancy detected.**

**THERAPEUTIC CLASS:** Angiotensin II receptor antagonist

**INDICATIONS:** Treatment of hypertension (HTN) alone or in combination with other antihypertensives. Treatment of diabetic nephropathy with an elevated serum creatinine and proteinuria (>300mg/day) in patients with type 2 diabetes and hypertension.

**DOSAGE:** *Adults:* HTN: Initial: 150mg qd. Titrate: May increase to 300mg qd. A low-dose diuretic may be added if BP is not controlled. Intravascular Volume/Salt Depletion: Initial: 75mg qd. Nephropathy: Maint: 300mg qd.
*Pediatrics:* HTN: ≥17 yrs: Initial: 150mg qd. Titrate: May increase to 300mg qd. Intravascular Volume/Salt Depletion: Initial: 75mg qd.

**HOW SUPPLIED:** Tab: 75mg, 150mg, 300mg

**WARNINGS/PRECAUTIONS:** Symptomatic hypotension may occur in volume and/or salt depleted patients; correct volume depletion prior to therapy and monitor closely. Changes in renal function may occur; caution with renal artery stenosis, severe CHF. Increases in SrCr or BUN reported with renal artery stenosis.

**ADVERSE REACTIONS:** Diarrhea, fatigue, orthostatic hypotension, dizziness.

**PREGNANCY:** Category C (1st trimester) and D (2nd and 3rd trimesters), not for use in nursing.

**MECHANISM OF ACTION:** Angiotensin II receptor antagonist; blocks vasoconstrictor and aldosterone-secreting effects of angiotensin II by selectively binding to $AT_1$ angiotensin II receptor.

**PHARMACOKINETICS: Absorption:** Rapid and complete, absolute bioavailability (60-80%); $T_{max}$=1.5-2 hrs. **Distribution:** $V_d$=53-93L; plasma protein binding (90%); crosses placenta; excreted in breast milk. **Metabolism:** CYP2C9 (oxidation), glucuronide conjugation. **Elimination:** Urine, feces; $T_{1/2}$=11-15 hrs.

## NURSING CONSIDERATIONS

**Assessment:** Assess for pregnancy/nursing status, renal impairment, and volume/salt depletion.

**Monitoring:** Monitor renal function periodically. Monitor for signs/symptoms of hypotension, hypersensitivity reactions, hyperkalemia, and renal dysfunction.

**Patient Counseling:** Inform of pregnancy risks. Advise to seek medical attention if symptoms of hypotension or hypersensitivity reactions occur. Inform that drug may be taken with/without food.

**Administration:** Oral route. **Storage:** 25°C (77°F); excursions permitted to 15-30°C (59-86°F).

# AVASTIN RX

bevacizumab (Genentech)

**Incidences of wound healing and surgical complications; d/c at least 28 days prior to elective surgery. Do not initiate for at least 28 days after surgery and until the surgical wound is fully healed. Severe or fatal hemorrhage including hemoptysis, GI bleeding, CNS hemorrhage, epistaxis, and vaginal bleeding have occurred; avoid with serious hemorrhage or recent hemoptysis. D/C if GI perforation or wound dehiscence develops.**

**THERAPEUTIC CLASS:** Vascular endothelial growth factor (VEGF) inhibitor

**INDICATIONS:** 1st- or 2nd-line treatment of metastatic colorectal cancer (mCRC), in combination with 5-fluorouracil (5-FU)-based chemotherapy. 1st-line treatment of unresectable, locally advanced, recurrent or metastatic non-squamous non-small cell lung cancer (NSCLC), in combination with carboplatin and paclitaxel. Treatment of patients who have not received chemotherapy for metastatic HER2-negative breast cancer (mBC), in combination with paclitaxel. Treatment of glioblastoma with progressive disease following prior therapy as a single agent. Treatment of metastatic renal cell carcinoma (mRCC), in combination with interferon alfa.

**DOSAGE:** *Adults:* mCRC: 5mg/kg or 10mg/kg q2 weeks (in combination with 5-FU). 5mg/kg q2 weeks (in combination with bolus IFL). 10mg/kg q2 weeks (in combination with FOLFOX4). NSCLC: 15mg/kg q3 weeks (in combination with carboplatin/paclitaxel). mBC: 10mg/kg q2 weeks (in combination with paclitaxel). Glioblastoma: 10mg/kg q2 weeks. mRCC: 10mg/kg q2 weeks (in combination with interferon alfa).

**HOW SUPPLIED:** Inj: 100mg/4mL, 400mg/16mL

**WARNINGS/PRECAUTIONS:** Serious and fatal non-GI fistula formation (eg, in tracheo-esophageal, bronchopleural, biliary, vaginal, renal, and bladder sites), hemorrhage (eg, hemoptysis, GI, hematemesis, CNS, epistaxis, vaginal), arterial thromboembolic events (eg, cerebral infarction, transient ischemic attacks, MI, angina), nephrotic syndrome may occur; d/c use if any occur. Increased incidence of severe HTN; monitor BP every 2-3 weeks during therapy and treat with appropriate antihypertensive agents. D/C use with hypertensive crisis and hypertensive encephalopathy. Reversible posterior leukoencephalopathy syndrome reported. Increased incidence and severity of proteinuria; monitor by urine analysis. Suspend treatment for ≥2g proteinuria/24 hrs and resume when proteinuria is <2g/24 hrs. Infusion reactions (eg, HTN, hypertensive crisis with neurologic signs and symptoms, wheezing, oxygen desaturation, hypersensitivity) reported; stop infusion for severe cases and administer appropriate medical therapy.

**ADVERSE REACTIONS:** Epistaxis, headache, hypertension, rhinitis, proteinuria, taste alteration, dry skin, rectal hemorrhage, lacrimation disorder, back pain, exfoliative dermatitis, polyserositis, pulmonary HTN, pancytopenia, dysphonia.

**INTERACTIONS:** Increased risk of arterial thromboembolic events when coadministered with chemotherapy. Serious or fatal pulmonary hemorrhage has occurred with chemotherapy in patients with NSCLC. May decrease paclitaxel exposure when coadministered.

**PREGNANCY:** Category C, not for use in nursing.

**MECHANISM OF ACTION:** Vascular endothelial growth factor (VEGF) inhibitor; binds VEGF and prevents interaction with receptors (Flt-1, KDR) on surface of endothelial cells, thereby inhibiting endothelial cell proliferation and new blood vessel formation.

**PHARMACOKINETICS: Absorption:** $T_{max}$=100 days. **Distribution:** $V_d$=3.25L (male) and 2.66L (female). **Elimination:** $T_{1/2}$=20 days.

## NURSING CONSIDERATIONS

**Assessment:** Assess for history of hemoptysis ( ≥1/2 tsp of red blood), HTN, hepatic/renal dysfunction (proteinuria, nephrotic syndrome), baseline urinalysis, BP, CBC, pregnancy/nursing status, and possible drug interactions.

**Monitoring:** Monitor CBC, BP every 2-3 weeks, and perform serial urinalysis. Monitor for signs/symptoms of GI perforation, fistula formation, wound-healing complications, serious hemorrhage, arterial thromboembolic events, hypertensive events (eg, crisis, encephalopathy), reversible posterior leukoencephalopathy syndrome, neutropenia, proteinuria, nephrotic syndrome, severe infusion reactions, CHF, and hypersensitivity reactions.

**Patient Counseling:** Inform of pregnancy risks and need to continue contraception for 6 months after therapy. Inform of risk for adverse events and instruct to seek medical attention if symptoms of the following occur: GI perforation (abdominal pain, constipation, vomiting), fistula formation, wound-healing complications, serious hemorrhage, arterial thromboembolic events, hypertensive events, reversible posterior leukoencephalopathy syndrome (headache, seizures, lethargy, confusion, blindness), neutropenia (fever, infection), proteinuria, nephrotic syndrome, and hypersensitivity reactions. Advise patient to undergo BP monitoring and contact health care provider if BP is elevated.

**Administration:** IV route. Do not administer as an IV push or bolus. Give as IV infusion over 90 min; if 1st infusion is well tolerated, give 2nd infusion over 60 min and subsequent doses over 30 min. **Storage**: 2-8°C (36-46°F). (Diluted): 2-8°C (36-46°F) for up to 8 hrs. Protect from light. Do not freeze or shake.

# AVELOX — RX

moxifloxacin HCl (Schering)

**Fluoroquinolones are associated with an increased risk of tendinitis and tendon rupture in all ages. Risk is further increased in patients >60 yrs, patients taking corticosteroid drugs, and patients with kidney, heart or lung transplants.**

**THERAPEUTIC CLASS:** Fluoroquinolone

**INDICATIONS:** Treatment of acute bacterial sinusitis, acute bacterial exacerbation of chronic bronchitis (ABECB), uncomplicated skin and skin structure infections (SSSI), community-acquired pneumonia (CAP), complicated intra-abdominal infections, and complicated SSSI caused by susceptible strains of microorganisms in adults ≥18 yrs.

**DOSAGE:** *Adults:* ≥18 yrs: Sinusitis: 400mg PO/IV q24h for 10 days. ABECB: 400mg PO/IV q24h for 5 days. Uncomplicated SSSI: 400mg PO/IV q24h for 7 days. Complicated SSSI: 400mg PO/IV q24h for 7-21 days. CAP: 400mg PO/IV q24h for 7-14 days. Complicated Intra-Abdominal Infections: 400mg PO/IV q24h for 5-14 days. For complicated intra-abdominal infections, therapy should usually be initiated IV.

**HOW SUPPLIED:** Inj: 400mg/250mL; Tab: 400mg

**WARNINGS/PRECAUTIONS:** Not for intra-arterial, IM, intrathecal, intraperitoneal, or SQ use. Avoid with known QT interval prolongation, and uncorrected hypokalemia. Caution with ongoing proarrhythmic conditions (eg, significant bradycardia, acute myocardial ischemia. QT-prolongation may be dose or infusion-rate dependent; do not exceed recommended dose. QT prolongation may increase risk of ventricular arrhythmias (eg, torsades de pointes). Caution in patients with mild, moderate, or severe liver cirrhosis. *Clostridium difficile*-associated diarrhea (CDAD) reported. Convulsions reported; caution with CNS disorders (eg, severe cerebral arteriosclerosis, epilepsy). Tendon ruptures and tendinitis reported. D/C if convulsions, CNS effects, hypersensitivity reaction, tendon rupture, phototoxicity occurs. Avoid excessive exposure to sun/UV light. Rare cases of peripheral neuropathy reported. Caution in elderly.

**ADVERSE REACTIONS:** Nausea, diarrhea.

**INTERACTIONS:** See Black Box Warning. Take oral formulation at least 4 hrs before or 8 hrs after aluminum-, magnesium-, or calcium-containing antacids, sucralfate, multivitamins with iron or zinc, and didanosine chewable/buffered tablets or oral solution. Avoid Class IA (eg, quinidine, procainamide) or Class III (eg, amiodarone, sotalol) antiarrhythmics. Caution with drugs that prolong the QT interval (eg, cisapride, erythromycin, antipsychotics, TCAs). NSAIDs may increase risk of CNS stimulation and convulsions. Monitor PT and INR with warfarin. Do not add other substances, additives, or medications to injection or infuse simultaneously through same IV line.

**PREGNANCY:** Category C, not for use in nursing.

**MECHANISM OF ACTION:** Fluoroquinolone; synthetic broad-spectrum antibiotic with activity against gram-positive and gram-negative microorganisms. Inhibits topoisomerase II (DNA gyrase) and topoisomerase IV, which are required for bacterial DNA replication, transcription, repair, and recombination.

**PHARMACOKINETICS: Absorption:** Well-absorbed; absolute bioavailability (90%). Single dose: (Oral) $C_{max}$=3.1mg/L, AUC=36.1mg•hr/L; (IV) $C_{max}$= 3.9mg/L, AUC=39.3mg•hr/L. Multiple dose: (Oral) $C_{max}$=4.5mg/L, AUC=48.0mg•hr/L; (IV) $C_{max}$= 4.2mg/L, AUC=38.0mg•hr/L. Refer to PI for further info. **Distribution:** $V_d$=1.7-2.7L/kg; plasma protein binding (30-50%); widely distributed. May be found in breast milk. **Metabolism:** Glucuronide and sulfate conjugation. **Elimination:** 45% unchanged; urine (20%), feces (25%); Single dose: $T_{1/2}$=11.5-15.6 hrs (oral), 8.2-15.4 hrs (IV). Multiple dose: $T_{1/2}$=12.7-1.9 hrs (oral), 14.8-2.2 hrs (IV).

## NURSING CONSIDERATIONS

**Assessment:** Assess for QT interval prolongation, uncorrected hypokalemia, patients receiving Class IA (eg, quinidine, procainamide) or Class III (eg, amiodarone, sotalol) antiarrhythmic agents, ongoing proarrhythmic conditions (eg, bradycardia, acute MI), CNS disorders (eg, severe cerebral arteriosclerosis, epilepsy), or risk factors that may predispose to seizures or lower seizure threshold. Assess pregnancy/nursing status and possible drug interactions.

**Monitoring:** Monitor ECG and lab changes (eg, CBC, PT, INR, Ca, glucose, bilirubin, and amylase). Monitor for signs/symptoms of anaphylactic reactions (eg, fever, rash, toxic epidermal necrolysis, Stevens-Johnson syndrome, allergic pneumonitis, interstitial nephritis, hepatitis, anemia, and vasculitis), prolongation of QT interval, ventricular arrhythmia/torsades de pointes, CNS events (eg, dizziness, confusion, tremors, hallucinations, depression, suicidal thoughts or acts, and seizures), drug resistance, CDAD that ranges from mild diarrhea to fatal colitis, peripheral neuropathy (eg, paresthesia, hypoesthesia, dysesthesia, weakness), tendon rupture (eg, shoulder, hand, achilles, or other tendons), and photosensitivity.

**Patient Counseling:** Notify healthcare provider if experience symptoms of pain, swelling, or inflammation of a tendon, or weakness or inability to move joints; rest and refrain from exercise and d/c therapy. Inform that drug treats bacterial, not viral, infections. Inform that drug may produce ECG (QTc prolongation) changes. Take exactly as directed; skipping doses or not completing full course may decrease effectiveness and increase resistance. Inform that moxifloxacin tablets may be taken with or without meals, and drink fluids liberally. Inform about potential benefits/risks. D/C and notify physician if allergic reaction, skin rash, and watery and bloody stools (with or without stomach cramps and fever) occur. Notify physician if experiencing palpitations or fainting spells. Notify if pregnant/nursing or taking antiarrhythmics, OTC drugs, multivitamins, antacids, or sucralfate. Use caution while performing hazardous tasks (eg, operating machinery/driving). Avoid excessive exposure to sunlight and wear protective clothes. Contact physician if sunburn-like reaction occurs.

**Administration:** Oral, IV routes. Avoid rapid or bolus IV infusion. Inspect visually for particulate matter in vial prior to administration. **Storage:** 25°C (77°F); excursions permitted to 15-30°C (59-86°F). Avoid high humidity. Do not refrigerate.

## AVINZA

morphine sulfate (King)

CII

**Swallow capsules whole or sprinkle contents on applesauce. Do not crush, chew, or dissolve capsule beads. Avoid alcohol and alcohol-containing medications; consumption of alcohol may result in the rapid release and absorption of potentially fatal dose of morphine.**

**THERAPEUTIC CLASS:** Opioid analgesic

**INDICATIONS:** Relief of moderate to severe pain requiring continuous opioid therapy for an extended period of time.

**DOSAGE:** *Adults:* Conversion from other oral morphine products: Give total daily dose as a single dose q24h. Conversion from parenteral morphine: Initial: Give about 3x the previous daily parenteral requirement. Conversion from other parenteral or oral non-morphine opioids: Initial: Give 1/2 of estimated daily requirement q24h. Supplement with immediate-release morphine or short-acting analgesics if needed. Titrate: Adjust dose as frequently as every other day. Non-opioid tolerant: 30mg q24h. Titrate: Increase by increments ≤30mg every 4 days. The 45, 60, 90, and 120mg caps are for opioid-tolerant patients. Max: 1600mg/day. Doses >1600mg/day contain a quantity of fumaric acid, which may cause renal toxicity. Elderly: Start at low end of dosing range.

**HOW SUPPLIED:** Cap, Extended-Release: 30mg, 45mg, 60mg, 75mg, 90mg, 120mg

**CONTRAINDICATIONS:** Respiratory depression in the absence of resuscitative equipment, acute or severe bronchial asthma, paralytic ileus.

**WARNINGS/PRECAUTIONS:** Abuse potential. Extreme caution with COPD, cor pulmonale, decreased respiratory reserve (eg, severe kyphoscoliosis), hypoxia, hypercapnia, pre-existing respiratory depression, increased ICP, head injury. May cause orthostatic hypotension, syncope, severe hypotension with depleted blood volume. Caution with circulatory shock, biliary tract disease, severe renal/hepatic insufficiency, Addison's disease, hypothyroidism, prostatic hypertrophy, urethral stricture, elderly or debilitated; consider dose reduction. Caution with CNS depression, toxic psychosis, acute alcoholism, delirium tremens, seizure disorders. Avoid with GI obstruction. Avoid abrupt withdrawal. Tolerance and physical dependence may develop. Potential for severe constipation; use laxatives, stool softeners at onset of therapy. May impair mental/physical abilities. Not for use as a prn or postoperative analgesic.

**ADVERSE REACTIONS:** Constipation, N/V, somnolence, dehydration, headache, peripheral edema, diarrhea, abdominal pain, infection, UTI, flu syndrome, back pain, rash, sweating, depression.

**INTERACTIONS:** See Black Box Warning. Additive effects with alcohol, other opioids, illicit drugs that cause CNS depression. Reduce dose with other CNS depressants (eg, sedatives, hypnotics, general anesthetics, antiemetics, phenothiazines, tranquilizers, alcohol); caution when coadministering. May enhance neuromuscular blocking action of skeletal muscle relaxants. Increased risk of respiratory depression with muscle relaxants. Avoid with mixed agonist/antagonists (eg, pentazocine, nalbuphine, butorphanol) and within 14 days of MAOI use. Risk of precipitate apnea, confusion, muscle twitching reported with cimetidine; monitor for respiratory and CNS depression.

**PREGNANCY:** Category C, not for use in nursing.

**MECHANISM OF ACTION:** Opioid analgesic; pure opioid agonist that is relatively selective for μ-receptor but may interact with other opioid receptors at higher doses. Analgesic effects not established. Specific CNS opiate receptors (eg, μ-receptors) and endogenous compounds with morphine-like activity are found throughout brain and spinal cord and are likely to play a role in analgesic effects.

**PHARMACOKINETICS: Absorption:** $C_{max}$=18.65ng/mL; AUC=273.25ng/mL•h. **Distribution:** Plasma protein binding (20-35%), $V_d$=1-6L/kg, distributed to skeletal muscle, kidneys, liver, GI tract, lung, spleen, and brain. Small quantities cross the blood-brain barrier. Found in placental membranes and human breast milk. **Metabolism:** Hepatic conjugation; 3-glucuronide (M3G) (metabolite); 6-glucuronide (M6G) (active metabolite). **Elimination:** Urine (major M3G/M6G, 10% unchanged), feces (7-10%), bile (small); (IV) $T_{1/2}$=2 hrs (IV) and 15 hrs (PO).

## NURSING CONSIDERATIONS

**Assessment:** Assess for respiratory depression, GI obstruction (eg, paralytic ileus), acute or severe bronchial asthma, COPD, presence of head injury or increased ICP, biliary tract disease, acute pancreatitis, Addison's disease, hypothyroidism, prostatic hypertrophy, urethral stricture, CNS depression, toxic psychosis, seizure disorders, acute alcoholism, hepatic/renal function, age, nursing/pregnancy status, and possible drug interactions.

**Monitoring:** Monitor for signs/symptoms of respiratory depression, orthostatic hypotension, syncope, drug dependence and tolerance, and withdrawal syndrome (eg, restlessness, lacrimation, rhinorrhea, myalgia, mydriasis). Monitor for signs of increased ICP with head injuries.

**Patient Counseling:** May take with/without food. Instruct to swallow whole (not to chew, crush, or dissolve) or open and sprinkle onto small amount of applesauce. Instruct not to consume alcohol during therapy, including Rx/OTC drugs containing alcohol. Notify physician of all concurrent medications and avoid use of other CNS depressants. Caution when performing hazardous tasks (eg, operating machinery/driving). Do not adjust dose or abruptly d/c medication without consulting physician. Advise that medication has potential for abuse. Instruct to keep out of reach of children. Advise to dispose of any unused medication via toilet. Counsel about severe constipation; take appropriate laxatives or stool softeners at start of therapy.

**Administration:** Oral route. **Storage:** 25°C (77°F); excursions permitted to 15-30°C (59-86°F). Protect from light and moisture; dispense in a tight, light-resistant container.

# AVODART RX

dutasteride (GlaxoSmithKline)

**THERAPEUTIC CLASS:** Type I and II 5 alpha-reductase inhibitor (2nd generation)

**INDICATIONS:** Treatment of symptomatic benign prostatic hyperplasia (BPH) in men with an enlarged prostate, either as monotherapy or in combination with the α-blocker tamsulosin.

**DOSAGE:** *Adults:* Monotherapy: 0.5mg qd. Combination Therapy with Tamsulosin: 0.5mg qd and tamsulosin 0.4mg qd.

**HOW SUPPLIED:** Cap: 0.5mg

**CONTRAINDICATIONS:** Pregnancy, women of childbearing potential, and pediatric patients.

**WARNINGS/PRECAUTIONS:** Risk to male fetus; should not be handled by pregnant women or women who may become pregnant. Rule out prostate cancer and other urological diseases prior to treatment. Monitor for obstructive uropathy in patients with a large residual urinary volume and/or severely diminished urinary flow; these patients may not be good candidates for therapy with dutasteride. Avoid donating blood until 6 months after last dose. May decreases serum PSA levels by about 40-50%; obtain a new baseline PSA concentration after 3-6 months of treatment. To interpret an isolated PSA value in a man treated for ≥6 months, double the PSA value for comparison with normal values.

**ADVERSE REACTIONS:** Impotence, decreased libido, breast disorders, ejaculation disorders, dizziness.

**INTERACTIONS:** Caution with potent CYP3A4 inhibitors (eg, ritonavir, ketoconazole, verapamil, diltiazem, cimetidine, ciprofloxacin); may increase blood levels.

**PREGNANCY:** Category X, not for use in nursing.

**MECHANISM OF ACTION:** Type I, II 5α-reductase inhibitor; inhibits conversion of testosterone to dihydrotestosterone (DHT), the androgen primarily responsible for development and enlargement of the prostate gland.

**PHARMACOKINETICS: Absorption:** Absolute bioavailability (60%); $T_{max}$=2-3 hrs. **Distribution:** $V_d$=300-500L; plasma protein binding (99%). **Metabolism:** CYP3A4, 3A5. Major active metabolites: 4'-hydroxydutasteride, 1,2-dihydroxydutasteride, 6-hydroxydutasteride. **Elimination:** Feces (5% unchanged, 40% metabolites), urine (<1%); $T_{1/2}$=5 weeks.

## NURSING CONSIDERATIONS

**Assessment:** Assess for hepatic impairment, large residual urinary volume or severely diminished urinary flow, and for possible drug interactions. Rule out prostate cancer and other urologic diseases.

**Monitoring:** Monitor for signs/symptoms of prostate cancer and other urological diseases and for hepatic dysfunction. Obtain new baseline PSA after 3-6 months of treatment.

**Patient Counseling:** Advise not to donate blood for at least 6 months after d/c therapy. Inform females who are pregnant, or intend to become pregnant, not to handle drug due to potential risk to fetus; inform that if contact is made, to wash area immediately with soap and water. Advise to swallow cap whole. Inform that may take with or without food.

**Administration:** Oral route. **Storage:** 25°C (77°F); excursions permitted to 15-30°C (59-86°F).

# AXERT RX

almotriptan malate (Ortho-McNeil/Janssen)

**THERAPEUTIC CLASS:** 5-$HT_{1B/1D}$ agonist

**INDICATIONS:** Acute treatment of migraine attacks with a history of migraine with or without aura in adults. Acute treatment of migraine headache pain with a history of migraine attacks with or without aura usually lasting ≥4 hrs in adolescents 12-17 yrs.

**DOSAGE:** *Adults:* Initial: 6.25-12.5mg at onset of headache. May repeat after 2 hrs. Max: 25mg/day. Hepatic/Renal Impairment: 6.25mg at onset of headache. Max: 12.5mg/24 hrs. Elderly: Start at lower end of dosing range.
*Pediatrics:* 12-17 yrs: Initial: 6.25-12.5mg at onset of headache. May repeat after 2 hrs. Max: 25mg/day. Hepatic/Renal Impairment: 6.25mg at onset of headache. Max: 12.5mg/24 hrs.

**HOW SUPPLIED:** Tab: 6.25mg, 12.5mg

**CONTRAINDICATIONS:** Ischemic heart disease, coronary artery vasospasm, other significant CVD, cerebrovascular syndromes (eg, stroke, transient ischemic attacks), peripheral vascular disease (eg, ischemic bowel disease), uncontrolled HTN, hemiplegic or basilar migraine. Avoid use within 24 hrs of another 5-$HT_1$ agonist (eg, triptans) or ergotamine-containing or ergot-type medications (eg, dihydroergotamine, ergotamine tartrate, methysergide).

**WARNINGS/PRECAUTIONS:** Confirm diagnosis. Supervise first dose and monitor cardiac function in those at risk of CAD (eg, HTN, hypercholesterolemia, smoker, obesity, diabetes, CAD family history, postmenopausal women, males >40 yrs). Monitor cardiovascular function with long-term intermittent use. May cause vasospastic reactions or cerebrovascular events. Serotonin syndrome symptoms (eg, mental status changes, autonomic instability, neuromuscular aberrations, and GI symptoms) reported. Sensations of tightness, pain, presure, and heaviness in the precordium, throat, neck, and jaw reported. May bind to melanin in the eye. Caution with renal or hepatic dysfunction. Caution with known hypersensitivity to sulfonamides. Caution in elderly.

**ADVERSE REACTIONS:** N/V, dizziness, somnolence, headache, paresthesia, coronary artery vasospasm, MI, ventricular tachycardia, ventricular fibrillation, transient myocardial ischemia and dry mouth.

**INTERACTIONS:** See Contraindications. Additive vasospastic reactions with ergotamines. Selective serotonin reuptake inhibitors (SSRIs) may cause weakness, hyperreflexia, and incoordination. Life-threatening serotonin syndrome reported with combined use of SSRIs or serotonin norepinephrine reuptake inhibitors (SNRIs). Clearance may be decreased by MAOIs (eg, moclobemide). Increased levels possible with CYP3A4 inhibitors (eg, ketoconazole).

**PREGNANCY:** Category C, caution in nursing.

**MECHANISM OF ACTION:** Selective 5-$HT_{1B/1D}$ receptor agonist; binds with high affinity to 5-$HT_{1B/1D}$ receptors on extracerebral, intracranial blood vessels that become dilated during migraine attack and on nerve terminal in trigeminal system. Activation of these receptors results in cranial nerve constriction, inhibition of neuropeptide release, and reduced transmission in trigeminal pain pathways.

**PHARMACOKINETICS: Absorption:** Absolute bioavailability (70%); $T_{max}$=1-3 hrs. **Distribution:** $V_d$=180-200L; plasma protein binding (35%). **Metabolism:** Monoamine oxidase (MAO)-mediated oxidative deamination and CYP450-mediated oxidation (major pathways), flavin monooxygenase (minor pathway); indoleacetic acid, gamma-aminobutyric acid (inactive metabolites). **Elimination:** Urine (75%, 40% unchanged), feces (13%, unchanged and metabolite); $T_{1/2}$=3-4 hrs.

## NURSING CONSIDERATIONS

**Assessment:** Confirm diagnosis of migraine before therapy. Assess for cluster headache, ischemic heart disease (eg, angina pectoris, Prinzmetal's variant angina, MI or documented silent MI), HTN, hemiplegic or basilar migraine, presence of risk factors (eg, hypercholesterolemia, smoking, obesity, DM, strong family history of CAD, female with surgical or physiological menopause, or male >49 yrs), ECG changes, hepatic/renal impairment, hypersensitivity to the drug and to sulfonamides, pregnancy/nursing status, and possible drug interactions.

**Monitoring:** Administration of 1st dose should be in physician's office or medically staffed and equipped facility as cardiac ischemia may occur in absence of clinical symptoms; ECG should be obtained immediately during interval in those with risk factors. Monitor for signs/symptoms of cardiac events (eg, coronary vasospasm, acute MI, arrhythmia, ECG changes, follow-up coronary angiography), cerebrovascular events (eg, hemorrhage, stroke, TIAs), peripheral vascular ischemia, colonic ischemia with bloody diarrhea and abdominal pain, serotonin syndrome (eg, mental status changes, autonomic instability, neuromuscular aberrations and/or GI symptoms), ophthalmic effects, hypersensitivity reactions, and increased BP.

**Patient Counseling:** Inform about potential risks (eg, serotonin syndrome manifestations such as confusion, hallucinations, fast heartbeat, fever, sweating, muscle spasm, and diarrhea), especially if taken with SSRIs or SNRIs. Instruct to report adverse reactions to physician. Advise to take exactly as directed. Counsel to use caution during hazardous tasks (eg, driving/operating machinery). Instruct to notify if pregnant/nursing or planning to become pregnant.

**Administration:** Oral route. **Storage:** 25°C (77°F); excursions permitted to 15-30°C (59-86°F).

# AXID RX

nizatidine (GlaxoSmithKline)

**OTHER BRAND NAMES:** Axid Oral Solution (Braintree)

**THERAPEUTIC CLASS:** $H_2$-blocker

**INDICATIONS:** Short term treatment of active duodenal ulcer (DU) and benign gastric ulcer (GU). Maintenance therapy for duodenal ulcers. Treatment of endoscopically diagnosed esophagitis, including erosive and ulcerative esophagitis, and heartburn due to GERD.

**DOSAGE:** *Adults:* Active DU/Active Benign GU: Usual: 300mg qhs or 150mg bid up to 8 weeks. Healed DU: Maint: 150mg qhs, up to 1 year. GERD: 150mg bid up to 12 weeks. Renal Impairment: Treatment: CrCl 20-50mL/min: 150mg/day. CrCl <20mL/min: 150mg every other day. Maint: CrCl 20-50mL/min: 150mg every other day. CrCl <20mL/min: 150mg every 3 days. *Pediatrics:* ≥12 yrs: (Sol) Erosive Esophagitis/GERD: 150mg bid up to 8 weeks. Max: 300mg/day. Renal Impairment: Treatment: CrCl 20-50mL/min: 150mg/day. CrCl <20mL/min: 150mg every other day. Maint: CrCl 20-50mL/min: 150mg every other day. CrCl <20mL/min: 150mg every 3 days.

**HOW SUPPLIED:** Cap: 150mg, 300mg; Sol: 15mg/mL

**WARNINGS/PRECAUTIONS:** Caution with renal dysfunction; reduce dose. Symptomatic response does not preclude the presence of gastric malignancy. False positive tests for urobilinogen with Multistix.

**ADVERSE REACTIONS:** Headache, abdominal pain, pain, asthenia, diarrhea, NV, flatulence, dyspepsia, rhinitis, pharyngitis, dizziness.

**INTERACTIONS:** May elevate serum salicylate levels with high dose ASA.

**PREGNANCY:** Category B, not for use in nursing.

**MECHANISM OF ACTION:** $H_2$ receptor antagonist; competitive, reversible inhibitor of histamine at the histamine $H_2$ receptors, particularly those in gastroparietal cells.

**PHARMACOKINETICS: Absorption:** Absolute bioavailability (>70%); (150mg, 300mg) $C_{max}$=700-1800mcg/L, 1400-3600mcg/L; $T_{max}$=0.5-3 hrs. (12-18 yrs, 150mg) $C_{max}$=1422.9ng/mL; $T_{max}$=1.3 hrs; AUC=3764ng•hr/mL. **Distribution:** (Adult) $V_d$=0.8-1.5L/kg; (12-18 yrs) $V_d$=71.4L. Plasma protein binding (35%); found in breast milk. **Metabolism:** $N_2$-monodesmethylnizatidine (major). **Excretion:** Urine (90%, 60% unchanged); feces (6%). (Adult) $T_{1/2}$=1-2 hrs; (12-18 yrs) $T_{1/2}$=1.2 hrs.

## NURSING CONSIDERATIONS

**Assessment:** Assess for hypersensitivity to other $H_2$ receptor antagonists, renal dysfunction, presence of gastric malignancy, pregnancy/nursing status, and possible drug interactions.

**Monitoring:** Monitor for signs/symptoms of hepatocellular injury (eg, elevation in liver enzymes), hematological effects (eg, anemia), hypersensitivity reactions (eg, anaphylaxis), and for signs of clinical improvement. If treatment is for active duodenal ulcer, monitor for signs of healing after 4 weeks and for complete healing by 8 weeks.

**Patient Counseling:** Advise if taking single dosing, take at bedtime. Contact physician if hypersensitivity reaction develops. Notify pregnant/nursing females about risks of use.

**Administration:** Oral route. **Storage:** Dispense in tightly closed container. Cap: 20-25° (68-77°F). Sol: 25° (77°F); excursions permitted to 15-30°C (59-86°F).

# AYGESTIN RX

norethindrone acetate (Duramed)

**THERAPEUTIC CLASS:** Progestogen

**INDICATIONS:** Treatment of secondary amenorrhea, endometriosis, and abnormal uterine bleeding due to hormonal imbalance in the absence of organic pathology.

**DOSAGE:** *Adults:* Assume interval between menses is 28 days. Secondary Amenorrhea/Abnormal Uterine Bleeding: 2.5-10mg qd for 5-10 days during second half of menstrual cycle. Endometriosis: Initial: 5mg qd for 2 weeks. Titrate: Increase by 2.5mg qd every 2 weeks until 15mg/day. Continue for 6-9 months or until breakthrough bleeding demands temporary termination.

**HOW SUPPLIED:** Tab: 5mg* *scored

**CONTRAINDICATIONS:** Pregnancy, thrombophlebitis, thromboembolic disorders, cerebral apoplexy, liver impairment, breast carcinoma, undiagnosed vaginal bleeding, missed abortion, use as a pregnancy diagnostic test.

**WARNINGS/PRECAUTIONS:** D/C with migraine, vision loss, proptosis, diplopia, papilledema, or retinal vascular lesions. May cause thrombophlebitis, pulmonary embolism, and fluid retention. Caution with epilepsy, migraine, psychic depression, asthma, cardiac or renal dysfunction, depression, DM, and hyperlipidemia. May mask onset of climacteric. Not for use during the first trimester of pregnancy; risk to the fetus.

**ADVERSE REACTIONS:** Breakthrough bleeding, spotting, change in menstrual flow, amenorrhea, edema, weight changes, cervical changes, cholestatic jaundice, rash, melasma, chloasma, depression.

**PREGNANCY:** Category X, safety in nursing is not known.

**MECHANISM OF ACTION:** Progestogen; induces secretory changes in estrogen-primed endometrium.

**PHARMACOKINETICS: Absorption:** Rapid; $C_{max}$=26.19ng/mL; $T_{max}$=1.83 hrs; AUC=166.9ng/mL•hr. **Distribution:** $V_d$=4L/kg; sex hormone binding globulin (SHBG) (36%); albumin binding (61%); found in breast milk. **Metabolism:** Extensive, via reduction; sulfate and glucuronide conjugation. **Elimination:** Urine, feces (metabolites); $T_{1/2}$=9 hrs.

## NURSING CONSIDERATIONS

**Assessment:** Assess for known/suspected pregnancy, vaginal bleeding, presence or history of breast cancer, DVT, PE, active or recent (within past yr) arterial thromboembolic disease (eg, stroke, MI), and impaired renal/hepatic function. Assess use in nursing females, history of depression, and those at risk for arterial vascular disease (eg, presence of HTN, hypercholesterolemia, DM, obesity, tobacco use) and for VTE (eg, family history, obesity, SLE). Assess for possible lab interactions.

**Monitoring:** Monitor for signs/symptoms of cardiovascular disorders (eg, thromboembolic events), visual abnormalities (eg, loss of vision, proptosis, diplopia), fluid retention, and breakthrough bleeding. Monitor for signs of worsening depression in patients with previous history. Monitor with hyperlipidemias and DM for changes in lipid and carbohydrate metabolism.

**Patient Counseling:** Counsel to contact physician if breast lumps, dizziness or faintness, changes in speech, severe headaches, chest pain, SOB, leg pain, or changes in vision occur. Advise to have annual breast exam and mammography unless otherwise directed by physician. Counsel to avoid using tobacco.

**Administration:** Oral route. **Storage:** 20-25°C (68-77°F).

## AZACTAM — RX

aztreonam (Elan)

**THERAPEUTIC CLASS:** Monobactam

**INDICATIONS:** Treatment of septicemia and lower respiratory tract (eg, pneumonia, bronchitis) infections, skin and skin-structure infections (eg, postoperative wounds, ulcers, burns), complicated/uncomplicated urinary tract infections (UTI) including pyelonephritis and initial/recurrent cystitis, gynecologic infections (eg, endometritis, pelvic cellulitis), and intra-abdominal (eg, peritonitis) infections caused by susceptible microorganisms. Adjunct therapy to surgery for management of infections caused by susceptible microorganisms (eg, abscesses, hollow viscus perforation infections, cutaneous infections, infections of serous surfaces).

**DOSAGE:** *Adults:* UTI: 500mg-1g IM/IV q8-12h. Moderately Severe Systemic Infections: 1-2g IM/IV q8-12h. Severe Systemic/Life-Threatening Infections/ *Pseudomonas aeruginosa*: 2g IV q6-8h. Max: 8g/day. CrCl 10-30mL/ min/1.73m²: Initial: LD: 1 or 2g. Maint: 50% of usual dose. CrCl <10mL/ min/1.73m²: Initial: LD: 500mg, 1g or 2g. Maint: 25% of usual initial dose at usual intervals of 6, 8 or 12 hrs. Serious/Life-Threatening Infections: In addition to maint dose, give 1/8 initial dose after each hemodialysis session. IV

route recommended for single doses >1g or for bacterial septicemia, localized parenchymal abscess (eg, intra-abdominal abscess), peritonitis, or other severe systemic or life-threatening infections. Continue for at least 48 hrs after patient is asymptomatic or evidence of bacterial eradication. Elderly: Start at lower end of dosing range.
*Pediatrics:* 9 months-16 yrs: Mild-Moderate Infections: 30mg/kg IV q8h. Moderate-Severe Infections: 30mg/kg IV q6-8h. Max: 120mg/kg/day. In patients with cystic fibrosis, higher doses may be warranted.

**HOW SUPPLIED:** Inj: 1g, 2g, 1g/50mL, 2g/50mL

**WARNINGS/PRECAUTIONS:** Caution with hypersensitivity to other β-lactams (eg, penicillins, cephalosphorins, carbapenems) or allergens; d/c if occurs. *Clostridium difficile*-associated diarrhea (CDAD) reported. May promote overgrowth of nonsusceptible organisms; take appropriate measures if superinfection develops. Toxic epidermal necrolysis (TEN) reported (rarely) in bone marrow transplant with multiple risk factors including sepsis and radiation therapy. Increased risk of development of drug-resistant bacteria in the absence of a proven or strongly suspected bacterial infection or a prophylactic indication. Monitor patients with impaired renal or hepatic function. If using concomitantly with an aminoglycoside, renal function should be monitored because of the potential nephrotoxicity and ototoxicity of aminoglycosides. Caution in the elderly.

**ADVERSE REACTIONS:** Phlebitis/thrombophlebitis, discomfort/swelling at injection site, diarrhea, N/V, rash, abdominal cramps, vaginal candidiasis, hypersensitivity reaction.

**INTERACTIONS:** TEN reported (rarely) in bone marrow transplant (BMT) patients who were receiving concomitant therapy with other drugs associated with TEN. Avoid concomitant use with beta-lactamase inducing antibiotics (eg, cefoxitin, imipinem).

**PREGNANCY:** Category B, not for use in nursing.

**MECHANISM OF ACTION:** Monobactam; synthetic bactericidal antibiotic. Inhibits bacterial cell-wall synthesis due to high affinity of aztreonam for penicillin-binding protein 3 (PBP3).

**PHARMACOKINETICS: Absorption:** $C_{max}$=90μ/mL (1g dose), 204μ/mL (2g dose); $T_{max}$=1 hr. **Distribution:** $V_d$=12.6L; crosses placenta; found in breast milk. **Metabolism:** Hydrolysis. **Elimination:** Urine (60-70%), feces (12%); $T_{1/2}$=1.7 hr.

## NURSING CONSIDERATIONS

**Assessment:** Assess for proven/strongly suspected bacterial infection, hypersensitivity to any allergens, history of hypersensitivity to other beta-lactams (eg, penicillins, cephalosporins, carbapenems), hepatic/renal impairment, pregnancy/nursing status, and for possible drug interactions. Assess use in patients undergoing BMT with multiple risk factors (eg, sepsis, radiation therapy).

**Monitoring:** Monitor for signs/symptoms of hypersensitivity reactions, CDAD, overgrowth of non-susceptible organisms, development of drug resistance, and for superinfection. Monitor for signs/symptoms of TEN in patients undergoing BMT. Monitor hepatic/renal function.

**Patient Counseling:** Inform about potential benefits/risks of therapy. Advise that drug treats bacterial, not viral, infections. Instruct to take exactly as directed; inform that skipping doses or not completing full course may decrease effectiveness and increase bacterial resistance. Instruct to d/c therapy and notify physician if allergic reactions, watery/bloody diarrhea (with/without stomach cramps) occur (may occur as late as 2 or more months after therapy). Instruct to notify physician if pregnant/nursing.

**Administration:** IM/IV routes. Refer to PI for preparation instructions and compatibility information. **Storage:** Prior to Reconstitution: Store at room Temperature; avoid excessive heat. Refer to PI for storage information of reconstituted solution.

## AZASITE RX
azithromycin (Inspire)

**THERAPEUTIC CLASS:** Macrolide

**INDICATIONS:** Treatment of bacterial conjunctivitis caused by susceptible strains of microorganisms.

**DOSAGE:** *Adults:* Initial: 1 drop bid, 8 to 12 hrs apart, for first 2 days. Maint: 1 drop qd for next 5 days.
*Pediatrics:* ≥1 yr: Initial: 1 drop bid, 8 to 12 hrs apart, for first 2 days. Maint: 1 drop qd for next 5 days.

**HOW SUPPLIED:** Sol: 1% [2.5mL]

**WARNINGS/PRECAUTIONS:** Not for injection; do not give systemically, inject subconjunctivally or into chamber of eye. Caution may cause hypersensitivity reactions. Growth of resistant organisms including fungi may occur with prolonged use. Avoid contact lens use.

**ADVERSE REACTIONS:** Eye irritation, burning, stinging and irritation upon instillation, contact dermatitis, corneal erosion, dry eye, dysgeusia, nasal congestion, ocular discharge, punctate keratitis, sinusitis.

**PREGNANCY:** Category B, caution in nursing.

**MECHANISM OF ACTION:** Macrolide; binds to the 50S ribosomal subunit of susceptible microorganisms and interferes with microbial protein synthesis.

**PHARMACOKINETICS: Absorption:** $C_{max}$≤10ng/mL.

### NURSING CONSIDERATIONS

**Assessment:** Assess proper diagnosis of causative bacteria.

**Monitoring:** Monitor for signs/symptoms of anaphylaxis (angioedema, Stevens-Johnson syndrome), development of growth of resistant organisms, and eye irritation.

**Patient Counseling:** Advise patients with signs/symptoms of bacterial conjuctivitis to avoid wearing contact lenses. Instruct not to allow applicator tip to touch the eye, fingers, or other sources. Take exactly as directed. Advise if doses are skipped or medication is stopped early, treatment effectiveness will be decreased and bacteria may develop resistance. Direct to d/c and contact physician if signs of allergic reaction occur.

**Administration:** Ocular route. **Storage:** Store unopened bottle under refrigeration at 2-8°C (36-46°F). Once bottle is opened, store at 2-25°C (36-77°F) for up to 14 days. Discard after 14 days.

## AZELEX RX
azelaic acid (Allergan)

**THERAPEUTIC CLASS:** Dicarboxylic acid antimicrobial

**INDICATIONS:** Mild to moderate inflammatory acne vulgaris.

**DOSAGE:** *Adults:* Wash and dry skin. Massage gently into affected area bid (am and pm).
*Pediatrics:* ≥12 yrs: Wash and dry skin. Massage gently into affected area bid (am and pm).

**HOW SUPPLIED:** Cre: 20% [30g, 50g]

**WARNINGS/PRECAUTIONS:** Avoid mouth, eyes, mucous membranes, and occlusive dressings.

**ADVERSE REACTIONS:** Pruritus, burning, stinging, tingling, hypopigmentation.

**PREGNANCY:** Category B, caution in nursing.

**MECHANISM OF ACTION:** Dicarboxylic acid antimicrobial; not established. Possesses antimicrobial activity that may be attributable to inhibition of microbial cellular protein synthesis. A normalization of keratinization leading to an anticomedonal effect of azelaic acid may also contribute to clinical activity.

**PHARMACOKINETICS: Absorption:** Penetrates stratum corneum (3-5%), up to 10% of dose found in dermis and epidermis; systemic absorption (4%); $C_{max}$=20-80ng/mL. **Metabolism:** Cutaneous (negligible), beta-oxidation. **Elimination:** Urine (mainly unchanged); $T_{1/2}$=12 hrs (after topical dosing).

## NURSING CONSIDERATIONS

**Assessment:** Assess proper diagnosis of acne vulgaris. Assess use in nursing females.

**Monitoring:** Monitor for signs/symptoms of hypopigmentation (especially in patients with dark complexions), sensitivity reactions, and severe skin irritation.

**Patient Counseling:** Counsel to use medication for the full prescribed treatment period. Instruct to avoid using occlusive dressings with medication. Advise to keep medication away from mouth, eyes, and mucous membranes. If contact occurs with eyes, instruct to wash eyes with large amounts of water and consult physician if problem persists. Instruct that temporary skin irritation may occur when applied to broken or inflamed skin; if irritation persists, consult physician immediately. Counsel patients with dark complexions to notify physician if they notice pigment changes.

**Administration:** Topical. **Storage:** 15-30°C (59-86°F). Protect from freezing.

# AZILECT RX

rasagiline mesylate (Teva)

**THERAPEUTIC CLASS:** Monoamine oxidase inhibitor (Type B)

**INDICATIONS:** Treatment of signs and symptoms of idiopathic Parkinson's disease as initial monotherapy and adjunct therapy to levodopa.

**DOSAGE:** *Adults:* Monotherapy: 1mg qd. Adjunctive Therapy: Initial: 0.5mg qd. Titrate: May increase to 1mg qd. Adjust dose of levodopa with concomitant use. Concomitant Ciprofloxacin or Other CYP1A2 Inhibitors/Hepatic Impairment: 0.5mg qd. May be taken with or without food.

**HOW SUPPLIED:** Tab: 0.5mg, 1mg

**CONTRAINDICATIONS:** Concomitant use with meperidine, tramadol, methadone, propoxyphene, dextromethorphan, St. John's wort, cyclobenzaprine, during or within 14 days of other MAOI use.

**WARNINGS/PRECAUTIONS:** May increase incidence of melanoma. Concomitant use with levodopa may potentiate dopaminergic side effects and exacerbate pre-existing dyskinesia. Orthostatic/postural hypotension reported. Restrict dietary tyramines and avoid amine-containing medications for 2 weeks after d/c. Caution with serotonin syndrome and neuroleptic malignant syndrome. Hallucinations may develop, and may cause or exacerbate psychotic-like behavior.

**ADVERSE REACTIONS:** Headache, arthralgia, dyspepsia, depression, fall, flu syndrome, dyskinesia, accidental injury, N/V, weight loss, constipation, postural hypotension, dry mouth.

**INTERACTIONS:** See Contraindications. Concomitant use with SSRIs, SNRIs, tricyclic, tetracyclic and triazolopyridine antidepressants is not recommended due to severe CNS toxicity. Increased plasma concentrations up to 2-fold with concomitant ciprofloxacin and other CYP1A2 inhibitors. Severe hypertensive reactions reported with concomitant use of sympathomimetics, and other MAOIs.

**PREGNANCY:** Category C, caution in nursing.

**MECHANISM OF ACTION:** MAO-B inhibitor; suspected to inhibit MAO type B, which causes an increase in extracellular dopamine levels in the striatum and increases dopaminergic activity.

**PHARMACOKINETICS: Absorption**: Rapid. Absolute bioavailability (36%); $T_{max}$=1 hr. **Distribution**: $V_d$=87L; plasma protein binding (88-94%). **Metabolism**:

N-dealkylation, hydroxylation; CYP1A2: 1-aminoindan (AI), 3-hydroxy-N-propargyl-1 aminoindan (3-OH-PAI) and 3-hydroxy-1-aminoindan (3-OH-AI). **Elimination**: Urine (62% over 7 days), (84% over 38 days), (<1% unchanged), feces (7%); $T_{1/2}$=3 hrs.

## NURSING CONSIDERATIONS

**Assessment:** Assess LFTs, renal function tests, and dyskinesia. Note other diseases/conditions and drug therapies.

**Monitoring:** Monitor LFTs, renal function test, BP, signs of melanoma, hallucinations, postural hypotension, diarrhea, weight loss, rash, dyskinesia.

**Patient Counseling:** Instruct about the risks of therapy and to take meds with/without food. Restrict tyramine-rich foods (aged cheeses). Instruct to take as prescribed and not to double dose if a dose is missed. Report adverse side effects.

**Administration:** Oral route. **Storage**: 25°C (77°F); excursions permitted to 15-30°C (59-86°F).

# AZMACORT RX

triamcinolone acetonide (Abbott)

**THERAPEUTIC CLASS:** Corticosteroid

**INDICATIONS:** Maintenance treatment of asthma as prophylactic therapy in patients ≥6 yrs; to reduce or eliminate the need for oral corticosteroidal therapy.

**DOSAGE:** *Adults:* 2 inh (150mcg) tid-qid or 4 inh (300mcg) bid. Severe Asthma: Initial: 12-16 inh/day. Max: 16 inh/day (1200mcg). Rinse mouth after use.
*Pediatrics:* >12 yrs: 2 inh (150mcg) tid-qid or 4 inh (300mcg) bid. Severe Asthma: Initial: 12-16 inh/day. Max: 16 inh/day (1200mcg). 6-12 yrs: 1-2 inh (75-150mcg) tid-qid or 2-4 (150-300mcg) inh bid. Max: 12 inh/day (900mcg). Rinse mouth after use.

**HOW SUPPLIED:** MDI: 75mcg/inh [20g]

**CONTRAINDICATIONS:** Primary treatment of status asthmaticus or other acute asthma attacks.

**WARNINGS/PRECAUTIONS:** Deaths due to adrenal insufficiency have occurred with transfer from systemic corticosteroids to inhaled corticosteroids. Resume oral corticosteroids during stress or severe asthma attack. Observe for adrenal insufficiency, systemic corticosteroid withdrawal effects, hypercorticoidism and growth suppression (children). More susceptible to infections. Not for acute bronchospasm. D/C if bronchospasm occurs after dosing. Caution with TB of respiratory tract; untreated systemic fungal, bacterial, viral or parasitic infections; or ocular herpes simplex. *Candida* infection of mouth and pharynx reported.

**ADVERSE REACTIONS:** Pharyngitis, sinusitis, headache, flu syndrome.

**INTERACTIONS:** Caution with prednisone.

**PREGNANCY:** Category C, caution in nursing.

**MECHANISM OF ACTION:** Corticosteroid; not established. Inhaled route makes possible to provide local anti-inflammatory activity.

**PHARMACOKINETICS: Absorption:** $T_{max}$=1.5-2 hrs. **Distribution:** $V_d$=99.5L; plasma protein binding (68%). **Elimination:** Urine (40%), feces (60%); $T_{1/2}$=88 min.

## NURSING CONSIDERATIONS

**Assessment:** Assess for concomitant diseases such as status asthmaticus, active or quiescent pulmonary TB, untreated systemic fungal, bacterial, parasitic or viral infections, and possible drug interactions (prednisone).

**Monitoring:** Monitor for localized oral infections with *Candida albicans*, body height in children, adrenal insufficiency, paradoxical bronchospasm, and hypersensitivity reactions.

**Patient Counseling:** Inform not for relief of acute bronchospasm. Advise that drug may unmask allergies (rhinitis, conjunctivitis, eczema). Instruct to track use of drug and dispose canister after 240 actuations since reliable dose delivery not assured after 240 doses. Warn to avoid exposure to chickenpox or measles. Advise to seek medical attention if exposed to chickenpox or measles, symptoms do not improve or worsen, during periods of stress or severe asthmatic attack, paradoxical bronchospasm or hypersensitivity reaction occurs. Counsel to avoid spraying in eyes and shake well before each use.

**Administration:** Oral inhalation. **Storage:** 20-25°C (68-77°F). Do not puncture, use, or store near heat or open flame; do not freeze.

## AZOPT RX
brinzolamide (Alcon)

**THERAPEUTIC CLASS:** Carbonic anhydrase inhibitor

**INDICATIONS:** Open-angle glaucoma. Ocular hypertension.

**DOSAGE:** *Adults:* 1 drop tid. Space dosing with other ophthalmic drugs by 10 min.

**HOW SUPPLIED:** Sus: 1% [5mL, 10mL, 15mL]

**WARNINGS/PRECAUTIONS:** Systemically absorbed. Avoid with sulfonamide allergy or severe renal impairment. Caution with hepatic impairment. Not studied in acute angle-closure glaucoma.

**ADVERSE REACTIONS:** Blurred vision, taste disturbances, blepharitis, dermatitis, dry eye, foreign body sensation, headache, hyperemia, ocular discharge, ocular discomfort, ocular keratitis, ocular pain, ocular pruritus, rhinitis.

**INTERACTIONS:** Caution with high-dose salicylates. Acid-base disturbances with oral carbonic anhydrase inhibitors. Avoid oral carbonic anhydrase inhibitors due to additive effects. Wait 10 min before using another ophthalmic drug.

**PREGNANCY:** Category C, not for use in nursing.

**MECHANISM OF ACTION:** Carbonic anhydrase II inhibitor; inhibits aqueous humor formation and reduces elevated IOP.

**PHARMACOKINETICS: Distribution:** Plasma protein binding (60%). **Elimination:** Urine (unchanged).

### NURSING CONSIDERATIONS

**Assessment:** Assess for allergy to sulfonamides, hepatic/renal function prior to therapy, and possible drug interactions.

**Monitoring:** Monitor for signs/symptoms of Stevens-Johnson syndrome, toxic epidermal necrolysis, fulminant hepatic necrolysis, agranulocytosis, aplastic anemia, and other blood dyscrasias.

**Patient Counseling:** Advise to contact physician if any serious or unusual ocular or systemic reactions occur while on medication. Instruct to avoid touching container tip to the eye or any other surfaces. Instruct if having ocular surgery or if an intercurrent ocular condition (eg, trauma, infection) develops, to contact physician prior to using present multidose container. Instruct to remove contact lenses prior to administration; wait 15 min after administration to wear contact lenses. Advise that if using more than 1 topical ophthalmic medication, separate medication by at least 10 min.

**Administration:** Ocular route. **Storage:** 4-30°C (39-86°F).

## AZOR RX
amlodipine besylate - olmesartan medoxomil (Daiichi Sankyo)

**When used in pregnancy during 2nd and 3rd trimesters, drugs that act directly on the renin-angiotensin system can cause injury and even death to developing fetus. When pregnancy is detected, d/c therapy asap.**

**THERAPEUTIC CLASS:** ARB/Calcium channel blocker (dihydropyridine)

**INDICATIONS:** Treatment of hypertension, alone or with other antihypertensive agents. Initial therapy in patients likely to need multiple antihypertensive agents to achieve their BP goals.

**DOSAGE:** *Adults:* Replacement Therapy: May substitute for individually titrated components for patients on amlodipine and olmesartan. When substituting for individual components, the dose of 1 or both components may be increased if needed. Add-On Therapy: May be used to provide additional BP lowering when not adequately controlled on amlodipine or olmesartan alone. Initial Therapy: Initiate at 5mg-20mg qd. Titrate: May increase dose after 1-2 weeks to maximum dose of 10mg-40mg qd as needed to control BP. Max: 10mg-40mg qd.

**HOW SUPPLIED:** Tab: (Amlodipine-Olmesartan) 5mg-20mg, 5mg-40mg, 10mg-20mg, 10mg-40mg

**WARNINGS/PRECAUTIONS:** Hypotension, especially in volume- or salt-depleted patients, may occur with treatment initiation; monitor closely. Caution with severe aortic stenosis and HF. Increased risk of severe obstructive coronary artery disease (CAD), angina, or MI with CCBs may occur with dosage initiation or increase. Changes in renal function, oliguria, progressive azotemia, or acute renal failure may occur. Avoid initial therapy in patients ≥75 yrs or in patients with hepatic impairment

**ADVERSE REACTIONS:** Edema, dizziness, headache, palpitations.

**PREGNANCY:** Category C (1st trimester) and D (2nd and 3rd trimester), not for use in nursing.

**MECHANISM OF ACTION:** Amlodipine: Calcium channel receptor blocker (dihydropyridine); inhibits transmembrane influx of calcium ions into vascular smooth muscle and cardiac muscle. Olmesartan: Angiotensin II receptor blocker; blocks vasoconstrictor effect of angiotensin II.

**PHARMACOKINETICS: Absorption:** Amlodipine: $T_{max}$=6-12 hrs, absolute bioavailability (64-90%). Olmesartan: Rapid and complete, absolute bioavailability (26%), $T_{max}$=1-2 hrs. **Distribution:** Amlodipine: Plasma protein binding (93%). Olmesartan: $V_d$=17L, plasma protein binding (99%), crosses placental barrier; excreted in breast milk. **Metabolism:** Amlodipine: Liver. Olmesartan: Ester hydrolysis. **Elimination:** Amlodipine: Urine (60%); $T_{1/2}$=30-50 hrs. Olmesartan: Urine (35-50%), feces; $T_{1/2}$=13 hrs.

## NURSING CONSIDERATIONS

**Assessment:** Assess for severe obstructive CAD, CHF, severe aortic stenosis, volume/salt depletion, renal/hepatic impairment and pregnancy/nursing status.

**Monitoring:** Monitor for signs/symptoms of hypotension, hypersensitivity reactions, renal/hepatic dysfunction. Monitor for symptoms of severe obstructive CAD, angina or MI after dosage initiation or increase.

**Patient Counseling:** Inform of pregnancy risks. Notify physician if pregnant/intend to become pregnant, or if breastfeeding. Advise to seek medical attention if symptoms of hypotension or hypersensitivity reactions occur.

**Administration:** Oral route. **Storage:** 25°C (77°F); excursions permitted to 15-30°C (59-86°F).

# AZULFIDINE RX

sulfasalazine (Pharmacia & Upjohn)

**THERAPEUTIC CLASS:** 5-Aminosalicylic acid derivative/sulfapyridine

**INDICATIONS:** Treatment of mild to moderate ulcerative colitis. Adjunct therapy in severe ulcerative colitis. To prolong remission period between acute attacks of ulcerative colitis.

**DOSAGE:** *Adults:* Initial: 3-4g/day in evenly divided doses not >8-hr interval. May initiate at 1-2g/day to reduce GI intolerance. Maint: 2g/day. Response to therapy can be evaluated by clinical criteria (eg, presence of fever, weight changes, degree and frequency of diarrhea and bleeding, sigmoidoscopy, evaluation of biopsy samples). When endoscopic examination confirms satisfactory improvement, dosage should be reduced to maintenance level. If diarrhea recurs, dosage should be increased to previously effective levels. If symptoms of GI intolerance occur after 1st few doses, reduce dose in 1/2, then gradually increase. If GI intolerance persists, d/c for 5-7 days, then reintroduce at a lower dose.

*Pediatrics:* ≥6 yrs: 40-60mg/kg/day divided into 3-6 doses. Maint: 30mg/kg/day divided into 4 doses. Response to therapy can be evaluated by clinical criteria (eg, presence of fever, weight changes, degree and frequency of diarrhea and bleeding, sigmoidoscopy, evaluation of biopsy samples). When endoscopic examination confirms satisfactory improvement, dosage should be reduced to maintenance level. If diarrhea recurs, dosage should be increased to previously effective levels. If symptoms of GI intolerance occur after 1st few doses, reduce dose in 1/2, then gradually increase. If GI intolerance persists, d/c for 5-7 days, then reintroduce at a lower dose.

**HOW SUPPLIED:** Tab: 500mg* *scored

**CONTRAINDICATIONS:** Intestinal or urinary obstruction, porphyria, hypersensitivity to sulfonamides, salicylates.

**WARNINGS/PRECAUTIONS:** Caution with hepatic/renal impairment, blood dyscrasias, severe allergy, and bronchial asthma. Monitor patients with glucose 6-phosphate dehydrogenase deficiency for signs of hemolytic anemia. Deaths reported from hypersensitivity reactions, agraunulocytosis, aplastic anemia, other blood dyscrasias, renal and liver damage, irreversible neuromuscular and CNS changes, and fibrosing alveolitis. Presence of sore throat, fever, pallor, purpura, or jaundice may be the indications of serious blood disorder or hepatotoxicity. Monitor CBC including differential WBC, LFTs, at baseline, every 2nd week for 1st 3 months, monthly for next 3 months, and every 3 months thereafter. D/C while awaiting the results of blood tests. Monitor urinalysis and renal function periodically. Maintain adequate fluid intake to prevent crystalluria and stone formation. D/C if hypersensitivity or toxic reaction occurs. Oligospermia and infertility reported in males.

**ADVERSE REACTIONS:** Anorexia, headache, N/V, gastric distress, reversible oligospermia.

**INTERACTIONS:** Reduces absorption of folic acid, digoxin.

**PREGNANCY:** Category B, caution in nursing.

**MECHANISM OF ACTION:** 5-aminosalicylic acid (5-ASA) derivative/sulfapyridine (SP); not established, may be related to anti-inflammatory and/or immunomodulatory properties of sulfasalazine (SSZ) or its metabolites (5-ASA and SP), its affinity for connective tissue, and/or to relatively high concentration reached in serous fluids, the liver, and intestinal walls.

**PHARMACOKINETICS: Absorption:** SSZ: $C_{max}$=6µg/mL, $T_{max}$=6 hrs; Absolute bioavailability=<15%. 5-ASA, SP: $T_{max}$=10 hrs. SP: Well absorbed from colon. 5-ASA: Much less well absorbed from GI tract. **Distribution:** SSZ: $V_d$=7.5L; Plasma protein binding (>99.3%). SP: Plasma protein binding (70%). AcSP: Plasma protein binding (90%). **Metabolism:** Intestinal bacteria to 5-ASA and SP (metaolites); liver (acetylation). Found in breast milk. **Elimination:** Urine (37%), feces. SSZ: $T_{1/2}$=7.6 hrs (IV); SP: $T_{1/2}$=10.4 hrs (fast acetylators), 14.8 hrs (slow acetylators).

## NURSING CONSIDERATIONS

**Assessment:** Assess for intestinal or urinary obstruction, porphyria, blood dyscrasias, renal/liver damage, severe allergy or bronchial asthma, glucose 6-phosphate dehydrogenase deficiency, pregnancy/nursing status, and for possible drug interactions. Obtain baseline CBC, including differential WBC, LFTs.

**Monitoring:** Monitor for signs/symptoms of hypersensitivity reactions, agranulocytosis, aplastic anemia or other blood dyscrasias, renal and liver damage, neuromuscular and CNS changes, and for fibrosing alveolitis. Monitor for signs of hemolytic anemia in patients with glucose-6 phosphate dehydrogenase deficiency. Perform CBC, including differential WBC, and LFTs before start of therapy, every 2 weeks during the first 3 months of therapy, every month for second 3 months of therapy, then every 3 months during treatment. Perform periodic monitoring of serum SP levels, urinalysis, and renal function.

**Patient Counseling:** Advise about the possibility of adverse reactions and of the need for careful medical supervision. Instruct to seek medical attention if develop sore throat, fever, pallor, purpura, or jaundice. Inform that ulcerative colitis rarely remits completely and that risk of relapse can be substantially reduced by continued administration at a maintenance dosage. Instruct to take in evenly divided doses, preferably after meals. Advise that orange-yellow discoloration of urine or skin may occur.

**Administration:** Oral route. **Storage:** 25°C (77°F); excursions permitted to 15-30°C (59-86°F).

## AZULFIDINE EN **RX**

sulfasalazine (Pharmacia & Upjohn)

**THERAPEUTIC CLASS:** 5-Aminosalicylic acid derivative/sulfapyridine

**INDICATIONS:** Treatment of mild to moderate ulcerative colitis. Adjunct treatment of severe ulcerative colitis. To prolong the remission period between acute attacks of ulcerative colitis. Treatment of rheumatoid arthritis and pediatric patients with polyarticular-course juvenile rheumatoid arthritis that have responded inadequately to salicylates or other NSAIDs.

**DOSAGE:** *Adults:* Ulcerative Colitis: Initial: 3-4g/day in evenly divided doses at intervals not >8 hrs. May initiate at 1-2g/day to reduce GI intolerance. Maint: 2g/day. Rheumatoid Arthritis: Initial: 0.5-1g/day. Maint: 2g/day given bid. Swallow tabs whole after meals.
*Pediatrics:* ≥6 yrs: Ulcerative Colitis: Initial: 40-60mg/kg/day in 3-6 divided doses. Maint: 30mg/kg/day in 4 divided doses. Juvenile Rheumatoid Arthritis: 30-50mg/kg/day in 2 divided doses. To reduce GI effects give 1/4 to 1/3 initial dose; increase weekly for 1 month. Max: 2g/day. Swallow tabs whole after meals.

**HOW SUPPLIED:** Tab, Delayed-Release: 500mg

**CONTRAINDICATIONS:** Intestinal or urinary obstruction, porphyria, hypersensitivity to sulfonamides or salicylates.

**WARNINGS/PRECAUTIONS:** Caution with hepatic or renal impairment, blood dyscrasias, severe allergy, bronchial asthma or glucose 6-phosphate dehydrogenase deficiency. Monitor CBC, WBC, and LFTs prior to therapy and every 2nd week for the 1st 3 months, once monthly for next 3 months, then every 3 months thereafter. D/C while awaiting the result of blood tests. Monitor urinalysis and renal function periodically. Maintain adequate fluid intake to prevent crystalluria and stone formation. D/C if tabs pass undisintegrated, hypersensitivity or toxic reactions occur. Oligospermia and infertility reported in males.

**ADVERSE REACTIONS:** Anorexia, headache, N/V, gastric distress, reversible oligospermia, rash, pruritus, fever, dyspepsia, abdominal pain, dizziness, stomatitis, abnormal LFT, leukopenia.

**INTERACTIONS:** Reduces absorption of folic acid and digoxin. Increased incidence of GI adverse events with combination of sulfasalazine (2g/day) and methotrexate (7.5mg/week).

**PREGNANCY:** Category B, caution in nursing.

**MECHANISM OF ACTION:** 5-aminosalicylic acid (5-ASA) derivative/sulfapyridine (SP); not established, may be related to the anti-inflammatory and/or immunomodulatory properties of sulfasalazine (SSZ) or its metabolites (5-ASA and SP), its affinity for connective tissue, and/or to relatively high concentration reached in serous fluids, liver and intestinal wall.

**PHARMACOKINETICS: Absorption:** SSZ: $C_{max}$=6µg/mL, $T_{max}$=6 hrs; Absolute bioavailability=<15%. 5-ASA, SP: $T_{max}$=10 hrs. SP: Well absorbed from colon, estimated bioavailability=60%. 5-ASA: Much less well absorbed from GI tract, estimated bioavailability=10-30%. **Distribution:** SSZ: $V_d$=7.5L; plasma protein binding=>99.3%. SP: Plasma protein binding=70%. AcSP: plasma protein binding=90%. **Metabolism:** Intestinal bacteria to 5-ASA and SP; liver (acetylation).

Found in breast milk. **Elimination:** Urine (37%), feces. SSZ: $T_{1/2}$=7.6 hrs (IV), SP: $T_{1/2}$=10.4 hrs (fast acetylators), 14.8 hrs (slow acetylators).

## NURSING CONSIDERATIONS

**Assessment:** Assess for intestinal or urinary obstruction, porphyria, blood dyscrasias, renal/liver damage, severe allergy or bronchial asthma, pregnancy/nursing status, glucose 6-phosphate dehydrogenase deficiency and drug interactions. Obtain baseline CBC, including WBC, LFTs.

**Monitoring:** Perform CBC, including differential WBC and LFTs before start, every 2 weeks during the first 3 months, every month for second 3 months, then every 3 months. Monitor serum SP levels, urinalysis and renal function test periodically. Monitor for signs/symptoms of serious blood disorder (sore throat, fever, pallor, purpura, jaundice), hypersensitivity/allergic reactions, renal/hepatic dysfunction.

**Patient Counseling:** Inform that ulcerative colitis rarely remits completely and that risk of relapse can be substantially reduced by continued administration at maintenance dosage. Inform patient that rheumatoid arthritis rarely remits and that patients should follow up with their physician to determine the need for continued therapy. Instruct take in evenly divided doses after meals and to swallow tablet whole. Orange-yellow discoloration of urine or skin may occur. Inform to seek medical attention if sore throat, fever, pallor, purpura, or jaundice, allergic reactions or hypersensitivity occur.

**Administration:** Oral route. **Storage:** 25°C (77°F); excursions permitted to 15-30°C (59-86°F).

# BACLOFEN — RX

baclofen (Various)

**OTHER BRAND NAMES:** Kemstro (Schwarz)

**THERAPEUTIC CLASS:** GABA analog

**INDICATIONS:** Treatment of spasticity associated with multiple sclerosis. May be effective in spinal cord injuries and other spinal cord diseases.

**DOSAGE:** *Adults:* Initial: 5mg tid for 3 days. Titrate: May increase dose by 5mg tid every 3 days. Usual: 40-80mg/day. Max: 80 mg/day (20mg qid). Renal Impairment: Reduce dose.
*Pediatrics:* ≥12 yrs: Initial: 5mg tid for 3 days. Titrate: May increase dose by 5mg tid every 3 days. Usual: 40-80mg/day. Max: 80 mg/day (20mg qid). Renal Impairment: Reduce dose.

**HOW SUPPLIED:** Tab: (Generic) 10mg, 20mg; Tab, Disintegrating (ODT): (Kemstro) 10mg, 20mg

**WARNINGS/PRECAUTIONS:** Caution with psychosis, schizophrenia, confused states; may exacerbate conditions. Caution with bladder sphincter hypertonia, peptic ulceration, seizures, elderly, cerebrovascular disorder, respiratory failure, hepatic or renal failure. Abnormal AST, alkaline phosphatase and blood glucose reported. Caution when used to maintain locomotion or to obtain increased function. Decreased alertness with operating machinery. Has not significantly benefited stroke patients. Avoid abrupt discontinuation; reduce dose slowly over 1-2 weeks.

**ADVERSE REACTIONS:** Drowsiness, dizziness, weakness, fatigue, confusion, daytime sedation, headache, insomnia, hypotension, nausea, constipation, urinary frequency.

**INTERACTIONS:** May potentiate antihypertensives. May increase CNS depressant effects with MAO inhibitors. Potentiated by TCAs. Mental confusion, hallucinations and agitation with levodopa plus carbidopa therapy. May increase blood glucose and require dosage adjustment of antidiabetic agents. Synergistic effects with magnesium sulfate and other neuromuscular blockers. Additive CNS effects with alcohol and other CNS depressants.

**PREGNANCY:** Category C, caution in nursing.

**MECHANISM OF ACTION:** A GABA analog; muscle relaxant/antispastic agent; not fully known; capable of inhibiting both monosynaptic and polysynaptic reflexes at the spinal level, possibly by hyperpolarization of afferent terminals, although actions at supraspinal sites may also occur and contribute to its clinical effect.

## NURSING CONSIDERATIONS

**Assessment:** Assess for renal dysfunction, pregnancy/nursing status, epilepsy, and possible drug interactions.

**Monitoring:** Monitor for CNS depression, deterioration of seizure control, EEG changes, and ovarian cysts.

**Patient Counseling:** Caution against performing hazardous tasks (eg, operating machinery/driving). Notify if pregnant/nursing; not for use by children.

**Administration:** Oral route. **Storage:** 20-25°C (68-77°F); excursions permitted to 15-30°C (59-86°F); avoid moisture.

# BACTRIM RX

sulfamethoxazole - trimethoprim (AR Scientific)

**OTHER BRAND NAMES:** Bactrim DS (AR Scientific)

**THERAPEUTIC CLASS:** Sulfonamide/tetrahydrofolic acid inhibitor

**INDICATIONS:** Treatment of urinary tract infection (UTI), acute otitis media, acute exacerbation of chronic bronchitis (AECB), traveler's diarrhea, shigellosis. Treatment and prophylaxis against *Pneumocystis carinii* pneumonia (PCP) in immunosuppressed and those at increased risk.

**DOSAGE:** *Adults:* UTI/Shigellosis: 800mg-160mg or 2 tabs of 400mg-80mg q12h for 10-14 days (UTI) or 5 days (Shigellosis). AECB: 800mg-160mg or 2 tabs of 400mg-80mg q12h for 14 days. Traveler's Diarrhea: 800mg-160mg or 2 tabs of 400mg-80mg q12h for 5 days. PCP Treatment: 75-100mg/kg SMX and 15-20mg/kg TMP per 24 hrs given in equally divided doses q6h for 14-21 days. PCP Prophylaxis: 800mg-160mg qd. Renal Impairment: CrCl 15-30mL/min: 1/2 of usual dose. CrCl <15mL/min: Not recommended.
*Pediatrics:* ≥2 months: UTI/Otitis Media/Shigellosis: 40mg/kg SMX and 8mg/kg TMP per 24 hrs given in 2 divided doses q12h for 10 days (UTI/Otitis Media) or 5 days (Shigellosis). PCP Treatment: 75-100mg/kg SMX and 15-20mg/kg TMP per 24 hrs given in equally divided doses q6h for 14-21 days. PCP Prophylaxis: 750mg/m$^2$/day SMX and 150mg/m$^2$/day TMP given in equally divided doses bid, on 3 consecutive days/week. Max: 1600mg SMX and 320mg TMP/day. Renal Impairment: CrCl 15-30mL/min: 1/2 of usual dose. CrCl <15mL/min: Not recommended.

**HOW SUPPLIED:** (Sulfamethoxazole [SMX]-Trimethoprim [TMP]) Tab: 400mg-80mg*; Tab, DS: 800mg-160mg* *scored

**CONTRAINDICATIONS:** Megaloblastic anemia due to folate deficiency, pregnancy, nursing, infants <2 months, marked hepatic damage, severe renal insufficiency when renal status cannot be monitored.

**WARNINGS/PRECAUTIONS:** Fatal hypersensitivity reactions (eg, Stevens-Johnson syndrome, toxic epidermal necrolysis, fulminant hepatic necrosis, agranulocytosis, aplastic anemia and other blood dyscrasias) may occur; d/c at first appearance of skin rash or any sign of adverse reaction. *Clostridium difficile*-associated diarrhea (CDAD), cough, SOB, and pulmonary infiltrates reported. Thrombocytopenia reported; risk of fatal hemorrhage may occur. Monitor CBC frequently; d/c if with significant reduction in any formed blood element. Avoid with group A β-hemolytic streptococcal infections. Hemolysis may occur in glucose-6-phosphate dehydrogenase (G6PD)-deficient patients. Cases of hypoglycemia seen rarely. Caution with hepatic/renal impairment, elderly, possible folate deficiency (eg, chronic alcoholics, anticonvulsants, malabsorption, malnutrition), bronchial asthma and severe allergies. Increased incidence of adverse events (eg, hyperkalemia, mild intolerance) in AIDS patients; re-evaluate therapy if develops skin rash or any sign of adverse reactions. Hyperkalemia reported; caution in patients receiving high doses of

TMP and with underlying disorders of $K^+$ metabolism. Ensure adequate fluid intake and urinary output to prevent crystalluria. Slow acetylators more prone to idiosyncratic reactions to sulfonamides. Caution with porphyria or thyroid dysfunction. TMP may impair phenylalanine metabolism.

**ADVERSE REACTIONS:** N/V, anorexia, rash, urticaria.

**INTERACTIONS:** Increased incidence of thrombocytopenia with purpura in elderly patients with diuretics (primarily thiazides). May prolong PT with warfarin. Increased effects of phenytoin and oral hypoglycemics. Increased plasma levels of methotrexate and digoxin in elderly. Marked but reversible nephrotoxicity reported with cyclosporine in renal transplant recipients. May develop megaloblastic anemia with pyrimethamine >25mg/week. Increased SMX levels with indomethacin. May decrease efficacy of TCAs. Single case of toxic delirium with amantadine. Potentiate effects of oral hypoglycemics. May cause hyperkalemia in elderly patients with ACE inhibitors.

**PREGNANCY:** Category C, not for use in nursing.

**MECHANISM OF ACTION:** SMX: Inhibits bacterial synthesis of dyhydrofolic acid by competing with PABA. TMP: Blocks the production of tetrahydrofolic acid from dihydrofolic acid by binding to and reversibly inhibiting the required enzyme, dihydrofolate reductase.

**PHARMACOKINETICS: Absorption:** Rapid; $T_{max}$=1-4 hrs. **Distribution:** SMX: Plasma protein binding (70%); TMP: Plasma protein binding (44%). Crosses placenta, found in breast milk. **Metabolism:** SMX: $N_4$-acetylation; TMP: 1- and 3-oxides, 3'-4'-hydroxy derivatives (principal metabolites). **Elimination:** Urine (84.5% total sulfonamide), (66.8%, free TMP); $T_{1/2}$=10 hrs (SMX), 8-10 hrs (TMP).

## NURSING CONSIDERATIONS

**Assessment:** Assess for hypersensitivity reaction to drug components, documented megaloblastic anemia due to folate deficiency (eg, malabsorption syndrome, chronic alcoholic, malnutrition status, elderly, receiving anticonvulsant therapy), hepatic/renal insufficiency, severe allergies, bronchial asthma, G6PD deficiency, phenylketonurics, porphyria or thyroid dysfunction, underlying disorders of $K^+$ metabolism, slow acetylators, pregnancy/nursing status and possible drug interactions. Obtain baseline CBC.

**Monitoring:** Monitor for severe allergic reactions (eg, SJS, TEN, fulminant hepatic necrosis, agranulocytosis, aplastic anemia and other blood dyscrasias) and their clinical signs (eg, rash, sore throat, fever, arthralgia, pallor, purpura or jaundice), CDAD (mild diarrhea to fatal colitis), development of drug resistance, overgrowth of nonsusceptible microorganisms, hypersensitivity reactions of respiratory tract (eg, cough, SOB, pulmonary infiltrates), kernicterus if given to infants, hypogylcemia, signs of bone marrow depression after chronic use and interference with serum methotrexate assay and with the Jaffe alkaline picrate reaction assay for creatinine. Periodically monitor CBC, renal function, LFTs and $K^+$ levels and perform urinalysis with careful microscopic exam.

**Patient Counseling:** Inform about potential benefits/risks of therapy. Inform that drug only treats bacterial, not viral, infections. Instruct to take exactly as directed; skipping doses or not completing full course may decrease effectiveness and increase bacterial resistance. D/C and notify physician if allergic reaction, watery/bloody diarrhea (with/without stomach cramps) occur (may occur up to ≥2 months after treatment). Counsel to drink adequate fluids to prevent crystalluria and stone formation. Notify physician if pregnant/nursing or planning to become pregnant. Instruct medication is not recommended for use in pediatrics <2 months of age.

**Administration:** Oral route. **Storage:** 20-25°C (68-77°F). Dispense in tight, light-resistant container.

# BACTROBAN — RX

mupirocin (GlaxoSmithKline)

**THERAPEUTIC CLASS:** Bacterial protein synthesis inhibitor

**INDICATIONS:** (Oint) Topical treatment of impetigo due to *S. aureus* and *S. pyogenes*. (Cre) Treatment of secondarily infected traumatic skin lesions (up to 10cm in length or 100cm$^2$) due to *S. aureus* and *S. pyogenes*.

**DOSAGE:** *Adults:* (Oint) Apply tid. (Cre) Apply tid for 10 days. May cover with gauze. Re-evaluate if no response within 3-5 days.
*Pediatrics:* (Oint) 2 months -16 yrs: Apply tid. (Cre) 3 months-16 yrs: Apply tid for 10 days. May cover with gauze. Re-evaluate if no response within 3-5 days.

**HOW SUPPLIED:** Cre: 2% [15g, 30g]; Oint: 2% [22g]

**WARNINGS/PRECAUTIONS:** Avoid eyes. D/C if sensitization or irritation occurs. May cause superinfection with prolonged use. Caution with oint in renal dysfunction. Avoid mucosal surfaces. Avoid open wounds or damaged skin with oint.

**ADVERSE REACTIONS:** Burning, pain, pruritus, headache, rash, nausea.

**PREGNANCY:** Category B, caution in nursing.

**MECHANISM OF ACTION:** Bacterial protein synthesis inhibitor; inhibits bacterial protein synthesis by reversibly and specifically binding to bacterial isoleucyl transfer-RNA synthetase. Active against a wide range of gram-positive bacteria including methicillin-resistant *Staphylococcus aureus* (MRSA). Also active against certain gram-negative bacteria.

**PHARMACOKINETICS: Absorption:** Minimal percutaneous absorption. **Metabolism:** Rapid. Monic acid (inactive metabolite). **Elimination:** Renal (metabolite).

## NURSING CONSIDERATIONS

**Assessment:** Perform proper diagnosis of skin infection. Assess use in pregnant/nursing females.

**Monitoring:** Monitor for sensitization or severe local irritation of the skin. In patients on prolonged therapy, monitor for possible overgrowth of nonsusceptible microorganisms, including fungi.

**Patient Counseling:** Inform that medication is for external use only and to avoid contact of medication with the eyes. Counsel that treated area can be covered with a gauze dressing. Advise to contact physician and d/c medication if any signs of local adverse reactions (eg, irritation, severe itching, rash) develop. Notify if no clinical improvement is seen within 3-5 days.

**Administration:** Topical. **Storage:** Store at or below 25°C (77°F). Do not freeze.

# BACTROBAN NASAL RX

mupirocin calcium (GlaxoSmithKline)

**THERAPEUTIC CLASS:** Antibacterial agent

**INDICATIONS:** Eradication of nasal colonization of MRSA in adults and health-care workers in certain institutional settings during outbreaks of MRSA.

**DOSAGE:** *Adults:* Apply 1/2 of the single-use tube into each nostril bid for 5 days. Spread oint by pressing together and releasing the sides of the nose repetitively for 1 min. Do not re-use tube.
*Pediatrics:* ≥12 yrs: Apply 1/2 of the single-use tube into each nostril bid for 5 days. Spread oint by pressing together and releasing the sides of the nose repetitively for 1 min. Do not re-use tube.

**HOW SUPPLIED:** Oint: 2% [1g pkt]

**WARNINGS/PRECAUTIONS:** Avoid eyes. D/C if sensitization or irritation occur. May cause superinfection with prolonged use.

**ADVERSE REACTIONS:** Headache, rhinitis, respiratory disorder, pharyngitis, taste perversion.

**INTERACTIONS:** Avoid use with other intranasal products.

**PREGNANCY:** Category B, caution in nursing.

**MECHANISM OF ACTION:** Antibacterial agent; inhibits protein synthesis by reversibly and specifically binding to bacterial isoleucyl transfer-RNA synthetase.

**PHARMACOKINETICS: Absorption:** Significant in neonates and premature infants. **Elimination:** Urine.

## NURSING CONSIDERATIONS

**Assessment:** Assess for drug hypersensitivity, high-risk health care workers during institutional outbreaks of methicillin-resistant *S.aureus,* possible drug interactions.

**Monitoring:** Monitor for sensitization, severe local irritation, tearing, and for overgrowth of nonsusceptible microorganisms (eg, fungi).

**Patient Counseling:** Avoid contact with eyes. Consult physician if sensitization or severe irritation occurs.

**Administration:** Intranasal route. Apply approximately half of ointment from single-use tube directly into 1 nostril and other half into other nostril; discard tube after using. Press sides of nose together and gently massage after application to spread ointment throughout inside of nostril. **Storage:** 20-25°C (68-77°F); excursions permitted to 15-30°C (59-86°F). Do not refrigerate.

# BANZEL RX

rufinamide (Eisai)

**THERAPEUTIC CLASS:** Triazole derivative

**INDICATIONS:** Adjunctive treatment of seizures associated with Lennox-Gastaut syndrome in adults and children ≥4 yrs.

**DOSAGE:** *Adults:* Initial: 400-800mg/day in two equally divided doses. Titrate: May increase by 400-800mg/day every two days until max of 3200mg/day, given in two equally divided doses. Max: 3200mg/day. Take with food. May give as whole tabs, half-tabs, or crushed. Elderly: Start at the low end of the dosing range.
*Pediatrics:* ≥4 yrs: Initial: 10mg/kg/day in two equally divided doses. Titrate: May increase by 10mg/kg increments every other day to target dose of 45mg/kg/day or 3200mg/day, whichever is less, given in two equally divided doses. Max: 45mg/kg/day or 3200mg/day. Take with food. May give as whole tabs, half-tabs, or crushed.

**HOW SUPPLIED:** Tab: 200mg*, 400mg* *scored

**CONTRAINDICATIONS:** Familial short QT syndrome.

**WARNINGS/PRECAUTIONS:** May increase risk of suicidal thoughts or behavior; monitor for emergence or worsening of depression, or any unusual changes in mood or behavior. Associated with CNS-related adverse effects (somnolence/fatigue, coordination abnormalities, dizziness, gait disturbance and ataxia). QT interval shortening reported. Multi-organ hypersensitivity syndrome reported; d/c if signs and symptoms (fever, rash) develop. Withdraw gradually to minimize risk of precipitating seizures, seizure exacerbation, or status epilepticus. Avoid with severe hepatic impairment. Caution with mild to moderate hepatic impairment and elderly.

**ADVERSE REACTIONS:** Somnolence, N/V, headache, fatigue, dizziness, tremor, nystagmus, nasopharyngitis, rash, ataxia, diplopia, bronchitis, blurred vision.

**INTERACTIONS:** Potent CYP450 inducers (eg, carbamazepine, phenytoin, primodone, phenobarbital) may increase clearance of rufinamide. Valproate may reduce clearance and increase levels; initiate valproate at low dose and titrate to clinically effective dose. Decreases lamotrigine concentration by 7-13%. May decrease levels of hormonal contraceptives; additional forms of contraception are recommended during coadministration. May decrease levels of drugs that are substrates of CYP3A4 (eg, triazolam). May increase plasma levels of drugs that are substrates of CYP2E1 (eg, chlorzoxazone). Caution with other drugs that shorten QT interval. May increase clearance with carboxylesterase inducer. May decrease metabolism with carboxylesterase inhibitors. Other CNS-acting medications and alcohol may cause additive CNS effects.

**PREGNANCY:** Category C, not for use in nursing.

**MECHANISM OF ACTION:** Triazole derivative; mechanism not established. Suspected to modulate activity of sodium channels and, in particular, prolongation of the inactive state of the channel. Slows channel recovery from inactivation after prolonged prepulse in cultured cortical neurons, and limited sustained repetitive firing of sodium-dependent action potentials (in-vitro studies).

**PHARMACOKINETICS: Absorption:** Well-absorbed, $T_{max}$=4-6 hrs. **Distribution:** Plasma protein binding (34%); $V_d$=50L (3200mg/day); found in breast milk. **Metabolism:** Via hydrolysis; CGP 47292, CYP2E1 (weak inhibitor), CYP3A4 (weak inducer). **Elimination:** Urine (2%, unchanged); $T_{1/2}$=6-10 hrs.

## NURSING CONSIDERATIONS

**Assessment:** Assess for history of depression, familial short QT syndrome, ventricular arrhythmias, hepatic dysfunction, possible drug interactions, and pregnancy/nursing status.

**Monitoring:** Monitor for emergence or worsening of depression, suicidal thoughts, change in behavior, QT interval shortening and other arrhythmias, seizures, rash associated with fever, and for pregnancy during therapy.

**Patient Counseling:** Inform patients, caregivers, and families of the high risk of suicidal thoughts and behavior and to be alert for emergence or worsening of signs/symptoms of depression, unusual changes in mood or behavior, suicidal thoughts and behavior, and thoughts of self-harm. Instruct to take only as prescribed and to avoid alcohol. Counsel about potential somnolence or dizziness. Advise not to drive or operate machinery until gaining sufficient experience to gauge whether therapy adversely affects mental and/or motor performance. Notify physician if pregnant or intend to become pregnant, and if breastfeeding or intend to breastfeed. Encourage patients to enroll in North American Antiepileptic Drug (NAAED) Pregnancy Registry by calling 888-233-2334 or go to www.aedpregnancyregistry.org. Instruct to seek consultation if rash with fever occurs. Tabs are scored on both sides and may be cut in half for dosing flexibility; swallow as whole, as half tabs or crushed.

**Administration:** Oral route. **Storage:** Store at 25°C (77°F); excursions permitted to 15°-30°C (59°F-86°F). Protect from moisture.

# BARACLUDE RX

entecavir (Bristol-Myers Squibb)

**Lactic acidosis and severe, possibly fatal, hepatomegaly with steatosis reported. Reports of severe acute exacerbations of hepatitis B upon discontinuation of therapy. Follow-up liver function monitoring required. Limited clinical experience suggests there is a potential for the development of resistance to HIV nucleoside reverse transcriptase inhibitors if Entecavir is used to treat chronic hepatitis B virus infection in patients with HIV infection that is not being treated. Not recommended for HIV/HBV coinfected who are not receiving highly active antiretroviral therapy (HAART).**

**THERAPEUTIC CLASS:** Guanosine nucleoside analogue

**INDICATIONS:** Treatment of chronic hepatitis B virus (HBV) infection with active viral replication and persistent elevations in serum aminotransferases (ALT or AST) or histologically active disease.

**DOSAGE:** *Adults:* Nucleoside-Treatment-Naive: 0.5mg qd. CrCl 30 to <50mL/min: 0.25mg qd or 0.5mg q48h. CrCl 10 to <30mL/min: 0.15mg qd or 0.5mg q72h. CrCl <10mL/min: 0.05mg qd or 0.5mg q7 days. Receiving Lamivudine or Known Lamivudine Resistance Mutation: 1mg qd. CrCl 30 to <50mL/min: 0.5mg qd or 1mg q48h. CrCl 10 to <30mL/min: 0.3mg qd or 1mg q72h. CrCl <10mL/min: 0.1mg qd or 1mg q7 days. Take on empty stomach. *Pediatrics:* ≥16 yrs: Nucleoside-Treatment-Naive:0.5mg qd. CrCl 30 to <50mL/min: 0.25mg qd or 0.5mg q48h. CrCl 10 to <30mL/min: 0.15mg qd or 0.5mg q72h. CrCl <10mL/min: 0.05mg qd or 0.5mg q7 days. Receiving Lamivudine or Known Lamivudine Resistance Mutation: 1mg qd. CrCl 30 to <50mL/min: 0.5mg qd or 1mg q48h. CrCl 10 to <30mL/min: 0.3mg qd or 1mg q72h. CrCl <10mL/min: 0.1mg qd or 1mg q7 days. Take on empty stomach.

**HOW SUPPLIED:** Sol: 0.05mg/mL; Tab: 0.5mg, 1mg

**WARNINGS/PRECAUTIONS:** Reduce dose in renal dysfunction (CrCl <50mL/min) including patients on hemodialysis or continuous ambulatory peritoneal dialysis (CAPD). Exacerbations of hepatitis after discontinuation of treatment. Caution with known risk factors of liver disease. D/C with lactic acidosis and hepatotoxicity.

**ADVERSE REACTIONS:** Headache, fatigue, dizziness, nausea, hyperglycemia, ALT >5.0 X ULN, lipase ≥2.1 X ULN, glycosuria, hematuria, anaphylactoid reactions, alopecia, rash, acute hepatitis exacerbation after d/c of entecavir, lactic acidosis, and severe hepatomegaly with steatosis.

**INTERACTIONS:** May increase serum concentrations of entecavir or coadministered drug with drugs that reduce renal function or compete for active tubular secretion.

**PREGNANCY:** Category C, not for use in nursing.

**MECHANISM OF ACTION:** Guanosine nucleoside analogue; inhibits base priming, reverse transcription of negative strand from pregenomic mRNA, and synthesis of positive strand of HBV DNA.

**PHARMACOKINETICS: Absorption:** (0.5mg) $C_{max}$=4.2ng/mL; $T_{max}$=0.5-1.5 hrs. (1.0mg) $C_{max}$=8.2ng/mL. **Distribution:** Extensively into tissues, human protein binding (13% in vitro). **Metabolism:** Hepatic (minor). **Elimination:** Kidneys; urine (62-73% unchanged); $T_{1/2}$=128-149 hrs.

## NURSING CONSIDERATIONS

**Assessment:** Assess for hepatic/renal impairment, HIV antibody testing, pregnancy/nursing status and possible drug interactions.

**Monitoring:** Periodic monitoring of hepatic/renal function is recommended during treatment and for those who d/c anti-hepatitis B therapy for at least several months.

**Patient Counseling:** Advise to read Patient Information before taking entecavir and with each refill. Advise to take on an empty stomach ( ≥2 hrs pc and 2 hrs before next meal). Inform that deterioration of liver disease may occur in some cases if treatment is discontinued, and should discuss any change in regimen. Counsel on serious side effects (eg, lactic acidosis. hepatotoxicity). Inform that treatment has not shown to reduce risk of transmission of HBV. Advise to remain under care of physician; discuss new symptoms or concurrent medications. Offer HIV antibody testing before starting therapy. Instruct to take a missed dose as soon as remembered but not to take two doses at the same time.

**Administration:** Oral route. For oral solution, hold dosing spoon in a vertical position and fill gradually to the mark corresponding to prescribed dose. **Storage:** 25°C (77°F); excursion permitted between 15-30°C (59-86°F). Protect from light. Do not store in a damp place.

# BAYER ASPIRIN — OTC

aspirin (Bayer Healthcare)

**OTHER BRAND NAMES:** Genuine Bayer Aspirin (Bayer Healthcare) - Bayer Aspirin Regimen (Bayer Healthcare) - Bayer Aspirin Regimen with Calcium (Bayer Healthcare) - Bayer Aspirin Children's (Bayer Healthcare)

**THERAPEUTIC CLASS:** Salicylate

**INDICATIONS:** To reduce the risk of death and nonfatal stroke with previous ischemic stroke or transient ischemia of the brain. To reduce risk of vascular mortality with suspected acute MI. To reduce risk of death and nonfatal MI with previous MI or unstable angina. To reduce risk of MI and sudden death in chronic stable angina pectoris. For patients who have undergone revascularization procedures with a pre-existing condition for which ASA is indicated.

B

Relief of signs of rheumatoid arthritis (RA), juvenile rheumatoid arthritis (JRA), osteoarthritis (OA), spondyloarthropathies, arthritis, and pleurisy associated with systemic lupus erythematosus (SLE). For minor aches and pains.

**DOSAGE:** *Adults:* Ischemic Stroke/TIA: 50-325mg qd. Suspected Acute MI: Initial: 160-162.5mg qd as soon as suspect MI. Maint: 160-162.5mg qd for 30 days post-infarction, consider further therapy for prevention/recurrent MI. Prevention or Recurrent MI/Unstable Angina/Chronic Stable Angina: 75-325mg qd. CABG: 325mg qd, start 6 hrs post-surgery. Continue for 1 yr. PTCA: Initial: 325mg, 2 hrs pre-surgery. Maint: 160-325mg qd. Carotid Endarterectomy: 80mg qd to 650mg bid, start pre-surgery. RA: Initial: 3g qd in divided doses. Increase for anti-inflammatory efficacy to 150-300mcg/mL plasma salicylate level. Spondyloarthropathies: Up to 4g/day in divided doses. OA: Up to 3g/day in divided doses. Arthritis/SLE Pleurisy: Initial: 3g/day in divided doses. Increase for anti-inflammatory efficacy to 150-300mcg/mL plasma salicylate level. Pain: 325-650mg q4-6h. Max: 4g/day.
*Pediatrics:* JRA: Initial: 90-130mg/kg/day in divided doses. Increase for anti-inflammatory efficacy to 150-300mcg/mL plasma salicylate level. Pain: ≥12 yrs: 325-650mg q4-6h. Max: 4g/day.

**HOW SUPPLIED:** Tab: (Genuine Bayer Aspirin) 325mg; Tab: (Bayer Aspirin Regimen with Calcium) 81mg; Tab, Chewable: (Bayer Aspirin Children's) 81mg; Tab, Delayed-Release: (Bayer Aspirin Regimen) 81mg, 325mg

**CONTRAINDICATIONS:** NSAID allergy, viral infections in children or teenagers, syndrome of asthma, rhinitis, and nasal polyps.

**WARNINGS/PRECAUTIONS:** Increased risk of bleeding with heavy alcohol use ( ≥3 drinks/day). May inhibit platelet function; can adversely affect inherited (hemophilia) or acquired (hepatic disease, vitamin K deficiency) bleeding disorders. Monitor for bleeding and ulceration. Avoid in history of active peptic ulcer, severe renal failure, severe hepatic insufficiency, and sodium-restricted diets. Associated with elevated LFTs, BUN, and SrCr; hyperkalemia; proteinuria; and prolonged bleeding time. Avoid 1 week before and during labor.

**ADVERSE REACTIONS:** Fever, hypothermia, dysrhythmias, hypotension, agitation, cerebral edema, dehydration, hyperkalemia, dyspepsia, GI bleed, hearing loss, tinnitus, problems in pregnancy.

**INTERACTIONS:** Diminished hypotensive and hyponatremic effects of ACE inhibitors. May increase levels of acetazolamide, valproic acid. Increased bleeding risk with heparin, warfarin. Decreased levels of phenytoin. Decreased hypotensive effects of β-blockers. Decreased diuretic effects with renal or cardiovascular disease. Decreased methotrexate clearance; increased risk of bone marrow toxicity. Avoid NSAIDs. Increased effects of hypoglycemic agents. Antagonizes uricosuric agents.

**PREGNANCY:** Avoid in 3rd trimester of pregnancy and nursing.

**MECHANISM OF ACTION:** Provides temporary relief from arthritis pain and arthritis inflammation.

## NURSING CONSIDERATIONS

**Assessment:** Assess for hypersensitivity, stomach problems, bleeding problems, ulcers, history of chickenpox or flu symptoms, and possible drug interactions.

**Monitoring:** Monitor for Reye's syndrome, allergic reactions include hives, facial swelling, asthma (wheezing) and shock.

**Patient Counseling:** Instruct to immediately report worsening of any adverse effects.

**Administration:** Oral route. **Storage:** Room temperature.

# BECONASE AQ RX

beclomethasone dipropionate (GlaxoSmithKline)

**THERAPEUTIC CLASS:** Corticosteroid

**INDICATIONS:** Relief of symptoms of seasonal or perennial allergic and nonallergic rhinitis. Prevention of nasal polyp recurrence following surgical removal.

**DOSAGE:** *Adults:* 1-2 sprays per nostril bid. Max: 2 sprays per nostril bid. *Pediatrics:* >12 years: 1-2 sprays per nostril bid. 6-12 yrs: Initial: 1 spray per nostril bid. Titrate: May increase to 2 sprays per nostril. Decrease to 1 spray per nostril bid once adequate control achieved. Max: 2 sprays per nostril bid.

**HOW SUPPLIED:** Spray: 42mcg/spray [25g]

**WARNINGS/PRECAUTIONS:** Risk of adrenal insufficiency and withdrawal symptoms when replacing systemic corticosteroids with topical corticosteroids. Caution with active or quiescent tuberculous (TB), ocular herpes simplex, or untreated bacterial, fungal and systemic viral or parasitic infections. Avoid with recent nasal trauma/surgery or septum ulcers. Risk for more severe/fatal course of infections (eg, chickenpox, measles) and for *Candida* infections of nose and pharynx. Potential for reduced growth velocity in pediatrics. Rare cases of nasal septum perforation, wheezing, cataracts, glaucoma, increased intraocular pressure reported. Hypersensitivity reactions may occur. D/C if nasopharyngeal irritation persists. Caution in elderly.

**ADVERSE REACTIONS:** Nasopharyngeal irritation, sneezing, headache, nausea, lightheadedness, irritated/dry nose and throat, unpleasant taste/smell.

**INTERACTIONS:** Concomitant systemic corticosteroids increase risk of hypercorticism and/or HPA axis suppression.

**PREGNANCY:** Category C, caution in nursing.

**MECHANISM OF ACTION:** Corticosteroid; mechanism not established; anti-inflammatory and vasoconstrictor effects.

**PHARMACOKINETICS: Absorption:** Absolute bioavailability (44%) (for the active metabolite B-17-MP). $C_{max}$<50pg/mL. **Distribution:** $V_d$=20L (parent drug); $V_d$=424L (B-17-MP). Plasma protein binding (87%). **Metabolism:** B-17-MP (active metabolite) via esterase enzymes. **Elimination:** Urine (12% metabolites), feces (60% metabolites). $T_{1/2}$=0.5 hrs (parent drug), 2.7 hrs (B-17-MP).

## NURSING CONSIDERATIONS

**Assessment:** Assess for associated asthma with history of long-term therapy with systemic steroids, active or quiescent TB of upper respiratory tract, untreated local or systemic fungal or bacterial infections, systemic viral or parasitic infections, ocular herpes simplex, nasal polyps or recent nasal septal ulcers, nasal surgery/trauma, and possible drug interactions.

**Monitoring:** Monitor for reduced growth velocity (in pediatrics), nasal septum perforation, localized infection, *Candida* infection, exacerbation of infections, nasopharyngeal irritation, signs of adrenal insufficiency, and symptoms of hypercorticism.

**Patient Counseling:** Instruct to take as directed at regular intervals and to avoid exposure to chickenpox or measles. Consult physician immediately if exposed to infection or symptoms do not improve, if the condition worsens, or if sneezing or nasal irritation occurs. Advise to avoid spraying in the eyes.

**Administration:** Intranasal route. **Storage:** 15-30°C (59-86°F).

# BENICAR — RX

olmesartan medoxomil (Daiichi Sankyo)

**Avoid use in pregnancy; may cause death/injury to developing fetus.**

**THERAPEUTIC CLASS:** Angiotensin II receptor antagonist

**INDICATIONS:** Treatment of hypertension alone or in combination with other antihypertensives.

**DOSAGE:** *Adults:* Individualized dosing. Monotherapy Without Volume Depletion: Initial: 20mg qd. Titrate: May increase to 40mg qd after 2 weeks if needed. May add diuretic if BP not controlled. Intravascular Volume Depletion (eg, with diuretics, impaired renal function): Lower initial dose; monitor closely.

B

*Pediatrics:* 6-16yrs: Individualized dosing. 20-<35kg: Usual: 10mg qd. Titrate: May increase to 20 mg qd after 2 weeks if needed. ≥35kg: Usual: 20mg qd. Titrate: May increase to 40mg qd after 2 weeks if needed. If Cannot Swallow Tablets: Refer to PI for preparation of suspension; follow same dose as tablets.

**HOW SUPPLIED:** Tab: 5mg, 20mg, 40mg

**WARNINGS/PRECAUTIONS:** Symptomatic hypotension may occur in volume- and/or salt-depleted patients; correct volume depletion prior to therapy and monitor closely. Changes in renal function may occur; caution in renal artery stenosis and severe CHF. Increase in SrCr or BUN reported with renal artery stenosis.

**ADVERSE REACTIONS:** Dizziness.

**PREGNANCY:** Category C (1st trimester) and D (2nd and 3rd trimesters), not for use in nursing.

**MECHANISM OF ACTION:** Angiotensin II receptor antagonist; blocks vasoconstrictor effects of angiotensin II by selectively blocking binding of angiotensin II to $AT_1$ receptor in vascular smooth muscle.

**PHARMACOKINETICS: Absorption:** Rapid, complete. Absolute bioavailability (26%); $T_{max}$=1-2 hrs. **Distribution:** $V_d$=17L; plasma protein binding (99%). **Metabolism:** Ester hydrolysis. **Elimination:** Urine (35-50%), feces; $T_{1/2}$=13 hrs.

## NURSING CONSIDERATIONS

**Assessment:** Assess for pregnancy/nursing status, volume/salt depletion, and renal/hepatic impairment.

**Monitoring:** Monitor LFTs and renal function periodically. Monitor for signs/symptoms of hypotension, renal/hepatic dysfunction.

**Patient Counseling:** Inform of pregnancy risks. Advise to seek medical attention if symptoms of hypotension occur. Inform that drug may be taken with/without food.

**Administration:** Oral route. **Storage:** 20-25°C (68-77°F).

# Benicar HCT RX

olmesartan medoxomil - hydrochlorothiazide (Daiichi Sankyo)

**Can cause death/injury to developing fetus during 2nd and 3rd trimesters. Stop therapy if pregnancy detected.**

**THERAPEUTIC CLASS:** Angiotensin II receptor antagonist/thiazide diuretic

**INDICATIONS:** Hypertension. Not for initial therapy.

**DOSAGE:** *Adults:* If BP not controlled with olmesartan alone: Add HCTZ 12.5mg qd. May titrate to 25mg qd if BP uncontrolled after 2-4 weeks. If BP not controlled with HCTZ alone: Add olmesartan 20mg qd. May titrate to 40mg qd if BP uncontrolled after 2-4 weeks. Intravascular Volume Depletion (eg, with diuretics, impaired renal function): Lower initial dose; monitor closely. Elderly: Start at lower end of dosing range.

**HOW SUPPLIED:** Tab: (Olmesartan-HCTZ) 20mg-12.5mg, 40mg-12.5mg, 40mg-25mg

**CONTRAINDICATIONS:** Sulfonamide hypersensitivity.

**WARNINGS/PRECAUTIONS:** Can cause fetal injury/death. Correct volume or salt depletion before therapy or monitor closely. Caution with hepatic or severe renal dysfunction, progressive liver disease, history of allergies or asthma, renal artery stenosis, severe CHF. Avoid if CrCl ≤30mL/min. May exacerbate or activate SLE. Monitor serum electrolytes. Hyperuricemia, hyperglycemia, hypercalcemia, hypomagnesemia may occur. May increase cholesterol and triglyceride levels.

**ADVERSE REACTIONS:** Dizziness, upper respiratory tract infection, hyperuricemia, NV, asthenia, angioedema, hyperkalemia, rhabdomyolysis, ARF, alopecia, urticaria.

**INTERACTIONS:** Potentiates orthostatic hypotension with alcohol, barbiturates, or narcotics. May need to adjust antidiabetics. Potentiates other antihypertensives. Impaired absorption with cholestyramine, colestipol. Corticosteroids, ACTH deplete electrolytes. May decrease response to pressor amines. May potentiate non-depolarizing skeletal muscle relaxants. Risk of lithium toxicity. NSAIDs decrease diuretic effects.

**PREGNANCY:** Category C (1st trimester) and D (2nd and 3rd trimesters), not for use in nursing.

**MECHANISM OF ACTION:** Olmesartan: Angiotensin II receptor antagonist; blocks vasoconstrictor effects of angiotensin II by selectively blocking binding of angiotensin II to $AT_1$ receptor in vascular smooth muscle. HCTZ: Thiazide diuretic; affects renal tubular mechanism of electrolyte reabsorption, directly increasing excretion of $Na^+$ and $Cl^-$ and indirectly reducing plasma volume.

**PHARMACOKINETICS: Absorption:** Olmesartan: Rapid, complete; absolute bioavailability (26%); $T_{max}$=1-2 hrs. **Distribution:** Olmesartan: $V_d$=17 L; plasma protein binding (99%). Crosses placenta; excreted in breast milk. HCTZ: Crosses placenta; excreted in breast milk. **Metabolism:** Olmesartan: Ester hydrolysis. **Elimination:** Olmesartan: Urine (35-50%), feces; $T_{1/2}$=13 hrs. HCTZ: Kidney (61%); $T_{1/2}$=5.6-14.8 hrs.

## NURSING CONSIDERATIONS

**Assessment:** Assess for pregnancy status, possible drug interactions, volume/salt depletion, SLE, DM, anuria, sulfonamide hypersensitivity, history of allergy or bronchial asthma, hepatic/renal impairment.

**Monitoring:** Monitor serum electrolytes periodically. Monitor for signs/symptoms of electrolyte imbalance, exacerbation or activation of systemic lupus erythematosus (SLE), hypotension, hyperglycemia, hyperuricemia or precipitation of gout, hypersensitivity reactions, renal/hepatic dysfunction.

**Patient Counseling:** Inform of pregnancy risks. Advise that inadequate fluid intake or loss of fluids may result in drop of BP, leading to lightheadedness or syncope. Advise to seek medical attention if syncope, symptoms of electrolyte imbalance (dry mouth, thirst, weakness, lethargy), or hypersensitivity reactions occur.

**Administration:** Oral route. **Storage:** 20-25°C (68-77°F).

# BENTYL — RX

dicyclomine HCl (Axcan Scandipharm)

**THERAPEUTIC CLASS:** Anticholinergic

**INDICATIONS:** Treatment of functional bowel/irritable bowel syndrome.

**DOSAGE:** *Adults:* (Tab/Syrup) Initial: 20mg qid. Usual: 40mg qid if tolerated. Discontinue if no improvement after 2 weeks or if doses ≥80mg/day are not tolerated. (Inj) 20mg IM qid for 1-2 days, followed by oral dicyclomine. Not for IV use.

**HOW SUPPLIED:** Cap: 10mg; Inj: 10mg/mL; Syrup: 10mg/5mL; Tab: 20mg

**CONTRAINDICATIONS:** GI tract obstruction, obstructive uropathy, severe ulcerative colitis, reflux esophagitis, glaucoma, myasthenia gravis, unstable cardiovascular status and in acute hemorrhage, nursing mothers, infants <6 months of age.

**WARNINGS/PRECAUTIONS:** Caution in autonomic neuropathy, hepatic/renal impairment, ulcerative colitis, hyperthyroidism, HTN, CHF, cardiac tachyarrhythmia, coronary heart disease, hiatal hernia, and prostatic hypertrophy. Heat prostration may occur in high environmental temperature. Monitor for diarrhea, may be the early symptom of intestinal obstruction. Psychosis reported. Serious respiratory symptoms, seizures, syncope and death reported in infants.

**ADVERSE REACTIONS:** Dry mouth, NV, blurred vision, dizziness, drowsiness, nervousness, mental confusion/excitement (especially in the elderly), mydriasis, increased ocular tension, urinary retention, dyspnea, apnea, tachycardia, decreased sweating, lactation suppression, impotence.

B

**INTERACTIONS:** Potentiated by amantadine, Class I antiarrhythmics (eg, quinidine), antihistamines, antipsychotics (eg, phenothiazines), benzodiazepines, MAOIs, narcotic analgesics (eg, meperidine), nitrates/nitrites, sympathomimetics, TCAs. Antagonizes the effects of antiglaucoma agents; do not give with corticosteroid eye drops. Antagonizes the effect of metoclopramide. May effect the GI absorption of delayed release digoxin. Decreased absorption with antacids. Antagonized by drugs treating achlorhydria and those used to test gastric secretion.

**PREGNANCY:** Category B, contraindicated in nursing.

**MECHANISM OF ACTION:** Dicyclomine anticholinergic and antispasmodic agent; relieves smooth muscle spasm of the GI tract, and antagonizes bradykinin- and histamine-induced spasms.

**PHARMACOKINETICS: Absorption:** Rapidly absorbed; $T_{max}$=60-90 mins. **Distribution:** $V_d$=approximately 3.65L/Kg (extensive); excreted in breast milk **Elimination:** Urine (79.5%), feces (8.4%); $T_{1/2}$=1.8 hrs.

## NURSING CONSIDERATIONS

**Assessment:** Assess for glaucoma, obstructive uropathy, obstructive disease of GI tract, paralytic ileus, ulcerative colitis, myasthenia gravis, hiatal hernia associated with reflux esophagitis, renal/hepatic dysfunction, hyperthyroidism, cardiac disorders.

**Monitoring:** Monitor for heat prostration, drowsiness, blurred vision, increased HR, constipation, diarrhea, urinary hesitancy/retention, hypersensitivity reactions.

**Patient Counseling:** Review side effects and report if any develop. Exercise caution while operating machinery/driving. Avoid high environmental temperatures.

**Administration:** PO, IM. IM form should not be used for more than 2 days. **Storage:** Cap/Tab/Syrup/Inj: Room temperature below 30°C (86°F). Syrup: Protect from excessive heat. Inj: Protect from freezing.

# BenzaClin — RX

clindamycin phosphate - benzoyl peroxide (Dermik)

**THERAPEUTIC CLASS:** Antibacterial/keratolytic

**INDICATIONS:** Topical treatment of acne vulgaris.

**DOSAGE:** *Adults:* Wash face and pat dry. Apply bid (am and pm). *Pediatrics:* ≥12 yrs: Wash face and pat dry. Apply bid (am and pm).

**HOW SUPPLIED:** Gel: (Clindamycin-Benzoyl Peroxide) 1%-5% [25g, 35g, 50g]

**CONTRAINDICATIONS:** History of regional enteritis, ulcerative colitis, or antibiotic-associated colitis.

**WARNINGS/PRECAUTIONS:** Diarrhea, bloody diarrhea, and colitis (including pseudomembranous colitis) reported; d/c if significant diarrhea occurs. Avoid contact with eyes and mucous membranes. May cause an overgrowth of nonsuceptible organisms, including fungi; d/c use and treat appropriately.

**ADVERSE REACTIONS:** Dry skin, application-site reaction, pruritus, peeling, erythema, sunburn, allergic reactions.

**INTERACTIONS:** Antiperistaltic agents (eg, opiates, diphenoxylate with atropine) may prolong and/or worsen diarrhea. Cumulative irritancy possible with other topical acne agents. Avoid use with erythromycin agents.

**PREGNANCY:** Category C, not for use in nursing.

**MECHANISM OF ACTION:** Antibacterial/keratolytic; acts against *Propionibacterium acnes*.

**PHARMACOKINETICS: Distribution:** Orally and parenterally administered clindamycin has been reported to appear in breast milk.

## NURSING CONSIDERATIONS

**Assessment:** Assess for hypersensitivity to lincomycin, a history of regional enteritis, ulcerative or antibiotic-associated colitis, pregnancy/nursing status, and for possible drug interactions.

**Monitoring:** Monitor signs and symptoms of diarrhea, bloody diarrhea, colitis (including pseudomembranous colitis), overgrowth of nonsusceptible organisms (eg, fungi), and for allergic reactions.

**Patient Counseling:** Advise to use as directed, for external use only, to avoid contact with eyes, inside nose, mouth, and mucous membranes. Inform that therapy may bleach hair or colored fabric. Inform to minimize or avoid exposure to natural/artificial sunlight. Instruct to contact physician if develop any adverse reactions. Counsel to d/c use if develop severe allergic symptoms (eg, severe swelling, shortness of breath). Prior to use, instruct to wash skin gently, then rinse with warm water and pat dry.

**Administration:** Topical. **Storage:** 25°C (77°F). Do not freeze. Keep tightly closed. Keep out of reach of children. Discard unused product after 3 months.

# BENZTROPINE — RX

benztropine mesylate (Various)

**OTHER BRAND NAMES:** Cogentin (Lundbeck)

**THERAPEUTIC CLASS:** Anticholinergic

**INDICATIONS:** Adjunct in all forms of parkinsonism. Control of drug-induced extrapyramidal disorders.

**DOSAGE:** *Adults:* Individulaize dose. Titrate: May increase by 0.5mg/day q 5-6 days. Idiopathic Parkinsonism: Initial: 0.5-1mg qhs. Postencephalitic Parkinsonism: 2mg/day given in 1 or more doses. Extrapyramidal Disorders: 1-4mg/day given qd-bid. D/C and re-evaluate necessity after 1-2 weeks; may reinstitute if disorders recur. (Inj) Acute Dystonic Reactions: 1-2mg IM/IV. *Pediatrics:* >3 yrs: Individulaize dose. Titrate: May increase by 0.5mg/day q 5-6 days. Idiopathic Parkinsonism: Initial: 0.5-1mg qhs. Postencephalitic Parkinsonism: 2mg/day given in 1 or more doses. Extrapyramidal Disorders: 1-4mg/day given qd-bid. D/C and re-evaluate necessity after 1-2 weeks; may reinstitute if disorders recur. (Inj) Acute Dystonic Reactions: 1-2mg IM/IV.

**HOW SUPPLIED:** Inj: 1mg/mL; Tab: 0.5mg*, 1mg*, 2mg* *scored

**CONTRAINDICATIONS:** Patients <3 yrs.

**WARNINGS/PRECAUTIONS:** May produce anhidrosis, caution in hot weather. Muscle weakness and dysuria may occur. Caution in pediatrics >3 years of age. Not recommended for tardive dyskinesia. Avoid with angle-closure glaucoma. Caution with CNS disease, mental disorders, tachycardia, prostatic hypertrophy, alcoholics, chronically ill, those exposed to hot environments. May impair mental/physical abilities.

**ADVERSE REACTIONS:** Tachycardia, paralytic ileus, constipation, vomiting, nausea, dry mouth, confusion, blurred vision, urinary retention, heat stroke, hyperthermia, fever.

**INTERACTIONS:** Paralytic ileus, hyperthermia and heat stroke reported with phenothiazines and TCAs. Caution with other atropine-like agents.

**PREGNANCY:** Safety in pregnancy and nursing not known.

**MECHANISM OF ACTION:** Anticholinergic agent; controls extrapyramidal symptoms in parkinsonism.

## NURSING CONSIDERATIONS

**Assessment:** Assess for tachycardia, prostatic hypertrophy, anhidrosis, TD. Note other diseases/conditions and drug therapy.

**Monitoring:** Monitor for tachycardia, prostatic hypertrophy, anhidrosis, hyperthermia, constipation, urinary retention, paralytic ileus, toxic psychosis.

**Patient Counseling:** Caution during hot weather, especially when given concomitantly with other atropine-like drugs to the chronically ill, alcoholics, those who have CNS disease, and those who do manual labor in a hot environment. Caution while operating machinery/driving.

**Administration:** IV/IM, Oral route. **Storage:** 15-30°C. Dispense in well-closed container.

## BERINERT RX

c1 inhibitor (human) (CSL Behring)

**THERAPEUTIC CLASS:** C1 inhibitor

**INDICATIONS:** Treatment of acute abdominal or facial attacks of hereditary angioedema (HAE) in adults and adolescents.

**DOSAGE:** *Adults:* 20 U/kg. Administer at a rate of 4mL/min.
*Adolescents:* 20 U/kg. Administer at a rate of 4mL/min.

**HOW SUPPLIED:** Inj: 500 U

**WARNINGS/PRECAUTIONS:** Severe hypersensitivity reactions (eg, hives, generalized urticaria, chest tightness, wheezing, hypotension, and/or anaphylaxis) may occur; d/c therapy immediately. Have epinephrine available. Thrombotic events at high doses reported (animal studies). May carry a risk of transmitting infectious agents (eg, viruses, Creutzfeldt-Jakob (CJD) agent). Report all infections transmitted by the product to the manufacturer.

**ADVERSE REACTIONS:** Headache, abdominal pain, N/V, muscle spasms, pain, diarrhea, dysgeusia.

**PREGNANCY:** Category C, caution in nursing.

**MECHANISM OF ACTION:** C1 esterase inhibitor; regulates the activation of the complement and intrinsic coagulation (contact system) pathway, the fibrinolytic system, and coagulation cascade; regulation is performed through the formation of complexes between the proteinase and the inhibitor.

**PHARMACOKINETICS: Absorption: Adults:** AUC =27.5hr•IU/mL (unadjusted for baseline), 12.8hr•IU/mL (adjusted for baseline); **Pediatrics:** 25.45hr•IU/mL (unadjusted for baseline), 9.78hr•IU/mL (adjusted for baseline). **Elimination: Adults:** $T_{1/2}$=21.9hrs (unadjusted for baseline), 18.4hrs (adjusted for baseline); **Pediatrics:** 22.4hrs (unadjusted for baseline), 16.7hrs (adjusted for baseline).

### NURSING CONSIDERATIONS

**Assessment:** Assess signs and symptoms of hypersensitivity reactions, known risk factors for thrombotic events, and pregnancy/nursing status.

**Monitoring:** Monitor for hypersensitivity reactions and thrombotic events.

**Patient Counseling:** Counsel about the risks and benefits of C1 inhibitor prior to treatment. Inform that medication is made from human plasma and may contain infectious agents that can cause disease (eg, viruses, CJD agent). Inform patients to report signs and symptoms of allergic hypersensitivity reactions and thrombosis immediately. Advise female patients to inform their physician if pregnant or plan to become pregnant. Advise patients to consult with their healthcare provider prior to travel.

**Administration:** IV route. Refer to PI for preparation and handling/detailed reconstitution and administration information. **Storage:** 2-25°C (36-77°F); up to 30 months. Do not freeze. Protect from light.

## BETAGAN RX

levobunolol HCl (Allergan)

**THERAPEUTIC CLASS:** Nonselective beta-blocker

**INDICATIONS:** Treatment of elevated IOP in chronic open-angle glaucoma and ocular hypertension.

**DOSAGE:** *Adults:* (0.5%) 1-2 drops qd; bid for more severe or uncontrolled glaucoma. (0.25%): 1-2 drops bid.

**HOW SUPPLIED:** Sol: 0.25% [5mL, 10mL], 0.5% [2mL, 5mL, 10mL, 15mL]

**CONTRAINDICATIONS:** Bronchial asthma, COPD, overt cardiac failure, sinus bradycardia, 2nd- and 3rd-degree AV block, cardiogenic shock.

**WARNINGS/PRECAUTIONS:** Caution with cardiac failure, diabetes mellitus (DM), COPD, cerebral insufficiency, pulmonary disease, bronchospastic disease, surgery and hepatic impairment. May mask symptoms of hypoglycemia and thyrotoxicosis. Contains sodium metabisulfite. Follow with a miotic in angle-closure glaucoma. Potentiates muscle weakness (eg, diplopia, ptosis).

**ADVERSE REACTIONS:** Ocular burning, ocular stinging, decreased heart rate, decreased blood pressure.

**INTERACTIONS:** Mydriasis with epinephrine. Additive effects with catecholamine-depleting drugs (eg, reserpine) and systemic β-blockers. AV conduction disturbance with calcium antagonists and digitalis. Left ventricular failure and hypotension with calcium antagonists also. Additive hypotensive effects with phenothiazine-related drugs. Risk of hypoglycemia with insulin and oral hypoglycemic agents.

**PREGNANCY:** Category C, caution in nursing.

**MECHANISM OF ACTION:** Noncardioselective β-adrenoceptor blocking agent; equipotent at both $\beta_1$ and $\beta_2$ receptors. Responsible for reducing cardiac output, increasing airway resistance, and lowering elevated as well as normal IOP. Presumed to lower IOP through decreasing production of aqueous humor.

**PHARMACOKINETICS: Absorption**: $T_{max}$=2 and 6 hrs.

## NURSING CONSIDERATIONS

**Assessment:** Assess for active or history of bronchial asthma, severe COPD, sinus bradycardia, 2nd- and 3rd- degree AV block, overt cardiac failure, and cardiogenic shock. Assess for possible sulfite allergy prior to therapy. Assess use in patients who have DM, hyperthyroidism, diminished pulmonary function, cerebrovascular insufficiencies, patients undergoing major elective surgery, and in pregnant/nursing females. Assess that patients with angle-closure glaucoma are not using this drug as monotherapy. Assess for possible drug interactions.

**Monitoring:** Monitor for signs/symptoms of muscle weakness (eg, diplopia, ptosis), severe respiratory and cardiac reactions, and anaphylactic reactions. Monitor for occurrence of a thyroid storm in patients who have thyrotoxicosis and withdraw abruptly from medication. Monitor for signs/symptoms of acute hypoglycemia with DM.

**Patient Counseling:** Counsel to notify physician immediately if any signs of anaphylactic reaction, cardiac or respiratory symptoms develop while on medication. Counsel patients with DM medication may mask symptoms of hypoglycemia.

**Administration:** Ocular route. **Storage:** 15-25°C (59-77°F), protect from light.

# BETAPACE RX

sotalol HCl (Bayer Healthcare)

**To minimize risk of arrhythmia, for a minimum of 3 days, place patients initiated or reinitiated on therapy in a facility that can provide ECG monitoring and cardiac resuscitation. Perform CrCl before therapy. Betapace is not approved for atrial fibrillation or atrial flutter; do not substitute for Betapace AF.**

**THERAPEUTIC CLASS:** Beta-blocker (group II/III antiarrhythmic)

**INDICATIONS:** Treatment of documented life-threatening ventricular arrhythmias.

**DOSAGE:** *Adults:* Initial: 80mg bid. Titrate: Increase to 120-160mg bid if needed. Allow 3 days between dose increases. Usual: 160-320mg/day given bid-tid. Refractory Patients: 480-640mg/day. CrCl 30-59mL/min: Dose q24h. CrCl 10-29mL/min: Dose q36-48h. CrCl <10mL/min: Individualize dose. May increase dose with renal impairment after at least 5-6 doses.
*Pediatrics:* ≥2 yrs: Initial: 30mg/m² tid. Titrate: Wait at least 36 hrs between dose increases. Guide dose by response, HR and QTc. Max: 60mg/m².

<2 yrs: See dosing chart in PI. Reduce dose or d/c if QTc >550msec. Renal Impairment: Reduce dose or increase interval.

**HOW SUPPLIED:** Tab: 80mg*, 120mg*, 160mg* *scored

**CONTRAINDICATIONS:** Bronchial asthma, sinus bradycardia, 2nd- and 3rd-degree AV block (unless a functioning pacemaker is present), congenital or acquired long QT syndromes, cardiogenic shock, uncontrolled CHF.

**WARNINGS/PRECAUTIONS:** May provoke new or worsen existing ventricular arrhythmias. Torsades de pointes reported; incidence is dose-related and risk increases with prolongation of QT interval, HR reduction, serum $K^+$ reduction, female gender, and history of cardiomegaly or CHF. Avoid with hypokalemia, hypomagnesemia, excessive QT interval prolongation (>550msec). Caution with heart failure controlled by digitalis and/or diuretics, left ventricular dysfunction, sick sinus syndrome, renal impairment, and 2 weeks post-myocardial infarction (MI). Correct electrolyte imbalances before therapy. Avoid abrupt withdrawal, use in patients with bronchospastic disease. May mask hypoglycemia, hyperthyroidism symptoms. Use in surgery is controversial.

**ADVERSE REACTIONS:** Dyspnea, fatigue, dizziness, bradycardia, chest pain, palpitation, asthenia, abnormal ECG, hypotension, headache, light-headedness, edema, N/V, pulmonary problem.

**INTERACTIONS:** May block epinephrine effects. Avoid with Class Ia (eg, disopyramide, quinidine and procainamide) and Class III (eg, amiodarone) antiarrhythmics; potential to prolong refractoriness. Additive Class II effects with β-blockers. Caution with drugs that prolong the QT interval (eg, Class I and III antiarrhythmics, phenothiazines, TCAs, bepridil, certain quinolones and oral macrolides, astemizole). Avoid within 2 hrs of aluminum- or magnesium-containing antacids. Potentiates rebound HTN with clonidine withdrawal. May potentiate bradycardia or hypotension with catecholamine-depleting drugs (eg, reserpine and guanethidine); and hypotension with calcium-blocking agents. Insulin and antidiabetic agents may need adjustment. $\beta_2$-agonists (eg, salbutamol, terbutaline and isoprenaline) may need dose increase. Proarrhythmic events were more common with digoxin. Caution with diuretics/digitalis. Severe hypotension and difficulty in restoring and maintaining normal cardiac rhythm after anesthesia reported in patients receiving β-blockers.

**PREGNANCY:** Category B, not for use in nursing.

**MECHANISM OF ACTION:** Antiarrhythmic drug (Class II and III properties); has both β-adrenoreceptor-blocking and cardiac action potential duration prolongation properties.

**PHARMACOKINETICS: Absorption:** Bioavailability (90-100%); $T_{max}$=2.5-4 hrs. **Distribution:** Crosses blood-brain barrier (poor); found in breast milk. **Elimination:** Urine (unchanged); $T_{1/2}$=12 hrs.

## NURSING CONSIDERATIONS

**Assessment:** Establish CrCl prior to dosing. Assess for bronchial asthma, sinus bradycardia/tachycardia, sick sinus syndrome, second- and third-degree heart block, patients with functioning pacemaker, congenital/acquired long QT syndromes, cardiogenic shock, left ventricular dysfunction or uncontrolled CHF, recent MI, ischemic heart disease, hypokalemia or hypomagnesemia, history of chronic bronchitis and emphysema, DM, episodes of hypoglycemia, upcoming major surgery, hyperthyroidism, renal impairment, nursing status, and for possible drug interactions.

**Monitoring:** After initiation, stay at least 3 days where continuous ECG monitoring and resuscitation are available if needed. Monitor ECG changes, proarrhythmia (eg, ventricular tachycardia/or fibrillation and torsades de pointes), HR and CrCl, asystole, new arrhythmias, signs/symptoms of depressed myocardial contractility and more severe HF, anaphylaxis, bronchospasm, MI, hypotension, masking of hypoglycemic signs, signs of electrolyte imbalance, exacerbation of hyperthyroidism symptoms and thyroid storm.

**Patient Counseling:** Do not d/c without consulting physician. Inform of benefits/risks of drug. Report any adverse reactions to physician. Inform that drug is not for use by nursing women.

**Administration:** Oral route. Preparation of 5mg/mL Oral solution: Add five 120mg tabs to 120mL simple syrup in a 6oz plastic, amber bottle. Shake well to wet all tabs. Allow tabs to hydrate for 2 hrs then shake bottle intermittently over 2 hrs until tabs are completely disintegrated. Shake well before administration. **Storage:** 25°C (77°F); excursions permitted to 15-30°C (59-86°F). Solution remains stable when stored at room temperature and ambient humidity for 3 months.

## Betapace AF RX

sotalol HCl (Bayer Healthcare)

**To minimize risk of arrhythmia, for a minimum of 3 days, place patients initiated or reinitiated on therapy in a facility that can provide CrCl, ECG monitoring, and cardiac resuscitation. Do not substitute Betapace for Betapace AF.**

**THERAPEUTIC CLASS:** Beta-blocker (group II/III antiarrhythmic)

**INDICATIONS:** Maintenance of normal sinus rhythm with symptomatic atrial fibrillation/atrial flutter (AFIB/AFL) in patients who are currently in sinus rhythm.

**DOSAGE:** *Adults:* Initiate with continuous ECG monitoring. Give dose qd for CrCl 40-60mL/min and bid for CrCl >60mL/min. Initial: 80mg. Monitor QT 2-4hrs after each dose. Reduce dose or d/c if QT ≥500msec. If QT <500msec after 3 days (after 5th or 6th dose if receiving qd dosing), discharge on current treatment. Alternatively, may increase dose to 120mg during hospitalization, and follow for 3 days with bid dose and for 5 or 6 doses if receiving qd dose. Max: 160mg qd or bid depending on CrCl.
*Pediatrics:* ≥2 yrs: Initial: 30mg/m² tid. Titrate: Wait at least 36 hrs between dose increases. Guide dose by response, HR and QTc. Max: 60mg/m².
<2 yrs: See dosing chart in PI. Reduce dose or d/c if QTc >550msec. Renal Impairment: Reduce dose or increase interval.

**HOW SUPPLIED:** Tab: 80mg*, 120mg*, 160mg* *scored

**CONTRAINDICATIONS:** Sinus bradycardia (<50bpm during waking hrs), sick sinus syndrome or 2nd- or 3rd-degree AV block (unless a functioning pacemaker is present), congenital or acquired long QT syndromes, baseline QT interval >450msec, cardiogenic shock, uncontrolled heart failure, hypokalemia (<4meq/L), CrCl <40mL/min, bronchial asthma.

**WARNINGS/PRECAUTIONS:** Can cause serious ventricular arrhythmias, primarily torsades de pointes. Incidence is dose-related and risk increases with sustained ventricular tachycardia, history or cardiomegaly or CHF, reduced renal clearance and female gender. Avoid with hypokalemia, hypomagnesemia. Correct electrolyte imbalances before therapy. Bradycardia reported. Caution with heart failure controlled by digitalis and/or diuretics, sick sinus syndrome, left ventricular dysfunction, renal dysfunction, post-myocardial infarction (MI). Avoid abrupt withdrawal, use in bronchospastic disease. May mask hypoglycemia, hyperthyroidism symptoms. Use in surgery is controversial.

**ADVERSE REACTIONS:** Bradycardia, dyspnea, fatigue, dose-related QT interval prolongation, abnormal ECG, chest pain, abdominal pain, disturbance rhythm subjective, diarrhea, N/V, hyperhidrosis, dizziness, weakness, headache.

**INTERACTIONS:** May block epinephrine effects. Avoid Class 1A (eg, disopyramide, quinidine and procainamide) and Class III (eg, amiodarone) antiarrhythmics; potential to prolong refractoriness. Not recommended with drugs that prolong the QT interval (eg, many antiarrhythmics, phenothiazines, TCAs, bepridil, and oral macrolides). Avoid within 2 hrs of aluminum- or magnesium-containing antacids. Potentiates rebound HTN with clonidine withdrawal. May potentiate bradycardia or hypotension with catecholamine-depleting drugs (eg, reserpine and guanethidine); hypotension with calcium-blocking drugs. Insulin and antidiabetic agents may need adjustment. β2-agonists (eg, salbutamol, terbutaline and isoprenaline) may need dose increase. Proarrhythmic events more common with digoxin. Caution with diuretics and digitalis. Severe

B

hypotension and difficulty in restoring and maintaining normal cardiac rhythm after anesthesia have been reported in patients receiving β-blockers.

**PREGNANCY:** Category B, not for use in nursing.

**MECHANISM OF ACTION:** Antiarrhythmic drug (Class II and III properties); has both β-adrenoreceptor blocking and cardiac action potential duration prolongation properties.

**PHARMACOKINETICS: Absorption:** Bioavailability (90-100%); $T_{max}$=2.5-4 hrs. **Distribution:** Crosses blood brain barrier (poor); found in breast milk. **Elimination**: Urine (unchanged); $T_{1/2}$=12 hrs.

## NURSING CONSIDERATIONS

**Assessment:** Calculate CrCl prior to dosing. Assess for structural heart disease, pre-existing long-QT syndrome, implanted pacemaker, other conduction defects, CHF, renal/hepatic dysfunction, recent MI, ischemic heart disease, history of chronic bronchitis and emphysema, DM, episodes of hypoglycemia, undergoing major surgery, hyperthyroidism, nursing status, medication history and possible drug/diet interactions. Correct hypokalemia and hypomagnesemia before initiation of therapy.

**Monitoring:** After initiation monitor patient for at least 3 days. Continuous ECG monitoring and resuscitation should be done if necessary. Monitor ECG changes, HR, and CrCl, asystole, new arrhythmias, signs/symptoms of depressed myocardial contractility and more severe HF, anaphylaxis, bronchospasm, MI, hypotension, masking of hypoglycemic signs, renal function, exacerbation of hyperthyroidism symptoms, and signs of electrolyte imbalance.

**Patient Counseling:** Do not abruptly d/c without consulting physician. Inform of benefits/risks and report any signs of electrolyte imbalance (eg, diarrhea and vomiting). After initiation, patient should stay for 3 days where continuous ECG monitoring and resuscitation are available. May experience abnormal heartbeat. Inform physician if taking any other medications or OTC drugs. Instruct the need for compliance with recommended dosing. Instruct if a dose is missed do not double the next dose and should take the next dose at the usual time.

**Administration:** Oral route. Preparation of 5mg/mL Oral Solution: Add five 120mg tabs to 120mL simple syrup in a 6oz plastic, amber bottle. Shake bottle to wet all tabs. Allow tabs to hydrate for 2 hrs then shake bottle intermittently over 2 hrs until tabs are completely disintegrated. Shake before administration. **Storage:** 25°C (77°F); excursions permitted to 15-30°C (59-86°F). Solution remains stable when stored in room temperature and ambient humidity for 3 months.

## BETIMOL RX

timolol (Vistakon)

**THERAPEUTIC CLASS:** Nonselective beta-blocker

**INDICATIONS:** Treatment of elevated IOP in patients with open-angle glaucoma or ocular hypertension.

**DOSAGE:** *Adults:* Initial: 1 drop 0.25% bid. May increase to max of 1 drop 0.5% bid. Maint: If adequate control, may try 1 drop 0.25-0.5% qd.

**HOW SUPPLIED:** Sol: 0.25%, 0.5% [2.5mL, 5mL, 10mL, 15mL]

**CONTRAINDICATIONS:** Bronchial asthma, history of bronchial asthma, severe COPD, sinus bradycardia, 2nd- or 3rd-degree AV block, overt cardiac failure, cardiogenic shock.

**WARNINGS/PRECAUTIONS:** Caution with cardiac failure, diabetes mellitus (DM), cerebrovascular insufficiency. Severe cardiac and respiratory reactions reported. May mask symptoms of hypoglycemia and hyperthyroidism. Bacterial keratitis reported with contaminated containers. May reinsert contacts 5 min after applying drops. Avoid with COPD, bronchospastic disease. Not for use alone in angle-closure glaucoma. May potentiate muscle weakness. D/C if cardiac failure develops. Withdrawal before surgery is controversial.

B

**ADVERSE REACTIONS:** Burning/stinging on instillation, dry eyes, itching, foreign body sensation, eye discomfort, eyelid erythema, conjunctival injection, headache.

**INTERACTIONS:** May potentiate systemic β-blockers and catecholamine-depleting drugs (eg, reserpine). Oral/IV calcium antagonists can cause AV conduction disturbances, left ventricular failure, or hypotension. Digitalis can cause additive effects in prolonging AV conduction time. May antagonize epinephrine.

**PREGNANCY:** Category C, not for use in nursing.

**MECHANISM OF ACTION:** Nonselective β-adrenergic antagonist; blocks both $\beta_1$- and $\beta_2$-adrenergic receptors. Thought to reduce IOP through reducing production of aqueous humor.

**PHARMACOKINETICS: Elimination:** Urine (metabolites); $T_{1/2}$=4 hrs

## NURSING CONSIDERATIONS

**Assessment:** Assess for overt heart failure, cardiogenic shock, sinus bradycardia, 2nd-or 3rd-degree AV block, active or history of bronchial asthma, and severe COPD. Assess use in patients with cerebrovascular insufficiencies, undergoing elective surgery, with DM, with hyperthyroidism, and in pregnant/nursing females. Assess patients with angle-closure glaucoma are not on monotherapy with this drug. Assess for possible drug interactions.

**Monitoring:** Monitor for signs/symptoms of reduced cerebral blood flow, cardiac failure, muscle weakness, bacterial keratitis when using multi-dose container, severe anaphylactic reactions, and hypoglycemia in patients with DM. Monitor for occurrence of thyroid storm in patients who abruptly withdraw from medication and have thyrotoxicosis.

**Patient Counseling:** Counsel to immediately notify physician if signs of cardiac, respiratory, or anaphylactic symptoms develop while on medication. Instruct patients with DM that this medication may mask signs of hypoglycemia. To avoid contaminating solution, avoid touching container tip to the eye or surrounding structures. Counsel that if taking concomitant topical ophthalmic medications, to separate dosing by at least 5 min. Instruct patients who wear soft contact lenses to wait at least 5 min after administration before reinserting.

**Administration:** Ocular route. **Storage:** 15-25°C (59-77°F). Do not freeze. Protect from light.

# BETOPTIC S — RX

betaxolol HCl (Alcon)

**THERAPEUTIC CLASS:** Selective $beta_1$-blocker

**INDICATIONS:** Chronic open-angle glaucoma. Ocular hypertension.

**DOSAGE:** *Adults:* 1-2 drops bid.

**HOW SUPPLIED:** Sus: 0.25% [5mL, 10mL, 15mL]

**CONTRAINDICATIONS:** Sinus bradycardia, greater than 1st-degree AV block, cardiogenic shock or overt cardiac failure.

**WARNINGS/PRECAUTIONS:** May be absorbed systemically. Caution with cardiac failure, heart block, diabetes mellitus (DM), asthma. May mask hypoglycemic symptoms and signs of hyperthyroidism. May potentiate muscle weakness. D/C before general anesthesia. Avoid abrupt withdrawal. Caution in patients with cerebrovascular insufficiency.

**ADVERSE REACTIONS:** Transient ocular discomfort, blurred vision, corneal punctate keratitis, foreign body sensation, photophobia, tearing, itching, dryness of eye, erythema, inflammation, discharge, ocular pain, decreased visual acuity, crusty lashes.

**INTERACTIONS:** May potentiate systemic β-blockers and catecholamine-depleting drugs (eg, reserpine). May be potentiated by systemic β-blockers. May antagonize adrenergic psychotropics. May increase risk of hypoglycemia with insulin or oral hypoglycemic drugs.

B

**PREGNANCY:** Category C, caution with nursing.

**MECHANISM OF ACTION:** It is a cardioselective (β-1-adrenergic) receptor inhibitor. Responsible for reducing intraocular pressure through a reduction of aqueous production.

**PHARMACOKINETICS: Absorption:** $T_{max}$=2 hrs.

## NURSING CONSIDERATIONS

**Assessment:** Assess for sinus bradycardia, >1st-degree atrioventricular block, cardiogenic shock, and overt cardiac failure. Assess use with history of cardiac failure or heart block, cerebrovascular insufficiencies, a history of hypoglycemia or DM, hyperthyroidism, patients undergoing elective surgery, patients with excessive restriction of pulmonary function, and in pregnant/nursing females. Assess that patients with angle-closure glaucoma are not on monotherapy with this drug. Assess for possible drug interactions.

**Monitoring:** Monitor for signs/symptoms of respiratory reactions, cardiac failure, muscle weakness, reduced cerebral blood flow, and anaphylaxis. Monitor for occurrence of a thyroid storm in patients who have thyrotoxicosis and withdraw abruptly from medication. Monitor for signs/symptoms of acute hypoglycemia with DM. Monitor for development of bacterial keratitis in patients who are using multidose containers. Monitor for occurrence of choroidal detachment.

**Patient Counseling:** Counsel that if any type of cardiac, respiratory, or anaphylactic reactions develop, to contact physician immediately. Advise patients with DM that medication may mask symptoms of hypoglycemia. Instruct to avoid allowing tip of dispensing container to contact the eye or surrounding structures. Advise if solution handled improperly, may become contaminated and cause bacterial infections. Advise if having ocular surgery or if an intercurrent ocular condition develops, to contact physician before continuing to use the multidose container they were previously using. Patients on concomitant topical ophthalmic medication should be instructed to administer medications at least 10 min apart.

**Administration:** Ocular route. 1) Wash hands prior to use. 2) Invert container and shake once before use. 3) Tilt head back and position bottle above affected eye. 4) With opposite hand, place finger under eye and gently pull down, creating a "V" pocket between eye and lower lid. 5) With hand holding the bottle, place index finger on bottom of bottle. Push bottom of bottle to dispense 1 drop. Do not squeeze sides of bottle. **Storage**: Store upright at room temperature.

# Bexxar RX

iodine I 131 tositumomab - tositumomab (GlaxoSmithKline)

**Hypersensitivity reactions, including anaphylaxis, and prolonged and severe cytopenias reported. Can cause fetal harm if given during pregnancy. Contains radioactive component.**

**THERAPEUTIC CLASS:** Monoclonal antibody/CD20-blocker

**INDICATIONS:** Treatment of CD20-positive, follicular, non-Hodgkin's lymphoma (NHL), with and without transformation, in patients refractory to rituximab and who have relapsed following chemotherapy.

**DOSAGE:** *Adults:* Premedication: Day 1: Begin thyro-protective regimen of either SSKI (4 drops po tid), Lugol's sol (20 drops po tid), or potassium iodide (130mg po qd). Continue until 14 days post-therapeutic dose. Day 0: APAP 650mg and diphenhydramine 50mg. Dosimetric Step: IV: 450mg tositumomab over 60 min followed by 5mCi Iodine I 131 tositumomab (35mg) over 20 min. Day 0 + Day 2, 3, or 4 + Day 6 or 7: Whole body dosimetry and biodistribution. Day 6 or 7: Calculation of patient-specific activity of iodine I 131 tositumomab to deliver 75cGy total body irradiation or 65cGy if platelets ≥100,000 but <150,000 platelets/$mm^3$. Day 7 (up to Day 14): Premedicate with APAP and diphenhydramine. Therapeutic Step: IV: Do not administer if biodistribution is altered. 450mg tositumomab over 60 min followed by prescribed therapeutic dose of iodine I 131 tositumomab (35mg) over 20 min.

**HOW SUPPLIED:** Inj: For Dosimetric Dosing: Tositumomab: 225mg [2 single-use vials], 35mg [1 single-use vial]; Iodine I 131 Tositumomab: 1 single-use vial. For Therapeutic Dosing: Tositumomab: 225mg [2 single-use vials], 35mg [1 single-use vial]; Iodine I 131 Tositumomab: 1 or 2 single-use vials.

**CONTRAINDICATIONS:** Pregnant women.

**WARNINGS/PRECAUTIONS:** Obtain CBCs weekly for 10-12 weeks. Safety not established with >25% lymphoma marrow involvement, platelet <100,000 cells/$mm^3$, or neutrophil count <1500 cells/$mm^3$. Secondary malignancies reported. May cause hypothyroidism; monitor TSH prior to initiation and then annually. Thyroid blocking agents must be used; initiate at least 24 hrs before dosimetric dose and continue until 14 days after therapeutic dose. Caution with impaired renal function. Effective contraceptive methods should be used during, and for 12 months following treatment. Increased risk of serious allergic reactions if positive for human anti-murine antibodies (HAMA).

**ADVERSE REACTIONS:** Neutropenia, thrombocytopenia, anemia, asthenia, fever, infection, cough, pain, chills, headache, GI effects, myalgia, arthralgia, pharyngitis, dyspnea, rash.

**INTERACTIONS:** Weigh risks vs benefits of concomitant agents that interfere with platelet function and/or anticoagulation.

**PREGNANCY:** Category X, not for use in nursing.

**MECHANISM OF ACTION:** Monoclonal antibody; possibly induces apoptosis, complement-dependent cytotoxicity, antibody-dependent cellular cytotoxicity mediated by the antibody; cell death associated with ionizing radiation from radioisotope. Tositumomab; murine IgG2a lambda monoclonal antibody directed against CD20 antigen found on surface of B lymphocytes. Iodine I 131 tositumomab; radio-iodinated derivative of tositumomab, covalently linked to Iodine-131.

**PHARMACOKINETICS: Elimination:** (Iodine-131): Decay (β and gamma emissions). Physical $T_{1/2}$=8.04 days. Excreted in urine; (Iodine I 131 Tositumomab): Urine; $T_{1/2}$=67 hrs.

## NURSING CONSIDERATIONS

**Assessment:** Assess for known hypersensitivity to murine proteins, lymphoma marrow involvement, impaired bone marrow reserve, renal function, pregnancy status, use of thyroid-blocking agent. Screen for human anti-mouse antibody (prior murine protein use) and possible drug interactions. Obtain baseline CBC, SrCr, TSH, and platelet count

**Monitoring:** Monitor CBC weekly for 10-12 weeks. Monitor renal function (periodically) and TSH (annually). Monitor for signs/symptoms of thrombocytopenia, neutropenia, anemia, secondary malignancies, hypersensitivity reaction (bronchospasm and angioedema), and hypothyroidism.

**Patient Counseling:** Inform of pregnancy risks and to d/c nursing. Instruct to use effective contraceptive methods during treatment and for 12 months after completion. Advise on importance of compliance with thyroid-blocking agents and need for lifelong monitoring. Seek medical attention if symptoms of thrombocytopenia, neutropenia, anemia, secondary malignancies, hypersensitivity reaction (bronchospasm and angioedema), and hypothyroidism occur.

**Administration:** IV infusion. Do not administer therapeutic dose if biodistribution is altered. Same IV tubing set and filter must be used throughout all steps. Changes in filter can result in loss of drug. Refer to Full PI for detailed administration. **Storage:** tositumomab: 2-8°C (36-46°). Do not freeze or shake. Protect from strong light. (Diluted): Stable for 24 hrs if refrigerated 2-8°C (36-46°F); stable for 8 hrs at room temperature. Do not freeze. Iodine I 131 tositumomab: Frozen in original lead pots at -20°C or below. (Thawed): Stable for 8 hrs at 2-8°C (36-46°), or room temperature. (Diluted): Refrigerate 2-8°C (36-46°).

B

# BIAXIN

RX

clarithromycin (Abbott)

**THERAPEUTIC CLASS:** Macrolide

**INDICATIONS:** Treatment of the following infections caused by susceptible strains of microorganisms: (Adults) Pharyngitis/tonsillitis, acute maxillary sinusitis, acute bacterial exacerbation of chronic bronchitis (ABECB), community-acquired pneumonia (CAP), uncomplicated skin and skin structure infections (SSSI), and disseminated mycobacterial infections. Combination therapy for *H.pylori* infection with duodenal ulcers. MAC prophylaxis in advanced HIV. (Pediatrics) Pharyngitis/tonsillitis, CAP, acute maxillary sinusitis, acute otitis media, uncomplicated SSSI, disseminated mycobacterial infections. MAC prophylaxis in advanced HIV.

**DOSAGE:** *Adults:* Pharyngitis/Tonsillitis: 250mg q12h for 10 days. Sinusitis: 500mg q12h for 14 days. ABECB: 250-500mg q12h for 7-14 days. SSSI/CAP: 250mg q12h for 7-14 days. MAC Prophylaxis/Treatment: 500mg bid. CrCl <30mL/min: Give 50% dose or double the dosing interval. *H.pylori:* Triple Therapy: 500mg + amoxicillin 1g + omeprazole 20mg, all q12h for 10 days (give additional omeprazole 20mg qd for 18 days with active ulcer); or 500mg + amoxicillin 1g + lansoprazole 30mg, all q12h for 10-14 days. Dual Therapy: 500mg q8h + omeprazole 40mg qd for 14 days (give additional omeprazole 20mg qd for 14 days with active ulcer); or 500mg q8h or q12h + ranitidine bismuth citrate 400mg q12h for 14 days (give additional ranitidine bismuth citrate 400mg bid for 14 days with active ulcer). May be taken with or without food.

*Pediatrics:* ≥6 months: Usual: 15mg/kg/day q12h for 10 days. MAC Prophylaxis/Treatment: ≥20 months: 7.5mg/kg bid, up to 500mg bid. CrCl <30mL/min: Give 50% dose or double the dosing interval. Refer to PI for pediatric dosage guidelines.

**HOW SUPPLIED:** Sus: 125mg/5mL, 250mg/5mL [50mL, 100mL]; Tab: 250mg, 500mg

**CONTRAINDICATIONS:** Concomitant use with cisapride, pimozide, astemizole, terfenadine, ergotamine or dihydroergotamine.

**WARNINGS/PRECAUTIONS:** Avoid in pregnancy. *Clostridium difficile*-associated diarrhea (CDAD) reported. Adjust dose with severe renal impairment. Use in the absence of a proven or strongly suspected bacterial infection or a prophylactic indication is unlikely to provide benefit and increases the risk of development of drug resistant bacteria. May exacerbate symptoms of myasthenia gravis; new onset of symptoms of myasthenic syndrome reported.

**ADVERSE REACTIONS:** Diarrhea, N/V, abnormal taste, dyspepsia, abdominal pain, headache, rash.

**INTERACTIONS:** See Contraindications. Increases serum levels of theophylline, carbamazepine, omeprazole, ranitidine bismuth citrate, digoxin, drugs metabolized by CYP3A, HMG-CoA reductase inhibitors, and tolterodine. Hypotension, bradyarrhythmias, and lactic acidosis observed with CCBs (eg, verapamil). Decreases zidovudine plasma levels. Potentiates oral anticoagulant effects. Decreased clearance of triazolam and midazolam; avoid coadministration of oral midazolam and monitor IV closely to allow dose adjustment. Somnolence and confusion may occur with concomitant use of triazolam; monitor for additive CNS effects. Concomitant use with strong inducers of CYP450 (eg, efavirenz, nevirapine, rifampicin, rifabutin, rifapentine) may decrease plasma levels of clarithromycin. Occurrence of torsades de pointes with antiarrhythmics (eg, quinidine, disopyramide) reported. Increased phosphodiesterase inhibitor exposure with sildenafil, tadalafil, or vardenafil. Avoid ranitidine bismuth citrate if CrCl <25mL/min or history of porphyria. Reduce dose with ritonavir if CrCl ≤60mL/min. Increased levels with fluconazole. Reduce dose with atazanavir if CrCl ≤60ml/min; doses of clarithromycin >1000mg/day should not be coadministered with protease inhibitors. Concomitant use with colchicine may increase colchicine exposure; colchicine toxicity reported with concomitant use, especially in elderly. Concomitant use with itraconazole may increase levels of itraconazole and clarithromycin.

Rare cases of rhabdomyolysis reported with HMG-CoA reductase inhibitors (eg, lovastatin, simvastatin). Interaction may occur when concomitantly used with cyclosporine, tacrolimus, alfentanil, methylprednisolone, cilostazol, bromocriptine, vinblastine, hexobarbital, phenytoin, or valproate.

**PREGNANCY:** Category C, caution in nursing.

**MECHANISM OF ACTION:** Semi-synthetic macrolide antibiotic; exerts antibacterial action by binding to the 50S ribosomal subunit of susceptible microorganisms, resulting in inhibition of protein synthesis. Active against aerobic and anaerobic gram-positive and gram-negative microorganisms.

**PHARMACOKINETICS: Absorption:** Rapid; (250 mg tab) absolute bioavailability (50%); $C_{max}$=1-2mcg/mL (250mg tab), 3-4mcg/mL (500mg tab), 2mcg/mL (sus); $T_{max}$=2-3 hrs. **Distribution:** Body tissues, fluids. **Metabolism:** 14-OH clarithromycin (active metabolite). **Elimination:** Urine: 20% (250mg tab), 30% (500mg tab), 40% (250mg sus), 10-15% (14-OH). Parent drug; $T_{1/2}$=3-4 hrs (250mg tab, sus), 5-7 hrs (500mg tab). 14-OH: $T_{1/2}$=5-6 hrs (250mg tab, sus), 7-9 hrs (500mg tab).

## NURSING CONSIDERATIONS

**Assessment:** Assess for hepatic/renal impairment, myasthenia gravis, pregnancy/nursing status, a history of acute porphyria, and for possible drug interactions.

**Monitoring:** Monitor for anaphylactic reactions (eg, Stevens-Johnson syndrome, toxic epidermal necrolysis), development of drug-resistant bacteria, CDAD ranging from mild diarrhea to fatal colitis, overgrowth of nonsusceptible microorganisms, cardiac arrhythmia if taken concurrently with cisapride, pimozide, astemizole, or terfenadine. Monitor for exacerbation of myasthenia gravis and new onset of symptoms of myasthenic syndrome. Monitor for colchicine toxicity if taken concurrently with colchicine, especially in elderly, and lab changes of LFTs, CBC, PT, and renal function. Monitor for additive CNS effects when coadministered with triazolam.

**Patient Counseling:** Advise of potential benefits/risks of therapy. Inform that drug only treats bacterial, not viral, infections. Instruct to take exactly as directed; inform that skipping doses or not completing full course may decrease effectiveness and increase antibiotic resistance. Advise that may take with or without food. Instruct to notify physician if watery/bloody diarrhea (with/without stomach cramps) develop (may occur up to 2 or more months after treatment) or if pregnant/nursing. Advise to notify physician of all medications currently taking. Inform that suspension is not to be refrigerated.

**Administration:** Oral route. **Storage:** (250 mg tab) 15-30°C (59-86°F). Protect from light. (500 mg tab) 20-25°C (68-77°F). (Sus) 15-30°C (59-86°F). Do not refrigerate.

# BIAXIN XL — RX

clarithromycin (Abbott)

**THERAPEUTIC CLASS:** Macrolide

**INDICATIONS:** Treatment of acute maxillary sinusitis, community-acquired pneumonia (CAP), and acute bacterial exacerbation of chronic bronchitis (ABECB) in adults.

**DOSAGE:** *Adults:* Sinusitis: 1000mg qd for 14 days. ABECB/CAP: 1000mg qd for 7 days. CrCl <30mL/min: Give 50% dose or double the dosing interval. Swallow whole; do not chew, break, or crush. Take with food.

**HOW SUPPLIED:** Tab, Extended-Release: 500mg [PAC 14[s]]

**CONTRAINDICATIONS:** Concomitant use with cisapride, pimozide, astemizole, terfenadine, ergotamine or dihydroergotamine.

**WARNINGS/PRECAUTIONS:** Avoid in pregnancy. *Clostridium difficile*-associated diarrhea (CDAD) reported. Adjust dose with severe renal impairment. Use in the absence of a proven or strongly suspected bacterial infection or a prophylactic indication is unlikely to provide benefit and increases the risk of development of drug-resistant bacteria. May exacerbate symptoms of myasthenia gravis; new onset of symptoms of myasthenic syndrome reported.

**ADVERSE REACTIONS:** Diarrhea, abnormal taste, nausea.

**INTERACTIONS:** See Contraindications. Increases serum levels of theophylline, carbamazepine, omeprazole, ranitidine bismuth citrate, digoxin, drugs metabolized by CYP3A, HMG-CoA reductase inhibitors, and tolterodine. Hypotension, bradyarrhythmias, and lactic acidosis observed with CCBs (eg, verapamil). Concomitant use with itraconazole may increase levels of itraconazole and clarithromycin. Decreases zidovudine plasma levels. Potentiates oral anticoagulant effects. Decreased clearance of triazolam and midazolam. Avoid coadministration of oral midazolam; monitor IV closely to allow dose adjustment. Somnolence and confusion may occur with concomitant use of triazolam; monitor for additive CNS effects. Concomitant use with strong inducers of CPY450 (eg, efavirenz, nevirapine, rifampicin, rifabutin, rifapentine) may decrease plasma levels of clarithromycin. Occurrence of torsades de pointes with antiarrythmics (eg, quinidine, disopyramide) reported. Increased phosphodiesterase inhibitor exposure with sildenafil, tadalafil, or vardenafil. Avoid ranitidine bismuth citrate if CrCl <25 mL/min or history of porphyria. Reduce dose with ritonavir if CrCl ≤60 mL/min. Increased levels with fluconazole. Concomitant use with colchicine may increase colchicine exposure; colchicine toxicity reported with concomitant use, especially in elderly. Reduce dose with atazanavir if CrCl ≤60ml/min; doses of clarithromycin >1000mg/day should not be coadministered with protease inhibitors. Rare cases of rhabdomyolysis reported with HMG-CoA reductase inhibitors (eg, lovastatin, simvastatin). Interaction may occur when concomitantly used with cyclosporine, tacrolimus, alfentanil, methylprednisolone, cilostazol, bromocriptine, vinblastine, hexobarbital, phenytoin, or valproate.

**PREGNANCY:** Category C, caution in nursing.

**MECHANISM OF ACTION:** Semi-synthetic macrolide antibiotic; exerts antibacterial action by binding to 50S ribosomal subunit of susceptible microorganisms resulting in inhibition of protein synthesis. Active against aerobic and anaerobic gram-positive and gram-negative microorganisms.

**PHARMACOKINETICS: Absorption:** Rapid. (2 x 500mg dose): (parent drug) $C_{max}$=2-3mcg/mL, $T_{max}$=5-8 hrs.(14-OH) $C_{max}$=0.8mcg/mL, $T_{max}$=6-9 hrs. (1 x 500mg dose): (parent drug) $C_{max}$=1-2mcg/mL, $T_{max}$=5-6 hr; (14-OH) $C_{max}$=0.6mcg/mL, $T_{max}$=6 hrs. **Distribution:** Body tissues, fluids. **Metabolism:** 14-OH clarithromycin (active metabolite). **Elimination:** Urine (30%).

## NURSING CONSIDERATIONS

**Assessment:** Assess for hepatic/renal impairment, myasthenia gravis, pregnancy/nursing status, a history of acute porphyria, and for possible drug interactions.

**Monitoring:** Monitor for anaphylactic reactions (eg, Stevens-Johnson syndrome, toxic epidermal necrolysis), development of drug-resistant bacteria, CDAD ranging from mild diarrhea to fatal colitis, overgrowth of nonsusceptible microorganisms, cardiac arrhythmia if taken concurrently with cisapride, pimozide, astemizole, or terfenadine. Monitor for exacerbation of myasthenia gravis and new onset of symptoms of myasthenic syndrome. Monitor for colchicine toxicity if taken concurrently with colchicine, especially in elderly, and lab changes to LFTs, CBC, PT, and renal function. Monitor for additive CNS effects when coadministered with triazolam.

**Patient Counseling:** Inform about potential benefits/risks of therapy. Counsel that drug treats bacterial, not viral, infections. Instruct to take exactly as directed; inform that skipping doses or not completing full course may decrease effectiveness and increase antibiotic resistance. Instruct to swallow tab whole; do not chew, break, or crush. Advise to take with food. Intruct to notify physician if watery/bloody diarrhea (with/without stomach cramps) develop (may occur as late as 2 or more months after treatment). Advise to notify physician if pregnant/nursing and all medications currently taking.

**Administration:** Oral route. Swallow whole with food; do not chew, crush, or break. **Storage:** 20-25°C (68-77°F); excursions permitted 15-30°C (59-86°F).

# BONIVA RX

ibandronate sodium (Roche)



**THERAPEUTIC CLASS:** Bisphosphonate

**INDICATIONS:** (Inj) Treatment of osteoporosis in postmenopausal women. (PO) Treatment and prevention of postmenopausal osteoporosis.

**DOSAGE:** *Adults:* Inj: 3mg IV over 15-30 sec every 3 months. PO: 150mg once monthly on the same date each month. Swallow whole with 6-8 oz water. Do not lie down for 60 min after dose. Take at least 60 min before 1st food, drink (other than water), medication, or supplementation. Must not take 2 tablets within the same week.

**HOW SUPPLIED:** Inj: 3mg/3mL; Tab: 150mg

**CONTRAINDICATIONS:** (Inj, PO) Hypocalcemia. (PO) Inability to stand or sit upright for at least 60 min and abnormalities of the esophagus which delay esophageal emptying (eg, stricture or achalasia).

**WARNINGS/PRECAUTIONS:** (Inj, PO) Not recommended in severe renal impairment (CrCl <30mL/min). Reports of osteonecrosis, primarily in the jaw, and severe, incapacitating bone, joint, and/or muscle pain. Caution with risk factors for jaw osteonecrosis (ONJ) including invasive dental procedures, cancer diagnosis, concomitant therapies (chemotherapy, radiotherapy, corticosteroids), and comorbid disorders (eg, anemia, coagulopathy, infection, and pre-existing dental disease). Treat hypocalcemia and other bone and mineral disturbance prior to therapy; hypocalcemia reported. Give supplemental calcium and vitamin D if dietary intake is inadequate. (PO) May cause local irritation of upper GI mucosa. Caution with upper GI problems (eg, Barrett's esophagus, dysphagia, esophageal diseases, gastritis, duodenitis or ulcer). D/C if dysphagia, odynophagia, retrosternal pain or new or worsening heartburn develops.

**ADVERSE REACTIONS:** (Inj) Influenza, nasopharyngitis, cystitis. (PO) Back pain, extremity pain, infection, dyspepsia, diarrhea, hypercholesterolemia, myalgia, headache, upper respiratory infection, bronchitis, pneumonia, UTI.

**INTERACTIONS:** (PO) Calcium and other multivalent cations (eg, aluminum, magnesium, iron) may interfere with absorption. Ibandronate should be taken at least 60 min before any oral medication, including medications containing multivalent cations (eg, antacids, supplements, vitamins). Caution when used concomitantly with NSAIDS or aspirin. May interfere with bone-imaging agents.

**PREGNANCY:** Category C, caution in nursing.

**MECHANISM OF ACTION:** Bisphosphonate; has affinity for hydroxyapatite, a component of the mineral matrix of the bone. Inhibits osteoclast activity and reduces bone resorption and turnover. In postmenopausal women, it reduces the elevated rate of bone turnover, leading to, on average, net gain in bone mass.

**PHARMACOKINETICS: Absorption:** (PO): $T_{max}$=0.5-2 hrs. **Distribution:** $V_d$=90L; serum protein binding (90.9-99.5%). **Elimination:** (IV, PO) Kidney (50-60%); (PO) Feces (unabsorbed dose); (PO)(150mg): $T_{1/2}$=37-157 hrs; (IV, 2mg): $T_{1/2}$=6.6-15.3 hrs; (IV, 4mg): $T_{1/2}$=5-25.5 hrs.

## NURSING CONSIDERATIONS

**Assessment:** (IV, PO) Assess for hypocalcemia and other disturbances of bone and mineral metabolism, severe renal impairment (eg, CrCl<30mL/min), risk of osteonecrosis, pregnancy/nursing status, and possible drug interactions. Obtain baseline serum calcium, CrCl. PO: Assess for abnormalities of the esophagus and ability to stand or sit upright for at least 60 min.

**Monitoring:** (IV, PO) Monitor for signs/symptoms of ONJ, musculoskeletal pain, hypocalcemia and renal toxicity. PO: Monitor for signs/symptoms of upper GI disorders (eg, dysphagia, esophagitis, esophageal or gastric ulcer)

**Patient Counseling:** (PO) Counsel to take at least 60 min before first food or drink (other than water) and before taking other oral medication or supplementation. Instruct to swallow whole with full glass of plain water (6 to 8 oz) while standing or sitting in upright position; avoid lying down for 60 min following administration of drug. Inform not to chew or suck medication. Take supplemental calcium and vitamin D if dietary intake is inadequate; should be delayed by at least 60 min following administration of ibandronate. If taking 2.5mg tab, take at the same time each day. If dose is missed, instruct to skip and return to normal schedule on the next day. If taking 150mg tab, take on the same date each month. If dose is missed and next scheduled dose is >7 days away, instruct to take one tab in the morning following the date it is remembered. If next dose is 1-7 days away, instruct to wait for next scheduled day to take tab. Instruct to d/c treatment and seek medical attention if signs of esophageal reaction develop during therapy. (IV): Must receive intravenously, only by healthcare professional, once every 3 months.

**Administration:** Oral or IV route. **Storage:** 25°C (77°F); excursions permitted to 15-30°C (59-86°F).

## Boostrix RX

pertussis vaccine, acellular - diphtheria toxoid - tetanus toxoid

(GlaxoSmithKline)

**THERAPEUTIC CLASS:** Vaccine/toxoid combination

**INDICATIONS:** Active booster immunization against tetanus, diphtheria, and pertussis as a single dose in individuals 10-64 yrs of age.

**DOSAGE:** *Adults:* >18-64 yrs: 0.5mL IM into the deltoid muscle. For minor and uncomplicated wounds, give a booster dose only if individuals have not received tetanus toxoid within the preceeding 10 years.
*Pediatrics:* 10-18 yrs: 0.5mL IM into the deltoid muscle. For minor and uncomplicated wounds, give a booster dose only if individuals have not received tetanus toxoid within the preceeding 10 years.

**HOW SUPPLIED:** Inj: (Diphtheria-Pertussis-Tetanus) 2.5LF-18.5mcg-5LF/0.5mL [vial]

**CONTRAINDICATIONS:** Encephalopathy (eg, coma, decreased level of consciousness, prolonged seizures) within 7 days of administration of a previous pertussis antigen-containing vaccine.

**WARNINGS/PRECAUTIONS:** Caution if Guillain-Barre syndrome and brachial neuritis within 6 weeks of previous tetanus toxoid vaccine. Defer Tdap vaccination if progressive neurologic disorder, uncontrolled epilepsy, progressive encepalopathy or unstable neurological conditions (eg, cerebrovascular events, acute encephalopathy) occur; caution in giving pertussis antigen-containing vaccine. Do not give Td, Tdap, or emergency dose of Td more frequently than every 10 yrs if patient has experienced previous Arthus-type reaction. May cause allergic reactions in latex-sensitive patients. May not obtain expected immune response in immunosuppressed individuals. Hypersensitivity reaction possible; epinephrine injection (1:1000) should be readily available.

**ADVERSE REACTIONS:** Local: pain, redness, swelling, increased arm circumference (>5mm). Systemic: headache, fatigue, fever, nausea, vomiting, diarrhea, abdominal pain.

**INTERACTIONS:** Concomitant with influenza virus vaccine lowers geometric mean antibody concentrations for antibodies to the pertussis antigens filamentous hemagglutinin and pertactin. Avoid mixing with other vaccines in the same syringe or vial. May give tetanus immune globulin on separate site, syringe, and needle. Immunosuppressive therapies, including irradiation, antimetabolites, alkylating agents, cytotoxic drugs, and corticosteroids may reduce the immune response to vaccines.

**PREGNANCY:** Category C, caution in nursing.

**MECHANISM OF ACTION:** Stimulates immune system to elicit immune response, which produces neutralizing antibodies that may protect against tetanus, diphtheria, and pertussis.

B

## NURSING CONSIDERATIONS

**Assessment:** Assess immunization history and current health/medical status, previous hypersensitivity, immunization-related complications such as Guillain-Barre syndrome and brachial neuritis, and possible drug interactions. Assess for uncontrolled epilepsy, progressive encephalopathy and neurological disorders, and pregnancy/nursing status.

**Monitoring:** Monitor for local adverse events (eg, pain, redness, swelling at injection site), increase in arm circumference, and GI symptoms.

**Patient Counseling:** Inform about benefits/risks; report any adverse reactions to physician. Advise patient, parent or guardian should acquire vaccine information statements given by the national childhood vaccine injury act of 1986 prior to immunization.

**Administration:** IM (deltoid muscle). **Storage:** Refrigerate at 2-8°C (36-46°F). Do not freeze. Discard if vaccine has been frozen.

# BREVIBLOC RX

esmolol HCl (Baxter)

**THERAPEUTIC CLASS:** Selective beta$_1$-blocker

**INDICATIONS:** For rapid control of ventricular rate in atrial fibrillation or atrial flutter in perioperative, postoperative, or other emergent circumstances. For noncompensatory sinus tachycardia. Treatment of tachycardia and hypertension that occur during induction and tracheal intubation, during surgery, on emergence from anesthesia, and in the postoperative period.

**DOSAGE:** *Adults:* Supraventricular Tachycardia: Titrate dose based on ventricular rate. Load: 0.5mg/kg over 1 min. Maint: 0.05mg/kg/min for next 4 min. May increase by 0.05mg/kg/min at intervals of 4 min or more up to 0.2mg/kg/min. Rapid slowing of ventricular response: Repeat 0.5mg/kg load over 1 min, then 0.1mg/kg/min for 4 min. If needed, another (final) load of 0.5mg/kg over 1 min, then 0.15mg/kg/min for 4 min up to 0.2mg/kg/min. May continue infusions for 24-48hrs. Intraoperative/Postoperative Tachycardia and/or HTN: Immediate Control: Initial: 80mg bolus over 30 sec. Maint: 0.15mg/kg/min. May titrate up to 0.3mg/kg/min. Gradual Control: Initial: 0.5mg/kg over 1 min. Maint: 0.05mg/kg/min for 4 min. Then, if needed, may repeat load and increase to 0.1mg/kg/min.

**HOW SUPPLIED:** Inj: 10mg/mL [10mL, 250mL], 20mg/mL [5mL, 100mL]

**CONTRAINDICATIONS:** Sinus bradycardia, heart block greater than first degree, cardiogenic shock or overt heart failure.

**WARNINGS/PRECAUTIONS:** Hypotension may occur; monitor BP and reduce dose or d/c if needed. May cause cardiac failure; withdraw at 1st sign of impending cardiac failure. Caution with supraventricular arrhythmias when patient is compromised hemodynamically or is taking other drugs that decrease peripheral resistance, myocardial filling/contractility, and/or electrical impulse propagation in the myocardium. Not for HTN associated with hypothermia. Caution in bronchospastic diseases; titrate to lowest possible effective dose and terminate immediately in the event of bronchospasm. Caution in diabetics; may mask tachycardia occurring with hypoglycemia. Caution in impaired renal function. Avoid concentrations >10mg/mL and infusions into small veins or through butterfly catheters. Sloughing of skin and necrosis reported with infiltration and extravasation. Use caution when discontinuing infusion in CAD patients.

**ADVERSE REACTIONS:** Hypotension, dizziness, diaphoresis, somnolence, confusion, headache, agitation, bronchospasm, nausea, infusion-site reactions.

**INTERACTIONS:** Additive effects with catecholamine-depleting agents (eg, reserpine); monitor for hypotension or bradycardia. Levels increased by warfarin or morphine; titrate with caution. May increase digoxin levels; titrate with caution. May prolong effects of succinylcholine; titrate with caution. Caution when using with verapamil in depressed myocardial function; fatal cardiac arrest may occur. Do not use to control supraventricular tachycardia with vasoconstrictive and inotropic agents (eg, dopamine, epinephrine, norepinephrine) because of the danger of blocking cardiac contractility when systemic vascular resistance is high. Patients with a history of severe anaphylactic reaction may be more reactive to repeated challenge and unresponsive to the usual doses of epinephrine used to treat allergic reaction.

**PREGNANCY:** Category C, caution in nursing.

**MECHANISM OF ACTION:** Selective $\beta_1$ blocker; inhibits $\beta_1$ receptors located chiefly in cardiac muscle, and at higher doses begins to inhibit $\beta_2$ receptors located chiefly in the bronchial and vascular musculature.

**PHARMACOKINETICS: Distribution:** Plasma protein binding (55%). **Metabolism:** Rapid. Through hydrolysis of the ester linkage in red blood cells to methanol and free acid. **Elimination:** Urine (73-88% unchanged); $T_{1/2}$=9 min (Brevibloc), and 3.7 hrs (acid metabolites).

## NURSING CONSIDERATIONS

**Assessment:** Assess for sinus bradycardia, heart block greater than first degree, cardiogenic shock or overt heart failure, hypotension, HTN associated with hypothermia, bronchospastic disease, DM, renal impairment, and possible drug interactions (verapamil).

**Monitoring:** Monitor BP, HR. Monitor for signs/symptoms of impending cardiac failure, hypotension (eg, diaphoresis or dizziness), postoperative tachycardia/HTN, bronchospasm, and masking signs of hypoglycemia.

**Patient Counseling:** Inform about benefits/risks. Report any adverse reactions to physician.

**Administration:** IV route. Prediluted to provide ready-to-use vials. Do not introduce additives to vials. **Storage:** Store at 25°C (77°F); excursions permitted to 15-30°C (59-86°F). Protect from freezing.

# BREVOXYL — RX

benzoyl peroxide (Stiefel)

**THERAPEUTIC CLASS:** Antibacterial/keratolytic

**INDICATIONS:** Topical treatment of mild to moderate acne vulgaris.

**DOSAGE:** *Adults:* (Gel) Apply qd-bid to clean affected area. (Creamy Wash) Shake well. Wet affected area, apply creamy wash, work to a full lather, rinse thoroughly and pat dry; wash qd for 1st week, then bid thereafter if tolerated. *Pediatrics:* ≥12 yrs: (Gel) Apply qd-bid to clean affected area. (Creamy Wash) Shake well. Wet affected area, apply creamy wash, work to a full lather, rinse thoroughly and pat dry; wash qd for 1st week, then bid thereafter if tolerated.

**HOW SUPPLIED:** Gel: 4%, 8% [42.5g]; Creamy Wash: 4%, 8% [170.1g]

**WARNINGS/PRECAUTIONS:** Avoid contact with hair, eyes, mucous membranes, carpeting, and fabrics. Avoid intensive sun bathing or UV radiation.

**ADVERSE REACTIONS:** Contact sensitization reactions, erythema, peeling, skin irritation, burning, dryness, pruritus, dermatitis, allergic contact dermatitis, face edema.

**PREGNANCY:** Category C, caution in nursing.

**MECHANISM OF ACTION:** Antibacterial/keratolytic agent; not established; demonstrated activity against *Propionibacterium acnes.* Has also shown to have a mild keratolytic effect.

**PHARMACOKINETICS: Absorption:** Absorbed by skin. **Metabolism:** Metabolized in skin to benzoic acid. **Elimination:** Urine (benzoate; metabolite).

## NURSING CONSIDERATIONS

**Assessment:** Assess proper diagnosis of acne vulgaris. Assess use in pregnant/nursing patients.

**Monitoring:** Monitor for adequate clinical response and development of contact sensitization reactions, and adverse reactions.

**Patient Counseling:** Cleanse affected areas prior to application of medication. Inform that clinically visible improvement will normally occur by third week of therapy and maximum lesion reduction may be expected after approximately 8-12 weeks of use. Avoid contact with eyes and mucous membranes. Avoid medication coming in contact with hair, fabrics, or carpeting to prevent bleaching. Avoid intensive sunbathing or UV radiation.

**Administration:** Topical. For external use only. **Storage:** Store at controlled room temperature; 15-30°C (59-86°F).

## BROVANA RX

arformoterol tartrate (Sepracor)

**Long-acting $\beta_2$-adrenergic agonists may increase the risk of asthma-related death.**

**THERAPEUTIC CLASS:** Beta$_2$-agonist

**INDICATIONS:** Long-term maintenance treatment of bronchoconstriction in patients with COPD, including chronic bronchitis and emphysema.

**DOSAGE:** *Adults:* Usual: 15mcg bid (am and pm). Max: 30mcg/day. Administer via nebulizer.

**HOW SUPPLIED:** Sol, Inhalation: 15mcg/2mL [30$^s$, 60$^s$]

**CONTRAINDICATIONS:** Hypersensitivity to racemic formoterol

**WARNINGS/PRECAUTIONS:** Not indicated for treatment of acute episodes of bronchospasm. Should not be initiated or used in children or patients with acutely deteriorating COPD. Fatalities reported with excessive use of inhaled sympathomimetics, avoid use with other long-acting $\beta_2$-agonists. D/C regular use of short acting $\beta_2$-agonists (eg, qid) before initiating therapy. May produce life-threatening paradoxical bronchospasm. Caution in patients with convulsive disorders, thyrotoxicosis, cardiovascular disorders especially coronary insufficiency, cardiac arrhythmias, and HTN. Immediate hypersensitivity reactions may occur.

**ADVERSE REACTIONS:** Pain, chest pain, back pain , diarrhea, sinusitis, leg cramps, dyspnea, rash, flu syndrome, peripheral edema.

**INTERACTIONS:** Sympathetic effects may be potentiated with concomitant use of additional adrenergic agonists. Concomitant use with methylxanthines, steroids, or diuretics may potentiate hypokalemia. Caution with co-administration with non-potassium sparing diuretics may cause ECG changes. Use extreme caution in patients being treated with MAOIs, TCAs, or any drugs known to prolong the QTc interval. Caution with β-blockers.

**PREGNANCY:** Category C, caution in nursing.

**MECHANISM OF ACTION:** $\beta_2$-adrenergic agonist; stimulates intracellular adenyl cyclase, which catalyzes conversion of ATP to cAMP to produce relaxation of bronchial smooth muscle and inhibition of release of mediators of immediate hypersensitivity from cells (mast cells).

**PHARMACOKINETICS: Absorption:** $C_{max}$=4.3pg/mL, $T_{max}$=30 min, AUC=34.5pg•hr/mL. **Distribution:** Plasma protein binding (52-65%). **Metabolism:** Glucuronidation (major) via uridine diphosphoglucuronosyltransferase (UGT) isoenzymes, O-demethylation (minor) via CYP2D6, CYP2C19. **Elimination:** Urine (1%); $T_{1/2}$=26 hrs.

### NURSING CONSIDERATIONS

**Assessment:** Assess for hepatic impairment, acute deteriorating COPD, CVD (coronary insufficiency, cardiac arrhythmias, HTN), convulsive disorders, thyrotoxicosis, and possible drug interactions. D/C inhaled, short-acting $\beta_2$-agonists (if using on regular basis) before therapy.

**Monitoring:** Monitor for signs/symptoms of acute deteriorating COPD, cardiovascular effects (increased BP, palpitations), worsening of symptoms, paradoxical bronchospasm, and hypersensitivity reactions (anaphylactic, urticaria, angioedema, rash, bronchospasm).

**Patient Counseling:** To be used by nebulizer only, instruct not to inject or swallow. If taking inhaled, short-acting $\beta_2$-agonists on regular basis, instruct to d/c before therapy. Inform not for relief of acute respiratory symptoms. Caution drug may increase risk of asthma-related death. Seek medical attention if symptoms of deterioration of COPD, worsening of symptoms, therapy becomes less effective, need more inhalation from short-acting $\beta_2$-agonist than usual, paradoxical bronchospasms, and hypersensitivity (anaphylactic, urticaria, angioedema, rash, bronchospasm) occur.

**Administration:** Oral inhalation. **Storage:** Refrigerate; 2-8°C (36-46°F) or store at 20-25°C (68-77°F) for up to 6 weeks. Use immediately once opened; discard if colored. Protect from light and excessive heat.

# BUMETANIDE — RX

bumetanide (Various)

**Can lead to profound water and electrolyte depletion with excessive use.**

**OTHER BRAND NAMES:** Bumex (Roche Labs)

**THERAPEUTIC CLASS:** Loop diuretic

**INDICATIONS:** Treatment of edema associated with CHF, hepatic disease, and renal disease including nephrotic syndrome.

**DOSAGE:** *Adults:* ≥18 yrs: PO: Usual: 0.5-2mg qd. Maint: May give every other day or every 3-4 days. Max: 10mg/day. IV/IM: Initial: 0.5-1mg over 1-2 min, may repeat every 2-3 hrs for 2-3 doses. Max: 10mg/day. Elderly: Start at low end of dosing range.

**HOW SUPPLIED:** Inj: 0.25mg/mL; Tab: 0.5mg*, 1mg*, 2mg* *scored

**CONTRAINDICATIONS:** Anuria, hepatic coma, severe electrolyte depletion.

**WARNINGS/PRECAUTIONS:** Monitor for volume/electrolyte depletion, hypokalemia, blood dyscrasias, hepatic damage. Elderly are prone to volume/electrolyte depletion. Caution in elderly, hepatic cirrhosis and ascites. Associated with ototoxicity, hypocalcemia, thrombocytopenia, hypomagnesemia, hypokalemia, and hyperuricemia. Hypersensitivity with sulfonamide allergy. D/C if marked increase in BUN or creatinine or if develop oliguria with progressive renal disease.

**ADVERSE REACTIONS:** Muscle cramps, dizziness, hypotension, headache, nausea, hyperuricemia, hypokalemia, hyponatremia, hyperglycemia, azotemia, increased serum creatinine.

**INTERACTIONS:** Avoid aminoglycosides, ototoxic and nephrotoxic drugs, indomethacin. Lithium toxicity. Probenecid reduces effects. Potentiates antihypertensives.

**PREGNANCY:** Category C, not for use in nursing.

**MECHANISM OF ACTION:** Loop diuretic; inhibits sodium reabsorption in ascending loop of Henle.

**PHARMACOKINETICS: Absorption:** (IV) $T_{max}$=15-30 min. (Tab) $T_{max}$=1-2 hrs. **Distribution:** Plasma protein binding (94-96%). **Metabolism:** Oxidation. **Elimination:** Urine, bile (2%); $T_{1/2}$=1-1.5 hrs.

## NURSING CONSIDERATIONS

**Assessment:** Assess for progressive renal disease, severe electrolyte depletion, anuria, oliguria, risk for vetricular arrhythmia, possible drug interactions, DM, impaired GI absorption, CHF, sulfonamide allergy, and liver disease (hepatic coma).

**Monitoring:** Periodically monitor serum potassium, serum electrolytes, CBC, blood glucose, and renal function. Monitor for signs/symptoms of ototoxicity, hypersensitivity reactions, hyperuricemia, oliguria, and thrombocytopenia.

**Patient Counseling:** Advise to seek medical attention if symptoms of ototoxicity, oliguria, hypersensitivity reactions, or thrombocytopenia occur.

**Administration:** Oral route. **Storage:** IV: 20-25°C (68-77°F). Protect from light. Tab: 15-30°C (59-86°F).

# BUPRENEX

CIII

B

buprenorphine HCl (Reckitt Benckiser)

**THERAPEUTIC CLASS:** Opioid analgesic

**INDICATIONS:** Relief of moderate to severe pain.

**DOSAGE:** *Adults:* 0.3mg IM/IV q6h prn. Repeat if needed, 30-60 min after initial dose and then prn. High Risk Patients/Concomitant CNS depressants: Reduce dose by approximately 50%. May use single doses ≤0.6mg IM if not at high-risk.
*Pediatrics:* ≥13 yrs: 0.3mg IM/IV q6h prn. Repeat if needed, 30-60 min after initial dose and then prn. High Risk Patients/Concomitant CNS depressants: Reduce dose by approximately 50%. May use single doses ≤0.6mg IM if not at high-risk. 2-12 yrs: 2-6mcg/kg IM/IV q4-6h.

**HOW SUPPLIED:** Inj: 0.3mg/mL

**WARNINGS/PRECAUTIONS:** Significant respiratory depression reported; caution with compromised respiratory function. May increase CSF pressure; caution with head injury, intracranial lesions. Caution with debilitated, BPH, biliary tract dysfunction, myxedema, hypothyroidism, urethral stricture, acute alcoholism, Addison's disease, CNS disease, coma, toxic psychoses, delirium tremens, elderly, pediatrics, kyphoscoliosis or hepatic/renal/pulmonary impairment. May impair mental or physical abilities. May precipitate withdrawal in narcotic-dependence. May lead to psychological dependence.

**ADVERSE REACTIONS:** Sedation, NV, dizziness, sweating, hypotension, headache, miosis, hypoventilation.

**INTERACTIONS:** Caution with MAOIs, CNS and respiratory depressants. Respiratory and cardiovascular collapse reported with diazepam. Increased CNS depression with other narcotic analgesics, general anesthetics, antihistamines, benzodiazepines, phenothiazines, other tranquilizers, sedative-hypnotics. Decreased clearance with CYP3A4 inhibitors (eg, macrolides, azole antifungals, protease inhibitors). Increased clearance with CYP3A4 inducers (eg, rifampin, carbamazepine, phenytoin).

**PREGNANCY:** Category C, not for use in nursing.

**MECHANISM OF ACTION:** Opioid analgesic; high affinity binding to μ-opiate receptors in CNS. Possesses slow rate of dissociation from its receptor. Also possesses narcotic antagonist activity.

**PHARMACOKINETICS: Absorption:** $T_{max}$=1 hr. **Distribution:** Found in breast milk. **Metabolism:** Liver. **Elimination:** $T_{1/2}$=1.2-7.2 hrs.

## NURSING CONSIDERATIONS

**Assessment:** Assess for compromised respiratory function (eg, COPD, hypoxia), head injury, intracranial lesions, age of patient, hepatic/renal function, myxedema or hypothyroidism, adrenal cortical insufficiencies (eg, Addison's disease), CNS depression or coma, toxic psychosis, prostatic hypertrophy or urethral stricture, acute alcoholism, delirium tremens, kyphoscoliosis, biliary tract dysfunction, pregnancy/nursing, and possible drug interactions.

**Monitoring:** Monitor for signs/symptoms of respiratory depression, CNS depression, elevation of CSF pressure, increased intracholedochal pressure, drug dependence, and withdrawal effects.

**Patient Counseling:** Inform that medication may impair mental/physicial abilities; use caution when performing dangerous tasks (eg, operating machinery/driving). Advise to notify physician of all medications currently taken. Instruct to avoid use of other CNS depressants and alcohol during therapy. Advise that medication may lead to dependence. Counsel to not exceed prescribed dosage. Advise to avoid abruptly discontinuing medication. Counsel to contact physician if signs/symptoms of respiratory depression develop.

**Administration:** Deep IM or slow IV route. **Storage:** Avoid excessive heat (over 40°C or 104°F ). Protect from prolonged exposure to light.

B

# BuSpar RX

## buspirone HCl (Bristol-Myers Squibb)

**THERAPEUTIC CLASS:** Atypical anxiolytic

**INDICATIONS:** Management of anxiety disorders, short-term relief of anxiety symptoms.

**DOSAGE:** *Adults:* Usual: 7.5mg bid. Titrate: May increase by 5mg/day every 2-3 days. Usual: 20-30mg/day. Max: 60mg/day. Use low dose with potent CYP3A4 inhibitors (eg, 2.5mg qd with nefazodone). Take consistently with or without food; bioavailability increased with food.

**HOW SUPPLIED:** Tab: 5mg*, 10mg*, 15mg*, 30mg* *scored

**WARNINGS/PRECAUTIONS:** Avoid with hepatic or renal impairment.

**ADVERSE REACTIONS:** Dizziness, nausea, headache, nervousness, lightheadedness, excitement, dystonia, fatigue, parkinsonism, akathisia, restless legs syndrome, restlessness.

**INTERACTIONS:** Avoid MAOIs and alcohol. Withdraw other CNS depressants gradually before therapy. Caution with psychotropics. Elevated liver transaminases reported with trazodone. Increases haloperidol levels. Verapamil, diltiazem, grapefruit juice, nefazodone, itraconazole, cimetidine, erythromycin increase plasma levels. May increase levels of both drugs with nefazodone; decrease dose of buspirone. Decreased plasma levels and effects with rifampin; may need to adjust buspirone dose. CYP3A4 inhibitors may increase plasma levels and CYP3A4 inducers may increase metabolism of buspirone; may need dose adjustment. Presystemic clearance may be decreased with food. May displace digoxin.

**PREGNANCY:** Category B, not for use in nursing.

**MECHANISM OF ACTION:** Atypical antianxiety agent; not fully established. Binds with high affinity to serotonin receptors (5-$HT_{1A}$) and moderate affinity to dopamine receptors ($D_2$); may have indirect effects on other neurotransmitter systems.

**PHARMACOKINETICS: Absorption:** Rapid; $C_{max}$=1-6ng/mL; $T_{max}$=40-90 min. **Distribution:** Plasma protein binding (86%). **Metabolism:** CYP3A4; oxidation and hyroxylation; 1-pyrimidinylpiperazine (active metabolite). **Elimination:** Urine (29-63%), feces (18-38%); $T_{1/2}$=2-3 hrs.

### NURSING CONSIDERATIONS

**Assessment:** Assess for hypersensitivity, hepatic/renal functions, and possible drug interactions (eg, MAOIs).

**Monitoring:** Monitor BP, CNS disturbances, withdrawal symptoms (eg, irritability, anxiety, agitation, insomnia, tremor, abdominal cramps/muscle cramps, vomiting, sweating, flu-like symptoms w/o fever, and seizures), pseudo-parkinsonism, akathisia, TD, dystonia.

**Patient Counseling:** Counsel to avoid hazardous tasks (eg, operating machinery/driving), ingesting large amounts of grapefruit juice. Advise to notify physician of current medications, alcohol use, and pregnancy status.

**Administration:** Oral route. **Storage:** 25°C (77°F); excursions permitted to 15-30°C (59-86°F). Dispense in tight, light-resistant container.

# Byetta RX

## exenatide (Amylin/Lilly)

**THERAPEUTIC CLASS:** Incretin mimetic

**INDICATIONS:** Adjunct to diet and exercise to improve glycemic control in adults with type 2 diabetes mellitus (DM).

**DOSAGE:** *Adults:* Initial: 5mcg SQ bid, at anytime within 60 mins before am & pm meals (or before the two main meals of day approx. 6 hrs or more apart). Titrate: May increase to 10mcg bid after 1 month. CrCl 30-50mL/min: Caution when initiating or escalating doses from 5mcg to 10mcg. Reduction of sulfonylurea dose may be considered to reduce risk of hypoglycemia.

**HOW SUPPLIED:** Inj: 5mcg/dose, 10mcg/dose [60-dose prefilled pen]

**WARNINGS/PRECAUTIONS:** Not a substitute for insulin. Should not be used in the treatment of type 1 diabetes or for the treatment of diabetic ketoacidosis. Acute pancreatitis reported; d/c if suspected. Increased SrCr, renal impairment, worsened chronic renal failure, and acute renal failure reported; avoid with severe renal impairment (CrCl <30mL/min) or end stage renal disease (ESRD). Avoid with severe GI disease or a history of pancreatitis. Caution with renal transplantation. May develop immunogenicity; consider alternative antidiabetic therapy if there is worsening glycemic control or failure to achieve targeted glycemic control. Hypersensitivity reactions reported. Caution in elderly.

**ADVERSE REACTIONS:** N/V, immunogenicity, diarrhea, feeling jittery, dizziness, headache, dyspepsia, asthenia, gastroesophageal reflux disease, hyperhidrosis, hypoglycemia.

**INTERACTIONS:** Caution with oral medications with narrow therapeutic index or require rapid GI absorption. Drugs dependent on threshold concentrations for efficacy (eg, contraceptives, antibiotics) should be taken 1 hr before. Caution with concomitant use of warfarin; may increase INR with associated bleeding. Increase risk of hypoglycemia when used in combination with sulfonylureas and with other glucose-independent insulin secretagogues (eg, meglitinides). May decrease concentrations of acetaminophen, digoxin, lovastatin. Concurrent use with insulin has not been studied and cannot be recommended.

**PREGNANCY:** Category C, caution in nursing.

**MECHANISM OF ACTION:** Incretin-mimetic agent, GLP-1 receptor agonist; enhances glucose-dependent insulin secretion by the pancreatic β-cell, suppresses inappropriately elevated glucagon secretion, and slows gastric emptying.

**PHARMACOKINETICS: Absorption:** (SQ) $C_{max}$=211pg/mL, AUC=1036pg•h/mL, $T_{max}$=2.1 hrs. **Distribution:** $V_d$=28.3L. **Elimination:** $T_{1/2}$=2.4 hrs.

## NURSING CONSIDERATIONS

**Assessment:** Assess for type 1 diabetes, diabetic ketoacidosis, history of pancreatitis, renal impairment, severe GI disease, pregnancy/nursing status, and for possible drug interactions. Assess glucose and $HbA_{1c}$ levels.

**Monitoring:** Monitor for signs/symptoms of acute pancreatitis (eg, severe abdominal pain, vomiting), hypoglycemia, GI events (eg, nausea, vomiting, diarrhea), immunogenicity, and for hypersensitivity reactions. Monitor renal function, glucose levels, and $HbA_{1c}$ levels.

**Patient Counseling:** Advise of the potential risks and benefits of therapy. Instruct to never share injection pen with another patient. Inform about self-management practices (eg, proper storage of drug, injection technique, timing of dosage and concomitant oral drugs, adherence to meal planning, regular physical activity). Instruct to administer within 60-min period before morning and evening meals. Advise to not administer after a meal. Inform that if a dose is missed, treatment regimen should be resumed as prescribed with the next scheduled dose. Advise to inform physician if pregnant or intend to become pregnant. Instruct to contact physician if signs/symptoms suggestive of acute pancreatitis (eg, severe abdominal pain), renal dysfunction, or hypersensitivity develop.

**Administration:** SQ injection (thigh, abdomen, or upper arm). **Storage:** Prior to first use, keep at 2-8°C (36-46°F). After first use, can be kept at ≤25°C (77°F). Do not freeze. Protect from light. Discard pen 30 days after the first use, even if some drug remains.

B

# BYSTOLIC RX

nebivolol HCl (Forest)

**THERAPEUTIC CLASS:** Selective $beta_1$-blocker

**INDICATIONS:** Treatment of hypertension alone or in combination with other antihypertensive agents.

**DOSAGE:** *Adults:* Initial: 5mg qd. Titrate: May increase dose if needed at 2-week intervals. Max: 40mg qd. Hepatic Impairment/CrCl <30mL/min: 2.5mg qd; upward titration may be performed cautiously.

**HOW SUPPLIED:** Tab: 2.5mg, 5mg, 10mg, 20mg

**CONTRAINDICATIONS:** Severe bradycardia, heart block >1st degree, cardiogenic shock, decompensated cardiac failure, sick sinus syndrome (unless permanent pacemaker in place), severe hepatic impairment (Child-Pugh >B).

**WARNINGS/PRECAUTIONS:** Exacerbation of angina and occurrence of MI and ventricular arrhythmias reported in patients with coronary artery disease (CAD) following abrupt withdrawal; taper over 1-2 weeks when possible. Avoid with bronchospastic disease. Caution with compensated CHF; d/c if heart failure worsens. Caution with peripheral vascular disease (PVD) and severe renal/moderate hepatic impairment. May mask signs/symptoms of hypoglycemia or hyperthyroidism. Abrupt withdrawal may also exacerbate symptoms of hyperthyroidism or precipitate a thyroid storm. Caution with history of severe anaphylactic reactions. Patients with known/suspected pheochromocytoma should initially receive an α-blocker prior to use of any β-blocker.

**ADVERSE REACTIONS:** Headache, fatigue, dizziness, diarrhea, nausea.

**INTERACTIONS:** CYP2D6 inhibitors (eg, fluoxetine, quinidine, propafenone, paroxetine, cimetidine) may increase levels; monitor and consider dosage adjustment. Sildenafil may decrease levels. May depress myocardial function with anesthetic agents (eg, ether, cyclopropane, trichloroethylene); monitor closely. May potentiate hypoglycemic effect of glucose-lowering agents (eg, insulin, oral hypoglycemic agents); use with caution. Caution with calcium antagonists (particularly verapamil and diltiazem type) or antiarrhythmic agents (eg, disopyramide). Excessive reduction of sympathetic activity may occur with catecholamine-depleting drugs (eg, reserpine, guanethidine); monitor closely. D/C for several days before gradually tapering clonidine.

**PREGNANCY:** Category C, not for use in nursing.

**MECHANISM OF ACTION:** β-adrenergic receptor blocking agent; not established. Possible factors include decreased HR, myocardial contractility, diminution of tonic sympathetic outflow to the periphery from cerebral vasomotor centers, suppression of renin activity, vasodilation, and decreased peripheral resistance.

**PHARMACOKINETICS: Absorption:** $T_{max}$=1.5-4 hrs. **Distribution:** Plasma protein binding (98%). **Metabolism**: N-dealkylation and oxidation via CYP2D6. **Elimination**: Urine (38%), feces (44%); $T_{1/2}$=12 hrs (CYP2D6 extensive metabolizers), 19 hrs (poor metabolizers).

## NURSING CONSIDERATIONS

**Assessment:** Assess for severe bradycardia, heart block, cardiogenic shock, cardiac failure, sick sinus syndrome, angina, MI, severe hypotension, severe hepatic impairment, hypersensitivity, pregnancy/nursing status, and possible drug interactions.

**Monitoring:** Monitor diastolic BP, ECG, HR, renal clearance, serum glucose level, difficulty breathing, and weight gain.

**Patient Counseling:** Advise patient with CAD not to abruptly d/c therapy. Use caution with severe renal impairment. Inform that drug can be taken with/without food and if a dose is missed, take the next scheduled only. Advise to consult a physician if any difficulty in breathing occurs or signs and symptoms of worsening CHF develop. Instruct not to interrupt or d/c therapy without consulting physician.

**Administration:** Oral route. **Storage:** 20-25°C (68-77°F).

# CADUET RX

atorvastatin calcium - amlodipine besylate (Pfizer)

C

**THERAPEUTIC CLASS:** Calcium channel blocker/HMG-CoA reductase inhibitor

**INDICATIONS:** When treatment with both amlodipine and atorvastatin is appropriate. (Amlodipine) Treatment of HTN, chronic stable or vasospastic angina (Prinzmetal's or variant angina), recently documented coronary artery disease (CAD). (Atorvastatin) To reduce the risk of MI, stroke, revascularization procedures, and angina in adults without clinically evident CHD but with multiple risk factors for CHD. To reduce the risk of MI and stroke in patients with type 2 DM, and without clinically evident CHD, but with multiple risk factors for CHD. In patients with clinically evident CHD to reduce the risk of non-fatal MI, fatal and non-fatal stroke, revascularization procedures, hospitalization for CHF, and angina. Adjunct to diet to reduce total cholesterol (total-C), LDL-C, TG, and Apo B levels, and to increase HDL-C in primary hypercholesterolemia (heterozygous familial and nonfamilial) and mixed dyslipidemia (Types IIa and IIb). Adjunct to diet for elevated serum TG levels (Type IV). Treatment of primary dysbetalipoproteinemia (Type III) inadequately responding to diet. Adjunct to other lipid-lowering treatments or if treatments are unavailable, to reduce total-C and LDL-C in homozygous familial hypercholesterolemia. Adjunct to diet to lower total-C, LDL-C, and Apo B in boys and postmenarchal girls, 10-17 yrs of age, with heterozygous familial hypercholesterolemia.

**DOSAGE:** *Adults:* Individualized dosing. (Amlodipine): HTN: Initial: 5mg qd. Titrate over 7-14 days according to patient's need. Max: 10mg qd. Small, Fragile, or Elderly/Hepatic Dysfunction/Concomitant Antihypertensive Therapy: Initial: 2.5mg qd. Angina/CAD: 5-10mg qd. (Atorvastatin): Hypercholesterolemia/Mixed Dyslipidemia: Initial: 10-20mg qd (or 40mg qd for LDL-C reduction >45%). Titrate: Adjust dose if needed at 2-4 week intervals. Usual: 10-80mg qd. Homozygous Familial Hypercholesterolemia: 10-80mg qd. Concomitant with Cyclosporine: 10mg qd. Concomitant with Clarithromycin/Itraconazole/Ritonavir plus Saquinavir or Lopinavir: 20mg qd. Replacement Therapy: May substitute for individually titrated components. *Pediatrics:* 6-17 yrs: (Amlodipine): HTN: 2.5-5mg qd. 10-17 yrs (Postmenarchal): (Atorvastatin): Heterozygous Familial Hypercholesterolemia: Initial: 10mg/day. Titrate: Adjust dose if needed at intervals of ≥4 weeks. Max: 20mg/day.

**HOW SUPPLIED:** Tab: (Amlodipine-Atorvastatin) 2.5mg-10mg, 2.5mg-20mg, 2.5mg-40mg, 5mg-10mg, 5mg-20mg, 5mg-40mg, 5mg-80mg, 10mg-10mg, 10mg-20mg, 10mg-40mg, 10mg-80mg

**CONTRAINDICATIONS:** Active liver disease, unexplained persistent elevations of serum transaminases, pregnancy, nursing mothers.

**WARNINGS/PRECAUTIONS:** May rarely increase angina or MI with severe obstructive CAD. Monitor LFTs prior to therapy, at 12 weeks after initiation, with dose elevation, and periodically thereafter. Reduce dose or withdraw if AST or ALT >3x ULN persists. Caution with heavy alcohol use and/or history of hepatic disease, severe aortic stenosis, and CHF. D/C if markedly elevated CPK levels occur, if myopathy is diagnosed or suspected, or if predisposition to renal failure secondary to rhabdomyolysis. Increased risk of hemorrhagic stroke in patients with recent stroke or TIA. Caution in elderly.

**ADVERSE REACTIONS:** Headache, edema, palpitations, dizziness, fatigue, infection, diarrhea, rash, arthralgia, asthenia, abdominal pain.

**INTERACTIONS:** (Atorvastatin) May increase levels when used with strong CYP3A4 inhibitors (eg, clarithromycin, HIV protease inhibitors, itraconazole) and grapefruit juice (>1.2L/day). Inhibitors of OATP1B1 (eg, cyclosporine) may increase bioavailability. Inducers of CYP 3A4 (eg, rifampin, efavirenz) decrease atorvastatin level. Coadministration with digoxin may increase digoxin levels; monitor appropriately. Coadministration with oral contraceptives increases AUC of norethindrone and ethinyl estradiol. Cyclosporine, fibric acid derivatives, niacin, erythromycin, immunosupressive drugs, and azole antifungals may increase the risk of myopathy. Caution with drugs that decrease levels and activity of endogenous steroid hormones (eg, ketoconazole, spirinolactone, cimetidine). Decreases level with Maalox TC, colestipol. Increases level with diltiazem.



**PREGNANCY:** Category X, not for use in nursing

## NURSING CONSIDERATIONS

**Assessment:** Assess for severe aortic stenosis, CHF, liver disease, obstructive CAD, alcoholism, pregnancy/nursing status and possible drug interactions. Obtain baseline LFTs.

**Monitoring:** Monitor LFTs at 12 weeks following initiation of therapy and any drug dose elevation, then periodically thereafter. Monitor for signs/symptoms of hypotension, hypersensitivity reaction, angina, and myopathy. Monitor LFTs, CPK.

**Patient Counseling:** Advise to seek medical attention if symptoms of hypotension, hypersensitivity reaction, angina, or myopathy (eg, unexplained muscle pain, tenderness, fever, malaise) occur. Instruct to avoid alcohol consumption.

**Administration:** Oral route. **Storage:** 25°C (77°F); excursions permitted to 15-30°C (59-86°F).

# CALAN — RX

verapamil HCl (G.D. Searle)

**THERAPEUTIC CLASS:** Calcium channel blocker (nondihydropyridine)

**INDICATIONS:** Treatment of essential hypertension and vasospastic, unstable, and chronic stable angina. Control of ventricular rate at rest and during stress in patients with chronic atrial flutter and/or atrial fibrillation (A-Fib), in association with digitalis. Prophylaxis of repetitive paroxysmal supraventricular tachycardia (PSVT).

**DOSAGE:** *Adults:* HTN: Individualize dosing by titration. Initial: 80mg tid. Usual: 360-480mg qd. Elderly/Small Stature: Initial: 40mg tid. Angina: Usual: 80-120mg tid. Patients with Increased Response to Verapamil (eg, Elderly, Decreased Hepatic Function): Initial: 40mg tid. Titrate: Increase daily or weekly. A-Fib (Digitalized): Usual: 240-320mg qd given tid-qid. PSVT Prophylaxis (Non-Digitalized): 240-480mg/day given tid-qid. Max: 480mg qd. Severe Hepatic Dysfunction: Give 30% of normal dose.

**HOW SUPPLIED:** Tab: 40mg, 80mg*, 120mg* *scored

**CONTRAINDICATIONS:** Severe left ventricular dysfunction, hypotension and cardiogenic shock. Sick-sinus syndrome and 2nd- or 3rd-degree AV block (except with functioning ventricular pacemaker). A-Fib/Flutter with an accessory bypass tract (eg, Wolff-Parkinson-White, Lown-Ganong-Levine syndromes).

**WARNINGS/PRECAUTIONS:** Avoid with moderate to severe cardiac failure, and ventricular dysfunction if taking a β-blocker. May cause hypotension, CHF, pulmonary edema, AV block, transient bradycardia, PR interval prolongation. Monitor LFTs periodically; hepatocellular injury reported. Caution with hypertrophic cardiomyopathy, renal or hepatic dysfunction. May decrease neuromuscular transmission in patients with Duchenne's muscular dystrophy; reduce dose with decreased neuromuscular transmission.

**ADVERSE REACTIONS:** Constipation, dizziness, heart failure, hypotension, elevated liver enzymes, AV block, and rapid ventricular response.

**INTERACTIONS:** Additive effects on HR, AV conduction, and contractility with β-blockers. Coadministration with other antihypertensives will have additive effect on BP lowering. May increase digoxin, carbamazepine, theophylline, cyclosporine, and alcohol levels. Avoid disopyramide within 48 hrs before or 24 hrs after verapamil. Additive negative inotropic effects and AV conduction prolongation with flecainide. Avoid quinidine with hypertrophic cardiomyopathy. Increased sensitivity to effects of lithium when used concomitantly; monitor carefully. Increased clearance with phenobarbital. Rifampin may reduce oral bioavailability. May potentiate neuromuscular blockers; both agents may need dose reduction. Careful titration is needed when concomitantly used with inhalation anesthetics to avoid excessive CV depression. Concurrent use with telithromycin may cause hypotension and bradyarrhythmias. May produce asymptomatic bradycardia with timolol eyedrops. Decrease metoprolol and propranolol clearance while variable effect with atenolol. Excessive reduction in BP with prazosin.

**PREGNANCY:** Category C, not for use in nursing.

**MECHANISM OF ACTION:** Calcium channel blocker; modulates influx of ionic calcium across cell membrane of arterial smooth muscle, and in conductile and contractile myocardial cells.

**PHARMACOKINETICS: Absorption:** Bioavailability (20-35%), $T_{max}$=1-2 hrs. **Distribution:** Plasma protein binding (90%); found in CSF and breast milk. **Metabolism:** Liver (extensive); norverapamil (metabolite). **Elimination:** Urine (70%, metabolite) (3-4%, unchanged), feces (16%); $T_{1/2}$=4.5-12 hrs.

## NURSING CONSIDERATIONS

**Assessment:** Assess for severe left ventricular dysfunction, Duchenne's muscular dystrophy, hypertrophic cardiomyopathy, cardiac failure, cardigenic shock, hypotension, sick sinus syndrome, AV block, A-Fib/Flutter with accessory bypass tract (WPW), hepatic/renal impairment, hypersensitivity, pregnancy/nursing status, and possible drug interactions.

**Monitoring:** Monitor LFTs and renal function periodically. Monitor for abnormal PR interval prolongation for toxicity; signs/symptoms of hepatotoxicity, renal dysfunction, CV events (hypotension), and hypersensitivity reactions.

**Patient Counseling:** Advise to seek medical attention if symptoms of hepatotoxicity (malaise, fever, right upper quadrant pain), CV events (hypotension), or hypersensitivity reactions occur. Counsel not to breastfeed and to report immediately if pregnant.

**Administration:** Oral route. **Storage:** 15-25°C (59-77°F). Protect from light. Dispense in tight, light-resistant containers.

# CALAN SR — RX

verapamil HCl (Pharmacia & Upjohn)

**THERAPEUTIC CLASS:** Calcium channel blocker (nondihydropyridine)

**INDICATIONS:** Management of essential hypertension.

**DOSAGE:** *Adults:* ≥18 yrs: Initial: 180mg qam. Titrate: If inadequate response, increase to 240mg qam, then 180mg bid; or 240mg qam plus 120mg qpm, then 240mg q12h. Elderly/Small Stature: Initial: 120mg qam. Take with food.

**HOW SUPPLIED:** Tab, Extended-Release: 120mg, 180mg*, 240mg* *scored

**CONTRAINDICATIONS:** Severe left ventricular dysfunction, hypotension, cardiogenic shock, sick sinus syndrome or 2nd- or 3rd-degree AV block (except with functioning ventricular pacemaker), atrial fibrillation/flutter (A-Fib/Flutter) with an accessory bypass tract (eg, Wolff-Parkinson-White, Lown-Ganong-Levine syndromes).

**WARNINGS/PRECAUTIONS:** Avoid with moderate to severe cardiac failure, and ventricular dysfunction if taking a β-blocker. May cause hypotension, CHF, pulmonary edema, AV block, transient bradycardia, PR interval prolongation. Monitor LFTs periodically; hepatocellular injury reported. Caution with hypertrophic cardiomyopathy, renal or hepatic dysfunction. Decrease dose with decreased neuromuscular transmission.

**ADVERSE REACTIONS:** Constipation, dizziness, nausea, hypotension, headache, edema, CHF, fatigue, elevated liver enzymes, bradycardia, AV block, heart failure.

**INTERACTIONS:** Additive effects on HR, AV conduction, and contractility with β-blockers. Potentiates other antihypertensives. May increase digoxin, carbamazepine, theophylline, cyclosporine, and alcohol levels. Avoid disopyramide within 48 hrs before or 24 hrs after verapamil. Additive negative inotropic effects and AV conduction prolongation with flecainide. Avoid quinidine with hypertrophic cardiomyopathy. Inceased sensitivity to effects of lithium; monitor carefully. Increased clearance with phenobarbital. Rifampin may reduce oral bioavailability. May potentiate neuromuscular blockers; both agents may need dose reduction. Careful titration is needed with inhalation anesthetics to avoid excessive cardiovascular depression. May produce asymptomatic bradycardia with timolol eyedrops. Decrease metoprolol and propranolol clearance.



**PREGNANCY:** Category C, not for use in nursing.

**MECHANISM OF ACTION:** Calcium channel blocker; modulates influx of ionic calcium across cell membrane of arterial smooth muscle and in conductile and contractile myocardial cells.

**PHARMACOKINETICS: Absorption:** Absolute bioavailability (20-35%); $T_{max}$=7.7 hrs; $C_{max}$=79ng/mL; AUC=841ng•h/mL. **Distribution:** Plasma protein binding (90%). **Metabolism:** Biotransformation; norverapamil (metabolite). **Elimination:** Urine (70%, metabolites), (3-4%, unchanged); feces (16%); $T_{1/2}$=4.5-12 hrs.

## NURSING CONSIDERATIONS

**Assessment:** Assess for severe left ventricular dysfunction, Duchenne's muscular dystrophy, severe heart failure, hypotension, sick sinus syndrome, AV block, atrial flutter/fibrillation with accessory bypass tract (eg, Wolff-Parkinson-White), hypertrophic cardiomyopathy, hepatic/renal impairment, hypersensitivity, pregnancy/nursing status, and possible drug interactions.

**Monitoring:** Monitor LFTs and renal function periodically; abnormal PR-interval prolongation for toxicity. Monitor for signs/symptoms of hepatotoxicity, renal dysfunction, CV events (hypotension), and hypersensitivity reactions.

**Patient Counseling:** Advise to seek medical attention if symptoms of hepatotoxicity (malaise, fever, right upper quadrant pain), cardiovascular events (hypotension), or hypersensitivity reactions occur.

**Administration:** Oral route. **Storage:** 15-25°C (59-77°F). Protect from light and moisture. Dispense in tight, light-resistant containers.

# CAMPATH — RX

alemtuzumab (Bayer Healthcare)

**Serious cytopenias including fatal pancytopenia/marrow hypoplasia, autoimmune idiopathic thrombocytopenia, and autoimmune hemolytic anemia may occur; avoid single doses >30mg or cumulative doses >90mg/week. Serious, including fatal, infusion reactions may occur; gradually escalate dose to prevent. Serious, including fatal, bacterial, viral, fungal, and protozoan infections can occur; administer prophylaxis against *Pneumocystis jirovecii* pneumonia (PCP) and herpes virus infections.**

**THERAPEUTIC CLASS:** Monoclonal antibody/CD52-blocker

**INDICATIONS:** Treatment of B-cell chronic lymphocytic leukemia (B-CLL).

**DOSAGE:** *Adults:* Administer as IV infusion over 2 hours. Initial: 3mg IV qd until tolerated, then increase to 10mg IV qd. Continue until tolerated, then increase to maint dose of 30mg (escalation to 30mg usually takes 3-7 days). Maint: 30mg/day IV 3x/week on alternate days up to 12 weeks. Max: 30mg single dose or 90mg/week. Refer to PI for recommended concomitant medications and dose modifications for neutropenia or thrombocytopenia.

**HOW SUPPLIED:** Inj: 30mg/mL.

**WARNINGS/PRECAUTIONS:** Premedicate with oral antihistamine, acetaminophen to avoid infusion reactions. Monitor BP, hypotensive symptoms in ischemic heart disease, with antihypertensives. If serious infection occurs, withhold treatment until infection resolves. Monitor CBC, platelets weekly during therapy and CD4 counts after therapy. D/C for autoimmune or severe hematologic adverse reactions. Severe, including fatal, autoimmune anemia and thrombocytopenia, and prolonged myelosuppression reported. Hemolytic anemia, pure red cell aplasia, bone marrow aplasia, and hypoplasia reported. D/C for autoimmune cytopenias. Severe and prolonged lymphopenias with increased incidence of opportunistic infections reported. Administer PCP and herpes viral prophylaxis for a minimum of 2 months after completion or until CD4+ count is ≥200 cells/µL and monitor for cytomegalovirus (CMV) infection during and for at least 2 months after completion of treatment. Administer only irradiated blood products to avoid transfusion-associated graft versus host disease (TAGVHD), unless emergent circumstances dictate immediate transfusion.

**ADVERSE REACTIONS:** Cytopenias, infusion reactions, CMV and other infections, immunosuppression, nausea, emesis, abdominal pain, insomnia, anxiety.

**INTERACTIONS:** Avoid live viral vaccines.

**PREGNANCY:** Category C, not for use in nursing.

**MECHANISM OF ACTION:** Monoclonal antibody/CD52-blocker; binds to CD52 on surfaces of B and T lymphocytes, monocytes, macrophages, NK cells, granulocytes and bone marrow cells, causing antibody-dependent cellular-mediated cell death.

**PHARMACOKINETICS: Distribution:** $V_d$=0.18L/kg. **Elimination:** (1st dose) $T_{1/2}$=11 hrs. (Last dose) $T_{1/2}$=6 days.

## NURSING CONSIDERATIONS

**Assessment:** Assess pregnancy status. Obtain baseline CBC, CD4, and platelet count.

**Monitoring:** Monitor CBC and platelet counts weekly; CD4 count after therapy until recovery to >200cells/mL; for CMV infections during therapy and 2 months following completion. Monitor for signs/symptoms of autoimmune anemia, thrombocytopenia, myelosuppression, hemolytic anemia, pure red cell aplasia, bone marrow aplasia, hypoplasia, infusion reactions (eg, pyrexia, chills/rigors, nausea, hypotension, urticaria, dyspnea, rash, emesis, bronchospasm), immunosuppression, and exacerbation of infection.

**Patient Counseling:** Instruct to administer only irradiated blood products to avoid TAGVHD, unless emergent circumstances dictate immediate transfusion. Use effective contraceptive methods during treatment and at least 6 months following therapy. Inform should not be immunized with live vaccines if recently treated. Counsel on importance of need to take premedications and prophylactic anti-infectives as prescribed. Advise to seek medical attention if symptoms of bleeding, easy bruising, petechiae/purpura, pallor, weakness, fatigue, infusion reactions, or infections occur.

**Administration:** IV infusion. Refer to PI for complete administration technique. **Storage:** 2-8°C (36-46°F). Do not freeze. If frozen, thaw at 2-8°C before administration. Protect from direct sunlight.

# CAMPRAL — RX

acamprosate calcium (Forest)

**THERAPEUTIC CLASS:** GABA analog

**INDICATIONS:** Maintenance of abstinence from alcohol in patients with alcohol dependence who are abstinent at treatment initiation.

**DOSAGE:** *Adults:* 2 tabs tid. CrCl 30-50mL/min: 1 tab tid.

**HOW SUPPLIED:** Tab: 333mg

**CONTRAINDICATIONS:** Severe renal impairment (CrCl ≤30mL/min).

**WARNINGS/PRECAUTIONS:** Use does not eliminate or diminish withdrawal symptoms. Dose reduction required with renal impairment (CrCl ≤30-50mL/min). Suicidal events reported.

**ADVERSE REACTIONS:** Accidental injury, asthenia, pain, anorexia, diarrhea, flatulence, nausea, anxiety, depression, dizziness, dry mouth, insomnia, paresthesia, pruritus, sweating.

**INTERACTIONS:** Naltrexone may increase levels. Weight gain/weight loss may occur with antidepressants.

**PREGNANCY:** Category C, caution in nursing.

**MECHANISM OF ACTION:** GABA analogue; not completely understood; suspected to interact with glutamate and GABA neurotransmitter systems centrally, hypothesized that the drug restores this balance.

**PHARMACOKINETICS: Absorption:** Absolute bioavailability (11%); $C_{max}$=350ng/mL; $T_{max}$=3-8 hrs. **Distribution:** $V_d$=72-109L. **Elimination:** Urine; $T_{1/2}$=20-33 hrs.



## NURSING CONSIDERATIONS

**Assessment:** Assess for renal impairment.

**Monitoring:** Monitor for emergence of symptoms of depression and suicidality.

**Patient Counseling:** Caution while performing hazardous tasks (operating machinery/driving). Notify if pregnant/nursing or planning to become pregnant. Alert families/caregivers to look for symptoms of suicidality or depression.

**Administration:** Oral route. **Storage:** 25°C (77°F); excursions permitted to 15-30°C (59-86°F).

# CAMPTOSAR RX

irinotecan HCl (Pharmacia & Upjohn)

**Early and/or late forms of diarrhea, severe myelosuppression may occur. Interrupt and reduce subsequent doses if severe diarrhea occurs. Carefully monitor with diarrhea; give fluid/electrolyte replacement if dehydrated or give antibiotics if ileus, fever, or severe neutropenia develop.**

**THERAPEUTIC CLASS:** Topoisomerase I inhibitor

**INDICATIONS:** First-line therapy in combination with 5-fluorouracil (5-FU) and leucovorin (LV) for metastatic colon or rectal carcinomas, and for disease that has progressed or recurred following initial 5-FU therapy.

**DOSAGE:** *Adults:* Combination Therapy (5-FU/LV, see PI for dosage): 125mg/m² IV over 90 min on Days 1, 8, 15, 22 for 6 weeks; or 180mg/m² IV over 90 min on Days 1, 15, and 29 for 6 weeks. Both regimens: Begin next cycle on Day 43. Single Therapy: 125mg/m² IV over 90 min on Days 1, 8, 15, 22 followed by a 2 week rest; or 350mg/m² IV over 90 min once every 3 weeks. Premedicate with antiemetics at least 30 min prior to therapy. Dose modifications for reduced UGT1A1 activity, neutropenia, diarrhea, and other toxicities: See PI. All dose modifications should be based on worst preceding toxicity.

**HOW SUPPLIED:** Inj: 20mg/mL

**WARNINGS/PRECAUTIONS:** Due to increased toxicity, avoid use of irinotecan with the "Mayo Clinic" regimen of 5-FU/LV (given 4-5 days every 4 weeks). Treat/prevent early diarrhea with atropine IV/SQ and late diarrhea (occurring >24 hrs after dose) with loperamide PO. If late diarrhea occurs, delay therapy until return of pretreatment bowel function for at least 24 hrs without antidiarrheals; decrease subsequent doses if late diarrhea is Grade 2, 3, or 4. Deaths due to sepsis reported following severe neutropenia. Temporarily hold therapy if neutropenic fever occurs or if neutrophils <1000/mm³. Increased risk for neutropenia in patients homozygous for the UGT1A1 28 allele. Consider reduced initial dose. Heterozygous patients may also have increased risk. Hypersensitivity reactions, colitis, ileus, and renal impairment/failure, thromboembolic events reported. May cause fetal harm during pregnancy. Monitor for extravasation at infusion site. Consider atropine for cholinergic symptoms. Caution with modestly elevated baseline bilirubin levels (eg, 1-2mg/dL), abnormal glucuronidation of bilirubin, hepatic insufficiency, elderly with comorbidities, previous pelvic/abdominal irradiation. Careful monitoring of WBC with differential, Hgb, and platelets is recommended before each dose. Avoid in severe bone marrow failure, and fructose intolerant patients.

**ADVERSE REACTIONS:** N/V, diarrhea, abdominal pain, blood dyscrasias, asthenia, mucositis, anorexia, alopecia, fever, pain, constipation, infection, dyspnea, increased bilirubin.

**INTERACTIONS:** Exacerbated myelosuppression and diarrhea with antineoplastic agents having similar adverse effects. Avoid concurrent irradiation therapy. Possible hyperglycemia and lymphocytopenia with dexamethasone. Akathisia reported with prochlorperazine. Laxatives may worsen diarrhea. Consider withholding diuretics with irinotecan therapy. Decreased levels with

CYP3A4 inducing anticonvulsants and St. John's wort. Consider substituting non-enzyme inducing anticonvulsants 2 weeks prior to and during treatment. Increased levels with ketoconazole. Discontinue ketoconazole at least 1 week prior to and during therapy.



**PREGNANCY:** Category D, not for use in nursing.

**MECHANISM OF ACTION:** Topoisomerase I inhibitor; binds to topoisomerase I-DNA complex and prevents religation of single-strand breaks induced by the enzyme to relieve torsional strain in DNA.

**PHARMACOKINETICS: Absorption:** Irinotecan: (125mg/m$^2$); $C_{max}$=1660ng/mL; $AUC_{0-24}$=10200ng•h/mL. (340mg/m$^2$); $C_{max}$=3392ng/mL; $AUC_{0-24}$=20604ng•h/mL. SN-38: (125mg/m$^2$) $C_{max}$=26.3ng/mL; $AUC_{0-24}$=229ng•h/mL. (340mg/m$^2$) $C_{max}$=56ng/mL; $AUC_{0-24}$=474ng•h/mL. **Distribution:** Irinotecan: (125mg/m$^2$) $V_d$=110L/m$^2$. (340mg/m$^2$) $V_d$=234L/m$^2$. Plasma protein binding (30-68%). SN-38: Plasma protein binding (95%). **Metabolism:** Liver via carboxyl esterase. Metabolite (SN-38 ). **Elimination:** Irinotecan: Urine (11-20%). (125mg/m$^2$) $T_{1/2}$=5.8 hrs. (340mg/m$^2$) $T_{1/2}$=11.7 hrs. SN-38: Urine (<1%). (125mg/m$^2$) $T_{1/2}$=10.4 hrs. (340mg/m$^2$) $T_{1/2}$=21 hrs

## NURSING CONSIDERATIONS

**Assessment:** Assess for severe bone marrow failure, bowel obstruction, hereditary fructose intolerance, reduced UDP-glucuronosyl transferase 1A1 activity, pregnancy status, DM, glucose intolerance, pelvic/abdominal radiation. Assess in elderly patients with comorbid conditions. Assess for deficient glucuronidation of bilirubin (Gilbert's syndrome), possible drug interactions, renal/hepatic function. Assess WBC with differential, Hgb, platelet count.

**Monitoring:** Monitor WBC with differential, Hgb, platelet count before each dose. Monitor for toxicity before each dose. Assess need to premedicate with antiemetics. Monitor for signs/symptoms of renal impairment, colitis/ileus, severe neutropenia (complications, fever), severe myelosuppression, inflammation of infusion site, thromboembolism, early and late form diarrhea (may lead to dehydration, electrolyte imbalance, sepsis), rhinitis, increased salivation, miosis, lacrimation, diaphoresis, flushing, intestinal hyperperistalsis, and anaphylactic reactions.

**Patient Counseling:** Instruct to avoid vaccinations with live vaccines. Inform of pregancy risks. Inform of toxic effects (GI complications). Instruct not to use with laxative properties and to have loperamide ready to use for treatment of late diarrhea occurring >24 hrs after infusion at 1st episode of poorly formed or loose stool. Inform loperamide not recommended for >48 hrs (risk of paralytic ileus). Premedication of loperamide not recommended. Seek medical attention for symptoms of diarrhea (first time during treatment), black or bloody stools, dehydration (lightheadedness, dizziness, faintness), inability to take fluids by mouth due to NV, inability to get diarrhea under control within 24 hrs, fever, evidence of infection, toxicity, or anaphylactic reactions. Caution dizziness or visual disturbances may occur within 24 hrs; may impair physical/mental abilities.

**Administration:** IV route. Dilute in 5% Dextrose or 0.9% NaCl to final concentration range of 0.12-2.8mg/mL. **Storage:** 25°C (stable for 24 hrs); 2-8°C (stable for 48 hrs). (Diluted): 15-30°C (59-86°F); (stable for 6 hrs). Protect from light.

# CANASA **RX**

mesalamine (Axcan Scandipharm)

**THERAPEUTIC CLASS:** Anti-inflammatory Agent

**INDICATIONS:** Treatment of active ulcerative proctitis.

**DOSAGE:** *Adults:* 1000mg rectally qhs. Retain suppository for at least 1-3 hrs.

**HOW SUPPLIED:** Sup: 1000mg

**CONTRAINDICATIONS:** Hypersensitivity to suppository vehicle (eg, saturated vegetable fatty acid esters) or salicylates.

C

**WARNINGS/PRECAUTIONS:** D/C if acute intolerance syndrome develops (eg, cramping, bloody diarrhea, abdominal pain, headache); consider sulfasalazine hypersensitivity. If rechallenge is considered, perform under careful observation. Caution with sulfasalazine hypersensitivity. Carefully monitor with renal dysfunction. Pancolitis, pericarditis (rare) reported.

**ADVERSE REACTIONS:** Dizziness, rectal pain, fever, acne, colitis, rash, hair loss.

**PREGNANCY:** Category B, caution in nursing.

**MECHANISM OF ACTION:** Not fully established; anti-inflammatory drug appears to act topically rather than systemically. Postulated to have a role as free radical scavenger or inhibitor of tumor necrosis factor.

**PHARMACOKINETICS: Absorption:** Variable; $C_{max}$=361ng/mL. **Metabolism:** Extensively metabolized to N-acetyl-5-ASA. **Elimination:** Urine; $T_{1/2}$=7 hrs.

## NURSING CONSIDERATIONS

**Assessment:** Assess for hypersensitivity to the suppository vehicle, sulfa allergy, pre-existing renal disease, history of pancreatitis, and pericarditis. Obtain baseline renal function (BUN, creatinine, urinalysis).

**Monitoring:** Monitor renal function (BUN, creatinine, urinalysis) periodically, signs/symptoms of pericarditis, pancreatitis, acute intolerance syndrome (cramping, abdominal pain, bloody diarrhea), renal dysfunction, hypersensitivity, and allergic reactions.

**Patient Counseling:** Inform may cause stains. Advise to empty rectum before use and not to handle too much. If miss dose, use as soon as possible, unless almost time for next dose. Do not use 2 doses at once. Seek medical attention if chest pain, SOB, cramping, abdominal pain, bloody diarrhea, hypersensitivity, and allergic reactions occur. Inform to d/c if rash or fever occur.

**Administration:** Rectal route. 1) Remove plastic wrapper. 2) Avoid excessive handling. 3) Insert completely into rectum. 4) Lubricant may be used to assist insertion. **Storage:** 25°C (77°F), do not freeze. Keep away from direct heat, light or humidity, and out of reach of children.

# CANCIDAS RX

caspofungin acetate (Merck)

**THERAPEUTIC CLASS:** Glucan synthesis inhibitor

**INDICATIONS:** For adults and pediatric patients ( ≥3 months): Empirical therapy for presumed fungal infections in febrile, neutropenic patients. Treatment of candidemia and the following *Candida* infections: intra-abdominal abscesses, peritonitis, and pleural space infections. Treatment of esophageal candidiasis. Treatment of invasive aspergillosis in patients refractory to or intolerant of other therapies (eg, amphotericin B, itraconazole).

**DOSAGE:** *Adults:* ≥18 yrs: LD: 70mg IV on Day 1. Maint: 50mg IV qd. Empirical Therapy: Should be continued until resolution of neutropenia. If with fungal infections, treat for ≥14 days; continue for at least 7 days after both neutropenia and clinical symptoms resolved. Increase to 70mg if needed. Candidemia/Candida Infections: Duration based on patient's clinical and microbiological response. In general, treat for ≥14 days after the last positive culture. Persistently neutropenic may require longer therapy. Esophageal Candidiasis: 50mg IV qd for 7-14 days. LD not studied for this indication. Consider PO suppressive therapy with HIV patients. Invasive Aspergillosis: Duration of treatment based on severity of underlying disease, recovery from immunosuppression and clinical response. Moderate Hepatic Insufficiency (Child-Pugh Score 7-9): Maint: 35mg IV qd. Concomitant Rifampin/Nevirapine/Efavirenz/Carbamazepine/Dexamethasone/Phenytoin: Maint: 70mg IV qd.
*Pediatrics:* 3 months-17 yrs: For all indications: LD: 70mg/m² IV on Day 1. Maint: 50mg/m² IV qd. Dose can be increased to 70mg/m² qd if needed. Dosing is based on the patient's body surface area (BSA). Max: 70mg/day. Concomitant Rifampin/Nevirapine/Efavirenz/Carbamazepine/Dexamethasone/Phenytoin: 70mg/m² IV qd. Max: 70mg/day.

C

**HOW SUPPLIED:** Inj: 50mg, 70mg

**WARNINGS/PRECAUTIONS:** LFT abnormalities may be seen; if abnormal LFTs develop, monitor for evidence of worsening hepatic function and re-evaluate.

**ADVERSE REACTIONS:** Fever, chills, hypotension, diarrhea, N/V, abdominal pain, edema, headache, rash, pneumonia, cough, erythema, respiratory failure, tachycardia, septic shock.

**INTERACTIONS:** Reduces blood levels of tacrolimus. Efavirenz, nevirapine, phenytoin, rifampin, dexamethasone, carbamazepine may decrease levels. Increased levels with cyclosporine; use only when benefits outweigh risks.

**PREGNANCY:** Category C, caution in nursing.

**MECHANISM OF ACTION:** Glucan synthesis inhibitor; inhibits the synthesis of β (1,3)-D-glucan, an essential component of the cell wall of susceptible species.

**PHARMACOKINETICS: Absorption:** Administration to different age group resulted in different parameters. **Distribution:** Plasma protein binding (97%). **Metabolism:** Hydrolysis and N-acetylation (slowly). **Elimination:** Urine (41%), feces (35%).

## NURSING CONSIDERATIONS

**Assessment:** Assess use in patients who are on concomitant therapy with cyclosporine. Assess hepatic function prior to therapy, pregnancy/nursing status and possible drug interactions.

**Monitoring:** Monitor for histamine-related and anaphylaxis reactions (eg, rash, facial swelling, bronchospasm) when administering. Monitor LFTs and CBC while on therapy.

**Patient Counseling:** Counsel patients that treatment should continue for at least 7 days after both neutropenia and clinical symptoms are resolved. Inform that there have been isolated reports of serious hepatic effects, and that therapy can cause hypersensitivity reactions (eg, rash, facial swelling, puritis, sensation of warmth, or broncospasm).

**Administration:** IV route. Administer by slow IV infusion over approximately 1hr. Do not mix or co-infuse with other medications. Do not use diluents containing dextrose. Refer to full prescribing information for preparation instructions. **Storage:** Vial: 2-8°C (36-46°F). Reconstituted: ≤25°C (≤77°F) for 1 hr prior to preparation of patient infusion solution. Final infusion in IV bag or bottle: ≤25°C (≤77°F) for 24 hrs or 2-8°C (36-46°F) for 48 hours.

# CAPOZIDE RX

hydrochlorothiazide - captopril (Par)

**ACE inhibitors can cause death/injury to developing fetus during 2nd and 3rd trimesters. Stop therapy if pregnancy detected.**

**THERAPEUTIC CLASS:** ACE Inhibitor/thiazide diuretic

**INDICATIONS:** Treatment of hypertension.

**DOSAGE:** *Adults:* Initial: 25mg-15mg tab qd. Titrate: Adjust dose at 6-week intervals. Max: 150mg captopril/50mg HCTZ per day. Replacement Therapy: Substitute combination for titrated components. Renal Impairment: Decrease dose or increase interval. Take 1 hr before meals.

**HOW SUPPLIED:** Tab: (Captopril-HCTZ) 25mg-15mg*, 25mg-25mg*, 50mg-15mg*, 50mg-25mg* *scored

**CONTRAINDICATIONS:** History of ACE inhibitor-associated angioedema, anuria, sulfonamide hypersensitivity.

**WARNINGS/PRECAUTIONS:** D/C if angioedema, jaundice, or marked LFT elevation occurs. Risk of hyperkalemia with DM, renal dysfunction may occur. Monitor WBCs in renal or collagen vascular disease. Anaphylactoid reactions reported. Fetal/neonatal morbidity and death reported. Monitor for hypotension in high-risk patients (heart failure, surgery/anesthesia, severe volume/

salt depletion, on dialysis, etc.) Caution with CHF, renal or hepatic dysfunction, and renal artery stenosis. May exacerbate or activate SLE. Monitor serum electrolytes. Hypercalcemia, hypomagnesemia, hyperuricemia may occur. Neutropenia with myeloid hypoplasia, persistent nonproductive cough, anaphylactoid reactions, proteinuria reported. Enhanced effects in post-sympathectomy. Avoid with severe renal impairment.



**ADVERSE REACTIONS:** Anaphylactoid reactions, tachycardia, chest pain, dysguesia, rash, pruritis, fever, arthralgia, eosinophilia.

**INTERACTIONS:** Increased risk of hyperkalemia with $K^+$-sparing diuretics, $K^+$ supplements, or $K^+$-containing salt substitutes. Caution with agents affecting sympathetic activity. D/C vasodilators before therapy. Caution and decrease vasodilator dose if resumed during therapy. Potentiates orthostatic hypotension with alcohol, barbiturates, and narcotics. Adjust other antihypertensives, anticoagulants, antidiabetic, or antigout drugs. Reduced absorption with cholestyramine, colestipol. Amphotericin B, corticosteroids, ACTH deplete electrolytes. May decrease methenamine effects. May decrease response to pressor amines. May potentiate non-depolarizing skeletal muscle relaxants, anesthetics. Risk of lithium toxicity. NSAIDs (eg, indomethacin) reduce effects. Enhanced hypotensive effects with MAOIs. Probenecid, sulfinpyrazone may need dose increase. Diazoxide enhances hyperglycemic, hyperuricemic, and antihypertensive effects. Monitor serum calcium levels with calcium salts. Monitor potassium levels with cardiac glycosides.

**PREGNANCY:** Category C (1st trimester) and D (2nd and 3rd trimesters), not for use in nursing.

**MECHANISM OF ACTION:** Captopril: ACE inhibitor; not established. Effects appear to result from suppression of renin-angiotensin-aldosterone system. HCTZ: Thiazide diuretic. Affects renal tubular mechanism of electrolyte reabsorption.

**PHARMACOKINETICS: Absorption:** Captopril: Rapid; $T_{max}$=1 hr. **Distribution:** Captopril: Plasma protein binding (25-30%). **Elimination:** Captopril: Urine (40-50%); $T_{1/2}$≤2 hrs. HCTZ: Kidney; $T_{1/2}$=2.5 hrs.

## NURSING CONSIDERATIONS

**Assessment:** Assess volume/salt depletion, SLE, DM, anuria, sulfonamide hypersensitivity, history of allergy, angioedema or bronchial asthma, collagen vascular disease, CHF, hepatic/renal impairment. Obtain baseline serum electrolytes, renal function, and WBC with differential (impaired renal function), pregnancy/nursing status and possible drug interactions.

**Monitoring:** Monitor serum electrolytes and renal function periodically. If impaired renal function or collagen vascular disease, monitor WBC with differential before therapy, at 2-week intervals for 3 months, and then periodically during therapy. Monitor for signs/symptoms of electrolyte imbalance, exacerbation or activation of systemic lupus erythematosus (SLE), hypotension, hyperuricemia or precipitation of gout, anaphylactoid or hypersensitivity reactions, head/neck and intestinal angioedema, infection and neutropenia/agranulocytosis.

**Patient Counseling:** Instruct to take 1 hr before meal. Inform of pregnancy risks. Advise that inadequate fluid intake or loss of fluids may lead to drop in BP, resulting in lightheadedness or syncope. Instruct not to interrupt or d/c therapy without consulting physician; may cause withdrawal symptoms (eg, angina). Advise to seek medical attention if symptoms of angioedema (head/neck; intestinal; abdominal pain with/without NV), infection (eg, sore throat, fever), syncope, edema, hypersensitivity reactions, or electrolyte imbalance (eg, dry mouth, thirst, lethargy) occur.

**Administration:** Oral route. **Storage:** Below 30°C (86°F).

# CAPTOPRIL RX

captopril (Various)

**ACE inhibitors can cause death/injury to developing fetus during 2nd and 3rd trimesters. D/C if pregnancy detected.**

**OTHER BRAND NAMES:** Capoten (Par)

**THERAPEUTIC CLASS:** ACE inhibitor

**INDICATIONS:** Treatment of hypertension alone or in combination with other antihypertensive agents (eg, thiazide-type diuretics) and CHF in combination with diuretics and digitalis. To improve survival in stable post-MI patients with left ventricular dysfunction and to reduce the incidence of overt heart failure or hospitalizations for CHF in these patients. Treatment of diabetic nephropathy (proteinuria >500mg/day) in patients with type I diabetes mellitus (DM) and retinopathy.

**DOSAGE:** *Adults:* Take 1 hr before meals. HTN: If possible, d/c recent antihypertensive drug for 1 week prior to therapy. Initial: 25mg bid-tid. Titrate: May increase to 50mg bid-tid after 1-2 weeks. With Concomitant Diuretic Therapy: Range: 25-150mg bid-tid. Max: 450mg qd. CHF: Initial: 25mg tid. Titrate: May increase to 50-100mg tid. With Risk of Hypotension or Salt/Volume Depletion: Initial: 6.25mg or 12.5mg tid. Max: 450mg qd. Left Ventricular Dysfunction Post-MI: Initial: 6.25mg single dose, then 12.5mg tid. Titrate: Increase to 25mg tid over next several days, then to 50mg tid over next several weeks. Usual: 50mg tid. Diabetic Nephropathy: 25mg tid. Significant Renal Dysfunction: Decrease initial dose and titrate slowly.

**HOW SUPPLIED:** Tab: 12.5mg*, 25mg*, 50mg*, 100mg *scored

**CONTRAINDICATIONS:** History of ACE inhibitor-associated angioedema.

**WARNINGS/PRECAUTIONS:** Persistent nonproductive cough, anaphylactoid reactions, angioedema (face, tongue, larynx), and neutropenia/agranulocytosis with myeloid hypoplasia reported. D/C if jaundice or marked LFT elevation occurs. Risk of hyperkalemia with DM, renal dysfunction. Fetal/neonatal morbidity and death reported. Monitor for hypotension in high-risk patients (surgery/anesthesia, dialysis, heart failure, volume/salt depletion, etc). Caution with CHF, renal dysfunction, renal artery stenosis, collagen vascular disease (especially with renal dysfunction). Monitor WBC before therapy, then every 2 weeks for 3 months, then periodically. Less effective on BP and higher rates of angioedema reported in blacks than nonblacks.

**ADVERSE REACTIONS:** Rash, fever, arthralgia, eosinophilia, loss of taste.

**INTERACTIONS:** May increase lithium levels. NSAIDs (eg, aspirin) and indomethacin may decrease antihypertensive effects. Hypotension risk with diuretics. Increased risk of hyperkalemia with $K^+$-sparing diuretics, $K^+$-containing salt substitutes, or $K^+$ supplements. Caution with vasodilators or agents affecting sympathetic activity. Augmented effect by antihypertensives that cause renin release (eg, thiazides). Nitritoid reactions (eg, facial flushing, NV, hypotension) reported rarely with injectable gold.

**PREGNANCY:** Category C (1st trimester) and D (2nd and 3rd trimesters), not for use in nursing.

**MECHANISM OF ACTION:** ACE inhibitor; not established. Effects appear to result from suppression of renin-angiotensin-aldosterone system.

**PHARMACOKINETICS: Absorption:** Rapid; $T_{max}$=1 hr. **Distribution:** Plasma protein binding (25-30%). **Elimination:** Urine (40-50%) unchanged; $T_{1/2}$=<2 hrs.

## NURSING CONSIDERATIONS

**Assessment:** Assess for pregnancy status, possible drug interactions, volume/salt depletion, DM, collagen vascular disease, CHF, aortic stenosis, hepatic/renal impairment. Obtain baseline BP, renal function, and WBC with differential (impaired renal function).

**Monitoring:** Monitor renal function periodically and BP in first 2 weeks and whenever dosage changes. If renal function is impaired, monitor WBC with differential before therapy, at 2-week intervals for 3 months, and then periodically during therapy. Monitor for signs/symptoms of hypotension, anaphylactoid or hypersensitivity reactions, head/neck and intestinal angioedema, infection, and neutropenia/agranulocytosis.

C

**Patient Counseling:** Inform of pregnancy risks; inadequate fluid intake or loss of fluids may lead to drop in BP resulting in lightheadedness or syncope. Instruct not to interrupt or d/c therapy without consulting physician; may cause withdrawal symptoms (eg, angina). Advise to seek medical attention if symptoms of angioedema (eg, swelling of extremities, lips, face, tongue; difficulty swallowing or breathing; intestinal/abdominal pain with/without N/V), infection (eg, sore throat, fever), syncope, edema, or hypersensitivity reactions occur. Caution patients against excessive perspiration and dehydration to avoid excessive fall in BP.

**Administration:** Oral route. Take 1 hr before meals. **Storage:** 20-25°C (68-77°F). Protect from moisture. Keep bottles tightly closed.

## CARBATROL RX

carbamazepine (Shire)

**Serious and fatal dermatologic reactions, including toxic epidermal necrolysis (TEN), Stevens-Johnson syndrome (SJS) reported; increased risk with presence of HLA-B*1502 allele; screen prior to initiation of therapy. Aplastic anemia and agranulocytosis reported. Obtain complete pretreatment hematological testing as a baseline. D/C if evidence of bone marrow depression develops.**

**THERAPEUTIC CLASS:** Carboxamide

**INDICATIONS:** Treatment of partial seizures with complex symptomatology, generalized tonic-clonic seizures, and mixed seizure patterns of these or other partial or generalized seizures. Treatment of pain associated with trigeminal or glossopharyngeal neuralgia.

**DOSAGE:** *Adults:* Epilepsy: Initial: 200mg bid. Titrate: May increase weekly by 200mg/day. Maint: 800-1200mg/day. Max: 1600mg/day. Combination Therapy: When added to existing anticonvulsant therapy, may be added gradually while other anticonvulsants are maintained or gradually decreased, except phenytoin, which may be increased. Trigeminal Neuralgia: Initial (Day 1): 200mg qd. Titrate: May increase by 200mg/day q12h. Maint: 400-800mg/day. Max: 1200mg/day. Re-evaluate every 3 months.
*Pediatrics:* Epilepsy: >12 yrs: Initial: 200mg bid. Titrate: May increase weekly by 200mg/day. Max: 12-15 yrs: 1000mg/day. >15 yrs: 1200mg/day. <12 yrs: May convert immediate-release dose ≥400mg/day to equal daily dose using bid regimen. Usual/Max: ≤35mg/kg/day.

**HOW SUPPLIED:** Cap, Extended-Release: 100mg, 200mg, 300mg

**CONTRAINDICATIONS:** History of bone marrow depression, MAOI use within 14 days, sensitivity to TCAs (eg, amitriptyline, desipramine, imipramine, protriptyline, nortriptyline).

**WARNINGS/PRECAUTIONS:** Increased risk of suicidal thoughts or behavior reported. May cause fetal harm with pregnancy. Withdraw gradually to minimize potential increase in seizure frequency. Caution in patients with history of cardiac conduction disturbance; cardiac, hepatic, or renal damage; history of adverse hematologic reactions to other drugs; increased IOP; mixed seizure disorder; previously interrupted course of carbamazepine. AV heart block, slight elevations in LFTs, rare cases of liver failure reported. May cause activation of latent psychosis and, in the elderly, confusion or agitation. May impair physical/mental abilities. Start on lower doses and increase slowly to avoid side effects.

**ADVERSE REACTIONS:** Dizziness, drowsiness, unsteadiness, nausea, vomiting, bone marrow depression, multi-organ hypersensitivity, SIADH, CHF, SJS, TEN.

**INTERACTIONS:** See Contraindications. CYP3A4 inhibitors (eg, azole antifungals, cimetidine, erythromycin, protease inhibitors) and epoxide hydrolase inhibitors increase plasma level. CYP3A4 inducers (eg, cisplatin, doxorubicin, rifampin) decrease plasma level. May decrease plasma level of CYP1A2 and

CYP3A4 substrates (eg, acetaminophen, oral contraceptives, trazodone, warfarin). May increase plasma levels of clomipramine, primidone. May increase or decrease plasma level of phenytoin. Increased risk of neurotoxic side effects with lithium. Reduced thyroid function with other anticonvulsants. Antimalarial drugs (eg, chloroquine, mefloquine) may antagonize activity of carbamazepine. Caution with other centrally acting drugs and alcohol. Coadministration with delavirdine may lead to loss of virologic response and possible resistance to NNRTIs.

**PREGNANCY:** Category D, not for use in nursing.

**MECHANISM OF ACTION:** Carboxamide; anticonvulsant: reduces polysynaptic response and blocks post-tetanic potentiation. Neuralgia: depresses thalamic potential and bulbar and polysynaptic reflexes.

**PHARMACOKINETICS: Absorption:** $C_{max}$=1.9mcg/mL (200mg), $C_{max}$=11mcg/mL (800mg); $T_{max}$=19 hrs (200mg), $T_{max}$=5.9 hrs (800mg). **Distribution:** Plasma protein binding (76%); crosses the placenta; found in breast milk. **Metabolism:** Liver via CYP3A4 to carbamazepine-10,11-epoxide (active metabolite). **Elimination:** Urine (72%), feces (28%); $T_{1/2}$=35-40 hrs (single dose), 12-17 hrs (multiple doses).

## NURSING CONSIDERATIONS

**Assessment:** Perform detailed history and physical exam prior to treatment. Assess for history of mixed seizure disorders, adverse hematologic reaction to any drug, bone marrow depression, sensitivity to TCAs, hypersensitivity, and possible drug interactions. Assess cardiac, hepatic, renal function and pregnancy status. Screen for HLA-B*1502 allele in suspected population. Obtain baseline CBC with platelets and differential, serum iron, LFTs, urinalysis, BUN, lipid profile, and eye exam. Assess pregnancy/nursing status.

**Monitoring:** Monitor for dermatologic reactions (eg, rash), signs of bone marrow depression, emergence or worsening of depression, suicidal ideation or behavior, unusual changes in mood or behavior, and hypersensitivity reactions. Monitor WBC, platelet count, liver function, kidney function, carbamazepine blood level, thyroid function, and serum sodium. Do periodic eye examination.

**Patient Counseling:** Instruct to report toxic signs/symptoms of potential hematologic problems (fever, sore throat, rash, ulcers in mouth, easy bruising, petechial or purpuric hemorrhage). Caution while operating machinery/driving. Notify physician if suicidal thoughts or behavior emerge. Instruct to take exactly as directed; do not crush or chew cap. Avoid abrupt d/c. Notify physician if pregnant or intend to become pregnant. Encourage patients to enroll in North American Antiepileptic Drug (NAAED) Pregnancy Registry by calling 888-233-2334 or go to www.aedpregnancyregistry.org.

**Administration:** Oral route. **Storage:** 25°C (77°F); excursions permitted to 15-30°C (59-86°F). Protect from light and moisture.

# CARDENE IV — RX

nicardipine HCl (EKR)

**THERAPEUTIC CLASS:** Calcium channel blocker (dihydropyridine)

**INDICATIONS:** Short-term treatment of hypertension when oral therapy is not feasible or desirable.

**DOSAGE:** *Adults:* IV: Individualized dose; Administer by slow continuous infusion at a concentration of 0.1mg/mL. Gradual Reduction: Initial: 50mL/hr (5mg/hr). Titrate: May increase by 25mL/hr (2.5mg/hr) q15 min. Max: 150mL/hr (15mg/hr). Rapid BP Reduction: Initial 50mL/hr (5mg/hr). Titrate: 25mL/hr (2.5mg/hr) q5 min. Max 150mL/hr (15mg/hr). Decrease rate to 30mL/hr (3mg/hr) after BP reduction is achieved. Equiv. PO/IV Dose: 20mg q8h=0.5mg/hr, 30mg q8h=1.2mg/hr, 40mg q8h=2.2mg/hr.

**HOW SUPPLIED:** Inj: 2.5mg/mL

**CONTRAINDICATIONS:** Advanced aortic stenosis.

C

**WARNINGS/PRECAUTIONS:** May induce or exacerbate angina. Caution with CHF, significant left ventricular dysfunction, or pheochromocytoma. To reduce possibility of venous thrombosis, phlebitis, local irritation, swelling, extravasation, and the rare occurrence of vascular impairment, administer drug through large peripheral or central veins. Change IV site every 12 hrs to minimize risk of peripheral venous irritation. Monitor BP during administration. Caution in hepatic/renal impairment or reduced hepatic blood flow.

**ADVERSE REACTIONS:** Headache, hypotension, tachycardia, NV.

**INTERACTIONS:** Monitor with other antihypertensive agents. Caution with β-blockers in CHF. Increased levels with cimetidine. Monitor digoxin levels. Caution with fentanyl anesthesia. May increase cyclosporine levels.

**PREGNANCY:** Category C, not for use in nursing.

**MECHANISM OF ACTION:** $Ca^{2+}$ channel blocker; inhibits transmembrane influx of $Ca^{2+}$ ions into cardiac muscle and smooth muscles without changing serum $Ca^{2+}$ concentration.

**PHARMACOKINETICS: Distribution:** $V_d$=8.3L/kg; plasma protein binding (>95%). **Metabolism:** Liver. **Elimination:** Urine, feces; $T_{1/2}$=14.4 hrs.

## NURSING CONSIDERATIONS

**Assessment:** Assess for advanced aortic stenosis, CHF, left ventricular dysfunction, possible drug interactions, pheochromocytoma, acute cerebral infarction or hemorrhage, portal HTN, liver/renal impairment.

**Monitoring:** Monitor BP during administration. Monitor for signs/symptoms of hypotension, angina, infusion-site reaction, hypersensitivity reactions, liver/renal dysfunction.

**Patient Counseling:** Advise to seek medical attention if symptoms of hypotension, angina, infusion-site reaction, or hypersensitivity reactions occur.

**Administration:** IV infusion. **Storage:** 20-25°C (68-77°F). Avoid elevated temperatures. Protect from light. Diluted: At room temperature, stable for 24 hrs.

# CARDENE SR — RX

nicardipine HCl (PDL BioPharma)

**THERAPEUTIC CLASS:** Calcium channel blocker (dihydropyridine)

**INDICATIONS:** Treatment of hypertension.

**DOSAGE:** *Adults:* Initial: 30mg bid. Usual: 30-60mg bid. Adjust according to BP response.

**HOW SUPPLIED:** Cap, Sustained-Release: 30mg, 45mg, 60mg

**CONTRAINDICATIONS:** Advanced aortic stenosis.

**WARNINGS/PRECAUTIONS:** Increased angina reported in patients with angina. Caution with CHF when titrating dose. Caution in hepatic/renal impairment, or reduced hepatic blood flow. May cause symptomatic hypotension. Monitor BP during initial administration and dose titration.

**ADVERSE REACTIONS:** Headache, pedal edema, vasodilation, palpitations, NV, dizziness, asthenia, postural hypotension, increased urinary frequency, pain, rash, increased sweating.

**INTERACTIONS:** Increased levels with cimetidine. Elevates cyclosporine levels. With β-blocker withdrawal, gradually reduce over 8-10 days. Monitor digoxin levels. Severe hypotension reported with fentanyl anesthesia.

**PREGNANCY:** Category C, not for use in nursing.

**MECHANISM OF ACTION:** $Ca^{2+}$ channel blocker; inhibits transmembrane influx of $Ca^{2+}$ ions into cardiac muscle and smooth muscle without changing serum $Ca^{2+}$ concentration.

**PHARMACOKINETICS: Absorption:** Complete; bioavailability (35%); $C_{max}$=13.4ng/mL (30mg), 34.0ng/mL (45mg), 58.4ng/mL (60mg); $T_{max}$=1-4 hrs. **Distribution:** Plasma protein binding (>95%). **Metabolism:** Liver. **Elimination:** Urine (<1%, intact), feces; $T_{1/2}$=8.6 hrs.

## NURSING CONSIDERATIONS

**Assessment:** Assess for advanced aortic stenosis, CHF, acute cerebral infarction or hemorrhage, liver/renal impairment, pregnancy/nursing status, and possible drug interactions. Obtain baseline BP.

**Monitoring:** Monitor BP initially and during titration. Monitor for signs/symptoms of angina, hypersensitivity reactions, hypotension, liver/renal dysfunction.

**Patient Counseling:** Advise to seek medical attention if symptoms of hypotension, angina, or hypersensitivity reactions occur.

**Administration:** Oral route. **Storage:** 15-30°C (59-86°F); keep in light-resistant container.

# CARDIZEM RX

diltiazem HCl (Biovail)

**THERAPEUTIC CLASS:** Calcium channel blocker (nondihydropyridine)

**INDICATIONS:** Management of chronic stable angina or angina due to coronary artery spasm.

**DOSAGE:** *Adults:* Initial: 30mg qid (before meals and qhs). Adjust at 1-2 day intervals. Usual: 180-360mg/day.

**HOW SUPPLIED:** Tab: 30mg, 60mg*, 90mg*, 120mg* *scored

**CONTRAINDICATIONS:** Sick sinus syndrome and 2nd- or 3rd-degree AV block (except with functioning pacemaker), hypotension (<90mmHg systolic), acute MI, pulmonary congestion.

**WARNINGS/PRECAUTIONS:** Caution in renal, hepatic, or ventricular dysfunction. Monitor LFTs and renal function with prolonged use. D/C if persistent rash occurs. Symptomatic hypotension may occur. Acute hepatic injury reported.

**ADVERSE REACTIONS:** Headache, dizziness, asthenia, flushing, 1st-degree AV block, edema, nausea, bradycardia, rash.

**INTERACTIONS:** Increased levels of propranolol, digoxin, carbamazepine, cyclosporine, lovastatin, quinidine; monitor closely. Increased levels of diltiazem with cimetidine. Potentiates depression of cardiac contractility, conductivity, automaticity and vascular dilation with anesthetics. Additive cardiac conduction effects with digitalis or β-blockers. Potential additive effects with agents known to affect cardiac contractility and/or conduction. May increase levels of midazolam/triazolam. Avoid with CYP3A4 inducers (eg, rifampin). Enhanced effects and increased toxicity of buspirone.

**PREGNANCY:** Category C, not for use in nursing.

**MECHANISM OF ACTION:** Calcium channel blocker; still being delineated; believed to be potent dilator of coronary arteries both epicardial and subendocardial. Inhibits spontaneous and ergonovine-induced coronary artery spasm. Increases exercise tolerance by its ability to reduce myocardial oxygen demand; accomplished via reduction in heart rate and systemic BP.

**PHARMACOKINETICS: Absorption:** Well absorbed, absolute bioavailability (40%). $T_{max}$=2-4 hrs. **Distribution:** Plasma protein bound (70-80%); found in breast milk. **Metabolism:** Liver (extensive). **Elimination:** Urine (2-4% unchanged), bile.

## NURSING CONSIDERATIONS

**Assessment:** Assess for cardiac conduction disorders (eg, sick sinus syndrome, second- or third-degree AV block and presence of a functioning ventricular pacemaker), presence of Prinzmetal's angina, hypotension, acute MI, pulmonary congestion documented by x-ray, CHF, hepatic/renal impairment, pregnancy/nursing status, and for possible drug interactions as additive effects on cardiac conduction if taken with digoxin or β-blockers.

**Monitoring:** Monitor LFTs and renal function regularly. Monitor heart rhythm, BP, dermatological events (eg, skin eruptions which may progress to erythema multiform and/or exfoliative dermatitis).

C

**Patient Counseling:** Inform about benefits/risks of drug and to report any adverse reactions to physician. Caution about the additive effects on cardiac conduction. Careful titration is needed in those receiving the drug concomitantly with agents known to affect cardiac contractility and/or conduction. Not for use by nursing women. Only use in pregnant women if benefit outweighs risk.

**Administration:** Oral route. **Storage:** 25°C (77°F), excursions permitted to 15-30°C (59-86°F).

## CARDIZEM CD

diltiazem HCl (Biovail)

**RX**

**OTHER BRAND NAMES:** Cartia XT (Watson) - Cardizem LA (Abbott)

**THERAPEUTIC CLASS:** Calcium channel blocker (nondihydropyridine)

**INDICATIONS:** Treatment of hypertension. Management of chronic stable angina (LA) or angina due to coronary artery spasm.

**DOSAGE:** *Adults:* HTN: (CD, Cartia XT) Initial (monotherapy): 180-240mg qd. Titrate: Adjust at 2-week intervals. Usual: 240-360mg qd. Max: 480mg qd. (LA) Initial: 180-240mg qd. Adjust at 2-week intervals. Max: 540mg qd. Angina: (CD, Cartia XT) Initial: 120-180mg qd. Adjust at 1-2 week intervals. Max: 480mg/day. (LA) Initial: 180mg qd. Adjust at 1-2 week intervals.

**HOW SUPPLIED:** Cap, Extended-Release: (Cardizem CD, Cartia XT) 120mg, 180mg, 240mg, 300mg, (Cardizem CD) 360mg; Tab, Extended-Release: (Cardizem LA) 120mg, 180mg, 240mg, 300mg, 360mg, 420mg

**CONTRAINDICATIONS:** Sick sinus syndrome and 2nd- or 3rd-degree AV block (except with functioning pacemaker), hypotension (<90mmHg systolic), acute MI, pulmonary congestion.

**WARNINGS/PRECAUTIONS:** Caution in renal, hepatic, or ventricular dysfunction. Monitor LFTs and renal function with prolonged use. D/C if persistent rash occurs. Symptomatic hypotension may occur. Acute hepatic injury reported.

**ADVERSE REACTIONS:** Headache, dizziness, asthenia, flushing, 1st-degree AV block, edema, nausea, bradycardia, rash.

**INTERACTIONS:** May require dosage adjustment with concomitant CYP3A4 substrates. Increased levels of propranolol, digoxin, carbamazepine, lovastatin. Increased levels of diltiazem with cimetidine. May increase effects of benzodiazepines. Monitor digoxin, cyclosporine. Potentiates the depression of cardiac contractility, conductivity, automaticity, and vascular dilation with anesthetics. Avoid concurrent use with CYP3A4 inducers (eg, rifampin). Additive cardiac conduction effects with digitalis or β-blockers. Potential additive effects with agents known to affect cardiac contractility and/or conduction.

**PREGNANCY:** Category C, not for use in nursing.

**MECHANISM OF ACTION:** Calcium channel blocker; inhibits influx of $Ca^{2+}$ ions during membrane depolarization of cardiac and vascular smooth muscle.

**PHARMACOKINETICS: Absorption:** CD: Absolute bioavailability (40%); $T_{max}$=10-14 hrs. LA: $T_{max}$=11-18 hrs. **Distribution:** Plasma protein binding (70-80%). **Elimination:** CD: Urine (2-4%); $T_{1/2}$=5-8 hrs; LA: $T_{1/2}$=6-9 hrs.

### NURSING CONSIDERATIONS

**Assessment:** Assess for sick sinus syndrome, hypotension, AV block, acute MI, pulmonary congestion, pre-existing impairment of ventricular function, possible drug interactions, renal/hepatic impairment.

**Monitoring:** Monitor renal function and LFTs periodically. Monitor for signs/symptoms of worsening CHF, hypotension, hypersensitivity reactions, renal/hepatic dysfunction.

**Patient Counseling:** Advise to seek medical attention if symptoms of worsening CHF, hypotension, or hypersensitivity reactions occur.

**Administration:** Oral route. **Storage:** 25°C (77°F); excursions permitted to 15-30°C (59-86°F). Avoid excessive humidity and temperature.

## CARDURA RX

doxazosin mesylate (Pfizer)

C

**THERAPEUTIC CLASS:** $Alpha_1$-blocker (quinazoline)

**INDICATIONS:** Treatment of hypertension and/or treatment of both the urinary outflow obstruction and obstructive and irritative symptoms associated with benign prostatic hyperplasia (BPH).

**DOSAGE:** *Adults:* HTN: Initial: 1mg qd. Monitor BP 2-6 hrs and 24 hrs after 1st dose. Titrate: Increase stepwise to 2mg, 4mg, 8mg, or 16mg qd prn. Max: 16mg/day. BPH: Initial: 1mg qd (am or pm). Titrate: Increase stepwise to 2mg, 4mg, and 8mg in 1-2 week intervals. Max: 8mg/day.

**HOW SUPPLIED:** Tab: 1mg*, 2mg*, 4mg*, 8mg* *scored

**WARNINGS/PRECAUTIONS:** Syncope and orthostatic hypotension (eg, dizziness, light-headedness, vertigo) can occur with 1st dose and dose increase. Caution with hepatic dysfunction. Rule out prostate cancer. Priapism (rare) and leukopenia/neutropenia reported. Intraoperative floppy iris syndrome observed during cataract surgery in patients treated with $alpha_1$ blockers.

**ADVERSE REACTIONS:** Dizziness, headache, fatigue/malaise, somnolence, edema, nausea, rhinitis.

**INTERACTIONS:** Caution with additional antihypertensive agents and drugs known to influence hepatic metabolism. Concomitant use with PDE-5 inhibitors may result in additive BP-lowering effects and symptomatic hypotension.

**PREGNANCY:** Category C, caution with nursing.

**MECHANISM OF ACTION:** $Alpha_1$-blocker; (BPH) antagonizes phenylephrine-induced contractions in prostate; (HTN) competitively antagonizes pressor effects of phenylephrine and systolic pressor effect of norepinephrine.

**PHARMACOKINETICS: Absorption:** Absolute bioavailability (65%); $T_{max}$=2-3 hrs. **Distribution:** Plasma protein binding (98%). **Metabolism:** Hepatic; O-demethylation or hydroxylation. **Elimination:** Feces (63%, 4.8% unchanged), urine (9%, trace amounts unchanged); $T_{1/2}$=22 hrs.

### NURSING CONSIDERATIONS

**Assessment:** Assess for liver impairment and possible drug interactions. Rule out prostate cancer.

**Monitoring:** Monitor BP periodically. Monitor for signs/symptoms of hypotension, priapism, liver dysfunction, and hypersensitivity reactions.

**Patient Counseling:** Inform of possibility of syncope and orthostatic symptoms, especially at initiation of therapy; urge to avoid driving or hazardous tasks for 24 hrs after first dose, dosage increase, and interruption of therapy when treatment is resumed. Caution to avoid situations where injury could result should syncope occur. Advise to sit or lie down when symptoms of low BP occur. Inform of possibility of priapism; advise to seek medical attention if priapism occurs.

**Administration:** Oral route. If drug use discontinued for several days, restart using the initial dosing regimen. **Storage:** 25°C (77°F); excursions permitted to 15-30°C (59-86°F).

## CARDURA XL RX

doxazosin mesylate (Pfizer)

**THERAPEUTIC CLASS:** $Alpha_1$-blocker (quinazoline)

**INDICATIONS:** Treatment of the signs and symptoms of benign prostatic hyperplasia (BPH).

**DOSAGE:** *Adults:* Initial: 4mg qd with breakfast. Titrate: May increase to 8mg after 3-4 weeks. Max: 8mg.

**HOW SUPPLIED:** Tab, Extended-Release: 4mg, 8mg

**WARNINGS/PRECAUTIONS:** Postural hypotension with or without symptoms (eg, dizziness, syncope) may develop; caution with symptomatic hypotension or hypotensive response to other medications. Rule out prostate cancer. Intraoperative floppy iris syndrome has been observed during cataract surgery in some patients on, or previously treated with, alpha$_1$ blockers. Caution with pre-existing severe GI narrowing (pathologic or iatrogenic). Caution with mild or moderate hepatic dysfunction; avoid with severe hepatic dysfunction. D/C with worsening of or new-onset angina pectoris symptoms.

**ADVERSE REACTIONS:** Dizziness, dyspnea, asthenia, headache, hypotension, postural hypotension, somnolence, respiratory tract infection, backache.

**INTERACTIONS:** Caution with potent CYP3A4 inhibitors (eg, atazanavir, clarithromycin, indinavir, itraconazole, ketoconazole, nefazodone, nelfinavir, ritonavir, saquinavir, telithromycin, voriconazole). Caution with drugs known to influence hepatic metabolism. Increased systemic exposure with drugs that reduce GI motility (eg, anticholinergics).

**PREGNANCY:** Category C, not for use in nursing.

**MECHANISM OF ACTION:** Alpha$_1$-blocker; antagonizes $\alpha_1$-agonist-induced contractions, decreasing urethral resistance, which may relieve BPH symptoms and improve urine flow.

**PHARMACOKINETICS: Absorption:** (4mg) $C_{max}$=10.1ng/mL, $T_{max}$=8 hrs, AUC=183ng•hr/mL. (8mg) $C_{max}$=25.8ng/mL, $T_{max}$=9 hrs, AUC=472ng-hr/mL. **Distribution:** Plasma protein binding (98%). **Metabolism:** Liver (extensive) via CYP3A4 (major) and CYP2D6, CYP2C19 (minor). **Elimination:** $T_{1/2}$=15-19 hrs.

## NURSING CONSIDERATIONS

**Assessment:** Assess for hepatic impairment, symptomatic hypotension, severe GI narrowing (chronic constipation), coronary insufficiency, and possible drug interactions. Rule out prostate cancer.

**Monitoring:** Monitor for signs/symptoms of postural hypotension, coronary insufficiency, and hypersensitivity reactions.

**Patient Counseling:** Instruct to take with breakfast; swallow whole; do not chew, divide, cut, or crush. Advise symptoms related to postural hypotension (eg, dizziness, syncope) may occur; caution about driving, operating machinery, and performing hazardous tasks. Advise to avoid situations where injury could result if syncope occurs. Caution not to be alarmed if the capsule is noticed in the stool. Instruct to inform ophthalmologist of drug use prior to cataract surgery.

**Admininistration:** Oral route. Swallow whole; do not chew, divide, cut, or crush. **Storage:** 25°C (77°F); excursions permitted to 15-30°C (59-86°F).

# CASODEX RX

bicalutamide (AstraZeneca)

**THERAPEUTIC CLASS:** Nonsteroidal antiandrogen

**INDICATIONS:** Treatment of stage $D_2$ metastatic carcinoma of the prostate in combination with a luteinizing hormone-releasing hormone (LHRH) analogue.

**DOSAGE:** *Adults:* 50mg qd at same time. Initiate with LHRH analogue therapy.

**HOW SUPPLIED:** Tab: 50mg

**CONTRAINDICATIONS:** Women, pregnancy.

**WARNINGS/PRECAUTIONS:** Rare cases of death or hospitalization due to severe liver injury reported. Hepatitis and marked increases in liver enzymes leading to drug d/c have occurred. Caution with moderate-severe hepatic impairment; serum transaminase levels should be measured prior to starting treatment, at regular intervals for first 4 months, then periodically. Monitor PSA regularly to assess therapy. For patients who have objective progression of disease together with elevated PSA, a treatment-free period of antiandrogen, while continuing LHRH analogue, may be considered. Gynecomastia, breast pain reported with single agent. Risk of hyperglycemia or loss of glucose control with pre-existing DM due to glucose tolerance.

**ADVERSE REACTIONS:** Hot flushes, pain, back pain, asthenia, constipation, pelvic pain, infection, nausea, dyspnea, peripheral edema, diarrhea, nocturia, urticaria, pneumonitis, pulmonary fibrosis, and hyperglycemia.

**INTERACTIONS:** Can displace coumarin anticoagulants, such as warfarin, from their protein-binding sites; monitor PT. Concomitant use of LHRH agonist may reduce glucose tolerance. Caution with CYP3A4 substrates (eg, midazolam).

**PREGNANCY:** Category X, not for use in nursing.

**MECHANISM OF ACTION:** Nonsteroidal antiandrogen; inhibits the action of androgens by binding to cytosol androgen receptors in target tissue.

**PHARMACOKINETICS: Absorption:** Well-absorbed, $C_{max}$=0.768mcg/mL, $T_{max}$=31.3 hrs. **Distribution:** Plasma protein binding (96%). **Metabolism:** Liver via oxidation and glucuronidation. **Elimination:** Urine, feces; $T_{1/2}$=5.8 days.

## NURSING CONSIDERATIONS

**Assessment:** Assess for hepatic impairment, pregnancy status, and CBC. Note other diseases/conditions and drug therapies.

**Monitoring:** Monitor LFTs, CBC, PSA, BP, PT, kidney function, blood glucose level, hot flushes, hypersensitivity reactions, hyperuricemia, and dyspnea.

**Patient Counseling:** Do not interrupt or d/c without consulting physician. Start treatment at the same time as treatment with an LHRH analogue. Take with/without food. Caution against driving or operating machinery. Counsel about the risks of DM or that loss of glycemic control with pre-existing DM may occur during therapy.

**Administration:** Oral route. **Storage:** 20-25°C (68-77°F).

# CATAFLAM — RX

diclofenac potassium (Novartis)

**NSAIDs may cause an increased risk of serious cardiovascular thrombotic events, MI, stroke, and serious GI adverse events including bleeding, ulceration, and perforation of the stomach or intestines. Contraindicated for the treatment of perioperative pain in the setting of coronary artery bypass graft (CABG) surgery.**

**THERAPEUTIC CLASS:** NSAID

**INDICATIONS:** Relief of signs and symptoms of osteoarthritis (OA) and rheumatoid arthritis (RA). Treatment of primary dysmenorrhea and relief of mild to moderate pain.

**DOSAGE:** *Adults:* OA: 100-150mg/day in divided doses, 50mg bid or tid. RA: 150-200mg/day in divided doses, 50mg tid or qid. Pain/Primary Dysmenorrhea: Initial: 50mg tid or 100mg on 1st dose, then 50mg on subsequent doses.

**HOW SUPPLIED:** Tab: 50mg

**CONTRAINDICATIONS:** ASA or other NSAID allergy that precipitates asthma, urticaria, or allergic reactions. Treatment of perioperative pain in the setting of CABG surgery.

**WARNINGS/PRECAUTIONS:** May lead to onset of new HTN or worsening of pre-existing HTN; monitor BP closely. Fluid retention and edema reported; caution in patients with fluid retention or heart failure. Caution with history of ulcer disease or GI bleeding. Caution in patients with considerable dehydration. Renal papillary necrosis and other renal injury reported after long-term use. Renal toxicity also reported in patients in whom renal prostaglandins have a compensatory role in the maintenance of renal perfusion; caution with impaired renal function, heart failure, liver dysfunction, and the elderly. Not recommended for use with advanced renal disease; if therapy must be initiated, monitor renal function. May cause elevations of LFTs; d/c if liver disease develops or systemic manifestations occur. Anaphylactoid reactions may occur. May cause serious skin adverse events (eg, exfoliative dermatitis, Stevens-Johnson syndrome, toxic epidermal necrolysis). Avoid in late pregnancy; may cause premature closure of ductus arteriosis. Not a substitute for corticosteroids or for the treatment of corticosteroid insufficiency. Anemia may occur; with long-term use, monitor Hgb/Hct if signs or symptoms of anemia develop. May inhibit platelet aggregation and prolong bleeding time; monitor with coagulation disorders. Caution with asthma and avoid with ASA-sensitive asthma.

**ADVERSE REACTIONS:** Dyspepsia, constipation, diarrhea, GI ulceration/perforation, n/v, flatulence, abnormal renal function, anemia, dizziness, edema, elevated liver enzymes, headache, increased bleeding time, rash, tinnitus.

**INTERACTIONS:** Avoid use with ASA. May enhance methotrexate toxicity; caution when co-administering. May increase nephrotoxicity of cyclosporine; caution when co-administering. May diminish antihypertensive effect of ACE-inhibitors. May reduce natriuretic effect of furosemide and thiazides; monitor for renal failure. May increase lithium levels; monitor for toxicity. Synergistic effects on GI bleeding with warfarin. Caution with hepatotoxic drugs (eg, antibiotics, anti-epileptics). Increase risk for GI bleeding with concomitant oral corticosteroids, anticoagulants, or alcohol. ACE inhibitors and diuretics may increase the risk of overt renal decompensation.

**PREGNANCY:** Category C, not for use in nursing.

**MECHANISM OF ACTION:** NSAID (benzeneacetic acid derivative); suspected to inhibit prostaglandin synthetase.

**PHARMACOKINETICS: Absorption:** Absolute bioavailabilty (55%), $T_{max}$=1 hr. **Distribution**: $V_d$=1.3L/kg; serum protein binding (>99%). **Metabolism**: Metabolites: 4'-hydroxy-, 5-hydroxy-, 3'-hydroxy-, 4',5-dihydroxy-, and 3'-hydroxy-4'-methoxy diclofenac. **Elimination:** Urine (65%), bile (35%); $T_{1/2}$=2 hrs.

## NURSING CONSIDERATIONS

**Assessment:** Assess for history of a hypersensitivity reaction to aspirin or other NSAIDS, asthma, cardiovascular disease (eg, pre-existing HTN, CHF) or risk factors for CVD, risk factors for a GI event (eg, prior history of ulcer disease or GI disease, smoking), fluid retention, renal/hepatic dysfunction, coagulation disorders, pregnancy/nursing status, and for possible drug interactions. Assess baseline LFTs, renal function, and CBC. Assess that use is not for the treatment of perioperative pain in the setting of CABG surgery.

**Monitoring:** Monitor for signs/symptoms of CV thrombotic events, new onset or worsening of pre-existing HTN, GI events (eg, inflammation, bleeding, ulceration, perforation), fluid retention and edema, renal effects (eg, renal papillary necrosis), hepatic effects (eg, jaundice, liver necrosis, liver failure), anaphylactoid reactions, skin reactions (eg, exfoliative dermatitis, Stevens-Johnson syndrome, toxic epidermal necrolysis), hematological effects (eg, anemia, prolongation of bleeding time), and for bronchospasm. Monitor BP. Perform periodic monitoring of CBC, renal function, and LFTs.

**Patient Counseling:** Instruct to seek medical attention for symptoms of hepatotoxicity (eg, nausea, fatigue, jaundice), anaphylactic reactions (eg, difficulty breathing, swelling of the face/throat), rash, CV events (eg, chest pain, SOB, weakness, slurring of speech), or if unexplained weight gain or edema occur. Inform of risks if used during pregnancy.

**Administration:** Oral route. **Storage:** Do not store above 30°C (86°F). Dispense in tight container.

# CATAPRES — RX

clonidine HCl (Boehringer Ingelheim)

**OTHER BRAND NAMES:** Catapres-TTS (Boehringer Ingelheim)

**THERAPEUTIC CLASS:** Central alpha-adrenergic agonist

**INDICATIONS:** Treatment of hypertension, alone or with other antihypertensives.

**DOSAGE:** *Adults:* (Patch) Apply to hairless, intact area of upper outer arm or chest weekly. Each new patch applied on different skin site from previous location. Taper previous antihypertensive gradually. Initial: 0.1mg/24 hr weekly. Titrate: May increase after 1-2 weeks if the desired reduction in BP is

C

not achieved. Max: 0.6mg/24 hr. (Tab) Initial: 0.1mg bid, am and pm. Titrate: May increase by 0.1mg weekly. Usual: 0.2-0.6mg/day in divided doses. Max: 2.4mg/day. Elderly: May benefit from lower initial dose. (Patch, Tab) Renal Impairment: Adjust according to degree of impairment.

**HOW SUPPLIED:** Patch, Extended-Release (TTS): 0.1mg/24 hr, 0.2mg/24 hr, 0.3mg/24 hr [4[s]]. Tab: 0.1mg, 0.2mg, 0.3mg

**WARNINGS/PRECAUTIONS:** Avoid abrupt discontinuation; reduce dose gradually over 2 to 4 days. Rare instances of hypertensive encephalopathy, cerebrovascular accidents (CVA) and death reported after withdrawal. Caution with severe coronary insufficiency, conduction disturbances, recent myocardial infarction (MI), cerebrovascular disease, or chronic renal failure. Substitution to PO may cause rash and may elicit allergic reaction if patient had localized contact sensitization and allergic reaction to clonidine transdermal system. (Tabs) Continue within 4 hrs of surgery and resume as soon as possible thereafter. (Patch) Do not remove during surgery, monitor BP and additional measures to control BP should be available. Remove before defibrillation or cardioversion due to the potential risk of altered electrical conductivity or MRI due to the occurrence of burns. Loss of BP control reported. May impair mental/physical abilities. Caution in elderly.

**ADVERSE REACTIONS:** Dry mouth, drowsiness, dizziness, constipation, sedation, localized skin reactions (patch).

**INTERACTIONS:** May potentiate CNS depression with alcohol, barbiturates, or other sedatives. Additive bradycardia and AV block with agents that affect sinus node function or AV nodal conduction (eg, digitalis, calcium channel blockers, and β-blockers). Hypotensive effect reduced by tricyclic antidepressants. Serious adverse events, including death, reported with methylphenidate.

**PREGNANCY:** Category C, caution in nursing.

**MECHANISM OF ACTION:** Central acting α-agonist; stimulates α-adrenoreceptor in brain stem, reducing sympathetic outflow from CNS and decreasing HR, BP, peripheral and renal vascular resistance.

**PHARMACOKINETICS: Absorption:** $T_{max}$=3-5 hrs. **Distribution:** Found in breast milk. **Metabolism:** Liver. **Elimination:** Urine (40-60%, unchanged); $T_{1/2}$=12-16 hrs.

## NURSING CONSIDERATIONS

**Assessment:** Assess for severe coronary insufficiency, conduction disturbances, recent MI, cerebrovascular disease, renal impairment, contact sensitization/allergic reaction to clonidine transdermal system, hypersensitivity reactions, pregnancy/nursing status, and possible drug interactions.

**Monitoring:** Monitor BP and renal function periodically. Monitor for withdrawal signs/symptoms (eg, hypertensive encephalopathy, CVA) and hypersensitivity reactions.

**Patient Counseling:** Caution against interruption of therapy without physician's advice. Instruct to consult a physician about possible need to remove patch due to adverse skin reactions. Inform that if patch begins to loosen, place adhesive cover directly over to ensure adhesion for 7 days. Instruct to avoid alcohol and drugs that may potentiate CNS depression. Caution in engaging hazardous activities (eg, operating machinery or driving). Inform that medication may cause dryness of eyes; caution with contact lenses. Inform to remove patch before MRI. Advise to keep used and unused patch out of reach of children.

**Administration:** Oral; transdermal route. **Storage:** (Tab) 25°C (77°F); excursions permitted to 15-30°C (59-86°F). Dispense in tight, light-resistant container. (Patch) Below 30°C (86°F).

# CEFACLOR

cefaclor (Various) **RX**

**THERAPEUTIC CLASS:** Cephalosporin (2nd generation)

**INDICATIONS:** Treatment of otitis media, pharyngitis, tonsillitis, lower respiratory tract, urinary tract, and skin and skin structure infections caused by susceptible strains of microorganisms.

**DOSAGE:** *Adults:* Usual: 250mg q8h. Severe Infections/Pneumonia: 500mg q8h. Treat β-hemolytic strep for 10 days.
*Pediatrics:* ≥1 month: Usual: 20mg/kg/day given q8h. Otitis Media/Serious Infections/Infections Caused by Less Susceptible Organisms: 40mg/kg/day. Max: 1g/day. May administer q12h for otitis media and pharyngitis. Treat β-hemolytic strep for 10 days.

**HOW SUPPLIED:** Cap: 250mg, 500mg; Sus: 125mg/5mL [75mL, 150mL], 250mg/5mL [75mL, 150mL], 375mg/5mL [50mL, 100mL]

**WARNINGS/PRECAUTIONS:** Cross-sensitivity to PCNs and other cephalosporins may occur. CDAD reported. Positive direct Coombs' test reported. Caution with markedly impaired renal function, history of GI disease. False (+) for urine glucose with Benedict's, Fehling's solution, and Clinitest tabs.

**ADVERSE REACTIONS:** Hypersensitivity reactions, diarrhea, eosinophilia, genital pruritus and vaginitis, serum-sickness-like reactions.

**INTERACTIONS:** Renal excretion inhibited by probenecid. May potentiate warfarin and other anticoagulants; monitor PT/INR.

**PREGNANCY:** Category B, caution in nursing.

**MECHANISM OF ACTION:** Cephalosporin; bactericidal agent, inhibits cell-wall synthesis.

**PHARMACOKINETICS: Absorption:** Well-absorbed; (Fasting): $C_{max}$=7mcg/mL (250mg), 13mcg (500mg), 23mcg (1g); $T_{max}$=30-60 min. **Elimination:** Urine (60-85% unchanged); $T_{1/2}$= 0.6-0.9 hrs.

## NURSING CONSIDERATIONS

**Assessment:** Assess for hypersensitivity reactions to cephalosporins, PCNs and other drugs, pregnancy/nursing status, renal impairment, and possible drug interactions.

**Monitoring:** Monitor for anaphylactic reactions, CDAD, superinfection, drug resistance, positive Coombs' test, increased anticoagulant effect when used concomitantly with anticoagulants, false (+) reaction for urinary glucose when using Benedict's and Fehling's solutions, and Clinitest tablets.

**Patient Counseling:** Inform drug only treats bacterial, not viral, infections. Take exactly as directed; skipping doses or not completing full course may decrease effectiveness and increase resistance. Inform about potential benefits/risks. D/C and notify physician if allergic reaction or watery/bloody diarrhea (with/without muscle cramps and fever) occur (as late as 2 months after treatment end). Notify if pregnant/nursing.

**Administration:** Oral route. **Storage:** 20-25°C (68-77°F).

# CEFACLOR ER — RX

cefaclor (Various)

**THERAPEUTIC CLASS:** Cephalosporin (2nd generation)

**INDICATIONS:** Treatment of acute bacterial exacerbation of chronic bronchitis (ABECB), secondary bacterial infections of acute bronchitis, pharyngitis, tonsillitis, and uncomplicated skin and skin structure infections (SSSI) caused by susceptible strains of microorganisms.

**DOSAGE:** *Adults:* ABECB/Acute Bronchitis: 500mg q12h for 7 days. Pharyngitis/Tonsillitis: 375mg q12h for 10 days. SSSI: 375mg q12h for 7-10 days. Take with meals. Do not crush, cut, or chew tab.
*Pediatrics:* ≥16 yrs: ABECB/Acute Bronchitis: 500mg q12h for 7 days. Pharyngitis/Tonsillitis: 375mg q12h for 10 days. SSSI: 375mg q12h for 7-10 days. Take with meals. Do not crush, cut, or chew tab.

**HOW SUPPLIED:** Tab, Extended-Release: 500mg

**WARNINGS/PRECAUTIONS:** Cross-sensitivity to PCNs and other cephalosporins may occur. *Clostridium difficile*-associated diarrhea (CDAD) reported.

Positive direct Coombs' test reported. Caution with markedly impaired renal function, history of GI disease. False (+) for urine glucose with Benedict's, Fehling's solution, and Clinitest tabs.

**ADVERSE REACTIONS:** Headache, rhinitis, diarrhea, nausea, vaginitis, abdominal pain, pharyngitis, increased cough, pruritus, back pain, serum-sickness-like reactions, superinfection (prolonged use).

**INTERACTIONS:** Decreased absorption with aluminum or magnesium hydroxide-containing antacids; space dose by 1 hr. Potentiated by probenecid. May potentiate warfarin, and other anticoagulants; monitor PT/INR.

**PREGNANCY:** Category B, caution in nursing.

**MECHANISM OF ACTION:** Cephalosporin; bactericidal, inhibits cell-wall synthesis.

**PHARMACOKINETICS: Absorption:** Fed: (375mg) $C_{max}$=3.7mcg/mL, $T_{max}$=2.7 hr, AUC=9.9mcg•hr/mL. (500mg) $C_{max}$=4.2mcg/mL, $T_{max}$=2.5 hr, AUC=18.1mcg•hr/mL. Fasting: $C_{max}$=5.4, $T_{max}$=1.5 hrs, AUC=14.8mcg•hr/mL.

## NURSING CONSIDERATIONS

**Assessment:** Assess for hypersensitivity reactions to cephalosporins, PCNs, and other drugs, pregnancy/nursing status, renal impairment, and possible drug interactions.

**Monitoring:** Monitor for anaphylactic reactions, pseudomembranous colitis, CDAD, superinfection, drug resistance, and false (+) reaction for urinary glucose when using Benedict's/Fehling's solution or Clinitest tab. Monitor for lab events for CBC, LFTs, renal function tests, and blood chemistry.

**Patient Counseling:** Inform drug only treats bacterial, not viral, infections. Take exactly as directed; skipping doses or not completing full course may decrease effectiveness and increase resistance. Inform about benefits/risks; d/c and notify physician if allergic reaction or diarrhea occurs. Notify if pregnant/nursing.

**Administration:** Oral route. Take with food. **Storage:** 20-25°C (68-77°F); store in tightly-closed, light-resistant container.

# CEFADROXIL — RX

cefadroxil monohydrate (Various)

**THERAPEUTIC CLASS:** Cephalosporin (1st generation)

**INDICATIONS:** Treatment of skin and skin structure (SSSI) and urinary tract infections (UTI), pharyngitis, and tonsillitis caused by susceptible strains of microorganisms.

**DOSAGE:** *Adults:* Uncomplicated Lower UTI: 1-2g/day given qd or bid. Other UTI: 2g in divided doses (bid). SSSI: 1g qd or 500mg bid. Group A β-hemolytic Strep Pharyngitis/Tonsillitis: 1g qd or 500mg bid for 10 days. CrCl ≤50mL/min: Initial: 1g. Maint: CrCl 25-50mL/min: 500mg q12h; CrCl 10-25mL/min: 500mg q24h; CrCl 0-10mL/min: 500mg q36h.
*Pediatrics:* UTI/SSSI: 15mg/kg q12h. Pharyngitis/Tonsillitis/Impetigo: 30mg/kg qd or 15mg/kg q12h. Treat β-hemolytic strep infections for at least 10 days.

**HOW SUPPLIED:** Cap: 500mg; Sus: 250mg/5mL [100mL], 500mg/5mL [75mL, 100mL]; Tab: 1g

**WARNINGS/PRECAUTIONS:** Caution in patients with PCN allergy, cross-sensitivity among β-lactam antibiotics may occur. D/C if an allergic reaction occurs. *Clostridium difficile*-associated diarrhea (CDAD) reported. Caution with renal impairment (CrCl <50mL/min/1.73 $m^2$); careful observation and appropriate laboratory studies should be made prior to and during therapy in patients with known or suspected renal impairment. If superinfection occurs, appropriate measures should be taken. Caution with history of colitis or other GI diseases. Positive Coomb's test reported.

**ADVERSE REACTIONS:** Diarrhea, hypersensitivity reactions, hepatic dysfunction, genital moniliasis, vaginitis, fever, superinfection (prolonged use).

**PREGNANCY:** Category B, caution in nursing.

**MECHANISM OF ACTION:** Cephalosporin; bactericidal due to inhibition of cell-wall synthesis.

**PHARMACOKINETICS: Absorption:** Rapid; $C_{max}$(500, 1000mg)=16mcg/mL, 28mcg/mL. **Elimination:** Urine (90% unchanged).

C

## NURSING CONSIDERATIONS

**Assessment:** Assess for history of hypersensitivity to PCNs, renal impairment, history of GI disease, and pregnancy/nursing status. Document indications for therapy, culture, and susceptibility testing.

**Monitoring:** Monitor for signs/symptoms of a hypersensitivity reaction, CDAD, and for superinfection. Monitor renal function and perform culture and susceptibility tests during therapy.

**Patient Counseling:** Inform drug only treats bacterial, not viral infections. Instruct to take exactly as directed; skipping doses or not completing full course may decrease effectiveness and increase resistance. Advise that may develop diarrhea during therapy; instruct to contact physician if watery/bloody stools, superinfection, or hypersensitivity reactions occur.

**Administration:** Oral route. **Storage:** 20-25°C (68-77°F). (Sus): Following reconstitution: Store in refrigerator; discard after 14 days. Shake well before use. Keep container tightly closed.

# CEFAZOLIN RX

cefazolin sodium (Various)

**THERAPEUTIC CLASS:** Cephalosporin (1st generation)

**INDICATIONS:** Treatment of respiratory tract, urinary tract (UTI), skin and skin structure, biliary tract, bone and joint, and genital infections, septicemia, and endocarditis caused by susceptible strains of microorganisms. Perioperative prophylaxis for surgical procedures classified as contaminated or potentially contaminated.

**DOSAGE:** *Adults:* Moderate-Severe Infections: 500mg-1g q6-8h. Mild Gram-Positive Cocci Infection: 250-500mg q8h. Acute, Uncomplicated UTI: 1g q12h. Pneumococcal Pneumonia: 500mg q12h. Severe Life-Threatening Infection (eg, Endocarditis, Septicemia): 1-1.5g q6h; Max: 12g/day (rare). Perioperative Prophylaxis: 1g IV 0.5-1 hr before surgery. For Procedures ≥2 hrs: 500mg-1g IV during surgery. Maint: 500mg-1g IV q6-8h for 24 hrs post-op. Continue for 3-5 days post-op for devastating procedures (eg, open-heart surgery, prosthetic arthroplasty). Renal Impairment: CrCl 35-54mL/min or SrCr of 1.6-3mg/dL: Full dose q8h. CrCl 11-34mL/min or SrCr of 3.1-4.5mg/dL: 1/2 usual dose q12h. CrCl ≤10mL/min or SrCr of ≥4.6mg/dL: 1/2 usual dose q18-24h. Apply reduced dosage recommendations after initial LD is given.
*Pediatrics:* Mild to Moderately Severe Infections: 25-50mg/kg/day, given tid or qid. Titrate: May increase to 100mg /kg/day for severe infections. Renal Impairment: CrCl 40-70mL/min: 60% of normal daily dose given in equally divided doses every 12 hrs. CrCl 20-40mL/min: 25% of normal daily dose given in equally divided doses every 12 hrs. CrCl 5-20mL/min: 10% of normal daily dose every 24 hrs. Apply reduced dosage recommendations after initial LD is given.

**HOW SUPPLIED:** Inj: 500mg, 1g, 10g, 20g

**WARNINGS/PRECAUTIONS:** Caution with PCN allergy; possible cross-hypersensitivity among β-lactam antibiotics. D/C if an allergic reaction develops. *C.difficile* associated diarrhea (CDAD) reported. Prolonged use may result in overgrowth of nonsusceptible organisms. Lower doses are required in patients with low urinary output due to renal impairment; seizures may occur if inappropriate high doses are administered to patients with renal impairment. Caution with history of colitis or other GI diseases. Safety in premature infants and neonates not established. Positive Coombs tests reported. False positive reaction for glucose in the urine may occur with Benedict's solution, Fehling's solution, or with Clinitest tabs. May cause a fall in prothrombin activity; caution in patients with renal/hepatic impairment, patients on protracted course of antimicrobial therapy, and in patients previously stabilized on anticoagulant therapy; monitor PT and administer Vit K as indicated.

**ADVERSE REACTIONS:** Diarrhea, oral candidiasis, N/V, stomach cramps, anorexia, allergic reactions, blood dyscrasias, renal failure, transient rise in AST/ALT/BUN/SrCr/alkaline phosphatase, genital and anal pruritus.

**INTERACTIONS:** Decreased renal tubular secretion with probenecid.

**PREGNANCY:** Category B, caution in nursing.

**MECHANISM OF ACTION:** Cephalosporin; inhibits cell wall synthesis.

**PHARMACOKINETICS: Absorption:** $C_{max}$=185mcg/mL. **Distribution:** Crosses placenta; found in breast milk. **Elimination:** Urine (unchanged); $T_{1/2}$=1.8 hrs.

## NURSING CONSIDERATIONS

**Assessment:** Assess for hypersensitivity to PCN, renal/hepatic impairment, history of GI disease (eg, colitis), nutritional status, pregnancy/nursing status, and for possible drug interactions.

**Monitoring:** Monitor for signs/symptoms of a hypersensitivity reaction, CDAD, drug resistance or superinfection. Monitor PT in patients at risk of a fall in prothrombin activity. Monitor for seizures in patients with renal dysfunction.

**Patient Counseling:** Inform drug only treats bacterial, not viral infections. Instruct to take as directed; skipping doses or not completing full course may decrease effectiveness and increase resistance. Advise to d/c therapy and notify physician if an allergic reaction or diarrhea occurs. Instruct to notify if pregnant/nursing.

**Administration:** IV route. **Storage**: -20°C (-4°F). Do not force thaw by immersion in water baths or by microwave irridiation. Thawed solution is stable for 30 days under refrigeration 5°C (41°F) and for 48 hrs at 25°C (77°F). Do not refreeze thawed antibiotics.

# CEFOXITIN RX

cefoxitin sodium (Various)

**OTHER BRAND NAMES:** Mefoxin (Merck)

**THERAPEUTIC CLASS:** Cephalosporin (2nd generation)

**INDICATIONS:** Treatment of lower respiratory tract, urinary tract, intra-abdominal, gynecological, skin and skin structure, and bone and joint infections, and septicemia caused by susceptible strains of microorganisms. Prophylaxis of infection in patients undergoing uncontaminated GI surgery, abdominal/vaginal hysterectomy, or cesarean section.

**DOSAGE:** *Adults:* Usual: 1-2g IV q6-8h. Uncomplicated Infections: 1g IV q6-8h. Moderate-Severe: 1g IV q4h or 2g IV q6-8h. Gas Gangrene/Other Infections Requiring Higher Dose: 2g IV q4h or 3g IV q6h. Renal Insufficiency: LD: 1-2g IV. Maint: CrCl 30-50mL/min: 1-2g IV q8-12h. CrCl 10-29mL/min: 1-2g IV q12-24h. CrCl 5-9mL/min: 0.5-1g IV q12-24h. CrCl <5mL/min: 0.5-1g IV q24-48h. Hemodialysis: LD: 1-2g IV after dialysis. Maint: See renal insufficiency doses above. Prophylaxis: Uncontaminated GI Surgery/Hysterectomy: 2g IV 0.5-1 hr prior to surgery (1/2-1 hr before initial incision), then 2g IV q6h after 1st dose up to 24 hrs. C-Section: 2g IV single dose as soon as umbilical cord is clamped, or 2g IV as soon as umbilical cord is clamped, followed by 2g IV at 4 and 8 hrs after initial dose.

*Pediatrics:* ≥3 months: 80-160mg/kg/day divided into 4-6 equal doses. Max: 12g/day. Prophylaxis: Uncontaminated GI Surgery/Hysterectomy: 30-40mg/kg IV 0.5-1 hr prior to surgery, then 30-40mg/kg IV q6h after first dose for up to 24 hrs.

**HOW SUPPLIED:** Inj: 1g, 1g/50mL, 2g, 2g/50mL, 10g

**WARNINGS/PRECAUTIONS:** Possible cross-sensitivity between PCNs and cephalosporins. *Clostridium difficile*-associated diarrhea (CDAD) reported. Caution with allergies, GI disease, particularly colitis. Prolonged use may result in overgrowth of nonsusceptible organisms. Monitor renal, hepatic, hematopoietic functions, especially with prolonged therapy. False (+) for urine glucose with Clinitest tabs.

**ADVERSE REACTIONS:** Thrombophlebitis, rash, pseudomembranous colitis, pruritus, fever, dyspnea, hypotension, diarrhea, blood dyscrasias, elevated LFTs, changes in renal function tests, exacerbation of myasthenia gravis.



**INTERACTIONS:** Increased nephrotoxicity with concomitant aminoglycosides.

**PREGNANCY:** Category B, caution in nursing.

**MECHANISM OF ACTION:** 2nd-generation cephalosporin; inhibits bacterial cell-wall synthesis.

**PHARMACOKINETICS: Metabolism:** Passes pleural and joint fluids; found in bile and breast milk. **Elimination:** Urine (85% unchanged); $T_{1/2}$=41-59 min.

## NURSING CONSIDERATIONS

**Assessment:** Assess for previous hypersensitivity reactions to cephalosporins, PCNs, or other drugs, renal/hepatic impairment, GI tract disease (particularly colitis), DM or carbohydrate intolerance, pregnancy/nursing status, and possible drug interactions.

**Monitoring:** Periodically monitor renal function, LFTs, and hematopoietic functions. Monitor for CDAD (may range from mild diarrhea to fatal colitis), development of superinfections or drug resistance, allergic reactions (eg, toxic epidermal necrolysis or exfoliative dermatitis). May interfere with lab test measurements of serum/urinary creatinine levels by Jaffe reaction (do not analyze creatinine if drawn within 2 hrs of administration). May interfere with measurement of urinary 17-hydroxy-corticosteroid by Porter-Silber reaction, and may cause false (+) reaction for urinary glucose using Clinitest.

**Patient Counseling:** Inform drug only treats bacterial, not viral, infections. Take exactly as directed; skipping doses or not completing full course may decrease effectiveness and increase resistance. Inform about potential benefits/risks. D/C therapy and notify physician if allergic reactions, watery/bloody diarrhea (with/without muscle cramps), or fever occurs. May occur up to 2 months or more after therapy. Notify if pregnant/nursing.

**Administration:** IV route; in DUPLEX container, keep container in folded position to avoid inadvertent activation. Do not use plastic containers in series connections to avoid air embolism. **Storage:** Unactivated unit at 20-25°C (68-77°F); excursions permitted to 15-30°C (59-86°F); use reconstituted product within 12 hrs if stored at room temperature or within 7 days if refrigerated. Can darken depending on storage conditions; do not freeze; discard if leak detected.

# CEFTAZIDIME — RX

ceftazidime (Various)

**THERAPEUTIC CLASS:** Cephalosporin (3rd generation)

**INDICATIONS:** Treatment of lower respiratory tract (eg, pneumonia), skin and skin structure (SSSI), bone and joint, gynecologic, CNS (eg, meningitis), intra-abdominal, and urinary tract infections (UTI), and septicemia caused by susceptible strains of microorganisms. For use in sepsis.

**DOSAGE:** *Adults:* Usual: 1g IM/IV q8-12h. Uncomplicated UTI: 250mg IM/IV q12h. Complicated UTI: 500mg IM/IV q8-12h. Bone and Joint Infection: 2g IV q12h. Uncomplicated Pneumonia/SSSI: 500mg-1g IM/IV q8h. Gynecological/Intra-Abdominal/Meningitis/Severe Life-Threatening Infection: 2g IV q8h. Lung Infection caused by *Pseudomonas* spp. in Cystic Fibrosis (normal renal function): 30-50mg/kg IV q8h. Max: 6g/day. CrCl 31-50mL/min: 1g q12h. CrCl 16-30mL/min: 1g q24h. CrCl 6-15mL/min: 500mg q24h. CrCl <5mL/min: 500mg q48h. For severe infections (6g/day), increase renal impairment dose by 50% or increase dosing interval. Apply reduced dosage recommendations after initial 1g LD is given. Hemodialysis: Give 1g before then 1g after each hemodialysis. Intra-Peritoneal Dialysis/Continuous Ambulatory Peritoneal Dialysis: Give 1g followed by 500mg q24h.
*Pediatrics:* ≥12 yrs: Usual: 1g IM/IV q8-12h. Uncomplicated UTI: 250mg IM/IV q12h. Complicated UTI: 500mg IM/IV q8-12h. Bone and Joint Infection: 2g IV q12h. Uncomplicated Pneumonia/SSSI: 500mg-1g IM/IV q8h. Gynecological/

Intra-Abdominal/Meningitis/Severe Life-Threatening Infection: 2g IV q8h. Lung Infection caused by *Pseudomonas* spp. in Cystic Fibrosis (normal renal function): 30-50mg/kg IV q8h. Max: 6g/day. CrCl 31-50mL/min: 1g q12h. CrCl 16-30mL/min: 1g q24h. CrCl 6-15mL/min: 500mg q24h. CrCl <5mL/min: 500mg q48h. For severe infections (6g/day), increase renal impairment dose by 50% or increase dosing interval. Apply reduced dosage recommendations after initial 1g LD is given. Hemodialysis: Give 1g before then 1g after each hemodialysis. Intra-Peritoneal Dialysis/Continuous Ambulatory Peritoneal Dialysis: Give 1g followed by 500mg q24h.

**HOW SUPPLIED:** Inj: 1g, 2g, 6g

**WARNINGS/PRECAUTIONS:** Monitor renal function; potential for nephrotoxicity. Prolonged use may result in overgrowth of nonsusceptible organisms. Possible cross-sensitivity between PCNs, cephalosporins, and other β-lactam antibiotics. Pseudomembranous colitis and *Clostridium difficile*-associated diarrhea (CDAD) reported. Elevated levels with renal insufficiency can lead to seizures, encephalopathy, asterixis, coma, and neuromuscular excitability. Possible decrease in PT; caution with renal or hepatic impairment, poor nutritional state; monitor PT and give vitamin K if needed. Caution with colitis and other GI diseases. Distal necrosis can occur after inadvertent intra-arterial administration. Continue therapy for 2 days after the signs and symptoms of infection have disappeared, but in complicated infections longer therapy may be required. False (+) for urine glucose with Benedict's, Fehling's solution, and Clinitest tabs.

**ADVERSE REACTIONS:** Phlebitis and inflammation at injection site, pruritus, rash, fever, diarrhea.

**INTERACTIONS:** Nephrotoxicity reported with aminoglycosides or potent diuretics (eg, furosemide). Avoid with chloramphenicol; may decrease effect of β-lactam antibiotics.

**PREGNANCY:** Category B, not for use in nursing.

**MECHANISM OF ACTION:** Broad spectrum, β-lactam antibiotic; exerts effects by inhibiting enzymes responsible for cell-wall synthesis.

**PHARMACOKINETICS: Absorption:** (IV) $C_{max}$=45mcg/mL (500mg), 90mcg/mL (1g). (IM) $C_{max}$=17mcg/mL (500mg), 39mcg/mL (1g), $T_{max}$=1 hr. **Distribution:** Plasma protein binding (<10%); found in breast milk. **Elimination:** Urine, (80-90% unchanged). $T_{1/2}$=1.9 hrs (IV), 2 hrs (IM).

## NURSING CONSIDERATIONS

**Assessment:** Assess for previous hypersensitivity to cephalosporins/PCNs or other drugs, renal/hepatic insufficiency, nutritional status, history of GI disease, pregnancy/nursing status, and possible drug interactions.

**Monitoring:** Periodically monitor PT, with vitamin K administration if indicated. Monitor for allergic reactions (eg, Stevens-Johnson syndrome), signs/symptoms of pseudomembranous colitis or CDAD, seizures, encephalopathy, coma, asterixis, neuromuscular excitability, and myoclonia, development of superinfection or drug resistance, renal function tests/urine output for daily dosage, LFTs, hematopoietic function, and lab test interactions.

**Patient Counseling:** Inform that drug only treats bacterial, not viral, infections. Take exactly as directed; skipping doses or not completing full course may decrease effectiveness and increase resistance. Inform about potential benefits/risks. D/C and notify physician if allergic reactions, watery/bloody diarrhea (with/without muscle cramps), or fever occurs. Notify if pregnant/nursing.

**Administration:** IV/IM routes. Do not use plastic containers for series connections to avoid development of air embolism. **Storage**: Dry state at 15-30°C (59-86°F); protect from light. As premixed solution not >-20°C; do not force thaw by immersion in water baths or by microwave irradiation; store thawed solutions for up to 24 hrs at room temperature or for 7 days in a refrigerator. Do not refreeze thawed solution.

# CEFTIN

**RX**

cefuroxime axetil (GlaxoSmithKline)

C

**THERAPEUTIC CLASS:** Cephalosporin (2nd generation)

**INDICATIONS:** Treatment of the following infections caused by susceptible strains of microorganisms: (Sus/Tab) Pharyngitis/tonsillitis and acute otitis media. (Sus) Impetigo. (Tab) Uncomplicated skin and skin structure infections (SSSI), uncomplicated urinary tract infections (UTI), uncomplicated gonorrhea, early Lyme disease, acute bacterial maxillary sinusitis, acute bacterial exacerbations of chronic bronchitis (ABECB), and secondary bacterial infections of acute bronchitis.

**DOSAGE:** *Adults:* (Tab) Pharyngitis/Tonsillitis/Sinusitis: 250mg bid for 10 days. ABECB/SSSI: 250-500mg bid for 10 days. Acute Bronchitis: 250-500mg bid for 5-10 days. UTI: 250mg bid for 7-10 days. Gonorrhea: 1000mg single dose. Lyme Disease: 500mg bid for 20 days.
*Pediatrics:* ≥13 yrs: (Tab) Pharyngitis/Tonsillitis/Sinusitis: 250mg bid for 10 days. ABECB/SSSI: 250-500mg bid for 10 days. Acute Bronchitis: 250-500mg bid for 5-10 days. UTI: 250mg bid for 7-10 days. Gonorrhea: 1000mg single dose. Lyme Disease: 500mg bid for 20 days. 3 months-12 yrs: (Sus) Pharyngitis/Tonsillitis: 20mg/kg/day divided bid for 10 days. Max: 500mg/day. Otitis Media/Sinusitis/Impetigo: 30mg/kg/day divided bid for 10 days. Max: 1000mg/day. (Tab-if can swallow whole) Otitis Media/Sinusitis: 250mg bid for 10 days.

**HOW SUPPLIED:** Sus: 125mg/5mL [100mL], 250mg/5mL [50mL, 100mL]; Tab: 250mg, 500mg

**WARNINGS/PRECAUTIONS:** Tabs are not bioequivalent to sus. Caution in patients with previous hypersensitivity to penicillins or other drugs; cross-sensitivity may occur in patients with a history of penicillin allergy. D/C if an allergic reaction occurs. Watery, bloody stools (with or without stomach cramps and fever) may develop after starting treatment. *Clostridium difficile*-associated diarrhea (CDAD) reported and may range in severity from mild diarrhea to fatal colitis. Caution with a history of colitis. Prolonged administration may result in overgrowth of nonsusceptible organisms; take appropriate measures if superinfection occurs. Safety and efficacy not established in patients with GI malabsorption. May cause fall in PT; those at risk include patients previously stable on anticoagulants, patients receiving protracted course of antibiotics, patients with renal/hepatic impairment, and in patients with a poor nutritional state. Monitor PT and give vitamin K as needed. Use in the absence of a proven or strongly suspected bacterial infection or a prophylactic indication may increase the risk of the development of drug-resistant bacteria. Safety and efficacy not established in patients with renal failure. False (+) for urine glucose with Benedict's, Fehling's solution, and Clinitest tabs. (Sus) Contains phenylalanine.

**ADVERSE REACTIONS:** Diarrhea, N/V, vaginitis, (suspension) dislike of taste, diaper rash.

**INTERACTIONS:** Probenecid increases plasma levels. Lower bioavailability with drugs that lower gastric acidity. Caution with agents causing adverse effects on renal function (diuretics). May lower estrogen reabsorption and reduced the efficacy of combined oral estrogen/progesterone contraceptives.

**PREGNANCY:** Category B, not for use in nursing.

**MECHANISM OF ACTION:** 2nd-generation cephalosporin; binds to essential target proteins and the resultant inhibition of cell-wall synthesis.

**PHARMACOKINETICS: Absorption:** Absolute bioavailability (37% before food), (52% after food). PO administration of variable doses resulted in different parameters. **Distribution:** Plasma protein binding (50%); found in breast milk. **Metabolism:** Rapid hydrolysis, via nonspecific esterases in the intestinal mucosa and blood. **Elimination:** Urine (50% unchanged).

## NURSING CONSIDERATIONS

**Assessment:** Assess for previous hypersensitivity reactions to cephalosporins/PCNs or other drugs, renal/hepatic impairment, nutritional state, history of colitis, GI malabsorption, pregnancy/nursing status, and for possible drug interactions. For patients planning on using sus formulation, assess for phenylketonuria.

**Monitoring:** Monitor signs/symptoms of an allergic reaction, pseudomembranous colitis or CDAD, superinfection, and lab test interactions. Monitor PT and renal function.

**Patient Counseling:** Advise of potential benefits/risks of therapy. Inform that drug only treats bacterial, not viral infections. Instruct to take exactly as directed; inform that skipping doses or not completing full course may decrease effectiveness and increase resistance. Counsel to d/c and notify physician if an allergic reaction or if watery/bloody diarrhea (with/without stomach cramps or fever) develop. Instruct to notify physician if pregnant/nursing. Inform caregivers of pediatric patients that if cannot swallow tab whole, should receive oral sus. Advise that crushed tab, has a strong/persistent bitter taste. Inform that tab may be administered without regard to meals but oral sus must be administered with food.

**Administration:** Oral route. Tab and sus not bioequivalent and not substitutable on mg-per-mg basis. Refer to prescribing information for reconstitution instructions for sus. Shake sus well before use. **Storage:** Tab: Store at 15-30°C (59-86°F). Sus Powder: Store at 2-30°C (36-86°F). Reconstituted Sus: Store at 2-8°C (36-46°F) in a refrigerator; discard after 10 days.

# CEFTRIAXONE — RX

ceftriaxone sodium (Various)

**OTHER BRAND NAMES:** Rocephin (Roche)

**THERAPEUTIC CLASS:** Cephalosporin (3rd generation)

**INDICATIONS:** Treatment of lower respiratory tract infections, skin and skin structure infections, bone and joint infections, intra-abdominal infections, urinary tract infections, acute otitis media, uncomplicated gonorrhea, pelvic inflammatory disease, bacterial septicemia, and meningitis caused by susceptible strains of microorganisms. Surgical prophylaxis during surgical procedures classified as contaminated or potentially contaminated.

**DOSAGE:** *Adults:* Usual: 1-2g/day IV/IM given qd or bid in equally divided doses depending on the type and severity of infection. Max: 4g/day. Gonorrhea: 250mg IM single dose. Surgical Prophylaxis: 1g IV 1/2-2 hrs before surgery. Usual duration of therapy is 4-14 days; complicated infections may require longer therapy.

*Pediatrics:* Skin/skin structure infections: 50-75mg/kg/day IV/IM given qd or in equally divided doses bid. Max: 2g/day. Otitis Media: 50mg/kg (up to 1g) IM single dose. Serious Infections: 50-75mg/kg IV/IM given bid q12h. Max: 2g/day. Meningitis: Initial: 100mg/kg (up to 4g) IV/IM, then 100mg/kg/day IV/IM given qd or in equally divided doses q12h for 7-14 days. Max: 4g/day.

**HOW SUPPLIED:** Inj: (Rocephin) 500mg, 1g; (Generic) 250mg, 500mg, 1g, 2g

**CONTRAINDICATIONS:** Hyperbilirubinemic neonates (≤28 days), especially if premature; calcium-containing IV solutions, including continuous calcium-containing infusions such as parenteral nutrition used in neonates.

**WARNINGS/PRECAUTIONS:** Caution in penicillin-sensitive patients and in patients who have demonstrated any form of an allergy. Serious acute hypersensitvity reactions may require the use of SQ epinephrine and other emergency measures. *Clostridium difficile*-associated diarrhea (CDAD) reported. Increased risk of drug-resistant bacteria if used in the absence of a proven or strongly suspected bacterial infection or a prophylactic indication. Transient BUN and SrCr elevations may occur. Caution in patients with both hepatic and significant renal disease, do not exceed a dose of 2g/day. May alter PT; monitor with impaired vitamin K synthesis or low vitamin K stores during treatment. May result in overgrowth of nonsusceptible organisms; take appropriate measures if superinfection develops. Caution with history of GI disease, especially colitis. D/C if gallbladder disease develops. Pancreatitis reported rarely. Anaphylactic shock may occur.

C

**ADVERSE REACTIONS:** Injection-site reactions (eg, warmth, tightness, induration), eosinophilia, thrombocytosis, AST elevation, ALT elevation.

**INTERACTIONS:** See Contraindications. Incompatible with vancomycin, amsacrine, aminoglycosides, and fluconazole; when administered concomitantly by intermittent IV infusion, give sequentially, with thorough flushing of the intravenous lines between administrations. Avoid physically mixing with or piggybacking with solutions containing antimicrobial drugs.

**PREGNANCY:** Category B, caution in nursing.

**MECHANISM OF ACTION:** 3rd-generation cephalosporin; bactericidal activity results from inhibition of cell-wall synthesis.

**PHARMACOKINETICS: Absorption:** (Adults) Complete; $T_{max}$=2-3 hrs. (Pediatrics) Bacterial meningitis: $C_{max}$=216mcg/mL (50mg/kg), 275mcg/mL (75mg/kg). Middle ear fluid: $C_{max}$=35mcg/mL; $T_{max}$=24 hrs. **Distribution:** Found in breast milk and crosses blood placenta barrier; plasma protein binding (95%) (<25mcg/mL), (85%) (300mcg/mL); (Adults) $V_d$=5.78-13.5L. (Pediatrics) Bacterial meningitis: $V_d$=338mL/kg (50mg/kg), 373mL/kg (75mg/kg). **Elimination:** Urine (33-67%, unchanged), feces. (Adults) $T_{1/2}$=5.8-8.7 hrs. (Pediatrics) Bacterial meningitis: $T_{1/2}$=4.6 hrs (50mg/kg), 4.3 hrs (75mg/kg); Middle ear fluid: $T_{1/2}$=25 hrs.

## NURSING CONSIDERATIONS

**Assessment:** Assess for presence of hyperbilirubinemia in neonates, hypersensitivity to penicillins or other drugs, presence of both hepatic dysfunction and significant renal disease, impaired vitamin K synthesis or low vitamin K stores, history of GI disease (eg, colitis), nursing status, and for possible drug interactions.

**Monitoring:** Monitor for signs/symptoms of hypersensitivity reactions, CDAD, overgrowth of nonsusceptible organisms (eg, superinfection), gallbladder disease, and pancreatitis. Periodically monitor BUN and SrCr levels. Monitor PT levels in patients with low impaired vitamin K synthesis or in patients with low vitamin K stores (eg, chronic hepatic disease, malnutrition).

**Patient Counseling:** Inform that therapy only treats bacterial, not viral, infections (eg, common cold). Instruct to take as directed; skipping doses or not completing full course may decrease drug effectiveness and increase risk of bacteria developing resistance. Inform that diarrhea (watery/bloody stools) may be experienced as late as 2 months or more after last dose.

**Administration:** IV/IM route. Refer to PI for reconstitution directions. **Storage:** 20°- 25°C (68°- 77°F). Protect from light. Refer to PI for storage requirements following reconstitution. Do not refreeze.

# CEFZIL RX

cefprozil (Bristol-Myers Squibb)

**THERAPEUTIC CLASS:** Cephalosporin (2nd generation)

**INDICATIONS:** Treatment of mild to moderate pharyngitis/tonsillitis, otitis media, acute sinusitis, secondary bacterial infection of acute bronchitis, acute bacterial exacerbation of chronic bronchitis (ABECB), and uncomplicated skin and skin structure infections (SSSI) caused by susceptible strains of microorganisms.

**DOSAGE:** *Adults:* Pharyngitis/Tonsillitis: 500mg q24h for 10 days. Acute Sinusitis: 250-500mg q12h for 10 days. ABECB/Acute Bronchitis: 500mg q12h for 10 days. SSSI: 250-500mg q12h or 500mg q24h for 10 days. CrCl <30mL/min: 50% of standard dose.

*Pediatrics:* ≥13 yrs: Use adult dose. 2-12 yrs: Pharyngitis/Tonsillitis: 7.5mg/kg q12h for 10 days. SSSI: 20mg/kg q24h for 10 days. 6 months-12 yrs: Otitis Media: 15mg/kg q12h for 10 days. Acute Sinusitis: 7.5-15mg/kg q12h for 10 days. Do not exceed adult dose. CrCl <30mL/min: 50% of standard dose.

**HOW SUPPLIED:** Sus: 125mg/5mL [50mL, 75mL, 100mL], 250mg/5mL [50mL, 75mL, 100mL]; Tab: 250mg, 500mg

**WARNINGS/PRECAUTIONS:** Cross-sensitivity with cephalosporins and PCNs. False (+) direct Coombs' tests reported. *Clostridium difficile*-associated diarrhea (CDAD) reported. Caution with GI disease, renal impairment, elderly. False (+) for urine glucose with Benedict's, Fehling's solution, and Clinitest tabs. Sus contains phenylalanine.

**ADVERSE REACTIONS:** Diarrhea, nausea, hepatic enzyme elevations, eosinophilia, genital pruritus, vaginitis, superinfection (prolonged use).

**INTERACTIONS:** Nephrotoxicity with aminoglycosides reported. Probenecid may increase plasma levels. Caution with agents causing adverse effects on renal function (diuretics).

**PREGNANCY:** Category B, caution in nursing.

**MECHANISM OF ACTION:** 2nd-generation cephalosporin; inhibits bacterial cell-wall synthesis.

**PHARMACOKINETICS: Absorption:** $C_{max}$=6.1mcg/mL (250mg), 10.5mcg/mL (500mg), 18.3mcg/mL(1g); $T_{max}$=1.5 hrs (adults), 1-2 hrs (peds). Plasma concentration (peds) at 7.5, 15, and 30mg/kg doses similar to those observed within same time frame in normal adults at 250, 500, and 1000mg doses, respectively. **Distribution:** $V_d$=0.23L/kg; plasma protein binding (36%); found in breast milk. **Elimination:** Urine (60%); $T_{1/2}$=1.3 hrs (adults), 1.5 hrs (peds).

## NURSING CONSIDERATIONS

**Assessment:** Assess for previous hypersensitivity reactions to PCNs/cephalosporins or other drugs, renal/hepatic impairment, pregnancy/nursing status, and possible drug interactions. Perform renal function tests prior to and during therapy.

**Monitoring:** Periodically monitor renal function tests, LFTs and hematopoietic functions. Monitor for allergic reactions (eg, Stevens-Johnson syndrome), signs/symptoms of CDAD(may range between mild diarrhea to fatal colitis), development of drug resistance or superinfection, nephrotoxicity if given concurrently with aminoglycosides and for lab test interactions (eg, positive Coombs' test, false (+) for urinary glucose if copper reduction tests used, false negative in ferricyanide test for blood glucose; no interference in plasma/urinary creatinine by alkaline picrate method).

**Patient Counseling:** Inform drug only treats bacterial, not viral, infections. Take exactly as directed; skipping doses or not completing full course may decrease effectiveness and increase resistance. Inform about potential benefits/risks. D/C and notify physician if allergic reactions, watery/bloody diarrhea (with/without muscle cramps), or fever occur (up to 2 months after therapy). Notify if pregnant/nursing.

**Administration:** Oral route. Shake sus well before use. **Storage:** Tab: 15-30°C (59-86°F); prior to reconstitution at 15-25°C (59-77°F), refrigerate after mixing; discard after 14 days.

# CELEBREX — RX

celecoxib (G.D. Searle)

**NSAIDs may cause an increased risk of serious cardiovascular thrombotic events, MI, stroke and serious GI adverse events including bleeding, ulceration, and perforation of the stomach or intestines, which can be fatal. These events can occur at any time during use without warning symptoms. Contraindicated for the treatment of perioperative pain in the setting of coronary artery bypass graft (CABG) surgery. Elderly patients are at greater risk for serious gastrointestinal events.**

**THERAPEUTIC CLASS:** COX-2 inhibitor

**INDICATIONS:** Relief of signs and symptoms of rheumatoid arthritis (RA) in adults, osteoarthritis (OA), and ankylosing spondylitis (AS). Management of acute pain in adults. Treatment of primary dysmenorrhea. Adjunct to usual care (eg, surgical endoscopic surveillance) to reduce the number of adenomatous colorectal polyps in familial adenomatous polyposis (FAP). Relief of signs and symptoms of juvenile rheumatoid arthritis (JRA) in patients ≥2 yrs.

C

**DOSAGE:** *Adults:* ≥18 yrs: OA: 200mg qd or 100mg bid. RA: 100-200mg bid. AS: 200mg qd or 100mg bid. Titrate: May increase to 400mg/day after 6 weeks. FAP: 400mg bid with food. Acute Pain/Primary Dysmenorrhea: Day 1: 400mg, then 200mg if needed. Maint: 200mg bid prn. Moderate Hepatic Insufficiency: Reduce daily dose by 50%. Poor Metabolizers of CYP2C9 Substrates: Half the lowest recommended dose.
*Pediatrics:* JRA: ≥2 yrs: 10-25kg: 50mg bid. >25kg: 100mg bid.

**HOW SUPPLIED:** Cap: 50mg, 100mg, 200mg, 400mg

**CONTRAINDICATIONS:** Asthma, urticaria, or allergic-type reactions after ASA, NSAID, or sulfonamide use. Treatment of perioperative pain in the setting of CABG surgery.

**WARNINGS/PRECAUTIONS:** May lead to onset of new HTN or worsening of pre-existing HTN; monitor BP closely. Fluid retention and edema reported; caution with fluid retention or heart failure. Renal papillary necrosis and other renal injury reported after long-term use. Not recommended for use with advanced renal disease; if therapy must be initiated, monitor renal function. Anaphylactoid reactions may occur. May cause serious skin adverse events (eg, exfoliative dermatitis, Stevens-Johnson syndrome, and toxic epidermal necrolysis). Avoid in late pregnancy; may cause premature closure of ductus arteriosus. May cause elevations of LFTs; d/c if liver disease develops or systemic manifestations occur. Anemia may occur; with long-term use, monitor Hgb/Hct if signs or symptoms of anemia or blood loss develop. Caution with asthma and avoid with ASA-sensitive asthma. Caution in pediatric patients with systemic onset JRA due to increased possibility of disseminated intravascular coagulation. Caution in patients to be known or suspected poor CYP2C9 metabolizers based on previous history/experience with other CYP2C9 substrates (eg, warfarin, phenytoin). Caution in elderly.

**ADVERSE REACTIONS:** Dyspepsia, diarrhea, abdominal pain, nausea, dizziness, headache, sinusitis, upper respiratory infection, rash, fever, cough, arthralgia, HTN, insomnia, pharyngitis.

**INTERACTIONS:** Monitor anticoagulant activity in patients also on warfarin or similar agents; reports of serious bleeding, some fatal. Decreased effects of ACE-inhibitors, angiotensin II antagonists, furosemide, thiazides, and loop diuretics; increased risk for renal toxicity. Increased levels with fluconazole. Monitor lithium. Caution with CYP2C9 inhibitors and drugs metabolized by CYP2D6. Celecoxib is not a substitute for ASA for CV prophylaxis; may use with low-dose ASA but may increase GI complications. Avoid with nonaspirin NSAID. Reduction in plasma celecoxib concentrations with aluminum- and magnesium-containing antacids.

**PREGNANCY:** Category C and D ( ≥30 weeks' gestation), caution in nursing.

**MECHANISM OF ACTION:** NSAID; inhibits prostaglandin synthesis primarily via inhibition of COX-2.

**PHARMACOKINETICS: Absorption:** $C_{max}$=705ng/mL, $T_{max}$=2.8 hrs. **Distribution:** $V_d$=429L; plasma protein binding (97%). **Metabolism:** CYP2C9. Primary alcohol, carboxylic acid, glucuronide conjugate (metabolites). **Elimination:** Urine (27%), feces (57%); $T_{1/2}$=11.2 hrs.

## NURSING CONSIDERATIONS

**Assessment:** Assess for risk of CV thrombotic events (eg, MI, stroke), CABG surgery, renal/hepatic insufficiency, HTN, history of peptic ulcer disease and/or GI bleeding, allergic-type reactions to sulfonamides, pre-existing asthma, and urticaria.

**Monitoring:** Monitor renal function, LFTs, chemistries, and CBC periodically. Monitor for signs and symptoms of CV thrombotic events, GI events (bleeding, ulceration, perforation), HTN, fluid retention, edema, CHF, hypersensitivity reactions, renal and hepatic dysfunction.

**Patient Counseling:** Inform of risk for MI or stroke, and GI adverse reactions; d/c and report immediately if rash develops. Seek medical attention if symptoms of unexplained weight gain or edema, anaphylactoid reactions (eg, difficulty in breathing, swelling of the face or throat), hepatotoxicity (eg, nausea, fatigue, lethargy, pruritus, jaundice, RUQ tenderness and "flu-like" symptoms), or signs/symptoms of chest pain, SOB, weakness, slurring of speech occur.

Inform that the drug can lead to the onset of new HTN or worsening of preexisting HTN. Inform of pregnancy risks.

**Administration:** Oral route. For patients with difficulty swallowing, capsule contents may be added to applesauce and ingested with water. **Storage:** 25°C (77°F); excursions permitted to 15-30°C (59-86°F).



## Celexa RX

citalopram hbr (Forest)

**Antidepressants increased the risk of suicidal thinking and behavior (suicidality) in short-term studies in children, adolescents, and young adults with major depressive disorder (MDD) and other psychiatric disorders. Citalopram is not approved for use in pediatric patients.**

**THERAPEUTIC CLASS:** Selective serotonin reuptake inhibitor

**INDICATIONS:** Treatment of depression.

**DOSAGE:** *Adults:* Initial: 20mg qd, in the am or pm. Titrate: Increase by 20mg at intervals of no less than 1 week. Max: 40mg/day (non-responders may require 60mg/day). Elderly/Hepatic Impairment: 20mg/day. Titrate: Increase to 40mg/day in nonresponders.

**HOW SUPPLIED:** Sol: 10mg/5mL [240mL]; Tab: 10mg, 20mg*, 40mg* *scored

**CONTRAINDICATIONS:** Concomitant use of MAOI or pimozide.

**WARNINGS/PRECAUTIONS:** Avoid abrupt withdrawal. May increase risk of bleeding events. Activation of mania/hypomania, SIADH, hyponatremia reported. Caution with history of mania or seizures, hepatic impairment, severe renal impairment, conditions that alter metabolism or hemodynamic responses. May impair judgment, thinking, or motor skills. Serotonin syndrome or neuroleptic malignant syndrome (NMS)-like reactions may occur. Monitor for clinical worsening and/or suicidality, especially at initiation of therapy or dose changes.

**ADVERSE REACTIONS:** N/V, dyspepsia, diarrhea, dry mouth, somnolence, insomnia, increased sweating, ejaculation disorder, rhinitis, anxiety, anorexia, tremor, and agitation.

**INTERACTIONS:** See Contraindications. Avoid alcohol, tryptophan. Caution with other centrally acting drugs, SSRIs, SNRIs, TCAs, lithium, carbamazepine, cimetidine. Increased risk of bleeding with warfarin, ASA, NSAIDs. Rare reports of weakness, hyperreflexia, incoordination with SSRIs and sumatriptan. Clearance may be decreased with potent CYP3A4 (eg, ketoconazole, itraconazole, fluconazole, erythromycin) and CYP2C19 (eg, omeprazole) inhibitors. May increase metoprolol levels, which leads to decreased cardioselectivity. Concomitant use of serotonergic drugs and with drugs that impair metabolism of serotonin may cause serotonin syndrome. Caution with other agents that may affect serotonergic neurotransmitter systems (eg, triptans, linezolid, tramadol, or St. John's wort).

**PREGNANCY:** Category C, not for use in nursing.

**MECHANISM OF ACTION:** SSRI; inhibits CNS neuronal reuptake of serotonin.

**PHARMACOKINETICS: Absorption:** Absolute bioavailability (80%); $T_{max}$=4 hrs. **Distribution:** $V_d$=12L/kg. **Metabolism:** Hepatic (biotransformation: N-demethylation) via CYP3A4 and CYP2C19 . **Elimination:** Urine (10%); $T_{1/2}$=35 hrs.

### NURSING CONSIDERATIONS

**Assessment:** Assess for risk for bipolar disorder, history of mania, history of seizures, disease/condition that alters metabolism or hemodynamic response, hepatic/renal impairment, pregnancy/nursing status, and possible drug interactions.

**Monitoring:** Monitor for signs/symptoms of clinical worsening (suicidality, unusual changes in behavior), serotonin syndrome/NMS-like reactions, abnormal bleeding, hyponatremia, seizures, cognitive and motor impairment, and hepatic/renal dysfunction. If therapy is abruptly d/c, monitor for symptoms of dysphoric mood, irritability, agitation, dizziness, sensory disturbances, anxiety, confusion, headache, lethargy, emotional lability, insomnia, and hypomania.

**Patient Counseling:** Advise to avoid alcohol. Seek medical attention for symptoms of serotonin syndrome (mental status changes, tachycardia, hyperthermia, NV, diarrhea, incoordination), abnormal bleeding (particularly if using NSAID or ASA), hyponatremia, activation of mania, seizures, clinical worsening (suicidal ideation, unusual changes in behavior) and discontinuation of symptoms (irritability, agitation, dizziness, anxiety, headache, insomnia). Caution against hazardous tasks (eg, operating machinery and driving). May notice improvement in 1-4 weeks; continue therapy as directed. Notify physician if pregnant/intend to become pregnant, or breastfeeding. Counsel about benefits and risks of therapy. Inform physician if taking, or plan to take any over-the-counter prescriptions.

**Administration:** Oral route. **Storage:** 25°C (77°F); excursions permitted to 15-30°C (59-86°F).

## CellCept — RX

mycophenolate mofetil (Roche Labs)

**Immunosuppression may lead to increased susceptibility to infection and possible development of lymphoma. Only physicians experienced in immunosuppressive therapy and management of renal, cardiac or hepatic transplant patients should use mycophenolate mofetil. Women of childboaring potential must use contraception; use during pregnancy is associated with increased risk of pregnancy loss and congenital malformations.**

**THERAPEUTIC CLASS:** Inosine monophosphate dehydrogenase inhibitor

**INDICATIONS:** Prophylaxis of organ rejection in allogeneic renal, cardiac, or hepatic transplants; used concomitantly with cyclosporine and corticosteroids.

**DOSAGE:** *Adults:* Renal Transplant: 1g IV/PO bid. Cardiac Transplant: 1.5g IV/PO bid. Hepatic Transplant: 1g IV bid or 1.5g PO bid. Start PO as soon as possible after transplant. Start IV within 24 hrs after transplant; can continue for up to 14 days. IV infusion should not last <2 hrs. Switch to oral when tolerated. Give on an empty stomach.

*Pediatrics:* 3 months-18 yrs: Renal Transplant: (Sus) 600mg/m$^2$ PO bid. Max: 2g/day (10 mL/day). (Cap) BSA 1.25m$^2$ to 1.5m$^2$: 750mg PO bid. (Cap/Tab) BSA >1.5m$^2$: 1g PO bid.

**HOW SUPPLIED:** Cap: 250mg; Tab: 500mg; Inj: 500mg/20mL; Sus: 200mg/mL

**CONTRAINDICATIONS:** (Inj) Hypersensitivity to Polysorbate 80 (TWEEN).

**WARNINGS/PRECAUTIONS:** Do not administer by rapid or bolus IV injection. Risk of lymphomas and other malignancies, especially of the skin. Limit exposure to sunlight to decrease risk of skin cancer. May cause fetal harm; must have negative serum/urine pregnancy test within 1 week before therapy. Two reliable forms of contraception required before and during therapy, and 6 weeks following discontinuation. Severe neutropenia reported; if ANC <1.3 x 10$^3$/µL, d/c or reduce dose. Monitor for bone marrow suppression. Risk of GI ulceration, hemorrhage, and perforation; caution with active digestive system disease. Caution with delayed renal graft function post-transplant. Oral suspension contains phenylalanine; caution with phenylketonurics. Monitor CBC weekly during the 1st month, twice monthly for the 2nd and 3rd months, and then monthly through 1st year. Avoid with rare hereditary deficiency of hypoxanthine-guanine phosphoribosyl-transferase (eg, Lesch-Nyhan and Kelley-Seegmiller syndromes). Increased susceptibility to infections/sepsis. Cases of pure red cell aplasia reported when used with other immunosuppressive agents. Activation of latent viral infections, including progressive multifocal leukoencephalopathy (PML) and BK virus-associated nephropathy (BKVAN) in immunosuppressed; reduce dose in patients who develop evidence of BKVAN. Cases of PML, sometimes fatal, reported. Caution in elderly.

**ADVERSE REACTIONS:** Infections, diarrhea, leukopenia, sepsis, N/V, HTN, peripheral edema, constipation, pain, abdominal pain, fever, headache, asthenia, back pain, anemia.

**INTERACTIONS:** Additive bone marrow suppression with azathioprine; avoid use. Reduced efficacy with drugs that interfere with enterohepatic recirculation (eg, cholestyramine); avoid concomitant use. Avoid live attenuated vaccines. Increased levels with probenecid. Increased levels of both drugs with acyclovir, ganciclovir. Decreased levels with sevelamer and other calcium-free phosphate binders, magnesium- and aluminum-containing antacids, space dosing. Decreased levels of oral contraceptives; caution and consider additional birth control. Decreased exposure with rifampin; concomitant use not recommended unless benefit outweighs risk. May decrease levels with ciprofloxacin or amoxicillin plus clavulanic acid. Decreased exposure with combination of norfloxacin and metronidazole; avoid concomitant use. Other drugs that compete for renal tubular secretion may raise levels of both drugs.

**PREGNANCY:** Category D, not for use in nursing.

**MECHANISM OF ACTION:** Inosine monophosphate dehydrogenase inhibitor; inhibits the de novo pathway of guanosine nucleotide synthesis without incorporation into DNA.

**PHARMACOKINETICS: Absorption:** Oral: Rapid and complete, absolute bioavailability (94%). **Distribution:** $V_d$=3.6L/kg (IV), 4L/kg (oral); plasma protein binding of MPA (97%), MPAG (82%). **Metabolism:** MPA (active metabolite) metabolized by glucuronyl transferase to MPAG, which is converted to MPA via entrohepatic recirculation. **Elimination:** Oral: Urine (93%), feces (6%). Urine: MPA (<1%) and MPAG (87%). MPA: (Oral) $T_{1/2}$=17.9 hrs. (IV) $T_{1/2}$=16.6 hrs. **Pediatrics:** Oral administration in different age groups ranging between 1-18 years results in different pharmacokinetics.

## NURSING CONSIDERATIONS

**Assessment:** Assess for drug hypersensitivity, hepatic/renal impairment, phenylketonuria, hereditary deficiency of HGPRT such as Lesch-Nyhan and Kelley-Seegmiller syndromes, and active digestive disease. Assess vaccination history, pregnancy/nursing status, and possible drug interactions.

**Monitoring:** Monitor for signs of delayed graft rejection (eg, anemia, thrombocytopenia, and hyperkalemia), lymphomas, skin cancer, GI bleeding/perforation, peptic/duodenal ulcers, infections (including opportunistic infections, latent viral infections, herpes, sepsis), unexpected bruising, bleeding, or any signs of bone marrow suppression. Monitor CBC weekly during the 1st month, twice monthly for the 2nd and 3rd months, and then monthly through the 1st year. Monitor pregnancy status and enroll patient in the National Transplantation Pregnancy Registry if patient becomes pregnant while on medication.

**Patient Counseling:** Counsel on importance of following dosage instructions and having periodic laboratory tests. Inform about increased risk of malignancies and infection, and reduced efficacy of concurrent vaccines; notify physician for any signs of infection, bruising, and/or bleeding. Advise to avoid prolonged exposure to sunlight. Not for use in pregnant/nursing women or those planning to become pregnant; inform of need for highly effective contraception before, during, and after therapy. Take on an empty stomach.

**Administration:** Oral route and slow IV infusion route. **Storage:** 25°C (77°F); excursions permitted to 15-30°C (59-86°F). Constituted sus: Stable up to 60 days and may be refrigerated at 2-8°C (36-46°F). Do not freeze.

# CENESTIN — RX

conjugated estrogens (Duramed)

**Estrogens increase risk of endometrial cancer. Estrogens, with or without progestins, should not be used for the prevention of cardiovascular disease. Increased risks of MI, stroke, invasive breast cancer, PE, and DVT in postmenopausal women reported.**

**THERAPEUTIC CLASS:** Estrogen

**INDICATIONS:** (0.45mg, 0.625mg, 0.9mg, 1.25mg) Treatment of moderate to severe vasomotor symptoms associated with menopause. (0.3mg) Treatment of vulvar and vaginal atrophy.



**DOSAGE:** *Adults:* Vasomotor Symptoms: Initial: 0.45mg/day. Adjust dose based on response. Discontinue or taper at 3-6 month intervals. Vulvar/ Vaginal Atrophy: 0.3mg qd.

**HOW SUPPLIED:** Tab: 0.3mg, 0.45mg, 0.625mg, 0.9mg, 1.25mg

**CONTRAINDICATIONS:** Pregnancy, undiagnosed abnormal genital bleeding, breast cancer, estrogen-dependent neoplasia, DVT/PE, active or recent (eg, within past year) arterial thromboembolic disease (eg, stroke, MI), liver dysfunction or disease.

**WARNINGS/PRECAUTIONS:** May increase risk of cardiovascular events (eg, MI, stroke), venous thrombosis, and PE; d/c immediately if any of these events occur or are suspected. May increase risk of breast/endometrial cancer, and gallbladder disease. May lead to severe hypercalcemia with breast cancer and bone metastases; monitor and d/c if hypercalcemia occurs. Retinal vascular thrombosis reported; monitor and d/c if papilledema or retinal vascular lesions occur. Consider addition of a progestin if no hysterectomy. May elevate BP; monitor at regular intervals. May cause elevations of plasma triglycerides with pre-existing hypertriglyceridemia. Caution with history of cholestatic jaundice associated with past estrogen use or with pregnancy; d/c with recurrence. May lead to increased thyroid-binding globulin levels; monitor thyroid function. May cause fluid retention; caution with cardiac/renal dysfunction. Caution with severe hypocalcemia. May increase risk of ovarian cancer. May exacerbate endometriosis, asthma, DM, epilepsy, migraine, porphyria, SLE, and hepatic hemangiomas; use with caution.

**ADVERSE REACTIONS:** Abdominal pain, back pain, pain, headache, infection, vomiting, leg cramps, paresthesia, breast pain, metrorrhagia, endometrial thickening, vaginitis.

**INTERACTIONS:** CYP3A4 inducers (eg, St. John's wort, phenobarbital, carbamazepine, rifampin) may decrease levels which may decrease therapeutic effects and/or change uterine bleeding profile. CYP3A4 inhibitors (eg, erythromycin, clarithromycin, ketoconazole, itraconazole, ritonavir, grapefruit juice) may increase levels which may result in side effects.

**PREGNANCY:** Contraindicated in pregnancy; caution in nursing.

**MECHANISM OF ACTION:** Estrogen; binds to nuclear receptor in estrogen-responsive tissues. Modulates pituitary secretion of gonadotropins, luteinizing hormone (LH) and follicle stimulating hormone (FSH), through negative feedback mechanism.

**PHARMACOKINETICS: Absorption:** Well-absorbed; conjugated and unconjugated estrogens had altered parameters. **Distribution:** Estrogens found in breast milk; largely bound to sex hormone binding globulin (SHBG) and albumin. **Metabolism:** Liver, to estrone (metabolite); estriol (major urinary metabolite); enterohepatic recirculation, via sulfate and glucuronide conjugation; biliary secretion of conjugates into the intestine; hydrolysis in gut; reabsorption; CYP3A4 (partial). **Elimination:** Urine.

## NURSING CONSIDERATIONS

**Assessment:** Assess for genital bleeding, presence or history of breast cancer, estrogen-dependent neoplasia, DVT, PE, active or recent (within past yr) arterial thromboembolic disease (eg, stroke, MI), liver dysfunction/disease, hypocalcemia, and known/suspected pregnancy. Assess use in nursing females and in patients ≥65 yrs. Assess for drug and lab interactions.

**Monitoring:** Monitor for signs/symptoms of cardiovascular disorders (eg, MI, stroke, venous thrombosis, PE), malignant neoplasms (eg, cancers of endometrium, breast, ovaries), dementia, gallbladder disease, hypercalcemia, visual abnormalities (eg, retinal vascular thrombosis), cholestatic jaundice, elevated BP, hypertriglyceridemia, hypothyroidism, fluid retention, exacerbation of endometriosis, and exacerbation of other conditions (eg, asthma, DM, epilepsy, migraines or porphyria, SLE, and hepatic hemangiomas). Monitor thyroid function in patients on thyroid hormone replacement therapy. If abnormal genital bleeding occurs, perform proper diagnostic measures (eg, endometrial sampling) to rule out malignancy. Re-evaluate every 3-6 months to evaluate need for therapy.

**Patient Counseling:** Inform that medication increases risk for uterine cancer and may increase risk for heart attack, stroke, breast cancer, blood clots, and dementia. Advise to notify physician if signs/symptoms of unusual vaginal bleeding, dizziness/faintness, changes in speech, severe headaches, CP, SOB, leg pain, visual changes, or vomiting develop.

**Administration:** Oral route. **Storage:** 20-25°C (68-77°F); excursions permitted 15-30°C (59-86°F).

C

## CEPHALEXIN RX

cephalexin (Various)

**OTHER BRAND NAMES:** Keflex (Middlebrook)

**THERAPEUTIC CLASS:** Cephalosporin (1st generation)

**INDICATIONS:** Treatment of otitis media and skin and skin structure (SSSI), bone, genitourinary tract, and respiratory tract infections caused by susceptible strains of microorganisms.

**DOSAGE:** *Adults:* Usual: 250mg q6h. Streptococcal Pharyngitis/SSSI/Uncomplicated Cystitis (>15yrs): 500mg q12h. Treat cystitis for 7-14 days. Max: 4g/day.
*Pediatrics:* Usual: 25-50mg/kg/day in divided doses. Streptococcal Pharyngitis (>1 yr)/SSSI: May divide dose and give q12h. Otitis Media: 75-100mg/kg/day in 4 divided doses. Administer for at least 10 days in β-hemolytic streptococcal infections. In severe infections, the dosage may be doubled.

**HOW SUPPLIED:** (Keflex) Cap: 250mg, 500mg, 750mg; (Generic) Cap: 250mg, 500mg; Tab: 250mg, 500mg; Sus: 125mg/5mL [60mL, 100mL, 200mL], 250mg/5mL [100mL, 200mL]

**WARNINGS/PRECAUTIONS:** Caution in penicillin sensitive patients, cross-hypersensivity reactions may occur. Caution in patients with any type of allergy. D/C use if an allergic reaction occurs. *Clostridium difficile*-associated diarrhea (CDAD) reported. Use in the absence of a proven or strongly suspected bacterial infection or prophylactic indication is unlikely to provide benefit and increases the risk of the development of drug-resistant bacteria. Prolonged use may result in overgrowth of nonsusceptible bacteria; take appropriate measures if superinfection occurs. Indicated surgical procedures should be performed in conjunction with antibiotic therapy. Caution in patients with markedly impaired renal function, history of GI disease. Positive direct Coombs' tests reported. False (+) for urine glucose with Benedict's, Fehling's solution, and Clinitest tabs. May cause a fall in PT; monitor PT in patients at risk (eg, hepatic/renal impairment, protracted course of antimicrobial therapy) and administer vitamin K as indicated.

**ADVERSE REACTIONS:** Diarrhea, allergic reactions, dyspepsia, gastritis, abdominal pain.

**INTERACTIONS:** Probenecid inhibits excretion. Concomitant use with metformin may increase concentrations of metformin and produce adverse effects; monitor patient closely and adjust dose of metformin accordingly. Patients previously stabilized on anticoagulants may be at risk for a fall in PT; monitor PT and administer vitamin K as indicated.

**PREGNANCY:** Category B, caution in nursing.

**MECHANISM OF ACTION:** Cephalosporin; bactericidal due to inhibition of cell-wall synthesis.

**PHARMACOKINETICS: Absorption:** Rapid; oral administration of variable doses resulted in different parameters. $T_{max}$=1 hr. **Distribution:** Found in breast milk. **Elimination:** Urine (90% unchanged).

## NURSING CONSIDERATIONS

C

**Assessment:** Assess for history of hypersensitivity to cephalosporins/PCNs, pregnancy/nursing status, renal impairment, history of GI disease, and for possible drug interactions. Document indications for therapy, culture and susceptibility testing. Perform indicated surgical procedures in conjunction with antibiotic therapy when indicated.

**Monitoring:** Monitor for signs/symptoms of hypersensitivity reactions (eg, anaphylaxis), CDAD, superinfection, seizures, and aplastic anemia. Monitor renal function, and LDH. Monitor PT in patients at risk for a decrease in PT (eg, hepatic/renal impairement, poor nutritional state, protracted course of antimicrobial therapy).

**Patient Counseling:** Inform drug only treats bacterial, not viral, infections. Instruct to take exactly as directed; skipping doses or not completing full course may decrease effectiveness and increase bacterial resistance. Inform patient may experience diarrhea. Instruct to contact physician if watery/bloody stools, superinfection, or hypersensitivity reactions occur.

**Administration:** Oral route. Sus: Refer to label for reconstitution instructions. Shake well before use. **Storage:** 20°-25°C (68°-77°F). Store sus in refrigerator after mixing.

# CEREBYX RX

fosphenytoin sodium (Parke-Davis)

**THERAPEUTIC CLASS:** Hydantoin

**INDICATIONS:** Short-term (up to 5 days) parenteral administration when other means of phenytoin administration are unavailable, inappropriate, or less advantageous, including to control general convulsive status epilepticus, prevent or treat seizures during neurosurgery, or as a short-term substitute for oral phenytoin.

**DOSAGE:** *Adults:* Doses, concentration in dosing solutions, and infusion rates are expressed as phenytoin sodium equivalents (PE). Status Epilepticus: LD: 15-20 PE/kg IV at 100-150mg PE/min then switch to maintenance dose. Non-Emergent Cases: LD: 10-20mg PE/kg IV (max 150mg PE/min) or IM. Maint: Initial: 4-6mg PE/kg/day. May substitute for oral phenytoin sodium at the same total daily dose. Elderly: Lower and less frequent dosing required.

**HOW SUPPLIED:** Inj: 50mg PE/mL (2mL, 10mL)

**CONTRAINDICATIONS:** Sinus bradycardia, sino-atrial block, 2nd- and 3rd-degree AV block, Adams-Stokes syndrome.

**WARNINGS/PRECAUTIONS:** Avoid abrupt discontinuation. Not for use in absence seizures. Hypotension and severe cardiovascular reactions and fatalities reported especially after IV administration at high doses and rates; continuously monitor ECG, BP, and respiration during and for at least 20 min after IV infusion and monitor phenytoin levels at least 2 hrs after IV infusion or 4 hrs after IM injection. Caution with severe myocardial insufficiency, porphyria, hepatic/renal dysfunction, hypoalbuminemia, elderly, and diabetes. Acute hepatotoxicity, lymphadenopathy, hemopoietic complications, hyperglycemia reported. D/C if rash or acute hepatotoxicity occurs. Severe sensory disturbances (eg, burning, itching, paresthesia) reported. Neonatal postpartum bleeding disorder, congenital malformations, and increased seizure frequency reported with use during pregnancy. Avoid use with seizures caused by hypoglycemia or other metabolic causes. Caution with phosphate restriction because of phosphate load (0.0037mmol phosphate/mg PE).

**ADVERSE REACTIONS:** Nystagmus, dizziness, pruritus, paresthesia, headache, somnolence, ataxia, tinnitus, stupor, nausea, hypotension, vasodilation, tremor, incoordination, dry mouth.

**INTERACTIONS:** Increased levels with acute alcohol intake, amiodarone, chloramphenicol, chlordiazepoxide, cimetidine, diazepam, dicumarol, disulfiram, estrogens, ethosuximide, fluoxetine, $H_2$-antagonists, halothane, isoniazid, methylphenidate, phenothiazines, phenylbutazone, salicylates, succinimides, sulfonamides, tolbutamide, trazodone. Decreased levels with carbamazepine, chronic alcohol abuse, reserpine. Decreases efficacy of anticoagulants, corticosteroids, coumarin, digitoxin, doxycycline, estrogens, furosemide, oral contraceptives, rifampin, quinidine, theophylline, vitamin D. Variable effects (increased or decreased levels) with phenobarbital, valproic acid, and sodium valproate. Caution with drugs highly bound to serum albumin. TCAs may precipitate seizures. May lower folate levels.

**PREGNANCY:** Category D, not for use in nursing.

**MECHANISM OF ACTION:** Anticonvulsant; prodrug of phenytoin. Modulates voltage-dependent sodium and calcium channels of neurons, inhibits calcium flux across neuronal membranes, and enhances sodium-potassium ATPase activity of neurons and glial cells.

**PHARMACOKINETICS: Absorption:** Fosphenytoin is completely converted to phenytoin. (IM) $T_{max}$=30 min. **Distribution:** Plasma protein binding (95-99%); $V_d$=4.3-10.8L. **Metabolism:** Phosphatases (conversion to phenytoin); liver (phenytoin metabolism). **Elimination:** Urine (1-5% phenytoin and metabolites); $T_{1/2}$=15 min (fosphenytoin), 12-28.9 hrs (phenytoin).

## NURSING CONSIDERATIONS

**Assessment:** Assess LFTs, renal function, CBC with platelets and differential, hypoalbuminemia, porphyria, cardiac conduction defects, pregnancy status, and phosphate levels. Note other diseases/conditions and drug therapies.

**Monitoring:** Careful cardiac monitoring is needed when administering IV loading doses. Monitor LFTs, renal function, CBC with differential and platelets, hypersensitivity reactions, myasthenia, pneumonia, and hypokalemia.

**Patient Counseling:** Instruct patient to call a physician if skin rash develops. Inform patient about the importance of adhering strictly to prescribed dosage regimen and not to abruptly d/c medication. Advise patient of possible risk to fetus during pregnancy. Encourage patients to enroll in North American Antiepileptic Drug (NAAED) Pregnancy Registry by calling 888-233-2334 or go to www.aedpregnancyregistry.org.

**Administration:** IM/IV route. Should be prescribed in phenytoin sodium equivalent units (PE). Rate of IV administration should not exceed 150mg PE/min. **Storage:** Refrigerate at 2-8°C (36-46°F). Do not store at room temperature for more than 48 hours.

# CERVARIX — RX

## human papillomavirus recombinant vaccine, bivalent (GlaxoSmithKline)

**THERAPEUTIC CLASS:** Vaccine

**INDICATIONS:** Prevention of the following diseases caused by oncogenic human papillomavirus (HPV) types 16 and 18 in females 10-25 yrs: Cervical cancer, cervical intraepithelial neoplasia (CIN) grade 2 or worse and adenocarcinoma *in situ,* and CIN grade 1.

**DOSAGE:** *Adults:* ≤25 yrs: Give 3 separate doses of 0.5mL IM in deltoid region of the upper arm at 0,1 and 6 months.
*Pediatrics:* ≥10 yrs: Give 3 separate doses of 0.5mL IM in deltoid region of the upper arm at 0,1 and 6 months

**HOW SUPPLIED:** Inj: 0.5mL

**WARNINGS/PRECAUTIONS:** Syncope may occur, sometimes resulting in falling with injury and may be associated with tonic-clonic movements and other seizure-like activity; observe for 15 minutes after administration. If anaphylactic reaction occurs, appropriate medical treatment and supervision should be readily available. Not for intradermal, IV or SQ administration. Does not protect against disease due to all HPV types, and disease from vaccine and non-vaccine HPV types to which a woman has been previously exposed to through sexual activity. Vaccination may not result in protection in all vaccine recipients. Tip cap and rubber plunger contain latex; caution in latex sensitive individuals.

C

**ADVERSE REACTIONS:** Local site reactions (eg, pain, redness, swelling), fatigue, headache, myalgia, gastrointestinal symptoms, arthralgia, fever, rash, urticaria, nasopharyngitis, influenza.

**INTERACTIONS:** Avoid mixing with any other vaccine in the same syringe or vial. Immunosuppressive therapies, including irradiation, antimetabolites, alkylating agents, cytotoxic drugs, and corticosteroids (used in greater than physiologic doses) may reduce immune response.

**PREGNANCY:** Category B, caution in nursing.

**MECHANISM OF ACTION:** Vaccine; may mediate the development of IgG neutralizing antibodies directed against HPV-L1 capsid proteins generated as a result of vaccination.

## NURSING CONSIDERATIONS

**Assessment:** Assess immunity and current health status, age of patient, hypersensitivity reactions, pregnancy/nursing status, latex hypersensitivity and possible drug interactions.

**Monitoring:** Monitor for signs and symptoms of syncope, tonic-clonic movements, seizure like activity and anaphylactic reactions. Monitor for any adverse events.

**Patient Counseling:** Inform of potential benefits and risks of immunization. Inform that vaccine does not substitute for routine cervical cancer screening. Advise that vaccine does not provide protection against disease and non-vaccine HPV types to which a woman has previously been exposed through sexual activity. Counsel that syncope may develop following vaccination. Inform about importance of completing immunization series unless contraindicated. Advise to report any adverse events to healthcare provider. Inform vaccine is not recommended during pregnancy.

**Administration:** IM in the deltoid muscle of the upper arm. Shake well before withdrawal and use. Inspect for particulate matter and discoloration; do not give if these conditions exist. **Storage:** 2-8°C (36-46°F). Do not freeze. Discard if frozen.

# CESAMET

**CII**

nabilone (Meda)

**THERAPEUTIC CLASS:** Cannabinoid

**INDICATIONS:** Treatment of N/V associated with cancer chemotherapy when conventional treatment has failed.

**DOSAGE:** *Adults:* Usual: 1 or 2mg bid. On the day of chemotherapy, administer initial dose 1-3 hrs before giving the chemotherapeutic agent. Start with lower dose and increase as necessary. 1 or 2mg the night before may be useful to minimize side effects. Max: 6mg/day given in divided doses tid. May be given bid or tid during the chemotherapy cycle and for 48 hrs after the last dose of each cycle, if needed.

**HOW SUPPLIED:** Cap: 1mg

**WARNINGS/PRECAUTIONS:** Patients should remain under the supervision of a responsible adult during treatment, especially during initial use and dose adjustments. Caution when initiating therapy with HTN, heart disease, elderly, current or previous psychiatric disorders (including manic depressive illness, depression, and schizophrenia) and with history of substance abuse. May impair mental/physical abilities. May cause dizziness, drowsiness, euphoria, ataxia, anxiety, disorientation, depression, hallucinations, psychosis, tachycardia and orthostatic hypotension. Adverse psychiatric reactions can persist for 48-72 hrs following cessation of treatment. Not intended for use on prn basis or as first antiemetic product prescribed.

**ADVERSE REACTIONS:** Drowsiness, vertigo, dry mouth, euphoria, ataxia, headache, concentration difficulties, nausea, dysphoria, sleep/visual disturbance, asthenia, anorexia, depression, hypotension, sedation.

C

**INTERACTIONS:** Additive HTN, tachycardia, possibly cardiotoxicity may occur with amphetamines, cocaine, other sympathomimetics. Additive or super-additive tachycardia, drowsiness may occur with atropine, scopolamine, antihistamines, other anticholinergics. Additive tachycardia, HTN, drowsiness may occur with TCAs. Additive drowsiness and CNS depression may occur with barbiturates, benzodiazepines, ethanol, lithium, opioids, buspirone, antihistamines, muscle relaxants, other CNS depressants. Hypomanic reaction reported with disulfiram, fluoxetine. May decrease clearance of antipyrine, barbiturates. May increase metabolism of theophylline. Cross-tolerance and mutual potentiation with opioids. Effects may be enhanced by opioid receptor blockade. Alcohol may increase the positive subjective mood effects. Avoid with alcohol, sedatives, hypnotics, or other psychoactive drugs. Impaired psychomotor function with diazepam. Change in dosage requirements with highly protein-bound drugs.

**PREGNANCY:** Category C, not for use in nursing.

**MECHANISM OF ACTION:** Cannabinoid; interacts with the cannabinoid receptor system (CB [1] receptor that has been discovered in neural tissues).

**PHARMACOKINETICS: Absorption:** (GI) Complete, $C_{max}$=2ng/mL, $T_{max}$=2.0 hrs. **Distribution:** $V_d$=12.5L/kg. **Metabolism:** Liver (extensive), via stereospecific enzymes and multiple P450 enzyme isoforms. Isomeric carbinol (metabolite). **Elimination:** Feces (60%), urine (24%); $T_{1/2}$=2 hrs (identified metabolite), 35 hrs (unidentified metabolite).

## NURSING CONSIDERATIONS

**Assessment:** Assess for heart disease, HTN, previous/current psychiatric disorders, alcohol intake or substance abuse, hepatic/renal impairment, pregnancy/nursing status, and possible drug interactions.

**Monitoring:** Monitor for adverse psychiatric reactions or unmasking of symptoms of psychiatric disorders, signs/symptoms of CNS effects (eg, dizziness, drowsiness, euphoria, ataxia, anxiety, disorientation, depression, hallucinations and psychosis), postural hypotension. Monitor BP and HR. Monitor for signs of excessive use, abuse and misuse. Monitor for signs and symptoms of hypersensitivity reactions.

**Patient Counseling:** Caution against performing hazardous tasks such as driving or operating machinery and inform of possibility of psychological or physical dependence. Avoid concomitant use of alcohol and other CNS depressants; remain under supervision of responsible adult during therapy. To avoid panic instruct patient to be aware of possible changes in mood and other adverse behavioral effects.

**Administration:** Oral route. **Storage:** 25°C (77°F); excursions permitted to 15-30°C (59-86°F).

# CHANTIX RX

varenicline tartrate (Pfizer)

**Serious neuropsychiatric events, including, but not limited to, depression, suicidal ideation, attempted/completed suicide reported. Monitor for symptoms such as changes in behavior, hostility, agitation, depressed mood, and suicide-related events, which may occur with or without pre-existing psychiatric illness. D/C immediately if agitation, hostility, depressed mood, or changes in behavior/thinking that are not typical are observed, or if patient develops suicidal ideation/behavior.**

**THERAPEUTIC CLASS:** Nicotinic Acetylcholine Receptor Agonist

**INDICATIONS:** Aid to smoking cessation treatment.

**DOSAGE:** *Adults:* ≥18 yrs: Days 1-3: 0.5mg qd. Days 4-7: 0.5mg bid. Day 8 to End of Treatment: 1mg bid. Duration: 12 weeks with additional 12 weeks after successful completion to ensure long-term abstinence. Severe Renal Impairment: Initial: 0.5mg qd. Titrate: Max: 0.5mg bid. End-Stage Renal Disease with hemodialysis: Max: 0.5mg qd. Take after eating and with a full glass of water.

**HOW SUPPLIED:** Tab: 0.5mg, 1mg

C

**WARNINGS/PRECAUTIONS:** Changes in mood, psychosis, hallucinations, paranoia, delusions, homicidal ideation, hostility, agitation, anxiety, suicidality reported; d/c if these symptoms appear. Hypersensitivity reactions including angioedema, rare but serious skin reactions (Stevens-Johnson syndrome [SJS] and erythema multiforme) reported. D/C and contact healthcare provider immediately at first appearance of skin rash with mucosal lesions, or any other signs of hypersensitivity. Nausea, sometimes persistent over several months, reported; consider dose reduction for patients with intolerable nausea. Traffic accidents, near-miss accidents, or accidental injuries reported. Use caution when driving or operating machinery until the effects of therapy are known. Physiological changes resulting from smoking cessation may alter pharmacokinetics or pharmacodynamics of some drugs (eg, theophylline, warfarin, insulin). Risk of toxic reactions with impaired renal function. Caution in elderly.

**ADVERSE REACTIONS:** N/V, sleep disturbances (insomnia, abnormal dreams), constipation, flatulence, abdominal pain, dyspepsia, dry mouth, headache, dysgeusia, somnolence, upper respiratory disorder, increased appetite, rash, depression, suicidal ideation.

**INTERACTIONS:** Reduced renal clearance and increased exposure with cimetidine. Increased incidence of adverse events (eg, nausea, headache, vomiting, dizziness, dyspepsia, fatigue) with Nicotine Replacement Therapy (NRT).

**PREGNANCY:** Category C, not for use in nursing.

**MECHANISM OF ACTION:** Nicotinic acetylcholine receptor agonist; binds with high affinity and selectivity at α4β2 neuronal nicotinic acetylcholine receptors, producing agonist activity while simultaneously blocking the ability of nicotine to activate these receptors and thus to stimulate the central nervous mesolimbic dopamine system.

**PHARMACOKINETICS: Absorption:** $T_{max}$=3-4 hrs. **Distribution:** Plasma protein binding (≤20%). **Metabolism:** Minimal. **Elimination:** Urine (92% unchanged); $T_{1/2}$=24 hrs.

## NURSING CONSIDERATIONS

**Assessment:** Assess for pre-existing psychiatric illness and impaired renal function. Assess pregnancy/nursing status and possible drug interactions.

**Monitoring:** Monitor for neuropsychiatric symptoms (eg, changes in behavior, agitation, depressed mood, suicidal ideation/behavior), worsening of pre-existing psychiatric illness, nausea, and insomnia. Monitor for hypersensitivity reactions. Monitor renal function especially in elderly. Monitor for altered pharmacokinetics or pharmacodynamics of some drugs (eg, theophylline, warfarin, insulin); dosage adjustments may be necessary.

**Patient Counseling:** Instruct to set a date to quit smoking, and start treatment 1 week before this date. Inform about the possibility of vivid, unusual, or strange dreams. Inform about side effects such as nausea and insomnia, and to report these, if persistent, to physician. Advise to d/c and contact healthcare provider immediately if agitation, hostility, depressed mood, or changes in behavior/thinking that are not typical occur, or if suicidal ideation or behavior develop. Inform to d/c and immediately seek medical care if hypersensitivity reactions including angioedema (swelling of face, mouth, extremities, neck) occur. Inform to d/c and contact healthcare provider immediately at the first appearance of rash with mucosal lesions. Caution about performing hazardous tasks (eg, operating machinery/driving). Counsel about risks/benefits of smoking cessation with varenicline when intending to become pregnant or planning to breastfeed. Counsel patients who do not succeed in stopping smoking during 12 weeks of initial therapy, or who relapse after treatment, to make another attempt at cessation once factors contributing to the failed attempt have been identified and addressed.

**Administration:** Oral route. Take pc and with a full glass of water. **Storage:** 25°C (77°F); excursions permitted to 15-30°C (59-86°F).

## CIALIS RX

tadalafil (Lilly)



**THERAPEUTIC CLASS:** Phosphodiesterase type 5 inhibitor

**INDICATIONS:** Treatment of erectile dysfunction (ED).

**DOSAGE:** *Adults:* Prn Use: Initial: 10mg prior to sexual activity. May increase to 20mg or decrease to 5mg based on efficacy and tolerability. Renal Impairment: CrCl 31-50mL/min: Initial: 5mg. Max: 10mg/48 hrs. CrCl <30mL/min/Hemodialysis: Max: 5mg/72 hrs. Mild/Moderate Hepatic Impairment: Max: 10mg qd. With Alpha Blockers: Initial: Use lowest recommended dose. With Potent CYP3A4 Inhibitors (eg, ketoconazole, ritonavir): Max: 10mg/72 hrs. Once-Daily Use: Initial: 2.5mg qd, taken at the same time every day. Titrate: May increase to 5mg qd based on efficacy and tolerability. With Alpha Blockers: Initial: Use lowest recommended dose. With Potent CYP3A4 Inhibitors (eg, ketoconazole, ritonavir): Max: 2.5mg.

**HOW SUPPLIED:** Tab: 2.5mg, 5mg, 10mg, 20mg

**CONTRAINDICATIONS:** Any form of organic nitrate, either regularly and/or intermittently used.

**WARNINGS/PRECAUTIONS:** Avoid in men for whom sexual activity is inadvisable due to underlying CV status. Avoid with MI (within last 90 days), unstable angina or angina occurring during sexual intercourse, NYHA Class 2 or greater heart failure (in the last 6 months), uncontrolled arrhythmias, hypotension (<90/50mmHg), or uncontrolled HTN (>170/100mmHg), and stroke within the last 6 months. May cause transient decrease in BP. Increased sensitivity to vasodilatory effect with left ventricular outflow obstruction and severely impaired autonomic control of BP. Rare reports of prolonged erections (>4 hrs ) and priapism; caution in conditions predisposing to priapism (eg, sickle cell anemia, multiple myeloma, leukemia), anatomical deformation of the penis (eg, angulation, cavernosal fibrosis, Peyronie's disease). Non-arteritic anterior ischemic optic neuropathy (NAION) reported; d/c if sudden loss of vision is experienced in one or both eyes. Sudden decrease or loss of hearing reported with tinnitus and dizziness; d/c if occurs. Avoid prn use in severe renal insufficiency (CrCl<30mL/min and on hemodialysis). Avoid use with hepatic impairment (Child-Pugh Class C), hereditary degenerative retinal disorders including retinal pigmentosa. Caution with mild to moderate hepatic insufficiency, bleeding disorders or significant peptic ulceration.

**ADVERSE REACTIONS:** Headache, dyspepsia, back pain, myalgia, nasal congestion, flushing, limb pain, nasopharyngitis, upper respiratory tract infection, gastroenteritis (viral), influenza, cough, gastroesophageal reflux disease, myalgia, HTN.

**INTERACTIONS:** See Contraindications. Avoid concomitant use with nitrates within 48 hrs. Additive hypotensive effects with alcohol, α-adrenergic blockers (eg, doxazosin, alfuzosin, tamsulosin), antihypertensives (eg, amlodipine, angiotensin II receptor blockers, bendrofluazide, enalapril, metoprolol). Increased tadalafil exposure with ritonavir and possibly other HIV protease inhibitors. CYP3A4 inhibitors (eg, ketoconazole, itraconazole, erythromycin, grapefruit juice) may result in increased exposure of tadalafil. CYP3A4 inducers (eg, rifampin, carbamazepine, phenytoin, phenobarbital) may result in decreased tadalafil exposure. Antacids (magnesium hydroxide/aluminum hydroxide) shown to reduce rate of absorption. Avoid concomitant use with Adcirca or other PDE5 inhibitors. A small increase in heart rate seen with theophylline.

**PREGNANCY:** Category B, not for use in nursing.

**MECHANISM OF ACTION:** Phosphodiesterase type 5 inhibitor; increases amount of cGMP that causes smooth muscle relaxation and increased blood flow into the corpus cavernosum.

**PHARMACOKINETICS: Absorption:** $T_{max}$=2hrs. **Distribution:** $V_d$=63L; plasma protein binding (94%). **Metabolism:** Via CYP3A4 to a catechol metabolite which undergoes extensive methylation and glucuronidation; methylcatechol glucuronide (major metabolite). **Elimination:** Urine (36%), feces (61%); $T_{1/2}$=17.5 hrs.

C

## NURSING CONSIDERATIONS

**Assessment:** Assess for CVD, long QT syndrome, retinitis pigmentosa, bleeding disorders, active peptic ulceration, anatomical deformation of the penis or presence of conditions that would predispose to priapism (eg, sickle cell anemia, multiple myeloma, leukemia), renal/hepatic impairment, contraindications for sexual activity. Assess for potential underlying causes of erectile dysfunction and for possible drug interactions.

**Monitoring:** Monitor for signs/symptoms of decreases in BP, prolonged erection, NAION, hearing loss, and for hypersensitivity reactions. Monitor therapeutic effect when used in combination with other drugs.

**Patient Counseling:** Instruct to seek medical assistance if erection persists >4 hrs. Advise of potential BP-lowering effect of α-blockers, other antihypertensive medications, alcohol, and cardiac risk of sexual activity. Counsel about the protective measures necessary to guard against STDs, including HIV. Inform about drug's contraindication with organic nitrates and potential interactions with other medications. Instruct to d/c and contact physician if sudden loss of vision or hearing occur. Counsel to take as prescribed.

**Administration:** Oral route. 1) For prn use, take at least 30 min before anticipated sexual activity. 2) For qd use, take one tablet at the same time of day.
**Storage:** 25°C (77°F); excursions permitted to 15-30°C (59-86°F).

# CILOXAN RX

ciprofloxacin HCl (Alcon)

**THERAPEUTIC CLASS:** Fluoroquinolone

**INDICATIONS:** Bacterial conjunctivitis and corneal ulcers.

**DOSAGE:** *Adults:* Bacterial Conjunctivitis: (Sol) 1-2 drops q2h while awake for 2 days, then 1-2 drops q4h while awake for 5 days. (Oint) 1/2 inch tid for 2 days, then bid for 5 days. Corneal Ulcer: (Sol) 2 drops every 15 min for 1st 6 hrs, then 2 drops every 30 min for rest of Day 1, then 2 drops every hr on Day 2, then 2 drops q4h on Days 3-14. May continue if re-epithelialization has not occurred.
*Pediatrics:* Bacterial Conjunctivitis: ≥1 yr: (Sol) 1-2 drops q2h while awake for 2 days, then 1-2 drops q4h while awake for 5 days. ≥2 yrs: (Oint) 1/2 inch tid for 2 days, then bid for 5 days. Corneal Ulcer: (Sol) ≥1 yr: 2 drops every 15 min for 1st 6 hrs, then 2 drops every 30 min for rest of Day 1, then 2 drops every hr on Day 2, then 2 drops q4h on Days 3-14. May continue if re-epithelialization has not occurred.

**HOW SUPPLIED:** Oint: 0.3% [3.5g]; Sol: 0.3% [2.5mL, 5mL, 10mL]

**WARNINGS/PRECAUTIONS:** Not for injection into eye. Superinfection may result with prolonged use. Fatal hypersensitivity reactions reported after 1st dose of systemic quinolone therapy. Avoid allowing tip of container to contact eye or surrounding structures. Avoid contact lenses with conjunctivitis. Risk of crystalline precipitate in cornea. Ointment may slow corneal healing and cause visual blurring.

**ADVERSE REACTIONS:** Local burning, white crystalline precipitants, lid margin crusting, crystals/scales, foreign body sensation, itching, conjunctival hyperemia, bad taste.

**INTERACTIONS:** Systemic quinolone therapy may increase theophylline levels, interfere with caffeine metabolism, enhance warfarin effects, and elevate serum creatinine with cyclosporine.

**PREGNANCY:** Category C, caution in nursing.

**MECHANISM OF ACTION:** Fluoroquinolone antibacterial agent; bactericidal, interferes with the enzyme DNA gyrase which is needed for synthesis of bacterial DNA.

**PHARMACOKINETICS: Absorption:** $C_{max}$≤5ng/mL.

C

## NURSING CONSIDERATIONS

**Assessment:** Assess for proper diagnosis of causative organisms and for hypersensitivity to other quinolones. Assess for possible drug interactions.

**Monitoring:** During prolonged use, monitor for overgrowth (eg, superinfection) of nonsusceptible organisms, including fungi. Monitor for signs of hypersensitivity or anaphylactic reaction (eg, cardiovascular collapse, loss of consciousness, pharyngeal or facial edema, dyspnea, and urticaria). Monitor for development of precipitate in the superficial portion of the corneal defect.

**Patient Counseling:** Instruct not to touch dropper tip to any surface; may contaminate solution. Advise to contact physician if any hypersensitivity reaction occurs (eg, rash). Instruct to remove contact lenses prior to therapy.

**Administration:** Ocular route. **Storage:** 2-25°C (36-77°F). Protect from light.

# CIMZIA — RX

certolizumab pegol (UCB)

**Increased risk for developing serious infections (eg, tuberculosis [TB], TB reactivation, invasive fungal infection, bacterial/viral infection due to opportunistic pathogens) that may lead to hospitalization or death. Concomitant use of immunosuppresants (eg, methotrexate [MTX] or corticosteroids) may develop these infections. Evaluate for latent TB and treat prior to initiation of therapy. Empiric antifungal therapy should be considered in patients at risk for invasive fungal infection who develop severe systemic illness. Monitor for development of infection during and after treatment. D/C if serious infection or sepsis develops. Lymphoma and other malignancies reported in children and adolescents.**

**THERAPEUTIC CLASS:** TNF-receptor blocker

**INDICATIONS:** Reducing signs and symptoms of Crohn's disease and maintaining clinical response in adults with moderately to severely active disease who have had an inadequate response to conventional therapy. Treatment of moderate to severely active rheumatoid arthritis (RA) in adults.

**DOSAGE:** *Adults:* Crohn's disease: Initial: 400mg SQ initially and at Weeks 2 and 4. Maint: 400mg SQ every 4 weeks. RA: Initial: 400mg SQ initially and at Weeks 2 and 4, followed by 200mg every other week. Maint: 400mg SQ every 4 weeks. Concomitant MTX: 200mg every other week.

**HOW SUPPLIED:** Inj: 200mg/mL

**WARNINGS/PRECAUTIONS:** Avoid with active infection. Caution in patients with history of recurrent infections, underlying conditions predisposing to infections, and with exposure to TB or those who travel in areas where TB and mycoses are endemic. Monitor hepatitis B virus (HBV) carriers; if reactivation occurs, d/c and start antiviral therapy. Anaphylaxis or serious allergic reactions may occur. Caution with pre-existing or recent onset CNS demyelinating disorders. Rare cases of pancytopenia, including aplastic anemia, reported; d/c if significant hematologic abnormalities occur. May cause or exacerbate congestive heart failure; monitor patients closely. May cause autoimmune antibodies; d/c if lupus-like syndrome develops. Caution in elderly. May affect host defenses against infections and malignancies.

**ADVERSE REACTIONS:** Upper respiratory tract infection, rash, urinary tract infections (UTI), headache, HTN, nasopharyngitis, back pain, pyrexia, pharyngitis, acute bronchitis, fatigue.

**INTERACTIONS:** Avoid combination treatment with anakinra, abatacept, rituximab, natalizumab, and biological disease-modifying antirheumatic drugs (DMARDS). Do not give live vaccines concurrently.

**PREGNANCY:** Category B, not for use in nursing

**MECHANISM OF ACTION:** TNF-blocker; binds to TNF-α and selectively neutralizes and inhibits its central role in inflammatory processes.

**PHARMACOKINETICS: Absorption:** Bioavailability (80%). **Distribution:** $V_d$=6-8L. **Elimination:** $T_{1/2}$=14 days.

C

## NURSING CONSIDERATIONS

**Assessment:** Assess for localized or chronic infections, heart disease, hematologic disorders, HBV infection, pre-existing or recurrent CNS demyelinating disorders, pregnancy/nursing status, and possible drug interactions. Assess for active TB and inactive (latent) TB infection; perform TB skin test prior to therapy.

**Monitoring:** Monitor for signs/symptoms suggestive of development of new infection, TB, worsening CHF, HBV infection, neurologic disorders (eg, seizures, optic neuritis, peripheral neuropathy), hematologic reactions (eg, aplastic anemia, pancytopenia), anaphylactic (eg, angioedema, dyspnea, rash) and injection-site reactions.

**Patient Counseling:** Inform about risks/benefits of therapy. Inform that drug may lower ability to fight infections; seek medical attention if any severe allergic reactions occur. Report any signs of new or worsening medical conditions such as heart disease; neurological or autoimmune disorders; symptoms such as bruising, bleeding or persistent fever, peristent cough, weight loss; or if any symptoms of TB, histoplasmosis, or HBV develop. Counsel about possible risk of lymphoma and other malignancies.

**Administration:** SQ route. Rotate injection sites; avoid tender, bruised, red, or hard areas of the skin. **Storage:** 2-8°C (36-46°F). Do not freeze. Protect from light.

# CINRYZE — RX

c1 inhibitor (human) (Viro Pharma)

**THERAPEUTIC CLASS:** C1 inhibitor

**INDICATIONS:** Prophylaxis for angioedema attacks in adolescent and adult patients with Hereditary Angioedema (HAE).

**DOSAGE:** *Adults:* 1,000 U IV every 3 or 4 days. Infusion Rate: Initial/Maintenance: 1mL/min (10 mins).

**HOW SUPPLIED:** Inj: 500 U

**WARNINGS/PRECAUTIONS:** Severe hypersensitivity reactions (eg, hives, urticaria, chest tightness, wheezing, hypotension, and/or anaphylaxis) may occur; d/c therapy immediately. Have epinephrine available. Thrombotic events at high doses reported (animal studies). May carry a risk of transmitting infectious agents [eg, viruses, Creutzfeldt-Jakob (CJD) agent].

**ADVERSE REACTIONS:** Upper respiratory tract infection, sinusitis, rash, and headache.

**PREGNANCY:** Category C, caution in nursing.

**MECHANISM OF ACTION:** C1 inhibitor; regulates the activation of the complement and intrinsic coagulation (contact system) pathway and regulates the fibrinolytic system; increases plasma levels of C1 inhibitor activity.

**PHARMACOKINETICS: Absorption:** $C_{max}$=0.68 U/mL (single dose), 0.85 U/mL (double dose); $T_{max}$=3.9 hrs; $AUC_{(0-t)}$=74.5 U*hr/mL (single dose), 95.9 U*hr/mL (double dose). **Elimination:** $T_{1/2}$=56 hrs.

## NURSING CONSIDERATIONS

**Assessment:** Assess signs and symptoms of hypersensitivity reactions, known risk factors for thrombotic events, and pregnancy/nursing status.

**Monitoring:** Monitor for hypersensitivity reactions and thrombotic events.

**Patient Counseling:** Counsel about the risks and benefits of C1 inhibitor prior to treatment. Inform that medication is made from human plasma and may contain infectious agents that can cause disease (eg, viruses, CJD agent).

**Administration:** IV route. Cinryze must be administered at room temperature within 3 hrs after reconstitution. Use aseptic technique. See PI for detailed reconstitution information. **Storage:** Store at 2-25°C (36-77°F). Do not freeze, mix with other materials, and/or use after expiration date. Protect from light prior to reconstitution.

## Cipro HC — RX

ciprofloxacin HCl - hydrocortisone (Alcon)

**THERAPEUTIC CLASS:** Antibacterial/corticosteroid combination

**INDICATIONS:** Acute otitis externa in adults and pediatric patients ≥1 year.

**DOSAGE:** *Adults:* 3 drops into affected ear bid for 7 days. Warm bottle in hand for 1-2 min to avoid dizziness. Shake well before use.
*Pediatrics:* ≥1 yr: 3 drops into affected ear bid for 7 days. Warm bottle in hand for 1-2 min to avoid dizziness. Shake well before use.

**HOW SUPPLIED:** Sus: (Ciprofloxacin-Hydrocortisone) 0.2%-1% [10mL]

**CONTRAINDICATIONS:** Perforated tympanic membrane, viral infections of external ear canal (eg, varicella and herpes simplex infections).

**WARNINGS/PRECAUTIONS:** D/C if hypersensitivity reaction occurs. Re-evaluate if no improvement after 1 week.

**ADVERSE REACTIONS:** Headache, pruritus.

**PREGNANCY:** Category C, not for use in nursing.

**MECHANISM OF ACTION:** Broad-spectrum anti-inflammatory antibiotic; exerts antimicrobial activity against gram-positive and gram-negative bacteria.

### NURSING CONSIDERATIONS

**Assessment:** Assess for history of hypersensitivity to hydrocortisone or quinolones, perforated tympanic membrane, and viral infection of the external canal.

**Monitoring:** Monitor for possible occurrence of superinfection, ear pain, fungal dermatitis, headache, hypersensitivity reactions, and pruritus.

**Patient Counseling:** Inform that if rash or allergic reactions occur, d/c and contact physician immediately. Counsel to use as directed. Advise to avoid contact with eyes to avoid contaminating dropper. Protect from light, shake well before use, and discard unused portion after completion.

**Administration:** Otic route. **Storage:** Below 25°C (77°F). Avoid freezing. Protect from light.

## Cipro IV — RX

ciprofloxacin (Bayer/Schering)

**Fluoroquinolones are associated with an increased risk of tendinitis and tendon rupture in all ages. Risk further increased in patients >60 yrs, patients taking corticosteroid drugs, and patients with kidney, heart or lung transplants.**

**THERAPEUTIC CLASS:** Fluoroquinolone

**INDICATIONS:** Treatment of skin and skin structure (SSSI), bone and joint, complicated intra-abdominal infections, lower respiratory tract infections (LRTI), urinary tract infections (UTI), nosocomial pneumonia, acute sinusitis, chronic bacterial prostatitis, postexposure inhalational anthrax, empirical therapy for febrile neutropenia, complicated UTI and pyelonephritis in pediatrics caused by susceptible strains of microorganisms.

**DOSAGE:** *Adults:* ≥18 yrs: IV: UTI: Mild-Moderate: 200mg q12h for 7-14 days. Complicated/Severe: 400mg q12h for 7-14 days. LRTI/SSSI: Mild-Moderate: 400mg q12h for 7-14 days. Complicated/Severe: 400mg q8h for 7-14 days. Bone and Joint: Mild-Moderate: 400mg q12h for ≥4-6 weeks. Complicated/Severe: 400mg q8h for ≥4-6 weeks. Nosocomial Pneumonia: 400mg q8h for 10-14 days. Complicated Intra-Abdominal: 400mg q12h (w/metronidazole) for 7-14 days. Acute Sinusitis: 400mg q12h for 10 days. Chronic Bacterial Prostatitis: 400mg q12h for 28 days. Febrile Neutropenia: 400mg q8h (w/piperacillin 50mg/kg q4h) for 7-14 days. Max: 24g/day. Inhalational Anthrax: 400mg q12h for 60 days. Administer over 60 min. CrCl 5-29mL/min: 200-400mg q18-24h.
*Pediatrics:* <18 yrs: Inhalational Anthrax: 10mg/kg PO q12h for 60 days. Max:

400mg/dose. 1-17 yrs: Complicated UTI/Pyelonephritis: 6-10mg/kg PO q8h for 10-21 days. Max: 400mg/dose.

**HOW SUPPLIED:** Inj: (Vial) 200mg/20ml, 400mg/40mL; (Flexible container) 200mg/100mL, 400mg/200mL



**CONTRAINDICATIONS:** Concomitant administration with tizanidine.

**WARNINGS/PRECAUTIONS:** Increased ICP, convulsions, and toxic psychosis reported. Caution with CNS disorders or if predisposed to seizures. Severe, fatal hypersensitivity reactions may occur. *Clostridium difficile*-associated diarrhea (CDAD), Achille's and other tendon ruptures reported. D/C at first sign of rash/hypersensitivity or if pain, inflammation, or ruptured tendon occur. May permit overgrowth of *Clostridia*. Maintain hydration; avoid alkalinizing urine. Avoid excessive sunlight and UV light. Monitor renal, hepatic, and hematopoietic function with prolonged use. Caution in patients with risk factors for torsades de pointes (eg, known QT prolongation, uncorrected hypokalemia). Adjust dose with renal dysfunction. Caution in elderly.

**ADVERSE REACTIONS:** N/V, diarrhea, CNS disturbances, local IV site reactions, abnormal LFTs, eosinophilia, headache, restlessness, rash.

**INTERACTIONS:** See Contraindications. May increase theophylline and caffeine levels and prolong effects. May alter serum levels of phenytoin. Severe hypoglycemia with glyburide (rare). Potentiated by probenecid. Transient SrCr elevations with cyclosporine. May enhance oral anticoagulant effects. Caution with drugs that lower seizure threshold. Severe tendon disorder risks are increased with concomitant corticosteroid therapy. Caution with drugs (eg, class IA or class III antiarrhythmics) that may result in prolongation of QT interval.

**PREGNANCY:** Category C, not for use in nursing.

**MECHANISM OF ACTION:** Fluoroquinolone; inhibits the enzymes topoisomerase II (DNA gyrase) and topoisomerase IV, which are required for bacterial DNA replication, transcription, repair, and recombination.

**PHARMACOKINETICS: Absorption:** Absolute bioavailability (70-80%); $C_{max}$=0.1, 0.2mcg/mL (200mg, 400mg, after 12 hrs). **Distribution:** Plasma protein binding (20-40%). **Metabolism:** CYP1A2. **Elimination:** Bile (unchanged), urine (50-70%, unchanged), feces (15%). $T_{1/2}$=5-6 hrs.

## NURSING CONSIDERATIONS

**Assessment:** Assess renal function tests, LFTs, history of seizures, pregnancy/nursing status, and possible drug interactions. Note other diseases/conditions and drug therapies.

**Monitoring:** Monitor for cardiac arrest, seizures, status epilepticus, respiratory failure, CDAD, renal function tests, LFTs, CBC, tendinitis and tendon rupture, peripheral neuropathy, and hypersensitivity reactions.

**Patient Counseling:** Notify healthcare provider if symptoms of pain, swelling, or inflammation of a tendon, or weakness or inability to move joints; rest and refrain from exercise; and d/c therapy. Inform that drug treats bacterial, not viral, infections. Take exactly as directed; skipping doses or not completing full course may decrease effectiveness and increase antibiotic resistance. Inform about potential benefits/risks. D/C and notify physician if skin rash, other allergic reactions, and watery and bloody stools (with or without stomach cramps, and fever) occur. Inform to use caution in any activity requiring mental alertness and coordination. Avoid excessive sun exposure and wear protective clothes.

**Administration:** IV route. Slow infusion over a period of 1 hr after reconstitution. **Storage:** Vial: 5-30°C (41-86°F). Flexible container: 5-25°C (41-77°F). Protect from light, avoid excessive heat, protect from freezing.

# CIPRO ORAL — RX

ciprofloxacin HCl (Bayer/Schering)



**Fluoroquinolones are associated with an increased risk of tendinitis and tendon rupture in all ages. Risk further increased in patients >60 yrs, patients taking corticosteroid drugs, and patients with kidney, heart or lung transplants.**

**THERAPEUTIC CLASS:** Fluoroquinolone

**INDICATIONS:** Treatment of lower respiratory tract (LRTI), complicated intra-abdominal, skin and skin structure (SSSI), bone and joint, and urinary tract infections (UTI), acute exacerbations of chronic bronchitis, acute sinusitis, acute uncomplicated cystitis in females, chronic bacterial prostatitis, infectious diarrhea, typhoid fever, postexposure inhalational anthrax, uncomplicated cervical and urethral gonorrhea, complicated UTI and pyelonephritis in pediatrics.

**DOSAGE:** *Adults:* ≥18 yrs: Acute Sinusitis/Typhoid Fever: 500mg q12h for 10 days. LRTI/SSSI: Mild-Moderate: 500mg q12h for 7-14 days. Severe/Complicated: 750mg q12h for 7-14 days. Cystitis/Acute Uncomplicated UTI: 250mg q12h for 3 days. Mild-Moderate UTI: 250mg q12h for 7-14 days. Severe/Complicated UTI: 500mg q12h for 7-14 days. Chronic Bacterial Prostatitis: 500mg q12h for 28 days. Intra-Abdominal: 500mg q12h (w/ metronidazole) for 7-14 days. Bone and Joint: Mild-Moderate: 500mg q12h for ≥4-6 weeks. Severe/Complicated: 750mg q12h for ≥4-6 weeks. Infectious Diarrhea: 500mg q12h for 5-7 days. Uncomplicated Urethral/Cervical Gonococcal Infections: 250mg single dose. Inhalational Anthrax: 500mg q12h for 60 days. CrCl 30-50mL/min: 250-500mg q12h. CrCl 5-29mL/min: 250-500mg q18h. Hemodialysis/Peritoneal Dialysis: 250-500mg q24h (after dialysis). Administer at least 2 hrs before or 6 hrs after magnesium- or aluminum-containing antacids, sucralfate, Videx (didanosine) chewable/buffered tablets or pediatric powder, or other products containing calcium, iron, or zinc. *Pediatrics:* <18 yrs: Inhalational Anthrax: 15mg/kg q12h for 60 days. Max: 500mg/dose. 1-17 yrs: Complicated UTI/Pyelonephritis: 10-20mg/kg q12h for 10-21 days. Max: 750mg/dose.

**HOW SUPPLIED:** Sus: 250mg/5mL, 500mg/5mL [100mL]; Tab: 250mg, 500mg, 750mg

**CONTRAINDICATIONS:** Concomitant administration with tizanidine.

**WARNINGS/PRECAUTIONS:** Convulsions, increased ICP, and toxic psychosis reported. Caution with CNS disorders or if predisposed to seizures. Severe, fatal hypersensitivity reactions may occur. *Clostridium difficile*-associated diarrhea (CDAD), colitis, achilles and other tendon ruptures reported. D/C at first sign of rash or if pain, inflammation, or ruptured tendon occurs. Maintain hydration; avoid alkaline urine. Avoid excessive sunlight and UV light. Do not give via feeding tube. Monitor renal, hepatic, and hematopoietic function with prolonged use. Adjust dose with renal dysfunction. Caution with concomitant drugs that may result in prolongation of the QT interval or in patients with risk factors for torsades de pointes. Caution in elderly taking corticosteroids.

**ADVERSE REACTIONS:** Nausea, dizziness, headache, CNS disturbances, vomiting, diarrhea, rash, abdominal pain/discomfort, pain, swelling, tendinitis, tendon tears.

**INTERACTIONS:** See Contraindications. Increases theophylline and caffeine levels and prolongs effects. Fatal reactions have occurred with theophylline. Magnesium- or aluminum-containing antacids, sucralfate, Videx (didanosine) chewable/buffered tablets or pediatric powder, and products containing calcium, iron, or zinc decrease serum and urine levels; space doses at least 2 hrs before or 6 hrs after administration. Altered serum levels of phenytoin. Severe hypoglycemia with glyburide (rare). Potentiated by probenecid. Transient serum creatinine elevations with cyclosporine. Enhances oral anticoagulant effects; monitor PT. Caution with drugs that lower seizure threshold. Severe tendon disorder risks increased with concomitant corticosteroid therapy. Caution with concomitant drugs that may result in prolongation of the QT interval.

**PREGNANCY:** Category C, not for use in nursing.

**MECHANISM OF ACTION:** Synthetic broad-spectrum antimicrobial agent; inhibits enzymes topoisomerase II (DNA gyrase) and topoisomerase IV, which are required for bacterial DNA replication.



**PHARMACOKINETICS: Absorption:** Rapid, well absorb (GIT); absolute bioavailability (70%); $C_{max}$=0.1, 0.2, 0.4mcg/mL (250mg, 500mg, 750mg, after 12 hrs); $T_{max}$=1-2 hrs. **Distribution:** Plasma protein binding (20-40%). **Metabolism:** CYP1A2. **Elimination:** Urine (40-50%); $T_{1/2}$=4 hrs.

## NURSING CONSIDERATIONS

**Assessment:** Assess renal function tests, LFTs, history of seizures, pregnancy/nursing status, and possible drug interactions. Note other diseases/conditions and drug therapies.

**Monitoring:** Monitor for cardiac arrest, seizure, status epilepticus, respiratory failure, *Clostridium difficile*-associated diarrhea, renal function tests, LFTs, CBC, tendinitis, tendon rupture, peripheral neuropathy.

**Patient Counseling:** Notify healthcare provider if symptoms of pain, swelling, or inflammation of a tendon, or weakness or inability to move joints; rest and refrain from exercise; and d/c therapy. Inform that drug treats bacterial, not viral, infections. Take exactly as directed; skipping doses or not completing full course may decrease effectiveness and increase resistance. Inform to take with or without food, and to drink fluids. Inform about potential benefits/risks. D/C and notify physician if skin rash, other allergic reaction, and watery and bloody stools (with or without stomach cramps and fever) occur. Notify if pregnant/nursing or taking antacids or sucralfate. Use caution in activity requiring mental alertness and coordination. Avoid sun exposure. Take full course as prescribed.

**Administration:** Oral route. **Storage:** Below 30°C (86°F). Microcapsules and diluent should be stored below 25°C (77°F). Protect from freezing.

# Cipro XR — RX

ciprofloxacin (Bayer/Schering)

**Fluoroquinolones are associated with an increased risk of tendinitis and tendon rupture in all ages. Risk further increased in patients >60 yrs, patients taking corticosteroid drugs, and patients with kidney, heart, or lung transplants.**

**THERAPEUTIC CLASS:** Fluoroquinolone

**INDICATIONS:** Treatment of urinary tract infections (UTI), including uncomplicated (acute cystitis) and complicated UTI, and acute uncomplicated pyelonephritis caused by susceptible strains of microorganisms.

**DOSAGE:** *Adults:* ≥18 yrs: Uncomplicated UTI: 500mg qd for 3 days. Complicated UTI/Acute Uncomplicated Pyelonephritis: 1000mg qd for 7-14 days. CrCl <30mL/min: 500mg qd. Dialysis: Give after procedure is completed. May switch from ciprofloxacin IV to extended release at discretion of physician. Administer at least 2 hrs before or 6 hrs after magnesium- or aluminum-containing antacids, sucralfate, didanosine chewable/buffered tablets or pediatric powder, metal cations (eg, iron), multivitamins with zinc. Space calcium intake (>800mg) by at least 2 hrs when coadministering.

**HOW SUPPLIED:** Tab, Extended-Release: 500mg, 1000mg

**CONTRAINDICATIONS:** Concomitant administration with tizanidine.

**WARNINGS/PRECAUTIONS:** Strenuous physical activity, renal failure, and previous tendon disorders (eg, rheumatoid arthritis) may independently increase risk of tendon rupture; d/c if experience pain, swelling, inflammation or rupture of a tendon. May cause cartilage erosion of weight bearing joints and other signs of arthropathy Increased intracranial pressure (ICP), convulsions, toxic psychosis, and other CNS events reported. D/C if CNS event occurs. Caution with CNS disorders or risk factors that may predispose to seizures or lower seizure threshold. Severe, sometimes fatal, hypersensitivity reactions reported; d/c at the first appearance of skin rash, jaundice, or any other sign of hypersensitivity. *Clostridium difficile*-associated diarrhea (CDAD) reported. Rare cases of sensory or sensorimotor axonal polyneuropathy affecting small and/or large axons resulting in paresthesias, hypoesthesias, dysesthesias, and weakness reported; d/c if occurs. Crystalluria (rare) reported; maintain hydration and avoid alkalinizing urine. Moderate to severe photosensitivity/phototoxicity reactions may occur; d/c if phototoxicity occurs. Avoid excessive sunlight and UV light. Not interchangeable with immediate-release tablets. Caution in elderly.

**ADVERSE REACTIONS:** N/V, headache, diarrhea, dizziness, vaginal moniliasis, dyspepsia.

**INTERACTIONS:** See Contraindications. Increase in plasma concentration of drugs metabolized by CYP1A2 (eg, theophylline, methylxanthines, tizanidine) when co-administered. Serious and fatal reactions reported with concurrent administration of theophylline. May reduce clearance of caffeine. Concurrent administration with multivalent containing products such as magnesium-or aluminum- containing antacids, sucralfate, didanosine chewable/buffered tablets or pediatric powder, other highly buffered drugs and products containing calcium, iron, or zinc may decrease serum and urine levels; administer at least 2 hrs before or 6 hrs after antacids containing magnesium or aluminum, sucralfate, didanosine chewable/buffered tablets or pediatric powder, other highly buffered drugs, metal cations (eg, iron), and multivitamins containing zinc. Slightly diminished absorption with omeprazole. May alter serum levels of phenytoin. Severe hypoglycemia with glyburide (rare). Transient elevations in serum creatinine with cyclosporine. Enhances the oral anticoagulant effects of warfarin and its derivatives; monitor PT and other suitable coagulation tests closely. Increased levels with probenecid. Increased methotrexate levels and may increase risk of toxic reactions. Accelerated absorption with metoclopramide. NSAIDs (except for acetyl salicylic acid) in combination with very high doses of quinolones shown to provoke convulsions in pre-clinical studies. Caution with drugs that lower seizure threshold. Caution with drugs that may result in prolongation of the QT interval (eg, class IA or class III antiarrhythmics). Avoid concomitant administration with dairy products alone, or with calcium-fortified products.

**PREGNANCY:** Category C, not for use in nursing.

**MECHANISM OF ACTION:** Fluoroquinolone; inhibits topoisomerase II (DNA gyrase) and topoisomerase IV, which are required for bacterial DNA replication, transcription, repair and recombination.

**PHARMACOKINETICS: Absorption:** (500mg): $C_{max}$=1.59mg/L; $T_{max}$=1.5 hrs; $AUC_{0-24h}$=7.97mg•h/L. (1000mg): $C_{max}$=3.11mg/L; $T_{max}$=2 hrs; $AUC_{0-24h}$=16.83mg•h/L. **Distribution:** (IV) $V_d$=2.1-2.7L/kg; plasma protein binding (20-40%); found in breast milk. **Metabolism:** Primary metabolites: oxociprofloxacin (M3) and sulfociprofloxacin (M2). **Elimination:** Urine (35%, unchanged).

## NURSING CONSIDERATIONS

**Assessment:** Assess for risk factors for developing tendinitis and tendon rupture (eg, age, kidney/heart/lung transplant, renal failure, previous tendon disorders), CNS disorders or risk factors that may predispose to seizure or lower seizure threshold, pregnancy/nursing status, and for possible drug interactions.

**Monitoring:** Monitor for signs/symptoms of tendinitis, tendon rupture, hypersensitivity reactions, CDAD, peripheral neuropathy, crystalluria, CNS events, and for photosensitivity/phototoxicity reactions. Monitor renal function, CBC, and LFTs.

**Patient Counseling:** Inform about potential benefits and risks of therapy. Instruct to notify healthcare provider if symptoms of pain, swelling, or inflammation of a tendon, or weakness or inability to move joints occur; instruct to rest and refrain from exercise and d/c therapy. Inform that drug treats bacterial, not viral, infections. Advise to take exactly as directed; inform that skipping doses or not completing full course may decrease effectiveness and increase antibiotic resistance. Counsel to drink fluids liberally and may take with or without food. Advise that if miss a dose at usual time, may take dose later in the day. Counsel to not take more than one tab per day, even if miss a dose. Instruct to d/c therapy and notify if skin rash, other allergic reaction, watery and bloody stools (with or without stomach cramps and fever), or symptoms of peripheral neuropathy (eg, pain, burning, tingling, numbness, weakness) occur. Instruct to notify if pregnant/nursing. Advise to notify healthcare provider of all prescription, nonprescription, and supplements currently taking. Inform that therapy may cause dizziness and lightheadedness and to use caution in activities requiring mental alertness and coordination. Advise to minimize or avoid exposure to natural or artificial sunlight.

**Administration:** Oral route. Swallow tab whole; do not split, crush, or chew. **Storage**: 25°C (77°F), excursions permitted to 15-30°C (59-86°F).

## CIPRODEX RX

dexamethasone - ciprofloxacin (Alcon)

**THERAPEUTIC CLASS:** Antibacterial/corticosteroid combination

**INDICATIONS:** Acute otitis media in pediatric patients with tympanostomy tubes. Acute otitis externa.

**DOSAGE:** *Adults:* Acute Otitis Externa: 4 drops in affected ear(s) bid for 7 days. Warm bottle in hand for 1-2 min to avoid dizziness. Shake well before use.
*Pediatrics:* ≥6 months: 4 drops in affected ear(s) bid for 7 days. Warm bottle in hand for 1-2 min to avoid dizziness. Shake well before use.

**HOW SUPPLIED:** Sus: (Ciprofloxacin-Dexamethasone) 0.3%-0.1% [5mL, 7.5mL]

**CONTRAINDICATIONS:** Viral infections of external ear canal including herpes simplex infections.

**WARNINGS/PRECAUTIONS:** D/C if hypersensitivity reaction occurs. Re-evaluate if no improvement after one week.

**ADVERSE REACTIONS:** Ear pain/discomfort/pruritus.

**PREGNANCY:** Category C, not for use in nursing.

**MECHANISM OF ACTION:** Fluoroquinolone, corticosteroid; antibacterial/anti-inflammatory; bactericidal action results from interference with the enzyme (DNA gyrase), which is needed for the synthesis of bacterial DNA.

**PHARMACOKINETICS: Absorption:** Ciprofloxacin: $C_{max}$=1.39ng/mL; $T_{max}$=15 min-2 hrs. Dexamethasone: $C_{max}$=1.14ng/mL; $T_{max}$=15 min-2 hrs.

### NURSING CONSIDERATIONS

**Assessment:** Assess for history of drug hypersensitivity and viral infection of the external canal, including herpes simplex virus infection.

**Monitoring:** Monitor for anaphylactic reactions, skin rash, overgrowth of non-susceptible organisms (eg, fungi and yeast) in large doses, lesions or erosions of cartilage in weight-bearing joints, and other signs of arthropathy.

**Patient Counseling:** Inform drug is for otic use only. Avoid touching dropper tip to ear material or any other surface. D/C if rash or allergic reaction occurs. Instruct to keep infected ear dry and clean. Take as prescribed.

**Administration:** Otic route. Warm suspension by holding bottle in hand for 1-2 min. Lie with affected ear up, then instill drops. Maintain position for 60 sec and repeat, if necessary, with opposite ear. **Storage:** Store at 15-30°C (59-86°F). Protect from light; avoid freezing.

## CLARINEX RX

desloratadine (Schering)

**OTHER BRAND NAMES:** Clarinex RediTabs (Schering) - Clarinex Syrup (Schering)

**THERAPEUTIC CLASS:** $H_1$-antagonist

C

**INDICATIONS:** Relief of perennial allergic rhinitis and chronic idiopathic urticaria in patients ≥6 months. Relief of seasonal allergic rhinitis in patients ≥2 yrs.

**DOSAGE:** *Adults:* 5mg qd. Hepatic/Renal Impairment: 5mg every other day. Dissolve RediTabs on tongue with or without water.
*Pediatrics:* Tabs: ≥12 yrs: 5mg qd. 6-11 yrs: 2.5mg qd. Syrup: ≥12 yrs: 10mL (5mg) qd. 6-11 yrs: 5mL (2.5mg) qd. 12 months-5 yrs: 2.5mL (1.25mg) qd. 6-11 months: 2mL (1mg) qd. Dissolve RediTabs on tongue with or without water.

**HOW SUPPLIED:** Tab: 5mg; Tab, Disintegrating: (RediTabs) 2.5mg, 5mg; Syrup: 0.5mg/mL

**WARNINGS/PRECAUTIONS:** Adjust dose with renal or hepatic impairment. Caution in elderly.

**ADVERSE REACTIONS:** Pharyngitis, dry mouth, headache, fever, diarrhea, cough, upper respiratory tract infection, irritability, somnolence, bronchitis, otitis media, N/V, fatigue.

**INTERACTIONS:** Erythromycin, ketoconazole increases plasma levels.

**PREGNANCY:** Category C, not for use in nursing.

**MECHANISM OF ACTION:** Long-acting tricyclic histamine antagonist with selective $H_1$-receptor histamine antagonist activity; inhibits histamine release from human mast cells.

**PHARMACOKINETICS: Absorption:** $T_{max}$=3 hrs., $C_{max}$=4ng/mL, AUC=56.9ng•hr/mL. **Distribution:** Found in breast milk; plasma protein binding (82-87% of desloratadine), (85-89% of 3-hydroxydesloratadine). **Metabolism:** Extensive. Desloratadine (major metabolite), 3-hydroxydesloratadine (active metabolite): **Elimination:** Urine and feces (metabolites); $T_{1/2}$=27 hrs.

## NURSING CONSIDERATIONS

**Assessment:** Assess for renal/hepatic impairment and for possible drug interactions.

**Monitoring:** Monitor for hypersensitivity reactions.

**Patient Counseling:** Take drug as directed, without regard to meals. Do not increase dose or dosing frequency.

**Administration:** Oral route. **Storage:** 25°C (77°F); excursions permitted to 15-30°C (59-86°F).

# CLARINEX-D RX

pseudoephedrine sulfate - desloratadine (Schering)

**THERAPEUTIC CLASS:** $H_1$-antagonist/sympathomimetic amine

**INDICATIONS:** Relief of nasal and non-nasal symptoms of seasonal allergic rhinitis, including nasal congestion in adults and adolescents ≥12 yrs.

**DOSAGE:** *Adults:* 2.5mg-120mg tab bid or 5mg-240mg tab qd w/ or w/o food. Hepatic Impairment: 12-Hour/24-Hour: Avoid use. Renal Impairment: 12-Hour/24-Hour: Avoid use.
*Pediatrics:* ≥12 yrs: 2.5mg-120mg tab bid or 5mg-240mg tab qd w/ or w/o food. Hepatic Impairment: 12-Hour/24-Hour: Avoid use. Renal Impairment: 12-Hour/24-Hour: Avoid use.

**HOW SUPPLIED:** Tab, Extended-Release: (Desloratadine-Pseudoephedrine) (12-Hr) 2.5mg-120mg, (24-Hr) 5mg-240mg

**CONTRAINDICATIONS:** Narrow-angle glaucoma, urinary retention, MAOI therapy or within 14 days of discontinuation, severe HTN, severe CAD.

**WARNINGS/PRECAUTIONS:** Cardiovascular (eg, CV collapse with hypotension) and CNS (eg, CNS stimulation, convulsions) effects reported; caution in patient with CV disorder. Caution in patient with DM and hyperthyroidism. Caution in patient with prostatic hypertrophy or increased IOP; urinary retention and narrow angle glaucoma may occur. Hypersensitivity reactions reported; d/c if any occur. Avoid in patients with hepatic and/or renal impairment. Caution in elderly.

C

**ADVERSE REACTIONS:** Dry mouth, headache, insomnia, fatigue, pharyngitis, somnolence.

**INTERACTIONS:** See Contraindications. Antihypertensive effects of β-adrenergic blocking agents, methyldopa, and reserpine may be reduced by sympathomimetics (eg, pseudoephedrine). Increased ectopic pacemaker activity with digitalis. Increased plasma concentrations with CYP450 3A4 inhibitors (eg, ketoconazole, erythromycin, azithromycin), cimetidine and fluoxetine.

**PREGNANCY:** Category C, not for use in nursing.

**MECHANISM OF ACTION:** Desloratadine: Long-acting tricyclic histamine antagonist with selective $H_1$-receptor antagonist activity. Inhibits histamine release from human mast cells *in vitro*. Pseudoephedrine: Orally active sympathomimetic amine, which exerts a decongestant action on nasal mucosa.

**PHARMACOKINETICS: Absorption:** Desloratadine: (24 hr) $C_{max}$=1.79ng/mL; $T_{max}$=6-7 hrs, AUC=61.1ng•hr/mL. (12 hr) $C_{max}$=1.09ng/mL; $T_{max}$=4-5 hrs, AUC=31.6ng•hr/mL. Pseudoephedrine: (24 hr) $C_{max}$=328ng/mL, $T_{max}$=8-9 hrs, AUC=6438ng•hr/mL. (12 hr) $C_{max}$=263ng/mL, $T_{max}$=6-7 hrs, AUC=4588ng•hr/mL. **Distribution:** Desloratadine: Found in breast milk, plasma protein binding (82-87%), 3-hydroxydesloratadine (85-89%). **Metabolism:** Desloratadine (major metabolite): extensive, 3-hydroxydesloratadine (active metabolite) and glucuronidation pathway. Pseudoephedrine: Liver (incomplete), through N-demethylation. **Elimination:** Desloratadine: (24 hr) $T_{1/2}$=24 hrs, (12 hr) $T_{1/2}$=27 hrs. Pseudoephedrine: Urine (55-96% unchanged). If urinary pH=5, ($T_{1/2}$=3-6 hrs); if urinary pH=8, ($T_{1/2}$=9-16 hrs).

## NURSING CONSIDERATIONS

**Assessment:** Assess for drug hypersensitivity, hepatic/renal impairment, increased IOP, narrow-angle glaucoma, prostatic hypertrophy, urinary retention, HTN, CAD, ischemic heart disease, DM, hyperthyroidism, possible drug interaction (eg, MAO inhibitors).

**Monitoring:** Monitor idiosyncratic effects (eg, insomnia, dizziness, weakness, tremor, arrhythmias), BP, IOP, cardiac function, somnolence, CNS stimulation effects with convulsions, CV collapse with hypotension, liver enzymes, renal function.

**Patient Counseling:** Inform patients that it may cause CV or CNS effects such as insomnia, dizziness, tremor or arrhythmias. Advise not to increase the dose or dosing frequency. Advise not to use other antihistamines, decongestants, and MAO inhibitors. Instruct to inform physician of present illness such as severe HTN, severe CAD, narrow angle glaucoma, or urinary retention prior to treatment. Not to be taken during nursing/pregnancy.

**Administration:** Oral route. Do not break or chew, swallow tab whole. **Storage:** 25°C (77°F); excursions permitted to 15-30°C (59-86°F). Heat sensitive. Avoid exposure at or above 30°C (86°F). Protect from excessive moisture. Protect from light.

# CLEOCIN RX

clindamycin HCl - clindamycin phosphate (Pharmacia & Upjohn)

***Clostridium difficile*-associated diarrhea (CDAD) reported and may range in severity from mild diarrhea to fatal colitis. Not for use with nonbacterial infections. CDAD must be considered in all patients with diarrhea following antibiotic use. If CDAD is suspected or confirmed, ongoing antibiotic use not directed against *C.difficile* may need to be d/c. Appropriate fluid and electrolyte management, protein supplementation, antibiotic treatment of *C.difficile* and surgical evaluation may be instituted as clinically indicated.**

**THERAPEUTIC CLASS:** Lincomycin derivative

**INDICATIONS:** Treatment of serious infections caused by susceptible anaerobes, streptococci, pneumococci and staphylococci.

**DOSAGE:** *Adults:* Serious Infection: 150-300mg PO q6h or 600-1200mg/day IM/IV given bid-qid. More Severe Infections: 300-450mg PO q6h or 1200-2700mg/day IM/IV given bid-qid. Life-Threatening Infections: Up to 4800mg/day IV. Max: 600mg per IM injection. Alternatively may administer as a single rapid infusion for the first dose followed by continuous IV infusion; see PI for dosing. Treat β-hemolytic strep for at least 10 days.
*Pediatrics:* PO: Serious Infections: (Cap) 8-16mg/kg/day given tid-qid or (Sol) 8-12mg/kg/day tid-qid. Severe Infection: (Sol) 13-16mg/kg/day tid-qid. More Severe Infections: (Cap) 16-20mg/kg/day given tid-qid or (Sol) 17-25mg/kg/day tid-qid . ≤10kg: 1/2 tsp (37.5mg) tid should be the minimum recommended dose. IM/IV: 1 month-16 yrs: 20-40mg/kg/day tid-qid; use the higher dose for more severe infections. Alternatively may give 350mg/m²/day for serious infections and 450mg/m²/day for more severe infections. <1 month: 15-20mg/kg/day tid-qid. Treat β-hemolytic strep for at least 10 days.

**HOW SUPPLIED:** Cap: (HCl) 75mg, 150mg, 300mg; Inj: (Phosphate) 150mg/mL [2mL, 4mL, 6mL, 60mL] 300mg/50mL, 600mg/50mL, 900mg/50mL; Sol (Palmitate): 75mg/5mL [100mL]

**WARNINGS/PRECAUTIONS:** Due to association with severe colitis, use should be reserved for serious infections where less toxic agents are inappropriate. Use in the absence of a proven or strongly suspected infection is unlikely to provide benefit and may increase the risk of development of drug-resistant bacteria. May cause overgrowth of nonsusceptible organisms. Not for treatment of meningitis. Caution with patients with liver disease; perform periodic liver enzyme determinations in patients with severe liver disease. Caution with atopic patients, renal disease, patients wih a history of GI disease (eg, colitis), and the elderly. Perform periodic monitoring of blood counts, hepatic and renal function with long-term use. Do not give injection undiluted as bolus. The 75mg and 150mg caps contain tartrazine, which may cause allergic-type reactions. Inj contains benzyl alcohol which has been associated with "gasping syndrome" in premature infants.

**ADVERSE REACTIONS:** Abdominal pain, colitis, esophagitis, N/V, diarrhea, maculopapular skin rash, jaundice, pruritus, vaginitis.

**INTERACTIONS:** Antagonism may occur with erythromycin. May potentiate neuromuscular blockers.

**PREGNANCY:** Category B, not for use in nursing.

**MECHANISM OF ACTION:** Lincomycin-derivative antibiotic; inhibits bacterial protein synthesis by binding to the 50s subunit of the ribosome.

**PHARMACOKINETICS: Absorption:** Cap: Rapid, complete; $C_{max}$=2.5mcg/mL, $T_{max}$=45 min. Inj: $C_{max}$=10.8mcg/mL (adults, 600mg IV q8h), 9mcg/mL (adults, 600 mg IM q12h), 10mcg/mL (peds, 5-7mg/kg IV in 1 hr), 8mcg/mL (peds, 5-7mg/kg IM); $T_{max}$=3 hrs (adults, IM), 1 hr (peds, IM). **Distribution:** Wide; body fluids, tissues, and bones; found in breast milk. **Elimination:** Cap: Urine (10% unchanged), feces (3.6% unchanged); $T_{1/2}$=2.4 hr. Inj: $T_{1/2}$=3 hrs (adults), 2.5 hrs (peds). Sol: $T_{1/2}$=2 hrs.

## NURSING CONSIDERATIONS

**Assessment:** Assess for previous sensitivities to drugs and other allergens, history of GI disease (eg, colitis), renal/hepatic impairment, pregnancy/nursing status, presence of meningitis, upcoming surgical procedures, and for possible drug interactions. Assess use in atopic patients and in elderly patients with severe illness.

**Monitoring:** Monitor for CDAD, overgrowth of nonsuspectible organisms, and for anaphylactoid reactions. Monitor for changes in bowel frequency in older patients. When culture and susceptibility information is available, consider modifying antibacterial therapy. If on prolonged therapy, perform periodic liver and kidney function tests and blood counts. Perform periodic liver enzyme determinations in patients with severe liver disease.

**Patient Counseling:** Inform about potential benefits/risks of use. Inform that therapy only treats bacterial, not viral infections. Instruct to take exactly as directed; skipping doses or not completing full course may decrease effectiveness and increase antibiotic resistance. Instruct to contact physician if an allergic reaction develops. Advise that watery and bloody stools may occur as late as 2 months after therapy. Instruct to notify physician if pregnant/nursing.

**Administration:** Oral/IM/IV route. See PI for proper preparation and administration. **Storage:** 20-25°C (68-77°F). (Sol) Do not refrigerate the reconstituted solution; stable at room temperature for 2 weeks.



## CLEOCIN T — RX

clindamycin phosphate (Pharmacia & Upjohn)

**THERAPEUTIC CLASS:** Lincomycin derivative

**INDICATIONS:** Acne vulgaris.

**DOSAGE:** *Adults:* Apply thin film bid.
*Pediatrics:* ≥12 yrs: Apply thin film bid. May use more than 1 pledget.

**HOW SUPPLIED:** Gel: 1% [30g, 60g]; Lot: 1% [60mL]; Sol: 1% [30mL, 60mL]; Swab (Pledgets): 1% [60$^{s}$]

**CONTRAINDICATIONS:** History of regional enteritis, ulcerative colitis, or antibiotic-associated colitis.

**WARNINGS/PRECAUTIONS:** Avoid eyes, abraded skin, mucous membranes, and mouth. Caution in atopic patients. D/C if significant diarrhea occurs.

**ADVERSE REACTIONS:** Dryness, oily skin, erythema, peeling, burning, itching, pseudomembranous colitis (rare).

**INTERACTIONS:** May potentiate neuromuscular blockers.

**PREGNANCY:** Category B, not for use in nursing.

**MECHANISM OF ACTION:** Inhibits growth of *Propionibacterium acnes* and decreases free fatty acids on the skin surface.

**PHARMACOKINETICS: Absorption:** Following topical administration of multiple doses, serum levels of clindamycin were measured at 0-3ng/mL. **Distribution:** Orally and parenterally administered clindamycin has been found in breast milk. **Metabolism:** Hydrolysis. **Elimination:** Urine (≤0.2% found as clindamycin).

### NURSING CONSIDERATIONS

**Assessment:** Assess proper diagnosis of acne vulgaris. Assess for history of hypersensitivity to lincomycin; regional, ulcerative, or antibiotic-associated colitis. Assess use in pregnant/nursing patients. Assess for possible drug interactions.

**Monitoring:** Monitor for signs/symptoms of diarrhea, bloody diarrhea, and colitis (eg, pseudomembranous colitis). Monitor for occurrence of severe abdominal cramps, blood, and mucus discharge. If significant diarrhea occurs, consider large bowel endoscopy, stool culture, and stool assay.

**Patient Counseling:** Inform that medication contains alcohol base that will cause burning and irritation if contact with eye occurs. If accidental contact with sensitive surfaces (eg, eye, abraded skin, mucous membranes) occurs, bathe affected areas with copious amounts of cold water. Medication has unpleasant taste. Use caution when applying around mouth. Notify physician immediately if any signs of abdominal pain or GI disturbances (eg, diarrhea) occur.

**Administration:** Topical. **Storage:** 20-25°C (68-77°F). Protect from freezing. Keep all liquid dosage forms in containers tightly closed.

## CLEOCIN VAGINAL — RX

clindamycin phosphate (Pharmacia & Upjohn)

**OTHER BRAND NAMES:** Cleocin Vaginal Ovules (Pharmacia & Upjohn) - Clindamax Vaginal (PharmaDerm)

**THERAPEUTIC CLASS:** Lincomycin derivative

**INDICATIONS:** (Cre) Treatment of bacterial vaginosis in non-pregnant women and pregnant women during the 2nd and 3rd trimester. (Sup) Treatment of bacterial vaginosis in non-pregnant women.

**DOSAGE:** *Adults:* (Cre) 1 applicatorful intravaginally qhs. Treat non-pregnant females for 3 or 7 days and pregnant females for 7 days. (Sup) 1 suppository intravaginally qhs for 3 days.
*Pediatrics:* Post-Menarchal: (Sup) 1 suppository intravaginally qhs for 3 days.

**HOW SUPPLIED:** Cre: 2% [40g]; Sup, Vaginal: (Ovules) 100mg [3[s]]

**CONTRAINDICATIONS:** Hypersensitivity to lincomycin, history of regional enteritis, ulcerative colitis, or a history of antibiotic-associated colitis.

**WARNINGS/PRECAUTIONS:** (Cre, Sup) Diarrhea, bloody diarrhea, and colitis (including pseudomembranous colitis) reported with oral, parenteral, and topical formulations of clindamycin; onset of pseudomembranous colitis may occur during or after antimicrobial treatment. Use may result in overgrowth of nonsusceptible organisms in the vagina. Cre formulation contains an oleaginous base and sup formulation contains mineral oil which may weaken latex or rubber products (eg, condoms, vaginal contraceptive diaphragms), use of such products within 72 hrs following treatment is not recommended. (Cre) Burning and irritation of the eye may occur with accidental contact.

**ADVERSE REACTIONS:** Vaginitis, vulvovaginal disorder, moniliasis.

**INTERACTIONS:** May potentiate neuromuscular blocking agents.

**PREGNANCY:** Category B, not for use in nursing.

**MECHANISM OF ACTION:** Lincomycin derivative; inhibits bacterial protein synthesis at the level of the bacterial ribosome. Binds preferentially to the 50S ribosomal subunit and affects the process of peptide chain initiation.

**PHARMACOKINETICS: Absorption:** (Cre) $C_{max}$=13ng/ml (Day 1); 16ng/mL (Day 7), $T_{max}$=14 hrs (women with bacterial vaginosis). (Sup) AUC=3.2µg•hr/mL; $C_{max}$=0.27µg/mL (Day 3); $T_{max}$=5 hrs (healthy volunteers). **Elimination:** (Cre) $T_{1/2}$=1.5-2.6 hrs (women with bacterial vaginosis). (Sup) $T_{1/2}$=11 hrs (healthy volunteers).

## NURSING CONSIDERATIONS

**Assessment:** Assess for clinical diagnosis of bacterial vaginosis, history of drug hypersensitivity, history of regional enteritis, ulcerative colitis, history of antibiotic-associated colitis, pregnancy/nursing status, and for possible drug interactions.

**Monitoring:** Monitor for signs/symptoms of pseudomembranous colitis, overgrowth of nonsusceptible organisms, and for anaphylactoid reactions.

**Patient Counseling:** (Cre, Sup) Instruct not to engage in vaginal intercourse or use other vaginal products (eg, tampons, douches) during therapy. Inform that product contains components that may weaken latex or rubber products (eg, condoms, diaphragms); instruct not to use such products within 72 hrs following treatment. (Cre) Instruct to rinse eye with copius amounts of water if accidental eye contact occurs.

**Administration:** Intravaginal. Refer to PI for administration instructions.
**Storage:** (Cre) 20-25°C (68-77°F); (Sup) 25° (77°F); excursions permitted to 15-30°C (59-86°F).

# CLEVIPREX — RX

clevidipine butyrate (The Medicines Company)

**THERAPEUTIC CLASS:** Calcium channel blocker (dihydropyridine)

**INDICATIONS:** Reduction of BP in patients when oral therapy is not desirable or feasible.

**DOSAGE:** *Adults:* IV use only: Individualize dose. Initial: 1-2mg/hr. Titrate: Double dose at 90 second intervals initially and then dose adjustments should be less than double every 5-10 min. Maint: 4-6mg/hr. Max: 16mg/hr. Due to lipid load restrictions, no more than 1000mL or an average of 21mg/hr is recommended/24 hrs. Transition to Oral Therapy: D/C or titrate downward until oral therapy is established. Consider lag time of oral agent's effect and monitor BP until desired effect is reached.

**HOW SUPPLIED:** Inj: 0.5mg/mL [50mL, 100mL]

**CONTRAINDICATIONS:** Allergy to soybeans, soy products, eggs, or egg products. Severe aortic stenosis, defective lipid metabolism (eg, pathologic hyperlipidemia, lipoid nephrosis, or acute pancreatitis accompanied with hyperlipidemia).

**WARNINGS/PRECAUTIONS:** Discard unused portions, including product being infused, within 4 hrs of stopper puncture. Systemic hypotension and reflex tachycardia may occur; decrease dose. Lipid intake restrictions may be necessary with significant disorders of lipid metabolism. May produce negative inotropic effects and exacerbation of heart failure; monitor heart failure patients. Does not lower HR and does not protect against effects of abrupt beta-blocker withdrawal. Monitor for rebound hypertension for at least 8 hrs after withdrawal.

**ADVERSE REACTIONS:** Headache, N/V, myocardial infarction, cardiac arrest, syncope, dyspnea, hypotension, reflex tachycardia.

**PREGNANCY:** Category C, safety not known in nursing.

**MECHANISM OF ACTION:** Calcium channel blocker (dihydropyridine); mediates the influx of calcium in arterial smooth muscle and reduces mean arterial blood pressure by decreasing systemic vascular resistance; does not reduce pre-load.

**PHARMACOKINETICS: Distribution:** $V_d$=0.17L/kg; plasma protein binding (>99.5%). **Metabolism:** Hydrolysis, glucuronidation, oxidation; carboxylic acid and formaldehyde (primary metabolites). **Excretion:** $T_{1/2}$=15 mins; urine (63-74%); feces (7-22%).

## NURSING CONSIDERATIONS

**Assessment:** Assess BP and HR, history of allergy to soy and egg products, defective lipid metabolism disorders, history of beta-blocker usage, and pregnancy/nursing status. Obtain baseline parameters (eg, BP, lipid profile).

**Monitoring:** Monitor BP and HR, hypotension, reflex tachycardia, rebound HTN (at least 8 hrs after the last dose), and heart failure.

**Patient Counseling:** Advise that underlying HTN requires follow up and continuation of oral antihypertensive medications as prescribed. Report any signs of new hypertensive emergency such as neurological symptoms, visual changes, or heart failure to healthcare provider immediately.

**Administration:** IV route. Refer to PI for details on administration. **Storage:** 2-8°C (36-46°F). Do not freeze. May be transferred to 25°C (77°F) for a period not to exceed 2 months. Do not return to refrigerated storage after exposing to room temperature. Protect from light.

# CLIMARA RX

estradiol (Bayer Healthcare)

**Estrogens increase the risk of endometrial cancer. Estrogens, with or without progestins, should not be used for the prevention of cardiovascular disease or dementia. Increased risk of MI, stroke, invasive breast cancer, PE, and DVT in postmenopausal women (50-79 yrs of age) reported. Increased risk of developing probable dementia in postmenopausal women ≥65 yrs of age reported.**

**THERAPEUTIC CLASS:** Estrogen

**INDICATIONS:** Treatment of moderate to severe vasomotor symptoms and/or vulvar/vaginal atrophy associated with menopause. Treatment of hypoestrogenism due to hypogonadism, castration, or primary ovarian failure. Prevention of postmenopausal osteoporosis.

**DOSAGE:** *Adults:* Apply 1 patch weekly to lower abdomen or upper area of buttocks (avoid breasts and waistline). Rotate application sites. Vasomotor Symptoms: Initial: 0.025mg/day patch once weekly. Titrate: Adjust dose as needed. Wait 1 week after withdrawal of oral therapy before initiating patch.

D/C or taper at 3-6 month intervals. Osteoporosis Prevention: Minimum Effective Dose: 0.025mg/day once weekly.

**HOW SUPPLIED:** Patch: 0.025mg/day, 0.0375mg/day, 0.05mg/day, 0.06mg/day, 0.075mg/day, 0.1mg/day [4[s]]

**CONTRAINDICATIONS:** Pregnancy, undiagnosed abnormal genital bleeding, breast cancer (or history of), estrogen-dependent neoplasia, deep vein thrombosis (or history of), pulmonary embolism (or history of), active or recent (eg, within 1 year) arterial thromboembolic disease (eg, stroke, MI), liver dysfunction or disease.

**WARNINGS/PRECAUTIONS:** May increase risk of cardiovascular events (eg, MI, stroke), venous thrombosis, and PE; d/c immediately if any of these events occur or are suspected. May increase risk of breast/endometrial cancer, and gallbladder disease. Retinal vascular thrombosis reported; monitor and d/c if papilledema or retinal vascular lesions occur. May increase risk of dementia. May cause severe hypercalcemia in patients with breast cancer and bone metastases; d/c if severe hypercalcemia occurs. Consider addition of a progestin if no hysterectomy. May elevate BP; monitor at regular intervals. May cause elevations of plasma triglycerides with pre-existing hypertriglyceridemia. Caution with history of cholestatic jaundice associated with past estrogen use or with pregnancy; d/c with recurrence. May lead to increased thyroid-binding globulin levels; monitor thyroid function in patients dependent on thyroid replacement therapy. May cause fluid retention; caution with cardiac/renal dysfunction. Caution with severe hypocalcemia. May increase risk of ovarian cancer. May exacerbate endometriosis, asthma, DM, epilepsy, migraine, porphyria, systemic lupus erythematosus (SLE), hepatic hemangiomas; use with caution.

**ADVERSE REACTIONS:** Headache, arthralgia, edema, abdominal pain, flatulence, depression, breast pain, leukorrhea, upper respiratory tract infection, sinusitis, rhinitis, pruritus.

**INTERACTIONS:** CYP3A4 inducers (eg, St. John's wort, phenobarbital, carbamazepine, rifampin) may decrease levels, which may decrease therapeutic effects and/or change uterine bleeding profile. CYP3A4 inhibitors (eg, erythromycin, clarithromycin, ketoconazole, itraconazole, ritonavir, grapefruit juice) may increase levels, which may result in side effects.

**PREGNANCY:** Contraindicated in pregnancy, caution in nursing.

**MECHANISM OF ACTION:** Estrogen; binds to nuclear receptors in estrogen-responsive tissues. Modulates pituitary secretion of gonadotropins, luteinizing hormone (LH), and follicle stimulating hormone (FSH), through negative feedback mechanism.

**PHARMACOKINETICS: Absorption:** Transdermal administration of different doses resulted in different parameters. **Distribution**: Estrogens are found in breast milk. Wide; largely bound to sex hormone binding globulin (SHBG) and albumin. **Metabolism:** Liver to estrone (metabolite); estriol (major urinary metabolite); enterohepatic recirculation via sulfate and glucuronide conjugation; biliary secretion of conjugates into the intestine; hydrolysis in the gut; and reabsorbtion. **Elimination:** Urine.

## NURSING CONSIDERATIONS

**Assessment:** Assess for abnormal genital bleeding, presence or history of breast cancer, deep vein thrombosis or history of, pulmonary embolism or history of, presence of estrogen-dependent neoplasia, active or recent (within past yr) arterial thromboembolic disease (eg, stroke, MI), liver dysfunction/disease, known/suspected pregnancy. Assess use in patients ≥65 yrs, nursing females, hypocalcemia, asthma, DM, epilepsy, migraine or porphyria, SLE, and hepatic hemangiomas. Assess for drug and lab interactions.

**Monitoring:** Monitor for signs/symptoms of cardiovascular disorders (eg, MI, stroke, venous thrombosis, PE), malignant neoplasms (eg, cancers of endometrium, breast, ovaries), dementia, gallbladder disease, hypercalcemia, visual abnormalities (eg, retinal vascular thrombosis), cholestatic jaundice, increased BP, hypertriglyceridemia, hypothyroidism, hypocalcemia, exacerbation of endometriosis and other conditions (eg, asthma, DM, epilepsy, migraine or porphyria, SLE, and hepatic hemangiomas). Monitor thyroid function in patients on thyroid replacement therapy. Perform proper diagnostic testing (eg, endometrial sampling) to rule out malignancy when undiagnosed, persistent or recurring, abnormal vaginal bleeding occurs. Perform periodic evaluation every 3-6 months to determine need for therapy.



**Patient Counseling:** Inform that medication increases risk for uterine cancer and may increase chances for heart attack, stroke, breast cancer, and blood clots. Advise to contact physician if breast lumps, unusual vaginal bleeding, dizziness or faintness, changes in speech, severe headaches, chest pain, SOB, leg pain, visual changes, or vomiting occur. Inform once in place, transdermal system should not be exposed to sun for prolonged periods of time. Removal of system should be done carefully and slowly to avoid skin irritation. If patch falls off during dosing interval, apply new patch for remainder of the 7-day period.

**Administration:** Transdermal application. Site of application should not be oily, damaged, or irritated. Apply patch after opening pouch and removing protective liner. Ensure patch sticks completely, especially around edges.
**Storage:** Do not store above 30°C (86°F). Do not store unpouched. Keep out of reach of children.

## CLIMARA PRO — RX

levonorgestrel - estradiol (Bayer Healthcare)

**Estrogens and progestins should not be used for the prevention of cardiovascular disease or dementia. Increased risks of MI, stroke, invasive breast cancer, PE, and DVT in postmenopausal women (50-79 yrs of age) reported. Increased risk of developing probable dementia in postmenopausal women ≥65 yrs of age reported.**

**THERAPEUTIC CLASS:** Estrogen/progestogen combination

**INDICATIONS:** Treatment of moderate to severe vasomotor symptoms associated with menopause. Prevention of postmenopausal osteoporosis.

**DOSAGE:** *Adults:* Apply 1 patch weekly to lower abdomen or upper area of buttocks (avoid breasts and waistline). Rotate application site; allow 1 week between same site. Re-evaluate periodically (3-6 month intervals).

**HOW SUPPLIED:** Patch: (Estradiol-Levonorgestrel): 0.045mg-0.015mg/day [4[s]]

**CONTRAINDICATIONS:** Pregnancy, undiagnosed abnormal genital bleeding, breast cancer, estrogen-dependent neoplasia, DVT/PE, active or recent (eg, within 1 yr) thromboembolic disease (eg, stroke, MI), liver dysfunction or disease.

**WARNINGS/PRECAUTIONS:** May increase risk of cardiovascular events (eg, MI, stroke), venous thrombosis, and PE; d/c immediately if any of these events occur or are suspected. May increase risk of breast/endometrial cancer, and gallbladder disease. Retinal vascular thrombosis reported; monitor and d/c if papilledema or retinal vascular lesions occur. Consider addition of a progestin if no hysterectomy. May elevate BP; monitor at regular intervals. May cause elevations of plasma triglycerides with pre-existing hypertriglyceridemia. Caution with history of cholestatic jaundice associated with past estrogen use or with pregnancy; d/c with recurrence. May lead to increased thyroid-binding globulin levels; monitor thyroid function. May cause fluid retention; caution with cardiac/renal dysfunction. Caution with severe hypocalcemia. May increase risk of ovarian cancer. May exacerbate endometriosis, asthma, DM, epilepsy, migraine, porphyria; use with caution.

**ADVERSE REACTIONS:** Application-site reaction, vaginal bleeding, breast pain, upper respiratory infection, back pain, headache, depression, arthralgia, flu syndrome, abdominal pain.

**INTERACTIONS:** CYP3A4 inducers (eg, St. John's wort, phenobarbital, carbamazepine, rifampin) may decrease levels which may decrease therapeutic effects and/or change uterine bleeding profile. CYP3A4 inhibitors (eg, erythromycin, clarithromycin, ketoconazole, itraconazole, ritonavir, grapefruit juice) may increase levels which may result in side effects.

**PREGNANCY:** Contraindicated in pregnancy, caution in nursing.

C

**MECHANISM OF ACTION:** Estradiol: Estrogen. Binds to nuclear receptors in estrogen-responsive tissue. Modulates pituitary secretion of gonadotropins, luteinizing hormone (LH) and follicle stimulating hormone, through negative feedback mechanism. Levonorgestrel: Progestogen. Inhibits gonadotropin production resulting in retardation of follicular growth and inhibition of ovulation. Counteracts proliferative effects of estrogens in endometrium.

**PHARMACOKINETICS: Absorption:**(Single dose): Estradiol: $C_{max}$=54.3pg/mL, $T_{max}$=42 hrs, AUC=6340pg•hr/mL; Estrone (metabolite): $C_{max}$=43.9pg/mL, $T_{max}$=84 hrs, AUC=6890pg•hr/ mL; Levonorgestrel: $C_{max}$=138pg/mL, $T_{max}$=90 hrs, AUC=22900pg•hr/mL. **Distribution:** Estrogens and progestin found in breast milk. Estradiol: Widely distributed; largely bound to sex hormone binding globulin (SHBG) and albumin. Levonorgestrel: Bound to SHBG and albumin. **Metabolism:** Estradiol: Hepatic, to estrone (metabolite); estriol (major urinary metabolite); enterohepatic recirculation, via sulfate and glucuronide conjugation; biliary secretion of conjugates into intestine; hydrolysis in gut, reabsorption. CYP3A4 (partial). Levonorgestrel: Reduction, hydroxylation, conjugation. **Elimination:** Estradiol, estrone, estriol: Urine. Estradiol: $T_{1/2}$=3 hrs. Levonorgestrel: Urine; $T_{1/2}$=28 hrs.

## NURSING CONSIDERATIONS

**Assessment:** Assess for abnormal genital bleeding, presence or history of breast cancer, estrogen-dependent neoplasia, DVT or PE, active or recent (within past yr) arterial thromboembolic disease (eg, stroke, MI), liver dysfunction/disease, and known/suspected pregnancy. Assess use in patients undergoing surgery associated with thromboembolism, patients with prolonged immobilization, nursing females, patients ≥65 yrs, presence of hypocalcemia, presence of asthma, DM, epilepsy, migraines or porphyria, SLE, or presence of hepatic hemangiomas. Assess for drug/lab test interactions.

**Monitoring:** Monitor for signs/symptoms of cardiovascular disorders (eg, stroke, MI, venous thrombosis, pulmonary embolism), malignant neoplasms (eg, cancers of endometrium, breast, ovaries), dementia, gallbladder disease, hypercalcemia, visual abnormalities (eg, retinal vascular thrombosis), elevated BP, hypertriglyceridemia, cholestatic jaundice, hypothyroidism, fluid retention, hypocalcemia, exacerbation of endometriosis and other conditions (eg, asthma, DM, epilepsy, migraines or porphyria, SLE, and hepatic hemangiomas). Periodically monitor BP and thyroid function in patients on thyroid replacement therapy. Periodically reassess use of therapy (every 3-6 months). If abnormal genital bleeding occurs, perform proper diagnostic measures (eg, endometrial sampling) to rule out malignancy.

**Patient Counseling:** Inform that drug may increase risk for heart attack, stroke, breast cancer, blood clots, and dementia. Instruct to report breast lumps, unusual vaginal bleeding, dizziness/faintness, changes in speech, severe headaches, chest pain, or SOB. Inform once transdermal system is in place, it should not be exposed to sun for prolonged periods of time. Counsel that if patch falls off, may reapply same patch or place new patch on different area. Remove patch carefully and slowly to avoid skin irritation.

**Administration:** Transdermal route. Site of application should not be oily, damaged, or irritated. Apply patch immediately after opening pouch and removing protective liner. Ensure that patch sticks, especially around edges. **Storage:** 20-25°C (68-77°F); excursions permitted to 15-30°C (59-86°F). Do not store above 30°C (86°F). Keep out of reach of children. Do not store unpouched.

# CLINDAGEL — RX

clindamycin phosphate (Galderma)

**OTHER BRAND NAMES:** Clindagel Inactive (Galderma)

**THERAPEUTIC CLASS:** Lincomycin derivative

**INDICATIONS:** Acne vulgaris.

**DOSAGE:** *Adults:* Apply thin film once daily.
*Pediatrics:* ≥12 yrs: Apply thin film once daily.

C

**HOW SUPPLIED:** Gel: 1% [40mL, 75mL]

**CONTRAINDICATIONS:** Hypersensitivity to lincomycin. History of regional enteritis, ulcerative colitis, or antibiotic-associated colitis.

**WARNINGS/PRECAUTIONS:** D/C if significant diarrhea occurs. Caution in atopic individuals.

**ADVERSE REACTIONS:** Peeling, pruritus, pseudomembranous colitis (rare).

**INTERACTIONS:** May potentiate neuromuscular blockers.

**PREGNANCY:** Category B, not for use in nursing.

**MECHANISM OF ACTION:** Lincomycin derivative; inhibits bacteria protein synthesis at ribosomal level by binding to the 50S ribosomal subunit and affecting the process of peptide chain initiation.

**PHARMACOKINETICS: Absorption:** $C_{max}$≤5.5ng/mL. **Distribution:** Orally and parenterally administered clindamycin appears in breast milk. **Excretion:** Urine (<0.4% of total dose).

## NURSING CONSIDERATIONS

**Assessment:** Assess for hypersensitivity to lincomycin, history of regional or ulcerative colitis, antibiotic-associated colitis, nursing status. Assess use in atopic individuals and for possible drug interactions.

**Monitoring:** Monitor for signs/symptoms of colitis (pseudomembranous colitis), diarrhea, and bloody diarrhea. In patients with diarrhea, consider stool culture for *C.difficile* and stool assay for *C.difficile* toxin. In patients with significant diarrhea, consider large bowel endoscopy.

**Patient Counseling:** Instruct to notify physician of significant diarrhea during therapy or up to several weeks following therapy end.

**Administration:** Topical application. **Storage:** Controlled room temperature, 20-25°C (68-77°F); excursions permitted to 15-30°C (59-86°F). Keep container tightly closed, out of direct sunlight.

# CLOBEVATE RX

clobetasol propionate (Stiefel)

**THERAPEUTIC CLASS:** Corticosteroid

**INDICATIONS:** Inflammatory and pruritic manifestations of corticosteroid-responsive dermatoses.

**DOSAGE:** *Adults:* Apply thin layer bid. Limit treatment to 2 consecutive weeks. Max: 50g/week. Avoid with occlusive dressings.
*Pediatrics:* ≥12 yrs: Apply thin layer bid. Limit treatment to 2 consecutive weeks. Max: 50g/week. Avoid with occlusive dressings.

**HOW SUPPLIED:** Gel: 0.05% [45g]

**WARNINGS/PRECAUTIONS:** May produce reversible HPA axis suppression, manifestations of Cushing's syndrome, hyperglycemia, and glucosuria. Pediatrics may be more susceptible to systemic toxicity. D/C if irritation occurs. Use appropriate antifungal or antibacterial with concomitant skin infections; d/c if infection does not clear. Should not be used to treat rosacea or perioral dermatitis. Avoid use on face, groin, or axillae.

**ADVERSE REACTIONS:** Burning, stinging, irritation, pruritus, erythema, folliculitis, cracking and fissuring of the skin, numbness of fingers, skin atrophy, telangiectasia.

**PREGNANCY:** Category C, caution in nursing.

**MECHANISM OF ACTION:** Corticosteroid; not established. Has anti-inflammatory, antipruritic, and vasoconstrictive properties. Anti-inflammatory not established; thought to induct phospholipase $A_2$ inhibitory proteins called lipocortins. Lipocortins control the biosynthesis of potent mediators of inflammation (eg, prostaglandins, leukotrienes) through inhibition of their common precursor, arachidonic acid. Arachidonic acid is released from membrane phospholipids by phospholipase $A_2$.

**PHARMACOKINETICS: Absorption:** Absorbed through skin. Occlusive dressings ≤24 hrs, no effect. Occlusive dressings at 96 hrs, markedly enhances penetration. **Distribution:** Systemically administered corticosteroids appear in breast milk.

## NURSING CONSIDERATIONS

**Assessment:** Assess use in patients who are <12 years old, and in pregnant/nursing females. Prior to therapy, assess patient is not using medication for treatment of rosacea or perioral dermatitis. Assess medication is not for use on the face, groin, or axillae areas.

**Monitoring:** Monitor for signs of HPA axis suppression, Cushing's syndrome, hyperglycemia, and glucosuria. In patients on high doses of corticosteroids, perform periodic monitoring for HPA-axis suppression using the ACTH stimulation, AM plasma cortisol, and urinary free cortisol tests. Monitor for signs of skin irritation and allergic contact dermatitis (eg, failure to heal). Monitor and treat if signs of concomitant skin infection develops (eg, fungal, bacterial).

**Patient Counseling:** Counsel to use medication exactly as directed. Instruct medication for external use only and to avoid contact with eyes. Inform not to use occlusive dressings with medication. Instruct to notify physician if any type of skin reaction or infection develops or if surgery is being contemplated while on medication.

**Administration:** Topical. Treatment should be limited to 2 consecutive weeks, and not to exceed ≥50g per week. **Storage:** Store between 15-30°C (59-86°F). Do not refrigerate.

# CLOBEX — RX

clobetasol propionate (Galderma)

**THERAPEUTIC CLASS:** Corticosteroid

**INDICATIONS:** (Lot) Relief of corticosteroid responsive dermatoses. Treatment of moderate to severe plaque psoriasis (<10% BSA). (Shampoo) Treatment of moderate to severe scalp psoriasis. (Spray) Treatment of moderate to severe plaque psoriasis affecting up to 20% BSA.

**DOSAGE:** *Adults:* ≥18 yrs: (Lot) Apply bid for up to 2 consecutive weeks. Psoriasis: Reassess after 2 weeks; may repeat for additional 2 weeks. Max: 50g/week or 50mL/week. (Shampoo) Apply thin film daily to dry scalp for up to 4 consecutive weeks. Leave in place for 15 mins before lathering and rinsing. (Spray) Spray on affected area(s) bid. Rub in gently and completely. Reassess after 2 weeks; may repeat for additional 2 weeks. Limit treatment to 4 weeks. Max: 50g/week.

**HOW SUPPLIED:** Lot: 0.05% [59mL, 118mL]; Shampoo: 0.05% [118mL]; Spray: 0.05% [59mL, 125mL]

**WARNINGS/PRECAUTIONS:** Not for use on the face, groin, axillae, eyes, lips, or for the treatment of rosacea or perioral dermatitis. May produce reversible HPA axis suppression, manifestations of Cushing's syndrome, hyperglycemia, and glucosuria. D/C if irritation occurs. Use appropriate antifungal or antibacterial agent with dermatological infections.

**ADVERSE REACTIONS:** Burning/stinging, pruritus, folliculitis, skin dryness, skin atrophy, telangiectasia.

**PREGNANCY:** Category C, caution in nursing.

**MECHANISM OF ACTION:** Corticosteroid; not fully established. Contains anti-inflammatory, antipruritic, and vasoconstrictive properties. Corticosteroids thought to act by induction of phospholipase $A_2$ inhibitory proteins, called lipocortins. Lipocortins control the biosynthesis of potent mediators of inflammation (eg, prostaglandins, leukotrienes) through inhibiting the release of their precursor, arachidonic acid. Arachidonic acid is released from membrane phospholipids by phospholipase $A_2$.

**PHARMACOKINETICS: Absorption:** Use of occlusive dressings ≥24 hrs, no change in drug penetration; use of occlusive dressings for up to 96 hrs, markedly increased drug penetration. **Distribution:** Systemically administered corticosteroids are found in breast milk. **Metabolism:** Liver **Elimination:** Kidneys, bile.



## NURSING CONSIDERATIONS

**Assessment:** Assess that the medication is not being used for the treatment of rosacea or perioral dermatitis or for the treatment on the face, groin, or underarm areas. Assess for hypersensitivity to other corticosteroids and conditions that increase systemic absorption of the medication. Assess use in pregnancy/nursing.

**Monitoring:** Monitor for signs/symptoms of HPA-axis suppression, Cushing's syndrome, hyperglycemia, and glucosuria. Monitor for signs of skin irritation, allergic contact dermatitis (eg, failure to heal), and skin infections (eg, bacterial, fungal); treat accordingly.

**Patient Counseling:** Use as directed; do not exceed the use of drug longer than the prescribed time period. Advise to not bandage, cover, or wrap treated area unless directed to do so. Instruct that drug is for external use only; do not use on face, underarms, groin area, or lips. Instruct to wash hands after applying medication. Advise to notify physician if any signs of local or systemic adverse effects develop, if no improvement is seen within 2 weeks, or if contemplating surgery while on medication.

**Administration:** Topical application. Do not use >50g per week. **Storage:** 20-25°C (68-77°F). Avoid freezing.

# CLODERM **RX**

clocortolone pivalate (Healthpoint)

**THERAPEUTIC CLASS:** Topical corticosteroid

**INDICATIONS:** Corticosteroid-responsive dermatoses.

**DOSAGE:** *Adults:* Apply tid. Use with occlusive dressing for management of psoriasis or recalcitrant conditions.
*Pediatrics:* Apply TID. Use with occlusive dressing for management of psoriasis or recalcitrant conditions.

**HOW SUPPLIED:** Cre: 0.1% [15g, 45g, 90g]

**WARNINGS/PRECAUTIONS:** May produce reversible HPA axis suppression, manifestations of Cushing's syndrome, hyperglycemia, glucosuria. Caution when applied to large surface areas or under occlusive dressings. Use appropriate antifungal or antibacterial agent with dermatological infections. D/C if infection is not adequately controlled or if irritation develops.

**ADVERSE REACTIONS:** Burning, itching, irritation, dryness, folliculitis, hypertrichosis, acneiform eruptions, hypopigmentation, perioral/allergic contact dermatitis, secondary infection, skin atrophy.

**PREGNANCY:** Category C, caution in nursing.

**MECHANISM OF ACTION:** Topical corticosteroid; mechanism not established. Possesses anti-inflammatory, anti-pruritic, and vasoconstrictive actions.

**PHARMACOKINETICS: Absorption:** Percutaneous; occlusion, inflammation, and other skin diseases increase absorption. **Distribution:** Bound to plasma protein to varying degrees. Systemically administered corticosteroids found in breast milk. **Metabolism:** Liver. **Elimination:** Kidney and bile.

## NURSING CONSIDERATIONS

**Assessment:** Assess use in pregnant/nursing females and in pediatric patients.

**Monitoring:** Monitor for signs/symptoms of HPA-axis suppression, Cushing's syndrome, hyperglycemia, and glucosuria. In patients on large doses of medication or using occlusive dressings, perform periodic testing for HPA-axis suppression by using the urinary free cortisol and ACTH stimulation tests. Monitor for systemic toxicity in pediatric patients. Monitor for signs of skin irritation, dermatological infections (eg, bacterial, fungal), and treat appropriately.

**Patient Counseling:** Counsel to use as directed; avoid contact with eyes. Advise not to bandage or wrap treated skin areas unless directed. Instruct to report any signs of local adverse reactions. Instruct caregivers of pediatric patients to avoid using tight-fitting diapers or plastic pants on treatment area.

**Administration:** Topical application. **Storage:** Store at 15-30°C (59-86°F). Avoid freezing.

## CLOLAR — RX

clofarabine (Genzyme)

**THERAPEUTIC CLASS:** Antimetabolite

**INDICATIONS:** Treatment of pediatric patients 1-21 years old with relapsed or refractory acute lymphoblastic leukemia after at least 2 prior regimens.

**DOSAGE:** *Pediatrics:* 1-21 yrs: 52mg/m$^2$ IV over 2 hours daily for 5 consecutive days. Treatment cycles are repeated following recovery or return to baseline organ function, approximately every 2-6 weeks. Provide supportive care such as IV fluids, allopurinol, and alkalinize urine throughout 5 days of therapy. Consider prophylactic anti-emetic medications. D/C if hypotension develops during 5 days of therapy. D/C if a Grade 4 noninfectious nonhematologic toxicity occurs. The use of prophylactic steroids (eg, 100mg/m$^2$ hydrocortisone on Days 1-3) may be of benefit in preventing signs and symptoms of systemic inflammatory response syndrome (SIRS) or capillary leak. If develop signs and symptoms of SIRS or capillary leak, d/c therapy and provide appropriate supportive measures. Monitor renal and hepatic function during 5 days of therapy. Monitor cardiac function. Dose Modifications and Reinitiation: Hematologic Toxicity: Subsequent cycles should not be earlier than 14 days from the first day of previous cycle with ANC ≥0.75 x 10$^9$/L. Grade 4 Neutropenia (ANC <0.5 x 10$^9$/L) ≥4 weeks: Reduce dose by 25% for the next cycle. Non-Hematologic Toxicity: Withhold if clinically significant infection develops, restart at full dose if infection is clinically controlled. Grade 3 Noninfectious Nonhematological Toxicity: Withhold therapy. Re-institute at a 25% dose reduction if resolution or return to baseline occurs. Grade 3 or Higher Increases in Creatinine or Bilirubin: D/C administration. Reinstitute when patient is stable and organ function has returned to baseline, generally with a 25% dose reduction.

**HOW SUPPLIED:** Inj: 1mg/mL

**WARNINGS/PRECAUTIONS:** Monitor CBC and platelet count during therapy. Anticipate suppression of bone marrow function. Severe bone marrow depression including neutropenia, anemia, and thrombocytopenia have been observed. Increased risk of infection, including severe sepsis is possible. Monitor for signs and symptoms of infection and treat promptly. Administration may result in a rapid reduction of peripheral leukemia cells; evaluate and monitor for signs and symptoms of tumor lysis syndrome. Provide IV infusion fluids throughout 5 days of administration to reduce effects of tumor lysis and other adverse events. Administer allopurinol if hyperuricemia is expected. Evaluate and monitor for cytokine release that could develop into SIRS, capillary leak syndrome, and organ dysfunction. D/C immediately if SIRS or capillary leak syndrome develop. Elevated hepatobiliary enzymes reported. Caution in patients with renal or hepatic dysfunction.

**ADVERSE REACTIONS:** N/V, diarrhea, anemia, leukopenia, thrombocytopenia, febrile neutropenia, headache, rash, pruritus, pyrexia, fatigue, palmar-plantar erythrodysesthesia syndrome, anxiety, flushing, and mucosal inflammation.

**INTERACTIONS:** High risk of hepatotoxicity with etoposide and cyclophosphamide. Consider avoiding concomitant administration of nephrotoxic and hepatotoxic drugs. Monitor during concomitant administration of medications known to affect blood pressure. Stevens-Johnson syndrome (SJS) and toxic epidermal necrolysis (TEN) reported in patients receiving clofarabine and other medications (eg, antibiotics, allopurinol) known to cause these syndromes.

**PREGNANCY:** Category D, not for use in nursing.

**MECHANISM OF ACTION:** Antimetabolite; clofarabine is sequentially metabolized intracellularly to the 5'-monophosphate metabolite by deoxycytidine kinase and mono- and di-phospho-kinases to the active 5'-triphophate metabolite. Clofarabine inhibits DNA synthesis by decreasing cellular deoxynucleotide triphosphate pools through an inhibitory action on ribonucleotide reductase, and by terminating DNA chain elongation and inhibiting repair through incorporation into DNA chain by competitive inhibition of DNA polymerases. Clofarabine 5'-triphosphate also disrupts the integrity of mitochondrial membrane leading to release of the pro-apoptotic mitochondrial proteins, cytochrome C and apoptosis-inducing factor, leading to programmed cell death.

**PHARMACOKINETICS: Distribution:** $V_d$=172L/$m^2$; plasma protein binding (47%). **Elimination:** Urine (49-60%, unchanged); $T_{1/2}$=5.2 hrs.

## NURSING CONSIDERATIONS

**Assessment:** Assess for hepatic/renal dysfunction, CBC with platelet count and differential, pregnancy/nursing status, and possible drug interactions. Assess for other diseases/conditions that patient has.

**Monitoring:** Monitor for signs and symptoms of infection including sepsis, bone marrow suppression, neutropenia, anemia, thrombocytopenia, hypotension, tumor lysis syndrome, SIRS, capillary leak syndrome, and organ dysfunction. Monitor CBC, platelet counts, BP, LFTs, cardiac function, respiratory function, and kidney function.

**Patient Counseling:** Advise patient to return for regular blood counts and to report any symptoms associated with hematological toxicity (eg, weakness, fatigue, pallor, shortness of breath, easy bruising, purpura, fever). Advise about signs or symptoms of infection (eg, fever) and to report if they occur. Inform about signs or symptoms of SIRS (eg, fever, tachycardia, tachypnea). Instruct to avoid any medications, including OTC herbal medications, that may be hepatotoxic or nephrotoxic, during 5 days of clofarabine administration. Advise to use effective contraceptive measures to prevent pregnancy and female patients to avoid breastfeeding during treatment.

**Administration:** IV route. Filter drug through a 0.2µm syringe filter, then dilute with D5W or 0.9% NS prior to infusion to a final concentration between 0.15mg/mL and 0.4mg/mL. Admixture must be used within 24 hrs. **Storage:** Undiluted Vial: 25°C (77°F); excursions permitted to 15-30°C (59-86°F). Diluted: Store at room temperature (15-30°C).

# CLORPRES — RX

clonidine HCl - chlorthalidone (Mylan)

**THERAPEUTIC CLASS:** Central alpha-agonist/monosulfamyl diuretic

**INDICATIONS:** Treatment of hypertension. Not for initial therapy.

**DOSAGE:** *Adults:* Determine dose by individual titration. 0.1mg clonidine-15mg chlorthalidone tab qd-bid. Max: 0.6mg clonidine-30mg chlorthalidone/day.

**HOW SUPPLIED:** Tab: (Clonidine-Chlorthalidone) 0.1mg-15mg*, 0.2mg-15mg*, 0.3mg-15mg* *scored

**CONTRAINDICATIONS:** Anuria, sulfonamide hypersensitivity.

**WARNINGS/PRECAUTIONS:** Caution with severe renal disease, hepatic dysfunction, asthma, severe coronary insufficiency, recent MI, cerebrovascular disease. May develop allergic reaction to oral clonidine if sensitive to clonidine patch. Avoid abrupt withdrawal. Continue therapy to within 4 hrs of surgery and resume after. Monitor for fluid/electrolyte imbalance. Hyperuricemia, hypokalemia, hyponatremia, hypochloremic alkalosis, and hyperglycemia may occur.

**ADVERSE REACTIONS:** Drowsiness, dizziness, constipation, sedation, fatigue, dry mouth, NV, orthostatic symptoms.

**INTERACTIONS:** Potentiates other antihypertensives. May increase response to tubocurarine. May decrease arterial response to norepinephrine. Antidiabetic agents may need adjustment. Risk of lithium toxicity. TCAs may reduce effects of clonidine. Amitriptyline may enhance ocular toxicity. Enhanced CNS-depressive effects of alcohol, barbiturates, or other sedatives. Orthostatic hypotension aggravated by alcohol, barbiturates, narcotics. D/C β-blockers several days before the gradual withdrawal of clonidine in patients taking both.

**PREGNANCY:** (Clonidine) Category C, caution in nursing. (Chlorthalidone) Category B, not for use in nursing.

**MECHANISM OF ACTION:** Clonidine: Imidazoline derivative; stimulates α-adrenoceptor in brain stem, resulting in reduced sympathetic outflow from CNS and decrease in peripheral resistance, renal vascular resistance, HR, and BP. Chlorthalidone: Monosulfamyl diuretic; increases excretion of $Na^+$ and $Cl^-$; decreases extracellular fluid volume, plasma volume, cardiac output, total exchangeable sodium, glomerular filtration rate, and renal plasma flow.

**PHARMACOKINETICS: Absorption:** Clonidine: $T_{max}$=3-5 hrs. **Distribution:** Chlorthalidone: Plasma protein binding (75%). **Metabolism:** Clonidine: Liver (50%). **Elimination:** Clonidine: Urine (40-60% unchanged); $T_{1/2}$=12-16 hrs; $T_{1/2}$ in severe renal impairment=41 hrs. Chlorthalidone: Urine (unchanged); $T_{1/2}$=40-60 hrs.

## NURSING CONSIDERATIONS

**Assessment:** Assess for anuria, sulfonamide hypersensitivity, coronary insufficiency, recent MI, cerebrovascular disease, history of allergy or bronchial asthma, systemic lupus erythematosus (SLE), DM, renal/hepatic impairment, pregnancy/nursing status, and possible drug interactions. Perform and obtain serum and urine electrolytes.

**Monitoring:** Monitor blood pressure. Periodically monitor serum and urine electrolytes, serum PBI level, serum $K^+$ levels, and renal function. Monitor for signs/symptoms of electrolyte imbalance, hypokalemia, possible exacerbation or activation of SLE, hyperglycemia, withdrawal symptoms, hyperuricemia or precipitation of gout, hypersensitivity reactions, renal/hepatic dysfunction.

**Patient Counseling:** Caution that drug may impair physical/mental abilities. Inform to avoid alcohol. Instruct not to interrupt or d/c therapy without consulting physician. Seek medical attention if symptoms of electrolyte imbalance (dry mouth, thirst, weakness), hypokalemia (thirst, tiredness, restlessness), withdrawal (nervousness, agitation, headaches), or hypersensitivity reactions occur.

**Administration:** Oral route. **Storage:** 15-30°C (59-86°F). Avoid excessive humidity.

# CLOTRIMAZOLE TOPICAL — RX

clotrimazole (Various)

**THERAPEUTIC CLASS:** Azole antifungal

**INDICATIONS:** Topical treatment of candidiasis due to *Candida albicans* and tinea versicolor due to *Malassezia furfur.*

**DOSAGE:** *Adults:* Apply bid (am and pm). Re-evaluate if no improvement after 4 weeks.
*Pediatrics:* Apply bid (am and pm). Re-evaluate if no improvement after 4 weeks.

**HOW SUPPLIED:** Cre: 1% [15g, 30g, 45g]; Sol: 1% [10mL, 30mL]

**WARNINGS/PRECAUTIONS:** Not for ophthalmic use. D/C if irritation or sensitivity occurs. If lack of a response, appropriate microbiological studies should be repeated to confirm diagnosis and rule out other pathogens before instituting another course of antimycotic therapy.

**ADVERSE REACTIONS:** Erythema, stinging, blistering, peeling, edema, pruritus, urticaria, burning, irritation.

**PREGNANCY:** Category B, caution in nursing.

**MECHANISM OF ACTION:** Broad spectrum antifungal agent; primary action is against dividing and growing organisms. Causes leakage of intracellular phosphorus compounds into the ambient medium with concomitant breakdown of cellular nucleic acids and accelerated potassium efflux.

**PHARMACOKINETICS: Absorption:** Minimally absorbed. **Elimination:** Urine (≤0.5%).



## NURSING CONSIDERATIONS

**Assessment:** Assess for proper diagnosis and pregnancy/nursing status.

**Monitoring:** Monitor for signs/symptoms of irritation or sensitivity at treatment site. Monitor for clinical response; if lack of response, repeat appropriate microbiological studies to confirm diagnosis.

**Patient Counseling:** Advise to use medication for full treatment period even if symptoms improve. Instruct to contact physician if no improvement seen after 4 weeks of therapy. Counsel to inform physician if treatment area shows signs of increased irritation (eg, redness, itching, burning, blistering, swelling, oozing). Advise to avoid sources of infection or reinfection. (Cre) Instruct to avoid the use of occlusive dressings or wrappings.

**Administration:** Topical route. **Storage:** Cre: 2-30°C (36-86°F). Sol: 2-30°C (36-86°F).

# CLOZAPINE RX

clozapine (Various)

**Risk of agranulocytosis, seizures, myocarditis, and other adverse cardiovascular and respiratory effects. Conduct baseline WBC and differential before therapy, then regularly, and 4 weeks after d/c. Elderly patients with dementia-related psychosis treated with atypical antipsychotic drugs are at an increased risk of death; most appeared to be cardiovascular (eg, heart failure, sudden death) or infectious (eg, pneumonia) in nature. Clozapine is not approved for the treatment of patients with dementia-related psychosis.**

**OTHER BRAND NAMES:** Clozaril (Novartis)

**THERAPEUTIC CLASS:** Dibenzapine derivative

**INDICATIONS:** Management of severe schizophrenia when response to standard schizophrenia treatment fails. To reduce the risk of recurrent suicidal behavior with schizophrenia or schizoaffective disorder.

**DOSAGE:** *Adults:* Initial: 12.5mg qd-bid. Titrate: Increase by 25-50mg/day, up to 300-450mg/day by end of 2nd week, then increase weekly or bi-weekly by up to 100mg. Usual: 100-900mg/day given tid. Max: 900mg/day. If at risk of suicidal behavior then treat for at least 2 yrs then assess; reassess thereafter at regular intervals. To d/c, gradually reduce dose over 1-2 weeks. Monitor for psychotic symptoms if abrupt d/c warranted (eg, leukopenia). To restart after brief interval off clozapine, reinitiate with 12.5 mg qd-bid and if well tolerated, may increase back to therapeutic dose more quickly than recommended for initial treatment.

**HOW SUPPLIED:** Tab: (Clozapine) 12.5mg, 25mg, 100mg; (Clozaril) 25mg*, 100mg* *scored

**CONTRAINDICATIONS:** Myeloproliferative disorders, uncontrolled epilepsy, paralytic ileus, history of clozapine induced agranulocytosis or severe granulocytopenia, severe CNS depression, coma, with agents with potential to cause agranulocytosis or suppress bone marrow function.

**WARNINGS/PRECAUTIONS:** Reserve treatment for severely ill patients unresponsive to other schizophrenia therapies. Monitor for hyperglycemia, worsening of glucose control with DM, FBG levels with diabetes risk. Significant risk of orthostatic hypotension, and tachycardia. May impair alertness with initial doses. May cause high fever, hyperglycemia, or pulmonary embolism. Cardiomyopathy reported; d/c unless benefit outweighs risk. Caution with prostatic enlargement; narrow-angle glaucoma; and renal, hepatic, or cardiac/pulmonary disease. NMS and tardive dyskinesia reported. Acquire WBC and ANC at baseline, then weekly for 1st 6 months of therapy, then every 2 weeks for 6 months, and then every 4 weeks thereafter if WBCs and ANC are acceptable. Avoid initiation of treatment if WBCs <3500/mm$^3$, ANC <2000/mm$^3$, history of myeloproliferative disorder, previous clozapine-induced agranulocytosis or granulocytopenia. D/C treatment if WBCs <3000/mm³, ANC <1500/mm³, eosinophils >4000/mm³, or if myocarditis develops. D/C over 1-2 weeks. Varying degrees of intestinal peristalsis impairment (eg, constipation, intestinal obstruction, paralytic ileus), ECG changes reported.



**ADVERSE REACTIONS:** Drowsiness, vertigo, headache, tremor, salivation, sweating, dry mouth, visual disturbances, tachycardia, hypotension, syncope, constipation, NV, weight gain, fever.

**INTERACTIONS:** See Contraindications. Avoid with bone-marrow suppressants, epinephrine, and carbamazepine. Caution with CNS-active drugs, anesthesia, alcohol, paroxetine, sertraline, fluoxetine, fluvoxamine, benzodiazepines, other psychotropics, inhibitors/inducers of CYP1A2, 2D6, 3A4. Potentiates hypotensive effects of antihypertensives and anticholinergic effects of atropine-type drugs. Decrease dose with drugs metabolized by CYP2D6. Caution with general anesthesia. CYP450 inducers (eg, phenytoin, nicotine, rifampin) decrease plasma levels. CYP450 inhibitors (eg, cimetidine, caffeine, erythromycin, ciprofloxacin, citalopram) increase plasma levels.

**PREGNANCY:** Category B, not for use in nursing.

**MECHANISM OF ACTION:** Atypical antipsychotic agent; interferes with binding of dopamine at $D_1$, $D_2$, $D_3$, and $D_5$ receptors. Has high affinity for $D_4$ receptor. Also acts as antagonist at adrenergic, cholinergic, histaminergic, and serotonergic receptors.

**PHARMACOKINETICS: Absorption:** $C_{max}$=319ng/mL; $T_{max}$=2.5 hrs. **Distribution:** Plasma protein binding (97%). **Elimination:** Urine (50%), feces (30%); $T_{1/2}$=8 hrs (after single dose), $T_{1/2}$=12 hrs (after multiple doses).

## NURSING CONSIDERATIONS

**Assessment:** Assess if patient has severe schizophrenic disorder and has failed at least 2 other trials with 2 other standard drugs, schizophrenic disorder and is at risk for suicidal behavior, dementia-related psychosis, myeloproliferative disorders, uncontrolled epilepsy, paralytic ileus, history of clozapine-induced agranulocytosis or severe granulocytopenia, or severe CNS depression prior to therapy. Assess for possible drug interactions. Assess baseline WBC counts and ANC prior to treatment. Assess fasting blood glucose levels in patients who have DM or are at risk for hyperglycemia.

**Monitoring:** Monitor for clinical response to treatment, WBC counts and ANC during therapy and for at least 4 weeks following discontinuation. Refer to PI for specific scheduling parameters. Monitor for agranulocytosis, myocarditis, other cardiovascular complications (eg, orthostatic hypotension, cardiomyopathy, cardiac arrest), respiratory complications, seizures, NMS, TD, fever, pulmonary embolism, and hepatitis.

**Patient Counseling:** Inform of need for regular monitoring of WBC counts and ANC. Advise to report immediately any lethargy, weakness, fever, sore throat, or any signs/symptoms of infection during therapy. Inform that drug have significant risk of seizure; avoid driving and other potentially hazardous activity. Counsel to avoid alcohol and notify if taking alcohol or any other OTC and prescription drugs. Advise to contact physician if more than 2 days of doses are missed. Counsel females to avoid pregnancy/nursing.

**Administration:** Oral route. **Storage:** Do not exceed 30°C (86°F). Dispense in tight, light-resistant container with child-resistant closure.

# COLAZAL RX

balsalazide disodium (Salix)

**THERAPEUTIC CLASS:** Anti-inflammatory Agent

**INDICATIONS:** Treatment of mild-to-moderate active ulcerative colitis in patients ≥5 yrs.

**DOSAGE:** *Adults:* 3 caps tid for up to 8 weeks (or 12 weeks if needed). May open cap and sprinkle on applesauce.
*Pediatrics:* 5-17 yrs: 1 or 3 caps tid for 8 weeks. May open cap and sprinkle on applesauce.

C

**HOW SUPPLIED:** Cap: 750mg

**CONTRAINDICATIONS:** Hypersensitivity to salicylates.

**WARNINGS/PRECAUTIONS:** May exacerbate symptoms of colitis. Prolonged gastric retention with pyloric stenosis. Caution with renal dysfunction or history of renal disease.

**ADVERSE REACTIONS:** Headache, abdominal pain, diarrhea, NV, respiratory problems, arthralgia, rhinitis, insomnia, fatigue, rectal bleeding, flatulence, fever, dyspepsia.

**INTERACTIONS:** Oral antibiotics may interfere with the release of mesalamine in the colon.

**PREGNANCY:** Category B, caution in nursing.

**MECHANISM OF ACTION:** Not established; a prodrug enzymatically cleaved in colon to produce mesalamine (5-ASA), an anti-inflammatory drug that acts locally to block production of arachidonic acid metabolites in the colon.

**PHARMACOKINETICS: Absorption:** Different dosing conditions (fasted, fed, sprinkled) resulted in variable parameters. **Distribution:** Plasma protein binding ( ≥99%). **Metabolism:** Key metabolites: 5-ASA and N-acetyl-5-ASA. **Elimination:** Urine, feces.

## NURSING CONSIDERATIONS

**Assessment:** Assess for pyloric stenosis, possible drug interactions, history of renal/hepatic disease.

**Monitoring:** Monitor renal function, LFTs, and CBC, signs/symptoms of prolonged gastric retention with pyloric stenosis, worsening of colitis symptoms, and hypersensitivity.

**Patient Counseling:** Inform can take with/without food or sprinkle on applesauce. Teeth and/or tongue may get stained when using sprinkle form with food. Seek medical attention if diagnosed with pyloric stenosis or renal dysfunction, experience worsening of colitis symptoms or hypersensitivity (eg, anaphylaxis, bronchospasm, skin reaction).

**Administration:** Oral route. **Storage:** 20-25°C (68-77°F); excursions permitted to 15-30°C (59-86°F).

# COLCHICINE — RX

colchicine (Various)

**THERAPEUTIC CLASS:** Miscellaneous gout agent

**INDICATIONS:** Treatment and prophylaxis of acute gouty arthritis.

**DOSAGE:** *Adults:* Acute Treatment: Initial: 1-1.2mg, followed by 0.5-0.6mg q1h, or 1-1.2mg q2h or 0.5-0.6mg q2-3h until pain relief, GI discomfort or diarrhea ensues. Usual: 4-8mg/attack. Wait 3 days before retreatment. Prophylaxis: <1 attack/yr: 0.5-0.6mg/day given 3-4x/week. >1 attack/yr: 0.5-0.6mg qd. Severe Cases: 2-3 tabs of 0.5mg or 0.6mg daily. Surgical Gout Prophylaxis: 0.5-0.6mg tid 3 days before and 3 days after surgery.

**HOW SUPPLIED:** Tab: 0.5mg, 0.6mg

**CONTRAINDICATIONS:** Serious GI, renal, hepatic or cardiac disorders, and blood dyscrasias.

**WARNINGS/PRECAUTIONS:** Caution in elderly, debilitated, or with GI, renal, hepatic, cardiac and hematologic disorders. D/C if nausea, vomiting, or diarrhea occurs. Monitor blood counts periodically with long-term therapy. May adversely affect spermatogenesis. Elevates SGOT and alkaline phosphatase. May cause false (+) for urine RBC and Hgb.

**ADVERSE REACTIONS:** Bone marrow depression, peripheral neuritis, purpura, myopathy, alopecia, dermatoses, reversible azoospermia, nausea, vomiting, diarrhea.

**INTERACTIONS:** Inhibited by acidifying agents. Potentiated by alkalinizing agents. Potentiates sympathomimetics and CNS depressants.

**PREGNANCY:** Category C, caution in nursing.

**MECHANISM OF ACTION:** Colchicum alkaloid; not established, but involves reduction in lactic acid production by leukocytes, resulting in a decrease in uric acid deposition and reduction in phagocytosis, abating inflammatory response.

**PHARMACOKINETICS: Absorption:** Rapid. **Elimination:** Biliary and renal excretion.

## NURSING CONSIDERATIONS

**Assessment:** Assess for serious GI tract, renal/hepatic or cardiac disorders, blood dyscrasias, debilitation, and possible drug interactions.

**Monitoring:** Monitor blood counts periodically.

**Patient Counseling:** Inform to learn dose needed and to keep at hand for use at first sign of attack. Advise to d/c if symptoms of NV and diarrhea occur.

**Administration:** Oral route. **Storage:** 15-30°C (59-86°F). Protect from light.

# COLCHICINE/PROBENECID RX

probenecid - colchicine (Various)

**THERAPEUTIC CLASS:** Uricosuric

**INDICATIONS:** Chronic gouty arthritis complicated by frequent, recurrent acute gout attacks.

**DOSAGE:** *Adults:* Initial: 1 tab qd for 1 week, then 1 tab bid. Titrate: May increase by 1 tab/day every 4 weeks. Max: 4 tabs/day. May reduce dose by 1 tab every 6 months if acute attacks have been absent ≥6 months. Decrease dose with gastric intolerance. Renal Impairment: May need to increase dose. May not be effective if CrCl ≤30mL/min.

**HOW SUPPLIED:** Tab: (Colchicine-Probenecid) 0.5mg-500mg

**CONTRAINDICATIONS:** Blood dyscrasias, uric acid kidney stones, children <2 yrs and pregnancy. Do not use in acute gout attack.

**WARNINGS/PRECAUTIONS:** Exacerbation of gout may occur. Use APAP if analgesic needed. Severe allergic reaction and anaphylaxis reported (rare). D/C if hypersensitivity occurs. Caution with peptic ulcer. Monitor for glycosuria. Determine benefit/risk ratio with long-term therapy. Maintain liberal fluid intake and alkalization of urine.

**ADVERSE REACTIONS:** Headache, dizziness, hepatic necrosis, vomiting, nausea, anorexia, sore gums, uric acid stones, renal colic, anaphylaxis, fever, pruritus, blood dyscrasias, peripheral neuritis, muscular weakness, abdominal pain, diarrhea, alopecia, dermatitis.

**INTERACTIONS:** Probenecid increases plasma levels of penicillin and other β-lactams; psychic disturbances reported. Salicylates and pyrazinamide antagonize uricosuric effects. Increased plasma levels of methotrexate, sulfonamides, sulfonylureas, thiopental or ketamine-induced anesthesia, some NSAIDs (eg, indomethacin, naproxen), lorazepam, APAP, and rifampin. Possible false high plasma levels of theophylline.

**PREGNANCY:** Contraindicated in pregnancy; safety in nursing not known.

**MECHANISM OF ACTION:** Probenecid: Uricosuric/renal tubular blocking agent; inhibits tubular reabsorption of urate, increasing urinary excretion of uric acid and decreasing serum urate levels. Colchicine: Colchicum alkaloid; not been established, has prophylactic, suppressive effect helping to reduce incidence of acute attacks and relieve residual pain and mild discomfort.

## NURSING CONSIDERATIONS

**Assessment:** Assess for known blood dyscrasias, uric acid kidney stones, acute vs chronic attack, history of peptic ulcer, and possible drug interactions.

**Monitoring:** Monitor for signs/symptoms of gout exacerbation, allergic reactions, hematuria, renal colic, costovertebral pain, and uric acid stone formation.

**Patient Counseling:** Instruct on importance of liberal fluid intake. Advise to seek medical attention if symptoms of allergic reaction, hematuria, renal colic, or costovertebral pain occur.

C

**Administration:** Oral route. **Storage:** 20-25°C (68-77°F). Protect from light.

## COLESTID RX

colestipol HCl (Pharmacia & Upjohn)

**THERAPEUTIC CLASS:** Bile acid sequestrant

**INDICATIONS:** Adjunct to diet, to reduce elevated serum total and LDL-C in primary hypercholesterolemia.

**DOSAGE:** *Adults:* Initial: Tab: 2g qd-bid. Granules: 1 pkt or 1 scoopful qd-bid. Titrate: Tab: Increase by 2g qd or bid at 1- to 2-month intervals. Granules: May increase at an increment of one dose/day (1 pkt or level tsp of granules) at 1-2 month intervals. Usual: 2-16g/day (tab) or 1-6 pkts or scoopfuls (granules) qd or in divided doses. Always mix granules with liquid. Take 1 tab at a time and swallow tabs whole with plenty of liquid.

**HOW SUPPLIED:** Granules: 5g/pkt [30$^s$ 90$^s$], 5g/scoopful [300g, 500g]; Tab: 1g

**WARNINGS/PRECAUTIONS:** Exclude secondary causes of hypercholesterolemia and obtain a lipid profile prior to therapy. May interfere with normal fat absorption. Chronic use may increase bleeding tendency due to vitamin K deficiency. Monitor cholesterol and TG based on NCEP guidelines. May cause hypothyroidism. May produce or worsen constipation. Avoid constipation with symptomatic CAD. Constipation associated with colestipol may aggravate hemorrhoids. May produce hyperchloremic acidosis with prolonged use. (Granules) Flavored form contains phenylalanine. Always mix granules with water or other fluids before ingesting.

**ADVERSE REACTIONS:** Constipation, abdominal discomfort, indigestion, musculoskeletal pain, headache, AST elevation, ALT elevation, alkaline phosphatase elevation, headache, chest pain, rash, anorexia, fatigue, tachycardia, SOB.

**INTERACTIONS:** May interfere with absorption of folic acid, fat-soluble vitamins (eg, A, D, K), oral phosphate supplements, hydrocortisone. May delay or reduce absorption of concomitant oral medication; take other drugs 1 hr before or 4 hrs after colestipol. Reduces absorption of chlorothiazide, tetracycline, furosemide, penicillin G, HCTZ, and gemfibrozil. Caution with digitalis agents, propranolol.

**PREGNANCY:** Safety in pregnancy not known, caution in nursing.

**MECHANISM OF ACTION:** Bile acid sequestrant; binds bile acids in the intestine, forming a complex that is excreted in the feces, leading to increased fecal loss of bile acids and increased oxidation of cholesterol to bile acids, a decrease in β lipoprotein or LDL, and a decrease in serum cholesterol levels.

**PHARMACOKINETICS: Elimination:** Feces.

### NURSING CONSIDERATIONS

**Assessment:** Assess for secondary causes of hypercholesterolemia (eg, hypothyroidism, DM, nephrotic syndrome, dysproteinemia, obstructive liver disease, alcoholism), pre-existing constipation, pregnancy/nursing status, and for possible drug interactions. Determine baseline lipid profile.

**Monitoring:** Monitor for signs/symptoms of vitamin K deficiency (eg, tendency for bleeding), constipation, hypothyroidism, and for hyperchloremic acidosis. Monitor serum cholesterol, lipoprotein and TG levels

**Patient Counseling:** Instruct to take as prescribed. Advise to take other medications at least 1 hr before or 4 hrs after taking colestipol. Inform about benefits/risks of therapy. Instruct to report any adverse reactions to physician. (Tab) Instruct to take tab one at a time, with plenty of water. Counsel not to cut, crush, or chew tab. (Granules) Advise to mix with water or other fluids before ingesting.

**Administration:** Oral route. **Storage:** 20-25°C (68-77°F).

## COMBIGAN RX

timolol maleate - brimonidine tartrate (Allergan)



**THERAPEUTIC CLASS:** Alpha$_2$-agonist/beta-blocker

**INDICATIONS:** Reduction of elevated intraocular pressure (IOP) in patients with glaucoma or ocular hypertension who require adjunctive or replacement therapy due to inadequately controlled IOP.

**DOSAGE:** *Adults:* 1 drop in affected eye(s) bid approximately 12 hrs apart. Instill other topical ophthalmic products at least 5 min apart.
*Pediatrics:* ≥2 yrs: 1 drop in affected eye(s) bid approximately 12 hrs apart. Instill other topical ophthalmic products at least 5 min apart.

**HOW SUPPLIED:** Sol: (Brimonidine-Timolol) 2mg-5mg/mL

**CONTRAINDICATIONS:** Bronchial asthma, history of bronchial asthma, severe COPD, sinus bradycardia, second- or third-degree AV block, overt cardiac failure, cardiogenic shock.

**WARNINGS/PRECAUTIONS:** Systemic absorption, leading to adverse reactions (including severe respiratory reactions) may occur. Caution with cardiac failure; d/c if cardiac failure develops. Avoid with bronchospastic disease and/or mild-to-moderate COPD. May potentiate syndromes associated with vascular insufficiency; caution with depression, cerebral or coronary insufficiency, Raynaud's phenomenon, orthostatic hypotension, or thromboangiitis obliterans. May increase reactivity to allergens. May potentiate muscle weakness consistent with certain myasthenic symptoms. May mask signs/symptoms of acute hypoglycemia; caution in patients subject to spontaneous hypoglycemia or diabetic patients receiving insulin or hypoglycemic agents. May mask signs of hyperthyroidism. Bacterial keratitis reported with use of multiple-dose containers of topical ophthalmic products. May need to gradually withdraw β-blocking agents in patients undergoing elective surgery.

**ADVERSE REACTIONS:** Allergic conjunctivitis, conjunctival folliculosis, conjunctival hyperemia, eye pruritus, ocular burning/stinging.

**INTERACTIONS:** May reduce BP; caution with antihypertensives and/or cardiac glycosides. Monitor with concomitant oral β-blockers; avoid concomitant use of 2 topical β-blocking agents. Caution with concomitant oral or IV calcium antagonists; avoid concomitant use with impaired cardiac function. Monitor closely with concomitant catecholamine-depleting drugs (eg, reserpine). Possibility of additive or potentiating effect with CNS depressants (eg, alcohol, barbiturates, opiates, sedatives, anesthetics). Concomitant use of β-blockers with digitalis and/or calcium antagonists may have additive effects in prolonging AV-conduction time. Potentiated systemic β-blockade reported with CYP2D6 inhibitors and timolol. Caution with TCAs and/or MAOIs.

**PREGNANCY:** Category C, not for use in nursing.

**MECHANISM OF ACTION:** Decreases elevated IOP. Brimonidine: Selective α-2 adrenergic receptor. Timolol: Nonselective β-blocker.

**PHARMACOKINETICS: Absorption:** Brimonidine: $C_{max}$=30pg/mL; $T_{max}$= 1-4 hrs. Timolol: $C_{max}$=400pg/mL; $T_{max}$=1-3 hrs. **Distribution:** Timolol: Plasma protein binding (60%). **Metabolism:** Brimonidine: Liver (extensive). Timolol: Liver (partial). **Elimination:** Brimonidine: Urine (74%); $T_{1/2}$=3 hrs. Timolol: Excreted mainly by kidney; $T_{1/2}$=7 hrs.

### NURSING CONSIDERATIONS

**Assessment:** Assess for ocular infection; signs/symptoms of systemic absorption of β-adrenergic blockers (eg, potentiation of bronchial asthma, COPD, cerebral or coronary insufficiency, cardiac failure).

**Monitoring:** Monitor IOP, vital signs, renal function, LFTs, and adverse reactions (eg, allergic conjunctivitis, conjunctival folliculosis, conjunctival hyperemia, eye pruritis, ocular burning and stinging).

**Patient Counseling:** To avoid ocular infection, avoid contact of container tip to affected eye. If more than 1 ophthalmic drug is being used, administer at least 5 min apart. Remove contact lenses prior to administration; may be reinserted after 15 min.

**Administration:** Ocular route. **Storage:** 15-25°C (59-77°F). Protect from light.

## CombiPatch RX

norethindrone acetate - estradiol (Novartis)

**Estrogens and progestins should not be used for prevention of cardiovascular disease or dementia. Increased risks of MI, stroke, invasive breast cancer, PE, and DVT in postmenopausal women (50-79 yrs of age) reported. Increased risk of developing probable dementia in postmenopausal women ≥65 yrs of age reported.**

**THERAPEUTIC CLASS:** Estrogen/progestogen combination

**INDICATIONS:** In women with an intact uterus, for the treatment of moderate to severe vasomotor symptoms associated with menopause, vulvar/vaginal atrophy. Treatment of hypoestrogenism due to hypogonadism, castration, or primary ovarian failure.

**DOSAGE:** *Adults:* Continuous Combined Regimen: Apply 0.05mg/0.14mg patch on lower abdomen (avoid breasts and waistline). Apply twice weekly during 28-day cycle. Continuous Sequential Regimen: Wear estradiol-only patch for 1st 14 days of 28-day cycle, replace twice weekly. Apply 0.05mg/0.14mg patch for remaining 14 days, replace twice weekly. For both regimens, use 0.05mg/0.25mg patch if additional progestin required. Re-evaluate at 3-6 month intervals. Rotate sites; allow 1 week between same site.

**HOW SUPPLIED:** Patch: (Estradiol-Norethindrone) 0.05-0.14mg/day, 0.05-0.25mg/day [8[s], 24[s]]

**CONTRAINDICATIONS:** Undiagnosed abnormal genital bleeding, breast cancer, estrogen-dependent neoplasia, DVT, PE, arterial thromboembolic disorder (eg, stroke, MI), liver dysfunction or disease.

**WARNINGS/PRECAUTIONS:** May increase risk of cardiovascular events (eg, MI, stroke), venous thrombosis, and PE; d/c immediately if any of these events occur or are suspected. May increase risk of breast/endometrial cancer, and gallbladder disease. May lead to severe hypercalcemia with breast cancer and bone metastases; monitor and d/c if hypercalcemia occurs. Retinal vascular thrombosis reported; monitor and d/c if papilledema or retinal vascular lesions occur. May elevate BP; monitor at regular intervals. May cause elevations of plasma triglycerides with pre-existing hypertriglyceridemia. Caution with history of cholestatic jaundice associated with past estrogen use or with pregnancy; d/c with recurrence. May lead to increased thyroid-binding globulin levels; monitor thyroid function. May cause fluid retention; caution with cardiac/renal dysfunction. Caution with severe hypocalcemia. May increase risk of ovarian cancer. May exacerbate endometriosis, asthma, DM, epilepsy, migraine, porphyria, SLE, and hepatic hemangiomas; use with caution.

**ADVERSE REACTIONS:** Abdominal pain, back pain, asthenia, flu syndrome, application site reaction, nausea, nervousness, pharyngitis, respiratory disorder, breast pain, dysmenorrhea, menstrual disorder, vaginitis.

**INTERACTIONS:** CYP3A4 inducers (eg, St. John's wort, phenobarbital, carbamazepine, rifampin) may decrease levels which may decrease therapeutic effects and/or change uterine bleeding profile. CYP3A4 inhibitors (eg, erythromycin, clarithromycin, ketoconazole, itraconazole, ritonavir, grapefruit juice) may increase levels which may result in side effects.

**PREGNANCY:** Contraindicated in pregnancy, caution in nursing.

**MECHANISM OF ACTION:** Estrogen/progestogen. Acts by binding to nuclear receptors in estrogen-responsive tissues. Modulates pituitary secretion of gonadotropins, luteinizing hormone and follicle stimulating hormone, through negative feedback mechanism.

**PHARMACOKINETICS: Absorption:** Estradiol: Well-absorbed. Administration of various doses led to altered parameters. Norethindrone: Well-absorbed.

Administration of various doses led to altered parameters. **Distribution:** Estrogens and progestins found in breast milk. Estradiol: Largely bound to sex hormone binding globulin (SHBG) and albumin. Norethindrone: 90% to SHBG and albumin. **Metabolism:** Liver, to estrone (metabolite); estriol (major urinary metabolite); enterohepatic recirculation, via sulfate and glucuronide conjugation; biliary secretion of conjugates in the intestine; hydrolysis in gut; reabsorption; CYP 3A4 (partial). Norethindrone: Liver. **Elimination:** Estradiol, estrone, estriol: Urine; $T_{1/2}$=2-3 hrs. Norethindrone: $T_{1/2}$=6-8 hrs.

## NURSING CONSIDERATIONS

**Assessment:** Assess for abnormal genital bleeding, presence or history of breast cancer, DVT or PE, estrogen-dependent neoplasias, active or recent (within past yr) arterial thromboembolic disease (eg, stroke, MI), liver dysfunction, and known/suspected pregnancy. Assess use in nursing females, patients ≥65 yrs, presence of severe hypocalcemia, asthma, DM, epilepsy, migraines or porphyria, SLE, or presence of hepatic hemangiomas. Assess for drug or lab interactions.

**Monitoring:** Monitor for signs/symptoms of cardiovascular events (eg, MI, stroke, venous thromboembolism, pulmonary embolism), malignant neoplasms (eg, endometrial, breast, ovarian cancer), dementia, gallbladder disease, hypercalcemia, visual abnormalities (eg, retinal vascular thrombosis), elevated BP, fluid retention, hypertriglyceridemia, cholestatic jaundice, hypothyroidism, exacerbation of endometriosis and other conditions (eg, asthma, DM, epilepsy, migraines or porphyria, SLE, and hepatic hemangiomas). Periodically monitor BP levels and thyroid function in patients on thyroid replacement therapy. Perform periodic assessment (eg, every 3-6 months) to evaluate need for therapy. If abnormal genital bleeding occurs, perform proper diagnostic measures (eg, endometrial sampling) to rule out malignancies.

**Patient Counseling:** Inform that drug may increase risk for heart attack, stroke, breast cancer, blood clots, and dementia. Report any breast lumps, unusual vaginal bleeding, dizziness or faintness, changes in speech, chest pain, SOB, leg pain, changes in vision, and vomiting. Counsel that if patch falls off, reapply same patch to different area of lower abdomen or use new patch.

**Administration:** Transdermal route. **Storage:** Prior to dispensing: Store refrigerated at 2-8°C (36-46°F). After dispensed: May be stored at room temperature below 25°C (77°F). Do not store in areas where extreme temperatures may occur.

# COMBIVENT — RX

## ipratropium bromide - albuterol sulfate (Boehringer Ingelheim)

**THERAPEUTIC CLASS:** $Beta_2$-agonist/anticholinergic

**INDICATIONS:** Treatment of patients with chronic obstructive pulmonary disease (COPD) on a regular aerosol bronchodilator who continue to have evidence of bronchospasm and who require a second bronchodilator.

**DOSAGE:** *Adults:* 2 inh qid. Max: 12 inh/24 hrs.

**HOW SUPPLIED:** MDI: (Albuterol-Ipratropium) 0.09mg-0.018mg/inh [14.7g]

**CONTRAINDICATIONS:** History of hypersensitivity to soya lecithin or related food products (eg, soybeans, peanuts).

**WARNINGS/PRECAUTIONS:** Paradoxical bronchospasm and rare occurrences of myocardial ischemia reported. Hypersensitivity reactions reported. Caution with coronary insufficiency, arrhythmias, narrow-angle glaucoma, prostatic hyperplasia, bladder-neck obstruction, HTN, DM, hyperthyroidism, convulsive disorders, renal or hepatic insufficiency and in those unusually responsive to sympathomimetic amines. May produce transient hypokalemia. Fatalities reported with excessive use.

**ADVERSE REACTIONS:** Headache, cough, upper respiratory tract infection, dyspnea, bronchitis.

**INTERACTIONS:** Potential additive interactions with other anticholinergic drugs. Increased risk of adverse CV effects with other sympathomimetics.

β-blockers and albuterol inhibit effects of each other. ECG changes and/or hypokalemia may occur with non-$K^+$-sparing diuretics. Action of albuterol on CV system maybe potentiated with MAOIs and TCAs or within 2 weeks of d/c of these drugs.



**PREGNANCY:** Category C, not for use in nursing.

**MECHANISM OF ACTION:** Ipratropium: Anticholinergic bronchodilator; inhibits vagally-mediated reflexes by antagonizing the action of acetylcholine. Albuterol: Selective $\beta_2$-adrenergic bronchodilator; activates $\beta_2$-receptors on airway smooth muscle, leading to activation of adenylyl cyclase and increase of intracellular cyclic AMP concentrations. This leads to activation of protein kinase A, which inhibits phosphorylation of myosin and lowers intracellular ionic calcium concentrations, resulting in relaxation.

**PHARMACOKINETICS: Absorption:** Ipratropium: Not readily absorbed. Albuterol: Rapid, complete; $C_{max}$=492pg/mL; $T_{max}$=3 hrs. **Distribution:** Ipratropium: Plasma protein binding (0-9%). **Metabolism:** Ipratopium: Partial; ester hydrolysis. Albuterol: Conjugation; albuterol 4'-O-sulfate (metabolite). **Elimination:** Ipratropium: Urine (50% unchanged); $T_{1/2}$=2 hrs. Albuterol: Urine (unchanged); $T_{1/2}$=3.9 hrs.

## NURSING CONSIDERATIONS

**Assessment:** Assess for known history of hypersensitivity to soya lecithin or related food products (eg, soybeans, peanuts). Assess for concomitant diseases (eg, narrow-angle glaucoma, prostatic hyperplasia, convulsive disorders, hyperthyroidism, DM, hepatic/renal insufficiency, CVD). Assess pregnancy/nursing status, potassium levels and possible drug interactions.

**Monitoring:** Monitor for hypersensitivity reactions, parodoxical bronchospasm, MI, CV effects such as flattening of the T wave, prolongation of the QT interval, and ST segment depression, unexpected development of severe acute asthmatic crisis and hypoxia.

**Patient Counseling:** Advise to avoid spraying into eyes, to not exceed recommended dose, and to shake canister vigorously for at least 10 seconds before use. Discard canister after labeled number of actuations have been used. Advise not to puncture, not to use or store near heat or open flame, and to never throw inhaler into fire or incinerator; exposure to temperature >120°C may cause bursting.

**Administration:** Inhalation route. 1) Insert metal canister into end of mouthpiece. 2) Remove orange dust cap and shake. Test spray into the air 3x before using for the first time or in cases when aerosol has not been used for 24 hrs. 3) Shake canister for 10 sec. 4) Inhale and exhale through mouth and at the same time spray product into mouth. 5) Hold breath for 10 sec and remove mouth piece. 6) Wait for 2 min before next spray. 7) Replace cap and keep mouthpiece clean. 8) Keep track of the number of sprays used and discard after 200 sprays. **Storage:** 25°C (77°F); excursions permitted to 15-30°C (59-86°F). Keep out of reach of children. Store the canister at room temperature before use and avoid excessive humidity. Do not store near heat or open flame.

# COMBIVIR — RX

zidovudine - lamivudine (GlaxoSmithKline)

**Zidovudine has been associated with hematologic toxicity (eg, neutropenia, anemia), especially with advanced HIV disease. Symptomatic myopathy reported with prolonged use. Lactic acidosis and severe, fatal hepatomegaly with steatosis reported with nucleoside analogues; suspend treatment if these occur. Acute exacerbations of hepatitis B reported in patients co-infected with hepatitis B virus (HBV) and HIV who discontinued lamivudine; monitor hepatic function closely for at least several months after discontinuation and initiate anti-hepatitis B therapy if needed.**

**THERAPEUTIC CLASS:** Nucleoside analog combination

**INDICATIONS:** Treatment of HIV-1 infection in combination with other antiretrovirals.

**DOSAGE:** *Adults:* ( ≥30 kg): 1 tab bid
*Pediatrics:* ( ≥30 kg): 1 tab bid

**HOW SUPPLIED:** Tab: (Lamivudine-Zidovudine) 150mg-300mg* *scored

**WARNINGS/PRECAUTIONS:** Caution in patients with granulocyte count <1000cells/mm$^3$ or Hgb <9.5g/dL; monitor blood counts frequently with advanced HIV and periodically with asymptomatic or early HIV. Caution in patients with known risk factors for liver disease and pancreatitis; d/c if signs and symptoms of hepatotoxicity and pancreatitis occur. Lamivudine-resistant HBV reported. Possible redistribution or accumulation of body fat. Immune reconstitution syndrome reported. Caution in elderly. Do not use in patients with reduced renal function (CrCl < 50ml/min), pediatric patients weighing <30 kg patients with hepatic impairment, or patients experiencing dose-limiting adverse reactions. Myopathy and myositis associated with prolonged use of zidovudine.

**ADVERSE REACTIONS:** Headache, malaise, fatigue, fever, chills, nausea, diarrhea, anorexia, abdominal pain/cramps, neuropathy, insomnia, dizziness, nasal signs and symptoms, cough, musculoskeletal pain.

**INTERACTIONS:** Should not be administered concomitantly with other lamivudine-, zidovudine- or, emtricitabine-containing products. Nelfinavir may increase lamivudine concentration and decrease zidovudine concentration. Lamivudine: Hepatic decompensation may occur in HIV/HCV co-infected patients receiving combination antiretroviral therapy for HIV-1 and interferon alfa with or without ribavirin; monitor for treatment-associated toxicities. Trimethoprim/sulfamethoxazole may increase lamivudine concentrations. Zidovudine: Avoid use with zalcitabine; may inhibit phosphorylation of lamuvidine. Avoid with stavudine, doxorubin, and nucleoside analogues affecting DNA replication such as ribavirin. Co-administration of ganciclovir, bone marrow suppressive or cytotoxic agents may increase the hematologic toxicity of zidovudine. Atovaqoune, fluconazole, methadone, probenecid, and valproic acid may increase zidovudine concentrations. Rifampin and ritonavir may decrease zidovudine concentrations.

**PREGNANCY:** Category C, not for use in nursing.

**MECHANISM OF ACTION:** Nucleoside analog combination; inhibits reverse transcriptase via DNA chain termination.

**PHARMACOKINETICS: Absorption:** Lamivudine: Rapid. Absolute bioavailabilty (86%). Zidovudine: Rapid. Absolute bioavailability (64%). **Distribution:** Lamivudine: $V_d$=1.3L/kg; plasma protein binding (<36%). Zidovudine: $V_d$=1.6L/kg; plasma protein binding (<38%). **Metabolism:** Zidovudine: Hepatic. 3'-azido-3'-deoxy-5'-*O*-β-*D*-glucopyranurosylthymidine (major metabolite). **Elimination:** Lamivudine: Urine (70%, unchanged), $T_{1/2}$=5-7 hrs. Zidovudine: Urine (14% unchanged, 74% metabolite); $T_{1/2}$=0.5-3 hrs.

## NURSING CONSIDERATIONS

**Assessment:** Assess for advanced symptomatic HIV disease, bone marrow supression, liver function and risk factors for liver disease, hepatitis B infection, history of pancreatitis and risk factors for its development, renal function, hypersensitivity to drug, pregnancy/nursing status, and possible drug interaction.

**Monitoring:** Monitor CBC, platelet counts, renal/liver function, and amylase level. Monitor signs/symptoms that suggest pancreatitis, lactic acidosis, or hepatotoxicity including hepatomegaly with steatosis, peripheral neuropathy, myopathy and myositis, exacerbations of hepatitis, immune reconstitution syndrome, redistibution/accumulation of body fat, and hypersensitivity reactions. May enroll patients in the Antiretroviral Pregnancy Registry if they become pregnant while on treatment.

**Patient Counseling:** Advise patients that they may continue to experience illnesses associated with HIV-1 while on therapy and that risk of transmission to others is not reduced. Inform that deterioration of liver disease can occur when drug is discontinued. Advise of zidovudine-related toxicities, such as neutropenia and anemia. Educate about redistribution/accumulation of fat that may occur. Counsel to seek medical attention if symptoms of lactic acidosis, anemia, infection, or myopathy occur. Inform about potential drug interactions.

**Administration:** Oral route. Take w/ or w/o food. **Storage:** 2-30°C (36-86°F).



## COMBUNOX

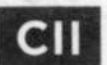

oxycodone HCl - ibuprofen (Forest)

**NSAIDs may cause an increased risk of serious cardiovascular thrombotic events, MI, stroke, and serious GI adverse events including bleeding, ulceration, and perforation of the stomach or intestines. Contraindicated for the treatment of perioperative pain in the setting of coronary artery bypass graft (CABG) surgery.**

**THERAPEUTIC CLASS:** Opioid analgesic

**INDICATIONS:** Short term (<7 days) management of acute, moderate to severe pain.

**DOSAGE:** *Adults:* 1 tab/dose. Do not exceed 4 tabs/day and 7 days.

**HOW SUPPLIED:** Tab: (Oxycodone-Ibuprofen) 5mg-400mg

**CONTRAINDICATIONS:** Significant respiratory depression, acute or severe bronchial asthma, hypercarbia, paralytic ileus, or in patients who have experienced asthma, urticaria, allergic-type reactions after taking ASA or NSAIDs. Treatment of perioperative pain in the setting of CABG surgery.

**WARNINGS/PRECAUTIONS:** May cause drug dependence and tolerance; potential for abuse. Risk of dose-related respiratory depression. May cause severe hypotension. Can lead to HTN or worsening of pre-existing HTN. Fluid retention and edema reported. Capacity to elevate CSF pressure may be exaggerated with head injury, other intracranial lesions or pre-existing increase in ICP. May obscure diagnosis or clinical course with head injuries or acute abdominal conditions. Risk of anaphylactoid reactions. NSAIDs can cause exfoliative dermatitis, Stevens-Johnson syndrome, and toxic epidermal necrolysis (TEN). Caution with severe hepatic impairment, pulmonary or renal dysfunction, hypothyroidism, Addison's disease, acute alcoholism, convulsive disorders, CNS depression or coma, delirium tremens, kyphoscoliosis associated with respiratory depression, toxic psychosis, prostatic hypertrophy, urethral stricture, biliary tract disease, anemia, pre-existing asthma, elderly or debilitated, aseptic meningitis.

**ADVERSE REACTIONS:** N/V, somnolence, dizziness, asthenia, fever, headache, vasodilation, constipation.

**INTERACTIONS:** (Oxycodone) Respiratory depression, hypotension and profound sedation with other CNS depressants (eg, narcotics, tranquilizers, sedatives, anesthetics, phenothiazines, alcohol). Concurrent use with anticholinergics may produce paralytic ileus. Mixed agonist/antagonist analgesics may reduce the analgesic effect and/or cause withdrawal. Do not use with or within 14 days of d/c MAOIs. May enhance skeletal muscle relaxant effects and increase respiratory depression. (Ibuprofen) May diminish antihypertensive effect of ACE inhibitors. Use caution with anticoagulants, such as warfarin. May enhance methotrexate toxicity. May decrease natriuretic effect of furosemide and thiazides. Avoid with ASA. May decrease lithium clearance; monitor for toxicity.

**PREGNANCY:** Category C, caution in nursing.

**MECHANISM OF ACTION:** Oxycodone: Opioid analgesic; not established. Suspected to be related to binding to opiate receptors in the CNS. Also may produce sedation and respiratory depression. Ibuprofen: Nonsteroidal anti-inflammatory agent; not established. Possesses analgesic and antipyretic activity. Inhibits cyclooxygenase activity and prostaglandin synthesis, and is a peripherally acting analgesic.

**PHARMACOKINETICS: Absorption:** Oxycodone: Rapid; $C_{max}$=9.8-11.7ng/mL; $T_{max}$=1.3-2.1 hrs. Ibuprofen: Rapid; $C_{max}$=18.5-34.3mcg/mL; $T_{max}$=1.6-3.1 hrs. **Distribution:** Oxycodone: Plasma protein binding (45%). Ibuprofen: Plasma protein binding (99%). **Metabolism:** Oxycodone: Liver via CYP2D6 (N-demethylation, O-demethylation, 6-ketoreduction, glucuronidation);

oxymorphone (active metabolite). Ibuprofen: Undergoes interconversion in plasma from R- to S-isomer: (+)-2-4'-(2-hydroxy-2-methyl-propyl) phenyl propionic acid, (+)-2-4'-(carboxypropyl) phenylpropionic acid (primary metabolites). **Elimination:** Oxycodone: Urine (4% unchanged); $T_{1/2}$=3.1-3.7 hrs. Ibuprofen: Urine (≤0.2% unchanged); $T_{1/2}$=1.8-2.6 hrs.

## NURSING CONSIDERATIONS

**Assessment:** Assess for respiratory depression, acute or severe bronchial asthma, hypercarbia, paralytic ileus, hypersensitivity to ASA (eg, asthma, urticaria), HTN, fluid retention, heart failure, circulatory shock, previous history of ulcer disease or GI bleeding, presence of head injury, intracranial lesions, pre-existing increase in ICP, acute abdominal conditions, renal dysfunction, liver dysfunction, biliary tract disease, acute pancreatitis, hypothyroidism, Addison's disease, acute alcoholism, convulsive disorders, CNS depression or coma, delirium tremens, toxic psychosis, prostatic hypertrophy, urethral stricture, nursing/pregnancy status, and possible drug interactions. Obtain baseline BP.

**Monitoring:** Monitor for signs/symptoms of cardiovascular thrombotic effects, HTN, GI effects (eg, ulceration, bleeding, perforation), abuse and dependence, respiratory depression, hypotension, anaphylactoid reactions, renal papillary necrosis, skin reactions (eg, exfoliative dermatitis, Stevens-Johnson syndrome), hematological effects (eg, anemia), liver dysfunction, and aseptic meningitis. Monitor Hgb and Hct in patients previously treated with NSAIDs and currently exhibiting signs/symptoms of anemia. Perform periodic monitoring of BP. For patients on long-term therapy, perform periodic monitoring of CBC and chemistry profile.

**Patient Counseling:** Inform that drug may impair mental/physical abilities; use caution when performing dangerous tasks (eg, operating machinery/driving). Advise to avoid using other CNS depressants and alcohol during therapy. Counsel that medication has abuse potential; only take for prescribed duration and dose. Notify physician if develop any serious cardiovascular effects (eg, chest pain, SOB), GI effects (eg, ulcers, bleeding), serious skin reactions (eg, exfoliative dermatitis, Stevens-Johnson syndrome), weight gain or edema, hepatotoxicity (eg, nausea, fatigue, jaundice), or anaphylactoid reactions (eg, difficulty breathing, facial swelling).

**Administration:** Oral route. **Storage:** 25°C (77°F); excursions permitted to 15-30°C (59-86°F).

# COMTAN — RX

entacapone (Novartis)

**THERAPEUTIC CLASS:** COMT inhibitor

**INDICATIONS:** Adjunct to levodopa/carbidopa for treatment of idiopathic Parkinson's disease if experience signs of end-of-dose "wearing-off."

**DOSAGE:** *Adults:* 200mg with each levodopa/carbidopa dose. Max: 1600mg/day. Withdraw slowly for d/c.

**HOW SUPPLIED:** Tab: 200mg

**WARNINGS/PRECAUTIONS:** Hypotension/syncope, diarrhea, hallucinations, dyskinesia reported. Rhabdomyolysis, hyperpyrexia, confusion, and fibrotic complications may occur due to increased dopaminergic activity. Caution with hepatic impairment, biliary obstruction. Neuroleptic malignant syndrome reported. Avoid rapid withdrawal or abrupt dose reduction. May impair mental/physical abilities. May increase risk of melanoma; monitor frequently. May cause renal toxicity.

**ADVERSE REACTIONS:** Back pain, dyskinesia, hyperkinesia, hypokinesia, N/V, diarrhea, abdominal pain, urine discoloration, dizziness, constipation, dry mouth, fatigue, dyspnea.

**INTERACTIONS:** Avoid non-selective MAOIs (eg, phenelzine, tranylcypromine). Caution with drugs metabolized by Catechol-O-methyltransferase (COMT) (eg, isoproterenol, epinephrine, norepinephrine, dopamine, dobutamine, α-methyldopa, apomorphine, isoetherine, bitolterol); increased HR, arrhythmias, and BP changes may occur. Additive sedative effects may occur with CNS depressants. Caution with concomitant use of drugs known to interfere with biliary excretion, glucuronidation, and intestinal β-glucuronidase such as probenecid, cholestyramine, and some antibiotics (eg, erythromycin, rifamipicin, ampicillin, chloramphenicol).

**PREGNANCY:** Category C, caution with nursing.

**MECHANISM OF ACTION:** COMT inhibitor; selectively and reversibly inhibits catechol-O-methyltransferase (COMT), and alters the plasma pharmacokinetics of levodopa.

**PHARMACOKINETICS: Absorption:** (PO) Rapid; absolute bioavailability (35%); $C_{max}$=1.2mcg/mL; $T_{max}$=1 hr. **Distribution:** Plasma protein binding (98%); (IV): $V_d$=20L. **Metabolism:** Isomerization to *cis*-isomer, and direct glucuronidation. **Elimination:** Urine 10% (0.2% unchanged), feces (90%); $T_{1/2}$ $(\beta_{-phase})$=0.4-0.7 hrs; $T_{1/2(gamma-phase)}$=2.4 hrs.

## NURSING CONSIDERATIONS

**Assessment:** Assess for dyskinesia, biliary obstruction, hepatic impairment, hypotension, pregnancy/nursing status, and possible drug interactions. Note other disease/conditions and drug therapies.

**Monitoring:** Monitor for signs and symptoms of orthostatic hypotension, diarrhea, hallucinations, dyskinesia, rhadomyolysis, Neuroleptic Malignant Syndrome (eg, elevated temperature, muscular rigidity, altered consciousness), fibrotic complications (eg, retroperitoneal fibrosis, pulmonary infiltrates, pleural effusion), renal toxicity. Monitor BP, LFTs, and renal function tests. Monitor for signs of melanoma frequently; perform periodic skin examinations.

**Patient Counseling:** Take only as prescribed. Inform that postural hypotension, hallucinations, nausea, increase dyskinesia, and change in urine color may occur. Caution against rising rapidly after sitting or lying, especially during initiation of treatment. Instruct to avoid driving a car or operating other complex machinery until aware of how medication effects mental and/or motor performance. Instruct to use caution when discontinuing treatment. Advise to inform physician if experiencing new or increased gambling, sexual and other urges.

**Administration:** Oral route. **Storage:** 25°C (77°F); excursions permitted to 15-30°C (59-86°F).

# CONCERTA CII

methylphenidate HCl (Ortho-Mcneil/Janssen)

**Caution with history of drug dependence or alcoholism. Marked tolerance and psychological dependence with varying degrees of abnormal behavior may occur with chronic abusive use. Careful supervision is necessary during withdrawal from abusive use to avoid severe depression.**

**THERAPEUTIC CLASS:** Sympathomimetic amine

**INDICATIONS:** Treatment of attention deficit hyperactivity disorder (ADHD) in patients ≥6-65 yrs.

**DOSAGE:** *Adults:* Methylphenidate-Naive or Receiving Other Stimulant: Initial: 18mg or 36mg qam. Titrate: Adjust dose at weekly intervals. Max: 72mg/day. Previous Methylphenidate Use: Initial: 18mg qam if previous dose 10-15mg/day; 36mg qam if previous dose 20-30mg/day; 54mg qam if previous dose 30-45mg/day; 72mg qam if previous dose 40-60mg/day. Initial conversion should not exceed 72mg/day. Titrate: Adjust dose at weekly intervals. Max: 72mg/day. Reduce dose or d/c if paradoxical aggravation of symptoms occurs. D/C if no improvement after appropriate dosage adjustments over 1 month. May be taken with or without food. Swallow whole with liquids. Do not crush, chew, or divide.

*Pediatrics:* ≥6 yrs: Methylphenidate-Naive or Receiving Other Stimulant: Initial: 18mg qam. Titrate: Adjust dose at weekly intervals. Max: 6-12 yrs: 54mg/day; 13-17 yrs: 72mg/day not to exceed 2mg/kg/day. Previous Methylphenidate

Use: Initial: 18mg qam if previous dose 10-15mg/day; 36mg qam if previous dose 20-30mg/day; 54mg qam if previous dose 30-45mg/day; 72mg qam if previous dose 40-60mg/day. Initial conversion should not exceed 72mg/day. Titrate: Adjust dose at weekly intervals. Max: 72mg/day. Reduce dose or d/c if paradoxical aggravation of symptoms occurs. D/C if no improvement after appropriate dosage adjustments over 1 month. May be taken with or without food. Swallow whole with liquids. Do not crush, chew, or divide.

**HOW SUPPLIED:** Tab, Extended-Release: 18mg, 27mg, 36mg, 54mg

**CONTRAINDICATIONS:** Patients with marked anxiety, tension, agitation, glaucoma, motor tics or family history or diagnosis of Tourette's syndrome. Treatment with or within 14 days of monoamine oxidase inhibitor (MAOI) use.

**WARNINGS/PRECAUTIONS:** Monitor growth during treatment in children. Difficulties with accommodation and blurred vision reported. May exacerbate symptoms of behavior disturbance and thought disorder in psychotic patients. Avoid with severe GI narrowing (eg, esophageal motility disorders, small bowel inflammatory disease, short-gut syndrome). May lower seizure threshold, especially in known EEG abnormalities. Caution with HTN, conditions affected by BP or HR elevation, history of drug abuse or alcoholism. Monitor during withdrawal from abusive use. Monitor CBC, differential, and platelets with prolonged use. Caution when using stimulants to treat patients with comorbid bipolar disorder because of concern for possible induction of mixed/manic episode in such patients. Stimulants at usual dose can cause treatment emergent psychotic or manic symptoms (eg, hallucinations, delusional thinking, mania) in children and adolescents without prior history of psychotic illness. Aggressive behavior or hostility reported in clinical trials and postmarketing experience of some medications indicated for the treatment of ADHD. Sudden death, stroke, MI reported; avoid with known structural cardiac abnormalities or other serious cardiac problems.

**ADVERSE REACTIONS:** Loss of appetite, headache, dry mouth, nausea, insomnia, nervousness, anxiety, dizziness, weight reduction, irritability, upper abdominal pain, hyperhidrosis, tachycardia, and palpitations.

**INTERACTIONS:** See Contraindications. Caution with vasopressor agents. May inhibit metabolism of coumarin anticoagulants, anticonvulsants (eg, phenobarbital, phenytoin, primidone), and some antidepressants (eg, tricyclics, selective serotonin reuptake inhibitors). Serious adverse events reported with clonidine.

**PREGNANCY:** Category C, caution in nursing.

**MECHANISM OF ACTION:** Sympathomimetic amine; CNS stimulant that blocks reuptake of norepinephrine and dopamine into presynaptic neuron and increases release of these monoamines into extraneuronal space.

**PHARMACOKINETICS: Absorption:** (PO) Readily absorbed; $C_{max}$=3.7ng/mL; AUC=41.8ng•h/mL; $T_{max}$=6-10 hrs. **Metabolism:** De-esterification; α-phenylpiperidine acetic acid (metabolite). **Elimination:** Urine (90%); $T_{1/2}$=3.5 hrs.

## NURSING CONSIDERATIONS

**Assessment:** Assess for agitation, glaucoma, tics, family history of Tourette's syndrome, CV conditions (eg, HTN, angina pectoris, cardiac arrhythmias, HF, recent MI), hyperthyroidism or thyrotoxicosis, bipolar disorder, history of drug dependence or alcoholism, severe GI narrowing (eg, esophageal motility disorders, small bowel inflammatory disease, and short-gut syndrome), hypersensitivity, pregnancy/nursing status, and possible drug interactions.

**Monitoring:** Monitor for cardiac abnormalities, exacerbations of behavior disturbances and thought disorder, bipolar disorder, aggression, seizures, visual disturbances, and hypersensitivity reactions. Monitor periodic CBC, differential and platelet count, LFTs, and height and weight in children.

**Patient Counseling:** Inform about risks of therapy, appropriate use, and drug abuse/dependence. Counsel to swallow tablet whole, do not crush or chew. May impair mental/physical abilities.

**Administration:** Oral route. **Storage:** 25°C (77°F); excursions permitted to 15-30°C (59-86°F). Protect from humidity.

## COPAXONE RX
### glatiramer acetate (Teva Neuroscience)

C

**THERAPEUTIC CLASS:** Immunomodulatory agent

**INDICATIONS:** To reduce frequency of relapses in patients with relapsing-remitting multiple sclerosis (RRMS), including patients who have experienced a first clinical episode and have magnetic resonance imaging (MRI) features of MS.

**DOSAGE:** *Adults:* 20mg SQ qd.

**HOW SUPPLIED:** Inj: 20mg/mL

**CONTRAINDICATIONS:** Hypersensitivity to mannitol.

**WARNINGS/PRECAUTIONS:** Not for IV use. Immediate post-injection reaction (eg, flushing, palpitations, dyspnea, urticaria, anxiety, throat constriction), chest pain, lipoatrophy, skin necrosis (rare) reported. May interfere with normal functioning of immune system.

**ADVERSE REACTIONS:** Injection-site reactions, vasodilation, chest pain, dyspnea, rash, asthenia, infection, pain, nausea, arthralgia, anxiety, hypertonia, depression, tachycardia, and tremor.

**PREGNANCY:** Category B, caution in nursing.

**MECHANISM OF ACTION:** Immunomodulatory agent; not fully established. Presumed to modify immune processes in MS.

### NURSING CONSIDERATIONS

**Assessment:** Assess for mannitol therapy, clinical episodes of MS, MRI.

**Monitoring:** Monitor for immediate post-injection reactions (eg, flushing, chest pain, palpitations, anxiety, dyspnea, constriction of throat, urticaria), hypersensitivity, pregnancy/nursing status.

**Patient Counseling:** Notify physician if pregnant/nursing or planning to become pregnant. Counsel about transient and self-limiting symptoms of adverse reactions (eg, flushing, chest pain, palpitations, anxiety, dyspnea, throat constriction, and urticaria). Inform to seek medical consultation if chest pain of unusual duration or intensity occurs. Instruct to follow proper injection technique and rotate injection sites on a daily basis. Use aseptic technique.

**Administration:** SQ route. **Storage:** 2-8°C (36-46°F); 15-30°C (59-86°F) for 1 month. Do not expose to high temperatures and intense light.

## COPEGUS RX
### ribavirin (Genentech)

**Not for monotherapy treatment of chronic hepatitis C. Primary toxicity is hemolytic anemia. Avoid with significant or unstable cardiac disease. Contraindicated in pregnancy and male partners of pregnant women. Use 2 forms of contraception during therapy and for 6 months after discontinuation.**

**THERAPEUTIC CLASS:** Nucleoside analogue

**INDICATIONS:** Treatment of chronic hepatitis C, in combination with Pegasys, in adults with compensated liver disease not previously treated with interferon alpha. Patients in whom efficacy was demonstrated included patients with compensated liver disease and histological evidence of cirrhosis (Child-Pugh class A) and patients with HIV disease that is clinically stable.

**DOSAGE:** *Adults:* HCV: Give bid in divided doses. Treat for 24-48 weeks with Pegasys 180mcg. Genotypes 1 and 4: <75kg: 1000mg/day for 48 weeks. ≥75kg: 1200mg/day for 48 weeks. Genotypes 2 and 3: 800mg/day for 24 weeks. HCV/HIV: 800mg qd. Treat for 48 weeks with Pegasys 180mcg. Dose Modifications: Reduce to 600mg/day if Hgb <10g/dL with no cardiac history, or if Hgb decreases by ≥2g/dL during a 4-week period with stable cardiac disease. D/C if Hgb <8.5g/dL with no cardiac history or if Hgb <12g/dL after 4 weeks of dose reduction with stable cardiac disease. After dose modification, may restart at 600mg/day, then may increase to 800mg/day. CrCl <50mL/min: Avoid use.

**HOW SUPPLIED:** Tab: 200mg

**CONTRAINDICATIONS:** Pregnancy, male partners of pregnant women, hemoglobinopathies (eg, thalassemia major, sickle cell anemia). Autoimmune hepatitis, and hepatic decompensation (Child-Pugh score greater than 6, Class B and C) in cirrhotic CHC patients, and in cirrhotic CHC patients co-infected with HIV before or during treatment when used in combination with Pegasys.

**WARNINGS/PRECAUTIONS:** D/C with hepatic decompensation, confirmed pancreatitis, and hypersensitivity reaction. Severe depression, suicidal ideation, hemolytic anemia, bone marrow suppression, autoimmune and infectious disorders, pancreatitis, and diabetes reported. Pulmonary symptoms reported; monitor closely with evidence of pulmonary infiltrates or pulmonary function impairment and d/c if appropriate. Assess for underlying cardiac disease (obtain EKG); fatal and nonfatal MI reported with anemia. Caution with cardiac disease, d/c if cardiovascular status deteriorates. Hemolytic anemia reported; monitor Hgb or Hct initially then at week 2 and 4 (or more if needed) of therapy. Suspend therapy if symptoms of pancreatitis arise. Avoid if CrCl <50mL/min. Obtain negative pregnancy test prior to initiation then monthly, and for 6 months post-therapy.

**ADVERSE REACTIONS:** Injection-site reaction, fatigue/asthenia, pyrexia, rigors, N/V, neutropenia, anorexia, myalgia, headache, irritability/anxiety/nervousness, insomnia, alopecia.

**INTERACTIONS:** Avoid concomitant use with didanosine and zidovudine. Hepatic decompensation can occur with concomitant use of NRTIs and Pegasys/ribavirin.

**PREGNANCY:** Category X, not for use in nursing.

**MECHANISM OF ACTION:** Nucleotide analogue; not established.

**PHARMACOKINETICS: Absorption:** $C_{max}$=2748ng/mL; $T_{max}$=2 hrs; AUC=25361ng•hr/mL. **Elimination:** $T_{1/2}$=120-170 hrs.

## NURSING CONSIDERATIONS

**Assessment:** Assess for known hypersensitivity, history of hemoglobinopathies (eg, thalassemia major or sickle cell anemia), cardiac disease, hepatic/renal dysfunction, DM, pulmonary dysfunction/disease, pancreatitis, pregnancy status (including female partners of male patients), and possible drug interactions. Assess baseline LFTs, renal function, CBC, ECG, thyroid function, Hgb, Hct, and CD4 count in HIV/AIDS.

**Monitoring:** Pregnancy testing should occur at initiation, monthly during therapy, and for 6 months after therapy (including female partners of male patients). Monitor for significant events including severe depression, suicidal ideation, hemolytic anemia, suppression of bone marrow function, autoimmune/infection disorder, pulmonary dysfunction, pancreatitis and DM. Monitor Hct and Hgb (before treatment, Weeks 2 and 4, and more if needed). Appropriately monitor ECG with pre-existing cardiac disease for deterioration of cardiac function. Monitor for signs/symptoms of pancreatitis, hepatic decompensation, hypersensitivity reaction, anemia, and pulmonary dysfunction (including exacerbation of sarcoidosis).

**Patient Counseling:** Inform of pregnancy risks; use 2 forms of effective contraception. Seek medical attention if symptoms of pancreatitis, hypersensitivity reaction, anemia, hepatic decompensation, deterioration of cardiac function, and pulmonary dysfunction (dyspnea) occur. Caution against operating machinery/driving if symptoms of dizziness, confusion, somnolence, or fatigue occur. Counsel to take with food and to keep well-hydrated.

**Administration:** Oral route. **Storage:** 25°C (77°F); excursions permitted between 15-30°C (59-86°F). Keep bottle tightly closed.

# CORDARONE RX

amiodarone HCl (Wyeth)

C

**THERAPEUTIC CLASS:** Class III antiarrhythmic

**INDICATIONS:** Treatment of documented, life-threatening recurrent ventricular fibrillation and recurrent hemodynamically unstable ventricular tachycardia.

**DOSAGE:** *Adults:* Give LD in hospital. LD: 800-1600mg/day for 1-3 weeks. After control is achieved, 600-800mg/day for 1 month. Maint: 400mg/day; up to 600mg/day if needed. May be administered as a single dose, or in patients with severe GI intolerance, as a bid dose. Give in divided doses for total daily dose >1000mg. Use lowest effective dose. Take with meals. Elderly: Start at low end of dosing range.

**HOW SUPPLIED:** Tab: 200mg* *scored

**CONTRAINDICATIONS:** Severe sinus-node dysfunction causing marked sinus bradycardia, 2nd- and 3rd-degree AV block, when episodes of bradycardia have caused syncope (except when used with a pacemaker), cardiogenic shock, hypersensitivity to iodine.

**WARNINGS/PRECAUTIONS:** Only for life-threatening arrhythmias due to its substantial toxicity. Pulmonary toxicities include hypersensitivity pneumonitis and interstitial/alveolar pneumonitis; d/c if any of these occur and institute appropriate treatment. Can cause exacerbation of arrhythmia. Can cause either hypo- or hyperthyroidism. In patients with implanted defibrillators or pacemakers, pacing and defibrillation thresholds should be assessed before and during treatment. Amiodarone-induced hyperthyroidism may result in thyrotoxicosis and/or the possibility of arrhythmia breakthrough or aggravation. Liver injury is common but usually mild; d/c if LFTs are 3x ULN or if elevated baseline doubles; monitor LFTs regularly. Optic neuropathy, optic neuritis reported. Fetal harm in pregnancy. May develop reversible corneal microdeposits (eg, visual halos, blurred vision), photosensitivity, peripheral neuropathy (rare). Adult respiratory distress syndrome (ARDS) reported with surgery. Rare occurrences of hypotension reported upon discontinuation of cardiopulmonary bypass during open-heart surgery. Correct $K^+$ or magnesium deficiency before therapy. Caution in elderly.

**ADVERSE REACTIONS:** Pulmonary toxicity, malaise, fatigue, involuntary movements, abnormal gait, constipation, arrhythmia exacerbation, hepatic injury, tremor, poor coordination, paresthesia, N/V, anorexia, photosensitivity, CHF.

**INTERACTIONS:** Risk of interactions after d/c due to its long half-life. May increase sensitivity to myocardial depressant and conduction effects of halogenated inhalation anesthetics. D/C or reduce digoxin dose by 50%. Reduce warfarin dose by 1/3-1/2; monitor PTT closely. Avoid grapefruit juice. Hemodynamic and electrophysiologic interactions have been observed with propranolol, diltiazem, verapamil. Caution with β-blockers, CCBs, lidocaine. May increase levels of cyclosporine, MTX, dextromethorphan, quinidine, procainamide, phenytoin, flecainide. Initiate added antiarrhythmic drug at 50% of usual dose. Quinidine and procainamide doses should be reduced by 1/3 if coadministered. Caution with loratadine, trazadone, disopyramide, fluoroquinolones, macrolides, azoles; QT prolongation reported. Decreased levels with cholestyramine, rifampin, phenytoin, St. John's wort. Rhabdomyolysis/myopathy reported with HMG-CoA reductase inhibitors that are CYP3A4 substrates (eg, simvastatin, atorvastatin); consider lower starting or maintenance doses of these drugs. Ineffective inhibition of platelet aggregation with clopidogrel. Fentanyl may cause hypotension, bradycardia, and decreased cardiac output. Increased levels with protease inhibitors; monitor for toxicity. Inhibits P-glycoprotein, CYP1A2, CYP2C9, CYP2D6, CYP3A4 and may increase levels of their substrates. Interactions reported with CYP3A4 inducers. CYP2C8 and CYP3A4 (eg, cimetidine) inhibitors may increase amiodarone levels.

**PREGNANCY:** Category D, not for use in nursing.

C

**MECHANISM OF ACTION:** Class III antiarrhythmic; prolongs myocardial cell-action potential duration and refractory period, and causes noncompetitive α- and β-adrenergic inhibition.

**PHARMACOKINETICS: Absorption:** Slow and variable; $T_{max}$=3-7 hrs; absolute bioavailability (35%-65%). **Distribution:** $V_d$=60L/kg; plasma protein binding (96%); found in breast milk. **Metabolism:** CYP3A4, 2C8; desethylamiodarone (major metabolite). **Elimination:** Bile, urine; $T_{1/2}$=58 days, 36 days (metabolite).

## NURSING CONSIDERATIONS

**Assessment:** Assess for life-threatening arrhythmias, ventricular arrhythmia, optic neuropathy or optic neuritis, hepatic impairment, pregnancy/nursing status, thyroid function, pre-existing pulmonary disease, recent MI, and possible drug interactions. Assess to determine failure of prior therapy. Correct hypokalemia and hypomagnesemia prior to initiation.

**Monitoring:** Monitor for pulmonary toxicities (eg, hypersensitivity pneumonitis, or interstitial/alveolar pneumonitis) manifested by cough, progressive dyspnea and accompanied by functional, radiological, gallium-scan, and pathological data. Perform history, physical exam, and chest X-ray every 3-6 months. Monitor for sinus bradycardia, sinus arrest, and heart block. Monitor induced hyperthyroidism/thyrotoxicosis, hepatic failure, optic neuritis/neuropathy, corneal microdeposits, vision loss, fetal harm, peripheral neuropathy, photosensitivity, LFTs, $T_4$, $T_3$ and reverse $T_3$. Perioperative monitoring for hypotension and ARDS recommended.

**Patient Counseling:** Advise to notify physician if pregnant/nursing. Inform about benefits/risks, including possibility of vision impairment, thyroid abnormalities, peripheral neuropathy, and photosensitivity. Report any adverse reactions to physician. Counsel to take as directed. Do not take with grapefruit juice. Avoid prolonged sunlight exposure. Advise that corneal refractive laser surgery is contraindicated with concurrent use.

**Administration:** Oral route. **Storage:** 20-25°C (68-77°F). Protect from light. Dispense in a tight, light-resistant container.

# CORDRAN — RX

flurandrenolide (Watson)

**OTHER BRAND NAMES:** Cordran SP (Watson)

**THERAPEUTIC CLASS:** Corticosteroid

**INDICATIONS:** Treatment of corticosteroid-responsive dermatoses.

**DOSAGE:** *Adults:* (Cre, Lot) Apply qd-qid depending on severity. For moist lesions, apply cream bid-tid. Apply lotion bid-tid. (Tape) Clean and dry skin. Shave or clip hair. Apply tape q12-24h.
*Pediatrics:* (Cre, Lot) Apply qd-qid depending on severity. For moist lesions, apply cream bid-tid. Apply lotion bid-tid. (Tape) Clean and dry skin. Shave or clip hair. Apply tape q12-24h.

**HOW SUPPLIED:** Cre (SP): 0.05% [15g, 30g, 60g]; Lot: 0.05% [15mL, 60mL]; Tape: 4mcg/$cm^2$ [60cm x 7.5cm, 200cm x 7.5cm]

**CONTRAINDICATIONS:** (Tape) Not for lesions exuding serum or in intertriginous areas.

**WARNINGS/PRECAUTIONS:** Systemic absorption may produce reversible HPA axis suppression, manifestations of Cushing's syndrome, hyperglycemia, and glucosuria. Application of more potent steroids, use on large surfaces, prolonged use, or occlusive dressings may augment systemic absorption. Evaluate periodically for HPA suppression if large dose applied to large area or with occlusive dressings. Pediatrics are more susceptible to toxicity. D/C if irritation develops. May use occlusive dressing for psoriasis or recalcitrant conditions.

**ADVERSE REACTIONS:** Burning, itching, irritation, dryness, folliculitis, hypertrichosis, acneiform eruptions, hypopigmentation, dermatitis. Occlusive dressing may cause skin maceration, secondary infection, skin atrophy, miliaria.

**PREGNANCY:** Category C, caution in nursing.

**MECHANISM OF ACTION:** Corticosteroid; possesses anti-inflammatory, antipruritic, and vasoconstrictive properties. Suspected to stabilize cellular and lysosomal membranes, thereby preventing release of proteolytic enzymes, and consequently reducing inflammation.

C

**PHARMACOKINETICS: Absorption:** Extent of percutaneous absorption depends on integrity of skin, vehicle, and use of occlusive dressings. **Distribution:** Plasma protein binding (variable). **Metabolism:** Liver. **Elimination:** Kidney (major), bile.

## NURSING CONSIDERATIONS

**Assessment:** Assess pregnancy/nursing status.

**Monitoring:** Monitor for signs/symptoms of reversible hypothalamic-pituitary-adrenal (HPA) axis suppression, Cushing's syndrome, hyperglycemia, glucosuria, skin irritation, and for development of dermatological infections (eg, bacterial, fungal). In patients on large doses or using occlusive dressings, perform periodic testing for HPA-axis suppression by using urinary free cortisol, and ACTH stimulation tests. Following d/c of therapy, monitor for signs/symptoms of steroid withdrawal. In pediatric patients, monitor for systemic toxicity, HPA-axis suppression, Cushing's syndrome, and intracranial HTN.

**Patient Counseling:** Inform to use exactly as directed, externally. Avoid contact with eyes. Counsel not to bandage or wrap treated skin unless directed by physician. (Tape) Cleanse treatment area and allow it to dry for 1 hour prior to application. Report adverse reactions. Instruct parents of pediatric patients to avoid using tight-fitting diapers or plastic pants on children receiving treatment in diaper area.

**Administration:** Topical. Application of Tape: 1) Clean treatment area so that scales, crusts, dried exudates, and previously used ointments or creams are removed. Use germicidal soap or cleanser to prevent odor from developing under tape. Shave or clip hair in treatment area. If shower or tub bath is to be taken, complete before application of tape. Dry skin prior to application. 2) Apply tape, keeping skin smooth; press tape into place. **Storage:** 15-30°C (59-86°F).

# Coreg CR — RX

carvedilol phosphate - carvedilol (GlaxoSmithKline)

**OTHER BRAND NAMES:** Coreg (GlaxoSmithKline)

**THERAPEUTIC CLASS:** Alpha$_1$/Beta-blocker

**INDICATIONS:** Treatment of mild to severe chronic heart failure of ischemic or cardiomyopathic origin; Reduction of cardivascular mortality in clinically stable patients post myocardial infarction (MI) with left ventricular dysfunction (LVD); Treatment of essential hypertension.

**DOSAGE:** *Adults:* Individualize dose. Take with food. Monitor dose increases. For extended-release capsules, take in am and swallow whole. CHF: Tab: Initial: 3.125mg bid for 2 weeks. Titrate: May double dose every 2 weeks as tolerated. Max: 50mg bid if >85kg. Reduce dose if HR <55 beats/min. Cap, Extended-Release: Initial: 10mg qd for 2 weeks. Titrate: May double dose every 2 weeks as tolerated. Reduce dose if HR <55 beats/min. HTN: Tab: Initial: 6.25mg bid for 7-14 days. Titrate: May double dose at 7-14 day intervals. Max: 50mg/day. Cap, Extended-Release: Initial: 20mg qd for 7-14 days. Titrate: May double dose every 7-14 days as tolerated. Max: 80mg/day. LVD Post-MI: Tab: Initial: 6.25mg bid for 3-10 days. Titrate: May double dose every 3-10 days to target of 25mg bid. May begin with 3.125mg bid and slow up-titration rate if clinically indicated. Cap, Extended-Release: Initial: 20mg qd for 3-10 days. Titrate: May double dose every 3-10 days to target of 80mg qd. May begin with 10mg qd and slow up-titration if clinically indicated. Elderly: Start at the low end of dosing range.

**HOW SUPPLIED:** Tab: 3.125mg, 6.25mg, 12.5mg, 25mg; Cap, Extended-Release: 10mg, 20mg, 40mg, 80mg

**CONTRAINDICATIONS:** Bronchial asthma or related bronchospastic conditions, 2nd- or 3rd-degree AV block, sick sinus syndrome, severe bradycardia (without permanent pacemaker), cardiogenic shock, decompensated heart failure requiring IV inotropic therapy, severe hepatic impairment.

**WARNINGS/PRECAUTIONS:** Exacerbation of angina, MI, ventricular arrhythmias reported with abrupt discontinuation; taper over 1-2 weeks. Bradycardia reported; reduce dose if pulse rate drops <55 beats/min. Hypotension and syncope reported, most commonly during up-titration period; avoid driving or hazardous tasks. May mask signs of hypoglycemia and hyperthyroidism (eg tachycardia). Monitor renal function during up-titration with low BP (SBP <100mmHg), ischemic heart disease, diffuse vascular disease, and/or renal insufficiency. Worsening heart failure or fluid retention may occur with up-titration. Caution in pheochromocytoma, peripheral vascular disease, major surgery with anesthesia, Prinzmetal's variant angina, and bronchospastic disease. Caution with use in elderly.

**ADVERSE REACTIONS:** Bradycardia, fatigue, edema, hypotension, dizziness, headache, diarrhea, N/V, hyperglycemia, weight increase, increased cough, arthralgia, nasopharyngitis, syncope, rales

**INTERACTIONS:** CYP2D6 inhibitors (eg, quinidine, fluoxetine, paroxetine, propafenone) may increase levels. Monitor for hypotension and bradycardia with catecholamine-depleting agents (eg, reserpine, MAOIs). Clonidine may potentiate BP-and HR-lowering effects. Rifampin may reduce plasma levels. Cimetidine may increase AUC. Monitor ECG and BP with CCBs (eg, verapamil, diltiazem). Monitor with insulin, oral hypoglycemics, cyclosporine, and digoxin. Caution with anesthetic agents that may depress myocardial function (eg, cyclopropane, trichloroethylene). Digitalis glycosides and β-blockers slow atrioventricular conduction and decrease heart rate. Concomitant use can increase the risk of bradycardia. Amiodarone may increase plasma levels resulting in further slowing of the HR or cardiac conduction.

**PREGNANCY:** Category C, not for use in nursing.

**MECHANISM OF ACTION:** Nonselective β-adrenergic and $\alpha_1$ blocker.

**PHARMACOKINETICS: Absorption**: Rapid; absolute bioavailability (25-35%). Cap: $T_{max}$=5 hrs. **Distribution:** Plasma protein binding (>98%); $V_d$=115L. **Metabolism**: Oxidation and glucuronidation; CYP2D6, 2C9 (primary); CYP3A4, 2C19, 1A2, 2E1 (minor). **Elimination**: Urine (<2% unchanged); $T_{1/2}$=7-10 hrs.

## NURSING CONSIDERATIONS

**Assessment:** Assess for bronchial asthma, bronchospastic disease, AV block, sick sinus syndrome, severe bradycardia, cardiogenic shock, CHF, Prinzmetal's angina, CAD, DM, pheochromocytoma, peripheral vascular disease, hyperthyroidism, pregnancy/nursing status, possible drug interactions, hepatic/renal impairment. Obtain baseline blood glucose levels, LFTs, and renal function.

**Monitoring:** Monitor blood glucose during initiation/dosage adjustments, and upon d/c of therapy; LFTs and renal function periodically. Monitor for signs/symptoms of cardiac failure, hypo/hyperglycemia, thyrotoxicosis, withdrawal symptoms, precipitation or aggravation of arterial insufficiency, hypotension, and hypersensitivity reactions.

**Patient Counseling:** Instruct not to d/c or interrupt therapy without consulting physician and to avoid situations where injury could result should syncope occur. Contact lens wearers may experience decreased lacrimation; may mask signs of thyrotoxicosis or hypoglycemia. Caution drug may impair physical/mental abilities. Instruct to take with food; do not crush or chew. Advise to seek medical attention if symptoms of heart failure (difficulty breathing), hypotension (syncope), withdrawal symptoms (angina), or hypersensitivity reactions occur.

**Administration:** Oral route. **Storage:** Tab: Below 30°C (86°F). Protect from moisture. Cap, Extended-Release: 25°C (77°F); excursions permitted to 15-30°C (59-86°F). Dispense in a tight, light-resistant container.

## CORMAX RX

clobetasol propionate (Watson)



**OTHER BRAND NAMES:** Cormax Scalp (Watson)

**THERAPEUTIC CLASS:** Corticosteroid

**INDICATIONS:** Corticosteroid-responsive dermatoses.

**DOSAGE:** *Adults:* Apply bid. Limit treatment to 2 consecutive weeks. Max: 50g/week or 50mL/week.
*Pediatrics:* ≥12 yrs: (Cre, Sol) Apply bid. Limit treatment to 2 consecutive weeks. Max: 50g/week or 50mL/week.

**HOW SUPPLIED:** Cre: 0.05% [15g, 30g, 45g]; Oint: 0.05% [15g, 45g]; Sol (Scalp): 0.05% [25mL, 50mL]

**CONTRAINDICATIONS:** Primary infections of the scalp with solution.

**WARNINGS/PRECAUTIONS:** Not for treatment of rosacea or perioral dermatitis. May produce reversible HPA axis suppression, manifestations of Cushing's syndrome, hyperglycemia, and glucosuria. Reassess diagnosis if no improvement after 2 weeks. D/C if irritation occurs. Pediatrics may be more susceptible to systemic toxicity. Use appropriate antifungal or antibacterial agent with dermatological infections. Avoid occlusive dressings.

**ADVERSE REACTIONS:** Burning, stinging, pruritus, skin atrophy, cracking/fissuring of skin, irritation, (sol) tingling, (sol) folliculitis.

**PREGNANCY:** Category C, caution in nursing.

**MECHANISM OF ACTION:** Corticosteroid; possesses anti-inflammatory, antipruritic, and vasoconstrictive properties. Suspected to stabilize cellular and lysosomal membranes, thereby preventing release of proteolytic enzymes, and consequently reducing inflammation.

**PHARMACOKINETICS: Absorption:** Extent of percutaneous absorption depends on integrity of skin, vehicle, and use of occlusive dressings. **Distribution:** Plasma protein binding (variable). **Metabolism:** Liver. **Elimination:** Kidney (major), bile.

### NURSING CONSIDERATIONS

**Assessment:** Assess for known hypersensitivity to other corticosteroids. Assess that medication is not for treatment of rosacea, or perioral dermatitis. Assess use in treatment of acne, and pregnancy/nursing status.

**Monitoring:** Monitor for signs/symptoms of HPA-axis suppression, Cushing's syndrome, hyperglycemia, and glucosuria. In patients taking large doses, perform periodic monitoring for HPA-axis suppression by using the urinary free cortisol and ACTH stimulation tests. Monitor for signs of skin irritation and infection (eg, bacterial, fungal), and treat accordingly. In patients using the medication on the face, groin, or underarm areas, monitor for atrophic changes. In pediatric patients, monitor for signs of HPA-axis suppression (eg, linear growth retardation, delayed weight gain, low plasma cortisol levels, and absence of response to ACTH), Cushing's syndrome, and intracranial HTN.

**Patient Counseling:** Instruct to use as directed and avoid contact with eyes. Counsel not to bandage, cover, or wrap treated skin areas. Inform to report any signs of local adverse reactions.

**Administration:** Topical. Treatment must be limited to 2 consecutive weeks, and should not exceed >50g per week. Not to be used with occlusive dressings. **Storage**: 15-30°C (59-86°F).

## CORTEF RX

hydrocortisone (Pharmacia & Upjohn)

**THERAPEUTIC CLASS:** Corticosteroid

**INDICATIONS:** Steroid-responsive disorders.

C

**DOSAGE:** *Adults:* Initial: 20-240mg/day depending on disease. Adjust until a satisfactory response. Maint: Decrease in small amounts to lowest effective dose. Acute Exacerbations of Multiple Sclerosis: (Tab) Initial: 200mg/day of prednisolone for 1 week, then 80mg every other day for 1 month (20mg hydrocortisone=5mg prednisolone).
*Pediatrics:* Initial: 20-240mg/day depending on disease. Adjust until a satisfactory response. Maint: After favorable response, decrease in small amounts to lowest effective dose. Acute Exacerbations of Multiple Sclerosis: Initial: (Tab) 200mg/day of prednisolone for 1 week, then 80mg every other day for 1 month (20mg hydrocortisone=5mg prednisolone).

**HOW SUPPLIED:** Sus: (Hydrocortisone Cypionate) 10mg/5mL [120mL]; Tab: (Hydrocortisone) 5mg, 10mg, 20mg

**CONTRAINDICATIONS:** Systemic fungal infections.

**WARNINGS/PRECAUTIONS:** May need to increase dose before, during, and after stressful situations. May mask signs of infections. Avoid abrupt withdrawal. Prolonged use may produce glaucoma, optic nerve damage, secondary ocular infections. Increases BP, salt/water retention, potassium excretion. More severe/fatal course of infections reported with chickenpox, measles. Caution with TB, hypothyroidism, cirrhosis, ocular herpes simplex, HTN, diverticulitis, fresh intestinal anastomosis, ulcerative colitis, osteoporosis, myasthenia gravis, renal insufficiency, peptic ulcer disease. Growth and development of children on prolonged therapy should be monitored. Monitor for psychic disturbances. Kaposi's sarcoma reported.

**ADVERSE REACTIONS:** Fluid and electrolyte disturbances, HTN, osteoporosis, muscle weakness, cushingoid state, menstrual irregularities, nervousness, insomnia, impaired wound healing, DM, ulcerative esophagitis, excessive sweating, increased ICP, carbohydrate intolerance, glaucoma, cataracts.

**INTERACTIONS:** Reduced efficacy and increased clearance with hepatic enzyme inducers (eg, phenobarbital, phenytoin, and rifampin). Decreased clearance with ketoconazole and troleandomycin. Increases clearance of chronic high-dose ASA; caution with hypoprothrombinemia. Effects on oral anticoagulants are variable; monitor PT. Increased insulin and oral hypoglycemic requirements in DM. Avoid live vaccines with immunosuppressive doses. Possible decreased vaccine response with killed or inactivated vaccines with immunosuppressive doses.

**PREGNANCY:** Safety in pregnancy and nursing not known.

**MECHANISM OF ACTION:** Anti-inflammatory glucocorticoid; causes profound and varied metabolic effects and modifies the body's immune responses to diverse stimuli.

## NURSING CONSIDERATIONS

**Assessment:** Assess systemic fungal infections, current infections, active TB, vaccination history, ulcerative colitis, diverticulitis, peptic ulcer, renal/hepatic insufficiency, septic arthritis/unstable joint, HTN, osteoporosis, myasthenia gravis, thyroid status, psychotic tendencies, and possible drug interactions.

**Monitoring:** Monitor for adrenocortical insufficiency, occurrence of infections, psychic derangement, cataracts, acute myopathy, Kaposi's sarcoma, fluid retention, and measurement of serum electrolytes, TSH, LFTs, IOP, and BP. Monitor urinalysis, blood sugar, weight, chest X-ray, and upper GI X-ray (if ulcer history) regularly during prolonged therapy.

**Patient Counseling:** Inform that susceptibility to infections may increase. Avoid exposure to chickenpox and measles; report immediately if exposed. Do not d/c abruptly or without medical supervision. Dietary salt restriction and supplementation of potassium is advised.

**Administration:** Oral route. **Storage:** 20-25°C (68-77°F).

C

## CORTISPORIN-TC OTIC RX

hydrocortisone acetate - thonzonium bromide - neomycin sulfate - colistin sulfate (JHP Pharmaceuticals, LLC)

**THERAPEUTIC CLASS:** Antibacterial/corticosteroid combination

**INDICATIONS:** Treatment of infections of the external auditory canal, mastoidectomy and fenestration cavities.

**DOSAGE:** *Adults:* Clean and dry ear canal. Dropper: 5 drops (calibrated dropper) or 4 drops (dropper bottle) tid-qid. Alternate Regimen: Insert cotton wick into ear canal, then saturate cotton. Repeat q4h to keep cotton moist. Replace wick q24h.

*Pediatrics:* Clean and dry ear canal. Dropper: 4 drops (calibrated dropper) or 3 drops (dropper bottle) tid-qid. Alternate Regimen: Insert cotton wick into ear canal, then saturate cotton. Repeat q4h to keep cotton moist. Replace wick q24h.

**HOW SUPPLIED:** (Colistin-Hydrocortisone-Neomycin-Thonzonium) Sus: 3mg-10mg-3.3mg-0.5mg/mL [10mL]

**CONTRAINDICATIONS:** Herpes simplex and varicella infections.

**WARNINGS/PRECAUTIONS:** Caution with perforated eardrum, chronic otitis media. Prolonged use may result in secondary infection. Re-evaluate if no improvement after 1 week. D/C after 10 days.

**ADVERSE REACTIONS:** Cutaneous sensitization.

**PREGNANCY:** Safety in pregnancy and nursing not known.

**MECHANISM OF ACTION:** Colistin: Polypeptide antibiotic; penetrates into and disrupts bacterial cell membrane. Neomycin: Aminoglycoside antibiotic; inhibits protein synthesis, disrupting normal cycle of ribosomal function. Hydrocortisone: Corticosteroid hormone; thought to act by regulating rate of protein synthesis and controls inflammation. Thonzonium: Surfactant; promotes tissue contact by dispersion and penetration of the cellular debris and exudate.

### NURSING CONSIDERATIONS

**Assessment:** Assess for hypersensitivity, external auditory canal disorder due to cutaneous viral infection, perforated tympanic membrane, chronic otitis media, stasis dermatitis and pregnancy/nursing status.

**Monitoring:** Monitor for allergic cross-reactions, cutaneous sensitization as in chronic dermatoses manifested by low-grade reddening with swelling, dry scaling and itching, auditory function, ototoxicity, overgrowth of nonsusceptible organisms and fungi, and lab monitoring of eosinophils and urinary 17-hydroxycorticosteroids.

**Patient Counseling:** Avoid contaminating dropper with material from the ear or any other surface. D/C and contact physician if sensitization or irritation occurs. Do not use in eyes.

**Administration:** Otic route. Shake well before use. **Storage:** 20-25°C (68-77°F).

## CORVERT RX

ibutilide fumarate (Pharmacia & Upjohn)

**THERAPEUTIC CLASS:** Class III antiarrhythmic

**INDICATIONS:** For rapid conversion of atrial fibrillation or flutter (A-Fib/Flutter) of recent onset to sinus rhythm.

**DOSAGE:** *Adults:* ≥60kg: 1mg over 10 min. <60kg: 0.01mg/kg over 10 min. If arrhythmia still present within 10 min after the end of the initial infusion, repeat infusion 10 min after completion of 1st infusion.

**HOW SUPPLIED:** Inj: 0.1mg/mL

**WARNINGS/PRECAUTIONS:** Proarrhythmic; can cause potentially fatal arrhythmias. Administer in setting with continuous ECG monitoring and person able to treat acute ventricular arrhythmia. Adequately anticoagulate if A-Fib >2-3 days. Correct hypokalemia and hypomagnesemia before therapy. Caution in elderly.



**ADVERSE REACTIONS:** Sustained and nonsustained polymorphic ventricular tachycardia, sustained and nonsustained monomorphic ventricular tachycardia, bundle branch and AV block, ventricular and supraventricular extrasystoles, hypotension, bradycardia.

**INTERACTIONS:** Avoid Class IA (eg, disopyramide, quinidine, procainamide) and other Class III (eg, amiodarone, sotalol) antiarrhythmics with or within 4 hrs postinfusion of ibutilide. Increase proarrhythmia potential with drugs that prolong the QT interval (eg, phenothiazines, TCAs). Supraventricular arrhythmias may mask cardiotoxicity associated with excessive digoxin levels.

**PREGNANCY:** Category C, not for use in nursing.

**MECHANISM OF ACTION:** Class III antiarrhythmic agent; prolongs atrial and ventricular action potential duration and refractoriness. Delays repolarization by activation of a slow, inward current, rather than blocking outward potassium currents.

**PHARMACOKINETICS: Distribution:** $V_d$=11 L/kg; plasma protein binding (40%). **Metabolism:** Omega-oxidation and β-oxidation; omega-hydroxy metabolite (active). **Elimination:** Urine 82% (7% unchanged) feces (19%); $T_{1/2}$=6 hrs.

## NURSING CONSIDERATIONS

**Assessment:** Assess for arrhythmia, bradycardia, hypokalemia, renal/hepatic impairment, and possible drug interactions.

**Monitoring:** Monitor for worsening of induction of new ventricular arrhythmia, torsades de pointes (a polymorphic ventricular tachycardia), and HR.

**Patient Counseling:** Inform about benefits/risks. Report any adverse reactions to physician. Patients with chronic A-Fib of ≥2-3 days duration must be adequately anticoagulated for at least 2 weeks. May cause potentially fatal arrhythmia, particularly sustained polymorphic ventricular tachycardia.

**Administration:** IV route. **Storage:** 20-25°C (68-77°F).

# COSOPT — RX

dorzolamide HCl - timolol maleate (Merck)

**THERAPEUTIC CLASS:** Carbonic anhydrase inhibitor/nonselective beta-blocker

**INDICATIONS:** Treatment of ocular hypertension and open-angle glaucoma insufficiently responsive to β-blockers.

**DOSAGE:** *Adults:* 1 drop bid. Space dosing of other ophthalmic drugs by 10 min.

*Pediatrics:* ≥2 yrs: 1 drop bid. Space dosing of other ophthalmic drugs by 10 min.

**HOW SUPPLIED:** Sol: (Dorzolamide-Timolol) 2%-0.5% [5mL, 10mL]

**CONTRAINDICATIONS:** Bronchial asthma, history of bronchial asthma, severe COPD, sinus bradycardia, 2nd- or 3rd-degree AV block, overt cardiac failure, cardiogenic shock.

**WARNINGS/PRECAUTIONS:** Caution with sulfonamide allergy, cardiac failure, diabetes mellitus (DM), COPD, bronchospastic disease, surgery and hepatic impairment. May mask symptoms of hypoglycemia and thyrotoxicosis. Bacterial keratitis reported with contaminated containers. Avoid in severe renal impairment. D/C if hypersensitivity or ocular reactions occur. Reinsert contact lenses 15 min after applying drops.

**ADVERSE REACTIONS:** Taste perversion, ocular burning, conjunctival hyperemia, blurred vision, superficial punctate keratitis, eye itching.

C

**INTERACTIONS:** Avoid oral carbonic anhydrase inhibitors, oral β-blockers, or topical β-blockers due to potential additive effects. Oral/IV calcium antagonists can cause AV-conduction disturbances, left ventricular failure or hypotension. Potentiated systemic β-blockade with concomitant CYP2D6 inhibitors. Reserpine can cause additive effects, hypotension and/or bradycardia. AV conduction time prolonged with digitalis. Quinidine may potentiate β-blockade. Increased risk of hypoglycemia with insulin or oral hypoglycemic agents. Wait 10 min before using another ophthalmic drug.

**PREGNANCY:** Category C, not for use in nursing.

**MECHANISM OF ACTION:** Dorzolamide: Inhibitor of human carbonic anhydrase II; decreases aqueous humor secretion, presumably by slowing formation of bicarbonate ions with subsequent reduction in $Na^+$ and fluid transport. Timolol: $\beta_1$ and $\beta_2$ (non-selective) adrenergic receptor blocking agent; decrease elevated IOP by reducing aqueous humor secretion.

**PHARMACOKINETICS: Absorption:** Timolol: $C_{max}$=0.46ng/mL. **Distribution:** Dorzolamide: Plasma protein binding (33%). **Elimination:** Dorzolamide: Urine (unchanged).

## NURSING CONSIDERATIONS

**Assessment:** Assess for history of bronchial asthma, severe COPD, sinus bradycardia, 2nd- or 3rd-degree AV block, overt cardiac failure, and cardiogenic shock. Assess sulfonamide allergy, use when undergoing elective surgery, risk for hypoglycemia with DM, with hyperthyroidism, with acute angle-closure glaucoma, with severe renal impairment (CrCl <30mL/min), with hepatic impairment, in pregnancy/nursing, and for possible drug interactions.

**Monitoring:** Monitor for signs/symptoms of anaphylaxis, severe respiratory reactions, cardiac reactions, Stevens-Johnson syndrome, toxic epidermal necrolysis, fulminant hepatic necrosis, agranulocytosis, aplastic anemia and other blood system dyscrasias, muscle weakness, choroidal detachment, acute hypoglycemia with DM, occurrence of thyroid storm with thyrotoxicosis and abrupt withdrawal, primary conjunctivitis and lid reactions with chronic therapy, and bacterial keratitis with use of multi-dose containers.

**Patient Counseling:** Contact physician immediately if any type of cardiac, respiratory, or anaphylactic reactions occur. Advise to d/c and report if ocular reactions (eg, conjunctivitis, lid reactions) occur. Handle solution properly. Do not touch container tip to eye or surrounding structures; may become contaminated. Immediately contact physician concerning use of present multidose container if undergoing ocular surgery or develop a concomitant ocular condition (eg, trauma, infection). Remove contact lenses prior to administration; may be reinserted 15 min after. Inform to administer at least 10 min apart if using other ophthalmic medications.

**Administration:** Ocular route. 1) Tilt head back and pull lower eyelid down to form pocket between eyelid and eye. 2) Invert bottle and press lightly until single drop is released. **Storage:** 15-30°C (59-86°F). Protect from light.

# COUMADIN — RX

warfarin sodium (Bristol-Myers Squibb)

**May cause major or fatal bleeding; monitor INR regularly.**

**OTHER BRAND NAMES:** Jantoven (Upsher-Smith)

**THERAPEUTIC CLASS:** Vitamin K-dependent coagulation factor inhibitor

**INDICATIONS:** Prophylaxis and treatment of venous thrombosis, pulmonary embolism (PE), and thromboembolic complications associated with atrial fibrillation (AF) and/or cardiac valve replacement. To reduce risk of death, recurrent myocardial infarction (MI), and thromboembolic events (eg, stroke, systemic embolization) after MI.

**DOSAGE:** *Adults:* Individualize dose. Adjust dose based on PT/INR. Give IV as alternate to PO. Initial: 2-5mg qd. Maintenance: 2-10mg qd. Venous Thromboembolism (including DVT and PE): Target INR 2.5 (INR Range, 2-3).

Atrial Fibrillation: INR 2-3. Post-MI: INR 2.5-3.5. Mechanical/Bioprosthetic Heart Valve: St. Jude Medical Bileaflet Valve in the Aortic Position: Target INR: 2.5 (INR Range, 2-3). Tilting Disk Valves and Bileaflet Mechanical Valves in the Mitral Position: Target INR: 3 (INR Range, 2.5-3.5). Caged Ball or Caged Disk Valve: Target INR 3 (INR Range, 2.5-3.5) in combination with ASA, 75-100mg/day. Bioprosthetic Valves in the Mitral and Aortic Position: Target INR: 2.5 (INR Range, 2-3). Valvular Heart Disease Associated with Atrial Fibrillation/Mitral Stenosis/Recurrent Systemic Embolism of Unknown Etiology: INR 2-3. Elderly: Start at the low end of dosing range.

**HOW SUPPLIED:** Inj: (Coumadin) 5mg; Tab: (Coumadin, Jantoven) 1mg*, 2mg*, 2.5mg*, 3mg*, 4mg*, 5mg*, 6mg*, 7.5mg*, 10mg* *scored

**CONTRAINDICATIONS:** Pregnancy. Hemorrhagic tendencies or blood dyscrasias. Recent or contemplated surgery of the central nervous system, eye, or traumatic surgery resulting in large open surfaces. Bleeding tendencies associated with active ulceration or overt bleeding of GI, genitourinary, or respiratory tract, cerebrovascular hemorrhage, aneurysms-cerebral, dissecting aorta, pericarditis and pericardial effusions, bacterial endocarditis. Threatened abortion, eclampsia, and preeclampsia. Inadequate laboratory facilities. Unsupervised patients with senility, alcoholism, or psychosis or other lack of patient cooperation. Spinal puncture and other diagnostic or therapeutic procedures with potential for uncontrollable bleeding. Major regional, lumbar block anesthesia, and malignant hypertension.

**WARNINGS/PRECAUTIONS:** Monitor PT/INR; many endogenous and exogenous factors may affect PT/INR. Risk of necrosis and/or gangrene of the skin and other tissues which may result in death or permanent disability; perform careful diagnosis to determine whether necrosis is caused by underlying disease or warfarin therapy. D/C if warfarin suspected to be cause of necrosis. Individualize therapy. Caution when administered in the presence of any predisposing condition where added risk of hemorrhage, necrosis, and/or gangrene is present. D/C if systemic cholesterol microembolization ("purple toe syndrome") occurs. Caution in patients with heparin-induced thrombocytopenia and deep vein thrombosis; cases of venous limb ischemia, necrosis, and gangrene reported when heparin d/c and warfarin started or continued. Weigh benefits/risks of therapy with lactation, severe-moderate hepatic or renal insufficiency, infectious diseases, disturbances of the intestinal flora, trauma which may result in internal bleeding, surgery or trauma resulting in large exposed raw surfaces, indwelling catheters, severe-moderate hypertension (HTN), protein C deficiency, polycythemia vera, vasculitis, and severe diabetes. Caution in the elderly.

**ADVERSE REACTIONS:** Fatal or non-fatal hemorrhage from any tissue or organ, necrosis of the skin and other tissues, paralysis, paresthesia, headache, chest/abdomen/joint/muscle pain, dizziness, shortness of breath, difficulty breathing or swallowing, unexplained swelling, weakness, hypotension, unexplained shock.

**INTERACTIONS:** May interact with protein bound drugs, hepatic enzyme inducers and inhibitors. Caution with drugs that may cause hemorrhage (eg, NSAIDs, ASA), botanicals. Some botanicals (bromelains, danshen, garlic, Gingko biloba, ginseng, cranberry products) may increase coumadin effects, others (coenzyme $Q_{10}$, St. John's wort) may decrease effects. May potentiate hypoglycemic and anticonvulsant drugs. May interact with antihyperlipidemic drugs like ezetimibe, thrombolytics, and many other drug classes. Refer to PI for extensive list of drug interactions. Concomitant administration with ticlopidine may be associated with cholestatic hepatitis.

**PREGNANCY:** Category X, safety not known in nursing.

**MECHANISM OF ACTION:** Vitamin K-dependent coagulation factor inhibitor; interferes with clotting factor synthesis by inhibition of the C1 subunit of the vitamin K epoxide reductase enzyme complex, thereby reducing the regeneration of vitamin $K_1$ epoxide.

**PHARMACOKINETICS: Absorption:** (PO) Complete; $T_{max}$=4 hrs. **Distribution:** $V_d$=0.14 L/kg; plasma protein binding (99%); found in fetal plasma. **Metabolism:** Hepatic via CYP2C9, 2C19, 2C8, 2C18, 1A2, 3A4. **Elimination:** Urine (major, up to 92%)(metabolites), bile (metabolites); $T_{1/2}$=1 week.

C

## NURSING CONSIDERATIONS

**Assessment:** Assess pregnancy status, presence of hemorrhagic tendencies or blood dyscrasias, bleeding tendencies associated with active ulceration, overt bleeding (eg, genitourinary, cerebrovascular hemorrhage, pericarditis), senility (psychosis), alcoholism, eclampsia, preeclampsia, presence of major regional lumbar block anesthesia, and malignant HTN. Assess that patient is not undergoing spinal puncture or other diagnostic or therapeutic procedures with the potential for uncontrollable bleeding. Assess for recent or contemplated surgery of the CNS, eye, or traumatic surgery resulting in large open surfaces. Assess use in nursing females, severe to moderate hepatic/renal insufficiencies, presence of infectious diseases, disturbances in the intestinal flora, indwelling catheters, severe to moderate HTN, known or suspected deficiency in protein C-mediated anticoagulant response, presence of polycythemia vera, vasculitis, and severe DM. Assess for drug and drug-disease interactions. Assess INR/PT.

**Monitoring:** Monitor for signs/symptoms of bleeding, necrosis of the skin and other organs, and systemic atheroemboli or cholesterol microemboli (eg, "purple toe syndrome," livedo reticularis, rash). Periodically monitor INR/PT.

**Patient Counseling:** Counsel to maintain strict adherence to dosing regimen. Instruct to notify physician of all medications (OTC, herbals) currently taken. Advise not to start or stop other medications before contacting physician. Instruct to avoid any activity or sport that may result in traumatic injury. Inform females about risk during pregnancy. Instruct that regular prothrombin time tests are required. Advice patient to carry ID card stating drug is being taken. Inform that vitamin K in diet may affect medication. Instruct to eat normal, balanced diet; avoid drastic changes in diet such as eating large amounts of leafy green vegetables. Instruct to avoid alcohol consumption, cranberry juice, and cranberry products. Inform to contact physician if dose is missed. Instruct to take missed dose as soon as possible on the same day, but instruct to not take a double dose the next day to make up for missed doses. Advise to immediately report unusual bleeding.

**Administration:** Oral or IV route. IV: Reconstitute with 2.7mL of sterile water for Inj to yield 2mg/mL. Administer as slow bolus injection over 1-2 mins into a peripheral vein. Not for IM use. **Storage:** Tab: 15-30°C (59-86°F). Dispense in tight, light-resistant container. Inj: 15-30°C (59-86°F). Use within 4 hrs after reconstitution. Do not refrigerate. Discard any unused solution.

# COVERA-HS — RX

verapamil HCl (G.D. Searle)

**THERAPEUTIC CLASS:** Calcium channel blocker (nondihydropyridine)

**INDICATIONS:** Management of hypertension and angina.

**DOSAGE:** *Adults:* Initial: 180mg qhs. Titrate: May increase to 240mg qhs, then 360mg qhs, then 480mg qhs, if needed. Elderly: Start at the low end of the dosing range. Swallow whole; do not chew, break, or crush.

**HOW SUPPLIED:** Tab, Extended-Release: 180mg, 240mg

**CONTRAINDICATIONS:** Severe left ventricular dysfunction, hypotension (systolic pressure <90mm Hg), cardiogenic shock, sick sinus syndrome, 2nd- or 3rd-degree AV block (except with functioning ventricular pacemaker), A-fibrillation/flutter with an accessory bypass tract (eg, Wolff-Parkinson-White (WPW), Lown-Ganong-Levine syndromes).

**WARNINGS/PRECAUTIONS:** Avoid with moderate to severe cardiac failure, and ventricular dysfunction if taking a β-blocker. May cause dizziness, hypotension, CHF, pulmonary edema, AV block, transient bradycardia, PR interval prolongation. Increased transaminases and hepatocellular injury reported. Monitor LFTs and abnormal PR prolongation. Give 30% of normal dose with severe hepatic dysfunction. Caution with hypertrophic cardiomyopathy, pre-existing severe GI narrowing, renal or hepatic dysfunction. Decrease dose with attenuated neuromuscular transmission. Caution in elderly.

C

**ADVERSE REACTIONS:** Constipation, dizziness, nausea, hypotension, headache, edema, fatigue, bradycardia, AV block, and upper respiratory infection.

**INTERACTIONS:** Additive negative effects on HR, AV conduction, and contractility with β-blockers. Asymptomatic bradycardia (36 beats/min) with a wandering atrial pacemaker reported with timolol eyedrops. May decrease metoprolol and propranolol clearance when coadministered. Potentiates other oral antihypertensive agents (eg, vasodilators, ACE inhibitors, diuretics). May increase digoxin, carbamazepine, theophylline, cyclosporine, and alcohol levels. Avoid disopyramide within 48 hrs before or 24 hrs after administration. Additive negative inotropic effects and AV conduction prolongation with flecainide. Avoid quinidine with hypertrophic cardiomyopathy. Monitor lithium levels. CYP3A4 inhibitors (eg, erythromycin, ritonavir) and grapefruit juice may increase levels. CYP3A4 inducers (eg, rifampin, phenobarbital) may decrease levels. Increased bleeding time with aspirin. May potentiate neuromuscular blockers; both agents may need dose reduction. Caution with inhalation anesthetics. Hypotension and bradyarrhythmias observed with telithromycin.

**PREGNANCY:** Category C, not for use in nursing.

**MECHANISM OF ACTION:** Calcium channel blocker; inhibits transmembrane influx of calcium ions into arterial smooth muscle and conductile/contractile myocardial cells.

**PHARMACOKINETICS: Absorption:** $T_{max}$=11 hrs. R-Enantiomer: Bioavailability (33-65%). S-Enantiomer: Bioavailability (13-34%). Oral administration of variable doses resulted in different parameters. **Distribution:** R-Enantiomer: Plasma protein binding (94%). S-Enantiomer: Plasma protein binding (88%). **Metabolism:** Liver; norverapamil (active metabolite). **Elimination:** Urine (70% [metabolites] , 3-4% [unchanged]), feces (16%).

## NURSING CONSIDERATIONS

**Assessment:** Assess for left ventricular dysfunction, hypotension, sick sinus syndrome, AV block, atrial flutter/fibrillation with accessory bypass tract (eg, WPW), hypertrophic cardiomyopathy, severe GI narrowing, hepatic/renal impairment, hypersensitivity to drug, pregnancy/nursing status, and possible drug interactions.

**Monitoring:** Monitor LFTs and renal function, abnormal PR interval prolongation (toxicity), hepatotoxicity, renal dysfunction, CV events (eg, hypotension), and hypersensitivity reactions.

**Patient Counseling:** Instruct to swallow tab whole; do not chew, break, or crush. Advise to seek medical attention if symptoms of hepatotoxicity (malaise, fever, right upper quandrant pain), CV events (hypotension), or hypersensitivity reactions occur. Instruct that outer shell of tablet does not dissolve; may occasionally observe in stool.

**Administration:** Oral route. **Storage:** 20-25°C (68-77°F); keep in a light-resistant container.

# COZAAR — RX

losartan potassium (Merck)

**Can cause death/injury to developing fetus during 2nd and 3rd trimesters. D/C therapy if pregnancy detected.**

**THERAPEUTIC CLASS:** Angiotensin II receptor antagonist

**INDICATIONS:** Treatment of hypertension (HTN), alone or with other antihypertensives. Reduction of the risk of stroke in patients with HTN and left ventricular hypertrophy (LVH), but evidence shows this does not apply to black patients. Treatment of diabetic nephropathy with an elevated SrCr and proteinuria (urinary albumin to creatinine ratio ≥300mg/g) in patients with type 2 diabetes and HTN.

**DOSAGE:** *Adults:* HTN: Initial: 50mg qd. Usual: 25-100mg/day given qd-bid. Intravascular Volume Depletion/Hepatic Impairment: Initial: 25mg qd. HTN with LVH: Initial: 50mg qd. Add hydrochlorothiazide (HCTZ) 12.5mg qd and/

or increase losartan to 100mg qd, followed by an increase in HCTZ to 25mg qd based on BP response. Nephropathy: Initial: 50 mg qd. Titrate: Increase to 100mg qd based on BP response.



*Pediatrics:* ≥6 yrs: HTN: Initial: 0.7mg/kg qd (up to 50mg/day). Max: 1.4mg/kg qd (100mg qd). Avoid in pediatric patients with GFR <30mL/min/1.73m².

**HOW SUPPLIED:** Tab: 25mg, 50mg, 100mg

**WARNINGS/PRECAUTIONS:** Correct volume or salt depletion before therapy or start therapy at a lower dose. Caution with severe CHF and renal artery stenosis. Changes in renal function may occur. Consider dose adjustment with hepatic dysfunction. Angioedema reported.

**ADVERSE REACTIONS:** Dizziness, cough, upper respiratory infection, diarrhea, asthenia/fatigue, chest pain, fever, influenza-like disease, vascular disease, cataracts, anemia, hypoglycemia, back pain, bronchitis, hyperkalemia.

**INTERACTIONS:** Concomitant with $K^+$-sparing diuretics (eg, spironolactone, triamterene, amiloride), $K^+$ supplements, or $K^+$-containing salt substitutes may increase serum $K^+$. May reduce excretion of lithium; monitor lithium levels. Combination with NSAIDs, including COX-2 inhibitors, may lead to further deterioration of renal function and diminish antihypertensive effect. Increased levels with cimetidine, fluconazole. Decreased levels with phenobarbital, rifampin.

**PREGNANCY:** Category C (1st trimester) and D (2nd and 3rd trimesters), not for use in nursing.

**MECHANISM OF ACTION:** Angiotensin II receptor antagonist; blocks vasoconstrictor and aldosterone-secreting effects of angiotensin II by selectively blocking binding of angiotensin II to $AT_1$ receptor.

**PHARMACOKINETICS: Absorption:** Systemic bioavailability (33%). **Adults:** $C_{max}$=224ng/mL, $T_{max}$=0.9 hrs, AUC=442ng•h/mL. (Metabolite) $C_{max}$=212ng/mL, $T_{max}$=3.5 hrs, AUC= 1685 ng•h/mL. **Pediatrics:** $C_{max}$=141ng/mL, $T_{max}$=2 hrs, AUC=368ng•h/mL. (Metabolite) $C_{max}$=222ng/mL, $T_{max}$=4.1 hrs, AUC=1866ng•h/mL. **Distribution:** Plasma protein binding (98.7%; 99.8% metabolite). $V_d$=34L, 12L (metabolite). **Metabolism:** Liver via CYP2C9, 3A4; active carboxylic acid metabolite. **Elimination:** Urine (35%), feces (60%). **Adults:** $T_{1/2}$=2.1 hrs, 7.4 hrs (metabolite). **Pediatrics:** $T_{1/2}$=2.3 hrs, 5.6 hrs (metabolite).

## NURSING CONSIDERATIONS

**Assessment:** Assess volume/salt depletion status, CHF, DM, hepatic/renal impairment, pregnancy/nursing status and possible drug interactions.

**Monitoring:** Monitor serum electrolytes and renal function periodically. Monitor for signs/symptoms of electrolyte imbalance, hypotension, hypersensitivity reactions, renal/hepatic dysfunction.

**Patient Counseling:** Inform of pregnancy risks. Advise to seek medical attention if symptoms of electrolyte imbalance, hypotension, or hypersensitivity reactions (angioedema) occur.

**Administration:** Oral route. Refer to PI for preparation of suspension. **Storage:** Tab: 25°C (77°F); excursions permitted to 15-30°C (59-86°F). Protect from light. Sus: 2-8°C (36-46°F) for up to 4 weeks.

# CRESTOR RX

rosuvastatin calcium (AstraZeneca)

**THERAPEUTIC CLASS:** HMG-CoA reductase inhibitor

**INDICATIONS:** Adjunct to diet in primary hyperlipidemia and mixed dyslipidemia to reduce elevated total cholesterol (total-C), LDL, apolipoprotein (ApoB), non-HDL, and triglyceride (TG) levels and to increase HDL in adult patients. Adjunct to diet in adolescent boys and girls, 10-17 yrs old, who are at least one year post-menarche with heterozygous familial hypercholesterolemia to reduce total-C, LDL and ApoB levels. Adjunct to diet for the treatment of adult patients with hypertriglyceridemia. Adjunct to diet for the treatment of primary dysbetalipoproteinemia (Type III hyperlipoproteinemia). Adjunct to other lipid-lowering treatments (eg, LDL apheresis) or alone if such treatments are unavailable, to reduce LDL, total-C, and ApoB in adult patients with homozygous familial hypercholesterolemia. Adjunct to diet to slow the progression of atherosclerosis in adult patients as part of a treatment strategy to lower total-C and LDL to target levels. Reduces risk of MI, stroke, and arterial revascularization procedures in patients without clinically evident coronary heart disease, but with multiple risk factors.

**DOSAGE:** *Adults:* General: Dosing Range: 5-40 mg qd. Initial: 10-20mg. Titrate: Adjust dose if needed at 2-4 week intervals. Homozygous Familial Hypercholesterolemia: 20mg qd. Asian Patients: 5mg qd. Concomitant Cyclosporine: Max: 5mg qd. Concomitant Lopinavir/Ritonavir or Atazanavir/Ritonavir: Max 10mg qd. Concomitant with Niacin/Fenofibrate: Reduce dose. Concomitant Gemfibrozil: Max: 10mg qd. Severe Renal Impairment: CrCl <30mL/min/1.73m$^2$ (not on hemodialysis): Initial: 5mg qd. Max: 10mg qd. *Pediatrics:* 10-17yrs: Heterozygous Familial Hypercholesterolemia: Individualize dose. Usual: 5-20mg/day. Titrate: Adjust dose at intervals of ≥4 weeks. Max: 20mg/day.

**HOW SUPPLIED:** Tab: 5mg, 10mg, 20mg, 40mg

**CONTRAINDICATIONS:** Active liver disease, including unexplained persistent elevations of hepatic transaminase levels, pregnancy, nursing mothers.

**WARNINGS/PRECAUTIONS:** Cases of myopathy and rhabdomyolysis with acute renal failure secondary to myoglobinuria reported; increase risk at highest dose (40mg). Caution in patients with predisposing factors for myopathy (eg, ≥65 yrs old, inadequately treated hypothyroidism, renal impairment). D/C if markedly elevated creatine kinase (CPK) levels occur or myopathy is diagnosed or suspected. Withhold if patient has acute condition predisposing to the development of renal failure secondary to rhabdomyolysis (eg, sepsis, hypotension, dehydration, trauma, severe metabolic, endocrine and electrolyte disorders, uncontrolled seizures). Increases in serum transaminases (AST, ALT) reported. Monitor LFTs prior to therapy, at 12 weeks following initiation of therapy and any dose elevation, and periodically thereafter. Reduce dose or d/c if AST/ALT >3x ULN persists. Caution with heavy alcohol use and/or history of chronic liver disease. Dipstick-positive proteinuria and microscopic hematuria observed; consider dose reduction with unexplained proteinuria and/or hematuria. Increase in Hba1c and FPG levels reported. Caution in elderly, renal/hepatic impairment, Asian patients.

**ADVERSE REACTIONS:** Headache, myalgia, asthenia, nausea, dizziness, constipation, increased CPK, arthralgia.

**INTERACTIONS:** Increased risk of myopathy with lipid-lowering therapies (fibrates or niacin), gemfibrozil, cyclosporine, lopinavir/ritonavir, or atazanavir/ritonavir. Increases INR with coumarin anticoagulants (eg, warfarin); monitor INR before therapy and frequently enough during early therapy to ensure that no significant change in INR occurs. Caution with drugs that decrease levels or activity of endogenous steroid hormones (eg, ketoconazole, spironolactone, cimetidine). Increased levels with cyclosporine, oral contraceptives, warfarin, digoxin, fibrates (eg, gemfibrozil), and certain protease inhibitors given in combination with ritonavir. Avoid use with gemfibrozil. Aluminum and magnesium hydroxide combination antacids should be taken at least 2 hrs following rosuvastatin administration. Decreased plasma concentration of erythromycin.

**PREGNANCY:** Category X, not for use in nursing.

**MECHANISM OF ACTION:** HMG-CoA reductase inhibitor; increases the number of hepatic LDL receptors on the cell surface to enhance uptake and catabolism of LDL. Also, inhibits hepatic synthesis of VLDL, which reduces the total number of VLDL and LDL particles.

**PHARMACOKINETICS: Absorption:** Absolute bioavailability (20%). $T_{max}$=3-5 hrs. **Distribution:** $V_d$=134L, plasma protein binding (88%). **Metabolism:** CYP2C9; N-desmethyl rosuvastatin (major metabolite). **Elimination:** Feces (90%); $T_{1/2}$=19 hrs.

## NURSING CONSIDERATIONS

**Assessment:** Assess for active liver disease, unexplained persistent elevations of hepatic transaminase levels, pregnancy/nursing status, and for possible drug interactions. Assess use in patients who consume substantial quantities of alcohol and/or have a history of chronic liver disease and in patients with predisposing factors for myopathy (eg, ≥65yrs, inadequately treated hypothyroidism, renal impairment). Assess LFTs prior to therapy. If taking coumarin type anticoagulant, assess INR prior to therapy.

**Monitoring:** Monitor for signs/symptoms of myopathy, rhabdomyolysis, increases in serum transaminase levels, and for proteinuria and hematuria (via urinalysis). Monitor creatinine kinase levels. Monitor LFTs 12 weeks after treatment initiation or any dose elevation and then periodically thereafter.

**Patient Counseling:** Inform about potential risks/benefits of therapy. Instruct to notify physician if pregnant/nursing or planning to become pregnant. Counsel to report promptly any signs of unexplained muscle pain, tenderness or weakness, particularly if accompanied by malaise or fever. Counsel to take at least 2 hrs after antacids containing aluminum and magnesium hydroxide.

**Administration:** Oral route. **Storage:** 20-25°C (68-77°F). Protect from moisture.

## CRIXIVAN — RX

indinavir sulfate (Merck)

**THERAPEUTIC CLASS:** Protease inhibitor

**INDICATIONS:** Treatment of HIV infection in combination with other antiretrovirals.

**DOSAGE:** *Adults:* Usual: 800mg q8h on empty stomach. Hepatic Insufficiency or Concomitant Delavirdine, Itraconazole, Ketoconazole: Reduce to 600mg q8h. Concomitant Didanosine: Administer at least 1 hr apart. Concomitant Rifabutin: 1g q8h (reduce rifabutin dose by 1/2). Take without food but with water 1 hr before or 2 hrs after meals. Maintain adequate hydration (1.5L fluid/24 hrs).

**HOW SUPPLIED:** Cap: 100mg, 200mg, 400mg

**CONTRAINDICATIONS:** Concomitant with pimozide, cisapride, amiodarone, triazolam, oral midazolam, alprazolam, dihydroergotamine, ergonovine, ergotamine, methylergonovine.

**WARNINGS/PRECAUTIONS:** D/C or suspend during acute nephrolithiasis/urolithiasis. Tubulointerstitial nephritis seen with asymptomatic severe leukocyturia; monitor frequently with urinalyses. Consider discontinuation with severe leukocyturia. Immune reconstitution syndrome, hemolytic anemia, hyperglycemia, new onset of diabetes mellitus (DM), exacerbation of preexisting DM, indirect hyperbilirubinemia, hepatitis and liver failure reported. Spontaneous bleeding may occur with hemophilia A and B. Monitor hepatic function. Maintain adequate hydration. Possible redistribution or accumulation of body fat. Caution in elderly.

**ADVERSE REACTIONS:** Nephrolithiasis/urolithiasis, hyperbilirubinemia, abdominal pain, headache, N/V, diarrhea, dizziness, pruritus, asthenia/fatigue, acid regurgitation, anorexia, somnolence.

**INTERACTIONS:** See Contraindications. Increased risk of myopathy including rhabdomyolysis in combination with statin drugs. Avoid coadministration with atazanavir, lovastatin, simvastatin, or rosuvastatin. Caution with atorvastatin. Avoid with St. John's wort and rifampin; may lead to loss of virologic response and possible resistance. Substantially increases sildenafil, tadalafil, vardenafil plasma levels; increased risk of phosphodiesterase type 5 inhibitor-related adverse events (eg, hypotension, visual changes, priapism). Caution with parenteral midazolam; consider dose reduction. Decreased plasma concentrations when coadministered with efavirenz, nevirapine, anticonvulsants (carbamazepine, phenobarbital, phenytoin), venlafaxine. Increased concentrations with nelfinavir, ritonavir, clarithromycin. May increase plasma levels of saquinavir, CCBs (felodipine, nifedipine, nicardipine), immunosuppressants (cyclosporine, tacrolimus, sirolimus), trazadone, fluticasone. Caution with antiarrhythmics (bepridil, lidocaine, quinidine); monitoring concentrations is recommended.

**PREGNANCY:** Category C, not for use in nursing.

**MECHANISM OF ACTION:** Protease inhibitor; prevents cleavage of viral polyproteins, resulting in the formation of immature, noninfectious viral particles.

**PHARMACOKINETICS: Absorption:** Rapid; $C_{max}$=12617nM; $T_{max}$=0.8 hrs; AUC=30691nM•hr. **Distribution:** Plasma protein binding (60%). **Metabolism:** Hepatic via CYP3A4. **Elimination:** Urine (<20%); $T_{1/2}$=1.8 hrs.

## NURSING CONSIDERATIONS

**Assessment:** Assess for asymptomatic severe leukocyturia, hemophilia, hepatic/renal dysfunction, anemia, DM, pregnancy/nursing status, and possible drug interactions.

**Monitoring:** Monitor for possible indirect hyperbilirubinemia, increase in serum transaminase, immune reconstitution syndrome, nephrolithiasis/urolithiasis, hemolytic anemia, hepatitis, fat redistribution, exacerbation of DM (hyperglycemia). Monitor urinalyses frequently for patients with severe leukocyturia and for possible tubulointerstitial nephritis with medullary calcification and cortical atrophy.

**Patient Counseling:** Inform that therapy is not cure for HIV, does not reduce risk of transmission of HIV and that opportunistic infections may develop. Seek medical attention if symptoms of infection, nephrolithiasis/urolithiasis (flank pain, with or without hematuria), anemia, hepatitis, fat redistribution/accumulation and hyperglycemia occur. Advise not to modify or d/c treatment without consulting physician. Advise to keep well hydrated while on drug. Instruct not to take with amiodarone, dihydroergotamine, ergonivine, ergotamine, methylergonovine, oral midazolam, triazolam, alprazolam, cisapride, pimozide. Instruct to report use of any prescription, non-prescription/herbal medication, particularly St. John's wort, to physician. Instruct mothers to d/c nursing if taking drug.

**Administration:** Oral route. If a dose is missed, take the next dose at the regularly scheduled time; do not double dose. Take without food but with water (1 hr before or 2 hrs after a meal). **Storage:** 15-30°C (59-86°F). Store in a tightly closed container; protect from moisture.

# Cromolyn Sodium Inhalation — RX

cromolyn sodium (Various)

**THERAPEUTIC CLASS:** Mast cell stabilizer

**INDICATIONS:** Prophylactic treatment of bronchial asthma and of acute bronchoconstriction due to exercise, environmental agents, and known antigens.

**DOSAGE:** *Adults:* Asthma: 20mg nebulized qid. Acute Bonchospasm Prevention: 20mg nebulized shortly before exposure to precipitant. Renal/Hepatic Dysfunction: Decrease inhaler dose.
*Pediatrics:* Asthma: ≥2 yrs: 20mg nebulized qid. Acute Bronchospasm Prevention: ≥2 yrs: 20mg nebulized shortly before exposure to precipitant. Renal/Hepatic Dysfunction: Decrease inhaler dose.

**HOW SUPPLIED:** Sol: (Cromolyn, neb) 10mg/mL [2mL, $10^s$ $60^s$]

**WARNINGS/PRECAUTIONS:** Not for treatment of acute attack. Severe anaphylaxis may occur. D/C if eosinophilic pneumonia or pulmonary infiltrates with eosinophilia develop. May experience cough and/or bronchospasm. Decrease dose or d/c with renal/hepatic dysfunction.

**ADVERSE REACTIONS:** Throat irritation/dryness, bad taste, cough, nausea, bronchospasm, sneezing, wheezing.

**INTERACTIONS:** Avoid with isoproterenol during pregnancy.

**PREGNANCY:** Category B, caution in nursing.

**MECHANISM OF ACTION:** Mast cell stabilizer; inhibits sensitized mast cell degranulation, release of mediators from mast cells, and both immediate and non-immediate bronchoconstrictive reactions to inhaled antigen.

**PHARMACOKINETICS: Absorption:** 8% absorbed. **Elimination:** Urine, bile.

## NURSING CONSIDERATIONS

**Assessment:** Assess for drug hypersensitivity to cromolyn sodium, impaired renal/hepatic function, respiratory function, CVD.

**Monitoring:** Monitor LFTs, renal function, hypersensitivity reactions, eosinophilic pneumonia, CVD. Maintain close supervision of concomitant therapy to avoid exacerbation of asthma.

**Patient Counseling:** Advise that effect of therapy depends on administration at regular intervals. Take as directed. Take at least 10-15 min before exposure to precipitating factor.

**Administration:** Nebulization. **Storage:** Store between 15-30°C (59-86°F).

# CUBICIN RX

daptomycin (Cubist)

**THERAPEUTIC CLASS:** Cyclic lipopeptide

**INDICATIONS:** Susceptible complicated skin and skin structure infections (cSSSI). *Staphylococcus aureus* bloodstream infections (bacteremia).

**DOSAGE:** *Adults:* ≥18 yrs: Administer as IV infusion over 30 min. cSSSI: 4mg/kg q24h for 7-14 days. *S.aureus* Bacteremia: 6mg/kg q24h for minimum 2-6 weeks. Renal impairment: CrCl <30mL/min, HD, or CAPD: 4mg/kg (cSSSI) or 6mg/kg (*S.aureus* bacteremia) once q48h.

**HOW SUPPLIED:** Inj: 500mg

**WARNINGS/PRECAUTIONS:** *Clostridium difficile*-associated diarrhea reported. D/C if CDAD confirmed. Monitor CPK levels weekly; d/c with unexplained signs and symptoms of myopathy and CPK elevation >1000 U/L (~5x ULN), or with CPK levels ≥10x ULN. Persisting or relapsing *S.aureus* infection or poor clinical response should have repeat blood cultures.

**ADVERSE REACTIONS:** Constipation, NV, injection site reactions, headache, diarrhea, insomnia, rash, abnormal LFTs, superinfection, pharyngolaryngeal pain, pain in extremity and pulmonary eosinophilia.

**INTERACTIONS:** Caution with tobramycin; may affect levels. Monitor PT/INR for first several days with warfarin. Consider temporarily suspending statins. HMG-CoA reductase inhibitors may cause myopathy; consider suspending these agents with concomitant therapy.

**PREGNANCY:** Category B, caution in nursing.

**MECHANISM OF ACTION:** Cyclic lipopeptide; binds to bacterial membranes and causes a rapid depolarization of membrane potential, causing inhibition of protein, DNA, RNA synthesis, which results in bacterial cell death.

**PHARMACOKINETICS: Absorption:** (6mg/kg) $C_{max}$=93.9μg/mL, AUC=632μg•h/mL. **Distribution:** Plasma protein binding (90-93%); $V_d$=0.1L/kg. **Elimination:** Urine (78%), feces (5.7%); $T_{1/2}$=7.7-8.3 hrs.

## NURSING CONSIDERATIONS

**Assessment:** Assess renal fuction, LFTs, CBC and possible drug interactions with HMG-CoA reductase inhibitors.

**Monitoring:** Monitor renal function tests, CPK, fluid electrolyte balance, CBC, PT/INR evaluation, CDAD, neuropathy, myopathy.

**Patient Counseling:** Counsel to immediately report development of watery/bloody diarrhea (with/without stomach cramps) and fever, (may occur as late as 2 months after therapy).

**Administration:** Reconstituted solution should be further diluted with 0.9% NaCl injection to be administered by IV infusion over a period of 30 min. **Storage:** 2-8°C (36-46°F). Avoid excessive heat.

# CUTIVATE — RX
fluticasone propionate (PharmaDerm)



**THERAPEUTIC CLASS:** Corticosteroid

**INDICATIONS:** (Cre, Oint) Relief of the inflammatory and pruritic manifestations of corticosteroid-responsive dermatoses. Cream may be used with caution in pediatric patients ≥3 months of age. (Lot) Relief of the inflammatory and pruritic manifestations of atopic dermatitis in patients ≥1 yr of age.

**DOSAGE:** *Adults:* Atopic Dermatitis: (Cre) Apply qd-bid. (Lot) Apply qd. Other Dermatoses: (Cre) Apply bid. (Oint) Apply bid. (Cre, Lot, Oint) Avoid occlusive dressings and re-evaluate if no improvement after 2 weeks.
*Pediatrics:* ≥3 months: Atopic Dermatitis: (Cre) Apply qd-bid. Other Dermatoses: (Cre) Apply bid. Avoid in diaper area. ≥1 yr: Atopic Dermatitis: (Lot) Apply qd. (Cre, Lot): Avoid occlusive dressings and re-evaluate if no improvement after 2 weeks. Oint not approved in pediatrics.

**HOW SUPPLIED:** Cre: 0.05% [15g, 30g, 60g]; Lot: 0.05% [120mL]; Oint: 0.005% [15g, 30g, 60g]

**WARNINGS/PRECAUTIONS:** Caution with cream in pediatrics. May produce reversible hypothalamic-pituitary-adrenal (HPA) axis suppression, manifestations of Cushing's syndrome, hyperglycemia and glucosuria. Cosyntropin ($ACTH_{1-24}$) stimulation test may be helpful in evaluating HPA axis suppression. May cause cutaneous local adverse reactions. D/C if irritation occurs and if favorable response does not occur promptly. Use appropriate antifungal or antibacterial agent with dermatological infections. Pediatrics may be more susceptible to systemic toxicity. Caution when applied to large surface areas or areas under occlusion. Avoid with pre-existing skin atrophy and presence of infection at treatment site. Not for use in rosacea or perioral dermatitis.

**ADVERSE REACTIONS:** (Cre) Pruritus, dryness, numbness of fingers, burning. (Oint) Pruritus, burning, hypertrichosis, increased erythema, hives, irritation, light-headedness. (Lot) Burning, stinging, headache, common cold, upper respiratory tract infection, cough, fever.

**PREGNANCY:** Category C, caution in nursing.

**MECHANISM OF ACTION:** Corticosteroid; not fully established. Possesses anti-inflammatory, antipruritic, and vasoconstrictive properties. Suspected to act by the induction of phospholipase $A_2$ inhibitory proteins (lipocortins). Lipocortins control biosynthesis of potent mediators of inflammation (eg, prostaglandins, leukotrienes) by inhibiting release of common precursor, arachidonic acid.

**PHARMACOKINETICS: Absorption**: Extent of percutaneous absorption depends on skin integrity, vehicle, and use of occlusive dressings. **Distribution:** (IV) $V_d$=4.2L/kg; plasma protein binding (91%). **Metabolism:** Liver via CYP3A4 (hydrolysis). **Elimination:** (IV) $T_{1/2}$=7.2 hrs.

## NURSING CONSIDERATIONS

**Assessment:** Assess for proper diagnosis, pre-existing skin atrophy, presence of skin infection at treatment site, rosacea and perioral dermatitis. Assess use in pediatrics and in pregnant/nursing patients.

**Monitoring:** Monitor for signs/symptoms of HPA-axis suppression, Cushing's syndrome, hyperglycemia and glucosuria. With large doses or occlusive dressings, monitor for HPA-axis suppression by using the $ACTH_{1-24}$ stimulation, plasma cortisol and urinary free cortisol tests. Monitor for signs/symptoms of local cutaneous reactions and for allergic contact dermatitis (eg, failure to heal). Monitor for signs of skin infections (eg, bacterial, fungal) and treat accordingly. In pediatrics, monitor for signs/symptoms of HPA-axis suppression, Cushing's syndrome, linear growth retardation, delayed weight gain and intracranial HTN.

**Patient Counseling:** Counsel to use as directed, avoid contact with eyes, not to bandage or cover or wrap treated skin and avoid using on face, underarms or groin areas unless directed by physician. Advise to contact physician if any signs of adverse reactions or no clinical improvement within 2 weeks of therapy occurs.

**Administration:** Topical route. **Storage**: (Cre, Oint) 2-30°C (36-86°F). (Lot) 15 and 30°C (59 and 86°F). Do not refrigerate. Keep container tightly sealed.



## CYCLESSA RX

desogestrel - ethinyl estradiol (Organon)

**OTHER BRAND NAMES:** Velivet (Barr)

**THERAPEUTIC CLASS:** Estrogen/progestogen combination

**INDICATIONS:** Prevention of pregnancy.

**DOSAGE:** *Adults:* 1 tab qd for 28 days, then repeat. Start 1st Sunday after menses begin or 1st day of menses.

**HOW SUPPLIED:** Tab: (Ethinyl Estradiol-Desogestrel) 0.025mg-0.1mg, 0.025mg-0.125mg, 0.025mg-0.15mg

**CONTRAINDICATIONS:** Thrombophlebitis, DVT or thromboembolic disorders, pregnancy, cerebrovascular or coronary artery disease, undiagnosed abnormal genital bleeding, cholestatic jaundice of pregnancy or jaundice with prior pill use, hepatic adenomas or carcinomas, breast cancer or other estrogen-dependent neoplasia, hepatic tumors, active liver disease, and heavy smoking ( ≥15 cigarettes/day) and over age 35.

**WARNINGS/PRECAUTIONS:** Cigarette smoking increases risk of serious cardiovascular side effects; risk increases with age (especially >35 yrs) and heavy smoking. Increased risk of MI, vascular disease, thromboembolism, stroke and gallbladder disease. Retinal thrombosis, hepatic neoplasia, carcinoma of breast and reproductive organs reported. May cause glucose intolerance. May increase BP, elevate LDL levels or cause other lipid changes, fluid retention, breakthrough bleeding, and spotting. May cause or exacerbate migraine. May develop visual changes with contact lens. Increased risk of MI with HTN, hyperlipidemia, obesity, and diabetes. Increased risk of stroke with thrombophilias, hyperlipidemias, obesity, and migraine (especially with aura). D/C if jaundice, significant depression or ophthalmic irregularities develop. Perform annual physical exam. Use before menarche is not indicated. May affect certain endocrine, LFT and blood components. Should not be used if pregnant. Does not protect against STDs. Caution in nursing mothers and those with lipid disorders.

**ADVERSE REACTIONS:** Nausea, vomiting, breakthrough bleeding, spotting, amenorrhea, migraine headache, mood changes (including depression), vaginal candidiasis, edema, weight or appetite changes, and fluid retention.

**INTERACTIONS:** Reduced effects, increased breakthrough bleeding, and menstrual irregularities with some antibiotics, antifungals, anticonvulsants. Anti-HIV protease inhibitors may affect safety and efficacy. St. John's wort may induce hepatic enzymes and reduce effectiveness as well as resulting in breakthrough bleeding. Increased plasma concentrations of cyclosporine, prednisolone, and theophylline.

**PREGNANCY:** Category X, not for use in nursing.

**MECHANISM OF ACTION:** Triphasic oral contraceptive; acts by suppression of gonadotropins and inhibition of ovulation. Also causes changes in the cervical mucus and in the endometrium.

**PHARMACOKINETICS: Absorption:** Desogestrel and ethinyl estradiol: Rapid and complete. **Distribution:** Etonogestrel: Plasma protein binding (98%). **Metabolism:** Desogestrel: Liver; hydroxylation in intestinal mucosa; CYP3A4, 2C9; etonogestrel (active metabolite). Ethinyl estradiol: Hepatic conjugation. **Elimination:** Urine, bile, feces. Etonogestrel: $T_{1/2}$=37.1 hrs. Ethinyl estradiol: $T_{1/2}$=28.2 hrs.

### NURSING CONSIDERATIONS

**Assessment:** Assess for presence or history of thrombophlebitis, thromboembolic disorders, CVD, CAD, valvular heart disease with thrombogenic complications, severe HTN, DM with vascular involvement, headaches with focal neurological symptoms, major surgery with prolonged immobilization, known or suspected carcinoma of the breast/endometrium, undiagnosed genital bleeding, cholestatic jaundice of pregnancy or jaundice with prior pill use, hepatic tumors, active liver disease, and pregnancy prior to therapy. Assess for possible drug interactions and use with concurrent smoking.

**Monitoring:** Monitor for venous and arterial thrombotic and thromboembolic events (eg, MI, thromboembolism, stroke), hepatic neoplasia, gallbladder disease, HTN, development of ocular lesions, ocular changes in patients who wear contact lenses, signs of hepatotoxicity (eg, jaundice). Monitor serum glucose levels with DM, BP with history of HTN, onset or exacerbations of migraines or headaches, lipid levels with hyperlipidemia, signs of depression (with a previous history), and bleeding irregularities.

**Patient Counseling:** Counsel about possible side effects, and to avoid smoking while on therapy. Inform that medication does not protect against STDs, and to use other forms of contraception to protect against such diseases. Inform not to skip pills and to take at the same time everyday, and that there is a risk of pregnancy if pills are missed. If a dose is missed, take as soon as possible; take next dose at regular time, or may take two pills in one day. Instruct to continue taking medication, even if irregular vaginal bleeding occurs; notify physician if bleeding occurs in more than one cycle or lasts for more than a few days. Instruct to go for annual physical while on therapy.

**Administration:** Oral route. **Storage:** 25°C (77°F); excursions permitted to 15-30°C (59-86°F).

## CYMBALTA RX

duloxetine HCl (Lilly)

**Antidepressants increased the risk of suicidal thinking and behavior (suicidality) in short-term studies in children, adolescents, and young adults with major depressive disorder (MDD) and other psychiatric disorders. Monitor and observe closely for clinical worsening, suicidality, or unusual changes in behavior in patients who are on therapy. Not approved for use in pediatric patients.**

**THERAPEUTIC CLASS:** Serotonin and norepinephrine reuptake inhibitor

**INDICATIONS:** Treatment of MDD and of generalized anxiety disorder in adults. Management of neuropathic pain (DPNP) associated with diabetic peripheral neuropathy. Management of fibromyalgia (FM).

**DOSAGE:** *Adults:* MDD: Initial: 40mg/day (given as 20mg bid) to 60mg/day (given qd or as 30mg bid) or 30mg qd for 1 week before increasing to 60mg qd. Max: 120mg. Reassess periodically to determine need for maintenance therapy and appropriate dose. DPNP: 60mg/day given qd. May lower starting dose if tolerability a concern. Renal Impairment: Consider lower starting dose with gradual increase. GAD: Initial: 60mg qd or 30mg qd for 1 week to adjust before increasing to 60mg qd. Titrate: May increase by increments of 30mg qd if needed. Max: 120 mg qd. Reassess periodically to determine need for maintenance therapy and appropriate dose. FM: Initial: 60mg qd or 30mg qd for 1 week to adjust before increasing to 60mg qd. Max: 60mg qd. Swallow whole. Do not chew, crush, open, sprinkle on food or mix with liquids.

**HOW SUPPLIED:** Cap, Delayed-Release: 20mg, 30mg, 60mg

**CONTRAINDICATIONS:** Concomitant use of MAOIs, uncontrolled narrow-angle glaucoma.

**WARNINGS/PRECAUTIONS:** Monitor for emergence of agitation, irritability, unusual changes in behavior, as well as the emergence of suicidality. May cause hepatotoxicity. Not approved for treating bipolar depression. Cases of cholestatic jaundice with minimal elevation of transaminase levels reported. Avoid with chronic liver disease. May increase BP; obtain baseline and monitor periodically. Orthostatic hypotension and syncope reported. Avoid abrupt cessation and with severe renal impairment/ESRD or hepatic insufficiency. Caution with conditions that may slow gastric emptying, history of mania or seizures. May increase risk of mydriasis; caution in patients with controlled narrow-angle glaucoma. Hyponatremia reported. May affect urethral resistance. Serotonin syndrome or neuroleptic malignant syndrome (NMS)-like reactions reported; monitor and d/c if with signs/symptoms. Caution in elderly. May worsen glycemic control in some patients with diabetes. May increase risk of bleeding events.



**ADVERSE REACTIONS:** N/V, dry mouth, constipation, diarrhea, decreased appetite, fatigue, dizziness, somnolence, hyperhidrosis, headache, insomnia, asthenia.

**INTERACTIONS:** See Contraindications. Avoid within 14 days of MAOI therapy. Upon discontinuation, wait at least 5 days before starting MAOI therapy. Avoid thioridazine, CYP1A2 inhibitors (eg, fluvoxamine, some quinolone antibiotics), substantial alcohol use. Increased levels with potent CYP2D6 inhibitors (eg, paroxetine, fluoxetine, quinidine). Caution with drugs metabolized by CYP2D6 having a narrow therapeutic index (eg, TCAs, phenothiazines, type 1C antiarrhythmics), and CNS-active drugs. May increase free concentration levels of highly protein-bound drugs. Potential for interaction with drugs that affect gastric acidity. Caution with serotonergic drugs (eg, triptans, tramadol, lithium, or St. John's wort). Avoid with other SSRIs, SNRIs, or tryptophan. Increased risk of bleeding with warfarin, ASA, and NSAIDs.

**PREGNANCY:** Category C, not for use in nursing.

**MECHANISM OF ACTION:** Selective serotonin and norepinephrine reuptake inhibitor; mechanism not established. Actions may be related to potentiation of serotonergic and noradrenergic activity in the CNS.

**PHARMACOKINETICS: Absorption:** $T_{max}$=6 hrs. **Distribution:** $V_d$=1640L; plasma protein binding (>90%). **Metabolism:** Hepatic via CYP1A2, 2D6; oxidation and conjugation. **Elimination:** Urine 70% (<1% unchanged), feces (20%); $T_{1/2}$=12 hrs.

## NURSING CONSIDERATIONS

**Assessment:** Assess for bipolar disorder risk, history of mania, chronic liver disease, chronic alcohol use, history of seizures, disease/condition that slows gastric emptying (eg, DM), uncontrolled narrow-angle glaucoma, risk factors for hyponatremia, history of urinary retention, hepatic/renal impairment, pregnancy/nursing status, and possible drug interactions. Assess baseline BP, LFTs, renal function tests, and blood glucose. Ear and labyrinth disorders, nervous system disorders, polyuria, and sexual dysfunction, contact dermatitis (gastritis).

**Monitoring:** Perform periodic BP, LFTs, and renal function tests. Monitor for signs/symptoms of clinical worsening (suicidality, unusual changes in behavior), hepatotoxicity, serotonin syndrome or NMS-like reactions, abnormal bleeding, hyponatremia, seizures, orthostatic hypotension, decreased glycemic control, urinary hesitation/retention, mydriasis, cognitive/motor impairment, and hepatic/renal dysfunction. If abruptly d/c, monitor for symptoms of dysphoric mood, irritability, agitation, dizziness, sensory disturbances, anxiety, confusion, headache, lethargy, emotional lability, insomnia, and hypomania.

**Patient Counseling:** Counsel to swallow whole, and not to chew, crush, open, sprinkle on food or mix with liquid. Advise to avoid alcohol. Seek medical attention for symptoms of serotonin syndrome (mental status changes, tachycardia, hyperthermia, NV, diarrhea, incoordination), abnormal bleeding (particularly if using NSAIDs or ASA), hyponatremia, activation of mania, mydriasis, decreased glycemic control, orthostatic hypotension, hepatotoxicity, urinary hesitation/retention, seizures, clinical worsening (suicidal ideation, unusual changes in behavior), or discontinuation symptoms (irritability, agitation, dizziness, anxiety, headache, insomnia). Caution may impair physical/mental abilities. May notice improvement within 1-4 weeks; continue therapy as directed.

**Administration:** Oral route. **Storage:** 25°C (77°F); excursions permitted to 15-30°C (59-86°F).

## CYTOMEL RX

liothyronine sodium (King)

**THERAPEUTIC CLASS:** Thyroid replacement hormone

**INDICATIONS:** Hypothyroidism. As a pituitary TSH suppressant in the treatment and prevention of euthyroid goiters, including thyroid nodules, and Hashimoto's and multinodular goiter. Diagnostic agent in suppression tests to differentiate mild hyperthyroidism or thyroid gland autonomy.

**DOSAGE:** *Adults:* Mild Hypothyroidism: Initial: 25mcg qd. Titrate: May increase by up to 25mcg qd every 1-2 weeks. Maint: 25-75mcg qd. Myxedema: Initial: 5mcg qd. Titrate: May increase by 5-10mcg qd every 1-2 weeks up to 25mcg qd, then increase by 5-25mcg qd every 1-2 weeks. Maint: 50-100mcg/day. Goiter: Initial: 5mcg/day. Titrate: May increase by 5-10mcg qd every 1-2 weeks up to 25mcg qd, then by 12.5-25mcg qd every 1-2 weeks. Maint: 75mcg qd. Elderly/Coronary Artery Disease: Initial: 5mcg qd. Titrate: Increase by no more than 5mcg qd every 2 weeks. Thyroid Suppression Therapy: 75-100mcg qd for 7 days. Radioactive iodine uptake is determined before and after administration of hormone.
*Pediatrics:* Congenital Hypothyroidism: Initial: 5mcg qd. Titrate: Increase by 5mcg qd every 3-4 days until desired response. Maint: <1 yr: 20mcg qd. 1-3 yrs: 50mcg qd. >3 yrs: 25-75mcg/day.

**HOW SUPPLIED:** Tab: 5mcg, 25mcg*, 50mcg* *scored

**CONTRAINDICATIONS:** Uncorrected adrenal cortical insufficiency and untreated thyrotoxicosis.

**WARNINGS/PRECAUTIONS:** Do not use in the treatment of obesity; larger doses in euthyroid patients can cause serious or even life threatening toxicity. Caution with angina pectoris and elderly; use lower doses. Rule out hypogonadism and nephrosis prior to therapy. With prolonged and severe hypothyroidism supplement with adrenocortical steroids. May aggravate diabetes mellitus or insipidus and adrenocortical insufficiency. Add glucocorticoid with myxedema coma. Excessive doses may cause craniosynostosis in infants.

**ADVERSE REACTIONS:** Allergic skin reactions (rare).

**INTERACTIONS:** Hypothyroidism decreases and hyperthyroidism increases sensitivity to oral anticoagulants; monitor PT/INR. Monitor insulin and oral hypoglycemic requirements. Decreased absorption with cholestyramine; space dosing by 4-5 hrs. Large dose may cause life-threatening toxicities with sympathomimetic amines. Estrogens increase thyroxine-binding globulin; increase in thyroid dose may be needed. Additive effects of both agents with TCAs. HTN and tachycardia with ketamine. May potentiate digitalis toxicity. Increased adrenergic effects of catecholamines; caution with CAD.

**PREGNANCY:** Category A, caution in nursing.

**MECHANISM OF ACTION:** Synthetic thyroid hormone; not established, suspected to enhance oxygen consumption by tissues, increases the basal metabolic rate and metabolism of carbohydrates, lipids, and proteins.

**PHARMACOKINETICS: Elimination:** $T_{1/2}$=2.5 days.

### NURSING CONSIDERATIONS

**Assessment:** Assess for possible drug interactions, CV disease (eg, CAD, angina pectoris), DM, adrenal cortical insufficiency, thyrotoxicosis, myxedema, hypogonadism, and nephrosis.

**Monitoring:** Periodically monitor thyroid function and urinary glucose with DM. Monitor for signs/symptoms of precipitation of adrenocortical insufficiency, aggravation of DM and diabetes insipidus, hypoglycemia, toxicity, and hypersensitivity reactions.

**Patient Counseling:** Inform that replacement therapy is taken for life. Warn that partial hair loss may be seen in pediatrics. Instruct to seek medical attention if symptoms of toxicity (eg, CP, increased HR, palpitations, excessive sweating, heat intolerance, nervousness), hypoglycemia, aggravation of DM and diabetes insipidus, or hypersensitivity reactions occur.

**Administration:** Oral route. **Storage:** 15-30°C (59-86°F).

C

## CYTOXAN RX

cyclophosphamide (Bristol-Myers Squibb)

**THERAPEUTIC CLASS:** Nitrogen mustard alkylating agent

**INDICATIONS:** Treatment of malignant lymphomas, Hodgkin's disease, lymphocytic lymphoma, mixed-cell type or histiocytic lymphoma, Burkitt's lymphoma, multiple myeloma, chronic lymphocytic leukemia, chronic granulocytic leukemia, acute myelogenous and monocytic leukemia, acute lymphoblastic leukemia in children, mycosis fungoides, neuroblastoma, ovary adenocarcinoma, retinoblastoma, breast carcinoma. Treatment of biopsy proven "minimal change" nephrotic syndrome in children, but not as primary therapy.

**DOSAGE:** *Adults:* Malignant Diseases (Without Hematologic Deficiency): Monotherapy: Initial: 40-50mg/kg IV in divided doses over 2-5 days, or 10-15mg/kg IV given every 7-10 days, or 3-5mg/kg twice weekly. Oral Dosing: Initial/Maint: 1-5mg/kg/day PO. Adjust dose according to antitumor activity and/or leukopenia. May need to reduce dose when combined with other cytotoxic drugs.
*Pediatrics:* Malignant Diseases (Without Hematologic Deficiency): Monotherapy: Initial: 40-50mg/kg IV in divided doses over 2-5 days, or 10-15mg/kg IV given every 7-10 days, or 3-5mg/kg twice weekly. Oral Dosing: Initial/Maint: 1-5mg/kg/day PO. Adjust dose according to antitumor activity and/or leukopenia. May need to reduce dose when combined with other cytotoxic drugs. Nephrotic Syndrome: 2.5-3mg/kg/day PO for 60-90 days.

**HOW SUPPLIED:** Inj (Lyophilized): 500mg, 1g, 2g; Tab: 25mg, 50mg

**CONTRAINDICATIONS:** Severely depressed bone marrow function.

**WARNINGS/PRECAUTIONS:** Second malignancies, cardiac dysfunction, and hemorrhagic cystitis reported. May cause fetal harm in pregnancy. Serious, fatal infections may develop if severely immunosuppressed. Monitor for toxicity with leukopenia, thrombocytopenia, tumor cell infiltration of bone marrow, previous x-ray therapy or cytotoxic therapy, and impaired hepatic and/or renal function. Monitor hematologic profile for hematopoietic suppression. Examine urine for red blood cells. Anaphylactic reactions reported. Possible cross-sensitivity with other alkylating agents. May cause sterility. May interfere with normal wound healing. Consider dose adjustment with adrenalectomy.

**ADVERSE REACTIONS:** Impairment of fertility, amenorrhea, NV, anorexia, abdominal discomfort, diarrhea, alopecia, leukopenia, thrombocytopenia, hemorrhagic ureteritis, interstitial pneumonitis, malaise, asthenia, renal tubular necrosis.

**INTERACTIONS:** Chronic, high doses of phenobarbital increase metabolism and leukopenic activity. Potentiates succinylcholine chloride effects and doxorubicin-induced cardiotoxicity. Alert anesthesiologist if treated within 10 days of general anesthesia.

**PREGNANCY:** Category D, not for use in nursing.

**MECHANISM OF ACTION:** Nitrogen mustard alkylating agent; exerts action by cross linking of tumor cell DNA.

**PHARMACOKINETICS: Absorption:** Well absorbed; bioavailability ( ≥75%). **Distribution:** Plasma protein binding ( ≥60% as metabolites). **Metabolism:** Liver; active metabolites. **Elimination:** Urine (5-25% unchanged); $T_{1/2}$=3-12 hrs.

### NURSING CONSIDERATIONS

**Assessment:** Assess for severely depressed bone marrow function, leukopenia, thrombocytopenia, tumor cell infiltration of bone marrow, previous X-ray therapy, previous therapy with other cytotoxic agents, impaired hepatic/renal function.

**Monitoring:** Monitor for second malignancies, amenorrhea, sterility, ovarian fibrosis, oligospermia or azoospermia, hemorrhagic cystitis, cardiac dysfunction, infection, anaphylactic reactions, CBC with differential and platelets.

**Patient Counseling:** Counsel about possible side effects and required contraceptive methods while on therapy. Take in the morning and drink adequate fluids. Report adverse side effects.

**Administration:** Oral, IV, IM, intraperitoneal, intrapleural route. Inspect drug product visually for particulate matter and discoloration prior to parenteral administration. **Storage:** Vial: Below 25°C (77°F). Tab: Below 25°C (77°F); excursions permitted to 30°C (86°F); protect from temperatures above 30°C (86°F).



## D.H.E. 45 RX

dihydroergotamine mesylate (Valeant)

**Serious and life-threatening peripheral ischemia reported with potent CYP3A4 inhibitors (eg, protease inhibitors, macrolides). Elevated levels of dihydroergotamine increases risk of vasospasm leading to cerebral ischemia or ischemia of the extremities. Concomitant use with CYP3A4 inhibitors is contraindicated.**

**THERAPEUTIC CLASS:** Ergot alkaloid

**INDICATIONS:** Acute treatment of migraine with or without aura. Acute treatment of cluster headache episodes.

**DOSAGE:** *Adults:* 1mL IV/IM/SQ. May repeat at 1 hr intervals. Max: 3mL/24hrs IM/SC or 2mL/24hrs IV and 6mL/week.

**HOW SUPPLIED:** Inj: 1mg/mL

**CONTRAINDICATIONS:** Ergot alkaloids hypersensitivity, ischemic heart disease, coronary artery vasospasm (eg, Prinzmetal's variant angina), uncontrolled HTN, hemiplegic or basilar migraine, peripheral artery disease, sepsis, following vascular surgery, severe renal/hepatic dysfunction, pregnancy, nursing, with potent CYP3A4 inhibitors (eg, ritonavir, nelfinavir, indinavir, erythromycin, clarithromycin, troleandomycin, ketoconazole, itraconazole), concomitant peripheral and central vasoconstrictors, and within 24 hrs after taking 5-$HT_1$ agonists, methysergide, ergotamine-containing, or ergot-type agents.

**WARNINGS/PRECAUTIONS:** Confirm migraine diagnosis. Inform of risks of adverse cardiac, cerebrovascular, and vasospastic events and fatalities. Avoid with cardiac risk factors (eg, HTN, hypercholesterolemia, smoker, obesity, DM, strong family history of CAD, females who are surgically/physiologically postmenopausal, or males >40 yrs) unless cardiovascular evaluation is done. Perform cardiovascular monitoring with long-term use. Significant BP elevations reported.

**ADVERSE REACTIONS:** Vasospasm, angina, paresthesia, HTN, dizziness, anxiety, dyspnea, headache, flushing, diarrhea, rash, increased sweating.

**INTERACTIONS:** Potentiated BP elevation with peripheral and central vasoconstrictors. Additive coronary vasospastic effect with sumatriptan; avoid within 24 hrs of each other. Propranolol and nicotine may potentiate the vasoconstrictive action. Increased plasma levels and peripheral vasoconstriction with macrolides. Contraindicated with CYP3A4 inhibitors (eg, macrolides, protease inhibitors). Caution with less potent CYP3A4 inhibitors (eg, saquinavir, nefazodone, fluconazole, grapefruit juice, fluoxetine, fluvoxamine, zileuton, clotrimazole).

**PREGNANCY:** Category X, contraindicated in nursing.

**MECHANISM OF ACTION:** Ergotamine; binds with high affinity to 5-$HT_{1D}$ receptors on intracranial blood vessels, causing vasoconstriction, or activates 5-$HT_{1D}$ receptors on sensory nerve endings of trigeminal system, resulting in inhibition of proinflammatory neuropeptide release.

**PHARMACOKINETICS: Distribution:** $V_d$=800L; plasma protein binding (93%). **Metabolism:** Liver; 8'-β-hydroxydihydroergotamine (major metabolite). **Elimination:** Feces (major), urine (6-7%); $T_{1/2}$=9 hrs.

## NURSING CONSIDERATIONS

**Assessment:** Assess for ischemic heart disease (angina pectoris, history of MI, documented silent ischemia), coronary artery vasospasm, Prinzmetal's variant angina, uncontrolled HTN, hemiplegic or basilar migraine, peripheral arterial disease, sepsis, pregnancy/nursing status, possible drug interactions, CAD, renal/hepatic impairment.

D

**Monitoring:** Monitor for signs/symptoms of vasospastic reactions, HTN, fibrosis, CV events, and hypersensitivity reactions.

**Patient Counseling:** Advise to seek medical attention if numbness or tingling in fingers and toes, muscle pain in arms and legs, weakness in legs, pain in chest, temporary speeding or slowing of HR, swelling, or itching occur.

**Administration:** SQ, IV, IM route. **Storage:** Below 25°C (77°F). Do not refrigerate or freeze. Protect from light and heat.

# DACOGEN — RX

decitabine (Eisai)

**THERAPEUTIC CLASS:** DNA methyltransferase inhibitor

**INDICATIONS:** Treatment of myelodysplastic syndromes.

**DOSAGE:** *Adults*: Initial: 15mg/m$^2$ IV over 3 hrs q8h for 3 days. Repeat cycle every 6 weeks. Treat for ≥4 cycles. Adjust dose based on hematology lab values, renal function, and serum electrolytes.

**HOW SUPPLIED:** Inj: 50mg

**WARNINGS/PRECAUTIONS:** May cause fetal harm. Avoid pregnancy in women of childbearing potential. Men should be advised not to father a child while receiving treatment and for 2 months afterward. Neutropenia and thrombocytopenia may occur; monitor CBC and platelets periodically (at minimum, before each cycle). Caution with renal and hepatic dysfunction. Avoid with SrCr >2mg/dL, transaminase >2x normal, or serum bilirubin >1.5mg/dL.

**ADVERSE REACTIONS:** Neutropenia, thrombocytopenia, anemia, fatigue, pyrexia, nausea, cough, petechiae, constipation, diarrhea, hyperglycemia, febrile neutropenia, leukopenia, headache, insomnia.

**PREGNANCY:** Category D, not for use in nursing.

**MECHANISM OF ACTION:** DNA methyltransferase inhibitor. Inhibition of methyltransferase causes hypomethylation of DNA and cellular differentiation or apoptosis.

**PHARMACOKINETICS: Distribution:** Plasma protein binding (<1%). **Metabolism:** Deamination in liver, granulocytes, intestinal epithelium, and blood. **Elimination:** $T_{1/2}$=0.51 hrs.

## NURSING CONSIDERATIONS

**Assessment:** Assess CBC with platelets, renal/hepatic functions, pregnancy status. Note other diseases/condition and drug therapies.

**Monitoring:** Monitor hypersensitivity reactions, CBC with platelets, renal/hepatic impairment, cardiac disorders, infections and infestations, intracranial hemorrhage, mental status change, cholecystitis, and hyperglycemia.

**Patient Counseling:** Counsel about contraception while on treatment, to avoid crowds and those with active infections, and to report abnormal bleeding or bruising and any adverse effects.

**Administration:** IV route. Reconstitute aseptically with 10mL of SWFI. Dilute with 0.9% NS, D5W, or LR to final concentration of 0.1-1.0mg/mL. Unless used within 15 min of reconstitution, diluted sol must be prepared using cold (2-8°C) infusion fluids. **Storage**: 2-8°C (36-46°F) for up to a maximum of 7 hrs, until administration. Vials: 25°C (77°F); excursions permitted to 15-30°C (59-86°F). Diluted solution: 2-8°C (36-46°F) for up to maximum of 7 hrs, until administration.

## DALMANE

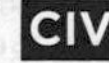


flurazepam HCl (Valeant)

**THERAPEUTIC CLASS:** Benzodiazepine

**INDICATIONS:** Treatment of insomnia.

**DOSAGE:** *Adults:* Usual: 15-30mg at bedtime. Elderly/Debilitated: Initial: 15mg at bedtime.
*Pediatrics:* ≥15 yrs: Usual: 15-30mg at bedtime.

**HOW SUPPLIED:** Cap: 15mg, 30mg

**CONTRAINDICATIONS:** Pregnancy.

**WARNINGS/PRECAUTIONS:** Caution in elderly, debilitated, severely depressed, those with suicidal tendencies, hepatic/renal impairment, respiratory disease. Ataxia and falls reported in elderly and debilitated. Withdrawal symptoms after d/c; avoid abrupt d/c. Rare cases of angioedema involving the tongue, glottis, or larynx reported. Complex behaviors (eg, sleep driving, preparing and eating food, making phone calls, having sex) reported. May impair mental/physical abilities.

**ADVERSE REACTIONS:** Confusion, dizziness, drowsiness, lightheadedness, ataxia, staggering, falling.

**INTERACTIONS:** Additive effects with alcohol and other CNS depressants.

**PREGNANCY:** Not for use in pregnancy or nursing.

**MECHANISM OF ACTION:** Benzodiazepine; hypnotic.

**PHARMACOKINETICS: Absorption:** Rapid; $C_{max}$=4.0ng/mL; $T_{max}$=1 hr. **Metabolism:** $N_1$-desalkyl-flurazepam (active metabolite); conjugation. **Elimination:** Urine; $T_{1/2}$=2.3 hrs, 47-100 hrs (active metabolite).

### NURSING CONSIDERATIONS

**Assessment:** Assess for primary psychiatric illness, impaired renal/hepatic function, chronic pulmonary insufficiency, depression, possible drug interactions, and history of drug abuse.

**Monitoring:** Monitor for anaphylactic and anaphylactoid reactions, worsening of insomnia, complex behaviors (eg, sleep driving), lab abnormalities (eg, LFTs).

**Patient Counseling:** Caution about hazardous tasks (eg, operating machinery/driving). Advise to consult physician before increasing dose or abruptly d/c, avoid concomitant alcohol consumption or other sedative-hypnotics, and do not take if pregnant.

**Administration:** Oral route. **Storage:** 25°C (77°F); excursions permitted to 15-30°C (59-86°F).

## DANTRIUM RX

dantrolene sodium (JHP Pharmaceuticals, LLC)

**Has potential for hepatotoxicity. Symptomatic/overt hepatitis, liver dysfunction reported. Risk of hepatic injury greater in females, patients >35 yrs, and patients taking other medications. Monitor hepatic function. D/C if no benefit after 45 days. Lowest possible effective dose should be prescribed.**

**THERAPEUTIC CLASS:** Direct acting skeletal muscle relaxant

**INDICATIONS:** To control manifestations of clinical spasticity from upper motor neuron disorders (eg, spinal cord injury, stroke, cerebral palsy, multiple sclerosis). Preoperatively to prevent or attenuate development of malignant hyperthermia, and after a malignant hyperthermia crisis.

**DOSAGE:** *Adults:* Chronic Spasticity: Individualize dose. Initial: 25mg qd for 7 days. Titrate: Increase to 25mg tid for 7 days, then 50mg tid for 7 days, then 100mg tid. Max: 100mg qid. If no further benefit at next higher dose, decrease to previous lower dose. Malignant Hyperthermia: Pre-Op: 4-8mg/kg/day given tid-qid for 1-2 days before surgery, with last dose given 3-4 hrs before surgery with minimum of water. Adjust dose within recommended dose range to avoid incapacitation or excessive gastrointestinal irritation. Post-Op Following Malignant Hyperthermia Crisis: 4-8mg/kg/day given qid for 1-3 days. *Pediatrics:* ≥5 yrs: Chronic Spasticity: Individualize dose. Initial: 0.5mg/kg qd for 7 days. Titrate: Increase to 0.5mg/kg tid for 7 days, then 1mg/kg tid for 7 days, then 2mg/kg tid. Max: 100mg qid. If no further benefit at next higher dose, decrease to previous lower dose.



**HOW SUPPLIED:** Cap: 25mg, 50mg, 100mg

**CONTRAINDICATIONS:** Active hepatic disease (eg, hepatitis, cirrhosis), where spasticity is utilized to sustain upright posture and balance in locomotion, when spasticity is utilized to obtain or maintain increased function.

**WARNINGS/PRECAUTIONS:** Not for treatment of skeletal muscle spasm resulting from rheumatic disorder. Brief withdrawal for 2 to 4 days may exacerbate manifestations of spasticity. Liver disorders (eg, idiosyncratic or hypersensitivity type) may occur. Monitor LFTs at baseline, then periodically. D/C if LFT abnormalities or jaundice appear. Caution with pulmonary dysfunction (eg, obstructive pulmonary disease), severely impaired cardiac function due to myocardial disease, and history of liver disease/dysfunction. Photosensitivity reaction may occur; limit sunlight exposure.

**ADVERSE REACTIONS:** Drowsiness, dizziness, weakness, malaise, fatigue, diarrhea, hepatitis, tachycardia, aplastic anemia, thrombocytopenia, depression, seizure.

**INTERACTIONS:** Increased drowsiness with CNS depressants (eg, sedatives, tranquilizers). Caution with estrogens; risk of hepatotoxicity especially in women >35 yrs. Increased risk of hepatic injury in patients taking other medications. Avoid with calcium channel blockers (CCBs); cardiovascular collapse with concomitant verapamil reported (rare). May potentiate vecuronium-induced neuromuscular block.

**PREGNANCY:** Category C, not for use in nursing.

**MECHANISM OF ACTION:** Direct-acting skeletal muscle relaxant; interferes with release of calcium ions from the sarcoplasmic reticulum.

**PHARMACOKINETICS: Absorption:** Incomplete/slow but consistent. **Metabolism:** Hepatic microsomal enzymes; 5-hydroxy and acetamido analog (major metabolites). **Elimination:** Urine; $T_{1/2}$=8.7 hrs.

## NURSING CONSIDERATIONS

**Assessment:** Assess for active hepatic disease (eg, hepatitis and cirrhosis), history of liver disease/dysfunction, skeletal muscle spasm from rheumatic disorders, pulmonary dysfunction, impaired cardiac function due to myocardial disease, pregnancy/nursing status, and possible drug interactions. Perform baseline LFTs to establish pre-existing liver disease. Assess use in patients >35 yrs due to increased risk of drug-induced hepatocellular disease.

**Monitoring:** Monitor for liver disorders, photosensitivity reactions, and signs/symptoms of hepatitis. Monitor LFTs (eg, SGOT, SGPT) regularly.

**Patient Counseling:** Inform about risks and benefits of therapy. Caution against performing hazardous tasks (eg, operating machinery/driving), and avoid prolonged sunlight exposure. Inform about other medications being taken. Notify if pregnant/nursing.

**Administration:** Oral route. **Storage:** Avoid excessive heat, over 40°C (104°F).

# DANTRIUM IV — RX

dantrolene sodium (Procter & Gamble Pharmaceuticals)

**THERAPEUTIC CLASS:** Direct acting skeletal muscle relaxant

**INDICATIONS:** Adjunct management of fulminant hypermetabolism of skeletal muscle characteristic of malignant hyperthermia crises. For pre- and post-operative use to prevent or attenuate development of malignant hyperthermia.

**DOSAGE:** *Adults:* Malignant Hyperthermia: Initial: Minimum 1mg/kg IV push. Continue until symptoms subside or max cumulative dose 10mg/kg. Pre-Op Malignant Hyperthermia Prophylaxis: 2.5mg/kg 1.25 hrs before anesthesia and infuse over 1 hr. May need additional therapy during anesthesia/surgery if symptoms arise. Post-Op Prophylaxis: Initial: 1mg/kg or more as clinical situation dictates.
*Pediatrics:* Malignant Hyperthermia: Initial: Minimum 1mg/kg IV push. Continue until symptoms subside or max cumulative dose 10mg/kg.

D

**HOW SUPPLIED:** Inj: 20mg

**WARNINGS/PRECAUTIONS:** Use with supportive therapies to treat malignant hyperthermia. Take steps to prevent extravasation. Fatal and non-fatal hepatic disorders reported. Do not operate automobile or engage hazardous activity for 48 hrs after therapy. Caution at meals on day of administration because difficulty in swallowing/choking reported. Monitor vital signs if receive preoperatively.

**ADVERSE REACTIONS:** Loss of grip strength, weakness in legs, drowsiness, dizziness, pulmonary edema, thrombophlebitis, urticaria, erythema.

**INTERACTIONS:** Plasma protein-binding reduced by warfarin and clofibrate, and increased by tolbutamide. Avoid with CCBs; possible risk of cardiovascular collapse. Caution with tranquilizers. Possible increased metabolism by drugs known to induce hepatic microsomal enzymes. May potentiate vecuronium-induced neuromuscular block.

**PREGNANCY:** Category C, safety in nursing not known.

**MECHANISM OF ACTION:** Direct acting skeletal muscle relaxant; interferes with release of calcium ions from sarcoplasmic reticulum.

**PHARMACOKINETICS: Distribution:** Found in breast milk. **Metabolism:** Hydrolysis and oxidation; 5-hydroxy dantrolene and acetylamino analog (major metabolites). **Elimination:** Urine; $T_{1/2}$=4-8 hrs.

## NURSING CONSIDERATIONS

**Assessment:** Assess for active hepatic disease (hepatitis and cirrhosis), pregnancy/nursing status, and possible drug interactions.

**Monitoring:** Monitor for vital signs, tissue necrosis, LFTs. Monitor for cardiovascular collapse if given concomitantly with CCBs.

**Patient Counseling:** Caution against performing hazardous tasks (eg, operating machinery/driving). Inform that at meals, on administration day, choking and difficulty swallowing have been reported. Inform about postop muscle weakness, reduced grip strength, and lightheadedness. Notify if pregnant/nursing.

**Administration:** IV route. **Storage:** 15-30°C (59-86°F); avoid prolonged light exposure.

# Darvocet A500 CIV

propoxyphene napsylate - acetaminophen (Xanodyne)

**Numerous cases of accidental/intentional overdose with propoxyphene products either alone or in combination with CNS depressants, including alcohol, have been reported. Many of the propoxyphene-related deaths occurred in patients with histories of emotional disturbances or suicidal ideation/attempts and/or concomitant administration of sedatives, tranquilizers, muscle relaxants, antidepressants, or other CNS-depressant drugs. Avoid with suicidal or have a history of suicidal ideation. Propoxyphene may be altered by strong CYP3A4 inhibitors (eg, ritonavir, ketoconazole, itraconazole, troleadomycin, clarithromycin, nelfinavir, nefazadone, amiodarone, aprepitant, diltiazem, erythromycin, fluconazole, fosamprenavir, grapefruit juice, and verapamil) leading to enhanced propoxyphene plasma levels; monitor carefully and adjust dosage if warranted.**

**THERAPEUTIC CLASS:** Opioid analgesic

**INDICATIONS:** Relief of mild to moderate pain.

**DOSAGE:** *Adults:* Individualize dose. Usual: 1 tab q4h prn for pain. Max: 6 tabs/24 hrs. Hepatic/Renal Impairment: Reduce daily dose. Elderly: Start at the low

D

end of the dosing range. Cessation of Therapy: gradually d/c; decrease dose 25-50% per day with careful monitoring for withdrawal signs/symptoms. If occurs, raise dose to previous level and titrate down more slowly.

**HOW SUPPLIED:** Tab: (Propoxyphene-APAP) 100mg-500mg

**CONTRAINDICATIONS:** Significant respiratory depression (in unmonitored settings or the absence of resuscitative equipment), acute/severe asthma, hypercarbia, paralytic ileus.

**WARNINGS/PRECAUTIONS:** Drug dependence, misuse, abuse and addiction potential. Not for suicidal or addiction-prone patients. Respiratory depression may occur; caution in elderly/debilitated patients and extreme caution with significant COPD/cor pulmonale, with decreased respiratory reserve, hypoxia, hypercapnia, pre-existing respiratory depression. May cause severe hypotension and orthostatic hypotension; caution with circulatory shock. May obscure the clinical course of patients with head injuries. May impair mental/physical abilities. Abstinence syndrome may occur; avoid abrupt discontinuation. May cause spasm of the sphincter of Oddi; caution with biliary tract disease, including acute pancreatitis. May increase serum amylase level. Caution with hepatic/renal impairment.

**ADVERSE REACTIONS:** Dizziness, sedation, N/V, liver dysfunction.

**INTERACTIONS:** See Black Box Warning. (Propoxyphene) Additive CNS depressant and interactive effects resulting in respiratory depression, hypotension, profound sedation, or coma may result if taken with narcotic analgesics, general anesthetics, phenothiazines, alcohol and other CNS depressants. Respiratory depression may occur when given in conjunction with other agents that depress respiration. Severe hypotension may occur after concurrent administration with other agents which compromise vasomotor tone. Caution with mixed agonist/antagonist analgesics (eg, pentazocine, nalbuphine, butorphanol and buprenorphine); may reduce analgesic effect and/or precipitate withdrawal symptoms. Avoid with MAOIs or within 14 days of stopping treatment. Severe neurologic signs, including coma reported with carbamazepine. Increase risk of bleeding with warfarin-like agents. Enhanced metabolite levels with strong CYP3A4 inducers (eg, rifampin). May increase levels and increase adverse effects with substrate of CYP3A4 or CYP2D6. (APAP) Hepatotoxicity may occur with alcohol. Effect may be delayed or decreased by anticholinergics. May increase plasma clearance and decrease half-life with oral contraceptives. May increase pharmacological effects with propranolol. May decrease effects of loop diuretics and decrease therapeutic effects of lamotrigine and zidovudine. May increase therapeutic effects with probenecid. Avoid with other acetaminophen-containing products.

**PREGNANCY:** Category C, caution in nursing.

**MECHANISM OF ACTION:** Propoxyphene: Centrally acting narcotic analgesic; inhibit the voltage-gated potassium current carried by cardiac rapidly activating delayed rectifier (hERG) channels with approximately equal potency. Acetaminophen: Non-opiate, non-salicylate analgesic and antipyretic; mechanism for analgesic is not established, antipyretic effect is mediated through activity in the hypothalamic heat-regulating centers, also inhibits prostaglandin synthetase.

**PHARMACOKINETICS: Absorption:** Propoxyphene: $T_{max}$=2-2.5 hrs; (65mg) $C_{max}$=0.05-0.1mcg/mL, (norpropoxyphene) $C_{max}$=0.1-0.2µg/mL. **Distribution:** Found in breast milk, crosses the placenta. Propoxyphene: $V_d$=16L/kg; plasma protein binding (80%). APAP: Plasma protein binding (variable). **Metabolism:** Propoxyphene: Liver via CYP3A4 (N-demethylation); norpropoxyphene (active metabolite) APAP: Liver via UGT1A6 (conjugation, mainly glucuronidation). **Elimination:** Propoxyphene: Urine (20-25%); $T_{1/2}$=6-12 hrs, (norpropoxyphene) 30-36 hrs. APAP: Urine (85%); $T_{max}$=1.25-3 hrs.

## NURSING CONSIDERATIONS

**Assessment:** Assess for significant respiratory depression, acute/severe asthma, hypercarbia, paralytic ileus, head injuries, addiction prone patients, suicidal tendencies/ideation, emotional disturbances, hepatic/renal impairment, alcoholism, COPD/cor pulmonale, decreased respiratory reserve, hypoxia, hypercapnia, circulatory shock, biliary tract disease, hypersensitivity, pregnancy/nursing status, and possible drug interactions.

**Monitoring:** Monitor for signs/symptoms of CNS depression, respiratory depression, severe/orthostatic hypotension, drug dependence, hepatic/renal impairment and hypersensitivity reactions. Monitor serum amylase levels.

**Patient Counseling:** Advise to report pain and adverse experiences occurring during therapy. Advise not to adjust dose without consulting the prescribing professional. Caution performing hazardous task (eg, driving, operating machinery). Counsel not to take CNS depressants (eg, sleep aids, tranquilizers), consume alcoholic beverages, over-the-counter medications that contain alcohol, and acetaminophen-containing products while on therapy. Inform pregnancy risks. Advise potential for drug abuse. Advise not to abruptly discontinue medication due to risk of precipitating withdrawal symptoms.

**Administration:** Oral route. **Storage**: 20-25°C (68-77°F).

## DARVOCET-N CIV

propoxyphene napsylate - acetaminophen (Xanodyne)

**Numerous cases of accidental/intentional overdose with propoxyphene products either alone or in combination with CNS depressants, including alcohol, have been reported. Many of the propoxyphene-related deaths occurred in patients with histories of emotional disturbances or suicidal ideation/attempts and/or concomitant administration of sedatives, tranquilizers, muscle relaxants, antidepressants, or other CNS-depressant drugs. Avoid in patients who are suicidal or have a history of suicidal ideation. Propoxyphene may be altered by strong CYP3A4 inhibitors (eg, ritonavir, ketoconazole, itraconazole, troleadomycin, clarithromycin, nelfinavir, nefazadone, amiodarone, aprepitant, diltiazem, erythromycin, fluconazole, fosamprenavir, grapefruit juice, and verapamil) leading to enhanced propoxyphene plasma levels; monitor carefully and adjust dosage if warranted.**

**THERAPEUTIC CLASS:** Opioid analgesic

**INDICATIONS:** Relief of mild to moderate pain.

**DOSAGE:** *Adults:* (Darvocet-N 100): Usual: 1 tab q4h prn for pain. Max: 6 tabs/day. (Darvocet-N 50): Usual: 2 tabs q4h prn for pain. Max: 12 tabs/day. Elderly: Start at the low end of dosing range. Hepatic/Renal Impairment: Reduce daily dose. Cessation of Therapy: Gradually d/c; decrease dose 25-50% per day with careful monitoring for withdrawal signs/symptoms. If occurs, raise dose to previous level and titrate down more slowly.

**HOW SUPPLIED:** Tab: (Propoxyphene-APAP) 50mg-325mg, 100mg-650mg

**CONTRAINDICATIONS:** Significant respiratory depression (in unmonitored settings or the absence of resuscitative equipment), acute/severe asthma or hypercarbia, paralytic ileus.

**WARNINGS/PRECAUTIONS:** Drug dependence, misuse, abuse and addiction potential. Not for suicidal or addiction-prone patients. Respiratory depression may occur; caution in elderly/debilitated patients and extreme caution with significant COPD/cor pulmonale, with decreased respiratory reserve, hypoxia, hypercapnia, pre-existing respiratory depression. May cause severe hypotension and orthostatic hypotension; caution with circulatory shock. May obscure the clinical course of patients with head injuries. May impair mental/physical abilities. Abstinence syndrome may occur; avoid abrupt d/c. May cause spasm of the sphincter of Oddi; caution with biliary tract disease, including acute pancreatitis. May increase serum amylase levels. Caution with hepatic/renal impairment.

**ADVERSE REACTIONS:** Dizziness, sedation, N/V, liver dysfunction.

**INTERACTIONS:** See Black Box Warning. (Propoxyphene) Additive CNS depressant and interactive effects resulting in respiratory depression, hypotension, profound sedation, or coma may result if taken with narcotic analgesics, general anesthetics, phenothiazines, alcohol and other CNS depressants. Respiratory depression may occur when given in conjunction with other agents that depress respiration. Severe hypotension may occur after concurrent administration with other agents which compromise vasomotor tone. Caution with mixed agonist/antagonist analgesics (eg, pentazocine, nalbuphine, butorphanol and buprenorphine); may reduce analgesic effect and/or precipitate withdrawal symptoms. Avoid with MAOIs or within 14 days of stopping treatment. Severe neurologic signs, including coma reported with carbamazepine. Increased risk of bleeding with warfarin-like agents. Enhanced metabolite levels with strong CYP3A4 inducers (eg, rifampin). May increase levels and increase adverse effects with substrates of CYP3A4 or CYP2D6. (APAP) Hepatotoxicity may occur with alcohol. Effect may be delayed or decreased by anticholinergics. May increase plasma clearance and decrease half-life with oral contraceptives. May increase pharmacological effects with propranolol. May decrease effects of loop diuretics and decrease therapeutic effects of lamotrigine and zidovudine. May increase therapeutic effects with probenecid. Avoid with other acetaminophen-containing products.



**PREGNANCY:** Category C, caution in nursing.

**MECHANISM OF ACTION:** Propoxyphene: Centrally acting narcotic analgesic; inhibits the voltage-gated potassium current carried by cardiac rapidly activating delayed rectifier (hERG) channels with approximately equal potency. Acetaminophen: Non-opiate, non-salicylate analgesic and antipyretic; mechanism for analgesic is not established, antipyretic effect is mediated through activity in the hypothalamic heat-regulating centers, also inhibits prostaglandin synthetase.

**PHARMACOKINETICS: Absorption:** Propoxyphene: $T_{max}$=2-2.5 hrs; (65mg) $C_{max}$=0.05-0.1mcg/mL, (norpropoxyphene) $C_{max}$=0.1-0.2µg/mL. **Distribution:** Found in breast milk, crosses the placenta. Propoxyphene: $V_d$=16L/kg; plasma protein binding (80%). APAP: Plasma protein binding (variable). **Metabolism:** Propoxyphene: Liver via CYP3A4 (N-demethylation); norpropoxyphene (active metabolite) APAP: Liver via UGT1A6 (conjugation, mainly glucuronidation). **Elimination:** Propoxyphene: Urine (20-25%); $T_{1/2}$=6-12 hrs, (norpropoxyphene) 30-36 hrs. APAP: Urine (85%); $T_{max}$=1.25-3 hrs.

## NURSING CONSIDERATIONS

**Assessment:** Assess for significant respiratory depression, acute/severe asthma, hypercarbia, paralytic ileus, head injuries, addiction prone patients, suicidal tendencies/ideation, emotional disturbances, hepatic/renal impairment, alcoholism, COPD/cor pulmonale, decreased respiratory reserve, hypoxia, hypercapnia, circulatory shock, biliary tract disease, hypersensitivity, pregnancy/nursing status, and possible drug interactions.

**Monitoring:** Monitor for signs/symptoms of CNS depression, respiratory depression, severe/orthostatic hypotension, drug dependence, hepatic/renal impairment and hypersensitivity reactions. Monitor serum amylase levels.

**Patient Counseling:** Advise to report pain and adverse experiences occurring during therapy. Advise not to adjust dose without consulting the prescribing professional. Caution performing hazardous tasks (eg, driving, operating machinery). Counsel not to take CNS depressants (eg, sleep aids, tranquilizers), consume alcoholic beverages, over-the-counter medications that contain alcohol, and acetaminophen-containing products while on therapy. Inform of pregnancy risks and potential for drug abuse. Advise not to abruptly d/c medication due to risk of precipitating withdrawal symptoms.

**Administration:** Oral route. **Storage:** 25°C (77°F); excursions permitted to 15-30°C (59-86°F).

## DARVON

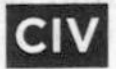


propoxyphene HCl (Xanodyne)

**THERAPEUTIC CLASS:** Opioid analgesic

**INDICATIONS:** Relief of mild to moderate pain.

**DOSAGE:** *Adults:* Usual: 65mg q4h as needed for pain. Max: 390mg/day. Elderly: Increase dosing interval. Hepatic/Renal Impairment: Reduce daily dose.

**HOW SUPPLIED:** Cap: 65mg

**WARNINGS/PRECAUTIONS:** Drug dependence potential. May impair mental/physical ability for operating machinery. Caution with hepatic or renal impairment and the elderly. Not for suicidal or addiction-prone patients. Do not exceed recommended dose.

**ADVERSE REACTIONS:** Dizziness, sedation, NV, liver dysfunction.

**INTERACTIONS:** Additive CNS-depressant effect with other CNS depressants, including alcohol. Increases plasma levels of antidepressants, anticonvulsants, and coumarins. Severe neurologic signs, including coma reported with carbamazepine. Caution with tranquilizers, antidepressants, and with excessive alcohol use.

**PREGNANCY:** Not for use in pregnancy, unknown use in nursing.

**MECHANISM OF ACTION:** Centrally acting narcotic analgesic agent.

**PHARMACOKINETICS: Absorption:** $C_{max}$=0.05-0.1mcg/mL; $T_{max}$=2-2.5 hrs. **Distribution:** Found in breast milk. **Metabolism:** Liver; norpropoxyphene (active metabolite). **Elimination:** $T_{1/2}$=6-12 hrs, 30-36 hrs (norpropoxyphene).

## NURSING CONSIDERATIONS

**Assessment:** Assess for suicidal tendencies, history of emotional disturbances, alcoholism, proneness to addiction, renal/hepatic impairment, age of patient, history of ulcers, pregnancy/nursing status, and possible drug interactions.

**Monitoring:** Monitor for signs/symptoms of CNS depression, drug dependence, and liver dysfunction. In cases of chronic overdosage, monitor for subacute painful myopathy.

**Patient Counseling:** Inform that drug may impair mental/physical abilities; use caution when performing hazardous tasks (eg, operating machinery/driving). Counsel to avoid using other CNS depressants and alcohol. Advise to notify physician of all medications currently taken. Inform that dependence may occur if higher than recommended doses taken for a long period of time. Advise to lie down and rest if any signs/symptoms of drowsiness, dizziness, or NV occur.

**Administration:** Oral route. **Storage:** 20-25°C (86-77° F); keep out of reach of children.

# DARVON-N

**CIV**

propoxyphene napsylate (Xanodyne)

**Accidental and intentional overdose with propoxyphene alone or with other CNS depressants, including alcohol reported. Propoxyphene-related deaths occured in patients with emotional disturbances or suicidal ideation/attempts and/or co-administration of sedatives, tranquilizers, muscle relaxants, antidepressants, or other CNS depressants. Do not prescribe to patients who are suicidal or with history of suicidal ideation. Careful monitoring in patients receiving propoxyphene and CYP3A4 inhibitors.**

**THERAPEUTIC CLASS:** Opioid analgesic

**INDICATIONS:** Relief of mild to moderate pain.

**DOSAGE:** *Adults:* Usual: 100mg q4h prn. Max: 600mg/day. Elderly: Start at the low end of dosing range. Hepatic/Renal Impairment: Reduce daily dose.

**HOW SUPPLIED:** Tab: 100mg

**CONTRAINDICATIONS:** Significant respiratory depression (in unmonitored settings or the absence of resuscitative equipment), acute/severe asthma or hypercarbia, paralytic ileus.

**WARNINGS/PRECAUTIONS:** Drug dependence potential. May impair mental/physical ability. Caution with hepatic or renal impairment and the elderly/debilitated patients. Not for suicidal or addiction-prone patients. Do not exceed recommended dose. Respiratory depression may occur; caution in patients with significant chronic obstructive pulmonary disease (COPD) or cor pulmonale, having substantially decreased respiratory reserve, hypoxia, hypercapnia, or pre-existing respiratory depression. May cause severe hypotension and orthostatic hypotension in ambulatory patients; caution to patients in circulatory shock. May obscure the clinical course of patients with head injuries. Abstinence syndrome may occur; avoid abrupt discontinuation. May cause spasm of the sphincter of Oddi and increase in serum amylase level; caution with biliary tract disease.



**ADVERSE REACTIONS:** Dizziness, sedation, NV, constipation, abdominal pain, skin rashes, lightheadedness, headache, weakness, euphoria, dysphoria, hallucinations, minor visual disturbances.

**INTERACTIONS:** See black box warning. Additive CNS-depressant effect with narcotic analgesics, general anesthetics, phenothiazines, other tranquilizers, sedative-hypnotics, or other CNS depressants, including alcohol. Severe neurologic signs, including coma, reported with carbamazepine. Caution with concomitant antidepressants, muscle relaxants. Increased risk of bleeding with warfarin-like agents. Reduced efficacy with CYP3A4 inducers. Caution with agonists/antagonist analgesics. Not recommended for patients taking MAOIs or within 14 days of stopping such treatment. Enhanced metabolite levels with rifampin. Enhanced plasma levels with strong CYP3A4 inhibitors. Increase pharmacologic or adverse effects of drugs that are CYP3A4 or CYP2D6 substrates.

**PREGNANCY:** Category C, caution in nursing.

**MECHANISM OF ACTION:** Centrally acting opioid analgesic agent; inhibits the voltage-gated potassium current carried by cardiac rapidly activating delayed rectifier (hERG) channels and sodium channels (local anesthetic effect).

**PHARMACOKINETICS: Absorption:** $C_{max}$=0.05-0.1µg/mL (propxyphene), 0.1-0.2µg/mL (norpropoxyphene); $T_{max}$=2-2.5 hrs. **Distribution:** $V_d$= 16L/kg; plasma protein binding=80%; crosses placenta, found in breast milk. **Metabolism:** Liver; norpropoxyphene (major; metabolite), CYP3A4 . **Elimination:** Urine (20-25%), $T_{1/2}$=6-12 hrs (propoxyphene), 30-36 hrs (norpropoxyphene).

## NURSING CONSIDERATIONS

**Assessment:** Assess for abuse potential, suicidal tendencies, previous history of emotional disorders, alcoholism, renal/hepatic function, age of patient, hypersensitivity, pregnancy/nursing status, and possible drug interactions.

**Monitoring:** Monitor for signs/symptoms of CNS depression, drug dependence, liver dysfunction, and hypersensitivity reactions. Monitor for subacute painful myopathy if chronic overdosage occurs.

**Patient Counseling:** Counsel that drug may impair mental/physical abilities; use caution when performing hazardous tasks (eg, operating machinery/driving). Advise to avoid using other CNS depressants and alcohol during therapy. Counsel to notify physician of all medications currently taken. Inform that dependence may occur if higher than recommended dose is taken for a longer period of time. Instruct not to consume alcoholic beverages including prescription and OTC meds that contain alcohol. Advice of pregnancy risks and potential drug abuse. Advice not to abruptly discontinue medication for risk of withdrawal symptoms and not to adjust dose without prior consult. Advise to report pain and adverse experiences occuring during therapy.

**Storage:** Oral route. **Storage:** 25°C (77°F); excursions permitted to 15-30°C (59-86°F).

# DAYTRANA

methylphenidate (Shire)

> **Give cautiously to patients with a history of drug dependence or alcoholism. Chronic abusive use may lead to marked tolerance and psychological dependence with varying degrees of abnormal behavior. Careful supervision required during withdrawal from abusive use to avoid severe depression.**

**THERAPEUTIC CLASS:** Sympathomimetic amine

**INDICATIONS:** Treatment of attention deficit hyperactivity disorder (ADHD).

**DOSAGE:** *Adults:* Individualize dose. Apply to hip area 2 hrs before effect is needed and remove 9 hrs after application. Recommended Titration Schedule:

Week 1: 10mg/9 hrs. Week 2: 15mg/9 hrs. Week 3: 20mg/9 hrs. Week 4: 30mg/9 hrs.
*Pediatrics:* ≥6 yrs: Individualize dose. Apply to hip area 2 hrs before effect is needed and remove 9 hrs after application. Recommended Titration Schedule: Week 1: 10mg/9 hrs. Week 2: 15mg/9 hrs. Week 3: 20mg/9 hrs. Week 4: 30mg/9 hrs.

**HOW SUPPLIED:** Patch: 10mg/9 hrs, 15mg/9 hrs, 20mg/9 hrs, 30mg/9 hrs [10[s], 30[s]]

D

**CONTRAINDICATIONS:** Marked anxiety, tension, and agitation; glaucoma; motor tics or family history or diagnosis of Tourette's syndrome; treatment with MAOIs and within minimum of 14 days following d/c.

**WARNINGS/PRECAUTIONS:** Avoid use with known structural cardiac abnormalities; sudden death reported. D/C if contact sensitization is suspected. Monitor growth during treatment. May exacerbate symptoms of behavior disturbance and thought disorder in psychotic patients. Caution when using stimulants to treat patients with comorbid bipolar disorder because of concern for possible induction of mixed/manic episode in such patients. Stimulants at usual doses can cause treatment emergent psychotic or manic symptoms (eg, hallucinations, delusional thinking, mania) in children and adolescents without prior history of psychotic illness. Aggressive behavior or hostility reported in clinical trials and postmarketing experience of some medications indicated for the treatment of ADHD. May lower convulsive threshold; d/c in the presence of seizures. Caution with HTN; monitor BP. Caution when underlying medical conditions might be compromised by increases in BP or HR (eg, pre-existing HTN, heart failure, recent MI, or hyperthyroidism). Visual disturbances reported. Caution with history of drug dependence or alcoholism. Avoid exposing application site to external heat sources (eg, heating pads, electric blankets, heated water beds, etc.). Monitor CBC, differential, and platelet counts during prolonged therapy.

**ADVERSE REACTIONS:** N/V, nasopharyngitis, weight decrease, anorexia, decreased appetite, affect lability, insomnia, tics, nasal congestion.

**INTERACTIONS:** See Contraindications. Caution with pressor agents. May decrease effectiveness of antihypertensive agents. May inhibit metabolism of coumarin anticoagulants, anticonvulsants (eg, phenobarbital, phenytoin, primidone), some tricyclic drugs (eg, imipramine, clomipramine, desipramine), and SSRIs. Monitor drug levels (or coagulation times with coumarin) and consider dose adjustments with concomitant use. Serious adverse events reported with concomitant clonidine use.

**PREGNANCY:** Category C, caution in nursing.

**MECHANISM OF ACTION:** Sympathomimetic amine; CNS stimulant. Suspected to block reuptake of norepinephrine and dopamine into presynaptic neuron and increase release of these monoamines into neuronal spaces.

**PHARMACOKINETICS: Absorption:** $C_{max}$=39ng/mL; $T_{max}$=7.5-10.5 hrs. **Distribution:** Plasma concentrations decline in biexponential manner due to continued distribution from skin after patch removal. **Metabolism:** De-esterification; ritalinic acid (metabolite). **Elimination:** $T_{1/2}$=3-4 hrs (*d*-methylphenidate); $T_{1/2}$=1.4-2.9 hrs (*l*-methylphenidate).

## NURSING CONSIDERATIONS

**Assessment:** Assess for marked anxiety, tension, agitation, known hypersensitivity to methylphenidate, glaucoma, motor tics, family history or diagnosis of Tourette's syndrome, behavior disturbances, thought disorder, bipolar disorder, depression, family history of suicide, pre-existing structural cardiac abnormalities, cardiomyopathy, heart rhythm abnormalities, CAD, HTN, heart failure, recent MI, psychiatric history, history of seizures, prior EEG abnormalities in absence of seizures, and patients without history of seizures and with no prior EEG evidence of seizures. Assess for history of drug dependence or alcoholism.

**Monitoring:** Monitor periodically for long-term usefulness, possible drug interactions, BP, HR, contact sensitization evidenced by erythema, edema, papules, vesicles, psychotic or manic symptoms such as hallucinations, delusional thinking, mania, confused state, crying, tics, headaches, irritability, anorexia, insomnia, infectious mononucleosis, and viral infection. Monitor for appearance of or worsening aggressive behavior or hostility. Perform follow-up weight and height in children 7-10 yrs. Periodic CBC, differential, and platelet counts are advised during prolonged therapy.



**Patient Counseling:** Counsel about drug abuse/dependence potential. Advise to avoid exposing application site to direct external heat sources while wearing the patch. Inform to apply patch to a clean, dry site on hip. Site of application must be alternated daily and patch should not be applied to waistline, where tight clothing may rub the patch. Encourage patient or caregiver to use administration chart to monitor application and removal time, and method of disposal. Patient or caregiver should avoid touching adhesive side of patch during application; if touched, wash hands after application. If any swelling or blistering occurs, remove patch; inform physician. Do not apply hydrocortisone or other solutions, creams, ointments, or emollients immediately prior to patch application. Inform of drug's side effects (heart-related problems, mental problems); notify physician if any occur.

**Administration:** Transdermal. Once tray is opened, use contents within 2 months. Apply patch immediately upon removal from protective pouch. If patch does not fully adhere to skin, or is partially or fully detached during wear time, discard patch and apply a new one. Inspect release liner to ensure no adhesive-containing medication has transferred to liner; if adhesive transfer has occurred, discard patch. If a patch is replaced, total recommended wear time for the day should remain 9 hrs. Peel patches off slowly. Patches should not be applied or re-applied with dressings, tape, or other common adhesives. **Storage:** Store at 25°C (77°F); excursions permitted to 15-30°C (59-86°F). Do not store patches unpouched. Do not refrigerate or freeze patches.

## DDAVP — RX

desmopressin acetate (Sanofi-Aventis)

**OTHER BRAND NAMES:** DDAVP Rhinal Tube (Sanofi-Aventis) - DDAVP Nasal Spray (Sanofi-Aventis)

**THERAPEUTIC CLASS:** Synthetic vasopressin analog

**INDICATIONS:** (Tab) Management of primary nocturnal enuresis. (Inj/Nasal Spray/Rhinal Tube/Tab) As antidiuretic replacement therapy in management of central (cranial) diabetes insipidus. Management of temporary polyuria and polydipsia following head trauma or surgery in the pituitary region. (Inj) Hemophilia A with factor VIII coagulant activity levels >5% and mild to moderate classic von Willebrand's disease (Type I) with factor VIII levels >5%.

**DOSAGE:** *Adults:* Diabetes Insipidus: (Tab) Initial: 0.05mg bid. Titrate: May increase/decrease to the range of 0.1-1.2mg/day given bid-tid. Maint: 0.1-0.8mg/day in divided doses. (Spray/Tube) Usual: 0.1-0.4mL/day given qd-tid. (Inj) 0.5-1mL/day IV/SQ given bid. Hemophilia A/von Willebrand's Disease: (Inj) 0.3mcg/kg IV over 15-30 min. Add 50mL diluent. If used pre-op, give 30 min before procedure. Primary Nocturnal Enuresis: (Tab) Initial: 0.2 mg hs. Titrate: May increase up to 0.6mg. Fluid restriction should be observed and fluid intake should be limited to a minimum from 1 hr before administration, until the next morning, or at least 8 hrs after administration. Elderly: Caution in dose selection.

*Pediatrics:* Diabetes Insipidus: (Tab) ≥4 yrs: Initial: 0.05mg bid. Titrate: May increase/decrease to the range of 0.1-1.2mg/day given bid-tid. Maint: 0.1-0.8mg/day in divided doses. (Spray/Tube) 3 months-12 yrs: Usual: 0.05-0.3mL/day given qd-bid. (Inj) ≥12 yrs: 0.5-1mL/day IV/SQ given bid. Hemophilia A/von Willebrand's Disease: (Inj) ≥3 months: 0.3mcg/kg IV over 15-30 min. Add 50mL diluent (>10kg) or 10mL diluent (≤10kg). If used pre-op, give 30 min before procedure. Primary Nocturnal Enuresis: (Tab) ≥6 yrs: Initial: 0.2 mg hs. Titrate: May increase up to 0.6mg. Fluid restriction should be observed and fluid intake should be limited to a minimum from 1 hr before administration, until the next morning, or at least 8 hrs after administration.

**HOW SUPPLIED:** Inj: 4mcg/mL; Nasal Spray: 10mcg/inh [5mL]; Tab: 0.1mg*, 0.2mg*; Rhinal Tube: 0.01% [2.5mL] *scored

**CONTRAINDICATIONS:** Moderate to severe renal impairment (CrCL<50mL/min), hyponatremia, or history of hyponatremia.

**WARNINGS/PRECAUTIONS:** Particularly in pediatric and geriatric patients fluid restriction should be decreased to decrease risk of water intoxication and hyponatremia; monitor for signs/symptoms of hyponatremia (eg, headache, N/V, weight gain, restlessness, fatigue, disorientation, depressed reflexes, abnormal mental status). Nasal Spray/Rhinal Tube should only be used in patients where orally administered formulations are not feasible. Use injectable form if intranasal route is compromised or patient consciousness is impaired. Caution in patients with habitual or psychogenic polydipsia, conditions associated with fluid and electrolyte imbalance (eg, CF, HF, renal disorders), coronary artery insufficiency, and hypertensive CVD. Allergic reactions rarely reported. Anaphylaxis rarely reported with IV and intranasal administration. Caution with IV use if history of thrombus formation. For diabetes insipidus, dosage must be adjusted according to diurnal pattern of response; estimate response by adequate duration of sleep and adequate, not excessive, water turnover. (Inj) Should not be used to treat Type IIB von Willebrand's disease. Not indicated for the treatment of hemophilia A with factor VIII coagulant activity levels ≤5% or for the treatment of hemophilia B, or in patients who have factor VIII antibodies.

**ADVERSE REACTIONS:** Inj: Headache, nausea, abdominal cramps, vulval pain, injection-site reactions, facial flushing, BP changes. Nasal Spray/ Rhinal Tube: Headache, nasal congestion, flushing, rhinitis, epistaxis. Tab: Nausea, flushing, abdominal cramps, headache, increased AST.

**INTERACTIONS:** Caution with other pressor agents. Caution with the concomitant administration of drugs that may increase the risk of water intoxication with hyponatremia (eg, TCA, SSRIs, chlorpromazine, opiate analgesics, NSAIDs, lamotrigine, carbamazepine).

**PREGNANCY:** Category B, caution in nursing.

**MECHANISM OF ACTION:** Synthetic vasopressin analog; antidiuretic affecting renal water conservation.

**PHARMACOKINETICS: Absorption:** (Inj) Rapid, $T_{max}$=90 min-2 hrs. (Tab, Nasal) Rapid, $T_{max}$=0.9-1.5 hrs. **Elimination:** Urine; (Inj, Nasal) $T_{1/2}$=3 hrs; (Tab) 1.5-2.5 hrs.

## NURSING CONSIDERATIONS

**Assessment:** Assess for hyponatremia or history of hyponatremia, habitual or psychogenic polydipsia, coronary artery insufficiency, hypertensive CVD, electrolyte imbalance disorders (eg, CF, HF, renal disorders), risk factors for thrombus formation, pregnancy/nursing status, and for possible drug interactions. Obtain baseline renal function. In patients with diabetes insipidus or post-surgical or head trauma-related polyuria and polydipsia, obtain baseline urine volume and osmolality. (Inj) Assess for hemophilia A with factor VIII coagulant activities ≤5% and for the presence of factor VIII antibodies. Assess not for the treatment of hemophilia B. In patients with hemophilia A, obtain baseline levels of factor VIII coagulant, factor VIII antigen, factor VIII ristocetin cofactor, and activated partial thromboplastin time. In patients with von Willebrand's disease, obtain baseline levels of factor VIII coagulant activity, factor VIII ristocetin cofactor activity, and factor VIII von Willebrand factor antigen. (Nasal, Rhinal Tube) Assess for factors against nasal insufflation (eg, nasal congestion, blockage, discharge, atrophy, severe rhinitis, impaired level of consciousness).

**Monitoring:** Monitor for signs/symptoms of hyponatremia (eg, headache, N/V, weight gain, restlessness, fatigue, loss of appetite), water intoxication, and for allergic reactions. In patients with diabetes insipidus or post-surgical or head trauma-related polyuria and polydipsia, monitor urine volume and osmolality. Monitor renal function. (Nasal) Monitor for elevations in BP, anaphylaxis, and for changes in the nasal mucosa. (Inj) Monitor for thrombotic events and for anaphylaxis. In patients with hemophilia A, monitor factor VIII coagulant levels, factor VIII antigen levels, factor VIII ristocetin cofactor levels, and partial thromboplastin time. In patients with von Willebrand's disease, monitor levels of factor VIII coagulant activity, factor VIII ristocetin cofactor activity, and factor VIII von Willebrand factor antigen.

**Patient Counseling:** Counsel to seek medical attention if signs of hyponatremia (eg, headache, N/V, weight gain, fatigue, disorientation) or if an allergic reaction occurs. If using nasal spray or rhinal tube, inform that administration should be under adult supervision to control dose intake, and to contact physician if symptoms of nasal blockage, discharge, or congestion occur.



**Administration:** Intranasal/IV/SQ/Oral routes. Refer to PI for specific administration techniques. **Storage:** Inj: 2-8°C (36-46°F). Tab: 20-25°C (68-77°F); avoid exposure to excessive light or heat. Nasal Spray: 20-25°C (68-77°F) in upright position. Rhinal Tube: 2-8°C (36-46°F); closed bottles stable for 3 weeks at 20-25°C (68-77°F). Keep out of the reach of children.

## DEMADEX RX

torsemide (Meda)

**THERAPEUTIC CLASS:** Loop diuretic

**INDICATIONS:** Treatment of edema associated with congestive heart failure (CHF), renal disease, chronic renal failure or hepatic disease. Treatment of hypertension, alone or with other antihypertensive agents.

**DOSAGE:** *Adults:* CHF: Initial: 10-20mg qd. Titrate: Double dose until desired diuretic response is obtained. Max: 200mg single dose. Chronic Renal Failure: Initial: 20mg qd. Titrate: Double dose until desired diuretic response is obtained. Max: 200mg single dose. Hepatic Cirrhosis: Initial: 5-10mg qd with aldosterone antagonist or $K^+$-sparing diuretic. Titrate: Double dose until desired diuretic response is obtained. Max: 40mg single dose. HTN: Initial: 5mg qd. Titrate: May increase to 10mg qd in 4-6 weeks, then may add additional antihypertensive agent.

**HOW SUPPLIED:** Tab: 5mg*, 10mg*, 20mg*, 100mg* *scored

**CONTRAINDICATIONS:** Anuria.

**WARNINGS/PRECAUTIONS:** Caution with cirrhosis and ascites in hepatic disease. Tinnitus and hearing loss (usually reversible) reported. Avoid excessive diuresis, especially in elderly. Caution with brisk diuresis, inadequate oral intake of electrolytes, and cardiovascular disease (CVD), especially if receiving digitalis glycosides. Monitor for electrolyte/volume depletion. Hyperglycemia, hypokalemia, hypermagnesemia, hypercalcemia and gout reported. May increase cholesterol and TG.

**ADVERSE REACTIONS:** Headache, excessive urination, dizziness, cough, ECG abnormality, asthenia, rhinitis, diarrhea.

**INTERACTIONS:** Caution with high-dose salicylates, aminoglycosides, lithium and digitalis glycoside. Indomethacin partially inhibits natriuretic effect. Avoid simultaneous cholestyramine administration. Probenecid decreases effects. Reduces spironolactone clearance. Risk of hypokalemia with ACTH, corticosteroids. Possible renal dysfunction with NSAIDs.

**PREGNANCY:** Category B, caution in nursing.

**MECHANISM OF ACTION:** Pyridine-sulfonylurea diuretic; acts within lumen of thick ascending part of loop of Henle, inhibiting $Na^+/K^+/2Cl^-$ carrier system.

**PHARMACOKINETICS: Absorption:** Absolute bioavailability (80%); $T_{max}$=1 hr. **Distribution:** $V_d$=12-15L; plasma protein binding (>99%). **Metabolism:** Liver; Carboxylic acid (major metabolite). **Elimination:** Urine (20%); $T_{1/2}$=3.5 hrs.

### NURSING CONSIDERATIONS

**Assessment:** Assess for sulfonamide hypersensitivity, anuria, CVD, renal/hepatic impairment, nursing status and possible drug interactions.

**Monitoring:** Monitor serum electrolytes, serum $K^+$ levels and renal function. Monitor for signs/symptoms of hypokalemia, electrolyte imbalance, arrhythmias, ototoxicity, hypersensitivity reactions and renal/hepatic dysfunction.

**Patient Counseling:** Discuss risks and benefits of therapy. Advise to seek medical attention if symptoms of hypokalemia, electrolyte imbalance, hypersensitivity reactions, hearing loss or tinnitus occur.

**Administration:** Oral route. **Storage:** 15-30°C (59-86°F). Do not freeze.

# DEMEROL INJECTION

CII



meperidine HCl (Hospira)

**THERAPEUTIC CLASS:** Opioid analgesic

**INDICATIONS:** For relief of moderate to severe pain. For preoperative medication, anesthesia support, and obstetrical analgesia.

**DOSAGE:** *Adults:* Pain: Usual: 50-150mg IM/SQ q3-4h prn. Preoperative: Usual: 50-100mg IM/SQ 30-90 min before anesthesia. Anesthesia Support: Use repeated slow IV inj of fractional doses (eg, 10mg/mL) or continuous IV infusion of a more dilute solution (eg, 1mg/mL). Titrate as needed. Obstetrical Analgesia: Usual: 50-100mg IM/SQ when pain is regular, may repeat at 1- to 3-hr intervals. Elderly: Start at lower end of dosage range and observe. With Phenothiazines/Other Tranquilizers: Reduce dose by 25 to 50%. IM method preferred with repeated use. For IV injection: Reduce dose and administer slowly, preferably using diluted solution.

*Pediatrics:* Pain: Usual: 0.5-0.8mg/lb IM/SQ, up to 50-150mg, q3-4h prn. Preoperative: Usual: 0.5-1mg/lb IM/SQ, up to 50-100mg, 30-90 min before anesthesia. With Phenothiazines/Other Tranquilizers: Reduce dose by 25 to 50%. IM method preferred with repeated use. For IV injection: Reduce dose and administer slowly, preferably using diluted solution.

**HOW SUPPLIED:** Inj: 25mg/mL, 50mg/mL, 75mg/mL, 100mg/mL

**CONTRAINDICATIONS:** MAOIs during or within 14 days of use.

**WARNINGS/PRECAUTIONS:** May develop tolerance and dependence; abuse potential. Extreme caution with head injury, increased ICP, intracranial lesions, acute asthmatic attack, chronic COPD or cor pulmonale, decreased respiratory reserve, respiratory depression, hypoxia, and hypercapnia. Rapid IV infusion may result in increased adverse reactions. Caution with acute abdominal conditions, atrial flutter, supraventricular tachycardias. May aggravate convulsive disorders. Caution and reduce initial dose with elderly or debilitated, renal/hepatic impairment, hypothyroidism, Addison's disease, prostatic hypertrophy or urethral stricture. Severe hypotension may occur post-op or if depleted blood volume. Orthostatic hypotension may occur. May impair mental/physical abilities. Not for use in pregnancy prior to labor. May produce depression of respiration and psychophysiologic functions in newborn when used as an obstetrical analgesic.

**ADVERSE REACTIONS:** Lightheadedness, dizziness, sedation, NV, sweating, respiratory/circulatory depression.

**INTERACTIONS:** See Contraindications. Caution and reduce dose with other CNS depressants (eg, narcotics, anesthetics, phenothiazines, tranquilizers, sedative-hypnotics, TCAs, alcohol).

**PREGNANCY:** Safety in pregnancy and nursing not known.

**MECHANISM OF ACTION:** Narcotic analgesic; produces actions similiar to morphine. Principle actions involve the CNS and organs composed of smooth muscle. Produces analgesic and sedative effects.

**PHARMACOKINETICS: Distribution:** Crosses placental barrier; found in breast milk.

## NURSING CONSIDERATIONS

**Assessment:** Assess for presence of head injury, intracranial lesions, presence of elevated intracranial pressure, nursing/pregnancy status, presence of acute asthmatic attack, COPD or cor pulmonale, respiratory depression, hypotension, atrial flutter and other supraventricular tachycardias, convulsive disorders, acute abdominal conditions, hepatic/renal impairment, hypothyroidism, Addison's disease, prostatic hypertrophy or urethral stricture, and drug interactions (eg, MAO inhibitors).

**Monitoring:** Monitor for signs/symptoms of drug dependence (eg, psychic dependence, physical dependence), respiratory depression, circulatory depression (eg, hypotension), and convulsions.

**Patient Counseling:** Inform that medication may impair mental/physical abilities; use caution when performing hazardous tasks (eg, operating machinery/driving). Advise to notify physician of all medications currently taken. Instruct patient cannot take medication if an MAO inhibitor was used within previous 14 days. Avoid using other CNS depressants and alcohol during medication. Advise about potential for dependence upon repeated administration. Inform women in labor that medication crosses placental barrier and can produce depression of respiration and psychophysiologic function in newborn.

**Administration:** SQ, IM, IV route. SQ route is suitable for occasional use, IM administration is preferred if repeated doses are required. IM injection should be injected well into the body of a large muscle. If IV route is required, dosage should be decreased and injection should be made very slowly, preferably using a diluted solution. Dosage should be adjusted according to severity of pain. **Storage:** 20-25°C (68-77°F).

## DEMEROL ORAL — CII

meperidine HCl (Sanofi-Aventis)

**THERAPEUTIC CLASS:** Opioid analgesic

**INDICATIONS:** Relief of moderate to severe pain.

**DOSAGE:** *Adults:* Usual: 50-150mg q3-4h prn. Concomitant Phenothiazines/Other Tranquilizers: Reduce dose by 25-50%.
*Pediatrics:* Usual: 1.1-1.8mg/kg, up to adult dose, q3-4h prn. Concomitant Phenothiazines/Other Tranquilizers: Reduce dose by 25-50%.

**HOW SUPPLIED:** Tab: 50mg*, 100mg* *scored

**CONTRAINDICATIONS:** During or within 14 days of MAOI use.

**WARNINGS/PRECAUTIONS:** May develop tolerance and dependence; abuse potential. Extreme caution with head injury, increased ICP, intracranial lesions, acute asthma attack, chronic COPD, cor pulmonale, decreased respiratory reserve, respiratory depression, hypoxia, and hypercapnia. Caution with sickle cell anemia, pheochromocytoma, acute alcoholism, Addison's disease, CNS depression or coma, delirium tremens, elderly or debilitated, kyphoscoliosis associated with respiratory depression, myxedema, hypothyroidism, acute abdominal conditions, epilepsy, atrial flutter and other supraventricular tachycardias, renal/hepatic impairment, prostatic hypertrophy, urethral stricture, drug dependencies, neonates, and young infants. Severe hypotension may occur post-op or if depleted blood volume. Orthostatic hypotension may occur. Not for use in pregnancy prior to labor. May impair mental/physical abilities.

**ADVERSE REACTIONS:** Lightheadedness, dizziness, sedation, N/V, sweating, respiratory depression.

**INTERACTIONS:** See Contraindications. Reduce dose with other CNS depressants (eg, narcotics, anesthetics, phenothiazines, tranquilizers, sedative-hypnotics, TCAs, alcohol). Mixed agonist/antagonist analgesics (eg, pentazocine, nalbuphine, butorphanol, buprenorphine) may reduce analgesic effects and/or precipitate withdrawal symptoms. Caution with acyclovir, cimetidine. Phenytoin may enhance hepatic metabolism. May enhance neuromuscular blocking action of skeletal muscle relaxants. Increased levels with ritonavir; avoid concomitant administration.

**PREGNANCY:** Category C, not for use in nursing.

**MECHANISM OF ACTION:** Narcotic analgesic; produces actions similiar to morphine. Principle actions involve the CNS and organs composed of smooth muscle. Produces analgesic and sedative effects.

**PHARMACOKINETICS: Distribution:** Crosses placental barrier; found in breast milk.

D

## NURSING CONSIDERATIONS

**Assessment:** Assess for abuse potential, head injury or intracranial lesions, presence of elevated ICP, presence of acute asthmatic attack, COPD, respiratory depression, hypotension, atrial flutter and other supraventricular tachycardias, pregnancy/nursing status, hepatic/renal impairment, sickle cell anemia, pheochromocytoma, acute alcoholism, adrenocortical insufficiency (eg, Addison's disease), CNS depression or coma, delirium tremens, convulsive disorders, presence of debilitation, myxedema or hypothyroidism, acute abdominal conditions, prostatic hypertrophy or urethral stricture, toxic psychosis, and possible drug interactions (eg, MAO inhibitors).

**Monitoring:** Monitor for signs/symptoms of tolerance or dependence, misuse or abuse, increase in CSF pressure, circulatory depression (eg, hypotension), respiratory depression, and convulsions.

**Patient Counseling:** Counsel to notify physician of all medications currently taking. Inform medication contains meperidine, a morphine-like substance. Caution to avoid with MAOI use within 14 days. Notify physician of any pain or adverse events during treatment. Do not adjust dosage or abruptly stop taking if on chronic therapy without consulting physician. Medication has potential for drug abuse; protect from theft and use by anyone other than the prescribed patient. Drug may impair mental/physical abilities; use caution when performing hazardous tasks (eg, operating machinery, driving). Avoid using other CNS depressants and alcohol. Inform pregnant women about effects of medication on pregnancy.

**Administration:** Oral route. **Storage:** 25°C (77°F); excursions permitted to 15-30°C (59-86°F).

# DENAVIR RX

penciclovir (Novartis)

**THERAPEUTIC CLASS:** Nucleoside analogue

**INDICATIONS:** Treatment of recurrent herpes labialis (cold sores) in adults and children ≥12 yrs.

**DOSAGE:** *Adults:* Apply q2h while awake for 4 days. Start with earliest sign or symptom.

*Pediatrics:* ≥12 yrs: Apply q2h while awake for 4 days. Start with earliest sign or symptom.

**HOW SUPPLIED:** Cre: 1% [1.5g]

**WARNINGS/PRECAUTIONS:** Only use on herpes labialis on the lips and face. Avoid mucous membranes or near the eyes. Effectiveness not established in immunocompromised patients.

**ADVERSE REACTIONS:** Headache, application-site reaction, local anesthesia, taste perversion, rash.

**PREGNANCY:** Category B, not for use in nursing.

**MECHANISM OF ACTION:** Antiviral agent; active against herpes simplex virus types 1 (HSV-1) and 2 (HSV-2). Inhibits HSV polymerase competitively with deoxyguanosine triphosphate. Consequently, herpes viral DNA synthesis and replication are selectively inhibited.

## NURSING CONSIDERATIONS

**Assessment:** Assess use in pregnancy/nursing.

**Monitoring:** Monitor lesions for clinical response. If lesions worsen or do not improve, monitor for secondary bacterial infection.

**Patient Counseling:** Counsel to avoid applying medication in or near eyes. Instruct to wash hands with soap and water after applying product. Advise females to notify physician if they become pregnant or are nursing.

**Administration:** Topical. **Storage**: 20-25°C (68-77°F).

# DEPACON RX

valproate sodium (Abbott)

D

**Fatal hepatic failure may occur, especially in children <2 yrs on multiple anticonvulsants, with congenital metabolic disorders, severe seizure disorders with mental retardation, and organic brain disease. Hepatotoxicity may be preceded by nonspecific symptoms such as malaise, weakness, lethargy, facial edema, anorexia, and vomiting, or loss of seizure control in patients with epilepsy. Monitor LFTs prior to therapy, frequently during 1st 6 months of treatment and at frequent intervals thereafter. Teratogenic effects (eg, neural tube defects), and life-threatening pancreatitis reported; d/c if pancreatitis diagnosed and initiate appropriate treatment.**

**THERAPEUTIC CLASS:** Valproate compound

**INDICATIONS:** Alternative when oral administration of valproate products is temporarily not feasible in the following conditions: monotherapy and adjunctive therapy for treatment of simple and complex absence seizures, and complex partial seizures; adjunctive therapy for multiple seizure types that include absence seizures.

**DOSAGE:** *Adults:* Simple/Complex Absence Seizure: Initial: 15mg/kg/day. Titrate: Increase weekly by 5-10mg/kg/day until optimal response. Max: 60mg/kg/day. Complex Partial Seizure/Conversion to Monotherapy/ Adjunctive Therapy: Initial: 10-15mg/kg/day. Titrate: Increase weekly by 5-10mg/kg/day until optimal response. Max: 60mg/kg/day. Elderly: Reduce initial dose and titrate slowly. Replacement Therapy: Give equivalent total daily dose as that of oral valproate. Administer as 60 min IV infusion, not >20mg/min. If dose >250mg/day, give in divided doses. Not for use >14 days; switch to oral route as soon as clinically feasible. Decrease dose or d/c if decreased food or fluid intake or if excessive somnolence occurs.
*Pediatrics:* ≥2 yrs: Simple/Complex Absence Seizure: Initial: 15mg/kg/day. Titrate: Increase weekly by 5-10mg/kg/day until optimal response. Max: 60mg/kg/day. ≥10 yrs: Complex Partial Seizure/Conversion to Monotherapy/ Adjunctive Therapy: Initial: 10-15mg/kg/day. Titrate: Increase weekly by 5-10mg/kg/day until optimal response. Max: 60mg/kg/day. Replacement Therapy: Give equivalent total daily dose as that of oral valproate. Administer as 60 min IV infusion, not >20mg/min. If dose >250mg/day, give in divided doses. Not for use >14 days; switch to oral route as soon as clinically feasible. Decrease dose or d/c if decreased food or fluid intake or if excessive somnolence occurs.

**HOW SUPPLIED:** Inj: 100mg/mL [5mL]

**CONTRAINDICATIONS:** Hepatic disease, significant hepatic dysfunction, known urea cycle disorders (UCD).

**WARNINGS/PRECAUTIONS:** Caution in hepatic disease; d/c if hepatic dysfunction suspected or apparent. Hyperammonemic encephalopathy in UCD patients; d/c if this occurs. Prior to therapy, evaluate for UCD in high-risk patients (eg, history of unexplained encephalopathy, coma, etc). If unexplained lethargy, vomiting, or mental status changes occur, measure ammonia levels. Caution in the elderly; monitor for fluid/nutritional intake, dehydration, somnolence. Dose-related thrombocytopenia and elevated liver enzymes reported. Monitor platelet and coagulation tests prior to therapy, then periodically. Altered thyroid function tests and urine ketone test. Avoid abrupt d/c. Multi-organ hypersensitivity reactions reported. May impair mental/physical abilities. Not for prophylaxis of post-traumatic seizures in acute head trauma. May stimulate replication of HIV and CMV.

**ADVERSE REACTIONS:** Dizziness, headache, N/V, elevated amylase, injection-site pain/reaction, somnolence, thrombocytopenia, ecchymosis.

**INTERACTIONS:** Drugs that affect the level of expression of hepatic enzymes (eg, phenytoin, carbamazepine, phenobarbital, primidone) may increase valproate clearance. Concomitant use with ASA decreases protein binding and metabolism of valproate. Carbapenem antibiotics (eg, meropenem, ertapenem, imipenem) may reduce serum valproic concentration to subtherapeutic levels. Rifampin increases oral clearance and may require valproate dosage adjustment. Concomitant use with felbamate leads to an increase in valproate $C_{max}$. Reduces the clearance of amitriptyline, nortriptyline, and lorazepam.

Induces metabolism of carbamazepine. Inhibits metabolism of diazepam, ethosuximide, phenobarbital and phenytoin; monitor drug serum concentrations and adjust dose appropriately. Breakthrough seizures reported with concomitant valproate and phenytoin use. Administration with clonazepam may induce absence status in patients with absence seizures. Increases $T_{1/2}$ of lamotrigine; serious skin reactions reported. Concomitant use with topiramate associated with hyperammonemia with or without encephalopathy. May displace protein-bound warfarin; monitor coagulation tests. Additive CNS depression with other CNS depressants (eg, alcohol). May decrease clearance of zidovudine in HIV-seropositive patients.



**PREGNANCY:** Category D, not for use in nursing.

**MECHANISM OF ACTION:** Anticonvulsant; has not been established. Proposed to increase GABA concentration in the brain.

**PHARMACOKINETICS: Distribution:** $V_d$=11L/1.73m$^2$; plasma protein binding (81.5%-90%); found in breast milk, CSF. **Metabolism:** Liver; glucuronidation, mitochondrial β-oxidation. **Elimination:** Urine (<3% unchanged); $T_{1/2}$=16 hrs.

## NURSING CONSIDERATIONS

**Assessment:** Assess LFTs, CBC with platelets, pancreatitis, plasma ammonia levels, other diseases/conditions, acute head injuries, pregnancy/nursing status, and possible drug interactions. Note other diseases/conditions and drug therapies.

**Monitoring:** Monitor LFTs, CBC with platelets, coagulation parameters, pancreatitis, hypersensitivity reactions, hyperammonemia, thyroid function tests.

**Patient Counseling:** Advise to avoid alcohol, sedatives, and other OTCs. Advise not to engage in hazardous activities (eg, driving/operating machinery). Counsel about signs/symptoms of pancreatitis, hepatotoxicity, hyperammonemia; notify physician if any symptoms or adverse effects occur. Instruct that a fever associated with other organ system involvement (rash, lymphadenopathy, etc.) may be drug-related and should be reported to physician immediately. Notify physician if pregnant or intend to become pregnant. Encourage patients to enroll in North American Antiepileptic Drug (NAAED) Pregnancy Registry by calling 888-233-2334 or go to www.aedpregnancyregistry.org.

**Administration:** IV route. Give as a 60-min infusion after diluting with at least 50mL of a compatible diluent. **Storage:** 15-30°C (59-86°F).

# DEPAKENE — RX

valproic acid (Abbott)

**Fatal hepatic failure may occur, especially in children <2 yrs on multiple anticonvulsants, with congenital metabolic disorders, severe seizure disorders with mental retardation, and organic brain disease. Hepatotoxicity may be preceded by nonspecific symptoms such as malaise, weakness, lethargy, facial edema, anorexia, and vomiting, or loss of seizure control in patients with epilepsy. Monitor LFTs prior to therapy, frequently during 1st 6 months of treatment and at frequent intervals thereafter. Teratogenic effects (eg, neural tube defects), and life-threatening pancreatitis reported; d/c if pancreatitis diagnosed and initiate appropriate treatment.**

**THERAPEUTIC CLASS:** Carboxylic acid derivative

**INDICATIONS:** Monotherapy and adjunctive therapy for treatment of simple and complex absence seizures, and complex partial seizures. Adjunctive therapy for multiple seizure types, which include absence seizures.

**DOSAGE:** *Adults:* Simple/Complex Absence Seizure: Initial: 15mg/kg/day. Titrate: Increase weekly by 5-10mg/kg/day until optimal response. Max: 60mg/kg/day. If dose >250mg/day, give in divided doses. Complex Partial Seizure: Monotherapy/Conversion to Monotherapy/Adjunctive Therapy: Initial: 10-15mg/kg/day. Titrate: Increase weekly by 5-10mg/kg/day until optimal response. If clinical response has not been achieved, plasma levels should be measured to determine whether they are in usually accepted therapeutic range (50-100μg/mL). Max: 60mg/kg/day. Concomitant AED dosage can ordinarily be reduced by approximately 25% q 2 weeks starting at initiation

of valproic acid or delayed 1-2 weeks if there is concern seizures are likely to occur. Elderly: Reduce initial dose and titrate slowly. Consider dose reduction or d/c in patients with decreased food or fluid intake and in patients with excessive somnolence. GI irritation: May benefit from administration of the drug with food or by slowly building up the dose from an initial low level.
*Pediatrics:* >2 yrs: Simple/Complex Absence Seizure: Initial: 15mg/kg/day. Titrate: Increase by 5-10mg/kg/day until optimal response. Max: 60 mg/kg/day. If dose >250mg/day, give in divided doses. ≥10 yrs: Complex Partial Seizure: Monotherapy/Conversion to Monotherapy/Adjunctive Therapy: Initial: 10-15mg/kg/day. Titrate: Increase weekly by 5-10mg/kg/day until optimal response. If clinical response has not been achieved, plasma levels should be measured to determine whether they are in usually accepted therapeutic range (50-100µg/mL). Max: 60mg/kg/day. Concomitant AED dosage can ordinarily be reduced by approximately 25% q 2 weeks starting at initiation of valproic acid or delayed 1-2 weeks if there is a concern that seizures are likely to occur. GI irritation: May benefit from administration of the drug with food or by slowly building up the dose from an initial low level.

**HOW SUPPLIED:** Cap: 250mg; Sol: 250mg/5mL

**CONTRAINDICATIONS:** Hepatic disease, significant hepatic dysfunction, known urea cycle disorders (UCD).

**WARNINGS/PRECAUTIONS:** Increased risk of suicidal thoughts or behavior; monitor for emergence or worsening of depression, suicidal thoughts or behaviors, and/or any unusual changes in mood or behavior. Hyperammonemic encephalopathy in UCD patients; d/c if this occurs. Prior to therapy, evaluate for UCD in high-risk patients (eg, history of unexplained encephalopathy, coma, etc.). Measure ammonia levels if develop unexplained lethargy, vomiting, or mental status changes. Caution in elderly; monitor for fluid/nutritional intake, dehydration, somnolence. Multi-organ hypersensitivity reactions and hypothermia, with or without hyperammonemia, reported. Monitor platelets and coagulation tests before therapy and periodically thereafter. Elevated liver enzymes and thrombocytopenia may be dose-related. May interfere with urine ketone and thyroid function tests. May impair mental/physical abilities. Caution with history of hepatic disease. May stimulate replication of HIV and CMV. Avoid abrupt d/c.

**ADVERSE REACTIONS:** Abdominal pain, amblyopia/blurred vision, alopecia, asthenia, diarrhea, diplopia, dizziness, headache, nystagmus, N/V, peripheral edema, somnolence, tremor, thrombocytopenia, weight gain.

**INTERACTIONS:** Carbapenem antibiotics may reduce serum valproic concentration to subtherapeutic levels, leading to loss of seizure control. Oral clearance increased by rifampin. Concomitant administration with clonazepam may induce absence status in patients with history thereof. Increases $T_{1/2}$ of lamotrigine; may result in serious skin reaction with lamotrigine. Reports of breakthrough seizures with the combination of valproate and phenytoin; monitor levels of both. Concomitant use with ASA decreases protein binding and metabolism of valproate. Reduces the clearance of amitriptyline, nortriptyline, zidovudine, and lorazepam. Induces metabolism of carbamazepine. Displaces protein-bound diazepam and decreases its $V_d$ and clearance. Inhibits metabolism and decreases clearance of ethosuximide. Concomitant use with felbamate leads to an increase in valproate $C_{max}$. Inhibits the metabolism of phenobarbital. Monitor for neurological toxicity when used with barbiturates. Displaces protein-bound tolbutamide, and warfarin; monitor coagulation tests. Concomitant use with topiramate has been associated with hyperammonemia with or without encephalopathy and hypothermia. Drugs that affect the level of expression of hepatic enzymes (eg, phenytoin, carbamazepine, phenobarbital, primidone) may increase valproate clearance. Additive CNS depression with other CNS depressants (eg, alcohol). Increased plasma level with chlorpromazine.

**PREGNANCY:** Category D, not for use in nursing.

**MECHANISM OF ACTION:** Carboxylic acid derivative; has not been established. Activity in epilepsy is proposed to be related to increased GABA concentration in the brain.

**PHARMACOKINETICS: Absorption:** Depakote:(Tab) $T_{max}$=4 hrs (fasting), 8 hrs (fed); (Cap) $T_{max}$=3.3 hrs (fasting), 4.8 hrs (fed). **Distribution:** $V_d$=11L/1.73m$^2$; plasma protein binding (10%-18.5%). **Metabolism:** Liver; glucuronidation, mitochondrial β-oxidation. **Elimination:** Urine (<3% unchanged); $T_{1/2}$=9-16 hrs.

## NURSING CONSIDERATIONS

**Assessment:** Assess LFTs, CBC with platelets, pancreatitis, plasma ammonia levels, hepatic dysfunction/disease, pregnancy/nursing status. Note other diseases/conditions and drug therapies. Prior to therapy, evaluate for UCD in high-risk patients (eg, history of unexplained encepalopathy, coma, etc.).

**Monitoring:** Monitor LFTs (at frequent intervals during first 6 months), CBC with platelets, coagulation parameters, pancreatitis, thyroid function tests, hypersensitivity reactions, hyperammonemia, ketone and thyroid function tests. Monitor for emergence of worsening of depression, suicidal thoughts or behavior, and/or unusual changes in mood or behavior.

**Patient Counseling:** Counsel to avoid alcohol, sedatives, OTCs. Caution while operating machinery/driving. Counsel about signs/symptoms of hepatotoxicity, pancreatitis, and hyperammonemic encephalopathy; notify physician if symptoms or adverse effects occur. Instruct that a fever associated with other organ system involvement (eg, rash, lympadenopathy, etc.) may be drug-related and should be reported to physician immediately. Notify physician if suicidal thoughts, behavior, or thoughts about self-harm emerge. Advise patients to enroll in the North American Antiepilepetic Drug (NAAED) Pregnancy Registry if they become pregnant. To enroll, call 888-233-2334 or go to www.aedpregnancyregistry.org.

**Administration:** Oral route. Swallow caps whole; do not chew. **Storage:** Cap: 15-25°C (59-77°F). Sol: Below 30°C (86°F).

# DEPAKOTE — RX

divalproex sodium (Abbott)

**Fatal hepatic failure may occur, especially in children <2 yrs on multiple anticonvulsants, with congenital metabolic disorders, severe seizure disorders with mental retardation, and organic brain disease. Hepatotoxicity may be preceded by nonspecific symptoms such as malaise, weakness, lethargy, facial edema, anorexia, and vomiting, or loss of seizure control in patients with epilepsy. Monitor LFTs prior to therapy, frequently during 1st 6 months of treatment and at frequent intervals thereafter. Teratogenic effects (eg, neural tube defects), and life-threatening pancreatitis reported; d/c if pancreatitis diagnosed and initiate appropriate treatment.**

**OTHER BRAND NAMES:** Depakote Sprinkle Capsules (Abbott)

**THERAPEUTIC CLASS:** Valproate compound

**INDICATIONS:** (Tab, Cap) Management of simple and complex absence seizures, complex partial seizures, and adjunctively with multiple seizure types including absence seizures. (Tab) Treatment of mania associated with bipolar disorder and migraine prophylaxis.

**DOSAGE:** *Adults:* (Cap/Tab) Complex Partial Seizures: Initial: 10-15mg/kg/day. Titrate: Increase by 5-10mg/kg/week. Max: 60mg/kg/day. Absence Seizures: Initial: 15mg/kg/day. Titrate: Increase weekly by 5-10mg/kg/day. Max: 60mg/kg/day. Give in divided doses if >250mg/day. Sprinkle capsules may be swallowed whole or contents may be sprinkled on soft food. Drug food mixture should be swallowed immediately; avoid chewing. (Tab) Migraine: Initial: 250mg bid. Max: 1000mg/day. Mania: 750mg daily in divided doses. Titrate: Increase dose rapidly to clinical effect. Max: 60mg/kg/day. Elderly: Reduce initial dose and titrate slowly. Decrease dose or d/c if decreased food or fluid intake or if excessive somnolence occurs.

*Pediatrics:* ≥16 yrs: (Tab) Migraine: Initial: 250mg bid. Max: 1000mg/day. ≥10 yrs: (Cap/Tab) Complex Partial Seizures: Initial: 10-15mg/kg/day. Titrate: Increase by 5-10mg/kg/week. Max: 60mg/kg/day. Absence Seizures: Initial: 15mg/kg/day. Titrate: Increase weekly by 5-10mg/kg/day. Max: 60mg/kg/day. Give in divided doses if >250mg/day. Sprinkle capsules may be swallowed whole or contents may be sprinkled on soft food. Drug food mixture should be swallowed immediately; avoid chewing.

**HOW SUPPLIED:** Cap, Delayed-Release: (Sprinkle) 125mg; Tab, Delayed-Release: 125mg, 250mg, 500mg

**CONTRAINDICATIONS:** Hepatic disease, significant hepatic dysfunction, known urea cycle disorders (UCD).

**WARNINGS/PRECAUTIONS:** Increased risk of suicidal thoughts or behavior; monitor for the emergence of worsening, and/or any unusual changes in mood or behavior. Hyperammonemic encephalopathy in UCD patients; d/c if this occurs. Prior to therapy, evaluate for UCD in high-risk patients (eg, history of unexplained encephalopathy, coma, etc). If unexplained lethargy, vomiting, or mental status changes occur, measure ammonia levels. Caution with hepatic disease; d/c if significant hepatic dysfunction suspected or apparent. Caution in the elderly; monitor fluid/nutritional intake, dehydration, and somnolence. Dose-related thrombocytopenia and elevated liver enzymes reported. Monitor platelet and coagulation tests prior to therapy, then periodically. Altered thyroid function tests and urine ketone tests. May stimulate replication of HIV and CMV. Avoid abrupt d/c. Multi-organ hypersensitivity reactions and hypothermia reported.

**ADVERSE REACTIONS:** Diarrhea, N/V, somnolence, dyspepsia, thrombocytopenia, asthenia, abdominal pain, tremor, headache, anorexia, diplopia, blurred vision, dizziness, weight gain, rash.

**INTERACTIONS:** Drugs that affect the level of expression of hepatic enzymes (eg, phenytoin, carbamazepine, phenobarbital, primidone) may increase valproate clearance. Concomitant use with ASA decreases protein binding and metabolism of valproate. Carbapenem antibiotics (eg, ertapenem, imipenem, meropenem) may reduce serum valproic concentration to subtherapeutic levels, resulting in loss of seizure control. Rifampin increases oral clearance and may requre valproate dosage adjustment. Concomitant use with felbamate leads to an increase in valproate $C_{max}$. Reduces the clearance of amitriptyline, nortriptyline, and lorazepam. Induces metabolism of carbamazepine. Inhibits metabolism of diazepam, ethosuximide, phenobarbital and phenytoin; monitor drug serum concentrations and adjust dose appropriately. Breakthrough seizures reported with concomitant valproate and phenytoin use. Administration with clonazepam may induce absence status in patients with absence seizures. Increases $T_{1/2}$ of lamotrigine; serious skin reactions reported. Concomitant use with topiramate associated with hyperammonemia, with or without encephalopathy, and hypothermia. May displace protein-bound warfarin; monitor coagulation tests. Additive CNS depression with other CNS depressants (eg, alcohol). May decrease clearance of zidovudine in HIV-seropositive patients.

**PREGNANCY:** Category D, not for use in nursing.

**MECHANISM OF ACTION:** Anticonvulsant; has not been established. Proposed to increases GABA concentrations in the brain.

**PHARMACOKINETICS: Absorption:** $T_{max}$=4-8 hrs (tab); $T_{max}$=3.3-4.8 hrs (cap). **Distribution:** Plasma protein binding (10%-18.5%). Found in breast milk. **Metabolism:** Liver; glucuronidation, mitochondrial β-oxidation. **Elimination:** Urine (<3% unchanged); $T_{1/2}$=9-16 hrs.

## NURSING CONSIDERATIONS

**Assessment:** Assess LFTs, CBC with platelets, pancreatitis, plasma ammonia levels, pregnancy status. Note other diseases/conditions and drug therapies.

**Monitoring:** Monitor LFTs, CBC with platelets, coagulation parameters, pancreatitis, hypersensitivity reactions, hyperammonemia, thyroid function tests.

**Patient Counseling:** Counsel to avoid alcohol, sedatives, OTC agents. Advise not to engage in hazardous activities (eg, driving/operating machinery). Counsel about signs/symptoms of pancreatitis, hepatotoxicity, hyperammonemia; notify physician if any symptoms or adverse effects occur. Instruct that a fever associated with other organ system involvement (eg, rash, lymphadenopathy, etc.) may be drug-related and should be reported to physician immediately. Notify physician if suicidal thoughts, behavior, or thoughts about self-harm emerge. Notify physician if pregnant or intend to become pregnant. Encourage patients to enroll in North American Antiepileptic

Drug (NAAED) Pregnancy Registry by calling 888-233-2334 or go to www.aedpregnancyregistry.org.

**Administration:** Oral route. **Storage:** Store below 30°C (86°F).

## DEPAKOTE ER RX

divalproex sodium (Abbott)



**Fatal hepatic failure may occur, especially in children <2 yrs on multiple anticonvulsants, with congenital metabolic disorders, severe seizure disorders with mental retardation, and organic brain disease. Hepatotoxicity may be preceded by nonspecific symptoms such as malaise, weakness, lethargy, facial edema, anorexia, and vomiting, or loss of seizure control in patients with epilepsy. Monitor LFTs prior to therapy, frequently during 1st 6 months of treatment and at frequent intervals thereafter. Teratogenic effects (eg, neural tube defects), and life-threatening pancreatitis reported; d/c if pancreatitis diagnosed and initiate appropriate treatment.**

**THERAPEUTIC CLASS:** Valproate compound

**INDICATIONS:** Migraine prophylaxis. Acute manic or mixed episodes associated with bipolar disorder. In adults and children ≥10 years, monotherapy and adjunctive therapy of complex partial seizures, and simple and complex absence seizures; an adjunct for multiple seizure types that include absence seizures.

**DOSAGE:** *Adults:* Migraine: Initial: 500mg qd for 1 week. Titrate: Increase to 1000mg qd. Max: 1000mg/day. Mania: Initial: 25mg/kg/day given qd. Titrate: Increase dose rapidly to achieve clinical effect. Max: 60mg/kg/day. Complex Partial Seizures: Monotherapy/Conversion to Monotherapy/Adjunctive Therapy: Initial: 10-15mg/kg/day. Titrate: Increase weekly by 5-10mg/kg/day until optimal response. Max: 60mg/kg/day. When converting to monotherapy, reduce concomitant antiepilepsy drug by 25% every 2 weeks starting at initiation or delay 1-2 weeks after start of therapy. Simple/Complex Absence Seizures: Initial: 15mg/kg/day. Titrate: Increase weekly by 5-10mg/kg/day until optimal response. Max: 60mg/kg/day. Conversion from Depakote: Administer dose 8-20% higher than total daily dose of Depakote. Refer to PI for dose conversion. If dose cannot be directly converted, consider increasing to next higher Depakote total daily dose before converting to appropriate total daily Depakote ER dose. Elderly: Reduce initial dose and titrate slowly. Decrease dose or d/c if decreased food or fluid intake or if excessive somnolence occurs. Swallow whole; do not crush or chew.
*Pediatrics:* ≥10yrs: Complex Partial Seizures: Monotherapy/Conversion to Monotherapy/Adjunctive Therapy: Initial: 10-15mg/kg/day. Titrate: Increase weekly by 5-10mg/kg/day until optimal response. Max: 60mg/kg/day. When converting to monotherapy, reduce concomitant antiepilepsy drug by 25% every 2 weeks starting at initiation or delay 1-2 weeks after start of therapy. Simple/Complex Absence Seizures: Initial: 15mg/kg/day. Titrate: Increase weekly by 5-10mg/kg/day until optimal response. Max: 60mg/kg/day. Conversion from Depakote: Administer dose 8-20% higher than total daily dose of Depakote. Refer to PI for dose conversion. If dose cannot be directly converted, consider increasing to next higher Depakote total daily dose before converting to appropriate total daily Depakote ER dose. Swallow whole; do not crush or chew.

**HOW SUPPLIED:** Tab, Extended-Release: 250mg, 500mg

**CONTRAINDICATIONS:** Hepatic disease, significant hepatic dysfunction, known urea cycle disorders (UCD).

**WARNINGS/PRECAUTIONS:** Increased risk of suicidal thoughts or behavior; monitor for the emergence of worsening, and/or any unusual changes in mood or behavior. Hyperammonemic encephalopathy in UCD patients; d/c if this occurs. Prior to therapy, evaluate for UCD in high-risk patients (eg, history of unexplained encephalopathy, coma, etc). If unexplained lethargy, vomiting, or mental status changes occur measure ammonia levels. Caution with hepatic disease; d/c if hepatic dysfunction suspected or apparent. Caution in the elderly; monitor fluid/nutritional intake, and for dehydration and somnolence. Dose-related thrombocytopenia and elevated liver enzymes reported. Monitor platelet and coagulation tests prior to therapy, then periodically. Altered thyroid function tests and urine ketone tests. May stimulate replication of HIV and CMV. Avoid abrupt d/c. Multi-organ hypersensitivity reactions and hypothermia reported. Developmental delay, autism and/or autism spectrum disorder in offspring of women exposed to valproate during pregnancy reported.



**ADVERSE REACTIONS:** N/V, dyspepsia, diarrhea, abdominal pain, asthenia, somnolence, headache, fever, anorexia, infection, dizziness, tremor, flu syndrome, alopecia.

**INTERACTIONS:** Drugs that affect the level of expression of hepatic enzymes (eg, phenytoin, carbamazepine, phenobarbital, primidone) may increase valproate clearance. Concomitant use with ASA decreases protein binding and metabolism. Carbapenem antibiotics (eg, ertapenem, imipenem, meropenem) may reduce serum concentration to subtherapeutic levels, resulting in loss of seizure control. Rifampin increases oral clearance and may require valproate dosage adjustment. Concomitant use with felbamate leads to an increase in valproate $C_{max}$. Reduces the clearance of amitriptylline, nortriptyline, and lorazepam. Induces metabolism of carbamazepine. Inhibits metabolism of diazepam, ethosuximide, phenobarbital and phenytoin; monitor drug serum concentrations and adjust dose appropriately. Breakthrough seizures reported with concomitant valproate and phenytoin use. Administration with clonazepam may induce absence status in patients with absence seizures. Increases $T_{1/2}$ of lamotrigine; serious skin reactions reported. Concomitant use with topiramate associated with hyperammonemia, with or without encephalopathy, and hypothermia. May displace protein-bound warfarin; monitor coagulation tests. Additive CNS depression with other CNS depressants (eg, alcohol). May decrease clearance of zidovudine in HIV-seropositive patients.

**PREGNANCY:** Category D, not for use in nursing.

**MECHANISM OF ACTION:** Anticonvulsant; has not been established. Proposed to increase GABA concentrations in the brain.

**PHARMACOKINETICS: Absorption:** Bioavailability (90%); $T_{max}$=4-17 hrs. **Distribution:** Plasma protein binding (10-18.5%). Found in breast milk, CSF. **Metabolism:** Liver; glucuronidation, mitochondrial β-oxidation. **Elimination:** Urine (<3% unchanged); $T_{1/2}$=9-16 hrs.

## NURSING CONSIDERATIONS

**Assessment:** Assess LFTs, CBC with platelets, pancreatitis, plasma ammonia levels, pregnancy status. Note other diseases/conditions and drug therapies.

**Monitoring:** Monitor LFTs, CBC with platelets, coagulation parameters, pancreatitis, hypersensitivity reactions, hyperammonemia, thyroid function tests. Monitor for emergence/worsening of depression, suicidality, unusual changes in behavior.

**Patient Counseling:** Counsel to avoid alcohol, sedatives, OTCs. Advise not to engage in hazardous activities (eg, driving/operating machinery). Counsel about signs/symptoms of pancreatitis, hepatotoxicity, hyperammonemia; notify physician if any symptoms or adverse effects occur. Instruct that a fever associated with other organ system involvement (eg, rash, lymphadenopathy, etc.) may be drug-related and should be reported to physician immediately. Notify physician if suicidal thoughts, behavior, or thoughts about self-harm emerge. Inform to take as prescribed and if dose is missed take as soon as possible; do not skip or double the dose. Notify physician if pregnant or intend to become pregnant. Encourage patients to enroll in North American Antiepileptic Drug (NAAED) Pregnancy Registry by calling 888-233-2334 or go to aedpregnancyregistry.org

**Administration:** Oral route. **Storage:** 25°C (77°F); excursions permitted to 15-30°C (59-86°F).

# DEPO-ESTRADIOL RX

estradiol cypionate (Pharmacia & Upjohn)

D

**Estrogens increase the risk of endometrial cancer. Estrogens, with or without progestins, should not be used for the prevention of cardiovascular disease or dementia. Increased risks of MI, stroke, invasive breast cancer, PE, and DVT in postmenopausal women (50-79 yrs of age) reported. Increased risk of developing probable dementia in postmenopausal women ≥65 yrs of age reported.**

**THERAPEUTIC CLASS:** Estrogen

**INDICATIONS:** Treatment of moderate to severe vasomotor symptoms associated with menopause and hypoestrogenism due to hypogonadism.

**DOSAGE:** *Adults:* Vasomotor Symptoms/Vaginal/Vulval Atrophy: 1-5mg IM every 3-4 weeks cyclically. Discontinue or taper at 3-6 month intervals. Hypoestrogenism: 1.5-2mg IM every month.

**HOW SUPPLIED:** Inj: 5mg/mL

**CONTRAINDICATIONS:** Pregnancy, undiagnosed abnormal genital bleeding, breast cancer, estrogen-dependent neoplasia, DVT/PE, active or recent (eg, within past year) arterial thromboembolic disease (eg, stroke, MI), liver dysfunction or disease.

**WARNINGS/PRECAUTIONS:** May increase risk of cardiovascular events (eg, MI, stroke), venous thrombosis, and PE; d/c immediately if any of these events occur or are suspected. May increase risk of breast/endometrial cancer, and gallbladder disease. May lead to severe hypercalcemia with breast cancer and bone metastases; monitor and d/c if hypercalcemia occurs. Retinal vascular thrombosis reported; monitor and d/c if papilledema or retinal vascular lesions occur. Consider addition of a progestin if no hysterectomy. May elevate BP; monitor at regular intervals. May cause elevations of plasma triglycerides with pre-existing hypertriglyceridemia. Caution with history of cholestatic jaundice associated with past estrogen use or with pregnancy; d/c with recurrence. May lead to increased thyroid-binding globulin levels; monitor thyroid function. May cause fluid retention; caution with cardiac/renal dysfunction. Caution with severe hypocalcemia. May increase risk of ovarian cancer. May exacerbate endometriosis, asthma, DM, epilepsy, migraine, porphyria, SLE, and hepatic hemangiomas; use with caution.

**ADVERSE REACTIONS:** Changes in vaginal bleeding pattern, breakthrough bleeding, vaginal candidiasis, breast tenderness/enlargement, NV, abdominal cramps, headache, migraine, dizziness, increase/decrease in weight.

**INTERACTIONS:** CYP3A4 inducers (eg, St. John's wort, phenobarbital, carbamazepine, rifampin) may decrease levels which may decrease therapeutic effects and/or change uterine bleeding profile. CYP3A4 inhibitors (eg, erythromycin, clarithromycin, ketoconazole, itraconazole, ritonavir, grapefruit juice) may increase levels which may result in side effects.

**PREGNANCY:** Contraindicated in pregnancy, caution in nursing.

**MECHANISM OF ACTION:** Estrogen; binds to nuclear receptors in estrogen-responsive tissues. Modulates pituitary secretion of gonadotropins, luteinizing hormone (LH) and follicle stimulating hormone (FSH), through negative feedback mechanism.

**PHARMACOKINETICS: Absorption:** Slow. **Distribution:** Wide; bound to sex hormone-binding globulin and albumin; found in breast milk. **Metabolism:** Liver via CYP3A4 (partial); estrone (active metabolite); estriol (major urinary metabolite); enterohepatic recirculation via sulfate and glucuronide conjugation. **Elimination:** Urine (estradiol, estrone, estriol, conjugates).

## NURSING CONSIDERATIONS

**Assessment:** Assess for abnormal genital bleeding, breast cancer, estrogen-dependent neoplasia, presence or history of DVT or PE, active or recent (within past yr) arterial thromboembolic disease (eg, stroke, MI), liver dysfunction/disease, known/suspected pregnancy. Assess use in patients undergoing surgeries associated with risk of thromboembolism, prolonged immobilization, presence of hypocalcemia, asthma, DM, epilepsy, migraines or porphyria,

SLE, presence of hepatic hemangiomas, nursing status, and in patients ≥65 yrs old. Assess for possible drug/lab test interactions.

**Monitoring:** Monitor for signs/symptoms of cardiovascular disorders (eg, MI, stroke), venous thrombosis, PE, malignant neoplasms (eg, endometrial, breast, ovarian cancer), dementia, gallbladder disease, hypercalcemia, visual abnormalities (eg, retinal vascular thrombosis), cholestatic jaundice, elevated BP, hypertriglyceridemia, hypothyroidism, fluid retention, exacerbation of endometriosis and other conditions (eg, asthma, DM, epilepsy, migraines or porphyria, SLE, and hepatic hemangiomas). Perform periodic BP monitoring. Monitor thyroid function in patients on thyroid replacement therapy. Perform annual breast exams. Perform periodic assessment (every 3-6 months) to determine therapy need. If abnormal genital bleeding occurs, perform proper diagnostic measures (eg, endometrial sampling) to rule out malignancies.

**Patient Counseling:** Inform that drug increases risk of uterine and breast cancer, heart attack, stroke, and blood clots. Advise to report breast lumps, unusual vaginal bleeding, dizziness or faintness, changes in speech, severe headaches, chest pain, SOB, leg pains, changes in vision, or vomiting. Instruct to perform monthly self breast exams.

**Administration:** IM route. **Storage:** 20-25°C (68-77°F).

## DEPO-MEDROL RX

methylprednisolone acetate (Pharmacia & Upjohn)

**THERAPEUTIC CLASS:** Glucocorticoid

**INDICATIONS:** Steroid-responsive disorders.

**DOSAGE:** *Adults:* Local Effect: Rheumatoid/Osteoarthritis: Large Joint: 20-80mg. Medium Joint: 10-40mg. Small Joint: 4-10mg. Administer intra-articularly into synovial space every 1-5 weeks or more depending on relief. Ganglion/Tendinitis/Epicondylitis: 4-30mg into cyst/area of greatest tenderness. May repeat if necessary. Dermatologic Conditions: Inject 20-60mg into lesion. Distribute 20-40mg doses by repeated injections into large lesions. Usual: 1-4 injections. Systemic Effect: Substitute for Oral Therapy: IM dose should equal total daily PO methylprednisolone dose q24h. Prolonged Therapy: Administer weekly PO dose as single IM injection. Androgenital Syndrome: 40mg IM every 2 weeks. Rheumatoid Arthritis: 40-120mg IM weekly. Dermatologic Lesions: 40-120mg IM weekly for 1-4 weeks. Acute Severe Dermatitis (Poison Ivy): 80-120mg IM single dose. Chronic Contact Dermatitis: May repeat injections every 5-10 days. Seborrheic Dermatitis: 80mg IM weekly. Multiple Sclerosis: 200mg/day prednisolone for 1 week, then 80mg every other day for 1 month (4mg methylprednisolone=5mg prednisolone). Asthma/Allergic Rhinitis: 80-120mg IM.
*Pediatrics:* Use lower adult doses. Determine dose by severity of condition and response.

**HOW SUPPLIED:** Inj: 20mg/mL, 40mg/mL, 80mg/mL

**CONTRAINDICATIONS:** Intrathecal administration, systemic fungal infections.

**WARNINGS/PRECAUTIONS:** Contains benzyl alcohol. Avoid contamination of multidose use of vials unless aseptic technique is observed. Injection may result in dermal/subdermal changes forming depressions in the skin at the injection site; do not exceed recommended doses. Avoid deltoid muscle injection. Anaphylactoid reactions reported. Do not use to treat traumatic brain injury. May cause elevation of BP, salt and water retention, and increased excretion of potassium; dietary salt restriction and potassium supplementation may be necessary. Caution with recent myocardial infarction. Hypothalamic-pituitary adrenal (HPA) axis suppression, Cushing's syndrome, and hyperglycemia reported; monitor prolonged use. Patients may be more susceptible to infections with any pathogen (viral, fungal, protozoan, or helminthic) when used alone or in combination with other immunosuppressive agents. May exacerbate systemic fungal infections. Latent disease due to certain pathogens may be activated or intercurrent infections exacerbated. Assess for latent or active amebiasis prior to therapy. Caution with known or suspected *Stronglyoides*, hypertension (HTN), congestive heart failure (CHF), renal insufficiency, active ocular herpes simplex, active or latent peptic ulcer, diverticulitis, fresh intestinal anastomoses, and non-specific ulcerative colitis. Chickenpox and measles may have more serious or fatal course in pediatric and adult patients. Metabolic clearance is decreased in hypothyroidism and increased in hyperthyroidism. Avoid injection into an infected site or a previously infected joint. May decrease bone formation and increase bone resorption. Acute myopathy reported with high doses. May elevate creatine kinase levels. Psychic derangements may appear during therapy (eg, euphoria, insomnia, mood swings, personality changes, and severe depression to frank psychotic manifestations).

D

**ADVERSE REACTIONS:** Anaphylactoid reaction, bradycardia, cardiac arrhythmias, cardiac enlargement, acne, erythema, sodium retention, abdominal distention, decreased carbohydrate and glucose tolerance, glycosuria, hirsutism, fluid retention, convulsions, depression.

**INTERACTIONS:** Cardiac enlargement and CHF reported when co-administered with amphotericin B. Macrolide antibiotics decrease clearance. Anticholinesterase agents should be withdrawn at least 24 hrs before initiating therapy. Serum concentrations of isoniazid may be decreased. Cholestyramine may increase clearance. Co-administration of digitalis glycosides increases risk of arrhythmias due to hypokalemia. Estrogens (eg, oral contraceptives) may decrease hepatic metabolism leading to increased effects. Hepatic enzyme inducers (eg, barbiturates, phenytoin, carbamazepine, and rifampin) enhance metabolism. Concomitant use with NSAIDs increases risks of GI side effects. The clearance of salicylates may be increased. Effects on oral anticoagulants are variable; monitor PT. Antidiabetic agents may require dosage adjustment. Patients on prolonged therapy may exhibit dimished response to vaccines; administration of vaccines should be deferred until therapy is discontinued. Mutual inhibition of metabolism with cyclosporine; convulsions reported. Ketoconazole decreases metabolism leading to increased risk of side effects.

**PREGNANCY:** Category C, not for use in nursing.

**MECHANISM OF ACTION:** Anti-inflammatory glucocorticoid; causes profound and varied metabolic effects and modifies the body's immune responses to diverse stimuli.

**PHARMACOKINETICS: Absorption:** $C_{max}$=11.8ng/mL; AUC=1286ng•hr/mL. **Elimination:** 139 hrs.

## NURSING CONSIDERATIONS

**Assessment:** Assess systemic fungal infections, current infections, active TB, vaccination history, ulcerative colitis, diverticulitis, peptic ulcer with impending perforation, renal/hepatic insufficiency, septic arthritis/unstable joint, HTN, osteoporosis, myasthenia gravis, thyroid status, psychotic tendencies, and possible drug interactions.

**Monitoring:** Monitor for adrenocortical insufficiency, occurrence of infections, psychic derangement, cataracts, acute myopathy, Kaposi's sarcoma, fluid retention, measurement of serum electrolytes, TSH, LFTs, IOP, and BP. Monitor urinalysis, blood sugar, weight, chest X-ray, and upper GI X-ray (if ulcer history) regularly during prolonged therapy.

**Patient Counseling:** Inform that susceptibility to infections may increase. Avoid exposure to chickenpox and measles; report immediately if exposed.

**Administration:** IM, intrasynovial, or intralesional. **Storage:** 20-25°C (68-77°F).

# DEPO-PROVERA — RX

medroxyprogesterone acetate (Pharmacia & Upjohn)

**THERAPEUTIC CLASS:** Progestogen

**INDICATIONS:** Adjunct and palliative treatment of inoperable, recurrent, and metastatic endometrial or renal carcinoma.

**DOSAGE:** *Adults:* Initial: 400-1000mg IM weekly. Maint: 400mg/month if disease stabilizes and/or improves within a few weeks or months.

**HOW SUPPLIED:** Inj: 400mg/mL [2.5mL]

**CONTRAINDICATIONS:** Pregnancy, undiagnosed vaginal bleeding, breast malignancy, thrombophlebitis, thromboembolic disorders, cerebral vascular disease, liver dysfunction.

**WARNINGS/PRECAUTIONS:** Avoid during first 4 months of pregnancy; risk of genital abnormalities in fetuses with exposure. May cause thromboembolic disorders, ocular disorders, fluid retention. Caution with history of depression; d/c if depression recurs to serious degree. Caution with family history of breast cancer or patients with breast nodules. Annual physical exam for all patients, with attention to BP, breasts, abdomen and pelvic organs. May mask the onset of climacteric.

**ADVERSE REACTIONS:** Menstrual irregularities, nervousness, dizziness, edema, weight and cervical changes, cholestatic jaundice, breast tenderness, galactorrhea, rash, acne, alopecia, hirsutism, depression, pyrexia, fatigue, insomnia, nausea.

**INTERACTIONS:** Aminoglutethimide may decrease serum levels.

**PREGNANCY:** Not recommended in pregnancy, caution in nursing.

## NURSING CONSIDERATIONS

**Assessment:** Physical exam of BP, breast, abdominal, pelvic exam, including cervical cytology and relevant lab tests should be done, with assessment of pregnancy status, vaginal bleeding, breast cancer, thromboembolic disorders/active thrombophlebitis and/or cerebrovascular disease, drug hypersensitivity, DM, mental depression, hepatic/renal impairment, and possible drug/lab test interactions.

**Monitoring:** Monitor for amenorrhea, menstrual irregularity, breast cancer risk, manifestations of thrombotic disorders (eg, thrombophlebitis, PE, cerebrovascular disorders, retinal thrombosis), ocular disorders (eg, partial/complete vision loss, proptosis, diplopia, migraine), anaphylaxis/anaphylactoid reaction, manifestations of fluid retentions, epilepsy, abdominal pain, weight changes. Lab monitoring of plasma/urinary steroid levels, gonadotropin level, sex hormone-binding globulin level, LFTs, glucose, lipid profile, and coagulation tests.

**Patient Counseling:** Counsel on risk/benefits. Notify if pregnant/nursing.

**Administration:** IM route. **Storage:** 20-25°C (68-77°F).

# DEPO-PROVERA CONTRACEPTIVE RX

medroxyprogesterone acetate (Pharmacia & Upjohn)

**May cause significant loss of bone mineral density (BMD); greater with increasing duration of use and may not be completely reversible. Should be used as long-term birth control (>2yrs) only if other birth control methods are inadequate. Unknown if use during adolescence or early adulthood will reduce peak bone mass and increase risk of osteoporotic fractures in later life.**

**THERAPEUTIC CLASS:** Progestogen

**INDICATIONS:** Prevention of pregnancy.

**DOSAGE:** *Adults:* 150mg IM every 3 months (13 weeks) in gluteal or deltoid muscle. Give 1st injection during 1st 5 days of menses; within 1st 5 days postpartum if not nursing; or 6 weeks postpartum if nursing.

**HOW SUPPLIED:** Inj: 150mg/mL

**CONTRAINDICATIONS:** Pregnancy, undiagnosed vaginal bleeding, breast malignancy, thrombophlebitis, thromboembolic disorders, cerebral vascular disease, liver dysfunction.

**WARNINGS/PRECAUTIONS:** Loss of BMD, may cause bleeding irregularities, cancer risk, thromboembolic disorders, ocular disorders, unexpected pregnancies, ectopic pregnancy, anaphylaxis and anaphylactoid reaction, fluid retention, return of fertility, decrease in glucose metabolism. Caution with CNS or convulsive disorders. D/C if jaundice develops.

**ADVERSE REACTIONS:** Menstrual irregularities, weight changes, abdominal pain, dizziness, headache, asthenia, nervousness, decreased libido, depression, nausea, insomnia, leukorrhea, acne, vaginitis, pelvic pain.

**INTERACTIONS:** Aminoglutethimide may decrease serum levels.

**PREGNANCY:** Category X, safety in nursing not known.

**MECHANISM OF ACTION:** Progestogen; inhibits secretion of gonadotropins, preventing follicular maturation and ovulation, resulting in endometrial thinning and producing a contraceptive effect.

**PHARMACOKINETICS: Absorption:** $C_{max}$=1-7ng/mL; $T_{max}$=3 weeks. **Distribution:** Found in breast milk. **Elimination**: $T_{1/2}$=50 days.

## NURSING CONSIDERATIONS

**Assessment:** Assess BP. Perform physical exam of breast, abdomen, pelvis, cervical cytology and relevant lab tests. Assess pregnancy status, vaginal bleeding, breast cancer, thromboembolic disorders, active thrombophlebitis and/or cerebrovascular disease, drug hypersensitivity, risk of osteoporosis (eg, metabolic bone disease, chronic alcohol or tobacco use, anorexia nervosa, strong family history of osteoporosis, and chronic use of anticonvulsants and/or corticosteroids), depression, DM, hepatic/renal impairment, CV disease, and possible drug/lab test interactions.

**Monitoring:** Monitor for amenorrhea, menstrual irregularity, breast cancer risk in women, manifestations of thrombotic disorders (eg, thrombophlebitis, PE, cerebrovascular disorders, and retinal thrombosis), ocular disorders (eg, partial/complete loss of vision, proptosis, diplopia, migraine), ectopic pregnancy, anaphylaxis/anaphylactoid reaction, manifestations of fluid retention, epilepsy, abdominal pain, weight changes, lab monitoring of bone minerals, densitometry for osteoporosis/osteoporotic fractures, plasma/urinary steroid levels, gonadotropin levels, sex hormone-binding globulin level, LFTs, glucose, lipid profile, and coagulation tests.

**Patient Counseling:** Counsel about risk/benefits of drug; inform drug does not protect against HIV infection and other STDs.

**Administration:** IM route. Gluteal or deltoid muscle; 1st injection must be given only during first 5 days of normal menstrual period or 5 days postpartum if not breast-feeding. If exclusively breast-feeding, give at 6th postpartum week. **Storage:** 20-25°C (68-77°F).

# DEPO-TESTOSTERONE

**CIII**

testosterone cypionate (Pharmacia & Upjohn)

**THERAPEUTIC CLASS:** Androgen

**INDICATIONS:** Testosterone replacement in males with primary hypogonadism and hypogonadotropic hypogonadism.

**DOSAGE:** *Adults:* Male Hypogonadism: 50-400mg IM every 2-4 weeks. Dose based on age, sex, and diagnosis. Adjust dose according to response and adverse reactions.
*Pediatrics:* ≥12 yrs: Male Hypogonadism: 50-400mg IM every 2-4 weeks. Dose based on age, sex, and diagnosis. Adjust dose according to response and adverse reactions.

**HOW SUPPLIED:** Inj: 100mg/mL, 200mg/mL

**CONTRAINDICATIONS:** Severe renal, hepatic and cardiac disease. Males with carcinoma of the breast or prostate gland. Pregnancy.

**WARNINGS/PRECAUTIONS:** May accelerate bone maturation without linear growth; monitor bone growth every 6 months. Risk of hepatic damage with long-term use. D/C if hypercalcemia occurs in immobilized patients. D/C with acute urethral obstruction, priapism, excessive sexual stimulation, or oligospermia; restart at lower doses. Risk of edema; caution with pre-existing cardiac, renal or hepatic disease. Caution in the elderly; increased risk of prostatic hypertrophy and prostatic carcinoma. Caution with BPH. Should not be used for enhancement of athletic performance. Do not administer IV. Monitor Hct, Hgb, cholesterol periodically.

**ADVERSE REACTIONS:** Gynecomastia, excessive frequency/duration of penile erections, male pattern baldness, increased/decreased libido, oligospermia, hirsutism, acne, fluid and electrolyte disturbances, nausea, hypercholesterolemia, clotting factor suppression, polycythemia, altered LFTs, priapism, anxiety, depression.



**INTERACTIONS:** May potentiate oral anticoagulants (eg, warfarin) and oxyphenbutazone. May decrease blood glucose and insulin requirements in diabetics.

**PREGNANCY:** Category X, not for use in nursing.

**MECHANISM OF ACTION:** Endogenous androgen; responsible for normal growth and development of male sex organs and for maintenance of secondary sex characteristics.

**PHARMACOKINETICS: Distribution:** Plasma protein binding (98%). **Elimination:** Urine (90%), feces (6%); $T_{1/2}$=8 days.

## NURSING CONSIDERATIONS

**Assessment:** Assess for known hypersensitivity to drug, males with carcinoma of the breast, males with known or suspected carcinoma of the prostate gland, hepatic/renal disease, delayed puberty, and benign prostatic hypertrophy.

**Monitoring:** Periodically monitor Hgb, Hct, LFTs, PSA, cholesterol and HDL, serum testosterone levels, serum calcium after initiation of therapy. Monitor for signs/symptoms of hypersensitivity reactions, edema with/without CHF, gynecomastia, prostatic hyperplasia/carcinoma, hepatocellular carcinoma. Assess bone development every 6 months in male adolescents.

**Patient Counseling:** Inform to contact physician if notice changes in body hair distribution, increase in acne, virilization, too frequent or persistent erections, changes in skin color, ankle swelling, unexplained NV, hypersensitivity reactions.

**Administration:** IM route, preferably gluteal muscle. **Storage:** Controlled temperature, 20-25°C (68-77°F). Protect from light.

# DESOGEN — RX

desogestrel - ethinyl estradiol (Organon)

**OTHER BRAND NAMES:** Apri (Barr)

**THERAPEUTIC CLASS:** Estrogen/progestogen combination

**INDICATIONS:** Prevention of pregnancy.

**DOSAGE:** *Adults:* Start 1st Sunday after onset of menstruation or 1st day of menstruation. 1 tab qd for 28 days continuously, then repeat.

**HOW SUPPLIED:** Tab: (Ethinyl Estradiol-Desogestrel) 0.03mg-0.15mg

**CONTRAINDICATIONS:** Thrombophlebitis, DVT or thromboembolic disorders, pregnancy, cerebrovascular or coronary artery disease (current or history), undiagnosed abnormal genital bleeding, cholestatic jaundice of pregnancy or jaundice with prior hormonal contraceptive use, hepatic adenomas or carcinomas, breast cancer or other estrogen-dependent neoplasia, valvular heart disease with thrombogenic complications, hepatic tumors (benign or malignant) or active liver disease, heavy smoking ( ≥ 15 cigarettes per day) and over age 35.

**WARNINGS/PRECAUTIONS:** Cigarette smoking increases risk of serious cardiovascular side effects. This risk increases with age (especially >35 yrs) and heavy smoking. Increased risk of MI, vascular disease, thromboembolism, stroke and gallbladder disease. Retinal thrombosis, hepatic neoplasia, carcinoma of breast and reproductive organs reported. May cause glucose intolerance. May increase BP, elevate LDL levels or cause other lipid changes, fluid retention, breakthrough bleeding, and spotting. May cause or exacerbate migraine. May develop visual changes with contact lenses. Increased risk of MI with HTN, hyperlipidemia, certain inherited or acquired thrombophilias, obesity, and diabetes. D/C if jaundice, significant depression or ophthalmic irregularities develop. Perform annual physical exam. Use before menarche is not indicated. May affect certain endocrine, LFTs and blood components. D/C if pregnancy is confirmed.

**ADVERSE REACTIONS:** NV, breakthrough bleeding, spotting, amenorrhea, migraine, mood changes including depression, vaginitis including candidiasis, edema, weight changes.

**INTERACTIONS:** Reduced effects, increased breakthrough bleeding, and menstrual irregularities with rifampin, barbiturates, phenylbutazone, phenytoin, and possibly with griseofulvin, ampicillin, and tetracyclines. Possible interaction with CYP2C9 substrates or inhibitors. St. John's wort may reduce the effectiveness of contraceptive steroids.

**PREGNANCY:** Category X, not for use in nursing.

**MECHANISM OF ACTION:** Estrogen/progestogen combination oral contraceptive; acts by suppression of gonadotropins. Also inhibits ovulation and causes changes in cervical mucus (increasing difficulty of sperm entry into uterus) and changes in endometrium (reducing likelihood of implantation) .

**PHARMACOKINETICS: Absorption:** Desogestrel: Rapid, complete; Etonogestrel: $C_{max}$=2805pg/mL (single dose), 5840pg/mL (multiple doses), $T_{max}$=1.4 hrs, AUC=33858pg/mL•hr (single dose), 52299pg/mL•hr (multiple doses). Ethinyl Estradiol: Rapid and complete, $C_{max}$=95pg/mL (single dose), 141pg/mL (multiple doses), $T_{max}$=1.5 hrs; AUC=1471pg/mL•hr (single dose), 1117pg/mL•hr (multiple doses). **Distribution:** Etonogestrel: Protein binding (98%). **Metabolism:** Desogestrel: Hepatic, hydroxylation in intestinal mucosa; CYP2C9, 3A4; Etonogestrel (major active metabolite). Ethinyl estradiol: Hepatic conjugation. **Elimination:** Urine, bile, feces. Desogestrel: $T_{1/2}$=38 hrs. Ethinyl Estradiol: $T_{1/2}$=26 hrs.

## NURSING CONSIDERATIONS

**Assessment:** Assess for current or history of thrombophlebitis or thromboembolic disorders, cerebral vascular disease, CAD, valvular heart disease with thrombogenic complications, severe HTN, DM with vascular involvement, headaches with focal neurological problems, recent major surgery with prolonged immobilization, known/suspected carcinoma of breast, endometrium or other known/suspected estrogen-dependent neoplasia, undiagnosed abnormal genital bleeding, cholestatic jaundice of pregnancy or jaundice with prior hormonal contraceptive use, hepatic tumors, active liver disease. Assess pregnancy status, use in patients >35 yrs old who smoke ≥15 cigarettes/day, and for possible drug interactions.

**Monitoring:** Monitor for venous and arterial thrombotic and thromboembolic events (eg, MI, thromboembolism, stroke), hepatic neoplasia, gallbladder disease, onset of headaches or migraines, HTN, fluid retention, ocular lesions, and bleeding irregularities. Refer patients with contact lenses to ophthalmologist if visual changes develop. Monitor serum glucose levels in DM and prediabetic patients, BP with history of HTN, lipid levels with history of hyperlipidemia. Monitor for signs/symptoms of liver dysfunction and worsening depression in patients with previous history.

**Patient Counseling:** Inform that drug does not protect against HIV infection and other STDs. Instruct not to smoke while using oral contraceptives. Advise to undergo annual physical exam while on medication. Inform may experience spotting or light bleeding, or may feel sick to stomach during first 1-3 packs of pill; advise this will usually subside and if not, to contact physician. Inform about pregnancy risk if pills are missed. Instruct to take same time every day. Instruct if one "active" pill is missed to take as soon as remembered; take next pill at regular time.

**Administration:** Oral route. **Storage:** 20-25°C (68-77°F).

## DesOwen — RX

desonide (Galderma)

D

**THERAPEUTIC CLASS:** Corticosteroid

**INDICATIONS:** Corticosteroid responsive dermatoses.

**DOSAGE:** *Adults:* Apply bid-tid, depending on severity. Reassess if no improvement after 2 weeks.

**HOW SUPPLIED:** Cre, Oint: 0.05% [15g, 60g]; Lot: 0.05% [60mL, 120mL]

**WARNINGS/PRECAUTIONS:** May produce reversible HPA axis suppression, manifestations of Cushing's syndrome, hyperglycemia, and glucosuria. D/C if irritation occurs. Use appropriate antifungal or antibacterial agent with dermatological infections. Peds may be more susceptible to systemic toxicity. Caution when applied to large surface areas. Avoid occlusive dressings.

**ADVERSE REACTIONS:** Stinging, burning, irritation, erythema, contact dermatitis, worsening condition, skin peeling, dryness/scaliness.

**PREGNANCY:** Category C, caution in nursing.

**MECHANISM OF ACTION:** Corticosteroid; possesses anti-inflammatory, antipruritic, and vasoconstrictive properties. Suspected to act by induction of phospholipase $A_2$ inhibitory proteins called lipocortins. Lipocortins control biosynthesis of potent mediators of inflammation (eg, prostaglandins, leukotrienes) by inhibiting the release of their common precursor, arachidonic acid.

**PHARMACOKINETICS: Absorption:** Extent of percutaneous absorption depends on skin integrity, vehicle, and use of occlusive dressings.

### NURSING CONSIDERATIONS

**Assessment:** Assess pregnancy/nursing status.

**Monitoring:** Monitor for signs/symptoms of reversible hypothalamic-pituitary-adrenal (HPA) axis suppression, Cushing's syndrome, hyperglycemia, and glucosuria. Following withdrawal of treatment, monitor for glucocorticosteroid insufficiency. In patients applying medication to a large surface area or using occlusive dressings, monitor for HPA-axis suppression through ACTH stimulation, AM plasma cortisol, and urinary free cortisol tests.

**Patient Counseling:** Instruct to use exactly as directed, externally, and to avoid contact with eyes. Instruct not to bandage, cover, or wrap treatment area so as to be occlusive, unless directed by physician. Counsel to report any local adverse reactions.

**Administration:** Topical. **Storage:** Lotion: 2-30°C (36-86°F). Ointment: Below 30°C (86°F), avoid freezing. Cream: 15-30°C (59-86°F).

## Desoxyn — CII

methamphetamine HCl (Ovation)

**High potential for abuse. Avoid prolonged therapy in obesity.**

**THERAPEUTIC CLASS:** Sympathomimetic amine

**INDICATIONS:** Attention deficit disorder with hyperactivity. Short-term adjunct to treat exogenous obesity.

**DOSAGE:** *Adults:* Obesity: 5mg, 1/2 hr before each meal. Do not exceed a few weeks of treatment.
*Pediatrics:* ADHD: ≥6 yrs: Initial: 5mg qd-bid. Titrate: Increase weekly by 5mg/day until optimum response. Usual: 20-25mg/day given bid. Obesity: ≥12 yrs: 5mg, 1/2 hr before each meal. Do not exceed a few weeks of treatment.

**HOW SUPPLIED:** Tab: 5mg

**CONTRAINDICATIONS:** Advanced arteriosclerosis, symptomatic cardiovascular disease, moderate to severe HTN, hyperthyroidism, glaucoma, agitated states, history of drug abuse, during or within 14 days of MAOI use.

**WARNINGS/PRECAUTIONS:** Tolerance to anorectic effect develops within a few weeks, do not exceed recommended dose to increase effect. Monitor growth in children. Caution with HTN. Do not use to combat fatigue or replace rest. Exacerbation of motor and phonic tics and Tourette's syndrome. May exacerbate behavior disturbance and thought disorder in psychotic pediatrics. Emergence of new psychotic symptoms may warrant d/c of therapy. Monitor for the appearance or worsening of aggressive behavior in children. Therapy may lower the convulsive threshold and cause blurred vision and difficulty with accommodation. Interrupt occasionally to determine if patient requires continued therapy. Misuse may cause sudden death and serious cardiovascular adverse events. Caution in patients with underlying cardiovascular conditions and comorbid bipolar disorder.

**ADVERSE REACTIONS:** BP elevation, tachycardia, palpitations, dizziness, insomnia, tremor, diarrhea, constipation, dry mouth, urticaria, impotence, changes in libido.

**INTERACTIONS:** May alter insulin requirements. May decrease hypotensive effect of guanethidine. Avoid MAOIs. Caution with TCAs and indirect acting sympathomimetic amines. Antagonized by phenothiazines.

**PREGNANCY:** Category C, not for use in nursing.

**MECHANISM OF ACTION:** Sympathomimetic amine; CNS stimulant. Peripheral actions involve elevation of BP, weak bronchodilation, and respiratory stimulant actions.

**PHARMACOKINETICS: Absorption:** Rapid. **Metabolism:** Liver; aromatic hydroxylation, N-dealkylation and deamination. **Elimination:** Urine (62%); $T_{1/2}$=4-5 hrs.

## NURSING CONSIDERATIONS

**Assessment:** Assess for agitation, glaucoma, tics, family history of Tourette's syndrome, cardiovascular conditions (eg, severe HTN, angina pectoris, cardiac arrhythmias, heart failure, recent MI), hyperthyroidism or thyrotoxicosis, bipolar illness, history of drug dependence or alcoholism.

**Monitoring:** Monitor for cardiac abnormalities, exacerbations of behavior disturbances and thought disorder, bipolar disorder, aggression, seizures, and visual disturbances. Height and weight follow-up in children.

**Patient Counseling:** Inform about risks of treatment, appropriate use, drug abuse/dependence. Caution while operating machinery/driving. Avoid late evening doses; insomnia may result.

**Administration:** Oral route. **Storage**: Store below 30°C (86°F). Protect from light.

# DETROL LA — RX

tolterodine tartrate (Pharmacia & Upjohn)

**OTHER BRAND NAMES:** Detrol (Pharmacia & Upjohn)

**THERAPEUTIC CLASS:** Muscarinic antagonist

**INDICATIONS:** Treatment of overactive bladder with symptoms of urinary frequency, urgency, or urge incontinence.

**DOSAGE:** *Adults:* (LA Cap) Usual: 4mg qd may lower to 2mg. (Tab) Initial: 2mg bid, may lower to 1mg bid. Titrate based on individual response and tolerability. Significant Hepatic/Renal Dysfunction/Concomitant Potent CYP3A4 Inhibitors: (Tab) 1mg bid, (LA Cap) 2mg qd.

**HOW SUPPLIED:** Cap, Extended-Release: 2mg, 4mg; Tab: 1mg, 2mg

**CONTRAINDICATIONS:** Urinary retention, gastric retention, uncontrolled narrow-angle glaucoma.

**WARNINGS/PRECAUTIONS:** Risk of urinary retention with clinically significant bladder outflow obstruction and risk of gastric retention with GI obstructive disorders. Caution with narrow-angle glaucoma, decreased GI motility (eg, intestinal atony), myasthenia gravis, known history of QT prolongation and hepatic/renal dysfunction. Not recommended in patients with severe hepatic impairment (Child-Pugh Class C) and CrCl <10mL/min.

**ADVERSE REACTIONS:** Dry mouth, dizziness, headache, abdominal pain, constipation, diarrhea, dyspepsia, fatigue, somnolence.

**INTERACTIONS:** May increase concentration with fluoxetine (potent CYP2D6 inhibitors) and ketoconazole (potent CYP3A4 inhibitor). Reduce dose with concomitant potent CYP3A4 inhibitors (eg, clarithromycin, ketoconazole, itraconazole, miconazole). May increase anticholinergic effects with concomitant anticholinergic agents. Caution with Class IA (eg, quinidine, procainamide) or Class III (eg, amiodarone, sotalol) antiarrhythmics and cholinesterase inhibitors.

D

**PREGNANCY:** Category C, not for use in nursing.

**MECHANISM OF ACTION:** Muscarinic receptor antagonist; competitive antagonist of acetylcholine at postganglionic muscarinic receptors mediating urinary bladder contraction and salivation.

**PHARMACOKINETICS: Absorption:** (Tab) Extensive metabolizers (EM): Multiple Dose: $C_{max}$=2.6mcg/L ; $T_{max}$=1.2 hrs; Single Dose: $C_{max}$=1.6mcg/L ; $T_{max}$=1.6 hrs. Poor metabolizers (PM): Multiple Dose: $C_{max}$=19mcg/L; $T_{max}$=1.9 hrs; Single Dose: $C_{max}$=10mcg/L; $T_{max}$=1.4 hrs.(Cap, Extended-Release) EM: Multiple Dose: $C_{max}$=3.4mcg/L; $T_{max}$=4 hrs; Single Dose: $C_{max}$=1.3mcg/L; $T_{max}$=4 hrs. PM: $C_{max}$=19mcg/L; $T_{max}$=4 hrs. **Distribution:** (IV) $V_d$=113L; high plasma protein binding. **Metabolism:** EM: CYP2D6 (oxidation); 5-hydroxymethyl (active metabolite). PM: CYP3A4 (dealkylation). **Elimination:** Urine (77% unchanged), feces (17% unchanged). (Tab) EM: $T_{1/2}$=2.2 hrs; PM: $T_{1/2}$=9.6 hrs. (Cap, Extended-Release) EM: $T_{1/2}$=6.9 hrs; PM: $T_{1/2}$=18 hrs.

## NURSING CONSIDERATIONS

**Assessment:** Assess for bladder outflow obstruction (urinary retention), GI obstructive disorder (gastric retention), narrow-angle glaucoma, myasthenia gravis, history of QT prolongation, hepatic/renal impairment, pregnancy/nursing status and possible drug interactions.

**Monitoring:** Monitor for signs/symptoms of urinary retention, gastric retention and hypersensitivity reactions. Monitor renal/hepatic function, QT prolongation and HR.

**Patient Counseling:** Inform may produce blurred vision, dizziness or drowsiness. Caution against potentially dangerous activities until drug effects have been determined. Notify physician if pregnant/nursing or planning to become pregnant. Do not change dose unless instructed by physician. Take capsule with water, tell your physician if difficulty swallowing. Can be taken with or without food. Do not take 2 doses at the same time. If miss a dose, take again the next day. Call your physician or poison control center if taken more than the prescribed dose.

**Administration:** Oral route. (Cap, extended release) Take with liquids and swallow whole. **Storage:** Tab: 25°C (77°F). Cap: 20-25°C (68-77°F); excursions permitted to 15-30°C (59-86°F). Protect from light.

# DEXAMETHASONE RX

dexamethasone (Various)

**THERAPEUTIC CLASS:** Glucocorticoid

**INDICATIONS:** (PO) Treatment of steroid-responsive disorders. (Inj) Treatment of steroid-responsive disorders when oral therapy not feasible.

**DOSAGE:** *Adults:* Individualize for disease and patient response. Withdraw gradually. (Tab) Initial: 0.75-9mg/day PO. Maint: Decrease in small amounts to lowest effective dose. Cushing's Syndrome Test: 1mg PO at 11pm; draw blood at 8am next morning. Or, 0.5mg PO q6h for 48 hrs; or 2mg (to distinguish if excess pituitary ACTH or other causes) PO q6h for 48 hrs; obtain 24-hr urine collections. (Inj) Initial: 0.5-9mg/day IV/IM. Cerebral Edema: Initial: 10mg IV, then 4mg IM q6h until edema subsides. Reduce dose after 2-4 days and gradually d/c over 5-7 days. Palliative Management of Recurrent/Inoperable

Brain Tumors: Maint: 2mg IV/PO bid-tid. Acute Allergic Disorders: 4-8mg IM on 1st day, then 1.5mg PO bid for 2 days, then 0.75mg PO bid for 1 day, then 0.75mg PO qd for 2 days. (Inj) Usual: 0.2-9mg. Maint: Decrease in small amounts to lowest effective dose. Intra-Articular/Intralesional/Soft Tissue Injection: Usual: 0.2-6mg once every 3-5 days to once every 2-3 weeks. See PI for Shock Treatment. Take tabs and oral Sol with meals and antacids to prevent peptic ulcer.

*Pediatrics:* Individualize for disease and patient response. Withdraw gradually. (Tab) Initial: 0.75-9mg/day PO. Maint: Decrease in small amounts to lowest effective dose. Cushing's Syndrome Test: 1mg PO at 11pm; draw blood at 8am next morning. Or, 0.5mg PO q6h for 48 hrs; or 2mg (to distinguish if excess pituitary ATCH or other causes) PO q6h for 48 hrs; obtain 24-hr urine collections. (Inj) Initial: 0.5-9mg/day IV/IM. Cerebral Edema: Initial: 10mg IV, then 4mg IM q6h until edema subsides. Reduce dose after 2-4 days and gradually d/c over 5-7 days. Palliative Management of Recurrent/Inoperable Brain Tumors: Maint: 2mg IV/PO bid-tid. Acute Allergic Disorders: 4-8mg IM on 1st day, then 1.5mg PO bid for 2 days, then 0.75mg PO bid for 1 day, then 0.75mg PO qd for 2 days. (Inj) Usual: 0.2-9mg. Maint: Decrease in small amounts to lowest effective dose. Intra-Articular/Intralesional/Soft Tissue Injection: Usual: 0.2-6mg once every 3-5 days to once every 2-3 weeks. See PI for shock treatment. Take tabs and oral Sol with meals and antacids to prevent peptic ulcer.

**HOW SUPPLIED:** Inj: (Dexamethasone Sodium Phosphate) 4mg/mL, 10mg/mL; Sol: (Dexamethasone) 0.5mg/5mL, 1mg/mL; Tab: (Dexamethasone) 0.5mg*, 0.75mg*, 1mg*, 1.5mg*, 2mg*, 4mg*, 6mg* *scored

**CONTRAINDICATIONS:** Systemic fungal infections.

**WARNINGS/PRECAUTIONS:** Increase dose before, during, and after stressful situations. Avoid abrupt withdrawal. May mask signs of infection, activate latent amebiasis, elevate BP, cause salt/water retention, increase excretion of potassium and calcium. Prolonged use may produce cataracts, glaucoma, secondary ocular infections. Caution with recent MI, ocular herpes simplex, emotional instability, nonspecific ulcerative colitis, diverticulitis, peptic ulcer, renal insufficiency, HTN, osteoporosis, myasthenia gravis, threadworm infection, active tuberculosis. Enhanced effect with hypothyroidism, cirrhosis. Consider prophylactic therapy if exposed to measles or chickenpox. Risk of glaucoma, cataracts, and eye infections. False negative dexamethasone suppression test with indomethacin.

**ADVERSE REACTIONS:** Fluid/electrolyte disturbances, muscle weakness, osteoporosis, peptic ulcer, pancreatitis, ulcerative esophagitis, impaired wound healing, headache, psychic disturbances, growth suppression (pediatrics), glaucoma, hyperglycemia, weight gain, nausea, malaise.

**INTERACTIONS:** Caution with ASA. Inducers of CYP3A4 (eg, phenytoin, phenobarbital, carbamazepine, rifampin) and ephedrine enhance clearance; increase steroid dose. Inhibitors of CYP3A4 (ketoconazole, macrolides) may increase plasma levels. Drugs that affect metabolism may interfere with dexamethasone suppression tests. Increased clearance of drugs metabolized by CYP3A4 (eg, indinavir, erythromycin). May increase or decrease phenytoin levels. Ketoconazole may inhibit adrenal corticosteroid synthesis and cause adrenal insufficiency during corticosteroid withdrawal. Antagonizes or potentiates coumarins. Hypokalemia with potassium-depleting diuretics. Live virus vaccines are contraindicated with immunosuppressive doses.

**PREGNANCY:** Category C, not for use in nursing.

**MECHANISM OF ACTION:** Adrenocortical steroid; produces anti-inflammatory effects.

**PHARMACOKINETICS: Distribution**: Found in breast milk. **Metabolism**: Liver; CYP3A4.

## NURSING CONSIDERATIONS

**Assessment:** Assess for hypersensitivity to drug, systemic fungal or current infections, active TB, vaccination, unusual stress, hypothyroidism, hepatic/renal impairment, ulcerative colitis, diverticulitis, peptic ulcer with/without impending perforation, fresh intestinal anastomoses, HTN, recent MI, osteoporosis, myasthenia gravis, unstable joints, septic arthritis, existing psychotic tendencies, and for possible drug interactions (eg, indomethacin).

**Monitoring:** Monitor for anaphylactoid reactions, appearance/exacerbation of infections, cataracts, fluid retention, psychic derangement. Monitor infants for hypoadrenalism and growth development. Monitor for fat embolism, adrenocortical insufficiency, LFTs, TSH, PT, glucose with IOP, BP, and ECG.



**Patient Counseling:** Inform that susceptibility to infection may increase. Avoid exposure to chickenpox or measles; report immediately if exposed. Advise to restrict dietary sodium and potassium supplements. Counsel not to overuse joint after intra-articular injection, and not to d/c abruptly without medical supervision.

**Administration:** Oral route. Parenteral: IM, IV, intra-articular, intralesional, and soft-tissue injection. **Storage:** Inj: 20-25°C (68-77°F); excursions permitted to 15-30°C (59-86°F).

## DEXEDRINE SPANSULES CII

dextroamphetamine sulfate (GlaxoSmithKline)

**High potential for abuse. Prolonged use may lead to drug dependence and must be avoided. Misuse may cause sudden death and serious cardiovascular adverse events.**

**THERAPEUTIC CLASS:** Sympathomimetic amine

**INDICATIONS:** Treatment of attention deficit disorder with hyperactivity (ADHD) and narcolepsy.

**DOSAGE:** *Adults:* Narcolepsy: Initial: 10mg/day. Titrate: May increase by 10mg/day at weekly intervals. Usual: 5-60mg/day in divided doses. May give once daily. Avoid late-evening doses.
*Pediatrics:* Narcolepsy: 6-12 yrs: Initial: 5mg qd. Titrate: May increase weekly by 5mg/day. ≥12 yrs: Initial: 10mg qd. Titrate: May increase by 10mg/day at weekly intervals. Usual: 5-60mg/day in divided doses. ADHD: ≥6 yrs: Initial: 5mg qd-bid. Titrate: May increase 5mg/day at weekly intervals. Max (usual): 40mg/day. May give once daily. Avoid late-evening doses.

**HOW SUPPLIED:** Cap, Sustained-Release: (Spansules) 5mg, 10mg, 15mg

**CONTRAINDICATIONS:** Advanced arteriosclerosis, symptomatic CV disease, moderate to severe hypertension (HTN), hyperthyroidism, glaucoma, agitated states, history of drug abuse, during or within 14 days of monoamine oxidase inhibitor (MAOI) use.

**WARNINGS/PRECAUTIONS:** Sudden death reported in children and adolescents with structural cardiac abnormalities or other serious heart problems. Sudden death, stroke, MI reported in adults. Avoid use with serious structural cardiac abnormalities, cardiomyopathy, serious heart rhythm abnormalities, CAD, or other serious cardiac problems. Caution with HTN. Prior to treatment, obtain a careful history and perform physical exam to assess for cardiac disease. May exacerbate symptoms of behavior disturbance and thought disorder in psychotic patients. May induce mixed/manic episode in patients with bipolar disorder. Use at usual doses can cause treatment-emergent psychotic or manic symptoms (eg, hallucinations, delusional thinking, mania) in children and adolescents without prior history of psychotic illness. Aggressive behavior or hostility reported in clinical trials and the postmarketing experience of some medications indicated for the treatment of ADHD. May cause long-term suppression of growth in children; monitor growth during treatment. D/C if seizures develop. Visual disturbances reported. May exacerbate motor and phonic tics and Tourette's syndrome.

**ADVERSE REACTIONS:** Palpitations, tachycardia, BP elevation, CNS overstimulation, restlessness, insomnia, dry mouth, GI disturbances, anorexia, urticaria, impotence.

**INTERACTIONS:** See Contraindications. GI acidifying agents (eg, guanethidine, reserpine, glutamic acid HCl, ascorbic acid, fruit juices) and urinary acidifying agents (eg, ammonium chloride, sodium acid, phosphate) decrease efficacy. Potentiated by GI alkalinizing agents (eg, sodium bicarbonate), urinary alkalinizing agents (eg, acetazolamide, some thiazides), and propoxyphene overdose. Urinary excretion of amphetamines is increased and efficacy is reduced by acidifying agents used in methenamine therapy. Potentiated effects of both agents with TCAs (eg, desipramine, protriptyline). May delay absorption of phenytoin, ethosuximide, phenobarbital. Potentiates meperidine, norepinephrine, phenobarbital, phenytoin. Antagonized by haloperidol, chlorpromazine, lithium. Antagonizes adrenergic blockers, antihistamines, antihypertensives, veratrum alkaloids (antihypertensive).



**PREGNANCY:** Category C, not for use in nursing.

**MECHANISM OF ACTION:** Amphetamine; noncatecholamine sympathomimetic amine with CNS stimulant activity. Peripheral actions include elevation of BP, weak bronchodilation, and respiratory stimulant actions.

**PHARMACOKINETICS: Absorption:** (15mg sustained release cap) $C_{max}$=23.5ng/mL, $T_{max}$=8 hrs. **Distribution:** Found in breast milk. **Elimination:** $T_{1/2}$=12 hrs.

## NURSING CONSIDERATIONS

**Assessment:** Assess for CV conditions (eg, advanced arteriosclerosis, moderate to severe HTN, cardiac structural abnormalities, cardiomyopthy, arrhythmias, heart failure, recent MI), hyperthyroidism, agitation, glaucoma, history of drug dependence or alcoholism, pre-existing psychosis, bipolar illness, prior history of seizures, pregnancy/nursing status, and for possible drug interactions. Assess for presence or family history of Tourette's syndrome.

**Monitoring:** Monitor for cardiac abnormalities, exacerbations of behavior disturbances and thought disorders, new psychotic or manic symptoms (eg, hallucinations, delusional thinking), aggression, seizures, and for visual disturbances. In children, perform periodic monitoring of height and weight. Monitor for signs/symptoms of mixed/manic episodes in patients with bipolar disorder.

**Patient Counseling:** Inform of benefits and risks of treatment. Advise on appropriate use of medication. Instruct that therapy may impair the ability to engage in potentially hazardous activities (eg, operating machinery or vehicles). Inform that late-evening doses should be avoided due to the risk of insomnia.

**Administration:** Oral route. **Storage:** 20-25°C (68-77°F). Dispense in a tight, light resistant container.

# DEXTROAMPHETAMINE SULFATE TABLET CII

dextroamphetamine sulfate (Shire)

**High potential for abuse. Avoid prolonged use.**

**THERAPEUTIC CLASS:** Sympathomimetic amine

**INDICATIONS:** Treatment of narcolepsy and attention deficit disorder with hyperactivity (ADHD).

**DOSAGE:** *Adults:* Narcolepsy: Initial: 10mg/day. Titrate: May increase by 10mg/day every week. Usual: 5-60mg/day. Give 1st dose upon awakening, and additional doses every 4-6 hrs.

*Pediatrics:* Narcolepsy: 6-12 yrs: Initial: 5mg/day. Titrate: Increase weekly by 5mg/day. ≥12 yrs: Initial: 10mg/day. Titrate: Increase weekly by 10mg/day. Usual: 5-60mg/day in divided doses. ADHD: 3-5 yrs: Initial: 2.5mg/day. Titrate: Increase weekly by 2.5mg/day until optimum response. 6-16 yrs: Initial 5mg qd-bid. Titrate: Increase weekly by 5mg/day until optimum response. Give 1st dose upon awakening, and additional doses q4-6h.

**HOW SUPPLIED:** Tab: 5mg*, 10mg* *scored

**CONTRAINDICATIONS:** Advanced arteriosclerosis, symptomatic cardiovascular disease, moderate to severe HTN, hyperthyroidism, glaucoma, agitated states, history of drug abuse, during or within 14 days of MAOI use.

**WARNINGS/PRECAUTIONS:** Caution in HTN. Contains tartrazine, may cause allergic reactions. Exacerbation of motor and phonic tics and Tourette's syndrome. May exacerbate behavior disturbance and thought disorder in psychotic pediatrics. Interrupt occasionally to determine if patient requires continued therapy. Monitor growth in children.

**ADVERSE REACTIONS:** BP elevation, tachycardia, palpitations, dizziness, insomnia, tremor, diarrhea, constipation, dry mouth, urticaria, impotence, changes in libido.

D

**INTERACTIONS:** GI acidifying agents (eg, guanethidine, reserpine, glutamic acid, etc.) and urinary acidifying agents (eg, ammonium chloride, etc.) decrease efficacy. MAOIs may cause hypertensive crisis. Potentiated by GI and urinary alkalinizers, propoxyphene overdose. Potentiated effects of both agents with TCAs. May delay absorption of phenytoin, ethosuximide, phenobarbital. Potentiates meperidine, norepinephrine, phenobarbital, phenytoin. Antagonized by haloperidol, chlorpromazine, lithium. Antagonizes adrenergic blockers, antihistamines, antihypertensives, veratrum alkaloids (antihypertensive).

**PREGNANCY:** Category C, not for use in nursing.

**MECHANISM OF ACTION:** Sympathomimetic amine; CNS stimulant activity. Peripheral actions involve elevation of BP, weak bronchodilation, and respiratory stimulant actions.

**PHARMACOKINETICS: Absorption:** $C_{max}$=29.2ng/mL, $T_{max}$=2 hrs. **Elimination:** Urine (45%); $T_{1/2}$=10.25 hrs.

## NURSING CONSIDERATIONS

**Assessment:** Assess for agitation, glaucoma, tics, family history of Tourette's syndrome, cardiovascular conditions (eg, severe HTN, angina pectoris, cardiac structural abnormalities, arrhythmias, HF, recent MI), hyperthyroidism or thyrotoxicosis, bipolar disorder, psychosis, history of drug dependence or alcoholism.

**Monitoring:** Monitor for cardiac abnormalities, exacerbations of behavior disturbances and thought disorder, bipolar disorder, aggression, seizures, and visual disturbances. Monitor growth in children.

**Patient Counseling:** Inform about risks of treatment, its appropriate use, drug abuse/dependence. Caution while operating machinery/driving. Avoid late evening doses to prevent insomnia.

**Administration:** Oral route. **Storage:** 25°C (77°F); excursions permitted to 15-30°C (59-86°F).

# DiaBeta — RX

glyburide (Sanofi-Aventis)

**THERAPEUTIC CLASS:** Sulfonylurea (2nd generation)

**INDICATIONS:** Adjunct to diet and exercise, to improve glycemic control in adults with type 2 diabetes mellitus (DM).

**DOSAGE:** *Adults:* Initial: 2.5-5mg qd with breakfast or first main meal; give 1.25mg if sensitive to hypoglycemia. Titrate: Increase by no more than 2.5mg/day at weekly intervals. Maint: 1.25-20mg given qd or in divided doses. May give bid with doses >10mg/day. Max: 20mg/day. Transfer From Other Oral Antidiabetic Agents: Initial: 2.5-5mg/day. Transfer From Maximum Dose of Other Sulfonylureas: Initial: 5mg qd. Switch From Insulin: If <20 U/day: 2.5-5mg qd. If 20-40 U/day: 5mg qd. If >40 U/day: Decrease insulin dose by 50% and give 5mg qd. Titrate: Progressive withdrawal of insulin and increase by 1.25-2.5mg/day every 2-10 days. Elderly/Debilitated/Malnourished/Renal or Hepatic Impairment/Adrenal or Pituitary Insufficiency: Initial: 1.25mg qd. Dose conservatively.

**HOW SUPPLIED:** Tab: 1.25mg*, 2.5mg*, 5mg* *scored

**CONTRAINDICATIONS:** Diabetic ketoacidosis with or without coma, treatment with bosentan.

**WARNINGS/PRECAUTIONS:** Increased risk of cardiovascular mortality. Risk of hypoglycemia, especially with renal and hepatic disease; elderly, debilitated, or malnourished patients; and those with adrenal or pituitary insufficiency.

May need to d/c and give insulin with stress (eg, fever, trauma). Secondary failure may occur. Hemolytic anemia may occur in patients with G6PD deficiency; caution during administration.

**ADVERSE REACTIONS:** Hypoglycemia, cholestatic jaundice, hepatitis, nausea, epigastric fullness, heartburn, allergic skin reactions (eg, pruritus, erythema, urticaria, morbilliform), disulfiram-like reactions (rarely), hyponatremia, LFT abnormalities, photosensitivity reactions, hematologic reactions (eg, leukopenia, agranulocytosis, thrombocytopenia), porphyria, cutanea tarda, and blurred vision.



**INTERACTIONS:** See Contraindications. Potentiate hypoglycemia with alcohol, NSAIDs, miconazole, fluoroquinolones, highly protein-bound drugs, salicylates, sulfonamides, chloramphenicol, probenecid, MAOIs, β-blockers, ACE inhibitors, disopyramide, fluoxetine, and clarithromycin. Risk of hyperglycemia and loss of glucose control with thiazides and other diuretics, corticosteroids, phenothiazines, thyroid products, estrogens, oral contraceptives, phenytoin, nicotinic acid, sympathomimetics, CCBs, and INH. Increased or decreased coumarin effects. Disulfiram-like reactions (rarely) with alcohol. Elevated liver enzymes reported with bosentan. May increase cyclosporine plasma levels and toxicity. May worsen glucose control with rifampin. β-blockers may mask signs of hyperglycemia.

**PREGNANCY:** Category C, not for use in nursing.

**MECHANISM OF ACTION:** Sulfonylurea; acts by stimulating the release of insulin from functioning β-cells in the pancreas.

**PHARMACOKINETICS: Absorption:** $T_{max}$=4 hrs. **Distribution:** Plasma protein binding (extensive). **Metabolism**: Hydroxylation. **Elimination:** Bile (50%), urine (50%); $T_{1/2}$=10 hrs.

## NURSING CONSIDERATIONS

**Assessment:** Assess for fasting blood glucose levels, glycosylated hemoglobin, type 1 DM, cardiovascular complications, hypoglycemia risk factors, renal/hepatic impairment, DM complications (eg, diabetic ketoacidosis), G6PD deficiency, pregnancy/nursing status, and possible drug interactions.

**Monitoring:** Monitor fasting blood glucose levels regularly and glycosylated hemoglobin periodically. Monitor GI, dermatologic, hematologic, metabolic, hypersensitivity reactions, and blurring of vision.

**Patient Counseling:** Stress importance of adherence to dietary instructions, regular exercise programs, and regular testing of blood glucose levels. Advise to take with breakfast or first meal. Inform patients for potential risks, advantages, and alternative modes of therapy. Counsel about the risks, symptoms, treatment, and conditions of hypoglycemia.

**Administration:** Oral route. **Storage:** 25°C (77°F); excursions permitted to 15-30°C (59-86°F).

# DIABINESE **RX**

chlorpropamide (Pfizer)

**THERAPEUTIC CLASS:** Sulfonylurea (1st generation)

**INDICATIONS:** Adjunct to diet and exercise to improve glycemic control in adults with type 2 diabetes mellitus.

**DOSAGE:** *Adults:* Take with breakfast. Divide dose with GI intolerance. Initial: 250mg qd. Titrate: After 5-7 days, adjust dose by 50-125mg/day every 3-5 days. Usual: 100-500mg qd. Max: 750mg/day. Switch From Insulin: If ≤40 U/day: D/C insulin; start 250mg qd. If >40 U/day: Reduce insulin dose by 50%; begin 250mg qd. Further insulin reductions depend on response. Elderly/Debilitated/Malnourished/Renal or Hepatic Impairment: Initial: 100-125mg qd. Dose conservatively.

**HOW SUPPLIED:** Tab: 100mg, 250mg

**CONTRAINDICATIONS:** Type 1 diabetes mellitus, diabetic ketoacidosis with or without coma.

**WARNINGS/PRECAUTIONS:** Increased risk of hypoglycemia with the elderly, debilitated, malnourished, renal and hepatic disease, adrenal or pituitary insufficiency. Increased risk of cardiovascular mortality reported. Loss of blood glucose control when exposed to stress (eg, fever, trauma, infection, or surgery); d/c therapy and start insulin. Secondary failure can occur over period of time. Treatment of patients with glucose 6-phosphate dehydrogenase (G6PD) deficiency with sulfonylurea agents can lead to hemolytic anemia. Caution in patients with G6PD deficiency and consider a non-sulfonylurea alternative. Hemolytic anemia reported in patients without G6PD deficiency. Caution in Elderly.

D

**ADVERSE REACTIONS:** Hypoglycemia, cholestatic jaundice, pruritus, photosensitivity reactions, skin eruptions, hepatic porphyria, disulfiram-like reactions, leukopenia, agranulocytosis, thrombocytopenia, hemolytic anemia, SIADH.

**INTERACTIONS:** Hypoglycemic effects potentiated by alcohol, NSAIDs, other highly protein-bound drugs, salicylates, sulfonamides, chloramphenicol, probenecid, coumarins, MAOIs, and β-blockers. Severe hypoglycemia reported with oral hypolycemics and oral miconazole. Alcohol may produce disulfiram-like reaction. Certain drugs have a tendency to cause hyperglycemia and may lead to loss of glycemic control including thiazides and other diuretics, corticosteroids, phenothiazines, thyroid products, estrogens, oral contraceptives, phenytoin, nicotinic acid, sympathomimetics, CCBs, and isoniazid. β-blockers may mask signs of hypoglycemia. May prolong the effects of barbiturates; use with caution.

**PREGNANCY:** Category C, not for use in nursing.

**MECHANISM OF ACTION:** Sulfonylurea; lowers blood glucose acutely by stimulating the release of insulin from the pancreas.

**PHARMACOKINETICS: Absorption:** Rapid; $T_{max}$=2-4 hrs. **Elimination:** Urine (80-90%); $T_{1/2}$=36 hrs.

## NURSING CONSIDERATIONS

**Assessment:** Assess cardiovascular risk factors prior to therapy. Assess for signs/symptoms of hyperglycemia, drug hypersensitivity, diabetic ketoacidosis with/without coma, type 1 DM, adrenal or pituitary insufficiency, pregnancy/nursing status and possible drug interactions.

**Monitoring:** Monitor blood glucose and $HbA_{1c}$ levels regularly. Monitor for hypoglycemia and other possible side effects.

**Patient Counseling:** Inform of importance of caloric restriction, weight loss, and regular exercise. Discuss primary and secondary therapy failure with patients. Counsel on signs/symptoms of cardiovascular mortality and hypoglycemia and its management. Instruct to take therapy once daily with breakfast. Promptly notify physician if symptoms of hypoglycemia or other adverse reactions occur.

**Administration:** Oral route. **Storage:** Below 30°C (86°F).

# DIASTAT

diazepam (Valeant)

**CIV**

**THERAPEUTIC CLASS:** Benzodiazepine

**INDICATIONS:** Management of selected, refractory patients with epilepsy, on stable regimens of anti-epileptic drugs, who require intermittent use to control bouts of increased seizure activity.

**DOSAGE:** *Adults:* Individualized: 0.2mg/kg rectally. Calculate amount and round upward to next available dose; refer to PI for acceptable weight ranges for each dose and age category. May give 2nd dose 4-12 hrs later. Max: ≤5 episodes/month and ≤1 episode every 5 days. Elderly/Debilitated patient: Adjust dosage downward.

*Pediatrics:* Individualized: ≥12 yrs: 0.2mg/kg. 6-11yrs: 0.3mg/kg. 2-5 yrs: 0.5mg/kg. Calculate amount and round upward to next available dose; refer to PI for acceptable weight ranges for each dose and age category. May give 2nd dose 4-12 hrs later. Max: ≤5 episodes/month and ≤1 episode every 5 days.

**HOW SUPPLIED:** Gel: 2.5mg, 10mg, 20mg

**CONTRAINDICATIONS:** Acute narrow angle-glaucoma, untreated open-angle glaucoma.

**WARNINGS/PRECAUTIONS:** Produces CNS depression; may impair mental/physical abilities. Caution with elderly, hepatic/renal dysfunction, compromised respiratory function, neurologic damage. Withdrawal symptoms reported with d/c; avoid abrupt d/c. Increase risk of congenital abnormalities; d/c if become or intent to become pregnant during therapy. May precipitate tonic status epilepticus in patients treated for petit mal seizures. Not recommended for chronic use.

**ADVERSE REACTIONS:** Somnolence, dizziness, headache, pain, abdominal pain, nervousness, vasodilation, diarrhea, ataxia, euphoria, incoordination, asthma, rhinitis, rash.

**INTERACTIONS:** Potentiated by phenothiazines, narcotics, barbiturates, valproate, MAOIs, and other antidepressants. Potential inhibitors of CYP450 2C19 (eg, cimetidine, quinidine, tranylcypromine) and CYP450 3A4 (eg, ketoconazole, troleandomycin, clotrimazole) may decrease elimination. CYP450 2C19 (eg, rifampin) and CYP450 3A4 (eg, carbamazepine, phenytoin, dexamethasone, phenobarbital) inducers could increase elimination. May interfere with metabolism of substrates for CYP450 2C19 (eg, omeprazole, propranolol, imipramine) and CYP450 3A4 (eg, cyclosporine, paclitaxel, terfenadine, theophylline, warfarin). Synergistic CNS-depressant effect with alcohol or other CNS depressants.

**PREGNANCY:** Category D, not for use in nursing.

**MECHANISM OF ACTION:** Benzodiazepine; unknown, suspected to suppress seizures through an interaction with GABA receptors (A-type). GABA acts at this receptor to allow entry of chloride ions, which causes an inhibitory potential that reduces the ability of neurons to depolarize to the threshold potential necessary to produce action potentials.

**PHARMACOKINETICS: Absorption:** Absolute bioavailability (90%); $T_{max}$=1.5 hrs. **Distribution:** $V_d$=1L/kg; plasma protein binding (95-98%); found in breast-milk. **Metabolism:** Hepatic (CYP3A4, CYP2C19) to form desmethyldiazepam (major active metabolite), temazepam and oxazepam (minor active metabolites). **Elimination:** $T_{1/2}$=46 hrs (15mg rectal).

## NURSING CONSIDERATIONS

**Assessment:** Assess for acute narrow-angle glaucoma, renal/hepatic and pulmonary function, pregnancy/nursing status and possible drug interactions. Note other diseases/conditions and drug therapies.

**Monitoring:** Monitor for hypersensitivity reactions, rebound or withdrawal symptoms, seizures, HR, insomnia, LFTs, renal and pulmonary function tests.

**Patient Counseling:** Advise to take as directed. Avoid alcohol and other sedatives; use caution while operating machinery/driving. Counsel about drug abuse/dependence, side effects, and report if any occur. Advise to inform physician of any new findings that are not typical of the patient's characteristic seizure episode. Advise to notify physician if become or intend to become pregnant during therapy. Encourage patients to enroll in North American Antiepileptic Drug (NAAED) Pregnancy Registry by calling 888-233-2334 or go to www.aedpregnancyregistry.org.

**Administration:** Rectal route. Refer to PI for proper administration. **Storage:** 25°C (77°F); excursions permitted to 15-30°C (59-86°F).

# Diazepam Injection

CIV

diazepam (Various)

**THERAPEUTIC CLASS:** Benzodiazepine

D

**INDICATIONS:** Management of anxiety disorders and short-term relief of anxiety symptoms. Symptomatic relief of acute alcohol withdrawal. Adjunct prior to endoscopic procedures, surgical procedures and cardioversion. Adjunct therapy in skeletal muscle spasm (eg, tetanus, etc), status epilepticus and severe recurrent convulsive disorders.

**DOSAGE:** *Adults:* Anxiety (moderate): 2-5mg IM/IV, may repeat in 3-4 hrs. Anxiety (severe): 5-10mg IM/IV, may repeat in 3-4 hrs. Alcohol Withdrawal (acute): 10mg IM/IV, then 5-10mg in 3-4 hrs if needed. Endoscopic Procedures: Usual: ≤10mg IV (up to 20mg) or 5-10mg IM 30 min prior to procedure. Muscle Spasm: 5-10mg IM/IV, then 5-10mg in 3-4 hrs if needed. Status Epilepticus/Severe Seizures: Initial: 5-10mg IV. Maint: May repeat at 10-15 min intervals. Max: 30mg. Preoperative: 10mg IM. Cardioversion: 5-15mg IV, 5-10 min prior to procedure. Elderly/Debilitated: Usual: 2-5mg.
*Pediatrics:* Tetanus: 30 days-5 yrs: 1-2mg IM/IV (slowly), may repeat every 3-4 hrs prn. ≥5 yrs: 5-10mg IM/IV, may repeat every 3-4 hrs. Status Epilepticus/Severe Seizures: 30 days-5 yrs: 0.2-0.5mg IV (slowly) every 2-5 min up to 5mg. ≥5 yrs: 1mg IV (slowly) every 2-5 min up to 10mg, may repeat in 2-4 hrs.

**HOW SUPPLIED:** Inj: 5mg/mL

**CONTRAINDICATIONS:** Acute narrow-angle glaucoma, untreated open-angle glaucoma.

**WARNINGS/PRECAUTIONS:** Inject slowly and avoid small veins with IV. Do not mix or dilute with other products in syringe or infusion flask. Extreme caution in elderly, severely ill and those with limited pulmonary reserve. Avoid if in shock, coma or acute alcohol intoxication with depressed vital signs. May impair mental/physical abilities. Increase in grand mal seizures reported. Caution with kidney or hepatic dysfunction. Not for obstetrical use. Withdrawal symptoms may occur. Hypotension and muscular weakness reported. Monitor blood counts and LFTs. Not for maintenance of seizures once controlled.

**ADVERSE REACTIONS:** Drowsiness, fatigue, ataxia, venous thrombosis and phlebitis (injection site).

**INTERACTIONS:** Phenothiazines, narcotics, barbiturates, MAOIs, and other antidepressants may potentiate effects. Delayed clearance with cimetidine. Reduce narcotic dose by at least one-third. Risk of apnea with concomitant barbiturates, alcohol, or other CNS depressants.

**PREGNANCY:** Not for use during pregnancy, safety in nursing unknown.

**MECHANISM OF ACTION:** Benzodiazepine/hypnotic agent; induces calming effect on parts of the limbic system, thalamus, and hypothalamus (animal study).

## NURSING CONSIDERATIONS

**Assessment:** Assess for acute narrow-angle glaucoma, open-angle glaucoma, acute alcoholic intoxication, shock, coma, cardiac arrest, apnea, hypotension, hypersensitivity, and for possible drug interactions.

**Monitoring:** Monitor injection site for thrombosis and phlebitis, tonic status epilepticus, drowsiness, fatigue, ataxia, CNS depression, and for habituation and dependence.

**Patient Counseling:** Caution against hazardous tasks (operating machinery/driving).

**Administration:** IV, IM route. **Storage:** 20-25°C (6°-77°F). Protect from light.

# DICLOXACILLIN — RX

dicloxacillin sodium (Various)

**THERAPEUTIC CLASS:** Penicillin (penicillinase-resistant)

**INDICATIONS:** Infections caused by penicillinase-producing staphylococci.

**DOSAGE:** *Adults:* Mild-Moderate Infection: 125mg q6h. Severe Infection: 250mg q6h for at least 14 days.
*Pediatrics:* <40kg: Mild-Moderate Infection: 12.5mg/kg/day in divided doses q6h. Severe Infection: 25mg/kg/day in divided doses q6h for at least 14 days.

**HOW SUPPLIED:** Cap: 250mg, 500mg

**WARNINGS/PRECAUTIONS:** Serious, fatal hypersensitivity reactions reported. Pseudomembranous colitis has been reported; toxin produced by *Clostridium difficile* is the primary cause. Caution with history of allergy and/or asthma. Monitor renal, hepatic, and hematopoietic function with prolonged use. Not for use as initial therapy with serious, life-threatening infections, or with nausea, vomiting, gastric dilation, cardiospasm, or intestinal hypermotility.

**ADVERSE REACTIONS:** Allergic reactions, NV, diarrhea, stomatitis, black or hairy tongue, superinfection (prolonged use), hepatotoxicity.

**INTERACTIONS:** Tetracycline may antagonize the bactericidal effects. Potentiated by probenecid.

**PREGNANCY:** Category B, caution in nursing.

**MECHANISM OF ACTION:** Penicillin (penicillinase-resistant); bactericidal against penicillin-susceptible microorganisms during state of active multiplication. Inhibits biosynthesis of bacterial cell-wall.

**PHARMACOKINETICS: Absorption:** Rapid, incomplete; $C_{max}$=1-1.5 hrs; $T_{max}$=10-17mcg/mL. **Distribution:** Serum protein binding (95%-99%); found in breast milk. **Elimination:** Urine (unchanged); $T_{1/2}$=0.7 hrs.

## NURSING CONSIDERATIONS

**Assessment:** Assess for comprehensive drug/allergy history (hypersensitivity to PCNs/cephalosporins, cephamycins and other 1-oxa-β-lactams, history of allergy or asthma), presence of severe illness or with NV, gastric dilation, cardiospasm and intestinal hypermotility, pregnancy/nursing status, and possible drug interactions. Perform blood cultures, WBC with differential prior to therapy and weekly thereafter.

**Monitoring:** Monitor for anaphylactic shock with collapse, pseudomembranous colitis or *C.difficile*-associated diarrhea (can range from mild diarrhea to fatal colitis), development of drug resistance, overgrowth of nonsusceptible organisms and lab monitoring for urine analysis, BUN, creatinine, SGOT, SGPT during therapy with dosage alteration if values elevated. Evaluate renal, hepatic, and hematopoietic functions during prolonged therapy.

**Patient Counseling:** Advise not to take drug if previous allergic reaction occurred. Counsel to take 1 hr before or 2 hrs after meal. Take exactly as prescribed to avoid developing drug resistance and to maintain effectiveness. Advise to notify physician if pregnant/nursing or experience SOB, wheezing, skin rash, mouth irritation, black tongue, sore throat, NV, diarrhea, fever, swollen joints, or any unusual bleeding or bruising. Instruct to notify if taking additional medications. Counsel that drug only treats bacterial, not viral, infections.

**Administration:** Oral route. **Storage:** 20-25°C (68-77°F).

# DIDRONEL — RX

etidronate disodium (Procter & Gamble)

**THERAPEUTIC CLASS:** Bisphosphonate

**INDICATIONS:** Treatment of Paget's disease. Treatment and prevention of heterotopic ossification following total hip replacement or due to spinal cord injury.

**DOSAGE:** *Adults:* Give as single dose (preferred) or in divided doses. Paget's Disease: Initial: 5-10mg/kg/day up to 6 months or 11-20mg/kg/day up to 3 months. May retreat after drug free-period of 90 days only if with evidence of active disease process. Heterotopic Ossification: Hip Replacement: 20mg/kg/day 1 month before and 3 months after surgery. Spinal Cord: 20mg/kg/day for 2 weeks, followed by 10mg/kg/day for 10 weeks.

**HOW SUPPLIED:** Tab: 400mg* *scored

**CONTRAINDICATIONS:** Overt osteomalacia, abnormalities of the esophagus which delay esophageal emptying (eg, stricture or achalasia).

**WARNINGS/PRECAUTIONS:** Therapy response in Paget's disease may be of slow onset and continue for months after stopping. Maintain adequate dietary intake of calcium and vitamin D. Diarrhea at higher doses, caution with enterocolitis. Monitor with renal impairment. Reduce dose with decreased GFR. Max dose (20mg/day) or long-term therapy (>6 months) may increase fracture risk. Rachitic syndrome reported in children at doses of 10mg/kg/day for prolonged periods (approaching or exceeding 1 yr). May cause local irritation of upper GI mucosa; caution with known Barretts esophagus, dysphagia, other esophageal diseases, gastritis, duodenitis or ulcers. Esophageal adverse event such as ulcers and erosion, rarely with bleeding and perforation, reported. D/C if with symptoms (eg, dysphagia, odynophagia, retrosternal pain, new or worsening heartburn). Caution in elderly. Osteonecrosis of the jaw reported.



**ADVERSE REACTIONS:** Diarrhea, nausea, increased bone pain in Paget's disease, alopecia, arthropathy, esophagitis, hypersensitivity reactions, osteomalacia, amnesia, confusion.

**INTERACTIONS:** Vitamins with mineral supplements or antacids that contain calcium, iron, aluminum, or magnesium reduce absorption (separate dosing by 2 hrs). Monitor PT with warfarin.

**PREGNANCY:** Category C, caution with nursing.

**MECHANISM OF ACTION:** Bone metabolism regulator; inhibits the formation, growth, and dissolution of hydroxyapatite crystals and their amorphous precursors by chemisorption to calcium phosphate surfaces.

**PHARMACOKINETICS: Metabolism:** Not metabolized. **Elimination:** Urine (50% of absorbed drug); feces (unabsorbed drug). **Elimination:** $T_{1/2}$=1-6 hrs.

## NURSING CONSIDERATIONS

**Assessment:** Assess for clinically overt osteomalacia, abnormalities of the esophagus, renal impairment, enterocolitis, presence of fractures, upcoming dental procedures, pregnancy/nursing status, and possible drug interactions.

**Monitoring:** Monitor for signs/symptoms of osteonecrosis (eg, jaw), musculoskeletal pain, osteomalacia and fractures, diarrhea, esophageal adverse experiences (eg, esophagitis, esophageal ulcers, esophageal erosions, followed by esophageal stricture or perforation), and hyperphosphatemia. Monitor renal function in patients with renal impairment. In patients with lytic lesions, monitor radiographically and biochemically to determine if responsive to therapy.

**Patient Counseling:** Counsel to maintain adequate nutritional status, particularly adequate intake of calcium and vitamin D. Advise food high in calcium, vitamins with mineral supplements, or antacids which are high in metals (eg, calcium, iron, magnesium, aluminum) should be separated from dose administration by 2 hrs. Advise dose may be divided if GI discomfort occurs. Instruct that a 90-day drug-free interval should be provided between therapy courses. Instruct to drink with full glass (6-8 oz) of water, and to avoid lying down after taking oral biphosphonates.

**Administration:** Oral route. **Storage:** 25°C (77°F); excursions permitted to 15-30°C (59-86°F).

# DIFFERIN — RX

adapalene (Galderma)

**THERAPEUTIC CLASS:** Naphthoic acid derivative (retinoid-like)

**INDICATIONS:** Topical treatment of acne vulgaris.

**DOSAGE:** *Adults:* Apply qhs after washing.
*Pediatrics:* ≥12 yrs: Apply qhs after washing.

**HOW SUPPLIED:** Cre: 0.1% [45g]; Gel: 0.1%, 0.3% [45g, 75g]

**WARNINGS/PRECAUTIONS:** Avoid contact with eyes, lips, paranasal creases, mucous membranes, cuts, abrasions, eczematous or sunburned skin. Minimize sun exposure. Extreme weather may increase skin irritation.

**ADVERSE REACTIONS:** Erythema, scaling, dryness, pruritus, burning, sunburn, acne flares.

**INTERACTIONS:** Caution with other topicals with strong drying effects, high concentration of alcohol, astringents, spices, or lime. Allow effects of sulfur, resorcinol, or salicylic acid to subside before use.

**PREGNANCY:** Category C, caution in nursing.

**MECHANISM OF ACTION:** Naphthoic acid derivative; not established. Suspected to normalize differentiation of follicular epithelial cells resulting in decreased microcomedone formation.

**PHARMACOKINETICS: Absorption:** Low. **Elimination:** Bile.

## NURSING CONSIDERATIONS

**Assessment:** Assess for sunburn. Assess use in pregnant/nursing patients and for possible drug interactions.

**Monitoring:** Monitor for sensitivity or chemical irritation, cutaneous signs/symptoms (eg, erythema, dryness, scaling, burning, or pruritus).

**Patient Counseling:** Instruct to avoid exposure to sunlight and sunlamps; use sunscreen and protective clothing over treated areas when exposed. Medication may also cause skin irritation when exposed to wind or cold. Avoid contact with eyes, lips, angles of the nose, and mucous membranes. Do not apply medication to cuts, abrasions, eczematous or sunburned skin.

**Administration:** Topical application. **Storage:** 20-25°C (68-77°F), excursions permitted to 15-30°C (59-86°F). Protect from freezing.

# DIFLUCAN RX

fluconazole (Pfizer)

**THERAPEUTIC CLASS:** Azole antifungal

**INDICATIONS:** Treatment of vaginal, oropharyngeal, and esophageal candidiasis, systemic *Candida* infections (eg, candidemia, disseminated candidiasis, pneumonia), peritonitis and UTI caused by *Candida,* and cryptococcal meningitis. Prophylaxis in patients undergoing bone marrow transplant.

**DOSAGE:** *Adults:* Vaginal Candidiasis: 150mg PO single dose. IV/PO: Oropharyngeal Candidiasis: 200mg on 1st day, then 100mg qd for at least 2 weeks. Esophageal Candidiasis: 200mg on 1st day, then 100mg qd for at least 3 weeks and for at least 2 weeks following resolution of symptoms. Max: 400mg/day. Systemic *Candida* Infections: Up to 400mg/day. UTI/Peritonitis: 50-200mg/day. Cryptococcal Meningitis: 400mg on 1st day, then 200mg qd for 10-12 weeks after negative CSF culture. Suppression of Cryptococcal Meningitis Relapse in AIDS: 200mg qd. Prophylaxis in bone marrow transplant: 400mg qd. Renal Impairment (Multiple Doses) CrCl≤50mL/min (no dialysis): Initial: LD 50-400mg. Maint: Give 50% of recommended dose. Dialysis: Give 100% of dose after each dialysis.

*Pediatrics:* IV/PO: Oropharyngeal Candidiasis: 6mg/kg on 1st day, then 3mg/kg/day for at least 2 weeks. Esophageal Candidiasis: 6mg/kg on 1st day, then 3mg/kg/day for at least 3 weeks and for at least 2 weeks following resolution of symptoms. Max: 12mg/kg/day. Systemic *Candida* Infections: 6-12mg/kg/day. Cryptococcal Meningitis: 12mg/kg 1st day, then 6mg/kg/day for 10-12 weeks after negative CSF culture. Suppression of Cryptococcal Meningitis Relapse in AIDS: 6mg/kg qd. Renal Impairment: CrCl ≤50mL/min (no dialysis): Initial: LD: 50-400mg. Maint: Give 50% of recommended dose. Dialysis: Give 100% of dose after each dialysis.

**HOW SUPPLIED:** Inj: 200mg/100mL, 400mg/200mL; Sus: 50mg/5mL, 200mg/5mL [35mL]; Tab: 50mg, 100mg, 150mg, 200mg

**CONTRAINDICATIONS:** Coadministration with cisapride or terfenadine (with multiple fluconazole doses of ≥400mg).

**WARNINGS/PRECAUTIONS:** Rarely associated with serious hepatic toxicity. Monitor LFTs. D/C if hepatic dysfunction develops. Exfoliative skin disorders rarely reported; monitor if rash develops during treatment and d/c if lesions progress. Anaphylaxis reported. Rare cases of QT prolongation and torsades de pointes reported; caution in patients with proarrhythmic conditions.

Consider risk vs. benefits of single PO tab dose therapy for the treatment of vaginal yeast infections.

**ADVERSE REACTIONS:** Headache, N/V, abdominal pain, diarrhea, skin rash.

**INTERACTIONS:** See Contraindications. Severe hypoglycemia with oral hypoglycemics. May increase PT with coumarin-type drugs. Increases levels of phenytoin, cyclosporine, cisapride, astemizole, zidovudine, rifabutin, tacrolimus, and theophylline. Rifampin enhances metabolism of fluconazole. Increases levels of midazolam; consider reducing dose of short-acting benzodiazepines that are metabolized by CYP P450 if given concomitantly with fluconazole. Cimetidine may decrease levels. HCTZ may increase levels. May increase or decrease levels of ethinyl estradiol- and levonorgestrel-containing oral contraceptives. Incidence of abnormality elevated serum transaminases was greater in patients taking fluconazole concomitantly with one or more following medications: rifampin, phenytoin, isoniazid, valproic acid, or oral sulfonylurea hypoglycemic agents.

**PREGNANCY:** Category C, not for use in nursing.

**MECHANISM OF ACTION:** Antifungal; inhibits fungal CYP450 dependent enzyme lanosterol 14-α-demethylase. This enzyme functions to convert lanosterol to ergosterol. Subsequent loss of normal sterol correlates with accumulation of 14 α-methyl sterols in fungi and may be responsible for its fungistatic activity.

**PHARMACOKINETICS: Absorption:** Oral: Absolute bioavailability (>90%); $C_{max}$=6.72mcg/mL (50-400mg), $T_{max}$=1-2 hrs (fasted). **Distribution:** Plasma protein binding (11-12%); found in breast milk. **Elimination:** Urine (80% unchanged and 11% metabolites); $T_{1/2}$=30 hrs. Refer to PI for pediatric and elderly pharmacokinetic parameters.

## NURSING CONSIDERATIONS

**Assessment:** Assess for renal impairment, proarrhythmic conditions, pregnancy/nursing status, and for possible drug interactions. Assess for proper clinical diagnosis of fungal infection.

**Monitoring:** Monitor for signs/symptoms of anaphylaxis and for exfoliative skin disorders. Monitor LFTs and for signs of hepatotoxicity. Monitor ECG for QT prolongation and torsades de pointes. Monitor renal function.

**Patient Counseling:** Instruct to contact physician if signs of hepatotoxicity, anaphylaxis, or rash develop. Advise to notify physician if pregnant/nursing and all medications currently taking.

**Administration:** IV infusion and oral route. IV infusion max rate is 200mg/hr. **Storage:** Tab: <86°F (30°C). Sus: Dry Powder: <86°F (30°C). Reconstituted: 86°F (30°C)-41°F (5°C); discard unused portion after 2 weeks. Protect from freezing. Inj in Glass Bottles: 86°F (30°C)-41°F (5°C), protect from freezing. Inj. in Viaflex Plus Plastic Container: 77°F (25°C)-41°F (5°C). Brief exposure up to 104°F (40°C) does not adversely affect the product. Protect from freezing.

# DIGIBIND RX

digoxin immune fab (ovine) (GlaxoSmithKline)

**THERAPEUTIC CLASS:** Antidote, digoxin toxicity

**INDICATIONS:** Treatment of life-threatening digoxin intoxication. Also has been successfully used to treat digitoxin overdose.

**DOSAGE:** *Adults:* Acute Ingestion of Unknown Amount: Usual: Administer 10 vials, observe response, then additional 10 vials if clinically indicated. Calculation: # vials = total digitalis body load (mg)/0.5mg of digitalis bound per vial. 1 vial will bind approximately 0.5mg of digoxin (or digitoxin). Steady-State Serum Digoxin Concentrations: # of vials = (serum dig conc in ng/mL) x (wt in kg)/100. Steady-State Digitoxin Concentrations: # of vials = (serum digitoxin conc in ng/mL) x (wt in kg)/1000. If toxicity not adequately reversed after several hrs or appears to recur, may need readministration. See PI for details.
*Pediatrics:* Acute Ingestion of Unknown Amount: Usual: Administer 10 vials,

observe response, then additional 10 vials if clinically indicated. Calculation: # vials = total digitalis body load (mg)/0.5mg of digitalis bound per vial. 1 vial will bind approximately 0.5mg of digoxin (or digitoxin). Steady-State Serum Digoxin Concentrations: Dose (mg) = (# vials) (38mg/vial). Steady-State Digitoxin Concentrations: # of vials = (serum digitoxin conc in ng/mL) x (wt in kg)/1000. If toxicity not adequately reversed after several hrs or appears to recur, may need readministration. See PI for details.

D

**HOW SUPPLIED:** Inj: 38mg

**WARNINGS/PRECAUTIONS:** Obtain digoxin level before initiation. Do not overlook possibility of multiple drug overdose. Risk of hypersensitivity is greater with allergies to papain, chymopapain, or other papaya extracts; skin testing may be appropriate for high-risk individuals. $K^+$ levels may drop rapidly after administration; monitor closely. Digitalis toxicity may recur with renal dysfunction; caution and monitor closely. Caution with cardiac dysfunction, further deterioration may occur from digoxin withdrawal. Consider additional support with inotropes or vasodilators. Monitor for volume overload in children. D/C if anaphylactoid reaction occurs and treat appropriately.

**ADVERSE REACTIONS:** Allergic reactions, exacerbation of low cardiac output, CHF, hypokalemia.

**PREGNANCY:** Category C, caution in nursing.

**MECHANISM OF ACTION:** Antidote; digoxin toxicity. Binds to molecules of digoxin, making them unavailable for binding at their site of action on cells.

**PHARMACOKINETICS: Elimination:** Urine; $T_{1/2}$=15-20 hrs.

## NURSING CONSIDERATIONS

**Assessment:** Assess for serum digoxin or digitoxin concentration, serum electrolytes, hypoxia, acid base disturbances, CVD, and renal functions. Note other diseases/conditions and drug therapies.

**Monitoring:** Monitor for serum potassium concentration, arrhythmias, and renal function.

**Patient Counseling:** Counsel about adverse effects.

**Administration:** IV route. Refer to PI for further information. **Storage:** 2-8°C (36-46°F). Unreconstituted vials can be stored at up to 30°C (86°F) for 30 days.

# Dilacor XR — RX

diltiazem HCl (Watson)

**OTHER BRAND NAMES:** Diltia XT (Andrx)

**THERAPEUTIC CLASS:** Calcium channel blocker (nondihydropyridine)

**INDICATIONS:** Treatment of hypertension alone or in combination with other antihypertensives and management of chronic stable angina.

**DOSAGE:** *Adults:* HTN: Initial: 180-240mg qd. Usual: 180-480mg qd. Max: 540mg qd. ≥60 yrs: Initial: 120mg qd. Angina: Initial: 120mg qd. Titrate: Adjust at 1-2 week intervals. Max: 480mg qd. Swallow whole on an empty stomach in the am.

**HOW SUPPLIED:** Cap, Extended-Release: 120mg, 180mg, 240mg

**CONTRAINDICATIONS:** Sick sinus syndrome, 2nd- or 3rd-degree AV block (except with functioning pacemaker), hypotension (<90mmHg systolic), acute MI, pulmonary congestion.

**WARNINGS/PRECAUTIONS:** Caution in renal, hepatic, or ventricular dysfunction, and pre-existing GI narrowing. Monitor LFTs and renal function with prolonged use. D/C if persistent rash occurs. Symptomatic hypotension may occur. Acute hepatic injury reported.

**ADVERSE REACTIONS:** Rhinitis, pharyngitis, increased cough, flu syndrome, peripheral edema, myalgia, NV, sinusitis, asthenia, vasodilation, headache, constipation, diarrhea, back pain, dyspepsia.

**INTERACTIONS:** Increased levels of propranolol and carbamazepine. Increased levels of diltiazem with cimetidine. Monitor digoxin, cyclosporine. Potentiates cardiac contractility, conductivity, and automaticity; and vascular dilation with anesthetics. Additive cardiac conduction effects with digitalis or β-blockers. Potential additive effects with agents known to affect cardiac contractility and/or conduction. Competitive inhibition of metabolism with agents that undergo biotransformation by CYP450 mixed function oxidase.



**PREGNANCY:** Category C, not for use in nursing.

**MECHANISM OF ACTION:** $Ca^{2+}$ channel blocker; inhibits influx of calcium ion during membrane depolarization of cardiac and vascular smooth muscle with resultant decrease in peripheral vascular resistance.

**PHARMACOKINETICS: Absorption:** Absolute bioavailability (41%); $T_{max}$=4-6 hrs. **Distribution:** Plasma protein binding (70-80%). **Metabolism:** Liver. Desacetyldiltiazem (major metabolite). **Elimination:** Urine (2-4%); $T_{1/2}$=5-10 hrs.

## NURSING CONSIDERATIONS

**Assessment:** Assess for sick sinus syndrome, hypotension, AV block, acute MI, pulmonary congestion, pre-existing impairment of ventricular function, pre-existing GI narrowing, renal/hepatic impairment, hypersensitivity to drug, pregnancy/nursing status, and possible drug interactions.

**Monitoring:** Monitor renal function and LFTs periodically. Monitor for signs/symptoms of worsening of CHF, hypotension, obstruction from strictures, hypersensitivity reactions, renal/hepatic dysfunction.

**Patient Counseling:** Instruct to take on empty stomach; not to open capsule; swallow whole, do not chew or crush. Advise to seek medical attention if symptoms of GI obstruction, worsening of CHF, hypotension, or hypersensitivity reactions occur.

**Administration:** Oral route. **Storage:** 20-25°C (68-77°F).

# DILANTIN RX

phenytoin sodium (Parke-Davis)

**OTHER BRAND NAMES:** Dilantin-125 (Parke-Davis) - Dilantin Kapseals (Parke-Davis)

**THERAPEUTIC CLASS:** Hydantoin

**INDICATIONS:** (CER, CTB) Control of generalized tonic-clonic (grand mal) and complex partial (psychomotor, temporal lobe) seizures. Prevention and treatment of neurosurgical induced seizures. (Sus) Control of tonic-clonic (grand mal) and psychomotor (temporal lobe) seizures.

**DOSAGE:** *Adults:* (CER) Individualized: Initial: 100mg tid. Titrate: May increase at 7- to 10-day intervals. Maint: 100mg tid-qid. Max: 200mg tid. May give once daily with 300mg extended-release capsules if controlled on 300mg daily. LD (clinic/hospital): 1g in 3 divided doses (400mg, 300mg, 300mg) given 2 hrs apart. Start maintenance 24 hrs later. (CTB) Initial: 100mg tid. Titrate: May increase at 7- to 10-day intervals. Usual: 300-400mg/day. Max: 600mg/day. May chew or swallow tab whole. Not for once-daily dosing. (Sus) Initial: 125mg tid. Titrate: May increase to 5 tsp (625mg) daily if necessary. Serum level determinations for optimal dosage adjustment.
*Pediatrics:* (CER, CTB, Sus) Individualized: Initial: 5mg/kg/day given bid-tid. Maint: 4-8mg/kg/day. Max: 300mg/day. >6 yrs: May require the minimum adult dose (300mg/day).

**HOW SUPPLIED:** Cap, Extended-Release (CER) [Capsule, Kapseals]: 30mg, 100mg; Sus: 125mg/5mL; Tab, Chewable (CTB): 50mg* *scored

**WARNINGS/PRECAUTIONS:** Avoid abrupt d/c; may precipitate status epilepticus. Increased risk of suicidal thoughts or behavior reported; monitor for worsening of depression and any unusual changes in mood or behavior. Caution with porphyria, hepatic dysfunction, elderly, seriously ill, diabetes, debilitated. Can cause serious skin adverse events such as exfoliative dermatitis, Stevens-Johnson syndrome, and toxic epidermal necrolysis; d/c if rash occurs.

Lymphadenopathy, anticonvulsant hypersensitivity syndrome (AHS), hyperglycemia, osteomalacia reported. Caution in pregnancy; increased seizure frequency, congenital malformation, bleeding disorder newborns reported. Give vitamin K to mother before delivery and to neonate after birth. Confused states referred to as delirium, psychosis, or encephalopathy reported with increased levels. Avoid use with seizures due to hypoglycemia or other metabolic causes.

**ADVERSE REACTIONS:** Nystagmus, ataxia, slurred speech, decreased coordination, confusion, dizziness, insomnia, transient nervousness, motor twitching, headaches, N/V, constipation, rash, hypersensitivity reactions.

**INTERACTIONS:** Increased levels with acute alcohol intake, amiodarone, chloramphenicol, chlordiazepoxide, cimetidine, diazepam, dicumarol, disulfiram, estrogens, ethosuximide, fluoxetine, $H_2$-antagonists, halothane, isoniazid, methylphenidate, phenothiazines, phenylbutazone, salicylates, succinimides, sulfonamides, ticlopidine, tolbutamide, trazodone. Decreased levels with chronic alcohol abuse, carbamazepine, reserpine, sucralfate. Decreases effects of corticosteroids, coumarin anticoagulants, digitoxin, doxycycline, estrogens, furosemide, oral contraceptives, paroxetine, quinidine, rifampin, theophylline, vitamin D. Phenobarbital, sodium valproate, valproic acid may increase or decrease levels. May increase or decrease levels of phenobarbital, sodium valproate, valproic acid. Calcium antacids decrease absorption; space dosing. Moban contains calcium ions that interfere with absorption. TCAs may precipitate seizures. Increased risk of phenytoin hypersensitivity with barbiturates, succinimides, oxazolidinediones. Avoid with enteral feeding preparations.

**PREGNANCY:** Pregnancy D, not for use in nursing.

**MECHANISM OF ACTION:** Anticonvulsant; inhibits seizure activity by promoting sodium efflux from neurons, stabilizing threshold against hyperexcitability caused by excessive stimulation of environmental changes capable of reducing membrane sodium gradient.

**PHARMACOKINETICS: Absorption:** (CTB, Sus) $T_{max}$=1.5-3 hrs; (CER) $T_{max}$=4-12 hrs. **Distribution:** Highly protein bound; found in breastmilk. **Metabolism:** Liver (hydroxylation). **Elimination:** Bile, urine; $T_{1/2}$=22 hrs.

## NURSING CONSIDERATIONS

**Assessment:** Assess that seizure is not due to hypoglycemia or other metabolic causes and that seizure is not an absence seizure. Assess use with impaired hepatic function and porphyria. Assess pregnancy/nursing status prior to therapy and for possible drug interactions. Assess for AHS.

**Monitoring:** Monitor for signs/symptoms of skin rash (Stevens-Johnson syndrome, toxic epidermal necrolysis), lymphadenopathy (benign lymph node hyperplasia, pseudolymphoma, Hodgkin's disease), and hyperglycemia in diabetic patients. Monitor serum phenytoin levels in pregnant women, occurrence of confused states (delirium, psychosis, encephalopathy), and osteomalacia.

**Patient Counseling:** Inform of importance of strictly adhering to prescribed dosage regimen. Caution on use of other drugs or alcoholic beverages without consulting physician. Instruct to immediately contact physician if skin rash develops. Instruct to maintain proper dental hygiene while on medication to minimize risk of gingival hyperplasia. Notify physician if suicidal thoughts or behavior emerge. Advise females about dangers of using medication during pregnancy. Inform pregnant women they will need to receive vitamin K prior to delivery. Encourage patients to enroll in the North American Antiepileptic Drug (NAAED) Pregnancy Registry if become pregnant by calling 888-233-2334 or go to www.aedpregnancyregistry.org.

**Administration:** Oral route. Dilantin Infatabs can either be chewed thoroughly before swallowing or swallowed whole. **Storage:** (Tab) 15-30°C (59-86°F); (Cap/Sus) 20-25°C (68-77°F). Preserve in tight, light-resistant containers. Protect from moisture.

# DILAUDID

CII

## hydromorphone HCl (Purdue Pharma)

D

**Contains hydromorphone, a potent Schedule II opioid agonist that has the highest potential for abuse and risk of producing respiratory depression. HP formulation is a highly concentrated solution of hydromorphone; do not confuse with standard parenteral formulations of hydromorphone or other opioids as overdose and death could result. Alcohol, other opioids, CNS depressants potentiate respiratory depressant effects, increasing risk of respiratory depression, which may result in death.**

**OTHER BRAND NAMES:** Dilaudid-HP (Purdue Pharma)

**THERAPEUTIC CLASS:** Opioid analgesic

**INDICATIONS:** Management of pain. (HP) Relief of moderate to severe pain in opioid-tolerant patients who require larger than usual doses of opioids to provide adequate pain relief.

**DOSAGE:** *Adults:* Individualize dose. Initial: 1-2mg SQ/IM/IV q4-6h prn. (HP) Range: 1-14mg IM/SQ; adjust dose based on response. (Sol) Usual: 2.5-10mg PO q3-6h prn. (Tab) Initial: 2-4mg PO q4-6h prn. Titrate: A grdaual increase in dose may be required if analgesia is inadequate, as intolerance develops or pain severity increases. Elderly: Start at lower end of dosing range.

**HOW SUPPLIED:** Inj: 1mg/mL, 2mg/mL, 4mg/mL, (HP) 10mg/mL. Sol: 1mg/mL. Tab: 2mg, 4mg, 8mg* *scored.

**CONTRAINDICATIONS:** Respiratory depression in the absence of resuscitative equipment, in status asthmaticus, obstetrical analgesia, labor and delivery. (HP) Not already receiving large amounts of opioids.

**WARNINGS/PRECAUTIONS:** Increased respiratory depression with head injury and/or increased ICP. May mask acute abdominal conditions. Caution with elderly/debilitated, COPD or cor pulmonale, decreased respiratory reserve, hypoxia, hypercapnia, preexisting respiratory depression, seizures, circulatory shock, biliary tract surgery, renal/hepatic impairment, hypothyroidism, Addison's disease, BPH, and urethral stricture; initial dose should be reduced in these patients. May suppress cough reflex. Potential for physical/psychological tolerance or dependence, especially in patients with alcoholism and drug dependencies; monitor closely. May impair mental/physical ability, produce orthostatic hypotension, cause spasm of the sphincter of Oddi and aggravate pre-existing convulsions. Seizures reported in compromised patients receiving high doses. Contains metabisulfite; may cause allergic type reactions (anaphylactic symptoms). Dilaudid-HP should only be used in patients already receiving large doses of opioids.

**ADVERSE REACTIONS:** Respiratory depression, apnea, circulatory depression, respiratory arrest, shock, cardiac arrest, lightheadedness, dizziness, sedation, N/V, sweating, flushing, dysphoria, euphoria.

**INTERACTIONS:** Additive CNS depression with other narcotic analgesics, neuromuscular blocking agents, general anesthetics, phenothiazines, tranquilizers, sedative hypnotics, skeletal muscle relaxants, alcohol, or other CNS depressants. Mixed agonist/antagonist analgesics (eg, pentazocine, nalbuphine, butorphanol, buprenorphine) may reduce the analgesic effect of hydromorphone and/or may precipitate withdrawal symptoms.

**PREGNANCY:** Category C, not for use in nursing.

**MECHANISM OF ACTION:** Opioid analgesic; not established. Suspected to bind to specific opiate receptors in the CNS to produce analgesia.

**PHARMACOKINETICS:** Absorption: (PO) Rapid; (Tab) $C_{max}$=5.5ng, $T_{max}$=0.74 hrs; (Sol) $C_{max}$=5.7ng, $T_{max}$=0.73 hrs. Distribution: Plasma protein binding (8-19%); (IV Bolus) $V_d$=302.9 L; crosses placenta, found in breast milk. Metabolism: Liver; glucuronidation (extensive); hydromorphone-3-glucuronide (metabolite). Elimination: Urine; (IV) $T_{1/2}$=2.3 hrs; (Tab) $T_{1/2}$=2.6 hrs; (Sol) $T_{1/2}$=2.8 hrs.

## NURSING CONSIDERATIONS

**Assessment:** Assess for respiratory depression, presence of status asthmaticus, COPD, potential for opioid abuse (eg, family history, mental illness), nursing/pregnancy status, age of patient, head injury, intracranial lesions, elevated intracranial pressure, circulatory shock, sulfite sensitivity, renal/hepatic impairment, myxedema or hypothyroidism, adrenocortical insufficiency (eg, Addison's disease), CNS depression or coma, toxic psychosis, convulsive disorder, prostatic hypertrophy or urethral stricture, gallbladder disease, upcoming surgery on the biliary tract, presence of acute abdominal conditions, acute alcoholism, delirium tremens, kyphoscoliosis, and possible drug interactions.

**Monitoring:** Monitor for signs/symptoms of respiratory depression, circulatory depression (eg, hypotension), misuse or abuse, addiction, tolerance or dependence, seizures, and for alleviation of pain.

**Patient Counseling:** Inform that medication may cause respiratory depression if not taken as directed. Instruct to report any adverse effects experienced. Instruct not to adjust dosage without physician's consent. Medication may impair mental/physical abilities; use caution when performing hazardous tasks (eg, operating machinery/driving). Avoid using other CNS depressants and alcohol. Inform pregnant women about effects of medication on pregnancy. Instruct to avoid abrupt withdrawal; dosage should be tapered. Educate that medication has abuse potential. Advise to keep out of reach of children and to dispose unused tablets via toilet.

**Administration:** Subcutaneous, IM, IV, oral, and rectal route. IV administration should be given slowly over at least 2-3 min, depending on dose. (Dilaudid HP) Reconstitute immediately prior to use with 25mL of Sterile Water for Injection to provide a sterile solution containing 10mg/mL. **Storage:** Parenteral and oral: 25°C (77°F); excursions permitted to 15-30° (59-86°F), protect from light.

# Diltiazem Injection — RX

diltiazem HCl (Various)

**THERAPEUTIC CLASS:** Calcium channel blocker (nondihydropyridine)

**INDICATIONS:** Temporary control of rapid ventricular rate in atrial fibrillation/flutter (A-Fib/Flutter). Rapid conversion of paroxysmal supraventricular tachycardia (PSVT) to sinus rhythm.

**DOSAGE:** *Adults:* Bolus: 0.25mg/kg IV over 2 min. If no response after 15 min, may give 2nd dose of 0.35mg/kg over 2 min. Continuous Infusion: 0.25-0.35mg/kg IV bolus, then 10mg/hr. Titrate: Increase by 5mg/hr. Max: 15mg/hr and duration up to 24 hrs.

**HOW SUPPLIED:** Inj: 5mg/mL

**CONTRAINDICATIONS:** Sick sinus syndrome and 2nd- or 3rd-degree AV block (except with functioning pacemaker), severe hypotension, cardiogenic shock, concomitant IV β-blockers or within a few hrs of use, A-Fib/Flutter associated with accessory bypass tract (eg, Wolff-Parkinson-White syndrome, short PR syndrome), ventricular tachycardia.

**WARNINGS/PRECAUTIONS:** Initiate in setting with resuscitation capabilities. Caution if hemodynamically compromised, and renal, hepatic, or ventricular dysfunction. Monitor ECG continuously and BP frequently. Symptomatic hypotension, acute hepatic injury reported. D/C if high-degree AV block occurs in sinus rhythm or if persistent rash occurs. Ventricular premature beats may be present on conversion of PSVT to sinus rhythm.

**ADVERSE REACTIONS:** Hypotension, injection-site reactions (eg, itching, burning), vasodilation (flushing), arrhythmias.

**INTERACTIONS:** Caution with drugs that decrease peripheral resistance, intravascular volume, myocardial contractility or conduction. Increased AUC of midazolam, triazolam, buspirone, quinidine, and lovastatin, which may require a dose adjustment due to increased clinical effects or increased adverse events. Elevates carbamazepine levels, which may result in toxicity.

Cyclosporine may need dose adjustment. Potentiates the depression of cardiac contractility, conductivity, automaticity and vascular dilation with anesthetics. Possible bradycardia, AV block, and contractility depression with oral β-blockers. Possible competitive inhibition of metabolism with drugs metabolized by CYP450. Avoid IV β-blockers and rifampin. Monitor for excessive slowing of HR and/or AV block with digoxin. Cimetidine increases peak diltiazem plasma levels and AUC.

D

**PREGNANCY:** Category C, not for use in nursing.

**MECHANISM OF ACTION:** Calcium channel blocker; inhibits influx of $Ca^{2+}$ ions during membrane depolarization of cardiac and vascular smooth muscle. Has ability to slow AV nodal conduction time and prolong AV nodal refractoriness, which has therapeutic benefits on supraventricular tachycardia. Decreases peripheral resistance, resulting in decreased systolic and diastolic BP.

**PHARMACOKINETICS: Distribution:** $V_d$=305-391L; plasma protein binding (70-80%); found in breast milk. **Metabolism:** Liver (extensive) via CYP450; deacetylation, N-demethylation, O-demethylation, and conjugation; N-monodesmethyldiltiazem and desacetyldiltiazem (major metabolites). **Elimination:** Urine and bile; $T_{1/2}$=3.4 hrs (single IV inj), 4.1-4.9 hrs (constant IV infusion).

## NURSING CONSIDERATIONS

**Assessment:** Assess for sick sinus syndrome and 2nd- or 3rd-degree AV block, presence of functioning pacemaker, severe hypotension, cardiogenic shock, A-Fib or atrial flutter associated with accessory bypass tract (eg, Wolff-Parkinson-White syndrome, short PR syndrome), ventricular tachycardia, wide complex tachycardia, AMI, CHF, pulmonary congestion documented by X-ray, hypertrophic cardiomyopathy, renal/hepatic impairment, pregnancy/nursing status, and possible drug interactions.

**Monitoring:** Initiation of therapy should be done in setting with monitoring and resuscitation capabilities, including DC cardioversion/defibrillation. Monitor BP, HR, LFTs, and ECG. Monitor for hemodynamic deterioration, ventricular fibrillation, cardiac conduction abnormalities (eg, 2nd- or 3rd-degree AV block), hypotension, bradycardia, ventricular premature beats, dermatologic events (erythema multiforme/exfoliative dermatitis), and acute hepatic injury.

**Patient Counseling:** Initiation of therapy should be done in a setting with monitoring and resuscitation capabilities, including DC cardioversion/defibrillation. Inform risks/benefits; report adverse reactions. Notify if pregnant/nursing.

**Administration:** IV. **Storage:** 2-8°C (36-46°F). Do not freeze. Room temperature for up to 1 month. Destroy after 1 month.

# DIOVAN RX

valsartan (Novartis)

**When used in pregnancy, drugs that act directly on the renin-angiotensin system can cause injury and even death to the developing fetus. D/C therapy when pregnancy is detected.**

**THERAPEUTIC CLASS:** Angiotensin II receptor antagonist

**INDICATIONS:** Treatment of hypertension alone or in combination with other antihypertensives. Treatment of heart failure (NYHA Class II-IV). Reduction of cardiovascular mortality in clinically stable patients with left ventricular failure or dysfunction following MI.

**DOSAGE:** *Adults:* HTN: Monotherapy Without Volume Depletion: Initial: 80mg or 160mg qd. Titrate: May increase to 320mg qd or add diuretic (greater effect than increasing dose >80mg). Max: 320mg/day. Heart Failure: Initial: 40mg bid. Titrate: May increase to 80mg or 160mg bid (use highest dose tolerated). Max: 320mg/day in divided doses. Post-MI: Initial: 20mg bid starting as soon as 12 hrs after MI. Titrate: May increase to 40mg bid within 7 days, with subsequent titrations up to 160mg bid. May take with or without food. *Pediatrics:* 6-16 yrs: HTN: Initial: 1.3mg/kg qd (up to 40mg total). Adjust dose according to BP response. Max: 2.7mg/kg (up to 160mg) qd. Use of a sus recommended for children who cannot swallow tabs, or children for whom calculated dosage (mg/kg) does not correspond to available tab strengths. Adjust dose accordingly when switching dosage forms.

**HOW SUPPLIED:** Tab: 40mg*, 80mg, 160mg, 320mg *scored

**WARNINGS/PRECAUTIONS:** Risk of hypotension; caution when initiating therapy in heart failure or post-MI. Symptomatic hypotension may occur in volume and/or salt-depleted patients; correct volume or salt depletion prior to therapy and monitor closely. Caution with renal/hepatic dysfunction (including obstructive biliary disorders). Changes in renal function may occur; caution with renal artery stenosis, severe CHF. Consider dose reduction and discontinuation of diuretic with renal dysfunction. Avoid use in pediatric patients with GFR <30mL/min/1.73m$^2$.

**ADVERSE REACTIONS:** Dizziness, viral infection, hypotension, diarrhea, arthralgia, fatigue and back pain.

**INTERACTIONS:** Co-administration of inhibitors of the hepatic uptake transporter OATP1B1 (eg, rifampin, cyclosporine) or the hepatic efflux transporter MRP2 (eg, ritonavir) may increase systemic exposure to valsartan. Concomitant use of $K^+$-sparing diuretics (eg, spironolactone, triamterene, amiloride), $K^+$ supplements, or salt substitutes containing $K^+$ may increase serum $K^+$ levels, and in heart failure patients increase in SrCr.

**PREGNANCY:** Category D, not for use in nursing.

**MECHANISM OF ACTION:** Angiotensin II receptor antagonist; blocks vasoconstrictor and aldosterone-secreting effects of angiotensin II by selectively blocking the binding of angiotensin II to the $AT_1$ receptor in many tissues, such as vascular smooth muscle and the adrenal gland.

**PHARMACOKINETICS: Absorption:** Absolute bioavailability (25%); $T_{max}$=2-4 hrs. **Distribution:** (IV) $V_d$=17L; plasma protein binding (95%). **Metabolism:** Valeryl 4-hydroxy valsartan (primary metabolite). **Elimination:** (Sus) Feces (83%), urine (13%); $T_{1/2}$=6 hrs.

## NURSING CONSIDERATIONS

**Assessment:** Assess for HTN, CHF, renal/hepatic impairment, obstructive biliary disorders, pregnancy/nursing status, and possible drug interactions. Assess for volume or salt depletion and correct before initiating therapy.

**Monitoring:** Monitor serum $K^+$, creatinine, and BUN periodically. Monitor for signs/symptoms of hypotension, and renal/hepatic dysfunction.

**Patient Counseling:** Inform that drug can cause serious problems to the fetus; d/c and consult physician when pregnancy is detected. Advise to seek medical attention if symptoms of hypotension occur. Counsel to inform physician of all medical conditions and medicines being taken. Take w/ or w/o food. If dose is missed, take as soon as remembered. If it is close to next dose, skip the missed dose and take the next dose at regular time.

**Administration:** Oral route. Refer to PI for instructions on preparation of oral sus for children who cannot swallow tablets. Shake sus for at least 10 sec prior to administration. **Storage:** Tab: 25°C (77°F); excursions permitted to 15-30°C (59-86°F). Protect from moisture. Sus: <30°C (86°F) for up to 30 days or refrigerate 2-8°C (35-46°F) for up to 75 days.

# DIOVAN HCT

RX

hydrochlorothiazide - valsartan (Novartis)

**When used in pregnancy, drugs that act directly on the renin-angiotensin system can cause injury and even death to the developing fetus. D/C therapy when pregnancy is detected.**

**THERAPEUTIC CLASS:** Angiotensin II receptor antagonist/thiazide diuretic

**INDICATIONS:** Treatment of hypertension in patients whose BP is uncontrolled on monotherapy and as initial therapy in patients who are likely to need multiple drugs to achieve BP goals.

D

**DOSAGE:** *Adults:* Uncontrolled with Valsartan (or another ARB) or HCTZ Alone: Initial: May be switched to valsartan-HCTZ. If dose-limiting adverse reactions are experienced on either component alone, switch to valsartan-HCTZ containing a lower dose of that component in combination with the other to achieve similiar BP reductions. Titrate: May increase after 3-4 weeks of therapy. Max: 320mg-25mg. Replacement Therapy: May be substituted for titrated components. Initial Therapy: 160mg-12.5mg qd. Titrate: May increase after 1-2 weeks of therapy. Max: 320mg-25mg qd. May be administered with or without food. Renal Impairment: CrCl≤30mL/min: Use not recommended. Hepatic Impairment: Start at low dose and titrate slowly.

**HOW SUPPLIED:** Tab: (Valsartan-HCTZ) 80mg-12.5mg, 160mg-12.5mg, 160mg-25mg, 320mg-12.5mg, 320mg-25mg

**CONTRAINDICATIONS:** Anuria, hypersensitivity to sulfonamides.

**WARNINGS/PRECAUTIONS:** Symptomatic hypotension may occur in volume and/or salt-depleted patients; correct volume or salt depletion before therapy and monitor closely. Caution with hepatic dysfunction or progressive liver disease, renal dysfunction, biliary obstructive disorders, renal artery stenosis, severe CHF, history of allergies, and asthma. May exacerbate or activate SLE. If progressive renal impairment becomes evident, consider withholding or d/c diuretic therapy. Avoid with CrCl ≤30mL/min. Hyponatremia, hypochloremic alkalosis, chloride deficit, hyperuricemia, hyperglycemia, hypokalemia, hypomagnesemia, and hypercalcemia may occur. Enhanced effects in post-sympathectomy patient. May increase cholesterol and triglyceride levels.

**ADVERSE REACTIONS:** Cough, headache, dizziness, nasopharyngitis.

**INTERACTIONS:** Alcohol, barbiturates, and narcotics may potentiate orthostatic hypotension. Insulin and oral antidiabetic agents may require dosage adjustment. May impair absorption of HCTZ with cholestyramine or colestipol. Corticosteroids and ACTH deplete electrolytes. May decrease response to pressor amines (eg, norepinephrine). Potentiates other antihypertensives. May increase responsiveness to nondepolarizing skeletal muscle relaxants (eg, tubocurarine). Risk of lithium toxicity; avoid concurrent use. NSAIDs may decrease diuretic effects; monitor closely. Coadministration with carbamazepine may lead to symptomatic hyponatremia.

**PREGNANCY:** Category D, not for use in nursing.

**MECHANISM OF ACTION:** Valsartan: Angiotensin II receptor antagonist; blocks vasoconstrictor and aldosterone-secreting effects of angiotensin II by selectively blocking binding of angiotensin II to $AT_1$ receptor in many tissues, such as vascular smooth muscle and the adrenal gland. HCTZ: Thiazide diuretic; affects renal tubular mechanisms of electrolyte reabsorption, directly increasing excretion of sodium and chloride and indirectly reducing plasma volume.

**PHARMACOKINETICS: Absorption:** Valsartan: Absolute bioavailability (25%); $T_{max}$=2-4 hrs. **Distribution:** Valsartan: $V_d$=17L (IV); plasma protein binding (95%). HCTZ: Crosses placenta; found in breast milk. **Metabolism:** Valsartan: Valeryl 4-hydroxy valsartan (primary metabolite). **Elimination:** Valsartan: Feces (83%), urine (13%) (oral solution); $T_{1/2}$=6 hrs. HCTZ: Urine (61%); $T_{1/2}$=5-15 hrs.

## NURSING CONSIDERATIONS

**Assessment:** Assess for volume/salt depletion, SLE, DM, anuria, hypersensitivity to sulfonamide or any component of the drug, history of allergies or bronchial asthma, hepatic/renal impairment, pregnancy/nursing status, and possible drug interactions.

**Monitoring:** Perform periodic measurements of serum electrolytes and renal function. Monitor for signs and symptoms of fluid or electrolyte imbalance, hypotension, hyperuricemia or precipitation of gout, exacerbation or activation of SLE, hypersensitivity reactions, hyperglycemia, increases in cholesterol and triglyceride levels, and renal/hepatic dysfunction.

**Patient Counseling:** Inform that drug can cause serious problems to the fetus; d/c and consult physician if pregnancy is detected. Advise that inadequate fluid intake, excessive perspiration, diarrhea or vomiting may result in drop of BP, leading to lightheadedness or syncope. Advise to seek medical attention if syncope, symptoms of electrolyte imbalance (eg, dry mouth, thirst, weakness), or hypersensitivity reactions occur.

**Administration:** Oral route. Take with or without food. **Storage:** 25°C (77°F); excursion permitted to 15-30°C (59-86°F). Protect from moisture.



## Diphenhydramine HCl Injection — RX

diphenhydramine HCl (Various)

**THERAPEUTIC CLASS:** Antihistamine

**INDICATIONS:** Amelioration of allergic reactions to blood or plasma. Adjunct to epinephrine in anaphylaxis. For other uncomplicated immediate-type allergic conditions when oral therapy is contraindicated. Treatment of motion sickness. For parkinsonism when oral therapy is not possible or contraindicated.

**DOSAGE:** *Adults:* Usual: 10-50mg IV or up to 100mg IM if needed. Max: 400mg/day.
*Pediatrics:* Usual: 5mg/kg/24 hrs or 150mg/m²/24 hrs IV/IM in 4 divided doses. Max: 300mg/day.

**HOW SUPPLIED:** Inj: 50mg/mL

**CONTRAINDICATIONS:** Neonates, premature infants, nursing, as a local anesthetic.

**WARNINGS/PRECAUTIONS:** Caution with narrow-angle glaucoma, stenosing peptic ulcer, pyloroduodenal obstruction, symptomatic prostatic hypertrophy, or bladder-neck obstruction. May cause excitation in pediatrics. Increased risk of dizziness, sedation, and hypotension in elderly. Caution with lower respiratory diseases, bronchial asthma, increased IOP, hyperthyroidism, CV disease, or HTN. Local necrosis with SQ or intradermal use.

**ADVERSE REACTIONS:** Sedation, drowsiness, dizziness, disturbed coordination, epigastric distress, thickening of bronchial secretions.

**INTERACTIONS:** Additive effects with alcohol and CNS depressants. MAOIs prolong and intensify anticholinergic effects.

**PREGNANCY:** Category B, contraindicated in nursing.

**MECHANISM OF ACTION:** Antihistamine; competes with histamine for cell receptor sites on effector cells.

**PHARMACOKINETICS: Metabolism:** Liver. **Elimination:** Urine.

### NURSING CONSIDERATIONS

**Assessment:** Assess for narrow-angle glaucoma, stenosing peptic ulcer, pyloroduodenal obstruction, prostatic hypertrophy, bladder-neck obstruction, history of bronchial asthma, increased IOP, hyperthyroidism, cardiovascular disease (HTN), lower respiratory disease, possible drug interactions, and nursing status.

**Monitoring:** Monitor for signs/symptoms of hypersensitivity reactions.

**Patient Counseling:** Caution may impair physical/mental abilities. Advise to seek medical attention if symptoms of hypersensitivity reactions occur.

**Administration:** IV, IM route **Storage:** 20-25°C (68-77°F). Protect from freezing and light.

## Diprolene — RX

betamethasone (augmented) dipropionate (Schering)

**OTHER BRAND NAMES:** Diprolene AF (Schering)

**THERAPEUTIC CLASS:** Corticosteroid

**INDICATIONS:** Relief of inflammatory and pruritic manifestations of corticosteroid-responsive dermatoses.

**DOSAGE:** *Adults:* (Lot) Apply qd-bid for no more than 2 weeks. Max: 50mL/week. (Cre, Oint) Apply qd-bid, up to 45g/week.
*Pediatrics:* ≥13 yrs: (Cre) Apply qd-bid for no more than 2 weeks. Limit to 45g/

week. ≥12 yrs: (Lot) Apply qd-bid for no more than 2 weeks. Limit to 50mL/week. (Oint) Apply qd-bid, up to 45g/week.

**HOW SUPPLIED:** Cre (AF), Oint: 0.05% [15g, 50g]; Lot: 0.05% [30mL, 60mL]

**WARNINGS/PRECAUTIONS:** May produce reversible HPA axis suppression, manifestations of Cushing's syndrome, hyperglycemia and glucosuria. D/C if irritation occurs. Use appropriate antifungal or antibacterial agent with dermatological infections. Pediatrics may be more susceptible to systemic toxicity. Caution when applied to large surface areas. Not for use with occlusive dressings. Gel is not for use in rosacea or perioral dermatitis or on the face, groin, or in the axillae.

**ADVERSE REACTIONS:** Stinging, burning, dry skin, pruritus, folliculitis, acneiform papules, irritation, hypopigmentation, skin maceration, secondary infection, skin atrophy, striae, miliaria.

**PREGNANCY:** Category C, (Cre, Lot) not for use in nursing; (Oint) caution in nursing.

**MECHANISM OF ACTION:** Corticosteroid; not established. Possesses anti-inflammatory, antipruritic, and vasoconstrictive actions.

**PHARMACOKINETICS: Absorption:** Percutaneous. Inflammation, use of occlusive dressings, and/or other disease states may increase absorption. **Distribution:** Systemically administered corticosteroids appear in breast milk. **Metabolism:** Liver. **Elimination:** Kidneys, bile.

## NURSING CONSIDERATIONS

**Assessment:** Assess for hypersensitivity to other corticosteroids. Assess use in pregnancy/nursing. Ensure medication is not being used for treatment of rosacea or perioral dermatitis or being used on face, groin, or in axillae.

**Monitoring:** Monitor signs/symptoms of HPA-axis suppression, Cushing's syndrome, hyperglycemia, and glucosuria. Perform periodic monitoring of HPA-axis suppression when using large doses, through use of urinary free cortisol and ACTH stimulation tests. Monitor for signs/symptoms of steroid withdrawal and treat accordingly. Monitor for signs of skin irritation and skin infection (eg, bacterial, fungal), and treat accordingly. In pediatric patients, monitor for systemic toxicity, HPA-axis suppression, Cushing's syndrome, and intracranial HTN.

**Patient Counseling:** Instruct to use externally, exactly as directed. Counsel to avoid contact with eyes. Inform not to bandage, cover, or wrap treated skin. Advise caregivers of pediatric patients not to use medication for treatment of diaper dermatitis and not to apply to diaper area. Advise to avoid using medication on face, underarms, or groin areas unless directed by physician. Instruct to contact physician if any signs of local adverse reactions develop or if there are no signs of clinical improvement within 2 weeks of initiating therapy.

**Administration:** Topical route. **Storage:** 25°C (77°F); excursions permitted to 15-30°C (59-86°F).

# DITROPAN XL — RX

oxybutynin chloride (Ortho-McNeil)

**OTHER BRAND NAMES:** Ditropan (Ortho-McNeil)

**THERAPEUTIC CLASS:** Anticholinergic

**INDICATIONS:** (All) Overactive bladder/bladder instability with symptoms of urge urinary incontinence, urgency, and frequency. (Tab, Extended-Release) Detrusor overactivity associated with a neurological condition in pediatrics ≥6 yrs.

**DOSAGE:** *Adults:* (Tab) Usual: 5mg bid-tid. Max: 5mg qid. Frail Elderly: 2.5mg bid-tid.(Tab, Extended-Release) Initial: 5 or 10mg qd. Titrate: May increase by 5mg weekly. Max: 30mg/day. Swallow XL whole with liquid; do not chew, divide, or crush tab.

*Pediatrics:* >5 yrs: (Tab) Usual: 5mg bid. Max: 5mg tid. ≥6 yrs: (Tab, Extended-

Release) Initial: 5mg qd. Titrate: May increase by 5mg weekly. Max: 20mg/day. Swallow XL whole with liquid; do not chew, divide, or crush tab.

**HOW SUPPLIED:** Tab: 5mg*; Tab, Extended-Release: 5mg, 10mg, 15mg
*scored

**CONTRAINDICATIONS:** Urinary retention, gastric retention and other severe decreased GI motility conditions, uncontrolled narrow-angle glaucoma, and in patients at risk for these conditions.

**WARNINGS/PRECAUTIONS:** Caution with hepatic or renal impairment, bladder outflow obstruction, GI obstruction/narrowing, ulcerative colitis, intestinal atony, gastroesophageal reflux disorder, myasthenia gravis, and pre-existing dementia. May aggravate symptoms of hyperthyroidism, CHD, CHF, arrythmias, hiatal hernia, tachycardia, HTN, myasthenia gravis, and prostatic hypertrophy. Reduce dose or d/c if anticholinergic CNS effects occur. Caution in frail elderly.

**ADVERSE REACTIONS:** Dry mouth, constipation, somnolence, headache, diarrhea, nausea, blurred vision, dyspepsia, pain, dizziness, UTI, memory impairment, QT interval prolongation, rash, impotence.

**INTERACTIONS:** Increased adverse effects with other anticholinergics. Increased drowsiness with alcohol. May alter GI absorption of other drugs due to GI motility effects. Increased levels with ketoconazole; caution with CYP3A4 inhibitors (eg, antimycotics, macrolides). Caution with bisphosphonates or other drugs that may exacerbate esophagitis.

**PREGNANCY:** Category B, caution in nursing.

**MECHANISM OF ACTION:** Antispasmodic/anticholinergic agent; inhibits muscarinic action of acetylcholine on smooth muscle exerting direct antispasmodic effect; relaxes smooth muscle of bladder.

**PHARMACOKINETICS: Absorption:** (Tab) Rapid; absolute bioavailability (6%). Refer to PI for pediatric, isomer, and metabolite parameters. **Distribution:** $V_d$=193L. **Metabolism:** Liver via CYP3A4; desethyloxybutynin (active metabolite). **Elimination:** Urine (<0.1% unchanged); $T_{1/2}$=2-3 hrs.

## NURSING CONSIDERATIONS

**Assessment:** Assess for bladder outflow obstruction (urinary retention), GI obstructive disorders (gastric retention), decreased GI motility conditions (UC, intestinal atony), GERD, GI narrowing, narrow-angle glaucoma, myasthenia gravis, hyperthyroidism, CAD, CHF, arrhythmias, hiatal hernia, HTN, prostatic hypertrophy, preexisting dementia, pregnancy/nursing status, possible drug interactions, and hepatic/renal impairment.

**Monitoring:** Monitor for aggravation of myasthenia gravis, hyperthyroidism, CAD, CHF, arrhythmias, hiatal hernia, HTN, prostatic hypertrophy symptoms, signs/symptoms of hypersensitivity reactions, GI narrowing (strictures), aggravation of dementia, and hepatic/renal impairment.

**Patient Counseling:** Inform heat prostration (fever, heat stroke due to decreased sweating), drowsiness, and blurred vision may occur. Instruct to avoid with alcohol. Swallow tab whole with liquid; do not chew, divide, or crush. Take approximately same time each day, with/without food. (Tab, Extended-Release) Inform that tablet shell may be excreted in the stool, and patient should not be concerned.

**Administration:** Oral route. **Storage:** (Tab): 15-30°C (59-86°F). (Tab, Extended-Release): 25°C (77°F); excursions permitted to 15-30°C (59-86°F). Protect from moisture and humidity.

# DOBUTAMINE — RX

dobutamine (Various)

**THERAPEUTIC CLASS:** Inotropic agent

**INDICATIONS:** Short-term treatment of cardiac decompensation due to depressed contractility resulting from organic heart disease or from cardiac surgical procedures.

**DOSAGE:** *Adults:* Initial: 0.5-1mcg/kg/min. Usual: 2-20mcg/kg/min. Max: 40mcg/kg/min (rare). Adjust rate and duration based on BP, urine flow, ectopic activity, HR, and when possible, cardiac output, central venous pressure, and/or pulmonary capillary wedge pressure.
*Pediatrics:* Initial: 0.5-1mcg/kg/min. Usual: 2-20mcg/kg/min. Max: 40mcg/kg/min (rare). Adjust rate and duration based on BP, urine flow, ectopic activity, HR, and when possible, cardiac output, central venous pressure, and/or pulmonary capillary wedge pressure.

**HOW SUPPLIED:** Inj: 12.5mg/mL

**CONTRAINDICATIONS:** Idiopathic hypertrophic subaortic stenosis (IHSS).

**WARNINGS/PRECAUTIONS:** May increase HR or BP, especially systolic pressure; caution with atrial fibrillation and HTN. May precipitate or exacerbate ventricular ectopic activity. Hypersensitivity reactions (eg, skin rash, fever, eosinophilia, bronchospasm) reported. Contains sulfites; caution in asthmatics. Monitor EKG, BP, pulmonary wedge pressure, and cardiac output. Correct hypovolemia prior to infusion. Caution in elderly. May decrease serum $K^+$ levels. Improvement may not be observed with marked mechanical obstruction (eg, severe valvular aortic stenosis).

**ADVERSE REACTIONS:** Increased HR, BP and ventricular ectopic activity, hypotension, infusion-site reactions, nausea, headache, anginal pain, palpitations, shortness of breath, decreased $K^+$ levels, nonspecific chest pain, phlebitis.

**INTERACTIONS:** Recent administration of β-blockers may reduce effectiveness and increase peripheral vascular resistance. Increased cardiac output and lower pulmonary wedge pressure with nitroprusside.

**PREGNANCY:** Category B, caution in nursing.

**MECHANISM OF ACTION:** Direct-acting inotropic agent; stimulates β-receptors of the heart while producing comparatively mild chronotropic, hypertensive, arrhythmogenic, and vasodilative effects.

**PHARMACOKINETICS: Metabolism**: Methylation of the catechol and conjugation. **Elimination**: Urine (the conjugates of dobutamine and 3-O-methyl dobutamine; inactive metabolite).

## NURSING CONSIDERATIONS

**Assessment:** Assess for IHSS, mechanical obstruction (eg, valvular aortic stenosis), HTN, atrial fibrillation, drug or sulfite hypersensitivity and pregnancy/nursing status. Prior to treatment, correct hypovolemia if present.

**Monitoring:** Continuous monitoring of ECG, BP, pulmonary wedge pressure, cardiac output. Monitor for HR and BP, hypersensitivity reactions (eg, skin rash, fever, eosinophilia, and bronchospasm), allergic-type reactions, including anaphylactic symptoms and life-threatening or less severe asthmatic episodes, ectopic activity or ventricular tachycardia, and serum potassium.

**Patient Counseling:** Inform that drug may increase HR and BP. Report if experience any reactions at infusion site, palpitations, or SOB.

**Administration:** IV route. Observe for particulate matter prior to administration. **Storage:** 15-30°C (59-86°F).

# DOLOPHINE

methadone HCl (Roxane)

**Only approved hospitals and pharmacies can dispense oral methadone for the treatment of narcotic addiction. Deaths, cardiac and respiratory, have been reported during initiation and conversion of pain in patients to methadone treatment from treatment with other opioid agonists. Respiratory depression is the main hazard associated with administration. QT interval prolongation and serious arrhythmias have been observed during treatment. Initiate treatment for analgesia in patients with acute or chronic pain only if benefits outweigh the risks.**

**OTHER BRAND NAMES:** Methadone (Various)

**THERAPEUTIC CLASS:** Opioid analgesic

D

**INDICATIONS:** Detoxification and maintenance treatment of opioid addiction (heroin or other morphine-like drugs). Treatment of moderate to severe pain not responsive to non-narcotic analgesics.

**DOSAGE:** *Adults:* Detoxification: Initial: 20-30mg single dose. Max: 30mg. Evaluate after 2-4 hrs. Give 5-10mg if withdrawal symptoms reappear. Total daily dose on 1st day of treatment should not exceed 40mg. Short-term Detoxification: Titrate to a total daily dose of 40mg in divided doses. Stabilize for 2-3 days, then may decrease every 1-2 days depending on symptoms. Maint: Titrate to a dose at which opioid symptoms are prevented for 24 hrs. Usual range: 80-120mg/day. Withdrawal after Maintenance Treatment: Reduce dose <10% of established tolerance q10-14 days. Pain (Opioid Non-Tolerant): Usual: 2.5-10mg q8-12h slowly titrated to effect. Conversion from Parenteral to Oral Methadone: Use 1:2 dose ratio initially. See PI for switching to methadone from other chronic opioids.

**HOW SUPPLIED:** Tab: 5mg, 10mg

**CONTRAINDICATIONS:** Acute bronchial asthma or hypercarbia, respiratory depression, with suspicion of a paralytic ileus.

**WARNINGS/PRECAUTIONS:** Extreme caution if narcotic antagonists used in patients physically dependent on narcotics. Incomplete cross-tolerance and iatrogenic overdose may occur. Can cause CSF pressure elevation. Caution with head injuries, acute asthma attacks, COPD, cor pulmonale, decreased respiratory reserve, pre-existing respiratory depression, hypoxia, or hypercapnia. Reduce initial dose in elderly, debilitated, severe hepatic or renal impairment, hypothyroidism, Addison's disease, prostatic hypertrophy, or urethral stricture. Drug tolerance, dependence, and abuse may occur. Infants born to opioid-dependent mothers may exhibit respiratory difficulties and withdrawal symptoms. Impairs physical and mental abilities. Ineffective in relieving anxiety. May mask symptoms and clinical course of acute abdominal conditions and head injuries. May produce hypotension. Incomplete cross-tolerance and iatrogenic overdose may occur as well as interactions with other CNS depressants, alcohol and other drugs of abuse.

**ADVERSE REACTIONS:** Lightheadedness, dizziness, sedation, sweating, N/V, asthenia, cardiomyopathy, ECG abnormalities, abdominal pain, agitation, seizures, confusion, hallucinations, respiratory depression.

**INTERACTIONS:** Concomitant use with other opioid analgesics, general anesthesia, phenothiazines, sedatives, hypnotics, and other CNS depressants (including alcohol) may experience respiratory depression, hypotension, profound sedation, or coma. Concomitant use with phenytoin, rifampin, opioid antagonists, mixed agonists/antagonists, and partial agonists may precipitate withdrawal symptoms. Decreased plasma levels with antiretrovirals. Increased AUC of zidovudine. Decreased AUC and peak levels of didanosine and stavudine. May precipitate severe reactions with monoamine oxidase inhibitors (MAOIs). Increased levels of desipramine. Caution with drugs known to prolong QT interval. Pharmacodynamic interaction may occur with class I and III antiarrhythmics, some neuroleptics, tricyclic antidepressants (TCAs), and calcium channel blockers (CCBs). Caution with drugs capable of inducing electrolyte imbalance (eg, diuretics, laxatives, mineralocorticoids). Decreased effects with CYP450 inducers while CYP450 inhibitors (eg, azole antifungals, macrolide antibiotics, SSRIs) may potentiate effects.

**PREGNANCY:** Category C, not for use in nursing.

**MECHANISM OF ACTION:** Opioid analgesic; μ-agonist. Produces many actions similiar to morphine. Acts prominently in the CNS and in organs composed of smooth muscle. Also acts as an antagonist at the N-methyl-D-aspartate (NMDA) receptor.

**PHARMACOKINETICS: Absorption:** Bioavailability (36-100%); $C_{max}$=124-1255ng/mL; $T_{max}$=1-7.5 hrs. **Distribution:** $V_d$=1.0-8.0L/kg; plasma protein binding (85-90%); found in saliva, breast milk, amniotic fluid, and umbilical cord plasma. **Metabolism:** Liver (N-demethylation) via CYP450 enzymes: 3A4 (primary), 2B6 (primary), 2C19 (primary); 2C9; 2D6. **Elimination:** Urine, feces; $T_{1/2}$=8-59 hrs.

D

## NURSING CONSIDERATIONS

**Assessment:** Assess for respiratory depression, acute bronchial asthma, hypercarbia, COPD, paralytic ileus, CNS depression or coma, age of patient, risk of QT prolongation (eg, cardiac hypertrophy, concomitant diuretic use, hypokalemia), potential for drug abuse, presence of head injury or other intracranial lesions, pre-existing elevation in ICP, hypotension, acute abdominal conditions, renal/hepatic impairment, hypothyroidism, Addison's disease, prostatic hypertrophy or urethral stricture, hypersensitivity, pregnancy/nursing status, and possible drug interactions.

**Monitoring:** Monitor for signs/symptoms of respiratory depression, QT prolongation and arrhythmia (eg, torsades de pointes), elevations in CSF pressure, hypotension, misuse or abuse, and tolerance or dependence, and hypersensitivity reactions.

**Patient Counseling:** Inform that drug may impair mental/physical abilities; use caution when performing hazardous tasks (eg, operating machinery/driving). Avoid use of other CNS depressants and alcohol during therapy. Instruct to notify physician if develop symptoms suggestive of arrhythmia (eg, palpitations, dizziness, lightheadedness, syncope). Medication may produce orthostatic hypotension. Avoid abrupt withdrawal from medication. Instruct that if using for treatment of opioid dependence, discontinuation may lead to relapse of illicit drug use.

**Administration:** Oral route. **Storage**: 25°C (77°F); excursions permitted to 15-30°C (59-86°F). Dispense in tight, light-resistant container.

## DONNATAL RX

hyoscyamine sulfate - atropine sulfate - scopolamine hydrobromide - phenobarbital (PBM Pharmaceuticals)

**OTHER BRAND NAMES:** Donnatal Extentabs (PBM Pharmaceuticals)

**THERAPEUTIC CLASS:** Anticholinergic/barbiturate

**INDICATIONS:** Adjunct therapy for irritable bowel syndrome, acute enterocolitis, duodenal ulcers.

**DOSAGE:** *Adults:* (Elixir/Tab) 1-2 tabs or 5-10mL tid-qid. (Extentabs) 1 tab q8-12h. Hepatic Disease: Use lower doses.
*Pediatrics:* (Elixir) 4.5kg: 0.5mL q4h or 0.75mL q6h. 9.1kg: 1mL q4h or 1.5mL q6h. 13.6kg: 1.5mL q4h or 2mL q6h. 22.7kg: 2.5mL q4h or 3.75mL q6h. 34kg: 3.75mL q4h or 5mL q6h. 45.4kg: 5mL q4h or 7.5mL q6h. Hepatic Disease: Use lower doses.

**HOW SUPPLIED:** (Atropine-Hyoscyamine-Phenobarbital-Scopolamine) Elixir: 0.0194mg-0.1037mg-16.2mg-0.0065mg/5mL; Tab: 0.0194mg-0.1037mg-16.2mg-0.0065mg; Tab, Extended-Release: (Extentabs) 0.0582mg-0.3111mg-48.6mg-0.0195mg

**CONTRAINDICATIONS:** Glaucoma, obstructive uropathy, obstructive GI disease, paralytic ileus, intestinal atony in elderly or debilitated, unstable cardiovascular status in acute hemorrhage, severe ulcerative colitis, myasthenia gravis, hiatal hernia with reflux esophagitis, intermittent porphyria, and for patients in whom phenobarbital produces restlessness and/or excitement.

**WARNINGS/PRECAUTIONS:** Inconclusive whether anticholinergic/antispasmodic drugs aid in duodenal ulcer healing, decrease recurrence rate, or prevent complications. Heat prostration can occur with high environmental temperatures. Avoid with intestinal obstruction. May be habit forming; caution with history of physical and/or psychological drug dependence. Caution with hepatic disease, renal disease, autonomic neuropathy, hyperthyroidism, coronary heart disease, CHF, arrhythmias, tachycardia, HTN. May delay gastric emptying. Diarrhea may be an early symptom of incomplete intestinal obstruction, especially with ileostomy or colostomy; treatment would be inappropriate.

**ADVERSE REACTIONS:** Xerostomia, urinary hesitancy/retention, blurred vision, tachycardia/palpitation, mydriasis, cycloplegia, increased ocular tension, loss of taste, headache, nervousness, drowsiness, weakness, dizziness, insomnia, nausea, vomiting, impotence, suppression of lactation, constipation, bloated feeling, musculoskeletal pain, allergic reaction/drug idiosyncrasies, decreased sweating.

**INTERACTIONS:** Phenobarbital may decrease anticoagulant effects; adjust dose.

**PREGNANCY:** Category C, caution in nursing.

**MECHANISM OF ACTION:** Anticholinergic/Barbiturate; drug combination provides peripheral anticholinergic, antispasmodic action and mild sedation.

## NURSING CONSIDERATIONS

**Assessment:** Assess for glaucoma, obstructive uropathy, obstructive disease of the GIT, paralytic ileus, ulcerative colitis, myasthenia gravis, hiatal hernia associated with reflux esophagitis, acute intermittent porphyria, renal/hepatic dysfunction, hyperthyroidism, cardiac disorders.

**Monitoring:** Monitor occurrence of heat prostration, drowsiness, blurred vision, HR, constipation, diarrhea, urinary hesitancy/retention, hypersensitivity reactions.

**Patient Counseling:** Counsel about side effects; report adverse effects. Counsel about drug abuse/dependence. Exercise caution while operating machinery/driving. Avoid high environmental temperatures.

**Administration:** Oral route. **Storage**: 20-25°C (68-77°F). Protect from light and moisture. Dispense in well-closed, light-resistant container using child-resistant closure.

# DOPAMINE RX

dopamine HCl (Various)

**OTHER BRAND NAMES:** Dopamine Hcl and 5% Dextrose (Baxter)

**THERAPEUTIC CLASS:** Inotropic agent

**INDICATIONS:** For correction of hemodynamic imbalances present in shock due to MI, trauma, endotoxic septicemia, open-heart surgery, renal failure, and chronic cardiac decompensation. (Dextrose); Hypotension due to inadequate cardiac output.

**DOSAGE:** *Adults:* Initial: 2-5mcg/kg/min. Use 5mcg/kg/min in seriously ill. Increase in 5-10mcg/kg/min increments, up to 20-50mcg/kg/min. (Dextrose): Avoid bolus administration. Elderly: Start at low end of dosing range. Drug additives should not be made.
*Pediatrics:* (Dextrose): Initial: 1-5mcg/kg/min. Max: 15-20mcg/kg/min, occasional ≥50mcg/kg/min.

**HOW SUPPLIED:** Inj: 40mg/mL, 80mg/mL, 160mg/mL. (Dopamine HCl and Dextrose) 800mcg/mL, 1600mcg/mL, 3200mcg/mL

**CONTRAINDICATIONS:** Pheochromocytoma, uncorrected tachyarrhythmias or ventricular fibrillation. (Dextrose); Allergy to corn or corn products.

**WARNINGS/PRECAUTIONS:** Contains sulfites. Monitor BP, urine flow, cardiac output and pulmonary wedge pressure. Correct hypovolemia, hypoxia, hypercapnia, and acidosis prior to use. Reduce infusion rate with increase in diastolic BP/marked decrease in pulse pressure; increase rate if hypotension occurs. D/C if hypotension persists. Reduce dose if increased ectopic beats occurs. Caution with history of occlusive vascular disease (eg, atherosclerosis, arterial embolism, Raynaud's disease, cold injury, diabetic endarteritis, and Buerger's disease); monitor for changes in skin color or temperature. Administer phentolamine if extravasation noted. Avoid abrupt withdrawal. (Dextrose): Do not add to any alkaline diluent solution. Do not administer at the same set as blood; pseudoagglutination or hemolysis may result. May cause fluid overloading. Caution in children and elderly. Avoid bolus administration.

**ADVERSE REACTIONS:** Tachycardia, palpitation, ventricular arrhythmia (high doses), dyspnea, nausea, vomiting, headache, anxiety, bradycardia, hypotension, HTN, vasoconstriction.

D

**INTERACTIONS:** If treated with MAOIs within 2-3 weeks prior to administration of dopamine, reduce initial dose of dopamine to not greater than 1/10th of usual dose. Potential additive or potentiating effects on urine flow with diuretics. TCAs may potentiate cardiovascular effects of adrenergic agents. Cardiac effects antagonized by β-blockers. Peripheral vasoconstriction antagonized by α-blockers. Butyrophenones (eg, haloperidol) and phenothiazines may suppress renal and mesenteric vasodilation. Extreme caution with cyclopropane or halogenated hydrocarbon anesthetics. Concomitant use with vasopressors, vasoconstricting agents (eg, ergonovine), some oxytocic drugs, and local anesthetics may result in severe HTN. Hypotension and bradycardia reported with phenytoin; consider alternatives.

**PREGNANCY:** Category C, caution in nursing.

**MECHANISM OF ACTION:** Catecholamine; produces positive chronotropic and inotropic effects on the myocardium, resulting in increased heart rate and cardiac contractility. Acts directly by exerting an agonist action on β-adrenoreceptor and indirectly by causing release of norepinephrine from storage sites in sympathetic nerve endings.

**PHARMACOKINETICS: Metabolism**: Liver, kidneys, and plasma via MAO and catechol-O-methyltransferase. **Elimination:** Urine (80%) as homovanillic acid and 3,4-dihydroxyphenylacetic acid.

## NURSING CONSIDERATIONS

**Assessment:** Assess for sulfite hypersensitivity, pheochromocytoma, uncorrected tachyarrhythmias/ventricular fibrillation, history of occlusive vascular disease (eg, atherosclerosis, arterial embolism, Raynaud's disease, cold injury, diabetic endarteritis, and Buerger's disease), pregnancy status, and possible drug interactions. Assess and correct prior to, or concurrently with, administration of therapy for hypovolemia, hypoxia, acidosis, and hypercapnia. Assess pregnancy/nursing status.

**Monitoring:** Close monitoring of urine flow, cardiac output, BP, and central venous pressure. Monitor for ventricular arrhythmias, decreased pulse pressure, hypotension, extravasation/peripheral ischemia; sloughing and necrosis of the surrounding tissue and allergic-type reactions, including anaphylactic symptoms and life-threatening or less severe asthmatic episodes. In occlusive vascular disease, monitor for changes in color or temperature of skin in extremities.

**Patient Counseling:** Inform about benefits/risks of therapy.

**Administration:** IV infusion route. Not for direct IV injection; drug must be diluted before administration to patient. Avoid injection to sodium bicarbonate or other alkaline and/or amphotericin B solutions. **Storage:** 15-30°C (59-86°F). (Dopamine Hcl and Dextrose): 25-40°C. Avoid excessive heat. Protect from freezing.

# DORIBAX — RX

doripenem (Ortho-McNeil)

**THERAPEUTIC CLASS:** Carbapenem

**INDICATIONS:** Treatment of complicated intra-abdominal and urinary tract infections, including pyelonephritis, caused by susceptible microorganisms.

**DOSAGE: Adults:** ≥18 yrs: 500mg IV q8h for 5-14 days (intra-abdominal) or 10 days (UTI). Infuse over 1 hour. Renal Impairment: CrCl: >50mL/min: No dose adjustment. CrCl 30-50mL/min: 250mg IV q8h. CrCl >10 to <30mL/min: 250mg IV q12h.

**HOW SUPPLIED:** Inj: 500mg

**CONTRAINDICATIONS:** Anaphylactic reactions to β-lactams.

**WARNINGS/PRECAUTIONS:** Serious hypersensitivity (anaphylactic) reactions reported. *Clostridium difficile*-associated diarrhea reported (ranging from mild diarrhea to fatal colitis); evaluate if diarrhea occurs. Consider alternative antibacterial therapies in patients receiving valproic acid or sodium valproate due to increased risk of breakthrough seizures. Increased risk of development of drug resistant bacteria in the absence of proven or strongly suspected bacterial infection. Do not administer via inhalation.

**ADVERSE REACTIONS:** Headache, nausea, diarrhea, rash, phlebitis, anemia, pruritus, anaphylaxis, neutropenia, leukopenia.

**INTERACTIONS:** May reduce serum valproic acid levels, which may increase risk of breakthrough seizures. Probenecid may increase levels; avoid co-administration.

**PREGNANCY:** Category B, caution in nursing.

**MECHANISM OF ACTION:** Broad-spectrum carbapenem; exerts bactericidal activity by inhibiting cell wall biosynthesis, resulting in cell death.

**PHARMACOKINETICS: Absorption:** $C_{max}$=23mcg/mL, AUC=36.3mcg•hr/mL. **Distribution:** $V_d$=16.8L; plasma protein binding (8.1%). **Metabolism:** Via dehydropeptidase-1. **Elimination:** Urine (70% unchanged and 15% metabolites), feces (<1%); $T_{1/2}$=1 hr.

## NURSING CONSIDERATIONS

**Assessment:** Assess for previous hypersensitivity reactions to other carbapenems, cephalosporins, PCNs, or other allergens. Assess for renal impairment and possible drug interactions. Document indications for therapy and culture and susceptibility testing.

**Monitoring:** Monitor for signs/symptoms of anaphylactoid/hypersensitivity reactions, CDAD, superinfection, seizures, anemia, phlebitis, rash.

**Patient Counseling:** Inform drug only treats bacterial, not viral, infections. Take exactly as directed; skipping doses or not completing full course may decrease effectiveness and increase resistance. May experience diarrhea; notify physician if taking valproic acid or if watery/bloody stools, hypersensitivity reactions, infection, or seizures occur.

**Administration:** IV route. **Storage:** Store at 25°C (77°F); excursions permitted to 15-30°C (59-86°F).

# DORYX RX

doxycycline hyclate (Warner Chilcott)

**THERAPEUTIC CLASS:** Tetracycline derivative

**INDICATIONS:** Treatment of the following infections: upper respiratory tract, respiratory tract, urinary tract, lymphogranuloma venereum, psittacosis, trachoma, uncomplicated urethral/endocervical/rectal, nongonococcal urethritis, relapsing fever, Rocky Mountain spotted fever, typhus fever and the typhus group, Q fever, rickettsialpox, tick fevers, inclusion conjunctivitis, tularemia, *Campylobacter* fetus infections, bartonellosis, granuloma inguinale, chancroid, plague, cholera, brucellosis, anthrax (including inhalational anthrax, post-exposure). When penicillin is contraindicated, treatment of syphilis, yaws, Vincent's infection, actinomycosis, and infections caused by *Clostridium* species. Adjunct therapy for acute intestinal amebiasis and severe acne. Prophylaxis of malaria due to *Plasmodium falciparum* in short-term travelers (<4 months) to areas with chloroquine and/or pyrimethamine-sulfadoxine resistant strains.

**DOSAGE:** *Adults:* Usual: 100mg q12h on 1st day, followed by 100mg/day (single dose or as 50mg q12h) or 100mg q12h for more severe infections (eg, chronic UTIs). *Streptococcus* Infection: Treat for 10 days. Uncomplicated Urethral, Endocervical, or Rectal Infection/ Nongonococcal Urethritis: 100mg bid for 7 days. Syphilis (Early): 100mg bid for 14 days. Syphilis (>1 yr): 100mg bid for 28 days. Acute Epididymo-orchitis: 100mg bid for ≥10 days. Inhalational Anthrax (post-exposure): 100mg bid for 60 days. Malaria Prophylaxis: 100mg qd, beginning 1-2 days before travel, continuing daily during travel and for 28 days after departure from malarious area. Elderly: Start at lower end of dosing range.

*Pediatrics:* >8 yrs: >100 lbs: Usual: 100mg q12h on 1st day, followed by 100mg/day (single dose or as 50mg q12h) or 100mg q12h for more severe infections (eg, chronic UTIs). *Streptococcus* Infection: Treat for 10 days.

D

Inhalational Anthrax (post-exposure): 100mg bid for 60 days. Malaria Prophylaxis: 100mg qd, beginning 1-2 days before travel, continuing daily during travel and for 28 days after departure from malarious area. Elderly: Start at lower end of dosing range. ≤100 lbs: Usual: 2mg/lb divided into 2 doses on 1st day, followed by 1mg/lb/day or up to 2mg/lb/day (single dose or divided into 2 doses) for more severe infections thereafter. *Streptococcus* Infection: Treat for 10 days. Inhalational Anthrax (post-exposure): 1mg/lb bid for 60 days. Malaria Prophylaxis: 2mg/kg qd, beginning 1-2 days before travel, continuing daily during travel and for 28 days after departure from malarious area. Max: 100mg/day

**HOW SUPPLIED:** Tab, Delayed-Release: 75mg*, 100mg*, 150mg* *scored

**WARNINGS/PRECAUTIONS:** *Clostridium difficile*-associated diarrhea (CDAD) reported. May decrease bone growth in premature infants, and cause fetal harm during pregnancy. May cause permanent discoloration of the teeth or enamel hypoplasia if used in last half of pregnancy, infancy or <8 yrs. Photosensitivity, increased BUN, false elevations of urinary catecholamines, and superinfection may occur. Bulging fontanels in infants and benign intracranial HTN in adults reported. Incision and drainage or other surgical procedures should be performed in conjunction when indicated. Those using doxycycline as a prophylaxis for malaria may transmit the infection to mosquitoes outside endemic areas. Use in the absence of the proper indication increases the risk of the development of drug-resistance. When coexistent syphilis is suspected, perform dark-field examination before treatment and blood serology repeatedly monthly for at least 4 months. Caution in elderly.

**ADVERSE REACTIONS:** Anorexia, N/V, diarrhea, dysphagia, enterocolitis, rash, inflammatory lesions in the anogenital area, exfoliative dermatitis, renal toxicity, hemolytic anemia, hypersensitivity reactions.

**INTERACTIONS:** May depress plasma PT, adjust anticoagulant dose with concomitant use. May interfere with bactericidal action of penicillin; avoid concurrent use when possible. Impaired absorption with bismuth subsalicylate and antacids containing aluminum, calcium or magnesium and iron-containing preparations. Decreased $T_{1/2}$ with barbiturates, carbamazepine and phenytoin. Fatal renal toxicity with methoxyflurane. May render oral contraceptives less effective.

**PREGNANCY:** Category D, not for use in nursing.

**MECHANISM OF ACTION:** Tetracycline; exert bacteriostatic effect by the inhibition of protein synthesis.

**PHARMACOKINETICS: Absorption:** Complete; $C_{max}$=2.6 mcg/mL; $T_{max}$=2 hrs. **Distribution:** Found in breast milk. **Metabolism:** Liver. **Elimination:** Urine and feces. $T_{1/2}$=18-22 hrs.

## NURSING CONSIDERATIONS

**Assessment:** Assess for hypersensitivity reactions, renal impairment, pregnancy/nursing status and possible drug interactions. Document indications for therapy, culture and susceptibility testing. Perform incision and drainage in conjunction with antibiotic therapy when indicated. When coexistent syphilis is suspected, perform dark-field examination before treatment and blood serology repeatedly monthly for at least 4 months.

**Monitoring:** Monitor for hypersensitivity reactions, photosensitivity, superinfection, CDAD, benign intracranial HTN. Monitor LFTs, hematopoietic values and renal function in long term therapy. When coexistent syphilis is suspected, perform blood serology repeatedly monthly for at least 4 months.

**Patient Counseling:** Inform of pregnancy risks and to avoid pregnancy. Counsel about photosensitivity reactions and to d/c at first sign of skin erythema. Advise to avoid excessive sunlight/UV light and wear sunscreen or sunblock. Take exactly as directed, skipping doses or not completing full course may decrease effectiveness and increase resistance. Avoid foods with calcium and drink fluids liberally to reduce risk of esophageal irritation or ulceration. Advise that may increase the incidence of vaginal candidiasis. Inform that drug only treats bacterial, not viral, infections. Diarrhea may occur; contact physician if watery/bloody stools, hypersensitivity reactions, superinfections, photosensitivity or benign intracranial HTN occurs. Counsel on malaria prophylaxis to begin therapy 2 days before travel; continue while in the malarious area and for 4 weeks after return. Therapy should not exceed 4 months. Counsel on appropriate way to take medicine, i.e. take with adequate amount of fluid, take with food or milk if gastric irritation occurs, and may sprinkle contents on a spoonful of applesauce to be swallowed without chewing followed by a glass of water.

**Administration:** Oral route. **Storage:** 25°C (77°F); excursions permitted to 15-30°C (59-86°F). Dispense in tight, light-resistant container.

D

## Dovonex RX

calcipotriene (Warner Chilcott)

**THERAPEUTIC CLASS:** Vitamin $D_3$ derivative

**INDICATIONS:** Treatment of plaque psoriasis.

**DOSAGE:** *Adults:* (Cream) Apply thin layer to affected skin bid and rub in gently and completely for up to 8 weeks. Wash hands after application.

**HOW SUPPLIED:** Cre: 0.005% [60g, 120g]

**CONTRAINDICATIONS:** Hypercalcemia or vitamin D toxicity. Do not use on the face.

**WARNINGS/PRECAUTIONS:** Avoid face and eyes. D/C if irritation or hypercalcemia occur; may continue once calcium levels are normal. Avoid excessive exposure to either natural or artificial sunlight.

**ADVERSE REACTIONS:** Local irritation, rash, pruritus, dermatitis, worsening of psoriasis.

**PREGNANCY:** Category C, caution in nursing.

**MECHANISM OF ACTION:** Vitamin $D_3$ derivative.

**PHARMACOKINETICS: Metabolism:** Liver. **Elimination:** Bile.

### NURSING CONSIDERATIONS

**Assessment:** Assess for drug hypersensitivity reactions, hypercalcemia, evidence of vitamin D toxicity, pregnancy/nursing status.

**Monitoring:** Monitor for serum calcium concentration, irritation of lesions and surrounding uninvolved skin.

**Patient Counseling:** Advise to take drug as prescribed; report signs of adverse reactions. Counsel to avoid excessive exposure to natural or artificial sunlight after application. For external use only; avoid contact with eyes or face. Advise to wash hands after application.

**Administration:** Topical route. **Storage:** 15-25°C (59-77°F). Do not freeze.

## Dovonex Scalp RX

calcipotriene (Warner Chilcott)

**THERAPEUTIC CLASS:** Vitamin $D_3$ derivative

**INDICATIONS:** Topical treatment of chronic, moderately severe psoriasis of the scalp.

**DOSAGE:** *Adults:* Comb hair to remove debris. After parting hair, apply and rub into affected area(s) bid for up to 8 weeks. Avoid uninvolved skin. Wash hands after application.

**HOW SUPPLIED:** Sol: 0.005% [60mL]

**CONTRAINDICATIONS:** Acute psoriatic eruptions, hypercalcemia, vitamin D toxicity.

**WARNINGS/PRECAUTIONS:** Avoid mucous membranes and eyes. D/C if irritation, sensitivity reaction, or hypercalcemia occur; may continue once calcium levels are normal. Avoid excessive exposure to either natural or artificial sunlight.

**ADVERSE REACTIONS:** Transient burning, stinging, tingling, rash, dry skin, irritation and worsening of psoriasis.

**PREGNANCY:** Category C, caution in nursing.

**MECHANISM OF ACTION:** Vitamin $D_3$ derivative; not understood. It is roughly equipotent to the natural vitamin in its effects on proliferation and differentiation of a variety of cell types.

D

**PHARMACOKINETICS: Metabolism:** Liver. **Elimination:** Bile.

## NURSING CONSIDERATIONS

**Assessment:** Assess for drug hypersensitivity, acute psoriatic eruptions, hypercalcemia, evidence of vitamin D toxicity, pregnancy/nursing status.

**Monitoring:** Monitor for irritation of both lesions of surrounding uninvolved skin, hypersensitivity reactions and serum calcium concentration.

**Patient Counseling:** Advise to use as directed and to d/c and contact physician if any adverse reactions occur. Avoid excessive exposure to natural or artificial sunlight after application. Counsel drug for external use only; avoid contact with face or eyes. Keep away from open flame.

**Administration:** Topical route. **Storage:** 15-25°C (59-77°F). Do not freeze. Avoid sunlight. Keep away from open flame.

# DOXIL — RX

doxorubicin HCl liposome (Ortho Biotech)

**Myocardial damage may lead to CHF when cumulative dose approaches 550mg/m². May lead to cardiac toxicity; consider prior use of anthracyclines or anthracenediones in cumulative dose calculations. Cardiac toxicity may occur at lower cumulative doses with prior mediastinal irradiation or concurrent cardiotoxic agents, such as cyclophosphamide. Acute infusion-associated reactions reported. Severe myelosuppression, myocardial toxicity may occur. Reduce dose with impaired hepatic function. Severe side effects reported with accidental substitution for doxorubicin HCl; do not substitute on mg-per-mg basis.**

**THERAPEUTIC CLASS:** Anthracycline

**INDICATIONS:** Treatment of ovarian cancer which has progressed or recurred after platinum-based chemotherapy. Treatment of AIDS-related Kaposi's sarcoma (KS) in patients with disease that has progressed on prior combination chemotherapy or in patients intolerant to such therapy. In combination with bortezomib for the treatment of multiple myeloma (MM) in patients who have not previously received bortezomib and have received at least one prior therapy.

**DOSAGE:** *Adults:* Administer as IV infusion at initial rate of 1mg/min to minimize risk of infusion-related reactions; if no reactions, may increase rate to complete infusion over 1 hr. Ovarian Cancer: 50mg/m² IV every 4 weeks for minimum of 4 courses. KS: 20mg/m² IV once every 3 weeks. MM: Give bortezomib 1.3mg/m² IV bolus on Days 1, 4, 8 and 11, every 3 weeks. Give doxorubicin 30mg/m² IV on Day 4 following bortezomib. May treat for up to 8 cycles depending on disease progression or unacceptable toxicity. Hepatic Dysfunction: If serum bilirubin 1.2-3mg/dL, give 50% of normal dose. If serum bilirubin >3mg/dL, give 25% of normal dose. Adjust dose based on toxicities (see PI).

**HOW SUPPLIED:** Inj: 2mg/mL

**CONTRAINDICATIONS:** Nursing mothers.

**WARNINGS/PRECAUTIONS:** Monitor cardiac function. Cardiac toxicity may occur after d/c. Recall of skin reaction due to radiotherapy reported. Myelosuppression may occur; obtain CBCs, including platelets frequently and at a minimum before each dose. Secondary AML reported with anthracyclines. Evaluate hepatic function before therapy. Avoid extravasation. Can cause fetal harm. Hand-foot syndrome and acute infusion-related reactions reported.

**ADVERSE REACTIONS:** Neutropenia, leukopenia, anemia, thromobocytopenia, stomatitis, fever, anorexia, fatigue, N/V, asthenia, rash, alopecia, diarrhea, constipation, hand-foot syndrome.

**INTERACTIONS:** See Black Box Warning. May potentiate toxicity of other anticancer therapies. May exacerbate cyclophosphamide-induced hemorrhagic cystitis. May enhance hepatotoxicity of 6-mercaptopurine. May increase radiation-induced toxicity of the myocardium, mucosa, skin, and liver. Hematological toxicity may be more severe with agents that cause bone-marrow suppression.

**PREGNANCY:** Category D, not for use in nursing.

**MECHANISM OF ACTION:** Anthracycline topoisomerase inhibitor; suspected to bind DNA and inhibit nucleic acid synthesis.

**PHARMACOKINETICS: Absorption:** (10mg/m²) $C_{max}$=4.12mcg/mL, AUC=277mcg/mL•h. (20mg/m²) $C_{max}$=8.34mcg/mL, AUC=590mcg/mL•h. **Distribution**: (10mg/m²) $V_d$=2.83L/m²; (20mg/m²) $V_d$=2.72L/m². **Metabolism:** Doxorubicinol (metabolite).

## NURSING CONSIDERATIONS

**Assessment:** Assess for history of CVD, radiotherapy, hepatic dysfunction, pregnancy/nursing status, and possible drug interactions. Obtain baseline WBC, neutrophil and platelet counts, Hgb/Hct, LFTs, and cardiac function.

**Monitoring:** Monitor CBCs including platelet counts, Hgb/Hct, LFTs, and cardiac function (EKG, multigated radionuclide scan) periodically. Signs and symptoms of hypersensitivity reaction, infusion reaction (flushing, SOB, facial swelling, headache, chills, back pain, tightness in chest or throat), severe myelosuppression (superinfection, neutropenic fever, hemorrhage), extravasation (stinging or burning sensation), recall reaction (radiotherapy), cardiotoxicity (CHF), impaired hepatic function, hand and foot syndrome (swelling, pain, erythema, and desquamation of skin of hands and feet), and stomatitis.

**Patient Counseling:** Inform that reddish-orange urine and other bodily fluids may occur. Inform of pregnancy risks. Advise to seek medical attention if symptoms of hypersensitivity reaction (rash), infusion reaction (flushing, SOB, facial swelling, headache, chills, back pain, tightness in chest or throat), infection, neutropenia, fever, hemorrhage, stinging or burning sensation, N/V, tiredness, weakness, mild hair loss, hand and foot syndrome (swelling, pain, erythema, and desquamation of skin of hands and feet), and stomatitis occur.

**Administration:** IV route. Do not administer as bolus injection or undiluted solution. Do not use with in-line filters. **Storage:** Refrigerate at 2-8°C (36-46°F). Avoid freezing.

# Doxorubicin HCl — RX

doxorubicin HCl (Various)

**To be administered only under supervision of a physician experienced in use of cancer chemotherapeutic agents. Severe local tissue necrosis will occur if extravasation occurs. Do not give IM/SC route. Myocardial toxicity may occur during or after therapy. Increased risk of CHF with high cumulative doses, previous anthracycline/anthracenedione therapy, pre-existing heart disease, radiotherapy to mediastinal/pericardial area, concomitant cardiotoxic drugs. Increased risk of delayed cardiotoxicity in pediatrics. Secondary acute myelogenous leukemia (AML) reported. Reduce dose in hepatic impairment. Severe myelosuppression may occur.**

**THERAPEUTIC CLASS:** Anthracycline

**INDICATIONS:** To produce regression in disseminated neoplastic conditions such as acute lymphoblastic and myeloblastic leukemias, Wilms' tumor, neuroblastoma, soft tissue/bone sarcomas, breast carcinoma, ovary, bladder and thyroid, gastric and bronchogenic carcinomas, Hodgkin's disease, malignant lymphoma in which the small-cell histologic type is the most responsive compared with other cell types. Adjuvant therapy in women with evidence of axillary lymph node involvement following resection of primary breast cancer.

**DOSAGE:** *Adults:* Monotherapy: 60-75mg/m² IV every 21 days. Use the lower dose with inadequate bone marrow reserves due to advanced age, prior therapy, or neoplastic marrow infiltration. Concomitant Chemotherapy: 40-60mg/m² IV every 21-28 days. Hyperbilirubinemia: Reduce dose by 50% if 1.2-3mg/dL; reduce dose by 75% if 3.1-5mg/dL.

*Pediatrics:* Monotherapy: 60-75mg/m² IV every 21 days. Use the lower dose with inadequate bone marrow reserves, prior therapy, or neoplastic marrow infiltration. Concomitant Chemotherapy: 40-60mg/m² IV every 21-28 days. Hyperbilirubinemia: Reduce dose by 50% if 1.2-3mg/dL; reduce dose by 75% if 3.1-5mg/dL.



**HOW SUPPLIED:** Inj: 2mg/mL

**CONTRAINDICATIONS:** Baseline neutrophil count <1500 cells/mm³, severe hepatic impairment, recent myocardial infarction, severe myocardial insufficiency, severe arrhythmias, and previous therapy with complete cumulative doses of doxorubicin, daunorubicin, idarubicin, or other anthracyclines and anthracenes.

**WARNINGS/PRECAUTIONS:** Acute life threatening arrhythmias reported. Enhanced toxicity with hepatic impairment; evaluate hepatic function before dosing. Risk of developing secondary acute myelogenous leukemia (AML) in pediatric patients. Urine may appear red for 1-2 days after administration. Extravasation with or without stinging or burning sensation may occur; immediately terminate and restart in another vein. May induce tumor lysis syndrome and hyperuricemia with rapidly growing tumors. Periodically monitor CBC, hepatic function, and radionuclide left ventricular ejection fraction (LVEF). May cause prepubertal growth failure and gonadal impairment. May cause fetal harm.

**ADVERSE REACTIONS:** Myelosuppression, cardiotoxicity, alopecia, N/V, mucositis, ulceration and necrosis of colon, anorexia, abdominal pain, fever, chills, urticaria, phlebosclerosis, facial flushing.

**INTERACTIONS:** May potentiate toxicity of other anticancer therapies. May exacerbate cyclophosphamide-induced hemorrhagic cystitis. May enhance hepatotoxicity of 6-mercaptopurine. May increase radiation-induced toxicity of the myocardium, mucosa, skin, and liver. Acute "recall" pneumonitis in pediatrics with actinomycin-D. Paclitaxel infused before doxorubicin may decrease clearance of doxorubicin and increase neutropenia and stomatitis episodes, than the reverse sequence of administration. Enhanced neutropenia and thrombocytopenia reported with concomitant IV progesterone. Cyclosporine may prolong and exacerbate hematologic toxicity. Phenobarbital increases elimination. May decrease phenytoin levels. Streptozocin may inhibit hepatic metabolism. Live vaccines may be hazardous in those undergoing cytotoxic chemotherapy. Necrotizing colitis reported with cytarabine. Seizures and coma reported with cyclosporine, cisplatin or vincristine. Possible increased risk of cardiotoxicity with CCBs. Increased risk of CHF with radiotherapy to mediastinal/pericardial area or cardiotoxic drugs.

**PREGNANCY:** Category D, not for use in nursing.

**MECHANISM OF ACTION:** Anthracycline antineoplastic agent; inhibits nucleotide replication and action of DNA and RNA polymerases.

**PHARMACOKINETICS: Distribution:** $V_d$=809-1214L/m². Plasma protein binding (74-76%), excreted in breast milk. **Metabolism:** Enzymatic reduction; doxorubicinol (major metabolite). **Elimination:** Bile (40%), urine (5-12%); $T_{1/2}$=20-48 hrs.

## NURSING CONSIDERATIONS

**Assessment:** Assess for recovery from previous acute toxicities from cytotoxic agents prior to start of therapy. Perform careful baseline assessment of blood counts (WBC, RBC, and platelets); serum levels of total bilirubin, AST, and creatinine; and cardiac function as measured by LVEF should be assessed before therapy. Note other diseases/conditions and drug therapies.

**Monitoring:** CBC with differential and platelet count, LFTs, cardiac function (LVEF), hyperuricemia, hypersensitivity reactions, creatinine level, secondary leukemias, injection-site reactions, and complications due to myelosuppression.

**Patient Counseling:** Inform about adverse effects, including GI symptoms and neutropenic complications. Consult physician if vomiting, dehydration, fever, evidence of infection, symptoms of CHF, or injection-site pain occur. Advise that alopecia will develop, and urine may appear red for 1-2 days after administration. Educate on risk of irreversible myocardial damage and treatment-related leukemia. Counsel men to use effective contraceptive methods while on treatment, and women that irreversible amenorrhea or premature menopause may occur.

**Administration:** IV route. **Storage:** Unreconstituted vial at 15-30°C (59-86°F). Refrigerate reconstituted solution at 2-8°C (36-46°F); stable for 7 days. Protect from light. Use appropriate handling and disposal techniques.



## Duac RX

### clindamycin - benzoyl peroxide (Stiefel)

**THERAPEUTIC CLASS:** Antibacterial/keratolytic

**INDICATIONS:** Topical treatment of inflammatory acne vulgaris.

**DOSAGE:** *Adults:* Wash face and pat dry. Apply qd in evening.
*Pediatrics:* ≥12 yrs: Wash face and pat dry. Apply qd in evening.

**HOW SUPPLIED:** Gel: (Clindamycin-Benzoyl Peroxide) 1%-5% [45g]

**CONTRAINDICATIONS:** History of regional enteritis, ulcerative colitis, pseudomembranous colitis, or antibiotic-associated colitis.

**WARNINGS/PRECAUTIONS:** Severe colitis reported with oral and parenteral clindamycin. Topical and systemic use of clindamycin may result in absorption of the antibiotic from the skin surface. Diarrhea, bloody diarrhea, and colitis (eg, pseudomembranous) reported; d/c if significant diarrhea occurs. Antiperistaltic agents (eg, opiates, diphenoxylate with atropine) may prolong and/or worsen condition. Avoid contact with eyes and mucous membranes. Minimize sun exposure after application.

**ADVERSE REACTIONS:** Erythema, peeling, dryness, and burning.

**INTERACTIONS:** Cumulative irritancy possible with other topical acne agents. Avoid erythromycin agents.

**PREGNANCY:** Category C, not for use in nursing.

**MECHANISM OF ACTION:** Clindamycin: Antibacterial; binds to 50S ribosomal subunits of susceptible bacteria and prevents elongation of peptide chains by interfering with peptidyl transfer, thereby suppressing protein synthesis. Benzoyl peroxide: Keratolytic; potent oxidizing agent.

**PHARMACOKINETICS: Distribution:** Orally and parenterally administered clindamycin found in breast milk.

### NURSING CONSIDERATIONS

**Assessment:** Assess for hypersensitivity to lincomycin, history of regional enteritis, ulcerative colitis, pseudomembranous colitis, antibiotic-associated colitis. Assess use in pregnancy and that females are not nursing. Assess for possible drug interactions.

**Monitoring:** Monitor for signs/symptoms of diarrhea, bloody diarrhea, and colitis (pseudomembranous colitis). Perform endoscopic exam to ID pseudomembranous colitis. If diarrhea occurs, perform stool culture for *Clostridium difficile* and stool assay for *Clostridium difficile* toxin. If severe diarrhea occurs, perform large bowel endoscopy. Monitor for overgrowth of nonsusceptible organisms (eg, fungi).

**Patient Counseling:** Inform to notify physician if diarrhea develops during therapy and up to several weeks after. Instruct to take medication exactly as directed, externally. Advise to avoid contact with eyes, inside nose, mouth, and all mucous membranes. Advise to avoid contact with hair or fabrics; drug causes bleaching. Advise to limit exposure to sunlight and to use protection (eg, hats, sunscreen) when exposed to sun.

**Administration:** Topical route. **Storage:** Prior to dispensing, 2-8°C (36-46°F). Do not freeze. After dispensing: Store up to 25°C (77°F). Do not freeze. Keep tube tightly closed.

# DUETACT RX

pioglitazone HCl - glimepiride (Takeda)

**Thiazolidinediones, including pioglitazone, may cause or exacerbate CHF in some patients. Duetact is not recommended in patients with symptomatic heart failure.**

D

**THERAPEUTIC CLASS:** Thiazolidinedione/sulfonylurea

**INDICATIONS:** Adjunct to diet and exercise to improve glycemic control in adults with type 2 diabetes already being treated with a thiazolidinedione and a sulfonylurea or who have inadequate glycemic control on a thiazolidinedione alone or sulfonylurea alone.

**DOSAGE:** *Adults:* Individualize dose. Base recommended starting dose on current regimen of pioglitazone and/or sulfonylurea. Give with 1st meal of day. Current Glimepiride Monotherapy or Switching from Combination Therapy of Pioglitazone plus Glimepiride as Separate Tablets: Initial: 30mg-2mg or 30mg-4mg qd. Current Pioglitazone or Different Sulfonylurea Monotherapy or Switching from Combination Therapy of Pioglitazone plus a Different Sulfonylurea: Initial: 30mg-2mg qd. Max: Once daily at any strength. Elderly/Debilitated/Malnourished/Renal or Hepatic Insufficiency (ALT ≤2.5x ULN): Initial: 1mg glimepiride prior to prescribing Duetact. Systolic Dysfunction: Initial: 15-30mg of pioglitazone; titrate carefully to lowest Duetact dose.

**HOW SUPPLIED:** Tab: (Pioglitazone-Glimepiride) 30mg-2mg, 30mg-4mg

**CONTRAINDICATIONS:** Established NYHA Class III or IV heart failure; diabetic ketoacidosis, with or without coma.

**WARNINGS/PRECAUTIONS:** Glimepiride: Increased CV mortality. May produce severe hypoglycemia, risk may be increased if debilitated, malnourished, with adrenal, pituitary, renal, or hepatic insufficiency, and after severe or prolonged exercise. Hypoglycemia may be masked in elderly patients and in patients taking β-adrenergic blocking drugs or sympatholytic agents. May lose blood glucose control with stress. Hemolytic anemia reported; use caution in patient with glucose-6-phosphate dehydrogenase (G6PD) deficiency and consider alternate non-sulfonylurea treatment. Pioglitazone: May cause fluid retention and exacerbation/initiation of heart failure; consider dose reduction or d/c therapy. Not indicated if NYHA Class III or IV cardiac status. Not for use in type 1 DM or diabetic ketoacidosis treatment. Caution with edema. Dose-related weight gain reported. Ovulation in premenopausal anovulatory patient may occur; risk of pregnancy with inadequate contraception. May decrease Hgb and Hct. Hepatitis and hepatic enzyme elevations >3x or more ULN reported and rarely hepatic failure reported. Avoid with active liver disease or if ALT levels >2.5x ULN. Check LFTs if hepatic dysfunction symptoms occur. D/C if ALT >3x ULN on therapy or if jaundice occurs. Macular edema reported; refer patients who develop any type of visual symptoms to an ophthalmologist. Increased incidence of bone fractures reported in female patients. Perform periodic measurements of FPG and $A_{1C}$ measurements to monitor glycemic control and therapeutic response. Measure LFTs prior to therapy and periodically thereafter.

**ADVERSE REACTIONS:** Hypoglycemia, upper respiratory tract infection, increased weight, lower limb edema/pain, headache, UTI, diarrhea, nausea, new onset or worsening diabetic macular edema with decreased visual acuity.

**INTERACTIONS:** Pioglitazone: May be at risk for hypoglycemia if used concomitantly with insulin or oral hypoglycemic agents; may require dose reduction of concomitant agent. May be a weak inducer of CYP3A4 substrates. CYP2C8 inhibitors (eg, gemfibrozil) may significantly increase the AUC levels of pioglitazone. CYP2C8 inducers (eg, rifampin) may significantly decrease the AUC levels of pioglitiazone. May decrease levels of midazolam and ethinyl estradiol levels. Glimepiride: Combined use with insulin, metformin, or when more than one glucose agent is used may increase the potential for hypoglycemia. Hypoglycemia more likely to occur when alcohol is ingested. Hypoglycemia may be potentiated with NSAIDs and other drugs that are highly protein bound (eg, salicylates, sulfonamides, chloramphenicol, coumarins, probenecid, MAOIs, β-blockers). Risk of severe hypoglycemia with oral miconazole. Risk of hyperglycemia with thiazides and other diuretics, corticosteroids, phenothiazines, thyroid products, estrogens, oral contraceptives, phenytoin, nicotinic acid, sympathomimetics, and isoniazid. Concomitant use with aspirin may decrease glimepiride concentrations. Concomitant use with propranolol may increase $C_{max}$, AUC, and $T_{1/2}$ of glimepiride. May interact with inhibitors (eg, fluconazole) and inducers (eg, rifampicin) of CYP 2C9.

D

**PREGNANCY:** Category C, not for use in nursing.

**MECHANISM OF ACTION:** Pioglitazone: Thiazolidinedione; insulin-sensitizing agent acts by enhancing peripheral glucose utilization. Glimepiride: Sulfonylurea; stimulates release of insulin from functional pancreatic β-cells.

**PHARMACOKINETICS: Absorption:** Administration of variable doses resulted in different parameters. Glimepiride: $T_{max}$=2-3 hrs. Pioglitazone: $T_{max}$=2 hrs. **Distribution:** Pioglitazone: $V_d$=0.63 L/kg, plasma protein binding (>99%). Glimepiride: (IV) $V_d$=8.8L, plasma protein binding (>99.5%). **Metabolism:** Pioglitazone: Extensive (hydroxylation & oxidation) via CYP2C8, CYP3A4, CYP1A1. M-II and M-III (hydroxy derivatives) and M-IV (keto derivatives) (active metabolites). Glimepiride: Oxidative biotransformation via CYP2C9. Cyclohexyl hydroxy methyl derivative (M1), carboxyl derivative (M2) (major metabolites). **Elimination:** Pioglitazone: Urine (15-30%), bile (unchanged), feces (metabolites); $T_{1/2}$=3-7 hrs (pioglitazone), 16-24 hrs (total pioglitazone). Glimepiride: Urine (60%), feces (40%).

## NURSING CONSIDERATIONS

**Assessment:** Assess for diabetic ketoacidosis, heart failure, macular edema, risk factors for developing heart failure, active liver disease, renal insufficiency, G6PD deficiency, pregnancy/nursing status, and for possible drug interactions. Assess LFTs and obtain CBC prior to therapy.

**Monitoring:** Monitor for signs and symptoms of heart failure, edema, hypoglycemia, weight gain, hematological changes (eg, decreases in Hgb and Hct), hepatic dysfunction (eg, N/V, abdominal pain, anorexia, dark urine, jaundice), macular edema, bone fractures, and for hemolytic anemia. Perform periodic monitoring of LFTs, FBG, and $A_{1C}$. Perform periodic eye exams.

**Patient Counseling:** Instruct to d/c with unexplained hyperventilation, myalgia, malaise, unusual somnolence symptoms. Counsel to report unexplained GI symptoms, rapid increase in weight or edema, SOB, N/V, abdominal pain, fatigue, anorexia, or dark urine. Advise to avoid excessive alcohol intake. Counsel females about use of reliable contraception. Inform about importance of adherence to meal planning, regular physical activity, regular blood glucose monitoring, periodic $HbA_{1c}$ testing, recognition and management of hypo- and hyperglycemia, and periodic assessment for diabetes complications. Inform that during periods of stress (eg, trauma, infection, surgery), medication requirements may change; seek prompt medical advice.

**Administration:** Oral route. **Storage:** Store at 25°C (77°F); excursions permitted to 15-30°C (59-86°F). Keep container tightly closed. Protect from moisture and humidity.

# DUONEB RX

ipratropium bromide - albuterol sulfate (Dey)

**THERAPEUTIC CLASS:** $Beta_2$ -agonist/anticholinergic

**INDICATIONS:** Treatment of bronchospasm in COPD in patients requiring more than one bronchodilator.

**DOSAGE:** *Adults:* 3mL qid via nebulizer. May give 2 additional doses/day.

**HOW SUPPLIED:** Sol, Inhalation: (Albuterol-Ipratropium) 3mg-0.5mg/3mL [3mL, 30[s] 60[s]]

**CONTRAINDICATIONS:** Hypersensitivity to atropine and its derivatives.

**WARNINGS/PRECAUTIONS:** Paradoxical bronchospasm and hypersensitivity reactions reported. Caution with cardiovascular disorders, convulsive disorders, hyperthyroidism, DM, narrow-angle glaucoma, prostatic hypertrophy, and bladder-neck obstruction.

**ADVERSE REACTIONS:** Pain, chest pain, diarrhea, dyspepsia, nausea, leg cramps, bronchitis, lung disease, pharyngitis, pneumonia, UTI.

**INTERACTIONS:** Additive interactions with anticholinergic agents. Increased risk of cardiovascular side effects with sympathomimetics. Use $\beta_1$-selective blockers with hyper-reactive airways. Caution within 2 weeks of discontinuation of MAOIs or TCAs.

D

**PREGNANCY:** Category C (albuterol) and B (ipratropium), not for use in nursing.

**MECHANISM OF ACTION:** Albuterol: $\beta_2$-adrenergic bronchodilator; stimulates adenyl cylase, enzyme that catalyzes formation of cAMP from ATP. Increased cAMP levels are associated with relaxation of bronchial smooth muscle and inhibition of release of mediators of immediate hypersensitivity. Ipratropium: Anticholinergic bronchodilator; blocks muscarinic receptors of acetylcholine. Prevents the increase in intracellular concentration of cGMP, resulting from interaction of acetylcholine with the muscarinic receptors of bronchial smooth muscle.

**PHARMACOKINETICS: Absorption:** Albuterol: $C_{max}$=4.65mg/mL; $T_{max}$=0.8 hrs; AUC=24.2ng•h/mL. **Distribution:** Ipratropium: Plasma protein binding (0-9%). **Metabolism:** Albuterol: Conjugation. Ipratropium: Ester hydrolysis. **Elimination:** Albuterol: Urine (8.4% unchanged). Ipratropium: Urine (3.9% unchanged); $T_{1/2}$=6.7 hrs.

## NURSING CONSIDERATIONS

**Assessment:** Assess for history of hypersensitivity to atropine or its derivatives. Assess for concomitant diseases such as narrow-angle glaucoma, prostatic hyperplasia, convulsive disorders, hyperthyroidism, DM, hepatic/renal insufficiency, CVD, and possible drug interactions.

**Monitoring:** Monitor serum potassium, pulse rate and BP, hypersensitivity reactions, parodoxical brochospasm, cardiovascular effects such as flattening of the T wave, prolongation of QT interval, and ST segment depression, severe acute asthmatic crisis, hypoxia, and adverse effects (eg, headache, cough, respiratory disorders, pain, dyspnea, and bronchitis). Monitor for anticholinergic effects.

**Patient Counseling:** Caution to avoid spraying aerosol into eyes; may cause precipitation or worsening of narrow-angle glaucoma, mydriasis, increased IOP, acute eye pain or discomfort, temporary blurring vision, visual halos or colored images. Advise not to exceed recommended dose. Report lack of response and adverse side effects.

**Administration:** Oral inhalation. 1) Remove vial and squeeze contents into nebulizer reservoir. 2) Connect nebulizer to mouthpiece and compressor. 3) Place mouthpiece in mouth or put on face mask and turn on compressor. 4) Breathe as calmly as possible through mouth until no more mist is formed (5-15 min). 5) Clean nebulizer. **Storage:** 2-30°C (36-86°F). Protect from light.

# DURAGESIC

CII

fentanyl (Ortho-McNeil)

**Life-threatening hypoventilation can occur. May be a target for abuse/diversion. Monitor for signs of misuse, abuse, or addiction. Avoid in patients <2 yrs. Only for use in patients who are already receiving opioid therapy, opioid-tolerant patients, and who require a total dose at least equivalent to 25mcg/h. Use in non-opioid tolerant patients may lead to fatal respiratory depression. Overestimating the fentanyl transdermal dose when converting patients from another opioid medication can result in fatal overdose with the first dose. Concomitant use with CYP3A4 inhibitors may increase plasma concentrations, which could increase or prolong adverse effects and cause fatal respiratory depression. For transdermal use only. Avoid exposing application site to direct external heat source (eg, heating pads, tanning lamps). There is a potential for temperature-dependent increase in fentanyl released, resulting to a possible overdose and death. Monitor patient with fever or exercise-induced increase in core body temperature for side effects and adjust dose if necessary.**

**THERAPEUTIC CLASS:** Opioid analgesic

**INDICATIONS:** Management of persistent, moderate to severe chronic pain in opioid-tolerant patients that requires continuous, around-the-clock opioid administration for an extended period of time, and cannot be managed by other means such as nonsteroidal analgesics, opioid combination products, or immediate-release opioids.

**DOSAGE:** *Adults:* Individualize dose. Determine dose based on opioid tolerance, previous analgesic requirement, and general condition and medical status of the patient. Minimum Initial Dose: 25mcg/hr for 72 hr. Titrate: Initial dose may be increased after 3 days; further increase in dosage should be made after the higher dose is worn through 2 applications. Dosage increments may be based on the daily dose of supplementary opioids using the ratio of 45mg/24 hrs of oral morphine to a 12.5mcg/h increase in dose. Some patients may not achieve adequate analgesia and may require systems to be applied q48h rather than q72h; an increase in dose should first be evaluated prior to changing the interval. Refer to PI for Dose Conversion Guidelines. Elderly/Debilitated/Cachetic/Renal/Hepatic impairment: Reduce dose.
*Pediatrics:* ≥2 yrs: Individualize dose. Determine dose based on opioid tolerance, previous analgesic requirement, and general condition and medical status of the patient. Minimum Initial Dose: 25mcg/hr for 72 hr. Titrate: Initial dose may be increased after 3 days; further increase in dosage should be made after the higher dose is worn through 2 applications. Dosage increments may be based on the daily dose of supplementary opioids using the ratio of 45mg/24 hrs of oral morphine to a 12.5mcg/h increase in dose. Refer to PI for Dose Conversion Guidelines.

**HOW SUPPLIED:** Patch: 12mcg/h (2.1mg), 25mcg/h (4.2mg), 50mcg/h (8.4mg), 75mcg/h (12.6mg), 100mcg/h (16.8mg). [5[s]].

**CONTRAINDICATIONS:** Opioid non-tolerant patients, management of acute pain or in patients who require opioid analgesia for a short period of time, post-operative pain, mild/intermittent pain. Diagnosis or suspicion of paralytic ileus, acute or severe bronchial asthma, significant respiratory depression especially in unmonitored settings where there is lack of resuscitative equipment.

**WARNINGS/PRECAUTIONS:** Do not use if seal is broken or patch is cut, damaged, or changed. Monitor patients with serious adverse events for at least 24 hrs after removal. Keep out of reach of children; death and other serious medical problems have occurred when people accidentally exposed to fentanyl (eg, transfer from adult's body to a child while hugging, accidentally sitting on patch). Hypoventilation may occur; caution with elderly, cachectic or debilitated patients, chronic pulmonary diseases or cor pulmonale, decreased respiratory reserve, hypoxia, hypercapnia, or pre-existing respiratory depression. May cause bradycardia; caution with bradyarrhythmias. Caution with brain tumors and renal/hepatic impairment. May cause spasm of the sphincter of Oddi; caution with biliary tract disease and pancreatic disease. May cause increases in serum amylase concentrations. Avoid with increased intracranial pressure, impaired consciousness, or coma. May obscure clinical course of head injury. Tolerance and physical dependence may occur. May impair mental/physical abilities. Withdrawal symptoms may occur; gradual downward titration is recommended.

**ADVERSE REACTIONS:** Hypoventilation, headache, fever, N/V, constipation, dry mouth, somnolence, confusion, asthenia, sweating, nervousness, pruritus, apnea, dyspnea.

**INTERACTIONS:** See Black Box Warning. Concomitant use with CNS depressants (eg, opioids, sedatives, hypnotics, tranquilizers, general anesthetics, phenothiazines, skeletal muscle relaxants, alcohol) may cause respiratory depression, hypotension, profound sedation, or potentially coma. Coadministration with CYP3A4 inducers may lead to reduced efficacy of fentanyl. Avoid use within 14 days of MAOI.

**PREGNANCY:** Category C, not for use in nursing.

**MECHANISM OF ACTION:** Opioid analgesic; interacts predominantly with the opioid μ-receptor in the brain, spinal cord and other tissues. Exerts principal pharmacological actions on CNS.

**PHARMACOKINETICS: Absorption:** $T_{max}$= 20-72 hrs. Transdermal administration of variable doses resulted in different parameters. **Distribution**: $V_d$=6 L/kg; found in breast milk; readily crosses placenta. **Metabolism**: Liver via CYP3A4; oxidative N-dealkylation to norfentanyl and other inactive metabolites. **Elimination**: Urine (75%), feces (9%); $T_{1/2}$= 20-27 hrs.



## NURSING CONSIDERATIONS

**Assessment:** Assess for opioid tolerance, level of pain intensity, type of pain (eg, postoperative pain, intermittent pain), patient's general condition and medical status, respiratory depression, acute or severe bronchial asthma, COPD, cor pulmonale, decreased respiratory reserve, hypoxia, hypercapnia, or pre-existing respiratory depression, brain tumors, abuse potential, evidence of increased intracranial pressure, impaired consciousness or coma, bradyarrhythmia, hepatic/renal disease, fever/increased in core body temperature, biliary tract disease, acute pancreatitis, presence of paralytic ileus, pregnancy/nursing status, and for possible drug interactions.

**Monitoring:** Monitor for signs/symptoms of respiratory depression, bradycardia, increases in serum amylase levels, abuse or misuse, addiction, and tolerance or physical dependence. Monitor for signs and symptoms of overdose especially when converting patient from another opioid.

**Patient Counseling:** Advise that patch contain fentanyl, an opioid pain medicine similar to morphine, hydromorphone, methadone, oxycodone, and oxymorphone. Advise to wear patch continuously for 72 hrs, and apply patch to different intact, nonirritated, and non irradiated on a flat surface of the skin (eg, chest, back, flank, upper arm), following removal of previous patch. Following use, advise to fold patch and flush down the toilet. Advise to apply immediately upon removal from the sealed package and after removal of the protective liner. Do not use broken, cut or damaged patch. Never adjust the dose or the number of patches applied to the skin without instruction from the healthcare professional. If cognitively impaired, advise to place on upper back, to decrease chance of removal. Clean with water and dry skin prior to application; avoid soaps, oils, lotions, or any skin irritants. Avoid exposing patch to direct external heat sources. Contact physician if fever develops and inform that may impair mental/physical abilities; instruct to use caution if performing hazardous tasks (eg, operating machinery/driving). Advise to notify physician of all medications currently taken. Counsel to avoid using other CNS depressants and alcohol. Inform that constipation may develop during therapy. Instruct to avoid abrupt withdrawal of medication; taper dose. Inform that medication has high potential for abuse. Instruct to place medication in secure place, away from children. Instruct that if patch sticks to a different person, remove patch and wash exposed area with water, and contact physician. Instruct if the gel from the drug reservoir accidentally contacts the skin the area should be washed clean with water. Advise that if patch falls off before 72 hours, a new patch should be applied to a different skin site.

**Administration:** Transdermal patch. Apply immediately after removal from individually sealed pouch. Do not use if the pouch seal is broken. Next patch should be applied to a different site. Apply to intact, nonirritated, and nonirradiated skin on flat surface such as the chest, back, flank or upper arm. In pediatric patient the upper back is the preferred. Refer to PI for further details on proper application. **Storage:** Store up to 25°C (77°F). Excursions permitted to 15-30°C (59-86°F). Store in original unopened pouch.

# Duramorph

morphine sulfate (Baxter)

**CII**

**THERAPEUTIC CLASS:** Opioid analgesic

**INDICATIONS:** Management of pain unresponsive to non-narcotic analgesics.

**DOSAGE:** *Adults:* IV: Initial: 2-10mg/70kg. Epidural Injection: Initial: 5mg in lumbar region. Titrate: If inadequate pain relief within 1 hr, increase by 1-2mg. Max: 10mg/24hrs. Continuous Epidural: Initial: 2-4mg/24hrs. Give additional

1-2mg if needed. Intrathecal: 0.2-1mg single dose, do not repeat; may follow with 0.6mg/hr naloxone infusion to reduce incidence of side effects.

**HOW SUPPLIED:** Inj: 0.5mg/mL, 1mg/mL, 5mg/mL

**CONTRAINDICATIONS:** Allergy to opiates, acute bronchial asthma, upper airway obstruction. Severe hypotension may occur in volume depleted patients or with concurrent administration of phenothiazines or general anesthetics.

**WARNINGS/PRECAUTIONS:** Have resuscitation equipment, oxygen, and antidote (eg, naloxone) available; severe respiratory depression may occur. Avoid rapid administration. May be habit-forming. Caution with head injury, increased intracranial/intraocular pressure, decreased respiratory reserve, hepatic/renal dysfunction, elderly, debilitated. High doses may cause seizures. Smooth muscle hypertonicity may cause biliary colic, urinary difficulty or retention. Orthostatic hypotension may occur with hypovolemia or myocardial dysfunction. Acute respiratory failure reported with COPD or acute asthmatic attack. Limit epidural/intrathecal route to lumbar area.

**ADVERSE REACTIONS:** Respiratory depression, convulsions, dysphoric reactions, pruritus, urinary retention, constipation, lumbar puncture-type headache, toxic psychoses.

**INTERACTIONS:** CNS depressants (eg, alcohol, sedatives, antihistamines) and psychotropics potentiate CNS depression. Neuroleptics may increase respiratory depression.

**PREGNANCY:** Category C, safety in nursing not known.

**MECHANISM OF ACTION:** Opioid analgesic; analgesic effects are produced via at least 3 areas of the CNS: the periaqueductal-periventricular gray matter, the ventromedial medulla, and the spinal cord. Interacts predominantly with μ-receptors which are found distributed in the brain, spinal cord, and in the trigeminal nerve.

**PHARMACOKINETICS: Absorption:** (Epidural): Rapid absorption; $C_{max}$=33-40ng/mL; $T_{max}$=10-15 min; (Intrathecal): $C_{max}$<1-7.8ng/mL; $T_{max}$=5-10 min. **Distribution:** Plasma protein binding (36%); Muscle tissue binding (54%). Readily passes into fetal circulation, found in breast milk. (IV): $V_d$=1.0-4.7L/kg. **Metabolism:** Hepatic glucuronidation. **Elimination:** Kidneys (major), urine (2-12% unchanged), feces (10%); (IV, IM) $T_{1/2}$=1.5-4.5 hrs; (epidural) $T_{1/2}$=39-249 min.

## NURSING CONSIDERATIONS

**Assessment:** Assess for acute bronchial asthma, upper airway obstruction, hypotension, infection at injection site, bleeding diathesis, seizure disorder, presence of head injury or increased intracranial pressure, age of patient, hepatic/renal dysfunction, biliary tract disorders or recent biliary surgery, urinary system disorders, impaired myocardial function, hypotension, nursing/pregnancy status, and possible drug interactions.

**Monitoring:** Monitor for signs/symptoms of respiratory depression and/or respiratory arrest, myoclonic events, seizures, dysphoric reactions, toxic psychoses, biliary colic, urinary retention, drug abuse, and drug dependence. If administered intrathecally or via epidural, monitor closely for 24 hrs for signs/symptoms of respiratory depression.

**Patient Counseling:** Counsel to notify physician immediately if develop signs/symptoms of respiratory depression. Instruct to avoid using other CNS depressants and alcohol during therapy. Inform that medication has potential for abuse and dependence. Counsel to avoid abrupt withdrawal of medication; withdrawal symptoms may occur. Instruct that if accidental skin contact occurs, wash affected area with water.

**Administration:** Intravenous, epidural, or intrathecal route. Proper placement of needle or catheter should be verified before epidural injection. **Storage:** 20-25°C (68-77°F); excursions permitted to 15-30°C (59-86°F). Protect from light. Do not freeze.

# DYAZIDE RX

## triamterene - hydrochlorothiazide (GlaxoSmithKline)

D

**THERAPEUTIC CLASS:** $K^+$-sparing diuretic/thiazide diuretic

**INDICATIONS:** For hypertension or edema if hypokalemia occurs on HCTZ alone, or when a thiazide diuretic is required and cannot risk hypokalemia.

**DOSAGE:** *Adults:* 1-2 caps qd.

**HOW SUPPLIED:** Cap: (Triamterene-HCTZ) 37.5mg-25mg

**CONTRAINDICATIONS:** Anuria, acute and chronic renal insufficiency or significant renal impairment, sulfonamide hypersensitivity, pre-existing elevated serum $K^+$, $K^+$-sparing agents (eg, spironolactone, amiloride, or other formulations containing triamterene), $K^+$ salt substitutes, $K^+$ supplements (except with severe hypokalemia).

**WARNINGS/PRECAUTIONS:** Risk of hyperkalemia ($K^+ \geq 5.5$mEq/L), especially with renal impairment, elderly, diabetes, and severely ill; monitor levels frequently. If hyperkalemia suspected, obtain ECG. D/C immediately if hyperkalemia is present. Avoid in severely ill in whom respiratory or metabolic acidosis may occur; if employed in these patients, perform frequent evaluations of acid-base balance and serum electrolytes. Caution in patients with diabetes, may cause hyperglycemia and glycosuria. May manifest diabetes mellitus (DM). Caution with hepatic dysfunction, may precipitate hepatic coma in patients with severe liver disease. Corrective measures must be taken if hypokalemia develops; d/c if serious hypokalemia develops ($K^+$<3.0 mEq/L). May cause hypochloremia. Dilutional hyponatremia may occur in edematous patients in hot weather. Caution with history of renal stones. May increase uric acid levels, BUN, and SrCr. May decrease PBI levels. D/C before parathyroid function tests. May potentiate electrolyte imbalance with heart failure, renal disease, cirrhosis.

**ADVERSE REACTIONS:** Muscle cramps, N/V, pancreatitis, weakness, blood dyscrasias, arrhythmia, impotence, dry mouth, jaundice, paresthesia, renal stones, hypersensitivity reactions, acute renal failure, hyperkalemia, hyponatremia.

**INTERACTIONS:** See Contraindications. May increase risk of hyperkalemia when used concomitantly with ACE inhibitors, blood from blood bank, low-salt milk, $K^+$-containing medications (eg, parenteral penicillin G potassium), salt substitutes. May increase risk of hyponatremia with concurrent use of chlorpropamide. Possible interaction resulting in acute renal failure when coadministered with NSAIDs (eg, indomethacin). Avoid concomitant use with lithium due to risk of lithium toxicity. Decreases arterial responsiveness to norepinephrine. Amphotericin B, corticosteroids, and corticotropin (ACTH) may intensify electrolyte depletion. Adjust oral anticoagulants and antigout drugs. May alter insulin requirements. Increases effects of nondepolarizing muscle relaxants (eg, tubocurarine), antihypertensives. Chronic or overuse of laxatives or use of exchange resins (eg, sodium polystyrene sulfonate) reduces $K^+$ levels. Reduces methenamine effects.

**PREGNANCY:** Category C, not for use in nursing.

**MECHANISM OF ACTION:** Triamterene: $K^+$-sparing diuretic; exerts diuretic effect on distal renal tubules to inhibit the reabsorption of $Na^+$ in exchange for $K^+$ and $H^+$ ions. HCTZ: thiazide diuretic; blocks reabsorption of $Na^+$ and $Cl^-$ ions and thereby increases the quantity of $Na^+$ transversing the distal tubule and the volume of water exceeded.

**PHARMACOKINETICS: Absorption:** Triamterene: $C_{max}$=46.4ng/mL; $T_{max}$=1.1 hrs; AUC=148.7ng•hrs/mL. HCTZ: $C_{max}$=135.1ng/mL; $T_{max}$=2 hrs; AUC=834ng•hrs/mL.

## NURSING CONSIDERATIONS

**Assessment:** Assess for anuria, renal/hepatic impairment, sulfonamide hypersensitivity, hyperkalemia, diabetes, history of renal stones, pregnancy/nursing status, and for possible drug interactions. Obtain baseline BUN, SrCr, and serum electrolytes.

**Monitoring:** Monitor for signs/symptoms of hyperkalemia, hypokalemia, hyperglycemia, hypochloremia, renal stones, hypersensitivity reactions, and for electrolyte imbalance. Monitor for hepatic coma in patients with severe liver disease. Monitor BUN, SrCr, and serum electrolytes.

**Patient Counseling:** Advise to seek medical attention if symptoms of hyperkalemia (eg, paresthesias, muscular weakness, fatigue), hypokalemia, hyperglycemia, renal stones, electrolyte imbalance (eg, dry mouth, thirst, weakness), or hypersensitivity reactions occur.

**Administration:** Oral route. **Storage:** 20-25°C (68-77°F); excursions permitted to 15-30°C (59-86°F). Protect from light. Dispense in a tight, light-resistant container.

## DYNACIN — RX

minocycline HCl (Medicis)

**THERAPEUTIC CLASS:** Tetracycline derivative

**INDICATIONS:** Treatment of rocky mountain spotted fever, typhus fever and the typhus group, Q fever, rickettsialpox, tick fevers, respiratory tract infections, lymphagranuloma venereum, psittacosis, trachoma, inclusion conjunctivitis, non-gonococcal urethritis, endocervical or rectal infections in adults, relapsing fever, chancroid, plague, tularemia, cholera, campylobacter fetus infections, brucellosis, bartonellosis and granuloma inguinale caused by susceptible strains of microorganisms. Treatment of infections caused by gram-negative microorganisms when bacteriologic testing indicates appropriate susceptibility to the drug (eg, respiratory tract and urinary tract infections) and gram-positive microorganisms (eg, upper respiratory tract, skin and skin structure infections). Alternative treatment in certain other infections (eg, uncomplicated urethritis in men, gonococcal infections, syphilis, yaws, listeriosis, anthrax, Vincent's infection, actinomycosis). Adjunctive therapy in acute intestinal amebiasis and severe acne. Treatment of *Mycobacterium marinum* and asymptomatic carriers of *Neisseria meningitidis*.

**DOSAGE:** *Adults:* Usual: 200mg initially, then 100mg q12h; alternative is 100-200mg initially, then 50mg qid. Uncomplicated Gonococcal Infection (Men, other than urethritis and anorectal infections): 200mg initially, then 100mg q12h for minimum 4 days, with post therapy cultures within 2-3 days. Uncomplicated Gonococcal Urethritis (Men): 100mg q12h for 5 days. Syphilis: Administer usual dose for 10-15 days. Meningococcal Carrier State: 100mg q12h for 5 days. *Mycobacterium marinum:* 100mg q12h for 6-8 weeks. Uncomplicated urethral, endocervical, or rectal infection: 100mg q12h for at least 7 days. Renal Dysfunction: Reduce dose and/or extend dose intervals. Take with plenty of fluids. Take 1 hr before or 2 hrs after meals.
*Pediatrics:* >8 yrs: 4mg/kg initially followed by 2mg/kg q12h. Take with plenty of fluids. Taken 1 hr before or 2 hrs after meals.

**HOW SUPPLIED:** Tab: 50mg, 75mg, 100mg

**WARNINGS/PRECAUTIONS:** May cause fetal harm during pregnancy. Use during tooth development (eg, last half of pregnancy, infancy, ≤8 yrs) may cause permanent discoloration of the teeth or enamel hypoplasia; avoid use during this period. Bulging fontanels in infants have been associated with use. May decrease bone growth in premature infants. Renal toxicity, hepatotoxicity, photosensitivity, increased BUN, superinfection, pseudotumor cerebri may occur; perform hematopoietic, renal and hepatic monitoring. May impair mental/physical abilities. Not for treatment of meningococcal infections.

**ADVERSE REACTIONS:** Anorexia, N/V, diarrhea, dysphagia, enterocolitis, pancreatitis, increased liver enzymes, maculopapular/erythematous rash, exfoliative dermatitis, Stevens-Johnson syndrome, skin and mucous membrane pigmentation, hemolytic anemia, headache.

**INTERACTIONS:** May require downward adjustments of anticoagulant dosage with concomitant use. May interfere with bactericidal action of penicillin; avoid concurrent use when possible. May decrease efficacy of oral contraceptives. Impaired absorption with antacids containing aluminum, calcium or magnesium and iron-containing products. Fatal renal toxicity with methoxyflurane has been reported.

**PREGNANCY:** Category D, not for use in nursing.

**MECHANISM OF ACTION:** Tetracycline derivative; bacteriostatic. Thought to inhibit protein synthesis.

D

**PHARMACOKINETICS: Absorption:** Rapid; $C_{max}$ = 758.29ng/mL; $T_{max}$ = 1.71 hrs. **Distribution:** Found in breast milk. **Elimination:** Urine and feces; $T_{1/2}$= 17.03 hrs, (hepatic dysfunction) 11-16 hrs, (renal dysfunction) 18-69 hrs.

## NURSING CONSIDERATIONS

**Assessment:** Assess for renal impairment, meningococcal infection, pregnancy/nursing status and possible drug interactions. Document indications for therapy, culture and susceptibility testing. Perform incision and drainage in conjunction with antibiotic therapy when indicated.

**Monitoring:** Monitor for signs/symptoms of hypersensitivity reactions, photosensitivity, superinfection, benign intracranial HTN, LFTs, renal function, CBC with platelet and differential count. In venereal disease with coexistent syphilis, conduct serologic test before treatment and after 3 months.

**Patient Counseling:** Inform of pregnancy risks and photosensitivity reactions (d/c at 1st sign of skin erythema). Avoid excessive sunlight/UV light and wear sunscreen/sunblock. Inform therapy treats bacterial, not viral, infections. Take as directed; skipping doses or not completing full course may decrease effectiveness and increase resistance. Notify physician if hypersensitivity reactions, superinfections, photosensitivity or benign intracranial HTN occur. Inform that concomitant use of tetracyclines may render oral contraceptives less effective.

**Administration:** Oral route. **Storage:** Store at 20-25°C (68-77°F). Protect from light, moisture and excessive heat.

# DynaCirc CR — RX

isradipine (Reliant)

**THERAPEUTIC CLASS:** Calcium channel blocker (dihydropyridine)

**INDICATIONS:** Management of hypertension alone or in combination with thiazide diuretics.

**DOSAGE:** *Adults:* Individualized dosing. Initial: 5mg qd alone or with a thiazide diuretic. Titrate: May adjust by 5mg/day at 2-4 week intervals. Max: 20mg/day. Swallow whole; do not bite or divide.

**HOW SUPPLIED:** Tab, Controlled-Release: 5mg, 10mg

**WARNINGS/PRECAUTIONS:** May produce symptomatic hypotension. Caution in patients with congestive heart failure (CHF), especially with concomitant β-blockers. Caution with pre-existing severe GI narrowing; obstructive symptoms reported. Dose-related, mild to moderate peripheral edema reported. Caution in elderly.

**ADVERSE REACTIONS:** Headache, edema, dizziness, constipation, fatigue, flushing, abdominal discomfort.

**INTERACTIONS:** Severe hypotension possible with fentanyl anesthesia and β-blockers; increased volume of circulating fluid might be required if such interaction occurred. May increases AUC and $C_{max}$, and may decrease $T_{max}$ of propranolol.

**PREGNANCY:** Category C, not for use in nursing.

**MECHANISM OF ACTION:** Dihydropyridine calcium channel blocker; binds to calcium channels with high infinity and specificity, and inhibits calcium flux into cardiac and smooth muscle.

**PHARMACOKINETICS: Absorption:** Bioavailability (15-24%); (10mg) $C_{max}$=3-4ng/mL; AUC=62-73ng•h/mL. **Distribution:** Plasma protein binding (95%). **Metabolism:** Oxidation, ester cleavage; CYP3A4. **Elimination:** Urine (60-65%), feces (25-30%).

## NURSING CONSIDERATIONS

**Assessment:** Assess for hypersensitivity, HTN, symptomatic hypotension, renal/hepatic impairment, CHF, pre-existing GI narrowing, ingestion of GITS products, pregnancy/nursing status, and possible drug interactions.

**Monitoring:** Monitor for signs/symptoms of hypotension (eg, syncope and dizziness), peripheral edema, obstruction from strictures, and hypersensitivity reactions.

**Patient Counseling:** Instruct to swallow tablet whole; do not bite or divide. Inform that tablet shell may be seen in stool.

**Administration:** Oral route. Swallow whole; do not bite or divide. **Storage:** Below 30°C (86°F). Store in a tight container, protected from moisture and humidity.

# DYRENIUM RX

triamterene (WellSpring)

**Abnormal elevation of serum K+ levels ( ≥5.5mEq/L) can occur with all K+-sparing agents, including triamterene. Hyperkalemia is more likely to occur with renal impairment and diabetes (even without evidence of renal impairment), and in the elderly, or severely ill. Monitor serum K+ at frequent intervals.**

**THERAPEUTIC CLASS:** $K^+$-sparing diuretic

**INDICATIONS:** Treatment of edema associated with congestive heart failure, liver cirrhosis, and nephrotic syndrome. Treatment of steroid induced edema, idiopathic edema, and edema due to secondary hyperaldosteronism.

**DOSAGE:** *Adults:* Initial: 100mg bid pc. Max: 300mg/day. Titrate dose to the needs of the individual patient.

**HOW SUPPLIED:** Cap: 50mg, 100mg

**CONTRAINDICATIONS:** Anuria, severe or progressive kidney disease or dysfunction (except with nephrosis), severe hepatic disease, hyperkalemia, $K^+$ supplements, $K^+$ salts or $K^+$ containing salt substitutes, $K^+$-sparing agents (eg, spironolactone, amiloride hydrochloride).

**WARNINGS/PRECAUTIONS:** Check ECG if hyperkalemia occurs. Isolated reports of hypersensitivity reactions; monitor for possible occurrence of blood dyscrasias, liver damage, or other idiosyncratic reactions. In cirrhotics with splenomegaly, may contribute to megaloblastosis in cases where folic stores have been depleted; perform periodic blood studies and observe for exacerbation of liver disease. Monitor BUN periodically. Caution with gouty arthritis; may elevate uric acid levels. May aggravate or cause electrolyte imbalances in CHF, renal disease, or cirrhosis. Caution with history of renal stones.

**ADVERSE REACTIONS:** Hypersensitivity reactions, hyper- or hypokalemia, azotemia, renal stones, jaundice, thrombocytopenia, megaloblastic anemia, N/V, diarrhea, weakness, dizziness.

**INTERACTIONS:** See Contraindications. Increased risk of hyperkalemia with ACE inhibitors. Indomethacin may cause renal failure; caution with NSAIDs. Risk of lithium toxicity. Hyperkalemia may occur when used concomitantly with blood from blood bank, low-salt milk, or potassium containing medications (eg, parenteral penicillin G potassium). May cause hyperglycemia; adjust antidiabetic agents. Chlorpropamide may increase risk of severe hyponatremia. May potentiate nondepolarizing muscle relaxants, antihypertensives, other diuretics, preanesthetics, and anesthetics.

**PREGNANCY:** Category C, not for use in nursing.

**MECHANISM OF ACTION:** $K^+$ sparing diuretic; inhibits reabsorption of $Na^+$ ions in exchange for $K^+$ and $H^+$ ions at segment of distal tubule under control of adrenal mineralocorticoids.

**PHARMACOKINETICS: Absorption:** Rapid; $C_{max}$=30ng/mL, $T_{max}$=3 hrs. **Distribution:** Plasma protein binding (67%); crosses placental barrier. **Metabolism:** Hydroxytriamterene (metabolite). **Elimination:** Urine (21%).

## NURSING CONSIDERATIONS

**Assessment:** Assess for anuria, CHF, DM, gout, hyperkalemia, history of kidney stones, liver/renal impairment, pregnancy/nursing status, and for possible drug interactions.

**Monitoring:** Monitor for signs/symptoms of electrolyte imbalance, exacerbation of gout, hypersensitivity reactions (eg, blood dyscrasias, liver damage), and for liver/renal dysfunction. Monitor for signs/symptoms of hyperkalemia and perform ECG if suspected. Monitor BUN, serum $K^+$ levels, and CBC periodically.

E

**Patient Counseling:** Advise to take after meals to avoid stomach upset. Inform that if single dose is prescribed, it may be preferable to take in a.m. to minimize frequency of urination during nighttime sleep. Instruct not to take more than prescribed dose at next dosing interval if dose missed. Seek medical attention if symptoms of hyperkalemia, electrolyte imbalance, or hypersensitivity reactions occur.

**Administration:** Oral route. **Storage:** 25°C (77°F); excursions permitted to 15-30°C (59-86°F). Dispense in tight, light-resistant container.

# EDLUAR

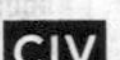


zolpidem tartrate (Meda)

**THERAPEUTIC CLASS:** Imidazopyridine hypnotic

**INDICATIONS:** Short-term treatment of insomnia, characterized by difficulties with sleep initiation.

**DOSAGE:** *Adults:* Individualize dose. 10mg SL qhs. Max: 10mg/day. Elderly/Debilitated Patients: 5mg SL qhs. Concomitant with CNS-Depressant Drugs: Require dose adjustment.

**HOW SUPPLIED:** Tab, Sublingual: 5mg, 10mg

**WARNINGS/PRECAUTIONS:** Evaluate for primary psychiatric and/or medical illness if insomnia fails to remit after 7-10 days of treatment. Severe anaphylactic and anaphylactoid reactions reported; do not rechallenge if patient develops reactions. Visual/auditory hallucinations, complex behavior (eg, sleep-driving), abnormal thinking and behavior changes reported. Worsening of depression, including suicidal thoughts and actions, have been reported in depressed patients. May impair mental/physical abilities. Caution with conditions that could affect metabolism or hemodynamic responses, sleep apnea, myasthenia gravis, and worsening depression. Signs and symptoms of withdrawal reported with abrupt d/c of sedative/hypnotics. Monitor elderly and debilitated patients for impaired motor and/or cognitive performance.

**ADVERSE REACTIONS:** Drowsiness, dizziness, diarrhea, headache, drugged feelings, dry mouth, back pain, allergy, sinusitis, and pharyngitis.

**INTERACTIONS:** CNS-active drugs may potentially enhance effects. Additive effects on psychomotor performance with alcohol/chlorpromazine. Decreased alertness observed with imipramine/chlorpromazine. Ketoconazole may enhance sedative effects. May decrease effects with rifampin.

**PREGNANCY:** Category C, caution in nursing.

**MECHANISM OF ACTION:** Imidazopyridine, non-benzodiazepine hypnotic; binds to GABA-BZ receptor complex at the α1/α5 subunits.

**PHARMACOKINETICS: Absorption:** Rapid; $C_{max}$=106ng/mL; $T_{max}$=82 min. **Distribution:** Plasma protein binding (92.5%). **Elimination:** Renal; (5mg) $T_{1/2}$=2.85 hrs, (10mg) $T_{1/2}$=2.65 hrs.

## NURSING CONSIDERATIONS

**Assessment:** Assess for primary psychiatric and/or medical illness, pre-existing respiratory impairment (eg, sleep apnea syndrome), myasthenia gravis, hypersensitivity reactions, hepatic impairment, history of alcohol, pregnancy/nursing status, and possible drug interactions.

**Monitoring:** Monitor for anaphylactic/anaphylactoid reactions, abnormal thinking, behavioral changes, complex behavior (eg, sleep-driving), hepatic impairment, and those on long-term treatment for drug abuse/dependence.

**Patient Counseling:** Instruct not to swallow or take with water. Tablet should be placed under the tongue. Should not to be given with or immediately after a meal. Inform to take just before bedtime. Advise not to take with alcohol. Caution against hazardous tasks (eg, driving/operating machines). Counsel about risks/benefits of use. Seek medical attention if severe anaphylactic and anaphylactoid reactions occur. Notify physician of all concomitant medications and any episodes of sleep-driving or complex behaviors.

**Administration:** Oral route. Tablet should be placed under the tongue.
**Storage:** 20-25°C (68-77°F). Protect from light and moisture.

## EFFEXOR — RX

venlafaxine HCl (Wyeth)

**Antidepressants increased the risk of suicidal thinking and behavior (suicidality) in children, adolescents, and young adults in short-term studies of major depressive disorder (MDD) and other psychiatric disorders. Not approved for use in pediatric patients.**

**THERAPEUTIC CLASS:** Serotonin and norepinephrine reuptake inhibitor

**INDICATIONS:** Treatment of major depressive disorder (MDD).

**DOSAGE:** *Adults:* Initial: 75mg/day given bid-tid with food. Titrate: Increase by 75mg/day at no less than 4-day intervals. Max: 375mg/day given tid. Hepatic Impairment (moderate): Reduce dose by 50%. Renal Impairment (mild to moderate): Reduce dose by 25%. Hemodialysis: Reduce dose by 50%.

**HOW SUPPLIED:** Tab: 25mg*, 37.5mg*, 50mg*, 75mg*, 100mg* *scored

**CONTRAINDICATIONS:** Concomitant use of MAOI or within 14 days of stopping an MAOI. At least 7 days must be allowed after stopping venlafaxine before starting an MAOI.

**WARNINGS/PRECAUTIONS:** Avoid abrupt withdrawal; monitor for new symptoms when d/c treatment and re-evaluate periodically. Monitor for clinical worsening, suicidality, and/or unusual behavioral changes, especially at initiation of therapy or dose changes. Assess bipolar disorder risk before initiating therapy. Serotonin syndrome or neuroleptic malignant syndrome (NMS)-like reactions reported; d/c immediately and monitor. May cause sustained increases in BP. Hyponatremia, syndrome of inappropriate antidiuretic hormone secretion (SIADH), treatment-emergent anxiety, nervousness, insomnia, anorexia, and activation of mania/hypomania reported. Caution with history of mania or seizures and conditions affecting hemodynamic responses or metabolism; d/c if seizures occur. Mydriasis may occur; monitor patients with increase of intraocular pressure (IOP) or risk of acute narrow-angle glaucoma. May increase risk of bleeding events. Elevation of cholesterol levels reported; monitor periodically. Caution with hyperthyroidism, heart failure, recent MI, renal or hepatic impairment. Interstitial lung disease and eosinophilic pneumonia reported rarely. Caution in elderly.

**ADVERSE REACTIONS:** Asthenia, sweating, N/V, headache, diarrhea, constipation, anorexia, insomnia, somnolence, dry mouth, dizziness, nervousness, anxiety, abnormal ejaculation/orgasm, and impotence in men.

**INTERACTIONS:** See Contraindications. Avoid alcohol, tryptophan. Increased risk of bleeding with ASA, NSAIDs, warfarin, and other anticoagulants. Caution with cimetidine in elderly, HTN, hepatic dysfunction. Altered coagulation effects with warfarin. Decreases clearance of haloperidol. Increases risperidone and desipramine plasma levels. Increase levels with ketoconazole. Caution with metoprolol, potent inhibitors of CYP3A4 and CYP2D6, CNS-active drugs, and serotonergic drugs (eg, triptans, SSRIs, other SNRIs, linezolid, lithium, tramadol, or St. John's wort). Dose-dependent weight loss reported; coadministration with weight-loss agents not recommended. Coadministration with tryptophan supplements is not recommended.

**PREGNANCY:** Category C, not for use in nursing.

**MECHANISM OF ACTION:** Serotonin and norepinephrine reuptake inhibitor; potentiates neurotransmitter activity of CNS activity by inhibiting neuronal serotonin and norephinephrine reuptake.

**PHARMACOKINETICS: Absorption:** Well absorbed; relative bioavailability (100%). **Distribution:** Venlafaxine: $V_d$=7.5L/kg; plasma protein binding (27%). ODV: $V_d$=5.7L/kg; plasma protein binding (30%). Found in breastmilk. **Metabolism:** Hepatic; metabolite: O-desmethylvenlafaxine (ODV). **Elimination:** Venlafaxine: Urine, unchanged (5%); $T_{1/2}$=5 hrs. ODV: Urine: unconjugated (29%), conjugated (26%); $T_{1/2}$=11 hrs.

E

## NURSING CONSIDERATIONS

**Assessment:** Assess for bipolar disorder risk, history of mania and drug abuse, hyperthyroidism, heart failure, recent MI, history of glaucoma, increased IOP, risk factors for acute-narrow angle glaucoma, pre-existing HTN, history of seizures, disease/condition that alters metabolism or hemodynamic response, cholesterol levels, hepatic/renal impairment, pregnancy/nursing status, and possible drug interactions.

**Monitoring:** Monitor HR, BP, LFTs, renal function, cholesterol, triglycerides (TG) and ECG changes, height and weight. Monitor for signs/symptoms of clinical worsening (suicidality, unusual changes in behavior), serotonin syndrome or NMS-like reactions, mydriasis, severe HTN, lung disease (progressive dyspnea, cough, chest discomfort), abnormal bleeding, allergic reactions (rash, hives), hyponatremia (headache, weakness, unsteadiness), seizures, cognitive/motor impairment, and hepatic/renal dysfunction. If abruptly d/c, monitor for symptoms of dysphoric mood, irritability, agitation, dizziness, sensory disturbances, anxiety, confusion, headache, lethargy, emotional lability, insomnia, and hypomania.

**Patient Counseling:** Advise to avoid alcohol. Seek medical attention for symptoms of serotonin syndrome (mental status changes, tachycardia, hyperthermia, NV, diarrhea, incoordination), abnormal bleeding (particularly if using NSAIDs or ASA), hyponatremia (headache, weakness, unsteadiness), mydriasis, severe HTN, lung disease (progressive dyspnea, cough, chest discomfort), activation of mania, allergic reaction (rash, hives), seizures, clinical worsening (suicidal ideation, unusual changes in behavior), or discontinuation symptoms (irritability, agitation, dizziness, anxiety, headache, insomnia). Notify physician if pregnant or breastfeeding, if rash, hives, or related allergic phenomenon develop. Notify healthcare provider of glaucoma history or an increase in IOP.

**Administration:** Oral route. **Storage:** 20-25°C (68-77°F) in a dry place.

# EFFEXOR XR — RX

venlafaxine HCl (Wyeth)

**Antidepressants increased the risk of suicidal thinking and behavior (suicidality) in children, adolescents, and young adults in short-term studies of major depressive disorder (MDD) and other psychiatric disorders. Not approved for use in pediatric patients.**

**THERAPEUTIC CLASS:** Serotonin and norepinephrine reuptake inhibitor

**INDICATIONS:** Treatment of major depressive disorder (MDD), generalized anxiety disorder (GAD), social anxiety disorder (SAD), and panic disorder (PD).

**DOSAGE:** *Adults:* Give qd, either in the qam or qpm. MDD/GAD/SAD: Initial: 75mg qd, or 37.5mg qd increase to 75mg qd after 4-7 days. Titrate: May increase by increments of up to 75mg/day at no less than 4-day intervals. Max: 225mg/day. PD: Initial: 37.5mg qd for 7 days. Titrate: May increase by increments of up to 75mg/day at no less than 7 day intervals. Max: 225mg/day. Switching from Effexor IR Tablets: Give the nearest equivalent dose (mg/day) qd. Individual dose adjustments may be necessary. Hepatic Impairment (Mild-Moderate): Reduce initial dose by 50%. Renal Impairment: Reduce total daily dose by 25-50%. Hemodialysis: Reduce total daily dose by 50%.

**HOW SUPPLIED:** Cap, Extended-Release: 37.5mg, 75mg, 150mg

**CONTRAINDICATIONS:** Concomitant use of MAOIs.

**WARNINGS/PRECAUTIONS:** Avoid abrupt withdrawal. Re-evaluate periodically. Monitor for clinical worsening, suicidality, and/or unusual behavioral changes, especially at initiation of therapy or dose changes. Serotonin syndrome or neuroleptic malignant syndrome (NMS)-like reactions reported; d/c immediately and monitor. May cause sustained increases in BP. Activation of mania/hypomania, mydriasis, hyponatremia, SIADH, altered platelet function, treatment-emergent nervousness, insomnia, and anorexia reported. Caution with history of mania or seizures, conditions affecting hemodynamic responses or metabolism; d/c if seizures occur. Monitor increase of intraocular pressure (IOP) or risk of acute narrow-angle glaucoma. May increase risk of bleeding events. Elevation of cholesterol levels reported; monitor periodically. Caution with hyperthyroidism, heart failure, recent MI, renal or hepatic impairment. Interstitial lung disease and eosinophilic pneumonia reported rarely. Caution in elderly.

**ADVERSE REACTIONS:** Asthenia, sweating, headache, N/V, constipation, anorexia, dry mouth, dizziness, insomnia, nervousness, somnolence, abnormal ejaculation, abnormal dreams, pharyngitis.

**INTERACTIONS:** See Contraindications. Avoid alcohol, tryptophan. Increased risk of bleeding with ASA, NSAIDs, warfarin, and other anticoagulants. Caution with cimetidine in elderly, HTN, hepatic dysfunction. Altered coagulation effects with warfarin. Decreases clearance of haloperidol. Increases risperidone and desipramine plasma levels. Increase levels with ketoconazole. Caution with metoprolol, potent inhibitors of CYP3A4 and CYP2D6, CNS-active drugs, and serotonergic drugs (eg, triptans, SSRIs, other SNRIs, linezolid, lithium, tramadol, or St. John's wort). Coadministration with tryptophan supplements and weight-loss agents are not recommended.

**PREGNANCY:** Category C, not for use in nursing.

**MECHANISM OF ACTION:** 5-HT and NE reuptake inhibitor; potentiates neurotransmitter activity of CNS by inhibiting neuronal serotonin and norephinephrine reuptake.

**PHARMACOKINETICS: Absorption:** Venlafaxine: Absolute bioavailability (45%), $C_{max}$=150ng/mL, $T_{max}$=5.5 hrs. ODV (metabolite): $C_{max}$=260ng/mL, $T_{max}$=9 hrs. **Distribution:** Venlafaxine: $V_d$=7.5L/kg; plasma protein binding (27%). ODV: $V_d$=5.7L/kg; plasma protein binding (30%). **Metabolism:** Hepatic via CYP2D6; Active metabolite: O-desmethylvenlafaxine (ODV). Found in breast milk. **Elimination:** Urine (5% unchanged). Venlafaxine: $T_{1/2}$=5 hrs. ODV: $T_{1/2}$=11 hrs.

## NURSING CONSIDERATIONS

**Assessment:** Assess for bipolar disorder risk, history of mania, hyperthyroidism, HF, recent MI, acute narrow-angle glaucoma, elevated IOP, HTN, seizures, hypersensitivity, concomitant use of MAOIs, serotonin syndrome, disease/condition that alters metabolism or hemodynamic response, cholesterol levels, hepatic/renal impairment, pregnancy/nursing status, and possible drug interactions.

**Monitoring:** Monitor HR, BP, LFTs, renal function, cholesterol, TG and ECG changes, signs/symptoms of clinical worsening (suicidality, unusual behavior), serotonin syndrome or NMS-like reactions (agitation, hallucinations, coma, uncoordination, tachycardia, hyperthermia, labile BP, N/V, diarrhea), mydriasis, severe HTN, lung disease (progressive dyspnea, cough, chest discomfort), abnormal bleeding, allergic reactions (rash, hives), hyponatremia (headache, weakness, unsteadiness), seizures, cognitive/motor impairment, and hepatic/renal dysfunction. If abruptly d/c, monitor for dizziness, sensory disturbances, anxiety, confusion, headache, lethargy, emotional lability, insomnia, and hypomania.

**Patient Counseling:** Advise to avoid alcohol; may impair physical/mental abilities. Seek medical attention for symptoms of serotonin syndrome (mental status changes, tachycardia, hyperthermia, N/V, diarrhea, incoordination), abnormal bleeding (particularly if using NSAIDs or ASA), hyponatremia (headache, weakness, unsteadiness), mydriasis, severe HTN, lung disease (progressive dyspnea, cough, chest discomfort), activation of mania, allergic reaction (rash, hives), seizures, clinical worsening (suicidal ideation, unusual changes in behavior), or discontinuation symptoms (irritability, agitation,

dizziness, anxiety, headache, insomnia). Caution that medication may impair physical/mental abilities. Notify a physician if a rash, hives, or related allergic phenomenon develop.
**Administration:** Oral route. Take with food; swallow whole without chewing or open cap and sprinkle on spoonful of applesauce followed with water.
**Storage:** 20-25°C (68-77°F).

E

## EFFIENT RX

prasugrel (Daiichi Sankyo/Eli Lilly)

**Prasugrel may cause significant, sometimes fatal, bleeding; risk factors include <60kg body weight, propensity to bleed, and concomitant use of medications that may increase bleeding. Do not use in patient with active pathological bleeding or history of transient ischemic attacks (TIA) or stroke. Not recommended in patients ≥75 yrs due to increased risk of fatal intracranial bleeding and uncertain benefits, except in diabetes or history of prior myocardial infarction (MI). Do not start in patients likely to undergo urgent coronary artery bypass graft surgery (CABG); d/c at least 7 days prior to surgery. Suspect bleeding in any patient who is hypotensive and has recently undergone coronary angiography, percutaneous coronary intervention (PCI), CABG, or other surgical procedures; if possible, manage bleeding without d/c. D/C in the first few weeks after acute coronary syndrome, increases the risk of subsequent CV events.**

**THERAPEUTIC CLASS:** Platelet aggregation inhibitor

**INDICATIONS:** Reduction of thrombotic CV events (eg, stent thrombosis) in patients with ACS (eg, unstable angina, non ST-elevation MI, ST-elevation MI) who are to be managed with percutaneous coronary intervention (PCI).

**DOSAGE:** *Adults:* LD: 60mg PO single dose. Maint: 10mg qd. ≤60 kg: Reduce to 5mg qd. Should be taken with ASA 75mg-325mg qd. Take with or without meals.

**HOW SUPPLIED:** Tab: 5mg, 10mg

**CONTRAINDICATIONS:** Active pathological bleeding (eg, peptic ulcer or intracranial hemorrhage), history of prior TIA or stroke.

**WARNINGS/PRECAUTIONS:** Witholding a dose will not be useful in managing a bleeding event or the risk of bleeding associated with an invasive procedure. CABG-related bleeding may be treated with blood transfusion (eg, packed red blood cells and platelets); platelet transfusion within 6 hrs of loading dose or 4 hrs of maintenance dose may be less effective. D/C if active bleeding, elective surgery, stroke or TIA occurs. Premature d/c of the therapy will be at increased risk for cardiac events. Lapses in therapy should be avoided; if therapy is temporarily d/c because of adverse events, should be restarted as soon as possible. Thrombotic thrombocytopenic purpura (TTP) reported, sometimes after brief exposure (<2 weeks); may require treatment (eg, plasmapheresis).

**ADVERSE REACTIONS:** CABG and Non-CABG-related bleeding, hypertension, hypercholesterolemia/hyperlipidemia, headache, back pain, dyspnea, nausea, dizziness, cough, hypotension, fatigue, non-cardiac chest pain.

**INTERACTIONS:** See Black Box Warning. May increase the risk of bleeding when coadministered with warfarin, heparin, fibrinolytic therapy and chronic use of NSAIDs.

**PREGNANCY:** Category B, caution in nursing.

**MECHANISM OF ACTION:** Platelet aggregation inhibitor; thienopyridine class. Inhibits activation and aggregation through irreversible binding of its active metabolite to the $P2Y_{12}$ ADP receptors on platelets.

**PHARMACOKINETICS: Absorption:** (Prodrug) Rapid ( ≥79%); $T_{max}$=30 mins. **Distribution:** Serum albumin (98%) $V_d$=112-166L/hr. **Metabolism:** Hydrolysis via CYP3A4 and CYP2B6 and to a lesser extent by CYP2C9 and CYP2C19 in the intestine to thiolactone (active metabolite). **Elimination:** Urine (68%), feces (27%); $T_{1/2}$= (active metabolite) 7 hrs.

### NURSING CONSIDERATIONS

**Assessment:** Assess for presence of active bleeding (eg, peptic ulcer, intracranial hemorrhage), history of prior TIA or stroke, ACS, concomitant use of medications that may increase bleeding (eg, warfarin, heparin, fibrinolytic therapy, NSAIDs), possible urgent CABG surgery, hepatic impairment, nursing/pregnancy status, and possible drug interactions. Assess use in patient ≥75 years of age and/or <60 kg. Obtain baseline hematologic parameters, including PT/PTT.

**Monitoring:** Monitor for signs/symptoms of hypotension, TTP (eg, thrombocytopenia) and for active bleeding. Patients who require premature d/c, monitor for cardiac events.

**Patient Counseling:** Counsel about benefits/risks of therapy. Instruct to take as prescribed. Encourage not to d/c therapy without discussing with physician who prescribed. Inform patients that they will bleed and bruise more easily, take longer time to stop bleeding. Instruct to report any unanticipated, prolonged, or excessive bleeding, or blood in urine or stool. Inform patients about signs and symptoms requiring medical attention such as TTP (rare). Notify healthcare provider if fever, weakness, extreme skin paleness, purple skin patches, yellowing of the skin or eyes, or neurological changes occur. Inform physician and dentist before invasive procedure. Notify physician of all prescription medications, OTC, or dietary supplements that are being taken or plan to take while on therapy. Advise patient not to take prasugrel if have abnormal bleeding such as stomach or intestinal bleeding; and have history of stroke or TIA.

**Administration:** Oral route. **Storage:** 25°C (77°F); excursions permitted to 15-30°C (59-86°F). Dispense and keep product in original container. Keep container closed and do not remove desiccant from bottle. Do not break the tablet.

## ELDEPRYL — RX

selegiline HCl (Somerset)

**THERAPEUTIC CLASS:** Monoamine oxidase inhibitor (Type B)

**INDICATIONS:** Adjunct in the management of Parkinsonian patients being treated with levodopa/carbidopa who exhibit deterioration in the quality of their response to this therapy.

**DOSAGE:** *Adults:* 5mg bid, at breakfast and lunch. Max: 10mg/day. May attempt to reduce levodopa/carbidopa after 2-3 days of therapy. Usual reduction of 10-30%; may reduce further with continued therapy.

**HOW SUPPLIED:** Cap: 5mg; Tab: 5mg

**CONTRAINDICATIONS:** Concomitant meperidine, or other opioids.

**WARNINGS/PRECAUTIONS:** Selegiline should not be used at doses exceeding 10 mg/day because of the risks associated with non-selective inhibition of MAO. Decrease levodopa/carbidopa by 10-30% to prevent exacerbation of levodopa-associated side effects. Patients with Parkinson's disease have higher risk of melanoma; monitor frequently for melanoma. There have been reports of patients experiencing intense urges to gamble, increased sexual urges, and other intense urges and the inability to control these urges while taking selegeline. Although it is not proved that the medications caused these events, these urges were reported to have stopped in some cases when the dose was reduced or the medication was stopped.

**ADVERSE REACTIONS:** Nausea, dizziness/lightheadedness/fainting, abdominal pain, confusion, hallucinations, dry mouth, vivid dreams, dyskinesias, headache.

**INTERACTIONS:** See Contraindications. Stupor, muscular rigidity, severe agitation, and elevated temperature reported with meperidine; avoid concomitant use. Avoid SSRIs and TCAs; severe toxicity reported. Allow 2 weeks between d/c of selegiline and initiation of TCAs or SSRIs. Allow 5 weeks between d/c of fluoxetine and initiation of selegiline due to long half-lives of fluoxetine and its active metabolite. Caution with sympathomimetics (eg, ephedrine), tyramine-containing food; hypertensive crises/reactions reported.

**PREGNANCY:** Category C, safety not known in nursing.

**MECHANISM OF ACTION:** Monoamine oxidase inhibitor (type B); mechanism accounting for the activity in Parkinson's disease is not fully understood. Irreversibly inhibits MAO type B (selectivity is dose-dependent) blocking the catabolism of dopamine. May also act through other mechanisms to increase dopaminergic activity.

**PHARMACOKINETICS: Absorption:** $C_{max}$=1ng/mL. **Metabolism:** Gut and liver (extensive). Metabolites: N-desmethylselegiline (active), L-amphetamine, L-methamphetamine. **Elimination:** $T_{1/2}$=2 hrs (single-dose), 10 hrs (steady-state)

E

## NURSING CONSIDERATIONS

**Assessment:** Assess BP, HR, dyskinesia. Note other conditions/diseases and drug therapies. Assess pregnancy/nursing status.

**Monitoring:** Monitor for hypersensitivity reactions, syncope, angina pectoris, hyperpyrexia, hypertensive crisis, hallucinations, myoclonic jerks, melanomas. Monitor for intense urges to gamble and for increased sexual urges.

**Patient Counseling:** Inform of the signs and symptoms of MAOI-induced hypertensive reactions. Instruct to avoid exceeding the recommended dose. Instruct to report adverse side effects (eg, severe headache, abnormal urges, loss of impulse control, etc.). Instruct to avoid tyramine-containing foods (eg, aged cheeses, pickled herring, yeast extract, air-dried meats) and beverages (certain red wines and beers).

**Administration:** Oral route. **Storage:** 20-25°C (68-77°F).

# ELESTAT RX

epinastine HCl (Inspire)

**THERAPEUTIC CLASS:** $H_1$-antagonist

**INDICATIONS:** Prevention of itching associated with allergic conjunctivitis.

**DOSAGE:** *Adults:* 1 drop in each eye bid.
*Pediatrics:* ≥3 yrs: 1 drop in each eye bid.

**HOW SUPPLIED:** Sol: 0.05% [5mL]

**WARNINGS/PRECAUTIONS:** Not for contact lens-related irritation. May reinsert contact lens 10 min after dosing if eye is not red.

**ADVERSE REACTIONS:** Burning sensation in the eye, folliculosis, hyperemia, pruritus, infection (cold symptoms and upper respiratory infections).

**PREGNANCY:** Category C, caution in nursing.

**MECHANISM OF ACTION:** $H_1$-receptor antagonist; inhibits histamine release from the mast cell; selective for the histamine $H_1$-receptor and has affinity for the histamine $H_2$-receptor and possesses affinity for the $\alpha_1$-$\alpha_2$ and 5-$HT_2$-receptors.

**PHARMACOKINETICS: Absorption:** $C_{max}$=0.04ng/ml; $T_{max}$=2 hrs. **Distribution:** Plasma protein binding (64%). **Metabolism:** Active tubular secretion. **Elimination:** Urine (55%, unchanged), feces (30%, unchanged); $T_{1/2}$=12 hrs.

## NURSING CONSIDERATIONS

**Assessment:** Assess for drug hypersensitivity.

**Monitoring:** Monitor adverse events such as burning sensation in the eye, folliculosis, hyperemia, pruritus, and infection (cold symptoms and upper respiratory infections).

**Patient Counseling:** Counsel not to wear contact lenses if eye is red; remove prior to instillation. Inform that medication is not for treatment of contact lens-related irritation. Instruct to avoid touching tip of container to eye or any other surface to avoid contamination.

**Administration:** Ocular route. **Storage:** 15-25°C (59-77°F). Keep tightly closed.

## ELIDEL RX

pimecrolimus (Novartis)

E

**THERAPEUTIC CLASS:** Macrolactam ascomycin derivative

**INDICATIONS:** Second-line therapy for the short-term and noncontinuous chronic therapy of mild to moderate atopic dermatitis in non-immunocompromised patients ≥ 2 yrs intolerant to or inadequately responsive to other topical prescription treatments.

**DOSAGE:** *Adults:* Apply thin layer to the affected area(s) bid until symptoms resolve. Re-evaluate if symptoms persist after 6 weeks.
*Pediatrics:* ≥2 yrs: Apply thin layer to the affected area(s) bid until symptoms resolve. Re-evaluate if symptoms persist after 6 weeks.

**HOW SUPPLIED:** Cre: 1% [30g, 60g, 100g]

**WARNINGS/PRECAUTIONS:** Long-term safety, beyond 1 year of noncontinuous use, has not been established. Rare cases of malignancy (eg, skin malignancies and lymphoma) reported with topical calcineurin inhibitors; therefore, continuous long-term use should be avoided and application limited to areas of involvement. If signs and symptoms persist beyond 6 weeks, re-examine to confirm diagnosis of atopic dermatitis. Avoid with malignant or pre-malignant skin conditions, Netherton's syndrome, or other skin conditions that may increase the potential for systemic absorption. Avoid in immunocompromised persons and children <2 yrs old. Resolve bacterial or viral infections at treatment sites before starting treatment. Increased risk of varicella zoster infection, herpes simplex virus infection or eczema herpeticum. Skin papilloma/warts reported; consider d/c if skin papillomas worsen or are unresponsive to conventional treatment. Lymphadenopathy reported; d/c if lymphadenopathy of uncertain etiology or acute infectious mononucleosis occurs. Minimize or avoid natural or artificial sunlight exposure.

**ADVERSE REACTIONS:** Application-site burning, application-site reaction, upper respiratory tract infection, headache, nasopharyngitis, influenza, abdominal pain, diarrhea, sore throat, hypersensitivity, pyrexia, cough, rhinitis, N/V.

**INTERACTIONS:** Caution with CYP3A4 inhibitors (eg, erythromycin, itraconazole, ketoconazole, fluconazole, CCBs, cimetidine) in patients with widespread and/or erythrodermic disease. Skin flushing associated with concomitant alcohol use has been reported.

**PREGNANCY:** Category C, not for use in nursing.

**MECHANISM OF ACTION:** Macrolactam ascomycin derivative; not fully established. Suspected to bind with high affinity to macrophilin-12 (FKBP-12) and inhibit the calcium-dependent phosphatase, calcineurin. Consequently, this inhibits T cell activation by blocking the transcription of early cytokines. In particular, pimecrolimus inhibits at nanomolar concentrations Interleukin-2 and interferon gamma (Th1-type) and Interleukin-4 and Interleukin-10 (Th2-type) cytokine synthesis in human T cells. In addition, pimecrolimus prevents the release of inflammatory cytokines and mediators from mast cells in vitro after stimulation by antigen/IgE.

**PHARMACOKINETICS: Absorption:** $C_{max}$=1.4ng/mL (adults), <2.6ng/mL (pediatrics). **Distribution:** Plasma protein binding (99.5%). **Metabolism:** Liver via CYP3A. **Elimination:** Feces (78.4% metabolites, <1% unchanged).

### NURSING CONSIDERATIONS

**Assessment:** Assess for malignant or premalignant skin conditions (eg, cutaneous-cell lymphoma), Netherton's syndrome or other skin diseases, viral or bacterial skin infections, generalized erythroderma, and possible drug interactions. Assess patient's age and pregnancy/nursing status.

**Monitoring:** Monitor for infections (eg, varicella virus infection, herpes simplex virus infection, eczema herpeticum), lymphomas, skin malignancies, local symptoms (eg, itching, rash, redness) and adverse reactions (eg, application-site reactions).

**Patient Counseling:** Inform not to use drug continuously for long periods of time. Advise to d/c medication when signs/symptoms of eczema subside (eg, itching, rash, and redness). Contact physician if symptoms get worse, a skin infection develops, or if symptoms do not improve after 6 weeks of treatment. Instruct to wash hands and dry skin before applying cream. Do not bathe, shower, or swim after applying cream. Instruct not to cover treated skin area with bandages, dressings, or wraps. Advise that is for external use only; avoid contact with eyes. Avoid natural or artificial sunlight exposure while on therapy.

**Administration:** Topical route. **Storage:** 25°C (77°F); excursions permitted to 15-30°C (59-86°F). Do not freeze.

E

## ELIGARD RX

leuprolide acetate (Sanofi-Aventis)

**THERAPEUTIC CLASS:** Synthetic gonadotropin releasing hormone analog

**INDICATIONS:** Palliative treatment of advanced prostate cancer.

**DOSAGE:** *Adults:* 7.5mg SQ monthly, 22.5mg SQ every 3 months, 30mg SQ every 4 months, or 45mg SQ every 6 months. Rotate injection sites.

**HOW SUPPLIED:** Inj: 7.5mg, 22.5mg, 30mg, 45mg

**CONTRAINDICATIONS:** Women, pregnancy, pediatric patients.

**WARNINGS/PRECAUTIONS:** Transient worsening of symptoms or onset of new signs/symptoms may occur during 1st few weeks of therapy. Closely monitor patients with metastatic vertebral lesions and/or urinary tract obstruction during first few weeks of therapy. Urethral obstruction and spinal cord compression reported. Monitor serum testosterone, PSA.

**ADVERSE REACTIONS:** Hot flashes, pain/burning/stinging/erythema/bruising at injection site, malaise/fatigue, atrophy of testes, weakness, gynecomastia, myalgia, dizziness, decreased libido, rigors, lethargy, dyspepsia, scanty urination, limb pain, insomnia, breast soreness, hypertension, clamminess, pituitary aplopexy.

**PREGNANCY:** Category X, safety in nursing not known.

**MECHANISM OF ACTION:** LH-RH agonist; acts as a potent inhibitor of gonadotropin secretion and suppresses testicular and ovarian steroidogenesis.

**PHARMACOKINETICS: Absorption**: (7.5mg, 1st inj) $C_{max}$=25.3ng/mL, $T_{max}$=5 hrs. (22.5mg; 1st inj, 2nd inj) $C_{max}$=127ng/mL, 107ng/mL, $T_{max}$=5 hrs. (30mg; 1st inj) $C_{max}$=150ng/mL, $T_{max}$=3.3 hrs. (45mg; 1st inj, 2nd inj): $C_{max}$=82ng/mL, 102ng/mL, $T_{max}$=4.5 hrs. **Distribution**: $V_d$=27L; plasma protein binding (43%-49%). **Metabolism**: Pentapeptide (major metabolite).

### NURSING CONSIDERATIONS

**Assessment:** Assess for metastatic vertebral lesions and urinary tract obstructions.

**Monitoring:** Monitor serum testosterone and PSA periodically and for signs/symptoms of worsening, spinal cord compression, renal impairment, and hypersensitivity reactions.

**Patient Counseling:** Inform may experience worsening of symptoms or onset of new symptoms during first weeks of treatment (bone pain, neuropathy, hematuria, or bladder outlet obstruction). Advise to seek medical attention if symptoms of worsening, spinal cord compression, or hypersensitivity reactions occur.

**Administration:** SQ. **Storage**: 2-8°C (36-46°F).

# ELLENCE RX

## epirubicin HCl (Pharmacia & Upjohn)

**Severe local tissue necrosis with extravasation. Not for IM/SQ administration. Myocardial toxicity manifested by congestive heart failure may occur during therapy or months to years after. May increase risk of cardiac toxicity with concomitant radiotherapy to the mediastinal/pericardial area, previous therapy with other anthracyclines or anthracenediones, or concomitant use of other cardiotoxic drugs. Secondary acute myelogenous leukemia (AML) reported in breast cancer treated patients. Occurrence of refractory secondary leukemia with DNA-damaging antineoplastics, heavy pretreatment with cytotoxic drugs, or escalated doses of anthracyclines. Reduce dose with hepatic dysfunction. Severe myelosuppression may occur. Administer only under supervision of a physician experienced with chemotherapeutic agents.**

**THERAPEUTIC CLASS:** Anthracycline

**INDICATIONS:** Component of adjuvant therapy in patients with evidence of axillary node tumor involvement following resection of primary breast cancer.

**DOSAGE:** *Adults:* Initial: 100-120mg/m², repeat at 3-4 week cycles. May give total dose on Day 1 of each cycle or divide equally on Days 1 and 8. Bone Marrow Dysfunction: Initial: 75-90mg/m². Hepatic Dysfunction: Bilirubin 1.2-3mg/dL or AST 2-4X ULN: Give 1/2 of initial dose. Bilirubin >3mg/dL or AST >4X ULN: Give 1/4 of initial dose. Severe Renal Dysfunction: Serum Creatinine >5mg/dL: Lower dose. Give prophylactic therapy with SMZ-TMP or fluoroquinolone with 120mg/m² regimen. Consider pretreatment with antiemetics. Adjust dose after 1st treatment cycle based on hematologic and nonhematologic toxicities; refer to PI for dosing. Administer by IV infusion.

**HOW SUPPLIED:** Inj: 2mg/mL [25mL, 100mL]

**CONTRAINDICATIONS:** Baseline neutrophils <1500 cells/mm³, severe myocardial insufficiency, recent MI, severe arrhythmias, previous anthracycline therapy with maximum cumulative dose, anthracenedione hypersensitivity, severe hepatic dysfunction.

**WARNINGS/PRECAUTIONS:** Increased risk of cardiotoxicity with active or dormant cardiovascular disease. Use extreme caution if exceeding cumulative dose of 900mg/m². Resolve acute toxicities from other cytotoxic agents prior to initiation. Monitor CBC, total bilirubin, AST, SrCr, and cardiac function before and during each cycle. May induce hyperuricemia. Potential for tumor lysis syndrome; monitor serum uric acid, potassium, calcium phosphate, and creatinine immediately after initial therapy. Thrombophlebitis, thromboembolic phenomena reported. Excessive rapid administration may cause facial flushing as well as local erythematous streaking along the vein.

**ADVERSE REACTIONS:** AML, tissue necrosis, myocardial toxicity, myelosuppression, hematologic abnormalities, amenorrhea, hot flashes, lethargy, fever, GI disturbances, infection, conjunctivitis/keratitis, alopecia, local toxicity, rash/itch.

**INTERACTIONS:** See Black Box Warning. Additive toxicity with other cytotoxic drugs. Cyclophosphamide and fluorouracil may cause severe leukopenia, neutropenia, thrombocytopenia, and anemia. Monitor closely with cardioactive compounds that could cause heart failure (eg, CCBs). Caution with agents that cause changes in hepatic function. AUC increased with cimetidine; stop cimetidine during therapy. Previous radiation therapy may induce inflammatory recall reaction at irradiation site. Administration of paclitaxel prior to therapy increase AUC levels.

**PREGNANCY:** Category D, not for use in nursing.

**MECHANISM OF ACTION:** Anthracycline; complexes with DNA by intercalating its planar rings between nucleotide base pairs, inhibiting nucleic acid (DNA and RNA) and protein synthesis, triggering DNA cleavage by topoisomerase II, inhibits DNA helicase activity, and generates free radicals.

**PHARMACOKINETICS: Absorption:** IV administration of variable doses resulted in different parameters. **Distribution:** Plasma protein binding (77%). **Metabolism:** Liver (extensive and rapid); reduction, conjugation, hydrolytic and redox process. Epirubicinol (metabolite). **Elimination:** Biliary (major), urine (minor).

## NURSING CONSIDERATIONS

**Assessment:** Assess for baseline neutrophil count >1500 cells/mm$^3$, CVD (insufficiency, MI, arrhythmias), acute toxicities (prior therapy), hepatic/renal dysfunction, risk factors for cardiac toxicities, pregnancy status, and possible drug interactions. Obtain baseline CBC, total bilirubin, AST, creatinine, and cardiac function (LVEF).

**Monitoring:** Monitor total and differential WBC, RBC, platelet count, AST, total bilirubin, and cardiac function (MUGA, ECHO) before and during each cycle. Assess need for antiemetics. Monitor for hypersensitivity reaction, CHF, liver dysfunction, myelosuppression, hyperuricemia (tumor lysis syndrome), extravasation, facial flushing or local erythematous streaking, and recall reaction (prior radiation).

**Patient Counseling:** Advise to seek medical attention if vomiting, dehydration, fever, evidence of infection, symptoms of CHF, or injection-site pain occur. Inform alopecia will develop. Inform urine may appear red for 1-2 days after administration. Inform of risk of irreversible myocardial damage. Instruct men to use effective contraceptive methods. Inform females may develop premature menopause.

**Administration:** IV route. Administer by IV infusion; see PI for administration technique. **Storage:** Refrigerate; 2-8°C (36-46°F). Do not freeze. Protect from light.

# ELMIRON RX

pentosan polysulfate sodium (Ortho-McNeil)

**THERAPEUTIC CLASS:** Anticoagulant

**INDICATIONS:** Relief of bladder pain/discomfort associated with interstitial cystitis.

**DOSAGE:** *Adults:* Take 1 hr before or 2 hrs after meals with water. 100mg tid for 3 months. Re-evaluate after 3 months; may continue for another 3 months. *Pediatrics:* ≥16 yrs: Take 1 hr before or 2 hrs after meals with water. 100mg tid for 3 months. Re-evaluate after 3 months; may continue for another 3 months.

**HOW SUPPLIED:** Cap: 100mg

**WARNINGS/PRECAUTIONS:** Bleeding complications (eg, rectal hemorrhage, ecchymosis, epistaxis, gum hemorrhage), alopecia reported. Caution with invasive procedures, coagulopathy, aneurysms, thrombocytopenia, hemophilia, GI ulcers, polyps, diverticula, history of heparin-induced thrombocytopenia, and hepatic impairment. Increases in PT/PTT, thrombocytopenia, and transient elevation of liver enzymes reported.

**ADVERSE REACTIONS:** Nausea, diarrhea, alopecia, headache, rash, dyspepsia, abdominal pain, rectal hemorrhage.

**INTERACTIONS:** Increased risk of bleeding with anticoagulants, heparin, t-PA, streptokinase, high-dose ASA, and NSAIDs.

**PREGNANCY:** Category B, caution in nursing.

**MECHANISM OF ACTION:** Not fully established; anticoagulant. Possesses anticoagulant and fibrinolytic effects.

**PHARMACOKINETICS: Absorption:** (300mg/450mg) $T_{max}$=0.6-120hrs. **Distribution:** Mainly into uroepithelium. **Metabolism:** Liver and spleen, partial desulfation; depolymerization in kidney. **Elimination:** Feces [(84%, unchanged) 300mg, (58%, unchanged) 450mg], Urine (6%, desulfated/depolymerized metabolites; 0.14%, intact); $T_{1/2}$=27hrs, 20hrs (300mg, 400mg) .

## NURSING CONSIDERATIONS

**Assessment:** Assess for upcoming surgery, pregnancy, liver function, and possible drug interactions (anticoagulants, aspirin, or anti-inflammatory drugs).

**Monitoring:** Monitor for tendency for bleeding, hair loss, diarrhea, nausea, blood in stool, and abnormal LFTs.

**Patient Counseling:** Instruct to take as prescribed and report any persistent side effects or presence of blood in stool.

**Administration:** Oral route. **Storage:** Store at 15-30°C (59-86°F).

## ELOCON RX

mometasone furoate (Schering)

**THERAPEUTIC CLASS:** Corticosteroid

**INDICATIONS:** Relief of inflammatory and pruritic manifestations of corticosteroid-responsive dermatoses.

**DOSAGE:** *Adults:* (Cre, Oint) Apply qd. (Lot) Apply a few drops qd. Re-assess if no improvement seen within 2 weeks.
*Pediatrics:* (Cre, Oint) ≥12 yrs: Apply qd. (Lot) ≥2yrs: Apply a few drops qd. Re-assess if no improvement seen within 2 weeks.

**HOW SUPPLIED:** Cre, Oint: 0.1% [15g, 45g]; Lot: 0.1% [30mL, 60mL]

**WARNINGS/PRECAUTIONS:** Systemic absorption may produce reversible hypothalamic-pituitary-adrenal (HPA) axis suppression, manifestations of Cushing's syndrome, hyperglycemia, and glucosuria. D/C if irritation occurs. Use appropriate antifungal or antibacterial agent with dermatological infections. Pediatric patients may be more susceptible to systemic toxicity. Lotion not recommended in children <12 yrs old. Caution when applied to large surface areas or with occlusive dressings.

**ADVERSE REACTIONS:** Burning, pruritus, skin atrophy, rosacea, acneiform reaction, tingling, stinging, furunculosis, folliculitis, hypertrichosis, hypopigmentation, perioral dermatitis, allergic contact dermatitis, striae, miliaria.

**PREGNANCY:** Category C, caution in nursing.

**MECHANISM OF ACTION:** Corticosteroid; possesses anti-inflammatory, antipruritic, and vasoconstrictive properties. Anti-inflammatory effects not established. Suspected to induce phospholipase $A_2$ inhibitory proteins, lipocortins. Lipocortins control biosynthesis of potent mediators of inflammation (eg, prostaglandins and leukotrienes) by inhibiting release of their precursor, arachidonic acid.

**PHARMACOKINETICS: Absorption:** Extent of absorption depends on skin integrity, vehicle, and use of occlusive dressing.

### NURSING CONSIDERATIONS

**Assessment:** Assess for hypersensitivity and use in pregnant/nursing patients.

**Monitoring:** Monitor for signs/symptoms of HPA axis suppression, glucocorticoid insufficiency, Cushing's syndrome, hyperglycemia, glucosuria, skin irritation, allergic contact dermatitis (eg, failure to heal), and skin infections. In patients applying medication to large surface areas or using occlusive dressings, perform periodic monitoring for HPA-axis suppression by using ACTH stimulation, AM plasma cortisol, and urinary free cortisol tests. In pediatric patients, monitor for systemic toxicity, HPA-axis suppression, Cushing's syndrome, linear growth retardation, delayed weight gain, and intracranial HTN.

**Patient Counseling:** Avoid contact with eyes, face, underarms, and groin. Do not wrap, cover, or bandage treated skin unless directed by physician. Instruct patients to report adverse reactions. Do not apply medication in diaper area. Contact physician if no improvement within 2 weeks. Notify physician before using other corticosteroid therapies.

**Administration:** Topical route. **Storage:** 25°C (77°F); excursions permitted to 15-30°C (59-86°F).

## ELOXATIN RX

oxaliplatin (Sanofi-Aventis)

**Anaphylactic-like reactions may occur within minutes of administration.**

**THERAPEUTIC CLASS:** Organoplatinum complex

**INDICATIONS:** Treatment of advanced metastatic carcinoma of colon or rectum and adjuvant treatment of Stage III colon cancer patients who have undergone complete resection of the primary tumor in combination with infusional 5-fluorouracil (5-FU) and leucovorin (LV).

**DOSAGE:** *Adults:* Advanced Colorectal Cancer: Day 1: 85mg/m$^2$ IV with LV 200mg/m$^2$; give over 120 min in separate bags using a Y-line; followed by 5-FU 400mg/m$^2$ bolus over 2-4 min, then 5-FU 600mg/m$^2$ as a 22-hr infusion. Day 2: LV 200mg/m$^2$ over 120 min; followed by 5-FU 400mg/m$^2$ bolus over 2-4 min, then 5-FU 600mg/m$^2$ as a 22-hr infusion. Repeat cycle every 2 weeks. Persistent Grade 2 Neurosensory Events: Reduce oxaliplatin to 65mg/m$^2$. Grade 3 Neurosensory Events: Consider d/c. After Recovery From Grade 3/4 GI or Grade 4 Hematologic Toxicity: Reduce oxaliplatin to 65mg/m$^2$ and 5-FU by 20%. Adjuvant Therapy Stage III Colon Cancer: Recommended cycle every 2 weeks for 6 months. Persistent Grade 2 Neurosensory Events: Reduce oxaliplatin to 75mg/m$^2$. Persistent Grade 3 Neurosensory Events: Consider d/c. After Recovery From Grade 3/4 GI or Grade 3/4 Hematologic Toxicity: Reduce oxaliplatin to 75mg/m$^2$ and 5-FU to 300mg/m$^2$ bolus and 500mg/m$^2$ 22-hr infusion.

**HOW SUPPLIED:** Inj: 50mg, 100mg, 200mg

**CONTRAINDICATIONS:** Hypersensitivity to platinum compounds.

**WARNINGS/PRECAUTIONS:** Acute and persistent neuropathy reported. Cold may exacerbate acute neurological symptoms; avoid ice for mucositis prophylaxis. Potentially fatal pulmonary fibrosis reported. If unexplained respiratory symptoms develop, d/c until interstitial lung disease or pulmonary fibrosis is ruled out. Monitor WBC with differential, Hgb, platelets, and blood chemistries (including ALT, AST, bilirubin, creatinine) before each cycle. Caution with preexisting renal impairment.

**ADVERSE REACTIONS:** Peripheral sensory neuropathy, fatigue, nausea, neutropenia, emesis, diarrhea, thrombocytopenia, anemia, increase in transaminases and alkaline phosphatase, stomatitis, transient vision loss, and other interstitial lung diseases.

**INTERACTIONS:** Increased 5-FU plasma levels with doses of 130mg/m$^2$ oxaliplatin dosed every 3 weeks; clearance may be decreased with nephrotoxic agents.

**PREGNANCY:** Category D, not for use in nursing.

**MECHANISM OF ACTION:** Organoplatinum complex; inhibits DNA replication and transcription.

**PHARMACOKINETICS: Absorption**: $C_{max}$=0.814mcg/mL. **Distribution**: $V_d$=440L; plasma protein binding (>90%). **Metabolism:** Rapid, nonenzymatic biotransformation. **Elimination**: Urine (54%), feces (2%).

## NURSING CONSIDERATIONS

**Assessment:** Assess for preexisting hepatic/renal impairment, pregnancy status, and possible drug interactions.

**Monitoring:** Monitor LFTs, WBC with differential, Hgb, platelet count, bilirubin, and creatinine periodically and before each dose. Monitor for signs/symptoms of anaphylactic reactions, neuropathy, neurosensory toxicity, portal HTN, liver/renal dysfunction, and pulmonary toxicity.

**Patient Counseling:** Inform of pregnancy risks. Inform of neurologic effects and persistent neurosensory toxicity that may be precipitated by exposure to cold or cold objects. Counsel to avoid cold drinks and ice. Cover exposed skin prior to exposure to cold temperature or cold objects. Advise to seek medical attention if persistent vomiting, diarrhea, fever, signs of dehydration or infection, cough, breathing difficulties, and allergic reactions (eg, rash, urticaria, erythema, pruritus, bronchospasm, and hypotension) occur. Vision abnormalities may impair ability to drive and use machinery; promptly report any vision problems to physician.

**Administration:** IV route. Infusion line should be flushed with D5W prior to administration of any concomitant medication. **Storage**: 25°C (77°F); excursions permitted to 15-30°C (59-86°F). Protect from light and do not freeze.

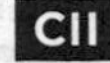

# EMBEDA

CII

naltrexone HCl - morphine sulfate (King)

**Contains morphine sulfate which may be abused in a manner similar to other opioid agonists, legal or illicit. Indicated for management of moderate-to-severe pain when a continuous, around-the-clock opioid analgesic is needed for an extended period of time. Not for use as a prn analgesic. Embeda 100mg/4mg is for use in opioid-tolerant patients only. Concomitant use of alcohol may result in an increase in plasma levels and potentially fatal overdose. Ingestion of capsules or pellets within the capsules may cause fatal respiratory depression when administered to patients not already tolerant to high doses of opioids. Swallow capsules whole or sprinkle contents on applesauce. Crushing, chewing, or dissolving capsules will result in the release of naltrexone, which may precipitate withdrawal in opioid-tolerant patients.**

E

**THERAPEUTIC CLASS:** Opioid agonist-antagonist analgesic

**INDICATIONS:** Management of moderate to severe pain when a continuous, aroung-the-clock opioid analgesic is needed for an extended period of time.

**DOSAGE:** *Adults:* Individualize dose. Chronic Pain: Initial: Start at the lowest dose. Titrate: Increase to qd or bid. Conversion from Other Oral Morphine: Give 50% of daily oral morphine dose q12h or give 100% oral morphine dose q24h. Do not give more frequently than q12h. Conversion from Parenteral Morphine: Oral morphine 3x the daily parenteral morphine dose may be sufficient in chronic use settings. Conversion from Other Parenteral or Oral Opioids: Initial: Give 50% of estimated daily morphine demand and supplement with immediate-release morphine.

**HOW SUPPLIED:** Cap, Extended-Release: (Morphine Sulfate-Naltrexone HCl) 20mg-0.8mg, 30mg-1.2mg, 50mg-2mg, 60mg-2.4mg, 80mg-3.2mg, 100mg-4mg

**CONTRAINDICATIONS:** Respiratory depression, acute or severe bronchial asthma, or hypercapnia in ummonitored settings or the absence of resuscitative equipment. Suspicion of paralytic ileus.

**WARNINGS/PRECAUTIONS:** Respiratory depression possible; caution in chronic obstructive pulmonary disease (COPD), cor pulmonale, or decreased respiratory reserve. Respiratory depressant effects and secondary elevations in cerbrospinal fluid pressure may be exaggerated in the presence of head injuries, intracranial lesions, or a pre-existing increase in intracranial pressure (ICP). May cause severe hypotension. Avoid with GI obstruction. Caution in biliary tract disease, elderly, debilitated, renal/hepatic insufficiency, Addison's disease, myxedema, hypothyroidism, prostatic hypertrophy, urethral stricture, CNS depression, toxic psychosis, acute alcoholism, delirium tremens, and convulsive disorders. D/C 24 hrs before procedure that interrupts pain transmission pathways (eg, cordotomy); give short-acting parenteral opioid. Physical dependence and tolerance are common during chronic therapy. Rare cases of anaphylaxis reported. May impair mental/physical abilities.

**ADVERSE REACTIONS:** Drowsiness, dizziness, constipation, N/V, diarrhea, dry mouth, fatigue, headache, somnolence, hyperhidrosis, pruritus.

**INTERACTIONS:** Increased risk of respiratory depression, hypotension, profound sedation or coma with CNS depressants (eg, sedatives, hypnotics, general anesthetics, antiemetics, phenothiazines, tranquilizers, alcohol); reduce initial dose of one or both agents by 50%. May enhance neuromuscular blocking action of skeletal relaxants. Mixed agonist/antagonist analgesics may reduce analgesic effects or precipitate withdrawal symptoms. Avoid MAOIs during or within 14 days of use. Confusion and severe respiratory depression on hemodialysis patients reported with coadministered cimetidine. May reduce diuretic effects. Anticholinergics or other medications with anticholinergic activity may result in increased risk of urinary retention or severe constipation which may lead to paralytic ileus. Caution when coadministered P-glycoprotein inhibitors.

**PREGNANCY:** Category C, not for use in nursing.

**MECHANISM OF ACTION:** Morphine: Opioid agonist; binds and activates opioid receptors at sites in the peri-aqueductal and peri-ventricular grey matter, the ventro-medial medulla, and the spinal cord to produce analgesia.

Naltrexone: Opioid antagonist; reverses the subjective and analgesic effects of mu-opioid receptor agonists by competitively binding at mu-opioid receptors.

**PHARMACOKINETICS: Absorption:** Various doses resulted in different parameters. **Distribution:** $V_d$=3-4 L/kg; plasma protein binding (30-35%); distributed to skeletal muscle, kidneys, liver, intestinal tract, lungs, spleen, brain; crosses the blood brain barrier (small amount); crosses placental membranes; found in breast milk. **Metabolism:** Morphine: Liver (conjugation and sulfonation); morphine-3-glucuronide, M3G; morphine-6-glucuronide, M6G. Naltrexone: 6-β-naltrexol (extensive). **Elimination:** Urine (major) (10% unchanged); bile (small amount); $T_{1/2}$=29 hrs.



## NURSING CONSIDERATIONS

**Assessment:** Assess for opioid tolerance, pain levels, abuse potential, severe bronchial asthma, COPD, circulatory shock, GI obstruction (paralytic ileus), presence of debilitation (elderly), hepatic/renal impairment, presence of head injury or other intracranial lesions, increased ICP, adrenocortical insufficiency (eg, Addison's disease), CNS depression or coma, toxic psychosis, prostatic hypertrophy or urethral stricture, acute alcoholism, delirium tremens, kyphoscoliosis, convulsive disorders, biliary tract disease (acute pancreatitis), pregnancy/nursing status, and drug interactions.

**Monitoring:** Monitor for signs/symptoms of respiratory depression, hypotension, anaphylaxis, convulsions, tolerance and physical dependence (eg, withdrawal symptoms), and signs of medication misuse or abuse. Monitor serum amylase levels.

**Patient Counseling:** Swallow medication whole (do not chew, crush, or dissolve) or open and sprinkle contents of capsule on small amount of applesauce. Instruct to rinse mouth after taking dose to ensure all pellets have been swallowed. Do not adjust dosing without physician's consent. Inform that drug may impair mental/physical abilities; use caution when performing hazardous tasks (eg, operating machinery/driving). Avoid alcohol and other CNS depressants. Do not abruptly d/c medication. May develop severe constipation during therapy; appropriate concomitant therapy should be given at start of treatment. Medication has potential for abuse.

**Administration:** Oral route. Refer to PI for alternative methods of administration. **Storage:** 25°C (77°F); excursion permitted between 15-30°C (59-86°F). Dispense in a sealed tamper-evident, childproof, light-resistant container.

# EMEND RX

aprepitant (Merck)

**THERAPEUTIC CLASS:** Substance P/neurokinin 1 receptor antagonist

**INDICATIONS:** In combination with other antiemetics for prevention of acute and delayed N/V associated with initial and repeat courses of highly emetogenic cancer chemotherapy (eg, high-dose cisplatin) and for moderately emetogenic cancer chemotherapy. For the prevention of postoperative nausea and vomiting (PONV).

**DOSAGE:** *Adults:* Prevention of Chemo-Induced N/V: Day 1: 125mg 1 hr prior to chemotherapy. Fosaprepitant Injection (115 mg IV over 15 min, 30 min prior to chemotherapy) may be substituted for PO therapy on Day 1 only. Days 2 and 3: 80mg qam. Regimen should include a corticosteroid and a 5-$HT_3$ antagonist. Refer to PI for dosing with corticosteroid (dexamethasone) and 5-$HT_3$ antagonist (ondansetron). Prevention of PONV: 40mg within 3 hrs prior to induction of anesthesia.

**HOW SUPPLIED:** Cap: 40mg, 80mg, 125mg; Tri-Pak: (one 125mg & two 80mg caps)

**CONTRAINDICATIONS:** Concurrent treatment with pimozide, terfenadine, astemizole, or cisapride.

**WARNINGS/PRECAUTIONS:** Chronic continuous use is not recommended. Caution with severe hepatic insufficiency.

**ADVERSE REACTIONS:** Asthenia/fatigue, N/V, constipation, diarrhea, hiccups, anorexia, headache, dizziness, dehydration, heartburn, pruritus, rash, urticaria, and anaphylactic reactions.

**INTERACTIONS:** See Contraindications. May increase levels of drugs metabolized by CYP3A4, including chemotherapeutic agents (eg, paclitaxel, etoposide, irinotecan, ifosfamide, imatinib, vinblastine, and vincristine), dexamethasone and methylprednisolone, certain benzodiazepines (eg, midazolam, alprazolam, triazolam). May reduce efficacy of oral contraceptives; use alternative contraception during treatment and for 1 month after last dose. May decrease levels of warfarin, tolbutamide, phenytoin or other drugs metabolized by CYP2C9. May increase plasma concentration with CYP3A4 inhibitors. Caution when used with strong/moderate inhibitors of CYP3A4 (eg, ketoconazole, itraconazole, nefazodone, troleandomycin, clarithromycin, ritonavir, nelfinavir, diltiazem). Decreased efficacy with CYP3A4 inducers (eg, rifampin, carbamazepine, phenytoin). Concomitant paroxetine may decrease levels of both drugs. Coadministration with warfarin may result in a clinically significant decrease in INR of prothrombin time.

**PREGNANCY:** Category B, not for use in nursing.

**MECHANISM OF ACTION:** Substance P/neurokinin 1 receptor antagonist; inhibits emesis induced by cytotoxic chemotherapeutic agents, such as cisplatin, via central actions.

**PHARMACOKINETICS: Absorption:** (40mg) AUC=7.8mcg•hr/mL, $C_{max}$=0.7mcg/mL, $T_{max}$=3 hrs. Refer to PI for detailed information. **Distribution:** $V_d$=70L; plasma protein binding (>95%); crosses blood-brain barrier. **Metabolism:** Liver (extensive) via CYP3A4, 1A2, 2C19. **Elimination:** Urine (57%), feces (45%); $T_{1/2}$=9-13 hrs.

## NURSING CONSIDERATIONS

**Assessment:** Assess if receiving concomitant medications primarily metabolized through CYP3A4. Assess other drug interactions, severe hepatic insufficiency, and pregnancy/nursing status.

**Monitoring:** Monitor INR in 2-week period (at 7-10 days if on chronic warfarin therapy). Monitor for hypersensitivity reactions.

**Patient Counseling:** Instruct to take drug as prescribed; first dose (125mg) 1 hr prior to chemotherapy treatment for prevention of chemotherapy-induced nausea and 40mg cap within 3 hrs prior to induction of anesthesia for prevention of PONV. Patients on chronic warfarin therapy should have clotting status closely monitored. Notify physician if using other Rx/OTC or herbal products. Instruct to d/c medication if allergic reactions (eg, hives, rash, itching, and difficulty in breathing or swallowing) occur; inform the physician immediately. Advise patient using hormonal contraceptives to use alternative or backup methods of contraceptives during therapy and for 1 month after the last dose of the regimen.

**Administration:** Oral route. **Storage:** 20-25°C (68-77°F).

# EMEND FOR INJECTION — RX

fosaprepitant dimeglumine (Merck)

**THERAPEUTIC CLASS:** Substance P/neurokinin 1 receptor antagonist

**INDICATIONS:** In combination with other antiemetics for prevention of acute and delayed N/V associated with initial and repeat courses of highly emetogenic cancer chemotherapy (eg, high-dose cisplatin) and moderately emetogenic cancer chemotherapy.

**DOSAGE:** *Adults:* 115mg IV over 15 min, 30 min prior to chemotherapy on Day 1 only of a 3-day regimen.

**HOW SUPPLIED:** Inj: 115mg/10mL

**CONTRAINDICATIONS:** Concurrent treatment with pimozide, terfenadine, astemizole, or cisapride.

**WARNINGS/PRECAUTIONS:** Chronic continuous use is not recommended. Caution with severe hepatic insufficiency (Child-Pugh score >9).

**ADVERSE REACTIONS:** Infusion-site pain, headache, asthenia/fatigue, dehydration, dizziness, constipation, diarrhea, N/V, gastritis, heartburn, anorexia, hiccups, neutropenia, alopecia, stomatitis.

**INTERACTIONS:** See Contraindications. May increase levels of drugs metabolized by CYP3A4, including chemotherapeutic agents (eg, paclitaxel, etoposide, irinotecan, ifosfamide, imatinib, vinblastine, and vincristine), dexamethasone and methylprednisolone, certain benzodiazepines (eg, midazolam, alprazolam, triazolam). May reduce efficacy of oral contraceptives; use alternative contraception during treatment and for 1 month after last dose. May decrease levels of warfarin, tolbutamide, phenytoin or other drugs metabolized by CYP2C9. May increase plasma concentration with CYP3A4 inhibitors. Caution when used with strong/moderate inhibitors of CYP3A4 (eg, ketoconazole, itraconazole, nefazodone, troleandomycin, clarithromycin, ritonavir, nelfinavir, diltiazem). Decreased efficacy with CYP3A4 inducers (eg, rifampin, carbamazepine, phenytoin). Concomitant paroxetine may decrease levels of both drugs. Coadministration with warfarin may result in a clinically significant decrease in INR of prothrombin time.

**PREGNANCY:** Category B, not for use in nursing.

**MECHANISM OF ACTION:** Substance P/neurokinin 1 receptor antagonist; inhibits emesis induced by cytotoxic chemotherapeutic agents, such as cisplatin, via central actions.

**PHARMACOKINETICS: Absorption:** AUC=31.7mcg•hr/mL, $C_{max}$=3.27mcg/mL. **Distribution:** $V_d$=70L; plasma protein binding (>95%); crosses blood-brain barrier. **Metabolism:** Liver (extensive) via CYP3A4, 1A2, 2C19. **Elimination:** Urine (57%), feces (45%); $T_{1/2}$=9-13 hrs.

## NURSING CONSIDERATIONS

**Assessment:** Assess if receiving concomitant medications primarily metabolized through CYP3A4. Assess other drug interactions, severe hepatic insufficiency, and pregnancy/nursing status.

**Monitoring:** Following initiation, monitor INR in 2-week period (particularly at 7-10 days) if on chronic warfarin therapy. Monitor for hypersensitivity reactions.

**Patient Counseling:** Instruct to notify physician and d/c if allergic reaction (eg, hives, rash, itching, and difficulty in breathing or swallowing) occurs. Inform physician about the use of any other Rx/OTC or herbal products. Patients on chronic warfarin therapy should have clotting status closely monitored. Advise patients using hormonal contraceptives to use alternative or backup methods of contraception during therapy and for 1 month after the last dose of the 3-day regimen.

**Administration:** IV route. **Storage**: 2-8°C (36-46°F). Reconstituted product is stable for 24 hrs at room temperature (at or below 25°C). Incompatible with any solutions containing divalent cations, including Lactated Ringer's Solution and Hartmann's Solution. Refer to PI for preparation of injection.

# EMLA — RX

prilocaine - lidocaine (APP Pharmaceuticals)

**THERAPEUTIC CLASS:** Acetamide local anesthetic

**INDICATIONS:** Topical anesthetic for use on normal intact skin. Topical anesthetic for genital mucous membranes for superficial minor surgery and as pretreatment for infiltration anesthesia.

**DOSAGE:** *Adults:* Apply thick layer of cream to intact skin and cover with occlusive dressing. Minor Dermal Procedure: Apply 2.5g over 20-25cm² of skin surface for at least 1 hr. Major Dermal Procedure: Apply 2g/10cm² of skin for 2 hrs. Adult Male Genital Skin: Apply 1g/10cm² of skin surface for 15 min. Female External Genitalia: Apply 5-10g for 5-10 min.
*Pediatrics:* 7-12 yrs and >20kg: Max: 20g/200cm² for up to 4 hrs. 1-6 yrs

and >10 kg: Max:10g/100cm² for up to 4 hrs. 3-12 months and >5 kg: Max: 2g/20cm² for up to 4 hrs. 0-3 months or <5kg: Max: 1g/10cm² for up to 1 hr. If >3 months and does not meet minimum weight requirement, max dose restricted to corresponding weight.

**HOW SUPPLIED:** Cre: (Lidocaine-Prilocaine) 2.5%-2.5%

**WARNINGS/PRECAUTIONS:** Application to larger areas or for longer than recommended times, may result in serious adverse effects. Should not be used where penetration or migration beyond the tympanic membrane into the middle ear is possible. Avoid with congenital or idiopathic methemoglobinemia and infants <12 months receiving treatment with methemoglobin-inducing agents. Very young or patients with glucose-6-phosphate dehydrogenase (G6PD) deficiency are more susceptible to methemoglobinemia. Reports of methemoglobinemia in infants and children following excessive applications. Monitor neonates and infants up to 3 months for Met-Hb levels before, during, and after application. Repeated doses may increase blood levels; caution in patients who may be more susceptible to systemic effects (eg, acutely ill, debilitated, elderly). Avoid eye contact and application to open wounds. Has been shown to inhibit viral and bacterial growth. Caution with severe hepatic disease and in patients with drug sensitivities.

**ADVERSE REACTIONS:** Erythema, edema, abnormal sensations, paleness (pallor or blanching), altered temperature sensations, burning sensation, itching, rash.

**INTERACTIONS:** Additive and potentially synergistic toxic effects with Class I antiarrhythmic drugs (eg, tocainide, mexiletine). May have additive cardiac effects with Class III antiarrhythmic drugs (eg, amiodarone, bretylium, sotalol, dofetilide). Avoid drugs associated with drug-induced methemoglobinemia (eg, sulfonamides, acetaminophen, acetanilid, aniline dyes, benzocaine, chloroquine, dapsone, naphthalene, nitrates/nitrites, nitrofurantoin, nitroglycerin, nitroprusside, phenobarbital, phenytoin, primaquine, pamaquine, para-aminosalicylic acid, phenacetin, quinine). Caution with other products containing lidocaine/prilocaine; consider the amount absorbed from all formulations.

**PREGNANCY:** Category B, caution in nursing.

**MECHANISM OF ACTION:** Amide-type local anesthetics; stabilizes neuronal membranes by inhibiting ionic fluxes required for initiation and conduction impulses, thereby effecting local anesthetic action.

**PHARMACOKINETICS: Absorption:** Lidocaine: (3 hrs 400cm²) $C_{max}$=0.12mcg/mL, $T_{max}$=4 hrs; (24 hrs 400cm²) $C_{max}$=0.28mcg/mL, $T_{max}$=10 hrs. Prilocaine: (3 hrs 400cm²) $C_{max}$=0.07mcg/mL, $T_{max}$=4 hrs; (24 hrs 400 cm²) $C_{max}$=0.14mcg/mL, $T_{max}$=10 hrs. **Distribution:** (IV) $V_d$=1.5L/kg (lidocaine), 2.6L/kg (prilocaine); (Cre) plasma protein binding 70% (lidocaine), 55% (prilocaine). Crosses placental and blood-brain barrier; found in breast milk. **Metabolism:** Lidocaine: Liver (rapid); monoethylglycinexylidide and glycinexylidide (active metabolites). Prilocaine: Liver and kidneys by amidases; ortho-toluidine and N-n-propylalanine (metabolites). **Elimination:** (IV) Lidocaine: Urine (>98%); $T_{1/2}$=110 min. Prilocaine: $T_{1/2}$=70 min.

## NURSING CONSIDERATIONS

**Assessment:** Assess for congenital or idiopathic methemoglobinemia, G6PD deficiency, hepatic disease, open wounds, presence of acute illness, presence of debilitation, history of drug sensitivities, pregnancy/nursing status, and for possible drug interactions. In neonates and infants ≤3 months, obtain Met-Hb levels prior to application.

**Monitoring:** Monitor for signs/symptoms of methemoglobinemia, ototoxicity, local skin reactions and for allergic/anaphylactoid reactions. Monitor Met-Hb levels in neonates and infants ≤3 months during and after application.

**Patient Counseling:** Inform about potential risks/benefits of drug. Advise to avoid inadvertent trauma to treated area. Instruct not to apply near eyes or on open wounds. Apply as directed by physician. Advise to notify physician if pregnant/nursing or planning to become pregnant. Instruct to remove cream and consult physician if child becomes very dizzy, excessively sleepy, or develops duskiness on the face or lips after application.

**Administration:** Topical route. Not for opthalmic use.**Storage:** 20-25°C (68-77°F). Keep tightly closed.

## Emsam RX

selegiline (Dey)

E

**Antidepressants increased the risk of suicidal thinking and behavior (suicidality) in short-term studies in children, adolescents, and young adults with major depressive disorder and other psychiatric disorders. Not approved for use in pediatric patients.**

**THERAPEUTIC CLASS:** Monoamine oxidase inhibitor (Type B)

**INDICATIONS:** Treatment of major depressive disorder.

**DOSAGE:** *Adults:* Initial/Target Dose: 6mg/24 hrs. Titrate: May increase in increments of 3mg/24 hrs at intervals no less than 2 weeks. Max: 12mg/24 hrs. Elderly: 6mg/24 hrs. Increase dose cautiously and monitor closely.

**HOW SUPPLIED:** Patch: 6mg/24 hrs, 9mg/24 hrs, 12mg/24 hrs [30[s]]

**CONTRAINDICATIONS:** Pheochromocytoma. Concomitant SSRIs (eg, fluoxetine, sertraline, paroxetine), dual serotonin and norepinephrine reuptake inhibitors (eg, venlafaxine, duloxetine), TCAs (eg, imipramine, amitriptyline), bupropion, buspirone, meperidine, analgesic agents (eg, tramadol, methadone, and propoxyphene), dextromethorphan, St. John's wort, mirtazapine, cyclobenzaprine, carbamazepine, oxcarbazepine, sympathetic amines (including amphetamines), cold products and weight-reducing preparations that contain vasoconstrictors (eg, pseudoephedrine, phenylephrine, phenylpropanolamine, ephedrine), oral selegiline, other MAOIs (eg, isocarboxazid, phenelzine, tranylcypromine), general anesthesia agents, cocaine, or local anesthesia-containing sympathomimetic vasoconstrictors. Dietary modifications required with 9mg/24 hrs and 12mg/24 hrs systems.

**WARNINGS/PRECAUTIONS:** Monitor for clinical worsening of depression, suicidality, and unusual changes in behavior, especially during the initial few months of therapy or at times of dose changes. Hypertensive crisis may occur with ingestion of foods with a high concentration of tyramine. Postural hypotension may occur; consider dosage adjustment with orthostatic symptoms. Activation of mania/hypomania may occur; caution with history of mania. Caution with disorders or conditions that can produce altered metabolism or hemodynamic responses. Avoid elective surgery requiring general anesthesia.

**ADVERSE REACTIONS:** Headache, diarrhea, dyspepsia, insomnia, dry mouth, pharyngitis, sinusitis, application-site reaction, rash, low systolic BP, orthostatic hypotension, weight change.

**INTERACTIONS:** See Contraindications. Avoid alcohol.

**PREGNANCY:** Category C, caution in nursing.

**MECHANISM OF ACTION:** MAOI: Mechanism of action as antidepressant not established; presumed to be linked to potentiation of monoamine neurotransmitter activity in the central nervous system (CNS) resulting from its inhibition of MAO activity.

**PHARMACOKINETICS: Absorption**: AUC=46.2ng•hr/mL. **Distribution**: Plasma protein binding (90%). **Metabolism**: Hepatic (N-dealkylation, N-depropargylation) via CYP2B6, 2C9, 3A4/5 (major), CYP2A6 (minor); N-desmethylselegiline, methamphetamine, amphetamine (metabolites). **Elimination**: Urine (10%), feces (2%); $T_{1/2}$=18-25 hrs.

### NURSING CONSIDERATIONS

**Assessment:** Assess for risk of bipolar disorder, history of mania, pre-existing orthostasis, and disease/condition that alters metabolism or hemodynamic response, pregnancy/nursing status, and possible drug interactions.

**Monitoring:** Monitor for signs/symptoms of clinical worsening (suicidality, unusual changes in behavior), hypertensive crises (occipital headaches, neck stiffness, N/V, sweating), postural hypotension, and cognitive and motor impairment.

**Patient Counseling:** Avoid concomitant use of alcohol, tyramine-containing foods/supplements/beverages (during and 2 weeks following d/c), and cough medicine containing dextromethorphan. Instruct to use only one patch at a time; do not cut patch into smaller portions. Seek medical attention for symptoms of hypertensive crises (occipital headaches, neck stiffness, N/V, sweating), postural hypotension, mania, and clinical worsening (suicidal ideation, unusual changes in behavior). May impair physical/mental abilities. Instruct to continue therapy as directed despite improvement. Avoid exposing application site to external sources of direct heat (heating pads, hot tubs). Advise to change position gradually if lightheaded, faint, or dizzy.

E

**Administration:** Transdermal route. Apply to dry, intact skin on the upper torso, upper thigh, or outer surface of upper arm once every 24 hrs. **Storage**: 20-25°C (68-77°F). Do not store outside sealed pouch.

## EMTRIVA RX

emtricitabine (Gilead)

**Lactic acidosis and severe hepatomegaly with steatosis, including fatal cases, reported with nucleoside analogs alone or with concomitant antiretrovirals. Not indicated for the treatment of chronic hepatitis B virus (HBV) infection; severe acute exacerbations of hepatitis B reported in patients coinfected with HBV and HIV upon discontinuation of emtricitabine.**

**THERAPEUTIC CLASS:** Nucleoside analogue

**INDICATIONS:** Treatment of HIV-1 infection in combination with other antiretroviral agents.

**DOSAGE:** *Adults:* ≥18 yrs: Cap: 200mg qd. CrCl 30-49mL/min: 200mg q48h. CrCl 15-29mL/min: 200mg q72h. CrCl <15mL/min (including hemodialysis): 200mg q96h. Sol: 240mg (24mL) qd. CrCl 30-49mL/min: 120mg (12mL) qd. CrCl 15-29mL/min: 80mg (8mL) qd. CrCl <15mL/min (including hemodialysis): 60mg (6mL) qd.
*Pediatrics:* 3 months-17 yrs: Cap: >33kg: 200mg qd. Sol: 6mg/kg qd. Max: 240mg (24mL). 0-3 months: Sol: 3mg/kg qd.

**HOW SUPPLIED:** Cap: 200mg; Sol: 10mg/mL [170mL]

**WARNINGS/PRECAUTIONS:** Test for chronic hepatitis B prior to initiating therapy; post-treatment exacerbations reported. Monitor hepatic function for several months in patients who d/c therapy and are coinfected with HIV and HBV. Reduce dose with renal dysfunction. Monitor changes in fasting cholesterol, serum amylase, creatinine kinase, and neutrophil count. Redistribution/accumulation of body fat reported. Immune reconstitution syndrome reported.

**ADVERSE REACTIONS:** Headache, diarrhea, nausea, fatigue, dizziness, depression, insomnia, abnormal dreams, rash, abdominal pain, asthenia, increased cough, rhinitis.

**INTERACTIONS:** Avoid coadministration with Atripla, Truvada, or lamivudine-containing products.

**PREGNANCY:** Category B, not for use in nursing.

**MECHANISM OF ACTION:** Nucleoside analog; inhibits the activity of HIV-1 reverse transcriptase by competing with the natural substrate deoxycytidine 5'-triphosphate and incorporating into nascent viral DNA, resulting in chain termination.

**PHARMACOKINETICS: Absorption:** Rapid and extensive. $C_{max}$=1.8mcg/mL, $T_{max}$=1-2 hrs, AUC=10.0mcg•hr/mL. (Cap) Absolute bioavailabilty (93%). (Sol) Absolute bioavailabilty (75%). **Distribution:** Plasma protein binding (<4%). **Metabolism:** Hepatic (conjugation and oxidation). Metabolites: 3'-sulfoxide diastereomers and 2'-O-glucuronide. **Elimination:** Urine (86%), feces (14%); $T_{1/2}$=10 hrs.

## NURSING CONSIDERATIONS

**Assessment:** Assess for impaired renal/hepatic function, HBV coinfection, risk factors for lactic acidosis, and possible drug interactions.

**Monitoring:** Monitor for signs/symptoms of lactic acidosis, hepatotoxicity (hepatomegaly and steatosis), peripheral neuropathy, myopathy, exacerbations of hepatitis, immune reconstitution syndrome, redistribution/accumulation of body fat. Closely monitor hepatic and renal function.

**Patient Counseling:** Advise patients that they may continue to experience illness associated with HIV-1 while on therapy and that risk of transmission to others is not reduced. Advise to seek medical attention if symptoms of lactic acidosis, hepatitis, myopathy, or infections occur. Educate about fat redistribution/accumulation that may occur. Inform to take with combination therapy as a regular dosing schedule and to avoid missing doses.

E

**Administration:** Oral route. **Storage:** (Cap): 25°C (77F°); excursions permitted to 15-30°C (59-86°F). (Sol): Refrigerated 2-8°C (36-46°F); if stored at 25°C (77°) use within 3 months; excursions permitted to 15-30°C (59-86°F).

## ENABLEX — RX

darifenacin (Novartis)

**THERAPEUTIC CLASS:** Muscarinic antagonist

**INDICATIONS:** Treatment of overactive bladder with symptoms of urge urinary incontinence, urgency and frequency.

**DOSAGE:** *Adults:* Initial: 7.5mg qd with liquid. Titrate: May increase up to 15mg qd after 2 weeks. Max: 15mg qd. Moderate Hepatic Impairment/Concomitant Potent CYP3A4 Inhibitors: Do not exceed 7.5mg/d. Severe Hepatic Impairment: Avoid use. Swallow whole; do not chew, divide, or crush.

**HOW SUPPLIED:** Tab, Extended-Release: 7.5mg, 15mg

**CONTRAINDICATIONS:** Urinary retention, gastric retention, uncontrolled narrow-angle glaucoma.

**WARNINGS/PRECAUTIONS:** Risk of urinary retention; caution with significant bladder outflow obstruction. Risk of gastric retention; caution with GI obstructive disorders. May decrease GI motility; caution with severe constipation, ulcerative colitis, and myasthenia gravis. Caution with moderate hepatic impairment and narrow-angle glaucoma. Avoid use with severe hepatic impairment. May produce blurred vision or dizziness.

**ADVERSE REACTIONS:** Dry mouth, constipation, dyspepsia, abdominal pain, nausea, diarrhea, UTI, dizziness, asthenia, dry eyes, hypersensitivity reactions (eg, angioedema), confusion and hallucinations, and palpitations.

**INTERACTIONS:** Do not exceed 7.5mg/day with concomitant potent CYP3A4 inhibitors. Caution with medications metabolized by CYP2D6. Additive effects with other anticholinergic agents.

**PREGNANCY:** Category C, caution in nursing.

**MECHANISM OF ACTION:** Muscarinic receptor antagonist; inhibits cholinergic muscarinic receptors, which mediate contractions of urinary bladder smooth muscle, and stimulation of salivary secretions.

**PHARMACOKINETICS: Absorption:** (7.5mg) Bioavailability (15%); extensive metabolizers (EM): $C_{max}$=2.01ng/mL, $T_{max}$=6.49 hrs, AUC=29.24ng•hr/mL. Poor metabolizers (PM): $C_{max}$=4.27ng/mL, $T_{max}$=5.2 hrs, AUC=67.56ng•hr/mL. (15mg) Bioavailability (19%); EM: $C_{max}$=5.76ng/mL, $T_{max}$=7.61 hrs, AUC=88.9ng•hr/mL. PM: $C_{max}$=9.99ng/mL, $T_{max}$=6.71 hrs, AUC=157.71ng•h/mL. **Distribution:** $V_d$=163L; plasma protein binding (98%). **Metabolism:** CYP2D6, 3A4 (monohydroxylation, ring opening, N-dealkylation). **Elimination:** Urine (3%); $T_{1/2}$=13-19 hrs.

### NURSING CONSIDERATIONS

**Assessment:** Assess for bladder outflow obstruction (urinary retention), GI obstructive disorders (gastric retention), narrow-angle glaucoma, possible drug interactions, severe constipation, ulcerative colitis, myasthenia gravis, and hepatic impairment.

**Monitoring:** Monitor for symptoms of urinary retention, gastric retention, hepatic impairment, and hypersensitivity reactions.

**Patient Counseling:** Advise may produce dizziness or blurred vision; caution may impair physical/mental abilities. Instruct take once daily with liquid, with/without food, swallow whole, do not chew, divide, or crush. Advise to seek medical attention if symptoms of constipation, retention, heat prostration (decreased sweating), or hypersensitivity reactions occur.

**Administration:** Oral route. **Storage:** 25°C (77°F); excursions permitted to 15-30°C (59-86°). Protect from light.



## ENBREL RX

etanercept (Amgen)

**Increased risk for developing serious infections (eg, tuberculosis [TB], TB reactivation, invasive fungal infection, bacterial/viral infection due to opportunistic pathogens) that may lead to hospitalization or death. Concomitant use of immunosuppresants (eg, methotrexate [MTX] or corticosteroids) may precipitate these infections. Evaluate for latent TB and treat prior to initiation of therapy. Empiric antifungal therapy should be considered in patients at risk for invasive fungal infection who develop severe systemic illness. Monitor for development of infection during and after treatment. D/C if serious infection or sepsis develops. Lymphoma and other malignancies reported in children and adolescents.**

**THERAPEUTIC CLASS:** TNF-receptor blocker

**INDICATIONS:** Reduce signs/symptoms, induce major clinical response, improve physical function, and inhibit progression of structural damage in moderate to severe rheumatoid arthritis (RA) (may be initiated in combination with methotrexate [MTX] or alone). Reduce signs/symptoms, inhibit progression of structural damage of active arthritis, and improve physical function in psoriatic arthritis (may be used with MTX in patients not responding to MTX alone). Reduce signs/symptoms of moderate to severe polyarticular juvenile idiopathic arthritis (JIA). Reduce signs/symptoms of active ankylosing spondylitis (AS). Treatment of chronic moderate to severe plaque psoriasis for candidates of systemic therapy or phototherapy.

**DOSAGE:** *Adults:* ≥18 yrs: RA/Psoriatic Arthritis/AS: 50mg SQ per week, given as one SQ injection. May continue MTX, glucocorticoids, salicylates, NSAIDs, or analgesics. Psoriasis: Initial: 50mg SQ twice weekly given 3 or 4 days apart for 3 months. May begin with 25-50mg/week. Maint: 50mg/week.
*Pediatrics:* 2-17 yrs: JIA: 0.8mg/kg SQ per week. Max: 50mg/week. May continue glucocorticoids, NSAIDs, or analgesics.

**HOW SUPPLIED:** Inj: (MDV) 25mg, (Syringe) 50mg/mL

**CONTRAINDICATIONS:** Sepsis.

**WARNINGS/PRECAUTIONS:** Avoid with active infections. Caution in patients with history or chronic/recurrent infection, underlying conditions predisposing to infections and with exposure to TB or who travel to areas where TB or mycoses are endemic. Caution with pre-existing or recent onset CNS demyelinating disorders. Rare cases of pancytopenia including aplastic anemia reported; d/c if significant hematologic abnormalities occur. Monitor hepatitis B virus (HBV) carriers; if reactivation occurs, d/c and start antiviral therapy. Caution in patients with moderate to severe alcoholic hepatitis or with heart failure; monitor closely. JIA patients should be brought up-to-date with current immunization guidelines prior to initiating therapy. D/C temporarily with significant varicella virus exposure and consider prophylaxis. Avoid with Wegener's granulomatosis. May cause autoimmune antibodies; d/c if lupus-like syndrome or autoimmune hepatitis develops. Needle cap on prefilled syringe and autoinjector contains dry natural rubber; caution with latex allergy. Caution in the elderly.

**ADVERSE REACTIONS:** (**Adults/Pediatrics**) Injection-site reactions, infections, headache, nausea, rhinitis, dizziness, pharyngitis. (Pediatrics) Varicella, gastroenteritis, vomiting, depression, cutaneous ulcer, esophagitis.

**INTERACTIONS:** Do not give live vaccines. Avoid with cyclophosphamide. May cause neutropenia and increased rate of infection with anakinra. Mild decrease in mean neutrophil count reported in patients who were on established therapy with sulfasalazine.

**PREGNANCY:** Category B, not for use in nursing.

**MECHANISM OF ACTION:** TNF-receptor blocker; binds specifically to tumor necrosis factor (TNF) and blocks its interaction with cell surface TNF-receptors.

**PHARMACOKINETICS: Absorption**: SQ administration of different doses resulted in different parameters.

## NURSING CONSIDERATIONS



**Assessment:** Assess for sepsis or localized or chronic infection, history of recurring infection, predisposition to infection (eg, DM), pre-existing or recent-onset CNS demyelinating disorders, history of significant hematological events, HBV infection, heart failure, pregnancy/nursing status, and possible drug interactions. Ensure patients with JIA are up-to-date with immunizations.

**Monitoring:** Monitor for signs/symptoms of infections (including sepsis), CNS demyelinating disorders, hematological events (eg, aplastic anemia), lymphoma, HBV reactivation, allergic reactions (eg, anaphylactoid reaction), CHF, lupus-like syndrome, and autoimmune hepatitis. Monitor pregnancy/nursing status.

**Patient Counseling:** Counsel about adverse events; seek immediate medical attention if signs/symptoms of infection or anaphylactic reaction develop. Inform that needle cap on prefilled syringe and on autoinjector contains dry natural rubber, a derivative of latex; use caution if there is sensitivity to latex. Instruct patient or caregiver of proper injection techniques, accurate measurement/administration of correct dose, proper syringe/needle disposal. Inform to avoid reuse of needles and syringes.

**Administration:** SQ route. Rotate sites for injection (thigh, abdomen, or upper arm). Avoid injecting into areas where skin is tender, bruised, red, or hard. Patient should not self-administer until receives proper training on how to prepare/administer correct dose. Before injection, medication may be allowed to reach room temperature. Multiple-use vial: 1) Reconstitute using 1 mL of Sterile Bacteriostatic Water for Inj, USP to solution of 1 mL containing 25mg of drug. **Storage**: Refrigerate at 2-8°C (36-46°F). Do not freeze. Keep in original carton; protect from light. Do not shake. Reconstituted: May be stored for up to 14 days if refrigerated at 2-8°C (36-46°F). Discard after 14 days. Keep out of reach of children.

# ENGERIX-B — RX

hepatitis B (recombinant) (GlaxoSmithKline)

**THERAPEUTIC CLASS:** Vaccine

**INDICATIONS:** Immunization against all known hepatitis B virus subtypes.

**DOSAGE:** *Adults:* >19 yrs: 20mcg/1mL IM (deltoid) at 0, 1, 6 months. Booster: 20mcg IM. Hemodialysis: 40mcg/2mL IM at 0, 1, 2, 6 months. Booster: 40mcg IM, given when antibody levels decline below 10 mIU/mL. Alternate Dosage and Administration Schedule: >19 yrs: 20mcg/1mL IM at 0, 1, 2, 12 months. Additional hepatitis B immune globulin (HBIG) should be given to unprotected individuals with known or presumed exposure to hepatitis B virus. *Pediatrics:* ≤10 yrs/Adolescents (11-19 yrs)/Infants born of HBsAg-positive/negative mothers: 10mcg/0.5mL IM (deltoid/anterolateral thigh) at 0, 1, 6 months. Booster: ≤10 yrs: 10mcg IM. Adolescents (11-19 yrs): 20mcg IM. Alternate Dosage and Administration Schedule: ≤10 yrs/Infants born of HBsAg-positive mothers: 10mcg/0.5mL IM at 0, 1, 2, 12 months. 5-10 yrs/11-16 yrs: 10mcg/0.5mL IM at 0, 12, 24 months. Adolescents (11-19 yrs): 20mcg/1mL IM at 0, 1, 6 months/0, 1, 2, 12 months. Additional HBIG should be given to unprotected individuals with known or presumed exposure to hepatitis B virus.

**HOW SUPPLIED:** Inj: 10mcg/0.5mL, 20mcg/mL

**CONTRAINDICATIONS:** Yeast hypersensitivity.

**WARNINGS/PRECAUTIONS:** Tip cap and the rubber plunger of the needleless prefilled syringes contain latex; may cause allergic reactions in latex-sensitive individuals. Will not prevent hepatitis A, C, and E virus infection. Vaccine may not prevent hepatitis B infection in individuals who had unrecognized hepatitis B infection at time of vaccine administration. May not prevent infection in individuals who do not achieve protective antibody titers. Delay vaccine with moderate or severe febrile illnesses. Expected immune response may not be obtained with immunosuppressed persons. Medical and immunization history should be reviewed prior to vaccination. Epinephrine injection (1:1000) and other appropriate agents should be immediately available if an acute anaphylactic reaction occurs. Avoid injection into a blood vessel. May exacerbate multiple sclerosis (rare). Caution with very premature infants (born ≤28 weeks of gestation).



**ADVERSE REACTIONS:** Injection-site soreness, erythema, swelling and induration, fatigue, fever, headache, dizziness.

**INTERACTIONS:** Expected immune response may not be obtained with immunosuppresants; defer vaccine ≥3 months after immunosuppressive therapy.

**PREGNANCY:** Category C, caution in nursing.

**MECHANISM OF ACTION:** Vaccine; may produce immune response for protection against infection caused by all known subtypes of hepatitis B virus.

## NURSING CONSIDERATIONS

**Assessment:** Assess presence of moderate or severe febrile illness and medical history, immunocompromised status, immunization history for possible vaccine sensitivity, previous vaccine-related adverse reactions, pregnancy/nursing status, and for possible drug interactions.

**Monitoring:** Monitor for injection-site reactions (eg, induration, erythema, swelling) and general reactions (eg, fever, headache, dizziness). Perform respiratory monitoring for 48-72 hrs in very premature infants.

**Patient Counseling:** Inform of potential benefits, risks, and the importance of completing the immunization series. Instruct to report any adverse reactions to healthcare provider where the vaccine was administered.

**Administration:** IM route. Inject IM in deltoid muscle for adults; and anterolateral thigh in neonates and infants who have smaller deltoid muscles. May give SQ if at risk for hemorrhage (eg, hemophiliacs). Shake well before withdrawal and use. Do not dilute to administer. **Storage:** Refrigerate between 2-8°C (36-46°F). Do not freeze; discard if frozen.

# ENJUVIA RX

conjugated estrogens (Teva)

**Estrogens increase the risk of endometrial cancer. Estrogens and progestins should not be used for the prevention of cardiovascular disease or dementia. Increased risks of MI, stroke, invasive breast cancer, PE, and DVT in postmenopausal women (50 to 79 yrs) reported. Increased risk of developing probable dementia in postmenopausal women ≥65 yrs reported.**

**THERAPEUTIC CLASS:** Estrogen

**INDICATIONS:** Treatment of moderate-severe vasomotor symptoms associated with menopause. Treatment of symptoms of vulvar and vaginal atrophy associated with menopause. Treatment of moderate-severe vaginal dryness and pain with intercourse; if used solely for this purpose, topical vaginal products should be considered.

**DOSAGE:** *Adults:* Individualize dosing. Initial: 0.3mg qd. Adjust dose based on response.

**HOW SUPPLIED:** Tab: 0.3mg, 0.45mg, 0.625mg, 0.9mg, 1.25mg

**CONTRAINDICATIONS:** Pregnancy, undiagnosed abnormal genital bleeding, breast cancer, estrogen-dependent neoplasia, DVT/PE, arterial thromboembolic disease (eg, stroke, MI), liver dysfunction.

**WARNINGS/PRECAUTIONS:** Increased risk of retinal vascular thrombosis, severe hypercalcemia in patients with breast cancer and bone metastases, gallbladder disease and breast and ovarian cancers. Elevated BP reported; monitor BP at regular intervals. May elevate plasma triglycerides resulting in pancreatitis. Caution in patients with impaired liver function or history of cholestatic jaundice. May increase TBG; monitor thyroid function of patients dependent on thyroid hormone replacement therapy and adjust dosage if needed. May cause fluid retention; caution with cardiac or renal dysfunction. Caution in individuals with severe hypocalcemia. May cause exacerbation of asthma, diabetes mellitus, epilepsy, migraine or porphyria, systemic lupus erythematosus, and hepatic hemangiomas.



**ADVERSE REACTIONS:** Abdominal pain, accidental injury, flu syndrome, headache, pain, flatulence, nausea, dizziness, paresthesia, bronchitis, rhinitis, sinusitis, breast pain, dysmenorrhea, vaginitis.

**INTERACTIONS:** CYP3A4 inducers (eg, St. John's wort, phenobarbital, carbamazepine, rifampin) may decrease levels, which may decrease therapeutic effects and/or uterine bleeding profile. CYP3A4 inhibitors (eg, erythromycin, clarithromycin, ketoconazole, itraconazole, ritonavir, grapefruit juice) may increase levels, which may result in side effects.

**PREGNANCY:** Category X, caution in nursing.

**MECHANISM OF ACTION:** Estrogen; binds to nuclear receptors in estrogen-responsive tissues. Circulating estrogens modulate pituitary secretion of the gonadotropins, luteinizing hormone and follicle stimulating hormone, through negative feedback mechanism. Reduces elevated levels of these hormones in postmenopusal women.

**PHARMACOKINETICS: Absorption:** Refer to package insert for conjugated and unconjugated estrogen parameters. **Distribution:** Largely bound to sex hormone binding globulin and albumin; found in breast milk. **Metabolism:** Liver to estrone (metabolite), estriol (major urinary metabolite); sulfate and glucuronide conjugation (liver); intestinal hydrolysis; CYP 3A4 (partial metabolism). **Elimination:** Urine (parent compound and metabolites); Conjugated estrone: $T_{1/2}$=14 hrs; Conjugated equilin: $T_{1/2}$=11 hrs.

## NURSING CONSIDERATIONS

**Assessment:** Assess for undiagnosed abnormal genital bleeding, presence or history of breast cancer, DVT, PE, estrogen-dependent neoplasia, liver dysfunction, history of cholestatic jaundice, pregnancy/nursing status, age of patient ( ≥65 yrs), hypertriglyceridemia, hypothyroidism, hypocalcemia, asthma, DM, epilepsy, migraine, porphyria, SLE, and possible drug interactions. Assess need for progestin therapy in patients who have not had a hysterectomy.

**Monitoring:** Monitor for signs/symptoms of cardiovascular disorders (eg, stroke, coronary heart disease, venous thromboembolism), malignant neoplasms (eg, endometrial, breast, or ovarian cancer), dementia, gallbladder disease, hypercalcemia, visual abnormalities (eg, retinal vascular thrombosis), elevations in BP, fluid retention, elevations in serum triglycerides, pancreatitis, hypothyroidism, hypocalcemia, exacerbation of endometriosis and other conditions (eg, asthma, DM, epilepsy, migraine, SLE). Monitor BP levels. Monitor thyroid function in patients on thyroid replacement therapy. If undiagnosed, persistent, or recurring abnormal vaginal bleeding occurs, perform proper diagnostic testing (eg, endometrial sampling) to rule out malignancy. Perform annual breast exam. Perform periodic monitoring (every 3-6 months) to determine therapy need.

**Patient Counseling:** Inform medication increases risk for uterine cancer. Report breast lumps, unusual vaginal bleeding, dizziness or faintness, changes in speech, severe headaches, chest pain, SOB, leg pains, changes in vision, or vomiting. Inform physician if planning surgery or prolonged immobilization. Perform monthly breast self-exams. Take with/without food. If a dose is missed, take as soon as possible; if almost time for next dose, skip missed dose and return to normal dosing schedule.

**Administration:** Oral route. **Storage:** 20-25°C (68-77°F). Dispense in tight container with child-resistant closure.

## ENTEREG RX

alvimopan (GlaxoSmithKline)

**Available only for short-term (15 doses) use in hospitalized patients. Only hospitals that have registered and met requirements for the Entereg Access Support and Education (E.A.S.E.) program may use drug.**

**THERAPEUTIC CLASS:** Opioid antagonist

**INDICATIONS:** Indicated to accelerate time to upper and lower GI recovery following partial large or small bowel resection surgery with primary anastomosis.

**DOSAGE:** *Adults:* ≥18 yrs: 12mg given 30 min to 5 hrs prior to surgery followed by 12mg bid beginning day after surgery for maximum of 7 days or until discharge. Max: 15 doses.

**HOW SUPPLIED:** Cap: 12mg

**CONTRAINDICATIONS:** Therapeutic doses of opioids for >7 consecutive days immediately prior to therapy.

**WARNINGS/PRECAUTIONS:** Caution in patients receiving >3 doses of opioids within week prior to surgery and in post-operative ileus. Avoid using in severe hepatic impairment, end-stage renal disease (ESRD), surgery for correction of complete bowel obstruction. Myocardial Infarction (MI) reported in patients treated with opioids for chronic pain.

**ADVERSE REACTIONS:** Anemia, constipation, dyspepsia, flatulence, hypokalemia, back pain, urinary retention.

**PREGNANCY:** Category B, caution in nursing.

**MECHANISM OF ACTION:** Selective antagonist of µ-opioid receptor; antagonizes the peripheral effects of opioids on GI motility and secretion by competitively binding to GI tract µ-opioid receptors.

**PHARMACOKINETICS: Absorption:** Absolute bioavailability (6%); Alvimopan: $T_{max}$=2 hrs; $C_{max}$=10.98ng/mL; Metabolite: $T_{max}$=36 hrs; $C_{max}$=35.73ng/mL. **Distribution:** $V_d$=30L. Plasma protein binding (80%, alvimopan; 94%, metabolite). **Elimination:** Renal excretion (35% of total clearance); Biliary (primary pathway); Alvimopan: $T_{1/2}$=10-17 hrs; Metabolite: $T_{1/2}$=10-18 hrs.

### NURSING CONSIDERATIONS

**Assessment:** Assess for hepatic/renal impairment, anemia, bowel obstruction, history of opioid use and pregnancy/nursing status.

**Monitoring:** Monitor for CBC, hepatic/renal function, signs/symptoms of possible side effects (eg, abdominal pain, nausea, vomiting, diarrhea) and MI.

**Patient Counseling:** Instruct to disclose long-term or intermittent opioid pain therapy, including any use of opioids in the week prior to receiving. Monitor for signs/symptoms of possible side effects (eg, abdominal pain, nausea, vomiting, diarrhea). Advise that therapy must be done in a hospital setting only for no more than 7 days after bowel resection. Inform that constipation, dyspepsia, and flatulence may occur.

**Administration:** Oral route. **Storage:** 25°C (77°F); excursions permitted to 15-30°C (59-86°F).

## ENTOCORT EC RX

budesonide (Prometheus)

**THERAPEUTIC CLASS:** Corticosteroid

**INDICATIONS:** Treatment of mild to moderate active Crohn's disease of the ileum and/or ascending colon. Maintenance of clinical remission of mild to moderate Crohn's disease of the ileum and/or ascending colon for up to 3 months.

**DOSAGE:** *Adults:* Usual: 9mg qd, in the am for up to 8 weeks. Recurring Episodes: Repeat therapy for 8 weeks. Maint: 6mg qd for 3 months, then taper to complete cessation. Moderate to Severe Hepatic Insufficiency/Concomitant CYP3A4 Inhibitors: Reduce dose. Swallow whole; do not chew or break.

**HOW SUPPLIED:** Cap, Delayed-Release: 3mg

**WARNINGS/PRECAUTIONS:** May reduce response of HPA axis to stress. Supplement with systemic glucocorticosteroids if undergoing surgery or other stressful situations. Increased risk of infection; avoid exposure to varicella/varicella zoster and measles. Caution with TB, HTN, DM, osteoporosis, peptic ulcer, glaucoma, cirrhosis, cataracts, family history of DM or glaucoma. Replacement of systemic glucocorticosteroids may unmask allergies. Chronic use may cause hypercorticism and adrenal suppression.

**ADVERSE REACTIONS:** Headache, respiratory infection, N/V, back pain, dyspepsia, dizziness, abdominal pain, diarrhea, flatulence, sinusitis, viral infection, arthralgia, benign intracranial HTN, signs/symptoms of hypercorticism

**INTERACTIONS:** Ketoconazole caused an eight-fold increase of systemic exposure to oral budesonide. Increased levels with CYP3A4 inhibitors (eg, ketoconazole, itraconazole, saquinavir, erythromycin, grapefruit, grapefruit juice); monitor for increased signs and symptoms of hypercorticism and reduce budesonide dose if coadministered.

**PREGNANCY:** Category C, not for use in nursing.

**MECHANISM OF ACTION:** Glucocorticosteroid.

**PHARMACOKINETICS: Absorption:** $C_{max}$=5nmol/L; $T_{max}$=30-600 min; AUC=30nmol•hr/L. Bioavailability=9-21%. **Distribution:** $V_d$=2.2-3.9L/kg; plasma protein binding (85-90%). **Metabolism:** Liver; CYP3A4. **Elimination:** Urine (60%); $T_{1/2}$=2-3.6 hrs.

## NURSING CONSIDERATIONS

**Assessment:** Assess for liver disease, history of chickenpox or measles, TB, HTN, osteoporosis, peptic ulcers, cataracts, history and/or family history of DM or glaucoma and possible drug interactions. Obtain baseline LFTs.

**Monitoring:** Monitor LFTs periodically and for signs/symptoms of hypercorticism and hypersensitivity reactions.

**Patient Counseling:** Advise to swallow whole; do not chew or break. Avoid consumption of grapefruit and grapefruit juice during therapy. Take particular care to avoid exposure to chickenpox or measles.

**Administration:** Oral route. **Storage:** 25° (77°F); excursions permitted to 15-30°C (59-86°F). Keep container tightly closed.

# EPIDUO RX

benzoyl peroxide - adapalene (Galderma)

**THERAPEUTIC CLASS:** Antibacterial/keratolytic

**INDICATIONS:** Topical treatment of acne vulgaris in patients ≥12 yrs.

**DOSAGE:** *Adults:* Apply a pea-sized amount to the affected areas of the face and/or trunk qd after washing.
*Pediatrics:* ≥12 yrs: Apply a pea-sized amount to the affected areas of the face and/or trunk once qd after washing.

**HOW SUPPLIED:** Gel: (Adapalene-Benzoyl Peroxide) 0.1%-2.5% [45g]

**WARNINGS/PRECAUTIONS:** Not for oral, ophthalmic, or intravaginal use. Minimize exposure to sunlight and sunlamps. Extreme weather may increase skin irritation. Avoid contact with eyes, lips, mucous membranes, cuts, abrasions, eczematous or sunburned skin. Erythema, scaling, dryness, stinging/burning may be experienced. Avoid concomitant use with potentially irritating topical products (eg, medicated/abrasive soaps/cleansers).

**ADVERSE REACTIONS:** Erythema, dry skin, scaling, stinging, burning, dryness, contact dermatitis, application-site burning/irritation, and skin irritation.

**INTERACTIONS:** Caution with concomitant sulfur, resorcinol, salicylic acid preparations, and topical acne therapy (eg, peeling, desquamatizing, or abrasive agents).

**PREGNANCY:** Category C, caution in nursing.

**MECHANISM OF ACTION:** Adapalene: Napthoic acid derivative; not established; binds to specific retinoic acid nuclear receptors. Benzoyl peroxide: Oxidizing agent with bacteriocidal and keratolytic effects.

**PHARMACOKINETICS: Absorption:** (Adapalene) $C_{max}$=0.21ng/mL; $AUC_{0-24h}$=1.99ng•h/mL. **Excretion:** (Adapalene) Bile. (Benzoic acid) Urine.

## NURSING CONSIDERATIONS

**Assessment:** Assess for sunburned skin, eczema, abrasion, skin cuts. Assess use in pregnancy/nursing patients and for possible drug interactions.

**Monitoring:** Monitor for sensitivity or chemical irritation, cutaneous signs/symptoms (eg, erythema, dryness, scaling, burning, stinging, application-site burning/irritation, and contact dermatitis).

**Patient Counseling:** Instruct to avoid exposure to sunlight and sunlamps; use sunscreen and protective clothing over treated areas when exposed. Medication may also cause skin irritation when exposed to wind or cold. Avoid contact with eyes, lips, and mucous membranes. Do not apply medication to cuts, abrasions, eczematous or sunburned skin.

**Administration:** Topical application. **Storage:** Store at 25°C; excursions permitted to 15-30°C (59-86°F). Protect from light. Keep away from heat. Keep tube tightly closed.

# EpiPen **RX**

epinephrine (Dey)

**OTHER BRAND NAMES:** EpiPen Jr. (Dey)

**THERAPEUTIC CLASS:** Sympathomimetic catecholamine

**INDICATIONS:** Immediate self-administered, emergency treatment of allergic reactions (Type I) including anaphylaxis to stinging insects (eg, order Hymenoptera, which includes bees, wasps, hornets, yellow jackets and fire ants) or biting insect (eg, triatoma, mosquitoes), allergen immunotherapy, foods, drugs, diagnostic testing substances (eg, radiocontrast media), and other allergens, as well as idiopathic or exercise-induced anaphylaxis.

**DOSAGE:** *Adults:* 15-30kg: 0.15mg (Epipen Jr) IM/SQ into anterolateral aspect of thigh. May repeat with severe anaphylaxis. ≥30 kg: 0.3mg (Epipen) IM/SQ into anterolateral aspect of thigh. May repeat with severe anaphylaxis. *Pediatrics:* 15-30kg: 0.15mg (Epipen Jr) IM/SQ into anterolateral aspect of thigh. May repeat with severe anaphylaxis. ≥30 kg: 0.3mg (Epipen) IM/SQ into anterolateral aspect of thigh. May repeat with severe anaphylaxis.

**HOW SUPPLIED:** Inj: (Epipen Jr) 0.5mg/mL, (Epipen) 1mg/mL

**WARNINGS/PRECAUTIONS:** Not intended as a substitute for immediate medical care. Do not inject into buttock; may not provide effective treatment of anaphylaxis. May result in loss of blood flow to the affected areas if accidentally injected into digits, hands or feet. Not for IV use; may cause cerebral hemorrhage due to sharp rise in BP if accidentally injected IV. Contains sodium metabisulfite; sulfite-sensitivity is not a contraindication in serious allergic or emergency situations. Caution with heart disease, including cardiac arrhythmias, coronary artery or organic heart disease, or hypertension. High risk of developing adverse reactions with hyperthyroidism, CVD, HTN, and DM, and in elderly, pregnant women, pediatrics <30kg using Epipen and pediatrics <15kg using Epipen Jr.

**ADVERSE REACTIONS:** Palpitations, sweating, N/V, respiratory difficulty, pallor, dizziness, weakness, tremor, headache, apprehensiveness, anxiety, restlessness, arrhythmias (including fatal ventricular fibrillation), angina, cerebral hemorrhage.

**INTERACTIONS:** Can counteract the marked pressor effects of epinephrine with rapidly acting vasodilators. Drugs that sensitize the heart to arrhythmias (eg, digitalis, diuretics, quinidine, or anti-arrhythmias) may precipitate or aggravate angina pectoris as well as produce ventricular arrhythmias.

Co-administration with TCAs, MAOIs, levothyroxine sodium, and certain antihistamines, including chlorpheniramine, tripelennamine and diphenhydramine, may lead to potentiation of epinephrine effects. Antagonized cardiostimulating and bronchodilating effects with beta-adrenergic blocking drugs, such as propranolol. Antagonized vasoconstricting and hypertensive effects with alpha-adrenergic blocking drugs such as phentoloamine. Ergot alkaloids may reverse pressor effects.

**PREGNANCY:** Category C, safety not known in nursing.

E

**MECHANISM OF ACTION:** Sympathomimetic catecholamine; acts on α receptors to lessen the vasodilation and increased vascular permeability that occurs during anaphylaxis, which can lead to loss of intravascular fluid volume and hypotension. Acts on β receptors to cause bronchial smooth muscle relaxation that helps alleviate bronchospasm, wheezing and dyspnea that may occur during anaphylaxis. Epinephrine also alleviates pruritus, urticaria, and angioedema and may be effective in relieving gastrointestinal and genitourinary symptoms associated with anaphylaxis because of its relaxer effects on the smooth muscle of the stomach, intestine, uterus, and urinary bladder.

## NURSING CONSIDERATIONS

**Assessment:** Assess for anaphylaxis.

**Monitoring:** Monitor for anginal pain, arrhythmia, BP, and cerebral hemorrhage (particularly in overdosage or inadvertent intravascular injection).

**Patient Counseling:** Inform about the signs and symptoms produced by the drug. Advise to go to nearest emergency room if accidentally injected into hands or feet; may result in loss of blood flow to affected area. Never inject into buttock or by IV route. Advise that epinephrine is not intended as a substitute for immediate medical care.

**Administration:** IM or SQ route. **Storage:** 25°C (77°F); excursions permitted to 15-30°C (59-86°F). Light sensitive; store in the tube provided. Do not refrigerate.

# EPIVIR RX

lamivudine (GlaxoSmithKline)

**Lactic acidosis and severe hepatomegaly with steatosis, including fatal cases, reported; suspend treatment if signs or symptoms of lactic acidosis or severe hepatotoxicity occur. Epivir tablets and solution, used to treat HIV, contain higher dose of lamivudine than Epivir-HBV, used to treat hepatitis B; only use appropriate dosing forms for HIV treatment. Severe acute exacerbations of hepatitis B reported in patients coinfected with hepatitis B virus and HIV who discontinued therapy; monitor hepatic function closely.**

**THERAPEUTIC CLASS:** Nucleoside analogue

**INDICATIONS:** Treatment of HIV-1 infection in combination with other antiretrovirals.

**DOSAGE:** *Adults/Adolescents:* >16 yrs: 150mg bid or 300mg qd, concomitantly with other antiretrovirals. Renal Impairment ( ≥ 30 kg): CrCl 30-49mL/min: 150mg qd. CrCl 15-29mL/min: 150mg first dose, then 100mg qd. CrCl 5-14mL/min: 150mg first dose, then 50mg qd. CrCl <5mL/min: 50mg first dose, then 25mg qd.

*Pediatrics:* Sol: 3 months-16 yrs: 4mg/kg bid, concomitantly with other antiretrovirals. Max: 150mg bid. Tab, Sc: 14-21kg: 1/2 tab (75mg) in am and 1/2 tab (75mg) in pm. >21-<30kg: 1/2 tab (75mg) in am and 1 tab (150mg) in pm. ≥30kg: 1 tab (150mg) in am and 1 tab (150mg) in pm. Renal Impairment ( ≥ 30 kg): CrCl 30-49mL/min: 150mg qd. CrCl 15-29mL/min: 150mg first dose, then 100mg qd. CrCl 5-14mL/min: 150mg 1st dose, then 50mg qd. CrCl <5mL/min: 50mg 1st dose, then 25mg qd.

**HOW SUPPLIED:** Sol: 10mg/mL [240mL]; Tab: 150mg*, 300mg *scored

**WARNINGS/PRECAUTIONS:** Caution in pediatric patients with history of prior antiretroviral nucleoside exposure, history of pancreatitis, or other significant risk factors for developing pancreatitis. D/C if pancreatitis develops. Reduce dose in renal dysfunction. Caution in elderly. Possible redistribution or accumulation of body fat. Immune reconstitution syndrome reported. Lamivudine resistance in patients coinfected with HIV-1/HBV associated with lamivudine-containing antiretroviral regimens has been reported.

**ADVERSE REACTIONS:** Lactic acidosis, severe hepatomegaly with steatosis, severe acute exacerbations of hepatitis B, headache, malaise, fatigue, N/V, diarrhea, nasal signs/symptoms, neuropathy, insomnia/sleep disorders, musculoskeletal pain, cough, fever, neutropenia.

**INTERACTIONS:** Hepatic decompensation occurred when used with interferon-α, w/ or w/o ribavirin. Avoid use with zalcitabine; may inhibit intracellular phosphorylation of drug. Avoid use with other lamivudine-containing products such as EPIVIR-HBV and fixed-dose combinations of abacavir, lamivudine, and zidovudine. Also avoid use with emtricitabine and fixed-dose combinations of emtricitabine, efavirenz, and tenofovir. Trimethoprim/Sulfamethoxazole may increase lamivudine levels. Drugs which are secreted via the organic cationic transport system may inhibit the elimination of lamivudine.

**PREGNANCY:** Category C, not for use in nursing.

**MECHANISM OF ACTION:** Nucleoside analogue; inhibits HIV-1 reverse transcriptase via DNA chain termination after incorporation into viral DNA.

**PHARMACOKINETICS: Absorption:** Rapid; Absolute bioavailability (tab: 86%, sol 87%); $C_{max}$=1.5mcg/mL (HIV); $T_{max}$=0.9 hrs (fasting), 3.2 hrs (fed). **Distribution:** $V_d$=1.3L/kg; plasma protein binding (<36%). **Metabolism:** Hepatic (minor). **Elimination:** Urine (71%, unchanged); $T_{1/2}$=5-7 hrs.

## NURSING CONSIDERATIONS

**Assessment:** Assess for impaired hepatic/renal function, risk factors for lactic acidosis, history of pancreatitis, HBV coinfection, DM, and possible drug interactions. Assess pregnancy/nursing status.

**Monitoring:** Monitor for signs/symptoms of pancreatitis, immune reconstitution syndrome, fat redistribution, lactic acidosis, hepatitis B exacerbation, hepatic/renal dysfunction. Monitor hepatic function closely for several months in patients with HIV/HBV coinfection who discontinue therapy. May enroll patients in the Antiretroviral Pregnancy Registry if they become pregnant while on treatment.

**Patient Counseling:** Instruct to take with combination therapy on regular dosing schedule; avoid missing doses. Advise to seek medical attention if symptoms of pancreatitis, hepatitis, exacerbation of HBV, infection, or fat redistribution occur. Inform diabetics that oral solution contains sucrose. Counsel that therapy does not reduce risk of HIV transmission through sexual contact or blood contamination. Instruct not to take concomitantly with emtricitabine-containing or other lamivudine-containing products.

**Administration:** Oral route. **Storage:** 25°C (77°F); excursions permitted to 15-30°C (59-86°F).

# EPIVIR-HBV RX

lamivudine (GlaxoSmithKline)

**Lactic acidosis and severe, possibly fatal, hepatomegaly reported. If prescribed for patients with unrecognized or untreated HIV infection, rapid emergence of HIV resistance is likely; Epivir-HBV contains a lower dose of lamivudine than Epivir, which is used to treat HIV. Severe acute exacerbations of hepatitis B reported upon discontinuation of therapy; monitor liver function closely.**

**THERAPEUTIC CLASS:** Nucleoside analogue

**INDICATIONS:** Treatment of chronic hepatitis B associated with evidence of viral replication and active liver inflammation.

**DOSAGE:** *Adults:* CrCl ≥ 50 mL/min: 100mg qd. CrCl 30-49mL/min: 100mg Day 1, then 50mg qd. CrCl: 15-29mL/min: 100mg Day 1, then 25mg qd. CrCl 5-14mL/min: 35mg Day 1, then 15mg qd. CrCl <5mL/min: 35mg Day 1,

then 10mg qd.
*Pediatrics:* 2-17 yrs: 3mg/kg qd. Max: 100mg/day.

**HOW SUPPLIED:** Sol: 5mg/mL [240mL]; Tab: 100mg

**WARNINGS/PRECAUTIONS:** This formulation is not appropriate for treatment of patients with both HBV and HIV infections. Pancreatitis reported, especially in HIV-infected pediatrics with prior nucleoside exposure. Suspend therapy if lactic acidosis or pronounced hepatotoxicity develops. Emergence of resistance-associated HBV mutations reported. Reduce dose in renal dysfunction. Caution in elderly. Monitor patient regularly during treatment, consider ALT and HBV DNA levels determination. Safety and efficacy of treatment after 1 yr is not known.



**ADVERSE REACTIONS:** Lactic acidosis, severe hepatomegaly with steatosis, post-treatment exacerbations of hepatitis, pancreatitis, malaise/fatigue, GI complaints, ear, nose, and throat infections, sore throat, elevated LFTs, arthralgia/myalgia.

**INTERACTIONS:** Avoid use with zalcitabine; may inhibit intracellular phosphorylation of lamivudine (3TC). TMP/SMX may increase 3TC levels. Do not take concurrently with other 3TC-containing products (eg, Epivir, Combivir, Epzicom or Trivizir).

**PREGNANCY:** Category C, not for use in nursing.

**MECHANISM OF ACTION:** Nucleoside analogue; phosphorylated to active 5'-triphosphate metabolite intracellularly; incorporation of monophosphate form into viral DNA by HBV reverse transcriptase results in DNA termination.

**PHARMACOKINETICS: Absorption:** Rapid; $C_{max}$=1.28mcg/mL (HBV), $C_{max}$=1.05mcg/mL (healthy); $T_{max}$=0.5-2.0 hrs; AUC=4.3mcg•h/mL (HBV), AUC=4.7mcg•h/mL (healthy). Tab: Absolute bioavailability (86%). Sol: Absolute bioavailability (87%). **Distribution:** Plasma protein binding (<36%); $V_d$=1.3L/kg. **Metabolism:** Hepatic (minor); trans-sulfoxide (metabolite). **Elimination:** Urine (unchanged); $T_{1/2}$=5-7 hrs.

## NURSING CONSIDERATIONS

**Assessment:** Assess for HIV infection, impaired liver/renal function, history of pancreatitis, risk factors for lactic acidosis, and possible drug interactions.

**Monitoring:** Monitor signs/symptoms of pancreatitis, lactic acidosis, renal dysfunction, hepatic decompensation/dysfunction (LFTs), exacerbations of hepatitis B, and fat redistribution. May enroll patients in the Antiretroviral Pregnancy Registry if they become pregnant while on treatment.

**Patient Counseling:** Advise to promptly report symptoms of pancreatitis, lactic acidosis, worsening of disease/emergence of resistant HBV, or fat redistribution/accumulation. Counsel on importance of HIV testing to avoid inappropriate therapy and development of resistant HIV. Offer HIV counseling and testing prior to initiation. Inform that therapy does not reduce risk of transmission of HBV through sexual contact or blood contamination. Inform diabetics that each 20mL of oral solution contains 4g of sucrose. Instruct not to take concurrently with other 3TC-containing products such as Epivir, Combivir, Epzicom or Trivizir.

**Administration:** Oral route. Take on the same time each day, with or without food. Do not skip doses. If a dose is missed, take immediately, but not 2 doses at one. **Storage:** Tab: 25°C (77°F); excursions permitted to 15-30°C (59-86°F). Sol: 20-25°C (68-77°F); store in tightly closed bottles.

# EPOGEN RX

epoetin alfa (Amgen)

**Increase mortality, serious CV events and stroke in CRF patient when administered to target Hgb levels of ≥13g/dL. Individualize dosing to achieve and maintain Hgb levels within range of 10-12g/dL. Shortened overall survival and/or increased risk of tumor progression or recurrence in patients with breast, non-small cell lung, head and neck, lymphoid, and cervical cancers. To decrease these risks, as well as risk of serious cardio- and thrombovascular events, use lowest dose needed to avoid RBC transfusions. Because of these risks, prescribers and hospitals must enroll in and comply with the ESA APPRISE Oncology Program to prescribe and/or dispense to patients with cancer. Use only for treatment of anemia due to concomitant myelosuppressive chemotherapy. Not indicated for patients receiving myelosuppressive therapy when anticipated outcome is cure. D/C following completion of chemotherapy course. Increased the rate of deep venous thromboses in patients not receiving prophylactic anticoagulation during surgery. Consider DVT prophylaxis.**

**THERAPEUTIC CLASS:** Erythropoiesis stimulator

**INDICATIONS:** Treatment of anemia of chronic renal failure (CRF); anemia related to therapy with zidovudine in HIV-infected patients; anemic patients (Hgb >10-≤13g/dL) who are at high risk for perioperative blood loss to reduce the need for allogeneic blood transfusions; anemia due to the effect of concomitantly administered chemotherapy based on studies that have shown a reduction in the need for RBC transfusions in patients with metastatic, non-myeloid malignancies receiving chemotherapy for minimum of 2 months.

**DOSAGE:** *Adults:* CRF: (IV/SQ) Initial: 50-100 U/kg TIW. IV route recommended in hemodialysis patients. Reduce dose by 25% when Hgb approaches 12g/dL or increases >1g/dL in any 2 week period. Increase dose by 25% if Hgb <10g/dL and has not increased by 1g/dL after 4 weeks of therapy or Hgb <10g/dL. Maint: Individually titrate for each patient on dialysis; Hgb levels between 10-12g/dL. Median Maint: (Hemodialysis) 75 U/kg TIW with the range of 12.5-525 U/kg TIW. To maintain Hct levels, 10% of the patients require <25 U/kg and approximately 10% of the patients required >200 U/kg TIW. Zidovudine-Treated HIV Patients: If serum erythropoietin ≤500 mU/mL and zidovudine ≤4200mg/week give 100 U/kg IV/SQ TIW for 8 weeks. Titrate: Increase by 50-100 U/kg TIW after 8 weeks if necessary. Max: 300 U/kg TIW. Maint: If Hgb >12g/dL, d/c until Hgb <11g/dL, then reduce dose by 25% when therapy is resumed. Surgery Patients: Initial: (Hgb >10-≤13g/dL) 300 U/kg/day SQ for 10 days before, on day of, and for 4 days after surgery; or 600 U/kg SQ once weekly on 21, 14, and 7 days before surgery. Cancer Patients on Chemotherapy: 150 U/kg SQ TIW or 40,000 U SQ weekly. Titrate: (TIW dosing) Increase to 300 U/kg TIW if response not satisfactory after 4 weeks to avoid need for RBC transfusion or (Weekly dosing) 60,000 U SQ weekly If Hgb is not increased by ≥1g/dL after 4 weeks. Reduce dose by 25% when Hgb reaches a level needed to avoid transfusion or increases >1g/dL in any 2 weeks. Withhold dose if Hgb exceeds a level needed to avoid transfusion and restart at 25% below the previous dose when Hgb approaches a level where transfusions may be required. D/C if no response after 8 weeks or if transfusions are still required.

*Pediatrics:* CRF: (IV/SQ) Initial: 50 U/kg TIW. Reduce dose by 25% if Hgb approaches 12g/dL or Hgb increases >1g/dL in any 2-week period. Increase dose by 25% if Hgb <10g/dL and has not increased by 1g/dL after 4 weeks of therapy or Hgb <10g/dL. Median Maint (Hemodialysis and Peritoneal dialysis): 167 U/kg/week (49-447 U/kg/week) and 76 U/kg/week (24-323 U/kg/week) in divided doses (TIW or BIW). If transferrin saturation is >20%, dose may be increased. Maintain Hgb levels between 10-12g/dL; 75-150 U/kg/week maintains the Hct of 36%-38% for 6 months. Cancer Patients on Chemotherapy: 600 U/kg IV weekly. Titrate: If Hgb is not increased by ≥1g/dL after 4 weeks increase to 900 U/kg IV weekly. Reduce dose by 25% when Hgb reaches a level needed to avoid transfusion or increases >1g/dL in any 2 weeks. Withhold dose if Hgb exceeds a level needed to avoid transfusion and restart at 25% below the previous dose when Hgb approaches a level where transfusions may be required. D/C if no response after 8 weeks. Max: 60,000 U.

**HOW SUPPLIED:** Inj: 2000 U/mL, 3000 U/mL, 4000 U/mL, 10,000 U/mL, 20,000 U/mL, 40,000 U/mL [1mL single dose]; 10,000 U/mL [2mL multidose]; 20,000 [1mL multidose]

**CONTRAINDICATIONS:** Uncontrolled HTN. Hypersensitivity to mammalian cell-derived products and albumin (human).

**WARNINGS/PRECAUTIONS:** Contains benzyl alcohol; increased incidence of neurological and other complications in premature infants have been reported. Pure red cell aplasia and severe anemia (with or without other cytopenias) may occur. Evaluate etiology if lack/loss of response occurs; test for presence of antibodies to erythropoietin; if present d/c permanently. Should not be switched to other ESAs as antibodies may cross-react. Formulation with albumin may carry risk for transmission of viral diseases. Do not use in patients with uncontrolled HTN. Closely monitor and aggressively control BP in those treated and adjust dose in CRF patients on dailysis with clinically evident ischemic heart disease or CHF. Seizures reported; presence of premonitory neurologic symptoms should be monitored. Avoid potentially hazardous activities such as driving or operating heavy machinery. Exacerbation of porphyria observed; caution in patients with known porphyria. Transient rashes occasionally observed. ESAs resulted in decreased locoregional control/progression-free survival and/or overall survival in patients with advanced head and neck cancer receiving radiation therapy, in patients receiving chemotherapy for metastatic breast cancer or lymphoid malignancy, and in patients with non-small cell lung cancer or various malignancies who were not receiving chemotherapy or radiotherapy. Functional iron deficiency may develop; evaluate iron stores prior to and during therapy. Monitor Hct, BP, iron levels, serum chemistry, and CBC. Menses may resume.

**ADVERSE REACTIONS:** HTN, headache, fatigue, arthralgias, N/V, diarrhea, edema, rash, pyrexia, clotted vascular access, respiratory congestion, dyspnea, asthenia, dizziness, seizures, thrombotic events.

**INTERACTIONS:** Adjust anticoagulant dose in dialysis patients.

**PREGNANCY:** Category C, caution in nursing.

**MECHANISM OF ACTION:** Erythropoiesis stimulator.

**PHARMACOKINETICS: Absorption:** (SC) $T_{max}$=5-24 hrs. **Elimination:** (IV) $T_{1/2}$=4-13 hrs.

## NURSING CONSIDERATIONS

**Assessment:** Assess for uncontrolled HTN, porphyria, history of HTN, cardiovascular disease (ischemic heart disease, CHF), renal failure, cancer, pure red cell aplasia, seizure, pregnancy/nursing status, possible drug interactions, hypersensitivity to mammalian cell-derived products and albumin. Obtain baseline BP measurements and iron status (transferrin saturation, serum ferritin).

**Monitoring:** Monitor BP, Hct, CBC with differential and platelet count, iron status (transferrin saturation, serum ferritin) regularly. CRF: Serum chemistries (BUN, uric acid, creatinine, phosphorus, $K^+$) regulary, Hgb twice weekly. HIV and cancer: Hgb once weekly. Monitor for signs/symptoms of CV events (MI, stroke, CHF), pure red cell aplasia, severe anemia, viral diseases, seizures, lack/loss of response to therapy, and hypersensitivity reactions.

**Patient Counseling:** Caution may impair physical/mental abilities. Advise to seek medical attention if symptoms of CV events, anemia, infections, seizures, or hypersensitivity reactions occur. Inform that it can increase the risk of having serious CV events, thromboembolic events and tumor progression or recurrence. Instruct for the proper dosage and administration. If use at home, inform about the proper disposal and cautioned against the reuse of needles, syringes or drug product. A puncture-resistant container should be available for disposal of used syringes and needles.

**Administration:** IV, SC route. **Storage:** 2-8°C (36-46°F). Do not freeze or shake. Protect from light.

# EPZICOM RX

abacavir sulfate - lamivudine (GlaxoSmithKline)

**Fatal hypersensitivity reactions reported with abacavir sulfate; d/c if hypersensitivity reaction suspected and do not restart. High risk of hypersensitivity reaction to abacavir in patients with HLA-B*5701 allele; screening is recommended prior to therapy. Lactic acidosis and severe hepatomegaly with steatosis, including fatal cases, reported with nucleoside analogs alone or in combination with other antivirals. Severe acute exacerbations of hepatitis B reported in patients coinfected with HBV and HIV and who have discontinued lamivudine.**

**THERAPEUTIC CLASS:** Nucleoside analog combination

**INDICATIONS:** Treatment of HIV infection in combination with other antiretrovirals.

**DOSAGE:** *Adults:* ≥18 yrs: CrCl >50mL/min: 1 tab qd.

**HOW SUPPLIED:** Tab: (Abacavir Sulfate-Lamivudine) 600mg-300mg

**CONTRAINDICATIONS:** Hepatic impairment.

**WARNINGS/PRECAUTIONS:** Serious hypersensitivity reactions reported. Suspend therapy if lactic acidosis or pronounced hepatotoxicity develops. Avoid use in patients with CrCl <50mL/min. Redistribution/accumulation of body fat and immune reconstitution syndrome reported. Hepatic decompensation has occurred in HIV/HCV coinfected patients receiving combination antiretroviral therapy for HIV and interferon α, w/ or w/o ribavirin. Consider discontinuation of lamivudine or dose reduction of concurrent drug therapy. Cross-resistance potential with nucleoside reverse transcriptase inhibitors (NRTIs) reported.

**ADVERSE REACTIONS:** Hypersensitivity, insomnia, depression, headache, fatigue, dizziness, nausea, diarrhea, rash, pyrexia, abdominal pain, abnormal dreams, anxiety.

**INTERACTIONS:** May increase methadone clearance. Decreased elimination with ethanol. TMP/SMX and/or nelfinavir may increase lamivudine exposure. Avoid with zalcitabine.

**PREGNANCY:** Category C, not for use in nursing.

**MECHANISM OF ACTION:** Abacavir: Carbocyclic nucleoside analogue. Inhibits HIV-1 reverse transcriptase (RT) by competing with natural substrate dGTP and incorporating into viral DNA. Lamivudine: Nucleoside analogue. Inhibits RT via DNA chain termination.

**PHARMACOKINETICS: Absorption:** Abacavir: Rapid, bioavailability (86%); $C_{max}$=4.26mcg/mL, AUC=11.95mcg•hr/mL. Lamivudine: Rapid, bioavailability (86%); $C_{max}$=2.04mcg/mL, AUC=8.87mcg•hr/mL. **Distribution:** Abacavir: $V_d$=0.86L/kg, plasma protein binding (50%). Lamivudine: $V_d$=1.3L/kg, plasma protein binding (70%). **Metabolism:** Abacavir: Via alcohol dehydrogenase. Lamivudine: Metabolite (trans-sulfoxide). **Elimination:** Abacavir: $T_{1/2}$=1.45 hrs. Lamivudine: (IV): Urine (70%); $T_{1/2}$=5-7 hrs.

## NURSING CONSIDERATIONS

**Assessment:** Assess for family history, hepatic/renal impairment, risk factors for lactic acidosis, acute respiratory disease, liver problems (including hepatitis B), smoking, high blood pressure, high cholesterol, pregnancy/nursing status, and possible drug interactions. Assess for HLA-B*5701 allele.

**Monitoring:** Monitor for signs/symptoms of lactic acidosis (eg, vomiting, diarrhea, abdominal pain), hepatic dysfunction (eg, decompensation, failure), immune reconstitution syndrome, fat redistribution, respiratory disorder (eg, dyspnea, cough), hypersensitivity reactions, and exacerbation of HBV. Monitor hepatic/renal function closely; observe for lab abnormalities (elevated LFTs, elevated CPK, elevated Cr, lymphopenia). Follow-up LFTs for several months after d/c therapy. May enroll patients in the Antiretroviral Pregnancy Registry if they become pregnant while on treatment.

**Patient Counseling:** Counsel regarding hypersensitivity reactions with abacavir (ABC); d/c if suspected. Do not restart or replace with any drug containing ABC following hypersensitivty reaction or treatment interruption for other reasons to avoid more serious symptoms (life-threatening hypotension) and possibly death. Advise to seek medical attention if symptoms of lactic acidosis (eg, vomiting, diarrhea, abdominal pain) hepatic dysfunction (eg, decompensation, failure), immune reconstitution syndrome, fat redistribution, respiratory disorder (eg, dyspnea, cough), hypersensitivity reactions (eg, fever, rash, NV), and exacerbation of HBV occur. Instruct not to take with other ABC- or lamivudine-containing agents.

**Administration:** Oral route. **Storage:** 25°C (77°F); excursions permitted to 15-30°C (59-86°F).



# EQUAGESIC

CIV

meprobamate - aspirin (Wyeth/Women First)

**THERAPEUTIC CLASS:** Carbamate derivative/salicylate

**INDICATIONS:** Adjunct in short-term treatment of pain accompanied by tension and/or anxiety in patients with musculoskeletal disease.

**DOSAGE:** *Adults:* 1-2 tabs tid-qid prn. Elderly/Debilitated: Use lowest effective dose.
*Pediatrics:* ≥12 yrs: 1-2 tabs tid-qid prn.

**HOW SUPPLIED:** Tab: (Meprobamate-ASA) 200mg-325mg* *scored

**CONTRAINDICATIONS:** Acute intermittent porphyria.

**WARNINGS/PRECAUTIONS:** Extreme caution with peptic ulcer, asthma, coagulation abnormalities, hypoprothrombinemia, or vitamin K deficiency. Abuse, physical and psychological dependence reported. Abrupt withdrawal after prolonged and excessive use may precipitate recurrence of pre-existing symptoms. May impair mental and physical abilities. Caution with hepatic or kidney dysfunction. May precipitate seizures in epileptic patients. Prescribe cautiously and in small amounts to suicidal patients.

**ADVERSE REACTIONS:** Epigastric discomfort, NV, drowsiness, ataxia, dizziness, slurred speech, headache, vertigo, weakness.

**INTERACTIONS:** Additive CNS suppression with alcohol or other psychotropic drugs. May antagonize uricosuric activity of probenecid and sulfinpyrazone. Extreme caution with anticoagulants. May enhance hypoglycemic effects of sulfonylureas.

**PREGNANCY:** Safety in pregnancy or nursing not known.

**MECHANISM OF ACTION:** Meprobamate: Carbamate derivative; affects multiple sites in CNS. ASA: Salicylate (non-narcotic analgesic); antipyretic and anti-inflammatory effects.

## NURSING CONSIDERATIONS

**Assessment:** Assess for history of peptic ulcer, abdominal conditions, Addison's disease, intracranial pressure, head injury, hypothyroidism, prostatic hypertrophy, uretheral stricture, acute intermittent porphyria, syndrome of asthma, rhinitis, and nasal polyps, viral infections, pregnancy status, suicidal tendencies, alcohol use, epilepsy, possible drug interactions, renal/hepatic impairment.

**Monitoring:** Monitor for GI ulceration and bleeding, Reye's syndrome, and hypersensitivity reactions.

**Patient Counseling:** Inform of pregnancy risks. Caution may impair physical/mental abilities. Seek medical attention if symptoms of GI bleeding or ulceration, Reye's syndrome, or hypersensitivity reactions occur.

**Administration:** Oral route. **Storage:** 20-25°C (68-77°F). Protect from moisture and light.

# EQUETRO

RX

carbamazepine (Validus)



**Serious and sometimes fatal dermatologic reactions, including toxic epidermal necrolysis (TEN) and Stevens-Johnson syndrome (SJS) reported; increased risk with presence of HLA-B*1502 allele. Patients with ancestry in genetically at-risk populations should be screened for presence of HLA-B*1502 prior to initiating treatment. Aplastic anemia and agranulocytosis reported. Obtain complete pretreatment hematological testing as baseline. D/C if evidence of bone marrow depression develops.**

**THERAPEUTIC CLASS:** Carboxamide

**INDICATIONS:** Treatment of acute manic and mixed episodes associated with bipolar I disorder.

**DOSAGE:** *Adults:* Initial: 400mg/day, given in divided doses, bid. Titrate: Adjust in increments of 200mg/day. Max: 1600mg/day.

**HOW SUPPLIED:** Cap, Extended-Release: 100mg, 200mg, 300mg

**CONTRAINDICATIONS:** History of previous bone marrow depression, MAOI use within 14 days, known sensitivity to any of the tricyclic compounds (eg, amitriptyline, desipramine, imipramine, protriptyline, nortriptyline).

**WARNINGS/PRECAUTIONS:** D/C at first sign of rash, unless rash is clearly not drug-related. Increased risk of suicidal thoughts or behavior; monitor for emergence or worsening of depression, suicidal thoughts and behavior, and/or any unusual changes in mood or behavior. May cause fetal harm if administered to a pregant woman. In patients with seizure disorder, avoid abrupt d/c; may precipitate status epilepticus. Mild anticholinergic activity may occur; observe closely with increased intraocular pressure (IOP). Caution in patients with a history of cardiac, hepatic, or renal damage, or interrupted courses of therapy. Previous adverse hematologic reaction to other drugs may increase risk of bone marrow depression. May activate latent psychosis. May cause confusion/agitation in elderly. May impair physical/mental ability. Before initiating therapy, obtain a detailed history and perform physical exam. Caution in patients who have had a history of interrupted courses of therapy with carbamazepine.

**ADVERSE REACTIONS:** Dizziness, somnolence, N/V, agranulocytosis, headache, infection, pain, rash, diarrhea, dyspepsia, asthenia, aplastic anemia, amnesia, TEN, SJS.

**INTERACTIONS:** See Contraindications. CYP3A4 and/or epoxide hydrolase inhibitors (eg, acetazolamide, azole antifungals, cimetidine, clarithromycin, protease inhibitors) may increase plasma levels. CYP3A4 inducers (eg, cisplatin, phenobarbital, phenytoin) may decrease plasma levels. May lower plasma levels of CYP1A2 substrates and CYP3A4 substrates (eg, acetaminophen, bupropion, clonazepam, doxycycline, oral contraceptives, warfarin). May decrease effectiveness and increase incidence of breakthrough bleeding with oral contraceptives. May increase or decrease plasma levels of phenytoin; monitor phenytoin levels. May reduce warfarin's anticoagulant effect. May increase plasma levels of clomipramine and primidone. Concomitant use with lithium, may increase the risk of neurotoxic side effects. May decrease levels of trazodone. Antimalarial drugs (eg, chloroquine, mefloquine) may antagonize the activity of carbamazepine. Caution with other centrally acting drugs and alcohol. Reduced thyroid function with other anticonvulsants. Coadministration with delavirdine may lead to loss of virologic response and possible resistance to NNRTIs.

**PREGNANCY:** Category D, not for use in nursing.

**MECHANISM OF ACTION:** Carboxamide; mechanism not established. Suspected to modulate sodium and calcium ion channels, receptor-mediated neurotransmitters, and intracellular signaling pathways.

**PHARMACOKINETICS: Absorption:** $C_{max}$=1.9mcg/mL (single dose), 11.0mcg/mL (multiple doses); $T_{max}$=19 hrs (single dose), 5.9 hrs (multiple doses). **Distribution:** Plasma protein binding (76%); found in breast milk. **Metabolism:** Liver, via CYP3A4; carbamazepine-10,11-epoxide (metabolite).

**Elimination:** Urine 72% (3% unchanged), feces (28%); $T_{1/2}$=35-40 hrs (single dose), 12-17 hrs (multiple doses).

## NURSING CONSIDERATIONS

E

**Assessment:** Assess use in patients with history of cardiac, hepatic or renal damage. Assess use in patients who have had a history of interrupted courses of therapy with carbamazepine and in patients who had a previous hematological reaction to other medications. Assess for history of bone marrow depression, sensitivity to any tricyclic compounds, presence of a seizure disorder, presence of increased IOP, pregnancy/nursing status, and for possible drug interactions. Assess for HLA-B*1502 allele in suspected patient populations. Prior to initiating therapy, obtain a detailed history and perform physical exam. Obtain baseline CBC, including reticulocyte count, serum iron levels, LFTs, urinalysis, BUN, and eye exam.

**Monitoring:** Monitor for signs/symptoms of dermatological reactions (eg, TEN, SJS), aplastic anemia, agranulocytosis, suicidal behavior or ideation, activation of latent psychosis, and for increased IOP. In elderly patients, monitor for signs/symptoms of agitation. Perform periodic monitoring of CBC including reticulocytes, serum iron levels, liver function, urinalysis, BUN, total cholesterol levels, LDL levels, HDL levels, thyroid function tests, and serum drug levels. Perform periodic eye exams, including slit-lamp examination, funduscopy, and tonometry.

**Patient Counseling:** Instruct to immediately report signs/symptoms of hematologic disorders (eg, fever, sore throat, rash, ulcers in the mouth, easy bruising, petechial or purpuric hemorrhage). Inform that therapy may increase the risk of suicidal throughts and behaviors; instruct to contact physician if symptoms of worsening depression develop or unusual changes in behavior or mood develop. Advise that dizziness or drowsiness may occur; caution against performing hazardous tasks (eg, operating machinery/driving). Inform that, if necessary, caps may be opened and contents sprinkled over food; instruct not to crush or chew caps. Advise to notify physician of all prescription, OTC, and herbal products currently taking.

**Administration:** Oral route; do not crush or chew. **Storage:** 25°C (77°F); excursions permitted to 15-30°C (59-86°F). Protect from light and moisture.

# ERAXIS RX

anidulafungin (Pfizer)

**THERAPEUTIC CLASS:** Echinocandin

**INDICATIONS:** Treatment of candidemia and other forms of *Candida* infections (intra-abdominal abscess and peritonitis); esophageal candidiasis.

**DOSAGE:** *Adults:* Candidemia/*Candida* Infections: LD: 200mg on Day 1. Follow with 100mg qd thereafter. Continue therapy for at least 14 days after last positive culture. Esophageal Candidiasis: LD: 100mg on Day 1. Follow with 50mg qd thereafter. Treat for minimum of 14 days and for at least 7 days after symptoms resolve.

**HOW SUPPLIED:** Inj: 50mg, 100mg

**WARNINGS/PRECAUTIONS:** Hepatic abnormalities (eg, hepatic dysfunction, hepatitis, or worsening hepatic failure)may occur; monitor hepatic function if abnormal LFTs develop during therapy.

**ADVERSE REACTIONS:** Diarrhea, hypokalemia, increased LFTs.

**INTERACTIONS:** Slightly increased levels with cyclosporine.

**PREGNANCY:** Category C, caution in nursing.

**MECHANISM OF ACTION:** Antifungal (Echinocandin); inhibits synthesis of 1, 3-β-D-glucan, an essential component of fungal cell walls.

**PHARMACOKINETICS: Absorption:** IV infusion of variable doses resulted in different parameters. **Distribution:** $V_d$=30-50L; plasma protein binding (>99%). **Elimination:** Urine (<1%), feces (30%); $T_{1/2}$=40-50 hrs.

## NURSING CONSIDERATIONS

**Assessment:** Assess cultures and other lab studies prior to therapy to properly identify causative organisms. Assess pregnancy/nursing status.

**Monitoring:** Monitor LFTs for possible hepatic dysfunction, hepatitis or worsening of hepatic failure, possible drug interactions, serum electrolytes ($K^+$), and signs of histamine-related reactions.

**Patient Counseling:** Inform of possible histamine-mediated symptoms including rash, urticaria, flushing, pruritus, dyspnea, and hypotension. Notify about signs/symptoms of hepatic dysfunction.

**Administration:** IV route. Refer to PI for preparation for administration. Rate of infusion should not exceed 1.1mg/min. **Storage:** 2°C-8°C (36°F-46°F); for up to 1 hr for reconstituted solution, and should be administered within 24 hrs for infusion solution. Do not freeze.



## ERBITUX — RX

cetuximab (Bristol-Myers Squibb)

**Severe infusion reactions have occurred; immediately interrupt and permanently d/c infusion if these reactions occur. Cardiopulmonary arrest and/or sudden death have occurred with squamous cell carcinoma of the head and neck treated with radiation therapy and cetuximab; closely monitor serum electrolytes during and after therapy.**

**THERAPEUTIC CLASS:** Epidermal growth factor receptor (EGFR) antagonist

**INDICATIONS:** In combination with irinotecan for the treatment of epidermal growth factor receptor (EGFR)-expressing, metastatic colorectal carcinoma in patients who are refractory to irinotecan-based chemotherapy. As monotherapy, for the treatment of EGFR-expressing, metastatic colorectal carcinoma in patients who are tolerant to irinotecan-based regimens or after failure of both irinotecan- and oxaliplatin-based regimens. In combination with radiation therapy for the initial treatment of locally or regionally advanced squamous cell carcinoma of the head and neck (SCCHN). As monotherapy, for the treatment of patients with recurrent or metastatic SCCHN for whom prior platinum-based therapy has failed.

**DOSAGE:** *Adults:* Premedication with $H_1$ antagonist (eg, 50mg diphenhydramine) IV 30-60 min prior to 1st dose is recommended. Colorectal Cancer: Initial: 400mg/m² IV infusion over 120 min. Maint: 250mg/m² IV infusion over 60 min once weekly. Max Infusion Rate: 10mg/min. Squamous Cell Carcinoma of Head and Neck: Combination Therapy: Initial: 400mg/m² IV over 120 min 1 week prior to initiation of a course of radiation treatment. Maint: 250mg/m² over 60 min weekly for duration of radiation therapy. Max Infusion Rate: 10mg/min. Recurrent/Metastatic Squamous Cell Carcinoma of Head and Neck: Monotherapy: Initial: 400mg/m² IV infusion over 120 min. Maint: 250mg/m² over 60 min weekly until disease progression or unacceptable toxicity. Dose Modifications: Grade 1 or 2/Non serious Grade 3 or 4 Infusion Reactions: Reduce rate by 50%. Severe Infusion Reactions: D/C. Development of Severe Acneform Rash (Grade 3 or 4): Delay infusion 1-2 weeks for 1st three occurrences. 1st Occurrence: If with improvement, continue at 250mg/m². 2nd Occurrence: If with improvement, reduce dose to 200mg/m². 3rd Occurrence: If with improvement, reduce dose to 150mg/m². 4th Occurrence/No Improvement After Delaying Therapy: D/C therapy.

**HOW SUPPLIED:** Inj: 2mg/mL [100mg/50mL, 200mg/100mL]

**WARNINGS/PRECAUTIONS:** Infusion reactions reported; observe closely for 1 hr following infusion. Permanently d/c therapy if serious infusion reactions develop. Caution when used in combination with radiation therapy in patients with history of coronary artery disease (CAD), congestive heart failure (CHF) or arrhythmias. Interstitial lung disease (ILD) reported; interrupt for acute onset or worsening of pulmonary symptoms and d/c if ILD confirmed. Dermatologic (eg, acneform rash, skin drying/fissuring, paronychial inflammation, and infectious sequelae) and hypertrichosis may occur; limit sun exposure during therapy. Monitor for hypomagnesemia, hypocalcemia, and hypokalemia, during and for at least 8 weeks following completion of therapy.

The safety of cetuximab in combination with radiation therapy and cisplatin has not been established; death and serious cardiotoxicity were observed. Not recommended for colorectal cancer treatment in patients with *KRAS* mutations in codon 12 or 13.

**ADVERSE REACTIONS:** Cutaneous reactions (eg, rash, pruritus, and nail changes), headache, diarrhea, infection, infusion reactions, cardiopulmonary arrest, dermatologic toxicity, radiation dermatitis, sepsis, renal failure, interstitial lung disease, and pulmonary embolus.

**INTERACTIONS:** Serious cardiotoxicity and death may occur with cetuximab, radiation therapy and cisplatin in patients with locally advanced SCCHN.

**PREGNANCY:** Category C, not for use in nursing.

**MECHANISM OF ACTION:** Epidermal growth factor receptor antagonist; binds specifically to EGFR on normal and tumor cells and inhibits binding of epidermal growth factor and other ligands, such as transforming growth factor-α.

**PHARMACOKINETICS: Absorption:** $C_{max}$=168-235µg/mL. **Distribution:** $V_d$=2-3L/m². **Elimination:** $T_{1/2}$=112 hrs.

## NURSING CONSIDERATIONS

**Assessment:** Assess for history of CAD, CHF, arrhythmias, hypersensitivity reactions and colorectal cancer with mutations. Assess pregnancy/nursing status and possible drug interactions. Obtain baseline serum electrolyte levels ($Mg^{2+}$, $K^+$, $Ca^{2+}$).

**Monitoring:** Monitor electrolytes ($Mg^{2+}$, $K^+$, $Ca^{2+}$) during and 8 weeks after drug administration. Monitor for signs/symptoms of hypomagnesemia, hypocalcemia, hypokalemia, acute onset or worsening of pulmonary symptoms, infusion reaction, dermatologic toxicities, and infectious sequelae.

**Patient Counseling:** Inform of pregnancy/nursing risks; advise to use effective contraceptive methods during and 6 months after therapy for both sexes. Advise to d/c nursing, limit sun exposure and apply sunscreen during and 2 months after therapy. Instruct to seek medical attention if symptoms of infusion reaction (eg, fever, chills, breathing problems), electrolyte imbalances, dermatologic toxicities (eg, acneform rash, skin drying), infectious sequelae (eg, cellulitis, abscess formation), acute onset or worsening of pulmonary symptoms occur.

**Administration:** IV infusion. Do not administer as IV push or bolus. Administer through low protein binding 0.22-µm in-line filter. Do not shake or dilute.
**Storage:** (Vials): Refrigerate; 2-8°C (36-46°F). Do not freeze. In infusion containers, stable for 12 hrs at 2-8°C (36-46°F), 8 hrs at 20-25°C (68-77°F).

# ERY-TAB RX

erythromycin (Abbott)

**THERAPEUTIC CLASS:** Macrolide

**INDICATIONS:** Treatment of mild to moderate upper/lower respiratory tract and skin and skin structure infections, listeriosis, pertussis, diphtheria, erythrasma, intestinal amebiasis, acute pelvic inflammatory disease (PID) (*N.gonorrhoeae*), primary syphilis (if PCN allergy), Legionnaires' disease, chlamydial infections (eg, newborn conjunctivitis, pneumonia of infancy, urogenital infections during pregnancy, or urethral, endocervical, or rectal infections when tetracyclines are contraindicated or not tolerated), and nongonococcal urethritis caused by susceptible strains of microorganisms. Prophylaxis of initial and recurrent attacks of rheumatic fever if PCN allergy.

**DOSAGE:** *Adults:* Usual: 250mg qid, 333mg q8h or 500mg q12h. Max: 4g/day. Do not take bid when dose is >1g/day. Treat strep infections for at least 10 days. Streptococcal Infection Long-Term Prophylaxis with Rheumatic Fever: 250mg bid. Chlamydial Urogenital Infection During Pregnancy: 500mg qid or 666mg q8h for at least 7 days, or 500mg q12h, 333mg q8h or 250mg qid for at least 14 days. Urethral/Endocervical/Rectal Chlamydial Infections and Nongonococcal Urethritis: 500mg qid or 666mg q8h for at least 7 days. Primary Syphilis: 30-40g in divided doses for 10-15 days. Acute PID: 500mg

(erythromycin lactobionate) IV q6h for 3 days, then 500mg PO q12h or 333mg q8h for 7 days. Intestinal Amebiasis: 500mg q12h, 333mg q8h or 250mg q6h for 10-14 days. Pertussis: 40-50mg/kg/day in divided doses for 5-14 days. Legionnaires' Disease: 1-4g/day in divided doses.
*Pediatrics:* Usual: 30-50mg/kg/day in divided doses. Severe Infections: May double dose. Max: 4g/day. Treat strep infections for at least 10 days. Streptococcal Infection Long-Term Prophylaxis with Rheumatic Fever: 250mg bid. Chlamydial Conjunctivitis of Newborns/Chlamydial Pneumonia in Infancy: 12.5mg/kg qid for 2 weeks and 3 weeks, respectively. Intestinal Amebiasis: 30-50mg/kg/day in divided doses for 10-14 days.



**HOW SUPPLIED:** Tab, Delayed-Release: 250mg, 333mg, 500mg

**CONTRAINDICATIONS:** Concomitant terfenadine, astemizole, pimozide, or cisapride.

**WARNINGS/PRECAUTIONS:** Pseudomembranous colitis, hepatic dysfunction reported. Caution with impaired hepatic function. May aggravate weakness of patients with myasthenia gravis. Erythromycin does not reach adequate concentrations in fetus to prevent congenital syphilis.

**ADVERSE REACTIONS:** NV, abdominal pain, diarrhea, anorexia, abnormal LFTs, allergic reactions, superinfection (prolonged use).

**INTERACTIONS:** See Contraindications. Rhabdomyolysis reported with lovastatin. May increase levels of theophylline, digoxin, drugs metabolized by CYP450 (eg, carbamazepine, cyclosporine, phenytoin, alfentanil, disopyramide, lovastatin, bromocriptine, valproate, etc). Increases effects of oral anticoagulants, triazolam, midazolam. Risk of acute ergot toxicity with ergotamine or dihydroergotamine. May increase AUC of sildenafil; consider dose reduction of sildenafil.

**PREGNANCY:** Category B, caution in nursing.

**MECHANISM OF ACTION:** Macrolide antibiotic; inhibits protein synthesis by binding 50*S* ribosomal subunits of susceptible organisms.

**PHARMACOKINETICS: Absorption:** (PO) readily absorbed. **Distribution:** Largely bound to plasma proteins. Crosses blood-brain barrier, placenta, and breast milk. Diffuses into most bodily fluids. **Elimination:** Biliary and urinary excretion (<5%).

## NURSING CONSIDERATIONS

**Assessment:** Assess history of impaired hepatic function, myasthenia gravis, hearing loss, arrhythmias. Note other diseases/conditions and drug therapies.

**Monitoring:** Monitor LFTs, renal function, CDAD, hearing loss, pancreatitis, arrhythmias, infantile hypertrophic pyloric stenosis, and hypersensitivity reactions.

**Patient Counseling:** Inform to take exactly as directed and to complete entire course of therapy. Instruct to take on empty stomach. Advise to report any adverse effects, lack of response, and prolonged/persistent diarrhea.

**Administration:** Oral route. **Storage:** 30°C (86°F).

# ERYTHROMYCIN BASE — RX

erythromycin (Various)

**THERAPEUTIC CLASS:** Macrolide

**INDICATIONS:** Treatment of mild to moderate upper/lower respiratory tract and skin and skin structure infections, listeriosis, pertussis, diphtheria, erythrasma, intestinal amebiasis, acute pelvic inflammatory disease (PID) (*N.gonorrhoeae*), primary syphilis (if PCN allergy), Legionnaires' disease, chlamydial infections (eg, newborn conjunctivitis, pneumonia of infancy, urogenital infections during pregnancy or urethral, endocervical, or rectal infections when tetracyclines are contraindicated or not tolerated), and nongonococcal urethritis caused by susceptible strains of microorganisms. Prophylaxis of initial and recurrent attacks of rheumatic fever if PCN allergy.

**DOSAGE:** *Adults:* Usual: 250mg qid or 500mg q12h without food. Max: 4g/day. Treat strep infections for at least 10 days. Streptococcal Infection Long-Term Prophylaxis of Rheumatic Fever: 250mg bid. Chlamydial Urogenital Infection During Pregnancy: 500mg qid for at least 7 days or 500mg q12h or 250mg qid for at least 14 days. Urethral/Endocervical/Rectal Chlamydial Infections and Nongonococcal Urethritis: 500mg qid for at least 7 days. Primary Syphilis: 30-40g in divided doses over 10-15 days. Acute PID: 500mg (erythromycin lactobionate) IV q6h for 3 days, then 500mg PO q12h for 7 days. Intestinal Amebiasis: 500mg q12h or 250mg q6h for 10-14 days. Pertussis: 40-50mg/kg/day in divided doses for 5-14 days. Legionnaires' Disease: 1-4g/day in divided doses.
*Pediatrics:* Usual: 30-50mg/kg/day in divided doses without food. Severe Infections: May double dose. Max: 4g/day. Treat strep infections for at least 10 days. Streptococcal Infection Long-Term Prophylaxis of Rheumatic Fever: 250mg bid. Chlamydial Conjunctivitis of Newborns/Chlamydial Pneumonia in Infancy: (Sus) 12.5mg/kg qid for 2 weeks and 3 weeks, respectively. Intestinal Amebiasis: 30-50mg/kg/day in divided doses for 10-14 days.

**HOW SUPPLIED:** Tab: 250mg, 500mg

**CONTRAINDICATIONS:** Concomitant terfenadine, astemizole, pimozide, or cisapride.

**WARNINGS/PRECAUTIONS:** Pseudomembranous colitis, hepatic dysfunction reported. Caution with impaired hepatic function. May aggravate weakness of patients with myasthenia gravis.

**ADVERSE REACTIONS:** Abdominal pain, N/V, diarrhea, anorexia, abnormal LFTs, allergic reactions, superinfection (prolonged use).

**INTERACTIONS:** See Contraindications. Rhabdomyolysis reported with lovastatin. May increase levels of theophylline, digoxin, drugs metabolized by CYP450 (eg, carbamazepine, cyclosporine, phenytoin, etc). Increases effects of oral anticoagulants, triazolam. Risk of acute ergot toxicity with ergotamine or dihydroergotamine. May increase AUC of sildenafil; consider dose reduction of sildenafil.

**PREGNANCY:** Category B, caution in nursing.

**MECHANISM OF ACTION:** Macrolide; inhibits protein synthesis by binding 50S ribosomal subunits of susceptible organisms.

**PHARMACOKINETICS: Absorption:** (PO) readily absorbed. **Distribution:** Largely bound to plasma proteins. Crosses blood-brain barrier, placenta, breast milk. Diffuses into most body fluids. **Elimination:** Bile, urine (<5% unchanged).

## NURSING CONSIDERATIONS

**Assessment:** Assess for history of impaired hepatic function, myasthenia gravis, hearing loss, arryhthmias. Note other diseases/conditions and drug therapies.

**Monitoring:** Monitor LFTs, renal function tests, CK, *C.difficile*-associated diarrhea, hearing loss, pancreatitis, arrhythmias, infantile hypertrophic pyloric stenosis, and hypersensitivity reactions.

**Patient Counseling:** Inform that therapy only treats bacterial infections. Instruct to take exactly as directed and to complete entire course of therapy. Take on an empty stomach. Advise to report any adverse effects, lack of response, or prolonged/persistent diarrhea.

**Administration:** Oral route. **Storage:** Below 30°C (86°F). Keep tightly closed.

# ERYTHROMYCIN DELAYED-RELEASE RX

erythromycin (Various)

**THERAPEUTIC CLASS:** Macrolide

**INDICATIONS:** Treatment of mild to moderate upper/lower respiratory tract and skin and skin structure infections, listeriosis, pertussis, diphtheria, erythrasma, intestinal amebiasis, acute pelvic inflammatory disease (PID)

(*N.gonorrhoeae*), primary syphilis (if PCN allergy), Legionnaires' disease, chlamydial infections (eg, newborn conjunctivitis, pneumonia of infancy, urogenital infections during pregnancy, or urethral, endocervical, or rectal infections when tetracyclines are contraindicated or not tolerated), and nongonococcal urethritis caused by susceptible strains of microorganisms Prophylaxis of initial and recurrent attacks of rheumatic fever if PCN allergy.

**DOSAGE:** *Adults:* Usual: 250mg q6h or 500mg q12h without food. Max: 4g/day. Treat strep infections for 10 days. Streptococcal Infection Prophylaxis with Rheumatic Heart Disease: 250mg bid. Primary Syphilis: 30-40g in divided doses over 10-15 days. Intestinal Amebiasis: 250mg q6h for 10-14 days. Legionnaires' Disease: 1-4g/day in divided doses. Chlamydial Urogenital Infection During Pregnancy: 500mg qid for 7 days or 250mg qid for 14 days. Urethral/Endocervical/Rectal Chlamydial Infections and Nongonococcal Urethritis: 500mg qid for at least 7 days. Pertussis: 40-50mg/kg/day in divided doses for 5-14 days. Acute PID: 500mg (erythromycin lactobionate) IV q6h for 3 days, then 250mg PO q6h for 7 days.
*Pediatrics:* Usual: 30-50mg/kg/day in divided doses without food. Severe Infections: May double dose. Max: 4g/day. Treat strep infections for 10 days. Streptococcal Infection Prophylaxis with Rheumatic Heart Disease: 250mg bid. Intestinal Amebiasis: 30-50mg/kg/day in divided doses for 10-14 days.

**HOW SUPPLIED:** Cap, Delayed-Release: 250mg

**CONTRAINDICATIONS:** Concomitant terfenadine, astemizole, pimozide, or cisapride.

**WARNINGS/PRECAUTIONS:** Hepatic dysfunction and pseudomembranous colitis reported. May aggravate weakness of patients with myasthenia gravis.

**ADVERSE REACTIONS:** Abdominal pain, N/V, diarrhea, anorexia, hepatic dysfunction, abnormal LFTs, superinfection (prolonged use).

**INTERACTIONS:** See Contraindications. Rhabdomyolysis reported with lovastatin. May increase levels of theophylline, digoxin, drugs metabolized by CYP450 (eg, carbamazepine, cyclosporine, phenytoin, etc). Increases effects of oral anticoagulants, triazolam. Risk of acute ergot toxicity with ergotamine or dihydroergotamine. Extreme caution with terfenadine.

**PREGNANCY:** Category B, caution in nursing.

**MECHANISM OF ACTION:** Macrolide; inhibits protein synthesis by binding 50S ribosomal subunits of susceptible organisms.

**PHARMACOKINETICS: Absorption:** (PO) readily absorbed; $C_{max}$=1.13-1.68mcg/mL; $T_{max}$=3 hrs. **Distribution:** Largely bound to plasma proteins; diffuses into most bodily fluids; crosses blood-brain barrier, placenta, and breast milk. **Elimination:** Bile, urine (<5% unchanged).

## NURSING CONSIDERATIONS

**Assessment:** Assess for history of impaired hepatic function, myasthenia gravis, hearing loss, arrhythmias. Note other diseases/conditions and drug therapies.

**Monitoring:** Monitor LFTs, renal function, CK, CDAD, hearing loss, pancreatitis, arrhythmias, infantile hypertrophic pyloric stenosis, and hypersensitivity reactions.

**Patient Counseling:** Inform therapy treats bacterial, not viral, infections. Take exactly as directed; complete entire course of therapy. Take medication on empty stomach. Advise to report adverse effects, lack of response, and prolonged/persistent diarrhea.

**Administration:** Oral route. **Storage:** Below 30°C (86°F). Protect from moisture and excessive heat.

# ESGIC — RX

acetaminophen - caffeine - butalbital (Forest)

**THERAPEUTIC CLASS:** Barbiturate/analgesic

**INDICATIONS:** Tension or muscle contraction headaches.

**DOSAGE:** *Adults:* 1-2 caps/tabs q4h prn. Max: 6 caps/tabs/day.
*Pediatrics:* ≥12 yrs: 1-2 caps/tabs q4h prn. Max: 6 caps/tabs/day.

**HOW SUPPLIED:** Cap/Tab: (Butalbital-APAP-Caffeine) 50mg-325mg-40mg*
*scored

**CONTRAINDICATIONS:** Porphyria.

**WARNINGS/PRECAUTIONS:** May be habit-forming; potential for abuse. Not for long-term use. Caution in elderly, debilitated, severe renal or hepatic impairment, acute abdominal conditions, suicidal tendencies, history of drug abuse.

E

**ADVERSE REACTIONS:** Drowsiness, lightheadedness, dizziness, sedation, SOB, N/V, abdominal pain, intoxicated feeling.

**INTERACTIONS:** Enhanced CNS effects with MAOIs. May enhance CNS depressant effects of other narcotic analgesics, alcohol, general anesthetics, tranquilizers, sedative hypnotics, or other CNS depressants.

**PREGNANCY:** Category C, not for use in nursing.

**MECHANISM OF ACTION:** Butalbital: Short- to intermediate-acting barbiturate. Acetaminophen: Nonopiate, nonsalicylate analgesic, antipyretic. Caffeine: CNS stimulant.

**PHARMACOKINETICS: Absorption:** APAP, caffeine: Rapid. **Distribution:** Butalbital: Plasma protein binding (45%); crosses placenta, found in breast milk. Caffeine: Found in breast milk. **Metabolism:** APAP: Conjugation. Caffeine: Biotransformation. **Elimination:** Butalbital: Urine (3.6%); $T_{1/2}$=35 hrs. APAP: Urine; $T_{1/2}$=1.25-3 hrs. Caffeine: Urine (3%); $T_{1/2}$=3 hrs.

## NURSING CONSIDERATIONS

**Assessment:** Assess for porphyria, possible drug interactions, history of drug abuse/dependence, acute abdominal conditions, renal/hepatic impairment.

**Monitoring:** Monitor LFTs and renal function periodically. Monitor for hypersensitivity reactions, abuse/dependence, renal/hepatic dysfunction.

**Patient Counseling:** Instruct to take as prescribed (amount, frequency); avoid alcohol use. Caution may impair physical/mental abilities. Seek medical attention if hypersensitivity reactions occur.

**Administration:** Oral route. **Storage:** 15-30°C (59-86°F).

# Esgic-Plus RX

acetaminophen - caffeine - butalbital (Forest)

**THERAPEUTIC CLASS:** Barbiturate/analgesic

**INDICATIONS:** Tension or muscle contraction headaches.

**DOSAGE:** *Adults:* 1 cap/tab q4h prn. Max: 6 caps/tabs/day.
*Pediatrics:* ≥12 yrs: 1 cap/tab q4h prn. Max: 6 caps/tabs/day.

**HOW SUPPLIED:** Cap/Tab: (Butalbital-APAP-Caffeine) 50mg-500mg-40mg*
*scored

**CONTRAINDICATIONS:** Porphyria.

**WARNINGS/PRECAUTIONS:** May be habit-forming; potential for abuse. Not for long-term use. Caution in elderly, debilitated, severe renal or hepatic impairment, acute abdominal conditions, suicidal tendencies, history of drug abuse.

**ADVERSE REACTIONS:** Drowsiness, lightheadedness, dizziness, sedation, SOB, N/V, abdominal pain, intoxicated feeling.

**INTERACTIONS:** Enhanced CNS effects with MAOIs. May enhance CNS depressant effects of other narcotic analgesics, alcohol, general anesthetics, tranquilizers, sedative hypnotics, or other CNS depressants.

**PREGNANCY:** Category C, not for use in nursing.

**MECHANISM OF ACTION:** Butalbital: Short- to intermediate-acting barbiturate. Acetaminophen: Nonopiate, nonsalicylate analgesic, antipyretic. Caffeine: CNS stimulant.

**PHARMACOKINETICS: Absorption:** APAP, caffeine: Rapid. **Distribution:** Butalbital: Plasma protein binding (45%); crosses placenta; found in breast milk. Caffeine: Found in breast milk. **Metabolism:** APAP: Conjugation. Caffeine: Biotransformation. **Elimination:** Butalbital: Urine (3.6%); $T_{1/2}$=35 hrs. APAP: Urine; $T_{1/2}$=1.25-3 hrs. Caffeine: Urine (3%); $T_{1/2}$=3 hrs.

## NURSING CONSIDERATIONS

**Assessment:** Assess for porphyria, possible drug interactions, history of drug abuse/dependence, acute abdominal conditions, renal/hepatic impairment.

**Monitoring:** Monitor LFTs and renal function periodically. Monitor for hypersensitivity reactions, abuse/dependence, renal/hepatic dysfunction.

**Patient Counseling:** Instruct to take as prescribed (amount, frequency); avoid alcohol use. Caution may impair physical/mental abilities. Seek medical attention if hypersensitivity reactions occur.

**Administration:** Oral route. **Storage:** 15-30°C (59-86°F).

# ESTRACE — RX

estradiol (Warner Chilcott)

**Estrogens increase risk of endometrial cancer in postmenopausal women. Avoid during pregnancy.**

**THERAPEUTIC CLASS:** Estrogen

**INDICATIONS:** (Cre/Tab) Treatment of vulval and vaginal atrophy. (Tab) Treatment of moderate to severe vasomotor symptoms associated with menopause. Treatment of hypoestrogenism due to hypogonadism, castration, or primary ovarian failure. Palliative treatment of metastatic breast cancer and advanced androgen-dependent prostate carcinoma. Prevention of osteoporosis.

**DOSAGE:** *Adults:* (Cre) Vulval/Vaginal Atrophy: Initial: 2-4g/day for 1-2 weeks, then decrease to 1-2g/day for 1-2 weeks. Maint: 1g, 1-3x/week. Discontinue or taper at 3-6 month intervals. (Tab) Vasomotor Symptoms/Vulval/Vaginal Atrophy: Initial: 1-2mg/day (3 weeks on, 1 week off). Maint: Minimum effective dose. Discontinue or taper at 3-6 month intervals. Hypoestrogenism: 1-2mg/day. Maint: Minimum effective dose. Metastatic Breast Cancer: 10mg tid for at least 3 months. Prostate Carcinoma: 1-2mg tid. Osteoporosis Prevention: 0.5mg qd cyclically (23 days on and 5 days off).

**HOW SUPPLIED:** Cre, Vaginal: 0.1mg/g [12g, 42.5g]; Tab: 0.5mg*, 1mg*, 2mg* *scored

**CONTRAINDICATIONS:** Pregnancy, undiagnosed abnormal genital bleeding, breast cancer unless being treated for metastatic disease, estrogen-dependent neoplasia, thrombophlebitis, or thromboembolic disorders.

**WARNINGS/PRECAUTIONS:** Risk of gallbladder disease, cardiovascular disease, endometrial and breast carcinoma, fetal congenital reproductive tract disorder, elevated BP, and hypercalcemia with breast cancer and bone metastases. Caution in liver dysfunction, asthma, epilepsy, migraine, and cardiac or renal dysfunction. Increase in HDL, triglycerides, thyroid binding globulin. Acceleration of PT, PTT. Hypercoagulability effects. Impaired glucose tolerance. Consider adding progestin in patient with intact uterus.

**ADVERSE REACTIONS:** Altered vaginal bleeding, vaginal candidiasis, breast tenderness/enlargement, GI effects, melasma, CNS effects, weight changes, edema, altered libido.

**PREGNANCY:** Category X, caution in nursing.

**MECHANISM OF ACTION:** Estrogen; binds to nuclear receptors in estrogen-responsive tissue. Circulating estrogens modulate pituitary secretion of gonadotropins, luteinizing hormone, and follicle stimulating hormone, through negative feedback mechanism. Reduces elevated levels of these hormones in postmenopausal women.

**PHARMACOKINETICS: Absorption**: (Cre) Absorbed through skin, mucous membranes, and GI tract. **Distribution**: Largely bound to sex hormone-binding globulin and albumin; found in breast milk. **Metabolism**: Liver to estrone (metabolite), estriol (major urinary metabolite); sulfate and glucuronide conjugation (liver); gut hydrolysis; CYP3A4 (partial metabolism). **Elimination**: Urine (parent compound and metabolites).

## NURSING CONSIDERATIONS

**Assessment:** Assess for undiagnosed abnormal genital bleeding, presence or history of breast cancer, DVT, PE, estrogen-dependent neoplasia, active or recent (within past yr) arterial thromboembolic disease (eg, stroke, MI), hepatic impairment, history of cholestatic jaundice, age ( ≥65 yrs old), hypertriglyceridemia, hypothyroidism, hypocalcemia, asthma, DM, epilepsy, migraine or porphyria, SLE, pregnancy/nursing status, and possible drug interactions. Assess need for progestin therapy in women who have not had a hysterectomy.

**Monitoring:** Monitor for signs/symptoms of cardiovascular disorders (eg, MI, stroke, venous thrombosis, pulmonary embolism), malignant neoplasms (eg, endometrial, breast, ovarian cancer), dementia, gallbladder disease, hypercalcemia, visual abnormalities (eg, retinal vascular thrombosis), elevations in BP, elevations in plasma triglycerides, pancreatitis, hypothyroidism, fluid retention, exacerbation of endometriosis and other conditions (eg, asthma, DM, epilepsy, migraine, SLE). For tablet formulation, monitor for hypersensitivity reactions. Monitor thyroid function in patients on thyroid replacement therapy. Monitor BP at regular intervals. If undiagnosed, persistent, or recurring abnormal vaginal bleeding occurs, perform proper diagnostic measures (eg, endometrial sampling) to rule out malignancy. Perform periodic monitoring (eg, every 3-6 months) to determine if treatment still required.

**Patient Counseling:** Inform medication increases chances of uterine cancer. Notify physician of upcoming surgery or need for prolonged bed rest. Contact physician if breast lumps, unusual vaginal bleeding, dizziness and faintness, changes in speech, severe headaches, chest pain, SOB, leg pains, changes in vision, or vomiting occur. Not for use during pregnancy. Perform monthly self breast exams.

**Administration:** Tab: Oral route. Cre: Intravaginal route. **Storage**: Tab: 20-25°C (68-77°F); dispense with child-resistant closure in a tight, light-resistant container. Cre: Store at room temperature; protect from temperatures >40°C (104°F). Keep out of reach of children.

# ESTRADERM RX

estradiol (Novartis)

**Estrogens increase the risk of endometrial cancer. Estrogens, with or without progestins, should not be used for the prevention of cardiovascular disease or dementia. Increased risks of MI, stroke, invasive breast cancer, PE, and DVT in postmenopausal women (50-79 yrs of age) reported. Increased risk of developing probable dementia in postmenopausal women ≥65 yrs of age reported.**

**THERAPEUTIC CLASS:** Estrogen

**INDICATIONS:** Treatment of moderate-to-severe vasomotor symptoms and/or vulvar/vaginal atrophy associated with menopause. Treatment of hypoestrogenism due to hypogonadism, castration, or primary ovarian failure. Prevention of postmenopausal osteoporosis.

**DOSAGE:** *Adults:* Apply to clean, dry area on trunk of body. Do not apply to breast or waistline. Replace twice weekly. Rotate application sites. May give continuously without intact uterus. May give cyclically (3 weeks on, 1 week off) with intact uterus. Vasomotor Symptoms/Vulvar/Vaginal Atrophy: Initial: Apply 0.05mg/day twice weekly. Discontinue/Taper at 3-6 month intervals. Start 1 week after discontinuing oral hormone therapy. Osteoporosis Prevention: Initial: 0.05mg/day.

**HOW SUPPLIED:** Patch: 0.05mg/24 hrs, 0.1mg/24 hrs [8[s], 24[s]]

**CONTRAINDICATIONS:** Pregnancy, undiagnosed abnormal genital bleeding, breast cancer unless being treated for metastatic disease, estrogen-dependent neoplasia, DVT/PE, active or recent (eg, within past year) arterial thromboembolic disease (eg, stroke, MI), liver dysfunction or disease.

**WARNINGS/PRECAUTIONS:** May increase risk of cardiovascular events (eg, MI, stroke), venous thrombosis, and PE; d/c immediately if any of these events occur or are suspected. May increase risk of breast/endometrial cancer, and gallbladder disease. May lead to severe hypercalcemia with breast cancer and bone metastases; monitor and d/c if hypercalcemia occurs. Retinal vascular thrombosis reported; monitor and d/c if papilledema or retinal vascular lesions occur. Consider addition of a progestin if no hysterectomy. May elevate BP; monitor at regular intervals. May cause elevations of plasma triglycerides with pre-existing hypertriglyceridemia. Caution with history of cholestatic jaundice associated with past estrogen use or with pregnancy; d/c with recurrence. May lead to increased thyroid-binding globulin levels; monitor thyroid function. May cause fluid retention; caution with cardiac/renal dysfunction. Caution with severe hypocalcemia. May increase risk of ovarian cancer. May exacerbate endometriosis, asthma, DM, epilepsy, migraine, porphyria, SLE, and hepatic hemangiomas; use with caution.

**ADVERSE REACTIONS:** Redness/irritation at application site, altered vaginal bleeding, vaginal candidiasis, breast tenderness/enlargement, GI effects, melasma, CNS effects, retinal vascular thrombosis, weight changes, edema, altered libido.

**INTERACTIONS:** CYP3A4 inducers (eg, St. John's wort, phenobarbital, carbamazepine, rifampin) may decrease levels resulting in decreased therapeutic effects and/or changes in uterine bleeding profile. CYP3A4 inhibitors (eg, erythromycin, clarithromycin, ketoconazole, itraconazole, ritonavir, grapefruit juice) may increase levels and result in side effects.

**PREGNANCY:** Category X, caution in nursing.

**MECHANISM OF ACTION:** Estrogen; binds to nuclear receptors in estrogen-responsive tissues. Modulates pituitary secretion of gonadotropins, luteinizing hormone and follicle stimulating hormone, through negative feedback mechanism. Reduces elevated levels of these hormones in postmenopausal women,

**PHARMACOKINETICS: Distribution**: Largely bound to sex hormone binding globulin and albumin; found in breast milk. **Metabolism**: Liver to estrone (metabolite) and estriol (major urinary metabolite); sulfate and glucuronide conjugation (liver), gut hydrolysis; CYP3A4 (partial metabolism). **Elimination**: Urine (parent compound and metabolites); $T_{1/2}$=1 hr.

## NURSING CONSIDERATIONS

**Assessment:** Assess for undiagnosed abnormal genital bleeding, presence or history of breast cancer, DVT, PE, estrogen-dependent neoplasia, active or recent (within past yr) arterial thromboembolic disease (eg, stroke, MI), pregnancy/nursing status, age of patient ( ≥65 yrs), hypertriglyceridemia, impaired liver function or history of cholestatic jaundice, hypothyroidism, hypocalcemia, asthma, DM, epilepsy, migraines or porphyria, SLE, and possible drug interactions. Assess need for progestin therapy in women who have not had a hysterectomy.

**Monitoring:** Monitor for signs/symptoms of cardiovascular events (eg, MI, stroke, venous thrombosis, PE), malignant neoplasms (eg, endometrial, breast, ovarian cancer), dementia, gallbladder disease, hypercalcemia, visual disorders (eg, retinal vascular thrombosis), elevations in BP, elevations in plasma triglycerides, pancreatitis, hypothyroidism, fluid retention, exacerbation of endometriosis and other conditions (eg, asthma, DM, epilepsy, migraines, SLE). Monitor thyroid function in patients on thyroid replacement therapy. Perform regular monitoring of BP levels, annual breast exam, and periodic evalution (every 3-6 months) to determine need for therapy. If undiagnosed, persistent, or recurring bleeding occurs, perform proper diagnostic testing (eg, endometrial sampling) to rule out malignancy.

**Patient Counseling:** Inform drug increases risk for uterine cancer. Report breast lumps, unusual vaginal bleeding, dizziness or faintness, changes in speech, severe headaches, chest pain, SOB, leg pains, changes in vision, or vomiting. Instruct to place medication system on clean, dry skin on the trunk (including buttocks and abdomen); site should not be exposed to sunlight;

area should not be oily, damaged, or irritated; do not apply to breasts. Rotate application sites. Apply immediately after opening pouch. If medication system falls off, reapply same system; if not able to, apply new system; continue with original treatment schedule. Notify physician if planning surgery or prolonged immobilization. Advise to perform monthly self breast exams.

**Administration:** Transdermal route. **Storage**: Do not store above 30°C (86°F). Do not store unpouched.



## Estrasorb RX

estradiol (Graceway)

**Estrogens increase the risk of endometrial cancer. Estrogens, with or without progestins, should not be used for the prevention of cardiovascular (CV) disease or dementia. Increased risks of MI, stroke, invasive breast cancer, pulmonary emboli (PE), and deep vein thrombosis (DVT) in postmenopausal women (50-79 yrs of age) reported. Increased risk of developing probable dementia in postmenopausal women ≥65 yrs of age reported.**

**THERAPEUTIC CLASS:** Estrogen

**INDICATIONS:** Treatment of moderate to severe vasomotor symptoms associated with menopause.

**DOSAGE:** *Adults:* Apply 2 pouches qam. Apply one pouch to each leg from the upper thigh to the calf. Rub in for 3 min until thoroughly absorbed.

**HOW SUPPLIED:** Emulsion, Topical: 4.35mg/1.74g (pouch)

**CONTRAINDICATIONS:** Undiagnosed abnormal genital bleeding, known/suspected/history of breast cancer, known/suspected history of estrogen-dependent neoplasia, DVT/PE, active or recent arterial thromboembolic disease (eg, stroke, MI), liver dysfunction or disease, pregnancy.

**WARNINGS/PRECAUTIONS:** Limit use to the shortest duration consistent with goals and risks; re-evaluate periodically. Increased risk of CV events (eg, MI, stroke, venous thromboembolism, PE), gallbladder disease, breast and endometrial cancer. D/C 4-6 weeks before surgery associated with an increased risk of thromboembolism or during prolonged immobilization. Possible increased risk of ovarian cancer. May lead to severe hypercalcemia in patients with breast cancer and bone metastases; monitor and d/c if hypercalcemia occurs. Consider adding progestin in patients with intact uterus to avoid endometrial hyperplasia. Increased thyroid-binding globulin levels (may need higher doses of thyroid hormone). May cause fluid retention; caution in cardiac or renal dysfunction. Retinal vascular thrombosis and elevated BP reported. May exacerbate endometriosis, asthma, diabetes mellitus (DM), epilepsy, migraine, porphyria, systemic lupus erythematosus (SLE), or hepatic hemangiomas; use with caution. Avoid use in close proximity to sunscreen application; may increase absorption. Potential for estradiol transfer through physical contact; wash application site 8 hrs post-application. May cause elevations of plasma triglycerides with pre-existing hypertriglyceridemia. Caution with history of cholestatic jaundice associated with past estrogen use or with pregnancy; d/c with recurrence.

**ADVERSE REACTIONS:** Headache, infection, sinusitis, pruritus, breast pain, endometrial disorder.

**INTERACTIONS:** CYP3A4 inducers (eg, St. John's wort, phenobarbital, carbamazepine, rifampin) may decrease levels, which may decrease therapeutic effects and/or change uterine bleeding profile. CYP3A4 inhibitors (eg, erythromycin, clarithromycin, ketoconazole, itraconazole, ritonavir, grapefruit juice) may increase levels, which may result in side effects. Increased abnormal mammogram results reported with estrogen plus progestin that requires further evaluation.

**PREGNANCY:** Contraindicated in pregnancy, caution in nursing.

**MECHANISM OF ACTION:** Estrogen; binds to nuclear receptors in estrogen-responsive tissues. Circulating estrogens modulate pituitary secretion of gonadotropins, LH and FSH, through negative feedback mechanism. Reduces elevated levels of these hormones in postmenopausal women.

**PHARMACOKINETICS: Distribution:** Largely bound to sex hormone binding globulin (SHBG) and albumin. **Metabolism:** Liver to estrone (metabolite), estriol (major urinary metabolite); sulfate and glucuronide conjugation (liver), gut hydrolysis; CYP 3A4 (partial metabolism). **Excretion:** Urine (parent compound and metabolites).

## NURSING CONSIDERATIONS

**Assessment:** Assess for undiagnosed abnormal genital bleeding, presence or history of breast cancer, DVT, PE, estrogen-dependent neoplasia, active or recent arterial thromboembolic disease (eg, MI, stroke), liver dysfunction, pregnancy/nursing status, familial hyperlipoproteinemia, age ( ≥65 yrs), hypothyroidism, hypocalcemia, asthma, DM, epilepsy, migraine, porphyria, SLE, and possible drug interactions. Assess need for progestin therapy in women who have not had a hysterectomy.

**Monitoring:** Monitor for signs/symptoms of CV events (eg, MI, stroke, venous thrombosis, PE), malignant neoplasms (eg, endometrial, breast, ovarian cancer), dementia, gallbladder disease, hypercalcemia, visual abnormalities (retinal vascular thrombosis), elevations in BP, elevations in plasma triglycerides, pancreatitis, hypothyroidism, fluid retention, exacerbation of endometriosis, and exacerbation of other conditions (eg, asthma, DM, epilepsy, migraines, SLE). Perform annual breast exam. Monitor thyroid function in patients on thyroid replacement therapy. Monitor BP levels at regular intervals. Perform proper diagnostic testing (eg, endometrial sampling) for abnormal, undiagnosed, persistent or recurring vaginal bleeding to rule out malignancy. Perform periodic evaluation (every 3-6 months) to determine need for therapy.

**Patient Counseling:** Inform that estrogens increase chances of developing uterine cancer. Contact physician if breast lumps, unusual vaginal bleeding, dizziness or faintness, changes in speech, severe headaches, chest pain, SOB, leg pains, changes in vision, or vomiting occur. Advise to open medication pouches just prior to use. Apply in the morning to clean, dry skin of both thighs and calves. Avoid applying medication to irritated or red skin. Sunscreen should not be applied to treatment area at same time; may interact with medication. Advise patients to have yearly breast examinations conducted by a healthcare provider and to perform monthly breast self-examinations.

**Administration:** Topical route. Refer to PI for proper application. **Storage:** 20-25°C (68-77°F); excursions permitted to 15-30°C (59-86°F).

# ESTRATEST — RX

esterified estrogens - methyltestosterone (Solvay)

**Estrogens increase risk of endometrial cancer in postmenopausal women. Avoid during pregnancy. Estrogens, with or without progestins, should not be used for the prevention of cardiovascular disease. Increased risks of MI, stroke, invasive breast cancer, PE, and DVT in postmenopausal women reported.**

**OTHER BRAND NAMES:** Estratest H.S. (Solvay)

**THERAPEUTIC CLASS:** Estrogen/androgen combination

**INDICATIONS:** Treatment of moderate-severe vasomotor symptoms associated with menopause, when not improved by estrogens alone.

**DOSAGE:** *Adults:* Vasomotor Symptoms: 0.625-1.25mg or 1.25-2.5mg qd cyclically (3 weeks on, 1 week off). Discontinue/taper at 3-6 month intervals.

**HOW SUPPLIED:** Tab: (Esterified Estrogens-Methyltestosterone) (Estratest HS) 0.625-1.25mg;(Estratest) 1.25-2.5mg

**CONTRAINDICATIONS:** Pregnancy, nursing, severe liver damage, undiagnosed abnormal genital bleeding, breast cancer except in selected patients treated for metastatic disease, estrogen-dependent neoplasia, and thrombophlebitis or thromboembolic disease (active disease or past history associated with estrogen use, except when used in treatment of breast malignancy).

**WARNINGS/PRECAUTIONS:** Risk of gallbladder disease, endometrial carcinoma, thromboembolic disease, hepatic dysfunction/adenoma/neoplasm, peliosis hepatis, elevated BP, impaired glucose tolerance, hypercalcemia with breast cancer and bone metastases. Caution with metabolic bone disease associated with hypercalcemia or renal insufficiency. May increase size of pre-existing uterine leiomyomata. Caution in liver dysfunction, family history of breast cancer, breast nodules, fibrocystic disease, abnormal mammograms, diabetes, asthma, epilepsy, migraine, depression, and cardiac or renal dysfunction. D/C if cholestatic hepatitis and/or jaundice occurs, or if LFTs are abnormal. D/C 4 weeks prior to surgery if prolonged immobilization required. Increased risk of jaundice with history of jaundice during pregnancy. May effect epiphyseal closure; caution in young patients. D/C if virilization occurs. Increase in triglycerides, thyroid binding globulin, PT.



**ADVERSE REACTIONS:** Breakthrough bleeding, amenorrhea, virilization, inhibition of gonadotropin secretion, breast tenderness and enlargement, nausea, hirsutism, abdominal cramps, bloating, altered libido, cholestatic jaundice, weight gain, edema.

**INTERACTIONS:** May decrease insulin and anticoagulant requirements. May increase levels of oxyphenbutazone.

**PREGNANCY:** Category X, contraindicated in nursing.

**MECHANISM OF ACTION:** Esterified estrogen: Binds to nuclear receptors in estrogen-responsive tissues. Circulating estrogens modulate pituitary secretion of gonadotropins, luteinizing hormone and follicle stimulating hormone, through negative feedback mechanism. Reduces elevated levels of these hormones in postmenopausal women. Methyltestosterone: An androgen; responsible for the normal growth and development of male sex hormones and for maintenance of secondary sex characteristics.

**PHARMACOKINETICS: Distribution:** Esterified estrogen: Largely bound to sex hormone-binding globulin and albumin; found in breast milk. Methyl testosterone: Bound to testosterone estradiol binding globulin (98%). **Metabolism:** Esterified estrogen: Liver to estrone (metabolite) and estriol (major urinary metabolite); sulfate and glucuronide conjugation (liver); gut hydrolysis, CYP3A4 (partial metabolism). Methyl testosterone: Liver. **Elimination:** Esterified estrogen: Urine (parent compound and metabolites). Methyltestosterone: Urine (90%), feces (6%); $T_{1/2}$=10-100 min.

## NURSING CONSIDERATIONS

**Assessment:** Assess for undiagnosed abnormal genital bleeding, presence or history of breast cancer, DVT or PE, estrogen-dependent neoplasia, active or recent (within past yr) arterial thromboembolic disease, liver disease, pregnancy/nursing status, age ( ≥65 yrs), DM, hypertriglyceridemia, hypothyroidism, asthma, epilepsy, migraines or porphyria, SLE, and possible drug interactions. Assess need for progestin therapy in females who have not had a hysterectomy. Assess for possible drug interactions.

**Monitoring:** Monitor for signs/symptoms of cardiovascular events (eg, MI, stroke, venous thrombosis, PE), malignant neoplasms (eg, breast, endometrial, ovarian cancer), dementia, gallbladder disease, glucose tolerance, hypercalcemia, visual abnormalities (eg, retinal vascular thrombosis), peliosis hepatitis, hepatic neoplasms, elevated BP, elevations in plasma triglycerides, hypothyroidism, fluid retention, exacerbation of endometriosis and other conditions (eg, asthma, DM, epilepsy, migraines, SLE), virilization, hypersensitivity reactions, and decreases in protein bound iodine. Perform annual breast exam. Monitor glucose levels with DM and thyroid function in patients on thyroid replacement therapy. Perform regular monitoring of BP levels and periodic LFTs. In females with disseminated breast carcinoma, perform frequent determinations of urine and serum calcium levels during course of androgen therapy. In patients on high doses of androgens, monitor for polycythemia by checking Hgb and Hct periodically. Monitor for undiagnosed persistent or recurring abnormal vaginal bleeding; perform adequate diagnostic testing (eg, endometrial sampling). Perform periodic evaluation (every 3-6 months) to determine need for therapy.

**Patient Counseling:** Inform drug increases chances of uterine cancer. Report any breast lumps, unusual vaginal bleeding, dizziness or faintness, changes in speech, severe headaches, chest pain, SOB, leg pains, changes in vision, vomiting, acne, changes in menstrual periods, increased facial hair, skin color changes, or ankle swelling. Counsel to perform self breast exams.

**Administration:** Oral route. **Storage:** 15-30°C (59-86°F). Keep out of reach of children.

## ESTRING RX

estradiol (Pharmacia & Upjohn)

**Adequate diagnostic measures should be undertaken to rule out malignancy in all cases of undiagnosed persistent or recurring abnormal vaginal bleeding. Estrogens with or without progestins should not be used for the prevention of cardiovascular disease or dementia. Increased risks of MI, stroke, invasive breast cancer, pulmonary embolism (PE), and deep vein thrombosis (DVT) in postmenopausal women (50-79 yrs of age) reported. Increased risk of developing probable dementia in postmenopausal women ≥65 yrs of age reported. Estrogens with or without progestins, should be prescribed at the lowest effective doses and for the shortest duration due to the associated risks.**

**THERAPEUTIC CLASS:** Estrogen

**INDICATIONS:** Treatment of moderate to severe urogenital symptoms due to postmenopausal atrophy of the vagina and/or the lower urinary tract.

**DOSAGE:** *Adults:* Insert ring deeply into upper 1/3 of vaginal vault. Remove and replace after 90 days. Reassess at 3 or 6 month intervals.

**HOW SUPPLIED:** Vaginal Ring: 0.0075mg/24 hrs [2mg]

**CONTRAINDICATIONS:** Undiagnosed abnormal genital bleeding; breast cancer or history of breast cancer, estrogen-dependent neoplasia, active or history of deep vein thrombosis (DVT), active or history of pulmonary embolism (PE), active or recent (within the past year) arterial thromboembolic disease (eg, stroke, MI), known liver dysfunction or disease, pregnancy.

**WARNINGS/PRECAUTIONS:** D/C immediately if stroke, DVT, PE, or MI occur or are suspected. May increase risk of breast/endometrial/ovarian cancer, and gallbladder disease. May lead to severe hypercalcemia with breast cancer and bone metastases; d/c if hypercalcemia occurs. Retinal vascular thrombosis reported; d/c if papilledema or retinal vascular lesions develop. May elevate BP; monitor at regular intervals. May cause elevations of plasma triglycerides with pre-existing hypertriglyceridemia; d/c if pancreatitis or other complications develop. Caution with hepatic impairment, history of cholestatic jaundice associated with past estrogen use or with pregnancy; d/c if recurrence occurs. May lead to increased thyroid-binding globulin levels; monitor thyroid function in patients on thyroid replacement therapy. May cause fluid retention; caution with cardiac/renal dysfunction. Caution with severe hypocalcemia. May exacerbate endometriosis, asthma, diabetes mellitus (DM), epilepsy, migraine or porphyria, systemic lupus erythematosus (SLE), and hepatic hemangiomas; use with caution. A narrow vagina, vaginal stenosis, prolapse, or a vaginal infection may make the vagina more susceptible to irritation or ulceration. If a vaginal infection develops, remove and reinsert after the infection is appropriately treated. May be expelled from the vagina, rinse with lukewarm water and reinsert if expelled.

**ADVERSE REACTIONS:** Headache, leukorrhea, back pain, genital moniliasis, sinusitis, vaginitis, vaginal discomfort, vaginal hemorrhage, arthritis, insomnia, abdominal pain, arthritis, N/V, upper respiratory tract infection, asymptomatic genital bacterial growth.

**INTERACTIONS:** CYP3A4 inhibitors (eg, erythromycin, clarithromycin, ketoconazole, itraconazole, ritonavir, grapefruit juice) may increase plasma concentrations.CYP3A4 inducers (eg, St. John's wort, phenobarbital, carbamazepine, rifampin) may decrease concentrations. May require increased doses of thyroid replacement therapy.

**PREGNANCY:** Not for use in pregnancy or nursing.

**MECHANISM OF ACTION:** Estrogen; binds to nuclear receptors in estrogen-responsive tissues. Circulating estrogens modulate the pituitary secretion of the gonadotropins, luteinizing hormone and follicle stimulating hormone through a negative feedback mechanism. Acts to reduce elevated levels of these hormones in postmenopausal women.

**PHARMACOKINETICS: Absorption:** Well absorbed; $C_{max}$=63.2pg/mL; $T_{max}$=0.5-1 hr. **Distribution:** Largely bound to sex hormone binding globulin and albumin; found in breast milk. **Metabolism:** Liver to estrone (metabolite) and estriol (major urinary metabolite); sulfate and glucuronide conjugation (liver); intestinal hydrolysis; CYP3A4 (partial metabolism). **Elimination:** Urine (parent compound and metabolites).



## NURSING CONSIDERATIONS

**Assessment:** Assess for undiagnosed abnormal genital bleeding, presence or history of breast cancer, estrogen-dependent neoplasia, active or history of DVT or PE, active or recent (within past yr) arterial thromboembolic disease (eg, stroke, MI), liver dysfunction or disease, pregnancy/nursing status, age ( ≥65 yrs), hypertriglyceridemia, hypothyroidism, hypocalcemia, asthma, DM, epilepsy, migraines or porphyria, SLE, and for possible drug interactions. Assess need of progestin in women who have not had a hysterectomy.

**Monitoring:** Monitor for signs/symptoms of cardiovascular events (eg, stroke, DVT, MI, PE), malignant neoplasms (eg, endometrial, breast, ovarian cancer), dementia, gallbladder disease, hypercalcemia, visual abnormalities (eg, retinal vascular thrombosis), elevations in BP, elevations in serum triglycerides, pancreatitis, hypothyroidism, fluid retention, exacerbation of endometriosis and other conditions (eg, asthma, DM, epilepsy, migraines, SLE). Monitor BP levels regularly. Perform annual breast exam. Monitor thyroid function in patients on thyroid replacement therapy. If undiagnosed, persistent, or recurring abnormal vaginal bleeding occurs, perform adequate diagnostic measures (eg, endometrial sampling) to rule out malignancy.

**Patient Counseling:** Inform that estrogens increase the risk of developing uterine cancer. Inform that therapy may increase the chance of getting a heart attack, stroke, breast cancer, and blood clots. Instruct to contact physician if develop breast lumps, unusual vaginal bleeding, dizziness and faintness, changes in speech, severe headaches, chest pain, SOB, leg pains, vision changes, vomiting, or yellowing of the skin, eyes, or nail beds. Advise to perform monthly self breast exams. Instruct to notify physician if pregnant/nursing or planning to become pregnant.

**Administration:** Intravaginal route. Wash and dry hands prior to handling medication. Remove medication ring from pouch and hold between thumb and index finger; press opposite sides of medication ring together and gently push compressed medication ring as far as possible, into upper one third of vagina. Should not feel anything once medication ring is properly in place. If there is discomfort, medication ring probably not far enough inside; push further into vagina. Medication ring should remain in place for 90 days. **Storage:** 15-30°C (59-86°F).

# ESTROGEL **RX**

estradiol (Ascend Therapeutics)

> **Estrogens increase the risk of endometrial cancer. Perform adequate diagnostic measures including directed or random endometrial sampling when indicated, to rule out malignancy in postmenopausal women with undiagnosed persistent or recurring abnormal genital bleeding. Do not use as monotherapy or concomitant with progestin for the prevention of cardiovascular (CV) disease or probable dementia. Increased risk of stroke, deep vein thrombosis (DVT), pulmonary embolism, myocardial infarction (MI), invasive breast cancer, and dementia in postmenopausal women. Should be prescribed at lowest effective doses and for shortest duration consistent with treatment goals and risks for individual women.**

**THERAPEUTIC CLASS:** Estrogen

**INDICATIONS:** Moderate to severe vasomotor symptoms and/or vulvar/vaginal atrophy associated with menopause.

**DOSAGE:** *Adults:* Apply one compression (1.25g) to one arm from wrist to shoulder once daily. Re-evaluate periodically.

**HOW SUPPLIED:** Gel: 0.06% [50g, 93g]

**CONTRAINDICATIONS:** Undiagnosed abnormal genital bleeding, breast cancer, estrogen-dependent neoplasia, DVT or PE, active or recent (within 1 yr) arterial thromboembolic disease (eg, stroke, MI), liver dysfunction or disease, pregnancy.

**WARNINGS/PRECAUTIONS:** May increase risk of breast cancer, endometrial cancer, ovarian cancer and gallbladder disease. May lead to severe hypercalcemia with breast cancer and bone metastases; monitor and d/c if hypercalcemia occurs. Retinal vascular thrombosis reported; monitor and d/c if papilledema or retinal vascular lesions occur. Consider addition of a progestin if patient has not had a hysterectomy. May elevate BP; monitor at regular intervals. May cause elevations of plasma triglycerides with pre-existing hypertriglyceridemia. Caution with history of cholestatic jaundice associated with past estrogen use or with pregnancy; d/c with recurrence. May lead to increased thyroid-binding globulin levels; monitor thyroid function. May cause fluid retention; caution with cardiac/renal dysfunction. Caution with severe hypocalcemia. May exacerbate endometriosis, asthma, DM, epilepsy, migraine, porphyria, SLE, and hepatic hemangiomas; use with caution. May affect endocrine and blood component in laboratories. Alcohol-based gels are flammable; avoid fire, flame, or smoking until the gel dries.

**ADVERSE REACTIONS:** Headache, infection, breast pain, vaginitis, abdominal pain, rash, nausea, pruritus, diarrhea, asthenia, flu syndrome, generalized pain, flatulence, back pain, suspicious pap smear.

**INTERACTIONS:** CYP3A4 inducers (eg, St. John's wort, phenobarbital, carbamazepine, rifampin) may decrease levels which may decrease therapeutic effects and/or change uterine bleeding profile. CYP3A4 inhibitors (eg, erythromycin, clarithromycin, ketoconazole, itraconazole, ritonavir, grapefruit juice) may increase levels which may result in side effects. May require higher doses of thyroid hormone. Use with progestin reported lowered incidence of endometrial hyperplasia but increased risk of breast cancer, low HDL, high LDL, and impaired glucose tolerance.

**PREGNANCY:** Contraindicated in pregnancy, caution in nursing.

**MECHANISM OF ACTION:** Estrogen; binds to nuclear receptors in estrogen-responsive tissues. Circulating estrogens modulate pituitary secretion of the gonadotropins, luteinizing hormone and follicle stimulating hormone, through negative feedback mechanism. Reduces elevated levels of these hormones in postmenopausal women

**PHARMACOKINETICS: Absorption:** $C_{max}$=46.4pg/mL. **Distribution:** Largely bound to sex hormone binding globulin and albumin; found in breast milk. **Metabolism:** Liver to estrone (metabolite) and estriol (major urinary metabolite); sulfate and glucuronide conjugation (liver); gut hydrolysis; CYP3A4 (partial metabolism). **Elimination:** Urine (parent compound and metabolites); $T_{1/2}$=36 hrs.

## NURSING CONSIDERATIONS

**Assessment:** Assess for undiagnosed abnormal genital bleeding, presence or history of breast cancer, DVT or PE, estrogen-dependent neoplasia, active or recent (within past yr) arterial thromboembolic disease (eg, stroke, MI), liver dysfunction, history of cholestatic jaundice, pregnancy/nursing status, age ( ≥65 yrs), gallbladder disease, hypertriglyceridemia, hypothyroidism, hypocalcemia, asthma, DM, epilepsy, migraines, porphyria, SLE, and possible drug interactions. Assess need for progestin therapy in women who have not had a hysterectomy.

**Monitoring:** Monitor for signs/symptoms of cardiovascular disorders (eg, MI, stroke, venous thrombosis, PE), malignant neoplasms (eg, endometrial, breast, ovarian cancer), dementia, gallbladder disease, hypercalcemia, visual abnormalities (eg, retinal vascular thrombosis), elevations in BP, elevations in plasma triglycerides, pancreatitis, hypothyroidism, fluid retention, exacerbation of endometriosis and other conditions (eg, asthma, DM, epilepsy, migraines, SLE). Monitor BP levels regularly and thyroid function in patients on thyroid replacement therapy. Perform annual breast exam. If undiagnosed persistent or recurring abnormal vaginal bleeding occurs, perform adequate diagnostic measures (eg, endometrial sampling) to rule out malignancy. Periodically evaluate (every 3-6 months) to determine therapy need.

**Patient Counseling:** Inform estrogens increase risk for uterine cancer. Report if breast lumps, unusual vaginal bleeding, dizziness and faintness, changes in speech, severe headaches, chest pain, SOB, leg pain, vision changes, or vomiting occur. Notify physician if planning surgery or prolonged bed rest. Instruct to perform monthly self breast exams and have annual gynecologic exam. Before using medication for first time, pump must be primed; fully depress pump 2 (90g medication pump) or 3 times (50g medication pump); discard unused medication. Apply at same time daily to clean, dry, unbroken skin. Apply to one arm, spreading medication as thinly as possible over entire area on inside and outside of arm, from wrist to shoulder. Do not apply to breast. Allow 5 min to dry before dressing; wash hands following application. Medication is alcohol-based and flammable; avoid fire, flame, or smoking until dry. Instruct if dose is missed and next dose is <12 hrs away, wait to apply medication at normal dosing time; if >12 hrs away until next dose, apply missed dose, and return to normal dosing schedule.

**Administration:** Topical route. **Storage:** 20-25°C (68-77°F); excursions permitted to 15-30°C (59-86°F).

## ESTROSTEP FE — RX

norethindrone acetate - ferrous fumarate - ethinyl estradiol (Warner Chilcott)

**THERAPEUTIC CLASS:** Estrogen/progestogen combination

**INDICATIONS:** Prevention of pregnancy. Treatment of acne vulgaris in females ≥15 yrs who want contraception (for at least 6 months), have achieved menarche, and are unresponsive to topical acne agents.

**DOSAGE:** *Adults:* Contraception/Acne: 1 tab qd for 28 days, then repeat. Start 1st Sunday after menses begin or the 1st day of menses.
*Pediatrics:* ≥15 yrs: Contraception (Postpubertal Adolescents)/Acne: 1 tab qd for 28 days, then repeat. Start 1st Sunday after menses begins or the 1st day of menses.

**HOW SUPPLIED:** Tab: (Ethinyl Estradiol-Norethindrone) 0.035mg-1mg, 0.030mg-1mg, 0.020mg-1mg and 75mg ferrous fumarate

**CONTRAINDICATIONS:** Thrombophlebitis, history of DVT, active or history of thromboembolic disorders, pregnancy, cerebrovascular disease, CAD, undiagnosed abnormal genital bleeding, cholestatic jaundice of pregnancy, jaundice with prior pill use, hepatic adenoma or carcinoma, breast carcinoma, endometrium or other estrogen-dependent neoplasia.

**WARNINGS/PRECAUTIONS:** Cigarette smoking increases risk of serious cardiovascular side effects. This risk increases with age (especially >35 yrs) and heavy smoking. Increased risk of MI, vascular disease, thromboembolism, stroke, and gallbladder disease. Retinal thrombosis, hepatic neoplasia reported. May cause glucose intolerance. May increase BP, elevate LDL levels or cause other lipid changes, fluid retention, breakthrough bleeding, and spotting. May cause or exacerbate migraine. May develop visual changes with contact lenses. Increased risk of MI with HTN, hyperlipidemia, obesity, and diabetes. D/C if jaundice, significant depression, or ophthalmic irregularities develop. Perform annual physical exam. Use before menarche is not indicated. May affect certain endocrine, LFTs, and blood components.

**ADVERSE REACTIONS:** NV, breakthrough bleeding, spotting, amenorrhea, migraine, depression, vaginal candidiasis, edema, weight changes.

**INTERACTIONS:** Reduced effects, increased breakthrough bleeding, and menstrual irregularities with rifampin, barbiturates, phenylbutazone, phenytoin, carbamazepine, St. John's wort, and possibly with griseofulvin, ampicillin, and tetracyclines. Increased plasma levels with atorvastatin. Ascorbic acid and APAP may increase plasma levels. Decreased plasma levels of APAP. Increased clearance of temazepam, salicylic acid, morphine, and clofibric acid. Increased plasma levels of cyclosporine, prednisolone, and theophylline.

**PREGNANCY:** Category X, not for use in nursing.

**MECHANISM OF ACTION:** Estrogen/progestogen oral contraceptive; acts by suppressing gonadotropins, inhibiting ovulation, and causing other alterations, including changes in the cervical mucus (increasing difficulty of sperm entry into uterus) and the endometrium (reducing likelihood of implantation).

**PHARMACOKINETICS: Absorption:** Rapid and complete. Absolute bioavailability: Norethindrone (64%), ethinyl estradiol (43%); $T_{max}$=1-2 hrs. **Distribution:** $V_d$=2-4L/kg; plasma protein binding (>95%). **Metabolism:** Norethindrone: Extensive; reduction, sulfate/glucuronide conjugation. Ethinyl estradiol: CYP3A4; oxidation, conjugation. **Elimination:** Norethindrone: $T_{1/2}$=13 hrs. Ethinyl estradiol: Urine, feces; $T_{1/2}$=19 hrs.

## NURSING CONSIDERATIONS

**Assessment:** Assess for current or history of thrombophlebitis or thromboembolic disorders, cerebrovascular or coronary artery disease, known or suspected carcinoma of the breast, endometrium or other known or suspected estrogen-dependent neoplasia, undiagnosed abnormal genital bleeding, history of cholestatic jaundice of pregnancy or jaundice with previous pill use, hepatic adenomas or carcinomas, known or suspected pregnancy. Assess for possible drug interactions.

**Monitoring:** Monitor for development of MI, thromboembolism, stroke, hepatic neoplasia, carcinoma of the reproductive organs and breasts, and gallbladder disease, signs/symptoms of hepatotoxicity (eg, jaundice), ocular lesions, visual changes in patients who wear contact lenses, blood glucose levels in prediabetic and diabetic patients, signs/symptoms of HTN, fluid retention, signs of worsening depression with a history, onset or exacerbation of migraines or development of headaches, cholesterol levels with a history of hyperlipidemia, and bleeding irregularities.

**Patient Counseling:** Counsel about possible side effects. Inform that medication does not protect against HIV and other STDs. Counsel to avoid smoking while on medication. Advise to take at the same time every day; if a dose is missed, take as soon as possible, then take next dose at regular time. Advise if spotting, light bleeding, or nausea develops during first 1-3 packs of pills, to continue taking medication, and to notify physician if symptoms do not subside. If NV or diarrhea occurs, instruct use of backup birth control method until physician is contacted. Counsel to go for an annual physical.

**Administration:** Oral route. **Storage:** Do not store above 25°C (77°F). Protect from light. Store tablets inside pouch when not in use.

# ETODOLAC — RX

etodolac (Various)

**NSAIDs may cause an increased risk of serious cardiovascular thrombotic events, MI, stroke and serious GI adverse events including bleeding, ulceration, and perforation of the stomach or intestines. Contraindicated for the treatment of perioperative pain in the setting of coronary artery bypass graft (CABG) surgery.**

**THERAPEUTIC CLASS:** NSAID

**INDICATIONS:** Management of osteoarthritis (OA), rheumatoid arthritis (RA), and acute pain.

**DOSAGE:** *Adults:* ≥18 yrs: Acute Pain: Usual: 200-400mg q6-8h. Max: 1000mg/day. OA/RA: Initial: 300mg bid-tid, or 400-500mg bid. May give 600mg/day for long-term use. Titrate: Lowest effective dose. Max: 1000mg/day.

**HOW SUPPLIED:** Cap: 200mg, 300mg; Tab: 400mg, 500mg

**CONTRAINDICATIONS:** ASA or other NSAID allergy that precipitates asthma, urticaria or other allergic type reactions. Treatment of perioperative pain in the setting of CABG surgery.

**WARNINGS/PRECAUTIONS:** May lead to onset of new HTN or worsening of pre-existing HTN; monitor BP closely. Fluid retention and edema reported; caution with fluid retention or heart failure. Renal papillary necrosis and other renal injury reported after long-term use. Not recommended for use with advanced renal disease; if therapy must be initiated, monitor renal function. Anaphylactoid reactions may occur. May cause serious skin adverse events (eg, exfoliative dermatitis, Stevens-Johnson syndrome, and toxic epidermal necrolysis). Avoid in late pregnancy; may cause premature closure of ductus arteriosis. May cause elevations of LFTs; d/c if liver disease develops or systemic manifestations occur. Caution in elderly. Anemia may occur; with long-term use, monitor Hgb/Hct if signs or symptoms of anemia develop. May inhibit platelet aggregation and prolong bleeding time; monitor with coagulation disorders. Caution with asthma and avoid with ASA-sensitive asthma. Risk of GI ulceration, bleeding, and perforation.



**ADVERSE REACTIONS:** Dyspepsia, abdominal pain, diarrhea, flatulence, nausea, constipation, gastritis, asthenia, malaise, dizziness, increased bleeding time, GI ulcers, GI bleeding/perforation, heartburn, abnormal renal function.

**INTERACTIONS:** May elevate digoxin, lithium, and methotrexate serum levels. May enhance nephrotoxicity associated with cyclosporine. Avoid with phenylbutazone and ASA. Increased adverse effect potential with ASA. Caution with warfarin. Diuretics may increase risk of renal toxicity. May diminish antihypertensive effects of ACE inhibitors.

**PREGNANCY:** Category C, not for use in nursing.

**MECHANISM OF ACTION:** NSAID; suspected to inhibit prostaglandin synthetase, exerts anti-inflammatory, analgesic, and antipyretic actions.

**PHARMACOKINETICS: Absorption:** Well absorbed. Bioavailability (100%); $C_{max}$=14-37mcg/mL, $T_{max}$=80 min. **Distribution:** $V_d$=390mL/kg; plasma protein binding (99%). **Elimination:** Urine, feces; $T_{1/2}$=6.4 hrs.

## NURSING CONSIDERATIONS

**Assessment:** Assess LFTs, renal function, CBC and coagulation profile. Assess for history of CABG surgery, asthma and allergic reactions to aspirin or other NSAIDs, active ulceration or chronic inflammation of GI tract, CVD, asthma, pregnancy status. Note other diseases/conditions and drug therapies.

**Monitoring:** Monitor for hypersensitivity reactions, cardiac complications, stroke, GI bleeding, asthma, skin side effects. Monitor BP, LFTs, renal function, CBC with differential and platelet count, coagulation profile, ocular effects and Reye's syndrome.

**Patient Counseling:** Counsel about side effects; seek medical attention if any occur. Tablet should be swallowed; not chewed or crushed. Advise to take as prescribed. Caution women against using medication late in pregnancy.

**Administration:** Oral route. **Storage:** 25-30°C (68-77°F). Protect from excessive heat and humidity.

# ETODOLAC EXTENDED-RELEASE — RX

etodolac (Various)

**NSAIDs may cause an increased risk of serious cardiovascular thrombotic events, MI, stroke and serious GI adverse events including bleeding, ulceration, and perforation of the stomach or intestines. Contraindicated for the treatment of perioperative pain in the setting of coronary artery bypass graft (CABG) surgery.**

**THERAPEUTIC CLASS:** NSAID

**INDICATIONS:** Relief of signs and symptoms of osteoarthritis (OA), rheumatoid arthritis (RA), and juvenile arthritis (JA).

**DOSAGE:** *Adults:* OA/RA: Initial: 400-1000mg qd. Titrate: Lowest effective dose.

*Pediatrics:* 6-16 yrs: JA: >60kg: 1000mg/day. 46-60kg: 800mg/day. 31-45kg: 600mg/day. 20-30kg: 400mg/day.

**HOW SUPPLIED:** Tab, Extended-Release: 400mg, 500mg, 600mg

**CONTRAINDICATIONS:** ASA or other NSAID allergy that precipitates asthma, urticaria, or allergic reaction. Treatment of perioperative pain in the setting of CABG surgery.

**WARNINGS/PRECAUTIONS:** May lead to onset of new HTN or worsening of pre-existing HTN; monitor BP closely. Fluid retention and edema reported; caution with fluid retention or heart failure. Renal papillary necrosis and other renal injury reported after long-term use. Not recommended for use with advanced renal disease; if therapy must be initiated, monitor renal function. Anaphylactoid reactions may occur. May cause serious skin adverse events (eg, exfoliative dermatitis, Stevens-Johnson syndrome, and toxic epidermal necrolysis). Avoid in late pregnancy; may cause premature closure of ductus arteriosus. May cause elevations of LFTs; d/c if liver disease develops or systemic manifestations occur. Caution in elderly. Anemia may occur; with long-term use, monitor Hgb/Hct if signs or symptoms of anemia develop. May inhibit platelet aggregation and prolong bleeding time; monitor with coagulation disorders. Caution with asthma and avoid with ASA-sensitive asthma.

E

**ADVERSE REACTIONS:** Dyspepsia, abdominal pain, diarrhea, flatulence, NV, constipation, GI ulcers, gross bleeding/perforation.

**INTERACTIONS:** May elevate digoxin, lithium, and methotrexate serum levels. May enhance nephrotoxicity associated with cyclosporine. Avoid with phenylbutazone. Increased adverse effect potential with ASA. Caution with warfarin. May decrease antihypertensive effects with ACE inhibitors. May reduce natriuretic effect of furosemide and thiazides.

**PREGNANCY:** Category C, not for use in nursing.

**MECHANISM OF ACTION:** NSAID; inhibits prostaglandin synthetase; exhibits anti-inflammatory, analgesic, and antipyretic activities.

**PHARMACOKINETICS: Absorption:** $T_{max}$=6 hrs. **Distribution:** $V_d$=566mL/kg; plasma protein binding (99%). **Metabolism:** Hydroxylation, glucuronidation. **Elimination:** Urine, feces; $T_{1/2}$=8.4 hrs.

## NURSING CONSIDERATIONS

**Assessment:** Assess LFTs, renal function, CBC and coagulation profile. Assess for history of CABG surgery, asthma and allergic reactions to aspirin or other NSAIDs, active ulceration or chronic inflammation of GI tract, CVD, pregnancy status, and for possible drug interactions.

**Monitoring:** Monitor for hypersensitivity reactions, cardiac complications, stroke, GI bleeding, asthma, skin side effects. Monitor BP, LFTs, renal function, CBC with differential and platelet count, and coagulation profile.

**Patient Counseling:** Counsel about potential side effects; seek medical attention if any occur. Instruct to take as prescribed. Caution women against using late in pregnancy. Advise to avoid alcohol and smoking during therapy.

**Administration:** Oral route. **Storage:** 25-30°C (68-77°F). Protect from excessive heat and humidity.

# ETOPOPHOS RX

etoposide phosphate (Bristol-Myers Squibb)

**Administer under supervision of qualified physician experienced in use of cancer chemotherapeutic agents. Severe myelosuppression with resulting infection or bleeding may occur.**

**THERAPEUTIC CLASS:** Podophyllotoxin derivative

**INDICATIONS:** Adjunct therapy for management of refractory testicular tumors. First-line combination therapy for management of small cell lung cancer (SCLC).

**DOSAGE:** *Adults:* Testicular Cancer: Range: 50-100mg/m²/day on Days 1-5 to 100mg/m²/day on Days 1, 3, and 5. SCLC: Range: 35mg/m²/day for 4 days to 50mg/m²/day for 5 days. After adequate recovery from toxicity, repeat course for either therapy at 3-4 week intervals. CrCl 15-50mL/min: 75% of dose.

**HOW SUPPLIED:** Inj: 100mg

**WARNINGS/PRECAUTIONS:** Observe for myelosuppression during and after therapy. Risk of anaphylactic reaction manifested by chills, fever, tachycardia, bronchospasm, dyspnea, and hypotension. Increased risk of toxicity with a low serum albumin. Perform CBC before each dose, during, and after therapy. May cause fetal harm in pregnancy. Caution with low serum albumin.

**ADVERSE REACTIONS:** Myelosuppression, leukopenia, neutropenia, thrombocytopenia, anemia, NV, anaphylactic-like reactions, BP changes, alopecia, anorexia, asthenia/malaise, chills, fever.

**INTERACTIONS:** Caution with drugs known to inhibit phosphatase activities (eg, levamisole). High-dose oral cyclosporine reduces clearance and increases exposure.

E

**PREGNANCY:** Category D, not for use in nursing.

**MECHANISM OF ACTION:** Podophyllotoxin derivative; induces DNA strand breaks by interacting with DNA-topoisomerase II or formation of free radicals.

**PHARMACOKINETICS: Absorption:** Rapid, complete; Etopophos 150mg/m$^2$: AUC=168.3μg•hr/mL, $C_{max}$=20μg/mL. **Distribution:** VePesid: $V_d$=7-17L/m$^2$; plasma protein binding (97%). **Metabolism:** VePesid: Liver via CYP3A4 (O-demethylation); hydroxy acid (metabolite). **Elimination:** VePesid: Biliary excretion, feces, urine; $T_{1/2}$=4-11 hrs.

## NURSING CONSIDERATIONS

**Assessment:** Assess for impaired renal function, pregnancy status, decreased serum albumin, and possible drug interactions. Obtain platelet, Hgb, and WBC with differential at start of therapy and before each cycle.

**Monitoring:** Monitor CBC and renal function periodically, for signs/symptoms of anaphylactic reaction, severe myelosuppression, and renal dysfunction.

**Patient Counseling:** Inform of pregnancy risks; avoid pregnancy. Advise to seek medical attention if symptoms of severe myelosuppression (infection or bleeding) or anaphylactic reaction (chills, fever, tachycardia, bronchospasm, dyspnea, hypotension) occur.

**Administration:** IV infusion. **Storage:** 2-8°C (36-46°F); refrigerate and protect from light. Reconstituted and diluted vials stable for 7 days refrigerated or 24 hrs at room temperature, 20-25°C (68-77°F).

# EUFLEXXA — RX

sodium hyaluronate (Ferring)

**THERAPEUTIC CLASS:** Hyaluronan

**INDICATIONS:** Treatment of pain in osteoarthritis of the knee in patients who have failed to respond adequately to conservative non-pharmacologic therapy and simple analgesics (eg, APAP).

**DOSAGE:** *Adults:* Inject 2mL intra-articularly into affected knee at weekly intervals for 3 weeks, for a total of 3 injections. Use strict aseptic injection procedures.

**HOW SUPPLIED:** Inj: 1% [2mL]

**CONTRAINDICATIONS:** Avoid with knee joint infections, infections or skin diseases in area of injection site.

**WARNINGS/PRECAUTIONS:** Avoid mixing with quaternary ammonium salts (eg, benzalkonium chloride); may result in formation of a precipitate. Avoid injecting intravascularly. Patients having repeated exposure have the potential for an immune response. Safety and effectiveness in joints other than the knee or in conjunction with other intra-articular injectables have not been established. Remove any joint effusion before injecting. Transient pain and/or swelling of the injected joint may occur. Avoid any strenuous activities or prolonged (eg, more than 1 hour) weight-bearing activities within 48 hours following injection. Safety and effectiveness have not been demonstrated in children.

**ADVERSE REACTIONS:** Arthralgia, nausea, back pain, rhinitis, BP increase, joint effusion/swelling, tendonitis, knee pain, skin irritation, headache, paresthesia.

**PREGNANCY:** Safety in pregnancy and nursing not known.

## NURSING CONSIDERATIONS

**Assessment:** Assess for knee joint infections, skin infections, or disease in the injection-site area.

**Monitoring:** Monitor for knee pain or swelling of joint.

**Patient Counseling:** Inform that drug may cause transient pain/swelling of injected joint. Avoid strenuous activities or prolonged weight-bearing activities (jogging, tennis) within 48 hrs following injection.

**Administration:** Intra-articular injection. **Storage:** 2-25°C (36-77°F). Protect from light. Remove from refrigeration at least 20-30 min before use. Do not freeze.

# EVISTA

**RX**

raloxifene HCl (Lilly)

**Increased risk of deep vein thrombosis (DVT) and pulmonary embolism (PE) reported. Avoid use in women with active or past history of venous thromboembolism. Increased risk of death due to stroke in postmenopausal women with documented coronary heart disease or at increased risk for major coronary events; consider risk-benefit balance in women at risk for stroke.**

**THERAPEUTIC CLASS:** Selective estrogen receptor modulator

**INDICATIONS:** Treatment and prevention of osteoporosis in postmenopausal women. Reduction in risk of invasive breast cancer in postmenopausal women with osteoporosis. Reduction in risk of invasive breast cancer in postmenopausal women at high risk for invasive breast cancer.

**DOSAGE:** *Adults:* 60mg qd. May be given at any time of day without regard to meals. Refer to PI for recommendations regarding calcium and vitamin D supplementation.

**HOW SUPPLIED:** Tab: 60mg

**CONTRAINDICATIONS:** Nursing, pregnancy, women who may become pregnant, active/past history of venous thromboembolism (VTE) (eg, DVT, PE, retinal vein thrombosis).

**WARNINGS/PRECAUTIONS:** Venous thromboembolism events including superficial venous thrombophlebitis reported; d/c at least 72 hrs prior to and during prolonged immobilization (eg, post-surgical recovery, prolonged bed rest); therapy should only be resumed after fully ambulatory. Caution in women at risk of thromboembolic disease. Should not be used for primary or secondary prevention of cardiovascular disease. Avoid in premenopausal women. Use not adequately studied in women with a history of breast cancer. Not recommended for use in men. May increase levels of triglycerides with pre-existing hypertriglyceridemia; monitor serum triglyceride levels in women with history of hypertriglyceridemia. Caution with hepatic impairment or with moderate or severe renal impairment. Monitor for unexplained uterine bleeding and breast abnormalites.

**ADVERSE REACTIONS:** DVT, pulmonary embolism, vaginal bleeding, hot flashes, leg cramps, arthralgia, infection, flu syndrome, headache, nausea, weight gain, sinusitis, rhinitis, cough increased, peripheral edema.

**INTERACTIONS:** Cholestyramine may decrease absorption; avoid concomitant administration with cholestyramine and other anion exchange resins. Monitor PT with warfarin and other warfarin derivatives. Caution with other highly protein-bound drugs (eg, diazepam, diazoxide, lidocaine). Avoid concomitant use with systemic estrogens.

**PREGNANCY:** Category X, contraindicated in nursing.

**MECHANISM OF ACTION:** Selective estrogen receptor modulator; binds to estrogen receptors. Binding results in activation of estrogenic pathways in some tissues and blockade of estrogenic pathways in others depending on extent of recruitment of coactivators and corepressors to estrogen receptor target gene promotors. Acts as an estrogen agonist in bone. Decreases bone resorption and bone turnover, increases bone mineral density, and decreases fracture incidence.

**PHARMACOKINETICS: Absorption:** Rapid; Absolute bioavailability (2%); Single dose: $C_{max}$=0.5(ng/mL)/(mg/kg); AUC=27.2(ng•hr/mL)/(mg/kg). Multiple doses: $C_{max}$=1.36(ng/mL)/(mg/kg); AUC=24.2(ng•hr/mL)/(mg/kg). **Distribution:** $V_d$=2348L/kg. Plasma protein binding (95%). **Metabolism:** Extensive; glucuronidation; raloxifene-4'-glucuronide, raloxifene-6-glucuronide, raloxifene-6',4'-diglucuronide (metabolites). **Elimination:** Feces (primary), urine (<0.2% unchanged); $T_{1/2}$=27.7 hrs (single dose); $T_{1/2}$=32.5 hrs (multiple doses).



## NURSING CONSIDERATIONS

**Assessment:** Assess for active or history of VTE (eg, DVT, PE, retinal vein thrombosis), CVD, risk factors for stroke, history of breast cancer, history of hypertriglyceridemia, prolonged immobilization, renal/hepatic impairment, pregnancy/nursing status, and for possible drug interactions.

**Monitoring:** Monitor for VTE (eg, DVT, PE, retinal vein thrombosis), stroke, unexplained uterine bleeding, and breast abnormalities. Monitor serum TG with history of hypertriglyceridemia.

**Patient Counseling:** For osteoporosis treatment/prevention, instruct to take supplemental calcium and/or vitamin D if intake is inadequate. Instruct to consider weight-bearing exercise and behavioral modification factors (eg, smoking, excessive alcohol consumption) for osteoporosis treatment/prevention. Advise to d/c therapy at least 72 hrs prior to and during prolonged immobilization. Instruct to avoid prolonged restrictions of movement during travel. Counsel that therapy may increase incidence of hot flashes or hot flashes may occur upon initiation of therapy. Inform that regular breast exams and mammography should be done before initiation of therapy and should continue during therapy. Instruct to read the medication guide before starting therapy.

**Administration:** Oral route. **Storage:** 20-25°C (68-77°F); excursions permitted to 15-30°C (59-86°F).

# EXELON RX

rivastigmine tartrate (Novartis)

**THERAPEUTIC CLASS:** Acetylcholinesterase inhibitor

**INDICATIONS:** Treatment of mild to moderate dementia of the Alzheimer's type and mild to moderate dementia associated with Parkinson's disease.

**DOSAGE:** *Adults:* Alzheimer's Dementia: Initial: 1.5mg bid. Titrate: May increase by 1.5mg bid every 2 weeks. Max: 12mg/day. If not tolerating, suspend therapy for several doses and restart at same or next lower dose. If interrupted longer than several days, reinitiate with lowest daily dose and titrate as above. Dementia Associated with Parkinson's Disease: Initial: 1.5mg bid. Titrate: May increase by 1.5mg every 4 weeks. Max: 12mg/day. Take with food in am and pm. May mix solution with water, cold fruit juice, or soda. Patch: Alzheimer's Dementia/Dementia Associated with Parkinson's Disease: Initial: Apply 4.6mg/24 hrs patch qd to clean, dry, hairless intact skin. Maint: Increase dose after 4 weeks. Max: 9.5mg/24 hrs if well tolerated. Switching from Capsules/Oral Sol: Total Oral Daily Dose <6mg: Switch to 4.6mg/24 hrs patch. Total Oral Daily Dose 6-12mg: Switch to 9.5mg/24 hrs patch. Apply 1st patch on day following last oral dose.

**HOW SUPPLIED:** Cap: 1.5mg, 3mg, 4.5mg, 6mg; Patch: 4.6mg/24 hrs, 9.5mg/24 hrs [30[s]]; Sol: 2mg/mL [120mL]

**CONTRAINDICATIONS:** Hypersensitivity to carbamate derivatives.

**WARNINGS/PRECAUTIONS:** Significant GI intolerance (eg, N/V, anorexia, and weight loss); always follow dosing guidelines. Vagotonic effect on HR (bradycardia), especially in "sick sinus syndrome" or supraventricular conduction abnormalities. May cause urinary obstruction and seizures. Monitor for peptic ulcers/GI bleeds. Caution in asthma and COPD. May exacerbate or induce extrapyramidal symptoms. (Patch) May impair mental/physical capabilities. Titrate dose with caution in patients with body weight below 50kg.

**ADVERSE REACTIONS:** N/V, abdominal pain, dyspepsia, constipation, somnolence, anorexia, asthenia, headache, dizziness, fatigue, diarrhea, tremor, depression.

**INTERACTIONS:** May block effects of anticholinergics. May be synergistic with succinylcholine, similar neuromuscular blockers, or cholinergic agonists (eg, bethanechol). May exaggerate succinylcholine-type muscle relaxation during anesthesia.

**PREGNANCY:** Category B, not for use in nursing.

**MECHANISM OF ACTION:** Reversible cholinesterase inhibitor; not fully established, suspected to enhance cholinergic function by increasing concentration of acetylcholine through reversible inhibition of its hydrolysis by cholinesterase.

**PHARMACOKINETICS: Absorption:** Patch: $T_{max}$=10-16 hrs. Cap, Sol: Rapid, complete; absolute bioavailability (36%); $T_{max}$=1 hr. **Distribution:** $V_d$=1.8-2.7L/kg; plasma protein binding (40%). **Metabolism:** Cholinesterase-mediated hydrolysis. **Elimination:** Urine (97%), feces (0.4%); $T_{1/2}$=1.5 hrs.

## NURSING CONSIDERATIONS

**Assessment:** Assess for history of ulcer disease, sick sinus syndrome, conduction defects, asthma or COPD, urinary obstruction, body weight, seizures, and possible drug interactions.

**Monitoring:** Monitor body weight and mental status; signs/symptoms of active or occult GI bleeding, extrapyramidal symptoms (EPS), and hypersensitivity reactions.

**Patient Counseling:** Inform to monitor for loss of weight or appetite, NV, anorexia, or diarrhea; may exacerbate or induce EPS. (Sol) Instruct to use provided syringe to withdraw prescribed amount. (Patch) Instruct to wash hands after application, and avoid contact with eyes; do not rub in or apply to area that is red, irritated, cut or to areas where cream, lotion, powder has recently been applied; replace every 24 hrs and consistent time of day; do not apply new patch to same spot for at least 14 days; can be used while bathing but avoid exposure to external heat sources (eg, excess sunlight, saunas, solariums). If dose is missed, apply new patch immediately, then continue scheduled dosage; do not apply 2 patches at once.

**Administration:** Oral, transdermal route. (Sol) Swallow directly from syringe or mix with small glass of water, juice or soda; stir before drinking. (Patch) Apply at upper or lower back. **Storage:** 25°C (77°F); excursions permitted to 15-30°C (59-86°F). Sol: Store in upright position and protect from freezing. Patch: Keep in sealed pouch until use.

# EXFORGE RX

## amlodipine besylate - valsartan (Novartis)

**D/C therapy when pregnancy is detected. Drugs that act directly on the renin-angiotensin system can cause injury and even death to the developing fetus.**

**THERAPEUTIC CLASS:** ARB/Calcium channel blocker (dihydropyridine)

**INDICATIONS:** Treatment of hypertension. May be used in patients whose BP is not adequately controlled on either monotherapy. May also be used as initial therapy in patients likely to need multiple drugs to achieve their BP goals.

**DOSAGE:** *Adults:* Initial Therapy: 5mg-160mg qd. Add-On/Replacement Therapy: May be substituted for titrated components. Titrate: If inadequate control, may increase after 1-2 weeks of therapy. Max: 10mg-320mg qd. Elderly: Initial: 2.5mg amlodipine.

**HOW SUPPLIED:** Tab: (Amlodipine-Valsartan) 5mg-160mg, 10mg-160mg, 5mg-320mg, 10mg-320mg

**WARNINGS/PRECAUTIONS:** May cause fetal harm, fetal/neonatal morbidity and mortality when taken by pregnant women. May cause excessive hypotension. May increase risk of angina and MI in patients with severe obstructive

CAD. Caution with CHF, severe hepatic impairment, renal dysfunction, renal artery stenosis, and in the elderly.

**ADVERSE REACTIONS:** Peripheral edema, vertigo, nasopharyngitis, upper respiratory tract infection, dizziness.

**INTERACTIONS:** $K^+$ supplements, $K^+$-sparing diuretics (eg, spironolactone, triamterene, amiloride), or salt substitutes containing $K^+$ may increase serum $K^+$ and SrCr in heart failure patients. Concomitant use with atenolol may potentiate antihypertensive effects.

E

**PREGNANCY:** Category D, not for use in nursing.

**MECHANISM OF ACTION:** Amlodipine: Calcium channel blocker (dihydropyridine); inhibits transmembrane influx of calcium ions into vascular smooth muscle and cardiac muscle. Valsartan: Angiotensin II receptor blocker; blocks vasoconstrictor and aldosterone-secreting effects of angiotensin II by selectively blocking binding of angiotensin II to $AT_1$ receptor.

**PHARMACOKINETICS: Absorption:** Amlodipine: Absolute bioavailability (64-90%); $T_{max}$=6-12 hrs. Valsartan: Absolute bioavailability (25%); $T_{max}$=2-4 hrs. **Distribution:** Amlodipine: $V_d$=21L; plasma protein binding (93%). Valsartan: $V_d$=17L (IV); plasma protein binding (95%). **Metabolism:** Amlodipine: Liver (90%). Valsartan: Valeryl 4-hydroxy valsartan (metabolite). **Elimination:** Amlodipine: Urine (10%); $T_{1/2}$=30-50 hrs. Valsartan: Feces, urine; $T_{1/2}$=6 hrs.

## NURSING CONSIDERATIONS

**Assessment:** Assess severe obstructive CAD, CHF, recent MI, severe aortic stenosis, pregnancy status, possible drug interactions, renal/hepatic impairment.

**Monitoring:** Monitor for signs/symptoms of hypotension, hypersensitivity reactions, renal/hepatic dysfunction, symptoms of angina or MI after dosage initiation or increase.

**Patient Counseling:** Inform of pregnancy risks. Advise to seek medical attention if symptoms of hypotension or hypersensitivity reactions occur.

**Administration:** Oral route. **Storage:** 25°C (77°F); excursions permitted to 15-30°C (59-86°F). Protect from moisture.

# EXFORGE HCT RX

amlodipine besylate - hydrochlorothiazide - valsartan (Novartis)

**D/C when pregnancy is detected. Drugs that act directly on the renin-angiotensin system can cause injury or even death to the developing fetus.**

**THERAPEUTIC CLASS:** ARB/Calcium channel blocker (dihydropyridine)/ Thiazide diuretic

**INDICATIONS:** Treatment of hypertension.

**DOSAGE:** *Adults:* CrCl >30mL/min:1 tab qd. Titrate: May increase after two weeks of therapy. Max: 10mg-25mg-320mg qd. Add-on/ Switch Therapy: May be switched to Exforge HCT containing a lower dose of that component if patient experiences dose-limiting adverse reactions to an individual component while on any dual combination. Replacement Therapy: May be substituted for the individually titrated components.

**HOW SUPPLIED:** Tab: (Amlodipine-HCTZ-Valsartan) 5mg-12.5mg-160mg, 5mg-25mg-160mg, 10mg-12.5mg-160mg, 10mg-25mg-160mg, 10mg-25mg-320mg

**CONTRAINDICATIONS:** Patients with anuria or hypersensitivity to other sulfonamide-derived drugs.

**WARNINGS/PRECAUTIONS:** Excessive hypotension, including orthostatic hypotension, reported; place patient in supine position and consider IV infusion of normal saline. Avoid in patients with aortic or mitral stenosis or obstructive hypertrophic cardiomyopathy. May increase frequency, duration or severity of angina or acute MI in patients with severe obstructive coronary artery disease (CAD). Avoid with severe hepatic impairment. Monitor for worsening of hepatic or renal function in patients with mild-moderate hepatic impairment and biliary obstructive disorders. May precipitate azotemia with renal disease. Avoid in patients with severe renal disease (CrCl≤30mL/min). Hypokalemia reported. (Amlodipine) Monitor fluid status, electrolytes, renal function, and BP in patients with heart failure. (Valsartan) May increase blood urea nitrogen (BUN), SrCr, and potassium levels. (HCTZ) Hypersensitivity reactions may occur in patients with or without a history of allergy or bronchial asthma. May cause exacerbation or activation of systemic lupus erythematosus.



**ADVERSE REACTIONS:** Dizziness, edema, headache, dyspepsia, fatigue, muscle spasms, back pain, nausea, nasopharyngitis, dry cough.

**INTERACTIONS:** (HCTZ) Potentiation of orthostatic hypotension may occur when co-administered with alcohol, barbiturates, or narcotics. Dosage adjustment of antidiabetic drug (eg, oral agents and insulin) may be required during co-administration. Additive effect or potentiation with other antihypertensive drugs. Anionic exchange resins may impair absorption. Cholestyramine (85%) or colestipol (43%) resins may reduce GI absorption. Hypokalemia reported with corticosteroid, ACTH. Decrease response to pressor amines may occur. Increase responsiveness to skeletal muscle relaxant, nondepolarizing (eg, tubocurarine) agents may occur. Avoid concomitant use of lithium; may reduce renal clearance adding risk of lithium toxicity. NSAIDS may reduce diuretic, natriuretic, and antihypertensive effects of loop, potassium-sparing and thiazide diuretics. May lead to symptomatic hyponatremia with carbamazepine. (Valsartan) $K^+$ supplements, $K^+$-sparing diuretics (eg, spironolactone, triamterene, amiloride), or salt substitutes containing $K^+$ may increase serum $K^+$ and SrCr in heart failure patients.

**PREGNANCY:** Category D, not for use in nursing.

**MECHANISM OF ACTION:** Amlodipine: Calcium channel blocker (dihydropyridine); inhibits transmembrane influx of calcium ions into vascular smooth muscle and cardiac muscle. HCTZ: Thiazide diuretic; directly increasing excretion of sodium and chloride in approximately equivalent amounts. Valsartan: Angiotensin II receptor blocker; blocks vasoconstrictor and aldosterone-secreting effects of angiotensin II by selectively blocking binding of angiotensin II to $AT_1$ receptor.

**PHARMACOKINETICS: Absorption:** Amlodipine: Absolute bioavailability (64-90%); $T_{max}$=6-12 hrs. Valsartan: Absolute bioavailability (25%); $T_{max}$=2-4 hrs. **Distribution:** Amlodipine: $V_d$=21 L; plasma protein binding (93%). HCTZ: Crosses the placental barrier and found in breast milk.Valsartan: $V_d$=17 L (IV); plasma protein binding (95%). **Metabolism:** Amlodipine: Liver (90%). HCTZ: found in breast milk. Valsartan: Valeryl 4-hydroxy valsartan (metabolite). **Elimination:** Amlodipine: Urine (10%, parent; 60%, inactive metabolites); $T_{1/2}$=30-50 hrs. HCTZ: Urine (61%, unchanged); $T_{1/2}$=5.8-18.9 hrs. Valsartan: Feces, urine; $T_{1/2}$=6 hrs.

## NURSING CONSIDERATIONS

**Assessment:** Assess for LFTs, renal function, severe renal/hepatic impairment, severe obstructive CAD, CHF, recent MI, aortic or mitral stenosis, obstructive hypertrophic cardiomyopathy, pregnancy/nursing status and possible drug interactions.

**Monitoring:** Monitor for signs/symptoms of hypotension, hypersensitivity reactions, renal/hepatic impairment , worsening of hepatic or renal function and adverse reactions, symptoms of angina or MI after dosage initiation or increase. Monitor BP, fluid and electrolytes status, BUN, SrCr, CrCl levels.

**Patient Counseling:** Inform of pregnancy risks and serious fetal problems (eg, low BP, poor skull bones development, kidney problems, and death) may occur. Notify physician if pregnant/planning to become pregnant or breastfeeding. Caution about lightheadedness, especially during the first days of therapy, and advise to report to physician. Instruct to d/c if syncope occurs. Caution about inadequate fluid intake, excessive perspiration, diarrhea, or vomiting may lead to an excessive fall in BP, with the same consequences of lightheadedness and possible syncope. Instruct to avoid potassium supplements or salt substitutes containing potassium without consulting a physician.

**Administration:** Oral route. **Storage:** 25°C (77°F); excursions permitted to 15-30°C (59-86°F). Protect from moisture.

## EXTAVIA RX

interferon beta-1b (Novartis)



**THERAPEUTIC CLASS:** Biological response modifier

**INDICATIONS:** Treatment in patients who have experienced a first clinical episode and have MRI features consistent with multiple sclerosis (MS). To reduce frequency of clinical exacerbations in patients with relapsing-remitting MS.

**DOSAGE:** *Adults:* Initial: 0.0625mg SQ every other day. Titrate: Increase over 6 weeks to 0.25mg SQ every other day. Refer to PI for Dose Titration schedule.

**HOW SUPPLIED:** Inj: 0.3mg/3mL [vial]

**CONTRAINDICATIONS:** Hypersensitivity to human albumin.

**WARNINGS/PRECAUTIONS:** Caution with depression; increased frequency of depression and suicide reported; d/c if develops. Injection-site reactions (eg, inflammation, pain, hypersensitivity, mass, edema, and necrosis) reported; d/c if multiple leisions occur. Monitor for signs and symptoms of anaphylaxis/allergic reactions (eg, dyspnea, bronchospasm, tongue edema, skin rash, and urticaria). Flu-like symptoms, leukopenia, and LFTs elevation (SGPT, SGOT) reported. Perform CBC, differential WBC, LFTs, and platelet count before therapy and periodically thereafter. Contains albumin; risk of viral disease transmission.

**ADVERSE REACTIONS:** Injection-site reactions/necrosis, flu-like symptoms, headache, lymphopenia, hypertonia, asthenia, pain, fever, chills, rash, insomnia, myalgia, abdominal pain, incoordination, urinary urgency.

**PREGNANCY:** Category C, not for use in nursing.

**MECHANISM OF ACTION:** Interferon β-1b: Not established; believed that interferon β-1b receptor binding induces expression of proteins that are responsible for pleiotropic bioactivities. Immunomodulatory effects include the enhancement of suppressor T cell activity, reduction of pro-inflammatory cytokine production, down-regulation of antigen presentation, and inhibition of lymphocyte trafficking into the CNS.

**PHARMACOKINETICS: Absorption:** $T_{max}$=1-8 hrs, $C_{max}$=40IU/mL. **Distribution:** $V_d$=0.25-2.88L/kg. **Elimination:** $T_{1/2}$=8 min-4.3 hrs.

### NURSING CONSIDERATIONS

**Assessment:** Assess for hypersensitivity, depression, leukopenia, myelosuppression, liver function, thyroid function, myelosupression, and pregnancy/nursing status.

**Monitoring:** Monitor for anaphylaxis, depression, suicidal ideation, injection-site reactions, injection-site necrosis, flu-like symptoms, and periodically monitor CBC, WBC, LFTs, thyroid function.

**Patient Counseling:** Inform about potential benefits/risks of drug. Advise not to change dose or schedule of administration. Inform that depression and suicidal ideation, injection-site reactions, injection-site necrosis at 1 or multiple sites, symptoms of allergic reactions and anaphylaxis may occur; d/c and notify physician if symptoms is experienced. Inform patients to take antipyretics and analgesics if with flu-like symptoms. Advise patients not to use the drug during pregnancy unless the potential benefit justifies the potential risk to the fetus.

**Administration:** SC; rotate injection sites. Do not take in 2 consecutive days. Refer to PI for reconstitution. **Storage:** 25°C (77°F); excursions permitted to 15-30°C (59-86°F). After reconstitution, if not used immediately, refrigerate and use within 3 hrs. Avoid freezing.

## EXTINA RX

ketoconazole (Stiefel)

**THERAPEUTIC CLASS:** Azole antifungal

**INDICATIONS:** Topical treatment of seborrheic dermatitis in immunocompetent patients ≥12 yrs of age.

**DOSAGE:** *Adults:* Apply to affected area(s) bid for 4 weeks. *Pediatrics:* ≥12 yrs: Apply to affected area(s) bid for 4 weeks.

**HOW SUPPLIED:** Foam: 2% [50g, 100g]

**WARNINGS/PRECAUTIONS:** May cause contact sensitization, including photoallergenicity. Contents are flammable. Avoid fire, flame, and/or smoking during and immediately following applications. Hepatitis, lowered testoterone and ACTH-induced corticosteroid serum levels reported with orally administered ketoconazole.

**ADVERSE REACTIONS:** Application-site burning, application-site reactions (eg, dryness, erythema, irritation, paresthesia, pruritus, rash, warmth), photoallergenicity, contact dermatitis.

**PREGNANCY:** Category C, caution in nursing.

**MECHANISM OF ACTION:** Azole antifungal; not established. Inhibits the synthesis of ergosterol, a key sterol in the cell membrane of *Malassezia furfur*.

### NURSING CONSIDERATIONS

**Assessment:** Assess pregnancy/nursing status.

**Monitoring:** Monitor for contact sensitization reactions, including photoallergenicity, improvement/worsening of symptoms.

**Patient Counseling:** Counsel to notify physician if any type of skin irritation or contact sensitization reaction develops; or if no improvement in 4 weeks of treatment. Inform medication is flammable; do not administer near fire, open flame, or direct heat. Instruct to wash hands well following administration. Advise on the proper way to apply the foam: 1.) Hold the can at an upright angle. 2.) Push the button to spray foam directly into the cap of the can or other cool surface. Spray only the amount that will be needed to cover the affected area. Do not spray directly onto the affected skin or into hands because the foam will begin to melt right away when it touches the skin. 3.) If fingers are warm, rinse them in cold water first. Be sure to dry them well before handling the foam. If the can seems warm or the foam seems runny, place the can under cool running water for a few minutes. 4.) Using fingertips, gently massage foam into the affected areas until the foam disappears. 5.) If treating skin with hair such as the scalp, move any hair away so that the foam can be applied to the affected skin.

**Administration:** Topical application. **Storage:** Room temperature 20-25°C (68-77°F). Do not store under refrigerated conditions or in direct sunlight. Do not expose containers to heat or store at temperatures above 49°C (120°F). Contents are flammable. Do not puncture and/or incinerate container. Keep out of reach of children.

## FACTIVE RX

gemifloxacin mesylate (Oscient)

**Fluoroquinolones are associated with an increased risk of tendinitis and tendon rupture in all ages. Risk further increased in patients >60 yrs, patients taking corticosteroid drugs, and patients with kidney, heart or lung transplants.**

**THERAPEUTIC CLASS:** Fluoroquinolone

**INDICATIONS:** Treatment of community-acquired pneumonia (CAP), including multi-drug resistant *Streptococcus pneumoniae* (MDRSP), and acute bacterial exacerbation of chronic bronchitis (ABECB).

**DOSAGE:** *Adults:* ≥18 yrs: ABECB: 320mg qd for 5 days. CAP: 320mg qd for 5 days (*S.pneumoniae*, *H.influenzae*, *M.pneumoniae*, or *C.pneumoniae*) or 7 days (MDRSP, *K.pneumoniae*, or *M.catarrhalis*). Renal Impairment: CrCl ≤40mL/min or Dialysis: 160mg qd. Take with fluids.

**HOW SUPPLIED:** Tab: 320mg

**WARNINGS/PRECAUTIONS:** May prolong QT interval; avoid in patients with a history of prolonged QTc interval, uncontrolled electrolyte disorders. Caution with proarrhythmic conditions, epilepsy, or if predisposed to convulsions. D/C at 1st sign of hypersensitivity (eg, rash). CNS effects, photosensitivity reactions, hypersensitivity reactions (some fatal) reported; d/c if any of these occur. *Clostridium difficile*-associated diarrhea (CDAD), Achilles and other tendon ruptures reported. D/C therapy if rash, pain, inflammation, or ruptured tendon occurs. Caution in elderly patients taking corticosteroids. Avoid excessive sunlight and UV light. Maintain hydration. Increases of International Normalized Ratio (INR), or prothrombin time (PT), and/or clinical episodes of bleeding have been noted with concurrent administration with warfarin or derivatives.

F

**ADVERSE REACTIONS:** Diarrhea, rash, N/V, headache, abdominal pain, dizziness, anaphylactic reaction, hemorrhage, peripheral edema, renal failure, syncope, transient ishemic attack, photosensitivity/phototoxicity reactions, tendinitis, tendon rupture.

**INTERACTIONS:** Magnesium- or aluminum-containing antacids, Videx® (didanosine) chewable/buffered tablets or pediatric powder, and products containing iron, and zinc, or other metal cations decrease absorption, space doses at least 3 hrs before or 2 hrs after administration. Space dosing of sucralfate by 2 hrs. Potentiated by probenecid. Monitor PT. Avoid Class IA (eg, quinidine, procainamide) or III (eg, amiodarone, sotalol) antiarrhythmics. Caution with drugs that prolong the QTc interval (eg, erythromycin, antipsychotics, TCAs).

**PREGNANCY:** Category C, not for use in nursing.

**MECHANISM OF ACTION:** Fluoroquinolone; synthetic broad-spectrum antimicrobial agent; inhibits enzymes topoisomerase II (DNA gyrase) and topoisomerase IV, which are required for bacterial DNA replication.

**PHARMACOKINETICS: Absorption:** Rapid; absolute bioavailability (71%); $T_{max}$=0.5-2 hrs; $C_{max}$=1.61µg/mL, AUC=8.36µg•hr/mL (respiratory infection, UTI). **Distribution:** $V_d$=4.18L/kg; plasma protein binding (55%-73%). **Metabolism:** Liver. **Elimination:** Feces (61%), urine (36%).

## NURSING CONSIDERATIONS

**Assessment:** Assess renal function, LFTs, pregnancy status, prolonged QT interval, history of seizures. Note other diseases/conditions and drug therapies.

**Monitoring:** Monitor for cardiac arrest, seizure, status epilepticus, respiratory failure, angioedema, hypersensitivity reactions, dermatological reactions (Stevens-Johnson syndrome), CDAD, LFTs, renal function, CBC with platelet and differential count, tendon rupture, peripheral neuropathy.

**Patient Counseling:** Notify healthcare provider if symptoms of pain, swelling, or inflammation of a tendon, or weakness or inability to move joints; rest and refrain from exercise; and d/c therapy. Inform that drug treats bacterial, not viral, infections. Take exactly as directed; skipping doses or not completing full course may decrease effectiveness and increase resistance. Inform to take with or without food, and to drink fluids. Inform about potential benefits/risks. D/C and notify physician if skin rash, other allergic reaction, and watery and bloody stools (with or without stomach cramps and fever) occur. Notify if pregnant/nursing or taking antacids or sucralfate. Use caution in activities requiring mental alertness and coordination. Avoid sun exposure. Take full course as prescribed. Instruct to swallow tablet whole.

**Administration:** Oral route. **Storage:** 25°C (77°F) excursions permitted to 15-30°C (59-86°F). Protect from light.

# FAMVIR **RX**

famciclovir (Novartis)

**THERAPEUTIC CLASS:** Nucleoside analogue

**INDICATIONS:** Treatment of acute herpes zoster (shingles). Treatment or suppression of recurrent genital herpes; or treatment of recurrent herpes labialis (cold sores) in immunocompetent patients. Treatment of recurrent mucocutaneous herpes simplex infections in HIV-infected patients.

**DOSAGE:** *Adults:* ≥18 yrs: Herpes Zoster: Usual: 500mg q8h for 7 days; start within 72 hrs after rash onset. CrCl ≥60mL/min: 500mg q8h. CrCl 40-59mL/min: 500mg q12h. CrCl 20-39mL/min: 500mg q24h. CrCl <20mL/min: 250mg q24h. Hemodialysis: 250mg following dialysis. Recurrent Genital Herpes: 1000mg bid for 1 day; start within 6 hrs of onset of symptom. CrCl ≥60mL/min: 1000mg q12h for 1 day. CrCl 40-59mL/min: 500mg q12h for 1 day. CrCl 20-39mL/min: 500mg as single dose. CrCl <20mL/min: 250mg as a single dose. Hemodialysis: 250mg single dose following dialysis. Suppression of Recurrent Genital Herpes: 250mg bid for up to 1 yr. CrCl ≥40mL/min: 250mg q12h. CrCl 20-39mL/min: 125mg q12h. CrCl <20mL/min: 125mg q24h. Hemodialysis: 125mg following dialysis. Recurrent Orolabial or Genital Herpes in HIV: 500mg bid for 7 days. CrCl ≥40mL/min: 500mg q12h. CrCl 20-39mL/min: 500mg q24h. CrCl <20mL/min: 250mg q24h. Hemodialysis: 250mg following dialysis. Recurrent Herpes Labialis: 1500mg as a single dose; CrCl 40-59mL/min: 750mg single dose. CrCl 20-39mL/min: 500mg single dose. CrCl ≥60mL/min: 1500mg single dose. CrCl <20mL/min: 250mg single dose. Hemodialysis: 250mg following dialysis

**HOW SUPPLIED:** Tab: 125mg, 250mg, 500mg

**CONTRAINDICATIONS:** Hypersensitivity to penciclovir cream.

**WARNINGS/PRECAUTIONS:** Dose adjustment in renal disease. Not indicated for initial episode of genital herpes infection, ophthalmic zoster, disseminated zoster or in immunocompromised patients with herpes zoster. Contain lactose; avoid with rare hereditary problems of galactose intolerance, severe lactase deficiency or glucose-galactose malabsorption.

**ADVERSE REACTIONS:** Headache, migraine, N/V, diarrhea, fatigue, urticaria, hallucinations, confusion, cholestatic jaundice, Stevens-Johnson syndrome, toxic epidermal necrolysis, abnormal LFTs, thrombocytopenia, dizziness, erythema multiforme, and somnolence.

**INTERACTIONS:** Increased plasma levels of penciclovir with probenecid and other drugs significantly eliminated by active renal tubular secretion. Potential interaction with drugs metabolized by aldehyde oxidase.

**PREGNANCY:** Category B, not for use in nursing.

**MECHANISM OF ACTION:** Nucleoside analogue; inhibits HSV-2 DNA polymerase competitively with deoxyguanosine triphosphate, inhibiting herpes viral DNA synthesis and replication.

**PHARMACOKINETICS: Absorption:** Penciclovir: Absolute bioavailability (77%). **Distribution:** Penciclovir (IV) $V_d$=1.08L/kg; plasma protein binding (<20%) **Metabolism**: Hepatic; deacetylation and oxidation; famciclovir (prodrug) converted to penciclovir. **Elimination:** Urine (73%), feces (27%). Penciclovir: Urine (94%); $T_{1/2}$=2-3 hrs.

## NURSING CONSIDERATIONS

**Assessment:** Assess for hepatic/renal dysfunction, galactose intolerance, severe lactase deficiency, or glucose-galactose malabsorption, hypersensitivity to drug, pregnancy/nursing status, and possibble drug interaction.

**Monitoring:** Monitor LFTs, total bilirubin, serum creatinine, CBC, amylase and lipase. Monitor maternal-fetal outcomes of pregnant women and hypersensitivity reactions.

**Patient Counseling:** Avoid contact with lesions or intercourse when lesions and/or symptoms are present to avoid infecting partners. Instruct to refrain from driving or operating machinery. Counsel to take without regard to meals. Encourage pregnancy registry to pregnant women.

**Administration:** Oral route. **Storage:** 25°C (77°F); excursions permitted to 15-30°C (59-86°F).

## FANAPT RX
iloperidone (Vanda)

**Elderly patients with dementia-related psychosis treated with antipsychotic drugs are at an increased risk of death; most appeared to be cardiovascular (eg, heart failure, sudden death) or infectious (eg, pneumonia) in nature. Iloperidone is not approved for the treatment of patients with dementia-related psychosis.**

F

**THERAPEUTIC CLASS:** Benzisoxazole derivative

**INDICATIONS:** Acute treatment of schizophrenia in adults.

**DOSAGE:** *Adults:* Initial: 1mg bid. Range: 6-12mg bid. Titrate: Must titrate dose slowly to avoid orthostatic hypotension. Day 2: 2mg bid. Day 3: 4mg bid. Day 4: 6mg bid. Day 5: 8mg bid. Day 6: 10mg bid. Day 7: 12mg bid. Max: 12mg bid (24mg/day). Concomitant Strong CYP2D6/CYP3A4 Inhibitors: Reduce dose by one-half. Upon withdrawal of CYP2D6/CYP3A4 inhibitors, iloperidone dose should be increased to previous dose. Maint: Responding patients should be continued beyond the acute response; reassess periodically to determine the need for maintenance treatment. Reinitiation of Treatment: Initial titration schedule to be followed when patients have had an interval off drug more than 3 days. Switching from Other Antipsychotics: Minimize overlapping period of antipsychotics.

**HOW SUPPLIED:** Tab: 1mg, 2mg, 4mg, 6mg, 8mg, 10mg, 12mg

**WARNINGS/PRECAUTIONS:** Avoid with hepatic impairment, congenital long QT syndrome, history of QT prolongation, recent acute myocardial infarction (MI), uncompensated heart failure, or cardiac arrhythmias. D/C if persistent QTc measurements >500 ms. Hyperglycemia, in some cases extreme and associated with ketoacidosis or hyperosmolar coma or death, has been reported; monitor diabetes mellitus (DM) patients regularly for worsening of glucose control and all patients for symptoms of hyperglycemia. Neuroleptic malignant syndrome (NMS), leukopenia/neutropenia, agranulocytosis, priapism and weight gain reported. D/C if signs/symptoms of tardive dyskinesia and severe neutropenia (absolute neutrophil count <1000/$mm^3$) occur. May induce orthostatic hypotension. May disrupt body's ability to reduce core body temperature and prolactin levels. Caution with history of seizures or conditions that lower seizure threshold (eg, Alzheimer's dementia), known cardiovascular (CV) disease (eg, heart failure, previous MI, ischemia), cerebrovascular disease, or conditions that predispose to hypotension (eg, dehydration, hypovolemia), and in patients at risk for aspiration pneumonia. Close supervision of high-risk patients should accompany drug therapy due to possibility of suicide attempt. May impair mental/physical abilities.

**ADVERSE REACTIONS:** Arthralgia, fatigue, tachycardia, nausea, dry mouth, diarrhea, nasopharyngitis, dizziness, somnolence, tremor, extrapyramidal disorder, nasal congestion, orthostatic hypotension, and weight gain.

**INTERACTIONS:** May increase levels with ketoconazole, fluoxetine and paroxetine. May increase total exposure of dextromethorphan with concomitant use. Avoid with Class IA (eg, quinidine, procainamide), Class III (eg, amiodarone, sotalol) antiarrhythmics, antipsychotics (eg, chlorpromazine, thiordazine), antibiotics (eg, gatifloxacin, moxifloxacin), or other drugs known to prolong QTc interval (eg, pentamidine, levomethadyl acetate, methadone). Caution with other centrally acting drugs and alcohol. May potentiate effects of antihypertensive agents. May increase levels with concomitant use of CYP2D6/CYP3A4 inhibitors.

**PREGNANCY:** Category C, not for use in nursing.

**MECHANISM OF ACTION:** Piperidinyl-benzisoxazole derivatives; mechanism not established. Proposed efficacy is mediated through combination of dopamine type 2 ($D_2$) and serotonin type 2 ($5\text{-}HT_2$) antagonisms.

**PHARMACOKINETICS: Absorption:** Well absorbed; bioavailability (96%); $T_{max}$=2-4 hrs. **Distribution:** $V_d$=1340-2800L; plasma protein binding (95%).

**Metabolism:** Liver via carbonyl reduction, hydroxylation, O-demethylation; predominant metabolites (P88 and P95). **Elimination:** Urine (58.2% in extensive metabolizers [EM] and 45.1% in poor metabolizers [PM]) and feces (19.9% in EM and 22.1% in PM). CYP2D6 extensive metabolizers: (Iloperidone) $T_{1/2}$=18 hrs; (P88, P95 metabolites) $T_{1/2}$=23 and 26 hrs. Poor metabolizers: (Iloperidone) $T_{1/2}$=33 hrs; (P88, P95 metabolites) $T_{1/2}$=31 and 37 hrs.

## NURSING CONSIDERATIONS

**Assessment:** Assess for dementia-related psychosis, significant CV disease, cerebrovascular disease, conditions that predispose to hypotension, risk factors for aspiration, history of seizures/conditons that lower seizure threshold, hepatic impairment, pre-existing low WBC count/history of drug-induced leukopenia/neutropenia, DM, hyperglycemia, significant electrolyte disturbances, suicidal tendency, pregnancy/nursing status, and possible drug interactions. Obtain baseline FPG, serum potassium and magnesium levels.

**Monitoring:** Monitor for orthostatic vital signs, body temperature, hyperglycemia, pneumonia, weight gain, seizures, leukopenia/neutropenia, agranulocytosis, priapism, fever and signs/symptoms of infection, hypersensitivity reactions (eg, pruritus, urticaria), tardive dyskinesia and NMS. Monitor for possibility of suicide attempt. Monitor WBC, CBC, blood glucose, serum potassium/magnesium levels.

**Patient Counseling:** Inform physician if taking, or plan to take, any prescription or OTC drugs that might cause QT prolongation and possible drug interactions. Advise NMS and orthostatic hypotension may occur. Notify physician if pregnant, intend to become pregnant, or breastfeeding. Instruct to avoid alcohol. Counsel about appropriate care to avoid dehydration. Caution against operating hazardous machinery (eg, automobiles).

**Administration:** Oral route. **Storage**: 25°C (77°F); excursions permitted to 15-30°C (59-86°F). Protect from light and moisture.

# FASLODEX — RX

fulvestrant (AstraZeneca)

**THERAPEUTIC CLASS:** Estrogen receptor antagonist

**INDICATIONS:** Treatment of hormone receptor positive metastatic breast cancer in postmenopausal women with disease progression following antiestrogen therapy.

**DOSAGE:** *Adults:* 250mg IM into buttock once monthly as either a single 5mL injection or two concurrent 2.5mL injections. Administer slowly.

**HOW SUPPLIED:** Inj: 50mg/mL [2.5mL, 5mL]

**CONTRAINDICATIONS:** Pregnancy.

**WARNINGS/PRECAUTIONS:** May cause fetal harm during pregnancy; women of childbearing age should be advised not to become pregnant and pregnancy should be ruled out prior to initiating therapy. Avoid in patients with bleeding diatheses or thrombocytopenia. Safety and efficacy have not been studied in patients with moderate or severe hepatic impairment.

**ADVERSE REACTIONS:** N/V, constipation, diarrhea, abdominal pain, headache, back pain, vasodilatation (hot flushes), pharyngitis, injection-site reactions, asthenia, pain, dyspnea, increased cough.

**INTERACTIONS:** Avoid with concurrent anticoagulants.

**PREGNANCY:** Category D, not for use in nursing.

**MECHANISM OF ACTION:** Estrogen receptor antagonist; binds to estrogen receptor and downregulates estrogen receptor protein in human breast cancer cells.

**PHARMACOKINETICS: Absorption:** $C_{max}$=8.5ng/mL; $T_{max}$=7 days; AUC=131ng•d/mL. **Distribution:** $V_d$=3-5L/kg; plasma protein binding (99%). **Metabolism:** CYP3A4; oxidation, aromatic hydroxylation, conjugation. **Elimination:** Feces (90%), urine (<1%); $T_{1/2}$=40 days.

## NURSING CONSIDERATIONS

**Assessment:** Assess for hypersensitivity, hepatic impairment, bleeding diatheses, thrombocytopenia, pregnancy/nursing status, and possible drug interactions.

**Monitoring:** Monitor for NV, constipation/diarrhea, abdominal pain, headache, back pain, hot flushes, pharyngitis, vasodilation, anemia, hypersensitivity reactions, bleeding diatheses, women of childbearing potential, and hepatic dysfunction.

**Patient Counseling:** Counsel about pregnancy/nursing risks; avoid pregnancy. Seek immediate medical attention if NV, constipation/diarrhea, abdominal pain, headache, back pain, hot flushes, pharyngitis, vasodilation, anemia, hypersensitivity reactions, or bleeding diatheses develops.

**Administration:** IM route. Refer to PI for full instructions. **Storage:** 2-8°C (36-46°F). Protect from light. Store in original carton until time of use.



# FAZACLO

RX

clozapine (Azur)

**Risk of potentially life-threatening agranulocytosis. Reserve use for severely ill patients with schizophrenia unresponsive to standard antipsychotic treatment or for patients with schizophrenia/schizoaffective disorder at risk for re-experiencing suicidal behavior. Obtain baseline WBC count and absolute neutrophil count (ANC) before initiation of treatment, regularly during treatment, and for at least 4 weeks after d/c. Seizures associated with use and with greater likelihood at higher doses; caution in patients with history of seizures or other predisposing factors. Increased risk of fatal myocarditis, especially during 1st month of treatment; d/c if suspected. Orthostatic hypotension, with or without syncope can occur. Rare reports of collapse accompanied by respiratory and/or cardiac arrest in patients taking benzodiazepines or any other psychotropic drugs. Elderly patients with dementia-related psychosis treated with an atypical antipsychotic are at an increased risk for death, which appeared to be either cardiovascular (eg, heart failure, sudden death) or infectious (eg, pneumonia) in nature. Not approved for the treatment of dementia-related psychosis.**

**THERAPEUTIC CLASS:** Dibenzapine derivative

**INDICATIONS:** Management of severely ill schizophrenic patients who fail to respond adequately to standard drug treatment for schizophrenia. Reduction of risk for suicidal behavior in patients with schizophrenia or schizoaffective disorder who are judged to be at chronic risk for reexperiencing suicidal behavior.

**DOSAGE:** *Adults:* Treatment-Resistant Schizophrenia: Initial: 12.5mg qd-bid. Titrate: Increase by 25-50mg/day, up to 300-450mg/day by end of 2 weeks; then increase weekly or bi-weekly in increments of ≤100mg. Usual range: 300-600mg/day given tid. Max: 900mg/day. To d/c, gradually reduce dose over 1-2 weeks. Monitor for psychotic symptoms if abrupt d/c warranted (eg, leukopenia). Re-initiation: Start with 12.5mg qd-bid and may titrate more quickly to therapeutic dose if initial dosing tolerated. Retitrate with extreme caution in those who experienced cardiac or respiratory arrest with initial dosing but successfully titrated to therapeutic dose. Do not restart in patients discontinued for WBC <2000mm$^3$ or ANC <1000mm$^3$. Reduction of Risk of Suicidal Behavior in Schizophrenia/Schizoaffective Disorder: May follow dosing recommendations for treatment-resistant schizophrenia. Usual range: 12.5-900mg/day (mean 300mg). To reduce the risk of suicidal behavior in patients who otherwise responded to therapy with another antipsychotic, treat for at least 2 years and then re-evaluate.

**HOW SUPPLIED:** Tab, Disintegrating: 12.5mg, 25mg, 100mg

**CONTRAINDICATIONS:** Myeloproliferative disorders, uncontrolled epilepsy, paralytic ileus, history of clozapine-induced agranulocytosis or severe granulocytopenia, CNS depression, comatose states from any cause, or with other agents with potential to cause agranulocytosis or otherwise suppress bone marrow function.

**WARNINGS/PRECAUTIONS:** Hyperglycemia, sometimes with ketoacidosis, hyperosmolar coma or death, reported. Monitor for worsening of glucose control with DM and FBG levels with diabetes risk or symptoms of hyperglycemia.

Tachycardia and cardiomyopathy reported; caution with known CV disease. D/C if cardiomyopathy confirmed unless benefits outweighs risk. May impair mental/physical abilities especially with initial doses. Neuroleptic malignant syndrome (NMS), tardive dyskinesia (TD), impaired intestinal peristalsis (eg, constipation, intestinal obstruction, paralytic ileus), pulmonary embolism, and ECG changes reported. Evaluate patients with fever; rule out infection, agranulocytosis and NMS. Potent anticholinergic effects warrants caution with prostatic enlargement and narrow-angle glaucoma. Caution with renal, hepatic, or pulmonary disease. Obtain WBC and ANC at baseline, then weekly for 1st six months of therapy, then every 2 weeks for next 6 months, and then every 4 weeks thereafter if counts are acceptable (WBCs ≥3500/mm³ or ANC ≥2000/mm³). Refer to PI for frequency of monitoring based on stage of therapy, WBC count and ANC. Avoid treatment if WBCs <3500/mm³ or ANC <2000/mm³. D/C treatment and do not rechallenge if WBCs <2000/mm³, ANC <1000/mm³, or if myocarditis develops. Interrupt therapy if eosinophilia (>4000/mm³) develops. D/C over 1-2 weeks. Contains aspartame (of which phenylalanine is a component), and not intended for use in infants.

**ADVERSE REACTIONS:** Drowsiness, vertigo, headache, tremor, salivation, sweating, dry mouth, visual disturbances, tachycardia, hypotension, syncope, constipation, nausea, fever.

**INTERACTIONS:** Avoid with bone marrow suppressants, epinephrine, and carbamazepine. Caution with CNS-active drugs, anesthesia, alcohol, paroxetine, fluoxetine, fluvoxamine, sertraline, benzodiazepines, other psychotropics, or inhibitors/inducers of CYP1A2, 2D6, 3A4. Dosage reduction may be needed with drugs metabolized by CYP2D6 (eg, antidepressants, phenothiazines, carbamazepine, Type 1C antiarrhythmics). May potentiate hypotensive effects of antihypertensives and anticholinergic effects of atropine-type drugs. Caution with general anesthesia. CYP450 inducers (eg, phenytoin, nicotine, carbamazepine, rifampin) may decrease plasma levels. CYP450 inhibitors (eg, cimetidine, caffeine, fluvoxamine, erythromycin) may increase plasma levels. NMS reported with lithium and other CNS-acting drugs.

**PREGNANCY:** Category B, not for use in nursing.

**MECHANISM OF ACTION:** Dibenzapine derivative; atypical antipsychotic agent. Interferes with the binding of dopamine specifically at the $D_1$, $D_2$, $D_3$, and $D_5$ receptors, and has a high affinity for $D_4$ receptor. Also acts as an antagonist at the adrenergic, cholinergic, histaminergic, and serotonergic receptors.

**PHARMACOKINETICS: Absorption:** $C_{max}$=413ng/mL, $T_{max}$=2.3 hrs. **Metabolism:** Demethylation, hydroxylation. Norclozapine (active metabolite) **Distribution:** Plasma protein binding (97%). **Elimination:** Urine (50%), feces (30%); $T_{1/2}$=8 hrs (initial dose), 12 hrs (multiple doses).

## NURSING CONSIDERATIONS

**Assessment:** Assess previous course of standard therapy prior to treatment. Assess for history of myeloproliferative disorders, uncontrolled epilepsy, paralytic ileus, clozapine-induced agranulocytosis or severe granulocytopenia, and severe CNS depression prior to therapy. Assess risk of seizure, dementia-related psychosis, narrow-angle glaucoma, male patients with prostrate enlargement, concomitant illnesses (eg, DM, hepatic, renal or cardiac/pulmonary disease). Perform baseline WBC count and ANC prior to treatment. Obtain baseline fasting blood glucose levels in patients at risk for hyperglycemia/DM. Assess for possible drug interactions (eg, agents with known potential to cause agranulocytosis or suppress bone marrow function, benzodiazepines and other pyschotropic drugs, etc.).

**Monitoring:** Monitor for clinical response to treatment, WBC counts and ANC while on therapy and for at least 4 weeks following d/c. Monitor for agranulocytosis, CV effects (myocarditis), tachycardia, severe respiratory effects, seizures, fever, pulmonary embolism, NMS, TD, and intestinal paralysis, signs/symptoms of hyperglycemia and check periodic fasting blood glucose levels in patients at risk for hyperglycemia, and for signs/symptoms of hepatitis while on therapy. Obtain LFTs if patient develops N/V and/or anorexia.

**Patient Counseling:** Inform that clozapine is available only through a program designed to ensure the required blood monitoring schedule. Counsel on risks of treatment (eg, agranulocytosis, seizures, orthostatic hypotension). Inform about signs/symptoms of agranulocytosis; advise to immediately report lethargy, weakness, fever, sore throat. Inform phenylketonuric patients drug contains phenylalanine. Medication may cause cognitive/motor impairment. Avoid hazardous activities (eg, operating machinery/driving), alcohol use. Advise females to avoid nursing while on medication. Advise drug can be taken with/without food. If a dose is missed for more than 2 days, consult physician before restarting medication. Advise that tablets are received in a blister and should be kept unopened until immediately prior to use.

**Administration:** Oral route. **Storage:** 25°C (77°F); excursions permitted to 15-30°C (59-86°F). Protect from moisture. Keep out of reach of children.



## FELBATOL — RX
felbamate (Meda)

**Associated with increased incidence of aplastic anemia; d/c if any evidence of bone marrow depression occurs. Acute liver failure reported; d/c if AST or ALT increased ≥2x ULN or if clinical signs and symptoms suggest liver failure. Monitor blood count and LFTs routinely. Avoid with history of hepatic dysfunction.**

**THERAPEUTIC CLASS:** Dicarbamate anticonvulsant

**INDICATIONS:** Monotherapy or adjunctive therapy in partial seizures, with and without generalization, in adults with epilepsy. Adjunctive therapy for partial and generalized seizures with Lennox-Gastaut syndrome in children.

**DOSAGE:** *Adults:* Initial Monotherapy: 300mg qid or 400mg tid. Titrate: Increase by 600mg every 2 weeks to 2.4g/day. Max: 3.6g/day. Initial Monotherapy Conversion/Adjunct Therapy: 300mg qid or 400mg tid while reducing present antiepileptic drugs (AED) (refer to PI). Titrate: Monotherapy Conversion: Increase at Week 2 to 2.4g/day, at Week 3 up to 3.6g/day. Adjunct Therapy: Increase by 1.2g/day every week up to 3.6mg/day. Renal Impairment: Initial/Maint: Reduce by one-half. Adjunct therapy: May need further dose reductions. Elderly: Start at lower end of dosing range. *Pediatrics:* ≥14 yrs: Initial Monotherapy: 300mg qid or 400mg tid. Titrate: Increase by 600mg every 2 weeks to 2.4g/day. Max: 3.6g/day. Initial Monotherapy Conversion/Adjunct Therapy: 300mg qid or 400mg tid while reducing present AED (refer to PI). Titrate: Monotherapy Conversion: Increase at Week 2 to 2.4g/day, at Week 3 up to 3.6g/day. Adjunct Therapy: Increase by 1.2g/day every week up to 3.6mg/day. Renal Impairment: Initial/Maint: Reduce by one-half. Adjunct therapy: May need further dose reductions. 2-14 yrs: Lennox-Gastaut Adjunct Therapy: Initial: 15mg/kg/day in 3-4 divided doses while reducing present AEDs by 20%. Titrate: Increase by 15mg/kg/day every week to 45mg/kg/day.

**HOW SUPPLIED:** Sus: 600mg/5mL [8oz, 32oz]; Tab: 400mg*, 600mg*
*scored

**CONTRAINDICATIONS:** History of blood dyscrasias or hepatic dysfunction.

**WARNINGS/PRECAUTIONS:** Not for first-line therapy. Avoid abrupt d/c. Increased risk of suicidal thoughts or behavior; monitor for emergence or worsening of depression, suicidal thoughts/behavior and any unusual changes in mood or behavior. Obtain full hematologic evaluations (eg, blood counts including platelets and reticulocytes) and LFTs before, during and after d/c. Caution with renal dysfunction. Caution in elderly.

**ADVERSE REACTIONS:** Anorexia, N/V, insomnia, headache, somnolence, dizziness, dyspepsia, constipation, fatigue, upper respiratory tract infection, diplopia, nervousness.

**INTERACTIONS:** Increases plasma concentrations of phenytoin, valproate, carbamazepine epoxide and phenobarbital. Decreases carbamazepine concentration. Decreased felbamate levels with phenytoin, carbamazepine and phenobarbital. Caution with oral contraceptives.

**PREGNANCY:** Category C, safety in nursing not known.

**MECHANISM OF ACTION:** Anticonvulsant; has not been established. Weak inhibitory effects on GABA-receptor binding and benzodiazepine receptor binding. Acts as an antagonist at the strychnine-insensitive glycine recognition site of the NMDA receptor-ionophore complex.

**PHARMACOKINETICS: Absorption:** Well-absorbed. **Distribution:** $V_d$=756mL/kg; plasma protein binding (22-25%); found in breastmilk. **Metabolism:** Parahydroxyfelbamate, 2-hydroxyfelbamate, felbamatemonocarbamate (metabolites). **Elimination:** Urine (90%, 40-50% unchanged); $T_{1/2}$=20-23 hrs.

## NURSING CONSIDERATIONS

**Assessment:** Assess for history of blood dyscrasias or hepatic dysfunction, depression and suicidal thoughts/behavior. Assess renal function and pregnancy/nursing status prior to therapy. Obtain baseline CBC (reticulocytes, platelets) and LFTs.

**Monitoring:** Monitor for signs/symptoms of hepatic failure, aplastic anemia (signs of infection, bleeding, anemia), bone marrow depression and seizures. Monitor for emergence or worsening of depression, suicidal thoughts/behavior and any unusual changes in mood or behavior. Monitor renal function. Monitor LFTs and CBC (platelets, reticulocytes) while on therapy and following treatment.

**Patient Counseling:** If signs of aplastic anemia (infection, bleeding, anemia) or liver dysfunction (jaundice, anorexia, gastrointestinal complaints, and malaise) occur, advise to contact physician immediately. Advise not to abruptly d/c medication. Inform of risk for hematological/hepatic complications following d/c; continued monitoring of CBC and LFTs required. Notify physician if emergence or worsening of depression, suicidal thoughts/behavior and any unusual changes in mood or behavior occur. If pregnant, encourage to enroll in the North American Antiepileptic Drug (NAAED) Pregnancy Registry. Call 888-233-2334 or go to aedpregnancyregistry.org. Inform of the need to obtain written, informed consent prior to therapy.

**Administration:** Oral route. Shake oral suspension well before using. **Storage:** 20-25°C (68-77°F). Dispense in tight container.

# FEMARA RX

letrozole (Novartis)

**THERAPEUTIC CLASS:** Nonsteroidal aromatase inhibitor

**INDICATIONS:** Adjuvant treatment of postmenopausal women with hormone-receptor positive early breast cancer. Extended adjuvant treatment of early breast cancer in postmenopausal women who have received 5 yrs of adjuvant tamoxifen therapy. First line treatment of hormone-receptor positive or hormone-receptor unknown locally advanced or metastic breast cancer in postmenopausal women. Treatment of advanced breast cancer with disease progression following antiestrogen therapy in postmenopausal women.

**DOSAGE:** *Adults:* 2.5mg qd. In advanced disease, continue until tumor progression is evident. Cirrhosis/Severe Liver Dysfunction: 2.5mg qod.

**HOW SUPPLIED:** Tab: 2.5mg

**CONTRAINDICATIONS:** Women of premenopausal endocrine status.

**WARNINGS/PRECAUTIONS:** May cause fetal harm. May cause fatigue and dizziness; caution when driving or using machinery. May decrease lymphocyte counts. Thrombocytopenia reported. May elevate LFTs and total cholesterol. May decrease bone density; monitor bone mineral density. Reduce dose in cirrhosis and severe liver dysfunction.

**ADVERSE REACTIONS:** Hot flashes/flushes, asthenia, edema, arthralgia/arthritis, myalgia, back pain, headache, dizziness, night sweats, constipation, nausea, hypercholesterolemia, bone fractures, weight increased, fatigue.

**INTERACTIONS:** Plasma levels lowered with tamoxifen.

**PREGNANCY:** Category D, caution in nursing.

**MECHANISM OF ACTION:** Nonsteroidal aromatase inhibitor; inhibits conversion of androgens to estrogens. Competitively binds to the heme of cytochrome P450 subunit of the enzyme, resulting in a reduction of estrogen biosynthesis in all tissues.

**PHARMACOKINETICS: Absorption:** Rapid and complete (GI tract). **Distribution:** $V_d$=1.9L/kg; weakly protein bound. **Metabolism:** Liver via CYP450 isoenzymes: 3A4, 2A6. **Elimination:** Urine (90%, 6% unchanged); $T_{1/2}$=2 days.

## NURSING CONSIDERATIONS

**Assessment:** Assess for premenopausal endocrine status, hepatic impairment, baseline bone mineral density, pregnancy/nursing status, and for possible drug interactions.

**Monitoring:** Monitor for signs/symptoms of fatigue, dizziness, decreased lymphocytes, thrombocytopenia, cardiovascular complications, hot flashes, and second malignancies. Monitor LFTs and bone mineral density.

**Patient Counseling:** Advise about possible fatigue, dizziness, and somnolence. Caution against operating machinery/driving. Counsel about side effects; seek medical attention if any develop.

**Administration:** Oral route. **Storage:** 25°C (77°F); excursions permitted to 15-30°C (59-86°F).

# FENTORA

CII

fentanyl citrate (Cephalon)

**Serious adverse events, including deaths, reported. Substitution for any other fentanyl product may result in fatal overdose. Indicated only for the management of breakthrough pain in cancer patients who are already receiving and who are tolerant to around-the-clock opioid therapy for their underlying persistent cancer pain. Not indicated for opioid non-tolerant patients. Life-threatening respiratory depression may occur in opioid non-tolerant patients. Special care must be used when dosing. Do not convert on a mcg-per-mcg basis from Actiq to Fentora. Contains fentanyl, an opioid analgesic with abuse potential similiar to other opioid analgesics. Must be kept out of the reach of children. Use only by healthcare professionals knowledgeable and skilled in the use of Schedule II opioids to treat cancer pain. Concomitant use with strong and moderate P450 3A4 inhibitors may result in increased fentanyl plasma concentrations and may cause potentially fatal respiratory depression.**

**THERAPEUTIC CLASS:** Opioid analgesic

**INDICATIONS:** Management of breakthrough pain in patients with cancer who are already receiving and who are tolerant to around-the-clock opioid therapy for their underlying persistent cancer pain.

**DOSAGE:** *Adults*: Initial: Breakthrough Pain: 100mcg. Max: 2 doses per breakthrough pain episode. Titration Above 100mcg: Use two 100mcg tabs (one on each side of mouth in the buccal cavity) with next breakthrough pain episode. If unsuccessful, use two 100mcg tabs on each side of mouth in the buccal cavity (total of four 100mcg tabs). Titration Above 400mcg: Use 200mcg increments. Max: Not more than 4 tabs simultaneously. Maint: Once titrated to an effective dose, use only one tab of the appropriate strength per breakthrough pain episode. If breakthrough pain not relieved after 30 min, may take only one additional dose of the same strength. Wait at least 4 hrs before treating another breakthrough pain episode. Re-evaluate maintenance (around the clock) opioid dose if >4 episodes of breakthrough pain per day. Refer to PI for information on conversion of dosing from Actiq to Fentora.

**HOW SUPPLIED:** Tab, Buccal: 100mcg, 200mcg, 300mcg, 400mcg, 600mcg, 800mcg

**CONTRAINDICATIONS:** Opioid non-tolerant patients and management of acute or postoperative pain including headache/migraine.

**WARNINGS/PRECAUTIONS:** Monitor for signs of abuse and addiction; appropriate measures should be taken to limit the incidence of abuse (eg, proper assessment of patient, proper prescribing practices, periodic re-evaluation of therapy, proper dispensing and storage). May cause physical dependence, which results in withdrawal symptoms when abruptly d/c therapy. May cause respiratory depression; caution with underlying respiratory disorders (eg,

COPD), elderly, debilitated patients, and in patients predisposed to respiratory depression. May impair physical or mental abilities. Extreme caution in patients who may be susceptible to the intracranial effects of $CO_2$ retention (eg, evidence of increased intracranial pressure or impaired consciousness). May obscure clinical course of a head injury. Application-site reactions (eg, paresthesia, ulceration, bleeding) reported. Caution in patients with renal/hepatic impairment, bradyarrhythmias, bipolar disorder, schizophrenia, and those at risk for suicide.

**ADVERSE REACTIONS:** Respiratory depression, headache, N/V, constipation, dizziness, dyspnea, somnolence, fatigue, anemia, neutropenia, asthenia, abdominal pain, dehydration, peripheral edema, diarrhea.

**INTERACTIONS:** See Black Box Warning. Carefully monitor for an extended period of time, patients receiving concomitant therapy with strong CYP3A4 inhibitors (eg, ritonavir, ketoconazole, itraconazole, troleandomycin, clarithromycin, nelfinavir, nefazadone) or moderate CYP3A4 inhibitors (eg, amprenavir, aprepitant, diltiazem, erythromycin, fluconazole, fosamprenavir, verapamil). Avoid concomitant use with grapefruit or grapefruit juice. CYP3A4 inducers may produce the opposite effects of CYP3A4 inhibitors. Concomitant use with other CNS depressants, including other opioids, sedatives, hypnotics, general anesthetics, phenothiazines, tranquilizers, skeletal muscle relaxants, sedating antihistamines, potent inhibitors of CYP450 A4 isoform (eg, erythromycin, ketoconazole, certain protease inhibitors), and alcoholic beverages may produce increased depressant effects. Withdrawal may be precipitated through administration of drugs with opioid antagonist activity (eg, naloxone, nalmefene) or mixed agonist/antagonist analgesics (eg, pentazocine, butorphanol, buprenorphine, nalbuphine). Avoid use within 14 days of MAOIs.

**PREGNANCY:** Category C, not for use in nursing.

**MECHANISM OF ACTION:** Pure opioid agonist; produces analgesia. Precise analgesic action not established; known to be μ opioid receptor agonist. Specific CNS opioid receptors with opioid-like activity are found throughout the brain and spinal cord and play a role in producing analgesic effects.

**PHARMACOKINETICS: Absorption:** Readily absorbed. Absolute bioavailability (65%); (400mcg) $C_{max}$=1.02ng.mL, $T_{max}$=46.8 mins, $AUC_{0\text{-}inf}$=6.48ng•hr/mL. **Distribution:** $V_d$=25.4 L/kg; plasma protein binding (80-85%); found in breast milk, readily passes across the placenta. **Metabolism:** Liver and intestinal mucosa via CYP3A4; norfentanyl (metabolite). **Elimination:** Urine (<7% unchanged), feces (1% unchanged); $T_{1/2}$=2.63 hrs (100mcg, healthy subjects), 11.70 hrs (800mcg, healthy subjects).

## NURSING CONSIDERATIONS

**Assessment:** Assess for pain intensity, opioid tolerance, abuse potential, respiratory depression, respiratory disorders (eg, COPD), presence of increased intracranial pressure, impaired consciousness, bradyarrhythmias, renal/hepatic impairment, risk of suicide, bipolar disorder, schizophrenia, pregnancy/nursing status, and for possible drug interactions.

**Monitoring:** Monitor for signs/symptoms of respiratory depression, drug abuse, physical dependence, application-site reactions, bradycardia, and for suicidality.

**Patient Counseling:** Advise to notify physician if signs/symptoms of respiratory depression develop. Inform that medication must be kept out of reach of children; may be fatal to child. Instruct not to swallow whole; effectiveness will be decreased if swallowed whole. Advise to contact physician if breakthrough pain is not alleviated or worsens. Counsel to avoid using concomitant therapy with other CNS depressants including alcohol. Inform that may cause mental/physical impairment; instruct to use caution during hazardous tasks (eg, operating machinery/driving). Advise to avoid abrupt withdrawal. Inform that medication has potential for abuse. Counsel to dispose of unused medication via toilet. Instruct not to take for acute pain, post-operative pain, pain from injuries, headache, migraine or any other short-term pain. Instruct not to share medication with anyone else; sharing may result in other individual's death due to overdose. Counsel to not take more than prescribed. Instruct to notify physician if pregnant, planning to become pregnant or if nursing.

**Administration:** Oral route. Do not substitute for other fentanyl products. Do not open blister package until ready for use. Do not attempt to push tablet through blister card. 1) Place tablet in buccal cavity (above a rear molar, between the upper cheek and gum). Do not attempt to split tablet. 2) Do not suck, chew or swallow. 3) Leave tablet between cheek and gum until disintegrated. 4) After 30 min, swallow remnants with glass of water. **Storage:** 20-25°C (68-77°F); excursions permitted to 15-30°C (59-86°F). Protect from freezing and moisture. Do not use if blister package has been tampered with. Keep out of reach of children.

F

## FERRLECIT RX

sodium ferric gluconate complex (Sanofi-Aventis)

**THERAPEUTIC CLASS:** Hematinic

**INDICATIONS:** Treatment of iron deficiency anemia in patients ≥6 yrs undergoing chronic hemodialysis and receiving supplemental epoetin therapy.

**DOSAGE:** *Adults:* 10mL (125mg) diluted in 100mL of 0.9% NaCl IV infusion over 1 hr or undiluted at a rate of up to 12.5mg/min. Most patients will require a minimum cumulative dose of 1g of elemental iron administered over 8 sessions at sequential dialysis sessions to achieve a favorable Hgb or Hct response. Elderly: Start at the low end of dosing range.
*Pediatrics:* ≥6 yrs: 0.12mL/kg (1.5mg/kg) diluted in 25mL 0.9% NaCl IV infusion over 1 hr at 8 sequential dialysis sessions. Max: 125mg/dose.

**HOW SUPPLIED:** Inj: 62.5mg elemental iron/5mL

**CONTRAINDICATIONS:** Anemia not associated with iron deficiency. Evidence of iron overload.

**WARNINGS/PRECAUTIONS:** Hypersensitivity reactions and hypotension reported. Iron overload is more common in patients with hemoglobinopathies and other refractory anemias; avoid in patients with iron overload. May cause hypotension; usually resolved with 1 to 2 hours. Contains benzyl alcohol; avoid in neonates. Do not mix with other medications or add parenteral nutritional solutions for IV infusion.Caution in elderly.

**ADVERSE REACTIONS:** Injection-site reactions, chest pain, pain, asthenia, headache, abdominal pain, cramps, dizziness, dyspnea, hypotension, HTN, N/V, diarrhea, pruritus, abnormal erythrocytes.

**INTERACTIONS:** May reduce absorption of concomitantly administered oral iron. Concomitant use with ACE inhibitors may increase the incidence of drug intolerance and suspected allergic events.

**PREGNANCY:** Category B, caution in nursing.

**MECHANISM OF ACTION:** Hematinic; used to replete the total body content of iron, which is critical for normal Hgb synthesis to maintain oxygen transport.

**PHARMACOKINETICS: Absorption: Adults:** Parameters varied by different dosage. (62.5mg) AUC=17.5mg-h/L; (125mg) $C_{max}$=19mg/L; $T_{max}$=7 min; AUC=35.6mg-h/L. **Pediatrics:** (1.5mg/kg) $C_{max}$=12.9mg/L; AUC=95mg•h/L. (3mg/kg) $C_{max}$=22.8mg/L; AUC=170.9mg•h/L. **Distribution:** $V_d$=6L. **Elimination: Adults:** $T_{1/2}$=1 hr. **Pediatrics:** (1.5mg/kg) $T_{1/2}$=2 hrs; (3mg/kg) $T_{1/2}$=2.5 hrs.

### NURSING CONSIDERATIONS

**Assessment:** Assess for evidence of iron overload, type of anemia, hypersensity, pregnancy/nursing status, and for possible drug interactions.

**Monitoring:** Monitor for signs/symptoms of hypersensitivity reactions, iatrogenic hemosiderosis, and hypotension.

**Patient Counseling:** Advise to seek medical attention if symptoms of a hypersensitivity reaction, hypotension (light-headedness, malaise, fatigue, weakness), or if hemosiderosis occur.

**Administration:** IV route. Do not mix with other medications or add to parenteral nutrition solutions. If diluted in saline, use immediately after dilution.

**Storage:** 20-25°C (68-77°F); excursions permitted to 15-30° (59-86°F). Do not freeze.

## FIBRICOR

RX

fenofibric acid (AR Scientific)

**THERAPEUTIC CLASS:** Fibric acid derivative

**INDICATIONS:** Adjunctive therapy to diet for treatment of severe hypertriglyceridemia ( ≥500mg/dL). Adjunctive therapy to diet to reduce elevated LDL-C, Total-C, TG, and Apo B, and to increase HDL-C in patients with primary hypercholesterolemia or mixed dyslipidemia.

**DOSAGE:** *Adults:* Severe Hypertriglyceridemia: Individualize dose. Initial: 35-105mg/day. Titrate: May adjust dose if necessary following repeat lipid determinations at 4-8 week intervals. Max: 105mg/day. Primary Hyperlipidemia or Mixed Dyslipidemia: 105mg/day. Max: 105mg/day. Mild-to-Moderate Renal Impairment: Initial: 35mg/day. Titrate: May increase dose after evaluation of effects on renal function and lipid levels. Elderly: Base dose selection on renal function. Monitor serum lipids periodically during initiation to establish lowest effective dose. Reduce dose if lipid levels significantly falls below target range. D/C if no adequate response after 2 months of treatment at max dose.

**HOW SUPPLIED:** Tab: 35mg, 105mg

**CONTRAINDICATIONS:** Severe renal impairment (including dialysis), active liver disease (including primary biliary cirrhosis and unexplained persistent liver function abnormalities), pre-existing gallbladder disease, and nursing mothers.

**WARNINGS/PRECAUTIONS:** May cause increases in serum transaminases (eg, AST, ALT); chronic active hepatocellular and cholestatic hepatitis reported; monitor LFTs, and d/c therapy if enzyme levels >3x ULN. May cause cholelithiasis; d/c if gallstones found. Increased risk of myopathy and associated rhabdomyolysis in elderly, diabetes, renal failure, or hypothyroidism; d/c therapy if myopathy or marked CPK elevation occurs. Elevation of serum creatinine reported; monitor renal function in patients with renal impairment and those at risk for renal insuffiency (eg, elderly, diabetes). Acute hypersensitivity reactions (including Stevens-Johnson syndrome [SJS], toxic epidermal necrolysis [TEN]) and pancreatitis reported. Decreased Hgb, Hct, WBCs, thrombocytopenia, and agranulocytosis reported. Pulmonary embolus (PE) and deep vein thrombosis (DVT) observed. Caution in elderly. Ascertain lipid abnormality before therapy. Place patient on lipid lowering diet prior and during therapy.

**ADVERSE REACTIONS:** Abdominal pain, back pain, headache, abnormal liver tests, increased ALT, increased creatinine phosphokinase, increased AST, respiratory disorder.

**INTERACTIONS:** May potentiate anticoagulant effects of coumarin anticoagulants; monitor PT/INR. Bile acid binding resins may bind other drugs given concurrently; take at least 1 hr before or 4-6 hrs after the resin. May impair renal function with immunosuppressants (eg, cyclosporine, tacrolimus) and other potentially nephrotoxic agents; use lowest effective dose and monitor renal function. Increased risk of rhabdomyolysis with HMG-CoA reductase inhibitors (statin). May decrease levels with atorvastatin, pravastatin, fluvastatin, simvastatin, glimepiride, metformin. May increase levels with ezetimibe and rosiglitazone. May decrease levels of atorvastatin, simvastatin, rosiglitazone, efavirenz. May increase levels of pravastatin, fluvastatin, ezetimibe, glimepiride, metformin. D/C medications known to exacerbate hypertriglyceridemia (β-blockers, estrogens, thiazides) prior to therapy.

**PREGNANCY:** Category C, not for use in nursing.

**MECHANISM OF ACTION:** Fibric acid derivative; activates peroxisome proliferator activated receptor α (PPARα). This causes an increase in lipolysis and elimination of triglyceride-rich particles from plasma by activating lipoprotein lipase and reducing production of apoprotein C-III (an inhibitor of lipoprotein lipase activity). Activation of PPARα also induces an increase in the synthesis of apoproteins A-I, A-II, and HDL cholesterol.

**PHARMACOKINETICS: Absorption:** $T_{max}$=2.5 hrs. **Distribution:** Plasma protein binding (99%). **Metabolism:** Conjugation with glucuronic acid. **Elimination:** Urine; $T_{1/2}$=20 hrs.

## NURSING CONSIDERATIONS

**Assessment:** Assess for severe renal impairment, active liver disease (eg, primary biliary cirrhosis, unexplained liver function abnormality), diabetes, hypothyroidism, pre-existing gallbladder disease, pregnancy/nursing status, and possible drug interactions. Obtain baseline LFTs (including ALT/AST), renal function, and lipid levels.

F

**Monitoring:** Monitor for signs/symptoms of active liver disease, cholelithiasis, pancreatitis, hypersensitivity reactions (eg, SJS, TEN), hematological changes (eg, agranulocytosis, thrombocytopenia), PE, DVT, myopathies, rhabdomyolysis, PE, DVT. Perform periodic monitoring of liver function (including ALT/AST) and blood counts. Perform periodic monitoring of serum lipid levels. If myopathy suspected, obtain CPK levels.

**Patient Counseling:** Inform of the potential benefits and risks of the drug. Inform of the medications that should not be taken in combination with the drug. Instruct that it may be taken once daily, with/without food, at the prescribed dose. Recommend to continue/follow an appropriate lipid-modifying diet during therapy. Instruct to notify physician of all medications, supplements, and herbal preparations taken and any changes in medical conditions. Instruct to notify physician of any muscle pain, tenderness, or weakness, onset of abdominal pain or if any other new symptoms develop.

**Administration:** Oral route. **Storage:** 20-25°C (68-77°F).

# FINACEA — RX

azelaic acid (Intendis)

**THERAPEUTIC CLASS:** Dicarboxylic acid antimicrobial

**INDICATIONS:** Topical treatment of inflammatory papules and pustules of mild to moderate rosacea.

**DOSAGE:** *Adults:* Wash and dry skin. Massage thin layer into affected areas on the face bid (am and pm). Reassess if no improvement observed after completing 12 weeks of therapy.

**HOW SUPPLIED:** Gel: 15% [50g]

**CONTRAINDICATIONS:** Hypersensitivity to propylene glycol.

**WARNINGS/PRECAUTIONS:** For dermatological use only; avoid contact with mouth, eyes, other mucous membranes. Hypopigmentation reported; monitor for hypopigmentation in patients with dark complexion. D/C if sensitivity or severe irritation occurs. Use only very mild soap or soapless cleansing lotion for facial cleansing. Wash hands following application. Avoid foods and beverages (eg, spicy foods, alcohol, thermally hot drinks) that may provoke erythema, flushing, and/or blushing. Avoid use of occlusive dressings or wrappings.

**ADVERSE REACTIONS:** Burning, stinging, tingling, pruritus, scaling, tightness, dry skin.

**INTERACTIONS:** Avoid alcoholic cleansers, tinctures, astringents, abrasives and peeling agents.

**PREGNANCY:** Category B, caution in nursing.

**MECHANISM OF ACTION:** Dicarboxylic acid antimicrobial; not established.

**PHARMACOKINETICS: Metabolism:** Cutaneous metabolism (negligible); β-oxidation to shorter chain dicarboxylic acids. **Elimination:** Urine (mainly unchanged).

## NURSING CONSIDERATIONS

**Assessment:** Assess use in nursing patients. Assess for possible drug interactions. Reassess if no improvement observed after completing 12 weeks of therapy.

**Monitoring:** Monitor for signs and symptoms of hypopigmentation and for sensitivity reactions or skin irritation (eg, pruritus, burning, stinging).

**Patient Counseling:** Instruct that medication is for external use only; avoid contact with eyes, mouth, and other mucous membranes. Inform that if contact with eyes occurs, wash with large amounts of water; consult physician if eye irritation persists. Instruct to cleanse affected areas with mild soap or soapless cleansing lotion and pat dry before applying medication. Advise to wash hands following administration of medication. Instruct to avoid occlusive dressings or wrappings on treatment site. Inform that cosmetics can be applied to treatment area after medication has dried. Advise that skin irritation (eg, pruritus, burning, stinging) may occur during first few weeks of treatment; if worsening occurs or persists, instruct to d/c therapy and contact physician. Instruct to avoid any foods and beverages that may provoke erythema, flushing, and blushing (eg, spicy food, alcoholic beverages, thermally hot drinks). Instruct to contact physician if abnormal changes in skin color occur.

**Administration:** Topical administration. **Storage:** 25°C (77°F); excursions permitted to 15-30°C (59-86°F).

## FIORICET **RX**

acetaminophen - caffeine - butalbital (Watson)

**THERAPEUTIC CLASS:** Barbiturate/analgesic

**INDICATIONS:** Tension or muscle contraction headaches.

**DOSAGE:** *Adults:* 1-2 tabs q4h prn. Max: 6 tabs/day. Not for extended use. *Pediatrics:* ≥12 yrs: 1-2 tabs q4h prn. Max: 6 tabs/day. Not for extended use.

**HOW SUPPLIED:** Tab: (Butalbital-APAP-Caffeine) 50mg-325mg-40mg

**CONTRAINDICATIONS:** Porphyria.

**WARNINGS/PRECAUTIONS:** May be habit-forming. Not for long-term use. Caution in elderly, debilitated, severe renal or hepatic impairment, acute abdominal conditions. Caution in mentally depressed and those with suicidal tendencies, history of drug abuse.

**ADVERSE REACTIONS:** Drowsiness, lightheadedness, dizziness, sedation, SOB, N/V, abdominal pain, intoxicated feeling.

**INTERACTIONS:** Enhanced CNS effects with MAOIs. May enhance CNS depressant effects of other narcotic analgesics, alcohol, general anesthetics, tranquilizers, sedative hypnotics, or other CNS depressants.

**PREGNANCY:** Category C, not for use in nursing.

**MECHANISM OF ACTION:** Butalbital: Short- to intermediate-acting barbiturate. APAP: Nonopiate, nonsalicylate analgesic, antipyretic. Caffeine: CNS stimulant.

**PHARMACOKINETICS: Absorption:** Well absorbed (butalbital), rapid (APAP, caffeine). **Distribution:** Butalbital: Plasma protein binding (45%); found in breast milk; crosses placenta. Caffeine: Found in CNS, placenta, and breast milk. **Metabolism:** APAP: Liver (conjugation). Caffeine: Hepatic; 1-methylxanthine, 1-methyluric acid. **Elimination:** Butalbital: Urine (59-88% unchanged or metabolite); $T_{1/2}$=35 hrs. APAP: Urine (85% metabolite, unchanged); $T_{1/2}$=1.25-3 hrs. Caffeine: Urine 70% (3% unchanged); $T_{1/2}$=3 hrs.

### NURSING CONSIDERATIONS

**Assessment:** Assess for porphyria, elderly/debilitated patients, renal/hepatic impairment, acute abdominal condition, alcohol intake, and possible drug interactions (eg, MAOIs).

**Monitoring:** Monitor for drug abuse/dependence. Monitor LFTs , renal function, false (+) test for urinary 5-hydroxyindoleacetic acid.

**Patient Counseling:** Advise to use caution during hazardous tasks (eg, operating machinery/driving). Instruct not to take with alcohol/other CNS depressants. Advise to take as directed. Inform drug may be habit-forming. Instruct to notify physician if pregnant/nursing.

**Administration:** Oral route. **Storage:** 30°C (86°F); tight container.

## FIORICET WITH CODEINE

CIII

codeine phosphate - acetaminophen - caffeine - butalbital (Watson)

**THERAPEUTIC CLASS:** Barbiturate/analgesic

**INDICATIONS:** Tension or muscle contraction headaches.

**DOSAGE:** *Adults:* 1-2 caps q4h prn. Max: 6 caps/day. Not for extended use.

**HOW SUPPLIED:** Cap: (Butalbital-APAP-Caffeine-Codeine) 50mg-325mg-40mg-30mg

F

**CONTRAINDICATIONS:** Porphyria.

**WARNINGS/PRECAUTIONS:** May be habit-forming. Not for extended use. Respiratory depression and CSF pressure enhanced with head injury or intracranial lesions. Caution in elderly, debilitated, severe renal or hepatic impairment, hypothyroidism, urethral stricture, Addison's disease, BPH, and history of drug abuse. May mask signs of acute abdominal conditions.

**ADVERSE REACTIONS:** Drowsiness, lightheadedness, dizziness, sedation, SOB, N/V, abdominal pain, intoxicated feeling.

**INTERACTIONS:** Enhanced CNS effects with MAOIs. May enhance CNS depressant effects of other narcotic analgesics, alcohol, general anesthetics, tranquilizers, sedative hypnotics, or other CNS depressants.

**PREGNANCY:** Category C, not for use in nursing.

**MECHANISM OF ACTION:** Codeine: Narcotic analgesic and antitussive. Butalbital: Short- to intermediate-acting barbiturate. Caffeine: CNS stimulant. APAP: Nonopiate, nonsalicylate analgesic and antipyretic. The role each component plays in relief of complex of symptoms known as tension headache is incompletely understood.

**PHARMACOKINETICS: Absorption:** Butalbital: Well absorbed. Codeine, caffeine, acetaminophen: Rapid. **Distribution:** Codeine: Crosses blood-brain barrier, found in fetal tissue, breast milk. Butalbital: Plasma protein binding (45%); found in breast milk; crosses placental barrier. Caffeine: Found in fetal tissue, CNS, breast milk. **Metabolism:** Caffeine: Hepatic biotransformation to 1-methylxanthine, 1-methyluric acid. APAP: Liver (conjugation). **Elimination:** Codeine: Urine (90%), feces; $T_{1/2}$=2.9 hrs. Butalbital: Urine (59-88% unchanged or metabolites); $T_{1/2}$=35 hrs. Caffeine: Urine (70%, only 3% unchanged); $T_{1/2}$=3 hrs. APAP: Urine (85% unchanged, conjugates); $T_{1/2}$=1.25-3 hrs.

### NURSING CONSIDERATIONS

**Assessment:** Assess for porphyria, renal/hepatic impairment, head injuries or other intracranial lesions, elevated intracranial pressure, acute abdominal conditions, elderly/debilitated patients, hypothyroidism, urethral stricture, Addison's disease, prostatic hypertrophy, pregnancy/nursing status, alcohol intake, individual with ultra-rapid metabolizers, and possible drug interactions.

**Monitoring:** Serial monitoring of LFTs, renal function. Monitor serum amylase levels, false (+) test results for urinary 5-hydroxyindoleacetic acid, drug abuse/dependence, CSF, and signs of CNS depression (eg, drowsiness, confusion, or shallow breathing).

**Patient Counseling:** Advise to use caution during hazardous tasks (eg, driving/operating machinery). Instruct not to take with other CNS depressants or alcohol. Advise to take as prescribed. Instruct to notify physician if pregnant/nursing or planning to become pregnant. Counsel that drug may be habit-forming.

**Administration:** Oral route. **Storage**: 30°C (86°F); tight container.

## FIORINAL

CIII

caffeine - aspirin - butalbital (Watson)

**THERAPEUTIC CLASS:** Barbiturate/analgesic

**INDICATIONS:** Tension or muscle contraction headache.

**DOSAGE:** *Adults:* 1-2 caps q4h prn. Max: 6 caps/day. Not for extended use.

**HOW SUPPLIED:** Cap: (Butalbital-ASA-Caffeine) 50mg-325mg-40mg

**CONTRAINDICATIONS:** Porphyria, peptic ulcer disease, serious GI lesions, hemorrhagic diathesis. Syndrome of nasal polyps, angioedema, and bronchospastic reactivity to ASA or NSAIDs.

**WARNINGS/PRECAUTIONS:** May be habit-forming. Not for extended use. Caution in elderly, debilitated, severe renal or hepatic impairment, hypothyroidism, urethral stricture, head injuries, elevated ICP, acute abdominal conditions, Addison's disease, prostatic hypertrophy, peptic ulcer, coagulation disorders. Avoid with ASA allergy. Risk of ASA hypersensitivity with nasal polyps and asthma. Caution in children with chickenpox or flu. Preoperative ASA may prolong bleeding time.

**ADVERSE REACTIONS:** Drowsiness, lightheadedness, dizziness, sedation, nausea, vomiting, flatulence.

**INTERACTIONS:** CNS effects enhanced by MAOIs. Additive CNS depression with alcohol, other narcotic analgesics, general anesthetics, tranquilizers (eg, chloral hydrate), sedatives/hypnotics, other CNS depressants. May enhance effects of anticoagulants. May cause hypoglycemia with oral antidiabetic agents and insulin. May cause bone marrow toxicity and blood dyscrasias with 6-MP and methotrexate. Increased risk of peptic ulceration and bleeding with NSAIDs. Decreased effects of uricosuric agents (eg, probenecid, sulfinpyrazone). Withdrawal of corticosteroids may cause salicylism with chronic ASA use.

**PREGNANCY:** Category C, not for use in nursing.

**MECHANISM OF ACTION:** Combines analgesic properties of ASA with anxiolytic and muscle relaxant properties of butalbital.

**PHARMACOKINETICS: Absorption:** ASA: $T_{max}$=40 min, $C_{max}$=8.8mcg/mL. Butalbital: Well-absorbed; $C_{max}$=202ng/mL, $T_{max}$=1.5 hrs. Caffeine: Rapid; $C_{max}$=1660ng/mL, $T_{max} \leq$1 hr. **Distribution:** ASA: Found in fetal tissue, breast milk, CNS; Plasma protein binding (50-80%). Butalbital: Crosses placenta, found in breast milk; Plasma protein binding (45%). Caffeine: Found in placenta, breast milk, CNS. **Metabolism:** ASA: Liver; salicyluric acid, phenolic/acyl glucuronides of salicylate, and gentisic and gentisuric acid (major metabolites). Caffeine: Liver; 1-methylxanthine and 1-methyluric acid (metabolites). **Elimination:** ASA: Urine; $T_{1/2}$=12 min (ASA), 3 hrs (salicylic acid/total salicylates). Butalbital: Urine (59-88%); $T_{1/2}$=35 hrs. Caffeine: Urine 70% (3% unchanged); $T_{1/2}$=3 hrs.

## NURSING CONSIDERATIONS

**Assessment:** Assess for hemorrhagic diathesis (eg, hemophilia, hypoprothrombinemia, von Willebrand's disease, thrombocytopenia, thrombasthenia and other ill-defined hereditary platelet dysfunctions, severe vitamin K deficiency and severe liver damage), syndrome of nasal polyps, angioedema and bronchospastic reactivity to aspirin and other NSAIDs, peptic ulcer, asthma, porphyria, renal/hepatic impairment, children with chickenpox or flu, head injuries, hypothyroidism, urethral stricture, elevated ICP, acute abdominal conditions, Addison's disease, prostatic hypertrophy, pregnancy/nursing status, and possible drug interactions.

**Monitoring:** Serial monitoring of LFTs and renal function. Monitor for anaphylactoid reactions, drug abuse/dependence, bleeding, prolongation of bleeding time, PT, urinary (glucose, 5-hydroxyindoleactic acid, Gerhardt ketone, VMA, uric acid, diacetic acid, spectrophotometric detection of barbiturates), Reye's syndrome, serum amylase, FBG, cholesterol, protein, and uric acid.

**Patient Counseling:** Advise not to take with ASA allergy. Instruct to take exactly as prescribed; do not take with alcohol or other CNS depressants. Advise to use caution during hazardous tasks (eg, operating machinery/driving). Counsel that drug may be habit-forming. Advise to notify physician if pregnant, nursing, or planning to become pregnant.

**Administration:** Oral route. **Storage:** 77°F (25°C); tight container.

# FIORINAL WITH CODEINE

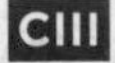

codeine phosphate - caffeine - aspirin - butalbital (Watson)

F

**OTHER BRAND NAMES:** Ascomp with Codeine (Breckenridge)

**THERAPEUTIC CLASS:** Barbiturate/analgesic

**INDICATIONS:** Tension or muscle contraction headache.

**DOSAGE:** *Adults:* 1-2 caps q4h prn. Max: 6 caps/day. Not for extended use.

**HOW SUPPLIED:** Cap: (Butalbital-ASA-Caffeine-Codeine) 50mg-325mg-40mg-30mg

**CONTRAINDICATIONS:** Porphyria, peptic ulcer disease, serious GI lesions, hemorrhagic diathesis. Syndrome of nasal polyps, angioedema and bronchospastic reactivity to ASA or NSAIDs.

**WARNINGS/PRECAUTIONS:** May be habit-forming. Not for extended use. Respiratory depression and CSF pressure may be enhanced with head injury or intracranial lesions. Caution in elderly, debilitated, severe renal or hepatic impairment, hypothyroidism, urethral stricture, head injuries, elevated ICP, acute abdominal conditions, Addison's disease, prostatic hypertrophy, peptic ulcer, coagulation disorders. Caution in children with chickenpox or flu. May obscure acute abdominal conditions. Preoperative ASA may prolong bleeding time. Avoid with ASA allergy. Risk of ASA hypersensitivity with nasal polyps and asthma.

**ADVERSE REACTIONS:** Drowsiness, lightheadedness, dizziness, sedation, SOB, N/V, abdominal pain, intoxicated feeling.

**INTERACTIONS:** CNS effects enhanced by MAOIs. Additive CNS depression with alcohol, other narcotic analgesics, general anesthetics, tranquilizers (eg, chloral hydrate), sedatives/hypnotics, other CNS depressants. May enhance effects of anticoagulants. May cause hypoglycemia with oral antidiabetic agents, insulin. May cause bone marrow toxicity, blood dyscrasias with 6-MP and methotrexate. Increased risk of peptic ulceration, bleeding with NSAIDs. Decreased effects of uricosuric agents (eg, probenecid, sulfinpyrazone). Withdrawal of corticosteroids may cause salicylism with chronic ASA use.

**PREGNANCY:** Category C, not for use in nursing.

**MECHANISM OF ACTION:** Butalbital: Short to intermediate acting barbiturate. ASA: Analgesic, antipyretic, and anti-inflammatory. Caffeine: Stimulates CNS. Codeine: Narcotic analgesic and antitussive. Role each component plays in relief of complex of symptoms known as tension headache is incompletely understood.

**PHARMACOKINETICS: Absorption:** Codeine: Rapid; $C_{max}$=198ng/mL, $T_{max}$=1 hr. Butalbital: Well-absorbed; $C_{max}$=2020ng/mL, $T_{max}$=1.5 hrs. Caffeine: Rapid; $C_{max}$=1660ng/mL, $T_{max}$≤1 hr. **Distribution:** ASA: Plasma protein binding (50-80%); found in fetal tissue, breast milk, CNS. Codeine: Crosses BBB, placenta, and breast milk. Butalbital: Plasma protein binding (45%); crosses placenta and breast milk. Caffeine: Fetal tissue, breast milk and CNS. **Metabolism:** ASA: Liver; salicyluric acid, phenolic/acyl glucuronides of salicylate, and gentisic and gentisuric acid (major metabolites). Codeine: Glucuronidation. Caffeine: Liver; 1-methylxanthine and 1-methyluric acid. **Elimination:** ASA: Urine; $T_{1/2}$=12 min (ASA), 3 hrs (salicylic acid/total salicylate). Codeine: Urine (90%), feces; $T_{1/2}$=2.9 hrs. Butalbital: Urine (59-88%); $T_{1/2}$=35 hrs. Caffeine: Urine 70% (3% unchanged); $T_{1/2}$=3 hrs.

## NURSING CONSIDERATIONS

**Assessment:** Assess for hemorrhagic diathesis (eg, hemophilia, hypoprothrombinemia, von Willebrand's disease, thrombocytopenia, thrombasthenia and other ill-defined hereditary platelet dysfunctions, severe vitamin K deficiency and severe liver damage), anticoagulant therapy, asthma, syndrome of nasal polyps, angioedema and bronchospastic reactivity to NSAIDs, peptic ulcer, porphyria, renal/hepatic impairment, hypothyroidism, urethral stricture, head injuries, elevated ICP, acute abdominal conditions, Addison's disease, prostatic hypertrophy, pregnancy/nursing status, children with chickenpox or flu, individuals with ultra-rapid metabolizers, alcohol intake, and possible drug interactions.

**Monitoring:** Serial monitoring of LFTs, renal function tests. Monitor for anaphylactoid reactions, symptoms of CNS depression (eg, drowsiness, confusion, shallow breathing), drug abuse/dependence, bleeding, prolongation of bleeding time, PT, urinary (glucose, 5-hydroxyindoleactic acid, Gerhardt ketone, VMA, uric acid, diacetic acid, spectrophotometric detection of barbiturates), Reye's syndrome, serum amylase, FBG, cholesterol, protein.

**Patient Counseling:** Advise not to take if patient has aspirin allergy. Take as prescribed; do not take with alcohol or other CNS depressants. Caution during hazardous tasks (eg, operating machinery/driving). Potential psychological dependence and for abuse. Notify if pregnant/nursing or planning to become pregnant. Inform about risks/benefits and to report any adverse reactions to physician.

**Administration:** Oral route. **Storage:** <25°C (77°F); tight container.

F

## FLAGYL RX

metronidazole (G.D. Searle)

**Metronidazole has been shown to be carcinogenic in mice and rats. Unnecessary use of the drug should be avoided.**

**THERAPEUTIC CLASS:** Nitroimidazole

**INDICATIONS:** Treatment of symptomatic/asymptomatic trichomoniasis, asymptomatic consorts, acute intestinal amebiasis, amebic liver abscess, and anaerobic bacterial infections (following IV metronidazole therapy for serious infections) caused by susceptible strains of microorganisms. Treatment of intra-abdominal, skin and skin structure, bone/joint, CNS, lower respiratory tract, and gynecologic infections, septicemia, and endocarditis caused by susceptible strains of microorganisms.

**DOSAGE:** *Adults:* Trichomoniasis (Female/Male Sex Partner): Seven-Day Treatment: (Cap/Tab) 375mg bid or 250mg tid for 7 days. One-Day Therapy: (Tab) 2g as single dose or in two divided doses of 1g each given in the same day. If repeat course needed, reconfirm diagnosis and allow 4-6 weeks between courses. Acute Intestinal Amebiasis: 750mg PO tid for 5-10 days. Amebic Liver Abscess: 500mg or 750mg PO tid for 5-10 days. Anaerobic Bacterial Infection: Usually IV therapy initially if serious. 7.5mg/kg PO q6h for 7-10 days or longer. Max: 4g/24 hrs. Elderly: Adjust dose based on serum levels. Hepatic Disease: Give lower dose cautiously; monitor levels.
*Pediatrics:* Amebiasis: 35-50mg/kg/24 hrs given tid for 10 days.

**HOW SUPPLIED:** Cap: 375mg; Tab: 250mg, 500mg

**CONTRAINDICATIONS:** Treatment during 1st trimester of pregnancy.

**WARNINGS/PRECAUTIONS:** Seizures and peripheral neuropathy reported. D/C if abnormal neurological signs occur. Caution with severe hepatic impairment, blood dyscrasias, or CNS diseases. Monitor leukocytes before and after therapy.

**ADVERSE REACTIONS:** Seizures, peripheral neuropathy, NV, headache, anorexia, urticaria, rash, metallic taste, dysuria, vaginal candidiasis, dizziness, leukopenia.

**INTERACTIONS:** Avoid alcohol during and for 3 days after use. Avoid within 2 weeks of disulfiram use; increased possibility of psychotic reactions. May potentiate anticoagulant effects of warfarin; monitor PT. Increased elimination with phenytoin, phenobarbital and other hepatic enzyme inducers. May impair phenytoin clearance. Potentiated by cimetidine and other hepatic enzyme inhibitors. May increase lithium levels.

**PREGNANCY:** Category B, not for use in nursing.

**MECHANISM OF ACTION:** Nitroimidazole antibacterial; exerts effect in anaerobic environment. Possesses bactericidal, amebicidal, and trichomonacidal activity.

**PHARMACOKINETICS: Absorption:** (PO) Well absorbed. PO administration of variable doses resulted in different parameters. **Distribution:** Plasma protein binding (<20%); excreted in breast milk. **Metabolism:** Side-chain oxidation and glucuronide conjugation. **Elimination:** Urine (60-80%), feces (6-15%); $T_{1/2}$=8 hrs.

## NURSING CONSIDERATIONS

**Assessment:** Assess for history of convulsions, peripheral neuropathy, candidiasis, renal function tests, LFTs, pregnancy status, and possible drug interactions.

**Monitoring:** Monitor CBC with differential count, LFTs, seizures, hypersensitivity reactions, peripheral neuropathy, candidiasis.



**Patient Counseling:** Instruct to avoid alcohol during therapy and for at least 3 days afterward. Counsel to take as directed and to complete entire prescription. Take with food to reduce GI upset; may cause metallic taste. Exercise caution while driving or operating machinery. During treatment for trichomoniasis, treat partner also and use condoms to prevent reinfection.

**Administration:** Oral route. **Storage:** Below 25°C (77°F). Protect from light.

# FLAGYL ER — RX

metronidazole (Pharmacia & Upjohn)

**Metronidazole has been shown to be carcinogenic in mice and rats. Unnecessary use of the drug should be avoided.**

**THERAPEUTIC CLASS:** Nitroimidazole

**INDICATIONS:** Treatment of bacterial vaginosis.

**DOSAGE:** *Adults:* 750mg qd for 7 days. Take 1 hr before or 2 hrs after meals. Elderly: Adjust dose based on serum levels. Hepatic Disease: Give lower dose cautiously; monitor levels.

**HOW SUPPLIED:** Tab, Extended-Release: 750mg

**CONTRAINDICATIONS:** Treatment during 1st trimester of pregnancy.

**WARNINGS/PRECAUTIONS:** Seizures and peripheral neuropathy reported. D/C if abnormal neurological signs occur. Caution with severe hepatic impairment, blood dyscrasias, or CNS diseases. Monitor leukocytes before and after therapy.

**ADVERSE REACTIONS:** Headache, vaginitis, NV, metallic taste, dizziness, seizures, peripheral neuropathy, leukopenia, urticaria, rash, dysuria, vaginal candidiasis.

**INTERACTIONS:** Avoid alcohol during and for 3 days after use. Avoid within 2 weeks of disulfiram; increased possibility of psychotic reactions. Potentiates anticoagulant effects of warfarin; monitor PT. Increased elimination with phenytoin, phenobarbital. May impair phenytoin clearance. Potentiated by cimetidine. Increased lithium levels.

**PREGNANCY:** Category B, not for use in nursing.

**MECHANISM OF ACTION:** Nitroimidazole antibacterial; exerts effect in anaerobic environment. Possesses bactericidal, amebicidal, and trichomonacidal activity.

**PHARMACOKINETICS: Absorption:** $C_{max}$=19.4µg/mL (fed), 12.5µg/mL (fasting); $T_{max}$=4 hrs (fed), 6.8 hrs (fasting); AUC=211µg/mL (fed), 198µg/mL (fasting). **Distribution:** Plasma protein binding (<20%). **Metabolism:** Side-chain oxidation and glucuronide conjugation. **Elimination:** Urine (60-80%), feces (6-15%); $T_{1/2}$=8 hrs.

## NURSING CONSIDERATIONS

**Assessment:** Assess for history of convulsions, peripheral neuropathy, candidiasis, hepatic/renal function, pregnancy status, and possible drug interactions.

**Monitoring:** Monitor CBC with differential, LFTs, seizures, hypersensitivity reactions, peripheral neuropathy, candidial proliferation.

**Patient Counseling:** Inform to avoid alcohol during therapy and for at least 3 days after. Counsel to take as directed and complete entire prescription. Take with food to reduce GI upset; may cause metallic taste. Exercise caution while driving or operating machinery. During treatment for trichomoniasis, treat partner also and use condoms to prevent reinfection.

**Administration:** Oral route. **Storage:** Dry place at 25°C (77°F); excursions permitted to 15-86°C (59-86°F). Dispense in a well-closed container.

## FLAGYL IV

metronidazole (Baxter)

RX



**Metronidazole has been shown to be carcinogenic in mice and rats. Use should be reserved only for conditions for which it is indicated.**

**THERAPEUTIC CLASS:** Nitroimidazole

**INDICATIONS:** Treatment of serious infections caused by susceptible anaerobic bacteria. Treatment of intra-abdominal, skin and skin structure, gynecologic, bone and joint, CNS, and lower respiratory tract infections caused by susceptible microorganisms; also treatment of bacterial septicemia and endocarditis caused by susceptible microorganisms. Prophylaxis of postoperative infection in contaminated or potentially contaminated colorectal surgery. Effective against *B. fragilis* infections resistant to clindamycin, chloramphenicol, and PCN.

**DOSAGE:** *Adults:* Anaerobic Infections: LD: 15mg/kg IV (infused over 1 hr). Maint: 7.5mg/kg IV (infused over 1 hr) q6h, starting 6 hrs after LD. Usual duration: 7-10 days, or longer. Max: 4g/24 hrs. Surgical Prophylaxis: 15mg/kg IV (infused over 30-60 min) given 1 hr before surgery, then 7.5mg/kg IV (infused over 30-60 min) given 6 hrs and 12 hrs after initial dose. Whole of initial infusion must be completed, approximately 1 hr before surgery.

**HOW SUPPLIED:** Inj: 500mg [100mL]

**WARNINGS/PRECAUTIONS:** Encephalopathy (associated with cerebellar toxicity and CNS lesions on MRI), peripheral neuropathy, convulsive seizures, aseptic meningitis reported; evaluate benefit/risk ratio of therapy if abnormal neurologic signs/symptoms occur. Caution with severe hepatic impairment, presence or history of blood dyscrasias, and in patients predisposed to edema. Sodium retention may occur due to $Na^+$ in solution. Monitor leukocytes before and after therapy. Candidiasis may present with more prominent symptoms; treat with candicidal agents. May interfere with serum chemistry values (eg, AST, ALT, LDH, triglycerides, hexokinase glucose). Do not use in absence of proven or strongly suspected infection due to susceptible organisms.

**ADVERSE REACTIONS:** Convulsive seizures, encephalopathy, aseptic meningitis, optic neuropathy, peripheral neuropathy (characterized by numbness/paresthesia of an extremity), N/V, diarrhea, leukopenia, erythematous rash, pruritus, fever, headache, syncope, Stevens-Johnson syndrome, thrombophlebitis.

**INTERACTIONS:** Avoid alcoholic beverages during therapy. Avoid within 2 weeks of disulfiram; increased possibility of psychotic reactions. Potentiates warfarin and other oral coumarin anticoagulants. Increased elimination with microsomal liver enzyme inducers (eg, phenytoin, phenobarbital). May impair phenytoin clearance. May prolong the half-life and decrease plasma clearance with microsomal liver enzyme inhibitors (eg, cimetidine). Caution with corticosteroids.

**PREGNANCY:** Category B, not for use in nursing.

**MECHANISM OF ACTION:** Nitroimidazole antibacterial; exerts effect in anaerobic environment. Possesses bactericidal, amebicidal, and trichomonacidal activity.

**PHARMACOKINETICS: Distribution:** Plasma protein binding (<20%); found in CSF, saliva and breast milk. **Metabolism:** Liver, via side-chain oxidation and glucuronide conjugation; 1-(β-hydroxyethyl)-2-hydroxymethyl-5-nitroimidazole and 2-methyl-5-nitroimidazole-1-yl-acetic acid (metabolites). **Elimination:** Urine (60-80%), feces (6-15%); $T_{1/2}$=8 hrs.

## NURSING CONSIDERATIONS

**Assessment:** Assess for evidence or history of a blood dyscrasia, hepatic impairment, predisposition to edema, pregnancy/nursing status, and for possible drug interactions. Obtain baseline LFTs and leukocyte count.

**Monitoring:** Monitor for signs/symptoms of encephalopathy, peripheral neuropathy, convulsive seizures, aseptic meningitis, and for candidiasis. Monitor LFTs and leukocyte counts.

**Patient Counseling:** Inform that drug treats bacterial infections, not viral infections. Instruct to take as directed and to not skip doses. Advise to report any symptoms of CNS toxicity or other adverse side effects.



**Administration:** IV route; via slow infusion. **Storage:** 15-30°C (59-86°F). Protect from light. Do not remove unit from overwrap until ready for use.

# FLEXERIL — RX

cyclobenzaprine HCl (McNeil Consumer)

**THERAPEUTIC CLASS:** Skeletal muscle relaxant (central-acting)

**INDICATIONS:** Relief of muscle spasm associated with acute, painful musculoskeletal conditions.

**DOSAGE:** *Adults:* Usual: 5mg tid. Titrate: May increase to 10mg tid. Mild Hepatic Dysfunction/Elderly: Initial: 5mg qd, then slowly increase. Moderate/Severe Hepatic Dysfunction: Avoid use. Treatment should not exceed 2-3 weeks.
*Pediatrics:* ≥15 yrs: Usual: 5mg tid. Titrate: May increase to 10mg tid. Mild Hepatic Dysfunction/Elderly: Initial: 5mg qd, then slowly increase. Moderate/Severe Hepatic Dysfunction: Avoid use. Treatment should not exceed 2-3 weeks.

**HOW SUPPLIED:** Tab: 5mg, 10mg

**CONTRAINDICATIONS:** Acute recovery phase of MI, arrhythmias, heart block or conduction disturbances, CHF, hyperthyroidism, MAOI use during or within 14 days.

**WARNINGS/PRECAUTIONS:** Caution with history of urinary retention, angle-closure glaucoma, increased IOP, hepatic dysfunction. Caution in elderly due to increased risk of CNS effects. May produce arrhythmias, sinus tachycardia and conduction time prolongation. May impair mental/physical abilities.

**ADVERSE REACTIONS:** Drowsiness, dry mouth, headache, fatigue.

**INTERACTIONS:** Enhances effects of alcohol, barbiturates, and other CNS depressants. May block antihypertensive action of guanethidine and similar compounds. May enhance seizure risk with tramadol. Contraindicated with MAOIs. Caution with anticholinergic medication.

**PREGNANCY:** Category B, caution in nursing.

**MECHANISM OF ACTION:** Centrally acting skeletal muscle relaxant; relieves skeletal muscle spasm of local origin without interfering with muscle function; reduces tonic somatic motor activity by influencing both gamma and α motor systems.

**PHARMACOKINETICS: Absorption**: Oral bioavailability (33-55%); $C_{max}$=25.9ng/mL; AUC=177ng•hr/mL. **Metabolism**: Extensive; through N-demethylation pathway. Via CYP3A4, 1A2, and 2D6. **Elimination**: Urine (glucuronides); $T_{1/2}$=18 hrs.

## NURSING CONSIDERATIONS

**Assessment:** Assess for hepatic impairment, seizures, hyperthyroidism, urinary retention, angle-closure glaucoma, IOP, recent MI, arrhythmias, heart block, CHF, alcohol intake, pregnancy/nursing status, and possible drug interactions (eg, MAOIs if concomitant use or within 14 days after d/c, and anticholinergic medications).

**Monitoring:** Monitor for cardiac arrhythmias, sinus tachycardia, MI, increased seizure risk, stroke, IOP, CBC, and LFTs.

**Patient Counseling:** Caution while performing hazardous tasks (eg, operating machinery/driving). Avoid alcohol or other CNS depressants. Notify if pregnant/nursing.

**Administration:** Oral route. **Storage**: 25°C (77°F); excursions permitted to 15-30°C (59-86°F).

## FLOMAX — RX

tamsulosin HCl (Boehringer Ingelheim/Astellas Pharma)



**THERAPEUTIC CLASS:** $\text{Alpha}_{1a}$-antagonist

**INDICATIONS:** Treatment of signs and symptoms of benign prostatic hyperplasia (BPH).

**DOSAGE:** *Adults:* Initial: 0.4mg qd, 30 min after same meal each day. Titrate: May increase to 0.8mg qd after 2-4 weeks. If therapy is interrupted, restart with 0.4mg qd.

**HOW SUPPLIED:** Cap: 0.4mg

**WARNINGS/PRECAUTIONS:** Screen for presence of prostate cancer prior to treatment and at regular intervals afterward. Orthostasis/syncope may occur. May cause priapism (rare). Intraoperative floppy iris syndrome (IFIS) has been observed during cataract surgery. Use with caution if sulfa allergy present. Not for use in treatment of HTN.

**ADVERSE REACTIONS:** Headache, dizziness, somnolence, diarrhea, asthenia, back pain, pharyngitis, rhinitis, abnormal ejaculation, chest pain, cough increased.

**INTERACTIONS:** Avoid use with other α-adrenergic blockers. Decreased clearance with cimetidine; caution with concomitant use, especially with doses higher than 0.4mg. Caution with warfarin. Avoid doses >0.4mg in combination with strong inhibitors of CYP3A4 (eg, ketoconazole); may increase plasma exposure. Caution in combination with moderate inhibitors of CYP3A4 (eg, erythromycin) in combination with strong (eg, paroxetine) or moderate (eg, terbinafine) inhibitors of CYP2D6 and known poor metabolizers of CYP2D6; avoid use with doses higher than 0.4mg. Caution with PDE5 inhibitors; may cause symptomatic hypotension.

**PREGNANCY:** Category B, not for use in nursing.

**MECHANISM OF ACTION:** $\alpha_{1A}$ antagonist; selective blockade of $\alpha_1$ receptors in the prostate result in relaxation of the smooth muscles of the bladder neck and prostate.

**PHARMACOKINETICS: Absorption:** Complete. (0.4mg) (light breakfast) $C_{max}$=10.1ng/mL, $T_{max}$=6 hrs, AUC=151ng•hr/mL; (fasting) $C_{max}$=17.1ng/mL, $T_{max}$=4 hrs, AUC=199ng•hr/mL . (0.8mg) (light breakfast) $C_{max}$=29.8ng/mL, $T_{max}$=7 hrs, AUC=440ng•hr/mL; (high-fat meal) $C_{max}$=29.1ng/mL, $T_{max}$=6.6 hrs, AUC=449ng•hr/mL; (fasting) $C_{max}$=41.6ng/mL, $T_{max}$=5 hrs, AUC=557ng•hr/mL. **Distribution:** (IV) $V_d$=16L, plasma protein binding (94-99%). **Metabolism:** Liver; CYP3A4, CYP2D6. **Elimination:** Urine (76%;<10% unchanged), feces (21%); $T_{1/2}$=9-13 hrs (healthy), 14-15 hrs.

### NURSING CONSIDERATIONS

**Assessment:** Assess for BPH, sulfa allergy, pregnancy/nursing status, and possible drug interactions. Rule out prostate cancer.

**Monitoring:** Monitor for signs/symptoms of orthostasis, priapism, IFIS, and allergic reactions.

**Patient Counseling:** Advise about possible occurrence of symptoms related to postural hypotension; caution may impair physical/mental abilities. Avoid situations where injury could result if syncope occurs. Take as prescribed. Do not crush, chew, or open capsule. Advise if considering cataract surgery to inform ophthalmologist of drug use. Advise about the possibility of priapism and to seek immediate medical attention if this occurs.

**Administration:** Oral route. **Storage:** 25°C (77°F); excursions permitted to 15-30°C (59-86°F).

## FLONASE RX

fluticasone propionate (GlaxoSmithKline)

**THERAPEUTIC CLASS:** Corticosteroid

**INDICATIONS:** Management of the nasal symptoms of seasonal and perennial allergic rhinitis, and nonallergic rhinitis.

**DOSAGE:** *Adults:* Initial: 2 sprays per nostril qd or 1 spray per nostril bid. Maint: 1 spray per nostril qd. May dose as 2 sprays per nostril qd as needed for seasonal allergic rhinitis.

F

*Pediatrics:* ≥4 yrs: Initial: 1 sprays per nostril qd. If inadequate response, may increase to 2 sprays per nostril. Maint: 1 spray per nostril qd. Max: 2 sprays per nostril/day. ≥12 yrs: May dose as 2 sprays per nostril qd as needed for seasonal allergic rhinitis.

**HOW SUPPLIED:** Spray: 50mcg/spray [16g]

**WARNINGS/PRECAUTIONS:** Risk of adrenal insufficiency and withdrawal symptoms when replacing systemic corticosteroids with topical corticosteroids. Caution with active or quiescent TB, ocular herpes simplex, or untreated bacterial, fungal and systemic viral infections. Avoid with recent nasal trauma, surgery or septum ulcers. Risk for more severe/fatal course of infections (eg, chickenpox, measles); avoid exposure in patients who have not had disease or been properly immunized. *Candida* infection of nose and pharynx reported (rare). Potential for reduced growth velocity in pediatrics. Excessive use may cause signs of hypercorticism or HPA suppression.

**ADVERSE REACTIONS:** Headache, pharyngitis, epistaxis, nasal burning/irritation, asthma symptoms, nausea/vomiting, cough.

**INTERACTIONS:** Caution with ketoconazole or other potent CYP3A4 inhibitors, may increase serum fluticasone levels. Concomitant inhaled corticosteroids increase risk of hypercorticism and/or HPA axis suppression. Increased levels with ritonavir; avoid use.

**PREGNANCY:** Category C, caution in nursing.

**MECHANISM OF ACTION:** Glucocorticosteroid; not established. Acts as anti-inflammatory agent with wide range of effects on multiple cell types (eg, mast cells, eosinophils, macrophages, and lymphocytes) and mediators (eg, histamine, eicosanoids, leukotrienes, and cytokines) involved in inflammation.

**PHARMACOKINETICS: Absorption:** Absolute bioavailability (<2%), $C_{max}$=50pg/mL.

### NURSING CONSIDERATIONS

**Assessment:** Assess for drug hypersensitivity, active or quiescent TB, untreated localized or systemic infections (eg, fungal, bacterial, systemic viral, parasitic), ocular herpes simplex, history of recent nasal septal ulcers, nasal surgery/trauma, concomitant use with other inhaled or systemic corticosteroids, and possible drug interactions.

**Monitoring:** Monitor acute adrenal insufficiency, hypercorticism and/or HPA-axis suppression, disseminated infections, chickenpox and measles, nasal or pharyngeal *Candida* infections, supression of growth velocity in children, hypersensitivity reactions or contact dermatitis, wheezing, nasal septum perforation, cataracts, glaucoma, and increased IOP.

**Patient Counseling:** Instruct to take as directed at regular intervals and to avoid exposure to chickenpox or measles and, consult physician immediately if exposed. Do not spray into eyes.

**Administration:** Intranasal route. **Storage:** 4-30°C (39-86°F).

## FLOVENT DISKUS RX

fluticasone propionate (GlaxoSmithKline)

**THERAPEUTIC CLASS:** Corticosteroid

**INDICATIONS:** Maintenance treatment of asthma as prophylactic therapy in patients ≥4 years and for patients requiring oral corticosteroid therapy for asthma.

**DOSAGE:** *Adults ( ≥12yrs):* Previous Bronchodilator Only: Initial: 100mcg bid. Max: 500mcg bid. Previous Inhaled Corticosteroid: Initial: 100-250mcg bid. Max: 500mcg bid. Previous Oral Corticosteroid: Initial: 500-1000mcg bid. Max: 1000mcg bid. Reduce PO prednisone no faster than 2.5mg/day weekly, beginning at least 1 week after starting fluticasone. Starting dosages >100mcg bid may be considered for patients with poorer asthma control or previous high-dose inhaled corticosteroid requirement.
*Pediatrics:* 4-11 yrs: Previous Bronchodilators Only: Initial: 50mcg bid. Max: 100mcg bid. Previous Inhaled Corticosteroid: Initial: 50mcg bid. Max: 100mcg bid. Reduce PO prednisone no faster than 2.5mg/day weekly, beginning at least 1 week after starting fluticasone. Starting dosages >50mcg bid may be considered for patients with poorer asthma control or previous high-dose inhaled corticosteroid requirement.

F

**HOW SUPPLIED:** Disk: 50mcg/inh, 100mcg/inh, 250mcg/inh [60 blisters]

**CONTRAINDICATIONS:** Primary treatment of status asthmaticus or other acute episodes of asthma.

**WARNINGS/PRECAUTIONS:** Deaths may occur due to adrenal insufficiency with transfer from systemic corticosteroids to inhaled corticosteroid. Resume oral corticosteroids during stress or severe asthma attack. Wean slowly from systemic corticosteroid therapy. Observe signs and symptoms of adrenal insufficiency (eg, fatigue, lassitude, weakness, nausea, vomiting, hypotension), systemic corticosteroid effects (eg, hypercorticism, adrenal suppression, adrenal crisis), reduction of growth rate in pediatric patients. Transfer from systemic corticosteroid therapy may unmask conditions previously suppressed (eg, rhinitis, conjunctivitis, eczema, arthritis, eosinophilic conditions). May increase susceptibility to infections (eg, chicken pox, measles). Avoid in acute bronchospasm. D/C and treat with fast-acting bronchodilator if bronchospasm occurs. Caution with tuberculosis, untreated systemic fungal, bacterial, viral, parasitic infection, ocular herpes simplex. *Candida albicans* infection of the pharynx reported. Glaucoma, increased intraocular pressure, and cataracts reported. Rare cases of eosinophilic conditions seen.

**ADVERSE REACTIONS:** Upper respiratory tract infection, throat irritation, headache, sinusitis/sinus infection, N/V, fever, rhinitis, GI discomfort and pain, viral GI infection, lower respiratory infection, cough, musculoskeletal pain.

**INTERACTIONS:** May increase levels and reduce serum cortisol levels with ritonavir; avoid concomitant use. Caution with ketoconazole and other CYP3A4 inhibitors; may increase levels and reduce plasma cortisol AUC.

**PREGNANCY:** Category C, not for use in nursing.

**MECHANISM OF ACTION:** Synthetic trifluorinated corticosteroid; potent anti-inflammatory activity, inhibits multiple cell types and mediates production or secretion involved in asthmatic response.

**PHARMACOKINETICS: Absorption:** Acts locally in lung, systemic bioavailability (18%); $C_{max}$=110pg/mL (500mg bid). **Distribution:** (IV) $V_d$=4.2 L/kg; plasma protein binding (91%). **Metabolism:** Liver via CYP3A4. **Elimination:** (IV) Feces, urine (≤5%); $T_{1/2}$=7.8 hrs.

## NURSING CONSIDERATIONS

**Assessment:** Assess for lung function, primary treatment of status asthmaticus or other acute asthma attacks, adrenal insufficiency in patients changing from systemic corticosteroids to inhaled corticosteroids, systemic corticosteroid therapy effects (eg, rhinitis, conjunctivitis, eczema, arthritis, eosinophilic conditions), reduction of growth rate in pediatric patients, infections, pregnancy/nursing status, and possible drug interactions. Assess for hepatic disease.

**Monitoring:** Monitor respiratory status and lung sounds, airflow changes, signs and symptoms of adrenal insufficiency, systemic corticosteroid effects, growth rate in pediatric patients, development of infections, hypersensitivity reactions. Patients with hepatic disease should be closely monitored for drug accumulation in the plasma.

**Patient Counseling:** Instruct to use Flovent Diskus at regular intervals as directed. Inform not to exceed recommended dose. Instruct not to use with a spacer device. Notify physician in patients who are pregnant or nursing. Inform to avoid exposure to chicken pox or measles; if exposed, seek medical consultation immediately. Instruct to read Patient's Instructions for proper use. Do not take the device apart.

**Administration:** Oral inhalation. **Storage:** 20°-25°C (68°-77°F). Protect from moisture, heat, and light. Device is not reusable. Discard diskus in 6 weeks (50mcg) or 2 months (100mcg and 250mcg) after removal from moisture-protective foil pouch or after all blisters have been used.

F

# FLOVENT HFA RX

## fluticasone propionate (GlaxoSmithKline)

**THERAPEUTIC CLASS:** Corticosteroid

**INDICATIONS:** Maintenance treatment of asthma as prophylactic therapy in patients ≥4 years; to reduce or eliminate the need for oral corticosteroidal therapy.

**DOSAGE:** *Adults:* Previous Bronchodilator Only: Initial: 88mcg bid. Max: 440mcg bid. Previous Inhaled Corticosteroids: Initial: 88-220mcg bid. Max: 440mcg bid. Previous Oral Corticosteroids: Initial: 440mcg bid. Max: 880mcg bid. Reduce PO prednisone no faster than 2.5 to 5mg/day weekly, beginning at least 1 week after starting fluticasone. Rinse mouth after use.
*Pediatrics:* ≥12 yrs: Previous Bronchodilator Only: Initial: 88mcg bid. Max: 440mcg bid. Previous Inhaled Corticosteroids: Initial: 88-220mcg bid. Max: 440mcg bid. Previous Oral Corticosteroids: Initial: 440mcg bid. Max: 880mcg bid. 4-11 yrs: Initial/Max: 88mcg bid. Reduce PO prednisone no faster than 2.5 to 5mg/day weekly, beginning at least 1 week after starting fluticasone. Rinse mouth after use.

**HOW SUPPLIED:** MDI: 44mcg/inh [10.6g], 110mcg/inh [12g], 220mcg/inh [12g]

**CONTRAINDICATIONS:** Primary treatment of status asthmaticus or other acute asthma attacks.

**WARNINGS/PRECAUTIONS:** Deaths due to adrenal insufficiency have occurred with transfer from systemic corticosteroids to inhaled corticosteroids. Resume oral corticosteroids during stress or severe asthma attack. Wean slowly from systemic corticosteroid therapy. Observe for adrenal insufficiency, systemic corticosteroid withdrawal effects, hypercorticism, adrenal suppression (including adrenal crisis), reduction in growth velocity (children and adolescents). May increase susceptibility to infections. Not for acute bronchospasm. D/C if bronchospasm occurs after dosing. Caution with TB of respiratory tract; untreated systemic fungal, bacterial, viral or parasitic infections; or ocular herpes simplex. *Candida* infection of mouth and pharynx reported. Glaucoma, increased IOP and cataracts reported. Rare cases of eosinophilic conditions.

**ADVERSE REACTIONS:** Upper respiratory tract infection, headache, throat irritation, sinusitis/sinus infection, candidiasis (mouth/throat and non-site specific), and cough.

**INTERACTIONS:** Increased levels with ritonavir; avoid use. Caution with ketoconazole and other potent CYP3A4 inhibitors; may increase serum fluticasone levels and reduced plasma cortisol AUC.

**PREGNANCY:** Category C, caution in nursing.

**MECHANISM OF ACTION:** Synthetic trifluorinated corticosteroid; possesses potent anti-inflammatory activity and inhibits multiple cell types involved in asthmatic response.

**PHARMACOKINETICS: Absorption:** Acts locally in lung. **Distribution:** $V_d$=4.2 L/kg; plasma protein binding (99%). **Metabolism:** Liver via CYP3A4. **Elimination:** Feces (primary), urine (<5%); $T_{1/2}$=7.8 hrs.

## NURSING CONSIDERATIONS

**Assessment:** Assess for primary treatment of status asthmaticus or other acute asthma attacks, lung function, adrenal insufficiency (eg, anorexia, nausea, weakness, fatigue, hypotension, hypoglycemia) in patients changing from systemic corticosteroids to inhaled corticosteroids, during initial therapy, and during times of stress.

**Monitoring:** Monitor respiratory status and lung sounds, withdrawal symptoms (eg, joint/muscular pain, lassitude, depression) during withdrawal from oral corticosteroids, growth rate in children, serum and urine glucose concentrations, adrenal function tests to assess degree of hypothalamic-pituitary-adrenal axis suppression in chronic therapy, and eosinophilic conditions.

**Patient Counseling:** Counsel patients to use drugs at regular intervals as directed. Notify physician if pregnant or intend to become pregnant, and nursing. Avoid exposure to chickenpox or measles and should consult physician immediately once exposed. Technique for administering drug to children should be similar to adult.

**Administration:** 1) Prime inhaler before using for first time by releasing 4 test sprays into air, away from face, shaking well for 5 seconds before each spray. If inhaler has not been used for >7 days, or when it has been dropped, prime inhaler again by shaking well before each spray and releasing 2 test sprays into air, away from face. 2) After inhalation, rinse mouth with water and spit out; do not swallow. Clean inhaler at least once a week after evening dose. Use only with actuator supplied with product. 3) Discard inhaler after 120 sprays have been used. **Storage:** 25°C (77°F); excursions permitted to 15-30°C (59-86°F). Store inhaler with mouthpiece down.

# FLOXIN RX

ofloxacin (Ortho-McNeil)

**Fluoroquinolones are associated with an increased risk of tendinitis and tendon rupture in all ages. Risk further increased in patients >60 yrs, patients taking corticosteroid drugs, and patients with kidney, heart or lung transplants.**

**THERAPEUTIC CLASS:** Fluoroquinolone

**INDICATIONS:** Treatment of complicated urinary tract infections (UTI), uncomplicated skin and skin structure infections (SSSI), acute bacterial exacerbation of chronic bronchitis (ABECB), community-acquired pneumonia (CAP), acute uncomplicated urethral and cervical gonorrhea, nongonococcal urethritis and cervicitis, mixed infections of urethra and cervix, acute pelvic inflammatory disease (PID), uncomplicated cystitis, and prostatitis caused by susceptible strains of microorganisms.

**DOSAGE:** *Adults:* ≥18 yrs: ABECB/CAP/SSSI: 400mg q12h for 10 days. Cervicitis/Urethritis: 300mg q12h for 7 days. Gonorrhea: 400mg single dose. PID: 400mg q12h for 10-14 days. Uncomplicated Cystitis: 200mg q12h for 3 days (*E.coli* or *K.pneumoniae*) or 7 days (other pathogens). Complicated UTI: 200mg q12h for 10 days. Prostatitis: *(E.coli)* 300mg q12h for 6 weeks. CrCl 20-50mL/min: Dose q24h. CrCl <20mL/min: After regular initial dose, give 50% of normal dose q24h. Severe Hepatic Impairment: Max: 400mg/day.

**HOW SUPPLIED:** Tab: 200mg, 300mg, 400mg

**WARNINGS/PRECAUTIONS:** Convulsions, increased ICP, toxic psychosis, CNS stimulation, and serious, sometimes fatal, hypersensitivity reactions reported; d/c if any occur. *Clostridium difficile*-associated diarrhea (CDAD) and ruptures of shoulder, hand, and Achilles tendon reported. Not shown to be effective for syphilis. Safety and efficacy unknown in patients <18 yrs old, pregnancy, and nursing. Maintain adequate hydration. Caution with renal or hepatic dysfunction, risk for seizures, CNS disorder with predisposition to seizures. Avoid excessive sunlight. Monitor blood, renal and hepatic function with prolonged therapy. Tendon ruptures reported. D/C immediately at the first appearance of skin rash, jaundice, or any other sign of hypersensitivity and supportive measures instituted. Drug therapy should be d/c if photosensitivity/phototoxicity occurs. Medications should be avoided in patients with known prolongation of the QT interval, patients with uncorrected hypokalemia, and patients receiving Class IA (quinidine, procainamide), or Class III (amiodarone, sotalol) antiarrhythmic agents. Caution in elderly taking corticosteroids.

**ADVERSE REACTIONS:** NV, insomnia, headache, dizziness, diarrhea, external genital pruritus in women, vaginitis.

**INTERACTIONS:** Decreased absorption with antacids, sucralfate, multivitamins, zinc, didanosine; separate dosing by 2 hrs. NSAIDs may increase risk of seizures. May potentiate theophylline, warfarin. May potentiate insulin, oral hypoglycemics; d/c if hypoglycemia occurs. May increase half-life of drugs metabolized by CYP450. Severe tendon disorder risks are increased with concomitant corticosteroid therapy.



**PREGNANCY:** Category C, not for use in nursing.

**MECHANISM OF ACTION:** Fluoroquinolone; synthetic broad-spectrum antimicrobial agent; inhibits topoisomerase II (DNA gyrase) and topoisomerase IV, which are required for bacterial DNA replication, transcription, repair, and recombination.

**PHARMACOKINETICS: Absorption:** Oral administration of variable doses resulted in different parameters; $T_{max}$=1-2 hrs; bioavailability (98%). **Elimination:** Biphasic ($T_{1/2}$=4-5 hrs, 20-25 hrs), renal.

## NURSING CONSIDERATIONS

**Assessment:** Assess renal function, LFTs, pregnancy/nursing status, history of seizures, QTc prolongation, and possible drug interactions.

**Monitoring:** Monitor for QTc prolongation, hematologic manifestations, glucosuria, hematuria, pulmonary edema, hypo/hyperglycemia, cardiac arrest, seizure, status epilepticus, respiratory arrest, CDAD, renal function, LFTs, CBC, tendon rupture, peripheral neuropathy, hypersensitivity reactions (toxic epidermal necrolysis, Stevens-Johnson syndrome).

**Patient Counseling:** Notify healthcare provider if symptoms of pain, swelling, or inflammation of a tendon, or weakness or inability to move joints; rest and refrain from excercise; and d/c therapy. Inform that drug treats bacterial, not viral, infections. Take exactly as directed; skipping doses or not completing full course may decrease effectiveness and increase resistance. Inform about potential benefits/risks. D/C and notify physician if skin rash, other allergic reaction, and watery and bloody stools (with or without stomach cramps, and fever) occur. Use caution in activities requiring mental alertness and coordination. Advise diabetic patients to use caution; hypoglycemia may develop during therapy. Inform to take with or without meals, and to drink fluids. Avoid sun exposure. Take full course as prescribed.

**Administration:** Oral route. **Storage**: 25°C (77°F), excursions permitted to 15-30°C (59-86°F).

# Floxin Otic — RX

ofloxacin (Daiichi Sankyo)

**OTHER BRAND NAMES:** Floxin Otic Singles (Daiichi Sankyo)

**THERAPEUTIC CLASS:** Fluoroquinolone

**INDICATIONS:** Otitis externa in patients ≥6 months. Chronic suppurative otitis media in patients ≥12 yrs with perforated tympanic membranes. Acute otitis media in patients ≥1 yr with tympanostomy tubes.

**DOSAGE:** *Adults:* Otitis Externa: 10 drops or 2 single-dispensing containers (SDCs) once daily for 7 days. Chronic Suppurative Otitis Media with Perforated Tympanic Membrane: 10 drops or 2 SDCs bid for 14 days. *Pediatrics:* Otitis Externa: 6 mos-13 yrs: 5 drops or 1 single-dispensing container (SDC) once daily for 7 days. ≥13 yrs: 10 drops or 2 SDCs once daily for 7 days. Chronic Suppurative Otitis Media with Perforated Tympanic Membrane: ≥12 yrs: 10 drops or 2 SDCs bid for 14 days. Acute Otitis Media with Tympanostomy Tubes: 1-12 yrs: 5 drops or 1 SDC bid for 10 days.

**HOW SUPPLIED:** Sol: 0.3% [5mL, 10mL], (Singles) 0.3% [20[s]]

**WARNINGS/PRECAUTIONS:** D/C if hypersensitivity reaction occurs. Re-evaluate if no improvement after one week.

**ADVERSE REACTIONS:** Pruritus, application site reaction, taste perversion.

**PREGNANCY:** Category C, not for use in nursing.

**MECHANISM OF ACTION:** Fluoroquinilone; exerts antibacterial activity; inhibits DNA gyrase (a bacterial topoisomerase), an essential enzyme which controls DNA topology and assists in DNA replication, repair, deactivation, and transcription.

**PHARMACOKINETICS: Absorption:** Perforated tympanic membrane; $C_{max}$=10ng/ml.

## NURSING CONSIDERATIONS

**Assessment:** Assess for drug hypersensitivity, pre-existing cholesteatoma, foreign body or tumor.

**Monitoring:** Monitor for anaphylactic reactions, cardiovascular collapse, loss of consciousness, angioedema, airway obstruction, dyspnea, urticaria and itching, overgrowth of non-susceptible organisms (fungi), erosions or lesions of cartilage of weight-bearing joints, signs of arthropathy, and for improvment/persistence of otorrhea.

**Patient Counseling:** Counsel to avoid touching applicator tip to fingers or other surfaces to avoid contamination. D/C and contact physician if signs of allergy occur. Not for ophthalmic use, nor for injection.

**Administration:** Otic route. Warm bottle by holding for 1-2 min, to avoid dizziness. **Storage:** 25°C (77°F); excursions permitted to 15-30°C (59-86°F).

# FLUARIX RX

influenza virus vaccine (GlaxoSmithKline)

**THERAPEUTIC CLASS:** Vaccine

**INDICATIONS:** Active immunization in persons ≥3 yrs for prevention of disease caused by influenza virus subtypes A and type B contained in the vaccine.

**DOSAGE:** *Adults:* 0.5mL IM as a single dose.
*Pediatrics:* 3-<9 yrs: Unvaccinated or vaccinated for first time last season with only 1 dose: Two 0.5mL IM doses, each 0.5mL dose should be administered at least 4 weeks apart. Vaccinated with 2 doses: 0.5mL IM as 1 dose. ≥9 yrs: 0.5mL IM as 1 dose.

**HOW SUPPLIED:** Inj: (Syringe) 0.5mL

**CONTRAINDICATIONS:** Hypersenstivity reactions to egg proteins or life-threatening reaction to previous administration of any influenza vaccine.

**WARNINGS/PRECAUTIONS:** Not for intradermal, IV or SQ administration. Do not inject in gluteal area or areas with major nerve trunk. Caution if Guillain-Barre syndrome has occurred within 6 weeks of receipt of prior influenza vaccine. Caution in patients with bleeding disorders (eg, hemophilia). Contains latex; may cause allergic reactions in latex-sensitive individuals. Immunosuppressed patients may have a lower immune response. Medical treatment and supervision must be available to manage possible anaphylactic reactions. May not protect all susceptible individuals.

**ADVERSE REACTIONS:** Local reaction (pain, redness, swelling), muscle aches, fatigue, headache, arthralgia, shivering, irritability, loss of appetite, drowsiness, fever.

**INTERACTIONS:** Caution with anticoagulants. Immunosuppressive therapies (eg, irradiation, antimetabolites, alkylating agents, cytotoxic drugs, corticosteroids [used in greater than physiological doses]) may reduce immune response to influenza virus vaccine. Do not mix with any other vaccine in the same syringe or vial.

**PREGNANCY:** Category B, caution in nursing.

**MECHANISM OF ACTION:** Vaccine; elicits the formation of antibodies that may protect against influenza virus subtypes A and B.

## NURSING CONSIDERATIONS

**Assessment:** Assess for hypersensitivity to egg proteins, hypersensitivity to latex, presence of immunosuppression, immunization history, bleeding disorders (eg, hemophilia), pregnancy/nursing status, and for possible drug interactions. Assess potential benefits and risks if Guillain-Barre syndrome occurred with previous influenza vaccination.

**Monitoring:** Monitor for allergic reactions, local injection-site reactions (eg, pain, redness, swelling), and for general adverse events (eg, headache, fatigue, muscle aches, arthralgia, fever).

F

**Patient Counseling:** Inform of potential benefits and risks of immunization. Counsel about potential adverse reactions. Instruct that vaccine contains noninfectious killed viruses and it cannot cause influenza. Advise that vaccine is intended to provide protection against illness due to influenza viruses only and cannot provide protection against all respiratory illnesses. Instruct to report any adverse events to healthcare provider. Inform that annual revaccination is recommended.

**Administration:** IM route; inject into deltoid muscle of upper arm. **Storage:** 2-8°C (36-46°F). Do not freeze. Discard if frozen. Store in original container and protect from light.

# FLUDROCORTISONE — RX

fludrocortisone acetate (Various)

**THERAPEUTIC CLASS:** Corticosteroid

**INDICATIONS:** Partial replacement therapy for adrenocortical insufficiency in Addison's disease. Treatment of salt-losing adrenogenital syndrome.

**DOSAGE:** *Adults:* Addison's Disease: Usual: 0.1mg/day with concomitant cortisone 10-37.5mg/day or hydrocortisone 10-30mg/day in divided doses. Dose Range: 0.1mg 3 times weekly to 0.2mg/day. If HTN develops, reduce to 0.05mg/day. Salt-Losing Adrenogenital Syndrome: 0.1-0.2mg/day.

**HOW SUPPLIED:** Tab: 0.1mg* *scored

**CONTRAINDICATIONS:** Systemic fungal infections.

**WARNINGS/PRECAUTIONS:** May increase dose before, during, and after stressful situations. Caution with hypothyroidism, cirrhosis, ocular herpes simplex, HTN, ulcerative colitis, diverticulitis, peptic ulcer, osteoporosis, myasthenia gravis, renal impairment, and elderly. May mask signs of infection or cause new infection. Avoid exposure to chickenpox or measles. Marked effect on sodium retention; monitor electrolytes. May need salt restriction and potassium supplements. Monitor for psychic disturbances. Risk of glaucoma, cataracts, and eye infections. Avoid abrupt withdrawal.

**ADVERSE REACTIONS:** HTN, CHF, edema, convulsions, hypokalemia, hypokalemic alkalosis, muscle weakness, impaired wound healing, menstrual irregularities, cataracts, suppression of growth, hyperglycemia, HPA-suppression, acne, rash.

**INTERACTIONS:** Decreases serum salicylate levels. Enhanced hypokalemia with amphotericin B and potassium-depleting diuretics (eg, furosemide, ethacrynic acid). Increased risk of digitalis toxicity and arrhythmias with hypokalemia. Decreased effects with rifampin, barbiturates, and hydantoins. Monitor PT with oral anticoagulants. Decreases effects of oral hypoglycemics, insulin. Enhanced edema with other anabolic steroids (eg, oxymethalone, norethandrolone). Adjust dose with initiation or termination of estrogen. Avoid live virus vaccines (including smallpox) and other immunizations. Caution with ASA.

**PREGNANCY:** Category C, caution in nursing.

**MECHANISM OF ACTION:** Synthetic adrenocortical steroid; acts on electrolyte balance and carbohydrate metabolism and on distal tubules of kidney to enhance reabsorption of sodium ions from tubular fluid into the plasma. Increases urinary excretion of both $K^+$ and hydrogen ions.

**PHARMACOKINETICS: Distribution**: Found in breast milk. **Metabolism:** Liver. **Elimination**: $T_{1/2}$=3.5 hrs (Plasma), 18-36 hr (Biological).

## NURSING CONSIDERATIONS

**Assessment:** Assess for hypersensitivity reactions to drug, systemic fungal infections, other current infections, active TB, vaccination, HTN, heart disease, renal/hepatic impairment, unusual stress, psychotic tendencies, thyroid function, hypoprothrombinemia, osteoporosis, myasthenia gravis, peptic ulcers with/without impending perforation, fresh intestinal anastomosis, diverticulitis/ulcerative colitis and possible drug/lab test interactions (eg, nitrobluetetrazolium test for bacterial infection).

**Monitoring:** Monitor for occurrence of infections, edema, weight gain, psychic derangement, cataracts, and frequent measuring of serum electrolytes, TSH, LFTs, glucose, IOP, and BP.

**Patient Counseling:** Inform drug increases susceptibility to infections. Instruct to avoid exposure to chickenpox or measles. Counsel to carry supply of medication for emergency use. Advise on the importance of regular follow-up visits and to use medication exactly as directed. Advise to notify physician of dizziness, severe or continuing headaches, swelling of feet or lower legs, or unusual weight gain. Not to be used while nursing.

**Administration:** Oral route. **Storage**: 15-30°C (59-86°F).

# FluLaval — RX

influenza virus vaccine (GlaxoSmithKline)

**THERAPEUTIC CLASS:** Vaccine

**INDICATIONS:** Active immunization of adults ( ≥18 yrs) against influenza disease caused by influenza virus subtypes A and type B contained in the vaccine.

**DOSAGE:** *Adults:* ≥18 yrs: 0.5mL IM in deltoid muscle.

**HOW SUPPLIED:** Inj: 15mcg/0.5mL [5mL]

**CONTRAINDICATIONS:** Hypersenstivity reactions to egg proteins (eg, eggs, egg products), chicken proteins, or life-threatening reaction to previous administration of any influenza vaccine.

**WARNINGS/PRECAUTIONS:** Do not administer IV, intradermal or SQ. Caution if Guillain-Barre syndrome has occurred within 6 weeks of receiving prior influenza vaccine. Caution with bleeding disorders (eg, hemophilia) or concomitant anticoagulants. May reduce immune response in immunocompromised. May not protect all susceptible individuals.

**ADVERSE REACTIONS:** Pain, redness, and/or swelling at injection site, headache, fatigue, myalgia, low-grade fever, malaise, sore throat, reddened eyes, cough, chills, chest tightness, and facial swelling.

**INTERACTIONS:** Do not mix with any other vaccine in same syringe or vial; administer other vaccines at different injection sites. Potential interaction with warfarin, theophylline, phenytoin. Immunosuppressive therapies (eg, irradiation, antimetabolites, alkylating agents, cytotoxic drugs, corticosteroids used in greater than physiologic doses) may reduce effectiveness. Caution with anticoagulants.

**PREGNANCY:** Category C, caution in nursing.

**MECHANISM OF ACTION:** Vaccine; elicits the formation of antibodies that may protect against influenza virus subtypes A and B.

## NURSING CONSIDERATIONS

**Assessment:** Assess immune status, possible drug interactions, known hypersensitivity reactions to egg and chicken proteins, bleeding, or current anticoagulation therapy. Assess potential benefits and risks if Guillain-Barre syndrome occurred with previous influenza vaccination.

**Monitoring:** Monitor hypersensitivity reactions, local injection-site reactions (eg, pain, redness, swelling), systemic adverse events (eg, headache, fatigue, myalgia, low-grade fever, malaise), bleeding tendencies.

**Patient Counseling:** Inform recipients and caregivers that vaccine provides protection against illness due to influenza viruses only and not against all respiratory diseases. Advise that annual revaccination is recommended. Instruct to report any severe or unusual adverse reactions. Give patient the Vaccine Information Statements.

**Administration:** IM. Administer at the deltoid muscle of the upper arm. Use ≥1-inch needle length. **Storage:** 2-8°C (36-46°F). Do not freeze. Store in package to protect from light. Discard vial after 28 days once entered.



## FLUMIST RX

influenza virus vaccine live (MedImmune)

**THERAPEUTIC CLASS:** Vaccine

**INDICATIONS:** Active immunization of individuals 2-49 yrs of age against influenza disease caused by influenza virus subtypes A and type B contained in the vaccine.

**DOSAGE:** *Adults:* ≤49 yrs: One 0.2mL (0.1mL per nostril) dose.
*Pediatrics:* ≥9 yrs: One 0.2mL (0.1mL per nostril) dose. 2-8 yrs: Not Previously Vaccinated With Influenza Vaccine: 0.2mL (0.1mL per nostril) for 2 doses at least 1 month apart. Previously Vaccinated With Influenza Vaccine: One 0.2mL (0.1mL per nostril) dose.

**HOW SUPPLIED:** Nasal Spray: 0.2mL [10s]

**CONTRAINDICATIONS:** Parenteral use. Hypersensitivity to eggs or egg products, gentamicin, gelatin, arginine. Children and adolescents 5-17 yrs of age receiving ASA or ASA-containing therapy.

**WARNINGS/PRECAUTIONS:** Avoid with history of asthma, active wheezing or children <5 yrs of age with recurrent wheezing. Have epinephrine available. Caution in individuals if Guillain-Barre syndrome has occurred within 6 weeks of any prior influenza vaccination, immunocompromised persons and those with underlying medical conditions predisposing to influenza complications.

**ADVERSE REACTIONS:** Runny nose, congestion, cough, irritability, headache, sore throat, fever, chills, muscle aches, vomiting, tiredness/weakness.

**INTERACTIONS:** See Contraindications. Avoid concurrent use with other vaccines and within 48 hrs after cessation of antiviral therapy; antiviral agents until 2 weeks after vaccination unless medically indicated; ASA or ASA-containing products in children and adolescents 5-17 yrs.

**PREGNANCY:** Category C, caution in nursing.

**MECHANISM OF ACTION:** Stimulates the immune system to produce antibodies (influenza-specific T cells) that may protect against influenza virus infection.

### NURSING CONSIDERATIONS

**Assessment:** Assess immune and current health status, history of asthma/recurrent wheezing, sensitivity to influenza vaccine, and possible drug interactions.

**Monitoring:** Monitor for anaphylactic reaction, wheezing, runny nose, fever, headache, myalagia, irritability, insomnia, otitis media, and GI or respiratory infections.

**Patient Counseling:** Inform patient or caregivers of benefits/risks. Report adverse reactions to physician. Inform that annual influenza vaccination is recommended.

**Administration:** Intranasal. **Storage:** 2-8°C (35-46°F). Do not freeze.

# FLUOCINOLONE ACETONIDE RX

fluocinolone acetonide (Various)

**THERAPEUTIC CLASS:** Corticosteroid

**INDICATIONS:** Relief of inflammatory and pruritic manifestations of corticosteroid-responsive dermatoses.

**DOSAGE:** *Adults:* Apply as a thin film to the affected area(s) tid-qid. May use occlusive dressing for psoriasis or recalcitrant conditions; d/c dressing if infection develops.
*Pediatrics:* Apply as a thin film to the affected area(s) tid-qid. May use occlusive dressing for psoriasis or recalcitrant conditions; d/c dressing if infection develops.

**HOW SUPPLIED:** Cre: 0.01%, 0.025% [15g, 60g]; Oint: 0.025% [15g, 60g]; Sol: 0.01% [60mL].

**WARNINGS/PRECAUTIONS:** May produce reversible hypothalamic-pituitary-adrenal (HPA) axis suppression, manifestations of Cushing's syndrome, hyperglycemia and glucosuria. Caution when applied to large surface areas or under occlusive dressings or for prolonged periods. Withdraw, reduce frequency or substitute to a less potent steroid if adrenal suppression noted. Infrequently, steroid withdrawal may occur, requiring supplemental systemic steroids. Use appropriate antifungal or antibacterial agent with dermatological infections; d/c until infection controlled. Pediatrics may be more susceptible to systemic toxicity and may interfere with their growth and development. HPA axis suppression (linear growth retardation, delayed weight gain, low plasma cortisol, no response to ACTH stimulation), Cushing's syndrome and intracranial HTN (bulging fontanelles, headache, bilateral papilledema) reported in pediatrics. Use smallest amount for effective treatment. Avoid eyes. D/C if irritation occurs.

**ADVERSE REACTIONS:** Burning, itching, irritation, dryness, folliculitis, hypertrichosis, acneiform eruptions, perioral dermatitis, hypopigmentation, allergic contact dermatitis, skin maceration, secondary infection, skin atrophy, striae.

**PREGNANCY:** Category C, caution with nursing.

**MECHANISM OF ACTION:** Corticosteroid; possesses anti-inflammatory, antipruritic and vasoconstrictive actions. Anti-inflammatory activity not established.

**PHARMACOKINETICS: Absorption:** Percutaneous; extent of absorption is determined by vehicle, integrity of the epidermal barrier and occlusive dressings. **Distribution:** Systemically administered corticosteroids are found in breast milk. **Metabolism:** Liver. **Excretion:** Kidneys and bile.

## NURSING CONSIDERATIONS

**Assessment:** Assess for hypersensitivity reactions, presence of concomitant skin infections and pregnancy/nursing status.

**Monitoring:** Monitor for signs/symptoms of HPA-axis suppression, Cushing's syndrome, hyperglycemia, glucosuria, treatment-site irritation and for development of dermatological infections (eg, bacterial, fungal). If on prolonged therapy, monitor for atrophy of skin and subcutaneous tissues. If on high doses or applying to large surface area, perform periodic monitoring for HPA-axis suppression using urinary free cortisol and ACTH stimulation tests. Monitor for signs/symptoms of systemic toxicity, HPA-axis suppression (eg, linear growth retardation, delayed weight gain) and intracranial HTN in pediatrics.

**Patient Counseling:** Instruct to use externally and exactly as directed; avoid contact with eyes. Counsel not to bandage or wrap treatment area unless directed by physician. Advise to report any local adverse reactions (eg, irritation). Instruct caregivers of pediatrics to avoid using tight-fitting diapers or plastic pants on treatment area.

**Administration:** Topical route. **Storage:** 15°-30°C (59°-86°F). Cre/Sol: Avoid excessive heat. Protect from freezing.

# FLUOROURACIL RX

fluorouracil (ICN)

**To be given under the supervision of a physician experienced in antineoplastic agents. Because of the possibility of severe toxic reactions, patients should be hospitalized at least during initial course of therapy.**

F

**THERAPEUTIC CLASS:** Antimetabolite

**INDICATIONS:** Palliative management of colon, rectum, breast, stomach, and pancreatic carcinomas.

**DOSAGE:** *Adults:* 12mg/kg IV qd for 4 days. Max: 800mg/day. If no toxicity, give 6mg/kg IV on 6th, 8th, 10th, and 12th days. Skip Days 5, 7, 9, and 11. Inadequate Nutritional State: 6mg/kg IV for 3 days. If no toxicity, give 3mg/kg IV on 5th, 7th, and 9th days. Max: 400mg/day. Skip Days 4, 6, and 8. Maint (Use Schedule 1 or Schedule 2): Schedule 1: If no toxicity, repeat 1st course every 30 days after last day of previous course. Schedule 2: When toxic signs from initial course subside, give 10-15mg/kg/week IV single dose; do not exceed 1g/week.

**HOW SUPPLIED:** Inj: 50mg/mL [10mL, 50mL, 100mL]

**CONTRAINDICATIONS:** Poor nutritional state, depressed bone marrow function, potentially serious infection.

**WARNINGS/PRECAUTIONS:** Extreme caution in poor risk patients with history of high-dose irradiation, previous use of alkylating agents, hepatic/renal dysfunction, widespread bone marrow involvement by metastatic tumors. Dipyrimidine dehydrogenase deficiency prolongs 5-FU clearance; can cause severe toxicity. May cause fetal harm in pregnancy. Other therapy interfering with nutrition or depressing bone marrow function increases toxicity. D/C with stomatitis, esophagopharyngitis, leukopenia, intractable vomiting, diarrhea, GI ulceration or bleeding, thrombocytopenia, or hemorrhage from any site. Palmar-plantar erythrodysesthesia syndrome (hand-foot syndrome) reported. Perform WBC with differential before each dose. Narrow margin of safety; monitor patients very closely.

**ADVERSE REACTIONS:** Stomatitis, esophagopharyngitis, diarrhea, anorexia, nausea, emesis, leukopenia, alopecia, dermatitis.

**INTERACTIONS:** Leucovorin calcium may enhance toxicity.

**PREGNANCY:** Category D, not for use in nursing.

**MECHANISM OF ACTION:** Antineoplastic antimetabolite; interferes with the synthesis of DNA and to a lesser extent inhibits the formation of RNA, which are essential for cell division and growth.

**PHARMACOKINETICS: Distribution:** Found in tumors, intestinal mucosa, bone marrow, liver; crosses the blood-brain barrier and found in brain tissue and cerebrospinal fluid. **Metabolism:** Liver. **Elimination:** Urine (7-20% unchanged); $T_{1/2}$=16 min.

## NURSING CONSIDERATIONS

**Assessment:** Assess nutritional state, bone marrow function or involvement of bone marrow by metastatic tumors, presence of serious infections, history of high-dose pelvic irradiation, previous use of alkylating agents, hepatic or renal impairment, dipyrimidine dehydrogenase deficiency, pregnancy/nursing status, and possible drug interactions. Assess WBC counts with differential before each dose.

**Monitoring:** Monitor for signs and symptoms of stomatitis, esophagopharyngitis, leukopenia (WBC count <3500), intractable vomiting, diarrhea, GI ulceration or bleeding, thrombocytopenia (platelet count <100,000), hemorrhage from any site, palmar-plantar erythrodysesthesia syndrome (eg, tingling sensation in hands and feet), alopecia, and dermatitis.

**Patient Counseling:** Counsel about possible effects of medication including NV and alopecia. Alopecia is usually a transient effect. Advise about risks of medication during pregnancy.

**Administration:** IV route; no dilution required. Should only be administered under the supervision of a physician experienced in cancer chemotherapy. Patient should be hospitalized during initial course of therapy. Avoid extravasation. **Storage:** 15-30°C (59-86°F). Protect from light. Retain in carton until time of use.

## FLUVOXAMINE RX

fluvoxamine maleate (Various)



**Antidepressants increased the risk of suicidal thinking and behavior (suicidality) in short-term studies in children, adolescents, and young adults with major depressive disorder (MDD) and other psychiatric disorders. Fluvoxamine is not approved for use in pediatric patients except for patients with obsessive compulsive disorder (OCD).**

**THERAPEUTIC CLASS:** Selective serotonin reuptake inhibitor

**INDICATIONS:** Treatment of OCD.

**DOSAGE:** *Adults:* Initial: 50mg qhs. Titrate: Increase by 50mg every 4-7 days, as tolerated, until maximum therapeutic response is achieved. Maint: 100-300mg/day. Give bid if total dose >100mg daily. Max: 300mg/day. Elderly/Hepatic Impairment: Modify initial dose and titration.
*Pediatrics:* 8-17 yrs: Initial: 25mg qhs. Titrate: Increase by 25mg every 4-7 days, as tolerated, until maximum therapeutic response is achieved. Maint: 50-200mg/day. Max: 8-11 yrs: 200mg/day. Adolescents 12-17 yrs: 300mg/day. Give bid if total dose >50mg daily.

**HOW SUPPLIED:** Tab: 25mg, 50mg*, 100mg* *scored

**CONTRAINDICATIONS:** Concomitant use of thioridazine, pimozide, alosetron, and tizanidine. During or within 14 days of MAOI therapy.

**WARNINGS/PRECAUTIONS:** Serotonin syndrome or neuroleptic malignant syndrome (NMS)-like reactions have been reported. Avoid abrupt withdrawal. May increase risk of bleeding events. Activation of mania/hypomania, SIADH, hyponatremia reported. Caution with history of seizures or mania, hepatic dysfunction, conditions that alter metabolism or hemodynamic responses. Decreased appetite and weight loss reported in children; monitor weight and growth. Consider tapering dose during the third trimester. May impair judgment, thinking, or motor skills. Monitor for clinical worsening and/or suicidality, especially at initiation of therapy or dose changes.

**ADVERSE REACTIONS:** N/V, somnolence, insomnia, asthenia, nervousness, dyspepsia, abnormal ejaculation, sweating, anorexia, tremor, anorgasmia, decreased libido, dry mouth, rhinitis, and agitation.

**INTERACTIONS:** See Contraindications. Avoid alcohol and diazepam. May potentiate metoprolol or propranolol. Increases serum levels of theophylline, warfarin, clozapine, carbamazepine, methadone, tacrine, amtriptyline, clomipramine, or imipramine. Risk of bradycardia with diltiazem. May enhance serotonergic effects with lithium or tryptophan. Risk of seizure with lithium reported. Caution with TCAs, lithium, or tryptophan. Severe vomiting reported with tryptophan. Reduces clearance of mexiletine and benzodiazepines metabolized by hepatic oxidation (eg, alprazolam, midazolam, triazolam). Rare reports of weakness, hyperreflexia, incoordination with SSRIs and sumitriptan. Concomitant use of serotonergic drugs and with drugs that impair metabolism of serotonin may cause serotonin syndrome. Caution with other agents that may affect serotonergic neurotransmitter systems (eg, triptans, linezolid, tramadol, or St. John's wort). Smoking increases metabolism. Avoid with ramelteon. Altered anticoagulation effects with warfarin.

**PREGNANCY:** Category C, not for use in nursing.

**MECHANISM OF ACTION:** SSRI; inhibits neuronal uptake of serotonin.

**PHARMACOKINETICS: Absorption:** Absolute bioavailability (53%). Administration of variable doses resulted in different parameters; $T_{max}$=3-8 hrs. **Distribution:** $V_d$=25L/kg; plasma protein binding (80%). **Metabolism:** Hepatic (oxidative demethylation and deamination). **Elimination:** Urine; $T_{1/2}$=15.6 hrs.

## NURSING CONSIDERATIONS

**Assessment:** Assess for risk for bipolar disorder, history of mania, history of seizures, disease/condition that alters metabolism or hemodynamic response, hepatic impairment, pregnancy/nursing status, and possible drug interactions.

**Monitoring:** Monitor for signs/symptoms of clinical worsening (suicidality, unusual changes in behavior), serotonin syndrome, NMS (muscle rigidity, hyperthermia, mental status changes), abnormal bleeding, hyponatremia, seizures, hepatic dysfunction, cognitive and motor impairment. If d/c therapy (particularly if abrupt), monitor for symptoms of dysphoric mood, irritability, agitation, dizziness, sensory disturbances, anxiety, confusion, headache, lethargy, emotional lability, insomnia, and hypomania.

**Patient Counseling:** Advise to avoid alcohol. Seek medical attention for symptoms of serotonin syndrome (mental status changes, tachycardia, hyperthermia, N/V, diarrhea, incoordination), NMS, allergic reactions (rash, hives), abnormal bleeding (particularly if using NSAIDs or ASA), hyponatremia, activation of mania, seizures, clinical worsening (suicidal ideation, unusual changes in behavior) and discontinuation symptoms (irritability, agitation, dizziness, anxiety, headache, insomnia). Caution against hazardous tasks (eg, operating machinery and driving). May notice improvement in 1-4 weeks; continue therapy as directed. Notify physician if pregnant, intend to become pregnant, or breastfeeding. Counsel about benefits and risks of therapy. Inform physician if taking or plan to take any over-the-counter prescriptions.

**Administration:** Oral route. **Storage:** 15-30°C (59-86°F). Protect from high humidity. Dispense in tight, light-resistant container with child-resistant closure.

# FLUZONE — RX

influenza virus vaccine (Sanofi Pasteur)

**OTHER BRAND NAMES:** Fluzone HD (Sanofi Pasteur)

**THERAPEUTIC CLASS:** Vaccine

**INDICATIONS:** Active immunization against influenza disease caused by influenza virus subtypes A and type B contained in the vaccine in persons (Fluzone) ≥6 months of age or (Fluzone HD) ≥65 years of age.

**DOSAGE:** *Adults:* (Fluzone) ≥18 yrs: 0.5mL IM in deltoid muscle; (Fluzone HD) ≥65 years: 0.5mL IM in deltoid muscle.
*Pediatrics:* Previously Unvaccinated or Incompletely Vaccinated for first time last season with only 1 dose: 3-8 yrs: Two 0.5mL IM doses, each 0.5mL dose should be 1 month apart. 6-35 months: Two 0.25mL IM doses, each 0.25mL dose should be 1 month apart. Vaccinated 2 doses last season or one or more doses at any time before last season: 3-8 yrs: 0.5mL IM as 1 dose. 6-35 months: 0.25mL IM as 1 dose. ≥9 yrs: 0.5mL IM as 1 dose. Administer in deltoid muscle in children (1-17 years) or anterolateral aspect of thigh muscle in infants (6-12 months).

**HOW SUPPLIED:** Inj: (Fluzone) 0.25mL, 0.5mL, 5mL; (Fluzone HD) 0.5mL

**CONTRAINDICATIONS:** Hypersensitivity reactions to egg proteins or life-threatening reactions after previous administration of any influenza vaccine.

**WARNINGS/PRECAUTIONS:** Caution if Guillain-Barre Syndrome (GBS) has occurred with 6 weeks of previous influenza vaccination. Immunosuppressed patients may have lower immune response. Medical treatment and supervision must be available to manage possible anaphylactic reactions. May not protect all susceptible individuals.

**ADVERSE REACTIONS:** Injection-site pain, erythema, swelling, myalgia, malaise, headache, fever

**INTERACTIONS:** Immunosuppressive therapies may reduce immune response.

**PREGNANCY:** Category C, caution in nursing.

**MECHANISM OF ACTION:** Stimulates the immune system to produce antibodies that may protect against influenza virus.

## NURSING CONSIDERATIONS

**Assessment:** Assess immunization and health/medical status, previous hypersensitivity or vaccination events (Guillain-Barre syndrome), pregnancy/nursing status, and possible drug interactions.

**Monitoring:** Monitor for hypersensitivity reactions, injection-site swelling or pain, fever, headache, myalgia, irritability, insomnia, and neurological complications.

**Patient Counseling:** Inform patients or caregivers of benefits/risks ratio; report any adverse reactions to physician. Inform patient or guardian that vaccine contains killed viruses, hence can't cause influenza. Advise that vaccine is intended to provide protection against illness due to influenza viruses only and cannot provide protection against all respiratory illnesses. Instruct to report any adverse events to healthcare provider. Inform that annual revaccination is recommended.

**Administration:** IM. Administer in deltoid muscle in children (1-17 years) or anterolateral aspect of thigh muscle in infants (6-12 months). Do not inject into gluteal region or areas where there may be a major nerve trunk. **Storage:** 2-8°C (35-46°F). Do not freeze. Discard if vaccine has been frozen.

F

# FML — RX

fluorometholone (Allergan)

**OTHER BRAND NAMES:** FML Forte (Allergan)

**THERAPEUTIC CLASS:** Corticosteroid

**INDICATIONS:** Treatment of inflammation of the palpebral and bulbar conjunctiva, cornea, and anterior segment of the globe.

**DOSAGE:** *Adults:* (Sus) 1 drop bid-qid or (Oint) apply 1/2 inch qd-tid. May give 0.1% q4h during initial 24-48 hrs. Re-evaluate after 2 days if no improvement. *Pediatrics:* ≥2 yrs: (Sus) 1 drop bid-qid or (Oint) apply 1/2 inch qd-tid. May give 0.1% q4h during initial 24-48 hrs. Re-evaluate after 2 days if no improvement.

**HOW SUPPLIED:** Oint: (S.O.P.) 0.1% [3.5g]; Sus: 0.1% [5mL, 10mL, 15mL]; (Forte) 0.25% [2mL, 5mL, 10mL, 15mL]

**CONTRAINDICATIONS:** Viral diseases of the cornea and conjunctiva including epithelial herpes simplex keratitis, vaccinia, and varicella. Mycobacterial infection and fungal diseases of the eye.

**WARNINGS/PRECAUTIONS:** Caution with glaucoma, herpes simplex, diseases causing thinning of cornea/sclera and other ocular viral infections. Prolonged use can cause glaucoma or secondary ocular infections (eg, fungal). Monitor IOP after 10 days of therapy. Re-evaluate if no response after 2 days. Ointment may retard corneal healing. May delay healing and increase incidence of bleb formation after cataract surgery. Avoid abrupt withdrawal with chronic use.

**ADVERSE REACTIONS:** Elevation of IOP, glaucoma, infrequent optic nerve damage, posterior subcapsular cataract formation, delayed wound healing, burning/stinging upon instillation, ocular irritation, taste perversion, visual disturbance.

**PREGNANCY:** Category C, not for use in nursing.

**MECHANISM OF ACTION:** Corticosteroid; suspected to act by induction of phospholipase $A_2$ inhibitory proteins called lipocortins, which control the biosynthesis of potent inflammation mediators (eg, prostaglandins, leukotrienes) by inhibiting release of their precursor, arachidonic acid.

## NURSING CONSIDERATIONS

**Assessment:** Assess for viral diseases of cornea and conjunctiva, dendritic keratitis, vaccinia, varicella, mycobacterial infection of eye, fungal disease of ocular structures, glaucoma, mustard gas keratitis, Sjogren's keratoconjuctivitis, thinning of corneal/scleral epithelium, hypersensitivity, and for cataract surgery.

**Monitoring:** Frequent measuring of IOP and slit lamp microscopy exam when appropriate, fluorescein staining for monitoring of glaucoma with damage to the optic nerve (with defects in visual acuity and fields of vision), posterior subcapsular cataract, delayed corneal healing, thinning of cornea and sclera, ulceration, perforation, and secondary ocular infections or masking of existing infections.

**Patient Counseling:** Advise to d/c and notify physician if symptoms persist or worsen. Instruct to wait 15 min after instillation to wear soft contact lenses. Counsel to avoid touching bottle tip to eyelids or any other surface.

**Administration:** Ocular route. **Storage:** Store between 2-25°C (36-77°F); protect from freezing.



# FML-S RX

## sulfacetamide sodium - fluorometholone (Allergan)

**THERAPEUTIC CLASS:** Sulfonamide/corticosteroid

**INDICATIONS:** Ocular inflammation associated with infection or risk of infection.

**DOSAGE:** *Adults:* 1 drop qid. Max: 20mL for initial prescription. Re-evaluate before refill.

**HOW SUPPLIED:** Sus: (Sulfacetamide-Fluorometholone) 10%-0.1% [5mL, 10mL]

**CONTRAINDICATIONS:** Viral diseases of the cornea and conjunctiva including epithelial herpes simplex keratitis, vaccinia, and varicella. Mycobacterial infection and fungal diseases of the eye.

**WARNINGS/PRECAUTIONS:** Caution with glaucoma, herpes simplex, diseases causing thinning of cornea/sclera and other ocular viral infections. Prolonged use can cause glaucoma or secondary ocular infections (eg, fungal). Monitor IOP after 10 days of therapy. Fatalities reported due to severe reactions to sulfonamides. Re-evaluate before renew prescription.

**ADVERSE REACTIONS:** Secondary infection, elevated IOP, delayed wound healing, allergic sensitization.

**INTERACTIONS:** Sulfacetamide preparations are incompatible with silver preparations.

**PREGNANCY:** Category C, not for use in nursing.

**MECHANISM OF ACTION:** Sulfonamide/corticosteroid. Fluorometholone: Corticosteroid; inhibits edema, fibrin deposition, capillary dilation, leukocyte migration, capillary proliferation, fibroblast proliferation, deposition of collagen, and scar formation associated with inflammation. May also inhibit body's defense mechanism against infection. Sulfacetamide: Anti-infective; provides activity against susceptible microorganisms.

### NURSING CONSIDERATIONS

**Assessment:** Assess proper diagnosis of patient (eg, slit lamp biomicroscopy, fluorescein staining). Assess patient does not have viral diseases of cornea and conjunctiva (epithelial herpes simplex keratitis, dendritic keratitis, vaccinia and varicella). Assess patient does not have mycobacterial infection of the eye or fungal disease of the ocular structures. Assess for hypersensitivity to sulfonamides and other corticosteroids. Assess use in pregnant/nursing females, patients with glaucoma, patients who underwent recent cataract surgery, and in patients with a history of herpes simplex.

**Monitoring:** Monitor for masking of acute purulent infections, Stevens-Johnson syndrome, toxic epidermal necrolysis, fulminant hepatic necrosis, agranulocytosis, aplastic anemia, and other blood dyscrasias. In patients on prolonged therapy, monitor for glaucoma with damage to the optic nerve, defects in visual acuity and fields of vision, posterior subcapsular cataract formation, secondary ocular infections (eg, fungal), and corneal and scleral thinning. In patients on therapy for 10 days or longer, monitor IOP. In patients with a history of herpes simplex, perform frequent slit lamp microscopy.

**Patient Counseling:** Instruct to notify physician if pain or inflammation persists for longer than 48 hrs. Instruct to avoid touching bottle tip to eyelids or any other surface to prevent contamination.

**Administration:** Ocular route. Shake well before use. **Storage:** 15-30°C (59-86°F). Protect from freezing and light. Keep out of reach of children.

## FOCALIN

CII

dexmethylphenidate HCl (Novartis)

F

**THERAPEUTIC CLASS:** Sympathomimetic amine

**INDICATIONS:** Treatment of attention deficit hyperactivity disorder (ADHD).

**DOSAGE:** *Adults:* Take bid at least 4 hrs apart. Methylphenidate-Naive: Initial: 2.5mg bid. Titrate: Increase weekly by 2.5-5mg/day. Max: 20mg/day. Currently on Methylphenidate: Initial: Take 1/2 of methylphenidate dose. Max: 20mg/day. Reduce or d/c if paradoxical aggravation of symptoms occur. D/C if no improvement after appropriate dosage adjustments over 1 month.
*Pediatrics:* ≥6 yrs: Take bid at least 4 hrs apart. Methylphenidate-Naive: Initial: 2.5mg bid. Titrate: Increase weekly by 2.5-5mg/day. Max: 20mg/day. Currently on Methylphenidate: Initial: Take 1/2 of methylphenidate dose. Max: 20mg/day. Reduce or d/c if paradoxical aggravation of symptoms occur. D/C if no improvement after appropriate dosage adjustments over 1 month.

**HOW SUPPLIED:** Tab: 2.5mg, 5mg, 10mg

**CONTRAINDICATIONS:** Marked anxiety, tension, and agitation; glaucoma; motor tics or family history or diagnosis of Tourette's syndrome; during or within 14 days of MAOI use.

**WARNINGS/PRECAUTIONS:** Stroke and myocardial infarction (MI) reported; avoid with known serious structural cardiac abnormalities, cardiomyopathy, serious heart rhythm abnormalities, coronary artery disease (CAD) or other serious cardiac problems. May cause modest increase in HR and BP; caution with HTN, heart failure, recent MI or ventricular arrhythmia. May exacerbate symptoms of behavior disturbance and thought disorder with pre-existing psychotic disorder. Caution when using stimulants to treat patients with comorbid bipolar disorder because of concern for possible induction of mixed/manic episodes. Stimulants at usual doses may cause treatment-emergent psychotic or manic symptoms (eg, hallucinations, delusional thinking, mania) in children and adolescents without prior history of psychotic illness or mania; d/c if occurs. Aggressive behavior or hostility reported in clinical trials and the postmarketing experience of some medications indicated for the treatment of ADHD. Suppression of growth reported with long-term use; monitor growth. May lower convulsive threshold; d/c in the presence of seizures. Visual disturbances reported. Monitor CBC, differential, and platelets with prolonged therapy. Give cautiously to patients with a history of drug dependence or alcoholism. Chronic abusive use may lead to marked tolerance and psychological dependence with varying degrees of abnormal behavior. Severe depression and unmasking of symptoms of underlying disorder may occur; careful supervision required during withdrawal from abusive use.

**ADVERSE REACTIONS:** Abdominal pain, fever, anorexia, nausea, nervousness, insomnia. (Pediatrics) Loss of appetite, weight loss, tachycardia.

**INTERACTIONS:** See Contraindications. May decrease the effectiveness of antihypertensives; caution with pressor agents. May inhibit metabolism of coumarin anticoagulants, anticonvulsants (eg, phenobarbital, phenytoin, primidone) and some antidepressants (eg, TCAs, SSRIs); adjust dose. Adverse events reported with clonidine.

**PREGNANCY:** Category C, caution in nursing.

**MECHANISM OF ACTION:** Sympathomimetic amine; blocks the reuptake of norepinephrine and dopamine into the presynaptic neuron and increases release of these monoamines into extraneuronal space.

**PHARMACOKINETICS: Absorption:** Readily absorbed; $T_{max}$=2.9 hrs (fed), 1.5 hrs (fasting). **Metabolism:** Via de-esterification (d-ritalinic acid; primary metabolite). **Elimination:** Urine (90%); $T_{1/2}$=2.2 hrs.

## NURSING CONSIDERATIONS

**Assessment:** Assess for marked anxiety, tension, agitation, glaucoma, motor tics, family history or diagnosis of Tourette's syndrome, cardiovascular conditions (eg, severe HTN, angina pectoris, cardiac structural abnormalities, arrhythmias, heart failure, recent MI), hyperthyroidism or thyrotoxicosis, bipolar disorder, seizures, LFTs, renal function, history of drug dependence or alcoholism, hypersensitivity, pregnancy/nursing status and possible drug interactions.

**Monitoring:** Monitor for cardiac abnormalities, exacerbations of behavior disturbances and thought disorder, bipolar disorder, aggression, seizures, visual disturbances and hypersensitivity reactions. Monitor HR, BP and LFTs. Periodically monitor LFTs, CBC, differential and platelet count. Follow up height and weight in children.

F

**Patient Counseling:** Inform about risks of treatment, appropriate use, drug abuse/dependence. Counsel about potential side effects and advise to report any. Inform physician if pregnant, planning to become pregnant or breast feeding. Inform of any other medications being taken. Advise to use as prescribed and not to give to others with similar condition unless advised.

**Administration:** Oral route. **Storage:** 25°C (77°F); excursions permitted to 15-30°C (59-86°F). Protect from light and moisture.

# FOCALIN XR

CII

dexmethylphenidate HCl (Novartis)

> **Give cautiously to patients with a history of drug dependence or alcoholism. Chronic abusive use may lead to marked tolerance and psychological dependence with varying degrees of abnormal behavior.**

**THERAPEUTIC CLASS:** Sympathomimetic amine

**INDICATIONS:** Treatment of attention deficit hyperactivity disorder (ADHD) in patients aged ≥6 yrs.

**DOSAGE:** *Adults:* Individualize dose: Methylphenidate-Naive: Initial: 10mg/day. Titrate: May adjust weekly by 10mg/day. Max: 40mg/day. Currently on Methylphenidate: Initial: Take 1/2 of methylphenidate dose. Max: 40mg/day. Currently on Dexmethylphenidate Immediate-Release: Switch to same daily dose of XR. Max: 40mg/day. Reduce or d/c if paradoxical aggravation of symptoms occurs. Swallow whole or sprinkle contents on applesauce. Contents should not be crushed, chewed or divided. D/C if no improvement after appropriate dosage adjustments over 1 month.
*Pediatrics:* ≥6 yrs: Individualize dose: Methylphenidate-Naive: Initial: 5mg/day. Titrate: May adjust weekly by 5mg/day. Max: 30mg/day. Currently on Methylphenidate: Initial: Take 1/2 of methylphenidate dose. Max: 30mg/day. Currently on Dexmethylphenidate Immediate-Release: Switch to same daily dose of XR. Max: 30mg/day. Reduce or d/c if paradoxical aggravation of symptoms occurs. Swallow whole or sprinkle contents on applesauce; contents should not be crushed, chewed or divided. D/C if no improvement after appropriate dosage adjustments over 1 month.

**HOW SUPPLIED:** Cap, Extended-Release: 5mg, 10mg, 15mg, 20mg, 30mg

**CONTRAINDICATIONS:** Marked anxiety, tension, and agitation; glaucoma; motor tics, or family history or diagnosis of Tourette's syndrome; during or within 14 days of MAOI use.

**WARNINGS/PRECAUTIONS:** Avoid with known serious structural cardiac abnormalities, cardiomyopathy, serious heart rhythm abnormalities, CAD, or other serious cardiac problems; sudden death reported in children and adolescents with structural cardiac abnormalities or other serious heart problems; sudden death, stroke, MI reported in adults. May cause modest increase in BP; caution with HTN, heart failure, recent MI, or ventricular arrhythmia. Prior to treatment perform a physical exam and medical history (including assessment for family history of sudden death or ventricular arrhythmia). Promptly evaluate if symptoms of cardiac disease develop during treatment. May exacerbate symptoms of behavior disturbance and thought disorder with pre-existing psychotic disorder. Caution when using stimulants to treat patients with comorbid bipolar disorder because of concern for possible induction of mixed/manic episodes in such patients. Stimulants at usual doses may cause treatment-emergent psychotic or manic symptoms (eg, hallucinations, delusional thinking, mania) in children and adolescents without prior history of psychotic illness or mania. Aggressive behavior or hostility reported in clinical trials and the postmarketing experience of some medications indicated for the treatment of ADHD. Suppression of growth reported with long-term use; monitor height and weight. May lower convulsive threshold; d/c in the presence of seizures. Visual disturbances reported. Monitor CBC, differential, and platelets with prolonged therapy. Psychotic episodes can occur, especially with parenteral abuse. Severe depression may occur during withdrawal from abusive use. Withdrawal following chronic therapeutic use may unmask symptoms of underlying disorder that may require follow-up.



**ADVERSE REACTIONS:** Nervousness, insomnia, dyspepsia, headache, anxiety. (Adults) dry mouth, pharyngolaryngeal pain, feeling jittery, dizziness. (Pediatrics) decreased appetite, abdominal pain, weight loss, loss of appetite, anorexia, tachycardia.

**INTERACTIONS:** See Contraindications. May decrease the effectiveness of antihypertensives. Caution with pressor agents. May inhibit metabolism of coumarin anticoagulants, anticonvulsants (eg, phenobarbital, phenytoin, primidone), and tricyclic drugs (eg, imipramine, clomipramine, desipramine); adjust dose. Antacids or acid supressants could alter the release of dexmethylphenidate. Serious adverse events reported with concomitant use of clonidine. May possibly interact with venlafaxine.

**PREGNANCY:** Category C, caution in nursing.

**MECHANISM OF ACTION:** Sympathomimetic amine; CNS stimulant. Mechanism in ADHD has not been established. Blocks reuptake of norepinephrine and dopamine into the presynaptic neuron and increases release of these monoamines into extraneuronal space.

**PHARMACOKINETICS: Absorption:** Bimodal plasma concentration. Absolute bioavailability (22-25%). $T_{max}$=1.5 hrs (first peak, range 1-4 hrs), 6.5 hrs (second peak, range 4.5-7 hrs). **Distribution:** (Racemic methylphenidate) Plasma protein binding (12-15%), $V_d$=2.65L/kg. **Metabolism:** Metabolized via de-esterification; d-ritalinic acid (metabolite). **Elimination:** Urine (approximately 90%, radiolabeled racemic methylphenidate); $T_{1/2}$=2-4.5 hrs (adults), 2-3 hrs (children).

## NURSING CONSIDERATIONS

**Assessment:** Assess for agitation, anxiety, tension, glaucoma, tics, family history of or diagnosis of Tourette's syndrome, cardiovascular conditions (eg, severe HTN, angina pectoris, cardiac arrhythmias, heart failure, recent MI), pre-existing psychotic disorders, seizure disorder, bipolar disorder, history of drug dependence or alcoholism, and possible drug interactions. Assess pregnancy/nursing status. Perform physical exam and obtain a medical history prior to therapy.

**Monitoring:** Monitor for cardiac abnormalities, exacerbations of behavior disturbances and thought disorder, bipolar disorder, aggression, seizures, and visual disturbances. Perform periodic monitoring of CBC, differential and platelet counts, and LFTs required. Height and weight follow-up required in children. Monitor BP and HR.

**Patient Counseling:** Inform about risks of therapy, appropriate use, drug abuse/dependence. Instruct to take once daily in the morning. Counsel to swallow tablet; never crush or chew. If unable to swallow, instruct to sprinkle over applesauce and swallow without chewing.

**Administration:** Oral route. **Storage:** 25°C (77°F), excursions permitted to 15-30° (59-86°F).

## FOLGARD RX 2.2 RX

vitamin B12 - vitamin B6 - folic acid (Upsher-Smith)

**THERAPEUTIC CLASS:** Folic acid/vitamin combination

**INDICATIONS:** For nutritional support and folic acid supplementation.

**DOSAGE:** *Adults:* 1 tab qd.

**HOW SUPPLIED:** Tab: Folic Acid 2.2mg-Vitamin $B_6$ 25mg-Vitamin $B_{12}$ 0.5mg*
*scored

**WARNINGS/PRECAUTIONS:** Folic acid >0.1mg/day may obscure pernicious anemia.

**ADVERSE REACTIONS:** Allergic sensitization.

**PREGNANCY:** Safety in pregnancy and nursing is not known.

**MECHANISM OF ACTION:** Folic acid/vitamin combination.

### NURSING CONSIDERATIONS

**Assessment:** Assess for pernicious anemia.

**Monitoring:** Monitor hematological parameters and for hypersensitivity reactions.

**Patient Counseling:** Report hypersensitivity reactions.

**Administration:** Oral route. **Storage:** 15-30°C (59-86°F). Protect from light and moisture. Dispense in tight container with child-resistant closure.

## FOLIC ACID RX

folic acid (Various)

**THERAPEUTIC CLASS:** Erythropoiesis agent

**INDICATIONS:** Treatment of megaloblastic anemia due to folic acid deficiency and in anemias of nutritional origin, pregnancy, infancy or childhood.

**DOSAGE:** *Adults:* Usual: Up to 1mg/day. Maint: 0.4mg qd. Pregnancy/Nursing: Maint: 0.8mg qd. Max: 1mg/day. Increase maintenance dose with alcoholism, hemolytic anemia, anticonvulsant therapy, chronic infection.
*Pediatrics:* Usual: Up to 1mg/day. Maint: Infants: 0.1mg qd. <4 yrs: 0.3mg qd. ≥4 yrs: 0.4mg qd.

**HOW SUPPLIED:** Inj: 5mg/mL; Tab: (OTC) 0.4mg, 0.8mg, (RX) 1mg

**WARNINGS/PRECAUTIONS:** Not for monotherapy in pernicious anemia and other megaloblastic anemias with $B_{12}$ deficiency. May obscure pernicious anemia in dosage >0.1 mg/day. Decreased $B_{12}$ serum levels with prolonged therapy.

**ADVERSE REACTIONS:** Allergic sensitization.

**INTERACTIONS:** Antagonizes phenytoin effects. Methotrexate, phenytoin, primidone, barbiturates, alcohol, alcoholic cirrhosis, nitrofurantoin, and pyrimethamine increase loss of folate. Increased seizures with phenytoin, primidone and phenobarbital reported. Tetracycline may cause false low serum and red cell folate due to suppression of *Lactobacillus casei*.

**PREGNANCY:** Category A, requirement increases during nursing.

**MECHANISM OF ACTION:** Acts as cofactor for transformylation reactions in biosynthesis of purines and thymidylates of nucleic acids; acts on megaloblastic bone marrow to produce normo-blastic marrow; required for nucleo-protein synthesis and maintenance of normal erythropoiesis.

**PHARMACOKINETICS: Absorption:** Rapid (small intestine); $T_{max}$=1 hr. **Distribution:** Excreted in breast milk. **Metabolism:** Liver via reduced diphospho-pyridine nucleotide and folate reductase. **Elimination:** Urine, feces.

### NURSING CONSIDERATIONS

**Assessment:** Assess for alcoholism, chronic infection, and pernicious, megaloblastic, and hemolytic anemias, and for possible drug interactions.

**Monitoring:** Monitor for allergic/hypersensitivity reactions.

**Patient Counseling:** Advise to seek medical attention if symptoms of allergic/hypersensitivity reaction occurs.

**Administration:** Oral route. **Storage**: 20-25°C (68-77°F).

## FOLTX RX
vitamin B12 - vitamin B6 - folic acid (PamLab)

**THERAPEUTIC CLASS:** Folic acid/vitamin combination

**INDICATIONS:** To supply nutritional requirements for those with end stage renal failure, dialysis, hyperhomocysteinemia, homocystinuria, nutrient malabsorption.

**DOSAGE:** *Adults:* 1-2 tabs qd.

**HOW SUPPLIED:** Tab: Folic Acid 2.5mg-Vitamin $B_6$ 25mg-Vitamin $B_{12}$ 2mg

**WARNINGS/PRECAUTIONS:** Folic acid >0.1mg/day may obscure pernicious anemia (may be alleviated by $B_{12}$ component).

**ADVERSE REACTIONS:** Allergic sensitization, paresthesia, somnolence, mild diarrhea, polycythemia vera, peripheral vascular thrombosis, itching, transitory exanthema, feeling of body swelling.

**INTERACTIONS:** Pyridoxine may antagonize levodopa; avoid concomitant use. May be used with carbidopa/levodopa. Decreases effect of phenytoin.

**MECHANISM OF ACTION:** Folic acid/vitamin combination.

### NURSING CONSIDERATIONS

**Assessment:** Assess for Leber's optic atrophy, pernicious anemia, and hyperhomocysteinemia. Note other diseases/conditions and drug therapies.

**Monitoring:** Monitor for polycythemia vera, headache, paresthesia, and hypersensitivity reactions.

**Patient Counseling:** Counsel about adverse effects; immediately report if any occur. Take as directed by physician.

**Administration:** Oral route. **Storage:** Room temperature, 15-30°C (59-86°F). Protect from light and moisture. Dispense in original light-resistant container with child-resistant closure.

## FORADIL RX
formoterol fumarate (Schering)

**Long-acting $\beta_2$-agonists may increase the risk of asthma-related death.**

**THERAPEUTIC CLASS:** Beta$_2$-agonist

**INDICATIONS:** Long-term maintenance treatment of asthma and prevention of bronchospasm with reversible obstructive airway disease (including nocturnal asthma) in patients who require regular treatment with inhaled short acting $\beta_2$-agonists. Maintenance treatment of bronchoconstriction in chronic obstructive pulmonary disease (COPD). Acute prevention of excercise-induced bronchospasm (EIB).

**DOSAGE:** *Adults:* Do not swallow cap; give only by inhalation with Aerolizer Inhaler. Asthma/COPD: 12mcg q12h. Max: 24mcg/day. EIB: 12mcg 15 min before exercise (do not give added dose if already on q12h dose).
*Pediatrics:* ≥5 yrs: Do not swallow cap; give only by inhalation with Aerolizer™ Inhaler. Asthma/COPD: 12mcg q12h. Max: 24mcg/day. ≥12 yrs: EIB: 12mcg 15 min before exercise (do not give added dose if already on q12h dose).

**HOW SUPPLIED:** Cap (Inhalation): 12mcg [12$^s$, 60$^s$]

**WARNINGS/PRECAUTIONS:** Do not d/c inhaled corticosteroids. Only use short-acting $\beta_2$-agonist inhaler for acute symptoms. D/C if paradoxical bronchospasm occurs. D/C if ECG changes, QT interval increases, or ST depression occurs. Caution with cardiovascular disorders (eg, HTN, arrhythmias), thyrotoxicosis and convulsive disorders. Anaphylactic and other allergic reactions reported. Not for use in acute asthmatic conditions. Should not be used with other long-acting $\beta_2$-agonist medications. May cause hypokalemia.

**ADVERSE REACTIONS:** Viral infection, dyspnea, chest pain, tremor, HTN, hypotension, tachycardia, arrhythmias, headache, nausea, vomiting, fatigue, hypokalemia, hyperglycemia, exacerbation of asthma.

**INTERACTIONS:** Potentiates other sympathomimetics. Hypokalemia potentiated by xanthine derivatives (eg, theophylline), steroids and non-potassium sparing diuretics. Extreme caution with MAOIs, TCAs, and drugs known to prolong QT interval. Antagonized effect with β-blockers.

**PREGNANCY:** Category C, caution in nursing.

**MECHANISM OF ACTION:** Long-acting selective $\beta_2$-adrenergic receptor agonist; acts as a bronchodilator, activates adenyl cyclase on airway smooth muscles and increases the intracellular concentration of cyclic AMP. Increased cAMP levels are associated with relaxation of bronchial smooth muscle and inhibition of release of mediators of immediate hypersensitivity.

**PHARMACOKINETICS: Absorption:** Healthy: $C_{max}$=92pg/mL, $T_{max}$=5 min. COPD patient: (12mcg) $C_{max}$=4.0-8.8, 8, 17.3pg/mL at 10 min, 2 hrs, 6 hrs, respectively. **Distribution:** Plasma protein binding (61-64%), serum albumin binding (31-38%). **Metabolism:** Glucuronidation, O-methylation via CYP450 enzymes 2D6, 2C19, 2CP, 2A6. **Elimination:** Healthy: Urine (59-62%), feces (32-34%). With asthma: Urine (10% unchanged). COPD: Urine (7%). $T_{1/2}$=10 hrs.

## NURSING CONSIDERATIONS

**Assessment:** Assess for convulsive disorders, hyperthyroidism, DM, CVD, and possible drug interactions.

**Monitoring:** Monitor pulse rate, BP, and ECG change, and for paradoxical bronchospasm and hypokalemia, hypersensitivity reactions, deterioration of asthma.

**Patient Counseling:** Inform that long-acting $\beta_2$-agonist may increase risk of asthma-related death. Take as directed. Report lack of response or adverse side effects. Capsule should not be swallowed.

**Administration:** Oral inhalation route. 1) Pull off aerolizer inhaler cover. 2) Twist mouthpiece in the direction of the arrow to open. 3) Make sure 4 pins can be seen in the capsule well. 4) Place capsule in capsule chamber and twist mouthpiece back to closed position. 5) Hold mouthpiece of inhaler upright and press both buttons at the same time. Only press once. A click should be heard as the capsule is being pierced. 6) Release the button and exhale. 7) Place the mouthpiece in mouth and breathe in quickly and deeply. 8) Remove inhaler from mouth and hold breath as long as possible and then exhale. 9) Open the inhaler to see if any powder is still in the capsule. If drug remains, repeat steps 7&8. 10) After use, open the inhaler, remove and discard the empty capsule. Close the mouthpiece and replace the cover. **Storage:** Prior to dispensing: 2-8°C (36-46°F). After dispensing: 20-25°C (68-77°F). Protect from heat and moisture. Capsule should always be stored in blister and only removed from blister before use.

# FORTAMET — RX

metformin HCl (Sciele)

**THERAPEUTIC CLASS:** Biguanide

**INDICATIONS:** Adjunct to diet and exercise, to improve glycemic control in type 2 diabetes mellitus.

**DOSAGE:** *Adults:* ≥17 yrs: Take with evening meal. Initial: 500-1000mg qd. With Insulin: Initial: 500mg qd. Titrate: May increase by 500mg/week. Max: 2500mg/day. Decrease insulin dose by 10-25% if FPG <120mg/dL. Elderly/Debilitated/Malnourished: Conservative dosing; do not titrate to max.

**HOW SUPPLIED:** Tab, Extended-Release: 500mg, 1000mg

**CONTRAINDICATIONS:** Renal disease/dysfunction (SrCr ≥1.5mg/dL [males], ≥1.4mg/dL [females], or abnormal CrCl), acute or chronic metabolic acidosis, including diabetic ketoacidosis. D/C temporarily (48 hrs) for radiologic studies with intravascular iodinated contrast materials.

**WARNINGS/PRECAUTIONS:** Lactic acidosis (rare) reported; may occur with pathophysiologic conditions, including DM, hypoperfusion, and hypoxemia. Increased risk with renal insufficiency (both intrinsic renal disease and renal hypoperfusion), CHF, and patient's age. Avoid use in patients ≥80 yrs unless renal function is not reduced. Should be promptly withheld with hypoxemia, dehydration, or sepsis. Caution against excessive alcohol intake. Lactic acidosis may be suspected in diabetic patient with metabolic acidosis lacking evidence of ketoacidosis (ketonuria and ketonemia). Immediately d/c with lactic acidosis; prompt hemodialysis is recommended to correct the acidosis and remove the accumulated metformin. Caution using concomitant medications that may affect renal function, or result in significant hemodynamic change, or interfere with the disposition of metformin (eg, cationic drugs eliminated by renal tubular secretion). Temporarily d/c prior to surgery (due to restricted food intake) and procedures requiring intravascular iodinated contrast materials. D/C in hypoxic states (eg, shock, CHF, acute MI). Avoid in patients with hepatic impairment. May decrease vitamin $B_{12}$ levels. Increased risk of hypoglycemia in elderly, debilitated/malnourished, adrenal or pituitary insufficiency, or alcohol intoxication. If loss of glycemic control occurs due to stress, temporarily withhold metformin and administer insulin. Reinstitute metformin after acute episode is resolved.

**ADVERSE REACTIONS:** Infection, diarrhea, nausea, accidental injury, headache, dyspepsia, and rhinitis.

**INTERACTIONS:** Furosemide, nifedipine, cimetidine, cationic drugs (eg, digoxin, amiloride, procainamide, quinidine, quinine, ranitidine, trimethoprim, vancomycin, triamterene, morphine) may increase metformin levels. Thiazides, other diuretics, corticosteroids, phenothiazines, thyroid products, estrogens, oral contraceptives, phenytoin, nicotinic acid, sympathomimetics, CCBs, and isoniazid may cause hyperglycemia. Risk of hypoglycemia with alcohol. Excess alcohol may increase potential for lactic acidosis. May decrease furosemide levels.

**PREGNANCY:** Category B, not for use in pregnancy or nursing.

**MECHANISM OF ACTION:** Biguanide; decreases hepatic glucose production, decreases intestinal absorption of glucose, and improves insulin sensitivity by increasing peripheral glucose uptake and utilization.

**PHARMACOKINETICS: Absorption:** $C_{max}$=2849ng/mL, $T_{max}$=6 hrs, AUC=26811ng•hr/mL. **Elimination:** Urine (90%); $T_{1/2}$=6.2 hrs (plasma), 17.6 hrs (blood).

## NURSING CONSIDERATIONS

**Assessment:** Assess for renal FPG, $HbA_{1c}$, renal function, LFTs, and CBC. Assess for CHF, septicemia, acute or chronic metabolic acidosis, adrenal or pituitary insufficiency, alcoholism, pregnancy status. Evaluate for other medical/surgical conditions and for possible drug interactions.

**Monitoring:** Monitor for infection, diarrhea, nausea, accidental injury, headache, dyspepsia, and rhinitis.

**Patient Counseling:** Inform of the potential risks and benefits of Fortamet and of alternative modes of therapy. Inform drug is adjunct to diet and exercise, and necessity of regular testing of blood glucose, glycosylated hemoglobin, renal function, and hematologic parameters. Temporarily d/c therapy prior to intravascular radiocontrast study or surgery. Report unexplained hyperventilation, myalgia, malaise, unusual somnolence, or other nonspecific symptoms. Counsel patient to avoid excessive alcohol intake, either acute or chronic. Drug alone does not cause hypoglycemia but can occur in conjunction with oral sulfonylureas and insulin. Instruct drug must be swallowed whole with a full glass of water and should not be chewed, cut, or crushed. Inactive ingredients may be eliminated in the feces as a soft mass.

**Administration:** Oral route. Must swallow whole with a full glass of water; do not crush or chew. **Storage:** 20-25°C (68-77°F); excursions permitted to 15-30°C (59-86°F). Keep tightly closed. Protect from light.

## FORTAZ RX

ceftazidime (GlaxoSmithKline)

F

**THERAPEUTIC CLASS:** Cephalosporin (3rd generation)

**INDICATIONS:** Treatment of lower respiratory tract (eg, pneumonia), skin and skin structure (SSSI), bone/joint, gynecologic, CNS (eg, meningitis), intra-abdominal, and urinary tract infections (UTI); and septicemia caused by susceptible strains of microorganisms. Treatment of sepsis.

**DOSAGE:** *Adults:* Usual: 1g IM/IV q8-12h. Uncomplicated UTI: 250mg IM/IV q12h. Complicated UTI: 500mg IM/IV q8-12h. Bone and Joint Infection: 2g IV q12h. Uncomplicated Pneumonia/SSSI: 500mg-1g IM/IV q8h. Gynecological/Intra-Abdominal/Meningitis/Severe Life-Threatening Infection: 2g IV q8h. Lung Infection Caused by *Pseudomonas* spp. in Cystic Fibrosis (Normal Renal Function): 30-50mg/kg IV q8h. Max: 6g/day. CrCl 31-50mL/min: 1g q12h. CrCl 16-30mL/min: 1g q24h. CrCl 6-15mL/min: 500mg q24h. CrCl <5mL/min: 500mg q48h. For severe infections (6g/day), increase renal impairment dose by 50% or increase dosing interval. Apply reduced dosage recommendations after initial 1g LD is given. Hemodialysis: Give 1g before, then 1g after each hemodialysis. Intra-Peritoneal Dialysis/Continuous Ambulatory Peritoneal Dialysis: Give 1g followed by 500mg q24h, or add to fluid at 250mg/2L. *Pediatrics:* 1 month-12 yrs: 30-50mg/kg IV q8h. Max: 6g/day. Neonates (0-4 weeks): 30mg/kg IV q12h. Higher doses for cystic fibrosis or meningitis. CrCl 31-50mL/min: 1g q12h. CrCl 16-30mL/min: 1g q24h. CrCl 6-15mL/min: 500mg q24h. CrCl <5mL/min: 500mg q48h. For severe infections (6g/day), increase renal impairment dose by 50% or increase dosing interval. Apply reduced dosage recommendations after initial 1g LD is given. Hemodialysis: Give 1g before, then 1g after each hemodialysis. Intra-Peritoneal Dialysis/Continuous Ambulatory Peritoneal Dialysis: Give 1g followed by 500mg q24h, or add to fluid at 250mg/2L.

**HOW SUPPLIED:** Inj: 500mg, 1g, 1g/50mL, 2g, 2g/50mL, 6g

**WARNINGS/PRECAUTIONS:** Monitor renal function; potential for nephrotoxicity. Prolonged use may result in overgrowth of nonsusceptible organisms. Possible cross-sensitivity between PCNs, cephalosporins, and other β-lactam antibiotics. *Clostridium difficile*-associated diarrhea (CDAD) reported and may range in severity from mild diarrhea to fatal colitis. Elevated levels with renal insufficiency can lead to seizures, encephalopathy, coma, asterixis, and neuromuscular excitability. Possible decrease in PT; caution with renal/hepatic impairment, poor nutritional state; monitor PT and give vitamin K if needed. Caution with colitis, other GI diseases, and elderly. Distal necrosis may occur after inadvertent intra-arterial administration. Continue therapy for 2 days after the signs and symptoms of infection have disappeared, but in complicated infections longer therapy may be required. False (+) for urine glucose with Benedict's solution, Fehling's solution, and Clinitest tabs.

**ADVERSE REACTIONS:** Phlebitis and inflammation at injection site, pruritus, rash, fever, diarrhea.

**INTERACTIONS:** Nephrotoxicity reported with aminoglycosides or potent diuretics (eg, furosemide). Avoid with chloramphenicol; may decrease effect of β-lactam antibiotics. Possible decrease in PT; caution with a protracted course of antimicrobial therapy; monitor PT and give vitamin K if needed. May reduce efficacy of oral contraceptives.

**PREGNANCY:** Category B, caution in nursing.

**MECHANISM OF ACTION:** 3rd-generation cephalosporin; bactericidal, inhibits cell-wall synthesis.

**PHARMACOKINETICS: Absorption:** (IV) Administration of variable doses resulted in different parameters. **Distribution:** Plasma protein binding (≤10%). **Elimination:** Urine (unchanged, 80-90%).

## NURSING CONSIDERATIONS

**Assessment:** Assess for history of hypersensitivity to cephalosporins/PCNs, pregnancy status, possible drug interactions, renal impairment. Document indications for therapy, culture and susceptibility testing. Incision and drainage should be performed in conjunction with antibiotic therapy when indicated.

**Monitoring:** Monitor for signs and symptoms of hypersensitivity reactions (anaphylaxis), CDAD, seizures, LDH, LFTs, renal function, PT, hemolytic anemia, superinfection.

**Patient Counseling:** Inform therapy only treats bacterial, not viral, infections. Take exactly as directed; skipping doses or not completing full course may decrease effectiveness and increase resistance. May experience diarrhea; notify physician if watery/bloody stools, superinfection, or hypersensitivity reactions occur.

**Administration:** IM/IV route. For direct intermittent IV administration, slowly inject into vein over period of 3-5 min or give through tubing of administration set while patient also receives compatible IV fluid. **Storage:** In dry state, store between 15-30°C (59-86°F) and protect from light. Frozen as premixed solution should not be stored above -20°C.

# FORTEO RX

teriparatide (Lilly)

**Increased incidence of osteosarcoma seen in rats. Only prescribe when benefits outweigh risks. Not for those at increased baseline risk for osteosarcoma, including Paget's disease or unexplained alkaline phosphatase elevations, open epiphyses, or prior radiation therapy involving the skeleton.**

**THERAPEUTIC CLASS:** Recombinant human parathyroid hormone

**INDICATIONS:** Treatment of postmenopausal women with osteoporosis at high risk for fracture. To increase bone mass in men with primary or hypogonadal osteoporosis at high risk for fracture. Treatment of men and women with glucocorticoid-induced osteoporosis at high risk for fracture.

**DOSAGE:** *Adults:* 20mcg qd SQ into thigh or abdominal wall. Administer initially under circumstances where patient can sit or lie down if symptoms of orthostatic hypotension occur. Discard pen after 28 days.

**HOW SUPPLIED:** Inj: 250mcg/mL [2.4, 3mL pen]

**WARNINGS/PRECAUTIONS:** Avoid in Paget's disease of the bone, pediatrics, prior external beam or implant radiation therapy, or with bone metastases, or history of skeletal malignancies, metabolic bone diseases other than osteoporosis, or pre-existing hypercalcemia (eg, primary hyperparathyroidism). Potential exacerbation of active or recent urolithiasis. Use with caution in patients with active urolithiasis or pre-existing hypercalciuria; consider determining baseline urinary calcium levels. May increase urinary calcium excretion and serum uric acid levels as well as transiently increase serum calcium levels. Transient episodes of symptomatic orthostatic hypotension reported. Use for >2 years during a patient's lifetime is not recommended.

**ADVERSE REACTIONS:** Pain, arthralgia, asthenia, nausea, rhinitis, dizziness, headache, HTN, increased cough, pharyngitis, constipation, diarrhea, dyspepsia, depression, insomnia.

**INTERACTIONS:** Hypercalcemia may predispose to digitalis toxicity; caution with concomitant use.

**PREGNANCY:** Category C; not for use in nursing.

**MECHANISM OF ACTION:** Recombinant human parathyroid hormone; binds to specific high-affinity cell-surface receptors. Stimulates new bone formation on trabecular and cortical bone surfaces by preferential stimulation of osteoblastic activity over osteoclastic activity. Produces an increase in skeletal mass, an increase in markers of bone formation and resorption, and an increase in bone strength.

**PHARMACOKINETICS: Absorption:** Rapidly absorbed; absolute bioavailability (95%); $T_{max}$=30 min. **Distribution:** (IV) $V_d$=0.12L/kg. **Metabolism:** Liver (nonspecific enzymatic mechanism). **Elimination:** Kidney.

## NURSING CONSIDERATIONS

**Assessment:** Assess for presence of risk factors for developing osteosarcoma (eg, Paget's disease of bone, unexplained elevations in alkaline phosphatase, age of patient or presence of open epiphyses, history of external beam or implant radiation therapy). Assess for presence of bone metastases or history of skeletal malignancies, metabolic bone disease other than osteoporosis, pre-existing hypercalcemia or presence of hypercalcemic disorder (eg, primary hyperparathyroidism), pre-existing hypercalciuria, active or recent urolithiasis, pregnancy/nursing status, and for possible drug interactions. If active urolithiasis or hypercalciuria is present, measure urinary calcium excretion.

**Monitoring:** Monitor for signs/symptoms of osteosarcoma, orthostatic hypotension, hypercalcemia (eg, N/V, constipation, muscle weakness).

**Patient Counseling:** Inform medication has been shown to cause osteosarcomas in animals (rats). Counsel to sit or lie down if lightheaded or develop palpitations following injection; if symptoms persist or worsen, contact physician before continuing treatment. Instruct to contact physician if develop signs of hypercalcemia (eg, N/V, constipation, muscle weakness). Counsel how to properly use delivery device, properly dispose of needles, and to avoid sharing injection pens. Inform each injection pen can be used for up to 28 days; discard after 28 days. Counsel not to use medication for more than 2 years. Advise about the roles of supplemental calcium and/or vitamin D, weight-bearing exercise, and behavior modification factors (eg, smoking/alcohol consumption). Encourage to enroll in the voluntary Forteo patient registry.

**Administration:** SQ route, into thigh or abdominal wall. **Storage:** 2-8°C (36-46°F). Recap pen when not in use to protect cartridge from physical damage and light. Minimize time out of refrigerator. Do not freeze; do not use if frozen.

# FORTICAL — RX

calcitonin-salmon (rdna origin) (Upsher-Smith)

**THERAPEUTIC CLASS:** Hormonal bone resorption inhibitor

**INDICATIONS:** Treatment of postmenopausal osteoporosis in females >5 yrs postmenopause in conjunction with an adequate calcium and vitamin D intake.

**DOSAGE:** *Adults:* 200 IU qd intranasally. Alternate nostrils daily.

**HOW SUPPLIED:** Nasal Spray: 200 IU/inh

**CONTRAINDICATIONS:** Clinical allergy to calcitonin-salmon.

**WARNINGS/PRECAUTIONS:** Possibility of systemic allergic reactions. Consider skin testing if sensitivity suspected. If nasal mucosa ulceration occurs, d/c until healed. D/C if severe ulceration of nasal mucosa occurs. Perform periodic nasal exams. Incidence of rhinitis, irritation, erythema, and excoriation higher in geriatric patients.

**ADVERSE REACTIONS:** Rhinitis, nasal symptoms, back pain, arthralgia, epistaxis, headache

**PREGNANCY:** Category C, not for use in nursing.

**MECHANISM OF ACTION:** Hormonal bone resorption inhibitor; not established. Calcitonin receptors are found in osteoclasts and osteoblasts. Single use produces transient inhibition of bone resorptive process; persistent use causes smaller decreases in rate of bone resorption. Inhibits osteoclast function with loss of ruffled osteoclast border.

**PHARMACOKINETICS: Absorption:** Rapid.

## NURSING CONSIDERATIONS

**Assessment:** Assess for sensitivity to calcitonin; perform skin testing if sensitivity suspected. Assess pregnancy/nursing status.

**Monitoring:** Monitor for signs/symptoms of allergic reaction (eg, anaphylactic shock, broncospasm, swelling of tongue or throat), nasal mucosal alterations, rhinitis, epitaxis, and sinusitis. Perform periodic nasal exams of nasal mucosa, turbinates, septum, and mucosal blood vessels. Perform periodic monitoring of urine sediment. Measure lumbar vertebral bone mass periodically to monitor for efficacy.

**Patient Counseling:** Counsel to notify physician of significant nasal irritation. Advise to store new, unassembled medication in refrigerator; do not freeze. Instruct that before priming pump and using new medication, allow to reach room temperature. Inform that after opening, store at room temperature, in upright position; discard unused medication 30 days after 1st use.

**Administration:** Intranasal route. **Storage:** Unopened: 2-8°C (36-46°F). Protect from freezing. Opened: 20-25°C (68-77°F); excursions permitted to 15-30°C (59-86°F). Store in upright position. Discard 30 days after 1st use.

F

## FOSAMAX RX

alendronate sodium (Merck)

**THERAPEUTIC CLASS:** Bisphosphonate

**INDICATIONS:** Treatment and prevention of osteoporosis in postmenopausal women. Treatment to increase bone mass in men with osteoporosis. Treatment of glucocorticoid-induced osteoporosis. Treatment of Paget's disease.

**DOSAGE:** *Adults:* Osteoporosis: Treatment: 70mg once weekly or 10mg qd. Prevention: 35mg once weekly or 5mg qd. Glucocorticoid-Induced: 5mg qd; 10mg qd for postmenopausal women not on estrogen. Paget's Disease: 40mg qd for 6 months. Take at least 30 min before the first food, beverage (other than water), or medication (Take tabs with 6-8 oz plain water or 2 oz with oral sol). Do not lie down for at least 30 min and until after 1st food of day.

**HOW SUPPLIED:** Sol: 70mg [75mL]; Tab: 5mg, 10mg, 35mg, 40mg, 70mg

**CONTRAINDICATIONS:** Esophagus abnormalities which delay esophageal emptying such as stricture or achalasia; inability to stand or sit upright for at least 30 min; hypocalcemia. Patients at risk of aspiration (oral solution).

**WARNINGS/PRECAUTIONS:** Caution with active upper GI problems. May cause local irritation of the upper GI mucosa. Esophageal adverse events (eg, esophagitis, esophageal ulcers/erosions) as well as postmarketing experience of severe gastric and duodenal ulcers with complications reported. D/C if esophageal reaction (eg, dysphagia, odynophagia, retrosternal pain, new or worsening heartburn) develop. Caution in patients with active upper GI problems (eg, dysphagia, esophageal diseases, gastritis, duodenitis, ulcers). Increased risk of esophageal adverse events if lie down after administration, if fail to swallow with recommended amount of water, and/or if continue to take after develop symptoms of esophageal irritation. Correct hypocalcemia or other mineral metabolism disturbances (eg, vitamin D deficiency) before initiating therapy; monitor serum calcium and for hypocalcemia during treatment. May cause asymptomatic decreases in serum calcium and phosphate. Supplement calcium and vitamin D if needed. Reports of severe, incapacitating bone, joint, and/or muscle pain; d/c if severe symptoms develop. Osteonecrosis of the jaw reported. Not recommended with renal insufficiency (CrCl <35mL/min). In patients with glucocorticoid induced osteoporosis, ascertain hormonal status and consider replacement therapy; perform BMD test at initiation and repeat after 6-12 months after alendronate and glucocorticoid treatment.

**ADVERSE REACTIONS:** Abdominal pain, nausea, dyspepsia, constipation, diarrhea, musculoskeletal pain (bone, muscle, or joint), acid regurgitation, flatulence, headache, abdominal distension, gastric ulcer, joint swelling.

**INTERACTIONS:** Calcium supplements and other multivalent cations, antacids, other oral medications may interfere with absorption; take at least one-half hour after alendronate. Increased GI irritation with ASA and alendronate >10mg. Caution with NSAIDs use. Reduced bioavailability when taken concomitantly with coffee, orange juice. Concomitant use with IV ranitidine may double bioavailibility of oral alendronate. Use with hormone replacement therapy (HRT) (estrogen +/- progestin) may significantly increase the degree of suppression of bone turnover.

**PREGNANCY:** Category C, caution in nursing.

**MECHANISM OF ACTION:** Bisphosphonate; binds to hydroxyapatite found in bone, specifically inhibits the osteoclast mediated bone resorption and reduces bone turnover.

**PHARMACOKINETICS: Distribution:** $V_d$=28L; plasma protein binding (78%). **Excretion:** Urine (50%), feces (little or none); $T_{1/2}$=>10 yrs.

F

## NURSING CONSIDERATIONS

**Assessment:** Assess for abnormalities of the esophagus which delay esophageal emptying (eg, stricture, achalsia), ability to stand or sit upright for at least 30 minutes, hypocalcemia, upper GI problems (dysphagia, esophageal diseases, gastritis, duodenitis, ulcers), risk of developing osteonecrosis of the jaw, renal impairment (eg, CrCl <35 mL/min), pregnancy/nursing status, and possible drug interactions. Assess for other causes of osteoporosis other than estrogen deficiency, aging, and glucocorticoid use. In patients with glucocorticoid-induced osteoporosis, assess the hormonal status and consider appropriate replacement therapy; obtain a baseline bone mineral density measurement if on concomitant therapy with glucocorticoids. Assess risk of aspiration if using alendronate oral solution.

**Monitoring:** Monitor for signs/symptoms of upper GI mucosal irritation, esophageal complications (eg, esophagitis, esophageal ulcers, esophageal erosions, esophageal stricture or perforation), gastric and duodenal ulcers, musculoskeletal pain, and osteonecrosis of the jaw. In patients with a history of hypocalcemia, monitor calcium levels and for signs/symptoms of hypocalcemia. If on concomitant therapy with glucocorticoids, monitor bone mineral density every 6-12 months.

**Patient Counseling:** Instruct to take supplemental calcium and vitamin D if daily dietary intake is inadequate. Counsel to consider weight-bearing exercise as well as modification of certain behavioral factors (eg, cigarette smoking, excessive alcohol consumption). Instruct to take medication with plain water in the morning (at least 30 min before the first food, beverage, or medication). Advise to swallow each tablet with a full glass of water (6-8 oz). If taking oral solution formulation, advise to take with at least 2 oz of water following administration of medication. Advise to avoid chewing or sucking on medication due to potential for oropharyngeal ulceration. Counsel not to take at bedtime or before rising for the day. Instruct to avoid lying down for at least 30 min following administration and until after first food of the day. Advise to d/c and contact physician if symptoms of esophageal disease (eg, difficulty swallowing, new or worsening heartburn) develop. Advise if the once-a-week dose is missed, take the following morning and return to taking dose on regularly scheduled day. Counsel to separate administration 30 min from other oral medications.

**Administration:** Oral route. **Storage:** Tab: 15-30°C (59-86°F); Oral sol: 25°C (77°F); excursions permitted to 15-30°C (59-86°F). Do not freeze.

# FOSAMAX PLUS D — RX

alendronate sodium - cholecalciferol (Merck)

**THERAPEUTIC CLASS:** Bisphosphonate/vitamin D analog

**INDICATIONS:** Treatment of osteoporosis in postmenopausal women. Treatment to increase bone mass in men with osteoporosis.

**DOSAGE:** *Adults:* 1 tab (70mg/5600 IU or 70mg/2800 IU) once weekly. Take with plain water (6-8 oz) at least 30 min before 1st food, beverage (other than water), or medication. Do not lie down for at least 30 min and until after 1st food of day.

**HOW SUPPLIED:** Tab: (Alendronate Sodium-Cholecalciferol) 70mg-2800 IU, 70mg-5600 IU

**CONTRAINDICATIONS:** Esophagus abnormalities which delay esophageal emptying such as stricture or achalasia; inability to stand or sit upright for at least 30 min; hypocalcemia.

**WARNINGS/PRECAUTIONS:** Caution with active upper GI problems. May cause local irritation of the upper GI mucosa. Esophageal adverse events (esophagitis, esophageal ulcers/erosions) as well as post-marketing experience of severe gastric and duodenal ulcers with complications reported. D/C if esophageal reaction (eg, dysphagia, odynophagia, retrosternal pain, new or worsening heartburn) develop. Correct hypocalcemia or other mineral metabolism disturbances before initiating therapy. May worsen hypercalcemia and/or hypercalciuria; monitor urine and serum calcium while on treatment. Supplement calcium if needed. Do not use to treat vitamin D deficiency. Not recommended with renal insufficiency (CrCl <35mL/min). Reports of severe, incapacitating bone, joint, and/or muscle pain; d/c if these develop. Osteonecrosis of the jaw may develop.



**ADVERSE REACTIONS:** Abdominal pain, nausea, dyspepsia, constipation, diarrhea, flatulence, acid regurgitation, musculoskeletal pain (bone, muscle, or joint).

**INTERACTIONS:** Alendronate: Calcium supplements, antacids, other oral medications may interfere with absorption; take at least one-half hour after alendronate. Increased GI irritation with ASA and alendronate >10mg. Caution with NSAIDs, other GI irritants. Bioavailability doubled by intravenous ranitidine. Reduced bioavailability when taken concomitantly with coffee, orange juice. Cholecalciferol: Olestra, mineral oils, orlistat, bile acid sequestrants may impair absorption of vitamin D while anticonvulsants, cimetidine, and thiazides may increase catabolism; consider supplementation.

**PREGNANCY:** Category C, caution in nursing.

**MECHANISM OF ACTION:** Alendronate: Bisphosphonate; binds to bone hydroxyapatite, specifically inhibits the activity of osteoclasts, reduces bone resorption with no direct effect on bone formation. Cholecalciferol: Vitamin D analog; increases intestinal absorption of calcium and phosphate; regulates excretion of serum calcium, renal calcium and phosphate, bone formation, and bone resorption.

**PHARMACOKINETICS: Absorption:** Cholecalciferol: $C_{max}$=4.0ng/mL; $T_{max}$=10.6 hrs; AUC=120.7ng•hr/mL. **Distribution:** Alendronate: $V_d$=28L; plasma protein binding (78%). Cholecalciferol: Found in breast milk. **Metabolism:** Cholecalciferol: Liver (rapid) (hydroxylation) to 25-hydroxyvitamin $D_3$ (major storage form metabolite); kidney to 1,25-dihydroxyvitamin $D_3$ (active metabolite). **Elimination:** Alendronate: Urine (50%), feces (little or none); $T_{1/2}$>10 years. Cholecalceferol: Urine (2.4%), feces (4.9%); $T_{1/2}$=14 hrs.

## NURSING CONSIDERATIONS

**Assessment:** Assess for esophageal abnormalities (eg, stricture, achalasia) or upper GI disorders (eg, dysphagia, gastritis, duodenitis, ulcers), GI malabsorption syndrome, ability to stand or sit upright for at least 30 min, risk of aspiration, hypocalcemia and other disorders affecting mineral metabolism (eg, vitamin D deficiency), risk of osteonecrosis of the jaw, renal insufficiencies (eg, CrCl<35mL/min), pregnancy/nursing status, and possible drug interactions.

**Monitoring:** Monitor for signs/symptoms of local upper GI mucosa irritation, esophageal complications (eg, esophagitis, esophageal ulcers, esophageal erosions), musculoskeletal pain, and osteonecrosis of the jaw. If patients have unregulated overproduction of 1,25 dihydroxyvitamin D (eg, leukemia, lymphoma), monitor urine and serum calcium levels. With history of hypocalcemia, monitor serum calcium levels and for signs/symptoms of hypocalcemia.

**Patient Counseling:** Instruct to take supplemental calcium if intake is inadequate. Instruct to take additional vitamin D if at risk for vitamin D deficiency (eg, >70 yrs, nursing home-bound, chronically ill); vitamin D needs increase with GI malabsorption syndromes. Counsel to consider weight-bearing exercise, behavioral modification (eg, cigarette smoking, excessive alcohol consumption). Take with full glass of water first thing in the morning (at least 30 min before first food/beverage or medication). Avoid lying down for 30 min following administration. Avoid chewing or sucking on medication; avoid taking medication at bedtime or before rising for the day. Advise to d/c and contact physician if signs of esophageal disease (eg, difficulty swallowing, new or worsening heartburn) develop. If a dose is missed, take the following morning; return to taking on regularly scheduled day.

**Administration:** Oral route. **Storage:** 20-25°C (68-77°F); excursions permitted to 15-30°C (59-86°F). Protect from moisture and light. Store in original blister package until use.



## FOSRENOL RX

lanthanum carbonate (Shire)

**THERAPEUTIC CLASS:** Phoshphate binder

**INDICATIONS:** Reduction of serum phosphate in patients with end-stage renal disease.

**DOSAGE:** *Adults:* Initial: 750-1500mg/day in divided doses. Titrate: Every 2-3 weeks in increments of 750mg/day until acceptable serum phosphate level is reached. Take with meals and chew tablets completely before swallowing. Usual range: 1500-3000mg/day. Usual max: 3750mg/day.

**HOW SUPPLIED:** Tab, Chewable: 250mg, 500mg, 750mg, 1000mg

**WARNINGS/PRECAUTIONS:** Caution with acute peptic ulcer, ulcerative colitis, Crohn's disease or bowel obstruction.

**ADVERSE REACTIONS:** Nausea, vomiting, dialysis graft occulsion, abdominal pain.

**INTERACTIONS:** Should not be taken within 2 hrs of antacids.

**PREGNANCY:** Category C, caution in nursing.

**MECHANISM OF ACTION:** Inhibits absorption of phosphate by forming highly insoluble lanthanum phosphate complexes, consequently reducing both serum phosphate and calcium product.

**PHARMACOKINETICS: Absorption:** $C_{max}$=1.0ng/mL. **Distribution:** Plasma protein binding (>99%). **Metabolism:** Not metabolized. **Elimination:** $T_{1/2}$=53 hrs, ($T_{1/2}$=2-3.6 yrs, from bone).

### NURSING CONSIDERATIONS

**Assessment:** Assess for acute peptic ulcer, ulcerative colitis, Crohn's disease, bowel obstruction, and pregnancy/nursing status.

**Monitoring:** Monitor for GI events and NV. Drug may appear as imaging agent in abdominal x-rays.

**Patient Counseling:** Take with or immediately after meals. Chew completely before swallowing. Do not swallow intact tablets.

**Administration:** Oral route. **Storage:** 25°C (77°F); excursions permitted to 15-30°C (59-86°F).

## FRAGMIN RX

dalteparin sodium (Eisai)

**Epidural or spinal hematomas resulting in long-term or permanent paralysis may occur in patients anticoagulated with low molecular weight heparins, heparinoids, or fondaparinux sodium and who are receiving neuraxial anesthesia or undergoing spinal puncture. Increased risk with indwelling epidural catheters, concomitant use of other drugs that affect hemostasis (eg, NSAIDs, platelet inhibitors, other anticoagulants), history of traumatic or repeated epidural or spinal puncture, or a history of spinal deformity or spinal surgery. Monitor frequently for signs/symptoms of neurologic impairment; if neurologic compromise noted, urgent treatment is necessary. Consider benefit and risks before neuraxial intervention in patients anticoagulated or to be anticoagulated for thromboprophylaxis.**

**THERAPEUTIC CLASS:** Low molecular weight heparin

**INDICATIONS:** Prophylaxis of ischemic complications in unstable angina and non-Q-wave MI in conjunction with ASA therapy. Prophylaxis of DVT in hip replacement surgery, abdominal surgery in patients who are at high risk for thromboembolic complications, and for those at risk for thromboembolic complications due to severely restricted mobility during acute illness. Extended treatment of symptomatic VTE (proximal DVT and/or PE) to reduce the recurrence of VTE in patients with cancer.



**DOSAGE:** *Adults:* Administer SQ. Unstable Angina/Non-Q-Wave MI: 120 IU/kg q12h in conjunction with ASA (75-165mg/day) for 5-8 days. Max: 10,000 IU q12h. Hip Surgery: Pre-Op Start: (if start 2 hrs pre-op): 2500 IU within 2 hrs pre-op, then 2500 IU 4-8 hrs post-op. (if start 10-14 hrs pre-op): 5000 IU 10-14 hrs pre-op, then 5000 IU 4-8 hrs post-op. Post-Op Start: 2500 IU 4-8 hrs post-op. Maint (for any starting dose): 5000 IU SQ qd for 5-10 days post-op (up to 14 days). Abdominal Surgery: 2500 IU 1-2 hrs pre-op. Maint: 2500 IU qd for 5-10 days post-op. Abdominal Surgery with High Risk: 5000 IU evening before surgery. Maint: 5000 IU qd for 5-10 days post-op. Abdominal Surgery with Malignancy: Initial: 2500 IU 1-2 hrs pre-op, then 2500 IU 12 hrs later. Maint: 5000 IU qd for 5-10 days post-op. Severely Restricted Mobility During Acute Illness: 5000 IU qd for 12-14 days. Symptomatic VTE in Cancer Patients: 200 IU/kg qd for first 30 days, then 150 IU/kg qd for months 2-6. Max: 18,000 IU/day. Platelet Count 50,000-100,000/$mm^3$: Reduce dose by 2500 IU until platelet count ≥100,000/$mm^3$. Platelet Count <50,000/$mm^3$: D/C therapy until platelet count >50,000/$mm^3$. Renal Impairment (CrCl <30mL/min): Monitor anti-Xa levels to determine appropriate dose.

**HOW SUPPLIED:** Inj: (Syringe) 2500 IU/0.2mL, 5000 IU/0.2mL, 7500 IU/0.3mL, 10,000 IU/0.4mL, 10,000 IU/1mL, 12,500 IU/0.5mL, 15,000 IU/0.6mL, 18,000 IU/0.72mL; (MDV) 10,000 IU/mL [9.5mL], 25,000 IU/mL [3.8mL]

**CONTRAINDICATIONS:** Active major bleeding or thrombocytopenia associated with positive in vitro tests for antiplatelet antibody in the presence of dalteparin sodium. Hypersensitivity to heparin or pork products. Patients undergoing regional anesthesia should not recieve dalteparin sodium for unstable angina or non-Q-wave MI. Patients with cancer undergoing regional anesthesia should not receive dalteparin sodium for extended treatment of symptomatic VTE.

**WARNINGS/PRECAUTIONS:** Not for IM injection. Cannot use interchangeably unit for unit with heparin or other low molecular weight heparins. Extreme caution in patients with increased risk of bleeding (severe uncontrolled HTN, bacterial endocarditis, congenital or acquired bleeding disorders, active ulceration and angiodyplastic GI disease, hemorrhagic stroke or shortly after brain, spinal or ophthalmological surgery). Bleeding and thrombocytopenia may occur. Use with extreme caution in patients who have a history of heparin-induced thrombocytopenia. Multi-dose vials contain benzyl alcohol; "Gasping Syndrome" in premature infants reported; caution in pregnant women. Perform periodic CBC including platelets, blood chemistry, and stool occult blood test. May use Anti-Factor Xa to monitor anticoagulant effect during therapy.

**ADVERSE REACTIONS:** Hemorrhage, elevation of serum transaminase (ALT, AST), injection-site pain, allergic reactions, thrombocytopenia.

**INTERACTIONS:** Caution with oral anticoagulants, platelet inhibitors, and thrombolytic agents due to increased risk of bleeding.

**PREGNANCY:** Category B, caution in nursing.

**MECHANISM OF ACTION:** Low molecular weight heparin; enhances inhibition of Factor Xa and thrombin by antithrombin, while only slightly affecting the activated partial thromboplastin time.

**PHARMACOKINETICS: Absorption:** Absolute bioavailability (87%). (2500 IU) $C_{max}$=0.19 IU/mL. (5000 IU) $C_{max}$= 0.41 IU/mL. (10,000 IU) $C_{max}$=0.82 IU/mL; $T_{max}$=4 hrs. **Distribution:** $V_d$=40-60mL/kg. **Elimination:** (40 IU/kg) (IV) $T_{1/2}$=2.1 hrs. (60 IU/kg) (IV) $T_{1/2}$=2.3 hrs; (SQ) $T_{1/2}$=3-5 hrs.

## NURSING CONSIDERATIONS

**Assessment:** Assess for active major bleeding, history of heparin-induced thrombocytopenia, conditions that may increase risk of hemorrhage (eg, severe uncontrolled HTN, bacterial endocarditis, congenital/acquired bleeding disorders, active ulceration, angiodysplastic GI disease, hypertensive or diabetic retinopathy and patients receiving neuraxial anesthesia or spinal puncture), pregnancy/nursing status, known hypersensitivity to heparin or pork products, and possible drug interactions. Assess use in patients with severe hepatic/renal insufficiencies.

**Monitoring:** Monitor for signs/symptoms of hemorrhage, thrombocytopenia, and allergic reactions. Monitor for signs/symptoms of spinal or epidural hematomas in patients on concomitant therapy with neuraxial anesthesia or spinal puncture. Perform periodic monitoring of CBC (platelet count), blood chemistry, and stool occult blood tests. In patients with severe renal impairment (CrCl <30mL/min) monitor anti-Xa levels.

F

**Patient Counseling:** Instruct to contact physician if any type of unusual bleeding or allergic reactions develop. Inform that periodic lab monitoring is required during medication. If pregnant, instruct to use preservative-free formulation. Counsel on the proper way to administer: do not mix with other injections or infusions; patient should be sitting or lying down; may be administered in U-shaped area around navel, upper outer side of thigh, or upper outer quadrangle of buttock; vary injection site daily; If area around navel or thigh is used, using thumb and forefinger, lift up fold of skin while giving injection; Insert at 45 to 90-degree angle.

**Administration:** SQ route. Do not mix with other injections or infusions. Patient should be sitting or lying down. May be administered in U-shaped area around navel, upper outer side of thigh, or upper outer quadrangle of buttock. Vary injection site daily. If area around navel or thigh is used, using thumb and forefinger, lift up fold of skin while giving injection. Insert at 45 to 90-degree angle. **Storage:** 20-25°C (68-77°F).

## FROVA — RX

frovatriptan succinate (Endo)

**THERAPEUTIC CLASS:** 5-$HT_{1B/1D}$ agonist

**INDICATIONS:** Acute treatment of migraine with or without aura.

**DOSAGE:** *Adults:* ≥18 yrs: 2.5mg with fluids. If headache recurs after initial relief, may repeat after 2 hrs. Max: 7.5mg/day. Safety of treating >4 headaches/30 days not known.

**HOW SUPPLIED:** Tab: 2.5mg

**CONTRAINDICATIONS:** Ischemic heart disease, coronary artery vasospasm (eg, Prinzmetal's angina), significant cardiovascular disease, cerebrovascular syndromes, peripheral vascular disease, uncontrolled HTN, hemiplegic or basilar migraine, use within 24 hrs of treatment with another 5-$HT_1$ agonist or ergot-type agent.

**WARNINGS/PRECAUTIONS:** Confirm diagnosis. Supervise 1st dose and monitor cardiac function in those at risk of CAD (eg, HTN, hypercholesterolemia, smoker, obesity, diabetes, CAD family history, postmenopausal women, males >40 yrs). Serious adverse cardiac events, cerebrovascular events, vasospastic reactions reported. May bind to melanin in the eye; possibility of long-term effects. Serotonin syndrome symptoms (eg, mental status changes, autonomic instability, neuromuscular aberrations, and GI symptoms) reported.

**ADVERSE REACTIONS:** Dizziness, headache, paresthesia, dry mouth, dyspepsia, fatigue, hot or cold sensation, chest pain, skeletal pain, and flushing.

**INTERACTIONS:** Prolonged vasospastic reactions reported with ergot-containing drugs; avoid use within 24 hrs. Avoid within 24 hrs of other 5-$HT_{1B/1D}$ agonists. Serotonin syndrome symptoms reported with concomitant use of SSRI or SNRI.

**PREGNANCY:** Category C, caution in nursing.

**MECHANISM OF ACTION:** Selective 5-$HT_1$ receptor agonist; binds with high affinity to 5-$HT_{1B/1D}$ receptors. Believed to act on extracerebral, intracranial blood vessels, and to inhibit excessive dilation of these vessels in migraine.

**PHARMACOKINETICS: Absorption:** Absolute bioavailability: (20%) male, (30%) female; $T_{max}$=2-4 hrs. **Distribution:** $V_d$=4.2L/kg (male), 3L/kg (female); plasma protein binding (15%). **Metabolism:** CYP1A2. **Elimination:** Feces (62%), urine (32%); $T_{1/2}$=26 hrs.

## NURSING CONSIDERATIONS

**Assessment:** Confirm diagnosis of migraine before initiating therapy. Assess for IHD (eg, angina pectoris, Prinzmetal's variant angina, MI or documented silent MI), HTN, hemiplegic/or basilar migraine, cerebrovascular syndromes (eg, stroke, TIAs), PVD, presence of risk factors of CAD (eg, hypercholesterolemia, smoking, obesity, DM, strong family history of CAD, female with surgical or physiological menopause, or male >49 yrs), ECG changes, hepatic/renal impairment, pregnancy/nursing status, and possible drug interactions.

**Monitoring:** Administration of 1st dose should be in physician's office or medically staffed and equipped facility as cardiac ischemia may occur in absence of clinical symptoms; ECG should be obtained immediately during interval in those with risk factors. Monitor for signs/symptoms of cardiac events (eg, coronary vasospasm, acute MI, arrhythmia, ECG changes, follow-up coronary angiography), cerebrovascular events (eg, hemorrhage, stroke, TIAs), peripheral vascular ischemia, colonic ischemia with bloody diarrhea and abdominal pain, serotonin syndrome (eg, mental status changes, autonomic instability, neuromuscular aberrations and/or GI symptoms), ophthalmic effects, and increased BP.

**Patient Counseling:** Instruct to read PI before use. Inform about potential risks (eg, serotonin syndrome manifestations), especially if taken with SSRIs or SNRIs. Report adverse reactions to physician. Advise to take as directed. Instruct to notify physician if pregnant/nursing or planning to become pregnant.

**Administration:** Oral route. **Storage**: 25°C (77°F); excursions permitted to 15-30°C (59-86°F). Protect from moisture.

# FUROSEMIDE RX

furosemide (Various)

**Can lead to profound water and electrolyte depletion with excessive use.**

**OTHER BRAND NAMES:** Lasix (Sanofi-Aventis)

**THERAPEUTIC CLASS:** Loop diuretic

**INDICATIONS:** (Inj, PO) Treatment of edema associated with CHF, liver cirrhosis, and renal disease including nephrotic syndrome. (PO) Treatment of hypertension. (Inj) Adjunct therapy for acute pulmonary edema.

**DOSAGE:** *Adults:* (PO) HTN: Initial: 40mg bid. Edema: Initial: 20-80mg PO. May repeat or increase by 20-40mg after 6-8 hrs. Max: 600mg/day. Alternative Regimen: Dose on 2-4 consecutive days each week. Closely monitor if on >80mg/day. (Inj) Edema: Initial: 20-40mg IV/IM. May repeat or increase by 20mg after 2 hrs. Acute Pulmonary Edema: Initial: 40mg IV. May increase to 80mg IV after 1 hr.
*Pediatrics:* Edema: (PO) Initial: 2mg/kg single dose. May increase by 1-2mg/kg after 6-8 hrs. Max: 6mg/kg. (Inj) Initial: 1mg/kg IV/IM single dose. May increase by 1mg/kg IV/IM after 2 hrs. Max: 6mg/kg.

**HOW SUPPLIED:** Inj: 10mg/mL; Sol: 10mg/mL, 40mg/5mL; Tab: 20mg, 40mg*, 80mg *scored

**CONTRAINDICATIONS:** Anuria.

**WARNINGS/PRECAUTIONS:** Monitor for fluid/electrolyte imbalance (eg, hypokalemia), renal or hepatic dysfunction. Initiate in hospital with hepatic cirrhosis and ascites. Tinnitus, hearing impairment, hyperglycemia, hyperuricemia reported. May activate SLE. Cross-sensitivity with sulfonamide allergy. Avoid excessive diuresis, especially in elderly.

**ADVERSE REACTIONS:** Pancreatitis, jaundice, anorexia, paresthesias, ototoxicity, blood dyscrasias, dizziness, rash, urticaria, photosensitivity, fever, thrombophlebitis, restlessness.

**INTERACTIONS:** Ototoxicity with aminoglycosides, ethacrynic acid. Caution with high-dose salicylates. Lithium toxicity. Antagonizes tubocurarine. Potentiates antihypertensives, succinylcholine, ganglionic or peripheral adrenergic blockers. Decreases arterial response to norepinephrine. Separate sucralfate dose by 2 hrs. Indomethacin may decrease effects. Hypokalemia with ACTH, corticosteroids. Renal changes with NSAIDs. Orthostatic hypotension may be aggravated by alcohol, barbiturates, or narcotics.



**PREGNANCY:** Category C, caution in nursing.

**MECHANISM OF ACTION:** Anthranilic acid derivative (diuretic); primarily inhibits reabsorption of $Na^+$ and $Cl^-$ in proximal and distal tubules and in loop of Henle.

**PHARMACOKINETICS: Distribution:** Plasma protein binding (91-99%). **Metabolism:** Biotransformation. Furosemide glucuronide (major metabolite). **Elimination:** Urine; $T_{1/2}$=2 hrs.

## NURSING CONSIDERATIONS

**Assessment:** Assess for anuria, sulfonamide hypersensitivity, DM, possible drug interactions, hepatic/renal impairment. Obtain baseline serum electrolytes, renal function, urine, and blood glucose.

**Monitoring:** Monitor serum electrolytes frequently in first few months, then periodically; renal function, urine, and blood glucose periodically. Monitor for signs/symptoms of electrolyte imbalance, blood dyscrasias, hyperglycemia, hyperuricemia or precipitation of gout, hypotension, ototoxicity, persistent PDA, and hypersensitivity reactions.

**Patient Counseling:** Advise to seek medical attention if symptoms of electrolyte imbalance (dry mouth, thirst, weakness), hypotension, ototoxicity (tinnitus, hearing impairment), or hypersensitivity reactions occur.

**Administration:** Oral, IV route. **Storage**: Tab, Sol: 25°C (77°F); excursions permitted to 15-30°C (59-86°F). IV: 15-30°C (59-86°F). Protect from light.

# FUZEON RX

enfuvirtide (Roche Labs)

**THERAPEUTIC CLASS:** Fusion inhibitor

**INDICATIONS:** In combination with other antiretroviral agents for the treatment of HIV-1 infection in treatment-experienced patients with evidence of HIV-1 replication despite ongoing antiretroviral therapy.

**DOSAGE:** *Adults:* 90mg SQ bid. Inject into upper arm, anterior thigh, or abdomen.
*Pediatrics:* 6-16 yrs: 2mg/kg SQ bid. Max: 90mg bid. Refer to PI for weight-based dosing chart. Inject into upper arm, anterior thigh, or abdomen.

**HOW SUPPLIED:** Inj: 90mg/mL [60[s]].

**WARNINGS/PRECAUTIONS:** 98% of subjects experienced at least one injection-site reaction during treatment in randomized, controlled, open-label, multicenter trials. Administration with Biojector 2000 may result in neuralgia and/or paresthesia, bruising and hematomas. Patients receiving anticoagulants or persons with hemophilia, or other coagulation disorders, may have a higher risk of post-injection bleeding. Monitor for signs and symptoms of pneumonia in HIV-infected patients, especially those predisposed to pneumonia (eg, low initial CD4 cell count, high initial viral load, intravenous drug use, smoking, and prior history of lung disease). Associated with systemic hypersensitivity reactions; d/c immediately upon signs and symptoms. Use in noninfected HIV patients may lead to anti-enfuvirtide antibody production which cross react with HIV gp41; false-positive HIV test with an ELISA assay may result. Patients treated with combination antiretroviral therapy may experience immune reconstitution syndrome requiring further evaluation and treatment.

**ADVERSE REACTIONS:** Diarrhea, local injection-site reactions, fatigue, nausea, decreased weight, sinusitis, abdominal pain, cough, herpes simplex, decreased appetite, pancreatitis, pneumonia, immune reconstitution syndrome, hypersensitivity reaction.

**INTERACTIONS:** Higher risk of post-injection bleeding with anticoagulants. Concomitant use with antiretrovirals.

**PREGNANCY:** Category B, not for use in nursing.

**MECHANISM OF ACTION:** Fusion inhibitor; interferes with the entry of HIV-1 into cells by inhibiting fusion of viral and cellular membranes; binds to the first heptad-repeat (HR1) in the gp41 subunit of the viral envelope glycoprotein and prevents the conformational changes required for the fusion of viral and cellular membranes.

**PHARMACOKINETICS: Absorption:** (Parameters when used in combination with other antiretrovirals) $C_{max}$=5mcg/mL; $T_{max}$=4-8 hrs; AUC=48.7mcg•hr/mL. (IV) Absolute bioavailabilty (84.3%). **Distribution:**$V_d$=5.5L; plasma protein binding (92%). **Metabolism:** Liver via hydrolysis; $M_3$ (metabolite). **Elimination:** $T_{1/2}$=3.8 hrs.

## NURSING CONSIDERATIONS

**Assessment:** Assess for risk factors for pneumonia (history of lung disease, decreased $CD4^+$ cell count, increased viral load, IV drug use, smoking), infections, hemophilia, history of coagulation disorders, hypersensitivity and pregnancy/nursing status.

**Monitoring:** Monitor for signs/symptoms of cellulitis or local injection-site reactions, immune reconstitution syndrome, post-injection bleeding, nerve pain/paresthesia, and hypersensitivity. Monitor for signs and symptoms of pneumonia (cough with fever, rapid breathing, SOB).

**Patient Counseling:** Inform patient that injection-site reactions occur in almost all patients. Advise to seek medical attention if symptoms of pneumonia, systemic hypersensitivity (eg, rash, fever, N/V, chills, rigors, hypotension), post-injection bleeding, cellulitis, and nerve pain (paresthesia) occur. Counsel that they may continue to contract illnesses associated with HIV-1 infection and may still transmit the infection through sexual contact or blood contamination. Inform that the drug must be taken as a part of a combination antiretroviral regimen. Instruct not to change dosage or schedule, or to stop drug without consulting physician. Instruct not to breastfeed. Advise to practice aseptic technique upon administration in order to avoid injection site infections.

**Administration:** SQ route. Refer to PI for proper administration. Do not inject into moles, scar tissue, bruises, navel, surgical scars, tattoos, burn sites, directly over a blood vessel, or areas where large nerves course close to the skin, preceding site or on current injection site reaction from an earlier dose. **Storage:** 25°C (77°F); excursions permitted to 15-30°C (59-86°F). Reconstituted Solution: 2-8°C (36-46°F). Use within 24 hrs.

# GABITRIL — RX

tiagabine HCl (Cephalon)

**THERAPEUTIC CLASS:** Nipecotic acid derivative

**INDICATIONS:** Adjunctive therapy in adults and children ≥12 yrs in the treatment of partial seizures.

**DOSAGE:** *Adults:* Induced (patients already taking enzyme-inducing antiepilepsy drugs [AEDs]): Initial: 4mg qd. Titrate: May increase weekly by 4-8mg until clinical response achieved. Refer to PI for typical dosing titration. Max: 56mg/day given bid-qid. Non-induced: Requires lower dose and slower titration. Hepatic Impairment: Requires lower initial/maint doses and longer dosing intervals.
*Pediatrics:* 12-18 yrs: Induced: Initial: 4mg qd. Titrate: May increase to 4mg qd at beginning of Week 2, then increase weekly by 4-8mg until clinical response achieved. Refer to PI for typical dosing titration. Max: 32mg/day.

Non-induced: Requires lower dose and slower titration. Hepatic Impairment: Requires lower initial/maint doses and longer dosing intervals.

**HOW SUPPLIED:** Tab: 2mg, 4mg, 12mg, 16mg

**WARNINGS/PRECAUTIONS:** New-onset seizures and status epilepticus in patients without epilepsy reported; d/c and evaluate for underlying seizure disorder. Increased risk of suicidal thoughts or behavior; monitor for emergence or worsening of depression, suicidal thoughts/behavior, and any unusual changes in mood or behavior. Avoid abrupt withdrawal. May impair mental/physical abilities. May exacerbate EEG abnormalities; caution with history of spike and wave discharges on EEG. Sudden unexpected death in epilepsy (SUDEP), incapacitating generalized weakness, and serious skin rash reported. Possibility of long-term ophthalmologic effects. Caution with hepatic impairment.



**ADVERSE REACTIONS:** Dizziness, asthenia, somnolence, N/V, nervousness, tremor, abdominal pain, abnormal thinking, depression, confusion, pharyngitis, rash.

**INTERACTIONS:** May reduce valproate concentrations. Increased clearance with carbamazepine, phenytoin, phenobarbital, and primidone. Additive effects with alcohol, triazolam, and CNS depressants. Reports of new-onset seizures and status epilepticus in patients without epilepsy with concomitant drugs that lower the seizure threshold (antidepressants, antipsychotics, stimulants, narcotics). Potential interactions with drugs that induce or inhibit hepatic metabolizing enzyme. May displace or be displaced by drugs that are highly protein bound, leading to higher free fractions of tiagabine or competing drugs.

**PREGNANCY:** Category C, caution in nursing.

**MECHANISM OF ACTION:** Nipecotic acid derivative; not established. May enhance activity of gamma aminobutyric acid (GABA), the major inhibitory neurotransmitter in the CNS. Binds to recognition sites associated with the GABA uptake carrier, thereby blocking GABA uptake into presynaptic neurons, permitting more GABA to be available for receptor binding on the surface of postsynaptic cells.

**PHARMACOKINETICS: Absorption:** Rapid; absolute bioavailability (90%). $T_{max}$=2.5 hrs (fed), $T_{max}$=45 min (fasting). **Distribution:** Plasma protein binding (96%). **Metabolism:** Liver via CYP3A; oxidation and glucuronidation. **Elimination:** Urine (25%; 2% unchanged), feces (63%); $T_{1/2}$=7-9 hrs (non-induced), 2-5 hrs (induced).

## NURSING CONSIDERATIONS

**Assessment:** Assess for underlying seizure disorder, history of status epilepticus and spike and wave discharges on EEG, depression, suicidal thoughts/behavior, hypersensitivity reactions, hepatic function, pregnancy/nursing status, and possible drug interactions.

**Monitoring:** Monitor for occurrence of new-onset seizures and status epilepticus in patients without a previous history of epilepsy, occurrence of seizures with abrupt discontinuation, cognitive and neuropsychiatric events (effects on thought processes, effects on levels of consciousness), EEG changes, rash (Stevens-Johnson syndrome), emergence or worsening of depression, suicidal thoughts/behavior, unusual changes in mood or behavior, generalized weakness, and possible ophthalmologic changes.

**Patient Counseling:** Inform of possible drowsiness or dizziness; avoid operating machinery/driving until adjusted to effects. Advise to contact physician if signs of rash develop. Instruct to take with food and not to abruptly d/c medication. If multiple doses are missed, contact physician before restarting. Notify physician if suicidal thoughts or behaviors emerge. Notify physician if pregnant or intend to become pregnant. Encourage patients to enroll in North American Antiepileptic Drug (NAAED) Pregnancy Registry by calling 888-233-2334 or go to aedpregnancyregistry.org.

**Administration:** Oral route. Take with food. **Storage:** 20-25°C (68-77°F). Protect from light and moisture.

# GANCICLOVIR — RX

ganciclovir sodium (Various)

**Risk of granulocytopenia, anemia, and thrombocytopenia. (PO) Risk of more rapid rate of CMV retinitis progression with caps; only use as maintenance treatment when the risk is balanced by the benefit of avoiding daily IV infusions. (IV) Use only for the treatment of retinitis in immunocompromised patients and for the prevention of cytomegalovirus (CMV) disease in transplant patients at risk for CMV disease.**

**OTHER BRAND NAMES:** Cytovene IV (Roche Labs)

**THERAPEUTIC CLASS:** Synthetic guanine derivative

**INDICATIONS:** (Caps) Prevention of CMV in solid organ transplant recipients and in advanced HIV patients at risk for CMV disease. Alternative to IV for maintenance treatment of CMV retinitis in immunocompromised patients, including patients with acquired immunodeficiency syndrome (AIDS) in whom retinitis is stable following appropriate induction therapy and for whom the risk of more rapid progression is balanced by the benefit associated with avoiding daily IV infusions. (IV) Treatment of CMV retinitis in immunocompromised patients, including patients with AIDS. Prevention of CMV disease in transplant recipients at risk for CMV disease.

**DOSAGE:** *Adults:* CMV Retinitis Treatment: Initial: 5mg/kg IV q12h for 14-21 days. Maint: 5mg/kg IV qd for 7 days or 6mg/kg IV qd for 5 days/week or 1000mg PO tid or 500mg PO 6 times daily q3h, while awake. CMV Retinitis Prevention in HIV Patients: 1000mg PO tid. CMV Retinitis Prevention in Transplant Patients: Initial: 5mg/kg IV q12h for 7-14 days. Maint: 5mg/kg IV qd for 7 days/week or 6mg/kg IV qd for 5 days/week or 1000mg PO tid. Renal Impairment: Refer to PI for Dosing. (PO) Take caps with food. (IV) Administer at constant rate over 1 hr.

**HOW SUPPLIED:** Cap: 250mg, 500mg; Inj: 500mg

**CONTRAINDICATIONS:** Hypersensitivity to acyclovir.

**WARNINGS/PRECAUTIONS:** Avoid if ANC <500 cells/µL or platelets <25,000 cells/µL. Caution in pre-existing cytopenias or history of cytopenic reactions to other drugs, chemicals, or irradiation. Reduce dose in renal impairment. High frequency of renal dysfunction in transplant recipients. May cause temporary or permanent inhibition of spermatogenesis and may suppress fertility in women. Mutagenic and teratogenic potential; women of childbearing potential should use effective contraception during treatment and men should practice barrier contraception during and for at least 90 days after therapy. Caution in elderly. CBC and platelet counts should be performed frequently and SrCr or CrCl should be monitored. (IV): Larger doses increase toxicity and more rapid infusions may increase toxicity. Administer adequate hydration. Phlebitis and/or pain may occur at infusion site. Administer into veins with adequate blood flow.

**ADVERSE REACTIONS:** Fever, diarrhea, anorexia, vomiting, leukopenia, anemia, sweating, infection, chills, thrombocytopenia, neutropenia, neuropathy, anemia, catheter infection.

**INTERACTIONS:** Concomitant use with zidovudine may increase AUC of zidovudine, decrease the AUC of ganciclovir, and increase the risk of neutropenia and anemia. Avoid imipenem-cilastatin; may precipitate seizures. Drugs that inhibit rapidly dividing cell populations such as bone marrow, spermatogonia and germinal layers of skin and GI mucosa (eg, dapsone, pentamidine, flucytosine, vincristine, vinblastine, adriamycin, amphotericin B, trimethoprim/sulfamethoxazole combinations, other nucleoside analogues) may have additive toxicity and should be administered only if benefits outweigh the risks. Concomitant use with probenecid may increase the AUC of ganciclovir and decrease the renal clearance of ganciclovir. (IV) Use with didanosine may increase the AUC and $C_{max}$ of didanosine. Increases in SrCr reported when used concomitantly with amphotercin B or cyclosporine; monitor renal function when concomitantly using nephrotoxic drugs. (PO) Use with didanosine may increase the AUC of didanosine. A decrease in the AUC of ganciclovir may occur when didanosine is administered two hours before ganciclovir.

**PREGNANCY:** Category C, not for use in nursing.

**MECHANISM OF ACTION:** Guanine derivative; inhibits viral DNA synthesis by competitively inhibiting viral DNA polymerases and incorporating into viral DNA, resulting in eventual termination of viral DNA elongation.

**PHARMACOKINETICS: Absorption:**(PO): Absolute bioavailability (5%) (fasted), (6-9%) (fed state); $AUC_{0-24}$=15.9µg•hr/mL, $C_{max}$=1.02µg/mL (500mg q 3 hrs, 6 times daily, fed state), $AUC_{0-24}$=15.4µg•hr/mL, $C_{max}$=1.18µg/mL (1000mg tid, fed state). (IV): $C_{max}$=8.27-9µg/mL; AUC=22.1-26.8µg•hr/mL. **Distribution:** Plasma protein binding (1-2%); (IV): $V_d$=0.74L/kg. **Elimination:** (IV): Urine (91.3%); $T_{1/2}$=3.5 hrs; (PO): $T_{1/2}$= 4.8 hrs.

## NURSING CONSIDERATIONS

G

**Assessment:** Assess for hypersensitivity to acyclovir, pregnancy/nursing status, renal impairment, and for possible drug interactions. Assess for preexisting cytopenias or a history of cytopenic reactions to other drugs, chemicals, or irradiation. Assess baseline renal function, absolute neutrophil count ( ≥500 cells/µL), and platelet count ( ≥25,000).

**Monitoring:** (IV, PO) Monitor for signs/symptoms of granulocytopenia, anemia, thrombocytopenia, and infertility. Perform frequent monitoring of CBC and platelet counts. Monitor SrCr or CrCl periodically. (IV): Monitor for infusion site reactions (eg, pain, phlebitis).

**Patient Counseling:** (IV, PO) Inform that the major toxicities of therapy are granulocytopenia (neutropenia), anemia, and thrombocytopenia. Advise that medication may increase SrCr levels. Inform that medication may decrease sperm production and cause infertility in men and women. Advise women of childbearing potential that medication should not be used during pregnancy and that effective contraception should be used and inform men that barrier contraception should be used during therapy and for at least 90 days following treatment. Inform that therapy may be a potential carcinogen. Advise immunocompromised patients with CMV retitinitis that medication is not a cure for CMV retinitis and that progression of retinitis may continue to occur during and after treatment; instruct to have opthalmologic follow-up examinations at a minimum of every 4-6 weeks during treatment. (PO): Instruct to take with food. (IV) Inform to keep well hydrated during therapy.

**Administration:** IV/Oral route. **Storage:** (IV) 25°C (77°F); excursions permitted to 15-30°C (59-86°F); (Cap): 20-25° (68-77°F); excursions permitted between 15-30°C (59-86°F).

# GARDASIL RX

human papillomavirus recombinant vaccine, quadrivalent (Merck)

**THERAPEUTIC CLASS:** Vaccine

**INDICATIONS:** Vaccination of girls and women 9-26 yrs old for the prevention of cervical, vulvar, and vaginal cancer caused by human papillomavirus (HPV) types 16 and 18, genital warts (condyloma acuminata) caused by HPV types 6 and 11, cervical intraepithelial neoplasia (CIN) grades 1 and 2/3, cervical adenocarcinoma *in situ* (AIS), vulvar intraepithelial neoplasia (VIN) grades 2 and 3, and vaginal intraepithelial neoplasia (VaIN) grades 2 and 3 caused by HPV types 6, 11, 16, and 18. Vaccination of boys and men 9-26 yrs old for the prevention of genital warts (condyloma acuminata) caused by HPV types 6 and 11.

**DOSAGE:** *Adults:* Give 3 separate 0.5mL IM doses in the deltoid region of upper arm or higher anterolateral area of the thigh. First dose: At elected date; second dose: 2 months after first dose; third dose: 6 months after first dose. *Pediatrics:* ≥9 yrs: Give 3 separate 0.5mL IM doses in the deltoid region of upper arm or higher anterolateral area of the thigh. First dose: At elected date; second dose: 2 months after first dose; third dose: 6 months after first dose.

**HOW SUPPLIED:** Inj: Vial/Syringe: 0.5mL

**WARNINGS/PRECAUTIONS:** Syncope may occur, sometimes resulting in falling with injury and may be associated with tonic-clonic movement and other seizure-like activity; observe for 15 minutes after administration. Immunological response to vaccine may be diminished in immunocompromised individuals. Appropriate medical treatment and supervision should be readily available in case of anaphylactic reactions following administration. Does not substitute for routine cervical screening. Does not protect against vaccine and non-vaccine HPV types previously exposed to through sexual activity. Not intended for treatment of active genital warts; cervical, vulvar, and vaginal cancers. Only protects against vulvar and vaginal cancers caused by HPV 16 and 18. Does not protect against genital disease not caused by HPV. Vaccination may not result in protection in all vaccine recipients. Not indicated for women ≥27 yrs old.

**ADVERSE REACTIONS:** Local site reactions (pain, swelling, erythema, pruritus, bruising), fever, falling, nausea, dizziness, diarrhea, syncope, headache, anaphylaxis.

**INTERACTIONS:** Immunosuppressive therapies, including irradiation, antimetabolites, alkylating agents, cytotoxic drugs, and corticosteroids (used in greater than physiologic doses) may reduce the immune responses to vaccines. May be administered concomitantly with Recombivax HB hepatitis B vaccine at a separate injection site.

**PREGNANCY:** Category B, caution in nursing.

**MECHANISM OF ACTION:** Vaccine; has not been established. Develops humoral immune response that may protect against human papillomavirus types 6, 11, 16, and 18 (animal studies).

## NURSING CONSIDERATIONS

**Assessment:** Assess current health and immune status, age of patient, hypersensitivity to drug and yeast, pregnancy/nursing status, and possible drug interactions.

**Monitoring:** Monitor for signs and symptoms of anaphylactic reactions and treat appropriately if occur. For 15 min following administration, monitor for signs and symptoms of syncope, tonic-clonic movements, and other seizure-like activity.

**Patient Counseling:** Inform patient or caregiver about benefits and risks associated with vaccine. Inform that vaccine does not substitute for routine cervical cancer screening. Advise that vaccine does not provide protection against disease from vaccine and non-vaccine HPV types to which an individual has previously been exposed to through sexual activity. Counsel may experience syncope following vaccination. Inform about importance of completing immunization series unless contraindicated. Advise that vaccine is not recommended during pregnancy. Enroll pregnant women exposed to vaccine in pregnancy registry to monitor maternal and fetal outcomes. Instruct to contact physician if develop any adverse events.

**Administration:** IM in the deltoid region of the upper arm or in the higher anterolateral area of the thigh. **Storage:** 2-8°C (36-46°F). Do not freeze. Protect from light.

# GEMZAR — RX

gemcitabine HCl (Lilly)

**THERAPEUTIC CLASS:** Nucleoside analogue antimetabolite

**INDICATIONS:** Combination with carboplatin for the treatment of advanced ovarian cancer that has relapsed at least 6 months after completion of platinum-based therapy. Combination with paclitaxel for 1st-line treatment of metastatic breast cancer after failure of prior anthracycline-containing adjuvant chemotherapy, unless anthracyclines were clinically contraindicated. Combination with cisplatin for 1st-line treatment of inoperable, locally advanced (Stage IIIA or IIIB), or metastatic (Stage IV) non-small cell lung cancer. 1st-line treatment of locally advanced (nonresectable Stage II or Stage III) or metastatic (Stage IV) adenocarcinoma of the pancreas; indicated for patients previously treated with 5-FU.

**DOSAGE:** *Adults:* Pancreatic Cancer: 1000mg/m² IV over 30 min once weekly for up to 7 weeks, then 1 week off. Give subsequent cycles as weekly infusions for 3 consecutive weeks out of every 4 weeks. Non-Small Cell Lung Cancer: 4-Week Cycle: 1000mg/m² IV over 30 min on Days 1, 8, and 15 of each 28-day cycle. Give cisplatin 100mg/m² IV on Day 1 after gemcitabine infusion. 3-Week Cycle: 1250mg/m² IV over 30 mins on Days 1 and 8 of each 21-day cycle. Give cisplatin 100mg/m² IV on Day 1 after gemcitabine infusion. Breast Cancer: 1250mg/m² IV over 30 mins on Days 1 and 8 of each 21-day cycle. Give paclitaxel 175mg/m² on Day 1 as 3-hr IV infusion before gemcitabine. Ovarian Cancer: 1000mg/m² IV over 30 min on Days 1 and 8 of each 21-day cycle. Give carboplatin AUC 4 on Day 1 after gemcitabine. Adjust dose based on hematologic toxicity. If marrow suppression is detected, modify or suspend according to guidelines; refer to PI for dosage reduction guidelines.



**HOW SUPPLIED:** Inj: 200mg, 1g

**WARNINGS/PRECAUTIONS:** Increased toxicity with infusion time >60 min and more than once-weekly dosing. Hemolytic Uremic Syndrome (HUS), hepatotoxicity, renal failure, bone marrow suppression reported. Myelosuppression is dose-limiting toxicity; monitor CBC with differential and platelet count prior to each dose. Adjust dose or d/c when marrow suppression is detected. Pulmonary toxicity reported; d/c if severe lung toxicity occurs and institute appropriate supportive care measures. Can cause fetal harm. Caution in patient with pre-existing renal impairment or hepatic insuffiency; monitor renal/hepatic function prior to initiation of therapy and periodically thereafter; d/c if severe renal/hepatic toxicity occur. Decreased clearance in women and the elderly. Greater tendency in women, especially older women to not proceed to next cycle and to experience Grade 3/4 neutropenia and thrombocytopenia. Concurrent and non-current use of gemcitabine with radiation therapy, may cause radiation toxicity.

**ADVERSE REACTIONS:** Myelosuppression, N/V, alopecia, stomatis, elevated serum transaminases, proteinuria, hematuria, fever, rash, dyspnea, edema, flu syndrome, infection, alopecia, paresthesia.

**INTERACTIONS:** Monitor SrCr, $K^+$, calcium, and magnesium with cisplatin. Serious hepatotoxicity, including liver failure and death, reported with hepatotoxic drugs.

**PREGNANCY:** Category D, not for use in nursing.

**MECHANISM OF ACTION:** Nucleoside analogue antimetabolite; exhibits cell cycle specificity, primarily killing cells undergoing DNA synthesis (S-phase); also blocks progression of cells through the G1/S-phase boundary.

**PHARMACOKINETICS: Absorption:** IV administration of variable doses resulted in different parameters. **Distribution:** Plasma protein binding (negligible). $V_d$=50L/m² (short-infusion), $V_d$=370L/m² (long-infusion). **Metabolism:** Intracellular by nucleoside kinases to the active diphosphate (dFdCDP) and triphosphate (dFdCTP) nucleosides. **Elimination:** Urine (92-98%)(<10% unchanged); $T_{1/2}$ (short infusion, long infusion)=42-94 min, 245-638 min.

## NURSING CONSIDERATIONS

**Assessment:** Assess for renal/hepatic impairment, pregnancy/nursing status, and for possible drug interactions. Obtain baseline renal and hepatic function. Obtain CBC with differential and platelet count prior to each dose.

**Monitoring:** Monitor for signs/symptoms of myelosuppression, pulmonary toxicity, HUS, renal failure, and hepatotoxicity including liver failure. Perform periodic monitoring of renal and hepatic function. Monitor SrCr, $K^+$, calcium, and magnesium when using concomitantly with cisplatin.

**Patient Counseling:** Advise of risks of therapy. Instruct to contact physician if develop any signs/symptoms suggestive of myelosuppression, pulmonary toxicity, or renal toxicity. Counsel to notify physician if pregnant or nursing and all medications currently taking.

**Administration:** IV route. Reconstitute with 5mL of 0.9% NaCl Inj (200mg vial) or 25mL of 0.9 NaCl Inj (1g vial). Avoid reconstitution at concentration >40mg/mL. Inspect reconstituted solution for particulates prior to administration. **Storage:** (Unopened vials) 20-25°C (68-77°F); excursions permitted to 15-30°C (59-86°F). (Reconstituted) 20-25°C (68-77°F) for 24 hrs. Discard unused portion. Do not refrigerate. Use gloves when handling and preparing. Avoid contact to skin.

## GEODON RX

ziprasidone HCl - ziprasidone mesylate (inj) (Pfizer)

**Elderly patients with dementia-related psychosis treated with antipsychotic drugs, including atypicals, are at an increased risk of death; most deaths appeared to be cardiovascular (eg, heart failure, sudden death) or infectious (eg, pneumonia) in nature. Not approved for the treatment of dementia-related psychosis.**

**OTHER BRAND NAMES:** Geodon for Injection (Pfizer)

**THERAPEUTIC CLASS:** Benzisoxazole derivative

**INDICATIONS:** (PO) Treatment of schizophrenia. Monotherapy for acute treatment of manic or mixed episodes associated with bipolar I disorder. Adjunct to lithium or valproate for maintenance treatment of bipolar I disorder. (IM) Treatment of acute agitation in schizophrenic patients who need IM medication for rapid control of agitation.

**DOSAGE:** *Adults:* Schizophrenia: (PO) Initial/Maint: 20mg bid with food. Titrate: May increase up to 80mg bid; adjust dose at intervals of not less than 2 days. Max: 100mg bid. Bipolar Mania: (PO) Initial: 40mg bid with food. Titrate: Increase to 60 or 80mg bid on 2nd day of treatment. Maint (as adjunct to lithium or valproate): 40-80mg bid. Agitation: (IM) Usual: 10mg q2h-20mg q4h. Max: 40mg/day for 3 days. Elderly: Start at lower end of dosing range.

**HOW SUPPLIED:** Cap: (HCl) 20mg, 40mg, 60mg, 80mg; Sus: (HCl) 10mg/mL [60mL, 240mL]; Inj: (Mesylate) 20mg/mL

**CONTRAINDICATIONS:** Concomitant dofetilide, sotalol, quinidine, Class Ia/III antiarrhythmics, mesoridazine, thioridazine, chlorpromazine, droperidol, pimozide, sparfloxacin, gatifloxacin, moxifloxacin, halofantrine, mefloquine, pentamidine, arsenic trioxide, levomethadyl acetate, dolasetron mesylate, probucol, tacrolimus and drugs that prolong QT interval. History of QT prolongation (including congenital long QT syndrome), recent acute MI and uncompensated heart failure.

**WARNINGS/PRECAUTIONS:** D/C if persistent QTc measurements >500 msec. Bradycardia, hypokalemia and/or hypomagnesemia may increase risk of QT prolongation and arrhythmia. Neuroleptic malignant syndrome (NMS), priapism and rash/urticaria reported. Tardive dyskinesia (TD), esophageal dysmotility and aspiration may occur. Monitor for hyperglycemia in patients with diabetes mellitus (DM) or at risk for DM. Caution with history of seizures or conditions that may lower seizure threshold (eg, Alzheimer's dementia). Leukopenia, neutropenia and agranulocytosis reported; d/c with severe neutropenia (ANC<1000/mm$^3$) or with significant decline in WBC in absence of other causes. May elevate prolactin levels. Orthostatic hypotension reported; caution with CV, cerebrovascular disease or conditions that predispose to hypotension (eg, dehydration, hypovolemia). May disrupt the body's ability to reduce core body temperature. Closely supervise high-risk patients for suicide attempt. May impair physical/mental abilities. Caution in elderly. Caution with IM use in renal dysfunction. Concomitant use of IM and oral preparations in schizophrenic patients not recommended.

**ADVERSE REACTIONS:** Asthenia, nausea, constipation, dyspepsia, diarrhea, dry mouth, extrapyramidal symptoms, somnolence, akathisia, dizziness, respiratory tract infection, rash, abnormal vision, chest pain.

**INTERACTIONS:** See Contraindications. Caution with centrally acting drugs. May enhance effects of antihypertensives. May antagonize effects of levodopa and dopamine agonists. Carbamazepine may decrease levels. CYP3A4 inhibitors (eg, ketoconazole) may increase levels.

**PREGNANCY:** Category C, not for use in nursing.

**MECHANISM OF ACTION:** Benzisoxazole derivative; psychotropic agent; mechanism not established. Actions are mediated through a combination of dopamine type 2 ($D_2$) and serotonin type 2 ($5HT_2$) antagonism.

**PHARMACOKINETICS: Absorption:** (PO) absolute bioavailability (60%); $T_{max}$=6-8 hrs. (IM) absolute bioavailability (100%); $T_{max}$=60 min. **Distribution:** (PO) $V_d$=1.5L/kg; plasma protein binding (>99%). **Metabolism:** (PO) Liver (extensive) via aldehyde oxidase (major), CYP3A4 (minor). **Elimination:** (PO) Urine (20%, <1% unchanged) and feces (66%, <4% unchanged); $T_{1/2}$=7 hrs. (IM) $T_{1/2}$=2-5 hrs.

## NURSING CONSIDERATIONS

**Assessment:** Assess for history of QT prolongation (congenital long QT syndrome), recent MI, uncompensated heart failure, cardiac arrhythmias, DM, conditions that predispose to hypotension and dementia-related psychosis. Perform baseline CBC and serum electrolytes ($K^+$, $Mg^+$) in patients at risk for QT prolongation. Replete serum electrolytes prior to treatment. Assess pregnancy/nursing status and possible drug interactions.

G

**Monitoring:** Monitor for QT prolongation, torsades de pointes, NMS, suicidal ideation, extrapyramidal symptoms, weight gain, and respiratory tract infections. Monitor prolactin levels, serum electrolytes ($K^+$, $Mg^+$) and CBC, especially for decline of WBC with signs/symptoms of infection.

**Patient Counseling:** Inform regarding the risks and benefits of therapy. Counsel on risk of orthostatic hypotension. Advise patient use may impair mental/physical abilities. Counsel to take with food, avoid alcohol and high temperatures or humidity; drug may interfere with body's ability to regulate temperature.

**Administration:** Oral, IM route. See PI for IM preparation. **Storage:** Cap: 25°C (77°F), excursions permitted to 15-30°C (59-86°F). Sus: 15-30°C (59-86°F). Inj: Dry form: 25°C (77°F); excursions permitted to 15-30°C (59-86°F). Reconstituted: 15-30°C (59-86°F) up to 24 hrs when protected from light or refrigerated at 2-8°C (36-46°F) for up to 7 days.

# GLEEVEC RX

## imatinib mesylate (Novartis)

**THERAPEUTIC CLASS:** Protein-tyrosine kinase inhibitor

**INDICATIONS:** (Adults) Treatment of newly diagnosed adult patients with Philadelphia chromosome positive (Ph+) chronic myeloid leukemia (CML) in chronic phase. Treatment of Ph+ CML in blast crisis, accelerated phase, or in chronic phase after failure of interferon-alpha therapy. Treatment of relapsed or refractory Ph+ acute lympoblastic leukemia (ALL). Treatment of myelodysplastic/myeloproliferative diseases (MDS/MPD) associated with platelet-derived growth factor receptor (PDGFR) gene rearrangements. Treatment of aggressive systemic mastocytosis (ASM) patients without the D816V c-Kit mutation or with unknown c-Kit mutational status. Treatment of hypereosinophilic syndrome (HES) and/or chronic eosinophilic leukemia (CEL) patients who have the FIP1L1-PDGFRα fusion kinase (mutational analysis or FISH demonstration of CHIC2 allele deletion) and for patients with HES and/or CEL who are FIP1L1-PDGFRα fusion kinase negative or unknown. Treatment of patients with unresectable, recurrent, and/or metastatic dermatofibrosarcoma protuberans (DFSP). Treatment of patients with Kit (CD117) positive unresectable and/or metastatic malignant gastrointestinal stromal tumors (GIST). Adjuvant treatment of patients following complete resection of Kit (CD117) positive GIST. (Pediatrics) Treatment of patients with Ph+ chronic phase CML in chronic phase who are newly diagnosed or whose disease has recurred after stem cell transplant or who are resistant to interferon-alpha therapy.

**DOSAGE:** *Adults:* CML: Chronic Phase: 400mg/d, may increase to 600mg qd. Accelerated Phase/Blast Crisis: 600mg/d, may increase to 400mg bid. Relapsed/Refractory Ph+ ALL: 600mg/d. MDS or MPD/ASM/HES and/or CEL: 400mg/d. ASM with Eosinophilia/HES or CEL with FIP1L1-PDGFRα: Initial: 100mg/d. Titrate: May increase up to 400mg/d in the absence of adverse reactions and insufficient response. DFSP: 800mg/d. GIST (Unresectable or Metastatic/Malignant): 400mg/d. Titrate: May increase up to 800mg (as 400mg bid) if clear signs/symptoms of disease progression and in the

absence of adverse reactions. Severe Hepatic Impairment: Reduce dose by 25%. Coadministration with Strong CYP3A4 Inducers: Avoid concomitant use, if necessary, increase dose by at least 50% and monitor carefully. Hepatotoxicity/Non-Hematologic Adverse Reaction: If bilirubin >3x ULN or transaminases >5x ULN, hold drug until bilirubin <1.5x ULN and transaminases <2.5x ULN. Continue at reduced dose. Moderate Renal Impairment (CrCl 20-39mL/min): Reduce starting dose by 50%. Titrate: As tolerated. Doses >400mg are not recommended. Mild Renal Impairment (40-59mL/min): Doses >600 mg are not recommended. Neutropenia/Thrombocytopenia: See PI for dosage adjustments. Take with food and plenty of water.
*Pediatrics:* CML: Newly Diagnosed: 340mg/m$^2$/d (not to exceed 600mg). Chronic Phase: 260mg/m$^2$/day given qd or split into 2 doses (morning and evening). Severe Hepatic Impairment: Reduce dose by 25%. Coadministration with Strong CYP3A4 Inducers: Avoid concomitant use, if necessary, increase dose by at least 50% and monitor carefully. Hepatotoxicity/Non-Hematologic Adverse Reaction: If bilirubin >3x ULN or transaminases >5x ULN, hold drug until bilirubin <1.5x ULN and transaminases <2.5x ULN. Continue at reduced dose. Moderate Renal Impairment (CrCl 20-39mL/min): Reduce starting dose by 50%. Titrate: As tolerated. Doses >400mg are not recommended. Mild Renal Impairment (40-59mL/min): Doses >600 mg are not recommended. Neutropenia/Thrombocytopenia: See PI for dosage adjustments. Take with food and plenty of water.

**HOW SUPPLIED:** Tab: 100mg, 400mg

**WARNINGS/PRECAUTIONS:** Fluid retention/edema (eg, pleural effusion, pericardial effusion, pulmonary edema, ascites) reported; monitor weight. Anemia/neutropenia/thrombocytopenia reported; monitor CBC weekly during 1st month, biweekly during 2nd month, and periodically thereafter. In pediatric patients, the most frequent toxicities observed were grade 3 and 4 cytopenias. May be hepatotoxic; monitor LFTs at baseline, then monthly or as needed. Severe CHF and left ventricular dysfunction reported; monitor patients with cardiac disease or risk factors for cardiac failure. Hemorrhages reported. May cause GI irritation; take with food and large glass of water. GI perforation reported rarely. In patients with hypereosinophilic syndrome and cardiac involvement, cardiogenic shock/left ventricular dysfunction reported. Bullous dermatological reactions (eg, erythema multiforme, Stevens-Johnson syndrome [SJS]) reported. Hypothyroidism reported in thyroidectomy patients undergoing levothyroxine treatment; monitor thyroid stimulating hormone (TSH) levels. Avoid becoming pregnant. Interrupt treatment if severe non-hematologic adverse reaction develops (eg, severe hepatotoxicity, severe fluid retention); resume if appropriate.

**ADVERSE REACTIONS:** N/V, edema, muscle cramps, musculoskeletal pain, diarrhea, rash, fatigue, headache, abdominal pain, nasopharyngitis, hemorrhage, dizziness, pyrexia, weight gain.

**INTERACTIONS:** Increased levels with CYP3A4 inhibitors, caution with strong CYP3A4 inhibitors (eg, ketoconazole, atazanavir, indinavir, nefazodone, nelfinavir, ritonavir, saquinavir, telithromycin, voriconazole, clarithromycin, itraconazole). Grapefruit juice may increase levels and should be avoided. Decreased levels with CYP3A4 inducers (eg, dexamethasone, phenytoin, carbamazepine, rifampin, phenobarbital); avoid concomitant use. Caution with CYP3A4 substrates with narrow therapeutic windows (eg, alfentanil, cyclosporine, diergotamine, ergotamine, fentanyl, quinidine, sirolimus, tacrolimus, cyclosporine, pimozide). Increases levels of drugs metabolized by CYP3A4 (eg, dihydropyridines, triazolo-benzodiazepines, HMG-CoA reductase inhibitors). Switch patients on warfarin to low molecular weight or standard heparin. Systemic exposure to acetaminophen and substrates of CYP2D6 are expected to increase. When concomitantly used with chemotherapy, liver toxicity reported; monitor hepatic function.

**PREGNANCY:** Category D, not for nursing.

**MECHANISM OF ACTION:** Protein-tyrosine kinase inhibitor; inhibits the bcr-abl tyrosine kinase, the constitutive abnormal tyrosine kinase created by the Philadelphia chromosome abnormality in CML. Also an inhibitor of the receptor tyrosine kinases for platelet-derived growth factor (PDGF) and stem cell factor (SCF), c-kit, and inhibits PDGF- and SCF-mediated cellular events. *In* *vitro* inhibits proliferation and induces apoptosis in GIST cells, which express an activating c-kit mutation.

**PHARMACOKINETICS: Absorption:** Absolute bioavailability (98%); $T_{max}$=2-4 hrs. **Distribution:** Plasma protein binding (95%); found in breast milk. **Metabolism:** Liver via CYP3A4 (major role), CYP1A2, CYP2D6, CYP2C9, CYP2C19 (minor roles). N-demethyl derivative (major active metabolite). **Elimination:** Urine, feces (predominant); $T_{1/2}$=18 hrs (imatinib), 40 hrs (active metabolite).

## NURSING CONSIDERATIONS

**Assessment:** Assess for renal/hepatic impairment, cardiac disease, hypereosinophilic syndrome, pregnancy/nursing status, and for possible drug interactions. Assess liver function prior to therapy.

G

**Monitoring:** Monitor for signs and symptoms of fluid retention, edema, congestive heart failure, left ventricular dysfunction, hepatotoxicity, hemorrhage, GI disorders (eg, GI irritation, GI perforation), and for bullous dermatological reactions (eg, erythema multiforme, SJS). Monitor for signs and symptoms of anemia, neutropenia, and thrombocytopenia; perform CBC weekly for the first month of therapy, biweekly for the second month of therapy, and periodically thereafter. Monitor liver function monthly or as clinically indicated. In patients with hypereosinophilic syndrome and cardiac involvement, monitor for cardiogenic shock/left ventricular dysfunction. In thyroidectomy patients, monitor TSH levels.

**Patient Counseling:** Instruct to take with a meal and large glass of water. Instruct to contact physician if pregnant. Counsel to not breastfeed while on therapy. Instruct to contact physician if any adverse effects develop while on therapy. Tablets should not be crushed; avoid direct contact of crushed tablets with skin or mucous membranes.

**Administration:** Oral route. If unable to swallow tablets, tablet may be dispersed in a glass of water or apple juice; required number of tablets should be placed in the appropriate volume of beverage (approximately 50mL for 100mg tablet and 200mL for a 400mg tablet); stir and administer suspension immediately after disintegration of tablets. **Storage:** 25°C (77°F); excursions permitted to 15-30°C (59-86°F). Protect from moisture.

# GLIPIZIDE RX

glipizide (Various)

**OTHER BRAND NAMES:** Glucotrol (Pfizer)

**THERAPEUTIC CLASS:** Sulfonylurea (2nd generation)

**INDICATIONS:** Adjunct to diet and exercise to improve glycemic control in adults with type 2 diabetes mellitus.

**DOSAGE:** *Adults:* Take 30 min before meals. Initial: 5mg qd before breakfast; give 2.5mg if sensitive to hypoglycemia (eg, elderly, hepatic impairment). Titrate: Increase by 2.5-5mg/day after several days. Divide doses with daily doses >15mg/day. Max: 40mg/day. Switch From Insulin: If ≤20 U/day: D/C insulin; start 5mg qd. If >20 U/day: Reduce insulin dose by 50%; begin 5mg qd. Further insulin reductions depend on response. Elderly/Debilitated/Malnourished/Renal or Hepatic Impairment: Dose conservatively.

**HOW SUPPLIED:** Tab: 5mg*, 10mg* *scored

**CONTRAINDICATIONS:** Type 1 diabetes mellitus, diabetic ketoacidosis with or without coma.

**WARNINGS/PRECAUTIONS:** Increased risk of hypoglycemia with the elderly, debilitated, malnourished, renal and hepatic disease, adrenal or pituitary insufficiency. Increased risk of cardiovascular mortality reported. Loss of blood glucose control when exposed to stress (eg, fever, trauma, infection, or surgery); d/c therapy and start insulin. Secondary failure can occur over period of time. Treatment of patients with glucose 6-phosphate dehydrogenase (G6PD) deficiency with sulfonylurea agents can lead to hemolytic anemia. Caution in patients with G6PD deficiency and consider a non-sulfonylurea alternative. Hemolytic anemia reported in patients without G6PD deficiency. Caution in elderly.

**ADVERSE REACTIONS:** Hypoglycemia, nausea, diarrhea, urticaria, pruritus, disulfiram-like reactions, hyponatremia, SIADH, dizziness, drowsiness, headache, leukopenia, thrombocytopenia, hemolytic anemia.

**INTERACTIONS:** Hypoglycemic effects potentiated by alcohol, NSAIDs, some azoles (eg, miconazole, fluconazole), other highly protein-bound drugs, salicylates, sulfonamides, chloramphenicol, probenecid, coumarins, MAOIs, and β-blockers. Severe hypoglycemia reported with oral hypolycemics and oral miconazole. Certain drugs have a tendency to cause hyperglycemia and may lead to loss of glycemic control including thiazides and other diuretics, corticosteroids, phenothiazines, thyroid products, estrogens, oral contraceptives, phenytoin, nicotinic acid, sympathomimetics, CCBs, and isoniazid. β-blockers may mask signs of hypoglycemia.

**PREGNANCY:** Category C, not for use in nursing.

**MECHANISM OF ACTION:** Sulfonylurea; lowers blood glucose acutely by stimulating the release of insulin from the pancreas.

**PHARMACOKINETICS: Absorption:** Rapid and complete; $T_{max}$=1-3 hrs. **Distribution:** $V_d$=11L; plasma protein binding (98-99%). **Metabolism**: Extensive via liver. **Elimination**: Urine (<10% unchanged); $T_{1/2}$=2-4 hrs.

## NURSING CONSIDERATIONS

**Assessment:** Assess FPG, $HbA_{1c}$, renal function, LFTs, pregnancy status, type 1 DM, ketoacidosis, GI disease, and for possible drug interactions.

**Monitoring:** Monitor blood and urine glucose, $HbA_{1c}$ every 3 months, renal function, LFTs, signs/symptoms of hypoglycemia, and for endocrine, metabolic, and hematologic reactions.

**Patient Counseling:** Take 30 min before meals. Inform about importance of adhering to dietary instructions, a regular exercise program, and regular testing of urine/blood glucose. Educate on risks/benefits of therapy; signs/symptoms, predisposing conditions, and treatment of hypoglycemia; primary and secondary failure.

**Administration:** Oral route. **Storage**: Below 30°C (86°F).

# GLUCAGON — RX

glucagon (Lilly)

**THERAPEUTIC CLASS:** Glucagon

**INDICATIONS:** Treatment for severe hypoglycemia. Diagnostic aid for radiologic examination of the stomach, duodenum, small bowel, and colon when diminished intestinal motility would be advantageous.

**DOSAGE:** *Adults:* Severe Hypoglycemia: ≥20kg: 1mg (1 U) SQ/IM/IV. May give another dose after 15 min if patient does not respond, but IV glucose is a better alternative. Use immediately after reconstitution, discard unused portion. After patient responds, give supplemental carbohydrate. Diagnostic Aid: Stomach/Duodenum/Small Bowel: 0.25-0.5mg (0.25-0.5 U) IV, or 1mg (1 U) IM, or 2mg (2 U) IV/IM before procedure. Higher incidence of N/V with 2mg dose. Colon: 2mg (2 U) IM 10 min before procedure. Elderly: Start at low end of dosing range.

*Pediatrics:* Severe Hypoglycemia: ≥20kg: 1mg (1 U) SQ/IM/IV. <20kg: 0.5mg (0.5 U) or dose equivalent to 20-30mcg/kg. May give another dose after 15 min if patient does not respond, but IV glucose would be a better alternative. Use immediately after reconstitution; discard unused portion. After patient responds, give supplemental carbohydrate.

**HOW SUPPLIED:** Inj: 1mg

**CONTRAINDICATIONS:** Pheochromocytoma.

**WARNINGS/PRECAUTIONS:** Caution with history suggestive of insulinoma and/or pheochromocytoma. In patients with insulinoma, IV glucagon may produce an initial increase in blood glucose and then subsequently cause hypoglycemia. In the presence of pheochromocytoma, may cause the tumor to release catecholamines, which may result in a sudden and marked increase in BP. Generalized allergic reactions reported including urticaria, respiratory distress, and hypotension. Effective in treating hypoglycemia only if sufficient liver glycogen is present. Not effective in states of starvation, adrenal insufficiency, or chronic hypoglycemia; use glucose to treat.

**ADVERSE REACTIONS:** N/V, allergic reactions, urticaria, respiratory distress, hypotension.

**INTERACTIONS:** Addition of an anticholinergic during diagnostic study may increase side effects.

**PREGNANCY:** Category B, caution in nursing.

**MECHANISM OF ACTION:** Polypeptide hormone; increases blood glucose levels and relaxes smooth muscle of the GI tract.

G

**PHARMACOKINETICS: Absorption:** (SQ) $C_{max}$=7.9ng/mL, $T_{max}$=20 min; (IM) $C_{max}$=6.9ng/mL, $T_{max}$=13 min. **Distribution:** $V_d$=0.25L/kg. **Metabolism:** Extensively degraded in liver, kidneys, plasma. **Elimination:** Urine; $T_{1/2}$=8-18 min.

## NURSING CONSIDERATIONS

**Assessment:** Assess for presence of pheochromocytoma, pregnancy/nursing status, and for possible drug interactions. Assess if patient is in a state of starvation, has adrenal insufficiencies, or has chronic hypoglycemia. Assess use in patients with a history suggestive of insulinoma and/or pheochromocytoma.

**Monitoring:** Monitor for occurrence of allergic reactions (eg, uticaria, respiratory distress, and hypotension). If pheochromocytoma, monitor for signs/symptoms of HTN and treat accordingly. In patients with insulinoma, monitor for signs/symptoms of hypoglycemia. Monitor blood glucose levels in patients with hypoglycemia until asymptomatic.

**Patient Counseling:** Instruct patient and family members, in event of emergency, how to properly prepare and administer glucagon. Inform about measures to prevent hypoglycemia; includes following a uniform regimen on a regular basis, careful adjustment of insulin program, frequent testing of blood or urine for glucose, and routinely carrying hyperglycemic agents to quickly elevate blood glucose levels (eg, sugar, candy, readily absorbed carbohydrates). Inform about symptoms of hypoglycemia and how to treat it appropriately. Inform caregivers that if patient is hypoglycemic, patient should be kept alert and hypoglycemia should be treated as quickly as possible to prevent CNS damage. Advise to inform physician when hypoglycemia occurs.

**Administration:** IM/IV/SQ routes. Accompanying diluent should be used only for parental injection. Glucagon should not be used in concentrations ≥1mg/mL (1 U/mL). Use reconstituted solution immediately and discard any unused portion. Inspect for particulate matter and discoloration prior to administration. Severe hypoglycemia should be treated initially with IV glucose. If not available, then dissolve lyophilized glucagon using accompanying diluent solution. 1) Wipe rubber stopper on bottle. Do not remove plastic clip from syringe. 2) Swirl bottle gently until glucagon dissolves completely. Do not use unless solution is clear and water-like consistency. 3) Hold bottle upside down, making sure needle tip remains in solution, gently withdrawing solution. 4) Cleanse injection site. 5) Insert needle into loose tissue. Apply light pressure at injection site, and withdraw needle. Press alcohol swab against injection site. **Storage:** Before reconstitution: 20-25°C (68-77°F); excursions allowed between 15-30°C (59-86°F). After reconstitution: Should be used immediately; discard any unused portion.

# GLUCOPHAGE XR — RX

metformin HCl (Bristol-Myers Squibb)

**OTHER BRAND NAMES:** Glucophage (Bristol-Myers Squibb) - Riomet (Ranbaxy)

**THERAPEUTIC CLASS:** Biguanide

**INDICATIONS:** Adjunct to diet and exercise, to improve glycemic control in type 2 diabetes mellitus (DM).

**DOSAGE:** *Adults:* (Sol, Tab) Individualize dose. Initial: 500mg bid or 850mg qd with meals. Titrate: Increase by 500mg/week or 850mg every 2 weeks, or may increase from 500mg bid to 850mg bid after 2 weeks. Max: 2550mg/day. Give in 3 divided doses with meals if dose is >2g/day. (Tab, Extended-Release) Initial: ≥17 yrs: 500mg qd with evening meal. Titrate: Increase by 500mg/week. Max: 2000mg/day. With Insulin: Initial: 500mg qd. Titrate: Increase by 500mg/week. Max: 2500mg/day and 2000mg/day (XR). Decrease insulin dose by 10-25% when FPG <120mg/dL. Elderly/Debilitated/Malnourished: Conservative dosing; do not titrate to max. (Tab, Extended-Release) Swallow tab whole; do not crush or chew.
*Pediatrics:* 10-16 yrs: (Sol, Tab) Individualize dose. Initial: 500mg bid with meals. Titrate: Increase by 500mg/week. Max: 2000mg/day.

G

**HOW SUPPLIED:** Sol: (Riomet) 500mg/5mL; Tab: 500mg, 850mg, 1000mg; Tab, Extended-Release: 500mg, 750mg

**CONTRAINDICATIONS:** Renal disease/dysfunction (eg, SrCr ≥1.5mg/dL [males], ≥1.4mg/dL [females], or abnormal CrCl), metabolic acidosis, diabetic ketoacidosis. D/C temporarily (48 hrs) for radiologic studies with intravascular iodinated contrast materials.

**WARNINGS/PRECAUTIONS:** Lactic acidosis reported (rare); increased risk with renal dysfunction, increased age, DM, CHF, and other conditions with risk of hypoperfusion and hypoxemia. Avoid use in patients ≥80 yrs unless renal function is normal. Monitor renal function, FPG, $HbA_{1c}$, and hematological parameters (eg, Hgb, Hct, red blood cell indices). Monitor for ketoacidosis and metabolic acidosis. Avoid in renal/hepatic impairment. D/C therapy in the presence of hypoxemia (eg, acute CHF, acute MI, cardiovascular collapse), dehydration, sepsis, or if loss of blood glucose occurs due to stress (give insulin). Temporarily d/c therapy prior to any surgical procedure (except minor procedures not associated with restricted intake of food and fluids). May decrease serum vitamin $B_{12}$ levels. Increased risk of hypoglycemia in elderly, debilitated/malnourished, adrenal or pituitary insufficiency, or alcohol intoxication.

**ADVERSE REACTIONS:** Lactic acidosis, diarrhea, N/V, flatulence, asthenia, abdominal discomfort, hypoglycemia, dizziness, dyspnea, taste disorder, chest discomfort, flu syndrome, palpitations, indigestion, headache.

**INTERACTIONS:** See contraindications. Furosemide, nifedipine, cimetidine, cationic drugs (eg, digoxin, amiloride, procainamide, quinidine, quinine, ranitidine, trimethoprim, vancomycin, triamterene, morphine) may increase metformin levels. Thiazides, other diuretics, corticosteroids, phenothiazines, thyroid products, estrogens, oral contraceptives, phenytoin, nicotinic acid, sympathomimetics, CCBs, and isoniazid may cause hyperglycemia. Risk of hypoglycemia with alcohol. Alcohol potentiates the effect on lactate metabolism. May interact with highly protein-bound drugs (eg, salicylates, sulfonamides, chloramphenicol, probenecid). May decrease furosemide levels. Caution with drugs that may affect renal function or result in significant hemodynamic change or may interfere with the disposition of metformin. Hypoglycemia may occur with concomitant use of other glucose-lowering agents (eg, sulfonylureas, insulin).

**PREGNANCY:** Category B, not for use in nursing.

**MECHANISM OF ACTION:** Biguanide; decreases hepatic glucose production, decreases intestinal absorption of glucose, and improves insulin selectivity by increasing peripheral glucose uptake and utilization.

**PHARMACOKINETICS: Absorption:** Absolute bioavailability (50-60%); $T_{max}$=7 hrs. **Distribution:** $V_d$=654L. **Elimination:** Urine (90%); $T_{1/2}$=6.2 hrs (plasma), 17.6 hrs (blood).

## NURSING CONSIDERATIONS

**Assessment:** Assess for renal/hepatic impairment, acute or chronic metabolic acidosis, presence of a hypoxic state (eg, CHF, acute MI, cardiovascular collapse), dehydration, sepsis, alcoholism, nutritional status, adrenal or pituitary insufficiency, pregnancy/nursing status, and for possible drug interactions.

Assess baseline renal function, FPG, $HbA_{1c}$, and hematological parameters (Hct, Hgb, red blood cell indices).

**Monitoring:** Monitor for lactic acidosis, hypoglycemia, hypoxemia (eg, cardiovascular collapse, acute CHF, acute MI), prerenal azotemia, and for decreases in Vitamin $B_{12}$ levels. Monitor FPG, $HbA_{1c}$, renal function (eg, SrCr), and hematological parameters (eg, Hgb, Hct, red blood cell indices).

**Patient Counseling:** Inform about the importance of adherence to dietary instructions and a regular exercise program. Inform of the risk of developing lactic acidosis during therapy; advise to d/c therapy immediately and contact physician if unexplained hyperventilation, myalgia, malaise, unusual somnolence, or other nonspecific symptoms occur. Instruct to avoid excessive alcohol intake. Inform that regular follow up is needed. Counsel to take with meals. Instruct that if taking the extended-release tablet, that tablet must be swallowed whole and not crushed or chewed.



**Administration:** Oral route. **Storage:** 20-25°C (68-77°F); excursions permitted to 15-30°C (59-86°F). Dispense in light-resistant containers.

## GLUCOTROL XL RX

glipizide (Pfizer)

**OTHER BRAND NAMES:** Glipizide ER (Various)

**THERAPEUTIC CLASS:** Sulfonylurea (2nd generation)

**INDICATIONS:** Adjunct to diet and exercise, to improve glycemic control in adults with type 2 diabetes mellitus (DM).

**DOSAGE:** *Adults:* Do not chew, divide, or crush. Initial: 5mg qd with breakfast; use lower doses if sensitive to hypoglycemics. Usual: 5-10mg qd. Max: 20mg/day. Combination Therapy: Initial: 5mg qd. Switch From Insulin: If ≤20 U/day: D/C insulin; start 5mg qd. If >20 U/day: Reduce insulin dose by 50%; begin 5mg qd. Further insulin reductions depend on response. Elderly/Debilitated/Malnourished/Renal or Hepatic Impairment: Dose conservatively.

**HOW SUPPLIED:** Tab, Extended-Release: 2.5mg, 5mg, 10mg

**CONTRAINDICATIONS:** Type 1 diabetes mellitus, diabetic ketoacidosis with or without coma.

**WARNINGS/PRECAUTIONS:** Increased risk of hypoglycemia with the elderly, debilitated, malnourished, renal and hepatic disease, adrenal or pituitary insufficiency. Increased risk of cardiovascular mortality. Loss of blood glucose control when exposed to stress (eg, fever, trauma, infection, or surgery); d/c therapy and start insulin. Secondary failure can occur over a period of time. May influence the pharmacokinetics and hence the clinical efficacy. Treatment of patients with glucose 6-phosphate dehydrogenase (G6PD) deficiency with sulfonylurea agents can lead to hemolytic anemia. Caution in patients with G6PD deficiency and consider a non-sulfonylurea alternative. Hemolytic anemia reported in patients without G6PD deficiency.

**ADVERSE REACTIONS:** Hypoglycemia, asthenia, headache, dizziness, nervousness, tremor, diarrhea, flatulence.

**INTERACTIONS:** Hypoglycemic effects potentiated by alcohol, NSAIDs, other highly protein-bound drugs, salicylates, sulfonamides, chloramphenicol, probenecid, coumarins, MAOIs, and β-blockers. Severe hypoglycemia reported with oral hypolycemics and oral miconazole. Certain drugs have a tendency to cause hyperglycemia and may lead to loss of glycemic control including thiazides and other diuretics, corticosteroids, phenothiazines, thyroid products, estrogens, oral contraceptives, phenytoin, nicotinic acid, sympathomimetics, CCBs, and isoniazid. β-blockers may mask signs of hypoglycemia.

**PREGNANCY:** Category C, not for use in nursing.

**MECHANISM OF ACTION:** Sulfonylurea; lowers blood glucose acutely by stimulating the release of insulin from the pancreas.

**PHARMACOKINETICS: Absorption:** Rapid and complete; bioavailability (100%); $T_{max}$=6-12 hrs. **Distribution:** $V_d$=10L; plasma protein binding (98-99%).

**Metabolism**: Liver; aromatic hydroxylation. **Elimination**: Urine (80%), feces (10%), unchanged (<10%); $T_{1/2}$=2-5 hrs.

## NURSING CONSIDERATIONS

**Assessment:** Assess FPG, $HbA_{1c}$, renal function, LFTs, pregnancy status, type 1 DM, ketoacidosis, GI disease, and for possible drug interactions.

**Monitoring:** Monitor blood and urine glucose, $HbA_{1c}$ every 3 months, renal function, LFTs, signs/symptoms of hypoglycemia, and for endocrine, metabolic, and hematologic reactions.

**Patient Counseling:** Counsel to swallow whole with breakfast, not to chew, divide, or crush. Inform about importance of adhering to dietary instructions, a regular exercise program, and regular testing of urine/blood glucose. Educate on risks/benefits of therapy; signs/symptoms, predisposing conditions, and treatment of hypoglycemia; primary and secondary failure.

**Administration:** Oral route. **Storage**: 15-30°C (59-86°F). Protect from moisture and humidity.

G

# GLUCOVANCE RX

metformin HCl - glyburide (Bristol-Myers Squibb)

**THERAPEUTIC CLASS:** Sulfonylurea/biguanide

**INDICATIONS:** Adjunct to diet and exercise to improve glycemic control in adults with type 2 diabetes mellitus (DM).

**DOSAGE:** *Adults:* Inadequate Glycemic Control on Diet/Exercise Alone: Initial: 1.25mg-250mg qd-bid with meals. If $HbA_{1c}$ >9% or fasting plasma glucose (FPG) >200mg/dL, give 1.25mg-250mg bid (with morning and evening meals). Titrate: Increase by 1.25mg-250mg/day q2 weeks. Do not use 5mg-500mg for initial therapy. Inadequate Glycemic Control on Sulfonylurea or Metformin/ Switching from previously treated combination therapy of Glyburide (or another Sulfonylurea) plus Metformin: Initial: 2.5mg-500mg or 5mg-500mg bid with meals. Starting dose should not exceed daily doses of glyburide or metformin already being taken. Titrate: Increase by no more than 5mg-500mg/day. Max: 20mg-2000mg/day. With Concomitant Thiazolidinediones (TZDs): Initiate and titrate TZD as recommended. If hypoglycemia occurs, reduce glyburide component. Elderly/Debilitated/Malnourished: Do not titrate to maximum dose.

**HOW SUPPLIED:** Tab: (Glyburide-Metformin) 1.25mg-250mg, 2.5mg-500mg, 5mg-500mg

**CONTRAINDICATIONS:** Renal disease or dysfunction (SrCr ≥1.5mg/dL [males], ≥1.4mg/dL [females], or abnormal CrCl), metabolic acidosis, including diabetic ketoacidosis. D/C temporarily for radiologic studies involving intravascular iodinated contrast materials.

**WARNINGS/PRECAUTIONS:** Lactic acidosis reported (rare); increased risk with increased age, DM with renal insufficiency, congestive heart failure (CHF), and conditions with risk of hypoperfusion and hypoxemia. Avoid use in patients ≥80 yrs unless renal function is normal. Increased risk of cardiovascular mortality. Increased risk of hypoglycemia in elderly, debilitated, malnourished, adrenal or pituitary insufficiency or alcohol intoxication. D/C with any condition associated with hypoxemia, dehydration, or sepsis. Monitor renal function and for metabolic acidosis. Avoid in renal/hepatic impairment. May decrease serum vitamin $B_{12}$ levels. D/C if cardiovascular collapse (shock), acute CHF, or acute MI occur. Temporarily suspend therapy before any surgical procedure, and do not restart until oral intake has resumed and renal function returns to normal. Caution in patients with glucose-6-phosphate dehydrogenase (G6PD) deficiency; may lead to hemolytic anemia.

**ADVERSE REACTIONS:** Upper respiratory infection, NV, abdominal pain, headache, dizziness, diarrhea.

**INTERACTIONS:** Furosemide, nifedipine, and cimetidine may increase metformin levels. Hypoglycemia is potentiated by alcohol, ciprofloxacin, miconazole, thiazolidinedione, salicylates, sulfonamides, chloramphenicol, probenecid, coumarins, MAOIs, and β-blockers. Thiazides and other diuretics, corticosteroids, phenothiazines, thyroid products, estrogens, oral contraceptives, phenytoin, nicotinic acid, sympathomimetics, CCBs, and isoniazid may cause hyperglycemia. Alcohol potentiates the effect of metformin on lactate metabolism. Monitor LFTs and weight gain with TZD and rosiglitazone. May compete for common renal tubular transport systems with cationic drugs (eg, amiloride, digoxin, morphine, procainamide, quinidine, ranitidine, triamterene, trimethoprim, or vancomycin).

**PREGNANCY:** Category B, not for use in nursing.

**MECHANISM OF ACTION:** Glyburide: Sulfonylurea; stimulates release of insulin from the pancreas. Metformin: Biguanide; decreases hepatic glucose production and intestinal absorption of glucose, and improves insulin sensitivity by increasing peripheral glucose uptake.

G

**PHARMACOKINETICS: Absorption:** Glyburide: $T_{max}$=4 hrs. Metformin: absolute bioavailability (50-60%). **Distribution:** Glyburide: plasma protein binding (extensive); found in breast milk. Metformin: $V_d$=654L. **Metabolism:** Glyburide: metabolites: 4-trans-hydroxy (major) and 3-cis hydroxyl derivatives. **Elimination:** Glyburide: bile, urine (50% each route); $T_{1/2}$=10 hrs. Metformin: renal excretion (90%); $T_{1/2}$=6.2 hrs (plasma), 17.6 hrs (blood).

## NURSING CONSIDERATIONS

**Assessment:** Assess FPG, $HbA_{1c}$ levels, renal function, LFTs, CBC. Assess for CHF, septicemia, acute or chronic metabolic acidosis, adrenal or pituitary insufficiency, G6PD deficiency, and alcoholism. Assess pregnancy/nursing status and hypersensitivity to drug. Evaluate for other medical conditions and for possible drug interactions.

**Monitoring:** Monitor for hypoglycemia, lactic acidosis, prerenal azotemia, CHF, cardiovascular disease, and hypersensitivity reactions. Monitor FPG, $HbA_{1c}$, renal function, LFTs, CBC.

**Patient Counseling:** Inform about potential risks and benefits of drug and alternative modes of therapy. Inform that drug is adjunct to diet and exercise to control diabetes. Inform about importance of adherence to dietary instructions, regular excercise programs, and regular testing of blood glucose, glycosylated Hgb, renal function, and hematologic parameters. Report unexplained hyperventilation, myalgia, malaise, N/V, and somnolence. Explain risk of lactic acidosis, its signs/symptoms, and conditions that predispose its development. Explain risk of hypoglycemia. Counsel against excessive alcohol intake.

**Administration:** Oral route. **Storage:** ≤25°C (77°F). Dispense in light-resistant container.

# GLUMETZA RX

metformin HCl (Depomed)

**THERAPEUTIC CLASS:** Biguanide

**INDICATIONS:** Adjunct to diet and exercise or with a sulfonylurea or insulin, to improve glycemic control in type 2 diabetes mellitus.

**DOSAGE:** *Adults:* ≥18 yrs: Take with evening meal. Initial: 1000mg qd. With Insulin: Initial: 500mg qd. Titrate: May increase by 500mg/week. Max: 2000mg/day. Decrease insulin dose by 10-25% if FPG <120mg/dL. Elderly/Debilitated/Malnourished: Conservative dosing; do not titrate to max. Swallow whole; do not crush or chew.

**HOW SUPPLIED:** Tab, Extended-Release: 500mg, 1000mg

**CONTRAINDICATIONS:** Renal disease or dysfunction (SrCr ≥1.5mg/dL [males], ≥1.4mg/dL [females], or abnormal CrCl), CHF, metabolic acidosis, including diabetic ketoacidosis. D/C temporarily (48 hrs) for radiologic studies with intravascular iodinated contrast materials.

**WARNINGS/PRECAUTIONS:** Lactic acidosis reported (rare); increased risk with renal dysfunction, increased age, DM, CHF, and other conditions with risk of hypoperfusion and hypoxemia. Avoid use in patients ≥80 yrs unless renal function is normal. Monitor renal function and for ketoacidosis and metabolic acidosis. Avoid in renal/hepatic impairment. D/C in hypoxic states (eg, CHF, shock, acute MI), loss of blood glucose control due to stress (give insulin), acidosis, dehydration, sepsis. Temporarily d/c prior to surgery (due to restricted food/fluid intake) or procedures requiring intravascular iodinated contrast materials. May decrease serum vitamin $B_{12}$ levels. Increased risk of hypoglycemia in elderly, debilitated/malnourished, adrenal or pituitary insufficiency, or alcohol intoxication.

**ADVERSE REACTIONS:** Hypoglycemia, diarrhea, nausea.

**INTERACTIONS:** Furosemide, nifedipine, cimetidine, cationic drugs (eg, digoxin, amiloride, procainamide, quinidine, quinine, ranitidine, trimethoprim, vancomycin, triamterene, morphine) may increase metformin levels. Thiazides, other diuretics, corticosteroids, phenothiazines, thyroid products, estrogens, oral contraceptives, phenytoin, nicotinic acid, sympathomimetics, CCBs, isoniazid may cause hyperglycemia. Risk of hypoglycemia with alcohol. Excess alcohol may increase potential for lactic acidosis. May decrease furosemide levels.



**PREGNANCY:** Category B, not for use in nursing.

**MECHANISM OF ACTION:** Biguanide; decreases hepatic glucose production, decreases intestinal absorption of glucose, and improves insulin selectivity by increasing peripheral glucose uptake and utilization.

**PHARMACOKINETICS: Absorption:** Administration of variable doses resulted in different absorption parameters. $T_{max}$=7-8 hrs. **Distribution:** $V_d$=654L. **Elimination:** Urine (90%); $T_{1/2}$=6.2 hrs (plasma), 17.6 hrs (blood).

## NURSING CONSIDERATIONS

**Assessment:** Assess FPG, $HbA_{1c}$, renal function, LFTs, CBC. Assess for CHF, septicemia, acute or chronic metabolic acidosis, adrenal or pituitary insufficiency, alcoholism, pregnancy status. Evaluate for other medical/surgical conditions and for possible drug interactions.

**Monitoring:** Monitor for hypoglycemia, lactic acidosis, prerenal azotemia, CHF, CVD. Monitor FPG, $HbA_{1c}$, renal function, LFTs, CBC.

**Patient Counseling:** Inform drug is adjunct to diet and exercise. Temporarily d/c therapy prior to intravascular radiocontrast study or surgery. Advise that excessive alcohol intake increases hypoglycemia risk. Report unexplained hyperventilation, myalgia, malaise, NV, and somnolence. Not recommended for use during pregnancy. Counsel about adverse effects; seek medical attention if any develop. Regular follow-ups needed; take as prescribed with evening meals.

**Administration:** Oral route. Must swallow whole; do not crush or chew. **Storage:** 20-25°C (68-77°F). Excursions permitted to 15-30°C (59-86°F).

# GLYNASE PRESTAB — RX

glyburide (Pharmacia & Upjohn)

**THERAPEUTIC CLASS:** Sulfonylurea (2nd generation)

**INDICATIONS:** Adjunct to diet and exercise, to improve glycemic control in adults with type 2 diabetes mellitus (DM).

**DOSAGE:** *Adults:* Initial: 1.5-3mg qd with breakfast or first main meal; give 0.75mg if sensitive to hypoglycemia. Titrate: Increase by no more than 1.5mg at weekly intervals. Maint: 0.75-12mg qd or in divided doses. Max: 12mg/day. Transfer from Other Oral Antidiabetic Agents: Initial: 1.5-3mg/day. Switch From Insulin: If <20 U/day, substitute with 1.5-3mg qd. If 20-40 U/day, give 3mg qd. If >40 U/day, decrease insulin dose by 50% and give 3mg qd. Titrate: Progressive withdrawal of insulin and increase by 0.75-1.5mg every 2-10 days. Elderly/Debilitated/Malnourished/Renal or Hepatic Impairment/Adrenal or Pituitary Insufficiency: Initial: 0.75mg qd.

**HOW SUPPLIED:** Tab: 1.5mg*, 3mg*, 6mg* *scored

**CONTRAINDICATIONS:** Diabetic ketoacidosis with or without coma, and Type I DM.

**WARNINGS/PRECAUTIONS:** Risk of hypoglycemia, especially with renal or hepatic insufficiency, elderly patients, debilitated patients, malnourished patients, and in patients with adrenal or pituitary insufficiency. Increased risk of cardiovascular mortality reported. Loss of blood glucose control may occur when exposed to stress (eg, fever, trauma, infection, surgery); d/c therapy and start insulin. Secondary failure can occur over period of time. Retitrate when transferring from other glyburide products or oral hypoglycemic agents. Treatment of patients with glucose 6-phosphate dehydrogenase (G6PD) deficiency with sulfonylurea agents can lead to hemolytic anemia; consider a non-sulfonylurea alternative. Therapeutic response should be monitored by frequent urine glucose tests and periodic blood glucose tests.

**ADVERSE REACTIONS:** Hypoglycemia, liver function abnormalities, GI disturbances, leukopenia, agranulocytosis, thrombocytopenia, hemolytic anemia, aplastic anemia, pancytopenia, hyponatremia, changes in accomodation, blurred vision, allergic reactions.



**INTERACTIONS:** Hypoglycemic effects may be potentiated by NSAIDs and other drugs that are highly protein bound, ciprofloxacin, salicylates, sulfonamides, chloramphenicol, probenecid, coumarins, monoamine oxidase inhibitors, and beta adrenergic blocking agents. Severe hypoglycemia reported with oral hypolycemics and oral miconazole. Certain drugs have a tendency to cause hyperglycemia and may lead to loss of glycemic control including thiazides and other diuretics, corticosteroids, phenothiazines, thyroid products, estrogens, oral contraceptives, phenytoin, nicotinic acid, sympathomimetics, calcium channel blockers, and isoniazid.

**PREGNANCY:** Category B, not for use in nursing.

**MECHANISM OF ACTION:** Sulfonylurea; lowers blood glucose acutely by stimulating the release of insulin from the pancreas.

**PHARMACOKINETICS: Absorption:** $C_{max}$=106ng/mL (3mg); AUC=568ng•hr/mL (3mg); $T_{max}$=2-3 hrs. **Distribution:** Plasma protein binding (extensive). **Metabolism:** 4-trans-hydroxy derivative (major metabolite). **Elimination:** Bile (50%), urine (50%); $T_{1/2}$=4 hrs.

## NURSING CONSIDERATIONS

**Assessment:** Assess for diabetic ketoacidosis, type 1 DM, renal or hepatic insufficiency, presence of debilitation or malnourishment, adrenal or pituitary insufficiency, G6PD deficiency, pregnancy/nursing status, and for possible drug interactions. Assess FPG and $HbA_{1c}$ levels.

**Monitoring:** Monitor for signs/symptoms of hypoglycemia and for hemolytic anemia. Monitor FPG, $HbA_{1c}$, and urine glucose.

**Patient Counseling:** Inform of the potential risks and advantages of therapy and about alternative modes of therapy. Instruct to take with breakfast or first main meal. Advise about the importance of adhering to dietary instructions, a regular exercise program, and regular testing of urine and/or blood glucose. Counsel on increased risk of cardiovascular mortality. Inform of risks of hypoglycemia, its symptoms and treatment, and conditions that predispose to its development. Counsel about primary and secondary failure.

**Administration:** Oral route. **Storage:** 20-25°C (68-77°F). Keep container tightly closed.

# GLYSET — RX

miglitol (Pharmacia & Upjohn)

**THERAPEUTIC CLASS:** Alpha-glucosidase inhibitor

**INDICATIONS:** Adjunct to diet and exercise, to improve glycemic control in type 2 diabetes mellitus. May use in combination with a sulfonylurea.

**DOSAGE:** *Adults:* Initial: 25mg tid. May give 25mg qd (to minimize GI side effects) and gradually increase to tid. Titrate: After 4-8 weeks, increase to 50mg tid up to 3 mos. Maint: 50mg tid. May increase to 100mg tid if needed. Max: 100mg tid. Take with first bite of each main meal.

**HOW SUPPLIED:** Tab: 25mg, 50mg, 100mg

**CONTRAINDICATIONS:** Diabetic ketoacidosis, inflammatory bowel disease, colonic ulceration, partial intestinal obstruction or if predisposed to intestinal obstruction. Chronic intestinal diseases with digestion or absorption disorders/conditions may deteriorate with increased gas formation in the intestine.

**WARNINGS/PRECAUTIONS:** Use glucose (dextrose) not sucrose (cane sugar) to treat mild-moderate hypoglycemia. Temporary insulin therapy may be necessary at times of stress such as fever, trauma, infection, or surgery. Not recommended with renal impairment (SrCr >2mg/dL).

**ADVERSE REACTIONS:** Flatulence, diarrhea, abdominal pain, skin rash, low serum iron.

**INTERACTIONS:** Intestinal absorbents (eg, charcoal) and digestive enzyme preparations (eg, amylase, pancreatin) may reduce effects. May reduce bioavailability of ranitidine and propranolol. May interact with glyburide, and digoxin.

**PREGNANCY:** Category B, not for use in nursing.

**MECHANISM OF ACTION:** α-glucosidase inhibitor; inhibits membrane-bound intestinal α-glucosidase hydrolase enzymes.

**PHARMACOKINETICS: Absorption:** Complete, $T_{max}$=2-3 hrs. **Distribution:** $V_d$=0.18 L/kg; plasma protein binding (<4.0%). **Elimination**: Urine (95% unchanged); $T_{1/2}$=2 hrs.

## NURSING CONSIDERATIONS

**Assessment:** Assess for diabetic ketoacidosis, inflammatory bowel disease, colonic ulceration, partial intestinal obstruction, chronic intestinal disease, renal function, pregnancy status.

**Monitoring:** Monitor for hypoglycemia, FPG, $HbA_{1c}$, renal function, diabetic ketoacidosis, GI symptoms, skin rash, serum iron.

**Patient Counseling:** Inform that drug is adjunct to diet and exercise. Counsel about adverse effects. Advise on need for regular follow-ups and to take drug as prescribed. During periods of stress (fever, trauma, infection, or surgery), medication requirements may change; patients should seek medical advice promptly.

**Administration:** Oral route. **Storage**: 25°C (77°F); excursions permitted to 15-30°C (59-86°F).

# GRIFULVIN V — RX

griseofulvin (Ortho Neutrogena)

**THERAPEUTIC CLASS:** *Penicillium*-derived antifungal

**INDICATIONS:** Management of tinea capitis, tinea corporis, tinea pedis, tinea unguium, tinea barbae, and tinea cruris. Inhibits the growth of fungi that commonly cause ringworm infections of hair, skin, and nails.

**DOSAGE:** *Adults:* T. capitis: 500mg qd for 4-6 weeks. T. corporis: 500mg qd for 2-4 weeks. T. pedis: 1g qd for 4-8 weeks. T. cruris: 500mg qd. T. unguium: 1g qd for at least 4 months (fingernail) or at least 6 months (toenails). *Pediatrics:* Usual: 5mg/lb/day. 30-50lb: 125-250mg qd. >50lb: 250-500mg qd. T. capitis: Treat for 4-6 weeks. T. corporis: Treat for 2-4 weeks. T. pedis: Treat for 4-8 weeks. T. unguium: Treat for at least 4 months (fingernail) or at least 6 months (toenails).

**HOW SUPPLIED:** Sus: 125mg/5mL [120mL]; Tab: 250mg, 500mg

**CONTRAINDICATIONS:** Porphyria, hepatocellular failure, pregnancy.

**WARNINGS/PRECAUTIONS:** Confirm diagnosis. Not for prophylactic use. Monitor renal, hepatic, and hematopoietic functions periodically with prolonged therapy. Cross-sensitivity with PCN may exist. Photosensitivity reported. D/C if granulocytopenia occurs.

**ADVERSE REACTIONS:** Rash, urticaria, oral thrush, N/V, epigastric distress, diarrhea, headache, dizziness, insomnia, mental confusion.

**INTERACTIONS:** Oral anticoagulants may need adjustment. Barbiturates decrease effects. Decreases effects of oral contraceptives; may increase incidence of breakthrough bleeding.

**PREGNANCY:** Not for use in pregnancy or nursing.

**MECHANISM OF ACTION:** Acts systemically to inhibit the growth of *Trichophyton, Microsporum*, and *Epidermophyton* genera of fungi. Fungistatic amounts deposit in keratin, which is gradually exfoliated and replaced by noninfected tissue.

**PHARMACOKINETICS: Absorption:** $C_{max}$=0.5g; $T_{max}$=4 hrs.

## NURSING CONSIDERATIONS

**Assessment:** Assess for proper diagnosis of infecting fungi. Assess for possible drug interactions and drug allergies (possible PCN cross-sensitivity).

G

**Monitoring:** Monitor for photosensitivity reactions. Periodically monitor organ system function, including renal, hepatic, and hematopoietic. Monitor for signs/symptoms of lupus erythematosus.

**Patient Counseling:** Counsel females to use additional forms of contraception while taking medication and for 1 month following cessation of therapy. Counsel males to use contraception while on treatment and for 6 months following. Warn patients to avoid exposure to intense natural or artificial sunlight. Counsel females to avoid use during pregnancy.

**Administration:** Oral route. **Storage:** Store at room temperature.

# GRIS-PEG RX

griseofulvin (Pedinol)

**THERAPEUTIC CLASS:** *Penicillium*-derived antifungal

**INDICATIONS:** Treatment of t. capitis, t. corporis, t. pedis, t. unguium, t. barbae, and t. cruris.

**DOSAGE:** *Adults:* T. capitis: 375mg qd in single or divided doses for 4-6 weeks. T. corporis: 375mg qd in single or divided doses for 2-4 weeks. T. pedis: 375mg bid for 4-8 weeks. T. cruris: 375mg qd in single or divided doses. T. unguium: 375mg bid for at least 4 months (fingernail) or at least 6 months (toenails).
*Pediatrics:* Usual: 3.3mg/lb/day. 35-60lb: 125-187.5mg qd. >60lb: 187.5-375mg qd. T. capitis: Treat for 4-6 weeks. T. corporis: Treat for 2-4 weeks. T. pedis: Treat for 4-8 weeks. T. unguium: Treat for at least 4 months (fingernail) or at least 6 months (toenails).

**HOW SUPPLIED:** Tab: 125mg*, 250mg* *scored

**CONTRAINDICATIONS:** Porphyria, hepatocellular failure, pregnancy.

**WARNINGS/PRECAUTIONS:** Not for prophylactic use. Periodically monitor renal, hepatic, and hematopoietic functions in prolonged therapy. Cross-sensitivity with PCN may exist. Photosensitivity reported. D/C if granulocytopenia occurs.

**ADVERSE REACTIONS:** Rash, urticaria, oral thrush, N/V, epigastric distress, diarrhea, headache, dizziness, insomnia, mental confusion.

**INTERACTIONS:** Oral anticoagulants may need dose adjustments. Decreased effects with barbiturates. Decreased effects of oral contraceptives. Increased alcohol effects.

**PREGNANCY:** Not for use in pregnancy and in nursing.

**MECHANISM OF ACTION:** Fungistatic agent. Active against various species of *Microsporum*, *Epidermophyton* and *Trichophyton*. Has greater affinity for depositing in keratin precursor cells of diseased tissue. Tightly binds to new keratin, which then becomes highly resistant to fungal invasions.

**PHARMACOKINETICS: Absorption:** $C_{max}$=600ng/mL; $T_{max}$=4 hrs; AUC=8618ng•hr/mL.

## NURSING CONSIDERATIONS

**Assessment:** Assess for ID of fungi responsible for infection (eg, cultures, microscopic exam). Assess pregnancy status prior to therapy.

**Monitoring:** Periodic monitoring of renal, hepatic, and hematopoietic functions should be performed with sustained therapy. Monitor for hypersensitivity reactions (eg, skin rashes, urticaria, and erythema multiform-like reactions). Monitor for signs/symptoms of lupus erythematosus or lupus-like syndrome and possible drug interactions while on therapy.

**Patient Counseling:** Counsel to avoid intense natural or artificial sunlight while on medication. Avoid alcohol. Instruct to take proper hygienic precautions to prevent spread of infection. Inform that medication may be swallowed whole or crushed; sprinkled into 1 tbl. of applesauce and swallowed immediately without chewing. Counsel about signs/symptoms of agranulocytosis. Advise females drug may interfere with oral contraceptives and to avoid pregnancy while on medication.

**Administration:** Oral route. **Storage:** Store at controlled room temperature 15-30°C (59-86°F) in tight, light-resistant containers.



# HALCION

**CIV**

triazolam (Pharmacia & Upjohn)

**THERAPEUTIC CLASS:** Benzodiazepine

**INDICATIONS:** Short-term treatment of insomnia.

**DOSAGE:** *Adults:* 0.25mg qhs. Max: 0.5mg. Elderly/Debilitated: Initial: 0.125mg. Max: 0.25mg.

**HOW SUPPLIED:** Tab: 0.125mg, 0.25mg* *scored

**CONTRAINDICATIONS:** Pregnancy. With ketoconazole, itraconazole, nefazodone, medications that impair CYP3A.

**WARNINGS/PRECAUTIONS:** Worsening or failure of response after 7-10 days may indicate other medical conditions. Increased daytime anxiety, abnormal thinking, and behavioral changes have occurred. May impair mental/physical abilities. Anterograde amnesia reported with therapeutic doses. Caution with baseline depression, suicidal tendencies, history of drug dependence, elderly/debilitated, renal/hepatic impairment, chronic pulmonary insufficiency, and sleep apnea. Withdrawal symptoms after d/c; avoid abrupt withdrawal.

**ADVERSE REACTIONS:** Drowsiness, dizziness, lightheadedness, headache, N/V, coordination disorders, ataxia.

**INTERACTIONS:** See Contraindications. Avoid the concomitant use with CYP3A inhibitors (eg, ketoconazole, itraconazole, all azole-type antifungals, nefazodone). Potentiated by the coadministration of isoniazid, oral contraceptives, grapefruit juice, ranitidine. Caution with fluvoxamine, diltiazem, verapamil, cimetidine, ergotamine, cyclosporine, amiodarone, nicardipine, nifedipine, sertraline, paroxetine, macrolides. Additive CNS depression with psychotropics, anticonvulsants, antihistamines, and alcohol.

**PREGNANCY:** Category X, not for use in nursing.

**MECHANISM OF ACTION:** Triazolobenzodiazepine hypnotic agent.

**PHARMACOKINETICS: Absorption:** $C_{max}$=1-6ng/mL, $T_{max}$=2 hrs. **Metabolism:** Hydroxylation via CYP3A. **Elimination:** Urine (79.9%), $T_{1/2}$=1.5-5.5 hrs.

## NURSING CONSIDERATIONS

**Assessment:** Assess for primary psychiatric and/or medical illness, chronic pulmonary insufficiency (sleep apnea, COPD), renal/hepatic function, and possible drug interactions.

**Monitoring:** Monitor worsening of insomnia, suicidality, severe sedation, complex behaviors (sleep-driving), abnormal thinking/behavioral changes (aggressiveness, hallucinations, and bizzare behavior), anterograde amnesia, paradoxical reactions.

**Patient Counseling:** Inform of benefits/risks of therapy and potential for physical/psychological dependence. Caution against hazardous tasks (operating machinery/driving). Do not increase dose or d/c before consulting physician. Avoid alcohol consumption. Notify if pregnant or planning to become pregnant.

**Administration:** Oral route. **Storage:** 20-25°C (68-77°F).

## HalfLytely RX

polyethylene glycol 3350 - sodium bicarbonate - potassium chloride - sodium chloride - bisacodyl (Braintree)

**THERAPEUTIC CLASS:** Bowel cleanser/stimulant laxative

**INDICATIONS:** Bowel cleansing prior to colonoscopy.

H

**DOSAGE:** *Adults:* Consume only clear liquids on day of preparation. Swallow all 4 bisacodyl tabs at noon (do not chew or crush). After 1st bowel movement (or max of 6 hrs) begin drinking sol, 240mL every 10 min (approx. 8 glasses). Drink all sol.

**HOW SUPPLIED:** Kit: Tab, Delayed-Release: (Bisacodyl) 5mg [4[s]]. Sol: (Polyethylene Glycol 3350-Potassium Chloride-Sodium Bicarbonate-Sodium Chloride) 210g-0.74g-2.86g-5.60g [2000mL].

**CONTRAINDICATIONS:** Ileus, GI obstruction, gastric retention, bowel perforation, toxic colitis, toxic megacolon.

**WARNINGS/PRECAUTIONS:** Do not add additional ingredients (eg, flavorings). Caution with severe ulcerative colitis, ileus or gastric retention. Monitor with impaired gag reflex, prone to regurgitation or aspiration. Slow administration or temporarily d/c if severe bloating, distention, or abdominal pain develops. Avoid large quantities of water during or after preparation or colonoscopy. Monitor closely with impaired water handling. Generalized tonic-clonic seizures, hives and skin rashes reported.

**ADVERSE REACTIONS:** NV, abdominal fullness, cramping, overall discomfort.

**INTERACTIONS:** Oral medications taken within 1 hr of start of administration start may not be absorbed from GI tract. Avoid bisacodyl delayed release tablets within 1 hr of taking an antacid.

**PREGNANCY:** Category C, caution in nursing.

**MECHANISM OF ACTION:** Stimulant laxative that induces diarrhea.

**PHARMACOKINETICS: Metabolism:** Hydrolysis by intestinal brush border enzymes and colonic bacteria to form bis-(hydroxyphenyl) pyridyl-2 methane (active metabolite).

### NURSING CONSIDERATIONS

**Assessment:** Assess for known allergy to polyethylene glycol, GI obstruction, bowel perforation, toxic colitis, toxic megacolon, renal impairment, and seizures.

**Monitoring:** Perform baseline and post-colonoscopy lab tests with known/suspected hyponatremia. D/C use if severe bloating, abdominal distention, or abdominal pain occur. Monitor for hypersensitivity reactions, aspiration, asystole, ischemic colitis, and seizures.

**Patient Counseling:** Do not drink large quantities of clear liquids. Oral medication administered within 1 hr of start of administration of sol may be flushed from GI tract, hence not absorbed. Instruct to take exactly as directed.

**Administration:** Oral route. **Storage:** 20-25°C (68-77°F); excursions permitted to 15-30°C (59-86°F). Use the reconstituted solution, which may be refrigerated, within 48 hrs.

## HALOPERIDOL RX

haloperidol (Various)

**Elderly patients with dementia-related psychosis treated with atypical antipsychotic drugs are at an increased risk of death; most appeared to be cardiovascular (eg, heart failure, sudden death) or infectious (eg, pneumonia) in nature. Haloperidol is not approved for the treatment of patients with dementia-related psychosis.**

**OTHER BRAND NAMES:** Haldol Decanoate (Ortho-McNeil) - Haldol (Ortho-McNeil) - Haloperidol Lactate (Teva)

**THERAPEUTIC CLASS:** Butyrophenone

**INDICATIONS:** (Immediate-Release) Treatment of psychosis, schizophrenia, Tourette's disorder, severe childhood behavioral problems. Short-term treatment of hyperactivity in children. (Decanoate) Prolonged management of psychosis.

**DOSAGE:** *Adults:* (Immediate-Release) PO: Moderate Symptoms/Elderly/Debilitated: 0.5-2mg bid-tid. Severe Symptoms/Resistant Patients: 3-5mg bid-tid. Max: 100mg/day. IM: Acute Agitation: 2-5mg every 4-8 hrs or hourly as needed for moderately severe or very severe symptoms. Max: 100mg/day. (Decanoate) For IM inj only. Give every 4 weeks or monthly. Initial:10-20 times daily oral dose up to 100mg. Give remainder of dose 3-7 days later if initial dose >100mg. Usual: 10-15 times daily oral dose. Max: 450mg/month. Elderly/Debilitated: Initial: 10-15 times daily oral dose.
*Pediatrics*: 3-12 yrs: (15-40kg): PO: Psychosis: Initial: 0.05-0.15mg/kg/day given bid-tid. Nonpsychotic Disorder/Tourette's: 0.05-0.075mg/kg/day given bid-tid. Max: 6mg/day.

**HOW SUPPLIED:** Inj: 5mg/mL; Inj: (Decanoate) 50mg/mL, 100mg/mL; Sol: 2mg/mL; Tab: 0.5mg*, 1mg*, 2mg*, 5mg*, 10mg*, 20mg* *scored

**CONTRAINDICATIONS:** Comatose states, severe toxic CNS depression, Parkinson's disease.

**WARNINGS/PRECAUTIONS:** Risk of tardive dyskinesia, especially in elderly. Neuroleptic malignant syndrome (NMS), hyperpyrexia, heat stroke, bronchopneumonia reported. Decreased cholesterol, cutaneous and/or ocular changes may occur. Neurotoxicity may occur with thyrotoxicosis. Caution with CV disease, seizures, EEG abnormalities, QT-prolonging conditions, elderly. Do not administer IV. Cases of sudden death and torsade de pointes reported. Leukopenia, neutropenia, and agranulocytosis reported. D/C if absolute neutrophil count (ANC) <1000/mm$^3$. Galactorrhea, amenorrhea, gynecomastia, and impotence reported.

**ADVERSE REACTIONS:** Extrapyramidal symptoms, tardive dyskinesia, tardive dystonia, ECG changes, QT prolongation, ventricular arrhythmias, tachycardia, hypotension, HTN, N/V, constipation, diarrhea, dry mouth, blurred vision, urinary retention.

**INTERACTIONS:** Caution with rifampin, anticonvulsants, anticoagulants, anticholinergics, antiparkinson agents. May potentiate CNS depression with alcohol, opiates, anesthetics, and other CNS depressants. Antagonizes epinephrine. Monitor for neurological toxicity with lithium. Avoid concomitant alcohol use.

**PREGNANCY:** Category C, not for use in nursing.

**MECHANISM OF ACTION:** Butyrophenone; not established, suspected to block effects of dopamine and increase turnover rate.

**PHARMACOKINETICS: Absorption:** $T_{max}$=6 days (IM). **Elimination:** $T_{1/2}$=3 weeks (IM).

## NURSING CONSIDERATIONS

**Assessment:** Assess for severe toxic CNS depression or Parkinson's disease prior to treatment. Assess use of haloperidol in patients who have severe cardiovascular disorders, are on anticonvulsant medications, with a history of seizures, on CNS depressants, and on concomitant lithium therapy. Assess for hypersensitivity to drug, pregnancy/nursing status, and possible drug interactions.

**Monitoring:** Monitor for signs/symptoms of NMS, EPS, TD, and bronchopneumonia. Monitor for neurotoxicity in patients with thyrotoxicosis. Monitor for cardiovascular effects (eg, torsade de pointes, QT prolongation) after receiving IM formulation. Monitor CBC, hypersensitivity reactions, and signs and symptoms of infection.

**Patient Counseling:** Drug may impair mental/physical abilities. Avoid alcohol use with drug due to possible additive effects and hypotension. Counsel not to abruptly d/c medication.

**Administration:** Oral route, IM. **Storage:** (Tab/Sus) 20-25°C (68-77°F), (Inj) 15-30°C (59-86°F). Do not freeze. Protect from light.

H

## HAVRIX RX

hepatitis A vaccine (inactivated) (GlaxoSmithKline)

**THERAPEUTIC CLASS:** Vaccine

**INDICATIONS:** Active immunization against disease caused by hepatitis A virus (HAV) in persons ≥12 months of age.

**DOSAGE:** *Adults:* 1mL IM, then 1mL IM booster after 6-12 months. Administer in the deltoid region.
*Pediatrics:* 1-18 yrs: 0.5mL IM, then 0.5mL IM booster after 6-12 months. Administer in the anterolateral aspect of the thigh in infants and young children and in the deltoid muscle of the upper arm in older children.

**HOW SUPPLIED:** Inj: 720 EL U/0.5mL, 1440 EL U/mL [TIP-LOK®, vial]

**CONTRAINDICATIONS:** Previous allergic reaction to neomycin.

**WARNINGS/PRECAUTIONS:** Tip cap and rubber plunger of needleless prefilled syringe contain latex; may cause allergic reactions in latex-sensitive individuals. Immunocompromised persons may have a diminished immune response. May not prevent hepatitis A in patients who have an unrecognized hepatitis A infection at time of vaccination. May not prevent infection in individuals who do not achieve protective antibody titers. Medical treatment and supervision must be available to manage possible anaphylactic reactions. Do not administer in the gluteal region.

**ADVERSE REACTIONS:** Injection-site reactions (eg, induration, soreness, redness, swelling, tenderness), headache, irritability, fever, fatigue, malaise, anorexia, nausea.

**INTERACTIONS:** Immunosuppressive therapies including irradiation, antimetabolites, alkylating agents, cytotoxic drugs, and corticosteroids (used in greater than physiological doses) may reduce immune respone.

**PREGNANCY:** Category C, caution in nursing.

**MECHANISM OF ACTION:** Vaccine; may produce immune response for protection against hepatitis A virus infection.

### NURSING CONSIDERATIONS

**Assessment:** Assess for hypersensitivity to neomycin and latex. Assess for presence of immunosuppression, immunization history, pregnancy/nursing status, and for possible drug interactions.

**Monitoring:** Monitor for signs/symptoms of an allergic reaction and for injection-site reactions (eg, pain, redness, swelling).

**Patient Counseling:** Inform of potential benefits and risks of immunization. Counsel about potential adverse reactions. Instruct to report any adverse events to healthcare provider where the vaccine was administered.

**Administration:** IM route. Shake well before withdrawal and use. Do not dilute to administer. Concomitant administration of other vaccines or immune globulin should be given at different injection site; do not mix with any other vaccine or product in the same syringe or vial. **Storage:** 2-8°C (36-46°F). Do not freeze. Discard if frozen.

# HELIDAC RX

tetracycline HCl - bismuth subsalicylate - metronidazole (Prometheus)

**Metronidazole has been shown to be carcinogenic in mice and rats. Unnecessary use of the drug should be avoided. Its use may be reserved for the eradication of *H.pylori* for treatment of patients with *H.pylori* infection and duodenal ulcer disease.**

**THERAPEUTIC CLASS:** *H.pylori* treatment combination

**INDICATIONS:** In combination with an $H_2$ antagonist for eradication of *H.pylori* for treatment of patients with *H.pylori* infection and duodenal ulcer disease (active or history of duodenal ulcer).

**DOSAGE:** *Adults:* (Bismuth) (2 tabs) 525mg + (Metronidazole) 250mg + (Tetracycline) 500mg, all qid for 14 days with an $H_2$ antagonist taken as directed. Missed Dose: Continue normal dosing schedule until medication is gone. Do not take double doses. If >4 doses missed, contact the prescriber. Take at meals and hs. Chew and swallow bismuth tablets. Take metronidazole and tetracycline with a full glass of water; swallow whole.

**HOW SUPPLIED:** Cap: (Tetracycline) 500mg; Tab: (Metronidazole) 250mg; Tab, Chewable: (Bismuth Subsalicylate) 262.4mg

**CONTRAINDICATIONS:** Pregnancy, nursing, pediatrics, renal/hepatic impairment, known allergy to aspirin (ASA).

**WARNINGS/PRECAUTIONS:** Use in the absence of a proven or strongly suspected bacterial infection or prophylactic indication is unlikely to provide benefit and increases the risk of development of drug-resistant bacteria. Caution in elderly. (Bismuth subsalicylate) Do not use to treat nausea and vomiting in children or teenagers who have or are recovering from chickenpox or flu. Rare reports of neurotoxicity with excessive doses. May cause temporary and harmless darkening of the tongue and/or black stool. (Metronidazole) Encephalopathy, peripheral neuropathy, convulsive seizures, aseptic meningitis reported; d/c if abnormal neurological signs develop. Caution in patients with CNS disease. May produce teratogenic effects. Mild leukopenia reported; caution with evidence of or history of blood dyscrasias. Known or previously unrecognized candidiasis may present more prominent symptoms. (Tetracycline) May cause permanent discoloration of the teeth during tooth development (Last half of pregnancy, infancy, and childhood up to 8 yrs). Enamel hypoplasia reported. May cause fetal harm. Photosensitivity manifested by an exaggerated sunburn reaction reported; d/c at first evidence of skin erythema. May increase BUN which may lead to azotemia, hyperphosphatemia, and acidosis in patients with significant renal impairment. May result in overgrowth of nonsusceptible organisms (eg, fungi); d/c if superinfection occurs. Pseudotumor cerebri (benign intracranial hypertension) in adults reported.

**ADVERSE REACTIONS:** Nausea, diarrhea, abdominal pain, melena.

**INTERACTIONS:** (Bismuth subsalicylate) Increased risk of bleeding when administered with anticoagulant therapy. May enhance hypoglycemic effect of antidiabetic agents. Caution with ASA, probenecid, and sulfinpyrazone. (Tetracycline) Depressed plasma prothrombin activity with anticoagulants. Impaired absorption with antacids containing aluminum, calcium, or magnesium; preparations containing iron, zinc, or sodium bicarbonate; or milk or dairy products. Possible reduced absorption with bismuth or calcium carbonate. May interfere with bactericidal action of penicillin; avoid concomitant use. May render oral contraceptives less effective; breakthrough bleeding reported. Fatal renal toxicity with methoxyflurane reported. (Metronidazole) Potentiates anticoagulant effect of warfarin and other oral coumarin anticoagulants. May prolong the half-life and decrease the plasma clearance when used concomitantly with drugs that decrease microsomal liver enzyme activity (eg, cimetidine). Accelerated elimination leading to reduced plasma levels of metronidazole when used concomitantly with drugs that induce microsomal liver enzymes (eg, phenytoin, phenobarbital). May impair phenytoin clearance. May increase lithium levels which may lead to toxicity. Avoid alcohol during and at least 1 day after therapy. Psychotic reactions reported in alcoholics with concomitant disulfiram; metronidazole should not be given to patients who have taken disulfiram within the last 2 weeks.

**PREGNANCY:** Category D, not for use in nursing.

**MECHANISM OF ACTION:** Antimicrobial; combination therapy with activity against *H.pylori*.

**PHARMACOKINETICS: Absorption**: (Salicylic acid, 525mg) $C_{max}$=13.1mcg/mL. (Metronidazole, 250mg) Well-absorbed; $C_{max}$=6mcg/mL; $T_{max}$=1-2 hrs. (Tetracycline) Readily absorbed. **Distribution**: (Bismuth) Plasma protein binding (>90%). (Salicylic acid) $V_d$=170mL/kg; plasma protein binding (90%). (Metronidazole) Plasma protein binding (<20%), appears in the CSF, saliva, breast milk. (Tetracycline) Crosses placenta, found in fetal tissues, secreted in breast milk. **Metabolism**: (Salicyclic acid) Extensive. (Metronidazole) Side chain oxidation, glucuronide conjugation; 2-hydroxymethyl (metabolite). **Elimination**: (Bismuth) Urine, bile; $T_{1/2}$=21-72 days. (Salicylic, 525mg) Urine (10%, unchanged); $T_{1/2}$=2-5 hrs. (Metronidazole) Urine (60-80%), feces (6-15%); $T_{1/2}$=8 hrs. (Tetracycline) Urine, feces.

H

## NURSING CONSIDERATIONS

**Assessment:** Assess for proper diagnosis, age of patient, renal/hepatic impairment, hypersensitivity to ASA or salicylates, chickenpox, flu, candidiasis, CNS diseases, presence or history of blood dyscrasias, pregnancy/nursing status, and for possible drug interactions.

**Monitoring:** Monitor for signs/symptoms of encephalopathy, peripheral neuropathy, convulsive seizures, aseptic meningitis, neurotoxicity, photosensitivity, darkening of the tongue or black stools, increases in BUN, leukopenia, candidiasis, overgrowth of nonsusceptible organisms, and for pseudotumor cerebri.

**Patient Counseling:** Instruct to take 4 times a day, at meal times and bedtime. Instruct to chew and swallow bismuth subsalicylate tabs. Instruct to swallow tetracycline cap and metronidazole tab whole, with a full glass of water. Advise to take tetracycline with an adequate amount of fluid, particularly at bedtime, to help prevent esophageal irritation and ulceration. Inform if a dose is missed, continue normal dosing until medication is done, do not double up doses. Counsel to continue therapy for full treatment period to prevent development of bacterial resistance. Inform that ringing in the ears may occur when taken with ASA; advise to consult prescriber regarding d/c ASA until treatment is complete. Inform that therapy may make oral contraceptives less effective; advise to use a different or an additional form of contraception. Instruct to contact physician if breakthrough bleeding occurs. Advise to notify prescriber if pregnancy occurs while on therapy. Instruct to avoid alcohol while on medication and for 1 day after d/c. Counsel to avoid exposure to sun/sun lamps. Inform may develop darkening of tongue or stool. Instruct to avoid pregnancy/nursing during therapy.

**Administration:** Oral route. **Storage**: 20-25°C (68-77°F).

# HEPARIN SODIUM RX

heparin sodium (Various)

**THERAPEUTIC CLASS:** Glycosaminoglycan

**INDICATIONS:** Prophylaxis and treatment of venous thrombosis and its extension; PE in atrial fibrillation; and peripheral arterial embolism. Prevention of postoperative DVT and PE. Diagnosis and treatment of acute and chronic consumptive coagulopathies; and prevention of clotting in arterial and cardiac surgery.

**DOSAGE:** *Adults:* Based on 68kg: Initial: 5000 U IV, then 10,000-20,000 U SQ. Maint: 8000-10,000 U q8h or 15,000-20,000 U q12h. Intermittent IV Injection: Initial: 10,000 U. Maint: 5000-10,000 U q4-6h. Continuous IV Infusion: Initial: 5000U. Maint: 20,000-40,000 U/24 hrs. Adjust to coagulation test results. See PI for details in specific disease states.

*Pediatrics:* Initial: 50 U/kg IV drip. Maint: 100 U/kg IV drip q4h or 20,000 U/$m^2$/24 hrs continuously.

**HOW SUPPLIED:** Inj: 1000 U/mL, 5000 U/mL, 10,000 U/mL, 20,000 U/mL

**CONTRAINDICATIONS:** Severe thrombocytopenia, if cannot perform appropriate blood-coagulation tests (with full-dose heparin), uncontrollable active bleeding state (except in DIC).

**WARNINGS/PRECAUTIONS:** Not for IM use. Fatal hemorrhage reported in pediatrics due to medication errors (eg, confused with "catheter lock flush" vials). Hemorrhage can occur at any site; caution with increased danger of hemorrhage (severe HTN, bacterial endocarditis, surgery, etc.). Monitor blood coagulation tests frequently. Thrombocytopenia, HIT and HITT reported, even up to several weeks after discontinuation of therapy. D/C if platelets <100,000$mm^3$ or if recurrent thrombosis develops. Monitor platelets, Hct, and occult blood in the stool. Increased heparin resistance with fever, thrombosis, thrombophlebitis, infections with thrombosing tendencies, MI, cancer, and post-op. Higher bleeding incidence in women >60 yrs. Hyperaminotransferasemia reported.

**ADVERSE REACTIONS:** Hemorrhage, local irritation, erythema, mild pain, hematoma, chills, fever, urticaria, asthma, lacrimation, NV, anaphylactoid reactions, thrombocytopenia, HIT, and HITT.

**INTERACTIONS:** Wait ≥5 hrs after last IV dose or 24 hrs after last SQ dose before measure PT for dicumarol or warfarin. Platelet inhibitors (eg, ASA, dextran, phenylbutazone, ibuprofen, indomethacin, dipyridamole, hydroxychloroquine) may induce bleeding. Digitalis, tetracyclines, nicotine, or antihistamines may counteract anticoagulant action.

**PREGNANCY:** Category C, safe in nursing.

**MECHANISM OF ACTION:** Glycosaminoglycan; inhibits reactions that lead to blood clotting and the formation of fibrin clots. Acts at multiple sites in the normal coagulation system.

**PHARMACOKINETICS: Absorption:** (SC) $T_{max}$=2-4 hrs. **Metabolism:** Liver and reticulo-endothelial system. **Elimination:** $T_{1/2}$=10 min.

## NURSING CONSIDERATIONS

**Assessment:** Assess for severe thrombocytopenia, pregnancy status, and drug interactions. Assess use in disease states at risk for hemorrhage (eg, subacute bacterial endocarditis, severe HTN) and use in older patients (>60 yrs). Assess that suitable coagulation tests (eg, whole blood clotting time, partial thromboplastin time) can be performed at appropriate intervals in patients on full-dose heparin. Assess for thrombocytopenia, heparin-induced thrombocytopenia (HIT), and heparin-induced thrombocytopenia and thrombosis (HITT).

**Monitoring:** Monitor for signs/symptoms of hemorrhage, thrombocytopenia, heparin resistance, hypersensitivity reactions, and hyperaminotransferasemia. Perform periodic monitoring of platelet counts, Hct, and tests for occult blood in stool. If given therapeutically, perform frequent coagulation tests. If given by continuous IV infusion, monitor coagulation time every 4 hrs during early stages of treatment. If given intermittently by IV inj, monitor coagulation tests before each inj during the initial phase of treatment and then at appropriate intervals thereafter.

**Patient Counseling:** Counsel about increased risk of bleeding tendencies while on medication. Instruct to notify physician if any type of unusual bleeding or hypersensitivity reaction occurs. Advise that periodic lab monitoring is required during treatment.

**Administration:** IV/SQ routes. If added to infusion solution for continuous IV administration, container should be inverted 6 times to ensure adequate mixing and prevention of heparin pooling in the solution. **Storage:** 20-25°C (68-77°F).

# HEPSERA RX

adefovir dipivoxil (Gilead Sciences)

**Discontinuation may result in severe acute exacerbations of hepatitis. Chronic use may result in nephrotoxicity in patients at risk of or having underlying renal dysfunction. HIV resistance may occur with unrecognized or untreated HIV infection. Lactic acidosis and severe hepatomegaly with steatosis, including fatal cases reported with the use of nucleoside analogs alone or in combination with other antiretrovirals.**

**THERAPEUTIC CLASS:** Acyclic nucleotide analog

**INDICATIONS:** Treatment of chronic hepatitis B in patients ≥12 yrs with evidence of active viral replication and either evidence of persistent elevations in serum aminotransferases (ALT or AST) or histologically active disease.

**DOSAGE:** *Adults:* 10mg qd. Renal Impairment: CrCl 30-49mL/min: 10mg q48h. CrCl 10-29mL/min: 10mg q72h. Hemodialysis Patients: 10mg every 7 days following dialysis.
*Pediatrics:* ≥12 yrs: 10mg qd.

H

**HOW SUPPLIED:** Tab: 10mg

**WARNINGS/PRECAUTIONS:** Hepatic function should be monitored with both clinical and laboratory follow-up for at least several months following discontinuation; if appropriate, resumption of anti-hepatitis B therapy may be warranted. Chronic administration may result in delayed nephrotoxicity; calculate CrCl in all patients prior to therapy. Monitor renal function in all patients; adjust dose as appropriate. Caution with use in adolescents with underlying renal dysfunction and monitor renal function closely in these patients. May require HIV antibody testing prior to treatment. Caution with use in patients with known risk factors for liver disease. Suspend treatment if clinical or laboratory findings suggestive of lactic acidosis or pronounced hepatotoxicity develop. Resistance to the drug can result in viral load rebound which may result in exacerbation of hepatitis B, leading to liver decompensation and possible fatal outcome. To reduce risk of resistance in patients with lamivudine resistant HBV, adefovir dipivoxil should be used in combination with lamivudine and not as monotherapy. In order to reduce the risk of resistance in all patients receiving monotherapy, a modification of treatment should be considered if serum HBV DNA remains above 1000 copies/mL with continued treatment. Caution in elderly.

**ADVERSE REACTIONS:** Nephrotoxicity, asthenia, headache, abdominal pain, nausea, flatulence, diarrhea, dyspepsia, increased creatinine, hypophosphatemia.

**INTERACTIONS:** Co-administration with drugs that reduce renal function or compete for active tubular secretion may increase concentrations of adefovir or the co-administered drugs; monitor closely for adverse events when used concomitantly with drugs that are excreted renally or with other drugs known to affect renal function. Avoid concomitant administration with tenofovir disoproxil fumarate (TDF) or TDF-containing products, including emtricitabine-TDF combination, and efavirenz-emtricitabine-TDF combination.

**PREGNANCY:** Category C, not for use in nursing.

**MECHANISM OF ACTION:** Acyclic nucleotide analog; inhibits HBV DNA polymerase by competing with natural substrate deoxyadenosine triphosphate and by causing DNA chain termination after incorporation into viral DNA.

**PHARMACOKINETICS: Absorption:** $C_{max}$=18.4ng/mL; $T_{max}$=1.75 hrs; AUC=220ng•h/mL. CrCl 50-80mL/min: $C_{max}$=22.4ng/mL; AUC=266ng•h/mL. CrCl 30-49mL/min: $C_{max}$=28.5ng/mL; AUC=455ng•h/mL., CrCl 10-29mL/min: $C_{max}$=51.6ng/mL; AUC=1240ng•h/mL. **Pediatrics:** $C_{max}$=23.3ng/mL; AUC=248.8ng•h/mL. **Distribution:** $V_d$=392mL/kg (IV, 1mg/kg/day), 352mL/kg (IV, 3mg/kg/day); plasma protein binding (≤4%). **Elimination:** Urine (45%); $T_{1/2}$=7.48 hrs.

## NURSING CONSIDERATIONS

**Assessment:** Assess for renal dysfunction, risk factors for liver disease (eg, obesity), pregnancy/nursing status, and for possible drug interactions.

Perform HIV antibody testing prior to therapy and assess CrCl prior to therapy.

**Monitoring:** Monitor for signs/symptoms of nephrotoxicity; monitor renal function. Monitor for signs and symptoms of acute exacerbations of hepatitis following d/c of therapy. Monitor for signs/symptoms of lactic acidosis, hepatomegaly with steatosis, and for clinical resistance.

**Patient Counseling:** Inform of risks and benefits of therapy. Instruct to immediately report any severe abdominal pain, muscle pain, yellowing of eyes, dark urine, pale stools, and/or loss of appetite. Instruct to not d/c therapy without first informing physician. Advise that routine laboratory monitoring and follow-up is important during therapy. Inform that obtaining HIV antibody testing prior to starting therapy is important. Inform childbearing women about risks during pregnancy. Instruct lamivudine-resistant patients to use as combination therapy with lamivudine and not as monotherapy.

**Administration:** Oral route. **Storage:** 25°C (77°F); excursions permitted to 15-30°C (59-86°F).



## HERCEPTIN RX

trastuzumab (Genentech)

**Use may result in cardiac failure manifesting as congestive heart failure (CHF) and decreased left ventricular ejection fraction (LVEF). Increased incidence/severity of left ventricular cardiac dysfunction in combination with anthracycline-containing chemotherapy regimens. Evaluate LVEF prior to and during therapy; d/c with significant decrease in left ventricular function or cardiomyopathy. Serious infusion reactions and pulmonary toxicity may occur. Interrupt infusion if dyspnea or clinically significant hypotension develops. D/C if anaphylaxis, angioedema, interstitial pneumonitis, or acute respiratory distress syndrome occurs.**

**THERAPEUTIC CLASS:** Monoclonal antibody/HER2-blocker

**INDICATIONS:** Adjuvant treatment of HER2-overexpressing node-positive or node-negative breast cancer. 1st-line treatment of HER2-overexpressing metastatic breast cancer in combination with paclitaxel. Single agent for treatment of HER2-overexpressing breast cancer in patients who received one or more chemotherapy regimens for metastatic disease.

**DOSAGE:** *Adults:* Adjuvant treatment: during and following paclitaxel, docetaxel, or docetaxel/carboplatin for 52 weeks total: Initial: 4mg/kg over 90 min. Maint: 2mg/kg weekly over 30 min for the first 12 weeks (paclitaxel or docetaxel) or 18 weeks (docetaxel/carboplatin). 1 week following the last weekly dose: 6mg/kg IV over 30-90 min q3 weeks. Following completion of multimodality, anthracycline-based regimens: Initial: 8mg/kg IV over 90 min. Maint: 6mg/kg over 30-90 min q3 weeks. Metastatic breast cancer: Alone or with paclitaxel: Initial: 4mg/kg over 90 min. Maint: 2mg/kg weekly over 30 min until disease progression. Cardiomyopathy: Assess LVEF and withhold for at least 4 weeks when there is ≥16% absolute decrease in LVEF from pretreatment values or LVEF below institutional limits of normal and ≥10% absolute decrease in LVEF from pretreatment values. Resume treatment within 4-8 weeks when LVEF returns to normal limits and the absolute decrease from baseline is ≤15%. D/C permanently for persistent (>8 weeks) LVEF decline or for suspension of dosing on >3 occasions for cardiomyopathy.

**HOW SUPPLIED:** Inj: 440mg

**WARNINGS/PRECAUTIONS:** May cause left ventricular cardiac dysfunction, arrhythmias, HTN, disabling cardiac failure, cardiomyopathy, and cardiac death. Obtain baseline cardiac assessment (eg, history, physical, LVEF). Monitor LVEF prior to initiation, every 3 months during, and every 6 months following completion for at least 2 yrs. Fatal pulmonary toxicity may occur. May exacerbate chemotherapy-induced neutropenia. Detection of HER2 protein overexpression is necessary for selection of patients appropriate for therapy as these are the only patients for whom benefit has been shown. May cause severe infusion reactions; interrupt infusion and intervene with medical therapy. May cause fetal harm when administered to pregnant women; increased risk of oligohydramnios during second and third trimesters.

**ADVERSE REACTIONS:** Fever, N/V, infusion reactions, diarrhea, infections, increased cough, headache, fatigue, dyspnea, rash, neutropenia, anemia, myalgia, headache, nasopharyngitis.

**INTERACTIONS:** Paclitaxel may increase serum levels. Concomitant anthracycline-containing chemotherapy regimens may increase incidence/severity of cardiac dysfunction.

**PREGNANCY:** Category D, not for use in nursing.

**MECHANISM OF ACTION:** Monoclonal antibody/HER2 blocker; inhibits the proliferation of human tumor cells that overexpress HER2.

**PHARMACOKINETICS: Absorption:** $C_{max}$=337mcg/mL (500mg). **Distribution:** $V_d$=44mL/kg. **Elimination:** $T_{1/2}$=2 days (10mg), $T_{1/2}$=12 days (500mg).

## NURSING CONSIDERATIONS

H

**Assessment:** Assess cardiac function including history and physical exam and baseline LVEF by echocardiogram or MUGA scan. Assess for HER2 overexpression and HER2 gene amplification. Assess CBC with differential and platelets, pregnancy/nursing status, and possible drug interactions.

**Monitoring:** Monitor for cardiac failure and CHF. LVEF must be measured every 3 months during and upon completion of therapy and every 6 months for 2 yrs following completion. Monitor for cardiomyopathy, infusion reactions, pulmonary reactions/toxicity, exacerbation of chemotherapy-induced neutropenia, and other serious adverse events. May enroll patients who become pregnant while on treatment in the Herceptin Pregnancy Registry.

**Patient Counseling:** Contact health care professional if there is new onset or worsening shortness of breath, cough, swelling of ankles/legs or face, palpitations, weight gain of more than 5 lbs in 24 hrs, dizziness, or loss of consciousness. Advise females to use effective contraceptive methods during and at least 6 months following therapy.

**Administration:** IV route. Do not administer as IV push or bolus. See PI for proper reconstitution. **Storage:** 2-8°C (34-46°F). Diluted infusion solution may be stored at 2-8°C (34-46°F) for no longer than 24 hrs prior to use. Do not freeze.

# HUMALOG — RX

insulin lispro (Lilly)

**THERAPEUTIC CLASS:** Insulin

**INDICATIONS:** Treatment of diabetes mellitus for the control of hyperglycemia.

**DOSAGE:** *Adults:* Individualize dose. Inject SQ within 15 min before or immediately after a meal. May need to reduce/adjust dose with renal/hepatic impairment. May use with external insulin pump; do not dilute or mix with other insulins when used with pump.

*Pediatrics:* ≥3 yrs: Individualize dose. Inject SQ within 15 min before or immediately after a meal. May need to reduce/adjust dose with renal/hepatic impairment. May use with external insulin pump; do not dilute or mix with other insulins when used with pump.

**HOW SUPPLIED:** Cartridge: 100 U/mL [3mL]; Inj: 100 U/mL [3mL, 10mL]; Pen: 100 U/mL [3mL]

**CONTRAINDICATIONS:** During episodes of hypoglycemia.

**WARNINGS/PRECAUTIONS:** Any change in insulin should be made cautiously. Changes in strength, manufacturer, type or method of manufacture may result in the need for a change in dosage. Hypoglycemia, hypokalemia, lipodystrophy or hypersensitivity may occur. An infection or illness may alter insulin requirements. With type 1 DM a longer-acting insulin is usually required to maintain glucose control. Caution with patients who are fasting or having autonomic neuropathy. Monitor glucose levels and adjust dose with hepatic impairment. Hyperglycemia or ketosis may occur; prompt identification and correction of the cause is necessary. May be used in an external insulin pump.

Reduce requirements with renal impairment. Antibody production reported. Not for IV use.

**ADVERSE REACTIONS:** Hypoglycemia, hypokalemia, allergic reactions, injection-site reactions, lipodystrophy, pruritus, rash.

**INTERACTIONS:** Increased insulin requirements with corticosteroids, isoniazid, niacin, estrogens, oral contraceptives, phenothiazines, thyroid replacement therapy. Decreased insulin requirements with oral antidiabetic drugs, salicylates, sulfa antibiotics, MAOIs, ACEIs, ARBs, β-blockers, octreotide, and alcohol. β-blockers may mask symptoms of hypoglycemia. Caution with potassium-lowering drugs or drugs sensitive to serum potassium levels.

**PREGNANCY:** Category B, caution in nursing.

**MECHANISM OF ACTION:** Insulin lispro (rDNA origin); regulates glucose metabolism.

**PHARMACOKINETICS: Absorption:** (0.1-0.2 U/kg dose) Absolute bioavailability (55-77%); (0.1-0.4 U/kg dose)$T_{max}$=30-90 min. **Distribution:** $V_d$=0.26-0.36L/kg. **Elimination:** $T_{1/2}$=1 hr.

H

## NURSING CONSIDERATIONS

**Assessment:** Assess renal function, LFTs, FPG, $HbA_{1c}$, hypokalemia, pregnancy status, autonomic neuropathy, and possible drug interactions.

**Monitoring:** Monitor blood glucose, potassium levels, and $HbA_{1c}$ levels regularly. Monitor for antibody production, allergic reactions (eg, redness, swelling, or itching at injection-site), SOB, wheezing, reduction in BP, rapid pulse or sweating, anaphylactic reactions, pruritus, lipodystrophy.

**Patient Counseling:** Inform about the potential risks and advantages of the drug and alternative therapies. Instruct that infusion set (reservoir syringe, tubing, and catheter), Disetronic D-TRON or D-TRON plus cartridge adapter, and Humalog in the external insulin pump reservoir should be replaced and a new infusion site selected every 48 hrs or less. Inform of the importance of proper insulin storage, injecting techniques, timing of dosage, adherence to meal planning, regular physical activity, regular blood glucose monitoring, periodic $HbA_{1c}$ testing, recognition and management of hypo/hyperglycemia, and periodic assessment for diabetes complications. Infrom physician if pregnant or intend to become pregant. Instruct or train on how to use the device.

**Administration:** SQ route. **Storage:** Refrigerate at 2-8°C (36-46°F). Do not use if frozen. Unrefrigerated [below 30°C (86°F)] must be used within 28 days or be discarded. Protect from direct heat and sunlight.

# HUMALOG MIX 75/25 RX

insulin lispro protamine - insulin lispro (Lilly)

**THERAPEUTIC CLASS:** Insulin

**INDICATIONS:** Treatment of diabetes mellitus for the control of hyperglycemia.

**DOSAGE:** *Adults:* Individualize dose. Inject SQ within 15 min before a meal. May need to reduce/adjust dose with renal/hepatic impairment.

**HOW SUPPLIED:** (Insulin Lispro Protamine, Human-Insulin Lispro, Human) Inj: 75 U-25 U/mL [10mL]; Pen: 75 U-25 U/mL [3mL]

**CONTRAINDICATIONS:** During episodes of hypoglycemia.

**WARNINGS/PRECAUTIONS:** Any change in insulin should be made cautiously. Changes in strength, manufacturer, type or method of manufacture may result in the need for a change in dosage. Hypoglycemia, hypokalemia, lipodystrophy or hypersensitivity may occur. An infection or illness may alter insulin requirements. With type 1 DM a longer-acting insulin is usually required to maintain glucose control. Caution with patients who are fasting or having autonomic neuropathy. Monitor glucose levels and adjust dose with hepatic impairment. Reduced requirements with renal impairment. Antibody production reported. Not for IV use.

**ADVERSE REACTIONS:** Hypoglycemia, hypokalemia, allergic reactions, injection-site reactions, lipodystrophy, pruritus, rash.

**INTERACTIONS:** Increased insulin requirements with corticosteroids, isoniazid, niacin, estrogens, oral contraceptives, phenothiazines, thyroid replacement therapy. Decreased insulin requirements with oral antidiabetic drugs, salicylates, sulfa antibiotics, MAOIs, ACEIs, ARBs, β-blockers, octreotide, and alcohol. β-blockers may mask symptoms of hypoglycemia. Caution with potassium-lowering drugs or drugs sensitive to serum potassium levels.

**PREGNANCY:** Category B, caution in nursing.

**MECHANISM OF ACTION:** Insulin; regulates glucose metabolism

**PHARMACOKINETICS: Absorption:** (0.3 U/kg dose) $T_{max}$ = 30-240 mins, 60 mins (median).

## NURSING CONSIDERATIONS

**Assessment:** Assess renal function, LFTs, FPG, $HbA_{1c}$, hypokalemia, pregnancy status, autonomic neuropathy, and possible drug interactions.

**Monitoring:** Monitor blood glucose, potassium levels, and $HbA_{1c}$ levels regularly. Monitor for antibody production, allergic reactions (eg, redness, swelling, or itching at injection site), SOB, wheezing, reduction in BP, rapid pulse or sweating, anaphylactic reactions, pruritus, lipodystrophy.

**Patient Counseling:** Inform about the potential risks and advantages of drugs and alternative therapies. Inform of the importance of proper insulin storage, injecting techniques, timing of dosage, adherence to meal planning, regular physical activity, regular blood glucose monitoring, periodic $HbA_{1c}$ testing, recognition and management of hypo/hyperglycemia, and periodic assessment for diabetes complications. Infrom physician if pregnant or intend to become pregant. Instruct how to use the device.

**Administration:** SQ route (15 min before meals). **Storage:** Refrigerate at 2-8°C (36-46°F). Do not use if frozen. Unrefrigerated [below 30°C (86°F)] must be used within 28 days (vials), within 10 days (pens and kwikpens) or be discarded. Protect from direct heat and light.

# HUMATROPE RX

somatropin (Lilly)

**THERAPEUTIC CLASS:** Human growth hormone

**INDICATIONS:** Treatment of pediatric patients who have growth failure due to inadequate secretion of endogenous growth hormone (GH), short stature associated with Turner syndrome, idiopathic short stature (ISS), short stature or growth failure in children with short stature homeobox-containing gene (SHOX) deficiency, and for growth failure in children born small for gestational age (SGA) who fail to demonstrate catch-up growth by 2-4 yrs. Replacement of endogenous GH in adults with adult-onset or childhood-onset GF deficiency.

**DOSAGE:** *Adults:* GHD: Non-Weight Based: Initial: 0.2mg/day (range, 0.15-0.30 mg/day) SQ. Titrate: Every 1-2 months in increments of 0.1-0.2mg/day based on clinical response and serum insulin-like growth factor I (IGF-I) concentrations. Weight Based: Initial: Not more than 0.006mg/kg/day SQ. Titrate: Increase dose based on individual requirement. Dose adjustment based on clinical response, side effects, and determination of age- and gender-adjusted serum insulin-like growth factor I (IGF-I) concentrations. Max: 0.0125mg/kg/day. Elderly: Lower starting dose and smaller dose increments. *Pediatrics:* SQ: Individualize dose. GHD: 0.026-0.043mg/kg/day (0.18-0.30mg/kg/week). Turner Syndrome: Up to 0.054mg/kg/day (0.375mg/kg/week). Idiopathic Short Stature: Up to 0.053mg/kg/day (0.37mg/kg/week). SHOX Deficiency: 0.050mg/kg/day (0.35mg/kg/week). SGA: Up to 0.067mg/kg/day (0.47mg/kg/week). Refer to PI for further details.

**HOW SUPPLIED:** Inj: 5mg (vial); 6mg, 12mg, 24mg (cartridge)

**CONTRAINDICATIONS:** Pediatrics with closed epiphyses. Active proliferative or severe non-proliferative diabetic retinopathy. Active malignancy.

Hypersensitivity to metacresol or glycerin. Acute critical illness due to complications following open heart or abdominal surgery, multiple accidental trauma, or acute respiratory failure. Prader-Willi syndrome with severe obesity, with history of upper airway obstruction or sleep apnea, or with severe respiratory impairment. Not indicated for patients who have growth failure due to genetically confirmed Prader-Willi syndrome.

**WARNINGS/PRECAUTIONS:** Cartridges should not be used if allergy to metacresol or glycerin exists. Increased mortality reported in patients with acute critical illness due to complications following open heart surgery, abdominal surgery or multiple accidental trauma, or those with acute respiratory failure. Fatalities reported in pediatrics with Prader-Willi syndrome who had severe obesity, h/o upper airway obstruction or sleep apnea, or unidentified respiratory tract infection; interrupt treatment if signs of upper airway obstruction or new onset sleep apnea develop; monitor for signs of respiratory infection and for weight control in patients with Prader-Willi syndrome. In patients with pre-existing tumors or GH deficiency secondary to intracranial lesion, monitor for progression/recurrence of underlying disease. Increased risk of second neoplasm reported in childhood cancer survivors. Monitor for malignant transformation of skin lesions. Impaired glucose tolerance and diabetes mellitus (DM) may be unmasked; monitor glucose levels; caution with DM. Intracranial HTN reported; fundoscopic exam should be performed routinely before initiation if therapy and periodically during treatment; d/c if papilledema occurs. Caution in patients with hypopituitarism and/or hypothyroidism. Perform periodic thyroid function tests and adjust thyroid hormone replacement therapy. Increased risk of ear/hearing disorders and CV disorders in patients with Turner syndrome. Pancreatitis reported. Fluid retention, slipped capital femoral epiphysis, progression of preexisting scoliosis, tissue atrophy, and local or systemic allergic reactions may occur. Serum levels of inorganic phosphorus, alkaline phosphatase, parathyroid hormone and IGF-I may increase after therapy. Caution in the elderly.



**ADVERSE REACTIONS:** Injection-site reactions, hypersensitivity to the diluent, hypothyroidism, edema, arthralgia, myalgia, carpal tunnel syndrome, paraesthesias, hyperglycemia, scoliosis, otitis media, hyperlipidemia, rhinitis, flu syndrome, headache.

**INTERACTIONS:** Use with glucocorticoid therapy may attenuate growth-promoting effects of somatropin in children; glucocorticoid replacement dosing should be carefully adjusted in children during concomitant use. May inhibit 11β-hydroxysteroid dehydrogenase type 1 (11βHSD-1), resulting in reduced serum cortisol concentrations; glucocorticoid replacement therapy may be required or adjustments in glucocorticoid therapy doses may be required. May alter clearance of compounds metabolized by CYP450 liver enzymes (eg, corticosteroids, sex steroids, anticonvulsants, antipyrine, cyclosporine). May require larger dose with oral estrogen replacement. Adjust dose of insulin and/or oral hypoglycemic agents in diabetic patients.

**PREGNANCY:** Category C, caution in nursing.

**MECHANISM OF ACTION:** Human growth hormone; GH binds to dimeric GH receptors located within the cell membranes of target tissue cells, resulting in intracellular signal transduction and subsequent induction of transcription and translation of GH-dependent proteins, including IGF-1, IGF BP-3, and acid labile subunit. GH has direct tissue and metabolic effects, including stimulation of chondrocyte differentiation, stimulation of lipolysis and stimulation of hepatic glucose output. Some effects including stimulation of protein synthesis and chondrocyte proliferation are mediated indirectly by insulin-like growth factor-I (IGF-I).

**PHARMACOKINETICS: Absorption:** (SQ) Absolute bioavailabilty (75%). (IM) Absolute bioavailabilty (63%). **Distribution:** (IV) $V_d$=0.07L/kg. **Metabolism:** Liver and kidney (protein catabolism). **Elimination:** Urine: (IV) $T_{1/2}$=0.36 hrs. (SQ) $T_{1/2}$=3.8 hrs. (IM) $T_{1/2}$=4.9 hrs.

## NURSING CONSIDERATIONS

**Assessment:** Assess for hypersensitivity to either metacresol or glycerin, closed epiphyses (pediatrics), diabetic retinopathy, active malignancy, acute critical illness (complications following open heart surgery or abdominal surgery, multiple accidental trauma, or acute respiratory failure), pre-existing type 1, type 2 DM or impaired glucose tolerance, history of scoliosis, hypothyroidism, hypopituitarism, pregnancy/nursing status, and for possible drug interactions. Assess for pre-existing papilledema; perform funduscopic examination prior to treatment. In patients with Prader-Willi syndrome, assess for the presence of severe obesity, history of upper airway obstruction or sleep apnea, or for the presence of severe respiratory impairment. In patients with Turner syndrome, assess for presence of otitis media or other ear disorders and for CV disorders before initiation of therapy.

**Monitoring:** Monitor for signs/symptoms of malignant transformation of skin lesions, fluid retention, tissue atrophy at the injection site, allergic reactions, and for pancreatitis. Monitor for signs/symptoms of slipped capital femoral epiphysis and for the progression of pre-existing scioliosis in pediatric patients. Monitor for signs symptoms of hypothyroidism; perform periodic monitoring of thyroid function tests. Monitor for signs/symptoms of glucose intolerance; perform periodic monitoring of glucose levels. In patients with Turner syndrome, monitor for signs/symptoms of ear disorders (eg, otitis media) and CV disorders. In patients with Prader-Willi syndrome, monitor weight of the patient and monitor for signs/symptoms of upper airway obstruction and for respiratory infections. In patients with pre-existing tumors or GH deficiency secondary to an intracranial lesion, monitor for progression or recurrence of underlying disease process. In patients with hypopituitarism, monitor other hormonal replacement therapy during treatment. Monitor for increases in serum levels of inorganic phosphorus, alkaline phosphatase, parathyroid hormone, and insulin-like growth factor-I (IGF-I).

**Patient Counseling:** Inform patients of the potential benefits/risks of therapy. Instruct that cartridges should be reconstituted only with supplied diluent and should not be used if allergic to metacresol or glycerin. Inform patients/caregivers to receive training/instructions of proper administration. Instruct thoroughly as to proper usage and disposal, and caution against any reuse of needles and syringes. Instruct to seek medical attention if symptoms of slipped capital femoral epiphysis (eg, onset of limp, hip or knee pain), hypersensitivity/allergic reactions, respiratory infections (Prader-Willi syndrome), ear disorders or CV disorders (Turner syndrome), or if progression of scoliosis occurs.

**Administration:** SQ route. Refer to PI for proper reconstitution procedure. (Vial) May be reconstituted with Bacteriostatic Water for injection or Sterile Water for Injection, if sensitivity to the diluent occurs. (Cartridge) Reconstitute only with diluent supplied. Rotate injection site. **Storage:** Refrigerate at 2-8°C (36-46°F). Avoid freezing. (Reconstituted with Diluent or Bacteriostatic water): Refrigerate; stable up to 14 days. (Reconstituted with Sterile water): Refrigerate; use within 24 hrs. (Cartridges: Reconstituted): Refrigerate; stable for 28 days; store injection device without the needle attached.

## HUMIRA — RX

adalimumab (Abbott)

**Increased risk for developing serious infections (eg, tuberculosis [TB], TB reactivation, invasive fungal infection, bacterial/viral infection due to opportunistic pathogens) that may lead to hospitalization or death. Concomitant use of immunosuppresants (eg, methotrexate [MTX] or corticosteroids) may precipitate these infections. Evaluate for latent TB and treat prior to initiation of therapy. Empiric antifungal therapy should be considered in patients at risk for invasive fungal infection who develop severe systemic illness. Monitor for development of infection during and after treatment. D/C if serious infection or sepsis develops. Lymphomas and other malignancies reported in children and adolescents.**

**THERAPEUTIC CLASS:** Monoclonal antibody/TNF-blocker

**INDICATIONS:** Reduce signs and symptoms, induce major clinical response, inhibit structural damage progression, and improve physical function in moderately to severely active rheumatoid arthritis (RA). Reduce signs and symptoms of moderately to severely active polyarticular juvenile idiopathic arthritis in patients ≥4 yrs. Reduce signs and symptoms of active arthritis, inhibit the progression of structural damage, and improve physical function in patients with psoriatic arthritis (PA). Reduce signs and symptoms of active ankylosing spondylitis (AS). Reduce signs and symptoms and induce and maintain clinical remission of moderately to severely active Crohn's disease in patients who have had an inadequate response to conventional therapy. Reduce signs and symptoms and induce clinical remission in patients who have lost response to or are intolerant to infliximab. Treatment of moderate to severe chronic plaque psoriasis in patients who are candidates for systemic therapy or phototherapy.

**DOSAGE:** *Adults:* (RA/PA/AS): 40mg SQ every other week. Some patients with RA not taking concomitant MTX may derive additional benefit from increasing to 40mg every week. Crohn's Disease: Initial: 160mg (may be given as 4 injections on Day 1, or 2 injections/day for 2 consecutive days); then 80mg after 2 weeks (Day 15). Maint: 40mg every other week beginning at Week 4 (Day 29). Plaque Psoriasis: Initial: 80mg. Maint: 40mg every other week starting 1 week after initial dose.
*Pediatrics:* Juvenile Idiopathic Arthritis: (4-17 yrs) 15kg-to-<30kg: 20mg every other week; ≥30kg: 40mg every other week.

H

**HOW SUPPLIED:** Inj: 20mg/0.4mL, 40mg/0.8mL [Prefilled glass syringe]; 40mg/0.8mL [Prefilled pen]

**WARNINGS/PRECAUTIONS:** Do not initiate with an active infection. Caution in patients with history of chronic/recurrent infections, underlying conditions predisposing to infections, and with exposure to TB or who travel in areas where TB and mycoses (eg, histoplasmosis, coccidioidomycosis, blastomycosis) are endemic. Monitor hepatitus B virus (HBV) carriers as reactivation may occur; if reactivation occurs, d/c and start antiviral therapy. Caution with pre-existing or recent-onset CNS demyelinating disorders. Rare possibility of anaphylaxis and pancytopenia including aplastic anemia. May cause CHF or worsen pre-existing disease. May result in autoantibody formation; d/c if lupus-like syndrome develops. May affect host defenses against infections and malignancies.

**ADVERSE REACTIONS:** Upper respiratory tract infections, injection-site pain/reactions, headache, rash, sinusitis, nausea, urinary tract infections, flu syndrome, abdominal pain, hyperlipidemia, hypercholesterolemia, back pain, hematuria, HTN, malignancy, immunogenicity.

**INTERACTIONS:** Do not give concurrently with live vaccines. Reduced clearance with methotrexate (MTX). Do not use concurrently with anakinra due to increased risk of serious infections and neutropenia.

**PREGNANCY:** Category B, not for use in nursing.

**MECHANISM OF ACTION:** Monoclonal antibody/TNF-blocker; binds specifically to TNF-α and blocks its interaction with p55 and p75 cell surface TNF receptors. Lyses surface TNF-expressing cells in the presence of complement. Modulates biological responses that are induced or regulated by TNF. In plaque psoriasis, reduces the epidermal thickness and infiltration of inflammatory cells.

**PHARMACOKINETICS: Absorption:** Absolute bioavailability (64%); $C_{max}$=4.7mcg/mL; $T_{max}$=131 hrs. **Distribution:** $V_d$=4.7-6L. **Elimination:** $T_{1/2}$=2 weeks.

## NURSING CONSIDERATIONS

**Assessment:** Assess for active infection (eg, chronic or localized infection), history of chronic/recurrent infection, predisposition to infection (eg, disease states), TB risk factors, risk of reactivation of HBV, demyelinating disease, CHF, pregnancy/nursing status, and possible drug interactions. Obtain test for latent TB.

**Monitoring:** Monitor for signs/symptoms of infections (eg, sepsis, TB, opportunistic infections), malignancies (eg, lymphoma), hypersensitivity reactions (eg, anaphylaxis, angioneurotic edema), HBV reactivation, demyelinating disease, hematological reactions (eg, thrombocytopenia, leukopenia, aplastic anemia), worsening CHF, lupus-like syndrome, immunosuppression.

**Patient Counseling:** Inform about risks/benefits of therapy. Medication may lower the ability of immune system to fight infection; instruct to contact physician if any symptoms of infection, including TB and reactivation of HBV, occur. Counsel about risk of lymphoma and other malignancies while on therapy. Seek immediate medical attention if signs of severe allergic reactions (eg, anaphylaxis) develop. Advise to report any new or worsening medical conditions (eg, heart disease, neurological disease, autoimmune disorder) or any symptoms suggestive of a cytopenia (eg, bleeding, bruising, or persistent fever). Counsel about proper injection technique.

**Administration:** SQ route. Rotate injection sites. Avoid injecting into areas where skin is tender, bruised, red, or hard. If using pen formulation or prefilled syringe, inject full amount of syringe. **Storage:** 2-8°C (36-46°F). Do not freeze. Protect prefilled syringe from exposure to light. Store in original carton until time of administration. Keep out of reach of children.

H

## HUMULIN OTC

insulin human, rdna origin - insulin, human isophane - insulin, human regular (Lilly)

**OTHER BRAND NAMES:** Humulin R (Lilly) - Humulin N (Lilly)

**THERAPEUTIC CLASS:** Insulin

**INDICATIONS:** To control hyperglycemia in diabetes. (Humulin R U-500) Treatment of diabetic patients with marked insulin resistance.

**DOSAGE:** *Adults:* Individualize dose.
*Pediatrics:* Individualize dose.

**HOW SUPPLIED:** Inj: 100 U/mL (Humulin N, Humulin R), 500 U/mL (Humulin R U-500); Pen: 100 U/mL (Humulin N).

**CONTRAINDICATIONS:** (Humulin R U-500) Hypoglycemia.

**WARNINGS/PRECAUTIONS:** Human insulin differs from animal-source insulin. Any change of insulin should be made cautiously. Changes in strength, manufacturer, type or method of manufacture may result in the need for a change in dosage. Hypoglycemia may occur with taking too much insulin, missing or delaying meals, exercising or working more than usual. Illness (especially with nausea or vomiting), pregnancy, exercise and travel may change insulin requirements. Administration of insulin SQ can result in lipoatrophy.

**ADVERSE REACTIONS:** Hypoglycemia, sweating, dizziness, palpitations, tremor, hunger, restlessness, lightheadedness, inability to concentrate, headache, injection-site reaction, allergic reaction.

**INTERACTIONS:** Increased insulin requirements with oral contraceptives, corticosteroids, or thyroid replacement therapy. Reduced insulin requirements with oral hypoglycemics, salicylates, sulfa antibiotics, and certain antidepressants. Alcoholic beverages may change insulin requirements. β-blockers may mask symptoms of hypoglycemia. (Humulin R U-500) Increased insulin requirements with isoniazid, certain lipid lowering drugs (eg, niacin), estrogen, phenothiazine. Reduced insulin requirements with MAOI, angiotensin II receptor blocking agents, and inhibitors of pancreatic function (eg, octreotide).

**PREGNANCY:** Pregnancy category is not known.

**MECHANISM OF ACTION:** Insulin; regular insulin human injection of rDNA origin that helps in maintenance of blood glucose at near normal level.

### NURSING CONSIDERATIONS

**Assessment:** Assess FPG, $HbA_{1c}$, renal function, LFTs, pregnancy/nursing status, infections, alcohol consumption, exercise routines, travel plans, adrenal or thyroid or pituitary diseases, and possible drug interactions.

**Monitoring:** Monitor FPG, $HbA_{1c}$, renal function, diabetic ketoacidosis, lipodystrophy, allergic reactions (eg, SOB, hypotension, tachycardia). Monitor for signs of hypoglycemia (eg, sweating, palpitations, seizures, disorientation, tremors).

**Patient Counseling:** Advise to never share needles and syringes. Vial must be shaken gently to completely mix the insulin; should look uniformly cloudy or milky before administration. Do not use if solid particles stick to the bottom or there are clumps in the insulin after mixing. Instruct to always carry a quick source of sugar (hard candy or glucose tablets). Local reactions may be expected (redness, swelling, itching at injection site that usually clears up in a few days). Counsel about signs/symptoms of hypoglycemia, importance of frequent monitoring of blood glucose levels, and need for eating a balanced diet and exercising regularly. Advise to keep extra/spare supply of syringes and needles on hand and always wear diabetic identification.

**Administration:** SQ route (abdomen, thigh, and arms). Refer to PI for proper administration. **Storage:** (Not-in use) Refrigerate. Do not freeze. (In-use): Below 30°C (86°F), away from heat and light. Do not use after the stamped expiration date.

## HUMULIN 70/30 — OTC

insulin human, rdna origin - insulin, human (isophane/regular) (Lilly)

**THERAPEUTIC CLASS:** Insulin

**INDICATIONS:** To control hyperglycemia in diabetes.

**DOSAGE:** *Adults:* Individualize dose. Administer SQ.
*Pediatrics:* Individualize dose. Administer SQ.

**HOW SUPPLIED:** (Isophane-Regular) Inj: (Humulin 70/30) 70 U-30 U/mL.

**WARNINGS/PRECAUTIONS:** Human insulin differs from animal-source insulin. Make any change of insulin cautiously. Changes in strength, manufacturer, type, or method of manufacture may result in the need for a change in dosage. In cases where patients are required for change in dosage from that used with other insulin, adjustment should be done with the first dose, or during the first several weeks or months. Hypoglycemia may occur with too much insulin, missing or delaying meals, exercising, or working more than usual. Infection or illness (especially with diarrhea or vomiting) may change insulin requirements. Administration of insulin SQ can result in lipoatrophy.

**ADVERSE REACTIONS:** Hypoglycemia, anxiety, sweating, dizziness, palpitations, tremor, hunger, restlessness, drowsiness, lightheadedness, inability to concentrate, headache, injection-site reaction, allergic reaction.

**INTERACTIONS:** Increased insulin requirements with oral contraceptives, corticosteroids, or thyroid replacement therapy. Reduced insulin requirements with oral hypoglycemics, salicylates, sulfa antibiotics, and certain antidepressants. Alcoholic beverages may change insulin requirements. β-blockers may mask symptoms of hypoglycemia.

**PREGNANCY:** Pregnancy category is not known.

**MECHANISM OF ACTION:** Insulin; lowers blood glucose levels by stimulating peripheral glucose uptake, especially by skeletal muscle and fat, and by inhibiting hepatic glucose production. Inhibits lipolysis and proteolysis, and enhances protein synthesis.

### NURSING CONSIDERATIONS

**Assessment:** Assess FPG, $HbA_{1c}$, renal function, LFTs, pregnancy status, infections, alcohol consumption, exercise routines, diet, work schedule, travel plans, adrenal or thyroid or pituitary diseases, and for possible drug interactions.

**Monitoring:** Monitor FPG, $HbA_{1c}$, renal function, diabetic ketoacidosis, lipodystrophy, allergic reactions, hypotension, tachycardia. Monitor proper dosaging and dose preparation. Monitor for signs of hypoglycemia (sweating, palpitation, seizures, disorientation, tremors).

**Patient Counseling:** Advise to always wash hands before preparing the dose. Advise never to share needles or syringes. Vial must be carefully shaken to completely mix insulin; should look uniformly cloudy or milky before administration. Do not use if solid particles stick to bottom or there are clumps in insulin after mixing. Instruct to always carry a quick source of sugar (hard candy or glucose tablets). Counsel that local reactions may be expected (redness, swelling, itching at injection site) which usually clear up in a few days. Educate about signs/symptoms of hypoglycemia, importance of frequent monitoring of blood glucose levels, and need for eating a balanced diet and exercising regularly. Advise to keep an extra/spare supply of syringes and needles and to always wear diabetic identification.

**Administration:** SQ route (alternate sites: abdomen, thigh, arms). Use syringe marked for U-100 insulin. **Storage:** Refrigerate unopened bottles. Do not freeze. Keep unopened bottles unrefrigerated at 30°C (86°F). Protect from heat and light.

## HYALGAN — RX

sodium hyaluronate (Sanofi-Aventis)

**THERAPEUTIC CLASS:** Hyaluronan

**INDICATIONS:** Treatment of pain in osteoarthritis of the knee in patients who have failed to respond adequately to conservative nonpharmacologic therapy, and to simple analgesics (eg, APAP).

**DOSAGE:** *Adults:* Administer 2mL by intra-articular injection once a week for a total of 5 injections. Some patients may experience benefit with 3 injections given at weekly intervals.

**HOW SUPPLIED:** Inj: 2mL

**CONTRAINDICATIONS:** Intra-articular injections are contraindicated in cases of infections or skin disease in the area of the injection site.

**WARNINGS/PRECAUTIONS:** Avoid disinfectants containing quaternary ammonium salts for skin preparation; hyaluronic acid can precipitate in their presence. Anaphylactoid and allergic reactions reported. Transient increases in inflammation in the injected knee in some patients with inflammatory arthritis such as rheumatoid arthritis or gouty arthritis have been reported. Safety and effectiveness in joints other than the knee or concomitantly with other intra-articular injectables have not been established. Caution in patients who are allergic to avian proteins, feathers, and egg products. Avoid any strenuous activities or prolonged (eg, >1 hr) weight-bearing activities within 48 hrs following the intra-articular injection. Remove any joint effusion before injecting. Safety and effectiveness have not been demonstrated in children.

**ADVERSE REACTIONS:** GI complaints, injection-site pain, headache, local skin reactions (rash, ecchymosis), local joint pain, pruritus (local), knee swelling/effusion.

**PREGNANCY:** Safety in pregnancy and nursing not known.

### NURSING CONSIDERATIONS

**Assessment:** Assess for knee joint infection, skin infection, or disease around injection site.

**Monitoring:** Monitor for anaphylactic and allergic reactions, injection-site pain, local skin reaction, and joint swelling/effusion.

**Patient Counseling:** Inform that drug may cause transient pain/swelling of injected joint. Avoid strenuous activities or prolonged weight-bearing activities (jogging, tennis) within 48 hrs following injection.

**Adminstration:** Intra-articular injection. Use strict aseptic technique. Inject full 2mL in one knee only. If treatment is bilateral, a separate vial should be used for each knee. **Storage**: Below 25°C (77°F). Do not freeze. Discard any used portions.

## HYDRALAZINE — RX

hydralazine HCl (Various)

**THERAPEUTIC CLASS:** Vasodilator

**INDICATIONS:** Management of HTN.

**DOSAGE:** *Adults:* Initial: 10mg qid for 2-4 days. Titrate: Increase to 25mg qid for the rest of the week, then increase to 50mg qid. Maint: Use lowest effective dose. Resistant Patients: 300mg/day or titrate to lower dose combined

with thiazide diuretic and/or reserpine, or β-blocker.
*Pediatrics:* Initial: 0.75mg/kg/day given qid. Titrate: Increase gradually over 3-4 weeks to a max of 7.5mg/kg/day or 200mg/day.

**HOW SUPPLIED:** Inj: 20mg/mL; Tab: 10mg, 25mg, 50mg, 100mg

**CONTRAINDICATIONS:** CAD and mitral valvular rheumatic heart disease.

**WARNINGS/PRECAUTIONS:** D/C if SLE symptoms occur. May cause angina and ECG changes of MI. Caution with suspected CAD, CVA, advanced renal impairment. May increase pulmonary artery pressure in mitral valvular disease. Postural hypotension reported. Add pyridoxine if peripheral neuritis develops. Monitor CBC and ANA titer before and periodically during therapy.

**ADVERSE REACTIONS:** Headache, anorexia, NV, diarrhea, tachycardia, angina.

**INTERACTIONS:** Caution with MAOIs. Profound hypotension with potent parenteral antihypertensives (eg, diazoxide). May reduce pressor response to epinephrine.

**PREGNANCY:** Category C, safety in nursing not known.

**MECHANISM OF ACTION:** Vasodilator; not established. Apparently lowers BP by direct relaxation of vascular smooth muscle; interferes with calcium movement within vascular smooth muscle responsible for initiating or maintaining contraction.

**PHARMACOKINETICS: Absorption:** Rapid; $T_{max}$=1-2 hrs. **Distribution:** Plasma protein binding (87%). **Metabolism:** Acetylation. **Elimination:** Urine; $T_{1/2}$=3-7 hrs.

## NURSING CONSIDERATIONS

**Assessment:** Assess for CAD, mitral valvular rheumatic heart disease, cerebral vascular accidents, renal disease, and possible drug interactions. Obtain baseline CBC and ANA.

**Monitoring:** Monitor CBC and ANA periodically. Monitor for signs/symptoms of peripheral neuritis, hypotension, blood dyscrasias, SLE-like symptoms, and hypersensitivity reactions.

**Patient Counseling:** Advise to seek medical attention if symptoms of peripheral neuritis (paresthesia, numbness, tingling), hypotension, blood dyscrasias, SLE-like symptoms, or hypersensitivity reactions occur.

**Administration:** Oral route. **Storage:** 15-30°C (59-86°F).

# HYDROCHLOROTHIAZIDE RX

hydrochlorothiazide (Various)

**THERAPEUTIC CLASS:** Thiazide diuretic

**INDICATIONS:** Management of HTN. Tab: Adjunct therapy in edema associated with CHF, hepatic cirrhosis, corticosteroid and estrogen therapy, renal dysfunction.

**DOSAGE:** *Adults:* Cap: Initial: 12.5mg qd. Max: 50mg/day. Elderly: Start at the low end of dosing range. Tab: Edema: 25-100mg qd or in divided doses. May give every other day or 3-5 days/week. HTN: Initial: 25mg qd. Titrate: May increase to 50mg/day.
*Pediatrics:* Tab: Diuresis/HTN: 1-2mg/kg/day given qd-bid. Max: Infants up to 2 yrs: 37.5mg/day. 2-12 yrs: 100mg/day. <6 months: Up to 3mg/kg/day given bid may be required.

**HOW SUPPLIED:** Cap: 12.5mg; Tab: 12.5mg, 25mg*, 50mg* *scored

**CONTRAINDICATIONS:** Anuria, sulfonamide hypersensitivity.

**WARNINGS/PRECAUTIONS:** Caution in severe renal disease, liver dysfunction, electrolyte/fluid imbalance. Can precipitate hepatic coma with severe liver disease, and azotemia with renal dysfunction. Latent diabetes mellitus may become manifest. Monitor electrolytes. Hyperuricemia, hyperglycemia, hypokalemia, hyponatremia, hypomagnesemia, hypercalcemia, hypophosphatemia may occur. Increases in cholesterol and triglyceride levels reported.

May exacerbate systemic lupus erythematosus (SLE). Sensitivity reactions reported. D/C prior to parathyroid test. Parathyroid pathology reported with prolonged use. Enhanced effects in post-sympathectomy patients.

**ADVERSE REACTIONS:** Weakness, hypotension (including orthostatic hypotension), pancreatitis, jaundice, diarrhea, vomiting, blood dyscrasias, rash, photosensitivity, electrolyte imbalance, impotence, renal dysfunction/failure, interstitial nephritis.

**INTERACTIONS:** May potentiate orthostatic hypotension with alcohol, barbiturates, narcotics. Adjust dose of concomitant antidiabetic drugs. Possible decreased response to pressor amines. Concomitant corticosteroids, ACTH increase electrolyte depletion. May potentiate nondepolarizing skeletal muscle relaxants, antihypertensives. Lithium toxicity possible; avoid concomitant use. NSAIDs decrease effects. Decreased PO absorption with cholestyramine, colestipol resins.

**PREGNANCY:** Category B, not for use in nursing.



**MECHANISM OF ACTION:** Thiazide diuretic; affects renal tubular mechanism of electrolyte reabsorption, increasing excretion of $Na^+$ and $Cl^-$.

**PHARMACOKINETICS: Absorption:** $C_{max}$=70-490ng/mL; $T_{max}$= 1-5 hrs. **Distribution:** Crosses placenta; found in breast milk; plasma protein binding (40%-68%). **Elimination:** Urine (55%-77%), unchanged (>95%); $T_{1/2}$(cap)=6-15 hrs, (tab)=5.6-14.8 hrs.

## NURSING CONSIDERATIONS

**Assessment:** Assess for anuria, SLE, DM, sulfonamide hypersensitivity, history of allergy or bronchial asthma, possible drug interactions, hepatic/renal impairment. Assess for pregnancy/nursing status.

**Monitoring:** Monitor serum electrolytes periodically. Monitor for signs/symptoms of electrolyte imbalance, exacerbation or activation of SLE, hyperglycemia, hyperuricemia or precipitation of gout, hypersensitivity reactions, renal/hepatic dysfunction.

**Patient Counseling:** Advise to seek medical attention if symptoms of electrolyte imbalance (dry mouth, thirst, weakness) or hypersensitivity reactions occur. Advise to avoid taking with food.

**Administration:** Oral route. **Storage:** 20-25°C (68-77°F). Cap: Protect from light, moisture, freezing.

# HYDROXYZINE HCL — RX

hydroxyzine HCl (Various)

**THERAPEUTIC CLASS:** Piperazine antihistamine

**INDICATIONS:** (PO) Symptomatic relief of anxiety and tension associated with psychoneurosis and as adjunct in organic disease states in which anxiety is manifest. As a sedative when used as premedication and following general anesthesia. Management of pruritus due to allergic conditions and histamine-mediated pruritus. (Inj) Management of anxiety, tension, and psychomotor agitation in conditions of emotional stress. Management of acutely disturbed or hysterical patients or acute/chronic alcoholics with anxiety withdrawal symptoms or delirium tremens. As pre-/postoperative and pre-/postpartum adjunctive medication to permit reduction in narcotic dosage, allay anxiety, and control emesis. To control nausea and vomiting, excluding pregnancy.

**DOSAGE:** *Adults:* PO: Anxiety: 50-100mg qid. Pruritus: 25mg tid-qid. Sedation: 50-100mg. IM: Nausea/Vomiting, Pre-/Postoperative and Pre-/Postpartum Adjunct: 25-100mg. Psychiatric/Emotional Emergencies: 50-100mg q4-6h prn.

*Pediatrics:* PO: Anxiety/Pruritus: ≥6 yrs: 50-100mg/day in divided doses. <6 yrs: 50mg/day in divided doses. Sedation: 0.6mg/kg. IM: Nausea/Vomiting, Pre-/Postoperative Adjunct: 0.5mg/lb.

**HOW SUPPLIED:** Inj: 25mg/mL [1mL], 50mg/mL [1mL, 2mL, 10mL]; Syrup: 10mg/5mL [118mL, 473mL, 3785mL]; Tab: 10mg, 25mg, 50mg

**CONTRAINDICATIONS:** Early pregnancy. Injection is intended only for IM administration and should not, under any circumstances, be injected subcutaneously, intra-arterially, or IV. (Inj) Inadvertent SQ injection may result in significant tissue damage.

**WARNINGS/PRECAUTIONS:** Caution in elderly. May impair mental/physical abilities. Effectiveness as an antianxiety agent for long-term use (>4 months) has not been established.

**ADVERSE REACTIONS:** Dry mouth, drowsiness, involuntary motor activity.

**INTERACTIONS:** Potentiates CNS depression with other CNS depressants (eg, narcotics, non-narcotic analgesics, barbiturates, alcohol); rare cases of cardiac arrest and death have been reported following the combined use of the injection and other CNS depressants. May increase alcohol effects. Counteracts pressor action of epinephrine.

**PREGNANCY:** Not safe in pregnancy.

**MECHANISM OF ACTION:** Piperazine antihistamines; believed to suppress activity in key regions of subcortical area of CNS; shown to have primary skeletal muscle relaxation, bronchodilator, antihistaminic, and analgesic effects.

**PHARMACOKINETICS: Absorption:** Rapid (GIT).

H

## NURSING CONSIDERATIONS

**Assessment:** Assess pregnancy/nursing status and possible drug interactions. Obtain baseline renal function.

**Monitoring:** Monitor for hypersensitivity reactions and renal dysfunction.

**Patient Counseling:** Caution may impair physical/mental abilities. Advise to avoid alcohol and other CNS depressants.

**Administration:** Oral route. **Storage:** Tab: 20-25°C (68-77°F). Dispense in a tight container. Syrup: 15-30°C (59-86°F). Protect from freezing. Protect from light. Dispense in a tight, light-resistant container. (Inj) 15-30°C (59-86°F). Protect from light.

# HYDROXYZINE PAMOATE — RX

hydroxyzine pamoate (Various)

**OTHER BRAND NAMES:** Vistaril (Pfizer)

**THERAPEUTIC CLASS:** Piperazine antihistamine

**INDICATIONS:** Relief of anxiety. Allergic pruritus. For sedation as premedication and following anesthesia.

**DOSAGE:** *Adults:* Anxiety: 50-100mg qid. Pruritus: 25mg tid-qid. Sedation: 50-100mg.
*Pediatrics:* Anxiety/Pruritus: >6 yrs: 50-100mg/day in divided doses. <6 yrs: 50mg/day in divided doses. Sedation: 0.6mg/kg.

**HOW SUPPLIED:** Cap: 25mg, 50mg, 100mg

**CONTRAINDICATIONS:** Early pregnancy.

**WARNINGS/PRECAUTIONS:** Caution in elderly. May impair mental/physical abilities. Effectiveness as an antianxiety agent for long-term use (>4 months) has not been established.

**ADVERSE REACTIONS:** Dry mouth, drowsiness, involuntary motor activity.

**INTERACTIONS:** Potentiated by CNS depressants (eg, narcotics, non-narcotic analgesics, barbiturates); reduce dose.

**PREGNANCY:** Safety unknown in pregnancy and is contraindicated in early pregnancy, not for use in nursing.

**MECHANISM OF ACTION:** Believed to suppress activity in key regions of subcortical area of CNS; shown to have primary skeletal muscle relaxation, bronchodilator, antihistaminic, and analgesic effects.

**PHARMACOKINETICS: Absorption:** Rapid.

## NURSING CONSIDERATIONS

**Assessment:** Assess for pregnancy/nursing status and possible drug interactions. Obtain baseline renal function.

**Monitoring:** Monitor for hypersensitivity reactions and renal dysfunction.

**Patient Counseling:** Caution may impair physical/mental abilities. Advise to avoid alcohol and other CNS depressants; seek medical attention if hypersensitivity reactions occur.

**Administration:** Oral route. **Storage:** Cap: Below 30°C (86°F). Susp: Shake vigorously until resuspended.

# HYOSCYAMINE SULFATE RX

hyoscyamine sulfate (Various)

H

**THERAPEUTIC CLASS:** Anticholinergic

**INDICATIONS:** Adjunct treatment of peptic ulcer, irritable bowel syndrome, neurogenic bladder, and neurogenic bowel disturbances. To reduce symptoms of functional intestinal disorders (eg, mild dysenteries, diverticulitis). To control gastric secretion, visceral spasm, and hypermotility in spastic colitis, spastic bladder, cystitis, pylorospasm, and associated abdominal cramps. Symptomatic relief of biliary and renal colic with concomitant morphine or other narcotics. "Drying agent" for symptomatic relief of acute rhinitis. To reduce rigidity and tremors of Parkinson's disease and control associated sialorrhea and hyperhidrosis. For anticholinesterase poisoning.

**DOSAGE:** *Adults:* 0.125-0.25mg q4h or prn. Max: 1.5mg/24hrs. Take with or without water.

*Pediatrics:* ≥12 yrs: 0.125-0.25mg q4h or prn. Max: 1.5mg/24hrs. 2 to <12 yrs: 0.0625-0.125mg q4h or prn. Max: 0.75mg/24hrs. Take with or without water.

**HOW SUPPLIED:** Tab, Disintegrating: 0.125mg

**CONTRAINDICATIONS:** Glaucoma, obstructive uropathy, GI tract obstruction, paralytic ileus; intestinal atony of elderly/debilitated, unstable cardiovascular status in acute hemorrhage, toxic megacolon complicating ulcerative colitis, myasthenia gravis.

**WARNINGS/PRECAUTIONS:** Risk of heat prostration with high environmental temperature. Avoid activities requiring mental alertness. Psychosis has been reported in sensitive patients. Caution with diarrhea, autonomic neuropathy, hyperthyroidism, coronary heart disease, CHF, arrhythmias/tachycardia, HTN, renal disease, and hiatal hernia associated with reflux esophagitis. Contains phenylalanine.

**ADVERSE REACTIONS:** Anticholinergic effects, drowsiness, headache, nervousness.

**INTERACTIONS:** Additive effects with other antimuscarinics, amantadine, haloperidol, phenothiazines, MAOIs, TCAs, and some antihistamines. Antacids interfere with absorption; take ac and antacids pc.

**PREGNANCY:** Category C, caution in nursing.

**MECHANISM OF ACTION:** Belladonna alkaloid; inhibits action of acetylcholine on structures innervated by postganglionic cholinergic nerves and on smooth muscle that respond to acetylcholine but lack cholinergic innervation, inhibiting GI propulsive motility, decreasing gastric acid secretion, and controlling excess pharyngeal, tracheal, and bronchial secretions.

**PHARMACOKINETICS: Absorption:** Complete. **Distribution:** Crosses placenta and BBB. **Metabolism:** Partial hydrolysis; tropic acid, tropine (metabolites). **Elimination:** Urine (primarily unchanged); $T_{1/2}$=2-3.5 hrs.

## NURSING CONSIDERATIONS

**Assessment:** Assess for possible drug interactions, bladder neck obstruction, prostatic hypertrophy, achalasia, pyloroduodenal stenosis, paralytic ileus, intestinal atony, CV status, UC, myasthenia gravis, autonomic neuropathy, hyperthyroidism, CAD, CHF, PKU, HTN, arrhythmias, renal disease, hiatal hernia, and glaucoma.

**Monitoring:** Monitor for signs/symptoms of heat prostration, incomplete intestinal obstruction, psychosis, and hypersensitivity reactions.

**Patient Counseling:** Caution may impair physical/mental abilities; hot environments may cause heat prostration (fever and heat stroke) due to decreased sweating. If on antacids, take drug before meals and antacids after meals. Seek medical attention if symptoms of incomplete intestinal obstruction (diarrhea), psychosis (confusion, disorientation, memory loss), or hypersensitivity reactions occur. Inform phenylketonurics that orally disintegrating tablets contain 0.5mg of phenylalanine/tablet.

**Administration:** Oral route. **Storage:** 25°C (77°F); excursions permitted to 15-30°C (59-86°F). Protect from moisture.

## HYZAAR — RX

losartan potassium - hydrochlorothiazide (Merck)

H

**Can cause death/injury to developing fetus during 2nd and 3rd trimesters. D/C if pregnancy detected.**

**THERAPEUTIC CLASS:** Angiotensin II receptor antagonist/thiazide diuretic

**INDICATIONS:** Treatment of HTN. Initial treatment of severe HTN only when the value of achieving prompt BP control exceeds the risk. Reduction of risk of stroke in patients with HTN and left ventricular hypertrophy (may not apply to Black patients).

**DOSAGE:** *Adults:* HTN: Usual: 50mg-12.5mg qd; maximal effect attained in 3 weeks. Uncontrolled BP on Losartan Monotherapy, HCTZ Alone or Controlled with HCTZ 25mg/day but Hypokalemic: Switch to 50mg-12.5mg qd with reduction of HCTZ dose. Uncontrolled BP on Losartan 100mg Monotherapy: Switch to 100mg-12.5mg qd. Titrate/Max: If uncontrolled after 3 weeks, increase to 100mg-25mg qd. Severe HTN: Initial: 50mg-12.5mg qd. Titrate/Max: If inadequate response after 2-4 weeks, increase to 100mg-25mg qd. HTN with Left Ventricular Hypertrophy: Initial: Losartan 50mg qd. If BP reduction inadequate, add HCTZ 12.5mg or substitute losartan/HCTZ 50mg-12.5mg. If additional BP reduction is needed, losartan 100mg and HCTZ 12.5mg or losartan/HCTZ 100mg-12.5mg may be substituted, followed by losartan 100mg and HCTZ 25mg or losartan/HCTZ 100mg-25mg. Patients with Renal Impairment: Usual regimens of therapy if CrCl >30mL/min. Replacement therapy: Combination may be substituted for titrated components.

**HOW SUPPLIED:** Tab: (Losartan-HCTZ) 50mg-12.5mg, 100mg-12.5mg, 100mg-25mg

**CONTRAINDICATIONS:** Anuria, sulfonamide hypersensitivity.

**WARNINGS/PRECAUTIONS:** Can cause fetal and neonatal injury/death. Correct volume or salt depletion before therapy. Caution with hepatic or renal dysfunction, renal artery stenosis, severe CHF, history of allergies, asthma. May exacerbate or activate systemic lupus erythematosus (SLE). Monitor serum electrolytes. Avoid if CrCl ≤30mL/min. Observe for signs of fluid or electrolyte imbalance. May precipitate hyperuricemia or gout. Hyperglycemia, hypomagnesemia, and hypercalcemia may occur. Enhanced effects in post-sympathectomy patient. May increase cholesterol, TG levels. Angioedema reported. Not recommended with hepatic dysfunction requiring losartan titration.

**ADVERSE REACTIONS:** Dizziness, upper respiratory infection, cough, chest pain, diarrhea, anemia, weakness, hypotension, malaise, hepatitis, hyperkalemia, hyponatremia, rhabdomyolysis, angioedema, erythroderma.

**INTERACTIONS:** May reduce renal clearance of lithium; monitor for toxicity. NSAIDS, including COX-2 inhibitors, may decrease effects of diuretics and ACE-inhibitors and may further deteriorate renal function. Losartan: Decreased levels with rifampin. Increased levels with fluconazole. Avoid $K^+$-sparing diuretics (eg, spironolactone, triamterene, amiloride), $K^+$ supplements, $K^+$-containing salt substitutes. HCTZ: Potentiates orthostatic hypotension with alcohol, barbiturates, narcotics. Adjust insulin, antidiabetic drugs.

Cholestyramine, colestipol impair absorption. Corticosteroids, ACTH deplete electrolytes. May decrease response to pressor amines (eg, norepinephrine). Potentiates other antihypertensives, skeletal muscle relaxants (eg, tubocurarine). Thiazides may cause hypokalemia which may lead to cardiac arrhythmia and sensitize or exaggerate the response of the heart to the toxic effects of digitalis.

**PREGNANCY:** Category C (1st trimester) and D (2nd and 3rd trimesters), not for use in nursing.

**MECHANISM OF ACTION:** Losartan: Angiotensin II receptor antagonist; inhibits vasoconstrictor and aldosterone-secreting effects of angiotensin II by selectively blocking binding of angiotensin II to $AT_1$ receptor. HCTZ: Thiazide diuretic; affects renal tubular mechanism of electrolyte reabsorption, directly increasing excretion of $Na^+$ and $Cl^-$ and indirectly reducing plasma volume.

**PHARMACOKINETICS: Absorption:** Losartan: Well absorbed, bioavailability (33%); $T_{max}$=1 hr, 3-4 hrs (metabolite). **Distribution:** Losartan: $V_d$=34L, 12L (metabolite); plasma protein binding (1.3%, 0.2% [metabolite]). HCTZ: Crosses placenta; found in breast milk. **Metabolism:** Losartan: CYP2C9, 3A4; carboxylic acid metabolite (active metabolite). **Elimination:** Losartan: Urine (4%, 6% [metabolite]); $T_{1/2}$=2 hrs, 6-9 hrs (metabolite). HCTZ: Kidney (61%); $T_{1/2}$=5.6-14.8 hrs.

## NURSING CONSIDERATIONS

**Assessment:** Assess for volume/salt depletion, SLE, DM, anuria, sulfonamide hypersensitivity, history of allergy or bronchial asthma, hepatic/renal impairment, pregnancy/nursing status, and possible drug interactions.

**Monitoring:** Monitor serum electrolytes and renal function periodically. Monitor for signs/symptoms of electrolyte imbalance, exacerbation or activation of SLE, hypotension, hyperglycemia, hypomagnesemia, hypercalcemia, hyperuricemia, or precipitation of gout, hypersensitivity reactions, hepatic/renal dysfunction.

**Patient Counseling:** Inform of pregnancy risks. Advise that inadequate fluid intake or loss of fluids may result in drop of BP, leading to lightheadedness or syncope. Instruct not to use $K^+$ supplements or salt substitutes without consulting physician. Advise to seek medical attention if syncope, symptoms of electrolyte imbalance (dry mouth, thirst, weakness, lethargy), or hypersensitivity reactions occur. Take with or without food.

**Administration:** Oral route. **Storage:** 25°C (77°F); excursions permitted to 15-30°C (59-86°F). Keep container tightly closed and protect from light.

# IFEX — RX

ifosfamide (Bristol-Myers Squibb)

**Risk of urotoxic side effects, especially hemorrhagic cystitis, and CNS toxicities (eg, confusion, coma); may require discontinuation of therapy. Severe myelosuppression reported. Administer only under supervision of a physician experienced in the use of antineoplastic agents.**

**OTHER BRAND NAMES:** Ifex/Mesnex (Bristol-Myers Squibb)

**THERAPEUTIC CLASS:** Cyclophosphamide analog

**INDICATIONS:** Third line chemotherapy of germ cell testicular cancer. Use in combination with prophylactic agent for hemorrhagic cystitis (eg, mesna).

**DOSAGE:** *Adults:* 1.2g/m²/day slow IV infusion over a minimum of 30 min for 5 consecutive days. Repeat treatment every 3 weeks or after recovery from hematologic toxicity (platelets ≥100,000/μL, WBC ≥4000/μL). Give with extensive hydration (eg, 2L fluid/day) and protector (eg, mesna) to prevent bladder toxicity/hemorrhagic cystitis.

**HOW SUPPLIED:** Inj (Ifosfamide): 1g, 3g; (Ifosfamide-Mesna) 1g-1g; 3g-1g

**CONTRAINDICATIONS:** Severely depressed bone marrow function.

**WARNINGS/PRECAUTIONS:** Hemorrhagic cystitis reported; obtain urinalysis before each dose. Withhold dose until complete resolution of microscopic hematuria. Monitor WBCs, platelets, Hgb before each dose and at appropriate intervals. Avoid with WBC <2000/µL and/or platelets <50,000/µL. D/C if somnolence, confusion, hallucinations, and/or coma occur. Caution with impaired renal function, compromised bone marrow reserve, prior radiation therapy. May interfere with normal wound healing.

**ADVERSE REACTIONS:** Myelosuppression, alopecia, NV, hematuria, CNS toxicity, infection, renal impairment, liver dysfunction, increased liver enzymes/bilirubin.

**INTERACTIONS:** Severe myelosuppression with other chemotherapeutic agents. Caution with other cytotoxic agents.

**PREGNANCY:** Category D, not for use in nursing.

**MECHANISM OF ACTION:** Chemotherapeutic agent; requires metabolic activation by microsomal liver enzymes and produces active metabolites that interact with DNA.

**PHARMACOKINETICS: Metabolism:** Extensive; 4-carboxyifosfamide, thiodiacetic acid, cysteine conjugates of chloroacetic acid (major metabolites). **Elimination:** (3.8-5g/m$^2$): Urine (61%), $T_{1/2}$=15 hrs. (1.6-2.4g/m$^2$/day): Urine (12-18%), $T_{1/2}$=7 hrs.

## NURSING CONSIDERATIONS

**Assessment:** Assess for severely depressed bone marrow function, leukopenia, granulocytopenia, extensive bone marrow metastases, prior radiation or cytotoxic agent therapy, renal dysfunction, and possible drug interactions. Obtain baseline WBC, platelet count, Hgb, and urinalysis.

**Monitoring:** Monitor WBC, platelet count, Hgb, and urinalysis prior to each dose and periodically throughout. Monitor for signs/symptoms of hemorrhagic cystitis, confusion, coma, severe myelosuppression, renal dysfunction, and hypersensitivity reaction.

**Patient Counseling:** Educate that alopecia may occur. Advise to keep well hydrated and to seek medical attention if symptoms of hemorrhagic cystitis, confusion, coma, severe myelosuppression, renal dysfunction, or hypersensitivity reaction occur.

**Administration:** IV infusion. **Storage:** 20-25°C (68-77°F). Protect from temperatures above 30°C (86°F). (Constituted/Diluted): Refrigerate; stable for 24 hrs.

# IMDUR RX

isosorbide mononitrate (Schering)

**THERAPEUTIC CLASS:** Nitrate vasodilator

**INDICATIONS:** Prevention of angina pectoris. Not for acute attack.

**DOSAGE:** *Adults:* Initial: 30-60mg qd in am. Titrate: May increase after several days to 120mg/day. Swallow whole with fluids. Elderly: Start at lower end of dosing range.

**HOW SUPPLIED:** Tab, Extended-Release: 30mg*, 60mg*, 120mg *scored

**WARNINGS/PRECAUTIONS:** Not for use with acute MI or CHF. Severe hypotension may occur; caution with volume depletion and hypotension. Hypotension may increase angina pectoris. May aggravate angina caused by hypertrophic cardiomyopathy. Monitor for tolerance. May interfere with cholesterol test.

**ADVERSE REACTIONS:** Headache, dizziness, hypotension.

**INTERACTIONS:** Severe hypotension with sildenafil. Orthostatic hypotension with CCBs. Additive vasodilation with other vasodilators (eg, alcohol).

**PREGNANCY:** Category B, caution with nursing.

**MECHANISM OF ACTION:** Nitrate vasodilator; relaxes vascular smooth muscle, and consequent dilatation of peripheral arteries and veins, especially the latter. Dilatation of veins leads to reducing the left ventricular end diastolic pressure and pulmonary capillary wedge pressure (preload). Arteriolar relaxation reduces systemic vascular resistance, systolic arterial pressure, and mean arterial pressure (afterload). It also dilates the coronary artery.

**PHARMACOKINETICS: Absorption:** Imdur: (60mg) $C_{max}$=557-572ng/mL, $T_{max}$=2.9-4.2 hrs, AUC=6625-7555ng•hr/mL. (120mg) $C_{max}$=1151-1180ng/mL, $T_{max}$=3.1-3.2 hrs, AUC=14241-16800ng•hr/mL. Absolute bioavailability (100%). **Distribution:** $V_d$=0.6-0.7L/kg; plasma protein binding (5%). **Metabolism:** Liver. Cleared through denitration and glucuronidation pathways. **Elimination:** Urine (96%), feces (1%). (60mg) $T_{1/2}$=6.2-6.3 hrs. (120mg) $T_{1/2}$=6.2-6.4 hrs.

## NURSING CONSIDERATIONS

**Assessment:** Assess for severe hypotension, volume-depleted patients, angina caused by hypertrophic cardiomyopathy, pregnancy status, alcohol intake, and possible drug interactions.

**Monitoring:** Careful clinical or hemodynamic monitoring for hypotension and tachycardia. Monitor for paradoxical bradycardia and increased angina pectoris, headaches and lightheadedness on standing, manifestation of true physical dependence (chest pain, acute MI). Monitor for the interference with Zlatkis-Zak color reaction, causing false low readings in cholesterol levels and for manifestations of methemoglobinemia.

I

**Patient Counseling:** Counsel to carefully follow dosing regimen. Inform about headaches (markers of drug activity) and lightheadedness on standing. Avoid alcohol consumption.

**Administration:** Oral route. Swallow tab with glass of water; do not crush or chew. **Storage:** 25°C (77°F); excursions permitted to 15-30°C (59-86°F).

# IMITREX RX

sumatriptan succinate - sumatriptan (GlaxoSmithKline)

**THERAPEUTIC CLASS:** $5\text{-}HT_1$-agonist

**INDICATIONS:** (Inj, Spray, Tab) Acute treatment of migraine attacks with or without aura in adults. (Inj) Acute treatment of cluster headache episodes.

**DOSAGE:** *Adults:* ≥18 yrs: (Inj) Initial: 6mg SQ. Max: Two 6mg inj/24 hrs. Injections must be separated by at least 1 hr. (Spray) 5mg, 10mg, or 20mg single dose; may repeat after 2 hrs. Max: 40mg/24 hrs. (Tab) Initial: 25-100mg; may repeat after 2 hrs. Max: 200mg/24 hrs. If headache returns after initial treatment with inj dose, may give additional single tabs, up to 100mg/day of tabs, with an interval of at least 2 hrs between tab doses. Hepatic Disease: Max: 50mg/single dose. Safety of treating >4 headaches/30 days not known.

**HOW SUPPLIED:** Inj: 4mg/0.5mL, 6mg/0.5mL; Tab: 25mg, 50mg, 100mg [9[s]]; Nasal Spray: 5mg, 20mg [0.1mL 6[s]]

**CONTRAINDICATIONS:** (Inj, Spray, Tab) History, symptoms, or signs of ischemic cardiac syndromes (eg, angina pectoris, MI, silent myocardial ischemia), cerebrovascular syndromes (eg, strokes, transient ischemic attacks), and peripheral vascular disease (eg, ischemic bowel disease). Other significant CVD, uncontrolled HTN, hemiplegic or basilar migraine, severe hepatic impairment, within 24 hrs of ergotamine-containing or ergot-type medications, or other $5\text{-}HT_1$ agonists. (Inj) IV administration. (Spray, Tab) Concurrent administration of MAO-A inhibitors or use within 2 weeks of d/c of an MAO-A inhibitor.

**WARNINGS/PRECAUTIONS:** Caution in patients with risk factors for coronary artery disease (CAD); evaluate CV status before use and administer first dose with supervision and subsequent ECG monitoring. Serious adverse cardiac events (eg, acute MI, life-threatening arrhythmias), cerebrovascular events (eg, cerebral hemorrhage, subarachnoid hemorrhage, stroke) and vasospastic reactions (eg, coronary vasospasm, peripheral vascular ischemia, colonic ischemia) reported. Serotonin syndrome, elevation in BP, including hypertensive crisis, and hypersensitivity may occur. Chest, jaw, and neck tightness reported. Avoid in elderly. Caution with diseases that may alter the absorption, metabolism, or excretion of drugs (eg, hepatic or renal impairment). Rare reports of seizures; caution in patients with a history of epilepsy or conditions associated with a lower seizure threshold. Caution in patients with brain lesions and in patients with controlled HTN. Possible long-term ophthalmic effects. Reconsider diagnosis before 2nd dose. (Inj) Should only be used when a clear diagnosis of migraine or cluster headache has been established. (Spray, Tab) Should only be used with a clear diagnosis of migraine headache has been established. (Spray) May cause irritation in the nose and throat.

**ADVERSE REACTIONS:** (Inj) Atypical sensations, flushing, chest discomfort, tightness in chest, throat discomfort, injection-site reaction. (Spray) Nasal cavity/sinuses disorder/discomfort; N/V, bad/unusual taste. (Tab): Atypical sensations, pain sensation, pressure sensation, malaise/fatigue, weakness, neck pain/stiffness, dizziness/vertigo.

**INTERACTIONS:** (Inj, Spray, Tab) See Contraindications. Serotonin syndrome reported with combined use of an SSRI or SNRI. (Inj) Use with an MAO-A is not recommended; if clinically warranted, suitable dose adjustment is advised.

**PREGNANCY:** Category C, caution in nursing.

**MECHANISM OF ACTION:** Selective $5\text{-}HT_1$ receptor subtype agonist; activates vascular $5\text{-}HT_1$ receptors, which are located on cranial arteries, on the basilar artery, and in the vasculature of human dura matter. Responsible for mediating vasoconstriction.

**PHARMACOKINETICS: Absorption:** Intranasal, 5mg: $C_{max}$=5ng/mL; Intranasal, 20mg: $C_{max}$= 16ng/mL; SQ, 6mg: (Deltoid) $C_{max}$=74ng/mL, $T_{max}$=12 min. (Thigh) $C_{max}$=52ng/mL; (PO, 25mg) $C_{max}$=18ng/mL; (PO, 100mg) $C_{max}$=51ng/mL. **Distribution:** (PO) $V_d$=2.4L/kg, (SQ) $V_d$=50 L; plasma protein binding (14-21%); found in breast milk following SQ administration. **Metabolism:** Via monoamine oxidase. **Elimination:** (SQ) Urine (22% unchanged and 38% as indole acetic acid), $T_{1/2}$=115 min; (Nasal Spray) Urine (3% unchanged and 42% as metabolites), $T_{1/2}$=2 hrs. (Oral) Urine (60%), feces (40%), $T_{1/2}$=2.5 hrs.

## NURSING CONSIDERATIONS

**Assessment:** Assess for presence/history of cardiac ischemic syndrome, cerebrovascular syndrome, or peripheral vascular syndrome, uncontrolled HTN, presence of hemiplegic or basilar migraines, presence of diseases that may alter the absorption, metabolism or excretion of drugs (eg, hepatic or renal impairment), history of epilepsy or conditions which lower seizure threshold, pregnancy/nursing status, and for possible drug interactions. Assess proper diagnosis of migraine headaches.

**Monitoring:** Monitor for signs/symptoms of cardiac events (eg, MI, cardiac rhythm disturbances, peripheral vascular ischemia, hypertensive crisis, chest tightness), colonic ischemia, bloody diarrhea, serotonin syndrome (eg, mental status changes), hypersensitivity reactions, jaw/neck tightness, seizures, exacerbation of headache, ophthalmic changes (eg, corneal opacities), and clinical response. In patients on long-term therapy and in patients with CAD risk factors, perform periodic monitoring of cardiovascular function. If clinical response does not occur following administration of first dose, reassess diagnosis.

**Patient Counseling:** Inform about possible adverse events (eg, cardiovascular effects, serotonin syndrome); instruct to consult physician if symptoms (eg, chest tightness, abdominal pain, SOB, confusion, hallucinations, flushing) of any adverse event occur. Advise to notify physician of all medications currently taking and if pregnant or nursing.

**Administration:** Oral, SQ, or nasal route. **Storage:** Injection: 2-30°C (36-86°F). Protect from light. Tab, Nasal Spray: 2-30°C (36-86°F).

# IMURAN RX

azathioprine (Prometheus)

**Increased risk of neoplasia with chronic immunosuppression. Physician should be familiar with this risk as well as mutagenic potential and possible hematologic toxicities.**

**THERAPEUTIC CLASS:** Purine antagonist antimetabolite

**INDICATIONS:** Adjunct for prevention of rejection in renal homotransplantation. Management of active rheumatoid arthritis (RA) to reduce signs and symptoms.

**DOSAGE:** *Adults:* Renal Homotransplantation: Individualize dose. Initial: 3-5mg/kg/day, start at time of transplant. Usually given as a single dose on the day of, and minority of cases 1-3 days before transplantation. Maint: 1-3mg/kg/day. Rheumatoid Arthritis: Initial: 1mg/kg/day given qd-bid. Titrate: Increase by 0.5mg/kg/day after 6-8 weeks, then at 4-week intervals. Max: 2.5mg/kg/day. Maint: Lowest effective dose. Decrease by 0.5mg/kg/day or 25mg/day every 4 weeks. If no response by Week 12, then consider refractory. Renal Dysfunction: Lower dose.

**HOW SUPPLIED:** Tab: 50mg* *scored; Inj (azathioprine sodium): 100mg/20mL

**CONTRAINDICATIONS:** Pregnancy in RA treatment. Patients with RA previously treated with alkylating agents (eg, cyclophosphamide, chlorambucil, melphalan) may increase risk of neoplasia.

**WARNINGS/PRECAUTIONS:** Severe leukopenia, thrombocytopenia, macrocytic anemia, pancytopenia, and severe bone marrow suppression may occur. Monitor CBCs, including platelets, weekly during the 1st month, twice monthly for the 2nd and 3rd months, then monthly or more frequently if dose/therapy changes. Serious infections including fungal, viral, bacterial, and protozoal may occur and may be fatal; reduce dose and/or consider use of other drugs. The risk of post-transplant lymphoma may be increased in patient who receive aggressive treatment with immunosuppressive drugs. May cause fetal harm. Gastrointestinal hypersensitivity reactions (severe nausea and vomiting) associated with diarrhea, rash, fever, malaise, myalgias, elevated liver enzymes, and hypotension may develop.

**ADVERSE REACTIONS:** Leukopenia, thrombocytopenia, infections, N/V, hepatotoxicity, bone marrow suppression, GI hypersensitivity, skin rashes, alopecia, fever, arthralgia, diarrhea, steatorrhea, negative nitrogen balance, interstial pneumonitis.

**INTERACTIONS:** Caution with concomitant aminosalicylates (eg, sulphasalazine, mesalazine, olsalazine); may inhibit TPMT. Reduce dose to approximately 1/3-1/4 of the usual dose with allopurinol. Drugs affecting leukocyte production (eg, co-trimoxazole) may exaggerate leukopenia. ACE inhibitors may induce anemia, severe leukopenia. Inhibits anticoagulant effects of warfarin.

**PREGNANCY:** Category D, not for use in nursing.

**MECHANISM OF ACTION:** Immunosuppressive antimetabolite; an imidazolyl derivative of 6-mercaptopurine (6-MP). In homograft survival, it suppresses hypersensitivities of the cell-mediated type and causes variable alterations in antibody production. Immuno-inflammatory response mechanisms not established; suppresses disease manifestation and underlying pathology in autoimmune disease.

**PHARMACOKINETICS: Absorption:** (PO) Well absorbed; $T_{max}$=1-2 hrs. **Distribution:** Plasma protein binding (30%); crosses placenta; found in breast milk. **Metabolism:** Liver and erythrocytes (extensive); 6-MP activated to 6-thioguanine nucleotides (major metabolites); inactivated via thiol methylation by thiopurine S-methyltransferase (TPMT) and oxidation by xanthine oxidase. **Elimination:** Urine; $T_{1/2}$=5 hrs.

## NURSING CONSIDERATIONS

**Assessment:** Assess for renal/hepatic dysfunction, previous treatment of rheumatoid arthritis with alkylating agents, pregnancy/nursing status, and for possible drug interactions. Conduct TPMT genotyping/phenotyping to identify absent or reduced enzymatic activity. Obtain baseline CBC with platelets.

**Monitoring:** Monitor for signs/symptoms of bone marrow suppression, malignancies (eg, skin cancer, reticulum cell or lymphomatous tumors), serious infections (eg, fungal, viral, bacterial, protozoal), and for GI hypersensitivity reactions. Monitor CBC, including platelet counts.

**Patient Counseling:** Inform about necessity of periodic CBC while on therapy. Instruct to report any unusual bleeding or bruising or signs of infections. Inform about risk of malignancy. Educate about careful dosage instructions, especially with impaired renal function or concomitant use with allopurinol. Advise to notify physician if pregnant or nursing.

**Administration:** IV and oral routes. **Storage:** 15-25°C (59-77°F). Protect from light. Store tablets in a dry place.

## INDERAL RX

propranolol HCl (Wyeth)

**THERAPEUTIC CLASS:** Nonselective beta-blocker

**INDICATIONS:** (Tab) Management of hypertension, angina pectoris, hypertrophic subaortic stenosis, atrial fibrillation, MI, and familial or hereditary essential tremor. Migraine prophylaxis. (Inj/Tab) For cardiac arrhythmias (supraventricular, ventricular tachycardia, tachyarrhythmia of digitalis intoxication, resistant tachyarrhythmia), reduction of cardiovascular mortality post-MI, essential tremor, and pheochromocytoma.

**DOSAGE:** *Adults:* HTN: (Tab) Initial: 40mg bid. Titrate: Increase gradually. Maint: 120-240mg/day. Angina: (Tab) 80-320mg/day, given bid-qid. Arrhythmia: (Inj) 1-3mg IV at 1 mg/min. (Tab) 10-30mg tid-qid ac and qhs. MI: (Tab) 180-240mg/day, given bid-tid. Migraine: (Tab) Initial: 80mg/day in divided doses. Usual: 160-240mg/day in divided doses. Tremor: (Tab) Initial: 40mg bid. Maint: 120mg/day. Max: 320mg/day. Hypertrophic Subaortic Stenosis: (Tab) 20-40mg tid-qid, ac and qhs. Pheochromocytoma: (Tab) 60mg/day in divided doses for 3 days before surgery with α-blocker. Inoperable Tumor: (Tab) 30mg/day in divided doses.
*Pediatrics:* HTN (Tab): Initial: 1mg/kg/day PO. Usual: 1-2mg/kg bid. Max: 16mg/kg/day.

**HOW SUPPLIED:** Inj: 1mg/mL; Tab: 10mg*, 20mg*, 40mg*, 60mg*, 80mg* *scored

**CONTRAINDICATIONS:** Cardiogenic shock, sinus bradycardia and >1st-degree block, bronchial asthma, CHF (unless failure is secondary to tachyarrhythmia treatable with propranolol).

**WARNINGS/PRECAUTIONS:** Reports of angina exacerbation and MI following abrupt d/c. Hypersensitivity including anaphylactic/anaphylactoid reactions reported. Caution with well-compensated cardiac failure, nonallergic bronchospasm, Wolff-Parkinson-White (WPW) syndrome, hepatic or renal dysfunction. Withdrawal before surgery is controversial. May mask hypoglycemia or hyperthyroidism symptoms. Avoid abrupt discontinuation. May reduce IOP. Can cause cardiac failure. Both digitalis glycosides and β-blockers slow atrioventricular conduction and decrease HR. Concomitant use can increase risk of bradycardia. Caution in elderly.

**ADVERSE REACTIONS:** Bradycardia, CHF, hypotension, lightheadedness, mental depression, N/V, allergic reactions, agranulocytosis.

**INTERACTIONS:** Increased propranolol levels/toxicity with CYP2D6 inhibitors (eg, amiodarone, cimetidine, fluoxetine, paroxetine, quinidine, ritonavir), CYP1A2 inhibitors (eg, imipramine, cimetidine, ciprofloxacin, fluvoxamine, isoniazid, ritonavir, theophylline, zileuton, zolmitriptan, rizatriptan), and CYP2C19 inhibitors (eg, fluconazole, cimetidine, fluoxetine, fluvoxamine, teniposide, tolbutamide). Decreased blood levels with hepatic enzyme inducers (eg, rifampin, ethanol, phenytoin, phenobarbital, cigarette smoking). Propafenone levels increased with concurrent administration. Lidocaine metabolism is inhibited with coadministration. Increased levels with concurrent nisoldipine and nicardipine. Zolmitriptan and rizatriptan concentrations increased with concurrent administration. Decreased theophylline clearance with concurrent administration. Increased concentrations of diazepam and its metabolites with coadministration. Increased thioridazine plasma concentrations with concurrent administration of doses ≥160mg/day. Increased plasma concentrations with chlorpromazine. Aluminum hydroxide gel may decrease plasma concentrations. Decreased plasma concentrations with coadministration of cholestyramine or colestipol. Concurrent administration increases warfarin levels and PT. Increased risk of bradycardia with concomitant digitalis glycosides. Caution with ACE Inhibitors. Avoid alcohol intake.

**PREGNANCY:** Category C, caution in nursing.

**MECHANISM OF ACTION:** Nonselective β-adrenergic receptor blocker; not established, proposed to decrease cardiac output, inhibit renin release and lessen tonic sympathetic nerve outflow from vasomotor centers in the brain.

**PHARMACOKINETICS: Absorption:** $T_{max}$=1-4 hrs. **Distribution:** $V_d$=4 L/kg; plasma protein binding (90%). Crosses placenta; found in breast milk. **Metabolism:** CYP2D6 (hydroxylation), CYP1A2, 2D6 (oxidation), N-dealkylation, glucuronidation. Propranolol glucuronide, naphthyloxylactic acid, glucuronic acid, sulfate conjugates (major metabolites). **Elimination:** $T_{1/2}$=3-6 hrs.

## NURSING CONSIDERATIONS

**Assessment:** Assess for bronchial asthma, sinus bradycardia, AV heart block, cardiogenic shock, CHF, bronchospastic disease, hyperthyroidism, DM, possible drug interactions, WPW syndrome, history of heart failure, hepatic/renal impairment.

**Monitoring:** Monitor for signs/symptoms of cardiac failure, hypoglycemia, decreased IOP, thyrotoxicosis, withdrawal symptoms (angina, MI), and hypersensitivity reactions.

**Patient Counseling:** Instruct not to interrupt or d/c therapy without consulting physician. Inform may interfere with glaucoma screening test. Drug may mask signs of thyrotoxicosis and hypoglycemia. Advise to contact physician if symptoms of heart failure, withdrawal (angina), or hypersensitivity reactions occur.

**Administration:** Oral route. **Storage:** 20-25°C (68-77°F); excursions permitted to 15-30°C (59-86°F).

# INDERAL LA — RX

propranolol HCl (Akrimax)

**THERAPEUTIC CLASS:** Nonselective beta-blocker

**INDICATIONS:** Management of hypertension, angina pectoris due to coronary atherosclerosis, and hypertrophic subaortic stenosis. Migraine prophylaxis.

**DOSAGE:** *Adults:* HTN: Initial: 80mg qd. Maint: 120-160mg qd. Angina: Initial: 80mg qd. Titrate: Increase gradually every 3-7 days. Maint: 160mg qd. Max: 320mg qd. Migraine: Initial: 80mg qd. Maint: 160-240mg qd. D/C gradually if unsatisfactory response within 4-6 weeks. Hypertrophic Subaortic Stenosis: Usual: 80-160mg qd.

**HOW SUPPLIED:** Cap, Extended-Release: 60mg, 80mg, 120mg, 160mg

**CONTRAINDICATIONS:** Cardiogenic shock, sinus bradycardia and >1st-degree block, bronchial asthma.

**WARNINGS/PRECAUTIONS:** Reports of angina exacerbation and myocardial infarction (MI) following abrupt d/c. Gradually reduce dose over at least a few weeks if discontinuance of therapy. Hypersensitivity reactions, including anaphylactic/anaphylactoid reactions, reported. Caution with well-compensated cardiac failure, nonallergic bronchospasm, Wolff-Parkinson-White (WPW) syndrome, hepatic or renal dysfunction. Withdrawal before surgery is controversial. May mask hypoglycemia or hyperthyroidism symptoms. May reduce IOP. Can cause cardiac failure. Stevens-Johnson syndrome, toxic epidermal necrolysis, exfoliative dermatitis, erythema multiforme, and urticaria reported. Caution in elderly. Not indicated for treatment of hypertensive emergencies.

**ADVERSE REACTIONS:** Bradycardia, CHF, hypotension, lightheadedness, mental depression, N/V, allergic reactions, agranulocytosis, dry eyes, alopecia, SLE-like reactions, male impotence, Peyronie's disease.

**INTERACTIONS:** Increased propranolol levels/toxicity with CYP2D6 inhibitors (eg, amiodarone, cimetidine, fluoxetine, paroxetine, quinidine, ritonavir), CYP1A2 inhibitors (eg, imipramine, cimetidine, ciprofloxacin, fluvoxamine, isoniazid, ritonavir, theophylline, zileuton, zolmitriptan, rizatriptan), and

CYP2C19 inhibitors (eg, fluconazole, cimetidine, fluoxetine, fluvoxamine, teniposide, tolbutamide). Decreased blood levels with hepatic enzyme inducers (eg, rifampin, ethanol, phenytoin, phenobarbital, cigarette smoking). Propafenone levels increased with concurrent administration. Lidocaine metabolism is inhibited with coadministration. Increased levels with concurrent nisoldipine and nicardipine. Nifedipine levels increased with coadministration. Zolmitriptan and rizatriptan concentrations increased with concurrent administration. Decreased theophylline clearance with concurrent administration. Increased concentrations of diazepam and its metabolites with coadministration. Increased thioridazine plasma concentrations with concurrent administration of doses ≥160mg/day. Increased plasma concentrations with chlorpromazine. Aluminum hydroxide gel may decrease plasma concentrations. Decreased plasma concentrations with coadministration of cholestyramine or colestipol. Propranolol given with lovastatin or pravastatin may decrease levels of both drugs. Concurrent administration increases warfarin levels and PT. Caution with ACE inhibitors, clonidine, terasozin/doxazosin, reserpine, inotropic agents, dobutamine/isoproterenol, NSAIDs, MAO inhibitors/TCA, methoxyflurane/trichloroethylene, neuroleptic drugs, and thyroxine. Avoid alcohol intake.

**PREGNANCY:** Category C, caution in nursing.

**MECHANISM OF ACTION:** Nonselective β-adrenergic receptor blocker; not fully established. Proposed to decrease cardiac output, inhibit renin release, and lessen tonic sympathetic nerve outflow from vasomotor centers in the brain.

**PHARMACOKINETICS: Absorption:** Complete; $T_{max}$=6 hrs. **Distribution:** $V_d$=4L/kg; plasma protein binding (90%); crosses placenta, blood-brain barrier; found in breast milk. **Metabolism:** CYP2D6 (hydroxylation and oxidation), CYP1A2, 2D6 (oxidation), N-dealkylation, glucuronidation. Propranolol glucuronide, naphthyloxylactic acid, glucuronic acid, sulfate conjugates (major metabolites). **Elimination:** $T_{1/2}$=10 hrs.

## NURSING CONSIDERATIONS

**Assessment:** Assess for sinus bradycardia, AV heart block, cardiogenic shock, overt CHF, bronchial asthma, bronchospastic disease, hyperthyroidism, DM, WPW syndrome, history of heart failure, possible drug interactions, hepatic/renal impairment.

**Monitoring:** Monitor for signs/symptoms of cardiac failure, hypoglycemia, decreased IOP, thyrotoxicosis, withdrawal symptoms (eg, angina, MI), and hypersensitivity reactions.

**Patient Counseling:** Instruct not to interrupt or d/c therapy without consulting physician. Inform drug may mask signs of thyrotoxicosis and hypoglycemia. Inform may interfere with glaucoma screening test. Advise to contact physician if symptoms of heart failure, withdrawal (eg, angina), or hypersensitivity reactions occur.

**Administration:** Oral route. **Storage:** 20-25°C (68-77°F); excursions permitted to 15-30°C (59-86°F). Protect from light, moisture, freezing, and excessive heat.

# INDERIDE — RX

propranolol HCl - hydrochlorothiazide (Wyeth)

**THERAPEUTIC CLASS:** Nonselective beta-blocker/thiazide diuretic

**INDICATIONS:** Management of hypertension. Not for initial therapy.

**DOSAGE:** *Adults:* Initial: 80-160mg propranolol/day; 25-50mg HCTZ/day. Max: (propranolol-HCTZ) 160mg-50mg/day. Elderly: Start at low end of dosing range. Do not substitute mg-for-mg of extended-release cap for immediate-release tab plus HCTZ. Dose tab bid and extended-release cap qd.

**HOW SUPPLIED:** (Propranolol-HCTZ) Tab: (Inderide) 40mg-25mg*, 80mg-25mg* *scored

**CONTRAINDICATIONS:** Cardiogenic shock, sinus bradycardia and >1st-degree block, bronchial asthma, CHF (unless failure is secondary to tachyarrhythmia treatable with propranolol), anuria, sulfonamide hypersensitivity.

**WARNINGS/PRECAUTIONS:** Caution with well-compensated cardiac failure, nonallergic bronchospasm, Wolff-Parkinson-White syndrome, hepatic or renal dysfunction. Withdrawal before surgery is controversial. May mask hypoglycemia or hyperthyroidism symptoms. Avoid abrupt discontinuation. May reduce IOP. Can cause cardiac failure, hypokalemia, hyperuricemia, hypercalcemia, hypophosphatemia. May exacerbate or activate SLE. Monitor for fluid/electrolyte imbalance. May manifest latent DM. Enhanced effect in postsympathectomy patient. Concomitant use with alcohol may increase plasma levels of propranolol.

**ADVERSE REACTIONS:** Bradycardia, CHF, hypotension, lightheadedness, mental depression, N/V, allergic reactions, blood dyscrasias, pancreatitis.

**INTERACTIONS:** Bradycardia/hypotension with catecholamine-depleting drugs. Potentiated by chlorpromazine, cimetidine. Antagonized by NSAIDs, phenytoin, phenobarbital, rifampin. May increase cardiac effects of CCBs. Reduces clearance of antipyrine, lidocaine, and theophylline. Aluminum hydroxide gel reduces intestinal absorption. Alcohol decreases absorption rate. May block epinephrine, thyroxine effects. Hypotension and cardiac arrest reported with haloperidol. May increase response to tubocurarine. May decrease arterial response to norepinephrine. Insulin dose may need adjustment. Risk of hypokalemia with corticosteroids, ACTH. Alcohol, barbiturates, or narcotics may aggravate orthostatic hypotension. Monitor digoxin. Potentiation with ganglionic or peripheral adrenergic-blockers. Concomitant use with alcohol may increase plasma levels of propranolol.

**PREGNANCY:** Category C, not for use in nursing. Intrauterine growth retardation, small placenta, and congenital abnormalities have been reported in neonates whose mothers received propranolol during pregnancy. Neonates whose mothers received propranolol at parturition have exhibited bradycardia, hypoglycemia, and/or respiratory depression.

**MECHANISM OF ACTION:** Propranolol: Nonselective β-adrenergic receptor blocker; not established, proposed to decrease cardiac output, inhibit renin release, and lessen tonic sympathetic nerve outflow. HCTZ: Thiazide diuretic; not established, affects renal tubular mechanism of electrolyte reabsorption.

**PHARMACOKINETICS: Absorption:** Propranolol: $T_{max}$=1-1.5 hrs. **Metabolism:** Propranolol: Liver. **Elimination:** Propranolol: $T_{1/2}$=4 hrs. HCTZ: Kidney.

## NURSING CONSIDERATIONS

**Assessment:** Assess for sinus bradycardia, AV heart block, cardiogenic shock, overt CHF, bronchospastic disease, hyperthyroidism, WPW syndrome, history of heart failure, SLE, DM, anuria, sulfonamide hypersensitivity, possible drug interactions, history of allergy or bronchial asthma, hepatic/renal impairment.

**Monitoring:** Monitor serum electrolytes and renal function periodically. Monitor for signs/symptoms of cardiac failure, hypoglycemia, decreased IOP, thyrotoxicosis, withdrawal (angina, MI), electrolyte imbalance, exacerbation or activation of SLE, hyperglycemia, hyperuricemia or precipitation of gout, hypersensitivity reactions, hepatic/renal dysfunction.

**Patient Counseling:** Instruct not to interrupt or d/c therapy without consulting physician. Inform may mask signs of thyrotoxicosis and hypoglycemia. Inform may interfere with glaucoma screening test. Advise to contact physician if symptoms of heart failure, withdrawal (angina), hypersensitivity reactions, or electrolyte imbalance (dry mouth, thirst, weakness) occur.

**Administration:** Oral route. **Storage:** 20-25°C (68-77°F); excursions permitted to 15-30°C (59-86°F). Protect from moisture, freezing, and excessive heat.

# INDOCIN I.V. RX

indomethacin sodium trihydrate (Lundbeck)

**THERAPEUTIC CLASS:** NSAID

**INDICATIONS:** To close hemodynamically significant patent ductus arteriosus in premature infants weighing between 500 - 1750g after 48 hrs of ineffective medical management. Clear-cut clinical evidence should be present (eg, respiratory distress, a continuous murmur, hyperactive precordium, cardiomegaly and pulmonary plethora on chest x-ray).

**DOSAGE:** *Pediatrics:* Neonates 500-1750g: Therapy includes 3 doses at 12- to 24-hr intervals. <48 hrs old: 0.2mg/kg IV followed by 0.1mg/kg IV then 0.1mg/kg IV. 2-7 days old: 0.2mg/kg IV for 3 doses. >7 days old: 0.2mg/kg IV followed by 0.25mg/kg IV then 0.25mg/kg IV. If anuria or marked oliguria (urinary output <0.6mL/kg/hr) occurs at scheduled time of 2nd or 3rd dose, hold doses until renal function normalizes. No further doses are necessary if ductus arteriosus closes or reduced in size after 48 hrs interval. May repeat course if ductus arteriosus reopens. Surgery may be needed if unresponsive after 2 courses. D/C if severe adverse reactions occur.

**HOW SUPPLIED:** Inj: 1mg

**CONTRAINDICATIONS:** Untreated infection, bleeding (active intracranial hemorrhage or GI bleeding), thrombocytopenia, coagulation defects, necrotizing enterocolitis, significant renal impairment, congenital heart disease when patency of ductus arteriosus is necessary for pulmonary or systemic blood flow (eg, pulmonary atresia, severe tetralogy of Fallot, severe coarctation of aorta).

**WARNINGS/PRECAUTIONS:** Risk of minor GI bleeding, intraventricular bleeding. May reduce urine output, CrCl, and GFR; may increase creatinine, BUN. May cause renal insufficiency, including acute renal failure; caution with extracellular volume depletion, CHF, sepsis, hepatic dysfunction. Monitor renal function and serum electrolytes. May mask signs of infection. D/C if liver disease develops. Administer carefully to avoid extravascular injection or leakage; may irritate tissue. May inhibit platelet aggregation; premature infants should be observed for signs of bleeding.

**ADVERSE REACTIONS:** Intracranial bleeding, GI bleeding, hyponatremia, elevated serum potassium, retrolental fibroplasia.

**INTERACTIONS:** May prolong half-life of digitalis; monitor ECG and serum digitalis levels. May elevate gentamicin and amikacin levels. May decrease natriuretic effect of furosemide. Increased risk of renal insufficiency with nephrotoxic drugs. Increased risk of bleeding with anticoagulants. Concomitant administration with anticoagulant may produce hypoprothrombinemia. Coadministration with ACE inhibitors or angiotensin II antagonists may result in further deterioration of renal function, including possible acute renal failure.

**PREGNANCY:** Safety in pregnancy or nursing not known.

**MECHANISM OF ACTION:** NSAID; not fully established, believed to inhibit prostaglandin synthesis.

**PHARMACOKINETICS: Metabolism:** Enterohepatic circulation. **Distribution:** Bound to protein plasma. **Elimination:** Renal, biliary; half-life varies with age and weight.

## NURSING CONSIDERATIONS

**Assessment:** Assess for bleeding (active intracranial hemorrhage, GI bleeding), thrombocytopenia, necrotizing enterocolitis, renal impairment, infection, coagulation defects, congenital heart disease (patent ductus arteriosus), and possible drug interactions. Obtain baseline CBC, serum electrolytes, and renal function.

**Monitoring:** Monitor renal function, serum electrolytes, and CBC periodically. Monitor for signs/symptoms of infection, liver disease, bleeding (intraventricular hemorrhage, GI bleeding), renal dysfunction, necrotizing enterocolitis, and hypersensitivity reactions. Monitor urine output.

**Patient Counseling:** Advise to seek medical attention if symptoms of infection, liver disease, renal impairment, bleeding, necrotizing enterocolitis, or hypersensitivity reactions occur.

**Administration:** IV route. **Storage:** 20-25°C (68-77°F). Protect from light. Store container in carton until contents have been used.

# INDOMETHACIN RX

indomethacin (Various)

**NSAIDs may cause an increased risk of serious cardiovascular thrombotic events, MI, stroke and serious GI adverse events including bleeding, ulceration, and perforation of the stomach or intestines. Contraindicated for the treatment of perioperative pain in the setting of coronary artery bypass graft (CABG) surgery.**

**OTHER BRAND NAMES:** Indocin (Merck)

**THERAPEUTIC CLASS:** NSAID

**INDICATIONS:** Management of moderate to severe rheumatoid arthritis (RA), ankylosing spondylitis, osteoarthritis (OA), acute painful shoulder (bursitis and/or tendinitis) and/or acute gouty arthritis.

**DOSAGE:** *Adults:* RA/Ankylosing Spondylitis/OA: Initial: 25mg PO bid-tid. Titrate: May increase by 25-50mg/day at weekly intervals. Max: 200mg/day. Bursitis/Tendinitis: 75-150mg/day given tid-qid for 7-14 days. Acute Gouty Arthritis: 50mg PO tid until pain is tolerable, then d/c. Take with food. *Pediatrics:* ≥14 yrs: RA/Ankylosing Spondylitis/OA: Initial: 25mg PO bid-tid. Titrate: May increase by 25-50mg/day at weekly intervals. Max: 200mg/day. Bursitis/Tendinitis: 75-150mg/day given tid-qid for 7-14 days. Acute Gouty Arthritis: 50mg PO tid until pain is tolerable, then d/c. 2-14 yrs (safety and effectiveness not established): Initial: 1-2mg/kg/day in divided doses. Max: 3mg/kg/day or 150-200mg/day. Take with food.

**HOW SUPPLIED:** Cap: 25mg, 50mg; Sus: 25mg/5mL [237mL]

**CONTRAINDICATIONS:** ASA or other NSAID allergy that precipitates acute asthmatic attack, urticaria, or rhinitis. Do not give suppositories with history of proctitis or recent rectal bleeding. Treatment of perioperative pain in the setting of CABG surgery.

**WARNINGS/PRECAUTIONS:** May lead to onset of new HTN or worsening of pre-existing HTN; monitor BP closely. Fluid retention and edema reported; caution with fluid retention or heart failure. Renal papillary necrosis and other renal injury reported after long-term use. Not recommended for use with advanced renal disease; if therapy must be initiated, monitor renal function. Anaphylactoid reactions may occur. May cause serious skin adverse events (eg, exfoliative dermatitis, Stevens-Johnson syndrome, and toxic epidermal necrolysis). Avoid in late pregnancy; may cause premature closure of ductus arteriosis. May cause elevations of LFTs; d/c if liver disease develops or systemic manifestations occur. Caution in elderly. Anemia may occur; with long-term use, monitor Hgb/Hct if signs or symptoms of anemia develop. May inhibit platelet aggregation and prolong bleeding time; monitor with coagulation disorders. Caution with asthma and avoid with ASA-sensitive asthma. Corneal deposits and retinal disturbances reported with prolonged therapy; perform eye exams at periodic intervals during prolonged therapy. May aggravate depression or other psychiatric disturbances, epilepsy, and parkinsonism; use with caution. D/C if severe CNS adverse reactions develop. May impair mental/physical abilities.

**ADVERSE REACTIONS:** Headache, dizziness, NV, dyspepsia, diarrhea, abdominal pain, constipation, vertigo, somnolence, depression, fatigue.

**INTERACTIONS:** Avoid salicylates, diflunisal, other NSAIDs, and triamterene. Potassium-sparing diuretics may cause hyperkalemia. Increase toxicity of methotrexate, cyclosporine, lithium, and digoxin. Probenecid increases levels. Caution with antihypertensives and anticoagulants. May decrease effects of diuretics, β-blockers, captopril.

**PREGNANCY:** Category C, not for use in nursing.

**MECHANISM OF ACTION:** NSAID; not established; exhibits antipyretic, analgesic, and anti-inflammatory properties. Potent inhibitor of prostaglandin synthesis; decreases prostaglandins in peripheral tissues, suppresses inflammation in RA, and diminishes basal and $CO_2$-stimulated cerebral blood flow.

**PHARMACOKINETICS: Absorption:** Readily absorbed. Bioavailability (100%); $C_{max}$=1-2mcg/mL; $T_{max}$=2 hrs. **Distribution:** Plasma protein binding (99%); crosses blood-brain barrier and placenta; found in breast milk. **Metabolism:**

Desmethyl, desbenzoyl, desmethyldesbenzoyl (metabolites). **Elimination:** Urine (60% as drug/metabolites), feces (33% as drug); $T_{1/2}$=4.5 hrs.

## NURSING CONSIDERATIONS

**Assessment:** Assess for history of asthma, urticaria or allergic-type reaction after previous use of NSAIDs, perioperative pain in setting of CABG surgery, CVD or risk factors for CVD, HTN, fluid retention or HF, hyponatremia, ulcer disease or GI bleeding, coagulation disorders or anticoagulant therapy, renal/hepatic impairment, rhinitis with or without nasal polyps, pregnancy/nursing status, depression or other psychiatric disturbances, epilepsy, parkinsonism, and possible drug interactions.

**Monitoring:** Monitor BP during initiation of therapy and thereafter. Monitor platelet function, CBCs, LFTs, dexamethasone suppression tests, renal function, and chemistry profile. Monitor signs/symptoms of anaphylactic/anaphylactoid reactions, adverse skin events (eg, exfoliative dermatitis, Stevens-Johnson syndrome, toxic epidermal necrolysis), eosinophilia, rash, corneal deposits and retinal disturbances with periodic ophthalmic exam, CNS effects, aggravation of depression or other psychiatric disturbances, GI bleeding/ulceration and perforation, anemia, CV thrombotic events, MI, stroke, new or worsening HTN, renal toxicity, renal papillary necrosis, other renal injury, and hyperkalemia.

**Patient Counseling:** Inform about potential serious side effects (eg, CV side effects such as MI or stroke); seek medical attention if signs/symptoms of chest pain, SOB, weakness, slurred speech, skin rash, blisters or fever, GI effects, bleeding, ulceration and perforation, signs of anaphylactic/anaphylactoid reaction, or hepatic toxicity occurs. Caution while performing hazardous tasks (eg, operating machinery/driving). Advise to notify physician if pregnant, nursing, planning to become pregnant, or if weight gain/edema occurs.

**Administration:** Oral route. **Storage:** 20-25°C (68-77°F); tight, light-resistant container.

# INFERGEN — RX

interferon alfacon-1 (Valeant)

**May cause or aggravate fatal or life-threatening neuropsychiatric, autoimmune, ischemic, and infectious disorders. Monitor closely with periodic clinical and laboratory evaluations.**

**THERAPEUTIC CLASS:** Biological response modifier

**INDICATIONS:** Treatment of chronic hepatitis C virus (HCV) with compensated liver disease in patients with anti-HCV antibodies and/or presence of HCV RNA.

**DOSAGE:** *Adults:* ≥18 yrs: 9mcg 3x/week (TIW) SQ for 24 weeks, wait 48 hrs between doses. If No Response or Relapse: 15mcg TIW for up to 48 weeks. Hold dose temporarily in severe adverse effects and reduce to 7.5mcg.

**HOW SUPPLIED:** Inj: 9mcg/0.3mL, 15mcg/0.5mL

**CONTRAINDICATIONS:** Decompensated hepatic disease, autoimmune hepatitis.

**WARNINGS/PRECAUTIONS:** Severe psychiatric adverse events (eg, depression, suicidal ideation, suicide attempt) may occur. Avoid in decompensated hepatic disease. Monitor CBC, platelets, and clinical chemistry tests before therapy and periodically thereafter. D/C if severe decrease in neutrophils or platelets, or serious hypersensitivity reaction occurs. Caution with cardiac disease, history of endocrine disorders, or low peripheral blood cell counts. Decrease/loss of vision and retinopathy reported; perform eye examination at baseline, if any ocular symptoms develop, and periodically with pre-existing disorder. May exacerbate autoimmune disorders. Neutropenia, thrombocytopenia, hypertriglyceridemia, and thyroid disorders reported. Caution in elderly. Pancreatitis, pneumonia, interstitial pneumonitis, colitis reported; d/c when signs and symptoms develop.

**ADVERSE REACTIONS:** Flu-like symptoms, depression, leukopenia, granulocytopenia, hot flushes, malaise, insomnia, dizziness, headache, myalgia, abdominal pain, N/V, diarrhea, anorexia, thrombocytopenia, nervousness.

**INTERACTIONS:** Caution with agents that cause myelosuppression or are metabolized by CYP450.

**PREGNANCY:** Category C, caution in nursing.

**MECHANISM OF ACTION:** Type-I interferon; binds interferon to the cell-surface receptor, leading to the production of several interferon-stimulated gene products.

## NURSING CONSIDERATIONS

**Assessment:** Assess for neuropsychiatric, autoimmune disease (ITP, RA, psoriasis), liver dysfunction (autoimmune hepatitis, decompensation, HBV), renal dysfunction, ophthalmologic disorders, endocrine disorders (thyroidism, DM), history of pulmonary disease, bone marrow suppression, immunocompromised, history of cardiac disease and possible drug interactions. Obtain baseline CBC, ANC, SrCr, LFTs, triglycerides, TFTs, Hgb, Hct, and eye exam.

I

**Monitoring:** Periodic monitoring of LFTs, CrCl, CBC, Hgb, platelet count, TFTs (baseline, 2 weeks after, and during therapy). Monitor for signs/symptoms of depression (suicidal ideation), cardiovascular and cerebrovascular events, ophthalmologic toxicity, pancreatitis, colitis, bone marrow toxicities, hyperglycemia, exacerbation of autoimmune disorders, renal impairment, worsening of liver disease/failure, respiratory, and hypersensitivity reactions.

**Patient Counseling:** Warn not to change brands of interferon or reduce dosage without consulting physician. Seek medical attention for symptoms of depression (suicidal ideation), chest pain, ocular symptoms, pancreatitis, colitis, fever, worsening of liver disease/failure (jaundice), respiratory, hyperglycemia and hypersensitivity reactions.

**Administration:** SQ route. **Storage:** In refrigerator, 2-8°C (36-46°F). Do not freeze; avoid vigorous shaking and exposure to direct sunlight.

# INFUMORPH

**CII**

morphine sulfate (Baxter)

**THERAPEUTIC CLASS:** Opioid analgesic

**INDICATIONS:** Treatment of intractable chronic pain in microinfusion devices.

**DOSAGE:** *Adults:* Lumbar Intrathecal: Opioid Intolerant: 0.2-1mg/day. Opioid Tolerant: 1-10mg/day. Max: Must be individualized. Caution with >20mg/day. Epidural: Opioid Intolerant: 3.5-7.5mg/day. Opioid Tolerant: 4.5-10mg/day. May increase to 20-30mg/day. Max: Must be individualized. Starting dose must be based on in-hospital evaluation of response to serial single-dose intrathecal/epidural bolus injections of regular morphine sulfate.

**HOW SUPPLIED:** Inj: 10mg/mL (200mg), 25mg/mL (500mg)

**CONTRAINDICATIONS:** For neuraxial analgesia: Infection at injection site, anticoagulants, uncontrolled bleeding diathesis, any therapy or condition that may render intrathecal or epidural administration hazardous.

**WARNINGS/PRECAUTIONS:** Have resuscitation equipment, oxygen, and antidote (eg, naloxone) available; severe respiratory depression may occur. Use only if less invasive means of controlling pain fail. Not for single-dose IV, IM, or SQ administration. May be habit-forming. Observe patient for 24 hours following test dose, and for 1st several days after catheter implantation. Caution with determining refill frequency. Make sure needle is properly placed in the filling port of device. Myoclonic-like spasm of the lower extremities reported if dose >20mg/day; may need detoxification. Caution with head injury, increased ICP, decreased respiratory reserve, hepatic/renal dysfunction (epidural injection), elderly. Avoid with chronic asthma, upper airway obstruction, other chronic pulmonary disorders. Biliary colic reported. May cause micturition disturbances especially with BPH. Increased risk of orthostatic hypotension with reduced circulating blood volume and impaired myocardial function. Avoid abrupt withdrawal. Risk of withdrawal in patients maintained on parenteral/oral narcotics. Not for routine use in obstetric labor/delivery.

**ADVERSE REACTIONS:** Respiratory depression, myoclonus convulsions, dysphoric reactions, pruritus, urinary retention, constipation, lumbar puncture-type headache, peripheral edema, orthostatic hypotension.

**INTERACTIONS:** Depressant effect may be potentiated by CNS depressants (eg, alcohol, sedatives, antihistamines, psychotropics). Increased risk of respiratory depression with neuroleptics. Contraindicated with anticoagulants. Risk of withdrawal with narcotic antagonists. Increased risk of orthostatic hypotension with sympatholytic drugs.

**PREGNANCY:** Category C, safety in nursing not known.

**MECHANISM OF ACTION:** Opioid analgesic; analgesic effects are produced via at least 3 areas of the CNS: the periaqueductal-periventricular gray matter, the ventromedial medulla, and the spinal cord. Interacts predominantly with µ-receptors which are found distributed in the brain, spinal cord, and in the trigeminal nerve.

**PHARMACOKINETICS: Absorption:** (Epidural): Rapid absorption; $C_{max}$=33-40ng/mL, $T_{max}$=10-15 min; (Intrathecal): $C_{max}$≤1-7.8ng/mL, $T_{max}$=5-10 mins. **Distribution:** Plasma protein binding (36%); Muscle tissue binding (54%). Readily passes into fetal circulation, found in breast milk. (IV):$V_d$=1.0-4.7L/kg. **Metabolism:** Hepatic glucuronidation. **Elimination:** Kidneys (major), urine (2-12% unchanged), feces (10%); $T_{1/2}$=1.5-4.5 hrs.

## NURSING CONSIDERATIONS

**Assessment:** Assess for acute bronchial asthma, upper airway obstruction, hypotension, infection at injection site, bleeding diathesis, seizure disorder, presence of head injury or increased intracranial pressure, age of patient, hepatic/renal dysfunction, biliary tract disorders or recent biliary surgery, urinary system disorders, impaired myocardial function, hypotension, pregnancy/nursing status, and possible drug interactions.

**Monitoring:** Monitor for signs/symptoms of respiratory depression and/or respiratory arrest, myoclonic events, seizures, dysphoric reactions, toxic psychoses, biliary colic, urinary retention, drug abuse and dependence. If administered intrathecally or via epidural, closely monitor for 24 hrs for signs/symptoms of respiratory depression.

**Patient Counseling:** Counsel to notify physician immediately if develop signs/symptoms of respiratory depression. Advise to avoid using other CNS depressants and alcohol during therapy. Medication has potential for abuse and dependence. Avoid abrupt withdrawal of medication; withdrawal symptoms may occur. Instruct that if accidental skin contact occurs, wash affected area with water.

**Administration:** IV, epidural, or intrathecal route. Proper placement of needle or catheter should be verified before epidural injection. **Storage:** 20-25°C (68-77°F); excursions permitted to 15-30°C (59-86°F). Protect from light. Do not freeze.

# INNOHEP RX

tinzaparin sodium (Celgene)

**Epidural or spinal hematomas resulting in long-term or permanent paralysis may occur in patients anticoagulated with low molecular weight heparins, heparinoids, or fondaparinux sodium and who are receiving neuraxial anesthesia or undergoing spinal puncture. Increased risk with indwelling epidural catheters, concomitant use of other drugs that affect hemostasis (eg, NSAIDs, platelet inhibitors, other anticoagulants), history of traumatic or repeated epidural or spinal puncture, or a history of spinal deformity or spinal surgery. Monitor frequently for signs/symptoms of neurologic impairment; if neurologic compromise noted, urgent treatment is necessary. Consider benefit and risks before neuraxial intervention in patients anticoagulated or to be anticoagulated for thromboprophylaxis.**

**THERAPEUTIC CLASS:** Low molecular weight heparin

**INDICATIONS:** Treatment of acute symptomatic deep vein thrombosis (DVT) with or without pulmonary embolism (PE) in conjunction with warfarin.

**DOSAGE:** *Adults:* 175 anti-Xa IU/kg SQ qd for at least 6 days and until anticoagulated with warfarin (INR ≥2 for 2 consecutive days). Begin warfarin within 1-3 days of therapy. Refer to PI for dosing chart.

**HOW SUPPLIED:** Inj: 20,000 anti-Xa IU/mL [2mL]

**CONTRAINDICATIONS:** Hypersensitivity to heparin, sulfite, benzyl alcohol, or pork. Active major bleeding, or in patients with history of heparin-induced thrombocytopenia (HIT).

**WARNINGS/PRECAUTIONS:** Not for IM/IV injection. Cannot use interchangeably unit for unit with heparin or other low molecular weight heparins. Increased risk for death in elderly patients with renal insufficiency; consider alternative therapy. Extreme caution in patients with increased risk of bleeding (severe uncontrolled hypertension, bacterial endocarditis, congenital or acquired bleeding disorders, active or recent ulceration and angiodyplastic GI disease, hemorrhagic stroke, diabetic retinopathy, or shortly after brain, spinal or ophthalmological surgery). Bleeding and thrombocytopenia may occur during therapy. D/C if severe hemorrhage occurs or if platelets <100,000/mm$^3$. Sulfite sensitivity, especially in asthmatic patients, reported. Priapism reported (rare). Contains benzyl alcohol; gasping syndrome in premature infants reported; caution in pregnant women. Periodic CBC including platelets, hct and hgb and stool occult blood test recommended.

**ADVERSE REACTIONS:** Bleeding, injection-site hematoma, asymptomatic increase in AST and ALT, and urinary tract infection.

**INTERACTIONS:** Prior to initiation of therapy, d/c agents that may enhance the risk of hemorrhage (eg, anticoagulants, platelet inhibitors, thrombolytics) unless the agents are essential; if coadministration is necessary, monitor closely for hemorrhage.

**PREGNANCY:** Category B, caution use in nursing.

**MECHANISM OF ACTION:** Low molecular weight heparin; inhibits reactions that lead to blood clotting, including the formation of fibrin clots. Acts as a potent co-inhibitor of several activated coagulation factors, including Factors Xa and IIa (thrombin). Primary inhibitory activity mediated through plasma protease inhibitor, antithrombin.

**PHARMACOKINETICS: Absorption:** (4,500 IU, Single Dose) $C_{max}$=0.25 IU/mL, $T_{max}$=3.7 hrs, AUC=2.0 IU•hr/mL. (175 IU/kg, Day 1) $C_{max}$=0.87 IU/mL, $T_{max}$=4.4 hrs, AUC=9.0 IU•hr/mL. (175 IU/kg, Day 5) $C_{max}$=0.93 IU/mL, $T_{max}$=4.6 hrs, AUC=9.7 IU•hr/mL; absolute bioavailability (86.7%). **Distribution:** $V_d$=3.1-5.0L. **Metabolism:** Partially metabolized by desulphation and depolymerization. **Elimination:** Renal; $T_{1/2}$=3-4 hrs.

## NURSING CONSIDERATIONS

**Assessment:** Assess for signs of active major bleeding; presence or history of heparin-induced thrombocytopenia; severe renal impairment; hypersensitivity to heparin, sulfites, benzyl alcohol or pork products; pregnancy/nursing status, and possible drug interactions. Assess use in conditions with increased risk of hemorrhage (eg, bacterial endocarditis, severe uncontrolled HTN, congenital or acquired bleeding disorders, in presence of spinal/epidural anesthesia or spinal puncture, with bleeding diathesis, uncontrolled HTN, history of GI ulceration, diabetic retinopathy, and hemorrhage).

**Monitoring:** Monitor for signs/symptoms of bleeding (eg, decreases in Hct, Hgb, BP), thrombocytopenia, hypersensitivity reactions, and priapism. If concomitant therapy with neuraxial anesthesia, monitor for epidural or spinal hematomas and for neurological impairment. Perform periodic monitoring of CBC including platelet count, Hgb/Hct, and stool test for occult blood.

**Patient Counseling:** Advise about increased risk of bleeding during therapy. Instruct to notify physician if unusual bleeding or hypersensitivity reaction occurs. During pregnancy, advise risk of gasping syndrome. Counsel on the proper way to administer: patients should be lying down or sitting when administering SQ Injection; alternate between left and right anterolateral and posterolateral abdominal wall; hold skin fold between thumb and forefinger;

insert whole length of needle into skin; to minimize bruising, do not rub injection site after administration.

**Administration:** SQ route. Patients should be lying down or sitting when administering SQ Injection. Alternate between left and right anterolateral and posterolateral abdominal wall. **Storage:** Store at 25°C (77°F); excursions permitted to 15-30°C (59-86°F). Keep out of the reach of children.

## InnoPran XL RX

propranolol HCl (GlaxoSmithKline)

**THERAPEUTIC CLASS:** Nonselective beta-blocker

**INDICATIONS:** For the management of hypertension; may use alone or combination with other antihypertensive agents.

**DOSAGE:** *Adults:* ≥18 yrs: Initial: 80mg qhs (approximately 10 PM) consistently either on empty stomach or with food. Titrate: Based on response may titrate to dose of 120mg.

**HOW SUPPLIED:** Cap, Extended-Release: 80mg, 120mg

**CONTRAINDICATIONS:** Cardiogenic shock, sinus bradycardia, sick sinus syndrome and >1st-degree heart block (unless a permanent pacemaker is in place), bronchial asthma.

**WARNINGS/PRECAUTIONS:** Caution with well-compensated cardiac failure, nonallergic bronchospasm (eg, chronic bronchitis, emphysema), Wolff-Parkinson-White syndrome, hepatic or renal dysfunction, or with history of severe anaphylactic reactions. Withdrawal before surgery is controversial. May mask hypoglycemia or hyperthyroidism symptoms. Avoid abrupt discontinuation, exacerbation of angina and MI reported. May reduce IOP. Can cause cardiac failure. Caution in patients with impaired hepatic or renal function. Not for treatment of hypertensive emergencies. Patients with history of severe anaphylactic reactions may be more reactive; treat reaction with epinephrine. Hypertensive patients has been associated with increase serum potassium, serum transaminase, alkaline phosphate; patients with heart failure may increase the BUN.

**ADVERSE REACTIONS:** Fatigue, dizziness (except vertigo), constipation.

**INTERACTIONS:** Caution with drugs that effect CYP2D6, 1A2, or 2C19; or those that slow down AV conduction (eg, digitalis, lidocaine, CCBs). ACE inhibitors can cause hypotension and may increase bronchial hyperactivity. May antagonize clonidine effects; caution when withdrawing from clonidine. Potentiated by α-blockers (eg, prazosin, terazosin, doxazosin), antiarrhythmics (eg, propafenone, quinidine, amiodarone), CYP2D6 substrates or inhibitors (eg, cimetidine, delavudin, fluoxetine, paroxetine, quinidine, ritonavir), CYP1A2 substrates or inhibitors (eg, imipramine, cimetidine, ciprofloxacin, fluvoxamine, isoniazid, theophylline, zileuton, zolmitriptan, rizatriptan), CYP2C19 substrates or inhibitors (eg, fluconazole, fluoxetine, fluvoxamine, teniposide, tolbutamide). Severe bradycardia, asystole, and heart failure associated with concomitant disopyramide. Decreases clearance of lidocaine and theophylline. Uncontrolled HTN may develop with concurrent epinephrine. Closely monitor for excessive reduction of resting sympathetic nervous activity (eg, hypotension, bradycardia, vertigo, orthostatic hypotension, syncope) with concurrent reserpine; reserpine may also potentiate depression. Anesthetics (eg, methoxyflurane, trichloroethylene) may depress myocardial contractility. Effects may be reversed by β-agonists (eg, dobutamine, isoproterenol). May exacerbate hypotensive effects of MAOIs or TCAs. Hypotension and cardiac arrest reported with haloperidol. Antagonized by NSAIDs. May result in lower than expected $T_3$ levels with concomitant thyroxine. Increases level of warfarin, diazepam, zolmitriptan, rizatriptan, thioridazine. Decreased levels with aluminum hydroxide gel (1200mg), cholestyramine, colestipol, rifampin, ethanol, and cigarette smoking. Co-administration with chlorpromazine may increase levels of both drugs. Decreases levels of lovastatin and pravastatin.

**PREGNANCY:** Category C; caution in nursing.

**MECHANISM OF ACTION:** β-adrenergic receptor blocker; not established, proposed to decrease cardiac output, to inhibit renin release by the kidneys, and to diminish tonic sympathetic nerve outflow from vasomotors in the brain.

**PHARMACOKINETICS: Absorption:** $T_{max}$=12-14 hrs. **Distribution:** $V_d$=4L; plasma protein binding (90%). **Metabolism:** CYP2D6 (hydroxylation), CYP1A2, 2D6 (oxidation), N-dealkylation, glucuronidation. Propranolol glucuronide, napthyloxylactic acid, glucuronic acid, sulfate conjugates (major metabolites). **Elimination:** $T_{1/2}$=8 hrs.

## NURSING CONSIDERATIONS

**Assessment:** Assess for pregnancy state, sinus bronchial asthma, bradycardia, AV heart block, cardiogenic shock, overt CHF, bronchospastic disease, hyperthyroidism, DM, possible drug interactions, WPW syndrome, history of heart failure, hepatic/renal impairment. Assess for serum potassium, serum transaminase, alkaline phosphate and BUN.

**Monitoring:** Monitor for signs/symptoms of cardiac failure, hypoglycemia, decreased IOP, thyrotoxicosis, withdrawal symptoms (angina, MI), and hypersensitivity reactions. Monitor for blood pressure changes, thyroid-function test and possible drug interactions.

I

**Patient Counseling:** Instruct not to interrupt or d/c therapy without consulting physician. Inform may mask signs of thyrotoxicosis and hypoglycemia. Drug may interfere with glaucoma screening test. Advise to contact physician if symptoms of heart failure, withdrawal (angina), or hypersensitivity reactions occur.

**Administration:** Oral route. **Storage:** 25°C (77°F), excursions permitted to 15-30°C (59-86°F). Keep tightly closed.

# INSPRA RX

eplerenone (Pfizer)

**THERAPEUTIC CLASS:** Aldosterone blocker

**INDICATIONS:** Improve survival of stable patients with left ventricular systolic dysfunction and congestive heart failure (CHF) post-MI. Treatment of hypertension, alone or with other antihypertensives.

**DOSAGE:** *Adults:* CHF Post-MI: Initial: 25mg qd. Titrate: Increase to 50mg qd within 4 weeks. Maint: 50mg qd. Adjust dose based on $K^+$ level: See table in PI. HTN: Initial: 50mg qd. May increase to 50mg bid if effect on BP is inadequate. Max: 100mg/day. With Moderate CYP3A4 Inhibitors: Initial: 25mg qd.

**HOW SUPPLIED:** Tab: 25mg, 50mg

**CONTRAINDICATIONS:** All Indications: Serum $K^+$ >5.5mgEq/L at initiation, CrCl ≤30mL/min, concomitant potent CYP3A4 inhibitors (eg, ketoconazole, itraconazole, nefazodone, troleandomycin, clarithromycin, ritonavir, nelfinavir). When treating HTN: Type 2 diabetes with microalbuminuria, SrCr >2mg/dL (males) or >1.8mg/dL (females), CrCl <50mg/min, concomitant $K^+$ supplements or $K^+$-sparing diuretics (eg, amiloride, spironolactone, triamterene).

**WARNINGS/PRECAUTIONS:** Minimize risk of hyperkalemia (>5.5mEq/L) with proper patient selection and monitoring. Patients with CHF post-MI, with SrCr >2mg/dL (males) or >1.8mg/dL (females), CrCl ≤50mL/min, or are diabetic (especially those with proteinuria) should be treated cautiously. Increased risk of hyperkalemia with decreased renal function.

**ADVERSE REACTIONS:** Headache, dizziness, hyperkalemia, increased SrCr/TG/GGT, angina/MI, hypokalemia, diarrhea, coughing, fatigue, flulike symptoms.

**INTERACTIONS:** See Contraindications. Increased levels with other CYP3A4 inhibitors (eg, erythromycin, verapamil, saquinavir, fluconazole). In HTN, use caution with ACE inhibitors and angiotensin II receptor antagonists; increased risk of hyperkalemia, especially with diabetics with microalbuminuria. Monitor lithium levels. Monitor antihypertensive effect with NSAIDs.

**PREGNANCY:** Category B, not for use in nursing.

**MECHANISM OF ACTION:** Aldosterone blocker; binds to mineralocorticoid receptor and blocks binding of aldosterone.

**PHARMACOKINETICS: Absorption:** Absolute bioavailability (69%); $T_{max}$=1.5 hrs. **Distribution:** $V_d$=43-90L; plasma protein binding (50%). **Metabolism:** CYP3A4. **Elimination:** Urine (67%, <5% unchanged), feces (32%, <5% unchanged); $T_{1/2}$=4-6 hrs.

## NURSING CONSIDERATIONS

**Assessment:** Assess serum $K^+$, SrCr. Assess for type 2 DM with microalbuminuria, proteinuria, impaired renal function, pregnancy/nursing status, and possible drug interactions.

**Monitoring:** Monitor serum $K^+$, BP, and renal function tests periodically. Monitor for signs/symptoms of hyperkalemia and hypersensitivity reactions.

**Patient Counseling:** Advise against use of $K^+$ supplements or salt substitutes containing $K^+$, and strong CYP3A4 inhibitors. Advise to seek medical attention if symptoms of hyperkalemia, dizziness, diarrhea, vomiting, rapid or irregular heartbeat, lower extremity edema, difficulty breathing, or hypersensitivity reactions occur.

**Administration:** Oral route. **Storage:** 25°C (77°F); excursions permitted to 15-30°C (59-86°F).

# INTEGRILIN RX

eptifibatide (Schering)

**THERAPEUTIC CLASS:** Glycoprotein IIb/IIIa inhibitor

**INDICATIONS:** Treatment of acute coronary syndrome (ACS) in patients being medically managed or undergoing percutaneous coronary intervention (PCI) including intracoronary stenting.

**DOSAGE:** *Adults:* ACS: 180mcg/kg IV bolus, then 2mcg/kg/min IV infusion until discharge or initiation of CABG, up to 72 hrs. If undergoing PCI, continue until discharge or 18-24 hrs post-PCI. CrCl <50mL/min: 180mcg/kg IV bolus, then 1mcg/kg/min IV infusion. PCI: 180mcg/kg IV bolus immediately before PCI, then 2mcg/kg/min IV infusion. Give 2nd bolus of 180mcg/kg 10 min after 1st bolus. Continue until discharge or 18-24 hrs post-PCI. CrCl <50mL/min: 180mcg/kg IV bolus immediately before PCI, then 1mcg/kg/min IV infusion. Give 2nd bolus of 180mcg/kg 10 min after 1st bolus. See PI for concomitant ASA and heparin doses.

**HOW SUPPLIED:** Inj: 20mg, 75mg, 200mg

**CONTRAINDICATIONS:** Active abnormal bleeding, history of bleeding diathesis, or stroke within past 30 days. Severe HTN uncontrolled with antihypertensives, major surgery within preceding 6 weeks, history of hemorrhagic stroke, current or planned concomitant parenteral glycoprotein IIb/IIIa inhibitor, renal dialysis dependency.

**WARNINGS/PRECAUTIONS:** Bleeding reported; mostly from arterial access site for cardiac catheterization, GI tract, or GU tract. Caution with renal dysfunction, platelets <100,000$mm^3$, femoral access site in PCI. Minimize vascular and other trauma. D/C if thrombocytopenia occurs. Monitor Hct/Hgb, platelets, SrCr, and PT/aPTT before therapy (and activated clotting time before PCI). D/C before CABG surgery.

**ADVERSE REACTIONS:** Bleeding (eg, intracranial hemorrhage, hematuria, hematemsis), thrombocytopenia, hypotension.

**INTERACTIONS:** Caution with other drugs that affect hemostasis (eg, thrombolytics, anticoagulants, NSAIDs, dipyridamole). Avoid other glycoprotein IIb/IIIa inhibitors. Cerebral, pulmonary, GI hemorrhage reported with ASA and heparin.

**PREGNANCY:** Category B, caution in nursing.

**MECHANISM OF ACTION:** Glycoprotein IIb/IIIa inhibitor; reversibly inhibits platelet aggregation by preventing the binding of fibrinogen, von Willebrand factor, and other adhesive ligands to glycoprotein IIb/IIIa.

**PHARMACOKINETICS: Absorption:** $T_{max}$=4-6 hrs. **Metabolism:** Deaminated eptifibatide (polar metabolite). **Distribution:** Plasma protein binding (25%). **Elimination:** Urine (50%; unchanged, metabolites); $T_{1/2}$=2.5 hrs.

## NURSING CONSIDERATIONS

**Assessment:** Assess for history of bleeding diathesis, evidence of bleeding within previous 30 days, severe HTN, major surgery within the previous 6 weeks, history of any stroke, concomitant use of another GP IIb/IIIa inhibitor, dependency on renal dialysis, and for drug interactions. Assess use if platelet count is <100,000/mm³. Obtain baseline Hgb, Hct, platelet count, SrCr, and PT/aPTT. In patients undergoing PCI, obtain activated clotting time (ACT). Assess pregnancy/nursing status and for possible drug interactions.

**Monitoring:** Monitor for signs/symptoms of bleeding (eg, intracranial bleeding), and thrombocytopenia (eg, platelet count <100,000/mm³). Periodically monitor aPTT and ACT. Monitor for hypersensitivity reactions.

I

**Patient Counseling:** Inform about bleeding tendency during therapy and instruct to contact physician if signs of unusual bleeding develop.

**Administration:** IV route. Do not administer in same line with furosemide. Refer to PI for proper administration. **Storage:** 2-8°C (36-46°F). May be stored at 25°C (77°F) for a period not exceeding 2 months with excursions permitted to 15-30°C (59-86°F) . Protect from light and discard any unused portion in the vial.

# INTELENCE — RX

etravirine (Tibotec)

**THERAPEUTIC CLASS:** Non-nucleoside reverse transcriptase inhibitor

**INDICATIONS:** In combination with other antiretrovirals for treatment of HIV-1 infection in antiretroviral treatment-experienced adult patients, who have evidence of viral replication and HIV-1 strains resistant to a non-nucleoside reverse transcriptase inhibitor (NNRTI) and other antiretrovirals.

**DOSAGE:** *Adults:* 200mg (two 100mg tabs) bid following a meal.

**HOW SUPPLIED:** Tab: 100mg

**WARNINGS/PRECAUTIONS:** Severe and life-threatening skin reactions (eg, Stevens-Johnson syndrome, hypersensitivity reaction, toxic epidermal necrolysis, and erythema multiforme) reported; d/c use and treat accordingly if severe hypersensitivity or rash with systemic symptoms and liver transaminase elevations develop. May cause body fat redistribution or accumulation (eg, central obesity, dorsocervical fat enlargement, peripheral wasting, facial wasting, breast enlargement, cushingoid appearance). Immune reconstitution syndrome reported with combination therapy. Caution in elderly.

**ADVERSE REACTIONS:** Rash, peripheral neuropathy.

**INTERACTIONS:** Coadministration of drugs that induce, inhibit or are substrates of CYP3A4, CYP2C9 and CYP2C19, or are transported by P-glycoprotein may alter therapeutic effect and adverse reaction profile. Concomitant use with NNRTIs (eg, efavirenz, nevirapine, delavirdine) and protease inhibitors (eg, atazanavir (ATV), fosamprenavir (FPV), nelfinavir, indinavir) administered without low-dose ritonavir (RTV) are not recommended. RTV 600mg bid decreases plasma levels and should not be coadministered. Do not administer with tipranavir/RTV, FPV/RTV, ATV/RTV. May decrease levels of antiarrhythmics; caution when coadministered; monitor drug levels. May increase warfarin concentration; monitor INR. Do not use in combination with CYP450 inducers (eg, carbamazepine, phenobarbital, phenytoin, rifampin, rifapentine, rifabutin). Adjust dose with antifungals (eg, itraconazole, ketoconazole, posaconazole). Consider alternatives to clarithromycin such as azithromycin for treatment of MAC. May decrease levels of lovastatin and simvastatin. May increase levels of fluvastatin. Caution when used with systemic dexamethasone and consider alternative therapy. May increase levels of diazepam. Caution with immunosuppressants (eg, cyclosporine, sirolimus, tacrolimus). Monitor for withdrawal symptoms when coadministered with methadone. May need to alter sildenafil dose. Caution when coadministered with lopinavir/RTV. Avoid concomitant use with St. John's wort.

**PREGNANCY:** Category B, not for use in nursing.

**MECHANISM OF ACTION:** Non-nucleoside reverse transcriptase inhibitor of HIV-1; binds directly to reverse transcriptase and blocks the RNA-dependent and DNA-dependent DNA polymerase activities, disrupting the enzyme's catalytic site.

**PHARMACOKINETICS: Absorption:** $T_{max}$=2.5-4 hrs. **Distribution:** Plasma protein binding (99.9%). **Metabolism:** Liver via CYP3A4, CYP2C9 and CYP2C19; (methyl hydroxylation). **Elimination:** Feces (93.7%); urine (1.2%); $T_{1/2}$=41 hrs.

## NURSING CONSIDERATIONS

**Assessment:** Assess treatment history, pregnancy/nursing status, and possible drug interactions. Perform resistance testing where possible.

**Monitoring:** Monitor for signs/symptoms of severe skin reactions (eg, Stevens-Johnson syndrome, hypersensitivity reactions [eg, rash, hepatic failure], toxic epidermal necroysis, erythema multiforme); if severe rash and elevations of liver transaminase develops, d/c treatment. Monitor for increase levels of liver transaminase. Monitor for clinical response (eg, viral load, CD4 count), fat redistribution (eg, central obesity, dorsocervical peripheral wasting, facial wasting), and immune reconstitution syndrome. May enroll patients in the Pregnancy Antiretroviral Registry if they become pregnant while on treatment.

**Patient Counseling:** Counsel that medication does not cure HIV and may continue to develop opportunistic infections and other complications of HIV disease. Medication does not reduce risk of HIV transmission to others; take precaution to avoid transmission (eg, safe sex practices). Take following a meal, twice a day as prescribed; swallow whole. If unable to swallow, disperse medication into glass of water; mix well and drink immediately; rinse glass several times with water; swallow each rinse to ensure full dose is taken. Avoid altering or stopping therapy without consulting physician. If a dose is missed within 6 hrs of time usually taken, take as soon as possible with a meal; if scheduled time exceeds 6 hrs, do not take missed dose; resume normal dosing schedule. Notify physician of all Rx or OTC medications and herbal products currently taking. D/C and notify if severe rash develops. Advise patient that redistribution or accumulation of body fat may occur. Inform mothers to avoid nursing to reduce risk of transmission.

**Administration:** Oral route. **Storage:** 25°C (77°F); excursions permitted to 15-30° C (59-86°F). Store in the original bottle. Keep bottle tightly closed to protect from moisture. Do not remove desiccant pouches.

# INTRON A — RX

interferon alfa-2b (Schering)

**May cause or aggravate fatal or life-threatening neuropsychiatric, autoimmune, ischemic, and infectious disorders. Monitor closely with periodic clinical and laboratory evaluations.**

**THERAPEUTIC CLASS:** Biological response modifier

**INDICATIONS:** Treatment of hairy cell leukemia, malignant melanoma, follicular lymphoma, condylomata acuminata, AIDS-related Kaposi's sarcoma, chronic hepatitis C and B.

**DOSAGE:** *Adults:* ≥18 yrs: Hairy Cell Leukemia: 2 MIU/m² IM/SQ 3x/week up to 6 months. Reduce dose by 50% or stop therapy with severe reactions. Malignant Melanoma: Initial: 20 MIU/m² IV for 5 consecutive days/week for 4 weeks. Maint: 10 MIU/m² SQ 3x/week for 48 weeks. Follicular Lymphoma: 5 MIU SQ 3x/week up to 18 months. Condylomata Acuminata: 1 MIU into lesion 3x/week alternating days for 3 weeks. Max: 5 lesions/course. Kaposi's Sarcoma: 30 MIU/m² 3x/week IM/SQ. Hepatitis C: 3 MIU IM/SQ 3x/week for

18-24 months. Hepatitis B: IM/SC: 5 MIU qd or 10 MIU IM/SQ 3x/week for 16 weeks. Dose adjust according to severe adverse reactions and laboratory abnormalities (See PI for more information).
*Pediatrics:* ≥1 yr: Hepatitis B: 3 MIU/$m^2$ SQ 3x/week for 1 week, then 6 MIU/$m^2$ 3x/week for total therapy of 16-24 weeks. Max: 10 MIU/$m^2$ 3x/week. Reduce dose by 50% or stop therapy with severe reactions. Adjust based on WBC, granulocyte, and/or platelet counts. Dose adjust according to severe adverse reactions and laboratory abnormalities (See PI for more information).

**HOW SUPPLIED:** Inj: 10 MIU, 18 MIU, 50 MIU, 10 MIU/mL, 3 MIU/0.2mL, 5 MIU/0.2mL, 10 MIU/0.2mL

**CONTRAINDICATIONS:** Autoimmune hepatitis, decompensated liver disease.

**WARNINGS/PRECAUTIONS:** Do not give IM if platelet count is less than 50,000 cells/$mm^3$. Hepatotoxicity, retinal hemorrhages, autoimmune diseases, pulmonary infiltrates, pneumonitis, thyroid abnormalities and pneumonia reported. Avoid with immunosuppressed transplant, autoimmune disorders, decompensated liver disease. Caution with cardiac disease, coagulation disorders, severe myelosuppression, pulmonary disease, thyroid disorders, or diabetes mellitus (DM) prone to ketoacidosis. Avoid with pre-existing psychiatric condition; depression, suicidal behavior, and aggressive behavior; monitor during treatment and in the 6 month follow-up period. D/C if psychiatric symptoms worsen or suicidal ideation is identified. Cases of encephalopathy observed in elderly treated with higher doses. Dental and periodontal disorders have been reported with ribavirin and interferon combination therapy. May exacerbate psoriasis or sarcoidosis. Do not interchange brands.

**ADVERSE REACTIONS:** Fever, headache, chills, fatigue, myalgia, GI disturbances, alopecia, dyspnea, depression.

**INTERACTIONS:** Increases theophylline levels by 100%. Caution with myelosuppressive agents (eg, zidovudine). Antidiabetics and thyroid agents may need adjustments. Increased risk of hemolytic anemia when coadministered with ribavirin. Risk of aplastic anemia and pure red cell aplasia with Rebetol.

**PREGNANCY:** Category C, Category X when used with ribavirin, not for use in nursing.

**MECHANISM OF ACTION:** α-interferon; binds to specific membrane receptors on cell surface initiating induction of enzymes, suppression of cell proliferation, immunomodulating activities, and inhibition of virus replication.

**PHARMACOKINETICS: Absorption:** (IM, SQ) $C_{max}$=18-116 IU/mL, $T_{max}$=3-12 hrs; (IV) $C_{max}$=135-273 IU/mL, $T_{max}$=30 min. **Elimination:** (IM, SQ) $T_{1/2}$=2-3 hrs; (IV) $T_{1/2}$=2 hrs.

## NURSING CONSIDERATIONS

**Assessment:** Assess for neuropsychiatric conditions, autoimmune disease (psoriasis), liver dysfunction, ischemic, ophthalmologic and infectious disorders, preexisting thyroid abnormalities, hemoglobinopathies (thalassemia major, sickle cell anemia), DM, history of pulmonary disease (eg, COPD, sarcoidosis), coagulation disorders (thrombophlebitis, PE), severe myelosuppression, history of cardiovascular disease (MI, arrhythmic disorder), and possible drug interactions. Obtain baseline CBC and platelet counts, LFTs, electrolytes, TSH, Hgb/Hct, ECG, CXR.

**Monitoring:** Periodic monitoring of LFTs, CrCl, CBC, Hgb, platelet count, PT, alkaline phosphatase, albumin, bilirubin, TSH, ECG, CXR. CBC and platelet count should be repeated 1-2 weeks following initiation of therapy, and monthly thereafter. Serum ALT should be evaluated at approximately 3-month intervals to assess response to therapy. Monitor for signs/symptoms of depression (suicidal ideation), cardiovascular and cerebrovascular events, ophthalmologic toxicity pancreatitis, colitis, cytopenia, worsening of liver disease/failure, respiratory, and hypersensitivity reactions.

**Patient Counseling:** Instruct on proper use of product. Seek medical attention for symptoms of depression (suicidal ideation), cardiovascular (chest pain) and cerebrovascular events, ophthalmologic toxicity (eg, decreased/loss of vision), pancreatitis and colitis (eg, abdominal pain, N/V), cytopenia (eg, fever, bruising, dyspnea), worsening of liver disease/failure (eg, jaundice), respiratory (eg, fever, cough, dyspnea), and hypersensitivity reactions. Keep well hydrated.

**Administration:** IM, SQ, IV, and intralesional administration. **Storage:** 2-8°C (36-46°F). After reconstitution use immediately, store up to 24 hrs.

## INTUNIV RX
guanfacine (Shire)

**THERAPEUTIC CLASS:** Alpha$_2$-agonist

**INDICATIONS:** Treatment of attention deficit hyperactivity disorder (ADHD).

**DOSAGE:** *Pediatrics:* 6-17 yrs: Initial: 1mg/day. Titrate: Adjust dose by increments of ≤1mg/week. Maint: 1-4mg/day based on clinical response and tolerability. Range: 0.05-0.08mg/kg/day. Efficacy increased with increasing weight-adjusted dose. If well tolerated, doses up to 0.12mg/kg/day may provide additional benefit. Max: 4mg/day. D/C: Taper off in decrements of ≤1mg every 3-7 days. Reinitiation: Consider titration of dose based on patient tolerability. Renal/Hepatic Impairment: Consider dose adjustment.

**HOW SUPPLIED:** Tab, Extended-Release: 1mg, 2mg, 3mg, 4mg

**WARNINGS/PRECAUTIONS:** Hypotension and bradycardia may occur. Syncope reported in pediatric patients. Caution with history of syncope or condition(s) that predispose to syncope such as hypotension, orthostatic hypotension, bradycardia, or dehydration. Somnolence and sedation reported. May impair mental/physical abilities. Caution with history of hypotension, heart block, bradycardia, or CV disease; assess HR, BP prior to initiation of therapy and monitor periodically.

**ADVERSE REACTIONS:** Hypotension, bradycardia, syncope, somnolence/sedation, headache, fatigue, abdominal pain, N/V, lethargy, dizziness, irritability, dry mouth, constipation, weight increase.

**INTERACTIONS:** Caution with ketoconazole and other strong CYP3A4/5 inhibitors. CYP3A4 inducers (eg, rifampin) may decrease exposure levels. May increase valproic acid concentrations. Additive effects with antihypertensives and CNS depressants (eg, alcohol, sedative/hypnotics, benzodiazepines, barbiturates, and antipsychotics); caution during coadministration. High-fat meals may increase levels.

**PREGNANCY:** Category B, caution with nursing.

**MECHANISM OF ACTION:** $\alpha_{2A}$-adrenergic agonist; mechanism not established. Known as an antihypetensive agent. Reduces sympathetic nerve impulses from the vasomotor center to the heart and blood vessels, resulting in decreased peripheral vascular resistance and reduction in heart rate.

**PHARMACOKINETICS: Absorption: Adults:** $C_{max}$=1ng/mL; AUC= 32ng•h/mL; $T_{max}$=6 hrs. Children (6-12 yrs): $C_{max}$=10ng/mL; AUC= 162ng•h/mL. Adolescents (13-17 yrs): $C_{max}$=7ng/mL; AUC= 116ng•h/mL. **Pediatrics:** $T_{max}$=5 hrs. **Distribution:** Plasma protein binding (70%). **Metabolism:** Liver, via CYP3A4/5. **Elimination:** $T_{1/2}$=18 hrs.

### NURSING CONSIDERATIONS

**Assessment:** Assess HR, BP. Assess for history of syncope, hypotension, orthostatic hypotension, bradycardia, dehydration, heart block, CV disease, possible drug interactions. Assess pregnancy/nursing status.

**Monitoring:** Monitor HR, BP. Monitor for orthostatic hypotension, somnolence, sedation.

**Patient Counseling:** Instruct to swallow whole with small amount of water, milk, or other liquid; do not crush, chew, or break before swallowing. Inform that taking drug with high-fat meal raises blood levels. Instruct caregiver to supervise the child or adolescent during therapy. Inform of the adverse reactions that may occur. Caution against operating heavy equipment or driving. Advise patients to avoid becoming dehydrated or overheated.

**Administration:** Oral route. **Storage:** 25°C (77°F); excursions permitted to 15-30°C (59-86°F).

# INVANZ — RX

## ertapenem sodium (Merck)

**THERAPEUTIC CLASS:** Carbapenem

**INDICATIONS:** Treatment of complicated intra-abdominal infections, complicated skin and skin structure infections (cSSSI) including diabetic foot infections without osteomyelitis, community-acquired pneumonia (CAP), complicated urinary tract infections (UTI) including pyelonephritis, and acute pelvic infections (including postpartum endomyometritis, septic abortion, and post-surgical gynecologic infections) caused by susceptible strains of microorganisms. Prophylaxis of surgical-site infection following elective colorectal surgery.

**DOSAGE:** *Adults:* 1g IM/IV qd. Duration: Intra-Abdominal Infections: 5-14 days. cSSSI: 7-14 days. CAP/UTI: 10-14 days. Acute Pelvic Infections: 3-10 days. Max: IV: 14 days. IM: 7 days. Prophylaxis Following Colorectal Surgery: 1g IV as single dose given 1 hr prior to surgical incision. CrCl ≤30mL/min/1.73m$^2$: 500mg IM/IV qd. Hemodialysis: Give 150mg IM/IV after dialysis only if 500mg dose was given within 6 hrs prior to dialysis.
*Pediatrics:* ≥13 yrs: 1g IM/IV qd. 3 months-12 yrs: 15mg/kg IM/IV bid. Max: 1g/day. Duration: Intra-Abdominal Infections: 5-14 days. cSSSI: 7-14 days. CAP/UTI: 10-14 days. Acute Pelvic Infections: 3-10 days. Max: IV: 14 days. IM: 7 days.

**HOW SUPPLIED:** Inj: 1g

**CONTRAINDICATIONS:** Hypersensitivity to local anesthetics of the amide type (due to lidocaine diluent) if administered IM.

**WARNINGS/PRECAUTIONS:** Serious, sometimes fatal, hypersensitivity reported with β-lactam therapy. *Clostridium difficile*-associated diarrhea (CDAD) reported; d/c if CDAD confirmed. Seizures and CNS adverse events reported. Increased risk of seizures with CNS disorders and/or compromised renal function. Monitor renal, hepatic, hematopoietic functions during prolonged therapy. Prolonged use may result in overgrowth of non-susceptible organisms. Caution with IM administration; avoid inadvertent injection into blood vessel. Not for treatment of viral infections (eg, common cold).

**ADVERSE REACTIONS:** Diarrhea, infused vein complication, N/V, anemia, headache, edema/swelling, fever, abdominal pain, constipation, altered mental status, insomnia, wound infection, ALT and AST increased.

**INTERACTIONS:** Decreased clearance with probenecid. May decrease serum levels of valproic acid or divalproex sodium when coadministered.

**PREGNANCY:** Category B, caution in nursing.

**MECHANISM OF ACTION:** Carbapenem; inhibits cell wall synthesis and is mediated through binding to penicillin binding proteins.

**PHARMACOKINETICS: Absorption:** Administration of different doses resulted in different parameters. (IM): Absolute bioavailability (90%); $T_{max}$=2.3 hrs. **Distribution:** $V_d$=0.12L/kg (adult); 0.2L/kg (3 months-12 yrs); 0.16L/kg (13-17 yrs). Plasma protein binding (95%); found in breast milk. **Metabolism:** Liver via hydrolysis of the β-lactam ring. **Elimination:** (Adults, 13-17 yrs) $T_{1/2}$=4 hrs. (3 months-12 years) $T_{1/2}$=2.5 hrs; Urine (38% unchanged, 37% metabolite), feces (10%).

## NURSING CONSIDERATIONS

**Assessment:** Assess for β-lactam/amide hypersensitivity, history of seizure or brain lesions, bacterial meningitis, renal impairment, pregnancy/nursing status, and possible drug interactions. Periodic assessment of organ system function, including renal, hepatic, and hematopoietic.

**Monitoring:** Monitor for signs/symptoms of anaphylactoid or hypersensitivity reactions, CDAD, superinfections, and seizures. Monitor renal, hepatic, hematopoietic functions.

**Patient Counseling:** Inform that drug only treats bacterial, not viral, infections. Instruct to take as directed; skipping doses or not completing full course may decrease effectiveness and increase resistance. May experience diarrhea; notify physician if watery/bloody stools, hypersensitivity reactions, infection, or seizures occur.

**Administration:** IV/IM routes. Refer to labeling for administration procedures. **Storage:** Before reconstitution: <25°C (77°F). Reconstituted and infusion solutions: Room temperature (25°C) and use within 6 hrs, or store for 24 hrs under refrigeration (5°C) and use within 4 hrs after removal from refrigeration. Do not freeze.

## INVEGA RX

paliperidone (Ortho-Mcneil/Janssen)

**Elderly patients with dementia-related psychosis treated with antipsychotic drugs are at an increased risk of death; most deaths appeared to be cardiovascular (eg, heart failure, sudden death) or infectious (eg, pneumonia) in nature. Paliperidone is not approved in patients with dementia-related psychosis.**

**THERAPEUTIC CLASS:** Benzisoxazole derivative

**INDICATIONS:** Acute and maintenance treatment of schizophrenia. Acute treatment of schizoaffective disorder as monotherapy or as an adjunct to mood stabilizers and/or antidepressants.

**DOSAGE:** *Adults:* Schizophrenia: 6mg qd in am. Titrate: May increase by 3mg/day at intervals >5 days. Max: 12mg/day. Schizoaffective Disorder: 6mg qd in am. Usual range: 3-12mg/day. Titrate: Increase by 3mg/day at intervals >4 days. Max: 12mg/day. Renal Impairment/Elderly: Individualize dose. CrCl ≥50 to <80mL/min: Initial: 3mg qd. Max: 6mg qd. CrCl ≥10 to <50mL/min: Initial: 1.5mg qd. Max: 3mg qd.

**HOW SUPPLIED:** Tab, Extended-Release: 1.5mg, 3mg, 6mg, 9mg

**CONTRAINDICATIONS:** Known hypersensitivity to risperidone.

**WARNINGS/PRECAUTIONS:** Neuroleptic malignant syndrome (NMS) reported. Causes a modest increase in QTc interval; avoid use in patients with risk factors for prolonged QT interval. Tardive dyskinesia may occur. Hyperglycemia, in extreme cases associated with ketoacidosis or hyperosmolar coma or death, has been reported; monitor for hyperglycemia and perform fasting blood glucose testing at the beginning of therapy and periodically during treatment in patients at risk for diabetes mellitus (DM). Elevates prolactin levels. Obstructive symptoms may result in patients with GI narrowing. May induce orthostatic hypotension and syncope; caution with history of CV, cerebrovascular disease and conditions that predispose to hypotension. Leukopenia, neutropenia and agranulocytosis reported. Monitor CBC during the first few months of therapy and d/c at the first signs of a clinically significant decline in WBC in absence of other causative factors. D/C in cases of severe neutropenia (ANC<1000/mm$^3$). May impair mental/physical abilities. Seizures reported; caution with history of seizures or conditions that lower the seizure threshold. Esophageal dysmotility and aspiration reported; caution with increased risk of aspiration pneumonia. Possibility of suicide attempt is inherent in patients with bipolar mania and schizophrenia. Rare cases of priapism reported. May cause thrombotic thrombocytopenic purpura (TTP). May disrupt body temperature regulation; caution when exposed to extreme temperature. May have antiemetic effects that may mask the signs and symptoms of overdosage with certain drugs or of conditions such as intestinal obstruction, Reye's syndrome, and brain tumor. Patients with Parkinson's disease or dementia with Lewy bodies are reported to have an increased sensitivity to antipsychotic medications. Caution with diseases/conditions affecting metabolism or hemodynamic responses, renal/hepatic impairment and in elderly.

**ADVERSE REACTIONS:** Extrapyramidal symptoms, tachycardia, bundle branch block, upper abdominal pain, dry mouth, akathisia, somnolence, dyspepsia, dizziness, nasopharyngitis, headache, nausea, hyperkinesia, constipation, weight gain.

**INTERACTIONS:** Caution with other CNS drugs and alcohol. May antagonize the effect of levodopa and other dopamine agonists. Additive effect observed when administered with other agents that cause orthostatic hypotension.

Avoid concomitant use with other drugs known to prolong QTc interval, including Class 1A (eg, quinidine, procainamide) or Class III (eg, amiodarone, sotalol) antiarrhythmics, antipsychotics (eg, chlorpromazine, thioridazine), antibiotics (eg, gatifloxacin, moxifloxacin). Concomitant use with carbamazepine may decrease levels. Divalproex sodium may increase plasma levels by 50%. Consider dose adjustment of paliperidone when administering with valproate (reduce) and carbamazepine (increase). Additive exposure with oral risperidone. Increased $C_{max}$ and AUC with high-fat/high-caloric meal.

**PREGNANCY:** Category C, caution in nursing.

**MECHANISM OF ACTION:** Benzisoxazole derivative; not established. Proposed to be mediated through a combination of central dopamine Type 2 ($D_2$) and serotonin Type 2 ($5HT_{2A}$) receptor antagonism.

**PHARMACOKINETICS: Absorption**: Absolute bioavailability (28%); $T_{max}$=24 hrs. **Distribution**: $V_d$=487L; plasma protein binding (74%); found in breast milk. **Metabolism**: CYP2D6, 3A4 (limited). **Elimination**: Urine (80%, 59% unchanged), feces (11%); $T_{1/2}$=23 hrs.

## NURSING CONSIDERATIONS

**Assessment:** Assess for dementia-related psychosis, Parkinson's disease, dementia, known CV disease (eg, heart failure, MI or ischemia, conduction abnormalities), cerebrovascular disease or conditions that predispose to hypotension such as dehydration and hypovolemia. Assess use in patients with pre-existing severe GI narrowing, history of seizures, known drug allergy to risperidone, renal function prior to administration, fasting blood glucose levels in patients at risk for hyperglycemia, pregnancy/nursing status and possible drug interactions.

**Monitoring:** Monitor for cerebrovascular adverse events in the elderly population, signs/symptoms of NMS, EPS, QT prolongation, TD, hyperglycemia, hyperprolactinemia, GI obstructions, orthostatic hypotension, seizures, attempted suicide, priapism and thrombotic thrombocytopenic purpura. Perform periodic monitoring of fasting blood glucose levels in patients with DM.

**Patient Counseling:** Advise risk of orthostatic hypotension during initiating/re-initiating treatment or dose increase. Caution when operating machinery/driving. Avoid concomitant use of alcohol. Instruct to inform physician if taking/plan to take any prescription/OTC drugs or if become/intend to become pregnant. Caution in nursing woman. Inform medication may impair body's ability to regulate temperatures; take appropriate measures when exposed to increased temperatures. Inform patient that medication must be swallowed whole with liquids; tablets should not be chewed, divided or crushed. Tablet shell along with insoluble core components may be found in stool.

**Administration:** Oral route. May be taken with or without food. Swallow tab whole with liquids; do not chew, divide or crush. **Storage**: 25°C (77°F); excursions permitted to 15-30°C (59-86°F). Protect from moisture.

# INVEGA SUSTENNA RX

paliperidone palmitate (Ortho-Mcneil/Janssen)

**Elderly patients with dementia-related psychosis treated with antipsychotic drugs, including atypicals, are at an increased risk of death; most deaths appeared to be cardiovascular (eg, heart failure, sudden death) or infectious (eg, pneumonia) in nature. Not approved in patients with dementia-related psychosis.**

**THERAPEUTIC CLASS:** Benzisoxazole derivative

**INDICATIONS:** Acute and maintenance treatment of schizophrenia in adults.

**DOSAGE:** (IM) Initial: 234mg on treatment Day 1 and 156mg after 1 week, administered in the deltoid muscle. Maint: 117mg/month. Range: 39mg-234mg based on clinical response. To avoid missing doses, the second initiation dose should be given 7±2 days after the first dose. The recommended injection cycle is monthly; doses may be given up to 7 days before or after the monthly scheduled dose. Maintenance Therapy: Continue at the lowest dose as necessary. Reassess periodically to determine need for continued treatment. CrCl ≥50-<80mL/min/Elderly with Decreased Renal Function; Initial: 156mg on Day 1 and 117mg after 1 week in deltoid muscle. Thereafter, follow with monthly injections of 78mg in either deltoid or gluteal muscle. Switching from Oral Antipsychotics: See PI for conversion. D/C oral antipsychotics when initiating IM therapy. Switching from Long-Acting Injectable Antipsychotics: Initiate treatment in place of the next scheduled injection and continue at monthly intervals. Re-evaluate periodically. For missed dosing instructions, please refer to the PI.

**HOW SUPPLIED:** Injectable Suspension, Extended-Release: 39mg, 78mg, 117mg, 156mg, 234mg

**WARNINGS/PRECAUTIONS:** May increase QTc interval; avoid with congenital long QT syndrome and with a history of cardiac arrhythmias. Neuroleptic malignant syndrome (NMS) and tardive dyskinesia (TD) may occur. Increased sensitivity in patients with Parkinson's disease or dementia with Lewy bodies. Monitor for hyperglycemia; perform fasting blood glucose testing if symptoms develop or with risk factors for diabetes mellitus (DM). Cerebrovascular events (eg, stroke, TIA) reported in elderly with dementia-related psychosis. May induce priapism, orthostatic hypotension and syncope; monitor those vulnerable to hypotension. Significant weight gain has been reported. Leukopenia, neutropenia, agranulocytosis reported; D/C if absolute neutrophil count <1000/mm$^3$. Caution with history of seizures or other conditions that may lower seizure threshold. May elevate prolactin levels. May cause esophageal dysmotility and aspiration; caution in those at risk for aspiration pneumonia. May disrupt body's ability to reduce core body temperature; caution in conditions that may contribute to an elevation in core body temperature. Caution with known suicidal tendencies, CV disease, elderly, and renal impairment. Antiemetic effect may occur and mask the signs/symptoms of overdosage with certain drugs/conditions (eg, intestinal obstruction, Reye's syndrome, brain tumor). May impair mental/physical abilities. Avoid in patients with CrCl<50mL/min.

**ADVERSE REACTIONS:** Upper abdominal pain, constipation, dry mouth, N/V, injection-site reactions, nasopharyngitis, weight gain, dizziness, extrapyramidal disorder, headache, somnolence/sedation, agitation, anxiety, insomnia, akathisia.

**INTERACTIONS:** Caution with other CNS drugs and alcohol. May antagonize the effect of levodopa and other dopamine agonists. An additive effect may be observed when administered with other agents that cause orthostatic hypotension. Avoid in combination with other drugs known to prolong QTc interval, including Class 1A (eg, quinidine, procainamide) or Class III (eg, amiodarone, sotalol) antiarrhythmics, antipsychotics (eg, chlorpromazine, thioridazine), antibiotics (eg, gatifloxacin, moxifloxacin). Concomitant use with carbamazepine may decrease levels.

**PREGNANCY:** Category C, not for use in nursing.

**MECHANISM OF ACTION:** Benzisoxazole derivative; not established. Proposed to be mediated through a combination of central dopamine Type 2 ($D_2$) and serotonin Type 2 ($5HT_{2A}$) receptor antagonism.

**PHARMACOKINETICS: Absorption:** $T_{max}$=13 days. **Distribution:** $V_d$=391L; plasma protein binding (74%). **Metabolism:** CYP2D6, 3A4 (limited). **Elimination:** Urine (80%, 59% unchanged), feces (11%); $T_{1/2}$=25 days.

## NURSING CONSIDERATIONS

**Assessment:** Assess for dementia-related psychosis, Parkinson's disease, dementia, known CV disease (eg, heart failure, MI or ischemia, conduction abnormalities), cerebrovascular disease or conditions that predispose to hypotension such as dehydration and hypovolemia. Assess use in patients with pre-existing severe GI narrowing, history of seizures, known drug allergy to risperidone, renal function prior to administration, fasting blood glucose levels in patients at risk for hyperglycemia, pregnancy/nursing status, and possible drug interactions.

**Monitoring:** Monitor for cerebrovascular adverse events in the elderly population, signs/symptoms of NMS, EPS, QT prolongation, TD, hyperglycemia, hyperprolactinemia, orthostatic hypotension, seizures, attempted suicide, priapism, and thrombotic thrombocytopenic purpura. Perform periodic monitoring of fasting blood glucose levels in patients with DM.

**Patient Counseling:** Caution when operating machinery/driving. Advise patients with the risk of orthostatic hypotension. Avoid concomitant use of alcohol. Instruct to inform physician if taking, or plan to take, any prescription or OTC drugs, or if become or intend to become pregnant. Advise not to breastfeed during treatment. Inform medication may impair body's ability to regulate temperatures; take appropriate measures when exposed to increased temperatures. Avoid overheating and dehydration.

**Administration:** IM route. Inject slowly, deep into the deltoid muscle. Avoid injecting into a blood vessel. Do not administer dose in divided injections. Refer to PI for proper instructions for use. **Storage:** 25°C (77°F); excursions permitted to 15-30°C (59-86°F).

## INVIRASE RX

saquinavir mesylate (Roche Labs)

I

**THERAPEUTIC CLASS:** Protease inhibitor

**INDICATIONS:** Treatment of HIV infection in combination with other antiretrovirals.

**DOSAGE:** *Adults:* >16yrs: 1000mg bid with ritonavir 100mg bid. Take within 2 hrs after a full meal. Concomitant therapy with lopinavir/ritonavir: 1000mg bid.

**HOW SUPPLIED:** Cap: 200mg; Tab: 500mg

**CONTRAINDICATIONS:** Concomitant amiodarone, bepridil, flecainide, propafenone, quinidine, rifampin, pimozide, terfenadine, cisapride, astemizole, triazolam, midazolam, lovostatin, simvastatin, ergot derivatives. Contraindicated with severe hepatic impairment when coadministered with ritonavir.

**WARNINGS/PRECAUTIONS:** New onset diabetes mellitus (DM), exacerbation of pre-existing DM, hyperglycemia, ketoacidosis may occur. Caution with hepatic/renal impairment. Spontaneous bleeding may occur with hemophilia A and B. Possible redistribution or accumulation of body fat. Elevated cholesterol and/or triglyceride levels observed. May develop pancreatitis with marked increase in triglycerides; monitor levels prior to treatment. Interrupt therapy if serious toxicity occurs. Immune reconstitution syndrome reported. Varying degrees of cross-resistance have been observed. Contains lactose in amounts that should not induce specific symptoms of intolerance.

**ADVERSE REACTIONS:** Diarrhea, abdominal pain, pruritus, fever, rash, N/V, fatigue, pneumonia, lipodystrophy

**INTERACTIONS:** Use atorvastatin or rosuvastatin at lowest possible dose. Avoid lovastatin, simvastatin, St. John's wort, garlic capsules, tipranavir, trazodone, fluticasone. Decreased plasma levels with nevirapine. Consider alternatives to CYP3A4 inducers (eg, phenobarbital, phenytoin, dexamethasone, carbamazepine). Ritonavir increases adverse effects. May elevate plasma levels of substrates of CYP3A4 (eg, calcium CCBs, clindamycin, dapsone, quinidine, triazolam). Delavirdine increases plasma levels; monitor LFTs frequently. Saquinavir/ritonavir increases digoxin levels; monitor digoxin serum concentration and reduce dose if needed. See Contraindications and PI for detailed information.

**PREGNANCY:** Category B, not for use in nursing.

**MECHANISM OF ACTION:** HIV protease inhibitor; binds to the protease active site and inhibits activity of the enzyme, preventing cleavage of the viral polyproteins and resulting in formation of immature, noninfectious virus particles.

**PHARMACOKINETICS: Absorption:** Administration of variable doses and combinations resulted in different parameters. **Distribution:** Plasma protein binding (98%). (IV): $V_d$=700L. **Metabolism:** Hepatic via CYP3A4. **Elimination:** (PO): Urine (1%), feces (88%). (IV): Urine (3%), feces (81%).

## NURSING CONSIDERATIONS

**Assessment:** Assess for renal/hepatic impairment, history of DM, hemophilia, lipid disorder, and possible drug interactions. Perform clinical chemistry tests (eg, triglycerides and cholesterol levels), viral load, and CD4 count prior to therapy.

**Monitoring:** Periodically monitor triglyceride levels, viral load, CD4 count, and other relevant clinical chemistry tests. Monitor for signs/symptoms of hyperlipidemia, spontaneous bleeding, immune reconstitution syndrome, fat redistribution/accumulation, hyperglycemia, infections, hepatic/renal function. May enroll patients in the Antiretroviral Pregnancy Registry if they become pregnant while on treatment.

**Patient Counseling:** Inform that the drug is not a cure for HIV and that they may continue to acquire illness associated with advanced HIV infection, including opportunistic infections. Advise to report use of other Rx, OTC, or herbal products (eg, St. John's wort). Infom that drug therapy has not been shown to reduce the isk of transmitting HIV to others through sexual contact or bloo contamination. Instruct to use in combination with ritonavir. Inform that redistribution or accumulation of body fat may occur and long-term effects of these conditions are not known this time. Take drug within 2 hrs of meals; do not alter or d/c therapy without consulting physician. Advise to take medication everyday, as prescribed, to achieve maximum benefit. If dose is missed, take as soon as possible; do not double next dose. Seek medical attention if symptoms of hyperlipidemia, spontaneous bleeding, immune reconstitution syndrome, fat redistribution/accumulation, hyperglycemia, infections, or hepatic/renal dysfunction occur.

**Administration:** Oral route. **Storage:** 25°C (77°F); excursions permitted to 15-30°C (59-86°F). Dispense in tightly closed bottles.

## IQUIX — RX

levofloxacin (Vistakon)

**THERAPEUTIC CLASS:** Fluoroquinolone

**INDICATIONS:** Bacterial corneal ulcer.

**DOSAGE:** *Adults:* Days 1-3: 1-2 drops q30min-2h while awake and 4-6 hrs after retiring. Days 4-completion: 1-2 drops q1-4h while awake.
*Pediatrics:* ≥6 yrs: Days 1-3: 1-2 drops q30min-2h while awake and 4-6 hrs after retiring. Days 4-completion: 1-2 drops q1-4h while awake.

**HOW SUPPLIED:** Sol: 1.5% [5mL]

**WARNINGS/PRECAUTIONS:** D/C if hypersensitivity or superinfection occurs. Avoid contact lenses with corneal ulcer.

**ADVERSE REACTIONS:** Headache, taste disturbance.

**INTERACTIONS:** Systemic quinolone therapy increases theophylline levels, interferes with caffeine metabolism, enhances warfarin effects, and may elevate SrCr with cyclosporine.

**PREGNANCY:** Category C, caution in nursing.

**MECHANISM OF ACTION:** Fluoroquinolone; antibacterial active against a broad spectrum of gram-positive and gram-negative ocular pathogens. Responsible for inhibition of bacterial topoisomerase IV and DNA gyrase, enzymes required for DNA replication, transcription, repair, and recombination.

**PHARMACOKINETICS: Absorption:** $C_{max}$=3.22ng/mL (initial dose), 10.9ng/mL (multiple doses).

## NURSING CONSIDERATIONS

**Assessment:** Assess proper diagnosis (eg, slit lamp biomicroscopy, fluorescein staining), hypersensitivity to other quinolones, and for possible drug interactions. Assess use in pregnant/nursing females.

**Monitoring:** Monitor for signs/symptoms of hypersensitivity or anaphylactic reactions (eg, cardiovascular collapse, loss of consciousness, angioedema, airway obstruction, dyspnea, urticaria, and itching). In patients on prolonged therapy, monitor for overgrowth of non-susceptible organisms (eg, fungi), and for the development of superinfection. Perform periodic monitoring of patient using the aid of magnification (eg, slit-lamp biomicroscopy, fluorescein staining).

**Patient Counseling:** Instruct to avoid contaminating applicator tip with material from the eye, fingers, or other sources. Caution not to wear contact lenses if there are signs/symptoms of a corneal ulcer. Advise to d/c medication and contact physician if any signs/symptoms of a hypersensitivity reaction (eg, rash) develop.

**Administration:** Ocular route. Do not inject subconjunctivally or introduce directly into anterior chamber of eye. **Storage:** 15-25°C (59-77°F).

## ISENTRESS — RX

raltegravir potassium (Merck)

I

**THERAPEUTIC CLASS:** HIV-integrase strand transfer inhibitor

**INDICATIONS:** Use in combination with other antiretroviral agents for treatment of HIV-1 infection in adults.

**DOSAGE:** *Adults:* 400mg bid. Coadministration with Rifampin: 800mg bid. Take with or without food.

**HOW SUPPLIED:** Tab: 400mg

**WARNINGS/PRECAUTIONS:** May develop immune reconstitution syndrome, an inflammatory response to indolent or residual opportunistic infections (eg, *Mycobacterium avium* complex, cytomegalovirus, *Pneumocystis jiroveci* pneumonia, *Mycobacterium* tuberculosis, or reactivation of varicella zoster virus), which may necessitate further evaluation and treatment. Caution in elderly.

**ADVERSE REACTIONS:** Headache, insomnia, neutropenia, hyperglycemia, thrombocytopenia, LFT elevation.

**INTERACTIONS:** Strong inducers of uridine diphosphate glucuronosyltransferase (UGT) 1A1 (eg, rifampin) may reduce plasma levels; dose should be increased. Efavirenz, etravirine, tipranavir/ritonavir combination may reduce plasma concentrations. Drugs that inhibit UGT1A1 (eg, atazanavir, atazanavir/ritonavir) may increase levels of raltegravir. Coadministration with drugs that increase gastric pH (eg, omeprazole) may increase levels. Caution with drugs that causes myopathy or rhabdomyolysis.

**PREGNANCY:** Category C, not for use in nursing.

**MECHANISM OF ACTION:** HIV-1 integrase strand transfer inhibitor; inhibits the catalytic activity of HIV-1 integrase (an HIV-1 encoded enzyme that is required for viral replication) preventing the formation of HIV-1 provirus, resulting in the prevention of propagation of the viral infection.

**PHARMACOKINETICS: Absorption:** $T_{max}$=3 hrs (fasting); variable doses resulted in different parameters. **Distribution:** Plasma protein binding (83%). **Metabolism:** Glucuronidation via UGT1A1. **Elimination:** Urine (32%), feces (51%); $T_{1/2}$=9 hrs.

### NURSING CONSIDERATIONS

**Assessment:** Assess for indolent or residual opportunistic infections, pregnancy/nursing status, and possible drug interactions.

**Monitoring:** Monitor for inflammatory response to indolent or residual opportunistic infections (immune reconstitution syndrome). May enroll patients in the Antiretroviral Pregnancy Registry if they become pregnant while on treatment.

**Patient Counseling:** Inform that therapy is not cure for HIV, does not reduce risk of transmission of HIV and that opportunistic infections may develop. Advise to practice safe sex by using latex or polyurethane condoms, or other barrier methods. If a dose is missed, take as soon as remembered; if not remembered until next dose, instruct to skip missed dose and go back to regular schedule. Do not take two tablets at same time. Instruct patients to read the Patient Package Insert before and during therapy. Advise to report development of unusual symptoms.

**Administration:** Oral route. **Storage:** 20-25°C (68-77°F); excursions permitted to 15-30°C (59-86°F).

## ISONIAZID RX

isoniazid (Various)

**Severe, fatal hepatitis may develop. Monitor LFTs monthly.**

**THERAPEUTIC CLASS:** Isonicotinic acid hydrazide

**INDICATIONS:** Prevention and treatment of TB.

**DOSAGE:** *Adults:* Active TB: 5mg/kg as a single dose. Max: 300mg/day or 15mg/kg 2 to 3 times/week. Max: 900mg/day. Use with other antituberculosis agents. Prevention: 300mg qd single dose.
*Pediatrics:* Active TB: 10-15mg/kg as a single dose. Max: 300mg qd or 20-40mg/kg 2 to 3 times/week. Max: 900mg/day. Use with other antituberculosis agents. Prevention: 10mg/kg qd single dose. Max: 300mg qd.

**HOW SUPPLIED:** Inj: 100mg/mL; Syrup: 50mg/5mL; Tab: 100mg, 300mg

**CONTRAINDICATIONS:** Severe hypersensitivity reactions including drug-induced hepatitis, previous INH-associated hepatic injury, severe adverse effects to INH (eg, drug fever, chills, arthritis), acute liver disease.

**WARNINGS/PRECAUTIONS:** D/C if hypersensitivity occurs. Monitor closely with liver or renal disease. Take with vitamin $B_6$ in malnourished and those predisposed to neuropathy.

**ADVERSE REACTIONS:** Peripheral neuropathy, NV, epigastric distress, elevated serum transaminases, bilirubinemia, jaundice, hepatitis, skin eruptions, pyridoxine deficiency.

**INTERACTIONS:** Alcohol is associated with hepatitis. May increase phenytoin, theophylline, and valproate serum levels. Do not take with food. Severe acetaminophen toxicity reported. Decreases carbamazepine metabolism and AUC of ketoconazole. Avoid tyramine- and histamine-containing foods.

**PREGNANCY:** Category C, caution in nursing.

**MECHANISM OF ACTION:** Inhibits mycoloic acid synthesis and acts against actively growing tuberculosis bacilli.

**PHARMACOKINETICS: Distribution**: Passes through placental barrier and into milk. **Metabolism**: Acetylation and dehydrazination. **Elimination**: Urine (50-70%).

### NURSING CONSIDERATIONS

**Assessment:** Assess for previous isoniazid-associated hepatic injury, acute liver disease, HIV status, pregnancy status, and drug interactions. Document reasons for therapy, culture and susceptibility.

**Monitoring:** Prior to therapy and periodically thereafter, measure hepatic enzymes (AST, ALT). D/C at first sign of hypersensitivity reaction. Monitor for peripheral neuropathy, convulsions, NV, agranulocytosis, hemolytic anemia, SLE-like syndrome, metabolic and endocrine reactions (hyperglycemia, pyridoxine deficiency, pellagra).

**Patient Counseling:** Immediately report signs/symptoms consistent with liver damage or other adverse events (unexplained anorexia, NV, dark urine, icterus, rash, persistent paresthesias of the hands and feet, persistent fatigue, weakness or fever of >3 days duration, and/or abdominal tenderness). Drug should not be taken with food; take as prescribed. Take pyridoxine tablets if peripheral neuropathy develops.

**Administration:** Oral and IM route. **Storage**: Store tab at 20-25°C (68-77°F) and syr at 15-30°C (59-86°F). Protect from light and moisture. Dispense in tight, light-resistant container with child-resistant closure. Store inj at 20-25°C (68-77°F). Protect from light. If vial contents crystallize, warm vial to room temperature to redissolve crystals before use.

## ISOSORBIDE DINITRATE RX
isosorbide dinitrate (Various)

**OTHER BRAND NAMES:** Isordil (Biovail) - Isordil Titradose (Biovail)

**THERAPEUTIC CLASS:** Nitrate vasodilator

**INDICATIONS:** Prevention of angina pectoris due to coronary artery disease.

**DOSAGE:** *Adults:* Prevention: Initial: 5-20mg bid-tid. Maint: 10-40mg bid-tid. Allow a dose-free interval of at least 14 hrs for both formulations. Elderly: Start at low end of dosing range.

**HOW SUPPLIED:** Tab: 5mg*, 10mg*, 20mg*, 30mg*; Tab, Extended-Release: 40mg; Tab, Sublingual: 2.5mg *scored

**WARNINGS/PRECAUTIONS:** Not for use with acute MI or CHF. Severe hypotension may occur. May aggravate angina caused by hypertrophic cardiomyopathy. Caution with volume depletion, hypotension, elderly. Monitor for tolerance.

I

**ADVERSE REACTIONS:** Headache, lightheadedness, hypotension, syncope, rebound HTN.

**INTERACTIONS:** Severe hypotension with sildenafil. Additive vasodilation with other vasodilators (eg, alcohol).

**PREGNANCY:** Category C, caution in nursing.

**MECHANISM OF ACTION:** Nitrate vasodilator; relaxes vascular smooth muscle, dilates peripheral arteries and veins, especially the latter. Dilatation of veins reduces left ventricular end diastolic pressure and pulmonary capillary wedge pressure (preload). Arteriolar relaxation reduces systemic vascular resistance, systolic arterial pressure, and mean arterial pressure (afterload). It also dilates the coronary artery.

**PHARMACOKINETICS: Absorption:** $T_{max}$=1 hr. **Distribution:** $V_d$=2-4L/kg. **Metabolism:** Liver; extensive first-pass metabolism; 2-mononitrate, 5-mononitrate (active metabolites). **Elimination:** $T_{1/2}$=5 hrs (5-mononitrate), 2 hrs (2-mononitrate).

### NURSING CONSIDERATIONS

**Assessment:** Assess for severe hypotension, volume-depleted patients, angina caused by hypertrophic cardiomyopathy, alcohol intake, and possible drug interactions.

**Monitoring:** Careful clinical or hemodynamic monitoring for hypotension and tachycardia. Monitor for paradoxical bradycardia, increased angina pectoris, hemodynamic rebound, decreased exercise tolerance, headaches, lightheadedness on standing, manifestation of true physical dependence (chest pain, acute MI) and methemoglobinemia.

**Patient Counseling:** Counsel carefully follow dosing regimen. Inform about headaches (markers of drug activity) and lightheadedness on standing. Avoid alcohol consumption.

**Administration:** Oral route. **Storage:** 25°C (77°F).

## IXEMPRA RX
ixabepilone (Bristol-Myers Squibb)

**Contraindicated in combination with capecitabine in patients with AST/ALT >2.5x ULN or bilirubin >1x ULN due to increased toxicity and neutropenia-related death.**

**THERAPEUTIC CLASS:** Antimicrotubule agent

**INDICATIONS:** In combination with capecitabine for treatment of patients with metastatic or locally advanced breast cancer resistant to treatment with an anthracycline and a taxane, or whose cancer is taxane resistant and for whom further anthracycline therapy is contraindicated. As monotherapy for treatment of metastatic or locally advanced breast cancer in patients whose tumors are resistant or refractory to anthracyclines, taxanes, and capecitabine.

**DOSAGE:** *Adults:* 40mg/m² IV infusion over 3 hrs every 3 weeks. Patients with BSA >2.2m² should be dosed based on 2.2m². Adjust dose based on toxicities (see PI). Patient should not begin a new cycle of treatment unless the neutrophil count is at least 1500 cells/min³, the platelet count is at least 100,000 cell/mm³, and nonhematologic toxicities have improved to grade 1 (mild) or resolved. Hepatic Impairment: Combination Therapy: AST or ALT ≤2.5x ULN and Bilirubin ≤1x ULN: 40mg/m². Monotherapy: Mild: AST and ALT ≤2.5x ULN and Bilirubin ≤1x ULN: 40mg/m². AST or ALT ≤10x ULN and Bilirubin ≤1.5x ULN: 32mg/m². Moderate (AST and ALT ≤10x ULN and Bilirubin >1.5 to ≤3x ULN): 20-30mg/m². Strong CYP3A4 Inhibitors: Avoid or reduce dose to 20mg/m². Premedicate all patients with $H_1$-antagonist (eg, diphenhydramine 50mg PO) and $H_2$-antagonist (eg, ranitidine 150-300mg PO) approximately 1 hr before infusion. Premedicate with corticosteroids (eg, dexamethasone 20mg, IV 30 min before infusion or PO 60 min before infusion) if prior hypersensitivity reaction experienced.

**HOW SUPPLIED:** Inj: 15mg, 45mg

I

**CONTRAINDICATIONS:** Neutrophil count <1500 cells/mm³ or platelet count <100,000 cells/mm³. In combination with capecitabine patients with AST or ALT >2.5x ULN or bilirubin >1x ULN. History of severe (CTC Grade 3/4) hypersensitivity reaction to Cremophor EL or derivatives (eg, polyoxyethylated castor oil).

**WARNINGS/PRECAUTIONS:** Peripheral neuropathy may occur; monitor for symptoms and manage by dose adjustment, dose delays or d/c. Caution with DM or pre-existing peripheral neuropathy. Myelosuppression, primarily neutropenia, may occur and is dose-dependent; monitor with frequent peripheral blood cell counts and adjust dose as needed. Hypersensitivity reactions may occur; premedicate all patients with $H_1$- and $H_2$-antagonists 1 hr before treatment; d/c and institute aggressive supportive treatment if hypersensitivity occurs. May cause fetal harm; avoid during pregnancy. Caution with history of cardiac disease. D/C if cardiac ischemia or impaired cardiac function develops. Caution with hepatic impairment in monotherapy treated patients; avoid therapy if AST or ALT >10x ULN or bilirubin >3x ULN and use caution if AST or ALT >5x ULN. Potential cognitive impairment may occur from excipients (eg, dehydrated alcohol USP).

**ADVERSE REACTIONS:** Peripheral neuropathy, fatigue/asthenia, myalgia/arthralgia, alopecia, N/V, stomatitis/mucositis, diarrhea, musculoskeletal pain, palmar-plantar erythrodysesthesia (hand-foot) syndrome, anorexia, abdominal pain, nail disorder, hepatic toxicity, neutropenia.

**INTERACTIONS:** CYP3A4 inhibitors may increase levels; avoid or reduce dose with strong CYP3A4 inhibitors (eg, ketoconazole, itraconazole, clarithromycin, atazanavir, nefazodone, saquinavir, telithromycin, ritonavir, amprenavir, indinavir, nelfinavir, delavirdine, voriconazole, grapefruit juice); use caution with mild/moderate CYP3A4 inhibitors (eg, erythromycin, fluconazole, verapamil), and monitor all patients closely for acute toxicities. Strong CYP3A4 inducers (eg, dexamethasone, phenytoin, carbamazepine, rifampin, rifampicin, rifabutin, phenobarbital) may decrease levels; consider alternative agents. St. John's wort may decrease levels and should be avoided.

**PREGNANCY:** Category D, not for use in nursing.

**MECHANISM OF ACTION:** Microtubule inhibitor; binds directly to β-tubulin subunits on microtubules, leading to suppression of microtubule dynamics. Blocks the mitotic phase of cell division, leading to cell death.

**PHARMACOKINETICS: Absorption:** $C_{max}$=252ng/mL; $T_{max}$=3 hrs; AUC=2143ng•hr/mL. **Distribution:** $V_d$= >1000L. **Metabolism:** Liver (oxidation) via CYP3A4. **Elimination:** Urine (21%, 5.6% unchanged), feces (65%, 1.6% unchanged); $T_{1/2}$=52 hrs.

## NURSING CONSIDERATIONS

**Assessment:** Assess for hypersensitivity to Cremophor EL or polyoxyethylated castor oil, DM, preexisting peripheral neuropathy, history of cardiac disease, renal dysfunction, hepatic impairment, pregnancy/nursing status, and possible drug interactions. Obtain baseline LFTs and peripheral blood cell count.

**Monitoring:** Monitor LFTs and peripheral blood cell count periodically. Monitor for signs/symptoms of neuropathy, myelosuppression, fever/neutropenia, cardiac adverse reactions, hepatic toxicity, and hypersensitivity reactions.

**Patient Counseling:** Advise to seek medical attention if symptoms of peripheral neuropathy (eg, numbness, tingling in hands or feet), fever/neutropenia (eg, chills, cough, burning or pain urinating), hypersensitivity reaction (eg, urticaria, pruritus, rash, flushing, swelling, chest tightness, dyspnea), or cardiac events (eg, chest pain, difficulty breathing, palpitations, unusual weight gain) occur. Instruct to avoid grapefruit juice. Inform of pregnancy/nursing risks; advise to use effective contraceptive methods and not to nurse.

**Administration:** IV infusion. Refer to PI for proper instructions of preparation and administration. **Storage**: 2-8°C (36-46°F). Protect from light. (Constituted) Store for maximum 1 hr at room temperature and room light. (Diluted) Stable at room temperature and room light for maximum of 6 hrs.

## JANUMET RX

metformin HCl - sitagliptin (Merck)

**Lactic acidosis may occur due to metformin accumulation; risk increases with conditions such as sepsis, dehydration, excess alcohol intake, hepatic insufficiency, renal impairment, and acute congestive heart failure (CHF). May present with nonspecific symptoms and cause low pH, increased anion gap, and elevated blood lactate. If suspected, d/c drug and hospitalize patient immediately.**

**THERAPEUTIC CLASS:** Dipeptidyl peptidase-4 inhibitor/biguanide

**INDICATIONS:** Adjunct to diet and exercise to improve glycemic control in adult patients with type 2 diabetes mellitus (DM).

**DOSAGE:** *Adults:* Individualize dosing. Inadequate Control with Metformin Monotherapy: Initial: 100mg/day (50mg bid) of sitagliptin and current metformin dose. For patients on metformin 850mg BID, start with 50mg-1000mg bid. Inadequate Control with Sitagliptin Monotherapy or with Diet and Exercise: Initial: 50mg-500mg bid. Titrate: Gradual increase to 50mg-1000mg bid. Max: 100mg sitagliptin and 2000mg metformin. Switching from Coadministration of Sitagliptin/Metformin: Initiate dose of sitagliptin/metformin already being taken. Take with meals.

**HOW SUPPLIED:** Tab: (Metformin-Sitagliptin) 500mg-50mg, 1000mg-50mg

**CONTRAINDICATIONS:** Renal disease (SrCr ≥1.5mg/dL [males], ≥1.4mg/dL [females], or abnormal CrCl), metabolic acidosis (eg, diabetic ketoacidosis).

**WARNINGS/PRECAUTIONS:** Assess renal function prior to initiation and during treatment. Avoid with renal/hepatic impairment. May decrease vitamin $B_{12}$ levels; monitor hematologic parameters. May cause hypoglycemia in elderly, debilitated/malnourished, adrenal/pituitary insufficiency, or alcohol intoxication. D/C in hypoxic states (eg, CHF, shock, acute MI), prior to surgical procedures (due to restricted food and fluid intake), and procedures requiring use of intravascular iodinated contrast materials.

**ADVERSE REACTIONS:** (Metformin) Diarrhea, NV, flatulence, abdominal pain/discomfort, indigestion, asthenia, headache, upper respiratory tract infection. (Sitagliptin) Nasopharyngitis, angioedema, cutaneous vasculitis, exfoliative skin conditions, pancreatitis, hepatic enzyme elevation.

**INTERACTIONS:** Monitor with digoxin. (Metformin) Furosemide, nifedipine, and cationic drugs (eg, digoxin, amiloride, procainamide, quinidine, quinine, ranitidine, trimethoprim, vancomycin, triamterene, morphine) may increase levels. Thiazides and other diuretics, corticosteroids, phenothiazines, thyroid products, estrogens, oral contraceptives, phenytoin, nicotinic acid, sympathomimetics, calcium channel blockers, and isoniazid may cause hyperglycemia. Alcohol may potentiate effect on lactate metabolism. May decrease furosemide levels. (Sitagliptin) May cause hypoglycemia with insulin secretagogues (eg, sulfonylurea, meglitinide); may require dose adjustment of insulin secretagogue.

**PREGNANCY:** Category B, caution in nursing.

**MECHANISM OF ACTION:** Sitagliptin: Dipeptidyl peptidase-4 inhibitor; acts by slowing the inactivation of incretin hormones. Metformin: Biguanide; decreases hepatic glucose production, decreases intestinal absorption of glucose, and improves insulin selectivity by increasing peripheral glucose uptake and utilization.

**PHARMACOKINETICS: Absorption**: Sitagliptin: Absolute bioavailability (87%). Metformin: Absolute bioavailability (50-60%). **Distribution**: Sitagliptin: $V_d$=198L; plasma protein binding (38%). Metformin: $V_d$=654L; plasma protein binding (>90%) . **Metabolism:** Sitagliptin: CYP3A4 and CYP2C8. **Elimination**: Sitagliptin: Feces (13%), urine (87%); $T_{1/2}$=12.4 hrs. Metformin: Urine (90%); $T_{1/2}$=6.2 hrs (plasma), 17.6 hrs (blood).

## NURSING CONSIDERATIONS

**Assessment:** Assess fasting plasma glucose (FPG), $HbA_{1c}$ levels, renal function, LFTs, CBC, and type 1 DM. Assess for CHF, septicemia, acute or chronic metabolic acidosis, adrenal or pituitary insufficiency, alcoholism, pregnancy status. Evaluate for other medical/surgical conditions and for possible drug interactions.

**Monitoring:** Monitor for hypoglycemia, lactic acidosis, prerenal azotemia, CHF, CV disease, hypersensitivity reactions (eg, anaphylaxis), angioedema, exfoliative skin conditions (eg, Stevens-Johnson syndrome). Check FPG, $HbA_{1c}$, CBC, renal function, and LFTs periodically.

**Patient Counseling:** Inform that drug is adjunct to diet and exercise and to take with meals. Advise that excessive alcohol intake increases the risk of hypoglycemia and lactic acidosis. Report unexplained hyperventilation, myalgia, malaise, NV, and somnolence. Counsel about adverse effects and to seek medical attention if any develop. Advise on the importance of adherence to dietary instructions, regular exercise, periodic blood glucose monitoring, $A_{1C}$ testing, recognition/management of hypoglycemia/hyperglycemia, and assessment of diabetic complications. Instruct to seek medical opinion during periods of stress (eg, fever, trauma, infection, surgery) as medication needs may change.

**Administration:** Oral route. **Storage:** 20-25°C (68-77°F); excursions permitted to 15-30°C (59-86°F).

# JANUVIA — RX

sitagliptin (Merck)

**THERAPEUTIC CLASS:** Dipeptidyl peptidase-4 inhibitor

**INDICATIONS:** Adjunct to diet and exercise to improve glycemic control in patients with type 2 diabetes mellitus (DM).

**DOSAGE:** *Adults:* 100mg qd. CrCl ≥30 to <50mL/min: 50mg qd. End-stage renal disease/CrCl: <30mL/min: 25mg qd.

**HOW SUPPLIED:** Tab: 25mg, 50mg, 100mg

**WARNINGS/PRECAUTIONS:** Assess renal function prior to initiation of treatment. Hypersensitivity reactions including anaphylaxis, angioedema, and exfoliative skin conditions reported. Caution in the elderly; evaluate renal function.

**ADVERSE REACTIONS:** Upper respiratory tract infection, nasopharyngitis, headache, hypoglycemia, diarrhea, anaphylaxis, angioedema, rash, urticaria, cutaneous vasculitis, exfoliative skin conditions, hepatic enzyme elevation, pancreatitis.

**INTERACTIONS:** May slightly increase digoxin levels; monitor appropriately. May require lower dose of sulfonylurea to reduce risk of hypoglycemia when used in combination.

**PREGNANCY:** Category B, caution in nursing.

**MECHANISM OF ACTION:** Dipeptidyl peptidase-4 inhibitor; suspected to exert action by slowing the inactivation of incretin hormones.

**PHARMACOKINETICS: Absorption:** Rapidly absorbed; absolute bioavailability (87%); $T_{max}$=1-4 hrs; AUC=8.52μM•hr; $C_{max}$=950nM. **Distribution:** $V_d$=198L; plasma protein binding (38%). **Metabolism:** Via CYP3A4 and CYP2C8 (minor). **Elimination:** Feces (13%), urine (87%, 79% unchanged); $T_{1/2}$=12.4 hrs.

## NURSING CONSIDERATIONS

**Assessment:** Assess fasting plasma glucose (FPG), $HbA_{1c}$ levels, renal function, pregnancy status, type 1 DM. Evaluate for other medical/surgical conditions and for possible drug interactions.

**Monitoring:** Monitor FPG, $HbA_{1c}$, renal function. Monitor for diabetic ketoacidosis, infection, nasopharyngitis, and hypersensitivity reactions (eg, anaphylaxis, angioedema, exfoliative skin conditions, including Stevens-Johnson syndrome).

**Patient Counseling:** Inform that therapy is an adjunct to diet and exercise. Counsel about adverse effects. Advise on the importance of adherence to dietary instructions, regular exercise, periodic blood glucose monitoring, A1C testing, recognition/management of hypoglycemia/hyperglycemia, and assessment of diabetic complications. Instruct to seek medical opinion during periods of stress (eg, fever, trauma, infection, surgery) as medication needs may change.

**Administration:** Oral route. **Storage:** 20-25°C (68-77°F); excursions permitted to 15-30°C (59-86°F).



# KADIAN

**CII**

morphine sulfate (Actavis)

**Contains morphine sulfate, an opioid agonist and Schedule II controlled substance, with an abuse liability similar to other opioid analgesics. Indicated for management of moderate-to-severe pain when a continuous, around-the-clock opioid analgesic is needed for an extended period of time. Not for use as a prn analgesic. The 100mg and 200mg capsules are for use in opioid-tolerant patients only. Swallow capsules whole or sprinkle contents on applesauce. Do not crush, chew, or dissolve pellets in capsules.**

**THERAPEUTIC CLASS:** Opioid analgesic

**INDICATIONS:** Management of moderate to severe pain when continuous around-the-clock opioid analgesia is needed.

**DOSAGE:** *Adults:* Individualize dose. Not for initial opioid analgesic; it is advisable to begin treatment using IR formulation. Conversion from Other Oral Morphine: Give 50% of daily oral morphine dose q12h or give 100% oral morphine dose q24h. Do not give more frequently than q12h. Conversion from Parenteral Morphine: Oral morphine 3x the daily parenteral morphine dose may be sufficient in chronic-use settings. Conversion from Other Parenteral or Oral Opioids: Initial: Give 50% of estimated daily morphine demand and supplement with IR morphine. 1st dose may be taken with the last dose of any IR morphine. Conversion from Other Non-Opioids and Intermittent Use of Moderate or Strong Opioids: Give 50% (of estimated total daily oral morphine dose) q12h or q24h. Titrate: No more frequently than qod to stabilize before escalating the dose. Breakthrough Pain: Give < 20% of daily dose of short acting analgesic. Switch to bid dosing after excessive sedation to qd dosing or inadequate analgesia before next dose. Opioid Non-Tolerant: Should only be started on 10-20mg. Titrate: Increase not >20mg qod. May sprinkle contents on small amount of applesauce or in water for gastrostomy tube (see PI for complete instructions). Do not chew, crush or dissolve pellets. Do not administer through NG-tube. Elderly: Start at low end of dosing range.

**HOW SUPPLIED:** Cap, Extended-Release: 10mg, 20mg, 30mg, 50mg, 60mg, 80mg, 100mg, 200mg

**CONTRAINDICATIONS:** Respiratory depression in the absence of resuscitative equipment, acute or severe bronchial asthma or hypercarbia, paralytic ileus.

**WARNINGS/PRECAUTIONS:** Do not administer pre-op for the management of post-op pain in patients not previously taking the drug. Respiratory depression possible; caution in COPD, cor pulmonale, decreased respiratory reserve. May obscure neurologic signs in head injuries, intracranial lesions, or a pre-existing increase in ICP. May cause severe hypotension. Avoid with GI obstruction. Caution in biliary tract disease (including pancreatitis), elderly, debilitated, renal/hepatic insufficiency, Addison's disease, myxedema, hypothyroidism, prostatic hypertrophy, urethral stricture, CNS depression, toxic psychosis, acute alcoholism, delirium tremens, kyphoscoliosis, inability to swallow and convulsive disorders. May impair mental/physical abilities. Depresses cough reflex. Decreases gastric, biliary, and pancreatic secretions. D/C 24 hrs before procedure that interrupts pain transmission pathways (eg, cordotomy); give short-acting parenteral opioid.

**ADVERSE REACTIONS:** Drowsiness, dizziness, constipation, nausea, anxiety.

**INTERACTIONS:** Increased risk of respiratory depression, hypotension, profound sedation or coma with CNS depressants (eg, sedatives, hypnotics, general anesthetics, antiemetics, phenothiazines, tranquilizers, alcohol); reduce initial dose of one or both agents by 50%. May enhance neuromuscular blocking action of skeletal relaxants. Mixed agonist/antagonist analgesics may reduce analgesic effects or precipitate withdrawal symptoms. Avoid MAOIs during or within 14 days of use. May reduce diuretic effects. Avoid concomitant use with cimetidine; confusion and severe respiratory depression reported.

**PREGNANCY:** Category C, not for use in nursing.

**MECHANISM OF ACTION:** Opioid analgesic; principal actions are analgesia and sedation. Precise mechanism of analgesic effects not established. Acts as a pure agonist, binding with and activating opioid receptors at sites in the peri-aqueductal and periventricular gray matter, the ventromedial medulla, and the spinal cord to produce analgesia.

**PHARMACOKINETICS: Absorption:** Various doses resulted in different parameters. **Distribution:** $V_d$=3-4 L/kg; plasma protein binding (30-35%); distributed to skeletal muscle, kidneys, liver, intestinal tract, lungs, spleen, brain; crosses the blood brain barrier (small amount); crosses placental membranes; found in breast milk. **Metabolism:** Liver (conjugation) to glucuronide metabolites; morphine-3-glucuronide, morphine-6-glucuronide. **Elimination:** Urine (10% unchanged); bile (small amount); feces (7-10%); $T_{1/2}$=2-4 hrs.

## NURSING CONSIDERATIONS

**Assessment:** Assess for opioid tolerance, pain levels, abuse potential, severe bronchial asthma, COPD, circulatory shock, GI obstruction (paralytic ileus), presence of debilitation (elderly), hepatic/renal impairment, presence of head injury or other intracranial lesions, increased intracranial pressure, adrenocortical insufficiency (eg, Addison's disease), CNS depression or coma, toxic psychosis, prostatic hypertrophy or urtheral stricture, acute alcoholism, delirium tremens, kyphoscoliosis, convulsive disorders, biliary tract disease (acute pancreatitis), pregnancy/nursing status, and drug interactions.

**Monitoring:** Monitor for signs/symptoms of respiratory depression, hypotension, anaphylaxis, convulsions, tolerance and physical dependence (eg, withdrawal symptoms), and signs of medication misuse or abuse. Monitor serum amylase levels.

**Patient Counseling:** Swallow medication whole (do not chew, crush, or dissolve) or open and sprinkle contents of capsule on small amount of applesauce (at room temperature or cooler). Instruct to rinse mouth after taking dose to ensure all pellets have been swallowed. Capsule may be administered through a French 16 gastrostomy tube if there is difficulty swallowing. Do not adjust dosing without physician's consent. Inform drug may impair mental/physical abilities; use caution when performing hazardous tasks (eg, operating machinery/driving). Avoid alcohol and other CNS depressants. Do not abruptly d/c medication. May develop severe constipation during therapy; appropriate concomitant therapy should be given at start of treatment. Medication has potential for abuse. Instruct to keep out of reach of children. If treatment is complete, dispose unused capsules via toilet.

**Administration:** Oral route. **Storage:** 25°C (77°F); excursions permitted to 15-30°C (59-86°F). Protect from light and moisture. Dispense in a sealed tamper-evident, childproof, light-resistant container.

## KALBITOR RX

ecallantide (Dyax Corp.)

**Anaphylaxis reported. Should be administered only by a healthcare professional with appropriate medical support. Healthcare professionals should be aware of the similarity of symptoms between hypersensitivity and HAE; monitor closely.**

**THERAPEUTIC CLASS:** Plasma kallikrein inhibitor

**INDICATIONS:** Treatment of acute attacks of hereditary angioedema (HAE) in patients ≥16 yrs.

**DOSAGE:** *Adults:* Usual: 30mg (3mL) SQ. If attack persists, additional 30mg may be administered within a 24hr period. Elderly: Start at low end of dosing range.

*Pediatrics:* ≥16 yrs: Usual: 30mg (3mL) SQ. If attack persists, additional 30mg may be administered within 24hr period.

**HOW SUPPLIED:** Inj: 10mg/mL

**WARNINGS/PRECAUTIONS:** Serious hypersensitivity reactions (eg, chest discomfort, flushing, pharyngeal edema, pruritus, rhinorrhea, sneezing, nasal congestion, throat irritation, urticaria, wheezing, and hypotension) including anaphylaxis may occur within the first hour after dosing. Caution in elderly.

K

**ADVERSE REACTIONS:** Anaphylaxis, headache, NV, fatigue, diarrhea, upper respiratory tract infection, injection-site reactions, nasopharyngitis, pruritus, upper abdominal pain, pyrexia, immunogenicity.

**PREGNANCY:** Category C, caution in nursing.

**MECHANISM OF ACTION:** Human plasma kallikrein inhibitor; binds to plasma kallikrein and blocks the binding site, inhibiting the conversion of HMW kininogen to bradykinin.

**PHARMACOKINETICS: Absorption:** $C_{max}$=586ng/mL; $T_{max}$=2-3 hrs; AUC=3017ng•hr/mL. **Distribution**: $V_d$= 26.4L. **Elimination:** $T_{1/2}$=2 hrs.

### NURSING CONSIDERATIONS

**Assessment:** Assess HAE and hypersensitivity reactions, and pregnancy/nursing status.

**Monitoring:** Monitor for anaphylaxis and hypersensitivity reactions such as chest discomfort, flushing, pharyngeal edema, pruritus, rhinorrhea, sneezing, nasal congestion, throat irritation, urticaria, wheezing, and hypotension.

**Patient Counseling:** Advise that it may cause anaphylaxis and other hypersensitivity reactions and must be administered by a healthcare professional with appropriate medical support to manage the reactions. Instruct patients not to receive additional doses with known hypersensitivity to the drug. Advise to consult Medication Guide for additional information regarding the risk of anaphylaxis and other hypersensitivity reactions.

**Administration:** SQ route.Refer to PI for preparation and handling/detailed reconstitution and administration information. **Storage:** 2°-8°C (36-46°F). Vials removed from refrigeration: store below 30°C (86°F) and use within 14 days or return to refrigeration until use. Protect from light.

## KALETRA RX

ritonavir - lopinavir (Abbott)

**THERAPEUTIC CLASS:** Protease inhibitor

**INDICATIONS:** Treatment of HIV infection in combination with other antiretrovirals.

**DOSAGE:** *Adults:* Therapy-Naive: 400/100mg (2 tabs or 5mL) bid or 800/200mg qd (4 tabs or 10mL). Therapy-Experienced: 400/100mg (2 tabs or 5mL) bid. Concomitant Therapy With Efavirenz, Nevirapine, (Fos)amprenavir, Nelfinavir: 500/125mg (2 tabs 200/50mg-1 tab 100/25mg) bid or 533/133mg (6.5mL) bid.
*Pediatrics:* 14 days-6 months: 16/4mg/kg or 300/75mg/$m^2$ bid.
6 months-18 yrs: 230/57.5mg/$m^2$ bid. <15 kg: 12/3mg/kg bid. ≥15-40kg: 10/2.5mg/kg bid. 15-25kg: 200/50mg (2 tabs 100/25 mg) bid. >25-35kg: 300/75mg (3 tabs 100/25 mg) bid. >35kg: 400/100mg (2 tabs 200/50 mg) bid. Concomitant Therapy With Efavirenz, Nevirapine, (Fos)amprenavir, or Nelfinavir: Treatment-Naive and Treatment-Experienced: <15kg: 13/3.25mg/kg bid. ≥15-45kg: 11/2.75mg/kg bid. 15-20kg: 200/50mg (2 tabs 100/25 mg) bid. >20-30kg: 300/75mg (3 tabs 100/25 mg) bid. >30-45 kg: 400/100mg (4 tabs 100/25 mg or 2 tabs 200/50 mg) bid.

**HOW SUPPLIED:** Tab: (Lopinavir-Ritonavir) 200mg-50mg, 100mg-25mg; Sol: 80mg-20mg/mL [160mL]

**CONTRAINDICATIONS:** Concomitant intake of drugs that induce or are highly dependent on CYP3A for metabolism (eg, rifampin, St. John's wort, lovastatin, simvastatin, ergot derivatives, cisapride, pimozide, midazolam, triazolam). Coadministration with CYP3A inducers may significantly reduce lopinavir levels and result in potential loss of virologic response and HIV resistance; coadministration with drugs metabolized extensively by CYP3A may result in serious/life-threatening reactions.



**WARNINGS/PRECAUTIONS:** May elevate TG and total cholesterol levels; monitor levels at baseline then periodically. Possible redistribution/accumulation of body fat. D/C if symptoms of pancreatitis occur. May exacerbate diabetes mellitus (DM) or cause hyperglycemia. Caution in hepatic impairment. Risk of further transaminase elevation or hepatic decompensation in patients with underlying hepatitis B or C or marked transaminase elevation prior to treatment; monitor ALT/AST more frequently during first several months of therapy. Hepatic dysfunction reported. Increased bleeding may occur with hemophilia A and B. Prolonged PR interval may occur; caution with underlying structural heart disease, pre-existing conduction system abnormalities, ischemic heart disease or cardiomyopathies. Increased risk for developing cardiac conduction abnormalities reported. Avoid use in patients with congenital long QT syndrome, hypokalemia, and with other drugs that prolong QT interval. Immune reconstitution syndrome reported with combination therapy. Caution in elderly.

**ADVERSE REACTIONS:** Asthenia, diarrhea, N/V, dysgeusia, hepatotoxicity, pancreatitis.

**INTERACTIONS:** See Contraindications. CYP3A inhibitors may increase lopinavir (LPV) levels. May increase levels of antiarrhythmics (eg, amiodarone, bepridil, systemic lidocaine, quinidine), dihydropyridine CCBs (eg, felodipine, nifedipine, nicardipine), immunosuppressants (eg, cyclosporine, tacrolimus, rapamycin); monitoring recommended. May increase levels of trazodone; use with caution and consider dose reduction. May increase levels of fluticasone; coadministration not recommended. May increase levels of amprenavir, indinavir, saquinavir. May increase levels of clarithromycin with renal impairment; reduce clarithromycin dose by 50% if CrCl 30-60mL/min and by 75% if CrCl <30mL/min. Decreased effect with dexamethasone, carbamazepine, phenobarbital, phenytoin. Monitor PT/INR with warfarin. Space dosing with didanosine; give 1 hr before or 2 hrs after LPV/ritonavir (RTV). Increased levels with delavirdine. Efavirenz, nevirapine, and tipranavir may decrease levels; adjust dose. May increase levels of ketoconazole or itraconazole; avoid ketoconazole or itraconazole doses >200mg/day. May increase rifabutin levels; reduce usual rifabutin dose by 75%. Decreases atovaquone levels. Oral solution contains alcohol; disulfiram-like reaction may occur with disulfiram or metronidazole. May increase sildenafil, tadalafil, vardenafil levels; reduce dose of sildenafil (eg, 25mg q48h); reduce dose of tadalafil (eg, 10mg q72h); reduce dose of vardenafil (eg, 2.5mg q72h). May decrease methadone levels; may need to increase methadone dose. May decrease ethinyl estradiol levels; alternative contraception is recommended. Increased atorvastatin levels; use lowest atorvastatin or rosuvastatin dose or consider alternate HMG-CoA reductase inhibitors (eg, pravastatin, fluvastatin). Increases tenofovir levels. May increase nelfinavir levels; dosage adjustments needed. Do not administer with tipranivir coadministered with RTV.

**PREGNANCY:** Category C, not for use in nursing.

**MECHANISM OF ACTION:** Lopinavir: HIV-1 protease inhibitor; prevents cleavage of the Gag-Pol polyprotein, resulting in the production of immature, noninfectious viral particles. Ritonavir: CYP3A inhibitor; inhibits metabolism of lopinavir, increasing its plasma levels.

**PHARMACOKINETICS: Absorption:** Lopinavir: $C_{max}$=9.8mcg/mL, $T_{max}$=4 hrs, AUC=92.6mcg•h/mL. **Distribution:** Lopinavir: Plasma protein binding (98-99%). **Metabolism:** Lopinavir: Hepatic via CYP3A. Ritonavir: Induces own metabolism. **Elimination:** Urine (2.2%), feces (19.8%).

## NURSING CONSIDERATIONS

**Assessment:** Assess for hepatitis B or C, DM or hyperglycemia, hemophilia type A or B, CV diseases, renal/hepatic impairment, history of pancreatitis, pregnancy/nursing status, and possible drug interactions.

**Monitoring:** Monitor LFTs, lipid profile, glucose, total bilirubin, serum lipase and amylase. Monitor for signs/symptoms of pancreatitis, hyperglycemia, hepatoxicity, infections, and fat redistribution.

**Patient Counseling:** Instruct that tablet may be taken with/without food, swallowed whole and solution must be taken with food. If missed dose, take dose as soon as possible and return to normal schedule; do not double next dose. Seek medical attention if symptoms of pancreatitis (N/V, abdominal pain), hyperglycemia, or fat redistribution occur.

K

**Administration:** Oral route. **Storage:** (Tab): 20-25°C (68-77°F); excursions permitted to 15-30°C (59-86°F). (Sol): 2-8°C (36-46°F). Avoid exposure to excessive heat. If stored at 25°C (77°F), solution should be used within 2 months.

# KAPIDEX — RX

dexlansoprazole (Takeda)

**THERAPEUTIC CLASS:** Proton pump inhibitor

**INDICATIONS:** Healing of all grades of erosive esophagitis (EE) for up to 8 weeks. Maintain healing of EE for up to 6 months. Treatment of heartburn associated with non-erosive gastroesophageal reflux disease (GERD) for 4 weeks.

**DOSAGE:** *Adults:* EE: 60mg qd for up to 8 weeks. Maint: 30mg qd for up to 6 months. Symptomatic Non-Erosive GERD: 30mg qd for 4 weeks. Moderate Hepatic Impairment (Child-Pugh Class B): Max: 30mg qd. Swallow whole or may open cap and sprinkle intact granules on 1 tbsp of applesauce; swallow immediately.

**HOW SUPPLIED:** Cap, Delayed-Release: 30mg, 60mg

**WARNINGS/PRECAUTIONS:** Symptomatic response does not preclude the presence of gastric malignancy.

**ADVERSE REACTIONS:** Diarrhea, abdominal pain, N/V, upper respiratory tract infection, flatulence.

**INTERACTIONS:** May reduce plasma levels of atazanavir; avoid concurrent use. May interfere with the absorption of other drugs where gastric pH is an important determinant of oral bioavailability (eg, ampicillin esters, digoxin, iron salts, ketoconazole). Concomitant use with warfarin may increase INR and PT; monitor PT and INR. May increase whole blood levels of tacrolimus. $C_{max}$ may increase with food.

**PREGNANCY:** Category B, not for use in nursing.

**MECHANISM OF ACTION:** Proton pump inhibitor; suppressess gastric acid secretion by specific inhibition of the ($H^+$,$K^+$) -ATPase in the gastric parietal cell. By acting specifically on the proton pump, it blocks the final step on acid production.

**PHARMACOKINETICS: Absorption:** $T_{max}$ = 1-2 hrs (1st peak ) and 4-5 hrs (2nd peak). (60mg) $C_{max}$=1397ng/mL, $AUC_{24}$=6529ng•h/mL. (30mg) $C_{max}$=658ng/mL, $AUC_{24}$=3275ng•h/mL. **Distribution:** $V_d$=40.3L; plasma protein binding (96.1%-98.8%). **Metabolism:** Liver (extensive) via CYP3A4 and CYP2C19. **Elimination:** Urine (50.7%) (metabolites), feces (47.6%); $T_{1/2}$=1-2 hrs.

## NURSING CONSIDERATIONS

**Assessment:** Assess for presence of gastric malignancy, hepatic impairment, pregnancy/nursing status, and for possible drug interactions.

**Monitoring:** Monitor for signs and symptoms of hypersensitivity (anaphylaxis) and for hepatic impairment. Monitor LFTs. In patients on warfarin, monitor INR and PT.

**Patient Counseling:** Inform that may swallow capsule whole without regard to food or may open capsule and sprinkle intact granules into one tablespoon of applesauce and swallow immediately. Instruct to notify physician if pregnant or intend to become pregnant, breastfeeding, or have liver problems.

**Administration:** Oral route. **Storage:** Store at 25°C (77°F); excursions permitted to 15-30°C (59-86°F).

# KAYEXALATE RX

sodium polystyrene sulfonate (Sanofi-Aventis)

K

**THERAPEUTIC CLASS:** Cation-exchange resin

**INDICATIONS:** Treatment of hyperkalemia.

**DOSAGE:** *Adults:* PO: 15g qd-qid. Rectal Enema: 30-50g q6h.
*Pediatrics:* Use 1g per 1mEq of $K^+$ as basis of calculation. Avoid PO administration in neonates.

**HOW SUPPLIED:** Powder: 453.6g [Jar]

**CONTRAINDICATIONS:** Hypokalemia, obstructive bowel disease, neonates with reduced gut motility (post-op or drug-induced), oral administration in neonates.

**WARNINGS/PRECAUTIONS:** Cases of colonic necrosis and other serious GI adverse events (eg, bleeding, ischemic colitis, perforation) reported. Hypokalemia may occur. May be insufficient for emergency correction of hyperkalemia. Monitor for electrolyte disturbances. Caution in those intolerant to sodium increases (eg, severe CHF or HTN, or marked edema). Follow full aspiration precautions when administering. Caution in premature infants or low birth weight infants. If clinically significant constipation occurs d/c until normal bowel movement is resumed.

**ADVERSE REACTIONS:** Anorexia, N/V, constipation, hypokalemia, hypocalcemia, sodium retention, diarrhea, fecal impaction, gastric irritation, colonic necrosis, intestinal obstruction.

**INTERACTIONS:** Avoid nonabsorbable cation-donating antacids and laxatives; systemic alkalosis may occur (eg, magnesium hydroxide, aluminum carbonate). Hypokalemia exaggerates toxic effects of digitalis. Intestinal obstruction reported with aluminum hydroxide. May decrease absorption of lithium and thyroxine. Concomitant use with sorbitol has been implicated in cases of colonic necrosis; avoid use.

**PREGNANCY:** Category C, caution in nursing.

**MECHANISM OF ACTION:** Cation exchange resin; partially releases sodium ions and replaced by $K^+$ ions.

## NURSING CONSIDERATIONS

**Assessment:** Assess for hypokalemia, obstructive bowel disease, neonates with reduced gut motility, CHF, HTN, marked edema, prematurity, history of intestinal disease or surgery, hypovolemia, renal insufficiency and failure, pregnancy/nursing status, and for possible drug interactions.

**Monitoring:** Monitor for signs/sympoms of colonic necrosis or other GI events (eg, bleeding, ischemic colitis, perforation), hypokalemia, cardiac arrhythmias, electrolyte disturbances, systemic alkalosis, and constipation. Monitor ECG and serum electrolytes.

**Patient Counseling:** Counsel about potential side effects and advise to seek medical attention if signs/symptoms develop.

**Administration:** Oral/Rectal routes. Follow full aspiration precautions during administration. Refer to PI for administration. **Storage:** 25°C (77°F); excursions permitted to 15-30°C (59-86°F). Suspension should be freshly prepared and not stored beyond 24 hrs.

## K-Dur RX

potassium chloride (Schering)

**THERAPEUTIC CLASS:** $K^+$ supplement

**INDICATIONS:** (For those unable to tolerate liquid or effervescent potassium preparations). Treatment and prevention of hypokalemia with or without metabolic alkalosis. Treatment of digitalis intoxication and hypokalemic familial periodic paralysis.

**DOSAGE:** *Adults:* Prevention: 20mEq/day. Hypokalemia: 40-100mEq/day. Divide dose if >20mEq. Take with meals and a full glass of water or liquid. Tab can be broken in half or dissolved in water.

**HOW SUPPLIED:** Tab, Extended-Release: 10mEq, 20mEq* *scored

K

**CONTRAINDICATIONS:** Hyperkalemia, esophageal ulceration, delay in GI passage (from structural, pathological, pharmacologic causes), cardiac patients with esophageal compression due to enlarged left atrium.

**WARNINGS/PRECAUTIONS:** Potentially fatal hyperkalemia may occur. Extreme caution with acidosis, cardiac and renal disease; monitor ECG and electrolytes. Hypokalemia with metabolic acidosis should be treated with an alkalinizing potassium salt (eg, potassium bicarbonate, potassium citrate). May produce ulcerative or stenotic GI lesions.

**ADVERSE REACTIONS:** Hyperkalemia, GI effects (obstruction, bleeding, ulceration), nausea, vomiting, abdominal pain, flatulence, diarrhea.

**INTERACTIONS:** Risk of hyperkalemia with ACE inhibitors (eg, captopril, enalapril), $K^+$-sparing diuretics and $K^+$ supplements. Contraindicated with anticholinergic agents due to possible delay in tablet passage through GI tract.

**PREGNANCY:** Category C, safe for use in nursing.

**MECHANISM OF ACTION:** $K^+$ supplement (electrolyte replenisher); potassium ions participate in maintenance of intracellular tonicity, transmission of nerve impulses, contraction of cardiac, skeletal, and smooth muscle, and maintenance of normal renal function.

### NURSING CONSIDERATIONS

**Assessment:** Assess for chronic renal disease, conditions which impair $K^+$ excretion, esophageal compression due to enlarged left atrium, structural/pathologic cause for arrest/delay in passing through GI (diabetic gastroparesis), and possible drug interactions. Obtain baseline serum $K^+$ levels and renal function test.

**Monitoring:** Monitor serum $K^+$ levels, renal function, ECG, and acid-base balance. Monitor for hyperkalemia, signs of acute metabolic acidosis, acute dehydration, GI ulcerations, and hypersensitivity reactions.

**Patient Counseling:** Instruct to report symptoms of GI bleeding (tarry stools), ulcerations/perforations (severe vomiting, abdominal pain, distention), trouble swallowing, or tablet sticking in throat. Take with meals and full glass of water; swallow whole, do not crush, chew, or suck. If difficulty swallowing whole tablet; break tablet in half. Take each half separately with glass of water or place whole tab in 1/2 glass of water and allow 2 min to disintegrate, stir for half min after disintegration, swirl suspension and drink content. Add another 1oz of water, swirl, and drink immediately and repeat once more.

**Administration:** Oral route. **Storage:** 25°C (77°F); excursions permitted to 15-30°C (59-86°F). Keep tightly closed.

## KENALOG **RX**

triamcinolone acetonide (Apothecon)

**THERAPEUTIC CLASS:** Corticosteroid

**INDICATIONS:** Corticosteroid responsive dermatoses

**DOSAGE:** *Adults:* (Cre, Lot, Oint) Apply 0.025% bid-qid. Apply 0.1% or 0.5% bid-tid. (Spray) Apply tid-qid. May use occlusive dressings for psoriasis or recalcitrant conditions. D/C dressings if infection develops.

**HOW SUPPLIED:** Cre: 0.1% [15g, 60g, 80g], 0.5% [20g]; Lot: 0.025%, 0.1% [60mL]; Oint: 0.1% [15g, 60g]; Spray: 0.147mg/g [63g]

**WARNINGS/PRECAUTIONS:** May produce reversible HPA axis suppression, manifestations of Cushing's syndrome, hyperglycemia, and glucosuria. D/C if irritation occurs. Pediatric patients may be more susceptible to systemic toxicity. Monitor for HPA suppression if applied to large surface areas or under occlusive dressings. Avoid eyes.

**ADVERSE REACTIONS:** Burning, itching, irritation, dryness, folliculitis, hypertrichosis, acneiform eruptions, hypopigmentation, perioral dermatitis, allergic contact dermatitis.

**PREGNANCY:** Category C, caution in nursing.

**MECHANISM OF ACTION:** Corticosteroid; possesses anti-inflammatory, antipruritic, and vasoconstrictive actions. Anti-inflammatory action not established.

**PHARMACOKINETICS: Absorption:** Percutaneous; inflammation, other disease states, and use of occlusive dressings may increase absorption. **Distribution:** Systemically administered corticosteroids found in breast milk. **Metabolism:** Liver. **Excretion:** Kidneys, bile.

### NURSING CONSIDERATIONS

**Assessment:** Assess pregnancy/nursing status.

**Monitoring:** Monitor for signs/symptoms of reversible HPA-axis suppression, Cushing's syndrome, hyperglycemia, glucosuria, thermal homeostasis impairment, treatment-site irritation, sensitivity reactions, and presence of dermatological infections (eg, fungal, bacterial). Monitor for withdrawal symptoms following d/c of therapy. If applying high doses of medication to large surface area or if using occlusive dressings, monitor for HPA-axis suppression by using urinary free cortisol and ACTH stimulation tests. (Pediatrics) Monitor for signs/symptoms of systemic toxicity, HPA-axis suppression (eg, linear growth retardation, delayed weight gain), Cushing's syndrome, and intracranial HTN.

**Patient Counseling:** Instruct to use externally and exactly as directed; avoid contact with eyes. Counsel not to bandage or wrap treated skin areas unless directed by physician. Advise to report any local adverse reactions. Advise caregivers of pediatric patients to avoid using tight fitting diapers or plastic pants on treatment area.

**Administration:** Topical route. **Storage:** Room temperature; avoid freezing.

## KEPIVANCE **RX**

palifermin (Amgen)

**THERAPEUTIC CLASS:** Keratinocyte growth factor

**INDICATIONS:** To decrease the incidence and duration of severe oral mucositis in patients with hematologic malignancies receiving myelotoxic therapy requiring hematopoietic stem cell support.

**DOSAGE:** *Adults:* 60mcg/kg/day IV bolus 3 consecutive days before and after myelotoxic therapy for a total of 6 doses.

**HOW SUPPLIED:** Inj: 6.25mg

**CONTRAINDICATIONS:** Known hypersensitivity to *E. Coli*-derived proteins.

K

**WARNINGS/PRECAUTIONS:** Potential for stimulation of tumor growth. Safety and efficacy have not been established in patients with nonhematologic malignancies.

**ADVERSE REACTIONS:** Rash, erythema, edema, fever, pruritus, dysesthesia, tongue discoloration, tongue thickening, alteration of taste, pain arthralgias.

**INTERACTIONS:** Do not administer 24 hrs before, during infusion, or 24 hrs after administration of myelotoxic chemotherapy due to risk of increased severity and duration of oral mucositis. May interact with unfractionated as well as low molecular weight heparins; if heparin is used to maintain IV line, use saline to rinse prior to and after administration.

**PREGNANCY:** Category C, caution in nursing.

**MECHANISM OF ACTION:** Keratinocyte growth factor; binds to the KGF receptor, which results in proliferation, differentiation, and migration of the epithelial cells.

**PHARMACOKINETICS: Elimination:** $T_{1/2}$=4.5 hrs.

## NURSING CONSIDERATIONS

**Assessment:** Assess for hypersensitivity to *E. coli*-derived proteins, pregnancy/nursing status, and for possible drug interactions.

**Monitoring:** Monitor for signs and symptoms of tumor growth, hypersensitivity reactions, rash, erythema, edema, pruritis, dysesthesia, tongue discoloration or thickening, taste alterations, and arthralgias.

K

**Patient Counseling:** Counsel about possible adverse effects, including mucocutaneous adverse effects. Instruct to seek medical attention if rash, erythema, edema, pruritus, oral/perioral dysesthesia, tongue discoloration, tongue thickening, or if taste alterations develop. Inform that use may stimulate tumor growth.

**Administration:** IV bolus for 3 consecutive days before and after myelotoxic therapy. **Storage:** Powder: 2-8°C (36-46°F). Reconstituted Sol: 2-8°C (36-46°F) for up to 24 hrs. May be allowed to reach room temperature for a maximum of one hour. Do not freeze. Protect from light.

# KEPPRA RX

levetiracetam (UCB)

**THERAPEUTIC CLASS:** Pyrrolidine derivative

**INDICATIONS:** (PO) Adjunctive therapy for partial onset seizures in adults and children ≥4 yrs. Adjunctive therapy in the treatment of myoclonic seizures in adults and children ≥12 yrs with juvenile myoclonic epilepsy (JME). Adjunctive therapy in the treatment of primary generalized tonic-clonic (PGTC) seizures in adults and children ≥6 yrs with idiopathic generalized epilepsy. (Inj) Alternative for patients ≥16 yrs when oral administration is temporarily not feasable in the adjunctive therapy of partial onset seizures, myoclonic seizures with JME and PGTC with idiopathic generalized epilepsy.

**DOSAGE:** *Adults:* Inj/PO: Initial: 500mg bid. Titrate: Increase by 1000mg/day every 2 weeks. Max: 3000mg/day. Inj: Replacement Therapy: Initial total daily dosage and frequency should equal total daily dosage and frequency of oral therapy. Dilute injection in 100mL of compatible diluent and give as 15-min IV infusion. Switching to PO: switch at equivalent daily dosage and frequency of the IV administration. Individualize dose: CrCl >80mL/min: 500mg-1500mg q12h. CrCl 50-80mL/min: 500mg-1000mg q12h. CrCl 30-50mL/min: 250mg-750mg q12h. CrCl <30mL/min: 250mg-500mg q12h. ESRD with Dialysis: 500-1000mg q24h. A supplemental dose of 250mg-500mg after dialysis is recommended. Elderly: Start at lower end of dosing range.
*Pediatrics:* PO: Partial Onset Seizures/PGTC: ≥16 yrs or Myoclonic Seizures with JME: ≥12 yrs: Initial: 500mg bid. Titrate: Increase by 1000mg/day every 2 weeks. Max: 3000mg/day. Partial Onset Seizures: 4 to <16 yrs or PGTC: 6-16 yrs: Initial: 10mg/kg bid: Titrate: Increase by 20mg/kg/day every 2 weeks. Max: 60mg/kg/day. Use oral sol for patients ≤20kg. (Inj): Partial Onset Seizures/Myoclonic Seizures with JME/PGTC: ≥16 yrs: Initial: 500mg

bid. Titrate: Increase by 1000mg/day every 2 weeks. Max: 3000mg/day. Replacement Therapy: Initial total daily dosage and frequency should equal total daily dosage and frequency of oral therapy. Dilute injection in 100mL of compatible diluent and give as 15-min IV infusion. Switching to PO: switch at equivalent daily dosage and frequency of the IV administration. Individualize dose: CrCl >80mL/min: 500mg-1500mg q12h. CrCl 50-80mL/min: 500mg-1000mg q12h. CrCl 30-50mL/min: 250mg-750mg q12h. CrCl <30mL/min: 250mg-500mg q12h. ESRD with Dialysis: 500mg-1000mg q24h. A supplemental dose of 250mg-500mg after dialysis is recommended.

**HOW SUPPLIED:** Inj: 500mg/5mL; Sol: 100mg/mL; Tab: 250mg*, 500mg*, 750mg*, 1000mg* *scored

**WARNINGS/PRECAUTIONS:** Increased risk of suicidal thoughts or behavior reported; monitor for emergence or worsening of depression, suicidal thoughts/behavior and any unusual changes in mood or behavior. Associated with somnolence, fatigue, coordination difficulties and behavioral abnormalities (eg, psychotic symptoms, suicidal ideation and other abnormalities). Avoid abrupt withdrawal. Hematologic abnormalities reported. May impair physical/mental abilities. Caution with moderate to severe renal impairment and hemodialysis. Caution in elderly.

**ADVERSE REACTIONS:** Somnolence, asthenia, headache, infection, pain, anorexia, dizziness, nervousness, vertigo, ataxia, pharyngitis, rhinitis, irritability, vomiting, diarrhea.

**INTERACTIONS:** (PO) Increased clearance with enzyme-inducing antiepileptic drugs in pediatrics.

**PREGNANCY:** Category C, not for use in nursing.

**MECHANISM OF ACTION:** Pyrrolidine derivative; not established. Proposed to inhibit burst firing without affecting normal neuronal excitability, suggesting that it may selectively prevent hypersynchronization of epileptiform burst firing and propagation of seizure activity.

**PHARMACOKINETICS: Absorption:** Rapid; absolute bioavailability (100%); $T_{max}$=1 hr. **Distribution:** Plasma protein binding (<10%); found in breast milk. **Metabolism:** Enzymatic hydrolysis (not extensive); ucbL057 (metabolite). **Elimination:** Urine (66%, unchanged); $T_{1/2}$=7 hrs.

## NURSING CONSIDERATIONS

**Assessment:** Assess for renal impairment, depression, suicidal thoughts/behavior, pregnancy/nursing status and possible drug interactions prior to therapy.

**Monitoring:** Monitor for CNS adverse effects such as somnolence, fatigue, coordination difficulties (ataxia, incoordination), behavioral abnormalities (agitation, anger, emotional lability), suicide ideation, emergence or worsening of depression, suicidal thoughts/behavior and any unusual changes in mood or behavior. Monitor renal function and hematological changes (RBCs, WBCs).

**Patient Counseling:** Instruct to take drug exactly as directed. Advise not to drive or operate heavy machinery until accustomed to the effects of medication. Monitor for changes in behavior (eg, aggression, anxiety, apathy, depression, irritability), psychotic symptoms and/or suicidal ideation. Notify if pregnant or intend to become pregnant. Encourage patients to enroll in North American Antiepileptic Drug (NAAED) Pregnancy Registry by calling 888-233-2334 or at UCB AED Pregnancy Registry by calling 888-537-7734 or go to aedpregnancyregistry.org.

**Administration:** Oral/IV route. Injection must be diluted prior to administration. Dilute in 100mL of compatible diluent (see PI). **Storage:** 25°C (77°F); excursions permitted to 15-30°C (59-86°F). Following IV dilution: Stable for 24 hrs at controlled room temperature 15-30°C (59-86°F).

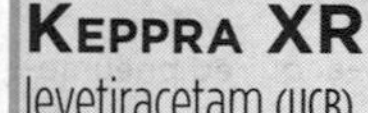

# KEPPRA XR

levetiracetam (UCB)

RX

**THERAPEUTIC CLASS:** Pyrrolidine derivative

**INDICATIONS:** Adjunct therapy for the treatment of partial onset seizures in patients ≥16 years with epilepsy.

**DOSAGE:** *Adults:* Initial: 1000mg qd. Titrate: Dose adjusted in increments of 1000mg q2 weeks. Max: 3000mg. CrCl >80mL/min: 1000-3000mg q24h. CrCl 50-80mL/min: 1000-2000mg q24h. CrCl 30-50mL/min: 500-1500mg q24h. CrCl <30mL/min: 500-1000 q24h. Elderly: Start at the lower end of dosing range.
*Pediatrics:* ≥16 yrs: Initial: 1000mg qd. Titrate: Dose adjusted in increments of 1000mg q2weeks. Max: 3000mg.

**HOW SUPPLIED:** Tab, Extended-Release: 500mg, 750mg

**WARNINGS/PRECAUTIONS:** Increased risk of suicidal thoughts or behavior reported; monitor for emergence or worsening of depression, suicidal thoughts/behavior, and any unusual changes in mood or behavior. May cause somnolence, dizziness, fatigue, coordination difficulties, and behavioral abnormalities (eg, psychotic symptoms, suicidal ideation, and other abnormalities). Withdraw gradually to minimize the potential of increased seizure frequency. Hematologic abnormalities and changes in LFTs may occur. May impair mental/physical abilities. Caution in renal impairment, hemodialysis, and elderly.

**ADVERSE REACTIONS:** Somnolence, influenza, nasopharyngitis, irritability, dizziness, nausea, asthenia, headache, infection, pain, anorexia, depression, nervousness, ataxia, vertigo.

**PREGNANCY:** Category C, not for use in nursing.

K

**MECHANISM OF ACTION:** Pyrrolidine derivative; not established. Proposed to inhibit burst firing without affecting normal neuronal excitability, suggesting that it may selectively prevent hypersynchronization of epileptiform burst firing and propagation of seizure activity.

**PHARMACOKINETICS: Absorption:** Complete. $T_{max}$=4 hrs. **Distribution:** Plasma protein binding (<10%); found in breast milk. **Metabolism:** Enzymatic hydrolysis (not extensive); ucbL057 (metabolite). **Elimination:** Urine (66%, unchanged); $T_{1/2}$=7 hrs.

## NURSING CONSIDERATIONS

**Assessment:** Assess for seizures, renal impairment, depression, suicidal thoughts/behavior, hematologic disorders, pregnancy/nursing status and possible drug interactions prior to therapy.

**Monitoring:** Monitor for CNS adverse effects such as somnolence, fatigue, coordination difficulties (ataxia, incoordination), behavioral abnormalities (agitation, anger, emotional lability), suicidal ideation. Monitor for hematological changes (RBC, WBC), changes in LFTs and renal function.

**Patient Counseling:** Instruct to take drug exactly as directed. Advise not to drive or operate heavy machinery until accustomed to the effects of medication. Monitor for changes in behavior (eg, aggression, anxiety, apathy, depression, irritability), psychotic symptoms and/or suicidal ideation. Notify physician if pregnant or intend to become pregnant. Encourage patients to enroll in North American Antiepileptic Drug (NAAED) Pregnancy Registry by calling 888-233-2334 or go to aedpregnancyregistry.org.

**Administration:** Oral route. Swallow whole; do not chew, break, or crush.
**Storage:** Store at 25°C (77°F); excursions permitted to 15-30°C (59-86°F).

# KETEK RX

telithromycin (Sanofi-Aventis)

**Contraindicated with myasthenia gravis.**

**THERAPEUTIC CLASS:** Ketolide antibiotic

**INDICATIONS:** Treatment of mild to moderate community-acquired pneumonia (CAP) due to susceptible strains of microorganisms.

**DOSAGE:** *Adults:* 800mg qd for 7-10 days. Severe Renal Impairment (CrCl <30mL/min): 600mg qd. Hemodialysis: Give after dialysis session on dialysis days. Severe Renal Impairment (CrCl <30mL/min) with Hepatic Impairment: 400mg qd.

**HOW SUPPLIED:** Tab: 300mg, 400mg

**CONTRAINDICATIONS:** Myasthenia gravis. History of hepatitis and/or jaundice associated with use of telithromycin or any macrolide antibiotic. Hypersensitivity to macrolide antibiotics. Concomitant use with cisapride or pimozide.

**WARNINGS/PRECAUTIONS:** Acute hepatic failure and severe liver injury, including fulminant hepatitis and hepatic necrosis reported; monitor closely and d/c if any signs/symptoms of hepatitis occur. Visual disturbances and loss of consciousness reported; minimize hazardous activities such as driving and operating heavy machinery. May prolong QTc interval; avoid with congenital prolongation, ongoing proarrhythmic conditions (eg, uncorrected hypokalemia or hypomagnesemia), significant bradycardia. Torsades de pointes reported. *Clostridium difficile*-associated diarrhea (CDAD) reported. Reduce dose with severe renal impairment (CrCl <30mL/min).

**ADVERSE REACTIONS:** Diarrhea, N/V, headache, dizziness, visual disturbances.

**INTERACTIONS:** See Contraindications. Increases levels of drugs metabolized by the CYP450 system (eg, carbamazepine, cyclosporine, tacrolimus, sirolimus, hexobarbital, phenytoin, triazolam, metoprolol), especially CYP3A4. Avoid cisapride, pimozide, simvastatin, lovastatin, atorvastatin, rifampin, ergot alkaloid derivatives, Class IA (eg, quinidine, procainamide) or Class III (eg, dofetilide) antiarrhythmics. Increased levels with itraconazole, ketoconazole. Monitor with midazolam, digoxin. Decreased effects with CYP3A4 inducers (eg, phenytoin, carbamazepine, phenobarbital). Decreases levels of sotalol. Space dosing of theophylline by 1 hr to reduce GI effects. Concomitant administration with oral anticoagulants may potentiate effects of the oral anticoagulants.

**PREGNANCY:** Category C, caution in nursing.

**MECHANISM OF ACTION:** Ketolide; blocks protein synthesis by binding to domains II and V of 23S rRNA of 50S ribosomal subunit. May also inhibit assembly of nascent ribosomal units.

**PHARMACOKINETICS: Absorption:** Absolute bioavailability (57%); $C_{max}$=2mcg/mL; $T_{max}$=1hr. **Distribution:** $V_d$=2.9L/kg; plasma protein binding (60-70%). **Metabolism:** Metabolized via CYP3A4 dependent and independent pathways. **Elimination:** Urine (13% unchanged); feces (7% unchanged); $T_{1/2}$=10 hrs.

## NURSING CONSIDERATIONS

**Assessment:** Assess for myasthenia gravis, LFTs, QTc prolongation, pregnancy/nursing status, and possible drug interactions. Document indications for therapy, culture, and susceptibility testing.

**Monitoring:** Monitor LFTs; ECG; QTc prolongation; visual disturbances including blurred vision, difficulty focusing, diplopia; loss of consciousness associated with vagal syndrome; renal impairment; *C. difficile*-associated diarrhea; pancreatitis; allergic reactions (angioedema, anaphylaxis).

**Patient Counseling:** Inform that therapy treats bacterial, not viral, infections. Take as directed; skipping doses or not completing full course may decrease effectiveness and increase antibiotic resistance. Notify physician if watery/bloody stools, superinfection, or hypersensitivity reactions occur. Counsel about signs/symptoms of hepatic failure (jaundice, malaise, anorexia). Advise against operating machinery or driving if visual difficulties or loss of consciousness is experienced.

**Administration:** Oral route. Can be given with/without food. Swallow tablet whole. **Storage:** 25°C (77°F); excursions permitted to 15-30°C (59-86°F). Keep out of reach of children.

K

## Ketoconazole Topical RX

ketoconazole (Various)

**THERAPEUTIC CLASS:** Azole antifungal

**INDICATIONS:** (Cre) Tinea corporis, tinea cruris, tinea pedis, tinea versicolor, cutaneous candidiasis, seborrheic dermatitis. (Shampoo) Tinea versicolor.

**DOSAGE:** *Adults:* (Cre) Cutaneous candidiasis, *T.corporis*, *T.cruris*, *T.versicolor*: Apply qd for 2 weeks. T.pedis: Apply qd for 6 weeks. Seborrheic Dermatitis: Apply bid for up to 4 weeks. Re-evaluate if no improvement after treatment period. (Shampoo) Apply to damp skin and lather. Rinse with water after 5 min. One application should be sufficient.

**HOW SUPPLIED:** Cre: 2% [15g, 30g, 60g]; Shampoo: 2% [120mL]

**WARNINGS/PRECAUTIONS:** (Cre) contains sulfites. (Shampoo) may remove curl from permanently waved hair. Avoid eyes.

**ADVERSE REACTIONS:** (Cre) Irritation, pruritus, stinging. (Shampoo) Abnormal hair texture, scalp pustules, mild skin dryness, pruritus, increase in normal hair loss, oily or dry scalp and hair.

**PREGNANCY:** Category C, (Cre) not for use in nursing, (Shampoo) caution in nursing.

**MECHANISM OF ACTION:** Azole antifungal; impairs synthesis of ergosterol, vital component of fungal cell membranes. Broad spectrum antifungal.

K

### NURSING CONSIDERATIONS

**Assessment:** Assess for sulfite hypersensitivity. Assess use in pregnant/nursing patients.

**Monitoring:** Monitor for signs/symptoms of sensitivity reactions or chemical irritation and for clinical response following treatment end. Reassess diagnosis if no response.

**Patient Counseling:** Instruct to report sensitivity or chemical irritation. Counsel that ketoconazole shampoo may irritate mucous membranes of the eyes; avoid contact. Ketoconazole shampoo may remove curls from permanently waved hair.

**Administration:** Topical route. **Storage:** Store below 25°C (77°F). Protect from light.

## Ketorolac RX

ketorolac tromethamine (Various)

**For short-term use only (≤5 days). Contraindicated with peptic ulcer disease, GI bleeding/perforation, perioperative pain in coronary artery bypass graft (CABG) surgery, advanced renal impairment, risk of renal failure due to volume depletion, cerebrovascular bleeding, hemorrhagic diathesis, incomplete hemostasis, high-risk of bleeding, intrathecal/epidural use, labor and delivery, nursing, and with concurrent ASA or NSAIDs. Greater risk of GI events with elderly patients. May cause an increased risk of cardiovascular (CV) thrombotic events (MI, stroke). Contraindicated in pediatric patients and for minor or chronic painful conditions.**

**OTHER BRAND NAMES:** Toradol (Roche Labs)

**THERAPEUTIC CLASS:** NSAID

**INDICATIONS:** Short-term (≤5 days) management of moderately severe acute pain that requires analgesia at the opioid level.

**DOSAGE: Adults:** >16 yrs to <65 yrs: Single-Dose: 60mg IM or 30mg IV. Multiple-Dose: 30mg IM/IV q6h. Max: 120mg/day. Transition from IM/IV to PO: 20mg PO single dose, then 10mg PO q4-6h prn. Max: 40mg/24 hrs. ≥65 yrs/Renal Impairment/<50kg: Single-Dose: 30mg IM or 15mg IV. Multiple-Dose: 15mg IM/IV q6h. Max: 60mg/day. Transition from IM/IV to PO: 10mg PO q4-6h prn. Max: 40mg/24 hrs.

**HOW SUPPLIED:** Inj: 15mg/mL, 30mg/mL; Tab: 10mg

**CONTRAINDICATIONS:** History or currently active peptic ulcer, recent GI bleeding/perforation, treatment of perioperative pain in CABG surgery, advanced renal impairment or risk of renal failure due to volume depletion, labor/delivery, nursing mothers, ASA or NSAID allergy, use as prophylactic analgesia before surgery, cerebrovascular bleeding, hemorrhagic diathesis, incomplete hemostasis, high risk of bleeding, neuraxial (epidural or intrathecal) administration, and concomitant ASA, NSAIDs, probenecid, or pentoxifylline.

**WARNINGS/PRECAUTIONS:** Do not exceed 5 days of therapy. Risk of GI ulcerations, bleeding, and perforation. Caution with renal/hepatic dysfunction, dehydration, HTN, CHF, coagulation disorders, pre-existing asthma. Preoperative use prolongs bleeding. CV thrombotic events, fluid retention, edema, NaCl retention, oliguria, anaphylactic reactions, elevated BUN and SrCr, anemia reported. Correct hypovolemia before therapy. Caution in elderly.

**ADVERSE REACTIONS:** Nausea, dyspepsia, abdominal pain, diarrhea, edema, headache, drowsiness, dizziness.

**INTERACTIONS:** May increase risk of serious bleeding with anticoagulants. May reduce diuretic response to furosemide and thiazide diuretics. Increased serum levels with salicylates. Avoid ASA, NSAIDs, and probenecid. Increased lithium and methotrexate levels. May increase risk of renal impairment with ACE-inhibitors/angiotension receptor angtagonist. May increase seizures with phenytoin and carbamazepine. Hallucinations reported with fluoxetine, thiothixene, and alprazolam. May cause apnea with nondepolarizing muscle relaxants.

**PREGNANCY:** Category C, not for use in nursing.

**MECHANISM OF ACTION:** NSAID; suspected to inhibit prostaglandin synthetase; exerts anti-inflammatory, analgesic, and antipyretic actions.

**PHARMACOKINETICS: Absorption**: Absolute oral bioavailability (100%). **Distribution:** $V_d$=13L; plasma protein binding (99%); enters breast milk. **Metabolism:** Liver; hydroxylation, conjugation. **Elimination:** Urine (92%; 40% metabolites, 60% unchanged), feces (6%); $T_{1/2}$=5-6 hrs.

## NURSING CONSIDERATIONS

**Assessment:** Assess LFTs, renal function, CBC, and coagulation profile. Assess for history of asthma and allergic reactions to aspirin or other NSAIDs, active ulceration or chronic inflammation of GI tract, CVD, pregnancy status. Note other diseases/conditions and drug therapies.

**Monitoring:** Monitor for hypersensitivity reactions, cardiac complications, stroke, GI bleeding, asthma, dermatological side effects. Monitor BP, LFTs, renal function, CBC with differential and platelet count, coagulation profile, and ophthalmic exams.

**Patient Counseling:** Counsel about side effects; seek medical attention if any occur. Avoid alcohol and smoking during treatment. Advise to take exactly as prescribed. Notify physician if signs of CV side effects (chest pain, SOB, weakness), GI bleeding (epigastric pain, dyspepsia), skin rash, unexplained weight gain, hepatotoxicity (nausea, fatigue) occur. Caution women against using late in pregnancy. Inform that drug is used as continuation treatment following IM or IV dosing and should not exceed 5 days.

**Administration:** IM/IV/Oral routes. **Storage:** 15-30°C (59-86°F).

# KINERET — RX

anakinra (Amgen)

**THERAPEUTIC CLASS:** Interleukin-1 receptor antagonist

**INDICATIONS:** Reduce the signs/symptoms and slow the progression of structural damage in moderately to severely active rheumatoid arthritis (RA), in patients 18 years of age or older who have failed 1 or more disease modifying antirheumatic drugs (DMARDs). Can be used alone or in combination with DMARDs other than TNF blocking agents.

**DOSAGE:** *Adults:* ≥18 yrs: 100mg SQ qd at approximately same time every day. CrCl <30mL/min: 100mg SQ qod.

**HOW SUPPLIED:** Inj: 100mg/0.67mL

**CONTRAINDICATIONS:** Hypersensitivity to *E.coli*-derived proteins.

**WARNINGS/PRECAUTIONS:** Increased incidence of serious infections alone and in combination with etanercept. D/C if serious infection or if a hypersensitivity reaction occurs. Do not initiate with active infection. Decrease in neutrophil count may be experienced; obtain neutrophil count before therapy, monthly for 3 months, and thereafter quarterly for up to 1 year. Needle cover of prefilled syringe contains dry latex rubber; caution in patients who are sensitive to latex. Caution in elderly.

**ADVERSE REACTIONS:** Serious infections, neutropenia, injection-site reactions, headache, nausea, diarrhea, infections, malignancy, worsening RA, abdominal pain, sinusitis, arthralgia, flu-like symptoms, URI.

**INTERACTIONS:** Neutropenia and higher rate of infections reported with etanercept; use with Tumor Necrosis Factor (TNF) blocking agents is not recommended. Avoid concomitant use with live vaccines.

**PREGNANCY:** Category B, caution in nursing.

**MECHANISM OF ACTION:** Interleukin-1 receptor antagonist; blocks biologic activity of IL-1 by competitively inhibiting IL-1 binding to the interleukin-1 type I receptor (IL-1RI), which is expressed in a wide variety of tissues and organs.

**PHARMACOKINETICS: Absorption:** Absolute bioavailability (95%); $T_{max}$=3-7 hrs. **Elimination:** $T_{1/2}$=4-6 hrs.

K

## NURSING CONSIDERATIONS

**Assessment:** Assess for known hypersensitivity to *E.coli*-derived proteins, active infection, immunosuppression, severe renal insufficiency or end-stage renal disease, pregnancy/nursing status, and possible drug interactions. Obtain neutrophil count.

**Monitoring:** Monitor for signs/symptoms of serious infections (eg, cellulitis, pneumonia, bone and joint infections), hypersensitivity reactions, neutropenia, and malignancies (eg, lymphomas). Monitor neutrophil count monthly for 3 months, and quarterly thereafter for up to a year.

**Patient Counseling:** Advise to avoid receiving live vaccines while on therapy. Counsel about proper dosage, administration, and disposal of medication; caution against reuse of needles, syringes, and drug product. Not be taken in combination with TNF-blocking agents. Counsel about signs/symptoms of allergic and adverse drug reactions. If severe hypersensitivity reaction occurs, d/c medication and start appropriate therapy. Advise that needle cover of prefilled syringe contains dry natural rubber, which may cause allergic reactions in latex-sensitive individuals.

**Administration:** SQ route. **Storage:** 2-8°C (36-46°F). Do not freeze or shake. Protect from light.

# KINRIX — RX

acellular pertussis, adsorbed - poliovirus vaccine, inactivated - diphtheria toxoid - tetanus toxoid (GlaxoSmithKline)

**THERAPEUTIC CLASS:** Vaccine/toxoid combination

**INDICATIONS:** Active immunization against diphtheria, tetanus, pertussis, and poliomyelitis as the fifth dose in the diphtheria, tetanus and acellular pertussis (DTaP) vaccine series and the fourth dose in the inactivated poliovirus vaccine (IPV) series in children 4-6 yrs whose previous DTaP vaccine doses have been with Infanrix® and/or Pediarix® for the first 3 doses and Infanrix® for the fourth dose.

**DOSAGE:** *Pediatrics:* 4-6 yrs: 0.5mL IM to the deltoid muscle. May be used for the fifth dose in the DTaP immunization series and the fourth dose in IPV immunization series.

**HOW SUPPLIED:** Inj: 0.5mL [TIP-LOK, vial]

**CONTRAINDICATIONS:** Encephalopathy within 7 days of administration of a previous pertussis-containing vaccine that is not attributable to another identifiable cause. Progressive neurologic disorders including infantile spasms, uncontrolled epilepsy or progressive encephalopathy. Previous allergic reaction to neomycin or polymyxin B.

**WARNINGS/PRECAUTIONS:** Not for IV, intradermal, or SQ use. Re-evaluate need if Guillain-Barre syndrome occurs within 6 weeks of receipt of a prior tetanus toxoid-containing vaccine. Weigh benefits and risks if any of the following occur in temporal relation to receipt of a pertussis-containing vaccine: temperature ≥40.5°C (105°F) within 48 hrs; collapse or shock-like state occuring within 48 hrs; hypotonic-hyporesponsive episode; persistent, inconsolable crying lasting ≥3 hrs occuring within 48 hrs; or if seizures (with or without fever) occur within 3 days. For children with a higher risk for seizures, administer an antipyretic at the time of vaccination to reduce the possibility of post-vaccination fever. May cause allergic reactions in latex sensitive individuals. Have epinephrine and other appropriate agents used for the control of immediate allergic reactions available.

**ADVERSE REACTIONS:** Local injection-site reactions (eg, pain, redness, increase in arm circumference, swelling), drowsiness, fever, loss of appetite.

**INTERACTIONS:** Immunosuppressive therapies (eg, irradiation, antimetabolites, alkylating agents, cytotoxic drugs, and corticosteroids) may reduce immune response. Do not mix with any other vaccine in the same syringe or vial.

**PREGNANCY:** Category C, safety in nursing not known.

**MECHANISM OF ACTION:** Vaccine/toxoid combination; provides active immunization by producing antibodies against diphtheria, tetanus, pertussis, and poliovirus.

## NURSING CONSIDERATIONS

**Assessment:** Review immunization history for possible vaccine sensitivity and previous vaccination-related adverse reactions. Assess for hypersensitivity to neomycin, polymyxin B, encephalopathy (eg, coma, decreased level of consciousness, prolonged seizures), progressive neurologic disorders (eg, infantile spasms, uncontrolled epilepsy, progressive encephalopathy), development of Guillain-Barre syndrome following a prior dose of tetanus toxoid, adverse events following pertussis vaccination (fever, collapse or shock-like state, persistent inconsolable crying, seizures), age of patient and possible drug interactions.

**Monitoring:** Monitor for signs/symptoms of Guillan-Barre syndrome, collapse or shock-like state, hypotonic/hyporesponsive episode, persistent inconsolable crying, fever, convulsions, hypersensitivity reactions, and local injection-site reactions.

**Patient Counseling:** Inform of potential benefits and risks of immunization. Counsel about potential adverse reactions. Instruct to report any adverse events to healthcare provider where the vaccine was administered. Inform that Vaccine Information Statements are available free of charge on the CDC website.

**Administration:** IM route. Prior to administration, shake vigorously to obtain homogenous, turbid, white suspension. Do not use if resuspension does not occur with vigorous shaking. Inspect visually for particulate matter, discoloration, cracks in the vial or syringe prior to administration; if any of these conditions exist, do not administer. Any remaining vaccine should be discarded after removal of the dose. **Storage:** 2-8°C (36-46°F). Do not freeze. Discard if frozen.

# KLONOPIN

clonazepam (Roche Labs)

CIV

**OTHER BRAND NAMES:** Klonopin Wafers (Roche Labs)

**THERAPEUTIC CLASS:** Benzodiazepine

K

**INDICATIONS:** Adjunct or monotherapy in the treatment of Lennox-Gastaut syndrome, akinetic and myoclonic seizures. May be useful in the treatment of absence seizures refractory to succinimides. Treatment of panic disorder with or without agoraphobia.

**DOSAGE:** *Adults:* Seizure Disorders: Initial: Not to exceed 1.5mg/day given tid. Titrate: May increase by 0.5-1mg every 3 days. Max: 20mg qd. Panic Disorder: Initial: 0.25mg bid. Titrate: Increase to 1mg/day after 3 days, then may increase by 0.125-0.25mg bid every 3 days. Max: 4mg/day. Elderly: Start at low end of dosing range.
*Pediatrics:* <10 yrs or 30kg: Seizure Disorders: Initial: 0.01-0.03mg/kg/day up to 0.05mg/kg/day given bid-tid. Titrate: Increase by no more than 0.25-0.5mg every 3 days. Maint: 0.1-0.2mg/kg/day.

**HOW SUPPLIED:** Tab: 0.5mg*, 1mg, 2mg; Tab, Disintegrating: (Wafer) 0.125mg, 0.25mg, 0.5mg, 1mg, 2mg *scored

**CONTRAINDICATIONS:** Significant liver disease, acute narrow-angle glaucoma.

**WARNINGS/PRECAUTIONS:** May impair physical/mental abilities. May increase risk of suicidal thoughts or behavior; monitor for emergence or worsening of depression and any unusual changes in mood or behavior. Caution with use in pregnancy, women of childbearing potential, renal dysfunction, and chronic respiratory distress. May increase incidence or precipitate generalized tonic-clonic seizures; addition of anticonvulsants or increased dosage may be required. Monitor blood counts and LFTs periodically with long-term therapy. Avoid abrupt withdrawal. Hypersalivation reported.

K

**ADVERSE REACTIONS:** Somnolence, depression, ataxia, upper respiratory tract infection, fatigue, dizziness, sinusitis, colpitis, behavioral problems, abnormal coordination, memory disturbance, nervousness, influenza, dysmenorrhea.

**INTERACTIONS:** Decreased serum levels with CYP450 inducers (eg, phenytoin, carbamazepine, phenobarbital), and propantheline. Caution with CYP3A inhibitors (eg, oral antifungals). Alcohol, narcotics, barbiturates, nonbarbiturate hypnotics, antianxiety agents, phenothiazines, thioxanthene and butyrophenone antipsychotics, MAOIs, TCAs and other anticonvulsant drugs potentiate CNS-depressant effects.

**PREGNANCY:** Category D, not for use in nursing.

**MECHANISM OF ACTION:** Benzodiazepine; not established, suspected to enhance activity of GABA, the major inhibitory neurotransmitter in the CNS.

**PHARMACOKINETICS: Absorption:** Rapid and complete. Absolute bioavailability (90%), $T_{max}$=1-4 hrs. **Distribution:** Plasma protein binding (85%). **Metabolism:** Liver via CYP450, then acetylation, hydroxylation, and glucuronidation. **Elimination:** Urine (<2% unchanged); $T_{1/2}$=30-40 hrs.

## NURSING CONSIDERATIONS

**Assessment:** Assess renal/hepatic function prior to therapy, significant liver disease, acute narrow-angle glaucoma, and possible drug interactions. Assess use with open-angle glaucoma and chronic respiratory diseases.

**Monitoring:** Monitor periodic blood counts and LFTs with prolonged therapy. Monitor for worsening of seizures, status epilepticus with abrupt withdrawal, and renal function in patients with a history of renal impairment.

**Patient Counseling:** Advise medication may cause CNS depression; avoid operating machinery/driving. Avoid abrupt withdrawal, alcohol use, and the use of other CNS depressants. Take at bedtime to avoid somnolence. Counsel females about possible risks if used during pregnancy. Encourage patients to enroll in North American Antiepileptic Drug (NAAED) Pregnancy Registry if they become pregnant by calling 888-233-2334 or go to aedpregnancyregistry.org.

**Administration:** Oral route. Disintegrating Tablet: 1) After opening pouch, peel back foil on blister. Do not push tablet through foil. 2) Using dry hands, place tablet in mouth. 3) Dissolve in mouth with or without water. **Storage:** 25°C (77°F); excursions permitted to 15-30°C (59-86°F).

## K-LOR RX
potassium chloride (Abbott)

**THERAPEUTIC CLASS:** $K^+$ supplement

**INDICATIONS:** Treatment and prevention of hypokalemia with or without metabolic alkalosis. Treatment of digitalis intoxication and hypokalemic familial periodic paralysis.

**DOSAGE:** *Adults:* Prevention: 20mEq/day. Hypokalemia: 40-100mEq/day. Divide dose if >20mEq. Dissolve each 20mEq in 4oz of cold water or juice.

**HOW SUPPLIED:** Pow: 20mEq

**CONTRAINDICATIONS:** Hyperkalemia.

**WARNINGS/PRECAUTIONS:** Potentially fatal hyperkalemia may occur. Extreme caution with acidosis, cardiac and renal disease; monitor ECG and electrolytes. Hypokalemia with metabolic acidosis should be treated with an alkalinizing potassium salt (eg, potassium bicarbonate, potassium citrate).

**ADVERSE REACTIONS:** Hyperkalemia, N/V, flatulence, abdominal pain, diarrhea.

**INTERACTIONS:** Risk of hyperkalemia with ACE inhibitors (eg, captopril, enalapril), $K^+$-sparing diuretics and $K^+$ supplements.

**PREGNANCY:** Category C, safe for use in nursing.

**MECHANISM OF ACTION:** $K^+$ supplement (electrolyte replenisher); helps in maintenance of intracellular tonicity, transmission of nerve impulses, contraction of cardiac, skeletal, and smooth muscles, and maintenance of normal renal function.

### NURSING CONSIDERATIONS

**Assessment:** Assess for chronic renal disease, conditions which impair $K^+$ excretion, and possible drug interactions. Obtain baseline serum $K^+$ levels and renal function test.

**Monitoring:** Monitor serum $K^+$ levels, renal function, ECG, and acid-base balance. Monitor for hyperkalemia, signs of acute metabolic acidosis, acute dehydration, and hypersensitivity reactions.

**Patient Counseling:** Instruct to report any adverse reactions. Dissolve in 1/2 glass of cold water or juice; take after a meal.

**Administration:** Oral route. **Storage:** Below 30°C (86°F).

## KLOR-CON M RX
potassium chloride (Upsher-Smith)

**OTHER BRAND NAMES:** Klor-Con (Upsher-Smith)

**THERAPEUTIC CLASS:** $K^+$ supplement

**INDICATIONS:** Treatment of hypokalemia with or without metabolic alkalosis, in digitalis intoxication, and in patients with hypokalemic familial periodic paralysis. Prevention of hypokalemia in patients at risk (eg, digitalized patients, cardiac arrhythmias).

**DOSAGE:** *Adults:* Individualize dose. Prevention: 20mEq/day. Hypokalemia: 40-100mEq/day. Divide dose if >20mEq. Elderly: Start at low end of dosing range. Take with meals and fluids. (Klor-Con Extended-Release Tab): Swallow tab whole; do not crush, chew, or suck. (Klor-Con M) May break Klor-Con M in half or mix with 4 oz of water.

**HOW SUPPLIED:** (Klor-Con M) Tab, Extended-Release: 10mEq, 15mEq, 20mEq; (Klor-Con) Pow: 20mEq, 25mEq; Tab, Extended-Release: 8mEq, 10mEq

**CONTRAINDICATIONS:** (Tab, ER) Hyperkalemia, cardiac patients with esophageal compression due to an enlarged left atrium. Structural, pathological (eg, diabetic gastroparesis) or pharmacological (eg, use of anticholinergic agents

K

or other agents with anticholinergic properties) cause for arrest or delay through the GI tract with all solid dosage forms. (Powder) Hyperkalemia.

**WARNINGS/PRECAUTIONS:** (Tab, Extended-Release; Powder) Potentially fatal hyperkalemia and cardiac arrest may occur; monitor serum $K^+$ levels and adjust dose appropriately. Extreme caution with acidosis or cardiac and renal disease; monitor ECG and electrolytes. Hypokalemia with metabolic acidosis should be treated with an alkalinizing $K^+$ salt (eg, $K^+$ bicarbonate, $K^+$ citrate). (Tab, Extended-Release) Solid oral dosage forms may produce ulcerative and/or stenotic lesions of the GI tract; d/c use if severe vomiting, abdominal pain, distention or GI bleeding occurs. Reserve use of ER preparations for those who cannot tolerate, cannot comply, or refuse to take liquid or effervescent preparations. Caution in elderly.

**ADVERSE REACTIONS:** (Tab, Extended-Release) Hyperkalemia, GI effects (eg, obstruction, bleeding, ulceration), N/V, abdominal pain/discomfort, flatulence, diarrhea. (Powder) Hyperkalemia, N/V, abdominal discomfort, diarrhea.

**INTERACTIONS:** (Tab, Extended-Release) See Contraindications. Risk of hyperkalemia with ACE inhibitors (eg, captopril, enalapril). (Tab, Extended-Release; Powder) Risk of hyperkalemia with $K^+$-sparing diuretics (eg, spironolactone, triamterene, amiloride).

**PREGNANCY:** Category C, (Tab, Extended-Release) Safe for use in nursing, (Powder) Not for use in nursing.

**MECHANISM OF ACTION:** $K^+$ supplement (electrolyte replenisher); participates in a number of essential physiological processes, including the maintenance of intracellular tonicity, the transmission of nerve impulses, the contraction of cardiac, skeletal, and smooth muscle, and the maintenance of normal renal function.

K

**PHARMACOKINETICS: Absorption:** (Klor-Con, Extended-Release Tablet) GI tract. **Elimination:** (Klor-Con, Extended-Release Tablet) Urine and feces.

## NURSING CONSIDERATIONS

**Assessment:** Assess for hyperkalemia, chronic renal failure, systemic acidosis (eg, diabetic acidosis), acute dehydration, extensive tissue breakdown (eg, severe burns, adrenal insufficiency), pregnancy/nursing status, and for possible drug interactions. If using ER tab formulation, assess cardiac patients for esophageal compression due to an enlarged left atrium and assess for for structural or pathological causes for arrest or delay in tablet passage through the GI tract (eg, diabetic gastroparesis). Prior to administration of an ER tab formulation, assess if patient cannot tolerate, refuses to take, or cannot comply with taking liquid or effervescent $K^+$ preparations. Assess baseline serum $K^+$ levels and renal function.

**Monitoring:** Monitor for signs/symptoms of hyperkalemia, serum $K^+$ levels, and renal function. In patients taking solid oral dosage forms, monitor for signs/symptoms of GI lesions. In patients with cardiac disease, acidosis, or renal disease, monitor acid-base balance and perform appropriate monitoring of serum electrolytes, ECG, and the clinical status of the patient.

**Patient Counseling:** (Klor-Con, Klor-Con M) Instruct to report to physician if develop any type of GI symptoms. (Tab): Instruct to contact physician if develop difficulty swallowing or if the tablets are sticking in the throat. (Klor-Con): Instruct to swallow tablets whole and to take with meals and full glass of water or other liquid. Counsel to not crush, chew, or suck tablets. (Klor-Con M): Instruct to take each dose with meals and with full glass of water or other liquid. Instruct to take dose without crushing, chewing, or sucking tablets. Inform that may break tablets in half or make an oral aqueous suspension with tablets and 4 ounces of water.

**Administration:** Oral route. **Storage:** (Klor-Con): 15-30°C (59-86°F). (Klor-Con M): 20-25°C (68-77°F); excursions permitted to 15-30°C (59-86°F).

## KRISTALOSE **RX**

lactulose (Cumberland)

**THERAPEUTIC CLASS:** Osmotic laxative

**INDICATIONS:** Treatment of constipation.

**DOSAGE:** *Adults:* 10-20g/day. Max 40g/day. Dissolve pkt contents in 4oz of water.

**HOW SUPPLIED:** Powder (crystals for suspension): 10g/pkt, 20g/pkt [1[s], 30[s]]

**CONTRAINDICATIONS:** Patients who require a low galactose diet.

**WARNINGS/PRECAUTIONS:** Caution in DM due to galactose and lactose content. Monitor electrolytes periodically in elderly or debilitated if used for >6 months. Potential for explosive reaction with electrocautery procedures during proctoscopy or colonoscopy.

**ADVERSE REACTIONS:** Flatulence, intestinal cramps, diarrhea, N/V.

**INTERACTIONS:** Nonabsorbable antacids may decrease effects.

**PREGNANCY:** Category B, caution in nursing.

**MECHANISM OF ACTION:** Osmotic laxative; increases osmotic pressure and slight acidification of the colonic contents.

**PHARMACOKINETICS: Absorption:** Poorly absorbed from GI tract. **Elimination:** Urine (≤3%).

### NURSING CONSIDERATIONS

**Assessment:** Assess for DM, patients requiring a low-galactose diet.

**Monitoring:** Monitor serum electrolytes (potassium, sodium, chloride, carbon dioxide), diarrhea, vomiting.

**Patient Counseling:** May be diluted with fruit juice, water, or milk. Report any potential adverse effects.

**Administration:** Oral route. Dissolve contents of packet in 4 ounces of water. **Storage:** Store 15-30°C (59-86°F).

## K-TAB **RX**

potassium chloride (Abbott)

**OTHER BRAND NAMES:** Klotrix (Apothecon)

**THERAPEUTIC CLASS:** $K^+$ supplement

**INDICATIONS:** (For those unable to tolerate liquid or effervescent potassium preparations). Treatment and prevention of hypokalemia with or without metabolic alkalosis. Treatment of digitalis intoxication and hypokalemic familial periodic paralysis.

**DOSAGE:** *Adults:* Prevention: 20mEq/day. Hypokalemia: 40-100mEq/day. Divide dose if >20mEq. Take with meals and full glass of water or liquid. Do not cut, crush or chew tab.

**HOW SUPPLIED:** Tab, Extended-Release: 10mEq

**CONTRAINDICATIONS:** Hyperkalemia, esophageal ulceration, delay in GI passage (from structural, pathological, pharmacologic causes), cardiac patients with esophageal compression due to enlarged left atrium.

**WARNINGS/PRECAUTIONS:** Potentially fatal hyperkalemia may occur. Extreme caution with acidosis, cardiac and renal disease; monitor ECG and electrolytes. Hypokalemia with metabolic acidosis should be treated with an alkalinizing potassium salt (eg, potassium bicarbonate, potassium citrate). May produce ulcerative or stenotic GI lesions. Use with caution in elderly due to decreased renal function, start dose at low end of dosing range.

**ADVERSE REACTIONS:** Hyperkalemia, GI effects (obstruction, bleeding, ulceration), nausea, vomiting, abdominal pain, flatulence, diarrhea.

**INTERACTIONS:** Risk of hyperkalemia with ACE inhibitors (eg, captopril, enalapril), potassium-sparing diuretics and potassium supplements.

Contraindicated with anticholinergic agents due to possible delay in tablet passage through GI tract.

**PREGNANCY:** Category C, safe for use in nursing.

**MECHANISM OF ACTION:** $K^+$ supplement (electrolyte replenisher). Slows release of $K^+$, so likelihood of high localized concentrations of $K^+$ within GI is reduced.

## NURSING CONSIDERATIONS

**Assessment:** Assess for chronic renal disease, conditions that impair $K^+$ excretion, esophageal compression due to enlarged left atrium, structural/pathologic cause for arrest/delay in passing through GI tract (eg, diabetic gastroparesis), and possible drug interactions. Obtain baseline serum $K^+$ levels and renal function test.

**Monitoring:** Monitor serum $K^+$ levels, renal function, ECG, and acid-base balance. Monitor for hyperkalemia, signs of acute metabolic acidosis, acute dehydration, GI ulcerations, and hypersensitivity reactions.

**Patient Counseling:** Instruct to report symptoms of GI bleeding (tarry stools), ulcerations/perforations (severe vomiting, abdominal pain, distention), trouble swallowing, or tablet sticking in throat. Take with meals and full glass of water. Swallow whole; do not crush, chew, or suck.

**Administration:** Oral route. **Storage:** Below 30°C (86°F).

K

# KYTRIL RX

granisetron HCl (Roche Labs)

**THERAPEUTIC CLASS:** 5-$HT_3$ receptor antagonist

**INDICATIONS:** (Inj, PO) Prevention of N/V associated with initial and repeated courses of emetogenic cancer therapy (eg, high-dose cisplatin). (Inj) Prevention and treatment of postoperative nausea and vomiting (PONV) in adults. (PO) Prevention of N/V associated with radiation (eg, total body irradiation and fractionated abdominal radiation).

**DOSAGE:** *Adults:* Emetogenic Chemotherapy: (PO) 2mg tab or 10mL sol qd up to 1 hr before chemotherapy or 1mg tab or 5mL sol bid up to 1 hr before chemotherapy and 12 hrs later. (IV) 10mcg/kg, undiluted over 30 sec or diluted (with 0.9% NaCl or 5% dextrose) over 5 min, within 30 min before chemotherapy. Prevention of N/V with Radiation: (PO) 2mg tab or 10mL sol qd within 1 hr of radiation. Prevention of PONV: (IV) 1mg undiluted over 30 sec before induction of anesthesia or immediately before anesthesia reversal. Treatment of PONV: (IV) 1mg undiluted over 30 sec.
*Pediatrics:* 2-16 yrs: Emetogenic Chemotherapy: 10mcg/kg IV within 30 min before chemotherapy.

**HOW SUPPLIED:** Inj: 0.1mg/mL [1mL single-use vial], 1mg/mL [1mL single-use vial, 4mL multi-use vial]; Sol: 2mg/10mL [30mL]; Tab: 1mg

**WARNINGS/PRECAUTIONS:** Does not stimulate gastric or intestinal peristalsis; do not use instead of nasogastric suction. May mask progressive ileus or gastric distension. Hypersensitivity reactions may occur in patients who exhibited hypersensitivity to other selective 5-$HT_3$ receptor antagonists. Granisetron 1mg/mL contains benzyl alcohol; neonatal adverse events (eg, gasping syndrome) reported. QT prolongation reported; caution if with preexisting arrhythmias, cardiac conduction disorders, cardiac disease, or cardiotoxic chemotherapy and electrolyte abnormalities.

**ADVERSE REACTIONS:** Headache, asthenia, somnolence, diarrhea, constipation, abdominal pain, dizziness, insomnia, dyspepsia, anemia, fever, alopecia, increased hepatic enzymes, bradycardia, leukocytosis.

**INTERACTIONS:** Hepatic CYP450 enzyme inducers or inhibitors may alter clearance and $T_{1/2}$. Avoid use with drugs known to prolong QT interval and/or arrhythmogenic drugs.

**PREGNANCY:** Category B, caution in nursing.

**MECHANISM OF ACTION:** 5-$HT_3$ receptor antagonist; blocks serotonin stimulation and subsequent vomiting after emetogenic stimuli.

**PHARMACOKINETICS: Absorption:** $C_{max}$=63.8ng/mL (IV, 40mcg/kg), 5.99ng/mL (PO, 1mg bid). **Distribution:** Plasma protein binding (65%). $V_d$=3.07L/kg (IV, 40mcg/kg), 2.42L/kg (IV, 1mg bid). **Metabolism:** CYP3A4; N-demethylation, aromatic ring oxidation, conjugation. **Elimination:** (PO) Urine (11% unchanged, 48% metabolites), feces (38% metabolites). (IV) Urine (12% unchanged, 49% metabolites), feces (34% metabolites); $T_{1/2}$=8.95 hrs (IV, 40mcg/kg), 8.63 hrs (IV, 1mg).

## NURSING CONSIDERATIONS

**Assessment:** Assess for N/V (chemotherapy-induced and post-operative), pre-existing arrhythmias, cardiac conduction disorders, cardiac disease, cardio-toxic chemotherapy, electrolyte abnormalities, hypersensitivity reactions, pregnancy/nursing status and possible drug interactions.

**Monitoring:** Monitor for progressive ileus, gastric distention, QT prolongation and hypersensitivity reactions.

**Patient Counseling:** Discuss risks and benefits of therapy. Advise patients to report any adverse events to their healthcare provider.

**Administration:** Oral, IV route. **Storage:** (Tab)15-30°C (59-86°F). Keep container tightly closed. Protect from light. (Sol/Inj) 25°C (77°F); excursions permitted to 15-30°C (59-86°F). Protect from light. (Inj) Once the multi-use vial is penetrated, its contact should be used within 30 days. Do not freeze. (Sol) Keep bottle tightly closed in an upright position.

# LABETALOL RX

labetalol HCl (Various)

**THERAPEUTIC CLASS:** Nonselective beta-blocker/alpha, blocker

**INDICATIONS:** (Tab) Management of hypertension. (Inj) Management of severe hypertension.

**DOSAGE:** *Adults:* (Tab) HTN: Initial: 100mg bid. Titrate: 100mg bid every 2-3 days. Maint: 200-400mg bid. Severe HTN: 1200-2400mg/day given bid-tid. Increments should not exceed 200mg bid for titration. (Inj) Severe HTN: Administer in supine position. Repeated IV Infusion: Initial: 20mg over 2 min. Titrate: Give additional 40-80mg at 10 min intervals if needed. Max: 300mg. Slow Continuous Infusion: 200mg at rate of 2mg/min. May adjust dose according to BP. Switch to tabs when BP is stable while in hospital. Initial: 200mg, then 200-400mg 6-12 hrs later on Day 1. Titrate: May increase at 1-day interval.

**HOW SUPPLIED:** Inj: 5mg/mL; Tab: 100mg*, 200mg*, 300mg *scored

**CONTRAINDICATIONS:** Bronchial asthma, obstructive airway disease, overt cardiac failure, >1st-degree heart block, cardiogenic shock, severe bradycardia, other conditions associated with severe and prolonged hypotension.

**WARNINGS/PRECAUTIONS:** Severe hepatocellular injury reported; caution with hepatic dysfunction. Monitor LFTs periodically; d/c at 1st sign of hepatic injury. Caution with well-compensated heart failure. Can cause heart failure. Exacerbation of ischemic heart disease with abrupt withdrawal. Caution in nonallergic bronchospasm patients refractory to or intolerant to other antihypertensives. May mask hypoglycemia symptoms. Withdrawal before surgery is controversial. Paradoxical HTN may occur with pheochromocytoma. Death reported during surgery. Avoid injection with low cardiac indices and elevated systemic vascular resistance.

**ADVERSE REACTIONS:** Fatigue, dizziness, dyspepsia, nausea, nasal stuffiness.

**INTERACTIONS:** Increased tremors with TCAs. Potentiated by cimetidine. Blunts reflex tachycardia of NTG without preventing hypotensive effect. Caution with calcium antagonists. Antagonizes bronchodilator effect of β-agonists. Antidiabetic agents may need dose adjustment. May block epinephrine effects. (Inj) Synergistic with halothane; do not use ≥3% halothane.

**PREGNANCY:** Category C, caution in nursing.

**MECHANISM OF ACTION:** α-1 and nonselective β-adrenergic receptor blocker; produces dose-related falls in BP without reflex tachycardia and significant reduction in heart rate.

**PHARMACOKINETICS: Absorption:** Complete; $T_{max}$=1-2 hrs. **Distribution:** Plasma protein binding (50%); crosses placenta. **Metabolism:** Conjugation. **Elimination**: Urine, feces; (Tab) $T_{1/2}$=6-8 hrs, (IV) $T_{1/2}$=5.5 hrs.

## NURSING CONSIDERATIONS

**Assessment:** Assess for bronchial asthma, bronchospastic disease, AV block, severe bradycardia, cardiogenic shock, overt CHF, DM, pheochromocytoma, possible drug interactions, hepatic impairment, severe or prolonged hypotension, history of obstructive airway disease, and history of heart failure.

**Monitoring:** Monitor LFTs periodically. Monitor for signs/symptoms of cardiac failure, hypoglycemia, withdrawal symptoms (angina, MI), hypersensitivity reactions, and hepatic dysfunction.

**Patient Counseling:** Instruct not to d/c or interrupt therapy without consulting physician. Inform of possible transient tingling of scalp. Advise to seek medical attention if symptoms of cardiac failure, hepatic dysfunction (pruritis, dark urine, anorexia, jaundice), or hypersensitivity reactions occur.

**Administration:** Oral, IV route. **Storage**: Tab: 15-30°C (59-86°F). IV: 2-30°C (36-86°F). Protect from light and freezing.

L

# LACTULOSE RX

lactulose (Various)

**OTHER BRAND NAMES:** Enulose (Alpharma) - Generlac (Morton Grove) - Constulose (Actavis)

**THERAPEUTIC CLASS:** Osmotic laxative

**INDICATIONS:** Treatment of constipation. Prevention and treatment of portal-systemic encephalopathy, including stages of hepatic pre-coma and coma.

**DOSAGE:** *Adults:* Constipation: 15-30mL qd. Max 60mL/day. May mix with fruit juice, water, or milk. Portal-Systemic Encephalopathy: 30-45mL tid-qid. Adjust dose every 1 or 2 days to produce 2-3 soft stools daily. Rectal Use: Reversal of Coma: Mix 300mL with 700mL of water or saline and retain for 30-60 min. May repeat q4-6h. Oral doses should be started before completely stopping enema.
*Pediatrics:* Portal-Systemic Encephalopathy: Older Children/Adolescents: 40-90mL/day divided tid-qid adjusted to produce 2-3 soft stools daily. *Infants:* 2.5-10mL in divided doses to produce 2-3 soft stools daily.

**HOW SUPPLIED:** Sol: 10g/15mL

**CONTRAINDICATIONS:** Patients who require a low galactose diet.

**WARNINGS/PRECAUTIONS:** Caution in DM due to galactose and lactose content. Monitor electrolytes periodically in elderly or debilitated if used >6 months. Potential for explosive reaction with electrocautery procedures during proctoscopy or colonoscopy.

**ADVERSE REACTIONS:** Flatulence, intestinal cramps, diarrhea, NV.

**INTERACTIONS:** Decreased effect with nonabsorbable antacids.

**PREGNANCY:** Category B, caution in nursing.

**MECHANISM OF ACTION:** Synthetic disaccharide; broken down primarily to lactic acid, by the action of colonic bacteria, resulting in increased osmotic pressure and slight acidification of colonic content, causing an increase in stool water content and softens the stool. In portal-systemic encephalopathy, acidification of colonic contents results in retention of ammonia in colon as ammonium ion; ammonia then migrates from blood into colon to form ammonium ion, which traps and prevents absorption of ammonia; finally, laxative actions expels trapped ammonium ion from colon.

**PHARMACOKINETICS: Absorption:** Poor. **Elimination:** Urine (≤3%).

## NURSING CONSIDERATIONS

**Assessment:** Assess for DM. Assess patients requiring a low-galactose diet and those requiring electrocautery procedures.

**Monitoring:** Monitor serum electrolytes (potassium, sodium, chloride, carbon dioxide) periodically, diarrhea, vomiting.

**Patient Counseling:** Drug may be diluted with fruit juice, water, or milk. Report potential adverse effects.

**Administration:** Oral route. **Storage:** 25°C (77°F); excursions permitted to 15-30°C (59-86°F). Dispense in tight, light-resistant container with child-resistant closure.

# LAMICTAL RX

lamotrigine (GlaxoSmithKline)

**Serious life-threatening rash, including Stevens-Johnson syndrome, toxic epidermal necrolysis, and/or rash-related death, reported. Occurs more often in pediatrics than adults. D/C at first sign of rash. Potential increased risk with concomitant VPA, exceeding the recommended initial dose, or exceeding the recommended dose escalation.**

**OTHER BRAND NAMES:** Lamictal CD (GlaxoSmithKline) - Lamictal ODT (GlaxoSmithKline)

**THERAPEUTIC CLASS:** Phenyltriazine

**INDICATIONS:** Adjunctive therapy in patients ( ≥2 yrs) with partial seizures, primary generalized tonic-clonic seizures and for generalized seizures of Lennox-Gastaut syndrome. For conversion to monotherapy in adults ( ≥16 yrs) with partial seizures receiving a single enzyme-inducing antiepileptic drug (EIAED) (carbamazepine, phenytoin, phenobarbital, primidone) or valproate (VPA). Maintenance treatment of bipolar I disorder to delay the time to occurrence of mood episodes (depression, mania, hypomania, mixed episodes) in patients ( ≥18 yrs) treated for acute mood episodes with standard therapy.

**DOSAGE:** *Adults:* Epilepsy: Concomitant VPA: Weeks 1 and 2: 25mg qod. Weeks 3 and 4: 25mg qd. Week 5 Onward: Increase every 1-2 weeks by 25-50mg/day. Maint: 100-200mg/day with VPA alone or 100-400mg/day in 1 or 2 divided doses with VPA and Other Enzyme-Inducing Drugs (EIDs). Concomitant AEDs other than EIAEDs or VPA: Weeks 1 and 2: 25mg qd. Weeks 3 and 4: 50mg qd. Week 5 Onward: Increase every 1-2 weeks by 50mg/day. Maint: 225-375mg/day in 2 divided doses. Concomitant EIAEDs without VPA: Weeks 1 and 2: 50mg/day. Weeks 3 and 4: 100mg/day in 2 divided doses. Week 5 Onward: Increase every 1-2 weeks by 100mg/day. Maint: 300-500mg/day in 2 divided doses. Conversion to Monotherapy: See PI. Bipolar Disorder: Patients Not Taking Other EIDs or VPA: Weeks 1 and 2: 25mg qd. Weeks 3 and 4: 50mg qd. Week 5: 100mg qd. Weeks 6 and 7: 200mg qd. Concomitant VPA: Weeks 1 and 2: 25mg qod. Weeks 3 and 4: 25mg qd. Week 5: 50mg qd. Weeks 6 and 7: 100mg qd. Concomitant EIDs without VPA: Weeks 1 and 2: 50mg qd. Weeks 3 and 4: 100mg qd. Week 5: 200mg qd. Week 6: 300mg qd. Week 7: Up to 400mg qd. Take in divided daily doses Weeks 3-7. D/C of Psychotropic Drugs Excluding VPA, Carbamazepine (CBZ), or Other EIDs: Maintain current dose. D/C of VPA with Current Dose of Lamotrigine 100mg qd: Week 1: 150mg qd. Week 2 Onward: 200mg qd. D/C of CBZ or Other EIDs with Current Dose of Lamotrigine 400mg qd: Week 1: 400mg qd. Week 2: 300mg qd. Week 3 Onward: 200mg qd. Concomitant/Starting/Stopping Estrogen-Containing Oral Contraceptives: See PI. Hepatic Impairment: Moderate and Severe: Reduce by 25%. Severe with Ascites: Reduce by 50%. Adjust maint and escalation doses based on clinical response. Elderly: Start at lower end of dosing range.
*Pediatrics:* Lennox-Gastaut/Partial/Generalized Tonic-Clonic Seizures: ≥12 yrs: Same as adults. 2-12 yrs: Give in 1-2 divided daily doses. Concomitant VPA: Weeks 1 and 2: 0.15mg/kg/day. Weeks 3 and 4: 0.3mg/kg/day. Week 5 Onward: Increase every 1-2 weeks by 0.3mg/kg/day. Maint: 1-3mg/kg/day with VPA alone or 1-5mg/kg/day. Max: 200mg/day. Concomitant AEDs Other Than EIAEDs or VPA: Weeks 1 and 2: 0.3mg/kg/day. Weeks 3 and 4:

0.6mg/kg/day. Week 5 Onward: Increase every 1-2 weeks by 0.6mg/kg/day. Maint: 4.5-7.5mg/kg/day. Max: 300mg/day. Concomitant EIAEDs without VPA: Weeks 1 and 2: 0.6mg/kg/day. Weeks 3 and 4: 1.2 mg/kg/day. Week 5 Onward: Increase every 1-2 weeks by 1.2mg/kg/day. Maint: 5-15mg/kg/day. Max: 400mg/day. <30kg: May increase maint dose by up to 50%. ≥16 yrs: Conversion to Monotherapy: See PI.

**HOW SUPPLIED:** Tab: 25mg*, 100mg*, 150mg*, 200mg*; Tab, Chewable: (CD) 2mg, 5mg, 25mg; Tab, Disintegrating: (ODT) 25mg, 50mg, 100mg, 200mg *scored

**WARNINGS/PRECAUTIONS:** Risk of serious life-threatening rash; d/c if rash occurs. Multiorgan failure, sudden unexplained death, hypersensitivity reactions and blood dyscrasias reported. Increased risk of suicidal thoughts or behavior; monitor for the emergence or worsening of depression, and unusual changes in mood or behavior. Avoid abrupt withdrawal in patients with epilepsy. May cause ophthalmic toxicity. Medication errors reported. Do not exceed recommended initial dose and dose escalations. Caution with renal, hepatic or cardiac functional impairment and in elderly.

**ADVERSE REACTIONS:** Ataxia, abdominal pain, blurred vision, diplopia, dizziness, fatigue, flu syndrome, headache, insomnia, N/V, pharyngitis, rhinitis, serious rash, somnolence, xerostomia.

**INTERACTIONS:** Decreased levels with phenytoin, carbamazepine, phenobarbital, primidone, rifampin and estrogen-containing oral contraceptives. May decrease levels of levonorgestrel. Increased levels with VPA. Inhibits dihydrofolate reductase. Higher incidence of headache, dizziness, nausea and somnolence with oxcarbazepine. May affect clearance with drugs known to induce or inhibit glucuronidation.

L

**PREGNANCY:** Category C, not for use in nursing.

**MECHANISM OF ACTION:** Phenyltriazine; mechanism not established. Suspected to inhibit voltage-sensitive sodium channels, thereby stabilizing neuronal membranes and consequently modulating presynaptic transmitter release of excitatory amino acids.

**PHARMACOKINETICS: Absorption:** Rapid and complete; absolute bioavailability (98%). $T_{max}$=1.4-4.8 hrs. **Distribution:** $V_d$=0.9-1.3L/kg; plasma protein binding (55%); found in breast milk. **Metabolism:** Liver via glucuronic acid conjugation, 2-N-glucuronide conjugate (major metabolite, inactive). **Elimination:** Urine (94%), feces (2%). Refer to PI for pediatric parameters.

## NURSING CONSIDERATIONS

**Assessment:** Assess renal/hepatic function prior to therapy. Assess use in patients with concomitant illnesses (renal/hepatic or cardiac impairment). Evaluate use in pediatric patients who have a history of major depressive disorder or other psychiatric disorder. Assess for hypersensitivity to drug, pregnancy/nursing status and possible drug interactions.

**Monitoring:** Monitor for signs/symptoms of rash (eg, Stevens-Johnson syndrome, toxic epidermal necrosis), hypersensitivity reaction, multiorgan failure, blood dyscrasias, status epilepticus, and ophthalmological changes. Monitor for emergence or worsening depressive symptoms and symptoms of suicidal ideation in patients with bipolar disorder, occurrence of seizures in patients who abruptly d/c medication. Monitor drug levels with concomitant medications or if dosage adjustments are being made.

**Patient Counseling:** Instruct to notify physician immediately if rash, signs/symptoms of hypersensitivity reaction, blood dyscrasias, multiorgan failure, worsening depression or suicide ideation occur. Inform CNS depression may occur; avoid operating machinery/driving until adjusted to effects. Advise females to notify physician if plan to start or stop oral contraceptives or other hormonal preparations or experience changes in menstruation. Encourage patients to enroll in North American Antiepileptic Drug (NAAED) Pregnancy Registry if they become pregnant: 1-888-233-2334 or www.aedpregnancyregistry.org. Do not abruptly d/c therapy; if therapy is stopped, notify physician before restarting.

**Administration:** Oral route. Round dose down to the nearest whole tab. Chewable dispersible tablets may be swallowed whole, chewed, dispersed in water or diluted in fruit juice. If tablets are chewed, consume a small amount of water or diluted fruit juice to aid in swallowing. When dispersing in water or diluted fruit juice, add tablets to small amount of liquid (1 tsp or enough to cover tablets) and approximately 1 min later, swirl solution and consume entire quantity immediately. Orally disintegrating tablets may be placed onto the tongue and moved around in the mouth. May disintegrate rapidly, swallow with or without water and may be taken with or without food. **Storage:** (Tab/ Tab, Chewable) 25°C (77°F); excursions permitted to 15-30°C (59-86°F), in a dry place, protected from light. (Tab, Disintegrating) 20-25°C (68-77°F); with excursions permitted between 15-30°C (59-86°F).

## LAMISIL **RX**

terbinafine HCl (Novartis)

**THERAPEUTIC CLASS:** Allylamine antifungal

**INDICATIONS:** (Granules) Treatment of tinea capitis in patients ≥4 yrs. (Tabs) Treatment of onychomycosis of toenail or fingernail due to dermatophytes (tinea unguium).

**DOSAGE:** *Adults:* Tabs: Fingernail: 250mg qd for 6 weeks. Toenail: 250mg qd for 12 weeks. Granules: Take qd with food for 6 weeks. <25kg: 125mg/day. 25-35kg: 187.5mg/day. >35kg: 250mg/day.

*Pediatrics:* ≥4 yrs: Granules: Take qd with food for 6 weeks. <25kg: 125mg/day. 25-35kg: 187.5mg/day. >35kg: 250mg/day.

**HOW SUPPLIED:** Granules: 125mg/pkt, 187.5mg/pkt; Tab: 250mg

**WARNINGS/PRECAUTIONS:** Liver disease and serious skin reactions reported; d/c therapy if these develop. Avoid with liver disease or renal impairment (CrCl ≤50 mL/min). Check serum transaminases before therapy. Monitor CBC if immunocompromised and taking terbinafine >6 weeks. Severe neutropenia reported; d/c therapy if neutrophil count ≤1,000 cells/mm³. Changes in ocular lens and retina reported (unknown significance).

**ADVERSE REACTIONS:** (Granules) Nasopharyngitis, headache, pyrexia, cough, vomiting, upper respiratory tract infection, upper abdominal pain, diarrhea, liver enzyme abnormalities, rash. (Tabs) Headache, diarrhea, dyspepsia, abdominal pain, liver enzyme abnormalities, rash.

**INTERACTIONS:** Increased clearance of cyclosporine. May potentiate levels of drugs metabolized by CYP2D6 (eg, TCAs, β-blockers, SSRIs, MAOIs-type B). Decreased clearance of IV caffeine. Clearance increased by rifampin and decreased by cimetidine.

**PREGNANCY:** Category B, not for use in nursing.

**MECHANISM OF ACTION:** Allylamine antifungal; acts by inhibiting squalene epoxidase, thus blocking biosynthesis of ergosterol, an essential component of fungal-cell membranes.

**PHARMACOKINETICS: Absorption:** (Tab) Well-absorbed (>70%), absolute bioavailability (40%); (250mg) $C_{max}$=1mcg/mL; $T_{max}$=2 hrs; AUC =4.56mcg.h/mL. **Distribution:** Plasma protein binding (>99%). **Metabolism:** Extensive, CYP2D6. **Elimination:** Urine (70%); $T_{1/2}$=200-400 hrs.

## NURSING CONSIDERATIONS

**Assessment:** Prior to treatment, conduct LFTs and obtain appropriate nail specimens for lab testing (KOH preparation, fungal culture, or nail biopsy) to diagnose onychomycosis. Assess for pre-existing liver disease.

**Monitoring:** Monitor for signs of hepatoxicity, occurrence of progressive skin rash (Stevens-Johnson syndrome), and signs/symptoms of lupus erythematosus. Perform CBC, LFTs, and renal function tests (CrCl) during therapy.

**Patient Counseling:** Inform that taste disturbances may occur while on medication. Counsel females to avoid nursing.

**Administration:** Oral route. **Storage**: Below 25°C (77°F). Dispense in a tight, light-resistant container.

## LANOXIN RX

digoxin (GlaxoSmithKline)

**OTHER BRAND NAMES:** Lanoxicaps (GlaxoSmithKline) - Digitek (Mylan Bertek) - Digoxin oral solution (Various)

**THERAPEUTIC CLASS:** Cardiac glycoside

**INDICATIONS:** Treatment of mild to moderate heart failure and to control ventricular response rate with chronic atrial fibrillation.

**DOSAGE:** *Adults:* Rapid Digitalization: LD: (Cap/Inj) 0.4-0.6mg PO/IV or (Tab) 0.5-0.75mg PO, may give additional (Cap/Inj) 0.1-0.3mg or (Tab) 0.125-0.375mg at 6-8 hr intervals until clinical effect. Maint: (Tab) 0.125-0.5mg qd. Elderly (>70 yrs)/Renal Dysfunction: Initial: 0.125mg qd. Marked Renal Dysfunction: Initial: 0.0625mg qd. Titrate: Increase every 2 weeks based on response. A-Fib: Titrate to minimum effective dose for desired response. (Sol) Recommended Initial: 3mcg/kg/day. Refer to PI for Usual Daily Maintenance Requirements (mcg) for estimated peak body stores of 10mcg/kg in adults and Daily Dose in Milliliters. Elderly: Start at low end of dosing range. *Pediatrics:* (Ped Sol) Oral Digitalizing Dose: Premature Infants: 20-30mcg/kg. Full-Term Infants: 25-35mcg/kg. 1-24 months: 35-60mcg/kg. 2-5 yrs: 30-40mcg/kg. 5-10 yrs: 20-35mcg/kg. >10 yrs: 10-15mcg/kg. Maint: Premature Infants: 20-30% of PO digitalizing dose/day. Full-Term Infants to >10 yrs: 25-35% of PO digitalizing dose. (Ped Inj) IV Digitalizing Dose: Premature Infants: 15-25mcg/kg. Full-Term Infants: 20-30mcg/kg. 1-24 months: 30-50mcg/kg. 2-5 yrs: 25-35mcg/kg. 5-10 yrs: 15-30mcg/kg. >10 yrs: 8-12mcg/kg. Maint: Premature Infants: 20-30% of IV digitalizing dose. Full-Term Infants to >10 yrs: 25-35% of IV digitalizing dose/day. (Cap) Oral Digitalizing Dose: 2-5 yrs: 25-35mcg/kg. 5-10 yrs: 15-30mcg/kg. >10 yrs: 8-12mcg/kg. Maint: ≥2 yrs: 25-25% of PO or IV digitalizing dose. (Tab) Maint: 2-5 yrs: 10-15mcg/kg. 5-10 yrs: 7-10mcg/kg. >10 yrs: 3-5mcg/kg. A-Fib: Titrate to minimum effective dose for desired response. (Generic Sol) Children >2yrs and Prepubertal Children: Recommended Initial: 10mcg/kg/day. Renal dysfunction: Start at the low end of dosing range.

**HOW SUPPLIED:** Cap: (Lanoxicaps) 0.1mg, 0.2mg; Inj: (Pediatric Inj) 0.1mg/mL, 0.25mg/mL; Sol: 50mcg/mL, (Pediatric Sol) 0.05mg/mL [60mL]; Tab: 0.125mg*, 0.25mg* *scored

**CONTRAINDICATIONS:** Ventricular fibrillation.

**WARNINGS/PRECAUTIONS:** May cause severe sinus bradycardia or sinoatrial block with pre-existing sinus node disease. May cause advanced or complete heart block with pre-existing incomplete AV block. May cause very rapid ventricular response or ventricular fibrillation. Caution with thyroid disorders, AMI, hypermetabolic states, restrictive cardiomyopathy, constrictive pericarditis, amyloid heart disease, elderly, acute cor pulmonale, and hypertrophic cardiomyopathy, and Wolff-Parkinson White syndrome. Caution with renal dysfunction; high risk for toxicity. Caution with hypokalemia, hypomagnesemia, or hypercalcemia; toxicity may occur. Hypocalcemia can nullify effects of digoxin. Monitor electrolytes and renal function periodically. Risk of ventricular arrhythmia with electrical cardioversion. Bioavailability is different between dosage forms.

**ADVERSE REACTIONS:** Heart block, rhythm disturbances, anorexia, N/V, diarrhea, visual disturbances, headache, weakness, dizziness, mental disturbances.

**INTERACTIONS:** Risk of toxicity with $K^+$-depleting corticosteroids and diuretics. Increased risk of arrhythmias with calcium, sympathomimetics, and succinylcholine. Increased serum levels with quinidine, verapamil, amiodarone, propafenone, indomethacin, itraconazole, alprazolam, and spironolactone; monitor for toxicity. Increased absorption with propantheline, diphenoxylate, macrolides, and tetracycline; monitor for toxicity. Decreased intestinal absorption with propantheline and diphenoxylate. Decreased serum levels with rifampin. Increased digoxin dose requirement with thyroid supplements. Additive effects on AV node conduction with β-blockers or CCBs. Caution with drugs that deteriorate renal function. (Generic Sol) May interfere with digoxin absorption with activated charcoal, kaolin-pectin, sulfasalazine, neomycin, cholestyramine, certain anticancer drugs, metoclopramide, meals high in bran, sucralfate, lansoprazole, esomeprazole, and omeprazole. Potential digoxin pharmacokinetics alteration with P-glycoprotein inducers/inhibitors. Monitor digoxin levels when initiating, adjusting, and discontinuing with diltiazem, nifedipine, nitrendipine, and telmisartan. Increased serum concentration with carvedilol, epoprostenol, diclofenac, indomethacin, ketoconazole, itraconazole, rabeprazole, azithromycin, erythromycin, tetracycline, gatifloxacin, and clarithromycin. Decreased serum concentration with rifampin, acarbose, miglitol, cyclosporine, albuterol, salbutamol, and St. John's wort. Colestipol bind digoxin. Digoxin toxicity reported with tramadol. May compete for common renal tubular transport systems with metformin. Higher rate of Torsade de pointes with dofetilide. Increase in PR interval and QRS duration with moricizine. Caution with teriparatide. May produce arrhythmias with calcium, sympathomimetics, and succinylcholine. Additive AV node conduction effect with β-adrenergic and calcium-channel blockers.

**PREGNANCY:** Category C, not for use in nursing.

**MECHANISM OF ACTION:** Cardiac glycoside; inhibits $Na^+$-$K^+$ ATPase, leading to increase in intracellular concentration of $Ca^+$.

**PHARMACOKINETICS: Absorption:** (Tab) Absolute bioavailability (60%-80%), $T_{max}$=1-3 hrs. (Sol) Absolute bioavailability (70-85%), $T_{max}$=30-90mins. (Lanoxicaps) Absolute bioavailability (90-100%). (Inj) Absolute bioavailability (100%). **Distribution:** Plasma protein binding (25%), crosses placenta; found in breastmilk. **Metabolism:** Hydrolysis, oxidation, and conjugation. **Elimination:** Urine (50%-70%); $T_{1/2}$=1.5-2 days. (Generic Sol) $T_{1/2}$= Children (18-26 hrs), adults (36-48 hrs), anuric patients (3.5-5 days).

## NURSING CONSIDERATIONS

**Assessment:** Assess for possible drug interactions, thyroid and electrolyte disorders, hypermetabolic states, sinus node disease, incomplete AV block, renal impairment, ventricular fibrillation, atrial fibrillation/flutter with accessory AV pathway (WPW syndrome), restrictive cardiomyopathy, constrictive pericarditis, amyloid heart disease, acute cor pulmonale, IHSS, and pregnancy/nursing status.

**Monitoring:** Monitor serum electrolytes and renal function periodically. Monitor for signs/symptoms of sinoatrial block, severe sinus bradycardia, complete AV block, electrolyte imbalances, and hypersensitivity reactions. Monitor serum digoxin levels.

**Patient Counseling:** Advise to seek medical attention if symptoms of hypersensitivity, electrolyte imbalance, or CV events occur.

**Administration:** Oral, IV route. **Storage:** 25°C (77°F); excursions permitted to 15-30°C (59-86°F). Store in dry place and protect from light.

# LANTUS — RX

insulin glargine, human (Sanofi-Aventis)

**THERAPEUTIC CLASS:** Insulin

**INDICATIONS:** Treatment of adults and pediatrics with type 1 diabetes mellitus. Treatment of adults with type 2 diabetes mellitus who require basal (long-acting) insulin.

**DOSAGE:** *Adults:* Individualize dose. For SQ injection only. Administer qd at same time each day. Insulin naive patients on oral antidiabetic drugs, start with 10 U qd. Switching from once-daily NPH or Ultralente does not require initial dose change. Switching from bid NPH, reduce initial dose by 20%. Maint: 2-100 U/day.

*Pediatrics:* ≥6 yrs: Individualize dose. For SQ injection only. Administer qd at same time each day. Insulin naive patients on oral antidiabetic drugs, start with 10 U qd. Switching from once-daily NPH or Ultralente does not require initial dose change. Switching from bid NPH, reduce initial dose by 20%. Maint: 2-100 U/day.

**HOW SUPPLIED:** Inj: 100 U/mL; OptiClik: 100 U/mL

**WARNINGS/PRECAUTIONS:** Human insulin differs from animal source insulin. Any change of insulin should be made cautiously. Changes in strength, manufacturer, type or method of manufacture may result in the need for a change in dosage. Hypoglycemia may occur with taking too much insulin, missing or delaying meals, exercising or working more than usual. An infection or illness (especially with diarrhea or vomiting) may change insulin requirements. Administration of insulin SQ can result in lipodystrophy. Not for IV use. Do not mix with other insulins. May cause sodium retention and edema. Caution in patients with renal and hepatic dysfunction.

**ADVERSE REACTIONS:** Hypoglycemia, allergic reactions, injection-site reactions, lipodystrophy, pruritus, rash.

**INTERACTIONS:** Increased glucose-lowering effects with ACE inhibitors, disopyramide, fibrates, fluoxetine, MAOIs, propoxyphene, salicylates, somatostatin analog, sulfonamide antibiotics, and other antidiabetic agents. Decreased blood glucose lowering effects with corticosteroids, danazol, diuretics, sympathomimetic amines, isoniazid, phenothiazine derivatives, somatropin, thyroid hormones, estrogens, progestogens, protease inhibitors, and atypical antipsychotics. Pentamidine may cause hypoglycemia, followed by hyperglycemia. β-blockers, clonidine, lithium salts, and alcohol may potentiate or weaken glucose lowering effect. β-blockers, clonidine, guanethidine, and reserpine may reduce or mask signs of hypoglycemia.

**PREGNANCY:** Category C, caution in nursing.

**MECHANISM OF ACTION:** Insulin glargine (rDNA origin); regulates glucose metabolism by stimulating peripheral glucose uptake by skeletal muscle and fat, inhibits hepatic glucose production, lipolysis in the adipocyte, proteolysis, and enhances protein synthesis.

**PHARMACOKINETICS: Absorption:** Slow, prolonged, and relatively constant. **Metabolism:** Partly metabolized into 2 active metabolites [M1 ($21^A$-Gly-insulin) and M2 ($21^A$-Gly-des-$30^B$-Thr-insulin)].

## NURSING CONSIDERATIONS

**Assessment:** Assess FPG, $HbA_{1c}$, renal function, LFTs, pregnancy status, infections, alcohol consumption, exercise routines, and possible drug interactions.

**Monitoring:** Monitor FPG, $HbA_{1c}$, renal function, diabetic ketoacidosis, lipodystrophy, allergic reactions. Monitor for signs of hypoglycemia (sweating, palpitations, seizures, disorientation, tremors).

**Patient Counseling:** Use only if the solution is clear and colorless, with no visible particles. Do not dilute or mix with other insulins or solutions. Counsel about signs/symptoms of hypoglycemia, hyperglycemia, diabetic ketoacidosis, the importance of frequent monitoring of blood glucose levels, the need for eating a balanced diet and exercising regularly. Advise to avoid excessive alcohol. During periods of stress (eg, trauma, infection, surgery), insulin requirements may be changed; advise patients to seek prompt medical advice. Counsel on proper administration techniques.

**Administration:** SQ route only. 1) Inspect solution for particles and discoloration before administration. 2) Do not mix with other solutions. 3) Alternate injection sites (upper arm, thigh, abdomen). 4) Leave needle in skin for 10 seconds after injection. The number in the dose window should read zero. 5) Gently press the spot injected; do not rub the area. **Storage:** Unopened: 2-8°C (36-46°F). Do not freeze. In-use: Below 30°C (86°F).

# Lescol XL **RX**

fluvastatin sodium (Novartis)

**OTHER BRAND NAMES:** Lescol (Novartis)

**THERAPEUTIC CLASS:** HMG-CoA reductase inhibitor

**INDICATIONS:** Adjunct to diet, to reduce total cholesterol (total-C), LDL, TG, and apolipoprotein B (Apo B) levels, and to increase HDL in primary hypercholesterolemia and mixed dyslipidemia (Types IIa and IIb) when response to nonpharmacological measures is inadequate. To slow coronary atherosclerosis progression in coronary heart disease by lowering total-C and LDL. To reduce risk of undergoing coronary revascularization procedures in patients with coronary heart disease. Adjunct to diet, to reduce Total-C, LDL-C, and Apo B levels in adolescent boys and postmenarchal girls, 10-16 yrs of age, with heterozygous familial hypercholesterolemia when response to dietary restriction is inadequate and LDL-C remains ≥190mg/dL, or if LDL-C remains ≥160mg/dL and there is positive family history of premature CV disease or 2 or more other CV disease risk factors are present.

**DOSAGE:** *Adults:* ≥18 yrs: (For LDL-C reduction of ≥25%) Initial: 40mg cap qpm or 80mg XL tab at any time of day or 40mg cap bid. (For LDL-C reduction of <25%) Initial: 20mg cap qpm. Range: 20-80mg/day. Severe Renal Impairment: Caution with dose >40mg/day.
*Pediatrics:* 10-16 yrs ( ≥1 year post menarche): Heterozygous Familial Hypercholesterolemia: Initial: One 20mg cap. Titrate: Adjust dose at 6-week intervals. Max: 40mg cap bid or 80mg XL tab qd.

**HOW SUPPLIED:** Cap: (Lescol) 20mg, 40mg; Tab, Extended-Release: (Lescol XL) 80mg

**CONTRAINDICATIONS:** Active liver disease or unexplained, persistent elevations of serum transaminases, pregnancy, nursing mothers.

**WARNINGS/PRECAUTIONS:** Monitor LFTs prior to therapy, at 12 weeks, and with dose elevation. D/C if AST or ALT ≥3x ULN on 2 consecutive occasions. Risk of myopathy and/or rhabdomyolysis reported. D/C if markedly elevated CPK levels occur, if myopathy is diagnosed or suspected, or if predisposition to renal failure secondary to rhabdomyolysis. Less effective with homozygous familial hypercholesterolemia. Caution with heavy alcohol use and/or history of hepatic disease. Evaluate if endocrine dysfunction develops.

**ADVERSE REACTIONS:** Dyspepsia, abdominal pain, headache, sinusitis, nausea, diarrhea, myalgia, flu-like symptoms, abnormal LFTs.

**INTERACTIONS:** Increases levels of glyburide, diclofenac, and phenytoin. Rifampicin significantly decreases serum levels. Glyburide, phenytoin, cimetidine, ranitidine, omeprazole, fluconazole, cyclosporine and digoxin increase levels of fluvastatin. Caution with drugs that decrease levels of endogenous steroid hormones (eg, ketoconazole, spironolactone, cimetidine). Avoid fibrates. Cyclosporine, colchicine, gemfibrozil, erythromycin, or niacin may increase risk of myopathy/rhabdomyolysis. Immediate-release fluvastatin given within 4 hrs of cholestyramine leads to decreased serum levels of fluvastatin but has additive effects when given 4 hrs after cholestyramine. Monitor PT of patients on warfarin-type anticoagulants.

**PREGNANCY:** Category X, not for use in nursing.

**MECHANISM OF ACTION:** HMG-CoA reductase inhibitor; inhibits conversion of HMG-CoA to mevalonate (precursor of sterols, including cholesterol). Inhibition of cholesterol biosynthesis reduces cholesterol in hepatic cells, which stimulates the synthesis of LDL receptors, thereby increasing uptake of LDL particles, resulting in reduction of plasma cholesterol concentration.

**PHARMACOKINETICS: Absorption:** Oral administration of variable doses resulted in different parameters. Cap: Rapid and complete, absolute bioavailability (24%); $T_{max}$=<1 hr. Tab: relative bioavailability (relative to cap) (29%); $T_{max}$=3 hrs (fasting), 2.5 hrs (Low-fat meal), 6 hrs (High-fat meal). **Distribution:** $V_d$=0.35L/kg, plasma protein binding (98%). **Metabolism:** Liver via CYP2C9, 2C8 and 3A4 through hydroxylation, N-dealkylation, and β-oxidation pathways. **Elimination:** Feces (90% metabolites, <2% unchanged), urine (5%); Tab: $T_{1/2}$=9 hrs.

## NURSING CONSIDERATIONS

**Assessment:** Assess for active liver disease or unexplained, persistent elevations in serum transaminase, pregnancy/nursing status, alcohol intake, homozygous familial hypercholestrolemia, renal impairment, DM, and possible drug interactions. Perform LFTs prior to therapy and at 12 weeks thereafter. Control hypercholesterolemia through appropriate diet, exercise, and weight reduction prior to therapy.

**Monitoring:** Monitor LFTs, CPK, thyroid functions. Monitor for signs/symptoms of myopathy (eg, diffuse muscle pain, tenderness or weakness, and fever or malaise), rhabdomyolysis, renal failure, endocrine dysfunction, and CNS toxicity or CNS vascular lesions (eg, hemorrhage and edema).

**Patient Counseling:** Inform about potential risks/benefits of therapy. Report promptly unexplained muscle pain, tenderness, or weakness, changes in urine or skin color, stomach pain, N/V, and malaise or fever. Notify physician if pregnant/nursing or planning to become pregnant.

**Administration:** Oral route. **Storage:** 25°C (77°F); excursions permitted to 15-30°C (15-86°F). Dispense in a tight container. Protect from light.

## Letairis — RX

ambrisentan (Gilead)

**May cause serious liver injury. Elevated ALT, AST to at least 3x ULN reported; monitor liver aminotransferases monthly and d/c if >5x ULN or if elevations are accompanied by bilirubin >2x ULN or by signs and symptoms of liver dysfunction. Contraindicated in pregnancy. May cause fetal harm; obtain monthly pregnancy tests. Available only through the Letairis Education and Access Program (LEAP).**

**THERAPEUTIC CLASS:** Endothelin receptor antagonist

**INDICATIONS:** Treatment of pulmonary arterial hypertension (WHO Group 1) in patients with WHO class II or III symptoms to improve exercise capacity and delay clinical worsening.

L

**DOSAGE:** *Adults:* Initial: 5mg qd. May increase to 10mg qd if 5mg is tolerated. Max: 10mg qd. May be taken with or without food. Do not split, crush, or chew tablets.

**HOW SUPPLIED:** Tab: 5mg, 10mg

**CONTRAINDICATIONS:** Pregnancy.

**WARNINGS/PRECAUTIONS:** Monitor LFTs before initiation and at least every month thereafter. Avoid therapy if elevated aminotransferase levels (>3x ULN) at baseline. If confirmed aminotransferase level is >3x ULN and ≤5x ULN, reduce daily dose or interrupt treatment and continue to monitor every 2 weeks until levels are <3x ULN. If aminotransferase elevations >5x ULN and ≤8x ULN, d/c and continue monitoring until levels are <3x ULN; may then reinitiate with more frequent monitoring. If aminotransferase elevations >8x ULN, d/c and avoid reinitiation. May cause peripheral edema; if clinically significant fluid retention develops, with or without weight gain, further evaluate to determine cause, such as heart failure and possible need for treatment. May decrease Hgb and Hct; measure Hgb prior to initiation, at 1 month, then periodically thereafter. D/C if significant decrease in Hgb is observed and other causes have been excluded. May decrease sperm count. Pregnancy must be excluded before initiation of treatment and prevented during treatment by using 2 acceptable methods of contraception unless the patient has had tubal sterilization or chooses to use a copper T 380A IUD or LNg 20 IUS, in which no additional contraception is needed.

**ADVERSE REACTIONS:** Peripheral edema, headache, nasal congestion, palpitations, flushing, constipation, dyspnea, sinusitis, nasopharyngitis, abdominal pain.

**PREGNANCY:** Category X, not for use in nursing.

**MECHANISM OF ACTION:** Endothelin receptor antagonist; not established.

**PHARMACOKINETICS: Absorption:** Rapid; $T_{max}$=2 hrs. **Distribution:** Plasma protein binding (99%). **Metabolism:** via CYP3A, CYP2C19 and uridine 5'-diphosphate glucuronosyltransferases (UGTs) 1A9S, 2B7S and 1A3S. **Elimination:** $T_{1/2}$=9 hrs.

### NURSING CONSIDERATIONS

**Assessment:** Assess for hepatic impairment and pregnancy/nursing status. Obtain baseline LFT, Hgb/Hct tests.

**Monitoring:** Obtain LFT, Hgb/Hct, and pregnancy tests monthly. Monitor for signs/symptoms of hepatotoxicity, peripheral edema, and hypersensitivity reactions.

**Patient Counseling:** Advise to enroll in LEAP and re-enroll after the first 12 months of treatment and annually thereafter. Inform that drug may cause fetal harm and instruct to use 2 forms of contraception during and 1 month after therapy. If IUD or tubal sterilization is used, additional contraception not needed. Notify healthcare professional if pregnancy is suspected. Inform of the importance of monthly Hgb and LFTs. Advise to seek medical attention if symptoms of liver injury (eg, NV, fever, malaise, itching) occur. Report peripheral edema or hypersensitivity reactions.

**Administration:** Oral route. Do not split, crush or chew tablets. **Storage:** 25°C (77°F); excursions permitted to 15-30°C (59-86°F).

## LEUKERAN — RX

chlorambucil (GlaxoSmithKline)

**Risk of severe bone marrow suppression. Potentially carcinogenic, mutagenic, and teratogenic. Produces human infertility.**

**THERAPEUTIC CLASS:** Nitrogen mustard alkylating agent

**INDICATIONS:** Treatment of chronic lymphatic (lymphocytic) leukemia (CLL), malignant lymphomas, and Hodgkin's disease.

**DOSAGE:** *Adults:* Usual: 0.1-0.2mg/kg qd for 3-6 weeks. Adjust according to response; reduce with abrupt WBC decline. Lymphocytic Infiltration of Bone Marrow/Hypoplastic Bone Marrow: Max: 0.1mg/kg/day. Caution within 4 weeks of full course of radiation or chemotherapy.

**HOW SUPPLIED:** Tab: 2mg

**CONTRAINDICATIONS:** Prior resistance to therapy.

**WARNINGS/PRECAUTIONS:** Convulsions, infertility, leukemia and secondary malignancies observed. Shown to cause chromatid or chromosome damage and sterility. Skin rash progressing to erythema multiforme, toxic epidermal necrolysis, or Stevens-Johnson syndrome reported. Avoid becoming pregnant. Lymphopenia reported, usually returns to normal upon completion. Monitor Hgb, leukocyte count and differential, platelet counts weekly. Avoid live vaccines in the immunocompromised.

**ADVERSE REACTIONS:** Bone marrow suppression, NV, diarrhea, tremors, muscular twitching, confusion, agitation, ataxia, urticaria, angioneurotic syndrome, pulmonary fibrosis, hepatotoxicity, jaundice.

**INTERACTIONS:** Cross-hypersensitivity may occur with other alkylating agents.

**PREGNANCY:** Category D, not for use in nursing.

**MECHANISM OF ACTION:** Nitrogen mustard alkylating agent.

**PHARMACOKINETICS: Absorption:** Rapid and complete. (0.6-1.2 mg/kg) $T_{max}$=1 hr; (0.2mg/kg) $C_{max}$=492ng/mL, $T_{max}$=0.83 hrs, AUC=883ng•h/mL; (Phenylacetic acid mustard) $C_{max}$=306ng/mL, $T_{max}$=1.9 hrs; AUC=1204ng•h/mL. **Distribution:** Plasma protein binding (99%); crosses placenta. **Metabolism:** Liver (rapid). Phenylacetic acid mustard (major metabolite). **Elimination:** Low urinary excretion; $T_{1/2}$=1.5 hrs (0.6-1.2mg/kg); $T_{1/2}$=1.3 hrs (0.2mg/kg); $T_{1/2}$=1.8 hrs (phenylacetic acid mustard).

### NURSING CONSIDERATIONS

**Assessment:** Assess for prior resistance, history of seizure disorder or head trauma, and possible drug interactions. Obtain baseline WBC and platelet count.

**Monitoring:** Monitor Hgb, WBC with differential and platelet count weekly. During first 3-6 weeks of therapy, obtain WBC levels 3 or 4 days after each weekly blood count. Monitor for signs/symptoms of myelosuppression, hypersensitivity reaction, secondary malignancies, and skin reactions.

**Patient Counseling:** Inform of pregnancy risks; avoid pregnancy. Advise to avoid vaccinations with live vaccines. Inform that major toxicities are related to hypersensitivity, drug fever, myelosuppression, hepatotoxicity, infertility, seizures, GI toxicity, and secondary malignancies. Instruct not to take without medical supervision; consult physician if skin rash, bleeding, fever, jaundice, persistent cough, seizures, or unusual lumps/masses occur.

**Administration:** Oral route. **Storage:** Refrigerate; 2-8°C (36-46°F).

## LEUKINE RX

sargramostim (Berlex)

**THERAPEUTIC CLASS:** Granulocyte-macrophage colony stimulating factor

**INDICATIONS:** Acute myelogenous leukemia (AML) following induction chemotherapy in older adults ( ≥55 yrs) to shorten time to neutrophil recovery and to reduce incidence of severe and life-threatening infections and infections resulting in death. For mobilization of hematopoietic progenitor cells into peripheral blood for collection by leukopheresis. Myeloid recovery after autologous bone marrow transplantation (BMT) in non-Hodgkin's lymphoma (NHL), acute lymphoblastic leukemia (ALL), and Hodgkin's disease. Myeloid recovery after allogeneic BMT. BMT (allogeneic or autologous) failure or engraftment delay.

**DOSAGE:** *Adults:* ≥55 yrs: Neutrophil Recovery Post-Chemo in AML: Hypoplastic Bone Marrow with <5% Blasts: 250mcg/m$^2$/day IV over 4 hrs starting on Day 11 or 4 days after completion of induction chemo. If 2nd cycle of induction chemo needed, give 4 days after completion of chemo. Continue until ANC >1500 cells/mm$^3$ for 3 consecutive days or max of 42 days. D/C immediately if leukemic regrowth occurs; reduce dose by 50% or temporarily d/c if severe adverse reaction occurs. Mobilization of Peripheral Blood Progenitor Cells (PBPC): 250mcg/m$^2$/day IV over 24 hrs or SC once daily. Continue through PBPC collection period. Reduce dose by 50% if WBC >50,000 cells/mm$^3$. Post Peripheral Blood Progenitor Cell Transplant: 250mcg/m$^2$/day IV over 24 hrs or SC once daily. Begin immediately after infusion of progenitor cells and continue until ANC >1500 cells/mm$^3$ for 3 consecutive days. Myeloid Reconstitution After BMT: 250mcg/m$^2$/day IV over 2 hrs 2-4 hrs post bone marrow infusion and not less than 24 hrs after last dose of chemo- or radiotherapy. Do not give until ANC <500 cells/mm$^3$. Continue until ANC >1500 cells/mm$^3$ for 3 consecutive days. May reduce dose by 50% or temporarily d/c if severe adverse reaction occurs. D/C immediately if blast cells appear or disease progression occurs. BMT Failure/Engraftment Delay: 250mcg/m$^2$/day IV over 2 hrs for 14 days. May repeat after 7 days if needed. Give 3rd course after another 7 days of 500mcg/m$^2$/day IV for 14 days if needed. May reduce dose by 50% or temporarily d/c if severe adverse reaction occurs. D/C immediately if blast cells appear or disease progression occurs. Reduce dose by 50% or interrupt treatment if ANC >20,000 cells/mm$^3$.

**HOW SUPPLIED:** Inj: 250mcg/vial, 500mcg/mL

**CONTRAINDICATIONS:** Excessive leukemic myeloid blasts in bone marrow or peripheral blood ( ≥10%), concomitant chemotherapy or radiotherapy.

**WARNINGS/PRECAUTIONS:** Contains benzyl alcohol; avoid use in neonates. Caution with pre-existing fluid retention, pulmonary infiltrate, CHF, hypoxia, cardiac disease, renal/hepatic dysfunction, or myeloid malignancies. Monitor CBC twice weekly and renal/hepatic function every other week with pre-existing dysfunction.

**ADVERSE REACTIONS:** Fever, N/V, diarrhea, alopecia, rash, headache, stomatitis, anorexia, mucous membrane disorder, asthenia, malaise, abdominal pain, edema, HTN.

**INTERACTIONS:** Caution with drugs that may potentiate myeloproliferative effects (eg, lithium, corticosteroids).

**PREGNANCY:** Category C, caution in nursing.

**MECHANISM OF ACTION:** Recombinant human granulocyte-macrophage colony stimulating factor (GM-CSF); stimulates proliferation and differentiation of hematopoietic progenitor cells.

**PHARMACOKINETICS: Absorption:** IV: (liquid) $C_{max}$=5ng/mL, AUC=640ng/mL•min; (lyophilized) $C_{max}$=5.4ng/mL, AUC=677ng/mL•min. SC: $C_{max}$=1.5ng/mL, $T_{max}$=1-3 hrs; (liquid) AUC=549ng/mL•min; (lyophilized) AUC=501ng/mL•min. **Elimination:** $T_{1/2}$=60 min (IV); 162 min (SC).

## NURSING CONSIDERATIONS

**Assessment:** Assess for excessive leukemic myeloid blasts in bone marrow or peripheral blood ( ≥10%), hypersensitivity to yeast, chemotherapy and radiotherapy use, pre-existing fluid retention, pulmonary infiltrates, CHF, lung disease, hypoxia, pre-existing pleural or pericardial effusion, malignancy with myeloid characteristics, pre-existing cardiac disease (arrhythmias), renal/hepatic dysfunction, pregnancy status, and possible drug interactions. Obtain baseline renal function, CBC with differential, body weight, and LFTs.

**Monitoring:** Monitor CBC with differential and exam for blast cells twice weekly; LFTs and renal function once every other week; body weight and hydration status periodically. Monitor for signs/symptoms of edema, capillary leak syndrome, hypersensitivity reactions, pleural/pericardial effusion, dyspnea or other respiratory symptoms, transient supraventricular arrhythmias, and syndrome characterized by respiratory distress, flushing, hypoxia, hypotension, syncope, and tachycardia.

**Patient Counseling:** Inform of pregnancy risks. Advise to seek medical attention for symptoms of hypersensitivity reactions, effusion, arrhythmias, dyspnea or other respiratory symptoms.

**Administration:** IV/SQ routes. Refer to PI for preparation. **Storage:** 2-8°C (36-46°F). Do not freeze or shake.

# LEVAQUIN — RX

levofloxacin (Ortho-McNeil)

**Fluoroquinolones are associated with an increased risk of tendinitis and tendon rupture in all ages. Risk is further increased with patients >60 yrs, concomitant corticosteroid drugs, or kidney, heart, or lung transplants.**

**THERAPEUTIC CLASS:** Fluoroquinolone

**INDICATIONS:** Treatment of uncomplicated and complicated skin and skin structure infections (SSSI), urinary tract infections (UTI), acute bacterial sinusitis, acute bacterial exacerbation of chronic bronchitis (ABECB), community-acquired pneumonia (CAP) including multi-drug resistant *Streptococcus pneumoniae*, nosocomial pneumonia, chronic bacterial prostatitis (CBP), and acute pyelonephritis caused by susceptible strains of microorganisms. To reduce the incidence or progression of disease of inhalational anthrax following exposure to *Bacillus anthracis*.

**DOSAGE:** *Adults:* ≥18 yrs: IV/PO: ABECB: 500mg qd for 7 days. CAP: 500mg qd for 7-14 days or 750mg qd for 5 days. Sinusitis: 500mg qd for 10-14 days or 750mg qd for 5 days. CBP: 500mg qd for 28 days. Uncomplicated SSSI: 500mg qd for 7-10 days. Complicated SSSI/Nosocomial Pneumonia: 750mg qd for 7-14 days. Inhalational Anthrax (Post-Exposure): 500mg qd for 60 days. Complicated SSSI/Nosocomial Pneumonia/CAP/Sinusitis: CrCl 20-49mL/min: 750mg, then 750mg q48h. CrCl 10-19mL/min/Hemodialysis/CAPD: 750mg, then 500mg q48h. ABECB/CAP/Sinusitis/Uncomplicated SSSI/CBP/Inhalational Anthrax (Post-Exposure): CrCl 20-49mL/min: 500mg, then 250mg q24h. CrCl 10-19mL/min/Hemodialysis/CAPD: 500mg, then 250mg q48h. Complicated UTI/Acute Pyelonephritis: 250mg qd for 10 days or 750mg qd for 5 days. CrCl 10-19mL/min: 250mg, then 250mg q48h or 750mg, then 500mg q48h. Hemodialysis: 750mg, then 500mg q48h. Uncomplicated UTI: 250mg qd for 3 days.

*Pediatrics:* IV/PO: Inhalational anthrax: ≥ 6 Months: >50kg: 500mg q24h for 60 days. <50kg: 8mg/kg q12h for 60 days. Max: 250mg/dose.

**HOW SUPPLIED:** Inj: 25mg/mL [vial], 5mg/mL [pre-mixed solution]; Sol: 25mg/mL; Tab: 250mg, 500mg, 750mg

**WARNINGS/PRECAUTIONS:** Convulsions, toxic psychoses, increased intracranial pressure, CNS stimulation reported; d/c if any occur. Caution with CNS disorders that may predispose seizures or lower seizure threshold (eg, epilepsy, renal insufficiency, drug therapy). Moderate to severe photosensitivity/phototoxicity reactions can occur. Serious/fatal hypersensitivity reactions reported; some reactions may be accompanied by cardiovascular collapse, hypotension/shock, seizures, loss of consciousness, angioedema, airway obstruction, and serious skin reactions. Severe dermatological reactions (eg, toxic epidermal necrolysis [TEN], Stevens-Johnson syndrome [SJS]) reported; d/c at first sign of rash. *Clostridium difficile*-associated diarrhea (CDAD) and colitis reported. Liver toxicities, hematologic toxicities (including agranulocytosis, thrombocytopenia), and renal toxicities may occur. Caution in renal insufficiency. Severe hepatotoxicity (eg, acute hepatitis) reported; d/c if signs and symptoms of hepatitis occur. QT prologation, arrhythmias, peripheral neuropathy, hyper- and hypoglycemia reported. Increased susceptibility to QT interval prolongation in elderly.

**ADVERSE REACTIONS:** N/V, diarrhea, constipation, headache, insomnia, dizziness, abdominal pain, dyspepsia, rash.

**INTERACTIONS:** (Sol, Tab) Decreased levels with antacids, sucralfate, didanosine, metal cations (eg, iron), and multivitamins with zinc; separate dosing by 2 hrs. (Inj, Sol, Tab) Concomitant NSAIDs may increase seizure risk and CNS stimulation. Blood glucose changes with concomitant antidiabetic agents; hyperglycemia or hypoglycemia may occur with insulin or oral hypoglycemics. May increase theophylline levels; monitor closely. May increase PT and cause bleeding episodes with warfarin; monitor closely. Risk of severe tendon disorders is increased with concomitant corticosteroid therapy. Caution with concomitant drugs that may result in prolongation of the QT interval (eg, Class IA antiarrhythmics and Class III antiarrhythmics).



**PREGNANCY:** Category C, not for use in nursing.

**MECHANISM OF ACTION:** Fluoroquinolone; inhibits bacterial topoisomerase IV and DNA gyrase, which are enzymes required for bacterial DNA replication, transcription, repair, and recombination.

**PHARMACOKINETICS: Absorption:** Rapid and complete; $T_{max}$=1-2 hrs. **Distribution:** $V_d$=74-112L; plasma protein binding (approximately 24-38%). **Metabolism:** Limited. **Elimination:** Urine, $T_{1/2}$=6-8 hrs.

## NURSING CONSIDERATIONS

**Assessment:** Assess for history of seizures, QT prolongation, history of tendon or joint-related problems. Assess renal function, LFTs, pregnancy/nursing status, and possible drug interactions.

**Monitoring:** Monitor for QT prolongation and other cardiac disorders, hematologic manifestations, edema, hypo- or hyperglycemia, seizures, musculoskeletal disorders (especially tendinitis and tendon rupture), photosensitivity/phototoxicity, respiratory problems, CDAD, renal function, peripheral neuropathy, hypersensitivity reactions (including TEN and SJS), and possible drug interactions. Monitor LFTs, CBC.

**Patient Counseling:** Instruct to notify healthcare provider if symptoms of pain, swelling, or inflammation of a tendon, or weakness or inability to move joints develop; must rest and refrain from excercise, and d/c therapy. Inform that drug treats bacterial, not viral, infections. Instruct that skipping doses or not completing full course may decrease effectiveness and increase bacterial resistance to drug. Inform to d/c use and notify physician if allergic reaction, skin rash, or watery/bloody stools occur. Counsel on possible drug interactions. Caution in activities requiring mental alertness and coordination. Advise to avoid excessive sun exposure. Advise diabetic patients to use caution; hypo- or hyperglycemia may develop.

**Administration:** IV, oral route. **Storage:** (Tab) 15-30°C (59-86°F), in tightly closed containers. (Sol) 25°C (77°F), excursions permitted to 15-30°C (59-86°F). (Inj) Single-use vials: Controlled room temperature, and protected from light. Pre-mixed solution: 25°C (77°F) or below; brief exposure up to 40°C (104°F) does not adversely affect product.

## LEVBID RX

hyoscyamine sulfate (Alaven)

**OTHER BRAND NAMES:** Levsin (Alaven) - Levsinex (Alaven)

**THERAPEUTIC CLASS:** Anticholinergic

**INDICATIONS:** Adjunct treatment of peptic ulcer, irritable bowel syndrome, neurogenic bladder, and neurogenic bowel disturbances. Management of functional intestinal disorders (eg, mild dysenteries, diverticulitis). To control gastric secretion, visceral spasm, and hypermotility in spastic colitis, spastic bladder, cystitis, pylorospasm, and associated abdominal cramps. Symptomatic relief of biliary and renal colic with concomitant morphine or other narcotics. Drying agent for symptomatic relief of acute rhinitis. To reduce rigidity and tremors of Parkinson's disease and control associated sialorrhea and hyperhidrosis. For anticholinesterase poisoning. To reduce pain and hypersecretion in pancreatitis. For certain cases of partial heart block associated with vagal activity. (Elixir, Drops) Treatment of infant colic. (Inj) Facilitates GI diagnostic procedures. Reduces pain and hypersecretion in pancreatitis, in cases of partial heart block associated with vagal activity, and as antidote for anticholinesterase poisoning. In anesthesia as a pre-op antimuscarinic. In urology to improve radiologic visibility of kidneys.

**DOSAGE:** *Adults:* May also chew or swallow SL tab. (Drops, Elixir, Tab, and Tab, SL) 0.125-0.25mg q4h or prn. Max: 1.5mg/24 hrs. (Cap and Tab, Extended-Release) 0.375-0.75mg q12h; or 1 cap q8h. Max: 1.5mg/24 hrs. Do not crush or chew. (Inj) GI Disorders: 0.25-0.5mg IM/IV/SQ as single dose or up to qid at 4-hr intervals. Diagnostic Procedures: 0.25-0.5mg IV 5-10 min before procedure. Anesthesia: 5mcg/kg IM/IV/SQ 30-60 min before anesthesia or with narcotic/sedative administration. GI Disorders: 0.25-0.5mg IM/IV/SQ as single dose; may require bid-qid administration at 4-hr intervals. Diagnostic Procedures: 0.25-0.5mg IV 5-10 min prior. Drug-Induced Bradycardia (Surgery): Increments of 0.25mL IV; repeat prn. Neuromuscular Blockade Reversal: 0.2mg for every 1mg neostigmine or equal dose of physostigmine or pyridostigmine.

*Pediatrics:* May also chew or swallow SL tab. ≥12 yrs: (Drops, Elixir, Tab, and Tab, SL) 0.125-0.25mg q4h or prn. Max: 1.5mg/24 hrs. (Cap and Tab, Extended-Release) 0.375-0.75mg q12h; or 1 cap may be given q8h. Max: 1.5mg/24 hrs. Do not crush or chew. 2 to <12 yrs: (Tab and Tab, SL) 0.0625-0.125mg q4h or prn. Max: 0.75mg/24 hrs. (Elixir) Give q4h or prn. 10kg: 1.25mL. 20kg: 2.5mL. 40kg: 3.75mL. 50kg: 5mL. Max: 30mL/24 hrs. (Drops) 0.25-1mL q4h or prn. Max: 6mL/24 hrs. <2 yrs: (Drops) Give q4h or prn. 3.4kg: 4 drops. Max: 24 drops/24 hrs. 5kg: 5 drops. Max: 30 drops/24 hrs. 7kg: 6 drops. Max: 36 drops/24 hrs. 10kg: 8 drops. Max: 48 drops/24 hrs. >2 yrs: Anesthesia: (Inj) 5mcg/kg IM/IV/SQ 30-60 min before anesthesia or with narcotic/sedative administration.

**HOW SUPPLIED:** (Levbid) Tab, Extended-Release: 0.375mg. (Levsin) Drops: 0.125mg/mL [15mL]; Elixir: 0.125mg/5mL [473mL]; Inj: 0.5mg/mL; Tab: 0.125mg*; Tab, SL: 0.125mg*. (Levsinex) Cap, Extended-Release: 0.375mg
*scored

**CONTRAINDICATIONS:** Glaucoma, obstructive uropathy, GI tract obstruction, paralytic ileus; intestinal atony of elderly/debilitated, unstable CV status in acute hemorrhage, toxic megacolon complicating ulcerative colitis, myasthenia gravis.

**WARNINGS/PRECAUTIONS:** Risk of heat prostration with high environmental temperature. Avoid activities requiring mental alertness. Psychosis has been reported. Caution with diarrhea, autonomic neuropathy, hyperthyroidism, coronary heart disease, CHF, arrhythmias/tachycardia, HTN, renal disease, and hiatal hernia associated with reflux esophagitis. D/C if diarrhea occurs.

**ADVERSE REACTIONS:** Anticholinergic effects, drowsiness, headache, nervousness.

**INTERACTIONS:** Additive effects with other antimuscarinics, amantadine, haloperidol, phenothiazines, MAOIs, TCAs, and some antihistamines. Antacids interfere with absorption; take ac and antacids pc.

**PREGNANCY:** Category C, caution in nursing.

**MECHANISM OF ACTION:** Anticholinergic/antipasmodic; inhibits specifically the actions of acetylcholine on structures innervated by postganglionic cholinergic nerves and on smooth muscles that respond to acetylcholine but lack cholinergic innervation.

**PHARMACOKINETICS: Absorption:** Complete. **Distribution:** Crosses blood-brain barrier and placental barrier. **Metabolism:** Hydrolyzed partially to tropic acid. **Elimination:** Urine (unchanged); $T_{1/2}$=2-3.5 hrs.

## NURSING CONSIDERATIONS

**Assessment:** Assess for glaucoma, obstructive uropathy, GI obstruction, paralytic ileus, intestinal atony, unstable CV status in acute hemorrhage, severe ulcerative colitis, toxic megacolon complicating ulcerative colitis, myasthenia gravis, and possible drug interactions.

**Monitoring:** Monitor for diarrhea, drowsiness, dizziness or blurred vision, psychosis, and CNS signs/symptoms including confusion, disorientation, short-term memory loss, hallucinations, dysarthria, ataxia, euphoria, anxiety, fatigue, insomnia, agitation, and unusual mannerisms.

**Patient Counseling:** Warn not to engage in activities requiring mental alertness (eg, operating a motor vehicle or other machinery), or to perform hazardous work while on treatment. Inform that decreased sweating resulting in heat prostration, fever or heat stroke may occur; caution if febrile, or exposed to high environmental temperatures. Counsel that extended-release tab/cap may not completely disintegrate and may be excreted.

**Administration:** Oral, IV, IM, SQ routes. **Storage:** 15-30°C (59-86°F).



# LEVEMIR RX

insulin detemir, rdna origin (Novo Nordisk)

**THERAPEUTIC CLASS:** Insulin

**INDICATIONS:** Treatment of adults and pediatrics with type 1 diabetes or adults with type 2 diabetes who require basal (long-acting) insulin for the control of hyperglycemia.

**DOSAGE:** *Adults:* Individualize dose. Administer SQ qd or bid. Once-Daily Dosing: Administer with evening meal or bedtime. Twice-Daily Dosing: Administer evening dose with evening meal, at bedtime, or 12 hrs after morning dose. Type 1/Type 2 Diabetes on Basal-Bolus Treatment or Patients Only on Basal Insulin: Change on a unit-to-unit basis. Insulin-Naive with Type 2 Diabetes Inadequately Controlled on Oral Antidiabetics: Initial: 0.1-0.2 U/kg in evening or 10 U qd or bid.
*Pediatrics:* Individualize dose. Administer SQ qd or bid. Once-Daily Dosing: Administer with evening meal or bedtime. Twice-Daily Dosing: Administer evening dose with evening meal, at bedtime, or 12 hrs after morning dose. Type 1 Diabetes on Basal-Bolus Treatment or Patients Only on Basal Insulin: Change on a unit-to-unit basis.

**HOW SUPPLIED:** Inj: 100 U/mL [3mL, 10mL]

**WARNINGS/PRECAUTIONS:** Monitor glucose; may cause hypoglycemia. Not for use in an insulin infusion pump. Should not be diluted or mixed with any other insulin preparations. May cause lipodystrophy or hypersensitivity. Dose adjustment may be needed in renal or hepatic impairment and during intercurrent conditions such as illness, emotional disturbances, or other stresses.

**ADVERSE REACTIONS:** Allergic reactions, inj site reactions, lipodystrophy, pruritus, rash, hypoglycemia, weight gain.

**INTERACTIONS:** Avoid mixing with other insulins. Increased glucose lowering effects with ACE inhibitors, disopyramide, fibrates, fluoxetine, MAOIs, propoxyphene, salicylates, somatostatin analog, sulfonamide antibiotics, and other antidiabetic agents. Decreased blood glucose lowering effects with corticosteroids, danazol, diuretics, sympathomimetic agents, isoniazid, phenothiazine derivatives, somatotropin, thyroid hormones, estrogens, progestogens. Pentamidine may cause hypoglycemia, followed by hyperglycemia. β-blockers, clonidine, lithium salts, and alcohol may potentiate or weaken glucose lowering effect. β-blockers, clonidine, guanethidine, and reserpine may reduce or mask signs of hypoglycemia.

**PREGNANCY:** Category C, caution in nursing.

**MECHANISM OF ACTION:** Insulin detemir (rDNA origin); regulates glucose metabolism and lowers blood glucose by facilitating cellular uptake and inhibiting the glucose output from the liver.

**PHARMACOKINETICS: Absorption:** Slow, prolonged; absolute bioavailability (60%); $T_{max}$=6-8 hrs. **Distribution:** $V_d$=0.1L/kg; plasma protein binding ( ≥98%). **Metabolism:** Liver. **Elimination:** $T_{1/2}$=5-7 hrs.

## NURSING CONSIDERATIONS

**Assessment:** Assess FPG, $HbA_{1c}$, renal function, LFTs, pregnancy status, infections, alcohol consumption, exercise routines, and possible drug interactions.

**Monitoring:** Monitor FPG, $HbA_{1c}$, hypokalemia, renal function, diabetic ketoacidosis, vision changes, lipodystrophy, allergic reactions. Monitor for signs of hypoglycemia (sweating, palpitations, seizures, disorientation, tremors).

**Patient Counseling:** Use only if the solution is clear and colorless with no visible particles. Do not dilute or mix with other insulins or solutions. Counsel about signs/symptoms of hypoglycemia, hyperglycemia, diabetic ketoacidosis, the importance of frequent monitoring of blood glucose levels, the need for eating a balanced diet and exercising regularly. Advise to avoid excessive alcohol. During periods of stress (eg, trauma, infection, surgery), insulin requirements may be changed; advise patients to seek prompt medical advice. Counsel on proper administration techniques.

**Administration:** SQ route (thigh, abdominal wall, or upper arm). **Storage:** 2-8°C (36-46°F). Do not use if frozen.

L

# LEVITRA RX

vardenafil HCl (Schering-Plough)

**THERAPEUTIC CLASS:** Phosphodiesterase type 5 inhibitor

**INDICATIONS:** Treatment of erectile dysfunction (ED).

**DOSAGE:** *Adults:* Initial: 10mg 1hr prior to sexual activity up to once daily. Titrate: May decrease to 5mg or increase to max of 20mg based on response. Elderly: ≥65 yrs: Initial: 5mg. Moderate Hepatic Impairment: Initial: 5mg; Max: 10mg. Concomitant Ritonavir: Max: 2.5mg/72 hrs. Concomitant Indinavir/Saquinavir/Atazanavir/Clarithromycin/Ketoconazole 400mg daily/ Itraconazole 400mg daily: Max: 2.5mg/24 hrs. Concomitant Ketoconazole 200mg daily/Itraconazole 200mg daily/Erythromycin: Max: 5mg/24 hrs. Concomitant Stable Alpha-blocker: Initial: 5mg; 2.5mg when used with certain CYP3A4 inhibitors.

**HOW SUPPLIED:** Tab: 2.5mg, 5mg, 10mg, 20mg

**CONTRAINDICATIONS:** Concomitant nitrates or nitric oxide donors.

**WARNINGS/PRECAUTIONS:** Avoid when sexual activity is inadvisable due to underlying cardiovascular (CV) status. Increased sensitivity to vasodilation effects with left ventricular outflow obstruction. Decrease in supine BP reported. Avoid with unstable angina, hypotension (SBP<90 mmHg), uncontrolled HTN( >170/100 mmHg), recent history of stroke, life-threatening arrhythmia, myocardial infarction (MI) within last 6 months, severe cardiac failure, severe hepatic impairment (Child-Pugh C), end-stage renal disease (ESRD) requiring dialysis, hereditary degenerative retinal disorders including retinitis pigmentosa, congenital QT prolongation. Caution with bleeding disorders, peptic ulcers, anatomical deformation of the penis or predisposition to priapism. Rare reports of non-arteritic anterior ischemic optic neuropathy

(NAION) with phosphodiesterase type 5 (PDE5) inhibitors. Sudden decrease or loss of hearing accompanied by tinnitus and dizziness reported.

**ADVERSE REACTIONS:** Headache, flushing, rhinitis, dyspepsia, sinusitis, flu syndrome, dizziness, nausea.

**INTERACTIONS:** See Contraindications. Avoid use with Class IA (eg, quinidine, procainamide) or Class III (eg, amiodarone, sotalol) antiarrhythmics and other agents for ED Increased levels with CYP3A4 inhibitors (eg, ritonavir, indinavir, saquinavir, atazanavir, ketoconazole, itraconazole, clarithromycin, erythromycin). Additive hypotensive effect, which may lead to symptomatic hypotension when used with α-blockers. Reduced clearance with CYP3A4 and CYP2C9 inhibitors.

**PREGNANCY:** Category B, not for use in nursing.

**MECHANISM OF ACTION:** PDE5 inhibitor; enhances the effect of nitric oxide by inhibiting PDE5, which is responsible for the degradation of cGMP in the corpus cavernosum.

**PHARMACOKINETICS: Absorption:** Rapid, absolute bioavailability (15%); $T_{max}$=30 min. **Distribution:** $V_d$=208L; plasma protein binding (95%). **Metabolism:** Via CYP3A4, CYP3A5, CYP2C. M1 (major metabolite). **Elimination:** Feces (91%), urine (2%); $T_{1/2}$=4 hrs.

## NURSING CONSIDERATIONS

**Assessment:** Assess for CV disease, long QT syndrome, retinitis pigmentosa, bleeding disorders, active peptic ulceration, anatomical deformation of the penis, renal/hepatic impairment. Assess potential underlying causes of erectile dysfunction, pregnancy/nursing status and for possible drug interactions.

**Monitoring:** Monitor potential for cardiac risk due to sexual activity, postural hypotension, color vision changes or other eye adverse events (eg, NAION), hypersensitivity reactions, stomach ulcers and hearing impairment. Monitor therapeutic effect when used in combination with other drugs.

**Patient Counseling:** Discuss risks and benefits of therapy. Seek medical assistance if erection persists >4 hrs or if with painful erection >6 hrs. Inform that possibility of postural hypotension may occur. Advise of potential BP-lowering effect of α-blockers and antihypertensive medications, and cardiac risk of sexual activity. Counsel about protective measures necessary to guard against STDs, including HIV. D/C and inform doctor if sudden loss of vision, color vision or hearing occur. Counsel to take as prescribed.

**Administration:** Oral route. **Storage:** 25°C (77°F); excursions permitted to 15-30° (59-86°F).

# LEVOTHROID RX

levothyroxine sodium (Forest)

**THERAPEUTIC CLASS:** Thyroid replacement hormone

**INDICATIONS:** Hypothyroidism. As a pituitary TSH suppressant for nonendemic goiter and for chronic lymphocytic thyroiditis. Diagnostic agent in suppression tests to differentiate mild hyperthyroidism or thyroid gland autonomy. Adjunct therapy with antithyroid drugs to treat thyrotoxicosis. Adjunct to surgery and radioiodine therapy for TSH-dependent thyroid cancer.

**DOSAGE:** *Adults:* Hypothyroidism: Usual: 100-200mcg/day. Endocrine/Cardiovascular Complications: Initial: 50mcg/day. Titrate: Increase by 50mcg/day every 2-4 weeks until euthyroid. Hypothyroid with Angina: Initial: 25mcg/day. Titrate: Increase by 25-50mcg every 2-4 weeks until euthyroid. *Pediatrics:* Hypothyroidism: >12 yrs: Usual: 100-200mcg/day. 6-12 yrs: 4-5mcg/kg/day. 1-5 yrs: 5-6mcg/kg/day. 6-12 months: 6-8mcg/kg/day. 0-6 months: 10-15mcg/kg/day. May crush tab and sprinkle over food (applesauce) or mix with 5-10mL water, formula (non-soy), or breast milk.

**HOW SUPPLIED:** Tab: 25mcg*, 50mcg*, 75mcg*, 88mcg*, 100mcg*, 112mcg*, 125mcg*, 137mcg*, 150mcg*, 175mcg*, 200mcg*, 300mcg* *scored

**CONTRAINDICATIONS:** Untreated thyrotoxicosis, acute MI, and uncorrected adrenal insufficiency.

**WARNINGS/PRECAUTIONS:** Do not use in the treatment of obesity; larger doses in euthyroid patients can cause serious or even life-threatening toxicity. Caution with cardiovascular disease, HTN. May aggravate diabetes mellitus or insipidus and adrenal cortical insufficiency. Excessive doses in infants may produce craniosynostosis. Add glucocorticoid with myxedema coma.

**ADVERSE REACTIONS:** Lactose hypersensitivity, transient partial hair loss in children.

**INTERACTIONS:** Monitor insulin and oral hypoglycemic requirements. May potentiate anticoagulant effects of warfarin; adjust warfarin dose and monitor PT/INR. Increased adrenergic effects of catecholamines; caution with CAD. Decreased absorption with cholestyramine and colestipol; space dosing by 4-5 hrs. Estrogens increase thyroxine-binding globulin; increase in thyroid dose may be needed. Large dose may cause life-threatening toxicities with sympathomimetic amines. Avoid mixing crushed tabs with foods/formula with large amounts of iron, soybean or fiber.

**PREGNANCY:** Category A, caution in nursing.

**MECHANISM OF ACTION:** Thyroid hormone; not understood, suspected to control DNA transcription and protein synthesis. Regulates multiple metabolic processes.

**PHARMACOKINETICS: Distribution:** Plasma protein binding (99%). **Metabolism:** Deiodination (major pathway), conjugation (minor pathway) in liver (mainly), kidneys, and other tissues. **Elimination:** Urine; $T_4$ (feces 20% unchanged); $T_{1/2}$=6-7 days; $T_{1/2}$≤2 days ($T_3$).

## NURSING CONSIDERATIONS

**Assessment:** Assess for drug hypersensitivity, CV disease, angina pectoris, acute MI, suppressed serum TSH level with normal $T_3$ and $T_4$ levels, overt thyrotoxicosis, DM, clotting disorder, adrenal/pituitary gland problems, malabsorption, autoimmune polyglandular syndrome, undergoing surgery, and possible drug and test interactions. Assess infants with congenital hypothyroidism for other congenital anomalies.

**Monitoring:** Requires frequent lab tests and clinical evaluation of thyroid function by TSH levels, and also glucose/lipid metabolism, urinary glucose in diabetics, and clotting status. Monitor for CV signs such as arrhythmia and coronary insufficiency, growth/development, bone metabolism, cognitive function, emotional state, GI function, reproductive function, partial hair loss in children, and signs/symptoms of thyrotoxicosis.

**Patient Counseling:** Counsel to take 1 hr before breakfast, and not to to use as part of weight control regimen. Inform that replacement therapy is essential for life, except in cases of transient hypothyroidism. Advise to notify physician if pregnant/nursing or intend to become pregnant. Advise to notify if taking any other drugs. Counsel to not d/c or change dosage. Instruct to report signs/symptoms of thyroid toxicity.

**Administration:** Oral route. **Storage:** 25°C (77°F); excursions permitted to 15-30°C (59-86°F). Protect from light and moisture.

## LEVOXYL — RX

levothyroxine sodium (King)

**THERAPEUTIC CLASS:** Thyroid replacement hormone

**INDICATIONS:** As replacement or supplemental therapy in congenital or acquired hypothyroidism of any etiology, except transient hypothyroidism during the recovery phase of subacute thyroiditis. In the treatment or prevention of various types of euthyroid goiters, including thyroid nodules, subacute or chronic lymphocytic thyroiditis, multinodular goiter and as an adjunct to surgery and radioiodine therapy for thyrotropin-dependent well-differentiated thyroid cancer.

**DOSAGE:** *Adults:* Take in the AM at least one-half hour before food. Take at least 4 hrs apart from drugs that are known to interfere with the absorption of levothyroxine. Hypothyroidism: Usual: 1.7mcg/kg/day. Doses >200mcg/day seldom required. >50 yrs/<50 yrs with Cardiac Disease: Initial: 25-50mcg/day. Titrate: Increase by 12.5-25mcg/day every 6-8 weeks until euthyroid. Elderly with Cardiac Disease: Initial: 12.5-25mcg/day. Titrate: Increase by 12.5-25mcg/day every 4-6 weeks until euthyroid. Severe Hypothyroidism: Initial: 12.5-25mcg/day. Titrate: Increase by 25mcg/day every 2-4 weeks until euthyroid. Pregnancy: May increase dose requirements. Subclinical Hypothyroidism: A lower doses may be adequate to normalize the TSH level. TSH Suppression in Well-differentiated Thyroid Cancer and Thyroid Nodules: Dose should be individualized based on the specific disease and the patient being treated. Refer to PI for further details.

*Pediatrics:* Take in the AM at least one-half hour before food. Take at least 4 hrs apart from drugs that are known to interfere with the absorption of levothyroxine. Hypothyroidism: 0-3 months: 10-15mcg/kg/day. 3-6 months: 8-10mcg/kg/day. 6-12 months: 6-8mcg/kg/day. 1-5 yrs: 5-6mcg/kg/day. 6-12 yrs: 4-5mcg/kg/day. >12 yrs: 2-3mcg/kg/day. Growth/Puberty Complete: 1.7mcg/kg/day. Infants at Risk for Cardiac Failure: Use lower dose. Titrate: Increase dose every 4-6 weeks as needed based until euthyroid. Infants with Serum $T_4$ <5mcg/dL: Initial: 50mcg/day. Chronic/Severe Hypothyroidism: Children: Initial: 25mcg/day. Titrate: Increase by 25mcg/day every 2-4 weeks until desired effect is achieved. Minimize Hyperactivity in Older Children: Initial: Give 1/4 of full replacement dose. Titrate: Increase on a weekly basis by an amount equal to 1/4 the full recommended replacement dose until the full recommended replacement dose is reached. May crush tab and mix with 5-10mL of water.

L

**HOW SUPPLIED:** Tab: 25mcg, 50mcg, 75mcg, 88mcg, 100mcg, 112mcg, 125mcg, 137mcg, 150mcg, 175mcg, 200mcg

**CONTRAINDICATIONS:** Untreated subclinical or overt thyrotoxicosis of any etiology, acute MI, and uncorrected adrenal insufficiency.

**WARNINGS/PRECAUTIONS:** Do not use in the treatment of obesity or weight loss; larger doses in euthyroid patients can cause serious or even life-threatening toxicity. Should not be used in the treatment of male or female infertility unless associated with hypothyroidism. Caution with nontoxic diffuse goiter or nodular thyroid disease. Carefully titrate dose to avoid over or under treatment. May decrease bone mineral density with long term use; give minimum dose necessary to achieve desired clinical and biochemical response. Caution with cardiovascular disorders and the elderly with risk of occult cardiac disease. If cardiac symptoms develop or worsen, reduce or withhold dose for one week and then restart at lower dose. May produce CV effects (eg, increase HR, increase in cardiac wall thickness, increase in cardiac contractility, precipitation of angina or arrhythmias). Monitor patients with CAD closely during surgical procedures, may precipitate cardiac arrhythmias. Caution with nontoxic diffuse goiter or nodular thyroid disease and in patients with adrenal insuffiency.

**ADVERSE REACTIONS:** Fatigue, increased appetite, weight loss, heat intolerance, headache, hyperactivity, irritability, insomnia, palpitations, arrhythmias, dyspnea, hair loss, menstrual irregularities, pseudotumor cerebri (children), slipped capital femoral epiphysis (children).

**INTERACTIONS:** Sympathomimetics may increase risk of coronary insufficiency with CAD. Upward dose adjustments may be needed for insulin and oral hypoglycemic agents. May decrease absorption with soybean flour (infant formula), cottonseed meal, walnuts, and dietary fiber. May potentiate oral anticoagulant effects; adjust dose and monitor PT. May decrease levels and effects of digitalis glycosides. Reduced TSH secretion with dopamine/dopamine agonists, glucocorticoids, octreotide. Decreased thyroid hormone secretion with aminoglutethimide, amiodarone, iodine (including iodine-containing radiographic contrast agents), lithium, methimazole, propylthiouracil (PTU), sulfonamides, tolbutamide. May increase thyroid hormone secretion with amiodarone and iodide. May decrease $T_4$ absorption with antacids (aluminum & magnesium hydroxides), simethicone, bile acid sequestrants (cholestyramine, colestipol), calcium carbonate, cation exchange resins (kayexalate), ferrous sulfate, orlistat, and sucralfate. May increased serum TBG concentration with clofibrate, estrogen-containing oral contraceptives, oral estrogens, heroin/methadone, 5-FU, mitotane, and tamoxifen. May decrease serum TBG concentration with androgens/anabolic steroids, asparaginase, glucocorticoids, and slow-release nicotinic acid. May cause protein-binding site displacement with furosemide (>80mg IV), heparin, hydantoins, NSAIDS (fenamates, phenylbutazone), and salicylates (>2g/day). May alter $T_4$ and $T_3$ metabolism with carbamazepine, hydantoins, phenobarbital, and rifampin. May decrease $T_4$ 5'-deiodinase activity with amiodarone, β-adrenergic antagonists (eg, propranolol >160mg/day), glucocorticoids (eg, dexamethasone >4mg/day), and PTU. Concurrent use with tri/tetracyclic antidepressants may increase the therapeutic and toxic effects of both drugs. Coadministration with sertraline in patients stabilized on levothyroxine, may result in increased levothyroxine requirements. Interferon-α may cause development of antithyroid microsomal antibodies causing transient hypothyroidism, hyperthyroidism, or both. Interleukin-2 has been associated with transient painless thyroiditis. Excessive use with growth hormones may accelerate epiphyseal closure. Ketamine may produce marked HTN and tachycardia. May reduce uptake of iodine-containing radiographic contrast agents. Decreased theophylline clearance may occur in hypothyroid patients. Altered levels of thyroid hormone and/or TSH level with choral hydrate, diazepam, ethionamide, lovastatin, metoclopramide, 6-mercaptopurine, nitroprusside, para-aminosalicylate sodium, perphenazine, resorcinol (excessive topical use), and thiazide diuretics.

**PREGNANCY:** Category A, caution in nursing.

**MECHANISM OF ACTION:** Thyroid hormone; not established. Suspected that principal effects are exerted through control of DNA transcription and protein synthesis.

**PHARMACOKINETICS: Distribution:** Plasma protein binding (99%); found in breast milk. **Metabolism:** Deiodination and conjugation in liver (mainly), kidneys, and other tissues. **Elimination:** Urine, feces (20% unchanged); ($T_4$) $T_{1/2}$=6-7days; ($T_3$) $T_{1/2}$≤2 days.

## NURSING CONSIDERATIONS

**Assessment:** Assess for untreated subclinical or overt thyrotoxicosis, presence of acute MI, uncorrected adrenal insuffiency, CV disorders, nontoxic diffuse goiter, nodular thyroid disease, DM, pregnancy/nursing status, and for possible drug interactions. In patients with secondary or tertiary hypothyroidism, assess for additional hypothalmic/pituitary hormone deficiencies. Assess that therapy is not for the treatment of obesity or for weight loss. In infants with congenital hypothyroidism, assess for other congenital anomalies.

**Monitoring:** Monitor for cardiovascular effects (eg, increase in heart rate, increase in cardiac wall thickness, angina, arrhythmias). In patients on long-term therapy, monitor for signs/symptoms of decreased bone mineral density. In patients with nontoxic diffuse goiter or nodular thyroid disease, monitor for precipitation of thyrotoxicosis. In adults with primary hypothyroidism, perform periodic monitoring of serum TSH levels. In pediatric patients with congenital hypothyroidism, perform periodic monitoring of serum TSH levels and total or free $T_4$ levels. In patients with secondary and tertiary hypothyroidism, perform periodic monitoring of serum free $T_4$ levels.

**Patient Counseling:** Instruct to notify physician if allergic to any foods or medicines, pregnant or planning to become pregnant, breastfeeding or taking any other drugs, including prescriptions and over-the-counter preparations. Advise to notify physician of any other medical conditions particularly heart disease, diabetes, clotting disorders, and adrenal or pituitary gland problems. Instruct to not d/c or change dose unless directed by physician. Instruct to take on empty stomach, with a full glass of water, at least 1/2 hour before eating any food. Advise that partial hair loss may occur during the first few months of therapy, but is usually temporary. Instruct to notify physician or dentist prior to surgery, that taking levothyroxine. Inform that should not use as a primary or adjunctive therapy in a weight control program.

**Administration:** Oral route. **Storage:** 20°-25°C (68-77°F); excursions permitted to 15-30°C (59-86°F).

# LEXAPRO

RX

escitalopram oxalate (Forest)

**Antidepressants increased the risk of suicidal thinking and behavior (suicidality) in short-term studies in children, adolescents, and young adults with major depressive disorder (MDD) and other psychiatric disorders. Escitalopram is not approved for use in pediatric patients <12 yrs of age.**

**THERAPEUTIC CLASS:** Selective serotonin reuptake inhibitor

**INDICATIONS:** Acute and maintenance treatment of major depressive disorder (MDD) in adults and adolescents aged 12-17 years. Acute treatment of generalized anxiety disorder (GAD) in adults.

**DOSAGE:** *Adults:* MDD: Initial: 10mg qd, in am or pm. Titrate: May increase to 20mg after 1 week. Max: 20mg qd. GAD: Initial: 10mg qd, in am or pm. Titrate: May increase to 20mg after 1 week. Elderly/Hepatic Impairment: 10mg qd. Re-evaluate periodically.
*Pediatrics:* 12-17 yrs: MDD: Initial: 10mg qd, in am or pm. Titrate: May increase to 20mg after 3 weeks. Max: 20mg qd. Re-evaluate periodically.

**HOW SUPPLIED:** Sol: 5mg/5mL [240mL]; Tab: 5mg, 10mg*, 20mg* *scored

**CONTRAINDICATIONS:** Concomitant use of MAOI or pimozide therapy.

**WARNINGS/PRECAUTIONS:** Avoid abrupt withdrawal. May increase the risk of bleeding events. Activation of mania/hypomania, hyponatremia reported. SIADH reported with citalopram. Caution with history of mania or seizures, hepatic impairment, severe renal impairment, and conditions that alter metabolism or hemodynamic responses. May impair mental/physical abilities. Serotonin syndrome or NMS-like reactions reported. Manage with immediate d/c and monitor.

**ADVERSE REACTIONS:** Nausea, insomnia, ejaculation disorder, increased sweating, somnolence, fatigue, diarrhea.

**INTERACTIONS:** See Contraindications. Avoid alcohol, citalopram, or within 14 days of MAOI therapy. Caution with other CNS drugs, lithium, carbamazepine, cimetidine, drugs metabolized by CYP2D6 (eg, desipramine). Increased risk of bleeding with NSAIDs, ASA, warfarin. May increase metoprolol levels, which leads to decreased cardioselectivity. Rare reports of weakness, hyperreflexia, incoordination with an SSRI and sumatriptan. Serotonin syndrome reported with linezolid.

**PREGNANCY:** Category C, caution in nursing.

**MECHANISM OF ACTION:** SSRI; inhibits CNS neuronal reuptake of serotonin.

**PHARMACOKINETICS: Absorption:** $T_{max}$=5 hrs. **Distribution:** Plasma protein binding (56%). **Metabolism:** Hepatic (biotransformation: N-demethylation) via CYP3A4, 2C19. **Elimination:** Urine (8%); $T_{1/2}$=27-36 hrs.

## NURSING CONSIDERATIONS

**Assessment:** Assess for risk of bipolar disorder, history of mania, possible drug interactions, history of seizures, disease/condition that alters metabolism or hemodynamic response, hepatic/renal impairment.

**Monitoring:** Monitor for signs/symptoms of clinical worsening (suicidality, unusual changes in behavior), serotonin syndrome, abnormal bleeding, hyponatremia, seizures, cognitive and motor impairment, and hepatic/renal dysfunction. If abruptly d/c therapy, monitor for symptoms of dysphoric mood, irritability, agitation, dizziness, sensory disturbances, anxiety, confusion, headache, lethargy, emotional lability, insomnia, and hypomania. Monitor for serotonin syndrome and NMS.

**Patient Counseling:** Advise to avoid alcohol. Seek medical attention for symptoms of serotonin syndrome (mental status changes, tachycardia, hyperthermia, NV, diarrhea, incoordination), abnormal bleeding (particularly if using NSAIDs or ASA), hyponatremia, activation of mania, seizures, clinical worsening (suicidal ideation, unusual changes in behavior) and discontinuation symptoms (irritability, agitation, dizziness, anxiety, headache, insomnia). Caution against operating hazardous machinery, including automobiles, until they are reasonably certain that Lexapro therapy does not affect their ability to engage in such activities. Inform may notice improvement in 1-4 weeks; continue therapy as directed.

**Administration:** Oral route. **Storage:** 25°C (77°F); excursions permitted to 15-30°C (59-86°F).

## LEXIVA RX

fosamprenavir calcium (GlaxoSmithKline)

**THERAPEUTIC CLASS:** Protease inhibitor

**INDICATIONS:** Treatment of HIV-1 infection in combination with other antiretroviral agents.

**DOSAGE:** *Adults:* Therapy-Naive: 1400mg bid or 1400mg qd + ritonavir (RTV) 200mg qd or 1400mg qd + RTV 100mg qd or 700mg bid + RTV 100mg bid. Protease Inhibitor (PI)-Experienced: 700mg bid + RTV 100mg bid. Mild Hepatic Impairment (Child-Pugh score 5-6): Therapy-Naive: 700mg bid. Therapy-Naive/PI-Experienced: 700mg bid + RTV 100mg qd. Moderate Hepatic Impairment (Child-Pugh score 7-9): Therapy-Naive: 700mg bid. Therapy-Naive/PI-Experienced: 450mg bid + RTV 100mg qd. Severe Hepatic Impairment (Child-Pugh score 10-15): Therapy-Naive: 350mg bid. Therapy-Naive/PI-Experienced: 300mg bid + RTV 100mg qd. Elderly: Caution in dosing.

*Pediatrics:* 2-18 yrs: Calculate based on body weight (kg). Dose should not exceed recommended adult dose. Therapy-Experienced: ≥6 yrs: 18mg/kg + RTV 3mg/kg bid, not to exceed 700mg + RTV 100mg bid. Therapy-Naive: ≥6 yrs: 30mg/kg bid, not to exceed 1400mg bid or 18mg/kg + RTV 3mg/kg bid, not to exceed 700mg + RTV 100mg bid. Therapy-Naive: 2-5 yrs: 30mg/kg bid, not to exceed 1400mg/kg bid. When used without ritonavir: Adult regimen of 1400mg bid may be used in patients ≥47kg. When administered with RTV: May be used for patients ≥39kg, RTV caps may be used in patients ≥33kg.

**HOW SUPPLIED:** Sus: 50mg/mL [225mL], Tab: 700mg

**CONTRAINDICATIONS:** Concomitant drugs dependent on CYP3A4 for clearance and for which elevated plasma concentrations are associated with serious and/or life-threatening events including St. John's wort, flecainide, propafenone, rifampin, delavirdine, lovastatin, simvastatin, ergot derivatives (eg, dihydroergotamine, ergonovine, ergotamine, methylergonovine), cisapride, pimozide, midazolam, and triazolam.

**WARNINGS/PRECAUTIONS:** Severe and life-threatening skin reactions (including Stevens-Johnson syndrome [SJS]) reported; d/c if severe or life-threatening reactions occur or if moderate rashes occur that are accompanied by systemic symptoms. Use with RTV at higher than recommended doses may result in transaminase elevations and should not be used. Patients with underlying hepatitis B or C or marked elevations in serum transaminases prior to treatment may be at increased risk for developing or worsening transaminase elevations. Monitor serum transaminases prior to therapy and during treatment. Acute hemolytic anemia, new onset or exacerbation of diabetes mellitus (DM), hyperglycemia, diabetic ketoacidosis, and immune reconstitution syndrome reported. Caution with known sulfonamide allergy. Spontaneous bleeding reported with hemophilia A and B. Redistribution/accumulation of body fat observed. Increased triglycerides (TG) and cholesterol levels may occur; assess TG and cholesterol levels prior to therapy and periodically thereafter. Cases of nephrolithiasis reported; if signs and symptoms occur, interrupt or d/c. Caution in elderly.

**ADVERSE REACTIONS:** Diarrhea, N/V, headache, rash, increased AST/ALT.

**INTERACTIONS:** See Contraindications. Use with CYP3A4 inducers may decrease amprenavir concentrations and reduce its therapeutic effect. Use with CYP3A4 inhibitors may increase amprenavir concentrations and increase the incidence of adverse effects. Use of fosamprenavir/ritonavir (RTV) with CYP2D6 substrates may cause an interaction. Concurrent nevirapine without RTV is not recommended. Indinavir and nelfinavir may increase levels. Concurrent use with lopinavir/RTV may decrease levels of lopinavir and amprenavir. Use of fosamprenavir/RTV with atazanavir may decrease atazanavir levels. Use with saquinavir may decrease amprenavir levels. Concomitant use with phenytoin may decrease amprenavir levels. Use of fosamprenavir/RTV may increase amprenavir levels and decrease phenytoin levels. Concomitant use of paroxetine with fosamprenavir/RTV may decrease paroxetine levels. Decrease levels with efavirenz; add 100mg/day of RTV (max 300mg) when efavirenz is administered with fosamprenavir/RTV qd. Decrease levels with carbamazepine, phenobarbital, dexamethasone, cimetidine, famotidine, nizatidine, and ranitidine; use with caution. Concomitant use with ethinyl estradiol may decrease amprenavir and ethinyl estradiol levels; consider alternate methods of non-hormonal contraception. Decrease levels with methadone; monitor opiate withdrawal symptoms. Increases levels of antiarrhythmics (eg, amiodarone, bepridil, systemic lidocaine, quinidine), calcium channel blockers (eg, diltiazem, felodipine, nifedipine, nicardipine, nimodipine, verapamil, amlodipine, nisoldipine, isradipine), immunosuppressants (eg, cyclosporine, tacrolimus, rapamycin), tricyclic antidepressants (eg, amitriptyline, imipramine); monitor therapeutic concentrations. Increase levels of benzodiazepines (eg, alprazolam, clorazepate, diazepam, flurazepam), trazodone; reduce dose. Increases levels of ketoconazole, itraconazole; monitor adverse events and reduce dose for patient's receiving 400mg of ketoconazole or itraconazole. High doses of ketoconazole, itraconazole >200mg/day are not recommended with fosamprenavir and ritonavir. Increases levels of rifabutin; reduce dose by at least 75% of the usual dose of 300mg/day (max: 150mg qod or 3 times/week). Increases levels with atorvastatin, rosuvastatin; use the lowest possible dose or consider fluvastatin or pravastatin. Increase levels of fluticasone; consider alternatives. May increase esomeprazole levels. Concomitant use with zidovudine may increase the AUC of amprenavir and increase zidovudine levels. Use with Maalox TC may decrease amprenavir levels. Increases levels of sildenafil, tadalafil, vardenafil; may increase PDE5 inhibitor-associated adverse events. Use with clarithromycin may increase amprenavir levels and decrease clarithromycin levels. May affect warfarin levels; monitor INR.



**PREGNANCY:** Category C, not for use in nursing.

**MECHANISM OF ACTION:** HIV protease inhibitor; prodrug that is rapidly hydrolyzed to amprenavir. Binds to active site of HIV-1 protease and thereby prevents the processing of viral Gag and Gag-Pol polyprotein precursors, resulting in the formation of immature noninfectious viral particles.

**PHARMACOKINETICS: Absorption:** Oral administration of variable doses resulted in different parameters. **Distribution:** Amprenavir: Plasma protein binding (90%). **Metabolism:** Gut, rapidly via hydrolysis to amprenavir and inorganic phosphate. Amprenavir: Liver via CYP3A4. **Elimination**: Amprenavir: Urine (14%, metabolites), (<1%, unchanged), Feces (75%, metabolites); $T_{1/2}$=7.7 hrs.

## NURSING CONSIDERATIONS

**Assessment:** Assess for sulfonamide allergy, hepatitis B or C or hepatic dysfunction, DM, hemophilia, pregnancy/nursing status, and for possible drug interactions. Assess serum transaminases, TG, and cholesterol levels.

**Monitoring:** Monitor for signs/symptoms of severe skin reactions (eg, SJS), hepatic toxicity, exacerbation of pre-existing DM and hyperglycemia, immune reconstitution syndrome, redistribution/accumulation of body fat, lipid elevations, nephrolithiasis, and hemolytic anemia. In patients with hemophilia, monitor for spontaneous bleeding events. Perform periodic monitoring of glucose, TG, cholesterol, and Sr transaminase levels. May enroll patients in the Antiretroviral Pregnancy Registry if they become pregnant while on treatment.

**Patient Counseling:** Inform that therapy is not cure for HIV, does not reduce risk of transmission of HIV and that opportunistic infections may develop. Instruct to take medication as prescribed by physician; do not alter dose or d/c therapy unless consulted physician. Inform that if a dose is missed, take dose as soon as possible and then return to normal schedule. Instruct to not double the next dose. If taking hormonal contraceptives, use an alternative contraceptive measure. Advise to notify physician of any sulfa allergy. Inform that redistribution or accumulation of body fat may occur during therapy.

**Administration:** Oral route. (Sus): Shake vigorously before use. **Storage:** Tab: 25°C (77°F); excursions permitted to 15-30°C (59-86°F). Keep tightly closed. Sus: 5-30°C (41-86°F). Do not freeze.

## LIALDA RX

mesalamine (Shire)

**THERAPEUTIC CLASS:** Anti-inflammatory Agent

**INDICATIONS:** Induction of remission in adult patients with active, mild to moderate ulcerative colitis.

**DOSAGE:** *Adults:* 2-4 tabs qd with meals for up to 8 weeks. Max: 2.4g or 4.8g per day.

**HOW SUPPLIED:** Tab, Delayed-Release: 1.2g

**WARNINGS/PRECAUTIONS:** Patients with pyloric stenosis may have prolonged gastric retention, which could delay mesalamine release in the colon. Caution with sulfasalazine allergy. May cause acute intolerance syndrome, if suspected prompt withdrawal is required. Cardiac hypersensitivity reactions (myocarditis, pericarditis) reported; caution in patients with conditions predisposing to the development of myocarditis or pericarditis. Renal impairment, including minimal change nephropathy, and acute or chronic interstitial nephritis reported; caution with known renal dysfunction. Monitor renal function prior to therapy and periodically after. Caution with hepatic impairment.

**ADVERSE REACTIONS:** Headache, flatulence.

**INTERACTIONS:** Concurrent use with nephrotoxic agents (eg, NSAIDs) may increase risk of renal reactions. Concurrent use with azathioprine or 6-mercaptopurine can increase potential for blood disorders.

**PREGNANCY:** Category B, caution in nursing.

**MECHANISM OF ACTION:** Anti-inflammatory agent; not established; suspected to diminish inflammation by blocking cyclooxygenase and inhibiting prostaglandin production in colon.

**PHARMACOKINETICS: Absorption:** PO administration of variable doses resulted in different parameters. **Distribution:** Plasma protein binding (43%); found in breast milk; crosses placental barrier. **Metabolism:** Liver and intestinal mucosa (acetylation), N-acetyl-5-aminosalicylic acid (major metabolite). **Elimination:** Urine (<8% unchanged, >13% N-acetyl-5-aminosalicylic acid); (2.4g) $T_{1/2}$=7-9 hrs; (4.8g) $T_{1/2}$=8-12 hrs

### NURSING CONSIDERATIONS

**Assessment:** Assess for pyloric stenosis, sensitivity to sulfasalazine, renal dysfunction, hepatic impairment, conditions predisposing to development of myo- and pericarditis, pregnancy/nursing status, and for possible drug interactions. Obtain baseline renal function, cardiac function and LFTs.

**Monitoring:** Monitor for signs/symptoms of acute intolerance syndrome (eg, cramping, acute abdominal pain, bloody diarrhea), prolonged gastric retention (pyloric stenosis), cardiac hypersensitivity reactions (eg, myocarditis, pericarditis), and for renal impairment (eg, nephropathy, acute or chronic interstitial nephritis). Monitor renal function periodically.

**Patient Counseling:** Instruct to swallow tablet whole, taking care not to break the outer coating. Instruct to seek medical attention if symptoms of acute intolerance syndrome (cramping, acute abdominal pain, bloody diarrhea), prolonged gastric retention (pyloric stenosis), or if hypersensitivity reactions occur.

**Administration:** Oral route. **Storage:** 15-25°C (59-77°F); excursions permitted to 30°C (86°F).

# LIBRAX

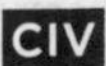

chlordiazepoxide HCl - clidinium bromide (Valeant)

**THERAPEUTIC CLASS:** Benzodiazepine/anticholinergic

**INDICATIONS:** Adjunct treatment of irritable bowel syndrome (IBS), acute enterocolitis, and peptic ulcer.

**DOSAGE:** *Adults:* Usual/Maint: 1-2 caps tid-qid ac and hs. Elderly/Debilitated: Initial: 2 caps/day and increase gradually, if needed.

**HOW SUPPLIED:** Cap: (Chlordiazepoxide-Clidinium) 5mg-2.5mg

**CONTRAINDICATIONS:** Glaucoma, prostatic hypertrophy, benign bladder neck obstruction.

**WARNINGS/PRECAUTIONS:** Risk of congenital malformations during first trimester of pregnancy; avoid use. Avoid abrubt withdrawal. Paradoxical reactions reported in psychiatric patients. Caution with depression, renal or hepatic dysfunction, the elderly. Inhibition of lactation may occur.

**ADVERSE REACTIONS:** Drowsiness, ataxia, confusion, skin eruptions, extrapyramidal symptoms, dry mouth, nausea, constipation, altered libido, blood dyscrasias, jaundice, hepatic dysfunction.

**INTERACTIONS:** Avoid with other psychotropics; if combination is indicated, use caution especially with MAOIs and phenothiazines. Caution with alcohol, other CNS depressants. Altered coagulation effects with oral anticoagulants.

**PREGNANCY:** Not for use in pregnancy; safety in nursing is not known.

**MECHANISM OF ACTION:** Anticholinergic/spasmolytic and antianxiety agent.



## NURSING CONSIDERATIONS

**Assessment:** Assess for glaucoma, prostatic hypertrophy, benign bladder neck obstruction, renal/hepatic dysfunction, alcohol intake, and for possible drug interactions (eg, MAOIs).

**Monitoring:** Monitor for ataxia, oversedation, confusion, paradoxical reactions (eg, excitement, stimulation, acute rage), and for possible physical and psychological dependence.

**Patient Counseling:** Inform that psychological and physical dependence may develop, to avoid performing hazardous tasks (eg, operating machinery/driving), and to consult physician before increasing dose or abruptly d/c.

**Administration:** Oral route.

# LIBRIUM

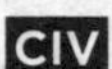

chlordiazepoxide HCl (Valeant)

**THERAPEUTIC CLASS:** Benzodiazepine

**INDICATIONS:** Management of anxiety disorders and short-term relief of anxiety symptoms, withdrawal symptoms of acute alcoholism, and preoperative apprehension and anxiety.

**DOSAGE:** *Adults:* Mild-Moderate Anxiety: 5-10mg tid-qid. Severe Anxiety: 20-25mg tid-qid. Alcohol Withdrawal: 50-100mg; repeat until agitation controlled. Max: 300mg/day. Preoperative Anxiety: 5-10mg PO tid-qid on days prior to surgery. Elderly/Debilitated: 5mg bid-qid.
*Pediatrics:* ≥6 yrs: 5mg bid-qid. May increase to 10mg bid-tid.

**HOW SUPPLIED:** Cap: 5mg, 10mg, 25mg

**WARNINGS/PRECAUTIONS:** Avoid in pregnancy. Paradoxical reactions reported in psychiatric patients and in hyperactive aggressive pediatrics. Caution with porphyria, renal or hepatic dysfunction. Reduce dose in elderly, debilitated. Avoid abrupt withdrawal after extended therapy. May impair mental/physical abilities.

**ADVERSE REACTIONS:** Drowsiness, ataxia, confusion, skin eruptions, edema, nausea, constipation, extrapyramidal symptoms, libido changes, EEG changes.

**INTERACTIONS:** Additive effects with CNS depressants and alcohol. Avoid other psychotropic agents.

**PREGNANCY:** Not for use in pregnancy, safety in nursing not known.

**MECHANISM OF ACTION:** Not established; has antianxiety, sedative, appetite stimulating, and weak analgesic actions; suspected to block EEG arousal from stimulation of brain stem reticular formation.

**PHARMACOKINETICS: Elimination:** Urine (1-2% unchaged, 3-6% as conjugates); $T_{1/2}$=24-48 hrs.

## NURSING CONSIDERATIONS

**Assessment:** Assess for pregnancy status, hepatic/renal function, and possible drug interactions.

**Monitoring:** Monitor geriatric patients for ataxia and oversedation, drowsiness, confusion; paradoxical reactions in psychiatric patients and in hyperactive aggressive pediatric patients. Periodic blood counts and LFTs are advisable when treatment is protracted.

**Patient Counseling:** Inform that psychological/physical dependence may result; consult physician before increasing dose or abruptly d/c drug. May impair mental/physical abilities; caution while operating machinery/driving. May impair mental alertness in children. Avoid alcohol and other CNS depressant drugs.

**Administration:** Oral route. **Storage:** 25°C (77°F); excursions permitted to15-30°C (59-86°F).

# LIDOCAINE OINTMENT RX

lidocaine (Fougera)

L

**THERAPEUTIC CLASS:** Acetamide local anesthetic

**INDICATIONS:** Production of anesthesia of accessible mucous membranes of the oropharynx. Anesthetic lubricant for intubation. Temporary relief of pain associated with minor burns, abrasions, and insect bites.

**DOSAGE:** *Adults:* Apply up to 5g (6 inches)/application. Max: 17-20g/day of ointment.

*Pediatrics:* Determine dose by age and weight. Max: 4.5mg/kg.

**HOW SUPPLIED:** Oint: 5% [35g]

**WARNINGS/PRECAUTIONS:** Avoid excessive dosage or too frequent administration; may result in serious adverse effects requiring resuscitative measures. Extreme caution in the presence of sepsis or if mucosa is traumatized in the area of application; risk of rapid systemic absorption. Debilitated, elderly, acutely ill, and children should be given reduced doses commensurate with their age and physical condition. Caution with heart block and severe shock. Caution in patients with known drug sensitivities. Monitor for the development of malignant hyperthermia and promptly d/c triggering agent and institute approprlate therapy (eg, oxygen therapy) if it develops.

**ADVERSE REACTIONS:** Lightheadedness, nervousness, confusion, euphoria, dizziness, drowsiness, blurred vision, tremors, convulsions, respiratory depression, bradycardia, hypotension, urticaria, edema, anaphylactoid reactions.

**INTERACTIONS:** CNS stimulants and depressants affect CNS levels of lidocaine.

**PREGNANCY:** Category B, caution in nursing.

**MECHANISM OF ACTION:** Local anesthetic; stabilizes neuronal membrane by inhibiting ionic fluxes required for the initiation and conduction of impulses.

**PHARMACOKINETICS: Absorption:** Rapid (after intratracheal administration). **Distribution:** Plasma protein binding (60-80%); crosses placenta and blood brain barriers. **Metabolism:** Hepatic (biotransformation); monoethylglycinexylidide, glycinexylidide (active metabolites). **Elimination:** Urine. (IV): $T_{1/2}$=1.5-2 hrs.

## NURSING CONSIDERATIONS

**Assessment:** Assess for sepsis, severely traumatized mucosa in the area of application, severe shock, heart block, drug sensitivities, renal/hepatic dysfunction, and for possible drug interactions.

**Monitoring:** Monitor for signs/symptoms of drug toxicity and for malignant hyperthermia (eg, tachycardia, tachypnea, labile BP). Monitor renal/hepatic function.

**Patient Counseling:** Inform that if medication is used in the mouth, swallowing may be impaired and enhance the danger of aspiration. Advise that food should not be ingested for 60 min following use of preparation in mouth or throat area. Inform that numbness of tongue or buccal mucosa may increase danger of biting trauma. Instruct to avoid chewing gum while mouth or throat is anesthetized. Instruct to strictly follow recommended dosage and administration instructions. Counsel to seek medical attention if symptoms of malignant hyperthermia (tachycardia, tachypnea) develop.

**Administration:** Topical route. Refer to PI for administration guidelines.
**Storage:** 15-30°C (59-86° F).

# Lidoderm Patch RX

lidocaine (Endo)

**THERAPEUTIC CLASS:** Acetamide local anesthetic

**INDICATIONS:** Relief of pain associated with post-herpetic neuralgia.

**DOSAGE:** *Adults:* Apply to intact skin, cover most painful area. Apply up to 3 patches, once for up to 12 hrs within 24-hr period. May cut patches into smaller sizes before removal of the release liner. Debilitated/Impaired Elimination: Treat smaller areas. Remove if irritation or burning occurs; may reapply when irritation subsides.

**HOW SUPPLIED:** Patch: 5% [30[s]]

**WARNINGS/PRECAUTIONS:** Serious adverse events may occur in children or pets if ingested. Increased risk of toxicity in severe hepatic disease. Avoid broken or inflamed skin, eye contact, larger area or longer duration than recommended. Increased levels with application of >3 patches, small patients.

**ADVERSE REACTIONS:** Application site reactions such as: erythema, edema, bruising, papules, vesicles, discoloration, depigmentation, burning sensation, pruritus, dermatitis, petechia, blisters, exfoliation, abnormal sensation, irritation, allergic reactions (rare).

**INTERACTIONS:** Additive toxic effects with concomitant Class I antiarrhythmics (eg, tocainide, mexiletine). Consider total amount absorbed from all formulations with other local anesthetics.

**PREGNANCY:** Category B, caution in nursing.

**MECHANISM OF ACTION:** Local anesthetic; stabilizes neuronal membranes by inhibiting ionic fluxes required for initiation and conduction of impulses.

**PHARMACOKINETICS: Absorption:** $C_{max}$=0.13mcg/mL; $T_{max}$=11 hrs.
**Distribution:** $V_d$=1.5L/kg; plasma protein binding (70%); crosses placenta.
**Metabolism:** Hepatic, monoethylglycinexylidide, glycinexylidide (metabolites).
**Elimination:** Kidneys; $T_{1/2}$=81-149 min.

## NURSING CONSIDERATIONS

**Assessment:** Assess for hepatic disease and possible drug interactions.

**Monitoring:** Monitor liver function, pain intensity, and pain relief scores periodically for 12 hrs.

**Patient Counseling:** Instruct if irritation or burning sensation occurs during application, to remove patch and not to reapply until irritation subsides. If eye contact occurs, immediately wash with water or saline and protect eye until sensation returns.

**Administration:** Transdermal route. **Storage:** Store at 25°C (77°F); excursions permitted to 15-30°C (59-86°F).

# LIPITOR RX

atorvastatin calcium (Parke-Davis/Pfizer)

**THERAPEUTIC CLASS:** HMG-CoA reductase inhibitor

**INDICATIONS:** Adjunct to diet, to reduce total cholesterol (total-C), LDL, TG, and apolipoprotein B (Apo B) levels, and to increase HDL in primary hypercholesterolemia (heterozygous familial and nonfamilial) and mixed dyslipidemia (Types IIa and IIb). Adjunct to diet for elevated serum TG levels (type IV). Treatment of primary dysbetalipoproteinemia (Type III) inadequately responding to diet. Adjunct to other lipid-lowering treatments or if treatments are unavailable, to reduce total-C and LDL in homozygous familial hypercholesterolemia. Adjunct to diet to lower total-C, LDL, and Apo B in boys and postmenarchal girls, 10 to 17 years of age, with heterozygous familial hypercholesterolemia. To reduce the risk of MI, stroke, revascularization procedures, and angina in adults without clinically evident CHD but with multiple risk factors for CHD. To reduce the risk of MI and stroke in patients with Type II DM, and without clinically evident CHD, but with multiple risk factors for CHD. In patients with clinically evident CHD to reduce the risk of non-fatal MI, fatal and non-fatal stroke, revascularization procedures, hospitalization for CHF, and angina.

**DOSAGE:** *Adults:* Hyperlipidemia (Heterozygous Familial and Nonfamilial)/ Mixed Dyslipidemia: Initial: 10-20mg qd (or 40mg qd for LDL reduction >45%). Titrate: Adjust dose if needed at 2-4 week intervals. Usual: 10-80mg qd. Homozygous Familial Hypercholesterolemia: 10-80mg qd. With Cyclosporine: 10 mg qd. With Clarithromycin, Itraconazole, or Combination of Ritonavir Plus Saquinavir or Lopinavir Plus Ritonavir: Caution in doses >20 mg qd; the lowest dose necessary should be used.
*Pediatrics:* 10-17 yrs: Heterozygous Familial Hypercholesterolemia: Initial: 10mg/day. Titrate: Adjust dose if needed at intervals of ≥4 weeks. Max: 20mg/day.

**HOW SUPPLIED:** Tab: 10mg, 20mg, 40mg, 80mg

**CONTRAINDICATIONS:** Active liver disease which may include unexplained persistent elevations of serum transaminases, pregnancy or nursing mothers.

**WARNINGS/PRECAUTIONS:** May cause biochemical abnormalities of liver function; monitor LFTs prior to therapy, at 12 weeks or with dose elevation, and periodically thereafter. Reduce dose or withdraw if AST or ALT ≥3x ULN persists. Caution with heavy alcohol use and/or history of hepatic disease. Rare cases of rhabdomyolysis with acute renal failure secondary to myoglobinuria reported. Monitor for skeletal muscle effects in patients with history of renal impairment. D/C if markedly elevated CPK levels occur, if myopathy is diagnosed or suspected, or if there are risk factors predisposing renal failure secondary to rhabdomyolysis. May affect endocrine function or cause CNS toxicity. Caution in patients with recent stroke or TIA. Caution in elderly.

**ADVERSE REACTIONS:** Nasopharyngitis, arthralgia, diarrhea, dyspepsia, nausea, pain in extremity, urinary tract infection, myalgia, muscle spasms, musculoskeletal pain, fatigue, hepatic enzyme elevation, rhabdomyolysis, myopathy, peripheral neuropathy.

**INTERACTIONS:** May increase levels when used with strong CYP3A4 inhibitors (eg, clarithromycin, HIV protease inhibitors, itraconazole), and grapefruit juice (>1.2L/day). Inhibitors of OATP1B1 (eg, cyclosporine) may increase bioavailability of atorvastatin. Coadministration with digoxin may increase digoxin levels; monitor appropriately. Inducers of CYP3A4 (eg, efavirenz, rifampin) may decrease atorvastatin levels. Coadministration with oral contraceptives increases AUC of norethindrone and ethinyl estradiol. Increased risk of myopathy with cyclosporine, fibric acid derivatives, erythromycin, clarithromycin, combination of ritonavir plus saquinavir or lopinavir plus ritonavir, niacin, and azole antifungals. Caution with drugs that decrease the levels or activity of endogenous steroid hormones (eg, ketoconazole, spironolactone, cimetidine). Diltiazem may increase the AUC of atorvastatin. Amlodipine may increase the AUC of atorvastatin and decrease the $C_{max}$ of atorvastatin. Colestipol may decrease the $C_{max}$ of atorvastatin. Maalox TC may decrease the AUC and $C_{max}$

L

of atorvastatin. Coadministration with antipyrine may increase the AUC and decrease the $C_{max}$ of antipyrine.

**PREGNANCY:** Category X, not for use in nursing.

**MECHANISM OF ACTION:** HMG-CoA reductase inhibitor; inhibits conversion of HMG-CoA to mevalonate (precursor of sterols, including cholesterol).

**PHARMACOKINETICS: Absorption:** Rapid; absolute bioavailability (14%); $T_{max}$=1-2 hrs. **Distribution:** $V_d$=381L; plasma protein binding (≥98%); found in breast milk. **Metabolism:** Extensive; via CYP3A4; ortho- and parahydroxylated derivatives and various β-oxidation products (metabolites). **Elimination:** Bile (drug, metabolites), urine (<2%); $T_{1/2}$=14 hrs.

## NURSING CONSIDERATIONS

**Assessment:** Assess for active or history of liver disease, unexplained and persistent elevations in serum transaminase levels, pregnancy/nursing status, alcohol intake, renal impairment, recent stroke or TIA, and for possible drug interactions. Assess for risk factors predisposing to the development of renal failure secondary to rhabdomyolysis (eg, severe acute infection, hypotension, major surgery, trauma, uncontrolled seizures). Perform LFTs prior to therapy. Try to control hypercholesterolemia through appropriate diet, exercise, and weight reduction prior to therapy.

**Monitoring:** Monitor for signs/symptoms of rhabdomyolysis with acute renal failure, myopathy (eg, muscle aches, muscle weakness, CPK elevations), liver dysfunction, endocrine dysfunction, and CNS toxicity. Monitor LFTs 12 weeks following initiation of therapy, with any elevation of dose, and periodically (eg, semiannually) thereafter.

**Patient Counseling:** Inform about potential risks/benefits of therapy. Instruct to follow standard cholesterol-lowering diet and regular exercise program as appropriate. Counsel to promptly report any signs of myopathy (eg, unexplained muscle pain, tenderness, weakness). Instruct to notify physician if pregnant/nursing or planning to become pregnant.

**Administration:** Oral route. **Storage:** 20-25°C (68-77°F).

# LITHIUM CARBONATE RX

lithium carbonate (Roxane)

**Lithium toxicity is related to serum lithium levels and can occur at doses close to therapeutic levels.**

**THERAPEUTIC CLASS:** Antimanic agent

**INDICATIONS:** Treatment of manic episodes of bipolar disorder and maintenance treatment of bipolar disorder.

**DOSAGE:** *Adults:* Acute Mania: 600mg tid to achieve effective serum levels of 1-1.5mEq/L; monitor levels twice a week until stabilized. Maint: 300mg tid-qid to maintain serum levels of 0.6-1.2 mEq/L; monitor levels every 2 months. Elderly: Reduce dose.

*Pediatrics:* ≥12 yrs: Acute Mania: 600mg tid. Effective serum levels are 1-1.5mEq/L; monitor levels twice a week until stabilized. Maint: 300mg tid-qid to maintain serum levels of 0.6-1.2mEq/L; monitor levels every 2 months.

**HOW SUPPLIED:** Cap: 150mg, 300mg, 600mg; Tab: 300mg

**CONTRAINDICATIONS:** Renal or cardiovascular disease, severe debilitation or dehydration, sodium depletion, and diuretic use.

**WARNINGS/PRECAUTIONS:** May cause fetal harm; if possible withdraw for at least the 1st trimester of pregnancy. Caution in the elderly. Maintain normal diet, adequate salt/fluid intake. Assess kidney function prior to and during therapy. May impair mental/physical abilities. Reduce dose or d/c with sweating, diarrhea, infection with elevated temperatures. Caution with thyroid disorders; monitor thyroid function. Chronic therapy associated with diminution of renal concentrating ability (eg, diabetes insipidus), glomerular and interstitial fibrosis, and nephron atrophy.

**ADVERSE REACTIONS:** Fine hand tremor, polyuria, mild thirst, incoordination, diarrhea, N/V, drowsiness, muscular weakness.

**INTERACTIONS:** Risk of encephalopathic syndrome (eg, weakness, lethargy, fever, tremulousness, confusion, EPS) with haloperidol and other antipsychotics; d/c therapy if such signs occur. May prolong effects of neuromuscular blockers. Increased levels with indomethacin, piroxicam and other NSAIDs. Increased risk of toxicity due to decreased clearance with diuretics and ACE inhibitors; contraindicated with diuretics.

**PREGNANCY:** Category D, not for use in nursing.

**MECHANISM OF ACTION:** Mood-stabilizing agent; mechanism not established. Suspected to alter sodium transport in nerve and muscle cells and effect a shift toward intraneuronal metabolism of catecholamines.

**PHARMACOKINETICS: Distribution**: Found in breast milk. **Elimination**: Urine (primary), feces; $T_{1/2}$=24 hrs.

## NURSING CONSIDERATIONS

**Assessment:** Assess use with significant renal or cardiovascular disease, severe debilitation or dehydration, sodium depletion, diuretics, drug interactions (eg, neuromuscular blocking agents), pregnancy status, baseline renal function (SrCr, urinalysis), and thyroid function.

**Monitoring:** Monitor for diminution of renal concentrating ability (eg, nephrogenic diabetes insipidus), glomerular and interstitial fibrosis and nephron atrophy, renal function and thyroid function while on therapy. Monitor serum lithium levels twice weekly during acute phase and until serum lithium level and condition of patient stabilized. Monitor for signs/symptoms of lithium toxicity (eg, diarrhea, vomiting, tremor, mild ataxia, drowsiness, muscular weakness).

**Patient Counseling:** Counsel about early signs of lithium toxicity (eg, diarrhea, vomiting, tremor, mild ataxia, drowsiness, muscle weakness) and activities requiring mental alertness. Counsel females to avoid pregnancy/nursing while on medication. Advise to maintain normal diet, including salt, and adequate fluid intake (2500-3000mL), at least during initial stabilization period. Counsel to contact physician if diarrhea or concomitant infection with elevated temperatures develop; may require change in dosing.

**Administration:** Oral route. **Storage**: 25°C (77°F); excursions permitted to 15-30°C (59-86°F). Protect from moisture. Dispense in a tight container.

# LITHOBID — RX

lithium carbonate (JDS)

**Lithium toxicity is related to serum levels, and can occur at doses close to therapeutic levels. Facilities for prompt and accurate serum lithium determination should be available before initiating therapy.**

**THERAPEUTIC CLASS:** Antimanic agent

**INDICATIONS:** Treatment of manic episodes of manic-depressive illness. Maintenance treatment for bipolar disorder.

**DOSAGE:** *Adults:* Acute Mania: Initial: 900mg bid or 600mg tid to achieve effective serum levels of 1-1.5mEq/L; monitor levels twice weekly until stabilized. Maint: 900-1200mg/day, given bid-tid to maintain serum levels of 0.6-1.2mEq/L; monitor levels every 2 months. Elderly: Lower dose to achieve therapeutic serum levels.

*Pediatrics:* ≥12 yrs: Acute Mania: Initial: 900mg bid or 600mg tid to achieve effective serum levels of 1-1.5mEq/L; monitor levels twice weekly until stabilized. Maint: 900-1200mg/day, given bid-tid to maintain serum levels of 0.6-1.2 mEq/L; monitor levels every 2 months.

**HOW SUPPLIED:** Tab, Extended-Release: 300mg, (Generic) 450mg* **scored*

**WARNINGS/PRECAUTIONS:** Avoid with significant renal or CV disease, severe debilitation, dehydration, or sodium depletion. Assess kidney function prior to and during therapy. Risk of encephalopathic syndrome (eg, weakness, lethargy, fever, tremulousness, confusion, EPS); d/c therapy. May impair mental/physical abilities. Reduce dose or d/c with sweating, diarrhea, infection with elevated temperatures. Caution with hypothyroidism; may need supplemental therapy. Chronic therapy associated with diminution of renal concentrating ability, glomerular and interstitial fibrosis, and nephron atrophy. Transient syndrome of acute dystonia and hyperreflexia reported in a <15kg child who ingested 300mg. May cause sodium depletion; maintain normal diet, including salt, and adequate fluid intake. Caution in elderly.

**ADVERSE REACTIONS:** Fine hand tremor, polyuria, mild thirst, general discomfort, diarrhea, N/V, drowsiness, muscular weakness, lack of coordination, ataxia, giddiness, tinnitus, blurred vision, large output of dilute urine.

**INTERACTIONS:** Avoid diuretics and ACE inhibitors; risk of lithium toxicity due to reduced renal clearance. May prolong effects of neuromuscular blockers. Decreased levels with acetazolamide, urea, xanthine preparations, and alkalinizing agents. May produce hypothyroidism with iodide preparations. Increased plasma levels with indomethacin, piroxicam, other NSAIDs. Increased risk of neurotoxic effects with carbamazepine and CCBs. Reduced renal clearance with metronidazole. Fluoxetine may increase and/or decrease lithium levels. (Generic) May increase plasma levels with angiotensin-converting enzyme inhibitors, such as enalapril and captopril, and angiotensin II receptor antagonists, such as losartan; reduce dosage and monitor serum levels periodically. Diarrhea, confusion, tremor, dizziness, and agitation reported with selective serotonin reuptake inhibitors; caution when coadministering. May interact with methyldopa and phenytoin.

**PREGNANCY:** Category D, not for use in nursing.

**MECHANISM OF ACTION:** Not established; suspected to alter sodium transport in nerve and muscle cells and effects a shift toward intraneuronal metabolism of catecholamines.

**PHARMACOKINETICS: Distribution:** Found in breast milk. **Elimination:** Urine (primary), feces (insignificant). $T_{1/2}$=24hrs.

## NURSING CONSIDERATIONS

**Assessment:** Assess use with significant renal dysfunction, cardiovascular disease, severe debilitation, dehydration, sodium depletion, concomitant therapy with either ACE inhibitors or diuretics. Assess renal function (urinalysis, SrCr) prior to therapy. Assess thyroid function with history of thyroid disease, pregnancy/nursing status, and possible drug interactions.

**Monitoring:** Monitor for diminution of renal concentrating ability (eg, nephrogenic diabetes insipidus), glomerular and interstitial fibrosis, and nephron atrophy in patients on long-term therapy, encephalopathic syndrome, renal function while on therapy, thyroid function in patients with a history of hypothyroidism, serum lithium levels, signs of lithium toxicity (eg, diarrhea, vomiting, tremor).

**Patient Counseling:** Instruct to maintain a normal diet, including proper sodium and fluid intake (2500mL-3500mL). Instruct to notify physician if protracted sweating or diarrhea, or concomitant infection with elevated temperatures develops; may require dose adjustment. Counsel to d/c therapy and notify physician if clinical signs of lithium toxicity (eg, diarrhea, vomiting, tremor, muscular weakness) occur. Inform may impair mental/physical abilities; use caution with activities requiring alertness.

**Administration:** Oral route. **Storage:** 15-30°C (59-86°F). Protect from moisture. Dispense in tight, light- and child-resistant containers.

## LIVALO **RX**

pitavastatin (Kowa)

**THERAPEUTIC CLASS:** HMG-CoA reductase inhibitor

**INDICATIONS:** Adjunctive therapy to diet to reduce elevated total cholesterol (TC), low-density lipoprotein cholesterol (LDL-C), apolipoprotein B (Apo

B), triglycerides (TG), and to increase high-density lipoprotein cholesterol (HDL-C) in adults with primary hyperlipidemia or mixed dyslipidemia.

**DOSAGE:** *Adults:* Initial: 2mg qd. Max: 4mg. Usual range: 1-4mg PO qd. Individualize according to goals of therapy and response. Upon initiation/titration, analyze for lipid levels after 4 weeks and adjust dosage accordingly. Moderate Renal Insufficiency (GFR 30 to <60mL/min/1.73m$^{2}$)/End-Stage Renal Disease: Initial: 1mg qd. Max: 2mg qd. Concomitant Erythromycin: Max: 1mg qd. Concomitant Rifampin: Max: 2mg qd.

**HOW SUPPLIED:** Tab: 1mg, 2mg, 4mg

**CONTRAINDICATIONS:** Active liver disease including unexplained persistent elevations of hepatic transaminase levels, pregnancy/nursing mothers, and coadministration with cyclosporine.

**WARNINGS/PRECAUTIONS:** Myopathy and rhabdomyolysis with acute renal failure secondary to myoglobinuria reported. Caution with predisposing factors for myopathy including advanced age, renal impairment, and inadequately treated hypothyroidism; d/c if elevated creatine kinase (CK) levels occur or myopathy is diagnosed or suspected. Transient increased serum transaminases reported; d/c or reduce dose if AST/ALT >3x ULN persists. Monitor LFTs prior to therapy, at 12 weeks, or with dose elevation. Caution with heavy alcohol use, renal impairment, and history of liver disease.

**ADVERSE REACTIONS:** Back pain, constipation, myalgia.

**INTERACTIONS:** See Contraindications. May increase levels with protease inhibitors (eg, lopinavir/ritonavir), erythromycin, and rifampin. Caution with other fibrates or gemfibrozil; increased risk of myopathy. Enhanced risk of skeletal effects in combination with niacin. Monitor PT and INR with warfarin coadministration.

**PREGNANCY:** Category X, not for use in nursing.

**MECHANISM OF ACTION:** HMG-CoA reductase inhibitor; inhibits cholesterol synthesis in the liver.

**PHARMACOKINETICS: Absorption:** $T_{max}$=1 hr; Absolute bioavailability (51%). **Distribution:** Plasma protein binding (>99%); $V_d$=148L. **Metabolism:** Conjugation; CYP2C9; uridine 5'-diphosphate (UDP) glucuronosyltransferase (UGT1A3 and UGT2B7) (active metabolites). **Elimination:** Urine (15%), feces (79%); $T_{1/2}$=12 hrs.

## NURSING CONSIDERATIONS

**Assessment:** Assess for active liver disease or unexplained elevations in serum transaminase levels, pregnancy/nursing status, renal impairment, and possible drug interactions. Obtain baseline lipid profile and LFTs prior to therapy. Assess use in patients who consume substantial quantities of alcohol and/or have a past history of liver disease.

**Monitoring:** Monitor signs/symptoms of myopathy, rhabdomyolysis, acute renal failure, and hypersensitivity reactions. Perform periodic monitoring of lipid profile, CK levels, and LFTs. Monitor PT and INR when using wafarin.

**Patient Counseling:** Advise to notify physician immediately if unexplained muscle pain, tenderness, or weakness occur. Notify physician of all concurrently taken medications, both prescription and over the counter. Counsel women of childbearing age to use effective method of birth control to prevent pregnancy during therapy. Notify physician if pregnant or breastfeeding.

**Administration:** Oral route. Take at any time of the day. **Storage:** 15-30°C (59-86°F). Protect from light.

# Lo/Ovral — RX

norgestrel - ethinyl estradiol (Wyeth)

**OTHER BRAND NAMES:** Low-Ogestrel (Watson) - Cryselle (Duramed)

**THERAPEUTIC CLASS:** Estrogen/progestogen combination

**INDICATIONS:** Prevention of pregnancy.

L

**DOSAGE:** *Adults:* Start 1st Sunday after menses begins or the 1st day of menses. *21-day:* 1 tab qd for 21 days, stop 7 days, then repeat. *28-day:* 1 tab qd for 28 days, then repeat.

**HOW SUPPLIED:** Tab: (Ethinyl Estradiol-Norgestrel) 0.03mg-0.3mg

**CONTRAINDICATIONS:** Thrombophlebitis, DVT or thromboembolic disorders, pregnancy, cerebrovascular or coronary artery disease, undiagnosed abnormal genital bleeding, cholestatic jaundice of pregnancy or jaundice with prior pill use, hepatic adenomas or carcinomas, breast cancer or other estrogen-dependent neoplasia, thrombogenic valvulopathies, thrombogenic rhythm disorders, diabetes with vascular involvement, uncontrolled HTN, endometrium carcinoma, active liver disease if liver function has not returned to normal.

**WARNINGS/PRECAUTIONS:** Cigarette smoking increases risk of serious cardiovascular side effects; risk increases with age (especially >35 yrs) and heavy smoking. Increased risk of MI, vascular disease, thromboembolism, stroke and gallbladder disease. Retinal thrombosis, hepatic neoplasia reported. May cause glucose intolerance. May increase BP, elevate LDL levels or cause other lipid changes, fluid retention, breakthrough bleeding, and spotting. May cause or exacerbate migraine. May develop visual changes with contact lens. Increased risk of MI with HTN, hyperlipidemia, obesity, and diabetes. D/C if jaundice, significant depression or ophthalmic irregularities develop. Perform annual physical exam. Use before menarche is not indicated. May affect certain endocrine, LFTs and blood components.

**ADVERSE REACTIONS:** N/V, breakthrough bleeding, spotting, amenorrhea, migraine, depression, vaginal candidiasis, edema, weight changes.

**INTERACTIONS:** Reduced effects, increased breakthrough bleeding, and menstrual irregularities with rifampin, rifabutin, barbiturates, phenylbutazone, phenytoin, griseofulvin, topiramate, some protease inhibitors, modafinil and possibly with St. John's wort, some penicillins, ampicillin and tetracylines. Increased levels with ascorbic acid and acetaminophen, indinavir, fluconazole, troleandomycin, and atorvastatin. May affect cyclosporine, theophylline and corticosteroid levels.

**PREGNANCY:** Category X, not for use in nursing.

**MECHANISM OF ACTION:** Estrogen/progestogen combination oral contraceptive; acts by suppressing gonadotropins. Primarily acts by inhibiting ovulation. Also responsible for causing changes in cervical mucus (increases difficulty of sperm entry into uterus) and in endometrium (reduces likelihood of implantation).

## NURSING CONSIDERATIONS

**Assessment:** Assess for current or history of thrombophlebitis or thromboembolic disorders, CVD or CAD, thrombogenic valvulopathies, thrombogenic rhythm disorders, major surgery with prolonged immobilization, DM with vascular involvement, headaches with focal neurological symptoms, uncontrolled HTN, known/suspected or history of carcinoma of breast, endometrium or other known/suspected estrogen-dependent neoplasia, undiagnosed abnormal genital bleeding, cholestatic jaundice of pregnancy or jaundice with prior pill use, hepatic adenomas or carcinomas, active liver disease with abnormal liver function, and known/suspected pregnancy. Assess use with HTN, hyperlipidemia, obesity, DM, women >35 yrs who smoke ≥15 cigarettes/day, or for possible drug interactions.

**Monitoring:** Monitor for venous and arterial thrombotic and thromboembolic events (eg, MI, stroke), hepatic neoplasia, gallbladder disease, and HTN, signs of fluid retention, onset or exacerbation of migraines or headaches, bleeding irregularities, development of ocular lesions. Monitor serum glucose levels in DM or prediabetic patients, lipid levels with history of hyperlipidemia, BP with history of HTN. Refer patients with contact lenses to ophthalmologist if visual changes occur. Monitor liver function, signs of depression with previous history, and signs of GI upset (eg, diarrhea, vomiting). Perform annual physical exam while on therapy.

**Patient Counseling:** Counsel about possible adverse effects of drug. Advise to avoid smoking while on medication. Inform that drug does not protect against HIV infection and other STDs. Instruct women to use additional method of birth control until after first 7 days of administration in initial cycle. Instruct to take medication at same time every day and at intervals not exceeding 24 hrs. Inform that if dose missed, take next pill as soon as possible, then take next dose at regular time. If patient skips 2 or more doses, advise to use another method of contraception until patient has taken medication for 7 consecutive days. Counsel that if spotting or breakthrough bleeding occurs, continue taking medication; notify physician if bleeding is persistent or prolonged.

**Administration:** Oral route. **Storage:** Store at controlled room temperature 20-25°C (68-77°F).

## LOCOID — RX
hydrocortisone butyrate (Ferndale)

**THERAPEUTIC CLASS:** Corticosteroid

**INDICATIONS:** (Cre, Oint) Corticosteroid-responsive dermatoses. (Sol) Seborrheic dermatitis.

**DOSAGE:** *Adults:* (Cre, Oint) Apply bid-tid. May use occlusive dressings for psoriasis or recalcitrant conditions. D/C dressings if infection develops. (Sol) Apply bid-tid.
*Pediatrics:* (Cre, Oint) Apply bid-tid. May use occlusive dressings for psoriasis or recalcitrant conditions. D/C dressings if infection develops. (Sol) Apply bid-tid. Use least amount effective for condition.

**HOW SUPPLIED:** Cre, Oint: 0.1% [15g, 45g]; Sol: 0.1% [20mL, 60mL]

**WARNINGS/PRECAUTIONS:** May produce reversible HPA axis suppression, manifestations of Cushing's syndrome, hyperglycemia, and glucosuria. D/C if irritation occurs. Use appropriate antifungal or antibacterial agent with dermatological infections. Pediatric patients may be more susceptible to systemic toxicity. Caution when applied to large surface areas. Avoid contact with eyes. Limit to smallest amount compatible with an effective therapeutic regimen. Chronic corticosteroid therapy may interfere with the growth and development of children, use least amount effective for condition.

**ADVERSE REACTIONS:** Burning, itching, irritation, dryness, folliculitis, hypertrichosis, acneiform eruptions, hypopigmentation, perioral dermatitis, allergic dermatitis, skin maceration, secondary infection, skin atrophy, striae, miliaria.

**PREGNANCY:** Category C, caution in nursing.

**MECHANISM OF ACTION:** Corticosteroid; possesses anti-inflammatory, anti-pruritic, and vasoconstrictive properties. Anti-inflammatory actions not established.

**PHARMACOKINETICS: Absorption:** Percutaneous; inflammation, other disease states, and occlusive dressings may increase absorption. **Distribution:** Bound to plasma proteins to varying degrees. Systemically administered corticosteroids found in breast milk. **Metabolism:** Liver. **Elimination:** Renal (major), bile.

### NURSING CONSIDERATIONS

**Assessment:** Assess use in pregnant/nursing patients.

**Monitoring:** Monitor for signs/symptoms of reversible HPA-axis suppression, Cushing's syndrome, hyperglycemia, glucosuria, dermatological infections (eg, fungal, bacterial), and steroid withdrawal. For patients on large doses or in patients using occlusive dressings, perform periodic monitoring for HPA-axis suppression using urinary free cortisol and ACTH stimulation tests. (Pediatrics) Monitor for signs/symptoms of systemic toxicity, HPA-axis suppression (eg, linear growth retardation, delayed weight gain), Cushing's syndrome, and intracranial HTN.

**Patient Counseling:** Counsel to use externally and exactly as directed; avoid contact with eyes. Report signs of adverse reactions; do not bandage, cover or wrap treated skin area. Inform caregivers of pediatric patients to avoid using tight-fitting diapers or plastic pants on treatment area.

**Administration:** Topical route. **Storage:** Cream: 15-25°C (59-77°F), Ointment: 2-30°C (36-86°F), Solution: 5-25°C (41-77°F).

## LOESTRIN RX

### norethindrone acetate - ethinyl estradiol - ferrous fumarate (Warner Chilcott)

**OTHER BRAND NAMES:** Loestrin 1/20 (Duramed/Warner Chilcott) - Loestrin 1.5/30 (Duramed/Warner Chilcott) - Loestrin Fe 1/20 (Duramed/Warner Chilcott) - Loestrin Fe 1.5/30 (Duramed/Warner Chilcott) - Microgestin Fe 1.5/30 (Watson) - Microgestin Fe 1/20 (Watson) - Junel Fe 1.5/30 (Barr) - Junel Fe 1/20 (Barr) - Junel 1/20 (Barr) - Junel 1.5/30 (Barr) - Gildess Fe 1.5/30 (Qualitest) - Gildess Fe 1/20 (Qualitest)

**THERAPEUTIC CLASS:** Estrogen/progestogen combination

**INDICATIONS:** Prevention of pregnancy.

**DOSAGE:** *Adults:* Start 1st Sunday after menses begin or the 1st day of menses. *21-day:* 1 tab qd for 21 days, stop 7 days, then repeat. *28-day:* 1 tab qd for 28 days, then repeat.

**HOW SUPPLIED:** Tab:(Ethinyl Estradiol-Norethindrone) (1/20) 20mcg-1mg, (1.5/30) 30mcg-1.5mg; (Fe 1/20) 20mcg-1mg and 75mg ferrous fumarate, (Fe 1.5/30) 30mcg-1.5mg and 75mg ferrous fumarate

**CONTRAINDICATIONS:** Thrombophlebitis, DVT or thromboembolic disorders, pregnancy, cerebrovascular or coronary artery disease, undiagnosed abnormal genital bleeding, cholestatic jaundice of pregnancy or jaundice with prior pill use, hepatic adenomas or carcinomas, breast cancer or other estrogen-dependent neoplasia.

L

**WARNINGS/PRECAUTIONS:** Cigarette smoking increases risk of serious cardiovascular side effects. This risk increases with age (especially >35 yrs) and heavy smoking. Increased risk of MI, vascular disease, thromboembolism, stroke, and gallbladder disease. Retinal thrombosis, hepatic neoplasia, carcinoma of breast and reproductive organs reported. May cause glucose intolerance. May increase BP, elevate LDL levels or cause other lipid changes, fluid retention, breakthrough bleeding, and spotting. May cause or exacerbate migraine. May develop visual changes with contact lens. Increased risk of MI with HTN, hyperlipidemia, obesity, and diabetes. D/C if jaundice, significant depression or ophthalmic irregularities develop. Perform annual physical exam. Use before menarche is not indicated. May affect certain endocrine, LFTs, and blood components.

**ADVERSE REACTIONS:** NV, breakthrough bleeding, spotting, amenorrhea, migraine, depression, vaginal candidiasis, edema, weight changes.

**INTERACTIONS:** Reduced effects, increased breakthrough bleeding, and menstrual irregularities with rifampin, barbiturates, phenylbutazone, phenytoin, carbamazepine, and possibly with griseofulvin, ampicillin, and tetracyclines. Increased levels with atorvastatin, ascorbic acid, and APAP. Increased plasma levels of cyclosporine, prednisolone, and theophylline. Decreased levels of APAP. Increased clearance of temazepam, salicylic acid, morphine, and clofibric acid. Troglitazone reduces plasma levels of hormones.

**PREGNANCY:** Category X, not for use in nursing.

**MECHANISM OF ACTION:** Estrogen/progestogen combination oral contraceptive; acts by suppression of gonadotropins. Primarily inhibits ovulation. Causes changes in cervical mucus (increasing difficulty of sperm entry into uterus) and endometrium (reducing likelihood of implantation).

**PHARMACOKINETICS: Absorption:** Rapid and complete. Norethindrone Acetate: Absolute bioavailability (64%); Single dose: $C_{max}$=8420pg/mL, $T_{max}$=1.0 hr, AUC=33390pg/mL•hr; Multiple doses: $C_{max}$=16400pg/mL, $T_{max}$=1.3 hrs, AUC=88160pg/mL•hr. Ethinyl Estradiol: Absolute bioavailability (43%); Single dose: $C_{max}$=64.5pg/mL, $T_{max}$=1.3 hrs, AUC=465.4pg/mL•hr. Multiple doses: $C_{max}$=81.9pg/mL, $T_{max}$=1.7 hrs, AUC=701.3pg/mL•hr. **Distribution:** $V_d$=2-4L/kg; plasma protein binding ( ≥95%). **Metabolism:** Norethindrone: Reduction, (sulfate-glucuronide conjugation). Ethinyl Estradiol: 1st-pass metabolism,

CYP3A4 (oxidation). **Elimination:** Urine, feces. Norethindrone: $T_{1/2}$=8 hrs. Ethinyl Estradiol: $T_{1/2}$=14 hrs.

## NURSING CONSIDERATIONS

**Assessment:** Assess current or history of thrombophlebitis or thromboembolic disorder, CVD or CAD, valvular heart disease with thrombogenic complications, severe HTN, DM with vascular involvement, headaches with focal neurological symptoms, major surgery with prolonged immobilization, known/suspected carcinoma of breast, endometrium or other known or suspected estrogen-dependent neoplasia, undiagnosed abnormal genital bleeding, cholestatic jaundice of pregnancy or jaundice with prior pill use, hepatic adenomas or carcinomas, active liver disease, or known/suspected pregnancy. Assess use in women ≥35 yrs who smoke ≥15 cigarettes/day, and for possible drug interactions.

**Monitoring:** Monitor for venous and arterial thrombotic and thromboembolic events (eg, MI, stroke), hepatic neoplasia, gallbladder disease, ocular lesions, HTN, fluid retention, onset or exacerbation of migraines or headaches, bleeding irregularities (eg, breakthrough bleeding, spotting). Monitor blood glucose levels in DM and prediabetic women, BP with history of HTN, lipid levels with history of hyperlipidemia, for signs/symptoms of hepatotoxicity (eg, jaundice), and for signs of worsening depression with previous history. Refer patients with contact lenses to opthalmologist if visual changes develop. Perform annual physical exam while on therapy.

**Patient Counseling:** Counsel about potential adverse effects. Inform that drug does not protect against HIV infection and other STDs. Instruct to use additional method of birth control for first 7 days of administration. Instruct to take exactly as directed and at intervals not exceeding 24 hrs. Advise that if dose missed, take as soon as remembered, then take next dose at regularly scheduled time. Counsel to take with/without food. Advise to continue regimen if spotting or breakthrough bleeding occurs; notify physician if prolonged or persists. Instruct to avoid smoking while on medication.

**Administration:** Oral route. **Storage:** Store at 25°C (77°F); excursions permitted to 15-30°C (59-86°F).

# LOFIBRA — RX

fenofibrate (Gate)

**THERAPEUTIC CLASS:** Fibric acid derivative

**INDICATIONS:** Adjunct to diet, for treatment of adult patients with hypertriglyceridemia (Fredrickson Types IV and V hyperlipidemia). Adjunct to diet, for reduction of LDL-C, Total-C, TG, and Apo B in adult patients with primary hypercholesterolemia or mixed dyslipidemia (Fredrickson Types IIa and IIb). (Tab) Adjunct to diet, for to increase HDL-C in adult patients with primary hypercholesterolemia or mixed dyslipidemia (Fredrickson Types IIa and IIb).

**DOSAGE:** *Adults.* Primary Hypercholesterolemia/Mixed Hyperlipidemia: Initial: Cap: 200mg qd. Tab: 160mg qd. Hypertriglyceridemia: Initial: Cap: 67-200mg/day. Tab: 54-160mg qd. Titrate: Adjust if needed after repeat lipid levels at 4-8 week intervals. Max: Cap: 200mg/day. Tab: 160mg/day. Renal Dysfunction/Elderly: Initial: Cap: 67mg/day. Tab: 54mg/day. Take with meals.

**HOW SUPPLIED:** Cap: 67mg, 134mg, 200mg; Tab: 54mg, 160mg

**CONTRAINDICATIONS:** Hepatic or severe renal dysfunction (including primary biliary cirrhosis and unexplained persistent liver function abnormality), pre-existing gallbladder disease.

**WARNINGS/PRECAUTIONS:** Hepatocellular, chronic active and cholestatic hepatitis and cirrhosis (rare) reported. Increases in serum transaminases reported; monitor LFTs regularly; d/c if >3x ULN. May cause cholelithiasis; d/c if gallstones found. May cause myositis, myopathy, or rhabdomyolysis; d/c if myopathy or marked CPK elevation occurs. Prior to therapy attempt to control serum lipids with appropriate diet, exercise, and weight loss in obese patients and attempt to control any medical problems (eg, diabetes mellitus [DM]), hypothyroidism) that are contributing to lipid abnormalities. Measure lipid levels prior to therapy and during initial treatment; d/c if inadequate response after 2 months on maximum dose of 200mg/day (caps) or 160 mg/day (tabs). Acute hypersensitivity reactions (rare) and pancreatitis reported. Decreased Hgb/Hct, WBCs, thrombocytopenia, and agranulocytosis reported; perform periodic monitoring of CBC during the first 12 months of therapy. Minimize dose in severe renal impairment. Caution in elderly.

**ADVERSE REACTIONS:** Abdominal pain, back pain, headache, abnormal LFTs, increased creatine phosphokinase, increased ALT, increased AST, respiratory disorder.

**INTERACTIONS:** Caution with anticoagulants because may potentiate coumarin anticoagulants; reduce anticoagulant dose to maintain desirable PT/INR. Avoid HMG-CoA reductase inhibitors unless benefits outweigh risks. Bile acid sequestrants may impede absorption; take at least 1 hr before or 4-6 hrs after bile acid binding resin. Evaluate benefits/risks with immunosuppressants (eg, cyclosporine) and other nephrotoxic agents; use lowest effective dose. Prior to therapy, d/c or change if possible, medications that are known to exacerbate hypertriglyceridemia (eg, beta-blockers, thiazides, estrogens). Caution with drugs that are substrates of CYP2C19, CYP2A6, or CYP2C9.

**PREGNANCY:** Category C, not for use in nursing.

**MECHANISM OF ACTION:** Fibric acid derivative; activates peroxisome proliferator activated receptor α (PPARα), increasing lipolysis and elimination of triglyceride-rich particles from plasma by activating lipoprotein lipase and reducing production of apoprotein C-III. Decreased triglycerides produces an alteration in the size and composition of LDL particles. LDL particles then have a greater affinity for cholesterol receptors and are catabolized rapidly. Activation of PPARα also induces an increase in the synthesis of apoproteins A-I, A-II, and HDL cholesterol. Also reduces serum uric acid levels in hyperuricemic and normal individuals by increasing the urinary excretion of uric acid.

**PHARMACOKINETICS: Absorption:** Well absorbed; $T_{max}$=6-8 hrs. **Distribution:** Plasma protein binding (99%). **Metabolism:** Rapid, via hydrolysis by esterases to fenofibric acid (active metabolite), conjugation. **Elimination:** Urine (60%), feces (25%); $T_{1/2}$=20 hrs.

## NURSING CONSIDERATIONS

**Assessment:** Assess for hepatic impairment including primary biliary cirrhosis, renal dysfunction, pre-existing gallbladder disease, pregnancy/nursing status, and for possible drug interactions. Prior to therapy, attempt to control serum lipids with appropriate diet, exercise, and weight loss in obese patients and attempt to control any medical problems (eg, DM, hypothyroidism) that are contributing to lipid abnormalities. Measure lipid levels and LFTs prior to therapy.

**Monitoring:** Monitor for signs/symptoms of myositis, myopathy, and rhabdomyolysis; measure CPK levels if myopathy is suspected. Monitor for signs/symptoms of increases in serum transaminases, hepatocellular, chronic active and cholestatic hepatitis, and for cirrhosis; perform periodic monitoring of LFTs. Monitor for signs/symptoms of cholelithiasis; perform gallbladder studies if cholelithiasis is suspected. Monitor for signs/symptoms of pancreatitis, hypersensitivity reactions (eg, skin rashes), Monitor for hematological changes (eg, agranulocytosis, thrombocytopenia); perform periodic blood counts. Measure lipid levels periodically.

**Patient Counseling:** Inform of risks/benefits of therapy. Instruct to take with meals. Advise to immediately contact physician if unexplained muscle pain, tenderness, or weakness, with malaise or fever occur. Recommend appropriate lipid-lowering diet.

**Administration:** Oral route. **Storage:** 20-25°C (68-77°F). Protect from moisture.

## LOMOTIL

**CV**

diphenoxylate HCl - atropine sulfate (Pharmacia & Upjohn)

**OTHER BRAND NAMES:** Lonox (Sandoz)

**THERAPEUTIC CLASS:** Opioid/anticholinergic

**INDICATIONS:** Adjunctive therapy for management of diarrhea.

**DOSAGE:** *Adults:* Initial: 2 tabs or 10mL qid. Titrate: Reduce dose after symptoms are controlled. Maint: 2 tabs or 10mL qd. Max: 20mg/day diphenoxylate. D/C if symptoms not controlled after 10 days at max dose of 20mg/day (diphenoxylate).
*Pediatrics:* 2-12 yrs: Initial: 0.3-0.4mg/kg/day of solution given qid. 13-16 yrs: Initial: 2 tabs or 10mL tid. Titrate: Reduce dose after symptoms are controlled. Maint: 25% of initial dose. D/C if no improvement within 48 hrs.

**HOW SUPPLIED:** (Diphenoxylate-Atropine) Sol: 2.5mg-0.025/5mL [60mL]; Tab: 2.5mg-0.025mg

**CONTRAINDICATIONS:** Obstructive jaundice, diarrhea associated with pseudomembranous enterocolitis or enterotoxin-producing bacteria.

**WARNINGS/PRECAUTIONS:** May induce toxic megacolon in ulcerative colitis; d/c if abdominal distention occurs. May cause intestinal fluid retention. Avoid with diarrhea associated with organisms that penetrate the intestinal mucosa, and with pseudomembranous enterocolitis. Caution in pediatrics, especially with Down's syndrome. Extreme caution advanced hepatorenal disease and liver dysfunction. Do not use with severe dehydration or electrolyte imbalance until corrective therapy is initiated.

**ADVERSE REACTIONS:** Numbness of extremities, dizziness, anaphylaxis, hyperthermia, tachycardia, urinary retention, flushing, drowsiness, toxic megacolon, nausea, vomiting.

**INTERACTIONS:** May potentiate barbiturates, tranquilizers and alcohol. MAOIs may precipitate hypertensive crisis.

**PREGNANCY:** Category C, caution in nursing.

**MECHANISM OF ACTION:** Diphenoxylate: Antidiarrheal. Atropine: Anticholinergic.

**PHARMACOKINETICS: Absorption:** (4 tabs): $C_{max}$=163ng/mL; $T_{max}$=2 hrs. **Metabolism:** Rapid and extensive metabolism through ester hydrolysis to diphenoxylic acid (major metabolite). **Elimination:** Urine (14%, 6% conjugate), feces (49%). $T_{1/2}$=12-14 hrs (diphenoxylic acid).

### NURSING CONSIDERATIONS

**Assessment:** Assess renal function test, LFTs, ulcerative colitis, Down's syndrome, diarrhea caused by *E coli*, salmonella, shigella, obstructive jaundice, pseudomembranous enterocolitis.

**Monitoring:** Monitor for severe dehydration and electrolyte imbalance, LFTs, renal function test, toxic megacolon in ulcerative colitis, pancreatitis.

**Patient Counseling:** Take as directed. Dosing to be accompanied by adequate fluids and electrolytes. Exercise caution while operating machinery/driving. Should not be used in children under 2 years. Report lack of response or adverse effects. Avoid alcohol and other CNS depressants.

**Administration:** Oral route. Plastic dropper should be used when measuring liquid for administration to children. **Storage:** Dispense liquids in original container.

## LOPID

**RX**

gemfibrozil (Parke-Davis)

**THERAPEUTIC CLASS:** Fibric acid derivative

**INDICATIONS:** Treatment of Types IV and V hyperlipidemia with risk of pancreatitis not responding to dietary management (usually TG >2000mg/dL).

May consider therapy if TG 1000-2000mg/dL with history of pancreatitis or recurrent abdominal pain typical of pancreatitis. Risk reduction of CAD in Type IIb patients without history or symptoms of existing coronary heart disease inadequately responding to weight loss, dietary therapy, exercise, other pharmacologic agents; with triad of low HDL, and elevated LDL and TG levels.

**DOSAGE:** *Adults:* 600mg bid. Give 30 min before morning and evening meals.

**HOW SUPPLIED:** Tab: 600mg* *scored

**CONTRAINDICATIONS:** Hepatic or severe renal dysfunction including primary biliary cirrhosis, pre-existing gallbladder disease, combination therapy with repaglinide.

**WARNINGS/PRECAUTIONS:** Cholelithiasis reported. Associated with myositis. Abnormal LFTs reported; monitor periodically. D/C if myositis and gallstones suspected/diagnosed or if abnormal LFTs persist. Only use if indicated and d/c if significant lipid response not obtained. Severe anemia, leukopenia, thrombocytopenia, and bone marrow hypoplasia (rare) reported. Monitor blood counts periodically during first 12 months. May worsen renal insufficiency.

**ADVERSE REACTIONS:** Dyspepsia, abdominal pain, diarrhea, fatigue, bacterial and viral infections, musculoskeletal symptoms, abnormal LFTs, hematologic changes, hypesthesia, paresthesia, taste perversion.

**INTERACTIONS:** See contraindications. Increased risk for severe hypoglycemia with repaglinide. Caution with anticoagulants; reduce dose and monitor PT. Increased risk of myopathy and rhabdomyolysis with HMG-CoA reductase inhibitors. Benefit with concomitant statins does not outweigh risks. Reduced bioavailability with resin-granule drugs (eg, colestipol); spaced dosing required.

L

**PREGNANCY:** Category C, not for use in nursing.

**MECHANISM OF ACTION:** Fibric acid derivative; not established. Suspected to inhibit peripheral lipolysis, decrease hepatic extraction of free fatty acids, thus reducing hepatic TG production and inhibiting synthesis and increasing clearance of VLDL carrier apolipoprotein B, leading to decreased VLDL production.

**PHARMACOKINETICS: Absorption:** Complete; $T_{max}$=1-2 hr. **Metabolism:** Oxidation to hydroxymethyl and carboxyl metabolites. **Elimination:** Urine (70% glucoronide conjugate) (<2% unchanged), feces (6%).

## NURSING CONSIDERATIONS

**Assessment:** Assess for hepatic/renal dysfunction, primary biliary cirrhosis, persistent abnormal levels of lipids, gallbladder disease, DM, hypothyroidism, pregnancy/nursing status, coronary heart disease, hypersensitivity to drug, and possible drug interactions (eg, anticoagulants). Control serum lipids with appropriate diet, exercise, and weight loss in obese patients prior to therapy.

**Monitoring:** Monitor lipids periodically and for LFTs, CPK, CBC, creatinine, INR, PT. Monitor for signs of myopathy (eg, unexplained muscle pain, weakness, or tenderness with fever or malaise), hypersensitivity reactions, cholelithiasis, cataracts, malignancy, abdominal pain leading to appendectomy, and noncoronary mortality.

**Patient Counseling:** Inform about potential risks/benefits of therapy. Report signs of myopathy (eg, unexplained muscle pain, tenderness, or weakness with fever or malaise). Notify physician if pregnant/nursing or planning to become pregnant.

**Administration:** Oral route. **Storage:** 20-25°C (68-77°F). Protect from light and moisture.

# LOPRESSOR RX

metoprolol tartrate (Novartis)

**THERAPEUTIC CLASS:** Selective $beta_1$-blocker

**INDICATIONS:** (Tab) Treatment of hypertension alone or in combination with other anti-hypertensives. Long-term treatment of angina pectoris. (Tab/inj) To reduce cardiovascular mortality in hemodynamically stable patients with definite or suspected acute myocardial infarction.

**DOSAGE:** *Adults:* HTN: Individualize dosing. Take with meals. Initial: 100mg/day PO in single or divided doses given alone or with a diuretic. Titrate: May increase at weekly (or longer) intervals until optimum BP reduction is achieved. Usual: 100-450mg/day. Max: 450mg/day. Angina: Individualize dosing. Take with meals. Initial: 100mg/day PO in two divided doses. Titrate: Increase weekly until optimum clinical response is achieved or pronounced slowing of HR. Usual: 100-400mg/day. Max: 400mg/day. MI (Early Phase): 5mg IV every 2 mins for 3 doses (monitor BP, HR, and ECG). If tolerated, give 50mg PO q6h for 48 hrs. Maint: 100mg bid. If not tolerated, give 25-50mg PO q6h. If severe intolerance d/c. Initiate PO dose 15 min after last IV dose. MI (Late Phase): 100mg bid for at least 3 months.

**HOW SUPPLIED:** Inj: 1mg/mL [5mL]; Tab: 50mg*, 100mg* *scored

**CONTRAINDICATIONS:** (HTN, Angina) Sinus bradycardia, >1st-degree heart block, cardiogenic shock, overt cardiac failure, sick sinus syndrome, severe peripheral arterial circulatory disorders. (MI) HR <45 beats/min, 2nd- and 3rd-degree heart block, significant 1st-degree heart block, systolic blood pressure (SBP) <100mmHg, moderate to severe cardiac failure.

**WARNINGS/PRECAUTIONS:** Caution with ischemic heart disease; avoid abrupt withdrawal, taper over 1-2 weeks. Caution in hypertensive and angina patients who have congestive heart failure (CHF) controlled by digitalis and diuretics. Continued myocardial depression may lead to cardiac failure; at first sign/symptom, digitalize and/or give diuretic. Avoid with bronchospastic diseases. Withdrawal prior to major surgery is controversial; difficulty in restarting and maintaining heart beat reported. May mask tachycardia occurring with hypoglycemia; caution in diabetics. May cause paradoxical increase in BP with pheochromocytoma if administered alone; always initiate an alpha blocker before starting therapy. May mask clinical signs of hyperthyroidism; if suspected to develop thyrotoxicosis, avoid abrupt withdrawal. May decrease sinus HR, slow AV conduction, produce significant heart block and hypotension (SBP ≤90mmHg); d/c if heart block and hypotension occurs. Caution with impaired hepatic function and in elderly.

**ADVERSE REACTIONS:** Bradycardia, tiredness, dizziness, depression, SOB, diarrhea, pruritus, rash, heart block, heart failure, hypotension.

**INTERACTIONS:** Additive effects with catecholamine-depleting drugs (eg, reserpine). May block epinephrine effects. Caution with digitalis; both agents slow AV conduction and decrease HR. May enhance cardiodepressant effect with some inhalational anesthetics. Potent CYP2D6 inhibitors may increase levels; caution when coadministering. When given concomitantly with clonidine, d/c several days before clonidine is withdrawn.

**PREGNANCY:** Category C, caution in nursing.

**MECHANISM OF ACTION:** β-blocker; not established. Proposed to competitively antagonize catecholamines at peripheral adrenergic-neuronal sites, has central effect leading to reduced sympathetic outflow to periphery and suppression of renin activity.

**PHARMACOKINETICS: Absorption:** Rapid and complete. **Distribution:** Serum albumin binding (12%); found in breast milk. **Metabolism:** Liver via CYP2D6 (oxidation). **Elimination:** PO: Urine (<5%, unchanged), IV: Urine (10%, unchanged); $T_{1/2}$=2.8 hrs (extensive metabolizers); $T_{1/2}$=7.5 hrs (poor metabolizers).

## NURSING CONSIDERATIONS

**Assessment:** Assess for sinus bradycardia, heart block, cardiogenic shock, history of or overt CHF, cardiac failure, ischemic heart disease, bronchospastic diseases, hyperthyroidism, DM, sick sinus syndrome, severe peripheral arterial circulatory disorders, pheochromocytoma, hepatic impairment, hypersensitivity, pregnancy/nursing status, and possible drug interactions. Perform baseline BP, heart rate, and ECG.

**Monitoring:** Monitor BP, HR, ECG and hemodynamic status periodically. Monitor for signs/symptoms of cardiac failure, hypoglycemia, thyrotoxicosis, withdrawal symptoms (angina, MI), hypotension, and hypersensitivity reactions.

**Patient Counseling:** Instruct to take regularly and continuously, as directed, with or immediately following meals. If dose is missed, take next dose at scheduled time (without doubling). Do not d/c without consulting physician. May impair physical/mental abilities. Advise to contact physician before any surgery or if symptoms of heart failure (difficulty breathing), withdrawal (angina) or hypersensitivity occur. Inform that signs of thyrotoxicosis and hypoglycemia may be masked.

**Administration:** Oral, IV route. **Storage:** 25°C (77°F); excursions permitted to 15-30°C (59-86°F). (Tab) Protect from moisture. (Inj) Protect from light.

## LOPRESSOR HCT RX

metoprolol tartrate - hydrochlorothiazide (Novartis)

**THERAPEUTIC CLASS:** Selective beta$_1$-blocker/thiazide diuretic

**INDICATIONS:** Management of hypertension. Not for initial therapy.

**DOSAGE:** *Adults:* Initial: 100mg metoprolol daily in single or divided dose. Usual: 100-450mg metoprolol/day and 12.5-50mg HCTZ/day. Max: 450mg metoprolol/day and 50mg HCTZ/day. Elderly: Start at the low end of the dosing range.

L

**HOW SUPPLIED:** Tab: (Metoprolol-HCTZ) 50mg-25mg*, 100-25mg*, 100mg-50mg* *scored

**CONTRAINDICATIONS:** Sinus bradycardia, >1st-degree heart block, cardiogenic shock, overt cardiac failure, sick-sinus syndrome, severe peripheral arterial circulatory disorders, anuria, sulfonamide hypersensitivity.

**WARNINGS/PRECAUTIONS:** Exacerbations of angina pectoris and MI reported following abrupt cessation of therapy. Withdrawal before surgery is controversial; difficulty in restarting heart and maintaining heartbeat reported. May mask hyperthyroidism and hypoglycemia symptoms. May precipitate severe cardiac failure. Caution with hepatic dysfunction, CHF controlled by digitalis, severe renal disease, allergy or asthma history. May precipitate azotemia with renal disease. Avoid in bronchospastic disease. Monitor for fluid/electrolyte imbalance. May manifest latent DM. Hypokalemia, hyperuricemia, hypercalcemia, hypophosphatemia, and hypomagnesemia may occur. May exacerbate SLE. Enhanced effects in post-sympathectomy patient. Paradoxical increase in blood pressure due to beta-mediated vasodilation in the setting of pheochromocytoma reported; alpha blocker should be given in combination before initiating therapy in this setting. Caution in elderly.

**ADVERSE REACTIONS:** Fatigue, dizziness, flu syndrome, drowsiness, hypokalemia, headache, bradycardia, tiredness, diarrhea, depression, lethargy, vertigo, shortness of breath.

**INTERACTIONS:** (Metoprolol) Potent CYP2D6 inhibitors (eg, antidepressants, antipsychotics, antiarrhythmics, antiretrovirals, antihistamines, antimalarials, antifungals, cimetidine) may increase drug levels. Additive effects with catecholamine-depleting drugs (eg, reserpine). May block epinephrine effects. Caution with digitalis; both agents slow AV conduction. Increased risk for rebound hypotension following clonidine withdrawal; stop metoprolol several days before clonidine d/c when both agents given concurrently. Inhalational anesthetics may enhance cardiodepressant effects. (Hydrochlorothiazide) Corticosteroids, ACTH may increase risk of hypokalemia. Risk of lithium toxicity. NSAIDs may reduce diuretic effects. Insulin may need adjustment. Impaired absorption with cholestyramine, colestipol. May increase responsiveness to tubocurarine. May decrease arterial responsiveness to norepinephrine. Alcohol, barbiturates, and narcotics may potentiate orthostatic hypotension. Rare reports of hemolytic anemia with methyldopa. May potentiate other antihypertensive drugs (eg, ganglionic or peripheral adrenergic blocking drugs).

**PREGNANCY:** Category C, not for use in nursing.

**MECHANISM OF ACTION:** Metoprolol: β-adrenergic receptor blocker; not established, proposed to competitively antagonize catecholamines at peripheral adrenergic-neuronal sites, have central effect leading to reduced sympathetic outflow to periphery and suppression of renin activity. HCTZ: Thiazide diuretic; affects renal tubular mechanism of electrolyte reabsorption.

**PHARMACOKINETICS: Absorption:** Metoprolol: Rapid and complete. HCTZ: Rapid; $T_{max}$=1-2.5 hrs. **Distribution:** Found in breast milk. Metoprolol: Plasma protein binding (12%). HCTZ: $V_d$=3.6-7.8L/kg; plasma protein binding (67.9%). **Metabolism:** Metoprolol: CYP2D6 (oxidation). **Elimination:** Metoprolol: Urine (<5%); $T_{1/2}$=2.8 hrs (extensive metabolizers), 7.5 hrs (poor metabolizers). HCTZ: Urine (72-97%); $T_{1/2}$=10-17 hrs.

## NURSING CONSIDERATIONS

**Assessment:** Assess for history of allergy or bronchial asthma, sinus bradycardia, AV block, cardiogenic shock, overt CHF, bronchospastic disease, SLE, hyperthyroidism, DM, sick sinus syndrome, severe peripheral arterial circulatory disorders, pheochromocytoma, history of CHF, anuria, sulfonamide hypersensitivity, hepatic/renal impairment. Obtain baseline serum electrolyte levels. Assess pregnancy/nursing status and for possible drug interactions.

**Monitoring:** Monitor serum electrolytes periodically. Monitor for signs/symptoms of electrolyte imbalance, hypoglycemia, thyrotoxicosis, withdrawal (eg, angina, MI), cardiac failure, hypersensitivity reactions, exacerbation or activation of SLE, hyperuricemia or precipitation of gout, renal/hepatic dysfunction.

**Patient Counseling:** Instruct to take regularly and continuously, as directed, with or immediately following meals. If dose is missed, take next dose at scheduled time (without doubling); do not d/c without consulting physician. Caution may impair physical/mental abilities. Advise to contact physician before any surgery, or if symptoms of heart failure (eg, difficulty breathing), hypersensitivity reactions, withdrawal (angina), or electrolyte imbalance (eg, dry mouth, thirst, weakness) occur. Inform may mask signs of thyrotoxicosis and hypoglycemia.

**Administration:** Oral route. **Storage:** 25°C (77°F); excursions permitted to 15-30°C (59-86°F). Protect from moisture. Dispense in tight, light-resistant container.

# LOPROX — RX

ciclopirox (Medicis)

**OTHER BRAND NAMES:** Loprox TS (Medicis)

**THERAPEUTIC CLASS:** Broad-spectrum antifungal

**INDICATIONS:** (Cre/Sus) Topical treatment of dermal infections of tinea pedis, tinea cruris, tinea corporis, cutaneous candidiasis and tinea versicolor. (Gel) Topical treatment of interdigital tinea pedis and tinea corporis. (Gel/Shampoo) Topical treatment of seborrheic dermatitis of the scalp.

**DOSAGE:** *Adults:* (Cre/Gel/Sus) Massage affected and surrounding areas bid (am and pm). (Shampoo) Apply about 5mL (up to 10mL for long hair) to wet scalp. Lather and rinse off after 3 min. Repeat twice weekly for 4 weeks, at least 3 days apart. If no improvement after 4 weeks reassess treatment. *Pediatrics:* ≥16 yrs: (Gel): ≥10 yrs: (Cre/Sus) Massage affected and surrounding areas bid (am and pm) up to 4 weeks. ≥16 yrs: (Shampoo) Apply about 5mL (up to 10mL for long hair) to wet scalp. Lather and rinse off after 3 min. Repeat twice weekly for 4 weeks, at least 3 days apart. If no improvement after 4 weeks reassess treatment.

**HOW SUPPLIED:** Cre: 0.77% [15g, 30g, 90g]; Gel: 0.77% [30g, 45g, 100g]; Shampoo: 1% [120mL]; Sus: (Loprox TS) 0.77% [30mL, 60mL]

**WARNINGS/PRECAUTIONS:** Not for ophthalmic, oral, or intravaginal use. D/C if sensitization or chemical irritation occurs. Avoid eyes; if contact occurs, rinse thoroughly with water. (Shampoo) Hair discoloration reported in patients with lighter hair color.

**ADVERSE REACTIONS:** Pruritus, burning. (Gel) Contact dermatitis. (Shampoo) Itching, erythema.

**PREGNANCY:** Pregnancy B, caution in nursing.

**MECHANISM OF ACTION:** Broad-spectrum antifungal; acts by chelation of polyvalent cations ($Fe^{3+}$or $Al^{3+}$) resulting in the inhibition of the metal-dependent enzymes that are responsible for degradation of peroxides in the fungal cell wall. Inhibits the growth of pathogenic dermatophytes, yeasts, and *Malassezia furfur.*

**PHARMACOKINETICS: Absorption:** (Cre) (5g) $C_{max}$=18.62ng/mL. (Gel) (5g) $C_{max}$=25.02ng/mL. (15g) $C_{max}$=100ng/mL. **Elimination:** (Cre/Sus) Urine (0.01%), feces; $T_{1/2}$=1.7 hrs. (Gel) Urine (3%), $T_{1/2}$=5.5 hrs. (Shampoo) Urine (0.5%).

## NURSING CONSIDERATIONS

**Assessment:** Assess proper diagnosis of causative organisms. Assess for hypersensitivity and use in pregnant/nursing patients.

**Monitoring:** Monitor for signs/symptoms of sensitivity or chemical irritation reactions.

**Patient Counseling:** Instruct to use medication as directed by physician. Counsel to continue therapy for the full treatment time even if symptoms improve. Instruct to notify physician if there are no signs of improvement after 4 weeks of therapy or if signs of increased irritation (eg, redness, itching, blistering, oozing) develop at the application site. Instruct to avoid occlusive wrappings or dressings. Advise that burning or itching may occur when using the gel formulation on the scalp. Advise patients with lighter hair color that the shampoo formulation may discolor hair.

L

**Administration:** Topical route. (Sus) Shake vigorously before use. **Storage:** (Cre/Gel/Shampoo) 15-30°C (59-86°F). (Sus) 5-25°C (41-77°F).

# Lorcet

CIII

hydrocodone bitartrate - acetaminophen (Forest)

**OTHER BRAND NAMES:** Lorcet Plus (Forest) - Lorcet 10/650 (Forest)

**THERAPEUTIC CLASS:** Opioid analgesic

**INDICATIONS:** Relief of moderate to moderately severe pain.

**DOSAGE:** *Adults:* (Plus, 10/650) Usual: 1 cap/tab q4-6h prn pain. Max: 6 tabs or caps/day.

**HOW SUPPLIED:** (Hydrocodone-APAP) Tab: (Plus) 7.5mg-650mg*, (10/650) 10mg-650mg* *scored

**WARNINGS/PRECAUTIONS:** May produce dose-related respiratory depression. May obscure acute abdominal conditions or head injuries. Caution in elderly, debilitated, severe hepatic or renal dysfunction, hypothyroidism, Addison's disease, prostatic hypertrophy, urethral stricture, pulmonary disease and postoperative use. May be habit-forming. Suppresses cough reflex.

**ADVERSE REACTIONS:** Dizziness, drowsiness, NV, dysphoria, urinary retention, urethral spasm, dyspnea, SOB, rash.

**INTERACTIONS:** May potentiate CNS depression with narcotics, alcohol, antianxiety agents, antihistamines, antipsychotics, other CNS depressants. Increased effect of antidepressant or hydrocodone with MAOIs or TCAs.

**PREGNANCY:** Category C, not for use in nursing.

**MECHANISM OF ACTION:** Hydrocodone: Narcotic analgesic; not established. Suspected to be related to existence of opiate receptors in the CNS. APAP: Nonopiate, nonsalicylate analgesic and antipyretic. Mechanism of analgesic actions not established; involves peripheral influences. Antipyretic activity is mediated through hypothalamic heat regulating centers. Inhibits prostaglandin synthetase.

**PHARMACOKINETICS: Absorption:** Hydrocodone: $C_{max}$=23.6ng/mL; $T_{max}$=1.3 hrs. APAP: Rapidly absorbed. **Distribution:** APAP: Found in breast milk. **Metabolism**: Hydrocodone: O-demethylation, N-demethylation, and 6-keto reduction. APAP: Liver (conjugation). **Elimination**: Hydrocodone: $T_{1/2}$=3.8 hrs. APAP: Urine (85%); $T_{1/2}$=1.25-3 hrs.

## NURSING CONSIDERATIONS

**Assessment:** Assess for impaired hepatic/renal function, presence of head injury or other intracranial lesions, elevations in ICP, acute abdominal conditions, presence of debilitation (elderly), hypothyroidism, Addison's disease, prostatic hypertrophy or urethral stricture, pulmonary disease, pregnancy/nursing status, and possible drug interactions.

**Monitoring:** Monitor for signs/symptoms of respiratory depression, elevated CSF pressure, dependence on medication, and abuse. Monitor serial hepatic/renal function tests in with severe hepatic/renal disease.

**Patient Counseling:** Advise that medication may impair mental/physical abilities; use caution when performing hazardous tasks (eg, operating machinery/driving). Advise to avoid using alcohol and other CNS depressants during therapy. Inform that medication may be habit-forming; counsel to take only as long as prescribed, in amounts prescribed, and not more frequently than prescribed.

**Administration:** Oral route. **Storage:** 20-25°(68-77°); excursions permitted to 15-30°C (59-86°F). Dispense in tight, light-resistant container.

# LORTAB

hydrocodone bitartrate - acetaminophen (UCB)

CIII

**THERAPEUTIC CLASS:** Opioid analgesic

**INDICATIONS:** Relief of moderate to moderately severe pain.

**DOSAGE:** *Adults:* (2.5/500, 5/500) 1-2 tabs q4-6h prn. Max: 8 tabs/day. (7.5/500, 10/500) 1 tab q4-6h prn. Max: 6 tabs/day. (Sol) 15mL q4-6h prn. Max: 90mL/day.

*Pediatrics:* ≥2 yrs: (Sol) 12-15kg: 3.75mL. 16-22kg: 5mL. 23-31kg: 7.5mL. 32-45kg: 10mL. ≥46kg: 15mL. May repeat q4-6h prn.

**HOW SUPPLIED:** (Hydrocodone-APAP) Sol: 7.5mg-500mg/15mL; Tab: 2.5mg-500mg*, 5mg-500mg*, 7.5mg-500mg*, 10mg-500mg* *scored

**WARNINGS/PRECAUTIONS:** May produce dose-related respiratory depression. May obscure acute abdominal conditions or head injuries. Caution in elderly, debilitated, severe hepatic or renal dysfunction, hypothyroidism, Addison's disease, prostatic hypertrophy, urethral stricture, pulmonary disease, postoperative use. May be habit-forming. Suppresses cough reflex.

**ADVERSE REACTIONS:** Lightheadedness, dizziness, sedation, N/V.

**INTERACTIONS:** Additive CNS depression with other narcotics, antihistamines, antipsychotics, antianxiety agents, alcohol, CNS depressants. Increased effect of antidepressant or hydrocodone with MAOIs or TCAs.

**PREGNANCY:** Category C, not for use in nursing.

**MECHANISM OF ACTION:** Hydrocodone: Narcotic analgesic and antitussive; not established. Suspected to be related to existence of opiate receptors in CNS. APAP: Nonopioid, nonsalicylate analgesic, and antipyretic. Analgesic action involves peripheral influences; specific mechanism not established. Antipyretic activity is mediated through hypothalamic heat-regulating centers. Inhibits prostaglandin synthetase.

**PHARMACOKINETICS: Administration:** Hydrocodone: $C_{max}$=23.6ng/mL; $T_{max}$=1.3 hrs. APAP: Rapidly absorbed. **Distribution:** Hydrocodone: Crosses placental barrier. APAP: Found in breast milk. **Metabolism:** Hydrocodone: O-demethylation, N-demethylation and 6-keto reduction. APAP: Liver (conjugation). **Elimination:** Hydrocodone: $T_{1/2}$=3.8 hrs; APAP: Urine (85%); $T_{1/2}$=1.25-3 hrs.

## NURSING CONSIDERATIONS

**Assessment:** Assess for pulmonary disease, renal/hepatic impairment, presence of debilitation (elderly), hypothyroidism, Addison's disease, prostatic

L

hypertrophy or urethral stricture, presence of acute abdominal conditions, head injury or other intracranial lesions, increased ICP, pregnancy/nursing status, and possible drug interactions.

**Monitoring:** Monitor for signs/symptoms of respiratory depression, elevations in CSF pressure, drug dependence, and drug abuse. Monitor serial hepatic/renal function tests in patients with severe hepatic/renal disease.

**Patient Counseling:** Inform that medication may impair mental/physical abilities; use caution when performing hazardous tasks (eg, operating machinery/driving). Avoid the use of alcohol and other CNS depressants while on medication. Inform that medication may be habit forming; instruct to only take amount prescribed for duration of time prescribed.

**Administration:** Oral route. **Storage:** (2.5mg/500mg): 15-30°C (59-86°F); (5 mg/500mg, 10mg/500mg, 7.5mg/500mg, (Sol) 7.5mg-500mg/15mL): 20-25°C (68-77°F). Dispense in tight, light-resistant container with child-resistant closure.

## LOSEASONIQUE — RX

ethinyl estradiol - levonorgestrel (Duramed)

**Cigarette smoking increases the risk of serious CV events from combination oral contraceptive (COC) use. This risk increases with age and with number of cigarettes smoked. Women who are >35 yrs and smoke should not use COCs.**

**THERAPEUTIC CLASS:** Estrogen/progestogen combination

**INDICATIONS:** Prevention of pregnancy.

**DOSAGE:** *Adults:* 1 tablet qd for 91 days. Begin taking on first Sunday after the onset of menstruation. If menses begin on Sunday, start on that day. Use non-hormonal back-up method of contraception (eg, condoms, spermicide) until levonorgestrel-ethinyl estradiol tablet has been taken daily for 7 consecutive days. Begin next and all subsequent 91 day cycles without interruption on same day of week (Sunday) upon which first course began, following the same schedule. Postpartum women should start COC no earlier than 4-6 weeks postpartum.

**HOW SUPPLIED:** Tab: (Ethinyl Estradiol-Levonorgestrel) 0.02mg-0.1mg; Tab: (Ethinyl Estradiol) 0.01mg.

**CONTRAINDICATIONS:** Patients with high risk of arterial or venous thrombotic diseases (eg, women who smoke, if over age 35; presence or history of deep vein thrombosis or pulmonary embolism; cerebrovascular or coronary artery disease; thrombogenic valvular or thrombogenic rhythm diseases of the heart; hypercoagulopathies; uncontrolled hypertension; diabetes with vascular disease; headaches with focal neurological symptoms or migraine headaches with or without aura if over age 35), presence or history of breast cancer or other estrogen or progestin sensitive cancer, liver tumors (benign or malignant) or liver disease, and pregnancy.

**WARNINGS/PRECAUTIONS:** Increases the risk of venous thromboembolism, arterial thromboses (eg, stroke, MI); d/c if arterial or deep venous thrombotic event occurs. D/C if unexplained loss of vision, proptosis, diplopia, papilledema, or retinal vascular lesions occur; evaluate for retinal vein thrombosis. May increase risk of cervical cancer or intraepithelial neoplasia. D/C if jaundice develops. Increases risk of hepatic adenomas, hepatocellular carcinoma, and gallbladder disease. Oral contraceptive cholestasis may occur in women with history of pregnancy related cholestasis. May cause HTN; d/c if BP rises significantly in women with history of well controlled HTN. May decrease glucose tolerance; monitor prediabetic and diabetic women. May affect lipid levels; consider alternate therapy in patients with uncontrolled dyslipidemias. Breakthrough bleeding and spotting may occur, especially during the first 3 months; if bleeding persists, check for causes. Amenorrhea may occur during use; check for pregnancy. Amenorrhea or oligomenorrhea may occur after d/c therapy. May change the results of some laboratory tests (eg, coagulation factors, lipids, glucose tolerance, binding proteins). May need to increase dose of thyroid hormone in patients on thyroid hormone replacement therapy.

**ADVERSE REACTIONS:** Headaches, irregular and/or heavy uterine bleeding, dysmenorrhea, N/V, backpain, breast tenderness, mood changes, acne, and weight gain.

**INTERACTIONS:** Use with drugs or herbal products that induce enzymes, including CYP3A4, that metabolize contraceptive hormones, may decrease the plasma concentrations of contraceptive hormones and may decrease the effectiveness of the hormonal contraceptive or cause breakthrough bleeding; counsel to use additional contraception or a different method of contraception. Barbiturates, bosentan, carbamazepine, felbamate, griseofulvin, oxcarbazepine, phenytoin, rifampin, St. John's wort, and topiramate may decrease contraceptive effectiveness. HIV protease inhibitors may increase or decrease levels. Reports of pregnancy with antibiotic use. Increased levels with atorvastatin, ascorbic acid, acetaminophen, and CYP3A4 inhibitors (eg, itraconazole, ketoconazole). Decreases levels of lamotrigine and may reduce seizure control; may require dosage adjustment of lamotrigine.

**PREGNANCY:** Safety not known in pregnancy, caution in nursing.

**MECHANISM OF ACTION:** Estrogen/progestogen combination oral contraceptive; primarily suppresses ovulation. Also responsible for causing changes in cervical mucus (increases difficulty in sperm entry into uterus) and endometrium (reduces likelihood of implantation).

**PHARMACOKINETICS: Absorption:** Rapid; Levonorgestrel: Absolute bioavailability (nearly 100%); $T_{max}$=1.6 hrs; $C_{max}$ = 6.0ng/mL; AUC=76.5ng•hr/mL. Ethinyl estradiol: Absolute bioavailability (43%); $T_{max}$=1.8 hrs; $C_{max}$=122.8pg/mL; AUC=1335.8pg•hr/mL. **Distribution:** Found in breast milk; Levonorgestrel: $V_d$=1.8L/kg; plasma protein binding (97.5%-99%). Ethinyl estradiol: $V_d$=4.3L/kg; plasma protein binding (95%-97%). **Metabolism:** Levonorgestrel: Sulfate and glucuronide conjugates. Ethinyl estradiol: 1st past metabolism in gut wall, Hepatic, via CYP3A4 (hydroxylation), methylation, conjugation. **Elimination:** Levonorgestrel: Urine (45%), feces (32%); $T_{1/2}$=28.5 hrs. Ethinyl estradiol: Urine, feces; $T_{1/2}$=17.5 hrs.

## NURSING CONSIDERATIONS

**Assessment:** Assess for risk of arterial or venous thrombotic diseases (eg, smokers over 35, presence or history of deep vein thrombosis or pulmonary embolism, cerebrovascular disease, coronary artery disease, thrombogenic valvular or thrombogenic rhythm diseases of the heart, hypercoagulopathies, uncontrolled HTN, DM with vascular disease, headaches with focal neurological symptoms or migraine headaches with or with out aura and over the age of 35), presence or history of breast cancer, presence or history of estrogen or progestin sensitive cancer, benign or malignant liver tumors or liver disease), pregnancy/nursing status, history of pregnancy-related cholestasis, uncontrolled dyslipidemias, and for possible drug interactions.

**Monitoring:** Monitor for signs/symptoms of venous thromboembolism, arterial thromboses (eg, stroke, MI), cervical cancer or intraepithelial neoplasia, retinal vein thrombosis (eg, loss of vision, proptosis, diplopia, papilledema, retinal vascular lesions), jaundice, hepatic adenomas, hepatocellular carcinoma, gallbladder disease, headaches, bleeding irregularities, and for interference with laboratory tests. Monitor glucose levels in DM or prediabetic patients. Monitor for HTN; monitor BP in women with well controlled HTN and d/c therapy if BP rises significantly. Monitor for cholestasis in women who have a history of pregnancy related cholestasis.

**Patient Counseling:** Inform that drug does not protect against HIV infection (AIDS) and other STDs. Advise not to smoke while on medication. Instruct to take medication by mouth at the same time everyday, and what to do in the event pills are missed. Counsel to use back-up or alternative method of contraception when enzyme inducers are used with COCs. Counsel COCs may reduce breast milk production. Counsel any patient who uses COCs postpartum, and have not yet had a period, to use an additional method of contraception until she has taken a levonorgestrel-ethinyl estradiol tablet for 7 consecutive days.

**Administration:** Oral route. **Storage:**20-25°C (68-77°F).

## LOTEMAX

loteprednol etabonate (Bausch & Lomb)

RX

**THERAPEUTIC CLASS:** Corticosteroid

**INDICATIONS:** Treatment of inflammation of the palpebral and bulbar conjunctiva, cornea and anterior segment of the globe. Management of postoperative inflammation.

**DOSAGE:** *Adults:* Steroid-Responsive Disease: 1-2 drops qid, may increase up to 1 drop every hr within the 1st week of treatment. Re-evaluate after 2 days if no improvement. Postoperative: 1-2 drops qid starting 24 hrs post-op and continue for 2 weeks.

**HOW SUPPLIED:** Sus: 0.5% [2.5mL, 5mL, 10mL, 15mL]

**CONTRAINDICATIONS:** Viral diseases of the cornea and conjunctiva including epithelial herpes simplex keratitis, vaccinia, and varicella. Mycobacterial infection and fungal diseases of the eye.

**WARNINGS/PRECAUTIONS:** Caution with glaucoma, history of herpes simplex, and diseases causing thinning of cornea/sclera. Prolonged use can cause glaucoma, optic nerve damage, defects in visual acuity and fields of vision, cataracts, or secondary ocular infections (eg, fungal). Monitor IOP after 10 days of therapy. Re-evaluate if no response after 2 days. May delay healing and increase incidence of bleb formation after cataract surgery. May mask or enhance existing infection in acute, purulent conditions.

**ADVERSE REACTIONS:** Elevated IOP, abnormal vision, chemosis, discharge, dry eyes, burning on instillation, epiphora, itching, photophobia, foreign body sensation, optic nerve damage, visual field defects.

L

**PREGNANCY:** Category C, caution in nursing.

**MECHANISM OF ACTION:** Glucocorticoid; anti-inflammatory agent, no accepted explanation for MOA; suspected to inhibit edema, fibrin deposition, capillary dilation and deposition of collagen and scar formation by the induction of phospholipase $A_2$ inhibitory proteins, lipocortins.

### NURSING CONSIDERATIONS

**Assessment:** Assess for viral diseases of cornea and conjunctiva, dendritic keratitis, vaccinia, varicella, mycobacterial infection, fungal disease of ocular structures, glaucoma, thinning of corneal/scleral epithelium, hypersensitivity, cataract surgery.

**Monitoring:** Frequent measuring of IOP and slit lamp microscopy exam where appropriate, fluorescein staining for monitoring of glaucoma with damage to optic nerve with defects in visual acuity and fields of vision, posterior subscapsular cataract, delayed corneal healing, thinning of cornea and sclera, ulceration, perforation, secondary ocular infections or masking of existing infections.

**Patient Counseling:** Advise to d/c drug and notify physician if symptoms persist or worsen. Instruct to not wear soft contact lenses during treatment. Counsel to avoid touching bottle tip to eyelids or any other surface.

**Administration:** Ocular route. Shake vigorously before using. **Storage:** 15-25°C (59-77°F). Do not freeze.

## LOTENSIN

benazepril HCl (Novartis)

RX

**When used in pregnancy, ACE inhibitors can cause injury and even death to the developing fetus. D/C therapy when pregnancy detected.**

**THERAPEUTIC CLASS:** ACE inhibitor

**INDICATIONS:** Treatment of hypertension. May be used alone or in combination with thiazide diuretics.

**DOSAGE:** *Adults:* If possible, d/c diuretic 2-3 days prior to initiation of therapy. Initial: 10mg qd or 5mg with concomitant diuretic. Maint: 20-40mg/day given qd-bid. Resume diuretic if BP not controlled. Max: 80mg/day. CrCl <30mL/min/1.73m²: Initial: 5mg qd. Max: 40mg/day.
*Pediatrics:* ≥6 yrs: Initial: 0.2mg/kg qd. Max: 0.6mg/kg or 40mg/day.

**HOW SUPPLIED:** Tab: 5mg, 10mg, 20mg, 40mg

**CONTRAINDICATIONS:** History of angioedema.

**WARNINGS/PRECAUTIONS:** D/C if angioedema, jaundice or if marked LFT elevation occurs. Less effective on BP in blacks and more reports of angioedema than nonblacks. Risk of hyperkalemia with diabetes mellitus (DM), renal dysfunction. Persistent nonproductive cough reported. May cause agranulocytosis and bone marrow depression; monitor WBC in patients with renal and collagen vascular disease. May increase BUN and SrCr levels. Anaphylactoid reactions reported. Monitor for hypotension in high-risk patients (eg, surgery/anesthesia, prolonged diuretic therapy, heart failure, volume and/or salt depletion, dialysis, diarrhea, vomiting). Caution with congestive heart failure (CHF), renal dysfunction and renal artery stenosis.

**ADVERSE REACTIONS:** Cough, dizziness, headache, fatigue.

**INTERACTIONS:** May increase lithium levels; risk of lithium toxicity. Hypotension risk with diuretics. Increased risk of hyperkalemia with $K^+$-sparing diuretics, $K^+$-containing salt substitutes, or $K^+$ supplements. Nitritoid reactions (eg, facial flushing, N/V, hypotension) reported when used concomitantly with injectable gold (sodium aurothiomalate). Hypoglycemia may develop with concomitant use with oral anti-diabetics or insulin in diabetics.

**PREGNANCY:** Category D, not for use in nursing.

**MECHANISM OF ACTION:** ACE inhibitor; effects appear to result from suppression of renin-angiotensin-aldosterone system. Inhibition results in decreased plasma angiotensin II, which leads to decreased vasopressor activity and to decreased aldosterone secretion.

**PHARMACOKINETICS: Absorption:** Benazepril: $T_{max}$ = 0.5-1 hr; absolute bioavailability (37%). Benazeprilat: $T_{max}$ =1-2 hrs (fasting), 2-4 hrs (nonfasting). **Distribution:** Plasma protein binding (96.7%, benazepril) (95.3%, benazeprilat); excreted in breast milk. **Metabolism:** Liver, cleavage of ester group; benazeprilat (active metabolite). **Elimination:** Benazepril: Urine (trace). Benazeprilat: Urine (20%), biliary (11-12%); $T_{1/2}$= 10-11 hrs (adults), 5 hrs (pediatrics).

## NURSING CONSIDERATIONS

**Assessment:** Assess for pregnancy/nursing status, volume/salt depletion, collagen vascular disease (SLE, scleroderma), CHF, DM, renal/hepatic impairment, history of angioedema or hypersensitivity reactions, and possible drug interactions.

**Monitoring:** Monitor renal function for 1st few weeks, LFTs, WBC (collagen vascular disease) and serum electrolytes periodically. Monitor for signs/symptoms of hypotension, anaphylactoid or hypersensitivity reactions, head/neck and intestinal angioedema, jaundice, agranulocytosis, bone marrow depression, hyperkalemia and renal/hepatic dysfunction.

**Patient Counseling:** Inform of pregnancy risks. Inform that inadequate fluid intake or fluid loss may lead to drop in BP resulting in lightheadedness or syncope; avoid $K^+$ supplements or salt substitutes. Advise to seek medical attention if symptoms of hypotension (syncope), anaphylactoid or hypersensitivity reactions, angioedema (head/neck; abdominal pain with/without N/V), infection (eg, sore throat, fever), hyperkalemia, or hepatic dysfunction occur.

**Administration:** Oral route. **Storage:** ≤30°C (86°F). Protect from moisture. Dispense in a tight container.

L

# LOTENSIN HCT RX

benazepril HCl - hydrochlorothiazide (Novartis)

**When used in pregnancy, ACE inhibitors can cause injury and even death to the developing fetus. D/C therapy if pregnancy detected.**

**THERAPEUTIC CLASS:** ACE inhibitor/thiazide diuretic

**INDICATIONS:** Treatment of hypertension.

**DOSAGE:** *Adults:* Initial (if not controlled on benazepril monotherapy): 10mg-12.5mg or 20mg-12.5mg. Titrate: May increase after 2-3 weeks. Initial (if controlled on 25mg HCTZ/day with hypokalemia): 5mg-6.25mg. Replacement Therapy: Substitute combination for titrated components. Renal Impairment: Avoid use if CrCl ≤30mL/min/1.73m$^2$.

**HOW SUPPLIED:** Tab: (Benazepril-HCTZ) 5mg-6.25mg*, 10mg-12.5mg*, 20mg-12.5mg*, 20mg-25mg* *scored

**CONTRAINDICATIONS:** Anuria, sulfonamide hypersensitivity, history of angioedema.

**WARNINGS/PRECAUTIONS:** Not for initial therapy. Anaphylactoid reactions during desensitization and membrane exposure, intestinal angioedema and angioedema of the head and neck reported. Higher incidence of angioedema reported in blacks than nonblacks. D/C if angioedema occurs. Symptomatic hypotension may occur; caution in patients who are volume/salt depleted and in patients undergoing surgery or anesthesia. Caution in patients with congestive heart failure (CHF); hypotension, oliguria, azotemia, acute renal failure and death (rare) may occur in patients with CHF. Enhanced effects may occur in postsympathectomy patients. May increase BUN and SrCr levels. Caution in patients with renal dysfunction, renal artery stenosis, impaired hepatic function or liver disease. May precipitate azotemia in patients with renal disease. May cause agranulocytosis and bone marrow depression; monitor WBC in patients with renal and collagen-vascular disease. Associated with syndrome of cholestatic jaundice that progresses to fulminant hepatic necrosis and sometimes death; d/c use if jaundice or marked elevations in hepatic enzymes develop. May exacerbate or activate systemic lupus erythematosus (SLE). Increased risk of hyperkalemia in patients with diabetes mellitus (DM) and renal insufficiency; monitor electrolytes. May cause hyponatremia, hypokalemia, hypochloremic alkalosis, hypercalcemia, hypophosphatemia and hypomagnesemia. May reduce glucose tolerance and increase cholesterol, triglycerides (TG) and serum uric acid levels. Persistent, nonproductive cough reported.

**ADVERSE REACTIONS:** Dizziness/postural dizziness, headache, fatigue, cough, angioedema.

**INTERACTIONS:** Increased risk of hyperkalemia with $K^+$ supplements, $K^+$-sparing diuretics (eg, spironolactone, amiloride, triamterene), or $K^+$-containing salt substitutes. May increase lithium levels; risk of lithium toxicity. Nitritoid reactions reported when used concomitantly with injectable gold (sodium aurothiomalate). May increase responsiveness to tubocurarine. NSAIDs reduces effects. Cholestyramine, colestipol decreases absorption. Insulin requirements in diabetics may need adjustment. May decrease arterial responsiveness to norepinephrine. May potentiate other antihypertensives, especially ganglionic or peripheral adrenergic blocking drugs. Risk of hypokalemia with use, which may sensitize or exaggerate the response of the heart to the toxic effects of digitalis. Increased risk of hypokalemia when used concomitantly with corticosteroids or ACTH. Orthostatic hypotension may be potentiated by alcohol, barbiturates or narcotics. Symptomatic hypotension may occur in patients undergoing anesthesia. Absorption of HCTZ is increased by agents that reduce GI motility.

**PREGNANCY:** Category D, not for use in nursing.

**MECHANISM OF ACTION:** Benazepril: ACE inhibitor; inhibition results in decreased plasma angiotensin II, which leads to decreased vasopressor activity and to decreased aldosterone secretion. HCTZ: Thiazide diuretic; affects renal tubular mechanisms of electrolyte reabsorption, directly increasing excretion of $Na^+$ and $Cl^-$. Mechanism of antihypertensive effect is unknown.

**PHARMACOKINETICS: Absorption:** Benazepril: $T_{max}$ = 0.5-1 hr; absolute bioavailability (37%). Benazeprilat: $T_{max}$=1-2 hrs (fasting), 2-4 hrs (nonfasting). HCTZ: $T_{max=}$1-2.5 hrs; absolute bioavailability (50-80%). **Distribution:** Benazepril: Plasma protein binding (96.7%). Benazeprilat: Plasma protein binding (95.3%). Trace amounts found in breast milk. HCTZ: Plasma protein binding (67.9%); $V_d$= 3.6-7.8 L/Kg; crosses placenta; found in breast milk. **Metabolism**: Benazepril: Cleavage of ester group (primarily in liver); benazeprilat (active metabolite). **Elimination:** Benazepril: Urine (trace). Benazeprilat: Urine (20%), biliary (11-12%); $T_{1/2}$= 10-11 hrs. HCTZ: Kidney; $T_{1/2}$= 5-15 hrs.

## NURSING CONSIDERATIONS

**Assessment:** Assess for anuria, pregnancy/nursing status, history of angioedema, sulfonamide hypersensitivity, history of allergy or bronchial asthma, volume/salt depletion, CHF, renal artery stenosis, collagen vascular disease (eg, SLE, scleroderma), hepatic dysfunction or progressive liver disease, DM and for possible drug interactions. Assess baseline renal function and electrolyte levels.

**Monitoring:** Monitor for signs and symptoms of hypotension, anaphylactoid or hypersensitivity reactions, head/neck and intestinal angioedema, agranulocytosis and bone marrow depression, gout, exacerbation or activation of SLE, hepatic dysfunction, persistent non-productive cough, reduced glucose tolerance and for raised serum cholesterol and triglyceride levels. Perform periodic monitoring of renal function and electrolyte levels. Monitor WBC in patients with collagen vascular disease.

**Patient Counseling:** Inform of pregnancy risks. Advise that inadequate fluid intake or fluid loss may lead to drop in BP resulting in lightheadedness or syncope. Instruct to avoid $K^+$ supplements or salt substitutes. Advise to seek medical attention if symptoms of hypotension (eg, syncope), angioedema (eg, swelling of face, eyes, lips, tongue) or infection (eg, sore throat, fever) occur.

**Administration:** Oral route. **Storage**: ≤30°C (86°F). Protect from moisture and light. Dispense in a tight, light-resistant container.

# LOTREL — RX

## benazepril HCl - amlodipine besylate (Sandoz)

**ACE inhibitors can cause death/injury to the developing fetus. D/C if pregnancy detected.**

**THERAPEUTIC CLASS:** Calcium channel blocker (dihydropyridine)/ACE inhibitor

**INDICATIONS:** Treatment of hypertension. Fixed combination drug is not for initial therapy.

**DOSAGE:** *Adults:* Usual: 2.5-10mg amlodipine and 10-80mg benazepril qd. Titrate: Dosage must be guided by clinical response. Small/Elderly/Frail/Hepatic Impairment: Initial: 2.5mg amlodipine. Not recommended in patients with severe renal impairment (CrCl <30mL/min/1.73m²). Replacement Therapy: May be substituted for individual components.

**HOW SUPPLIED:** Cap: (Amlodipine-Benazepril) 2.5mg-10mg, 5mg-10mg, 5mg-20mg, 5mg-40mg, 10mg-20mg, 10mg-40mg.

**CONTRAINDICATIONS:** History of angioedema, with or without previous ACE inhibitor treatment.

**WARNINGS/PRECAUTIONS:** D/C if laryngeal stridor, angioedema (face, tongue, glottis), jaundice, or if marked LFT elevation occurs. Risk of hyperkalemia with DM, renal dysfunction. Persistent nonproductive cough reported. Monitor WBCs in collagen vascular disease. Anaphylactoid reactions reported. Monitor for hypotension in high-risk patients (heart failure, surgery/anesthesia, volume and/or salt depletion, etc). Caution with CHF, severe hepatic or renal dysfunction, severe aortic stenosis, and renal artery stenosis. Intestinal angioedema reported. Avoid if CrCl ≤30mL/min. Caution in elderly. Increased angina/MI with severe obstructive CAD reported. May increase risk of birth defects when used in 1st trimester of pregnancy.

**ADVERSE REACTIONS:** Cough, headache, dizziness, edema, angioedema.

**INTERACTIONS:** May increase lithium levels; if coadministered monitor lithium levels and signs/symptoms of toxicity. Hypotension risk with diuretics, anesthesia. Increased risk of hyperkalemia with $K^+$-sparing diuretics, $K^+$ supplements, or $K^+$-containing salt substitutes. Caution with other peripheral vasodilators.

**PREGNANCY:** Category D, not for use in nursing.

**MECHANISM OF ACTION:** Amlodipine: $Ca^{2+}$ channel blocker (dihydropyridine); inhibits transmembrane influx of $Ca^{2+}$ ions into vascular smooth muscle and cardiac muscle. Benazepril: ACE inhibitor; decreases plasma angiotensin II, which leads to decreased vasopressor activity and to decreased aldosterone secretion.

**PHARMACOKINETICS: Absorption:** Amlodipine: Absolute bioavailability (64-90%); $T_{max}$=6-12 hrs. Benazepril: Absolute bioavailability ( ≥37%); $T_{max}$=0.5-2 hrs, 1.5-4 hrs (metabolite). **Distribution:** Amlodipine: $V_d$=21 L/kg; plasma protein binding (93%). Benazepril: $V_d$=0.7 L/kg; plasma protein bound; found in breast milk (minimal amounts). **Metabolism:** Amlodipine: Liver. Benazepril: Liver, cleavage of ester group; benazeprilat (active metabolite). **Elimination:** Amlodipine: Urine (10% parent compound, 60% metabolites); $T_{1/2}$=2 days. Benazepril: Urine (trace), biliary (11-12%). Benazeprilat: Urine (20%); $T_{1/2}$=10-11 hrs.

## NURSING CONSIDERATIONS

**Assessment:** Assess for history of angioedema, severe aortic stenosis, CHF, severe obstructive CAD, pregnancy/nursing status, volume/salt depletion, collagen vascular disease (lupus, scleroderma), DM, unilateral or bilateral renal artery stenosis, and hepatic/renal impairment. Check for hypersensitivity to other ACE inhibitors and possible drug interactions.

L

**Monitoring:** Monitor renal function for the first few weeks in patients with renal artery stenosis. Monitor WBC, blood potassium level and serum electrolytes periodically. Monitor for signs/symptoms of hypotension, anaphylactoid or hypersensitivity reactions, head/neck and intestinal angioedema, agranulocytosis, hyperkalemia, renal/hepatic dysfunction. Monitor for symptoms of angina or MI after dosage initiation or increase.

**Patient Counseling:** Inform of pregnancy risks. Advise to seek medical attention if symptoms of hypotension, anaphylactoid or hypersensitivity reactions, angioedema (head/neck, intestinal), infection, hyperkalemia, or hepatic dysfunction occur. Advise patient to take missed dose as soon as remembered; if more than 12 hrs, just take the next dose at regular time.

**Administration:** Oral route. **Storage:** 25°C (77°F); excursions permitted to 15-30°C (59-86°F). Protect from moisture. Dispense in tight container.

# LOTRISONE RX

betamethasone dipropionate - clotrimazole (Schering)

**THERAPEUTIC CLASS:** Corticosteroid/azole antifungal

**INDICATIONS:** Topical treatment of symptomatic inflammatory tinea pedis, tinea cruris, and tinea corporis caused by *Trichophyton rubrum*, *Trichophyton mentagrophytes*, and *Epidermophyton floccosum* in patients ≥17 yrs.

**DOSAGE:** *Adults:* ≥17 yrs: Massage sufficient amount into affected skin area(s) bid (am and pm). Do not use for >2 weeks for the treatment of tinea cruris and tinea corporis or for >4 weeks for the treatment of tinea pedis. Amounts of cream >45g/week or of lotion >45mL/week should not be used.

**HOW SUPPLIED:** (Betamethasone Dipropionate-Clotrimazole) Cre: 0.643mg/g-10mg/g [15g, 45g]; Lot: 0.643mg/g-10mg/g [30mL]

**WARNINGS/PRECAUTIONS:** Systemic absorption of corticosteroids may produce reversible HPA axis suppression, Cushing's syndrome, hyperglycemia, and glucosuria. Use over large surface areas, prolonged use, and use under occlusive dressings augment systemic absorption. Not for use with occlusive dressing. D/C if irritation develops. Pediatrics may be more susceptible to systemic toxicity. Not recommended for patients <17 yrs or patients with diaper dermatitis.

**ADVERSE REACTIONS:** Cre, Lot: Itching, irritation, folliculitis, hypertrichosis, acneiform eruptions, hypopigmentation. Cre: Paresthesia, rash, edema, secondary infection. Lot: Burning, dry skin, stinging.

**PREGNANCY:** Category C, caution in nursing.

**MECHANISM OF ACTION:** Corticosteroid/azole antifungal agent. Clotrimazole: Imidazole antifungal agent; inhibits 14-α-demethylation of lanosterol in fungi by binding to 1 of the CYP450 enzymes. Leads to accumulation of 14-α-methylsterols and reduced concentrations of ergosterol, a sterol essential for a normal fungal cytoplasmic membrane. The methylsterols may affect the electron transport system, thereby inhibiting growth of fungi. Betamethasone: Corticosteroid; has been shown to have topical systemic pharmacologic and metabolic effects characteristic of this class of drugs.

**PHARMACOKINETICS: Metabolism:** Liver. **Elimination:** Renal, biliary.

## NURSING CONSIDERATIONS

**Assessment:** Assess for hypersensitivity to other corticosteroids or imidazoles. Assess use in pediatric patients. Assess pregnancy/nursing status.

**Monitoring:** Monitor for signs/symptoms of HPA-axis suppression, Cushing's syndrome, hyperglycemia, glucosuria, glucocorticosteroid insufficiencies, and skin irritation. When used on large surface areas and/or with occlusive dressings, perform periodic monitoring for HPA-axis suppression using ACTH test, morning plasma cortisol test, and urinary free-cortisol level test. (Pediatrics) Monitor for systemic toxicity, HPA-axis suppression, Cushing's syndrome, delayed weight gain, and intracranial HTN.

**Patient Counseling:** Counsel to use exactly as directed for fully prescribed treatment period. Advise to avoid contact with eyes, mouth, or intravaginally. Inform to contact physician if no improvement after 1 week of treatment for tinea cruris or tinea corporis, or 2 weeks for tinea pedis. Instruct to avoid using occlusive dressings or tight-fitting clothing on treated areas and not to use with other corticosteroids. Counsel the patient to use only for 2 weeks if the affected area is the groin and notify physician if condition persists after 2 weeks. Advise that the medication should be used only for the disorder for which it was prescribed. Counsel on adverse events.

**Administration:** Topical route. Shake lotion well before each use. **Storage:** 25C°(77°F), excursions permitted to 15-30°C (59-86°F). Store lotion in upright position.



# LOTRONEX — RX

alosetron HCl (Prometheus)

**Serious GI adverse events, some fatal, reported (eg, ischemic colitis, serious constipation complications). Physicians must enroll in the Prescribing Program for Lotronex and patients must sign the Patient-Physician Agreement. Discontinue immediately if constipation or symptoms of ischemic colitis develop (rectal bleeding, bloody diarrhea, abdominal pain); do not resume therapy.**

**THERAPEUTIC CLASS:** 5-$HT_3$ receptor antagonist

**INDICATIONS:** Treatment for women with severe diarrhea-predominant IBS who have chronic symptoms (>6 months), exclusion of anatomic or biochemical abnormalities of GI tract, failure to respond to conventional therapy, frequent and severe abdominal pain/discomfort, frequent bowel urgency/fecal incontinence, and disability/restriction of daily activities due to IBS.

**DOSAGE:** *Adults:* Initial: 0.5mg bid for 4 weeks. Titrate: If tolerated and IBS symptoms not controlled, may increase to 1mg bid. D/C after 4 weeks if symptoms not controlled on 1mg bid.

**HOW SUPPLIED:** Tab: 0.5mg, 1mg

**CONTRAINDICATIONS:** Current constipation. History of chronic/severe constipation or sequelae of constipation, intestinal obstruction/stricture, toxic megacolon, GI perforation/adhesions, ischemic colitis, impaired intestinal circulation, thrombophlebitis, hypercoagulable state, Crohn's disease, ulcerative colitis, diverticulitis, severe hepatic impairment. Inability to understand/comply with Patient-Physician Agreement.

**WARNINGS/PRECAUTIONS:** Increased risk of constipation and ischemic colitis. Caution with mild or moderate hepatic impairment.

**ADVERSE REACTIONS:** Constipation, abdominal discomfort/pain, nausea, GI discomfort/pain.

**INTERACTIONS:** Increased risk of constipation with medications that decrease GI motility. CYP Inducers and inhibitors (especially CYP1A2) drug-metabolizing enzymes may change the clearance of alosetron. Fluvoxamine increases AUC, concomitant administration is contraindicated. Avoid with quinolone antibiotics and cimetidine. Caution with ketoconazole, clarithromycin, telithromycin, protease inhibitors, voriconazole, itraconazole.

**PREGNANCY:** Category B, caution in nursing.

**MECHANISM OF ACTION:** 5-$HT_3$ receptor antagonist.

**PHARMACOKINETICS: Absorption:** Rapidly absorbed, absolute bioavailability (50-60%), $C_{max}$=5ng/mL (male), 9ng/mL (female); $T_{max}$=1 hr. **Distribution:** $V_d$=65-95L, plasma protein binding (82%). **Metabolism:** Extensively metabolized. **Elimination:** Urine (73%), feces (24%); $T_{1/2}$=1.5 hrs.

## NURSING CONSIDERATIONS

**Assessment:** Assess history of chronic or severe constipation, intestinal obstruction, stricture, toxic megacolon, GI perforation or adhesion, ischemic colitis, impaired intestinal circulation, thrombophlebitis or hypercoagulable state, Crohn's disease, ulcerative colitis, diverticulitis, severe hepatic impairment.

**Monitoring:** Monitor LFTs, signs/symptoms of ischemic colitis and serious complications of constipation, hypersensitivity reactions.

**Patient Counseling:** Review side effects and advise to report if any develop. Inform that tab may be taken with or without meals. Instruct to d/c treatment and seek medical attention if no response after 4 weeks.

**Administration:** Oral route. **Storage:** 25°C (77°F); excursions permitted to 15-30°C (59-86°F). Protect from light and moisture.

# LOVAZA RX

omega-3-acid ethyl esters (GlaxoSmithKline)

**THERAPEUTIC CLASS:** Lipid-regulating agent

**INDICATIONS:** Adjunct to diet to reduce triglyceride (TG) levels in adults with severe ( ≥500mg/dL) hypertriglyceridemia.

**DOSAGE:** *Adults:* 4 caps qd or 2 caps bid. Swallow whole. Do not break open, crush, dissolve, or chew.

**HOW SUPPLIED:** Cap: 1g

**WARNINGS/PRECAUTIONS:** Contains ethyl esters of omega-3 fatty acids (EPA and DHA) obtained from the oil of several fish sources; unknown whether patients allergic to fish and/or shellfish are at an increased risk of an allergic reaction. Possible increase in alanine aminotransferase levels without a concurrent increase in aspartate aminotransferase levels. May increase LDL levels. Monitor LFTs, LDL and TG periodically during therapy.

**ADVERSE REACTIONS:** Eructation, infection, flu-syndrome, dyspepsia.

**INTERACTIONS:** Possible prolongation of bleeding time with concomitant anticoagulants (eg, ASA, NSAIDs, warfarin, coumarin, clopidogrel); monitor periodically.

**PREGNANCY:** Category C, caution in nursing.

**MECHANISM OF ACTION:** Lipid-regulating agent; not established. Inhibits acyl CoA:1,2-diacylglycerol acyltransferase, increases mitochondrial and peroxisomal β-oxidation in the liver, decreases lipogenesis in the liver, and increases plasma lipoprotein lipase activity. May reduce the synthesis of triglycerides in the liver because EPA and DHA are poor substrates for the enzymes responsible for TG synthesis, and EPA and DHA inhibit esterification of other fatty acids.

## NURSING CONSIDERATIONS

**Assessment:** Assess for persistent abnormal TG levels, DM, thyroid conditions, pregnancy/nursing status, and for possible drug interactions (eg, anticoagulants). Attempt to control serum TG levels with appropriate diet, exercise, and weight loss in obese patients before instituting therapy. Assess for sensitivity/allergy.

**Monitoring:** Periodic monitoring of TG, LFTs, LDL-C, PT, and INR (during concomitant use with drugs affecting coagulation). Monitor for possible adverse effects.

**Patient Counseling:** Caution patients with known sensitivity or allergy to fish and/or shellfish. Advise that the use of lipid-regulating agents does not reduce the importance of adhering to diet. Advise not to alter capsules in any way and to ingest intact capsules only. Advise to take exactly as prescribed. Do not change and stop dose or if miss a dose, take as soons as remember; do not double the dose. Advise to swallow whole, do not break, open, crush, dissolve or chew.

**Administration:** Oral route. **Storage:** 25°C (77°F); excursions permitted to 15-30°C (59-86°F). Do not freeze.

# LOVENOX — RX

enoxaparin sodium (Sanofi-Aventis)

**Epidural or spinal hematomas resulting in long-term or permanent paralysis may occur in patients anticoagulated with low molecular weight heparins, heparinoids, or fondaparinux sodium and who are receiving neuraxial anesthesia or undergoing spinal puncture. Increased risk with indwelling epidural catheters, concomitant use of other drugs that affect hemostasis (eg, NSAIDs, platelet inhibitors, other anticoagulants), history of traumatic or repeated epidural or spinal puncture, or a history of spinal deformity or spinal surgery. Monitor frequently for signs/symptoms of neurologic impairment; if neurologic compromise noted, urgent treatment is necessary. Consider benefit and risks before neuraxial intervention in patients anticoagulated or to be anticoagulated for thromboprophylaxis.**

**THERAPEUTIC CLASS:** Low molecular weight heparin

**INDICATIONS:** Prophylaxis of deep vein thrombosis (DVT) in abdominal surgery, hip replacement surgery, knee replacement surgery, or medical patients with severely restricted mobility during acute illness. Inpatient treatment of acute DVT with or without pulmonary embolism in conjunction with warfarin. Outpatient treatment of acute DVT without pulmonary embolism in conjunction with warfarin. Prophylaxis of ischemic complications of unstable angina and non-Q-wave myocardial infarction (MI) when administered with ASA. Treatment of acute ST-segment elevation myocardial infarction (STEMI) managed medically or with subsequent percutaneous coronary intervention (PCI) when administered with ASA.

**DOSAGE:** *Adults:* DVT Prophylaxis: Abdominal Surgery: 40mg SQ qd, starting 2 hrs pre-op, for 7-10 days. Knee Surgery: 30mg SQ q12h, starting 12-24 hrs post-op for 7-10 days. Hip Surgery: 30mg SQ q12h, starting 12-24 hrs post-op for 7-10 days, or 40mg SQ qd starting 12 hrs pre-op for 3 weeks. Acute Medical Illness: 40mg SQ qd for 6-11 days. DVT Treatment: Outpatient, without PE: 1mg/kg SQ q12h. Inpatient, with or without PE: 1mg/kg SQ q12h, or 1.5mg/kg SQ qd, administered at the same time daily. Initiate concomitant warfarin therapy as soon as possible, usually within 72 hrs. Continue treatment with enoxaparin for at least 5 days and until a therapeutic anticoagulant effect is established (INR=2-3). Unstable Angina/Non-Q-Wave MI: 1mg/kg SQ q12h in conjunction with ASA therapy (100-325mg/day) for a minimum of 2 days. Acute STEMI: <75 yrs: 30mg single IV bolus plus a 1mg/kg SQ dose, followed by 1mg/kg SQ q12h (maximum 100mg for the first 2 doses only, followed by 1mg/kg dosing for the remaining doses). ≥75 yrs: Do not use initial IV bolus. 0.75mg/kg SQ q12h (maximum 75mg for the first 2 doses only, followed by 0.75mg/kg dosing for the remaining doses). In Conjunction with Thrombolytic: Give enoxaparin dose between 15 min before and 30 min after start of fibrinolytic therapy. PCI: Give IV bolus of 0.3mg/kg of enoxaparin if last enoxaparin SQ dose >8 hrs before balloon inflation. Severe Renal Impairment (<30mL/min): Refer to prescribing information.

**HOW SUPPLIED:** Inj: (MDV) 300mg/3mL; (Syringe) 30mg/0.3mL, 40mg/0.4mL, 60mg/0.6mL, 80mg/0.8mL, 100mg/mL, 120mg/0.8mL, 150mg/mL

**CONTRAINDICATIONS:** Active major bleeding, thrombocytopenia associated with a positive in vitro test for antiplatelet antibody in the presence of enoxaparin sodium, hypersensitivity to heparin or pork products, hypersensitivity to benzyl alcohol (only with the multi-dose formulation).

**WARNINGS/PRECAUTIONS:** Not for IM injection. Cannot be compared with activities of heparin or low molecular weight heparins. Extreme caution in conditions with an increased risk of hemorrhage (eg, congenital or acquired bleeding disorders, active ulcerative and angiodysplastic GI disease, hemorrhagic stroke, uncontrolled arterial HTN, diabetic retinopathy, shortly after brain, spinal, or ophthalmological surgery). To minimize the risk of bleeding during PCI, it is important to obtain hemostasis at the puncture site before sheath removal. Use with extreme caution in patients who have a history of heparin-induced thrombocytopenia. Thrombocytopenia reported; d/c if platelets <100,000/mm$^3$. Perform routine CBC (including platelet count), SrCr, and stool occult blood tests during treatment. Pregnant women with mechanical prosthetic heart valves and their fetuses may be at increased risk and may need more frequent monitoring and dosage adjustment. Multi-dose vial contains benzyl alcohol which crosses the placenta and has been associated with fatal "gasping syndrome" in premature neonates; use only when clearly needed in pregnant women.

**ADVERSE REACTIONS:** Hemorrhage, thrombocytopenia, local reactions (ecchymosis, erythema), anemia, dyspnea.

**INTERACTIONS:** Prior to initiation of therapy, d/c agents that may enhance the risk of hemorrhage unless the agents are essential; if coadministration is necessary, monitor closely for hemorrhage.

**PREGNANCY:** Category B, caution in nursing.

**MECHANISM OF ACTION:** Low molecular-weight heparin with antithrombotic properties.

**PHARMACOKINETICS: Absorption:** (1mg/kg bid) Cmax=1.2 IU/mL. **Distribution:** Vd=4.3L. **Metabolism:** Desulfation and/or depolymerization in liver. **Elimination:** Urine; T1/2=4.5 hrs (single dose); 4.5 hrs (single dose), 7 hrs (multiple doses).

## NURSING CONSIDERATIONS

**Assessment:** Assess for renal/hepatic impairment, presence of active major bleeding, bacterial endocarditis, history of heparin-induced thrombocytopenia, weight of patient, conditions which increase the risk of hemorrhage (eg, congenital or acquired bleeding disorders, active ulcerative and angiodysplastic GI disease, hemorrhagic stroke, uncontrolled arterial HTN, diabetic retinopathy), hypersensitivity to heparin or pork products, hypersensitivity to benzyl alcohol, nursing/pregnancy status, and for possible drug interactions.

**Monitoring:** Monitor for signs/symptoms of hemorrhage and thrombocytopenia. Monitor for epidural or spinal hematomas, and for neurological impairment if used concomitantly with spinal/epidural anesthesia or spinal puncture. Periodically monitor CBC including platelet count, stool occult blood tests. If bleeding occurs, monitor anti-factor Xa.

**Patient Counseling:** Inform of instructions for injecting if therapy is to continue after discharge: Lie down during administration; do not expel air bubble before injection; alternate administration sites between left and right anterolateral and posterolateral abdominal wall; the entire length of the needle should be introduced into skin fold held between thumb and forefinger; skin fold should be held throughout injection. To minimize bruising, do not rub injection site. Advise that bleeding time may be extended during therapy and bruising and bleeding may occur more easily. Instruct to report any unusual bleeding, bruising, or signs of thrombocytopenia to physician. Advise pregnant females about risk of gasping syndrome with use of multiple-dose vials. Inform to watch for signs and symptoms of spinal or epidural hematoma (tingling, numbness, muscular weakness). Advise that it will take longer than usual to stop bleeding; may bruise and/or bleed more easily when treated with enoxaparin. Inform health practitioners when taking enoxaparin and/or product known to affect bleeding before any surgery or new drug is taken.

**Administration:** SC or IV (bolus) injection route. **Storage:** 25°C (77°F); excursions permitted to 15-30°C (59-86°F). Do not store multiple-dose vials for >28 days after first use.

## LUCENTIS RX

ranibizumab (Genentech)

**THERAPEUTIC CLASS:** Monoclonal antibody/VEGF-A blocker

**INDICATIONS:** Treatment of patients with neovascular (wet) age-related macular degeneration.

**DOSAGE:** *Adults:* Administer 0.5mg (0.05mL) by intravitreal injection once a month (approximately q28 days). May reduce to 1 injection every 3 months after the first 4 injections if monthly injections are not feasible.

**HOW SUPPLIED:** Inj: 10mg/mL

**CONTRAINDICATIONS:** Ocular or periocular infections.

**WARNINGS/PRECAUTIONS:** Intravitreal injections have been associated with endophthalmitis and retinal detachments; use proper aseptic injection technique. Increases in IOP have been noted within 60 min of intravitreal injection. Risk of arterial thromboembolic events.

**ADVERSE REACTIONS:** Injection procedure reactions (eg, endophthalmitis, rhegmatogenous retinal detachments, traumatic cataracts), conjunctival hemorrhage, eye pain, vitreous floaters/detachment, increased IOP, intraocular inflammation, cataract, nasopharyngitis, foreign body sensation in the eyes, eye irritation, lacrimation increased.

**INTERACTIONS:** May develop serious intraocular inflammation when used adjunctively with Verteporfin photodynamic therapy (PDT); incidence reported when drug was administered 7 days after Verteporfin PDT.

**PREGNANCY:** Category C, caution in nursing.

**MECHANISM OF ACTION:** Monoclonal antibody/human vascular endothelial growth factor A (VEGF-A) blocker; binds to receptor binding site of VEGF-A; prevents the interaction of VEGF-A with its receptors (VEGFR1 and VEGFR2) on the surface of endothelial cells, thereby reducing endothelial cell proliferation, vascular leakage, and new blood vessel formation.

**PHARMACOKINETICS: Absorption:** $C_{max}$=1.5ng/mL; $T_{max}$=1 day. **Elimination:** $T_{1/2}$=9 days.

### NURSING CONSIDERATIONS

**Assessment:** Assess for ocular or periocular infections, hypersensitivity to drug, and pregnancy/nursing status.

**Monitoring:** Monitor for signs/symptoms of endophthalmitis, retinal detachments, cataracts, elevated IOP, arterial thromboembolic events, and hypersensitivity reactions. Monitor perfusion of the optic nerve head. Perform tonometry 30 min following injection and biomicroscopy between 2 and 7 days after injection.

**Patient Counseling:** Inform about risks of developing endophthalmitis, rhegmatogenous retinal detachments, or traumatic cataracts following administration of the injection. Notify physician if eye becomes red, sensitive to light, painful, or a change in vision develops.

**Administration:** Ophthalmic intravitreal injection. **Storage:** 2-8°C (36-46°F). Do not freeze. Protect from light and store in the original carton until time of use.

## LUMIGAN — RX
bimatoprost (Allergan)

**THERAPEUTIC CLASS:** Prostaglandin analog

**INDICATIONS:** Reduction of elevated intraocular pressure (IOP) in open-angle glaucoma. Ocular hypertension if intolerant or unresponsive to other IOP therapies.

**DOSAGE:** *Adults:* Usual: 1 drop in affected eye(s) qd in pm. Max: Once-daily dosing. Space dosing with other ophthalmic drugs by at least 5 min.

**HOW SUPPLIED:** Sol: 0.03% [2.5mL, 5mL]

**WARNINGS/PRECAUTIONS:** Changes to pigmented tissues, including increased pigmentation of iris (may be permanent), eyelids and eyelashes (may be reversible), and growth of eyelashes. Macular edema reported. May change eye color and eyelashes. Do not administer with contact lenses. Caution with intraocular inflammation, renal or hepatic impairment. Caution with active intraocular inflammation, aphakic patients, pseudophakic patients with a torn posterior lens capsule, patients at risk of macular edema, and renal or hepatic impairment. Not for the treatment of angle closure, inflammatory, or neovascular glaucoma.

**ADVERSE REACTIONS:** Conjunctival hyperemia, ocular pruritus, growth of eyelashes, ocular dryness, visual disturbances, eye burning, foreign body sensation, eye pain, periocular skin pigmentation, blepharitis, cataracts, eyelid erythema, eyelash darkening, superficial punctate keratitis.



**INTERACTIONS:** Space dosing of other ophthalmics by 5 min.

**PREGNANCY:** Category C, caution in nursing.

**MECHANISM OF ACTION:** Prostaglandin analog: selectively mimics the effects of naturally occurring substances, prostamides. Believed to lower IOP by increasing outflow of aqueous humor through both the trabecular meshwork and uveoscleral routes.

**PHARMACOKINETICS: Absorption:** $C_{max}$=0.08ng/mL; $T_{max}$=10 min; AUC=0.09ng•hr/mL. **Distribution:** $V_d$=0.67L/kg. **Metabolism:** Via oxidation, N-de-ethylation and glucuronidation. **Elimination:** Urine (67%), feces (25%); $T_{1/2}$=45 min.

### NURSING CONSIDERATIONS

**Assessment:** Assess use in aphakic patients, pseudophakic patients with a torn posterior lens capsule, patients at risk for macular edema, pregnant/nursing females, and patients with angle-closure, inflammatory, or neovascular glaucoma.

**Monitoring:** Monitor for increased iris pigmentation, changes in the periorbital tissue (eyelid), changes in eyelashes or growth of eyelashes, macular edema (eg, cystoid macular edema), and bacterial keratitis.

**Patient Counseling:** Inform about risk of brown pigmentation of the iris, which may be permanent; darkening of eyelid skin; eyelashes and vellus hair changes. Instruct to avoid touching container tip to the eye, surrounding structures, fingers, or any other surface to avoid contamination. Inform to contact physician if an intercurrent ocular condition (eg, trauma or infection) or any type of ocular reaction (eg, conjunctivitis, eyelid reaction) develop while on medication. Instruct to remove contact lenses prior to instillation; reinsert 15 min after administration. Administer at least 5 min apart of using >1 topical ophthalmic drug.

**Administration:** Ocular route. **Storage:** Store in original container at 2-25°C (36-77°F).

## LUNESTA 
eszopiclone (Sepracor)

**THERAPEUTIC CLASS:** Nonbenzodiazepine hypnotic agent

**INDICATIONS:** Treatment of insomnia.

**DOSAGE:** *Adults:* Initial: 2mg qhs. Max: 3mg qhs. Elderly: Difficulty Falling Asleep: Initial: 1mg qhs. Max: 2mg qhs. Difficulty Staying Asleep: Initial/Max: 2mg qhs. Avoid high-fat meals.

**HOW SUPPLIED:** Tab: 1mg, 2mg, 3mg

**WARNINGS/PRECAUTIONS:** Abnormal thinking and behavioral changes reported. Amnesia and other neuropsychiatric symptoms may occur. Worsening of depression including suicidal thinking reported in primarily depressed patients. Avoid rapid dose decrease or abrupt d/c. Should only be taken immediately prior to bed or after going to bed and experiencing difficulty falling asleep. Avoid hazardous occupations. Caution in elderly, debilitated, or conditions affecting metabolism or hemodynamic responses. Reduce dose with severe hepatic impairment or concurrent use of potent CYP3A4 inhibitors. Caution with signs and symptoms of depression or suicidal tendencies.

**ADVERSE REACTIONS:** Headache, unpleasant taste, somnolence, dry mouth, dizziness, infection, rash, chest pain, peripheral edema, migraine.

**INTERACTIONS:** Possible additive effect on psychomotor performance with ethanol. Coadministration with olanzapine produced a decrease in DSST score. Strong inhibitors of CYP3A4 may significantly increase the AUC of eszopiclone.

**PREGNANCY:** Category C, caution in nursing.

**MECHANISM OF ACTION:** Not established. Pyrrolopyrazine derivative; suspected to interact with GABA-receptor complexes at binding domains located close to or allosterically coupled to benzodiazepine receptor.

**PHARMACOKINETICS: Absorption:** Rapidly absorbed; $T_{max}$=1 hr. **Distribution:** Plasma protein binding (52-59%). **Metabolism:** Liver (extensive); oxidation and demethylation pathways via CYP3A4 and CYP2E1. Primary metabolites: (S)-zopiclone-N-oxide and (S)-N-desmethyl zopiclone. **Elimination:** Urine (75% metabolite), (<10% parent drug); $T_{1/2}$=6 hrs, 9 hrs (elderly).

## NURSING CONSIDERATIONS

**Assessment:** Assess for psychiatric or physical illness, diseases/conditions that could affect metabolism or hemodynamic response. Assess for depression, suicidal ideations, respiratory function, hepatic/renal impairment, hypersensitivity reactions, drug interactions (eg, other CNS depressants), and pregnancy/nursing status.

**Monitoring:** Anaphylactic/anaphylactoid reactions, insomnia, severe sedation, memory disorders, abnormal thinking/behavioral changes (eg, aggressiveness or extraversion that seem out of character), complex/bizarre behavior (eg, hallucinations, agitation, sleep-driving), worsening of depression including suicidal thoughts, physical/psychological dependence, respiratory depression, motor or cognitive performance in elderly, withdrawal-emergent anxiety, and rebound insomnia.

**Patient Counseling:** Inform about potential benefits/risks of drug and possibility of physical/psychological dependence. Counsel to take immediately before bed when patient can dedicate 8 hrs to sleep. Do not take with alcohol or other sedating drugs; notify physician if pregnant. Avoid hazardous tasks (eg, operating machinery/driving).

**Administration:** Oral route. **Storage:** 25°C (77°F), excursions permitted to 15-30°C (59-86°F).

# LUPRON — RX

leuprolide acetate (TAP)

**THERAPEUTIC CLASS:** Synthetic gonadotropin releasing hormone analog

**INDICATIONS:** Palliative treatment of advanced prostate cancer.

**DOSAGE:** *Adults:* 1mg SQ qd. Rotate injection sites.

**HOW SUPPLIED:** Inj: 5mg/mL

**CONTRAINDICATIONS:** Pregnancy.

**WARNINGS/PRECAUTIONS:** Transient worsening of symptoms may occur during 1st few weeks of therapy. Closely monitor patients with metastatic vertebral lesions and/or urinary tract obstruction during 1st few weeks of therapy; may cause neurological problems or increase obstruction. Monitor serum testosterone, acid phosphatase levels. Contains benzyl alcohol.

**ADVERSE REACTIONS:** General pain, headache, hot flashes, urinary disorders, dizziness/vertigo, ECG changes/ischemia, peripheral edema, HTN, asthenia, constipation, anorexia, insomnia, myocardial infarction, diabetes, respiratory problems.

**PREGNANCY:** Category X, not for use in nursing.

**MECHANISM OF ACTION:** LH-RH agonist; acts as a potent inhibitor of gonadotropin secretion resulting in suppression of testicular and ovarian steroidogenesis.

**PHARMACOKINETICS: Absorption:** (M-1): $T_{max}$=2-6 hrs. **Distribution:** $V_d$=27L, plasma protein binding (43-49%). **Metabolism:** M-I (major metabolite). **Elimination:** Urine (<5%); $T_{1/2}$=3 hrs.

## NURSING CONSIDERATIONS

**Assessment:** Assess pregnancy status, metastatic vertebral lesions, urinary tract obstruction, and possible drug interactions. Obtain baseline serum testosterone and PSA levels.

**Monitoring:** Monitor serum testosterone and PSA levels periodically and for signs/symptoms of anaphylactoid reactions, transient worsening of symptoms, and injection-site reaction.

L

**Patient Counseling:** Inform of pregnancy risks. Advise not to d/c therapy even if feeling better. If need alternative syringe, may use low-dose insulin syringes. Advise not to attempt to get every last drop in vial. Seek medical attention if symptoms of hot flushes, transient worsening of symptoms (bone pain, increased difficulty in urinating, onset or aggravation of nerve symptoms), injection-site reaction (burning, itching, swelling), or anaphylactoid reactions occur.

**Administration:** SQ route. **Storage:** 25°C (77°F). Do not freeze. Protect from light.

# LUPRON DEPOT (ONCOLOGY) RX

leuprolide acetate (TAP)

**OTHER BRAND NAMES:** Lupron Depot 4-Month (TAP) - Lupron Depot 3-Month 22.5 mg (TAP) - Lupron Depot 7.5mg (Abbott)

**THERAPEUTIC CLASS:** Synthetic gonadotropin releasing hormone analog

**INDICATIONS:** Palliative treatment of advanced prostate cancer.

**DOSAGE:** *Adults:* 7.5mg IM as single dose monthly, 22.5mg IM single dose every 3 months, or 30mg IM single dose every 4 months. Rotate injection site.

**HOW SUPPLIED:** Inj: (1-month) 7.5mg, (3-month) 22.5mg, (4-month) 30mg

**CONTRAINDICATIONS:** Pregnancy.

**WARNINGS/PRECAUTIONS:** Transient worsening of symptoms may occur during 1st few weeks of therapy. Closely monitor patients with metastatic vertebral lesions and/or urinary tract obstruction during 1st few weeks of therapy. Monitor serum testosterone, PSA. (7.5mg, 30mg): Temporary increase in bone pain. Ureteral obstruction and spinal cord compression reported; caution during initial weeks of therapy in patients with metastatic vertebral lesions and/or urinary tract obstruction. May initiate with SQ formulation for 1st 2 weeks to facilitate withdrawal if needed.

**ADVERSE REACTIONS:** Injection-site reactions, general pain, headache, hot flushes, sweating, edema, urinary disorders, respiratory disorders, dizziness/vertigo, asthenia, GI disorders, impotence.

**PREGNANCY:** Category X, safety in nursing not known.

**MECHANISM OF ACTION:** LH-RH agonist; acts as a potent inhibitor of gonadotropin secretion, resulting in suppression of testicular and ovarian steroidogenesis.

**PHARMACOKINETICS: Absorption:** (22.5mg): $C_{max}$= 48.9ng/mL, $T_{max}$=4 hrs. **Distribution:** $V_d$=27L; plasma protein binding (43-49%). **Metabolism:** M-1 (Major metabolite). **Elimination:** $T_{1/2}$=3 hrs. (3.75mg): Urine (<5%).

## NURSING CONSIDERATIONS

**Assessment:** Assess pregnancy status, metastatic vertebral lesions, urinary tract obstruction, and possible drug interactions. Obtain baseline serum testosterone and PSA levels.

**Monitoring:** Monitor serum testosterone and PSA levels periodically. Monitor for signs/symptoms of anaphylactoid reactions, transient worsening of symptoms, and injection-site reactions.

**Patient Counseling:** Inform of pregnancy risks. Advise to seek medical attention if symptoms of hot flushes, transient worsening of symptoms (eg, bone pain, increased difficulty in urinating, onset or aggravation of nerve symptoms), injection-site reactions (eg, burning, itching, swelling), or anaphylactoid reactions occur.

**Administration:** IM route. **Storage:** 25°C (77°F); excursions permitted to 15-30°C (59-86°F).

# LUPRON PEDIATRIC RX

leuprolide acetate (TAP)

**OTHER BRAND NAMES:** Lupron Depot-Ped (TAP)

**THERAPEUTIC CLASS:** Synthetic gonadotropin releasing hormone analog

**INDICATIONS:** Treatment of central precocious puberty.

**DOSAGE:** *Pediatrics:* Initial: 50mcg/kg/d as single SQ dose or (depot) 0.3mg/kg every 4 weeks (minimum 7.5mg) as single IM dose. Depot Start Dose: ≤25kg: 7.5mg; >25-37.5kg: 11.25mg; >37.5kg: 15mg. Titrate: Increase by 10 mcg/kg/day SQ or (depot) 3.75mg IM every 4 weeks if downregulation not achieved. Maint: Dose that produces adequate downregulation. Verify adequate downregulation with significant weight increase.

**HOW SUPPLIED:** Inj: 5mg/mL, (Depot) 7.5mg, 11.25mg, 15mg

**CONTRAINDICATIONS:** Pregnancy.

**WARNINGS/PRECAUTIONS:** Monitor hormonal effects after 1-2 months of therapy. Measure bone age every 6-12 months. Increase in clinical signs and symptoms may occur in early phase of therapy due to rise in gonadotropins and sex steroids. D/C before age 11 in females and age 12 in males.

**ADVERSE REACTIONS:** Initial exacerbation of signs and symptoms, injection site reactions, pain, acne/seborrhea, rash, urogenital bleeding/discharge, vaginitis.

**PREGNANCY:** Category X, not for use in nursing.

**MECHANISM OF ACTION:** A GnRH agonist; initially stimulates gonadotropins. Chronic stimulation results in reversible suppression of ovarian and testicular steroidogenesis.

**PHARMACOKINETICS: Absorption:** $C_{max}$=20ng/mL; $T_{max}$=4 hrs. **Distribution:** $V_d$=27L, plasma protein binding (43-49%). **Metabolism:** M-I (major metabolite). **Elimination:** Urine (<5% parent and metabolite); $T_{1/2}$=3 hrs.

## NURSING CONSIDERATIONS

**Assessment:** Assess pregnancy status prior to therapy.

**Monitoring:** Monitor GnRH stimulation test, sex steroid levels, pituitary gonadotropic and gonadal functions and Tanner staging. GnRH stimulation tests and sex steroid levels should be monitored 1-2 months following initiation of therapy. Monitor measurements of bone age for advancement every 6-12 months.

**Patient Counseling:** Counsel about importance of adherence to 4-week drug administration schedule. Inform females that menses or spotting may occur during first 2 months of therapy. Report any irritation at injection site and any unusual signs/symptoms immediately. D/C of medication should be considered before age 11 in females and age 12 for males.

**Administration:** IM route. 1) Visually inspect powder. 2) Gently mix powder thoroughly to form uniform suspension. 3) Administered IM. Discard suspension if unused. **Storage:** 25°C (77°F); excursions permitted to 15-30°C (59-86°F).

# Luvox CR

RX

fluvoxamine maleate (Jazz Pharmaceuticals, Inc.)

**Antidepressants increased the risk of suicidal thinking and behavior (suicidality) in short-term studies in children, adolescents, and young adults with major depressive disorder (MDD) and other psychiatric disorders. Monitor appropriately and observe closely for clinical worsening, suicidality, or unusual changes in behavior. Fluvoxamine is not approved for use in pediatric patients.**

**THERAPEUTIC CLASS:** Selective serotonin reuptake inhibitor

**INDICATIONS:** Treatment of social anxiety disorder, also known as social phobia and obsessive compulsive disorder.

**DOSAGE:** *Adults:* Initial: 100mg qhs. Titrate: May increase by 50mg every week, as tolerated, until maximum therapeutic response is achieved. Maint: 100-300mg/day. Max: 300mg/day. Maint/Continuation of Extended Treatment: Adjust dose to maintain the lowest effective dosage and reassess periodically to determine the need for continued treatment. Switching to/from MAOI: Space by at least 14 days between d/c and initiation of therapy. Elderly/Hepatic Impairment: Titrate slowly following initial dose. Do not crush or chew.

L

**HOW SUPPLIED:** Cap, Extended-Release: 100mg, 150mg

**CONTRAINDICATIONS:** Concomitant use of alosetron, tizanidine, thioridazine, or pimozide. During or within 14 days of MAOI therapy.

**WARNINGS/PRECAUTIONS:** Serotonin syndrome or neuroleptic malignant syndrome (NMS)-like reactions have been reported. Avoid abrupt withdrawal. May increase risk of bleeding events. Caution with history of convulsive disorders; d/c if seizures occur or if seizure frequency increases. Avoid with unstable epilepsy and monitor patients with controlled epilepsy. Caution with history of mania, hepatic dysfunction, conditions that alter metabolism or hemodynamic responses. Hyponatremia may occur; caution in elderly and d/c with symptomatic hyponatremia. Consider potential risks and benefits of treatment during third trimester of pregnancy; may consider tapering in the third trimester. May impair judgment, thinking, or motor skills. Monitor for clinical worsening and/or suicidality, especially at initiation of therapy or dose changes.

**ADVERSE REACTIONS:** Headache, asthenia, N/V, diarrhea, anorexia, dyspepsia, insomnia, somnolence, nervousness, dizziness, anxiety, dry mouth, tremor, abnormal ejaculation.

**INTERACTIONS:** See Contraindications. Avoid alcohol, diazepam, ramelteon, tryptophan and with other SSRIs or SNRIs. Caution with metoprolol or propranolol; reduce the initial β-blocker dose and titrate cautiously. Serotonin syndrome or NMS-like reactions reported with concomitant use of serotonergic drugs that impair metabolism of serotonin (including MAOIs), or with antipsychotics or other dopamine antagonists. Caution when coadministered with other drugs that may affect the serotonergic neurotransmitter systems (eg, triptans, linezolid, lithium, tramadol, St. John's wort). Rare reports of weakness, hyperreflexia, and incoordination with concomitant use of sumatriptan. Risk of bleeding with concomitant use of NSAIDs, ASA, warfarin, or other drugs that affect coagulation. Monitor PT with concomitant oral anticoagulants; adjust anticoagulant dose accordingly. Monitor plasma levels closely if used concomitantly with drugs eliminated via oxidative metabolism and has a narrow therapeutic window (eg, warfarin, theophylline, certain benzodiazepines, phenytoin). If used with alprazolam, initial alprazolam dosage should be halved and titrated to the lowest effective dose. If used with theophylline, reduce theophylline dose to one-third of the usual daily maintenance dose and monitor plasma concentrations of theophylline. Reduced clearance with benzodiazepines. Monitor serum mexiletine levels with concomitant use. Monitor patients closely when used concurrently with clozapine. Caution with TCAs; monitor plasma TCA concentrations and may need to reduce TCA dose. Smoking increases fluvoxamine metabolism.

**PREGNANCY:** Category C, not for use in nursing.

**MECHANISM OF ACTION:** SSRI; inhibits neuronal uptake of serotonin.

**PHARMACOKINETICS: Absorption:** $C_{max}$ (at doses 100mg, 200mg, 300mg) =47ng/mL, 161ng/mL, 319ng/mL. **Distribution:** $V_d$=25L/kg; plasma protein binding (80%); found in breast milk. **Metabolism:** Extensive via liver. **Elimination:** Urine (94%), $T_{1/2}$ =16.3 hrs.

## NURSING CONSIDERATIONS

**Assessment:** Assess for MDD, risk for bipolar disorder, history of mania, history of seizures, unstable epilepsy, disease/condition that alters metabolism or hemodynamic response, hepatic impairment, suicidality, pregnancy/nursing status and possible drug interactions.

**Monitoring:** Monitor for signs/symptoms of clinical worsening (suicidality, unusual changes in behavior), serotonin syndrome, NMS-like reactions (muscle rigidity, hyperthermia, mental status changes), abnormal bleeding, hyponatremia, seizures, hepatic dysfunction, cognitive and motor impairment. If d/c therapy (particularly if abrupt), monitor for symptoms of dysphoric mood, irritability, agitation, dizziness, sensory disturbances, anxiety, confusion, headache, lethargy, emotional lability, insomnia, and hypomania.



**Patient Counseling:** Advise to avoid alcohol. Instruct to seek medical attention for symptoms of serotonin syndrome (eg, mental status changes, tachycardia, hyperthermia, N/V, diarrhea, incoordination), NMS, allergic reactions (eg, rash, hives), abnormal bleeding (particularly if using NSAIDs or ASA), hyponatremia, activation of mania, seizures, clinical worsening (eg, suicidal ideation, unusual changes in behavior) and discontinuation symptoms (eg, irritability, agitation, dizziness, anxiety, headache, insomnia). Instruct not to crush or chew; may be taken with or without food. Caution against hazardous tasks (eg, operating machinery and driving). May notice improvement in 1-4 weeks; continue therapy as directed. Notify physician if pregnant, intend to become pregnant, or breastfeeding. Counsel about benefits and risks of therapy. Inform physician if taking or plan to take any OTC medications.

**Administration:** Oral route. **Storage:** Store at 25°C (77°F); excursions permitted to 15°-30°C (59°-86°F). Avoid exposure to temperatures above 30°C (86°F). Protect from high humidity.

# Luxiq — RX

betamethasone valerate (Stiefel)

**THERAPEUTIC CLASS:** Corticosteroid

**INDICATIONS:** Relief of the inflammatory/pruritic manifestations of corticosteroid-responsive dermatoses of the scalp.

**DOSAGE:** *Adults:* Place foam onto saucer or other cool surface first, then apply in small amounts to scalp. Gently massage into affected area bid (am and pm) until foam disappears. Reassess if no improvement after 2 weeks.

**HOW SUPPLIED:** Foam: 0.12% [50g, 100g, 150g]

**WARNINGS/PRECAUTIONS:** May produce reversible HPA axis suppression, manifestations of Cushing's syndrome, hyperglycemia, and glucosuria; pediatric patients are at greater risk. Caution when applied to large surface areas, for prolonged use, or under occlusive dressings; evaluate periodically for HPA suppression. D/C if irritation develops. Use appropriate antifungal or antibacterial agent with dermatological infections; if infection does not clear, d/c until infection is controlled. Administration to children should be limited to smallest amount compatible with an effective therapeutic regimen; may interfere with growth and development. Flammable; avoid fire, flame, or smoking during and immediately after application.

**ADVERSE REACTIONS:** Burning, stinging, pruritus, paresthesia, acne, alopecia, conjunctivitis.

**PREGNANCY:** Category C, caution in nursing.

**MECHANISM OF ACTION:** Corticosteroid; possesses anti-inflammatory, antipruritic, and vasoconstrictive properties. Anti-inflammatory mechanism not established. Suspected to induce phospholipase $A_2$ inhibitory proteins, lipocortins. Lipocortins control biosynthesis of potent mediators of inflammation (eg, prostaglandins, leukotrienes) by inhibiting release of their precursor, arachidonic acid.

**PHARMACOKINETICS: Absorption:** Percutaneous; occlusion, inflammation, and other diseases may increase absorption. **Distribution:** Systemically administered corticosteroids are found in breast milk. **Metabolism:** Liver. **Elimination:** Renal (major), bile.

## NURSING CONSIDERATIONS

**Assessment:** Assess for hypersensitivity to corticosteroids and pregnancy/nursing status.

**Monitoring:** Monitor for signs/symptoms of HPA-axis suppression, Cushing's syndrome, hyperglycemia, glucosuria, local skin irritation, allergic contact dermatitis (eg, failure to heal), and for the development of dermatological infections (eg, fungal, bacterial). Monitor for signs of glucocorticoid insufficiency following withdrawal from treatment. In patients on high doses or using occlusive dressings, perform periodic monitoring for HPA-axis suppression using ACTH stimulation, A.M. plasma cortisol, and urinary free cortisol tests. In pediatric patients, monitor for signs/symptoms of systemic toxicity, HPA-axis suppression, Cushing's syndrome, linear growth retardation, delayed weight gain, and intracranial HTN.

**Patient Counseling:** Inform to use exactly as directed; avoid contact with eyes. Instruct not to bandage, cover, or wrap treated scalp area unless directed by physician. Contact physician if no improvement within 2 weeks of starting therapy or if adverse reactions develop. Avoid fire, flame, or smoking during and immediately following drug application.

**Administration:** Administered topically on scalp. Invert can for proper dispensing of foam. **Storage:** 20-25°C (68-77°F). Do not expose to heat or store at temperatures above 49°C (120°F). Do not puncture or incinerate container. Contents under pressure.

# LYBREL — RX

ethinyl estradiol - levonorgestrel (Wyeth)

**THERAPEUTIC CLASS:** Estrogen/progestogen combination

**INDICATIONS:** Prevention of pregnancy.

**DOSAGE:** *Adults:* 1 tab qd. Start Day: No Current Contraceptive Therapy: Day 1 of menstrual cycle. 21- or 28-day Regimen: Day 1 of withdrawal bleed (at the latest 7 days after last active tablet). Progestin-Only Pill: Day after taking progestin-only pill. Implant: Day of implant removal. Inj: Day next inj due. Use nonhormonal back-up method of birth control for 1st 7 days of therapy when initiating after progestin-only pill, implant, or inj.

**HOW SUPPLIED:** Tab: (Ethinyl Estradiol-Levonorgestrel) 20mcg-90mcg

**CONTRAINDICATIONS:** Thrombophlebitis, deep vein thrombosis (DVT) or thromboembolic disorders, cerebrovascular or coronary artery disease (CAD), valvular heart disease with thrombogenic complications, thrombogenic rhythm disorders, hereditary or acquired thrombophilias, major surgery with prolonged immobilization, diabetes mellitus (DM) with vascular involvement, headaches with focal neurological symptoms, uncontrolled HTN, breast cancer, endometrial carcinoma or other estrogen-dependent neoplasia, undiagnosed abnormal genital bleeding, cholestatic jaundice of pregnancy or jaundice with prior pill use, hepatic adenomas or carcinomas, active liver disease, pregnancy.

**WARNINGS/PRECAUTIONS:** Cigarette smoking increases risk of serious cardiovascular (CV) side effects; risk increases with age (especially >35 yrs) and extent of smoking. Increased risk of venous and arterial thrombotic and thromboembolic events (eg, MI, thromboembolism, stroke, TIA), hepatic neoplasia, gallbladder disease, and HTN. May increase risk of breast and cervical cancer. Retinal thrombosis reported; d/c if unexplained loss of vision. May worsen existing gallbladder disease. May cause glucose intolerance; monitor prediabetic and diabetic patients. May cause fluid retention and increase BP; monitor closely with HTN and d/c if significant elevation of BP occurs. May cause onset or exacerbation of migraine or development of headaches. Weigh benefit of fewer planned menses against inconvenience of unscheduled breakthrough bleeding and spotting. Ectopic or intrauterine pregnancy may occur. Monitor closely with hyperlipidemias. D/C if jaundice develops. Monitor closely with depression and d/c if depression recurs to serious degree. May develop visual changes with contact lenses. Perform annual physical exam. Use before menarche is not indicated.

**ADVERSE REACTIONS:** Acne, Budd-Chiari syndrome, change in cervical erosion and secretion, dizziness, edema/fluid retention, focal nodular hyperplasia, GI symptoms (eg, abdominal pain, cramps, and bloating), hirsutism, infertility, lactation, persistent melasma/chloasma, N/V, pancreatitis, rash (allergic), and loss of scalp hair.

**INTERACTIONS:** Reduced effects, increased breakthrough bleeding with rifampin, rifabutin, barbiturates, phenylbutazone, primidone, dexamethasone, phenytoin, carbamazepine, felbamate, oxcarbazepine, griseofulvin, topiramate, St. Johns wort, modafinil, and possibily with ampicillin and tetracyclines. Atorvastatin, ascorbic acid, acetaminophen, CYP3A4 inhibitors (eg, itraconazole, ketoconazole) may increase hormone levels. Troleandomycin may increase risk for intrahepatic cholestasis. Anti-HIV protease inhibitors may increase or decrease levels. May increase levels of cyclosporine, theophylline, prednisolone, and other corticosteroids. May decrease levels of acetaminophen and lamotrigine. Increases clearance of temazepam, salicylic acid, morphine, clofibric acid.

**PREGNANCY:** Category X, not for use in nursing.

**MECHANISM OF ACTION:** Estrogen/progesterone combination oral contraceptive. Acts by suppression of gonadotropins. Primarily inhibits ovulation. Also responsible for changes in cervical mucus (increasing difficulty of sperm entry into uterus) and in endometrium (reducing likelihood of implantation).

**PHARMACOKINETICS: Absorption:** Oral administration on variable days resulted in different parameters. Levonorgestrel: Rapid and completely absorbed, absolute bioavailability (100%); Ethinyl estradiol: Rapid and completely absorbed, absolute bioavailability (38%). **Distribution:** Levonorgestrel: Sex hormone-binding globulin (SHBG). Ethinyl Estradiol: Plasma protein binding (97%). **Metabolism:** Levonorgestrel: Reduction, hydroxylation and conjugation. Ethinyl Estradiol: Hepatic via CYP3A4 (hydroxylation, sulfation, glucuronidation). **Elimination:** Levonorgestrel: Urine (40%), feces (16%); $T_{1/2}$=36 hrs. Ethinyl Estradiol: Urine, feces; $T_{1/2}$=21 hrs.

## NURSING CONSIDERATIONS

**Assessment:** Assess for current/past history of thrombophlebitis or thromboembolic disorders, CVD, CAD, valvular heart disease with thrombogenic complications, thrombogenic rhythm disorder, hereditary or acquired thrombophilias, major surgery with prolonged immobilization, DM with vascular involvement, headache with focal neurological symptoms, uncontrolled HTN, known/suspected carcinoma (breast, endometrium or other known/suspected estrogen-dependent neoplasia), abnormal genital bleeding, cholestatic jaundice of pregnancy or jaundice with prior pill use, hepatic adenomas or carcinomas, and known/suspected pregnancy. Assess for possible drug interactions, use in patients >35 years old who smoke ≥15 cigarettes/day.

**Monitoring:** Monitor for venous and arterial thrombotic and thromboembolic events (eg, MI, stroke), hepatic neoplasia, gallbladder disease, ocular lesions, HTN, fluid retention, bleeding irregularities, and onset or exacerbation of headaches or migraines. Monitor blood glucose levels with history of DM or in prediabetic patients, BP with history of HTN, lipid levels with a history of hyperlipidemia. Monitor for signs/symptoms of liver toxicity (eg, jaundice), GI upset (eg, diarrhea, vomiting), and signs of worsening depression with previous history. Refer patients with contact lenses to ophthalmologist if ocular changes develop. Perform annual physical exam.

**Patient Counseling:** Instruct that medication does not protect against HIV infection (AIDS) and other STDs. Inform may experience spotting/bleeding; continue therapy and notify physician if persists. Advise to avoid smoking. Instruct to take pill at same time every day. Inform that if 1 pill missed, take as soon as remembered; take next pill at next regular scheduled time. Advise that pregnancy can occur if patient has sexual intercourse during 7 days after restarting pills; use nonhormonal birth control method during that time.

**Administration:** Oral route. **Storage:** 25°C (77°F); excursions permitted to 15-30°C (59-86°F).

## LYRICA

CV

pregabalin (Pfizer)

**THERAPEUTIC CLASS:** GABA analog

**INDICATIONS:** Management of neuropathic pain associated with diabetic peripheral neuropathy. Management of post-herpetic neuralgia. Adjunct therapy for adult patients with partial onset seizures. Management of fibromyalgia.

**DOSAGE:** *Adults:* Neuropathic Pain: Initial: 50mg tid (150mg/day). Titrate: May increase to 300mg/day within 1 week based on efficacy and tolerability. Max: 100mg tid (300mg/day). Postherpetic Neuralgia: Initial: 150mg/day divided bid or tid. Titrate: May increase to 300mg/day within 1 week based on efficacy and tolerability. May increase again to up to 600mg/day divided bid or tid if patient does not experience sufficient pain relief following 2 to 4 weeks of treatment with 300mg/day. Max: 600mg/day divided bid or tid. Epilepsy: Initial: 150mg/day divided bid-tid. Max: 600mg/day. Fibromyalgia: Initial: 75mg bid (150mg/day). Titrate: May increase to 150mg bid (300mg/day) within 1 week based on efficacy and tolerability. May further increase to 225mg bid (450mg/day) if needed. Max: 450mg/day. Renal Impairment: CrCl 15-30 mL/min: 25-150mg/day divided qd or bid. CrCl <15mL/min: 25-75mg/day given qd. Give supplemental dose (25-150mg) immediately after every 4-hr hemodialysis treatment. Refer to prescribing information for further details. D/C: Taper over minimum of 1 week.

**HOW SUPPLIED:** Cap: 25mg, 50mg, 75mg, 100mg, 150mg, 200mg, 225mg, 300mg. Sol: 20mg/mL.

**WARNINGS/PRECAUTIONS:** Avoid abrupt withdrawal; gradually taper over 1 week. Increased risk of suicidal thoughts or behavior. Possible tumorigenic potential. May impair physical/mental abilities. May cause weight gain, blurred vision/ophthalmological effects, peripheral edema. Caution in congestive heart failure. May elevate creatine kinase, d/c if myopathy or markedly elevated creatine kinase levels occur. Associated with decrease in platelet count and mild PR-interval prolongation. Postmarketing reports of angioedema (eg, swelling of face, mouth, and neck) and hypersensitivity (eg, skin redness, blisters, hives, rash, dyspnea, and wheezing); d/c if with symptoms.

**ADVERSE REACTIONS:** Somnolence, dizziness, dry mouth, edema, blurred vision, weight gain, abnormal thinking (difficulty with concentration/attention), headache, constipation, asthenia, infection, neuropathy, ataxia.

**INTERACTIONS:** Additive CNS side effects with CNS depressants (eg, opiates, benzodiazepines). May potentiate the impairment of motor skills and sedation of alcohol; avoid consumption of alcohol during therapy. Increased risk of angioedema with other drugs associated with angioedema (eg, ACE inhibitors). Additive effects on cognitive and gross motor functioning with oxycodone, lorazepam, or ethanol. Caution with thiazolidinedione class of antidiabetic drugs.

**PREGNANCY:** Category C, not for use in nursing.

**MECHANISM OF ACTION:** Gamma-aminobutyric acid derivative; not fully established. Suspected to bind to the alpha$_2$-delta site (an auxillary subunit of voltage-gated calcium channels) in CNS tissues. In vitro, shown to reduce calcium-dependent release of several neurotransmitters, possibly by modulation of calcium channel function.

**PHARMACOKINETICS: Absorption:** Well absorbed; $T_{max}$=1.5 hrs (fasting), 3 hrs (fed); bioavailability ( ≥90%). **Distribution:** $V_d$=0.5L/kg. **Metabolism:** Negligible metabolism; N-methylated derivative (major metabolite). **Elimination:** Urine (90% unchanged); $T_{1/2}$=6.3 hrs.

## NURSING CONSIDERATIONS

**Assessment:** Assess for impaired renal function, history of drug abuse, history of depression, previous episode of angioedema, pregnancy/nursing status, hypersensitivity reactions and for possible drug interactions.

**Monitoring:** Monitor for the emergence or worsening of depression, suicidal thoughts or behavior, and/or unusual changes in mood or behavior. Monitor creatine kinase, platelet count, and renal function. Monitor for angioedema, hypersensitivity reactions, weight gain, peripheral edema, ophthalmic changes, myopathy, seizures, dizziness, somnolence, and possible drug interactions. Monitor for PR interval prolongation and possible seizures when withdrawing therapy.

**Patient Counseling:** Inform that drug may cause physical/mental impairment; use with caution when operating machinery/driving. Instruct to report unexplained muscle pain, tenderness, or weakness, particularly if these symptoms are accompanied by malaise or fever. Avoid consuming alcohol. Take with/without food. Inform about signs/symptoms of angioedema, and not to abruptly d/c; taper dose over a week. Advise to be alert of the emergence or worsening of symptoms of depression, any unusual changes in mood or behavior, or the emergence of suicidal thoughts, behavior or thoughts about self-harm. Instruct to notify physician if pregnant, tend to become pregnant, breast feeding or intend to breast feed. Encourage to enroll in the North American Antiepileptic Drug (NAAED) Pregnancy Registry. Inform men of risk of male-mediated teratogenicity. Instruct diabetic patients to watch for the development of skin ulcers. Inform that a Medication Guide is available and should be read before taking the drug.

**Administration:** Oral route. **Storage:** 25°C (77°F); excursions permitted to 15-30°C (59-86°F). (Sol) Use within 45 days of first opening the bottle.

M

# MACROBID — RX

nitrofurantoin monohydrate (Procter & Gamble)

**THERAPEUTIC CLASS:** Imidazolidinedione antibacterial

**INDICATIONS:** Treatment of acute uncomplicated urinary tract infections (acute cystitis).

**DOSAGE:** *Adults:* 100mg q12h for 7 days. Take with food.
*Pediatrics:* >12 yrs: 100mg q12h for 7 days. Take with food.

**HOW SUPPLIED:** Cap: 100mg

**CONTRAINDICATIONS:** Anuria, oliguria, CrCl <60mL/min, pregnancy at term (38-42 weeks gestation), labor and delivery, and neonates <1 month of age, and previous history of cholestatic jaundice or hepatic dysfunction.

**WARNINGS/PRECAUTIONS:** Acute, subacute, or chronic pulmonary reactions have occurred. Anemia, diabetes mellitus (DM), renal dysfunction, electrolyte imbalance, vitamin B deficiency, and debilitating disease may enhance occurrence of peripheral neuropathy. D/C with acute and chronic pulmonary reactions, hepatic disorders, hemolysis, or peripheral neuropathy. Monitor renal function, LFTs, and pulmonary function periodically during long-term therapy.

Optic neuritis and hepatic reactions reported. *Clostridium difficile*-associated diarrhea (CDAD) has been reported.

**ADVERSE REACTIONS:** Pulmonary disorders, hepatic damage, peripheral neuropathy, nausea, headache, flatulence, diarrhea, dizziness, alopecia, exfoliative dermatitis, Stevens-Johnson syndrome, anaphylaxis, aplastic anemia.

**INTERACTIONS:** Antacids, especially magnesium trisilicate, decrease rate and extent of absorption. Uricosuric drugs (eg, probenecid and sulfinpyrazone) increase nitrofurantoin levels.

**PREGNANCY:** Category B, not for use in nursing.

**MECHANISM OF ACTION:** Imidazolidinedione antibacterial; inhibits protein synthesis, aerobic energy metabolism, DNA, RNA, and cell-wall synthesis.

**PHARMACOKINETICS: Absorption:** $C_{max}$ ≤1mcg/mL. **Elimination:** Urine (20-25% unchanged).

## NURSING CONSIDERATIONS

**Assessment:** Assess for anuria, oliguria, renal impairment (CrCl <60mL/min or significant SrCr elevation), glucose 6 phosphate dehydrogenase deficiency, DM, anemia, hypersensitivity, and drug interactions.

**Monitoring:** Monitor for acute/chronic pulmonary reactions (eg, diffuse interstitial pneumonitis, fibrosis), hepatic reactions (eg, hepatitis, cholestatic jaundice, chronic active hepatitis, and hepatic necrosis), peripheral neuropathy, optic neuritis, hematologic manifestations, CDAD, renal function, LFTs, benign intracranial HTN, Stevens-Johnson syndrome, cyanosis (methemoglobinemia).

**Patient Counseling:** Advise to take with food to enhance tolerance and improve drug absorption. Advise not to use antacids containing magnesium trisilicate and uricosuric drugs. Inform that therapy treats bacterial, not viral, infections. Take exactly as directed; skipping doses or not completing full course may decrease effectiveness and increase bacterial resistance. Inform may experience diarrhea; notify physician if watery/bloody stools, hypersensitivity reactions, or benign intracranial HTN develops.

**Administration:** Oral route. **Storage:** 15-30°C (59-86°F).



# MACRODANTIN RX

nitrofurantoin macrocrystals (Procter & Gamble)

**THERAPEUTIC CLASS:** Imidazolidinedione antibacterial

**INDICATIONS:** Treatment of urinary tract infection.

**DOSAGE:** *Adults:* 50-100mg qid for at least 7 days. Take with food. Long-term Suppressive Use: 50-100mg at bedtime.
*Pediatrics:* ≥1 month: 5-7mg/kg/day given qid for at least 7 days. Take with food. Long-term Suppressive Use: 1mg/kg/day given qd-bid.

**HOW SUPPLIED:** Cap: 25mg, 50mg, 100mg

**CONTRAINDICATIONS:** Anuria, oliguria, CrCl <60mL/min, pregnancy at term (38-42 weeks gestation), labor and delivery, neonates <1 month of age.

**WARNINGS/PRECAUTIONS:** Acute, subacute or chronic pulmonary reactions have occurred. Anemia, diabetes mellitus, renal dysfunction, electrolyte imbalance, vitamin B deficiency, and debilitating disease enhance occurrence of peripheral neuropathy. Stop therapy with acute and chronic pulmonary reactions, hepatic disorders, hemolysis, or peripheral neuropathy. Monitor renal function, LFTs and pulmonary function periodically during long-term therapy. Optic neuritis and hepatic reactions reported. False (+) reaction for glucose in urine may occur with Benedict's and Fehling's solution.

**ADVERSE REACTIONS:** Pulmonary disorders, hepatic damage, peripheral neuropathy, nausea, emesis, anorexia, dizziness, alopecia, exfoliative dermatitis, Stevens-Johnson syndrome, anaphylaxis, headache, drowsiness, asthenia, vertigo.

**INTERACTIONS:** Antacids, especially magnesium trisilicate, decrease rate and extent of absorption. Uricosuric drugs (eg, probenecid and sulfinpyrazone) increase nitrofurantoin levels.

**PREGNANCY:** Category B, not for use in nursing

**MECHANISM OF ACTION:** Imidazolidinedione antibacterial; inhibits protein synthesis, aerobic energy metabolism, DNA, RNA, and cell-wall synthesis.

## NURSING CONSIDERATIONS

**Assessment:** Assess for anuria, oliguria, renal impairment (CrCl <60mL/min, significant SrCr elevation), glucose 6 phosphate dehydrogenase deficiency, DM, anemia, hypersensitivity, and drug interactions.

**Monitoring:** Monitor for acute/chronic pulmonary reactions (eg, diffuse interstitial pneumonitis or fibrosis), hepatic reactions (eg, hepatitis, cholestatic jaundice, chronic active hepatitis, and hepatic necrosis), peripheral neuropathy, optic neuritis, hematologic manifestations, CDAD, renal function, LFTs, benign intracranial HTN, Stevens-Johnson syndrome, cyanosis (methemoglobinemia).

**Patient Counseling:** Advise to take with food to enhance tolerance and improve drug absorption. Advise not to use antacids containing magnesium trisilicate and uricosuric drugs. Inform that therapy treats bacterial, not viral, infections. Take exactly as directed; skipping doses or not completing full course may decrease effectiveness and increase resistance. Inform may experience diarrhea; notify physician if watery/bloody stools, hypersensitivity reactions, or benign intracranial HTN develops.

**Administration:** Oral route.

# MACUGEN RX

pegaptanib sodium (Eyetech/Pfizer)

**THERAPEUTIC CLASS:** Vascular endothelial growth factor (VEGF) inhibitor

**INDICATIONS:** Treatment of neovascular (wet) age-related macular degeneration.

**DOSAGE:** *Adults*: 0.3mg by intravitreous injection once every 6 weeks.

**HOW SUPPLIED:** Inj: 0.3mg

**CONTRAINDICATIONS:** Ocular or periocular infections.

**WARNINGS/PRECAUTIONS:** Rare post-marketing cases of anaphylaxis/anaphylactoid reactions, including angioedema, reported. Endophthalmitis associated with intravitreous injections. Use proper aseptic injection technique. Monitor for increased IOP. For ophthalmic intravitreal injection only.

**ADVERSE REACTIONS:** Anterior chamber inflammation, blurred vision, cataract, conjunctival hemorrhage, corneal edema, eye discharge, eye irritation, eye pain, HTN, increased IOP, ocular discomfort, punctate keratitis, reduced visual acuity, visual disturbance, vitreous floaters, and vitreous opacities.

**PREGNANCY:** Category B, caution in nursing.

**MECHANISM OF ACTION:** Selective vascular endothelial growth factor (VEGF) antagonist; inhibits VEGF, which is responsible for inducing angiogenesis, increasing vascular permeability and inflammation. VEGF has also been implicated in blood retinal barrier breakdown and pathological ocular neovascularization.

**PHARMACOKINETICS: Absorption:** Slowly into circulation from eye. $C_{max}$=80ng/mL. AUC=25mcg•hr/mL. **Distribution:** Vitreous fluid, retina, aqueous fluid. Metabolism: Via endo- and exonucleases. **Elimination:** Urine; $T_{1/2}$=10 days.

## NURSING CONSIDERATIONS

**Assessment:** Prior to therapy, assess for ocular or periocular infections. Assess medical history for hypersensitivity reactions.

**Monitoring:** Monitor for signs/symptoms of elevated IOP, endophthalmitis, anaphylaxis reactions (eg, angioedema), retinal detachment, and iatrogenic traumatic cataract. Monitor perfusion of optic nerve immediately, perform tonometry within 30 min and biomicroscopy between 2 and 7 days following injection.

**Patient Counseling:** Advise about risk of developing endophthalmitis following administration. Instruct to seek immediate care with ophthalmologist if eye becomes red, sensitive to light, painful, or if change in vision develops.

**Administration:** Ophthalmic intravitreal injection. Injection procedure should be carried out under controlled aseptic conditions, including sterile gloves, sterile drape, and sterile eyelid speculum. Adequate anesthesia and a broad-spectrum microbicide should be given prior to injection. **Storage:** 2-8°C (36-46°F). Do not freeze or shake vigorously.

## MALARONE RX

proguanil HCl - atovaquone (GlaxoSmithKline)

**OTHER BRAND NAMES:** Malarone Pediatric (GlaxoSmithKline)

**THERAPEUTIC CLASS:** Pyrimidine synthesis inhibitor

**INDICATIONS:** Prophylaxis or treatment of acute, uncomplicated malaria caused by *P. falciparum.*

**DOSAGE:** *Adults:* Prevention: Begin 1-2 days before entering endemic area, continue during stay and for 7 days after return. 250mg-100mg qd. Treatment: 1000mg-400mg qd for 3 days. Repeat dose, in the event of vomiting within 1 hr after dosing. Take at the same time each day with meal or milky drink.

*Pediatrics:* Prevention: Begin 1-2 days before entering endemic area, continue during stay and for 7 days after return. 11-20kg: 62.5mg-25mg qd. 21-30kg: 125mg-50mg qd. 31-40kg: 187.5mg-75mg qd. >40kg: 250mg-100mg qd. Treatment: Treat for 3 consecutive days. 5-8kg: 125mg-50mg qd. 9-10kg: 187.5mg-75mg qd. 11-20kg: 250mg-100mg. 21-30kg: 500mg-200mg qd. 31-40kg: 750mg-300mgs. >40kg: 1000mg-400mg qd. Repeat dose, in the event of vomiting within 1 hr after dosing. May be taken at the same time each day with meal or milky drink. May crush and mix with condensed milk just prior to administration for children who may have difficulty swallowing tablets.

M

**HOW SUPPLIED:** Tab: (Atovaquone-Proguanil) 62.5mg-25mg, 250mg-100mg

**CONTRAINDICATIONS:** Prophylaxis in patients with severe renal impairment (CrCl <30mL/min).

**WARNINGS/PRECAUTIONS:** Use not evaluated for cerebral malaria or other severe manifestations of complicated malaria, including hyperparasitemia, pulmonary edema, or renal failure. Patients with severe malaria are not candidates for PO therapy. Rare cases of hepatitis and elevated LFTs reported with prophylactic use. Diarrhea or vomiting may reduce absorption; monitor for parasitemia and consider use of an antiemetic in patients who are vomiting. Alternative therapy may be required with severe or persistent diarrhea or vomiting. Parasite relapse occured commonly when used as monotherapy to treat *P. vivax.* Caution for the treatment of malaria in patients with severe renal impairment. Use a different blood schizoticide in the event of recrudescent P. falciparum infections or failure of chemoprophylaxis with Malarone.

**ADVERSE REACTIONS:** Abdominal pain, headache, vomiting, pruritus, diarrhea, nausea, elevated LFTs, hepatitis (rare), asthenia, anorexia, dizziness.

**INTERACTIONS:** Concomitant use of rifampin, rifabutin, tetracycline may decrease levels. Reduced bioavailability with metoclopramide. Caution with indinavir; may decrease trough levels of indinavir. May potentiate anticoagulant effect of warfarin and similar anticoagulants; caution when initiating and withdrawing Malarone therapy.

**PREGNANCY:** Category C, caution in nursing.

**MECHANISM OF ACTION:** Pyramidine synthesis inhibitor. Atovaquone: Antiparasitic agent that acts as a selective inhibitor of parasite mitochondrial electron transport. Proguanil: Antiparasitic agent that acts via its metabolite, cycloguanil, which inhibits dihydrofolate reductase in the malaria parasite, resulting in disruption of deoxythymidylate synthesis.

**PHARMACOKINETICS: Absorption:** Atovaquone: Absolute bioavailability (23% with food). Proguanil: Extensively absorbed. **Distribution:** Atovaquone: $V_d$=8.8L/kg; plasma protein binding ( ≥99%). Proguanil: $V_d$=1617-2502L (adult and pediatric patients ≥15 yrs with body weight 31-110kg), $V_d$=462-966L (pediatric patients ≤15 yrs with body weight 11-56kg). Plasma protein binding (75%). **Metabolism:** Proguanil: Cycloguanil (active metabolite) via CYP2C19. **Elimination:** Atovaquone: Feces (94 unchanged), urine (<0.6%). $T_{1/2}$=2-3 days (adult). Proguanil: Urine (40-60%); $T_{1/2}$=12-21 hrs (adult and pediatric patients).

## NURSING CONSIDERATIONS

**Assessment:** Assess for uncomplicated *P.falciparum* malaria, renal impairment, cerebral malaria, hyperparasitemia, pulmonary edema, diarrhea, vomiting, decreased hepatic/renal function, pregnancy/nursing status, and possible drug interactions. Note other diseases/conditions and drug therapies.

**Monitoring:** Monitor for parasitemia and parasite relapse. Monitor for adverse reactions.

**Patient Counseling:** Take tablet at the same time each day with food or a milky drink; repeat dose if vomiting occurs within 1 hr after dosing. If dose is missed, take as soon as possible and then return to normal dosing schedule. Do not double dose if dose is skipped. Use protective clothing, insect repellant, and bednets for malaria prophylaxis. There are rare but serious side effects with the use of Malarone. Consult physician for any febrile illness that occurs during or after return from a malaria-endemic area. Pregnant/nursing women anticipating travel to malarious areas should inform physician.

**Administration:** Oral route. Take with food. **Storage:** 25°C (77°F); excursions permitted to 15-30°C (59-86°F).

# MARINOL

CIII

dronabinol (Solvay)

**THERAPEUTIC CLASS:** Cannabinoid

**INDICATIONS:** Treatment of anorexia associated with weight loss in AIDS patients and N/V associated with chemotherapy when conventional treatment has failed.

**DOSAGE:** *Adults:* Appetite Stimulation: Initial: 2.5mg bid before lunch and supper or 2.5mg qpm or qhs if 5mg/day is intolerable. Max: 20mg/day in divided doses. Antiemetic: Initial: 5mg/m² given 1-3 hrs before chemotherapy, then q2-4h after chemotherapy, up to 4-6 doses/day. Titrate: May increase by 2.5mg/m² increments. Max: 15mg/m²/dose.

**HOW SUPPLIED:** Cap: 2.5mg, 5mg, 10mg

**WARNINGS/PRECAUTIONS:** Do not engage in any hazardous activity until ability to tolerate drug is established. Seizure and seizure-like activity reported; caution in patients with history of seizure disorders; d/c if seizures develop. Caution with cardiac disorders due to possible HTN/hypotension, syncope, tachycardia. Caution with history of substance abuse. Caution and monitor in patients with mania, depression, schizophrenia; may exacerbate illness. Caution in elderly due to increased sensitivity to the psychoactive, neurological, and postural hypotensive effects. Initial dose and adjustments should be supervised by a responsible adult.

**ADVERSE REACTIONS:** Euphoria, dizziness, paranoid reaction, somnolence, abnormal thinking, abdominal pain, N/V.

**INTERACTIONS:** Highly protein-bound drugs may require dosage changes. Additive effects with alcohol, sedatives, hypnotics, or other psychoactive drugs. Additive HTN, tachycardia, and possible cardiotoxicity with amphetamines, cocaine, and sympathomimetics. Increased tachycardia, and drowsiness with anticholinergic agents. Potentiates effects of TCAs and CNS depressants (eg, benzodiazepines). Additive drowsiness and CNS depression with lithium, opioids, buspirone, antihistamines and muscle relexants. Coadministration with theophylline in patients who smoked marijuana/tobacco has resulted in an increase in theophylline metabolism. Coadministration with disulfiram and fluoxetine in patients who smoked marijuana has resulted to hypomanic reactions. Decreasedclearance of antipyrine and barbiturates.

**PREGNANCY:** Category C, not for use in nursing.

**MECHANISM OF ACTION:** Cannabinoid; has complex effects on the CNS, including central sympathomimetic activity.

**PHARMACOKINETICS: Absorption:** Complete (90-95%); (2.5mg bid) $C_{max}$=1.32ng/mL, $T_{max}$=1 hr, AUC=2.88ng•hr/mL; (5mg bid) $C_{max}$=2.96ng/mL, $T_{max}$=2.5 hr, AUC=6.16ng•hr/mL; (10mg bid) $C_{max}$=7.88ng/mL, $T_{max}$=1.5 hr, AUC=15.2ng•hr/mL. **Distribution:** $V_d$=10L/kg; plasma protein binding (97%). Found in breast milk. **Metabolism:** Liver via microsomal hydroxylation; 11-OH-delta-9-THC (active metabolite). **Elimination:** Urine (10-15%), bile/feces (50%, <5% unchanged); $T_{1/2}$=25-36 hrs.

## NURSING CONSIDERATIONS

**Assessment:** Assess for hypersensitivity, especially to sesame oil, seizure/cardiac disorders, history of substance abuse (including alcohol abuse/dependence), mania, depression, schizophrenia, pregnancy/nursing status, hepatic/renal impairment, and possible drug interactions.

**Monitoring:** Monitor for psychiatric illness exacerbation, abdominal pain, N/V, dizziness, euphoria, paranoid reaction, somnolence, abnormal thinking, hypotension or HTN, syncope, tachycardia, and for psychological and physiological dependence.

**Patient Counseling:** Do not drink alcohol or take other CNS depressants. Use caution while performing hazardous tasks (eg, operating machinery/driving) until well tolerated. Inform of mood changes and other behavioral effects that may occur during therapy. Must be under constant supervision during initial use. Immediately report any adverse effects to physician.

**Adminisration:** Oral route. **Storage:** 8-15°C (46-59°F). Could be stored in a refrigerator. Protect from freezing.

M

# MAVIK — RX

trandolapril (Abbott)

**ACE inhibitors can cause death/injury to developing fetus during 2nd and 3rd trimesters. D/C if pregnancy detected.**

**THERAPEUTIC CLASS:** ACE inhibitor

**INDICATIONS:** Treatment of hypertension alone or in combination with other antihypertensives. Treatment of CHF post MI or left-ventricular dysfunction post MI.

**DOSAGE:** *Adults:* HTN: If possible, d/c diuretic 2-3 days before therapy. Initial: 1mg qd in non-black patients; 2mg qd in black patients; 0.5mg with concomitant diuretic. Titrate: Adjust at 1-week intervals. Usual: 2-4mg qd. Resume diuretic if not controlled. Max: 8mg/day. Post-MI: Initial: 1mg qd. Titrate: Increase to target dose of 4mg qd as tolerated. CrCl <30mL/min/Hepatic Cirrhosis for HTN or Post-MI: Initial: 0.5mg qd.

**HOW SUPPLIED:** Tab: 1mg*, 2mg, 4mg *scored

**CONTRAINDICATIONS:** History of ACE inhibitor-associated angioedema.

**WARNINGS/PRECAUTIONS:** D/C if angioedema or jaundice occurs. Anaphylactoid reactions and angioedema of the face, extremities, lips, tongue, glottis, larynx, intestines has been reported. Risk of hyperkalemia with DM, renal dysfunction. Monitor WBCs in renal impairment and/or collagen vascular disease. Fetal/neonatal morbidity and death reported. Monitor for hypotension in high-risk patients (heart failure, surgery/anesthesia, prolonged diuretic therapy, volume and/or salt depletion, etc). Caution with CHF, renal dysfunction, and renal artery stenosis. Hyperkalemia, persistent non-productive cough, and light-headedness reported. More reports of angioedema in blacks than nonblacks.

**ADVERSE REACTIONS:** Cough, dizziness, diarrhea, hypotension, elevated serum uric acid, elevated BUN, elevated creatinine, cardiogenic shock, syncope, hyperkalemia, angioedema.

**INTERACTIONS:** May increase lithium levels. Hypotension risk with diuretics. Increased risk of hyperkalemia with $K^+$-sparing diuretics, $K^+$-containing salt substitutes, or $K^+$ supplements. Nitritoid reactions (eg, facial flushing, N/V, hypotension) reported rarely with injectable gold.

**PREGNANCY:** Category C (1st trimester) and D (2nd and 3rd trimesters), not for use in nursing.

**MECHANISM OF ACTION:** ACE inhibitor; reduces angiotensin II formation, decreases vasoconstriction and aldosterone secretion, and increases plasma renin.

**PHARMACOKINETICS: Absorption:** Parent, metabolite: Absolute bioavailability (10%, 70%); $T_{max}$=1 hr, 4-10 hrs. **Distribution:** $V_d$=18L; plasma protein binding (80%). **Metabolism:** Cleavage of ester group; trandolaprilat (metabolite). **Elimination:** Urine (33%), feces (66%); $T_{1/2}$=6 hrs.

## NURSING CONSIDERATIONS

**Assessment:** Assess for pregnancy status, volume/salt depletion, collagen vascular disease (SLE, scleroderma), CHF, DM, possible drug interactions, ischemic heart disease, aortic stenosis, cerebrovascular disease, renal/hepatic impairment.

**Monitoring:** Monitor renal function for 1st few weeks; WBC (collagen vascular disease) periodically. Monitor for nitritoid reactions, hypotension, anaphylactoid or hypersensitivity reactions, head/neck and intestinal angioedema, agranulocytosis, hyperkalemia, renal/hepatic dysfunction.

**Patient Counseling:** Inform of pregnancy risks. Inform that inadequate fluid intake or fluid loss may lead to drop in BP resulting in lightheadedness or syncope; avoid $K^+$ supplements or salt substitutes. Advise to seek medical attention if symptoms of hypotension (syncope), anaphylactoid or hypersensitivity reactions, angioedema (head/neck, intestinal), infection (sore throat, fever), hyperkalemia, or hepatic dysfunction occur.

**Administration:** Oral route. **Storage:** 20-25°C (68-77°F).

M

# MAXAIR — RX

pirbuterol acetate (Graceway)

**OTHER BRAND NAMES:** Maxair Autohaler (Graceway)

**THERAPEUTIC CLASS:** $Beta_2$-agonist

**INDICATIONS:** Prevention and reversal of bronchospasm in reversible bronchospasm (eg, asthma).

**DOSAGE:** *Adults:* 1-2 inh q4-6h. Max: 12 inh/day.
*Pediatrics:* ≥12 yrs: 1-2 inh q4-6h. Max: 12 inh/day.

**HOW SUPPLIED:** Autohaler: 0.2mg/inh [14g, 25.6g]; MDI: 0.2mg/inh [14g]

**WARNINGS/PRECAUTIONS:** Caution with cardiovascular disorders, (eg, ischemic heart disease, HTN, arrhythmias), hyperthyroidism, diabetes, convulsive disorders. Fatalities reported with excessive use. Can produce paradoxical bronchospasm. Monitor BP.

**ADVERSE REACTIONS:** Nervousness, tremor, headache, dizziness, palpitations, tachycardia, cough, nausea.

**INTERACTIONS:** Avoid other aerosol $\beta_2$ agonists. Vascular effects may be potentiated by MAOIs, TCAs, and sympathomimetics. ECG changes and/or hypokalemia may occur with non-potassium sparing diuretics. Decreased effect with β-blockers.

**PREGNANCY:** Category C, caution in nursing.

**MECHANISM OF ACTION:** $\beta_2$-adrenergic bronchodilator; activates adenyl cyclase on airway smooth muscles and increases intracellular concentration of cyclic AMP. Increased cAMP levels are associated with relaxation of bronchial smooth muscle and inhibition of release of mediators of immediate hypersensitivity.

**PHARMACOKINETICS: Elimination:** Urine; $T_{1/2}$=2 hrs.

## NURSING CONSIDERATIONS

**Assessment:** Assess for history of hypersensitivity to drug. Assess for convulsive disorders, hyperthyroidism, DM, CVD, and possible drug interactions.

**Monitoring:** Monitor pulse rate, BP, ECG changes, for paradoxical bronchospasm and hypokalemia, hypersensitivity reactions, deterioration of asthma.

**Patient Counseling:** Take as directed. Report lack of response or adverse side effects.

**Administration:** Oral inhalation administration. **Storage:** 15-30°C (59-86°F). Shake well before use. Do not puncture. Do not use or store near heat or open flame. Keep out of reach of children.

# MAXALT RX

rizatriptan benzoate (Merck)

**OTHER BRAND NAMES:** Maxalt-MLT (Merck)

**THERAPEUTIC CLASS:** 5-$HT_{1B/1D}$ agonist

**INDICATIONS:** Acute treatment of migraine attacks with or without aura.

**DOSAGE:** *Adults:* ≥18 yrs: 5-10mg, may repeat q2h. Max: 30mg/24 hrs. Safety of treating >4 headaches/30 days not known. MLT: Dissolve on tongue without water. Concomitant Propranolol: 5mg, up to 3 doses/24 hrs.

**HOW SUPPLIED:** Tab: 5mg, 10mg; Tab, Disintegrating: (MLT) 5mg, 10mg

**CONTRAINDICATIONS:** Ischemic heart disease, coronary artery vasospasm (eg, Prinzmetal's angina), uncontrolled HTN, significant cardiovascular disease, hemiplegic or basilar migraine, MAOI use within 14 days, other 5-$HT_1$ agonist or ergot-type agent use within 24 hrs.

M

**WARNINGS/PRECAUTIONS:** Confirm diagnosis. Supervise 1st dose and monitor cardiac function in those at risk of CAD (eg, HTN, hypercholesterolemia, smoker, obesity, diabetes, CAD family history, postmenopausal women, males >40 yrs). Serious adverse cardiac events, cerebrovascular events, vasospastic reactions, hypertensive crisis, and fatalities reported with 5-$HT_1$ agonists. Disintegrating tabs contain phenylalanine. Caution with renal dialysis and hepatic dysfunction. Serotonin syndrome may occur; symptoms may include mental status changes, autonomic instability, neuromuscular aberrations, and GI symptoms.

**ADVERSE REACTIONS:** Paresthesia, dry mouth, nausea, dizziness, somnolence, asthenia/fatigue.

**INTERACTIONS:** Increased plasma levels with propranolol. Prolonged vasospastic reactions with ergot-type agents and other 5-$HT_1$ agonists. Serotonin syndrome reported with combined use of an SSRI or SNRI. Avoid MAOIs during or within 14 days.

**PREGNANCY:** Category C, caution in nursing.

**MECHANISM OF ACTION:** 5-$HT_{1B/1D}$ receptor agonist; binds with high affinity to 5-$HT_{1B/1D}$ receptors on the extracerebral, intracranial blood vessels that become dilated during migraine attack; activation of these receptors results in cranial vessel constriction, inhibition of neuropeptide release, and reduced transmission in trigeminal pain pathways.

**PHARMACOKINETICS: Absorption:** Complete; absolute bioavailability (45%); $T_{max}$=1-1.5 hrs. **Distribution:** $V_d$=140L (male), 110L (female); plasma protein binding (14%). **Metabolism:** Oxidative deamination via MAO-A. N-monodesmethyl-rizatriptan (active metabolite). **Elimination:** Urine (82%), (14% unchanged, 51% indole acetic acid metabolite), feces (12%); $T_{1/2}$=2-3 hrs.

## NURSING CONSIDERATIONS

**Assessment:** Confirm the diagnosis of migraine before instituting therapy. Assess for history of IHD (eg, angina pectoris, MI or documented silent ischemia), coronary artery vasospasm (eg, Prinzmetal's variant angina), HTN, hemiplegic or basilar migraine, presence of risk factors for CAD (eg, HTN, hypercholesterolemia, smoker, obesity, DM, strong family history of CAD, female with surgical or physiological menopause, or male >40 years of age), hepatic/

renal impairment, phenylketonuria, pregnancy/nursing status, ECG changes, and possible drug interactions.

**Monitoring:** Administration of first dose should be in physician's office or medically staffed and equipped facility as cardiac ischemia may occur in absence of clinical symptoms; ECG should be obtained immediately during interval in those with risk factors. Monitor for signs/symptoms of cardiac events (eg, coronary vasospasm, acute MI, arrhythmia, ECG changes, follow-up coronary angiography), cerebrovascular events (eg, hemorrhage, stroke, TIAs), peripheral vascular ischemia, colonic ischemia with bloody diarrhea and abdominal pain, serotonin syndrome (eg, mental status changes, autonomic instability, neuromuscular aberrations and/or GI symptoms), ophthalmic effects, and increased BP.

**Patient Counseling:** Caution during hazardous tasks (eg, operating machinery/driving). Warn of risk of serotonin syndrome, especially if combined with SSRIs or SNRIs. Instruct to read patient package insert before taking. Notify physician if pregnant/nursing or planning to become pregnant.

**Administration:** Oral route. Disintegrating Tabs: Just prior to dosing, remove blister from outer pouch with dry hands, place on tongue to be dissolved and swallow. **Storage:** 15-30°C (59-86°F); tight container.

## MAXIPIME — RX

cefepime HCl (Elan)

**THERAPEUTIC CLASS:** Cephalosporin (4th generation)

**INDICATIONS:** Treatment of uncomplicated/complicated urinary tract (UTI) including pyelonephritis, uncomplicated skin and skin structure (SSSI), complicated intra-abdominal infections, and pneumonia caused by susceptible strains of microorganisms. Empiric therapy for febrile neutropenia.

**DOSAGE:** *Adults:* Moderate-Severe Pneumonia: 1-2g IV q12h for 10 days. Febrile Neutropenia Empiric Therapy: 2g IV q8h for 7 days or until neutropenia resolved. Mild-Moderate UTI: 0.5-1g IM/IV q12h for 7-10 days; IM only indicated for mild to moderate UTI due to *E.coli* when IM route is more appropriate. Severe UTI/Moderate-Severe SSSI: 2g IV q12h for 10 days. Complicated Intra-Abdominal Infections: 2g IV q12h for 7-10 days in combination with metronidazole. Renal Impairment (CrCl ≤60mL/min): Initial (except for hemodialysis): Normal dose. Maint: CrCl 30-60mL/min: 500mg-2g q24h or 2g q12h. CrCl 11-29mL/min: 500mg-2g q24h. CrCl <11mL/min: 250mg-1g q24h. CAPD: 500mg-2g q48h. Hemodialysis: 1g on Day 1, then 500mg q24h or 1g q24h. *Pediatrics:* 2 months-16 yrs: ≤40kg: UTI/SSSI/Pneumonia: 50mg/kg IV q12h. IM injection only indicated for mild to moderate UTI due to *E.coli* when IM route is more appropriate. Febrile Neutropenia: 50mg/kg IV q8h. Give for the same duration as adults. Max: Do not exceed adult dose.

**HOW SUPPLIED:** Inj: 500mg, 1g, 2g

**CONTRAINDICATIONS:** Hypersensitivity to penicillins (PCNs) or other β-lactam antibiotics.

**WARNINGS/PRECAUTIONS:** Caution with PCN sensitivity; cross hypersensitivity may occur. D/C use if an allergic reaction occurs. Caution with renal impairment (CrCl ≤60mL/min) or history of GI disease, especially colitis. Encephalopathy, myoclonus, and seizures reported; most cases reported in patients with renal impairment who exceeded recommended dosing schedule. *Clostridium difficile*-associated diarrhea (CDAD) reported. Use in the absence of a proven or strongly suspected bacterial infection or prophylactic indication is unlikely to provide benefit and may increase risk of drug-resistant bacteria. Prolonged use may result in overgrowth of nonsusceptible organisms. May alter glucose values or elevate serum $K^+$ levels. Associated with a fall in PT; monitor PT in patients with renal or hepatic impairment, or poor nutritional state, and in patients on a protracted course of antimicrobials; give vitamin K as indicated. Associated with (+) direct Coombs' test. False (+) for urine glucose with Clintest tabs.

**ADVERSE REACTIONS:** Local reactions (eg, phlebitis), rash, diarrhea, (+) Coombs' test (without hemolysis).

**INTERACTIONS:** Increased risk of nephrotoxicity and ototoxicity with aminoglycosides. Risk of nephrotoxicity with potent diuretics (eg, furosemide).

**PREGNANCY:** Category B, caution in nursing.

**MECHANISM OF ACTION:** 4th generation cephalosporin; acts by inhibiting cell wall synthesis.

**PHARMACOKINETICS: Absorption:** Refer to PI for IM and IV parameters. **Distribution:** $V_d$=18L; plasma protein binding (20%); found in human breast milk. **Metabolism:** Metabolized to N-methylpyrrolidine (NMP), which is rapidly converted to N-oxide (NMP-N-oxide). **Elimination:** Urine, (85% unchanged, <1% NMP, 6.5% NMP-N-oxide); $T_{1/2}$=2hrs.

## NURSING CONSIDERATIONS

**Assessment:** Assess for PCN allergy, pregnancy/nursing status, renal/hepatic impairment, nutritional status, history of GI disease, and for possible drug interactions. Document indications for therapy with culture and susceptibility testing.

**Monitoring:** Monitor for signs/symptoms of hypersensitivity reactions (anaphylaxis), CDAD, encephalopathy, myoclonus, seizures, superinfection, a fall in prothrombin activity, changes in glucose metabolism, and for elevations in serum $K^+$ levels. Monitor PT in patients at risk for a fall in prothrombin activity (eg, renal/hepatic impairment, poor nutritional state, protracted course of antimicrobial therapy).

**Patient Counseling:** Inform that therapy only treats bacterial, not viral infections. Instruct to take as directed; skipping doses or not completing full course of therapy may decrease effectiveness and increase bacterial resistance. Advise that diarrhea may occur. Instruct to notify physician if watery/bloody stools (with/without stomach cramps and fever), hypersensitivity reactions, neurological signs/symptoms including encephalopathy (disturbance of consciousness including confusion, hallucinations, and coma), myoclonus, or seizures occur.

**Administration:** IV/IM routes; give IV over 30 min. See PI for administration instructions. **Storage:** Dry State: 2-25°C (36-77°F). Protect from light.

# MAXZIDE RX

triamterene - hydrochlorothiazide (Mylan Bertek)

**OTHER BRAND NAMES:** Maxzide-25 (Mylan Bertek)

**THERAPEUTIC CLASS:** $K^+$-sparing diuretic/thiazide diuretic

**INDICATIONS:** For hypertension or edema if hypokalemia occurs on HCTZ alone, or when a thiazide diuretic is required and cannot risk hypokalemia.

**DOSAGE:** *Adults:* (37.5mg-25mg tab) 1-2 tabs qd. (75mg-50mg tab) 1 tab qd.

**HOW SUPPLIED:** (Triamterene-HCTZ) Tab: (Maxzide) 75mg-50mg*, (Maxzide-25) 37.5mg-25mg* *scored

**CONTRAINDICATIONS:** Hyperkalemia, anuria, acute or chronic renal insufficiency, sulfonamide hypersensitivity, diabetic neuropathy, $K^+$-sparing agents (eg, diuretics), $K^+$ supplements, $K^+$ salt substitutes, $K^+$-rich diet.

**WARNINGS/PRECAUTIONS:** Risk of hyperkalemia ( ≥5.5mEq/L) especially with renal impairment, elderly, DM or severely ill; monitor levels frequently. Check ECG if hyperkalemia occurs. Caution with history of renal lithiasis, hepatic dysfunction. Monitor BUN and creatinine periodically. D/C if azotemia increases. May contribute to megaloblastosis in folic acid deficiency. Hyperuricemia, hypercalcemia, hypophosphatemia, hypokalemia may occur. May manifest latent DM. May decrease serum PBI levels. Monitor for fluid/electrolyte imbalance.

**ADVERSE REACTIONS:** Jaundice, pancreatitis, NV, taste alteration, drowsiness, dry mouth, depression, anxiety, tachycardia, blood dyscrasias, electrolyte disturbances.

**INTERACTIONS:** May potentiate other antihypertensives. Risk of lithium toxicity. Indomethacin may cause renal failure; caution with NSAIDs. Increased risk of hyperkalemia with ACE inhibitors. May increase responsiveness to tubocurarine. May decrease arterial responsiveness to norepinephrine. May alter insulin requirements. Alcohol, barbiturates, or narcotics may potentiate orthostatic hypotension.

**PREGNANCY:** Category C, not for use in nursing.

**MECHANISM OF ACTION:** HCTZ: Thiazide diuretic; blocks renal tubular absorption of $Na^+$ and $Cl^-$ ions. This natriuresis and diuresis is accompanied by a secondary loss of $K^+$ and bicarbonate. Triamterene: Potassium-sparing diuretic; acts on the distal renal tubule to inhibit the reabsorption of $Na^+$ in exchange for $K^+$ and $H^+$, thus increases $Na^+$ excretion and reduces excessive loss of $K^+$ and $H^+$ associated with HCTZ.

**PHARMACOKINETICS: Absorption:** HCTZ: $T_{max}$=2 hrs. Triamterene: Rapid, $T_{max}$=1 hr. **Metabolism:** Triamterene: Liver; sulfate conjugation; hydroxytriamterene (metabolite). **Elimination**: HCTZ: Urine (unchanged).

## NURSING CONSIDERATIONS

**Assessment:** Assess for hyperkalemia, anuria, acute or chronic renal insufficiency, hepatic impairment or progressive liver disease, diabetic neuropathy, DM, risk for respiratory or metabolic acidosis, history of renal lithiasis, SLE, history of allergy or bronchial asthma, and possible drug interactions.

**Monitoring:** Monitor serum potassium levels, ECG, serum and urine electrolytes, folic acid levels, parathyroid function, BUN, creatinine (frequent intervals), signs of hyperkalemia (eg, paresthesias, muscular weakness, fatigue, flaccid paralysis of the extremities, bradycardia, and shock), electrolyte imbalance (eg, dry mouth, thirst, drowsiness, restlessness, oliguria, tachycardia, GI disturbance), folic acid deficiency or megaloblastosis, renal stone formation, hyperuricemia or acute gout, metabolic and endocrine effects, dilutional hyponatremia, hypokalemia, pathological changes in the parathyroid gland with hypercalcemia/hypophosphatemia and hepatic coma.

**Patient Counseling:** Inform about warning signs of hyperkalemia, and importance of periodic monitoring of serum potassium levels and ECG. Notify if pregnant/nursing.

**Administration:** Oral route. **Storage:** 20-25°C (68-77°F); in tight, light-resistant container.

# MEDROL — RX

methylprednisolone (Pharmacia & Upjohn)

**OTHER BRAND NAMES:** Medrol Dosepak (Pharmacia & Upjohn)

**THERAPEUTIC CLASS:** Glucocorticoid

**INDICATIONS:** Steroid-responsive treatment for acute control of severe intractable allergic conditions, rheumatic, collagen, dermatologic, respiratory, acute regional enteritis and ulcerative colitis, allergic and edematous states, tuberculous meningitis with subarachnoid block when used with antituberculous chemotherapy, and trichinosis with neurologic/myocardial involvement. For the short-term adjunct treatment of synovitis, osteoarthritis (OA), rheumatoid arthritis (RA), bursitis, acute gouty arthritis, epicondylitis and acute nonspecific tenosynovitis.

**DOSAGE:** *Adults:* Initial: 4-48mg/day depending on disease and response. Maint: Decrease dose by small amounts to lowest effective dose. MS: Initial: 160mg/day for 1 week. Maint: 64mg every other day for 1 month. Alternate Day Therapy: Twice the usual dose qod for long-term therapy.

**HOW SUPPLIED:** Tab: 2mg, 4mg, 8mg, 16mg, 32mg; (Dosepak) 4mg [21[s]]

**CONTRAINDICATIONS:** Systemic fungal infections.

**WARNINGS/PRECAUTIONS:** May need to increase dose before, during, and after stressful situations. May mask signs of infection or cause new infections. Prolonged use may produce glaucoma, optic nerve damage, secondary ocular infections. Increases BP, salt/water retention, potassium excretion. More severe/fatal course of infections reported with chickenpox, measles.

Caution with strongyloides, latent TB, hypothyroidism, cirrhosis, ocular herpes simplex, HTN, diverticulitis, fresh intestinal anastomoses, ulcerative colitis, osteoporosis, myasthenia gravis, renal insufficiency, peptic ulcer disease. Kaposi's sarcoma reported. Growth and development of children on prolonged therapy should be monitored. Monitor for psychic disturbances. Avoid abrupt withdrawal.

**ADVERSE REACTIONS:** Fluid and electrolyte disturbances, HTN, osteoporosis, muscle weakness, cushingoid state, menstrual irregularities, nervousness, insomnia, impaired wound healing, DM, ulcerative esophagitis, excessive sweating, increased ICP, carbohydrate intolerance, glaucoma, cataracts, weight gain, nausea, malaise.

**INTERACTIONS:** Reduced efficacy with hepatic enzyme inducers (eg, phenobarbital, phenytoin, and rifampin). Increases clearance of chronic high-dose ASA. Caution with ASA in hypoprothrombinemia. Effects on oral anticoagulants are variable; monitor PT. Increased insulin and oral hypoglycemic requirements in DM. Avoid live vaccines with immunosuppressive doses. Possible decreased vaccine response with killed or inactivated vaccines with immunosuppressive doses. Mutual inhibition of metabolism with cyclosporine; convulsions reported. Potentiated by ketoconazole and troleandomycin.

**PREGNANCY:** Safety in pregnancy and nursing not known.

**MECHANISM OF ACTION:** Anti-inflammatory glucocorticoid; causes profound and varied metabolic effects and modifies the body's immune responses to diverse stimuli.

**PHARMACOKINETICS: Absorption:** Readily absorbed from GI tract.

## NURSING CONSIDERATIONS

**Assessment:** Assess for systemic fungal infections, current infections, active TB, vaccination history, ulcerative colitis, diverticulitis, peptic ulcer with impending perforation, renal/hepatic insufficiency, septic arthritis/unstable joint, HTN, osteoporosis, myasthenia gravis, thyroid status, psychotic tendencies, and possible drug interactions.

**Monitoring:** Monitor for adrenocortical insufficiency, occurrence of infection, psychic derangement, cataracts, acute myopathy, Kaposi's sarcoma, fluid retention, measurement of serum electrolytes, TSH, LFTs, IOP, and BP. Monitor urinalysis, blood sugar, weight, chest X-ray, and upper GI X-ray (if ulcer history) regularly during prolonged therapy.

**Patient Counseling:** Inform that susceptibility to infections may increase. Avoid exposure to chickenpox or measles; report immediately if exposed. Dietary salt restriction and supplementation of $K^+$ is advised.

**Administration:** Oral route. **Storage:** 20-25°C (68-77°F).

## MEFLOQUINE HCL — RX

mefloquine HCl (Various)

**THERAPEUTIC CLASS:** Quinolinemethanol derivative

**INDICATIONS:** Treatment and prophylaxis of mild to moderate acute malaria caused by *P.falciparum* or *P.vivax*.

**DOSAGE:** *Adults:* Treatment: 1250mg single dose. Take with at least 8oz (240 mL) of water. Prophylaxis: 250mg weekly. Start 1 week before arrival in endemic malarial area and continue weekly (always on the same day each week). Continue for 4 weeks after leaving the area.

*Pediatrics:* ≥20kg: Treatment: Usual: 20-25mg/kg, split in 2 doses. Take 6-8 hrs apart. If vomiting occurs <30 min after dose, give a 2nd full dose. If vomiting occurs 30-60 min after dose, give additional half-dose. If vomiting continues, start alternative treatment. Prophylaxis: 5mg/kg weekly. >45kg: 1 tab weekly. 30-45kg: 3/4 tab weekly. 20-30kg: 1/2 tab weekly.

**HOW SUPPLIED:** Tab: 250mg* *scored

**CONTRAINDICATIONS:** Use as prophylaxis in patients with active or recent history of depression, generalized anxiety disorder, psychosis, schizophrenia, or other major psychiatric disorders, or with a history of convulsions.

**WARNINGS/PRECAUTIONS:** In life-threatening malaria infection due to *P.falciparum*, use IV antimalarials. High risk of relapse seen with acute *P.vivax*; after initial treatment, subsequently treat with 8-aminoquinoline (eg, primaquine). May cause psychiatric symptoms. During prophylaxis, d/c if symptoms of acute anxiety, depression, restlessness, or confusion occur. In long-term therapy, monitor LFTs and perform ophthalmic exams. May impair mental/physical abilities. Increased risk of convulsions in epileptic patients. Caution with cardiac disease, psychiatric disturbances, hepatic dysfunction, and the elderly. Should not be administered with halofantrine or ketoconazole within 15 weeks of the last dose of mefloquine due to fatal QTc interval prolongation risk.

**ADVERSE REACTIONS:** N/V, myalgia, fever, dizziness, headache, syncope, sleep disorders, chills, diarrhea, abdominal pain, fatigue, tinnitus, pruritus, skin rash, and vertigo.

**INTERACTIONS:** Avoid halofantrine and ketoconazole; may prolong QTc interval. Concomitant administration with other related compounds (eg, quinine, quinidine, chloroquine) may cause ECG abnormalities and increased risk of convulsions; delay mefloquine dose for 12 hrs after last dose of these drugs. Avoid propranolol; cardiopulmonary arrest reported. Drugs that may alter cardiac conduction (eg, anti-arrhythmic or β-blockers, CCBs, antihistamines, $H_1$-blockers, TCAs, and phenothiazines) may prolong $QT_c$ interval. May lower plasma levels of anticonvulsants (eg, valproic acid, carbamazepine, phenobarbital, phenytoin); monitor blood levels and adjust dosage accordingly. Complete vaccinations with live, attenuated vaccines (eg, typhoid vaccine) at least 3 days before mefloquine therapy. Caution with anticoagulants, antidiabetic agents, rifampin. May increase/decrease mefloquine plasma concentration with CYP450 inhibitors or inducers.

**PREGNANCY:** Category C, not for use in nursing.

**MECHANISM OF ACTION:** Quinolinemethanol derivative; suspected to act as blood schizonticide. Exact mechanism of action is not established.

**PHARMACOKINETICS: Absorption:** $C_{max}$=1000-2000mcg/L; $T_{max}$=6-24 hrs. **Distribution:** $V_d$=20L/kg; plasma protein binding (98%); crosses placenta; found in breast milk. **Metabolism:** Extensive. Liver via CYP3A4. **Elimination:** Bile/feces, urine (9% unchanged, 4% metabolite); $T_{1/2}$=2-4 weeks.

## NURSING CONSIDERATIONS

**Assessment:** Assess LFTs, ECG. Assess for history of depression, epilepsy, pregnancy status, and possible drug interactions. Note other diseases/conditions and drug therapies.

**Monitoring:** Monitor for psychiatric symptoms, convulsions, QTc interval prolongation, and for possible drug interactions. Monitor CBC, platelet count, LFTs, and ECG periodically. Monitor anticonvulsant blood level when taking antiseizure medications concomitantly. Periodic ophthalmic exams recommended.

**Patient Counseling:** Inform that malaria can be a life-threatening infection. Report any adverse reactions and seek medical attention for any febrile illness that occurs after return from a malarious area. Advise that no chemoprophylactic regimen is 100% effective; use of protective clothing, insect repellants, and bednets are important components of malaria prophylaxis. Advise females to use effective birth control during treatment. Caution with activities requiring alertness and fine motor coordination (eg, driving, piloting aircraft, operating machinery, and deep-sea diving). Advise that when used as prophylaxis, the first dose should be taken 1 week prior to arrival in an endemic area. Advise not to take on an empty stomach; administer with at least 8oz (240mL) of water.

**Administration:** Oral route. Tablets may be crushed and suspended in a small amount of water, milk or other beverages for those who are unable to swallow the tablet. **Storage:** 25°C (77°F); excursions permitted to 15-30°C (59-86°F).

M

## Megace ES

**RX**

megestrol acetate (Par)

**OTHER BRAND NAMES:** Megace Suspension (Bristol-Myers Squibb)

**THERAPEUTIC CLASS:** Progesterone

**INDICATIONS:** Management of anorexia, cachexia, or unexplained significant weight loss in AIDS patients.

**DOSAGE:** *Adults:* (Megace) Initial: 800mg/day (20mL/day). Usual: 400-800mg/day. Shake well before use. Elderly: Start at lower end of dosing range. (Megace ES) Initial/Usual: 625mg/day (5mL/day).

**HOW SUPPLIED:** Sus: 40mg/mL [240mL], (ES) 125mg/mL [150mL]

**CONTRAINDICATIONS:** Pregnancy.

**WARNINGS/PRECAUTIONS:** May cause fetal harm; avoid in pregnancy. New onset or exacerbation of diabetes or Cushing's syndrome reported. Risk of adrenal suppression if taking or withdrawing from chronic therapy; monitor for hypotension, N/V, dizziness, or weakness. Caution with history of thromboembolic diseases. Use in HIV-infected women has been limited. Do not use as prophylaxis to avoid weight loss.

**ADVERSE REACTIONS:** Diarrhea, rash, flatulence, N/V, HTN, asthenia, insomnia, anemia, fever, decreased libido, dyspepsia, headache, hyperglycemia, and pneumonia.

**INTERACTIONS:** May increase insulin requirements. Decrease in pharmacokinetic parameters of indinavir; higher dose should be considered.

**PREGNANCY:** Category X, not for use in nursing.

**MECHANISM OF ACTION:** Progesterone; not established; has appetite-enhancing property.

**PHARMACOKINETICS: Absorption:** PO administration of variable doses resulted in different parameters. **Elimination:** Urine (major), feces.

### NURSING CONSIDERATIONS

**Assessment:** Assess for pre-existing DM, history of thromboembolic disease, renal dysfunction, treatable causes of weight loss, pregnancy status/nursing status, and possible drug interactions.

**Monitoring:** Monitor for adrenal insufficiency, hypoadrenalism (N/V, dizziness, hypotension, weakness), breakthrough bleeding, renal function, and hypersensitivity reactions.

**Patient Counseling:** Inform of pregnancy risks; avoid becoming pregnant. Advise to seek medical attention if symptoms of adrenal insufficiency, hypoadrenalism (N/V, dizziness, hypotension, weakness), breakthrough bleeding, or hypersensitivity reactions occur.

**Administration:** Oral route. **Storage:** 15-25°C (59-77°F). Protect from heat.

## Meperidine/Promethazine

**CII**

meperidine HCl - promethazine HCl (Ethex)

**OTHER BRAND NAMES:** Meprozine (Vintage)

**THERAPEUTIC CLASS:** Opioid analgesic/phenothiazine

**INDICATIONS:** Management of moderate pain and sedation for postoperative and postpartum use, and pain associated with malignancies.

**DOSAGE:** *Adults:* 1 cap q4-6h prn.

**HOW SUPPLIED:** Cap: (Meperidine-Promethazine) 50mg-25mg

**CONTRAINDICATIONS:** During or within 14 days of MAOIs.

**WARNINGS/PRECAUTIONS:** May cause tolerance and dependence; potential for abuse. Extreme caution with head injury, increased ICP, intracranial lesions, acute asthma, COPD, cor pulmonale, decreased respiratory reserve, respiratory depression, hypoxia, hypercapnia. Severe hypotension may occur with depleted blood volume. Orthostatic hypotension may occur. Caution with atrial flutter and other supraventricular tachycardias. May obscure diagnosis or clinical course of acute abdominal conditions. Reduce initial dose in elderly, debilitated, severe hepatic or renal dysfunction, hypothyroidism, Addison's disease, prostatic hypertrophy, urethral stricture. May aggravate seizure disorders. Not for use in pregnant women prior to labor.

**ADVERSE REACTIONS:** Lightheadedness, dizziness, sedation, NV, sweating.

**INTERACTIONS:** See Contraindications. Additive sedative effects with CNS depressants (eg, narcotics, anesthetics, phenothiazines, tranquilizers, sedative-hypnotics, TCAs, alcohol). Reduce analgesic depressant dose by 25-50% and dose of barbiturates by 50%. Severe hypotension possible with concurrent phenothiazines, certain anesthetics.

**PREGNANCY:** Safety in pregnancy and nursing not known.

**MECHANISM OF ACTION:** Meperidine: Narcotic analgesic. Promethazine: Phenothiazine derivative; has antiemetic, sedative, antihistaminic actions.

## NURSING CONSIDERATIONS

**Assessment:** Assess for hypothyroidism, Addison's disease, seizure disorder, urethral stricture, prostatic hypertrophy, acute abdominal conditions, increased ICP, head injury, intracranial lesions, asthma, COPD, cor pulmonale, decreased respiratory reserve, respiratory depression, hypoxia, hypercapnia, atrial flutter, SVT, possible drug interactions, renal/hepatic impairment.

**Monitoring:** Monitor for signs/symptoms of seizures, respiratory depression, hypotension, tachycardia, and hypersensitivity reactions.

**Patient Counseling:** Caution may impair physical/mental abilities. Advise to seek medical attention if symptoms of seizures, respiratory depression, hypotension, tachycardia, or hypersensitivity reactions occur.

**Administration:** Oral route. **Storage:** 25°C (77°F). Protect from light.

M

# MEPRON — RX

atovaquone (GlaxoSmithKline)

**THERAPEUTIC CLASS:** Napthoquinone antiprotozoal

**INDICATIONS:** Prevention and acute treatment of mild to moderate *Pneumocystis carinii* pneumonia (PCP) in those intolerant to trimethoprim-sulfamethoxazole.

**DOSAGE:** *Adults:* Prevention: 1500mg qd. Treatment: 750mg bid for 21 days. Take with food

*Pediatrics:* 13-16 yrs: Prevention: 1500mg qd. Treatment: 750mg bid for 21 days. Take with food.

**HOW SUPPLIED:** Sus: 750mg/5mL [5mL, $42^{s}$; 210mL]

**WARNINGS/PRECAUTIONS:** Hepatitis, elevated LFTs, and fatal liver failure reported; caution use with severe hepatic impairment and monitor closely. Absorption significantly increased with food. GI disorders may limit absorption. Consider parenteral therapy in patients with difficulty taking the drug with food.

**ADVERSE REACTIONS:** Rash, nausea, GI effects, increased cough, rhinitis, asthenia, infection, dyspnea, insomnia, asthenia, pruritus.

**INTERACTIONS:** Significantly decreased plasma levels with rifampin and rifabutin. Decrease levels of trimethoprim-sulfamethoxazole. Increase levels of zidovudine. Caution with other highly protein-bound drugs.

**PREGNANCY:** Category C, caution in nursing.

**MECHANISM OF ACTION:** Naphthoquinone antiprotozoal; site of action appears to be cytochrome $bc_1$ complex, which is linked to mitochondrial electron transport. Inhibition of electron transport by atovaquone will result in indirect inhibition of these enzymes, resulting in nucleic acid and ATP synthesis inhibition.

**PHARMACOKINETICS: Absorption:** Absolute bioavailability (47%); dependent on formulation and diet. **Distribution:** $V_d$=0.6L/kg; plasma protein binding (99.9%). **Elimination:** Feces ( ≥94%, unchanged), urine (≤0.6%).

## NURSING CONSIDERATIONS

**Assessment:** Assess CBC with differential and platelets, renal/hepatic functions. Assess pregnancy/nursing status and possible drug interactions.

**Monitoring:** Monitor for hypersensitivity reactions (eg, rash, fever, allergic reaction), GI events (eg, NV, diarrhea), bronchospasm. Monitor CBC, LFTs (ALT, AST, alkaline phosphatase, amylase), renal function tests.

**Patient Counseling:** Instruct to take as prescribed, daily, with meals. Counsel about potential side effects; seek medical attention if any develop.

**Administration:** Oral route. Shake bottle gently before use. **Storage:** 15-25°C (59-77°F). Do not freeze.

# MERIDIA CIV

sibutramine HCl monohydrate (Abbott)

**THERAPEUTIC CLASS:** Dopamine/norepinephrine/serotonin reuptake inhibitor

**INDICATIONS:** Management of obesity, including weight loss and maintenance of weight loss, and should be used in conjunction with a reduced-calorie diet. Recommended for obese patients with an initial BMI ≥30kg/m² or ≥27kg/m² with risk factors (eg, HTN, diabetes, dyslipidemia).

**DOSAGE:** *Adults:* Initial: 10mg qd. Titrate: May increase after 4 weeks to 15mg qd. Max: 15mg/day. Use 5mg/day in patients unable to tolerate 10mg/day. May continue for up to 2 yrs.

M

**HOW SUPPLIED:** Cap: 5mg, 10mg, 15mg.

**CONTRAINDICATIONS:** Concomitant use of MAOIs or centrally acting weight-loss drugs, eating disorders (eg, anorexia/bulimia nervosa).

**WARNINGS/PRECAUTIONS:** May increase BP and/or pulse rate. Avoid with uncontrolled or poorly controlled HTN, CAD, CHF, arrhythmias, stroke, severe hepatic or renal dysfunction. Monitor BP and pulse rate before therapy and regularly thereafter. Potentially life-threatening serotonin syndrome, or neuroleptic malignant syndrome (NMS)-like reactions, reported. Caution with narrow angle glaucoma, mild to moderate renal impairment, if predisposed to bleeding, and history of HTN. D/C if seizures develop. Exclude organic causes of obesity before prescribing. Gallstone formation precipitated with weight loss. May impair physical/mental abilities. Caution in elderly. Cases of depression, psychosis, mania, suicidal ideation, and suicide reported rarely.

**ADVERSE REACTIONS:** Headache, anorexia, constipation, dry mouth, insomnia, rhinitis, increased appetite, back pain, flu syndrome, dizziness, nausea, arthralgia, nervousness, dyspepsia, rash, psychiatric issues.

**INTERACTIONS:** Avoid excess alcohol, CNS-active drugs, other serotonergic agents (eg, SSRIs, migraine therapy agents, certain opioids), within 14 days of MAOI use. Concomitant use with antipsychotics, other dopamine antagonists, agents for migraine therapy (eg sumatriptan, dihydroergotamine), and certain opioids may cause serotonin syndrome or NMS-like reactions. Caution with drugs affecting hemostasis or platelet function; ephedrine, pseudoephedrine; and other agents that increase BP, heart rate. Possible decreased metabolism with ketoconazole and erythromycin.

**PREGNANCY:** Category C, not for use in nursing.

**MECHANISM OF ACTION:** Inhibits norepinephrine, serotonin, and dopamine reuptake.

**PHARMACOKINETICS: Absorption:** Rapid; $T_{max}$=1.2 hrs; (15mg Dose, $M_1$, $M_2$) $C_{max}$=4ng/mL, 6.4ng/mL; $T_{max}$=3.6 hrs, 3.5 hrs; AUC=25.5ng•h/mL, 92.1ng•h/mL. **Distribution:** Plasma protein binding (97%); $M_1$, $M_2$ (94%). **Metabolism:** Liver via CYP3A4; $M_1$ and $M_2$ (active metabolites). **Elimination:** Urine (77%), feces; $T_{1/2}$=1.1 hrs.

## NURSING CONSIDERATIONS

**Assessment:** Assess for renal/hepatic impairment, anorexia nervosa, bulimia nervosa, history of HTN, history of CAD, CHF, arrhythmias, stroke, narrow-angle glaucoma, seizures, hypothyroidism, hypersensitivity and possible drug interactions. Obtain baseline BP and pulse rate. Evaluate for history of drug abuse.

**Monitoring:** Monitor BP and pulse rate periodically. Monitor for signs/symptoms of mydriasis, HTN, seizures, bleeding events, gallstone formation, psychomotor or cognitive performance, serotonin syndrome, and hypersensitivity reactions. If ≥4 lbs not lost in first 4 weeks, consider reevaluation of therapy.

**Patient Counseling:** Advise to notify physician if taking any prescription (eg, lithium, sumatriptan, antidepressants, dihydroergotamine) or OTC drugs (eg, decongestants, cough suppressants), if breastfeeding, or if allergic reactions, seizures, bleeding events, signs/symptoms of serotonin syndrome or visual disturbances develop. Regular BP and pulse monitoring recommended.

**Administration:** Oral route. **Storage:** 25°C (77°F); excursions permitted to 15-30°C (59-86°F). Protect from heat and moisture.

# MERREM — RX

meropenem (AstraZeneca)

**THERAPEUTIC CLASS:** Carbapenem

**INDICATIONS:** Treatment of intra-abdominal infections, bacterial meningitis, and complicated skin and skin structure infections (cSSSI) caused by susceptible strains of microorganisms.

**DOSAGE:** *Adults:* IV: Intra-Abdominal Infections: CrCl ≥ 51mL/min: 1g q8h. CrCl 26-50mL/min: 1g q12h. CrCl 10-25mL/min: 500mg q12h. CrCl <10mL/min: 500mg q24h. cSSSI: CrCl ≥ 51mL/min: 500mg q8h. CrCl 26-50mL/min: 500mg q12h. CrCl 10-25mL/min: 250mg q12h. CrCl <10mL/min: 250mg q24h. Administer as infusion over 15-30 min; doses of 1g may also be administered as bolus injection (5-20mL) over 3-5 min.
*Pediatrics:* IV: ≥3 months: >50kg: Intra-Abdominal Infections: 1g q8h. Meningitis: 2g q8h. cSSSI: 500mg q8h. ≤50kg: Intra-Abdominal Infections: 20mg/kg q8h. Max: 1g q8h. Meningitis: 40mg/kg q8h. Max: 2g q8h. cSSSI: 10mg/kg q8h. Max: 500mg q8h. Administer as infusion over 15-30 min, or as bolus injection (5-20mL) over 3-5 min.

**HOW SUPPLIED:** Inj: 500mg, 1g

**CONTRAINDICATIONS:** Hypersensitivity to β-lactams.

**WARNINGS/PRECAUTIONS:** Severe and fatal hypersensitivity reactions reported; increased risk with PCN sensitivity; d/c immediately if allergic reaction occurs, and institute emergency treatment for serious anaphylactic reaction(s). *Clostridium difficile*-associated diarrhea reported; if CDAD is suspected, d/c therapy. Seizures and other CNS effects reported, particularly with pre-existing CNS disorders, bacterial meningitis, and renal dysfunction. Thrombocytopenia reported with severe renal impairment. Prolonged use may result in superinfection.

**ADVERSE REACTIONS:** Diarrhea, N/V, rash. (Adults) Headache, constipation, sepsis, pruritus, shock, apnea, anemia, pain, inflammation at injection site. (Pediatrics) Oral moniliasis, glossitis.

**INTERACTIONS:** Probenecid inhibits renal excretion; avoid concomitant use. May reduce valproic acid levels, thereby increasing risk of breakthrough seizures; if concomitant administration is necessary, consider supplemental anticonvulsant therapy.

**PREGNANCY:** Category B, caution in nursing.

**MECHANISM OF ACTION:** Broad-spectrum carbapenem; penetrates bacterial cells and interferes with synthesis of vital cell wall components, resulting in cell death.

**PHARMACOKINETICS: Absorption:** 30 min infusion: $C_{max}$=23mcg/mL (500mg); 49mcg/mL (1g). 5-min bolus injection: $C_{max}$=45mcg/mL (500mg);

112mcg/mL (1g). **Distribution:** Plasma protein binding (2%). **Elimination:** Urine (70%); $T_{1/2}$=1 hr (in patients ≥2 yrs), 1.5 hrs (in pediatrics [3 months-2 yrs]).

## NURSING CONSIDERATIONS

**Assessment:** Assess for β-lactam hypersensitivity, history of seizure or brain lesions, bacterial meningitis, renal impairment, and possible drug interactions. Assess pregnancy/nursing status.

**Monitoring:** Monitor for signs/symptoms of anaphylactic/hypersensitivity reactions, CDAD, superinfections, and seizures.

**Patient Counseling:** Inform that drug only treats bacterial, not viral, infections. Instruct to take as directed; skipping doses or not completing full course may decrease effectiveness and increase antibiotic resistance. Inform that diarrhea may occur; advise to contact physician if watery/bloody stools, hypersensitivity reactions, infection, or seizures occur. Counsel to inform physician if taking valproic acid or divalproex sodium.

**Administration:** IV route. Infusion over 15-30 mins, or as bolus injection (5-20mL) over 3-5 mins. Refer to PI for preparation of solution and stability parameters. **Storage:** 20-25°C (68-77°F).

# METADATE CD

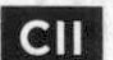

methylphenidate HCl (UCB)

**Give cautiously to patients with a history of drug dependence or alcoholism. Chronic abusive use may lead to marked tolerance and psychological dependence with varying degrees of abnormal behavior. Careful supervision required during withdrawal from abusive use.**

**THERAPEUTIC CLASS:** Sympathomimetic amine

**INDICATIONS:** Treatment of attention deficit hyperactivity disorder (ADHD).

**DOSAGE:** *Pediatrics:* ≥6 yrs: Usual: 20mg qam before breakfast. Titrate: Increase weekly by 20mg depending on tolerability/efficacy. Max: 60mg/day. Reduce dose or discontinue if paradoxical aggravation of symptoms occur. D/C if no improvement after appropriate dose adjustments over 1 month. Swallow whole with liquids or open and sprinkle on 1 tbs applesauce followed by water. Do not crush, chew, or divide.

**HOW SUPPLIED:** Cap, Extended-Release: 10mg, 20mg, 30mg, 40mg, 50mg, 60mg

**CONTRAINDICATIONS:** Marked anxiety, tension, and agitation; glaucoma; motor tics, family history or diagnosis of Tourette's syndrome, severe HTN, angina pectoris, cardiac arrhythmias, heart failure, recent MI, hyperthyroidism or thyrotoxicosis; during or within 14 days of MAOI use.

**WARNINGS/PRECAUTIONS:** Monitor growth in children. Not for severe depression or fatigue. May exacerbate symptoms of behavior disturbance and thought disorder in psychotic patients. Caution when using stimulants to treat patients with comorbid bipolar disorder because of concern for possible induction of mixed/manic episode in such patients. Stimulants at usual doses can cause treatment emergent psychotic or manic symptoms (eg, hallucinations, delusional thinking, mania) in children and adolescents without prior history of psychotic illness. Aggressive behavior or hostility reported in clinical trials and postmarketing experience of some medications indicated for the treatment of ADHD. May lower seizure threshold, especially in known EEG abnormalities. Caution with HTN, conditions affected by BP or HR elevation, history of drug abuse or alcoholism. Monitor during withdrawal from abusive use. Visual disturbances may occur (rare). Monitor CBC, differential, and platelets with prolonged use. Avoid with serious structural cardiac abnormalities, cardiomyopathy, serious heart rhythm abnormalities, CAD, or other serious cardiac problems.

**ADVERSE REACTIONS:** Headache, abdominal pain, anorexia, insomnia.

**INTERACTIONS:** See Contraindications. Potentiates anticoagulants, anticonvulsants (eg, phenobarbital, phenytoin, primidone), TCAs, and SSRIs. Caution with α-agonist (eg, clonidine) and pressor agents.

**PREGNANCY:** Category C, caution in nursing.

**MECHANISM OF ACTION:** CNS stimulant; not established, thought to block reuptake of norepinephrine and dopamine into presynaptic neuron and increase release of these monoamines into extraneuronal space.

**PHARMACOKINETICS: Absorption:** (PO) Readily absorbed. Administration of variable doses resulted in different parameters. **Metabolism:** Via de-esterification. Metabolite: α-phenyl-piperidine acetic acid (ritalinic acid). **Elimination:** $T_{1/2}$=6.8 hrs.

## NURSING CONSIDERATIONS

**Assessment:** Assess for agitation, glaucoma, tics, family history of Tourette's syndrome, cardiovascular conditions (eg, severe HTN, angina pectoris, cardiac abnormalities, arrhythmias, heart failure, recent MI), hyperthyroidism or thyrotoxicosis, bipolar illness, history of drug dependence or alcoholism.

**Monitoring:** Monitor for cardiac abnormalities, exacerbations of behavior disturbances and thought disorder, bipolar illness, aggression, seizures, and visual disturbances. Periodic monitoring of CBC, differential and platelet count, LFTs. Height and weight follow-up in children.

**Patient Counseling:** Inform about risks of therapy, appropriate use, and drug abuse/dependence. Must swallow tablet; never crush or chew. Take last dose before 6 pm to avoid insomnia.

**Administration:** Oral route. **Storage:** 25°C (77°F); excursions permitted to 15-30°C (59-86°F).

# METADATE ER

CII

methylphenidate HCl (UCB)

M

**Give cautiously to patients with a history of drug dependence or alcoholism. Chronic abusive use may lead to marked tolerance and psychological dependence with varying degrees of abnormal behavior. Careful supervision required during withdrawal from abusive use.**

**THERAPEUTIC CLASS:** Sympathomimetic amine

**INDICATIONS:** Treatment of attention deficit disorder (ADHD) and narcolepsy.

**DOSAGE:** *Adults:* (Immediate-Release Methylphenidate) 10-60mg/day given bid-tid 30-45 min ac. Take last dose before 6 pm if insomnia occurs. (Tab, Extended-Release) May use in place of immediate-release tabs when the 8-hr dose corresponds to the titrated 8-hr immediate-release dose. Swallow whole; do not chew or crush.
*Pediatrics:* ≥6 yrs: (Immediate-Release Methylphenidate) Initial: 5mg bid before breakfast and lunch. Titrate: Increase gradually by 5-10mg weekly. Max: 60mg/day. (Tab, Extended-Release) May use in place of immediate-release tabs when the 8-hr dose corresponds to the titrated 8-hr immediate-release dose. Swallow whole; do not chew or crush. Reduce dose or d/c if paradoxical aggravation of symptoms occur. D/C if no improvement after appropriate dose adjustment over 1 month.

**HOW SUPPLIED:** Tab, Extended-Release: 10mg, 20mg

**CONTRAINDICATIONS:** Marked anxiety, tension, and agitation; glaucoma; motor tics or family history or diagnosis of Tourette's syndrome; during or within 14 days of MAOI use.

**WARNINGS/PRECAUTIONS:** Caution with comorbid bipolar disorder. Monitor growth in children. Not for severe depression or fatigue. May exacerbate symptoms of behavior disturbance and thought disorder in psychotic children. Treatment emergent psychotic/manic symptoms in children and adolescents may occur. Aggressive behavior or hostility observed. May lower seizure threshold, especially in known EEG abnormalities. Caution with HTN, emotionally unstable patients. Monitor during withdrawal. Visual disturbances may occur (rare). Monitor CBC, differential, and platelets with prolonged use. Periodically d/c to assess condition.

**ADVERSE REACTIONS:** Nervousness, insomnia, hypersensitivity reactions, anorexia, nausea, dizziness, palpitations, headache, dyskinesia, drowsiness, BP and pulse changes, tachycardia, angina, arrhythmia, abdominal pain.

**INTERACTIONS:** See Contraindications. May decrease hypotensive effect of guanethidine. Caution with pressor agents. Potentiates anticoagulants, anticonvulsants (eg, phenobarbital, phenytoin, primidone), phenylbutazone, TCAs (eg, imipramine, clomipramine, desipramine).

**PREGNANCY:** Category C, caution in nursing.

**MECHANISM OF ACTION:** Not established, suspected to have sympathomimetic activity in the brain stem arousal system and cortex.

**PHARMACOKINETICS: Absorption:** Slowly absorbed. $T_{max}$=1.3-8.2 hrs (sustained-release tab), 0.3-4.4 hrs (immediate release tab).

## NURSING CONSIDERATIONS

**Assessment:** Assess for agitation, hereditary problems of galactose intolerance, Lapp lactase deficiency or glucose-galactose malabsorption, glaucoma, tics, family history of Tourette's syndrome, cardiovascular conditions (severe HTN, angina pectoris, cardiac arrhythmias, heart failure, recent MI), hyperthyroidism or thyrotoxicosis, bipolar illness, history of drug dependence or alcoholism.

**Monitoring:** Monitor for cardiac abnormalities, exacerbations of behavior disturbances and thought disorder, bipolar illness, aggression, seizures, and visual disturbances. Periodic monitoring of CBC, differential and platelet count, LFTs. Height and weight follow-up in children.

**Patient Counseling:** Inform about potential risks of therapy, appropriate use, drug dependence/abuse. Must swallow, never crush or chew. Take last dose before 6 pm to avoid insomnia.



**Administration:** Administer PO, preferably 30-45 min before meals. **Storage:** 20-25°C (77°F); excursions permitted to 15-30°C (59-86°F). Keep tightly closed. Protect from moisture.

## Metaglip RX

metformin HCl - glipizide (Bristol-Myers Squibb)

**THERAPEUTIC CLASS:** Sulfonylurea/biguanide

**INDICATIONS:** Adjunct to diet and exercise to improve glycemic control in adults with type 2 diabetes mellitus.

**DOSAGE:** *Adults:* Individualize dose. Inadequate glycemic control on diet/exercise alone: Initial: 2.5mg-250mg with a meal qd. If fasting plasma glucose (FPG) 280-320mg/dL, give 2.5mg-500mg bid. Titrate: Increase by 1 tab/day q2 weeks. Max: 10mg-1000mg/day or 10mg-2000mg/day in divided doses. Inadequate glycemic control on sulfonylurea or metformin: Initial: 2.5mg-500mg or 5mg-500mg bid (with morning and evening meals). Starting dose should not exceed daily dose of metformin or glipizide already being taken. Titrate: Increase by no more than 5mg-500mg/day. Max: 20mg-2000mg/day.

**HOW SUPPLIED:** Tab: (Glipizide-Metformin) 2.5mg-250mg, 2.5mg-500mg, 5mg-500mg

**CONTRAINDICATIONS:** Renal disease/dysfunction (SrCr ≥1.5mg/dL [males], ≥1.4mg/dL [females], abnormal CrCl), metabolic acidosis including diabetic ketoacidosis. D/C temporarily (48 hrs) for radiologic studies involving intravascular iodinated contrast materials.

**WARNINGS/PRECAUTIONS:** Lactic acidosis reported (rare); increased risk with increased age, DM with renal insufficiency, congestive heart failure (CHF), and other conditions with risk of hypoperfusion and hypoxemia. Avoid use in patients ≥80 yrs unless renal function is normal. Increased risk of cardiovascular mortality. Increased risk of hypoglycemia in elderly, debilitated, malnourished, adrenal or pituitary insufficiency, or alcohol intoxication. D/C in hypoxic states (eg, CHF, shock, acute MI) and prior to surgical procedures (due to restricted food intake). Avoid in renal/hepatic impairment. May decrease serum vitamin $B_{12}$ levels. Impaired renal and/or hepatic function may slow excretion. Withhold with any condition associated with hypoxemia, dehydration, or sepsis. Monitor renal function. Caution in patients with glucose-6-phosphate dehydrogenase (G6PD) deficiency; may lead to hemolytic anemia. Hemolytic anemia reported in patients without G6PD deficiency.

**ADVERSE REACTIONS:** Upper respiratory tract infection, HTN, headache, diarrhea, dizziness, musculoskeletal pain, N/V, abdominal pain, hypoglycemia.

**INTERACTIONS:** Furosemide, nifedipine, cimetidine, and cationic drugs (eg, digoxin, procainamide, quinidine, quinine, ranitidine, trimethoprim, vancomycin, triamterene, morphine) may increase metformin levels. Temporarily d/c metformin before and for 48 hrs after intravascular contrast studies with iodinated materials. Hypoglycemia is potentiated by alcohol, NSAIDs, some azoles, and other highly protein-bound drugs, salicylates, sulfonamides, chloramphenicol, probenecid, coumarins, MAOIs, and β-blockers. Severe hypoglycemia reported with concomitant oral miconazole. Thiazides and other diuretics, corticosteroids, phenothiazines, thyroid products, estrogens, oral contraceptives, phenytoin, nicotinic acid, sympathomimetics, CCBs, and isoniazid may cause hyperglycemia. Alcohol potentiates the effect of metformin on lactate metabolism. May decrease furosemide levels.

**PREGNANCY:** Category C, not for use in nursing.

**MECHANISM OF ACTION:** Glipizide: Sulfonylurea; stimulates release of insulin from the pancreas. Metformin: Biguanide; decreases hepatic glucose production and intestinal absorption of glucose and improves insulin sensitivity by increasing peripheral glucose uptake and utilization.

**PHARMACOKINETICS: Absorption:** Glipizide: Rapid, complete; $T_{max}$=1-3 hrs. Metformin: Absolute bioavailability (50-60%). **Distribution:** Glipizide: Plasma protein binding (98-99%); $V_d$=11L (IV). Metformin: $V_d$=654L (PO). **Metabolism:** Glipizide: Liver (extensive). **Elimination:** Glipizide: Urine; $T_{1/2}$=2-4 hrs. Metformin: Urine (90% [PO], unchanged [IV]); $T_{1/2}$=6.2 hrs (plasma), 17.6 hrs (blood).

## NURSING CONSIDERATIONS

**Assessment:** Assess FPG, $HbA_{1c}$, renal function (eg, SrCr), LFTs, hematologic parameters (eg, Hgb/Hct, CBC). Assess for CHF, septicemia, acute or chronic metabolic acidosis, adrenal or pituitary insufficiency, alcoholism, other medical conditions, hypersensitivity, pregnancy/nursing status, and possible drug interactions.

**Monitoring:** Monitor for hypoglycemia, lactic acidosis, prerenal azotemia, CHF, cardiovascular disease, and hypersensitivity reactions. Monitor FPG, $HbA_{1c}$, renal function (eg, SrCr), LFTs, hematologic parameters (eg, Hgb/Hct, CBC).

**Patient Counseling:** Inform about potential risks and benefits of drug and alternative modes of therapy. Inform that drug is adjunct to diet and exercise to control diabetes. Inform about importance of adherence to dietary instructions, regular excercise programs, and regular testing of blood glucose, glycosylated Hgb, renal function, and hematologic parameters. Report unexplained hyperventilation, myalgia, malaise, N/V, and somnolence. Explain risk of lactic acidosis, its signs/symptoms, and conditions that predispose to its development. Explain risk of hypoglycemia. Counsel against excessive alcohol intake.

**Administration:** Oral route. **Storage:** 20-25°C (68-77°F); excursions permitted to 15-30°C (59-86°F).

# METHADOSE

**CII**

methadone HCl (Mallinckrodt)

**Deaths due to cardiac and respiratory effects reported during initiation and conversion from other opioid agonists. Respiratory depression and QT prolongation observed. Only certified/approved opioid treatment programs can dispense oral methadone for treatment of narcotic addiction. Use as analgesic should be initiated only if benefits outweigh risks.**

**THERAPEUTIC CLASS:** Opioid analgesic

**INDICATIONS:** Detoxification and maintenance treatment of opioid addiction (heroin or other morphine-like drugs) in conjunction with appropriate social and medical services. Tab: Treatment of moderate to severe pain not responsive to non-narcotic analgesics.

**DOSAGE:** *Adults:* Detoxification: Initial/Induction: 20-30mg/day. Give 5-10mg 2-4 hrs later if needed. Max: 40mg on first day. Adjust dose to control withdrawal symptoms over 1st week. Short Term Detoxification: Titrate to 40mg/day given in divided doses to achieve adequate stabilizing level. Stabilization can continue for 2-3 days, then may decrease every 1-2 days depending on symptoms. Maintenance: Titrate to a dose at which symptoms prevented for 24 hrs. Usual: 80-120mg/day. Pain in Opioid Non-Tolerant: Usual: 2.5-10mg q8-12h, slowly titrated to effect. Conversion From Parenteral: Initial: Use a 1:2 dose ratio parenteral to oral. Switching From Other Chronic Opioids: Use caution; see PI for dosing details.

**HOW SUPPLIED:** Oral Concentrate: 10mg/mL; Tab: 5mg*, 10mg*; Tab, Dispersible: 40mg *scored

**CONTRAINDICATIONS:** Respiratory depression. Acute bronchial asthma or hypercarbia. Paralytic ileus.

**WARNINGS/PRECAUTIONS:** Do not inject agent. Extreme caution if using narcotic antagonists in patients physically dependent on narcotics. Can cause respiratory depression and elevate CSF pressure. Caution with head injuries, acute asthma attacks, COPD, cor pulmonale, decreased respiratory reserve, pre-existing respiratory depression, hypoxia, or hypercapnia. Reduce initial dose in elderly, debilitated, severe hepatic or renal impairment, hypothyroidism, Addison's disease, prostatic hypertrophy, or urethral stricture. Risk of tolerance, dependence, and abuse may occur. Impairs physical and mental abilities. Ineffective in relieving anxiety. May mask symptoms of acute abdominal conditions. May produce hypotension. Caution in patients with risk of prolonged QT interval (eg, cardiac hypertrophy, hyponatremia, hypomagnesemia, diuretic use).

M

**ADVERSE REACTIONS:** Lightheadedness, dizziness, sedation, sweating, N/V.

**INTERACTIONS:** Concurrent μ-agonists (eg, pentazocine, nalaxone, buprenorphine), St. John's wort, phenobarbital, carbamazepine may precipitate withdrawal. Decreased levels with CYP3A4 inducers (eg, rifampin). Increased levels with CYP3A4 inhibitors, such as azole antifungals (eg, ketoconazole), macrolide antibiotics (eg, erythromycin), some SSRIs (eg, sertraline, fluvoxamine). Caution and reduce dose with CNS depressants (eg, tranquilizers, sedative-hypnotics, phenothiazines, TCAs, alcohol). Caution with drugs that may prolong QT interval (eg, class I and III antiarrhythmics, neuroleptics, calcium channel blockers). MAOIs may cause severe reactions. May increase levels of desipramine.

**PREGNANCY:** Category C, not for use in nursing.

**MECHANISM OF ACTION:** Synthetic opioid analgesic; μ-agonist. Produces actions similiar to morphine; acts on CNS and organs composed of smooth muscle. May also act as N-methyl-D-aspartate (NMDA) receptor antagonist.

**PHARMACOKINETICS: Absorption:** Bioavailability (36-100%); $C_{max}$=124-1255ng/mL; $T_{max}$=1-7.5 hrs. **Distribution:** $V_d$=1-8 L/kg; bound to $\alpha_1$-acid glycoprotein (85-90%); secreted in saliva, breast milk, amniotic fluid, and umbilical cord plasma. **Metabolism:** Hepatic N-demethylation; CYP3A4, 2B6, 2C19 (major); 2C9, 2D6 (minor). **Elimination**: Urine, feces; $T_{1/2}$=8-59 hrs.

## NURSING CONSIDERATIONS

**Assessment:** Assess for respiratory depression, acute bronchial asthma or hypercarbia, COPD, myxedema, kyphoscoliosis, CNS depression or coma, paralytic ileus, history of cardiac conduction abnormalities, hypokalemia, hypomagnesemia, head injury or other intracranial lesions, increased ICP, acute abdominal conditions, volume depletion, hepatic/renal impairment, presence of debilitation (eg, elderly), hypothyroidism, Addison's disease, prostatic hypertrophy or urethral stricture, hypersensitivity to drug, pregnancy/nursing status, and possible drug interactions.

**Monitoring:** Monitor for signs/symptoms of respiratory depression, QT prolongation and arrhythmias (eg, torsade de pointes), misuse or abuse of medication, physical dependence and tolerance, elevations in CSF pressure, hypotension, and hypersensitivity reactions.

**Patient Counseling:** Inform that medication may impair mental/physical abilities; use caution when performing hazardous tasks (eg, operating machinery/driving). Advise to avoid using alcohol and other CNS depressants. Instruct to seek immediate medical care if develop signs/symptoms of arrhythmia (eg, palpitations, dizziness, syncope) or if develop difficulty in breathing; orthostatic hypotension may occur. Instruct to keep out of reach of children. Advise to avoid abrupt withdrawal; taper dosing. Inform patients treated for opioid dependence that d/c may lead to relapse of illicit drug use. Educate on potential for abuse and to protect from theft.

**Administration:** Oral route. **Storage:** 20-25°C (68-77°F); dispense in tight container, protected from light.

## METHOTREXATE RX

methotrexate (Various)

**Should only be used by physicians whose knowledge and experience includes the use of antimetabolite therapy. Only for life-threatening neoplastic diseases, or with severe, recalcitrant, disabling disease not adequately responsive to other forms of therapy. Fetal death/congenital anomalies reported. Elimination reduced with impaired renal function, ascites, or pleural effusions; monitor carefully. Severe, sometimes fatal, bone marrow suppression and GI toxicity reported with concomitant NSAIDs. May cause hepatotoxicity, fibrosis, and cirrhosis (usually after prolonged use). Lung disease, malignant melanomas, and potentially fatal opportunistic infections may occur. Interrupt therapy if diarrhea or ulcerative colitis occur. May induce tumor lysis syndrome. Severe, occasionally fatal, skin reactions reported. Concomitant radiotherapy may increase risk of soft tissue necrosis and osteonecrosis.**

**OTHER BRAND NAMES:** Rheumatrex (Stada)

**THERAPEUTIC CLASS:** Dihydrofolic acid reductase inhibitor

**INDICATIONS:** (Inj/PO) Treatment of neoplastic diseases (eg, acute lymphocytic leukemia, gestational choriocarcinoma, chorioadenoma destruens, hydatidiform mole, breast cancer, epidermoid cancer of the head and neck, advanced mycosis fungoides, lung cancer, advanced stage non-Hodgkin's lymphomas). Prophylaxis and treatment of meningeal leukemia, and maintenance with other chemotherapeutics. For prolonging relapse-free survival in non-metastatic osteosarcoma followed by leucovorin. Symptomatic control of severe, recalcitrant, disabling psoriasis. (PO) Management of rheumatoid arthritis (RA) or polyarticular-course juvenile rheumatoid arthritis (JRA) unresponsive to other therapies.

**DOSAGE:** *Adults:* Choriocarcinoma/Trophoblastic Disease: 15-30mg qd PO/IM for 5 days. May repeat 3-5 times as required with rest period of ≥1 week. Leukemia: Induction: 3.3mg/m² with prednisone 60mg/m² qd. Remission Maintenance: 15mg/m² PO/IM twice weekly or 2.5mg/kg IV every 14 days. Burkitt's Tumor: Stages I-II: 10-25mg/day PO for 4-8 days. Administer several courses with rest periods of 7-10 days in between. Lymphosarcoma: Stage III: 0.625-2.5mg/kg/day with other antitumor agents. Mycosis Fungoides: 5-50mg once weekly. If poor response, give 15-37.5mg twice weekly. Adjust dose based on response and hematologic monitoring. Osteosarcoma: Initial: 12g/m² IV, increase to 15g/m² if peak serum levels of 1000 micromolar not reached at end of infusion. Meningeal Leukemia: Dilute preservative free MTX to 1mg/mL. Give 12mg intrathecally at 2-5 day intervals. Psoriasis: Initial: 10-25mg PO/IM/IV weekly until response or use divided oral dose schedule, 2.5mg at 12 hr intervals for 3 doses. Titrate: Increase gradually until optimal response. Maint: Reduce to lowest effective dose. Max: 30mg/week. Rheumatoid Arthritis: Initial: 7.5mg PO once weekly, or 2.5mg q12h for 3 doses given as a course once weekly. Titrate: Gradual increase. Max: 20mg weekly. After response, reduce dose to lowest effective amount of drug.
*Pediatrics:* Meningeal Leukemia: Dilute preservative free MTX to 1mg/mL. <1 yr: 6mg. 1 yr: 8mg. 2 yrs: 10mg. ≥3yrs: 12mg. Give intrathecally at 2-5 day intervals. JRA: 2-16 yrs: Initial: 10mg/m² once weekly. Adjust dose gradually to achieve optimal response.

**HOW SUPPLIED:** Inj: (Generic) (Methotrexate Sodium) 25mg/mL, 1g; Tab: (Generic) (Methotrexate) 2.5mg*; Tab: (Rheumatrex) (Methotrexate) 2.5mg* [Dose Pack 15mg, 4 x 6 tabs; 12.5mg, 4 x 5 tabs; 10mg, 4 x 4 tabs; 7.5mg, 4 x 3 tabs; 5mg, 4 x 2 tabs] *scored

**CONTRAINDICATIONS:** Pregnant women with psoriasis or RA (should be used in treatment of pregnant women with neoplastic diseases only when potential benefit outweighs risk), nursing mothers. Psoriasis or RA patients with alcoholism, alcoholic liver disease, chronic liver disease, immunodeficiency syndromes, and pre-existing blood dyscrasias (eg, bone marrow hypoplasia, leukopenia, thrombocytopenia, significant anemia).

**WARNINGS/PRECAUTIONS:** Monitor closely; toxicity may be related to dose and frequency of administration. When reactions do occur, doses should be reduced or discontinued and corrective measures should be taken. Avoid pregnancy if either partner is receiving therapy. Avoid intrathecal administration or high-dose therapy. Injection contains benzyl alcohol; avoid use in neonates (<1 month), may cause gasping syndrome.

**ADVERSE REACTIONS:** Ulcerative stomatitis, leukopenia, nausea, abdominal distress, malaise, fatigue, chills, fever, dizziness, decreased resistance to infection, anemia, photosensitivity, rash, pruritus, hepatotoxicity.

**INTERACTIONS:** See Black Box Warning. Avoid NSAIDs with high doses. Caution with nephrotoxic agents (eg, cisplatin), NSAIDs, probenecid, and highly protein bound drugs (eg, sulfonamides, phenytoin, phenylbutazone, salicylates). Oral antibiotics (eg, tetracycline, chloramphenicol) may decrease absorption or interfere with enterohepatic circulation. Penicillins may decrease clearance. Closely monitor with hepatotoxins (eg, azathioprine, retinoids, sulfasalazine). Folic acid may decrease response to MTX. TMP/SMZ may increase bone marrow suppression. May decrease theophylline clearance.

**PREGNANCY:** Category X, contraindicated in nursing.



**MECHANISM OF ACTION:** Dihydrofolic acid reductase inhibitor; interferes with DNA synthesis, repair, and cellular replication. MOA in rheumatoid arthritis not established; may affect immune function.

**PHARMACOKINETICS:** Absorption: (PO, Healthy) $T_{max}$=1-2 hrs. (IM) $T_{max}$=30-60 min. Oral administration resulted in different parameters according to disease state and dosing; refer to PI for further information. **Distribution:** (IV, Initial) $V_d$=0.18L/kg; (Steady state) $V_d$=0.4-0.8L/kg; plasma protein binding (50%); found in breast milk. **Metabolism:** Hepatic and intracellular; 7-hydroxymethotrexate (metabolite). **Elimination:** Renal (primary route), bile (≤10%). (Psoriasis, rheumatoid arthritis, low-dose chemotherapy at <30mg/m$^2$) $T_{1/2}$=3-10 hrs; (High dose) $T_{1/2}$=8-15 hrs.

## NURSING CONSIDERATIONS

**Assessment:** Assess pregnancy/nursing status, alcoholism, alcoholic or other chronic liver disease, immunodeficiency, active infection, blood dyscrasias (eg, bone marrow hypoplasia, leukopenia, thrombocytopenia), impaired renal function, ascites, pleural effusions, debility, and possible drug interactions. Obtain baseline CBC with differential and platelet counts, hepatic enzymes, renal function tests, and chest X-ray.

**Monitoring:** Monitor for signs/symptoms of bone marrow suppression, hematological effects, GI toxicity (eg, vomiting, diarrhea, stomatitis), hepatotoxicity, fibrosis, cirrhosis, lung disease (eg, dry, nonproductive cough), malignant lymphomas, opportunistic infections, neurotoxicity (eg, seizures, leukoencephalopathy), nephrotoxicity, and skin reactions (eg, toxic epidermal necrolysis, Stevens-Johnson syndrome). Monitor for tumor lysis syndrome in patients with rapidly growing tumors. If given concomitantly with radiotherapy, monitor for soft-tissue necrosis and osteonecrosis. For psoriasis treatment, monitor CBC with differential and platelet counts monthly; renal/liver functions every 1-2 months. Perform more frequent monitoring of lab parameters during antineoplastic therapy. If drug-induced lung disease is suspected, perform pulmonary function tests. For psoriatic patients on long-term therapy, perform periodic liver biopsies.

**Patient Counseling:** Counsel about risks/benefits of therapy, effects on reproduction in both males and females. Advise about early signs/symptoms of toxicity; contact physician immediately. Periodic laboratory tests necessary during therapy. If taking oral dose for rheumatoid arthritis or psoriasis, dose is taken weekly.

**Administration:** Oral, IM, IV, intra-arterial, or intrathecal route. **Storage:** Tablet: 20-25°C (68-77°F); excursions permitted to 15-30°C (59-86°F), protect from light. Injection: 15-30°C (59-86°F), protect from light.

## METHYLDOPA RX

methyldopa (Various)

**THERAPEUTIC CLASS:** Central alpha-adrenergic agonist

**INDICATIONS:** Treatment of hypertension.

**DOSAGE:** *Adults:* Initial: 250mg bid-tid for 48 hrs. Adjust dose at intervals of not less than 2 days. Maint: 500mg-2g/day given bid-qid. Max: 3g/day. Concomitant Antihypertensives (other than thiazides): Initial: Limit to 500mg/day. Renal Impairment: May respond to lower doses.
*Pediatrics:* Initial: 10mg/kg/day given bid-qid. Max: 65mg/kg/day or 3g/day, whichever is less.

**HOW SUPPLIED:** Tab: 125mg, 250mg, 500mg

**CONTRAINDICATIONS:** Active hepatic disease, history of methyldopa associated liver disorder, concomitant MAOIs.

**WARNINGS/PRECAUTIONS:** Positive Coombs' test, hemolytic anemia, and liver disorders may occur. Fever reported within the first 3 weeks of therapy. HTN has recurred after dialysis. Caution with liver disease or dysfunction. D/C if signs of heart failure, or involuntary choreoathetotic movements develop. Edema and wt gain reported. Blood count, Coombs' test and LFTs prior to therapy and periodically thereafter.

**ADVERSE REACTIONS:** Sedation, headache, asthenia, edema/wt gain, hepatic disorders, vomiting, diarrhea, nausea, sore or "black" tongue, blood dyscrasias, BUN increase, gynecomastia, impotence.

**INTERACTIONS:** See Contraindications. May potentiate other antihypertensives. Anesthetics may need dose reduction. Monitor for lithium toxicity. Ferrous sulfate and ferrous gluconate may decrease bioavailability; avoid coadministration.

**PREGNANCY:** Category B, caution in nursing.

**MECHANISM OF ACTION:** Aromatic-aminoacid decarboxylase inhibitor; not established, antihypertensive effect probably due to metabolism to α-methylnorepinephrine, which lowers arterial pressure by stimulation of central inhibitory α-adrenergic receptors, false neurotransmission, and reduction of plasma renin activity.

**PHARMACOKINETICS: Distribution:** Crosses placenta, found in breast milk. **Metabolism:** Extensive. **Elimination:** Urine; $T_{1/2}$=105 min.

### NURSING CONSIDERATIONS

**Assessment:** Assess for active hepatic disease (eg, acute hepatitis, active cirrhosis), other liver disorders, pheochromocytoma, severe bilateral cerebrovascular disease, and possible drug interactions. Obtain baseline blood count (Hct, Hgb, RBC), direct Coombs' test, and LFTs.

**Monitoring:** Monitor LFTs for 1st 6-12 weeks of therapy or if unexplained fever occurs; direct Coombs' test at 6 and 12 months after therapy, and blood count periodically. Monitor for signs/symptoms of hemolytic anemia, progressive edema, heart failure, hypersensitivity reactions, and hepatic dysfunction.

**Patient Counseling:** Advise to seek medical attention if symptoms of hemolytic anemia, progressive edema, heart failure, hypersensitivity reactions, or hepatic dysfunction occurs.

**Administration:** Oral route. **Storage:** 20-25°C (68-77°F). Protect from light.

# Methyldopa/HCTZ RX

methyldopa - hydrochlorothiazide (Various)

**Not for initial therapy of HTN.**

**THERAPEUTIC CLASS:** Central alpha-adrenergic agonist/thiazide diuretic

**INDICATIONS:** Treatment of HTN. Not for initial treatment.

**DOSAGE:** *Adults:* Initial: 250mg-15mg tab bid-tid, 250mg-25mg tab bid, or 500mg-30mg qd. Max: 50mg HCTZ/day or 3g methyldopa/day.

**HOW SUPPLIED:** Tab: (HCTZ-Methyldopa) 15mg-250mg, 25mg-250mg

**CONTRAINDICATIONS:** Active hepatic disease, anuria, sulfonamide allergy, concomitant MAOIs, history of methyldopa associated liver disorder.

**WARNINGS/PRECAUTIONS:** Positive Coombs' test, hemolytic anemia, liver disorders, sensitivity reactions, hypokalemia, hyperuricemia, hyperglycemia, hypomagnesemia, hypercalcemia may occur. Fever reported within first 3 weeks of therapy. HTN has recurred after dialysis. Caution with liver disease or dysfunction, severe renal disease. D/C if signs of heart failure, progressive renal dysfunction, or involuntary choreoathetotic movements develop. Edema and wt gain reported. Blood count, Coombs' test, and LFTs before therapy and periodically thereafter. Monitor electrolytes. May exacerbate or activate SLE. May increase cholesterol and TG levels. Enhanced effects in postsympathectomy patient.

**ADVERSE REACTIONS:** Weakness, asthenia, headache, pancreatitis, diarrhea, NV, constipation, blood dyscrasias, rash, electrolyte imbalance, renal failure, impotence, vertigo.

**INTERACTIONS:** See Contraindications. Potentiates orthostatic hypotension with alcohol, barbiturates, narcotics. Lithium toxicity. Adjust antidiabetic drugs. NSAIDs decrease diuretic effects. Reduce dose of anesthetics. Ferrous sulfate and ferrous gluconate may decrease bioavailability; avoid coadministration. May potentiate nondepolarizing skeletal muscle relaxants, antihypertensives. May decrease response to pressor amines. Corticosteroids, ACTH intensify electrolyte depletion. Impaired absorption with cholestyramine, colestipol.

**PREGNANCY:** Category C, not for use in nursing.

**MECHANISM OF ACTION:** Methyldopa: Central α-adrenergic agonist. Aromatic-amino-acid decarboxylase inhibitor; lowers arterial pressure by stimulating central inhibitory α-adrenergic receptor, false neurotransmission, and/or reduction of plasma renin activity. HCTZ: Thiazide diuretic; affects renal tubular mechanism of electrolyte reabsorption, directly increasing excretion of sodium salt and chloride.

**PHARMACOKINETICS: Distribution:** Methyldopa: Crosses placental barrier, appears in breast milk and cord blood. HCTZ: Crosses placenta, excreted in breast milk. **Metabolism:** Methyldopa: Extensive. **Elimination:** Methyldopa: Urine (70%); $T_{1/2}$=105 min; HCTZ: Urine (61% unchanged); $T_{1/2}$=5.6-14.8 hrs.

## NURSING CONSIDERATIONS

**Assessment:** Assess LFTs, renal functions, CBC with platelet and differential count, Coombs' test, PT time, serum electrolytes. Assess for sulfite allergy, SLE, pregnancy status, bronchial asthma, and possible drug interactions.

**Monitoring:** Monitor BP, Hct, serum electrolytes, LFTs, bilirubin, PT time, Coombs' test, CBC with differential, BUN, lipid profile. Monitor for arrhythmias, pancreatitis, aggravation of angina, CHF, orthostatic hypotension, hyperprolactinemia, hyperuricemia, hyperglycemia, renal function, bone marrow depression, hypersensitivity (myocarditis, pericarditis, vasculitis), toxic epidermal necrolysis, xanthopsia.

**Patient Counseling:** Instruct that fixed combination drug not indicated for initial therapy of HTN and patient re-evaluation required as conditions warrant. Advise to contact physician if any adverse events occur.

**Administration:** Oral route. **Storage:** 15-30°C (59-86°F). Protect from light, moisture, freezing -20°C (-4°F). Keep container tightly closed.

## METHYLIN

CII

methylphenidate HCl (Mallinckrodt)

**OTHER BRAND NAMES:** Methylin ER (Mallinckrodt)

**THERAPEUTIC CLASS:** Sympathomimetic amine

**INDICATIONS:** Treatment of attention deficit disorder (ADHD) and narcolepsy.

**DOSAGE:** *Adults:* (Sol/Tab/Tab, Chewable) 10-60mg/day given bid-tid 30-45 min ac. Take last dose before 6 pm if insomnia occurs. (Tab, Extended-Release) May used in place of immediate-release tabs when 8-hr dose corresponds to titrated 8-hr immediate release dose. Swallow whole; do not chew or crush.
*Pediatrics:* ≥6 yrs: (Sol/Tab/Tab, Chewable) Initial: 5mg bid before breakfast and lunch. Titrate: Increase gradually by 5-10mg weekly. Max: 60mg/day. (Tab, Extended-Release) May be used in place of immediate-release tabs when 8-hr dose corresponds to titrated 8-hr immediate release dose. Swallow whole; do not chew or crush. Reduce dose or d/c if paradoxical aggravation of symptoms occur. D/C if no improvement after appropriate dose adjustment over 1 month.

**HOW SUPPLIED:** Sol: 5mg/5mL [500mL], 10mg/5mL [500mL]; Tab: 5mg, 10mg, 20mg; Tab, Chewable: 2.5mg, 5mg, 10mg; Tab, Extended-Release: 10mg, 20mg

**CONTRAINDICATIONS:** Marked anxiety, tension, and agitation; glaucoma; motor tics or family history or diagnosis of Tourette's syndrome; during or within 14 days of MAOI use. (Methylin ER) Severe hypertension, angina pectoris, cardiac arrhythmias, heart failure, recent myocardial infarction (MI), hyperthyroidism, thyrotoxicosis.

**WARNINGS/PRECAUTIONS:** Give cautiously to patients with a history of drug dependence or alcoholism. Chronic abusive use may lead to marked tolerance and psychological dependence with varying degrees of abnormal behavior. Careful supervision required during withdrawal from abusive use. Monitor growth in children. Not for severe depression or fatigue. May exacerbate symptoms of behavior disturbance or thought disorder in psychotic children. Caution when using stimulants to treat patients with comorbid bipolar disorder because of concern for possible induction of mixed/manic episode in such patients. Stimulants at usual doses can cause treatment emergent psychotic or manic symptoms (eg, hallucinations, delusional thinking, mania) in children and adolescents without prior history of psychotic illness. Aggressive behavior or hostility has been reported in clinical trials and the postmarketing experience of some medications indicated for the treatment of ADHD. May lower seizure threshold, especially in known EEG abnormalities. Monitor during withdrawal. Visual disturbances may occur (rare). Monitor CBC, differential, and platelets with prolonged use. Periodically d/c to assess condition. Sudden death reported in association with CNS stimulant treatment in children and adolescents with pre-existing cardiac abnormalities or problems while sudden death, MI, and stroke are reported in adults. Monitor heart rate and BP. Assess cardiac status before initiating therapy. Avoid with serious structural abnormalities, cardiomyopathy or other serious cardiac problems.

**ADVERSE REACTIONS:** Nervousness, insomnia, hypersensitivity reactions, anorexia, nausea, dizziness, palpitations, headache, dyskinesia, drowsiness, BP and pulse changes, tachycardia, angina, arrhythmia, abdominal pain.

**INTERACTIONS:** May decrease hypotensive effect of guanethidine. Caution with pressor agents. Avoid during or within 14 days of MAOI use. Potentiates anticoagulants, anticonvulsants (eg, phenobarbital, diphenylhydantoin, primidone), phenylbutazone, TCAs (eg, imipramine, clomipramine, desipramine). Caution with $\alpha_2$-agonists (eg, clonidine); serious adverse reactions reported with concurrent use. May decrease the effectiveness of antihypertensives.

**PREGNANCY:** Category C, caution in nursing.

M

**MECHANISM OF ACTION:** CNS stimulant; activates the brain-stem arousal system and cortex to produce its stimulant effect. Blocks the reuptake of norepinephrine and dopamine into the presynaptic neuron and increases release of monoamines into extraneuronal space.

**PHARMACOKINETICS: Absorption:** (20mg, Sol) $C_{max}$=9ng/mL, $T_{max}$=1-2 hrs. **Metabolism:** Deesterification to α-phenyl-piperidine acetic acid. **Elimination:** Urine (90%), $T_{1/2}$=2.7 hrs (sol), 3 hrs (chewable), 2.8 hrs (extended-release).

## NURSING CONSIDERATIONS

**Assessment:** Assess for agitation, history of depression, glaucoma, tics, family history of Tourette's syndrome, cardiovascular status and conditions (eg, severe HTN, angina pectoris, cardiac arrhythmias, heart failure, recent MI), hyperthyroidism or thyrotoxicosis, bipolar illness, history of drug dependence or alcoholism.

**Monitoring:** Monitor BP, cardiac abnormalities, exacerbations of behavior disturbances and thought disorders, bipolar illness, aggression, seizures, and visual disturbances. Periodic monitoring of CBC, differential and platelet count, and LFTs. Height and weight follow-up in children.

**Patient Counseling:** Inform about risks of treatment, its appropriate use, drug abuse/dependence. Inform to take last dose before 6pm to avoid insomnia. Advise not to take chewable tablets if having difficulty swallowing. Seek medical attention if chest pain, vomiting, or difficulty swallowing or breathing occur. Swallow ER tablets whole; never crush or chew. Advise to notify physician if new or worsening mental symptoms or problems occur.

**Administration:** Oral route. **Storage:** 20-25°C (68-77°F).

M

# METOCLOPRAMIDE RX

metoclopramide HCl (Various)

**D/C if signs/symptoms of tardive dyskinesia develop; avoid ≥12 weeks of therapy.**

**OTHER BRAND NAMES:** Reglan (Alaven) - Reglan Injection (Baxter) - Metozolv ODT (Salix)

**THERAPEUTIC CLASS:** Dopamine antagonist/prokinetic

**INDICATIONS:** (PO) Symptomatic treatment of gastroesophageal reflux disease (GERD) in patients who fail to respond to conventional therapy. (Inj, PO) Symptomatic relief of diabetic gastroparesis. (Inj) Prevention of post-op or chemo-induced nausea/vomiting. Diagnostic aid during radiological examination and facilitates intubation of small intestine.

**DOSAGE:** *Adults:* GERD: 10-15mg PO qid 30 min ac and hs. Elderly: 5 mg qid. Max: 12 weeks of therapy. Intermittent Symptoms: Up to 20mg as single dose prior to provoking situation. Gastroparesis: 10mg PO qid30 min ac and hs for 2-8 weeks. Diabetic Gastroparesis: May give same doses IV/IM over 1-2 mins for up to 10 days if needed. Antiemetic: (Post-op) 10-20mg IM near end of surgery. (Chemotherapy-Induced) 1-2mg/kg 30 min before chemotherapy then q2h for 2 doses, then q3h for 3 doses. Give 2mg/kg for highly emetogenic drugs for initial 2 doses. Small Bowel Intubation/Radiological Exam: 10mg IV as single dose. CrCl <40mL/min: 50% of normal dose. Elderly: (Inj) Start at the low end of dosing range.

*Pediatrics:* Small Bowel Intubation: >14 yrs: 10 mg IV single dose. 6-14 yrs: 2.5-5mg IV single dose. <6 yrs: 0.1mg/kg IV single dose. CrCl <40mL/min: 50% of normal dose.

**HOW SUPPLIED:** Inj: 5mg/mL; Syr: 5mg/5mL; Tab: 5mg, 10mg* *scored; Tab, Disintegrating: 5mg,10mg

**CONTRAINDICATIONS:** Where GI mobility stimulation is dangerous (eg, perforation, obstruction, hemorrhage), pheochromocytoma, seizure disorder, and concomitant drugs that cause EPS effects (eg, antidepressants, antipsychotics, neuroleptics).

**WARNINGS/PRECAUTIONS:** Caution with HTN, Parkinson's disease, depression and renal impairment. EPS, acute dystonic reactions, tardive dyskinesia

(TD), Parkinsonian-like symptoms, and neuroleptic malignant syndrome (rare) reported. Risk of developing fluid retention and volume overload, especially with cirrhosis or CHF; d/c if these occur. May increase pressure on suture lines. Caution in elderly. D/C if signs/symptoms of tardive dyskinesia develop.

**ADVERSE REACTIONS:** Headache, N/V, fatigue, somnolence, acute dystonic reactions, restlessness, lassitude.

**INTERACTIONS:** See Contraindications. May decrease gastric absorption of drugs (eg, digoxin) and increase intestinal absorption of drugs (eg, APAP, tetracycline, levodopa, ethanol, and cyclosporine). Additive sedation with alcohol, hypnotics, narcotics, or tranquilizers. Caution with MAOIs. Antagonized by anticholinergics and narcotics. Insulin dose or timing of dose may need adjustment to prevent hypoglycemia. Rare cases of hepatotoxicity with drugs with hepatotoxic potential.

**PREGNANCY:** Category B, caution with nursing.

**MECHANISM OF ACTION:** Dopamine antagonist/promotility agent; not established, stimulates motility of upper GI tract, increases tone of gastric contractions, relaxes pyloric sphincter and duodenal bulb, increases peristalsis of duodenum and jejunum resulting in increased gastric emptying and intestinal transit, increases resting tone of LES, antagonizes central and peripheral dopamine receptors blocking stimulation of CTZ.

**PHARMACOKINETICS: Absorption:** Rapid; absolute bioavailability (80%). (Peds) $C_{max}$ at 10th dose=56.8mcg/L, $T_{max}$=2.2 hrs. (Adults) $T_{max}$=1-2 hrs. **Distribution:** Plasma protein binding (30%); (adults)$V_d$=3.5L/kg; (peds) $V_d$ =4.4L/kg. **Elimination:** Urine; (adults) $T_{1/2}$=5-6 hrs, (peds) $T_{1/2}$=4.1 hrs.

## NURSING CONSIDERATIONS

**Assessment:** Assess for GI hemorrhage, mechanical obstruction or perforation, CHF, cirrhosis, pheochromocytoma, depression, Parkinson's disease, TD, epilepsy, hypersensitivity, pregnancy/nursing status, and possible drug interactions.

**Monitoring:** Monitor for signs/symptoms of depression, EPS, NMS, TD, HTN, fluid retention, volume overload, exacerbation of Parkinson's disease, and hypersensitivity reactions.

**Patient Counseling:** Caution while operating machinery/driving. Seek medical attention if symptoms of depression, EPS (involuntary movements of limbs, facial grimacing, torticollis), TD (involuntary movements of tongue, face, mouth), NMS (hyperthermia, muscle rigidity, altered consciousness), HTN, fluid retention, volume overload, or hypersensitivity reactions occur.

**Administration:** Oral, IV/IM route. Administer IV injection slowly (1-2 mins). Refer to PI for IV admixture compatibilities. **Storage:** Tab, Inj, Sol: 20-25°C (68-77°F). Inj: Protect from light. Diluted; stable for 24 hrs. Sol: Protect from freezing.

# METROGEL — RX

metronidazole (Galderma)

**OTHER BRAND NAMES:** MetroCream (Galderma) - MetroLotion (Galderma)

**THERAPEUTIC CLASS:** Imidazole antibiotic

**INDICATIONS:** Treatment of inflammatory papules and pustules of rosacea.

**DOSAGE:** *Adults:* (Cre, Gel 0.75%, Lot) Wash affected area(s) then apply bid, am and pm. (Gel 1%) Wash affected area(s) then apply qd.

**HOW SUPPLIED:** Cre: 0.75% [45g]; Gel: 0.75%, 1% [45g]; Lot: 0.75% [59mL]

**WARNINGS/PRECAUTIONS:** Avoid eye contact. Decrease frequency or d/c if skin irritation occurs. Caution with blood dyscrasias.

**ADVERSE REACTIONS:** Burning, skin irritation, dryness, redness, metallic taste, tingling/numbness of extremities, nausea.

**INTERACTIONS:** Oral metronidazole may potentiate warfarin; unknown effect with topical formulation.

**PREGNANCY:** Category B, not for use in nursing.

**MECHANISM OF ACTION:** Imidazole antibiotic; not established. Suspected to have an anti-inflammatory effect.

**PHARMACOKINETICS: Absorption:** (1g of 1% Gel) $C_{max}$=32ng/mL; $T_{max}$=6-10 hrs; $AUC_{0-24}$=595ng•hr/mL. (1g of 0.75% Lot) $C_{max}$=96ng/mL; $AUC_{0-24}$=962ng•hr/mL.

## NURSING CONSIDERATIONS

**Assessment:** Assess nursing status, use with evidence/history of blood dyscrasias, and for possible drug interactions.

**Monitoring:** Monitor for tearing of eyes and local skin irritation reactions.

**Patient Counseling:** Instruct to use medication exactly as directed (for external use only, avoid contact with eyes, and cleanse affected area(s) before applying). Advise to report adverse reactions, and use less frequently or d/c if local skin irritation develops. May use cosmetics following application.

**Administration:** Topical application only. Wash areas to be treated with mild cleanser before application. **Storage:** 20-25°C (68-77°F).

# MetroGel-Vaginal RX

metronidazole (Graceway)

**THERAPEUTIC CLASS:** Imidazole antibacterial

**INDICATIONS:** Treatment of bacterial vaginosis.

**DOSAGE:** *Adults:* Insert 1 applicatorful intravaginally qd-bid for 5 days. For once daily dosing, administer hs.

**HOW SUPPLIED:** Gel: 0.75% [70g]

**CONTRAINDICATIONS:** Hypersensitivity to other nitroimidazole derivatives.

**WARNINGS/PRECAUTIONS:** Caution with CNS or severe hepatic disease. D/C if abnormal neurologic signs appear. Avoid vaginal intercourse during therapy. May develop *Candida* vaginitis. May interfere with lab tests (ALT, SGPT, AST, SGOT, LDH, triglycerides, and glucose hexokinase).

**ADVERSE REACTIONS:** *Candida* cervicitis/vaginitis, vaginal discharge, pelvic discomfort, nausea, vomiting, headache, vulva/vaginal irritation, GI discomfort, change in WBC count.

**INTERACTIONS:** May potentiate warfarin, other anticoagulants, and lithium. Cimetidine may potentiate metronidazole. Avoid alcohol; possible disulfiram-like reaction may occur. Do not administer gel within 2 weeks of discontinuing disulfiram therapy.

**PREGNANCY:** Category B, not for use in nursing.

**MECHANISM OF ACTION:** Antibacterial/antiprotozoal agent; not established, suspected that 5-nitro group of metronidazole is reduced by metabolically active anaerobes and the reduced form of the drug interacts with bacterial DNA.

**PHARMACOKINETICS: Absorption:** $C_{max}$=237ng/mL; $T_{max}$=6-12 hrs. **Distribution:** Found in breast milk and crosses placental barrier.

## NURSING CONSIDERATIONS

**Assessment:** Assess for hypersensitivity to drug, hepatic impairment, CNS diseases, vaginal candidiasis, alcohol intake, for possible drug/lab test interactions (eg, disulfiram).

**Monitoring:** Monitor for convulsive seizures and peripheral neuropathy, psychotic reactions, disulfiram-like reaction, *Candida* vaginitis, lab tests for AST, ALT, LDH, TG, glucose hexokinase, and WBCs.

**Patient Counseling:** Instruct not to engage in vaginal intercourse or drink alcohol during treatment. Avoid contact with eyes; rinse with cool tap water if occurs.

**Administration:** Intravaginal route. Insert applicator into vagina, push plunger to deposit gel, and then withdraw applicator. **Storage:** 15-30°C (59-86°F). Protect from freezing.

# Mevacor

RX

lovastatin (Merck)

**THERAPEUTIC CLASS:** HMG-CoA reductase inhibitor

**INDICATIONS:** To reduce risk of MI, unstable angina, and coronary revascularization procedures in patients without symptomatic coronary disease, average to moderately elevated total-C and LDL-C, and below average HDL-C. To slow progression of coronary atherosclerosis in patients with coronary heart disease to reduce total-C and LDL-C. Adjunct to diet to lower total-C and LDL-C in primary hypercholesterolemia (Types IIa and IIb). Adjunct to diet to lower total-C, LDL, and Apo B in boys and postmenarchal girls, 10 to 17 years of age, with heterozygous familial hypercholesterolemia.

**DOSAGE:** *Adults:* (For LDL-C reduction of ≥20%) Initial: 20mg qd with evening meal. Titrate: Adjust every 4 weeks. Usual: 10-80mg/day given qd or bid. Max: 80mg/day. (For LDL-C reduction of <20%) Initial: 10mg/day. Concomitant Cyclosporine/Danazol: Initial: 10mg/day. Max: 20mg/day. Concomitant Fibrates/Niacin ( ≥1g/day): Max: 20mg/day. Concomitant Amiodarone/ Verapamil: Max: 40mg/day. CrCl <30mL/min: Caution with doses >20mg/day. *Pediatrics:* 10-17 yrs: Heterozygous Familial Hypercholesterolemia: (For LDL-C reduction of ≥20%) Initial: 20mg qd with evening meal. Titrate: Adjust every 4 weeks. Usual: 10-40mg/day given qd or bid. Max: 40mg/day. (For LDL-C reduction of <20%) Initial: 10mg/day. Concomitant Cyclosporine/Danazol: Initial: 10mg/day. Max: 20mg/day. Concomitant Fibrates/Niacin ( ≥1g/day): Max: 20mg/day. Concomitant Amiodarone/Verapamil: Max: 40mg/day. CrCl <30mL/min: Caution with doses >20mg/day.

**HOW SUPPLIED:** Tab: 20mg, 40mg

**CONTRAINDICATIONS:** Active liver disease, unexplained persistent elevations of serum transaminases, pregnancy, nursing mothers.

M

**WARNINGS/PRECAUTIONS:** May increase serum transaminases and CPK levels; consider in differential diagnosis of chest pain. D/C if AST or ALT ≥3x ULN persists, or if myopathy diagnosed or suspected. Monitor LFTs prior to therapy when appropriate then periodically or with dose elevation. Caution with heavy alcohol use and/or history of hepatic disease. Caution with dose escalation in renal insufficiency. Less effective with homozygous familial hypercholesterolemia. Rhabdomyolysis (rare), myopathy reported. D/C a few days before elective major surgery and when any major acute medical or surgical condition supervenes.

**ADVERSE REACTIONS:** Headache, constipation, flatulence, CK elevations.

**INTERACTIONS:** Increased risk of myopathy with CYP3A4 inhibitors (eg, cyclosporine, itraconazole, ketoconazole, erythromycin, clarithromycin, telithromycin, protease inhibitors, nefazodone, >1 quart/day of grapefruit juice), verapamil, amiodarone, fibrates (eg, gemfibrozil), danazol, and ≥1g/day of niacin. Monitor PT with warfarin-type anticoagulants. Caution with drugs that diminish levels or activity of steroid hormones (eg, ketoconazole, spironolactone, cimetidine).

**PREGNANCY:** Category X, not for use in nursing.

**MECHANISM OF ACTION:** HMG-CoA reductase inhibitor; inhibits conversion of HMG-CoA to mevalonate (precursor of sterols, including cholesterol).

**PHARMACOKINETICS: Absorption:** $T_{max}$=2-4 hrs. **Distribution:** Plasma protein binding (>95%). **Metabolism:** Liver (first pass) via CYP3A4. β-hydroxyacid, 6'-hydroxy derivative (major active metabolites). **Elimination:** Urine (10%), feces (83%).

## NURSING CONSIDERATIONS

**Assessment:** Assess for secondary causes of hypercholesterolemia (eg, poorly controlled DM, hypothyroidism, nephrotoxic syndrome, dysproteinemias, obstructive liver disease, other drug therapy, alcoholism), presence of active liver disease or unexplained elevations of serum transaminases, and pregnancy/ nursing status. Assess lipid profile (total-C, HDL-C, and TG) and LFTs prior to therapy. Assess use in presence of homozygous familial hypercholesterolemia or renal insufficiencies and for possible drug interactions.

**Monitoring:** Monitor for signs/symptoms of myopathy (eg, muscle pain, tenderness, weakness), rhabdomyolysis, elevations of creatine kinase, liver dysfunction, endocrine dysfunction, and CNS toxicity (eg, optic nerve degeneration, CNS vascular lesions). Perform periodic monitoring of cholesterol levels, CK levels, and LFTs (eg, ALT, AST).

**Patient Counseling:** Inform about possible drug interactions and possible interaction with grapefruit juice. Advise to report any signs/symptoms of unexplained muscle pain, tenderness, or weakness immediately. Inform that periodic blood testing is required to evaluate cholesterol levels and liver function. Counsel females about risks of use during pregnancy/nursing.

**Administration:** Oral route. **Storage:** 20-25°C (68-77°F). Protect from light and store in a well-closed, light-resistant container.

## MIACALCIN RX

calcitonin-salmon (Novartis)

**THERAPEUTIC CLASS:** Hormonal bone resorption inhibitor

**INDICATIONS:** (Inj) Treatment of Paget's disease of bone and hypercalcemia. (Inj/Spray) Treatment of postmenopausal osteoporosis in females >5 yrs postmenopause.

**DOSAGE:** *Adults:* (Inj) Paget's Disease: Usual: 100 IU IM/SQ qd. Maint: 50 IU IM/SQ qd or qod. Maintain higher dose with serious deformity and neurological involvement. Hypercalcemia: Initial: 4 IU/kg IM/SQ q12h. Titrate: May increase to 8 IU/kg q12h after 1-2 days, then to 8 IU/kg q6h after 2 days if unsatisfactory response. Postmenopausal Osteoporosis: (Inj) 100 IU IM/SQ qod. If >2mL, use IM injection. (Spray) 200 IU qd intranasally. Alternate nostrils daily. Take with supplemental calcium (1.5g calcium carbonate qd) and vitamin D (400 IU qd) for postmenopausal osteoporosis.

**HOW SUPPLIED:** Inj: 200 IU/mL; Nasal Spray: 200 IU/inh

**WARNINGS/PRECAUTIONS:** Serious allergic-type reactions (eg, bronchospasm, swelling of tongue or throat, anaphylactic shock) reported. May lead to hypocalcemic tetany; provisions for parenteral calcium should be available on the first several administration of calcitonin. Monitor urine sediment periodically with chronic use. (Spray) D/C if severe ulceration (ulcers >1.5mm diameter, penetrating below mucosa or if with heavy bleeding) of the nasal mucosa occurs. Perform periodic nasal exams.

**ADVERSE REACTIONS:** (Inj) N/V, injection-site inflammation, flushing of face or hands, nocturia, ear lobe pruritus, poor appetite, abdominal pain. (Spray) Nasal symptoms, rhinitis, back pain, headache, arthralgia, epistaxis.

**INTERACTIONS:** Concomitant use with lithium may lead to reduced plasma lithium; lithium dose may nee to be adjusted. Prior diphosphonate use with Paget's disease may reduce antiresorptive response.

**PREGNANCY:** Category C, not for use in nursing.

**MECHANISM OF ACTION:** Hormonal bone resorption inhibitor; actions on bone not fully established. Calcitonin receptors have been found in osteoclasts and osteoblasts. Initially causes a marked transient inhibition of the ongoing bone resorptive process. Prolonged use causes a smaller decrease in the rate of bone resorption. Thought to be associated with decrease in number of osteoclasts as well as decrease in resorptive activity.

**PHARMACOKINETICS: Absorption:** (Intranasal): Bioavailability (3-5%), $T_{max}$=13 min; (Inj): Absolute bioavailability (66% IM), (71% SQ), $T_{max}$=23 min (SQ). **Distribution:** $V_d$=0.15-0.3L/kg. **Metabolism:** Kidney, blood, peripheral tissues. **Elimination:** Urine; (Intranasal): $T_{1/2}$=18 mins; (Inj): $T_{1/2}$=58 mins (IM), $T_{1/2}$=59-64 mins (SQ).

## NURSING CONSIDERATIONS

**Assessment:** Assess for hypersensitivity to medication; consider skin testing. Assess pregnancy/nursing status. If using intranasal formulation, obtain baseline nasal exam (eg, visualization of the nasal mucosa, turbinates, septum, and mucosal blood vessel status). If using parenteral formulation and treating osteoporosis, obtain baseline measurement of bone resorption/turnover and bone mineral density.

**Monitoring:** Monitor for signs/symptoms of allergic reaction (eg, bronchospasm, swelling of tongue or throat, anaphylactic shock). Perform periodic exams of urine sediment. If using intranasal formulation, monitor for nasal mucosal alterations, transient nasal conditions, and ulceration of nasal mucosa; perform periodic nasal exams. For intranasal formulation, perform periodic measurements of lumbar vertebral bone. If using parenteral formulation, monitor for hypocalcemic tetany. For parenteral administration in treatment of Paget's disease, perform periodic measurement of serum alkaline phosphatase and 24-hr urinary hydroxyproline. For parenteral administration in treatment of osteoporosis, monitor biochemical markers of bone resorption/turnover and bone mineral density.

**Patient Counseling:** Intranasal formulation: Instruct how to assemble and prime pump, and introduce medication in the nasal passages. Advise to contact physician if allergic reaction or nasal irritation occur. Inform that new, unassembled bottles should be refrigerated and protected from freezing. Allow medication to reach room temperature before priming pump and using a new bottle. Store opened bottle upright at room temperature for up to 35 days. Parenteral formulation: Advise to use sterile injection technique.

**Administration:** Intranasal/IM/SQ routes. **Storage:** (Intranasal) Unopened: 2-8°C (36-46°F). Protect from freezing. Used: 15-30°C (59-86°F) in upright position for up to 35 days. (Inj) 2-8°C (36-46°F).

M

# MICARDIS — RX

telmisartan (Boehringer Ingelheim)

**Drugs that act directly on renin-angiotensin system may cause death/injury to the developing fetus when used in pregnancy. D/C immediately if pregnancy is detected.**

**THERAPEUTIC CLASS:** Angiotensin II receptor antagonist

**INDICATIONS:** Treatment of HTN, alone or with other antihypertensives. Reduction of risk of myocardial infarction (MI), stroke, or death from cardiovascular causes in patients ≥55 yrs who are unable to take ACE inhibitors.

**DOSAGE:** *Adults:* HTN: Initial: 40mg qd. Usual: 20-80mg/day. May add diuretic if additional BP reduction is desired. Cardiovascular Risk Reduction: 80mg qd. Monitor BP and adjust dose of medications that lower BP if needed.

**HOW SUPPLIED:** Tab: 20mg, 40mg, 80mg

**WARNINGS/PRECAUTIONS:** May cause fetal/neonatal injury (including hypotension, skull hypoplasia, anuria, renal failure, oligohydramnios). Correct volume or salt depletion before therapy; hypotension may occur in volume- and/or salt-depleted patients. Changes in renal function may occur. Reduced clearance with biliary obstructive disorders or hepatic insufficiency; use with caution. Hyperkalemia may occur; consider periodic monitoring of serum electrolytes to detect possible imbalances.

**ADVERSE REACTIONS:** Upper respiratory tract infection, back pain, sinusitis, diarrhea, hyperkalemia, MI, headache, dizziness, asthenia, coughing, nausea, fatigue, weakness, edema, urticaria.

**INTERACTIONS:** May increase digoxin levels; monitor digoxin levels during concurrent use. May decrease warfarin levels. May increase lithium levels/toxicity; monitor lithium levels during concurrent use. Increased levels of ramipril/ramiprilat noted during concomitant use, whereas telmisartan levels are decreased; possible additive effects with ramipril. Dual blockade of the renin-angiotensin-aldosterone system with ACE inhibitors.

**PREGNANCY:** Category C (1st trimester) and D (2nd and 3rd trimesters), not for use in nursing.

**MECHANISM OF ACTION:** Angiotensin II receptor antagonist; blocks vasoconstrictor and aldosterone-secreting effects of angiotensin II by selectively blocking the binding of angiotensin II to the $AT_1$ receptor in many tissues, such as vascular smooth muscle and adrenal gland.

**PHARMACOKINETICS: Absorption:** Absolute bioavailability (40mg, 160mg)=42%, 58%; $T_{max}$=0.5-1 hr. **Distribution:** $V_d$=500L; plasma protein binding (>99.5%). **Metabolism:** Conjugation; acyl glucuronide (only metabolite identified in human plasma and urine). **Elimination**: Feces (>97%, unchanged), urine (0.91% [IV administration]; 0.49% [oral administration]); $T_{1/2}$=24 hrs.

## NURSING CONSIDERATIONS

**Assessment:** Assess LFTs, renal function, BP, pregnancy/nursing status, and possible drug interactions.

**Monitoring:** Monitor BP, LFTs, renal function, CBC (with platelet and differential count), serum potassium levels. Monitor for MI, CHF, angioneurotic edema, hypersensitivity reactions, diarrhea, sinusitis.

**Patient Counseling:** Counsel about signs/symptoms of adverse effects, and advise to seek prompt medical attention if any occur. Inform about fetal risks if taken during pregnancy; instruct to report pregnancy immediately if detected.

**Administration:** Oral route. **Storage:** 25°C (77°F); excursions permitted to 15-30°C (59-86°F).

# MICARDIS HCT **RX**

telmisartan - hydrochlorothiazide (Boehringer Ingelheim)

**Can cause death/injury to the fetus during 2nd and 3rd trimesters. D/C immediately if pregnancy is detected.**

**THERAPEUTIC CLASS:** Angiotensin II receptor antagonist/thiazide diuretic

**INDICATIONS:** Treatment of hypertension. Not for initial therapy.

**DOSAGE:** *Adults:* Uncontrolled BP on 80mg Telmisartan, or Uncontrolled BP on 25mg/day of HCTZ, or Controlled BP on 25mg/day of HCTZ But With Decreased Serum $K^+$: Initial: 80mg-12.5mg tab qd. Alternative (For Those With Uncontrolled BP on 25mg/day of HCTZ): Initial: 80mg-25mg tab qd. Titrate/Max: Increase to 160mg-25mg if BP uncontrolled after 2-4 weeks. Biliary Obstruction/Hepatic Insufficiency: Initial: 40mg-12.5mg tab qd; monitor closely.

**HOW SUPPLIED:** Tab: (Telmisartan-HCTZ) 40mg-12.5mg, 80mg-12.5mg, 80mg-25mg

**CONTRAINDICATIONS:** Anuria, sulfonamide hypersensitivity.

**WARNINGS/PRECAUTIONS:** May cause fetal/neonatal injury (eg, hypotension, skull hypoplasia, anuria, renal failure, oligohydramnios). Correct volume or salt depletion before therapy due to risk of hypotension. (HCTZ) Caution with impaired hepatic function, liver disease, and severe renal disease. May exacerbate or activate systemic lupus erythematosus (SLE). Hypersensitivity reactions may occur; more likely with history of allergy or bronchial asthma. Hyponatremia (including dilutional hyponatremia), hypokalemia, hypochloremic alkalosis, hyperuricemia, hyperglycemia, decreased urinary calcium excretion, and increased urinary magnesium excretion may occur; monitor for serum electrolytes. (Telmisartan) Caution with biliary obstructive disorders, and unilateral or bilateral renal artery stenosis. Changes in renal function (including acute renal failure) reported.

**ADVERSE REACTIONS:** Fatigue, influenza-like symptoms, dizziness, diarrhea, sinusitis, upper respiratory tract infection.

**INTERACTIONS:** (HCTZ) Potentiation of orthostatic hypotension with alcohol, barbiturates, or narcotics. Adjust dose of insulin and oral antidiabetic drugs. Additive effect or potentiation with other antihypertensive drugs. Impaired absorption with cholestyramine and colestipol resins. Intensified electrolyte depletion (particularly leading to hypokalemia) with corticosteroids and ACTH. Decreased response to pressor amines (eg, norepinephrine). Increased responsiveness to non-depolarizing skeletal muscle relaxants (eg, tubocurarine). Avoid lithium; risk of toxicity. Reduced diuretic, natriuretic, and antihypertensive effects of diuretics, with NSAIDs. Thiazide-induced hypokalemia may sensitize or exaggerate response of heart to toxic effects of digitalis. (Telmisartan) May increase digoxin levels; monitor digoxin levels. May increase lithium levels/toxicity; avoid concomitant use. Possible additive effects with ramipril. May decrease warfarin levels. Dual blockade of the renin-angiotensin-aldosterone system with ACE inhibitors.

**PREGNANCY:** Category C (1st trimester) and D (2nd and 3rd trimesters), not for use in nursing.

**MECHANISM OF ACTION:** Telmisartan: Angiotensin II receptor antagonist; blocks the vasoconstrictor and aldosterone-secreting effects of angiotensin II by selectively blocking the binding of angiotensin II to the $AT_1$ receptor in vascular smooth muscle and adrenal gland. HCTZ: Thiazide diuretic; affects renal tubular mechanisms of electrolyte reabsorption, directly increasing excretion of sodium salt and chloride in approximately equivalent amounts.

**PHARMACOKINETICS: Absorption:** Telmisartan: $T_{max}$=0.5-1 hr; Absolute bioavailability =42% (40mg), 58% (160mg). **Distribution:** Telmisartan: Plasma protein binding (>99.5%); $V_d$= 500L. **Metabolism:** Telmisartan: Conjugation. **Elimination:** Telmisartan: Feces (>97%), urine (0.91% [IV administration]; 0.49% [oral administration]); $T_{1/2}$=24 hrs. HCTZ: Urine (61%, unchanged); $T_{1/2}$=5.6-14.8 hrs.

## NURSING CONSIDERATIONS

**Assessment:** Assess LFTs, renal function, BP, SLE, asthma, serum electrolytes, cirrhosis, pregnancy/nursing status, and possible drug interactions.

**Monitoring:** Monitor BP, LFTs, renal function, CBC with platelet and differential count, serum electrolytes, hyperuricemia, lipid profile. Monitor for MI, CHF, angioneurotic edema, hypersensitivity reactions, upper respiratory tract infection, diarrhea, sinusitis, pancreatitis, Stevens-Johnson syndrome (SJS), xanthopsia.

**Patient Counseling:** Counsel about the signs and symptoms of potential adverse effects, and advise to seek prompt medical attention if any occur. Inform about fetal risks if taken during pregnancy; instruct to report pregnancy immediately if detected. Instruct to inform physician if lightheadedness occurs, d/c if syncope occurs. Warn against inadequate fluid intake and concurrent vomiting/diarrhea/excessive perspiration. Advise against use of $K^+$ supplements/salt substitutes without consulting physician.

**Administration:** Oral route. **Storage:** 25°C (77°F); excursions permitted to 15-30°C (59-86°F).

# MICRO-K RX

potassium chloride (Ther-Rx)

**THERAPEUTIC CLASS:** $K^+$ supplement

**INDICATIONS:** (For those unable to tolerate liquid or effervescent potassium preparations). Treatment and prevention of hypokalemia with or without metabolic alkalosis. Treatment of digitalis intoxication and hypokalemic familial periodic paralysis.

**DOSAGE:** *Adults:* Prevention: 20mEq/day. Hypokalemia: 40-100mEq/day. Divide dose if >20mEq. Take with meal and full glass of water or liquid. May sprinkle on soft food; swallow without chewing.

**HOW SUPPLIED:** Cap, Extended-Release: 8mEq, 10mEq

**CONTRAINDICATIONS:** Hyperkalemia, esophageal ulceration, delay in GI passage (from structural, pathological, pharmacologic causes), cardiac patients with esophageal compression due to enlarged left atrium.

**WARNINGS/PRECAUTIONS:** Potentially fatal hyperkalemia may occur. Extreme caution with acidosis, cardiac and renal disease; monitor ECG and electrolytes. Hypokalemia with metabolic acidosis should be treated with an alkalinizing potassium salt (eg, potassium bicarbonate, potassium citrate). May produce ulcerative or stenotic GI lesions.

**ADVERSE REACTIONS:** Hyperkalemia, GI effects (obstruction, bleeding, ulceration), NV, abdominal pain, diarrhea.

**INTERACTIONS:** Risk of hyperkalemia with ACE inhibitors (eg, captopril, enalapril), $K^+$-sparing diuretics, and $K^+$ supplements. Contraindicated with anticholinergic agents due to possible delay in tablet passage through GI tract.

**PREGNANCY:** Category C, safe for use in nursing.

**MECHANISM OF ACTION:** $K^+$ supplement; helps in maintenance of intracellular tonicity, transmission of nerve impulses, contraction of cardiac, skeletal, and smooth muscle, and maintenance of normal renal function.

## NURSING CONSIDERATIONS

**Assessment:** Assess for conditions that impair excretion of $K^+$, hyperkalemia, esophageal compression due to enlarged left atrium, conditions causing arrest or delay in passage through GI, renal insufficiency, DM, and possible drug interactions.

**Monitoring:** Monitor serum $K^+$ levels regularly; renal function, ECG, and acid-base balance. Monitor for GI ulceration/obstruction/perforation, hyperkalemia, renal dysfunction, and hypersensitivity reactions.

**Patient Counseling:** Instruct to take with meals; swallow with full glass of water or other suitable liquid. Do not crush, chew, or suck. Seek medical attention if symptoms of GI ulceration, obstruction, perforation (vomiting, abdominal pain, distention, GI bleeding), hyperkalemia, or hypersensitivity reactions occur.

M

**Administration:** Oral route. **Storage:** 20-25°C (68-77°F).

# MICRONASE RX

glyburide (Pharmacia & Upjohn)

**THERAPEUTIC CLASS:** Sulfonylurea (2nd generation)

**INDICATIONS:** Adjunct to diet and exercise, to improve glycemic control in type 2 diabetes mellitus (DM).

**DOSAGE:** *Adults:* Initial: 2.5-5mg qd with breakfast or 1st main meal; give 1.25mg if sensitive to hypoglycemia. Titrate: Increase by no more than 2.5mg/day at weekly intervals. Maint: 1.25-20mg given qd or in divided doses. Max: 20mg/day. May give bid with >10mg/day. Renal or Hepatic Disease/ Elderly/Debilitated/Malnourished/Adrenal or Pituitary Insufficiency: Initial: 1.25mg qd. Transfer From Other Oral Antidiabetic Agents: Initial: 2.5-5mg/day. Switch From Insulin: If <20 U/day: 2.5-5mg qd. If 20-40 U/day: 5mg qd. If >40 U/day, decrease dose by 50% and give 5mg qd. Titrate: Progressive withdrawal of insulin, and increase by 1.25-2.5mg/day every 2-10 days. Concomitant Metformin: Add glyburide gradually to max dose of metformin monotherapy after 4 weeks if needed.

**HOW SUPPLIED:** Tab: 1.25mg*, 2.5mg*, 5mg* *scored

**CONTRAINDICATIONS:** Diabetic ketoacidosis with or without coma and type 1 DM.

**WARNINGS/PRECAUTIONS:** Increased risk of cardiovascular mortality. Risk of hypoglycemia, especially with renal and hepatic disease, elderly, debilitated or malnourished patients, and those with adrenal or pituitary insufficiency. May need to d/c and give insulin with stress (eg, fever, trauma, infection or surgery). Secondary failure may occur. May cause hemolytic anemia; caution in patients with or without G6PD deficiency and consider a non-sulfonylurea alternative treatment.

**ADVERSE REACTIONS:** Hypoglycemia, nausea, epigastric fullness, heartburn, allergic skin reactions, hepatic porphyria and disulfiram-like reactions (rarely), hyponatremia, liver function abnormalities, photosensitivity reactions, angioedema, arthralgia, myalgia, vasculitis, leukopenia, and agranulocytosis.

**INTERACTIONS:** Hypoglycemia potentiated by alcohol, NSAIDs, miconazole, fluoroquinolones, highly protein-bound drugs, salicylates, sulfonamides, chloramphenicol, probenecid, coumarins, MAOIs, and β-blockers. Risk of hyperglycemia with diuretics, corticosteroids, phenothiazines, thyroid products, estrogens, oral contraceptives, phenytoin, nicotinic acid, sympathomimetics, CCBs, and INH. β-blockers may mask hypoglycemia. Disulfiram-like reactions (rarely) with alcohol.

**PREGNANCY:** Category B, not for use in nursing.

**MECHANISM OF ACTION:** Sulfonylurea; lowers blood glucose acutely by stimulating the release of insulin from the pancreas.

**PHARMACOKINETICS: Absorption:** $T_{max}$=4 hrs. **Distribution:** Serum protein binding (extensive). **Metabolism:** 4-trans-hydroxy derivative (major metabolite), 3-cishydroxy derivative (second metabolite). **Elimination:** Bile (50%), urine (50%); $T_{1/2}$=10 hrs.

## NURSING CONSIDERATIONS

**Assessment:** Assess FPG, $HbA_{1c}$, renal function, LFTs, type 1 DM, ketoacidosis, GI disease, pregnancy status, and possible drug interactions.

**Monitoring:** Monitor hypoglycemia, diabetic ketoacidosis, asthenia, tremors, nervousness, metabolic reactions (eg, SIADH), and dermatologic reactions; FPG, $HbA_{1c}$, renal function tests, LFTs, CBC with differential and platelet count.

**Patient Counseling:** Counsel to take with breakfast or first main meal. Inform about importance of adhering to dietary instructions, regular exercise program, and regular testing of urine and blood glucose. Educate on signs/symptoms of hypoglycemia, its treatment, and predisposing conditions; primary and secondary failure; risks/benefits of therapy.

**Administration:** Oral route. **Storage:** 20-25°C (68-77°F). Dispense in well-closed containers with safety closures.

M

# MICRONOR — RX

norethindrone (Ortho-McNeil)

**OTHER BRAND NAMES:** Errin (Barr) - Camila (Barr)

**THERAPEUTIC CLASS:** Progestogen

**INDICATIONS:** Prevention of pregnancy.

**DOSAGE:** *Adults:* 1 tab qd without interruption (continuous regimen) on 1st day of menstrual period. If fully nursing, start 6 weeks postpartum. If partially nursing, start 3 weeks postpartum.

**HOW SUPPLIED:** Tab: 0.35mg

**CONTRAINDICATIONS:** Pregnancy, breast carcinoma, undiagnosed abnormal genital bleeding, benign or malignant liver tumors, acute liver disease.

**WARNINGS/PRECAUTIONS:** Avoid smoking. Perform annual physical exam. Not for use before menarche. May affect certain endocrine tests (eg, sex hormone binding globulin, thyroxine binding globulin). Monitor glucose tolerance in prediabetics and diabetics. May alter lipid metabolism. May increase risk of breast cancer and hepatic adenomas. May cause irregular menstrual patterns. Delayed follicular atresia/ovarian cysts and ectopic pregnancy may occur. D/C with recurrent migraines or severe headaches.

**ADVERSE REACTIONS:** Menstrual irregularities, frequent or irregular bleeding, headache, breast tenderness, nausea, dizziness, androgenic effects (rare).

**INTERACTIONS:** Reduced efficacy with hepatic enzyme inducers (eg, rifampin, phenytoin, carbamazepine, barbiturates).

**PREGNANCY:** Not for use in pregnancy, caution in nursing.

**MECHANISM OF ACTION:** Progestogen oral contraceptive; suppresses ovulation. Thickens cervical mucus to inhibit sperm penetration, lowers midcycle

LH and FSH peaks, slows movement of ovum through fallopian tubes, and alters endometrium.

**PHARMACOKINETICS: Absorption:** $T_{max}$=2 hrs. **Distribution:** Rapid.

## NURSING CONSIDERATIONS

**Assessment:** Assess for pregnancy, carcinoma of breast, undiagnosed abnormal genital bleeding, benign/malignant liver tumor, and acute liver disease. Assess use in smokers and for possible drug interactions.

**Monitoring:** Monitor for ectopic pregnancy, delayed follicular atresia, ovarian cysts, irregular genital bleeding, and hepatic neoplasias. Perform annual physical exam while on medication. Monitor serum glucose levels with DM and prediabetic patients, lipid levels while on medication, and for onset or exacerbation of migraine or development of severe headaches.

**Patient Counseling:** Counsel about possible adverse effects. Inform that drug does not protect against HIV infection (AIDS) or other STDs. Advise to avoid smoking while on medication. Instruct to take at same time daily. Instruct that if dose missed or taken 3 hrs past scheduled time, use backup form of contraception for next 48 hrs.

**Administration:** Oral route. **Storage:** 25°C (77°F); excursions permitted to 15-30°C (59-86°F). Keep out of reach of children.

# MICROZIDE RX

hydrochlorothiazide (Watson)

M

**THERAPEUTIC CLASS:** Thiazide diuretic

**INDICATIONS:** Management of hypertension.

**DOSAGE:** *Adults:* Initial: 12.5mg qd. Max: 50mg/day.

**HOW SUPPLIED:** Cap: 12.5mg

**CONTRAINDICATIONS:** Anuria, sulfonamide hypersensitivity.

**WARNINGS/PRECAUTIONS:** Caution in severe renal disease, liver dysfunction, electrolyte/fluid imbalance. Monitor electrolytes. Hyperuricemia, hyperglycemia, hypokalemia, hyponatremia, hypomagnesemia, hypercalcemia may occur. Increases in cholesterol and triglyceride levels reported. May exacerbate SLE. Sensitivity reactions reported. D/C prior to parathyroid test. Enhanced effects in post-sympathectomy patient.

**ADVERSE REACTIONS:** Weakness, hypotension, pancreatitis, jaundice, diarrhea, vomiting, blood dyscrasias, rash, photosensitivity, electrolyte imbalance, impotence.

**INTERACTIONS:** May potentiate orthostatic hypotension with alcohol, barbiturates, narcotics. Adjust antidiabetic drugs. Possible decreased response to pressor amines. Corticosteroids, ACTH increase electrolyte depletion. May potentiate nondepolarizing skeletal muscle relaxants, antihypertensives. Lithium toxicity. NSAIDs decrease effects. Decreased PO absorption with cholestyramine, colestipol.

**PREGNANCY:** Category B, not for use in nursing.

**MECHANISM OF ACTION:** Thiazide diuretic; affects renal tubular mechanism of electrolyte reabsorption, directly increasing excretion of $Na^+$ and $Cl^-$.

**PHARMACOKINETICS: Absorption:** Well absorbed (65-75%); $C_{max}$=70-490ng/mL; $T_{max}$=1-5 hrs. **Distribution:** Plasma protein binding (40-68%). **Elimination:** Urine (unchanged), $T_{1/2}$=6-15 hrs.

## NURSING CONSIDERATIONS

**Assessment:** Assess for anuria, known hypersensitivity to sulfonamide-derived drugs, DM, hypoglycemia, impaired renal/hepatic function, serum electrolytes, parathyroid disease, pregnancy status, and possible drug interactions.

**Monitoring:** Monitor BP, hyperuricemia or acute gout, signs/symptoms of electrolyte imbalance, serum glucose, lipid profile, pancreatitis, Stevens-Johnson syndrome, xanthopsia, impotence.

**Patient Counseling:** Counsel about signs/symptoms of electrolyte imbalance (dryness of mouth, thirst, weakness, lethargy, drowsiness, restlessness, muscle pains or cramps, muscular fatigue, hypotension, oliguria, tachycardia, and GI disturbance such as NV) and advise to seek prompt medical attention.

**Administration:** Oral route. **Storage:** 20-25°C (68-77°F). Protect from light, moisture, freezing -20°C (-4°F). Keep container tightly closed.

## MIDAZOLAM INJECTION — CIV

midazolam HCl (Various)

**Associated with respiratory depression and respiratory arrest especially when used for sedation in noncritical care settings. Use only in hospital or ambulatory care settings that provide continuous monitoring of respiratory and cardiac function. For deeply sedated pediatric patients, a dedicated individual, other than the practitioner performing the procedure should monitor the patient throughout the procedure. The initial IV dose for sedation in normal, healthy adults should not exceed 2.5mg. Lower doses are necessary for older (>60 yrs) patients or debilitated patients and in patients receiving concomitant narcotic or other CNS depressants. Initial and all subsequent doses should always be titrated slowly. Doses for pediatrics must be calculated on a mg/kg basis. Do not administer by rapid injection to neonates.**

**THERAPEUTIC CLASS:** Benzodiazepine

**INDICATIONS:** For sedation, anxiolysis, and amnesia induction pre-op, prior to or during diagnostic, therapeutic, or endoscopic procedures, either alone or in combination with other CNS depressants. For induction of general anesthesia. For sedation of intubated and ventilated patients.

**DOSAGE:** *Adults:* Sedation/Anxiolysis/Amnesia Induction: <60 yrs: Initial: 1-2.5mg IV over 2 min. Titrate: In small increments at 2 min intervals if needed. Max: 5mg IV. Concomitant Narcotics/Other CNS Depressants: Reduce dose by 30%. ≥60 yrs/Debilitated/Chronically Ill: Initial: 1-1.5mg IV over 2 min. Titrate: In small increments at 2-min intervals if needed. Max: 3.5mg IV. Concomitant Narcotics/Other CNS Depressants: Reduce dose by 50%. Maint: 25% of sedation dose by slow titration. Preoperative Sedation/Anxiolysis/Amnesia: <60 yrs: 0.07-0.08mg/kg IM up to 1 hr before surgery. ≥60 yrs/Debilitated: 1-3mg IM. Anesthesia Induction: Unpremedicated: <55 yrs: Initially: 0.3-0.35mg/kg IV over 20-30 seconds. May give additional doses of 25% of initial dose to complete induction. ≥55 yrs: Initial: 0.3mg/kg IV. Debilitated: Initial: 0.15-0.25mg/kg IV. Premedicated: <55 yrs: Initial: 0.25mg/kg IV over 20-30 seconds. ≥55 yrs: Initial: 0.2mg/kg IV. Debilitated: 0.15mg/kg IV. Continuous Infusion: LD: 0.01-0.05mg/kg IV. May repeat dose at 10-15 min intervals until adequate sedation is achieved. Maint: 0.02-0.1mg/kg/hr. Infusion rate should be adjusted up or down by 25-50% of the initial infusion rate so as to assure adequate titration of sedation level. Infusion rate should be decreased 10-25% every few hrs to find minimum effective infusion rate.
*Pediatrics:* Sedation/Anxiolysis/Amnesia Induction: IV by Intermittent Inj: <6 months: Limited information; titrate with small increments and monitor. 6 months-5 yrs: Initial: 0.05-0.1mg/kg IV over 2-3 min, up to 0.6mg/kg IV if needed. Max: 6mg IV. 6-12 yrs: Initial: 0.025-0.05mg/kg IV over 2-3 min, up to 0.4mg/kg IV if needed. Max: 10mg IV. 12-16 yrs: Should be dosed as adults. Max: 10mg IV. Continuous Infusion for Sedation/Anxiolysis/Amnesia in Critical Care Settings: LD: 0.05-0.2mg/kg IV over 2-3 min. Maint: 0.06-0.12mg/kg/hr IV. May adjust dose by 25%. Continuous IV Infusion for Sedation in Critical Care: Neonatal Dose: <32 weeks: Initial: 0.03mg/kg/hr IV. >32 weeks: Initial: 0.06mg/kg/hr IV. Adjust to lowest effective dose. IM (Non-Neonatal) Preoperative Sedation/Anxiolysis/Amnesia: 0.1-0.15mg/kg IM, up to 0.5mg/kg IM if needed. Max: 10mg IM.

**HOW SUPPLIED:** Inj: 1mg/mL, 5mg/mL

**CONTRAINDICATIONS:** Acute narrow-angle glaucoma, untreated open-angle glaucoma, intrathecal or epidural use.

M

**WARNINGS/PRECAUTIONS:** Must never be used without individualization of dosage. Agitation, involuntary movements, hyperactivity, and combativeness reported. Caution with CHF, chronic renal failure, pulmonary disease, uncompensated acute illnesses (eg, severe fluid or electrolyte disturbances), and in elderly or debilitated. Pediatric and adult patients undergoing procedures involving the upper airway are particularly vulnerable to episodes of desaturation and hypoventilation. Avoid use with shock or coma, or in acute alcohol intoxication with depression of vital signs. Precautions against unintended intra-arterial injection should be taken. Administer IM or IV only. Should not operate hazardous machinery or a motor vehicle until effects of drug have subsided or until one full day after anesthesia or surgery, whichever is longer. May increase risk of congenital malformations and cause withdrawal symptoms in infants if used during pregnancy. Neonates may be vulnerable to profound and/or prolonged respiratory effects. Contains benzyl alcohol. Does not protect against the increase in intracranial pressure or against the HR rise and/or BP rise associated with endotracheal intubation under light anesthesia.

**ADVERSE REACTIONS:** Decreased tidal volume and/or respiratory rate, BP/HR variations, desaturation, local effects at injection site, apnea, hiccoughs.

**INTERACTIONS:** Prolonged sedation with CYP3A4 inhibitors (eg, erythromycin, diltiazem, verapamil, ketoconazole, itraconazole, cimetidine). Increased sedative effects with morphine, meperidine, fentanyl, secobarbital, droperidol, or other CNS depressants. May require a moderate reduction in induction dosage requirements of thiopental when used concomitantly with IM midazolam. IV midazolam may decrease the minimum alveolar concentration (MAC) of halothane required for general anesthesia. May cause severe hypotension with concomitant use of fentanyl in neonates. Concomitant use of barbiturates, alcohol, or other CNS depressants may increase the risk of hypoventilation, airway obstruction, desaturation, or apnea and may contribute to profound and/or prolonged drug effect. Narcotic premedication depresses the ventilatory response to carbon dioxide stimulation.

M

**PREGNANCY:** Category D, caution in nursing.

**MECHANISM OF ACTION:** Benzodiazepine; short-acting CNS depressant.

**PHARMACOKINETICS: Absorption:** (IM) Absolute bioavailability (>90%), $C_{max}$=90ng/mL, $T_{max}$=0.5 hr. (1-hydroxy-midazolam) $C_{max}$=8 ng/ml, $T_{max}$=1 hr. **Distribution:** Crosses placenta, found in breast milk and CSF. $V_d$=1.0-3.1L/kg; plasma protein binding (97%). **Metabolism:** Liver via CYP450-3A4;1-hydroxy-midazolam (major metabolite). **Elimination:** Urine; (0.5% unchanged, 45%-57% as 4-hydroxy-midazolam); $T_{1/2}$= 3 hrs.

## NURSING CONSIDERATIONS

**Assessment:** Assess for acute narrow angle glaucoma, untreated open-angle glaucoma, COPD, renal/hepatic impairment, CHF, shock, presence of a comatose state, uncompensated acute illnesses (eg, fluid or electrolyte disturbances), pregnancy/nursing status, and for possible drug interactions.

**Monitoring:** Monitor for signs/symptoms of cardiorespiratory complications (eg, respiratory depression, airway obstruction, oxygen desaturation, apnea, respiratory arrest, cardiac arrest), hypotension, agitation, involuntary movements, hyperactivity, and for combativeness. Monitor vital signs.

**Patient Counseling:** Advise of possible effects that medication may produce including sedation and amnesia. Inform that patient must use caution when engaging in activities requiring mental alertness (eg, driving, operating heavy machinery). Instruct to inform physician about any alcohol consumption and all medications currently taking. Counsel to notify physician if pregnant, planning to become pregnant, or if nursing. Advise that if receiving therapy over an extended period of time, may experience symptoms of withdrawl if abruptly d/c therapy.

**Administration:** IM/IV route. **Storage:** 20-25°C (68-77°F); excursions permitted to 59°-86°F.

## MIDRIN

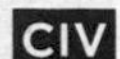


isometheptene mucate - dichloralphenazone - acetaminophen (Women First)

**OTHER BRAND NAMES:** Amidrine (Amide) - Duradrin (Duramed) - Migquin (Qualitest) - Migrazone (Various)

**THERAPEUTIC CLASS:** Analgesic/sedative/sympathomimetic

**INDICATIONS:** Relief of tension and vascular headaches. FDA has classified this agent as "possibly" effective in the treatment of migraine headache.

**DOSAGE:** *Adults:* Migraine: 2 caps, then 1 cap every hr until relieved. Max: 5 caps/12hrs. Tension Headache: 1-2 caps q4h. Max: 8 caps/day.

**HOW SUPPLIED:** Cap: (APAP-Dichloralphenazone-Isometheptene) 325mg-100mg-65mg

**CONTRAINDICATIONS:** Glaucoma, severe renal disease, HTN, organic heart disease, hepatic disease, concomitant MAOI therapy.

**WARNINGS/PRECAUTIONS:** Caution with HTN, peripheral vascular disease, or recent cardiovascular attacks.

**ADVERSE REACTIONS:** Transient dizziness, skin rash.

**PREGNANCY:** Safety in pregnancy and nursing are not known.

**MECHANISM OF ACTION:** Isometheptene: Sympathomimetic amine; acts by constricting dilated cranial and cerebral arterioles, reducing stimuli. Dichloralphenazone: Mild sedative; reduces emotional reaction to pain. Acetaminophen: Non-salicylate; raises threshold to painful stimuli exerting analgesic effect.

### NURSING CONSIDERATIONS

**Assessment:** Assess for glaucoma, severe renal disease, HTN, organic heart disease, peripheral vascular disease, recent cardiovascular attack, hepatic disease, and possible drug interactions.

**Monitoring:** Monitor for hypersensitivity reaction.

**Patient Counseling:** Advise to reduce dose if hypersensitivity reaction (transient dizziness, skin rash) occurs.

**Administration:** Oral route. **Storage:** 15-30°C (59-86°F); protect from light and moisture.

## MIGRANAL

RX

dihydroergotamine mesylate (Valeant)

**Serious and life-threatening peripheral ischemia reported with potent CYP3A4 inhibitors (eg, protease inhibitors, macrolides). Elevated levels of dihydroergotamine increases risk of vasospasm leading to cerebral ischemia or ischemia of the extremities. Concomitant use with CYP3A4 inhibitors is contraindicated.**

**THERAPEUTIC CLASS:** Ergot alkaloid

**INDICATIONS:** Acute treatment of migraine headache with or without aura.

**DOSAGE:** *Adults:* 1 spray per nostril, repeat in 15 min. Max: 6 sprays/24 hrs or 8 sprays/week.

**HOW SUPPLIED:** Nasal Spray: 0.5mg/spray [3.5mL]

**CONTRAINDICATIONS:** Ischemic heart disease (angina, history of MI, documented silent ischemia), coronary artery vasospasm (Prinzmetal's variant angina), uncontrolled HTN, known peripheral artery disease, sepsis, following vascular surgery, severe renal or hepatic dysfunction, hemiplegic or basilar migraine, pregnancy or nursing, with potent CYP3A4 inhibitors (eg, ritonavir, nelfinavir, indinavir, erythromycin, clarithromycin, troleandomycin, ketoconazole, itraconazole). Do not use with peripheral and central vasoconstrictors or within 24 hrs of 5-$HT_1$ agonists, ergot-type drugs, or methysergide.

**WARNINGS/PRECAUTIONS:** Confirm diagnosis. Monitor and consider ECG with 1st dose in patients with CAD risk factors (eg, HTN, hypercholesterolemia, smoker, obesity, DM, strong family history, postmenopausal women, men >40 yrs). Risk of elevated BP, MI, and other adverse cardiac or vasospastic effects. Monitor cardiovascular function with intermittent long-term use. Fibrotic complications (eg, pleural and retroperitoneal fibrosis) reported.

**ADVERSE REACTIONS:** Rhinitis, altered taste, application-site reactions, dizziness, N/V, pharyngitis, somnolence.

**INTERACTIONS:** Potentiated BP elevation with peripheral and central vasoconstrictors. Additive coronary vasospastic effect with sumatriptan; avoid within 24 hrs of each other. Propranolol and nicotine may potentiate the vasoconstrictive action. Increased plasma levels and peripheral vasoconstriction with macrolides. Contraindicated with CYP3A4 inhibitors (eg, macrolides, protease inhibitors). Caution with less potent CYP3A4 inhibitors (eg, saquinavir, nefazodone, fluconazole, grapefruit juice, fluoxetine, fluvoxamine, zileuton, clotrimazole).

**PREGNANCY:** Category X, not for use in nursing.

**MECHANISM OF ACTION:** Ergotamine; binds with high affinity to 5-$HT_{1D}$ receptors on intracranial blood vessels, causing vasoconstriction, or activates 5-$HT_{1D}$ receptors on sensory nerve endings of trigeminal system, inhibiting proinflammatory neuropeptide release.

**PHARMACOKINETICS: Absorption:** Bioavailability (32%). **Distribution:** $V_d$=800L; plasma protein binding (93%). **Metabolism:** 8-β-hydroxydihydroergotamine (major metabolite). **Elimination:** Bile (major), urine (2%).

## NURSING CONSIDERATIONS

**Assessment:** Assess for ischemic heart disease (angina pectoris, MI, silent ischemia), coronary artery vasospasm, Prinzmetal's variant angina, CAD or risk factors, HTN, peripheral arterial disease, sepsis, s/p vascular surgery, possible drug interaction, hemiplegic or basilar migraine, renal/hepatic impairment. Obtain baseline cardiac evaluation.

M

**Monitoring:** Perform periodic cardiac evaluations. Monitor for signs/symptoms of vasospasm, vasoconstriction, CV effects, and hypersensitivity reactions.

**Patient Counseling:** Once applicator prepared, discard after 8 hrs. Advise to seek medical attention immediately if numbness or tingling in fingers and toes, muscle pain in arms and legs, weakness in legs, chest pain, speeding or slowing of HR, swelling, or itching occur.

**Administration:** Intranasal. Prime (squeeze 4 times) before use. Spray once into each nostril; do not tilt back or sniff through nose while spraying or immediately after; wait 15 min; spray once again into each nostril. **Storage:** Below 25°C (77°F). Do not refrigerate, freeze, or keep opened vial for more than 8 hrs. Keep away from heat and light.

# MINIPRESS — RX

prazosin HCl (Pfizer)

**THERAPEUTIC CLASS:** $Alpha_1$-blocker (quinazoline)

**INDICATIONS:** Treatment of hypertension either alone or in combination with other antihypertensive drugs.

**DOSAGE:** *Adults:* Initial: 1mg bid-tid. Titrate: Slowly increase to 20mg/day in divided doses. Maint: 6-15mg qd in divided doses. Max: 40mg/day. Concomitant with Diuretic/Antihypertensive Agent: Reduce to 1-2mg tid, then retitrate.

**HOW SUPPLIED:** Cap: 1mg, 2mg, 5mg

**WARNINGS/PRECAUTIONS:** Syncope with sudden loss of consciousness may occur, usually after initial dose or dose increase; Patient should be placed in the recumbent position and treated with supportive care. Due to excessive postural hypotensive effect, caution to avoid situations where injury could result should syncope occur during initiation of therapy. Always start on 1mg cap. Possible adverse effects (eg, dizziness, lightheadedness) may occur. Intraoperative Floppy Iris Syndrome (IFIS) may occur during cataract surgery. False (+) for pheochromocytoma may occur. D/C with elevated urinary VMA levels and retest after 1 month.

**ADVERSE REACTIONS:** Dizziness, headache, drowsiness, lack of energy, weakness, palpitations, NV, edema, orthostatic hypotension, dyspnea, syncope, depression, urinary frequency, diarrhea, and blurred vision.

**INTERACTIONS:** Additive hypotensive effects with diuretics, PDE5 inhibitors, β-blockers, or other antihypertensives. Dizziness or syncope may occur with alcohol.

**PREGNANCY:** Category C, caution in nursing.

**MECHANISM OF ACTION:** $\alpha_1$ blocker, quinazoline derivative; not established. Blocks the postsynaptic α-adrenoreceptors resulting in vasodilation and reduction in total peripheral resistance.

**PHARMACOKINETICS: Absorption:** $T_{max}$=3 hrs. **Distribution:** Plasma protein binding (highly bound). Found in breast milk. **Metabolism:** Demethylation and conjugation. **Elimination:** Bile and feces; $T_{1/2}$=2-3 hrs.

## NURSING CONSIDERATIONS

**Assessment:** Assess BP, LFTs, urinary VMA levels, hypersensitivity, pregnancy/nursing status, and for possible drug interactions.

**Monitoring:** Monitor BP, LFTs, HR, urinary VMA levels. Monitor for orthostatic hypotension, edema, epistaxis, lichen planus, angina pectoris and hypersensitivity reactions.

**Patient Counseling:** Inform that dizziness or drowsiness may occur after first dose; avoid driving or performing hazardous tasks for first 24 hrs. Dizziness, lightheadedness or fainting may occur; get up slowly when rising from a lying or sitting position. Instruct to be careful in the amount of alcohol taken. Counsel to use extra care during exercise or hot weather, or if standing for long periods.

**Administration:** Oral route. **Storage:** Below 30°C (86°F)

# MINOXIDIL — RX

minoxidil (Mutual Pharmaceutical Co Inc)

**May cause pericardial effusion, occasionally progressing to tamponade, and may exacerbate angina pectoris. Only for nonresponders to maximum therapeutic doses of two other antihypertensives and a diuretic. Administer under supervision with a β-blocker and diuretic. Monitor in hospital for a decrease in BP in those receiving guanethidine with malignant hypertension.**

**THERAPEUTIC CLASS:** Peripheral vasodilator

**INDICATIONS:** Treatment of hypertension that is symptomatic or associated with target organ damage and is not manageable with maximum therapeutic doses of diuretic plus 2 other antihypertensive drugs.

**DOSAGE:** *Adults:* Initial: 5mg qd. Titrate: Increase daily dose to 10mg, 20mg and then to 40mg in single or divided doses. Usual: 10-40mg/day. Max: 100mg/day. Frequency: Give qd if diastolic BP is reduced to <30mmHg and if reduced to >30mmHg give bid. Give with a diuretic (eg, HCTZ 50mg bid; chlorthalidone 50-100mg qd; furosemide 40mg bid) and a β-blocker (equivalent to propranolol 80-160mg/day) or methyldopa (250-750mg bid starting 24 hrs before therapy) or clonidine (0.1-0.2mg bid). Renal Failure/Dialysis: Reduce dose.

*Pediatrics:* >12 yrs: Initial: 5mg qd. Titrate: Increase daily dose to 10mg, 20mg and then to 40mg in single or divided doses. Usual: 10-40mg/day. Max: 100mg/day. Frequency: Give qd if diastolic BP is reduced to <30mmHg and if reduced to >30mmHg give bid. Give with a diuretic (eg, HCTZ 50mg bid; chlorthalidone 50-100mg qd; furosemide 40mg bid) and a β-blocker (equivalent to propranolol 80-160mg/day) or methyldopa (250-750mg bid starting 24 hrs before therapy) or clonidine (0.1-0.2mg bid). <12 yrs: 0.2mg/kg qd.

Titrate: May increase by 50-100% increments. Usual: 0.25-1mg/kg/day. Max: 50mg/day. Renal Failure/Dialysis: Reduce dose.

**HOW SUPPLIED:** Tab: 2.5mg*, 10mg* *scored

**CONTRAINDICATIONS:** Pheochromocytoma.

**WARNINGS/PRECAUTIONS:** Refractory fluid retention may require d/c of therapy. Monitor for pericardial disorder and consider d/c of minoxidil if pericardial effusion persists. With renal failure or dialysis, reduce dose to prevent renal failure exacerbation and precipitation of cardiac failure. Avoid rapid control with severe HTN. Monitor body weight, fluid and electrolyte balance. Extreme caution with post-MI. Hypersensitivity reactions reported.

**ADVERSE REACTIONS:** Salt and water retention, pericarditis, pericardial effusion, tamponade, hypertrichosis.

**INTERACTIONS:** See BlackBox Warning. Severe orthostatic hypotension with guanethidine.

**PREGNANCY:** Category C, not for use in nursing.

**MECHANISM OF ACTION:** Antihypertensive peripheral vasodilator; reduces systolic and diastolic BP by decreasing peripheral vascular resistance.

**PHARMACOKINETICS: Absorption:** Almost complete (90%); $T_{max}$=1 hr. **Distribution:** Found in breast milk. **Metabolism:** Glucuronide conjugation. **Elimination:** Urine; $T_{1/2}$=4.2 hrs.

## NURSING CONSIDERATIONS

**Assessment:** Assess for hypersensitivity, pheochromocytoma, MI, CHF, BP, pregnancy/nursing status, renal dysfunction, and possible drug interactions.

**Monitoring:** Monitor fluid and electrolyte balance, body weight, HR, BP, pericarditis, cerebrovascular episodes, orthostatic effects, hypertrichosis, Stevens-Johnson syndrome, renal functions, ECG, EKG, chest x-ray, urinalysis, for thrombocytopenia, leukopenia, and N/V. Observe for signs/symptoms of pericardial disorder.



**Patient Counseling:** Instruct to take as directed; do not d/c without consulting physician. Do not skip doses. If dose is missed, wait until time for next dose and continue with regular schedule. Advise to immediately report any adverse effects (eg, N/V, rash, change in HR or body weight, headache, fatigue, breast tenderness, chest pain, dizziness, difficulty breathing). Inform that body hair may grow darker or longer on certain parts of the body within 3-6 weeks from start and will disappear within 1-6 months after completion.

**Administration:** Oral route. **Storage:** 20°-25°C (68°-77°F). Dispense in tight, child-resistant container.

# MiraLax — OTC

polyethylene glycol 3350 (Schering-Plough)

**THERAPEUTIC CLASS:** Osmotic laxative

**INDICATIONS:** Treatment of occasional constipation.

**DOSAGE:** *Adults:* Stir and dissolve 17g in 4-8 oz of beverage and drink qd. Use no more than 7 days.
*Pediatrics:* ≥17 yrs: Stir and dissolve 17g in 4-8 oz of beverage and drink qd. Use no more than 7 days.

**HOW SUPPLIED:** Powder: 17g/dose [119g, 238g]

**WARNINGS/PRECAUTIONS:** Avoid in kidney disease.

# Mirapex — RX

pramipexole dihydrochloride (Boehringer Ingelheim)

**THERAPEUTIC CLASS:** Non-ergot dopamine agonist

**INDICATIONS:** Treatment of signs and symptoms of idiopathic Parkinson's disease. Treatment of moderate-to-severe primary Restless Legs Syndrome (RLS).

**DOSAGE:** *Adults:* Parkinson's: Initial: 0.125mg tid. Titrate: May increase every 5-7 days (eg, Week 2: 0.25mg tid; Week 3: 0.5mg tid; Week 4: 0.75mg tid; Week 5: 1mg tid; Week 6: 1.25mg tid; Week 7: 1.5mg tid). Maint: 0.5-1.5mg tid. Max: 1.5mg tid. CrCl >60mL/min: Initial: 0.125mg tid. Max: 1.5mg tid. CrCl 35-59mL/min: Initial: 0.125mg bid. Max: 1.5mg bid. CrCl 15-34mL/min: Initial: 0.125mg qd. Max: 1.5mg qd. RLS: Initial: 0.125mg once daily, 2-3 hours before bedtime. Titrate: May double dose every 4-7 days up to 0.5mg/day.

**HOW SUPPLIED:** Tab: 0.125mg, 0.25mg*, 0.5mg*, 0.75mg, 1mg*, 1.5mg*
*scored

**WARNINGS/PRECAUTIONS:** Somnolence, symptomatic hypotension, hallucinations and rhabdomyolysis reported. Caution with renal insufficiency. May potentiate dyskinesia. May cause retinal pathology, fibrotic complications, withdrawal-emergent hyperpyrexia and confusion. Consider d/c if significant daytime sleepiness or sudden onset of sleep occurs during daily activities. Cases of pathological gambling, hypersexuality, and compulsive eating reported. Rebound and augmentation in RLS reported. Falling asleep during activities of daily living. Melanoma reported; monitor regularly.

**ADVERSE REACTIONS:** Nausea, dizziness, somnolence, insomnia, constipation, asthenia, hallucinations, vision abnormalities, peripheral edema, arthritis, dry mouth, postural hypotension, chest pain, malaise.

**INTERACTIONS:** Cimetidine, ranitidine, diltiazem, triamterene, verapamil, quinidine, and quinine may decrease clearance. Dopamine antagonists (eg, phenothiazines, butyrophenones, thioxanthenes, metoclopramide) may decrease effects.

**PREGNANCY:** Category C, not for use in nursing.

**MECHANISM OF ACTION:** Non-ergot dopamine agonist; suspected to stimulate dopamine receptors on the striatum.

**PHARMACOKINETICS: Absorption:** Rapid, absolute bioavailability (>90%), $T_{max}$=2 hrs. **Distribution:** $V_d$=500L; plasma protein binding (15%). **Elimination:** Urine (90% unchanged); $T_{1/2}$=12hrs (elderly).

## NURSING CONSIDERATIONS

**Assessment:** Assess for symptomatic hypotension, sleep disorders, renal function test, dyskinesia, retinal exam. Note other diseases/conditions and drug therapies.

**Monitoring:** Monitor BP, renal function test, signs/symptoms of rhabdomyolysis, NMS, melanomas, fibrotic complications, hallucinations, impulse control behaviors/compulsive behaviors.

**Patient Counseling:** Instruct to take with/without food. Caution while operating machinery/driving. Counsel about impulse control disorders/compulsive behaviors; avoid concomitant use of alcohol; report side effects. Notify physician if intense urge to gamble, increased sexual urges, and other intense urges occur.

**Administration:** Oral route. **Storage:** 25°C (77°F); excursions permitted to 15-30°C (59-86°F). Protect from light.

# MIRCETTE RX

desogestrel - ethinyl estradiol (Duramed)

**OTHER BRAND NAMES:** Kariva (Barr)

**THERAPEUTIC CLASS:** Estrogen/progestogen combination

**INDICATIONS:** Prevention of pregnancy.

**DOSAGE:** *Adults:* Start 1st Sunday after menses begin or 1st day of menses. 28-day: 1 tab qd for 28 days, then repeat.

**HOW SUPPLIED:** Tab: (Ethinyl Estradiol-Desogestrel) 0.02mg-0.15mg and 0.01mg-NA

**CONTRAINDICATIONS:** Thrombophlebitis, DVT or thromboembolic disorders, pregnancy, cerebrovascular or coronary artery disease, undiagnosed abnormal genital bleeding, cholestatic jaundice of pregnancy or jaundice with prior pill use, hepatic adenomas or carcinomas, breast cancer or other estrogen-dependent neoplasia.

**WARNINGS/PRECAUTIONS:** Cigarette smoking increases risk of serious cardiovascular side effects. This risk increases with age (especially >35 yrs) and heavy smoking. Increased risk of MI, vascular disease, thromboembolism, stroke and gallbladder disease. Retinal thrombosis, hepatic neoplasia, carcinoma of breast and reproductive organs reported. May cause glucose intolerance. May increase BP, elevate LDL levels or cause other lipid changes, fluid retention, breakthrough bleeding, and spotting. May cause or exacerbate migraine. May develop visual changes with contact lens. Increased risk of MI with HTN, hyperlipidemia, obesity, and diabetes. D/C if jaundice, significant depression, or ophthalmic irregularities develop. Perform annual physical exam. Use before menarche is not indicated. May affect certain endocrine, LFTs and blood components.

**ADVERSE REACTIONS:** NV, breakthrough bleeding, spotting, amenorrhea, migraine, depression, vaginal candidiasis, edema, weight changes.

**INTERACTIONS:** Reduced effects, increased breakthrough bleeding, and menstrual irregularities with rifampin, barbiturates, phenylbutazone, phenytoin, carbamazepine, and possibly with griseofulvin, ampicillin, and tetracyclines.

**PREGNANCY:** Category X, not for use in nursing.

**MECHANISM OF ACTION:** Oral contraceptive combination; supresses gonadotropins, inhibits ovulation, increases difficulty of sperm entry into uterus, and reduces likelihood of implantation by producing changes in cervical mucus and endometrium, respectively.

M

**PHARMACOKINETICS: Absorption:** Desogestrel: Rapid, complete; relative bioavailability (100%). Ethinyl estradiol: Rapid, complete; absolute bioavailability (93-99%). **Distribution:** Desogestrel: Sex hormone-binding globulin (99%, metabolite). Ethinyl estradiol: Plasma protein binding (98.3%). **Metabolism:** Desogestrel: Hydroxylation in intestinal mucosa; etonogestrel (metabolite). Ethinyl estradiol: Conjugation. **Elimination:** Urine, bile, feces. Desogestrel: $T_{1/2}$=27.8 hrs (metabolite). Ethinyl estradiol: $T_{1/2}$=23.9 hrs.

## NURSING CONSIDERATIONS

**Assessment:** Assess for history or recent DVT or thromboembolic disorders, thrombophlebitis, CVD, CAD, breast cancer, endometrium or other estrogen-dependent neoplasia, abnormal genital bleeding, cholestatic jaundice of pregnancy or jaundice with prior pill use, hepatic adenomas or carcinomas, and pregnancy. Obtain complete medical history and physical exam with special reference to BP, breasts, abdomen and pelvic organs, cervical cytology, and relevant lab tests.

**Monitoring:** Monitor for thromboembolic disorders and other vascular problems, malignant neoplasms, MI, stroke, hepatic neoplasia, jaundice, emotional disorders, ocular lesions, gallbladder disease, carbohydrate and lipid metabolic effects, elevated BP, bleeding irregularities, migraine headaches, lipid profile (HDL, LDL, TG), LFTs, PT, TBG, $T_3$ and $T_4$, blood glucose, and serum folate levels.

**Patient Counseling:** Strongly advise not to smoke; increases risk of cardiovascular side effects. Instruct to take daily at same time as directed. Counsel that light bleeding is possible. Inform that drug does not protect against HIV infections/AIDS and other STDs. Caution that some drugs decrease efficacy, and to consult with physician before use to determine appropriate back-up contraceptive method. Advise to immediately report sharp chest pains, coughing of blood, sudden SOB, pain in calf, severe headache and vomiting, dizziness or fainting, disturbances of vision or speech, severe pain or tenderness in stomach area, difficulty sleeping, weakness, changes in mood, and jaundice.

**Administration:** Oral route. **Storage:** 20-25°C (68-77°F).

# MIRENA RX

levonorgestrel (Bayer Healthcare)

**THERAPEUTIC CLASS:** Progestogen

**INDICATIONS:** Intrauterine contraception up to 5 yrs. Treatment of heavy menstrual bleeding in women who choose to use intrauterine contraception as their method of contraception.

**DOSAGE:** *Adults:* Initial release rate is 20mcg/day. Replace every 5 yrs. Initial insertion into uterine cavity is recommended within 7 days of the onset of mentruation or immediately after a first trimester abortion. Replacement may be done at any time during menstrual cycle. May insert 6 weeks postpartum or until involution of uterus is complete. If involution is substantially delayed, consider waiting until 12 weeks postpartum. Re-examine and evaluate 4 to 12 weeks after insertion, and once a year thereafter. To be inserted by a trained healthcare provider using strong aseptic technique.

**HOW SUPPLIED:** Intrauterine Insert: 52mg

**CONTRAINDICATIONS:** Pregnancy, congenital or acquired uterine anomaly, acute or history of PID, postpartum endometritis, infected abortion in the past 3 months, uterine or cervical neoplasia or unresolved, abnormal Pap smear, genital bleeding of unknown etiology, untreated acute cervicitis or vaginitis including bacterial vaginosis or other lower genital tract infections until infections is controlled, acute liver disease, liver tumor, conditions associated with increased susceptibility to pelvic infections, previously inserted IUD that is not removed, breast carcinoma.

**WARNINGS/PRECAUTIONS:** Recommended for women with at least one child. Replace after 5 yrs for continued use. Risk of ectopic pregnancy and glucose intolerance. Pregnancy with IUD in place may increase the risk of septic abortion, congenital anomalies, premature labor and delivery, and miscarriage. Increased risk of PID, sepsis, ovarian cysts. Can alter bleeding patterns and result in spotting, irregular bleeding, heavy bleeding, oligomenorrhea, and amenorrhea. Partial penetration or embedment in myometrium may decrease effectiveness. May perforate the uterus or cervix during insertion; increased risk in women with fixed retroverted uteri, during lactation, and postpartum. Partial or complete expulsion may occur. May cause enlarged ovarian follicles. Persistent enlarged follicles should be evaluated. Post marketing reports of breast cancer reported. Caution in patients with increased risk of infective endocarditis (eg, valvular or congenital heart disease, surgically constructed systemic pulmonary shunts), coagulopathy, migraines, focal migraines with asymmetrical visual loss or other symptoms indicating transient cerebral ischemia, severe headaches, marked increase in blood pressure, and/or severe arterial disease (eg, stroke, MI). Observe strict aseptic technique and careful sounding of the uterus prior to insertion. Fundal positioning important. If decrease in pulse, perspiration or pallor develops, remain in supine position until resolved. Insertion associated with some pain, bleeding, syncope, bradycardia or other neurovascular episodes.

**ADVERSE REACTIONS:** Uterine/vaginal bleeding alterations, amenorrhea, intramenstrual bleeding, spotting, abdominal/pelvic pain, ovarian cysts, headache/migraine, acne, depressed/altered mood, menorrhagia, vaginal discharge, IUD expulsion.

**INTERACTIONS:** May decrease serum concentrations of progestins with drugs or herbal products that induce enzymes such as CYP3A4 (barbiturates, bosentan, carbamazepine, felbamate, griseofulvin, oxcarbamazepine, phenytoin, rifampin, St. John's wort, topiramate). Significant changes (increase or decrease) in serum concentrations of progestin with HIV protease inhibitors. Monitor for infection if receiving chronic corticosteroid therapy or insulin. Caution if receiving anticoagulants.

**PREGNANCY:** Category X, not for use in nursing.

**MECHANISM OF ACTION:** Progestogen; not conclusively demonstrated. Thickening of cervical mucus, preventing passage of sperm into uterus, inhibition of sperm capacitation or survival, and alteration of endometrium.

**PHARMACOKINETICS: Absorption**: $C_{max}$(20mcg/day)=150-200pg/mL. **Distribution:** $V_d$=1.8L/kg, plasma protein binding (97.5-99%). Found in breast milk. **Metabolism:** Sulfate and glucuronide conjugates. **Excretion:** Urine (45%), feces (32%); $T_{1/2}$=17 hrs.

## NURSING CONSIDERATIONS

**Assessment:** Perform complete medical and social history (including that of partner), physical exam including a pelvic exam, ultrasonography of uterus to assess patency of endocervical canal and congenital or acquired uterine anomalies (eg, fibroids and endometriosis), pap smear, and tests for STDs. Assess for presence or history of pelvic inflammatory disease (PID), conditions associated with increased susceptibility to pelvic infections, pregnancy status including presence of ectopic pregnancy, nursing status, postpartum endometritis, previous history of infected abortion, cervical/uterine neoplasia, genital bleeding, cervicitis/vaginitis, hepatic diseases or tumors, cardiovascular diseases, coagulopathy, immune status, previous IUD insertion, breast cancer, and possible drug interactions.

**Monitoring:** Monitor for ectopic pregnancy, intrauterine pregnancy, miscarriage, septic abortion, premature labor, premature delivery, congenital anomalies, Group A streptococcal sepsis, PID, irregular bleeding/amenorrhea, embedment in the myometrium, perforation or penetration of uterine wall or cervix, partial or complete expulsion of drug device, development of breast cancer, ovarian cysts, and blood glucose in diabetics.

**Patient Counseling:** Advise that drug does not protect against HIV infection (AIDS) and other STDs. Inform of risks/benefits of the drug device. Advise to immediately report any symptoms of PID (eg, menstrual disorders, unusual vaginal discharge, abdominal/pelvic pain/tenderness, dyspareunia, chills, fever) and if partner becomes HIV-positive or acquires an STD. Inform that some bleeding (eg, irregular or prolonged bleeding, spotting), cramps, pain, decrease in pulse, perspiration, pallor, syncope, bradycardia and other neurovascular episodes may occur after insertion. Instruct to contact physician if symptoms continue or are severe. Instruct to contact healthcare provider if experiencing stroke or heart attack, develops very severe or migraine headaches, unexplained fever, yellowing of the skin or whites in the eyes, pelvic pain or pain during sex, HIV positive, exposed to STD, genital sores, severe vaginal bleeding. Instruct how to check after menstrual period that threads still protrude from cervix and caution not to pull on threads and displace drug device. Inform that there is no contraceptive protection if drug device is displaced or expelled. Advise that prescribing information is available upon request.



**Administration:** Administered into the uterine cavity. Refer to PI for insertion instructions. **Storage**: 25°C (77°F); excursions permitted to 15-30°C (59-86°F).

# M-M-R II RX

## rubella vaccine live - measles vaccine live - mumps vaccine live (Merck)

**THERAPEUTIC CLASS:** Vaccine

**INDICATIONS:** Vaccination against measles, mumps, and rubella.

**DOSAGE:** *Adults:* 0.5mL SQ into outer aspect of upper arm.
*Pediatrics:* 12-15 months: 0.5mL SQ into outer aspect of upper arm. Repeat before entering elementary school. If vaccinated at 6-12 months due to measles outbreak, give another dose between 12-15 months and then before entering elementary school.

**HOW SUPPLIED:** Inj: 0.5mL

**CONTRAINDICATIONS:** Pregnant females and avoid pregnancy for 3 months after vaccine, anaphylactic reaction to neomycin, febrile/active respiratory illness, immunosuppressive therapy (except corticosteroids as replacement therapy), blood dyscrasias, leukemia, lymphoma, malignant neoplasms affecting bone marrow or lymphatic system, immunodeficiency states and family history of congenital or hereditary immunodeficiency.

**WARNINGS/PRECAUTIONS:** Caution with egg allergy, cerebral injury, and individual/family history of convulsions. Avoid conditions that cause stress due to fever. Defer vaccination for 3 months after blood or plasma transfusions or administration of human immune globulin. Avoid pregnancy for 3 months after vaccination. May worsen thrombocytopenia. Contains albumin, remote risk of viral infection transmission. Have epinephrine (1:1000) available.

**ADVERSE REACTIONS:** Atypical measles, fever, syncope, headache, dizziness, malaise, diarrhea, local reactions, vomiting, nausea, arthralgia, pneumonitis, sore throat, Stevens-Johnson syndrome.

**INTERACTIONS:** Do not give with immune globulin. May depress TB skin sensitivity, administer test either simultaneously or before. Do not give <1 month before or after other live viral vaccines. Do not give simultaneously with DTP or oral poliovirus vaccine.

**PREGNANCY:** Category C, caution in nursing.

**MECHANISM OF ACTION:** May induce antibodies that may protect against measles, mumps, and rubella.

## NURSING CONSIDERATIONS

**Assessment:** Assess for immune and current health/medical status, history of blood dyscrasias, previous sensitivity/vaccination history, family history of neurological or immunodeficiency disorders, and possible drug interactions.

**Monitoring:** Monitor for anaphylactoid reactions, panniculitis, atypical measles, fever, syncope, headache, dizziness, malaise, irritability, vasculitis, pancreatitis, DM, diarrhea, NV, thrombocytopenia, encephalitis, optic neuritis, and orchitis.

**Patient Counseling:** Inform patients or caregivers of benefits/risks ratio; report any adverse reactions. Do not take during pregnancy or with active untreated TB.

**Administration:** SQ route. **Storage:** 2-8°C (36-46°F). Do not freeze.

M

# MOBIC — RX

meloxicam (Boehringer Ingelheim)

**NSAIDs may cause an increased risk of serious cardiovascular thrombotic events, MI, stroke and serious GI adverse events including bleeding, ulceration, and perforation of the stomach or intestines. Contraindicated for the treatment of perioperative pain in the setting of coronary artery bypass graft (CABG) surgery.**

**THERAPEUTIC CLASS:** NSAID

**INDICATIONS:** Relief of signs and symptoms of osteoarthritis (OA) and rheumatoid arthritis (RA). Relief of the signs and symptoms of pauciarticular or polyarticular course juvenile rheumatoid arthritis (JRA) in patients ≥2 yrs.

**DOSAGE:** *Adults:* ≥18 yrs: OA/RA: Initial/Maint: 7.5mg qd. Max: 15mg/day. *Pediatrics:* >2 yrs: JRA: 0.125mg/kg qd. Max: 7.5mg/day.

**HOW SUPPLIED:** Sus: 7.5mg/5mL; Tab: 7.5mg, 15mg

**CONTRAINDICATIONS:** ASA or other NSAID allergy that precipitates asthma, urticaria, or allergic-type reactions. Treatment of perioperative pain in the setting of CABG surgery.

**WARNINGS/PRECAUTIONS:** May lead to onset of new HTN or worsening of pre-existing HTN; monitor BP closely. Fluid retention and edema reported; caution with fluid retention, HTN, or heart failure. Renal papillary necrosis, renal insufficiency, acute renal failure, and other renal injury reported after long-term use. Not recommended for use with advanced renal disease; if therapy must be initiated, monitor renal function. Anaphylactoid reactions may occur. May cause serious skin adverse events (eg, exfoliative dermatitis, Stevens-Johnson syndrome, and toxic epidermal necrolysis). Avoid in late pregnancy; may cause premature closure of ductus arteriosis. May cause elevations of LFTs; d/c if liver disease develops or systemic manifestations occur. Caution with considerable dehydration and in elderly. Anemia may occur; with long-term use, monitor Hgb/Hct if signs or symptoms of anemia develop. May inhibit platelet aggregation and prolong bleeding time; monitor with coagulation disorders. Caution with asthma and avoid with ASA-sensitive asthma.

**ADVERSE REACTIONS:** Abdominal pain, constipation, diarrhea, dyspepsia, NV, headache, anemia, arthralgia, insomnia, upper respiratory tract infection, UTI.

**INTERACTIONS:** May decrease antihypertensive effects of ACE inhibitors. Potentiates GI bleeds with ASA; avoid concomitant use. Increased clearance with cholestyramine. May decrease natriuretic effects of furosemide, thiazides. Decreased lithium clearance/increased serum levels. Monitor PT/INR with warfarin. Caution with methotrexate.

**PREGNANCY:** Category C, not for use in nursing.

**MECHANISM OF ACTION:** NSAIDs; unknown, may inhibit prostaglandin synthetase.

**PHARMACOKINETICS: Absorption:** Absolute bioavailability (89%), $C_{max}$=1.05mcg/mL, $T_{max}$=4.9 hrs. **Distribution:** $V_d$=10 L/kg, plasma protein binding (99.4%). **Metabolism:** Hepatic (oxidation) via CYP2C9 (major), CYP3A4 (minor). **Elimination:** Urine (0.2%), feces (1.6%); $T_{1/2}$=20.1 hrs. Significant biliary and/or enteral secretion.

## NURSING CONSIDERATIONS

**Assessment:** Assess for history of asthma, cardiovascular disease (pre-existing HTN, CHF) or risk factors for disease, fluid retention, edema, increased risk of serious cardiovascular thrombotic events, stroke, pregnancy status, risk factors for GI events (bleeding, ulceration, perforation), possible drug interactions, renal/hepatic dysfunction.

**Monitoring:** Monitor CBC, LFTs, renal function, and chemistries periodically. Monitor for signs/symptoms of GI events (bleeding, ulceration, perforation), CV thrombotic events, CHF, HTN, salt depletion, renal/liver dysfunction.



**Patient Counseling:** Seek medical attention if symptoms of hepatotoxicity (nausea, fatigue, pruritus), anaphylactic reaction (difficulty breathing, swelling of face/throat), hypersensitivity reaction (rash), CV events (chest pain, SOB, weakness, slurring of speech), GI ulceration and bleeding (epigastric pain, dyspepsia, melena, hematemesis), weight gain, or edema occur. Inform of pregnancy risks. Caution may impair physical/mental abilities if experience drowsiness, dizziness, vertigo, or depression during therapy.

**Administration:** Oral route. **Storage:** (Tab; Sus): 25°C (77°F); excursions permitted to 15-30°C (59-86°F).

# MONODOX RX

doxycycline monohydrate (Watson)

**THERAPEUTIC CLASS:** Tetracycline derivative

**INDICATIONS:** Treatment of rocky mountain spotted fever, typhus fever and the typhus group, Q fever, rickettsialpox, ticks fever, respiratory tract infections, urinary tract infections, skin and skin structure infections, inclusion conjunctivitis, uncomplicated urethral/endocervical/rectal infections caused by *C.trachomatis*, nongonococcal urethritis caused by *C.trachomatis* and *U.urealyticum*, relapsing fever, lymphogranuloma, psittacosis, trachoma, tularemia, campylobacter fetus, chancroid, plague, cholera, brucellosis, bartonellosis, granuloma inguinale, and anthrax. Treatment of infections caused by *E.coli, Enterobacter aerogenes, Shigella species,* and *Acinetobacter species.* Treatment of uncomplicated gonorrhea, syphilis, yaws, listeriosis, Vincent's infection, actinomycosis, and *Clostridium* species infections when PCN is contraindicated. Adjunct therapy for amebicides and severe acne.

**DOSAGE:** *Adults:* Usual: 100mg q12h or 50mg q6h for 1 day, then 100mg/day. Severe Infection: 100mg q12h. Uncomplicated Gonococcal Infections (Except Anorectal Infections in Men): 100mg bid for 7 days or 300mg stat, then repeat in 1 hr. Acute Epididymo-Orchitis caused by *N.gonorrhoeae* or *C.trachomatis:* 100mg bid for at least 10 days. Primary/Secondary Syphilis: 300mg/day in divided doses for at least 10 days. Uncomplicated Urethral/Endocervical/

Rectal Infection caused by *C.trachomatis:* 100mg bid for at least 7 days. Nongonococcal Urethritis caused by *C.trachomatis* and *U.urealyticum:* 100mg bid for at least 7 days. Inhalational Anthrax (Post-Exposure): 100mg bid for 60 days. Take with full glass of water. Take with food if GI upset occurs. *Pediatrics:* >8 yrs: ≤100 lbs: 2mg/lb divided in 2 doses for 1 day, then 1mg/lb daily in single or 2 divided doses. Severe Infection: ≤100 lbs: May use up to 2mg/lb/day. >100 lbs: Use usual adult dose. Inhalation Anthrax (Post-Exposure): <100 lbs: 1mg/lb bid for 60 days. ≥100 lbs: 100mg bid for 60 days. Take with full glass of water. Take with food if GI upset occurs.

**HOW SUPPLIED:** Cap: 50mg, 75mg, 100mg

**WARNINGS/PRECAUTIONS:** Avoid direct sunlight or UV light. May cause permanent tooth discoloration during tooth development (last half of pregnancy and children <8 years). Enamel hypoplasia reported. Monitor renal/hepatic function, and blood with long-term therapy. In venereal disease when coexistent syphilis is suspected, a dark field examination should be done before treatment is started and the blood serology repeated monthly for at least four months. A decrease in fibula growth rate may occur if given to prematures. May cause fetal harm. May increase BUN. Photosensitivity, pseudotumor cerebri reported. D/C if superinfection occurs. Bulging fontanels in infants and intracranial HTN in adults reported. *Clostridium difficile*-associated diarrhea reported. Use in the absence of proven or strongly suspected bacterial infection is unlikely to provide benefit and increases the risk of drug resistant bacteria.

**ADVERSE REACTIONS:** GI effects, photosensitivity, rash, blood dyscrasias, hypersensitivity reactions.

**INTERACTIONS:** Carbamazepine, barbiturates, phenytoin decrease half-life of doxycycline. May decrease PT; adjust anticoagulants. Avoid concomitant use with penicillin. May decrease effects of oral contraceptives. Aluminum-, calcium-, iron-, and magnesium-containing products and bismuth subsalicylate impair absorption. Fatal renal toxicity may occur with methoxyflurane. Absorption may be decreased when taken with food.

**PREGNANCY:** Category D, not for use in nursing.

**MECHANISM OF ACTION:** Tetracycline; bacteriostatic, thought to inhibit protein synthesis.

**PHARMACOKINETICS: Absorption:** $C_{max}$=3.61mcg/mL; $T_{max}$=2.6 hrs. **Distribution:** Found in breast milk. **Elimination**: Urine, feces; $T_{1/2}$=16.33 hrs.

## NURSING CONSIDERATIONS

**Assessment:** Assess for renal impairment, pregnancy/nursing status, and for possible drug interactions. In venereal disease, when coexistent syphilis is suspected, perform a dark-field examination before treatment.

**Monitoring:** Monitor for signs/symptoms of hypersensitivity reactions, photosensitivity, superinfection, *C. difficile*-associated diarrhea, vaginal candidiasis, and benign intracranial HTN. In long-term therapy, perform periodic laboratory evaluation of organ systems, including hematopoietic, renal, and hepatic studies. In venereal disease, when coexistent syphilis is suspected, repeat blood serology for at least four months.

**Patient Counseling:** Inform of pregnancy risks. Instruct to avoid excessive sunlight or artificial UV light and to d/c therapy if phototoxicity (eg, skin eruptions) occur. Instruct to wear sunscreen or sunblock. Instruct to drink fluids liberally to reduce risk of esophageal irritation or ulceration. Inform therapy treats bacterial, not viral, infections. Counsel to take as directed; skipping doses or not completing full course may decrease effectiveness and increase antibiotic resistance. Inform that may experience diarrhea. Instruct to notify physician if watery/bloody stools, hypersensitivity reactions, superinfections, photosensitivity, or benign intracranial HTN occur.

**Administration:** Oral route. **Storage**: 20-25°C (68-77°F).

# MONOPRIL RX

fosinopril sodium (Bristol-Myers Squibb)

**ACE inhibitors can cause death/injury to developing fetus during 2nd and 3rd trimesters. D/C therapy if pregnancy detected.**

**THERAPEUTIC CLASS:** ACE inhibitor

**INDICATIONS:** Treatment of hypertension (HTN), may be used alone or with thiazide diuretics. Adjunct therapy for heart failure (HF).

**DOSAGE:** *Adults:* Hypertension: If possible, d/c diuretic 2-3 days before therapy. Initial: 10mg qd, monitor carefully if cannot d/c diuretic. Maint: 20-40mg qd. Resume diuretic if BP not controlled. Max: 80mg qd. Heart Failure: Initial: 10mg qd, 5mg with moderate to severe renal failure or vigorous diuresis. Titrate: Increase over several weeks. Maint: 20-40mg qd. Max: 40mg qd. Elderly: Start at low end of dosing range.
*Pediatric >50kg:* Hypertension: 5-10mg qd.

**HOW SUPPLIED:** Tab: 10mg*, 20mg, 40mg *scored

**CONTRAINDICATIONS:** History of ACE inhibitor associated angioedema.

**WARNINGS/PRECAUTIONS:** Head, neck, and intestinal angioedema reported; d/c if laryngeal stridor or angioedema of the face, lips, mucous membranes, tongue, glottis, or extremities occur. Anaphylactoid reactions during desensitization and during membrane exposure reported. Monitor for hypotension in high-risk patients (eg, heart failure, volume and/or salt depletion, surgery/anesthesia). May cause agranulocytosis; consider monitoring WBCs in patients with collagen vascular disease, especially if associated with renal impairment. Fetal/neonatal morbidity and death reported. Rarely associated with cholestatic jaundice that progresses to fulminant hepatic necrosis and sometimes death; d/c if jaundice or if marked elevations of hepatic enzymes occur. May cause changes in renal function; caution in patients with severe CHF, renal artery stenosis, and in patients with pre-existing renal impairment. May cause hyperkalemia; caution in patients with risk factors for hyperkalemia (eg, diabetes mellitus (DM), renal dysfunction). Persistent non-productive cough reported. Caution in patients with impaired liver function. Less effective on BP in blacks and more reports of angioedema than nonblacks. Caution in elderly.

M

**ADVERSE REACTIONS:** Dizziness, cough, hypotension, musculoskeletal pain, headache, fatigue, diarrhea, n/v.

**INTERACTIONS:** May increase lithium levels. Hypotension risk with diuretics. Increased risk of hyperkalemia with $K^+$-sparing diuretics (eg, spironolactone, amiloride, triamterene), $K^+$-containing salt substitutes, or $K^+$ supplements. Decreased absorption with antacids; space dosing by 2 hrs. Nitritoid reactions (eg, facial flushing, NV, hypotension) reported rarely with injectable gold.

**PREGNANCY:** Category C (1st trimester) and D (2nd and 3rd trimesters), not for use in nursing.

**MECHANISM OF ACTION:** ACE inhibitor; inhibition results in decreased plasma angiotensin II, which leads to decreased vasopressor activity and decreased aldosterone secretion.

**PHARMACOKINETICS: Absorption:** Slow; $T_{max}$=3 hrs. **Distribution**: Plasma protein binding (99.4%); found in breast milk. **Metabolism:** Hepatic; glucuronidation; fosinoprilat (active metabolite). **Elimination:** Urine, feces; (HTN) $T_{1/2}$=11.5 hrs. (HF) $T_{1/2}$=14 hrs.

## NURSING CONSIDERATIONS

**Assessment:** Assess for history of ACE inhibitor associated angioedema. Assess for volume and/or salt depletion, renal artery stenosis, CHF, pregnancy/nursing status, renal/hepatic function, hypersensitivity to drug, and for possible drug interactions. Assess for risk factors for developing hyperkalemia (eg, DM).

**Monitoring:** Monitor for signs/symptoms of head/neck and intestinal angioedema, anaphylactoid reactions, hypotension, agranulocytosis, hepatic failure, renal impairment, hyperkalemia, and for persistent non-productive cough.

Monitor renal function. In patients with collagen vascular disease, consider monitoring WBC count.

**Patient Counseling:** Inform that angioedema including laryngeal edema can occur; instruct to immediately report to physician and d/c therapy if any signs or symptoms of angioedema (eg, swelling of face, eyes, lips, tongue, extremities; difficulty swallowing or breathing) occur. Advise that lightheadedness may occur, instruct to d/c therapy if syncope occurs until physician has been contacted. Inform that inadequate fluid intake or excessive perspiration, diarrhea, or vomiting can lead to an excessive fall in BP. Instruct to avoid using potassium supplements or salt substitutes containing potassium unless physician has been notified. Counsel to report any signs of infection (eg, sore throat, fever). Inform of potential risks of therapy if used during pregnancy.

**Administration:** Oral route. **Storage:** 25°C (77°F); excursions permitted to 15-30°C (59-86°F). Protect from moisture; keep bottle tightly closed.

## MONOPRIL HCT — RX

fosinopril sodium - hydrochlorothiazide (Bristol-Myers Squibb)

**ACE inhibitors can cause death/injury to developing fetus during 2nd and 3rd trimesters. Stop therapy if pregnancy detected.**

**THERAPEUTIC CLASS:** ACE inhibitor/thiazide diuretic

**INDICATIONS:** Treatment of hypertension.

**DOSAGE:** *Adults:* Initial (if not controlled with fosinopril/HCTZ monotherapy): 12.5mg-10mg tab or 12.5mg-20mg tab qd.

**HOW SUPPLIED:** Tab: (Fosinopril-HCTZ) 10mg-12.5mg, 20mg-12.5mg

**CONTRAINDICATIONS:** Anuria, sulfonamide hypersensitivity.

**WARNINGS/PRECAUTIONS:** D/C if angioedema, jaundice, or marked LFT elevation occurs. Risk of hyperkalemia with DM, renal dysfunction. Persistent nonproductive cough reported. Monitor WBCs in renal and collagen vascular disease. Anaphylactoid reactions reported. Fetal/neonatal morbidity and death reported. Monitor for hypotension in high-risk patients (eg, surgery/anesthesia, volume/salt depletion). Caution with CHF, renal or hepatic dysfunction. More reports of angioedema in blacks than nonblacks. May exacerbate or activate SLE. Monitor electrolytes. Avoid if CrCl ≤30mL/min/1.7m². May increase cholesterol, TG. Hypercalcemia, hypomagnesemia, hyperuricemia may occur.

**ADVERSE REACTIONS:** Headache, cough, fatigue, dizziness.

**INTERACTIONS:** Increased risk of hyperkalemia with $K^+$-sparing diuretics, $K^+$ supplements, or $K^+$-containing salt substitutes. Risk of lithium toxicity. Antacids may impair absorption; separate dose by 2 hrs. May alter insulin requirements. May increase responsiveness to tubocurarine. NSAIDs reduce effects. May decrease effects of methenamine. Reduced absorption with cholestyramine, colestipol. Caution with other antihypertensives. May decrease response to norepinephrine. Nitritoid reactions (eg, facial flushing, NV, hypotension) reported rarely with injectable gold. Potentiate effects of ganglionic or peripheral adrenergic-blocking agents.

**PREGNANCY:** Category C (1st trimester) and D (2nd and 3rd trimesters), not for use in nursing.

**MECHANISM OF ACTION:** ACE inhibitor; inhibition results in decreased plasma angiotensin II, which leads to decreased vasopressor activity and decreased aldosterone secretion. Thiazide diuretic; affects renal tubular mechanism of electrolyte reabsorption directly increasing excretion of sodium salt and chloride.

**PHARMACOKINETICS: Absorption:** Fosinopril: Slow, $T_{max}$=3 hrs; HCTZ: $T_{max}$=1-2.5 hrs. **Distribution**: Fosinopril: Plasma protein binding (95%). HCTZ: $V_d$ =3.6-7.8L; plasma protein binding (67.9%). **Metabolism:** Hepatic, glucuronidation. **Elimination:** Fosinopril: Renal, $T_{1/2}$=11.5 hrs. HCTZ: Renal; $T_{1/2}$=5-15 hrs.

## NURSING CONSIDERATIONS

**Assessment:** Assess BP, LFTs, renal function, CHF, renal artery stenosis, SLE, serum electrolytes, pregnancy status, history of allergy to sulfonamides, bronchial asthma, parathyroid disorders, and for possible drug interactions.

**Monitoring:** Monitor BP, LFT, renal functions, CBC with platelet and differential count, serum electrolytes. Monitor for MI, CHF, angioedema of head/neck and intestines, anaphylactoid reactions, hepatic failure, hyperuricemia, hyperglycemia, hypersensitivity reactions, cough, NV, dizziness, nitritoid reactions.

**Patient Counseling:** Inform about fetal risks if taken during pregnancy. Caution that inadequate fluid intake, excessive perspiration, diarrhea, or vomiting can lead to excessive fall in BP, with the same consequences of lightheadedness and possible syncope. Advise not to use salt or $K^+$ supplements. Counsel about signs/symptoms of neutropenia (infections), angioedema, electrolyte imbalance (thirst, weakness, lethargy), and other adverse effects; advise to seek prompt medical attention.

**Administration:** Oral route. **Storage:** 25°C (77°F); excursions permitted to 15-30°C (59-86°F). Protect from moisture by keeping bottle tightly closed.

# MORPHINE SULFATE ORAL SOLUTION AND TABLETS

CII

morphine sulfate (Various)

**(Sol, 100mg/5mL) concentration is indicated for use in opioid-tolerant patients only. Use caution when prescribing, dispensing, and administering to avoid dosing errors due to confusion between different concentrations and between mg and mL, which could result in accidental overdose and death. Ensure the proper dose is communicated and dispensed. Keep out of reach of children. Seek medical help in case of accidental ingestion.**

M

**THERAPEUTIC CLASS:** Opioid analgesic

**INDICATIONS:** (Sol/Tab) Relief of moderate to severe acute chronic pain where use of an opioid analgesic is appropriate. (Sol, 100mg/5mL) Relief of moderate to severe acute chronic pain in opioid-tolerant patients.

**DOSAGE:** *Adults:* Individualize dose: Initial: (Sol): 10-20mg q4h prn for pain. (Tab): 15-30mg q4h prn for pain. Titrate: Based upon the individual patient's response. Use 100mg/5mL only for patients who have already been titrated to a stable analgesic regimen using lower strengths and who can benefit from use of a smaller volume of oral sol; always use the enclosed calibrated oral syringe. Conversion from Parenteral to Oral Morphine Sulfate: Anywhere from 3-6mg to provide pain relief equivalent to 1mg of parenteral morphine. Conversion from Parenteral Oral Non-Morphine Opioids to Oral Morphine Sulfate/Oral Controlled-Release to Oral Morphine Sulfate: Refer to published relative potency information. Close observation and dose adjustment is recommended. Periodically reassess the continued need for opioid analgesic use. Taper dose gradually. Elderly: Start at the low end of dosing range.

**HOW SUPPLIED:** Sol: 10mg/5mL [5mL, 100mL, 200mL], 20mg/5mL [100mL, 500mL], 100mg/5mL [30mL, 120mL]; Tab: 15mg*, 30mg* *scored

**CONTRAINDICATIONS:** Diagnosis or suspicion of paralytic ileus, acute or severe bronchial asthma or hypercarbia, respiratory depression in absence of lack of resuscitative equipment.

**WARNINGS/PRECAUTIONS:** Increased risk of respiratory depression in elderly, debilitated patients, those suffering from conditions accompanied by hypoxia, hypercapnia, or upper airway obstruction. Morphine sulfate is a Schedule II controlled substance with an abuse liability similar to other opioids. Respiratory depression and potential to elevate CSF pressure may be markedly exaggerated in the presence of head injury, other intracranial lesions; may obscure signs of increased intracranial pressure. May cause orthostatic hypotension and syncope; increased risk of hypotension with compromised ability to maintain blood pressure. Avoid in patients with gastrointestinal obstruction, especially paralytic ileus; may obscure diagnosis of acute abdominal conditions. Caution in patients with biliary tract disease; may cause spasm of the sphincter of Oddi and diminish biliary/pancreatic secretions. Use with caution and in reduced dosages in patients with severe renal/hepatic impairment, Addison's disease, hypothyroidism, prostatic hypertrophy, or urethral stricture, elderly, CNS depression, toxic psychosis, acute alcoholism and delirium tremens, may aggravate or induce seizures. May impair mental/ physical abilities.

**ADVERSE REACTIONS:** Respiratory depression, lightheadedness, dizziness, constipation, somnolence, N/V, sweating.

**INTERACTIONS:** Caution with CNS depressants (including sedatives, hypnotics, general anesthetics, antiemetics, phenothiazines, TCAs, other opioids, illicit drugs, alcohol); may increase the risk of respiratory depression, hypotension, profound sedation, or coma. May enhance the neuromuscular blocking action of skeletal muscle relaxants. Avoid with mixed agonist/antagonist analgesics (eg, pentazocine, nalbuphine, and butorphanol). Precipitates apnea, confusion, and muscle twitching with cimetidine. Potentiated by MAOIs; allow at least 14 days after stopping MAOIs before initiating treatment. May result in increased risk of urinary retention/severe constipation, which may lead to paralytic ileus with anticholinergics or other medications with anticholinergic activity. Caution with P-glycoprotein (PGP) inhibitors.

**PREGNANCY:** Category C, not for use in nursing.

**MECHANISM OF ACTION:** Opioid analgesic; precise mechanism unknown. Binds to CNS opiate receptors, producing analgesic effects. Also produces respiratory depression by direct action on brain stem respiratory centers, and depresses cough reflex by direct action on cough center in the medulla.

**PHARMACOKINETICS: Absorption:** Bioavailability (<40%); $C_{max}$ = 78ng/mL (Tab), 58ng/mL (Sol). **Distribution:** $V_d$=1-6L/kg; plama protein binding (20-35%); crosses placenta; found in breast milk. **Metabolism:** Liver via conjugation; 3- and 6- glucuronide (metabolite). **Elimination:** Urine (10% unchanged), feces (7-10%), bile; $T_{1/2}$=2-15 hrs (IV).

## NURSING CONSIDERATIONS

**Assessment:** Assess for pre-existing respiratory depression, COPD, cor pulmonale, acute or severe bronchial asthma, hypercarbia, paralytic ileus, severe hepatic/renal impairment, head injury, increased ICP, intracranial lesions, patients in circulatory shock, hypothyroidism, Addison's disease, CNS depression, toxic psychosis, prostatic hypertrophy or urethral stricture, acute alcoholism, delirium tremens, kyphoscoliosis, convulsive disorders, acute pancreatitis, biliary tract disease, pregnancy/nursing status, and for possible drug interactions.

**Monitoring:** Monitor for signs/symptoms of respiratory/CNS depression and development of psychological and physical dependence. Monitor for hypersensitivity reactions.

**Patient Counseling:** Advise to take only as directed by physician. Advise not to adjust dose without consulting a physician. Inform physician if pregnant, become pregnant, or planning to become pregnant prior to therapy. Instruct to safely taper dose upon discontinuing. Advise of the potential for severe constipation; appropriate laxatives/stool softeners should be initiated. Inform that therapy may produce physical or psychological dependence. Caution against performing hazardous tasks (eg, operating machinery/driving). Avoid alcohol or CNS depressants during therapy. Instruct to keep in a secure place out of reach of children.

**Administration:** Oral route. **Storage:** 15-30°C (59-86°F). Protect from moisture.

# MOTRIN RX

ibuprofen (McNeil Consumer)

**NSAIDs may cause an increased risk of serious cardiovascular thrombotic events, MI, stroke, and serious GI adverse events including bleeding, ulceration, and perforation of the stomach or intestines. Contraindicated for the treatment of perioperative pain in the setting of coronary artery bypass graft (CABG) surgery.**

**THERAPEUTIC CLASS:** NSAID

**INDICATIONS:** (Sus, Tab): For the relief of the signs and symptoms of rheumatoid arthritis (RA) and osteoarthritis (OA) and for the treatment of primary dysmenorrhea in adults. (Sus): For the reduction of fever in patients aged 6 months up to 2 yrs of age. For the relief of mild to moderate pain in patients aged 6 months up to 2 yrs of age. For the relief of signs and symptoms of juvenile arthritis (JA) in pediatrics. (Tab) For the relief of mild to moderate pain in adults.

**DOSAGE:** *Adults:* Pain: 400mg q 4-6 hrs prn. Max: 3200mg/day. Dysmenorrhea: 400mg q 4 hrs prn. Max: 3200mg/day. RA/OA: 300mg qid or 400mg, 600mg, or 800mg tid or qid. Max: 3200mg/day. If GI complaints occur, take tab with meals or milk.

*Pediatrics:* Fever: 6 months-2 yrs: 5mg/kg for temp <102.5°F; 10mg/kg if temp ≥102.5°F q6-8h. Max: 40mg/kg/day. Pain: 6 months-2 yrs: 10mg/kg q6-8 hrs. Max: 40mg/kg/day. JA: 30-40mg/kg/day divided into 3 or 4 doses. Milder disease may use 20mg/kg/day.

**HOW SUPPLIED:** Sus: 100mg/5mL; Tab: 400mg, 600mg, 800mg

**CONTRAINDICATIONS:** Treatment of perioperative pain in the setting of CABG surgery. Asthma, urticaria, or allergic-type reactions after taking ASA or other NSAIDs.

**WARNINGS/PRECAUTIONS:** May lead to onset of new HTN or worsening of pre-existing HTN; monitor BP closely. Fluid retention and edema reported; caution in patients with fluid retention or heart failure. Caution with history of ulcer disease or GI bleeding. Renal papillary necrosis and other renal injury reported after long-term use. Renal toxicity also reported in patients in whom renal prostaglandins have a compensatory role in the maintenance of renal perfusion; caution with impaired renal function, heart failure, liver dysfunction, and the elderly. Not recommended for use with advanced renal disease; if therapy must be initiated, monitor renal function. Anaphylactoid reactions may occur. May cause serious skin adverse events (eg, exfoliative dermatitis, Stevens-Johnson syndrome, toxic epidermal necrolysis). Avoid in late pregnancy; may cause premature closure of ductus arteriosis. Not a substitute for corticosteroids or for the treatment of corticosteroid insufficiency. May cause elevations of LFTs; d/c if liver disease develops or systemic manifestations occur. Anemia may occur; with long-term use, monitor Hgb/Hct if signs or symptoms of anemia develop. May inhibit platelet aggregation and prolong bleeding time; monitor with coagulation disorders. Caution with asthma and avoid with ASA-sensitive asthma. D/C if visual disturbances occur. Aseptic meningitis with fever and coma reported. Suspension contains sucrose and calories; caution with diabetic patients.

**ADVERSE REACTIONS:** Anemia, abnormal renal function, dizziness, edema, elevated liver enzymes, abdominal pain, bloating, constipation, diarrhea, dyspepsia, flatulence, heartburn, N/V, pruritus, rashes.

**INTERACTIONS:** May enhance methotrexate toxicity. May decrease natriuretic effect of furosemide and thiazides. Avoid use with ASA. May decrease lithium clearance; monitor for toxicity. Concomitant use with ACE inhibitors may diminish the antihypertensive effect of ACE inhibitors. Synergistic GI bleeding effects when used concomitantly with warfarin. May increase risk of serious GI bleeding when used concomitantly with oral corticosteroids, anticoagulants, or alcohol. ACE inhibitors and diuretic may increase risk of overt renal decompensation.

**PREGNANCY:** Category C, not for use in nursing.

**MECHANISM OF ACTION:** NSAID; suspected to inhibit prostaglandin synthetase.

**PHARMACOKINETICS: Absorption:** (Tab) Rapid; $T_{max}$=1-2 hrs. (Susp) **Adults:** $C_{max}$=19µg/mL; $T_{max}$=0.79 hrs; AUC=64µg•h/mL. Febrile children: $C_{max}$= 55µg/mL; $T_{max}$=0.97 hrs; AUC=155µg•h/mL. **Distribution:** (Susp): Plasma protein binding (>99%). **Adults:** $V_d$=0.12L/kg; febrile children: $V_d$=0.2L/kg. **Metabolism:** Hepatic. **Elimination:** Urine. (Tab): $T_{1/2}$=1.8-2 hrs. (Sus): $T_{1/2}$=2 hrs.

## NURSING CONSIDERATIONS

**Assessment:** Assess for history of hypersensitivity reaction to aspirin or other NSAIDs, asthma, cardiovascular disease (eg, pre-existing HTN, CHF) or risk factors for CVD, risk factors for a GI event (eg, prior history of ulcer disease or GI bleeding, smoking), fluid retention, SLE, connective tissue diseases, renal/hepatic dysfunction, coagulation disorders, pregnancy/nursing status, and for possible drug interactions. Assess that use is not for the treatment of perioperative pain in the setting of CABG surgery. Assess baseline LFTs, CBC, and renal function. If planning to use sus formulation, assess for DM.

**Monitoring:** Monitor for signs/symptoms of CV thrombotic events, new onset or worsening of pre-existing HTN, fluid retention and edema, GI events (eg, bleeding, ulceration, perforation), renal effects (eg, renal papillary necrosis), anaphylactoid reactions, skin reactions (eg, exfoliative dermatitis, Stevens-Johnson syndrome, toxic epidermal necrolysis), hepatic effects (eg, jaundice, liver necrosis, hepatic failure), hematological effects (eg, anemia, prolongation of bleeding time), bronchospasm, and for aseptic meningitis. Perform periodic monitoring of BP, CBC, LFTs, and renal function. If using sus formulation, monitor blood glucose levels in patients with DM.

**Patient Counseling:** Instruct to seek medical attention for symptoms of hepatotoxicity (eg, nausea, fatigue, jaundice), anaphylactic reactions (eg, difficulty breathing, swelling of face/throat), rash, CV events (eg, chest pain, SOB, weakness, slurring of speech), GI ulceration and bleeding (eg, epigastric pain, dyspepsia, melena, hematemesis), and unexplained weight gain or edema. Inform of risks if used during pregnancy.

**Administration:** Oral route. **Storage:** (Sus): 15-30°C (59-86°F). Shake before use. (Tab): 20-25°C (68-77°F).



## MoviPrep RX

ascorbic acid - sodium ascorbate - polyethylene glycol 3350 - potassium chloride - sodium chloride - sodium sulfate (Salix)

**THERAPEUTIC CLASS:** Bowel cleanser

**INDICATIONS:** Colon cleansing as a preparation for colonoscopy in adults ≥18 yrs of age.

**DOSAGE:** *Adults:* ≥18 yrs: Split-Dose Regimen: 8oz every 15 min (first liter) followed by 0.5 liters of clear liquid the evening prior, then another liter over 1 hr followed by 0.5 liters of clear liquid in the morning at least 1 hr prior to colonoscopy. Evening-Only Regimen: Around 6 pm take 8oz every 15 min (first liter), then 1.5 hrs later take second liter over one hour, additionally take 1 liter of clear liquid.

**HOW SUPPLIED:** Pow: (PEG 3350-Sodium Sulfate-Sodium Chloride-Potassium Chloride-Ascorbic Acid-Sodium Ascorbate) 100g-7.5g-2.69g-1.015g-4.7g-5.9g

**WARNINGS/PRECAUTIONS:** Rare reports of generalized tonic-clonic seizures with use of PEG colon preparations. Caution with concomitant medications that increase risk of electrolyte abnormalities (eg, diuretics, ACEIs) or in patients with hyponatremia; consider baseline and post-colonoscopy lab tests (eg, sodium, potassium, calcium, creatinine, BUN).

**ADVERSE REACTIONS:** Abdominal distension, anal discomfort, thirst, NV, abdominal pain, sleep disorder, rigors, hunger, malaise, dizziness.

**INTERACTIONS:** Oral medications given within 1 hour of administration may be flushed from GI and may not be absorbed.

**PREGNANCY:** Category C, caution in nursing.

**MECHANISM OF ACTION:** Laxative/evacuant; produces watery stool leading to cleansing of colon.

## NURSING CONSIDERATIONS

**Assessment:** Assess for electrolyte abnormalities, seizures, ileus, GI obstruction, gastric retention, bowel perforation, toxic colitis or toxic megacolon, severe ulcerative colitis, phenylalanine levels.

**Monitoring:** Perform baseline and post-colonoscopy lab tests with known or suspected hyponatremia. D/C use if severe bloating, abdominal distention, or abdominal pain. Monitor for hypersensitivity reactions. Exercise caution while administering to patients prone to aspirate.

**Patient Counseling:** Advise to adequately hydrate before, during, and after use. Inform that may have clear soup and/or plain yogurt for dinner, finishing evening meal at least 1 hr prior to start of treatment until after the colonoscopy. Advise that if severe abdominal discomfort occurs, stop drinking temporarily, or drink at longer intervals until symptoms disappear. Instruct to take exactly as directed.

**Administration:** Oral route. **Storage**: 25°C (77°F); excursions permitted to 15-30°C (59-86°F). When reconstituted, store upright and keep refrigerated. Use within 24 hrs.

# MS Contin

CII

morphine sulfate (Purdue Pharma)

M

**Contains morphine sulfate with an abuse liability similar to other opioid analgesics. Not intended for use as a prn analgesic. MS Contin 100mg and 200mg tablets are for use in opioid-tolerant patients only. Tablets are to be swallowed whole; do not break, crush, chew, or dissolve.**

**THERAPEUTIC CLASS:** Opioid analgesic

**INDICATIONS:** Management of moderate to severe pain when a continuous, around-the-clock opioid analgesic is needed for an extended period of time.

**DOSAGE:** *Adults:* Conversion from Immediate-Release Oral Morphine: Give 1/2 of patient's 24-hr requirement as MS Contin q12h or give 1/3 of daily requirement as MS Contin q8h. Conversion from Parenteral Morphine: Initial: If daily morphine dose ≤120mg/day, give MS Contin 30mg. Titrate: Switch to 60mg or 100mg MS Contin. Swallow whole; do not crush, chew, or break. Taper dose; do not d/c abruptly.

**HOW SUPPLIED:** Tab, Extended-Release: 15mg, 30mg, 60mg, 100mg, 200mg

**CONTRAINDICATIONS:** Paralytic ileus, respiratory depression in the absence of resuscitative equipment, acute or severe bronchial asthma.

**WARNINGS/PRECAUTIONS:** Extreme caution with COPD, cor pulmonale, decreased respiratory reserve, hypoxia, hypercapnia, respiratory depression. Caution with elderly, debilitated, head injury, increased ICP, circulatory shock, severe hepatic/renal/pulmonary dysfunction, myxedema, hypothyroidism, adrenocortical insufficiency, CNS depression, coma, toxic psychosis, prostatic hypertrophy, urethral stricture, alcoholism, delirium tremens, kyphoscoliosis, inability to swallow, convulsive disorder, acute abdominal problems, biliary tract surgery, acute pancreatitis secondary to biliary tract disease. May cause hypotension and drug dependence. Reserve 200mg tabs for opioid-tolerant patients requiring ≥400mg/day of morphine. May cause neonatal withdrawal syndrome.

**ADVERSE REACTIONS:** Constipation, lightheadedness, dizziness, sedation, N/V, sweating, dysphoria, euphoria, respiratory depression.

**INTERACTIONS:** Additive depressant effects with other CNS depressants (eg, sedatives, hypnotics, general anesthetics, phenothiazines, tranquilizers, alcohol). Enhances neuromuscular blocking effects and increases respiratory depression with skeletal muscle relaxants. Avoid agonist/antagonist analgesics (eg, pentazocine, nalbuphine, butorphanol, buprenorphine); may reduce analgesic effect or cause withdrawal symptoms. Risk of hypotension with phenothiazines or general anesthetics.

**PREGNANCY:** Category C, not for use in nursing.

**MECHANISM OF ACTION:** Opioid analgesic; pure opioid agonist whose principal therapeutic action is analgesia. Precise mechanism of analgesic action not established. Specific CNS opiate receptors for endogenous compounds with opioid-like activity are found throughout the brain and spinal cord and are likely to play a role in analgesic effects.

**PHARMACOKINETICS: Distribution:** $V_d$ = 4L/kg; found in skeletal muscle, kidneys, liver, intestinal tract, lungs, spleen, and brain; crosses placental membranes; found in breast milk. **Metabolism:** Liver to glucuronide metabolites, M3G (major metabolite), M6G (active metabolite). **Elimination:** Renal (primary), bile; (IV): $T_{1/2}$=2-4 hrs.

## NURSING CONSIDERATIONS

**Assessment:** Assess for opioid tolerance, respiratory depression, acute or severe bronchial asthma or hypercapnia, COPD, paralytic ileus, head injury or other intracranial lesions, presence of increased ICP, circulatory shock, presence of debilitation, hepatic/renal impairment, myxedema or hypothyroidism, adrenocortical insufficiency (eg, Addison's disease), CNS depression or coma, toxic psychosis, prostatic hypertrophy or urethral stricture, acute alcoholism, delirium tremens, kyphoscoliosis, acute abdominal conditions, biliary tract disease, acute pancreatitis, ability to swallow, pregnancy/nursing status, drug abuse potential, and possible drug interactions.

**Monitoring:** Monitor for signs/symptoms of respiratory depression, elevations in CSF pressure, hypotension, convulsions, tolerance and physical dependence, and misuse or abuse.

**Patient Counseling:** Instruct to swallow medication whole (do not break, chew, dissolve, or crush). Advise not to adjust dosing without consulting physician. Counsel to report episodes of breakthrough pain or adverse events (eg, respiratory depression). Advise that drug may cause mental/physical impairment; use caution if performing hazardous tasks (eg, operating machinery/driving). Instruct to avoid alcohol or other CNS depressants. Avoid abrupt withdrawal if on medication more than few weeks; taper dosing. Advise medication has drug abuse potential; protect from theft. Inform patient may see empty matrix of tablet in stool. Keep out of reach of children.

**Administration:** Oral route. **Storage:** Store at 25°C (77°F); excursions permitted to between 15-30°C (59-86°F).

M

# MULTAQ — RX

dronedarone (Sanofi-Aventis)

**Dronedarone is contraindicated in patients with NYHA Class IV heart failure, or NYHA Class II-III heart failure with a recent decompensation requiring hospitalization or referral to a specialized heart failure clinic.**

**INDICATIONS:** Reduces risk of cardiovascular hospitalization in patients with paroxysmal or persistent atrial fibrillation (AF) or atrial flutter (AFL), with a recent episode of AF/AFL and associated cardiovascular risk factors (eg, age >70, hypertension, diabetes, prior cerebrovascular accident, left atrial diameter ≥50mm or left ventricular ejection fraction [LVEF] <40%), who are in sinus rhythm or who will be cardioverted.

**DOSAGE:** *Adult:* ≥18 yrs: 400mg bid. Take 1 tab with morning and evening meals.

**HOW SUPPLIED:** Tab: 400mg

**CONTRAINDICATIONS:** See Black Box Warning. Second- or third-degree atrioventricular (AV) block or sick sinus syndrome (except when used in conjunction with a functioning pacemaker), bradycardia <50 bpm, concomitant use of strong CYP3A inhibitors (eg, ketoconazole, itraconazole, voriconazole, cyclosporine, telithromycin, clarithromycin, nefazodone, ritonavir), concomitant use of drugs or herbal products that prolong the QT interval and might increase the risk of Torsade de Pointes (eg, phenothiazine anti-psychotics, tricyclic antidepressants, certain oral macrolide antibiotics, Class I and III antiarrhythmics), QTc Bazett interval ≥500 ms or PR interval >280 ms, severe hepatic impairment, pregnancy/nursing.

**WARNINGS/PRECAUTIONS:** D/C if heart failure develops or worsens. May induce moderate QT interval prolongation; d/c if the QTc Bazett interval is ≥500 ms. Increased serum creatinine levels by about 0.1 mg/dL reported. Premenopausal women who have not undergone a hysterectomy or oophorectomy must use effective contraception while on therapy.

**ADVERSE REACTIONS:** Diarrhea, NV, abdominal pain, asthenia, bradycardia, rashes, pruritus, eczema, dermatitis.

**INTERACTIONS:** See Contraindications. Hypokalemia or hypomagnesemia may occur with potassium-depleting diuretics. May potentiate electrophysiologic effects with digoxin; reduce digoxin dose by half and monitor levels closely. Calcium channel blockers (eg, verapamil, diltiazem) may potentiate conduction and increase dronedarone exposure. Bradycardia reported with concomitant use of beta-blockers. Seventeen-fold increase in drug levels and 9-fold increase on $C_{max}$ reported when used concomitantly with ketoconazole. Avoid grapefruit juice, rifampin, or other CYP3A inducers (eg, phenobarbital, carbamazepine, phenytoin, St. John's wort). May increase simvastatin/simvastatin acid, digoxin and other P-glycoprotein substrates, propranolol, metoprolol and other CYP 2D6 substrates (eg, tricyclic antidepressants, SSRIs), and calcium channel blocker exposure. Increased plasma levels of tacrolmus, sirolimus, and other CYP3A substrates.

**PREGNANCY:** Category X, not for use in nursing.

**MECHANISM OF ACTION:** Benzofuran derivative; mechanism not established. Antiarrhythmic properties belong to all four Vaughan-Williams classes.

M

**PHARMACOKINETICS: Absorption:** Absolute bioavailability (4% no food, 15% with high fat meal); $T_{max}$=3-6 hrs. **Distribution:** (In vitro) Plasma protein binding (>98%); $V_d$=1400 L. **Metabolism:** Extensive via CYP3A; N-debutylation and oxidative deamination; N-debutyl metabolite (active). **Elimination:** Urine (6%, metabolites), feces (84%, metabolites); $T_{1/2}$=13-19 hrs.

## NURSING CONSIDERATIONS

**Assessment:** Assess for AF, AFL, cardiovascular risk factors, NYHA Class II, III, and IV heart failure, AV block, sick sinus syndrome, bradycardia, severe hepatic impairment, Class I or III antiarrhythmics (eg, amiodarone, flecainide, propafenone, quinidine, disopyramide, dofetilide, sotalol), concomitant use of strong CYP3A inhibitors (eg, ketoconazole, itraconazole, voriconazole, cyclosporine, telithromycin, clarithromycin, nefazodone, ritonavir), drugs or herbal products that prolong the QT interval and might increase the risk of Torsade de Pointes, pregnancy/nursing status, and possible drug interactions. Determine baseline serum potassium levels.

**Monitoring:** Monitor for signs or symptoms of worsening heart failure, bradycardia, serum potassium and magnesium levels, ECG abnormalities (eg, QT interval prolongation).

**Patient Counseling:** Instruct to avoid grapefruit juice during therapy. Advise to take with meals. Inform to take the next dose at the regularly scheduled time and not to double the dose if missed. Notify physician if signs/symptoms of worsening heart failure such as acute weight gain, dependent edema, or increasing shortness of breath. Advise to inform physician of any history of heart failure, rhythm disturbance other than AF or AFL, or predisposing conditions such as uncorrected hypokalemia. Advise to report use of any other prescription, non-prescription medication, or herbal products, particularly St. John's wort. Counsel women of childbearing potential about appropriate contraceptive choices while on therapy.

**Administration:** Oral route. Take 1 tab with morning and evening meals. **Storage:** 25°C (77°F); excursions permitted to 15-30°C (59-86°F).

## MYCAMINE RX
micafungin sodium (Astellas)

**THERAPEUTIC CLASS:** Glucan synthesis inhibitor

**INDICATIONS:** Treatment of candidemia, acute disseminated candidiasis, *Candida* peritonitis, abscesses, and esophageal candidiasis. Prophylaxis of *Candida* infections in patients undergoing hematopoietic stem cell transplantation (HSCT).

**DOSAGE:** *Adults:* Candidemia/Acute Disseminated Candidiasis/*Candida* Peritonitis/Abscesses: 100mg IV qd (usual range 10-47 days). Esophageal Candidiasis: 150mg IV qd (usual range 10-30 days). *Candida* Infection Prophylaxis in HSCT: 50mg IV qd (usual range 6-51 days). Do not mix or co-infuse with other drugs.

**HOW SUPPLIED:** Inj: 50mg, 100mg

**WARNINGS/PRECAUTIONS:** Reports of serious hypersensitivity reactions (eg, anaphylaxis, anaphylactoid, shock); d/c drug and administer appropriate treatment. LFT abnormalities, monitor for evidence of worsening. Reports of significant renal dysfunction, acute renal failure, and elevations in BUN and creatinine. Reports of acute intravascular hemolysis, hemolytic anemia and hemoglobinuria.

**ADVERSE REACTIONS:** Hyperbilirubinemia, neutropenia, headache, rash, phlebitis, N/V, diarrhea, pyrexia, hypokalemia, thrombocytopenia.

**INTERACTIONS:** Monitor for sirolimus, nifedipine, or itraconazole toxicity; reduce dose if toxicity occurs. May precipitate when mixed or co-infused with other drugs.

**PREGNANCY:** Category C, caution in nursing.

**MECHANISM OF ACTION:** Antifungal agent; inhibits the synthesis of 1,3-β-D-glucan, a component of fungal cell walls.

**PHARMACOKINETICS: Absorption:** IV infusion of variable doses resulted in different parameters. **Distribution:** $V_d$=0.39±0.11L/kg (terminal phase); plasma protein binding ( ≥99%). **Metabolism:** Metabolized to M-1 (catechol form) by arylsulfatase and further metabolized to M-2 (methoxy form) by catechol-O-methyltransferase. Catalyzed by CYP450 isoenzymes. **Elimination:** Urine and feces (major route).

### NURSING CONSIDERATIONS

**Assessment:** Assess cultures and other diagnostic tests prior to therapy and for possible drug interactions.

**Monitoring:** Monitor for hypersensitivity and anaphylaxis reaction (shock), LFTs for possible hepatic dysfunction, hepatitis or hepatic failure, elevations in BUN and creatinine, and signs/symptoms of renal dysfunction or acute renal failure. Monitor for hematological effects (hemolysis, hemoglobinuria).

**Patient Counseling:** Instruct to notify physician if signs/symptoms of hypersensitivity or anaphylaxis reactions, hematological reactions, hepatic complications, or renal complications develop.

**Administration:** IV infusion. 1) Aseptically add 5mL of 0.9% NaCl Inj, USP (without bacteriostatic agent) to each 50mg or 100mg vial to yield a preparation containing 10mg, 20mg micafungin/mL. 2) To minimize foaming, gently dissolve the powder by swirling the vial. Do not vigorously shake vial. **Storage:** Unopened vial: Stored at room temperature, 25°C (77°F); excursions permitted to 15-30°C (59-86°F). Reconstitituted, diluted infusions: May be stored at room temperature 25°C (77°F) for up to 24 hrs.

## MYCELEX TROCHE RX
clotrimazole (Ortho-McNeil)

**THERAPEUTIC CLASS:** Azole antifungal

**INDICATIONS:** Local treatment of oropharyngeal candidiasis. Prophylactically to reduce the incidence of oropharyngeal candidiasis in immunocompromised conditions (eg, chemotherapy, radiotherapy, steroid therapy).

**DOSAGE:** *Adults:* Treatment: Slowly dissolve 1 troche in mouth 5 times/day for 14 days. Prophylaxis: Slowly dissolve 1 troche in mouth tid for duration of chemotherapy or until steroids reduced to maint levels.
*Pediatrics:* ≥3 yrs: Treatment: Slowly dissolve 1 troche in mouth 5 times/day for 14 days. Prophylaxis: Slowly dissolve 1 troche in mouth tid for duration of chemotherapy or until steroids reduced to maint levels.

**HOW SUPPLIED:** Tab: 10mg

**WARNINGS/PRECAUTIONS:** Not for systemic mycoses. May cause abnormal LFTs; monitor hepatic function. Only use in patients mentally and physically able to dissolve the troche. Confirm diagnosis by KOH smear and/or culture.

**ADVERSE REACTIONS:** Abnormal LFTs, N/V, unpleasant mouth sensations, pruritus.

**PREGNANCY:** Category C, safety in nursing is not known.

**MECHANISM OF ACTION:** Broad-spectrum antifungal agent; inhibits growth of pathogenic yeasts by altering cell membrane permeability.

**PHARMACOKINETICS: Absorption:** $C_{max}$=4.98ng/mL (30 min), 3.23ng/mL (60 min).

## NURSING CONSIDERATIONS

**Assessment:** Assess for proper diagnosis of oropharyngeal candidiasis prior to therapy (KOH smear or culture).

**Monitoring:** Periodically monitor for LFTs. Monitor for NV, pruritus, and unpleasant mouth sensations.

**Patient Counseling:** Counsel to allow lozenge to dissolve slowly in mouth; report adverse reactions.

**Administration:** Oral route. **Storage:** Store below 30°C (86°F). Avoid freezing.

M

# MYFORTIC — RX

mycophenolic acid (Novartis)

**Immunosupression may lead to increased susceptibility to infection and possible development of lymphoma and other neoplasms. Only physicians experienced in immunosuppressive therapy and management of organ transplant recipients should prescribe mycophenolic acid. Women of childbearing potential must use contraception. Increased risk of pregnancy loss and congenital malformations.**

**THERAPEUTIC CLASS:** Inosine monophosphate dehydrogenase inhibitor

**INDICATIONS:** Prophylaxis of organ rejection in patients receiving allogeneic renal transplants, administered in combination with cyclosporine and corticosteroids.

**DOSAGE:** *Adults:* 720mg bid on empty stomach, 1 hr before or 2 hrs after food intake. Elderly: Max: 720mg bid. Do not crush, chew or cut.
*Pediatrics:* 400mg/m² bid. Max: 720mg bid. BSA 1.19-1.58m²: 540mg bid. BSA >1.58m²: 720mg bid. BSA <1.19m²: cannot be accurately administered with current formulations.

**HOW SUPPLIED:** Tab, Delayed-Release: 180mg, 360mg

**WARNINGS/PRECAUTIONS:** Risk of lymphomas and other malignancies, particularly of the skin. Avoid sunlight, wear protective clothing and use sunscreen to decrease risk of skin cancer. Increased susceptibility to infections (eg, opportunistic, fatal infections, and sepsis). Increased risk of opportunistic infections, including activation of latent viral infections such as progressive multifocal leukoencephalopathy (PML), BK virus-associated nephropathy, sometimes fatal, and pure red cell aplasia (PRCA). Monitor for neutropenia and bone marrow suppression. Risk of GI ulceration (eg, duodenal ulcer), hemorrhage, and perforation; caution with active digestive system disease. Caution with delayed renal graft function post-transplant. Avoid with rare hereditary deficiency of hypoxanthine-guanine phosphoribosyl-transferase (eg, Lesch-Nyhan and Kelley-Seegmiller syndrome). May cause fetal harm during pregnancy; increased risk of pregnancy loss and congenital malformations. Must have negative serum/urine pregnancy test within 1 week before therapy. Two reliable forms of contraception are required before and during therapy, and 6 weeks following discontinuation. Avoid with live vaccine. Caution in elderly.

**ADVERSE REACTIONS:** Constipation, diarrhea, leukopenia, N/V, anemia, dyspepsia, CMV infection, urinary tract infection, insomnia, postoperative pain, cough, edema, dehydration, depression.

**INTERACTIONS:** Avoid concomitant use with azathioprine and mycophenolate mofetil. Reduced efficacy with drugs that interfere with enterohepatic recirculation (eg, cholestyramine) and drugs that bind bile acids (eg, bile acid sequestrants, and oral activated charcoal). Decreased effects of live attenuated vaccines. Increased levels of both drugs with acyclovir, ganciclovir. Decreased levels with magnesium- and aluminum-containing antacids; space dosing. Decreased effects of oral contraceptives.

**PREGNANCY:** Category D, not for use in nursing.

**MECHANISM OF ACTION:** Inosine monophosphate dehydrogenase inhibitor; inhibits the de novo pathway of guanosine nucleotide synthesis without incorporation to DNA.

**PHARMACOKINETICS: Absorption:** Absolute bioavailability (72%); $T_{max}$=1.5-2.75 hrs. **Distribution:** $V_d$=54L (steady state); plasma protein binding: >98% (mycophenolic acid (MPA), 82% (mycophenolic acid glucuronide (MPAG). **Metabolism:** (MPA) metabolized by glucuronyl transferase to MPAG (major metabolite). **Elimination:** Urine: >60% (MPAG), 3% (unchanged), and bile; $T_{1/2}$=8-16 hrs (MPA), 13-17 hrs (MPAG).

## NURSING CONSIDERATIONS

**Assessment:** Assess for drug hypersensitivity, hepatic/renal impairment, pregnancy status, vaccination history, inherited deficiency of HGPRT such as Lesch-Nyhan and Kelley-Seegmiller syndromes, and possible drug interactions.

**Monitoring:** Monitor for signs of delayed graft rejection (eg, anemia, thrombocytopenia, and hyperkalemia), lymphomas, skin cancer, GI bleeding/perforation, infection or opportunistic infection (eg, herpes virus, fatal infection, sepsis). Monitor unexpected bruising, bleeding, or signs of bone marrow suppression with periodic CBCs. Monitor CBC weekly during the 1st month, twice monthly for the 2nd and 3rd months, and then monthly through 1st year.

**Patient Counseling:** Counsel to take on an empty stomach, to swallow tab whole; do not crush, chew, or cut. Instruct to avoid prolonged exposure to sunlight and UV light by wearing protective clothing and using sunscreen. Inform medication is not to be used by women who are pregnant/nursing or planning to become pregnant. Advise to follow dosage instructions and have periodic laboratory tests performed. Inform about increased risk for malignancies and infections.

**Administration:** Oral route. **Storage:** 25°C (77°F); excursions permitted to 15-30°C (59-86°F). Protect from moisture. Dispense in a tight container.

# MYLERAN RX

busulfan (GlaxoSmithKline)

**Do not use unless CML diagnosis is established. May induce severe bone marrow hypoplasia; reduce dose or d/c if unusual depression of bone marrow function occurs.**

**THERAPEUTIC CLASS:** Alkylating agent

**INDICATIONS:** Palliative treatment of chronic myelogenous leukemia (CML).

**DOSAGE:** *Adults:* 60mcg/kg/day or 1.8mg/m²/day. Range: 4-8mg/day. Reserve dose >4mg/day for the most compelling symptoms.

*Pediatrics:* 60mcg/kg/day or 1.8mg/m²/day. Range: 4-8mg/day. Reserve dose >4mg/day for the most compelling symptoms.

**HOW SUPPLIED:** Tab: 2mg

**CONTRAINDICATIONS:** Lack of definitive diagnosis of CML.

**WARNINGS/PRECAUTIONS:** Induction of bone marrow failure resulting in severe pancytopenia reported. Bronchopulmonary dysplasia with pulmonary fibrosis, cellular dysplasia, malignant tumors, acute leukemias, hepatic veno-occlusive disease reported. Ovarian suppression and amenorrhea with menopausal symptoms have occurred. Cardiac tamponade in patients with thalassemia and seizures reported. Caution with compromised bone marrow reserve from prior irradiation/chemotherapy. Seizures reported.

**ADVERSE REACTIONS:** Myelosuppression, pulmonary fibrosis, cardiac tamponade, hyperpigmentation, weakness, fatigue, weight loss, nausea, vomiting, melanoderma, hyperuricemia, myasthenia gravis, hepatic veno-occlusive disease.

**INTERACTIONS:** Additive myelosuppression with myelosuppressive drugs. Additive pulmonary toxicity with myelotoxic drugs. Increased clearance of cyclophosphamide and busulfan with phenytoin pretreatment. Decreased clearance with concomitant cyclophosphamide alone. Reduced clearance with itraconazole; monitor for signs of toxicity. Concurrent thioguanine was associated with portal HTN and esophageal varices with abnormal LFTs; caution with long-term therapy.

**PREGNANCY:** Category D, not for use in nursing.

**MECHANISM OF ACTION:** Bifunctional alkylating agent.

**PHARMACOKINETICS: Absorption**: (IV, PO) Absolute bioavailability (adults 80%, children 68%); $C_{max}$(2mg, 4mg)=30ng/mL, 68ng/mL; $T_{max}$=0.9 hrs; AUC (4mg) =269ng•hr/mL **Distribution**: Plasma protein binding (32%); crosses blood-brain barrier. **Metabolism**: Liver (extensive); 3-hydroxytetrahydrothiopene-1, 1-dioxide (major metabolite). **Elimination**: Urine (>2% unchanged); $T_{1/2}$=2.69 hrs.

M

## NURSING CONSIDERATIONS

**Assessment:** Assess for chronic myelogenous leukemia, history of seizure disorder, head trauma, if receiving other potentially epileptogenic drugs, pregnancy status. Note other diseases/conditions and drug therapies.

**Monitoring:** Periodically measure serum transaminases, alkaline phosphatase, and bilirubin for early detection of hepatotoxicity, and evaluate weekly Hgb/Hct, total WBC count and differential, quantitative platelet count, and bone marrow exam for evaluation of marrow status. Monitor for signs/symptoms of busulfan toxicity and bronchopulmonary dysplasia with pulmonary fibrosis, secondary malignancies, chromosomal aberrations.

**Patient Counseling:** Counsel about need for periodic blood counts and to report unusual bleeding, fever, breathing difficulty, anorexia, weight loss, or melanoderma.

**Administration:** Oral route. **Storage**: 25°C (77°F); excursions permitted to 15-30°C (59-86°F).

# MYLOTARG — RX

gemtuzumab ozogamicin (Wyeth)

**Administer under the supervision of physicians experienced in the treatment of acute leukemia and in facilities equipped to monitor and treat leukemia patients. Use only as a single agent chemotherapy. Severe myelosuppression, severe hypersensitivity reactions (eg, anaphylaxis, pulmonary events), and infusion-related reactions may occur. Consider leukoreduction with hydroxyurea or leukapheresis with high peripheral blood counts. Hepatotoxicity, including severe hepatic veno-occlusive disease (VOD) reported; monitor for symptoms including rapid weight gain, right upper quadrant pain, hepatomegaly, ascites, elevations in bilirubin and/or liver enzymes.**

**THERAPEUTIC CLASS:** $IgG_4$ kappa antibody/calicheamicin conjugate

**INDICATIONS:** Treatment of patients with CD33 positive acute myeloid leukemia (AML) in 1st relapse patients ≥60 yrs who are not candidates for chemotherapy.

**DOSAGE:** *Adults:* ≥60 yrs: 9mg/m² IV over 2 hrs. Give 2 doses with 14 days between doses. Premedicate 1 hr prior with diphenhydramine 50mg PO and APAP 650-1000mg PO (may give additional APAP dose q4h for 2 doses as needed).

**HOW SUPPLIED:** Inj: 5mg

**WARNINGS/PRECAUTIONS:** See BlackBox Warning. D/C if anaphylaxis, pulmonary edema, or acute respiratory distress syndrome develops. May produce post-infusion symptom complex of fever, chills, hypotension, and dyspnea during the first 24 hrs after administration. Monitor vital signs during infusion and 4 hrs after. May be at high risk of severe pulmonary reactions with symptomatic intrinsic lung disease. Increased risk of severe veno-occlusive disease (VOD) if used before or after hematopoietic stem-cell transplant, underlying hepatic disease, abnormal liver function, or with combination chemotherapy. Renal failure secondary to tumor lysis syndrome (TLS) reported. Not for IV push or bolus use. Monitor for electrolytes, LFTs, CBCs, and platelet counts.

**ADVERSE REACTIONS:** Chills, fever, NV, headache, hypotension, HTN, hypoxia, dyspnea, hyperglycemia, antibody formation, severe myelosuppression, anemia, thrombocytopenia, sepsis, pneumonia.

**INTERACTIONS:** Potential for interactions with drugs affected by CYP450 enzymes.

**PREGNANCY:** Category D, not for use in nursing.

**MECHANISM OF ACTION:** IgG4 kappa antibody/calicheamicin conjugate; binds to CD33 antigen, resulting in formation of a complex that is internalized. Upon internalization, the calicheamicin derivative is released inside lysosomes of myeloid cell, which then binds to DNA in the minor groove, resulting in DNA double strand breaks and cell death.

**PHARMACOKINETICS: Elimination:** $T_{1/2}$=41 hrs (total), 143 hrs (unconjugated).

## NURSING CONSIDERATIONS

**Assessment:** Assess for history of liver disease or hematopoietic stem cell transplant (HSCT). Consider leukoreduction with hydroxyurea or leukapheresis to reduce peripheral WBC count to <30,000/uL.

**Monitoring:** Monitor for symptoms of hepatotoxicity, veno-occlusive disease (VOD), tumor lysis syndrome, hyperglycemia, infections, severe hypersensitivity reactions, and other infusion-related reactions including severe pulmonary events. Monitor vital signs (during infusion and 4 hrs following infusion), electrolytes, LFTs, CBC, with differential and platelet counts.

**Patient Counseling:** Instruct to seek medical attention if signs/symptoms of potential adverse effects occur such as fever, chills, difficulty breathing, or rapid weight gain.

**Administration:** IV route. Refer to PI on instructions for reconstitution, dilution, administration, use, handling, and disposal. **Storage**: 2-8°C (36-46°F). Protect from light.

# NABUMETONE — RX

nabumetone (Various)

**NSAIDs may cause an increased risk of serious cardiovascular thrombotic events, MI, stroke and serious GI adverse events including bleeding, ulceration, and perforation of the stomach or intestines. Contraindicated for the treatment of perioperative pain in the setting of coronary artery bypass graft (CABG) surgery.**

**THERAPEUTIC CLASS:** NSAID

**INDICATIONS:** Relief of signs and symptoms of osteoarthritis and rheumatoid arthritis.

**DOSAGE:** *Adults:* Initial: 1000mg qd. Max: 2000mg/day.

**HOW SUPPLIED:** Tab: 500mg, 750mg

**CONTRAINDICATIONS:** Allergy to ASA or other NSAID that precipitates asthma, urticaria, or other allergic-type reaction. Treatment of perioperative pain in the setting of CABG surgery.

**WARNINGS/PRECAUTIONS:** May lead to onset of new HTN or worsening of pre-existing HTN; monitor BP closely. Fluid retention and edema reported; caution with fluid retention or heart failure. Renal papillary necrosis and other renal injury reported after long-term use. Not recommended for use with advanced renal disease; if therapy must be initiated, monitor renal function. Anaphylactoid reactions may occur. May cause serious skin adverse events (eg, exfoliative dermatitis, Stevens-Johnson syndrome, and toxic epidermal necrolysis). Avoid in late pregnancy; may cause premature closure of ductus arteriosis. May cause elevations of LFTs; d/c if liver disease develops or systemic manifestations occur. Caution in elderly. Anemia may occur; with long-term use, monitor Hgb/Hct if signs or symptoms of anemia develop. May inhibit platelet aggregation and prolong bleeding time; monitor with coagulation disorders. Caution with asthma and avoid with ASA-sensitive asthma. May induce photosensitivity. Risk of GI ulceration, bleeding, and perforation.

**ADVERSE REACTIONS:** Diarrhea, dyspepsia, abdominal pain, constipation, flatulence, nausea, positive stool guaiac, dizziness, headache, pruritus, rash, tinnitus, edema.

**INTERACTIONS:** Caution with warfarin, other protein bound drugs. Nephrotoxicity risk with diuretics. May elevate lithium and methotrexate levels. May diminish antihypertensive effect of ACE inhibitors. Avoid concomitant ASA.

**PREGNANCY:** Category C, not for use in nursing.

**MECHANISM OF ACTION:** NSAID (napthylalkanone derivative); suspected to inhibit prostaglandin synthetase, exerts anti-inflammatory, analgesic, and antipyretic actions.

N

**PHARMACOKINETICS: Absorption:** Well-absorbed (GIT). PO administration of variable doses resulted in different parameters. **Distribution:** Plasma protein binding ( ≥99%). **Metabolism:** Liver (extensive biotransformation), 6-methoxy-2-naphthylacetic acid (active metabolite). **Elimination:** Urine (approximately 75%), feces; $T_{1/2}$=24 hrs.

## NURSING CONSIDERATIONS

**Assessment:** Assess LFTs, renal function, CBC and coagulation profile. Assess for history of CABG surgery, asthma and allergic reactions to aspirin or other NSAIDs, active ulceration or chronic inflammation of GI tract, CVD, asthma, pregnancy status. Note other diseases/conditions and drug therapies.

**Monitoring:** Monitor for hypersensitivity reactions, cardiac complications, stroke, GI bleeding, asthma, skin adverse effects. Monitor BP, LFTs, renal function, CBC with differential and platelet count, coagulation profile, ocular effects, photosensitivity.

**Patient Counseling:** Counsel about potential side effects; seek medical attention if any develop. Take as prescribed. Advise women not to use late in pregnancy.

**Administration:** Oral route. **Storage:** Controlled room temperature 15-30°C (59-86°F). Dispense in tight, light-resistant container.

# NADOLOL — RX

nadolol (Various)

**OTHER BRAND NAMES:** Corgard (King)

**THERAPEUTIC CLASS:** Nonselective beta-blocker

**INDICATIONS:** Long-term management of angina pectoris. Management of hypertension; may be used alone or in combination with other antihypertensive agents, especially thiazide type diuretics.

**DOSAGE:** *Adults:* Angina Pectoris: Initial: 40mg qd. Titrate: Increase by 40-80mg every 3-7 days. Usual: 40-80mg qd. Max: 240mg/day. HTN: Initial: 40mg qd. Titrate: Increase in 40-80mg increments. Usual: 40-80mg qd. Max: 320mg/day. Renal Dysfunction: CrCl 31-50mL/min: Dose q24-36h. CrCl 10-30mL/min: Dose q24-48h. CrCl <10mL/min: Dose q40-60h.

**HOW SUPPLIED:** Tab: 20mg*, 40mg*, 80mg* *scored

**CONTRAINDICATIONS:** Bronchial asthma, sinus bradycardia and >1st-degree conduction block, cardiogenic shock, overt cardiac failure.

**WARNINGS/PRECAUTIONS:** May lead to incidence or worsening of cardiac failure. Exacerbation of angina, myocardial infarction reported upon abrupt discontinuation of therapy. Avoid in patients with bronchospastic disease. Impairs ability of heart to respond to β-adrenergically mediated stimuli, but d/c prior to surgery is controversial. May prevent appearance of signs and symptoms of acute hypoglycemia (eg, tachycardia, and BP changes). May mask clinical signs of hyperthyroidism; may precipitate thyroid storm with abrupt withdrawal. Caution in elderly and patients with renal dysfunction.

**ADVERSE REACTIONS:** Paresthesias, sedation, change in behavior, nausea, diarrhea, anorexia, abdominal discomfort, rash, pruritus, weight gain, blurred vision, peripheral vascular insufficiency, cardiac failure, rhythm/conduction disturbances.

**INTERACTIONS:** Additive hypotension and/or bradycardia with catecholamine-depleting drugs (eg, reserpine) and digitalis glycoside. Reduces insulin release in response to hyperglycemia and may prevent premonitory signs/symptoms of acute hypoglycemia; adjust antidiabetic agents accordingly. General anesthetics may exaggerate hypotension. May reduce effects of epinephrine.

**PREGNANCY:** Category C, not for use in nursing.

**MECHANISM OF ACTION:** Nonselective β-blocker; has not been established. Suspected to competitively antagonize catecholamines at peripheral adrenergic neuron sites, leading to decreased cardiac output; a central effect leading to reduced sympathetic outflow to the periphery and suppression of renin activity.

**PHARMACOKINETICS: Absorption:** $T_{max}$=3-4 hrs. **Distribution:** Plasma protein binding (30%). **Elimination:** Kidney, excreted unchanged; $T_{1/2}$=20-40 hrs.

## NURSING CONSIDERATIONS

**Assessment:** Assess for bronchial asthma, sinus bradycardia, AV block, cardiogenic shock, CHF, bronchospastic disease, CAD, hyperthyroidism, DM, renal impairment, possible drug interactions, pregnancy/nursing status.

**Monitoring:** Monitor renal function periodically. Monitor for signs/symptoms of cardiac failure, hypoglycemia, thyrotoxicosis, withdrawal symptoms, renal dysfunction, and hypersensitivity reactions.

**Patient Counseling:** Warn against interruption or d/c of therapy without consulting physician. Inform drug may mask signs of thyrotoxicosis and hypoglycemia. Advise to seek medical attention if symptoms of heart failure, withdrawal (angina, tremulousness, sweating, headache) or hypersensitivity reactions occur.

**Administration:** Oral route. **Storage:** Room temperature; avoid excessive heat. Protect from light. Keep bottle tightly closed.

# NALBUPHINE — RX

nalbuphine HCl (Various)

**THERAPEUTIC CLASS:** Agonist-antagonist analgesic

**INDICATIONS:** Relief of moderate to severe pain. Adjunct to balanced anesthesia for pre- and postoperative analgesia, and for obstetrical analgesia during labor and delivery.

**DOSAGE:** *Adults:* ≥18 yrs: Pain: Initial: 10mg/70kg IV/IM/SQ q3-6h prn. Adjust according to severity, physical status, and concomitant agents. Max:

20mg/dose or 160mg/day. Anesthesia Adjunct: Induction: 0.3-3mg/kg IV over 10-15 min. Maint: 0.25-0.5mg/kg IV.

**HOW SUPPLIED:** Inj: 10mg/mL, 20mg/mL

**WARNINGS/PRECAUTIONS:** Increased risk of respiratory depression with head injury, intracranial lesions, or pre-existing increased ICP. Only for use by specifically trained persons. Naloxone, resuscitative and intubation equipment, and oxygen should be readily available. Caution with emotionally unstable patients, narcotic abuse, impaired respiration, MI with nausea and vomiting, biliary tract surgery. May impair ability to drive or operate machinery. Caution with renal or hepatic dysfunction; reduce dose. Caution during labor and delivery; monitor newborns for respiratory depression, apnea, bradycardia, and arrhythmias.

**ADVERSE REACTIONS:** Sedation, sweating, N/V, dizziness/vertigo, dry mouth, headache, injection-site reactions.

**INTERACTIONS:** Possible additive effects with narcotic analgesics, general anesthetics, phenothiazines, tranquilizers, sedatives, hypnotics, or other CNS depressants. Incompatible with nafcillin and ketorolac.

**PREGNANCY:** Category B, caution in nursing.

**MECHANISM OF ACTION:** Opioid agonist-antagonist analgesic; kappa agonist/partial mu antagonist analgesic.

**PHARMACOKINETICS: Metabolism:** Liver. **Elimination:** Urine; $T_{1/2}$=5 hrs.

## NURSING CONSIDERATIONS

**Assessment:** Assess for emotional instability, history of opioid abuse, head injury, intracranial lesions, increased ICP, possible drug interactions, respiratory, renal and hepatic impairment.

**Monitoring:** Monitor for signs/symptoms of respiratory depression, hypersensitivity reactions, increased ICP, and withdrawal symptoms.

**Patient Counseling:** May impair physical/mental abilities. Advise to seek medical attention if symptoms of respiratory depression, hypersensitivity reactions, increased ICP, or withdrawal symptoms (upon abrupt d/c) occur.

**Administration:** SC, IM, or IV. **Storage:** 25°C (77°F); excursions permitted to 15-30°C (59-86°F). Protect from excessive light.



# NALOXONE — RX

naloxone HCl (Various)

**THERAPEUTIC CLASS:** Opioid antagonist

**INDICATIONS:** For complete or partial opioid depression reversal induced by natural and synthetic opioids. Diagnosis of suspected opioid tolerance or acute opioid overdose. Adjunct in management of septic shock to increase blood pressure.

**DOSAGE:** *Adults:* Opioid Overdose: Initial: 0.4-2mg IV every 2-3 min up to 10mg. IM/SQ if IV route not available. Post-op Opioid Depression: 0.1-0.2mg IV every 2-3 min to desired response. May repeat in 1-2 hr intervals. Elderly: Start at the low end of dosing range. Supplemental IM doses last longer. *Pediatrics:* Opioid Overdose: Initial: 0.01mg/kg IV. Inadequate Response: repeat 0.1mg/kg once. IM/SQ in divided doses if IV route not available. Post-op Opioid Depression: 0.005-0.01mg IV every 2-3 min to desired response. May be diluted with sterile water for injection prn. Supplemental IM doses last longer. Neonates: Opioid-induced Depression: 0.01mg/kg IV/IM/SQ, every 2-3 min until desired response. May repeat in 1-2 hr intervals.

**HOW SUPPLIED:** Inj: 0.4mg/mL, 1mg/mL

**WARNINGS/PRECAUTIONS:** Caution in patients including newborns of mothers known or suspected of opioid physical dependence. May precipitate acute withdrawal syndrome. Have other resuscitative measures available. Caution with cardiac, renal, or hepatic disease. Monitor patients satisfactorily responding due to extended opioid duration of action. Abrupt postoperative opioid depression reversal may result in serious adverse effects leading to death. Not effective against respiratory depression due to non-opioid drugs. Caution in elderly.

**ADVERSE REACTIONS:** HTN, hypotension, ventricular tachycardia and fibrillation, dyspnea, pulmonary edema, cardiac arrest, N/V, sweating, seizures, body aches, fever, nervousness, weakness, diarrhea.

**INTERACTIONS:** Caution using drugs with potential adverse cardiac effects. Reversal of buprenorphine-induced respiratory depression may be incomplete. Methohexital appears to block the acute onset of withdrawal symptoms in opiate addicts.

**PREGNANCY:** Category C, caution in nursing.

**MECHANISM OF ACTION:** Narcotic antagonist; prevents or reverses effects of opioids, including respiratory depression, sedation, and hypotension, by competing for same receptor sites. Also reverses psychotomimetic and dysphoric effects of agonist-antagonists (eg, pentazocine).

**PHARMACOKINETICS: Distribution:** Rapid; crosses the placenta. Plasma protein binding (weak). **Metabolism:** Liver; via glucuronide conjugation; naloxone-3-glucuronide (major metabolite). **Elimination:** Urine (25-40% in 6 hrs, 50% in 24 hrs, 60-70% in 72 hrs); $T_{1/2}$=30-81 mins (adults), 3.1 hrs (neonates).

## NURSING CONSIDERATIONS

**Assessment:** Assess for hypersensitivity, history of drug dependency, presence of resuscitative measures (eg, free airway, artificial ventilation, cardiac massage, vasopressors), hypo/hypertension, ventricular tachycardia and fibrillation, pulmonary edema, and cardiac arrest.

**Monitoring:** Monitor for signs/symptoms of opioid withdrawal (eg, body aches, diarrhea, tachycardia, fever, runny nose, sneezing, piloerection, sweating, yawning, NV, nervousness, restlessness, irritability, shivering or trembling, abdominal cramps, weakness, increase BP), and satisfactory response.

**Administration:** IM/IV/SQ routes. **Storage:** 20-25°C (68-77°F). Protect from light.

N

# NAMENDA RX

memantine HCl (Forest)

**THERAPEUTIC CLASS:** NMDA receptor antagonist

**INDICATIONS:** Treatment of moderate to severe dementia of the Alzheimer's type.

**DOSAGE:** *Adults:* Initial: 5mg qd. Titrate: Increase at intervals of at least one week to 5mg bid, then 5mg and 10mg as separate doses, then to 10mg bid. Severe Renal Impairment: (5-29mL/min): Target Dose: 5mg bid.

**HOW SUPPLIED:** Sol: 2mg/mL; Tab: 5mg, 10mg; Titration-Pak: 5mg [28s], 10mg [21s].

**WARNINGS/PRECAUTIONS:** Use not evaluated with seizure disorders. Alkalinized urine (eg, renal tubular acidosis, severe urinary tract infections) may increase levels. Reduce dose with severe renal impairment. Should be administered with caution to patients with severe hepatic impairment.

**ADVERSE REACTIONS:** Dizziness, confusion, headache, constipation, coughing, HTN, pain, vomiting, somnolence, hallucinations.

**INTERACTIONS:** Caution with other NMDA antagonists (eg, amantadine, ketamine, dextromethorphan), urinary alkalinizers (eg, carbonic anhydrase inhibitors, sodium bicarbonate). Other renally-excreted drugs (eg, HCTZ, triamterene, metformin, cimetidine, ranitidine, quinidine, nicotine) may alter levels of both agents.

**PREGNANCY:** Category B, caution in nursing.

**MECHANISM OF ACTION:** NMDA receptor antagonist; postulated to exert effect by binding to NMDA receptor-operated cation channels.

**PHARMACOKINETICS: Absorption:** $T_{max}$=3-7 hrs. **Distribution:** $V_d$=9-11L/kg; plasma protein binding (45%). **Metabolism:** Hepatic (partial). **Elimination:** Urine (48%); $T_{1/2}$=60-80 hrs.

## NURSING CONSIDERATIONS

**Assessment:** Assess for conditions that raise urine pH (carbonic anhydrase inhibitors, $NaHCO_3$, RTA, severe UTI), possible drug interactions, renal/hepatic function.

**Monitoring:** Monitor renal/hepatic function.

**Patient Counseling:** Inform can be taken with/without food.

**Administration:** Oral route. **Storage**: 25°C (77°F); excursions permitted to 15-30°C (59-86°F).

# NAPRELAN RX

naproxen sodium (Elan)

**NSAIDs may cause an increased risk of serious cardiovascular (CV) thrombotic events, myocardial infarction (MI), stroke, and serious GI adverse events including bleeding, ulceration, and perforation of the stomach or intestines. Contraindicated for the treatment of perioperative pain in the setting of coronary artery bypass graft (CABG) surgery.**

**THERAPEUTIC CLASS:** NSAID

**INDICATIONS:** Treatment of rheumatoid arthritis (RA), osteoarthritis (OA), ankylosing spondylitis (AS), tendinitis, bursitis, primary dysmenorrhea, and acute gout. Relief of mild to moderate pain.

**DOSAGE:** *Adults:* RA/OA/AS: Initial: 750mg-1g qd. Max: 1.5g/day. Pain/ Primary Dysmenorrhea/Tendinitis/Bursitis: 1g/day or 1.5g for a limited period. Max: 1g/day thereafter. Acute Gout: Initial: 1-1.5g qd for 1 day, Maint: 1g qd until attack subsides. Elderly/Renal/Hepatic Impairment: Start at lower end of dosing range.

N

**HOW SUPPLIED:** Tab, Controlled-Release: 375mg, 500mg, 750mg

**CONTRAINDICATIONS:** History of asthma, urticaria, allergic/anaphylactic type reactions with aspirin (ASA), or other NSAIDs. Treatment of perioperative pain in the setting of CABG surgery.

**WARNINGS/PRECAUTIONS:** Patients with known CV disease or risk factors for CV disease may be at greatest risk for thrombotic events, MI, or stroke; use lowest effective dose for the shortest duration possible. May lead to onset of new HTN or worsening of pre-existing HTN; monitor BP closely. Caution in patients with fluid retention or heart failure. Renal papillary necrosis and other renal injury reported after long-term use. Not recommended for use with advanced renal disease; if therapy must be initiated, monitor renal function. Anaphylactoid reactions may occur. May cause serious skin adverse events (eg, exfoliative dermatitis, Stevens-Johnson syndrome (SJS), and toxic epidermal necrolysis (TEN)). Avoid in late pregnancy; may cause premature closure of ductus arteriosis. May cause elevations of LFTs; d/c if liver disease develops or systemic manifestations occur. Caution in elderly. Anemia may occur; monitor Hgb/Hct if signs or symptoms of anemia develop with long-term use. May inhibit platelet aggregation and prolong bleeding time; monitor with coagulation disorders. Caution with asthma and avoid with ASA-sensitive asthma. Not intended to substitute for corticosteroids or treat corticosteroid insufficiency.

**ADVERSE REACTIONS:** Headache, dyspepsia, flu syndrome, pain, infection, nausea, diarrhea, constipation, tinnitus, heartburn, drowsiness, edema, skin rash, ecchymoses, pharyngitis.

**INTERACTIONS:** Avoid concomitant use with other products containing naproxen and ASA. May inhibit natriuretic effect of furosemide and thiazides. May diminish antihypertensive effect of angiotensin converting enzyme (ACE) inhibitors. May increase lithium levels; monitor for lithium toxicity. May enhance methotrexate toxicity. Synergistic effect with warfarin.

**PREGNANCY:** Category C, not for use in nursing.

**MECHANISM OF ACTION:** NSAID; not fully established, suspected to inhibit prostaglandin synthetase.

**PHARMACOKINETICS: Absorption:** Rapid, complete; bioavailability (95%); $C_{max}$=94mcg/mL; $T_{max}$=5 hrs; AUC=1448mcg•hr/mL. **Distribution:** $V_d$=0.16L/kg; plasma protein binding (>99%). **Metabolism:** Hepatic; 6-O-desmethyl naproxen (metabolite). **Elimination:** Urine, feces (≤5%); $T_{1/2}$=15 hrs.

## NURSING CONSIDERATIONS

**Assessment:** Assess for CVD (HTN, CHF) or risk factors for disease, history of ulcer disease, asthma, pregnancy status, risk factors for GI events (bleeding, ulceration, perforation), possible drug interactions, renal and hepatic dysfunction.

**Monitoring:** Monitor BP, CBC, LFTs, renal function, and blood chemistries periodically. Monitor for signs/symptoms of GI events (bleeding, ulceration, perforation), hypersensitivity reaction (eosinophilia, rash), renal/liver dysfunction.

**Patient Counseling:** Advise to seek medical attention if symptoms of hepatotoxicity (eg, nausea, fatigue, lethargy, pruritus, jaundice, right upper quadrant tenderness, and flu-like symptoms), anaphylactic reaction (difficulty breathing, swelling of face/throat), hypersensitivity reaction (eg, rash, blisters, itching), fever, exfoliative dermatitis, SJS, TEN, CV events (eg, MI, stroke, chest pain, SOB, weakness, slurring of speech), GI ulceration and bleeding (eg, epigastric pain, dyspepsia, melena, hematemesis), weight gain, or edema occur. Inform of pregnancy risks.

**Administration:** Oral route. **Storage:** 20-25°C (68-77°F).

# NAPROSYN **RX**

naproxen (Roche Labs)

**NSAIDs may cause an increased risk of serious cardiovascular thrombotic events, MI, stroke, and serious GI adverse events including bleeding, ulceration, and perforation of the stomach or intestines. Contraindicated for the treatment of perioperative pain in the setting of coronary artery bypass graft (CABG) surgery.**

**OTHER BRAND NAMES:** EC-Naprosyn (Roche Labs)

**THERAPEUTIC CLASS:** NSAID

**INDICATIONS:** (Naprosyn, EC-Naprosyn) Relieves signs and symptoms of rheumatoid arthritis (RA), osteoarthritis (OA), ankylosing spondylitis, and juvenile arthritis (JA). (Naprosyn) Relieves signs and symptoms of tendinitis, bursitis, and acute gout. Management of pain and primary dysmenorrhea. EC-Naprosyn not recommended for initial treatment of acute pain.

**DOSAGE:** *Adults:* RA/OA/Ankylosing Spondylitis: Naprosyn: 250, 375, or 500mg bid; EC-Naprosyn: 375 or 500mg bid. Max: 1500mg/day. Acute Gout: Naprosyn: 750mg followed by 250mg q8h until attack subsides. Pain/Dysmenorrhea/Tendinitis/Bursitis: Naprosyn: 500mg followed by 500mg q12h or 250mg q6-8h prn. EC-Naprosyn should not be chewed, crushed, or broken.

*Pediatrics:* ≥2 yrs: JA: (Sus) 5mg/kg bid. Max: 10mg/kg/day.

**HOW SUPPLIED:** (Naprosyn) Sus: 25mg/mL; Tab: 250mg*, 375mg, 500mg*; (EC-Naprosyn) Tab, Delayed-Release: 375mg, 500mg *scored

**CONTRAINDICATIONS:** Asthma, urticaria, or other allergic-type reactions with aspirin (ASA) or other NSAIDs. Treatment of perioperative pain in the setting of CABG surgery.

**WARNINGS/PRECAUTIONS:** May lead to onset of new HTN or worsening of pre-existing HTN; monitor BP closely. Fluid retention, edema, and peripheral edema reported; caution with fluid retention, HTN, or heart failure. Renal papillary necrosis and other renal injury reported after long-term use. Not recommended for use with advanced renal disease; if therapy must be initiated, monitor renal function closely. Anaphylactoid reactions may occur. May cause serious skin adverse events (eg, exfoliative dermatitis, Stevens-Johnson syndrome, toxic epidermal necrolysis). Avoid in late pregnancy; may

N

cause premature closure of ductus arteriosis. Monitor for visual changes or disturbances. May cause elevations of LFTs; d/c if liver disease develops or systemic manifestations occur. Caution with high doses in chronic alcoholic liver disease and elderly. Anemia may occur with long-term use; monitor Hgb/Hct if signs or symptoms of anemia develop or if initial Hgb ≤10g. May inhibit platelet aggregation and prolong bleeding time; monitor with coagulation disorders. Caution with asthma and avoid with ASA-sensitive asthma.

**ADVERSE REACTIONS:** Edema, drowsiness, dizziness, constipation, heartburn, abdominal pain, nausea, headache, tinnitus, dyspnea, pruritus, skin eruptions, ecchymoses.

**INTERACTIONS:** (Naprosyn, EC-Naprosyn) Avoid with other products containing naproxen. Potential for increased effects with ASA. May reduce tubular secretion of methotrexate; monitor for toxicity. May increase nephrotoxicity of cyclosporine; caution when coadministering. May diminish antihypertensive effect and potentiate renal disease with ACE inhibitors. May reduce natriuretic effect of furosemide and thiazides; monitor for renal failure. May increase lithium levels; monitor for toxicity. Increased risk of GI bleeding with SSRIs. Synergistic effects on GI bleeding with warfarin. Observe for dose adjustment with hydantoins, sulfonamides, or sulfonylureas. May reduce antihypertensive effects of propranolol and other β-blockers. Probenecid increases half-life significantly. (EC-Naprosyn) Avoid with $H_2$-blockers, sucralfate, or intensive antacid therapy.

**PREGNANCY:** Category C, not for use in nursing.

**MECHANISM OF ACTION:** NSAID; unknown, related to prostaglandin synthetase inhibition.

**PHARMACOKINETICS: Absorption:** Rapid and complete. Bioavailability (95%), $C_{max}$=97.4mcg/mL; $T_{max}$=2-4 hrs; $AUC_{0-12h}$=767mcg•hr/mL. (Tab, Delayed-Release) $C_{max}$=94.9mcg/mL; $T_{max}$=4 hrs; $AUC_{0-12h}$=845mcg•hr/mL. (Sus) $T_{max}$=1-4 hrs. **Distribution:** $V_d$=0.16L/kg; plasma protein binding (>99%). **Metabolism:** Hepatic. Metabolite (6-O-desmethyl naproxen). **Elimination:** Urine (95%), feces (≤3%); $T_{1/2}$=12-17 hrs.



## NURSING CONSIDERATIONS

**Assessment:** Assess for history of asthma, CV thrombotic events, CABG surgery, stroke, MI, CV disease (pre-existing HTN, CHF) or risk factors for disease, fluid retention, edema, pregnancy status, risk factors for GI events (bleeding, ulceration, perforation), possible drug interactions, renal/hepatic dysfunction.

**Monitoring:** Monitor BP, CBC, LFTs, renal function, and chemistries periodically. Monitor for signs/symptoms of GI events (bleeding, ulceration, perforation), CV thrombotic events, CHF, HTN, anemia, salt depletion, renal/liver dysfunction.

**Patient Counseling:** Seek medical attention if symptoms of hepatotoxicity (nausea, fatigue, pruritus), anaphylactic reaction (difficulty breathing, swelling of face/throat), hypersensitivity reaction (rash), CV events (chest pain, SOB, weakness, slurring of speech), GI ulceration and bleeding (epigastric pain, dyspepsia, melena, hematemesis), weight gain, and edema occur. Inform of pregnancy risks. Caution should be exercised if drowsiness, dizziness, vertigo or depression is experienced during therapy.

**Administration:** PO. **Storage:** (Sus): 15-30°C (59-86°); avoid excessive heat, above 40°C (104°F). Dispense in light-resistant containers. Shake before use. (Tab, Delayed-Release): 15-30° (59-86°F) in tightly closed containers; dispense in light-resistant containers. (Tab): 15-30°C (59-86°F) in tightly closed containers.

# NARDIL RX

phenelzine sulfate (Parke-Davis)

**Antidepressants increased the risk of suicidal thinking and behavior (suicidality) in short-term studies in children, adolescents, and young adults with major depressive disorder (MDD) and other psychiatric disorders. Phenelzine is not approved for use in pediatric patients.**

**THERAPEUTIC CLASS:** Monoamine oxidase inhibitor

**INDICATIONS:** Treatment of atypical, nonendogenous or neurotic depression not responsive to other antidepressants.

**DOSAGE:** *Adults:* Initial: 15mg tid. Titrate: Increase to 60-90mg/day at a fairly rapid pace until maximum benefit. Maint: Reduce slowly over several weeks to 15mg qd or 15mg every other day.

**HOW SUPPLIED:** Tab: 15mg

**CONTRAINDICATIONS:** Pheochromocytoma, CHF, history of liver disease, abnormal LFTs, severe renal impairment or renal disease, meperidine, MAOIs, dextromethorphan, CNS depressants, alcohol, certain narcotics, sympathomimetic drugs (eg, amphetamines, cocaine, methylphenidate, dopamine, epinephrine, norepinephrine), or related compounds (eg, methyldopa, L-dopa, L-tryptophan, L-tyrosine, phenylalanine), high tyramine-containing food (eg, cheese, pickled herring, beer, wine, yeast extract, salami, yogurt), excessive caffeine and chocolate, dextromethorphan, CNS depressants, buspirone, serotoninergic agents (eg, dexfenfluramine, fluoxetine, fluvoxamine, paroxetine, sertraline, venlafaxine), bupropion, guanethidine.

**WARNINGS/PRECAUTIONS:** Hypertensive crisis, postural hypotension reported; monitor BP frequently. Caution with epilepsy, asthma, DM, or psychosis. D/C if palpitations or headache occur. Excessive stimulation in schizophrenics. D/C 10 days prior to elective surgery. Avoid abrupt withdrawal.

**ADVERSE REACTIONS:** Dizziness, headache, drowsiness, sleep disturbances, constipation, dry mouth, GI disturbances, elevated serum transaminases, weight gain, edema, sexual disturbances.

**INTERACTIONS:** See Contraindications. Hypertensive crisis with other MAOIs, sympathomimetics, high tyramine-containing foods. Allow 10 days between starting another MAOI, or antidepressant or buspirone. Serious reactions reported with serotoninergic agents. Allow 5 weeks after d/c fluoxetine before starting therapy. Allow 2 weeks after d/c therapy before starting bupropion. Avoid cocaine and local, general, and spinal anesthesia. Reduce dose of barbiturates. Caution with rauwolfia alkaloids. Exaggerated hypotensive effects with antihypertensives. Excitation, seizures, delirium, hyperpyrexia, circulatory collapse, coma, and death have been reported with meperidine.

**PREGNANCY:** Safety in pregnancy and nursing not known.

**MECHANISM OF ACTION:** MAOI; inhibits MAO activity.

**PHARMACOKINETICS: Absorption:** (30mg): $C_{max}$=19.8ng/mL, $T_{max}$=43 mins. **Metabolism:** Oxidation via MAO. Acetylation (minor). **Elimination:** (30mg): $T_{1/2}$=11.6 hrs.

## NURSING CONSIDERATIONS

**Assessment:** Assess for DM, pheochromocytoma, CHF, history of liver disease, possible drug interactions, risk for bipolar disorder, history of mania or seizures or schizophrenia, pregnancy/nursing status, severe renal/hepatic impairment.

**Monitoring:** Monitor BP, renal/hepatic function, for signs/symptoms of clinical worsening (suicidality, unusual changes in behavior), hypertensive crisis (occipital headaches, neck stiffness, NV, sweating), seizures, liver dysfunction, postural hypotension, hypoglycemia, increased psychosis, and activation of mania.

**Patient Counseling:** Instruct to avoid concomitant use of alcohol, tyramine-containing foods/supplements/beverages (during and 2 weeks following d/c), and any cough medicine containing dextromethorphan. Seek medical attention for symptoms of hypertensive crisis (occipital headaches, neck

N

stiffness, NV, sweating), hypoglycemia, increased psychosis, seizures, postural hypotension, mania, clinical worsening (suicidal ideation, unusual changes in behavior), and liver dysfunction. Advise to change position gradually if lightheaded, faint, or dizzy. Counsel about pregnancy risks.

**Administration:** Oral route. **Storage:** 15-30°C (59-86°F).

## NAROPIN RX

ropivacaine HCl (Abraxis)

**THERAPEUTIC CLASS:** Local anesthetic

**INDICATIONS:** Production of local or regional anesthesia in surgery. Management of acute pain.

**DOSAGE:** *Adults:* Dose may vary by procedure, area to be anesthetized, tissue vascularity, duration and depth of anesthesia needed. Administer test dose of 3-5mL before induction of complete block. Surgical: Lumbar Epidural: Usual: 75-200mg in 15-30mL. Thoracic Epidural for Surgery: 25-113mg in 5-15mL. Lumbar Epidural in Cesarean: 100-150mg in 15-30mL. Major Nerve Block: 75-300mg in 10-50mL. Field Block: 5-200mg in 1-40mL Labor: Lumbar Epidural: Initial: 20-40mg. Maint: 12-28mg/h. Postoperative: Lumbar/Thoracic Epidural: 12-28mg/hr. Infiltration: 2-200mg in 1-100mL.

**HOW SUPPLIED:** Inj: 2mg/mL, 5mg/mL, 7.5mg/mL, 10mg/mL

**WARNINGS/PRECAUTIONS:** Administer in incremental doses. High risk of arrhythmias, circulatory arrest, and death reported in pregnant patients. Not for production of obstetrical paracervical block, retrobulbar block, or spinal anesthesia. Use lowest effective dose. Perform syringe aspiration to avoid extravasation and subarachnoid injection. Administer test dose with epidural anesthesia. Anxiety, dizziness, blurred vision, tremors, depression, and tinnitus are early signs of CNS toxicity. Caution in hepatic impairment, cardiovascular disorders, hypotension, hypovolemia, heart block. Should cardiac arrest occur, prolonged resuscitative efforts may be required to improve the probability of a successful outcome.



**ADVERSE REACTIONS:** Hypotension, bradycardia, N/V, paresthesia, back pain, fever, chills, headache, pain, urinary retention, dizziness, pruritus, HTN, anemia.

**INTERACTIONS:** Caution with other local anesthetics, amide-type anesthetics; additive toxic effects may occur. Caution with class III antiarrhythmics. Increased levels with inhibitors of CYP450 1A2 (eg, fluvoxamine) and CYP450 3A4 (eg, ketoconazole).

**PREGNANCY:** Category B, caution in nursing.

**MECHANISM OF ACTION:** Amino amide local anesthetic; blocks the generation and conduction of nerve impulses, presumably by increasing the threshold for electrical excitation in the nerve by slowing the propagation of the nerve impulse and by reducing the rate of rise of the action potential.

**PHARMACOKINETICS: Absorption:** Complete and biphasic absorption (epidural space). Systemic concentration of drug is dependent on total dose, concentration, and route of administration; refer to PI for more information. **Distribution:** $V_d$=41L (IV); plasma protein binding (94%); crosses placenta; excreted in breast milk. **Metabolism:** Liver (extensive); aromatic hydroxylation, CYP4501A; 3-hydroxyropivacaine. **Elimination:** Urine: IV (86%), (1% unchanged); $T_{1/2}$=1.8 hrs and 4.2 hrs (epidural).

### NURSING CONSIDERATIONS

**Assessment:** Assess for drug hypersensitivity, hepatic disease, impaired cardiovascular function, hypotension, hypovolemia or heart block or taking class III antiarrhythmic drugs (eg, amiodarone), pregnancy/nursing status, and possible drug interactions.

**Monitoring:** Monitor HR, BP and ECG, for allergic reactions, test dose reactions (eg, palpitations, nervousness and circumoral pallor), signs of CNS toxicity (eg, anxiety, light headedness, blurred vision, dizziness, and tremors), signs of unintended intrathecal administration, cardiovascular/respiratory vital signs, state of consciousness, and malignant hyperthermia.

**Patient Counseling:** Inform may experience temporary loss of sensation and motor activity in the anesthetized part of the body.

**Administration:** Epidural, IV route. **Storage:** 20-25°C (68-77°F).

# NASACORT AQ RX

triamcinolone acetonide (Sanofi-Aventis)

**THERAPEUTIC CLASS:** Corticosteroid

**INDICATIONS:** Treatment of the nasal symptoms of seasonal and perennial allergic rhinitis in adults and children ≥2 yrs.

**DOSAGE:** *Adults:* Initial/Max: 2 sprays per nostril qd. With improvement, may reduce dose to 1 spray per nostril qd.
*Pediatrics:* ≥12 yrs: Initial/Max: 2 sprays per nostril qd. With improvement, may reduce dose to 1 spray per nostril qd. 6-12 yrs: Initial: 1 spray per nostril qd. Max: 2 sprays per nostril qd. 2-5 yrs: Initial/Max: 1 spray per nostril qd.

**HOW SUPPLIED:** Spray: 55mcg/spray [16.5g]

**WARNINGS/PRECAUTIONS:** Glaucoma and/or cataracts may occur. Risk of adrenal insufficiency and withdrawal symptoms when replacing systemic corticosteroid with topical corticosteroids. Caution with active or quiescent TB, ocular herpes simplex, or untreated bacterial, fungal and systemic viral infections. Avoid with recent nasal trauma, surgery or septum ulcers. Risk for more severe/fatal course of infections (eg, chickenpox, measles) and for *Candida* infections of nose and pharynx. Potential for reduced growth velocity in pediatrics. Epistaxis and nasal septal perforation reported.

**ADVERSE REACTIONS:** Pharyngitis, epistaxis, increased cough, flu syndrome, bronchitis, dyspepsia, tooth disorder, headache, pharyngolaryngeal pain, nasopharyngitis, upper abdominal pain, diarrhea, asthma, and rash.

**PREGNANCY:** Category C, caution in nursing.

**MECHANISM OF ACTION:** Corticosteroid; not established; anti-inflammatory action.

**PHARMACOKINETICS: Absorption:** $C_{max}$=0.5ng/mL; $T_{max}$=1.5 hrs; AUC (110mcg, 400mcg)=1.4ng•hr/mL, 4.7ng•hr/mL. **Distribution:** $V_d$=99.5L. **Elimination:** $T_{1/2}$=3.1 hrs.

## NURSING CONSIDERATIONS

**Assessment:** Assess for hypersensitivity, active or quiescent TB, untreated local or systemic fungal or bacterial infections, systemic viral or parasitic infections, ocular herpes simplex, nasal polyps or recent nasal septal ulcers, nasal surgery/trauma, concomitant use with other inhaled or systemic corticosteroids, and possible drug interactions.

**Monitoring:** Monitor for acute adrenal insufficiency, withdrawal symptoms, joint and/or muscular pain, lassitude and depression, hypercorticism and/or HPA-axis suppression, disseminated infections (eg, chickenpox and measles), nasal or pharyngeal *Candida* infections, hypoadrenalism in infants whose mothers received corticosteroids during pregnancy, suppression of growth velocity in children, nasal septal perforation or nasal septum discomfort, epistaxis, glaucoma, and cataracts.

**Patient Counseling:** Instruct to take as directed at regular intervals. Avoid exposure to chickenpox or measles; immediately notify physician if exposed, if symptoms worsen or do not improve, or if sneezing or nasal irritation occurs. Avoid spraying into eyes.

**Administration:** Intranasal. **Storage:** 20-25°C (68-77°F).

## NASONEX RX

mometasone furoate monohydrate (Schering)

**THERAPEUTIC CLASS:** Corticosteroid

**INDICATIONS:** Treatment of the nasal symptoms of seasonal and perennial allergic rhinitis. Prophylaxis of the nasal symptoms of seasonal allergic rhinitis. Treatment of nasal polyps in patients 18 years of age and older.

**DOSAGE:** *Adults:* Allergic Rhinitis: Treatment/Prophylaxis: 2 sprays per nostril qd. For prophylaxis, start 2-4 weeks before allergy season. Nasal Polyps: 2 sprays per nostril bid.
*Pediatrics:* ≥12 yrs: Treatment/Prophylaxis: 2 sprays per nostril qd. For prophylaxis, start 2-4 weeks before allergy season. 2-11 yrs: Treatment: 1 spray per nostril qd.

**HOW SUPPLIED:** Spray: 50mcg/spray [17g]

**WARNINGS/PRECAUTIONS:** Risk of adrenal insufficiency and withdrawal symptoms when replacing systemic corticosteroids with topical corticosteroids. Caution with active or quiescent TB, ocular herpes simplex, or untreated bacterial, fungal and systemic viral infections. Avoid with recent nasal trauma, surgery or septum ulcers. Risk for more severe/fatal course of infections (eg, chickenpox, measles) and for *Candida* infections of nose and pharynx. Potential for reduced growth velocity in pediatrics.

**ADVERSE REACTIONS:** Headache, viral infection, pharyngitis, epistaxis, cough, upper respiratory tract infection, dysmenorrhea, myalgia, sinusitis.

**PREGNANCY:** Category C, caution with nursing.

**MECHANISM OF ACTION:** Corticosteroid; not established; demonstrates anti-inflammatory properties, shown to have a wide range of effects on multiple cell types (eg, mast cells, eosinophils, neutrophils, macrophages, lymphocytes) and mediators (eg, histamine, eicosanoids, leukotrienes, cytokines) involved in inflammation.



**PHARMACOKINETICS: Distribution:** Plasma protein binding (98-99%). **Metabolism:** Liver (extensive) via CYP3A4. **Elimination:** Bile (as metabolites); $T_{1/2}$=5.8 hrs.

### NURSING CONSIDERATIONS

**Assessment:** Assess for active or quiescent TB, untreated localized or systemic viral, fungal or bacterial infections, history of glaucoma or cataracts, history of nasal polyps, recent nasal septal ulcers, nasal surgery/trauma, and possible drug interactions.

**Monitoring:** Monitor for acute adrenal insufficiency, hypercorticism and/or HPA-axis suppression, nasal or pharyngeal *Candida* infections, suppression of growth velocity in children, hypersensitivity reactions or contact dermatitis, wheezing, nasal septum perforation, changes in vision, increased IOP.

**Patient Counseling:** Take as directed at regular intervals; do not increase prescribed dosage to increase effectiveness. Avoid exposure to chickenpox or measles; immediately consult physician if exposed or experience episodes of epistaxis. Contact physician if symptoms worsen or do not improve. Avoid spraying into eyes or directly onto nasal septum.

**Administration:** Intranasal route. **Storage:** 25°C (77°F); excursions permitted to 15-30°C.

## NATRECOR RX

nesiritide (Scios Inc.)

**THERAPEUTIC CLASS:** Human B-type natriuretic peptide

**INDICATIONS:** Treatment of acutely decompensated congestive heart failure with dyspnea at rest or with minimal activity.

**DOSAGE:** *Adults:* 2mcg/kg IV bolus over 60 seconds, then 0.01mcg/kg/min IV infusion.

**HOW SUPPLIED:** Inj: 1.5mg

**CONTRAINDICATIONS:** Primary therapy with cardiogenic shock or systolic BP <90mmHg.

**WARNINGS/PRECAUTIONS:** Avoid with low cardiac filling pressures. Use precautions for parenteral administration of protein pharmaceuticals or *E.coli*-derived products; may cause allergic or untoward reaction. Avoid when vasodilators are inappropriate (eg, significant valvular stenosis, restrictive/obstructive cardiomyopathy, constrictive pericarditis, pericardial tamponade, conditions where cardiac output is dependent on venous return). May affect renal function; azotemia reported. Monitor BP closely; hypotension reported. Caution with BP <100mmHg at baseline. Reduce dose or d/c if hypotension occurs.

**ADVERSE REACTIONS:** Hypotension, ventricular tachycardia, ventricular extrasystoles, headache, back pain, dizziness, anxiety, nausea, abdominal pain, insomnia.

**INTERACTIONS:** Increased risk of hypotension with drugs that cause hypotension, such as oral ACE inhibitors. Do not coadminister through the same IV catheter with heparin, insulin, ethacrynate sodium, bumetanide, enalaprilat, hydralazine, furosemide, or injectable drugs containing sodium metabisulfite; flush catheter between use with incompatible drugs.

**PREGNANCY:** Category C, caution in nursing.

**MECHANISM OF ACTION:** Human B-type natriuretic peptide; binds to the particulate guanylate cyclase receptor of vascular smooth muscle and endothelial cells, leading to increased intracellular concentrations of cGMP and smooth muscle relaxation.

**PHARMACOKINETICS: Distribution:** $V_d$=0.19L/kg. **Elimination:** Renal; $T_{1/2}$=18 min.

## NURSING CONSIDERATIONS

**Assessment:** Assess for cardiogenic shock or with SBP ≤90mmHg, significant valvular stenosis, restrictive or obstructive cardiomyopathy, constrictive pericarditis, pericardial tamponade, low cardiac filling pressure, and known hypersensitivity to drug or any of its components.

**Monitoring:** Monitor renal function test, BP, symptoms of hypotension, cardiac index/status, and hemodynamic monitoring, HR, VT, bradycardia, N/V.

**Patient Counseling:** Counsel about potential adverse effects of drug.

**Administration:** (IV) Infusion bag preparation: 1) Reconstitute one 1.5mg vial by adding 5mL of diluent. 2) Do not shake the bottle. Rock the vial gently so that all surfaces, including the stopper, are in contact with the diluent to ensure complete reconstitution. 3) Withdraw the entire contents of the reconstituted vial and add to the 250mL plastic IV bag. The IV bag should be inverted several times to ensure complete mixing. 4) Use reconstituted solution within 24 hrs and store at 2-25°C (36-77°F). **Storage:** Store below 25°C. Do not freeze. Protect from light.

# NAVANE — RX

thiothixene (Pfizer)

> **Elderly patients with dementia-related psychosis treated with atypical antipsychotic drugs are at an increased risk of death; most deaths appeared to be cardiovascular (eg, heart failure, sudden death) or infectious (eg, pneumonia) in nature. Treatment with conventional antipsychotic drugs may similarly increase mortality. Thiothixene is not approved for the treatment of patients with dementia-related psychosis.**

**THERAPEUTIC CLASS:** Thioxanthene

**INDICATIONS:** Management of schizophrenia.

**DOSAGE:** *Adults:* Mild Condition: Initial: 2mg tid. Titrate: May increase to 15mg/day. Severe Condition: Initial: 5mg bid. Usual: 20-30mg/day. Max: 60mg/day.
*Pediatrics:* ≥12 yrs: Mild Condition: Initial: 2mg tid. Titrate: May increase to

15mg/day. Severe Condition: Initial: 5mg bid. Usual: 20-30mg/day. Max: 60mg/day.

**HOW SUPPLIED:** Cap: 1mg, 2mg, 5mg, 10mg, 20mg

**CONTRAINDICATIONS:** Circulatory collapse, comatose states, CNS depression, and blood dyscrasias.

**WARNINGS/PRECAUTIONS:** May cause tardive dyskinesia (TD); consider d/c. May cause neuroleptic malignant syndrome (NMS); d/c if develops. May impair mental/physical abilities. May mask symptoms of overdose of toxic drugs. May obscure conditions such as intestinal obstruction and brain tumor. May lower seizure threshold. Monitor for pigmentary retinopathy and lenticular pigmentation. Caution with CV disease, extreme heat exposure, activities requiring alertness. May elevate prolactin levels. May cause leukopenia/neutropenia/agranulocytosis; d/c with severe neutropenia (ANC<1000/mm³), consider d/c at first sign of clinically significant decline in WBC in absence of other causes.

**ADVERSE REACTIONS:** NMS, TD, tachycardia, hypotension, lightheadedness, syncope, drowsiness, restlessness, agitation, insomnia, extrapyramidal symptoms, cerebral edema, CSF abnormalities, allergic reactions, hematologic effects (eg, leukopenia/leucocytosis).

**INTERACTIONS:** Possible additive effects (eg, hypotension) with hypotensive agents, CNS depressants, and alcohol. Increased clearance with hepatic microsomal enzyme inducers (eg, carbamazepine). Caution with atropine or related drugs. Paradoxical effects with pressor agents (eg, epinephrine).

**PREGNANCY:** Safety in pregnancy and nursing not known.

**MECHANISM OF ACTION:** Thioxanthene derivative.

## NURSING CONSIDERATIONS

**Assessment:** Assess for history of CV disorders, CNS depression or coma, blood dyscrasias, convulsive disorders, alcohol intake, and possible drug interactions.

N

**Monitoring:** Monitor for hypersensitivity reactions, TD, clinical manifestations of NMS, CV effects, visual disturbances, extrapyramidal symptoms. Monitor liver enzymes, bilirubin, CBC, prolactin, and blood glucose.

**Patient Counseling:** Advise about risk of chronic use of drug. Use caution when performing hazardous tasks (operating machinery/driving). Warn about possible additive effects (eg, hypotension) when drug is combined with hypotensive agents, with CNS depressants and/or alcohol.

**Administration:** Oral route.

# NAVELBINE — RX

vinorelbine tartrate (Pierre Fabre Pharmaceuticals Inc.)

**For IV use only; fatal if given intrathecally. Severe granulocytopenia may occur; granulocyte counts should be ≥1000cells/mm³ prior to administration. Use extreme caution to prevent extravasation (can cause local tissue necrosis and/or thrombophlebitis). Administer only under supervision of a physician experienced in the use of antineoplastic agents. Extremely important to properly position IV needle or catheter before injection.**

**THERAPEUTIC CLASS:** Vinca alkaloid

**INDICATIONS:** Single agent or in combination with cisplatin for 1st-line treatment of unresectable, advanced nonsmall cell lung cancer (NSCLC), including Stage IV NSCLC. For use in combination with cisplatin for Stage III NSCLC .

**DOSAGE:** *Adults:* Single-Agent: 30mg/m² IV weekly over 6-10 min. With Cisplatin: 25mg/m² weekly with cisplatin 100mg/m² every 4 weeks, or 30mg/m² weekly with cisplatin 120mg/m² on Days 1 and 29, then every 6 weeks. Adjustments Based on Granulocytes: If 1000-1499cells/mm³ give 50% starting dose. If <1000cells/mm³, hold dose and repeat count in 1 week. D/C if hold 3 consecutive weekly doses because granulocyte <1000cells/mm³. If fever and/or sepsis occurs while granulocytopenic or if hold 2 consecutive weekly doses due to granulocytopenia; give 75% of the starting dose if granulocytes ≥1500cells/mm$^3$, and 37.5% of the starting dose if granulocytes 1000-1499cells/mm$^3$. Hepatic Insufficiency: (bilirubin 2.1-3mg/dL) 50% of starting dose or (bilirubin >3mg/dL) 25% of starting dose. If both hematologic toxicity and hepatic insufficiency, use lowest dose. Neurotoxicity: D/C if Grade ≥2 develops.

**HOW SUPPLIED:** Inj: 10mg/mL

**CONTRAINDICATIONS:** Pretreatment granulocytes <1000cells/mm$^3$.

**WARNINGS/PRECAUTIONS:** Monitor for myleosuppression during and after therapy, and for infection and/or fever with developing severe granulocytopenia. Interstitial pulmonary changes, acute respiratory distress syndrome (ARDS), acute shortness of breath and severe bronchospasm reported. Extreme caution with compromised bone marrow reserve due to prior irradiation or chemotherapy. Radiation recall reactions may occur. Monitor for new or worsening signs/symptoms of neuropathy. Avoid contact with skin, mucosa, and eyes. Avoid pregnancy. May cause severe constipation, paralytic ileus, intestinal obstruction, necrosis, and/or perforation. Caution with severe hepatic injury or impairment.

**ADVERSE REACTIONS:** Granulocytopenia, leukopenia, thrombocytopenia, anemia, asthenia, injection site reactions/pain, phlebitis, peripheral neuropathy, NV, diarrhea, severe constipation, dyspnea, alopecia, chest pain, fatigue.

**INTERACTIONS:** Risk of acute pulmonary reactions with mitomycin. Increased incidence of granulocytopenia with cisplatin. Monitor for signs/symptoms of neuropathy with paclitaxel, either concomitantly or sequentially. Radiosensitizing effects may occur with prior or concomitant radiation therapy. Caution with CYP450 3A inhibitors, or with hepatic dysfunction; earlier onset and/or increased severity of side effects may occur.

**PREGNANCY:** Category D, not for use in nursing.

**MECHANISM OF ACTION:** Vinca alkaloid; antitumor activity thought to be due primarily to inhibition of mitosis at metaphase through its interaction with tubulin. Also interferes with amino acid, cyclic AMP, and glutathione metabolism; calmodulin-dependent $Ca^{++}$-transport ATPase activity; cellular respiration; and nucleic acid and lipid biosynthesis.

N

**PHARMACOKINETICS: Distribution**: $V_d$=25.4-40.1L/kg, plasma protein binding (79.6%-91.2%). **Metabolism**: CYP450, 3A4: deacetylvinorelbine (major metabolite), vinorelbine N-oxide. **Elimination**: Feces (46%), urine (18%); $T_{1/2}$=27.7-43.6 hrs.

## NURSING CONSIDERATIONS

**Assessment:** Assess CBC with differential, LFTs, pulmonary function. Assess for history of prior irradiation or chemotherapy, neuropathy, CVD, pregnancy status.

**Monitoring:** Monitor CBC with differential, LFTs, pulmonary function, constipation, paralytic ileus, injection-site reactions, chest pain.

**Patient Counseling:** Inform about major acute toxicities (bone marrow toxicity, specifically granulocytopenia with increased susceptibility to infection). Immediately report fever or chills, SOB, cough, other new pulmonary symptoms, abdominal pain, or constipation. Advise women to avoid pregnancy. D/C nursing.

**Administration:** IV route. **Storage:** Refrigerate vials at 2-8°C (36-46°F) in the carton. Protect from light; do not freeze.

# NEORAL **RX**

cyclosporine (Novartis)

**Should only be prescribed by experienced physicians in management of systemic immunosuppressive therapy for indicated disease. Patients should be managed at equipped and staffed facilities with adequate laboratory and supportive medical resources. Increased susceptibility to infection, development of neoplasia, HTN, and nephrotoxicity may result. Monitor blood levels to avoid toxicity or low concentration. Not bioequivalent to Sandimmune; not interchangeable without physician supervision. Caution in switching from Sandimmune. Risk of skin malignancies if previously treated with radiation therapy, UVB, coal tar, radiation, MTX, or other immunosuppressives. Caution with renal dysfunction including structural kidney damage; monitor renal function during therapy.**

**THERAPEUTIC CLASS:** Cyclic polypeptide immunosuppressant

**INDICATIONS:** Prophylaxis of organ rejection in kidney, liver, and heart allogeneic transplants. Treatment of severe active, rheumatoid arthritis (RA) unresponsive to methotrexate (MTX). Treatment of nonimmunocompromised adults with severe, recalcitrant, plaque psoriasis unresponsive to at least 1 systemic therapy (eg, PUVA, retinoids, MTX) or when other systemic therapies are contraindicated/not tolerated.

**DOSAGE:** *Adults:* Transplant: Give initial oral dose 4-12 hrs before transplant or post-op. Dose bid. Initial: Renal Transplant: 9 ± 3mg/kg/day. Liver Transplant: 8±4mg/kg/day. Heart Transplant: 7 ± 3mg/kg/day. Give with corticosteroids initially. Conversion from Sandimmune: 1:1 dose conversion. Monitor blood levels every 4-7 days while adjusting to trough levels. RA: Initial: 1.25mg/kg bid. Titrate: May increase by 0.5-0.75mg/kg/day after 8 weeks, again after 12 weeks. Max: 4mg/kg/day. Discontinue if no benefit by Week 16. Psoriasis: Initial: 1.25mg/kg bid for 4 weeks. Titrate: May increase by 0.5mg/kg/day every 2 weeks. Max: 4mg/kg/day. Decrease dose by 25-50% to control adverse events. Discontinue if no benefit by Week 6 at max dose, dose reduction not effective or adverse events severe. Take at the same time every day. Elderly: Start at lower end of dosing range.

N

**HOW SUPPLIED:** Cap: 25mg, 100mg; Sol: 100mg/mL [50mL]

**CONTRAINDICATIONS:** Abnormal renal function, uncontrolled HTN, malignancies. PUVA or UVB therapy, MTX, other immunosuppressants, coal tar, or radiation in psoriasis patients.

**WARNINGS/PRECAUTIONS:** Risk of hepatotoxicity and nephrotoxicity. Caution in elderly. Hyperkalemia, hyperuricemia, thrombocytopenia, microangiopathic hemolytic anemia, and encephalopathy reported in transplant patients. Monitor CBC and LFTs monthly with MTX. HTN may occur and persist which may require antihypertensive therapy; monitor for drug interactions. Make careful physical and dermatological examination prior to therapy in RA or psoriasis patients. Monitor BP and renal function before therapy, every 2 weeks during 1st 3 months, then monthly if stable with RA or psoriasis. Monitor SCr after initiation or increases in NSAID dose for RA. Monitor CBC, uric acid, $K^+$, lipids and magnesium every 2 weeks during 1st 3 months, then monthly if stable in RA. Monitor LFTs repeatedly. Monitor CBC, SCr with transplants. Transplant patients are at increased risk of serious infection with fatal outcome. Increased risk of opportunistic infections, including activation of latent viral infections such as BK virus-associated nephropathy in patients receiving immunosuppressants.

**ADVERSE REACTIONS:** Renal dysfunction, HTN, hirsutism/hypertrichosis, tremor, headache, gingival hyperplasia, diarrhea, N/V, paresthesia, dyspepsia, stomatitis, hypomagnesemia, BK virus-associated nephropathy.

**INTERACTIONS:** See Contraindications. Phenytoin, phenobarbital, rifampin, nafcillin, carbamazepine, orlistat, ticlopidine, octreotide, St. John's wort, oxcarbazepine, sulfinpyrazone, terbinafine and bosentan decrease cyclosporine levels. Concomitant use may increase MTX and repaglinide levels. Clarithromycin, diltiazem, fluconazole, erythromycin, itraconazole, ketoconazole, voriconazole, verapamil, nicardipine, quinupristin/dalfopristin, allopurinol, bromocriptine, danazol, metoclopramide, colchicine, amiodarone, azithromycin, methyprednisolone, imatinib, nefazodone, oral contraceptives, grapefruit and grapefruit juice increase cyclosporine levels. Aminoglycosides, ciprofloxacin, vancomycin, SMZ/TMP, melphalan, ketoconazole, NSAIDs, colchicine, cimetidine, ranitidine, tacrolimus, amphotericin B, bezafibrate, fenofibrate, methotrexate, gentamicin, tobramycin and azapropazon may potentiate renal dysfunction. Digitalis toxicity reported. Myotoxicity with statins, frequent gingival hyperplasia with nifedipine and convulsions with high-dose methylprednisolone reported. Decreased clearance of prednisolone, digoxin, and lovastatin. Avoid $K^+$ sparing diuretics. Caution with HIV protease inhibitors, $K^+$ sparing drugs (eg, ACEIs, angiotensin II receptor blockers), $K^+$ containing drugs and $K^+$ rich diets. Increased SrCr with sirolimus. Decreased effects of vaccinations; avoid live attenuated vaccines.

**PREGNANCY:** Category C, not for use in nursing.

**MECHANISM OF ACTION:** Immunosuppressive agent; inhibits immunocompetent lymphocytes in the $G_0$-and $G_1$ phase of cell cycle, preferentially T-lymphocytes (mainly T-helper cells). Also inhibits lymphokine production and release, including interleukin-2.

**PHARMACOKINETICS: Absorption:** Incomplete; $T_{max}$=1.5-2 hrs. Pharmacokinetic parameters varied with different indications (renal, liver, rheumatoid arthritis and/or psoriasis). **Distribution:** $V_d$=3L/kg (IV); plasma protein binding (90%); found in breast milk. **Metabolism:** (extensive) Via CYP3A, in liver, GI tract, kidneys. Major metabolites (M1, M9, and M4N); oxidation and demethylation pathways. **Elimination:** Bile (primary), urine (6% unchanged and metabolites); $T_{1/2}$=8.4 hrs.

## NURSING CONSIDERATIONS

**Assessment:** Baseline lab assessment for CBC, SrCr, BUN, BP, serum magnesium, $K^+$, uric acid, bilirubin, liver enzymes, and lipids. Assess for occult infections, malignancies, skin lesions, RA/psoriasis and immunosuppressive agents, vaccination history, pregnancy/nursing status, and possible drug interactions.

**Monitoring:** Routinely monitor blood levels, CBC, $K^+$, uric acid, lipids, bilirubin, liver enzymes, magnesium, microangiopathic hemolytic anemia, vasculopathy, BP, lymphoproliferative and skin malignancies, convulsions, encephalopathy, impaired consciousness, graft-versus-host disease, infections (eg, BK virus-associated nephropathy), symptoms/signs of graft rejection or nephrotoxicity, kidney biopsies for renal tubular atrophy, and interstitial fibrosis.

**Patient Counseling:** Counsel not to administer concurrently with UVB or other radiation therapy/immunosuppressive agents. Inform of necessity for repeated lab tests for renal and liver functions. Instruct to take exactly as directed. Advise regarding potential risks during pregnancy, increased risk of neoplasia, HTN, and renal dysfunction.

**Administration:** Oral route. (Dilute only with orange or apple juice, not grapefruit juice). **Storage:** Cap/Sol: 20-25°C (68-77°F). Sol: Do not refrigerate. Use within 2 months upon opening. At <20°C (68°F) may form gel, light flocculation, or formation of light sediment; warm at 25°C (77°C) to reverse changes.

# NEOSPORIN OPHTHALMIC RX

polymyxin B sulfate - neomycin sulfate - gramicidin (Monarch Pharmaceuticals Inc.)

**THERAPEUTIC CLASS:** Antibacterial combination

**INDICATIONS:** Treatment of superficial infections of the external eye and its adnexa caused by susceptible infection; including conjunctivitis, keratitis and keratoconjunctivitis, blepharitis and blepharoconjunctivitis.

**DOSAGE:** *Adults:* (Oint) Apply q3-4h for 7-10 days. (Sol) Instill 1-2 drops q4h for 7-10 days. Severe Infection: 2 drops q1h.

**HOW SUPPLIED:** Oint: (Bacitracin-Neomycin-Polymyxin B) 400U-3.5mg-10,000U/g [3.5g]; Sol: (Gramicidin-Neomycin-Polymyxin B) 0.025mg-1.75mg-10,000U/mL [10mL]

**WARNINGS/PRECAUTIONS:** Not for injection into the eye. Do not directly introduce into the anterior chamber of the eye or inject subconjunctivally. May cause cutaneous sensitization; manifested by itching, reddening and edema of the conjunctiva and eyelid; may subside quickly when medications are withdrawn. Prolonged use may result in overgrowth of nonsuceptible organisms (eg, fungi); initiate appropriate measures if superinfection develops. Bacterial resistance may develop. D/C if purulent discharge, inflammation or pain becomes aggravated. Bacterial keratitis reported. Allergic-cross reactions may occur which could prevent use of any or all of the following: kanamycin, paromomycin, streptomycin, and possibly gentamycin.

**ADVERSE REACTIONS:** Itching, swelling, conjunctival erythema, local irritation, superinfection.

**PREGNANCY:** Category C, caution in nursing.

**MECHANISM OF ACTION:** Antibacterial combination. Neomycin: aminoglycoside antibiotic; inhibits protein synthesis by binding with ribosomal RNA and causing misreading of the bacterial genetic code. Polymyxin B: increases permeability of the bacterial cell membrane by interacting with the phospholipid components of the membrane. Gramicidin: increases permeability of bacterial cell membrane to inorganic cations by forming network of channels through normal lipid bilayer of membrane. Bacitracin: interferes with bacterial cell wall synthesis by inhibition of the regeneration of phospholipid receptors involved in peptidoglycan synthesis.

## NURSING CONSIDERATIONS

**Assessment:** Assess for proper diagnosis of causative organisms and pregnancy/nursing status.

**Monitoring:** Monitor for signs/symptoms of cutaneous sensitization (eg, itching, reddening, edema of the conjunctiva or eyelid, failure to heal) and for bacterial resistance (eg, purulent discharge, inflammation). For patients on prolonged therapy, monitor for overgrowth of nonsusceptible organisms (eg, fungi) and development of superinfection. Monitor for bacterial keratitis in patients using multiple-dose containers.

**Patient Counseling:** Instruct to avoid allowing tip of dispensing container to contact the eye, eyelid, fingers, or any other surfaces. Advise that use of product by more than one person, may spread infection. Inform that ocular products, if handled improperly, can cause ocular infections. Advise if condition persists or gets worse, or if rash or allergic reaction occurs, to stop use and notify physician. Inform not to use product if have allergy to any of the ingredients. Instruct to keep medication container tightly closed when not using and to keep out of reach of children.

**Administration:** Ocular route. Do not inject into eye. **Storage:** 15-25°C (59-77°F). Protect from light.

# NEULASTA — RX

pegfilgrastim (Amgen)

**THERAPEUTIC CLASS:** Granulocyte colony stimulating factor

**INDICATIONS:** To decrease the incidence of infection, as manifested by febrile neutropenia, in patients with nonmyeloid malignancies receiving myelosuppressive anticancer drugs associated with a clinically significant incidence of febrile neutropenia.

**DOSAGE:** *Adults:* 6mg SQ once per chemotherapy cycle. Do not administer in the period between 14 days before and 24 hrs after cytotoxic chemotherapy.

**HOW SUPPLIED:** Inj: 6mg/0.6mL

**WARNINGS/PRECAUTIONS:** May cause splenic rupture; evaluate for enlarged spleen or splenic rupture in patients with left upper abdominal and/or shoulder pain. May cause acute respiratory distress syndrome (ARDS); evaluate patients who develop fever and lung infiltrates or respiratory distress; d/c if ARDS develops. Serious allergic reactions (eg, anaphylaxis) reported; d/c permanently if it occurs. May cause fatal sickle cell crises in patients with sickle cell disorders. May act as a growth factor for any tumor type including myeloid malignancies and myelodysplasia; not approved for myeloid malignancies and myelodysplasia. Needle cover on prefilled syringe contains latex; avoid use with latex allergy.

**ADVERSE REACTIONS:** Splenic rupture, ARDS, allergic reactions, bone pain, pain in extremity.

**PREGNANCY:** Category C, caution in nursing.

**MECHANISM OF ACTION:** Pegylated granulocyte colony stimulating factor; acts on hematopoietic cells by binding to specific cell surface receptors, thereby stimulating proliferation, differentiation, commitment, and end cell functional activation.

**PHARMACOKINETICS: Elimination:** (SQ) $T_{1/2}$=15-80 hrs.

## NURSING CONSIDERATIONS

**Assessment:** Assess for myeloid malignancies, myelodysplasia, history of hypersensitivity to the drug, latex allergy, sickle cell disorders, and pregnancy/nursing status.

**Monitoring:** Monitor for signs/symptoms of an allergic reaction, splenic rupture, ARDS (eg, fever, lung infiltrates), and for tumor growth. Monitor for signs/symptoms of sickle cell crises in patients with sickle cell disorders.

**Patient Counseling:** Discuss signs/symptoms of an allergic drug reaction and advise appropriate actions. Counsel on importance of compliance with treatment. Caution patient and caregivers against reuse of needles, syringes, or drug product, and thoroughly instruct in their proper disposal. Advise to report if LUQ abdominal or shoulder pain, SOB, signs/symptoms of sickle cell crisis, signs/symptoms of infection, flushing, dizziness, or rash occur.

**Administration:** SQ route. Inspect for particulate matter and discoloration prior to administration. **Storage:** Refrigerate at 2-8°C (36-46°F) in the carton to protect from light. Do not shake. Discard syringes stored at room temperature for >48hrs. Avoid freezing; if frozen, thaw in the refrigerator before administration. Discard if frozen more than once.



# NEUMEGA RX

oprelvekin (Wyeth)

**Allergic or hypersensitivity reactions, including anaphylaxis, reported; permanently d/c if an allergic or hypersensitivity reaction develops.**

**THERAPEUTIC CLASS:** Thrombopoietic agent

**INDICATIONS:** Prevention of severe thrombocytopenia and reduction of the need for platelet transfusions following myelosuppressive chemotherapy in nonmyeloid malignancy patients at high risk.

**DOSAGE:** *Adults:* 50mcg/kg qd SQ. Severe renal impairment (CrCl<30mL/min) 25mcg/kg qd SQ.Initiate 6-24 hrs after chemotherapy completion. Monitor platelets to assess optimal duration of therapy. Continue therapy until post-nadir platelets ≥50,000 cells/mcL. D/C at least 2 days before next chemotherapy cycle. Max: 21 days of therapy.

**HOW SUPPLIED:** Inj: 5mg

**WARNINGS/PRECAUTIONS:** Fluid retention reported; caution in CHF and patients receiving aggressive hydration. Capillary leak syndrome, pleural/pericardial effusion, renal failure, visual disturbances, papilledema, stroke, and rash reported. Monitor fluid and electrolyte balance with chronic diuretic therapy. Permanently d/c if significant allergic reactions occur. Moderate decreases in Hgb/Hct and RBCs reported. Caution with history of atrial arrhythmias. May develop antibodies to therapy. Obtain CBC before therapy, then regularly. Monitor platelets during expected nadir time and until adequate recovery.

**ADVERSE REACTIONS:** Edema, dyspnea, tachycardia, conjunctival injection, palpitations, atrial arrhythmias, pleural effusions, syncope, pneumonia, neutropenic fever, headache, N/V, fever, mucositis, diarrhea.

**PREGNANCY:** Category C, not for use in nursing.

**MECHANISM OF ACTION:** Thrombopoietic agent; stimulates megakaryocytopoiesis and thrombopoiesis.

**PHARMACOKINETICS: Absorption:** Absolute bioavailability (>80%); $C_{max}$=17.4ng/mL; $T_{max}$=3.2 hrs. **Elimination:** Kidneys (animal studies); $T_{1/2}$=6.9 hrs.

## NURSING CONSIDERATIONS

**Assessment:** Assess pregnancy status, bone marrow transplant, fluid retention or overload, capillary leak syndrome, pleural/pericardial effusion, CHF, aggressive hydration, history of papilledema or tumors of CNS, renal failure, prior myeloablative chemotherapy, history of atrial arrhythmias, and history of stroke or transient ischemic attack. Obtain baseline CBC including platelet count.

**Monitoring:** Periodically monitor CBC including platelet counts, fluid balance, fluid and electrolyte status (chronic diuretics). Monitor for signs/symptoms of hypersensitivity reactions, papilledema, fluid retention, pleural/pericardial effusion, atrial arrhythmias, and anemia.

**Patient Counseling:** Inform of pregnancy risks. Advise to seek medical attention if symptoms of hypersensitivity reactions (edema, SOB, wheezing, chest pain, hypotension), worsening of dyspnea (CHF, pleural effusion), atrial arrhythmias, anemia, or papilledema (blurred vision, blindness) occur.

**Administration:** SQ route; thigh, abdomen, or hip (upper arm if not self-injecting). **Storage:** 2-8°C (36-46°F). Protect from light; do not freeze. Reconstituted: 2-8°C (36-46°F) or room temperature, 25°C (77°F); stable for 3 hrs. Do not freeze or shake.

# NEUPOGEN RX

filgrastim (Amgen)

N

**THERAPEUTIC CLASS:** Granulocyte colony stimulating factor

**INDICATIONS:** To decrease incidence of infection, as manifested by febrile neutropenia in patients with nonmyeloid malignancies receiving myelosuppressive anti-cancer drugs associated with significant incidence of severe neutropenia with fever. To reduce the time to neutrophil recovery and duration of fever, following consolidation chemotherapy treatment of adults with acute myeloid leukemia (AML). To reduce the duration of neutropenia and neutropenia-related clinical sequelae in patients with nonmyeloid malignancies undergoing myeloablative chemotherapy followed by marrow transplantation. For mobilization of hematopoietic progenitor cells into peripheral blood for collection by leukapheresis. For chronic administration to reduce incidence and duration of sequelae of neutropenia in symptomatic patients with congenital neutropenia, cyclic neutropenia, or idiopathic neutropenia.

**DOSAGE:** *Adults:* Myelosuppressive Chemotherapy: Initial: 5mcg/kg qd SQ bolus, short IV infusion, or continuous SQ/IV infusion. Titrate: Increase 5mcg/kg for each chemotherapy cycle according to duration and severity of ANC nadir. Avoid 24 hrs before through 24 hrs after cytotoxic chemotherapy. Continue therapy after chemotherapy until the post nadir ANC =10,000/mm³. BMT: 10mcg/kg/day by IV infusion of 4 or 24 hrs or by continuous 24-hr SQ infusion. First dose at least 24 hrs after chemotherapy and at least 24 hrs after bone marrow infusion. Dose Adjustment: If ANC >1000/mm³ for 3 days, 5mcg/kg/day; increase to 10mcg/kg/day if ANC <1000/mm³. If ANC >1000/mm³ for 3 more days, stop therapy. If ANC drops to <1000/mm³, resume 5mcg/kg/day. Peripheral blood progenitor cell collection: 10mcg/kg/day bolus or continuous SQ 4 days before and for 6-7 days with leukapheresis on days 5, 6, and 7. Monitor neutrophils after 4 days and adjust if WBC >100,000/mm³. Chronic Neutropenia: Congenital Neutropenia: Initial: 6mcg/kg SQ bid. Idiopathic or Cyclic Neutropenia: Initial: 5mcg/kg SQ qd. Adjust dose based on clinical course and ANC.

**HOW SUPPLIED:** Inj: 300mcg/0.5mL, 300mcg/mL, 480mcg/0.8mL, 480mcg/1.6mL

**CONTRAINDICATIONS:** Hypersensitivity to *E. coli*-derived proteins.

**WARNINGS/PRECAUTIONS:** Allergic-type reactions reported. Splenic rupture reported, some fatal. Evaluate for enlarged spleen or splenic rupture if complaints of left upper abdominal and/or shoulder tip pain. Acute respiratory distress syndrome reported; d/c until resolved. Alveolar hemorrhage manifesting as pulmonary infiltrates and hemoptysis requiring hospitalization reported. Severe sickle cell crises reported with sickle cell disorders. Take care to confirm diagnosis of severe chronic neutropenia prior to therapy. Avoid simultaneous use with chemotherapy and radiation therapy. CBC monitoring is recommended twice a week during therapy to avoid potential complications of excessive leukocytosis. Potential for immunogenicity. Avoid premature d/c of therapy prior to time of recovery from expected neutrophil nadir. Cutaneous vasculitis reported; continue therapy at a reduced dose.

**ADVERSE REACTIONS:** N/V, skeletal pain, alopecia, diarrhea, neutropenic fever, mucositis, fever, fatigue, anorexia, dyspnea, headache, cough, skin rash, chest pain, generalized weakness.

**INTERACTIONS:** Caution with drugs that may potentiate the release of neutrophils (eg, lithium). Transient positive bone imaging changes have been associated with increased hematopoietic activity of the bone marrow in response to growth factor therapy.

**PREGNANCY:** Category C, caution in nursing.

**MECHANISM OF ACTION:** Granulocyte colony-stimulating factor (G-CSF); acts on hematopoietic cells by binding to specific cell surface receptors. Stimulates proliferation, differentiation commitment, and some end-cell functional activation.

**PHARMACOKINETICS: Absorption**: (IV, 20mcg/kg over 24 hrs): $C_{max}$=48ng/mL; (SQ, 3.45mcg/kg, 11.5mcg/kg): $C_{max}$=4ng/mL, 49ng/mL; $T_{max}$=2-8 hrs. **Distribution**: $V_d$=150mL/kg. **Elimination**: $T_{1/2}$=3.5 hrs, (IV) $T_{1/2}$=231 min (34.5mcg/kg), (SQ) $T_{1/2}$=210 min (3.45mcg/kg).

N

## NURSING CONSIDERATIONS

**Assessment:** Obtain CBC and platelet count. Assess for severe chronic neutropenia, history of chemotherapy/radiation therapy, history of hypersensitivity to *E. coli*-derived proteins, pregnancy/nursing status, and possible drug interactions.

**Monitoring:** Monitor CBC with differential and platelet count twice weekly. Perform annual bone marrow and cytogenetic evaluations throughout treatment for patients with congenital neutropenia. Monitor for hypersensitivity reactions, splenic rupture, ARDS, alveolar hemorrhage and hemoptysis, and sickle cell crises (in patients with sickle cell disease).

**Patient Counseling:** Counsel about potential adverse effects; seek medical attention if any develop. Advise to report any left upper abdominal or shoulder tip pain. Refer patients to Information for Patients and Caregivers included with package insert in each dispensing pack, as it provides information about neutrophils, neutropenia, and safety/efficacy of the drug.

**Administration:** SQ/IV route. Refer to PI for details. **Storage:** 2-8°C (36-46°F). Avoid shaking.

# Neurontin — RX

gabapentin (Parke-Davis)

**THERAPEUTIC CLASS:** GABA analog

**INDICATIONS:** Adjunct therapy for partial seizures with or without secondary generalization in patients ≥12 yrs. Adjunct therapy for partial seizures in pediatrics 3-12 yrs. Management of postherpetic neuralgia (PHN) in adults.

**DOSAGE:** *Adults:* Epilepsy: Initial: 300mg tid. Titrate: Increase up to 1800mg/day. The maximum time between doses in the TID schedule should not exceed 12 hrs. PHN: 300mg single dose on Day 1, then 300mg bid on Day 2, and 300mg tid on Day 3. Titrate: Increase prn for pain up to 1800mg (divided TID). Renal Impairment: CrCl ≥60mL/min: 900-3600mg/day. CrCl 30-59mL/min: 400-1400mg/day. CrCl 15-29mL/min: 200-700mg/day. CrCl 15mL/min: 100-300mg/day. CrCl <15mL/min: Reduce dose in proportion to CrCl. Hemodialysis: Maint: Base on CrCl. Give supplemental dose (125-350mg) after 4 hrs of hemodialysis. Refer to PI for dose adjustment. Elderly: Start at the low end of the dosing range.

*Pediatrics:* Epilepsy: >12 yrs: Initial: 300mg tid. Titrate: Increase up to 1800mg/day. The maximum time between doses in the TID schedule should not exceed 12 hrs. 3-12 yrs: Initial: 10-15mg/kg/day given tid. Titrate: Increase over 3 days. Usual: ≥5 yrs: 25-35mg/kg/day given tid. 3-4 yrs: 40mg/kg/day given tid. Max: 50mg/kg/day. Renal Impairment: ≥12 yrs: CrCl ≥60mL/min: 900-3600mg/day. CrCl 30-59mL/min: 400-1400mg/day. CrCl 15-29mL/min: 200-700mg/day. CrCl 15mL/min: 100-300mg/day. CrCl <15mL/min: Reduce dose in proportion to CrCl. Hemodialysis: Maint: Base on CrCl. Give supplemental dose (125-350mg) after 4 hrs of hemodialysis. Refer to PI for dose adjustment.

**HOW SUPPLIED:** Cap: 100mg, 300mg, 400mg; Sol: 250mg/5mL [470mL]; Tab: 600mg*, 800mg* *scored

**WARNINGS/PRECAUTIONS:** Avoid abrupt withdrawal. Possible tumorigenic potential. Sudden and unexplained deaths reported. Neuropsychiatric adverse events in pediatrics (3-12 yrs). Increased risk of suicidal thoughts or behavior reported; monitor for worsening of depression, any unusual changes in mood or behavior, or thoughts about self-harm. May impair physical/mental abilities. Caution in elderly.

**ADVERSE REACTIONS:** Somnolence, dizziness, peripheral edema, ataxia, nystagmus, fatigue, tremor, rhinitis, weight gain, N/V, infection.

**INTERACTIONS:** Decreased levels when taken with antacids (Maalox); take 2 hrs following antacid. Increased levels with controlled-release morphine, naproxen sodium. Hydrocodone increases gabapentin AUC values while gabapentin decreases hydrocodone $C_{max}$ and AUC in dose-dependent manner.

N

**PREGNANCY:** Category C, caution in nursing.

**MECHANISM OF ACTION:** GABA analog; not established. Anticonvulsant activity: Suspected to bind to different areas of the brain including neocortex and hippocampus. Analgesic effects: Prevents allodynia and hyperalgesia.

**PHARMACOKINETICS: Absorption:** PO administration of variable doses resulted in different parameters. **Distribution:** $V_d$=58L; plasma protein binding (<3%); found in breast milk. **Metabolism:** Not appreciably metabolized. **Elimination:** Renal excretion (unchanged); $T_{1/2}$=5-7 hrs.

## NURSING CONSIDERATIONS

**Assessment:** Assess renal function, hypersensitivity, pregnancy/nursing status, and possible drug interactions.

**Monitoring:** Monitor for neuropsychiatric events (emotional lability, hostility, thought disorders, and hyperkinesia) in pediatric patients. Monitor for withdrawal-precipitated seizures, status epilepticus, and the emergence of tumors while on medication, emergence or worsening of depression, suicidal thoughts, changes in behavior, adverse reactions, and hypersensitivity reactions.

**Patient Counseling:** Instruct that medication may be taken with or without food. Caution against operating machinery/driving until accustomed to effects of medication. Counsel about signs/symptoms of CNS depression. Instruct not to abruptly d/c drug or skip doses. Counsel that if taking Maalox, separate dosing by 2 hrs. Encourage patients to enroll in North American Antiepileptic Drug (NAAED) Pregnancy Registry if they become pregnant. Advise patients to be alert for and to contact physician if they have any increase of suicidal thoughts, worsening of depression, or any unusual changes in mood or behavior.

**Administration:** Oral route. Advise that scored tabs can be broken in half. The remaining half tab should be administered at next dose, or discard if unused after several days. **Storage:** Cap/Tab: 25°C (77°F); excursions permitted to 15-30°C (59-86°F). Oral Solution: 2-8°C (36-46°F).

## NEVANAC — RX

nepafenac (Alcon)

**THERAPEUTIC CLASS:** NSAID

**INDICATIONS:** Treatment of pain and inflammation associated with cataract surgery.

**DOSAGE:** *Adults:* 1 drop tid, start 24 hrs prior to surgery, continue to 2 weeks post-op.

**HOW SUPPLIED:** Sus: 0.1% [3mL]

**WARNINGS/PRECAUTIONS:** Possible cross-sensitivity to acetylsalicylic acid, phenylacetic acid derivatives, and other NSAIDs. May cause increased bleeding of ocular tissue; slowed or delayed healing; keratitis. With continued use, may cause epithelial breakdown, corneal thinning, erosion, ulceration, perforation. Caution with bleeding tendencies and in complicated ocular surgeries, corneal denervation, corneal epithelial defects, diabetes mellitus, ocular surface diseases, rheumatoid arthritis, or repeat ocular surgeries.

**ADVERSE REACTIONS:** Capsular opacity, decreased visual acuity, foreign body sensation, increased IOP, and sticky sensation.

**PREGNANCY:** Category C, caution in nursing.

**MECHANISM OF ACTION:** NSAID; inhibits the cyclo-oxygenase that is essential for the biosynthesis of prostaglandins.

### NURSING CONSIDERATIONS

**Assessment:** Assess for hypersensitivity or cross-sensitivity with some drugs (eg, acetylsalicylic acid), history of complicated or repeated ocular surgeries, corneal denervation, corneal epithelial defects, DM, ocular surface diseases (eg, dry eye syndrome), RA, bleeding tendencies, and history of concomitant use of medications that may prolong bleeding time or delay wound healing.

**Monitoring:** Monitor for hypersensitivity reactions, wound healing problems, keratitis, corneal thinning, corneal erosion, corneal ulceration or perforation, increased bleeding time, and bleeding of ocular tissues (hyphemas) in conjunction with ocular surgery.

**Patient Counseling:** Instruct not to administer suspension while wearing contact lenses.

**Administration:** Intraocular route. **Storage:** 2-25°C (36-77°F).

N

## NEXAVAR — RX

sorafenib (Bayer/Onyx)

**THERAPEUTIC CLASS:** Multikinase inhibitor

**INDICATIONS:** Treatment of advanced renal cell carcinoma or unresectable hepatocellular carcinoma.

**DOSAGE:** *Adults:* 400mg bid without food (1 hr before or 2 hrs after eating). Continue until no clinical benefit or unacceptable toxicity. Temporary interruption or dose reduction to 400mg qd or qod may be necessary if serious adverse events suspected.

**HOW SUPPLIED:** Tab: 200mg

**WARNINGS/PRECAUTIONS:** Risk of ischemia and/or infarction occured; temporary or permanent discontinuation may be necessary. Increased risk of bleeding may occur; consider discontinuation if bleeding necessitates medical intervention. HTN reported; monitor BP weekly during first 6 weeks and periodically thereafter. Hand-foot skin reaction and rash may occur; may require topical treatment, temporary treatment interruption, dose modification, or permanent discontinuation. D/C if GI perforation occurs. Temporary interruption of therapy recommended when undergoing surgical procedures. May cause fetal harm; women of childbearing potential should avoid becoming pregnant during therapy. Hepatic impairment may reduce plasma levels. Caution when co-administered with docetaxel and doxorubicin.

**ADVERSE REACTIONS:** HTN, fatigue, wt loss, rash/desquamation, hand-foot skin reaction, alopecia, pruritus, diarrhea, N/V, anorexia, constipation, hemorrhage, dyspnea, abdominal pain, liver dysfunction, cardiac ischemia.

**INTERACTIONS:** Caution with compounds metabolized/eliminated predominantly by the UGT1A1 pathway (eg, irinotecan); systemic exposure to substrates of UGT1A1 and UGT1A9 may increase with co-administration. May increase AUC of docetaxel and doxorubicin; co-administer with caution. May alter AUC of fluorouracil; co-administer with caution. Systemic exposure to substrates of CYP2B6 and CYP2C8 may increase with co-administration. CYP3A4 inducers may increase metabolism and decrease levels of sorafenib. May increase INR; monitor with concomitant warfarin.

**PREGNANCY:** Category D, not for use in nursing.

**MECHANISM OF ACTION:** Multikinase inhibitor; inhibits multiple intracellular and cell surface kinases which are thought to be involved in tumor cell signaling, angiogenesis, and apoptosis.

**PHARMACOKINETICS: Absorption**: Relative bioavailability (38-49%), $T_{max}$=3 hrs. **Distribution**: Plasma protein binding (99.5%). **Metabolism**: Liver via oxidation and glucuronidation; CYP3A4, UGT1A9: Pyridine N-oxide. **Elimination**: Feces (77%, 51% unchanged), urine (19% as glucuronidated metabolites); $T_{1/2}$=25-48 hrs.

## NURSING CONSIDERATIONS

**Assessment:** Assess for CVD, bleeding problems, HTN, renal/hepatic dysfunction, pregnancy status. Note other diseases/conditions and drug therapies.

**Monitoring:** Monitor BP, changes in PT, INR, or clinical bleeding episodes. Monitor for risks of cardiac ischemia or infarction, hemorrhage, HTN, dermatologic toxicities, GI perforation, hypophosphatemia, LFTs, depression.



**Patient Counseling:** Counsel about possible side effects; report any episodes of chest pain, bleeding, or any other adverse effects. Both males and females should use effective birth control during treatment to avoid conception. Tablet should be swallowed and taken without food.

**Administration:** Oral route, taken without food (at least 1 hr before or 2 hrs after a meal). **Storage**: 25°C (77°F); excursions permitted to 15-30°C (59-86°F). Store in dry place. Keep out of reach of children.

# NEXIUM — RX

esomeprazole magnesium (AstraZeneca)

**THERAPEUTIC CLASS:** Proton pump inhibitor

**INDICATIONS:** Symptomatic treatment of GERD; healing and maintenance treatment of erosive esophagitis. Reduction in occurrence of gastric ulcers associated with continuous NSAID therapy in patients at risk for developing gastric ulcers. Adjunct therapy (with amoxicillin and clarithromycin) for *H.pylori* eradication to reduce the risk of duodenal ulcer recurrence. Long-term treatment of pathological hypersecretory conditions including Zollinger-Ellison syndrome.

**DOSAGE:** *Adults:* Erosive Esophagitis: Healing: 20mg or 40mg qd for 4-8 weeks; may extend treatment for 4-8 weeks if not healed. Maint: 20mg qd for up to 6 months. Symptomatic GERD: 20mg qd for 4 weeks; may extend treatment for 4 weeks if symptoms do not resolve. Risk Reduction of NSAID-Associated Gastric Ulcer: 20mg or 40mg qd for up to 6 months. *H.pylori:* Triple Therapy: 40mg qd + amoxicillin 1000mg bid + clarithromycin 500mg bid, all for 10 days. Zollinger-Ellison Syndrome: 40mg bid. Severe Hepatic Dysfunction: Max: 20mg/day. Take 1 hr before meals. Swallow capsule whole. Contents may be mixed with soft food (eg, applesauce, yogurt) that does not require chewing.

*Pediatrics:* GERD: 12-17 yrs: 20mg or 40mg qd for up to 8 weeks. 1-11 yrs: 10mg qd for up to 8 weeks. Erosive Esophagitis: 1-11 yrs: ≥20kg: 10mg or 20mg qd for 8 weeks. <20kg: 10mg qd for 8 weeks. Severe Hepatic Dysfunction: Max: 20mg/day. Take 1 hr before meals. Swallow capsule whole. Contents may be mixed with soft food (eg, applesauce, yogurt) that does not require chewing.

**HOW SUPPLIED:** Cap, Delayed-Release: 20mg, 40mg; Sus, Delayed-Release: 10mg, 20mg, 40mg (granules/pkt).

**CONTRAINDICATIONS:** Hypersensitivity to substituted benzimidazoles.

**WARNINGS/PRECAUTIONS:** Atrophic gastritis may occur. Symptomatic response does not preclude gastric malignancy.

**ADVERSE REACTIONS:** Headache, diarrhea, abdominal pain, constipation, nausea, flatulence, dry mouth, agranulocytosis, pancytopenia, pancreatitis, myalgia, taste disturbance, gynecomastia, bronchospasm, alopecia.

**INTERACTIONS:** Potentiates diazepam. May alter absorption of pH-dependent drugs (eg, ketoconazole, digoxin, iron salts) and antiretroviral drugs. May reduce atazanavir and nelfinavir levels. May increase saquinavir levels; monitor for possible toxicity. Increased levels with amoxicillin and clarithromycin. Concomitant use with warfarin may increase INR and PT. Concomitant use with CYP2C19 and CYP3A4 inhibitors (eg, voriconazole) may result in doubling of plasma exposure.

**PREGNANCY:** Category B, safety not known in nursing.

**MECHANISM OF ACTION:** Proton pump inhibitor; suppresses gastric acid secretion by specific inhibition of the $H^+/K^+$-ATPase in the gastric parietal cell.

**PHARMACOKINETICS: Absorption:** (40 mg) $C_{max}$=4.7µmol/L; $T_{max}$=1.6 hrs; AUC=12.6µmol•hr/L. (20mg) $C_{max}$=2.1µmol/L; $T_{max}$=1.6 hrs; AUC=4.2µmol•hr/L. **Distribution:** $V_d$=16L; plasma protein binding (97%). **Metabolism:** Liver (extensive) via CYP2C19, CYP3A4. **Elimination:** Urine (80%), feces; $T_{1/2}$=1-1.5 hrs. For pediatric parameters, refer to full PI.

## NURSING CONSIDERATIONS

**Assessment:** Assess for hypersensitivity to other proton pump inhibitors, presence of gastric malignancy, severe hepatic impairment, pregnancy/nursing status, and possible drug interactions.

**Monitoring:** Monitor for signs/symptoms of atrophic gastritis, and hypersensitivity reactions (eg, anaphylaxis, angioedema). Monitor for possible toxicity with saquinavir.

**Patient Counseling:** Counsel to contact physician if signs/symptoms of hypersensitivity reaction occur. May take antacids while on therapy. Advise to take 1 hr before meals and to swallow capsules whole. If difficulty swallowing, open capsules and empty granules into applesauce, which should not be warm. For oral suspension, empty packet of medication into container containing 1 tbsp of water (15mL); stir contents, let stand for 2-3 min to thicken; drink solution within 15 min. If contents of solution remain, add more water, stir, and drink immediately.

**Administration:** Oral route. **Storage:** 25°C (77°F); excursions permitted to 15-30°C (59-86°F). Dispense in tightly closed container.

# NEXIUM IV — RX

esomeprazole sodium (AstraZeneca)

**THERAPEUTIC CLASS:** Proton pump inhibitor

**INDICATIONS:** Short-term treatment (up to 10 days) of GERD with history of erosive esophagitis when oral therapy not possible or appropriate.

**DOSAGE:** *Adults:* 20mg or 40mg qd IV injection (no less than 3 min) or infusion (10-30 min). D/C as soon as patient able to resume oral therapy. Severe Hepatic Dysfunction: Max: 20mg/day.

**HOW SUPPLIED:** Inj: 20mg, 40mg

**WARNINGS/PRECAUTIONS:** Atrophic gastritis may occur. Symptomatic response does not preclude gastric malignancy. D/C and convert to oral therapy as soon as possible.

**ADVERSE REACTIONS:** Headache, flatulence, dyspepsia, nausea, abdominal pain, diarrhea, and dry mouth.

**INTERACTIONS:** Potentiates diazepam. May alter absorption of gastric pH-dependent drugs (eg, ketoconazole, iron salts, digoxin). Concomitant warfarin therapy may increase INR and PT. May reduce plasma levels of atazanavir and nelfinavi; avoid with these drugs. Concomitant CYP2C19 and CYP3A4 inhibitor (eg, voriconazole) may double plasma levels.

**PREGNANCY:** Category B, not for use in nursing.

**MECHANISM OF ACTION:** Proton pump inhibitor. Suppresses gastric acid secretion by specific inhibition of the $H^+/K^+$-ATPase in the gastric parietal cell.

**PHARMACOKINETICS: Absorption:** (20mg): AUC=5.11μmol•hr/L; $C_{max}$=3.86μmol/L; (40mg): AUC=16.21μmol•hr/L. **Distribution**: $V_d$= 16L; plasma protein binding (97%). **Metabolism:** Liver (extensive) via CYP2C19, 3A4. **Elimination**: Urine (primary), (<1% unchanged), feces; $T_{1/2}$=1.1-1.4 hrs.

## NURSING CONSIDERATIONS

**Assessment:** Assess for hypersensitivity to other proton pump inhibitors, presence of gastric malignancy, severe hepatic insufficiency, pregnancy/nursing status, and possible drug interactions.

**Monitoring:** Monitor for signs/symptoms of atrophic gastritis.

**Patient Counseling:** Instruct to contact physician if any adverse events develop.

**Administration:** IV injection or infusion route. Injection: Reconstitute vial with 5mL of 0.9% NaCl and inject. Infusion: 1) Reconstitute vial with 5mL of compatible solution (eg, 0.9% NaCl, Lactated Ringer's, or 5% Dextrose). 2) Further dilute to final volume of 50mL. Should not be administered concomitantly with any other medications through same IV site or tubing. Always flush IV line both prior to and after administration. IV formulation should be switched to oral formulation as soon as possible. **Storage:** Vial: 25°C (77°F); excursions permitted to 15-30°C (59-86°F). Protect from light. Store in carton until time of use. Reconstituted: 30°C (86°F); administer within 12 hrs. Infusion: Up to 30°C (86°F); if reconstituted with 0.9% NaCl or Lactated Ringer's, use within 12 hrs; 5% Dextrose, use within 6 hrs.



# NIASPAN — RX

niacin (Abbott)

**THERAPEUTIC CLASS:** Nicotinic acid

**INDICATIONS:** To reduce total cholesterol (TC), LDL-C, TG, and Apo B levels, and to increase HDL-C in primary hyperlipidemia (heterozygous familial and nonfamilial) and mixed dyslipidemia (Types IIa and IIb). With concomitant lovastatin or simvastatin, in primary hyperlipidemia (heterozygous familial and nonfamilial) and mixed dyslipidemia (Types IIa and IIb) when treatment with monotherapy is considered inadequate. To reduce the risk of recurrent nonfatal MI with history of MI and hyperlipidemia. With concomitant bile acid binding resin, to slow progression/promote regression of atherosclerotic disease in patients with history of CAD and hyperlipidemia. With concomitant bile acid binding resin to reduce TC and elevated LDL-C levels in adult patients with primary hyperlipidemia (Type IIa). Adjunct for treatment of adult patients with severe hypertriglyceridemia (Type IV and Type V hyperlipidemia) with risk of pancreatitis and who do not respond adequately to diet. Therapy is indicated as an adjunct to diet.

**DOSAGE:** *Adults:* Take qhs after low-fat snack. Individualize dose. Initial: 500mg qhs. Titrate: Increase by 500mg every 4 weeks. Maint: 1-2g qhs. Max: 2g/day. With Lovastatin: Initial Lovastatin: 20mg qd. Max: 2000mg niacin/40 mg lovastatin qd. With Simvastatin: Initial Simvastatin: 20mg qd. Max: 2000mg niacin/40 mg qd simvastatin. May take ASA (up to 325mg) 30 min before to reduce flushing. Do not chew, crush, or break; swallow whole. Women may respond to lower doses than men. If d/c therapy for an extended period of time, reinstitution should include titration phase.

**HOW SUPPLIED:** Tab, Extended-Release: 500mg, 750mg, 1000mg

**CONTRAINDICATIONS:** Active liver disease or unexplained persistent elevations in hepatic transaminases, active peptic ulcer disease, arterial bleeding.

**WARNINGS/PRECAUTIONS:** Do not substitute with equivalent doses of immediate-release niacin (severe hepatic toxicity may occur). Caution with heavy alcohol use and/or past history of liver disease, renal impairment, unstable angina, and acute phase of MI. Associated with abnormal LFTs; monitor LFTs before therapy, every 6-12 weeks during 1st yr, and periodically thereafter. D/C if transaminase levels show signs of progression, particularly of >3x ULN and are persistent or are associated with symptoms of nausea, fever, and/or malaise. Monitor for rhabdomyolysis. Observe closely with history of jaundice, hepatobiliary disease, or peptic ulcer. May cause a dose-related increase in glucose intolerance in diabetic patients. Perform frequent monitoring of glucose levels. Elevated uric acid levels reported, caution in patients predisposed to gout. May reduce platelet levels and phosphorus levels. May increase PT, caution in patients undergoing surgery. May produce false elevations in some fluorometric determinations of plasma or urinary catecholamines and may give false-positive reactions with cupric sulfate solution in urine glucose tests.

**ADVERSE REACTIONS:** Flushing episodes (eg, warmth, itching, tingling), dizziness, tachycardia, SOB, sweating, chills, edema, diarrhea, N/V, increased cough, pruritus, rash.

**INTERACTIONS:** Rhabdomyolysis may occur with HMG-CoA reductase inhibitors; consider performing periodic monitoring of CPK and $K^+$ levels. May potentiate effects of ganglionic blocking agents and vasoactive drugs. Separate dosing from bile acid-binding resins by at least 4-6 hrs. Concomitant aspirin use may decrease metabolic clearance of nicotinic acid. Concurrent use with vitamins or other nutritional supplements containing large doses of niacin or related compounds (eg, nicotinamide) may potentiate adverse effects of niacin. Avoid ingestion of alcohol, hot drinks, or spicy foods around time of administration; may increase flushing and pruritus. Caution with anticoagulants, monitor platelet counts and PT. Caution with unstable angina or acute phase MI and vasoactive drugs (eg, nitrates, calcium channel blockers, adrenergic blockers). Antidiabetic agents may need adjustment.

**PREGNANCY:** Category C, not for use in nursing.

**MECHANISM OF ACTION:** Nicotinic acid; not established. May partially inhibit release of free fatty acids from adipose tissue, and increase lipoprotein lipase activity, which may increase the rate of chylomicron triglyceride removal from plasma. Decreases the rate of hepatic synthesis of VLDL and LDL.

**PHARMACOKINETICS: Absorption:** $T_{max}$=5 hrs. **Distribution:** Found in breast milk. **Metabolism:** Liver rapid and extensive to nicotinamide adenine dinucleotide (NAD) and other metabolites; conjugation to nicotinuric acid (NUA) (metabolite). **Elimination:** Urine; parent and metabolites (60-76%), (12%, unchanged).

## NURSING CONSIDERATIONS

**Assessment:** Assess for presence or history of liver disease, unexplained persistent elevations in hepatic transaminases, presence or history of a peptic ulcer, arterial bleeding, unstable angina or acute MI, renal impairment, history of hepatobiliary disease, alcohol abuse, DM, gout, upcoming surgery, pregnancy/nursing status, and for possible drug interactions. Assess LFTs and lipid levels prior to therapy. Assess that patient is on cholesterol-lowering diet prior to therapy.

**Monitoring:** Monitor for signs/symptoms of hepatotoxicity (eg, fulminant hepatic necrosis), rhabdomyolysis (eg, muscle pain, tenderness, weakness), decreases in platelet counts, increases in prothrombin time, and for increased uric acid levels. Monitor phosphorus levels in patients at risk for hypophosphatemia. Monitor LFTs (eg, AST, ALT) every 6-12 weeks during first year and periodically thereafter. Perform periodic monitoring of fasting lipid levels.

**Patient Counseling:** Counsel to take at bedtime after a low-fat snack. Inform that flushing may occur but may subside after several weeks of therapy. Advise not to break, crush, or chew; swallow whole. Inform that aspirin 30 min before dosing may minimize flushing. Instruct to avoid ingestion of alcohol or hot drinks with administration to prevent flushing. Instruct to contact physician if discontinuing drug for extended period of time, taking vitamins or other nutritional supplements, or if dizziness occurs. Instruct diabetic patients to contact physician if changes in blood glucose levels occur. Advise to discontinue use and contact physician if become pregnant or if currently breastfeeding.

**Administration:** Oral route. **Storage:** 20-25°C (68-77°F).

## NIFEDIPINE RX

nifedipine (Various)

**OTHER BRAND NAMES:** Procardia (Pfizer)

**THERAPEUTIC CLASS:** Calcium channel blocker (dihydropyridine)

**INDICATIONS:** Management of vasospastic angina and chronic stable angina.

**DOSAGE:** *Adults:* >18 yrs: Initial: 10mg tid. Usual: 10-20mg tid or 20-30mg tid-qid with evidence of coronary artery spasm. Titrate: Over a 7-14 day period. If symptoms warrant (eg, activity level, attack frequency, SL nitroglycerin consumption) dose may be increased from 10mg tid to 20mg tid then 30mg tid over a 3-day period. Hospitalized patients may increase in 10mg increments over 4-6 hr periods. Doses above 120mg qd are rarely necessary. Max: 180mg qd.

**HOW SUPPLIED:** Cap: 10mg, 20mg

**WARNINGS/PRECAUTIONS:** May cause hypotension; monitor BP initially or with titration. May exacerbate angina from β-blocker withdrawal. CHF risk, especially with aortic stenosis or β-blockers. Peripheral edema reported. Not for acute reduction of BP or essential HTN. May increase angina or MI with severe obstructive CAD. Avoid with acute coronary syndrome or within 1-2 weeks of MI. Caution in elderly.

N

**ADVERSE REACTIONS:** Dizziness, lightheadedness, giddiness, flushing, heat sensation, heartburn, muscle cramps, tremor, headache, weakness, nausea, peripheral edema, nervousness/mood changes, palpitation.

**INTERACTIONS:** β-blockers may increase risk of CHF, severe hypotension, or angina exacerbation. Possible hypotension with fentanyl. Potentiates digoxin. Monitor quinidine, coumarin, digitalis. Potentiated by cimetidine and grapefruit juice. Avoid grapefruit juice.

**PREGNANCY:** Category C, caution in nursing.

**MECHANISM OF ACTION:** Calcium channel blocker; inhibits the transmembrane influx of calcium ions into cardiac muscle and smooth muscle. Angina: MOA not fully determined; believed to act by relaxation and prevention of coronary artery spasm, and reduction of oxygen utlilization.

**PHARMACOKINETICS: Absorption:** Rapid and full; $T_{max}$=30 min. **Distribution:** Plasma protein binding (92-98%). **Metabolism:** Liver, via biotransformation. **Elimination:** Urine (80%).

### NURSING CONSIDERATIONS

**Assessment:** Assess for CHF, aortic stenosis, hepatic/renal impairment, essential HTN, recent MI, β-blocker withdrawal syndrome with increased angina, and possible drug interactions.

**Monitoring:** Monitor for hypotension and/or increased fluid volume requirements, increased angina and/or MI, HF, peripheral edema, allergic hepatitis, cholestatsis with/without jaundice. Monitor BP, LFTs, BUN, SrCr, decreased platelet aggregation, increased bleeding time, positive direct Coombs' test with/without hemolytic anemia.

**Patient Counseling:** Not to be used for acute reduction of BP. Do not take with grapefruit juice. Inform about potential risks/benefits of drug.

**Administration:** Oral route. Swallow whole. **Storage:** 15-25°C (59-77°F). Avoid freezing. Protect from light and moisture.

## NILANDRON RX
nilutamide (Sanofi-Aventis)

**THERAPEUTIC CLASS:** Nonsteroidal antiandrogen

**INDICATIONS:** Treatment of metastatic prostatic cancer (Stage $D_2$) in combination with surgical castration.

**DOSAGE:** *Adults:* Initial: 300mg/day for 30 days beginning on the day of, or on the day after, surgical castration. Maint: 150mg qd.

**HOW SUPPLIED:** Tab: 150mg

**CONTRAINDICATIONS:** Severe hepatic impairment, respiratory insufficiency.

**WARNINGS/PRECAUTIONS:** Not for use in women. Interstitial pneumonitis reported; d/c if symptoms occur. Hepatotoxicity reported; d/c if jaundice or ALT >2x ULN develop. May cause aplastic anemia. Patients whose disease progresses while on therapy may experience clinical improvement with discontinuation. Delayed adaptation to dark reported; wearing tinted glasses may alleviate effect.

**ADVERSE REACTIONS:** Hot flushes, decreased libido, abnormal vision, increased LFTs, dyspnea, dizziness, HTN, anemia, testicular atrophy, gynecomastia, pain, NV, constipation, impaired adaptation to dark.

**INTERACTIONS:** Inhibits CYP450 *in vitro* and may reduce the metabolism of their substrates. May, thus, potentiate vitamin K antagonists, phenytoin, and theophylline leading to toxicity. May cause intolerance to alcohol (eg, hypotension, malaise).

**PREGNANCY:** Category C, safety not known in nursing.

**MECHANISM OF ACTION:** Nonsteroidal antiandrogen; acts by blocking effects of testosterone at the androgen receptor sites.

**PHARMACOKINETICS: Absorption**: Rapid and complete. **Distribution:** Plasma protein binding (Moderate). **Metabolism:** Extensive, via oxidation. **Elimination**: Urine (62%, <2% unchanged), feces (1.4%-7%); $T_{1/2}$=38-59.1 hrs (100mg-300mg single dose).

### NURSING CONSIDERATIONS

**Assessment:** Mesaure baseline hepatic enzymes, chest x-ray, and pulmonary function test. Assess comorbidities and possible drug interactions.

**Monitoring:** Prior to treatment and periodically thereafter, measure baseline hepatic enzymes, routine chest x-ray, and pulmonary function tests. Monitor for occurrence of interstitial pneumonitis, hepatotoxicity, hypersensitivity reactions.

**Patient Counseling:** Instruct to report new or worsening SOB, NV, abdominal pain, or jaundice. Inform to start on day of or day after surgical castration; do not interrupt or d/c dosing without consulting physician. Advise to avoid taking with alcohol. Instruct patients to wear tinted glasses to alleviate the delayed adaptation to dark; caution about driving at night and through tunnels.

**Administration:** Oral route. **Storage**: 25°C (77°F); excursions permitted to 15-30°C (59-86°F). Protect from light.

## NIMODIPINE RX
nimodipine (Various)

**Do not administer IV or by other parenteral routes. Deaths and serious, life-threatening adverse events have occurred when contents of capsules injected parenterally.**

**OTHER BRAND NAMES:** Nimotop (Bayer Healthcare)

**THERAPEUTIC CLASS:** Calcium channel blocker

N

**INDICATIONS:** Improvement of neurological outcome in patients with subarachnoid hemorrhage (SAH) from ruptured intracranial berry aneurysms regardless of their post-ictus neurological condition.

**DOSAGE:** *Adults:* 60mg q 4 hrs for 21 days, 1 hr before or 2 hrs after meals. Hepatic Cirrhosis: 30mg q 4 hrs for 21 days. Start therapy within 96 hrs of SAH. If cannot swallow cap, extract contents into syringe and empty into NG tube, then flush with 30mL of 0.9% NaCl.

**HOW SUPPLIED:** Cap: 30mg

**WARNINGS/PRECAUTIONS:** Carefully monitor BP. Monitor BP and HR closely with hepatic dysfunction. Do not administer IV or by other parenteral routes.

**ADVERSE REACTIONS:** Decreased BP, headache, rash, diarrhea, bradycardia, nausea, abnormal LFTs.

**INTERACTIONS:** May enhance cardiovascular effects of other CCBs. Increased serum levels with cimetidine. May intensify effects of antihypertensives.

**PREGNANCY:** Category C, not for use in nursing.

**MECHANISM OF ACTION:** Calcium channel blocker; not established; suspected to inhibit calcium ion transfer into smooth muscle cells, thereby inhibiting contractions of vascular smooth muscle.

**PHARMACOKINETICS: Absorption:** Rapid; $T_{max}$=1 hr. **Distribution:** Plasma protein binding ( ≥95%). Crosses blood-brain barrier. **Elimination:** Urine (≤1% unchanged); $T_{1/2}$=8-9 hrs.

## NURSING CONSIDERATIONS

**Assessment:** Assess for hepatic impairment and possible drug interactions.

**Monitoring:** Carefully monitor BP and pulse rate. Monitor for serious adverse effects when administering IV (eg, death, cardiac arrest, cardiovascular collapse, hypotension, and bradycardia).

**Patient Counseling:** Inform about potential risks/benefits of drug. Do not take with grapefruit juice. Regular BP monitoring recommended.

N

**Administration:** Oral route. **Storage:** Store at 25°C (77°F); excursions permitted to 15-30°C (59-86°F). Avoid light and freezing.

# NIRAVAM

CIV

alprazolam (Schwarz)

**THERAPEUTIC CLASS:** Benzodiazepine

**INDICATIONS:** Management of anxiety disorders and short-term relief of anxiety symptoms. Treatment of panic disorder with or without agoraphobia.

**DOSAGE:** *Adults:* Anxiety: Initial: 0.25-0.5mg tid. Titrate: May increase every 3-4 days. Max: 4mg/day. Panic Disorder: Initial: 0.5mg tid. Titrate: Increase by no more than 1mg/day every 3-4 days; slower titration if ≥4mg/day. Usual: 1-10mg/day. Decrease dose slowly (no more than 0.5mg every 3 days). Elderly/Advanced Liver Disease/Debilitated: Initial: 0.25mg bid-tid. Titrate: Increase gradually as tolerated.

**HOW SUPPLIED:** Tab, Orally Disintegrating: 0.25mg*, 0.5mg*, 1mg*, 2mg*
*scored

**CONTRAINDICATIONS:** Acute narrow-angle glaucoma, untreated open-angle glaucoma, concomitant ketoconazole or itraconazole.

**WARNINGS/PRECAUTIONS:** Risk of dependence. Withdrawal symptoms, including seizure, reported with dose reduction or abrupt d/c; avoid abrupt withdrawal. Risk of CNS depression and impaired performance. May cause fetal harm. Caution with impaired renal, hepatic, or pulmonary function, severe depression, obesity, elderly and debilitated. Hypomania/mania reported with depression. Weak uricosuric effect.

**ADVERSE REACTIONS:** Drowsiness, fatigue/tiredness, impaired coordination, irritability, memory impairment, cognitive disorder, dysarthria, decreased libido, confusional state, lightheadedness, dry mouth, hypotension, increased salivation.

**INTERACTIONS:** Avoid with potent CYP3A inhibitors (eg, azole antifungals). Potentiated by nefazodone, fluvoxamine, cimetidine, fluoxetine, oral contraceptives. Decreased plasma levels with propoxyphene and carbamazepine. Caution with diltiazem, isoniazid, macrolides, grapefruit juice, sertraline, paroxetine, ergotamine, cyclosporine, amiodarone, nicardipine, nifedipine and other CYP3A inhibitors. Increases levels of imipramine and desipramine. Additive CNS depressant effects with psychotropic agents, anticonvulsants, antihistamines, ethanol.

**PREGNANCY:** Category D, not for use in nursing.

**MECHANISM OF ACTION:** Benzodiazepine; not established, CNS depressant, believed to exert its effects by binding at stereo specific receptor at several sites within the CNS.

**PHARMACOKINETICS: Absorption:** Readily absorbed; $C_{max}$=8-37ng/mL; $T_{max}$=1.5-2 hrs. **Distribution:** Plasma protein binding (80%). **Metabolism:** Metabolized (extensively), hydroxylation, 4-hydroxyalprazolam and α-hydroxyalprazolam (major metabolites). **Elimination:** Urine, $T_{1/2}$=12.5 hrs.

## NURSING CONSIDERATIONS

**Assessment:** Assess for known sensitivity to drug, open-angle and acute-closed glaucoma, renal/hepatic impairment, pulmonary function insufficiency, and possible drug interactions. Assess for risk of dependence among panic disorder patients.

**Monitoring:** Monitor early morning anxiety and emergence of anxiety symptoms, CNS depression, physical/psychological dependence, suicidality, mania/hypomania, uricosuric effects, acute renal failure, seizures and status epilepticus. Monitor blood counts, urinalysis, and blood chemistry analysis.

**Patient Counseling:** Inform of benefits/risks and possibilty of physical/psychological dependence. Caution against hazardous tasks (eg, operating machinery/driving). Avoid alcohol. Notify physician if pregnant or planning to become pregnant or before increasing dose or d/c the drug.

**Administration:** Oral route. Remove tablets from bottle just before dosing. Can be swallowed with/without water. **Storage:** 20-25°C (68-77°F); excursions permitted to 15-30°C (59-86°F). Protect from moisture. Dispense in tight container.

# NITRO-DUR — RX

nitroglycerin (Schering)

**OTHER BRAND NAMES:** Minitran (Graceway) - Nitrek (Mylan Bertek)

**THERAPEUTIC CLASS:** Nitrate vasodilator

**INDICATIONS:** Prevention of angina pectoris. Not for acute attack.

**DOSAGE:** *Adults:* Initial: 0.2-0.4mg/hr for 12-14 hrs. Remove for 10-12 hrs.

**HOW SUPPLIED:** Patch: (Minitran) 0.1mg/hr, 0.2mg/hr, 0.4mg/hr, 0.6mg/hr [30$^s$]; (Nitrek) 0.2mg/hr, 0.4mg/hr, 0.6mg/hr [30$^s$]; (Nitro-Dur) 0.1mg/hr, 0.2mg/hr, 0.3mg/hr, 0.4mg/hr, 0.6mg/hr, 0.8mg/hr [30$^s$]

**CONTRAINDICATIONS:** Allergy to adhesives in NTG patches.

**WARNINGS/PRECAUTIONS:** Severe hypotension may occur; caution with volume depletion or hypotension. Vasodilatory effects with phosphodiesterase inhibitors (eg, sildenafil) can result in severe hypotension. May aggravate angina caused by hypertrophic cardiomyopathy. Tolerance to other nitrate forms may decrease effects. Monitor with acute MI or CHF. Do not discharge defibrillator/cardioverter through the patch.

**ADVERSE REACTIONS:** Headache, lightheadedness, hypotension, syncope.

**INTERACTIONS:** Additive vasodilating effects with other vasodilators (eg, alcohol). Marked orthostatic hypotension reported with CCBs. Severe hypotension with sildenafil.

**PREGNANCY:** Category C, caution in nursing.

**MECHANISM OF ACTION:** Nitrate vasodilator; relaxes vascular smooth muscle, and consequent dilatation of peripheral arteries and veins, especially the latter. Dilatation of veins leads to reduced left ventricular end-diastolic pressure and pulmonary capillary wedge pressure (preload). Arteriolar relaxation reduces systemic vascular resistance, systolic arterial pressure, and mean arterial pressure (afterload). It also dilates the coronary artery.

**PHARMACOKINETICS: Absorption:** $T_{max}$=2 hrs. **Distribution:** $V_d$=3L/kg. **Metabolism:** Extrahepatic metabolism (RBC and vascular walls). Inorganic nitrate and the 1,2- and 1,3- dinitroglycerols. Dinitrates are metabolized to mononitrates and to glycerol and $CO_2$. **Elimination:** $T_{1/2}$=3 min.

## NURSING CONSIDERATIONS

**Assessment:** Assess for severe hypotension or volume depleted patients, angina caused by hypertrophic cardiomyopathy, alcohol intake and possible drug interactions.

**Monitoring:** Careful clinical or hemodynamic monitoring for hypotension and tachycardia. Monitor for paradoxical bradycardia and increased angina pectoris, decreased exercise tolerance and hemodynamic rebound, headaches and lightheadedness on standing, manifestation of true physical dependence (chest pain, acute MI), and methemoglobinemia.

**Patient Counseling:** Counsel to carefully follow dosing regimen. Inform about headaches (markers of drug activity) and lightheadedness on standing. Avoid alcohol consumption.

**Administration:** Transdermal route. **Storage:** 15-30°C (59-86°F).

# NITROLINGUAL SPRAY — RX

nitroglycerin (Sciele)

N

**OTHER BRAND NAMES:** NitroMist (NovaDel Pharma)

**THERAPEUTIC CLASS:** Nitrate vasodilator

**INDICATIONS:** For acute relief of an attack or prophylaxis of angina pectoris due to coronary artery disease.

**DOSAGE:** *Adults:* Acute: 1-2 sprays at onset of attack onto or under tongue. May be repeated every 3-5 mins prn. Max: 3 sprays/15 min. Prophylaxis: 1-2 sprays onto or under tongue 5-10 min before activity that may cause acute attack. The spray should not be inhaled. Do not expectorate medication or rinse mouth for 5-10 min after administration.

**HOW SUPPLIED:** Spray: 400mcg/spray

**CONTRAINDICATIONS:** Use with certain drugs for erectile dysfunction (phosphodiesterase inhibitors), as their concomitant use can cause severe hypotension.

**WARNINGS/PRECAUTIONS:** Severe hypotension may occur; caution with volume depletion or hypotension. May aggravate angina caused by hypertrophic cardiomyopathy. Tolerance and cross-tolerance to other nitrates/nitrites may occur. Monitor during early days of AMI. (Nitrolingual Spray) Physical dependence may occur.

**ADVERSE REACTIONS:** Headache, hypotension, flushing, dizziness, weakness, rash, exfoliative dermatitis.

**INTERACTIONS:** See Contraindications. Alcohol may cause hypotension. Decreased or increased effect with other agents that depend on vascular smooth muscle. Concomitant use with calcium channel blockers may cause orthostatic hypotension. (NitroMist) Increased hypotensive effects with β-adrenergic blockers (eg, labetolol). ASA may increase levels. May decrease anticoagulant effect of heparin. Avoid ergotamine. Caution with tissue-type plasminogen activator.

**PREGNANCY:** Category C, caution in nursing.

**MECHANISM OF ACTION:** Nitrate vasodilator; relaxation of vascular smooth muscle, producing a vasodilator effect on both peripheral arteries and veins with more prominent effects on the latter.

**PHARMACOKINETICS: Absorption:**(Nitrolingual Spray) $C_{max}$=1041pg/mL•min, $T_{max}$=7.5min, AUC=12769pg/mL•min. **Metabolism:** Rapid, liver via reductase enzyme to glycerol nitrate metabolites and inorganic nitrates; hydrolysis to 1,2- and 1,3-dinitroglycerols (active metabolites)

## NURSING CONSIDERATIONS

**Assessment:** Assess for angina pectoris, hypotension, presence of volume-depletion, angina caused by hypertrophic cardiomyopathy, pregnancy/nursing status, and possible drug interactions.

**Monitoring:** Monitor for hypotension with paradoxical bradycardia and increased angina, tolerance development and physical dependence. Monitor for methemoglobinemia and signs of impaired oxygen delivery despite of adequate arterial $O_2$.

**Patient Counseling:** Inform about side effects of the drug (eg, headache, lightheadness). Inform to not take drug concomitantly with drugs used for erectile dysfunction. Instruct patient to use 5-10 minutes prior to engaging in activities which might provoke an acute attack. Do not open the bottle forcibly or use near open flame. Avoid alcohol consumption. Instruct how to prime device prior to use and if device has not been used within 6 weeks.

**Administration:** Spray on or under the tongue. **Storage:** 25°C (77°F); excursions permitted to 15-30°C (59-85°F).

# NITROSTAT RX

nitroglycerin (Parke-Davis)

**OTHER BRAND NAMES:** Nitroquick (Ethex)

**THERAPEUTIC CLASS:** Nitrate vasodilator

**INDICATIONS:** For acute relief of angina attack. Prophylaxis of angina pectoris.

**DOSAGE:** *Adults:* Treatment: 1 tab SL or in buccal pouch at onset of attack. May repeat in 5 min. Max: 3 tabs in 15 min. Prophylaxis: Take 5-10 min before activity that may cause acute attack. Administer in sitting position.

**HOW SUPPLIED:** Tab, Sublingual: 0.3mg, 0.4mg, 0.6mg

**CONTRAINDICATIONS:** Early MI, severe anemia, increased ICP, concomitant sildenafil.

**WARNINGS/PRECAUTIONS:** Do not swallow tabs. Severe hypotension may occur; caution with volume depletion or hypotension. May aggravate angina caused by hypertrophic cardiomyopathy. D/C if develop blurred vision or dry mouth. May interfere with cholesterol test. Monitor with acute MI or CHF. Tolerance to other nitrate forms may decrease effects. Caution in elderly.

**ADVERSE REACTIONS:** Headache, vertigo, dizziness, weakness, palpitation, syncope, flushing, postural hypotension, drug rash, exfoliative dermatitis.

**INTERACTIONS:** Additive hypotension with alcohol, β-blockers, phenothiazines, CCBs, other antihypertensives. Avoid ergotamine (related drugs), sildenafil. Vasodilatory and hemodynamic effects potentiated by ASA. Caution with alteplase. TCAs, anticholinergics may make sublingual dissolution difficult. Long-acting nitrates may decrease effects.

**PREGNANCY:** Category C, caution in nursing.

**MECHANISM OF ACTION:** Nitrate vasodilator; relaxes the vascular smooth muscle; activates guanylate cyclase, resulting in an increase of guanosine 3'5' monophosphate in smooth muscle and other tissues, resulting in vasodilatation.

**PHARMACOKINETICS: Absorption:** (SL) rapid, absolute bioavailability (40%). (0.3mg) $C_{max}$=2.3ng/mL, $T_{max}$=6.4 min, AUC=14.9ng•mL/min; (0.6mg) $C_{max}$=2.1ng/mL, $T_{max}$=7.2 min, AUC=14.9ng•mL/min. **Distribution:** $V_d$=3.3 L/kg, plasma protein binding (60%). **Metabolism:** Liver via reductase, extrahepatic (red cells and vascular wall). 1,2- and 1,3-dinitroglycerin (major metabolites). **Elimination:** (0.3mg) $T_{1/2}$=2.8 min, (0.6mg) 2.6 min.

## NURSING CONSIDERATIONS

**Assessment:** Assess for hypotension, volume depletion, severe anemia, angina caused by hypertrophic cardiomyopathy, and possible drug interactions.

**Monitoring:** Careful clinical or hemodynamic monitoring for hypotension and tachycardia. Monitor for paradoxical bradycardia, increased angina pectoris, headache and lightheadedness on standing, manifestation of true physical dependence (chest pain, acute MI), and methemoglobinemia.

**Patient Counseling:** Use smallest dose to relieve acute attacks to prevent developing dependence. Inform about side effects of drug (eg, headaches, lightheadedness on standing, burning or tingling sensation when administered SL). Avoid alcohol.

**Administration:** Sublingual route. **Storage:** 20-25°C (68-77°F).

# NIZORAL — RX

ketoconazole (Janssen)

**Risk of fatal hepatotoxicity. Concomitant terfenadine, astemizole and cisapride are contraindicated due to serious cardiovascular adverse events.**

**THERAPEUTIC CLASS:** Azole antifungal

**INDICATIONS:** Treatment of the following systemic fungal infections: candidiasis, chronic mucocutaneous candidiasis, oral thrush, candiduria, blastomycosis, coccidioidomycosis, histoplasmosis, chromomycosis, and paracoccidioidomycosis. Treatment of severe recalcitrant cutaneous dermatophyte infections not responsive to topical therapy or oral griseofulvin. Not for treatment of fungal meningitis.

**DOSAGE:** *Adults:* Initial: 200mg qd. Max: 400mg qd.
*Pediatrics:* >2 yrs: 3.3-6.6mg/kg/day.

**HOW SUPPLIED:** Tab: 200mg* *scored

**CONTRAINDICATIONS:** Concomitant terfenadine, astemizole, cisapride or oral triazolam.

**WARNINGS/PRECAUTIONS:** Hepatotoxicity reported. Monitor LFTs prior to therapy and periodically thereafter. Serum testosterone levels may be lowered. Hypersensitivity reactions reported. Tablets require acidity for dissolution. Not for use in children unless benefit outweighs risk.

**ADVERSE REACTIONS:** N/V, abdominal pain, pruritus.

**INTERACTIONS:** See Contraindications. Give antacids, anticholinergics, and $H_2$ blockers 2 hrs after ketoconazole. May potentiate midazolam, triazolam, oral hypoglycemics. May enhance anticoagulant effect of coumarin-like drugs. Avoid rifampin, isoniazid. Monitor digoxin, phenytoin. May alter metabolism of cyclosporine, tacrolimus, methylprednisolone and drugs metabolized by CYP3A4.

**PREGNANCY:** Category C, not for use in nursing.

**MECHANISM OF ACTION:** Azole antifungal; impairs synthesis of ergosterol, a vital component of fungal cell membranes.

**PHARMACOKINETICS: Absorption:** $C_{max}$=3.5mcg/mL; $T_{max}$=1-2 hrs.
**Distribution**: Plasma protein binding (99%). **Metabolism**: Via oxidation, degradation of imidazole and piperazine rings, oxidative dealkylation and aromatic hydroxylation. CYP3A4 inhibitor. **Elimination:** Biphasic. $T_{1/2}$=2 hrs (during first 10 hrs); $T_{1/2}$=8 hrs (thereafter); bile (major), urine (13%).

## NURSING CONSIDERATIONS

**Assessment:** Assess for lab, as well as clinical, documentation of infection prior to therapy. Assess LFTs and possible drug interactions (eg, terfenadine, astemizole) prior to therapy.

**Monitoring:** Monitor LFTs, signs/symptoms of hepatotoxicity and anaphylaxis. Monitor for cardiovascular events if using concomitant therapy with terfenadine or astemizole.

**Patient Counseling:** Counsel females to avoid nursing while on medication. Advise to report any signs/symptoms of liver dysfunction (eg, fatigue, anorexia, NV, jaundice, dark urine, or pale stools). If concomitant antacids, anticholinergics and $H_2$-blockers are needed, give at least 2 hrs after administration of drug. Continue treatment until tests indicate infection subsided.

**Administration:** Oral route. In cases of achlorhydria, instruct to dissolve each tab in 4mL aqueous solution of 0.2 N HCl. Use drinking straw to avoid contact with teeth. Follow administration with cup of water. **Storage**: Oral; store at controlled room temperature 15-25°C (59-77°F). Protect from moisture. Keep out of reach of children.

## Nizoral Shampoo — RX

ketoconazole (Ortho-McNeil)

**THERAPEUTIC CLASS:** Azole antifungal

**INDICATIONS:** Treatment of tinea (pityriasis) versicolor caused by or presumed to be caused by *Pityrosporum orbiculare* (also known as *Malassezia furfur* or *M. orbiculare*).

**DOSAGE:** *Adults:* Apply to the damp skin of the affected area and a wide margin surrounding this area. Lather, leave in place for 5 min, and then rinse with water. One application should be sufficient.

**HOW SUPPLIED:** Shampoo: 2% [4oz]

**WARNINGS/PRECAUTIONS:** Severe hypersensitivity reactions, including anaphylaxis, reported; d/c if a reaction suggesting sensitivity or chemical irritation occur. Avoid contact to eyes. Hair discoloration and abnormal hair texture, removal of the curl from permanently waved hair, itching, skin-burning sensation and contact dermatitis, hypersensitivity, alopecia, rash, urticaria, skin irritation, dry skin, and application-site reactions reported. Caution in pregnant and nursing women.

**ADVERSE REACTIONS:** Abnormal hair texture, scalp pustules, mild skin dryness, itching, oily or dry scalp and hair, pruritus, application-site reactions.

**PREGNANCY:** Category C, caution in nursing.

**MECHANISM OF ACTION:** Azole antifungal; impairs synthesis of ergosterol, a vital component of fungal membranes.

### NURSING CONSIDERATIONS

**Assessment:** Assess for drug hypersensitivity. Assess for pregnancy/nursing status.

**Monitoring:** Monitor for sensitivity or chemical irritation and adverse reactions such as hair loss, abnormal hair texture, scalp pustules, mild dryness of skin and hair and scalp, itching, oiliness, hair discoloration.

**Patient Counseling:** Inform that shampoo may be irritating to mucous membranes of eyes; avoid contact with eyes. Advise that hair discoloration and abnormal hair texture, removal of the curl from permanently waved hair, itching, skin-burning sensation and contact dermatitis, hypersensitivity, alopecia, rash, urticaria, skin irritation, dry skin, and application-site reactions have been reported after usage. Exercise caution when administering to nursing women.

**Administration:** Topical route. **Storage:** ≤25°C (77°F). Protect from light.

## Norco — CIII

hydrocodone bitartrate - acetaminophen (Watson)

**OTHER BRAND NAMES:** Maxidone (Watson)

**THERAPEUTIC CLASS:** Opioid analgesic

**INDICATIONS:** Relief of moderate to moderately severe pain.

**DOSAGE:** *Adults:* Usual: 1 tab q4-6h prn pain (or 2 tabs of 5-325mg). (Norco) Max: 6 tabs/day. (Maxidone) 5 tabs/day. Elderly: Start at lower end of dosing range.

**HOW SUPPLIED:** Tab: (Hydrocodone bitartrate-APAP): (Norco) 5mg-325mg*, 7.5mg-325mg*, 10mg-325mg*. (Maxidone) 750mg-10mg* *scored

**WARNINGS/PRECAUTIONS:** May produce dose-related respiratory depression. Respiratory depressant effects and elevation of CSF pressure may be exaggerated in the presence of head injury, intracranial lesions, or pre-existing increase in intracranial pressure. May obscure diagnosis or clinical course of acute abdominal conditions or head injuries. Caution in elderly, debilitated, severe hepatic or renal dysfunction, hypothyroidism, Addison's disease, prostatic hypertrophy, urethral stricture, pulmonary disease, and postoperative use. May be habit-forming. Suppresses cough reflex. May produce false-positive results for urinary 5-hydroxyindoleacetic acid.

**ADVERSE REACTIONS:** Lightheadedness, dizziness, sedation, N/V, rash, drowsiness, thrombocytopenia, agranulocytosis, allergic reactions.

**INTERACTIONS:** Additive CNS depression with narcotics, antipsychotics, antihistamines, antianxiety agents, alcohol, or other CNS depressants. Increased effect of antidepressants or hydrocodone with MAOIs or TCAs.

**PREGNANCY:** Category C, not for use in nursing.

**MECHANISM OF ACTION:** Hydrocodone: Opioid analgesic; most effects involve the CNS and smooth muscles. Precise MOA not established; suspected to relate to existence of opiate receptors in the CNS. Acetaminophen (APAP): Nonopiate, nonsalicylate analgesic and antipyretic. Analgesic activity involves peripheral influences; mechanism not established. Antipyretic activity is mediated through hypothalmic heat regulating-centers; inhibits prostaglandin synthetase.

**PHARMACOKINETICS: Absorption:** Hydrocodone: $C_{max}$=23.6ng/mL; $T_{max}$=1.3 hrs. APAP: Rapidly absorbed. **Distribution:** APAP: Excreted in breast milk. **Metabolism:** Hydrocodone: O-demethylation, N-demethylation, and 6-ketoreduction; APAP: Liver via conjugation. **Elimination:** Hydrocodone: $T_{1/2}$=3.8 hrs. APAP: Urine (85%, glucoronide conjugate). $T_{1/2}$=1.25-3 hrs.

N

## NURSING CONSIDERATIONS

**Assessment:** Assess for head injury, intracranial lesions, elevations in intracranial pressure, acute abdominal conditions, presence of debilitation (eg, elderly), hepatic/renal impairment, hypothyroidism, Addison's disease, prostatic hypertrophy or urethral stricture, pulmonary disease, nursing/pregnancy status, and possible drug interactions.

**Monitoring:** Monitor for signs/symptoms of respiratory depression, elevations in CSF pressure, medication dependence or tolerance, and medication abuse or misuse. Monitor serial hepatic/renal function tests with severe hepatic/renal disease.

**Patient Counseling:** Inform that medication may impair mental/physical abilities; use caution if performing hazardous tasks (eg, operating machinery/driving). Advise to avoid alcohol and other CNS depressants. Inform that medication may be habit-forming; only take for as long as prescribed, in amounts prescribed, and no more frequently than prescribed.

**Administration:** Oral route. **Storage:** 15-30°C (59-86°F). Store in tight, light-resistant container with child-resistant closure.

# NORDETTE-28 RX

ethinyl estradiol - levonorgestrel (Duramed)

**OTHER BRAND NAMES:** Levora (Watson) - Portia (Barr)

**THERAPEUTIC CLASS:** Estrogen/progestogen combination

**INDICATIONS:** Prevention of pregnancy.

**DOSAGE:** *Adults:* 1 tab qd for 28 days, then repeat. Start 1st Sunday after menses begin.

**HOW SUPPLIED:** Tab: (Ethinyl Estradiol-Levonorgestrel) 0.03mg-0.15mg

**CONTRAINDICATIONS:** Thrombophlebitis, DVT or thromboembolic disorders, pregnancy, cerebrovascular or coronary artery disease, undiagnosed abnormal genital bleeding, cholestatic jaundice of pregnancy or jaundice with prior pill use, hepatic adenomas or carcinomas, breast cancer or other estrogen-dependent neoplasia.

**WARNINGS/PRECAUTIONS:** Cigarette smoking increases risk of serious cardiovascular side effects; risk increases with age (especially >35 yrs) and heavy smoking. Increased risk of MI, vascular disease, thromboembolism, stroke and gallbladder disease. Retinal thrombosis, hepatic neoplasia, carcinoma of breast and reproductive organs reported. May cause glucose intolerance. May increase BP, elevate LDL levels or cause other lipid changes, fluid retention, breakthrough bleeding, and spotting. May cause or exacerbate migraine. May develop visual changes with contact lens. Increased risk of MI with HTN, hyperlipidemia, obesity, and diabetes. D/C if jaundice, significant depression or ophthalmic irregularities develop. Perform annual physical exam. Use before menarche is not indicated. May affect certain endocrine, LFTs and blood components.

**ADVERSE REACTIONS:** NV, breakthrough bleeding, spotting, amenorrhea, migraine, depression, vaginal candidiasis, edema, weight changes.

**INTERACTIONS:** Reduced effects, increased breakthrough bleeding, and menstrual irregularities with rifampin, barbiturates, phenylbutazone, phenytoin, griseofulvin, topiramate, some protease inhibitors, modafinil, and possibly St. John's wort, penicillins, and tetracyclines. Increased plasma levels with ascorbic acid, APAP, indinavir, fluconazole, troleandomycin, and atorvastatin. May affect cyclosporine, theophylline, and corticosteroid levels.

**PREGNANCY:** Category X, not for use in nursing.

**MECHANISM OF ACTION:** Estrogen/progestogen oral contraceptive; acts by suppressing gonadotropins. Primarily responsible for inhibiting ovulation. Also causes changes in cervical mucus (increases difficulty of sperm entry into uterus) and endometrium (reduces likelihood of implantation).

**PHARMACOKINETICS: Distribution:** Found in breast milk.



## NURSING CONSIDERATIONS

**Assessment:** Assess for current or history of thrombophlebitis or thromboembolic disorders, cerebrovascular or coronary artery disease, known/suspected carcinoma of the breast, endometrium, or other suspected estrogen-dependent neoplasia, undiagnosed abnormal genital bleeding, cholestatic jaundice of pregnancy or jaundice with prior pill use, hepatic adenomas, hepatic carcinomas, benign liver tumors, and known/suspected pregnancy. Assess use in patients ≥35 yrs who smoke ≥15 cigarettes/day. Assess use with history of HTN, DM, hyperlipidemias, hypercholesterolemia, increased age, obesity, and possible drug interactions.

**Monitoring:** Monitor for MI, thromboembolism, stroke, hepatic neoplasia, ocular lesions, onset or exacerbation of headaches or migraines, bleeding irregularities, fluid retention, and gallbladder disease. Monitor serum glucose levels with DM or prediabetic patients, lipid levels with history of hyperlipidemia, BP with history of HTN. Monitor for signs of liver toxicity (eg, jaundice) while on therapy and for signs of worsening depression with previous history. Refer patients with contact lenses to ophthalmologist if visual changes develop. Perform annual physical exam.

**Patient Counseling:** Inform that drug does not protect against HIV infection (AIDS) and other STDs. Advise to take exactly as directed at intervals not exceeding 24 hrs. Counsel to use an additional form of contraception until after first 7 days of administration in initial cycle of medication. Instruct if pill missed, take as soon as possible; take next dose at regularly scheduled time. Advise to continue to take medication if spotting or breakthrough bleeding occur; notify physician if it persists. Instruct not to smoke while on therapy.

**Administration:** Oral route. **Storage:** 15-25°C (59-77°F).

# NORDITROPIN RX

somatropin (Novo Nordisk)

**OTHER BRAND NAMES:** Norditropin Nordiflex (Novo Nordisk) - Norditropin FlexPro (Novo Nordisk)

**THERAPEUTIC CLASS:** Human growth hormone

**INDICATIONS:** (Adults) Replacement of endogenous growth hormone deficiency who meet either of the following criteria: (1) adult-onset patients with growth hormone deficiency (GHD), either alone or associated with multiple hormone deficiencies (hypopituitarism), as a result of pituitary disease, hypothalamic disease, surgery, radiation therapy, or trauma; or (2) childhood-onset patients who were growth hormone deficient during childhood as a result of congenital, genetic, acquired, or idiopathic causes. (Pediatrics) Treatment of children with growth failure due to inadequate growth hormone secretion. Treatment of children with short stature associated with Noonan syndrome and Turner syndrome. Treatment of children with short stature born small for gestational age (SGA) with no catch-up growth by age 2-4 yrs.

**DOSAGE:** *Adults:* Initial: No more than 0.004mg/kg/day. Increase to no more than 0.016mg/kg/day after 6 weeks. Alternative: Initial: 0.2mg/day (range, 0.15-0.30mg/day). May increase gradually every 1-2 months by increments of 0.1-0.2mg/day based on clinical response and serum IGF-I concentrations. *Pediatrics:* GHD: 0.024-0.034mg/kg 6-7x/week. Noonan Syndrome: Dose up to 0.066mg/kg/day. Turner Syndrome/SGA: Dose up to 0.067mg/kg/day. Carefully monitor growth response and adjust the recombinant human growth hormone (rhGH) dose as necessary.

**HOW SUPPLIED:** Inj: (Norditropin (cartridge) and Norditropin Nordiflex (prefilled pen) 5mg/1.5mL, 15mg/1.5mL; (prefilled pen), 10mg/1.5mL, 30mg/3mL

**CONTRAINDICATIONS:** Acute critical illness due to complications following open heart surgery, abdominal surgery or multiple accidental trauma, or acute respiratory failure; Prader-Willi syndrome with severe obesity, a history of upper airway obstruction or sleep apnea, or severe respiratory impairment; presence of active malignancy; active proliferative or severe non-proliferative diabetic retinopathy; pediatric patients with closed epiphyses.



**WARNINGS/PRECAUTIONS:** Increased mortality reported in patients with acute critical illness; weigh benefits vs. risks of therapy. Reports of fatalities after initiating therapy in Prader-Willi syndrome; evaluate Prader-Willi patients for signs of upper airway obstruction and sleep apnea before treatment and interrupt therapy if occurs during treatment. In patients with pre-existing tumors or GHD secondary to an intracranial lesion, monitor for progression or recurrence of underlying disease. Monitor for potential malignant transformation of skin lesions. May decrease insulin sensitivity; monitor blood sugar. Intracranial HTN reported; perform funduscopic examination before therapy and during therapy. Fluid retention may occur. Undiagnosed/untreated hypothyroidism may prevent optimal response; perform periodic thyroid function tests. Slipped capital femoral epiphysis may occur. Progression of scoliosis may occur in patients with rapid growth. Increased occurrence of otitis media in patients with Turner syndrome. Monitor for CV disorders in patients with Turner syndrome. Patients with epiphyseal closure who were treated in childhood should be reevaluated before continuation of therapy as adults. Tissue atrophy may occur with repeated administration at same site. Allergic reactions may occur. Serum levels of inorganic phosphorus, alkaline phosphatase, parathyroid hormone, and IGF-I may increase.

**ADVERSE REACTIONS:** (Pediatrics): Glucose intolerance, unmasking of latent central hypothyroidism, infection, arthralgia, headache, increased sweating, gynecomastia, injection-site reactions. (Adults): Glucose intolerance, unmasking of latent central hypothyroidism, injection-site reactions, edema, arthralgia, infection, paresthesia, skeletal pain, headache.

**INTERACTIONS:** May impact metabolism of cortisol and cortisone; use of glucocorticoid replacement therapy for previously undiagnosed hypoadrenalism may require an increase in maintenance or stress doses, especially with cortisone acetate or prednisone. Excessive glucocorticoid therapy may attenuate growth-promoting effects of somatotropin in children; glucocorticoid therapy may need to be adjusted in children. May alter the clearance of compounds metabolized by CYP450 liver enzymes (eg, corticosteroids, sex steroids, anticonvulsants, cyclosporine). Use with oral estrogen replacement therapy may require a larger dose. May require dosage adjustment of insulin or oral hypoglycemic agents.

**PREGNANCY:** Category C, caution in nursing.

**MECHANISM OF ACTION:** Human growth hormone; binds to dimeric GH receptor in cell membrane of target cells, resulting in intracellular signal transduction and a host of pharmacodynamic effects.

**PHARMACOKINETICS: Absorption**: $T_{max}$=4-5 hrs; (4mg): $C_{max}$=13.8ng/mL; (8mg): $C_{max}$=17.1ng/mL. **Elimination**: $T_{1/2}$=7-10 hrs.

## NURSING CONSIDERATIONS

**Assessment:** Assess for acute critical illness, active malignancy, diabetic retinopathy, presence of closed epiphyses in pediatric patients, pre-existing type 1 or type 2 DM or impaired glucose tolerance, presence of scoliosis, hypopituitarism, pregnancy/nursing status, and possible drug interactions. Assess for intracranial HTN; perform baseline funduscopic examination to identify pre-existing papilledema. Assess for hypothyroidism; perform baseline thyroid function tests. In Prader-Willi syndrome, assess for signs of upper airway obstruction and sleep apnea. In patients with Turner syndrome, evaluate for otitis media, other ear disorders, and CV disorders. In patients with epiphyseal closure who were treated with somatotropin replacement therapy in childhood, reevaluate before continuing therapy as adults.

**Monitoring:** Monitor for signs and symptoms of malignant transformation of skin lesions, fluid retention, slipped capital femoral epiphysis, progression of scoliosis, tissue atrophy at injection site, allergic reactions, and increases in serum levels of inorganic phosphorus, alkaline phosphatase, parathyroid hormone, and IGF-I. Monitor for intracranial HTN; perform periodic funduscopic examinations. Monitor for glucose intolerance; perform periodic measurements of glucose levels. Monitor for hypothyroidism; perform periodic thyroid function tests. In Prader-Willi syndrome patients, monitor for signs of upper airway obstruction, proper weight control, and for signs of respiratory infection. In patients with pre-existing tumors or GHD secondary to an intracranial lesion, monitor for progression of underlying disease process. In patients with Turner's syndrome, monitor for signs/symptoms of otitis media and for CV disorders.

**Patient Counseling:** Inform about benefit/risks of therapy. Instruct on proper usage and disposal, and caution against reuse of needles and syringes. Advise to seek medical attention if symptoms of allergic reactions, slipped capital femoral epiphysis (onset of limp, hip or knee pain), respiratory infections (eg, otitis media or ear or CV disorders) and/or progression of scoliosis occur.

**Administration:** SQ. **Storage**: Unused: 2-8°C (36-46°F); do not freeze; avoid direct light. In-use: 5mg, 10mg: 2-8°C (36-46°F) and use within 4 weeks or store up to 25°C (77°F) for up to 3 weeks. Discard unused portion. 15mg, 30 mg: 2-8°C (36-46°F) and use within 4 weeks; discard unused portion after 4 weeks.

N

# Norinyl 1/50 — RX

norethindrone - mestranol (Watson)

**OTHER BRAND NAMES:** Necon 1/50 (Watson) - Brevicon (Watson)

**THERAPEUTIC CLASS:** Estrogen/progestogen combination

**INDICATIONS:** Prevention of pregnancy.

**DOSAGE:** *Adults:* 1 tab qd for 28 days, then repeat. Start 1st Sunday after menses begins or 1st day of menses.

**HOW SUPPLIED:** Tab: (Mestranol-Norethindrone) 0.05mg-1mg

**CONTRAINDICATIONS:** Thrombophlebitis, DVT or thromboembolic disorders, pregnancy, cerebrovascular or coronary artery disease, undiagnosed abnormal genital bleeding, cholestatic jaundice of pregnancy or jaundice with prior pill use, hepatic adenomas or carcinomas, breast cancer or other estrogen-dependent neoplasia.

**WARNINGS/PRECAUTIONS:** Cigarette smoking increases risk of serious cardiovascular side effects. This risk increases with age (especially >35 yrs) and heavy smoking. Increased risk of MI, vascular disease, thromboembolism, stroke, and gallbladder disease. Retinal thrombosis, hepatic neoplasia, carcinoma of breast and reproductive organs reported. May cause glucose intolerance. May increase BP, elevate LDL levels or cause other lipid changes, fluid retention, breakthrough bleeding, and spotting. May cause or exacerbate migraine. May develop visual changes with contact lens. Increased risk of MI with HTN, hyperlipidemia, obesity, and diabetes. D/C if jaundice, significant depression, or ophthalmic irregularities develop. Perform annual physical exam. Use before menarche is not indicated. May affect certain endocrine, LFTs, and blood components.

**ADVERSE REACTIONS:** N/V, breakthrough bleeding, spotting, amenorrhea, migraine, depression, vaginal candidiasis, edema, weight changes.

**INTERACTIONS:** Reduced effects, increased breakthrough bleeding, and menstrual irregularities with rifampin, barbiturates, phenylbutazone, phenytoin, carbamazepine, griseofulvin, topiramate, St. John's wort, and possibly with ampicillin and tetracyclines.

**PREGNANCY:** Category X, not for use in nursing.

**MECHANISM OF ACTION:** Estrogen/progestogen combination oral contraceptive; acts by suppressing gonadotropin, inhibiting ovulation, causing changes in cervical mucus (increasing difficulty of sperm entry into uterus) and endometrium (reducing likehood of implantation).

**PHARMACOKINETICS: Distribution:** Found in breast milk.

## NURSING CONSIDERATIONS

N

**Assessment:** Assess for current or history of thrombophlebitis or thromboembolic disorder, cerebrovascular disease, CAD, known/suspected carcinoma of breast, endometrium or other known/suspected estrogen-dependent neoplasia, undiagnosed abnormal genital bleeding, cholestatic jaundice of pregnancy or jaundice with prior pill use, hepatic adenomas or carcinomas, benign liver tumors, and known/suspected pregnancy. Assess use in patients with hyperlipidemia, hypercholesterolemia, HTN, obesity, DM, and in patients ≥35 yrs who smoke ≥15 cigarettes/day. Assess for possible drug interactions.

**Monitoring:** Monitor for MI, thromboembolism, stroke, hepatic neoplasia, ocular lesions, bleeding irregularities, fluid retention, onset or exacerbation of headaches or migraines, vascular disease, HTN, hypertriglyceridemia, and gallbladder disease. Monitor glucose levels in DM or prediabetic patients, BP with history of HTN, and lipid levels with history of hyperlipidemia, for signs of liver dysfunction (eg, jaundice), and signs of worsening depression with previous history. Perform annual physical exam while on therapy.

**Patient Counseling:** Inform that drug does not protect against HIV infection and other STDs. When initiating treatment, instruct to use additional form of contraception until after 7 days on therapy. Instruct to take 1 pill at same time daily at intervals not exceeding 24 hrs. If dose missed, take as soon as possible, then take next dose at regularly scheduled time. Instruct to continue medication if spotting or breakthrough bleeding occur; notify physician if symptoms persist. Inform that missing a pill can cause spotting or light bleeding. Advise not to smoke while on therapy.

**Administration:** Oral route. **Storage:** 15-25°C (59-77°F).

# NORPACE — RX

disopyramide phosphate (Pharmacia & Upjohn)

**OTHER BRAND NAMES:** Norpace CR (Pharmacia & Upjohn)

**THERAPEUTIC CLASS:** Class I antiarrhythmic

**INDICATIONS:** Treatment of documented life-threatening ventricular arrhythmias.

**DOSAGE:** *Adults:* Usual: 400-800mg/day in divided dose. Recommended: 150mg q6h immediate-release (IR) or 300mg q12h extended-release (CR). Adjust dose with anticholinergic effects. Weight <110lbs/Moderate Hepatic or Renal Insufficiency (CrCl >40mL/min): 100mg q6h IR or 200mg q12h CR. Severe Renal Insufficiency (with or without initial 150mg LD): CrCl 30-40mL/min: 100mg q8h IR. CrCl 30-15mL/min: 100mg q12h IR. CrCl <15mL/min: 100mg q24h IR. Rapid Control of Ventricular Arrhythmia: LD: 300mg IR (200mg if <110lbs). Follow with maint dose. Cardiomyopathy/Cardiac Decompensation: Initial: 100mg q6-8h IR. Adjust gradually. See PI if no response or toxicity occurs. Elderly: Start at low end of dosing range. *Pediatrics:* <1 yr: 10-30mg/kg/day. 1-4 yrs: 10-20mg/kg/day. 4-12 yrs: 10-15mg/kg/day. 12-18 yrs: 6-15mg/kg/day. Give in equally divided doses q6h. Hospitalize patient during initial therapy. Start dose titration at lower end of range.

**HOW SUPPLIED:** Cap: (Norpace) 100mg, 150mg; Cap, Extended-Release: (Norpace CR) 100mg, 150mg

**CONTRAINDICATIONS:** Cardiogenic shock, 2nd- or 3rd-degree AV block (if no pacemaker present), congenital QT prolongation.

**WARNINGS/PRECAUTIONS:** Proarrhythmic; reserve for life-threatening ventricular arrhythmias. May cause or worsen CHF and produce hypotension due to negative inotropic properties. Reduce dose if 1st-degree heart block occurs. Avoid with urinary retention, glaucoma, and myasthenia gravis unless adequate overriding measures taken. Atrial flutter/fibrillation; digitalize first. Monitor closely or withdraw if QT prolongation >25% occurs and ectopy continues. D/C if QRS widening >25% occurs. Avoid LD with cardiomyopathy or cardiac decompensation. Correct $K^+$ abnormalities before therapy. Reduce dose with renal/hepatic dysfunction; monitor ECG. Avoid CR formulation with CrCl ≤40mL/min. Caution with sick sinus syndrome, Wolff-Parkinson-White syndrome, bundle branch block, or elderly. May significantly lower blood glucose.

**ADVERSE REACTIONS:** Dry mouth, urinary retention/frequency/urgency, constipation, blurred vision, GI effects, dizziness, fatigue, headache.

**INTERACTIONS:** Avoid type IA and IC antiarrhythmics, and propranolol except in unresponsive, life-threatening arrhythmias. Hepatic enzyme inducers may lower levels. Avoid within 48 hrs before or 24 hrs after verapamil. Possible fatal interactions with CYP3A4 inhibitors. Monitor blood glucose with β-blockers, alcohol.

**PREGNANCY:** Category C, not for use in nursing.

**MECHANISM OF ACTION:** Type I antiarrhythmic; decreases rate of diastolic depolarization in cells with augmented automaticity, decreases upstroke velocity, and increases action potential duration of normal cardiac cells. Decreases disparity in refractoriness between infracted and adjacent normally perfused myocardium and has no effect on α- or β-adrenergic receptors.

**PHARMACOKINETICS: Absorption:** Rapid and complete; $C_{max}$=2.22mcg/mL, $T_{max}$=4.5 hrs. **Distribution:** Plasma protein binding (50-65%). **Metabolism:** Liver. **Elimination:** Urine (50% unchanged), (20% mono-N-dealkylated metabolite), (10% other metabolite); $T_{1/2}$=11.65 hrs.

## NURSING CONSIDERATIONS

**Assessment:** Prior to therapy, patients with atrial flutter or AF should be digitalized and potassium abnormalities should be corrected. Assess for cardiogenic shock, pre-existing 2nd- or 3rd-degree HB, presence of functioning pacemaker, sick sinus syndrome (bradycardia/tachycardia syndrome), Wolff-Parkinson-White syndrome, bundle branch block, congenital QT prolongation, MI, life-threatening arrhythmia, CHF, cardiomyopathy or myocarditis, chronic malnutrition, hepatic/renal impairment, alcohol intake, glaucoma, myasthenia gravis, urinary retention or BPH, pregnancy/nursing status, and possible drug interactions.

**Monitoring:** Monitor for hypotension, HF, PR interval prolongation, widening of QRS, hypoglycemia, HB, urinary retention, and myasthenia crisis.

**Patient Counseling:** Inform about risks/benefits; report adverse reactions. Notify if pregnant/nursing.

**Administration:** Oral route. **Storage:** 25°C (77°F); excursions permitted to 15-30°C (59-86°F).

## NORPLANT II — RX

levonorgestrel (Population Council)

**OTHER BRAND NAMES:** Jadelle (Population Council)

**THERAPEUTIC CLASS:** Progestogen

**INDICATIONS:** Long-term (up to 5 yrs) prevention of pregnancy.

**DOSAGE:** *Adults:* Implant 150mg (2 implants) in midportion of upper arm during 1st 7 days of onset of menses. Place in a "V" shape 30° apart. Replace by end of 5th year.

**HOW SUPPLIED:** Implant: 75mg

**CONTRAINDICATIONS:** Active thrombophlebitis or thromboembolic disorders, undiagnosed abnormal genital bleeding, pregnancy, acute live disease or liver tumors, carcinoma of the breast, and idiopathic intracranial HTN.

**WARNINGS/PRECAUTIONS:** Complications related to insertion and removal of capsules reported. Bleeding irregularities have occurred. Retinal thrombosis leading to partial or complete loss of vision, hepatic neoplasia, carcinoma of breast and reproductive organs reported. Risk of thromboembolic and thrombotic diseases, MI, ectopic pregnancy, ovarian cysts, breast cancer, gall bladder and autoimmune diseases, cerebrovascular diseases. Cigarette smoking increases risk of serious cardiovascular side effects; risk increases with age (especially >35 yrs) and the extent of smoking. Idiopathic intracranial HTN and increases in BP reported. Caution with fluid retention. Vision changes reported; caution with contact lenses. Weight gain, thrombosis, and thrombophlebitis reported. May worsen depression, increase LDL levels. If jaundice develops, remove implants. Altered glucose tolerance; monitor diabetics. Rare reports of congenital anomalies with use during early pregnancy.

N

**ADVERSE REACTIONS:** Menorrhagia, amenorrhea, oligomenorrhea, irregular bleeding, pain/itching or infection at implant site, headache, nervousness, GI effects, dizziness, rash, acne, weight gain, cervicitis.

**INTERACTIONS:** Not recommended with chronic phenytoin, carbamazepine, phenobarbital, or oxcarbazepine use; decreased effectiveness. Back-up method of contraception with short-term therapy with CYP450 inducers. Rifampicin and St. John's wort may decreases levels and effectiveness.

**PREGNANCY:** Use in pregnancy not known, caution in nursing.

**MECHANISM OF ACTION:** Progestin; inhibits ovulation and thickens cervical mucus.

**PHARMACOKINETICS: Absorption:** $C_{max}$=722pg/mL (day 2), $T_{max}$=2-3 days. **Distribution:** Highly bound to sex-hormone-binding globulin. **Metabolism:** β-hydroxylation. **Excretion:** Urine (40-68%), feces (16-48%); $T_{1/2}$=13-18 hrs

### NURSING CONSIDERATIONS

**Assessment:** Perform physical exam of implant site, breast, abdomen, and pelvis. Assess cervical cytology and relevant lab tests, pregnancy status, breast cancer, vaginal bleeding, thromboembolic disorders/active thrombophlebitis and/or cerebrovascular diseases, osteoporosis, history of depression, DM, hepatic/renal impairment, CV disease, HTN, and possible drug/lab test interactions.

**Monitoring:** Monitor for insertion and removal complications, amenorrhea, menstrual irregularity, manifestations of thromboembolic disorders (eg, thrombophlebitis, PE, cerebrovascular disorders, retinal thrombosis), ocular disorders, manifestations of fluid retention, epilepsy, abdominal pain, weight changes. Lab monitoring of bone mineral density for osteoporosis/osteoporotic fractures, LFTs, TFTs, glucose, lipid profile, and coagulation tests.

**Patient Counseling:** Inform of potential benefits/risks of therapy and insertion/removal procedure. Inform drug does not protect against HIV infection/AIDS or other STDs. Advise to avoid smoking while on therapy.

**Administration:** Subdermal implantation. Refer to PI for full instructions on insertion/removal. **Storage:** 15-30°C (59-86°F).

## Norvasc RX

amlodipine besylate (Pfizer)

**THERAPEUTIC CLASS:** Calcium channel blocker (dihydropyridine)

**INDICATIONS:** Treatment of hypertension and coronary artery disease (CAD) including chronic stable or vasospastic angina (Prinzmetal's or Variant Angina) alone or in combination with other antihypertensives/antianginals. To reduce risks of hospitalization due to angina and to reduce risk of coronary revascularization procedure in patients with recently documented CAD by angiography and without heart failure (ejection fraction <40%).

**DOSAGE:** *Adults:* HTN: Initial: 5mg qd. Titrate over 7-14 days. Max: 10mg qd. Small, Fragile, or Elderly Individuals/Hepatic Dysfunction/Concomitant Antihypertensive: 2.5mg qd. Angina: Usual dose: 5-10mg qd. CAD: 5-10mg qd. *Pediatrics:* 6-17 yrs: HTN: Usual range: 2.5-5mg qd.

**HOW SUPPLIED:** Tab: 2.5mg, 5mg, 10mg

**WARNINGS/PRECAUTIONS:** Symptomatic hypotension possible with sever aortic stenosis. May increase angina or acute MI with severe obstructive CAD. Caution with severe hepatic impairment and in elderly

**ADVERSE REACTIONS:** Edema, palpitation, dizziness, headache, fatigue, somnolence, flushing, nausea.

**PREGNANCY:** Category C, not for use in nursing.

**MECHANISM OF ACTION:** Dihydropyridine calcium antagonist (calcium ion antagonist or slow-channel blocker): Inhibits transmembrane influx or calcium ions into vascular smooth muscle and cardiac muscle; binds to both dihydropyridine and nondihydropyridine binding sites resulting in peripheral arterial vasodilation and reduction in BP.

**PHARMACOKINETICS: Absorption:** Absolute bioavailability (64-90%); $T_{max}$=6-12 hrs. **Distribution:** Plasma protein binding (93%). **Metabolism:** Hepatic. **Elimination:** Urine (10% parent compound; 60% inactive metabolites), $T_{1/2}$=30-50 hrs.

### NURSING CONSIDERATIONS

**Assessment:** Assess for CAD, severe aortic stenosis, CHF, LFTs, BP, and pregnancy/nursing status.

**Monitoring:** Monitor BP, LFTs. Check for adverse events (eg. edema, flushing, palpitations, headache, fatigue, jaundice, MI).

**Patient Counseling:** Counsel about potential adverse effects; advise to seek medical attention if any develop. Instruct to take as prescribed.

**Administration:** Oral route. **Storage:** 15-30°C (59-86°F); store in tight, light-resistant container.

## Norvir RX

ritonavir (Abbott)

**Coadministration with sedative hypnotics, antiarrhythmics, or ergot alkaloids may result in potentially serious and/or life-threatening adverse events.**

**THERAPEUTIC CLASS:** Protease inhibitor

**INDICATIONS:** Treatment of HIV infection in combination with other antiretrovirals.

**DOSAGE:** *Adults:* Initial: 300mg bid. Titrate: Increase every 2-3 days by 100mg bid. Maint: 600mg bid. Max: 600mg bid. Elderly: Start at low end of dosing

N

range. Take with meals.
*Pediatrics:* >1 month: Initial: 250mg/m$^2$ bid. Titrate: Increase by 50mg/m$^2$ every 2-3 days. Maint: 350-400mg/m$^2$ bid or highest tolerated dose. Max: 600mg bid. Take with meals. Refer to PI for pediatric dosage guideline.

**HOW SUPPLIED:** Cap: 100mg; Tab: 100mg; Sol: 80mg/mL [240mL]

**CONTRAINDICATIONS:** Co-administration with drugs highly dependent on CYP3A for clearance and for which elevated plasma concentrations are associated with serious and/or life-threatening events. Co-administration with drugs that significantly reduce ritonavir. These drugs are alfuzosin HCl, amiodarone, bepridil, flecainide, propafenone, quinidine, voriconazole, ergot derivatives (dihydroergotamine, ergonovine, ergotamine, methylergonovine), St. John's wort, lovastatin, simvastatin, pimozide, sildenafil (only when used for treatment of pulmonary arterial hypertension), oral midazolam, triazolam and cisapride.

**WARNINGS/PRECAUTIONS:** Allergic reaction (eg, urticaria, mild skin eruptions, bronchospasm and angioedema) may occur. D/C if signs and symptoms of pancreatitis, anaphylaxis, Steven-Johnson syndrome occur. New onset/exacerbation of pre-existing diabetes mellitus (DM), hyperglycemia, and immune reconstitution syndrome reported. Caution with pre-existing liver disease, liver enzyme abnormalities, or hepatitis; hepatic transaminase elevations, clinical hepatitis and jaundice reported. Monitor LFT's, especially first 3 months. Prolonged PR interval may occur; caution with underlying structural heart disease, pre-existing conduction system abnormalities, ischemic heart disease and cardiomyopathies. May elevate TG and total cholesterol levels; monitor levels at baseline then periodically. Increased bleeding may occur with hemophilia A and B. Possible redistribution or accumulation of body fat. May increase likelihood of cross-resistance to other protease inhibitors. Caution in elderly.

**ADVERSE REACTIONS:** Diarrhea, anorexia, N/V, abdominal pain, asthenia, headache, malaise, vasodilation, constipation, dizziness, taste perversion, circumoral/peripheral paresthesia, insomnia, sweating.

N

**INTERACTIONS:** See Contraindications. Neurologic and cardiac events reported with disopyramide, mexiletine, nefazodone, fluoxetine, and β-blockers. May decrease ritonavir levels with rifampin; may lead to loss of virologic response. Concomitant use with tipranavir may cause hepatitis and hepatic decompensation. May increase levels of clarithromycin with renal impairment; reduce clarithromycin dose by 50% if CrCl 30-60mL/min and by 75% if CrCl<30mL/min. May increase ketoconazole/itraconazole levels; avoid ketoconazole/itraconazole doses >200mg/day. May increase tadalafil, vardenafil and sildenafil levels; monitor for adverse events. May increase levels of tramadol, propoxyphene, antiarrhythmics (disopyramide, lidocaine, mexiletene), anticonvulsants (carbamazepine, clonazepam, ethosuximide), antidepressants (nefazodone, SSRIs, TCAs), dronabinol, quinine, metoprolol, β-blockers (metoprolol, timolol), CCBs (diltiazem, nifedipine, verapamil), atorvastatin, rosuvastatin, immunosuppressants (cyclosporine, tacrolimus, sirolimus), neuroleptics (perphenazine, risperidone, thioridazine), sedative/hypnotics (buspirone, clorazepate, diazepam, estazolam, flurazepam, zolpidem), fluticasone, methamphetamine, maraviroc, anticancer agents (vincristine, vinblastine), digoxin, salmeterol, saquinavir, atazanavir, darunavir, fosamprenavir, desipramine, indinavir, rifabutin and parenteral midazolam. Reduce dose with dexamethasone, prednisone. May increase levels of trazodone; use with caution and consider lower trazodone dose. May increase levels with delavirdine. May decrease levels of phenytoin, divalproex, lamotrigine, bupropion, atovaquone, meperidine, theophylline, and methadone. Separate dosing with didanosine by 2.5 hrs. May increase plasma levels of drugs metabolized by CYP3A or CYP2D6. May decrease ethinyl estradiol levels; use alternative contraceptive measures. Decreases warfarin levels; monitor INR. Solution contains alcohol; may produce disulfiram-like reactions with disulfiram, metronidazole.

**PREGNANCY:** Category B, not for use in nursing.

**MECHANISM OF ACTION:** HIV protease inhibitor; anti-viral; renders enzyme incapable of processing Gag-Pol polyprotein precursor, which leads to production of noninfectious immature HIV particles.

**PHARMACOKINETICS: Absorption:** $C_{max}$=11.2mcg/mL; $T_{max}$=2 hrs (fasting), 4 hrs (fed); AUC=121.7mcg•hr/mL (Cap), AUC=129mcg•hr/mL (Sol). **Distribution:** Plasma protein binding (98-99%). **Metabolism:** CYP3A, 2D6 (oxidation); isopropylthiazole (major metabolite). **Elimination:** Urine (11.3%, 3.5% unchanged), feces (86.4%, 33.8% unchanged); $T_{1/2}$=3-5 hrs.

## NURSING CONSIDERATIONS

**Assessment:** Assess for pre-existing liver disease or impairment (eg, enzyme abnormalities, hepatitis), DM, hemophilia A and B, underlying cardiac problems (eg, structural heart disease, ischemic heart disease, cardiomyopathies, conduction system abnormalities), pregnancy/nursing status and possible drug interactions. Obtain baseline ECG, ALT, AST, GGT, CPK, uric acid, TG and cholesterol levels.

**Monitoring:** Monitor LFTs periodically for first 3 months. Monitor for signs/symptoms of anaphylactoid/allergic reactions, new onset or exacerbation of DM, hyperglycemia, pancreatitis, immune reconstitution syndrome, fat redistribution or accumulation and hepatic dysfunction. Monitor ECG, ALT, AST, GGT, CPK, uric acid, TG and cholesterol levels. May enroll patients in the Antiretroviral Pregnancy Registry if they become pregnant while on treatment.

**Patient Counseling:** Discuss risks and benefits of therapy. Inform that drug does not cure HIV; may continue to develop opportunistic infections. Does not reduce risk of transmitting HIV. Instruct to take every day with food, if possible; do not alter dose or d/c without consulting physician. If miss dose, take next dose as soon as possible; do not double dose. Notify physician if using Rx/OTC or herbal products particularly St. John's wort. Seek medical attention if experience symptoms of PR interval prolongation (dizziness, lightheadedness, abnormal heart rhythm, or loss of consciousness), allergic reactions, pancreatitis (N/V, abdominal pain), infections, or fat redistribution/accumulation. Women taking estrogen-based hormonal contraceptives should use an additional/alternative method of birth control while on therapy.

**Administration:** Oral route. (Tab) Swallow whole, do not chew, break or crush. (Sol) May mix with chocolate milk within 1 hr of dosing. **Storage:** Cap: 2-8°C (36-46°F). Tab: 20-25°C (68-77°F) excursions permitted to 15-30°C (59-86°F) [Room Temperature]. Sol: 20-25°C (68-77°F). Do not refrigerate. Shake well before use. Avoid exposure to excessive heat.

# NOVOLIN — OTC

## insulin human, rdna origin - insulin, human isophane - insulin, human regular (Novo Nordisk)

**OTHER BRAND NAMES:** Novolin N (Novo Nordisk) - Novolin R (Novo Nordisk)

**THERAPEUTIC CLASS:** Insulin

**INDICATIONS:** To control hyperglycemia in diabetes.

**DOSAGE:** *Adults:* Individualize dose.
*Pediatrics:* Individualize dose.

**HOW SUPPLIED:** Inj: 100 U/mL (Novolin N, Novolin R)

**WARNINGS/PRECAUTIONS:** Human insulin differs from animal source insulin. Any change in insulin should be made cautiously. Changes in strength, manufacturer, type or method of manufacture may result in the need for a change in dosage. Hypoglycemia may occur with taking too much insulin, missing or delaying meals, exercising or working more than usual. An infection or illness (especially if accompanied by diarrhea or vomiting) may change insulin requirements. Administration of insulin SQ can result in lipoatrophy. Novolin R is not recommended for use in insulin pumps.

**ADVERSE REACTIONS:** Hypoglycemia, sweating, dizziness, palpitations, tremor, hunger, restlessness, lightheadedness, inability to concentrate, headache, injection-site reaction, allergic reaction.

**INTERACTIONS:** Increased insulin requirements with oral contraceptives, corticosteroids, or thyroid replacement therapy. Reduced insulin requirements with oral hypoglycemics, salicylates, sulfa antibiotics, and certain antidepressants. Alcoholic beverages may change insulin requirements. β-blockers may mask symptoms of hypoglycemia.

**PREGNANCY:** Pregnancy category is not known.

**MECHANISM OF ACTION:** Insulin (rDNA origin); regulates glucose metabolism, lowers blood glucose by facilitating cellular uptake of glucose and simultaneously inhibiting the glucose output from the liver.

## NURSING CONSIDERATIONS

**Assessment:** Assess FPG, $HbA_{1c}$, renal function, LFTs, pregnancy status, infections, alcohol consumption, exercise routines, and for possible drug interactions.

**Monitoring:** Monitor FPG, $HbA_{1c}$, hypokalemia, renal function, diabetic ketoacidosis, vision changes, lipodystrophy, allergic reactions. Monitor for signs of hypoglycemia (sweating, palpitations, seizures, disorientation, tremors).

**Patient Counseling:** Use only if solution is clear and colorless with no visible particles. Counsel about signs/symptoms of hypoglycemia, hyperglycemia, diabetic ketoacidosis, the importance of frequent monitoring of blood glucose levels, eating a balanced diet and exercising regularly. Advise to avoid excessive alcohol. During periods of stress (eg, trauma, infection, surgery), insulin requirements may be changed; advise patients to seek prompt medical advice. Counsel on proper administration techniques.

**Administration:** SQ route. Refer to labeling for administration techniques.
**Storage:** Below 30°C (86°F). Do not freeze. Protect from light.

# Novolin 70/30 — OTC

insulin human, rdna origin - insulin, human (isophane/regular) (Novo Nordisk)

N

**THERAPEUTIC CLASS:** Insulin

**INDICATIONS:** To control hyperglycemia in diabetes.

**DOSAGE:** *Adults:* Individualize dose. Administer SQ.
*Pediatrics:* Individualize dose. Administer SQ.

**HOW SUPPLIED:** (Isophane/Regular) Inj: 70 U-30 U/mL

**WARNINGS/PRECAUTIONS:** Human insulin differs from animal source insulin. Any change of insulin should be made cautiously. Changes in strength, manufacturer, type or method of manufacture may result in the need for a change in dosage. Hypoglycemia may occur with taking too much insulin, missing or delaying meals, exercising or working more than usual. An infection or illness (especially with diarrhea or vomiting) may change insulin requirements. Caution with diseases of adrenal, pituitary, or thyroid glands, or progression of kidney or liver disease. Administration of insulin SQ can result in lipodystrophy.

**ADVERSE REACTIONS:** Hypoglycemia, sweating, dizziness, palpitations, tremor, hunger, restlessness, lightheadedness, inability to concentrate, headache, injection-site reaction, allergic reaction.

**INTERACTIONS:** Increased insulin requirements with oral contraceptives, corticosteroids, or thyroid replacement therapy. Reduced insulin requirements with oral hypoglycemics, salicylates, sulfa antibiotics, and certain antidepressants. Alcoholic beverages may change insulin requirements. β-blockers may mask symptoms of hypoglycemia.

**PREGNANCY:** Pregnancy category is not known.

**MECHANISM OF ACTION:** Insulin (rDNA origin); has 70% NPH human insulin isophane suspension and 30% regular human insulin. Regulates glucose metabolism, lowers blood glucose by facilitating cellular uptake of glucose and simultaneously inhibiting the glucose output from the liver.

## NURSING CONSIDERATIONS

**Assessment:** Assess FPG, $HbA_{1c}$, renal function, LFTs, pregnancy status, infections, alcohol consumption, exercise routines, and for possible drug interactions.

**Monitoring:** Monitor FPG, $HbA_{1c}$, hypokalemia, renal function, diabetic ketoacidosis, vision changes, lipodystrophy, allergic reactions. Monitor for signs of hypoglycemia (sweating, palpitation, seizures, disorientation, tremors).

**Patient Counseling:** Use only if the solution is clear and colorless with no visible particles. Counsel about signs/symptoms of hypoglycemia, hyperglycemia, diabetic ketoacidosis, the importance of frequent monitoring of blood glucose levels, the need for eating a balanced diet and exercising regularly. Advise to avoid excessive alcohol. During periods of stress (eg, trauma, infection, surgery) insulin requirements may be changed; advise patients to seek prompt medical advice. Counsel on proper administration techniques.

**Administration:** SQ route. Refer to labeling for administration techniques.
**Storage:** Below 30°C (86°F). Do not freeze. Protect from light.

# Novolog RX

insulin aspart (Novo Nordisk)

**THERAPEUTIC CLASS:** Insulin

**INDICATIONS:** To improve glycemic control in adults and children with diabetes mellitus (DM).

**DOSAGE:** *Adults:* Individualize dose. (SQ) Inject immediately within 5-10 min before a meal. (External Pump) Change the reservoir at least every 6 days, change the infusion set, and the infusion set insertion site at least every 3 days. Do not use or mix with any other insulin or diluent in pump. (IV) Used at concentrations from 0.05 U/mL to 1.0 U/mL, insulin aspart in infusion systems using polypropylene infusion bags.
*Pediatrics:* ≥4 yrs: Individualize dose.(SQ) Injected immediately within 5-10 min before a meal. (External Pump) Change the reservoir at least every 6 days, change the infusion set, and the infusion set insertion site at least every 3 days. Do not use or mix with any other insulin or diluent in pump. (IV) Used at concentrations from 0.05 U/mL to 1.0 U/mL, insulin aspart in infusion systems using polypropylene infusion bags.

**HOW SUPPLIED:** Inj: 100 U/mL; FlexPen, PenFill: 3mL; Vial: 10mL.

**CONTRAINDICATIONS:** Hypoglycemia.

**WARNINGS/PRECAUTIONS:** Administer with meals. Any change of insulin should be made cautiously and under medical supervision. Glucose monitoring is recommended. Changes in strength, manufacturer, type, or method of manufacture may result in the need for a change in dosage. Hypoglycemia may occur with too much insulin, changes in food intake, exercising, and taking concomitant medication. IV-administered insulin requires close monitorig for hypoglycemia. Insulin mixtures should not be administered IV. May cause hypokalemia; caution in patients who are predisposed. May reduce dosage with hepatic/renal impairment. Dosage adjustment is needed during pregnancy. When used in an external SQ insulin infusion pump, it should not be mixed with any other insulin or diluent.

**ADVERSE REACTIONS:** Hypoglycemia, headache, N/V, diarrhea, hyporeflexia, onychomycosis, sensory disturbance, urinary tract infection, chest pain, lipodystrophy, hypersensitivity reaction, injection site reactions, pruritus, rash.

**INTERACTIONS:** Increased glucose-lowering effects with ACE inhibitors, disopyramide, fibrates, fluoxetine, MAOIs, propoxyphene, salicylates, somatostatin analog, sulfonamide antibiotics and other antidiabetic agents. Decreased blood glucose-lowering effects with corticosteroids, niacin, danazol, diuretics, sympathomimetic agents, isoniazid, phenothiazine derivatives, somatropin, thyroid hormones, estrogens, progestogens (eg, in oral contraceptives), atypical antipsychotics. Pentamidine may cause hypoglycemia followed by hyperglycemia. β-blockers, clonidine, lithium salts, and alcohol may potentiate or weaken glucose-lowering effect. Masked or reduced hypoglycemic symptoms with sympatholytic products such as β-blockers, clonidine, guanethidine, and reserpine.

**PREGNANCY:** Category B, caution in nursing.

**MECHANISM OF ACTION:** Insulin aspart (rDNA origin); regulates glucose metabolism, lowers blood glucose by facilitating cellular uptake of glucose and simultaneously inhibiting glucose output from the liver.

**PHARMACOKINETICS: Absorption:** $C_{max}$=82 mU/L; $T_{max}$=40-50 min. **Distribution:** Plasma protein binding (<10%). **Elimination:** $T_{1/2}$=81 min.

## NURSING CONSIDERATIONS

**Assessment:** Assess fasting plasma glucose (FPG), $HbA_{1c}$, renal function, LFTs, pregnancy status, infections, alcohol consumption, exercise routines, and possible drug interactions.

**Monitoring:** Monitor FPG, $HbA_{1c}$, hypokalemia, renal function, diabetic ketoacidosis, vision changes, lipodystrophy, allergic reactions. Monitor for signs of hypoglycemia (sweating, palpitations, seizures, disorientation, tremors).

**Patient Counseling:** Advise to use solution, only if it is clear and colorless with no visible particles. Counsel about signs/symptoms of hypoglycemia, hyperglycemia, diabetic ketoacidosis, the need to eat a balanced diet, and regular exercise. Inform about potential risks and benefits of taking insulin and possible adverse reactions. Counsel on proper administration techniques, lifestyle management, regular glucose monitoring, periodic glycosylated hemoglobin technique, hemoglobin testing, recognition and management of hypo- and hyperglycemia, complications of insulin therapy, timing of dose, instruction in the use of injection or SQ infusion device, and proper storage of insulin. Caution when driving or operating machinery. Check carefully when administering insulin to avoid medication errors.

**Administration:** IV, SQ route in abdominal wall, thigh, or upper arm. Give immediately within 5-10 min before a meal. Refer to labeling information for administration techniques. **Storage:** 2-8°C (36-46°F). Do not freeze and not to be used when frozen; should be discarded. Open vials can be refrigerated. Protect from excessive heat or sunlight. Store at room temperature <30°C (86°F) up to 28 days.

N

# Novolog Mix 70/30 RX

## insulin aspart protamine - insulin aspart (Novo Nordisk)

**THERAPEUTIC CLASS:** Insulin

**INDICATIONS:** To control hyperglycemia in diabetes.

**DOSAGE:** *Adults:* Individualize dose. For SQ inj only. Inject SQ bid within 15 min before breakfast and dinner. Do not mix with other insulins or use in insulin pumps.

**HOW SUPPLIED:** (Insulin Aspart Protamine-Insulin Aspart) Inj: 70 U-30 U/mL; PenFill: 70 U-30 U/mL; Prefilled: 70 U-30 U/mL

**CONTRAINDICATIONS:** Hypoglycemia.

**WARNINGS/PRECAUTIONS:** Any change of insulin should be made cautiously. Changes in strength, manufacturer, type or method of manufacture may result in the need for a change in dosage. Hypoglycemia and hypokalemia may occur; caution with fasting and autonomic neuropathy. Illness, stress, change in meals and exercise may change insulin requirements. Smoking, temperature, and exercise affect insulin absorption. Caution with liver or kidney disease. Administration of insulin SQ can result in lipoatrophy.

**ADVERSE REACTIONS:** Hypoglycemia, hypokalemia, lipodystrophy, hypersensitivity reaction, injection-site reactions, pruritus, rash.

**INTERACTIONS:** Increased glucose lowering effects with ACE inhibitors, disopyramide, fibrates, fluoxetine, MAOIs, propoxyphene, salicylates, somatostatin analog, sulfonamide antibiotics, and oral antidiabetics. Decreased blood glucose lowering effects with corticosteroids, niacin, danazol, diuretics, sympathomimetics, isoniazid, phenothiazine derivatives, somatropin, thyroid hormones, estrogens, progestogens. β-blockers, clonidine, lithium salts, and alcohol may potentiate or weaken glucose lowering effect. β-blockers, clonidine, guanethidine, and reserpine may reduce or mask signs of hypoglycemia. Do not mix with other insulin products. Caution with potassium-lowering drugs or drugs sensitive to serum potassium levels. Pentamidine may cause hypoglycemia, followed by hyperglycemia.

**PREGNANCY:** Category C, safety in nursing not known.

**MECHANISM OF ACTION:** Insulin; regulates glucose metabolism. Lowers blood glucose by facilitating cellular uptake of glucose, simultaneously inhibiting output of glucose from liver.

**PHARMACOKINETICS: Absorption:** (0.2, 0.3 U/kg): $C_{max}$=23.4, 61.3m U/L; $T_{max}$=60, 85 min. **Distribution:** Plasma protein binding (0-9%). **Elimination:** $T_{1/2}$=8-9 hrs.

## NURSING CONSIDERATIONS

**Assessment:** Assess FPG, $HbA_{1c}$, renal function, LFTs, pregnancy status, infections, alcohol consumption, exercise routines, and for possible drug interactions.

**Monitoring:** Monitor FPG, $HbA_{1c}$, hypokalemia, renal function, diabetic ketoacidosis, vision changes, lipodystrophy, allergic reactions. Monitor for signs and symptoms of hypoglycemia (eg, sweating, palpitation, seizures, disorientation, tremors).

**Patient Counseling:** Inform to use only if solution is clear and colorless with no visible particles, and not to dilute or mix with other insulins or solution. Counsel about the signs and symptoms of hypoglycemia, hyperglycemia, and diabetic ketoacidosis; importance of frequent monitoring of blood glucose levels, need for a balanced diet, and regular exercise. Advise to avoid excessive alcohol. Counsel that during periods of stress (eg, trauma, infection, surgery), insulin requirements may be changed; advise to seek prompt medical attention. Educate on proper administration techniques.

**Administration:** SQ route. Administer in abdominal wall, thigh, or upper arm. Give with meals. Refer to PI for administration techniques. **Storage**: 2-8°C (36-46°F). Do not freeze.



# NOXAFIL — RX

posaconazole (Schering)

**THERAPEUTIC CLASS:** Azole antifungal

**INDICATIONS:** Prophylaxis of invasive *Aspergillus* and *Candida* infections in patients ≥13 yrs who are at high risk of developing these infections due to being severely immunocompromised. Treatment of oropharyngeal candidiasis, including oropharyngeal candidiasis refractory to itraconazole and/or fluconazole.

**DOSAGE:** *Adults:* Prophylaxis of Invasive Fungal Infections: 200mg (5mL) tid. Base duration of therapy on recovery from neutropenia or immunosuppression. Oropharyngeal Candidiasis: LD: 100mg (2.5mL) bid on 1st day, then 100mg qd for 13 days. Oropharyngeal Candidiasis Refractory to Itraconazole and/or Fluconazole: 400mg (10mL) bid. Base duration of therapy on severity of underlying disease and clinical response. Give each dose with a full meal or nutritional supplement.

*Pediatrics:* ≥13 yrs: Prophylaxis of Invasive Fungal Infections: 200mg (5mL) tid. Base duration of therapy on recovery from neutropenia or immunosuppression. Oropharyngeal Candidiasis: LD: 100mg (2.5mL) bid on 1st day, then 100mg qd for 13 days. Oropharyngeal Candidiasis Refractory to Itraconazole and/or Fluconazole: 400mg (10mL) bid. Base duration of therapy on severity of underlying disease and clinical response. Give each dose with full meal or nutritional supplement.

**HOW SUPPLIED:** Susp: 40mg/mL

**CONTRAINDICATIONS:** Coadministration with ergot alkaloids, terfenadine, astemizole, cisapride, pimozide, halofantrine, quinidine, or sirolimus.

**WARNINGS/PRECAUTIONS:** Hepatic reactions (eg, mild to moderate elevations in ALT, AST, alkaline phosphatase, total bilirubin, and/or clinical hepatitis) reported; monitor LFTs at start of and during therapy. Caution with hepatic impairment. Monitor closely with severe renal impairment. Prolongation of QT interval reported; caution with potentially proarrhythmic conditions.

**ADVERSE REACTIONS:** Fever, headache, rigors, HTN, anemia, neutropenia, diarrhea, N/V, abdominal pain, constipation, hypokalemia, thrombocytopenia, coughing, dyspnea.

**INTERACTIONS:** See Contraindications. May elevate cyclosporine and tacrolimus levels; consider dose reduction and more frequent clinical monitoring when therapy is initiated. Avoid use with drugs that are known to prolong the QTc interval and are metabolized through CYP3A4. Avoid concurrent use of cimetidine, rifabutin, phenytoin, and efavirenz unless benefits outweigh risks. If concomitant phenytoin is required, monitor closely and consider phenytoin dose reduction. If concomitant rifabutin is required, monitor CBC and adverse events. Monitor adverse events with concomitant benzodiazepines metabolized through CYP3A4 (eg, midazolam); consider dose reduction of these benzodiazepines during coadministration. May increase levels of vinca alkaloids; consider dose adjustment of vinca alkaloid. Consider dose reduction of concomitant HMG-CoA reductase inhibitors metabolized through CYP3A4. Monitor for adverse events and toxicity with concomitant CCBs metabolized through CYP3A4, atazanavir, and ritonavir. Dose reduction of CCBs may be needed. Monitor for breakthrough fungal infection with esomeprazole and metoclopramide. May increase digoxin levels; monitor digoxin levels. Inhibitors or inducers of UDP glucuronidation or p-glycoprotein (P-gp) may affect posaconazole concentrations. May increase plasma concentrations of drugs metabolized by CYP3A4.

**PREGNANCY:** Category C, not for use in nursing.

**MECHANISM OF ACTION:** Triazole antifungal agent; blocks synthesis of ergosterol, a key component of fungal cell membrane, through inhibition of the enzyme lanosterol 14α-demethylase and accumulation of methylated sterol precursors.

N

**PHARMACOKINETICS: Administration:** Oral administration of variable doses resulted in different parameters. **Distribution:** $V_d$=1774L, plasma protein binding (>98%). **Metabolism:** Via UDP glucuronidation; CYP3A4 enzyme. **Elimination:** Feces (71%), urine (13%); $T_{1/2}$=35 hrs.

## NURSING CONSIDERATIONS

**Assessment:** Assess for severe renal impairment, pregnancy/nursing status, and for possible drug interactions (eg, ergot alkaloids, CYP3A4 substrates, cylosporine, QT prolonging medications). Assess use in patients with proarrhythmic conditions. Assess liver function (LFTs, bilirubin) prior to therapy.

**Monitoring:** Monitor for signs/symptoms of hepatic toxicity, QT prolongation, and arrhythmias. Monitor liver function (LFTs, bilirubin) while on therapy. In patients with severe renal impairment, monitor for breakthrough invasive fungal infections (IFIs).

**Patient Counseling:** Instruct to take medication with full meal or liquid nutritional supplement; maybe taken with acidic carbonated beverage. Instruct to inform physician if severe diarrhea or vomiting develop. Inform physician of all medications being taken.

**Administration:** Oral. **Storage**: 25°C (77°F); excursions permitted to 15-30°C (59-86°F). Do not freeze.

# NPLATE — RX

romiplostim (Amgen)

**THERAPEUTIC CLASS:** Thrombopoietin receptor agonist

**INDICATIONS:** Treatment of thrombocytopenia in patients with chronic immune (idiopathic) thrombocytopenic purpura (ITP) who have had an insufficient response to corticosteroids, immunoglobulins, or splenectomy.

**DOSAGE:** *Adults:* Initial: 1mcg/kg SQ based on actual body wt. Titrate: Adjust dose by increments of 1mcg/kg until platelet count is ≥50 x $10^9$/L. Max: 10mcg/kg/week. If platelet count <50 x $10^9$/L, increase dose by 1mcg/kg. If platelet count >200 x $10^9$/L x 2 consecutive weeks, reduce dose by 1mcg/kg. If platelet count >400 x $10^9$/L, do not dose; continue assessing platelet count weekly. If platelet count falls to <200 x $10^9$/L, resume therapy at a dose reduced by 1mcg/kg. D/C if platelet count does not increase to a sufficient level after 4 weeks of therapy; obtain CBCs and platelet counts weekly for 2 weeks.

**HOW SUPPLIED:** Inj: 250mcg, 500mcg

**WARNINGS/PRECAUTIONS:** May increase risk for development or progression of reticulin fiber deposition within bone marrow. Examine peripheral blood smear closely to establish baseline level of cellular morphological abnormalities; d/c treatment if new or worsening morphological abnormalities or cytopenia develop. Discontinuation may worsen thrombocytopenia and increase risk of bleeding. Excessive doses may result in thrombotic/thromboembolic complications. Assess patients for the formation of neutralizing antibodies if platelet counts decrease following an initial Nplate response. D/C if platelet count does not increase to a level sufficient to avoid bleeding after 4 weeks. May increase risk for hematologic malignancies. Monitor CBCs, including platelet counts, and peripheral blood smears prior to initiation, throughout, and following discontinuation of therapy. Caution in renal/hepatic impairment and elderly. Available only through restricted distribution program.

**ADVERSE REACTIONS:** Bone marrow reticulin deposition, worsening thrombocytopenia, headache, arthralgia, dizziness, insomnia, myalgia, pain in extremity, abdominal pain, shoulder pain, dyspepsia, and paresthesia.

**PREGNANCY:** Category C, not for use in nursing.

**MECHANISM OF ACTION:** Fc-peptide fusion protein; increases platelet production through binding and activation of the TPO receptor.

**PHARMACOKINETICS: Absorption:** $T_{max}$=7-50 hrs. **Elimination:** $T_{1/2}$=1-34 days.

## NURSING CONSIDERATIONS

**Assessment:** Assess for CBCs, platelet counts, peripheral blood smears, peripheral blood differential count, and pregnancy/nursing status.

**Monitoring:** Monitor for CBCs, platelet counts, peripheral blood smears (weekly during dose adjustment phase and then monthly after establishment of a stable dose) bone marrow reticulin deposition, worsening thrombocytopenia, headache, arthralgia, dizziness, insomnia, myalgia, pain in extremities, abdominal pain, shoulder pain, dyspepsia, and paresthesia. Obtain CBCs, platelet counts, peripheral smears during therapy and after d/c for at least 2 weeks.

**Patient Counseling:** Counsel patients about the risks and benefits of Nplate prior to therapy. Inform the risks associated with prolonged treatment of Nplate are not fully established and must enroll in Nplate NEXUS (Network of Experts Understanding and Supporting Nplate and Patients) program for proper use. Advise to monitor closely platelet counts weekly, and CBCs for at least 2 weeks after d/c therapy. Counsel about situations or medications that may increase risk for bleeding.

**Administration:** SQ route. Do not shake during reconstitution. Administer reconstituted within 24 hrs. **Storage:** Refrigerated at 2°-8°C (36°-46°F). Preservative free and sterile. Protect from light. Do not freeze.

# NUCYNTA

tapentadol (PRICARA)

**CII**

**THERAPEUTIC CLASS:** Opioid analgesic

**INDICATIONS:** Relief of moderate to severe acute pain in patients ≥18 yrs.

**DOSAGE:** *Adults:* ≥18 yrs: Individualize dose. Usual: 50mg, 75mg, or 100mg q4-6h depending upon pain intensity. Day 1: 2nd dose may be given 1 hr after the 1st dose, if pain relief inadequate. Max: 700mg on day 1, then 600mg/day thereafter. Moderate Hepatic Impairment: Initial: 50mg q8h or longer between doses. Max: 3 doses/24 hrs. Elderly: Start at low end of dosing range.

**HOW SUPPLIED:** Tab: 50mg, 75mg, 100mg

**CONTRAINDICATIONS:** Respiratory depression (unmonitored), acute or severe bronchial asthma or hypercapnia, paralytic ileus, and use within 14 days of taking MAOIs.

**WARNINGS/PRECAUTIONS:** Caution in respiratory depression, asthma, COPD or cor pulmonale, severe obesity, sleep apnea syndrome, myxedema, kyphoscoliosis, CNS depression, or coma. Caution with head injury, intracranial lesions or increased intracranial pressure, history of seizure disorder or risk of seizures, moderate hepatic impairment, and biliary tract disease (eg, acute pancreatitis). May be abused in a manner similar to other opioids; carefully monitor for signs of abuse and addiction. May impair physical/mental abilities. Serotonin syndrome reported. Avoid abrupt withdrawal.

**ADVERSE REACTIONS:** N/V, constipation, dry mouth, fatigue, headache, dizziness, somnolence, pruritus, hyperhidrosis.

**INTERACTIONS:** See Contraindications. May exhibit additive CNS depression with other opioid analgesics, general anesthetics, phenothiazines, antiemetics, other tranquilizers, sedatives, hypnotics, other CNS depressants including alcohol; consider dose reduction. Risk of serotonin syndrome may occur with serotonergic drugs such as SSRIs or SNRIs, TCAs, MAOIs and triptans, and drugs that may impair metabolism of serotonin.

**PREGNANCY:** Category C, not for use in nursing.

**MECHANISM OF ACTION:** Opioid analgesic; mechanism not established. Analgesic efficacy thought to be due to mu-opioid agonist activity and inhibition of norepinephrine reuptake.

**PHARMACOKINETICS: Absorption:** $T_{max}$=1.25 hrs; Absolute bioavailability (32%). **Distribution:** $V_d$=540L; Plasma protein binding (20%). **Metabolism:** Conjugation (extensive). **Elimination:** Kidneys (99%); urine (3% unchanged, 70% conjugated); $T_{1/2}$=4 hrs.

N

## NURSING CONSIDERATIONS

**Assessment:** Assess for respiratory depression, acute or severe bronchial asthma, hypercapnia, paralytic ileus, history of seizures, hepatic impairment, biliary tract disease, pregnancy/nursing status, and possible drug interactions.

**Monitoring:** Monitor for signs of abuse and addiction, CNS depression, respiratory depression, hypotension, sedation, coma, GI symptoms, and serotonin syndrome, including mental status change (eg, agitation, hallucinations, coma), autonomic instability (eg, tachycardia, labile BP, hyperthermia), neuromuscular aberrations (eg, hyperreflexia, incoordination), and/or GI symptoms (eg, N/V, diarrhea).

**Patient Counseling:** Instruct to report episodes of breakthrough pain and adverse experiences during therapy. Inform of potential for drug abuse. Advise that judgement, thinking, and motor skills when performing hazardous tasks (eg, operating machinery/driving) may be impaired. Notify physician if pregnant, intend to become pregnant, or if breastfeeding. Avoid MAOIs or serotonergic drugs, which may potentiate serotonin syndrome. Drug may increase seizure risk; notify physician of concomitant prescription or OTC drugs. Advise to avoid alcohol while on therapy.

**Administration:** Oral route. **Storage:** 25°C (77°F); excursions permitted to 15-30°C (59-86°F). Protect from moisture.

# NUTROPIN RX

somatropin (Genentech)

**OTHER BRAND NAMES:** Nutropin AQ (Genentech)

**THERAPEUTIC CLASS:** Human growth hormone

**INDICATIONS:** (Adults) Replacement of endogenous growth hormone (GH) in GH deficiency (GHD). (Pediatrics) Long-term treatment of growth failure due to lack of adequate endogenous GH secretion, in short stature associated with Turner syndrome, and in idiopathic short stature (ISS). Treatment of growth failure associated with chronic renal insufficiency (CRI) up to the time of renal transplantation.

**DOSAGE:** *Adults:* GHD: Initial: Up to 0.006mg/kg/day SQ. Max: <35 yrs: 0.025mg/kg qd. ≥35 yrs: 0.0125mg/kg/day. Alternatively may use 0.2mg/day (range: 0.15-0.30mg/day). Increase every 1-2 months by increments of 0.1-0.2mg qd. Elderly: Start at low end of dosing range.
*Pediatrics:* GHD: Usual: 0.3mg/kg/week divided into daily SQ doses. Pubertal Patients: Up to 0.7mg/kg/week divided into daily SQ doses. CRI: 0.35mg/kg/week divided into daily SQ doses. Continue until renal transplantation. Hemodialysis: Give qhs or 3-4 hrs post-dialysis. Chronic Cycling Peritoneal Dialysis: Give in am after dialysis. Chronic Ambulatory Peritoneal Dialysis: Give qhs during overnight exchange. Turner Syndrome: Up to 0.375mg/kg/week SQ in divided doses 3-7x/week. ISS: 0.3mg/kg/week divided into daily SQ doses.

**HOW SUPPLIED:** Inj: 5mg, 10mg, (AQ) 10mg/2mL, 20mg/2mL, (AQ NuSpin) 5mg/2mL, 10mg/2mL, 20mg/2mL

**CONTRAINDICATIONS:** Acute critical illness after serious surgeries (eg, open heart or abdominal surgery, accidental trauma, acute respiratory failure), closed epiphyses in pediatrics, active proliferative or severe nonproliferative diabetic retinopathy, active neoplasia, evidence of recurrence or progression of an intracranial tumor. Prader-Willi syndrome (unless also diagnosed with GH deficiency) with severe obesity or respiratory impairment.

**WARNINGS/PRECAUTIONS:** Caution with epiphyseal closure in adults treated with GH-replacement therapy in childhood. Recurrence/progression reported with intracranial lesions. Renal osteodystrophy may occur with growth failure secondary to renal impairment. Scoliosis and slipped capital femoral epiphysis may develop in rapid growth. Caution with Turner syndrome and ISS. Intracranial HTN with papilledema, visual changes, headache, N/V has been reported. Funduscopic exam should be done before and during treatment. Monitor for malignant transformation of skin lesions. Injecting SQ in same site over long period of time may cause tissue atrophy. May decrease insulin sensitivity; monitor blood sugar. Caution in elderly.

**ADVERSE REACTIONS:** Antibodies to the protein, leukemia, transient peripheral edema, arthralgia, carpal tunnel syndrome, malignant transformations, gynecomastia, pancreatitis.

**INTERACTIONS:** Decreased effects with glucocorticoids. May reduce insulin sensitivity; may need insulin adjustment. May need to increase dose in adult women on estrogen replacement.

**PREGNANCY:** Category C, caution in nursing.

**MECHANISM OF ACTION:** Human growth hormone; increases growth rate and serum insulin-like growth factor-I levels.

**PHARMACOKINETICS: Absorption:** (SQ) Absolute bioavailability (81%), $C_{max}$=71.1mcg/L, $T_{max}$=3.9 hrs, AUC=677 mcg•hr/L. **Distribution:** $V_d$=50mL/kg. **Metabolism:** Liver and kidneys. **Elimination:** (SQ) $T_{1/2}$=2.1 hrs. (IV) $T_{1/2}$=19.5 min.

## NURSING CONSIDERATIONS

**Assessment:** Assess for closed epiphyses (pediatric), proliferative diabetic retinopathy, active malignancy, acute critical illness due to complications of surgery, multiple accidental trauma, or acute respiratory failure, pre-existing type 1 or type 2 DM or impaired glucose tolerance, history of scoliosis, pre-existing papilledema, hypothyroidism, diagnostic imaging (rule out pituitary or intracranial tumor), hypopituitarism and possible drug interactions. Obtain baseline funduscopic exam. Chronic renal insufficiency (pediatrics): Baseline x-ray of hips. Prader-Willi syndrome: Evaluate for signs of upper airway obstruction or sleep apnea before initiation. Turner syndrome: Evaluate for otitis media or other ear disorders, and for CV disorders before initiation.

**Monitoring:** Monitor fasting blood glucose, and thyroid function tests periodically, periodic funduscopic exam, weight control (Prader-Willi), signs/symptoms of malignant transformation of skin lesions, intracranial HTN, renal osteodystrophy, slipped capital femoral epiphysis (onset of limp, hip or knee pain), hypersensitivity/allergic reactions, respiratory infections (Prader-Willi), otitis media or ear disorders, CV disorders (Turner syndrome), and progression of scoliosis.

**Patient Counseling:** Instruct thoroughly on proper usage, proper disposal, and caution against reuse of needles and syringes. Seek medical attention if symptoms of slipped capital femoral epiphysis (onset of limp, hip or knee pain), hypersensitivity/allergic reactions, respiratory infections (Prader-Willi), otitis media or ear disorders and CV disorders (Turner syndrome), and progression of scoliosis occur.

**Administration:** SQ route. Do not shake. Refer to PI for proper administration. **Storage:** Before and after reconstitution: 2-8°C (36-46°F) (under refrigeration). Avoid freezing. (AQ): Stable for 28 days after initial use. Protect from light. (Nutropin): Stable 14 days after reconstitution.

## NUVARING RX

etonogestrel - ethinyl estradiol (Organon)

**THERAPEUTIC CLASS:** Estrogen/progestogen combination

**INDICATIONS:** Prevention of pregnancy.

**DOSAGE:** *Adults:* Insert ring vaginally. Ring is to remain in place continuously for 3 weeks. It should be removed for 1 week break and then a new ring should be inserted on same day of week as the last ring was removed. No Hormonal Contraceptive Use in the Preceding Cycle: Insert ring on Day 1-5 of menstrual bleeding. If inserted on days 2-5 of cycle, use an additional barrier method of contraception (eg, condom, spermicide) for 1st 7 days. Changing from Combined Hormonal Contraceptive: May switch any day, but at the latest on the day following the usual hormone-free interval. Changing from Progestin-Only Method (minipill, implant, or injection) or from Progestogen-Releasing Intrauterine System (IUS): May switch on any day from the minipill. May switch from an implant or IUS on the day of its removal and from an injectable on the day when the next injection is due. In all cases, additional barrier method (eg, condom, spermicide) should be use for the 1st 7 days.

**HOW SUPPLIED:** Vaginal ring: (Ethinyl estradiol-Etonogestrel) 0.015mg-0.120mg/day

**CONTRAINDICATIONS:** Thrombophlebitis, history of deep vein thrombophlebitis, active or history of thromboembolic disorders, current or history of cerebral vascular disease, current or history of coronary artery disease, valvular heart disease with thrombogenic complications, severe HTN, diabetes with vascular involvement, headaches with focal neurological symptoms, major surgery with prolonged immobilization, breast carcinoma or history of breast carcinoma, carcinoma of the endometrium or other estrogen-dependent neoplasia, undiagnosed abnormal genital bleeding, cholestatic jaundice of pregnancy or jaundice with prior hormonal contraceptive use, hepatic tumors (benign or malignant) or active liver disease, pregnancy, heavy smoking ( ≥15 cigarettes per day) and >35 yrs.

**WARNINGS/PRECAUTIONS:** Cigarette smoking increases risk of serious cardiovascular side effects; this risk increases with age (especially >35 yrs) and heavy smoking. Increases risk of MI, thromboembolism, stroke, hepatic neoplasia, vascular disease, gallbladder disease, and hypertension. Increased risk of morbidity and mortality in certain inherited thrombophilias, HTN, hyperlipidemias, obesity, and diabetes. May increase risk of breast cancer and cancer of the reproductive organs. Retinal thrombosis reported; d/c if unexplained partial or complete loss of vision, onset of proptosis or diplopia, papilledema, or retinal vascular lesions develop. May cause decreased glucose tolerance, fluid retention, breakthrough bleeding, and spotting. May increase BP; d/c if significant elevation in BP occurs. May elevate LDL levels or cause other lipid changes. May cause or exacerbate migraine headaches; d/c if severe or recurrent headache or migraine develops. D/C if jaundice or if significant depression develops. May develop visual changes with contact lens. May be expelled while removing tampons on rare occasions. Toxic shock syndrome reported. Older women who take hormonal contraceptive should take the lowest possible dose formulation that is effective. Ectopic as well as intrauterine pregnancy may occur in contraceptive failures. Does not protect against HIV infection (AIDS) and other STDs. Vaginal/cervical erosion or ulceration rarely reported. Perform annual physical exam. May affect certain endocrine, LFTs, and blood components in laboratory tests.

**ADVERSE REACTIONS:** Vaginitis, headache, upper respiratory tract infection, vaginal secretion, sinusitis, weight gain, nausea.

**INTERACTIONS:** May reduce contraceptive effectiveness when co-administered with some anti-fungals, anticonvulsants, and other drugs that increase the metabolism of contraceptive steroids (eg, barbiturates, griseofulvin, rifampin, phenylbutazone, phenytoin, carbamazepine, felbamate, oxycarbazepine, topiramate, modafinil); use additonal form of contraception when taking such medications. HIV protease inhibitors may increase or decrease estrogen and progestin levels. St. John's wort may reduce contraceptive effectiveness and may cause breakthrough bleeding. Atorvastatin, ascorbic acid, acetaminophen, CYP3A4 inhibitors (eg, itraconazole, ketoconazole), vaginal miconazole nitrate may increase plasma hormone levels. May increase levels of cyclosporine, prednisolone, and theophylline. May decrease levels of acetaminophen and increase clearance of temazepam, salicylic acid, morphine, and clofibric acid.

**PREGNANCY:** Category X, not for use in nursing.

**MECHANISM OF ACTION:** Estrogen/progestogen combination; suppresses gonadotropins, leading to inhibition of ovulation, and increases difficulty of sperm entry into uterus and reduces likelihood of implantation by producing changes in cervical mucus and endometrium, respectively.

**PHARMACOKINETICS: Absorption:** Etonorgestrel: Rapid; bioavailability (100%); $C_{max}$=1716pg/mL; $T_{max}$=200.3 hrs. Ethinyl estradiol: Rapid; absolute bioavailability (56%); $C_{max}$=34.7pg/mL; $T_{max}$=59.3 hrs. **Distribution:** Found in breast milk. Etonorgestrel: Serum albumin binding (66%), sex hormone-binding globulin (32%). Ethinyl estradiol: Serum albumin binding (98.5%). **Metabolism:** Hepatic via CYP3A4. **Elimination:** Urine, bile, feces; Etonorgestrel: $T_{1/2}$=29.3 hrs; Ethinyl estradiol: $T_{1/2}$=44.7 hrs.

## NURSING CONSIDERATIONS

**Assessment:** Assess for thrombophlebitis or history of deep vein thrombophlebitis, presence of history of thromboembolic disorder, presence or history of cerebral vascular or coronary disease, valvular heart disease with thrombogenic complications, severe HTN, diabetes with vascular involvement, headaches with focal neurological symptoms, major surgery with prolonged immobilization, carcinoma of the breast or history of, carcinoma of the endometrium or other estrogen dependent neoplasia, undiagnosed abnormal genital bleeding, cholestatic jaundice of pregnancy or jaundice with prior hormonal contraceptive use, hepatic tumors (benign or malignant) or active liver disease, pregnancy/nursing status, and for possible drug interactions. Assess if a heavy smoker and over the age of 35. Assess use in patients who have inherited thrombophilias, hypertension, hyperlipidemias, obesity, or DM.

**Monitoring:** Monitor for signs and symptoms of MI, thromboembolism, stroke, hepatic neoplasia, gallbladder disease, ocular lesions, bleeding irregularities, carcinoma of the breast and reproductive organs, fluid retention, onset or exacerbation of a migraine headache, toxic shock syndrome, worsening depression, ectopic pregnancy, and for signs of liver dysfunction (eg, jaundice). Monitor lipid levels with history of hyperlipidemia; monitor BP if have history of HTN; monitor serum glucose levels in DM or prediabetic patients. Refer patients with contact lenses to an opthalmologist if visual changes or changes in lens tolerance occur. Perform annual physical exam.

**Patient Counseling:** Counsel that drug does not protect against HIV infection/AIDS or other STDs and to take as directed. Counsel about possibility of light spotting. Advise to avoid smoking to prevent cardiovascular side effects. Instruct to seek immediate medical attention if develop sharp chest pain, coughing blood, shortness of breath, pain in the calf, chest pain or chest heaviness, vision or speech abnormalities, severe headache, severe vomiting, severe dizziness, severe abdominal pain, sudden fever or sunburn rash, breast lumps, irregular vaginal bleeding or spotting, urination problems, swelling of fingers or ankles, or if develop sleeping disturbances or fatigue. Caution that some medications decrease efficacy and should not be used without physician instructions. Inform that if ring is accidentally expelled and left outside of the vagina for less than three hours, contraceptive efficacy is not reduced; ring can be rinsed with cool to lukewarm water and reinserted as soon as possible or a new ring can be inserted and the regimen should continue without alteration.

**Administration:** Intravaginal route. Refer to PI for specific instructions.

**Storage:** 2-8°C (36-46°F). After dispensing store up to 4 months at 25°C (77°F); excursions permitted to 15-30°C (59-86°F). Avoid direct sunlight or above 30°C (86°F).

## NUVIGIL

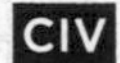


armodafinil (Cephalon)

**THERAPEUTIC CLASS:** Wakefulness-promoting agent

**INDICATIONS:** To improve wakefulness in patients with excessive daytime sleepiness associated with narcolepsy, obstructive sleep apnea/hypopnea syndrome (OSAHS), shiftwork sleep disorder (SWSD). As adjunct to standard treatment for underlying obstruction in OSAHS.

**DOSAGE:** *Adults:* OSAHS/Narcolepsy: 150mg or 250mg qd in AM. SWSD: 150mg qd 1 hr prior to work shift. Hepatic Dysfunction: Reduce dose. Elderly: Consider dose reduction.

**HOW SUPPLIED:** Tab: 50mg, 150mg, 250mg

**WARNINGS/PRECAUTIONS:** May cause serious rash, including Stevens-Johnson syndrome, anaphylactoid reactions, angioedema, and multi-organ hypersensitivity. May impair mental/physical abilities. Psychiatric adverse experiences reported; consider d/c treatment if psychiatric symptoms develop and use caution with history of psychosis, depression, or mania. Caution with history of MI or unstable angina. Avoid with history of left ventricular hypertrophy, ischemic ECG changes, chest pain, arrhythmia, or other manifestations of mitral valve prolapse with CNS stimulants. Monitor hypertensive patients.

**ADVERSE REACTIONS:** Headache, nausea, dizziness, insomnia, diarrhea, dry mouth, anxiety, depression, rash.

**INTERACTIONS:** Potent CYP3A4/5 inducers, (eg, carbamazepine, phenobarbital, rifampin) or inhibitors, (eg, ketoconazole, erythromycin) may alter plasma levels. Effectiveness of CYP3A substrates (eg, cyclosporine, ethinyl estradiol, midazolam, triazolam) may be reduced. May cause moderate inhibition of CYP2C19 activity; dosage reduction may be required for some CYP2C19 substrates (eg, omeprazole, diazepam, phenytoin, propranolol). Methylphenidate or dextroamphetamine may delay absorption. Caution with MAOIs. Monitor PT/INR with warfarin. Effectiveness of steroidal contraceptives may be reduced during and for 1 month after d/c of therapy; alternate or concomitant methods of contraception are recommended.

**PREGNANCY:** Category C, caution in nursing.

**MECHANISM OF ACTION:** Not known; suspected to bind to the dopamine transporter and inhibit dopamine reuptake.

**PHARMACOKINETICS: Absorption**: Readily absorbed. $T_{max}$=2 hrs (fasted), 2-4 hrs (fed). **Distribution**: $V_d$=42L; plasma protein binding (60%). **Metabolism**: Liver via amide hydrolysis with sulfone formation by CYP450, 3A4, 3A5: R-modafinil acid, modafinil sulfone. **Elimination**: Feces, urine; $T_{1/2}$=15 hrs.

### NURSING CONSIDERATIONS

**Assessment:** Perform complete evaluation of patient's excessive sleepiness, LFTs. Note other diseases/conditions and drug therapies.

**Monitoring:** Monitor for hypersensitivity reactions, psychiatric symptoms (depression, hallucination, suicidal ideations), cardiac abnormalities.

**Patient Counseling:** Avoid taking alcohol concurrently; exercise caution while driving, operating machinery, or performing other activities that require mental alertness. Potential increased risk of pregnancy when using steroidal contraceptives with drug and for 1 month after d/c therapy. Report adverse side effects, allergic reactions, psychiatric symptoms, chest pain.

**Administration:** Oral route. **Storage**: 20-25°C (68-77°F). Keep out of reach of children.

## NYSTATIN ORAL RX

nystatin (Various)

**THERAPEUTIC CLASS:** Polyene antifungal

**INDICATIONS:** (Sus) Treatment of oral candidiasis. (Tab) Treatment of non-esophageal mucous membrane GI candidiasis.

**DOSAGE:** *Adults:* Oral Candidiasis: (Sus) 2-3mL in each side of mouth qid. Retain in mouth as long as possible before swallowing. Non-Esophageal GI Candidiasis: (Tab) 1-2 tab tid.
*Pediatrics:* Oral Candidiasis: (Sus) 2-3mL in each side of mouth qid. Infants: 1mL in each side of mouth qid. Retain in mouth as long as possible before swallowing. Avoid feeding for 5 to 10 min after.

**HOW SUPPLIED:** Sus: 100,000 U/mL [60mL, 480mL]; Tab: 500,000 U

**WARNINGS/PRECAUTIONS:** Not for systemic mycoses; d/c if sensitization/irritation occurs. Continue for at least 48 hrs after symptons have disappeared to prevent relapses. Caution with renal insufficiency.

**ADVERSE REACTIONS:** Oral irritation, sensitization, diarrhea, NV, GI disturbances, rash, urticaria, Stevens-Johnson syndrome.

**PREGNANCY:** Category C, caution in nursing.

**MECHANISM OF ACTION:** Polyene antifungal; fungistatic and fungicidal agent. Binds to sterols in the cell membrane of susceptible *Candida* species with a resultant change in membrane permeability, allowing leakage of intracellular components.

**PHARMACOKINETICS: Absorption:** Insignificant. **Elimination:** Feces (unchanged).

### NURSING CONSIDERATIONS

**Assessment:** Assess for proper diagnosis of oral/non-esophageal GI candidiasis, renal insufficiency and pregnancy/nursing status.

**Monitoring:** Monitor for possible adverse reactions including oral irritation, hypersensitivity, diarrhea, nausea, vomiting, GI upset/disturbance, rash, Stevens-Johnson syndrome. Monitor renal function.

**Patient Counseling:** Discuss risks and benefits of therapy. Inform that it is not for treatment of systemic mycoses. D/C medication if sensitization or irritation occurs. Notify physician for any adverse reactions. Counsel to shake suspension well before use.

**Administration:** Oral route. **Storage:** (Sus) 20-25°C (68°-77°F); excursions permitted to 15-30°C (59-86°F). (Tab) 20°-25°C (68°-77°F).

## NYSTATIN VAGINAL RX

nystatin (Odyssey)

**THERAPEUTIC CLASS:** Polyene antifungal

**INDICATIONS:** Local treatment of vulvovaginal candidiasis.

**DOSAGE:** *Adults:* Insert 1 tablet vaginally qd for 2 weeks. Deposit tablets high in the vagina by means of the applicator.

**HOW SUPPLIED:** Tab, Vaginal: 100,000U [15$^s$]

**WARNINGS/PRECAUTIONS:** D/C if sensitization or irritation occurs. Confirm diagnosis by KOH smears and/or cultures.

**PREGNANCY:** Category A, safety in nursing not known.

**MECHANISM OF ACTION:** Antimycotic polyene antibiotic; fungistatic and fungicidal against yeast and yeast-like fungi; acts by binding to sterols in the cell membrane of fungus with a resultant change in membrane permeability allowing leakage of intracellular components.

**PHARMACOKINETICS: Absorption:** None from intact skin or mucous membrane.

## NURSING CONSIDERATIONS

**Assessment:** Assess for history of hypersensitivity, KOH smears, cultures, or other diagnostic method to rule out infection caused by other pathogens.

**Monitoring:** Monitor for possible allergic reaction, burning, itching, rash, eczema and pain, irritation or sensitization development; d/c and notify physician if occurs.

**Patient Counseling:** Instruct to use as directed; not for systemic, oral, or ophthalmic infections. Advise not to interrupt or d/c therapy until completed. Caution that therapeutic douches are unnecessary but may use cleansing douches if not pregnant. Counsel to promptly report any adverse effect (eg, irritation, sensitization) to physician.

**Administration:** Intravaginally. Refer to labeling for instruction on use. **Storage:** 20-25°C (68-77°F). Avoid excessive heat.

# Nystop RX

nystatin (Paddock)

**THERAPEUTIC CLASS:** Polyene antifungal

**INDICATIONS:** Treatment of cutaneous and mucocutaneous mycotic infections caused by susceptible *Candida* species.

N

**DOSAGE:** *Adults:* Apply to lesions bid-tid until healing is complete. For fungal infections of the feet, dust powder on feet and also in shoes.
*Pediatrics:* Neonates and Older: Apply to lesions bid-tid until healing is complete. For fungal infections of the feet, dust powder on feet and also in shoes.

**HOW SUPPLIED:** Powder, Topical: 100,000 U/g [15g, 30g, 60g]

**WARNINGS/PRECAUTIONS:** D/C if irritation or sensitization occurs. Confirm diagnosis. Not for systemic, oral, intravaginal, or ophthalmic use.

**ADVERSE REACTIONS:** Allergic reactions, burning, itching, rash, eczema, pain at application site.

**PREGNANCY:** Category C, caution in nursing.

**MECHANISM OF ACTION:** Polyene antifungal; binds sterols in the cell membrane of susceptible species causing a change in membrane permeability and subsequent leakage of intracellular components. Fungistatic and fungicidal.

**PHARMACOKINETICS: Absorption:** Not absorbed from intact skin or mucous membranes.

## NURSING CONSIDERATIONS

**Assessment:** Assess proper diagnosis of cutaneous or mucocutaneous candidiasis through use of KOH smears, cultures, or other diagnostic methods. Assess use in pregnancy/nursing.

**Monitoring:** Monitor for irritation or sensitization and therapeutic response. If no therapeutic response, reassess diagnosis (eg, KOH smears, cultures, other diagnostic methods).

**Patient Counseling:** Instruct to use exactly as directed and not to interrupt or d/c therapy even if symptom relief occurs within first few days of treatment. Notify physician if skin irritation develops.

**Administration:** Topical route. **Storage:** 15-30°C (59-86°F); avoid excessive heat 40°C (104°F).

## OCUFLOX — RX

ofloxacin (Allergan)

**THERAPEUTIC CLASS:** Fluoroquinolone

**INDICATIONS:** Management of bacterial infections in conjunctivitis and corneal ulcers.

**DOSAGE:** *Adults:* Conjunctivitis: 1-2 drops q2-4h for 2 days, then 1-2 drops qid for 5 days. Corneal Ulcer: 1-2 drops every 30 min while awake and 1-2 drops 4-6 hrs after retiring for 2 days, then 1-2 drops q1h while awake for 5-7 days, then 1-2 drops qid for 2 days or until treatment completion.
*Pediatrics:* ≥1 yr: Conjunctivitis: 1-2 drops q2-4h for 2 days, then 1-2 drops qid for 5 days. Corneal Ulcer: 1-2 drops every 30 min while awake and 1-2 drops 4-6 hrs after retiring for 2 days, then 1-2 drops q1h while awake for 5-7 days, then 1-2 drops qid for 2 days or until treatment completion.

**HOW SUPPLIED:** Sol: 0.3% [5mL, 10mL]

**WARNINGS/PRECAUTIONS:** Not for injection into eye. Do not inject subconjunctivally or into the eye's anterior chamber. Superinfection may result with prolonged use. Fatal hypersensitivity reactions reported after 1st dose of systemic quinolone therapy. Avoid allowing tip of container to contact fingers, eye or surrounding structures.

**ADVERSE REACTIONS:** Transient ocular burning or discomfort, stinging, redness, itching, keratitis, ocular periocular/facial edema, photophobia, blurred vision, tearing, dryness, eye pain.

**INTERACTIONS:** Systemic quinolone therapy may increase theophylline levels, interfere with caffeine metabolism, enhance warfarin effects, and elevate SrCr with cyclosporine.

**PREGNANCY:** Category C, not for use in nursing.

**MECHANISM OF ACTION:** Fluoroquinolone; exerts bactericidal effect on susceptible bacteria by inhibiting DNA gyrase, an essential bacterial enzyme that is a critical catalyst in duplication, transcription, and repair of bacterial DNA.

**PHARMACOKINETICS: Absorption:** $C_{max}$=1.1 ng/mL (Day 1, qid dosing), 1.9 ng/mL (Day 11, qid dosing). **Excretion:** Urine.

### NURSING CONSIDERATIONS

**Assessment:** Assess for proper diagnosis of causative organisms (eg, slit lamp biomicroscopy, fluorescein staining), allergies to other quinolones, use in pregnant/nursing females, and possible drug interactions.

**Monitoring:** Monitor for signs/symptoms of serious hypersensitivity or anaphylactic reactions (eg, cardiovascular collapse, loss of consciousness, angioedema, airway obstruction, dyspnea, urticaria, and itching), Stevens-Johnson syndrome and toxic epidermal necrosis. For patients on sustained therapy, monitor for overgrowth of nonsusceptible organisms (eg, fungal) and for development of superinfection. Monitor creatinine levels in patients receiving cyclosporine concomitantly.

**Patient Counseling:** Advise to avoid contaminating applicator tip with material from eye, fingers, or other sources. Instruct to immediately report first sign of a rash or allergic reaction.

**Administration:** Ocular route. Do not inject into eye. **Storage:** 15-25°C (59-77°F).

## OCUPRESS — RX

carteolol HCl (Novartis Ophthalmics)

**THERAPEUTIC CLASS:** Nonselective beta-blocker

**INDICATIONS:** Reduction of intraocular pressure (IOP) in chronic open-angle glaucoma and intraocular hypertension.

**DOSAGE:** *Adults:* 1 drop bid.

O

**HOW SUPPLIED:** Sol: 1% [5mL, 10mL, 15mL]

**CONTRAINDICATIONS:** Bronchial asthma, severe COPD, sinus bradycardia, 2nd- and 3rd-degree AV block, overt cardiac failure, cardiogenic shock.

**WARNINGS/PRECAUTIONS:** May be absorbed systemically. Caution with cardiac failure, bronchospasm, diminished pulmonary function, and diabetes mellitus (DM). May mask symptoms of hypoglycemia and hyperthyroidism. Not for use alone in angle-closure glaucoma. May potentiate muscle weakness. D/C if cardiac failure develops. Withdrawal before surgery is controversial.

**ADVERSE REACTIONS:** Eye irritation, burning, tearing, conjunctival hyperemia, conjunctival edema, photophobia, decreased night vision, ptosis, bradycardia, decreased BP, dyspnea, asthenia, headache, dizziness, taste perversion.

**INTERACTIONS:** May potentiate systemic effects with oral β-blockers. Possible hypotension and bradycardia with catecholamine-depleting drugs (eg, reserpine). May antagonize epinephrine.

**PREGNANCY:** Category C, caution in nursing.

**MECHANISM OF ACTION:** Nonselective β-adrenergic blocker; reduces normal and elevated levels of IOP. Exact mechanism of ocular hypotensive effect not definitely demonstrated. β-adrenergic blockers also associated with reducing cardiac output and increasing airway resistance in bronchi and bronchioles.

## NURSING CONSIDERATIONS

**Assessment:** Prior to therapy, assess for presence or history of bronchial asthma, severe COPD, sinus bradycardia, AV-block, overt cardiac failure, and cardiogenic shock. Assess use with DM (or patients subject to episodes of spontaneous hypoglycemia), non-allergic bronchospasm (eg, chronic bronchitis, emphysema), hyperthyroidism, undergoing elective surgery, angle-closure glaucoma, use in pregnant/nursing, and possible drug interactions.

**Monitoring:** Monitor for severe respiratory or cardiac reactions (eg, cardiac failure), muscle weakness, anaphylactic reactions, symptoms of hypoglycemia in patients with DM, and development of thyroid storm in patients with thyrotoxicosis who abruptly d/c medication.



**Patient Counseling:** Instruct to immediately notify physician if any respiratory, cardiac, or anaphylaxic reaction develops. Avoid touching dropper tip to eyelids or surrounding areas to prevent contamination.

**Administration:** Ocular route. **Storage:** 15-25°C (59-77°F). Protect from light. Keep bottle tightly closed.

# Olux — RX

clobetasol propionate (Stiefel)

**THERAPEUTIC CLASS:** Corticosteroid

**INDICATIONS:** Short-term treatment of inflammatory and pruritic manifestations of moderate to severe corticosteroid-responsive dermatoses of the scalp. Short-term treatment of mild to moderate plaque-type psoriasis of non-scalp regions excluding the face and intertriginous areas.

**DOSAGE:** *Adults:* Apply to affected area bid (am and pm). No more than 1.5 capfuls/application. Limit to 2 consecutive weeks. Avoid with occlusive dressings unless directed. Max 50g/week.

*Pediatrics:* ≥12 yrs: Apply to affected area bid (am and pm). No more than 1.5 capfuls/application. Limit to 2 consecutive weeks. Avoid with occlusive dressings unless directed. Max 50g/week.

**HOW SUPPLIED:** Foam: 0.05% [50g, 100g]

**WARNINGS/PRECAUTIONS:** May produce reversible hypothalamic-pituitary-adrenal (HPA) axis suppression, manifestations of Cushing's syndrome, hyperglycemia, and glucosuria. Caution when applied to large surface areas or under occlusive dressings. Withdraw, reduce frequency, or substitute to a less potent steroid if adrenal suppression noted. Use appropriate antifungal or antibacterial agent with dermatological infections; d/c until infection controlled. Pediatric patients may be more susceptible to systemic toxicity. Striae, adrenal suppression (low plasma cortisol, no response to ACTH stimulation), Cushing's syndrome, linear growth retardation, delayed weight gain, and intracranial HTN (bulging fontanelle, headache, bilateral papilledema) reported in pediatrics. Avoid eyes. D/C if irritation occurs. Avoid extensive or prolonged use in pregnant patients. Not recommended in pediatrics <12 yrs. Caution in elderly. Flammable; avoid fire, flame, or smoking during and immediately following application.

**ADVERSE REACTIONS:** Burning/stinging, pruritus, irritation, erythema, folliculitis, cracking/fissuring of skin, numbness of fingers, telangiectasia, skin atrophy, hypertrichosis, acneiform eruptions, hypopigmentation, maceration of the skin.

**PREGNANCY:** Category C, caution in nursing.

**MECHANISM OF ACTION:** Corticosteroid; possesses anti-inflammatory, antipruritic and vasoconstrictive properties. Anti-inflammatory effects not established; suspected to act by induction of phospholipase $A_2$ inhibitory proteins, lipocortins. Lipocortins control biosynthesis of inflammation mediators (eg, prostaglandins and leukotrienes) by inhibiting release of their common precursor, arachidonic acid.

**PHARMACOKINETICS: Absorption:** Percutaneous; occlusion, inflammation, and other disease states may increase absorption. **Distribution:** Systemically administered corticosteroids are found in breast milk. **Metabolism:** Liver. **Elimination**: Kidney (major), bile.

## NURSING CONSIDERATIONS

**Assessment:** Asses for hypersensitivity reactions, pregnancy/nursing status, and use in pediatric patients.

**Monitoring:** Monitor for signs/symptoms of reversible HPA-axis suppression, Cushing's syndrome, hyperglycemia, glucosuria, skin irritation, contact dermatitis (eg, failure to heal) and dermatological infections (eg, fungal, bacterial). In patients on high doses or using occlusive dressings, perform periodic monitoring for HPA-axis suppression using ACTH stimulation, A.M plasma cortisol, and urinary free cortisol tests. Following withdrawal from therapy, monitor for signs/symptoms of glucocorticosteroid insufficiency. Monitor for systemic toxicity, adrenal suppression, Cushing's syndrome, linear growth retardation, delayed weight gain, and intracranial HTN (bulging fontanel, headache, bilateral papilledema) in pediatrics.

**Patient Counseling:** Counsel patient on the signs/symptoms of adverse reactions and to contact physician if any occur. Counsel to use exactly as directed, externally, and not for >2 weeks. Propellant in this foam is flammable; avoid fire, flame, or smoking during and immediately following application. Advise not to bandage or wrap treated skin area, unless directed by physician. Advise to avoid contact with eyes or other mucous membranes and wash hands following use. Avoid extensive or prolonged use in pregnant patients.

**Administration:** Topical route. 1) Place small amount of medication into cap of medication container, onto a saucer, other cool surface or directly onto affected skin area. Do not use more than 1 1/2 capfuls. Do not squirt medication directly into the hands (unless hands are the treatment area); medication will melt in contact with warm skin. If fingers are warm, rinse in cold water and dry prior to application. If can is warm, run under cold water prior to administration. 2) Using fingertips, massage medication into treatment area. **Storage:** 20-25°C (68-77°F). Do not puncture or incinerate container. Do not expose to heat or store above 49°C (120°F).

# Olux-E — RX

clobetasol propionate (Stiefel)

**THERAPEUTIC CLASS:** Corticosteroid

**INDICATIONS:** Treatment of inflammatory and pruritic manifestations of corticosteroid-responsive dermatoses in patients ≥12 yrs.

**DOSAGE:** *Adults:* Apply thin layer to affected area bid (am and pm). Limit to 2 consecutive weeks; d/c when control achieved. Avoid with occlusive dressings unless directed. Max: 50g/week or 21 capfuls/week.
*Pediatrics:* ≥12 yrs: Apply thin layer to affected area bid (am and pm). Limit to 2 consecutive weeks; d/c when control achieved. Avoid with occlusive dressings unless directed. Max: 50g/week or 21 capfuls/week.

**HOW SUPPLIED:** Foam: 0.05% [50g, 100g]

**WARNINGS/PRECAUTIONS:** May produce reversible hypothalamic-pituitary-adrenal (HPA) axis suppression, manifestations of Cushing's syndrome, hyperglycemia, and glucosuria. Caution when applied to large surface areas or under occlusive dressings. Withdraw, reduce frequency, or substitute to a less potent steroid if adrenal suppression noted. Use appropriate antifungal or antibacterial agent with dermatological infections; d/c until infection controlled. Pediatrics may be more susceptible to systemic toxicity. Striae, HPA axis suppression (low plasma cortisol, no response to ACTH stimulation), Cushing's syndrome, linear growth retardation, delayed weight gain, and intracranial HTN (eg, bulging fontanelles, headache, bilateral papilledema) reported in pediatrics. D/C if irritation occurs. Not for treatment of rosacea or perioral dermatitis. Not recommended in pediatrics <12 yrs. Avoid eyes, face, groin, axillae or other intertriginous areas. If no improvement within 2 weeks, reassess diagnosis. Flammable; avoid fire, flame, or smoking during and immediately following application.

**ADVERSE REACTIONS:** Application-site atrophy, folliculitis, acneiform eruptions, hypopigmentation, perioral dermatitis, allergic contact dermatitis, secondary infection, irritation, striae, miliaria.

**PREGNANCY:** Category C, caution in nursing.

**MECHANISM OF ACTION:** Corticosteroid; possesses anti-inflammatory, antipruritic, and vasoconstrictive properties. Anti-inflammatory effect not established; suspected to act by induction of phospholipase $A_2$ inhibitory proteins called lipocortins. Lipocortins control biosynthesis of inflammation mediators (eg, prostaglandins and leukotrienes) by inhibiting release of their common precursor, arachidonic acid.

O

**PHARMACOKINETICS: Absorption:** Percutaneous; occlusion, inflammation, and other disease states may increase absorption; $C_{max}$=59pg/mL; $T_{max}$=5 hrs. **Distribution:** Systemically administered corticosteroids are found in breast milk. **Metabolism:** Liver. **Elimination**: Kidneys and bile.

## NURSING CONSIDERATIONS

**Assessment:** Assess for hypersensitivity reactions, perioral dermatitis or rosacea, presence of concomitant skin infections, pregnancy/nursing status, and use in pediatric patients.

**Monitoring:** Monitor for signs/symptoms of reversible adrenal suppression, Cushing's syndrome, hyperglycemia, glucosuria, treatment-site irritation, allergic contact dermatitis (eg, failure to heal) and development of skin infections (eg, fungal, bacterial). If applying to large surface area or to occluded areas, monitor for HPA-axis suppression using cosyntropin (ACTH) stimulation test. Following d/c of therapy, monitor for glucocorticosteroid insufficiency. Monitor for systemic toxicity, HPA axis suppression, Cushing's syndrome, linear growth retardation, delayed weight gain, and intracranial HTN (eg, bulging fontanel, headache, bilateral papilledema) in pediatrics. Monitor response to therapy; if no improvement within 2 weeks, reassess diagnosis.

**Patient Counseling:** Counsel to use externally and exactly as directed; avoid use on face, skin folds (eg, underarms, groin), contact with eyes or other mucous membranes. Wash hands following administration. Advise not to bandage or wrap treatment area, unless directed by physician. Counsel to contact physician if any local or systemic adverse events occur or if no improvement seen after 2 weeks. Inform that propellant in medication is flammable; avoid fire, flame, or smoking during and immediately following application.

**Administration:** Topical route. Shake can, hold upside down and depress the actuator. Dispense small amount and gently massage into affected area. **Storage:** 20-25°C (68-77°F). Do not puncture or incinerate container. Do not expose to heat or store above 49°C (120°F).

# OMNARIS RX

ciclesonide (Sepracor)

**THERAPEUTIC CLASS:** Non-halogenated glucocorticoid

**INDICATIONS:** Treatment of nasal symptoms associated with seasonal allergic rhinitis in adults and children ≥6 yrs. Treatment of nasal symptoms associated with perennial allergic rhinitis in adults and adolescents ≥12 yrs.

**DOSAGE:** *Adults:* Seasonal Allergic Rhinitis/Perennial Allergic Rhinitis: 2 sprays (50mcg/spray) each nostril qd.
*Pediatrics:* Seasonal Allergic Rhinitis: ≥6 yrs: 2 sprays (50mcg/spray) each nostril qd. Perennial Allergic Rhinitis: ≥12 yrs: 2 sprays (50mcg/spray) each nostril qd.

**HOW SUPPLIED:** Spray: 50mcg/spray [12.5g]

**WARNINGS/PRECAUTIONS:** Risk of acute adrenal insufficiency and withdrawal symptoms when replacing systemic corticosteroids with topical corticosteroids; monitor closely. Risk for more severe/fatal course of infections (eg, chickenpox, measles); avoid exposure in patients who have not had the disease or been properly immunized. May cause reduced growth velocity in pediatrics; routinely monitor growth of pediatrics. May impair wound healing; avoid in recent nasal septal ulcers, nasal surgery, or nasal trauma until healed. *Candida* infections of nose or pharynx may occur; examine periodically and treat accordingly. Caution with active or quiescent TB infections, untreated local or systemic fungal or bacterial infections, systemic viral or parasitic infections, or ocular herpes simplex. Taper dose if symptoms of hypercorticism occur. Caution with history of glaucoma and/or cataracts; monitor IOP accordingly.

**ADVERSE REACTIONS:** Headache, epistaxis, nasopharyngitis, ear pain, pharyngolaryngeal pain.

**INTERACTIONS:** Ketoconazole may increase levels of the pharmacologically active metabolite des-ciclesonide; coadminister with caution.

**PREGNANCY:** Category C, caution in nursing.

**MECHANISM OF ACTION:** Glucocorticoid has anti-inflammatory effect and other effects on multiple cell types (eg, mast cells, eosinophils, macrophages, and lymphocytes) and mediators (eg, histamine, eicosanoids, leukotrienes, and cytokines) involved in allergic inflammation.

**PHARMACOKINETICS: Absorption:** (50-800mcg) $C_{max}$<30pg/mL (adults); (25-200mcg) $C_{max}$<45pg/mL (pediatrics). **Metabolism:** Nasal mucosa estrases to des-ciclesonide (active metabolite) followed by liver CYP3A4, 2D6.

## NURSING CONSIDERATIONS

**Assessment:** Assess for drug hypersensitivity, active or quiescent TB, untreated localized or systemic fungal or bacterial infections, systemic viral infections, ocular herpes simplex, history of recent nasal septal ulcers, nasal surgery/trauma, concomitant use with other inhaled or systemic corticosteroids, withdrawal symptoms in event of replacing systemic with topical corticosteroids, and possible drug interactions.

**Monitoring:** Monitor for acute adrenal insufficiency, TB, local/systemic fungal or bacterial infections, systemic viral or parasitic infections, ocular herpes simplex, or other infections (chickenpox, measles). Monitor growth velocity in children, wound healing, hypercorticism (eg, menstrual irregularities, acneiform lesions, and cushingoid features), hypoadrenalism in infant born to mother receiving corticosteroids during pregnancy, hypersensitivity reactions, or contact dermatitis.

**Patient Counseling:** Avoid spraying in eyes or directly onto nasal septum. Counsel to take as directed at regular intervals; do not exceed prescribed dosage. Avoid exposure to chickenpox or measles; consult physician immediately if exposed or symptoms worsen.

**Administration:** Intranasal route, shake gently before use, spray tip into one nostril, and close other nostril with finger. **Storage:** 25°C (77°F); excursions permitted to 15-30°C (59-86°F). Do not freeze. Keep out of reach of children.

O

# OMNICEF — RX

cefdinir (Abbott)

**THERAPEUTIC CLASS:** Cephalosporin (3rd generation)

**INDICATIONS:** Community-acquired pneumonia (CAP), acute exacerbations of chronic bronchitis (AECB), acute maxillary sinusitis, pharyngitis/tonsillitis, and uncomplicated skin and skin structure infections (SSSIs) in adult and adolescent patients. Acute bacterial otitis media, pharyngitis/tonsillitis, and uncomplicated SSSIs in pediatric patients.

**DOSAGE:** *Adults:* (Cap) SSSI/CAP: 300mg q12h for 10 days. AECB/ Pharyngitis/Tonsillitis: 300mg q12h for 5-10 days or 600mg q24h for 10 days. Sinusitis: 300mg q12h or 600mg q24h for 10 days. CrCl <30mL/min: 300mg qd. Hemodialysis: Initial: 300mg or 7mg/kg qod. 300mg or 7mg/kg should be given at end of each hemodialysis session. Usual: 300mg or 7mg/kg qod. *Pediatrics:* (Sus) ≥43 kg: Max dose: 600mg/day. 6 months-12 yrs: Otitis Media/ Pharyngitis/Tonsillitis: 7mg/kg q12h for 5-10 days or 14mg/kg q24h for 10 days. Sinusitis: 7mg/kg q12h or 14mg/kg q24h for 10 days. SSSI: 7mg/kg q12h for 10 days. (Cap) ≥13 yrs: CAP/SSSI: 300mg q12h for 10 days. AECB/ Pharyngitis/Tonsillitis: 300mg q12h for 5-10 days or 600mg q24h for 10 days. Sinusitis: 300mg q12h or 600mg q24h for 10 days. CrCl <30mL/min/1.73m$^2$: 7mg/kg qd. Max: 300mg qd.

**HOW SUPPLIED:** Cap: 300mg; Sus: 125mg/5mL, 250mg/5mL [60mL, 100mL]

**WARNINGS/PRECAUTIONS:** Cross-sensitivity to PCNs and other cephalosporins may occur. D/C use if an allergic reaction occurs. *Clostridium difficile*-associated diarrhea (CDAD) has been reported. Use in the absence of a proven or strongly suspected bacterial infection or prophylactic indication is unlikely to provide benefit and increases risk of development of drug resistant bacteria. Prolonged treatment may result in emergence and overgrowth of resistant organisms; administer appropriate alternate therapy if superinfection develops. Reduce dose in patients with transient or persistent renal insufficiency (CrCl<30mL/min). Caution in patients with a history of colitis. Sus contains sucrose; caution in diabetes. Positive direct Coombs' tests may occur as well as false (+) for urine glucose with Clinitest and Benedict's or Fehling's solution. A false (+) reaction for ketones in the urine may occur with tests using nitroprusside.

O

**ADVERSE REACTIONS:** Diarrhea, vaginal moniliasis, nausea.

**INTERACTIONS:** Iron-fortified foods, iron supplements, and aluminum- or magnesium-containing antacids reduce absorption; separate doses by 2 hrs. Probenecid inhibits the renal excretion. Reddish stools reported with iron-containing products. Possible interaction between cefdinir and diclofenac.

**PREGNANCY:** Category B, safe in nursing.

**MECHANISM OF ACTION:** Extended-spectrum cephalosporin; bactericidal activity from inhibition of cell-wall synthesis.

**PHARMACOKINETICS: Absorption:** Cap: (300mg) $C_{max}$=1.6mcg/mL, $T_{max}$=2.9 hrs, AUC=7.05mcg•h/mL. (600mg) $C_{max}$=2.87mcg/mL, $T_{max}$=3 hrs, AUC=11.1mcg•h/mL. Sus: (7mg/kg)$C_{max}$=2.3mcg/mL, $T_{max}$=2.2 hrs, AUC=8.31mcg•h/mL. (14mg/kg) $C_{max}$=3.86mcg/mL, $T_{max}$=1.8 hrs, AUC=13.4mcg•h/mL. **Distribution:** $V_d$=0.35L/kg (adults), 0.67L/kg (pediatrics); plasma protein binding (60-70%). **Elimination:** (300mg) Urine (18.4% unchanged); (600mg) Urine (11.6% unchanged); $T_{1/2}$=1.7 hrs.

## NURSING CONSIDERATIONS

**Assessment:** Assess for allergy to other cephalosporins, PCN, or to other drugs. Assess for history of colitis, renal impairment, and for possible drug interactions. Assess for diabetes if planning to use sus formulation. Assess proper diagnosis of causative organisms.

**Monitoring:** Monitor for signs/symptoms of hypersensitivity reactions, CDAD, and for development of a superinfection.

**Patient Counseling:** Inform that therapy treats bacterial, not viral, infections. Instruct to take as directed; skipping doses or not completing full course may decrease effectiveness and increase bacterial resistance. Instruct to take 2 hrs before or after antacid or iron supplements. Inform diabetics that sus contains sucrose. Advise diarrhea may occur; notify physician if watery/bloody stools, superinfection, or hypersensitivity reactions occur.

**Administration:** Oral route. **Storage:** Cap/ Unsuspended Powder: 25°C (77°F); excursions permitted to 15-30°C (59-86°F). Reconstituted Sus: Can be stored at controlled room temperature for 10 days.

## OMNITROPE RX

somatropin (Sandoz)

**THERAPEUTIC CLASS:** Human growth hormone

**INDICATIONS:** Long-term treatment of pediatric patients who have growth failure due to an inadequate secretion of endogenous growth hormone. Long-term replacement therapy in adults with growth hormone deficiency (GHD) of either childhood- or adult-onset etiology.

**DOSAGE:** *Adults:* Individualize dose. GHD: ≤0.04mg/kg/week. May increase at 4-8 week intervals. Max: 0.08mg/kg/week. Divide dose into daily SQ injections (give preferably in the evening).
*Pediatrics:* Individualize dose. GHD: 0.16-0.24mg/kg/week. Divide dose into daily SQ injections (give preferably in the evening).

**HOW SUPPLIED:** Inj: 1.5mg, 5.8mg; Prefill: 5mg/1.5mL (15 IU), 10mg/1.5mL (30 IU)

**CONTRAINDICATIONS:** Evidence of neoplastic activity. Pediatrics with fused epiphyses. Acute critical illness due to complications after open heart or abdominal surgery, multiple accidental trauma, or with acute respiratory failure. Patients with Prader-Willi syndrome who are severely obese or have severe respiratory impairment.

**WARNINGS/PRECAUTIONS:** Contains benzyl alcohol; avoid use in newborns. Patients with GHD secondary to an intracranial lesion should be monitored closely for progression or recurrence of underlying disease process. Monitor closely for any malignant transformation of skin lesions, scoliosis progression, or gait abnormalities. Monitor closely with DM, glucose intolerance, hypopituitarism. Intracranial HTN reported. Funduscopic exam recommended at initiation, and periodically during course of therapy.

**ADVERSE REACTIONS:** Hypothyroidism, elevated $HbA_{1c}$, eosinophilia, hematoma, headache, hypertriglyceridemia, leg pain.

**INTERACTIONS:** Growth promoting effects may be inhibited by glucocorticoids. May alter clearance of CYP450 substrates (eg, corticosteroids, sex steroids, anticonvulsants, cyclosporine); monitor closely. May need insulin dose adjustment.

**PREGNANCY:** Category B, caution in nursing.

**MECHANISM OF ACTION:** Human growth hormone; binds to dimeric GH receptor in cell membrane of target cells resulting in intracellular signal transduction.

**PHARMACOKINETICS: Absorption:** $C_{max}$=72mcg/mL, $T_{max}$=4 hrs. **Elimination:** $T_{1/2}$=2.8 hrs.

## NURSING CONSIDERATIONS

**Assessment:** Assess for closed epiphyses, proliferative diabetic retinopathy, active malignancy, acute critical illness due to complications of surgery or multiple accidental trauma, acute respiratory failure, Prader-Willi syndrome (severely obese or severe respiratory failure), preexisting type 1 or type 2 DM or impaired glucose tolerance, history of scoliosis, pre-existing papilledema, hypothyroidism, undernutrition, advanced bone age, diagnostic imaging (rule out pituitary or intracranial tumor), hypopituitarism and possible drug interactions.

**Monitoring:** Monitor fasting blood glucose and thyroid function tests periodically. Periodic funduscopic exam. Signs/symptoms of malignant

O

transformation of skin lesions, intracranial HTN, slipped capital femoral epiphysis (onset of limp, hip or knee pain), hypersensitivity/allergic reactions, and progression of scoliosis.

**Patient Counseling:** Instruct thoroughly as to proper usage, proper disposal, and caution against any reuse of needles and syringes.

**Administration:** SQ route. **Storage:** 2-8°C (36-46°F ). Protect from light. Do not freeze. After 1[st] injection: Refrigerate, discard after 21 days. (Reconstitution): Diluent without preservative: refrigerate up to 24 hrs. Diluent with preservative: Use within 3 weeks.

## ONCASPAR RX

pegaspargase (Enzon)

**THERAPEUTIC CLASS:** Protein synthesis inhibitor

**INDICATIONS:** Acute lymphoblastic leukemia in patients who have developed hypersensitivity to the native forms of L-asparaginase. May be given as monotherapy if multi-agent therapy is inappropriate.

**DOSAGE:** *Adults:* Usual: 2500 IU/m² IM or IV every 14 days.
*Pediatrics:* 1-9 yrs: 2500 IU/m² IM on Day 3 of 4-Week induction phase and on Day 3 of each of two 8-Week delayed intensifications phases.

**HOW SUPPLIED:** Inj: 750 IU/mL [5mL]

**CONTRAINDICATIONS:** Pancreatitis. History of pancreatitis, significant hemorrhagic events, or serious thrombosis with prior L-asparaginase therapy.

**WARNINGS/PRECAUTIONS:** May be a contact irritant. Avoid inhalation or contact with skin or mucous membranes. Serious allergic reaction, pancreatitis, or glucose intolerance can occur. Increased prothrombin time, partial thromboplastin time, and hypofibrinogenemia can occur; monitor coagulation parameters. May predispose to infections, bleeding, thrombosis. D/C in patients with serious thrombotic event including sagittal sinus thrombosis.

**ADVERSE REACTIONS:** Allergic reactions (including anaphylaxis), CNS thrombosis, coagulopathy, elevated transaminases, hyperbilirubinemia, hyperglycemia, pancreatitis.

**PREGNANCY:** Category C, not for use in nursing.

**MECHANISM OF ACTION:** Protein synthesis inhibitor; selectively kills leukemic cells due to depletion of plasma asparagine.

**PHARMACOKINETICS: Elimination:** $T_{1/2}$=5.8 days.

### NURSING CONSIDERATIONS

**Assessment:** Assess for history of serious allergic reactions to L-asparginase, thrombosis, pancreatitis, and serious hemorrhagic events.

**Monitoring:** Monitor coagulation parameters at baseline and periodically during and after treatment. Monitor for occurrence of anaphylaxis, thrombosis, pancreatitis, glucose intolerance, and coagulopathy.

**Patient Counseling:** Advise to immediately report swelling, SOB, severe headache, chest pain, severe abdominal pain, excessive thirst, or any increase in volume or frequency of urination.

**Administration:** IM or IV. When administered IM, the volume at a single injection site should be limited to 2mL. If the volume to be administered is greater than 2 mL, multiple inj sites should be used. When administered IV, should be given over period of 1-2 hrs in 100mL of NaCl or dextrose inj 5%, through an already running infusion. **Storage**: Refrigerate at 2-8°C (36-46°F).

## ONGLYZA RX

saxagliptin (Bristol-Myers Squibb/ AstraZeneca)

**THERAPEUTIC CLASS:** Dipeptidyl peptidase-4 inhibitor

**INDICATIONS:** Adjunct to diet and exercise to improve glycemic control in adults with type 2 diabetes mellitus (DM).

**DOSAGE:** *Adults:* 2.5-5mg qd. Moderate or Severe Renal Impairment/End-Stage Renal Disease (CrCl ≤50mL/min)/Strong CYP3A4/5 Inhibitors: 2.5mg qd.

**HOW SUPPLIED:** Tab: 2.5mg, 5mg

**WARNINGS/PRECAUTIONS:** Assess renal function prior to initiation of treatment. Not for the treatment of type 1 DM or ketoacidosis. Caution in the elderly; evaluate renal function.

**ADVERSE REACTIONS:** Upper respiratory tract infection, urinary tract infection, headache, peripheral edema, hypersensitivity (eg, urticaria, facial edema), hypoglycemia.

**INTERACTIONS:** Increases in plasma levels with moderate CYP3A4/5 inhibitors (eg, diltiazem, amprenavir, aprepitant, fosamprenavir, erythromycin, fluconazole, grapefruit juice, verapamil). Significant increase with strong CYP3A4/5 inhibitors (eg, ketoconazole, atazanavir, clarithromycin, indinavir, itraconazole, nefazodone, nelfinavir, ritonavir, saquinavir, telithromycin); limit dose. Rifampin may decrease plasma concentration. Concomitant use with insulin secretagogues (eg, sulfonylureas) may increase risk of hypoglycemia; lower dose of insulin secretagogue may be required.

**PREGNANCY:** Category B, caution in nursing.

**MECHANISM OF ACTION:** Dipeptidyl peptidase-4 inhibitor; slows the activation of the incretin hormones and increases their bloodstream concentrations resulting in reduction of fasting and postprandial glucose concentrations in a glucose-dependent manner in type 2 DM.

**PHARMACOKINETICS: Absorption:** $C_{max}$= 24-47ng/mL, $T_{max}$ = 2-4 hrs. **Metabolism:** Via CYP3A4/5. **Elimination:** Feces (22%), urine (24% unchanged, 36% active metabolite); $T_{1/2}$= 2.5-3.1 hrs.

## NURSING CONSIDERATIONS

**Assessment:** Assess for type 1 DM, renal function prior to initiation, pregnancy/nursing status, and possible drug interactions.

**Monitoring:** Monitor for hypoglycemia if taken with other antidiabetic agents. Monitor for upper respiratory tract or urinary infections and other adverse effects. Monitor blood glucose, A1C levels, and renal function periodically.

**Patient Counseling:** Inform patients of the potential risk/benefits and alternative modes of therapy. Advise on the importance of adherence to dietary instructions, regular exercise, periodic blood glucose monitoring, A1C testing, recognition/management of hypoglycemia/hyperglycemia, and assessment of diabetic complications. Instruct to seek medical opinion during periods of stress (eg, fever, trauma, infection, surgery) as medication needs may change.

**Admistration:** Oral route. **Storage:** 20-25°C (68-77°F); excursions permitted to 15-30°C (59-86°F).

# ONSOLIS

fentanyl (Meda)

**CII**

**Contains fentanyl with abuse liability similar to other opioid analgesics. Must be used only in opioid-tolerant patients. Contraindicated for use in opioid non-tolerant patients and management of acute or postoperative pain. Life-threatening respiratory depression in opioid non-tolerant patients reported. Do not substitute for any other fentanyl. If breakthrough pain is not relieved, patients should wait at least 2 hrs for the next dose. Keep out of reach of children and dispose of unneeded films properly. Concomitant use with CYP3A4 inhibitors may cause fatal respiratory depression. Use only by knowledgeable/skilled Schedule II opioid specialists. Available only through restricted distribution program, called the FOCUS program.**

**THERAPEUTIC CLASS:** Opioid analgesic

**INDICATIONS:** Management of breakthrough pain in patients with cancer ( ≥18 yrs) who are already receiving and who are tolerant to opioid therapy for their underlying persistent cancer pain.

**DOSAGE:** *Adults:* Initial: 200mcg. Titrate: May titrate by using multiples of 200mcg (for doses of 400mcg, 600mcg, or 800mcg) if adequate pain relief is not achieved after initiation. Do not use more than 4 of 200mcg films simultaneously. If adequate pain relief is not achieved after 800mcg, and patient has tolerated the 800mcg dose, may treat next episode by using one 1200mcg film. Max: 1200mcg. Single doses should only be used once per episode, and should be separated by at least 2 hrs. If adequate pain relief is not achieved within 30 min, use a rescue medication prn. Limit to 4 or fewer doses/day. If >4 breakthrough pain episodes a day, increase around-the-clock opioid medicine used for persistent cancer pain. Switching From Another Oral Transmucosal Fentanyl: Initial: ≤200mcg. Do not switch on a mcg-per-mcg basis.

**HOW SUPPLIED:** Film, Buccal: 200mcg, 400mcg, 600mcg, 800mcg, 1200mcg

**CONTRAINDICATIONS:** Opioid non-tolerant patients and management of acute or postoperative pain including headache/migraine, dental pain, or use in the emergency room.

**WARNINGS/PRECAUTIONS:** May cause respiratory depression, especially in patients with underlying respiratory disorders, elderly or debilitated patients and in non-opioid tolerant patients following large initial doses. Caution with COPD, pre-existing medical conditions predisposing to hypoventilation, severe renal or hepatic disease and bradyarrhythmias. Extreme caution with evidence of increased intracranial pressure or impaired consciousness. May impair physical/mental abilities. Caution in elderly.

**ADVERSE REACTIONS:** Respiratory depression, circulatory depression, hypotension, shock, N/V, constipation, dehydration, dizziness, dyspnea, somnolence, asthenia, fatigue, decreased weight, confusional state.

**INTERACTIONS:** See Black Box Warning. Increased depressant effects with other CNS depressants (eg, other opioids, sedatives or hypnotics, general anesthetics, phenothiazines, tranquilizers, skeletal muscle relaxants, alcoholic beverages). CYP3A4 inducers (eg, barbiturates, carbamazepine, efavirenz, glucocorticoids, modafinil, nevirapine, oxcarbazepine, phenobarbital, phenytoin, pioglitazone, rifabutin, rifampin, St. John's wort, or troglitazone) decrease plasma concentration and may reduce efficacy. Avoid use within 14 days of MAOIs. Respiratory depression reported with other drugs that depress respiration.



**PREGNANCY:** Category C, not for use in nursing.

**MECHANISM OF ACTION:** Pure opioid agonist; produces analgesia. Precise analgesic action not established; known to be μ opioid receptor agonist. Specific CNS opioid receptors for endogenous compounds with opioid-like activity are found throughout the brain and spinal cord and are involved in producing analgesic effects.

**PHARMACOKINETICS: Absorption:** Rapid (buccal mucosa) and prolonged (GI tract) absorption. Absolute bioavailability (71%); (800mcg) $C_{max}$=1.67ng/mL, AUC=14.46hr•ng/mL, $T_{max}$=1 hr; (200mcg) $C_{max}$=0.38ng/mL, AUC=3.46hr•ng/mL; (600mcg) $C_{max}$=1.16ng/mL, AUC=11.72hr•ng/mL; (1200mcg) $C_{max}$=2.19ng/mL, AUC=20.43hr•ng/mL. **Distribution:** $V_d$=4 L/kg; plasma protein binding (80-85%). Rapidly distributed to brain, heart, lungs, kidneys, spleen; slowly to muscles and fat. **Metabolism:** Liver and intestinal mucosa via CYP3A4; norfentanyl (metabolite). **Elimination:** Urine (<7% unchanged), feces (1% unchanged); $T_{1/2}$=14 hrs.

## NURSING CONSIDERATIONS

**Assessment:** Assess pain intensity, opioid tolerance, respiratory disorders (eg, COPD), age of patient, drug abuse potential, presence of increased intracranial pressure or impaired consciousness, bradyarrhythmia, renal/hepatic impairment, pregnancy/nursing status, and possible drug interactions.

**Monitoring:** Monitor for signs/symptoms of respiratory depression, drug abuse, physical dependence, application-site reactions, bradycardia, opioid toxicity, signs of increased drug activity.

**Patient Counseling:** Advise to notify physician if signs/symptoms of respiratory depression develop. Keep out of reach of children. Notify physician if breakthrough pain is not alleviated or worsens. Counsel to avoid using concomitant therapy with other CNS depressants and alcohol. May cause mental/physical impairment. Medication has potential for abuse. Counsel to dispose of unused medication via toilet. Patients must enroll in FOCUS program by calling 1-877-466-7654 (1-877-4Onsolis) or visit online.

**Administration:** Oral (buccal) route. May be placed on both sides of the mouth not on top of each other when multiple films are used. Do not cut or tear prior to use. Refer to PI for proper administration. **Storage:** 20-25°C (68-77°F) excursions permitted between 15-30°C (59-86°F) until ready to use. Protect from freezing and moisture. Do not use if the foil package has been opened.

## OPANA ER

oxymorphone HCl (Endo)

**(Tab, Extended-Release) Abuse liability and potential. For continuous analgesia only; not intended for prn use. To be swallowed whole; not to be broken, chewed, dissolved, or crushed. Must not be taken with alcohol.**

**OTHER BRAND NAMES:** Opana (Endo)

**THERAPEUTIC CLASS:** Opioid analgesic

**INDICATIONS:** (Tab) Relief of moderate to severe acute pain. (Tab, Extended-Release) Relief of moderate to severe pain in patients requiring continuous, around-the-clock opioid treatment for extended period of time.

**DOSAGE:** *Adults:* Individualize dose. Opana: Opioid-Naive: Initial: 5-20mg q4-6h. Titrate based on response. Max: 20mg/dose. Conversion from Parenteral Oxymorphone: Give 10x total daily parenteral oxymorphone dose in 4 or 6 equally divided doses. Conversion from Other Oral Opioids: Give half of calculated total daily dose in 4-6 equally divided doses, q4-6h. Opana ER: Swallow whole; do not break, chew, crush, or dissolve. Opioid-Naive: Initial: 5mg q12h. Titrate based on response. Usual: Increase dose by 5-10mg q12h every 3-7 days. Conversion from Opana: Divide 24h Opana dose in half to obtain q12h dose. Conversion from Parenteral Oxymorphone: Give 10x total daily parenteral oxymorphone dose in 2 equally divided doses. Conversion from Other Oral Opioids: Divide calculated 24h Opana dose (refer to PI for conversion ratios) in half to obtain q12h dose. Mild Hepatic Impairment or Renal Impairment (CrCl <50mL/min): Start with lowest dose and titrate slowly while carefully monitoring side effects. With CNS Depressants: Start at 1/3 to 1/2 of usual dose. Elderly: Start at lower end of dosing range.

**HOW SUPPLIED:** Tab: (Opana) 5mg, 10mg; Tab, Extended-Release: (Opana ER) 5mg, 7.5mg, 10mg, 15mg, 20mg, 30mg, 40mg

**CONTRAINDICATIONS:** Respiratory depression (except in monitored settings with resuscitative equipment), acute/severe bronchial asthma or hypercarbia, paralytic ileus, moderate/severe hepatic impairment. (Opana ER) Not indicated for pain in immediate postoperative period (12-24 hrs following surgery) for patients not previously taking opioids or, if the pain is mild or not expected to persist for extended period of time.

**WARNINGS/PRECAUTIONS:** Schedule II controlled substance with abuse liability. Respiratory depression, hypotension, and profound sedation or coma may occur. Extreme caution with hypoxia, hypercapnia, or decreased respiratory reserve. With head injury, intracranial lesions or a pre-existing increase in ICP, possible respiratory depressant effects and potential to elevate CSF pressure may be markedly exaggerated; effects on pupillary response and consciousness may obscure neurologic signs of further increases in ICP with head injuries. May cause severe hypotension with compromised ability to maintain BP due to depleted blood volume. Caution in elderly or debilitated patients sensitive to CNS depressants. Caution with circulatory shock, acute alcoholism, adrenocortical insufficiency (eg, Addison's disease), CNS depression or coma, delirium tremens, kyphoscoliosis associated with respiratory depression, myxedema or hypothyroidism, prostatic hypertrophy or urethral stricture, severe impairment of pulmonary or renal function, mild/moderate hepatic impairment and toxic psychosis. May aggravate convulsions with convulsive disorders; may induce or aggravate seizures in some clinical settings. Monitor for decreased bowel motility in post-op patients. May cause spasm of the sphincter of Oddi; caution with biliary tract disease (including acute pancreatitis). May produce tolerance and dependence. Should not abruptly d/c, may cause abstinence syndrome in physically dependent patients.

**ADVERSE REACTIONS:** Constipation, N/V, pyrexia, somnolence, headache, dizziness, pruritus, increased sweating, xerostomia, sedation, diarrhea, insomnia, fatigue, tachycardia, miosis, biliary colic, hypotension.

**INTERACTIONS:** Additive CNS depression with other CNS depressants (eg, sedatives, hypnotics, tranquilizers, general anesthetics, phenothiazines, other opioids, alcohol); reduce dose of either/both agents. Caution with concomitant use of MAOIs; reduce dose of either/both agents. Anticholinergics may increase risk of urinary retention and/or severe constipation, which may lead to paralytic ileus. CNS toxicity (eg, confusion, disorientation, respiratory depression, apnea, seizures) reported with cimetidine. Avoid use with mixed agonist/antagonist opioid analgesics, may reduce effect and/or precipitate withdrawal symptoms.

**PREGNANCY:** Category C, caution with nursing.

**MECHANISM OF ACTION:** Opioid analgesic; an opioid agonist. Prescise action not established. However, specific CNS opioid receptors for endogenous compounds with opioid-like activity have been found throughout the brain and spinal cord and play a role in analgesic effects. Opioid receptors have also been found in the peripheral nervous system.

**PHARMACOKINETICS: Absorption:** Absolute bioavailability (10%); various doses led to altered parameters. **Distribution**: Plasma protein binding (10-12%); crosses placenta. **Metabolism:** Liver (conjugation) to form oxymorphone-3-glucuronide (major metabolite), 6-OH-oxymorphone (major active metabolite). **Elimination:** Urine (<1% unchanged), feces.

## NURSING CONSIDERATIONS

**Assessment:** Assess type and severity of pain, respiratory depression, acute or severe bronchial asthma or hypercarbia, COPD, myxedema or hypothyroidism, kyphoscoliosis, CNS depression or coma, head injury or intracranial lesions, presence of increased ICP, intraparalytic ileus, circulatory shock, presence of debilitation (eg, elderly), hepatic/renal impairment, cardiovascular disease, prostatic hypertrophy or urethral stricture, toxic psychosis, acute abdominal conditions, convulsive disorders, biliary tract disease, acute pancreatitis, pregnancy/nursing status, drug abuse potential, and possible drug interactions.

**Monitoring:** Monitor for signs/symptoms of respiratory depression, presence of elevated CSF pressure, hypotension, convulsions, spasms of sphincter of Oddi, physical dependence and tolerance, and abuse or misuse of medication.

**Patient Counseling:** Advise to swallow medication whole; do not break, chew, dissolve, or crush. If broken or chewed, contents of tab may release all at once and cause fatal overdose. Instruct to take on empty stomach, at least 1 hr prior to or 2 hrs after eating. Drug may impair physical/mental abilities; use caution if performing hazardous tasks (eg, operating machinery/driving). Counsel to avoid alcohol (eg, beverages, medications containing alcohol) and other CNS depressants during therapy. Advise to contact physician if episodes of breakthrough pain or adverse events (eg, respiratory depression) develop. Instruct not to adjust dosing without consulting physician. Inform that medication has potential for abuse; protect from theft. Inform that if on therapy for a few days to weeks, avoid abrupt withdrawal; taper dosing. Instruct to keep out of reach of children.

**Administration:** Oral route. **Storage**: 25°C (77°F); excursions permitted to 15-30°C (59-86°F). Dispense in tight container with child-resistant closure.

## OPTIVAR RX
azelastine HCl (Meda)

**THERAPEUTIC CLASS:** $H_1$-antagonist

**INDICATIONS:** Treatment of itching of the eye associated with allergic conjunctivitis.

**DOSAGE:** *Adults:* 1 drop bid.
*Pediatrics:* ≥3 yrs: 1 drop bid.

**HOW SUPPLIED:** Sol: 0.05% [6mL]

**WARNINGS/PRECAUTIONS:** Not for injection or oral use. Do not wear contact lens if the eye is red. Not for treatment of contact-lens irritation. Wait 10 min after instilling drops to insert contact lens.

**ADVERSE REACTIONS:** Transient eye burning/stinging, headaches, asthma, conjunctivitis, dyspnea, eye pain, fatigue, influenza-like symptoms, pharyngitis, pruritus, rhinitis, temporary blurring.

**PREGNANCY:** Category C, caution in nursing.

**MECHANISM OF ACTION:** Antihistaminic agent; relatively selective $H_1$-receptor antagonist; inhibits release of histamine and other mediators from cells (eg, mast cells) involved in the allergic response and decreases chemotaxis and activation of eosinophils.

**PHARMACOKINETICS: Metabolism:** N-desmethylazelastine (principle metabolite).

### NURSING CONSIDERATIONS

**Assessment:** Assess for drug hypersensitivity.

**Monitoring:** Monitor for transient burning/stinging, headaches, and bitter taste.

**Patient Counseling:** Counsel not to wear contact lenses if the eye is red. Avoid touching tip of dropper to eye or any other surface to avoid contamination. Wait 10 min after instillation to wear soft-contact lenses.

**Administration:** Ocular route. **Storage:** Store upright at 2-25°C (36-77°F).

O

## ORACEA RX
doxycycline (CollaGenex)

**THERAPEUTIC CLASS:** Tetracycline derivative

**INDICATIONS:** Treatment of only inflammatory lesions (papules and pustules) of rosacea in adult patients.

**DOSAGE:** *Adults:* 40mg qd in am. Take on empty stomach.

**HOW SUPPLIED:** Cap: 40mg

**WARNINGS/PRECAUTIONS:** May cause fetal harm during pregnancy. Use during tooth development (eg, last half of pregnancy, infancy, ≤8 yrs) may cause permanent discoloration of teeth or enamel hypoplasia. Pseudomembranous colitis and superinfection reported; caution in patients with history of or predisposition to candidiasis overgrowth. Bacterial resistance may develop; use only as indicated. May cause an increase in BUN; caution in patients with renal impairment. May cause photosensitivity, autoimmune syndromes, tissue hyperpigmentation, bulging fontanels in infants, and benign intracranial HTN in adults reported. Safety beyond 9 months of use has not been established.

**ADVERSE REACTIONS:** Nasopharyngitis, diarrhea, HTN.

**INTERACTIONS:** May require downward adjustment of anticoagulant dosage. May interfere with bactericidal action of penicillin; avoid concurrent use when possible. Concomitant use with methoxyflurane may result in fatal renal toxicity. Bismuth subsalicylate, proton pump inhibitors, antacids containing aluminum, calcium or magnesium and iron-containing preparations may impair absorption. May interfere with the effectiveness of oral contraceptives. Avoid concurrent use with oral retinoids (eg, isotretinoin, acitretin).

**PREGNANCY:** Category D, not for use in nursing.

**MECHANISM OF ACTION:** Tetracycline derivative. Antibacterial agent; does not produce any long-term effects on bacterial flora in the oral cavity, skin, intestinal tract, or vagina.

**PHARMACOKINETICS: Absorption:** Single dose: $C_{max}$=510ng/mL; $T_{max}$=3 hrs; AUC=9227ng•hr/mL. Multiple doses: $C_{max}$=600ng/mL; $T_{max}$=2 hrs; AUC=7543ng•hr/mL. **Distribution**: Plasma protein binding (>90%), crosses the placenta, excreted in breast milk. **Elimination**: Urine (unchanged), feces (unchanged); $T_{1/2}$=21.2 hrs (single dose), 23.2 hrs (multiple doses).

## NURSING CONSIDERATIONS

**Assessment:** Determine pregnancy/nursing status. Assess use in patients with renal impairment, history of or predisposition to candidiasis overgrowth, and those with gastric insufficiencies (eg, patients with gastrectomy, gastric bypass surgery, or in patients who are achlorhydric). Assess for possible drug interactions.

**Monitoring:** Monitor for signs/symptoms of pseudomembranous colitis, infection, autoimmune syndrome, bulging fontanels in infants, and benign intracranial HTN in adults. Monitor BUN level, LFTs, ANA, CBC. In patients with renal insufficiencies, monitor for signs/symptoms of azotemia, hyperphosphatemia, and acidosis. Perform periodic monitoring of drug serum levels in patients with renal impairment.

**Patient Counseling:** Take medication as directed (1 hr before or 2 hrs after meals with fluid); exceeding recommended dosage may increase incidence of side effects including the development of resistant microorganisms. Minimize or avoid exposure to natural or artificial sunlight (eg, tanning beds). Wear loose fitting-clothes that protect skin from sun exposure; d/c at first evidence of sunburn. Counsel medication may cause autoimmune disorders; contact physician if arthalgia, fever, rash, or malaise develop. Advise drug may cause discoloration of skin, scars, teeth, or gums. Inform females drug may render oral contraceptives less effective, and to avoid if pregnant or nursing or planning to conceive. Advise to use second form of contraceptive to avoid contraceptive failure.



**Administration:** Oral route. **Storage**: 15-30°C (59-86°F). Dispense in tight, light-resistant containers. Keep out of reach of children.

# ORAMORPH SR

CII

morphine sulfate (Xanodyne)

**This is a sustained-release tablet. Swallow tab whole; do not break in half, crush or chew.**

**THERAPEUTIC CLASS:** Opioid analgesic

**INDICATIONS:** Relief of pain in patients who require opioid analgesics for more than a few days.

**DOSAGE:** *Adults:* Conversion from Parenteral or Immediate Release Oral Morphine: Daily dose determined by daily requirement of immediate-release formulation. Single dose is 1/2 of daily requirement given q12h. Initial: 30mg is recommended if daily morphine requirement is ≤120mg. Use 15mg for low daily morphine requirements. Titrate: Increase to 60mg or 100mg after stable dose reached.

**HOW SUPPLIED:** Tab, Extended-Release: 15mg, 30mg, 60mg, 100mg

**CONTRAINDICATIONS:** Respiratory depression in the absence of resuscitative equipment, acute or severe bronchial asthma, paralytic ileus.

**WARNINGS/PRECAUTIONS:** Not for initial treatment. Caution with hepatic and renal dysfunction, increased ICP or with head injury, decreased respiratory reserve (eg, emphysema, severe obesity, kyphoscoliosis, or paralysis of the phrenic nerve), chronic asthma, upper airway obstruction, or in other chronic pulmonary disorders. Tolerance, psychological and physical dependence may develop. Avoid abrupt discontinuation. Not for pediatrics or use in women during or immediately before labor.

**ADVERSE REACTIONS:** Constipation, NV, dizziness, sedation, dysphoria, euphoria, and sweating, respiratory depression.

**INTERACTIONS:** Potentiated depressant effects with CNS depressants, alcohol, sedatives, antihistaminics, or psychotropics. Increased risk of respiratory depression, hypotension, sedation and coma with neuroleptics. Mixed agonist/antagonist opioid analgesics (eg, pentazocine, nalbuphine, butorphanol, or buprenorphine) may alter effect or precipitate withdrawal symptoms.

**PREGNANCY:** Category C, not for use in nursing.

**MECHANISM OF ACTION:** Opioid analgesic; interacts predominantly with μ-receptor. μ binding sites are found distributed in the brain, spinal cord, and in trigeminal nerve. Primary actions are analgesia and sedation.

**PHARMACOKINETICS: Absorption:** Absolute bioavailability (40%), oral administration of variable doses resulted in different parameters. **Distribution:** $V_d$=4L/kg; crosses placental membrane; found in breast milk. **Metabolism:** Liver to glucuronide metabolites; morphine-3-glucuronide (major metabolite), morphine-6-glucuronide (active metabolite). **Elimination:** Kidneys (major), feces (10%), bile (small amount); $T_{1/2}$=2-4 hrs.

## NURSING CONSIDERATIONS

**Assessment:** Assess for respiratory depression, acute or severe bronchial asthma, COPD, presence of debilitation (eg, elderly), paralytic ileus, ICP or head injury, hepatic/renal dysfunction, pregnancy/nursing status, and possible drug interactions.

**Monitoring:** Monitor for signs/symptoms of respiratory depression, elevations in CSF pressure, medication dependence and abuse.

**Patient Counseling:** Instruct to swallow medication whole; do not break, chew, or crush. Drug may cause psychological and/or physical dependence. Do not adjust dose without consulting physician. Avoid abrupt withdrawal of medication. Advise to avoid alcohol or other CNS depressants. Medication may impair mental/physical abilities; use caution if performing hazardous tasks (eg, operating machinery/driving).

**Administration:** Oral route. **Storage:** 25°C (77°F); excursions permitted to 15-30°C (59-86°F).

O

# ORAPRED RX

prednisolone sodium phosphate (Biomarin)

**OTHER BRAND NAMES:** Orapred ODT (Sciele)

**THERAPEUTIC CLASS:** Glucocorticoid

**INDICATIONS:** Steroid-responsive disorders.

**DOSAGE:** *Adults:* (Sol) Initial: 5-60mg/day depending on disease and response. (Tab) Initial: 10-60mg/day depending on disease and response. Maint: Decrease dose by small amounts to lowest effective dose. (Sol/Tab) MS Exacerbations: 200mg qd for 1 week, then 80mg qod for 1 month. *Pediatrics:* (Sol/Tab) Initial: 0.14-2mg/kg/day, depending on disease and response, given tid-qid. Nephrotic Syndrome: 20mg/m² tid for 4 weeks, then 40mg/m² qod for 4 weeks. Uncontrolled Asthma: 1-2mg/kg/day in single or divided doses until peak expiratory flow rate of 80% is achieved (usually 3-10 days).

**HOW SUPPLIED:** Sol: 15mg/5mL [237mL]; Tab, Orally Disintegrating: 10mg, 15mg, 30mg

**CONTRAINDICATIONS:** Systemic fungal infections.

**WARNINGS/PRECAUTIONS:** May produce reversible HPA axis suppression. Adjust dose during stress or change in thyroid status. May mask signs of infection or cause new infections. May activate latent amebiasis. Avoid with cerebral malaria. Avoid exposure to chickenpox or measles. Not for treatment of optic neuritis or active ocular herpes simplex. May cause elevation of BP or IOP, cataracts, glaucoma, optic nerve damage, Kaposi's sarcoma, psychic derangements, salt/water retention, increased excretion of potassium and/or calcium, osteoporosis, growth suppression in children, secondary ocular infections. Caution with strongyloides, CHF, diverticulitis, HTN, renal insufficiency, fresh intestinal anastomoses, active or latent peptic ulcer, ulcerative colitis. Enhanced effect in hypothyroidism or cirrhosis. Avoid abrupt withdrawal.

**ADVERSE REACTIONS:** Edema, fluid/electrolyte disturbances, osteoporosis, muscle weakness, pancreatitis, peptic ulcer, impaired wound healing, increased intracranial pressure, cushingoid state, hirsutism, menstrual irregularities, growth suppression in children, glaucoma, nausea, weight gain.

**INTERACTIONS:** Enhanced metabolism with barbiturates, phenytoin, ephedrine, and rifampin. Use with cyclosporine may increase activity of both drugs; convulsions reported with concomitant use. Decreased metabolism with estrogens or ketoconazole. May inhibit response to warfarin. Increased risk of GI side effects with ASA or other NSAIDs. May increase clearance of salicylates. High doses or concurrent neuromuscular drugs may cause acute myopathy. Enhanced possibility of hypokalemia when given with potassium-depleting agents. May produce severe weakness in myasthenia gravis patients on anticholinesterase agents. Avoid live vaccines with immunosuppressive doses. Possible diminished response with killed or inactivated vaccines. May increase blood glucose; adjust antidiabetic agents. May suppress reactions to skin tests.

**PREGNANCY:** Category C, caution in nursing.

**MECHANISM OF ACTION:** Synthetic adrenocorticoid steroid; promotes gluconeogenesis, increases deposition of glycogen in the liver, inhibits glucose utilization, increases catabolism of protein, lipolysis, glomerular filtration that leads to increased urinary excretion of urate and calcium.

**PHARMACOKINETICS: Absorption:** Readily absorbed from GI tract. **Distribution:** Plasma protein binding (70-90%); found in breast milk. **Metabolism:** Liver. **Elimination:** Urine (as sulfate and glucuronide conjugates), $T_{1/2}$=2-4 hrs.

## NURSING CONSIDERATIONS

O

**Assessment:** Assess for systemic fungal infection, other current infections, active TB, HTN, CHF, renal insufficiency, ophthalmic disease, osteoporosis, thyroid status, hepatic impairment, nonspecific ulcerative colitis, and possible drug interactions.

**Monitoring:** Monitor for adrenocortical insufficiency, occurrence of infections, psychic derangement, cataracts, acute myopathy, Kaposi's sarcoma, fluid retention, measurement of serum electrolytes, TSH, LFTs, glucose, IOP, and BP.

**Patient Counseling:** Advise not to d/c abruptly or without medical supervision. Avoid exposure to chickenpox or measles; report immediately if exposed. ODT tablets should be placed on tongue and allowed to dissolve in mouth, with/without water. Do not cut, split, or break tablets. Do not use partial tablets.

**Administration:** Oral route. **Storage:** (Sol) 2-8°C (36-46°F); (Tab) 20-25°C (68-77°F); protect from moisture.

# ORENCIA — RX

abatacept (Bristol-Myers Squibb)

**THERAPEUTIC CLASS:** Selective costimulation modulator

**INDICATIONS:** To reduce signs and symptoms, induce major clinical response, inhibit progression of structural damage, and improve physical function in adult patients with moderately to severely active rheumatoid arthritis (RA). May be used as monotherapy or concomitantly with disease-modifying antirheumatic drugs (DMARDs) other than TNF-antagonists. To reduce signs and symptoms in pediatric patients ≥6 yrs with moderately to severely active polyarticular juvenile idiopathic arthritis. May be used alone or in combination with methotrexate (MTX).

**DOSAGE:** *Adults:* Initial: <60kg: 500mg; 60-100kg: 750mg; >100kg: 1g IV over 30 min. Maint: Give at 2 and 4 weeks after initial infusion, then every 4 weeks thereafter.
*Pediatrics:* 6-17 yrs: ≥75 kg: Follow adult dosing regimen. Max: 1000mg; <75kg: Initial: 10mg/kg IV over 30 min. Maint: Give at 2 and 4 weeks after initial infusion, then every 4 weeks thereafter.

**HOW SUPPLIED:** Inj: 250mg/15mL

**WARNINGS/PRECAUTIONS:** Increased risk of infections and serious infections with concomitant TNF-antagonist therapy; concurrent use not recommended. Anaphylaxis or anaphylactoid reactions reported. Caution with history of recurrent infections, underlying conditions which may predispose to infections, chronic, latent, localized infections; d/c if serious infections develop. Screen for latent tuberculosis (TB) and viral hepatitis prior to initiation of therapy. Avoid live vaccines. Caution with COPD. Cases of lung cancer and lymphoma reported. Juvenile idiopathic arthritis patients should be brought up to date with all immunizations prior to therapy. Caution in elderly.

**ADVERSE REACTIONS:** Headache, nasopharyngitis, dizziness, cough, back pain, HTN, dyspepsia, urinary tract infection, rash, pain in extremities, upper respiratory tract infection, nausea, sinusitis, influenza, bronchitis, malignancies.

**INTERACTIONS:** Concomitant use with TNF antagonist may increase risk of serious infections. Concomitant use with anakinra not recommended. May falsely elevate blood glucose readings with glucose dehydrogenase pyrroloquinolonequinone-(GDH-PQQ) based monitors; use other test methods. Do not use live vaccines concurrently or within 3 months of discontinuation.

**PREGNANCY:** Category C, not for use in nursing.

**MECHANISM OF ACTION:** Selective costimulation modulator; inhibits T cell activation by binding to CD80 and CD86, thereby blocking interaction with CD28.

**PHARMACOKINETICS: Absorption:** $C_{max}$=292mcg/mL (Healthy subjects); $C_{max}$=295mcg/mL (RA patients); $C_{max}$=217 mcg/mL (Juvenile Idiopathic Arthritis patients). **Distribution:** $V_d$=0.09L/Kg (Healthy subjects); $V_d$=0.07L/Kg (RA patients). **Elimination:** $T_{1/2}$=16.7 days (Healthy subjects); $T_{1/2}$=13.1 days (RA patients)

O

## NURSING CONSIDERATIONS

**Assessment:** Assess for history of recurrent infections, chronic/latent/localized infections, disease states which may predispose to infection, and COPD. Screen for latent TB infection and viral hepatitis. Assess pregnancy/nursing status and for possible drug interactions.

**Monitoring:** Monitor for signs/symptoms of hypersensitivity, infection, immunosuppression, malignancies, and hepatitis B reactivation. If COPD present, monitor for COPD exacerbation, cough, rhonchi, and dyspnea. When monitoring blood glucose in diabetic patients, use methods not based on GDH-PQQ.

**Patient Counseling:** Instruct not to receive live vaccines during therapy or within 3 months following discontinuation. Immediately contact physician if hypersensitivity reaction (eg, anaphylaxis) occur. Discuss increased risk of infections when used concomitantly with TNF antagonist (eg, adalimunab, etanercept, and infliximab) and other biologic RA therapy (eg, anakinra), and potential risk for malignancies. Inform diabetic patients that the infusion contains maltose, which can give falsely elevated blood glucose readings on the day of administration; may need alternate monitoring method.

**Administration:** IV infusion route. Refer to PI for complete preparation instructions. Administer diluted solution over 30 min. Infusion must be completed within 24 hrs of reconstitution. **Storage:** Lypholized powder: 2-8°C (36-46°F). Do not use after expiration date. Protect vials from light; store in original package until time of use. Infusion solution: Room temperature, or 2-8°C (36-46°F); use within 24 hrs.

# ORTHO EVRA RX

ethinyl estradiol - norelgestromin (Ortho-McNeil)

**THERAPEUTIC CLASS:** Estrogen/progestogen combination

**INDICATIONS:** Prevention of pregnancy.

**DOSAGE:** *Adults:* Start on either 1st Sunday after menses begin or 1st day of menses. Apply patch every week on same day for 3 weeks. Week 4 is patch-free. Apply to clean, dry intact skin on buttock, abdomen, upper outer arm, or upper torso.

**HOW SUPPLIED:** Patch: (Ethinyl Estradiol-Norelgestromin): 0.75mg-6mg [1[s], 3[s]]

**CONTRAINDICATIONS:** Thrombophlebitis or history of deep vein thrombophlebitis, thromboembolic disorders (current or past history), known thrombophilic conditions, cerebrovascular or coronary artery disease (CAD) (current or past history), valvular heart disease with complications, persistent blood pressure values of ≥160mm Hg systolic or ≥100mm Hg diastolic, diabetes with vascular involvement, headaches with focal neurological symptoms, major surgery with prolonged immobilization, breast cancer (current or past history), carcinoma of the endometrium or other estrogen-dependent neoplasia, undiagnosed abnormal genital bleeding, cholestatic jaundice of pregnancy or jaundice with prior hormonal contraceptive use, acute/chronic hepatocellular disease with abnormal liver function, hepatic adenomas or carcinomas, pregnancy.

**WARNINGS/PRECAUTIONS:** Cigarette smoking increases risk of serious CV side effects; risk increases with age (especially >35 yrs) and heavy smoking ( ≥15 cigarettes/day). Increased risk of MI, vascular disease, thromboembolism, thrombotic disease, and stroke. Benign hepatic adenomas and hepatocellular carcinoma reported; d/c if jaundice develops. Retinal thrombosis reported; d/c if unexplained partial or complete loss of vision, onset of proptosis or diplopia, papilledema, or retinal vascular lesions develops. Should not be used to induce withdrawal bleeding as a test for pregnancy, or to treat threatened or habitual abortion during pregnancy. May increase the risk or worsen existing gallbladder disease. May cause glucose intolerance, elevations in LDL levels or other lipid level changes. May cause fluid retention and increase BP; d/c if persistent elevation of BP occurs ( ≥160mmHg systolic or ≥100mmHg diastolic). D/C if with onset or exacerbation of migraine headache occurs. May cause breakthrough bleeding and spotting. Ectopic and intrauterine pregnancies may occur with contraceptive failures. May be less effective in women with body weight ≥198 lbs. Caution in patient with history of depression; d/c if significant depression develops. Visual changes or changes in lens tolerance may develop with contact lens use. May affect certain endocrine, LFTs, and blood components in laboratory tests. Not indicated for use before menarche. May affect certain endocrine and LFTs and blood components. Does not protect against HIV infection (AIDS) and other sexually transmitted diseases.

**ADVERSE REACTIONS:** Breast symptoms (eg, breast discomfort, engorgement, pain), vaginal bleeding, dysmenorrhea, dizziness, diarrhea, headache, application-site disorder, N/V, mood, affect, and anxiety disorders, abdominal pain, vaginal yeast infection.

**INTERACTIONS:** May reduce the effectiveness or increase the incidence of breakthrough bleeding when used concomitantly with a drug that induces enzymes (eg, CYP3A4) that metabolize contraceptive hormones (eg, barbiturates, bosentan, carbamazepine, felbamate, griseofulvin, oxcarbazepine, phenytoin, rifampin, St. John's wort, topiramate); use additional contraception or a different method of contraception. Protease inhibitors and non-nucleoside reverse transcriptase inhibitors may alter estrogen and progestin levels. Pregnancy has been reported with use of hormonal contraceptives and antibiotics; refer to PI of specific antibiotic for possible interaction. HMG-CoA reductase inhibitors (atorvastatin, rosuvastatin), ascorbic acid, acetaminophen, and CYP3A4 inhibitors (eg, itraconazole, ketoconazole, voriconazole, fluconazole, grapefruit juice) may increase ethinyl estradiol levels. May increase levels of cyclosporine, prednisolone, and theophylline. May decrease levels of acetaminophen, clofibric acid, morphine, salicyclic acid, and temazepam. May decrease lamotrigine levels; dosage adjustment of lamotrigine may be necessary.

**PREGNANCY:** Category X, not for use in nursing.

**MECHANISM OF ACTION:** Estrogen/progestogen combination contraceptive; suppresses gonadotropins. Inhibits ovulation, promotes changes in cervical mucus (which increases difficulty of sperm entry into uterus) and in the endometrium (which reduce likelihood of implantation).

**PHARMACOKINETICS: Absorption:** Administration of doses during different dosing cycles led to altered parameters. **Distribution:** Found in breast milk. Ethinyl estradiol: Serum albumin binding (extensive). Norelgestromin: Serum protein binding (>97%). **Metabolism:** Ethinyl estradiol: Hydroxylated, glucuronide and sulfate conjugates. Norelgestromin: Hepatic, hydroxylated and conjugate metabolites, norgestrel (metabolite). **Elimination:** Ethinyl estradiol: Urine, feces; $T_{1/2}$=17 hrs. Norelgestromin: Urine, feces; $T_{1/2}$=28 hrs.

## NURSING CONSIDERATIONS

**Assessment:** Assess for current or history of thrombophlebitis or thromboembolic disorders, thrombophilic conditions, current or past history of cerebrovascular disease or CAD, valvular heart disease with complications, persistent BP ≥160 mm Hg systolic or ≥100 mm Hg diastolic, diabetes with vascular involvement, headaches with focal neurological symptoms, major surgery with prolonged immobilization, known/suspected carcinoma of the breast or history of breast cancer, carcinoma of the endometrium or other known or suspected estrogen dependent neoplasia, undiagnosed abnormal genital bleeding, cholestatic jaundice of pregnancy or jaundice with prior hormonal contraceptive use, acute or chronic hepatocellular disease with abnormal liver function, hepatic adenomas or carcinomas, pregnancy/nursing status, and for possible drug interactions. Assess use in patients with HTN, hyperlipidemias, obesity, diabetes, and in patients>35 yrs who smoke ≥15 cigarettes/day.

**Monitoring:** Monitor for signs/symptoms of thromboembolism, MI, stroke, vascular disease, hepatic neoplasia, carcinoma of the breast and reproductive organs, ocular lesions, gallbladder disease, onset or exacerbation of a migraine headache, breakthrough bleeding or spotting, ectopic pregnancy, liver dysfunction (eg, jaundice), fluid retention, and for signs of worsening depression in patients with previous history. Monitor for signs of hypertension; perform regular monitor of BP throughout duration of therapy. Monitor for changes in lipid levels; measure lipid levels periodically. Monitor serum glucose levels in prediabetic and diabetic patients. Refer patients with contact lenses to an ophthalmologist if visual changes or changes in lens tolerance develop. Perform annual physical exam.

**Patient Counseling:** Inform that drug does not protect against HIV infection (AIDS) and other STDs. Advise to avoid smoking. Inform about possible adverse effects. Instruct to have annual physical exam and medical evaluation while on therapy. Instruct to apply patch to clean, dry, intact healthy skin (on buttock, abdomen, upper outer arm, or upper torso) where it will not be rubbed by tight clothing. Inform that patch should not be placed on red, irritated, or cut skin, nor on the breasts. Advise that may have spotting, light bleeding, breast tenderness, or may feel sick in the stomach during use; do not d/c and if symptoms persist notify physician. Advise not to skip patches and to never have the patch off for more than 7 days in a row.

**Administration:** Transdermal route. **Storage:** 25°C (77°F); excursions permitted to 15-30°C (59-86°F). Do not store in refrigerator or freezer.

# ORTHO TRI-CYCLEN — RX

ethinyl estradiol - norgestimate (Ortho-McNeil)

**OTHER BRAND NAMES:** Tri-Sprintec (Barr) - Tri-Previfem (Teva) - Trinessa (Watson)

**THERAPEUTIC CLASS:** Estrogen/progestogen combination

**INDICATIONS:** Prevention of pregnancy. Treatment of acne vulgaris in females ≥15 yrs who want contraception, have achieved menarche, and are unresponsive to topical acne agents.

**DOSAGE:** *Adults:* Contraception/Acne: 28-day: 1 tab qd for 28 days, then repeat. Start 1st Sunday after menses begin or 1st day of menses.
*Pediatrics:* Contraception (postpubertal adolescents)/Acne: 28-day: 1 tab qd for 28 days, then repeat. Start 1st Sunday after menses begin or 1st day of menses.

**HOW SUPPLIED:** Tab: (Ethinyl Estradiol-Norgestimate) 0.035mg-0.18mg, 0.035mg-0.215mg, 0.035mg-0.25mg

**CONTRAINDICATIONS:** Thrombophlebitis or past history of deep vein thrombophlebitis, thromboembolic disorders (current or past history of), cerebral vascular or coronary artery disease (current or past history of), valvular heart disease with complications, severe hypertension, diabetes with vascular involvement, headaches with focal neurological symptoms, major surgery with prolonged immobilization, carcinoma of the breast (current or past history of), carcinoma of the endometrium or other known or suspected estrogen dependent neoplasia, undiagnosed abnormal genital bleeding, cholestatic jaundice of pregnancy or jaundice with prior pill use, acute or chronic hepatocellular disease with abnormal liver function, hepatic adenomas or carcinomas, pregnancy.

**WARNINGS/PRECAUTIONS:** Cigarette smoking increases risk of serious cardiovascular side effects; risk increases with age (especially >35 yrs) and heavy smoking. Increased risk of MI, vascular disease, thromboembolism, stroke, gallbladder disease, and hepatic neoplasia. May increase risk of breast cancer and cancer of the reproductive organs. Retinal thrombosis reported; d/c if unexplained partial or complete loss of vision, onset of proptosis or diplopia, papilledema, or retinal vascular lesions develop. May cause glucose intolerance, fluid retention, breakthrough bleeding, and spotting. May increase BP; d/c if significant elevations in BP occur. May elevate LDL levels or cause other lipid changes. May cause or exacerbate migraine headaches. May develop visual changes with contact lens. Increased risk of morbidity and mortality with HTN, hyperlipidemia, obesity, and DM. D/C if jaundice or if significant depression develops. Perform annual physical exam. Use before menarche is not indicated. Does not protect against HIV infection (AIDS) or other sexually transmitted diseases. May affect certain endocrine, LFTs, and blood components in laboratory tests.



**ADVERSE REACTIONS:** N/V, breakthrough bleeding, gastrointestinal symptoms (such as abdominal cramps, bloating), spotting, menstrual flow changes, amenorrhea, migraine, depression, vaginal candidiasis, edema, weight changes, cervical erosion and secretion.

**INTERACTIONS:** Reduced effects resulting in breakthrough bleeding or unintended pregnancy may occur when co-administered with antibiotics, anticonvulsants and other drugs that increase the metabolism of contraceptive steroids (eg, rifampin, barbiturates, phenylbutazone, phenytoin, carbamazepine, felbamate, oxcarbazepine, griseofulvin, topiramate, bosentan). HIV protease inhibitors may increase or decrease levels. St. John's Wort may reduce contraceptive effectiveness and may result in breakthrough bleeding. Atorvastatin, ascorbic acid, acetaminophen, CYP3A4 inhibitors (eg, itraconazole, ketoconazole) may increase hormone levels. Increases levels of cyclosporine, prednisolone, and theophylline. Decreases levels of acetaminophen. Increases clearance of temazepam, salicylic acid, morphine, and clofibric acid. May decrease plasma levels of lamotrigine; dosage adjustment of lamotrigine may be necessary.

**PREGNANCY:** Category X, not for use in nursing.

**MECHANISM OF ACTION:** Estrogen/progestogen combination oral contraceptive; acts by suppressing gonadotropins. Inhibits ovulation and produces changes in the cervical mucus (increases difficulty of sperm entry into uterus) and endometrium (reduces likelihood of implantation)

**PHARMACOKINETICS: Absorption:** Rapid. Oral administration on various days during dosing led to altered parameters. **Distribution:** Found in breast milk. Norgestimate: Albumin binding (>97%). Ethinyl estradiol: Albumin binding (>97%). **Metabolism:** Norgestimate: GI tract and/or liver (1st pass mechanism). Norelgestromin (primary active metabolite): Hepatic, norgestrel (active metabolite). Ethinyl estradiol: Hydroxylated, glucuronide, sulfate conjugates. **Elimination:** Norgestimate: Urine (47%), feces (37%).

## NURSING CONSIDERATIONS

**Assessment:** Assess for thrombophlebitis or past history of deep vein thrombophlebitis, current or history of thromboembolic disorders, current or history of cerebral vascular or coronary artery disease, valvular heart disease with complications, severe hypertension, diabetes with vascular involvement, headaches with focal neurological symptoms, major surgery with prolonged immobilization, presence of or history of carcinoma of the breast, carcinoma of the endometrium or other known or suspected estrogen dependent neoplasia, undiagnosed abnormal genital bleeding, cholestatic jaundice of pregnancy or jaundice with prior pill use, acute or chronic hepatocellular disease with abnormal liver function, hepatic adenomas or carcinomas, and pregnancy. Assess use in patients >35 who smoke ≥15 cigarettes/day. Assess use in patients with HTN, hyperlipidemias, obesity, and DM. Assess nursing status and for possible drug interactions.

**Monitoring:** Monitor for signs/symptoms of MI, thromboembolism, stroke, hepatic neoplasia, breast cancer and cancer or the reproductive organs, ocular lesions, bleeding irregularities, fluid retention, onset or exacerbation of migraine headaches, gallbladder disease, and ectopic pregnancy. Monitor serum glucose levels in DM and prediabetic patients. Monitor BP with history of HTN, lipid levels with history of hyperlipidemia, and for signs of worsening depression with previous history. Refer patients to an ophthalmologist if ocular changes develop. Perform annual physical exam while on therapy. Monitor liver function and for signs of liver toxicity (eg, jaundice).

**Patient Counseling:** Inform that drug does not protect against HIV infection (AIDS) and other STDs. Advise to avoid smoking while on medication. Counsel about potential adverse effects. Instruct to take as exactly as directed at intervals not exceeding 24 hrs. Advise about risk of pregnancy if dose is missed. Instruct that if one dose missed, take as soon as possible; take next pill at regularly scheduled time. Inform may experiece spotting, light bleeding, or stomach sickness during first 1-3 packs of pills; advise not to d/c medication and if symptoms persist, notify physician.

**Administration:** Oral route. **Storage:** 25°C (77°F); excursions permitted to 15-30°C (59-86°F). Protect from light.

O

# ORTHO TRI-CYCLEN LO — RX

ethinyl estradiol - norgestimate (Ortho-McNeil)

**OTHER BRAND NAMES:** Tr-Lo-Sprintec (Barr)

**THERAPEUTIC CLASS:** Estrogen/progestogen combination

**INDICATIONS:** Prevention of pregnancy.

**DOSAGE:** *Adults:* 1 tab qd for 28 days, then repeat. Start 1st Sunday after menses begin or 1st day of menses.

**HOW SUPPLIED:** Tab: (Ethinyl Estradiol-Norgestimate) 0.025mg-0.18mg, 0.025mg-0.215mg, and 0.025mg-0.25mg

**CONTRAINDICATIONS:** Thrombophlebitis or history of deep vein thrombophlebitis, thromboembolic disorders (current or past history), pregnancy, cerebrovascular or CAD (current or past history), valvular heart disease with complications, severe HTN, DM with vascular involvement, headaches with focal neurological symptoms, major surgery with prolonged immobilization, undiagnosed abnormal genital bleeding, cholestatic jaundice of pregnancy or jaundice with prior pill use, hepatic adenomas or carcinomas, breast cancer (current or past history), endometrial carcinoma or other estrogen-dependent neoplasia.

**WARNINGS/PRECAUTIONS:** Cigarette smoking increases risk of serious cardiovascular side effects; risk increases with age (especially >35 yrs) and heavy smoking. Increased risk of MI, vascular disease, thromboembolism, stroke, hepatic neoplasia, and gallbladder disease. May increase risk of breast cancer and cancer of the reproductive organs. Retinal thrombosis reported; d/c if unexplained partial or complete loss of vision, onset of proptosis or diplopia, papilledema, or retinal vascular lesions develop. May cause glucose intolerance, fluid retention, breakthrough bleeding, and spotting. May increase BP; d/c if significant elevations in BP occur. May elevate LDL levels or cause other lipid changes. May cause or exacerbate migraine headaches. May develop visual changes with contact lens. Increased risk of morbidity and mortality with HTN, hyperlipidemia, obesity, and DM. D/C if jaundice or if significant depression develops. Does not protect against HIV infection (AIDS) and other sexually transmitted infections. Perform annual physical exam. Use before menarche is not indicated. May affect certain endocrine, LFTs, and blood components in laboratory tests.

**ADVERSE REACTIONS:** N/V, breakthrough bleeding, spotting, amenorrhea, migraine, depression, vaginal candidiasis, edema, weight changes, melasma, breast changes, changes in cervical erosion and secretion, allergic reaction.

**INTERACTIONS:** Reduced effects resulting in pregnancy or breakthrough bleeding may occur when coadministered with antibiotics, anticonvulsants, and other drugs that increase the metabolism of contraceptive steroids (eg, rifampin, barbiturates, phenylbutazone, phenytoin, carbamazepine, felbamate, oxcarbazepine, griseofulvin, topiramate, ampicillin, tetracyclines). Concomitant use with St. John's wort may reduce effectiveness of contraceptive steroids and may result in breakthrough bleeding. Atorvastatin, ascorbic acid, acetaminophen (APAP), CYP3A4 inhibitors (eg, itraconazole, ketoconazole) may increase hormone levels. HIV protease inhibitors may increase or decrease levels. May increases levels of cyclosporine, prednisolone, theophylline. May decrease levels of APAP. May increase the clearance of temazepam, salicylic acid, morphine, and clofibric acid. May decrease plasma levels of lamotrigine which may reduce seizure control; dosage adjustments of lamotrigine may be necessary.

**PREGNANCY:** Category X, not for use in nursing.

O

**MECHANISM OF ACTION:** Estrogen/progestogen oral contraceptive; acts by suppressing gonadotropins. Inhibits ovulation and produces alterations in the cervical mucus (increases difficulty of sperm entry into uterus) and the endometrium (reduces likehood of implantation).

**PHARMACOKINETICS: Absorption:** Rapidly absorbed. Oral administration on various days during dosing schedule led to altered parameters. **Distribution:** Found in breast milk. Norgestimate: Serum protein binding (>97%). Ethinyl Estradiol: Serum albumin binding (>97%). **Metabolism:** Norgestimate: 1st pass metabolism, GI tract and/or liver. Norelgestromin (active major metabolite), norgestrel (active metabolite). Norelgestromin: Hepatic. Ethinyl Estradiol: Hydroxylated, glucuronide and sulfate congugates. **Elimination:** Urine, feces; $T_{1/2}$=28.1 hrs (norelgestromin), 36.4 hrs (norgestrel), 17.7 hrs (ethinyl estradiol).

## NURSING CONSIDERATIONS

**Assessment:** Assess for current or history of thrombophlebitis or thromboembolic disorders, current or history of cerebrovascular or coronary artery disease, valvular heart disease with complications, severe HTN, DM with vascular involvement, headaches with focal neurological symptoms, major surgery with prolonged immobilization, known/suspected carcinoma of breast or history of, carcinoma of the endometrium or other known or suspected estrogen-dependent neoplasia, undiagnosed abnormal genital bleeding, cholestatic jaundice of pregnancy or jaundice with prior pill use, and known or suspected pregnancy. Assess use in patients >35 yrs who smoke ≥15 cigarettes/day. Assess use in patients with HTN, hyperlipidemias, DM, and obesity. Assess nursing status and for possible drug interactions.

**Monitoring:** Monitor for signs/symptoms of MI, thromboembolism, stroke, hepatic neoplasia, ocular lesions, bleeding irregularities, fluid retention, onset or exacerbation of a migraine headache, gallbladder disease, carcinoma of the breast and reproductive organs, and ectopic pregnancy. Monitor BP if have history of HTN; monitor serum glucose levels in DM or prediabetic patients, lipid levels with history of hyperlipidemia, for signs/symptoms of liver dysfunction while on therapy (eg, jaundice), for signs of worsening depression with previous history. Refer patients with contact lenses to an ophthalmologist if ocular changes occur. Perform annual physical exam.

**Patient Counseling:** Inform that drug does not protect against HIV infection (AIDS) and other STDs. Advise to avoid smoking. Counsel about potential adverse effects. Instruct to take exactly as directed at intervals not exceeding 24 hrs. Instruct that if one dose missed, take as soon as possible; take next pill at regularly scheduled time. Inform may experience spotting, light bleeding, or nausea during first 1-3 packs of pills; advise not to d/c medication and if symptoms persist, notify physician.

**Administration:** Oral route. **Storage:** 25°C (77°F); excursions permitted to 15-30°C (59-86°F).

## ORTHO-CEPT — RX

desogestrel - ethinyl estradiol (Ortho-McNeil)

**THERAPEUTIC CLASS:** Estrogen/progestogen combination

**INDICATIONS:** Prevention of pregnancy.

**DOSAGE:** *Adults:* 1 tab qd for 28 days, then repeat. Start 1st Sunday after menses begin or 1st day of menses.

**HOW SUPPLIED:** Tab: (Ethinyl Estradiol-Desogestrel) 0.03mg-0.15mg

**CONTRAINDICATIONS:** Thrombophlebitis, DVT or thromboembolic disorders, pregnancy, cerebrovascular or coronary artery disease, undiagnosed abnormal genital bleeding, cholestatic jaundice of pregnancy or jaundice with prior pill use, hepatic adenomas or carcinomas, breast cancer or other estrogen-dependent neoplasia.

**WARNINGS/PRECAUTIONS:** Cigarette smoking increases risk of serious cardiovascular side effects. This risk increases with age (especially >35 yrs) and heavy smoking. Increased risk of MI, vascular disease, thromboembolism, stroke, and gallbladder disease. Retinal thrombosis, hepatic neoplasia, carcinoma of breast and reproductive organs reported. May cause glucose intolerance. May increase BP, elevate LDL levels or cause other lipid changes, fluid retention, breakthrough bleeding, and spotting. May cause or exacerbate migraine. May develop visual changes with contact lens. Increased risk of MI with HTN, hyperlipidemia, obesity, and diabetes. D/C if jaundice, significant depression, or ophthalmic irregularities develop. Perform annual physical exam. Use before menarche is not indicated. May affect certain endocrine, LFTs, and blood components.

**ADVERSE REACTIONS:** NV, breakthrough bleeding, spotting, amenorrhea, migraine, depression, vaginal candidiasis, edema, weight changes.

**INTERACTIONS:** Reduced effects, increased breakthrough bleeding, and menstrual irregularities with rifampin, barbiturates, phenylbutazone, phenytoin, carbamazepine, griseofulvin, topiramate, St. John's wort, and possibly with ampicillin and tetracyclines.

**PREGNANCY:** Category X, not for use in nursing.

**MECHANISM OF ACTION:** Estrogen/progestogen combination oral contraceptive; responsible for suppressing gonadotropins. Primarily inhibits ovulation. Also causes changes in cervical mucus (increases difficulty of sperm entry into uterus) and endometrium (reduces likehood of implantation).

**PHARMACOKINETICS: Absorption:** Desogestrel: Rapid, $C_{max}$=2,805pg/mL (single dose), 5840 (multiple doses), $T_{max}$=1.4 hrs (single dose), 1.4 hrs (after multiple doses); AUC=33,858pg/mL•hr (single dose), 52,299pg/mL•hr (after multiple doses); Ethinyl estradiol: $C_{max}$=95pg/mL (single dose), 141pg/mL (multiple doses), $T_{max}$=1.5 hrs (single dose), 1.4 hrs (multiple doses) AUC=1471pg/mL•hr. **Distribution:** Found in breast milk. **Metabolism:** Desogestrel: 3-keto-desogestrel (major active metabolite), conjugation into sulfates and glucuronides. Ethinyl estradiol: Phase I metabolism: 2-OH-ethinyl estradiol, 2-methoxy-ethinyl-estradiol (major metabolites), hepatic conjugation. **Elimination:** 3-ketodesogestrel: $T_{1/2}$=38 hrs; Ethinyl estradiol: $T_{1/2}$=26 hrs.

## NURSING CONSIDERATIONS

**Assessment:** Assess for current or history of thrombophlebitis or thromboembolic disorder, cerebrovascular or coronary artery disease, valvular heart disease with complications, severe HTN, DM with vascular involvement, headaches with focal neurological symptoms, major surgery with prolonged immobilization, known/suspected or history of breast cancer, carcinoma of endometrium or other known/suspected estrogen-dependent neoplasia, abnormal genital bleeding, cholestatic jaundice of pregnancy or jaundice with prior pill use, hepatic adenomas or carcinomas, and known/suspected pregnancy. Assess use in patients ≥35 yrs who smoke ≥15 cigarettes/day. Assess for possible drug interactions.

**Monitoring:** Monitor for MI, thromboembolism, stroke, hepatic neoplasia, gallbladder disease, headaches, bleeding irregularities, ocular lesions, hyperlipidemia, HTN, fluid retention, and ectopic pregnancy. Monitor blood glucose levels in DM or prediabetic patients, BP with history of HTN, lipid levels with history of hyperlipidemia, for signs of worsening depression with previous history, for signs/symptoms of liver dysfunction (eg, jaundice). Instruct patients with contact lenses to an ophthalmologist if ocular changes develop. Perform annual physical exam.

**Patient Counseling:** Inform that drug does not protect HIV infection (AIDS) and other STDs. Advise to avoid smoking while on drug. Instruct to take medication at same time daily. Inform that if dose missed, take as soon as possible; take next dose at regularly scheduled time. Inform may have spotting, light bleeding or nausea during first first 1-3 packs of pills; advise not to d/c medication and if symptoms persist, notify physician.

**Administration:** Oral route. **Storage:** 25°C (77°F); excursions permitted to 15-30°C (59-86°F).

## ORTHO-CYCLEN — RX

ethinyl estradiol - norgestimate (Ortho-McNeil)



**OTHER BRAND NAMES:** Sprintec (Barr) - MonoNessa (Watson)

**THERAPEUTIC CLASS:** Estrogen/progestogen combination

**INDICATIONS:** Prevention of pregnancy.

**DOSAGE:** *Adults:* 1 tab qd for 28 days, then repeat. Start 1st Sunday after menses begin or 1st day of menses.

**HOW SUPPLIED:** Tab: (Ethinyl Estradiol-Norgestimate) 0.035mg-0.25mg

**CONTRAINDICATIONS:** Thrombophlebitis or past history of deep vein thrombophlebitis, thromboembolic disorders (current or past history of), cerebral vascular or coronary artery disease (current or past history of), valvular heart disease with complications, severe hypertension, diabetes with vascular involvement, headaches with focal neurological symptoms, major surgery with prolonged immobilization, carcinoma of the breast (current or past history of), carcinoma of the endometrium or other known or suspected estrogen dependent neoplasia, undiagnosed abnormal genital bleeding, cholestatic jaundice of pregnancy or jaundice with prior pill use, acute or chronic hepatocellular disease with abnormal liver function, hepatic adenomas or carcinomas, known or suspected pregnancy.

**WARNINGS/PRECAUTIONS:** Cigarette smoking increases risk of serious cardiovascular side effects; risk increases with age (especially >35 yrs) and heavy smoking. Increased risk of MI, vascular disease, thromboembolism, stroke, gallbladder disease, and hepatic neoplasia. May increase risk of breast cancer and cancer of the reproductive organs. Retinal thrombosis reported; d/c if unexplained partial or complete loss of vision, onset of proptosis or diplopia, papilledema, or retinal vascular lesions develop. May cause glucose intolerance, fluid retention, breakthrough bleeding, and spotting. May increase BP; d/c if significant elevations in BP occur. May elevate LDL levels or cause other lipid changes. May cause or exacerbate migraine headaches. May develop visual changes with contact lens. Increased risk of morbidity and mortality with HTN, hyperlipidemia, obesity, and DM. D/C if jaundice or if significant depression develops. Perform annual physical exam. Use before menarche is not indicated. Does not protect against HIV infection (AIDS) or other sexually transmitted diseases. May affect certain endocrine, LFTs, and blood components in laboratory tests.

**ADVERSE REACTIONS:** N/V, breakthrough bleeding, gastrointestinal symptoms (such as abdominal cramps, bloating), spotting, menstrual flow changes, amenorrhea, migraine, depression, vaginal candidiasis, edema, weight changes, cervical erosion and secretion

**INTERACTIONS:** Reduced effects resulting in breakthrough bleeding or unintended pregnancy may occur when co-administered with antibiotics, anticonvulsants, and other drugs that increase the metabolism of contraceptive steroids (eg, rifampin, barbiturates, phenylbutazone, phenytoin, carbamazepine, felbamate, oxcarbazepine, griseofulvin, topiramate, bosentan). HIV protease inhibitors may increase or decrease levels. St. John's wort may reduce contraceptive effectiveness and may result in breaktrough bleeding. Atorvastatin, ascorbic acid, acetaminophen, CYP3A4 inhibitors (eg, itraconazole, ketoconazole) may increase hormone levels. Increases levels of cyclosporine, prednisolone, and theophylline. Decreases levels of acetaminophen. Increases clearance of temazepam, salicylic acid, morphine, and clofibric acid. May significantly decrease plasma levels of lamotrigine; dosage adjustment of lamotrigine may be necessary.

**PREGNANCY:** Category X, not for use in nursing.

**MECHANISM OF ACTION:** Estrogen/progestogen combination oral contraceptive; acts by suppression of gonadotropins. Inhibits ovulation and produces changes in cervical mucus (increases difficulty of sperm entry into uterus) and the endometrium (reduces likelihood of implantation).

**PHARMACOKINETICS: Absorption:** Rapid. Oral administration of various doses led to altered parameters. **Distribution:** Found in breast milk. Norgestimate: Albumin binding (>97%). Ethinyl estradiol: Albumin binding (>97%). **Metabolism:** Norgestimate: GI tract and/or liver (1st pass mechanism), hepatic. Norelgestromin (primary active metabolite): Hepatic, norgestrel (active metabolite). Ethinyl estradiol: Hydroxylated, glucuronide, sulfate conjugates. **Elimination:** Norgestimate: Urine (47%), feces (37%).

## NURSING CONSIDERATIONS

**Assessment:** Assess for thrombophlebitis or past history of deep vein thrombophlebitis, current or history of thromboembolic disorders, current or history of cerebral vascular or coronary artery disease, diabetes with vascular involvement, headaches with focal neurological symptoms, major surgery with prolonged immobilization, presence or history of carcinoma of the breast, carcinoma of the endometrium or other known or suspected estrogen dependent neoplasia, undiagnosed abnormal genital bleeding, cholestatic jaundice of pregnancy or jaundice with prior pill use, acute or chronic hepatocellular disease with abnormal liver function, hepatic adenomas or carcinomas, and pregnancy. Assess use in patients >35 yrs old who smoke ≥15 cigarettes/day. Assess use with history of HTN, hyperlipidemia, obesity, or DM. Assess nursing status and for possible drug interactions.

**Monitoring:** Monitor for signs/symptoms of MI, thromboembolism, stroke, hepatic neoplasia, breast cancer and cancer of the reproductive organs, ocular lesions, bleeding irregularities, fluid retention, onset or exacerbation of migraine headaches, gallbladder disease, and ectopic pregnancy. Monitor serum glucose levels in DM and prediabetic patients. Monitor BP with history of HTN, lipid levels with history of hyperlipidemia, and for signs of worsening depression with previous history. Refer patients to an ophthalmologist if ocular changes develop. Perform annual physical exam while on therapy. Monitor liver function and for signs of liver toxicity (eg, jaundice).

**Patient Counseling:** Inform that drug does not protect against HIV infection (AIDS) and other STDs. Advise to avoid smoking while on medication.Counsel about potential adverse effects. Instruct to take as exactly as directed at intervals not exceeding 24 hrs. Advise about risk of pregnancy if dose is missed. Instruct that if one dose missed, take as soon as possible; take next pill at regularly scheduled time. Inform may experience spotting, light bleeding, or

O

stomach sickness during first 1-3 packs of pills; advise not to d/c medication and if symptoms persist, notify physician.

**Administration:** Oral route. **Storage:** 25°C (77°F); excursions permitted to 15-30°C (59-86°F). Protect from light.

## ORTHO-NOVUM 1/35 RX

ethinyl estradiol - norethindrone (Ortho-McNeil)

**OTHER BRAND NAMES:** Necon 1/35 (Watson) - Norinyl 1/35 (Watson) - Nortrel 1/35 (Barr)

**THERAPEUTIC CLASS:** Estrogen/progestogen combination

**INDICATIONS:** Prevention of pregnancy.

**DOSAGE:** *Adults:* 1 tab qd for 28 days, then repeat. Start 1st Sunday after onset of menstruation or 1st day of menstruation.

**HOW SUPPLIED:** Tab: (Ethinyl Estradiol-Norethindrone) 0.035mg-1mg

**CONTRAINDICATIONS:** Thrombophlebitis or thromboembolic disorders or past history of deep vein thrombophlebitis or thromboembolic disorders, cerebral vascular disease or coronary artery disease (CAD), known or suspected carcinoma of the breast, carcinoma of the endometrium or other known or suspected estrogen-dependent neoplasia, undiagnosed abnormal genital bleeding, cholestatic jaundice of pregnancy or jaundice with prior pill use, hepatic adenomas or carcinomas, pregnancy. (Ortho-Novum 1/35) History of cerebrovascular disease or CAD, valvular heart disease with complications, severe HTN, diabetes with vascular involvement, headaches with focal neurological symptoms, major surgery with prolonged immobilization, acute or chronic hepatocellular disease with abnormal liver function. (Norinyl 1/35) Benign liver tumors.

**WARNINGS/PRECAUTIONS:** Cigarette smoking increases risk of serious cardiovascular side effects; risk increases with age (especially >35 yrs) and heavy smoking ( ≥15 cigarettes/day). Increased risk of myocardial infarction (MI), vascular disease, thromboembolism, stroke, gallbladder disease, and hepatic neoplasia. Increased risk of morbidity and mortality in patients with HTN, hyperlipidemias, obesity, and diabetes. Retinal thrombosis reported; d/c if unexplained partial or complete loss of vision, onset of proptosis or diplopia, papilledema, or retinal vascular lesions develop. May cause glucose intolerance, fluid retention, breakthrough bleeding, and spotting. May increase BP; d/c if significant elevations in BP occur. May develop visual changes with contact lenses. May elevate LDL levels or cause other lipid changes. May cause or exacerbate migraine headaches. D/C if jaundice or if significant depression develops. Perform annual physical exam. Use before menarche is not indicated. May affect certain endocrine, LFTs, and blood components. Ectopic and intrauterine pregnancies may occur with contraceptive failures. Does not protect against HIV infection (AIDS) or other sexually transmitted diseases.

**ADVERSE REACTIONS:** N/V, breakthrough bleeding, spotting, amenorrhea, migraine, depression, vaginal candidiasis, edema, weight changes, abdominal cramps/bloating, menstrual flow changes, melasma.

**INTERACTIONS:** Reduced effects, increased breakthrough bleeding, and menstrual irregularities with rifampin, barbiturates, phenylbutazone, phenytoin, griseofulvin, and possibly with ampicillin and tetracyclines. (Ortho-Novum 1/35) Reduced effects, increased breakthrough bleeding may occur when coadministered with antibiotics, anticonvulsants, and other drugs that increase the metabolism of contraceptive steroids (eg, carbamazepine, felbamate, oxcarbazepine, topiramate, bosentan), and St. John's wort. Significant changes in plasma levels of estrogen and progestin may occur with coadministration with anti-HIV protease inhibitors. Concomitant use with atorvastatin, ascorbic acid, and acetaminophen may increase plasma estradiol levels. Concomitant use with CYP3A4 inhibitors (eg, itraconazole, ketoconazole) may increase plasma hormone levels. May increase plasma concentrations of cyclosporine, prednisolone, and theophylline. May decrease plasma concentrations of acetaminophen and lamotrigine. May increase clearance of temazepam, salicylic acid, morphine, and clofibric acid.

**PREGNANCY:** Category X, not for use in nursing.

**MECHANISM OF ACTION:** Estrogen/progestogen combination oral contraceptive; acts by suppression of gonadotropins. Primarily inhibits ovulation. Also produces other alterations including changes in the cervical mucus (increasing difficulty of sperm entry into uterus) and the endometrium (reducing likelihood of implantation).

**PHARMACOKINETICS: Distribution:** Found in breast milk.

## NURSING CONSIDERATIONS

**Assessment:** Assess for thrombophlebitis or a past history of deep vein thrombophlebitis, thromboembolic disorders or a past history of thromboembolic disorders, cerebral vascular disease or CAD, known or suspected carcinoma of the breast, carcinoma of the endometrium or other known or suspected estrogen-dependent neoplasia, undiagnosed abnormal genital bleeding, cholestatic jaundice of pregnancy or jaundice with prior pill use, hepatic adenomas or carcinomas, pregnancy/nursing status, and for possible drug interactions. Assess use in patients ≥35 yrs who smoke ≥15 cigarettes/day. Assess use in patients with HTN, hyperlipidemia, obesity, or diabetes. (Ortho Novum 1/35) Assess for history of cerebral vascular disease or CAD, valvular heart disease with complications, severe HTN, diabetes with vascular involvement, headaches with focal neurological symptoms, major surgery with prolonged immobilization, and for acute or chronic hepatocellular disease with abnormal liver function. (Norinyl 1/35) Assess for benign liver tumors.

**Monitoring:** Monitor for signs/symptoms of MI, thromboembolism, stroke, vascular disease, hepatic neoplasia, breast cancer and cancer of the reproductive organs, ocular lesions, bleeding irregularities, fluid retention, HTN, onset or exacerbation of migraine headaches, gallbladder disease, hypertriglyceridemia, and ectopic pregnancy. Monitor BP, serum glucose levels in DM and prediabetic patients, lipid levels with history of hyperlipidemia, and for signs of worsening depression with previous history. Monitor LFTs and for signs of liver dysfunction (eg, jaundice). Refer patients with contact lenses to ophthalmologist if ocular changes develop. Monitor liver function for liver abnormalities (eg, jaundice). Perform annual history and physical exam.

**Patient Counseling:** Counsel about possible side effects. Inform that drug does not protect against HIV infection (AIDS) and other STDs. Advise not to smoke while on therapy. Instruct to take 1 pill at same time daily at intervals not exceeding 24 hrs. Counsel if dose missed, take as soon as possible; take next dose at regularly scheduled time. Inform may have spotting, light bleeding or nausea during first 1-3 packs of pills; advise not to d/c medication and if symptoms persist, notify physician. Counsel that if vomiting/diarrhea develop or if taking other medications (eg, antibiotics) efficacy may decrease; use backup method of contraception.

**Administration:** Oral route. **Storage:** 25°C (77°F); excursions permitted to 15-30°C (59-86°F). (Norinyl 1/35) 15-25°C (59-77°F).

# ORTHO-NOVUM 10/11 RX

ethinyl estradiol - norethindrone (Ortho-McNeil)

**OTHER BRAND NAMES:** Necon 10/11 (Watson)

**THERAPEUTIC CLASS:** Estrogen/progestogen combination

**INDICATIONS:** Prevention of pregnancy.

**DOSAGE:** *Adults:* 1 tab qd for 28 days, then repeat. Start 1st Sunday after menses begin or 1st day of menses.

**HOW SUPPLIED:** Tab: (Ethinyl Estradiol-Norethindrone) 0.035mg-0.5mg and 0.035mg-1mg

**CONTRAINDICATIONS:** Thrombophlebitis, DVT or thromboembolic disorders, pregnancy, cerebrovascular or coronary artery disease, undiagnosed abnormal genital bleeding, cholestatic jaundice of pregnancy or jaundice with prior pill use, hepatic adenomas or carcinomas, breast cancer or other estrogen-dependent neoplasia.

**WARNINGS/PRECAUTIONS:** Cigarette smoking increases risk of serious cardiovascular side effects; risk increases with age (especially >35 yrs) and heavy smoking. Increased risk of MI, vascular disease, thromboembolism, stroke, and gallbladder disease. Retinal thrombosis, hepatic neoplasia reported. May cause glucose intolerance. May increase BP, elevate LDL levels or cause other lipid changes, fluid retention, breakthrough bleeding, and spotting. May cause or exacerbate migraine. May develop visual changes with contact lens. Morbidity and mortality risk increased with HTN, hyperlipidemia, obesity, and diabetes. D/C if jaundice, significant depression, or ophthalmic irregularities develop. Perform annual physical exam. Use before menarche is not indicated. May affect certain endocrine, LFTs, and blood components.

**ADVERSE REACTIONS:** NV, breakthrough bleeding, spotting, amenorrhea, migraine, depression, vaginal candidiasis, edema, weight changes.

**INTERACTIONS:** Reduced effects, increased breakthrough bleeding, and menstrual irregularities with rifampin, barbiturates, phenylbutazone, phenytoin, carbamazepine, and possibly with griseofulvin, ampicillin, and tetracyclines.

**PREGNANCY:** Category X, not for use in nursing.

**MECHANISM OF ACTION:** Estrogen/progestogen combination oral contraceptive; acts by suppressing gonadotropins. Primarily inhibits ovulation. Also causes changes in cervical mucus (increases difficulty of sperm entry into uterus) and endometrium (reduces likelihood of implantation).

**PHARMACOKINETICS: Distribution:** Found in breast milk.

## NURSING CONSIDERATIONS

**Assessment:** Assess for current or history of thrombophlebitis or thromboembolic disorders, cerebrovascular disease, CAD, valvular heart disease with complications, severe HTN, DM with vascular involvement, headaches with focal neurological symptoms, major surgery with prolonged immobilization, known/suspected carcinoma of breast, endometrium or other known/suspected estrogen-dependent neoplasia, undiagnosed abnormal genital bleeding, cholestatic jaundice of pregnancy or jaundice with prior pill use, acute or chronic hepatocellular disease with abnormal liver function, hepatic adenoma or carcinoma, and known/suspected pregnancy. Assess use with HTN, hyperlipidemias, obesity, DM, or in patients ≥35 yrs who smoke ≥15 cigarettes/day). Assess for possible drug interactions.



**Monitoring:** Monitor for signs/symptoms of MI, thromboembolism, stroke, vascular disease, hepatic neoplasia, ocular lesions, bleeding irregularities, fluid retention, onset or exacerbation of migraines or headaches, gallbladder disease, hypertriglyceridemia, HTN, and ectopic pregnancy. Monitor serum glucose levels in DM and prediabetic patients, lipid levels with history of hyperlipidemia, for signs of liver dysfunction (eg, jaundice), for signs of worsening depression with previous history. Refer patients with contact lenses to ophthalmologist if ocular changes develop. Perform annual physical exam while on medication.

**Patient Counseling:** Inform that does not protect against HIV infection and other STDs. Advise to avoid smoking while on therapy. Instruct to take 1 pill at same time daily, at intervals not exceeding 24 hrs. Instruct if dose is missed, take as soon as possible, then take next dose at regularly scheduled time. Inform may have spotting, light bleeding, or stomach upset during first 1-3 packs of pills; advise not to d/c medication and notify physician if symptoms persist. Inform if vomiting, having diarrhea, or taking concomitant medications, efficacy of medication may be affected; use backup forms of contraception.

**Administration:** Oral route. **Storage:** 25°C (77°F); excursions permitted to 15-30°C (59-86°F).

# ORTHO-NOVUM 7/7/7 RX

ethinyl estradiol - norethindrone (Ortho-McNeil)

**OTHER BRAND NAMES:** Nortrel 7/7/7 (Barr)

**THERAPEUTIC CLASS:** Estrogen/progestogen combination

**INDICATIONS:** Prevention of pregnancy.

**DOSAGE:** *Adults:* 28-day regimen: 1 tab qd for 28 days, then repeat. Start 1st Sunday after onset of menstruation or 1st day of menstruation. 21-day Regimen: 1 tab qd for 21 days. No tabs for 7 days then a new course is started. Start 1st Sunday after onset of menstruation or 1st day of menstruation. For the first cycle of a Sunday start regimen, another method of contraception should be used until after the first 7 consecutive days of administration.

**HOW SUPPLIED:** Tab: (Ethinyl Estradiol-Norethindrone) 0.035mg-0.5mg, 0.035mg-0.75mg, 0.035mg-1mg. [Nortel 7/7/7, 21 tabs, 28 tabs; Ortho-Novum 7/7/7, 28 tabs].

**CONTRAINDICATIONS:** Thrombophlebitis or thromboembolic disorders or past history of deep vein thrombophlebitis or thromboembolic disorders, cerebral vascular disease or coronary artery disease (CAD), known or suspected carcinoma of the breast, carcinoma of the endometrium or other known or suspected estrogen-dependent neoplasia, undiagnosed abnormal genital bleeding, cholestatic jaundice of pregnancy or jaundice with prior pill use, hepatic adenomas or carcinoma, pregnancy. (Ortho-Novum 7/7/7) History of cerebral vascular or CAD, valvular heart disease with complications, severe HTN, diabetes with vascular involvement, headaches with focal neurological symptoms, major surgery with prolonged immobilization, acute or chronic hepatocellular disease with abnormal liver function.

**WARNINGS/PRECAUTIONS:** Cigarette smoking increases risk of serious cardiovascular side effects; risk increases with age (especially >35 yrs) and heavy smoking ( ≥15 cigarettes per day). Increased risk of myocardial infarction (MI), vascular disease, thromboembolism, stroke, gallbladder disease, and hepatic neoplasia. May increase risk of breast cancer or cancer of the reproductive organs. Increased risk of morbidity and mortality in patients with HTN, hyperlipidemias, obesity, and diabetes. Retinal thrombosis reported; d/c if unexplained partial or complete loss of vision, onset of proptosis or diplopia, papilledema, or retinal vascular lesions develop. May cause glucose intolerance, fluid retention, breakthrough bleeding, and spotting. May increase BP; d/c if significant elevations in BP occur. May develop visual changes with contact lenses. May elevate LDL levels or cause other lipid changes. May cause or exacerbate migraine headaches. D/C if jaundice or if significant depression develops. Perform annual physical exam. Use before menarche is not indicated. May affect certain endocrine, LFTs, and blood components. Ectopic and intrauterine pregnancies may occur with contraceptive failures. Does not protect against HIV infection (AIDS) or other sexually transmitted diseases.

**ADVERSE REACTIONS:** N/V, breakthrough bleeding, spotting, amenorrhea, migraine, depression, vaginal candidiasis, edema, weight changes, abdominal cramps/bloating, menstrual flow changes, melasma.

**INTERACTIONS:** Reduced effects, increased breakthrough bleeding, and menstrual irregularities may occur with concomitant use of rifampin, barbiturates, phenylbutazone, phenytoin, carbamazepine, griseofulvin, and possibly with ampicillin and tetracyclines. (Ortho-Novum 7/7/7) Reduced effects, increased breakthrough bleeding may occur when coadministered with antibiotics, anticonvulsants, and other drugs that increase the metabolism of contraceptive steroids (eg, felbamate, oxcarbazepine, topiramate, bosentan), and St. John's wort. Significant changes in plasma levels of estrogen and progestin may occur with coadministration with anti-HIV protease inhibitors. Concomitant use with atorvastatin, ascorbic acid, and acetaminophen may increase plasma estradiol levels. Concomitant use with CYP3A4 inhibitors (eg, itraconazole, ketoconazole) may increase plasma hormone levels. May increase plasma concentrations of cyclosporine, prednisolone, and theophylline. May decrease plasma concentrations of acetaminophen and lamotrigine. May increase clearance of temazepam, salicylic acid, morphine, and clofibric acid.

O

**PREGNANCY:** Category X, not for use in nursing.

**MECHANISM OF ACTION:** Estrogen/progestogen combination oral contraceptive; acts by suppression of gonadotropins. Primarily inhibits ovulation. Also produces other alterations including changes in the cervical mucus (increasing difficulty of sperm entry into uterus) and the endometrium (reducing likelihood of implantation).

**PHARMACOKINETICS: Distribution:** Found in breast milk.

## NURSING CONSIDERATIONS

**Assessment:** Assess for thrombophlebitis or a past history of deep vein thrombophlebitis, thromboembolic disorders or a past history of thromboembolic disorders, cerebral vascular disease or CAD, known or suspected carcinoma of the breast, carcinoma of the endometrium or other known or suspected estrogen-dependent neoplasia, undiagnosed abnormal genital bleeding, cholestatic jaundice of pregnancy or jaundice with prior pill use, hepatic adenomas or carcinomas, pregnancy/nursing status, and for possible drug interactions. Assess use in patients ≥35 yrs who smoke ≥15 cigarettes/day. Assess use in patients with HTN, hyperlipidemia, obesity, or diabetes. (Ortho-Novum 7/7/7) Assess for history of cerebral vascular disease or CAD, valvular heart disease with complications, diabetes with vascular involvement, headaches with focal neurological symptoms, major surgery with prolonged immobilization, and for acute or chronic hepatocelluular disease with abnormal liver function.

**Monitoring:** Monitor for signs/symptoms of MI, thromboembolism, stroke, vascular disease, hepatic neoplasia, breast cancer and cancer of the reproductive organs, ocular lesions, bleeding irregularities, fluid retention, HTN, onset or exacerbation of migraine headaches, gallbladder disease, hypertriglyceridemia, and ectopic pregnancy. Monitor BP, serum glucose levels in DM and prediabetic patients, lipid levels with history of hyperlipidemia, and for signs of worsening depression with previous history. Monitor LFTs and for signs of liver dysfunction (eg, jaundice). Refer patients with contact lenses to an ophthalmologist if ocular changes develop. Perform annual history and physical exam.

O

**Patient Counseling:** Counsel about possible side effects. Inform that drug does not protect against HIV infection (AIDS) and other STDs. Advise not to smoke while on therapy. Instruct to take 1 pill at same time daily at intervals not exceeding 24 hrs. Counsel if dose missed, take as soon as possible; take next dose at regularly scheduled time. Inform may have spotting, light bleeding, or nausea during first 1-3 packs of pills; advise not to d/c medication and if symptoms persist, notify physician. Counsel that if vomiting/diarrhea develop or if taking other medication (eg, antibiotics) efficacy may decrease; use backup method of contraception.

**Administration:** Oral route. **Storage**: 25°C (77°F); excursions permitted to 15-30°C (59-86°F).

# OSMOPREP RX

sodium phosphate (Salix)

**Rare reports of serious acute phosphate nephropathy. Some cases resulted in permanent renal impairment requiring long-term dialysis. Patients at increased risk of acute phosphate nephropathy may include those with increased age, hypovolemia, increased bowel transit time (eg, bowel obstruction), active colitis, or baseline kidney disease, and if using medicines that affect renal perfusion or function (eg, diuretics, angiotensin converting enzyme [ACE] inhibitors, angiotensin receptor blockers [ARBs], and possibly NSAIDs). Use the recommended dose and dosing regimen (pm/am split dose).**

**THERAPEUTIC CLASS:** Bowel cleanser

**INDICATIONS:** For cleansing the colon in preparation for colonoscopy in adults ≥18 years of age.

**DOSAGE:** *Adults:* ≥18 yrs: Evening Before Colonoscopy Procedure: 4 tabs with 8oz clear liquids q15min for a total of 20 tabs. Day of Colonoscopy Procedure:

Starting 3-5 hrs before procedure, 4 tabs with 8oz of clear liquids q15min for a total of 12 tabs. Drink only clear liquids. Adequately hydrate before, during, and after use. Do not use within 7 days of previous administration. Do not take any additional enema or laxative, particularly one containing sodium phosphate.

**HOW SUPPLIED:** Tab: (Sodium Phosphate Monobasic Monohydrate-Sodium Phosphate Dibasic Anhydrous) 1.102g-0.398g

**CONTRAINDICATIONS:** Patients with biopsy-proven acute phosphate nephropathy.

**WARNINGS/PRECAUTIONS:** Fatalities reported due to significant fluid shifts, severe electrolyte abnormalities, and cardiac arrhythmias. Adequately hydrate before, during, and after use. Inadequate fluid intake may lead to excessive fluid loss, hypovolemia, and dehydration. Caution with impaired renal function, congestive heart failure (CHF), ascites, unstable angina, acute bowel obstruction, bowel perforation, toxic megacolon, gastric retention, ileus, pseudo-obstruction of the bowel, severe chronic constipation, acute colitis, gastric bypass, stapling surgery, hypomotility syndrome, history of acute phosphate nephropathy, known or suspected electrolyte disturbances. Correct electrolyte abnormalities before treatment. Consider baseline and post-colonoscopy labs (phosphate, calcium, $K^+$, Na, SrCr , BUN) in those that may be at increased risk for serious adverse events and measure post colonoscopy labs in patients who develop signs of vomiting and/or dehydration. Rare reports of generalized tonic-clonic seizures and/or loss of consciousness in patients without prior history of seizures. Caution in patients with history of seizures and in patients at higher risk of seizures (eg, patients withdrawing from alcohol or benzodiazepines, patients with known or suspected hyponatremia). Rare reports of serious arrhythmias, caution in patients with high risk of arrthymias. Prolongation of QT interval reported. Consider pre-dose and post-colonscopy ECGs in patients with high risk of serious cardiac arrhythmias and in patients with known prolonged QT interval. May induce colonic mucosal aphthous ulcerations and exacerbate inflammatory bowel disease (IBD).

**ADVERSE REACTIONS:** Abdominal bloating, abdominal pain, N/V, renal impairment, acute phosphate nephropathy.

**INTERACTIONS:** See Black Box Warning. Medications administered in close proximity to sodium phosphate tablets may not be absorbed from the GI tract. Caution if taking medications that may effect electrolyte levels (eg, diuretics), with medications that may reduce seizure threshold (eg, tricyclic antidepressants), or if taking medications known to prolong QT interval. Do not administer additional laxative or purgative agents.

**PREGNANCY:** Category C, safety not known in nursing.

**MECHANISM OF ACTION:** Purgative; not established. Primary actions thought to be through the osmotic effect of Na, causing large amounts of water to be drawn into the colon, promoting colon evacuation.

## NURSING CONSIDERATIONS

**Assessment:** Assess if at increased risk of developing acute phosphate nephropathy or biopsy- proven acute phosphate nephropathy. Assess use in patients with severe renal insufficiency or renal impairment, CHF, ascites, unstable angina, gastric retention, ileus, acute bowel obstruction, pseudo-obstruction of the bowel, severe chronic constipation, bowel perforation, acute colitis, toxic megacolon, presence of chronic inflammatory bowel disease, gastric bypass or stapling surgery, hypomotility syndrome, history of acute phosphate nephropathy, known or suspected electrolyte disturbances, patients with history of seizures or patients at increased risk of seizures, and in patients with higher risk of arrhythmias. Consider baseline labs (phosphate, calcium, $K^+$, Na, SrCr, BUN) in patients who may be at increased risk for serious adverse events. Consider pre-dose ECG in patients with known prolonged QT or in patients with serious risk of cardiac arrhythmias. Assess pregnancy/nursing status and for possible drug interactions.

**Monitoring:** Monitor for signs and symptoms of acute phosphate nephropathy, fluid shifts, severe electrolyte abnormalities, cardiac arrhythmias, renal failure, nephrocalcinosis, generalized tonic-clonic seizures, loss of consciousness,

O

cardiac arrhythmias, QT prolongation, and colonic mucosal aphthous ulcerations. Consider performing post-colonscopy labs (phosphate, calcium, phosphate, Na, $K^+$, SrCr, BUN) in patients at increased risk for adverse events or if develop vomiting or signs of dehydration. Consider post colonoscopy ECG in patients with high risk of serious cardiac arrhythmias or in patients with known prolonged QT.

**Patient Counseling:** Stress importance of adequate hydration before, during, and after use. Instruct to drink 8oz of clear liquid with each 4-tab dose. Instruct to contact physician if experience symptoms of dehydration. Instruct not to use within 7 days of previous administration and to not to administer additional laxative or purgative agents, particularly additional sodium phosphate-based products. Instruct to contact physician if develop worsening of bloating, abdominal pain, N/V, or headache.

**Administration:** Oral route. **Storage:** 25°C (77°F); excursions permitted to 15-30°C (59-86°F). Discard any unused portion.

## OVACE — RX

sulfacetamide sodium (Healthpoint)

**THERAPEUTIC CLASS:** Sulfonamide

**INDICATIONS:** Topical application for seborrheic dermatitis, seborrhea sicca (dandruff). Treatment of secondary bacterial infections of the skin.

**DOSAGE:** *Adults:* Seborrheic Dermatitis/Dandruff: (Cre/Gel/Foam) Apply to affected area bid for 8-10 days. (Wash) Wash affected area bid for 8-10 days. To prevent recurrence, apply once or twice weekly, or every other week. Bacterial Infection: (Cre/Gel) Apply to affected area bid for 8-10 days. (Foam) Apply to affected area qd for 8-10 days. (Wash) Wash affected area qd for 8-10 days.

**HOW SUPPLIED:** Cre: 10% [30g, 60g]; Gel: 10% [30g, 60g]; Foam: 10% [50g, 100g]; Wash: 10% [170mL, 340mL]

**CONTRAINDICATIONS:** Hypersensitivity to sulfonamides.

O

**WARNINGS/PRECAUTIONS:** Stevens-Johnson syndrome in hypersensitive individuals, and systemic lupus erythematous reported with sulfonamides. May cause proliferation of nonsusceptible organisms. D/C if hypersensitivity or untoward reactions occur. Greater systemic absorption in application to large, infected, abraded, denuded or severely burned area.

**ADVERSE REACTIONS:** Irritation, hypersensitivity.

**INTERACTIONS:** Incompatible with silver preparations.

**PREGNANCY:** Category C, caution in nursing.

**MECHANISM OF ACTION:** Sulfonamide; exerts a bacteriostatic effect against susceptible gram-positive and gram-negative microorganisms. Acts by restricting the synthesis of folic acid required by bacteria for growth, through competition with paraminobenzoic acid (PABA).

### NURSING CONSIDERATIONS

**Assessment:** Assess for sulfonamide hypersensitivity. Assess use in pregnant/nursing females. Assess for possible drug interactions.

**Monitoring:** Monitor for signs/symptoms of hypersensitivity reactions, Stevens-Johnson syndrome, drug-induced systemic lupus erythematosus, overgrowth of nonsusceptible organism (eg, fungi). In patients applying medication to a large, infected, abraded, denuded, or severely burned area, monitor for increased occurrence of adverse drug events.

**Patient Counseling:** Counsel to d/c therapy and notify physician if condition worsens or if rash develops. Instruct to contact physician if any signs of arthritis, fever, or sores of the mouth develop while on medication.

**Administration:** Topical route. **Storage**: 20-25°C (68-77°F). Do not freeze. Keep out of reach of children.

# Ovcon-35 RX

ethinyl estradiol - norethindrone (Warner Chilcott)

**OTHER BRAND NAMES:** Ovcon-50 (Warner Chilcott) - Balziva (Barr)
**THERAPEUTIC CLASS:** Estrogen/progestogen combination
**INDICATIONS:** Prevention of pregnancy.

**DOSAGE:** *Adults:* 1 tab qd for 28 days, then repeat. Start 1st Sunday after menses begin or the 1st day of menses.
*Pediatrics:* Postpubertal adolescents ≥16 yrs: 1 tab qd for 28 days, then repeat. Start 1st Sunday after menses begin or the 1st day of menses.

**HOW SUPPLIED:** Tab: (Ethinyl Estradiol-Norethindrone) (Ovcon 35, Balziva) 0.035mg-0.4mg; (Ovcon 50) 0.05mg-1mg

**CONTRAINDICATIONS:** Thrombophlebitis or thromboembolic disorders, past history of deep vein thrombophlebitis or thromboembolic disorders, cerebrovascular or coronary artery disease (CAD), known or suspected carcinoma of the breast, endometrial carcinoma or other known or suspected estrogen-dependent neoplasia, undiagnosed abnormal genital bleeding, cholestatic jaundice of pregnancy or jaundice with prior pill use, hepatic adenomas or carcinomas, known or suspected pregnancy.

**WARNINGS/PRECAUTIONS:** Cigarette smoking increases risk of serious cardiovascular side effects; risk increases with age (especially >35 yrs) and heavy smoking (>15 cigarettes/day). Increased risk of myocardial infarction (MI), thromboembolism, cerebrovascular events, breast cancer, cancer of the reproductive organs, gallbladder disease, and hepatic neoplasia. Increased risk of morbidity and mortality in patients with HTN, hyperlipidemia, obesity, and diabetes mellitus (DM). Retinal thrombosis reported; d/c if unexplained partial or complete loss of vision, onset of proptosis or diplopia, papilledema, or retinal vascular lesions develop. May cause glucose intolerance; monitor prediabetic and diabetic patients. May cause fluid retention and increase BP; monitor closely with HTN and d/c if significant elevation of BP occurs. May cause onset or exacerbation of migraine or development of headaches. Breakthrough bleeding and spotting reported; rule out malignancy or pregnancy. Monitor closely with hyperlipidemias. D/C if jaundice develops. Monitor closely with depression and d/c if depression recurs to serious degree. May develop visual changes with contact lenses. Does not protect against HIV infection (AIDS) or other sexually transmitted diseases. Perform annual physical exam. Use before menarche is not indicated. May affect certain endocrine, LFTs, and blood components in laboratory tests. Should not be used to induce withdrawal bleeding as a test for pregnancy, or to treat threatened or habitual abortion during pregnancy.

**ADVERSE REACTIONS:** N/V, breakthrough bleeding, GI symptoms(such as abdominal cramps, bloating), spotting, menstrual flow changes, amenorrhea, migraine, depression, vaginal candidiasis, edema, weight changes, cervical erosion and secretion.

**INTERACTIONS:** Reduced effects, increased breakthrough bleeding, and menstrual irregularities with rifampin, barbiturates, phenylbutazone, phenytoin sodium, and possibly with griseofulvin, ampicillin, and tetracyclines.

**PREGNANCY:** Category X, not for use in nursing.

**MECHANISM OF ACTION:** Estrogen/progestogen combination oral contraceptive; acts by suppressing gonadotropins. Primarily inhibits ovulation. Also produces other alterations including changes in the cervical mucus (increases difficulty of sperm entry into uterus) and endometrium (reduces likelihood of implantation).

**PHARMACOKINETICS: Distribution**: Found in breast milk.

## NURSING CONSIDERATIONS

**Assessment:** Assess for thrombophlebitis or past history of DVT or thromboembolic disorders, cerebrovascular or CAD, known/suspected carcinoma of breast and endometrium or other known/suspected estrogen dependent-neoplasia, undiagnosed abnormal genital bleeding, cholestatic jaundice of

O

pregnancy or jaundice with prior pill use, hepatic adenomas or carcinomas, and known/suspected pregnancy. Assess use in patients ≥35 yrs who smoke ≥15 cigarettes/day, with HTN, hyperlipidemia, obesity, and DM.

**Monitoring:** Monitor for signs/symptoms of thromboembolism, stroke, MI, hepatic neoplasia, gallbladder disease, vascular disease, breast cancer and cancer of the reproductive organs, ocular lesions, onset or exacerbation of migraine headaches, HTN, hypertriglyceridemia, breakthrough bleeding, spotting, fluid retention, and jaundice. Monitor BP in patients with a history of HTN, HTN related disease, or renal disease. Monitor for signs of depression in patients with a history of depression. Perform annual history and physical exam. Monitor serum glucose levels in prediabetic and diabetic patients. Monitor lipid levels in patients with a history of hyperlipidemia. Refer patients with contact lenses to an ophthalmologist if visual changes or changes in lens tolerance develop.

**Patient Counseling:** Inform that medication does not protect against HIV/AIDS and other STDs. Counsel about possible serious side effects. Advise to avoid smoking while on therapy. Instruct to take 1 pill at same time daily. If dose missed, take as soon as remembered; take next dose at usual time. If spotting, light bleeding, or nausea occurs during first 1-3 packs of pills, advise not to d/c medication and if symptoms persist, notify physician. Inform if vomiting, diarrhea or taking other medications, efficacy may decrease; use backup method of contraception.

**Administration:** Oral route. **Storage:** (Ovcon 35, Balziva) 20-25°C (68-77°F). (Ovcon 50) Below 30°C (86°F).

## Ovcon-35 Fe — RX

ethinyl estradiol - ferrous fumarate - norethindrone (Warner Chilcott)

**THERAPEUTIC CLASS:** Estrogen/progestogen combination

**INDICATIONS:** Prevention of pregnancy.

**DOSAGE:** *Adults:* 1 tab qd for 28 days, then repeat. Start 1st Sunday after menses begin or the 1st day of menses.

**HOW SUPPLIED:** Tab, Chewable: (Ethinyl Estradiol-Norethindrone) 0.035mg-0.4mg [21[s]], (Ferrous Fumarate) 75mg [7[s]]

**CONTRAINDICATIONS:** Thrombophlebitis, DVT or thromboembolic disorders, pregnancy, cerebrovascular or coronary artery disease, valvular heart disease with thrombogenic complications, uncontrolled HTN, DM with vascular involvement, HA with focal neurological symptoms, major surgery with prolonged immobilization, undiagnosed abnormal genital bleeding, cholestatic jaundice of pregnancy or jaundice with prior pill use, hepatic adenomas or carcinomas, breast cancer, endometrial cancer or other estrogen-dependent neoplasia.

**WARNINGS/PRECAUTIONS:** Cigarette smoking increases risk of serious cardiovascular side effects; risk increases with age (especially >35 yrs) and heavy smoking. Increased risk of MI, vascular disease, thromboembolism, stroke and gallbladder disease. Retinal thrombosis, hepatic neoplasia, carcinoma of breast and reproductive organs reported. May cause glucose intolerance. May increase BP, elevate LDL levels or cause other lipid changes, fluid retention, breakthrough bleeding, and spotting. May cause or exacerbate migraine. May develop visual changes with contact lens. Increased risk of MI with HTN, hyperlipidemia, obesity, and diabetes. D/C if jaundice, significant depression, or ophthalmic irregularities develop. Perform annual physical exam. Use before menarche is not indicated. May affect certain endocrine, LFTs and blood components.

**ADVERSE REACTIONS:** N/V, breakthrough bleeding, spotting, amenorrhea, migraine, depression, vaginal candidiasis, edema, weight changes.

**INTERACTIONS:** Reduced effects, increased breakthrough bleeding, and menstrual irregularities with rifampin, barbiturates, phenylbutazone, phenytoin, carbamazepine, felbamate, oxcarbazepine, topiramate, griseofulvin, ampicillin, and tetracyclines. Anti-HIV PIs may change (increase or decrease) the levels of OCs. Herbal products, such as St. John's wort may reduce the levels of OCs and result in breakthrough bleeding. Atorvastatin, ascorbic acid, acetaminophen, CYP3A4 inhibitors (itraconazole or ketoconazole) may increase the levels of ethinyl estradiol. Increased levels of cyclosporine, prednisolone, theophylline reported. Decreased levels of acetaminophen and increased clearance of temazepam, salicylic acid, morphine, clofibric acid reported.

**PREGNANCY:** Category X, not for use in nursing.

**MECHANISM OF ACTION:** Estrogen/progestogen combination oral contraceptive; acts by suppressing gonadotropins. Primarily inhibits ovulation. Also causes changes in cervical mucus (increases difficulty of sperm entry ino uterus) and endometrium (reduces likehood of implantation).

**PHARMACOKINETICS: Absorption:** Rapid. Norethindrone: Absolute bioavailability (65%), $C_{max}$=4210.6pg/mL, $T_{max}$=1.24 hr, AUC=18034.9pg•h/mL. Ethinyl estradiol: Absolute bioavailability (43%), $C_{max}$=131.4pg/mL, $T_{max}$=1.44 hrs, AUC=1065.8pg•h/mL. **Distribution:** $V_d$=2-4L/kg; Norethindone: Sex hormone-binding globulin binding (36%), albumin binding (61%). Ethinyl estradiol: Albumin binding (98.5%). **Metabolism:** Norethindone: Reduction, sulfate, glucuronide conjugation. Ethinyl estradiol: CYP3A4, via oxidation (conjugation with sulfate and glucuronide), 2-hydroxy-ethinyl estradiol (primary oxidative metabolite). **Elimination:** Norethindrone: Urine (50%), feces (20-40%); $T_{1/2}$=9 hrs. Ethinyl Estradiol: Urine, feces; $T_{1/2}$=17 hrs.

## NURSING CONSIDERATIONS

**Assessment:** Assess for current or history of thrombophlebitis or thromboembolic disorder, cerebrovascular disease, CAD, valvular heart disease with thrombogenic complications, uncontrolled HTN, DM with vascular involvement, headaches with focal neurological problems, major surgery with prolonged immobilization, known/suspected carcinoma of breast, endometrium or other known/suspected estrogen-dependent neoplasia, abnormal genital bleeding, cholestatic jaundice, hepatic adenomas or carcinoma, and known/suspected pregnancy. Assess use with inherited thrombophilias, HTN, hyperlipidemias, obesity, DM, or in patients ≥35 yrs who smoke ≥15 cigarettes/day. Assess for possible drug/lab test interactions.

**Monitoring:** Monitor for venous and arterial thrombotic events (eg, MI, thromboembolism, stroke), hepatic neoplasias, ocular lesions, bleeding irregularities, fluid retention, onset or exacerbation of headaches or migraines, gallbladder disease, hypertriglyceridemia, and HTN. Monitor blood glucose levels in DM and prediabetic patients, BP with history of HTN, lipid levels with history of hyperlipidemia, for signs of liver dysfunction (eg, jaundice), and of worsening depression with previous history. Refer patients with contact lenses to an ophthalmologist if visual changes occur. Perform annual history and physical exam.

**Patient Counseling:** Advise about possible serious cardiovascular and respiratory effects. Inform that medication does not protect against HIV infection (AIDS) and other STDs. Advise to avoid smoking while on medication. Instruct to take medication at same time daily. Instruct if dose missed, take as soon as possible; take next pill at regularly scheduled time. Inform may have spotting, light bleeding, or stomach upset during first 1-3 packs of pills; advise not to d/c medication and if symptoms persist, notify physician. If vomiting, diarrhea, or taking other medications may alter efficacy; use backup forms of contraception. Perform regular physical exams.

**Administration:** Oral route. **Storage:** 25° (77°F); excursions permitted to 15-30°C (59-86°F).

# OxyContin

CII

oxycodone HCl (Purdue Pharma)

**For continuous analgesia. Not for prn analgesia. Abuse potential. 60mg and 80mg, or a single dose greater than 40mg tabs only for opioid-tolerant patients. A single dose of >40mg or total daily doses >80mg may cause fatal respiratory depression. Swallow tabs whole.**

O

**THERAPEUTIC CLASS:** Opioid analgesic

**INDICATIONS:** Management of moderate to severe pain when a continuous, around-the-clock analgesic is needed for an extended period of time. Only for postoperative use in patients already receiving the drug before surgery or those expected to have moderate-severe postoperative pain for an extended period of time.

**DOSAGE:** *Adults:* ≥18 yrs: Individualize dose. Opioid-Naive: 10mg q12h. Titrate: May increase the total daily dose by 25-50% of the current dose. Increase every 1-2 days. Conversion from Oxycodone: Divide 24-hr oxycodone dose in half to obtain q12h dose. Round down to appropriate tab strength. Refer to PI for conversion from other opioid analgesics. Opioid-Tolerant Patients: May use 60mg and 80mg, or a single dose >40mg. D/C other around-the-clock opioids. With CNS Depressants: Reduce dose by 1/3 or 1/2.

**HOW SUPPLIED:** Tab, Extended-Release: 10mg, 15mg, 20mg, 30mg, 40mg, 60mg, 80mg,

**CONTRAINDICATIONS:** Significant respiratory depression (in unmonitored settings or the absence of resuscitative equipment), acute or severe bronchial asthma, hypercarbia, or in any patient who has or is suspected of having paralytic ileus.

**WARNINGS/PRECAUTIONS:** Taking broken, chewed, or crushed tabs leads to rapid release and absorption of a potentially fatal dose. Extreme caution with COPD, cor pulmonale, decreased respiratory reserve, hypoxia, hypercapnia, pre-existing respiratory depression. The respiratory depressant effects of opioids may be markedly exaggerated in the presence of head injury, intracranial lesions, or other sources of pre-existing increased intracranial pressure. Caution with circulatory shock, delirium tremens, acute alcoholism, adrenocortical insufficiency, CNS depression, myxedema or hypothyroidism, BPH, severe hepatic/renal/pulmonary impairment, toxic psychosis, biliary tract disease, increased intracranial pressure (ICP) or head injury, elderly or debilitated. May cause severe hypotension; increased risk in patients with depleted blood volume. Has been reported as being abused by crushing, chewing, snorting, or injecting the dissolved product. May produce drug dependence; caution in known drug abuse. May aggravate convulsive disorders and mask abdominal disorders.



**ADVERSE REACTIONS:** Respiratory depression, apnea, respiratory arrest, circulatory depression, hypotension, shock, constipation, N/V, somnolence, dizziness, pruritus, headache, dry mouth, sweating, asthenia.

**INTERACTIONS:** Respiratory depression, hypotension, and profound sedation with other CNS depressants (eg, sedatives, tranquilizers, centrally acting antiemetics, anesthetics, phenothiazines, alcohol). Mixed agonist/antagonist analgesics may reduce the analgesic effect and/or cause withdrawal. Risk of severe hypotension with phenothiazines, or other agents that compromise vasomotor tone. May enhance skeletal muscle relaxant effects and increase respiratory depression. May interact with CYP2D6 inhibitors (eg, amiodarone, quinidine, polycyclic antidepressants). Caution with MAOIs. Increased plasma concentration with CYP3A4 inhibitors such as macrolide antibiotics (eg, erythromycin), azole-antifungal agents (eg, ketoconazole), and protease inhibitors (eg, ritonavir). Decreased plasma concentration with CYP450 inducers such as rifampin, carbamazepine, and phenytoin.

**PREGNANCY:** Category B, not for use in nursing.

**MECHANISM OF ACTION:** Opioid analgesic; pure agonist opioid whose principal therapeutic action is analgesia. Precise analgesic action not established. However, specific CNS opioid receptors for endogenous compounds with opioid-like activity have been found throughout the brain and spinal cord, and play a role in analgesic effects.

**PHARMACOKINETICS: Absorption:** Well absorbed, various doses resulted in altered parameters. Absolute bioavailability (60-87%). **Distribution:** $V_d$=2.6L/kg; plasma protein binding (45%); found in breast milk. **Metabolism:** Extensively to noroxycodone (major metabolite) via CYP3A4, oxymorphone (active metabolite) via CYP2D6, noroxymorphone via CYP2D6 and CYP3A4. **Elimination:** Urine (19% free oxycodone, 50% conjugated oxycodone, ≤14% conjugated oxymorphone); $T_{1/2}$=4.5 hrs.

## NURSING CONSIDERATIONS

**Assessment:** Before initiating therapy assess the general condition and medical status of the patient; their daily dose, potency, and kind of analgesic(s) they're been taking; their opioid exposure and opioid tolerance (if any). Assess for respiratory depression, type and level of pain, acute or severe bronchial asthma or hypercarbia, COPD or cor pulmonale, kyphoscoliosis, paralytic ileus, risk for drug misuse or abuse, head injury, intracranial lesions, increased ICP, circulatory shock, acute alcoholism, adrenocortical insufficiency (eg, Addison's disease), CNS depression or coma, delirium tremens, presence of debilitation (eg, elderly), myxedema or hypothyroidism, prostatic hypertrophy or urethral stricture, hepatic/renal impairment, presence of acute abdominal conditions, biliary tract disease, acute pancreatitis, toxic psychosis, convulsive seizures, pregnancy/nursing status, and possible drug interactions.

**Monitoring:** Monitor for signs/symptoms of respiratory depression, elevations in CSF pressure, hypotension, spasm of sphincter of Oddi, tolerance and physical dependence, and abuse/misuse of medication. Monitor serum amylase levels.

**Patient Counseling:** Instruct to swallow medication whole; do not break, chew, or crush. If broken or chewed, contents may release all at once and cause fatal overdose. Advise to report episodes of breakthough pain or adverse events (eg, respiratory depression). Do not adjust dosing without consulting physician. May impair mental/physical abilities; use caution if performing hazardous tasks (eg, operating machinery, driving). Avoid alcohol or other CNS depressants. Inform that medication has potential for abuse; protect from theft. Inform patient may pass empty matrix tablets via stool. If on medication for more than a few weeks, avoid abrupt withdrawal; taper dosing. Keep out of reach of children. Dispose of any unused medication via toilet.

**Administration:** Oral route. Swallow whole; do not break, crush, or chew. **Storage:** 25°C (77°F); excursions permitted to 15-30°C (59-86°F). Dispense in tight, light-resistant container.

# OxyIR

**CII**

oxycodone HCl (Purdue Pharma)

**THERAPEUTIC CLASS:** Opioid analgesic

**INDICATIONS:** Moderate to moderately severe pain.

**DOSAGE:** *Adults:* Usual: 5mg q6h prn for pain. May add to 30mL of juice or other liquid, applesauce, pudding, or other semi-solid foods.

**HOW SUPPLIED:** Cap: 5mg

**CONTRAINDICATIONS:** Respiratory depression, acute or severe bronchial asthma, hypercarbia, paralytic ileus, situations where opioids are contraindicated.

**WARNINGS/PRECAUTIONS:** Extreme caution with COPD, cor pulmonale, decreased respiratory reserve, hypoxia, hypercapnia, pre-existing respiratory depression. Caution with circulatory shock, delirium tremens, acute alcoholism, adrenocortical insufficiency, CNS depression, myxedema or hypothyroidism, BPH, severe hepatic/renal/pulmonary impairment, toxic psychosis, biliary tract disease, increased ICP, or head injury, elderly or debilitated. May cause severe hypotension. May produce drug dependence; caution in known drug abuse. May aggravate convulsive disorders and mask abdominal disorders. May impair mental/physical abilities.

**ADVERSE REACTIONS:** Lightheadedness, dizziness, NV, sedation.

**INTERACTIONS:** Respiratory depression, hypotension and profound sedation with other CNS depressants (eg, sedatives, anesthetics, phenothiazines, alcohol). Mixed agonist/antagonist analgesics may reduce the analgesic effect and/or cause withdrawal. Risk of severe hypotension with phenothiazines, or other agents that compromise vasomotor tone. May enhance skeletal muscle relaxant effects and increase respiratory depression. May interact with CYP2D6 inhibitors (eg, amiodarone, quinidine, polycyclic antidepressants). Caution with MAOIs.

**PREGNANCY:** Category B, not for use in nursing.

**MECHANISM OF ACTION:** Opioid analgesic; pure agonist opioid whose principle therapeutic effect is analgesia. Precise action not established. However, specific CNS opioid receptors for endogenous compounds with opioid-like activity are found throughout the brain and spinal cord and play a role in analgesic effects.

**PHARMACOKINETICS: Distribution:** Found in breast milk. **Metabolism:** Via CYP2D6 to oxymorphone (metabolite).

## NURSING CONSIDERATIONS

**Assessment:** Assess for respiratory depression, acute or severe bronchial asthma or hypercarbia, chronic obstructive pulmonary disease, paralytic ileus, circulatory shock, pregnancy/nursing status, acute alcoholism, adrenocortical insufficiency (eg, Addison's disease), CNS depression or coma, delirium tremens, presence of debilitation (eg, elderly), kyphoscoliosis associated with respiratory depression, myxedema or hypothyroidism, prostatic hypertrophy or urethral stricture, severe impairment of hepatic/renal function, toxic psychosis, convulsive disorders, biliary tract disease, acute pancreatitis, presence of head injury or other intracranial lesions, presence of increased ICP, acute abdominal condition, and possible drug interactions.

**Monitoring:** Monitor for signs/symptoms of respiratory depression, hypotension, convulsions, medication dependence and tolerance, medication abuse, sphincter of Oddi spasms, elevations in CSF pressure, and elevations in serum amylase levels.

**Patient Counseling:** Advise not to adjust dosing without consulting physician. Inform that medication may impair mental/physical abilities required for performing hazardous tasks (eg, operating machinery/driving). Counsel to avoid alcohol and other CNS depressants. Inform medication has potential for abuse; protect from theft. Advise not to abruptly d/c medication if on therapy for a few weeks; taper dosing.

**Administration:** Oral route. **Storage:** 25°C (77°F); excursions permitted to 15-30°C (59-86°F).



# OXYTROL RX

oxybutynin (Watson)

**THERAPEUTIC CLASS:** Anticholinergic

**INDICATIONS:** Treatment of overactive bladder with symptoms of urge urinary incontinence, urgency, and frequency.

**DOSAGE:** *Adults:* Apply 3.9mg qd system to dry, intact skin on the abdomen, hip, or buttock twice weekly (every 3-4 days). Rotate sites; avoid reapplication to same site for 7 days.

**HOW SUPPLIED:** Patch: 3.9mg qd [8[s]]

**CONTRAINDICATIONS:** Urinary retention, gastric retention, uncontrolled narrow-angle glaucoma, and in patients at risk for these conditions.

**WARNINGS/PRECAUTIONS:** Caution with hepatic or renal impairment, bladder outflow obstruction, GI obstructive disorders, ulcerative colitis, intestinal atony, myasthenia gravis, and gastroesophageal reflux disease (GERD). Heat prostration may occur when used in a hot environment.

**ADVERSE REACTIONS:** Application-site reactions, dry mouth, diarrhea, constipation, drowsiness, dizziness, blurred vision.

**INTERACTIONS:** Increased adverse events with other anticholinergics. Alcohol may enhance drowsiness effect. Caution with bisphosphonates or other drugs that may exacerbate esophagitis. May alter GI absorption of other drugs due to GI motility effects.

**PREGNANCY:** Category B, caution in nursing.

**MECHANISM OF ACTION:** Antispasmodic, anticholinergic agent; acts as competitive antagonist of acetylcholine at postganglionic muscarinic receptors, resulting in relaxation of bladder smooth muscle.

**PHARMACOKINETICS: Absorption:** (Single dose) $C_{max}$=3-3.4ng/mL; $T_{max}$=36-48 hrs. (Multiple dose) $C_{max}$=4.2-6.6ng/mL; $T_{max}$=10-28 hrs. **Distribution:** $V_d$=193L. **Metabolism:** Liver; CYP3A4, N-desethyloxybutynin (active metabolite). **Elimination:** Urine (<0.1% unchanged, <0.1% N-desethyloxybutynin); $T_{1/2}$=7-8 hrs.

## NURSING CONSIDERATIONS

**Assessment:** Assess for bladder outflow obstruction (urinary retention), GI obstructive disorders (gastric retention), narrow-angle glaucoma, possible drug interactions, GERD, esophagitis, ulcerative colitis, intestinal atony, myasthenia gravis, renal/hepatic impairment. Assess pregnancy/nursing status.

**Monitoring:** Monitor for signs/symptoms of gastric retention, urinary retention, decreased gastric motility, hypersensitivity reactions, renal/hepatic dysfunction.

**Patient Counseling:** Inform that heat prostration may occur in hot environment. Dizziness and blurred vision may also occur. Alcohol may enhance drowsiness. Instruct to apply to dry, intact skin on abdomen, hip, or buttocks. Avoid reapplication to same site for 7 days.

**Administration:** Transdermal route. **Storage:** 25°C (77°F); excursions permitted to 15-30°C (59-86°F). Protect from moisture and humidity. Do not store outside the sealed pouch. Apply immediately after removal from protective pouch.

# PACERONE — RX

amiodarone HCl (Upsher-Smith)

**THERAPEUTIC CLASS:** Class III antiarrhythmic

**INDICATIONS:** Treatment of documented, life-threatening recurrent ventricular fibrillation and recurrent hemodynamically unstable ventricular tachycardia when these conditions have not responded to available antiarrhythmics or other available agents.

**DOSAGE:** *Adults:* Give LD in hospital. LD: 800-1600mg/day in divided doses for 1-3 weeks. After control is achieved, then 600-800mg/day for 1 month. Maint: 400mg/day; up to 600mg/day if needed. Use lowest effective dose. Take with meals. Elderly: Start at low end of dosing range.

**HOW SUPPLIED:** Tab: 100mg, 200mg*, *scored

**CONTRAINDICATIONS:** Severe sinus-node dysfunction causing marked sinus bradycardia; 2nd- and 3rd-degree AV block; when episodes of bradycardia have caused syncope (except when used with a pacemaker); cardiogenic shock

**WARNINGS/PRECAUTIONS:** Only for life-threatening arrhythmias due to its substantial toxicity (eg, pulmonary toxicity, hepatic injury, arrhythmia exacerbation). Hospitalize when giving LD. May cause a clinical syndrome of cough and progressive dyspnea. D/C if LFTs are 3x ULN or if an elevated baseline doubles; monitor LFTs regularly. Optic neuropathy, optic neuritis reported. May develop reversible corneal microdeposits (eg, visual halos, blurred vision), photosensitivity, peripheral neuropathy (rare). Fetal harm in pregnancy; reports of congenital goiter/hypothyroidism and hyperthyroidism. May decrease $T_3$ levels, increase thyroxine levels, increase inactive reverse $T_3$ levels in clinically euthyroid patients and cause hyperthyroidism. Hyperthyroidism may result in thyrotoxicosis and/or arrhythmia breakthrough or aggravation. Adult Respiratory Distress Syndrome (ARDS) reported with surgery. Correct $K^+$ or magnesium deficiency before therapy. Caution in elderly. Assess threshold in patients with implanted pacemakers or defibrillators before initiation of treatment.

**ADVERSE REACTIONS:** Pulmonary toxicity (inflammation, fibrosis), arrhythmia exacerbation, hepatic injury, malaise, fatigue, tremor, poor coordination, paresthesis, N/V, constipation, anorexia, ophthalmic abnormalities.

**INTERACTIONS:** Risk of interactions after D/C due to long half-life. May increase sensitivity to myocardial depressant and conduction effects of halogenated inhalation anesthetics. Reports of sinus bradycardia with lidocaine, and hypotension, bradycardia and decreased cardiac output with fentanyl. CYP3A4 inhibitors may decrease metabolism and increase serum levels (eg, protease inhibitors, loratidine, cimetidine, trazodone, grapefruit juice). Monitor for amiodarone toxicity with protease inhibitors, and ECG changes with loratidine and trazodone. CYP3A4 inducers may accelerate metabolism and decrease levels, potentially decreasing efficacy (eg, St. John's wort, rifampin). Cholestyramine increases enterohepatic elimination resulting in decreased levels and $T_{1/2}$. May increase levels of CYP3A4 substrates (eg, cyclosporine, HMG CoA reductase inhibitors). Reports of elevated SrCr with cyclosporine and myopathy/rhabdomyolysis with atorvastatin and simvastatin. May impair dextromethorphan, methotrexate and phenytoin metabolism with chronic use (>2 wks). D/C or decrease digoxin dose by 50%. D/C or decrease warfarin dose by 1/3-1/2. Ineffective inhibition of platelet aggregation reported with clopidogrel. Caution with β-blockers, calcium channel blockers. May increase levels of quinidine, procainamide, flecainide, and phenytoin. D/C or decrease quinidine and procainamide doses by 1/3. QT prolongation reported with disopyramide, fluoroquinolones, macrolides and azoles.

**PREGNANCY:** Category D, not for use in nursing.

**MECHANISM OF ACTION:** Class III anti-arrhythmic; prolongs the myocardial cell-action potential duration and refractory period and noncompetitively inhibits α- and β-adrenergic receptors, which leads to decreased sinus rate, increased PR and QT interval, development of U-waves and changes in T-wave contour.

**PHARMACOKINETICS: Absorption:** Slow; bioavailability (50%); $T_{max}$=3-7 hrs. **Distribution:** $V_d$=60L/kg; protein binding (96%); found in breast milk. **Metabolism:** Liver via CYP3A4, 2C8; desethylamidarone (major metabolite). **Elimination:** Bile (major), urine; $T_{1/2}$=58 days, 36 days (metabolite).

## NURSING CONSIDERATIONS

**Assessment:** Assess for cardiogenic shock, severe sinus-node dysfunction, bradycardia, 2nd- or 3rd-degree heart block, life-threatening arrhythmias, optic neuropathy/neuritis, syncope, presence of functioning pacemaker, liver impairment, thyroid function, hypokalemia or hypomagnesemia, pregnancy/nursing status, and possible drug interactions. Perform baseline chest X-ray and pulmonary function tests, including diffusion capacity.

P

**Monitoring:** Monitoring of history, physical exam, chest X-ray, and pulmonary function should be repeated every 3-6 months and evaluated. Monitor for pulmonary toxicities (eg, hypersensitivity pneumonitis or interstitial/alveolar pneumonitis), worsening of arrhythmia, induced hyperthyroidism/thyrotoxicosis, hepatic failure, optic neuritis/neuropathy, corneal microdeposits, loss of vision, neonatal hypo/hyperthyroidism, peripheral neuropathy, and photosensitivity. Monitor LFTs regularly, $T_4$, $T_3$, and reverse $T_3$. Monitor for myocardial depression, hypotension and adult respiratory distress syndrome during and after surgery.

**Patient Counseling:** Inform that therapy should only be administered by physician experienced in treatment of life-threatening arrhythmia. Inform about risks/benefits; report adverse reactions. Avoid prolonged exposure to sunlight. Advise that corneal refractive laser surgery is contraindicated with concurrent use. Advise that manufacturers of corneal refractive surgery devices contraindicate the procedure in patients taking amiodarone. Counsel to take as directed and not to take with grapefruit juice. Notify if pregnant/nursing.

**Administration:** Oral route. **Storage:** 20-25°C (68-77°F); excursions permitted to 15-30°C (59-86°F). Protect from light.

## PAMELOR RX

nortriptyline HCl (Mallinckrodt)

**Antidepressants increased the risk of suicidal thinking and behavior (suicidality) in short-term studies in children, adolescents, and young adults with major depressive disorder (MDD) and other psychiatric disorders. Nortriptyline is not approved for use in pediatric patients.**

**THERAPEUTIC CLASS:** Tricyclic antidepressant

**INDICATIONS:** Relief of symptoms of depression.

**DOSAGE:** *Adults:* 25mg tid-qid. Max: 150mg/day. Total daily dose may be given once a day. Monitor serum levels if dose >100mg/day. Elderly/Adolescents: 30-50mg/day in single or divided doses.

**HOW SUPPLIED:** Cap: 10mg, 25mg, 50mg, 75mg; Sol: 10mg/5mL

**CONTRAINDICATIONS:** MAOI use within 14 days, acute recovery period following MI.

**WARNINGS/PRECAUTIONS:** MI, arrhythmia, strokes have occurred. Caution with cardiovascular disease, glaucoma, history of urinary retention, hyperthyroidism. May lower seizure threshold, exacerbate psychosis or activate schizophrenia, cause symptoms of mania in bipolar disease, or alter glucose levels. D/C several days prior to elective surgery.

**ADVERSE REACTIONS:** Arrhythmias, hypotension, HTN, tachycardia, MI, heart block, stroke, confusion, hallucination, insomnia, tremors, ataxia, anxiety, dry mouth, blurred vision, skin rash, extrapyramidal symptoms, photosensitivity, SIADH, anorexia.

**INTERACTIONS:** See Contraindications. May block guanethidine effects. Arrhythmia risk with thyroid agents. Alcohol may potentiate effects. "Stimulating" effect with reserpine. Monitor with anticholinergic and sympathomimetic drugs. Increased plasma levels with cimetidine. Hypoglycemia reported with chlorpropamide. SSRIs, antidepressants, phenothiazines, propafenone, flecainide and CYP2D6 inhibitors (eg, quinidine) may potentiate effects. Decreased clearance with quinidine.

**PREGNANCY:** Safety during pregnancy and nursing not known.

**MECHANISM OF ACTION:** Tricyclic antidepressant; inhibits activity of histamine, 5-hydroxytryptamine, and acetylcholine; increases pressor effect of NE, blocks pressor response of phenethylamine, and interferes with transport, release, and storage of catecholamine.

### NURSING CONSIDERATIONS

**Assessment:** Assess if acute recovery period after MI, for bipolar disorder risk, history of mania, unrecognized/history of schizophrenia, possible drug interactions, history of seizures, CVD, hyperthyroidism, DM, glaucoma, urinary retention, and history of agitation or overactivity.

**Monitoring:** Periodically monitor thyroid function and blood glucose. Monitor for signs/symptoms of clinical worsening (suicidality, unusual changes in behavior), mania, cardiovascular events, increasing psychosis, increasing anxiety/agitation, mydriasis, hypo/hyperglycemia, seizures, cognitive/motor impairment.

**Patient Counseling:** Advise to avoid alcohol. Seek medical attention for symptoms of activation of mania, seizures, clinical worsening (suicidal ideation, unusual changes in behavior), cardiovascular events, increasing psychosis, increasing anxiety/agitation, mydriasis, and hypo/hyperglycemia. Caution may impair physical/mental abilities.

**Administration:** Oral route. **Storage:** 20-25°C (68-77°F).

## PANDEL RX

hydrocortisone probutate (PharmaDerm)

**THERAPEUTIC CLASS:** Corticosteroid

**INDICATIONS:** Relief of the inflammatory and pruritic manifestations of corticosteroid-responsive dermatoses in patients ≥18 yrs.

**DOSAGE:** *Adults:* Apply thin film to affected area qd-bid depending on severity of condition. May use occlusive dressing for refractory lesions of psoriasis and other deep-seated dermatoses. D/C when control is achieved. Reassess diagnosis if no improvement within 2 weeks.

**HOW SUPPLIED:** Cre: 0.1% [15g, 45g, 80g]

**WARNINGS/PRECAUTIONS:** May produce reversible hypothalamic-pituitary-adrenal (HPA) axis suppression, manifestations of Cushing's syndrome, hyperglycemia, glucosuria; ACTH stimulation, AM plasma cortisol or urinary free cortisol tests may be done. Steroid withdrawal may occur. Allergic contact dermatitis may manifest as failure to heal. D/C if irritation occurs. Use appropriate antifungal or antibacterial agent with dermatological infections. Pediatrics may be more susceptible to systemic toxicity. Caution when applied to large surface areas or areas under occlusion. Avoid eyes.

**ADVERSE REACTIONS:** Burning, stinging, moderate paresthesia, itching, dryness, folliculitis, hypertrichosis, acneiform eruptions, hypopigmentation, perioral dermatitis, skin atrophy, secondary infections, striae, miliaria.

**PREGNANCY:** Category C, caution in nursing.

**MECHANISM OF ACTION:** Corticosteroid; has anti-inflammatory, anti-pruritic, and vasoconstrictive actions. Anti-inflammatory activity not established. Suspected to act by the induction of phospholipase $A_2$ inhibitory proteins, lipocortins. Lipocortins control the biosynthesis of potent mediators of inflammation (eg, prostaglandins, leukotrienes) by inhibiting the release of their common precursor, arachidonic acid.

**PHARMACOKINETICS: Absorption:** Percutaneous; inflammation, other disease states, or the use of occlusive dressings may increase absorption. Use of occlusive dressings ≤24 hrs does not increase penetration. Use of occlusive dressings ≥96 hrs markedly enhances penetration. **Distribution:** Systemically administered corticosteroids have been found in breast milk.

## NURSING CONSIDERATIONS

**Assessment:** Assess for proper diagnosis and use in pregnant/nursing females.

**Monitoring:** Monitor for signs/symptoms of reversible HPA-axis suppression, Cushing's syndrome, hyperglycemia, glucosuria, skin irritation, allergic contact dermatitis (eg, failure to heal) and for development of concomitant skin infections (eg, bacterial, fungal). In patients applying medication to a large body surface area or using occlusive dressings, perform periodic monitoring for HPA-axis suppression using ACTH stimulation, AM plasma cortisol or urinary free cortisol tests. Monitor for glucocorticosteroid insufficiencies following withdrawal of medication.

**Patient Counseling:** Instruct to use externally and exactly as directed; avoid contact with eyes, use on face, underarms or groin areas unless directed by physician. Advise not to bandage, cover or wrap treated skin area. Instruct to contact physician if any signs of local adverse reactions (eg, burning, itching, irritation) develop or if no clinical improvement is seen within 2 weeks of initiating therapy.

**Administration:** Topical route. **Storage:** 15-30°C (59-86°F).

# PARCOPA — RX

levodopa - carbidopa (Schwarz)

**THERAPEUTIC CLASS:** Dopa-decarboxylase inhibitor/dopamine precursor

**INDICATIONS:** Treatment of symptoms of idiopathic Parkinson's disease, postencephalitic parkinsonism, and symptomatic parkinsonism.

**DOSAGE:** *Adults:* ≥18yrs: 25mg-100mg tab: Initial: 1 tab tid. Titrate: Increase by 1 tab qd or qod until 8 tabs/day. 10mg-100mg tab: Initial: 1 tab tid-qid. Titrate: Increase 1 tab qd or qod until 2 tabs qid. 70-100mg/day carbidopa required.

Max 200mg/day carbidopa. Levodopa must be d/c 12 hrs before starting carbidopa-levodopa.

**HOW SUPPLIED:** Tab, Disintegrating: (Carbidopa-Levodopa) 10mg-100mg*, 25mg-100mg*, 25mg-250mg* *scored

**CONTRAINDICATIONS:** MAOIs during or within 14 days of use; narrow-angle glaucoma; suspicious, undiagnosed skin lesions; history of melanoma.

**WARNINGS/PRECAUTIONS:** Dyskinesias and mental disturbances may occur. Caution with severe CV or pulmonary disease, bronchial asthma, renal or hepatic disease, endocrine disease, chronic wide-angle glaucoma, peptic ulcer, and MI with residual arrhythmias. NMS reported during dose reduction or withdrawal. Dark color may appear in saliva, urine, or sweat. May cause false (+) ketonuria or false (-) glucosuria (glucose-oxidase method).

**ADVERSE REACTIONS:** Dyskinesias, choreiform, dystonia and other involuntary movements, nausea.

**INTERACTIONS:** See Contraindications. Risk of postural hypotension with antihypertensives, selegiline. HTN and dyskinesia may occur with TCAs. Reduced effects with dopamine $D_2$ antagonists (eg, phenothiazines, butyrophenones, risperidone), isoniazid. Antagonized by phenytoin, papaverine, metoclopramide. Reduced bioavailability with iron salts, high-protein diets.

**PREGNANCY:** Category C, caution in nursing

**MECHANISM OF ACTION:** Carbidopa: Inhibits decarboxylation of peripheral levodopa. Levodopa: Crosses blood-brain barrier, converting into dopamine and thereby increasing concentrations in the brain.

**PHARMACOKINETICS: Absorption:** Carbidopa: Bioavailability (99%). **Elimination:** Urine.

## NURSING CONSIDERATIONS

**Assessment:** Assess LFTs, renal function, CBC, glaucoma, dyskinesia, psychosis, depression, cardiovascular complications, melanomas, asthma, phenyl alanine levels.

**Monitoring:** Monitor for cardiac, hepatic/renal functions during initial dosage adjustment period, depression and suicidal ideation, worsening of dyskinesia, rhabdomyolysis, diarrhea, hallucinations, fibrotic complications, hyperpyrexia, melanomas, IOP, and hypersensitivity reactions.

**Patient Counseling:** Instruct to take as prescribed. Caution while operating machinery/driving. Discoloration of body fluids may occur. High-protein diet, excessive acidity, and iron salts reduce clinical effectiveness. Wearing-off effect may be seen at end of dosing interval. Report any adverse effects. Place tablet on tongue and dissolve with saliva.

**Administration:** Oral route. **Storage:** 20-25°C (68-77°F); excursions permitted to 15-30°C (59-86°F).

# PARLODEL RX

bromocriptine mesylate (Novartis)

**THERAPEUTIC CLASS:** Dopamine receptor agonist

**INDICATIONS:** Management of hyperprolactinemia including amenorrhea with or without galactorrhea, infertility, or hypogonadism. Treatment of prolactin-secreting adenomas, acromegaly, and symptoms of Parkinson's disease.

**DOSAGE:** *Adults:* Take with food. Parkinson's Disease: Initial: 1.25mg bid. Titrate: if needed, increase by 2.5mg/day every 2-4 weeks. Max: 100mg/day. Hyperprolactinemia: Initial: 1.25mg-2.5mg qd. Titrate: If needed, increase by 2.5mg every 2-7 days. Usual: 2.5-15mg/day. Acromegaly: Initial: 1.25-2.5mg qhs for 3 days. Titrate: Increase by 1.25-2.5mg every 3-7 days until optimal response. Usual: 20-30mg/day. Max: 100mg/day. Withdraw for 4-8 weeks every year in patients treated with pituitary irradiation.
*Pediatrics:* Take with food. 11-15 yrs: Prolactin-Secreting Pituitary Adenomas: Initial: 1.25-2.5mg/day. Titrate: Increase as tolerated. Usual: 2.5-10mg/day.

**HOW SUPPLIED:** Cap: 5mg; Tab: 2.5mg* *scored

**CONTRAINDICATIONS:** Uncontrolled HTN, ergot alkaloid sensitivity, postpartum with CVD unless withdrawal is medically contraindicated, pregnancy if treating hyperprolactinemia, HTN in pregnancy.

**WARNINGS/PRECAUTIONS:** Caution with renal or hepatic dysfunction, psychosis, CVD, peptic ulcer, dementia. D/C with macroadenomas associated with rapid regrowth of tumor and increased prolactin levels and if severe headache or HTN develops. Risk of pulmonary infiltrates, pleural effusion, thickening of pleura, and retroperitoneal fibrosis with long-term use. Not for prevention of physiological lactation. Monitor BP for symptomatic hypotension and HTN.

**ADVERSE REACTIONS:** Headache, dizziness, GI effects, orthostatic hypotension, fatigue, arrhythmia, insomnia, hallucinations, abnormal involuntary movements, depression, syncope.

**INTERACTIONS:** Decreased effects with dopamine antagonists (eg, butyrophenones, haloperidol, phenothiazines, pimozide, metoclopramide). Levodopa may cause hallucinations. Caution with antihypertensives. Alcohol may potentiate side effects. Not for use with other ergot alkaloids.

**PREGNANCY:** Category B, not for use in nursing.

**MECHANISM OF ACTION:** Dopamine receptor agonist; activates post-synaptic dopamine receptors and modulates prolactin secretion from anterior pituitary by secreting prolactin inhibitory factor.

**PHARMACOKINETICS: Absorption:** GI tract (28%); $C_{max}$=0.4652ng/mL (5mg); $T_{max}$=1-3 hrs. **Distribution:** Serum albumin binding (90-96%). **Metabolism:** Liver, via CYP3A and hydroxylation. **Elimination:** Liver and kidneys (6%); $T_{1/2}$=8-20 hrs.

## NURSING CONSIDERATIONS

**Assessment:** Assess for HTN, history of CAD, pituitary tumors, dementia, unexplained pleuropulmonary disorder, history of psychosis, hereditary problems such as galactose intolerance, severe lactase deficiency or glucose malabsorption, and pregnancy status.

**Monitoring:** Monitor for somnolence, sudden sleep onset, confusion, mental disturbances, seizures, visual disturbances, pleuropulmonary disorders, constrictive pericarditis, retroperitoneal fibrosis, BP, prolactin level, LFTs, renal function, CBC, BP, and CNS toxicities.

P

**Patient Counseling:** Advise to use caution while operating machinery/driving. Instruct to take exactly as prescribed with meals. Counsel to report lack of response or adverse effects.

**Administration:** Oral route. **Storage:** Store below 25°C (77°F); tight, light-resistant container.

# PARNATE — RX

tranylcypromine sulfate (GlaxoSmithKline)

**Antidepressants increased the risk of suicidal thinking and behavior (suicidality) in short-term studies in children, adolescents, and young adults with major depressive disorder and other psychiatric disorders. Monitor appropriately and observe closely for clinical worsening, suicidality, or unusual changes in behavior for all patients who are started on antidepressant therapy. Tranylcypromine is not approved for use in pediatric patients.**

**THERAPEUTIC CLASS:** Monoamine oxidase inhibitor

**INDICATIONS:** Treatment of major depressive episode without melancholia.

**DOSAGE:** *Adults:* Usual: 30mg/day in divided doses. Titrate: After 2 weeks, may increase by 10mg/day every 1-3 weeks depending on signs of improvement. Max: 60mg/day.

**HOW SUPPLIED:** Tab: 10mg

**CONTRAINDICATIONS:** Cardiovascular or cerebrovascular disorder, HTN, history of headache, pheochromocytoma. Concomitant MAOIs, dibenzazepine derivatives, sympathomimetics (including amphetamines and OTC drugs that contain vasoconstrictors), some CNS depressants (including narcotics and alcohol), antihypertensives, diuretics, antihistamines, sedatives, anesthetics, bupropion, buspirone, meperidine, SSRIs, SNRIs, dextromethorphan, foods with high tyramine content (cheese, sour cream, liqueurs, pickled herring, liver, dried fruits, bananas, avacados, chocolate, soy sauce, sauerkraut, fava beans, yogurt, meat tenderizers) and excessive quantities of caffeine. Elective surgery requiring general anesthesia. History of liver disease or abnormal LFTs. Caution with anti-parkinsonism drugs.

**WARNINGS/PRECAUTIONS:** Hypertensive crises, sometimes fatal, may occur; paradoxical increase in BP can cause intracranial bleeding; d/c if palpitations or frequent headaches occur. Hypotension, especially postural hypotension, reported; usually at dose above 30 mg. Drug dependency possible in doses excessive of the therapeutic range. May suppress anginal pain in myocardial ischemia. Caution with hyperthyroidism, renal dysfunction, diabetes, elderly. May aggravate depression symptoms. May lower seizure threshold; caution in epileptic patients. May precipitate mixed/manic episode in patients at risk for bipolar disorder; adequately screen patients to determine risk prior to initiating treatment. Inhibition of MAOI may persist up to 10 days after d/c.

**ADVERSE REACTIONS:** Restlessness, insomnia, weakness, drowsiness, nausea, diarrhea, tachycardia, anorexia, edema, tinnitus, muscle spasm, overstimulation, dizziness, dry mouth, blood dyscrasias.

**INTERACTIONS:** See Contraindications. Caution with disulfiram. Additive hypotensive effects with phenothiazines. Tryptophan may precipitate disorientation, memory impairment and other neurological and behavioral signs. Avoid metrizamide; d/c 48 hrs before myelography and may resume 24 hrs post-procedure.

**PREGNANCY:** Safety in pregnancy and nursing not known.

**MECHANISM OF ACTION:** Non-hydrazine MAOI; inhibits monoamine oxidase, increasing concentration of epinephrine, norepinephrine, and serotonin in storage sites throughout nervous system.

## NURSING CONSIDERATIONS

**Assessment:** Assess for DM, pheochromocytoma, HTN, history of headache, seizures, liver disease, possible drug interactions, risk for bipolar disorder, renal impairment, hyperthyroidism, Parkinson's disease, CV and cerebrovascular defects.

**Monitoring:** Monitor BP, renal function, and LFTs; signs/symptoms of clinical worsening (suicidality, unusual changes in behavior), hypertensive crisis (occipital headaches, neck stiffness, NV, sweating), seizures, liver dysfunction, postural hypotension, and hypoglycemia.

**Patient Counseling:** Inform risks and benefits of therapy. Counsel appropriate use. Instruct to avoid concomitant use of alcohol, tyramine-containing foods/supplements/beverages (during and 2 weeks following d/c), and cough medicine containing dextromethorphan. Advise to seek medical attention if symptoms of hypertensive crisis (occipital headaches, neck stiffness, NV, sweating), hypoglycemia, seizures, postural hypotension, clinical worsening (suicidal ideation, unusual changes in behavior), and liver dysfunction occur; change positions gradually if lightheaded, faint, or dizzy.

**Administration:** Oral route. **Storage:** 15-30°C (59-86°F).

# Paser — RX

aminosalicylic acid (Jacobus)

**THERAPEUTIC CLASS:** Hydroxybenzoic acid derivative

**INDICATIONS:** Treatment of TB in combination with other agents.

**DOSAGE:** *Adults:* 4g tid. Sprinkle on applesauce, yogurt, or mix with tomato or orange juice.
*Pediatrics:* Use correspondingly smaller doses to the adult dose. Sprinkle on applesauce, yogurt, or mix with tomato or orange juice.

**HOW SUPPLIED:** Pkt: 4g

**CONTRAINDICATIONS:** Severe renal disease.

**WARNINGS/PRECAUTIONS:** Monitor for rash, or signs of intolerance during 1st 3 months. D/C if hypersensitivity occurs. Can desensitize by administering small, gradually increasing doses.

**ADVERSE REACTIONS:** Diarrhea, NV, abdominal pain, fever, dermatitis, lymphoma-like syndrome, agranulocytosis, thrombocytopenia, anemia, jaundice, hepatitis, hypoglycemia.

**INTERACTIONS:** Reduces acetylation of isoniazid, especially in rapid acetylators. Decreases vitamin $B_{12}$ absorption; consider vitamin $B_{12}$ maintenance treatment. Decreases digoxin levels.

**PREGNANCY:** Category C, safety in nursing not known.

**MECHANISM OF ACTION:** Bacteriostatic agent; believed to inhibit folic acid synthesis and/or inhibition of synthesis of the cell-wall component, mycobactin, thus reducing iron uptake by *M.tuberculosis*.

**PHARMACOKINETICS: Absorption:** $C_{max}$=20mcg/mL; $T_{max}$=6 hrs. **Distribution:** Plasma protein binding (50-60%), CSF penetration occurs only if the meninges is inflamed. **Metabolism:** Via acetylation. **Excretion:** Urine (80%); aminosalicylic acid (metabolite); $T_{1/2}$=26.4 min.

## NURSING CONSIDERATIONS

**Assessment:** Assess renal function, LFTs, and possible drug interactions.

**Monitoring:** Monitor LFTs, renal functions, hepatomegaly, lymphadenopathy, diarrhea, leucocytosis, eosinophilia. Monitor for rash or signs of intolerance during first 3 months; desensitize by administering small, gradually increasing doses.

**Patient Counseling:** D/C if hypersensitivity (rash, fever, diarrhea) occurs. Inform that poor compliance in taking anti-TB drugs leads to treatment failure and resistance against organisms. Skeleton of the granules may be seen in stool. Sprinkle granules on acidic foods such as applesauce or yogurt or stir into a fruit drink and swirl to protect the coating from sinking. Store drug in refrigerator or freezer; do not use if the packets are swollen or the granules have lost their tan color and are dark brown or purple.

**Administration:** Oral route. **Storage:** Store below 15°C (59°F), refrigerate or freeze.



# PATANOL RX

olopatadine HCl (Alcon)

**THERAPEUTIC CLASS:** $H_1$-antagonist and mast cell stabilizer

**INDICATIONS:** Allergic conjunctivitis.

**DOSAGE:** *Adults:* 1 drop bid, q6-8h.
*Pediatrics:* ≥3 yrs: 1 drop bid, q6-8h.

**HOW SUPPLIED:** Sol: 0.1% [5mL]

**WARNINGS/PRECAUTIONS:** May re-insert contact lens 10 min after dosing if eye is not red.

**ADVERSE REACTIONS:** Headache, asthenia, blurred vision, burning, stinging, cold syndrome, dry eye, foreign body sensation, hyperemia, hypersensitivity, keratitis, lid edema, nausea, pharyngitis, pruritus, rhinitis, sinusitis, taste perversion.

**PREGNANCY:** Category C, caution in nursing.

**MECHANISM OF ACTION:** Antihistaminic drug; relatively selective histamine $H_1$-antagonist; inhibits the type 1 immediate hypersensitivity reaction, including inhibition of histamine induced effects on human conjunctival epithelial cells.

**PHARMACOKINETICS: Absorption:** $C_{max}$=0.5-1.3ng/mL; $T_{max}$=2 hrs. **Metabolism:** Metabolites: Mono-desmethyl and N-oxide. **Elimination:** Urine (60-70% parent drug).

## NURSING CONSIDERATIONS

**Assessment:** Assess for drug hypersensitivity.

**Monitoring:** Monitor for headache and other adverse reactions.

**Patient Counseling:** Counsel not to wear contact lenses if eye is red; wait at least 10 min after instillation to wear contact lenses. Instruct to avoid touching tip of container to eye or any other surface to avoid contamination.

**Administration:** Ocular route. **Storage:** 4-25°C (39-77°F). Keep bottle tightly closed.

## PAXIL — RX

paroxetine HCl (GlaxoSmithKline)

**Antidepressants increased the risk of suicidal thinking and behavior (suicidality) in short-term studies in children, adolescents, and young adults with major depressive disorder (MDD) and other psychiatric disorders. Paroxetine is not approved for use in pediatric patients.**

**THERAPEUTIC CLASS:** Selective serotonin reuptake inhibitor

**INDICATIONS:** Treatment of major depressive disorder (MDD), panic disorder with or without agoraphobia, obsessive compulsive disorder (OCD), social anxiety disorder (SAD), generalized anxiety disorder (GAD), and post-traumatic stress disorder (PTSD).

**DOSAGE:** *Adults:* Give qd, usually in the AM. MDD: Initial: 20mg/day. Max: 50mg/day. OCD: Initial: 20mg/day. Usual: 40mg qd. Max: 60mg/day. Panic Disorder: Initial: 10mg/day. Usual: 40mg/day. Max: 60mg/day. GAD: Initial: 20mg/day. Usual: 20-50mg/day. SAD: Initial/Usual: 20mg/day. Max: 60mg/day. PTSD: Initial: 20mg/day. Usual: 20-50mg/day. To titrate, may increase weekly by 10mg/day. Elderly/Debilitated/Severe Renal/Hepatic Impairment: Initial: 10mg/day. Max: 40mg/day.

**HOW SUPPLIED:** Sus: 10mg/5mL [250mL]; Tab: 10mg*, 20mg*, 30mg, 40mg *scored

**CONTRAINDICATIONS:** Concomitant use with MAOIs including linezolid or within 14 days of MAOI use. Concomitant use with thioridazine or pimozide.

**WARNINGS/PRECAUTIONS:** Monitor for clinical worsening, suicidality, and unusual changes in behavior, especially at initiation of therapy or dose changes. Not approved for treatment of bipolar depression. Potentially life-threatening serotonin syndrome or neuroleptic malignant syndrome (NMS)-like reactions reported. Increased risk of congenital malformations, particularly CV malformations reported in infants. May increase the risk of bleeding events. Activation of mania/hypomania reported; caution in patients with a history of mania. Caution with history of seizures; d/c if seizures occur. Akathisia may develop. Hyponatremia reported, caution in elderly and volume-depleted patients. May increase risk of bleeding events. Caution in disease/conditions that could affect metabolism or hemodynamic responses. Acute angle-closure glaucoma reported; caution with narrow-angle glaucoma. May impair judgment, thinking, or motor skills. Dysphoric mood, irritability, agitation, dizziness, sensory disturbances, anxiety, confusion, headache, lethargy, emotional lability, insomnia, and hypomania reported upon d/c; avoid abrupt withdrawal.

**ADVERSE REACTIONS:** Somnolence, headache, insomnia, nausea, asthenia, abnormal ejaculation, dry mouth, constipation, dizziness, diarrhea, decreased libido, sweating, decreased appetite, tremor, nervousness.

**INTERACTIONS:** See Contraindications. Serotonin syndrome or NMS-like reactions reported when used alone and in combination with serotonergic drugs, with drugs that impair serotonin metabolism, antipsychotics, and with dopamine antagonists. Caution with drugs that may affect serotonergic neurotransmitter systems such as triptans, lithium, tramadol, or St. John's wort. Use with other SSRIs, SNRIs, or tryptophan is not recommended. Avoid alcohol. Concomitant use with ASA, NSAIDs, warfarin, and other anticoagulants may increase risk of bleeding events. Use with diuretics may increase risk of developing hyponatremia. Metabolism and pharmacokinetics of paroxetine may be affected by induction or inhibition of drug-metabolizing enzymes. Increased levels with cimetidine. Caution with phenobarbital and phenytoin; elevated levels of phenytoin reported. Caution with drugs that are metabolized by CYP2D6 (eg, antidepressants, phenothiazines, risperidone, tamoxifen, Type 1C antiarrhythmics) and with drugs that inhibit CYP2D6 (eg, quinidine). May increase levels of risperidone. May increase levels of atomoxetine; may require dose adjustments. May reduce efficacy of tamoxifen. May impair metabolism of TCAs, caution with concomitant use. May shift concentrations when concomitantly used with highly protein-bound drugs. Caution with digoxin. May increase procyclidine levels; reduce dose if anticholinergic effects are seen. Severe hypotension reported when added to chronic metoprolol treatment. Monitor theophylline levels. Fosamprenavir/ritonavir may decrease levels.

**PREGNANCY:** Category D, caution in nursing.

**MECHANISM OF ACTION:** SSRI; inhibits CNS neuronal reuptake of serotonin.

**PHARMACOKINETICS: Absorption:** Complete; $C_{max}$=61.7ng/mL; $T_{max}$=5.2 hrs. **Distribution:** Plasma protein binding (95%); found in breast milk. **Metabolism:** Extensive; oxidation and methylation via CYP2D6. **Elimination:** Urine (62%) (metabolites), (2%) (parent compound); feces (36%) (metabolites), (<1%) (parent compound); $T_{1/2}$=21 hrs.

## NURSING CONSIDERATIONS

**Assessment:** Assess for history of seizures, history of mania, volume depletion, diseases/conditions that alter metabolism or hemodynamic responses, hepatic/renal impairment, narrow-angle glaucoma, pregnancy/nursing status, and for possible drug interactions. Assess for risk of bipolar disorder.

**Monitoring:** Monitor for signs/symptoms of clinical worsening (eg, suicidality, unusual changes in behavior), serotonin syndrome or NMS-like reactions, activation of mania/ hypomania, seizures, akathisia, hyponatremia, abnormal bleeding, mydriasis, acute angle closure glaucoma, cognitive/motor impairment, and for hepatic/renal dysfunction. Upon discontinuation, monitor for symptoms of dysphoric mood, irritability, agitation, dizziness, sensory disturbances, anxiety, confusion, headache, lethargy, emotional lability, insomnia, and hypomania.

**Patient Counseling:** Instruct to swallow whole, not to chew or crush. Advise to avoid alcohol. Instruct to notify physician of all prescription, nonprescription, and herbal products currently taking. Counsel to seek medical attention for symptoms of serotonin syndrome (eg, mental status changes, tachycardia, hyperthermia, NV, diarrhea, incoordination), abnormal bleeding (particularly if using NSAIDs or ASA), akathisia, hyponatremia (eg, headaches, unsteadiness), mydriasis, activation of mania, seizures, clinical worsening (eg, suicidal ideation, unusual changes in behavior), or discontinuation symptoms (irritability, agitation, dizziness, anxiety, headache, insomnia). Caution against hazardous tasks (eg, operating machinery, driving). Inform may notice improvement in 1-4 weeks; continue therapy as directed. Advise to notify physician if pregnant/intend to become pregnant, or breastfeeding. Counsel about benefits and risks of therapy.

**Administration:** Oral route. **Storage:** (Tab): 15-30°C (59-86°F). (Sol): At or below 25°C (77°F).

# PAXIL CR — RX

paroxetine HCl (GlaxoSmithKline)

**Antidepressants increased the risk of suicidal thinking and behavior (suicidality) in short-term studies in children, adolescents, and young adults with major depressive disorder (MDD) and other psychiatric disorders. Paroxetine is not approved for use in pediatric patients.**

**THERAPEUTIC CLASS:** Selective serotonin reuptake inhibitor

**INDICATIONS:** Treatment of major depressive disorder (MDD), panic disorder with or without agoraphobia, social anxiety disorder (SAD), and premenstrual dysphoric disorder (PMDD).

**DOSAGE:** *Adults:* Give qd, usually in the AM. MDD: Initial: 25mg/day. May increase weekly by 12.5mg/day. Max: 62.5mg/day. Panic Disorder: Initial: 12.5mg/day. May increase weekly by 12.5mg/day. Max: 75mg/day. SAD: Initial: 12.5mg/day. May increase weekly by 12.5mg/day. Max: 37.5mg/day. PMDD: Initial: 12.5mg/day throughout the menstrual cycle or limited to luteal phase of menstrual cycle. Dose changes should occur at intervals of at least 1 week. Elderly/Debilitated/Severe Renal/Hepatic Impairment: Initial: 12.5mg/day. Max: 50mg/day. Swallow whole; do not chew or crush.

**HOW SUPPLIED:** Tab, Controlled-Release: 12.5mg, 25mg, 37.5mg

**CONTRAINDICATIONS:** Concomitant use with MAOIs including linezolid or within 14 days of MAOI use. Concomitant use with thioridazine or pimozide.

**WARNINGS/PRECAUTIONS:** Monitor for clinical worsening and/or suicidality, especially at initiation of therapy or dose changes. Not approved for use in treating bipolar depression. Potentially life-threatening serotonin syndrome or neuroleptic malignant syndrome (NMS)-like reactions reported. Increased risk of congenital malformations, particularly CV malformations reported in infants. May increase risk of bleeding events. May activate mania/hypomania; caution in patients with a history of mania. Caution with a history of seizures; d/c if seizures develop. Dysphoric mood, irritability, agitation, dizziness, sensory disturbances, anxiety, confusion, headache, lethargy, emotional lability, insomnia, hypomania reported upon d/c; avoid abrupt withdrawal. Akathisia may develop. Hyponatremia reported; caution in elderly and volume-depleted patients. May increase risk of bleeding events. Caution with conditions that affect metabolism or hemodynamic responses. Acute angle-closure glaucoma may occur; caution in patients with narrow-angle glaucoma. May impair mental/physical abilities.

**ADVERSE REACTIONS:** Somnolence, insomnia, nausea, asthenia, abnormal ejaculation, dry mouth, constipation, dizziness, diarrhea, decreased libido, sweating, abnormal vision, headache, tremor.

**INTERACTIONS:** See Contraindications. Serotonin syndrome or NMS-like reactions reported alone and in combination with serotonergic drugs, drugs that impair serotonin metabolism, antipsychotics, and dopamine antagonists. Caution with drugs that may affect the serotonergic neurotransmitter systems such as triptans, lithium, tramadol, and St. John's wort. Use with other SSRIs, SNRIs, or tryptophan is not recommended. Avoid alcohol. Concomitant use with ASA, NSAIDs, warfarin, and other anticoagulants may increase risk of bleeding events. Use with diuretics may increase risk of hyponatremia. Metabolism and pharmacokinetics may be affected by induction or inhibition of drug-metabolizing enzymes. May increase levels when used concomitantly with cimetidine. Caution with concomitant use of phenobarbital and phenytoin; elevated phenytoin levels reported. Caution with drugs that are metabolized by CYP2D6 (eg, antidepressants, phenothiazines, risperidone, tamoxifen, Type 1C antiarrhythmics) and with drugs that inhibit CYP2D6 (eg, quinidine). May increase levels of risperidone. May increase levels of atomoxetine; dosage adjustments may be required and reduced initial atomoxetine dose. May reduce efficacy of tamoxifen. May impair TCA metabolism, caution with concomitant use. May shift concentrations when concomitantly used with highly protein-bound drugs. Caution with digoxin. May increase procyclidine levels; reduce dose of procyclidine if anticholinergic effects are seen. Severe hypotension reported when added to chronic metoprolol treatment. Monitor theophylline levels. Fosamprenavir/ritonavir may decrease levels.

**PREGNANCY:** Category D, caution in nursing.

**MECHANISM OF ACTION:** SSRI; inhibits CNS neuronal reuptake of serotonin.

**PHARMACOKINETICS: Absorption:** Complete; administration of variable doses resulted in different parameters; $T_{max}$=6-10 hrs. **Distribution:** Plasma protein binding (95%); found in breast milk. **Metabolism:** Extensive; oxidation and methylation via CYP2D6. **Elimination:** Urine (62%) (metabolites), (2%) (parent compound), feces (36%) (metabolites), (<1%) (parent compound); $T_{1/2}$=15-20 hrs.

P

## NURSING CONSIDERATIONS

**Assessment:** Assess for risk of bipolar disorder, history of mania, history of seizures, narrow-angle glaucoma, diseases/conditions that alter metabolism or hemodynamic responses, hepatic/renal impairment, pregnancy/nursing status, and for possible drug interactions.

**Monitoring:** Monitor for signs/symptoms of clinical worsening (suicidality, unusual changes in behavior), serotonin syndrome or NMS-like reactions, activation of mania/hypomania, seizures, akathisia, hyponatremia, abnormal bleeding, mydriasis, acute angle closure glaucoma, cognitive/motor impairment, and hepatic/renal dysfunction. Upon discontinuation, monitor for symptoms of dysphoric mood, irritability, agitation, dizziness, sensory disturbances, anxiety, confusion, headache, lethargy, emotional lability, insomnia, and hypomania.

**Patient Counseling:** Instruct to swallow whole, not to chew or crush. Advise to avoid alcohol. Instruct to notify physician of all prescription, nonprescription, and herbal products currently taking. Counsel to seek medical attention for symptoms of serotonin syndrome (eg, mental status changes, tachycardia, hyperthermia, N/V, diarrhea, incoordination), abnormal bleeding (particularly if using NSAIDs or ASA), akathisia, hyponatremia (eg, headaches, unsteadiness), mydriasis, activation of mania, seizures, clinical worsening (eg, suicidal ideation, unusual changes in behavior), or discontinuation symptoms (eg, irritability, agitation, dizziness, anxiety, headache, insomnia). Caution against hazardous tasks (eg, operating machinery, driving). Inform may notice improvement in 1-4 weeks; continue therapy as directed. Instruct to notify physician if pregnant/intend to become pregnant, or breastfeeding. Counsel about benefits and risks of therapy.

**Administration:** Oral route. **Storage:** Store at or below 25°C (77°F).

# PEDIAPRED RX

prednisolone sodium phosphate (Celltech)

**THERAPEUTIC CLASS:** Glucocorticoid

**INDICATIONS:** Steroid-responsive dermatoses.

P

**DOSAGE:** *Adults:* Initial: 5-60mg/day depending on disease and response. Maint: Decrease dose by small amounts to lowest effective dose. MS Exacerbations: 200mg qd for 1 week, then 80mg qod for 1 month. *Pediatrics:* Initial: 0.14-2mg/kg/day given tid-qid. Nephrotic Syndrome: 20mg/m$^2$ tid for 4 weeks, then 40mg/m$^2$ qod for 4 weeks. Uncontrolled Asthma: 1-2mg/kg/day in single or divided doses until peak expiratory rate of 80% is achieved (usually 3-10 days).

**HOW SUPPLIED:** Sol: 5mg/5mL [120mL]

**CONTRAINDICATIONS:** Systemic fungal infections.

**WARNINGS/PRECAUTIONS:** May produce reversible HPA axis suppression. Adjust dose during stress or change in thyroid status. May mask signs of infection or cause new infections. May activate latent amebiasis. Avoid with cerebral malaria. Avoid exposure to chickenpox or measles. Not for treatment of optic neuritis or active ocular herpes simplex. May cause elevation of BP or IOP, cataracts, glaucoma, optic nerve damage, Kaposi's sarcoma, psychic derangements, salt/water retention, increased excretion of potassium and/or calcium, osteoporosis, growth suppression in children, secondary ocular infections. Caution with strongyloides, CHF, diverticulitis, HTN, renal insufficiency, fresh intestinal anastomoses, active or latent peptic ulcer, ulcerative colitis. Enhanced effect in hypothyroidism or cirrhosis. Avoid abrupt withdrawal. Use with caution in elderly, increased risk of corticosteroid-induced side effects; start at low end of dosing range; monitor bone mineral density.

**ADVERSE REACTIONS:** Edema, fluid/electrolyte disturbances, osteoporosis, muscle weakness, pancreatitis, peptic ulcer, impaired wound healing, increased intracranial pressure, cushingoid state, hirsutism, menstrual irregularities, growth suppression in children, glaucoma, nausea, weight gain.

**INTERACTIONS:** Enhanced metabolism with barbiturates, phenytoin, ephedrine, and rifampin. Use with cyclosporine may increase activity of both drugs; convulsions reported with concomitant use. Decreased metabolism with estrogens or ketoconazole. May inhibit response to warfarin. Increased risk of GI side effects with ASA or other NSAIDs. May increase clearance of salicylates. High doses or concurrent neuromuscular drugs may cause acute myopathy. Enhanced possibility of hypokalemia when given with potassium-depleting agents. May produce severe weakness in myasthenia gravis patients on anticholinesterase agents. Avoid live vaccines with immunosuppressive doses. Possible diminished response with killed or inactivated vaccines. May increase blood glucose; adjust antidiabetic agents. May suppress reactions to skin tests.

**PREGNANCY:** Category C, caution in nursing.

**MECHANISM OF ACTION:** Synthetic adrenocorticoid steroid; promotes gluconeogenesis, increases deposition of glycogen in the liver, inhibits glucose utilization, increases catabolism of protein, lipolysis, glomerular filtration that leads to increased urinary excretion of urate and calcium.

**PHARMACOKINETICS: Absorption:** Rapidly absorbed from GI tract. **Distribution:** Plasma protein binding (70-90%); found in breast milk. **Metabolism:** Liver. **Elimination:** Urine (as sulfate and glucuronide congugates); $T_{1/2}$=2-4 hrs.

## NURSING CONSIDERATIONS

**Assessment:** Assess for systemic fungal/other infections, active TB, vaccination history, HTN, CHF, renal insufficiency, ophthalmic disease, osteoporosis, thyroid status, hepatic impairment, nonspecific ulcerative colitis, ulcers, and possible drug interactions.

**Monitoring:** Monitor for adrenocortical insufficiency, occurrence of infections, psychic derangement, cataracts, acute myopathy, Kaposi's sarcoma, fluid retention, and measurement of serum electrolytes, TSH, LFTs, glucose, IOP, and BP.

**Patient Counseling:** Advise not to d/c therapy abruptly or without medical supervision. Avoid exposure to chickenpox or measles; report immediately if exposed. Dietary salt restriction and $K^+$ supplementation is advised.

**Administration:** Oral route. **Storage:** 4-25°C (39-77°F).

# PEDIARIX RX

pertussis vaccine, acellular - hepatitis B (recombinant) - poliovirus vaccine, inactivated - diphtheria toxoid - tetanus toxoid (GlaxoSmithKline)

**THERAPEUTIC CLASS:** Vaccine/toxoid combination

**INDICATIONS:** Active immunization against diphtheria, tetanus, pertussis (whooping cough), all known subtypes of hepatitis B virus, and poliomyelitis (polioviruses Types 1, 2, and 3) in infants born of HBsAg negative mothers, beginning as early as 6 weeks of age.

**DOSAGE:** *Pediatrics:* ≥6 weeks-up to 7 yrs: 3 doses of 0.5mL IM at 6-8 week intervals (preferably 8 weeks). Start at 2 months old or as early as 6 weeks old if necessary. May be used to complete the first 3 doses of DTaP series in infants who have received 1 or 2 doses of Infanrix® and are scheduled to receive other components of Pediarix. May be used to complete first 3 doses of the IPV series in infants who have received 1 or 2 doses of IPV and are scheduled to receive other components of Pediarix. Not recommended for completion of the first 3 doses of the DTaP vaccination series initiated with a DTaP vaccine from a different manufacturer. No need to start the series again, regardless of the time elapsed between doses. The use of fractional doses is not recommended. Not indicated for use as a booster dose.

**HOW SUPPLIED:** Inj: 0.5mL [TIP-LOK®, vial]

**CONTRAINDICATIONS:** Encephalopathy (eg, coma, decreased level of consciousness, prolonged seizures) within 7 days of administration of a previous

P

pertussis-containing vaccine that is not attributable to another cause. Progressive neurologic disorder, including infantile spasms, uncontrolled epilepsy, or progressive encephalopathy. Hypersensitivity to yeast, neomycin, or polymyxin B.

**WARNINGS/PRECAUTIONS:** Re-evaluate need if Guillain-Barre syndrome occurs within 6 weeks of receipt of prior tetanus toxoid-containing vaccine. Risk of fever. Caution if any of the following occur in temporal relation to receipt of DTwP or a vaccine containing an acellular pertussis component: temperature ≥40.5°C (105°F) within 48 hrs not due to another identifiable cause; collapse or shock-like state (hypotonic-hyporesponsive episode) occurring within 48 hrs; persistent, inconsolable crying lasting ≥3 hrs occurring within 48 hrs; or seizures (with or without fever) occurring within 3 days. Caution with CNS disorders. For children with a higher risk for seizures, administer antipyretic at the time of vaccination to reduce the possibility of post-vaccination fever. Tip cap and rubber plunger of the needleless prefilled syringe contain latex which may cause an allergic reaction. Caution with bleeding disorders (eg, hemophilia, thrombocytopenia). Expected immune response may not be obtained in immunosuppressed persons. Prior to immunization, review immunization history for possible vaccine sensitivity; epinephrine and other appropriate agents should be immediately available for the control of immediate allergic reactions. Apnea following IM vaccine has been observed in premature infants. Avoid injection into a blood vessel. Decisions about when to administer IM vaccine to premature infants should be based on consideration of infant's medical status, and potential benefits and possible risks of vaccination.

**ADVERSE REACTIONS:** Local injection-site reactions (pain, redness, swelling), fever, fussiness, irritability, drowsiness, loss of appetite.

**INTERACTIONS:** Caution with anticoagulants. Immunosuppressive therapies including irradiation, antimetabolites, alkylating agents, cytotoxic drugs, and corticosteroids (when used in greater than physiologic doses) may reduce immune response.

**PREGNANCY:** Category C, safety in nursing not known.

**MECHANISM OF ACTION:** Vaccine/toxoid combination; stimulates immune system to elicit immune response, which produces antibodies that may protect against diphtheria, tetanus, pertussis, hepatitis B, and poliovirus infections.



## NURSING CONSIDERATIONS

**Assessment:** Review current health status, medical history and immunization history for possible vaccine sensitivity and previous vaccination-related adverse reactions. Assess for progressive neurologic disorder, including infantile spasms, uncontrolled epilepsy or progressive encephalopathy. Assess for history adverse events following administration of pertussis vaccination (eg, encephalopathy, temperature ≥105°F, collapse or shock-like state, persistent/inconsolable crying lasting ≥3 hrs, seizures with/without fever). Assess for history of Guillain-Barre syndrome occurring after tetanus toxoid administration. Assess for hypersensitivity to any component of the vaccine, including yeast, neomycin and polymyxin B and/or latex. Assess for CNS disorder, risk of seizure, bleeding disorders, immunosuppression, and for possible drug interactions. Assess use in premature infants.

**Monitoring:** Monitor for signs/symptoms of Guillain-Barre syndrome, collapse or shock-like state, hypotonic-hyporesponsive episode, persistent inconsolable crying, fever, seizures, hematoma, and for allergic reactions. Monitor for signs of apnea in premature infants.

**Patient Counseling:** Inform of potential benefits and risks of immunization, and of the importance of completing the immunization series. Counsel about potential adverse reactions. Instruct to report any adverse events to healthcare provider where the vaccine was administered. Advise that if at risk for developing seizures, an appropriate antipyretic should be taken at time of vaccination and for 24 hrs following administration.

**Administration:** IM route. Prior to administration, shake vial vigorously to obtain homogeneous, turbid, white suspension. Do not use if resuspension does not occur with vigorous shaking. Inspect visually for particulate matter, discoloration, cracks in the vial or syringe prior to administration; if any of these conditions exist, do not administer. Preferred administration site of <1 yr of age is anterolateral aspect of thigh; in older children, can administer via deltoid muscle. Do not inject in gluteal area or areas where there may be a major nerve trunk. Do not administer SQ or IV. Do not mix with any other vaccine in the same syringe or vial. **Storage:** 2-8°C (36-46°F). Do not freeze. Discard if frozen.

## PEGASYS — RX

peginterferon alfa-2a (Roche)

**May cause or aggravate fatal or life-threatening neuropsychiatric, autoimmune, ischemic, and infectious disorders. Monitor closely with periodic clinical and laboratory evaluations. D/C with persistently severe or worsening signs or symptoms of these conditions. When used with ribavirin, including Copegus, refer to the individual monograph.**

**THERAPEUTIC CLASS:** Pegylated virus proliferation inhibitor

**INDICATIONS:** Treatment of chronic hepatitis C, alone or in combination with Copegus, in adults with compensated liver disease not previously treated with interferon alpha. Treatment of HBeAg positive and HBeAg negative chronic hepatitis B in adults with compensated liver disease, evidence of viral replication, and liver inflammation.

**DOSAGE:** *Adults:* ≥18 yrs: HCV: Monotherapy: 180mcg SQ (in abdomen or thigh) once weekly for 48 weeks. Combination Therapy With Copegus: 180mcg SQ once weekly for 24 weeks with genotypes 2 and 3 or 48 weeks with genotypes 1 and 4. HCV w/ HIV: Monotherapy: 180mcg SQ once weekly for 48 weeks. Combination Therapy with Copegus: 180mcg SQ once weekly for 48 weeks, regardless of genotype. HBV: Monotherapy: 180mcg SQ once weekly for 48 weeks. Adjust dose based on hematological parameters and depression severity. (See PI for dose modifications).

**HOW SUPPLIED:** Inj: Prefilled syringe: 180mcg/0.5mL; Single-Dose Vial: 180mcg/mL

**CONTRAINDICATIONS:** Autoimmune hepatitis, hepatic decompensation (Child-Pugh score >6 [class B and C] in cirrhotic patients before or during treatment), hepatic decompensation with Child-Pugh score ≥6 in cirrhotic CHC patients coinfected with HIV before or during treatment, neonates and infants (contains benzyl alcohol). When used with Copegus, refer to the PI for additional contraindications.

**WARNINGS/PRECAUTIONS:** Life-threatening neuropsychiatric reactions may occur; extreme caution with history of depression; d/c immediately for severe cases. Serious and severe infections (bacterial, viral, fungal) reported. Risk of bone marrow suppression and may result in severe cytopenias; obtain CBCs prior to initiation and routinely thereafter. HTN, arrhythmias, chest pain, and MI reported; caution with pre-existing cardiac disease. Ischemic and hemorrhagic cerebrovascular events reported. Chronic hepatitis C patients with cirrhosis may be at risk for hepatic decompensation and death; monitor hepatic function and clinical status. Exacerbation of hepatitis B reported; monitor liver function. May cause or aggravate hypothyroidism or hyperthyroidism. Hypoglycemia, hyperglycemia, and diabetes mellitus (DM) reported. Development or exacerbation of autoimmune disorders reported. May induce or aggravate dyspnea, pulmonary infiltrates, pneumonia, bronchiolitis obliterans, interstitial pneumonitis, pulmonary HTN, and sarcoiditis; d/c if develop persistent or unexplained pulmonary infiltrates or pulmonary function impairment. Hypersensitivity reactions, ulcerative and hemorrhagic/ischemic colitis, and pancreatitis reported; d/c if any of these develop. Decrease/loss of vision and retinopathy reported as well as serous retinal detachment; perform eye exam at baseline (periodically with pre-existing disorder); d/c if patient develops new or worsening of ophthalmologic disorders. Monitor for signs/symptoms of toxicity with impaired renal function and caution with CrCl <50mL/min. Caution in elderly. Safety and efficacy has not been established in patients who have failed other alpha interferon treatments, liver or other organ transplant recipients, hepatitis b patients coinfected with HCV or

HIV, or in Hepatitis C patients coinfected with HBV or coinfected with HIV with a CD4+ count <100 cells/μL.

**ADVERSE REACTIONS:** Injection-site reaction, fatigue/asthenia, diarrhea, pyrexia, rigors, N/V, neutropenia, myalgia, headache, irritability/anxiety/nervousness, insomnia, depression, alopecia, pruritus, dermatitis.

**INTERACTIONS:** May inhibit CYP1A2 and increase theophylline AUC; monitor theophylline serum levels. Hepatic decompensation can occur with concomitant use of NRTIs and peginterferon alfa-2a/ribavirin. May increase methadone levels; monitor for methadone toxicity. Coadministration of Copegus with didanosine is not recommended. Concomitant use of peginterferon alfa-2a/ribavirin with zidovudine may cause severe neutropenia and severe anemia. Peripheral neuropathy reported in combination with telbivudine.

**PREGNANCY:** Category C (monotherapy) and Category X (with ribavirin), not for use in nursing.

**MECHANISM OF ACTION:** α-2a interferon; binds to specific receptors on the cell surface-initiating intracellular signaling leading to rapid activation of gene transcription.

**PHARMACOKINETICS: Absorption:** $T_{max}$=72-96 hrs. **Elimination:** $T_{1/2}$=160 hrs (chronic HCV).

## NURSING CONSIDERATIONS

**Assessment:** Assess for hepatic dysfunction (autoimmune hepatitis, decompensation, failure), history of depression, hypothyroidism, hyperthyroidism, DM, cardiac disease, autoimmune disorders, bone marrow suppression, ophthalmologic disorders, pulmonary disorders, renal impairment, pregnancy/nursing status, and for possible drug interactions. Obtain baseline CBC, SrCr, TFTs, LFTs, CD4+(HIV), Hgb, Hct, and eye examination. Obtain baseline pregnancy test in women of childbearing potential.

**Monitoring:** Monitor for signs/symptoms of neuropsychiatric disorders, bone marrow toxicities, CV disorders (HTN, supraventricular arrhythmias, chest pain, MI), cerebrovascular disorders, infectious disorders, hepatic failure, hepatitis exacerbations, hypersensitivity reactions, endocrine disorders (hypothyroidism, hyperthyroidism, DM), autoimmune disorders, pulmonary disorders, ulcerative and hemorrhagic/ischemic colitis, pancreatitis, and ophthalmologic disorders. Monitor hematological (weeks 2 and 4), biochemical tests (week 4), LFTs, TFTs. Perform periodic ophthalmologic exams in patients with pre-existing ophthalmologic disorders. Perform monthly pregnancy tests if on combination therapy with Copegus and for 6 months after d/c therapy.



**Patient Counseling:** Inform of how to properly use medication as well as risk/benefits of therapy. Inform patients using combination therapy with Copegus, that therapy must not be used by women who are pregnant or by men whose female partners are pregnant; inform female patients of child bearing potential and male patients with female partners of child bearing potential of the teratogenic/embryocidal risks and instruct to practice effective contraception during Copegus therapy and for 6 months post-therapy. Inform that laboratory evaluations are required before and during therapy. Advise to remain well hydrated. Counsel that it is not known if therapy will prevent transmission of HCV or HBV infection to others or prevent cirrhosis, liver failure, or liver cancer that might result from HCV or HBV infection. Advise that if develop dizziness, confusion, somnolence, or fatigue, that driving or operating machinery should be avoided.

**Administration:** SQ route. **Storage:** Refrigerate at 2-8°C (36-46°F). Do not freeze or shake. Protect from light.

## PEG-Intron RX
peginterferon alfa-2b (Schering)

**May cause or aggravate fatal or life-threatening neuropsychiatric, autoimmune, ischemic, and infectious disorders. Monitor closely with periodic clinical and laboratory evaluations. D/C with severe or worsening signs or symptoms of these conditions. When used with Rebetol, refer to the individual monograph.**

**THERAPEUTIC CLASS:** Pegylated virus proliferation inhibitor

**INDICATIONS:** Treatment of chronic hepatitis C (CHC) in combination with Rebetol in patients ≥3 yrs with compensated liver disease. Treatment of chronic hepatitis C alone in patients ≥18 yrs with compensated liver disease not previously treated with interferon-alpha.

**DOSAGE:** *Adults:* ≥18 yrs: Monotherapy: Administer 1mcg/kg/week for 1 yr. Combination Therapy With Rebetol: 1.5mcg/kg/week plus Rebetol 800-1400mg/day PO based on patient's body weight for 48 weeks in genotype 1, and 24 weeks genotype 2 and 3 patients. CrCl <50mL/min: D/C therapy. Adjust dose based on hematological parameters and depression severity (see PI for dose modifications). Renal Impairment: CrCl 30-50mL/min: Reduce dose by 25%. CrCl 10-29mL/min: Reduce dose by 50%. D/C if renal function decreases, >2 $\log_{10}$ drop or loss of HCV-RNA at 12 weeks, or HCV-RNA levels remain detectable after 24 weeks.
*Pediatrics:* 3-17 yrs: Combination Therapy With Rebetol: 60mcg/m²/week SQ plus Rebetol 15mg/kg/day in 2 divided doses for 48 weeks in genotype 1, and 24 weeks in genotype 2 and 3 patients. CrCl <50mL/min: D/C therapy. Adjust dose based on hematological parameters and depression severity (see PI for dose modifications). Renal Impairment: CrCl 30-50mL/min: Reduce dose by 25%. CrCl 10-29mL/min: Reduce dose by 50%. D/C if renal function decreases, HCV-RNA dropped <2 $\log_{10}$ at 12 weeks, or HCV-RNA levels remain detectable after 24 weeks.

**HOW SUPPLIED:** Inj: 50mcg/0.5mL, 80mcg/0.5mL, 120mcg/0.5mL, 150mcg/0.5mL

**CONTRAINDICATIONS:** Known hypersensitivity reactions (eg, urticaria, angioedema, bronchoconstriction, anaphylaxis, Stevens-Johnson syndrome, and toxic epidermal necrolysis), autoimmune hepatitis, hepatic decompensation (Child-Pugh score >6 [class B and C]) in cirrhotic CHC patients. When used with Rebetol, refer to the PI for additional contraindications.

**WARNINGS/PRECAUTIONS:** Life-threatening neuropsychiatric reactions may occur; caution with history of depression or psychiatric symptoms/disorders. Risk of bone marrow suppression; monitor CBCs and blood chemistry at initiation and periodically thereafter. Hypotension, arrhythmia, tachycardia, angina pectoris, MI reported; caution with CV disease. Conduct baseline eye exam in all patients and periodic exams with pre-existing ophthalmologic disorders; d/c if new or worsening ophthalmologic disorders occur. Caution with CrCl <50mL/min, and autoimmune disorders. D/C if persistent or unexplained pulmonary infiltrates, or pulmonary dysfunction, or hypersensitivity reaction occurs, or if hemorrhagic/ischemic colitis or pancreatitis, bone marrow toxicity (eg, severe decrease in neutrophil or platelet counts) develops. May cause or aggravate hypo/hyperthyroidism. Hyperglycemia and diabetes mellitus (DM) reported. Avoid if failed other interferon-alpha treatments, liver or other organ transplant recipients, or with HIV or HBV coinfection. May elevate triglyceride levels. Monitor renal impairment for toxicity, including increase in SrCr levels. Risk of hepatic decompensation and death in CHC patients with cirrhosis. Dental and periodontal disorders reported. Altered weight and height development. Caution in elderly.

**ADVERSE REACTIONS:** Headache, fatigue, rigors, dizziness, N/V, anorexia, depression, suicidal ideation, emotional lability/irritability, myalgia, injection-site inflammation/reaction, abdominal pain, neutropenia, pyrexia.

**INTERACTIONS:** Hemolytic anemia reported with ribavirin. May increase levels; monitor signs/symptoms of increased narcotic effect. Caution with medications metabolized by CYP2C8/9 (eg, warfarin and phenytoin) or CYP2D6 (eg, flecainide). Monitor treatment-associated toxicities (eg, hepatic

P

decompenstion, anemia) with ribavirin and nucleoside reverse transcriptase inhibitors (NRTIs). Increased methadone levels. Worsen clinical toxicities with didanosine.

**PREGNANCY:** Category C (monotherapy) and X (combination therapy), not for use in nursing.

**MECHANISM OF ACTION:** α-2b interferon. Binds to and activates the human type 1 interferon receptor. Upon binding, the receptor subunits dimerize and activate multiple intracellular signal transduction pathway.

**PHARMACOKINETICS: Absorption:** $T_{max}$=15-44 hrs. **Elimination:** $T_{1/2}$=approximately 40 hrs (HCV).

## NURSING CONSIDERATIONS

**Assessment:** Assess for neuropsychiatric conditions, autoimmune disease, liver dysfunction (autoimmune hepatitis, decompensation), renal dysfunction, bone marrow suppression, ophthalmologic disorders, endocrine disorders (thryoidism, DM), colitis, pancreatitis, pulmonary function, history of CVD, and possible drug interactions. Obtain baseline CBC and platelet counts, LFTs, bilirubin, uric acid, TSH, Hgb, Hct, and ECG.

**Monitoring:** Monitor periodically CBC (hemoglobin, neutrophil and platelet count), LFTs, renal function (SrCr), bilirubin and uric acid, TSH level, HCV RNA, TG levels, and complete eye exam. Signs/symptoms of autoimmune, ischemic, infectious disorders, neuropsychiatric events, bone marrow toxicity, hepatic failure, endocrine disorder, CV events, pulmonary disorders, colitis, pancreatitis, ophthalmic disorders, dental/periodontal disorders, and hypersensitivity.

**Patient Counseling:** Seek medical attention for symptoms of depression (suicidal ideation), CV (chest pain) and cerebrovascular events, ophthalmologic toxicity (decreased/loss of vision), pancreatitis and colitis (abdominal pain, N/V), worsening of liver disease/failure (jaundice); respiratory (fever, cough, dyspnea), hyperglycemia, and hypersensitivity reactions. Advise to take at bedtime to minimize flu-like symptoms. Advise to brush teeth thoroughly twice a day and have regular dental examinations. Keep well-hydrated.

**Administration:** SQ **Storage:** (Redipen) 2-8°C (36-46°F). Do not freeze. (Vials) 25°C (77°F); excursions permitted to 15-30°C (59-86°F). After reconstitution, use solution immediately, but may store up to 24 hrs at 2-8°C (36-46°F). Do not freeze.



# PENICILLIN VK — RX

penicillin V potassium (Various)

**OTHER BRAND NAMES:** Veetids (Sandoz)

**THERAPEUTIC CLASS:** Penicillin

**INDICATIONS:** Treatment of mild to moderately severe bacterial infections including conditions of the respiratory tract, oropharynx, skin and soft tissue caused by susceptible strains of microorganisms. Prevention of recurrence following rheumatic fever and/or chorea. May be useful as prophylaxis against bacterial endocarditis in patients with congenital heart disease or rheumatic or other acquired valvular heart disease who are undergoing dental procedures and surgical procedures of the upper respiratory tract.

**DOSAGE:** *Adults:* Usual: Streptococcal Infections (Scarlet Fever/Erysipelas/Upper Respiratory Tract): 125-250mg q6-8h for 10 days. Pneumococcal Infections (Otitis Media/Respiratory Tract): 250-500mg q6h until afebrile for at least 2 days. Staphylococcus Infections (Skin/Soft Tissue): 250-500mg q6-8h. Fusospirochetosis (Oropharnyx): 250-500mg q6-8h. Rheumatic Fever/Chorea Prevention: 125-250mg bid. Bacterial Endocarditis Prophylaxis: 2g 1 hr before procedure; 1g after 6 hrs.

*Pediatrics:* ≥12 yrs: Usual: Streptococcal Infections (Scarlet Fever/Erysipelas/Upper Respiratory Tract): 125-250mg q6-8h for 10 days. Pneumococcal Infections (Otitis Media/Respiratory Tract): 250-500mg q6h until afebrile for at least 2 days. Staphylococcus Infections (Skin/Soft Tissue): 250-500mg q6-

8h. Fusospirochetosis (Oropharnyx): 250-500mg q6-8h. Rheumatic Fever/Chorea Prevention: 125-250mg bid. Bacterial Endocarditis Prophylaxis: 2g or 1g (<60 lbs) 1 hr before procedure; 1g or 500mg (<60 lbs) after 6 hrs.

**HOW SUPPLIED:** Sus: 125mg/5mL, 250mg/5mL [100mL, 200mL]; Tab: 250mg, 500mg

**WARNINGS/PRECAUTIONS:** Not for severe pneumonia, empyema, bacteremia, pericarditis, meningitis and arthritis during the acute stage. Serious, fatal anaphylactic reactions reported. *Clostridium difficile*-associated diarrhea (CDAD) reported. Oral administration may not be effective with severe illnesses, nausea, vomiting, gastric dilatation, cardiospasm, or intestinal hypermotility. Cross-sensitivity with cephalosporins. Use in the absence of a proven or strongly suspected bacterial infection or prophylaxis indication, may increase risk of development of drug resistant bacteria. Prolonged use may promote overgrowth of nonsusceptible organisms (eg, fungi); take appropriate measures if superinfection develops. Caution with history of significant asthma and allergies. In streptococcal infections, perform culture following completion of treatment.

**ADVERSE REACTIONS:** Epigastric distress, N/V, diarrhea, hypersensitivity reactions, black hairy tongue, anaphylaxis, superinfection (prolonged use).

**PREGNANCY:** Safety in pregnancy/nursing is not known.

**MECHANISM OF ACTION:** Penicillin; exerts a bactericidal action against penicillin-sensitive microorganisms during the stage of active multiplication. Acts through inhibition of biosynthesis of cell-wall mucopeptide.

**PHARMACOKINETICS: Distribution:** Plasma protein binding (80%). **Elimination:** Urine.

## NURSING CONSIDERATIONS

**Assessment:** Assess for history of significant allergies or asthma, N/V, gastric dilatation, severe illness, cardiospasm, intestinal hypermotility, and pregnancy/nursing status. Obtain culture and sensitivity tests especially in suspected staphylococcal infections.

**Monitoring:** Monitor for signs/symptoms of hypersensitivity reactions, CDAD (mild diarrhea to fatal colitis), and for superinfections. Perform culture following completion of streptococcal treatment to ensure eradication.

**Patient Counseling:** Inform that therapy only treats bacterial, not viral infections. Instruct to take as directed. Advise that skipping doses or not completing full course of therapy may decrease effectiveness and increase resistance. Advise that may experience diarrhea; instruct to contact physician if watery and bloody stools or hypersensitivity reactions occur.

**Administration:** Oral route. **Storage:** 20-25°C (68-77°F). Keep tightly closed. Dispense in a tight container.



# Penlac RX

ciclopirox (Dermik)

**THERAPEUTIC CLASS:** Broad-spectrum antifungal

**INDICATIONS:** Mild to moderate onychomycosis of fingernails or toenails without lunula involvement due to *Trichophyton rubrum* (in immunocompetent patients).

**DOSAGE:** *Adults:* Apply qhs or 8 hrs before washing to nail bed, hyponychium, and under surface when it is free of nail bed. Apply daily over previous coat and remove with alcohol every 7 days. Repeat cycle up to 48 weeks.

**HOW SUPPLIED:** Sol: 8% [6.6mL]

**WARNINGS/PRECAUTIONS:** Only for use on nails and adjacent skin. Caution with removal of infected nail in insulin-dependent DM or diabetic neuropathy.

**ADVERSE REACTIONS:** Periungual erythema, erythema of proximal nail fold, nail shape change, nail irritation, ingrown toenail, nail discoloration.

**INTERACTIONS:** Avoid nail polish or other nail cosmetics on treated nails.

**PREGNANCY:** Category B, caution in nursing.

**MECHANISM OF ACTION:** Broad spectrum antifungal; acts by chelation of polyvalent cations ($Fe^{+3}$ or $Al^{+3}$), resulting in the inhibition of the metal-dependent enzymes responsible for degradation of peroxides within fungal cell.

**PHARMACOKINETICS: Absorption:** Serum levels range from 12-80ng/mL following topical administration. **Elimination:** Urine (<5% of applied topical dose).

## NURSING CONSIDERATIONS

**Assessment:** Assess use with insulin-dependent DM, diabetic neuropathy, and in pregnant/nursing females. Assess medication is only being used on nails or immediately adjacent skin.

**Monitoring:** Monitor for signs/symptoms of sensitivity reactions and chemical irritation. Perform frequent (eg, monthly) removal of unattached infected nails, trimming of onycholic nails, and filing of any excess horny material.

**Patient Counseling:** Advise to avoid bringing medication in contact with eyes and mucous membranes. Instruct to apply medication evenly over entire nail plate and 5mm of surrounding skin. Counsel to notify physician if signs of increased irritation at the application site develop (eg, redness, itching, burning, oozing, blistering). Inform to file away (with emery board) loose nail material and trim nails as required. Advise not to use nail polish or other nail cosmetic products on the treated nails. Instruct not to use medication near open flame. Inform that it may take up to 48 weeks of daily application of the medication (including monthly professional removal of unattached infected nails) before a clear or almost clear nail is seen.

**Administration:** Topical route. **Storage:** Between 15-30°C (59-86°F). Flammable; keep away from heat and flame.

# PENTASA RX

mesalamine (Shire)

**THERAPEUTIC CLASS:** Anti-inflammatory Agent

**INDICATIONS:** Induction of remission and for treatment of mild to moderate active ulcerative colitis.

P

**DOSAGE:** *Adults:* 1g qid. Can be given up to 8 weeks.

**HOW SUPPLIED:** Cap, Extended-Release: 250mg, 500mg

**CONTRAINDICATIONS:** Hypersensitivity to salicylates.

**WARNINGS/PRECAUTIONS:** Caution with hepatic and renal dysfunction; monitor closely. D/C if acute intolerance syndrome develops (eg, cramping, bloody diarrhea, abdominal pain, headache). If rechallenge is considered, perform under careful observation.

**ADVERSE REACTIONS:** Diarrhea, headache, nausea, abdominal pain.

**PREGNANCY:** Category B, caution in nursing.

**MECHANISM OF ACTION:** Unknown, suspected to act as anti-inflammatory agent for blocking cyclooxygenase and inhibiting prostaglandin in gastrointestinal use.

**PHARMACOKINETICS: Absorption:** $C_{max}$=1mcg/mL, $T_{max}$=3 hrs. (N-acetylmesalamine) $C_{max}$=1.8mcg/mL, $T_{max}$=3 hrs. **Metabolism:** N-acetylmesalamine (Metabolite). **Elimination:** Feces, N-acetylmesalamine: Urine (19-30%).

## NURSING CONSIDERATIONS

**Assessment:** Assess for pre-existing renal disease, hepatic/renal impairment. Obtain baseline LFTs, BUN, creatinine, and urinalysis (protein).

**Monitoring:** Monitor LFTs, BUN, creatinine, and urinalysis (protein) periodically. Monitor signs/symptoms of hepatotoxicity, acute intolerance syndrome (cramping, acute abdominal pain, bloody diarrhea), hypersensitivity, and allergic reactions.

**Patient Counseling:** Seek medical attention if symptoms of hepatotoxicity, acute intolerance syndrome (cramping, acute abdominal pain, bloody diarrhea), hypersensitivity and allergic reactions occur.

**Administration:** Oral route. **Storage:** 25°C (77°F); excursions permitted to 15-30°C (59-86°F).

## PEPCID
famotidine (Merck) **RX**

**THERAPEUTIC CLASS:** $H_2$-blocker

**INDICATIONS:** (PO/Inj) Short term treatment of active duodenal ulcer (DU), active benign gastric ulcer (GU), gastroesophageal reflux disease (GERD) and esophagitis due to GERD. Maintenance therapy for DU. Treatment of hypersecretory conditions (eg, Zollinger-Ellison syndrome). (Inj) For hospitalized patients with hypersecretory conditions or intractable ulcers. As an alternative in patients unable to take oral forms.

**DOSAGE:** *Adults:* (PO) Acute DU: 40mg qhs or 20mg bid for 4-8 weeks. Maint DU: 20mg qhs. GU: 40mg qhs. GERD: 20mg bid up to 6 weeks. GERD with Esophagitis: 20-40mg bid up to 12 weeks. Hypersecretory Conditions: Initial: 20mg q6h. Max: 160mg q6h. (Inj) 20mg IV q12h, hypersecretory conditions may require higher doses. CrCl <50mL/min: Reduce to 1/2 dose, or increase interval to q36-48h.
*Pediatrics:* 1-16 yrs: (PO) DU/GU: Usual: 0.5mg/kg/day qhs or divided bid. Max: 40mg/day. GERD With or Without Esophagitis: 0.5mg/kg PO bid. Max: 40mg bid. (Inj) 0.25mg/kg IV q12h up to 40mg/day. Base duration of therapy on clinical response, and/or pH, and endoscopy. (PO) GERD: 3 months-1yr: 0.5mg/kg bid for up to 8 weeks. <3 months: 0.5mg/kg qd for up to 8 weeks. CrCl <50mL/min: Reduce to 1/2 dose, or increase interval to q36-48h.

**HOW SUPPLIED:** Inj: 0.4mg/mL, 10mg/mL; Sus: 40mg/5mL [50mL]; Tab: 20mg, 40mg

**CONTRAINDICATIONS:** Hypersensitivity to other $H_2$ antagonists.

**WARNINGS/PRECAUTIONS:** CNS adverse effects reported with moderate to severe renal insufficiency; adjust dose. Disintegrating tabs contain phenylalanine; caution in phenylketonurics. Symptomatic response does not preclude the presence of gastric malignancy.

**ADVERSE REACTIONS:** Headache, dizziness, constipation, diarrhea, convulsions, interstitial pneumonia, Stevens-Johnson syndrome.

**INTERACTIONS:** May give with antacids.

**PREGNANCY:** Category B, not for use in nursing.

**MECHANISM OF ACTION:** Histamine $H_2$-receptor antagonist; inhibits both acid concentration and volume of gastric secretion.

**PHARMACOKINETICS: Absorption:** (Adults PO): Incompletely absorbed; $T_{max}$=1.3 hrs. (Adults, IV): $T_{max}$=20-30 min. **Distribution:** (Adult) Plasma protein binding (15-20%); excreted in breast milk. **Metabolism:** S-oxide (metabolite). **Elimination:** Renal (65-70%), (PO) 25-30% unchanged; (IV) 65-70% unchanged. Metabolic (65-70%); (Adults) $T_{1/2}$=2.5-3.5 hrs. Refer to package insert for pediatric parameters.

### NURSING CONSIDERATIONS

**Assessment:** Assess for hypersensitivity to other $H_2$ receptor antagonists, renal insufficiency, pregnancy/status.

**Monitoring:** If renal impairment present, monitor renal function. Monitor for signs/symptoms of hypersensitivity reactions (eg, anaphylaxis), GI effects (eg, constipation, diarrhea), and headache.

**Patient Counseling:** Instruct to contact physician if hypersensitivity or other adverse reactions develop. Inform may take antacids concomitantly. Avoid nursing while on medication.

**Administration:** Oral or IV route. **Storage:** Tablet: Controlled room temperature; preserve in well-closed, light-resistant containers. Injection: 2-8°C (36-

P

46°F); if solution freezes, bring to room temperature; allow sufficient time to solubilize all components. Premixed: 25°C (77°F); avoid exposure of premixed product to excessive heat.

## PERCOCET

CII

oxycodone HCl - acetaminophen (Endo)

**OTHER BRAND NAMES:** Endocet (Endo)

**THERAPEUTIC CLASS:** Opioid analgesic

**INDICATIONS:** Relief of moderate to moderately severe pain.

**DOSAGE:** *Adults:* (2.5mg-325mg): 1-2 tabs q6h prn. Max: 12 tabs/day. (5mg-325mg): 1 tab q6h prn. Max: 12 tabs/day. (7.5mg-500mg): 1 tab q6h prn. Max: 8 tabs/day. (10mg-650mg) 1 tab q6h prn. Max: 6 tabs/day. (7.5mg-325mg): 1 tab q6h prn. Max: 8 tabs/day. (10mg-325mg): 1 tab q6h prn. Max: 6 tabs/day. Do not exceed APAP 4g/day.

**HOW SUPPLIED:** Tab: (Oxycodone-APAP) 2.5mg-325mg, 5mg-325mg, 7.5mg-325mg, 7.5mg-500mg, 10mg-325mg, 10mg-650mg

**CONTRAINDICATIONS:** Oxycodone: Significant respiratory depression (in unmonitored settings or absence of resuscitative equipment), acute or severe bronchial asthma or hypercarbia, paralytic ileus.

**WARNINGS/PRECAUTIONS:** May cause drug dependence and tolerance; potential for abuse. Risk of respiratory depression. Capacity to elevate CSF pressure may be exaggerated with head injury, other intracranial lesions or a pre-existing increase in ICP. May obscure the diagnosis or clinical course with head injuries or with acute abdominal conditions. Caution with severe hepatic impairment, renal dysfunction, hypothyroidism, Addison's disease, prostatic hypertrophy, urethral stricture, the elderly or debilitated.

**ADVERSE REACTIONS:** Lightheadedness, dizziness, sedation, N/V, euphoria, dysphoria, constipation, skin rash, pruritus.

**INTERACTIONS:** Potentiates CNS depression with other opioid analgesics, general anesthetics, phenothiazines, tranquilizers, sedative-hypnotics, alcohol and other CNS depressants. Risk of paralytic ileus with anticholinergics.

**PREGNANCY:** Category C, caution in nursing.

P

**MECHANISM OF ACTION:** Oxycodone: Opioid analgesic; semisynthetic pure opioid agonist whose principal therapeutic action is analgesia. Other pharmacological effects include anxiolysis, euphoria, and feelings of relaxation. Effects mediated by CNS receptors (eg, μ and kappa) for endogenous opioid-like compounds (eg, endorphins, enkephalins). APAP: Nonopiate, nonsalicyclic analgesic, and antipyretic. Site and mechanism of analgesic effect not established. Antipyretic effect produced through inhibition of endogenous pyrogen action on the hypothalamic heat-regulating centers.

**PHARMACOKINETICS: Absorption:** Oxycodone: Absolute bioavailability (87%). APAP: Rapid absorption. **Distribution:** Oxycodone: Plasma protein binding (45%); (IV):$V_d$= 211.9L; found in breast milk. APAP: Plasma protein binding (20-50%) (variable). **Metabolism:** Oxycodone: N-dealkylation to noroxycodone (metabolite); CYP2D6 (O-demethylation) to oxymorphone (metabolite). Acetaminophen: Liver via cytochrome P450 (conjugation), NAPQI (toxic metabolite). **Elimination:** Oxycodone: Urine (parent compound and metabolites); $T_{1/2}$=3.51 hrs. APAP: Urine (90-100%).

### NURSING CONSIDERATIONS

**Assessment:** Assess for respiratory depression, acute or severe bronchial asthma or hypercarbia, COPD, paralytic ileus, potential for abuse, presence of debilitation (eg, elderly), head injury or other intracranial lesions, elevations in ICP, circulatory shock, acute abdominal condition, biliary tract disease, acute pancreatitis, hepatic/renal impairment, CNS depression, hypothyroidism, Addison's disease, prostatic hypertrophy, urethral stricture, acute alcoholism, delirium tremens, convulsive disorder, kyphoscoliosis with respiratory depression, myxedema, toxic psychosis, nursing/pregnancy status, medication abuse potential, and possible drug interactions.

**Monitoring:** Monitor for signs/symptoms of respiratory depression, elevations in CSF pressure, hypotension, hepatotoxicity, convulsions, anaphylactic reactions, decreased bowel motility, sphincter of Oddi spasms, increased serum amylase levels, tolerance and physical dependence, and medication abuse.

**Patient Counseling:** Instruct to keep out of reach of children. If accidental ingestion occurs, seek emergency medical care. Advise to flush unused medication down toilet. Counsel not to adjust dose without consulting physician. Inform drug may impair mental/physical abilities required to perform hazardous tasks (eg, operating machinery/driving). Advise to avoid alcohol or other CNS depressants. Instruct not to abruptly d/c if on for few weeks; taper dosing. Inform that medication has potential for abuse; protect from theft.

**Administration:** Oral route. **Storage:** 20-25°C (68-77°F). Dispense in tight, light-resistant container, with child-resistant closure.

## PERCODAN

oxycodone HCl - aspirin (Endo)

CII

**OTHER BRAND NAMES:** Endodan (Endo)

**THERAPEUTIC CLASS:** Opioid analgesic

**INDICATIONS:** Management of moderate to moderately severe pain.

**DOSAGE:** *Adults:* Usual: 1 tab q6h prn. Max: 12 tabs/day or ASA 4g/day.

**HOW SUPPLIED:** Tab: (Oxycodone HCl-ASA) 4.8355mg-325mg* *scored

**CONTRAINDICATIONS:** Oxycodone: Significant respiratory depression (in unmonitored settings or absence of resuscitative equipment), acute or severe bronchial asthma or hypercarbia, paralytic ileus. ASA: Hemophilia, viral infection in children/teens with or w/o fever, syndrome of asthma, rhinitis, and nasal polyps.

**WARNINGS/PRECAUTIONS:** May cause drug dependence and tolerance; potential for abuse. Risk of respiratory depression. Capacity to elevate CSF pressure may be exaggerated with head injury, other intracranial lesions or a pre-existing increase in ICP. May obscure the diagnosis or clinical course with head injuries or with acute abdominal conditions. Caution with severe hepatic impairment, renal dysfunction, hypothyroidism, Addison's disease, prostatic hypertrophy, urethral stricture, peptic ulcer, coagulation abnormalities, and the elderly or debilitated. May increase the risk of developing Reye's syndrome in children and teenagers. May impair mental/physical abilities.

**ADVERSE REACTIONS:** Lightheadedness, dizziness, sedation, N/V, euphoria, dysphoria, constipation, pruritus.

**INTERACTIONS:** Additive CNS depression with other opioid analgesics, general anesthetics, phenothiazines, tranquilizers, sedative-hypnotics, or other CNS depressants (including alcohol). ASA may enhance effect of anticoagulants and inhibit effects of uricosuric agents.

**PREGNANCY:** Category B (Oxycodone) and D (ASA), not for use in nursing.

**MECHANISM OF ACTION:** Oxycodone: Semisynthetic pure opioid agonist. Principle therapeutic effect is analgesia. Other effects include anxiolysis, euphoria, and feelings of relaxation. Effects mediated by CNS receptors (eg, μ, kappa) for endogenous opioid-like compounds (eg, endorphins, enkephalins). ASA: Inhibits prostaglandin production, including those involved in inflammation. (Prostaglandins cause pain sensation by stimulating muscle contractions and dilating blood vessels throughout body.) In CNS, works on hypothalamus heat-regulating center to reduce fever.

**PHARMACOKINETICS: Absorption:** Oxycodone: Absolute bioavailability (87%). ASA: Rapidly absorbed. **Distribution:** Oxycodone: Plasma protein binding (45%); found in breast milk; (IV) $V_d$=211.9L. ASA: Found in most body tissues, fluids (eg, fetal tissues, breast milk, CNS, liver, kidneys); variable serum protein binding. **Metabolism:** Oxycodone: N-dealkylation to noroxycodone (metabolite); CYP2D6 (O-demethylation) to oxymorphone (metabolite). ASA: Liver, hydrolysis to salicylate, salicyluric acid, salicyl phenolic glucuronide, salicyl acyl glucuronide, gentisic acid, gentisuric acid (major metabolites).

**Elimination:** Oxycodone: Urine (parent compound and metabolites); $T_{1/2}$=3.51 hrs. ASA: Urine (parent compound and metabolites) (80-100%); $T_{1/2}$=2-3 hrs.

## NURSING CONSIDERATIONS

**Assessment:** Assess for hemophilia, presence of viral infection if using in pediatrics, hypersensitivity to NSAIDS, asthma, rhinitis, nasal polyps, respiratory depression, hypercarbia, paralytic ileus, medication abuse potential, head injury or other intracranial lesions, presence of increased ICP, circulatory shock, inherited or acquired bleeding disorders (eg, hemophilia, vitamin K deficiency), active peptic ulcer disease, CNS depression, presence of debilitation (eg, elderly), hepatic/renal dysfunction, hypothyroidism, Addison's disease, prostatic hypertrophy, urethral stricture, acute alcoholism, delirium tremens, kyphoscoliosis with respiratory depression, myxedema, toxic psychosis, convulsive disorder, biliary tract disease, acute pancreatitis, pregnancy/nursing status, and possible drug interactions.

**Monitoring:** Monitor for signs/symptoms of respiratory depression, elevations in CSF pressure, hypotension, hemorrhage, GI effects (eg, stomach pain, heartburn, ulceration, GI bleeding), convulsions, anaphylactic reactions, decreased bowel motility, sphincter of Oddi spasms, tolerance, and physical dependence. Monitor for elevated hepatic enzymes, elevated BUN and SrCr, hyperkalemia, proteinuria, prolonged bleeding time, and increases in serum amylase levels. In pediatrics, monitor for Reye's syndrome.

**Patient Counseling:** Instruct to keep out of reach of children; if accidental ingestion occurs, seek medical attention. Advise to dispose of unused drug via toilet. Counsel to consult physician before adjusting dosing. Caution that drug may impair mental/physical abilities required for performing hazardous tasks (eg, operating machinery/driving). Instruct to avoid alcohol and other CNS depressants. Advise not to abruptly d/c if on medication for more than few weeks; taper dosing. Instruct to report adverse events (eg, respiratory depression). Inform that medication has potential for abuse; protect from theft.

**Administration:** Oral route. **Storage:** 25°C (77°F); excursions permitted to 15-30°C (59-86°F). Dispense in a tight, light-resistant container with child-resistant closure.

P

# PERFOROMIST RX

formoterol fumarate (Dey)

**Long-acting $\beta_2$-agonists may increase risk of asthma-related death.**

**THERAPEUTIC CLASS:** Beta$_2$-agonist

**INDICATIONS:** Long-term maintenance treatment of bronchoconstriction in patients with chronic obstructive pulmonary disease (COPD), including chronic bronchitis and emphysema.

**DOSAGE:** *Adults:* 20mcg q12h by nebulization. Max: 40mcg/day.

**HOW SUPPLIED:** Sol, Inhalation: 20mcg/2mL

**WARNINGS/PRECAUTIONS:** Only use short-acting $\beta_2$-agonist inhalers for acute symptoms. Should not be used with other long acting $\beta_2$-agonist medications. D/C if paradoxical bronchospasm occurs. D/C if ECG changes, QT interval increases, or ST depression occurs. Caution with cardiovascular (CV) disorders (eg, coronary insufficiency, arrythmias, and HTN), convulsive disorders, thyrotoxicosis, and DM. May cause hypokalemia and hyperglycemia.

**ADVERSE REACTIONS:** Diarrhea, nausea, nasopharyngitis, dry mouth, angina, HTN, hypotension, tachycardia, arrythmias, nervousness, headache, tremor, muscle cramps, palpitations, dizziness.

**INTERACTIONS:** Adrenergic drugs may potentiate effects. Xanthine derivatives, steroids, diuretics, or non-potassium sparing diuretics may potentiate hypokalemia or ECG changes; use with caution. MAOIs, TCAs, and drugs known to prolong QTc interval may potentiate effect on CV system; use with extreme caution. β-blockers may decrease effectiveness; use with caution.

**PREGNANCY:** Category C, caution in nursing.

**MECHANISM OF ACTION:** $\beta_2$-agonist; acts as bronchodilator, stimulates intracellular adenyl cyclase, the enzyme that catalyzes the conversion of ATP to cAMP. Increased cAMP levels cause relaxation of bronchial smooth muscle and inhibition of release of mediators of immediated hypersensitivity from cells such as mast cells.

**PHARMACOKINETICS: Absorption:** $C_{max}$=72pg/mL; $T_{max}$=12 min. **Distribution:** Plasma protein binding (61-64%). **Metabolism:** Glucuronidation, O-demethylation; CYP2D6, 2C19, 2A6. **Elimination:** Urine (unchanged); $T_{1/2}$=7 hrs.

## NURSING CONSIDERATIONS

**Assessment:** Assess for acute COPD, asthma, acute bronchospasm, CV disease (coronary insufficiency, cardiac arrhythmias, HTN), convulsive disorders, thyrotoxicosis, K+ levels, DM, ketoacidosis, pregnancy/nursing status, and possible drug interactions.

**Monitoring:** Monitor for serious asthma exacerbations, paradoxical bronchospasm, cardiovascular effects, hypokalemia, hyperglycemia, aggravation of DM, ketoacidosis, pulse rate, BP, and ECG changes (T-wave flattening, prolongation of QTc interval, ST segment depression).

**Patient Counseling:** Do not inhale more than prescribed. Excessive use may increase likelihood of CV side effects. Maximum daily dose is 1 vial twice daily. Use other inhaler (albuterol) only for acute symptoms, and consult with physician about use of other inhalers. Immediately report any side effects to physician (chest pain, rapid heart rate, headache, nervousness, dry mouth, muscle cramps, nausea, dizziness, fatigue, malaise, and BP changes). Always keep in foil patch; only remove for use and discard container and top right after use.

**Administration:** Oral inhalation. Only administered via a standard jet nebulizer connected to an air compressor with adequate airflow and equipped with a facemask or mouthpiece. **Storage:** Prior to dispensing: 2-8°C (36-46°F). After dispensing: 2-25°C (36-77°F) for up to 3 months. Protect from heat.

# PEXEVA — RX

paroxetine mesylate (Noven)

**Antidepressants increased the risk of suicidal thinking and behavior (suicidality) in short-term studies in children, adolescents, and young adults with major depressive disorder (MDD) and other psychiatric disorders. Paroxetine is not approved for use in pediatric patients.**

**THERAPEUTIC CLASS:** Selective serotonin reuptake inhibitor

**INDICATIONS:** Treatment of major depressive disorder (MDD), obsessive compulsive disorder (OCD), panic disorder with or without agoraphobia, and generalized anxiety disorder (GAD).

**DOSAGE:** *Adults:* Give qd, usually in the AM. MDD: Initial: 20mg/day. Max: 50mg/day. OCD: Initial: 20mg/day. Titrate: Increase by 10mg/day increments at intervals of at least 1 week. Usual: 40mg/day. Max: 60mg/day. Panic Disorder: Initial: 10mg/day. Titrate: 10mg/day increments at intervals of at least 1 week. Max: 60mg/day. GAD: Initial: 20mg/day. Titrate: Increase by 10mg/day increments at intervals of at least 1 week. Max: 50mg/day. Elderly/Debilitated/Severe Renal or Hepatic Impairment: Initial: 10mg/day. Max: 40mg/day.

**HOW SUPPLIED:** Tab: 10mg, 20mg*, 30mg, 40mg *scored

**CONTRAINDICATIONS:** Concomitant use of MAOIs, thioridazine, and pimozide.

**WARNINGS/PRECAUTIONS:** Serotonin syndrome and neuroleptic malignant syndrome (NMS)-like reactions reported. Avoid abrupt withdrawal. May increase risk of bleeding events. Caution with history of mania, seizures, conditions that affect metabolism or hemodynamic responses, narrow-angle glaucoma. D/C if seizures occur. Activation of mania/hypomania, altered platelet function, hyponatremia reported. May impair judgment, thinking, or motor skills. Serotonin syndrome may occur. Monitor for clinical worsening and/or suicidality, especially at initiation of therapy or dose changes.

**ADVERSE REACTIONS:** Asthenia, sweating, nausea, decreased appetite, somnolence, dizziness, insomnia, tremor, nervousness, abnormal ejaculation, dry mouth, constipation, decreased libido, impotence, headache, tinnitus.

**INTERACTIONS:** See Contraindications. Avoid alcohol, tryptophan. May shift concentrations with plasma-bound drugs. Caution with SSRIs, SNRIs, TCAs, lithium. Increased risk of bleeding with NSAIDS, ASA, warfarin. Rare reports of weakness, hyperreflexia, incoordination with SSRIs and a triptan. Monitor theophylline. Reduce procyclidine dose if anticholinergic effects occur. Increased levels with cimetidine. Caution with digoxin, drugs metabolized by CYP2D6 (eg, antidepressants, phenothiazines, Type 1C antiarrhythmics), or drugs that inhibit CYP2D6 (eg, quinidine). Fosamprenavir/ritonavir may decrease levels. Concomitant use of serotonergic drugs and drugs that impair metabolism of serotonin may cause serotonin syndrome. Caution with other agents that may affect serotonin neurotransmitter systems (eg, triptans, linezolid, tramadol, or St. John's wort).

**PREGNANCY:** Category D, caution in nursing.

**MECHANISM OF ACTION:** SSRI; inhibits CNS neuronal reuptake of serotonin.

**PHARMACOKINETICS: Absorption:** Complete; $C_{max}$=81.3ng/mL; $T_{max}$=8.1 hr. **Distribution:** Plasma protein binding (95%). **Metabolism:** Oxidation and methylation via CYP2D6. **Elimination:** Urine (2%), feces (<1%); $T_{1/2}$=33.2 hrs.

## NURSING CONSIDERATIONS

**Assessment:** Assess for bipolar disorder risk, history of mania, history of seizures, narrow-angle glaucoma, disease/condition that alters metabolism or hemodynamic response, hepatic/renal impairment, and possible drug interactions.

**Monitoring:** Monitor for signs/symptoms of clinical worsening (suicidality, unusual changes in behavior), serotonin syndrome, abnormal bleeding, activation of mania, mydriasis, akathisia, hyponatremia, seizures, cognitive/motor impairment, hepatic/renal dysfunction. If abruptly d/c, monitor for symptoms of dysphoric mood, irritability, agitation, dizziness, sensory disturbances, anxiety, confusion, headache, lethargy, emotional lability, insomnia, and hypomania.

**Patient Counseling:** Instruct to swallow whole, not to chew or crush. Advise to avoid alcohol. Seek medical attention for symptoms of serotonin syndrome (mental status changes, tachycardia, hyperthermia, NV, diarrhea, incoordination), abnormal bleeding (particularly if using NSAIDs or ASA), akathisia, hyponatremia (headaches, unsteadiness), mydriasis, activation of mania, seizures, clinical worsening (suicidal ideation, unusual changes in behavior), or d/c symptoms (irritability, agitation, dizziness, anxiety, headache, insomnia). Caution against hazardous tasks (eg, operating machinery and driving). Inform may notice improvement in 1-4 weeks; continue therapy as directed. Notify physician if pregnant/intend to become pregnant, or breastfeeding. Counsel about benefits and risks of therapy. Inform physician if taking, or plan to take any over-the-counter prescriptions.

**Administration:** Oral route. **Storage:** 25°C (77°F); excursions permitted to 15-30°C (59-86°F). Protect from humidity.

# PHENERGAN INJECTION — RX

promethazine HCl (Baxter)

**Do not use in pediatric patients <2 yrs because of potential for fatal respiratory depression. Caution when used in pediatrics ≥2 yrs. Injection may cause severe chemical irritation and damage to tissue regardless of the route of administration. Irritation and damage may result from perivascular extravasation, unintentional intra-arterial injection, or intraneuronal/perineuronal infiltration; surgical intervention may be required. Preferred route of administration is deep IM injection; SQ injection is contraindicated.**

**THERAPEUTIC CLASS:** Phenothiazine derivative

**INDICATIONS:** Amelioration of allergic reactions to blood or plasma. In anaphylaxis as an adjunct to epinephrine and other standard measures after acute symptoms have been controlled. For other uncomplicated allergic conditions of the immediate type when oral therapy is not possible or contraindicated. For sedation and relief of apprehension to produce light sleep. Active treatment of motion sickness. Prevention and control of nausea and vomiting associated with certain types of anesthesia and surgery. Adjunct to analgesics for the control of postoperative pain. Preoperative, postoperative, and obstetric (during labor) sedation. IV in special surgical situations such as repeated bronchoscopy, ophthalmic surgery, and poor-risk patients, with reduced amounts of meperidine or other narcotic analgesic as adjunct to anesthesia and analgesia.

**DOSAGE:** *Adults:* (IM/IV) IM route is preferred. Allergy: Initial: 25mg, may repeat within 2 hrs. Adjust to the smallest adequate amount to relieve symptoms. For continued therapy, oral route preferred. Sedation: 25-50mg qhs in hospitalized patients. Nausea/Vomiting: Usual: 12.5-25mg, not to be repeated more frequently than q4h. Preoperative/Postoperative Adjunct: 25-50mg. May be combined with appropriately reduced doses of analgesics and atropine-like drugs. Obstetrics: 50mg in early stages of labor, 25-75mg in established labor may be given with an appropriately reduced dose of any desired narcotic, may repeat once or twice q4h in normal labor. Max: 100mg/24 hrs of labor. Do not give IV administration >25mg/mL and at a rate >25mg/min. Elderly: Start at lower end of dosing range.
*Pediatrics:* ≥2 yrs: Dose should not exceed half of suggested adult dose. Premedication Adjunct: Usual: 1.1 mg/kg body weight in combination with an appropriately reduced dose of narcotic or barbiturate and appropriate dose of an atropine-like drug. Do not give IV administration >25mg/mL and at a rate >25mg/min.

**HOW SUPPLIED:** Inj: 25mg/mL, 50mg/mL

**CONTRAINDICATIONS:** Children <2 yrs, comatose states, intra-arterial or SQ injection.

**WARNINGS/PRECAUTIONS:** Not recommended for uncomplicated vomiting in pediatrics. May impair physical/mental ability. Fatal respiratory depression reported; avoid with compromised respiratory function or patients at risk of respiratory failure (eg, COPD, sleep apnea). May impair mental and/or physical abilities. May lower seizure threshold. Caution with bone marrow depression; leukopenia and agranulocytosis reported. Neuroleptic malignant syndrome (NMS) reported. Sulfite sensitivity may occur; caution especially in asthmatics. Inspect inj before use and discard if either color or particulate is observed. Avoid in pediatrics with Reye's syndrome or other hepatic diseases. Hallucinations and convulsions may occur in pediatrics. Increased susceptibility to dystonias in acutely ill pediatric patients with dehydration. May inhibit platelet aggregation in the newborn when used in pregnant women within two weeks of delivery. Caution with narrow-angle glaucoma, prostatic hypertrophy, stenosing peptic ulcer, bladder-neck or pyloroduodenal obstruction, cardiovascular (CV) disease, hepatic dysfunction. Cholestatic jaundice reported. May cause false interpretations of diagnostic pregnancy tests and may increase blood glucose. Caution in elderly.

**ADVERSE REACTIONS:** Respiratory depression, severe tissue injury, drowsiness, dizziness, tinnitus, blurred vision, dry mouth, increased or decreased BP, urticaria, N/V, blood dyscrasia, gangrene.

**INTERACTIONS:** Concomitant use with respiratory depressants in pediatric patients may result in death. May increase, prolong, or intensify sedation when used concomitantly with CNS depressants (eg, alcohol, sedative/hypnotics [including barbiturates], general anesthetics, narcotics, narcotic analgesics, TCAs, tranquilizers); avoid concomitant use or reduce dose. Reduce dose of barbiturates by at least 50% if given concomitantly. Reduce dose of narcotics by 25-50% if given concomitantly. Caution with drugs that alter seizure threshold (eg, narcotics, local anesthetics). Leukopenia and agranulocytosis reported when used with other known marrow-toxic agents. Do not use epinephrine for promethazine injection overdose. Caution with anticholinergics. Possible adverse reactions with MAOIs. NMS reported alone and in combination with antipsychotics.

**PREGNANCY:** Category C, not for use in nursing.

**MECHANISM OF ACTION:** Phenothiazine derivative/$H_1$ receptor antagonist; possesses antihistamine (does not block release of histamine), sedative, anti-motion sickness, antiemetic, and anticholinergic effects.

**PHARMACOKINETICS: Metabolism:** Liver; sulfoxides, N-desmethylpromethazine (metabolites). **Elimination:** Urine; $T_{1/2}$=9-16 hrs (IV), 9.8 hrs (IM).

## NURSING CONSIDERATIONS

**Assessment:** Assess for history of seizure disorder, compromised respiratory function or risk of respiratory failure (eg, COPD, sleep apnea), bone marrow depression, sulfite hypersensitivity, asthma, narrow-angle glaucoma, prostatic hypertrophy, stenosing peptic ulcer, pyloroduodenal obstruction, bladder-neck obstruction, CV disease, hepatic impairment, pregnancy/nursing status, and for possible drug interactions. Assess age of patient and presence of a comatose state. In pediatrics, assess for Reye's syndrome or presence of acute illness with dehydration.

**Monitoring:** Monitor for signs/symptoms of respiratory depression, seizures, leukopenia, agranulocytosis, NMS, cholestatic jaundice, injection-site reactions, and for hypersensitivity reactions. Monitor for hallucinations, convulsions, extrapyramidal symptoms and dystonia in pediatrics. In newborns, monitor platelet count, when used in pregnant women within 2 weeks of delivery.

**Patient Counseling:** Advise regarding risk of respiratory depression and risk of tissue injury. Caution patients that the medication may impair physical/mental abilities. Seek medical attention if symptoms of respiratory depression, seizures, infections, NMS (hyperpyrexia, muscle rigidity, autonomic instability), injection site reaction (burning, pain, erythema), or hypersensitivity reactions occur. Advise to avoid alcohol and certain other medications with possible interactions. Advise to avoid prolonged sun exposure.

**Administration:** IV, IM route. If pain occurs during IV injection, stop immediately and evaluate for possible arterial injection or perivascular extravasation. **Storage:** 20-25°C (68-77°F). Protect from light.

# PHENOBARBITAL

phenobarbital (Various)

CIV

P

**THERAPEUTIC CLASS:** Barbiturate

**INDICATIONS:** Treatment of generalized, tonic-clonic and cortical focal seizures. For relief of anxiety, tension and apprehension. Short-term treatment of insomnia.

**DOSAGE:** *Adults:* Sedation: 30-120mg/day given bid-tid. Max: 400mg/24h. Hypnotic: 100-200mg. Seizures: 60-200mg/day. Elderly/Debilitated/Renal or Hepatic Dysfunction: Reduce dosage.
*Pediatrics:* Seizures: 3-6mg/kg/day.

**HOW SUPPLIED:** Elixir: 20mg/5mL; Tab: 15mg, 30mg, 32.4mg, 60mg, 64.8mg, 100mg

**CONTRAINDICATIONS:** Respiratory disease with dyspnea or obstruction, porphyria, severe liver dysfunction. Large doses with nephritic patients.

**WARNINGS/PRECAUTIONS:** May be habit-forming. Avoid abrupt withdrawal. Caution with acute or chronic pain; may mask symptoms or paradoxical excitement may occur. Cognitive deficits reported in children with febrile seizures. May cause excitement in children; excitement, depression or confusion in elderly, debilitated. Caution with hepatic dysfunction, borderline hypoadrenal function, depression.

**ADVERSE REACTIONS:** Drowsiness, residual sedation, lethargy, vertigo, somnolence, respiratory depression, hypersensitivity reactions, N/V, headache.

**INTERACTIONS:** May be potentiated by MAOIs, antihistamines, alcohol, tranquilizers, sedative/hypnotics, other CNS depressants. Decreases effects of oral anticoagulants. Increases corticosteroid metabolism. Decreases effects of oral contraceptives. Decreases absorption of griseofulvin. Decreases half-life of doxycycline. May alter phenytoin metabolism. Increased levels with sodium valproate and valproic acid.

**PREGNANCY:** Category D, caution in nursing.

**MECHANISM OF ACTION:** Barbiturate; nonselective CNS depressant. Capable of producing all levels of CNS mood alteration. Responsible for depressing the sensory cortex, decreasing motor activity, altering cerebellar function, causing sedation and hypnosis.

**PHARMACOKINETICS: Distribution**: Distributed to all tissues and fluids. High concentrations found in the brain, liver, and kidneys. Found in breast milk. **Metabolism:** Hepatic. **Elimination:** Urine (primary), feces; $T_{1/2}$=79 hrs (adults), 110 hrs (children and newborns less than 48 hrs old).

## NURSING CONSIDERATIONS

**Assessment:** Assess for history of manifest or latent porphyria, hepatic impairment, or respiratory disease with evidence of dyspnea or obstruction. Assess use in children, pregnant women, history of drug abuse, elderly or debilitated patients, acute or chronic pain, borderline hypoadrenal function, and history of depression or suicidal tendencies. Assess for possible drug interactions.

**Monitoring:** For patients on prolonged therapy, perform periodic evaluations of hematopoietic, renal/hepatic function. Monitor for signs of psychological/physical dependence, cognitive deficits in children, signs/symptoms of CNS depression, acute intoxication of medication (eg, unsteady gait, slurred speech), signs of chronic intoxication (eg, confusion, insomnia), and for exfoliative dermatitis (eg, Stevens-Johnson syndrome, toxic epidermal necrosis). Monitor for withdrawal symptoms (eg, anxiety, muscle twitching, weakness, convulsions, delirium) after d/c medication.

**Patient Counseling:** Inform psychological/physical dependence may result. Instruct not to increase dosage without consulting physician. Inform medication may impair mental/physical abilities; use caution when performing hazardous tasks. Avoid alcohol or other CNS depressants while on medication. Notify physician if any type of rash develops.

**Administration:** Oral route. **Storage:** Store at controlled room temperature, 15-30°C (59-86°F).

# PHENYTEK — RX

phenytoin sodium (Mylan)

P

**THERAPEUTIC CLASS:** Hydantoin

**INDICATIONS:** Control of generalized tonic-clonic (grand mal) and complex partial (psychomotor, temporal lobe) seizures. Prevention and treatment of neurosurgically induced seizures.

**DOSAGE:** *Adults:* No Previous Treatment: Initial: 100mg tid. Titrate: May increase at 7- to 10-day intervals. Maint: 100mg tid-qid. May increase up to 200mg tid. Once Daily Dosing: 300mg qd may replace 100mg tid if seizures are controlled. LD (clinic/hospital): 1g in 3 divided doses (400mg, 300mg, 300mg) given 2 hrs apart. Start maintenance dose 24 hrs later. Avoid LD with renal and hepatic disease.

*Pediatrics:* Initial: 5mg/kg/day given in 2 or 3 equally divided doses. Titrate: May increase at 7- to 10-day intervals. Maint: 4-8mg/kg/day. Max: 300mg/day. >6 yrs: May require the minimum adult dose (300mg/day).

**HOW SUPPLIED:** Cap, Extended-Release: 200mg, 300mg

**WARNINGS/PRECAUTIONS:** Avoid abrupt withdrawal. D/C if rash occurs. Lymphadenopathy, with or without serum sickness (eg, fever, rash, liver involvement), reported; observe for an extended period and use alternative antiepileptic drugs. May exacerbate porphyria. Monitor levels. Confusional states reported with toxic levels. Caution with hepatic impairment, the elderly or if gravely ill. Reduce dose or d/c if symptoms persist. Hyperglycemia and osteomalacia reported. Not for seizures due to hypoglycemia or other metabolic causes. Birth defects, fetal hydantoin syndrome (eg, prenatal deficiency, microcephaly, and mental deficiency) and isolated cases of malignancies (eg, neuroblastoma) reported. Weigh benefits versus risks in treating women of childbearing potential. Neonatal coagulation defects may occur within first 24 hrs of birth; give vitamin K to mother before delivery and to neonate after birth. May alter protein-bound iodine, alkaline phosphatase, gamma glutamyl transeptidase levels and interfere with dexamethasone and metyrapone tests.

**ADVERSE REACTIONS:** Nystagmus, ataxia, slurred speech, decreased coordination, confusion, dizziness, insomnia, transient nervousness, motor twitchings, headaches, N/V, constipation, rash, hypersensitivity reactions.

**INTERACTIONS:** Increased levels with acute alcohol intake, amiodarone, chloramphenicol, chlordiazepoxide, diazepam, dicumarol, disulfiram, estrogens, ethosuximide, $H_2$-antagonists, halothane, isoniazid, methylphenidate, phenothiazines, phenylbutazone, salicylates, succinamides, sulfonamides, tolbutamide, trazodone. Decreased levels with chronic alcohol abuse, carbamazepine, reserpine, sucralfate. Decreases effects of corticosteroids, coumarin anticoagulants, digitoxin, doxycycline, estrogens, furosemide, oral contraceptives, quinidine, rifampin, theophylline, vitamin D. May increase or decrease levels of phenobarbital, sodium valproate, valproic acid. Calcium antacids decrease absorption; space dosing. Moban contains calcium ions that interfere with absorption. TCAs may precipitate seizures; adjust phenytoin dose. Increased risk of phenytoin hypersensitivity with barbiturates, succinamides, oxazolidinediones.

**PREGNANCY:** Safety not known in pregnancy, not for use in nursing.

**MECHANISM OF ACTION:** Anti-epileptic: primary site of action appears to be the motor cortex. Inhibits the spread of seizure activity possibly by promoting sodium efflux from neurons, stabilizing the threshold against hyperexcitability caused by excessive stimulation or environmental changes capable of reducing membrane sodium gradient. Also reduces the post-tetanic potentiation at synapses, which prevents cortical seizure foci from detonating adjacent cortical areas.

**PHARMACOKINETICS: Absorption:** $T_{max}$=4-12 hrs. **Metabolism:** Hepatic via hydroxylation. **Elimination:** Renal; bile (inactive metabolite) and urine; $T_{1/2}$=22 hrs.

## NURSING CONSIDERATIONS

P

**Assessment:** Assess for impaired liver function, porphyria, seizures due to hypoglycemic or other metabolic causes, nursing status, and possible drug interactions. Obtain baseline serum phenytoin levels.

**Monitoring:** Monitor serum phenytoin levels. Obtain levels to determine compliance and proper therapeutic efficacy just prior to patient's next scheduled dose. Monitor for skin rash (Stevens-Johnson syndrome), hyperglycemia, osteomalacia, phenytoin toxicity, which may produce confused states including delirium, psychosis, encephalopathy, development of lymphadenopathy.

**Patient Counseling:** Counsel to avoid alcohol while on medication. Instruct to notify physician if skin rash develops. Advise about importance of good dental hygiene to minimize development of gingival hyperplasia; importance of strictly adhering to prescribed dosage regimen, instruct not to abruptly d/c medication. Notify physician if pregnant or intend to become pregnant. Encourage patients to enroll in North American Antiepileptic Drug (NAAED) Pregnancy Registry by calling 888-233-2334 or go to www.aedpregnancyregistry.org.

**Administration:** Oral route. **Storage:** 20-25°C (68-77°F). Protect from light and moisture. Dispense in a tight, light-resistant container.

# PhosLo RX

calcium acetate (Fresenius)

**THERAPEUTIC CLASS:** Phoshphate binder

**INDICATIONS:** Control of hyperphosphatemia in end stage renal failure (ESRF). Does not promote aluminum absorption.

**DOSAGE:** *Adults:* Initial: 2 caps/tabs with each meal. Titrate: Increase gradually until serum phosphate <6mg/dL, as long as hypercalcemia does not develop. Maint: 3-4 caps/tabs with each meal.

**HOW SUPPLIED:** Cap: 667mg; Tab: 667mg

**CONTRAINDICATIONS:** Hypercalcemia.

**WARNINGS/PRECAUTIONS:** Increased risk of hypercalcemia when calcium given with meals in ESRF. Monitor serum calcium twice weekly during early dose adjustment period. If hypercalcemia develops, reduce dose or d/c depending on severity. Caution with arrhythmias.

**ADVERSE REACTIONS:** Hypercalcemia, constipation, anorexia, nausea, vomiting, confusion, delirium, stupor, coma.

**INTERACTIONS:** Decreased bioavailability of tetracyclines. Hypercalcemia may precipitate arrhythmia; avoid digitalis. Avoid other calcium supplements.

**PREGNANCY:** Category C, safety in nursing not known.

**MECHANISM OF ACTION:** Calcium acetate combines with dietary phosphate to form insoluble calcium phosphate, which is excreted in the feces.

## NURSING CONSIDERATIONS

**Assessment:** Assess for hypercalcemia, patients taking digitalis, pregnancy status, and possible drug interaction.

**Monitoring:** Monitor serum calcium level twice weekly: (CaXP) product ≤66. X-ray suspect anatomical region to detect soft tissue calcification. Monitor for cardiac arrhythmia and vascular calcification.

**Patient Counseling:** Inform about compliance with dosage and diet instructions. Avoid use of nonprescription antacids. Inform about symptoms of hypercalcemia.

**Administration:** Oral route, taken with meal. **Storage:** 25°C (77°F); excursions permitted to 15-30°C (59-86°F).

# PILOCARPINE RX

pilocarpine HCl (Various)

P

**OTHER BRAND NAMES:** Isopto Carpine (Alcon)

**THERAPEUTIC CLASS:** Cholinergic agent

**INDICATIONS:** To control IOP.

**DOSAGE:** *Adults:* 2 drops tid-qid or more if needed. Heavily pigmented irises may require higher strengths.

**HOW SUPPLIED:** Sol: 0.5%, 1%, 2%, 3%, 4%, 6% [15mL]

**CONTRAINDICATIONS:** Where constriction is undesirable (eg, acute iritis) or pupillary block glaucoma.

**WARNINGS/PRECAUTIONS:** Difficulty adapting in the dark. Caution while night driving and in poor illumination. Risk of retinal detachment.

**ADVERSE REACTIONS:** Local irritation, ciliary spasm, conjunctival vascular congestion, temporal or supraorbital headache, induced myopia, reduced visual acuity in poor illumination (elderly), lens opacity (prolonged use).

**PREGNANCY:** Category C, caution in nursing.

**MECHANISM OF ACTION:** Cholinergic agent; acts through direct stimulation of muscarinic neuroreceptors and smooth muscle such as iris and secretory glands. Produces miosis through contraction of iris sphincter, causing increased tension on scleral spur and opening of trabecular mesh work spaces to facilitate outflow of aqueous humor, thereby reducing outflow resistance and lowering IOP.

## NURSING CONSIDERATIONS

**Assessment:** Prior to initiation, assess for acute iritis and pupillary block glaucoma. Assess pregnancy/nursing status.

**Monitoring:** Monitor for possible miosis, retinal detachment, and lens opacity with prolonged therapy.

**Patient Counseling:** Advise that visual difficulties in dark environments may occur; use caution performing hazardous activities in poor light. Do not touch dropper tip to any surface to avoid contamination.

**Administration:** Ocular route. **Storage:** 8-27°C (46-80°F).

## PINDOLOL RX

pindolol (Various)

**THERAPEUTIC CLASS:** Nonselective beta-blocker

**INDICATIONS:** Management of hypertension.

**DOSAGE:** *Adults:* Initial: 5mg bid. Titrate: May increase by 10mg/day after 3-4 weeks. Max: 60mg/day.

**HOW SUPPLIED:** Tab: 5mg, 10mg

**CONTRAINDICATIONS:** Bronchial asthma, overt cardiac failure, cardiogenic shock, 2nd- and 3rd-degree heart block, severe bradycardia.

**WARNINGS/PRECAUTIONS:** Caution with well-compensated heart failure, nonallergic bronchospasm, renal or hepatic impairment. Can cause cardiac failure. Avoid abrupt withdrawal. Withdrawal before surgery is controversial. May mask hypoglycemia or hyperthyroidism symptoms.

**ADVERSE REACTIONS:** Dizziness, fatigue, insomnia, nervousness, dyspnea, edema, joint pain, muscle cramps/pain.

**INTERACTIONS:** Additive hypotension and/or bradycardia with catecholamine-depleting drugs. Both thioridazine and pindolol levels may increase when used concomitantly.

**PREGNANCY:** Category B, not for use in nursing.

**MECHANISM OF ACTION:** Nonselective β-blocker; inhibits β-andrenergic receptor with intrinsic sympathomimetic activity.

**PHARMACOKINETICS: Absorption:** Rapid; $T_{max}$=1 hr. **Distribution:** $V_d$=2L/Kg; plasma protein binding (40%). **Metabolism:** Metabolized to hydroxymetabolites, which are excreted as glucoronides and ethereal sulfates. **Elimination:** Urine (35-40%), feces (6-9%); $T_{1/2}$=approximately 3-4 hrs, $T_{1/2}$=8 hrs (metabolites).

P

### NURSING CONSIDERATIONS

**Assessment:** Assess for history of anaphylactic reaction, bronchial asthma, overt cardiac failure, cardiogenic shock, 2nd- or 3rd-degree heart block, severe bradycardia, bronchospastic disease, DM, thyrotoxicosis, LFTs, renal functions, pregnancy status, and possible drug interactions. D/C drug well before any surgeries.

**Monitoring:** Monitor for anaphylactic reactions, LFTs, dizziness, fatigue, edema, dyspnea, muscle pain, heart block, hypotension, claudication, visual disturbances, impotence, CBC with differential and platelet count, Peyronie's disease, CHF, bronchospasm.

**Patient Counseling:** Instruct not to interrupt or d/c therapy without consulting physician. Counsel about signs/symptoms of CHF, bronchospasm, and other adverse effects; seek prompt medical assistance if any develop.

**Administration:** Oral route. **Storage:** Below 30°C (86°F); tight, light-resistant container.

## PIPERACILLIN RX

piperacillin sodium (Various)

**THERAPEUTIC CLASS:** Broad-spectrum penicillin

**INDICATIONS:** Treatment of serious infections caused by susceptible strains of microorganisms in the following conditions: intra-abdominal, urinary tract, gynecologic, lower respiratory tract, skin and skin structure, bone/joint, and uncomplicated gonococcal urethritis, and septicemia. Perioperative surgical prophylaxis during certain procedures.

**DOSAGE:** *Adults:* Usual: 3-4g IM/IV q4-6h. Max: 24g/day; IM: 2g/site. Serious Infections: 200-300mg/kg/day IV divided q4-6h. Complicated UTI: 125-200mg/kg/day IV divided q6-8h. Uncomplicated UTI/CAP: 100-125mg/kg/day IM/IV divided q6-12h. Uncomplicated Gonorrhea: 2g IM single dose with 1g PO probenecid 1/2 hr before injection. Surgical Prophylaxis: 2g IV 20-30 min just prior to anesthesia (See PI for follow-up dosing). Renal Impairment: Uncomplicated/Complicated UTI: CrCl <20mL/min: 3g q12h. Complicated UTI: CrCl 20-40mL/min: 3g q8h. Serious Infection: CrCl 20-40mL/min: 4g q8h. CrCl <20mL/min: 4g q12h. Hemodialysis: Give 1g additional dose after each dialysis. Max: 2g q8h. Usual treatment is for 7-10 days; treat gynecologic infections for 3-10 days; treat *S.pyogenes* infections for at least 10 days.

*Pediatrics:* ≥12 yrs: Usual: 3-4g IM/IV q4-6h. Max: 24g/day; IM: 2g/site. Serious Infections: 200-300mg/kg/day IV divided q4-6h. Complicated UTI: 125-200mg/kg/day IV divided q6-8h. Uncomplicated UTI/CAP: 100-125mg/kg/day IM/IV divided q6-12h. Uncomplicated Gonorrhea: 2g IM single dose with 1g PO probenecid 1/2 hr before injection. Surgical Prophylaxis: 2g IV 20-30 min just prior to anesthesia (See PI for follow-up dosing). Renal Impairment: Uncomplicated/Complicated UTI: CrCl <20mL/min: 3g q12h. Complicated UTI: CrCl 20-40mL/min: 3g q8h. Serious Infection: CrCl 20-40mL/min: 4g q8h. CrCl <20mL/min: 4g q12h. Hemodialysis: Give 1g additional dose after each dialysis. Max: 2g q8h. Usual treatment is for 7-10 days; treat gynecologic infections for 3-10 days; treat *S.pyogenes* infections for at least 10 days.

**HOW SUPPLIED:** Inj: 2g, 3g, 4g

**CONTRAINDICATIONS:** Hypersensitivity to cephalosporins.

**WARNINGS/PRECAUTIONS:** Serious, sometimes fatal, hypersensitivity reactions reported with PCN therapy. *Clostridium difficile*-associated diarrhea reported. Cross-sensitivity to cephalosporins. Monitor renal, hepatic and hematopoietic functions with prolonged use. D/C if bleeding manifestations occur; increased risk with renal failure. Prolonged use may cause superinfections. May experience neuromuscular excitability or convulsions with higher than recommended doses. Contains 1.85mEq/g sodium; caution with salt restriction. Monitor electrolytes periodically with low potassium levels. Increased incidence of rash and fever in cystic fibrosis. Continue treatment for at least 48-72 hrs after patient becomes asymptomatic.

**ADVERSE REACTIONS:** Thrombophlebitis, erythema and pain at injection site, diarrhea, headache, dizziness, anaphylaxis, rash, superinfections.

**INTERACTIONS:** Do not mix with aminoglycoside in a syringe or infusion bottle; may cause inactivation of aminoglycoside. May prolong neuromuscular blockade of nondepolarizing muscle relaxants (eg, vecuronium). Increased risk of hypokalemia with cytotoxic therapy or diuretics. May reduce methotrexate clearance. Probenecid may increase levels. Monitor coagulation parameters closely with concomitant anticoagulants.

**PREGNANCY:** Category B, caution in nursing.

**MECHANISM OF ACTION:** Broad-spectrum penicillin; exerts bacterial activity by inhibiting both septum and cell wall synthesis; active against a variety of gram-positive and gram-negative aerobic and anaerobic bacteria.

**PHARMACOKINETICS: Absorption:** (2g) Rapid; $C_{max}$=36mcg/mL, $T_{max}$=30 min. **Distribution:** Plasma protein binding (16%). **Elimination:** Urine (60%-80%); (2g) $T_{1/2}$=54 min., (6g) 63 min.

## NURSING CONSIDERATIONS

**Assessment:** Assess for history of allergic reaction to betalactams, renal impairment, CF, history of bleeding disorder, and possible drug interaction.

**Monitoring:** Monitor CBC, renal function and serum electrolytes periodically. Monitor for signs/symptoms of electrolyte imbalance (hypokalemia), hypersensitivity reactions, *C. difficile*-associated diarrhea, superinfections,

P

leukopenia/neutropenia, bleeding maninfestations, neuromuscular excitability or convulsions, rash and fever in CF patients.

**Patient Counseling:** Inform drug only treats bacterial, not viral, infections. Take as directed; skipping doses or not completing full course may decrease effectiveness and increase resistance. May experience diarrhea; contact physician if develop watery/bloody stools or hypersensitivity reactions.

**Administration:** IM, IV. **Storage:** 20-25°C (68-77°F). Reconstituted: 20-25°C (68-77°F), stable for 24 hrs; refrigerated: 2-8°C (36-46°F), stable for 48 hrs.

## PLAQUENIL RX

hydroxychloroquine sulfate (Sanofi-Aventis)

**Be familiar with complete prescribing information before prescribing hydroxychloroquine.**

**THERAPEUTIC CLASS:** Quinine derivative

**INDICATIONS:** Suppression and treatment of acute attacks of malaria in adults and children. Treatment of discoid and systemic lupus erythematosus and rheumatoid arthritis (RA) in adults.

**DOSAGE:** *Adults:* Malaria Suppression: 400mg weekly. Begin 2 weeks before exposure and continue for 8 weeks after leaving endemic area. Give 400mg q6h for 2 doses if therapy is not begun before exposure. Acute Attack: 800mg, then 400mg 6-8 hrs later, then 400mg for 2 more days. RA: Initial: 400-600mg qd with food or milk; increase until optimum response. Maint: After 4-12 weeks, 200-400mg qd with food or milk. Lupus Erythematosus: Initial: 400mg qd-bid for several weeks depending on response. Maint: 200-400mg/day.

*Pediatrics:* Malaria Suppression: 5mg/kg (base) weekly, max 400mg/dose. Begin 2 weeks before exposure and continue for 8 weeks after leaving endemic area. Acute Attack: 10mg base/kg, max 800mg/dose; then 5mg base/kg, max 400mg/dose at 6, 24 and 48 hrs after 1st dose.

**HOW SUPPLIED:** Tab: 200mg (200mg tab=155mg base)

**CONTRAINDICATIONS:** Long term therapy in children or if retinal/visual field changes due to 4-aminoquinoline compounds.

P

**WARNINGS/PRECAUTIONS:** Caution with hepatic disease, G6PD deficiency, alcoholism, psoriasis, and porphyria. Perform baseline and periodic (3 months) ophthalmologic exams and blood cell counts with prolonged therapy. Test periodically for muscle weakness. D/C if blood disorders occur. Avoid if possible in pregnancy. D/C after 6 months if no improvement in RA.

**ADVERSE REACTIONS:** Headache, dizziness, diarrhea, loss of appetite, muscle weakness, nausea, abdominal cramps, bleaching of hair, dermatitis, ocular toxicity, visual field defects.

**INTERACTIONS:** Caution with hepatotoxic drugs.

**PREGNANCY:** Safety in pregnancy and nursing not known.

**MECHANISM OF ACTION:** Quinine derivative; has antimalarial action. Precise mechanism not established.

### NURSING CONSIDERATIONS

**Assessment:** Assess for retinal or visual field defects, psoriasis, hepatic disease, alcoholism, G-6-PD deficiency, chloroquine-resistant strains of *P. falciparum*, auditory damage, pregnancy status. Note other diseases/conditions and drug therapies.

**Monitoring:** Monitor CBC with differential and platelet count, dermatologic reactions, chloroquine retinopathy, psychosis, irritability, myopathy, abnormal nerve conduction, depression of deep tendon reflexes, and allergic reactions.

**Patient Counseling:** Counsel about adverse effects and to d/c drug and seek medical attention if any signs/symptoms develop. Advise about need for periodic follow-up.

**Administration:** Oral route. **Storage:** Room temperature up to 30°C (86°F).

# PLAVIX RX

clopidogrel bisulfate (Bristol-Myers Squibb/Sanofi-Aventis)

**THERAPEUTIC CLASS:** Platelet aggregation inhibitor

**INDICATIONS:** For reduction of atherothrombotic events in those with recent stroke or MI, or in patients with established peripheral arterial disease (PAD). For reduction of atherothrombotic events in patients with non-ST-segment elevation acute coronary syndrome (unstable angina/non-Q-wave MI) and in patients with ST-segment elevation acute myocardial infarction (STEMI).

**DOSAGE:** *Adults:* Recent MI/Stroke or PAD: 75mg qd. Acute Coronary Syndrome: Initial: LD: 300mg. Maint: 75mg qd. Take with 75-325mg ASA qd. STEMI: 75mg with ASA, qd, with or without thrombolytics. May be administered with or without a LD.

**HOW SUPPLIED:** Tab: 75mg, 300mg.

**CONTRAINDICATIONS:** Active pathological bleeding (eg, peptic ulcer, intracranial hemorrhage).

**WARNINGS/PRECAUTIONS:** Thrombotic thrombocytopenic purpura (TTP) rarely reported. Caution with risk of increased bleeding from trauma, surgery, or other pathological conditions. D/C 5 days before surgery if antiplatelet effect is not desired. Monitor blood cell count and other appropriate tests if symptoms of bleeding or undesirable hematological effects arise. Use caution with severe hepatic or renal impairment. Caution in those who have lesions with a propensity to bleed, such as ulcers. Avoid use with impaired CYP2C19 function due to known genetic variation.

**ADVERSE REACTIONS:** Upper respiratory tract infection, chest pain, headache, influenza-like symptoms, pain, arthralgia, dizziness, back pain, abdominal pain, purpura/bruising, dyspepsia, dyspnea, diarrhea, HTN, major bleeding.

**INTERACTIONS:** Potentiates effect of ASA on collagen-induced platelet aggregation. May increase risk of bleeding with warfarin and NSAIDs. Coadministration with naproxen may increase occult GI blood loss. Avoid drugs that inhibit CYP2C19 including omeprazole, esomeprazole, cimetidine, fluconazole, ketoconazole, voriconazole, etravirine, felbamate, fluoxetine, fluvoxamine and ticlopidine. Caution with phenytoin, tamoxifen, tolbutamide, warfarin, torsemide, fluvastatin and many NSAIDs.

**PREGNANCY:** Category B, not for use in nursing.

**MECHANISM OF ACTION:** Platelet aggregation inhibitor; selectively inhibits the binding of adenosine diphosphate (ADP) to its platelet $P2Y_{12}$ receptor and subsequent ADP-mediated activation of the glycoprotein GIIb/IIIa complex.

**PHARMACOKINETICS: Absorption:** Rapid. (75mg) $C_{max}$=2.2-2.5ng/mL; $T_{max}$=45 mins. **Distribution:** Plasma protein binding (98%); found in breast milk. **Metabolism:** Liver (extensive) via multiple CYP450 (active thiol metabolite) and hydrolysis. **Elimination:** Urine (50%), feces (46%); $T_{1/2}$=6 hrs.

## NURSING CONSIDERATIONS

**Assessment:** Assess for presence of active bleeding (eg, peptic ulcer, intracranial hemorrhage), hepatic/renal impairment, pregnancy/nursing status, reduced CYP2C19 function and for possible drug interactions. Assess use in patients at risk for increased bleeding (eg, undergoing surgery, recent trauma).

**Monitoring:** Monitor for signs/symptoms of TTP (eg, thrombocytopenia, microangiopathic hemolytic anemia) and for bleeding (eg, GI bleeding). Perform CBC and other appropriate tests when bleeding is suspected.

**Patient Counseling:** Advise that medication may prolong bleeding time and may bruise and/or bleed more easily; instruct to contact physician if any unusual bleeding occurs. Advise to notify other physicians or dentists when taking clopidogrel or before scheduling surgery and before any new drug is taken. Instruct patients to tell their physician about any concomitant medications, including OTC omeprazole.

**Administration:** Oral route. **Storage:** 25°C (77°F); excursions permitted to 15-30°C (59-86°F).

## Plendil RX
felodipine (AstraZeneca)

**THERAPEUTIC CLASS:** Calcium channel blocker (dihydropyridine)

**INDICATIONS:** Treatment of hypertension alone or concomitantly with other antihypertensive agents.

**DOSAGE:** *Adults:* Initial: 5mg qd. Titrate: Adjust at no less than 2-week intervals. Maint: 2.5-10mg qd. Elderly: Initial: 2.5mg qd. Take without food or with a light meal. Swallow tab whole.

**HOW SUPPLIED:** Tab, Extended-Release: 2.5mg, 5mg, 10mg

**WARNINGS/PRECAUTIONS:** May cause hypotension and syncope (rare). May lead to reflex tachycardia with precipitation of angina pectoris. Caution with heart failure or ventricular dysfunction, especially with concomitant β-blockers. Monitor dose adjustment with hepatic dysfunction or elderly. Caution in elderly. Peripheral edema reported. Maintain good dental hygiene; gingival hyperplasia reported.

**ADVERSE REACTIONS:** Peripheral edema, headache, flushing, dizziness, asthenia, dyspepsia, upper respiratory infection.

**INTERACTIONS:** CYP3A4 inhibitors (eg, itraconazole, ketoconazole, erythromycin, grapefruit juice, cimetidine) may increase plasma levels. Levels decreased with long-term anticonvulsant therapy. May increase metoprolol and tacrolimus levels.

**PREGNANCY:** Category C, not for use in nursing.

**MECHANISM OF ACTION:** Calcium channel blocker; reversibly competes with nitrendipine and/or other calcium channel blockers for dihydropyridine binding sites and blocks voltage-dependent calcium ion currents in vascular smooth muscle.

**PHARMACOKINETICS: Absorption:** Complete, systemic bioavailability (approximately 20%); $T_{max}$=2.5-5 hrs (oral). **Distribution:** $V_d$=10 L/kg; plasma protein binding (99%). **Elimination:** Urine (70%), feces (10%); $T_{1/2}$(immediate release)=11-16 hrs.

P

### NURSING CONSIDERATIONS

**Assessment:** Assess for hypotension, CHF, LFTs, pregnancy status, and for possible drug interactions.

**Monitoring:** Monitor BP, LFT, CBCs. Monitor for peripheral edema, CHF, palpitations, arrhythmias, angina.

**Patient Counseling:** Instruct to take tablet whole; do not crush or chew. Counsel about adverse side effects; notify physician if any develop. Inform that gingival hyperplasia (gum swelling) reported; maintain good dental hygiene.

**Administration:** Oral route. **Storage:** 30°C (86°F). Keep in tight, light-resistant container.

## Pletal RX
cilostazol (Otsuka America)

**Contraindicated with CHF of any severity due to possible decrease in survival.**

**THERAPEUTIC CLASS:** Phosphodiesterase III inhibitor

**INDICATIONS:** Reduction of symptoms with intermittent claudication.

**DOSAGE:** *Adults:* 100mg bid, 1/2 hr before or 2 hrs after breakfast and dinner. Concomitant CYP3A4 and CYP2C19 Inhibitors: Consider 50mg bid.

**HOW SUPPLIED:** Tab: 50mg, 100mg

**CONTRAINDICATIONS:** CHF of any severity. Haemostatic disorders or active pathologic bleeding (eg, peptic ulcer, intracranial bleeding).

**WARNINGS/PRECAUTIONS:** Risks not known in patients with severe underlying heart disease, moderate or severe hepatic impairment, or with long-term use. Rare cases of thrombocytopenia or leukopenia reported.

**ADVERSE REACTIONS:** Headache, palpitation, tachycardia, abnormal stool, diarrhea, peripheral edema, dizziness, infection, rhinitis, blood pressure increase, aplastic anemia.

**INTERACTIONS:** Caution with CYP3A4 inhibitors (eg, ketoconazole, diltiazem, erythromycin) or CYP2C19 inhibitors (eg, omeprazole); may increase cilostazol levels. Avoid grapefruit juice.

**PREGNANCY:** Category C, not for use in nursing.

**MECHANISM OF ACTION:** Phosphodiesterase III inhibitor; not established. Inhibits phosphodiesterase activity and suppresses cyclic AMP (cAMP) degradation. Results in an increase of cAMP in platelets and blood vessels. Leads to reversible inhibition of platelet aggregation and produces vasodilation.

**PHARMACOKINETICS: Distribution:** Plasma protein binding (95-98%). **Metabolism:** Liver via CYP450 3A4 (primary), 2C19; 3,4-dehydro-cilostazol, 4'-trans-hydroxy-cilostazol (major active metabolites). **Elimination:** Urine (74%), feces (20%); $T_{1/2}$=11-13 hrs.

## NURSING CONSIDERATIONS

**Assessment:** Assess for CHF, hemostatic disorders, presence of major bleeding (eg, peptic ulcer, intracranial bleeding), renal/hepatic function, pregnancy/nursing status, and drug interactions.
**Monitoring:** Monitor for signs/symptoms of thrombocytopenia, leukopenia, agranulocytosis, cardiovascular toxicity (eg, cardiovascular lesions), and headaches.

**Patient Counseling:** Advise to take at least 30 min before or 2 hours after food. Inform that benefits of medication may not be immediate; treatment required for up to 12 weeks before beneficial effect.

**Administration:** Oral route. **Storage:** 25°C (77°F); excursions permitted to 15-30°C (59-86°F).

# PNEUMOVAX 23 RX

pneumococcal vaccine polyvalent (Merck)

**THERAPEUTIC CLASS:** Vaccine
**INDICATIONS:** Immunization against pneumococcal disease caused by those pneumococcal types included in the vaccine.
**DOSAGE:** *Adults:* Usual: 0.5mL SQ/IM in deltoid muscle or lateral mid-thigh. Revaccination: 0.5 mL SQ/IM
*Pediatrics:* ≥2 yrs: 0.5mL SQ/IM in deltoid muscle or lateral mid-thigh. Revaccination: 0.5 mL SQ/IM
**HOW SUPPLIED:** Inj: 575mcg/0.5mL

**WARNINGS/PRECAUTIONS:** Should be given at least 2 weeks before elective splenectomy and immunosuppressive therapy. Vaccination during chemotherapy or radiation should be avoided. Suboptimal response may occur in immunocompromised patients. Intradermal administration may cause severe local reactions. Caution with severely compromised cardiovascular or pulmonary function where systemic reaction would be a significant risk. Delay vaccine with febrile respiratory illness or other active infection. Do not revaccinate immunocompetent patients. Patients ≥65yrs who have not received the vaccine in 5 years (and were <65yrs of age at the time of vaccination) should receive another dose. Continue prophylaxis with pneumococcal antibiotics. May not prevent pneumococcal meningitis with chronic CSF leakage.

**ADVERSE REACTIONS:** Local injection-site reactions (eg, soreness, warmth, erythema, swelling, induration), fever (≤102°F), asthenia, fatigue, myalgia, headache

**INTERACTIONS:** Immunosuppressive therapies may reduce immune response; administer vaccine at least 2 weeks prior to the initiation of chemotherapy or other immunosuppresive therapies.

**PREGNANCY:** Category C, caution in nursing.

**MECHANISM OF ACTION:** Vaccine; bacterial capsular polysaccharides induce antibodies primarily by T-cell-independent mechanisms that protect against pneumococcal infection.

## NURSING CONSIDERATIONS

**Assessment:** Assess current health status and previous vaccination history, reaction to previous pneumococcal vaccine, immune status, history of cardiovascular and pulmonary function. Assess timing in chemotherapy and immunosuppressive therapy patients.

**Monitoring:** Monitor patients with compromised cardiovascular and pulmonary function. Monitor injection site for erythema, swelling, and induration.

**Patient Counseling:** May not offer 100% protection from pneumococcal infection. Inform of benefits/risks; report any serious adverse reactions.

**Administration:** IM (preferably in deltoid muscle or lateral mid-thigh) and SQ only. **Storage:** 2-8°C (36-46°F).

# PONSTEL RX

mefenamic acid (Sciele)

**NSAIDs may cause an increased risk of serious cardiovascular thrombotic events, MI, stroke, and serious GI adverse events including bleeding, ulceration, and perforation of the stomach or intestines. Contraindicated for the treatment of perioperative pain in the setting of coronary artery bypass graft (CABG) surgery.**

**THERAPEUTIC CLASS:** NSAID

**INDICATIONS:** Relief of mild to moderate pain in patients ≥14 yrs, when therapy will not exceed 7 days. Treatment of primary dysmenorrhea.

**DOSAGE:** *Adults:* Acute Pain: Usual: 500mg, then 250mg q6h prn up to 1 week. Primary Dysmenorrhea: Usual: 500mg, then 250mg q6h up to 3 days. Take with food.

*Pediatrics:* ≥14 yrs: Acute Pain: Usual: 500mg, then 250mg q6h prn up to 1 week. Primary Dysmenorrhea: Usual: 500mg, then 250mg q6h up to 3 days. Take with food.

**HOW SUPPLIED:** Cap: 250mg

**CONTRAINDICATIONS:** Pre-existing renal disease, active ulceration or chronic inflammation of the GI tract. Allergic-type reactions, including asthma and urticaria, after taking ASA or other NSAIDs. Treatment of perioperative pain in the setting of CABG surgery.

**WARNINGS/PRECAUTIONS:** May lead to onset of new HTN or worsening of pre-existing HTN; monitor BP closely. Fluid retention and edema reported; caution with fluid retention or heart failure. Renal papillary necrosis and other renal injury reported after long-term use. Not recommended for use with advanced renal disease. Anaphylactoid reactions may occur. May cause serious skin adverse events (eg, exfoliative dermatitis, Stevens-Johnson syndrome, and toxic epidermal necrolysis). Avoid in late pregnancy; may cause premature closure of ductus arteriosis. May cause elevations of LFTs; d/c if liver disease develops or systemic manifestations occur. Caution in elderly. Anemia may occur; with long-term use, monitor Hgb/Hct if signs or symptoms of anemia develop. May inhibit platelet aggregation and prolong bleeding time; monitor with coagulation disorders. Caution with asthma and avoid with ASA-sensitive asthma.

**ADVERSE REACTIONS:** Abdominal pain, constipation, diarrhea, dyspepsia, flatulence, gross bleeding/perforation, heartburn, nausea, GI ulcers, vomiting, abnormal renal function, anemia, dizziness, edema, elevated liver enzymes, headache, increased bleeding time, pruritus, rash, tinnitus.

**INTERACTIONS:** Caution with CYP2C9 inhibitors. ASA may increase adverse effects; avoid use. Warfarin may increase GI bleeding. May prolong PT with oral anticoagulants. May enhance methotrexate toxicity. Decreases effects of ACE inhibitors, furosemide, and thiazides; monitor for renal toxicity. Increases lithium levels. Magnesium hydroxide may increase mefenamic acid levels. Enhances methotrexate toxicity; caution with concomitant use.

**PREGNANCY:** Category C, not for use in nursing.

**MECHANISM OF ACTION:** NSAID (fenamate derivative); suspected to inhibit prostaglandin synthetase, exerts anti-inflammatory, analgesic, and antipyretic actions.

**PHARMACOKINETICS: Absorption:** Rapid; $C_{max}$=10-20mcg/mL³, $T_{max}$=2-4 hrs. **Distribution:** $V_d$=1.06L/kg²; plasma protein binding (90%). **Metabolism**: Via CYP2C9. **Elimination:** Urine (52%), feces (20%); $T_{1/2}$=2 hrs.

## NURSING CONSIDERATIONS

**Assessment:** Assess LFTs, renal function, CBC and coagulation profile. Assess for history of CABG surgery, asthma and allergic reactions to aspirin or other NSAIDs, active ulceration or chronic inflammation of GI tract, CVD, pregnancy status. Note other diseases/conditions and drug therapies.

**Monitoring:** Monitor for hypersensitivity reactions, cardiac complications, stroke, GI bleeding, asthma, skin side effects. Monitor BP, LFT, renal functions, CBC with differential and platelet count and coagulation profile, hyperglycemia.

**Patient Counseling:** Counsel about side effects; seek medical attention if any develop. Avoid alcohol and smoking during treatment. Take drug as prescribed. Caution women against using medication late in pregnancy.

**Administration:** Oral route. **Storage:** 20-25°C (68-77°F); excursions permitted to 15-30°C (59-86°F).

# PRANDIMET RX

metformin HCl - repaglinide (Novo Nordisk)

**Lactic acidosis can occur due to metformin accumulation; increased risk with sepsis, dehydration, excess alcohol intake, hepatic impairment, renal impairment, and acute CHF. If acidosis suspected, d/c drug and hospitalize patient immediately.**

**THERAPEUTIC CLASS:** Biguanide/Meglitinide

**INDICATIONS:** Adjunct to diet and exercise to improve glycemic control in adults with type 2 diabetes mellitus who are already treated with a meglitinide and metformin HCl, or who have inadequate glycemic control on a meglitinide alone or metformin HCl alone.

**DOSAGE:** *Adults:* Individualize dose. Administer 2-3 times a day up to 4mg-1000mg/meal. Max Daily Dose: 10mg repaglinide-2500mg metformin. Patient Inadequately Controlled on Metformin Monotherapy: Initial: 1mg-500mg bid w/ meals. Titrate: Gradually escalate dose to reduce risk of hypoglycemia. Patient Inadequately Controlled w/ Meglitinide Monotherapy: Initial: 500mg metformin bid. Titrate: Gradually escalate dose to reduce GI side effects. Concomitant use of Repaglinide/Metformin: Initiate at dose of repaglinide and metformin similar to (not exceeding) current doses. Titrate to maximum daily dose as necessary. Always take with meals, either 15 mins before or 30 mins after.

**HOW SUPPLIED:** Tab: (Repaglinide-Metformin) 1mg-500mg, 2mg-500mg

**CONTRAINDICATIONS:** Renal impairment (eg, SrCr ≥1.5mg/dL [males], ≥1.4mg/dL [females], or abnormal CrCl). Acute or chronic metabolic acidosis, including diabetic ketoacidosis. Patients receiving both gemfibrozil and itraconazole.

**WARNINGS/PRECAUTIONS:** Assess renal function prior to initiation and annually thereafter; d/c if renal impairment is present. Avoid in hepatic impairment and excess alcohol intake. D/C in hypoxic states (eg, acute CHF, shock, acute MI), prior to surgical procedures or procedures requiring use of

P

intravascular iodinated contrast materials, and ketoacidosis. May cause hypoglycemia; caution in elderly, debilitated, or malnourished patients and those with adrenal or pituitary insuffiency or alcohol intoxication. Loss of glycemic control may occur in patients with fever, infection, trauma or surgery; d/c and shift to insulin temporarily. If change in clinical status occurs in patients with previously controlled Type 2 DM, promptly evaluate for evidence of lactic acidosis or ketoacidosis. May cause vitamin $B_{12}$ deficiency; measure hematologic parameters on an annual basis.

**ADVERSE REACTIONS:** Lactic acidosis, hypoglycemia, headache, diarrhea, nausea, and upper respiratory tract infection.

**INTERACTIONS:** See Contraindications. (Metformin) Cationic drugs (eg, amiloride, digoxin, morphine, procainamide, quinidine, quinine, ranitidine, triamterene, trimethoprim, vancomycin) may increase metformin levels. Increase levels with cimetidine, furosemide, nifedipine, ibuprofen. Decrease levels with propranolol. Alcohol potentiates effect of metformin. May decrease furosemide levels. Caution with drugs that may affect renal function or result in significant hemodynamic change or may interfere with the disposition of metformin. (Repaglinide) CYP2C8 inhibitors (eg, gemfibrozil, trimethoprim), CYP3A4 inhibitors (eg, itraconazole, ketaconazole), or CYP2C8/3A4 inducers (eg, rifampin) may alter the pharmacokinetics and pharmacodynamics of repaglinide. Not for use in combination with NPH insulin. May alter levels when used concomitantly with levonorgestrel/ethinyl estradiol. Increase levels with clarithromycin, ketoconazole, simvastatin, trimethoprim. Decrease levels with nifedipine, rifampin. May increase ethinyl estradiol levels.

**PREGNANCY:** Category C, not for use in nursing.

**MECHANISM OF ACTION: Metformin:** Biguanide; improves glucose tolerance by lowering both basal and post prandial plasma glucose. Decreases hepatic glucose production, decreases intestinal absorption of glucose, and improves insulin sensitivity by increasing peripheral glucose uptake and utilization. **Repaglinide:** Meglitinide; lowers blood glucose levels by stimulating the release of insulin from the pancreas.

**PHARMACOKINETICS: Absorption:** Metformin: Absolute bioavailabilty (50%-60%). Repaglinide: Absolute bioavailability (56%); $T_{max}$=1 hr. **Distribution:** Metformin: $V_d$=654L. Repaglinide: $V_d$=31L; Plasma protein binding (>98%). **Metabolism:** Repaglinide: CYP2C8, 3A4; oxidation and direct conjugation; oxidized dicarboxylic acid (M2), aromatic amine (M1), acyl glucuronide (M7) (major metabolites). **Elimination:** Metformin: Urine (90%); $T_{1/2}$=6.2 hrs (plasma), 17.6 hrs (blood). Repaglinide: Feces (90%), urine (8%); $T_{1/2}$=1 hr.

## NURSING CONSIDERATIONS

**Assessment:** Assess for acute or chronic metabolic acidosis, renal/hepatic impairment, CHF, septicemia, acute or chronic metabolic acidosis, presence of debilitation or malnourishment, adrenal or pituitary insufficiency, alcohol intoxication, pregnancy/nursing status, and for possible drug interactions. Assess if patient is planning to undergo any surgical procedure or is under any form of stress (eg, fever, infection, trauma). Obtain baseline FPG, $HbA_{1c}$, renal function, LFTs, and hematological parameters.

**Monitoring:** Monitor for signs/symptoms of hypoglycemia, lactic acidosis, decreased Vitamin $B_{12}$ levels, cardiovascular collapse, acute CHF, acute MI, and for pre-renal azotemia. Perform periodic monitoring of FPG, $HbA_{1c}$, and LFTs. Perform annual monitoring of renal function and hematological parameters.

**Patient Counseling:** Inform that drug is an adjunct to diet and exercise, and should be taken as prescribed with meals. Inform patient of importance of regular testing of blood glucose, $HbA_{1c}$, renal function, and hematologic parameters. Advise that during periods of stress (eg, fever, trauma, infection, or surgery), medication requirements may change. Inform about the risks of hypoglycemia, symptoms, treatment, and conditions that predispose development. Inform of risk of lactic acidosis, its symptoms and conditions which predispose to its development; advise to d/c immediately and contact physician if develop unexplained hyperventilation, myalgia, malaise, unusual somolence, or other nonspecific symptoms occur. Advise to notify physician of all medications currently taking and if pregnant or nursing.

**Administration:** Oral route. **Storage:** Do not store above 25°C (77°F).

## PRANDIN RX

repaglinide (Novo Nordisk)

**THERAPEUTIC CLASS:** Meglitinide

**INDICATIONS:** Adjunct to diet and exercise, to improve glycemic control in type 2 diabetes mellitus.

**DOSAGE:** *Adults:* Initial: Treatment-Naive or $HbA_{1c}$ <8%: 0.5mg with each meal. Previous Oral Therapy/Combination Therapy and $HbA_{1c}$ ≥8%: 1-2mg with each meal. Titrate: May double preprandial dose up to 4mg (bid-qid) at no less than 1 week intervals. Maint: 0.5-4mg with meals. Max: 16mg/day. If hypoglycemia with combination metformin or thiazolidinediones (TZDs) occurs, reduce repaglinide dose. Renal Dysfunction: CrCl 20-40mg/dL: Initial: 0.5mg with each meal; titrate carefully. Hepatic Dysfunction: Increase intervals between dose adjustments. Take within 15-30 min before meals.

**HOW SUPPLIED:** Tab: 0.5mg, 1mg, 2mg

**CONTRAINDICATIONS:** Diabetic ketoacidosis, type 1 diabetes, and coadministration of gemfibrozil.

**WARNINGS/PRECAUTIONS:** Hypoglycemia risk especially with renal/hepatic insufficiency, elderly, malnourished, and adrenal/pituitary insufficiency. Loss of blood glucose control when exposed to stress (fever, trauma, infection, or surgery); d/c therapy and start insulin. Secondary failure can occur over a period of time. Caution with hepatic and renal dysfunction.

**ADVERSE REACTIONS:** Hyperglycemia, hypoglycemia, upper respiratory infection, headache, rhinitis, sinusitis, bronchitis, arthralgia, back pain, N/V, diarrhea, dyspepsia, CV events, constipation, paresthesia.

**INTERACTIONS:** See Contraindications. Avoid coadministering with NPH-insulin. Increased metabolism with CYP3A4 inducers (eg, rifampin, barbiturates, carbamazepine). Ketoconazole, itraconazole, clarithromycin, and erythromycin (CYP3A4 inhibitors) and trimethoprim, gemfibrozil, and montelukast (CYP2C8 inhibitors) may inhibit metabolism. Increased levels with Organic Anion Transporting Protein (OATP1B1) inhibitors (eg, cyclosporine). Increased levels with gemfibrozil; caution and monitor levels if already on both drugs, avoid initiation of concurrent use. Avoid itraconazole if already on gemfibrozil and repaglinide; synergistic effect may occur. Potentiated hypoglycemia with alcohol, β-blockers, NSAIDs, and other highly protein-bound drugs, salicylates, sulfonamides, chloramphenicol, coumarins, probenecid, MAOIs. Risk of hyperglycemia with diuretics, corticosteroids, phenothiazines, thyroid products, estrogens, phenytoin, nicotinic acid, sympathomimetics, CCBs, and isoniazid. β-blockers may mask hypoglycemia. Increased levels of repaglinide and levonorgestrel/ethinyl estradiol combination during coadministration. Increased levels with simvastatin.

**PREGNANCY:** Category C, not for use in nursing.

**MECHANISM OF ACTION:** Meglitinide; lowers blood glucose levels by stimulating the release of insulin from the pancreas.

**PHARMACOKINETICS: Absorption:** Rapid and complete; bioavailability (56%); $T_{max}$=1 hr. **Distribution:** $V_d$=31L; plasma protein binding (98%). **Metabolism:** CYP2C8, 3A4; oxidation, glucuronidation. **Elimination:** Feces (90%), urine (8%); $T_{1/2}$=1 hr.

### NURSING CONSIDERATIONS

**Assessment:** Assess FPG, $HbA_{1c}$, renal function, LFTs, pregnancy status, diabetic ketoacidosis, type 1 DM, concomitant use of gemfibrozil, CV risk factors, pregnancy/nursing status, and possible drug interactions.

**Monitoring:** Monitor blood glucose levels, $HbA_{1c}$ every 3 months, hypo/hyperglycemia, hypersensitivity reactions, and severe adverse events.

**Patient Counseling:** Inform about importance of adherence to meal planning, regular physical activity, regular blood glucose monitoring, periodic $HbA_{1c}$

P

testing, recognition and management of hypo/hyperglycemia, and periodic assessment of diabetes complications. Educate about risks/benefits of therapy and primary and secondary failure. During periods of stress (eg, trauma, infection, surgery), medication requirements may change; seek prompt medical advice. Instruct to take before meals. Instruct to skip dose if skipping a meal and add dose if adding a meal.

**Administration:** Oral route. **Storage:** 25°C (77°F). Protect from moisture. Keep and dispense in tight containers with safety closures.

## PRAVACHOL RX

pravastatin sodium (Bristol-Myers Squibb)

**THERAPEUTIC CLASS:** HMG-CoA reductase inhibitor

**INDICATIONS:** In Primary Hypercholesterolemia and Mixed Dyslipidemia (Type IIa and IIb): Adjunct to diet; to reduce elevated total-C, LDL-C, Apo B, TG (Type IV) levels, and to increase HDL-C. In Primary Dysbetalipoproteinemia (Type III) with Inadequate Response to Diet: Treatment of. In Type IV Hyperlipidemia: Adjunct to diet, treatment of. In Heterozygous Familial Hypercholesterolemia in Patients ≥8 years-old: Adjunct to diet and lifestyle modifications if LDL-C remains ≥190mg/dL, or LDL-C remains ≥160mg/dL (with positive family history of premature cardiovascular disease (CVD), or 2 or more other CVD risk factors present). In Hypercholesterolemia without Coronary Heart Disease (CHD): Reduction of risk of MI, of undergoing myocardial revascularization procedures, and of cardiovascular mortality with no increase in death from non-cardiovascular causes. In Clinically Evident CHD: Reduction of risk of mortality by reducing coronary death, of undergoing myocardial revascularization procedures, and of MI, stroke, and transient ischemic attack (TIA); and to slow progression of coronary atherosclerosis.

**DOSAGE:** *Adults:* ≥18 yrs: Initial: 40mg qd. Perform lipid tests within 4 weeks and adjust according to response and guidelines. Titrate: May increase to 80mg qd if needed. Significant Renal/Hepatic Dysfunction: Initial: 10mg qd. Concomitant Immunosuppressives (eg, cyclosporine): Initial:10mg qhs. Max: 20mg/day.

*Pediatrics:* Heterozygous Familial Hypercholesterolemia: 14-18 yrs: Initial: 40mg qd. Max: 40mg/day. 8-13 yrs: 20mg qd. Max: 20mg/day. Concomitant Immunosuppressives (eg, cyclosporine): Initial: 10mg qhs. Max: 20mg/day.



**HOW SUPPLIED:** Tab: 10mg, 20mg, 40mg, 80mg

**CONTRAINDICATIONS:** Active liver disease, unexplained persistent elevations of LFTs, pregnancy, nursing mothers.

**WARNINGS/PRECAUTIONS:** May cause biochemical abnormalities of liver function; perform LFTs before therapy, before dose increases, and if clinically indicated. Risk of myopathy, myalgia, and rhabdomyolysis. D/C if AST or ALT ≥3x ULN persists, if elevated CPK levels occur, or if myopathy diagnosed or suspected. Less effective with homozygous familial hypercholesterolemia. Monitor for endocrine dysfunction. Closely monitor with heavy alcohol use, recent history or signs of hepatic disease, or renal dysfunction.

**ADVERSE REACTIONS:** Rash, NV, diarrhea, headache, chest pain, abdominal pain, dizziness, constipation, flatulence, fatigue, localized pain, common cold, rhinitis, dyspepsia/heartburn, musculoskeletal pain.

**INTERACTIONS:** Risk of myopathy with fibrates, niacin, cyclosporine, erythromycin. Increased levels with gemfibrozil, itraconazole. Avoid fibrates unless benefit outweighs drug combination risk. Decreased levels with concomitant cholestyramine/colestipol; take 1 hr before or 4 hrs after resins. Caution with drugs that diminish levels or activity of steroid hormones (eg, ketoconazole, spironolactone, cimetidine).

**PREGNANCY:** Category X, not for use in nursing.

**MECHANISM OF ACTION:** HMG-CoA reductase inhibitor; causes increased number of LDL-receptors on cell surfaces and enhanced receptor mediated catabolism and clearance of circulating LDL. Inhibits LDL production by inhibiting hepatic synthesis of VLDL, LDL precursor.

**PHARMACOKINETICS: Absorption:** Rapid. Absolute bioavailability (17%); $T_{max}$=1-1.5 hrs. **Distribution:** Plasma protein binding (50%). **Metabolism:** Liver. **Elimination:** Feces (70%), urine (20%); $T_{1/2}$=77 hrs.

## NURSING CONSIDERATIONS

**Assessment:** Prior to initiation, assess secondary causes of hypercholesterolemia (eg, poorly controlled DM, hypothyroidism, nephrotic syndrome, dysproteinemias, obstructive liver disease, other drug therapy, alcoholism), active liver disease, elevations in serum transaminases, pregnancy/nursing status, and possible drug interactions. Obtain baseline lipid profile and LFTs.

**Monitoring:** Monitor for signs/symptoms of active liver disease, rhabdomyolysis with acute renal failure, myoglobinuria, myopathies. Monitor CPK and LFTs periodically, and lipid levels every 4 weeks to evaluate response.

**Patient Counseling:** Advise to report signs/symptoms of unexplained muscle pain, tenderness, or weakness, particularly with malaise or fever. Recommend standard cholesterol-lowering diet prior to and during treatment. Educate about pregnancy/nursing risks. Counsel to take with/without food.

**Administration:** Oral route. **Storage:** 25°C (77°F); excursions permitted to 15-30°C (59-86°F). Keep tightly closed, protect from light and moisture.

# PRECOSE **RX**

acarbose (Bayer Healthcare)

**THERAPEUTIC CLASS:** Alpha-glucosidase inhibitor

**INDICATIONS:** Adjunct to diet and exercise, to improve glycemic control in type 2 diabetes mellitus.

**DOSAGE:** *Adults:* Initial: 25mg tid with first bite of each main meal. To minimize GI effects: 25mg qd, increase gradually to 25mg tid. Titrate: After reaching 25mg tid, may increase at 4-8 week intervals. Maint: 50-100mg tid. Max: ≤60kg: 50mg tid. >60kg: 100mg tid. If no further reduction in postprandial glucose or $HbA_{1c}$ with 100mg tid, consider reducing dose.

**HOW SUPPLIED:** Tab: 25mg, 50mg, 100mg

**CONTRAINDICATIONS:** Diabetic ketoacidosis, cirrhosis, inflammatory bowel disease, colonic ulceration, partial or predisposition to intestinal obstruction, chronic intestinal disease with marked disorders of digestion or absorption, and conditions that may deteriorate from increased intestinal gas formation.

**WARNINGS/PRECAUTIONS:** Avoid with significant renal dysfunction (SrCr >2mg/dL). May need to d/c and give insulin with stress (eg, fever, trauma). Dose-related elevated serum transaminase levels reported. Monitor serum transaminases every 3 months for first year, then periodically. Reduce dose or d/c if elevated serum transaminases persist. Use glucose (dextrose) instead of sucrose (sugar cane) to treat mild to moderate hypoglycemia.

**ADVERSE REACTIONS:** Flatulence, diarrhea, abdominal pain.

**INTERACTIONS:** Risk of hyperglycemia with diuretics, corticosteroids, phenothiazines, thyroid products, estrogens, oral contraceptives, phenytoin, nicotinic acid, sympathomimetics, CCBs, and isoniazid. Reduced effect with intestinal adsorbents (eg, charcoal) and digestive enzymes containing carbohydrate-splitting enzymes (eg, amylase, pancreatin); avoid concomitant use. May affect digoxin bioavailability; may require dose adjustment of digoxin. Monitor for hypoglycemia with insulin or sulfonylureas.

**PREGNANCY:** Category B, not for use in nursing.

**MECHANISM OF ACTION:** α-glucosidase inhibitor; reversibly inhibits pancreatic α-amylase and membrane-bound intestinal α-glucoside hydrolase enzymes.

**PHARMACOKINETICS: Absorption:** Poor; $T_{max}$=1 hr. **Metabolism:** GI tract by intestinal bacteria or digestive enzymes; 4-methylpyrogallol derivatives (major metabolites). **Elimination:** Urine (unchanged); $T_{1/2}$=2 hrs.

## NURSING CONSIDERATIONS

**Assessment:** Assess for renal dysfunction, cirrhosis, diabetic ketoacidosis, inflammatory bowel disease, colonic ulceration or partial intestinal obstruction, chronic intestinal disease, pregnancy status, and possible drug interactions.

**Monitoring:** Monitor for hypoglycemia, FPG, $HbA_{1c}$, LFTs, renal function, diabetic ketoacidosis, GI symptoms (eg, abdominal pain, diarrhea, flatulence), hypersensitivity reactions.

**Patient Counseling:** Instruct to take three times daily at the start of each meal. Counsel about signs/symptoms of hypoglycemia. Inform about importance of adhering to dietary instructions, a regular exercise program, and regular testing of urine and blood glucose.

**Administration:** Oral route. **Storage:** 25°C (77°F); protect from moisture; keep container tightly closed.

# PRED FORTE — RX

prednisolone acetate (Allergan)

**THERAPEUTIC CLASS:** Corticosteroid

**INDICATIONS:** Treatment of inflammation of the palpebral and bulbar conjunctiva, cornea and anterior segment of the globe.

**DOSAGE:** *Adults:* 1-2 drops bid-qid. May dose more frequently during initial 24-48 hrs. Re-evaluate after 2 days if no improvement.

**HOW SUPPLIED:** Sus: 1% [1mL, 5mL, 10mL, 15mL]

**CONTRAINDICATIONS:** Viral diseases of the cornea and conjunctiva including epithelial herpes simplex keratitis, vaccinia, and varicella. Mycobacterial infection and fungal diseases of the eye.

**WARNINGS/PRECAUTIONS:** Caution with glaucoma, herpes simplex, diseases causing thinning of cornea/sclera and other ocular viral infections. Prolonged use can cause glaucoma or secondary ocular infections (eg, fungal). Monitor IOP after 10 days of therapy. Re-evaluate if no response after 2 days. May delay healing and increase incidence of bleb formation after cataract surgery. Avoid abrupt withdrawal with chronic use. Contains sodium bisulfite.

P

**ADVERSE REACTIONS:** Elevation of IOP, glaucoma, infrequent optic nerve damage, posterior subcapsular cataract formation, delayed wound healing, burning/stinging upon instillation, ocular irritation, secondary infection, visual disturbance.

**PREGNANCY:** Category C, not for use in nursing.

**MECHANISM OF ACTION:** Glucocorticoid; anti-inflammatory agent; inhibits edema, fibrin deposition, capillary dilation, deposition of collagen, and scar formation.

## NURSING CONSIDERATIONS

**Assessment:** Assess for viral disease of cornea and conjunctiva, dendritic keratitis, vaccinia and varicella, mycobacterial infection and/or fungal disease of ocular structures, glaucoma, mustard gas keratitis, Sjogren's keratoconjuctivitis, thinning of corneal/scleral epithelium, hypersensitivity to sulfite, asthma, and cataract surgery.

**Monitoring:** Monitor for anaphylactic symptoms and asthma attacks. Frequent measuring of IOP and slit lamp microscopy exam where appropriate, fluorescein staining for monitoring of glaucoma with damage to the optic nerve with defects in visual acuity and fields of vision, posterior subcapsular cataract, delayed corneal healing, thinning of cornea and sclera, ulceration, perforation, and secondary ocular infections (or masking of existing infections).

**Patient Counseling:** Advise to d/c drug and consult physician if symptoms persist or worsen. Instruct to wait 15 min after instillation to wear soft contact lenses. Counsel to avoid touching bottle tip to eyelids or any other surface.

**Administration:** Ocular route. **Storage:** 25°C (77°F). Protect from freezing. Keep tightly closed.

## PRED MILD — RX

prednisolone acetate (Allergan)

**THERAPEUTIC CLASS:** Corticosteroid

**INDICATIONS:** Treatment of noninfectious ocular inflammation.

**DOSAGE:** *Adults:* 1-2 drops bid-qid. May dose more frequently during initial 24-48 hrs. Re-evaluate after 2 days if no improvement.

**HOW SUPPLIED:** Sus: 0.12% [5mL, 10mL]

**CONTRAINDICATIONS:** Viral diseases of the cornea and conjunctiva including epithelial herpes simplex keratitis, vaccinia, and varicella. Mycobacterial infection and fungal diseases of the eye.

**WARNINGS/PRECAUTIONS:** Caution with glaucoma, herpes simplex, diseases causing thinning of cornea/sclera and other ocular viral infections. Prolonged use can cause glaucoma or secondary ocular infections (eg, fungal). Monitor IOP after 10 days of therapy. Re-evaluate if no response after 2 days. May delay healing and increase incidence of bleb formation after cataract surgery. Avoid abrupt withdrawal with chronic use. Contains sodium bisulfite.

**ADVERSE REACTIONS:** Elevation of IOP, glaucoma, infrequent optic nerve damage, posterior subcapsular cataract formation, delayed wound healing, burning/stinging upon instillation, ocular irritation, secondary infection, visual disturbance.

**PREGNANCY:** Category C, not for use in nursing.

**MECHANISM OF ACTION:** Glucocorticoid; inhibits edema, fibrin disposition, capillary dilation, and phagocytic migration of acute inflammatory response as well as capillary proliferation, deposition of collagen and scar formation.

### NURSING CONSIDERATIONS

**Assessment:** Assess for viral diseases of the cornea and conjunctiva, dendritic keratitis, vaccinia, and varicella, mycobacterial infection and/or fungal diseases of ocular structures, and glaucoma.

**Monitoring:** Monitor for improvement of signs/symptoms; frequent measuring of IOP if using for >10 days.

**Patient Counseling:** Advise to d/c and notify physician if symptoms persist or worsen. Wait 15 min after instillation to wear soft contact lenses. Avoid touching bottle tip to eyelids or any other surface.

**Administration:** Intraocular route. **Storage:** 15-30°C (59-56°F). Protect from freezing. Keep tightly closed.



## PRED-G — RX

prednisolone acetate - gentamicin sulfate (Allergan)

**OTHER BRAND NAMES:** Pred-G S.O.P. (Allergan)

**THERAPEUTIC CLASS:** Aminoglycoside/corticosteroid

**INDICATIONS:** Ocular inflammation associated with infection or risk of infection.

**DOSAGE:** *Adults:* (Sus) 1 drop bid-qid. May increase dose to every hour during initial 24-48 hrs. Max: 20mL for initial prescription. (Oint) Apply 1/2 inch in conjunctival sac qd-tid. Max: 8g for initial prescription.

**HOW SUPPLIED:** (Gentamicin-Prednisolone) Oint: (S.O.P.) 0.3%-0.6% [3.5g]; Sus: 0.3%-1% [2mL, 5mL, 10mL]

**CONTRAINDICATIONS:** Viral diseases of the cornea and conjunctiva including epithelial herpes simplex keratitis, vaccinia, and varicella. Mycobacterial infection and fungal diseases of the eye.

**WARNINGS/PRECAUTIONS:** Not for injection into eye. Caution with glaucoma, herpes simplex, diseases causing thinning of cornea/sclera and other ocular viral infections. Prolonged use can cause glaucoma or secondary ocular infections (eg, fungal). Monitor IOP after 10 days of therapy. Re-evaluate if no response after 2 days. May delay healing and increase incidence of bleb formation after cataract surgery. Ocular irritation and punctate keratitis reported. Cataract formation and optic nerve damage with prolonged use.

**ADVERSE REACTIONS:** Elevation of IOP, glaucoma, infrequent optic nerve damage, posterior subcapsular cataract formation, delayed wound healing, irritation upon instillation, ocular discomfort, secondary infection, allergic sensitization, burning, stinging, eye irritation.

**PREGNANCY:** Category C, not for use in nursing.

**MECHANISM OF ACTION:** Aminoglycoside/corticosteroid. Gentamicin: Anti-infective component that provides action against susceptible organisms. Prednisolone: Corticosteroid that suppresses the inflammatory response and delays or slows healing.

## NURSING CONSIDERATIONS

**Assessment:** Prior to therapy, assess proper diagnosis of patient (eg, measurement of IOP, slit lamp biomicroscopy, fluorescein staining). Assess for hypersensitivity to other corticosteroids, viral diseases of the cornea and conjunctiva (eg, epithelial herpes simplex [dendritic keratitis], vaccina, and varicella), mycobacterial infection of the eye, and fungal diseases of the ocular structures. Assess use with glaucoma, history of herpes simplex, recent cataract surgery, and in pregnancy/nursing.

**Monitoring:** Monitor for masking of acute purulent infections, ocular irritation, and punctate keratitis. For patients on prolonged therapy, monitor for development of glaucoma with damage to the optic nerve, defects in visual acuity and fields of vision, posterior subcapsular cataract formation, corneal and scleral thinning, and secondary infections (eg, fungal, viral). Monitor IOP in patients on therapy for ≥10 days. Perform frequent slit lamp microscopy in patients with a history of herpes simplex.

**Patient Counseling:** Advise to d/c medication and consult physician if inflammation or pain persists longer than 48 hrs or becomes aggravated. Instruct to avoid touching bottle tip to the eyelids or other surfaces.

**Administration:** Ocular route. Do not inject into eye. Shake well before using. **Storage:** 15-25°C (59-77°F). Avoid excessive heat, 40°C (104°F) and above. Protect from freezing.



# PREDNISONE RX

prednisone (Roxane)

**THERAPEUTIC CLASS:** Glucocorticoid

**INDICATIONS:** Steroid-responsive disorders.

**DOSAGE:** *Adults:* Initial: 5-60mg/day depending on disease and response. Maint: Decrease dose by small amounts to lowest effective dose.
*Pediatrics:* Initial: 5-60mg/day depending on disease and response. Maint: Decrease dose by small amounts to lowest effective dose.

**HOW SUPPLIED:** Sol: 5mg/mL, 5mg/5mL; Tab: 1mg, 2.5mg, 5mg, 10mg, 20mg, 50mg

**CONTRAINDICATIONS:** Systemic fungal infections.

**WARNINGS/PRECAUTIONS:** May need to increase dose before, during, and after stressful situations. May mask signs of infection or cause new infections. Prolonged use may produce glaucoma, optic nerve damage, secondary ocular infections. Increases BP, salt/water retention, potassium excretion. More severe/fatal course of infections reported with chickenpox, measles. Caution with latent TB, hypothyroidism, cirrhosis, ocular herpes simplex, HTN, diverticulitis, fresh intestinal anastomosis, ulcerative colitis, osteoporosis, myasthenia gravis, renal insufficiency, peptic ulcer disease. Growth and development of children on prolonged therapy should be monitored. Monitor for psychic disturbances. Avoid abrupt withdrawal.

**ADVERSE REACTIONS:** Fluid and electrolyte disturbances, HTN, osteoporosis, muscle weakness, cushingoid state, menstrual irregularities, nervousness, insomnia, impaired wound healing, DM, ulcerative esophagitis, excessive sweating, increased ICP, carbohydrate intolerance, glaucoma, cataracts, weight gain, nausea, malaise.

**INTERACTIONS:** Increases clearance of high dose ASA; caution in hypoprothrombinemia. Increased insulin and oral hypoglycemic requirements in DM. Avoid smallpox vaccine, and live vaccines with immunosuppressive doses. Possible decreased vaccine response with killed or inactivated vaccines with immunosuppressive doses. Increased clearance with hepatic enzyme inducers. Decreased metabolism with troleandomycin, ketoconazole. Variable effect on oral anticoagulants.

**PREGNANCY:** Safety in pregnancy and nursing not known.

**MECHANISM OF ACTION:** Anti-inflammatory glucocorticoid; causes profound and varied metabolic effects and modifies the body's immune responses to diverse stimuli.

**PHARMACOKINETICS: Absorption:** Readily absorbed (GI tract).

## NURSING CONSIDERATIONS

**Assessment:** Assess unusual stress, fungal/other current infections, active TB, thyroid status, vaccination status, hepatic/liver impairment, hypoprothrombinemia, psychiatric tendencies, ulcerative colitis, diverticulitis, peptic ulcer with/without impending perforation, intestinal anastamoses, HTN, osteoporosis, myasthenia gravis, pregnancy status.

**Monitoring:** In pediatrics, monitor for hypoadrenalism, growth and development. Monitor for psychiatric derangements, infection, cataracts, fluid retention, adrenocortical insufficiency, intestinal perforation/peritoneal irritation, serum electrolytes, TSH, glucose, LFTs, BP, IOP.

**Patient Counseling:** Avoid exposure to chickenpox or measles; report immediately if exposed. Advise regarding dietary salt restriction and $K^+$ supplementaion.

**Administration:** Oral route. **Storage:** 25°C (77°F); excursions permitted to 15-30°C.

# PREMARIN TABLETS RX

conjugated estrogens (Wyeth)

P

**Estrogens increase the risk of endometrial cancer. Estrogens, with or without progestins, should not be used for the prevention of cardiovascular disease or dementia. Increased risks of MI, stroke, invasive breast cancer, PE, and DVT in postmenopausal women (50-79 yrs of age) reported. Increased risk of developing probable dementia in postmenopausal women ≥65 yrs of age reported.**

**THERAPEUTIC CLASS:** Estrogen

**INDICATIONS:** Treatment of moderate to severe vasomotor symptoms and/or vulvar/vaginal atrophy associated with menopause. Treatment of hypoestrogenism due to hypogonadism, castration, or primary ovarian failure. Palliative treatment of breast cancer in patients with metastatic disease and/or advanced androgen-dependent carcinoma of the prostate. Prevention of postmenopausal osteoporosis.

**DOSAGE:** *Adults:* Vasomotor Symptoms/Vulvar/Vaginal Atrophy: 0.3mg qd continuously or cyclically (eg, 25 days on, 5 days off). Adjust dose based on response. Re-evaluate at 3-6 month intervals. Osteoporosis Prevention: 0.3mg qd continuously or cyclically (eg, 25 days on, 5 days off). Female Hypogonadism: 0.3-0.625mg qd cyclically (eg, 3 weeks on, 1 week off). Titrate at 6-12 month intervals. Female Castration/Ovarian Failure: 1.25mg qd cyclically. Breast Cancer (palliation): 10mg tid for minimum 3 months. Prostate Cancer (palliation): 1.25-2.5mg tid.

**HOW SUPPLIED:** Tab: 0.3mg, 0.45mg, 0.625mg, 0.9mg, 1.25mg

**CONTRAINDICATIONS:** Pregnancy, undiagnosed abnormal genital bleeding, breast cancer unless being treated for metastatic disease, estrogen-dependent neoplasia, DVT/PE, active or recent (eg, within past year) arterial thromboembolic disease (eg, stroke, MI), liver dysfunction or disease.

**WARNINGS/PRECAUTIONS:** May increase risk of cardiovascular events (eg, MI, stroke), venous thrombosis, and PE; d/c immediately if any of these events occur or are suspected. May increase risk of breast/endometrial cancer, and gallbladder disease. May lead to severe hypercalcemia with breast cancer and bone metastases; monitor and d/c if hypercalcemia occurs. Retinal vascular thrombosis reported; monitor and d/c if papilledema or retinal vascular lesions occur. Consider addition of a progestin if no hysterectomy. May elevate BP; monitor at regular intervals. May cause elevations of plasma triglycerides with pre-existing hypertriglyceridemia. Caution with history of cholestatic jaundice associated with past estrogen use or with pregnancy; d/c with recurrence. May lead to increased thyroid-binding globulin levels; monitor thyroid function. May cause fluid retention; caution with cardiac/renal dysfunction. Caution with severe hypocalcemia. May increase risk of ovarian cancer. May exacerbate endometriosis, asthma, DM, epilepsy, migraine, porphyria, SLE, and hepatic hemangiomas; use with caution.

**ADVERSE REACTIONS:** Abdominal pain, back pain, headache, infection, pain, arthralgia, leg cramps, breast pain, vaginal hemorrhage, vaginitis.

**INTERACTIONS:** CYP3A4 inducers (eg, St. John's wort, phenobarbital, carbamazepine, rifampin) may decrease levels which may decrease therapeutic effects and/or change uterine bleeding profile. CYP3A4 inhibitors (eg, erythromycin, clarithromycin, ketoconazole, itraconazole, ritonavir, grapefruit juice) may increase levels which may result in side effects. Reduced response to metyrapone test.

**PREGNANCY:** Contraindicated in pregnancy, caution in nursing.

**MECHANISM OF ACTION:** Estrogen; binds to nuclear receptors in estrogen-responsive tissues. Circulating estrogens modulate pituitary secretion of the gonadotropins, luteinizing hormone and follicle stimulating hormone, through negative feedback mechanism. Reduces elevated levels of these hormones in postmenopausal women.

**PHARMACOKINETICS: Absorption:** Well absorbed; oral administration of variable doses resulted in different parameters. **Distribution:** Largely bound to sex hormone binding globulin and albumin; found in breast milk. **Metabolism:** Liver, to estrone (metabolite) and estriol (major urinary metabolite); sulfate and glucuronide conjugation (liver); gut hydrolysis; CYP3A4 (partial metabolism). **Elimination:** Urine (parent drug and metabolites).



## NURSING CONSIDERATIONS

**Assessment:** Assess for undiagnosed abnormal genital bleeding, presence or history of breast cancer, estrogen-dependent neoplasia, DVT or PE, active or recent (within past yr) arterial thromboembolic disease (eg, stroke, MI), liver dysfunction, history of cholestatic jaundice, pregnancy/nursing status, age ( ≥65 yrs), hypertriglyceridemia, hypothyroidism, hypocalcemia, asthma, DM, epilepsy, migraines or porphyria, SLE, and possible drug interactions. Assess need for progestin therapy in women who have not had a hysterectomy.

**Monitoring:** Monitor for signs/symptoms of cardiovascular disorders (eg, stroke, coronary heart disease, venous thromboembolism), malignant neoplasms (eg, endometrial, breast, ovarian cancer), dementia, gallbladder disease, hypercalcemia, visual abnormalities (eg, retinal vascular thrombosis), BP elevations, elevations in plasma triglycerides, pancreatitis, hypothyroidism, fluid retention, exacerbation of endometriosis and other conditions (eg, asthma, DM, epilepsy, migraines, SLE). Perform annual breast exam. Monitor BP levels regularly and thyroid function in patients on thyroid replacement therapy. Perform periodic evaluation (every 3-6 months) to determine treatment need. If undiagnosed persistent or recurring genital bleeding occurs, perform adequate diagnostic measures (eg, endometrial sampling) to rule out malignancy.

**Patient Counseling:** Inform that drug increases risk for uterine cancer, heart attack, stroke, breast cancer, blood clots, and dementia. Report any breast lumps, unusual vaginal bleeding, dizziness and faintness, changes in speech, severe headaches, chest pain, SOB, leg pains, changes in vision, or vomiting.

Advise to notify physician if planning surgery or bedrest. Instruct to take medication at same time daily and to perform monthly self breast exams. Counsel that if dose is missed, take as soon as possible; if almost time for next dose, skip dose, and go back to normal dosing schedule.

**Administration:** Oral route. **Storage:** 20-25°C (68-77°F); excursions permitted to 15-30°C (59-86°F); dispense in tightly closed container.

## PREMARIN VAGINAL RX

conjugated estrogens (Wyeth)

**Estrogens increase risk of endometrial cancer. Estrogens, with or without progestins, should not be used for the prevention of cardiovascular (CV) disease or dementia. Increased risks of MI, stroke, invasive breast cancer, pulmonary emboli (PE), and deep vein thrombosis (DVT) in postmenopausal women (50-79 yrs of age) reported. Increased risk of developing probable dementia in postmenopausal women ≥65 yrs of age reported. Estrogens with or without progestins should be prescribed at the lowest effective dose and for the shortest duration consistent with treatment goals and risks for the individual woman.**

**THERAPEUTIC CLASS:** Estrogen

**INDICATIONS:** Treatment of atrophic vaginitis, kraurosis vulvae, and moderate-to-severe dyspareunia.

**DOSAGE:** *Adults:* Atrophic Vaginitis/Kraurosis Vulvae: Usual: 0.5g intravaginally qd cyclically (3 weeks on, 1 week off). Titrate: 0.5-2g based on individual response. Moderate To Severe Dyspareunia: 0.5g intravaginally twice weekly (eg, Monday and Thursday) continuous regimen or cyclically (3 weeks on, 1 week off).

**HOW SUPPLIED:** Cre: 0.625mg/g [42.5g]

**CONTRAINDICATIONS:** Pregnancy, undiagnosed abnormal genital bleeding, breast cancer, estrogen-dependent neoplasia, DVT/PE, active or recent (eg, within past year) arterial thromboembolic disease (eg, stroke, MI), liver dysfunction or disease.

**WARNINGS/PRECAUTIONS:** May increase risk of breast/endometrial cancer, dementia and gallbladder disease. May lead to severe hypercalcemia with breast cancer and bone metastases; monitor and d/c if hypercalcemia occurs. Retinal vascular thrombosis reported; monitor and d/c if papilledema or retinal vascular lesions occur. Consider addition of a progestin if no hysterectomy. May elevate BP; monitor at regular intervals. May cause elevations of plasma triglycerides with pre-existing hypertriglyceridemia. Caution with history of cholestatic jaundice associated with past estrogen use or with pregnancy; d/c with recurrence. May lead to increased thyroid-binding globulin levels; monitor thyroid function. May cause fluid retention; caution with cardiac/renal dysfunction. Caution with severe hypocalcemia. May increase risk of ovarian cancer. May exacerbate endometriosis, asthma, diabetes mellitus (DM), epilepsy, migraine, porphyria, systemic lupus erythema (SLE), and hepatic hemangiomas; use with caution. May weaken and contribute to the failure of condoms, diaphragms, or cervical caps made of latex or rubber.

**ADVERSE REACTIONS:** Breakthrough bleeding, vaginal candidiasis, change in cervical secretion, breast tenderness and enlargement, N/V, abdominal cramps, bloating, chloasma, melasma, venous thromboembolism, pulmonary embolism, headache.

**INTERACTIONS:** CYP3A4 inducers (eg, St. John's wort, phenobarbital, carbamazepine, rifampin) may decrease levels, which may decrease therapeutic effects and/or change uterine bleeding profile. CYP3A4 inhibitors (eg, erythromycin, clarithromycin, ketoconazole, itraconazole, ritonavir, grapefruit juice) may increase levels, which may result in side effects.

**PREGNANCY:** Contraindicated in pregnancy, caution in nursing.

**MECHANISM OF ACTION:** Estrogen; binds to nuclear receptors in estrogen-responsive tissues. Circulating estrogens modulate pituitary secretion of the gonadotropins, luteinizing hormone and follicle stimulating hormone, through negative feedback mechanism. Reduces elevated levels of these hormones in postmenopausal women.

**PHARMACOKINETICS: Absorption:** Well-absorbed. **Distribution:** Largely bound to sex hormone binding globulin and albumin; found in breast milk. **Metabolism:** Liver to estrone (metabolite), estriol (major urinary metabolite); sulfate and glucuronide conjugation (liver); gut hydrolysis; CYP 3A4 (partial metabolism). **Elimination:** Urine (parent compound and metabolites).

## NURSING CONSIDERATIONS

**Assessment:** Assess for undiagnosed abnormal genital bleeding, presence or history of breast cancer, DVT or PE, estrogen-dependent neoplasia, active or recent (within past yr) arterial thromboembolic disease (eg, stroke, MI), liver dysfunction or past history of cholestatic jaundice, pregnancy/nursing status, age ( ≥65 yrs), hypertriglyceridemia, hypothyroidism, hypocalcemia, asthma, DM, epilepsy, migraines or porphyria, SLE, and possible drug interactions. Assess need for progestin therapy in women who have not had a hysterectomy.

**Monitoring:** Monitor for signs/symptoms of CV disorders (eg, stroke, CHD, venous thromboembolism), malignant neoplasms (eg, endometrial, breast, ovarian cancer), dementia, gallbladder disease, hypercalcemia, visual abnormalities (eg, retinal vascular thrombosis), BP elevations, elevations in plasma TG, pancreatitis, hypothyroidism, fluid retention, exacerbation of endometriosis and of other conditions (eg, asthma, DM, epilepsy, migraines, SLE). Perform annual breast exam. Monitor BP levels at regular intervals and thyroid function in patients on thyroid replacement therapy. Perform periodic evaluation (every 3-6 months) to determine treatment need. If undiagnosed persistent or recurring genital bleeding occurs, perform adequate diagnostic measures (eg, endometrial sampling) to rule out malignancy.

**Patient Counseling:** Inform that drug increases risk for uterine cancer, heart attack, stroke, breast cancer, blood clots, and dementia. Report any breast lumps, unusual vaginal bleeding, dizziness and faintness, changes in speech, severe headaches, chest pain, SOB, leg pain, changes in vision, and vomiting. Advise on proper administration of medication; applicator should be cleansed with mild soap and warm water following application; do not boil or use hot water. Instruct to perform monthly self breast exams. Inform that medication may weaken barrier contraceptives (eg, latex condoms, diaphragms, cervical caps).

**Administration:** Intravaginal route. **Storage:** 20-25°C (68-77°F); excursions permitted to 15-30°C (59-86°F).

P

# PREMPHASE RX

medroxyprogesterone acetate - conjugated estrogens (Wyeth)

**Estrogens and progestins should not be used for prevention of cardiovascular (CV) disease or dementia. Increased risks of myocardial infarction (MI), stroke, invasive breast cancer, pulmonary emboli (PE), and deep vein thrombosis (DVT) in postmenopausal women (50-79 yrs of age) reported. Increased risk of developing probable dementia in postmenopausal women ≥65 yrs of age reported. Estrogens, with or without progestins, should be prescribed at the lowest effective doses and for the shortest duration consistent with treatment goals.**

**THERAPEUTIC CLASS:** Estrogen/progestogen combination

**INDICATIONS:** Treatment of moderate to severe vasomotor symptoms and/or vulvar/vaginal atrophy associated with menopause and prevention of postmenopausal osteoporosis in women with intact uterus.

**DOSAGE:** *Adults:* Vasomotor Symptoms/Vulvar/Vaginal Atrophy/ Osteoporosis Prevention: 0.625mg tab qd on Days 1-14 and 0.625mg-5mg tab qd on Days 15-28. Re-evaluate after 3-6 months.

**HOW SUPPLIED:** Tab: 0.625mg (Estrogens, Conjugated) and 0.625mg-5mg (Estrogens, Conjugated-Medroxyprogesterone)

**CONTRAINDICATIONS:** Pregnancy, undiagnosed abnormal genital bleeding, breast cancer, estrogen dependent neoplasia, active or history of DVT/PE, active or recent (eg, within past year) arterial thromboembolic disease (eg, stroke, MI), liver dysfunction or disease.

**WARNINGS/PRECAUTIONS:** May increase risk of CV events (eg, MI, stroke), venous thrombosis, and PE; d/c immediately if any of these events occur or are suspected. May increase risk of breast/endometrial cancer and gallbladder disease. May increase risk of dementia in women ≥65 yrs. May lead to severe hypercalcemia in patients with breast cancer and bone metastases; monitor and d/c if hypercalcemia occurs. Retinal vascular thrombosis reported; monitor and d/c if papilledema or retinal vascular lesions occur. May elevate BP; monitor at regular intervals. May cause elevations of plasma triglycerides with pre-existing hypertriglyceridemia. Caution with history of cholestatic jaundice associated with past estrogen use or with pregnancy; d/c with recurrence. May lead to increased thyroid-binding globulin levels; monitor thyroid function. May cause fluid retention; caution with cardiac/renal dysfunction. Caution with severe hypocalcemia. May increase risk of ovarian cancer. May exacerbate endometriosis, asthma, diabetes mellitus (DM), epilepsy, migraine, porphyria, systemic lupus erythema (SLE), and hepatic hemangiomas; use with caution.

**ADVERSE REACTIONS:** Abdominal pain, asthenia, flu syndrome, leukorrhea, pharyngitis, dysmenorrhea, breast pain, nausea, arthralgia, headache, depression, back pain, infection, pain, rhinitis.

**INTERACTIONS:** CYP3A4 inducers (eg, St. John's wort, phenobarbital, carbamazepine, rifampin) may decrease levels which may decrease therapeutic effects and/or change uterine bleeding profile. CYP3A4 inhibitors (eg, erythromycin, clarithromycin, ketoconazole, itraconazole, ritonavir, grapefruit juice) may increase levels which may result in side effects. Concomitant aminoglutethimide may significantly depress bioavailability of medroxyprogesterone. Patients concomitantly receiving thyroid hormone replacement therapy and estrogens may require increased doses of their thyroid replacement therapy.

**PREGNANCY:** Contraindicated in pregnancy, not for use in nursing

**MECHANISM OF ACTION:** Conjugated Estrogens: Estrogen; binds to nuclear receptors in estrogen-responsive tissues. Circulating estrogens modulate pituitary secretion of the gonadotropins, luteinizing hormone and follicle stimulating hormone, through negative feedback. Medroxyprogesterone (MPA): Progesterone derivative; inhibits gonadotropin production which prevents follicular maturation and ovulation. Decreases nuclear estrogen receptors and suppresses epithelial DNA synthesis in endometrial tissue.

**PHARMACOKINETICS: Absorption**: Well-absorbed. Oral administration of various doses resulted in different parameters. **Distribution**: Found in breast milk. Estrogen: Largely bound to sex hormone binding globulin and albumin. Medroxyprogesterone (MPA): Plasma protein binding (90%). **Metabolism**: Estrogen: Liver, to estrone (metabolite) and estriol (major urinary metabolite); sulfate and glucuronide conjugation (liver); gut hydrolysis; CYP3A4 (partial metabolism). MPA: Liver, via hydroxylation, conjugation. **Elimination**: Estrogen: Urine (parent compound and metabolites); MPA: Urine (metabolites).

## NURSING CONSIDERATIONS

**Assessment:** Assess for undiagnosed abnormal genital bleeding, presence or history of breast cancer, DVT or PE, estrogen-dependent neoplasia, active or recent (within past yr) arterial thromboembolic disease (eg, stroke, MI), liver dysfunction, history of cholestatic jaundice, age ( ≥65 yrs), hypertriglyceridemia, hypothyroidism, hypocalcemia, asthma, DM, epilepsy, migraines, porphyria, SLE, cardiac/hepatic/renal impairment, smoking, and possible drug interactions. Assess pregnancy/nursing status.

**Monitoring:** Monitor for signs/symptoms of CV disorders (eg, stroke, coronary heart disease, venous thromboembolism), malignant neoplasms (eg, endometrial, breast, ovarian cancer), dementia, gallbladder disease, hypercalcemia, visual abnormalities (eg, retinal vascular thrombosis), BP elevations, elevations in plasma triglycerides, pancreatitis, hypothyroidism, fluid retention, exacerbation of endometriosis and other conditions (eg, asthma, DM, epilepsy, migraines, SLE). Perform annual breast exam. Monitor BP levels at regular intervals and thyroid function if on thyroid replacement therapy. Perform periodic evaluation (every 3-6 months) to determine treatment need. If undiagnosed persistent or recurring genital bleeding occurs, perform adequate diagnostic measures (eg, endometrial sampling) to rule out malignancy.

**Patient Counseling:** Inform of pregnancy risks. Advise to seek medical attention if symptoms of hepatic dysfunction (jaundice), hypercalcemia, visual abnormalities (partial/complete loss of vision, diplopia), migraines, abnormal vaginal bleeding, hypersensitivity reactions, HTN, thromboembolic disorders, fluid retention, exacerbation of diseases, CV events, or dementia occur. Inform of warning signs of serious side effects eg, breast lumps, dizziness and faintness, changes in vision/speech, chest pain and shortness of breath, leg pains, vomiting.

**Administration:** Oral route. **Storage**: 20-25°C (68-77°F); excursions permitted to 15-30°C (59-86°F).

## PREMPRO RX

medroxyprogesterone acetate - conjugated estrogens (Wyeth)

**Estrogens and progestins should not be used for prevention of cardiovascular (CV) disease or dementia. Increased risks of myocardial infarction (MI), stroke, invasive breast cancer, pulmonary emboli (PE), and deep vein thrombosis (DVT) in postmenopausal women (50-79 yrs of age) reported. Increased risk of developing probable dementia in postmenopausal women ≥65 yrs of age reported. Estrogens, with or without progestins, should be prescribed at the lowest effective doses and for the shortest duration consistent with treatment goals.**

**THERAPEUTIC CLASS:** Estrogen/progestogen combination

**INDICATIONS:** Treatment of moderate to severe vasomotor symptoms and/or vulvar/vaginal atrophy associated with menopause and prevention of postmenopausal osteoporosis in women with intact uterus.

**DOSAGE:** *Adults:* Vasomotor Symptoms/Vulvar/Vaginal Atrophy/Osteoporosis Prevention: Initial: 0.3mg-1.5mg qd. Adjust dose based on individual response. Re-evaluate after 3-6 months.

**HOW SUPPLIED:** Tab: (Estrogens, Conjugated-Medroxyprogesterone) 0.3mg-1.5mg, 0.45mg-1.5mg, 0.625mg-2.5mg, 0.625mg-5mg

**CONTRAINDICATIONS:** Pregnancy, undiagnosed abnormal genital bleeding, breast cancer, estrogen dependent neoplasia, active or history of DVT/PE, active or recent (eg, within past year) arterial thromboembolic disease (eg, stroke, MI), liver dysfunction or disease.



**WARNINGS/PRECAUTIONS:** May increase risk of CV events (eg, MI, stroke), venous thrombosis, and PE; d/c immediately if any of these events occur or are suspected. May increase risk of breast/endometrial cancer, and gallbladder disease. May increase risk of dementia in women ≥65 yrs. May lead to severe hypercalcemia in patients with breast cancer and bone metastases; monitor and d/c if hypercalcemia occurs. Retinal vascular thrombosis reported; monitor and d/c if papilledema or retinal vascular lesions occur. May elevate BP; monitor at regular intervals. May cause elevations of plasma triglycerides with pre-existing hypertriglyceridemia. Caution with history of cholestatic jaundice associated with past estrogen use or with pregnancy; d/c with recurrence. May lead to increased thyroid-binding globulin levels; monitor thyroid function. May cause fluid retention; caution with cardiac/renal dysfunction. Caution with severe hypocalcemia. May increase risk of ovarian cancer. May exacerbate endometriosis, asthma, diabetes mellitus (DM), epilepsy, migraine, porphyria, systemic lupus erythema (SLE), and hepatic hemangiomas; use with caution.

**ADVERSE REACTIONS:** Abdominal pain, flu syndrome, pharyngitis, pruritus, flatulence, sinusitis, vaginal moniliasis, breast pain, nausea, arthralgia, headache, depression, back pain, infection, pain.

**INTERACTIONS:** CYP3A4 inducers (eg, St. John's wort, phenobarbital, carbamazepine, rifampin) may decrease levels which may decrease therapeutic effects and/or change uterine bleeding profile. CYP3A4 inhibitors (eg, erythromycin, clarithromycin, ketoconazole, itraconazole, ritonavir, grapefruit juice) may increase levels which may result in side effects. Concomitant aminoglutethimide may significantly depress bioavailability of medroxyprogesterone.

Patients concomitantly receiving thyroid hormone replacement therapy and estrogens may require increased doses of their thyroid replacement therapy.

**PREGNANCY:** Contraindicated in pregnancy, not for use in nursing.

**MECHANISM OF ACTION:** Conjugated Estrogens: Estrogen; binds to nuclear receptors in estrogen-responsive tissues. Circulating estrogens modulate pituitary secretion of the gonadotropins, luteinizing hormone and follicle stimulating hormone, through negative feedback. Medroxyprogesterone (MPA): Progesterone derivative; inhibits gonadotropin production which prevents follicular maturation and ovulation. Decreases nuclear estrogen receptors and suppresses epithelial DNA synthesis in endometrial tissue.

**PHARMACOKINETICS: Absorption**: Well absorbed. Oral administration of various doses resulted in different parameters. **Distribution**: Found in breast milk. Estrogen: Largely bound to sex hormone binding globulin and albumin. Medroxyprogesterone (MPA): Plasma protein binding (90%). **Metabolism**: Estrogen: Liver, to estrone (metabolite) and estriol (major urinary metabolite); sulfate and glucuronide conjugation (liver); gut hydrolysis; CYP3A4 (partial metabolism). MPA: Liver, via hydroxylation, conjugation. **Elimination**: Estrogen: Urine (parent compound and metabolites). MPA: Urine (metabolites).

## NURSING CONSIDERATIONS

**Assessment:** Assess for undiagnosed abnormal genital bleeding, presence or history of breast cancer, DVT or PE, estrogen-dependent neoplasia, active or recent (within past yr) arterial thromboembolic disease (eg, stroke, MI), liver dysfunction, history of cholestatic jaundice, age ( ≥65 yrs), hypertriglyceridemia, hypothyroidism, hypocalcemia, asthma, DM, epilepsy, migraines, porphyria, SLE, cardiac/renal/hepatic impairment, smoking, and possible drug interactions. Assess pregnancy/nursing status.

**Monitoring:** Monitor for signs/symptoms of CV disorders (eg, stroke, coronary heart disease, venous thromboembolism), malignant neoplasms (eg, endometrial, breast, ovarian cancer), dementia, gallbladder disease, hypercalcemia, visual abnormalities (eg, retinal vascular thrombosis), BP elevations, elevations in plasma triglycerides, pancreatitis, hypothyroidism, fluid retention, exacerbation of endometriosis and other conditions (eg, asthma, DM, epilepsy, migraines, SLE). Perform annual breast exam. Monitor BP levels at regular intervals and thyroid function if on thyroid replacement therapy. Perform periodic evaluation (every 3-6 months) to determine treatment need. If undiagnosed persistent or recurring genital bleeding occurs, perform adequate diagnostic measures (eg, endometrial sampling) to rule out malignancy.

**Patient Counseling:** Inform of pregnancy risks. Advise to seek medical attention if symptoms of hepatic dysfunction (jaundice), hypercalcemia, visual abnormalities (partial/complete loss of vision, diplopia), migraines, abnormal vaginal bleeding, hypersensitivity reactions, HTN, thromboembolic disorders, fluid retention, exacerbation of diseases, CV events, or dementia occur. Inform of warning signs of serious side effects, eg, breast lumps, dizziness and faintness, changes in vision/speech, chest pain or shortness of breath, leg pains, vomiting.

**Administration:** Oral route. **Storage**: 20-25°C (68-77°F); excursions permitted to 15-30°C (59-86°F).

# PREVACID — RX

lansoprazole (Takeda)

**OTHER BRAND NAMES:** Prevacid Solutab (Takeda)

**THERAPEUTIC CLASS:** Proton pump inhibitor

**INDICATIONS:** (PO) Treatment of active duodenal ulcer (DU), active benign gastric ulcer (GU), erosive esophagitis, symptomatic GERD. Maintain healing of erosive esophagitis and duodenal ulcers. Treatment of pathological hypersecretory conditions (eg, Zollinger-Ellison syndrome). Combination therapy with amoxicillin +/- clarithromycin for *H.pylori* eradication in duodenal ulcer disease, to reduce risk of ulcer recurrence. Treatment and risk reduction in NSAID-induced gastric ulcer. (Inj) Short-term treatment of erosive esophagitis.

**DOSAGE:** *Adults:* >17 yrs: (PO) DU: 15mg qd for 4 weeks. Maint: 15mg qd. GU: 30mg qd up to 8 weeks. GERD: 15mg qd up to 8 weeks. Erosive Esophagitis: 30mg qd up to 8 weeks. May repeat for 8 weeks if needed. Maint: 15mg qd. NSAID-Induced GU: 30mg qd for 8 weeks. Reduce Risk of NSAID Induced GU: 15mg qd for 12 weeks. Hypersecretory Conditions: Initial: 60mg qd, then adjust. Max: 90mg bid. Divide dose if >120mg/day. *H.pylori*: Triple Therapy: 30mg + clarithromycin 500mg + amoxicillin 1000mg, all bid (q12h) for 10-14 days. Dual Therapy: 30mg + amoxicillin 1000mg both tid (q8h) for 14 days. Take before eating.

*Pediatrics:* 12-17 yrs: Short-Term Symptomatic GERD: 15mg qd for up to 8 weeks. Erosive Esophagitis: 30mg qd for up to 8 weeks. 1-11 yrs: Short-Term Symptomatic GERD/Erosive Esophagitis: ≤30kg: 15mg qd for up to 12 weeks. >30kg: 30mg qd for up to 12 weeks. Titrate: May increase up to 30mg bid after 2 weeks if symptomatic. Severe Hepatic Impairment: Adjust dose. Take before eating.

**HOW SUPPLIED:** Cap, Delayed-Release: 15mg, 30mg; Tab, Disintegrating (SoluTab): 15mg, 30mg.

**WARNINGS/PRECAUTIONS:** Symptomatic response does not preclude the presence of gastric malignancy. Adjust dose with hepatic impairment.

**ADVERSE REACTIONS:** Abdominal pain, constipation, diarrhea, and nausea.

**INTERACTIONS:** May alter absorption of pH-dependent drugs (eg, ketoconazole, ampicillin esters, digoxin, and iron salts). Give at least 30 min prior to sucralfate. Theophylline may need dose adjustment. Concomitant use with warfarin may increase INR and prothrombin time. Avoid with atazanavir; may decrease atazanavir levels.

**PREGNANCY:** Category B, not for use in nursing.

**MECHANISM OF ACTION:** Proton pump inhibitor; suppresses gastric acid secretion by specific inhibition of the $(H^+, K^+)$-ATPase enzyme system at the secretory surface of the gastric parietal cell.

**PHARMACOKINETICS: Absorption:** absolute bioavailability (>80%); $T_{max}$=1.7 hrs. **Distribution:** plasma protein binding (97%). **Metabolism:** Liver (extensive). **Elimination:** Urine (33%), feces (66%); $T_{1/2}$=1.5 hrs. Refer to package insert for pediatric parameters.



## NURSING CONSIDERATIONS

**Assessment:** Assess for gastric malignancy, severe hepatic insufficiency, pregnancy/nursing status, and possible drug interactions. Oral formulation: Assess for hypersensitivity to phenylketonurics.

**Monitoring:** Monitor for signs/symptoms of GI effects (eg, diarrhea, dyspepsia).

**Patient Counseling:** Instruct to contact physician if adverse events occur. Oral formulation: Instruct to take before eating; swallow whole, do not crush or chew. If difficulty swallowing, open capsule and sprinkle granules onto tablespoon of applesauce, pudding, cottage cheese, yogurt, or strained pears or into apple/orange/tomato juice; rinse glass with juice two or more times to ensure complete delivery of dose. Swallow completely.

**Administration:** Oral route. Refer to PI for all the different methods of administration. **Storage:** 25°C (77°F); excursions permitted to 15-30°C (59-86°F).

# PREVACID NAPRAPAC RX

lansoprazole - naproxen (TAP)

**NSAIDs may cause an increased risk of serious cardiovascular thrombotic events, MI, and stroke. Risk may increase with duration of use and in patients with cardiovascular disease or risk factors for cardiovascular disease. NSAIDs may cause an increased risk of serious GI events which may be fatal. Patients with history of gastric and/or duodenal ulcers (especially patients with history of bleeding or perforation) and geriatric patients are at greater risk for serious GI events. Contraindicated for the treatment of perioperative pain in the setting of coronary artery bypass graft (CABG) surgery.**

**THERAPEUTIC CLASS:** NSAID/Proton Pump Inhibitor

**INDICATIONS:** To reduce the risk of NSAID-associated gastric ulcers in patients with a history of documented gastric ulcers who require the use of an NSAID for treatment of rheumatoid arthritis, osteoarthritis, and ankylosing spondylitis.

**DOSAGE:** *Adults:* Take am dose before eating. Lansoprazole 15mg qam + naproxen 500mg bid in am and pm. Max: 1000mg naproxen/day. Swallow lansoprazole whole.

**HOW SUPPLIED:** Cap, Delayed-Release: (Naproxen-Lansoprazole): 500mg-15mg [14 tabs naproxen + 7 caps lansoprazole/weekly blister card; 4 cards/pkg]

**CONTRAINDICATIONS:** Presence or history of NSAID/ASA-related asthma, urticaria, or allergic-type reactions. Perioperative pain in the setting of CABG surgery.

**WARNINGS/PRECAUTIONS:** Risk of GI ulceration, bleeding, and perforation. Monitor for visual disturbances, fluid retention/edema, Hgb levels (if initial ≤10g), and LFTs with chronic use. Acute interstitial nephritis, hematuria, proteinuria, nephrotic syndrome and severe hepatic reactions reported. Caution with impaired renal (CrCl <20mL/min) or hepatic function, elderly, heart failure, and high doses with chronic alcoholic liver disease. NSAIDs can lead to onset or worsening of pre-existing HTN; monitor BP closely. Naproxen can cause exfoliative dermatitis, Stevens-Johnson syndrome, toxic epidermal necrolysis.

**ADVERSE REACTIONS:** Nausea, abdominal pain, constipation, heartburn, headache, dizziness, drowsiness, pruritus, skin eruptions, ecchymoses, tinnitus, edema, dyspnea.

**INTERACTIONS:** Avoid other forms of naproxen, ASA. May potentiate renal disease with ACE inhibitors. Naproxen may displace other albumin-bound drugs. Caution with warfarin. Monitor for toxicity with hydantoin, sulfonamide, or sulfonylureas. Decreased plasma levels with ASA. May antagonize natriuretic effect of furosemide and thiazides. Decreases renal clearance of lithium and methotrexate. May decrease antihypertensive effects of propranolol and other β-blockers. Increased levels and half-life with probenecid. Take lansoprazole 30 min prior to sucralfate. Lansoprazole may alter absorption of pH-dependent drugs (eg, ketoconazole, ampicillin, iron, digoxin).

**PREGNANCY:** Category C, not for use in nursing.

**MECHANISM OF ACTION:** Naproxen: NSAID; inhibits prostaglandin synthetase. Lansoprazole: PPI; inhibits gastric acid secretion by blocking proton pumps.

**PHARMACOKINETICS: Absorption:** Naproxen: Rapid, complete; bioavailability (95%); $T_{max}$=2-4 hrs. Lansoprazole: Rapid; bioavailability (80%); $T_{max}$=1.7 hrs. **Distribution:** Naproxen: $V_d$=0.16 L/kg; plasma protein binding ( ≥99%); found in breast milk. Lansoprazole: Plasma protein binding (97%). **Metabolism:** Naproxen: Hepatic; 6-O-desmethyl naproxen (metobolite). Lansoprazole: Hepatic. **Elimination:** Naproxen: Kidney; urine (95%), feces (≤3%); $T_{1/2}$=12-17 hrs. Lansoprazole: Biliary; $T_{1/2}$≤2 hrs.

## NURSING CONSIDERATIONS

**Assessment:** Assess for history of asthma, CVD (HTN, CHF) or risk factors for disease, fluid retention, edema, pregnancy status, risk factors for GI events

P

(bleeding, ulceration, perforation), possible drug interactions, renal/hepatic dysfunction.

**Monitoring:** Monitor CBCs, LFTs, renal function, and chemistries periodically. Monitor for signs/symptoms of GI events (bleeding, ulceration, perforation), CHF, HTN, salt depletion, renal/liver dysfunction.

**Patient Counseling:** Advise to seek medical attention if symptoms of hepatotoxicity (nausea, fatigue, pruritis), anaphylactic reactions (difficulty breathing, swelling of face/throat), hypersensitivity reactions (rash), CV events (chest pain, SOB, weakness, slurring of speech), GI ulceration and bleeding (epigastric pain, dyspepsia, melena, hematemesis), weight gain, or edema occurs. Inform of pregnancy risks. Caution may impair physical/mental abilities if experience drowsiness, dizziness, vertigo, or depression during therapy.

**Administration:** Oral route. **Storage:** 25°C (77°F); excursions permitted to 15-30°C (59-86°F).

## PREVNAR — RX

pneumococcal vaccine, diphtheria conjugate (Wyeth)

**OTHER BRAND NAMES:** Prevnar 13 (Wyeth)

**THERAPEUTIC CLASS:** Vaccine

**INDICATIONS:** Active immunization of infants and toddlers against invasive disease caused by *S.pneumoniae*. Active immunization of infants and toddlers against otitis media caused by serotypes included in the vaccine.

**DOSAGE:** *Pediatrics:* 6 weeks-2 months: 4 doses of 0.5mL IM. Give 3 doses at 2-month intervals and 4th dose at 12-15 months old. Unvaccinated Children: 7-11 months: 3 doses of 0.5mL IM. Give first 2 doses at least 4 weeks apart and 3rd dose after first birthday; separate from 2nd dose by at least 2 months. 12-23 months: 2 doses of 0.5mL IM at least 2 months apart. ≥24 months-9 yrs: 0.5mL IM single dose.

**HOW SUPPLIED:** Inj: 0.5mL (1 dose syringe)

**WARNINGS/PRECAUTIONS:** Will not protect against *S. pneumoniae* disease caused by serotypes unrelated to those in the vaccine. Avoid with thrombocytopenia or coagulation disorder. Postpone if patient has acute, severe, febrile illness. Impaired immune responses due to immunosuppressive therapy may cause reduced response. Not a substitute for diphtheria or 23-valent pneumococcal vaccinations. Have epinephrine (1:1000) or other agents available for control of immediate allergic reaction. Fever and rarely febrile seizures reported.

**ADVERSE REACTIONS:** Injection-site reactions, irritability, drowsiness, restless sleep, decreased appetite, vomiting, diarrhea, fever.

**INTERACTIONS:** Suboptimal response with immunosuppressants (eg, large amounts of corticosteroids, antimetabolites, alkylating agents, cytotoxic agents). Caution with anticoagulants.

**PREGNANCY:** Category C, not for use in nursing.

**MECHANISM OF ACTION:** Vaccine; elicits formation of antibodies that may protect against invasive pneumococcal disease and otitis media.

### NURSING CONSIDERATIONS

**Assessment:** Assess health/immunity status, history of febrile convulsions, bleeding disorders, previous sensitivity/vaccination history, family history, and possibility of drug interactions.

**Monitoring:** Monitor hypersensitivity reactions; injection site for redness, tenderness, and induration; fever; irritability; drowsiness; restless sleep; anorexia; vomiting; and diarrhea.

**Patient Counseling:** Inform patient/guardian of benefits/risks ratio, the importance of completing the immunization series, and to report any adverse reactions to physician.

**Administration:** IM, at the anterolateral aspect of thigh (infants) or deltoid region (toddlers and young children). **Storage:** 2-8°C (36-46°F). Do not freeze.

# PREVPAC RX

## amoxicillin - clarithromycin - lansoprazole (TAP)

**THERAPEUTIC CLASS:** *H.pylori* treatment combination

**INDICATIONS:** Treatment of *H.pylori* infection associated with active duodenal ulcer and to reduce the risk of duodenal ulcer recurrence.

**DOSAGE:** *Adults:* 1g amoxicillin, 500mg clarithromycin and 30mg lansoprazole, all bid (am and pm) before meals for 10 or 14 days. Swallow each pill whole. Renal Impairment (with or without hepatic impairment): Decrease clarithromycin dose or prolong intervals.

**HOW SUPPLIED:** Cap: (Amoxicillin) 500mg, Tab: (Clarithromycin) 500mg, Cap, Delayed-Release: (Lansoprazole) 30mg

**CONTRAINDICATIONS:** History of allergic reaction to any penicillins. Known hypersensitivity to clarithromycin, erythromycin, or any of the macrolide antibiotics and concomitant with cisapride, pimozide, astemizole, terfenadine, ergotamine or dihydroergotamine.

**WARNINGS/PRECAUTIONS:** Serious and occasional fatal hypersensitivity reactions reported in patients on penicillin therapy. Avoid if CrCl <30mL/min. Caution with cephalosporin/PCN allergy; anaphylactic reactions have been reported. Pseudomembranous colitis reported. D/C if superinfections occur. Caution in elderly. Clarithromycin may increase colchicine; monitor for toxicity. Do not use clarithromycin during pregnancy. Symptomatic response to lansoprazole does not preclude the presence of gastric malignancy. *Clostridium difficile*-associated diarrhea (CDAD) reported. D/C if confirmed. Avoid with CrCl <30mL/min. Exacerbation of symptoms with myasthenia gravis and new onset of myasthenic syndrome reported with clarithromycin.

**ADVERSE REACTIONS:** Diarrhea, taste perversion, headache, abdominal pain, dark stools, myalgia, confusion, respiratory disorders, skin reactions, vaginitis.

**INTERACTIONS:** See Contraindications. Lansoprazole: May interfere with absorption of drugs dependent on gastric pH for bioavailability (eg, atazanavir, ketoconazole, ampicillin esters, iron salts, digoxin). Monitor increase in INR and prothrombin time with concomitant use of warfarin. Amoxicillin: May decrease renal tubular secretion when coadministered with Probenecid. May interfere bactericidal effects of penicillin with chloramphenicol, macrolides, sulfonamides and tetracycline. Clarithromycin: May increase of theophylline and carbamazepine levels. Simultaneous administration with zidovudine resulted in decreased steady-state zidovudine levels in HIV-infected patients. Elevated digoxin levels in patients receiving concomitant digoxin. May lead to increased exposure to colchicine when coadministered. May increase or prolong both therapeutic and adverse effects with erythromycin. Torsades de pointes may occur with quinidine or disopyramide. May increase systemic exposure of sildenafil; consider dose reduction.

**PREGNANCY:** Category C, not for use in nursing.

**MECHANISM OF ACTION:** Lansoprazole: Substituted benzimidazole; inhibits gastric acid secretion. Amoxicillin: Semi-synthetic antibiotic; has broad spectrum of bactericidal activity against many gram-positive and gram-negative microorganisms. Clarithromycin: Semi-synthetic macrolide antibiotic.

**PHARMACOKINETICS: Absorption:** Lansoprazole: Rapidly absorbed; absolute bioavailability (80%); $T_{max}$=1.7 hrs. Amoxicillin: Rapidly absorbed. Clarithromycin: Rapidly absorbed; absolute bioavailability (50%); $T_{max}$=2-2.5 hrs. **Distribution:** Lansoprazole: Plasma protein binding (97%); found in breast milk. Amoxicillin: Plasma protein binding (approximately 20%). Clarithromycin: Found in breast milk. **Metabolism:** Lansoprazole: Liver (extensive). Clarithromycin: 14-OH clarithromycin (active metabolite). **Elimination:** Lansoprazole: Urine, feces; $T_{1/2}$=<2 hrs. Amoxicillin: Urine (60%); $T_{1/2}$=61.3 min. Clarithromycin: Urine (30%); $T_{1/2}$=5-7 hrs; (metabolite); $T_{1/2}$=7-9 hrs.

## NURSING CONSIDERATIONS

**Assessment:** Assess for hypersensitivity to other macrolides, PCNs, or cephalosporins. Assess for proper diagnosis of susceptible bacteria (eg, cultures),

P

pregnancy/nursing status, renal impairment, gastric malignancy, presence of bacterial infection, and possible drug interactions.

**Monitoring:** Monitor for signs/symptoms of drug interactions (eg, cardiac arrhythmias), hypersensitivity reactions (eg, anaphylaxis), pseudomembranous colitis and *Clostridium difficile,* and development of superinfections.

**Patient Counseling:** Instruct to take each dose twice per day before eating; swallow pill whole. Advise to notify physician of all medications currently taking. Inform that drug treats bacterial, not viral, infections. Take exactly as directed; skipping doses may decrease effectiveness and increase antibiotic resistance. Instruct to avoid pregnancy/nursing during therapy and contact physician if diarrhea occurs.

**Administration:** Oral route. **Storage:** 20-25°C (68-77°F). Protect from light and moisture.

## PREZISTA RX

darunavir (Tibotec)

**THERAPEUTIC CLASS:** Protease inhibitor

**INDICATIONS:** For use with ritonavir, and other antiretroviral agents, for the treatment of HIV-1 infection in adult and pediatric (>6 yrs) patients.

**DOSAGE:** *Adults:* Treatment-Naive: 800mg with ritonavir 100mg qd. Treatment-Experienced: 600mg with ritonavir 100mg bid. Take with food. *Pediatrics:* 6 to <18 yrs: ≥20-<30kg: 375mg with ritonavir 50mg bid. ≥30-<40kg: 450mg with ritonavir 60mg bid. ≥40kg: 600mg with ritonavir 100mg bid. Take with food.

**HOW SUPPLIED:** Tab: 75mg, 150mg, 300mg, 400mg, 600mg

**CONTRAINDICATIONS:** Concomitant ergot derivatives (eg, dihydroergotamine, ergonovine, ergotamine, methylergonovine), cisapride, pimozide, sedatives/hypnotics (eg, midazolam, triazolam), St. John's wort, HMG-CoA reductase inhibitors (lovastatin, simvastatin), and rifampin.

**WARNINGS/PRECAUTIONS:** Must be coadministered with ritonavir and food to achieve desired effect. Drug-induced hepatitis (eg, acute hepatitis, cytolytic hepatitis), including new or worsening liver dysfunction may occur; d/c therapy. Increased risk of liver injury reported with pre-existing liver dysfunction (eg, hepatitis B or C); avoid in patients with severe hepatic impairment. Severe skin rash, including Stevens-Johnson syndrome reported. Caution with sulfonamide allergy. New onset diabetes mellitus (DM), exacerbation of pre-existing DM, and hyperglycemia reported. Redistribution/accumulation of body fat reported. Immune reconstitution syndrome may occur. Increased bleeding (eg, spontaneous skin hematomas and hemarthrosis) in patients with hemophilia type A and B reported. Do not give to patients <3 yrs old. Caution in elderly.

**ADVERSE REACTIONS:** Diarrhea, N/V, headache, abdominal pain, rash, asthenia, fatigue.

**INTERACTIONS:** See Contraindications. Potential for serious reactions (eg, myopathy, rhabdomyolysis) with HMG-CoA reductase inhibitors. Concentrations of antiarrhythmics (eg, bepridil, lidocaine, quinidine, amiodarone) may be increased with concomitant use; caution is warranted and therapeutic concentration monitoring recommended. May increase digoxin, carbamazepine (monitor levels), trazodone, desipramine, clarithromycin, antifungals, rifabutin, β-blockers, midazolam, CCBs and neuroleptics. May decrease phenytoin and phenobarbital. Monitor INR with concomitant warfarin use. Therapeutic concentration monitoring recommended for concomitant immunosuppressants (eg, cyclosporine, tacrolimus, sirolimus). May decrease methadone concentrations. Monitoring is recommended if coadministered with buprenorphine or buprenorphine/naloxone. May decrease ethinyl estradiol levels; alternate methods of contraception are recommended. Refer to PI for a complete list of drug interactions.

**PREGNANCY:** Category C, not for use in nursing.

**MECHANISM OF ACTION:** Protease inhibitor; inhibits cleavage of HIV encoded Gag-Pol polyproteins in infected cells, preventing the formation of mature virus particles.

**PHARMACOKINETICS: Absorption:** Darunavir: Absolute bioavailability (37%). Darunavir/Ritonavir: Absolute bioavailability (82%); $T_{max}$=2.5-4 hrs. **Distribution:** Darunavir: Plasma protein binding (95%). **Metabolism:** Darunavir: Hepatic (oxidation) via CYP3A. **Elimination:** Darunavir: Feces (41.2%), urine (7.7%). Darunavir/Ritonavir: Feces (79.5%), urine (13.9%). Darunavir/Ritonavir: $T_{1/2}$=15 hrs.

## NURSING CONSIDERATIONS

**Assessment:** Assess for sulfonamide allergy, liver dysfunction (chronic active hepatitis), hemophilia, pre-existing DM, pregnancy/nursing status, and possible drug interactions.

**Monitoring:** Perform therapeutic drug monitoring for drug interactions as recommended. Monitor for signs/symptoms of severe skin reactions (eg, Stevens-Johnson syndrome), new onset DM, exacerbation of DM and hyperglycemia, LFT abnormalities, hemophilia, fat redistribution, immune reconstitution syndrome, lab abnormalities (biochemistry, hematology), and hepatic impairment. Enroll patients in the Antiretroviral Pregnancy Registry if they become pregnant while on treatment.

**Patient Counseling:** Inform that drug does not cure HIV and may continue to develop opportunistic infections and other complications associated with HIV. Sustained decrease in plasma HIV RNA associated with a reduced risk of progression to AIDS and death. Advise to take with food qd, to swallow tab whole, and not to alter dose or d/c without consulting physician. If a dose is missed by 6 hrs, take next dose at regularly scheduled time; do not double next dose. Report use of any other Rx, OTC or herbal medication (eg, St. John's wort). Instruct to use alternative contraceptive measures to estrogen-based contraceptive during therapy. Seek medical attention if symptoms of severe skin reactions (eg, erythema multiforme, Stevens-Johnson syndrome), exacerbation of DM and hyperglycemia, liver dysfunction, bleeding (unexplained), fat redistribution, immune reconstitution syndrome occur.

**Administration:** Oral route. **Storage:** 25°C (77°F); excursions permitted to 15-30°C (59-86°F).

P

# PRIALT RX

ziconotide acetate (Elan)

**Severe psychiatric symptoms and neurological impairment may occur during treatment. Patients with a pre-existing history of psychosis should not be treated with ziconotide. Monitor patients for evidence of cognitive impairment, hallucinations, or changes in mood or consciousness. Therapy can be interrupted or discontinued abruptly without evidence of withdrawal effects in the event of serious neurological or psychiatric signs or symptoms.**

**THERAPEUTIC CLASS:** N-type Calcium Channel Blocker

**INDICATIONS:** Management of severe chronic pain in patients for whom intrathecal (IT) therapy is warranted, and who are intolerant of or refractory to other treatment, such as systemic analgesics, adjunctive therapies, or IT morphine.

**DOSAGE:** *Adults*: Initial: No more than 2.4mcg/d IT (0.1mcg/hr). Titrate by 2.4mcg/d no more than 2-3x/week. Max: 19.2mcg/d (0.8mcg/hr) by Day 21.

**HOW SUPPLIED:** Sol: 25mcg/mL [20mL], 100mcg/mL [1mL, 2mL, 5mL]

**CONTRAINDICATIONS:** Pre-existing history of psychosis. Contraindications to the use of IT analgesia: presence of infection at the microinfusion injection site, uncontrolled bleeding diathesis, and spinal canal obstruction that impairs circulation of CSF.

**WARNINGS/PRECAUTIONS:** Caution against engaging in hazardous activity requiring complete mental alertness or motor coordination. Dosage adjustments may be necessary when combined with other CNS-depressants due to additive effects. Ziconotide is not an opiate and cannot prevent or relieve the symptoms associated with the withdrawal of opiates. Risk of meningitis due to inadvertent contamination of the microinfusion device. Monitor for signs and symptoms of meningitis. Reports of CNS-related adverse events: psychiatric symptoms, cognitive impairment, and decreased alertness/unresponsiveness. D/C if patient becomes unresponsive or stuporous. Monitor for elevations in serum creatine kinase levels.

**ADVERSE REACTIONS:** Dizziness, nausea, confusion, headache, somnolence, nystagmus, asthenia, pain, vertigo, blurred vision, constipation, dry mouth, anorexia.

**INTERACTIONS:** Coadministration with CNS depressants increases the risk of CNS adverse effects.

**PREGNANCY:** Category C, caution in nursing.

**MECHANISM OF ACTION:** Not established; suggested that it binds to N-type calcium channels, which leads to a blockade of excitatory neurotransmitter release from the primary afferent nerve terminals and antinociception.

**PHARMACOKINETICS: Absorption**: $C_{max}$=16.4-132ng/mL, $T_{max}$=1 hr, AUC=83.6-608ng•h/mL. **Distribution**: $V_d$=155mL; plasma protein binding (50%). **Metabolism:** Kidneys, liver, lungs, muscle via endopeptidases, exopeptidases and proteases. **Elimination**: $T_{1/2}$=4.6 hrs.

## NURSING CONSIDERATIONS

**Assessment:** Assess for pre-existing history of psychosis, presence of infection at injection site, uncontrolled bleeding diathesis, spinal cord obstruction, immunocompromised patients, and possible drug interactions.

**Monitoring:** Monitor serum CK periodically; every other week for first month and monthly thereafter. Monitor signs/symptoms of serious infection or meningitis (eg, fever, headache, stiff neck, altered mental status), psychiatric symptoms, cognitive impairment, decreased alertness/unresponsiveness, reduced level of consciousness, hallucinations, changes in mood, paranoid reactions, elevated CK, EMG finding, myopathy, rhabdomyolysis, and acute renal failure.

**Patient Counseling:** Caution against engaging in hazardous activities (eg, operating machinery/driving). Do not take other CNS depressants. Inform about signs/symptoms of serious infection or meningitis; d/c and consult physician immediately if any occur. Consult physician immediately if experience change in mental status or mood, symptoms of depression or suicidal ideation, seizures, new or worsening muscle pain, soreness, and weakness with/without darkened urine occur.



**Administration:** IT route. **Storage**: 2-8°C (36-46°F). Refrigerate during transit. Do not freeze. Store at 2-8°C for 24 hrs if diluted.

# PRILOSEC — RX

omeprazole magnesium - omeprazole (AstraZeneca)

**THERAPEUTIC CLASS:** Proton pump inhibitor

**INDICATIONS:** Short-term treatment of active duodenal ulcer and active benign gastric ulcer in adults. Treatment of heartburn and other symptoms associated with GERD in adults and pediatrics. Short-term treatment of erosive esophagitis and to maintain healing of erosive esophagitis in adults and pediatrics. Long-term treatment of pathological hypersecretory conditions (eg, Zollinger-Ellison syndrome, multiple endocrine adenomas, systemic mastocytosis) in adults. Combination therapy with clarithromycin +/- amoxicillin for *H.pylori* eradication in duodenal ulcer disease, and to reduce risk of ulcer recurrence, in adults.

**DOSAGE:** *Adults:* Duodenal Ulcer: 20mg qd for 4-8 weeks. Gastric Ulcer: 40mg qd for 4-8 weeks. GERD: 20mg qd up to 4 weeks without esophageal lesions. Treatment Erosive Esophagitis with GERD: 20mg qd for 4-8 weeks. Maint: 20mg qd. Hepatic Impairment/Asian Population: Consider dose reduction. Hypersecretory Conditions: Initial: 60mg qd, then adjust if needed. Divide dose if >80mg/day. Doses up to 120mg tid have been given. *H.pylori*

Triple Therapy: 20mg + clarithromycin 500mg + amoxicillin 1g, all bid for 10 days. Give additional 18 days of omeprazole 20mg every morning if ulcer present initially. Dual Therapy: 40mg qd + clarithromycin 500mg tid for 14 days. Give additional 14 days of omeprazole 20mg every morning if ulcer present initially. Do not crush or chew. Take before eating. Can add contents of caps to applesauce if difficulty swallowing; swallow immediately without chewing. *Pediatrics:* 1-16 yrs: GERD/Erosive Esophagitis: ≥20kg: 20mg qd. 10 to <20kg: 10mg qd. 5 to <10kg: 5mg qd. Do not crush or chew. Take before eating. Can add contents of caps to applesauce if difficulty swallowing; swallow immediately without chewing.

**HOW SUPPLIED:** Cap, Delayed-Release: 10mg, 20mg, 40mg; Sus, Delayed-Release: 2.5mg, 10mg granules/pkt

**WARNINGS/PRECAUTIONS:** Atrophic gastritis reported with long-term use. Symptomatic response does not preclude the presence of gastric malignancy.

**ADVERSE REACTIONS:** Headache, diarrhea, abdominal pain, flatulence, N/V, fever, respiratory disorders.

**INTERACTIONS:** May potentiate diazepam, warfarin, phenytoin, and drugs metabolized by oxidation. May alter absorption of pH-dependent drugs (eg, ketoconazole, ampicillin esters, iron salts). Monitor drugs metabolized by CYP450 (eg, cyclosporine, disulfiram, benzodiazepines). When used with clarithromycin, the levels of both drugs may be increased. May increase levels with voriconazole. May reduce plasma levels of atazanavir and nelfinavir. May increase levels of tacrolimus and saquinavir.

**PREGNANCY:** Category C, not for use in nursing.

**MECHANISM OF ACTION:** Proton pump inhibitor; suppresses gastric acid secretion by specific inhibition of the ($H^+/K^+$)-ATPase enzyme system at the secretory surface of the gastric parietal cell.

**PHARMACOKINETICS: Absorption:** Rapid; absolute bioavailability (30-40%); $T_{max}$=0.5-3.5 hrs. (Adult, single dose) $C_{max}$=668ng/mL; AUC=1220ng•hr/mL. (Children<20kg, 2-5yrs, 10mg single dose) $C_{max}$=288ng/mL; AUC=511ng•hr/mL. (Children >20kg, 6-16yrs, 20mg single dose) $C_{max}$=495ng/mL; AUC=1140ng•hr/mL. **Distribution:** Plasma protein binding (95%); found in breast milk. **Metabolism:** Hydroxyomeprazole and corresponding carboxylic acid (metabolites). **Elimination:** Urine (77%), feces; $T_{1/2}$=0.5-1 hr.

## NURSING CONSIDERATIONS

**Assessment:** Assess for gastric malignancy, hepatic impairment, hypersensitivity, pregnancy/nursing status, and for possible drug interactions. Assess dosing in Asian patients.

**Monitoring:** Monitor for signs/symptoms of atrophic gastritis, hypersensitivity reactions, and other GI effects (eg, abdominal pain, diarrhea, nausea). Monitor LFTs, INR and PT when given with warfarin.

**Patient Counseling:** Inform to take before eating; swallow whole, do not open, chew, or crush. May empty contents of capsule into one tablespoon of applesauce if cannot swallow whole. Mix with applesauce and swallow immediately with cool glass of water; do not chew or crush pellets.

**Administration:** Oral route. (Sus) Empty contents in water. Stir and leave 2-3 mins to thicken. Drink within 30 mins. If any material remaining, add more water, stir and drink immediately. **Storage:** (Cap) 15-30°C (59-86°F); protect from light and moisture. (Sus) 25°C (77°F); excursions permitted to 15-30°C (59-86°F).



# PRIMAXIN I.M. RX

cilastatin sodium - imipenem (Merck)

**THERAPEUTIC CLASS:** Thienamycin/dehydropeptidase I inhibitor

**INDICATIONS:** Treatment of lower respiratory tract (LRTI), skin and skin structure (SSSI), intra-abdominal, and gynecologic infections caused by susceptible strains of microorganisms.

**DOSAGE:** *Adults:* Dose according to imipenem. Mild to Moderate LRTI/SSSI/Gynecologic Infection: 500mg or 750mg IM q12h depending on severity. Intra-Abdominal Infection: 750mg IM q12h. Continue for at least 2 days after symptoms resolve. Elderly: Start at low end of dosing range. Continue for at least 2 days after symptoms resolve; do not treat >14 days. Max: 1500mg/day. Avoid if CrCl <20mL/min.
*Pediatrics:* ≥12 yrs: Dose according to imipenem. Mild to Moderate LRTI/SSSI/Gynecologic Infections: 500mg or 750mg IM q12h depending on severity. Intra-Abdominal Infection: 750mg IM q12h. Continue for at least 2 days after symptoms resolve; do not treat >14 days. Max: 1500mg/day. Avoid if CrCl <20mL/min.

**HOW SUPPLIED:** Inj: (Cilastatin-Imipenem) 500mg-500mg, 750mg-750mg

**CONTRAINDICATIONS:** Severe shock, heart block, hypersensitivity to local anesthetics of amide type (due to lidocaine diluent).

**WARNINGS/PRECAUTIONS:** Serious, sometimes fatal, hypersensitivity reactions reported with β-lactam therapy. *Clostridium difficile*-associated diarrhea (CDAD) reported. Prolonged use may result in overgrowth of nonsusceptible organisms. Avoid injection into blood vessel. Caution in elderly. CNS adverse events (eg, myoclonic activity, confusion, seizures) reported most commonly with CNS disorders and renal dysfunction; d/c if any occur. Positive Coomb's test reported.

**ADVERSE REACTIONS:** Injection-site pain, N/V, diarrhea, rash.

**INTERACTIONS:** Avoid probenecid. Do not mix or physically add with other antibiotics. May give concomitantly with other antibiotics, such as aminoglycosides. May decrease levels of valproic acid or divalproex sodium; may cause loss of seizure control.

**PREGNANCY:** Category C, caution in nursing.

**MECHANISM OF ACTION:** Imipenem: Thienamycin; inhibits cell-wall synthesis. Cilastatin: Dehydropeptidase I inhibitor; prevents renal metabolism of parent drug.

**PHARMACOKINETICS: Absorption:** Imipenem: Bioavailability (75%), $C_{max}$=10mcg/mL (500mg), 12mcg/mL (750mg); $T_{max}$=2 hrs. Cilastatin: Bioavailability (95%), $C_{max}$=24mcg/mL (500mg), 33mcg/mL (750mg); $T_{max}$=1 hr. **Distribution:** Imipenem: Plasma protein binding (20%). Cilastatin: Plasma protein binding (40%). **Metabolism:** Imipenem: Kidneys. **Elimination:** Imipinem: Urine (50%); $T_{1/2}$=2-3 hrs. Cilastatin: Urine (75%).

P

## NURSING CONSIDERATIONS

**Assessment:** Assess for hypersensitivity to local anesthetics (amide), penicillins, cephalosporins, other β-lactams, and other allergens. Assess for severe shock, heart block, CNS disorders (brain lesions, history of seizures), pregnancy/nursing status, and possible drug interactions.

**Monitoring:** Monitor for seizures, myoclonic activity, hypersensitivity reactions, CDAD, and superinfections.

**Patient Counseling:** Inform therapy only treats bacterial, not viral, infections. Take as directed; skipping doses or not completing full course may decrease effectiveness and increase resistance. Counsel to inform physician if they are taking valproic acid or divalproex sodium. May experience diarrhea; notify physician if watery/bloody stools, hypersensitivity reactions, superinfections, seizures, or myoclonic activity occur.

**Administration:** IM route; use within 1 hr of reconstitution. **Storage:** Below 25°C (77°F).

# PRIMAXIN I.V. RX

cilastatin sodium - imipenem (Merck)

**THERAPEUTIC CLASS:** Thienamycin/dehydropeptidase I inhibitor

**INDICATIONS:** Treatment of serious lower respiratory tract, urinary tract (UTI), intra-abdominal, gynecologic, skin and skin structure, bone and joint, septicemia, endocarditis, and polymicrobic infections caused by susceptible strains of microorganisms.

**DOSAGE:** *Adults:* ≥70kg and CrCl >70mL/min: Dose based on imipenem component. Uncomplicated UTI: 250mg q6h. Complicated UTI: 500mg q6h. Mild Infection: 250-500mg q6h. Moderate Infection: 500mg q6-8h or 1g q8h. Severe, Life-Threatening Infection: 500mg-1g q6h or 1g q8h. Max: 50mg/kg/day or 4g/day, whichever lower. Renal Impairment and/or <70kg: Refer to PI. CrCl 6-20mL/min: 125-250mg q12h. CrCl ≤5mL/min: Administer hemodialysis within 48 hrs of dose.
*Pediatrics:* ≥3 months: Dose based on imipenem component. Non-CNS Infections: 15-25mg/kg q6h. Max: 2g/day if susceptible or 4g/day if moderately susceptible. May use up to 90mg/kg/day in older cystic fibrosis children. 4 weeks-3 months and ≥1500g: 25mg/kg q6h. 1-4 weeks and ≥1500g: 25mg/kg q8h. <1 week and ≥1500g: 25mg/kg q12h. Not recommended with CNS infection, and <30kg with impaired renal function.

**HOW SUPPLIED:** Inj: (Imipenem-Cilastatin) 250mg-250mg, 500mg-500mg

**WARNINGS/PRECAUTIONS:** Serious, sometimes fatal, hypersensitivity reactions reported with β-lactam therapy. *Clostridium difficile*-associated diarrhea reported. Prolonged use may result in overgrowth of nonsusceptible organisms. CNS adverse events (eg, myoclonic activity, confusion, seizures) reported most commonly with CNS disorders and renal dysfunction.

**ADVERSE REACTIONS:** Phlebitis/thrombophlebitis, N/V, diarrhea, rash, fever, hypotension, seizures, dizziness, pruritus, urticaria, somnolence, hepatitis (including fulminant hepatitis), hepatic failure.

**INTERACTIONS:** Seizures reported with ganciclovir; avoid concomitant use. Avoid probenecid. Do not mix or physically add to other antibiotics. May give concomitantly with other antibiotics. May decrease levels of valproic acid.

**PREGNANCY:** Category C, caution in nursing.

**MECHANISM OF ACTION:** Imipenem: Thienamycin; inhibits cell-wall synthesis. Cilastatin: Dehydropeptidase I inhibitor; prevents renal metabolism of parent drug.

**PHARMACOKINETICS: Absorption:** Variable doses resulted in different parameters. **Distribution:** Imipenem: Plasma protein binding (20%). Cilastatin: Plasma protein binding (40%). **Metabolism:** Imipenem: Kidneys. **Elimination:** Imipenem: Urine (70%). Cilastatin: Urine (70%).

P

## NURSING CONSIDERATIONS

**Assessment:** Assess for CNS disorders (brain lesions, history of seizures), renal impairment, and possible drug interactions.
**Monitoring:** Monitor for seizures, myoclonic activity, confusional states, hypersensitivity reactions, *C. difficile*-associated diarrhea, and superinfections.
**Patient Counseling:** Inform therapy only treats bacterial, not viral, infections. Take as directed; skipping doses or not completing full course may decrease effectiveness and increase resistance. May experience diarrhea; notify physician if watery/bloody stools, hypersensitivity reactions, superinfections, seizures, myoclonic activity, or confusional states occur.
**Administration:** IV. **Storage:** Below 25°C (77°F). Reconstituted: refrigerate (5°C); stable for 24 hrs: room temperature; stable for 4 hrs.

# PRINIVIL RX

lisinopril (Merck)

**ACE inhibitors can cause death/injury to the fetus during 2nd and 3rd trimesters. D/C therapy if pregnancy is detected.**

**THERAPEUTIC CLASS:** ACE inhibitor

**INDICATIONS:** Treatment of hypertension used alone or with other antihypertensive agents. Adjunct therapy in heart failure if inadequately controlled by diuretics and digitalis. Adjunct therapy in stable patients within 24 hrs of acute myocardial infarction to improve survival.

**DOSAGE:** *Adults:* HTN: If possible, d/c diuretic 2-3 days prior to therapy. Initial: 10mg qd; 5mg qd with diuretic. Usual: 20-40mg qd. Resume diuretic if BP not controlled. Max: 80mg qd. CrCl 10-30mL/min: Initial: 5mg qd. Max: 40mg qd. CrCl <10mL/min: Initial: 2.5mg qd. Max: 40mg qd. Heart Failure: Initial: 5mg qd. Usual: 5-20mg qd. Hyponatremia or CrCl ≤30mL/min: Initial: 2.5mg qd. AMI: Initial: 5mg within 24 hrs, then 5mg after 24 hrs, then 10mg after 48 hrs, then daily. Use 2.5mg during first 3 days with low systolic BP. Maint: 10mg qd for 6 weeks, 2.5-5mg with hypotension. D/C with prolonged hypotension. Elderly/Renal Impairment: Caution with dose adjustment. *Pediatrics:* ≥6 yrs: HTN: Initial: 0.07mg/kg qd (up to 5mg total). Adjust dose based on BP response. Max: 0.61mg/kg qd (40mg qd).

**HOW SUPPLIED:** Tab: 5mg*, 10mg*, 20mg* *scored

**CONTRAINDICATIONS:** History of ACE inhibitor-associated angioedema and hereditary or idiopathic angioedema.

**WARNINGS/PRECAUTIONS:** Intestinal/head/neck angioedema reported. D/C if angioedema, jaundice, or marked LFT elevation occurs. Risk of hyperkalemia with DM, renal dysfunction. Persistent nonproductive cough reported. Monitor WBCs in renal and collagen vascular disease. Anaphylactoid reactions reported. Monitor for hypotension in high-risk patients (eg, heart failure with systolic BP <100mmHg, surgery/anesthesia, hyponatremia, high-dose diuretic therapy, severe volume and/or salt depletion). Caution with renal artery stenosis/artery stenosis/hypertrophic cardiomyopathy, CHF, renal dysfunction, or if obstruction to left ventricle outflow tract. Less effective on BP and higher rates of angioedema reported in blacks than nonblacks. Caution in hypoglycemia and leukopenia/neutropenia. Patients should report any indication of infection, which may be sign of leukopenia/neutropenia.

**ADVERSE REACTIONS:** Hypotension, diarrhea, headache, dizziness, cough, chest pain.

**INTERACTIONS:** May increase lithium levels. Hypotension risk with diuretics. May further decrease renal dysfunction with NSAIDs. Hyperkalemia with $K^+$-sparing diuretics, $K^+$-containing salt substitutes, or $K^+$ supplements. Nitritoid reactions have been reported rarely in patients on therapy with injectable gold and concomitant ACE inhibitor therapy. NSAIDs may diminish antihypertensive effects. Increase hypoglycemic risk with concomitant administration of antidiabetic meds (insulin, oral hypoglycemics). May attenuate $K^+$ loss with thiazide diuretics.

P

**PREGNANCY:** Category C (1st trimester) and D (2nd and 3rd trimesters), not for use in nursing.

**MECHANISM OF ACTION:** ACE inhibitor; inhibition results in decreased plasma angiotensin II, which leads to decreased vasopressor activity and aldosterone secretion.

**PHARMACOKINETICS: Absorption:** (Adults:) 25%; $T_{max}$=7 hrs. **Pediatrics:** $T_{max}$:=6 hrs. **Elimination:** (Adults:) Urine (unchanged); $T_{1/2}$=12 hrs. **Pediatrics:** Urine (28%).

## NURSING CONSIDERATIONS

**Assessment:** Assess for aortic stenosis, hypertrophic cardiomyopathy, renal function, MI, CHF, LFTs, renal artery stenosis, HTN, pregnancy status, history of angioedema, DM, and possible drug interactions.

**Monitoring:** Monitor for head/neck and intestinal angioedema, anaphylactoid reactions, MI. Monitor CBC with platelet count and differential, serum $K^+$, hypoglycemia, LFTs, renal function.

**Patient Counseling:** Counsel about fetal risks during pregnancy, signs/symptoms of angioedema (eg, laryngeal edema, tongue edema, abdominal pain), adverse effects (eg, anaphylaxis, cough, hypotension, hyperkalemia). Inform that periodic monitoring of electrolytes and blood counts is required.

**Administration:** Oral route. **Storage:** 15-30°C (59-86°F); protect from moisture. Dispense in a tight container.

## PRINZIDE RX

lisinopril - hydrochlorothiazide (Merck)

**ACE inhibitors can cause death/injury to developing fetus during 2nd and 3rd trimesters. D/C when pregnancy is detected.**

**THERAPEUTIC CLASS:** ACE inhibitor/thiazide diuretic

**INDICATIONS:** Treatment of hypertension. Not for initial therapy.

**DOSAGE:** *Adults:* Not Controlled with Lisinopril/HCTZ Monotherapy: Initial: 10mg-12.5mg tab or 20mg-12.5mg tab daily. Titrate: May increase after 2-3 weeks. Controlled on 25mg HCTZ/day with Hypokalemia: Initial: 10mg-12.5mg tab. Doses >80mg-50mg should not be used. Replacement Therapy: Substitute combination for titrated components.

**HOW SUPPLIED:** Tab: (Lisinopril-HCTZ) 10mg-12.5mg, 20mg-12.5mg*, 20mg-25mg *scored

**CONTRAINDICATIONS:** Anuria, history of ACE inhibitor associated angioedema and hereditary or idiopathic angioedema, hypersensitivity to other sulfonamide-derived drugs.

**WARNINGS/PRECAUTIONS:** D/C if angioedema, jaundice, or if marked LFT elevation occurs. Fetal and neonatal injury and death reported. Risk of hyperkalemia with DM, renal dysfunction. Persistent nonproductive cough reported. Agranulocytosis and bone marrow depression in renal impairment, especially with collagen vascular disease; monitor WBCs in renal disease and collagen vascular disease. Anaphylactoid reactions reported. Monitor for hypotension in high-risk patients (eg, surgery/anesthesia, volume/salt depletion). Caution with CHF, renal or hepatic dysfunction, obstruction to left ventricle outflow tract, renal artery stenosis, elderly. More reports of angioedema in blacks than nonblacks. May exacerbate or activate systemic lupus erythematosus (SLE). Monitor electrolytes. Avoid if CrCl ≤30mL/min/1.73m². May increase cholesterol, TG. Hypercalcemia, hyperglycemia, hypomagnesemia, hyperuricemia may occur. Enhanced effects with postsympathectomy patients.

**ADVERSE REACTIONS:** Dizziness, cough, fatigue, orthostatic effects, diarrhea, nausea, muscle cramps, angioedema, headache.

**INTERACTIONS:** Increase risk of hyperkalemia with $K^+$-sparing diuretics, $K^+$ supplements, or $K^+$-containing salt substitutes. Potentiates orthostatic hypotension with alcohol, barbiturates, and narcotics. Adjust antidiabetic drugs. Reduced absorption with cholestyramine, colestipol. Corticosteroids, ACTH deplete electrolytes. May decrease response to pressor amines. Potentiates other antihypertensives. May increase responsiveness to non-depolarizing skeletal muscle relaxants. Risk of lithium toxicity. NSAIDs reduce effects and worsen renal dysfunction. Nitritoid reactions have been reported rarely in patients on therapy with injectable gold and concomitant ACE inhibitor therapy. Patients on diuretics may experience an excessive reduction of blood pressure.

**PREGNANCY:** Category C (1st trimester) and D (2nd and 3rd trimesters), not for use in nursing.

**MECHANISM OF ACTION:** Lisinopril: ACE inhibitor. Inhibition results in decreased plasma angiotensin II, which leads to decreased vasopressor activity and decreased aldosterone secretion. HCTZ: Thiazide diuretic; affects renal tubular mechanism of electrolyte reabsorption, directly increasing excretion of sodium salt and chloride.

**PHARMACOKINETICS: Absorption:** Lisinopril: $T_{max}$=7 hrs. **Distribution:** Lisinopril: Crosses blood-brain barrier. HCTZ: Crosses placental barrier. **Elimination:** Lisinopril: Urine (unchanged); $T_{1/2}$=12 hrs. HCTZ: Renal (61% unchanged); $T_{1/2}$=5.6-14.8 hrs.

## NURSING CONSIDERATIONS

**Assessment:** Assess for aortic stenosis, hypertrophic cardiomyopathy, renal function, MI, CHF, LFTs, renal artery stenosis, HTN, history of angioedema,

P

serum electrolytes, DM, hypersensitivity to sulfonamide or any component of the drug, pregnancy/nursing status and possible drug interactions.

**Monitoring:** Monitor for angioedema (head/neck, intestinal), anaphylactoid reactions, MI, CBC with platelet count and differential, serum electrolytes, hypoglycemia, LFTs, renal function (BUN, SrCr), hyperuricemia, hypersensitivity reactions.

**Patient Counseling:** Inform about fetal risks if taken during pregnancy. Caution that inadequate fluid intake, excessive perspiration, diarrhea, or vomiting may lead to excessive fall in BP, with same consequences of lightheadedness and possible syncope. Advise not to use $K^+$ supplements or salt substitutes containing $K^+$ without consulting physician. Counsel about signs/symptoms of neutropenia (eg, infections), angioedema, electrolyte imbalance (eg, thirst, weakness, lethargy), and other adverse effects and to seek prompt medical attention. Inform about importance for periodic monitoring of electrolytes and blood counts.

**Administration:** Oral route. **Storage:** 15-30°C (59-86°F). Protect from excessive light and humidity. Dispense in a well-closed container, if product package is subdivided.

## PRISTIQ — RX

desvenlafaxine (Wyeth)

**Antidepressants increased the risk of suicidal thinking and behavior (suicidality) in short-term studies in children, adolescents, and young adults with major depressive disorder (MDD) and other psychiatric disorders. Not approved for use in pediatric patients.**

**THERAPEUTIC CLASS:** Serotonin and norepinephrine reuptake inhibitor

**INDICATIONS:** Treatment of major depressive disorder (MDD).

**DOSAGE:** *Adults:* ≥18 yrs: 50mg qd. Renal Impairment (CrCl<30mL/min) or ESRD: 50mg every other day. Supplemental doses should not be given to patients after dialysis. Doses should not be escalated in patients with moderate or severe renal impairment or ESRD. Hepatic Impairment: Usual: 50mg/day. Max: 100mg/day. May be taken with or without food; swallow whole with fluid. Take at same time each day.

P

**HOW SUPPLIED:** Tab, Extended-Release: 50mg, 100mg

**CONTRAINDICATIONS:** Concomitant use of MAOI or within 14 days of stopping an MAOI. At least 7 days must be allowed after stopping desvenlafaxine before starting an MAOI.

**WARNINGS/PRECAUTIONS:** Avoid abrupt withdrawal. Re-evaluate periodically. Monitor for clinical worsening, suicidality, and/or unusual behavior changes, especially at initiation of therapy or dose changes. Not approved for treatment of bipolar depression; prior to treatment, adequately screen for risk of bipolar disorder. Serotonin syndrome or neuroleptic malignant syndrome (NMS)-like reactions reported; d/c immediately and initiate supportive symptomatic treatment. Caution in patients with pre-existing HTN; pre-existing HTN should be controlled before initiating treatment. May cause sustained increases in BP; monitor BP regularly. May increase risk of bleeding events. Mydriasis reported; monitor patients with increased intraocular pressure (IOP) or if at risk of acute narrow-angle glaucoma. Activation of mania/hypomania, hyponatremia, and syndrome of inappropriate antidiuretic hormone secretion (SIADH) reported. Caution with history of mania/hypomania. Caution with CV, cerebrovascular disease, lipid metabolism disorder, and renal impairment. Seizures reported; caution in patients with a seizure disorder. May cause elevations in fasting serum total cholesterol, LDL, and TG levels; consider monitoring serum lipids during treatment. Consider the risks vs. benefits of therapy if treating a pregnant women during the third trimester. Discontinuation symptoms may occur; taper dose and monitor symptoms. Interstitial lung disease and eosinophilic pneumonia may occur.

**ADVERSE REACTIONS:** Headache, N/V, dry mouth, diarrhea, dizziness, insomnia, somnolence, hyperhidrosis, blurred vision, constipation, palpitations, anxiety, decreased appetite, male sexual disorders, fatigue.

**INTERACTIONS:** See Contraindications. Avoid concomitant use with alcohol, serotonin precursors (eg, tryptophan), and products containing venlafaxine. Increased risk of bleeding may occur with concomitant use of ASA, NSAIDs, warfarin, and other anticoagulants. May increase levels of desvenlafaxine when used concomitantly with potent CYP3A4 inhibitors (eg, ketoconazole). May increase levels of CYP2D6 substrates (eg, desipramine). May decrease levels of CYP3A4 substrates (eg, midazolam). Caution with CNS-active drugs and with other drugs that may affect the serotonergic neurotransmiter system (eg, triptans, drugs which impair the metabolism of serotonin, antipsychotics or other dopamine antagonists).

**PREGNANCY:** Category C, not for use in nursing.

**MECHANISM OF ACTION:** Selective serotonin and norepinephrine reuptake inhibitor; potentiates neurotransmitter activity of CNS activity by inhibiting neuronal serotonin and norephinephrine reuptake.

**PHARMACOKINETICS: Absorption:** Absolute oral bioavailability (80%); $T_{max}$=7.5 hrs. **Distribution:** Plasma protein binding (30%); $V_d$=3.4L/kg; found in human breast milk. **Metabolism:** Conjugation and via CYP3A4 mediated oxidation (minor). **Elimination:** Urine (45% unchanged); $T_{1/2}$= 11 hrs.

## NURSING CONSIDERATIONS

**Assessment:** Assess for HTN, increased IOP, risk factors for acute-narrow angle glaucoma, history or family history of mania, cardiovascular disorders, cerebrovascular disorders, lipid metabolism disorders, hepatic/ renal impairment, seizure disorders, pregnancy/nursing status, and for possible drug interactions. Prior to treatment, perform adequate screening for risk of bipolar disorder.

**Monitoring:** Monitor for signs and symptoms of clinical worsening, suicidality, unusual changes in behavior, serotonin syndrome or NMS-like reactions, HTN, abnormal bleeding, mydriasis, activation of mania/hypomania, increases in HR, elevated total cholesterol levels, elevated LDL levels, elevated triglyceride levels, seizures, hyponatremia, interstitial lung disease, eosinophilic pneumonia, and for allergic reactions (eg, rash, hives). If stopping therapy (particularly if abrupt), monitor for symptoms of dysphoric mood, irritability, agitation, dizziness, sensory disturbances, anxiety, confusion, headache, lethargy, emotional lability, insomnia, and hypomania. Monitor BP, LFTs, renal function, and serum lipid levels.

**Patient Counseling:** Advise to avoid alcohol. Instruct to seek medical attention for symptoms of serotonin syndrome (eg, mental status changes, tachycardia, hyperthermia, N/V, diarrhea, incoordination), abnormal bleeding, hyponatremia (eg, headache, weakness, unsteadiness), mydriasis, severe HTN, interstitial lung disease or eosinophilic pneumonia (eg, progressive dyspnea, cough, chest discomfort), activation of mania/hypomania, allergic reaction (eg, rash, hives), seizures, clinical worsening (eg, suicidal ideation, unusual changes in behavior) and or if symptoms occur upon discontinuation of therapy (eg, irritability, agitation, dizziness, anxiety, headache, insomnia). Inform that may impair physical/mental abilities. Advise that may notice an inert matrix tablet passing in the stool or via colostomy. Instruct to notify physician if pregnant or nursing or if become pregnant during therapy.

**Administration:** Oral route. Swallow tab whole; do not divide, crush, chew, or dissolve tab. **Storage:** 20-25°C (68-77°F); excursions permitted to 15-30° (59-86°F).

P

# ProAir HFA RX

albuterol sulfate (Teva)

**THERAPEUTIC CLASS:** $Beta_2$-agonist

**INDICATIONS:** Treatment or prevention of bronchospasm in patients ≥4 yrs with reversible obstructive airway disease. Prevention of exercise-induced bronchospasm (EIB) in patients ≥4 yrs.

**DOSAGE:** *Adults*: Treatment/Prevention of Bronchospasm: 2 inh q4-6h or 1 inh q4h. EIB: 2 inh 15-30 min before activity.
*Pediatrics:* ≥4 yrs: Treatment/Prevention of Bronchospasm: 2 inh q4-6h or 1 inh q4h. EIB: 2 inh 15-30 min before activity.

**HOW SUPPLIED:** MDI: 90mcg/inh [8.5g]

**WARNINGS/PRECAUTIONS:** May produce paradoxical bronchospasm; d/c therapy immediately. Monitor for worsening asthma. May produce clinically significant cardiovascular effects; caution with cardiovascular disorders, especially coronary insufficiency, cardiac arrhythmias, and HTN. Fatalities reported with excessive use. Immediate hypersensitivity reactions may occur. May need concomitant corticosteroids. Caution with convulsive disorders, hyperthyroidism, DM, and in patients unusually responsive to sympathomimetic amines. May cause significant hypokalemia and changes in blood glucose.

**ADVERSE REACTIONS:** Pharyngitis, headache, rhinitis, dizziness, pain, and tachycardia.

**INTERACTIONS:** Avoid use with other short-acting sympathomimetic aerosol bronchodilators. Caution with additional adrenergic drugs. Avoid β-blockers; if not possible, use cardioselective β-blockers with caution. Extreme caution with, or within 2 weeks of discontinuation of, MAOIs and TCAs. Monitor digoxin levels. May worsen ECG changes and/or hypokalemia with non-$K^+$-sparing diuretics; consider monitoring potassium levels.

**PREGNANCY:** Category C, not for use in nursing.

**MECHANISM OF ACTION:** $\beta_2$-adrenergic agonist; activates $\beta_2$-adrenergic receptors on airway smooth muscle. Activation of receptors leads to activation of adenylcyclase and increase in intracellular cyclic AMP (cAMP). Increased cAMP leads to activation of protein kinase A, which then leads to relaxation of smooth muscle of all airways, from the trachea to terminal bronchioles. Increased cAMP concentrations are also associated with inhibition of the release of mediators from mast cells in the airway.

**PHARMACOKINETICS: Absorption:** $C_{max}$=4100pg/mL; AUC=28,426pg•hr/mL. (Pediatrics) $C_{max}$=1100pg/mL; AUC=5120pg•hr/mL. **Metabolism:** GI tract by SULTIA3. **Elimination:** Renal excretion (80-100%), urine (unchanged), feces (<20%); $T_{1/2}$=6 hrs.(Pediatrics) $T_{1/2}$=166 min.

## NURSING CONSIDERATIONS

P

**Assessment:** Assess for convulsive disorders, hyperthyroidism, DM, CVD, possible drug interactions, and pregnancy/nursing status. Assess use in patients unusually responsive to sympathomimetic amines.

**Monitoring:** Monitor HR, BP, ECG changes, blood glucose, paradoxical bronchospasm, hypokalemia, hypersensitivity reactions, and deterioration of asthma.

**Patient Counseling:** Instruct on how to properly prime, clean, and use inhaler. Inform to take as directed and to report lack of response or adverse side effects.

**Administration:** Oral inhalation route. Shake well before use. Avoid spraying in eyes. 1) Prime inhaler before using for 1st time or if inhaler has not been used for 2 weeks by releasing 3 test sprays into air, away from face. 2) Clean mouthpiece at least once a week. Use only with actuator supplied with product. 3) Discard inhaler after 200 sprays. **Storage:** 15-25°C (59-77°F). Protect from freezing and prolonged exposure to direct sunlight.

# ProAmatine — RX

midodrine HCl (Shire)

**Can cause marked elevation of supine BP. Clinical benefits of improving ability to carry out activities of daily living have not been verified.**

**THERAPEUTIC CLASS:** $Alpha_1$-agonist

**INDICATIONS:** Treatment of symptomatic orthostatic hypotension.

**DOSAGE:** *Adults:* Initial: 10mg tid; at 3-4 hr intervals, while awake. Max: 30mg/day. To avoid supine HTN during sleep, do not give <4 hrs before bedtime or after evening meal. Renal Dysfunction: Initial: 2.5mg tid.

**HOW SUPPLIED:** Tab: 2.5mg*, 5mg*, 10mg* *scored

**CONTRAINDICATIONS:** Severe organic heart disease, acute renal disease, urinary retention, pheochromocytoma, thyrotoxicosis, persistent and excessive supine HTN.

**WARNINGS/PRECAUTIONS:** Risk of supine HTN; monitor for symptoms of supine HTN (eg, pounding in ears, headache, blurred vision) and supine and standing BP; d/c if supine HTN persists. Caution with urinary retention, diabetes, renal or hepatic dysfunction. May decrease HR due to vagal reflex. Monitor renal and hepatic function prior to therapy and subsequently as appropriate.

**ADVERSE REACTIONS:** Supine and sitting HTN, paresthesia, scalp pruritus, goosebumps, chills, urinary urge/retention/frequency.

**INTERACTIONS:** Caution with concomitant use of drugs that cause vasoconstriction (eg, phenylephrine, ephedrine, phenylpropanolamine, dihydroergotamine, pseudoephedrine); monitor BP. Fludrocortisone may potentiate supine HTN due to salt-retaining properties. OTC cold and diet products may potentiate pressor effects. Antagonized by alpha-blockers (eg, prazosin, terazosin, doxazosin). Metformin, cimetidine, ranitidine, procainamide, triamterene, flecainide, and quinidine may increase clearance. Caution with cardiac glycosides (eg, digitalis), psychopharmacologics, β-blockers, or other drugs that directly or indirectly reduce HR.

**PREGNANCY:** Category C, caution in nursing.

**MECHANISM OF ACTION:** Desglymidodrine; (major metabolite); $\alpha_1$-agonist; exerts its actions via activation of the α-adrenergic receptors of the arteriolar and venous vasculature, producing an increase in vascular tone and elevation of BP.

**PHARMACOKINETICS: Absorption:** Midodrine (prodrug): Rapid; absolute bioavailability (93%); $T_{max}$=1/2 hr. Desglymidodrine: $T_{max}$=1-2 hrs. **Distribution:** across blood-brain barrier. **Metabolism:** Liver via deglycination to desglymidodrine (major metabolite). **Elimination:** Urine (80%, metabolite); $T_{1/2}$=3-4 hrs (metabolite).

## NURSING CONSIDERATIONS

P

**Assessment:** Assess for severe organic heart disease, acute renal impairment, urinary retention, hepatic impairment, pheochromocytoma or thyrotoxicosis, orthostatic hypotension with DM, history of visual problems, pregnancy/nursing status, and for possible drug interactions. Evaluate baseline renal and LFTs.

**Monitoring:** Monitor for signs/symptoms of supine HTN (eg, cardiac awareness, pounding in the ears, headache, blurred vision) and for bradycardia (eg, pulse slowing, increased dizziness, syncope, cardiac awarness). Monitor supine and sitting BP, HR, and renal/hepatic function.

**Patient Counseling:** Inform that certain OTC products (eg, cold remedies, diet aids) can elevate BP and may potentiate the pressor effect of the drug. Inform about the signs/symptoms of supine HTN; instruct to not take dose if supine for any length of time.

**Administration:** Oral route. Take during daytime, not to be taken after evening meals or <4 hrs before bedtime. **Storage:** 25°C (77°F); excursions permitted to 15-30°C (59-86°F).

# PROBENECID RX

probenecid (Various)

**THERAPEUTIC CLASS:** Uricosuric

**INDICATIONS:** Treatment of hyperuricemia associated with gout and gouty arthritis. Adjunct to penicillin, ampicillin, methicillin, oxacillin, cloxacillin, or nafcillin for elevation and prolongation of plasma levels.

**DOSAGE:** *Adults:* Gout: Initial: 250mg bid for 1 week. Titrate: May increase by 500mg every 4 weeks. Maint: 500mg bid. Max: 2g/day. May reduce by 500mg every 6 months if acute attack has been absent ≥6 months and serum urate levels are normal. Renal Impairment: Usual: 1g/day. Adjunct Antibiotic Therapy: 500mg qid. Elderly/Renal Impairment: Reduce dose. Decrease dose with gastric intolerance. May not be effective if CrCl ≤30mL/min. *Pediatrics:* 2-14 yrs: Adjunct Antibiotic Therapy: Initial: 25mg/kg. Maint: 10mg/kg qid. ≥50kg: 500mg qid.

**HOW SUPPLIED:** Tab: 500mg

**CONTRAINDICATIONS:** Blood dyscrasias, uric acid kidney stones and children <2 yrs. Do not use in acute gout attack.

**WARNINGS/PRECAUTIONS:** Initiate therapy when acute gout attack subsides. Exacerbation of gout may occur; treat with colchicine. Use APAP if analgesic needed. Severe allergic reactions and anaphylaxis reported. D/C if hypersensitivity occurs. Caution with peptic ulcer. Monitor for glycosuria. Maintain liberal fluid intake and alkalization of urine.

**ADVERSE REACTIONS:** Headache, acute gouty arthritis, dizziness, hepatic necrosis, vomiting, nausea, anorexia, sore gums, nephrotic syndrome, uric acid stones, renal colic, costovertebral pain, urinary frequency, anaphylaxis, fever, urticaria, pruritus, blood dyscrasias, dermatitis, alopecia, flushing.

**INTERACTIONS:** Probenecid increases plasma levels of penicillin and other β-lactams; psychic disturbances reported. Avoid use with penicillin in the presence of renal impairment. Salicylates and pyrazinamide antagonize uricosuric effects. Increased plasma levels of methotrexate, sulfonamides, sulfonylureas, thiopental or ketamine-induced anesthesia, some NSAIDs (eg, indomethacin, naproxen), lorazepam, APAP, and rifampin. Possible false high plasma levels of theophylline.

**PREGNANCY:** Safety in pregnancy and nursing is not known.

**MECHANISM OF ACTION:** Uricosuric/renal tubular blocking agent; inhibits tubular reabsorption of urate, increasing urinary excretion of uric acid and decreasing serum urate levels.



## NURSING CONSIDERATIONS

**Assessment:** Assess for known blood dyscrasias, uric acid kidney stone, acute vs chronic attack, history of peptic ulcer, possible drug interactions, and renal impairment.

**Monitoring:** Monitor for signs/symptoms of gout exacerbation, allergic reactions, hematuria, renal colic, costovertebral pain, and uric acid stone formation.

**Patient Counseling:** Instruct on importance of liberal fluid intake. Advise to seek medical attention if symptoms of allergic reaction, hematuria, renal colic, or costovertebral pain occur.

**Administration:** Oral route. **Storage:** 20-25°C (68-77°F). Protect from light.

# PROCARDIA XL — RX

nifedipine (Pfizer)

**THERAPEUTIC CLASS:** Calcium channel blocker (dihydropyridine)

**INDICATIONS:** Management of vasospastic angina and chronic stable angina. Treatment of hypertension.

**DOSAGE:** *Adults:* Angina/HTN: Initial: 30-60mg qd. Titrate over 7-14 days. Max: 120mg qd. Caution if dose >90mg with angina.

**HOW SUPPLIED:** Tab, Extended-Release: 30mg, 60mg, 90mg

**WARNINGS/PRECAUTIONS:** May cause hypotension; monitor BP initially or with titration. May exacerbate angina from β-blocker withdrawal. CHF risk, especially with aortic stenosis or β-blockers. Peripheral edema reported. May increase angina or MI with severe obstructive CAD. Caution in pre-existing severe GI narrowing.

**ADVERSE REACTIONS:** Dizziness, lightheadedness, giddiness, flushing, heat sensation, heartburn, muscle cramps, tremor, headache, weakness, nausea, peripheral edema, nervousness/mood changes, palpitations.

**INTERACTIONS:** β-Blockers may increase risk of CHF, severe hypotension, or angina exacerbation. Possible hypotension with fentanyl. Potentiates digoxin. Monitor quinidine, coumarin. Potentiated by cimetidine and grapefruit juice. Monitor with digitalis.

**PREGNANCY:** Category C, unknown use in nursing.

**MECHANISM OF ACTION:** Calcium channel blocker; inhibits calcium ion influx into cardiac muscle and smooth muscle. Angina: MOA not fully determined; believed to act by relaxation and prevention of coronary artery spasm and reduction of oxygen utilization. HTN: Peripheral vasodilation and resulting reduction in peripheral resistance.

**PHARMACOKINETICS: Absorption:** Complete. **Distribution:** Plasma protein binding (92-98%). **Metabolism:** Hepatic biotransformation. **Elimination:** Urine, feces; $T_{1/2}$=2 hrs.

## NURSING CONSIDERATIONS

**Assessment:** Assess for aortic stenosis, CHF, hypotension, MI, angina (vasospastic, chronic stable), HTN, LFTs, GI narrowing, and possible drug interactions.

**Monitoring:** Monitor BP, left ventricular dysfunction, edema, GI obstructive symptoms, hypersensitivity reactions, hypotension, CHF, LFTs, bleeding time, Coombs' test, fatigue, dizziness.

**Patient Counseling:** Advise to take exactly as prescribed. Instruct to swallow tablet whole; do not crush or chew. Counsel about adverse effects; advise to report any.

**Administration:** Oral route. Swallow whole. Do not chew, divide or crush tablet. **Storage:** Below 30°C (86°F). Protect from moisture and humidity.

# PROCHLORPERAZINE — RX

prochlorperazine (Various)

P

**THERAPEUTIC CLASS:** Phenothiazine derivative

**INDICATIONS:** Control of severe nausea and vomiting. Management of psychotic disorders (eg, schizophrenia). Short-term treatment of generalized non-psychotic anxiety.

**DOSAGE:** *Adults:* N/V: (Tab) Usual: 5-10mg tid-qid. Max: 40mg/day. (IM) 5-10mg IM q3-4h prn. Max: 40mg/day. (IV) 2.5-10mg IV (not bolus). Max: 10mg single dose and 40mg/day. N/V with Surgery: 5-10mg IM 1-2 hrs or 5-10mg IV 15-30 min before anesthesia, or during or after surgery; repeat once if needed. Non-Psychotic Anxiety: (Tab) 5mg tid-qid; Psychosis: Mild/Outpatient: 5-10mg PO tid-qid. Moderate-Severe/Hospitalized: Initial: 10mg PO tid-qid. May increase in small increments every 2-3 days. Severe: (PO) 100-150mg/day. (IM) 10-20mg, may repeat q2-4 hrs if needed. Switch to oral after obtain control or if needed, 10-20mg IM q4-6h. Elderly: use lower dosing range and titrate more gradually.

*Pediatrics:* N/V: >2 yrs and >20 lbs: (PO/PR) 20-29 lbs: Usual: 2.5mg qd-bid. Max: 7.5mg/day. 30-39 lbs: 2.5mg bid-tid. Max: 10mg/day. 40-85 lbs: 2.5mg tid or 5mg bid. Max: 15mg/day. (IM) 0.06mg/lb, usually single dose for control. Psychosis: (PO/PR) 2-12 yrs: Initial: 2.5mg bid-tid, up to 10mg/day on 1st day. Max: 2-5 yrs: 20mg/day. 6-12 yrs: 25mg/day. (IM) <12 yrs: 0.06mg/lb single dose. Switch to oral after obtain control.

**HOW SUPPLIED:** Inj: (Edisylate) 5mg/mL; Supp: 5mg, 25mg; Tab: (Maleate) 5mg, 10mg

**CONTRAINDICATIONS:** Comatose states, concomitant large dose CNS depressants (eg, alcohol, barbiturates, narcotics), pediatric surgery, pediatrics <2 yrs or <20 lbs.

**WARNINGS/PRECAUTIONS:** Secondary extrapyramidal symptoms can occur. Tardive dyskinesia, NMS may develop. Caution with activities requiring alertness. May mask symptoms of overdose of other drugs. May obscure diagnosis of intestinal obstruction, brain tumor, and Reye's syndrome. May interfere with thermoregulation. Caution with glaucoma, cardiac disorders. Caution in children with dehydration or acute illness and the elderly. D/C 48 hrs before myelography; may resume after 24 hrs post-procedure.

**ADVERSE REACTIONS:** Drowsiness, dizziness, amenorrhea, blurred vision, skin reactions, hypotension, NMS, cholestatic jaundice.

**INTERACTIONS:** May decrease oral anticoagulant effects. May potentiate α-adrenergic blockade. Thiazide diuretics potentiate orthostatic hypotension. Increased levels of both drugs with propranolol. Anticonvulsants may need adjustment. Risk of encephalopathic syndrome with lithium. May antagonize antihypertensive effects of guanethidine and related compounds.

**PREGNANCY:** Safety in pregnancy is not known; caution in nursing.

**MECHANISM OF ACTION:** Phenothiazine derivative; antiemetic and antipsychotic.

## NURSING CONSIDERATIONS

**Assessment:** Assess for Reye's syndrome, TD, possible drug interactions, bone marrow depression, impaired CV system, and glaucoma.

**Monitoring:** Monitor for signs/symptoms of TD, NMS, hypotension, EPS, mydriasis, encephalopathic syndrome, and hypersensitivity reactions.

**Patient Counseling:** Caution may impair physical/mental abilities. Seek medical attention if symptoms of TD, NMS (hyperpyrexia, muscle rigidity, AMS), hypotension, mydriasis, encephalopathic syndrome (weakness, lethargy, fever), or hypersensitivity reactions occur.

**Administration:** IV, Oral route. **Storage:** Tab, inj: 20-25°C (68-77°F). Do not freeze. Protect from light.

P

# PROCRIT RX

epoetin alfa (Ortho Biotech)

**Increase mortality, serious CV events and stroke in CRF patient when administered to target Hgb levels of ≥13g/dL. Individualize dosing to achieve and maintain Hgb levels within range of 10-12g/dL. Shortened overall survival and/or increased risk of tumor progression or recurrence in patients with breast, non-small cell lung, head and neck, lymphoid, and cervical cancers. To decrease these risks, as well as risk of serious cardio- and thrombovascular events, use lowest dose needed to avoid RBC transfusions. Because of these risks, prescribers and hospitals must enroll in and comply with the ESA APPRISE Oncology Program to prescribe and/or dispense to patients with cancer. Use only for treatment of anemia due to concomitant myelosuppressive chemotherapy. Not indicated for patients receiving myelosuppressive therapy when anticipated outcome is cure. D/C following completion of chemotherapy course. Increased the rate of deep venous thromboses in patients not receiving prophylactic anticoagulation during surgery. Consider DVT prophylaxis.**

**THERAPEUTIC CLASS:** Erythropoiesis stimulator

**INDICATIONS:** Treatment of anemia of chronic renal failure (CRF); anemia related to therapy with zidovudine in HIV-infected patients; anemic patients (Hgb >10-≤13g/dL) who are at high risk for perioperative blood loss to reduce the need for allogeneic blood transfusions; anemia due to the effect of concomitantly administered chemotherapy based on studies that have shown a reduction in the need for RBC transfusions in patients with metastatic, nonmyeloid malignancies receiving chemotherapy for minimum of 2 months.

**DOSAGE:** *Adults:* CRF: (IV/SQ) Initial: 50-100 U/kg TIW. IV route recommended in hemodialysis patients. Reduce dose by 25% when Hgb approaches 12g/dL or increases >1g/dL in any 2 week period. Increase dose by 25% if Hgb <10g/dL and has not increased by 1g/dL after 4 weeks of therapy or

Hgb <10g/dL. Maint: Individually titrate for each patient on dialysis; Hgb levels between 10-12g/dL. Median Maint: (Hemodialysis) 75 U/kg TIW with the range of 12.5-525 U/kg TIW. To maintain Hct levels, 10% of the patients require <25 U/kg and approximately 10% of the patients required >200 U/kg TIW. Zidovudine-Treated HIV Patients: If serum erythropoietin ≤500 mU/mL and zidovudine ≤4200mg/week give 100 U/kg IV/SQ TIW for 8 weeks. Titrate: Increase by 50-100 U/kg TIW after 8 weeks if necessary. Max: 300 U/kg TIW. Maint: If Hgb >12g/dL, d/c until Hgb <11g/dL, then reduce dose by 25% when therapy is resumed. Surgery Patients: Initial: (Hgb >10-≤13g/dL) 300 U/kg/day SQ for 10 days before, on day of, and for 4 days after surgery; or 600 U/kg SQ once weekly on 21, 14, and 7 days before surgery. Cancer Patients on Chemotherapy: 150 U/kg SQ TIW or 40,000 U SQ weekly. Titrate: (TIW dosing) Increase to 300 U/kg TIW if response not satisfactory after 4 weeks to avoid need for RBC transfusion or (Weekly dosing) 60,000 U SQ weekly If Hgb is not increased by ≥1g/dL after 4 weeks. Reduce dose by 25% when Hgb reaches a level needed to avoid transfusion or increases >1g/dL in any 2 weeks. Withhold dose if Hgb exceeds a level needed to avoid transfusion and restart at 25% below the previous dose when Hgb approaches a level where transfusions may be required. D/C if no response after 8 weeks or if transfusions are still required.

*Pediatrics:* CRF: (IV/SQ) Initial: 50 U/kg TIW. IV route recommended in hemodialysis patients. Reduce dose by 25% if Hgb approaches 12g/dL or Hgb increases >1g/dL in any 2-week period. Increase dose by 25% if Hgb <10g/dL and has not increased by 1g/dL after 4 weeks of therapy or Hgb <10g/dL. Median Maint(Hemodialysis and Peritoneal dialysis): 167 U/kg/week (49-447 U/kg/week) and 76 U/kg/week (24-323 U/kg/week) in divided doses (TIW or BIW). If transferrin saturation is >20%, dose may be increased. Maintain Hgb levels between 10-12g/dL; 75-150 U/kg/week maintains the Hct of 36%-38% for 6 months. Cancer Patients on Chemotherapy: 600 U/kg IV weekly. Titrate: If Hgb is not increased by ≥1g/dL after 4 weeks increase to 900 U/kg IV weekly. Reduce dose by 25% when Hgb reaches a level needed to avoid transfusion or increases >1g/dL in any 2 weeks. Withhold dose if Hgb exceeds a level needed to avoid transfusion and restart at 25% below the previous dose when Hgb approaches a level where transfusions may be required. D/C if no response after 8 weeks. Max: 60,000 U.

**HOW SUPPLIED:** Inj: 2000 U/mL, 3000 U/mL, 4000 U/mL, 10,000 U/mL, 20,000 U/mL, 40,000 U/mL

**CONTRAINDICATIONS:** Uncontrolled HTN. Hypersensitivity to mammalian cell-derived products and albumin (human).

**WARNINGS/PRECAUTIONS:** Contains benzyl alcohol; increased incidence of neurological and other complications in premature infants have been reported. Pure red cell aplasia and severe anemia (with or without other cytopenias) may occur. Evaluate etiology if lack/loss of response occurs; test for presence of antibodies to erythropoietin; if present d/c permanently. Should not be switched to other ESAs as antibodies may cross-react. Formulation with albumin may carry risk for transmission of viral diseases. Do not use in patients with uncontrolled HTN. Closely monitor and aggressively control BP in those treated and adjust dose in CRF patients on dailysis with clinically evident ischemic heart disease or CHF. Seizures reported; presence of premonitory neurologic symptoms should be monitored. Avoid potentially hazardous activities such as driving or operating heavy machinery. Exacerbation of porphyria observed; caution in patients with known porphyria. Transient rashes occasionally observed. ESAs resulted in decreased locoregional control/progression-free survival and/or overall survival in patients with advanced head and neck cancer receiving radiation therapy, in patients receiving chemotherapy for metastatic breast cancer or lymphoid malignancy, and in patients with non-small cell lung cancer or various malignancies who were not receiving chemotherapy or radiotherapy. Functional iron deficiency may develop; evaluate iron stores prior to and during therapy. Monitor Hct, BP, iron levels, serum chemistry, and CBC. Menses may resume.

**ADVERSE REACTIONS:** HTN, headache, fatigue, arthralgias, N/V, diarrhea, edema, rash, pyrexia, constipation, respiratory congestion, dyspnea, asthenia, skin reaction.

P

**INTERACTIONS:** Adjust anticoagulant dose in dialysis patients.

**PREGNANCY:** Category C, caution in nursing.

**MECHANISM OF ACTION:** Erythropoiesis stimulator.

**PHARMACOKINETICS: Absorption:** (SQ) $T_{max}$=5-24 hrs. **Elimination:** (IV) $T_{1/2}$=4-13 hrs.

## NURSING CONSIDERATIONS

**Assessment:** Assess for uncontrolled HTN, porphyria, cardiovascular disease (ischemic heart disease, CHF), renal failure, possible drug interactions, hypersensitivity to mammalian cell-derived products and albumin. Obtain baseline BP measurements and iron status (transferrin saturation, serum ferritin).

**Monitoring:** Monitor BP, CBC with differential and platelet count, iron status (transferrin saturation, serum ferritin) regularly. CRF: Serum chemistries (BUN, uric acid, creatinine, phosphorus, $K^+$) regularly, Hgb twice weekly. HIV and cancer: Hgb once weekly. Monitor for signs/symptoms of CV events (MI, stroke, CHF), pure red cell aplasia, severe anemia, viral diseases, seizures, lack/loss of response to therapy, and hypersensitivity reactions.

**Patient Counseling:** Caution may impair physical/mental abilities. Seek medical attention if symptoms of CV events, anemia, infections, seizures, or hypersensitivity reactions occur.

**Administration:** IV, SC route. **Storage:** 2-8°C (36-46°F). Do not freeze or shake.

# PROGRAF — RX

tacrolimus (Astellas)

**Increased susceptibility to infection and development of lymphoma.**

**THERAPEUTIC CLASS:** Macrolide immunosuppressant

**INDICATIONS:** Prophylaxis of organ rejection in allogeneic liver, kidney, or heart transplants with concomitant adrenal corticosteroids. In heart transplant patients, azathioprine or mycophenolate mofetil coadministration is recommended.

P

**DOSAGE:** *Adults:* Initial (6 hrs after transplantation): 0.03-0.05mg/kg/day (liver, kidney) or 0.01mg/kg/day (heart) IV infusion if cannot tolerate PO. Hepatic Transplant: 0.05-0.075mg/kg PO q12h with grapefruit juice; start 8-12 hrs after last IV dose. Kidney Transplant: 0.1mg/kg PO q12h, 24 hrs after transplant or until renal function recovered. Heart Transplant: 0.0375mg/kg PO q12h; start 8-12 hrs after last IV dose. Renal/Hepatic Impairment: Give lowest recommended dose. Severe Hepatic Impairment (Pugh ≥10): May require lower doses. Wait at least 48 hrs with post-op oliguria.
*Pediatrics:* Liver Transplant: Initial: 0.03-0.05mg/kg/day IV or 0.15-0.2mg/kg/day PO. Severe Hepatic Impairment (Pugh ≥10): May require lower doses. .

**HOW SUPPLIED:** Cap: 0.5mg, 1mg, 5mg; Inj: 5mg/mL

**WARNINGS/PRECAUTIONS:** Insulin-dependent post-transplant DM, HTN, myocardial hypertrophy, neurotoxicity, hyperkalemia, nephrotoxicity reported. Monitor drug levels frequently to prevent organ rejection and/or reduce potential toxicity. Monitor for anaphylaxis with infusion. Monitor levels closely with hepatic impairment. Increased risk of latent viral infections with immunosupressed patients.

**ADVERSE REACTIONS:** BK nephropathy, posterior reversible encephalopathy syndrome, PML, interstitial lung disease, HTN, headache, insomnia, fever, pruritus, hyperglycemia, hyperkalemia, hypomagnesemia, diarrhea, NV, increased BUN.

**INTERACTIONS:** CYP450 3A inducers (eg, carbamazepine, phenobarbital, phenytoin, rifabutin, caspofungin, rifampin, St. John's wort, sirolimus, etc.) may decrease plasma levels. Caution with other nephrotoxic drugs (eg, aminoglycosides, amphotericin B, cisplatin). May affect drugs metabolized by CYP450 3A. Avoid grapefruit juice. CYP450 3A inhibitors (eg, diltiazem, nicardipine, nifedipine, verapamil, azole antifungals, macrolides, cisapride, metoclopramide, etc.) may increase plasma levels. Vaccination may be less effective. Avoid live vaccines, cyclosporine (when switching to tacrolimus, wait at least 24 hrs after last cyclosporine dose), $K^+$-sparing diuretics, and sirolimus. Caution with calcium-channel blocking agents.

**PREGNANCY:** Category C, not for use in nursing.

**MECHANISM OF ACTION:** Macrolide immunosuppressant; not established. Suspected to inhibit T-lymphocyte activation. Binds to intracellular protein (FKBP-12). Complex of tacrolimus-FKBP-12, calcium, calmodulin, and calcineurin is then formed and phosphatase activity of calcineurin inhibited. Effect may prevent dephosphorylation and translocation of nuclear factor of activated T cells (NF-AT), a nuclear component responsible for initiating gene transcription for the formation of lymphokines. Results in inhibition of T-lymphocyte activation.

**PHARMACOKINETICS: Absorption:** (PO) Incomplete and variable, absolute bioavailability (18%), $C_{max}$=29.7ng/mL, $T_{max}$=1.6 hrs, AUC=243ng•hr/mL; (IV) AUC=598ng•hr/mL. **Distribution:** Plasma protein binding (99%), appears in breast milk; (PO) $V_d$=1.94L/kg; (IV) $V_d$=1.91 L/kg. **Metabolism:** Hepatic, via CYP3A (demethylation and hydroxylation); 13-methyl tacrolimus (major metabolite); 31-demethyl (active metabolite). **Elimination:** (PO) Feces (92.6%), urine (2.3%); $T_{1/2}$=34.8 hrs. (IV) Feces (92.4%); $T_{1/2}$=34.2 hrs. Refer to PI for parameters in patients with renal, hepatic, and cardiac transplants.

## NURSING CONSIDERATIONS

**Assessment:** Assess for hypersensitivity to HCO-60 (polyoxyl 60 hydrogenated castor oil), impaired hepatic/renal function, and possible drug interactions. Assess use in pregnant/nursing females.

**Monitoring:** Monitor for signs/symptoms of insulin dependent post-transplant DM, neurotoxicity, nephrotoxicity, hyperkalemia, lymphomas and other malignancies (eg, skin), lymphoproliferative disorder, anaphylactic reactions, HTN, myocardial hypertrophy, and latent viral infections. Monitor with renal impairment for dose adjustments. Perform regular evaluation of SrCr, $K^+$, and fasting glucose. Monitor metabolic and hematologic systems as clinically warranted.

**Patient Counseling:** Inform that repeated lab testing required. Advise females about risks of use during pregnancy. Advise to avoid adjusting dose without consulting a physician. Inform about increased risk of neoplasia and DM. Instruct to contact physician if frequent urination, increased hunger, or thirst occur. Counsel to wear protective clothing, use sunscreen, and avoid exposure to sunlight/UV light to reduce risk of malignant skin changes.

**Administration:** Oral/IV routes. IV: Must be diluted with 0.9% NS or D5W to concentration between 0.004mg/mL and 0.02 mg/mL. Patients receiving IV formulation should be under continuous observation for at least first 30 min following start of infusion and at frequent intervals thereafter. **Storage:** Cap: 25°C (77°F); excursions permitted to 15-30°C (59-86°F). Inj: 5-25°C (41-77°F). Store diluted infusion in glass or polyethylene containers and discarded after 24 hrs.

# PROMACTA RX

eltrombopag (GlaxoSmithKline)

**May cause hepatotoxicity. Measure serum ALT, AST, and bilirubin prior to initiation, every 2 weeks during the dose-adjustment phase and monthly following establishment of a stable dose. If bilirubin is elevated, perform fractionation. Evaluate abnormal LFTs with repeat testing within 3 to 5 days. If the abnormalities are confirmed, monitor LFTs weekly until the abnormality(ies) resolves, stabilizes, or returns to baseline levels. D/C if ALT levels increase to ≥3X ULN and are: progressive, persistent for ≥4 weeks, accompanied by increased direct bilirubin, or accompanied by clinical symptoms of liver injury or evidence for hepatic decompensation. Available only through a restricted distribution program.**

**THERAPEUTIC CLASS:** Thrombopoietin receptor agonist

P

**INDICATIONS:** Treatment of thrombocytopenia in patients with chronic immune (idiopathic) thrombocytopenia purpura (ITP) who have had insufficient response to corticosteroids, immunoglobulins, or splenectomy.

**DOSAGE:** *Adults:* Initial: 50mg qd. East Asian Ancestry/Moderate or Severe Hepatic Impairment: Initial: 25mg qd. Titrate: Adjust daily dose to achieve and maintain platelet count ≥50 x $10^9$/L. Max: 75mg/day. Platelet Count <50 x $10^9$/L After ≥2 Weeks of Therapy: Increase daily dose by 25mg to maximum of 75mg/day. Platelet Count ≥200 x $10^9$/L to ≤400 x $10^9$/L at Any Time: Decrease daily dose by 25mg. Wait 2 weeks to assess effects of this and any subsequent dose adjustments. Platelet count >400 x $10^9$/L: D/C therapy; monitor platelet count twice weekly. Once platelet count falls to <150 x $10^9$/L, reinitiate therapy at dose reduced by 25mg. Platelet Count >400 x $10^9$/L After 2 Weeks of Therapy at Lowest Dose: D/C permanently. Take on empty stomach (1 hr before meal or 2 hrs after meal). Allow at least 4-hr interval between eltrombopag and other medications (eg antacids), calcium-rich food, or supplements containing polyvalent cations. Do not take >1 dose within any 24-hour period. D/C if no increase in platelet count after 4 weeks at max dose.

**HOW SUPPLIED:** Tab: 25mg, 50mg

**WARNINGS/PRECAUTIONS:** Use only in patients with ITP whose degree of thrombocytopenia and clinical condition increase the risk for bleeding; not to be used in an attempt to normalize platelet counts. Increases the risk for development or progression of reticulin fiber deposition within the bone marrow; monitor peripheral blood smear and CBC for worsening of morphological abnormalities or cytopenias; if the following develops d/c treatment and consider bone marrow biopsy. D/C may result in worsening of thrombocytopenia which may lead to increased risk of bleeding. Monitor weekly CBCs, including platelet counts for at least 4 weeks after d/c. Excessive doses may increase platelet counts to a level that produces thrombotic/thromboembolic complication; caution in patients with risk factor for thromboembolism. May increase the risk for hematological malignancies. Do not use for treatment of thrombocytopenia due to causes other than ITP. Monitor CBCs, including platelet counts and peripheral blood smears, weekly during the dose-adjustment phase of therapy and then monthly following establishment of a stable dose. Cataracts may develop or worsen during therapy; perform baseline ocular exam and regularly monitor for signs and symptoms of cataracts. Caution in patients with renal/hepatic impairment and the elderly.



**ADVERSE REACTIONS:** Worsening thrombocytopenia, N/V, menorrhagia, myalgia, paresthesia, cataracts, dyspepsia, ecchymosis, increased ALT/AST, conjunctival hemorrhage.

**INTERACTIONS:** Monitor for signs/symptoms of excessive exposure when concomitantly administered with moderate/strong inhibitors of CYP1A2 (eg, ciprofloxacin, fluvoxamine) or CYP2C8 (eg, gemfibrozil, trimethoprim). May increase systemic exposure of other drugs that are substrates of OATP1B1 (eg, benzylpenicillin, atorvastatin, fluvastatin, pravastatin, rosuvastatin, methotrexate, nateglinide, repaglinide, rifampin); use caution, monitor closely and consider dose reductions of these drugs with concomitant use. Polyvalent cations (eg, iron, calcium, aluminum, magnesium, selenium, zinc) may reduce absorption significantly; avoid within 4 hrs of foods, mineral supplements, and antacids which contain polyvalent cations. Eltrombopag is an inhibitor of UGT1A1, UGT1A3, UGT1A4, UGT1A6, UGT1A9, UGT2B7, UGT2B15, enzymes involved in the metabolism of multiple drugs (eg, APAP, narcotics, NSAIDs); monitor closely for signs/symptoms of excessive exposure to these drugs with concomitant use. Monitor for signs/symptoms of excessive exposure when concomitantly administered with moderate/strong inhibitors of UGT1A1 or UGT1A3.

**PREGNANCY:** Category C, not for use in nursing.

**MECHANISM OF ACTION:** Thrombopoietin-receptor agonist; interacts with human thrombopoietin-receptor and initiates signaling cascades that induce proliferation and differentiation of megakaryocytes from bone marrow progenitor cells.

**PHARMACOKINETICS: Absorption:** $T_{max}$=2-6 hrs, AUC= 91.9 mcg•hr/mL (50mg). **Distribution:** Plasma protein binding (>99%). **Metabolism:** Cleavage, oxidation (via CYP1A2, CYP2C8), and conjugation with glucuronic acid (via UGT1A1, UGT1A3), glutathione, or cysteine. **Elimination:** Urine (31%), feces (59%), $T_{1/2}$=26-35 hrs.

## NURSING CONSIDERATIONS

**Assessment:** Assess for degree of thrombocytopenia, risk factors for thromboembolism, pregnancy/nursing status, hepatic/renal disease and possible drug interactions. Obtain baseline CBC (including platelet counts, peripheral blood smears, peripheral blood differential count), LFTs and eye exam.

**Monitoring:** Monitor for bone marrow reticulin deposition, worsening thrombocytopenia, cataracts, and hematologic malignancies. Monitor LFTs every 2 weeks during dose-adjustment phase and monthly after establishment of stable dose. If bilirubin is elevated, perform fractionation. If LFT abnormalities, monitor LFTs weekly until abnormalities resolve, stabilize or return to baseline levels. Monitor CBC including platelet counts, peripheral smears during therapy (weekly during dose-adjustment phase and then monthly after establishment of a stable dose) and after d/c for at least 4 weeks.

**Patient Counseling:** Counsel patients about risks and benefits prior to therapy. Inform that the risks associated with prolonged treatment are unknown and that they must enroll in Promacta *CARES* program for proper use. Advise to closely monitor platelet counts weekly, and CBCs for at least 2 weeks after d/c therapy. Inform that thrombocytopenia and risk of bleeding may develop that is worse than that experienced prior to therapy following d/c. Advise to report signs and symptoms of a blot clot in the leg (swelling, pain, or tenderness in the leg). Counsel about situations or medications that may increase risk for bleeding. Inform that therapy may be associated with hepatobiliary laboratory abnormalities; monitor LFTs prior, during and after therapy. Advise to report any signs/symptoms of liver problem (eg, yellowing of the skin or the whites of the eyes, unusual darkening of the urine, unusual tiredness, right upper stomach area pain) to healthcare provider. Advise regarding the risk of reticulin fiber formation, progression of underlying hematologic malignancies. Advise to take on an empty stomach. Advise to space at least a 4-hour interval when taking other medications concomitantly. Notify physician if using other Rx/OTC, vitamins or herbal products.

**Administration:** Oral route. **Storage:** 25° (77°F); excursions permitted to 15-30°C (59-86°F).



# PROMETHAZINE RX

promethazine HCl (Various)

**OTHER BRAND NAMES:** Phenergan (Wyeth) - Promethegan (G & W Labs)

**THERAPEUTIC CLASS:** Phenothiazine derivative

**INDICATIONS:** Allergic and vasomotor rhinitis, allergic conjunctivitis, blood or plasma allergic reactions, dermographism, urticaria, angioedema. Pre- and postoperative sedation. Adjunct in anaphylaxis, postoperative pain. Prevention and control of nausea, vomiting, and motion sickness.

**DOSAGE:** *Adults:* Allergy: 25mg qhs or 12.5mg ac and hs. Motion Sickness: Initial: 25mg 30-60 min before travel, then 25mg 8-12 hrs later if needed. Maint: 25mg bid. Prevention/Control of N/V: 25mg initially, then 12.5-25mg q4-6h prn. Sedation: 25-50mg qhs. Preoperative: 50mg night before surgery, then 50mg preoperatively. Postoperative: 25-50mg.
*Pediatrics:* ≥2 yrs: Allergy: 25mg or 0.5mg/lb qhs or 6.25-12.5 tid. Motion Sickness: 12.5-25mg bid. Prevention/Control of N/V: 25mg or 0.5mg/lb initially then 12.5-25mg or 0.5mg/lb q4-6h prn. Sedation: 12.5-25mg hs. Preoperative: 12.5-25mg night before surgery, then 0.5mg/lb preoperatively. Postoperative: 12.5-25mg.

**HOW SUPPLIED:** Sup: (Promethegan, Phenergan, Promethazine)12.5mg, 25mg, 50mg; Tab: (Phenergan, Promethazine)12.5mg*, 25mg*, 50mg *scored

**CONTRAINDICATIONS:** Treatment of lower respiratory tract symptoms (eg, asthma). Pediatric patients <2 yrs.

**WARNINGS/PRECAUTIONS:** Potential for fatal respiratory depression in pediatric patients <2 yrs. Caution in patients ≥2 yrs. Avoid with compromised respiratory function (eg, COPD, sleep apnea). Caution with bone marrow depression, narrow-angle glaucoma, stenosing peptic ulcer, bladder or pyloroduodenal obstruction, prostatic hypertrophy, CVD, hepatic dysfunction. Cholestatic jaundice reported. Alters hCG pregnancy tests. May lower seizure threshold, increase blood glucose, cause sun sensitivity. May impair mental/physical abilities.

**ADVERSE REACTIONS:** Drowsiness, sedation, blurred vision, dizziness, increased or decreased blood pressure, urticaria, dry mouth, N/V.

**INTERACTIONS:** Additive sedative effects with CNS depressants (eg, alcohol, narcotic analgesics, sedatives, hypnotics, tranquilizers); reduce dose or eliminate these agents. Reduce barbiturate dose by one-half and analgesic depressant dose by one-quarter to one-half. Caution with drugs that alter seizure threshold (eg, narcotics, local anesthetics). Avoid sedatives and CNS depressants with sleep apnea.

**PREGNANCY:** Category C, not for use in nursing.

**MECHANISM OF ACTION:** Phenothiazine derivative; $H_1$ receptor-blocking agent. Also has sedative and antiemetic properties.

**PHARMACOKINETICS: Absorption:** GI tract (well absorbed). **Metabolism:** Liver. **Elimination:** Urine.

## NURSING CONSIDERATIONS

**Assessment:** Assess for compromised respiratory depression, bone-marrow depression, seizure, LFTs, narrow-angle glaucoma, prostatic hypertrophy, stenosing peptic ulcer, pyloroduodenal obstruction, bladder-neck obstruction, and cardiovascular disease. Note other diseases/conditions and drug therapies.

**Monitoring:** Monitor respiratory function, LFTs, CBC with differential and platelet count, renal function, blood glucose, BP, temperature and EKG. Monitor for neuroleptic malignant syndrome, raised intraocular pressure, and seizures.

**Patient Counseling:** Inform drug can cause drowsiness and impair mental or physical abilities required to perform potentially hazardous tasks (eg, operating machinery/driving). Counsel about side effects and to seek medical attention if any develop. Advise to avoid concomitant use of alcohol and other CNS depressants.

**Administration:** Oral route and rectal administration. **Storage:** (Tab) 20-25°C (68-77°F). Protect from light. Keep tightly closed. Dispense in light-resistant container. (Sup) Refrigerate 2-8°C (36-46°F).

P

# PROMETHAZINE DM — RX

dextromethorphan hbr - promethazine HCl (Various)

**THERAPEUTIC CLASS:** Phenothiazine derivative/antitussive

**INDICATIONS:** Temporary relief of coughs and upper respiratory symptoms associated with allergy or the common cold.

**DOSAGE:** *Adults:* 5mL q4-6h. Max: 30mL/24 hr. Elderly: Start at low doses. *Pediatrics:* ≥12 yrs: 5mL q4-6h. Max: 30mL/24hr. 6-<12 yrs: 2.5-5mL q4-6h. Max: 20mL/24hr. 2-<6 yrs: 1.25-2.5mL q4-6h. Max: 10mL/24hr.

**HOW SUPPLIED:** Syrup: (Dextromethorphan-Promethazine) 15mg-6.25mg/5mL

**CONTRAINDICATIONS:** Concomitant MAOIs, comatose states, treatment of lower respiratory tract symptoms (eg, asthma), pediatric patients <2 yrs.

**WARNINGS/PRECAUTIONS:** Caution in pediatrics ≥2 yrs because of potential for fatal respiratory depression. Avoid in pediatric patients whose signs and symptoms may suggest Reye's syndrome or other hepatic diseases. May impair mental/physical abilities. May lower seizure threshold; caution with seizure disorders. May lead to potentially fatal respiratory depression; avoid with compromised respiratory function (eg, COPD, sleep apnea). Caution with bone marrow depression; leukopenia and agranulocytosis reported. Neuroleptic malignant syndrome reported. Caution with narrow-angle glaucoma, prostatic hypertrophy, stenosing peptic ulcer, bladder neck or pyloroduodenal obstruction, cardiovascular disease, hepatic impairment, atopic children, sedated, elderly, or debilitated patients, and patients confined to supine position. Cholestatic jaundice reported. May alter HCG pregnancy test reading. May increase blood glucose. Avoid prolonged exposure to sunlight.

**ADVERSE REACTIONS:** Drowsiness, dizziness, sedation, GI disturbance, blurred vision, dry mouth, increased or decreased BP, rash, nausea, vomiting.

**INTERACTIONS:** See Contraindications. May increase, prolong, or intensify sedative action of other CNS depressants, such as alcohol, sedatives/hypnotics (including barbiturates), narcotics, narcotic analgesics, general anesthetics, TCAs, and tranquilizers; avoid such agents or administer in reduced dosages. Reduce barbiturate dose by at least one-half and narcotic analgesics by one-quarter to one-half. May reverse epinephrine's vasopressor effect. May lower seizure threshold; caution with concomitant medications which may also affect seizure threshold (eg, narcotics, local anesthetics). Avoid concomitant administration with other respiratory depressants in pediatrics. Caution with concomitant use of other agents with anticholinergic properties.

**PREGNANCY:** Category C, do not use in nursing.

**MECHANISM OF ACTION:** Dextromethorphan: Antitussive agent; acts centrally and elevates the threshold for coughing. Promethazine: Phenothiazine derivative, (antihistaminic); $H_1$ receptor blocking agent and provides clinically useful sedative and antiemetic effects.

**PHARMACOKINETICS: Absorption:** Dextromethorphan (rapid); Promethazine (well-absorbed). **Metabolism:** Promethazine: Liver. Dextromethorphan: Liver via O-demethylation, N-demethylation, and partial conjugation with glucuronic acid and sulfate. **Elimination:** Promethazine: Urine (sulfoxides and N-demethylpromethazine). Dextromethorphan: Urine.

## NURSING CONSIDERATIONS

**Assessment:** Assess for drug hypersensitivity, sedation, level of consciousness, compromised respiratory function (eg, COPD, sleep apnea), seizures, liver/renal function, bone marrow depression, atopic children, and for signs/symptoms of Reye's syndrome or encephalopathy, narrow-angle glaucoma, prostatic hypertrophy, stenosing peptic ulcer, pyloroduodenal obstruction, bladder neck obstruction, CVD, DM, pregnancy status, and potential drug/lab test interactions.

**Monitoring:** Monitor for CNS/respiratory depression and sleep apnea, signs/symptoms of NMS, seizures, cholestatic jaundice and other side effects. Monitor children for hallucinations, convulsions, extrapyramidal symptoms, and dystonias. Monitor false positive and false negative pregnancy tests, blood glucose, BP and CBCs.

**Patient Counseling:** Advise to use accurate measuring device when administering. Caution against any hazardous tasks (eg, operating machinery/driving). Instruct to report involuntary muscle movements. Avoid alcohol; limit sunlight exposure.

**Administration:** Oral route. **Storage:** 20-25°C (68-77°F). Protect from light. Keep bottle tightly closed.

# PROMETHAZINE VC — RX

phenylephrine HCl - promethazine HCl (Various)

**THERAPEUTIC CLASS:** Phenothiazine derivative/sympathomimetic

**INDICATIONS:** Temporary relief of upper respiratory symptoms including nasal congestion associated with allergy or the common cold.

**DOSAGE:** *Adults:* 5mL q4-6h. Max: 30mL/24 hr. Elderly: Start at low end of dosing range.

*Pediatrics:* ≥12 yrs: 5mL q4-6h. Max: 30mL/24 hr. 6-<12 yrs: 2.5-5mL q4-6h. Max: 30mL/24 hr. 2-<6 yrs: 1.25-2.5mL q4-6h.

**HOW SUPPLIED:** Syrup: (Promethazine-Phenylephrine) 6.25mg-5mg/5mL

**CONTRAINDICATIONS:** Concomitant use with monoamine oxidase inhibitors (MAOIs), comatose states, treatment of lower respiratory tract symptoms (eg, asthma), HTN, peripheral vascular insufficiency, pediatric patients <2 yrs, idiosyncratic reaction to other phenothiazines.

**WARNINGS/PRECAUTIONS:** Caution in pediatrics ≥2 yrs. Avoid in pediatric patients whose signs and symptoms may suggest Reye's syndrome or other hepatic diseases. May lead to potentially fatal respiratory depression; avoid with compromised respiratory function (eg, COPD, sleep apnea). May impair mental/physical abilities. May lower seizure threshold; caution with seizure disorders. May decrease cardiac output; caution in patients with arteriosclerosis and in patients with poor cerebral or coronary circulation. Hallucinations and convulsions may occur in pediatrics with therapeutic doses or overdoses. Acutely ill pediatric patients who are dehydrated, may have increased susceptibility to dystonias. Caution with bone marrow depression; leukopenia and agranulocytosis reported. Neuroleptic malignant syndrome (NMS), cholestatic jaundice reported. Should only be given to a pregnant women if clearly needed. Caution with narrow-angle glaucoma, benign prostatic hypertrophy, stenosing peptic ulcer, bladder neck or pyloroduodenal obstruction, cardiovascular disease, DM, thyroid disease, and in the elderly. May alter HCG pregnancy test reading. May increase blood glucose. Avoid prolonged exposure to sunlight.

**ADVERSE REACTIONS:** Drowsiness, dizziness, anxiety, jaundice, blurred vision, extrapyramidal symptoms, dermatitis, hyperexcitability, abnormal movements, increased or decreased blood pressure, n/v, respiratory distress, angioneurotic edema, nervousness, weakness.

**INTERACTIONS:** See Contraindications. Concomitant administration with other respiratory depressants may result in death in pediatric patients. Phenylephrine: Cardiac pressor response potentiated and possible hypertensive crisis with MAOIs. Pressor response increased with TCAs. Excessive rise in BP with ergot alkaloids. Tachycardia or other arrhythmias may occur with sympathomimetics. Reflex bradycardia blocked and pressor response enhanced with atropine sulfate. Cardiostimulating effects blocked with β-blockers. Pressor response decreased with α-adrenergic blockers. Synergistic adrenergic response with diet preparations (eg, amphetamines, phenylpropanolamine). Promethazine: Caution with concomitant use of medications which may affect seizure threshold (eg, narcotics, local anesthetics). May increase, prolong, or intensify the sedative action of other CNS depressants such as alcohol, sedatives/hypnotics (including barbiturates), narcotics, narcotic analgesics, general anesthetics, TCAs, and tranquilizers; avoid such agents or administer in reduced dosages. Reduce barbiturate dose by at least one-half and narcotic analgesics by one-quarter to one-half. Caution with concomitant use of other agents with anticholinergic properties. May reverse epinephrine's vasopressor effect. NMS reported alone or in combination with antipsychotic drugs.

**PREGNANCY:** Category C, caution in nursing.

**MECHANISM OF ACTION:** Promethazine: Phenothiazine derivative; $H_1$-receptor blocking agent. Phenylephrine: Sympathomimetic; α-receptor agonist with little effect on β-receptors of heart; increases resistance and decreases capacitance of blood vessels; has mild central stimulant effect.

**PHARMACOKINETICS: Absorption:** Promethazine: Well-absorbed (GI tract). Phenylephrine: Irregularly absorbed. **Metabolism:** Promethazine: Liver, sulfoxides and N-demethylpromethazine (metabolites). Phenylephrine: Liver and intestine via monoamine oxidase. **Elimination:** Promethazine: Urine (sulfoxides and N-demethylpromethazine).

## NURSING CONSIDERATIONS

**Assessment:** Assess for presence of a comatose state, lower respiratory tract symptoms (eg, asthma), HTN, peripheral vascular insuffiency, compromised respiratory function (eg, COPD, sleep apnea), seizure disorder, bone

P

marrow depression, thyroid diseases, DM, prostatic hypertrophy, narrow angle glaucoma, stenosing peptic ulcer, pyloroduodenal or bladder neck obstruction, CV disease, liver impairment, pregnancy/nursing status, and for possible drug interactions. Assess for Reye's Syndrome or encephalopathy in pediatric patients. Assess age of patient.

**Monitoring:** Monitor for signs/symptoms of CNS and respiratory depression, seizures, leukopenia, agranulocytosis, NMS, and for cholestatic jaundice. Monitor for urinary retention in men with benign prostatic hypertrophy. Monitor pediatric patients for hallucinations, convulsions, and for dystonias. Monitor for false positive and false negative pregnancy tests. Monitor blood glucose levels.

**Patient Counseling:** Inform that therapy may cause marked drowsiness or may impair mental and/or physical abilities required for performing hazardous tasks (eg, driving, operating machinery). Counsel to avoid the use of alcohol and other CNS depressants while on therapy. Advise to report any involuntary muscle movements. Instruct to avoid prolonged exposure to the sun.

**Administration:** Oral route. **Storage:** 20-25°C (68-77°F). Keep tighly closed. Protect from light. Dispense in a tight, light-resistant container with a child-resistant closure.

## PROMETHAZINE VC/CODEINE CV

phenylephrine HCl - promethazine HCl - codeine phosphate (Various)

**THERAPEUTIC CLASS:** Phenothiazine derivative/antitussive/sympathomimetic

**INDICATIONS:** Temporary relief of cough and upper respiratory symptoms (eg, nasal congestion) associated with allergy or the common cold.

**DOSAGE:** *Adults:* 5mL q4-6h. Max: 30mL/24hr.
*Pediatrics:* ≥16 yrs: 5mL q4-6h. Max: 30mL/24hr.

**HOW SUPPLIED:** Syrup: (Promethazine-Codeine-Phenylephrine) 6.25mg-10mg-5mg/5mL

**CONTRAINDICATIONS:** Concomitant MAOIs, comatose states, treatment of lower respiratory tract symptoms (eg, asthma), HTN, peripheral vascular insufficiency, pediatric patients <16 yrs.

**WARNINGS/PRECAUTIONS:** May cause or aggravate constipation. May lead to potentially fatal respiratory depression; avoid with compromised respiratory function (eg, COPD, sleep apnea). Caution in atopic children. May elevate CSF pressure; caution with head injury, intracranial lesions, or pre-existing increase in ICP. Avoid with asthma, acute febrile illness with chronic cough, or with chronic respiratory disease where interference with ability to clear tracheobronchial tree of secretions would have a deleterious effect on patient's respiratory function. May cause orthostatic hypotension. May impair mental/physical abilities. May lower seizure threshold; caution with seizure disorders. Caution with bone marrow depression; leukopenia and agranulocytosis reported. Neuroleptic malignant syndrome reported. Hallucinations and convulsions have occurred in pediatrics. Cholestatic jaundice reported. Caution with acute abdominal conditions, convulsive disorders, significant hepatic/renal impairment, fever, hypothyroidism, Addison's disease, ulcerative colitis, prostatic hypertrophy, recent GI or urinary tract surgery, elderly, debilitated, narrow-angle glaucoma, stenosing peptic ulcer, pyloroduodenal or bladder-neck obstruction, cardiovascular disease, thyroid disease, DM, heart disease. Urinary retention may occur with BPH. May decrease cardiac output; use extreme caution with arteriosclerosis, elderly, and patients with initially poor cerebral or coronary circulation. May alter HCG pregnancy test reading. May increase blood glucose. Avoid prolonged exposure to sunlight.

**ADVERSE REACTIONS:** Drowsiness, dizziness, sedation, tremor, anxiety, blurred vision, dry mouth, increased or decreased blood pressure, rash, nausea, vomiting, constipation, urinary retention.

**INTERACTIONS:** See Contraindications. May increase, prolong, or intensify the sedative action of other CNS depressants such as alcohol, sedatives/

hypnotics (including barbiturates), narcotics, narcotic analgesics, general anesthetics, TCAs, and tranquilizers. Reduce barbiturate dose by at least one-half and narcotic analgesics by one-quarter to one-half. Cardiac pressor response potentiated and acute hypertensive crisis may occur with MAOIs; consider small test dose. May reverse epinephrine's vasopressor effect. Caution with concomitant use of other agents with anticholinergic properties. Pressor response increased with TCAs. Excessive rise in BP with ergot alkaloids. Tachycardia or other arrhythmias may occur with other sympathomimetics. Cardiostimulating effects blocked with β-blockers. Reflex bradycardia blocked and pressor response enhanced with atropine. Pressor response decreased with α-adrenergic blockers. Synergistic adrenergic response with diet preparations (eg, amphetamines or phenylpropanolamine). Avoid concomitant administration with other respiratory agents in pediatrics. May lower seizure threshold; caution with concomitant medications which may also affect seizure threshold (eg, narcotics, local anesthetics).

**PREGNANCY:** Category C, caution in nursing.

**MECHANISM OF ACTION:** Promethazine: Phenothiazine derivative. Blocks $H_1$-receptor. Phenylephrine; sympathomimetic. Potent postsynaptic-α-receptor agonist with little effect on β-receptors of heart; increases resistance and decreases capacitance of blood vessels. Codeine: Narcotic analgesic/antitussive. Primary effects on central CNS and GI tract.

**PHARMACOKINETICS: Absorption:** Codeine: Well-absorbed. Promethazine: Well-absorbed (GI tract). Phenylephrine: Irregularly-absorbed. **Distribution:** Codeine: Found in breast milk. **Metabolism:** Promethazine: Liver. Phenylephrine: Liver and intestine, via monoamine oxidase. Codeine: Liver, via O-demethylation, N-demethylation, and partial conjugation with glucuronic acid. **Elimination:** Promethazine: Urine (sulfoxides and N-demethylpromethazine). Codeine: Urine (inactive metabolite and free/conjugated morphine), feces.

## NURSING CONSIDERATIONS

**Assessment:** Assess for drug hypersensitivity or idiosyncracy, acute abdominal conditions, convulsive disorders, hepatic/renal impairment, fever, thyroid diseases, Addison's disease, ulcerative colitis, prostatic hypertrophy, history of recent GI tract surgery, narrow-angle glaucoma, prostatic hypertrophy, stenosing peptic ulcer, pyloroduodenal obstruction, and bladder neck obstruction, CVD, BP, pregnancy/nursing status, and possible drug/lab test interactions.

P

**Monitoring:** Monitor for CNS and respiratory depression, bone marrow depression, cholestatic jaundice, seizures, signs/symptoms of NMS, BP, convulsions/hallucinations and dystonias in children, false positive and false negative interpretations in pregnancy tests, blood glucose, and CBC. Inform about orthostatic hypotension and overdose symptoms such as extreme sleepiness.

**Patient Counseling:** Advise to use caution during hazardous tasks (eg, operating machinery/driving). Counsel to report any involuntary muscle movements. Avoid alcohol; limit sunlight exposure. Inform not to be taken by nursing mothers.

**Administration:** Oral route. **Storage:** 20-25°C (68-77°F).

# PROMETHAZINE W/CODEINE CV

promethazine HCl - codeine phosphate (Various)

**THERAPEUTIC CLASS:** Phenothiazine derivative/antitussive

**INDICATIONS:** Temporary relief of coughs and upper respiratory symptoms associated with allergy or the common cold.

**DOSAGE:** *Adults:* 5mL q4-6h. Max: 30mL/24 hr.
*Pediatrics:* ≥12 yrs: 5mL q4-6h. Max: 30mL/24 hr. 6-<12 yrs: 2.5-5mL q4-6h. Max: 30mL/24 hr.

**HOW SUPPLIED:** Syrup: (Codeine-Promethazine) 10mg-6.25mg/5mL

**CONTRAINDICATIONS:** Comatose states, treatment of lower respiratory tract symptoms (eg, asthma), pediatric patients <6 yrs, known hypersensitivity or idosyncratic reactions to other phenothiazines.

**WARNINGS/PRECAUTIONS:** Do not increase dose if cough unresponsive; re-evaluate after 5 days or sooner if cough fails to respond. May lead to potentially fatal respiratory depression; avoid with compromised respiratory function (eg, COPD, sleep apnea). Caution in atopic children. Capacity to elevate CSF pressure and respiratory depressant effects may be markedly exaggerated in head injury, intracranial lesions, or with pre-existing increased ICP. May obscure clinical course in patients with head injuries. May produce orthostatic hypotension. May cause/aggravate constipation. May impair mental/physical abilities. May lower seizure threshold; caution with seizure disorders. Caution with bone marrow depression; leukopenia and agranulocytosis reported. Neuroleptic malignant syndrome (NMS), cholestatic jaundice reported. Excessively large doses in pediatric patients may cause sudden death. Hallucinations and convulsions have occurred in pediatrics with therapeutic doses and overdoses. Increased susceptibility to dystonias in pediatric patients who are acutely ill and who are dehydrated. Administer cautiously and with reduced initial dose in acute abdominal conditions, convulsive disorders, significant hepatic/renal impairment, fever, hypothyroidism, Addison's disease, ulcerative colitis, prostatic hypertrophy, recent GI or urinary tract surgery, and in the very young, elderly, or debilitated. Should only be given to a pregnant women if clearly needed. Caution with narrow-angle glaucoma, stenosing peptic ulcer, pyloroduodenal or bladder-neck obstruction, cardiovascular disease, and ultra-rapid metabolizers. May alter HCG pregnancy test reading. May increase blood glucose. Avoid prolonged exposure to sunlight.

**ADVERSE REACTIONS:** Drowsiness, dizziness, sedation, blurred vision, dry mouth, increased or decreased blood pressure, n/v, constipation, urinary retention, photosensitivity, leukopenia, agranulocytosis, respiratory depression, neuroleptic malignant syndrome.

**INTERACTIONS:** Codeine-Promethazine: Concomitant administration with other respiratory depressants may result in death in pediatric patients. Possible interaction with MAOIs; consider small test dose. Promethazine: Caution with concomitant medications which affect seizure threshold (eg, narcotics, local anesthetics). May increase, prolong, or intensify the sedative action of other CNS depressants such as alcohol, sedative/hypnotics (including barbiturates), general anesthetics, TCAs, and tranquilizers; avoid such agents or administer in reduced doses. Reduce barbiturate dose by at least one-half and narcotic analgesics by one-quarter to one-half. May reverse epinephrine's vasopressor effect. Caution with concomitant use of other agents with anticholinergic properties. NMS reported alone or in combination with antipsychotic drugs.

P

**PREGNANCY:** Category C, caution in nursing.

**MECHANISM OF ACTION:** Codeine: Narcotic analgesic and antitussive; primary effects are on CNS and GI tract. Promethazine: Phenothiazine derivative; blocks $H_1$ receptor (antihistaminic action) and provides sedative and antiemetic effects.

**PHARMACOKINETICS: Absorption:** Promethazine and codeine (well absorbed). **Distribution:** Codeine: Found in breast milk. **Metabolism:** Promethazine: Liver, sulfoxides and N-demethylpromethazine (metabolites). Codeine: Liver via O-demethylation, N-demethylation, and partial conjugation with glucuronic acid. **Elimination:** Promethazine: Urine (sulfoxides and N-demethylpromethazine). Codeine: Urine (inactive metabolites and free/conjugated morphine), feces (parent compound and metabolites).

## NURSING CONSIDERATIONS

**Assessment:** Assess for presence of a comatose state, lower respiratory tract symptoms (eg, asthma), head injury or increased intracranial pressure, acute abdominal conditions, hypothyroidism, Addison's disease, hypothyroidism, ulcerative colitis, recent GI or urinary tract surgery, presence of debilitation, fever, seizure disorder, bone marrow depression, narrow angle glaucoma, prostatic hypertrophy, stenosing peptic ulcer, pyloroduodenal obstruction, bladder neck obstruction, CV disease, hepatic or renal impairment, pregnancy/nursing status, and for possible drug interactions. Assess age of patient.

**Monitoring:** Monitor for signs/symptoms of CNS/respiratory depression, constipation, cholestatic jaundice, seizures, leukopenia, agranulocytosis, NMS, and for orthostatic hypotension. Monitor glucose levels. Reevaluate 5 days or sooner if cough is unresponsive to treatment.

**Patient Counseling:** Instruct to use accurate measuring device to measure out medication. Inform that therapy may cause drowsiness and may impair mental and/or physical abilities required for performing potentially hazardous tasks (eg, driving, operating machinery). Instruct to report any involuntary muscle movements. Advise to avoid prolonged exposure to the sun. Counsel to avoid the use of alcohol and other CNS depressants while on therapy. Advise to notify physician if pregnant or nursing.

**Administration:** Oral route. **Storage:** 20-25°C (68-77°F). Dispense in a tight, light-resistant container.

## PROPECIA RX

finasteride (Merck)

**THERAPEUTIC CLASS:** Type II 5 alpha-reductase inhibitor

**INDICATIONS:** Treatment of male pattern hair loss (androgenetic alopecia). For men only.

**DOSAGE:** *Adults:* 1mg qd. Continue use to sustain benefit.

**HOW SUPPLIED:** Tab: 1mg [ProPak, 3 x 30 tabs]

**CONTRAINDICATIONS:** Pregnancy or women who may potentially become pregnant.

**WARNINGS/PRECAUTIONS:** Caution with hepatic dysfunction. Consider doubling PSA level results in men >41 yrs of age, without BPH, who are undergoing PSA test. Women who are pregnant or may become pregnant should not handle crushed or broken tablets; potential risk to a male fetus. Do not use in pediatrics or women.

**ADVERSE REACTIONS:** Decreased libido, erectile dysfunction, decreased volume of ejaculate, breast tenderness, hypersensitivity reactions.

P

**PREGNANCY:** Category X, not for use in nursing.

**MECHANISM OF ACTION:** Competitive and specific inhibitor of type II 5-α reductase; blocks peripheral conversion of testosterone to DHT, resulting in significant decreases in serum and tissue DHT concentrations.

**PHARMACOKINETICS: Absorption:** $C_{max}$=9.2ng/mL; $T_{max}$=1-2 hrs; AUC=53ng•hr/mL. **Distribution:** $V_d$=76L; plasma protein binding (approximately 90%); crosses blood-brain barrier. **Metabolism:** Liver (extensive); via CYP3A4. **Elimination:** Urine (39%, metabolites), feces (57%); $T_{1/2}$=4.5 hrs.

### NURSING CONSIDERATIONS

**Assessment:** Assess for drug hypersensitivity, liver dysfunction, and pregnancy status.

**Monitoring:** Monitor for breast changes (eg, lumps, pain, nipple discharge, breast enlargement, tenderness, neoplasm). Interaction with interpretation of serum PSA levels in BPH.

**Patient Counseling:** Caution women who are pregnant/nursing or planning to become pregnant not to handle broken or crushed tabs. Inform about risks; promptly report breast changes.

**Administration:** Oral route. **Storage:** 15-30°C (59-86°F).

## PROPYLTHIOURACIL RX

propylthiouracil (Various)

**THERAPEUTIC CLASS:** Thiourea-derivative antithyroid agent

**INDICATIONS:** Treatment of hyperthyroidism.

**DOSAGE:** *Adults:* Initial: 300mg/day in 3 divided doses, q8h. Severe Hyperthyroidism/Very Large Goiters: Initial: 400mg/day in 3 divided doses; may give up to 600-900mg/day if needed. Maint: 100-150mg/day. *Pediatrics:* 6-10 yrs: Initial: 50-150mg/day. ≥10 yrs: Initial: 150-300mg/day. Maint: Determine by patient response.

**HOW SUPPLIED:** Tab: 50mg

**CONTRAINDICATIONS:** Nursing mothers.

**WARNINGS/PRECAUTIONS:** D/C with agranulocytosis, aplastic anemia, hepatitis, fever, or exfoliative dermatitis. Rare reports of severe hepatic reactions exist. D/C with significant hepatic abnormality, including transaminases >3x ULN. Caution with pregnancy, may cause fetal harm. Monitor PT and TFTs.

**ADVERSE REACTIONS:** Agranulocytosis, granulopenia, thrombocytopenia, aplastic anemia, drug fever, hepatitis, periarteritis, hypoprothrombinemia, skin rash, urticaria, NV, epigastric distress, arthralgia, paresthesias.

**INTERACTIONS:** May potentiate anticoagulant effects. Hyperthyroidism increases clearance of β-blockers; reduce β-blocker dose when patient becomes euthyroid. Increased digitalis glycoside levels when patient becomes euthyroid; reduce digitalis dose. Decreased theophylline clearance when patient becomes euthyroid; reduce theophylline dose. Caution with other drugs that cause agranulocytosis.

**PREGNANCY:** Category D, contraindicated in nursing.

**MECHANISM OF ACTION:** Antithyroid agent; inhibits synthesis of thyroid hormones.

**PHARMACOKINETICS: Absorption:** GI tract (readily absorbed). **Distribution:** Found in breast milk, crosses placental membranes. **Elimination:** Urine (35%); $T_{1/2}$=24 hrs.

## NURSING CONSIDERATIONS

**Assessment:** Assess for drug hypersensitivity, pregnancy/nursing status, and possible drug interactions.

**Monitoring:** Monitor for fever, sore throat, interstitial pneumonitis, exfoliative dermatitis, and ANCA-positive vasculitis. Requires frequent lab tests including CBC, PT , thyroid function, LFTs, and bone marrow function.

**Patient Counseling:** Instruct to inform physician if pregnant/nursing or planning to become pregnant. Advise to report signs/symptoms of illness (eg, fever, sore throat, skin eruptions, headache, general malaise).

**Administration:** Oral route. **Storage:** 15-30°C (59-86°F).

P

# ProQuad RX

varicella virus vaccine live - rubella vaccine live - measles vaccine live - mumps vaccine live (Merck)

**THERAPEUTIC CLASS:** Vaccine

**INDICATIONS:** Vaccination against measles, mumps, rubella, and varicella in children 12 months to 12 yrs of age.

**DOSAGE:** *Pediatrics:* 12 months-12 yrs: 0.5mL SQ. At least 1 month should elapse between dose of measles-containing vaccine and dose of ProQuad. If for any reason a 2nd dose of varicella-containing vaccine is required, at least 3 months should elapse between doses.

**HOW SUPPLIED:** Inj: 0.5mL

**CONTRAINDICATIONS:** Anaphylactic reactions to neomycin; hypersensitivity to gelatin; blood dyscrasias, leukemia, lymphomas, or other malignant neoplasms affecting the bone marrow or lymphatic system; immunosuppressive therapy; primary and acquired immunodeficiency states (e.g., AIDS/HIV); congenital or hereditary immunodeficiency; active untreated tuberculosis; active febrile illness with fever >101.3°F; pregnant. Disseminated varicella vaccine virus infection has been reported in children with underlying immunodeficiency disorders who were inadvertently vaccinated with a varicella-containing vaccine.

**WARNINGS/PRECAUTIONS:** Caution with egg allergy. May cause thrombocytopenia. Contains albumin, remote risk of viral infection transmission. Have epinephrine (1:1000) available. Caution with a history of cerebral injury, history of or active convulsions or any condition in which stress due to fever should be avoided.

**ADVERSE REACTIONS:** Injection Site: Pain/tenderness/soreness, erythema, swelling. Systemic: Fever, irritability, measles-like rash, herpes zoster and varicella infection, anaphylactic reaction, ataxia, convulsions, febrile seizure, pruritus.

**INTERACTIONS:** Do not give with immune globulin. Avoid use of salicylates for 6 weeks after vaccination. Avoid use of immunosuppressive doses of corticosteriods or other immunosuppressive drugs.

**PREGNANCY:** Category C, not for use in nursing.

**MECHANISM OF ACTION:** Vaccine; stimulates immune system to elicit immune response to produce antibodies that may protect against measles, mumps, rubella, and varicella disease.

## NURSING CONSIDERATIONS

**Assessment:** Assess for history of anaphylactic reactions to neomycin, hypersensitivity to gelatin or any other component of vaccine, congenital or hereditary immunodeficiency, health status, immunization history, and varicella. Assess for blood dyscrasias, leukemia, lymphoma or other malignant neoplasms affecting bone marrow or lymphatic system, active untreated TB, active febrile illness with fever, pregnancy status, and possible drug interactions.

**Monitoring:** Monitor for thrombocytopenia, Reye's syndrome, and adverse reactions at injection site (eg, pain, tenderness, soreness, erythema, swelling, ecchymosis, rash).

**Patient Counseling:** Inform of potential benefits/risk; report adverse reactions. Vaccine may not offer 100% protection. Inform to avoid use of salicylates for 6 weeks after vaccination, and to postpone pregnancy for 3 months after vaccination.

P

**Administration:** SQ route; 1) Inspect for particulate matter and discoloration before administration. 2) Inject SQ in outer aspect of deltoid region of upper arm or in higher anterolateral area of thigh. **Storage:** Refrigerate at 2-8°C (36-46°F) or store at room temperature, 20-25°C (68-77°F). Do not freeze. Discard within 30 min if not in use.

# PROQUIN XR — RX

ciprofloxacin HCl (Depomed)

> **Fluoroquinolones are associated with an increased risk of tendinitis and tendon rupture in all ages. Risk further increased in patients >60 yrs, patients taking corticosteroid drugs, and patients with kidney, heart or lung transplants.**

**THERAPEUTIC CLASS:** Fluoroquinolone

**INDICATIONS:** Treatment of uncomplicated urinary tract infections (acute cystitis) caused by *E.coli* and *K.pneumoniae*.

**DOSAGE:** *Adults:* 500mg qd with pm meal for 3 days. Administer at least 4 hrs before or 2 hrs after magnesium- or aluminum-containing antacids, sucralfate, Videx (didanosine) chewable/buffered tablets or pediatric powder, metal cations (eg, iron), multivitamins with zinc. Swallow whole; do not split, crush, or chew.

**HOW SUPPLIED:** Tab, Extended-Release: 500mg

**WARNINGS/PRECAUTIONS:** Convulsions, increased ICP, and toxic psychosis reported. D/C if dizziness, confusion, tremors, hallucinations, depression, or suicidal thoughts/acts occur. Caution in patients with CNS disorders or other risk factors that may predispose them to seizures or lower the seizure threshold (eg, severe cerebral arteriosclerosis, epilepsy, renal dysfunction). May cause CNS events (eg, nervousness, agitation, insomnia, anxiety, nightmares, paranoia). Severe, fatal hypersensitivity reactions may occur; d/c at first sign of rash, jaundice, or any other signs of hypersensitivity. *Clostridium difficile*-associated diarrhea (CDAD) and colitis reported. Achilles and other tendon ruptures reported; d/c if pain, swelling, inflammation, or rupture of a tendon occurs. D/C if symptoms of peripheral neuropathy occur. Crystalluria reported rarely; avoid alkalinizing urine. May cause moderate to severe photosensitivity/phototoxicity reactions; avoid excessive sunlight and UV light. Safety and efficacy in pediatric patients and adolescents (<18 yrs of age), pregnant women, and lactating women have not been established. Proquin XR is not interchangeable with other ciprofloxacin extended-release or immediate-release formulations. Caution in elderly. Caution in patients with risk factors for torsades de pointes (eg, known QT prolongation, uncorrected hypokalemia). Use in the absence of a strongly suspected bacterial infection is unlikely to benefit the patient and increases the risk of drug-resistant bacteria.

**ADVERSE REACTIONS:** Fungal infection, nasopharyngitis, headache, micturition urgency.

**INTERACTIONS:** See Black Box Warning. Increases theophylline and caffeine levels and prolongs effects. Serious/fatal reactions have occurred with theophylline. Magnesium- or aluminum-containing antacids, sucralfate, didanosine chewable/buffered tablets or pediatric powder, and products containing calcium, iron, or zinc decrease serum and urine levels; administer at least 4 hrs before or 2 hrs after these drugs. Altered serum levels of phenytoin. Severe hypoglycemia with glyburide (rare). Concomitant use with probenecid may increase ciprofloxacin levels. Transient SrCr elevations with cyclosporine. Enhances oral anticoagulant effects with warfarin or its derivatives; monitor prothrombin time or other suitable coagulation tests. May increase risk of methotrexate toxic reactions due to inhibition of renal tubular transport. High-dose quinolones shown to provoke convulsions with NSAIDs (not ASA). Caution with drugs that can result in prolongation of the QT interval (eg, class 1A or class III antiarrhythmics). Caution with concomitant use of drugs that may lower the seizure threshold.

**PREGNANCY:** Category C, not for use in nursing.

**MECHANISM OF ACTION:** Broad-spectrum fluoroquinolone; inhibits topoisomerase II (DNA gyrase) and topoisomerase IV (both type II topoisomerases), which are required for bacterial DNA replication, transcription, repair, and recombination.

**PHARMACOKINETICS: Absorption:** $C_{max}$=0.82mcg/mL; $T_{max}$=6.1 hrs; AUC=7.67mcg•hr/mL. **Distribution:** Plasma protein binding (9.9-36.6%). Found in human milk. **Metabolism:** Desethyleneciprofloxacin, sulfociprofloxacin, oxociprofloxacin and formylciprofloxacin (active metabolites). **Elimination:** Urine (26.9%, unchanged), feces (43%); $T_{1/2}$=4.5 hrs.

## NURSING CONSIDERATIONS

**Assessment:** Assess for risk factors for torsades de pointes (eg, known QT prolongation, uncorrected hypokalemia) and for factors that may predispose to seizures or lower the seizure threshold (eg, severe cerebral arteriosclerosis, epilepsy, renal dysfunction). Assess for pregnancy/nursing status and for possible drug interactions. Assess for proper diagnosis of causative organisms.

**Monitoring:** Monitor for signs/symptoms of tendinitis or tendon rupture, convulsions, increased ICP, toxic psychosis, dizziness, confusion, tremors, hallucinations, depression, suicidal thoughts or acts, nervousness, anxiety, agitation, insomnia, anxiety, nightmares, paranoia, CDAD, peripheral neuropathy, crystalluria, phototoxicity, and hypersensitivity reactions.

**Patient Counseling:** Inform that medication only treats bacterial infections. Instruct to take exactly as directed and to not skip doses. Advise to take with evening meal. Instruct to swallow whole, do not split, crush, or chew tablet. Instruct to contact physician and d/c treatment if experience pain, swelling, inflammation of a tendon, or weakness or inability to use a joint. Advise to avoid concomitant administration with aluminum- or magnesium-containing antacids, sucralfate, didanosine chewable buffered tablets or pediatric

P

powder, iron, calcium, and multivitamin preparations containing zinc; instruct to take 4 hrs before or 2 hrs after these products. Instruct to contact physician and d/c medication at first sign of a skin rash or if other allergic type reaction develops. Inform that medication may cause peripheral neuropathy; instruct to contact physician if symptoms of peripheral neuropathy develop (eg, pain, burning, tingling, numbness, weakness). Advise that therapy may cause photosensitivity or phototoxicity; instruct to minimize or avoid exposure to natural or artificial sunlight. Instruct to contact physician if symptoms do not improve or if develop fever or back pain while on therapy or after d/c therapy. Counsel that medication may cause dizziness and lightheadedness and to use caution in engaging in activities that require mental alertness or coordination. Instruct to contact physician if develop watery or bloody stools during therapy or after d/c therapy. Advise to notify physician if pregnant, nursing, or if have a history of convulsions.

**Administration:** Oral route. **Storage:** 25°C (77°F); excursions permitted to 15-30°C (59-86°F).

## PROSCAR RX

finasteride (Merck)

**THERAPEUTIC CLASS:** Type II 5 alpha-reductase inhibitor

**INDICATIONS:** Treatment of symptomatic benign prostatic hyperplasia (BPH) in men with an enlarged prostate to improve symptoms, reduce the risk of acute urinary retention, and reduce the risk of the need for surgery including transurethral resection of the prostate (TURP) and prostatectomy. To reduce the risk of symptomatic progression of BPH in combination with doxazosin.

**DOSAGE:** *Adults:* 5mg qd.

**HOW SUPPLIED:** Tab: 5mg

**CONTRAINDICATIONS:** Pregnancy.

**WARNINGS/PRECAUTIONS:** Not for use in pediatrics or women. Pregnant women should not handle crushed or broken tablets because of potential risk to a male fetus. Prior to therapy, identify other conditions that might mimic BPH (eg, infection, prostate cancer, stricture disease, hypotonic bladder or other neurogenic disorders). Carefully monitor patients with large residual urinary volume and/or severely diminished urinary flow for obstructive uropathy. Caution with liver dysfunction. Decreases serum PSA levels by ~50% in patients with BPH, even with prostate cancer; any sustained increase should be carefully evaluated.

**ADVERSE REACTIONS:** Impotence, decreased libido, decreased ejaculate volume, asthenia, postural hypotension, dizziness, somnolence, abnormal ejaculation, peripheral edema, abnormal sexual function.

**PREGNANCY:** Category X, not for use in nursing.

**MECHANISM OF ACTION:** Type II 5α-reductase inhibitor; inhibits type II 5α-reductase, which metabolizes testosterone to 5α-dihydrotestosterone (DHT), a potent androgen.

**PHARMACOKINETICS: Absorption:** Absolute bioavailability (63%); $C_{max}$=37ng/mL; $T_{max}$=1-2 hrs. **Distribution:** $V_d$=76L; plasma protein binding (90%). **Metabolism:** Liver (extensive) via CYP3A4. **Elimination:** Feces (57%), urine (39%, metabolites); $T_{1/2}$=8 hrs (age ≥70 yrs), 6 hrs (age 45-60 yrs).

### NURSING CONSIDERATIONS

**Assessment:** Assess for pregnancy status, conditions which may mimic BPH (eg, infection, prostate cancer, stricture disease, hypotonic bladder or other neurogenic disorder) and for liver function abnormalities. Obtain baseline PSA levels.

**Monitoring:** Monitor for signs/symptoms of hypersensitivity reaction and for breast changes. In patients with large residual urinary volume and/or severely diminished urinary flow, monitor for obstructive uropathy. Monitor PSA levels.

**Patient Counseling:** Instruct pregnant women not to handle crushed or broken tablets due to potential risk to male fetus. Inform males that the volume of ejaculate may decrease. Advise to notify physician if changes in breast (eg, lumps, pain, nipple discharge) or hypersensitivity reactions occur.

**Administration:** Oral route. **Storage:** Below 30°C (86°F). Protect from light and keep container tightly closed.

## PROTAMINE SULFATE — RX

protamine sulfate (Various)

**May cause severe hypotension, cardiovascular collapse, noncardiogenic pulmonary edema, catastrophic pulmonary vasoconstriction, and pulmonary HTN; risk factors include high dose/overdose, rapid/previous administration, repeated doses, and current/previous use of protamine-containing drugs. Risk to benefit of administration should be carefully considered with presence of any risk factors. Should not be given when bleeding occurs without prior heparin use.**

**THERAPEUTIC CLASS:** Heparin antagonist

**INDICATIONS:** Management of heparin overdose.

**DOSAGE:** *Adults:* Administer as very slow IV infusion over 10 min in doses not to exceed 50mg. Determine dose by blood coagulation studies. Each mg neutralizes not less than 100 USP heparin units.

**HOW SUPPLIED:** Inj: 10mg/mL [5mL, 25mL]

**WARNINGS/PRECAUTIONS:** May cause allergic reactions with fish hypersensitivity. Rapid administration may cause severe hypotensive and anaphylactoid-like reactions. Caution in cardiac surgeries; hyperheparinemia or bleeding reported. Previous exposure to protamine/protamine-containing insulin may induce humoral immune response; severe hypersensitivity reaction, including life-threatening anaphylaxis reported. Increased risk of antiprotamine antibodies in infertile or vasectomized men.

**ADVERSE REACTIONS:** Hypotension, bradycardia, transitory flushing/feeling of warmth, lassitude, dyspnea, N/V, back pain, anaphylaxis that causes severe respiratory distress, circulatory collapse, noncardiogenic pulmonary edema, acute pulmonary HTN.

**INTERACTIONS:** Incompatible with certain antibiotics, such as cephalosporins and penicillins. Concomitant or previous use of protamine-containing drugs (eg, NPH insulin, protamine zinc insulin, certain beta-blockers) is risk factor for severe adverse events; see Black Box Warning.

**PREGNANCY:** Category C, caution in nursing.

**MECHANISM OF ACTION:** Heparin antagonist; has anticoagulant effects when administered alone, however, when given in presence of heparin, a stable salt is formed and anticoagulant activity of both drugs is lost.

### NURSING CONSIDERATIONS

**Assessment:** Assess for fish allergy, previous vasectomy, previous exposure, severe left ventricular dysfunction, abnormal preoperative pulmonary hemodynamics, and possible drug interactions. Assess blood coagulation studies for appropriate dosage.

**Monitoring:** Monitor for hypersensitivity/allergic reactions, hypotension, CV collapse, pulmonary edema, and pulmonary HTN. Monitor blood coagulation studies.

**Administration:** Slow IV infusion. Large-size 25mL vials are designed for antiheparin treatment only when large doses of heparin have been given during surgery. **Storage:** 20-25°C (68-77°F). Do not freeze.

## PROTONIX — RX

pantoprazole sodium (Wyeth)

**OTHER BRAND NAMES:** Protonix IV (Wyeth)

**THERAPEUTIC CLASS:** Proton pump inhibitor

**INDICATIONS:** (PO) Short-term treatment (up to 8 weeks) of erosive esophagitis associated with GERD in adults and pediatric patients ≥5 yrs. Maintenance of healing of erosive esophagitis and reduction in relapse rate of daytime and nighttime heartburn symptoms associated with GERD in adults. Long-term treatment of pathological hypersecretory conditions (eg, Zollinger-Ellison syndrome). (Inj) Short-term treatment (7-10 days) of GERD with a history of erosive esophagitis. Treatment of pathological hypersecretory conditions associated with Zollinger-Ellison syndrome or other neoplastic conditions.

**DOSAGE:** *Adults:* (PO) Erosive Esophagitis Treatment: 40mg qd for up to 8 weeks. May repeat for 8 weeks if needed. Maint: 40mg qd. Hypersecretory Conditions: Initial: 40mg bid. Adjust to patient's needs. Max: 240mg/day. Do not split, crush, or chew. (Inj) GERD: 40mg IV qd for 7-10 days. Pathological Hypersecretory Conditions: 80mg IV q12h. May adjust up to 80mg IV q8h based on acid output<10mEq/h. Max: 240mg/day. Duration >6 days not studied. Administer IV over a period of 15 min at 7mL/min rate.
*Pediatrics:* ≥5yrs: Erosive Esophagitis (Short-term Treatment): ≥15kg-<40kg: 20mg qd for up to 8 weeks. ≥40kg: 40mg qd for up to 8 weeks. Do not split, crush, or chew. Administer oral suspension in 1 tsp of applesauce or apple juice 30 min prior to a meal.

**HOW SUPPLIED:** Inj: 40mg; Sus, Delayed-Release: 40mg (granules/pkt); Tab, Delayed-Release: 20mg, 40mg

**WARNINGS/PRECAUTIONS:** Symptomatic response does not preclude the presence of gastric malignancy. Atrophic gastritis has been noted with long-term therapy. Vitamin $B_{12}$ deficiency reported with long-term use (>3 yrs). False positive result for urine screening tests for tetrahydrocannabinol. (Inj) Anaphylaxis and injection-site reactions (eg, thrombophlebitis) reported. LFT elevation observed in clinical studies.

**ADVERSE REACTIONS:** (Inj) Abdominal pain, headache, constipation, dyspepsia, nausea, injection-site reactions. (PO) Headache, flatulence, diarrhea, abdominal pain, N/V, dizziness.

**INTERACTIONS:** May alter absorption of pH-dependent drugs (eg, ketoconazole, ampicillin esters, and iron salts). May substantially decrease atazanavir or nelginavir levels; avoid concomitant use. May increase INR and PT time with concomitant warfarin therapy. (Inj) Caution with other edetate disodium (EDTA) containing products; consider zinc supplementation.

P

**PREGNANCY:** Category B, not for use in nursing.

**MECHANISM OF ACTION:** Proton pump inhibitor; suppresses final step in gastric acid production by covalently binding to the $(H^+,K^+)$-ATPase enzyme system at the secretory surface of the gastric parietal cell. Leads to inhibition of both basal and stimulated gastric acid secretion irrespective of the stimulus.

**PHARMACOKINETICS: Absorption:** (PO) Absolute bioavailability (77%); $C_{max}$=2.52mcg/mL; $T_{max}$=2.5 hr; AUC=4.8mcg•hr/mL. (IV) $C_{max}$=5.52mcg/mL; AUC=5.4mcg•hr/mL. **Distribution:** $V_d$=11.0-23.6L; plasma protein binding (98%); found in breast milk. **Metabolism:** Liver (extensive) via CYP2C19 (demethylation), sulfation; CYP3A4 (oxidation). **Elimination:** Urine (71%), feces (18%); $T_{1/2}$=1 hr.

## NURSING CONSIDERATIONS

**Assessment:** Assess for gastric malignancy, hypersensitivity, pregnancy/nursing status, and possible drug interactions.

**Monitoring:** Monitor for signs/symptoms of GI tumors, vitamin $B_{12}$ deficiency, and atrophic gastritis. In patients using IV formulation, monitor for hypersensitivity reaction (eg, anaphylaxis), injection-site reactions (eg, thrombophlebitis), zinc deficiency, and hepatic effects (eg, elevations in transaminases).

**Patient Counseling:** If using IV formulation, switch treatment to oral formulation as soon as patient is able. Contact physician immediately if hypersensitivity or other adverse events occur. If taking oral formulation, swallow whole, with or without food in stomach; do not split, crush, or chew tablet. Concomitant administration of antacids does not effect absorption of tablets. If using suspension formulation, administer in applesauce or apple juice approximately 30 min before meal; do not place in water, other liquids, or food.

**Administration:** Oral and IV route. Do not divide the 40mg packet to create a 20 mg dosage for pediatric patients unable to take tablet. IV lines should be flushed prior to and after administration with either 5% Dextrose Inj, USP, 0.9% NaCl Inj USP, or Lactated Ringer's Inj, USP. **Storage:** 20-25°C (68-77°F); excursions permitted to 15-30°C (59-86°F). Protect injection vials from light; do not freeze.

## PROTOPIC — RX

tacrolimus (Astellas)

**THERAPEUTIC CLASS:** Macrolide immunosuppressant

**INDICATIONS:** Short-term and intermittent long-term therapy of moderate to severe atopic dermatitis intolerant or unresponsive to conventional therapy.

**DOSAGE:** *Adults:* (0.03% or 0.1%) Apply thin layer bid. Rub in gently. Stop use when signs and symptoms resolve.
*Pediatrics:* ≥16 yrs: (0.03% or 0.1%) Apply thin layer bid. Rub in gently. 2-15 yrs: (0.03%) Apply thin layer bid. Rub in gently. Stop use when signs and symptoms resolve.

**HOW SUPPLIED:** Oint: 0.03%, 0.1% [30g, 60g, 100g]

**WARNINGS/PRECAUTIONS:** Do not use with occlusive dressings. Increased risk of varicella zoster, herpes simplex, or eczema herpeticum. Lymphadenopathy reported; monitor closely. D/C if unknown etiology of lymphadenopathy or presence of acute infectious mononucleosis. Avoid in Netherton's syndrome. Minimize or avoid exposure to natural or artificial sunlight. Long-term safety not established. Rare cases of malignancy (eg, skin and lymphoma) reported with topical calcineurin inhibitors; therefore, continuous long-term use should be avoided and application limited to areas of involvement. Should not use in immunocompromised adults and children. Caution in patients predisposed to renal impairment. Not indicated for use in children <2 yrs. Only 0.03% oint is indicated for use in children 2-15 yrs.

**ADVERSE REACTIONS:** Skin burning, pruritus, flu-like symptoms, allergic reaction, skin erythema, headache, skin infection, fever, herpes simplex, rhinitis.

**INTERACTIONS:** Caution with CYP3A4 inhibitors (eg, erythromycin, itraconazole, ketoconazole, fluconazole, CCBs, cimetidine) in widespread and/or erythrodermic disease. Increased risk for lymphomas in transplant patients receiving other immunosuppressive therapy.

**PREGNANCY:** Category C, not for use in nursing.

**MECHANISM OF ACTION:** Macrolide immunosuppressant; not known in atopic dermatitis. Inhibits T-lymphocyte activation by first binding to an intracellular protein, FKBP-12. A complex of tacrolimus-FKBP-12, calcium, calmodulin, and calcineurin is then formed and the phosphate activity of calcineurin is inhibited. This has been shown to prevent the dephosphorylation and translocation of nuclear factor of activated T-cells.

**PHARMACOKINETICS: Absorption:** Absolute bioavailability (0.5%), $C_{max}$<2ng/mL (90% of population). **Distribution:** $V_d$=99%. **Metabolism:** CYP3A (extensive); demethylation and hydroxylation; 13-demethyl tacrolimus (major metabolite). **Elimination:** Feces (major).

### NURSING CONSIDERATIONS

**Assessment:** Assess for history of hypersensitivity to tacrolimus or any other component of the ointment, premalignant and malignant skin conditions, and renal impairment. Prior to initiation, resolve cutaneous bacterial or viral infections at treatment sites.

**Monitoring:** Monitor for varicella zoster virus infection (chickenpox or shingles), acute mononucleosis, lymphomas, skin malignancies (eg, cutaneous T-cell lymphoma), lymphadenopathy, and acute renal failure. Monitor improvement of signs/symptoms of atopic dermatitis within 6 weeks.

**Patient Counseling:** Advise to be re-examined if signs/symptoms of atopic dermatitis do not improve within 6 weeks. Instruct to d/c when signs/symptoms of eczema (eg, itching, rash and redness) occur; avoid ultraviolet therapy sun lamps and tanning beds during treatment. Advise to limit sun exposure, to wear loose-fitting clothing that protects treated area from the sun, and not to cover treated skin with bandages, dressings, or wraps.

**Administration:** Topical. **Storage:** 25°C (77°F); excursions permitted to 15-30°C (59-86°F).

# PROVENTIL HFA — RX

albuterol sulfate (Schering)

**THERAPEUTIC CLASS:** $Beta_2$-agonist

**INDICATIONS:** Prevention and treatment of bronchospasm with reversible obstructive airway disease; prevention of exercise-induced bronchospasm (EIB) in patients ≥4 yrs.

**DOSAGE:** *Adults:* Bronchospasm: 2 inh q4-6h or 1 inh q4h. EIB: 2 inh 15-30 min before activity.
*Pediatrics:* ≥4 yrs: Bronchospasm: 2 inh q4-6h or 1 inh q4h. EIB: 2 inh 15-30 min before activity.

**HOW SUPPLIED:** MDI: 90mcg/inh [6.7g]

**WARNINGS/PRECAUTIONS:** Hypersensitivity reactions reported. Monitor for worsening asthma. Fatalities reported with excessive use. Caution with cardiovascular disorders, especially coronary insufficiency, arrhythmias and HTN. May need concomitant corticosteroids. Can produce paradoxical bronschospasm. Caution with DM, hyperthyroidism, and seizures. May cause transient hypokalemia.

**ADVERSE REACTIONS:** Tachycardia, tremor, dizziness, nausea/vomiting, palpitations, rhinitis, upper respiratory tract infection, fever, inhalation site and taste sensation, back pain, and nervousness.

**INTERACTIONS:** Avoid other sympathomimetic agents. Extreme caution wtih MAOIs and TCAs. Monitor digoxin. May worsen ECG changes and/or hypokalemia with non-$K^+$-sparing diuretics. Antagonized by β-blockers.

**PREGNANCY:** Category C, not for use in nursing.

**MECHANISM OF ACTION:** $β_2$-adrenergic bronchodilator; stimulates adenyl cylase, the enzyme that catalyzes the formation of cAMP from ATP. Increased cAMP levels are associated with relaxation of bronchial smooth muscle and inhibition of release of mediators of immediate hypersensitivity.

## NURSING CONSIDERATIONS

**Assessment:** Assess for convulsive disorders, hyperthyroidism, DM, CVD, and possible drug interactions.

**Monitoring:** Monitor pulse rate, BP, ECG changes, for paradoxical bronchospasm and hypokalemia, hypersensitivity reactions, and deterioration of asthma.

**Patient Counseling:** Take as directed. Report lack of response or adverse side effects.

**Administration:** Oral inhalation. 1) Prime inhaler before using for first time or if inhaler has not been used for 2 weeks by releasing 4 test sprays into air, away from face. 2) Clean inhaler at least once a week. Use only with actuator supplied with product. 3) Discard inhaler after 200 sprays. **Storage:** 15-25°C (59-77°F).

# PROVERA RX

medroxyprogesterone acetate (Pharmacia & Upjohn)

**Estrogen and progestins should not be used for prevention of cardiovascular disease or dementia. Increased risk of myocadial infarction (MI), stroke, invasive breast cancer, pulmonary embolism (PE), and deep vein thrombosis (DVT) in postmenopausal women (50-79 yrs). Increased risk of developing probable dementia in postmenopausal women ( ≥65 yrs).**

**THERAPEUTIC CLASS:** Progestogen

**INDICATIONS:** Treatment of secondary amenorrhea and abnormal uterine bleeding due to hormonal imbalance in the absence of organic pathology, such as fibroids or uterine cancer. Reduce incidence of endometrial hyperplasia in non-hysterectomized postmenopausal women receiving 0.625mg conjugated estrogen.

**DOSAGE:** *Adults:* Secondary Amenorrhea: 5-10mg qd for 5-10 days. Abnormal Uterine Bleeding: 5-10mg qd for 5-10 days beginning on Day 16 or 21 of cycle. Endometrial Hyperplasia: 5-10mg qd for 12-14 consecutive days per month beginning on Day 1 or 16 of cycle.

**HOW SUPPLIED:** Tab: 2.5mg*, 5mg*, 10mg* *scored

**CONTRAINDICATIONS:** Undiagnosed abnormal genital bleeding, breast cancer, estrogen- or progesterone-dependent neoplasia, active or history of DVT/PE, arterial thromboembolic disease (eg, stroke, MI), liver dysfunction or disease, missed abortion, pregnancy, as a diagnostic test for pregnancy.

**WARNINGS/PRECAUTIONS:** D/C if thrombotic events, malignancy, papilledema, or retinal vascular lesions develop. D/C pending exam with sudden onset of proptosis, partial or complete loss of vision, diplopia, or migraine. May elevate BP; monitor at regular intervals. May lower HDL and raise LDL levels as well as impair glucose tolerance. May increase plasma TG with pre-existing hypertriglyceridemia. Caution in patients with history of cholestatic jaundice associated with past estrogen use or pregnancy and with severe hypocalcemia. May cause fluid retention; caution with cardiac/renal dysfunction. May exacerbate asthma, DM, epilepsy, migraine, prophyria, SLE, and hepatic hemangiomas; use with caution. Annual breast exam by physician and monthly self breast exam recommended.

**ADVERSE REACTIONS:** Abnormal uterine bleeding, breast tenderness, galactorrhea, urticaria, pruritus, edema, rash, thromboembolic phenomena, menstrual changes, change in weight, cervical changes, cholestatic jaundice, depression, insomnia, nausea, somnolence.

**INTERACTIONS:** Patients on thyroid replacement therapy may require higher doses of thyroid hormone.

**PREGNANCY:** Category X, not for use in nursing.

**MECHANISM OF ACTION:** Progesterone derivative; transforms proliferative into secretory endometrium.

**PHARMACOKINETICS: Absorption:** (10mg) Rapid; $C_{max}$=0.71ng/mL; $T_{max}$=2.83 hrs; AUC=6.01ng•h/mL. **Distribution:** $V_d$=40564L; plasma protein binding (90%); Found in breast milk. **Metabolism:** hydroxylation, conjugation. **Elimination:** $T_{1/2}$= 16.6 hrs; Urine.

## NURSING CONSIDERATIONS

**Assessment:** Assess for undiagnosed abnormal genital bleeding; known/suspected or history of breast cancer, estrogen- or progesterone-dependent neoplasia, pregnancy status, missed abortion, thromboembolic disease, CAD, asthma, DM, epilepsy, SLE, migraine, porphyria, hypocalcemia, cardiac or renal/hepatic impairment.

**Monitoring:** Monitor BP regularly; breast exam by physician yearly and self monthly; mammogram as required. Monitor for signs/symptoms of thromboembolic disease (eg, stroke, DVT, PE, MI), HTN, hypocalcemia, abnormal vaginal bleeding, dementia, visual abnormalities, hypersensitivity reactions, hepatic dysfunction, fluid retention, exacerbation of asthma, DM, epilepsy,

P

SLE, migraine, and porphyria. Monitor BP levels at regular intervals and thyroid function if on thyroid replacement therapy.

**Patient Counseling:** Inform of risks, including birth defects if exposed during 1st trimester, thromboembolic events, dementia and malignancy in postmenopausal use. Advise to seek medical attention if experience symptoms of hepatic dysfunction (jaundice), hypocalcemia, visual abnormalities (partial/complete loss of vision, diplopia, migraines), abnormal vaginal bleeding, hypersensitivity reactions, HTN, thromboembolic disease, fluid retention, exacerbation of diseases, or dementia.

**Administration:** Oral route. **Storage:** 20-25°C (68-77°F).

## PROVIGIL
modafinil (Cephalon)

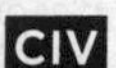

**THERAPEUTIC CLASS:** Wakefulness-promoting agent

**INDICATIONS:** To improve wakefulness in patients with excessive daytime sleepiness associated with narcolepsy, obstructive sleep apnea/hypopnea syndrome (OSAHS), shiftwork sleep disorder (SWSD). As adjunct treatment for underlying obstruction in OSAHS.

**DOSAGE:** *Adults:* 200mg qd. Narcolepsy/OSAHS: Take in AM. SWSD: Take 1 hr prior to start of work shift. Hepatic Dysfunction: 100mg qd. Elderly: Consider dose reduction.

**HOW SUPPLIED:** Tab: 100mg, 200mg* *scored

**WARNINGS/PRECAUTIONS:** Avoid in history of left ventricular hypertrophy, ischemic ECG changes, chest pain, arrhythmia or other manifestations of mitral valve prolapse with CNS stimulants. Caution if recent MI, unstable angina, history of psychosis. Monitor hypertensive patients. Rare cases of severe or life-threatening rash, including Stevens-Johnson syndrome (SJS), toxic epidermal necrolysis (TEN), and drug rash with eosinophilia and systemic symptoms (DRESS) have been reported with the use of modafinil. Angioedema and anaphylactoid reactions reported.

**ADVERSE REACTIONS:** Headache, infection, nausea, nervousness, anxiety, insomnia, rhinitis, diarrhea, back pain, dizziness, dyspepsia, hostility.

P

**INTERACTIONS:** Methylphenidate may delay absorption. May reduce efficacy of steroidal contraceptives up to 1 month after d/c. Caution with MAOIs. CYP3A4 inducers (eg, carbamazepine, phenobarbital, rifampin) may decrease levels. CYP3A4 inhibitors (eg, ketoconazole, itraconazole) may increase levels. May increase levels of drugs metabolized by CYP2C19 (eg, diazepam, propranolol, phenytoin) or CYP2C9 (eg, warfarin). Monitor for toxicity with phenytoin and PT with warfarin. May increase levels of clomipramine, desipramine. May decrease levels of drugs metabolized by CYP3A4 (eg, cyclosporine, steroidal contraceptives, theophylline). Avoid alcohol.

**PREGNANCY:** Category C, caution in nursing.

**MECHANISM OF ACTION:** Wakefulness promoting agent: Psychoactive and euphoric effects, alterations in mood, perception, thinking and feelings typical of other CNS stimulants: Modafinil binds to dopamine transporter, inhibits dopamine reuptake, and results in increased extracellular dopamine levels in some brain regions.

**PHARMACOKINETICS: Absorption:** $T_{max}$=2-4 hrs. **Distribution:** $V_d$=0.9L/kg; plasma protein binding (60%). **Metabolism:** Liver via hydrolytic deamination, S-oxidation, aromatic ring hydroxylation, and glucuronide conjugation through CYP3A4. **Elimination:** Urine, feces.

### NURSING CONSIDERATIONS

**Assessment:** Assess for hypersensitivity to modafinil, armodafinil or its components, hepatic impairment, history of psychosis, depression or mania, left ventricular hypertrophy, mitral valve prolapse. Use drug only in patients who have had complete evaluation of their excessive sleepiness, and in whom a diagnosis of either narcolepsy, OSAHS, and/or SWSD has been made in accordance with ICSD or DSM diagnostic criteria.

**Monitoring:** Monitor serious rash, Stevens-Johnson syndrome, toxic epidermal necrolysis, drug rash with eosinophilia and systemic symptoms (DRESS), angioedema, dysphagia, bronchospasm, multi-organ hypersensitivity reactions (myocarditis, hepatitis, LFT abnormalities, hematological abnormalities such as leukopenia and thrombocytopenia, pruritus, asthenia), psychiatric adverse symptoms such as anxiety, nervousness, insomnia, confusion, agitation, and depression. Also monitor BP, possible drug interactions, and adverse reactions such as headache, nausea, dizziness, chest pain.

**Patient Counseling:** Advise to d/c therapy and immediately report to physician any signs/symptoms suggesting angioedema or anaphylaxis (eg, swelling of face, eyes, lips, tongue or larynx; difficulty breathing or swallowing; hoarseness). Advise that level of wakefulness may not return to normal, thus caution to avoid driving or any other potentially dangerous activity. Contact physician if experience chest pain, rash, depression, anxiety, or signs of psychosis or mania; notify if breastfeeding, if intend to become pregnant, and if taking or plan to take any Rx or OTC drugs. Avoid alcohol.

**Administration:** Oral route. **Storage:** Store at room temperature 20-25°C (68-77°F). Keep out of reach of children.

## PROZAC — RX

fluoxetine HCl (Lilly)

**Antidepressants increased the risk of suicidal thinking and behavior (suicidality) in short-term studies in children, adolescents, and young adults with major depressive disorder (MDD) and other psychiatric disorders. Patients started on antidepressants should be monitored and observed for clinical worsening, suicidality or unusual changes in behavior. Prozac is approved for use in pediatric patients with MDD and obsessive compulsive disorder (OCD).**

**THERAPEUTIC CLASS:** Selective serotonin reuptake inhibitor

**INDICATIONS:** Treatment of major depressive disorder (MDD), obsessive compulsive disorder (OCD), bulimia nervosa, and panic disorder with or without agoraphobia. In combination with olanzapine, acute treatment of depressive episodes associated with Bipolar I disorder, and treatment resistant depression (MDD patients who failed to respond to 2 separate trials of different antidepressants) in adults.

**DOSAGE:** *Adults:* ≥18 yrs: MDD: Initial: 20mg qam; increase dose if no improvement after several weeks. Doses >20mg/day, give qam or bid (am and noon). Max: 80mg/day. OCD: Initial: 20mg qam; may increase dose if no significant improvement after several weeks. Maint: 20-60mg/day given qd-bid, am and noon. Max: 80mg/day. Bulimia Nervosa: 60mg qam. Max: 60mg/day. Panic Disorder: Initial: 10mg/day. May increase to 20mg/day after 1 week. May increase further after several weeks if no clinical improvement. Max: 60mg/day. Hepatic Impairment/Elderly: Use lower or less frequent dosage. Consider dose tapering for pregnant women during the third trimester. Combination with Olanzapine: Depressive Episodes Associated with Bipolar I Disorder/Treatment Resistant Depression: Initial: 20mg plus olanzapine 5mg qd in evening. Titrate: Adjust dose based on efficacy and tolerability. Usual: 25mg-50mg plus olanzapine 6mg-12mg (depressive episodes associated with Bipolar I disorder) or 6mg-18mg (treatment resistant depression). Predisposed to Hypotensive Reactions/Hepatic Impairment/Factors to Slow Metabolism of Olanzapine or Fluoxetine in Combination: 20mg plus olanzapine 2.5mg-5mg.

*Pediatrics:* MDD: ≥8 yrs: Higher Wt Peds: Initial: 10 or 20mg/day. After 1 week at 10mg/day, may increase to 20mg/day. Lower Wt Peds: Initial: 10mg/day. Titrate: May increase to 20mg/day after several weeks if clinical improvement is not observed. OCD: ≥7 yrs: Adolescents and Higher Wt Peds: Initial: 10mg/day. Titrate: Increase to 20mg/day after 2 weeks. Consider additional dose increases after several more weeks if clinical improvement is not observed. Usual: 20-60mg/day. Lower Wt Peds: Initial: 10mg/day. Titrate: Consider additional dose increases after several weeks if clinical improvement is not observed. Usual: 20-30mg/day. Max: 60mg/day.

**HOW SUPPLIED:** Cap: 10mg, 20mg, 40mg; Sol (Generic): 20mg/5mL

**CONTRAINDICATIONS:** During or within 14 days of MAOI therapy. Thioridazine during or within 5 weeks of d/c. Concomitant use of pimozide.

**WARNINGS/PRECAUTIONS:** Avoid abrupt withdrawal. Serotonin syndrome and neuroleptic malignant syndrome (NMS)-like reactions reported. May increase risk of bleeding events. Activation of mania/hypomania, SIADH, hyponatremia, anxiety, insomnia, nervousness reported. D/C if unexplained allergic reaction occurs. Caution with diseases or conditions that could affect hemodynamic responses or metabolism, altered glucose levels, history of seizures or mania, suicidal tendencies. Monitor height and weight periodically in children. Altered appetite and weight loss reported. Caution in third trimester of pregnancy due to risk of serious neonatal complications. Caution with hepatic impairment. May impair judgment, thinking, or motor skills. May precipitate mixed/manic episode in patients at risk for bipolar disorder. Fluoxetine monotherapy is not approved for use in treating bipolar depression.

**ADVERSE REACTIONS:** Abnormal dreams, abnormal ejaculation, anorexia, anxiety, asthenia, diarrhea, dry mouth, dyspepsia, flu syndrome, impotence, insomnia, decreased libido, nausea, nervousness, pharyngitis.

**INTERACTIONS:** See Contraindications. Caution with CYP2D6 substrates including antidepressants (eg, TCA), antipsychotics (eg, phenothiazines and most atypicals), and antiarrhythmics (eg, propafenone, flecainide). May increase levels of phenytoin, carbamazepine, haloperidol, clozapine, diazepam, imipramine, desipramine. Caution with CNS active drugs. May increase/decrease lithium levels; lithium toxicity and increased serotogenic effects reported. Caution with drugs that may affect serotogenic neurotransmitter systems (eg, triptans, linezolid, tramadol, lithium, St. John's Wort). Avoid with other selective serotonin reuptake inhibitors (SSRIs), serotonin-norepinephrine reuptake inhibitors (SNRIs), or tryptophan. May cause a shift in plasma concentration with drugs that are tightly bound to protein (eg, warfarin, digoxin) resulting in an adverse effect. Increased risk of bleeding events with aspirin, nonsteroidal anti-inflammatory drugs (NSAID), warfarin, and other anti-coagulants. Greater risk of hyponatremia with diuretics. Increased risk of NMS-like reactions with serotogenic drugs (eg, triptans), MAOIs, antipsychotics, other dopamine antagonists. Antidiabetic drugs may need adjustment. Rare reports of prolonged seizures with combined electroconvulsive therapy.

**PREGNANCY:** Category C, not for use in nursing.

P

**MECHANISM OF ACTION:** SSRI; not established. Presumed to be linked to inhibition of CNS neuronal reuptake of serotonin.

**PHARMACOKINETICS: Absorption:** $C_{max}$=15-55ng/mL, $T_{max}$=6-8 hrs. **Distribution:** Plasma protein binding (94.5%); excreted in breast milk. **Metabolism:** Liver (extensive) via demethylation, norfluoxetine (active metabolite). **Elimination:** Urine; $T_{1/2}$=1-3 days (fluoxetine), 4-16 days (norfluoxetine).

## NURSING CONSIDERATIONS

**Assessment:** Assess for risk of bipolar disorder, history of mania, history of seizures, disease/condition that alters metabolism or hemodynamic response, hepatic/renal impairment, MAOI, thioridazine, or pimozide therapy, pregnancy/nursing status, and possible drug interactions.

**Monitoring:** Monitor for signs/symptoms of clinical worsening, suicidality and unusual changes in behavior (especially during initial few months, and dosage changes), hypersensitivity reactions, serotonin syndrome, abnormal bleeding, altered appetite and weight, hyponatremia, seizures, hypo/hyperglycemia, and abrupt withdrawal symptoms

**Patient Counseling:** Advise to avoid alcohol. Seek medical attention for symptoms of serotonin syndrome (mental status changes, tachycardia, hyperthermia, N/V, diarrhea, incoordination), abnormal bleeding (particularly if using NSAIDs or ASA), akathisia, hyponatremia (headaches, unsteadiness), mydriasis, activation of mania, seizures, clinical worsening (suicidal ideation, unusual changes in behavior) and discontinuation symptoms (irritability, agitation, dizziness, anxiety, headache, insomnia). Caution against hazardous tasks (eg, operating machinery and driving). May notice improvement in 1-4 weeks; continue therapy as directed. Notify physician if pregnant/intend to become pregnant, or breastfeeding. Counsel about benefits and risks of therapy. Inform physician if taking, or plan to take any OTC prescriptions.

**Administration:** Oral route. **Storage:** 15-30°C (59-86°F). Protect from light.

## PROZAC WEEKLY RX

fluoxetine HCl (Lilly)

**Antidepressants increased the risk of suicidal thinking and behavior (suicidality) in short-term studies in children, adolescents, and young adults with major depressive disorder (MDD) and other psychiatric disorders. Patients started on antidepressants should be monitored and observed for clinical worsening, suicidality or unusual changes in behavior. Prozac is approved for use in pediatric patients with MDD and obsessive compulsive disorder (OCD).**

**THERAPEUTIC CLASS:** Selective serotonin reuptake inhibitor

**INDICATIONS:** Treatment of major depressive disorder (MDD).

**DOSAGE:** *Adults:* One 90mg cap every week starting 7 days after last daily dose of fluoxetine 20mg.

**HOW SUPPLIED:** Cap, Delayed-Release: 90mg

**CONTRAINDICATIONS:** During or within 14 days of MAOI therapy. Thioridazine during or within 5 weeks of discontinuation. Concomitant use of pimozide.

**WARNINGS/PRECAUTIONS:** Avoid abrupt withdrawal. Serotonin syndrome and neuroleptic malignant syndrome (NMS)-like reactions reported. May increase risk of bleeding events. Activation of mania/hypomania, SIADH, hyponatremia, anxiety, insomnia, nervousness reported. D/C if unexplained allergic reaction occurs. Caution with diseases or conditions that could affect hemodynamic responses or metabolism, altered glucose levels, history of seizures or mania, suicidal tendencies. Monitor height and weight periodically in children. Altered appetite and weight loss reported. Caution in third trimester of pregnancy due to risk of serious neonatal complications. Caution with hepatic impairment. May impair judgment, thinking, or motor skills. May precipitate mixed/manic episode in patients at risk for bipolar disorder. Fluoxetine monotherapy is not approved for use in treating bipolar depression.

**ADVERSE REACTIONS:** Abnormal dreams, abnormal ejaculation, anorexia, anxiety, asthenia, diarrhea, dry mouth, dyspepsia, flu syndrome, impotence, insomnia, decreased libido, nausea, nervousness, and pharyngitis.

**INTERACTIONS:** See Contraindications. Caution with CYP2D6 substrates including antidepressants (eg, TCA), antipsychotics (eg, phenothiazines and most atypicals), and antiarrhythmics (eg, propafenone, flecainide). May increase levels of phenytoin, carbamazepine, haloperidol, clozapine, diazepam, imipramine, desipramine. Caution with CNS active drugs. May increase/decrease lithium levels; lithium toxicity and increased serotogenic effects reported. Caution with drugs that may affect serotogenic neurotransmitter systems (eg, triptans, linezolid, tramadol, lithium, St. John's Wort). Avoid with other selective serotonin reuptake inhibitors (SSRIs), serotonin-norepinephrine reuptake inhibitors (SNRIs), or tryptophan. May cause a shift in plasma concentration with drugs that are tightly bound to protein (eg, warfarin, digoxin) resulting in an adverse effect. Increased risk of bleeding events with aspirin, nonsteroidal anti-inflammatory drugs (NSAID), warfarin, and other anti-coagulants. Greater risk of hyponatremia with diuretics. Increased risk of NMS-like reactions with serotogenic drugs (eg, triptans), MAOIs, antipsychotics, other dopamine antagonists. Antidiabetic drugs may need adjustment. Rare reports of prolonged seizures with combined electroconvulsive therapy.

**PREGNANCY:** Category C, not for use in nursing.

**MECHANISM OF ACTION:** SSRI; exact mechanism is not established. Believed to inhibit CNS neuronal reuptake of serotonin.

**PHARMACOKINETICS: Absorption:** Delayed onset by 1-2 hrs. **Distribution:** Plasma protein binding (94.5%). Excreted in breast milk. **Metabolism:** Liver (extensive) via demethylation, norfluoxetine (active metabolite). **Elimination:** Kidney. $T_{1/2}$=1-3 days (fluoxetine), 4-16 days (norfluoxetine).

## NURSING CONSIDERATIONS

**Assessment:** Assess for risk of bipolar disorder, history of mania, history of seizures, disease/condition that alters metabolism or hemodynamic response, hepatic/renal impairment, MAOI, thioridazine, or pimozide therapy, pregnancy/nursing status, and possible drug interactions.

**Monitoring:** Monitor for signs/symptoms of clinical worsening, suicidality and unusual changes in behavior (especially during initial few months, and dosage changes), hypersensitivity reactions, serotonin syndrome, abnormal bleeding, altered appetite and weight, hyponatremia, seizures, hypo/hyperglycemia, and abrupt withdrawal symptoms

**Patient Counseling:** Advise to avoid alcohol. Seek medical attention for symptoms of serotonin syndrome (mental status changes, tachycardia, hyperthermia, N/V, diarrhea, incoordination), abnormal bleeding (particularly if using NSAIDs or ASA), akathisia, hyponatremia (headaches, unsteadiness), mydriasis, activation of mania, seizures, clinical worsening (suicidal ideation, unusual changes in behavior) and d/c symptoms (irritability, agitation, dizziness, anxiety, headache, insomnia). Caution against hazardous tasks (eg, operating machinery and driving). May notice improvement in 1-4 weeks; continue therapy as directed. Notify physician if pregnant/intend to become pregnant, or breastfeeding. Counsel about benefits and risks of therapy. Inform physician if taking, or plan to take any over-the-counter prescriptions.

**Administration:** Oral route. **Storage:** 15-30°C (59-86°F). Protect from light.

# PULMICORT RX

budesonide (AstraZeneca)

**OTHER BRAND NAMES:** Pulmicort Flexhaler (AstraZeneca) - Pulmicort Respules (AstraZeneca)

**THERAPEUTIC CLASS:** Corticosteroid

**INDICATIONS:** (Flexhaler) Maintenance treatment of asthma as prophylactic therapy in patients ≥6 yrs and to reduce or eliminate the need for oral systemic corticosteroidal therapy. (Respules) Maintenance treatment of asthma and as prophylactic therapy in children 12 months to 8 yrs.

P

**DOSAGE:** *Adults:* (Flexhaler) Initial: 180-360mcg bid. Max: 720mcg bid. Individualize dose.

*Pediatrics:* (Flexhaler) ≥6 yrs: Initial: 180-360mcg bid. Max: 360mcg bid. Individualize dose. (Respules) Administer via compressed air driven jet nebulizer only; 1-8 yrs: Previous Bronchodilator Only: Initial: 0.5mg qd or 0.25mg bid. Max: 0.5mg/day. Previous Inhaled Corticosteroid: 0.5mg qd or 0.25mg bid. Max: 1mg/day. Taper to lowest effective dose once desired clinical effect achieved. Previous Oral Corticosteroid: 1mg qd or 0.5mg bid. Max: 1mg/day. Gradually reduce PO corticosteroid after 1 week of budesonide. Not responding to non-steroidal therapy: Initial: 0.25mg qd.

**HOW SUPPLIED:** Powder, Inhalation: (Flexhaler) 90mcg/dose, 180mcg/dose; Sus, Inhalation: (Respules) 0.25mg/2mL, 0.5mg/2mL, 1mg/2mL [2mL, 30$^s$]

**CONTRAINDICATIONS:** Primary treatment of status asthmaticus or other acute episodes of asthma where intensive measures are required.

**WARNINGS/PRECAUTIONS:** Deaths due to adrenal insufficiency have occurred with transfer from systemic corticosteroids to inhaled corticosteroids. Resume oral corticosteroids during stress or severe asthma attack. Transferring from systemic to inhalation therapy may unmask allergic conditions (eg, rhinitis, conjunctivitis, arthritis, eosinophilic conditions, eczema). Observe for adrenal insufficiency, systemic corticosteroid withdrawal effects, and growth suppression (children). Increased susceptibility to infections (eg, chickenpox, measles) which may lead to serious/fatal course; if exposed, prophylaxis/treatment considered. Not for acute bronchospasm. D/C if bronchospasm with immediate increase in wheezing occurs after dosing. Caution with TB, untreated systemic fungal, bacterial, viral or parasitic infections or ocular herpes simplex. *Candida* infection of mouth and pharynx reported; treat and/or d/c if needed. Patients requiring oral corticosteroids should be weaned slowly from systemic corticosteroid use. Glaucoma, increased intraocular pressure (IOP) and cataracts reported. (Respules) Hypersensitivity reactions including anaphylaxis, rash, contact dermatitis, urticaria, angioedema, and bronchospasm reported; d/c treatment if reactions occurs.

**ADVERSE REACTIONS:** Nasopharyngitis, pharyngitis, headache, fever, sinusitis, pain, bronchospasm, bronchitis, respiratory infection, moniliasis. (Respules) Respiratory infection, rhinitis, coughing, otitis media, viral infection.

**INTERACTIONS:** Oral ketoconazole increases plasma levels. CYP3A4 inhibitors (eg, itraconazole, clarithromycin, erythromycin) may inhibit metabolism and increase systemic exposure. (Respules) Slight decrease in clearance and increase in oral bioavailability with cimetidine.

**PREGNANCY:** (Flexhaler/Respules) Category B, caution in nursing

**MECHANISM OF ACTION:** Corticosteroid; not established. Shown to have inhibitory effects on multiple cell types (mast cells, eosinophils, neutrophils, macrophages and lymphocytes) and mediators (histamine, eicosanoids, leukotrienes and cytokines) involved in inflammatory and asthmatic response.

**PHARMACOKINETICS: Absorption:** Respules: (4-6 yrs) Absolute bioavailability (6%); $C_{max}$=2.6nmol/L, $T_{max}$=20 min. Turbuhaler: $T_{max}$=30 min. Flexhaler: (Adults) $T_{max}$=10 min, (180mg qd) $C_{max}$=0.6nmol/L. (360mg bid) $C_{max}$=1.6nmol/L. (Peds) $T_{max}$=15-30 min, (180mg qd) $C_{max}$=0.4nmol/L. (360mg bid) $C_{max}$=1.5nmol/L. **Distribution:** $V_d$=3L/kg; plasma protein binding (85-90%); found in breast milk (0.3-1%). **Metabolism:** Liver (extensive), via CYP3A4. **Elimination:** (Respules) Urine and feces (metabolites); $T_{1/2}$=2.3 hrs. (Turbuhaler, Flexhaler) $T_{1/2}$=2-3 hrs.

## NURSING CONSIDERATIONS

**Assessment:** Assess for concomitant diseases such as status asthmaticus, acute bronchospasm, other acute episodes of asthma, active or quiescent pulmonary TB, ocular herpes simplex, untreated systemic fungal, bacterial, parasitic or viral infections, hepatic dysfunction, pregnancy/nursing status, and possible drug interactions. Obtain baseline lung function and LFTs prior to therapy.

**Monitoring:** Monitor lung function periodically. Perform periodic eye exams; monitor for development of glaucoma, increased IOP and cataracts. Monitor for localized oral infections with *Candida albicans*, decreased bone mass, worsening or acutely deteriorating asthma (increased use of inhaled $\beta_2$-agonist, decreased lung function), asthma instability (serial objective measures of airflow), body height in children, development adrenal insufficiency (eg, fatigue, weakness, N/V, hypotension), paradoxical bronchospasm, and hypersensitivity reactions.

**Patient Counseling:** Do not increase dosage or d/c inhaler abruptly unless directed by physician. Instruct patients whose chronic systemic corticosteroids have been reduced or withdrawn to carry a warning card indicating the need for supplemental systemic corticosteroid during periods of stress or asthma attack not responsive to bronchodilators. Should not be used for sudden symptoms of SOB or acute bronchospasm. Inform that medication may cause reduction in growth rate (pediatrics) and may unmask allergies (eg, rhinitis, conjunctivitis, eczema). Advise to seek medical attention if exposed to chickenpox or measles, worsening of existing TB, infections or ocular herpes simplex. Also notify a healthcare provider if symptoms worsen or do not improve or if adrenal insufficiency (eg, fatigue, weakness, N/V, hypotension), paradoxical bronchospasm, or hypersensitivity reactions occur.

**Administration:** Oral inhalation route. **Storage:** (Turbuhaler, Flexhaler): 20-25°C (68-77°F). (Respules): 20-25°C (68-77°F). Protect from light. Do not freeze. After aluminum foil opened; stable for 2 weeks. Before use, shake using circular motion. Keep out of reach of children.

# PURINETHOL

mercaptopurine (Gate)

RX

**THERAPEUTIC CLASS:** Purine analog

**INDICATIONS:** Maintenance therapy of acute lymphatic (lymphocytic, lymphoblastic) leukemia as part of a combination therapy.

**DOSAGE:** *Adults:* Maint: Usual: 1.5-2.5mg/kg/day as single dose. Renal/Hepatic Impairment: Reduce dose. Concomitant Allopurinol: Reduce mercaptopurine dose by 1/3-1/4 of usual dose. TPMT Deficiency: Consider dose reduction. Elderly: Start at the low end of the dosing range.
*Pediatrics:* Maint: Usual: 1.5-2.5mg/kg/day as single dose. Renal/Hepatic Impairment: Reduce dose. Concomitant Allopurinol: Reduce mercaptopurine dose by 1/3-1/4 of usual dose. TPMT Deficiency: Consider dose reduction.

**HOW SUPPLIED:** Tab: 50mg* *scored

**CONTRAINDICATIONS:** Prior resistance to mercaptopurine.

**WARNINGS/PRECAUTIONS:** Not effective for prophylaxis or treatment of CNS leukemia. Not effective in acute myelogenous leukemia, chronic lymphatic leukemia, the lymphomas (including Hodgkins disease), or solid tumors. Risk of dose-related bone marrow suppression. Monitor weekly platelet counts, Hgb, Hct, total WBC with differential; increase monitoring frequency during induction phase. Life-threatening infections and bleeding reported; d/c at first sign on unexpectedly abnormal large fall in any formed elements of the blood not attributable to other drugs or disease process. Increased sensitivity to myelosuppressive effects with thiopurine-S-methyltransferase (TPMT) gene deficiency; consider TPMT testing with evidence of severe toxicity. Risk of hepatotoxicity, anorexia, diarrhea, jaundice, and ascites (especially with >2.5mg/kg dose). Hepatic encephalopathy reported. Monitor LFTs weekly initially, then monthly; monitor more frequently with pre-existing liver disease. D/C with deterioration of liver function, toxic hepatitis and biliary stasis. Risk of immunosuppression; may manifest decreased cellular hypersensitivities and decreased allograft rejection. May cause fetal harm. Monitor patient's clinical status and modify therapy depending on response and manifestations of toxicity. Caution in elderly, renal, and hepatic impairment.

**ADVERSE REACTIONS:** Bone marrow toxicity, hepatotoxicity, hyperuricemia, hyperuricosuria, intestinal ulceration, rash, hyperpigmentation, alopecia, oligospermia.

**INTERACTIONS:** Severe toxicity with allopurinol; reduce mercaptopurine dose to 1/3 to 1/4 of the usual dose. Reduce dose with other myelosuppressants. Enhanced bone marrow suppression reported with trimethoprim-sulfamethoxazole. Cross-resistance with thioguanine. Increased risk of bone marrow toxicity with coadministration of drugs that inhibit TPMT (eg, olsalazine, mesalazine, sulphasalazine). Inhibition of the anticoagulant effect of warfarin reported when used concomitantly with mercaptopurine. Perform careful clinical and biochemical monitoring of hepatic function when concomitantly using other hepatoxic agents. Hepatotoxicity reported with concomitant use of doxorubicin. Subnormal induction of immunity to vaccines may occur with concomitant use.

**PREGNANCY:** Category D, not for use in nursing.

**MECHANISM OF ACTION:** Purine analog; competes with hypoxanthine and guanine for hypoxanthine-guanine phosphoribosyltransferase and is converted to thioinosinic acid, which then inhibits glutamine-5-phosphoribosylpyrophosphate amidotransferase of the de novo pathway for purine ribonucleotide synthesis.

**PHARMACOKINETICS: Absorption:** Incomplete. **Distribution:** Plasma protein binding (19%). **Elimination:** (PO) Urine (46%). (IV) $T_{1/2}$=21 min (pediatric); 47 min (adult).

## NURSING CONSIDERATIONS

**Assessment:** Assess for CNS leukemia, acute myelogenous leukemia, chronic lymphatic leukemia, the lymphomas (including Hodgkins disease), solid

P

tumors, prior drug resistance, pre-existing liver/renal disease, TPMT gene defect, pregnancy/nursing status, and for possible drug interactions. Obtain baseline WBC with differential, Hgb/Hct, platelet count, serum transaminase levels, alkaline phosphatase levels, bilirubin levels, and renal function.

**Monitoring:** Monitor for signs/symptoms of bone marrow toxicity, hepatoxicity, and immunosuppression. Monitor WBC with differential, Hgb/Hct, and platelet count weekly. Monitor serum transaminase levels, alkaline phosphatase, and bilirubin levels weekly at beginning of therapy and then at monthly intervals thereafter. Perform bone marrow exam for evaluation of marrow status. Consider performing TPMT testing if evidence of severe bone marrow toxicity develops. Monitor patient clinical status and need to modify therapy based on response and manifestations of toxicity.

**Patient Counseling:** Inform of major toxicities related to therapy (eg, myelosuppression, hepatotoxicity, GI toxicity). Advise women of childbearing potential to avoid becoming pregnant while on therapy. Instruct to take under medical supervision. Advise to seek medical attention if symptoms of fever, sore throat, jaundice, N/V, signs of local infection, bleeding from any site, or if symptoms suggestive of anemia develop.

**Administration:** Oral route. **Storage:** 15-25°C (59-77°F) in a dry place.

## PYLERA RX

tetracycline HCl - bismuth subcitrate potassium - metronidazole (Axcan Scandipharm)

**Unnecessary use of the drug should be avoided. Reserved only for the treatment of** *Helicobacter pylori* **infection and duodenal ulcer disease.**

**THERAPEUTIC CLASS:** *H.pylori* treatment combination

**INDICATIONS:** Treatment *Helicobacter pylori* (*H. pylori*) infection and duodenal ulcer disease (in combination with omeprazole).

**DOSAGE:** *Adults:* Usual: 3 caps qid, after meals and at bedtime. Take with omeprazole 20mg bid after morning and evening meals for 10 days.

**HOW SUPPLIED:** Cap: (Bismuth Subcitrate Potassium-Metronidazole-Tetracycline HCl) 140mg-125mg-125mg [120].

**CONTRAINDICATIONS:** Pregnancy, nursing women, pediatric patients, and patients with renal or hepatic impairment.

**WARNINGS/PRECAUTIONS:** (Bismuth) Neurotoxicity (rare) associated with excessive doses reported. May interfere with x-ray diagnostics of the GI tract. (Metronidazole) Convulsive seizures and peripheral neuropathy, which is characterized by numbness or paresthesia of an extremity, reported. D/C if abnormal neurologic signs appear. Caution with CNS diseases, evidence or history of blood dyscrasia. Known or previously unrecognized candidiasis may present more prominent symptoms and requires treatment with an antifungal agent. (Tetracycline) May cause permanent discoloration (yellow-gray-brown) of the teeth during tooth development (last half of pregnancy, infancy, and childhood to the age of 8 yrs). Enamel hypoplasia reported; avoid in patients with enamel hypoplasia. Photosensitivity manifested by an exaggerated sunburn reaction, reported; d/c if skin erythema occurs. May increase blood urea nitrogen (BUN). Higher serum tetracycline levels may lead to azotemia, hyperphosphatemia, and acidosis in patients with renal impairment. May cause overgrowth of non-susceptible organisms, including fungi; d/c and appropriate therapy should be instituted. Pseudotumor cerebri (benign intracranial hypertension) reported.

**ADVERSE REACTIONS:** May cause temporary and harmless darkening of the tongue and/or black stools, diarrhea, dyspepsia, abdominal pain, nausea, headache, flu syndrome, taste perversion, asthenia, vaginitis, dizziness, pain, infection and pharyngitis.

**INTERACTIONS:** (Metronidazole) Increase lithium levels and signs of lithium toxicity with high doses of lithium and short term therapy. Avoid alcoholic beverages for at least 1 day during therapy. Psychotic reactions reported in alcoholic patients when co-administered with disulfiram. May potentiate anticoagulant effect of warfarin and other oral coumarin anticoagulant. Cimetidine, phenytoin, or phenobarbital may decrease microsomal liver enzyme activity, and may prolong half-life and decrease plasma clearance. (Tetracycline) Fatal renal toxicity reported when co-administered with methoxyflurane. Concomitant use of oral contraceptives may become less effective and breakthrough bleeding reported. Anticoagulants may depress plasma prothrombin activity monitor clotting times periodically and make appropriate dosage adjustment to anticoagulants. May interfere bactericidal effects of penicillin; avoid co-administration. Antiacids containing aluminum, calcium, or magnesium; preparations containing iron, zinc, or sodium bicarbonate; or milk and dairy products may impair absorption. Bismuth may reduce systemic absorption.

**PREGNANCY:** Category D, not for use in nursing.

**MECHANISM OF ACTION:** Antimicrobial agent. (Bismuth) Antibacterial action not well understood. (Metronidazole) Metabolized through reductive pathways into reactive intermediates that have cytotoxic action. (Tetracycline HCl) Interacts with 30S subunit of the bacterial ribosome and inhibits protein synthesis.

**PHARMACOKINETICS: Absorption:** Bismuth: AUC 56.5ng(hr)/mL, $C_{max}$=16.7ng/mL. Metronidazole: AUC 84413ng(hr)/mL, $C_{max}$=8666.3ng/mL. Tetracycline: AUC 9987ng(hr)/mL, $C_{max}$=773.8ng/mL. **Distribution:** Bismuth: Orally absorbed bismuth is distributed throughout the entire body and is 90% bound to plasma proteins. Metronidazole: <20% bound to plasma proteins, appears in CSF, saliva and breast milk in concentrations similar to the plasma. Tetracycline: Distributed into most body tissues and fluids. **Metabolism:** Metronidazole: Side chain oxidation and glucuronide conjugation. **Elimination:** Bismuth: $T_{1/2}$=5 days in blood and urine, elimination of bismuth is primarily through urinary biliary routes. Metronidazole: $T_{1/2}$=8 hrs, urine 60-80%, fecal 6-15%, approximately 20% is excreted unchanged. Tetracycline: $T_{1/2}$=6-11 hrs, concentrated by the liver in the bile and excreted in the urine and feces in a biologically active form.

## NURSING CONSIDERATIONS

**Assessment:** Assess for history of blood dyscrasia, known or previously unrecognized candidiasis, renal function, LFTs, BUN levels, pregnancy/nursing status, and possible drug interactions.

**Monitoring:** Monitor for BUN levels, renal/hepatic impairment, lithium levels in patients taking lithium, leucopenia, black stool, abnormal neurologic signs, skin erythema, candidiasis, photosensitivity, neuropathy, convulsive seizures, neurotoxicity, enamel hypoplasia, azotemia, hyperphosphatemia, and acidosis. Monitor for occult blood in stool if indicated.

**Patient Counseling:** Swallow capsules whole with full glass of water espically at bedtime to reduce the risk of esophagel irritation and ulceration. Co-administration with oral contraceptives may render birth control less effective; advise to use a different or additional form of contraception. Notify a physician immediately if pregnant/intend to become pregnant, or breastfeeding. Avoid exposure to sun or sun lamps. Avoid alcoholic beverages. Counsel about temporary and harmless darkening of the tongue and/or black stool. Stool darkening should not be confused with melena. Advise not to take double doses; missed doses may be made up by continuing normal dosing schedule until medication is gone.

**Administration:** Oral route. Swallow whole with a full glass of water (8 ounces). **Storage:** 20-25°C (68-77°F).

# QUESTRAN — RX

cholestyramine (Par)

**OTHER BRAND NAMES:** Questran Light (Par)

**THERAPEUTIC CLASS:** Bile acid sequestrant

**INDICATIONS:** Adjunct to reduce elevated cholesterol in primary hypercholesterolemia not responding to diet or to reduce LDL in hypertriglyceridemia. Relief of pruritus associated with partial biliary obstruction.

**DOSAGE:** *Adults:* Initial: 1 pkt or scoopful qd or bid. Maint: 2-4 pkts or scoopfuls/day, given bid. Titrate: Adjust at no less than 4 week intervals. Max: 6 pkts/day or 6 scoopfuls/day. May also give as 1-6 doses/day. Mix with fluid or highly fluid food.
*Pediatrics:* Usual: 240mg/kg/day of anhydrous cholestyramine resin in 2-3 divided doses. Max: 8g/day.

**HOW SUPPLIED:** Powder: 4g/pkt [60$^s$, 378g], (Light) 4g/scoopful [60$^s$, 268g]

**CONTRAINDICATIONS:** Complete biliary obstruction.

**WARNINGS/PRECAUTIONS:** May produce hyperchloremic acidosis with prolonged use. Caution in renal insufficiency, volume depletion, and with concomitant spironolactone. Chronic use may produce or worsen constipation. Avoid constipation with symptomatic CAD. May increase bleeding tendency due to vitamin K deficiency. Serum or red cell folate reduced with chronic use. Constipation may aggravate hemorrhoids. Light formulation contains phenylalanine. Measure cholesterol during 1st few months; periodically thereafter. Measure TG periodically.

**ADVERSE REACTIONS:** Constipation, heartburn, nausea, vomiting, abdominal pain, flatulence, diarrhea, anorexia, osteoporosis, rash, hyperchloremic acidosis (children), vitamin A and D deficiency, steatorrhea, hypoprothrombinemia (vitamin K deficiency).

**INTERACTIONS:** May interfere with absorption of fat-soluble vitamins (A, D, E, K), drugs that undergo enterohepatic circulation, and oral phosphate supplements. Take concomitant drugs 1hr before or 4-6 hrs after. Additive effects with HMG-CoA reductase inhibitors and nicotinic acid. Caution with spironolactone. May reduce or delay absorption of phenylbutazone, warfarin, thiazide diuretics, propranolol, tetracycline, penicillin G, phenobarbital, thyroid and thyroxine agents, estrogens, progestins, digitalis.

**PREGNANCY:** Category C, caution in nursing.

**MECHANISM OF ACTION:** Bile acid sequestrant; absorbs and combines with bile acids in intestine to form insoluble complex excreted in the feces, resulting in partial removal of bile acids from enterohepatic circulation by preventing their absorption. This leads to increased oxidation of cholesterol to bile acids and decreased plasma LDL and serum cholesterol levels.

**PHARMACOKINETICS: Elimination:** Feces.

## NURSING CONSIDERATIONS

**Assessment:** Prior to initiation, assess secondary causes of hypercholesterolemia (eg, poorly controlled DM, hypothyroidism, nephrotic syndrome, dysproteinemias, obstructive liver disease, other drug therapy, alcoholism), presence of biliary obstruction, pregnancy/nursing status, and possible drug interactions. Obtain baseline serum, cholesterol, and TG levels.

**Monitoring:** Monitor for signs/symptoms of increased bleeding tendencies (vitamin K deficiency), hyperchloremic acidosis, and worsening of pre-existing constipation. Monitor serum cholesterol and TGs periodically.

**Patient Counseling:** Advise to drink plenty of fluids and to mix each 9g dose of Questran in at least 2-6 oz of fluid or each 6.4g dose of Questran Light in at least 4-6 oz of fluid. Instruct not to sip or hold suspension in mouth for prolonged periods; may lead to changes on surface of teeth (eg, discoloration, erosion of enamel, or decay). Advise to maintain good oral hygiene.

**Administration:** Oral route. **Storage:** Room temperature.

# QUIXIN RX

levofloxacin (Vistakon)

**THERAPEUTIC CLASS:** Fluoroquinolone

**INDICATIONS:** Treatment of bacterial conjunctivitis.

**DOSAGE:** *Adults:* Days 1-2: 1-2 drops q2h while awake, up to 8x/day. Days 3-7: 1-2 drops q4h while awake, up to qid.
*Pediatrics:* ≥1 yr: Days 1-2: 1-2 drops q2h while awake, up to 8x/day. Days 3-7: 1-2 drops q4h while awake, up to qid.

**HOW SUPPLIED:** Sol: 0.5% [5mL]

**WARNINGS/PRECAUTIONS:** D/C if hypersensitivity or superinfection occurs. Avoid contact lenses with conjunctivitis.

**ADVERSE REACTIONS:** Transient ocular burning, decreased vision, fever, foreign body sensation, headache, ocular pain, pharyngitis, photophobia.

**INTERACTIONS:** Systemic quinolone therapy may increase theophylline levels, interfere with caffeine metabolism, enhance warfarin effects, and elevate SrCr with cyclosporine.

**PREGNANCY:** Category C, caution in nursing.

**MECHANISM OF ACTION:** Fluoroquinolone; antibacterial active against broad spectrum of gram-positive and gram-negative organisms. Responsible for inhibition of bacterial topoisomerase IV and DNA gyrase, enzymes required for DNA replication, transcription, repair, and recombination.

**PHARMACOKINETICS: Absorption:** $C_{max}$=0.94ng/mL (single dose), 2.15ng/mL (multiple doses).

## NURSING CONSIDERATIONS

**Assessment:** Assess for proper diagnosis (eg, slit-lamp biomicroscopy, fluorescein staining), hypersensitivity to other quinolones, possible drug interactions, and use in pregnant/nursing females.

**Monitoring:** Monitor for signs/symptoms of hypersensitivity or anaphylactic reaction (eg, cardiovascular collapse, loss of consciousness, angioedema, airway obstruction, dyspnea, uticaria, and itching). With prolonged therapy, monitor for overgrowth of nonsusceptible organisms (eg, fungi) and for development of superinfection. Perform periodic exam of patient using magnification (eg, slit-lamp biomicroscopy, fluorescein staining).

**Patient Counseling:** Instruct to avoid touching applicator tip to material from eye, fingers, or other sources to prevent contamination. Advise not to wear contact lenses if there are signs/symptoms of bacterial conjunctivitis. Instruct to d/c medication and contact physician if signs of hypersensitivity reaction (eg, rash) develop.

**Administration:** Ocular route. Do not inject subconjunctivally or introduce directly into anterior chamber of eye. **Storage:** 15-25°C (59-77°F). Keep out of reach of children.



# QVAR **RX**

beclomethasone dipropionate (Teva)

**THERAPEUTIC CLASS:** Corticosteroid

**INDICATIONS:** Maintenance treatment of asthma as prophylactic therapy in patients ≥5 yrs. To reduce or eliminate the need for systemic corticosteroids in asthma patients requiring systemic corticosteroids.

**DOSAGE:** *Adults:* Previous Bronchodilator Only: 40-80mcg bid. Max: 320mcg bid. Previous Inhaled Corticosteroid (CS) Therapy: 40-160mcg bid. Max: 320mcg bid. Maintained on Systemic CS: May attempt gradual reduction of systemic CS dose after 1 week on inhaled therapy. Elderly: Start at lower end of dosing range.
*Pediatrics:* Adolescents: Previous Bronchodilator Only: 40-80mcg bid. Max: 320mcg bid. Previous Inhaled Corticosteroid (CS) Therapy: 40-160mcg bid. Max: 320mcg bid. 5-11 yrs: Previous Bronchodilator Only or Inhaled CS Therapy: 40mcg bid. Max: 80mcg bid. Maintained on Systemic CS: May attempt gradual reduction of systemic CS dose after 1 week on inhaled therapy.

**HOW SUPPLIED:** MDI: 40 mcg/inh, 80 mcg/inh [7.3g]

**CONTRAINDICATIONS:** Primary treatment of status asthmaticus or other acute episodes of asthma where intensive measures are required.

**WARNINGS/PRECAUTIONS:** Deaths due to adrenal insufficiency have occurred with transfer from systemic corticosteroids to inhaled corticosteroids. Resume oral corticosteroids during stress or severe asthma attack. Risk of adrenal insufficiency and withdrawal symptoms when replacing systemic corticosteroids. May unmask allergic conditions previously suppressed by systemic steroid therapy. Caution with tuberculosis (TB), ocular herpes simplex, or untreated systemic bacterial, fungal, parasitic, or viral infections. May suppress growth in children. Exposure to chickenpox or measles requires prophylactic treatment. Not for rapid relief of bronchospasm. Rare cases of glaucoma, increased intraocular pressure (IOP), and cataract reported.

**ADVERSE REACTIONS:** Headache, pharyngitis, upper respiratory tract infection, rhinitis, increased asthma symptoms, sinusitis, dysphonia, dysmenorrhea, coughing.

**PREGNANCY:** Category C, not for use in nursing.

**MECHANISM OF ACTION:** Corticosteroid; shown to have inhibitory effects on multiple cell types (mast cells, eosinophils, neutrophils, macrophages and lymphocytes) and mediators (histamine, eicosanoids, leukotrienes and cytokines) involved in inflammatory and asthmatic response.

**PHARMACOKINETICS: Absorption:** $C_{max}$ = 88pg/mL, $T_{max}$ = 0.5 hr. **Metabolism:** Liver (biotransformation), via CYP3A4. **Elimination:** Feces, urine (<10%); $T_{1/2}$= 2.8 hrs.

## NURSING CONSIDERATIONS

**Assessment:** Assess for history of IOP, glaucoma, cataracts, concomitant diseases such as status asthmaticus, active or quiescent pulmonary TB, ocular herpes simplex, untreated systemic fungal, bacterial, parasitic or viral infections, pregnancy/nursing status, and possible drug interactions.

**Monitoring:** Monitor for localized oral infections, asthma instability (serial objective measures of airflow), body height in children, development of glaucoma, increased IOP, cataracts, adrenal insufficiency (eg, fatigue, weakness, NV, hypotension), paradoxical bronchospasm, and hypersensitivity reactions.

**Patient Counseling:** Advise that drug not intended for treatment of acute asthma (sudden symptoms of SOB or acute bronchospasm). Advise to rinse mouth after using inhaler. Inform that medication may cause reduction in growth rate (pediatrics) and may also unmask allergies (eg, rhinitis, conjunctivitis, eczema). Avoid exposure to chickenpox or measles. Advise to seek medical attention if exposed to chickenpox or measles, worsening of existing TB, infections, ocular herpes simplex, symptoms do not improve or worsen, during periods of stress or severe asthmatic attack, adrenal insufficiency (eg, fatigue, weakness, NV, hypotension), paradoxical bronchospasm or hypersensitivity reactions occur. Inform that the drug should be used at regular intervals as directed and should not be stopped abruptly.

**Administration:** Oral inhalation. Refer to PI for directions for use. **Storage:** 25°C (77°F); excursions permitted to 15-30° (59-86°F). For optimal results, canister should be at room temperature when used. Keep out of reach of children.

R

# RANEXA RX

ranolazine (CV Therapeutics)

**THERAPEUTIC CLASS:** Miscellaneous antianginal

**INDICATIONS:** Treatment of chronic angina; may coadminister with β-blockers, nitrates, calcium channel blockers, anti-platelet therapy, lipid-lowering therapy, ACE inhibitors, and angiotensin receptor blockers.

**DOSAGE:** *Adults:* Initial: 500mg bid. Titrate: May increase to 1000mg bid. Max: 1000mg bid. Concurrent With Diltiazem/Verapamil/Other Moderate CYP3A Inhibitors: 500mg bid. Concurrent With P-gp Inhibitors: Down titrate dose based on clinical response. Swallow whole; do not crush, break, or chew.

**HOW SUPPLIED:** Tab, Extended-Release: 500mg, 1000mg

**CONTRAINDICATIONS:** Strong CYP3A inhibitors (eg, ketoconazole, clarithromycin, saquinavir), CYP3A inducers (eg, rifampin, phenobarbital, carbamazepine), and hepatic dysfunction (Child-Pugh Classes A and B).

**WARNINGS/PRECAUTIONS:** May prolong QTc interval in a dose-related manner; avoid with known QT prolongation (including congenital long QT syndrome, uncorrected hypokalemia), known history of ventricular tachycardia, hepatic dysfunction. Monitor BP with severe renal impairment.

**ADVERSE REACTIONS:** Dizziness, nausea, asthenia, constipation, and headache.

**INTERACTIONS:** See Contraindications. Avoid with moderate CYP3A inhibitors, fluconazole, diltiazem, verapamil, macrolide antibiotics, HIV protease inhibitors, grapefruit juice or grapefruit-containing products. May increase levels of digoxin, simvastatin; consider dosage reduction of digoxin, simvastatin. Avoid with drugs that may prolong the QTc interval, such as Class Ia (eg, quinidine) and Class III (eg, dofetilide, sotalol) antiarrhythmics, and antipsychotics (eg, thioridazine, ziprasidone). May increase levels of drugs metabolized by CYP2D6 such as TCAs and some antipsychotics; consider dosage reduction of these drugs.

**PREGNANCY:** Category C, not for use in nursing.

**MECHANISM OF ACTION:** Not established; suspected to have antianginal and antiischemic effects that do not depend upon reductions of HR and BP.

**PHARMACOKINETICS: Absorption:** $C_{max}$=2569ng/mL, $T_{max}$=2-5 hrs. **Distribution:** Plasma protein binding (62%). **Metabolism:** Gut and liver (extensive), via CYP3A and CYP2D6. **Elimination:** Urine (75%), feces (25%), and (<5% unchanged); $T_{1/2}$=7 hrs.

## NURSING CONSIDERATIONS

**Assessment:** Assess for renal/hepatic impairment, pre-existing QT prolongation (eg, congenital long QT syndrome, uncorrected hypokalemia) or on QT-prolonging agents (eg, quinidine), ventricular tachycardia, and possible drug interactions (eg, diltiazem, potent CYP3A inhibitors, and digoxin).

**Monitoring:** Monitor SrCr, transient eosinophilia, ECG changes (eg, prolongation of the QTc interval), tumor formation, and progression to malignancy.

**Patient Counseling:** Inform about risks/benefits of drug and not to exceed recommended dose. Swallow tab whole; do not crush, break, or chew. If a dose is missed, take the prescribed dose at the next scheduled time; do not double the next dose. Do not take with grapefruit juice. Use caution while performing hazardous tasks (operating machinery/driving). Notify physician if concurrently taking any other medications.

**Administration:** Oral route. **Storage:** 25°C (77°F); excursions permitted to 15-30°C (59-86°F).



# RAPAFLO

silodosin (Watson)

RX

**THERAPEUTIC CLASS:** Alpha$_1$-antagonist

**INDICATIONS:** Treatment of the signs and symptoms of benign prostatic hyperplasia (BPH).

**DOSAGE:** *Adults:* 8mg qd with a meal. Moderate Renal Impairment (CrCl 30-50mL/min): 4mg qd with a meal.

**HOW SUPPLIED:** Cap: 4mg, 8mg

**CONTRAINDICATIONS:** Severe renal impairment (CrCl<30mL/min), severe hepatic impairment (Child-Pugh score ≥10), and concomitant administration with strong CYP3A4 inhibitors (eg, ketoconazole, clarithromycin, itraconazole, ritonavir).

**WARNINGS/PRECAUTIONS:** Postural hypotension and syncope may occur. May impair mental/physical abilities. Caution in patients with moderate renal impairment. Rule out prostrate cancer prior to therapy. Intraoperative floppy iris syndrome observed during cataract surgery in some patients on $\alpha_1$-blockers or previously treated with $\alpha_1$-blockers.

**ADVERSE REACTIONS:** Retrograde ejaculation, dizziness, diarrhea, orthostatic hypotension, headache.

**INTERACTIONS:** See Contraindications. Concomitant administration with moderate CYP3A4 inhibitors (eg, diltiazem, erythromycin, verapamil) may increase plasma concentrations. Caution with antihypertensives; monitor for possible adverse events. Avoid with strong P-gp inhibitors (eg, cyclosporine) and other α-blockers.

**PREGNANCY:** Category B, safety not known in nursing.

**MECHANISM OF ACTION:** $\alpha_1$-antagonist; blocks $\alpha_1$-adrenoreceptors, causing smooth muscle in bladder neck and prostate to relax, resulting in improved urine flow and decreased symptoms of BPH.

**PHARMACOKINETICS: Absorption:** Absolute bioavailability (32%), $C_{max}$=61.6ng/mL, $T_{max}$=2.6 hrs, $AUC_{ss}$=373.4ng•hr/mL. **Distribution:** $V_d$=49.5L; plasma protein binding (97%). **Metabolism:** Via glucuronidation (CYP3A4), KMD-3213G (main metabolite), KMD-3293 (second major metabolite). **Elimination:** Urine (33.5%), feces (54.9%); $T_{1/2}$=13.3 hrs.

## NURSING CONSIDERATIONS

**Assessment:** Assess for severe renal/hepatic impairment, prostate cancer, and possible drug interactions.

**Monitoring:** Monitor for signs/symptoms of postural hypotension, hypersensitivity reactions, and adverse reactions.

**Patient Counseling:** Counsel about possible symptoms of postural hypotension; caution about driving, operating machinery, or performing hazardous tasks. Inform that orgasm with reduced or no semen does not pose a safety concern and is reversible when drug is discontinued. Notify ophthalmologist about the use of silodosin before cataract surgery or other eye procedures, even if no longer taking silodosin.

**Administration:** Oral route. **Storage:** Store at 25°C (77°F); excursions permitted to 15-30°C (59-86°F). Protect from light and moisture.

# RAPAMUNE RX

sirolimus (Wyeth)

**Increased susceptibility to infection and possible development of lymphoma and other malignancies may result from immunosuppression. Only physicians experienced in immunosuppressive therapy and management of renal transplant patients should use sirolimus. Avoid use in liver or lung transplant patients as immunosuppressive therapy. Excess mortality and graft loss in combination with tacrolimus reported in liver transplant patients. Increased hepatic artery thrombosis (HAT) with cyclosporine or tacrolimus in liver transplant patients. Cases of bronchial anastomotic dehiscence, most fatal, reported in lung transplant patients.**

**THERAPEUTIC CLASS:** Macrocyclic lactone immunosuppressant

**INDICATIONS:** Prophylaxis of organ rejection in patients ≥13 yrs receiving renal transplants.

**DOSAGE:** *Adults:* Take initial dose as soon as possible after transplantation. Low-Moderate Immunologic Risk: Taken initially with cyclosporine and corticosteroids. LD: 6mg. Maint: 2mg qd. After cyclosporine is d/c at 2-4 months (d/c over 4-8 weeks), adjust dose to maintain blood trough concentration within target range. High-Immunologic Risk: Taken with cyclosporine and corticosteroids for the first 12 months. LD: up to 15mg on day 1 post-transplantation. Maint: 5mg/day beginning on day 2. Obtain trough level between Day 5 to 7 and adjust daily dose thereafter. Mild-Moderate Hepatic Impairment: Reduce maintenance dose by one-third. Severe Hepatic Impairment: Reduce maintenance dose by one-half. Take 4 hours after cyclosporine. Elderly: Start at low end of dosing range. Do not crush, chew or split.

*Pediatrics:* ≥13 yrs: Take initial dose as soon as possible after transplantation. Low-Moderate Immunologic Risk: Taken initially with cyclosporine and corticosteroids. LD: 6mg. Maint: 2mg qd. After cyclosporine is d/c at 2-4 months (d/c over 4-8 weeks), adjust dose to maintain blood trough concentration within target range. High-Immunologic Risk: Taken with cyclosporine and corticosteroids for the first 12 months. LD: up to 15mg on day 1 post-transplantation. Maint: 5mg/day beginning on day 2. Obtain trough level between Day 5 to 7 and adjust daily dose thereafter. ≥13 yrs and <40kg: LD: $3mg/m^2$ Maint: $1mg/m^2$/day. Mild-Moderate Hepatic Impairment: Reduce maintenance dose by one-third. Severe Hepatic Impairment: Reduce maintenance doase by one-half. Take 4 hrs after cyclosporine. Do not crush, chew or split.

**HOW SUPPLIED:** Sol: 1mg/mL; Tab: 1mg, 2mg

**WARNINGS/PRECAUTIONS:** May increase cholesterol and TG that may require treatment; monitor for hyperlipidemia. Proteinuria observed in maintenance renal transplant patients, periodic monitoring recommended. May delay recovery of renal function in patients with delayed graft function. Provide 1 year prophylaxis for *Pneumocystis carinii* pneumonia (PCP) and 3 months for cytomegalovirus (CMV) after transplant. Increased risk of skin cancer; limit exposure to sunlight and UV light. Interstitial lung disease reported. Impaired wound healing, lymphocele, wound dehiscence and fluid accumulation reported. Hypersensitivity reactions (eg, anaphylactic/anaphylactoid reactions, angioedema, exfoliative dermatitis, hypersensitivity vasculitis) reported. May activate latent viral infections (eg, BK virus-associated nephropathy). Effective contraception must be initiated before, during therapy and 12 weeks after d/c. Caution in elderly.

**ADVERSE REACTIONS:** Peripheral edema, hypertriglyceridemia, HTN, constipation, hypercholesterolemia, increased creatinine, abdominal pain, diarrhea, headache, fever, UTI, anemia, nausea, arthralgia and pain.

**INTERACTIONS:** CYP3A4 and P-gp inducers may decrease sirolimus concentrations. CYP3A4 and P-gp inhibitors may increase sirolimus concentrations. Caution with drugs that are modulators of CYP3A4 and P-gp. May increase levels with cyclosporine, bromocriptine, cimetidine, cisapride, clotrimazole, danazol, diltiazem, fluconazole, HIV-protease inhibitors (eg, ritonavir, indinavir), metoclopramide, nicardipine, troleandomycin, and verapamil. May decrease levels with carbamazepine, phenobarbital, phenytoin, rifapentine, St. John's wort. May increase verapamil concentration. Avoid with strong inhibitors (eg, ketoconazole, voriconazole, itraconazole, erythromycin, telithromycin, clarithromycin) and strong inducers (eg, rifampin, rifabutin) of CYP3A4 and P-gp. Do not dilute or take with grapefruit juice. Avoid live vaccines. Increased risk of angioedema with ACE inhibitors, rhabdomyolysis with HMG CoA reductase inhibitors/fibrates, and deterioration of renal function, serum lipid abnormalities, and urinary tract infections with calcineurin inhibitors and corticosteroids. Caution with other nephrotoxic drugs (eg, aminoglycosides, amphotericin B).

R

**PREGNANCY:** Category C, not for use in nursing.

**MECHANISM OF ACTION:** Immunosuppressant; inhibits T-lymphocyte activation and proliferation that occurs in response to antigenic and cytokine (interleukin [IL]-2, IL-4, and IL-15) stimulation by a mechanism distinct from that of other immunosuppressants. Also inhibits antibody production. Prolongs allograft survival and suppresses immune-mediated events (animal study).

**PHARMACOKINETICS: Absorption:** (Sol) AUC =194ng•h/mL, $C_{max}$=14.4ng/mL, $T_{max}$=2.1hrs, bioavailability=14%. (Tab) AUC =230ng•h/mL, $C_{max}$=15ng/mL, $T_{max}$=3.5hrs. **Distribution:** $V_d$=12L/kg; plasma protein binding (approximately 92%). **Metabolism:** CYP3A4 and P-gp, intestinal wall, liver (extensive) via O-demethylation and hydroxylation; hydroxy, demethyl and hydroxymethyl (major metabolites). **Elimination:** Feces (91%), urine (2.2%); $T_{1/2}$=62 hrs. Different pharmacokinetic data resulted from concentration-controlled trials of pediatric renal transplants.

## NURSING CONSIDERATIONS

**Assessment:** Assess for drug hypersensitivity, low-moderate immunologic risk or high immunological risk patients, hepatic impairment, body weight/body mass index, hyperlipidemia, risk of CMV infection, pregnancy/nursing status and possible drug interactions.

**Monitoring:** Monitor for infections including opportunistic infections such as TB, CMV, and PCP, fatal infections and sepsis, lymphoma, skin malignancy, anaphylactic/anaphylactoid reactions, angioedema, exfoliative dermatitis and hypersensitivity vasculitis, delayed wound healing and lymphocele, interstitial lung disease (eg, pneumonitis, bronchiolitis obliterans organizing pneumonia, and pulmonary fibrosis), and hyperlipidemia. Monitor for urinary protein excretion, renal/hepatic functions, cholesterol, TG, and BP.

**Patient Counseling:** Instruct to avoid prolonged exposure to sunlight and UV light. Instruct not to take during pregnancy/nursing. Instruct to use effective contraception prior to, during therapy and 12 weeks after therapy has been stopped. Inform to take with/without food, but do not crush, chew, or split.

**Administration:** Oral route. **Storage:** (Sol) 2-8°C (36-46°F), should be used within 1 month once opened. May store at temperatures up to 25°C (77°F) for a short period of time (eg, ≤15 days). (Tab) 20-25°C (68-77°F). Protect from light.

## Razadyne ER — RX

galantamine hbr (Ortho-McNeil)

**OTHER BRAND NAMES:** Razadyne (Ortho-McNeil)

**THERAPEUTIC CLASS:** Acetycholinesterase inhibitor

**INDICATIONS:** Treatment of mild to moderate dementia of the Alzheimer's type.

**DOSAGE:** *Adults:* (Sol, Tab) Initial: 4mg bid with am and pm meals. Titrate: Increase to 8mg bid after 4 weeks if tolerated, then increase to 12mg bid after 4 weeks if tolerated. Usual: 16-24mg/day. Max: 24mg/day. (Cap, ER) Initial: 8mg qd with am meal. Titrate: Increase to 16mg qd after 4 weeks, then increase to 24mg qd after 4 weeks if tolerated. Usual: 16-24mg/day. Max: 24mg/day. If therapy is interrupted, restart at lowest dose and increase to current dose. Moderate Renal/Hepatic Impairment (Child-Pugh: 7-9): Caution during dose titration. Max: 16mg/day. Avoid use with severe renal (CrCl <9mL/min) and severe hepatic impairment (Child-Pugh: 10-15).

**HOW SUPPLIED:** Sol: (Razadyne) 4mg/mL [100mL]; Tab: (Razadyne) 4mg, 8mg, 12mg. Cap, Extended-Release: (Razadyne ER) 8mg, 16mg, 24mg.

**WARNINGS/PRECAUTIONS:** Vagotonic effects; caution with supraventricular conduction disorder. May cause bradycardia and/or heart block. Caution with asthma or obstructive pulmonary disease. Monitor for active or occult GI bleeding and ulcers due to increased gastric acid secretion. Risk of generalized convulsions or bladder outflow obstruction. Ensure adequate fluid intake during treatment. Deaths reported with mild cognitive impairment.

**ADVERSE REACTIONS:** N/V, diarrhea, anorexia, weight loss, fatigue, dizziness, headache, depression, insomnia, abdominal pain, dyspepsia, UTI.

**INTERACTIONS:** Potential to interfere with anticholinergics. Synergistic effect with succinylcholine, other cholinesterase inhibitors, similar neuromuscular blockers, or cholinergic agonists (eg, bethanechol). Increased levels with cimetidine, ketoconazole, and paroxetine. Caution with drugs that slow heart rate due to vagotonic effects. Monitor for GI bleeding with NSAIDs.

**PREGNANCY:** Category B, not for use in nursing.

**MECHANISM OF ACTION:** Unknown; suspected to inhibit acetylcholinesterase-enhancing cholinergic function by increasing concentration of acetylcholine through reversible inhibition of its hydrolysis.

**PHARMACOKINETICS: Absorption:** Bioavailability: (90% rapid and complete), $T_{max}$=1 hr. **Distribution:** $V_d$=175L; plasma protein binding (18%). **Metabolism:** Liver (glucuronidation). CYP450 enzymes: 2D6, 3A4. **Elimination:** Urine (unchanged); $T_{1/2}$=7 hrs.

### NURSING CONSIDERATIONS

**Assessment:** Assess for drug hypersensitivity, cardiovascular conduction defects, GI bleeding, ulcer disease, severe asthma or COPD, renal/hepatic function, and possible drug interactions.

**Monitoring:** Monitor closely for symptoms of active or occult GI bleeding, and cardiac conduction defects. Monitor for common adverse events (eg, NV, anorexia, dizziness, syncope).

**Patient Counseling:** Take drug preferably with morning and evening meals. Ensure adequate fluid intake during treatment. If therapy has been interrupted for several days or longer, physician must restart patient at lowest dose and gradually increase to current dose. Report any adverse effects.

**Administration:** Oral route. **Storage:** 25°C (77°F); excursions permitted to 15-30°C (59-86°F). Do not freeze.

## REBETOL **RX**

ribavirin (Schering)

**Not for monotherapy treatment of chronic hepatitis C. Primary toxicity is hemolytic anemia. Avoid with significant or unstable cardiac disease. Contraindicated in pregnancy and male partners of pregnant women. Use 2 reliable forms of contraception during therapy and for 6 months after discontinuation.**

**THERAPEUTIC CLASS:** Nucleoside analogue

**INDICATIONS:** In combination with interferon alfa-2b (pegylated and nonpegylated) for treatment of chronic hepatitis C in patients ≥3 yrs with compensated liver disease.

**DOSAGE:** *Adults:* ≥18 yrs: With Intron A: ≤75kg: 400mg qam and 600mg qpm. >75kg: 600mg qam and 600mg qpm. Treat for 24-48 weeks interferon-naive; 24 weeks in relapse. With Peg-Intron: <40-65kg: 400mg qam and 400mg qpm. 66-80kg: 400mg qam and 600mg pm. 81-105kg: 600mg qam and 600mg qpm. >105kg: 600mg qam and 800mg qpm. Interferon-alpha naive: Genotype 1: Treat for 48 weeks. D/C if <2 $log_{10}$ drop or loss of HCV-RNA at 12 weeks or if HCV-RNA remain detectable after 24 weeks. Genotype 2 or 3: Treat for 24 weeks. Relapse: Treat for 48 weeks. D/C if with detectable HCV-RNA at week 12 or 24. Refer to PI for dose modification based on laboratory parameters. Elderly: Start at lower end of dosing range.
*Pediatrics:* ≥3 yrs: <47kg: 15mg/kg/day divided into two doses. 47-59kg: 400mg qam and 400mg qpm. 60-73kg: 400mg qam and 600mg qpm. >73: 600mg qam and 600mg qpm. May use sol regardless of body weight. Genotype 1: Treat for 48 weeks. D/C at 12 weeks if HCV-RNA dropped <2 $log_{10}$ compared to pretreatment or at 24 weeks if still with detectable HCV-RNA. Genotype 2 or 3: Treat for 24 weeks. If reached 18th birthday while receiving therapy, should remain on pediatric dosing. Refer to PI for dose modification based on laboratory parameters.

R

**HOW SUPPLIED:** Cap: 200mg; Sol: 40mg/mL [100mL]

**CONTRAINDICATIONS:** Pregnancy, male partners of pregnant women, autoimmune hepatitis, hemoglobinopathies (eg, thalassemia major, sickle cell anemia), CrCl <50mL/min, concomitant use with didanosine.

**WARNINGS/PRECAUTIONS:** Patients with the following characteristics are less likely to benefit from retreatment after failing a course of therapy: previous nonresponse, previous pegylated interferon treatment, significant bridging fibrosis or cirrhosis, and genotype 1 infection. Hemolytic anemia may occur with a significant initial drop in hemoglobin; hemoglobin or hematocrit should be obtained pretreatment and at weeks 2 and 4 of therapy or more frequently. Suspend therapy in patients with signs and symptoms of pancreatitis and d/c therapy in patients with confirmed cases of pancreatitis. Pulmonary symptoms, including dyspnea, pulmonary infiltrates, pneumonitis, pulmonary hypertension, and pneumonia, have been reported; if appropriate d/c combination therapy of ribavirin and alpha interferon. All patients should receive an examination at baseline; d/c combination therapy in patients who develop new or worsening ophthalmologic disorders. Severe decreases in neutrophil and platelet counts, and hematologic, endocrine (eg, TSH), and hepatic abnormalities; monitor labs at baseline, weeks 2, 4, 8, 12, and then at 6-week intervals or more frequently. Dental/periodontal disorders reported with combination therapy. Weight loss and growth inhibition reported with combination therapy in pediatric patients. There are significant adverse reactions caused by combination therapy, including severe depression and suicidal ideation, hemolytic anemia, suppression of bone marrow function, autoimmune and infectious disorders, pulmonary dysfunction, pancreatitis, and diabetes. Caution in elderly.

**ADVERSE REACTIONS:** Hemolytic anemia, headache, fatigue/asthenia, rigors, fever, N/V, anorexia, myalgia, arthralgia, insomnia, irritability, depression, neutropenia.

**INTERACTIONS:** See Contraindications. Closely monitor for toxicities (hepatic decompensation, anemia) with nucleoside reverse transcriptase inhibitors (NRTIs); d/c NRTI, reduce dose or d/c interferon, ribavirin or both with worsening toxicities. Caution with lamivudine, stavudine and zidovudine.

**PREGNANCY:** Category X, not for use in nursing.

**MECHANISM OF ACTION:** Nucleoside analog; not established. Has direct antiviral activity in tissue culture against many RNA viruses; increases mutation frequency in the genomes of several viruses and ribavirin triphosphate inhibits HCV polymerase in a biochemical reaction.

**PHARMACOKINETICS: Absorption:** Rapid; (Cap) $C_{max}$=782ng/mL, $T_{max}$=1.7 hrs, AUC=13400ng•h/mL; absolute bioavailability (64%). (Sol) $C_{max}$=872ng/mL, $T_{max}$=1 hr, AUC=14098ng•h/mL. **Distribution:** (Cap) $V_d$=2825L. **Metabolism:** Nucleated cells (phosphorylation); deribosylation and amide hydrolysis. **Elimination:** Urine (61%), feces (12%). (Cap) $T_{1/2}$=43.6 hrs.

## NURSING CONSIDERATIONS

**Assessment:** Assess for history of hemoglobinopathy (eg, thalassemia major, sickle-cell anemia, anemia), depression, hepatic/renal dysfunction (eg, autoimmune hepatitis), DM, autoimmune disorders, infections, bone marrow suppression, pancreatitis, pregnancy status (including female partners of male patients), ophthalmic disorders, cardiac and lung disease. Prior to initiation; conduct pregnancy test, hematologic test (CBC with differential, Hct, Hgb), chemistries (LFTs, TSH) and ECG.

**Monitoring:** Monitor CBC, LFTs, TSH, and ECG periodically. Monitor height and weight in pediatrics. Obtain Hct and Hgb (Week 2 and 4, more if needed). Perform pregnancy test monthly and 6 months after d/c of therapy (including female partners of male patients). Schedule regular dental exams. Perform periodic ophthalmologic exams. Monitor for signs/symptoms of anemia, pancreatitis, renal/hepatic dysfunction, cardiac deterioration, pulmonary impairment, dental/periodontal disorders, suicidal ideation and depression.

**Patient Counseling:** Counsel risk/benefits associated with treatment. Instruct to take with food and keep well hydrated; do not open, break or crush capsules before swallowing. Counsel that if dose missed, take as soon as possible during same day; do not double dose. Inform of pregnancy risks. Use 2 forms of contraception during therapy and 6 months after d/c of therapy (including female partners of male patients). Advise that to reduce damage to teeth and oral membranes from dry mouth, brush teeth bid and if vomiting is experienced, rinse mouth thoroughly. Seek medical attention if signs/symptoms of pancreatitis, hepatic dysfunction, depression (suicidal ideation), anemia, cardiac deterioration or pulmonary impairment occur.

**Administration:** Oral route. **Storage:** Cap: 25°C (77°F); excursions permitted to 15-30°C (59-86°F). Sol: 2-8°C (36-46°F) or 25°C (77°F); excursions permitted to 15-30°C (59-86°F).

# REBIF — RX

interferon beta-1a (EMD Serono)

**THERAPEUTIC CLASS:** Biological response modifier

**INDICATIONS:** Treatment of patients with relapsing forms of multiple sclerosis.

**DOSAGE:** *Adults:* Initial: 20% of prescribed dose SQ 3x/week; 4.4mcg for prescribed dose of 22mcg, 8.8mcg for prescribed dose of 44mcg. Titrate:

R

Increase over a 4-week period to either 22mcg or 44mcg SQ 3x/week. Maint: 22mcg or 44mcg SQ 3x/week. Refer to PI for full schedule for patient titration. Leukopenia/Elevated LFTs: Reduce dose until toxicity resolves. Administer dose at the same time every day (late afternoon, evening) on the same 3 days/week at least 48 hrs apart.

**HOW SUPPLIED:** Inj: 22mcg/0.5mL [12[s]], 44mcg/0.5mL [12[s]]; Titration Pack: 8.8mcg/0.2mL and 22mcg/0.5mL

**WARNINGS/PRECAUTIONS:** Caution with depression, alcohol abuse, active hepatic disease, increased serum SGPT (>2.5x ULN), history of significant hepatic disease, seizure disorder. Consider discontinuing therapy if depression, jaundice/hepatic dysfunction develops. Reduce dose if serum SGPT >5x ULN. Contains albumin; theoretical risk of viral disease transmission. Prolonged use may cause allergic reactions, some severe.

**ADVERSE REACTIONS:** Psychiatric disorders, injection-site disorders, influenza-like symptoms (eg, headache, fatigue, fever, rigors, chest pain), back pain, myalgia, abdominal pain, depression, elevation of liver enzymes, hematologic abnormalities.

**INTERACTIONS:** Monitor with myelosuppressive agents. Potential risk for increased hepatotoxicty with other hepatotoxic agents. The overall effectiveness of concomitant vaccination is unknown.

**PREGNANCY:** Category C, caution in nursing.

**MECHANISM OF ACTION:** Biological response modifier; binding of interferon beta to its receptors initiates a complex cascade of intracellular events that leads to the expression of numerous interferon-induced gene products and markers, including 2, 5-oligoadenylate synthetase, beta 2-microglobulin and neopterin, which may mediate some of the biological activities. The specific interferon-induced proteins and mechanisms by which interferon beta-1a exerts its effects in multiple sclerosis have not been fully defined.

**PHARMACOKINETICS: Absorption:** $C_{max}$=5.1 IU/mL, $T_{max}$=16 hrs, $AUC_{0-96}$=294 IU•h/mL. **Elimination:** $T_{1/2}$=69 hrs.

## NURSING CONSIDERATIONS

**Assessment:** Assess for drug hypersensitivity, depression, liver disease or increased serum glutamic pyruvic transaminase, alcohol abuse, thyroid dysfunction, preexisting seizure disorder, myelosuppression, pregnancy/nursing status, and possible drug interactions.

**Monitoring:** Monitor blood cell counts and LFTs at 1, 3, and 6 months after initiation, then periodically. Monitor thyroid function tests every 6 months with history of thyroid dysfunction. Monitor tests used for monitoring MS, depression, suicidal ideation, suicide attempts, hepatic dysfunction, jaundice, seizures, anaphylaxis, skin rash, urticaria, and Creutzfeldt-Jakob disease (CJD).



**Patient Counseling:** Do not change dosage or schedule without consulting physician. Inform about risks/benefits of drug; report any adverse reactions. Notify if pregnant/nursing or planning to become pregnant. Instruct on aseptic technique when administering drug and on importance of proper syringe disposal. Inform of the importance of rotating injection sites.

**Administration:** SQ route. Rotate site of injection. **Storage:** Refrigerate 2-8°C (36-46°F). Do not freeze. If refrigerator is not available, store at or below 25°C (77°F) up to 30 days, away from heat and light.

# RECLAST RX

zoledronic acid (Novartis)

**THERAPEUTIC CLASS:** Bisphosphonate

**INDICATIONS:** Treatment and prevention of osteoporosis in postmenopausal women. Treatment to increase bone mass in men with osteoporosis. Treatment and prevention of glucocorticoid-induced osteoporosis in men and women who are either initiating or continuing systemic glucocorticoids in a daily dosage equivalent to 7.5mg or greater of prednisone and who are expected to remain on glucocorticoids for at least 12 months. Treatment of Paget's disease of bone in men and women.

**DOSAGE:** *Adults:* Osteoporosis (Men/Postmenopausal Women): 5mg IV once a year over ≥15 mins at a constant infusion rate. Paget's disease: 5mg IV once a year over ≥15 mins at a constant infusion rate. Prevention of Osteoporosis (Postmenopausal Women): 5mg IV once every 2 years over ≥15 mins at a constant infusion rate. Treatment/Prevention of Glucocorticoid-Induced Osteoporosis: 5mg IV once a year over ≥15 mins at a constant infusion rate. CrCl ≥ 35mL/min: 5mg IV over ≥15 mins. CrCl <35mL/min: Avoid use. Recommended Intake of Calcium in Osteoporosis: 1200mg/day. Recommended Intake of Vitamin D in Osteoporosis: 800-1000 IU/day. Recommended Intake of Calcium in Paget's Disease: 1500mg/day in 2-3 divided doses. Recommended Intake of Vitamin D in Paget's Disease: 800 IU/day, particularly in 2 weeks following zoledronic acid administration. Hydrate prior to administration. Administration of acetaminophen following administration may reduce incidence of acute phase reaction symptoms.

**HOW SUPPLIED:** Sol: 5mg/100mL [100mL]

**CONTRAINDICATIONS:** Hypocalcemia.

**WARNINGS/PRECAUTIONS:** Prior to treatment, pre-existing hypocalcemia and disturbances of mineral metabolism (eg, hypoparathyroidism, thyroid surgery, parathyroid surgery, malabsorption syndromes) must be treated and serum calcium and mineral levels (phosphorus, magnesium) must be monitored during treatment for these patients. Increases risk of hypocalcemia; may need calcium and vitamin D supplements. Not recommended for use in patients with severe renal impairment (CrCl <35mL/min); monitor SrCr before each dose; carefully monitor renal function in elderly. Renal impairment may occur, especially with pre-existing renal compromise or other risk factors (eg, concomitant nephrotoxic medications, concomitant diuretic therapy, severe dehydration). May cause osteonecrosis of the jaw; routine oral exam needed prior to treatment; preventive dentistry should be considered prior to treatment in patients with history of concomitant risk factors (eg, cancer, chemotherapy, radiotherapy, corticosteroids, poor oral hygiene, pre-existing dental disease or infection, anemia, coagulopathy). Avoid during pregnancy. Musculoskeletal pain may occur; d/c if severe symptoms develop. Caution with aspirin-sensitive patients; may cause bronchoconstriction.

**ADVERSE REACTIONS:** Pain, chills, diarrhea, dizziness, osteoarthritis, fatigue, hypocalcemia, headache, HTN, influenza-like illness, myalgia, arthralgia, pyrexia, dyspepsia, N/V.

**INTERACTIONS:** Caution with aminoglycosides; may have an additive effect to lower serum calcium levels for prolonged periods. Caution when used in combination with loop diuretics; may increase risk of hypocalcemia. Caution with other nephrotoxic drugs (eg, NSAIDs). Avoid use in patients treated with Zometa, which contains same active ingredient. Exposure to concomitant medications that are primarily renally excreted (eg, digoxin) may increase in patients with renal impairment.

**PREGNANCY:** Category D, not for use in nursing.

**MECHANISM OF ACTION:** Bisphosphonate; acts primarily on bone. Inhibits osteoclast-mediated bone resorption.

**PHARMACOKINETICS: Distribution:** Plasma protein binding (28-53%). **Elimination:** Urine, feces (<3%), $T_{1/2}$=146 hrs.

## NURSING CONSIDERATIONS

**Assessment:** Assess for hypocalcemia and disturbances of mineral metabolism (eg, hypoparathyroidism, malabsorption syndromes). Assess for renal impairment and for risk factors for developing renal impairment (eg, dehydration); measure SrCr before each dose. Assess for presence of risk factors for developing osteonecrosis of the jaw (eg, poor oral hygeine, pre-existing dental disease or infection, cancer, anemia, coagulopathy); perform dental exam prior to treatment in patients with risk factors. Assess for aspirin sensitivity, pregnancy/nursing status, and for possible drug interactions.

**Monitoring:** Monitor for signs and symptoms of hypocalcemia; monitor calcium and mineral levels (phosphorus, magnesium) in patients with pre-existing hypocalcemia and mineral metabolism disturbances. Monitor for renal impairment; measure SrCr levels. Monitor for signs and symptoms of acute phase reactions (eg, fever, myalgia, flu like symptoms, headache, arthralgia), osteonecrosis of the jaw, bone/joint/muscle pain, and for bronchoconstriction.

**Patient Counseling:** Advise to take calcium in divided doses for a total of 1500mg/day, along with 800 IU/day of vitamin D in Paget's disease. Advise to take 1200mg/day of calcium with 800-1000 IU/day of vitamin D in osteoporosis. Instruct to notify physician if pregnant or nursing or if have an aspirin sensitivity. Advise on day of treatment to eat and drink normally and to drink at least 2 glasses of fluid (eg, water). Counsel about possible possible adverse effects; instruct to contact physician or dentist if develop persistent pain and/or non-healing sore of the mouth or jaw.

**Administration:** IV route. **Storage:** 25°C (77°F); excursions permitted to 15-30°C (59-86°F). Stable for 24 hrs at 2-8°C (36-46°F) after opening. If refrigerated, allow to reach room temperature before administration.

## RECOMBIVAX HB — RX

hepatitis B (recombinant) (Merck)

**OTHER BRAND NAMES:** Recombivax HB Pediatric/Adolescent (Merck) - Recombivax HB Dialysis (Merck) - Recombivax HB Adult (Merck)

**THERAPEUTIC CLASS:** Vaccine

**INDICATIONS:** Vaccination against hepatitis B virus.

**DOSAGE:** *Adults:* Give IM into deltoid muscle. Give SQ if risk of hemorrhage. ≥20 yrs: 3-Dose Regimen: 10mcg at 0,1,6 months. Predialysis/Dialysis (Dialysis Formulation): 40mcg at 0,1,6, months; consider booster if anti-HBs level <10MIU/mL.

*Pediatrics:* Give IM into anterolateral thigh in infants/young children. Give SQ if risk of hemorrhage. 0-19 yrs: 3-Dose Regimen (Pediatric/Adolescent Formulation) 5mcg at 0,1,6 months. 11-15 yrs: 2-Dose Regimen (Adult Formulation): 10mcg 1st dose, 10mcg 4-6 months later. Infants Born to HBsAg Positive/Unknown Status Mothers: Give 3-dose regimen vaccine and 0.5mL HBIG in opposite anterolateral thigh.

**HOW SUPPLIED:** Inj: (Pediatric/Adolescent-Preservative Free) 5mcg/0.5mL, (Adult) 10mcg/mL, (Dialysis) 40mcg/mL

**CONTRAINDICATIONS:** Yeast hypersensitivity.

**WARNINGS/PRECAUTIONS:** Do not continue therapy if hypersensitivity occurs after injection. May not prevent hepatitis B with unrecognized infection. Caution with severely compromised cardiopulmonary status and those where febrile or systemic reaction is a significant risk. May delay use with serious active infection (eg, febrile illness). Have epinephrine available. Do not give intradermally or IV.

**ADVERSE REACTIONS:** Irritability, fever, diarrhea, fatigue/weakness, diminished appetite, rhinitis, injection-site reactions.

**PREGNANCY:** Category C, caution in nursing.

**MECHANISM OF ACTION:** Stimulation of immune response to produce antibodies that may protect against all subtypes of hepatitis B virus infection.

### NURSING CONSIDERATIONS

**Assessment:** Assess current health status, medical history, previous vaccination history, possible drug interactions, and HBsAg status in pregnancy.

**Monitoring:** Monitor hypersensitivity reactions, injection site for pain, swelling, pruritus and erythema, fever, headache, nausea, diarrhea, fatigue/weakness, pharyngitis, and upper respiratory tract infection.

**Patient Counseling:** Inform of potential benefits/risks ratio; report any adverse reactions to physician.

**Administration:** IM. **Storage:** 2-8°C (36-46°F). Do not freeze.

R

# REFLUDAN RX

lepirudin (Bayer Healthcare)

**THERAPEUTIC CLASS:** Thrombin inhibitor

**INDICATIONS:** Anticoagulant for heparin-induced thrombocytopenia (HIT) and associated thromboembolic disease.

**DOSAGE:** *Adults:* LD: 0.4mg/kg (max 44mg) IV over 15-20 seconds. Initial: 0.15mg/kg/hr (max 16.5mg/hr) continuous infusion for 2-10 days. Adjust dose based on aPTT. If aPTT is above target range, stop infusion for 2 hrs and restart at 50% of previous rate. Check aPTT 4 hrs later. If aPTT is below target range, increase rate in steps of 20% and check aPTT 4 hrs later. Do not exceed 0.21mg/kg/hr. Renal Impairment: LD: 0.2mg/kg. Initial: CrCl 45-60 mL/min: 0.075mg/kg/hr. CrCl 30-44mL/min: 0.045mg/kg/hr. CrCl 15-29 mL/min: 0.0225mg/kg/hr. CrCl <15mL/min/Hemodialysis: Avoid or stop infusion. Concomitant Thrombolytic Therapy: LD: 0.2mg/kg. Initial: 0.1mg/kg/hr.

**HOW SUPPLIED:** Inj: 50mg

**WARNINGS/PRECAUTIONS:** Risk of bleeding. Weigh risks/benefits with recent puncture of large vessels or organ biopsy, anomaly of vessels or organs, recent CVA, stroke, intracerebral surgery or other neuraxial procedures, severe uncontrolled HTN, bacterial endocarditis, advanced renal impairment, hemorrhagic diathesis, recent major surgery or bleeding. Avoid with baseline aPTT ≥2.5. Monitor aPTT 4 hrs after initiating infusion and at least once daily. Liver injury may enhance anticoagulant effects. Antihirudin antibodies reported; may increase anticoagulant effects.

**ADVERSE REACTIONS:** Hemorrhagic events (eg, bleeding, anemia, hematoma, hematuria, epistaxis, hemothorax), fever, liver dysfunction, pneumonia, sepsis, allergic skin reactions, multiorgan failure.

**INTERACTIONS:** Thrombolytics increase risk of life-threatening intracranial bleeding or other bleeding complications and may enhance the effect on aPTT prolongation. Increased risk of bleeding with coumarin derivatives and other drugs that affect platelet function.

**PREGNANCY:** Category B, not for use in nursing.

**MECHANISM OF ACTION:** Thrombin inhibitor; binds to thrombin and thereby blocks its thrombogenic activity.

**PHARMACOKINETICS: Absorption:** $C_{max}$=1500ng/mL. **Distribution:** $V_d$=12.2L. **Metabolism:** Catabolic hydrolysis. **Elimination:** Urine(48%); $T_{1/2}$=1.3 hrs.

## NURSING CONSIDERATIONS

**Assessment:** Assess for bleeding risk (eg, recent puncture of large vessels, recent cerebrovascular accident, severe uncontrolled HTN, bacterial endocarditis, hemorrhagic diasthesis), presence of hepatic/renal dysfunction, nursing status, and drug interactions. Obtain baseline aPTT ratio.

**Monitoring:** Monitor for signs/symptoms of bleeding complications (eg, intracranial bleeding) and allergic reactions (eg, anaphylactic reactions). Monitor aPTT ratio 4 hours after start of infusion and perform once daily thereafter during treatment.

**Patient Counseling:** Instruct to notify physician immediately if develop any type of allergic reaction (eg, anaphylaxis). Advise about increased risk of bleeding during therapy. Laboratory monitoring is needed during therapy.

**Administration:** IV route. Do not mix with other drugs. Reconstitute: 1) Use Sterile Water for Inj, USP; or 0.9% for NaCl Inj, USP. 2) For rapid, complete reconstitution, inject 1mL of diluent into the vial and shake it gently. 3) Further dilute to final concentration of 5mg/mL. Dilute using 0.9% NaCl Inj USP, or 5% Dextrose Inj USP. 4) Warm to room temperature prior to administration. **Storage:** Unopened vials: 2-25°C (35.6-77°F). Reconstituted: Use immediately; will remain stable for 24 hrs at room temperature.

# RELENZA RX

zanamivir (GlaxoSmithKline)

**THERAPEUTIC CLASS:** Neuraminidase inhibitor

**INDICATIONS:** Treatment of uncomplicated acute illness due to influenza A and B virus in adults and pediatric patients (>7 yrs) symptomatic for ≤2 days. Prophylaxis of influenza in adults and pediatric patients >5 yrs.

**DOSAGE:** *Adults:* Treatment: Usual: 2 inh (10mg) q12h for 5 days. Take 2 doses on 1st day at least 2 hrs apart; then 12 hrs apart on subsequent days. Prophylaxis: Household Setting: 2 inh (10mg) qd for 10 days. Community Outbreaks: 2 inh (10mg) qd for 28 days. Administer at same time every day. *Pediatrics:* Treatment: ≥7 yrs: Usual: 2 inh (10mg) q12h for 5 days. Two doses should be taken on first day at least 2 hrs apart; then 12 hrs apart on subsequent days. Prophylaxis: ≥5 yrs: Household Setting: 2 inh (10mg) qd for 10 days. Community Outbreaks: 2 inh (10mg) qd for 28 days. Administer at same time every day.

**HOW SUPPLIED:** Disk: 5mg/inh [4 blisters]

**CONTRAINDICATIONS:** Allergy to lactose

**WARNINGS/PRECAUTIONS:** Not a substitute for annual influenza vaccination. Not recommended for use with underlying airways disease (eg, asthma, COPD). Serious cases of bronchospasm reported during treatment; d/c if bronchospasm or decline in respiratory function develops. D/C if allergic reaction occurs. Postmarketing neuropsychiatric events (eg, seizures, delirium, hallucinations) reported. Not shown to prevent complications secondary to flu-like or concurrent bacterial infections.

**ADVERSE REACTIONS:** Headaches, diarrhea, nausea, sinusitis, cough, ear/nose/throat infections, nasal symptoms, throat/tonsil discomfort and pain, muscle pain, musculoskeletal pain, malaise/fatigue, fever/chills, viral respiratory infection, decreased/increased appetite, anorexia.

**INTERACTIONS:** Avoid administration of live attenuated influenza vaccine within 2 weeks before or 48 hrs after.

**PREGNANCY:** Category C, caution in nursing.

**MECHANISM OF ACTION:** Neuraminidase inhibitor; inhibits influenza virus neuraminidase, affecting release of viral particles.

**PHARMACOKINETICS: Absorption:** Absolute bioavailability (4-17%); $C_{max}$=17-142ng/mL; $T_{max}$=1-2 hrs; AUC=111-1364ng•hr/mL. **Distribution:** Plasma protein binding (<10%). **Elimination**: Renal; $T_{1/2}$=2.5-5.1 hrs.

R

## NURSING CONSIDERATIONS

**Assessment:** Assess for history of allergic reaction to lactose (milk proteins) and airway diseases (asthma or COPD).

**Monitoring:** Monitor for signs/symptoms of bronchospasm (worsening wheezing, SOB), allergic-like reactions (oropharyngeal edema, serious skin rashes, anaphylaxis) and neuropsychiatric events (seizures, hallucinations, abnormal behavior). Respiratory function must be monitored in patients with underlying airway disease.

**Patient Counseling:** Advise to seek medical attention if symptoms of bronchospasm (worsening wheezing, SOB), allergic reaction (oropharyngeal edema, rash), or neuropsychiatric events (seizures, confusion, abnormal behavior) occur. Inform that the use of zanamavir does not reduce the risk of transmission. Use inhaled bronchodilator before therapy. Do not puncture any zanamavir blister until taking a dose using the diskhaler. Instruct on proper use of diskhaler.

**Administration:** Oral route. **Storage**: 25°C (77°F); excursions permitted to 15-30°C (59-86°F).

# Relpax RX

eletriptan hydrobromide (Pfizer)

**THERAPEUTIC CLASS:** 5-$HT_{1B/1D}$ agonist

**INDICATIONS:** Acute treatment of migraine with or without aura.

**DOSAGE:** *Adults:* ≥18 yrs: Initial: 20 or 40mg at onset of headache. If recurs after initial relief, may repeat after 2 hrs. Max: 40mg/dose or 80mg/day. Safety of treating >3 headaches/30 days not known. Severe Hepatic Impairment: Avoid use. Avoid within 72 hrs of potent CYP3A4 inhibitors.

**HOW SUPPLIED:** Tab: 20mg, 40mg

**CONTRAINDICATIONS:** Ischemic heart disease, coronary artery vasospasm (eg, Prinzmetal's angina) or other significant underlying cardiovascular disease, peripheral vascular disease, cerebrovascular syndromes, uncontrolled HTN, hemiplegic or basilar migraine, use within 24 hrs of other 5-$HT_1$ agonist or ergot-type agent (eg, dihydroergotamine, methysergide), severe hepatic impairment.

**WARNINGS/PRECAUTIONS:** Confirm diagnosis. Supervise 1st dose and monitor cardiac function in those at risk of CAD (eg, HTN, hypercholesterolemia, smoker, obesity, diabetes, CAD family history, postmenopausal women, males >40 yrs). Consider ECG during interval immediately following initial administration in patients with CAD risk factors. Monitor cardiac function in intermittent long-term users with CAD risk factors. Serious adverse cardiac events, increased BP, cerebrovascular events, vasospastic reactions reported. Serotonin syndrome symptoms (eg, mental status changes, autonomic instability, neuromuscular aberrations, and GI symptoms) reported. Caution in elderly. Possible long-term ophthalmic effects.

**ADVERSE REACTIONS:** Asthenia, chest tightness, dizziness, dry mouth, headache, nausea, paresthesia, somnolence, pain/pressure/heaviness in precordium/throat/jaw.

**INTERACTIONS:** Prolonged vasospastic reactions reported with ergot-containing drugs; avoid within 24 hrs of each other. Avoid within 72 hrs of potent CYP3A4 inhibitors (eg, ketoconazole, itraconazole, nefazodone, troleandomycin, clarithromycin, ritonavir, nelfinavir). Serotonin syndrome reported with combined use of an SSRI or SNRI. Avoid within 24 hrs of other 5-$HT_1$ agonists. Propranolol, erythromycin, verapamil, fluconazole may increase levels.

**PREGNANCY:** Category C, caution in nursing.

**MECHANISM OF ACTION:** Selective $5HT_{1D/1B}$ agonist; binds with high affinity to $5HT_{1D/1B/1F}$ receptors. Believed to activate receptors located on intracranial blood vessels, including those on arteriovenous ananstomoses, which leads to vasoconstriction and is correlated with relief of migraine headache. Activation of receptors located on sensory nerve endings in trigeminal system results in inhibition of pro-inflammatory neuropeptide release.

**PHARMACOKINETICS: Absorption:** Complete; absolute bioavailability (50%); $T_{max}$=1.5 hrs. **Distribution:** $V_d$=138L; plasma protein binding (85%). **Metabolism:** N-demethylated (active metabolite). **Elimination:** $T_{1/2}$= 4 hrs (parent drug), 13 hrs (metabolite).

## NURSING CONSIDERATIONS

**Assessment:** Confirm diagnosis of migraine before therapy. Assess for IHD (eg, angina pectoris, Prinzmetal's variant angina, MI or documented silent MI), cerebrovascular syndrome (eg, stroke, TIAs), HTN, hemiplegic or basilar migraine, PVD, presence of CAD risk factors (eg, hypercholesterolemia, smoking, obesity, DM, strong family history of CAD, female with surgical or physiological menopause, or male >49 yrs), ECG changes, hepatic/renal impairment, pregnancy/nursing status, and possible drug interactions.

**Monitoring:** Administration of 1st dose should be in physician's office or medically staffed and equipped facility as cardiac ischemia can occur in absence of clinical symptoms; ECG should be obtained immediately during interval in those with risk factors. Monitor for signs/symptoms of cardiac events (eg, coronary vasospasm, acute MI, arrhythmia, ECG changes, follow-up coronary

R

angiography), cerebrovascular events (eg, hemorrhage, stroke, TIAs), peripheral vascular ischemia, colonic ischemia with bloody diarrhea and abdominal pain, serotonin syndrome (eg, mental status changes, autonomic instability, neuromuscular aberrations and/or GI symptoms), ophthalmic effects, and increased BP.

**Patient Counseling:** Inform about potential benefits/risks (eg, symptoms of serotonin syndrome especially if taken with SSRIs or SNRIs). Advise to take exactly as prescribed. Instruct to notify physician if pregnant/nursing or planning to become pregnant.

**Administration:** Oral route. **Storage:** 25°C (77°F); excursions permitted to 15-30°C (59-86°F).

## REMERON RX

mirtazapine (Schering)

**Antidepressants increased the risk of suicidal thinking and behavior (suicidality) in short-term studies in children, adolescents, and young adults with major depressive disorder (MDD) and other psychiatric disorders. Mirtazapine is not approved for use in pediatric patients.**

**OTHER BRAND NAMES:** Remeron SolTab (Schering)

**THERAPEUTIC CLASS:** Piperazino-azepine

**INDICATIONS:** Treatment of major depressive disorder.

**DOSAGE:** *Adults:* Initial: 15mg qhs. Titrate: May increase every 1-2 weeks. Max: 45mg/day. Disintegrating tabs disintegrate rapidly on tongue and can be swallowed with saliva. Do not cut disintegrating tabs in half. Reassess periodically to determine the need for maintenance treatment. Switching to or from an MAOI: Observe 14-day interval between d/c of an MAOI and initiation of mirtazapine, and vice versa.

**HOW SUPPLIED:** Tab: 15mg*, 30mg*, 45mg; Tab, Disintegrating: 15mg, 30mg, 45mg *scored

**WARNINGS/PRECAUTIONS:** Risk of agranulocytosis. D/C if sore throat, fever, stomatitis, or other signs of infection, along with low WBC count, develop. Caution in patients with a history of seizures, mania/hypomania, hepatic or renal impairment, altered metabolic or hemodynamic conditions. Caution in elderly, with history of cerebrovascular or CV disease, or with conditions that predispose to hypotension (eg, dehydration, hypovolemia). Somnolence, dizziness reported. May impair judgment, thinking, or motor skills. Monitor closely for clinical worsening, suicidality, and behavior changes at start of therapy or when adjusting dose. Screen patients for bipolar disorder. Increased appetite and weight gain, elevation in cholesterol, TG, and ALT reported.

R

**ADVERSE REACTIONS:** Somnolence, appetite increase, weight gain, dizziness, dry mouth, constipation, asthenia, flu syndrome, abnormal dreams.

**INTERACTIONS:** Alcohol and diazepam increase cognitive and motor skill impairment. Reports of serious and fatal reactions with MAOIs; avoid within 14 days of use. Caution with antihypertensive medications; orthostatic hypotension observed infrequently. Metabolism and pharmacokinetics may be affected by drugs that induce or inhibit drug metabolizing enzymes.

**PREGNANCY:** Category C, caution in nursing.

**MECHANISM OF ACTION:** Piperazino-azepine group; the mechanism of action is unknown. Mirtazapine acts as an antagonist at central presynaptic $\alpha_2$ adrenergic inhibitory autoreceptors and heteroreceptors, an action that is potulated to result in an increase in central noradrenergic and serotonergic activity.

**PHARMACOKINETICS: Absorption:** Rapidly and completely absorbed; Absolute bioavailability (50%); $T_{max}$=2 hrs. **Distribution:** Plasma protein binding (85%). **Metabolism:** Demethylation and hydroxylation via CYP2D6, CYP1A2, and CYP3A followed by glucuronide conjugation. **Elimination:** Urine (75%), feces (15%); $T_{1/2}$=37 hrs (female), 26 hrs (male).

## NURSING CONSIDERATIONS

**Assessment:** Assess for seizures, major depressive disorder, bipolar disorder, cardiac arrhythmias, MI, pregnancy/nursing status. Note other diseases/conditions and drug therapies.

**Monitoring:** Monitor for worsening of depression and/or emergence of suicidal ideation or unusual changes in behavior, LFTs, renal function tests, CBC with differential, and lipid profile.

**Patient Counseling:** Warn about risk of developing agranulocytosis. Advise families and caregivers of the need for close observation of clinical worsening and suicidal risks. Advise to avoid alcohol, sedatives, and OTC agents. Caution against operating machinery/driving. Instruct to report adverse reactions and consult physician before taking any other medications. Instruct to inform physician if pregnant, trying to become pregnant or nursing.

**Administration:** Oral route. **Storage:** Store at 25°C (77°F); excursions permitted to 15-30°C (59-86°F). Protect from light and moisture.

# REMICADE RX

infliximab (Centocor)

**Increased risk for developing serious infections (eg, tuberculosis (TB), TB reactivation, invasive fungal infection, bacterial/viral infection due to opportunistic pathogens) that may lead to hospitalization or death. Concomitant use of immunosuppressants (eg, methotrexate [MTX] or corticosteroids) may precipitate these infections. Evaluate for latent TB and treat prior to initiation of therapy. Empiric antifungal therapy should be considered in patients at risk for invasive fungal infection who develop severe systemic illness. Monitor for development of infection during and after treatment. D/C if serious infection or sepsis develops. Lymphoma and other malignancies reported in children and adolescents.**

**THERAPEUTIC CLASS:** Monoclonal antibody/TNF-alpha receptor blocker

**INDICATIONS:** Reduce signs and symptoms, inhibit progression of structural damage and improve physical function in patients with moderately to severely active rheumatoid arthritis (RA) (in combination with MTX) and psoriatic arthritis. Reduce signs/symptoms, induce and maintain clinical remission of moderately to severely active Crohn's disease when response to conventional therapy is inadequate. Reduce the number of draining enterocutaneous and rectovaginal fistulas and maintain closure in fistulizing Crohn's disease. Reduce signs/symptoms of active ankylosing spondylitis. Reduce signs/symptoms, induce and maintain clinical remission and mucosal healing, and eliminate corticosteroid use in patients with moderately to severely active ulcerative colitis who have inadequate response to conventional therapy. Treatment of patients with chronic, severe plaque psoriasis who are candidates for systemic therapy and when other systemic therapies are medically less appropriate.

**DOSAGE:** *Adults:* RA (with MTX): 3mg/kg as IV infusion; repeat at 2 and 6 weeks. Maint: 3mg/kg every 8 weeks. Incomplete Response: May increase to 10mg/kg or give every 4 weeks. Crohn's Disease/Fistulizing Crohn's Disease: Induction Regimen: 5mg/kg IV at 0, 2 and 6 weeks. Maint: 5mg/kg every 8 weeks. Patients who Respond and Lose Their Response: may increase to 10mg/kg. Consider d/c if no response by Week 14. Ankylosing Spondylitis: 5mg/kg as IV infusion; repeat at 2 and 6 weeks. Maint: 5mg/kg every 6 weeks. Psoriatic Arthritis: 5mg/kg as IV infusion; repeat at 2 and 6 weeks. Maint: 5mg/kg every 8 weeks. May be used with or without MTX. Plaque Psoriasis: 5mg/kg IV infusion; repeat at 2 and 6 weeks. Maint: 5mg/kg every 8 weeks. Ulcerative Colitis: Induction Regimen: 5mg/kg at 0, 2 and 6 weeks. Maint: 5mg/kg every 8 weeks. Elderly: Start at lower end of dosing range. *Pediatrics:* ≥6 yrs: Crohn's Disease: Induction Regimen: 5mg/kg IV at 0, 2 and 6 weeks. Maint: 5mg/kg every 8 weeks.

**HOW SUPPLIED:** Inj: 100mg/20mL

**CONTRAINDICATIONS:** Hypersensitivity to murine proteins. Moderate or severe CHF (NYHA Class III/IV) with doses >5mg/kg.

**WARNINGS/PRECAUTIONS:** Do not initiate with an active infection. Caution in patients with chronic/recurrent infections, who have been exposed to TB, resided or traveled in areas of endemic TB or mycoses (eg, histoplasmosis, coccidiodomycosis, blastomycosis) or with underlying conditions that may predispose them to infection. Monitor for signs and symptoms of infection during and after therapy; d/c if serious infection develops. Hepatitis B virus (HBV) reactivation reported; caution in HBV carriers. Monitor for signs and symptoms of liver dysfunction; d/c if jaundice or marked elevations of liver enzymes develop. Caution in patients with heart failure; d/c if new or worsening symptoms develop. Blood dyscrasias (leukopenia, neutropenia, thrombocytopenia and pancytopenia) and hypersensitivity reactions reported. Associated with optic neuritis, seizure disorder, CNS demyelinating disorders such as multiple sclerosis (MS), CNS systemic vasculitis and peripheral demyelinating disorders such as Guillain-Barre Syndrome (GBS); d/c if with significant CNS adverse reaction. Lymphoma reported; caution in patients with history of malignancies and with chronic obstructive pulmonary disease (COPD). Cases of acute and chronic leukemia reported; increased risk in patients with RA. Monitor psoriasis patients for nonmelanoma skin cancer. May result in autoantibody formation; d/c if lupus-like syndrome develops. Update vaccination of pediatric patients with Crohn's disease prior to therapy. Caution in elderly.

**ADVERSE REACTIONS:** Nausea, infections, rash, infusion reactions, headache, sinusitis, pharyngitis, coughing, abdominal pain, diarrhea, bronchitis, dyspepsia, fatigue, rhinitis, arthralgia.

**INTERACTIONS:** See Black Box Warning. Do not give concurrently with live vaccines. May increase risk of serious infections and neutropenia with anakinra.

**PREGNANCY:** Category B, not for use in nursing.

**MECHANISM OF ACTION:** Monoclonal antibody/TNF-α receptor blocker; neutralizes biological activity of TNF-α by binding with high affinity to the soluble and transmembrane forms of TNF-α and inhibiting binding of TNF-α with its receptors.

**PHARMACOKINETICS: Elimination:** $T_{1/2}$=7.7-9.5 days.

## NURSING CONSIDERATIONS

**Assessment:** Assess for active/chronic/recurrent infection (eg, TB, HBV), TB exposure, recent travel in areas of endemic TB or mycoses, heart failure, pre-existing or recent onset of demyelinating disorder, seizure disorder, history of malignancy, moderate to severe COPD, pregnancy/nursing status and possible drug interactions. Assess that vaccination of pediatric patients with Crohn's disease are up-to-date. Perform test for latent TB and treat if necessary.

R

**Monitoring:** Monitor for signs/symptoms of serious infection (eg, sepsis, pneumonia, TB, invasive fungal infection), HVB reactivation, hepatotoxicity (eg, acute liver failure, autoimmune hepatitis, jaundice, cholestasis), hematological events (eg, leukopenia, neutropenia, thrombocytopenia, pancytopenia), hypersensitivity reactions (eg, urticaria, dyspnea, hypotension, serum sickness-like reactions), infusion reactions, neurologic events (eg, optic neuritis, seizures, CNS demyelinating disorders), malignancies (eg, lymphoma), and lupus-like syndrome. In adolescents/young adults with Crohn's disease, monitor for T-cell lymphoma. In patients with heart failure, monitor for worsening of symptoms.

**Patient Counseling:** Advise to immediately contact physician if experience signs/symptoms of infection (eg, fever, fatigue, cough, warm/red/painful skin), hypersensitivity reaction (eg, hives, difficulty breathing, chest pain, fever), lupus-like syndrome (eg, joint pain, shortness of breath), malignancies, worsening heart failure, liver injury (eg, jaundice, dark brown urine), hematological complications (eg, bruising, fever) or CNS disorders (eg, visual changes, weakness in arms or legs).

**Administration:** IV infusion route. Reconstitute: 1) Use 10mL of Sterile Water for Injection. 2) Further dilute to 250mL with 0.9% NaCl Inj. Infusion concentration ranges 0.4-4mg/mL. Infusion should begin within 3 hrs of preparation.

Infusion solution must be administered over a period of not less than 2 hrs. Do not store any unused portion. Prior to infusion, premedication may be administered (eg, antihistamines, acetaminophen, corticosteroids). Infusion reactions may improve by slowing or suspending infusion. Upon resolution of reaction, reinitiate at a slower rate. D/C if cannot tolerate reaction. **Storage:** Lyophilized powder: 2-8°C (36-46°F). Do not use beyond expiration date. Product contains no preservative.

## RENAGEL — RX

sevelamer HCl (Genzyme)

**THERAPEUTIC CLASS:** Phoshphate binder

**INDICATIONS:** Control of serum phosphorus in patients with chronic kidney disease (CKD) on dialysis.

**DOSAGE:** *Adults:* Not Taking Phosphate Binder: Usual: 800-1600mg with each meal. Initial: Based on Serum Phosphorus: >5.5 to <7.5mg/dL: 800mg tid. ≥7.5 to <9mg/dL: 1200-1600mg tid. ≥9mg/dL: 1600mg tid. Titrate: Serum Phosphorus >5.5mg/dL: Increase by 1 tab per meal at 2-week intervals. 3.5-5.5mg/dL: Maintain dose. <3.5mg/dL: Decrease 1 tab per meal at 2-week intervals. Switching from Calcium Acetate (667mg tab): Adjust according to calcium dose. Calcium acetate 1 tab per meal: 800mg per meal. Calcium acetate 2 tabs per meal: 1200-1600mg per meal. Calcium acetate 3 tabs per meal: 2000mg-2400mg per meal. Elderly: Start at lower end of dosing range.

**HOW SUPPLIED:** Tab: 400mg, 800mg

**CONTRAINDICATIONS:** Hypophosphatemia or bowel obstruction.

**WARNINGS/PRECAUTIONS:** Caution with dysphagia, swallowing disorders, severe GI motility, constipation or GI surgery. Monitor bicarbonate and chloride levels. May reduce vitamin D, E and K levels. Caution in elderly.

**ADVERSE REACTIONS:** N/V, abdominal pain, constipation, diarrhea, flatulence, dyspepsia, peritonitis, intestinal obstruction, ileus, fecal impaction, intestinal perforation.

**INTERACTIONS:** May decrease ciprofloxacin bioavailability by 50%. Very rare cases of increased thyroid stimulating hormone (TSH) levels reported when coadministered with levothyroxine; monitor TSH levels. May bind other drugs; give drugs with narrow therapeutic index 1 hr before or 3 hrs after sevelamer. Caution with antiarrhythmic or anti-seizure medications.

**PREGNANCY:** Category C, safety in nursing not known.

**MECHANISM OF ACTION:** Phosphate binder; binds to phosphate in the dietary tract, decreasing absorption and lowering its serum concentration.

### NURSING CONSIDERATIONS

**Assessment:** Assess for hypophosphatemia, bowel obstruction, dysphagia, swallowing disorders, severe GI motility disorders including severe constipation, major GI tract surgery, pregnancy status, peritoneal/hemodialysis patients and possible drug interactions.

**Monitoring:** Monitor serum chemistries (eg, bicarbonate and chloride levels), levels of vitamin D, E, and K (clotting factors) and folic acid, and for constipation.

**Patient Counseling:** Counsel to take with meals and adhere to prescribed diets. Dose separately from therapy if taken with concomitant medication. Report if new onset or worsening of existing constipation occurs.

**Administration:** Oral route. **Storage:** 25°C (77°F); excursions permitted to 15-30°C (59-86°F). Protect from moisture.

## RENOVA — RX

tretinoin (Ortho Neutrogena)

**OTHER BRAND NAMES:** Refissa (Spear Dermatology)

**THERAPEUTIC CLASS:** Retinoid

**INDICATIONS:** Adjunct to comprehensive skin care and sunlight avoidance programs, for mitigation of fine facial wrinkles.

**DOSAGE:** *Adults:* 18-71 yrs: Wash face with mild soap, pat skin dry, and wait 20-30 min before use. Apply once daily in evening. Max: 52 weeks of therapy. May apply cosmetics 1 hr later. Use moisturizer every morning to prevent dryness.

**HOW SUPPLIED:** Cre: 0.02% [40g]

**WARNINGS/PRECAUTIONS:** Avoid with sunburned skin, eczema, chronic skin conditions, and pregnancy. Larger amounts will not lead to better or faster results and may increase adverse effects. Avoid contact with eyes, mouth, paranasal creases, and mucous membranes. D/C if sensitivity, irritation, or systemic adverse reaction develops. Minimize sunlight exposure; avoid sunlamps. Wear protective clothing and use SPF ≥15. Causes photosensitivity. Extreme weather may increase skin irritation.

**ADVERSE REACTIONS:** Peeling, dry skin, burning, stinging, erythema, pruritus at the site of application.

**INTERACTIONS:** Caution with topical agents with strong drying effects, high concentration of alcohol, astringents, spices or lime, permanent wave solutions, electrolysis, hair depilatories, waxes or medicated or abrasive soaps, shampoos and cleansers. Increased phototoxicity with photosensitizers (eg, thiazides, tetracyclines, fluoroquinolones, phenothiazines, sulfonamides).

**PREGNANCY:** Category C, not for use in nursing.

**MECHANISM OF ACTION:** Endogenous retinoid metabolite of vitamin A; binds to intracellular receptors in the cytosol and nucleus. Activates three members of the retinoic acid (RAR) nuclear receptors (RARα, RARβ, RAR-gamma), which may act to modify gene expression, subsequent protein synthesis, and epithelial cell growth and differentiation.

## NURSING CONSIDERATIONS

**Assessment:** Assess for hypersensitivity reactions, skin eczema, pregnancy/nursing status, and possible drug interactions (eg, photosensitizing drugs such as thiazides and tetracyclines).

**Monitoring:** Monitor for irritation, erythema, pruritus, burning, stinging, and peeling at application site and for atypical changes in melanocytes, keratinocytes, and increased dermal elastosis.

**Patient Counseling:** Counsel to avoid prolonged exposure to sunlight; wear protective clothing. Inform that extreme weather such as wind or cold may cause irritation. Notify if pregnant/nursing or planning to become pregnant.

R

**Administration:** Topical application. **Storage:** 25°C (77°F); excursions permitted to 15-30°C (59-86°F).

# REOPRO **RX**

abciximab (Lilly)

**THERAPEUTIC CLASS:** Glycoprotein IIb/IIIa inhibitor

**INDICATIONS:** Adjunct to percutaneous coronary intervention (PCI) for prevention of cardiac ischemic complications in patients undergoing PCI or with unstable angina unresponsive to conventional therapy when PCI is planned within 24 hrs. Intended for use with aspirin and heparin.

**DOSAGE:** *Adults:* PCI: 0.25mg/kg IV bolus given 10-60 min before start PCI, followed by 0.125mcg/kg/min IV infusion (Max: 10mcg/min) for 12 hrs. Unstable Angina: 0.25mg/kg IV bolus followed by 10mcg/min infusion for 18-24 hrs, concluding 1 hr after PCI.

**HOW SUPPLIED:** Inj: 2mg/mL

**CONTRAINDICATIONS:** Active internal bleeding, recent (within 6 weeks) significant GI or GU bleeding, CVA within 2 yrs, CVA with significant residual neurological deficit, bleeding diathesis, oral anticoagulants within 7 days (unless PT ≤1.2x control), thrombocytopenia, recent (within 6 weeks) major surgery or trauma, intracranial neoplasm, arteriovenous malformation, aneurysm, severe uncontrolled HTN, history of vasculitis, IV dextran use before PCI or during an intervention. Hypersensitivity to murine proteins.

**WARNINGS/PRECAUTIONS:** Increased risk of bleeding. Monitor all potential bleeding sites (eg, catheter insertion sites, arterial and venous puncture sites, cutdown sites). Minimize vascular and other trauma. D/C if serious, uncontrollable bleeding, thrombocytopenia, or emergency surgery occurs. Anaphylaxis may occur. Antibody (HACA) formation may occur; risk of hypersensitivity, thrombocytopenia, decreased benefit with readministration. Monitor platelets, PT, APTT, ACT before infusion.

**ADVERSE REACTIONS:** Bleeding, thrombocytopenia, hypotension, bradycardia, NV, back/chest pain, headache.

**INTERACTIONS:** Caution with other drugs that affect hemostasis (eg, thrombolytics, heparin, oral anticoagulants, NSAIDs, dipyridamole, ticlopidine). Increased risk of bleeding with anticoagulants, thrombolytics, and antiplatelets. If have HACA titers, possible allergic reactions with monoclonal antibody agents.

**PREGNANCY:** Category C, caution in nursing.

**MECHANISM OF ACTION:** Glycoprotein IIb/IIIa inhibitor; binds to the GPIIb/IIIa receptor and inhibits platelet aggregation by preventing the binding of fibrinogen, von Willebrand factor, and other adhesive molecules to GPIIb/IIIa receptor sites on activated platelets. Also binds to vitronectin receptor, which mediates the procoagulant properties of platelets and the proliferative properties of vascular endothelial and smooth muscle cells.

**PHARMACOKINETICS: Elimination:** $T_{1/2}$=30 min.

## NURSING CONSIDERATIONS

**Assessment:** Assess for active internal bleeding, recent GI or genitourinary bleeding, history of cerebrovascular accident, bleeding diathesis, thrombocytopenia, recent major surgery or trauma, intracranial neoplasm, arteriovenous malformation, aneurysm, severe uncontrolled HTN, presence or history of vasculitis, pregnancy/nursing status, and drug interactions. Obtain baseline prothrombin time, ACT, aPTT, and platelet counts.

**Monitoring:** Monitor for signs/symptoms of bleeding; document and monitor vascular puncture sites. If hematoma develops, monitor for enlargement. Monitor for allergic reactions (eg, anaphylaxis) and thrombocytopenia. Check aPTT or ACT prior to arterial sheath removal; should not be removed unless aPTT ≤50 seconds or ACT ≤175 seconds. Monitor platelet counts 2-4 hrs following bolus dose and 24 hrs prior to discharge.

**Patient Counseling:** Counsel to contact physician if develop hypersensitivity reactions (eg, anaphylaxis). Inform may take longer than usual to stop bleeding and may bruise or bleed easier while on medication. Instruct to report any unusual bleeding to physician.

**Administration:** IV infusion. In case of hypersensitivity reaction, epinephrine, dopamine, theophylline, antihistamines, and corticosteroids should be available for immediate use. **Storage:** Store at 2-8°C (36-46°F). Do not freeze. Do not shake. Discard any unused portion left in vial.

# Requip — RX

ropinirole HCl (GlaxoSmithKline)

**OTHER BRAND NAMES:** Requip XL (GlaxoSmithKline)

**THERAPEUTIC CLASS:** Non-ergoline dopamine agonist

**INDICATIONS:** (Tab/Tab, Extended-Release) Treatment of signs and symptoms of idiopathic Parkinson's disease. (Tab) Treatment of moderate-to-severe primary Restless Legs Syndrome (RLS).

**DOSAGE:** *Adults:* Parkinson's: Tab: Initial: 0.25mg tid. Titrate: May increase weekly by 0.25mg tid (0.75mg/day) for 4 weeks. After week 4, may increase weekly by 1.5mg/day up to 9mg/day, then by 3mg/day weekly to 24mg/day.

Max: 24mg/day. Withdrawal: Decrease dose to bid for 4 days, then qd for 3 days. Tab, XL: Initial: 2mg qd for 1-2 weeks. Titrate: May increase by 2mg/day at ≥1 week intervals, depending on therapeutic response and tolerability. Max: 24mg/day. Swallow whole; do not chew, crush, or divide. Switching from Immediate-Release (IR) to XL: Initial dose should match total daily dose of IR formulation. Refer to PI for conversion from IR to XL. RLS: Tab: Initial: 0.25mg qd, 1-3 hours before bedtime. Titrate: 0.5mg qd days 3-7, 1mg qd week 2, then increase by 0.5mg weekly. Max: 4mg.

**HOW SUPPLIED:** Tab: 0.25mg, 0.5mg, 1mg, 2mg, 3mg, 4mg, 5mg; Tab, Extended-Release: (XL) 2mg, 4mg, 6mg, 8mg, 12mg

**WARNINGS/PRECAUTIONS:** (Tab/Tab, XL) Falling asleep during activities of daily living reported; if significant, d/c or warn patient to refrain from dangerous activities. Syncope, bradycardia, postural hypotension, and hallucinations reported. Caution with hepatic dysfunction. Symptom complex similar to neuroleptic malignant syndrome (NMS), fibrotic complications, and melanoma reported. (Tab, XL) May cause elevation of BP and changes in HR. May exacerbate psychosis.

**ADVERSE REACTIONS:** (Tab) Neuralgia, hallucinations, somnolence, vomiting, headache, edema, fatigue, syncope, orthostatic symptoms. (Tab, XL) Dyskinesia, nausea, dizziness, constipation, abdominal pain/discomfort, back pain.

**INTERACTIONS:** Adjust dose if CYP1A2 inhibitor or estrogen is stopped or started during treatment. Potentiated by ciprofloxacin. Decreased effects with dopamine antagonists (eg, phenothiazines, butyrophenones, thioxanthenes, metoclopramide). Caution with alcohol, CNS depressants, and sedatives which may increase drowsiness. May increase clearance with smoking. May potentiate dopaminergic side effects of L-dopa and cause or exacerbate pre-existing dyskinesia.

**PREGNANCY:** Category C, not for use in nursing.

**MECHANISM OF ACTION:** Non-ergoline dopamine agonist; believed to stimulate postsynaptic $D_2$-type receptors within the caudate-putamen in the brain.

**PHARMACOKINETICS: Absorption:** Rapid; absolute bioavailability (45-55%), $T_{max}$=1-2 hrs (IR), 6-10 hrs (XL). **Distribution:** $V_d$=7.5L/kg, plasma protein binding (40%). **Metabolism:** Liver via CYP1A2 (extensive); N-despropylation and hydroxylation. **Elimination:** Urine (<10%, unchanged), $T_{1/2}$=6 hrs.

## NURSING CONSIDERATIONS

**Assessment:** Assess for presence of sleep disorder, history of cardiovascular disease, dyskinesia, major psychotic disorder, pregnancy/nursing status and possible drug interactions. Assess LFTs, renal function tests, and CBC.



**Monitoring:** Perform dermatological screening periodically. Monitor eye exams and for symptoms of neuroleptic malignant syndrome, impulse control symptoms (eg, compulsive behaviors such as pathological gambling and hypersexuality), fibrotic complications, melanomas, signs/symptoms of postural hypotension, hallucinations.

**Patient Counseling:** Caution while operating machinery/driving. Counsel on potential for drowsiness, daytime sleepiness, falling asleep during activity; d/c if these events occurs. Risk of symptomatic hypotension. Take as prescribed; avoid alcohol or concurrent CNS depressants. Report lack of response or severe adverse effects. Notify physician if new or increased gambling urges, increased sexual urges, or other intense urges occur.

**Administration:** Oral route. **Storage:** (Tab) 20-25°C (68-77°F). Protect from light and moisture. (Tab, Extended-Release) 25°C (77°F); excursions permitted to 15-30°C (59-86°F).

# RESCRIPTOR — RX

delavirdine mesylate (Pfizer)

**THERAPEUTIC CLASS:** Non-nucleoside reverse transcriptase inhibitor

**INDICATIONS:** Treatment of HIV-1 infection in combination with other antiretrovirals.

**DOSAGE:** *Adults:* Usual: 400mg tid. May disperse 100mg tabs in ≥3 ounce of water (200mg tab is not dispersible). Take with acidic beverage (eg, orange juice) if achlorhydric.
*Pediatrics:* ≥16yrs: Usual: 400mg tid. May disperse 100mg tab in ≥3 ounce of water (200mg tab is not dispersible). Take with acidic beverage (eg, orange juice) if achlorhydric.

**HOW SUPPLIED:** Tab: 100mg, 200mg

**CONTRAINDICATIONS:** Concomitant use of astemizole, terfenadine, ergot derivatives, cisapride, pimozide, alprazolam, midazolam, triazolam.

**WARNINGS/PRECAUTIONS:** Severe rash (eg, erythema multiforme, Stevens-Johnson syndrome) reported; d/c use if occur. May cause immune reconstitution and fat redistribution. Caution with hepatic impairment. Caution in elderly. May confer cross-resistance to the other NNRTIs.

**ADVERSE REACTIONS:** Headache, fatigue, N/V, diarrhea, increased ALT and AST, rash, maculopapular rash, pruritus, erythema, insomnia, upper respiratory infection.

**INTERACTIONS:** See Contraindications. Antacids decrease absorption; separate doses by 1 hr. $H_2$-antagonists reduce absorption; avoid chronic use. CYP3A inducers (eg, carbamazepine, phenobarbital, phenytoin, rifabutin, rifampin) may decrease plasma levels; avoid concomitant use. Increased plasma levels of drugs metabolized by CYP3A and 2C9 and amprenavir. Certain nonsedating antihistamines, sedative hypnotics, antiarrhythmics, CCBs, ergot agents, amphetamines, cisapride, and sildenafil (max of 25mg/48hrs of sildenafil) may result in potentially serious and/or life-threatening adverse events. Avoid use with lovastatin, simvastatin and St. John's wort. Caution use with other HMG-CoA reductase inhibitors (eg, atorvastatin); increased risk of myopathy and rhabdomyolysis. Reduced effects of both delavirdine and didanosine; separate doses by 1 hr. Increase saquinavir levels; consider dose reduction. Increases indinavir plasma levels; reduce indinavir dose to 600mg tid. May increase levels of clarithromycin, warfarin, trazodone, amphetamines, immunosuppressants and methadone; adjust doses and perform therapeutic drug monitoring. See PI for complete information.

**PREGNANCY:** Category C, not for use in nursing.

**MECHANISM OF ACTION:** HIV-1 non-nucleoside reverse transcriptase inhibitor (NNRTI); binds directly to reverse transcriptase (RT) and blocks RNA-dependent and DNA-dependent DNA polymerase activities.

**PHARMACOKINETICS: Absorption:** Rapid; $C_{max}$=35µM, $T_{max}$=1 hr, AUC=180µM•hr. Bioavailability (85%). **Distribution:** Plasma protein binding (98%). **Metabolism:** Hepatic (N-desalkylation, pyridine hydroxylation) via CYP3A (major), 2D6. **Elimination:** Urine (<5%). $T_{1/2}$=5.8 hrs.

## NURSING CONSIDERATIONS

**Assessment:** Assess for hepatic dysfunction, allergic reactions, pregnancy/nursing status and possible drug interactions.

**Monitoring:** Monitor for signs/symptoms of hypersensitivity reactions, immune reconstitution syndrome, hepatic dysfunction, and fat redistribution. May enroll patients in the Antiretroviral Patient Registry if they become pregnant while on treatment.

**Patient Counseling:** Inform to take as prescribed, not to alter dose without consulting doctor. If a dose is missed, do not double next dose. Patients with achlorhydria should take with acidic beverage (orange/cranberry juice). Counsel to take at least 1 hr apart if taking antacids, and to take with/without food. Advise to seek medical attention if symptoms of hypersensitivity reaction (rash, fever, blistering, oral lesions, conjunctivitis, swelling, and muscle and joint aches), immune reconstitution syndrome, hepatic dysfunction, and fat redistribution occur.

**Administration:** Oral route. **Storage:** 20-25°C (68-77°F). Keep container tightly closed. Protect from high humidity.

## RESERPINE — RX

reserpine (Various)

**THERAPEUTIC CLASS:** Rauwolfia alkaloid

**INDICATIONS:** Treatment of mild essential hypertension and adjunct treatment of severe hypertension. Relief of symptoms in agitated psychotic states.

**DOSAGE:** *Adults:* HTN: Initial: 0.5mg/day for 1-2 weeks. Maint: reduce to 0.1-0.25mg/day. Psychotic Disorders: Initial: 0.5mg/day. Range: 0.1-1mg/day.

**HOW SUPPLIED:** Tab: 0.1mg, 0.25mg

**CONTRAINDICATIONS:** Active or history of mental depression, active peptic ulcer, ulcerative colitis, current electroconvulsive therapy.

**WARNINGS/PRECAUTIONS:** Caution with renal insufficiency. May cause depression; d/c at 1st sign. Caution with history of peptic ulcer, ulcerative colitis, or gallstones.

**ADVERSE REACTIONS:** GI effects, dry mouth, hypersecretion, arrhythmia, syncope, edema, dyspnea, muscle aches, dizziness, depression, nervousness, impotence, gynecomastia, rash.

**INTERACTIONS:** Avoid MAOIs or use extreme caution. Prolonged effect of direct-acting sympathomimetics (eg, epinephrine, isoproterenol). May inhibit effects of indirect-acting sympathomimetics (eg, ephedrine, tyramine). Risk of arrhythmia with quinidine or digoxin. Titrate carefully with other antihypertensives. Decreased effect with TCAs.

**PREGNANCY:** Category C, not for use in nursing.

**MECHANISM OF ACTION:** Rauwolfia alkaloid; antihypertensive, depletes stores of catecholamine and 5-hydroxytryptamine in many organs including brain and adrenal medulla, resulting in decreased HR and lowering of arterial BP.

**PHARMACOKINETICS: Absorption:** (0.5mg) Absolute bioavailability (50%); $C_{max}$=1.1ng/mL; $T_{max}$=2.5 hrs. **Distribution:** Plasma protein binding (95%); found in breast milk. **Metabolism:** Complete. **Elimination:** Urine (1% unchanged); $T_{1/2}$=200 hrs.

### NURSING CONSIDERATIONS

**Assessment:** Assess for hypersensivity, mental depression (suicidal tendencies), active peptic ulcer, ulcerative colitis, renal insufficiency, possible drug interactions, and pregnancy/nursing status.

**Monitoring:** Monitor for signs of mental depression (eg, despondency, early morning insomnia, loss of appetite, impotence, self-depreciation); d/c if any occur. Monitor BP, GI motility/secretion, and signs/symptoms of overdose (eg, flushing, pupilary constriction, hypotension, respiratory depression, impairment of consciousness, bradycardia).

**Patient Counseling:** Inform of possible adverse effects; immediately notify physician if any occur. Advise to take medication regularly and continuously as directed.

**Administration:** Oral route. **Storage:** 20-25°C (68-77°F). Protect from moisture. Preserve in tight, light-resistant container.



## RESTASIS — RX

cyclosporine (Allergan)

**THERAPEUTIC CLASS:** Topical immunomodulator

**INDICATIONS:** To increase tear production in patients with suppressed tear production due to ocular inflammation associated with keratoconjunctivitis sicca.

**DOSAGE:** *Adults:* 1 drop bid, q12h. Concomitant Artificial Tears: Space by 15 min.

*Pediatrics:* ≥16 yrs: 1 drop bid, q12h. Concomitant Artificial Tears: Space by 15 min.

**HOW SUPPLIED:** Emul: 0.05% [0.4mL, 32[s]]

**CONTRAINDICATIONS:** Active ocular infections.

**WARNINGS/PRECAUTIONS:** Not studied in patients with a history of herpes keratitis. Not to be given while wearing contact lenses; lenses may be reinserted 15 min following administration.

**ADVERSE REACTIONS:** Ocular burning, conjunctival hyperemia, discharge, epiphora, eye pain, foreign body sensation, pruritus, stinging, visual disturbance (eg, blurring).

**PREGNANCY:** Category C, caution in nursing.

**MECHANISM OF ACTION:** Topical immunomodulator; not established. Systemically acts as an immunosuppressive agent.

**PHARMACOKINETICS: Distribution:** Following systemic administration, found in breast milk.

## NURSING CONSIDERATIONS

**Assessment:** Assess for presence of active ocular infection. Assess use in pregnant/nursing females and in patients with a history of herpes keratitis.

**Monitoring:** Monitor for signs/symptoms of ocular burning.

**Patient Counseling:** Inform to use single-use vial immediately after opening and discard remaining contents following use. Instruct not to allow tip of vial to touch eye or any surface to avoid contamination. Advise to remove contact lenses prior to use; lenses may be reinserted 15 min following administration.

**Administration:** Ocular route. 1) Invert unit dose vial a few times to obtain uniform, white, opaque emulsion before using. 2) Instill 1 drop bid in each eye, approximately 12 hrs apart. May be used concomitantly with artificial tears, allowing 15 min interval between products. 3) Discard vial immediately after administration. **Storage:** 15-25°C (59-77°F).

# RESTORIL

**CIV**

temazepam (Mallinckrodt)

**THERAPEUTIC CLASS:** Benzodiazepine

**INDICATIONS:** Short-term treatment of insomnia (7-10 days).

**DOSAGE:** *Adults:* Usual: 15mg qhs. Range: 7.5-30mg qhs. Transient Insomnia: 7.5mg qhs. Elderly/Debilitated: Initial: 7.5mg qhs.

**HOW SUPPLIED:** Cap: 7.5mg, 15mg, 22.5mg, 30mg

**CONTRAINDICATIONS:** Pregnancy.

**WARNINGS/PRECAUTIONS:** Caution in elderly, debilitated, severely depressed, those with suicidal tendencies, hepatic/renal impairment, pulmonary insufficiency. Avoid abrupt d/c. If no improvement after 7-10 days, may indicate primary psychiatric and/or medical condition. May impair physical/mental abilities; complex behaviors such as sleep-driving (driving while not fully awake after ingestion of a sedative-hypnotic, with amnesia for event) have been reported. Amnesia and other neuro-psychiatric symptoms may occur unpredictable. Worsening of depression including suicidal thinking has been reported in primarily depressed patients. Rare cases of angioedema (eg, tongue, glottis, or larynx) that could lead to airway obstruction may occur and can be fatal.

**ADVERSE REACTIONS:** Headache, dizziness, drowsiness, fatigue, nervousness, nausea, lethargy.

**INTERACTIONS:** Additive CNS depressant effects with alcohol and CNS depressants. May be synergistic with diphenhydramine.

**PREGNANCY:** Category X, caution in nursing.

**MECHANISM OF ACTION:** Benzodiazepine hypnotic agent.

R

**PHARMACOKINETICS: Absorption:** Well-absorbed; $C_{max}$=666-982ng/mL; $T_{max}$=approximately 1.5 hrs. **Distribution:** Plasma protein binding (96% unchanged), crosses placenta. **Metabolism:** Conjugation (major metabolites): O-conjugate . **Elimination:** Urine (80-90%); $T_{1/2}$=8.8 hrs.

## NURSING CONSIDERATIONS

**Assessment:** Assess for primary physical and/or psychiatric illness, severe depression, impaired renal/hepatic function, chronic pulmonary insufficiency, hypersensitivity reactions, possible drug interactions, and alcohol use.

**Monitoring:** Worsening of insomnia, severe depresssion with suicidal ideation, oversedation, dizziness, drowsiness, headache, nervousness, lethargy, confusion and/or ataxia, emergence of new abnormalities of thinking or behavior, physical/psychological dependence, and withdrawal symptoms. Monitor LFTs and pulmonary functions.

**Patient Counseling:** Inform about the benefits/risks and possibility of physical/psychological dependence and memory problems (eg, sleep-driving). Caution against hazardous tasks (eg, operating machinery/driving). Never drink alcohol. Notify physician if pregnant or planning to become pregnant. Do not take any other drug, increase dose, or d/c without direction of physician.

**Administration:** Oral route. **Storage:** Store at 20-25°C (68-77°F). Dispense in a well-closed, light-resistant container with a child-resistant closure.

# RETAVASE RX

reteplase (PDL)

**THERAPEUTIC CLASS:** Thrombolytic agent

**INDICATIONS:** To improve ventricular function following acute myocardial infarction (AMI), reduce the incidence of congestive heart failure (CHF) and reduce the mortality associated with AMI.

**DOSAGE:** *Adults:* 10 U IV over 2 min. Repeat in 30 min.

**HOW SUPPLIED:** Inj: 10.4 U

**CONTRAINDICATIONS:** Active internal bleeding, history of CVA, recent intracranial or intraspinal surgery or trauma, intracranial neoplasm, arteriovenous malformation, aneurysm, bleeding diathesis, severe uncontrolled HTN.

**WARNINGS/PRECAUTIONS:** Weigh benefits/risks with recent major surgery, previous puncture of noncompressible vessels, cerebrovascular disease, recent GI or GU bleeding, recent trauma, HTN, left heart thrombus, acute pericarditis, subacute bacterial endocarditis, hemostatic defects, severe hepatic or renal dysfunction, pregnancy, diabetic hemorrhagic retinopathy or other hemorrhagic ophthalmic conditions, septic thrombophlebitis or occluded AV cannula at a seriously infected site, elderly, any other bleeding condition that is difficult to manage. Cholesterol embolism and internal/superficial bleeding reported. Arrhythmias may occur with reperfusion. Avoid IM injection, noncompressible arterial puncture, and internal jugular or subclavian venous puncture. Cholesterol embolism and internal/superficial bleeding reported.

**ADVERSE REACTIONS:** Bleeding, allergic reactions, dyspnea, hypotension.

**INTERACTIONS:** Increased risk of bleeding with heparin, vitamin K antagonists, and drugs that alter platelet function (eg, ASA, NSAIDs, dipyridamole, abciximab) before or after therapy. Weigh benefits/risks with oral anticoagulants.

**PREGNANCY:** Category C, caution in nursing.

**MECHANISM OF ACTION:** Thrombolytic agent; recombinant plasminogen activator that catalyzes the cleavage of endogenous plasminogen to generate plasmin. Plasmin, in turn, degrades the fibrin matrix of the thrombus, thereby exerting its thrombolytic action.

**PHARMACOKINETICS: Metabolism:** Liver. **Elimination:** Renal; $T_{1/2}$=13-16 min.

## NURSING CONSIDERATIONS

**Assessment:** Assess for active internal bleeding, history of cerebrovascular accident, recent intracranial or intraspinal surgery or trauma, intracranial neoplasm, arteriovenous malformation, aneurysm, known bleeding diathesis, severe uncontrolled HTN, renal/hepatic function, nursing/pregnancy status, and for drug interactions. Assess use in patients at risk for bleeding events (eg, recent major surgery, acute pericarditis, recent GI bleeding).

**Monitoring:** Monitor for signs/symptoms of bleeding (eg, intracranial, retroperitoneal, GI, genitourinary), cholesterol embolization (eg, livedo reticularis, "purple toe" syndrome, MI, cerebral infarction, HTN), and arrhythmias. Monitor all potential bleeding sites (eg, catheter insertion sites, sites of recent surgical intervention).

**Patient Counseling:** Counsel about increased risk of bleeding tendencies while on therapy. Instruct to contact physician if any unusual bleeding occurs. Avoid IM injections while on therapy.

**Administration:** IV route. Reconstitute. 1) Transfer 10mL of sterile water for injection into vial. 2) Swirl to dissolve drug, but do not shake. 2) Withdraw 10 mL of reconstituted solution into syringe. 3) Attach sterile needle; syringe is now ready for IV bolus dose. Reconstitute just prior to administration. Do not administer in the same IV line as heparin. **Storage:** Unused vial: 2-25°C (36-77°F). Box should remain sealed until use to protect the lyophilisate from exposure to light. Reconstituted: 2-30°C (36-86°F); use within 4 hrs.

# RETIN-A — RX

tretinoin (Ortho Neutrogena)

**OTHER BRAND NAMES:** Retin-A Micro (Ortho Neutrogena)

**THERAPEUTIC CLASS:** Retinoid

**INDICATIONS:** Topical treatment of acne vulgaris.

**DOSAGE:** *Adults:* Cleanse area thoroughly, then apply qhs. May temporarily d/c or reduce dosing frequency if irritation occurs.
*Pediatrics:* ≥12 yrs: (Gel: 0.04%, 0.1%) Cleanse area thoroughly, then apply qhs. May temporarily d/c or reduce dosing frequency if irritation occurs.

**HOW SUPPLIED:** (Retin-A) Cre: 0.025%, 0.05%, 0.1% [20g, 45g]; Gel: 0.01%, 0.025% [15g, 45g]; Sol: 0.05% [28mL]; (Retin-A Micro) Gel: 0.04%, 0.1% [20g, 45g]

**WARNINGS/PRECAUTIONS:** Avoid eyes, lips, paranasal creases, mucous membranes, and sunburned skin. Acne exacerbation during 1st weeks of therapy may occur. D/C if sensitivity or irritation occurs. Severe irritation with eczematous skin. Causes photosensitivity. Extreme weather (eg, cold, wind) may irritate skin.

**ADVERSE REACTIONS:** Local skin reactions (red, edematous, blistered, crusted), photosensitivity, temporary skin pigmentation changes.

**INTERACTIONS:** Caution with topical agents with strong drying effects, high concentration of alcohol, astringents, spices, or lime. Caution with sulfur, resorcinol, or salicylic acid; allow effects of these agents to subside before application of tretinoin.

**PREGNANCY:** Category C, caution in nursing.

**MECHANISM OF ACTION:** Retinoic acid derivative; not established. Responsible for decreasing cohesiveness of follicular epithelial cells with decreased microcomedo formation. Also stimulates mitotic activity and increases turnover of follicular epithelial cells, causing extrusion of comedones.

## NURSING CONSIDERATIONS

**Assessment:** Assess for presence of sunburn and eczematous skin, pregnancy/nursing status, and possible drug interactions.

**Monitoring:** Monitor for signs/symptoms of a skin sensitivity reaction (eg, red, edematous, blistered, or crusted skin) or chemical irritation.

**Patient Counseling:** Avoid exposure to sunlight/sunlamps during therapy. Advise using effective sunscreen when outdoors and protective clothing during extended sun exposure. If sunburn occurs, instruct to d/c until skin is recovered. Avoid excessive exposure to wind or cold. Medication is flammable; avoid fire, flame, or smoking during use. Keep away from eyes, mouth, angles of the nose, and mucous membranes. Inform to notify physician if severe skin irritation occurs (eg, excessively red, swollen, blistered, or crusted skin).

**Administration:** Topical administration. **Storage:** Retin A Liquid, Gel: Below 86°F; Retin A Cream: Below 80°F.

## RETROVIR RX

zidovudine (GlaxoSmithKline)

**Associated with hematologic toxicity (eg, neutropenia, severe anemia), especially with advanced HIV disease. Symptomatic myopathy associated with prolonged use. Lactic acidosis and severe hepatomegaly with steatosis, including fatal cases, reported.**

**THERAPEUTIC CLASS:** Nucleoside analogue

**INDICATIONS:** Treatment of HIV-1 infection in combination with other antiretrovirals. Prevention of maternal-fetal HIV-1 transmission.

**DOSAGE:** *Adults:* HIV-1 Infection: (Cap/Tab) 600mg/day in divided doses in combination with other antiretroviral agents. (Inj) 1mg/kg IV over 1 hr 5-6 times/day. Prevention of Maternal-Fetal HIV Transmission: >14 weeks pregnancy: Maternal Dosing: 100mg PO 5 times/day until start of labor. During Labor and Delivery: 2mg/kg IV over 1 hr followed by 1mg/kg/hr IV infusion until clamping of umbilical cord. End-Stage Renal Disease/Dialysis: 100mg PO q6-8h or 1mg/kg IV q6-8h. Severe Anemia/Neutropenia: May require dose interruption and adjunctive epoetin therapy. Mild to Moderate Hepatic Impairment: Monitor for hematologic toxicity and reduce dose if needed. *Pediatrics:* HIV-1 Infection: 4 wks to <18 yrs: BSA Based: 480mg/m²/day PO in divided doses (240mg/m² bid or 160mg/m² tid). Weight Based: 4 to <9kg: 12mg/kg bid or 8mg/kg tid. ≥9 to <30kg: 9mg/kg bid or 6mg/kg tid. ≥30kg: 300mg bid or 200mg tid. Prevention of Maternal-Fetal HIV Transmission: Neonates: 2mg/kg PO q6h or 1.5mg/kg IV over 30 min q6h, starting within 12 hrs after birth and continuing through 6 weeks of age. End-Stage Renal Disease/Dialysis: 100mg PO q6-8h or 1mg/kg IV q6-8h. Significant Anemia/Neutropenia: May require dose interruption and adjunctive epoetin therapy. Mild to Moderate Hepatic Impairment: Monitor for hematologic toxicity and reduce dose if needed.

**HOW SUPPLIED:** Cap: 100mg; Inj: 10mg/mL [20mL]; Syrup: 50mg/5mL [240mL]; Tab: 300mg



**WARNINGS/PRECAUTIONS:** Adverse reactions increase with disease progression. Caution with compromised bone marrow (granulocyte count<1,000cells/mm³ or Hgb<9.5g/dL) or in elderly. Monitor for hematologic toxicity; reduce dose or stop therapy. Caution with obesity and liver disease; increased risk of lactic acidosis and hepatomegaly with steatosis. Suspend treatment with clinical or laboratory findings suggestive of lactic acidosis or pronounced hepatotoxicity. Possible redistribution/accumulation of body fat. Immune reconstitution syndrome reported. Myopathy and myositis reported with prolonged use.

**ADVERSE REACTIONS:** Headache, N/V, malaise, anorexia, asthenia, constipation, anemia, neutropenia, abdominal pain, arthralgia, chills, dyspepsia, fatigue, insomnia.

**INTERACTIONS:** Hepatic decompensation has occurred in HIV/HCV coinfected patients receiving combination antiretroviral therapy for HIV and interferon-α w/ or w/o ribavirin; monitor for treatment-associated toxicities. Increased risk of hematologic toxicities with ganciclovir, interferon-α, ribavirin, bone marrow suppressives, and cytotoxic drugs. Possible increased levels with lamivudine, atovaquone, fluconazole, methadone, probenecid, and valproic acid. Possible decreased levels with nelfinavir, ritonavir, and rifampin. Avoid with stavudine, nucleoside analogues affecting DNA replication such as ribavirin, doxorubicin, and other combination products containing zidovudine. May decrease phenytoin levels.

**PREGNANCY:** Category C, not for use in nursing.

**MECHANISM OF ACTION:** Nucleoside analogue; inhibits reverse transcriptase via DNA chain termination.

**PHARMACOKINETICS: Absorption:** (PO): Rapid. Bioavailability (64%). $T_{max}$=0.5-1.5 hrs. (IV) $C_{max}$=1.06mcg/mL. **Distribution:** $V_d$=1.6L/kg; plasma protein binding (<38%); found in breastmilk. **Metabolism:** Hepatic. 3'-azido-3'-deoxy-5'-*O*-β-*D*-glucopyranuronosylthymidine (major metabolite). **Elimination:** (PO): Urine (14% unchanged, 74% metabolite). $T_{1/2}$=0.5-3 hrs. (IV): Urine (18% unchanged, 60% metabolite). $T_{1/2}$=0.5-2.9 hrs. Refer to full PI for pediatric parameters.

## NURSING CONSIDERATIONS

**Assessment:** Assess for advanced symptomatic HIV disease, anemia, myopathy, risk of liver disease, bone marrow suppression (neutropenia, pancytopenia), risk factors for lactic acidosis, renal dysfunction, hypersensitivity to drug, pregnancy/nursing status, and possible drug interactions.

**Monitoring:** Periodic monitoring of CBC, granulocyte, Hgb, renal/hepatic function tests. Monitor for signs/symptoms of hypersensitivity reactions, anemia, myopathy, liver dysfunction (decompensation, failure), bone marrow suppression (neutropenia, pancytopenia), lactic acidosis, immune reconstitution syndrome, fat redistribution and renal dysfunction. May enroll patients in the Antiretroviral Pregnancy Registry if they become pregnant while on treatment.

**Patient Counseling:** Inform that therapy is not cure for HIV, does not reduce risk of transmission of HIV and that opportunistic infections may develop. Seek medical attention if symptoms of lactic acidosis (weakness, SOB), hepatic dysfunction, anemia, myopathy, bone marrow suppression (neutropenia, pancytopenia), renal dysfunction, immune reconstitution syndrome, and fat redistribution occur. Consult physician if experience muscle weakness, SOB, symptoms of hepatitis or pancreatitis, or any other adverse events. Inform pregnant women that transmission may still occur despite therapy and not to breastfeed to prevent postnatal transmission.

**Administration:** IV or oral route. **Storage:** (Vial): 15-25°C (59-77°F); protect from light. (Diluted): Stable for 24 hrs at room temperature. Stable for 48 hrs when refrigerated at 2-8°C (36-46°F). (Cap, Tab, Syrup): 15-25°C (59-77°F); protect caps from moisture.

# REVATIO — RX

sildenafil citrate (Pfizer)

**THERAPEUTIC CLASS:** Phosphodiesterase type 5 inhibitor

**INDICATIONS:** Treatment of pulmonary arterial hypertension (PAH) (WHO Group I) to improve exercise ability and delay clinical worsening.

**DOSAGE:** *Adults:* Inj: 10mg IV bolus tid. Tab: 20mg tid, 4-6 hrs apart, with or without food.

**HOW SUPPLIED:** Inj: 10mg/12.5mL; Tab: 20mg

**CONTRAINDICATIONS:** Do not use with organic nitrates in any form, either regularly or intermittently.

**WARNINGS/PRECAUTIONS:** Caution with myocardial infaction (MI), stroke or life-threatening arrhythmia within last 6 months, coronary artery disease (CAD) causing unstable angina, and HTN (BP >170/110). Vasodilatory effects may advesely affect patients with resting BP <90/50, fluid depletion, severe left ventricular outflow obstruction, or autonomic dysfunction. Not recommended with pulmonary veno-occlusive disease (PVOD). Non-arteritic anterior ischemic optic neuropathy (NAION) reported; d/c if sudden loss of vision in one or both eyes occurs. Caution in retinitis pigmentosa. Sudden decrease or loss of hearing reported. Caution in patients with anatomical penile deformation (eg, angulation, cavernosal fibrosis, or Peyronie's disease) or with conditions predisposing risk to priapism (eg, sickle cell anemia, multiple myeloma, or leukemia). If erection persists >4 hrs, immediate medical attention is necessary; penile tissue damage and permanent loss of potency may result.

**ADVERSE REACTIONS:** Epistaxis, headache, flushing, dyspepsia, insomnia, erythema, dyspnea, rhinitis, diarrhea, myalgia, pyrexia, gastritis, sinusitis, paresthesia.

**INTERACTIONS:** See Contraindications. Reports of bleeding (epistaxis) with vitamin K antagonists. May potentiate anti-aggregatory effect of sodium nitroprusside. Increased levels with CYP3A4 inhibitors (eg, cimetidine, ketoconazole, itraconazole, erythromycin, saquinavir) and protease inhibitors (eg, ritonavir, saquinavir). CYP2C9 inhibitors may decrease sildenafil clearance. Concomitant use with CYP3A inducers (eg, bosentan) may decrease plasma levels. Administration with CYP3A substrates and/or β-blockers may reduce clearance or increase oral bioavalability of sildenafil. Additive BP-lowering effects with α-blockers. Additional reduction on supine BP with amlodipine reported. Avoid concomitant use with other PDE5 inhibitors (eg, Viagra®).

**PREGNANCY:** Category B, caution in nursing.

**MECHANISM OF ACTION:** Phosphodiesterase type-5 (PDE5) inhibitor; Increases cGMP within pulmonary vascular smooth muscle cells, resulting in relaxation. This can lead to vasodilation of pulmonary vascular bed and, to a lesser degree, vasodilation systemic circulation.

**PHARMACOKINETICS: Absorption:** Rapid; absolute bioavailability (41%); $T_{max}$=30-120 min. **Distribution:** $V_{ss}$=105L; plasma protein binding (96%). **Metabolism:** CYP3A4 (major route) and CYP2C9 (minor route) hepatic microsomal isoenzyme; through N-desmethylation. **Elimination:** Feces (80% metabolites), urine (13%); $T_{1/2}$=4 hrs.

## NURSING CONSIDERATIONS

**Assessment:** Assess resting BP and for fluid depletion, left ventricular outflow obstruction, autonomic dysfunction, or PVOD. Assess if MI, stroke or life-threatening arrhythmia within last 6 months, CAD causing unstable angina, HTN, retinitis pigmentosa, anatomical deformities of the penis (eg, Peyronie's disease, angulation, cavernosal fibrosis), conditions predisposing to priapism (eg, sickle cell anemia, multiple myeloma, or leukemia), stomach ulcer or any bleeding problems, and drug hypersensitivity. Check nursing/pregnancy status, use of organic nitrates and other possible drug interactions.

**Monitoring:** Monitor BP and for signs of pulmonary edema, decrease/sudden loss of vision or hearing, epistaxis, and priapism. Monitor for hypersensitivity reaction and drug interactions.

R

**Patient Counseling:** Inform about risks of drug and to consult physician if any adverse events occur. Inform that drug is also marketed as Viagra for male erectile dysfunction. Advise not to take Viagra or other PDE5 inhibitors during therapy. Counsel about the increased risk of NAION with patients who experienced NAION in one eye. Instruct to notify physician if sudden loss of vision or hearing occur. Advise to seek immediate medical assistance if erection persists >4 hrs.

**Administration:** Oral, IV route. **Storage:** 25°C (77°F); excursions permitted to 15-30°C (59-86°F).

# REVIA — RX

naltrexone HCl (Duramed)

**THERAPEUTIC CLASS:** Opioid antagonist

**INDICATIONS:** Treatment of alcohol dependence and to block effects of exogenously administered opioids.

**DOSAGE:** *Adults:* Alcoholism: 50mg qd up to 12 weeks. Opioid Dependence: Begin 7-10 days after opioid-free period and no signs or withdrawal. Initial: 25mg qd. Maint: 50mg qd. Naloxone Challenge Test: 0.2mg IV, observe for 30 sec, then 0.6mg IV, observe for 20 min; or 0.8mg SQ, observe for 20 min.

**HOW SUPPLIED:** Tab: 50mg* *scored

**CONTRAINDICATIONS:** Acute hepatitis or liver failure, failed naloxone challenge test or positive urine screen for opioids, opioid-dependent, concomitant opioid analgesics, acute opioid withdrawal.

**WARNINGS/PRECAUTIONS:** Hepatotoxicity with excessive doses; does not appear to be a hepatotoxin at recommended doses. Only treat patients opioid-free for 7-10 days. Attempting to overcome opiate blockade is very dangerous. More sensitive to lower doses of opioids after naltrexone is d/c. Safety in ultra-rapid opiate detoxification is not known. Increased risk of suicide in substance abuse patients. Severe opioid withdrawal syndromes reported with accidental ingestion in opioid-dependent patients. Monitor closely during blockade reversal. Caution in renal or hepatic impairment. Perform naloxone challenge test if question of opioid dependence.

**ADVERSE REACTIONS:** N/V, headache, dizziness, nervousness, fatigue, restlessness, insomnia, anxiety, somnolence.

**INTERACTIONS:** See Contraindications. Do not use with disulfiram unless benefits outweigh risk of hepatotoxicity. Lethargy and somnolence reported with thioridazine. Antagonizes opioid-containing cough and cold, antidiarrheal, and analgesic agents.

**PREGNANCY:** Category C, caution in nursing.

**MECHANISM OF ACTION:** Opioid antagonist; markedly attenuates or completely blocks (reversibly) the subjective effects of IV-administered opioids.

**PHARMACOKINETICS: Absorption:** Rapid and complete. Bioavailability (5-40%); $T_{max}$=1 hr. **Distribution:** $V_d$=1350L; plasma protein binding (21%). **Metabolism:** Liver , 6β-naltrexol (major metabolite). **Elimination:** Urine (2% unchanged), (43% conjugated); (naltrexone, β-naltrexol) $T_{1/2}$=4 hrs, 13 hrs.

## NURSING CONSIDERATIONS

**Assessment:** Start treatment only under medical judgment of prescribing physician, assess potential of opioid use within past 7-10 days. If question of occult opioid dependence, perform naloxone challenge test. Assess for acute hepatitis or liver failure and possible drug interactions.

**Monitoring:** Monitor LFTs, symptoms/signs of respiratory depression, hepatotoxicity, idiopathic thrombocytopenic purpura, suicide attempts, withdrawal symptoms in opioid-dependent patients.

**Patient Counseling:** Instruct to take as prescribed. Drug treats alcoholism or drug dependence. Carry identification card to alert medical personnel of naltrexone use and to ensure adequate treatment in a medical emergency. Caution against taking heroin or any other opioid drug with therapy; may lead to serious injury, including coma. Notify physician if pregnant/nursing.

**Administration:** Oral route. **Storage:** 20-25°C (68-77°F).

R

# REVLIMID RX

lenalidomide (Celgene)

**Lenalidomide is an analogue of thalidomide, a known human teratogen that causes severe life-threatening birth defects. Avoid pregnancy due to potential toxicity and to avoid fetal exposure. Effective contraception must be used by female patients of childbearing potential for at least 4 weeks before beginning therapy, during therapy and for 4 weeks following d/c of therapy. Females should have two negative pregnancy tests (sensitivity of at least 50mIU/mL). The 1st test should be performed within 10-14 days; the 2nd test within 24 hrs prior to prescribing. Negative pregnancy test must be verified by prescriber prior to any prescription. Continue pregnancy testing weekly during 1st 4 weeks of therapy, then repeat q 4 weeks if regular menstrual cycle; q 2 weeks for irregular cycles. Male patients must always use latex condom during sexual contact even if with vasectomy. Only available under RevAssist restricted distribution program. Associated with significant neutropenia and thrombocytopenia in patients with del 5q myelodysplastic syndromes (MDS). Monitor CBC weekly for the 1st 8 weeks of therapy and monthly thereafter. May require dose interruption and/or reduction and the use of blood products and/or growth factors. Increased risk of deep vein thrombosis (DVT) and pulmonary embolism (PE) in patients with multiple myeloma. Observe for signs and symptoms of thromboembolism.**

**THERAPEUTIC CLASS:** Thalidomide Analog

**INDICATIONS:** Treatment for transfusion-dependent anemia due to low- or intermediate-1-risk myelodysplastic syndromes associated with a deletion 5q cytogenetic abnormality with or without additional cytogenetic abnormalities. In combination with dexamethasone for the treatment of multiple myeloma in patients who have received at least 1 prior therapy.

**DOSAGE:** *Adults:* ≥18 yrs: Myelodysplastic Syndromes: 10mg qd with water. Renal Impairment: Moderate (CrCL <60mL/min): 5mg q24h. Severe without Dialysis (CrCL <30mL/min): 5mg q48h. End Stage Renal Disease (ESRD) with Dialysis (CrCL <30mL/min): 5mg 3 x a week following dialysis. Multiple Myeloma: 25mg qd with water. Administer as single dose on Days 1-21 of repeated 28-day cycles. Renal Impairment: Moderate (CrCL <60mL/mmin): 10mg q24h. Severe without Dialysis (CrCL <30mL/min): 15mg q48h. ESRD with Dialysis (CrCL <30mL/min): 5mg qd following dialysis. Refer to PI for dose adjustment based on platelet and/or neutrophil counts. For grade 3/4 toxicities, hold treatment and restart at next lower dose when toxicity resolved to ≤grade 2. Do not break, chew, or open caps.

**HOW SUPPLIED:** Cap: 5mg, 10mg, 15mg, 25mg

**CONTRAINDICATIONS:** Pregnancy.

**WARNINGS/PRECAUTIONS:** D/C if angioedema, Stevens-Johnson syndrome (SJS), grade 2-3 rash, exfoliative or bullous rash, and toxic epidermal necrolysis (TEN) occur. Caution with the prior history of grade 4 rash associated with thalidomide. Tumor lysis syndrome may occur; monitor closely. Caution with renal impairment.

**ADVERSE REACTIONS:** Thrombocytopenia, neutropenia, pruritus, rash, diarrhea, constipation, nausea, nasopharyngitis, fatigue, arthralgia, cough, pyrexia, peripheral edema, insomnia, asthenia.

**INTERACTIONS:** May increase digoxin levels; monitor periodically.

**PREGNANCY:** Category X, not for use in nursing.

**MECHANISM OF ACTION:** Thalidomide analog; not established, possesses antineoplastic, immunomodulatory and antiangiogenic properties. Inhibits secretion of pro-inflammatory cytokines and increases secretion of anti-inflammatory cytokines from peripheral blood mononuclear cells, inhibits cell proliferation, and inhibits growth of multiple myeloma cells by inducing cell cycle arrest and apoptosis.

**PHARMACOKINETICS: Absorption**: $T_{max}$=0.625-1.5 hrs (healthy), 0.5-4.0 hrs (multiple myeloma). **Distribution**: Plasma protein binding (30%). **Elimination**: Urine; $T_{1/2}$=3 hrs.

## NURSING CONSIDERATIONS

R

**Assessment:** Assess for pregnancy/nursing status, renal impairment, tumor lysis syndrome, history of grade 4 rash, and possible drug interactions. Obtain pregnancy test 10-14 days before and 24 hrs before initiating therapy. Confirm use of 2 forms of effective contraception for 4 weeks prior to therapy.

**Monitoring:** Perform pregnancy test weekly for 1st 4 weeks of use, repeat q 4 weeks with regular menstrual cycles and q 2 weeks with irregular menstrual cycles. Monitor CBC, including WBC count with differential, platelet count, Hgb, Hct weekly for 1st 8 weeks of therapy and monthly thereafter (MDS); q 2 weeks for 1st 3 months and monthly thereafter (multiple myeloma). Monitor for signs/symptoms of hypersensitivity reactions, thromboembolic disorders, neutropenia, thrombocytopenia, angioedema, grade 2-3 rash, exfoliative/bullous rash, SJS, TEN, and tumor lysis syndrome. Monitor renal function, especially in elderly.

**Patient Counseling:** Instruct not to break, chew, or open caps. Inform of pregnancy risks; avoid pregnancy during therapy. Use 2 effective contraceptive methods during therapy, during therapy interruptions, and for at least 4 weeks after completing therapy. Males receiving therapy must always use a latex condom during any sexual contact, even if with successful vasectomy. Men cannot donate semen or sperm during therapy. Seek medical attention if symptoms of thromboembolism (eg, SOB, chest pain, arm or leg swelling), hypersensitivity reactions, or infection occur. Avoid donating blood during therapy.

**Administration:** Oral route. **Storage**: 25°C (77°F); excursions permitted to 15-30°C (59-86°F). Dispense no more than a 28 day supply.

## REYATAZ RX

atazanavir sulfate (Bristol-Myers Squibb)

**THERAPEUTIC CLASS:** Protease inhibitor

**INDICATIONS:** Treatment of HIV-1 infection in combination with other antiretrovirals.

**DOSAGE:** *Adults:* Therapy-Naive: 300mg with ritonavir (RTV) 100mg qd. If intolerant to RTV, give atazanavir (ATV) 400mg qd. Therapy-Experienced: 300mg with RTV 100mg qd. Concomitant therapy with tenofovir, $H_2$-receptor antagonists, PPIs, and efavirenz require dose adjustment (see PI). Take with food.
*Pediatrics:* Therapy-Naive: ≥13 yrs and ≥39kg/Ritonavir (RTV) Intolerant: 400mg qd without RTV. Therapy-Naive: 6-<18 yrs: 15-<25kg: 150mg with RTV 80mg qd. 25-<32kg: 200mg with RTV 100mg qd. 32-<39kg: 250mg with RTV 100mg qd. ≥39kg: 300mg with RTV 100mg qd. Therapy-Experienced: 6-<18 yrs: 25-<32kg: 200mg with RTV 100mg qd. 32-<39kg: 250mg with RTV 100mg qd. ≥39kg: 300mg with RTV 100mg qd. Take with food.

**HOW SUPPLIED:** Cap: 100mg, 150mg, 200mg, 300mg

**CONTRAINDICATIONS:** Concomitant with (oral) midazolam, triazolam, ergot derivatives (eg, dihydroergotamine, ergotamine, ergonovine, methylergonovine), cisapride, pimozide, rifampin, irinotecan, St. John's wort, lovastatin, simvastatin, and indinavir.

**WARNINGS/PRECAUTIONS:** May prolong PR-interval; caution with pre-existing cardiac conduction system disease. New-onset diabetes mellitus (DM), exacerbation of pre-existing DM, hyperglycemia, hyperbilirubinemia, Stevens-Johnson syndrome, erythema multiforme, nephrolithiasis reported. Caution with hepatic impairment; avoid with severe hepatic insufficiency. D/C with severe rash, hyperbilirubinemia. Consider alternative antiretroviral therapy if jaundice or scleral icterus occurs. Immune reconstitution syndrome reported with combination therapy. Possible redistribution/accumulation of body fat. Increased risk of bleeding (eg, spontaneous skin hematomas and hemarthrosis) may occur with hemophilia A and B. Avoid in HIV-treatment-experienced patients with end-stage renal disease (ESRD) managed with hemodialysis. Various degrees of cross-resistance reported. Caution in elderly.

**ADVERSE REACTIONS:** Headache, N/V, abdominal pain, diarrhea, rash, myalgia, insomnia, jaundice/scleral icterus, hyperbilirubinemia, hypercholesterolemia, neutropenia, creatinine kinase elevation, peripheral neurologic symptoms, fever and depression.

**INTERACTIONS:** See Contraindications. Caution with drugs highly dependent on CYP2C8 with narrow therapeutic indices (eg, paclitaxel, repaglinide). Avoid nevirapine, voriconazole, other protease inhibitors with ATV/RTV therapy. May increase levels of drugs metabolized by CYP3A or UGT1A1 or prolong therapeutic and adverse effects. CYP3A inducers may decrease levels and reduce therapeutic effect. CYP3A inhibitors, voriconazole may increase levels. Decreased levels with buffered didanosine, tenofovir, efavirenz, antacids/buffered medications (give ATV 2 hrs before or 1 hr after), $H_2$-receptor antagonists (space dosing by 10 hrs). Increased levels of saquinavir, diltiazem (reduce dose by 50%), amiodarone, lidocaine (systemic), bepridil, quinidine, warfarin, TCAs, trazodone, rifabutin (reduce dose up to 75%), CCBs, oral contraceptives (use lowest possible dose), sildenafil/tadalafil/vardenafil (reduce dose), atorvastatin, rosuvastatin, cyclosporine, sirolimus, tacrolimus, clarithromycin (reduce dose by 50%; consider alternative therapy for infections other than MAC), immunosuppressants, fluticasone (use with caution). Increased levels with RTV (give ATV 300mg/day with RTV 100mg/day with food). Caution with high doses of ketoconazole, itraconazole with ATV/RTV therapy. ATV/RTV therapy may significantly increase plasma fluticasone propionate exposure resulting in significantly decreased serum cortisol concentrations; not recommended unless potential benefit outweighs risk of corticosteroid side effects. Avoid use of PPIs and efavirenz in treatment-experienced patients. Additive effect on PR interval when coadministered with diltiazem. See PI for complete information.

**PREGNANCY:** Category B, not for use in nursing.

**MECHANISM OF ACTION:** HIV-1 protease inhibitor; inhibits virus-specific processing of viral Gag-Pol polyproteins in HIV-1 infected cells, preventing formation of mature virions.

**PHARMACOKINETICS: Absorption:** Rapid. $T_{max}$=2.5 hrs. **Distribution:** Plasma protein binding (86%). **Metabolism:** Liver; biotransformation: mono- and dioxygenation via CYP3A. **Elimination:** Urine (7%), feces (20%); $T_{1/2}$=7 hrs.

## NURSING CONSIDERATIONS

**Assessment:** Assess for concomitant drugs that are highly dependent on CYP3A or UGT1A1 for clearance and increase plasma levels, known hypersensitivity (eg, Stevens-Johnson syndrome, erythema multiforme, or toxic skin eruptions), hepatic impairment, HBV or HCV infection, ESRD, DM, hemophilia, conduction system disease (1st- to 3rd-degree heart block), pregnancy/nursing status, and possible drug interactions. Assess LFTs, total bilirubin/cholesterol, creatinine kinase, neutrophil count, ECG.

**Monitoring:** Monitor for signs/symptoms of PR interval prolongation, exacerbation of DM and hyperglycemia, hyperbilirubinemia, rash, unexplained bleeding, nephrolithiasis, changes in body fat, immune reconstitution syndrome, hypercholesterolemia, neutropenia. Monitor hematologic tests, LFTs, CK, cholesterol profile, chemistries, total bilirubin, neutrophil count, ECG abnormalities. May enroll patients in the Antiretroviral Pregnancy Registry if they become pregnant while on treatment.

**Patient Counseling:** Inform that therapy is not cure for HIV, does not reduce risk of transmission of HIV and that opportunistic infections may develop. Inform that sustained decreases in plasma HIV RNA are associated with reduced risk of progression to AIDS and death. Take with food as prescribed. Do not alter dose or d/c without consulting physician. If miss dose, take as soon as possible and return to normal schedule; do not double next dose. Report use of any other medication (St. John's wort, PDE5 inhibitor). If taking antacids or didanosine, take capsule 2 hrs before or 1 hr after. Inform that mild rashes, asymptomatic elevations in indirect bilirubin, redistribution and accumulation of body fat may occur and may also produce changes in ECG. Seek medical attention if experience symptoms of PR interval prolongation (dizziness or lightheadedness), exacerbation of DM and hyperglycemia, hyperbilirubinemia (jaundice), rash, unexplained bleeding, nephrolithiasis, redistribution of body fat, and immune reconstitution syndrome. Instruct not to breastfeed when taking this drug.



**Administration:** Oral route. **Storage:** Store at 25°C (77°F); excursions permitted to 15-30°C (59-86°F).

## RHINOCORT AQUA — RX

budesonide (AstraZeneca)

**THERAPEUTIC CLASS:** Corticosteroid

**INDICATIONS:** Management of nasal symptoms of seasonal or perennial allergic rhinitis.

**DOSAGE:** *Adults*: 1 spray per nostril qd. Max: 4 sprays/nostril/day.
*Pediatrics*: ≥12 yrs: 1 spray per nostril qd. Max: 4 sprays/nostril/day. 6-11 yrs: 1 spray per nostril qd. Max: 2 sprays/nostril/day.

**HOW SUPPLIED:** Spray: 32mcg/spray [8.6g]

**WARNINGS/PRECAUTIONS:** Risk of adrenal insufficiency and withdrawal symptoms when replacing systemic corticosteroids with a topical corticosteroid. Transfer from systemic corticosteroids may unmask allergic or other immunologic conditions previously suppressed by systemic corticosteroid therapy (eg, rhinitis, conjunctivitis, eczema, arthritis). May be more susceptible to infections. Caution with active or quiescent TB, ocular herpes simplex, or untreated bacterial, fungal, and systemic viral infections. Avoid with recent nasal trauma, surgery, or septum ulcers. Risk of more severe/fatal course of infections (eg, chickenpox, measles) and for *Candida* infections of the nose and pharynx. Potential for reduced growth velocity in pediatrics; monitor growth routinely in pediatrics. Immediate and/or delayed hypersensitivity reactions may occur rarely. Larger than recommended doses should be avoided; may cause hypercorticism and adrenal suppression; d/c slowly if such changes occur. Caution with hepatic dysfunction. Rare reports of glaucoma, increased intraocular pressure, cataracts, wheezing, and nasal septum perforation.

**ADVERSE REACTIONS:** Pharyngitis, epistaxis, cough, bronchospasm, nasal irritation.

**INTERACTIONS:** Oral ketoconazole and cimetidine may increase plasma levels. CYP3A4 inhibitors (eg, itraconazole, clarithromycin, erythromycin) may inhibit metabolism and increase systemic exposure.

**PREGNANCY:** Category B, caution in nursing.

**MECHANISM OF ACTION:** Corticosteroid; mechanism not established. Possesses a wide range of inhibitory activities against multiple cell types (eg, mast cells, eosinophils, neutrophils, macrophages, lymphocytes) and mediators (eg, histamine, leukotrienes, ecosanoids, cytokines) involved in allergic-mediated inflammation.

**PHARMACOKINETICS: Absorption:** Well-absorbed, $T_{max}$=0.7 hr. **Distribution:** $V_d$=2-3L/Kg, plasma protein binding (85-90%), found in breastmilk. **Metabolism:** Liver (extensive), 16α-hydroxyprednisolone and 6β-hydroxybudesonide (major metabolites) via CYP3A4-catalyzed biotransformation. **Elimination:** Urine and feces; $T_{1/2}$(22R form)=2-3 hrs.

## NURSING CONSIDERATIONS

**Assessment:** Assess for active or quiescent TB, untreated localized/systemic fungal or bacterial infections, systemic viral infections, ocular herpes simplex, history of glaucoma, recent nasal septal ulcers, recent nasal surgery/trauma, hepatic impairment, pregnancy/nursing status, and for possible drug interactions.

**Monitoring:** Monitor for signs/symptoms of adrenal insufficiency, hypercorticism, chickenpox, measles, nasal/pharyngeal *Candida* infections, hypoadrenalism in infants born to mothers who received corticosteroids during pregnancy, suppression of growth velocity in children, hypersensitivity reactions, wheezing, nasal septum perforation, epistaxis, glaucoma, vision changes, cataracts, and for increased IOP.

**Patient Counseling:** Counsel to take as directed at regular intervals. Advise to avoid exposure to chickenpox or measles. Instruct to consult physician immediately if exposed to chickenpox or measles, if symptoms worsen, or if episodes of epistaxis or nasal discomfort occur. Instruct to avoid spraying into eyes. Advise that long-term use may increase risk of some eye problems. Counsel to notify physician of all current medications.

**Administration:** Intranasal route. Refer to PI for further administration instructions. **Storage:** Store at 20-25°C (68-77°F) with the valve up. Do not freeze. Protect from light.



# RIFADIN RX

rifampin (Sanofi-Aventis)

**THERAPEUTIC CLASS:** Rifamycin derivative

**INDICATIONS:** Treatment of all forms of TB. Treatment of asymptomatic carriers of *Neisseria meningitidis* to eliminate meningococci from nasopharynx.

**DOSAGE:** *Adults:* TB: 10mg/kg PO/IV qd. Max: 600mg/day. Meningococcal Carriers: 600mg bid for 2 days. Take 1 hr before or 2 hrs after a meal with a full glass of water.
*Pediatrics:* TB: 10-20mg/kg PO/IV qd. Max: 600mg/day. Meningococcal Carriers: ≥1 month: 10mg/kg q12h for 2 days. Max: 600mg/dose. <1 month: 5mg/kg q12h for 2 days. Take 1 hr before or 2 hrs after a meal with a full glass of water.

**HOW SUPPLIED:** Cap: 150mg, 300mg; Inj: 600mg

**WARNINGS/PRECAUTIONS:** May produce liver dysfunction. May cause hyperbilirubinemia. Not for treatment of meningococcal disease. May produce reddish coloration of the urine, sweat, sputum, and tears. May permanently stain soft contact lenses.

**ADVERSE REACTIONS:** GI distress, thrombocytopenia, visual disturbances, menstrual disturbances, edema of face and extremities, elevated BUN and serum uric acid levels.

**INTERACTIONS:** May accelerate elimination of drugs metabolized by CYP450 (eg, anticonvulsants, antiarrhythmics, anticoagulants, azole antifungals, barbiturates, β-blockers, CCBs, chloramphenicol, clarithromycin, corticosteroids, cyclosporine, cardiac glycosides, clofibrate, oral or systemic contraceptives, dapsone, diazepam, doxycycline, fluoroquinolones, haloperidol, oral hypoglycemics, levothyroxine, methadone, narcotics, nortriptyline, progestins, quinine, tacrolimus, theophylline, TCAs, and zidovudine). Give antacids at least 1 hr before rifampin. Increased hepatotoxicity with halothane or isoniazid. Increased serum levels with probenecid and cotrimoxazole. Caution with other hepatotoxic agents. Concomitant ketoconazole decreases both drug serum levels. Decreased levels of enalapril, atovaquone. Increased levels with atovaquone.

**PREGNANCY:** Category C, not for use in nursing.

**MECHANISM OF ACTION:** Rifamycin derivative; has bacterial activity against intracellular and extracellular *Mycobacterium tuberculosis*. Inhibits DNA-dependent RNA polymerase activity in susceptible cells. Interacts with bacterial RNA polymerase; does not inhibit the mammalian enzyme.

**PHARMACOKINETICS: Absorption:** Readily absorbed from GI tract. (PO, 600mg) $C_{max}$=7mcg/mL. (IV, 300mg, 600mg) $C_{max}$=9.0mcg/mL, 17.5mcg/mL. **Distribution:** (IV, 300mg, 600mg): $V_d$=0.66L/kg, 0.64L/kg; distributed in body fluids and cerebrospinal fluid; plasma protein binding 80%. **Metabolism:** Via deacetylation; 25-desacetyl-rifampin (major metabolite). **Elimination:** Urine (30%), bile; (600mg, 900mg) $T_{1/2}$=3.35 hrs, 5.08hrs.

## NURSING CONSIDERATIONS

**Assessment:** Assess for liver and renal function, DM, possible drug interactions. Document indications for therapy, culture and sensitivity.

**Monitoring:** Monitor LFTs (SGPT and SGOT, bilirubin or transaminase), SrCr, CBCs, and platelet count. Monitor for hematopoietic reactions (leukopenia, thrombocytopenia or acute hemolytic anemia), cutaneous reactions, hypersensitivity reactions (Stevens-Johnson syndrome, vasculitis, anaphylaxis), renal function, serum uric acid, convulsions, visual disturbances, flu-like syndrome.

R

**Patient Counseling:** Drug treats bacterial, not viral, infections. Inform that drug may produce reddish urine, sweat, sputum, and tears. Take drug 1 hr before or 2 hrs after meal with a full glass of water. Report immediately any fever, loss of appetite, malaise, N/V, darkened urine, yellowish discoloration of skin/eyes, and joint pain/swelling. Take full course of therapy, not missing doses. Reliability of oral contraceptives may be affected; use alternate contraceptive measures.

**Administration:** Oral and IV route. **Storage:** Avoid excessive heat (40-104°C). Protect from light.

# RIFAMATE RX

rifampin - isoniazid (Sanofi-Aventis)

**Isoniazid associated with severe and sometimes fatal hepatitis. Monitor LFTs on a monthly basis.**

**THERAPEUTIC CLASS:** Isonicotinic acid hydrazide/rifamycin derivative

**INDICATIONS:** For pulmonary TB. Not for initial therapy or prevention.

**DOSAGE:** *Adults:* 2 caps qd. Take 1 hr before or 2 hrs after meals. Give with pyridoxine in the malnourished, those predisposed to neuropathy (eg, alcoholics, diabetics), and adolescents.

**HOW SUPPLIED:** Cap: (Isoniazid-Rifampin) 150mg-300mg

**CONTRAINDICATIONS:** Previous isoniazid-associated hepatic injury, severe adverse reactions to isoniazid (eg, drug fever, chills, and arthritis), acute liver disease.

**WARNINGS/PRECAUTIONS:** Monitor LFTs before therapy, periodically thereafter. Not for intermittent therapy. Urine, feces, saliva, sputum, sweat, and tears may be colored red-orange; may stain soft contact lenses permanently. Caution with chronic liver disease or severe renal dysfunction. Perform periodic ophthalmoscopic exams.

**ADVERSE REACTIONS:** Headache, drowsiness, fatigue, ataxia, dizziness, confusion, visual disturbances, weakness, GI effects, peripheral neuropathy, pyridoxine deficiency, anorexia, nausea, renal or hepatic insufficiency, blood dyscrasias.

**INTERACTIONS:** Anticoagulants may need dose increase. May decrease activity of methadone, oral hypoglycemics, digitoxin, quinidine, disopyramide, dapsone, and corticosteroids. Higher incidence of isoniazid hepatitis with daily alcohol ingestion. Risk of phenytoin toxicity. Caution with other hepatotoxic agents and phenytoin. May decrease effects of oral contraceptives; use alternative measures.

**PREGNANCY:** Safety in pregnancy not known, caution in nursing.

**MECHANISM OF ACTION:** Isonicotinic acid hydrazide/rifamycin derivative. Isoniazid/Rifampin: Exhibits bacterial activity against intracellular and extracellular *Mycobacterium tuberculosis*. Inhibits DNA-dependent RNA polymerase activity in susceptible cells; interacts with bacterial RNA polymerase but does not inhibit the mammalian enzyme. Inhibits mycoloic acid synthesis and acts against actively growing tubercle bacilli.

**PHARMACOKINETICS: Absorption:** Rifampin: $C_{max}$=10mcg/mL, $T_{max}$=$1\frac{1}{2}$-3 hrs. Isoniazid: $T_{max}$=1-2 hrs. **Distribution:** Isoniazid: Diffuses into body fluids; crosses placental barrier and into milk. **Metabolism:** Isoniazid: Acetylation and dehydrazination. **Elimination:** Rifampin: Bile, urine; $T_{1/2}$=3 hrs.

## NURSING CONSIDERATIONS

**Assessment:** Assess for previous isoniazid-associated hepatic injury, acute liver disease, HIV status, pregnancy status, and drug interactions. Document reasons for therapy, culture and susceptibility.

**Monitoring:** Prior to therapy and periodically thereafter, measure hepatic enzymes (AST, ALT). D/C at first sign of hypersensitivity reactions (fever, skin eruptions, Stevens-Johnson syndrome, vasculitis, anaphylaxis). Monitor for peripheral neuropathy, convulsions, N/V, agranulocytosis, hemolytic anemia, SLE-like syndrome, metabolic and endocrine reactions (hyperglycemia, pyridoxine deficiency, pellagra), visual disturbances, serum uric acid levels.

**Patient Counseling:** Advise to immediately report signs/symptoms consistent with liver damage or other adverse events (eg, unexplained anorexia, N/V, dark urine, icterus, rash, persistent paresthesias of the hands and feet, persistent fatigue, weakness or fever of >3 days duration and/or abdominal tenderness). Counsel not to administer with food, take as prescribed, take pyridoxine tablets if peripheral neuropathy develops. Inform that drug may produce reddish urine, sweat, sputum, and tears. Periodic eye exams are recommended when visual symptoms occur.

**Administration:** Oral route. **Storage:** Keep tightly closed. Store in a dry place. Avoid excessive heat.

# RIFATER RX

pyrazinamide - rifampin - isoniazid (Sanofi-Aventis)

**Isoniazid associated with severe and sometimes fatal hepatitis. Monitor LFTs on a monthly basis.**

**THERAPEUTIC CLASS:** Isonicotinic acid hydrazide/rifamycin derivative/nicotinamide analogue

**INDICATIONS:** For initial phase of pulmonary TB treatment.

**DOSAGE:** *Adults:* ≤44kg: 4 tabs single dose qd. 45-54kg: 5 tabs single dose. ≥55kg: 6 tabs single dose. Give pyridoxine in malnourished, if predisposed to neuropathy (eg, alcoholics, diabetics), and adolescents. Take 1 hr before or 2 hrs after meals with full glass of water. Treatment usually lasts 2 months. *Pediatrics:* ≥15 yrs: ≤44kg: 4 tabs single dose qd. 45-54kg: 5 tabs qd single dose. ≥55kg: 6 tabs qd single dose. Give pyridoxine in malnourished, if predisposed to neuropathy (eg, alcoholics, diabetics), and adolescents. Take 1 hr before or 2 hrs after meals with full glass of water. Treatment usually lasts 2 months.

**HOW SUPPLIED:** Tab: (Isoniazid-Pyrazinamide-Rifampin) 50mg-300mg-120mg

**CONTRAINDICATIONS:** Severe hepatic damage, adverse reactions to isoniazid (eg, drug fever, chills, arthritis), acute liver disease, acute gout.

**WARNINGS/PRECAUTIONS:** Liver dysfunction, hyperbilirubinemia, and hyperuricemia with acute gouty arthritis reported. Caution in patient's with impaired liver function; monitor LFTs (every 2-4 weeks), serum uric acid. Perform regular ophthalmologic exams. Caution with DM, severe renal dysfunction. May produce reddish coloration of urine, sweat, sputum, and tears. May permanently stain soft contact lenses. Caution in elderly.

**ADVERSE REACTIONS:** Rifampin: heartburn, epigastric distress, thrombocytopenia, headache, fever, drowsiness, visual disturbances, elevation of BUN and uric acid. Isoniazid: peripheral neuropathy, N/V, epigastric distress. Pyrazinamide: hepatic reactions, N/V.

**INTERACTIONS:** Rifampin may accelerate metabolism of anticonvulsants (eg, phenytoin), antiarrhythmics (eg, disopyramide, mexiletine, quinidine, tocainide), anticoagulants, antifungals (eg, fluconazole, itraconazole, ketoconazole), barbiturates, β-blockers, CCBs (eg, diltiazem, nifedipine, verapamil), chloramphenicol, ciprofloxacin, corticosteroids, cyclosporine, cardiac glycosides, clofibrate, oral contraceptives, dapsone, diazepam, haloperidol, oral hypoglycemics (eg, sulfonylureas), methadone, narcotic analgesics, nortriptyline, progestins, theophylline. Antacids may reduce rifampin absorption. Avoid foods containing tyramine and histamine (eg, cheese, red wine, tuna). Anticoagulants may need dose increase. Higher incidence of isoniazid (INH) hepatitis with daily alcohol ingestion. Avoid halothane. INH inhibits certain CYP450 enzymes; monitor with anticonvulsants, benzodiazepines, haloperidol, ketoconazole, warfarin. Decreased levels with corticosteroids. Exaggerates CNS effects of meperidine, cycloserine, disulfiram. Excess catecholamine stimulation with L-dopa.

**PREGNANCY:** Category C, not for use in nursing.

**MECHANISM OF ACTION:** Rifampin: Inhibits DNA-dependent RNA polymerase activity in susceptible *Mycobacterium tuberculosis* organism. Interacts with bacterial RNA polymerase, but does not inhibit the mammalian enzyme. Isoniazid: Kills growing tubercle bacilli by inhibiting the biosynthesis of mycolic acids, which are major component of the cell wall of *Mycobacterium tuberculosis.* Pyrazinamide: Inhibits growth of *Mycobacterium tuberculosis.*

**PHARMACOKINETICS: Absorption:** Isoniazid: Bioavailability (100.6%), $C_{max}$=3.09mcg/mL, $T_{max}$=1-2 hrs. Rifampin: Bioavailability (88.8 %), $C_{max}$=11.04mcg/mL. Pyrazinamide: Bioavailability (96.8%), $C_{max}$=28.02mcg/mL. **Distribution:** Isoniazid: Passes through placental barrier and into milk. Pyrazinamide: Plasma protein binding (10%), distributed in liver, lungs, and CSF; found in breast milk. Rifampin: Protein binding (80%). **Metabolism:** Isoniazid: Acetylation and dehydrazination. Pyrazinamide: Liver, via

R

hydroxylation; pyrazinoic acid (major active metabolite). Rifampin: Via deacetylation; 25-desacetyl-rifampin (major metabolite). **Elimination:** Rifampin: Urine (30%), bile; $T_{1/2}$=3.35 hrs. Pyrazinamide: Urine (70%), (4-14% unchanged); $T_{1/2}$=9-10 hrs. Isoniazid: Urine (50-70%); $T_{1/2}$=1-4 hrs.

## NURSING CONSIDERATIONS

**Assessment:** Assess for previous isoniazid-associated hepatic injury, acute gout, HIV status, pregnancy status, DM, and drug interactions. Document reasons for therapy, culture and susceptibility.

**Monitoring:** Prior to therapy and periodically thereafter, measure hepatic enzymes (AST, ALT). D/C at first sign of hypersensitivity reactions (fever, skin eruptions, Stevens-Johnson syndrome, vasculitis, anaphylaxis). Monitor for peripheral neuropathy, convulsions, N/V, agranulocytosis, hemolytic anemia, SLE like syndrome, metabolic and endocrine reactions (hyperglycemia, pyridoxine deficiency, pellagra), visual disturbances, serum uric acid levels.

**Patient Counseling:** Immediately report signs/symptoms consistent with liver damage or other adverse events (unexplained anorexia, N/V, dark urine, icterus, rash, persistent paresthesias of hands and feet, persistent fatigue, weakness or fever of >3 days' duration and/or abdominal tenderness). Do not administer with food; take as prescribed. Take pyridoxine tablets if peripheral neuropathy develops. Drug may produce reddish urine, sweat, sputum, and tears. Periodic ophthalmoscopic examination is recommended when visual symptoms occur. Avoid tyramine- and histamine-containing foods. Effectiveness of oral contraceptives may be decreased; consider alternative contraceptive methods.

**Administration:** Oral route. **Storage:** 15-30°C (59-86°F). Protect from excessive humidity.

# RILUTEK RX

riluzole (Sanofi-Aventis)

**THERAPEUTIC CLASS:** Benzothiazole

**INDICATIONS:** Treatment of amyotrophic lateral sclerosis (ALS). Extends survival and/or time to tracheostomy.

**DOSAGE:** *Adults:* 50mg q12h. Take 1 hr before or 2 hrs after meals.

**HOW SUPPLIED:** Tab: 50mg

**WARNINGS/PRECAUTIONS:** Caution with hepatic impairment; monitor LFTs. D/C if ALT levels ≥5 x ULN or clinical jaundice develops. Clinical hepatitis reported. Neutropenia may occur; monitor WBC count with febrile illness. Interstitial lung disease reported; perform chest radiography if respiratory symptoms develop such as dry cough and/or dyspnea. May impair mental/physical abilities. Caution in elderly.

**ADVERSE REACTIONS:** Asthenia, N/V, dizziness, decreased lung function, diarrhea, abdominal pain, vertigo, circumonal paresthesia, anorexia, somnolence, headache, anorexia, rhinitis, HTN.

**INTERACTIONS:** Caution with concomitant use with potentially hepatotoxic drugs (eg, allopurinol, methyldopa, sulfasalazine). CYP1A2 inhibitors (eg, caffeine, phenacetin, theophylline, amitriptyline, quinolones) may decrease elimination. CYP1A2 inducers (eg, cigarette smoke, charcoal-broiled food, rifampicin, omeprazole) may increase elimination. Potential interaction may occur if riluzole is given concurrently with drugs metabolized by CYP1A2 (eg, theophylline, caffeine, tacrine).

**PREGNANCY:** Category C, not for use in nursing.

**MECHANISM OF ACTION:** Benzothiazole; mechanism not established. May inhibit the effect on glutamate release, inactivates voltage-dependent sodium channels, and interferes with intracellular events that follow transmitter binding at excitatory amino acid receptors.

**PHARMACOKINETICS: Absorption:** Well absorbed; absolute bioavailability (60%). **Distribution:** Plasma protein binding (96%). **Metabolism:** Extensive;

R

liver via CYP450 by hydroxylation and glucuronidation; N-hydroxyriluzole (major metabolite). **Elimination:** Urine (metabolites [90%], unchanged [2%]), feces (5%); $T_{1/2}$=12 hrs.

## NURSING CONSIDERATIONS

**Assessment:** Assess for hepatic impairment, pregnancy/nursing status, alcohol intake, hypersensitivity and possible drug interactions. Perform baseline LFTs.

**Monitoring:** Perform baseline LFTs before therapy, every month during first 3 months, every 3 months for the remainder of the first year, then periodically thereafter. Take WBC count and chest radiography if necessary. Monitor for signs/symptoms of febrile illness, liver toxicity, and hypersensitivity reactions.

**Patient Counseling:** Notify healthcare professional of any signs of febrile illness. Caution about hazardous tasks (eg, operating machinery/driving). Notify healthcare professional if cough or shortness of breath occur. Avoid use with excessive intake of alcohol. Instruct patient if a dose is missed take next tablet as originally planned.

**Administration:** Oral route. **Storage:** 20-25°C (68-77°F); protect from bright light.

# RISPERDAL — RX

risperidone (Ortho-Mcneil/Janssen)

**Elderly patients with dementia-related psychosis treated with atypical antipsychotic drugs are at an increased risk of death; most deaths appeared to be cardiovascular (eg, heart failure, sudden death) or infectious (eg, pneumonia) in nature. Risperidone is not approved for treatment of dementia-related psychosis.**

**OTHER BRAND NAMES:** Risperdal M-Tab (Ortho-Mcneil/Janssen)

**THERAPEUTIC CLASS:** Benzisoxazole derivative

**INDICATIONS:** Acute and maintenance treatment of schizophrenia in adults. Treatment of schizophrenia in adolescents 13-17 yrs. Short-term treatment of acute manic or mixed episodes associated with bipolar I disorder as monotherapy (adults and adolescents 10-17 yrs) or in combination with lithium or valproate (adults). Treatment of irritability associated with autistic disorder in children and adolescents 5-16 yrs, including symptoms of aggression toward others, deliberate self-injuriousness, temper tantrums, and quickly changing moods.

**DOSAGE:** *Adults:* Schizophrenia: Initial: 2mg/day qd or bid. Titrate: Adjust dose at intervals not <24 hrs, in increments of 1-2mg/day, as tolerated, to recommended dose of 4-8mg/day. Max: 16mg/day. Reinitiating Treatment: Follow initial titration schedule. Switching from Other Antipsychotics: Minimize overlapping period of antipsychotics when switching. When switching from depot antipsychotics, initiate therapy in place of next scheduled injection. Bipolar Mania: Initial: 2-3mg qd. Titrate: Adjust dose at intervals not <24 hrs and in increments/decrements of 1mg/day. Max: 6mg/day. If with persistent somnolence, give half the daily dose bid. Elderly/Debilitated/Hypotension/Severe Renal or Hepatic Impairment: Initial: 0.5mg bid. Titrate: Adjust dose in increments not >0.5mg bid. Increases to doses >1.5mg bid should occur at intervals of ≥1 week. If qd dosing regimen in elderly or debilitated is being considered, titrate bid regimen for 2-3 days at the target dose. Subsequent switches to a qd dosing regimen can be done thereafter. Periodically reassess to determine maintenance treatment. Titrate accordingly when coadministered with certain other medications.
*Pediatrics:* Schizophrenia: 13-17 yrs: Initial: 0.5mg qd in am or pm. Titrate: Adjust dose at intervals not <24 hrs in increments of 0.5 or 1mg/day, as tolerated, to recommended dose of 3mg/day. Max: 6mg/day. Reinitiating Treatment: Follow initial titration schedule. Switching from Other Antipsychotics: Minimize overlapping period of antipsychotics when switching. When switching from depot antipsychotics, initiate therapy in place of next scheduled injection. Bipolar Mania: 10-17 yrs: Initial: 0.5mg qd in am

or pm. Titrate: Adjust dose at intervals not <24 hrs in increments of 0.5 or 1mg/day, as tolerated, to recommended dose of 2.5mg/day. Max: 6mg/day. If with persistent somnolence, give half the daily dose bid. Irritability Associated with Autistic Disorder: 5-16 yrs: Initial: <20kg: 0.25mg/day qd or bid; ≥20kg: 0.5mg/day qd or bid. Titrate: After at least 4 days, may increase dose to 0.5mg/day (<20kg) or 1mg/day ( ≥20kg). Maint: Minimum of 14 days. Inadequate Response: Increase at ≥2-wk intervals: <20kg: Increase by 0.25mg/day; ≥20kg: Increase by 0.5mg/day. Caution in patients <15kg. Max: <20kg: 1mg/day; ≥20kg: 2.5mg/day; >45kg: 3mg/day. If with persistent somnolence, give qd dose hs or half the daily dose bid, or reduce dose. Titrate accordingly when co-administered with certain other medications.

**HOW SUPPLIED:** Sol: 1mg/mL [30mL]; Tab: 0.25mg, 0.5mg, 1mg, 2mg, 3mg, 4mg; Tab, Disintegrating: (M-Tab) 0.5mg, 1mg, 2mg, 3mg, 4mg.

**WARNINGS/PRECAUTIONS:** Neuroleptic malignant syndrome (NMS) reported. Tardive dyskinesia may occur. Hyperglycemia, in extreme cases associated with ketoacidosis or hyperosmolar coma or death, has been reported; monitor for hyperglycemia and perform fasting blood glucose testing at the beginning of therapy and periodically during treatment in patients at risk for diabetes mellitus (DM). Elevates prolactin levels. May induce orthostatic hypotension; caution with history of CV, cerebrovascular disease and conditions that predispose to hypotension. Leukopenia, neutropenia and agranulocytosis reported. Patients with a history of clinically significant low WBC or a drug-induced leukopenia/neutropenia should have their CBC monitored during the first few months of therapy and d/c at the first signs of a clinically significant decline in WBC in absence of other causative factors. D/C in cases of severe neutropenia (ANC<1000/mm$^3$). May impair mental/physical abilities. Seizures reported; caution with history of seizures. Esophageal dysmotility and aspiration reported; caution with increased risk of aspiration pneumonia. Rare cases of priapism reported. A single case of thrombotic thrombocytopenic purpura (TTP) reported. May disrupt body temperature regulation; caution when exposed to extreme temperatures. May have antiemetic effects that may mask the signs and symptoms of overdosage with certain drugs or of conditions such as intestinal obstruction, Reye's syndrome, and brain tumor. Possibility of suicide attempt is inherent in patients with bipolar mania and schizophrenia. Patients with Parkinson's disease or dementia with Lewy bodies are reported to have an increased sensitivity to antipsychotic medications. Caution with diseases/conditions affecting metabolism or hemodynamic responses, renal/hepatic impairment and in elderly.

**ADVERSE REACTIONS:** Somnolence, increased appetite, fatigue, N/V, coughing, urinary incontinence, constipation, fever, parkinsonism, abdominal pain, anxiety, dizziness, tremor, dyspepsia.

**INTERACTIONS:** Caution with other CNS drugs and alcohol. May potentiate hypotensive effects of other drugs with this potential (eg, antihypertensives). May antagonize effects of levodopa and dopamine agonists. Increased bioavailability with cimetidine and ranitidine. Decreased clearance with chronic use of clozapine. Increased valproate peak plasma concentration with concomitant use. Increased concentration with fluoxetine, paroxetine and CYP2D6 inhibitors. Carbamazepine and other enzyme inducers (eg, phenytoin, rifampin, phenobarbital) may decrease concentration. Increased mortality with furosemide in elderly patients with dementia-related psychosis.

**PREGNANCY:** Category C, not for use in nursing.

**MECHANISM OF ACTION:** Benzisoxazole derivative; exact mechanism unknown. Therapeutic activity is proposed to be mediated through a combination of dopamine Type 2 ($D_2$) and serotonin Type 2 ($5HT_2$) receptor antagonism.

**PHARMACOKINETICS: Absorption**: Well absorbed; absolute bioavailability (70%). Risperidone $T_{max}$=1 hr; 9-hydroxyrisperidone $T_{max}$=3hrs (extensive metabolizers), 17hrs (poor metabolizers) **Distribution**: $V_d$=1-2L/kg; plasma protein binding (risperidone 90%) (9-hydroxyrisperidone 77%); found in breast milk. **Metabolism**: Liver via CYP 2D6; hydroxylation, N-dealkylation; 9-hydroxyrisperidone (major metabolite). **Elimination**: Urine (70%), feces (14%); $T_{1/2}$=3 hrs (extensive metabolizers); 20 hrs (poor metabolizers).

R

## NURSING CONSIDERATIONS

**Assessment:** Assess patient for dementia-related psychosis, high-risk patients (suicidal), pre-existing low WBCs or drug-induced leukopenia/neutropenia, history of cardiovascular/cerebrovascular diseases, predisposition to hypotension, diseases/conditions affecting hemodynamic response, DM, seizures, risk of aspiration pneumonia, liver/renal impairment, pregnancy/nursing status, and possible drug interactions.

**Monitoring:** Monitor for TD, NMS, priapism, TTP, extrapyramidal symptoms, cerebrovascular events (eg, stroke, transient ischemic attacks), esophageal dysmotility, aspiration, orthostatic hypotension, hypoglycemia, body temperature lability, seizures, suicidal attempts, and cognitive/motor impairment. Perform periodic monitoring of fasting blood glucose levels in patients with DM or at risk for DM. Monitor for signs/symptoms of leukopenia, neutropenia, and agranulocytosis; perform frequent monitoring of CBC in patients with history of clinically significant low WBC or drug-induced. Monitor liver/renal function and prolactin levels.

**Patient Counseling:** Advise of risk of orthostatic hypotension and of nonpharmacologic interventions that help reduce its occurrence. Counsel to notify physician if taking any other medications and if intending to become pregnant or becomes pregnant during therapy. Advise to use caution while performing hazardous tasks (eg, operating machinery/driving). Do not breastfeed while on therapy. Advise to avoid alcohol. Disintegrating tab contains phenylalanine.

**Administration:** Oral route. Take with or without meals. Sol can be administered directly from the calibrated pipette or mixed with a compatible beverage. Do not split or chew tab. **Storage**: 15-25°C (59-77°F). Keep out of reach of children. (Sol)Protect from light and freezing. (Tab) Protect from light and moisture.

# Risperdal Consta — RX

risperidone (Ortho-Mcneil/Janssen)

**Elderly patients with dementia-related psychosis treated with atypical antipsychotic drugs are at an increased risk of death; most deaths appeared to be cardiovascular (eg, heart failure, sudden death) or infectious (eg, pneumonia) in nature. Risperidone is not approved for the treatment of patients with dementia-related psychosis.**

**THERAPEUTIC CLASS:** Benzisoxazole derivative

**INDICATIONS:** Treatment of schizophrenia. As monotherapy or adjunctive therapy to lithium or valproate for maintenance treatment of bipolar I disorder.

R

**DOSAGE:** *Adults:* Give 1st injection with oral dosage form or other oral antipsychotic. Continue for 3 weeks, then d/c oral therapy. Titrate: Increase at intervals of ≥4 weeks. Schizophrenia: 25mg IM q 2 weeks. Max: 50mg q 2 weeks. Bipolar I Disorder: Monotherapy/With Lithium or Valproate: 25mg IM q 2 weeks. If used for extended periods, re-evaluate periodically for long-term risks and benefits of therapy. Max: 50mg. Hepatic or Renal Impairment: Prior to initiating IM therapy, administer oral dosage, 0.5mg po bid during the 1st week. Titrate: May increase oral dosage to 1mg po bid or 2mg po qd during the 2nd week of therapy. If total daily dose of 2mg po is tolerated, may start at 12.5mg or 25mg IM q 2 weeks. Continue oral supplementation for 3 weeks. Elderly: 25mg IM q 2 weeks.

**HOW SUPPLIED:** Inj: 12.5mg, 25mg, 37.5mg, 50mg

**WARNINGS/PRECAUTIONS:** Neuroleptic malignant syndrome (NMS) reported. Tardive dyskinesia may occur. Hyperglycemia, in extreme cases associated with ketoacidosis or hyperosmolar coma or death, has been reported; monitor for hyperglycemia and perform fasting blood glucose testing at the beginning of therapy and periodically during treatment in patients at risk for diabetes mellitus (DM). Elevates prolactin levels. May induce orthostatic hypotension; caution with history of CV, cerebrovascular disease and conditions that predispose to hypotension. Leukopenia, neutropenia and agranulocytosis reported. Patients with a history of clinically significant low WBC or drug-induced leukopenia/neutropenia should have their CBC monitored during the first few months of therapy and d/c at the first signs of a clinically significant decline in WBC in absence of other causative factors. D/C in cases of severe neutropenia (ANC<1000/mm$^3$). May impair mental/physical abilities. Seizures reported; caution with history of seizures. Esophageal dysmotility and aspiration reported; caution with increased risk of aspiration pneumonia. Rare cases of priapism reported. A single case of thrombotic thrombocytopenic purpura (TTP) reported. May disrupt body temperature regulation; caution when exposed to extreme temperatures. May have antiemetic effects that may mask the signs and symptoms of overdosage with certain drugs or conditions such as intestinal obstruction, Reye's syndrome, and brain tumor. Possibility of suicide attempt is inherent in patients with bipolar mania and schizophrenia. Should be injected into the deltoid or gluteal muscle, avoiding inadvertent injection into a blood vessel. Patients with Parkinson's disease or dementia with Lewy bodies are reported to have an increased sensitivity to antipsychotic medications. Caution with diseases/conditions affecting metabolism or hemodynamic responses, renal/hepatic impairment and in elderly.

**ADVERSE REACTIONS:** Headache, dizziness, constipation, dyspepsia, akathisia, parkinsonism, weight increase, dry mouth, fatigue, pain in extremity, tremor, nausea.

**INTERACTIONS:** Caution with other CNS drugs and alcohol. May potentiate hypotensive effects of other drugs with this potential (eg, antihypertensives). May antagonize effects of levodopa and dopamine agonists. Increased bioavailability with cimetidine and ranitidine. Decreased clearance with chronic use of clozapine. Increased valproate peak plasma concentration with concomitant use. Increased concentration with fluoxetine, paroxetine and CYP2D6 inhibitors. Carbamazepine and other enzyme inducers (eg, phenytoin, rifampin, phenobarbital) may decrease concentration. Increased mortality with furosemide in elderly patients with dementia-related psychosis.

**PREGNANCY:** Category C, not for use in nursing.

**MECHANISM OF ACTION:** Benzisoxazole derivative; exact mechanism unknown. Therapeutic activity is proposed to be mediated through a combination of dopamine Type 2 ($D_2$) and serotonin Type 2 ($5HT_2$) receptor antagonism.

**PHARMACOKINETICS: Distribution**: $V_d$=1-2L/kg; plasma protein binding (risperidone: 90%), (9-hydroxyrisperidone: 77%); found in breast milk. **Metabolism**: Liver via CYP 2D6; hydroxylation, N-dealkylation; 9-hydroxyrisperidone (major metabolite). **Elimination**: Urine (70%), feces (14%); $T_{1/2}$=3-6 days.

## NURSING CONSIDERATIONS

**Assessment:** Assess patient for dementia-related psychosis, liver/renal impairment, history of seizures or conditions that may lower seizure threshold, cardiovascular disease (eg, history of MI or ischemia, heart failure, conduction abnormalities), cerebrovascular disease, conditions which predispose patient to hypotension (eg, dehydration, hypovolemia), risk of aspiration pneumonia, pregnancy/nursing status, and for possible drug interactions. Assess for DM or risk factors for DM (eg, obesity, family history of DM) and baseline fasting blood glucose in patients with DM.

**Monitoring:** Monitor signs/symptoms of tardive dyskinesia, NMS, hyperprolactinemia, cognitive and motor impairment, seizures, esophageal dysmotility, aspiration, priapism, TTP, disruption of body temperature regulation, and for suicide attempts. Monitor for signs and symptoms of hyperglycemia; perform periodic monitoring of fasting blood glucose levels in patients with DM or in patients at risk for DM. Monitor for signs/symptoms of orthostatic hypotension; monitor orthostatic vital signs in patients at risk for orthostatic hypotension. Monitor for signs/symptoms of leukopenia, neutropenia, and agranulocytosis; perform frequent monitoring of CBC in patients with history of clinically significant low WBC or drug-induced leukopenia/neutropenia.

**Patient Counseling:** Advise of risk of orthostatic hypotension and instruct about nonpharmacologic interventions that help reduce its occurrence. Counsel to notify physician of all medications currently taking and if intending to become pregnant or becomes pregnant during therapy. Instruct not to breastfeed during therapy. Advise to use caution while performing hazardous tasks (eg, operating machinery/driving). Instruct to avoid alcohol during treatment.

**Administration:** IM route. Deep IM into the gluteal or deltoid muscle every 2 weeks. Not for IV use. Do not combine two different dose strengths in a single administration. **Storage**: 2-8°C (36-46°F). Protect from light. If refrigeration is unavailable, store at temperatures not exceeding 25°C (77°F) for no more than 7 days prior to administration.

## RITALIN

methylphenidate HCl (Novartis)

CII

**OTHER BRAND NAMES:** Ritalin SR (Novartis) - Ritalin LA (Novartis)

**THERAPEUTIC CLASS:** Sympathomimetic amine

**INDICATIONS:** (Cap, Extended-Release, Tab, Extended-Release) Treatment of attention deficit disorders. (Tab, Extended-Release) Treatment of narcolepsy.

**DOSAGE:** *Adults:* (Tab) 10-60mg/day given bid-tid 30-45 min ac. Take last dose before 6 pm if insomnia occurs. (Tab, ER) May use in place of immediate-release (IR) when the 8-hr dose corresponds to the titrated 8-hr IR dose. (Cap, ER) Initial: 20mg qam. Titrate: Adjust weekly by 10mg. Max: 60mg qam. Swallow whole; do not chew or crush. Previous Methylphenidate Use: May use as qd in place of IR dosed bid or daily dose of methylphenidate SR. Swallow whole or sprinkle over spoonful of applesauce. Reduce dose or d/c if paradoxical aggravation of symptoms occur. D/C if no improvement after appropriate dose adjustment over 1 month.
*Pediatrics:* ≥6 yrs: (Tab) Initial: 5mg bid before breakfast and lunch. Titrate: Increase gradually by 5-10mg weekly. Max: 60mg/day. (Tab, ER) May use in place of immediate-release (IR) when the 8-hr dose corresponds to the titrated 8-hr IR dose. (Cap, ER) Initial: 20mg qam. Titrate: Adjust weekly by 10mg. Max: 60mg qam. Swallow whole; do not chew, crush, divide. Previous Methylphenidate Use: May use as qd in place of IR dosed bid or daily dose of methylphenidate SR. Swallow whole or sprinkle over spoonful of applesauce. Reduce dose or d/c if paradoxical aggravation of symptoms occurs. D/C if no improvement after appropriate dose adjustment over 1 month.

**HOW SUPPLIED:** Cap, Extended-Release (Ritalin LA): 10mg, 20mg, 30mg, 40mg; Tab (Ritalin): 5mg, 10mg*, 20mg*; Tab, Extended-Release (Ritalin SR): 20mg *scored



**CONTRAINDICATIONS:** Marked anxiety, tension, and agitation; glaucoma; motor tics or family history or diagnosis of Tourette's syndrome; during or within 14 days of MAOI use.

**WARNINGS/PRECAUTIONS:** Sudden death, stroke, and MI reported; avoid with known structural cardiac abnormalities or other serious cardiac problems. May cause increase in BP and HR; caution with pre-existing HTN, heart failure, MI, or ventricular arrhythmias. When symptoms suggestive of cardiac disease develop, prompt evaluation required. May exacerbate symptoms of behavior disturbance and thought disorder in patients with a pre-existing psychotic disorder. Care should be taken in using stimulants to treat patients with comorbid bipolar disorder because of concern for possible induction of mixed/manic episode in such patients. Stimulants at usual doses can cause treatment emergent psychotic or manic symptoms (hallucinations, delusional thinking, mania) in children and adolescents without prior history of psychotic illness. Aggressive behavior or hostility reported in clinical trials and the postmarketing experience of some medications indicated for the treatment of ADHD. Monitor growth during therapy; d/c if patient is not growing or gaining weight. May lower seizure threshold, especially with prior history of seizures or with prior EEG abnormalities; d/c if seizures occur. Visual disturbances may occur (rare). Caution with emotionally unstable patients or prior history of drug dependence or alcoholism; chronic use may lead to tolerance and psychological dependence. Monitor during withdrawal.

**ADVERSE REACTIONS:** Nervousness, insomnia, hypersensitivity reactions, anorexia, nausea, dizziness, headache, dyskinesia, drowsiness, BP and pulse changes, tachycardia, angina, arrhythmia.

**INTERACTIONS:** See Contraindications. Caution with $\alpha_2$-agonists (eg, clonidine) and pressor agents. May decrease effectiveness of antihypertensives. Potentiates anticoagulants, anticonvulsants (eg, phenobarbital, diphenylhydantoin, primidone), TCAs (eg, imipramine, clomipramine, desipramine); monitor plasma drug levels or PT/INR. (Cap, Extended-Release) Antacids or acid suppressants may alter release characteristics of cap. May decrease the effect of guanethidine.

**PREGNANCY:** Category C, caution in nursing.

**MECHANISM OF ACTION:** Sympathomimetic amine; CNS stimulant, blocks reuptake of norepinephrine and dopamine into presynaptic neuron and increases release of monoamines into extraneuronal space.

**PHARMACOKINETICS: Absorption:** Adult: (Cap, ER) $T_{max1}$=2 hrs, $C_{max1}$=5.3ng/mL, $T_{max2}$=5.5 hrs, $C_{max2}$=6.2ng/mL, AUC=45.8ng•h/mL. Peds: Absolute bioavailability (30%); (Cap, ER) $T_{max1}$=2 hrs, $C_{max1}$=5.3ng/mL, $T_{max2}$=6.6 hrs, $C_{max2}$=10.2ng/mL, AUC=102.4ng•h/mL. (Tab, ER) $T_{max}$=4.7 hrs. (Tab) $T_{max}$=1.9 hrs. **Distribution:** Plasma protein binding (10%-33%). (IV) $V_d$=6L/kg **Metabolism:** α-phenyl-2-piperidine acetic acid (major metabolite). **Elimination:** (Tab) Urine (78-97%), feces (1-3%). (Cap, ER) **Adults:** $T_{1/2}$=3.3 hrs; Children: $T_{max}$=2.4 hrs.

## NURSING CONSIDERATIONS

**Assessment:** Assess for agitation, glaucoma, tics, family history of Tourette's syndrome, cardiovascular conditions (eg, severe HTN, angina pectoris, cardiac structural abnormalities, arrhythmias, HF, recent MI), comorbid depression symptoms, bipolar disorder, psychosis, seizures, history of drug dependence or alcoholism, possible drug interactions.

**Monitoring:** Monitor cardiovascular status, exacerbations of behavior disturbances and thought disorders, bipolar disorder, aggression, seizures, visual disturbances, CBC with differential and platelet counts. Monitor growth in children. Periodically d/c drug to assess child's condition.

**Patient Counseling:** Inform about risks and benefits of treatment, appropriate use, drug abuse/dependence. Avoid afternoon dose; may cause insomnia. Counsel to take 30 min before food; swallow tablet whole, do not crush or chew.

**Administration:** Oral route. **Storage:** 25°C (77°F), excursion permitted 15-30°C (59-86°F). (Tab) Protect from light. Dispense in tight, light-resistant container. (Tab, ER) Protect from moisture. Dispense in tight, light-resistant container. (Cap, ER) Dispense in a tight container.



# RITUXAN RX

rituximab (Genentech/Biogen Idec)

**Serious, sometimes fatal, infusion reactions reported. Acute renal failure, sometimes fatal, reported in the setting of tumor lysis syndrome (TLS) following treatment of non-Hodgkin's lymphoma (NHL). Severe, including fatal, mucocutaneous reactions may occur. JC virus infection resulting in progressive multifocal leukoencephalopathy (PML) may occur.**

**THERAPEUTIC CLASS:** Monoclonal antibody/CD20-blocker

**INDICATIONS:** Treatment of NHL in patients with: 1) relapsed or refractory, low-grade or follicular, CD20-positive, B-cell NHL as a single agent; 2) previously untreated follicular, CD20-positive, B-cell NHL in combination with CVP chemotherapy; 3) nonprogressing (including stable disease), low-grade, CD20-positive, B-cell NHL, as a single agent, after 1st-line CVP chemotherapy; 4) previously untreated diffuse large B-cell, CD20-positive NHL in combination with CHOP or other anthracycline-based chemotherapy regimens. In combination with fludarabine and cyclophosphamide (FC), for the treatment with previously untreated and previously treated CD20-positive CLL. In combination with methotrexate in patients with moderately to severely active rheumatoid arthritis (RA) who have had inadequate response to one or more TNF-antagonist therapies.

**DOSAGE:** *Adults:* Premedicate before each infusion. Relapsed or Refractory, Low-Grade or Follicular, CD20-Positive, B-cell NHL: 375mg/m$^2$ once weekly for 4 or 8 doses. Retreatment: 375mg/m$^2$ once weekly for 4 doses. Previously Untreated, Follicular, CD20-Positive, B-cell NHL: 375mg/m$^2$ on Day 1 of each CVP chemotherapy cycle for up to 8 doses. Nonprogressing, Low-Grade, CD20-Positive, B-cell NHL: Following completion of 6-8 cycles of CVP chemotherapy, 375mg/m$^2$ once weekly for 4 doses at 6-month intervals to max of 16 doses. Diffuse Large B-cell NHL: 375mg/m$^2$ on Day 1 of each chemotherapy cycle for up to 8 infusions. CLL: 375mg/m$^2$ the day prior to initiation of FC chemotherapy, then 500mg/m$^2$ on Day 1 of cycles 2-6 (every 28 days). For dosing as a component of Zevalin® please refer to PI. RA: Give with methotrexate. Administer two 1000mg IV infusions separated by 2 weeks. Give methylprednisolone 100mg IV (or equivalent) 30 min prior to each infusion to reduce infusion reactions. May be administered q24 weeks or based on evaluation, but not >16 weeks on subsequent courses. Do not administer as IV push or bolus.

**HOW SUPPLIED:** Inj: 100mg/10mL, 500mg/50mL [single use vial]

**WARNINGS/PRECAUTIONS:** Severe infusion reactions (eg, urticaria, hypotension, angioedema, hypoxia, bronchospasm, pulmonary infiltrates, MI) may occur during the first infusion with time to onset of 30-120 min. D/C if severe reaction develops; may resume at a 50% rate reduction when symptoms subside. Hepatitis B virus (HBV) reactivation with fulminant hepatitis, hepatic failure, and death reported; d/c if viral hepatitis develops. Serious, including fatal, bacterial, fungal, and new or reactivated viral infections may occur during and up to one year following completion of therapy; d/c for serious infections and institute appropriate anti-infective therapy. D/C if serious cardiac arrhythmias occur. Severe renal toxicity reported; d/c if SrCr rises or oliguria occurs. Not recommended in patients with RA who have not had prior inadequate response to one or more TNF-antagonists and with severe active infections.

**ADVERSE REACTIONS:** Fever, chills, rash, asthenia, lymphopenia, leukopenia, neutropenia, headache, abdominal pain, night sweats, pruritus, infusion reactions, mucocutaneous reactions, TLS, JC virus infection.

**INTERACTIONS:** Renal toxicity reported with cisplatin. Vaccination with live-virus vaccines not recommended. Observe closely for signs of infection if biologic agents and/or DMARDs are used concomitantly. Combined use with chemotherapy may cause abdominal pain, bowel obstruction and perforation.

**PREGNANCY:** Category C, caution in nursing.

R

**MECHANISM OF ACTION:** Chimeric murine/human monoclonal $IgG_1$ kappa antibody/CD20 antigen blocker; binds to CD20 antigen on B lymphocytes and recruits immune effector functions to mediate B-cell lysis, possibly by complement-dependent cytotoxicity and antibody-dependent, cell-mediated cytotoxicity.

**PHARMACOKINETICS: Absorption:** RA: $C_{max}$=157mcg/mL (1st infusion), 183mcg/mL (2nd infusion), 318mcg/mL (2x500mg dose), 381mcg/mL (2x1000mg dose). **Distribution:** RA: $V_d$=3.1L. **Elimination:** NHL: $T_{1/2}$=22 days. RA: $T_{1/2}$=18 days. CLL: 32 days.

## NURSING CONSIDERATIONS

**Assessment:** Assess for pre-existing cardiac or pulmonary conditions, prior cardiopulmonary adverse events, high number of circulating malignant cells (>25,000/mm$^3$), history of arrhythmias or angina, high tumor burden, possible drug interactions, renal impairment. Screen for HBV infection prior to therapy.

**Monitoring:** Monitor serum electrolytes, renal function, fluid balance, CBC and platelet counts periodically; cardiac function (history of arrhythmias, angina), for signs/symptoms of HBV reactivation, infusion reaction, TLS, arrhythmias, viral infections, mucocutaneous reactions, PML, renal failure, cytopenias, bowel obstruction/perforation, and hypersensitivity reactions.

**Patient Counseling:** Inform that the drug is detectable in serum for up to 6 months following completion of therapy. Instruct to use effective contraception during treatment and for 12 months after therapy. Vaccinations with live vaccines are not recommended. Advise to seek medical attention if symptoms of arrhythmias, infusion reaction (urticaria, hypotension, angioedema), new onset of neurological symptoms, infection, bowel obstruction (abdominal pain), mucocutaneous reactions, or hypersensitivity reactions occur.

**Administration:** IV route. Administer as IV infusion only. Use appropriate aseptic technique. First infusion: Initiate rate of 50mg/hr; if no toxicity, increase by 50mg/hr increments every 30 min to max of 400mg/hr. Subsequent infusion: Initiate rate of 100mg/hr; if no toxicity, increase by 100mg/hr increments every 30 min to max of 400mg/hr. **Storage:** Vials: 2-8°C (36-46°F). Protect from direct sunlight. Do not freeze or shake. Sol for infusion: 2-8°C (36-46°F) for 24 hrs. Stable for additional 24 hrs at room temp.

## ROBAXIN — RX

methocarbamol (Schwarz)

**OTHER BRAND NAMES:** Robaxin Injection (Baxter) - Robaxin-750 (Schwarz)

**THERAPEUTIC CLASS:** Muscular analgesic (central-acting)

**INDICATIONS:** Adjunct for relief of acute, painful musculoskeletal conditions.

**DOSAGE:** *Adults:* (PO) Initial: (500mg tab) 1500mg qid for 2-3 days. Maint: 1000mg qid. Initial: (750mg tab) 1500mg qid for 2-3 days. Maint: 750mg q4h or 1500mg tid. Max: 6g/d for 2-3 days; 8g/d if severe. (Inj) Moderate Symptoms: 10mL IV/IM. IV Max Rate: 3mL undiluted drug/min. IM Max: 5mL into each gluteal region. Severe/Post-Op Condition: Max: 20-30mL/day up to 3 consecutive days. If feasible, continue with PO. Tetanus: 10-20mL up to 30mL. May repeat q6h until NG tube can be inserted. Continue with crushed tabs. Max: 24g/day PO.

*Pediatrics:* Tetanus: Initial: 15mg/kg or 500mg/$m^2$. Repeat q6h prn. Max: 1.8g/$m^2$ for 3 consecutive days. Administer by injection into tubing or IV infusion.

**HOW SUPPLIED:** Inj: 100mg/mL [10mL]; Tab: 500mg, 750mg

**CONTRAINDICATIONS:** (Inj) Renal pathology with injection due to propylene glycol content.

**WARNINGS/PRECAUTIONS:** May impair mental/physical abilities required for operating machinery or driving a motor vehicle. May cause color interference in certain screening tests for 5-hydroxy-indoleacetic acid (5-HIAA) and vanillylmandelic acid (VMA). Caution in epilepsy with the injection. Injection rate should not exceed 3mL/min. Avoid extravasation with injection. Avoid use of injection particularly during early pregnancy.

**ADVERSE REACTIONS:** Lightheadedness, dizziness, drowsiness, nausea, urticaria, pruritus, rash, conjunctivitis, nasal congestion, blurred vision, headache, fever, seizures, syncope, flushing.

**INTERACTIONS:** Additive adverse effects with alcohol and other CNS depressants. May inhibit effect of pyridostigmine; caution in patients with myasthenia gravis receiving anticholinergics.

**PREGNANCY:** Category C, caution in nursing.

**MECHANISM OF ACTION:** Carbamate derivative of guaifenesin; not established, suspected to have CNS depressant with sedative and musculoskeletal relaxant properties.

**PHARMACOKINETICS: Distribution:** Plasma protein binding (46-50%). **Distribution:** Found in breast milk. **Metabolism:** Via dealkylation, hydroxylation, and conjugation pathways. **Elimination:** Urine; $T_{1/2}$=1-2 hrs.

### NURSING CONSIDERATIONS

**Assessment:** Assess for renal/hepatic impairment, myasthenia gravis, seizures, pregnancy/nursing status, alcohol intake, and drug interactions.

**Monitoring:** Monitor for congenital and fetal abnormalities if taken during pregnancy, for color interference in certain screening tests for 5-HIAA using

R

nitrosonaphthol reagent and in screening tests for urinary VMA using Gitlow method.

**Patient Counseling:** Caution while performing hazardous tasks (operating machinery/driving). Avoid alcohol or other CNS depressants. Notify if pregnant/nursing or if planning to become pregnant.

**Administration:** Oral route, IV infusion, and IM; careful supervision of dose and rate of injection. **Storage:** 20-25°C (68-77°F), in tight container; excursions permitted to 15-30°C (59-86°F).

## ROCALTROL — RX

calcitriol (Validus)

**OTHER BRAND NAMES:** Calcitriol (Various)

**THERAPEUTIC CLASS:** Vitamin D analog

**INDICATIONS:** Management of secondary hyperparathyroidism and resultant metabolic bone disease with moderate to severe chronic renal failure (CrCl 15-55mL/min) in patients not yet on dialysis. Management of hypocalcemia and resultant metabolic bone disease in patients undergoing chronic renal dialysis. Management of hypocalcemia and its clinical manifestations in patients with postsurgical hypoparathyroidism, idiopathic hypoparathyroidism, and pseudohypoparathyroidism.

**DOSAGE:** *Adults:* Predialysis: Initial: 0.25mcg/day. Max: 0.5mcg/day. Hypoparathyroidism: Initial: 0.25mcg/day every am. Titrate: May increase at 2-4 week intervals. Usual: 0.5-2mcg/day. Dialysis: Initial: 0.25mcg/day. Titrate: May increase by 0.25mcg/day at 4-8 week intervals. Patients with normal or slightly reduced calcium levels may respond to 0.25mcg qod. Usual: 0.5-1mcg/day. Monitor serum calcium levels at least twice weekly during titration. D/C with hypercalcemia; when calcium levels return to normal, continue therapy and decrease daily dose by 0.25mcg. Elderly: Start at lower end of dosing range.

*Pediatrics:* Predialysis: ≥3 yrs: Initial: 0.25mcg/day. Max: 0.5mcg/day. <3yrs: Initial: 10-15ng/kg/day. Hypoparathyroidism: ≥6 yrs: Usual: 0.5-2mcg/day every am. 1-5yrs: Usual: 0.25-0.75mcg/day every am. Monitor serum calcium levels twice weekly during titration. D/C with hypercalcemia; when calcium levels return to normal, continue therapy and decrease daily dose by 0.25mcg.

**HOW SUPPLIED:** Cap: 0.25mcg, 0.5mcg; Sol: 1mcg/mL [15mL]

**CONTRAINDICATIONS:** Hypercalcemia or vitamin D toxicity.

**WARNINGS/PRECAUTIONS:** Administration in excess of daily requirements may cause hypercalcemia, hypercalciuria, and hyperphosphatemia; early in treatment during dosage adjustment, monitor calcium levels twice weekly. Chronic hypercalcemia can lead to generalized vascular calcification, nephrocalcinosis, and other soft tissue calcification. D/C immediately if hypercalcemia develops; monitor serum calcium and phosphate levels daily during periods of hypercalcemia; when normal levels attained, may resume treatment at a daily dose 0.25mcg lower than the previous dose. May increase inorganic phosphate levels in serum leading to ectopic calcification in renal failure; use non-aluminum phosphate binders and low phosphate diet to control serum phosphate in dialysis patients. Caution in elderly and immobilized patients. If treatment switched from ergocalciferol, may take several months for ergocalciferol level in blood to return to baseline. Avoid dehydration in patients with normal renal function. In patients with normal renal function, chronic hypercalcemia may be associated with an increase in SrCr. Maintain adequate calcium intake, at least 600mg/day. For dialysis patients, serum calcium, phosphorus, magnesium, and alkaline phosphatase should be monitored periodically. For hypoparathyroid patients, serum calcium, phosphorus, and 24-hour urinary calcium should be determined periodically. For predialysis patients, serum calcium, phosphorus, alkaline phosphatase, creatinine, and intact PTH (iPTH) should be determined initially; thereafter serum calcium, phosphorus, alkaline phosphatase, and creatinine should be determined monthly for a 6 month period and then periodically. iPTH should be determined periodically every 3-4 months.

**ADVERSE REACTIONS:** Weakness, N/V, dry mouth, constipation, muscle and bone pain, metallic taste, polyuria, polydipsia, weight loss, pancreatitis, photophobia, pruritus, decreased libido, hyperthermia, hypersensivity reactions.

**INTERACTIONS:** Avoid pharmacological doses of vitamin D products and derivatives during therapy. Avoid uncontrolled intake of additional calcium-containing preparations. Avoid concomitant administration with magnesium-containing preparations (eg, antacids) in patients on chronic renal dialysis because use may lead to hypermagnesemia. May reduce intestinal absorption with cholestyramine. May reduce endogenous plasma levels with phenytoin or phenobarbital. Concomitant use with thiazides may cause hypercalcemia. May reduce endogenous serum concentrations when used comcomitantly with ketoconazole. Hypercalcemia may precipitate cardiac arrhythmias in patients on digitalis. Functional antagonism with corticosteroids. Dose of the phosphate binding agent may be need to be adjusted when used concomitantly with calcitriol.

**PREGNANCY:** Category C, not for use in nursing.

**MECHANISM OF ACTION:** Synthetic vitamin D analog; regulates absorption of calcium from the GI tract and its utilization in the body.

**PHARMACOKINETICS: Absorption:** Rapidly absorbed (intestine). $T_{max}$=3-6 hrs (adult); $C_{max}$=116pmol/L (pediatrics). **Distribution:** Plasma protein binding (99.9%); found in breast milk. **Metabolism:** Liver via hydroxylation. 1,25R$(OH)_2$-26, 23S-lactone $D_3$ (major metabolite). **Elimination:** Urine (16%), feces (49%); $T_{1/2}$=5-8 hrs (adult), 27.4 hrs (pediatrics).

## NURSING CONSIDERATIONS

**Assessment:** Assess for hypercalcemia, evidence of vitamin D toxicity, renal dysfunction, presence of immobilization, pregnancy/nursing status, and for possible drug interactions. In predialysis patients, obtain baseline levels of serum calcium, phosphorus, alkaline phosphatase, creatinine, and iPTH.

**Monitoring:** Monitor for signs/symptoms of hypercalcemia, hypercalciuria, hyperphosphatemia, and for hypersensitivity reactions. If hypercalcemia develops d/c use and perform daily monitoring of serum calcium and phosphate levels. For dialysis patients, perform periodic monitoring of serum calcium, phosphorus, magnesium, and alkaline phosphatase. In hypoparathyroid patients, perform periodic monitoring of serum calcium, phosphorus, and 24-hr urinary calcium. In predialysis patients serum calcium, phosphorus, alkaline phosphatase and creatinine should be monitored monthly during the first 6 months of therapy and then periodically. Intact PTH (iPTH) should be evaluated every 3 to 4 months. During titration periods, serum calcium levels should be checked twice weekly.

**Patient Counseling:** Inform about compliance with dosage instructions, adherence to instructions about diet and calcium supplementation, and avoidance of the use of unapproved nonprescription drugs. Carefully inform about symptoms of hypercalcemia. Inform patients with normal renal function to avoid dehydration and maintain proper fluid intake during therapy. Advise to maintain adequate calcium intake, at least 600mg/day.

**Administration:** Oral route. **Storage:** 59-86°F (15-30°C) . Protect from light.

R

# ROMAZICON — RX

flumazenil (Roche Labs)

**THERAPEUTIC CLASS:** Benzodiazepine antagonist

**INDICATIONS:** Complete or partial reversal of sedative effects of benzodiazepines (BZDs) given with general anesthesia, or diagnostic and therapeutic procedures, and for the management of BZD overdose in adults. For reversal of BZD-induced conscious sedation in pediatrics (1-17 yrs old).

**DOSAGE:** *Adults:* Reversal of Conscious Sedation/General Anesthesia: Give IV over 15 seconds. Initial: 0.2mg. May repeat dose after 45 seconds and again at 60 second intervals up to a max of 4 additional times until reach desired level of consciousness. Max Total Dose: 1mg. In event of resedation, repeated doses may be given at 20-min intervals. Max: 1mg/dose (0.2mg/min) and 3mg/hr. BZD Overdose: Give IV over 30 seconds. Initial: 0.2mg. May repeat with 0.3mg after 30 seconds and then 0.5mg at 1-min intervals until reach desired level of consciousness. Max Total Dose: 3mg. In event of resedation, repeated doses may be given at 20-min intervals. Max: 1mg/dose (0.5mg/min); 3mg/hr. *Pediatrics*: >1yr: Give IV over 15 seconds. Initial: 0.01mg/kg (up to 0.2mg). May repeat dose after 45 seconds and again at 60-second intervals up to a max of 4 additional times until reach desired level of consciousness. Max Total Dose: 0.05mg/kg or 1mg, whichever is lower.

**HOW SUPPLIED:** Inj: 0.1mg/mL

**CONTRAINDICATIONS:** Patients given BZDs for life-threatening conditions (eg, control of ICP or status epilepticus), signs of serious cyclic antidepressant overdose.

**WARNINGS/PRECAUTIONS:** Caution in overdoses involving multiple drug combinations. Risk of seizures, especially with long-term BZD-induced sedation, cyclic antidepressant overdose, concurrent major sedative-hypnotic drug withdrawal, recent therapy with repeated doses of parenteral BZDs, myoclonic jerking or seizure prior to flumazenil administration. Monitor for resedation, respiratory depression, or other residual BZD effects (up to 2 hrs). Avoid use in the ICU; increased risk of unrecognized BZD dependence. Caution with head injury, alcoholism, and other drug dependencies. Does not reverse respiratory depression/hypoventilation or cardiac depression. May provoke panic attacks with history of panic disorder. Adjust subsequent doses in hepatic dysfunction. Not for use as treatment for BZD dependence or for management of protracted abstinence syndromes. May trigger dose-dependent withdrawal syndromes. Extravasation may occur; administer IV into a large vein.

**ADVERSE REACTIONS:** N/V, dizziness, injection-site pain, increased sweating, headache, abnormal or blurred vision, agitation.

**INTERACTIONS:** Avoid use until neuromuscular blockade effects are reversed. Toxic effects (eg, convulsions, cardiac dysrhythmias) may occur with mixed drug overdose (eg, cyclic antidepressants).

**PREGNANCY:** Category C, caution in nursing.

**MECHANISM OF ACTION:** Benzodiazepine receptor antagonist; inhibits activity at the benzodiazepine recognition site on the GABA/benzodiazepine receptor complex.

**PHARMACOKINETICS: Absorption:** $C_{max}$=24ng/mL; AUC=15ng•hr/mL. **Distribution:** $V_d$=1L/kg (steady state); plasma protein binding (50%). **Metabolism:** Complete (99%). **Elimination**: Urine (90-95%), feces (5-10%); $T_{1/2}$=54 min.

R

## NURSING CONSIDERATIONS

**Assessment:** Assess patients using benzodiazepine for control of potentially life-threatening condition, those showing signs of serious cyclic antidepressant overdose. Assess for head injury, history of convulsions, panic disorders, lung disease, hepatic impairment, and possible drug interactions.

**Monitoring:** Monitor for occurrence of seizure, re-sedation, respiratory depression, or other residual benzodiazepine effects, dizziness, injection-site pain, increased sweating, headache, and abnormal or blurred vision.

**Patient Counseling:** Advise not to engage in activities requiring complete alertness (eg, operating machinery/driving) during first 24 hrs after discharge. Advise not to take alcohol or non-prescription drugs first 24 hrs after flumazenil administration, or if effects of the benzodiazepine persist.

**Administration:** IV route. **Storage:** 25°C (77°F); excursions permitted to 15-30°C (59-86°F).

# RONDEC SYRUP RX

phenylephrine HCl - chlorpheniramine maleate (Sciele)

**THERAPEUTIC CLASS:** Antihistamine/decongestant

**INDICATIONS:** Symptomatic relief of seasonal and perennial allergic rhinitis and vasomotor rhinitis.

**DOSAGE:** *Adults:* 5mL q4-6h. Max: 30mL/24 hrs.
*Pediatrics:* ≥12 yrs: 5mL q4-6h. Max: 30mL/24 hrs. 6 to <12 yrs: 2.5mL q4-6h. Max: 15mL/24 hrs. 2 to <6 yrs: 1.25mL q4-6h. Max: 7.5mL/24 hrs.

**HOW SUPPLIED:** Syrup: (Chlorpheniramine-Phenylephrine) 4mg-12.5mg/5mL [20mL, 118mL, 473mL]

**CONTRAINDICATIONS:** Severe HTN or CAD, narrow-angle glaucoma, urinary retention, peptic ulcer, acute asthma attack, concurrent MAOI therapy.

**WARNINGS/PRECAUTIONS:** Caution in asthma, DM, HTN, heart disease, hyperthyroidism, increased IOP, prostatic hypertrophy, elderly. May cause excitability, especially in children.

**ADVERSE REACTIONS:** Sedation, dizziness, diplopia, N/V, diarrhea, dry mouth, headache, nervousness, convulsions, CNS stimulation, cardiac arrhythmias, respiratory difficulty, increased HR or BP.

**INTERACTIONS:** See Contraindications. May enhance effects of TCAs, benzodiazepines, barbiturates, alcohol, other CNS depressants. Increased sympathomimetic effects with MAOIs, β-blockers. May reduce antihypertensive effects of reserpine, veratrum alkaloids, methyldopa, mecamylamine.

**PREGNANCY:** Category C, not for use in nursing.

**MECHANISM OF ACTION:** Brompheniramine: $H_1$ antihistaminic activity with mild anticholinergic and sedative effects. Pseudoephedrine: Sympathomimetic; acts as decongestant to respiratory tract mucous membranes.

**PHARMACOKINETICS: Absorption:** Brompheniramine: $T_{max}$=5 hrs. **Metabolism:** Brompheniramine: Liver. **Elimination:** Brompheniramine: Urine. Pseudoephedrine: Urine; $T_{1/2}$=6-8 hrs.

## NURSING CONSIDERATIONS

**Assessment:** Assess for drug hypersensitivity, HTN, CAD, narrow-angle glaucoma, urinary retention, peptic ulcer, DM, hyperthyroidism, prostatic hypertrophy, asthma, and possible drug interaction (MAO inhibitors).

**Monitoring:** Monitor for CNS stimulation with convulsions, cardiovascular collapse with hypotension, excitability, nervousness, dizziness, or sleeplessness.

**Patient Counseling:** Counsel about risks and to avoid alcohol and other CNS depressants during therapy.

**Adminstration:** Oral route. **Storage:** 8-30°C (46-86°F).

# RotaTeq — RX

rotavirus vaccine, live (Merck)



**THERAPEUTIC CLASS:** Vaccine

**INDICATIONS:** Prevention of rotavirus gastroenteritis in infants and children caused by the serotypes G1, G2, G3, and G4 when administered as a 3-dose series to infants between the ages of 6-32 weeks. The first dose should be administered between 6-12 weeks of age.

**DOSAGE:** *Pediatrics:* Administer series of 3 doses orally starting at 6-12 weeks of age, with subsequent doses administered at 4-10 week intervals. Third dose should not be given after 32 weeks of age. Do not mix with any other vaccines or solutions. Do not reconstitute or dilute.

**HOW SUPPLIED:** Sus: 2mL

**WARNINGS/PRECAUTIONS:** Consider delaying use with febrile illness. Vaccination may not result in complete protection in all recipients. May increase risk of intussusception. Caution when administering to individuals with immunodeficient close contacts who may be at increased risk of acquiring and transmitting rotaviruses.

**ADVERSE REACTIONS:** Bronchiolitis, gastroenteritis, pneumonia, fever, UTI.

**INTERACTIONS:** Immunosuppressive therapies including irradiation, antimetabolites, alkylating agents, cytotoxic drugs, and corticosteroids (used in greater than physiologic doses) may reduce the immune response to vaccines.

**PREGNANCY:** Safety in pregnancy and nursing not known.

**MECHANISM OF ACTION:** Immunologic mechanism not established; may replicate in small intestine and induce immunity against rotavirus gastroenteritis.

### NURSING CONSIDERATIONS

**Assessment:** Assess immunity and current health status.

**Monitoring:** Monitor for hypersensitivity reactions, diarrhea, vomiting, otitis media, nasopharyngitis, bronchospasm, intussusception, hematochezia, and Kawasaki syndrome.

**Patient Counseling:** Inform of potential benefits/risks ratio; report any adverse reactions to physician.

**Administration:** Oral route. **Storage:** 2-8°C (36-46°F). Protect from light.

## ROWASA — RX

mesalamine (Alaven)

**OTHER BRAND NAMES:** SF Rowasa (Alaven)

**INDICATIONS:** Treatment of active mild to moderate distal ulcerative colitis, proctosigmoiditis or proctitis.

**DOSAGE:** *Adults:* Use 1 enema rectally qhs for 3-6 weeks. Retain for 8 hrs. Empty bowel prior to administration.

**HOW SUPPLIED:** Enema: 4g/60mL

**WARNINGS/PRECAUTIONS:** D/C if acute intolerance syndrome develops (eg, cramping, bloody diarrhea, abdominal pain, headache); consider sulfasalazine hypersensitivity. If rechallenge is considered, perform under careful observation. Caution with sulfasalazine hypersensitivity. Carefully monitor with renal dysfunction. Contains potassium metabisulfite; caution with sulfite sensitivity especially in asthmatics. Pancolitis, pericarditis (rare) reported.

**ADVERSE REACTIONS:** Abdominal problems, headache, flatulence, flu, fever, nausea, malaise/fatigue.

**PREGNANCY:** Category B, not for use in nursing.

**MECHANISM OF ACTION:** Unknown, possibly diminishes inflammation by blocking cyclooxygenase and inhibiting prostaglandin production in the colon.

**PHARMACOKINETICS: Absorption:** Colon: Poor. Extent dependent on retention time. **Metabolism:** Acetylation, N-acetyl-5-ASA (Metabolite). **Elimination:** Urine, feces, $T_{1/2}$=0.5-1.5 hrs.

### NURSING CONSIDERATIONS

**Assessment:** Assess for history of sulfasalazine intolerance, preexisting renal disease, and history of asthma or atopic allergies. Obtain baseline BUN, urinalysis, and creatinine.

**Monitoring:** Monitor BUN, urinalysis, and creatinine periodically. Signs/symptoms of acute intolerance syndrome (cramping, acute abdominal pain, bloody diarrhea), hypersensitivity or allergic reaction (rash, fever).

**Patient Counseling:** Best results achieved if bowel emptied immediately before. Seek medical attention if symptoms of acute intolerance syndrome (cramping, acute abdominal pain, bloody diarrhea), hypersensitivity or allergic reactions occur. If signs of rash or fever occur, d/c therapy.

**Administration:** Rectal. 1) Shake bottle well and remove sheath from tip. 2) Lie either on left side with left leg extended and right leg flexed or "knee-chest" position. 3) Gently insert lubricated tip into rectum, slightly toward navel; grasp firmly, tilt so nozzle aimed at back and squeeze slowly to instill drug. 4) Remain in position for 30 min to allow distribution. Retain all night if possible. **Storage:** 20-25°C (68-77°F).

# ROXANOL

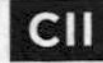


morphine sulfate (Xanodyne)

**Highly concentrated, check dose carefully.**

**OTHER BRAND NAMES:** Roxanol-T (Xanodyne)

**THERAPEUTIC CLASS:** Opioid analgesic

**INDICATIONS:** Relief of severe acute and chronic pain.

**DOSAGE:** *Adults:* Usual: 10-30mg q4h. During first effective pain relief, dose should be maintained for at least 3 days before any dose reduction, if respiratory activity and other vital signs are adequate. Elderly/Very Ill/Respiratory Problems/Severe Renal and Hepatic Impairment: Lower doses may be required.

**HOW SUPPLIED:** Sol, Concentrate: 20mg/mL (Roxanol) [30mL, 120mL, 240mL], (Roxanol-T) [30mL, 120mL]

**CONTRAINDICATIONS:** Respiratory insufficiency or depression, severe CNS depression, attack of bronchial asthma, heart failure secondary to chronic lung disease, cardiac arrhythmias, increased intracranial or cerebrospinal pressure, head injuries, brain tumor, acute alcoholism, delirium tremens, convulsive disorders, after biliary tract surgery, suspected surgical abdomen, surgical anastomosis, concomitantly with MAOIs or within 14 days of such treatment.

**WARNINGS/PRECAUTIONS:** May cause tolerance, psychological, and physical dependence; withdrawal may occur on abrupt discontinuation. Caution with head injury, increased ICP, acute asthmatic attack, COPD, cor pulmonale, decreased respiratory reserve, pre-existing respiratory depression, hypoxia, hypercapnia, elderly, debilitated, severe hepatic/renal impairment, hypothyroidism, Addison's disease, prostatic hypertrophy, or urethral stricture. May cause orthostatic hypotension in ambulatory patients, severe hypotension with depleted blood volume. May obscure diagnosis/clinical course of acute abdominal conditions. May impair mental/physical abilities.

**ADVERSE REACTIONS:** Respiratory depression, lightheadedness, dizziness, sedation, NV, sweating, constipation.

**INTERACTIONS:** See Contraindications. Potentiated by alkalizing agents and antagonized by acidifying agents. Analgesic effect potentiated by chlorpromazine, methocarbamol. Enhanced depressant effects with other CNS depressants such as anesthetics, hypnotics, barbiturates, phenothiazines, chloral hydrate, glutethimide, sedatives, MAOIs (eg, procarbazine), antihistamines, β-blockers (eg, propranolol), alcohol, furazolidone, other narcotics, tranquilizers, and TCAs. May increase anticoagulant activity of coumarin and other anticoagulants.

**PREGNANCY:** Category C, caution in nursing.

**MECHANISM OF ACTION:** Opioid analgesic; acts as agonist interacting with stereospecific and saturable binding sites or receptors in the brain and other tissues. Major effects are on CNS and bowel.

**PHARMACOKINETICS: Absorption:** $T_{max}$=60 min. **Distribution:** Crosses placenta; found in breast milk.

## NURSING CONSIDERATIONS

**Assessment:** Assess for respiratory depression, severe CNS depression, bronchial asthma attack, chronic obstructive pulmonary disease, heart failure secondary to chronic lung disease, cardiac arrhythmias, increased intracranial or CSF pressure, head injury, brain tumor, acute alcoholism, delirium tremens, convulsive disorder, recent biliary tract surgery, presence of surgical abdomen, surgical anastomosis, presence of debilitation (eg, elderly), hepatic/renal dysfunction, hypothyroidism, Addison's disease, prostatic hypertrophy or urethral stricture, pregnancy/nursing status, and possible drug interactions (eg, MAOIs).

**Monitoring:** Monitor for signs/symptoms of respiratory depression, hypotension, elevations in CSF pressure, tolerance, and dependence.

**Patient Counseling:** Instruct not to take medication if MAO inhibitors used within previous 14 days. Inform that drug may impair mental/physical abilities required to perform hazardous tasks (eg, operating machinery/driving). Advise to avoid alcohol and other CNS depressants while on medication. Counsel not to abruptly d/c medication. Instruct to contact physician if adverse events (eg, respiratory depression) develop.

**Administration:** Oral route. **Storage:** 25°C (77°F); excursions permitted to 15-30°C (59-86°F).

## Roxicet

CII

oxycodone HCl - acetaminophen (Roxane)

**THERAPEUTIC CLASS:** Analgesic combination

**INDICATIONS:** Relief of moderate to moderately severe pain.

**DOSAGE:** *Adults:* Usual: (5mg-325mg): 1 tab or 5mL sol q6h prn. (5mg-500mg): 1 tab q6h prn. Titrate: May need to exceed usual dose based on individual response, pain severity and tolerance. Max: 12 tabs/day or 60mL/day. Do not exceed Acetaminophen (APAP) 4g/day.

**HOW SUPPLIED:** (Oxycodone-Acetaminophen) Sol: 5mg-325mg/5mL [5mL; 500mL]; Tab: 5mg-325mg*, 5mg-500mg* *scored

**CONTRAINDICATIONS:** Oxycodone: Significant respiratory depression (in unmonitored settings or absence of resuscitative equipment), acute or severe bronchial asthma or hypercarbia, known/suspected paralytic ileus.

**WARNINGS/PRECAUTIONS:** May cause physical dependence and tolerance; d/c gradually to avoid withdrawal symptoms. Potential for misuse, abuse or diversion; monitor for prevention or early detection. May cause respiratory depression, induce or aggravate convulsions/seizures, produce severe hypotension in compromised patients and orthostatic hypotension in ambulatory patients. May decrease bowel motility; monitor for ileus in postoperative patients. May obscure the diagnosis or clinical course with head injuries or acute abdominal conditions. Caution with circulatory shock, head injury, other intracranial lesions, pre-existing increase in intracranial pressure (ICP), elderly, debilitated, CNS depression, non tolerant patients, hepatic, pulmonary or renal impairment, liver disease, hypothyroidism, Addison's disease, prostatic hypertrophy, urethral stricture, acute alcoholism, delirium tremens, kyphoscoliosis with respiratory depression, myxedema, toxic psychosis, biliary tract disease (eg, acute pancreatitis), prostatic hypertrophy, urethral stricture. Caution with acute asthma, chronic obstructive pulmonary disease (COPD), cor pulmonale, pre existing respiratory impairment; may decrease respiratory drive leading to apnea even at therapeutic doses. May increase serum amylase levels, cross react with assays for detection of cocaine or cannabinoids (eg, marijuana) in human urine. APAP may interfere with home blood glucose measurement system. Anaphylactic reactions reported.



**ADVERSE REACTIONS:** Respiratory depression, apnea, respiratory arrest, circulatory depression, hypotension, shock, lightheadedness, dizziness, sedation, nausea, vomiting, euphoria, dysphoria, constipation, pruritus.

**INTERACTIONS:** Oxycodone: May enhance neuromuscular-blocking action of skeletal muscle relaxants and produce an increase in the degree of respiratory depression. Additive CNS depression with other opioid analgesics, general anesthetics, centrally acting anti-emetics, phenothiazines, tranquilizers, sedatives-hypnotics, alcohol and other CNS depressants (eg, alcohol); reduce dose of one or both agents. Agonist/antagonist analgesics (eg, pentazocine, nalbuphine and butorphanol) may reduce analgesic effect of oxycodone and/or may precipitate withdrawal symptoms; administer with caution. May produce paralytic ileus with anticholinergics. APAP: Hepatotoxicity occured in chronic alcoholics. Onset of effect may be delayed or decreased slightly but ultimate pharmacological effect is not significantly affected with anticholinergics. Increase in glucuronidation, plasma clearance and decreased half-life with oral contraceptives. Activated charcoal reduces acetaminophen absorption when administered immediately after overdose. Increase in pharamacologic effects with propranolol. Decrease loop diuretic effects. Reduce serum lamotrigine concentrations producing decrease therapeutic effects. Increase therapeutic effectiveness with probenecid. Decrease zidovudine pharmacologic effects.

**PREGNANCY:** Category C, not for use in nursing.

**MECHANISM OF ACTION:** Oxycodone: Pure opioid agonist; principal therapeutic effect is analgesia. Other effects include anxiolysis, euphoria, and feelings of relaxation. Effects mediated by CNS receptors (eg, μ and kappa) for endogenous opioid-like compounds (eg, endorphins, enkephalins). APAP: Non-opiate, non-salicylate; site and mechanism for analgesic effect not established. Antipyretic effect occurs through inhibition of endogenous pyrogen action on the hypothalamic heat-regulating centers.

**PHARMACOKINETICS: Absorption:** Oxycodone: Absolute bioavailability (87%). APAP: Rapid and almost complete. **Distribution:** Oxycodone: Plasma protein binding (45%); (IV) $V_d$=211.9 L; found in breast milk. APAP: Plasma protein binding (20-50%) (variable); found in most body fluids, breast milk. **Metabolism:** Oxycodone: N-dealkylation to noroxycodone (metabolite); CYP2D6, O-demethylation to oxymorphone (metabolite). APAP: Liver via CYP450 (conjugation), N acetyl-pbenzoquinoneimine, N-acetylimidoquinone (NAPQI, toxic metabolite). **Excretion:** Oxycodone: Urine (parent compound and metabolites); $T_{1/2}$=3.51 hrs. APAP: Urine (90-100%).

## NURSING CONSIDERATIONS

**Assessment:** Assess for respiratory depression, anaphylactic reactions, acute or severe bronchial asthma or hypercarbia, paralytic ileus, decrease bowel motility, COPD, cor pulmonale, pre existing respiratory impairment, debilitation, presence of head injury or other intracranial lesions, elevated ICP, circulatory shock, acute abdominal conditions, hepatic/renal dysfunction, hypothyroidism, Addison's disease, prostatic hypertrophy, urethral stricture, acute alcoholism, delirium tremens, kyphoscoliosis with respiratory depression, myxedema, toxic psychosis, convulsive disorders, biliary tract disease, acute pancreatitis, pregnancy/nursing status and possible drug interactions.

**Monitoring:** Monitor for signs/symptoms of respiratory depression, anaphylactic reactions, elevations of CSF pressure, ileus, decrease bowel motility in postoperative patients, hypotension, hepatotoxicity, convulsions, anaphylactic reactions, sphincter of Oddi spasms, abuse, tolerance and physical dependence. Monitor serum amylase.

**Patient Counseling:** Instruct to keep out of reach of children. Counsel to dispose of unused drug down toilet. Advise not to adjust dosing without consulting physician. Inform that drug may impair mental/physical abilities required to perform hazardous tasks (eg, operating machinery/driving). Counsel to avoid alcohol and other CNS depressants. If on medication for more than a few weeks, consult physician for gradual d/c dose schedule. Inform that medication has potential for abuse; protect from theft. Inform that medication may interfere with home blood glucose measurement system and may cross react with assays for detection of cocaine or cannabinoids (eg, marijuana) in human urine.

**Administration:** Oral route. **Storage:** (Sol/Tab) 20-25°C (68-77°F); Dispense in a tight, light-resistant container. Protect from moisture.



# ROXICODONE CII

oxycodone HCl (Xanodyne)

**THERAPEUTIC CLASS:** Opioid analgesic

**INDICATIONS:** Management of moderate to severe pain.

**DOSAGE:** *Adults:* Individualize dose. Initial: Opioid-Naive: 5-15mg q4-6h prn. Titrate: Based on individual response. For chronic pain, give around-the-clock. For severe chronic pain, give q4-6h at lowest effective dose. Conversion from Fixed Ratio Opioid/Non-Opioid Analgesic: D/C non-opioid analgesic; titrate dose in response to level of analgesia and adverse effects. Continuing Concomitant Non-Opioid Analgesic: Initial dose based upon most recent dose of opioid as a baseline for further titration. Conversion from Different Opioid:

Consider potency of prior opioid in selection of total daily dose and adjust dosage based on patient's response. May administer supplemental analgesia for breakthrough or incident pain and titrate as needed. Re-assess the need for continued use. D/C gradually by decrements of 25-50% daily. If withdrawal symptoms occur, raise dose to previous level and titrate down more slowly.

**HOW SUPPLIED:** Sol: 5mg/5mL [500mL], 20mg/mL [30mL]; Tab: 5mg*, 15mg*, 30mg* *scored

**CONTRAINDICATIONS:** Significant respiratory depression (in unmonitored settings or the absence of resuscitative equipment), acute or severe bronchial asthma, hypercarbia, paralytic ileus.

**WARNINGS/PRECAUTIONS:** Potential for tolerance and physical dependence. May cause respiratory depression; caution in elderly/debilitated patients, significant chronic obstructive pulmonary disease (COPD), cor pulmonale, decreased respiratory drive, hypoxia, hypercapnia or pre-existing respiratory depression. May markedly exaggerate respiratory depressant effects in head injuries, other intracranial lesions or increased ICP. May obscure the clinical course of patients with head injuries and acute abdominal conditions. May cause severe hypotension if with compromised ability to maintain BP due to depleted volume and orthostatic hypotension. May aggravate convulsions and seizures. Caution with acute alcoholism, adrenocortical insufficiency (eg, Addison's disease), convulsive disorders, CNS depression or coma, delirium tremens, kyphoscoliosis associated with respiratory depression, myxedema or hypothyroidism, prostatic hypertrophy or urethral stricture, severe hepatic or renal impairment, toxic psychosis and biliary tract disease (eg, acute pancreatitis). May increase serum amylase. Avoid giving to women during and prior to labor. Withdrawal symptoms reported. May impair mental/physical abilities.

**ADVERSE REACTIONS:** Respiratory depression/arrest, circulatory depression, cardiac arrest, hypotension, shock, N/V, constipation, headache, pruritus, insomnia, dizziness, asthenia, somnolence.

**INTERACTIONS:** Additive CNS depression with narcotic analgesics, general anesthetics, phenothiazines, tranquilizers, sedative-hypnotics, alcohol, and other CNS depressants; reduce dose. Mixed agonist/antagonist analgesics may reduce analgesic effect and/or cause withdrawal symptoms. May enhance effect of neuromuscular blockers. May intensify effects with MAOIs; avoid within 14 days of stopping MAOIs. Severe hypotension may occur with phenothiazines or other agents that compromise vasomotor tone. Possible interaction with CYP2D6 inhibitors (eg, certain cardiovascular drugs, antidepressants).

**PREGNANCY:** Category B, not for use in nursing.

**MECHANISM OF ACTION:** Opioid analgesic; pure opioid agonist whose principal therapeutic effect is analgesia. Precise mechanism of analgesic effect has not been established. Specific CNS opioid receptors for endogenous compounds with opioid-like activity are found in the brain and spinal cord and play a role in analgesic effects.

**PHARMACOKINETICS: Absorption:** Various doses resulted to different parameters; refer to PI. **Distribution:** Plasma protein binding (45%), (IV): $V_d$=2.6L/kg; found in breast milk. **Metabolism:** Hepatic (extensively); noroxycodone (major metabolite); CYP2D6 to oxymorphone (metabolite) and glucuronides. **Elimination:** Urine(19% oxycodone, 50% conjugated oxycodone, ≤14% conjugated oxymorphone, free and conjugated noroxycodone); $T_{1/2}$=3.5-4 hrs.

## NURSING CONSIDERATIONS

**Assessment:** Assess for respiratory depression, acute or severe bronchial asthma or hypercarbia, COPD or cor pulmonale, paralytic ileus, circulatory shock, head injury or other intracranial lesions, presence of increased ICP, acute alcoholism, adrenocortical insufficiency (eg, Addison's disease), convulsive disorders, CNS depression or coma, delirium tremens, presence of debilitation, kyphoscoliosis associated with respiratory depression, myxedema or hypothyroidism, prostatic hypertrophy or urethral stricture, hepatic/renal impairment, toxic psychosis, acute abdominal conditions, biliary tract disease (eg, acute pancreatitis), pregnancy/nursing status and possible drug interactions.

**Monitoring:** Monitor for signs/symptoms of respiratory depression, hypotension, elevations in CSF pressure, convulsions/seizures, tolerance and physical dependence. Monitor serum amylase.

**Patient Counseling:** Instruct to report episodes of breakthrough pain and adverse events (eg, respiratory depression). Advise to avoid adjusting dose without consulting physician. Inform that drug may impair mental/physical abilities required to perform hazardous tasks (eg, operating machinery/driving). Instruct to avoid alcohol consumption and other CNS depressants. Advise drug has potential for abuse. Counsel that if on medication for more than a few weeks and need to d/c therapy, taper dosing to avoid abrupt withdrawal. Advise women of childbearing potential to consult physician regarding analgesic effects and other drug use during pregnancy.

**Administration:** Oral route. **Storage:** 25°C (77°F); excursions permitted to 15-30°C (59-86°F). (Tab): Dispense in a tight, light-resistant container. Protect from moisture.

## ROZEREM RX

ramelteon (Takeda)

**THERAPEUTIC CLASS:** Melatonin receptor agonist

**INDICATIONS:** Treatment of insomnia characterized by difficulty with sleep onset.

**DOSAGE:** *Adults:* 8mg within 30 min of bedtime. Do not take with or after high-fat meal.

**HOW SUPPLIED:** Tab: 8mg

**CONTRAINDICATIONS:** Avoid with fluvoxamine. Patients who develop angioedema after treatment should not be rechallenged with the drug.

**WARNINGS/PRECAUTIONS:** Severe anaphylactic and anaphylactoid reactions reported. Sleep disturbances may manifest as a physical and/or psychiatric disorder, symptomatic treatment of insomnia should be initiated after evaluation. Abnormal thinking, behavioral changes, hallucinations, complex behaviors (eg, sleep driving), worsening depression, suicidal ideation reported. D/C therapy if complex sleep behavior occurs. May impair physical/mental abilities. May affect reproductive hormones. Avoid with severe hepatic impairment and severe sleep apnea. Respiratory depressant effects in patients with COPD have not been determined. Caution in moderate hepatic impairment.

**ADVERSE REACTIONS:** Somnolence, fatigue, dizziness, nausea, exacerbated insomnia.

**INTERACTIONS:** See Contraindications. Fluvoxamine increases AUC for ramelteon. Decreased efficacy with strong CYP inducers (eg, rifampin). Caution with less strong CYP1A2 inhibitors, strong CYP3A4 inhibitors (eg, ketoconazole), strong CYP2C9 inhibitors (eg, fluconazole). Additive effect with alcohol and CNS depressants. Avoid taking with or directly after a high-fat meal.

**PREGNANCY:** Category C, caution in nursing.

**MECHANISM OF ACTION:** Melatonin receptor agonist; activity at receptors believed to contribute to sleep-promoting properties.

**PHARMACOKINETICS: Absorption:** Rapid; absolute bioavailabilty (1.8%); $T_{max}$=0.75 hr. **Distribution**: Plasma protein binding (82%); $V_d$=73.6 L(IV). **Metabolism**: Oxidation via CYP1A2 (major), CYP3A4 (minor). M-II (active metabolite). **Elimination**: Urine, feces (<0.1%); $T_{1/2}$=1-2.6 hrs, 2-5 hrs (M-II).

### NURSING CONSIDERATIONS

**Assessment:** Assess for manifestations of physical or psychiatric disorders, hepatic impairment, sleep apnea, depression, pregnancy/nursing status, and possible drug interactions.

**Monitoring:** Monitor for signs/symptoms of worsening of depression, suicidal ideations, exacerbations of insomnia, hypersensitivity reactions, emergence of cognitive behavioral abnormalities, and anaphylactic/anaphylactoid reactions.

**Patient Counseling:** Instruct to take just prior to bedtime on empty stomach. Caution against hazardous tasks (eg, operating machinery, driving). Seek medical attention if worsening of insomnia, symptoms of cognitive or behavioral abnormalities, hypersensitivity reactions, cessation of menses, galactorrhea, decreased libido, or infertility occur. Swallow tablet whole.

**Administration:** Oral route. **Storage**: 25°C (77°F); excursions permitted to 15-30°C (59-86°F). Protect from moisture and humidity.

## RYTHMOL **RX**

propafenone HCl (GlaxoSmithKline)

**THERAPEUTIC CLASS:** Class IC antiarrhythmic

**INDICATIONS:** To prolong the time to recurrence of paroxysmal atrial fibrillation/flutter (PAF) and paroxysmal supraventricular tachycardia (PSVT) associated with disabling symptoms in patients without structural heart disease. Treatment of life-threatening documented ventricular arrhythmias.

**DOSAGE:** *Adults:* Initial: 150mg q8h. Titrate: May increase at minimum 3-4 day intervals to 225mg q8h, then to 300mg q8h if needed. Max: 900mg/day. Elderly/Marked Myocardial Damage: Increase more gradually during initial phase. Hepatic Dysfunction: Reduce dose by 20%-30%.

**HOW SUPPLIED:** Tab: 150mg*, 225mg*, 300mg* *scored

**CONTRAINDICATIONS:** Uncontrolled congestive heart failure (CHF), cardiogenic shock, bradycardia, marked hypotension, bronchospastic disorders, electrolyte imbalance, and sinoatrial, atrioventricular (AV) and intraventricular disorders of impulse generation and/or conduction (eg, sick sinus node syndrome, AV block) in the absence of an artificial pacemaker.

**WARNINGS/PRECAUTIONS:** Avoid with non-life-threatening ventricular arrhythmias, bronchospastic disorders. May cause new or worsened arrhythmias. Caution with hepatic or renal dysfunction. Slows AV conduction and causes 1st-degree AV block. Patients with CHF should be fully compensated before receiving therapy. D/C if CHF worsens and, if indicated, restart at lower dose. Avoid in patients with sick sinus node syndrome. Agranulocytosis, myasthenia gravis exacerbation, positive ANA titers reported. May alter pacing and sensing thresholds of artificial pacemakers; monitor during therapy. Caution in elderly.



**ADVERSE REACTIONS:** Taste disturbances, nausea, vomiting, dizziness, constipation, headache, fatigue, blurred vision, first degree AV block, intraventricular conduction delay.

**INTERACTIONS:** Inhibitors of CYP2D6 (eg, desipramine, paroxetine, ritonavir, sertraline), CYP1A2 (eg, amiodarone), CYP3A4 (eg, ketoconazole, ritonavir, saquinavir, erythromycin, grapefruit juice) may increase levels; monitor closely. May increase levels of drugs metabolized by CYP2D6 (eg, desipramine, imipramine, haloperidol, venlafaxine). May increase CNS side effects of lidocaine. May increase levels of digoxin, propranolol, warfarin; monitor closely. Cimetidine, fluoxetine may increase plasma levels. Rifampin, orlistat may decrease plasma levels. Concurrent use of antiarrhythmic drugs (eg, quinidine and amiodarone) not recommended. Amiodarone can affect conduction and repolarization.

**PREGNANCY:** Category C, not for use in nursing.

**MECHANISM OF ACTION:** Class 1C antiarrhythmic; local anesthetic effects and direct stablizing action on myocardium. Reduces upstroke velocity (phase 0) of the monophasic action potential in Purkinje fibers, and to a lesser extent myocardial fibers, and reduces the fast inward current carried by Na ions. Reduces spontaneous automaticity and depresses triggered activity.

**PHARMACOKINETICS: Absorption:** Complete, absolute bioavailability (150mg) 3.4%, (300mg) 10.6%. $T_{max}$=3.5 hrs. **Metabolism:** Liver (rapid, extensive) via CYP3A4, 1A2 and 2D6. 5-hydroxypropafenone and N-depropylpropafenone (active metabolites). **Elimination:** $T_{1/2}$=2-10 hrs.

## NURSING CONSIDERATIONS

**Assessment:** Assess for CHF, cardiogenic shock, sinoatrial/trioventricular/intraventricular disorders of impulse generation and conduction (eg, sick sinus node syndrome, AV block), implanted functioning pacemaker, bradycardia, marked hypotension, bronchospastic disorders, electrolyte imbalance, renal/hepatic dysfunction, pregnancy/nursing status, and possible drug interactions.

**Monitoring:** Monitor LFTs, renal functions, ANA titers, CBC, BP, ECG. Monitor signs/symptoms of neuromuscular dysfunction and exacerbation of myasthenia gravis, convulsions, atrioventricular block and acute circulatory failure.

**Patient Counseling:** Inform about risks/benefits. Advise to report signs of infection or electrolyte imbalance or any adverse reactions to physician. Notify if pregnant/nursing.

**Administration:** Oral route. **Storage:** 25°C (77°F) excursions permitted to 15-30°C (59-86°F). Dispense in a tight, light-resistant container.

# RYTHMOL SR — RX

propafenone HCl (GlaxoSmithKline)

**THERAPEUTIC CLASS:** Class IC antiarrhythmic

**INDICATIONS:** To prolong the time to recurrence of symptomatic atrial fibrillation in patients without structural heart disease.

**DOSAGE:** *Adults:* Initial: 225mg q12h. Titrate: May increase at minimum 5-day intervals to 325mg q12h, then to 425mg q12h if needed. Hepatic Impairment/QRS Widening/2nd- or 3rd-degree AV Block: Reduce dose.

**HOW SUPPLIED:** Cap, Extended-Release: 225mg, 325mg, 425mg

**CONTRAINDICATIONS:** Congestive Heart Failure (CHF), cardiogenic shock, bradycardia, marked hypotension, bronchospastic disorders, electrolyte imbalance, and sinoatrial, atrioventricular (AV) and intraventricular disorders of impulse generation or conduction (eg, sick sinus node syndrome, AV block) in the absence of an artificial pacemaker.

**WARNINGS/PRECAUTIONS:** Avoid with non-life-threatening ventricular arrhythmias and bronchospastic disease. Should not be given with AV and intraventricular conduction defects in the absence of a pacemaker. May cause new or worsened arrhythmias; evaluate electrocardiographically prior to and during therapy. May provoke overt CHF. Caution with hepatic or renal dysfunction. 1st-degree AV block, agranulocytosis, positive ANA titers reported. May exacerbate myasthenia gravis. May alter pacing and sensing thresholds of artificial pacemakers.

**ADVERSE REACTIONS:** Dizziness, chest pain, palpitations, taste disturbance, dyspnea, N/V, constipation, anxiety, fatigue, upper respiratory tract infection, influenza, 1st-degree heart block, edema, bradycardia, headache.

**INTERACTIONS:** Avoid with drugs that prolong QT interval (eg, some phenothiazines, cisapride, bepridil, TCAs, oral macrolides, other antiarrhythmics). Concurrent use of Class Ia and III antiarrhythmics (eg, quinidine, amiodarone) not recommended. Amiodarone can affect conduction and repolarization. Inhibitors of CYP2D6 (eg, desipramine, paroxetine, ritonavir, sertraline), CYP1A2 (eg, amiodarone), CYP3A4 (eg, ketoconazole, ritonavir, saquinavir, erythromycin, grapefruit juice) may increase levels; monitor closely. May increase levels of drugs metabolized by CYP2D6 (eg, desipramine, imipramine, haloperidol, venlafaxine). May increase CNS side effects of lidocaine. May increase levels of digoxin, propranolol, warfarin; monitor closely. Cimetidine may increase plasma levels. Fluoxetine may increase levels. Rifampin, orlistat may decrease plasma levels.

**PREGNANCY:** Category C, caution in nursing.

**MECHANISM OF ACTION:** Class 1C antiarrhythmic drug with local anesthetic effects and direct stabilizing action on myocardial membranes. Reduces upstroke velocity (phase 0) of the monophasic action potential. In Purkinje fibers, and to a lesser extent myocardial fibers, propafenone reduces the fast inward current carried by Na ions. Diastolic exicitability is increased and effective refractory period is prolonged. Reduces spontaneous automaticity and depresses triggered activity.

**PHARMACOKINETICS: Absorption:** $T_{max}$=3-8 hrs. **Distribution:** $V_d$=252L; plasma protein binding (>95%); found in breast milk. **Metabolism:** Rapid, extensive, via CYP2D6, 3A4 and 1A2. 5-hydroxypropafenone and N-depropylpropafenone (active metabolites). **Elimination:** $T_{1/2}$=2-10 hrs.

## NURSING CONSIDERATIONS

**Assessment:** Assess for CHF, cardiogenic shock, sinoatrial, AV and intraventricular disorders of impulse generation or conduction (eg, sick sinus syndrome, AV block), implanted functioning pacemaker, bradycardia, marked hypotension, bronchospastic disorders, electrolyte imbalance, MI, supraventricular arrhythmias, renal/hepatic dysfunction, pregnancy/nursing status, and for possible drug interactions. Perform ECG prior to and therapy.

**Monitoring:** Monitor for proarrhythmic effects (eg, ventricular fibrillation, ventricular tachycardia, asystole, torsade de pointes). Monitor for signs/symptoms of conduction disturbances, agranulocytosis (eg, fever, chills, weakness, and neutropenia), electrolyte imbalance, impaired spermatogenesis, and for exacerbation of myasthenia gravis. Monitor artifical pacemakers during therapy and program accordingly. Perform ECG during therapy. Monitor ANA titers, CBC, LFTs, BUN, and SrCr.

**Patient Counseling:** Inform about risks/benefits of therapy. Instruct to to report any signs of infection or electrolyte imbalance. Advise to notify physician if pregnant/nursing, if recently hospitalized, and all prescription and over the counter medications currently taking.

**Administration:** Oral route. Dose should be titrated to individual's drug response and tolerance. Do not crush or further divide capsule contents. **Storage:** 25°C (77°F); excursions permitted to 15-30°C (59-86°F). Dispense in a tight container.

# Ryzolt RX

tramadol HCl (Purdue Pharma)

**THERAPEUTIC CLASS:** Central acting analgesic

**INDICATIONS:** Management of moderate to moderately severe chronic pain.

**DOSAGE:** *Adults:* Individualize dose: Initial: 100mg/day. Titrate: 100mg every 2-3 days to achieve adequate pain control and tolerability. For patients requiring 300mg/day, titration should take at least 4 days. Usual: 200-300mg/day. Max: 300mg/day. Patients Currently on Tramodol IR Products: Calculate 24 hr IR dose and initiate on a total daily dose rounded down to next lowest 100mg increment. Max: 300mg/day. Elderly: Start at low end of dosing range. Swallow whole with liquid; do not split, chew, dissolve or crush.

**HOW SUPPLIED:** Tab, Extended-Release: 100mg, 200mg, 300mg

**CONTRAINDICATIONS:** Significant respiratory depression in unmonitored settings, acute or severe bronchial asthma, and hypercapnia.

**WARNINGS/PRECAUTIONS:** Seizures and anaphylactoid reactions reported. Avoid in suicidal or addiction-prone patients. May increase risk of serotonin syndrome (eg, mental changes, autonomic instability, neuromuscular aberrations, and GIT symptoms). Caution if at risk for respiratory depression, or with increased ICP or head trauma. May impair mental or physical abilities. Do not d/c abruptly; withdrawal symptoms may occur. May complicate acute abdominal conditions. Avoid in severe renal or hepatic impairment.

**ADVERSE REACTIONS:** Dizziness, N/V, constipation, headache, somnolence, pruritus, sweating, dry mouth, fatigue, anorexia, vertigo, insomnia, arthralgia, anxiety, hot flushes.

**INTERACTIONS:** CYP2D6 inhibitors (eg, quinidine, fluoxetine, paroxetine, amitriptyline) and CYP3A4 inhibitors (eg, ketoconazole, erythromycin) may reduce clearance of tramadol and increase risk for serious adverse events (eg, seizures, serotonin syndrome). Serotinergic drugs (eg, SSRIs, SNRIs, MAOIs, triptans, $\alpha_2$-adrenergic blockers, linzeolid, lithium, St. John's wort) may increase risk of seizures and/or serotonin syndrome; monitor closely, especially during treatment initiation and dose increases. Avoid with carbamazepine. Rare reports of digoxin toxicity and altered warfarin effects. Caution and reduce dose with CNS depressants (eg, alcohol, opioids, anesthetics, phenothiazines, tranquilizers, sedative hypnotics). Additive effects with alcohol and CNS depressants may occur.

**PREGNANCY:** Category C, safety in nursing not known.

**MECHANISM OF ACTION:** Centrally acting synthetic opioid analgesic; not fully understood. Shown to inhibit reuptake of norepinephrine and serotonin.

**PHARMACOKINETICS: Absorption:** Bioavailability (95%); $T_{max}$=4 hrs (drug), 5 hrs (M1 metabolite); $C_{max}$=345ng/mL (drug), 71ng/mL (M1 metabolite); $AUC_{0-24}$=5991ng•h/mL (drug), 1361ng•h/mL (M1 metabolite). **Distribution:** $V_d$=2.6L/kg (male), 2.9L/kg (female); plasma protein binding (20%). **Metabolism:** Liver (extensive); through N-and O-demethylation and glucuronidation or sulfation pathways via CYP3A4, 2D6. M1 (active metabolite). **Elimination:** Urine (30% unchanged), (60% as metabolite); $T_{1/2}$=6.3 hrs (drug), 7.4 hrs (M1).

## NURSING CONSIDERATIONS

**Assessment:** Assess for significant respiratory depression, acute or severe bronchial asthma, hypercapnia, seizure risk, epilepsy, risk for respiratory depression, increased ICP, acute abdominal conditions, renal/hepatic impairment, pregnancy/nursing status, and possible drug interactions.

**Monitoring:** Monitor for anaphylactoid reactions (eg, pruritus, hives, bronchospasm, angioedema, toxic epidermal necrolysis, and Stevens-Johnson syndrome), respiratory/CNS symptoms, physical dependence/abuse, seizures, serotonin syndrome, withdrawal symptoms with abrupt d/c (eg, anxiety, sweating, insomnia, rigors, upper respiratory symptoms, diarrhea, piloerection, and, rarely, hallucinations).

**Patient Counseling:** Advise to use caution while performing hazardous tasks (eg, operating machinery, driving). Do not take with alcohol, tranquilizers, or hypnotics. Notify physician if pregnant/nursing or planning to become pregnant. Take as prescribed.

**Administration:** Oral route. **Storage:** Store at 25°C (77°F); excursions permitted between 15-30°C (59-86°F).

# SABRIL

RX

vigabatrin (Lundbeck)

**Causes permanent vision loss in a high percentage of infants, children, and adults; timing of onset unpredictable. Causes progressive and permanent bilateral concentric visual field constriction in a high percentage of adult patients; in some cases may damage central retina and may reduce visual acuity. Risk increases with dose and cumulative exposure; use lowest effective dose and shortest exposure. Risk may persist after d/c therapy. D/C in patients who fail to show clinical benefit within 2-4 weeks (peds) or 3 months (adults) of initiation, or as soon as treatment failure is obvious. Vision testing is required at baseline, while on therapy, and after d/c. Unless benefit clearly outweighs the risk, avoid use with other drugs associated with serious adverse ophthalmic effects (eg, retinopathy, glaucoma) and in patients with, or at high risk of, other types of irreversible vision loss. Available only through restricted distribution program (SHARE).**

**THERAPEUTIC CLASS:** GABA analog

**INDICATIONS:** (Powder) Monotherapy for pediatrics (1 month-2 yrs) with infantile spasms (IS) for whom the potential benefits outweigh the potential risk of vision loss. (Tab) Adjunctive therapy for adults with refractory complex partial seizures (CPS) who have inadequately responded to several alternative treatments and for whom the potential benefits outweigh the risk of vision loss.

S

**DOSAGE:** *Adults:* Refractory CPS: (Tab) Initial: 500mg bid (1g/day). Titrate: May increase in 500mg increments at weekly intervals depending on response. Maint: 1.5g bid (3g/day). Renal Impairment: CrCl >50 to 80mL/min: Decrease dose by 25%. CrCl >30 to 50mL/min: Decrease dose by 50%. CrCl >10 to <30mL/min: Decrease dose by 75%. Withdraw gradually to d/c therapy.
*Pediatrics:* 1 month-2 yrs: IS: (Powder) Initial: 50mg/kg/day in 2 divided doses. Titrate: May increase by 25-50mg/kg/day increments every 3 days. Max: 150mg/kg/day. Refer to PI for volume of individual doses. Renal Impairment: CrCl >50 to 80mL/min: Decrease dose by 25%. CrCl >30 to 50mL/min: Decrease dose by 50%. CrCl >10 to <30mL/min: Decrease dose by 75%. Withdraw gradually to d/c therapy.

**HOW SUPPLIED:** Powder: 500mg/pkt [50$^s$]; Tab: 500mg* *scored

**WARNINGS/PRECAUTIONS:** Vision testing required at baseline (no later than 4 weeks), at least every 3 months during therapy, and 3-6 months after stopping therapy. Abnormal MRI changes involving thalamus, basal ganglia, brain stem, and cerebellum observed in some infants. May increase risk of suicidal thoughts/behavior. Monitor for worsening/emergence of depression and unusual changes in mood/behavior; risk observed as early as 1 week after initiation. May cause anemia, somnolence, and fatigue. May impair mental/ physical abilities. May cause peripheral neuropathy, weight gain, and edema in adults. Should be withdrawn gradually when necessary. Enroll all patients in SHARE; may be dispensed only to patients enrolled in, and who meet all conditions of, SHARE (1-888-45-SHARE).

**ADVERSE REACTIONS:** Vision loss, headache, somnolence, fatigue, dizziness, convulsions, nasopharyngitis, weight gain, upper respiratory tract infection, visual field defects, depression, tremor, nystagmus, N/V, diarrhea.

**INTERACTIONS:** See Black Box Warning. Decreases phenytoin plasma levels, probably due to induction of CYP 450 2C enzymes. Increases $C_{max}$ and decreases $T_{max}$ of clonazepam.

**PREGNANCY:** Category C, not for use in nursing.

**MECHANISM OF ACTION:** GABA analog; precise mechanism not established; may be due to irreversible inhibition of GABA-T, which results in increased levels of GABA in the CNS.

**PHARMACOKINETICS: Absorption:** Complete; $T_{max}$=1 hr (Adults/Children), 2.5 hrs (Infants). **Distribution:** $V_d$=1.1L/kg. Found in breast milk. **Elimination:** Urine (95%); $T_{1/2}$=7.5 hrs (Adults), 5.7 hrs (Infants).

## NURSING CONSIDERATIONS

**Assessment:** Perform baseline vision test. Assess renal function, pregnancy/ nursing status, underlying suicidal behavior/ideation.

**Monitoring:** Monitor worsening vision/visual field changes. Perform vision testing q3 months during therapy and 3-6 months after d/c. Monitor for signs of hypersensitivity, signal changes on MRI, and any untoward effects (eg, suicidal thoughts/behavior, worsening/emergence of depression, thoughts of self-harm). Monitor CBC, Hgb, Hct, LFTs, renal function, weight, edema.

**Patient Counseling:** Inform patients of the risk of permanent vision loss and the need for vision monitoring. If changes in vision occur, instruct to notify healthcare provider. Advise that drug may increase the risk of suicidal thoughts and behavior. Behaviors of concern should be reported immediately to healthcare provider. Advise to not drive or operate complex machinery until familiar with effects of drug. Inform of the possibility of developing abnormal MRI signal changes. If pregnant or about to become pregnant, instruct to enroll in the North American Antiepileptic Drug (NAAED) Pregnancy Registry by calling 888-233-2334 or go to www.aedpregnancyregistry.org. Instruct caregivers to withdraw gradually during d/c of therapy.

**Administration:** Oral route. (Powder) Empty contents of pkt into empty cup and dissolve with 10mL of cold/room temperature water using oral syringe. Final solution concentration should be 50mg/mL. Prepare each dose immediately prior to administration. Refer to PI for dilution table. **Storage:** 20-25°C (68-77°F).

# SAMSCA RX

tolvaptan (Otsuka America)

**Initiate and re-initiate therapy in hospitalized patients only; monitor serum sodium levels closely. Risk of osmotic demyelination syndrome (eg, dysarthria, mutism, dysphagia, lethargy, affective changes, spastic quadriparesis, seizures, coma or death) may occur during rapid correction of hyponatremia (eg, >12mEq/L/24 hrs). Slow rate of correction in susceptible patients with severe malnutrition, alcoholism, or advanced liver disease is advised.**

**THERAPEUTIC CLASS:** Arginine vasopressin antagonist

**INDICATIONS:** Treatment of hypervolemic and euvolemic hyponatremia (eg, serum sodium <125mEq/L or less marked hyponatremia that is symptomatic and has resisted correction with fluid restriction), including patients with heart failure, cirrhosis, and Syndrome of Inappropraiate Antidiuretic Hormone (SIADH).

**DOSAGE:** *Adults:* Initial: 15mg qd. Titrate: May increase to 30mg qd after at least 24 hrs to maximum of 60mg qd until desired level of serum sodium is achieved. Max: 60mg qd. Monitor for changes in serum electrolytes and volume during initiation and titration.

**HOW SUPPLIED:** Tab: 15mg, 30mg

**CONTRAINDICATIONS:** Urgent need to increase serum sodium acutely, unable to auto-regulate fluid balance, risks associated with worsening hypovolemic, hyponatremia (eg, hypotension, renal failure), concomitant use of strong CYP3A inhibitors (eg, ketoconazole, clarithromycin, itraconazole, ritonavir, indinavir, nelfinavir, saquinavir, nefazodone, telithromycin), and anuria.

**WARNINGS/PRECAUTIONS:** D/C if patient develop rapid elevation of serum sodium, consider hypotonic fluid administration. Avoid fluid restriction during first 24 hrs of therapy. GI bleeding reported in patients with cirrhosis. Dehydration and hypovolemia may occur; interrupt or d/c therapy and provide supportive care with careful management of vital signs, fluid balance and electrolytes. Increased serum potassium levels reported.

**ADVERSE REACTIONS:** Thirsty, dry mouth, asthenia, constipation, pollakiuria, polyuria, hyperglycemia, pyrexia, anorexia.

**INTERACTIONS:** See Contraindications. Increase levels with ketoconazole or other strong CYP3A inhibitors (eg, ketoconazole, clarithromycin, itraconazole, telithromycin, saquinavir, nelfinavir, ritonavir, and nefazodone), grapefruit juice, and digoxin. Avoid with moderate CYP3A inhibitors (eg, erythromycin, fluconazole, aprepitant, dilitiazem, and verapamil). Dose reduction with P-gp inhibitors (eg, cyclosporine). Avoid with CYP3A inducers (eg, rifampin, rifabutin, barbiturates, phenytoin, carbamazepine, and St. John's wort). Avoid with concomitant use of hypertonic saline.

**PREGNANCY:** Category C, not for use in nursing.

**MECHANISM OF ACTION:** Selective Vasopressin $V_2$-receptor antagonist; antagonize the effect of vasopressin and cause increase in urine water excretion resulting in increase free water clearance (aquaresis), decrease urine osmolarity and increase serum sodium levels.

**PHARMACOKINETICS: Absorption:** $T_{max}$=2-4 hrs. **Distribution:** $V_d$=3L/kg; plasma protein binding (99%). **Metabolism:** Via CYP3A. **Elimination:** $T_{1/2}$=12 hrs.

## NURSING CONSIDERATIONS

**Assessment:** Assess for serum sodium levels, neurologic status, anuria, hypovolemia, possible complications of hypotension and renal failure, cirrhosis, pregnancy/nursing status, and possible drug interactions.

**Monitoring:** Monitor for serum potassium levels, neurologic status, changes in serum sodium/volume status, vital signs, fluid balance and electrolytes.

**Patient Counseling:** Avoid patients to continue fluid ingestion in response to thirst. Instruct fluid restriction within 24 hrs of therapy. Inform physician if they are taking or planning to take any prescription or over-the-counter drugs, use strong or moderate CYP3A inhibitors, and P-gp inhibitors. Advise nursing mothers not to breastfeed.

**Administration:** Oral route. **Storage:** 25°C(77°F), excursions permitted between 15-30°C (59-86°F).

## SANCTURA XR

RX

trospium chloride (Allergan)

**OTHER BRAND NAMES:** Sanctura (Allergan)

**THERAPEUTIC CLASS:** Muscarinic antagonist

**INDICATIONS:** Treatment of overactive bladder with symptoms of urge urinary incontinence, urgency, and urinary frequency.

**DOSAGE:** *Adults:* (Tab) 20mg bid. (Cap, Extended-Release) 60mg qam. Take at least 1 hr before meals on an empty stomach. (Tab) CrCl <30mL/min: 20mg qhs. Elderly ≥75 yrs: May titrate to 20mg qd based upon tolerability.

**HOW SUPPLIED:** Cap, Extended-Release: 60mg; Tab: 20mg

**CONTRAINDICATIONS:** Active or risk of urinary retention, gastric retention, and uncontrolled narrow-angle glaucoma.

**WARNINGS/PRECAUTIONS:** (Cap, Tab) Caution with significant bladder outflow obstruction, GI obstructive disorders, ulcerative colitis, intestinal atony, myasthenia gravis, moderate or severe hepatic dysfunction. Consider risks and benefits with controlled narrow-angle glaucoma. (Tab) Reduce dose with severe renal insufficiency. (Cap) Not recommended for use with severe renal impairment (CrCl <30mL/min). Consumption of alcohol within 2 hrs is not recommended.

**ADVERSE REACTIONS:** Dry mouth, constipation, urinary tract infection, headache.

**INTERACTIONS:** (Cap/Tab) Increased adverse effects with other anticholinergics. May alter GI absorption of other drugs due to GI motility effects. Monitor closely with other drugs eliminated by active renal tubular secretion (eg, procainamide, pancuronium, morphine, vancomycin, metformin, tenofovir). May enhance drowsiness if co-administered with alcohol. (Cap) An increase or decrease in trospium exposure with antacids containing aluminum hydroxide and magnesium carbonate.

**PREGNANCY:** Category C, caution in nursing.

**MECHANISM OF ACTION:** Antispasmodic, antimuscarinic agent; reduces tonus of smooth muscle in bladder by antagonizing effect of acetylcholine on muscarinic receptors.

**PHARMACOKINETICS: Absorption:** (Tab) Absolute bioavailability (9.6%); $C_{max}$=3.5ng/mL; $T_{max}$=5.3 hrs; AUC=36.4ng/mL•hr. (Cap) $C_{max}$=2ng/mL; $T_{max}$=5 hrs; AUC=18ng•hr/mL. **Distribution:** (Tab) Plasma protein binding (50-85%); $V_d$=395L. (Cap) Plasma protein binding (48-78%); $V_d$:>600L. **Metabolism:** Ester hydrolysis with subsequent conjugation. **Elimination:** Feces (85.2%), urine (5.8%). (Tab) $T_{1/2}$=18.3 hrs. (Cap) $T_{1/2}$=36 hrs.

S

### NURSING CONSIDERATIONS

**Assessment:** Assess for bladder outflow obstruction (urinary retention), GI obstructive disorders (gastric retention), narrow-angle glaucoma, ulcerative colitis, intestinal atony, myasthenia gravis, hepatic/renal impairment, hypersensitivity, pregnancy/nursing status and possible drug interactions.

**Monitoring:** Monitor for signs/symptoms of gastric retention, urinary retention, decreased gastric motility, hypersensitivity reactions and hepatic/renal dysfunction.

**Patient Counseling:** Inform that heat prostration may occur when used in hot environment, and dry mouth, constipation, trouble emptying the bladder, dizziness and blurred vision may also be experienced. Advise not to take if urinary and gastric retention and uncontrolled narrow-angle glaucoma are present. Advise that alcohol may enhance drowsiness effect. Instruct to take tab 1 hr prior to meals or on empty stomach. Inform that if dose is skipped, next dose should be taken 1 hr prior to next meal. Instruct to take cap in the am with water on empty stomach or 1 hr prior to meal. Counsel to avoid alcohol within 2 hrs of dosing of cap.

**Administration:** Oral route. **Storage:** Cap: 20-25°C (68-77°F); excursions permitted at 15-30°C. Tab: 20-25°C (68-77°F).

## SANCUSO RX

granisetron (Prostrakan)

**THERAPEUTIC CLASS:** 5-$HT_3$ receptor antagonist

**INDICATIONS:** Prevention of nausea and vomiting in patients receiving moderately and/or highly emetogenic chemotherapy for up to 5 consecutive days.

**DOSAGE:** *Adults:* Apply single patch to upper outer arm a minimum of 24 hrs before chemo. May be applied up to a maximum of 48 hrs before chemo. Remove patch a minimum of 24 hrs after completion of chemo. Patch can be worn for up to 7 days depending on duration of chemo regimen.

**HOW SUPPLIED:** Patch: 3.1mg/24 hrs

**WARNINGS/PRECAUTIONS:** May mask progressive ileus and/or gastric distention. Avoid placing on red, irritated, or damaged skin. Generalized skin reaction (eg, allergic rash, including erythematous, macular, papular rash, pruritis) may occur; d/c and remove patch immediately. Avoid direct natural or artificial sunlight. Cover application site in case of risk of exposure to sunlight throughout the period of wear and for 10 days following removal.

**ADVERSE REACTIONS:** Constipation, abdominal pain, diarrhea, HTN, hypotension, dizziness, insomnia, fever.

**PREGNANCY:** Category B, caution in nursing.

**MECHANISM OF ACTION:** 5-$HT_3$ receptor antagonist; blocks serotonin stimulation and subsequent vomiting after emetogenic stimuli such as cisplatin in animal studies.

**PHARMACOKINETICS: Absorption:** $T_{max}$=48 hrs. Mean $C_{max}$=5.0ng/mL. Mean $AUC_{0-168hr}$=527ng-hr/mL. **Distribution:** Plasma protein binding (65%). **Metabolism:** N-demethylation and aromatic ring oxidation mediated by hepatic CYP1A1 and CYP3A4. **Elimination:** Urine (12%, unchanged; 49%, metabolites), feces (34%).

### NURSING CONSIDERATIONS

**Assessment:** Assess skin condition and GI history.

**Monitoring:** Monitor for abdominal pain and/or swelling, generalized skin reactions, and adverse events.

**Patient Counseling:** Instruct to apply to clean, dry, intact healthy skin on upper outer arm. Do not place on skin that is red, irritated, or damaged. Instruct patient to tell physician if abdominal pain and swelling occurs. Advise patients to remove patch if severe skin or generalized skin reactions (eg, allergic rash, including erythematous macular, papular rash, or pruritus) occur. Instruct patients to cover patch application site when there is a risk of exposure to sunlight or sunlamps during the period of wear and for 10 days after removal. Patch should not be cut into pieces.

**Administration:** Topical route. Patch should be applied to clean, dry, intact healthy skin on the upper outer arm. **Storage:** Store at 20-25°C (68-77°F); excursions permitted between 15-30°C (59-86°F).



## SANDIMMUNE RX

cyclosporine (Novartis)

**Give with adrenal corticosteroids but not with other immunosuppressives. Increased susceptibility to infection and development of lymphoma. Sandimmune and Neoral are not bioequivalent. Monitor blood levels to avoid toxicity.**

**THERAPEUTIC CLASS:** Cyclic polypeptide immunosuppressant

**INDICATIONS:** Prophylaxis of organ rejection in kidney, liver, and heart allogeneic transplants with concomitant adrenal corticosteroids. Treatment of chronic rejection in patients previously treated with other immunosuppressives.

**DOSAGE:** *Adults:* Initial: PO: 15mg/kg single dose 4-12 hrs before transplant; continue same dose qd for 1-2 weeks. Usual: Taper by 5% per week until 5-10mg/kg/day. IV: 1/3 PO dose. Initial: 5-6mg/kg/day single dose; begin 4 to 12 hrs prior to transplantation. Maint: Continue single daily dose until PO forms are tolerated. Elderly: Start at lower end of dosing range.
*Pediatrics:* Initial: PO: 15mg/kg single dose 4-12 hrs before transplant; continue same dose qd for 1-2 weeks. Usual: Taper by 5% per week until 5-10mg/kg/day. IV: 1/3 PO dose. Initial: 5-6mg/kg/day single dose; begin 4 to 12 hrs prior to transplantation. Maint: Continue single daily dose until PO forms are tolerated.

**HOW SUPPLIED:** Cap: 25mg, 100mg; Inj: 50mg/mL; Sol: 100mg/mL [50mL]

**CONTRAINDICATIONS:** Hypersensitivity to Cremophor EL (polyoxyethylated castor oil).

**WARNINGS/PRECAUTIONS:** Due to risk of anaphylaxis, only use injection if unable to take oral agents. May cause hepatotoxicity and nephrotoxicity. Convulsions, elevated SrCr, and BUN levels reported. Thrombocytopenia and microangiopathic hemolytic anemia, hyperuricemia, hyperkalemia, encephalopathy may develop. Increases risk for development of lymphomas and other malignancies. Anaphylactic reactions reported rarely with IV administration; observe for 30 min after start of infusion and frequently thereafter. Caution with malabsorption. HTN may occur and persist which may require antihypertensive therapy. Increased risk of opportunistic infections including activation of latent viral infection such as BK virus-associated nephropathy in immunosuppressed patients receiving immunosuppressants. Caution in elderly.

**ADVERSE REACTIONS:** Renal dysfunction, tremor, hirsutism, HTN, gum hyperplasia, cramps, acne, convulsions, headache, diarrhea, hepatotoxity, abdominal discomfort, paresthesia, flushing, BK virus-associated nephropathy.

**INTERACTIONS:** Ciprofloxacin, gentamicin, tobramycin, vancomycin, SMZ/TMP, amphotericin B, ketoconazole, melphalan, diclofenac, azapropazon, sulindac, naproxen, colchicine, cimetidine, ranitidine, tacrolimus, bezafirate, fenofibrate may potentiate renal dysfunction. Diltiazem, nicardipine, colchicine, fluconazole, itraconazole, ketoconazole, verapamil, azithromycin, clarithromycin, erythromycin, quinupristin/dalfopristin, allopurinol, amiodarone, bromocriptine, danazol, imatinib, metoclopramide, oral contraceptives, methylprednisolone, grapefruit juice, HIV protease inhibitors may increase levels. St. John's wort, carbamazepine, phenobarbital, phenytoin, rifampin, sulfinpyrazone, octreotide, orlistat, terbinafine, ticlopidine, and naficillin may decrease levels. Avoid with potassium-sparing diuretics. Caution with ACEIs, angiotensin II blockers, NSAIDs. Digitalis toxicity reported. Myotoxicity with statins, frequent gingival hyperplasia with nifedipine, and convulsions with high dose methylprednisolone reported. Increased levels of sirolimus; give 4 hrs after cyclosporine. Avoid live vaccines during therapy.



**PREGNANCY:** Category C, not for use in nursing.

**MECHANISM OF ACTION:** Cyclic polypeptide immunosuppressant; not fully established. May cause specific and reversible inhibition of immunocompetent lymphocytes in the $G_0$- or $G_1$-phase of the cell cycle. T lymphocytes are preferentially inhibited with T-helper cell as main target while also possibly suppressing T-suppressor cells. Also inhibits lymphokine production and release (eg, interleukin-2, T-cell growth factor).

**PHARMACOKINETICS: Absorption:** Incomplete and variable. Absolute bioavailability (30%)(PO); $C_{max}$=1ng/mL/mg; $T_{max}$=3.5 hrs. **Distribution:** Plasma protein binding (90%). **Metabolism:** Extensively metabolized via hydroxylation, cyclic ether formation, and *N*-demethylation. **Elimination:** Urine (6%); $T_{1/2}$=19 hrs.

## NURSING CONSIDERATIONS

**Assessment:** Prior to IV administration, assess that patient cannot take oral formulations and is on concomitant therapy with adrenal corticosteroids.

Assess for hypersensitivity to Cremophor EL (polyoxyethylated castor oil), pregnancy/nursing status, possible drug interactions. Assess use of oral formulations in patients with malabsorption problems.

**Monitoring:** Patients receiving IV formulation should be under continuous observation for anaphylactic reactions for at least first 30 min following start of infusion and at frequent intervals thereafter. Monitor for signs/symptoms of hepatotoxicity, nephrotoxicity, thrombocytopenia, microangiopathic hemolytic anemia, HTN, hyperkalemia, glomerular capillary thrombosis, lymphomas, and other malignancies, convulsions, encephalopathy, and development of anaphylactic reactions (eg, facial flushing, non-cardiogenic pulmonary edema with acute respiratory distress, dyspnea, changes in blood pressure, and tachycardia). Frequently monitor cyclosporine blood levels, especially when converting from Neoral to Sandimmune, as well as renal/hepatic function (eg, BUN, SrCr, serum bilirubin, liver enzymes).

**Patient Counseling:** Instruct to contact a physician before changing formulations of cyclosporine, which may require dose change. Inform patients that repeated tests are required while on medication. Inform that the drug may cause increased risk of neoplasias. Advise females about risks of use during pregnancy. Instruct patients using the oral syringe, that syringe should not be washed before or after use as that will cause variation in dosage.

**Administration:** Oral/IV routes. IV concentrate should be administered by slow IV infusion over 2-6 hrs. **Storage:** Cap: 25°C (77°F); excursions permitted to 15-30°C (59-86°F). Oral Sol: Store in original container, below 30°C (86°F). Do not refrigerate. Protect from freezing. Once opened, use contents within 2 months. Injection: Below 30°C (86°F), protected from light. Discard diluted infusion after 24 hrs.

## SANDOSTATIN LAR — RX

octreotide acetate (Novartis)

**THERAPEUTIC CLASS:** Somatostatin analog

**INDICATIONS:** Long term maintenance therapy in acromegalic patients with inadequate response to surgery and/or radiotherapy or for whom surgery and/or radiotherapy is not an option. Long-term treatment of severe diarrhea and flushing associated with metastatic carcinoid tumors. Long-term treatment of profuse watery diarrhea associated with vasoactive intestinal peptide tumors (VIPomas).

**DOSAGE:** *Adults:* Administer intragluteally. Patients not currently receiving octreotide should begin therapy with Sandostatin Injection; please see PI for dosing. Acromegaly: Initial: 20mg IM every 4 weeks for 3 months. Titrate: See PI for dose adjustment based on growth hormone (GH), IGF-1, and/or clinical symptoms. Max: 40mg every 4 weeks. Withdraw yearly for 8 weeks to assess disease activity after pituitary irradiation. Carcinoid Tumors/VIPomas: Initial: 20mg IM every 4 weeks for 2 months. Continue with Sandostatin injection SQ for at least 2 weeks. Titrate: If symptoms not controlled, increase to 30mg every 4 weeks. If symptoms controlled at 20mg, reduce to 10mg. If symptoms recur increase dose to 20mg every 4 weeks. Max: 30mg every 4 weeks. For exacerbation of symptoms, give Sandostatin Injection SQ for at least 2 weeks. Patients must be considered responders and tolerate the injection before switching to the depot. Renal Failure Requiring Dialysis/Cirrhotic patients: Initial: 10mg every 4 weeks.

**HOW SUPPLIED:** Inj, Depot: 10mg, 20mg, 30mg

**WARNINGS/PRECAUTIONS:** May inhibit gallbladder contractility and decrease bile secretions; increased risk of gallbladder abnormalities. May alter balance between insulin, glucagon, and GH and lead to hypoglycemia or hyperglycemia; monitor glucose tolerance and antidiabetic treatment periodically. May cause hypothyroidism; monitor thyroid levels periodically. Cardiac conduction and other CV abnormalities may occur; caution in patients at-risk. Depressed vitamin $B_{12}$ levels, alteration in fat absorption and abnormal Schilling's test reported. Caution in the elderly and in patient on total parenteral nutrition (TPN).

**ADVERSE REACTIONS:** Diarrhea, N/V, abdominal discomfort, flatulence, constipation, hyperglycemia, injection-site pain, upper respiratory infection, flu-like symptoms, fatigue, dizziness, headache, malaise, fever.

**INTERACTIONS:** May alter absorption of orally administered drugs. May decrease cyclosporine effects. May need dose adjustments of insulin, oral hypoglycemics, and bradycardia-inducing drugs (eg, beta-blocker). Increased availability of bromocriptine. Caution in other drugs metabolized by CYP3A4 with a low therapeutic index (eg, quinidine, terfenadine).

**PREGNANCY:** Category B, caution in nursing.

**MECHANISM OF ACTION:** Somatostatin analog; long acting. Exerts similiar actions to natural hormone somatostatin, but is more potent in inhibiting GH, glucagon, and insulin. Like somatostatin, it also suppresses LH response to GnRH, decreases splanchnic blood flow and inhibits release of serotonin, gastrin, vasoactive intestinal peptide, secretin, motilin and pancreatic polypeptide.

**PHARMACOKINETICS: Absorption:** (SQ) Rapid, Complete. $C_{max}$=5.2ng/mL; $T_{max}$=0.4 hrs; Acromegaly: $C_{max}$=2.8ng/mL, $T_{max}$=0.7 hr. Distribution: $V_d$=13.6L; plasma protein binding (65%); Acromegaly: $V_d$=21.6L, plasma protein binding (41.2%). Elimination: Urine (32%, unchanged); $T_{1/2}$=1.7-1.9 hrs.

## NURSING CONSIDERATIONS

**Assessment:** Assess GH and IGF-I levels, baseline renal function. Obtain baseline thyroid function tests (TSH, total and/or free T4). Assess use with cardiac dysfunction, for glycemic control with DM, and for possible drug interactions.

**Monitoring:** Monitor for signs/symptoms of biliary tract abnormalities (eg, gallstones, biliary duct dilatation), hypo/hyperglycemia, hypothyroidism, cardiac conduction abnormalities, and pancreatitis. With acromegaly: Monitor GH and IGF-1 levels. With carcinoids: Monitor 5-HIAA (urinary 5-hydroxyindoleacetic acid), plasma serotonin levels, and plasma Substance P levels. With VIPoma: Monitor VIP levels. Monitor zinc levels if receiving TPN.

**Patient Counseling:** Advise patients with carcinoid tumors and VIPomas to adhere closely to scheduled return visits for reinjection to minimize exacerbation of symptoms. Advise patients with acromegaly to adhere to return visit schedule to help ensure steady control of GH and IGF-1 levels.

**Administration:** IM route. Do not directly inject diluent without preparing sus. Never administer via IV/SQ routes. Sandostatin LAR depot drug product kit should remain at room temperature for 30-60 min prior to preparation of drug sus. Administer sus immediately after preparation. **Storage:** Refrigerate between 2-8°C (36-46°F) and protect from light until time of use.

# SAPHRIS — RX

asenapine (Schering-Plough)

**Elderly patients with dementia-related psychosis are at an increased risk of death when treated with atypical antipsychotic drugs. Most deaths appeared to be either cardiovascular (eg, heart failure, sudden death) or infectious (eg, pneumonia) in nature. Asenapine is not approved for the treatment of patients with dementia-related psychosis.**

**THERAPEUTIC CLASS:** Dibenzapine derivative

**INDICATIONS:** Acute treatment of schizophrenia and of manic or mixed episodes associated with bipolar I disorder with or without psychotic features in adults.

**DOSAGE:** *Adults:* Schizophrenia: Usual: 5mg bid. Max: 10mg bid. Maint: Responding patients continue use beyond acute response. Bipolar Disorder: Usual: 10mg bid. Decrease to 5mg bid if there are adverse effects. Maint: Responding patients continue beyond acute response.

**HOW SUPPLIED:** Tab, SL: 5mg, 10mg

**WARNINGS/PRECAUTIONS:** Neuroleptic malignant syndrome (NMS) reported; d/c and instill symptomatic treatment and monitoring. Tardive dyskinesia (TD) reported; d/c therapy or use lowest dose and shortest treatment duration if using chronically. Hyperglycemia, in some cases extreme and associated with ketoacidosis or hyperosmolar coma or death, has been reported; monitor diabetes mellitus (DM) patients for symptoms of hyperglycemia. May cause weight gain. May induce orthostatic hypotension and syncope; caution with known CV disease, presence of cerebrovascular disease, conditions that predispose to hypotension (dehydration, hypovolemia and treatment with antihypertensive medications), and in elderly; monitor orthostatic vital signs if at risk of hypotension and consider dose reduction. Leukopenia, neutropenia, agranulocytosis reported; monitor CBC frequently during first few months and d/c at first decline of WBC patients with previous history. If severe neutropenia (absolute neutrophil count <1000/mm³), d/c and have WBC followed until recovery. May prolong $QT_c$ interval; avoid use if have history of cardiac arrhythmias or at increased risk of torsades de pointes. May cause hyperprolactinemia, which may lead to galactorrhea, amenorrhea, gynecomastia, impotence, and decreased bone density. Seizures reported; caution if history of seizures or conditions that lower seizure threshold. Somnolence reported; may impair mental/physical abilities. May disrupt body temperature regulation. Prescribe in smallest quantity to reduce risk of overdose and inherent risk of suicide. May cause dysphagia, esophageal dysmotility, and aspiration; do not use when at risk for aspiration pneumonia. Use not recommended with severe hepatic impairment (Child Pugh C).

**ADVERSE REACTIONS:** Somnolence, insomnia, headache, dizziness, extrapyramidal symptoms, akathisia, vomiting, oral hypoesthesia, constipation, weight increase, fatigue.

**INTERACTIONS:** Avoid use with other drugs known to prolong $QT_c$, including Class 1A antiarrhythmics (eg, quinidine, procainamide), Class 3 antiarrhythmics (eg, amiodarone, sotalol), antipsychotic medications (eg, ziprasidone, chlorpromazine, thioridazine), and antibiotics (eg, gatifloxacin, moxifloxacin). Caution with fluvoxamine, may increase concentrations. Coadministration with paroxetine may increase paroxetine exposure and may enhance inhibitory effects on its own metabolism. Caution with other centrally acting drugs, alcohol, and with drugs that are both substrates and inhibitors of CYP2D6. May enhance effects of antihypertensive agents. Concomitant use with medications with anticholinergic activity, may increase risk of elevating core body temperature.

**PREGNANCY:** Pregnancy C, not for use in nursing.

**MECHANISM OF ACTION:** Atypical antipsychotic; unknown. Suggested that may be mediated through a combination of antagonist activity at $D_2$ and $5\text{-}HT_{2A}$ receptors.

**PHARMACOKINETICS: Absorption:** Rapidly absorbed; absolute bioavailability (35%); $T_{max}$=0.5-1.5 hrs. **Distribution:** $V_d$=20-25L/kg; plasma protein binding (95%). **Metabolism:** Direct glucuronidation via UGT1A4 and oxidation via cytochrome P450 (predominantly CYP1A2). **Elimination:** Urine (50%), feces (40%); $T_{1/2}$=24 hrs.

S

## NURSING CONSIDERATIONS

**Assessment:** Assess for dementia-related psychosis, DM, history of seizures, conditions which lower seizure threshold (eg, Alzheimer's dementia), patients with suicide risk, aspiration pneumonia, hepatic impairment, pregnancy/nursing status, and possible drug interactions. In patients with DM and patients at risk for DM (eg, obesity, family history of DM), obtain baseline FPG. Assess if at increased risk of developing orthostatic hypotension or syncope (eg, patients with known CVD, cerebrovascular disease, dehydration, hypovolemia). Assess if at increased risk for leukopenia/neutropenia (eg, pre-existing low WBC, history of drug-induced leukopenia/neutropenia); perform baseline CBC if at risk for leukopenia/neutropenia. Assess if at increased risk of developing QT interval prolongation (eg, cardiac arrhythmias, bradycardia, hypokalemia, hypomagnesemia, presence of congenital prolongation of QT interval).

**Monitoring:** Monitor for signs and symptoms of NMS (eg, hyperpyrexia, muscle rigidity, altered mental status, autonomic instability), TD (eg, irreversible, involuntary, dyskinetic movements), hyperglycemia (eg, ketoacidosis, hyperosmolar coma, polydipsia, polyuria, polyphagia, weakness), leukopenia, neutropenia, agranulocytosis, QT prolongation, seizures, aspiration pneumonia, and dysphagia. In patients with DM, patients at risk for DM, or if develop hyperglycemia, perform periodic FBG measurements. In patients with preexisting low WBC or history of drug-induced leukopenia/neutropenia, monitor CBC frequently. If neutropenia present, monitor for fever and other signs of infection. Monitor for signs and symptoms of orthostatic hypotension; perform periodic monitoring of orthostatic vital signs. Monitor for ECG measurements.

**Patient Counseling:** Instruct not to remove tablet from packaging until ready to take. Inform to use dry hands when handling tablet. Advise that tablet should not be chewed, crushed, or swallowed. Inform that tablet should be placed under tongue and allowed to dissolve. Instruct to not eat or drink for 10 min after administration. Advise that medication may impair cognitive and motor performance; instruct to use caution when performing tasks requiring mental alertness (eg, operating hazardous machinery or motor vehicle). Inform about risk of developing NMS and counsel about signs and symptoms (eg, hyperpyrexia, muscle rigidity, autonomic instability). Inform about risk of developing orthostatic hypotension and instruct about nonpharmacological interventions to reduce occurence of orthostatic hypotension (eg, sitting on edge of bed before slowly rising). Instruct to inform physician if pregnant or nursing and all medications currently taking. Advise to avoid alcohol during use. Instruct to avoid conditions that would lead to overheating or dehydration.

**Administration:** SL. Place under tongue; dissolve completely. Do not eat or drink for 10 mins after administration. Do not crush, chew, or swallow.
**Storage:** 15-30°C (59-86°F).

## SAVELLA — RX

milnacipran HCl (Forest)

> **Increased risk of suicidal ideation, thinking and behavior in children, adolescents, and young adults taking antidepressants for major depressive disorder (MDD) and other psychiatric disorders. It is not approved for use in pediatric patients.**

**THERAPEUTIC CLASS:** Serotonin and norepinephrine reuptake inhibitor

**INDICATIONS:** Management of fibromyalgia.

**DOSAGE:** *Adults:* 100mg qd (50mg bid). Titrate: Day 1: 12.5mg qd. Days 2-3: 25mg qd (12.5mg bid). Days 4-7: 50mg qd (25mg bid). After Day 7: 100mg qd (50mg bid). May increase dose to 200mg qd (100mg bid) based on response. Max: 200mg/day. Severe Renal Impairment (CrCl =5-29mL/min): Reduce maintenance dose to 50mg qd (25mg bid). Titrate: May increase dose up to 100mg qd (50mg bid) based on response.

**HOW SUPPLIED:** Tab: 12.5mg, 25mg, 50mg, 100mg

S

**CONTRAINDICATIONS:** Uncontrolled narrow-angle glaucoma and concomitant use with monoamine oxidase inhibitors (MAOIs).

**WARNINGS/PRECAUTIONS:** Serotonin syndrome symptoms, increased BP, HR, liver enzymes, and severe liver injury reported. Caution with HTN or cardiac disease. BP should be measured prior to therapy and periodically. If sustained increase in BP occurs; reduce dose or d/c therapy. Caution with history of seizure disorder. D/C if jaundice or liver dysfunction occurs. Avoid with substantial alcohol use or chronic liver disease. Withdrawal and physical dependence reported; avoid abrupt discontinuation. Taper after long-term use. Hyponatremia may occur. Increased risk of bleeding events. Caution with history of mania. Caution with history of dysuria, prostatic hypertrophy, prostatitis, and other lower urinary tract obstructive disorders. Mydriasis reported; caution with controlled narrow-angle glaucoma. Caution with moderate renal and severe hepatic impairment.

**ADVERSE REACTIONS:** N/V, headache, constipation, dizziness, insomnia, hot flush, hyperhidrosis, palpitations, tachycardia, dry mouth, and HTN.

**INTERACTIONS:** See contraindications. Risk of serotonin syndrome with lithium, serotonergic drugs (eg, triptans and tramadol), and MAOIs. Concurrent use with epinephrine and norepinephrine may increase risks of paroxysmal

HTN and arrhythmia. Concomitant use with other serotonin reuptake inhibitors may result in HTN and coronary artery vasoconstriction. Digoxin may potentiate adverse hemodynamic effects. Risks of postural hypotension and tachycardia with IV digoxin. May inhibit clonidine effect. Switch from clomipramine may increase risk of euphoria and postural hypotension. Caution with other centrally acting drugs. Avoid with serotonin precursors (eg, tryptophan). Concurrent use of aspirin, nonsteroidal anti-inflammatory drugs, warfarin, and other anticoagulants may increase risk of bleeding events (eg, ecchymoses, hematomas, epistaxis, petechiae or life-threatening hemorrhages).

**PREGNANCY:** Category C, not for use in nursing.

**MECHANISM OF ACTION:** Serotonin and norepinephrine reuptake inhibition; exact mechanism of central pain inhibitory action and its ability to improve symptoms of fibromyalgia in humans are not established.

**PHARMACOKINETICS: Absorption:** Complete; absolute bioavailability (85%-90%); $T_{max}$=2-4 hrs. **Distribution:** $V_d$=400L; plasma protein binding (13%). **Metabolism:** Via liver; *l*-milnacipran carbamoyl-O-glucuronide (major metabolite). **Elimination:** Urine (unchanged, 55%), $T_{1/2}$=6-8 hrs (milnacipran); 8-10 hrs (*d*-milnacipran); 4-6 hrs (*l*-milnacipran).

## NURSING CONSIDERATIONS

**Assessment:** Assess for suicidality, worsening of depression, uncontrolled narrow-angle glaucoma, taking MAOIs, pre-existing tachyarrhythmias, other cardiac diseases, history of seizure disorder, pre-existing liver disease, pregnancy/nursing status, and possible drug interactions. Assess BP, HR, and LFTs (eg, AST, ALT).

**Monitoring:** Monitor BP, HR, LFTs, sodium levels. Monitor for emergence of agitation, irritability, unusual changes in behavior, serotonin syndrome (eg, mental status changes, autonomic instability, neuromuscular aberrations, GIT symptoms), withdrawal symptoms, physical dependence, hyponatremia, and abnormal bleeding.

**Patient Counseling:** Counsel patients, families, and caregivers about the risks and benefits of therapy. Instruct families and caregivers of patients to notify a healthcare provider if emergence of agitation, irritability, suicidality or unusual changes in behavior occur. Inform patients about the risk of serotonin syndrome with concomitant use of triptans, tramadol, or other serotonergic agents. Advise to monitor BP and PR periodically. Caution about the increased risk of abnormal bleeding with concomitant use of NSAIDs, aspirin, and other anticoagulation drugs. Caution against operating machinery or driving motor vehicles until effects of drug known. Avoid consumption of alcohol. Advise that withdrawal symptoms may occur with abrupt discontinuation. Notify physician if pregnant or intend to become pregnant, or if breastfeeding.

**Administration:** Oral route. **Storage:** Store at 25°C (77°F); excursions permitted to 15-30°C (59-86°F).



# SEASONALE RX

ethinyl estradiol - levonorgestrel (Duramed)

> **Cigarette smoking increases the risk of serious CV side effects. Risk increases with age (>35yrs) and with heavy smoking (>15 cigarettes/day). Women who use oral contraceptives should be strongly advised not to smoke.**

**OTHER BRAND NAMES:** Quasense (Watson)

**THERAPEUTIC CLASS:** Estrogen/progestogen combination

**INDICATIONS:** Prevention of pregnancy.

**DOSAGE:** *Adults:* 1 tab qd for 91 days, then repeat. Start 1st Sunday after menses begin or on 1st day of menses if menses begins on a Sunday.
*Pediatrics:* Postpubertal adolescents ≥16 yrs: 1 tab qd for 91 days, then repeat. Start 1st Sunday after menses begin or on 1st day of menses if menses begins on a Sunday.

**HOW SUPPLIED:** Tab: (Ethinyl Estradiol-Levonorgestrel) 0.03mg/0.15mg

**CONTRAINDICATIONS:** Thrombophlebitis or past history of deep vein thrombophlebitis, thromboembolic disorders or past history of thromboembolic disorders, current or history of cerebrovascular or coronary artery disease (CAD), valvular heart disease with thrombogenic complications, uncontrolled HTN, diabetes with vascular involvement, headaches with focal neurological symptoms, major surgery with prolonged immobilization, breast carcinoma (current or past history), carcinoma of the endometrium or other known or suspected estrogen-dependent neoplasia, undiagnosed abnormal genital bleeding, cholestatic jaundice of pregnancy or jaundice with prior pill use, hepatic adenomas or carcinomas or active liver disease, known or suspected pregnancy.

**WARNINGS/PRECAUTIONS:** Increased risk of MI, vascular disease, thromboembolism, stroke, HTN, and gallbladder disease, and hepatic neoplasia. May increase risk of breast cancer and cancer of the reproductive organs. Retinal thrombosis reported; d/c if unexplained partial or complete loss of vision, onset of proptosis or diplopia, papilledema, or retinal vascular lesions develop. May cause glucose intolerance, fluid retention, breakthrough bleeding, and spotting. May increase BP, elevate LDL levels or cause other lipid changes. May cause or exacerbate migraine headaches. Refer to an ophthalmologist if develop visual changes with contact lens or changes in lens tolerance. Increased risk of morbidity and mortality with certain inherited thrombophilias, HTN, hyperlipidemia, obesity, and diabetes. D/C if jaundice, significant depression, or recurrent/persistent new headache patterns develop. Perform periodic history and physical exam. Not for use before menarche. May affect certain endocrine, LFTs, and blood components. Does not protect against HIV infection (AIDS) or other sexually transmitted diseases. Weigh benefit of fewer planned menses against inconvenience of increased intermenstrual bleeding or spotting.

**ADVERSE REACTIONS:** N/V, breakthrough bleeding, gastrointestinal symptoms (such as abdominal cramps, bloating), spotting, amenorrhea, migraine, depression, vaginal candidiasis, edema, weight changes, changes in cervical erosion and secretion.

**INTERACTIONS:** Reduced effects resulting in breakthrough bleeding or unintended pregnancy may occur when co-administered with antibiotics, anticonvulsants and other drugs that increase the metabolism of contraceptive steroids (eg, rifampin, barbiturates, phenylbutazone, phenytoin, carbamazepine, felbamate, oxcarbazepine, griseofulvin, topiramate). Contraceptive failure and breakthrough bleeding may occur with concomitant use of ampicillin or tetracyclines. St. John's Wort may reduce contraceptive effectiveness and may result in breakthrough bleeding. Atorvastatin, ascorbic acid, acetaminophen (APAP), CYP3A4 inhibitors (eg, itraconazole, ketoconazole) may increase hormone levels. HIV protease inhibitors may increase or decrease levels. May increase levels of cyclosporine, prednisolone, theophylline. May decrease levels of acetaminophen. Increases clearance of temazepam, salicylic acid, morphine, clofibric acid. May significantly decrease plasma levels of lamotrigine; dosage adjustment of lamotrigine may be necessary.



**PREGNANCY:** Category X, not for use in nursing.

**MECHANISM OF ACTION:** Estrogen/progestogen combination oral contraceptive; acts by suppression of gonadotropins. Primarily inhibits ovulation. Also produces other alterations including changes in the cervical mucus (increases difficulty of sperm entry into uterus) and endometrium (reduces likelihood of implantation).

**PHARMACOKINETICS: Absorption:** Levonorgestrel: Rapid and complete. Absolute bioavailability (100%), $C_{max}$=5.6ng/mL, $T_{max}$=1.4 hrs, AUC=60.8ng•hr/mL. Ethinyl estradiol: Rapid. Absolute bioavailability (43%), $C_{max}$=145pg/mL, $T_{max}$=1.6 hrs, AUC=1307pg•hr/mL. **Distribution:** Found in breast milk. Levonorgestrel: $V_d$=1.8L/kg, plasma protein binding (97.5-99%). Ethinyl estradiol: $V_d$=4.3L/kg, plasma protein binding (95-97%). **Metabolism:** Levonogestrel: Sulfate and glucuronide conjugates. Ethinyl estradiol: First-pass metabolism, hepatic via CYP3A4 (hydroxylation), methylation, conjugation. **Elimination:** Levonogestrel: Urine (45%), feces (32%); $T_{1/2}$=30 hrs. Ethinyl estradiol: Urine, feces; $T_{1/2}$=15 hrs.

## NURSING CONSIDERATIONS

**Assessment:** Assess for presence or history of thrombophlebitis or thromboembolic disorders, presence or history of cerebrovascular disease, presence or history of CAD, valvular heart disease with thrombogenic complications, uncontrolled HTN, diabetes with vascular involvement, headache with focal neurological symptoms, major surgery with prolonged immobilization, history of or known/suspected carcinoma of breast, carcinoma of the endometrium or other known/suspected estrogen-dependent neoplasia, undiagnosed abnormal genital bleeding, cholestatic jaundice of pregnancy or jaundice with prior pill use, hepatic adenomas or carcinomas, active liver disease, pregnancy/nursing status, and for possible drug interactions. Assess use in patients ≥35 yrs who smoke ≥15 cigarettes/day.

**Monitoring:** Monitor for venous or arterial thrombotic or thromboembolic events (eg, MI, thromboembolism, stroke), hepatic neoplasia, ocular lesions, bleeding irregularities, fluid retention, onset or exacerbation of migraine headaches, gallbladder disease, HTN, and hypertriglyceridemia. Monitor glucose levels in DM and prediabetic patients, lipid levels with history of hyperlipidemia, signs of liver dysfunction (eg, jaundice), and signs of worsening depression with a history. Refer patients with contact lenses to ophthalmologist if visual changes occur. Perform periodic history and physical exam.

**Patient Counseling:** Inform that drug does not protect against HIV infection (AIDS) and other STDs. Counsel about potential adverse effects. Inform about possible serious cardiovascular and pulmonary effects. Advise to avoid smoking while on medication. Counsel to take medication at same time daily. Instruct that if miss 1 pill, take as soon as possible; take next dose at regular time. Advise that stomach upset, spotting, or light bleeding may develop when initiating therapy; continue taking medication. Advise to notify physician if bleeding lasts longer than 7 days. If vomiting, diarrhea, or taking other medications, advise may need backup form of contraception. Inform patient will have 4 menstrual periods per yr while on medication.

**Administration:** Oral route. 1) Take 1 pill at same time every day until last pill in dispenser taken. 2) After taking last white pill, start 1st pink pill from new extended-cycle tab dispenser the next day regardless of when period started. This should be on a Sunday. **Storage:** 20-25°C (68-77°F).

## SEASONIQUE — RX

ethinyl estradiol - levonorgestrel (Teva)

**THERAPEUTIC CLASS:** Estrogen/progestogen combination

**INDICATIONS:** Prevention of pregnancy.

**DOSAGE:** *Adults*: 1 tablet qd for 91 days, then repeat. During first cycle of medication, start on 1st Sunday after onset of menstruation. Begin next and all subsequent 91-day courses without interruption on same day of week (Sunday) upon which first course began, following the same schedule.

**HOW SUPPLIED:** Tab: (Ethinyl Estradiol-Levonorgestrel) 0.03mg-0.15mg; Tab: (Ethinyl Estradiol) 0.01mg

**CONTRAINDICATIONS:** Thrombophlebitis, DVT or thromboembolic disorders, cerebrovascular or coronary artery disease (CAD), valvular heart disease with thrombogenic complications, uncontrolled HTN, diabetes mellitus (DM) with vascular involvement, headaches with focal neurological symptoms, major surgery with prolonged immobilization, breast cancer, endometrial cancer or other estrogen-dependent neoplasia, undiagnosed abnormal genital bleeding, cholestatic jaundice of pregnancy or jaundice with prior pill use, hepatic adenomas or carcinomas, active liver disease, or pregnancy.

**WARNINGS/PRECAUTIONS:** Cigarette smoking increases risk of serious cardiovascular (CV) side effects. This risk increases with age (especially >35 yrs) and heavy smoking. Increased risk of myocardial infarction (MI), vascular disease, thromboembolism, stroke, HTN, and gallbladder disease. Retinal thrombosis, hepatic neoplasia, carcinoma of breast and reproductive organs reported. May cause glucose intolerance, fluid retention, breakthrough bleeding, and spotting. May increase BP, elevate LDL levels or cause other lipid changes. May cause or exacerbate migraine. May develop visual changes with contact lenses. Increased risk of morbidity and mortality with certain inherited thrombophilias, HTN, hyperlipidemia, obesity, and diabetes. D/C if jaundice, significant depression, recurrent/persistent new headache patterns, or ophthalmic irregularities develop. Perform annual physical exam. Not for use before menarche or with uncontrolled HTN. May affect certain endocrine, LFTs, and blood components. Weigh benefit of fewer planned menses against inconvenience of increased intermenstrual bleeding or spotting.

**ADVERSE REACTIONS:** N/V, breakthrough bleeding, spotting, amenorrhea, migraine, depression, vaginal candidiasis, edema, weight changes, thrombophlebitis, MI, hypertension, hepatic adenoma.

**INTERACTIONS:** Reduced effects, increased breakthrough bleeding, and menstrual irregularities with antibiotics, anticonvulsants, rifampin, barbiturates, phenylbutazone, phenytoin, carbamazepine, felbamate, oxcarbazepine, topiramate, hypericum perforatum, griseofulvin, ampicillin, and tetracyclines. Increased levels with atorvastatin, ascorbic acid, APAP, and CYP3A4 (eg, itraconazole, ketoconazole) inhibitors. Anti-HIV protease inhibitors may increase or decrease levels. May increase plasma levels of cyclosporine, prednisolone, and theophylline. May decrease levels of APAP. Increased clearance of temazepam, salicylic acid, morphine, and clofibric acid. Decreased plasma concentrations of lamotrigine; reduces seizure control.

**PREGNANCY:** Category X, not for use in nursing.

**MECHANISM OF ACTION:** Estrogen/progestogen combination oral contraceptive; acts by suppressing gonadotropins. Primarily inhibits ovulation. Also responsible for causing changes in cervical mucus (increases difficulty of sperm entry into uterus) and endometrium (reduces likelihood of implantation).

**PHARMACOKINETICS: Absorption:** Rapid; $T_{max}$=2 hrs; Levonorgestrel: Absolute bioavailability (100%). Ethinyl estradiol: Absolute bioavailability (43%). Oral administration of variable doses resulted in different parameters. **Distribution:** Levonorgestrel: $V_d$=1.8L/kg; plasma protein binding (97.5-99%). Ethinyl estradiol: $V_d$=4.3L/kg; plasma protein binding (95-97%). **Metabolism:** Levonogestrel: Sulfate and glucuronide conjugates. Ethinyl estradiol: 1st pass metabolism in gut wall, Hepatic, via CYP3A4 (hydroxylation), methylation, conjugation. **Elimination:** Levonorgestrel: Urine (45%), feces (32%); $T_{1/2}$=34 hrs. Ethinyl estradiol: Urine, feces; $T_{1/2}$=18 hrs.

## NURSING CONSIDERATIONS

**Assessment:** Assess for current or history of thrombophlebitis or thromboembolic disorders, CAD, cerebrovascular disease, valvular heart disease with thrombogenic complications, uncontrolled HTN, DM with vascular involvement, headache with focal neurological symptoms, major surgery with prolonged immobilization, known/suspected or history of carcinoma of breast, endometrium or other known/suspected estrogen-dependent neoplasia, undiagnosed abnormal genital bleeding, cholestatic jaundice of pregnancy or jaundice with prior pill use, hepatic adenomas or carcinomas or active liver disease, and known or suspected pregnancy. Assess use in patients ≥35yrs who smoke ≥15 cigarettes/day. Assess use in patients with inherited thrombophilias, HTN, hyperlipidemias, obesity, or DM. Assess for possible drug interactions.

**Monitoring:** Monitor for venous or arterial thrombotic and thromboembolic events (eg, MI, thromboembolism, stroke), vascular disease, hepatic neoplasia, ocular lesions, bleeding irregularities, fluid retention, onset or exacerbation of migraines or headaches, gallbladder disease, hypertriglyceridemia, and HTN. Monitor glucose levels in DM or prediabetic patients, lipid levels with history of hyperlipidemia, for signs/symptoms of liver dysfunction (eg, jaundice), and for signs of worsening depression with previous history. Perform annual physical exam. Refer patients who wear contact lenses to an ophthalmologist if visual changes develop.

**Patient Counseling:** Inform that drug does not protect against HIV infection (AIDS) and other STDs. Advise not to smoke while on medication. Inform about possible side effects of medication (eg, blood clots, HTN, liver tumors). Instruct patients will only have 4 menstrual cycles per yr while on medication. Instruct to take medication at same time daily and if dose is missed, take as soon as possible, then take next dose at regularly scheduled time. Inform may have nausea, spotting, or light bleeding when starting therapy; continue taking medication and notify physician if bleeding persists more than 7 days. If vomiting, diarrhea, or taking concomitant medications use backup form of contraception.

**Administration:** Oral route. **Storage:** 20-25°C (68-77°F).

## SECTRAL RX

acebutolol HCl (Reddy Pharm)

**THERAPEUTIC CLASS:** Selective beta$_1$-blocker

**INDICATIONS:** Management of hypertension alone or in combination with other antihypertensive agents (eg, thiazide diuretics). Management of ventricular premature beats.

**DOSAGE:** *Adults:* HTN: Mild-Moderate: Initial: 400mg/day, given qd-bid. Usual: 200-800mg/day. Severe: 1200mg/day, given bid. Ventricular Arrhythmia: Initial: 200mg bid. Maint: Increase gradually to 600-1200mg/day. CrCl <50mL/min: Decrease daily dose by 50%. CrCl <25mL/min: Decrease daily dose by 75%. Elderly: Start at low end of dosing range. Max: 800mg/day.

**HOW SUPPLIED:** Cap: 200mg, 400mg

**CONTRAINDICATIONS:** Persistently severe bradycardia, 2nd- and 3rd-degree heart block, overt cardiac failure, cardiogenic shock.

**WARNINGS/PRECAUTIONS:** Withdrawal before surgery is controversial. Caution with bronchospastic disease, peripheral vascular disease, hepatic or renal dysfunction. May mask hypoglycemia or hyperthyroidism symptoms. Avoid in overt cardiac failure. Exacerbation of ischemic heart disease (eg, angina pectoris, myocardial infarction [MI]) reported; avoid abrupt withdrawal. Risk of anaphylactic reaction may occur in patients with previous history of severe anaphylaxis to a variety of allergens. May develop antinuclear antibodies (ANA).

**ADVERSE REACTIONS:** Fatigue, dizziness, headache, constipation, diarrhea, dyspepsia, flatulence, nausea, dyspnea, micturition, insomnia.

**INTERACTIONS:** Possible additive effects with catecholamine-depleting drugs (eg, reserpine); monitor closely for hypotension and bradycardia. NSAIDs may reduce antihypertensive effects. Exaggerated hypertensive responses with alpha adrenergic stimulants. May antagonize epinephrine. May potentiate insulin-induced hypoglycemia. Digitalis glycosides increase risk of bradycardia. Use lowest possible dose with aneshetic agents that depress the myocardium (eg, ether, cyclopropane, trichlorethylene).

**PREGNANCY:** Category B, not for use in nursing.

**MECHANISM OF ACTION:** Cardioselective β-adrenoreceptor blocking agent; reduction in resting heart rate and decrease in exercise-induced tachycardia, reduction in cardiac output at rest and after exercise, reduction of systolic and diastolic BP at rest and post exercise, and inhibition of isoproterenol-induced tachycardia.

**PHARMACOKINETICS: Absorption:** Well-absorbed; absolute bioavailability (40%); $T_{max}$=2.5 hrs. **Distribution:** Plasma protein binding (26%); crosses placental barrier; secreted in breast milk. **Metabolism:** Diacetolol (major metabolite). **Elimination:** Renal (30-40%), nonrenal (50-60%). $T_{1/2}$=3-4 hrs (acebutolol), 8-13 hrs (diacetolol).

### NURSING CONSIDERATIONS

**Assessment:** Assess for bradycardia, cardiogenic shock, 2nd- and 3rd-degree heart block, overt cardiac failure, impaired hepatic/renal function, bronchospastic disease, PVD, DM, thyrotoxicosis, valvular heart disease, nursing status, and possible drug interactions.

S

**Monitoring:** Monitor for cardiac failure, HTN, renal dysfunction, exacerbation of ischemia following abrupt withdrawal, bronchospastic disease, PVD, ANA, anaphylactoid reactions, hypersensitivity reactions.

**Patient Counseling:** Instruct not to interrupt or d/c therapy without consulting physician. Advise to consult physician if signs/symptoms of impending CHF or unexplained respiratory symptoms develop. Inform about hypertensive reactions from concomitant use of α-adrenergic stimulants, such as nasal decongestants used in OTC cold preparations.

**Administration:** Oral route. **Storage:** 20-25°C (68-77°F). Protect from light.

## SELZENTRY RX

maraviroc (Pfizer)

**Hepatotoxicity reported; may be preceded by evidence of systemic allergic reaction. Evaluate patients immediately if exhibiting signs or symptoms of hepatitis or allergic reaction (eg, pruritic rash, eosinophilia, elevated IgE).**

**THERAPEUTIC CLASS:** CCR5 co-receptor antagonist

**INDICATIONS:** Combination antiretroviral treatment of adults infected with only CCR5-tropic HIV-1.

**DOSAGE:** *Adults:* Give in combination with other antiretrovirals as follows: With Potent CYP3A Inhibitors including protease inhibitors (except tipranavir/ritonavir), delavirdine, ketoconazole, itraconazole, clarithromycin: 150mg bid. With tipranavir/ritonavir, nevirapine, raltegravir, all NRTIs and enfuvirtide: 300mg bid. With potent CYP3A Inducers including efavirenz, rifampin, etravirine, carbamazepine, phenobarbital, and phenytoin: 600mg bid.

**HOW SUPPLIED:** Tab: 150mg, 300mg

**WARNINGS/PRECAUTIONS:** D/C if signs or symptoms of hepatitis or increased liver transaminases occur along with rash or other systemic symptoms. Caution with pre-existing liver dysfunction or coinfection with viral hepatitis B (HBV) or C (HCV). Caution in patients with increased risk for cardiovascular (CV) events especially with history of postural hypotension. Immune reconstitution syndrome reported. May increase risk of developing infections; monitor closely for evidence of infections. Caution with renal and hepatic impairment. Caution in elderly. May affect immune surveillance and may lead to increased risk of malignancy. Not for use with dual/mixed or CXCR4-tropic HIV-1.

**ADVERSE REACTIONS:** Cough, pyrexia, upper respiratory tract infections, rash, musculoskeletal disorder, dizziness, sleep disturbances, appetite disorders, herpes infection, sinusitis, bronchitis, constipation, pain/discomfort, paresthesias/dysesthesias.



**INTERACTIONS:** Decreased concentration with St. John's wort; concomitant use not recommended. Concomitant use with CYP3A inhibitor in patients with CrCl <50mL/min may increase levels and risk of dizziness and postural hypotension. Additive/synergistic effect with enfuvirtide. Dose adjustment may be required when coadministered with CYP3A inhibitors/inducers and Pgp inhibitors/inducers. Caution with concomitant medication known to lower BP.

**PREGNANCY:** Category B, not for use in nursing.

**MECHANISM OF ACTION:** CCR5 co-receptor antagonist; selectively binds to human chemokine receptor CCR5 present on cell membranes, preventing interaction of HIV-1 gp120 and CCR5 necessary for CCR5-tropic HIV-1 to enter cells.

**PHARMACOKINETICS: Absorption:** (1-1200mg) $T_{max}$=0.5 hr (100mg, 300mg) Absolute bioavailability (23%, 33%). **Distribution:** $V_d$=194L; plasma protein binding (76%). **Metabolism:** CYP3A; secondary amine (N-dealkylation metabolite). **Elimination:** Urine: 20% (8% unchanged), feces: 76% (25% unchanged); $T_{1/2}$=14 hrs.

## NURSING CONSIDERATIONS

**Assessment:** Assess for known liver dysfunction or coinfection with HBV or HCV, history of postural hypotension, risk of CV events, renal/hepatic impairment, pregnancy/nursing status and possible drug interactions. May conduct tropism testing to identify appropriate patients. Assess LFTs and renal function.

**Monitoring:** Monitor for signs/symptoms of hepatotoxicity, allergic reactions, immune reconstitution syndrome, CV events, infections, development of malignancy and renal/hepatic impairment.

**Patient Counseling:** Inform that therapy is not a cure for HIV, does not reduce risk of transmission of HIV and that opportunistic infections may develop. Caution with history of postural hypotension or concomitant medication that lowers BP; avoid driving/operating machinery if dizziness occurs. Seek medical attention if signs/symptoms of infections, CV events, hepatitis (yellow eyes/skin, dark urine, vomiting, abdominal pain) or allergic reactions (rash) occur. Instruct to take as prescribed; do not change dose or dosing schedule without consulting a physician. Notify physician if taking prescription, nonprescription, or herbal medications. When dose missed, instruct to take the next dose as soon as possible and take next scheduled dose at regular time. If <6 hrs before next scheduled dose, do not take missed dose and wait and take the next dose at regular time. Enroll patients in the Antiretroviral Pregnancy Registry if they become pregnant while on treatment.

**Administration:** Oral route. **Storage:** 25°C (77°F); excursions permitted 15-30°C (59-86°F). Shelf life is 24 months.

## SENSIPAR — RX

cinacalcet HCl (Amgen)

**THERAPEUTIC CLASS:** Calcimimetic agent

**INDICATIONS:** Treatment of secondary hyperparathyroidism in patients with chronic kidney disease (CKD) on dialysis. Treatment of hypercalcemia in patients with parathyroid carcinoma.

**DOSAGE:** *Adults:* Individualize dosing. Secondary Hyperparathyroidism with CKD: Initial: 30mg qd. Titrate: Increase no more frequently than every 2-4 weeks through sequential doses of 60, 90, 120, and 180mg qd to target iPTH of 150-300pg/mL. Serum Ca and serum phosphorus should be measured within 1 week and PTH should be measured 1-4 weeks after initiation or dose adjustment. Hypercalcemia with Parathyroid Carcinoma: Initial: 30mg bid. Titrate: Increase every 2-4 weeks through sequential doses of 30mg bid, 60mg bid, 90mg bid, and 90mg tid-qid prn to normalize serum Ca levels. Adjust based on serum Ca levels (see PI). May be used alone or in combination with vitamin D sterols and/or phosphate binders. Should be taken whole, with food or shortly after meal.

**HOW SUPPLIED:** Tab: 30mg, 60mg, 90mg

**WARNINGS/PRECAUTIONS:** Seizures reported; monitor serum Ca particularly in patients with history of seizure disorder. Hypotension, worsening heart failure, and/or arrhythmia reported in patients with impaired cardiac function. Monitor closely for hypocalcemia; manifestations may include paresthesia, myalgias, cramping, tetany, and convulsions. Do not initiate with serum Ca <8.4mg/dL. If serum Ca <8.4mg/dL but remains >7.5mg/dL, or if symptoms of hypocalcemia occur, calcium-containing phosphate binders and/or vitamin D sterols can be used to raise serum Ca. If serum Ca <7.5 mg/dL, or if symptoms of hypocalcemia persist and dose of vitamin D cannot be increased d/c therapy. After maintenance dose established, measure serum Ca monthly. In patients with CKD, on dialysis, measure serum Ca and phosphorus levels and intact parathyroid hormone levels (iPTH) before initiation and during therapy. Avoid use in patients with CKD not on dialysis. In patients with parathyroid carcinoma, measure serum Ca levels during therapy. Adynamic bone disease may develop with iPTH levels <100pg/mL; reduce dose or d/c therapy if iPTH levels decrease below recommended target range (150-300pg/mL). Monitor patients with moderate and severe hepatic impairment during treatment.

S

**ADVERSE REACTIONS:** N/V, diarrhea, myalgia, dizziness, HTN, asthenia, anorexia, chest pain (non-cardiac), access infection.

**INTERACTIONS:** Drugs metabolized by CYP2D6 (eg, metoprolol, carvedilol, flecainide, vinblastine, thioridazine, most TCAs) may require dose adjustment. Increased desipramine, amitriptyline, nortriptyline exposure in CYP2D6 extensive metabolizers. Increased exposure with strong CYP3A4 inhibitors (eg, ketoconazole, erythromycin, itraconazole); may require dose adjustments. PTH and serum Ca concentrations should be closely monitored if initiating or discontinuing therapy with a strong CYP3A4 inhibitor.

**PREGNANCY:** Category C, not for use in nursing.

**MECHANISM OF ACTION:** Calcimimetic agent; lowers PTH levels by increasing the sensitivity of the calcium-sensing receptor to extracellular calcium.

**PHARMACOKINETICS: Absorption:** $T_{max}$=2-6 hrs. **Distribution:** $V_d$=1000L; plasma protein binding (93-97%). **Metabolism:** Rapid and extensively metabolized. Liver via CYP450 enzymes 3A4, 2D6, and 1A2. Oxidation, conjugation, and glucuronidation. **Elimination**: Urine (80%), feces (15%); $T_{1/2}$=30-40 hrs.

## NURSING CONSIDERATIONS

**Assessment:** Assess for a history of seizure disorder, hepatic impairment, cardiac function impairment, pregnancy/nursing status, and possible drug interactions. Assess serum Ca levels prior to administration.

**Monitoring:** Monitor for seizures, signs/symptoms of hypocalcemia, and adynamic bone disease. Monitor hepatic function if patient has a history of hepatic insufficiency. In patients with impaired cardiac function, monitor for hypotension, worsening HF, and/or arrhythmias. For patients with CKD on dialysis, monitor serum Ca and phosphorus levels within 1 week after initiation of therapy or dose adjustment and iPTH levels within 1-4 weeks after initiation of therapy or dose adjustment. After maintenance dose reached, serum Ca and phosphorus levels should be measured monthly and PTH levels should be measured every 1-3 months. For patients with parathyroid carcinoma, measure serum Ca levels within 1 week after drug initiation or dose adjustment; measure serum Ca levels every 2 months after maintenance dose levels have been established. All patients on therapy require periodic monitoring of serum Ca levels. Monitor PTH/Ca levels with moderate and severe hepatic impairment.

**Patient Counseling:** Instruct to report any adverse reactions such as paresthesias, myalgias, cramping, tetany, and convulsions. Inform patients about the need for monitoring serum Ca, phosphorus, and PTH levels during treatment.

**Administration:** Oral route. Swallow whole; do not divide. **Storage:** 25°C (77°F); excursions permitted to 15-30°C (59-86°F).

S

# SEPTRA RX

sulfamethoxazole - trimethoprim (King)

**OTHER BRAND NAMES:** Septra DS (King) - Sulfatrim Pediatric (Alpharma)

**THERAPEUTIC CLASS:** Sulfonamide/tetrahydrofolic acid inhibitor

**INDICATIONS:** Treatment of urinary tract infections (UTI), acute otitis media, acute exacerbations of chronic bronchitis (AECB), *Pneumocystis carinii* pneumonia (PCP), traveler's diarrhea, and shigellosis caused by susceptible strains of microorganisms.

**DOSAGE:** *Adults:* UTI/Shigellosis: 800mg-160mg PO q12h for 10-14 days (UTI) or 5 days (shigellosis). AECB: 800mg-160mg PO q12h for 14 days. Traveler's Diarrhea: 800mg-160mg PO q12h for 5 days. PCP Treatment: 15-20mg/kg TMP and 75-100mg/kg SMX per 24 hrs given PO q6h for 14-21 days. PCP Prophylaxis: 800mg-160mg PO qd. Renal Impairment: CrCl 15-30mL/min: 50% usual dose. CrCl <15mL/min: Not recommended.
*Pediatrics:* ≥2 months: UTI/Otitis Media/Shigellosis: 4mg/kg TMP and 20mg/kg SMX q12h for 10 days (UTI/otitis media) or 5 days (shigellosis). PCP Treatment: 15-20mg/kg TMP and 75-100mg/kg SMX per 24 hrs given q6h

for 14-21 days. PCP Prophylaxis: 150mg/m²/day TMP and 750mg/m²/day SMX PO given bid, on 3 consecutive days per week. Max: 320mg TMP and 1600mg SMX per day. Renal Impairment: CrCl 15-30mL/min: 50% usual dose. CrCl <15mL/min: Not recommended.

**HOW SUPPLIED:** (Sulfamethoxazole [SMX]-Trimethoprim [TMP]) Sus: (Sulfatrim Pediatric, Septra) 200mg-40mg/5mL [100mL, 473mL]; Tab: (Septra) 400mg-80mg*; Tab, DS: (Septra DS) 800mg-160mg* *scored

**CONTRAINDICATIONS:** Megaloblastic anemia due to folate deficiency, pregnancy at term, nursing, infants <2 months old.

**WARNINGS/PRECAUTIONS:** Fatal hypersensitivity reactions (eg, Stevens-Johnson syndrome [SJS], toxic epidermal necrolysis [TEN], fulminant hepatic necrosis, agranulocytosis, aplastic anemia) may occur. Cough, SOB, and pulmonary infiltrates reported. Avoid with group A β-hemolytic streptococcal infections. *Clostridium difficile*-associated diarrhea reported. Caution with hepatic/renal impairment, elderly, folate deficiency (eg, chronic alcoholics, anticonvulsants, malabsorption, malnutrition), bronchial asthma, and other allergies. In G6PD deficiency, hemolysis may occur. Increased incidence of adverse events in AIDS patients. Maintain adequate fluid intake.

**ADVERSE REACTIONS:** Anorexia, N/V, rash, urticaria, cough, SOB, cholestatic jaundice, agranulocytosis, anemia, hyperkalemia, renal failure, interstitial nephritis, hyponatremia, convulsions.

**INTERACTIONS:** Increased risk of thrombocytopenia with purpura with diuretics (especially thiazides) in the elderly. Caution with warfarin; may prolong PT. Increased effects of phenytoin, methotrexate. Concomitant ACE inhibitor therapy may cause hyperkalemia.

**PREGNANCY:** Category C, not for use in nursing.

**MECHANISM OF ACTION:** Sulfamethoxazole: Inhibits bacterial synthesis of dihydrofolic acid by competing with para-aminobenzoic acid (PABA). Trimethoprim: Blocks production of tetrahydrofolic acid from dihydrofolic acid by binding to and reversibly inhibiting required enzyme, dihydrofolate reductase; thus drug blocks 2 consecutive steps in biosynthesis of nucleic acids and proteins essential to many bacteria.

**PHARMACOKINETICS: Absorption:** Rapid; $T_{max}$=1-4 hrs. **Distribution:** Trimethoprim: Plasma protein binding (44%); Sulfamethoxazole: Plasma protein binding (70%). Crosses placenta, found in breast milk. **Metabolism:** Sulfamethoxazole: $N_4$ acetylation. Trimethoprim: 1-and 3-oxide, 3'-and 4'-hydroxy derivative (principal metabolites). **Elimination:** Urine, trimethoprim (66.8%), sulfamethoxazole (84.5%; 30% as free and remaining as $N_4$ acetylated metabolite); $T_{1/2}$=10 hr (sulfamethoxazole), 8-10 hr (trimethoprim).

## NURSING CONSIDERATIONS

**Assessment:** Assess for previous drug hypersensitivity, megaloblastic anemia, renal/hepatic impairment, folate deficiency (eg, elderly, chronic alcoholics, patients on anticonvulsants, malabsorption syndrome, malnutrition states), glucose-6-phosphate-dehydrogenase-deficient individuals, severe allergy or bronchial asthma, pregnancy/nursing status, and possible drug interactions.

**Monitoring:** Monitor for severe reactions (eg, SJS, TEN, fulminant hepatic necrosis, agranulocytosis), *C.difficile*-associated diarrhea (may range from mild diarrhea to fatal colitis), development of drug resistance, superinfection, signs of bone marrow depression or specific decrease in platelets with or without pupura, hyperkalemia, hyponatremia, kernicterus, and clinical signs (eg, skin rash, sore throat, fever, arthralgia, pallor, jaundice) that may be early indications of serious reactions. Frequent monitoring of CBC; d/c if significant reduction is noted, perform urinalysis with careful microscopic exam and renal function tests (particularly for renal impairment).

**Patient Counseling:** Inform that drug only treats bacterial, not viral, infections. Take exactly as directed; skipping doses or not completing full course may decrease effectiveness and increase resistance. Instruct to maintain adequate fluid intake to prevent crystalluria and stone formation. Inform about potential benefits/risks of therapy. D/C and notify physician if skin rash, watery/bloody diarrhea (with/without muscle cramps), or fever occurs (may occur up to 2 months after therapy). Notify if pregnant/nursing.

**Administration:** Oral route. **Storage:** 15-25°C (59-77°F); protect from light.

## SEREVENT RX

salmeterol xinafoate (GlaxoSmithKline)

**Long-acting $\beta_2$-adrenergic agonists, such as salmeterol, may increase the risk of asthma-related deaths.**

**THERAPEUTIC CLASS:** Beta$_2$-agonist

**INDICATIONS:** Long-term maintenance treatment of asthma and COPD. Prevention of bronchospasm with reversible obstructive airway disease (including nocturnal asthma) when regular treatment with inhaled short-acting $\beta_2$-agonists is required. Prevention of exercise-induced bronchospasm (EIB).

**DOSAGE:** *Adults:* Asthma/COPD: 1 inh bid, am and pm (12 hrs apart). EIB Prevention: 1 inh 30 min before exercise (do not give preventive doses if already on bid dose).
*Pediatrics:* ≥4 yrs: Asthma: 1 inh bid, am and pm (12 hrs apart). EIB Prevention: 1 inh 30 min before exercise (do not give preventive doses if already on bid dose).

**HOW SUPPLIED:** Disk: 50mcg [28, 60 blisters]

**WARNINGS/PRECAUTIONS:** Avoid with significantly worsening or acutely deteriorating asthma. Not for acute treatment or substitute for oral/inhaled corticosteroids. Monitor for increasing use of inhaled $\beta_2$-agonists. QTc interval prolongation reported when recommended dose exceeded. D/C if paradoxical bronchospasm occurs. Immediate hypersensitivity and upper airway symptom reactions reported. Caution with cardiovascular disorder (eg, coronary insufficiency, arrhythmia, HTN), convulsive disorders, thyrotoxicosis, if usually unresponsive to sympathomimetic amines. May cause hypokalemia.

**ADVERSE REACTIONS:** Nasal/sinus congestion, pallor, rhinitis, headache, tracheitis/bronchitis, influenza, throat irritation.

**INTERACTIONS:** Caution with non-potassium-sparing diuretics. Extreme caution within 14 days of using MAOIs or TCAs. Avoid with β-blockers. Caution with >8 inhalations of short-acting $\beta_2$-agonists.

**PREGNANCY:** Category C, not for use in nursing.

**MECHANISM OF ACTION:** $\beta_2$-adrenergic agonist; increases cAMP levels causing relaxation of bronchial smooth muscles and inhibits the release of mediators of immediate hypersensitivity from mast cells.

**PHARMACOKINETICS: Absorption:** $C_{max}$=167pg/mL; $T_{max}$=20 min. **Distribution:** Plasma protein binding (96%). **Metabolism:** Liver (aliphatic oxidation) via CYP3A4. (Metabolite) α-hydroxysalmeterol. **Elimination:** $T_{1/2}$=5.5 hrs.

S

### NURSING CONSIDERATIONS

**Assessment:** Assess for CVD (coronary insufficiency, cardiac arrhythmia, HTN), convulsive disorder, thyrotoxicosis, DM, and possible drug interactions. Obtain baseline lung function before therapy.

**Monitoring:** Monitor lung function periodically. Monitor for upper airway symptoms (laryngeal spasm, irritation, swelling), worsening or acutely deteriorating asthma (increased use of inhaled $\beta_2$-agonist, decreased lung function), asthma instability (serial objective measures of airflow), paradoxical bronchospasm, and hypersensitivity reactions.

**Patient Counseling:** Inform drug may increase risk of asthma-related death. Do not use with a spacer device. Do not stop therapy unless directed by health provider. Never exhale into Diskus, never take Diskus apart. Activate and use in a level, horizontal position. Never wash mouthpiece or any part; keep dry. Inform not to use for sudden symptoms of SOB or acute bronchospasm. Advise to rinse mouth after inhalation. Seek medical attention if symptoms worsen or do not improve, severe asthmatic attack, paradoxical bronchospasm, or hypersensitivity reaction occur.

**Administration:** Oral inhaled route. 1) Hold with one hand and put thumb of other hand on thumb grip. Push thumb away from self until mouthpiece appears and snaps into position 2) Hold in level, flat position with mouthpiece toward self. Slide lever away from self until it clicks 3) Exhale fully, then put mouthpiece in lips and breath in quickly and deeply. Hold breath for 10 seconds or as long as comfortable. Breath out slowly. **Storage:** 20-25°C (68-77°F). Keep in dry place, away from heat or sunlight.

## SEROQUEL — RX

quetiapine fumarate (AstraZeneca)

**Elderly patients with dementia-related psychosis treated with atypical antipsychotic drugs are at an increased risk of death; most deaths appeared to be cardiovascular (eg, heart failure, sudden death) or infectious (eg, pneumonia) in nature. Quetiapine is not approved for the treatment of patients with dementia-related psychosis. Antidepressants increased the risk of suicidal thinking and behavior (suicidality) in short-term studies in children, adolescents, and young adults with major depressive disorder (MDD) and other psychiatric disorders. Increased risk of suicide with depression and certain psychiatric disorders. Monitor and observe for clinical worsening, suicidality, or unusual changes in behavior in patients who are started on antidepressant therapy. Quetiapine is not approved for use in pediatric patients <10 yrs.**

**THERAPEUTIC CLASS:** Dibenzapine derivative

**INDICATIONS:** Treatment of schizophrenia in adults and adolescents (13-17 yrs). Acute treatment of manic episodes associated with bipolar I disorder, both as monotherapy and as an adjunct therapy to lithium or divalproex in adults and pediatrics (10-17 yrs). Monotherapy for acute treatment of depressive episodes associated with bipolar disorder in adults. Maintenance treatment of bipolar I disorder as adjunct therapy to lithium or divalproex.

**DOSAGE:** *Adults:* Schizophrenia: Initial: 25mg bid. Titrate: Increase by 25-50mg bid-tid on the 2nd and 3rd day as tolerated to 300-400mg/day given bid-tid by the 4th day. Adjust doses by 25-50mg bid at intervals of at least 2 days if further adjustment is needed. Max: 800mg/day. Maint: Responding patients should continue beyond acute response at lowest dose to maintain remission. Periodically reassess to determine the need for maintenance treatment. Bipolar I Disorder: Manic Episodes: Monotherapy/Adjunct: Give bid. Day 1: 100mg/day, increase to 400mg/day on Day 4 in increments of up to 100mg/day and further adjust to 800mg/day by Day 6 in increments ≤200mg/day. Max: 800mg/day. Depressive Episodes: Give qd at hs. Day 1: 50mg/day. Day 2: 100mg/day. Day 3: 200mg/day. Day 4: 300mg/day. Maint (Bipolar I Disorder): 400-800mg/day given bid as adjunct therapy to lithium or divalproex. Hepatic Impairment: Initial: 25mg/day. Titrate: May increase by 25-50mg/day to an effective dose, depending on response and tolerability. Elderly/Debilitated/Predisposition to Hypotension: Consider slower rate of dose titration and lower target dose. Reinitiation of Treatment: If off >1 week: Follow initial titration schedule. If <1 week: No titration required, reinitiate the maintenance dose. Switching from Depot Antipsychotics: Initiate therapy in place of the next scheduled injection.
*Pediatrics:* Schizophrenia: 13-17 yrs: Administer bid or tid based on response and tolerability. Day 1: 50mg/day. Day 2: 100mg/day. Day 3: 200mg/day. Day 4: 300mg/day. Day 5: 400mg/day. Adjust dose based on response and tolerability within recommended range of 400-800mg/day with increments of ≤100mg/day. Max: 800mg/day. Bipolar I Disorder: Manic Episodes: 10-17 yrs: Administer bid or tid based on response and tolerability. Day 1: 50mg/day. Day 2: 100mg/day. Day 3: 200mg/day. Day 4: 300mg/day. Day 5: 400mg/day. After Day 5, adjust dose based on response and tolerability within recommended range of 400-600mg/day with increments of ≤100mg/day. Max: 600mg/day. Maint: Responding patients should continue beyond acute response at lowest dose to maintain remission. Periodically reassess to determine the need for maintenance treatment.

**HOW SUPPLIED:** Tab: 25mg, 50mg, 100mg, 200mg, 300mg, 400mg

**WARNINGS/PRECAUTIONS:** Hyperglycemia, in some cases extreme and associated with ketoacidosis or hyperosmolar coma or death, has been reported; monitor diabetes mellitus (DM) patients regularly for worsening of

S

glucose control and all patients for symptoms of hyperglycemia. Undesirable alterations in lipids and weight gain reported. Neuroleptic malignant syndrome (NMS) and priapism reported. Tardive dyskinesia (TD) may develop. May induce orthostatic hypotension; caution with cardiovascular (CV) or cerebrovascular disease or conditions that predispose to hypotension (eg, dehydration, hypovolemia). Leukopenia, neutropenia, and agranulocytosis reported; use caution with pre-existing low WBC count or history of drug-induced leukopenia/neutropenia and d/c if absolute neutrophil count (ANC) <1000/mm$^3$. Lenticular changes reported; lenticular examination at initiation and at 6-month intervals recommended. Decrease in total and free thyroxine ($T_4$) may occur. Asymptomatic, transient, and reversible elevations in serum transaminase, primarily ALT, have been reported. May impair mental/physical abilities. May disrupt body's ability to reduce core body temperature. May increase BP and prolactin levels. Close supervision of high-risk patients should accompany drug therapy due to possibility of suicide attempt. Acute withdrawal symptoms (eg, N/V, insomnia) may occur after abrupt cessation; gradual withdrawal is advised. Seizures reported; caution with history of seizures or with conditions that potentially lower the seizure threshold (eg, Alzheimer's dementia). Caution in patients at risk for aspiration, elderly and debilitated.

**ADVERSE REACTIONS:** Headache, somnolence, dizziness, dry mouth, constipation, dyspepsia, tachycardia, asthenia, agitation, pain, weight gain, ALT increased, abdominal pain, back pain, vomiting.

**INTERACTIONS:** Caution with other centrally acting drugs. Avoid with alcohol; may increase cognitive and motor effects. May antagonize effects of levodopa and dopamine agonists. May enhance hypotensive effects of antihypertensives. Increased clearance with thioridazine, phenytoin, and other hepatic enzyme inducers (eg, carbamazepine, barbiturates, rifampin, glucocorticoids). Increased concentration with divalproex. Caution with CYP3A inhibitors (eg, itraconazole, ketoconazole, fluconazole, protease inhibitors, erythromycin). Decreased clearance with cimetidine. Decreases clearance of lorazepam.

**PREGNANCY:** Category C, not for use in nursing.

**MECHANISM OF ACTION:** Dibenzothiazepine derivative; not established. Mediated through a combination of dopamine type 2 ($D_2$) and serotonin type 2 ($5HT_2$) antagonism.

**PHARMACOKINETICS: Absorption:** Rapid, $T_{max}$=1.5 hrs. **Distribution:** $V_d$=10L/kg; plasma protein binding (83%). **Metabolism:** Liver (extensive) via sulfoxidation and oxidation; CYP3A4. **Elimination:** Urine (73%), feces (20%); $T_{1/2}$=6 hrs.

## NURSING CONSIDERATIONS

**Assessment:** Assess for history of dementia-related psychosis, MDD, bipolar mania, DM, pre-existing low WBCs or drug-induced leukopenia/neutropenia, liver impairment, CV or cerebrovascular disease, conditions that predispose to hypotension, history of seizure or conditions that may lower seizure threshold (eg, Alzheimer's dementia), risk of aspiration pneumonia, high-risk patients (eg, suicidal), pregnancy/nursing status and possible drug interactions. Perform baseline BP, FPG, cholesterol, TG, WBC count, ophthalmologic examination and weight determination.



**Monitoring:** Monitor for signs/symptoms of TD, clinical manifestation of NMS, EPS, suicide attempts, orthostatic hypotension, body temperature, ECG changes, worsening depression, behavioral changes, agitation, irritability, priapism, esophageal dysmotility, and aspiration. Monitor BP especially in children and adolescents, weight, FPG, cholesterol, TG, CBC, liver enzymes (ALT), BUN, thyroid function (total and free $T_4$) and prolactin. Monitor for lenticular changes at 6-month intervals during chronic treatment. Monitor for acute withdrawal symptoms (eg, N/V, insomnia) with abrupt withdrawal.

**Patient Counseling:** Discuss risks and benefits of therapy. Advise of risk of orthostatic hypotension and DM. Counsel to avoid activities requiring mental alertness (eg, operating machinery/driving). Instruct to notify physician if taking other drugs, pregnant or intend to become pregnant, or if signs of NMS, overheating or dehydration occur. Instruct to avoid breastfeeding or alcohol intake. Advise to monitor for clinical worsening or suicide attempts;

notify physician if these occur. Advise the need for comprehensive treatment program.

**Administration:** Oral route. **Storage:** 25°C (77°F); excursions permitted to 15-30°C (59-86°F).

## SEROQUEL XR RX

quetiapine fumarate (AstraZeneca)

**Elderly patients with dementia-related psychosis treated with atypical antipsychotic drugs are at an increased risk of death; most deaths appeared to be cardiovascular (eg, heart failure, sudden death) or infectious (eg, pneumonia) in nature. Quetiapine is not approved for the treatment of patients with dementia-related psychosis. Antidepressants increased the risk of suicidal thinking and behavior (suicidality) in short-term studies in children, adolescents, and young adults with major depressive disorder (MDD) and other psychiatric disorders. Increased risk of suicide with depression and certain psychiatric disorders. Monitor and observe for clinical worsening, suicidality, or unusual changes in behavior in patients who are started on antidepressant therapy. Quetiapine is not approved for use in pediatric patients.**

**THERAPEUTIC CLASS:** Dibenzapine derivative

**INDICATIONS:** Treatment of schizophrenia. Acute treatment of manic or mixed episodes associated with bipolar I disorder, both as monotherapy and as an adjunct to lithium or divalproex. Acute treatment of depressive episodes associated with bipolar disorder. Maintenance treatment of bipolar I disorder as adjunct therapy to lithium or divalproex. Adjunctive therapy to antidepressants for treatment of major depressive disorder (MDD).

**DOSAGE:** *Adults:* Schizophrenia: Give qd in pm. Initial: 300mg/day. Titrate: Within range of 400-800mg/day depending on response and tolerance. Dose increases may be made at intervals as short as 1 day and in increments up to 300mg/day. Maint: 400-800mg/day for 16 weeks. Max: 800mg/day. Periodically reassess the need for maintenance treatment and the appropriate dose. Bipolar Disorder: Bipolar Mania: Monotherapy/Adjunct: Give qd in pm. Day 1: 300mg/day. Day 2: 600mg/day. Titrate: May adjust dose between 400-800mg beginning on Day 3 depending on response and tolerance. Depressive Episodes: Give qd in pm. Day 1: 50mg/day. Day 2: 100mg/day. Day 3: 200mg/day. Day 4: 300mg/day. Maint (Bipolar I Disorder): 400-800mg/day as adjunct therapy to lithium or divalproex. Periodically reassess the need for maintenance treatment and the appropriate dose. MDD, Adjunctive Therapy with Antidepressants: Initial: 50mg qd in pm. Increase dose to 150mg qd in pm on Day 3. Range: 150-300mg/day. Max: 300mg/day. Elderly/Hepatic Impairment: Initial: 50mg/day. Titrate: May increase in increments of 50mg/day depending on response and tolerance. Elderly/Debilitated/Predisposition to Hypotension: Consider slower rate of dose titration and lower target dose. Reinitiation of Treatment: If off >1 week: Follow initial dosing schedule. If <1 week: No dose escalation required, reinitiate the maintenance dose. Switching from Seroquel: May switch at equivalent total daily dose given qd. Switching from Depot Antipsychotics: Initiate in place of next scheduled injection. Swallow tab whole; do not split, crush, or chew. Take without food or with a light meal.

**HOW SUPPLIED:** Tab, Extended-Release: 50mg, 150mg, 200mg, 300mg, 400mg

**WARNINGS/PRECAUTIONS:** Hyperglycemia, in some cases extreme and associated with ketoacidosis or hyperosmolar coma or death, has been reported; monitor diabetes mellitus (DM) patients regularly for worsening of glucose control and all patients for symptoms of hyperglycemia. Undesirable alterations in lipids and weight gain reported. Neuroleptic malignant syndrome (NMS) and priapism reported. Tardive dyskinesia (TD) may develop. May induce orthostatic hypotension; caution with cardiovascular (CV) or cerebrovascular disease or conditions that predispose to hypotension (eg, dehydration, hypovolemia). Leukopenia, neutropenia, and agranulocytosis reported; caution with pre-existing low WBC count or history of drug-induced leukopenia/neutropenia and d/c if absolute neutrophil count (ANC) <1000/mm³. Lenticular changes reported; lenticular examination prior and

S

at 6-month intervals recommended. Decrease in total and free thyroxine ($T_4$) may occur. Asymptomatic, transient, and reversible elevations in serum transaminase, primarily ALT, have been reported. May impair mental/physical abilities. May disrupt body's ability to reduce core body temperature. May increase BP and prolactin levels. Close supervision of high-risk patients should accompany drug therapy due to possibility of suicide attempt. Acute withdrawal symptoms (eg, N/V, insomnia) may occur after abrupt cessation; gradual withdrawal is advised. Seizures reported; caution with history of seizures or with conditions that potentially lower the seizure threshold (eg, Alzheimer's dementia). Caution in patients at risk for aspiration, elderly and debilitated.

**ADVERSE REACTIONS:** Dry mouth, constipation, dyspepsia, somnolence, dizziness, orthostatic hypotension, weight gain, fatigue, dysarthria, nasal congestion, extrapyramidal symptoms, increased appetite, back pain, abnormal dreams, irritability.

**INTERACTIONS:** Caution with other centrally acting drugs. Avoid with alcohol; may increase cognitive and motor effects. May antagonize effects of levodopa and dopamine agonists. May enhance hypotensive effects of antihypertensives. Increased clearance with thioridazine, phenytoin, and other hepatic enzyme inducers (eg, carbamazepine, barbiturates, rifampin, glucocorticoids). Increased concentration with divalproex. Caution with CYP3A inhibitors (eg, itraconazole, ketoconazole, fluconazole, protease inhibitors, erythromycin). Decreased clearance with cimetidine. Decreases clearance of lorazepam.

**PREGNANCY:** Category C, caution in nursing.

**MECHANISM OF ACTION:** Dibenzothiazepine derivative; not established. Mediated through a combination of dopamine type 2 ($D_2$) and serotonin type 2A ($5HT_2A$) antagonism.

**PHARMACOKINETICS: Absorption:** $T_{max}$=6 hrs. **Distribution:** $V_d$=10L/kg; plasma protein bound (83%); found in breast milk. **Metabolism:** Liver (extensive) via sulfoxidation and oxidation; CYP3A4. **Elimination:** Urine (73%), feces (20%); $T_{1/2}$=7 hrs.

## NURSING CONSIDERATIONS

**Assessment:** Assess for history of dementia-related psychosis, MDD, bipolar mania, DM, pre-existing low WBCs or drug-induced leukopenia/neutropenia, liver impairment, CV or cerebrovascular disease, conditions that predispose to hypotension, history of seizure or conditions that may lower seizure threshold (eg, Alzheimer's dementia), risk of aspiration pneumonia, high-risk patients (eg, suicidal), pregnancy/nursing status and possible drug interactions. Perform baseline BP, FPG, cholesterol, TG, WBC count, ophthalmologic examination and weight determination.

**Monitoring:** Monitor for signs/symptoms of TD, clinical manifestation of NMS, EPS, suicide attempts, orthostatic hypotension, body temperature, ECG changes, worsening depression, behavioral changes, agitation, irritability, priapism, esophageal dysmotility, and aspiration. Monitor BP especially in children and adolescents, weight, FPG, cholesterol, TG, CBC, liver enzymes (ALT), BUN, thyroid function (total and free $T_4$) and prolactin. Monitor for lenticular changes at 6-month intervals during chronic treatment. Monitor for acute withdrawal symptoms (eg, N/V, insomnia) with abrupt withdrawal.

**Patient Counseling:** Discuss risks and benefits of therapy. Advise of risk of orthostatic hypotension and DM. Counsel to avoid activities requiring mental alertness (eg, operating machinery/driving). Instruct to notify physician if taking other drugs, pregnant or intend to become pregnant, or if signs of NMS, overheating or dehydration occur. Instruct to avoid breastfeeding or alcohol intake. Advise to monitor for clinical worsening or suicide attempts; notify physician if these occur.

**Administration:** Oral route. **Storage:** Store at 25°C (77°F); excursions permitted to 15-30°C (59-86°F).

## SEROSTIM — RX

somatropin (EMD Serono)

**THERAPEUTIC CLASS:** Human growth hormone

**INDICATIONS:** Treatment of AIDS wasting or cachexia.

**DOSAGE:** *Adults:* >55kg: 6mg SQ qhs. 45-55kg: 5mg SQ qhs. 35-44kg: 4mg SQ qhs. <35kg: 0.1mg/kg SQ qhs. Dose Reductions Due to Side Effects: Reduce total daily dose or number of doses/week. Rotate injection sites. Re-evaluate for infection if weight loss continues after 2 weeks of therapy.

**HOW SUPPLIED:** Inj: 4mg, 5mg, 6mg, 8.8mg

**CONTRAINDICATIONS:** Acute critical illness due to complications after open heart or abdominal surgery, accidental trauma, acute respiratory failure.

**WARNINGS/PRECAUTIONS:** Monitor malnutrition, malabsorption and hypogonadism; may contribute to catabolism. Maintain nucleoside analogue therapy throughout treatment. Carpal tunnel syndrome reported. Perform periodic funduscopic exams.

**ADVERSE REACTIONS:** Musculoskeletal discomfort, increased tissue turgor, edema, arthralgia, extremity pain, hypoesthesia, myalgia, hyperglycemia, arthrosis, diarrhea, headache, paresthesia, insomnia, upper respiratory tract infection.

**PREGNANCY:** Category B, caution in nursing.

**MECHANISM OF ACTION:** Human growth hormone; anabolic and anticatabolic agent exerting influence by interacting with specific receptors on variety of cell types.

**PHARMACOKINETICS: Absorption:** Absolute bioavailabilty (70-90%). **Distribution:** $V_d$=12.0L. **Metabolism:** Kidneys (major), liver (minor). **Elimination:** $T_{1/2}$=4.28 hrs.

### NURSING CONSIDERATIONS

**Assessment:** Assess for acute critical illness due to complications of surgery, multiple accidental trauma, acute respiratory failure, active malignancy, inadequate nutritional intake, malabsorption, hypogonadism, risk factors for glucose tolerance, preexisting DM, and possible drug interactions. Perform baseline fundoscopic exam.

**Monitoring:** Periodically perform fundoscopic exam. Monitor for signs/symptoms of carpal tunnel syndrome, increased tissue turgor, musculoskeletal discomfort, hypersensitivity/allergic reactions, and acute pancreatitis.

**Patient Counseling:** Instruct on proper disposal and how to rotate injection site. Seek medical attention if symptoms of carpal tunnel syndrome, swelling, musculoskeletal discomfort (pain, swelling, stiffness), hypersensitivity reactions, or pancreatitis occur.

**Administration:** SQ route. **Storage:** Before reconstitution: 15-30°C (59-86°F). After reconstitution: 2-8°C (36-46°F); stable for 14 days. Avoid freezing.

S

## SILVADENE — RX

silver sulfadiazine (Monarch Pharmaceuticals Inc.)

**OTHER BRAND NAMES:** SSD (Par)

**THERAPEUTIC CLASS:** Sulfonamide

**INDICATIONS:** Adjunct for prevention and treatment of wound sepsis in patients with 2nd- and 3rd-degree burns.

**DOSAGE:** *Adults:* Apply under sterile conditions qd-bid to thickness of approximately 1/16 inch. Re-apply if removed by patient activity. Continue until wound is healed.

**HOW SUPPLIED:** Cre: 1% [20g, 50g, 85g, 400g, 1000g]

**CONTRAINDICATIONS:** Late pregnancy, premature infants, newborns during first 2 months of life.

**WARNINGS/PRECAUTIONS:** Potential cross-sensitivity with other sulfonamides. Hemolysis may occur in G6PD deficient patients. Drug accumulation with hepatic and renal dysfunction. Monitor renal function and serum sulfa levels with extensive burns. Fungal proliferation, including superinfection, has been reported.

**ADVERSE REACTIONS:** Transient leukopenia, skin necrosis, erythema multiforme, skin discoloration, burning sensation, rash, interstitial nephritis, systemic sulfonamide reactions.

**INTERACTIONS:** May inactivate topical proteolytic enzymes. Leukopenia increased with cimetidine.

**PREGNANCY:** Category B, not for use in nursing.

**MECHANISM OF ACTION:** Topical antimicrobial of sulfonamide class; acts on cell membrane and cell wall of many gram-negative and gram-positive bacteria and yeast to produce bactericidal effect.

## NURSING CONSIDERATIONS

**Assessment:** Assess pregnancy status, patient is not premature infant or a newborn infant ≤2 months old, renal/hepatic dysfunction, glucose-6-phosphate dehydrogenase deficiency, and for possible drug interactions.

**Monitoring:** Monitor fungal proliferation, renal/hepatic function, urine to identify sulfa crystals, serum sulfa concentrations with wounds involving extensive body surface areas, and signs/symptoms of sulfonamide reaction (eg, agranulocytosis, aplastic anemia, thrombocytopenia, leukopenia, Stevens-Johnson syndrome, exfoliative dermatitis, hepatitis and hepatocellular necrosis, CNS reactions, and toxic nephrosis).

**Patient Counseling:** Instruct to clean wound with soap and water and dry thoroughly prior to application. Instruct patient to reapplyer to any areas from which the cream has been removed by patient's activity. Inform patients that dressings can be used if needed. Instruct patient to continue therapy until satisfactory healing has occurred, burn site is ready for graft, or serious adverse events occur.

**Administration:** Topical. **Storage:** At room temperature.

## SIMCOR — RX

simvastatin - niacin (Abbott)

**THERAPEUTIC CLASS:** HMG-CoA reductase inhibitor/Nicotinic acid

**INDICATIONS:** To reduce elevated total cholesterol, LDL, Apo B, non-HDL cholesterol, TG, or to increase HDL with primary hypercholesterolemia, mixed dyslipidemia (Types IIa and IIb). To reduce elevated TG with hypertriglyceridemia (Fredrickson type IV hyperlipidemia) when treatment with monotherapy components is inadequate.

S

**DOSAGE:** *Adults:* Patients not currently on niacin extended-release or switching from immediate-release niacin: Initial: 500mg/20mg qd hs, with a low-fat snack. Titrate: Adjust dose at ≥4 wks. Extended-release niacin should not be increased by more than 500mg daily every 4 wks. After Week 8, titrate to response and tolerance. Maint: 1000mg/20mg to 2000mg/40mg qd. Max: 2000mg/40mg qd. Do not break, crush, or chew before swallowing.

**HOW SUPPLIED:** Tab, Extended-Release: (Niacin-Simvastatin) 500mg-20mg, 750mg-20mg, 1000mg-20mg

**CONTRAINDICATIONS:** Active liver disease (unexplained persistent elevations of serum transaminases), active peptic ulcer disease, arterial bleeding, pregnancy, or nursing mothers.

**WARNINGS/PRECAUTIONS:** Do not substitute for equivalent dose of immediate-release niacin. Myopathy and rhabdomyolysis reported; monitor serum creatine kinase (CK) periodically. D/C therapy if myopathy is suspected or diagnosed, if transaminase levels increase ≥3 ULN persist, or prior to major surgery or when any major medical or surgical condition supervenes. Increased risk with higher doses, advanced age ( ≥65 yrs), hypothyroidism, renal impairment. Caution with heavy alcohol use, or history of liver disease; monitor LFTs prior to therapy, every 12 weeks for the first 6 months and periodically thereafter. Severe hepatic toxicity may occur in patients substituting sustained-release niacin for immediate-release niacin at equivalent doses. May increase serum glucose levels in diabetic or potentially diabetic patients, particularly in the first few months of therapy; adjust diet and/or hypoglycemic therapy or d/c if necessary. May reduce platelet count. Caution with those predisposed to gout.

**ADVERSE REACTIONS:** Flushing, headache, back pain, diarrhea, nausea, pruritus.

**INTERACTIONS:** Avoid use with concomitant CYP3A4 inhibitors including itraconazole, ketoconazole, and other antifungal azoles, erythromycin, clarithromycin, telithromycin, HIV protease inhibitors, nefazodone, grapefruit juice (>1 quart/day), cyclosporine, danazol, gemifibrozil, and fibrates; increased risk of myopathy/rhabdomyolysis. Max 20mg/day with amiodarone or verapamil. Concurrent use with propanolol decreases simvastatin levels. Potentiates effects of coumarin anticoagulants; monitor PT/INR. May increase digoxin levels; monitor appropriately. Concomitant use with aspirin decreases niacin levels. Colestipol and cholestyramine may increase niacin-binding capacity. Potentiates adverse effects with nutritional supplements containing large doses of niacin or related compounds. Concomitant use potentiates effects of ganglionic blocking agents and vasoactive drugs.

**PREGNANCY:** Category X, not for use in nursing.

**MECHANISM OF ACTION:** Niacin: Nicotinic acid; not well established. May partially inhibit release of free fatty acids from adipose tissue, and increases lipoprotein lipase activity, which increases rate of chylomicron triglyceride removal from plasma. Decreases rate of hepatic synthesis of VLDL and LDL. Simvastatin: HMG-CoA reductase inhibitor; lipid-lowering agent. Inhibits conversion of HMG-CoA to mevalonate. Also reduces VLDL, TG, and increases HDL.

**PHARMACOKINETICS: Absorption:** Niacin: $T_{max}$=4.6-4.9 hrs. Simvastatin: $T_{max}$=1.9-2.0 hrs. Simvastatin acid (active metabolite): $C_{max}$ =3.29ng/mL, $T_{max}$= 6.56 hrs, AUC =30.81 ng•hr/mL. **Metabolism:** Niacin: Rapid and extensive first-pass metabolism; conjugation. Simvastatin: Hydrolysis; β-hydroxyacid, 6'-hydroxy, 6'hydroxymethyl, 6'-exomethylene derivatives (active metabolites). **Elimination:** Niacin: Urine (54%). Simvastatin: Feces (60%), urine (13%), $T_{1/2}$ =4.2-4.9 hrs.

## NURSING CONSIDERATIONS

**Assessment:** Prior to initiation, assess for active liver disease or unexplained elevations in serum transaminases, renal dysfunction, active peptic ulcer disease, arterial bleeding, and pregnancy/nursing status. Obtain baseline lipid profile (total cholesterol, HDL, LDL, TG) and LFTs. Assess use in patients who consume substantial quantities of alcohol and/or have a past history of liver disease. Check for possible drug interactions.

**Monitoring:** Monitor for signs/symptoms of myopathy (eg, muscle pain, tenderness, weakness), rhabdomyolysis, decrease in platelet counts, increase in prothrombin time, and decrease in phosphorus levels. Perform periodic monitoring of lipid profile, CK, and blood glucose levels. Monitor LFTs every 12 weeks for the first 6 months and periodically every 6 months thereafter.

**Patient Counseling:** Counsel to take at bedtime after a low-fat snack. Inform that flushing may occur but should subside after several weeks of therapy; taking an NSAID 30 min prior may minimize. Instruct to avoid ingestion of alcohol or hot drinks with administration to prevent flushing. Advise not to break, crush, or chew, and to swallow whole. Instruct to contact physician if discontinuing drug for extended period of time, taking vitamins, other nutritional supplements, or if dizziness occurs. Notify diabetics that change in blood glucose may occur.

**Administration:** Oral route. Avoid on an empty stomach. **Storage:** 20-25°C (68-77°F).

S

# SIMPONI

golimumab (Centocor)

RX

**Increased risk for developing serious infections (eg, tuberculosis [TB], TB reactivation, invasive fungal infection, bacterial/viral infection due to opportunistic pathogens) that may lead to hospitalization or death. Most patients who developed these infections were taking concomitant immunosuppressants such as methotrexate (MTX) or corticosteroids. Evaluate for latent TB and treat prior to initiation of therapy. Empiric antifungal therapy should be considered in patients at risk for invasive fungal infection who develop severe systemic illness. Monitor for development of infection during and after treatment. D/C if serious infection or sepsis develops. Lymphoma and other malignancies reported in children and adolescents.**

**THERAPEUTIC CLASS:** Monoclonal antibody/TNF-alpha receptor blocker

**INDICATIONS:** Treatment of moderate to severe active rheumatoid arthritis (RA) in combination with methotrexate (MTX). Treatment of active psoriatic arthritis (PsA) alone or in combination with MTX. Treatment of active ankylosing spondylitis (AS).

**DOSAGE:** *Adults:* RA: 50mg SQ once a month in combination with MTX. PsA/AS: 50mg SQ once a month with or without MTX or other nonbiologic DMARDs. May continue corticosteroids, nonbiologic DMARDs and/or NSAIDs during treatment.

**HOW SUPPLIED:** Inj: 50mg/0.5mL

**WARNINGS/PRECAUTIONS:** Avoid with active infections, including localized infections. Caution in patients with chronic/recurrent infections, who have been exposed to TB, reside or traveled in areas of endemic TB or mycoses (eg, histoplasmosis, coccidiodomycosis, blastomycosis) or with underlying conditions that may predispose them to infection. Monitor for signs and symptoms of infection during and after therapy; d/c if serious infection, opportunistic infection, or sepsis develops. Monitor hepatitis B virus (HBV) carriers; if reactivation occurs, d/c and start antiviral therapy. Worsening congestive heart failure (CHF) and/or new onset CHF reported; monitor closely and d/c if new symptoms appear. Caution with pre-existing or recent-onset CNS demyelinating disorders such as multiple sclerosis (MS). Pancytopenia, leukopenia, neutropenia, aplastic anemia and thrombocytopenia reported; caution with significant cytopenias. Elevation of liver enzymes, formation of autoantibodies and new onset or exacerbation of psoriasis reported. Caution in elderly.

**ADVERSE REACTIONS:** Serious infections, upper respiratory tract infection, nasopharyngitis, elevated ALT/AST, injection-site erythema, HTN, development of antibodies.

**INTERACTIONS:** See Black Box Warning. Avoid with abatacept, anakinra and live vaccines. May cause neutropenia and increased rate of infection with anakinra. New onset/exacerbation of pre-existing psoriasis reported with concomitant immunosuppressants (eg, MTX, corticosteroids); d/c for severe cases. Caution with CYP450 substrates with a narrow therapeutic index; monitor effect (eg, warfarin) or drug concentration (eg, cyclosporine, theophylline) upon initiation or d/c of therapy. Dose adjustments may be needed.

**PREGNANCY:** Category B, not for use in nursing.

**MECHANISM OF ACTION:** Monoclonal antibody/TNFα receptor blocker; binds to both soluble and transmembrane bioactive forms of human TNFα preventing binding of TNFα to its receptors, thereby inhibiting the biological activity of TNFα.

**PHARMACOKINETICS: Absorption:** $C_{max}$=2.5µg/mL; $T_{max}$=2-6 days; absolute bioavailability (approximately 53%). **Distribution:** (IV) $V_d$=58-126mL/kg. **Elimination:** $T_{1/2}$=2 weeks (median).

## NURSING CONSIDERATIONS

**Assessment:** Assess for active/chronic/recurrent infection (eg, TB, HBV), TB exposure, recent travel in areas of endemic TB or mycoses, malignancy, heart failure, pre-existing or recent onset of demyelinating disorder (eg, MS), psoriasis, significant cytopenia, pregnancy/nursing status, and possible drug interactions. Perform test for latent TB and treat if necessary.

S

**Monitoring:** Monitor for signs/symptoms of infections (including sepsis), HBV reactivation, lymphoma, new or worsening CHF, hematological events (eg, aplastic anemia), formation of autoantibodies, lupus-like syndrome and severe psoriasis. Monitor effect or drug levels of concomitant CYP450 substrates with narrow therapeutic window.

**Patient Counseling:** Advise of potential risks and benefits of the drug. Instruct to read Medication Guide before initiation of therapy and each time the prescription is renewed. Inform that may lower ability of the immune system to fight infections. Instruct to contact doctor if they develop any symptoms of infection, including TB, invasive fungal infections, and hepatitis B reactivation. Counsel about the risk of lymphoma and other malignancies. Advise latex-sensitive patients that the needle cover contains dry natural rubber, a derivative of latex. Advise to report signs of new or worsening medical conditions such as CHF, demyelinating disorders, autoimmune disease, liver disease, cytopenias, or psoriasis.

**Administration:** SQ route. See PI for proper injection instructions. Rotate injection sites; avoid areas where skin is tender, bruised, red or hard. Do not use if discolored, cloudy or if with foreign particles present. **Storage:** Refrigerate at 2-8°C (36-46°F). Do not freeze. Do not shake. Protect from light.

## SIMULECT — RX

basiliximab (Novartis)

**Manage patient in facility with adequate lab and supportive resources. Prescribing physician should be experienced with immunosuppressives and transplantation. Physician should have complete information requisite for patient follow-up.**

**THERAPEUTIC CLASS:** Monoclonal antibody/IL-2R alpha (CD25) blocker

**INDICATIONS:** Prophylaxis of acute organ rejection in renal transplantation.

**DOSAGE:** *Adults:* 20mg within 2 hrs prior to transplant, repeat 4 days after transplant. Withhold 2nd dose if graft loss or complications occur.
*Pediatrics:* ≥35kg: 20mg within 2 hrs prior to transplant, repeat 4 days after transplant. <35kg: 10mg within 2 hrs prior to transplant, repeat 4 days after transplant. Withhold 2nd dose if graft loss or complications occur.

**HOW SUPPLIED:** Inj: 10mg, 20mg

**WARNINGS/PRECAUTIONS:** Only administer under qualified medical supervision. Increased risk of developing lymphoproliferative disorder and opportunistic infections. Anaphylaxis and other severe hypersensitivity reactions (eg, hypotension, cardiac failure, bronchospasm, respiratory failure, etc) reported and may necessitate discontinuation. Anti-idiotype antibodies may develop.

**ADVERSE REACTIONS:** GI effects, peripheral edema, fever, viral infection, hyperkalemia, hypokalemia, hyperglycemia, hypercholesterolemia, hypophosphatemia, hyperuricemia, UTI, dyspnea, upper respiratory infection, acne, HTN, headache, tremor, insomnia, anemia.

**PREGNANCY:** Category B, not for use in nursing.

**MECHANISM OF ACTION:** Monoclonal antibody/IL-2Rα (CD25) blocker; acts as an IL-2 receptor antagonist by binding to the IL-2 receptor complex and inhibiting IL-2 binding. Specifically targeted against IL-2Rα, which is selectively expressed on the surface of activated T-lymphocytes. Binding to IL-2Rα causes competitive inhibition of IL-2-mediated activation of lymphocytes, a critical pathway in the cellular immune response involved in allograft rejection.

**PHARMACOKINETICS: Absorption:** $C_{max}$=7.1ng/mL (adult). **Distribution:** $V_d$=8.6L (adult); 4.8L (1-11 yrs); 7.8L (12-16 yrs). **Elimination:** $T_{1/2}$=7.2 days (adult); 9.5 days (1-11 yrs); 9.1 days (12-16 yrs).

### NURSING CONSIDERATIONS

**Assessment:** Assess use in patients who were on previous therapy with this drug, and in pregnant/nursing females. Assess for possible drug interactions.

S

**Monitoring:** Monitor for signs/symptoms of lymphoproliferative disorders, opportunistic infections, and hypersensitivity reactions (eg, hypotension, tachycardia, cardiac failure, dyspnea, pulmonary edema, respiratory failure, urticaria, and rash).

**Patient Counseling:** Counsel about risks/benefits. Inform to contact physician immediately if signs/symptoms of hypersensitivity reaction (eg, dyspnea, uticaria, rash) occur. Instruct females of child-bearing potential to use effective form of contraceptive before starting therapy, during therapy, and for 4 months following d/c. Advise may experience NV during administration.

**Administration:** Central or peripheral IV administration. Reconstituted drug should be given as a bolus injection or diluted to a volume of 25mL (10mg vial) or 50mL (20mg vial) (normal saline or dextrose 5%). Administer as IV infusion over 20-30 min. **Storage**: Lyophilized Simulect: Under refrigerated condition, 2-8°C (36-46°F). Reconstituted: Use immediately. If not used immediately, store at 2-8°C (36-46°F) for 24 hrs or at room temperature for 4 hrs. Discard reconstituted solution if not used within 24 hrs.

## SINEMET CR — RX

levodopa - carbidopa (Bristol-Myers Squibb)

**OTHER BRAND NAMES:** Sinemet (Bristol-Myers Squibb)

**THERAPEUTIC CLASS:** Dopa-decarboxylase inhibitor/dopamine precursor

**INDICATIONS:** Treatment of symptoms of idiopathic Parkinson's disease, postencephalitic parkinsonism, and symptomatic parkinsonism.

**DOSAGE:** *Adults:* ≥18 yrs: Initial: (25mg-100mg tab) 1 tab tid. Titrate: Increase by 1 tab qd or every other day until 8 tabs/day. 10mg-100mg tab: Initial: 1 tab tid-qid. Titrate: Increase 1 tab qd or every other day until 2 tabs qid. 70-100mg/day carbidopa required. Max: 200mg/day carbidopa. Conversion from levodopa: <1500mg: (25mg-100mg) 1 tab tid or qid. >1500mg: (25mg-250mg) 1 tab tid or qid. (Tab, Extended-Release) No Prior Levodopa Use: Initial: 1 tab 50mg-200mg bid at intervals >6 hrs. Titrate: Increase or decrease dose or interval accordingly. Adjust dose every 3 days. Usual: 400-1600mg/day levodopa, given in 4-8 hr intervals while awake. Conversion to Extended-Release Tabs: See PI.

**HOW SUPPLIED:** Tab: (Carbidopa-Levodopa) 10mg-100mg*, 25mg-100mg*, 25mg-250mg*; Tab, Extended-Release: (Carbidopa-Levodopa) 25mg-100mg, 50mg-200mg* *scored

**CONTRAINDICATIONS:** MAOIs during or within 14 days of use, narrow-angle glaucoma, suspicious undiagnosed skin lesions, history of melanoma.

**WARNINGS/PRECAUTIONS:** D/C levodopa 12 hrs before initiating therapy. Dyskinesias and mental disturbances may occur. Caution with severe CV or pulmonary disease, bronchial asthma, renal or hepatic disease, endocrine disease, chronic wide-angle glaucoma, peptic ulcer, and MI with residual arrhythmias. NMS reported during dose reduction or withdrawal. Dark color may appear in saliva, urine, or sweat. May cause false (+) ketonuria or false (-) glucosuria (glucose-oxidase method). Melanoma reported; monitor frequently. Compulsive behaviors (eg, intense urges to gamble, increased sexual urges) reported.

**ADVERSE REACTIONS:** Dyskinesias, nausea, cardiac irregularities, hypotension, dark saliva, GI bleeding, psychotic episodes, NMS, confusion, agitation, dizziness, somnolence, dream abnormalities.

**INTERACTIONS:** See Contraindications. Risk of postural hypotension with antihypertensives, selegiline. HTN and dyskinesia may occur with TCAs. Reduced effects with dopamine $D_2$ antagonists (eg, phenothiazines, butyrophenones, risperidone), isoniazid. Antagonized by phenytoin, papaverine, metoclopramide. Reduced bioavailability with iron salts, high-protein diets.

**PREGNANCY:** Category C, caution in nursing.

**MECHANISM OF ACTION:** Dopa-decarboxylase inhibitor/dopamine precursor. Carbidopa: Inhibits decarboxylation of peripheral levodopa. Levodopa:

Rapidly decarboxylated to dopamine in extracerebral tissue so that only portion of a given dose is transported unchanged to the CNS.

**PHARMACOKINETICS: Absorption:** Levodopa: Absolute availability: 70-75%; $C_{max}$=1151ng/mL; $T_{max}$=2 hrs. Carbidopa: Absolute bioavailability (58%). **Elimination:** Levodopa and carbidopa: $T_{1/2}$ = 1.5 hrs.

## NURSING CONSIDERATIONS

**Assessment:** Assess LFTs, renal function, CBC, glaucoma, dyskinesia, psychosis, depression, CV complications, melanomas, and asthma.

**Monitoring:** Monitor LFTs, renal function, CBC, BP, biliary obstruction, depression and suicidal ideations, worsening of dyskinesia, rhabdomyolysis, diarrhea, hallucinations, fibrotic complications, hyperpyrexia, melanomas, IOP, hypersensitivity reactions, and compulsive behaviors (eg, pathological gambling, hypersexuality).

**Patient Counseling:** Instruct to take as prescribed. Caution while operating machinery/driving. Discoloration of bodily fluids may occcur. High-protein diet, excessive acidity, and iron salts reduce clinical effectiveness. Wearing-off effect may be seen at end of dosing interval. Report any adverse effects. Swallow tablet; do not chew or crush. Notify physician if new or increased gambling urges, increased sexual urges, or other intense urges occur.

**Administration:** Oral route. **Storage:** (Tab) 25°C (77°F), excursions permitted to 15-30°C (59-86°F). Protect from light. (Tab, extended-release) 30°C (86°F). Store in tightly closed container.

# SINGULAIR — RX

montelukast sodium (Merck)

**THERAPEUTIC CLASS:** Leukotriene receptor antagonist

**INDICATIONS:** Prophylaxis and chronic treatment of asthma ( ≥12 months). Relief of symptoms of seasonal allergic rhinitis ( ≥2 yrs) and perennial allergic rhinitis ( ≥6 months). Prevention of exercise-induced bronchoconstriction (EIB [ ≥15 yrs]).

**DOSAGE:** *Adults:* Asthma: 10mg qpm. Allergic Rhinitis: 10mg qd. EIB: 10mg 2 hrs before exercise. Do not take additional dose within 24 hrs of previous dose.

*Pediatrics:* Asthma: ≥15 yrs: 10mg qpm. 6-14 yrs: 5mg qpm. 6 months-5 yrs: 4mg qpm. Seasonal/Perennial Allergic Rhinitis: ≥15 yrs: 10mg qd. 6-14yrs: 5mg qd. 6 months-5 yrs: 4mg qd. EIB: ≥15 yrs: 10mg 2 hrs before exercise. Do not take additional dose within 24 hrs of previous dose. Granules may be mixed with applesauce, carrots, rice, or ice cream; give within 15 min of opening pkt.

**HOW SUPPLIED:** Granules: 4mg/pkt; Tab, Chewable: 4mg, 5mg; Tab: 10mg

**WARNINGS/PRECAUTIONS:** Not for treatment of acute asthma attacks, including status asthmaticus. Avoid abrupt substitution for inhaled or oral corticosteroids. Continue therapy during acute exacerbations of asthma. Systemic eosinophilic conditions reported (rare). Neuropsychiatric events (eg, agitation, aggressive behavior or hostility, anxiousness, depression, dream abnormalities, hallucinations, insomnia, irritability, restlessness, somnambulism, suicidal thinking and behavior, and tremor) reported.

**ADVERSE REACTIONS:** Headache, pharyngitis, influenza, fever, sinusitis, nausea, diarrhea, dyspepsia, otitis, viral infection, and increased bleeding tendency.

**INTERACTIONS:** Monitor with potent CYP450 inducers (eg, phenobarbital, rifampin). Avoid with known ASA sensitivity, and non-steroidal anti-inflammatory agents (NSAIDs).

**PREGNANCY:** Category B, caution in nursing.

**MECHANISM OF ACTION:** Leukotriene receptor antagonist; binds to cysteinyl leukotriene receptors found on airway smooth muscle cells and macrophages and other pro-inflammatory cells (eg, eosinophils); inhibits physiologic actions of leukotrienes.

**PHARMACOKINETICS: Absorption:** Rapid. (10mg) Bioavailability (64%) $T_{max}$=3-4 hrs. (5mg) $T_{max}$=2-2.5 hrs. Bioavailability (73%, fasted), (63%, fed). Fasted 2-5 yrs: (4mg Chewable) $T_{max}$=2 hrs. (4mg Granules) $T_{max}$=2.3 hrs (fasted), 6.4 hrs (fed). **Distribution:** $V_d$=8-11L; plasma protein binding (99%). **Metabolism:** Liver (extensive); CYP3A4, 2C9. **Elimination:** Biliary (major); $T_{1/2}$=2.7-5.5 hrs.

## NURSING CONSIDERATIONS

**Assessment:** Assess for hepatic dysfunction, history of phenylketonuria, bronchospasm (status asthmaticus), pregnancy/nursing status, and possible drug interactions. Obtain baseline LFTs.

**Monitoring:** Monitor for signs/symptoms of eosinophilia, vasculitic rash, worsening pulmonary symptoms, cardiac complications, neuropathy, neuropsychiatric events, and hypersensitivity reactions (eg, urticaria, angioedema, rash).

**Patient Counseling:** Inform not for treatment of acute asthma attacks and exercise-induced bronchoconstriction; appropriate rescue drug (eg, short acting $\beta_2$-agonist) should be available to prevent worsening. Advise to take daily as prescribed. Take directly or mix granules with applesauce, carrots, rice, or ice cream. Advise that chewable tablets contain phenylalanine with phenylketonuria. Instruct not to decrease dose or d/c other anti-asthma medications unless instructed by physician. Seek medical attention if symptoms of eosinophilia, vasculitic rash, worsening pulmonary symptoms, cardiac complications, neuropathy, neuropsychiatric events, and hypersensitivity reactions occur.

**Administration:** Oral route. **Storage:** 25°C (77°F); excursions permitted to 15-30°C (59-86°F). Protect from light and moisture.

# SKELAXIN RX

metaxalone (King)

**THERAPEUTIC CLASS:** Muscular analgesic (central-acting)

**INDICATIONS:** Adjunct to rest, physical therapy, and other measures for the relief of discomforts associated with acute, painful musculoskeletal conditions.

**DOSAGE:** *Adults:* 800mg tid-qid.
*Pediatrics:* >12 yrs: 800mg tid-qid.

**HOW SUPPLIED:** Tab: 800mg* *scored

**CONTRAINDICATIONS:** Tendency for drug-induced, hemolytic, and other anemias. Significant renal or hepatic impairment.

**WARNINGS/PRECAUTIONS:** Caution with pre-existing liver damage; serial liver function studies should be performed. False-positive Benedict's tests have been noted. May impair mental/physical abilities.

S

**ADVERSE REACTIONS:** N/V, GI upset, drowsiness, dizziness, headache, nervousness, leukopenia, hemolytic anemia, jaundice.

**INTERACTIONS:** Additive effects with food and other CNS depressants (eg, alcohol, benzodiazepines, opiods, tricyclic antidepressants). May increase exposure in the presence of high fat meal.

**PREGNANCY:** Not for use in pregnancy or nursing.

**MECHANISM OF ACTION:** Centrally acting muscular analgesic; not established; activity may be due to general depression of CNS.

**PHARMACOKINETICS: Absorption:** (400mg) $C_{max}$=983ng/mL, $T_{max}$= 3.3 hrs, AUC=7479ng•hr/mL. (800mg) $C_{max}$=1816ng/mL, $T_{max}$=3.0 hrs, AUC=15044ng•hr/mL. **Distribution:** $V_d$=800L; extensive in tissues. **Metabolism:** Liver. **Elimination**: Urine (metabolites); (400mg) $T_{1/2}$=9 hrs. (800mg) $T_{1/2}$=8 hrs.

## NURSING CONSIDERATIONS

**Assessment:** Assess for hemolytic or other anemia, renal/hepatic impairment, pregnancy/nursing status, alcohol intake, and possible drug interactions.

**Monitoring:** Perform frequent monitoring of LFTs. Monitor for signs/symptoms of CNS depression and lab test interactions (eg, false-positive Benedict's test).

**Patient Counseling:** Caution against performing hazardous tasks (operating machinery/driving). Advise to avoid alcohol or other CNS depressants. Instruct to notify if pregnant/nursing or planning to become pregnant.

**Administration:** Oral route; taking with food may enhance CNS depression. **Storage:** 15-30°C (59-86°F).

## SKELID RX

tiludronate disodium (Sanofi-Aventis)

**THERAPEUTIC CLASS:** Bisphosphonate

**INDICATIONS:** Treatment of Paget's disease when serum alkaline phosphatase is ≥2x ULN, or if symptomatic, or if at risk for future complications.

**DOSAGE:** *Adults:* 400mg qd for 3 months. After therapy, wait 3 months to assess response. Take with 6-8 oz of water. Take 2 hrs after food.

**HOW SUPPLIED:** Tab: 200mg

**WARNINGS/PRECAUTIONS:** May cause GI disorders (eg, dysphagia, esophagitis, esophageal or gastric ulcers). Maintain adequate vitamin D and calcium intake. Avoid in severe renal failure. May cause osteonecrosis, primarily in jaw, and musculoskeletal pain.

**ADVERSE REACTIONS:** Pain, headache, dizziness, paresthesia, diarrhea, N/V, dyspepsia, rhinitis, upper respiratory infection.

**INTERACTIONS:** Increased bioavailability with indomethacin; space dosing by 2 hrs. Decreased bioavailability with calcium supplements, ASA, and aluminum- or magnesium-containing antacids; space dosing by 2 hrs.

**PREGNANCY:** Category C, caution in nursing.

**MECHANISM OF ACTION:** Bisphosphonate; acts primarily on bone to inhibit osteoclastic activity, with a probable reduction in the enzymatic and transport processes that lead to resorption of mineralized matrix. Inhibits osteoclasts through inhibiting protein-tyrosine-phosphatase and through inhibition of the osteoclastic proton pump.

**PHARMACOKINETICS: Absorption:** Rapidly absorbed; $C_{max}$=3mg/L; $T_{max}$=2 hrs. **Distribution:** Plasma protein binding (90%). **Elimination:** Urine (60%); $T_{1/2}$=150 hrs.

### NURSING CONSIDERATIONS

**Assessment:** Assess for severe renal impairment (eg, CrCl <30mL/min), risk of osteonecrosis (eg, cancer, anemia, pre-existing dental disease), pregnancy/nursing status, and possible drug interactions.

**Monitoring:** Monitor for signs/symptoms of upper GI disorders (eg, dysphagia, esophagitis, esophageal ulcer, gastric ulcer), osteonecrosis (eg, jaw), and musculoskeletal pain.

**Patient Counseling:** Instruct to take with 6-8 oz of plain water. Do not take within 2 hrs of food. Maintain vitamin D and calcium intake. Do not take calcium supplements, aspirin, and indomethacin 2 hrs before or 2 hrs after medication. If aluminum- or magnesium-containing antacids are needed, take at least 2 hrs after medication. Medication should be taken for a period of 3 months, followed by another 3 months to assess response.

**Administration:** Oral route. **Storage:** 25°C (77°F); excursions permitted to 15-30°C (59-86°F). Do not remove tablets from foil strips until ready to be used.

S

# SOLIRIS RX

eculizumab (Alexion)

**Increases risk of meningococcal infections; may become fatal if not recognized and treated early. Vaccinate 2 weeks prior to receiving first dose; revaccinate according to current guidelines. Monitor for early signs of meningococcal infections, evaluate, and treat if necessary.**

**THERAPEUTIC CLASS:** Monoclonal antibody/Protein C5 blocker

**INDICATIONS:** Treatment of paroxysmal nocturnal hemoglobinuria (PNH) to reduce hemolysis.

**DOSAGE:** *Adults:* Initial: 600mg every 7 days for first 4 weeks, then 900mg as 5th dose 7 days later, then 900mg every 14 days thereafter. Do not administer as an IV push or bolus injection; administer by IV infusion over 35 min.

**HOW SUPPLIED:** Inj: 10mg/mL [30mL]

**CONTRAINDICATIONS:** Patients with unresolved serious *Neisseria meningitidis* infection and patients not vaccinated against it.

**WARNINGS/PRECAUTIONS:** Monitor for early signs and symptoms of meningococcal infections; d/c during treatment of serious meningococcal infections. Increased susceptibility to infection reported; caution in patients with systemic infection. Monitor for signs and symptoms of hemolysis (eg, LDH increase) for at least 8 weeks after discontinuation. Infusion reactions, including anaphylaxis and hypersensitivity, reported. Administration should be interrupted in patients experiencing severe infusion reaction and appropriate therapy administered.

**ADVERSE REACTIONS:** Meningococcal infections, headache, nasopharyngitis, back pain, nausea, fatigue, cough, herpes simplex infections, sinusitis, respiratory tract infection, constipation, myalgia, pain in extremities, influenza-like illness.

**PREGNANCY:** Category C, caution in nursing.

**MECHANISM OF ACTION:** Monoclonal antibody/protein C5 blocker; binds to the complement C5 with high affinity, thereby inhibiting its cleavage to C5a and C5b and preventing the generation of the terminal complement C5b-9. Inhibits terminal complement-mediated intravascular hemolysis in PNH patient.

**PHARMACOKINETICS: Absorption:** $C_{max}$ (week 26)=194mcg/mL; $C_{min}$ (week 26)=97mcg/mL. **Distribution:** $V_d$=7.7L. **Elimination:** $T_{1/2}$=272 hrs.

## NURSING CONSIDERATIONS

**Assessment:** Assess for signs and symptoms of *Neisseria meningitidis* infection and other serious infection; meningococcal vaccination status; pregnancy and nursing status. Obtain baseline serum LDH, Hgb, and SrCr.

S

**Monitoring:** Monitor for signs and symptoms of meningococcal infections; other serious infections; signs and symptoms of hemolysis (eg, LDH increased with any of the following: >25% absolute decrease in PNH clone size in ≤1 week, Hgb <5 gm/dL or decrease of >4 mg/dL in ≤1 week, angina, change in mental status, 50% increase in SrCr level); infusion reactions including anaphylaxis and hypersensitivity reaction.

**Patient Counseling:** Counsel about possible risks and benefits in particular the risk of meningococcocal infection. Inform patients they are required to receive meningococcal vaccination at least 2 weeks prior to receiving the first dose of eculizumab if not previously vaccinated and revaccinated according to current medical guidelines. Inform that vaccination may not prevent meningococcal infection. Educate about the signs and symptoms of meningococcal infection and advise to seek immediate medical attention if these signs or symptoms occur. Inform that there is a potential for serious hemolysis when discontinued and that they will be monitored for at least 8 weeks following discontinuation.

**Administration:** IV route. **Storage:** Refrigerate at 2-8°C (36-46°F) and protect from light. Do not freeze or shake.

# SOLODYN RX

minocycline HCl (Medicis)

**THERAPEUTIC CLASS:** Tetracycline derivative

**INDICATIONS:** Treatment of inflammatory lesions of non-nodular moderate to severe acne vulgaris in patients ≥12 yrs.

**DOSAGE:** *Adults:* 1mg/kg qd for 12 weeks. Reduce dose with renal impairment. Elderly: Start at the low end of the dosing range. Swallow tab whole, do not crush, chew, or split tab.
*Pediatrics:* ≥12 yrs: 1mg/kg qd for 12 weeks. Reduce dose with renal impairment. Swallow tab whole, do not crush, chew, or split tab.

**HOW SUPPLIED:** Tab, Extended-Release: 45mg, 65mg, 90mg, 115mg, 135mg.

**WARNINGS/PRECAUTIONS:** May cause fetal harm during pregnancy. Use during tooth development (last half of pregnancy, infancy, <8yrs) may cause permanent discoloration of the teeth or enamel hypoplasia; avoid use during this period. Reversible decrease in bone growth in premature infants reported. May cause pseudomembranous colitis; if it occurs, d/c therapy and treat appropriately. May cause an increase in BUN, resulting in azotemia, hyperphosphatemia and acidosis; caution in patients with renal impairment. CNS effects (eg, light-headedness, dizziness, vertigo) reported. Pseudotumor cerebri reported; permanent sequelae such as visual loss may occur. May develop drug resistant bacteria; use only as indicated. Use may result in overgrowth of drug-resistant bacteria; d/c if superinfection develops. Long-term use has been associated with development of autoimmune syndromes, including drug-induced lupus-like syndrome, autoimmune hepatitis and vasculitis; d/c if any of these occur. May induce tissue hyperpigmentation. Serious liver injury, anaphylaxis, serious skin reactions (eg, Stevens-Johnson syndrome, erythema multiforme), photosensitivity reported. Caution in elderly. No effect on non-inflammatory acne lesions. Safety beyond 12 weeks of use has not been established.

**ADVERSE REACTIONS:** Headache, fatigue, dizziness, pruritus, malaise, mood alteration.

**INTERACTIONS:** May require downward adjustments of anticoagulant dosage. May interfere with bactericidal action of penicillin; avoid concurrent use when possible. Concomitant use with methoxyflurane may result in fatal renal toxicity. Antacids containing aluminum, calcium or magnesium, and iron-containing preparations may impair absorption. May interfere with the effectiveness of oral contraceptives; female patients should use second form of contraception during treatment. Avoid concurrent use with isotretinoin.

**PREGNANCY:** Category D, not for use in nursing.

**MECHANISM OF ACTION:** Tetracycline derivative; not established.

**PHARMACOKINETICS: Absorption:** $C_{max}$=2.63mcg/mL; $T_{max}$=3.5-4 hrs; $AUC_{0-24}$=33.32mcg•hr/mL. **Distribution:** Crosses the placenta and found in breast milk.

S

## NURSING CONSIDERATIONS

**Assessment:** Assess pregnancy/nursing status, hepatic/renal impairment, hypersensitivity, and for possible drug interactions. Assess for visual disturbances. Obtain baseline BUN, LFTs, ANA and CBC.

**Monitoring:** Monitor for signs/symptoms of pseudomembranous colitis (eg, diarrhea), hepatoxicity, superinfection, development of drug-resistant bacteria, pseudotumor cerebri, photosensitivity, anaphylaxis, serious skin reactions (eg, Stevens-Johnson syndrome), tissue hyperpigmentation, CNS effects, and for autoimmune syndromes (eg, drug-induced lupus-like syndrome, autoimmune hepatitis, vasculitis). Perform periodic laboratory monitoring organ systems including hematopoetic, renal, and hepatic studies. In patients showing symptoms of an autoimmune syndrome, perform appropriate tests (eg, LFTs, ANA, CBC).

**Patient Counseling:** Inform that photosensitivity reactions (eg, exaggerated sunburn reaction) may occur; advise to minimize/avoid exposure to sunlight and to wear loose-fitting clothes when outdoors. Counsel about CNS symptoms (eg, dizziness, light-headedness); caution with driving or operating hazardous machinery. Advise to seek medical help if persistent headache/ blurred vision is experienced. Inform females that drug may render oral contraceptives less effective, and avoid if pregnant or nursing; use a second form of contraception during treatment. Instruct to avoid use if planning to conceive (male and female). Inform that autoimmune syndromes may occur; d/c therapy if symptoms (eg, arthalgia, fever, rash, and malaise) are experienced. Counsel that discoloration of skin, scars, teeth, or gums may arise during therapy. Advise that pseudomembranous colitis may occur; seek medical attention if watery/bloody stools develop. Counsel about possibility of hepatoxicity (eg, loss of appetite, fatigue, jaundice). Instruct to take exactly as directed; skipping doses or not taking as directed may decrease effectiveness of therapy and create bacterial resistance.

**Administration:** Oral route. **Storage:** 25°C (77°F); excursions permitted to 15-30°C(59-86°F). Dispense in tight, light, child-resistant container. Protect from light, moisture, excessive heat. Keep out of reach of children.

## SOLTAMOX RX

tamoxifen citrate (Savient)

**For women with ductal carcinoma in situ (DCIS) and women at high risk for breast cancer. Fatal uterine malignancies (eg, endometrial adenocarcinoma, uterine sarcoma), stroke, and PE reported with use in risk reduction setting. Discuss benefits/risks of events with this patient population. Benefits of tamoxifen outweigh risks in women already diagnosed with breast cancer.**

**THERAPEUTIC CLASS:** Antiestrogen

**INDICATIONS:** Treatment of metastatic breast cancer in women and men. Treatment of node-positive and axillary node-negative breast cancer in women following mastectomy, axillary dissection and breast irradiation. To reduce risk of invasive breast cancer in women with DCIS. Reduction of breast cancer incidence in high risk women. Use for up to 5 yrs.

**DOSAGE:** *Adults:* Breast Cancer Treatment: 20-40mg qd. Divide dosages >20mg into AM and PM doses. Breast Cancer Risk Reduction/DCIS: 20mg qd for 5 yrs.

**HOW SUPPLIED:** Sol: 10mg/5mL

**CONTRAINDICATIONS:** Reduction in breast cancer incidence in high risk women and women with DCIS who require coumarin-type anticoagulant therapy or have a history of DVT, PE.

**WARNINGS/PRECAUTIONS:** Hypercalcemia reported in patients with bone metastases. Increased incidence of uterine malignancies (eg, endometrial cancer, uterine sarcoma) and endometrial changes including hyperplasia and polyps reported. Increased incidence of thromboembolic events (eg, DVT, PE). Malignant and non-malignant effects on the liver and ocular disturbances reported. Leukopenia, anemia, thrombocytopenia, neutropenia, pancytopenia reported. Promptly evaluate abnormal vaginal bleeding if receiving or previously received tamoxifen. Patients receiving or previously received tamoxifen should have annual gynecological exam. Do not become pregnant within 2 months of therapy. May cause fetal harm during pregnancy. Does not cause infertility even with menstrual irregularity.

**ADVERSE REACTIONS:** (Females) Hot flashes, increased bone and tumor pain, vaginal discharge, irregular menses; (Males) loss of libido, impotence.

**INTERACTIONS:** Increases effects of coumarin-type anticoagulant; monitor PT. Increased risk of thromboembolic events with cytotoxic agents. Increased levels with bromocriptine. May decrease letrozole levels. Decreased levels with rifampin and aminoglutethimide. Decreased plasma levels of major metabolite, N-desmethyl tamoxifen with medroxyprogesterone.

**PREGNANCY:** Category D, not for use in nursing.

**MECHANISM OF ACTION:** Nonsteroidal antiestrogen; competes with estrogen for binding sites in target tissues.

**PHARMACOKINETICS: Absorption:** $C_{max}$=40mg/mL; $T_{max}$=5 hrs. N-desmethyl tamoxifen: $C_{max}$=15ng/mL. **Metabolism:** N-desmethyl tamoxifen (major metabolite). **Elimination:** Feces (primary); $T_{1/2}$=5-7 days.

## NURSING CONSIDERATIONS

**Assessment:** Assess for pregnancy status, history of DVT or PE, hepatic impairment, and possible drug interactions. Perform baseline breast and gynecologic exam; obtain baseline mammogram.

**Monitoring:** Monitor CBC with platelets and LFTs periodically; perform breast exams, mammograms, and gynecologic exams routinely. Monitor for signs/symptoms of hypercalcemia, strokes, PE, uterine malignancies, and hypersensitivity reactions.

**Patient Counseling:** Inform of pregnancy risks; advise to use nonhormonal contraception during therapy and for 2 months after d/c. Instruct to seek medical attention for symptoms of menstrual irregularities, abnormal vaginal bleeding, changes in vaginal discharge, pelvic pain or pressure, new breast lumps, leg swelling/tenderness, SOB, changes in vision, or hypersensitivity reactions.

**Administration:** Oral route. **Storage:** Below 25°C (77°F). Protect from light; use within 3 months of opening; do not freeze or refrigerate.

# SOLU-CORTEF RX

hydrocortisone sodium succinate (Pharmacia & Upjohn)

**THERAPEUTIC CLASS:** Corticosteroid

**INDICATIONS:** Steroid-responsive disorders.

**DOSAGE:** *Adults:* Dosage requirements are variable and must be individualized on basis of disease under treatment and response. Initial: 100-500mg IV/IM, depending on condition severity. May repeat dose at 2, 4, or 6 hrs based on clinical response. Acute Exacerbations of Mutliple Sclerosis: 800mg qd for 1 week followed by 320mg qod for 1 month.
*Pediatrics:* Dosage requirements are variable and must be individualized on basis of disease under treatment and response. Initial: 0.56-8mg/kg/day IV/IM in three or four divided doses (20-240mg/m²bsa/day).

**HOW SUPPLIED:** Inj: 100mg, 250mg, 500mg, 1g

**CONTRAINDICATIONS:** Premature infants, idiopathic thrombocytopenic purpura, intrathecal administration.

**WARNINGS/PRECAUTIONS:** Contains benzyl alcohol; potentially toxic when administered locally to neural tissue. Exercise caution; do not exceed recommended doses to minimize dermal or subdermal atrophy. Avoid injection into deltoid muscle. May need to increase dose before, during, and after stressful situations. High doses of systemic corticosteroids should not be used for the treatment of traumatic brain injury. May mask signs of infection or cause new infections. Prolonged use may produce glaucoma, optic nerve damage, secondary ocular infections. May elevate IOP; monitor IOP if steroid therapy >6 weeks. Increases BP, salt/water retention, potassium and calcium excretion. Not for use in cerebral malaria, active ocular herpes simplex, and optic neuritis. More severe/fatal course of infections reported with chickenpox, measles. Enhanced effect with hypothyroidism or cirrhosis. Caution with strongyloides, latent TB, ocular herpes simplex, HTN, CHF, diverticulitis, fresh intestinal anastomoses, ulcerative colitis, osteoporosis, myasthenia gravis, renal insufficiency, peptic ulcer disease. Kaposi's sarcoma reported. Monitor for psychic disturbances. Acute myopathy with high doses. Avoid abrupt withdrawal. Monitor growth and development of children on prolonged therapy. Hypernatremia may occur with high-dose therapy >48-72 hrs.

**ADVERSE REACTIONS:** Allergic or hypersensitivity reactions, bradycardia, HTN, CHF, pulmonary edema, tachycardia, syncope, acne, allergic dermatitis, decreased carbohydrate and glucose tolerance, hirsutism, hypertrichosis, glycosuria, fluid retention, $K^+$ loss, sodium retention, glaucoma, convulsions, weight gain, malaise.

**INTERACTIONS:** Aminoglutethimide may lead to a loss of corticosteriod-induced adrenal suppression. Concomitant use with potassium-depleting agents (eg, amphotericin B, diuretics) may cause hypokalemia. Reduced efficacy and increased clearance with hepatic enzyme inducers (eg, phenobarbital, phenytoin, rifampin). Increased plasma concentrations with hepatic enzyme inhibitors (eg, ketoconazole, erythromycin, troleandomycin). Increases clearance of chronic high dose ASA. Caution with ASA in hypoprothrombinemia. Effects on oral anticoagulants are variable; monitor PT/INR. Increased insulin and oral hypoglycemic requirements in DM. Avoid live vaccines with immunosuppressive doses. Possible decreased vaccine response with killed or inactivated vaccines with immunosuppressive doses. Concomitant use with anticholinesterase agents may produce weakness in patients with myasthenia gravis; withdraw 24 hrs prior to initiating corticosteroid therapy. May decrease serum concentrations of isoniazid. Cholestyramine may increase clearance. Concurrent use with cyclosporine may increase activity of both; convulsions reported.

**PREGNANCY:** Safety in pregnancy and nursing not known.

**MECHANISM OF ACTION:** Anti-inflammatory glucocorticoid; causes profound and varied metabolic effects and modifies the body's immune responses to diverse stimuli.

**PHARMACOKINETICS: Absorption:** (IM) Rapidly absorbed. $T_{max}$=1 hr. **Distribution:** Found in breast milk. **Elimination:** $T_{1/2}$=12 hrs.

## NURSING CONSIDERATIONS

**Assessment:** Assess for systemic fungal infections, other current infections, active TB, vaccination history, hypersensitivity to drug components, unusual stress, IOP, ulcerative colitis, diverticulitis, HTN, recent MI, fresh intestinal anastomoses, peptic ulcer with/without impending perforation, osteoporosis, myasthenia gravis, existing psychotic tendencies, hepatic/renal impairment, and for possible drug interactions.

**Monitoring:** Anaphylactoid reactions (gasping syndrome, kernicterus) in premature infants, growth/development in children, glucocorticosteroid insufficiency, fluid retention, hypokalemic alkalosis, intestinal perforation with/without hemorrhage, appearance of new or exacerbation of current infections, cataracts, osteoporosis, psychic derangements, Kaposi's sarcoma, acute myopathy. Perform frequent tests of LFTs, glucose, Ca, $K^+$, TSH, with BP and ECG.

**Patient Counseling:** Inform that susceptibility to infections may increase. Avoid exposure to chickenpox and measles; report immediately if exposed. Do not d/c abruptly or without medical supervision. Advise for dietary restriction of salt with $K^+$ supplementation.

**Administration:** IM and IV route. **Storage:** 20-25°C (68-77°F). Protect from light.

S

# SOLU-MEDROL RX

methylprednisolone sodium succinate (Pharmacia & Upjohn)

**THERAPEUTIC CLASS:** Glucocorticoid

**INDICATIONS:** Steroid-responsive disorders.

**DOSAGE:** *Adults:* Usual: Initial: 10-40mg IV over several min. May repeat IV/IM dose at intervals based on clinical response. High-Dose Therapy: 30mg/kg IV over at least 30 min, may repeat q4-6h for 48 hrs. High-dose therapy usually not >48-72 hrs. Give antacids prophylactically. Multiple Sclerosis: (4mg methylprednisolone=5mg prednisolone): 200mg/day prednisolone for 1 week, then 80mg qod for 1 month.
*Pediatrics:* Use lower adult doses. Determine dose by severity of condition and response. Dose should not be <0.5mg/kg q24h.

**HOW SUPPLIED:** Inj: 40mg, 125mg

**CONTRAINDICATIONS:** Premature infants (due to benzyl alcohol diluent) and systemic fungal infections.

**WARNINGS/PRECAUTIONS:** May need to increase dose before, during, and after stressful situations. May mask signs of infection or cause new infections. Prolonged use may produce cataracts, glaucoma, secondary ocular infections. Increases BP, salt/water retention, calcium/potassium excretion. More severe/fatal course of infections reported with chickenpox, measles. Caution with latent TB, hypothyroidism, cirrhosis, ocular herpes simplex, HTN, diverticulitis, fresh intestinal anastomoses, ulcerative colitis, osteoporosis, myasthenia gravis, renal insufficiency, peptic ulcer disease. Kaposi's sarcoma reported. Growth and development of children on prolonged therapy should be monitored. Monitor for psychic disturbances. Avoid abrupt withdrawal. Reports of cardiac arrhythmias, circulatory collapse, cardiac arrest following rapid administration of large IV doses. Effectiveness not established for the treatment of sepsis syndrome and septic shock. Bradycardia reported with high doses.

**ADVERSE REACTIONS:** Fluid and electrolyte disturbances, HTN, osteoporosis, muscle weakness, cushingoid state, menstrual irregularities, insomnia, impaired wound healing, DM, ulcerative esophagitis, excessive sweating, increased intracranial pressure, carbohydrate intolerance, glaucoma, cataracts, nausea.

**INTERACTIONS:** Reduced efficacy with hepatic enzyme inducers (eg, phenobarbital, phenytoin, and rifampin). Increases clearance of chronic high dose ASA. Caution with ASA in hypoprothrombinemia. Effects on oral anticoagulants are variable; monitor PT/INR. Increased insulin and oral hypoglycemic requirements in DM. Avoid live vaccines with immunosuppressive doses. Possible decreased vaccine response with killed or inactivated vaccines with immunosuppressive doses. Mutual inhibition of metabolism with cyclosporine; convulsions reported. Decreased clearance with ketoconazole and troleandomycin.

**PREGNANCY:** Safety in pregnancy and nursing not known.

**MECHANISM OF ACTION:** Anti-inflammatory glucocorticoid; causes profound and varied metabolic effects and modifies the body's immune responses to diverse stimuli.

## NURSING CONSIDERATIONS

**Assessment:** Assess for hypersensitivity to drug, unusual stress, infection, active TB, vaccination status, thyroid status, hepatic/renal impairment, HTN, ulcerative colitis, diverticulitis, intestinal anastomoses, hypoprothrombinemia, peptic ulcer with/without impending perforation, osteoporosis, myasthenia gravis, psychotic tendencies, glaucoma, and possible drug interactions.

**Monitoring:** Monitor for anaphylactic reactions. In pediatrics, monitor for gasping syndrome, hypoadrenalism, growth and development. Monitor for adrenocortical insufficiency, infection, intestinal perforation and hemorrhage, cataracts, acute myopathy, psychiatric derangement, Kaposi's sarcoma, creatinine kinase, BP, HR, serum electrolytes, IOP, TSH, LFTs, glucose, and ECG for cardiac arrhythmias and bradycardia.

**Patient Counseling:** Instruct to avoid exposure to chickenpox and measles; report immediately if exposed, or for fever/signs of infection. Advise regarding dietary salt restriction and $K^+$ supplementation.

**Administration:** IM/IV routes. **Storage:** 20-25°C (68-77°F) for unreconstituted product and solution. Use within 48 hrs after mixing.

## Soma — RX

carisoprodol (Meda)

**THERAPEUTIC CLASS:** Skeletal muscle relaxant (central-acting)

**INDICATIONS:** Relief of discomfort associated with acute, painful musculoskeletal conditions.

**DOSAGE:** *Adults:* ≤65 yrs: 250-350mg tid and hs for 2-3 weeks. *Pediatrics:* ≥16 yrs: 250-350mg tid and hs for 2-3 weeks.

**HOW SUPPLIED:** Tab: 250mg, 350mg

**CONTRAINDICATIONS:** History of acute intermittent porphyria.

**WARNINGS/PRECAUTIONS:** Sedative properties may impair physical/mental abilities. Cases of drug abuse, dependence, and withdrawal reported with prolonged use. Withdrawal symptoms reported following abrupt cessation after prolonged use. Seizures reported in postmarketing surveillance. Caution with hepatic or renal dysfunction and in addiction-prone patients.

**ADVERSE REACTIONS:** Drowsiness, dizziness, headache.

**INTERACTIONS:** Additive sedative effects with other CNS depressants (eg, alcohol, benzodiazepines, opioids, TCAs); caution when coadministering. Concomitant use with meprobamate not recommended. Increased exposure of carisoprodol and decreased exposure of meprobamate with CYP2C19 inhibitors (eg, omeprazole, fluvoxamine). Decreased exposure of carisoprodol and increased exposure of meprobamate with CYP2C19 inducers (eg, rifampin, St. John's wort).

**PREGNANCY:** Category C, caution in nursing.

**MECHANISM OF ACTION:** Centrally acting muscle relaxant; does not directly relax skeletal muscles. Action not been clearly identified. May be associated with altered interneuronal activity in the spinal cord and the descending reticular formation of the brain. Meprobamate, a metabolite, has anxiolytic and sedative properties.

**PHARMACOKINETICS: Absorption:** Carisoprodol: (250mg) $C_{max}$=1.2mcg/mL, $T_{max}$=1.5 hrs, AUC=4.5mcg•hr/mL; (350mg) $C_{max}$=1.8mcg/mL, $T_{max}$=1.7 hrs, AUC=7.0mcg•hr/mL. Meprobamate: (250mg) $C_{max}$=1.8mcg/mL, $T_{max}$= 3.6 hrs, AUC=32mcg•hr/mL; (350mg) $C_{max}$=2.5mcg/mL, $T_{max}$=4.5 hrs, AUC=46mcg•hr/mL. **Distribution:** Found in breast milk. **Metabolism:** Liver via CYP2C19. Meprobamate (metabolite). **Elimination:** Renal/Nonrenal route, Carisoprodol: $T_{1/2}$=1.7 hrs (250mg), 2.0 hrs (350mg). Meprobamate: $T_{1/2}$=9.7 hrs (250mg), 9.6 hrs (350mg).

## NURSING CONSIDERATIONS

**Assessment:** Assess for acute intermittent porphyria, renal/hepatic impairment, seizures, addiction-prone patients, use of alcohol/illegal drugs/drugs of abuse, pregnancy/nursing status, and possible drug interactions.

**Monitoring:** Monitor for signs/symptoms of CNS depression, drug abuse/dependence, and seizures.

**Patient Counseling:** Advise that drug may cause drowsiness and/or dizziness; caution in engaging in hazardous tasks (operating machinery/driving). Avoid alcohol, illegal drugs, drugs of abuse, or other CNS depressants. Notify if pregnant/nursing or planning to become pregnant. Drug is limited to acute use. Notify physician if musculoskeletal symptoms persist. Inform of drug dependence/abuse potential. Report any adverse reactions.

**Administration:** Oral route. **Storage:** 20-25°C (68-77°F).



# Somatuline Depot RX

lanreotide (Ipsen/Tercica)

**THERAPEUTIC CLASS:** Somatostatin analog

**INDICATIONS:** Long term treatment of acromegalic patients who have had inadequate response to surgery and/or radiotherapy, or for whom surgery and/or radiotherapy is not an option.

**DOSAGE: Adults:** Initial: 90mg deep SQ at 4 week intervals for 3 months. Titrate: Adjust dose based on IGF and GH levels. GH >1 to ≤2.5ng/mL, IGF-1 Normal and Controlled Clinical Symptoms: 90mg every 4 weeks. GH >2.5ng/mL, IGF-1 Elevated and/or Clinical Symptoms Uncontrolled: 120mg every 4 weeks. GH ≤1ng/mL, IGF-1 Normal and Clinical Symptoms Controlled: 60mg every 4 weeks. Moderate to Severe Renal/Hepatic Impairment: Initial: 60mg deep SQ at 4 week intervals for 3 months.

**HOW SUPPLIED:** Inj: 60mg, 90mg, 120mg

**WARNINGS/PRECAUTIONS:** May reduce gallbladder motility and lead to gallstone formation; monitor periodically. Hypo- and/or hyperglycemia may occur; monitor glucose levels. Decreased thyroid function reported. May decrease HR; caution with bradycardia.

**ADVERSE REACTIONS:** Diarrhea, abdominal pain, N/V, constipation, flatulence, loose stools, cholethiasis, injection-site reactions.

**INTERACTIONS:** May decrease cyclosporine levels. May reduce intestinal absorption of concomitant drugs. Dose adjustments for concomitant antidiabetic treatment and drugs that induce bradycardia may be needed. Caution with drugs metabolized by CYP3A4 (eg, quinidine, terfenadine) and have low therapeutic index. Drugs metabolized by liver may need dose reduction.

**PREGNANCY:** Category C, caution in nursing.

**MECHANISM OF ACTION:** Somatostatin analog; acts mainly at the human somatostatin receptors (SSTR) 2 and 5 to inhibit growth hormone. Like somatostatin, lanreotide is an inhibitor of various endocrine, neuroendocrine, exocrine, and paracrine functions.

**PHARMACOKINETICS: Absorption:** SQ administration of variable doses resulted in different parameters. **Elimination:** Urine (<0.5%), feces (<5% unchanged). Biliary excretion.

## NURSING CONSIDERATIONS

**Assessment:** Assess for cardiac disease, DM, impaired hepatic/renal function, and possible drug interactions.

**Monitoring:** Monitor for cholethiasis, gallbladder sludge, hyper/hypoglycemia, hypothyroidism, and cardiovascular abnormalities. Monitor blood glucose levels when dosages are adjusted. Monitor serum GH, and IGF-1 levels to assess effectiveness of treatment.

**Patient Counseling:** Instruct to report any adverse reactions or if condition persists or worsens. Rotate injection site between right and left side. Instruct to notify physician if dose is missed,

**Administration:** SQ. **Storage:** Refrigerate at 2-8°C (36-46°F). Protect from light in original package.

# SOMAVERT RX

pegvisomant (Pharmacia & Upjohn)

**THERAPEUTIC CLASS:** Growth hormone receptor antagonist

**INDICATIONS:** Treatment of acromegaly in those who have had an inadequate response to surgery and/or radiation therapy, and/or other medical therapies, or for whom these therapies are not appropriate.

**DOSAGE:** *Adults:* LD: 40mg SQ. Maint: 10mg SQ qd. Titrate: Adjust dose by 5mg increments/decrements, based on IGF-I levels, every 4-6 weeks. Max: 30mg/day. LFTs ≥3x/<5x ULN (without symptoms of liver dysfunction): Monitor LFTs weekly. LFTs ≥5x ULN/Transaminase Elevations ≥3x ULN: D/C immediately and evaluate. Do not initiate if baseline LFTs >3x ULN until cause is determined.

**HOW SUPPLIED:** Inj: 10mg, 15mg, 20mg

**WARNINGS/PRECAUTIONS:** May expand and cause serious complications of tumors that secrete GH; monitor with periodic imaging scans of the sella turcica. May increase glucose tolerance and risk of hypoglycemia in diabetics. May result in functional GH deficiency. AST/ALT elevations reported; obtain baseline ALT, AST, TBIL, and ALP levels prior to initiation. Monitor LFTs monthly for first 6 months, quarterly for next 6 months, then biannually; monitor more frequently if elevations occur. D/C if liver injury confirmed. Monitor IGF-I levels 4-6 weeks after initiation or dose adjustments; every 6 months after levels are normalized. Interferes with the measurement serum GH levels by commercially available GH assays; do not adjust dosage based on serum GH levels.

**ADVERSE REACTIONS:** Infection, abnormal LFTs, pain, injection site reactions, back pain, diarrhea, nausea, flu syndrome, chest pain, dizziness, paresthesia, HTN, sinusitis, peripheral edema.

S

**INTERACTIONS:** May need to reduce dosage of insulin and/or hypoglycemic agents. Concomitant opioids may increase dosage requirements of pegvisomant.

**PREGNANCY:** Category B; caution in nursing.

**MECHANISM OF ACTION:** Growth hormone receptor antagonist; selectively binds to growth hormone (GH) receptors on cell surfaces, where it blocks binding of endogenous GH and interferes with GH signal transduction. This decreases serum concentrations of insulin such as growth factor-I (IGF-I), as well as other GH-responsive proteins, including IGF binding protein-3 (IGFBP-3), and acid labile subunit (ALS).

**PHARMACOKINETICS: Absorption:** Absolute bioavailability (57%). **Distribution:** $V_d$=7L. **Elimination:** Urine (<1%); $T_{1/2}$=6 days.

## NURSING CONSIDERATIONS

**Assessment:** Assess for latex allergy before therapy (due to stopper on vial). Assess use with tumors that secrete growth hormone. Assess proper glucose control with DM prior to therapy. Obtain baseline serum liver tests (ALT, AST, TBIL, ALP). Assess for possible drug interactions.

**Monitoring:** Monitor for tumor growth in patients who have growth hormone-secreting tumors. Perform periodic image scans of the sella turcica. Monitor for increased glucose tolerance while on medication (hypoglycemia). Monitor for signs/symptoms of a GH-deficient state. Serum IGF-I concentrations should be evaluated 4-6 weeks after initiation of treatment, or when dose adjustments are made, and at least every 6 months after IGF-I levels have normalized. Monitor for signs/symptoms of liver dysfunction. Evaluate periodic serum levels of ALT, AST, TBIL, and ALP.

**Patient Counseling:** Counsel on signs/symptoms of liver dysfunction. Instruct that if jaundice develops, immediately contact physician and d/c therapy. Inform that serial monitoring of LFTs will be required. Instruct on how to properly administer drug. Inform patients will require periodic monitoring of serial IGF-I levels in order to adjust dosing.

**Administration:** SQ route. Reconstitute.1) Withdraw 1mL of SWFI and inject it into vial; 2) Roll vial; do not shake. Assess that solution is clear after reconstitution. Administer within 6 hrs after reconstitution. **Storage:** Refrigerate at 2-8°C (36-46°F). Protect from freezing.

# SONATA

zaleplon (King) **CIV**

**THERAPEUTIC CLASS:** Pyrazolopyrimidine (non-benzodiazepine)

**INDICATIONS:** Short-term treatment of insomnia.

S

**DOSAGE:** *Adults:* Insomnia: 10mg qhs. Low Weight Patients: Start with 5mg hs. Max: 20mg/day. Elderly/Debilitated/Concomitant Cimetidine: 5mg qhs. Max: 10mg/day. Mild to Moderate Hepatic Dysfunction: 5mg qhs. Take immediately prior to bedtime.

**HOW SUPPLIED:** Cap: 5mg, 10mg

**WARNINGS/PRECAUTIONS:** Monitor elderly/debilitated closely. Abnormal thinking and behavioral changes reported. Avoid abrupt withdrawal. Abuse potential exists. Caution in respiratory disorders, depression, conditions affecting metabolism or hemodynamic responses, and mild-to-moderate hepatic insufficiency. Not for use in severe hepatic impairment. May cause impaired coordination even the following day. Re-evaluate if no improvement of insomnia after 7-10 days of therapy. Contains tartrazine.

**ADVERSE REACTIONS:** Headache, asthenia, nausea, dizziness, amnesia, somnolence, eye pain, dysmenorrhea, abdominal pain.

**INTERACTIONS:** Potentiates CNS depression with psychotropics (eg, thioridazine, imipramine), anticonvulsants, antihistamines, alcohol and other CNS depressants. CYP3A4 inducers (eg, rifampin, phenytoin, carbamazepine and phenobarbital) decreases levels. Potentiated by cimetidine.

**PREGNANCY:** Category C, not for use in nursing.

**MECHANISM OF ACTION:** Pyrazolopyrimidine class; interacts with GABA-benzodiazepine receptor complex.

**PHARMACOKINETICS: Absorption:** Rapid and complete. $T_{max}$=1 hr. Absolute bioavailability (approximately 30%) (IV). **Distribution:** $V_d$=1.4L/kg; plasma protein binding (60%). **Metabolism:** Extensive, liver via aldehyde oxidase. **Elimination:** Urine (71%), feces (17%); $T_{1/2}$=1 hrs.

## NURSING CONSIDERATIONS

**Assessment:** Assess for primary psychiatric and/or medical illness; hypersensitivity to drug, compromised respiratory function (COPD, sleep apnea), depression, suicidal tendencies, hepatic/renal impairment, drug abuse/addiction, alcohol intake, and drug interactions.

**Monitoring:** Monitor for anaphylactic/anaphylactoid reactions, worsening of insomnia, abnormal thinking and behavior changes, complex behaviors (eg, sleep-driving), physical/psychological dependence, withdrawal symptoms, amnesia, headache, abdominal pain, asthenia, nausea and somnolence, hepatic and pulmonary functions.

**Patient Counseling:** Take drug immediately prior to bedtime. Caution against hazardous tasks (eg, operating machinery/driving). Inform about the benefits/risks, possibility of physical/psychological dependence and memory disturbances. Notify if pregnant/nursing or planning to become pregnant. Do not increase dose or d/c drug before consulting physician. Avoid alcohol.

**Administration:** Oral route. **Storage:** 20-25°C (68-77°F).

# SORIATANE — RX

acitretin (Stiefel)

**Avoid in pregnancy or becoming pregnant ≤3 yrs after discontinuation of therapy; use 2 reliable forms of contraception. Only use in females of reproductive potential with severe psoriasis unresponsive or contraindicated to other therapies, if receive warnings of therapy hazards and risk of contraception failure, if negative pregnancy test within 1 week before therapy, will begin therapy on the 2nd or 3rd day of next menstrual cycle, are capable of complying with contraceptive measures and are reliable. Repeat pregnancy testing and contraception counseling on a regular basis. The patient must have a negative result from a urine or serum pregnancy test. before receiving Soriatane prescription. It is not known whether residual acitretin in seminal fluid poses risk to fetus with male patients during or after therapy. Females should avoid ethanol during and 2 months after therapy. Severe birth defects reported.**

**THERAPEUTIC CLASS:** Retinoid

**INDICATIONS:** Treatment of severe psoriasis, including erythrodermic and generalized pustular types.

**DOSAGE:** *Adults:* Initial: 25-50mg single dose qd with main meal. Individualize dose based on intersubject variation in pharmacokinetics, clinical efficacy, and incidence of side effects. Maint: 25-50mg qd. Terminate therapy when lesions resolve. May treat relapses as outlined for initial therapy.

**HOW SUPPLIED:** Cap: 10mg, 25mg

**CONTRAINDICATIONS:** See Black Box Warnings. Pregnancy.

**WARNINGS/PRECAUTIONS:** Risk of hepatotoxicity, hyperostosis, pancreatitis, and pseudotumor cerebri. D/C if visual difficulties occur; decreased night vision and reduced tolerance to contact lenses reported. Bone abnormalities of the vertebral column, knees, and ankles reported. Increases TG and cholesterol and decreases HDL; perform lipid tests before therapy every 1-2 weeks until establish lipid response. Caution with severe hepatic/renal impairment. Transient worsening of psoriasis may occur initially. Do not donate blood during and for 3 yrs after therapy. Avoid sun lamps and excessive sun exposure. Depression and/or psychiatric symptoms (eg, aggressive feelings, thoughts of self-harm) reported. Thinning of the skin observed.

**ADVERSE REACTIONS:** Ophthalmologic effects, cheilitis, rhinitis, dry mouth, epistaxis, alopecia, dry skin, rash, skin peeling, nail disorder, pruritus, par-

S

esthesia, paronychia, skin atrophy, sticky skin, xerophthalmia, arthralgia, rash, acute myocardial infarction, stroke, vulvo-vaginitis.

**INTERACTIONS:** Caution with oral hypoglycemics. May increase risk of hepatotoxicity with methotrexate. Interferes with microdosed progestin "minipill" oral contraceptives. Females should avoid ethanol during and 2 months after therapy. Possible additive toxic effects with vitamin A doses that exceed minimum RDAs.

**PREGNANCY:** Category X, not for use in nursing.

**MECHANISM OF ACTION:** Retinoid antipsoriatic; not established.

**PHARMACOKINETICS: Absorption:** $C_{max}$=416ng/mL; $T_{max}$=2-5 hrs. **Distribution:** Plasma protein binding (99.9%); found in breast milk. **Metabolism:** Extensive; via isomerization to cis-acitretin; metabolized with the parent drug into chain-shortened breakdown metaboilites and conjugates. **Elimination:** Chain-shortened breakdown metabolites and conjugates; feces (34-54%), urine (16-53%). Acitretin: $T_{1/2}$=49 hrs. Cis-acitretin: $T_{1/2}$=63 hrs.

## NURSING CONSIDERATIONS

**Assessment:** Prior to therapy, must have had 2 negative urine or serum pregnancy tests. Assess for exclusion of pregnancy/nursing. Assess for renal/liver impairment, chronic abnormally elevated blood lipid values, DM, obesity, increased alcohol intake, or a familial history of these conditions, cardiovascular status, pre-existing abnormalities of the spine or knees or ankles, and possible drug interactions (eg, tetracyclines). Blood lipids and LFT levels should be evaluated prior to therapy and again at intervals of 1-2 weeks.

**Monitoring:** Monitor for hepatotoxicity, hyperostosis, hypertriglyceridemia, radiological changes of pre-exsiting abnormalities of the spine (eg, degenerative spurs, anterior bridging of spinal vertebrae, diffuse idiopathic skeletal hyperostosis, ligament calcification, and narrowing/destruction of the cervical disc space), MI or other thromboembolic events, pancreatitis, psychiatric problems, and signs/symptoms of pseudotumor cerebri (eg, headache, NV, visual disturbances, papilledema). Monitor the eye for dryness, lash loss, irritation, Bell's Palsy, blepharitis, blurred vision, cataracts, and papilledema. Careful monitoring for LFTs, lipids, and blood sugar. Pregnancy test must be repeated every month during therapy and for at least 3 yrs after d/c.

**Patient Counseling:** Inform about the Pregnancy Prevention Actively Required During and After Treatment (P.A.R.T) program and about the risks of therapy. Advise to use 2 effective forms of contraception at least 1 month prior to initiation of therapy. Do not donate blood during or at least 3 yrs following completion of therapy. Required by law that medication guide must be given to patient each time therapy is dispensed. Do not ingest beverages or products containing ethanol while taking therapy and for 2 months after d/c of therapy. Notify physician if nursing. Caution when driving or operating a vehicle at night. Advise against taking vitamin A supplements to avoid additive toxic effects. Avoid excessive exposure to sunlight.



**Administration:** Oral route. Take with food. **Storage:** 15-25°C (59-77°F). Avoid light or humidity exposure after opening bottle.

# SPIRIVA — RX

tiotropium bromide (Boehringer Ingelheim/Pfizer)

**THERAPEUTIC CLASS:** Anticholinergic bronchodilator

**INDICATIONS:** Long-term, once-daily maintenance treatment of bronchospasm associated with chronic obstructive pulmonary disease (COPD), including chronic bronchitis and emphysema. Reduction of exacerbations in COPD patients.

**DOSAGE:** *Adults:* 2 inhalations of the contents of 1 cap (18mcg) qd, with HandiHaler device.

**HOW SUPPLIED:** Cap, Inhalation: 18mcg

**CONTRAINDICATIONS:** Hypersensitivity to ipratropium.

**WARNINGS/PRECAUTIONS:** Not for initial treatment of acute episodes. D/C if hypersensitivity (eg, angioedema, itching, rash) or paradoxical bronchospasm occurs. Caution with narrow-angle glaucoma, prostatic hyperplasia, bladder-neck obstruction. New onset or worsening of glaucoma and urinary retention reported. Monitor for anticholinergic effects with moderate to severe renal impairment (CrCl ≤50mL/min). Contents of caps are for oral inhalation only and must not be swallowed.

**ADVERSE REACTIONS:** Dry mouth, arthritis, cough, flu-like symptoms, sinusitis, constipation, abdominal pain, urinary tract infection, upper respiratory tract infection, chest pain, edema, vomiting, myalgia, moniliasis, rash.

**INTERACTIONS:** Avoid with other anticholinergic-containing drugs (eg, ipratropium).

**PREGNANCY:** Category C, caution in nursing.

**MECHANISM OF ACTION:** Anticholinergic; inhibits $M_3$-receptors on smooth muscle leading to bronchodilation.

**PHARMACOKINETICS: Absorption:** Absolute bioavailability (19.5%); $T_{max}$=5 min. **Distribution:** $V_d$=32L/kg; plasma protein binding (72%). **Metabolism:** Liver (oxidation, conjugation) via CYP2D6, 3A4. **Elimination:** (Inhalation): Urine (14%); (IV): Urine (74%). $T_{1/2}$=5-6 days.

## NURSING CONSIDERATIONS

**Assessment:** Assess for hypersensitivity of atropine or its derivatives, narrow-angle glaucoma, prostatic hyperplasia, bladder-neck obstruction, renal impairment, and possible drug interactions.

**Monitoring:** Monitor for urinary retention, GI distress (diarrhea, N/V), paradoxical bronchospasm and allergic type-reaction (pruritus; angioedema of tongue, lips and face; urticaria; laryngospasm; anaphylaxis).

**Patient Counseling:** Inform that contents of capsule are for oral inhalation only and must not be swallowed. Advise not increase dose or frequency, or use in acute periods of bronchospasm. Seek medical attention if with symptoms of precipitation or worsening of narrow-angle glaucoma (increased IOP, acute eye pain/discomfort, blurring of vision, visual halos or colored images with red eyes from conjunctival, corneal congestion), or of prostatic hyperplasia or bladder neck obstruction (difficutly in passing urine, dysuria), with paradoxical bronchospasm, or allergic/hypersensitivity reactions.

**Administration:** Oral inhalation. 1) Press green piercing button to open cap; pull cap up to expose mouthpiece. Open mouthpiece by pulling ridge up. 2) Remove one cap immediately before use; insert in center chamber. 3) Close mouthpiece firmly until click is heard. 4) Hold device with mouthpiece up; press green piercing button against base and release. 5) Exhale (not into mouthpiece); put mouthpiece in lips; keep head upright, with device in horizontal position; breathe in slowly and deeply to hear or feel cap vibrate. Breathe in until lungs are full; hold breath as long as comfortable, and remove device from lips. 6) To ensure full dose, must breathe out again completely and inhale once again as described above. 7) After finished taking dose, open mouthpiece and tip out used cap and discard. 8) Clean mouthpiece once a month. **Storage:** 25°C (77°F); excursions permitted to 15-30°C (59-86°F). Do not expose cap to extreme temperatures or moisture. Do not store cap in Handihaler device.

S

# SPORANOX RX

itraconazole (Janssen/Ortho Biotech)

**Contraindicated with cisapride, pimozide, quinidine, dofetilide, or levacetylmethadol. Serious cardiovascular events (eg, QT prolongation, torsades de pointes, ventricular tachycardia, cardiac arrest, and/or sudden death) reported with cisapride, pimozide, quinidine, levacetylmethadol, and other CYP3A4 inhibitors. Do not use caps for onychomycosis with ventricular dysfunction. Reassess if signs/symptoms of CHF occur.**

**THERAPEUTIC CLASS:** Azole antifungal

**INDICATIONS:** (Cap) Onychomycosis of the toenail and fingernail in immunocompetent patients. Confirm diagnosis before therapy. (Cap/Inj) Treatment of blastomycosis and histoplasmosis (eg, chronic cavitary pulmonary disease, disseminated non-meningeal), and aspergillosis (eg, pulmonary and extrapulmonary) if refractory to or intolerant to amphotericin B in immunocompromised and non-immunocompromised patients. (Sol) Treatment of oropharyngeal and esophageal candidiasis. (Sol/Inj) Empiric therapy of febrile, neutropenic patients (ETFN) with suspected fungal infections.

**DOSAGE:** *Adults:* Cap: Take with full meal. If patient has achlorhydria or taking gastric acid suppressors, give with cola beverage. Onychomycosis: Toenail: 200mg qd for 12 consecutive weeks. Fingernail: 200mg bid for 1 week, skip 3 weeks, then repeat. Blastomycosis/Histoplasmosis: 200mg qd. May increase by 100mg increments if no improvement. Max: 400mg/day. Give bid if dose >200mg/day. Aspergillosis: 200-400mg/day. Life-Threatening Infections: LD: 200mg tid for 1st 3 days. Continue for at least 3 months and until infection subsides. Sol: Take on empty stomach. Swish 10mL at a time for several seconds, then swallow. Candidiasis: Oropharyngeal: 200mg/day for 1-2 weeks. If refractory to fluconazole, give 100mg bid (response in 2-4 weeks; may relapse shortly after d/c). Esophageal: 100-200mg/day for at least 3 weeks. Continue for 2 weeks after symptoms resolve. IV: ETFN: 200mg bid over 1 hr infusion for four doses, followed by 200mg qd for 14 days. Continue with oral solution 200mg bid until resolution of clinically significant neutropenia. Blastomycosis/Histoplasmosis/Aspergillosis: 200mg bid over 1 hr infusion for four doses, followed by 200mg qd. Continue for at least 3 months until active fungal infection subsides.

**HOW SUPPLIED:** Cap: 100mg [Blister, 3 x 10 caps], [PulsePak, 7 blisters x 4 caps]; Inj: 10mg/mL [25mL]; Sol: 10mg/mL [150mL]

**CONTRAINDICATIONS:** Concomitant with cisapride, oral midazolam, nisoldipine, pimozide, quinidine, dofetilide, triazolam, ergot alkaloids (eg, dihydroergotamine, ergometrine), and HMG-CoA reductase inhibitors metabolized by CYP3A4 (eg, lovastatin, simvastatin). (Cap) Treatment of onychomycosis if pregnant or contemplating pregnancy, and ventricular dysfunction (eg, CHF). (Inj) Patients with severe renal impairment. Concomitant use of sodium chloride injection.

**WARNINGS/PRECAUTIONS:** Rare cases of hepatotoxicity reported. Monitor LFTs; d/c if hepatic dysfunction develops. Avoid with liver disease. D/C if neuropathy or CHF occurs. Sol and caps not interchangeable. Consider alternative therapy if unresponsive in patients with cystic fibrosis. Avoid with ventricular dysfunction. Caution with ischemic/valvular disease, pulmonary disease, renal failure, hepatic impairment, and other edematous disorders. Avoid injection if CrCl <30mL/min. Transient or permanent hearing loss reported. Caution in elderly.

**ADVERSE REACTIONS:** N/V, diarrhea, abdominal pain, fever, cough, rash, increased sweating, headache, hypokalemia, vein disorder, and bilirubinemia.



**INTERACTIONS:** See Contraindications. Increased levels with cisapride, pimozide, quinidine, nisoldipine, levacetylmethadol, dofetilide, oral midazolam, triazolam, HMG-CoA reductase inhibitors. Increases levels of rifabutin, immunosuppressants, protease inhibitors, alfentanil, buspirone, methylprednisolone, trimetrexate, carbamazepine, HMG-CoA reductase inhibitors, digoxin, warfarin, busulfan, docetaxel, vinca alkaloids, astemizole, alprazolam, diazepam, oral midazolam, triazolam, dihydropyridine CCBs, verapamil, oral hypoglycemics. CYP3A4 inducers (eg, carbamazepine, phenobarbital, phenytoin, isoniazid, rifabutin, rifampin, nevirapine) decrease itraconazole levels. CYP3A4 inhibitors (eg, erythromycin, clarithromycin, indinavir, ritonavir) may increase itraconazole and hydroitraconazole levels. Severe hypoglycemia with oral hypoglycemics. Additive negative inotropic effects with CCBs. Edema reported with dihydropyridine CCBs; adjust dose. Decreased absorption of caps with antacids or gastric secretion suppressors. May increase digoxin levels. Caution with CCBs, halofantrine. Prolonged QT interval may occur with halofantrine. May increase or prolong fentanyl plasma levels. Fatal respiratory depression reported with fentanyl. May inhibit glucocorticosteroids (eg, budesonide, dexamethasone, fluticasone) and CCBs (eg, nifedipine, felodipine) metabolism.

**PREGNANCY:** Category C, not for use in nursing (HIV-infected women) and safety not known in nursing.

**MECHANISM OF ACTION:** Azole antifungal agent; inhibits the CYP450-dependent synthesis of ergosterol, which is a vital component of fungal cell membranes.

**PHARMACOKINETICS: Absorption:** (Cap/Sol) Absolute bioavailabilty (55%). Oral administration of variable doses resulted in different parameters. (IV) $C_{max}$=2856ng/mL; $T_{max}$=1.08 hr; AUC=30605ng.h/mL.**Metabolism:** Liver via CYP3A4; hydroxyitraconazole (major metabolite). **Distribution:** Plasma protein binding (99.8%); found in breast milk. (IV) $V_d$=796L. **Elimination:** Urine (40%), feces (3-18%) (inactive metabolites).

## NURSING CONSIDERATIONS

**Assessment:** Assess for proper diagnosis of fungal infection (eg, cultures, microscopic studies), cardiac function (eg, ventricular dysfunction, CHF) prior to administration. Assess pregnancy/nursing status prior to use.

**Monitoring:** Monitor for signs/symptoms of CHF including QT prolongation, torsade de pointes, ventricular tachycardia, cardiac arrest, and liver dysfunction, for possible drug interactions, and LFTs. Blood glucose concentrations should also be monitored when coadminstered with hypoglycemic agents. Monitor for signs of rash (Stevens-Johnson syndrome). Monitor for serum creatinine levels.

**Patient Counseling:** Instruct to take drug with a full meal. Counsel on signs/symptoms of CHF and liver dysfunction, which include unusual fatigue, anorexia, N/V, jaundice, dark urine or pale stools. Counsel females to avoid pregnancy while on medication and to remain on contraceptives for 2 months following completion of therapy. Notify physician if rash develops.

**Administration:** Oral/IV route. Not for IV bolus injection. **Storage:** (Cap): 15-25°C (59-77°F). Protect from light and moisture. (Sol): 25°C (77°F). Do not freeze. (Inj): 25°C (77°F). Protect from light and freezing.

# Sprycel **RX**

dasatinib (Bristol-Myers Squibb)

**THERAPEUTIC CLASS:** Kinase inhibitor

**INDICATIONS:** Treatment of adults with chronic, accelerated, or myeloid or lymphoid blast phase chronic myeloid leukemia (CML) with resistance or intolerance to prior therapy including imatinib. Treatment of Philadelphia chromosome-positive acute lymphoblastic leukemia (Ph+ ALL) with resistance or intolerance to prior therapy.

**DOSAGE:** *Adults:* Chronic Phase CML: Initial: 100mg qd. Titrate: If no response, increase to 140mg qd. Accelerated Phase CML/Myeloid or Lymphoid Blast Phase CML/Ph+ ALL: Initial: 140mg qd. Titrate: If no response, increase to 180mg qd. Concomitant Strong CYP3A4 Inducers: Consider dose increase. Concomitant Strong CYP3A4 Inhibitors: Consider dose decrease to 20mg if patients taking 100mg daily; and 40mg if patients taking 140mg daily. Refer to PI for dose adjustments for neutropenia and thrombocytopenia.

**HOW SUPPLIED:** Tab: 20mg, 50mg, 70mg, 100mg

**WARNINGS/PRECAUTIONS:** Severe thrombocytopenia, neutropenia, and anemia reported; monitor CBC weekly for first 2 months, then monthly thereafter. Severe CNS hemorrhages including fatalities, GI hemorrhage, and other severe hemorrhage cases reported. Pleural and pericardial effusion reported. Severe ascites, generalized edema, severe pulmonary edema reported; typically managed by supportive care. QT prolongation reported; caution in patients at risk (eg, hypokalemia or hypomagnesemia, congenital long QT syndrome). Correct hypokalemia or hypomagnesemia prior to administration. May cause fetal harm if used during pregnancy. Caution with hepatic impairment.

**ADVERSE REACTIONS:** Fluid retention, diarrhea, N/V, headache, abdominal pain, bleeding events, pyrexia, pleural effusion, neutropenia, thrombocytopenia, dyspnea, anemia, skin rash, fatigue.

**INTERACTIONS:** Increased levels with CYP3A4 inhibitors (eg, ketoconazole, itraconazole, voriconazole, clarithromycin, ritonavir, atazanavir, indinavir, nefazodone, nelfinavir, saquinavir, telithromycin). Grapefruit juice may also increase levels and should be avoided. Decreased levels with CYP3A4 inducers (eg, dexamethasone, phenytoin, carbamazepine, rifampin, rifabutin, phenobarbital). St. John's wort may decrease dasatinib levels unpredictably and should be avoided. Avoid antacids; if necessary, separate dose by 2 hrs. Concomitant use of $H_2$ blockers or PPIs not recommended. Caution with CYP3A4 substrates with narrow therapeutic windows (eg, alfentanil, astemizole, terfenadine, cisapride, cyclosporine, fentanyl, pimozide, quinidine, sirolimus, tacrolimus, or ergot alkaloids such as ergotamine and dihydroergotamine). Caution in patients on anticoagulants or on medications that inhibit platelet function. May increase risk of QT prolongation with concomitant antiarrhythmics or other QT-prolonging agents and cumulative high-dose anthracycline therapy.

**PREGNANCY:** Category D, not for use in nursing.

**MECHANISM OF ACTION:** Kinase inhibitor; inhibits BCR-ABL, SRC family, c-KIT, EPHA2, and PDGFRβ kinases.

**PHARMACOKINETICS: Absorption:** $T_{max}$=0.5-6 hrs. **Distribution:** $V_d$=2505L; plasma protein binding (96%). **Metabolism:** Extensive via CYP3A4. **Elimination:** Urine (4%), feces (85%); $T_{1/2}$=3-5 hrs.

## NURSING CONSIDERATIONS

**Assessment:** Assess for hepatic impairment, prolonged QTc, lactose intolerance, hypokalemia, and hypomagnesemia, pregnancy/nursing status and possible drug interactions. Obtain baseline CBC, LFTs, and electrolytes.

**Monitoring:** Monitor CBC weekly for first 2 months and monthly afterward and LFTs periodically. Monitor for signs/symptoms of hemorrhage, myelosuppression, pleural/pericardial effusion, fluid retention, QT prolongation, and hypersensitivity reactions. If symptoms of pleural effusion are present, perform chest X-ray.

**Patient Counseling:** Instruct to swallow whole; do not break, cut, or crush. Advise that may take with or without food in the morning or the evening. Inform of pregnancy risks and advise to avoid becoming pregnant during therapy. Instruct to not take with grapefruit juice. Counsel to avoid concomitant use with antacids; advise to separate antacids by at least 2 hrs. Advise to seek medical attention if experiencing symptoms of hemorrhage (eg, unusual bleeding, easy bruising), myelosuppression (eg, fever, infection), pleural effusion (eg, dyspnea, dry cough), fluid retention (eg, swelling, weight gain, SOB), QT prolongation, hypersensitivity reactions, significant N/V, diarrhea, headache, musculoskeletal pain, fatigue, or rash.



**Administration:** Oral route. Swallow whole; do not crush or cut. **Storage:** 25°C (77°F); excursions permitted between 15-30°C (59-86°F).

# STALEVO — RX

entacapone - levodopa - carbidopa (Novartis)

**THERAPEUTIC CLASS:** Dopa-decarboxylase inhibitor/dopamine precursor/ COMT inhibitor

**INDICATIONS:** Treatment of idiopathic Parkinson's disease; to substitute for equivalent doses of previously administered carbidopa/levodopa and entacapone or to substitute for those experiencing signs and symptoms of end-of-dose "wearing off" (only for those taking up to 600mg/day levodopa without experiencing dyskinesias).

**DOSAGE:** *Adults:* Currently Taking Carbidopa/Levodopa and Entacapone: May switch directly to corresponding strength of carbidopa/levodopa. Currently Taking Carbidopa/Levodopa but not Entacapone: First titrate individually with carbidopa/levodopa product and entacapone product then transfer to corresponding dose. Max: Stalevo 50/Stalevo 75/Stalevo 100/ Stalevo 125/Stalevo 150: 8 times/day. Stalevo 200: 6 times/day.

**HOW SUPPLIED:** Tab: (Carbidopa-Levodopa-Entacapone): Stalevo 50: 12.5mg-50mg-200mg; Stalevo 75: 18.75mg-75mg-200mg; Stalevo 100: 25mg-100mg-200mg; Stalevo 125: 31.25mg-125mg-200mg; Stalevo 150: 37.5mg-150mg-200mg; Stalevo 200: 50mg-200mg-200mg

**CONTRAINDICATIONS:** MAOIs during or within 14 days of use, narrow-angle glaucoma, undiagnosed skin lesions, history of melanoma.

**WARNINGS/PRECAUTIONS:** Dyskinesia, mental disturbances, hypotension/syncope, hallucinations, rhabdomyolysis, hyperpyrexia, confusion, and fibrotic complications reported. Caution with biliary obstruction, severe CV or pulmonary disease, bronchial asthma, renal/hepatic/endocrine disease, chronic wide-angle glaucoma, history of MI with residual arrhythmias, peptic ulcer. Neuroleptic malignant syndrome reported with dose reductions or withdrawal; observe carefully with rapid withdrawal or abrupt dose reduction. May elevate LFTs. May impair physical/mental abilities.

**ADVERSE REACTIONS:** Dyskinesia, hyperkinesia, hypokinesia, dizziness, diarrhea, abdominal pain, constipation, N/V, urine discoloration, back pain, fatigue, dry mouth, dyspnea.

**INTERACTIONS:** See Contraindications. Increased HR, arrhythmias, and BP changes with drugs metabolized by COMT (eg, isoproterenol, epinephrine, norepinephrine, dopamine, dobutamine, α-methyldopa, apomorphine, isoetherine, bitolterol). Probenecid, cholestyramine, and some antibiotics (eg, erythromycin, rifampicin, ampicillin, chloramphenicol) may interfere with biliary excretion. Risk of postural hypotension with antihypertensives and selegiline. HTN and dyskinesia may occur with TCAs. Reduced effect with phenytoin, papaverine, metoclopramide, isoniazid, dopamine $D_2$ antagonists (eg, phenothiazines, butyrophenones, risperidone). Reduced bioavailability with iron salts. Caution with highly protein-bound drugs (eg, warfarin, salicylic acid, phenylbutazone, diazepam).

**PREGNANCY:** Category C, caution in nursing.

**MECHANISM OF ACTION:** Dopa-decarboxylase inhibitor/dopamine precursor/COMT inhibitor. Carbidopa: Inhibits the decarboxylation of peripheral levodopa, making more levodopa available for transport to the brain. Levodopa: Crosses blood-brain barrier and presumably converted to dopamine in brain. Entacapone: Sustains plasma levels of levodopa, resulting in more constant dopaminergic stimulation in brain.

**PHARMACOKINETICS: Absorption:** Levodopa: Rapidly absorbed. (PO) Administration of variable doses resulted in different parameters. Entacapone: Rapidly absorbed; $C_{max}$=1200-1500ng/mL; $T_{max}$=0.8-1.2 hrs; AUC=1250-1750ng•hr/mL. Carbidopa: Slightly absorbed; $C_{max}$=40-225ng/mL; $T_{max}$=2.5-3.4 hrs; AUC=170-1200ng•hr/mL. **Distribution:** Levodopa: Plasma protein binding (10-30%). Entacapone: (98%). Carbidopa: (Approximately 36%). **Metabolism:** Levodopa: Extensive decarboxylation by dopa decarboxylase and O-methylation by catechol-O-methyltransferase. Entacapone: Completely metabolized. Carbidopa: Main metabolites: α-methyl-3-methoxy-4-hydroxyphenylpropionic acid, and α-methyl-3,4-dihydroxyphenylpropionic acid. **Elimination:** Levodopa: $T_{1/2}$=1.7 hrs. Entacapone: Feces (90%), urine (10%); $T_{1/2}$=0.8-1 hr. Carbidopa: Urine (30%, unchanged); $T_{1/2}$=1.6-2 hrs.

## NURSING CONSIDERATIONS

**Assessment:** Assess LFTs, renal function, CBC, chronic wide-angle glaucoma, dyskinesia, psychosis, depression, cardiovascular complications, biliary obstructions, skin lesions, history of melanoma, pregnancy/nursing status, and possible drug interactions.

**Monitoring:** Monitor LFTs, renal function, CBC, BP. Observe for biliary obstruction, mental disturbances, depression and suicidal ideations, worsening of dyskinesia, rhabdomyolysis, diarrhea, hallucinations, fibrotic complications, and hyperpyrexia.

**Patient Counseling:** Caution while operating machinery/driving until more experienced on therapy. Discoloration of bodily fluids may occur. High-protein diet, excessive acidity, and iron salts reduce clinical effectiveness. Wearing-off effect may be seen at end of dosing interval. Report any adverse effects. Inform that hallucinations, postural (orthostatic) hypotension, nausea, and increase in dyskinesia may occur. Notify physician if new or increased gambling, sexual, or other intense urges develop.

**Administration:** Oral route. **Storage:** Store at 25°C (77°F); excursions permitted to 15-30°C (59-86°F). Dispense in tight container.

## STARLIX **RX**

nateglinide (Novartis)

**THERAPEUTIC CLASS:** Hypoglycemic agent

**INDICATIONS:** Adjunct to diet and exercise, to improve glycemic control in adults with type 2 diabetes.

**DOSAGE:** *Adults:* Initial/Maint: 120mg tid before meals (with or without metformin or TZD). Take 1-30 min before meals. May use 60mg tid (with or without metformin or TZD) in patients near goal $HbA_{1c}$.

**HOW SUPPLIED:** Tab: 60mg, 120mg

**CONTRAINDICATIONS:** Type 1 diabetes, diabetic ketoacidosis.

**WARNINGS/PRECAUTIONS:** Caution in moderate to severe hepatic impairment. Transient loss of glucose control with trauma, surgery, fever, and infection; may need insulin therapy. Secondary failure may occur in prolonged therapy. Hypoglycemia risk in elderly, debilitated, malnourished, strenuous exercise, and with adrenal or pituitary insufficiency. Autonomic neuropathy may mask hypoglycemia.

**ADVERSE REACTIONS:** Upper respiratory infection, flu symptoms, dizziness, arthropathy, diarrhea, hypoglycemia, back pain, jaundice, cholestatic hepatitis, elevated liver enzymes.

**INTERACTIONS:** Potentiated hypoglycemia with alcohol, NSAIDs, salicylates, MAOIs, and non-selective β-blockers. Risk of hyperglycemia with thiazides, corticosteroids, thyroid products, and sympathomimetics. May potentiate tolbutamide. Peak plasma levels reduced with liquid meals. β-blockers may mask hypoglycemic effects. Caution with highly protein-bound drugs.

**PREGNANCY:** Category C, not for use in nursing.

**MECHANISM OF ACTION:** Meglitinide; lowers blood glucose levels by stimulating insulin secretion from the pancreas.

**PHARMACOKINETICS: Absorption:** Absolute bioavailability (73%); $T_{max}$=1 hr. **Distribution:** $V_d$=10L; plasma protein binding (98%). **Metabolism:** CYP2C9, 3A4; hydroxylation, glucuronide conjugation. **Elimination:** Urine (75%), feces; $T_{1/2}$=1.5 hrs.



### NURSING CONSIDERATIONS

**Assessment:** Assess FPG, $HbA_{1c}$, renal function, LFTs, diabetic ketoacidosis, pregnancy status, and for possible drug interactions.

**Monitoring:** Monitor FPG, $HbA_{1c}$, renal function, LFTs, uric acid levels, diabetic ketoacidosis, upper respiratory infection, back pain, flu symptoms, dizziness, arthropathy, diarrhea, accidental trauma, bronchitis, or coughing.

**Patient Counseling:** Inform about importance of adherence to meal planning, regular physical activity, regular blood glucose monitoring, periodic $HbA_{1c}$ testing, recognition and management of hypo/hyperglycemia, and periodic assessment for diabetes complications. During periods of stress (eg, trauma, infection, surgery) medication requirements may change; seek prompt medical advice. Instruct to take 30 min before meals.

**Administration:** Oral route. **Storage:** 25°C (77°F); excursions permitted to 15-30°C (59-86°F).

## STAVZOR — RX

valproic acid (Noven)

**Hepatotoxicity, including fatalities, usually during first 6 months of treatment. Children under the age of 2 years are at considerably higher risk of fatal hepatotoxicity. Monitor patients closely and perform liver function tests (LFTs) prior to therapy and at frequent intervals thereafter. Teratogenicity reported, including neural tube defects. Pancreatitis reported, including fatal hemorrhagic cases.**

**THERAPEUTIC CLASS:** Carboxylic acid derivative

**INDICATIONS:** Monotherapy and adjunctive therapy of complex partial seizures that occur in isolation or in association with other types of seizures in patients ≥10 yrs. Treatment of simple and complex absence seizures as sole and adjunctive therapy and adjunctively in patients with multiple seizure types that include absence seizures. Treatment of manic episodes associated with bipolar disorder. Prophylaxis of migraine headaches.

**DOSAGE:** *Adults*: Mania: Initial: 750mg/day in divided doses. Titrate: Increase dose rapidly to achieve clinical effect. Max: 60mg/kg/day. Complex Partial Seizures: Monotherapy/Conversion to Monotherapy/Adjunctive Therapy: Initial: 10-15mg/kg/day. Titrate: Increase weekly by 5-10mg/kg/day until optimal response. Max: 60mg/kg/day. When converting to monotherapy, reduce concomitant antiepilepsy drug by 25% every 2 weeks at the start of therapy or 1-2 weeks after. Simple and Complex Absence Seizures: Initial: 15mg/kg/day. Titrate: Increase weekly by 5-10mg/kg/day until optimal response. Max: 60mg/kg/day. If dose >250mg/day, give in 2-3 doses. Migraine: Initial: 250mg bid. Max: 1000mg/day. Elderly: Reduce initial dose and titrate slowly. Consider dose reduction or d/c in patients with decreased food or fluid intake or if excessive somnolence occurs.

*Pediatrics*: ≥10 yrs: Complex Partial Seizures: Monotherapy/Conversion to Monotherapy/Adjunctive Therapy: Initial: 10-15mg/kg/day. Titrate: Increase weekly by 5-10mg/kg/day until optimal response. Max: 60mg/kg/day. When converting to monotherapy, reduce concomitant antiepilepsy drug by 25% every 2 weeks at the start of therapy or 1-2 weeks after.

**HOW SUPPLIED:** Cap, Delayed-Release: 125mg, 250mg, 500mg

**CONTRAINDICATIONS:** Hepatic disease, significant hepatic dysfunction, and known urea cycle disorders (UCD).

**WARNINGS/PRECAUTIONS:** Increased risk of suicidal thoughts or behavior; monitor for the emergence of worsening and/or any unusual changes in mood or behavior. Hyperammonemic encephalopathy in UCD patients; d/c if this occurs. If unexplained lethargy, hypothermia, vomiting, or mental status changes occur, measure ammonia levels. Caution with hepatic disease; d/c if hepatic failure suspected or apparent. Caution in the elderly; monitor fluid/nutritional intake and for dehydration/somnolence. Dose-related thrombocytopenia and elevated liver enzymes reported. Monitor platelet and coagulation tests prior to therapy, then periodically. Altered thyroid function tests and urine ketone tests. May stimulate replication of HIV and CMV. Avoid abrupt d/c. Multi-organ hypersensitivity reactions and hypothermia reported.

**ADVERSE REACTIONS:** Headache, asthenia, rash, N/V, abdominal pain, dyspepsia, diarrhea, anorexia, somnolence, tremor, dizziness, diplopia, and flu syndrome.

**INTERACTIONS:** Drugs that affect level of expression of hepatic enzymes (eg, phenytoin, carbamazepine, phenobarbital, primidone) may increase valproate clearance. Concomitant use with ASA decreases protein binding and metabolism. Carbapenem antibiotics (eg, ertapenem, imipenem, meropenem) may reduce serum concentration to subtherapeutic levels, resulting in loss of seizure control. Rifampin increases oral clearance and may require valproate dosage adjustment. Concomitant use with felbamate leads to an increase in valproate $C_{max}$. Reduces the clearance of amitriptylline, nortriptyline, and lorazepam. Induces metabolism of carbamazepine. Inhibits metabolism of diazepam, ethosuximide, phenobarbital and phenytoin; monitor drug serum concentrations and adjust dose appropriately. Breakthrough seizures reported with concomitant valproate and phenytoin use. Administration with clonazepam

S

may induce absence status in patients with absence seizures. Increases $T_{1/2}$ of lamotrigine; serious skin reactions reported. Concomitant use with topiramate associated with hyperammonemia, with or without encephalopathy, and hypothermia. May displace protein-bound warfarin; monitor coagulation tests. Additive CNS depression with other CNS depressants (eg, alcohol). May decrease clearance of zidovudine in HIV-seropositive patients.

**PREGNANCY:** Category D, not for use in nursing.

**MECHANISM OF ACTION:** Carboxylic acid derivative; proposed to increase brain concentrations of GABA.

**PHARMACOKINETICS: Absorption:** $T_{max}$=2 hrs (fasting), 4.8 hrs (fed). **Distribution:** $V_d$=11L/1.73m², plasma protein binding (10% at 40mcg/mL and 18.5% at 130mcg/mL), CSF distribution (10%). Found in breast milk. **Metabolism:** Liver via glucuronidation, mitochondrial β-oxidation. **Elimination:** Urine (30-50% glucuronide conjugate, <3% unchanged); $T_{1/2}$=9-16 hrs.

## NURSING CONSIDERATIONS

**Assessment:** Assess LFTs prior to therapy, CBC with platelets, pancreatitis, plasma ammonia levels, hepatic dysfunction/disease, and pregnancy/nursing status. Note other diseases/conditions and drug therapies. Prior to therapy, evaluate for UCD in high-risk patients (eg, history of unexplained encephalopathy, coma, etc.).

**Monitoring:** Monitor LFTs (at frequent intervals during first 6 months), CBC with platelets, coagulation parameters, pancreatitis, ketone and thyroid function tests, plasma drug levels, hyperammonemia, and hypersensitivity reactions. Monitor for emergence/worsening of depression, suicidality, unusual changes in behavior.

**Patient Counseling:** Inform to take exactly as prescribed to get the most benefit and to reduce side effects. Instruct to swallow whole; do not chew. Counsel about signs/symptoms of hepatotoxicity, pancreatitis, and hyperammonemic encephalopathy. Avoid CNS depressants (eg, alcohol). Instruct that a fever associated with other organ system involvement (rash, lymphadenopathy, etc.) may be drug-related and should be reported to physician immediately. Advise not to engage in hazardous actvities (driving or operating machinery). Notify physician if suicidal thoughts, behavior, or thoughts about self harm emerge. Advise to enroll in North American Antiepileptic Drug (NAAED) Pregnancy Registry.

**Administration:** Oral route. **Storage:** 25°C (77°F); excursions permitted to 15-30°C (59-86°F).

# STELARA RX

ustekinumab (Centocor)

S

**THERAPEUTIC CLASS:** Monoclonal antibody

**INDICATIONS:** Treatment of adult patients ( ≥18 yrs) with moderate to severe plaque psoriasis who are candidates for phototherapy or systemic therapy.

**DOSAGE:** *Adults:* ≤100kg: Initial: 45mg SQ and 4 weeks later, followed by 45mg q12 weeks. >100kg: Initial: 90mg SQ and 4 weeks later, followed by 90mg q12 weeks.

**HOW SUPPLIED:** Inj: 45mg/0.5mL, 90mg/1mL

**WARNINGS/PRECAUTIONS:** May increase risk of infections, and reactivate latent infections and malignancy. Serious bacterial, fungal, and viral infections reported; includes cellulitis, diverticulitis, osteomyelitis, viral infections, gastroenteritis, pneumonia, and urinary tract infections. Should not be given with any important clinically active infection. Should not be administered until infection resolves or is adequately treated. Caution with chronic infection or history of recurrent infection. Caution in individuals who are interleukin (IL)-12/IL-23 deficient; disseminated infections from mycobacteria (including nontuberculous, environmental mycobacteria), salmonella (including nontyphi strains), and Bacillus Calmette-Guerin (BCG) vaccinations may occur. Evaluate for TB infection prior to initiation; monitor for signs and symptoms of active TB during and after treatment. Reversible posterior leukoencephalopathy syndrome (RPLS) reported; d/c if suspected. Needle cover on prefilled syringe contains dry natural rubber; caution in latex sensitive individuals. Caution when administering live vaccines to household contact of patients receiving this drug. May increase activity of immune system and increase the risk of certain type of cancers.

**ADVERSE REACTIONS:** Infection, malignancies, RPLS, nasopharyngitis, upper respiratory infection, headache, fatigue.

**INTERACTIONS:** Avoid with live vaccines; BCG vaccines should not be given during treatment or for 1 year prior to initiating treatment or 1 year following d/c of treatment. Non-live vaccinations received during a course of ustekinumab may not elicit an immune response sufficient to prevent disease. Monitor therapeutic effect (eg, warfarin) or drug concentration (eg, cyclosporine) with CYP450 substrates. Not evaluated with immunosuppressive agents or phototherapy.

**PREGNANCY:** Category B, caution in nursing.

**MECHANISM OF ACTION:** Human $IgG1_k$ monoclonal antibody; binds with high affinity and specificity to the p40 protein subunit used by both the IL-12 and IL-23 cytokines. May disrupt IL-12 and IL-23 mediated signaling and cytokine cascades by disrupting the interaction of these cytokines with a shared cell-surface receptor chain, IL-12 β1 (in vitro).

**PHARMACOKINETICS: Absorption:** (SQ): $T_{max}$=13.5 days (45mg) and 7 days (90mg). $C_{max}$=0.31mcg/mL (45mg); $C_{max}$=0.64mcg/mL (90mg). **Distribution:** (SQ) $V_d$=161mL/kg (45mg) and 179mL/kg (90mg). (IV) $V_d$=56.1-82.1mL/kg. Found in breast milk. **Elimination:** (SQ/IV) $T_{1/2}$=14.9-45.6 days.

## NURSING CONSIDERATIONS

**Assessment:** Assess for active/chronic infections, TB, history of recurrent infections, IL-12/IL-23 deficiency, BCG immunization, pregnancy/nursing status, and for possible drug interactions. Assess for symptoms of infection (eg, fever, sweats, chills, muscle aches etc.), cancer types, received vaccines, history of phototherapy, and any other medical conditions.

**Monitoring:** Monitor for serious of infection (eg, cellulitis, diverticulitis, osteomyelitis, viral infections, gastroenteritis, pneumonia, and urinary tract infections), reactivation of latent infections, TB, malignancies, and for RLPS (eg, headache, seizures, confusion, visual disturbances) and diagnostic test (eg, tissue culture and stool culture).

**Patient Counseling:** Instruct patient to seek medical advice if signs or symptoms suggestive of an infection occur. Inform of the risks and benefits of therapy. Inform that therapy may lower the ability of the immune system to fight infections. Counsel about the risk of malignancies while on therapy. Instruct patients of the importance of communicating any history of infections and contacting their physician if they develop any symptoms of infection. Advise latex-sensitive individuals not to handle the needle cover of prefilled syringe since it contains a derivative of latex. Instruct to read the Medication Guide before starting the therapy and to reread it each time the prescription is renewed.



**Administration:** SQ route. Administer each injection at different anatomic location (eg, upper arms, gluteal regions, thighs, or any quadrant abdomen) than the previous injection; not in the areas where skin is tender, bruised, erythematous or indurated. Use 27 gauge, 1/2 inch needle for single-use vial. For prefilled syringes, avoid touching the needle guard activation clip at any time during use to prevent premature activation of the needle safety guard and do not hold the plunger/plunger head while removing needle cover. Inject all the medications by pushing the plunger head in completely between the needle guard wings. Maintain the pressure on the plunger and remove the needle from the skin. **Storage:** Store upright and refrigerated at 2-8°C (36-46°F). Protect from light. Do not freeze or shake. Discard any unused portion.

# STRATTERA RX
atomoxetine HCl (Lilly)

**Increased risk of suicidal ideation in short-term studies in children or adolescents with ADHD. Closely monitor for suicidality, clinical worsening, or unusual changes in behavior. Close observation and communication with the prescriber by families and caregivers is advised. Not approved for major depressive disorder.**

**THERAPEUTIC CLASS:** Selective norepinephrine reuptake inhibitor

**INDICATIONS:** Treatment of attention-deficit hyperactivity disorder (ADHD).

**DOSAGE:** *Adults:* Initial: 40mg/day given qam or evenly divided doses in the am and late afternoon/early evening. Titrate: Increase after minimum of 3 days to target dose of about 80mg/day. After 2-4 weeks, may increase to 100mg/day. Max: 100mg/day. Hepatic Insufficiency: Moderate (Child-Pugh Class B): Reduce initial and target doses to 50% of normal dose. Severe (Child-Pugh Class C): Reduce initial and target doses to 25% of normal dose. Concomitant CYP2D6 Inhibitor (eg, paroxetine, fluoxetine, quinidine): Initial: 40mg/day. Titrate: Only increase to 80mg/day if symptoms fail to improve after 4 weeks.

*Pediatrics:* ≥6 yrs: ≤70kg: Initial: 0.5mg/kg/day given qam or evenly divided doses in the am and late afternoon/early evening. Titrate: Increase after minimum of 3 days to target dose of about 1.2mg/kg/day. Max: 1.4mg/kg/day or 100mg, whichever is less. >70kg: Initial: 40mg/day given qam or evenly divided doses in the am and late afternoon/early evening. Titrate: Increase after minimum of 3 days to target dose of about 80mg/day. After 2-4 weeks, may increase to 100mg/day. Max: 100mg/day. Hepatic Insufficiency: Moderate (Child-Pugh Class B): Reduce initial and target doses to 50% of the normal dose. Severe (Child-Pugh Class C): Reduce initial and target doses to 25% of normal dose. Concomitant CYP2D6 Inhibitor (eg, paroxetine, fluoxetine, quinidine): ≥6 yrs: ≤70kg: Initial: 0.5mg/kg/day. Titrate: Only increase to 1.2mg/kg/day if symptoms fail to improve after 4 weeks. >70kg: Initial: 40mg/day. Titrate: Only increase to 80mg/day if symptoms fail to improve after 4 weeks.

**HOW SUPPLIED:** Cap: 10mg, 18mg, 25mg, 40mg, 60mg, 80mg, 100mg

**CONTRAINDICATIONS:** During or within 14 days of MAOI use and narrow-angle glaucoma.

**WARNINGS/PRECAUTIONS:** Monitor for clinical worsening, emergence of suicidality, agitation, irritability, unusual changes in behavior. Reports of MI, stroke, and sudden death in adults. Avoid use with known structural cardiac abnormalities or other serious cardiac problems. Physical exam and evaluation of patient history is necessary. May increase BP and HR; caution with HTN, tachycardia, CV or cerebrovascular disease. Orthostatic hypotension and syncope reported; caution in any conditions that may predispose to hypotension or with abrupt HR or BP changes. May cause severe liver injury in rare cases; monitor liver enzymes and d/c with jaundice or laboratory evidence of liver injury. Stimulants at usual doses may cause treatment-emergent psychotic or manic symptoms (eg, hallucinations, delusional thinking, mania) in children and adolescents without prior history of psychotic illness. May increase urinary retention and hesitation. Rare cases of priapism reported. Monitor growth in children.

**ADVERSE REACTIONS:** Abdominal pain, N/V, fatigue, decreased appetite, somnolence, dizziness, headache, dry mouth, insomnia, constipation, hot flushes, urinary hesitation/retention, and decreased weight.

**INTERACTIONS:** See Contraindications. May potentiate the CV effects of systemically administered albuterol or other $\beta_2$ agonists. Caution with pressor agents (eg, dopamine, dobutamine). Increased levels with CYP2D6 inhibitors (eg, paroxetine, fluoxetine, quinidine); may need dose adjustment. Coadministration with midazolam increased the AUC of midazolam.

**PREGNANCY:** Category C, caution in nursing.



S

**MECHANISM OF ACTION:** Selective norepinephrine reuptake inhibitor; mechanism not established. May selectively inhibit the presynaptic norepinephrine transporter.

**PHARMACOKINETICS: Absorption:** Rapid; well absorbed; absolute bioavailability [extensive metabolizers (63%), poor metabolizers (94%)]; $T_{max}$=1-2 hrs. **Distribution:** $V_d$=0.85L/kg; plasma protein binding (98%). **Metabolism:** Via CYP2D6; 4-hydroxyatomoxetine (major metabolite). **Elimination:** Urine (>80% [4-hydroxyatomoxetine-O-glucuronide] and <3% [unchanged]), feces (<17%); $T_{1/2}$=5 hrs.

## NURSING CONSIDERATIONS

**Assessment:** Assess for BP, HR, renal function, LFTs, agitation, glaucoma, tics, family history of Tourette's syndrome, CV conditions (eg, severe HTN, cardiac abnormalities, arrhythmias, HF, recent MI), cerebrovascular disease, bipolar disorder, history of drug dependence or alcoholism, hypersensitivity, pregnancy/nursing status and possible drug interactions.

**Monitoring:** Monitor for cardiac abnormalities, bipolar disorder, suicidality, clinical worsening or unusual changes in behavior, seizures, and visual disturbances. Monitor height and weight in children, LFTs, hypersensitivity reactions (angioneurotic edema), urinary retention, and priapism.

**Patient Counseling:** Inform about risks of treatment and appropriate use. Encourage patients, their families and caregivers to be alert for the emergence of depression, suicidal ideation and other unusual changes in behavior. Advise to contact physician if symptoms of liver injury (eg, pruritus, dark urine, jaundice) or priapism occur. Drug is an occular irritant; avoid contact with eyes. Caution while operating machinery/driving. Avoid late evening doses to prevent insomnia.

**Administration:** Oral route. Take whole w/ or w/o food; do not open cap. **Storage:** 25°C (77°F); excursions permitted to 15-30°C (59-86°F).

# SUBLIMAZE CII

fentanyl citrate (Taylor)

**THERAPEUTIC CLASS:** Opioid analgesic

**INDICATIONS:** For analgesic action of short duration during the anesthetic periods, premedication, induction and maintenance, and in the immediate postoperative period (recovery room) as the need arises. For use as a narcotic analgesic supplement in general or regional anesthesia. For administration with a neuroleptic as an anesthetic premedication, for the induction of anesthesia and as an adjunct in the maintenance of general and regional anesthesia. For use as an anesthetic agent with oxygen in selected high-risk patients, such as those undergoing open heart surgery or certain complicated neurological or orthopedic procedures.

**DOSAGE:** *Adults:* Individualized: Premedication: 50-100mcg IM 30-60 min prior to surgery. Adjunct to General Anesthesia: Low-Dose: Total Dose: 2mcg/kg for minor surgery. Maint: 2mcg/kg. Moderate Dose: Total Dose: 2-20mcg/kg for major surgery. Maint: 2-20mcg/kg or 25-100mcg IM or IV if surgical stress or lightening of analgesia. High-Dose: Total Dose: 20-50mcg/kg for open heart surgery, complicated neurosurgery, or orthopedic surgery. Maint: 20-50mcg/kg. Additional dosage selected must be individualized, especially if the anticipated remaining operative time is short. Adjunct to Regional Anesthesia: 50-100mcg IM or slow IV over 1-2 min. Post-op: 50-100mcg IM, repeat q 1-2 hrs PRN. General Anesthetic: 50-100mcg/kg with oxygen and a muscle relaxant, up to 150mcg/kg may be used. Elderly/Debilitated patient: Start at low end of dosing range.
*Pediatrics:* 2-12 yrs: Individualized: Induction/Maint: 2-3mcg/kg.

**HOW SUPPLIED:** Inj: 50mcg/mL

**WARNINGS/PRECAUTIONS:** Administer only by persons specifically trained in the use of IV anesthetics and management of the respiratory effects of potent opioids. An opioid antagonist, resuscitative and intubation equipment and oxygen should be readily available. Fluids and other countermeasures to manage hypotension should be available when used with tranquilizers. Initial dose reduction recommended with narcotic analgesia for recovery. May cause muscle rigidity particularly with muscles used for respiration. Adequate facilities should be available for postoperative monitoring and ventilation. Caution in respiratory depression-susceptible patients (eg, comatose patients with head injury or brain tumor). May cause euphoria, miosis, bradycardia and bronchoconstriction and obscure the clinical course of patients with head injury. Reduce dose for elderly and debilitated patients. Caution with obstructive pulmonary disease, decreased respiratory reserve, liver and kidney dysfunction, cardiac bradyarrhythmias. Monitor vital signs routinely.

**ADVERSE REACTIONS:** Respiratory depression, apnea, rigidity, bradycardia.

**INTERACTIONS:** Severe and unpredictable potentiation by MAOIs has been reported. Appropriate monitoring and availability of vasodilators and β-blockers for the treatment of HTN is indicated. Additive or potentiating effects with other CNS depressants (eg, barbiturates, tranquilizers, narcotics, general anesthetics); reduce dose of other CNS depressants. Reports of CV depression with nitrous oxide. Alteration of respiration with certain forms of conduction anesthesia (eg, spinal anesthesia, some peridural anesthesia). Decreased pulmonary arterial pressure and hypotension with tranquilizers. May cause CV depression with diazepam. Elevated BP, with and without HTN, reported in combination with a neuroleptic; neuroleptic agents should be administered with extreme caution in the presence of risk factors for development of prolonged QT syndrome and torsades de pointes.

**PREGNANCY:** Category C, caution with nursing.

**MECHANISM OF ACTION:** Narcotic analgesic; produces analgesic and sedative effects. Alters respiratory rate and alveolar ventilation, which may last longer than analgesic effects.

**PHARMACOKINETICS: Distribution:** $V_d$=4L/kg. **Metabolism:** Liver. **Elimination:** Urine (75%, <10% unchanged), feces (9%); $T_{1/2}$=219 min.

## NURSING CONSIDERATIONS

**Assessment:** Assess the kind and duration of the surgery; the availability of opioid antagonist, resuscitative and intubation equipment and oxygen. Assess for intolerance to other opioid agonists, risk of respiratory depression (eg, comatose patients, presence of head injury, brain tumor), impaired respiration (eg, COPD), bradyarrhythmias, impaired hepatic or renal function, nursing/pregnancy status, and possible drug interactions. If combined with a neuroleptic, assess for risk of QT prolongation (eg, bradycardia, cardiac disease, electrolyte imbalance). Assess use in the elderly and debilitated patient.

**Monitoring:** Monitor for signs/symptoms of respiratory depression, muscle rigidity, medication abuse, and drug dependence. If given with nitrous oxide, monitor for CV depression. If administered with a tranquilizer, monitor for hypotension and hypovolemia. If combined with a neuroleptic, monitor for increases in BP; perform ECG monitoring. Monitor for severe and unpredictable potentiation by MAOIs if used within 14 days. Perform routine monitoring of vital signs.



**Patient Counseling:** Inform drug should be administered by persons specifically trained in use of IV anesthetics and management of respiratory effects of potent opioids. Inform patient to notify physician prior to surgery if with impaired respiration (eg. COPD), liver/kidney dysfunction, and CV problems (eg. bradyarrhythmias).

**Administration:** IM/IV route. **Storage:** 20-25°C (68-77°F). Protect from light. (Generic) Excursions permitted 15-30°C (59-86°F).

## SUBOXONE CIII

buprenorphine HCl - naloxone HCl dihydrate (Reckitt Benckiser)

**OTHER BRAND NAMES:** Subutex (Reckitt Benckiser)

**THERAPEUTIC CLASS:** Partial opioid agonist/opioid antagonist

**INDICATIONS:** Opioid dependence.

**DOSAGE:** *Adults:* Give either agent SL as a single daily dose in the range of 12-16mg/day. Hold tabs under tongue until dissolved; swallowing tabs reduces bioavailability. Induction: Subutex: Give at least 4 hrs after last short-acting opioid (eg, heroin) use or preferably when early signs of opioid withdrawal appear. Maint: Suboxone: Range: 4mg-24mg/day. Target dose: 16mg/day. Titrate: Adjust by 2mg or 4mg to a level that maintains treatment and suppresses opioid withdrawal effects. Hepatic Impairment: Adjust dose and observe for precipitated opioid withdrawal. Concomitant CNS Depressants: Consider dose reduction.

*Pediatrics:* ≥16 yrs: Give either agent SL as a single daily dose in the range of 12-16mg/day. Hold tabs under tongue until dissolved; swallowing tabs reduces bioavailability. Induction: Subutex: Give at least 4 hrs after last short-acting opioid (eg, heroin) use or preferably when early signs of opioid withdrawal appear. Maint: Suboxone: Range: 4mg-24mg/day. Target dose: 16mg/day. Titrate: Adjust by 2mg or 4mg to a level that maintains treatment and suppresses opioid withdrawal effects. Hepatic Impairment: Adjust dose and observe for precipitated opioid withdrawal. Concomitant CNS Depressants: Consider dose reduction.

**HOW SUPPLIED:** Suboxone (Buprenorphine-Naloxone) Tab, SL: 2mg-0.5mg, 8mg-2mg. Subutex (Buprenorphine) Tab, SL: 2mg, 8mg

**WARNINGS/PRECAUTIONS:** Significant respiratory depression reported with buprenorphine; caution with compromised respiratory function. Naloxone may not be effective in reversing any respiratory depression produced by buprenorphine. Cytolytic hepatitis and hepatitis with jaundice reported. Obtain LFTs prior to initiation and periodically thereafter. Acute and chronic hypersensitivity reactions reported. May increase CSF pressure; caution with head injury, intracranial lesions. May cause miosis, changes in level of consciousness, and orthostatic hypotension. Caution with elderly, debilitated, myxedema, hypothyroidism, acute alcoholism, Addison's disease, CNS depression or coma, toxic psychoses, prostatic hypertrophy, urethral stricture, delirium tremens, kyphoscoliosis, biliary tract dysfunction or severe hepatic/renal/pulmonary impairment. Suboxone may cause opioid withdrawal symptoms. May obscure diagnosis of acute abdominal conditions. May produce dependence.

**ADVERSE REACTIONS:** Headache, infection, pain (general, abdomen, back), withdrawal syndrome, constipation, nausea, insomnia, sweating, asthenia, anxiety, depression, rhinitis.

**INTERACTIONS:** May need dose reduction with CYP3A4 inhibitors (eg, azole antifungals, macrolides and HIV protease inhibitors). General anesthetics, other narcotic analgesics, benzodiazepines, phenothiazines, other tranquilizers, sedative/hypnotics or other CNS depressants (including alcohol) may increase risk of CNS depression; consider dose reduction of one or both agents. Monitor closely with CYP3A4 inducers (eg, phenobarbital, carbamazepine, phenytoin, rifampicin).

**PREGNANCY:** Category C, not for use in nursing.

**MECHANISM OF ACTION:** Buprenorphine: Partial agonist at the μ-opioid receptor, antagonist at the kappa-opioid receptor. Naloxone: Inhibits μ-opioid receptor activity.

**PHARMACOKINETICS: Absorption:** (Suboxone 16mg) $C_{max}$=5.95ng/mL, AUC=34.89 hr•ng/mL. (Subtex 16mg) $C_{max}$=5.47ng/mL, AUC=32.63 hr•ng/mL. Refer to PI for more detailed information. **Distribution:** Plasma protein binding 96% (buprenorphine), 45% (naloxone). **Metabolism:** Buprenorphine: Through N-dealkylation and glucuronidation pathways; norbuprenorphine (active metabolite). Naloxone: Through glucuronidation, N-dealkylation, and reduction. **Elimination:** Urine (30%), feces (69%); $T_{1/2}$=37 hrs (Buprenorphine), 1.1 hrs (Naloxone).

## NURSING CONSIDERATIONS

**Assessment:** Assess for hepatic/renal and pulmonary impairment, myxedema or hypothyroidism, Addison's disease, toxic psychosis, CNS depression or coma, prostatic hypertrophy or uretheral stricture, biliary tract dysfunction, acute abdominal conditions, pregnancy/nursing status, head injury or

S

intracranial lesions, increased CSF, alcohol intake, possible drug interactions. Perform LFTs prior to therapy and periodically thereafter.

**Monitoring:** Monitor LFTs. Monitor for signs/symptoms of respiratory/CNS depression, drug dependence, hepatitis, allergic reactions or anaphylactic shock, orthostatic hypotension, elevation of CSF.

**Patient Counseling:** Caution against hazardous tasks (eg, operating machinery/driving). Notify if pregnant/nursing. Concurrent administration of sedatives or alcohol may lead to serious overdose or death. Notify if taking or planning to take other medication.

**Administration:** Oral route. **Storage:** 25°C (77°F); excursions permitted to 15-30°C (59-86°F).

## SUFENTA

sufentanil citrate (Akorn)

CII

**THERAPEUTIC CLASS:** Opioid analgesic

**INDICATIONS:** Analgesic adjunct in the maintenance of balanced general anesthesia in patients who are intubated and ventilated. Primary anesthetic agent of the induction and maintenance of anesthesia with 100% oxygen in patients undergoing major surgical procedures who are intubated or ventilated, such as cardiovascular surgery or neurosurgical procedures in the sitting position, to provide favorable myocardial and cerebral oxygen balance or when extended postoperative ventilation is anticipated. For epidural administrations an analgesic combined with low dose bupivacaine, usually 12.5mg per administration during labor and vaginal delivery.

**DOSAGE:** *Adults:* ≥12 yrs: Individualize dose. Premedication: Based on patients needs. Analgesic: Total Dose: 1-8mcg/kg. Maint: Incremental: 10-50mcg. Infusion: Based on induction dose not to exceed 1mcg/kg/hr. Anesthetic: Total Dose: 8-30mcg/kg. Maint: Incremental 0.5-10mcg/kg. Infusion: Based on induction dose not to exceed 30mcg/kg. Epidural: 10-15mcg with 10mL bupivacaine 0.125% with or without epinephrine. May repeat for a total of 3 doses in not less than 1 hour intervals.
*Pediatrics:* Individualize dose. 10-25mcg/kg with 100% oxygen. Maint: 25-50mcg supplemental doses.

**HOW SUPPLIED:** Inj: 50mcg/mL

**WARNINGS/PRECAUTIONS:** Should only be administered by persons specifically trained in the use of IV and epidural anesthetics and management of the respiratory effects of potent opioids. An opioid antagonist, resuscitative and intubation equipment and oxygen should be readily available. Prior to catheter insertion, the physician should be familiar with patient conditions (such as infection at the injection site, bleeding diathesis, anticoagulation therapy) which call for special evaluation of the benefit versus risk potential. May cause muscle rigidity of the neck and extremities. Adequate facilities should be available for postoperative monitoring and ventilation. Monitor vital signs routinely. Reduce dose for elderly and debilitated patients. Caution with pulmonary disease, decreased respiratory reserve, liver and kidney dysfunction, cardiac bradyarrhythmias. Reports of bradycardia responsive to atropine. May obscure clinical course of patients with head injuries.



**ADVERSE REACTIONS:** Respiratory depression, skeletal muscle rigidity, bradycardia, HTN, hypotension, chest wall rigidity, somnolence, pruritus, N/V.

**INTERACTIONS:** Reports of cardiovascular depression with nitrous oxide. High doses of pancuronium may produce increase in heart rate. Reports of bradycardia and hypotension with other muscle relaxants. Greater incidence and degree of bradycardia and hypotension with chronic CCB and β-blocker therapy. Additive or potentiating effects with other CNS depressants (eg, barbiturates, tranquilizers, narcotics, general anesthetics). Reduce dose of either agent. Decrease in mean arterial pressure and systemic vascular resistance with benzodiazepines.

**PREGNANCY:** Category C, caution in nursing.

**MECHANISM OF ACTION:** An opioid analgesic.

**PHARMACOKINETICS: Distribution:** Plasma protein binding (healthy males: 93%, mothers: 91%, neonates: 79%). **Elimination:** $T_{1/2}$=164 min (adults), 97 min (neonates).

## NURSING CONSIDERATIONS

**Assessment:** Assess for pulmonary disease, decreased respiratory reserve, hepatic/renal dysfunction, cardiac bradyarrhythmias, head injury, and possible drug interactions.

**Monitoring:** Monitor for cardiovascular depression (eg, bradycardia and hypotension), respiratory depression, muscle rigidity of the neck and extremities, N/V, chills, arrhythmias, chest wall rigidity. Monitor vital signs routinely. Appropriate postoperative monitoring should ensure that adequate spontaneous breathing is established and maintained prior to discharging patient.

**Patient Counseling:** Counsel about side effects of drug and abuse potential.

**Absorption:** IV and epidural route. **Storage:** 20-25°C (68-77°F). Protect from light.

# SULAR RX

nisoldipine (Sciele)

**THERAPEUTIC CLASS:** Calcium channel blocker (dihydropyridine)

**INDICATIONS:** Treatment of hypertension alone or in combination with other antihypertensive agents.

**DOSAGE:** *Adults:* Initial: 17mg qd. Titrate: Increase by 8.5mg weekly or longer. Maint: 17-34mg qd. Max: 34mg/day. Elderly (>65 yrs)/Hepatic Dysfunction: Initial: Do not exceed 8.5mg/day. Take on an empty stomach (1 hr ac or 2 hrs pc). Swallow whole.

**HOW SUPPLIED:** Tab, Extended-Release: 8.5mg, 17mg, 25.5mg, 34mg

**WARNINGS/PRECAUTIONS:** May increase angina or MI in patients with severe obstructive coronary artery disease (CAD). May cause hypotension; monitor BP initially or with titration. Caution with heart failure or compromised ventricular function, especially with concomitant β-blockers. Caution with severe hepatic dysfunction or in elderly.

**ADVERSE REACTIONS:** Peripheral edema, headache, dizziness, pharyngitis, vasodilation, sinusitis, palpitations.

**INTERACTIONS:** Increased AUC and $C_{max}$ with cimetidine. Avoid phenytoin or CYP3A4 inducers and inhibitors. Decreased bioavailability with quinidine. Avoid high-fat meals as they increase peak drug levels. Avoid grapefruit juice.

**PREGNANCY:** Category C, not for use in nursing.

**MECHANISM OF ACTION:** Calcium channel antagonist (dihydropyridine); inhibits transmembrane influx of calcium into vascular smooth muscle and cardiac muscle resulting in dilation of arterioles and decreased peripheral vascular resistance.

**PHARMACOKINETICS: Absorption:** Well absorbed; absolute bioavailability (5%); $T_{max}$=9.2 hrs. **Metabolism:** CYP3A4 via hydroxylation. **Elimination:** Urine: (60-80%); $T_{1/2}$=13.7 hrs.

## NURSING CONSIDERATIONS

**Assessment:** Assess for CAD, CHF, LFTs, BP, pregnancy/nursing status, and possible drug interactions.

**Monitoring:** Monitor BP, LFTs. Monitor for peripheral edema, headache, dizziness, vasodilation, chest pain, rash, CBC with differential and platelet count, DM, thyroiditis, atrial fibrillation, hypokalemia, hematuria, sinusitis.

**Patient Counseling:** Instruct to swallow whole; do not chew, divide, or crush. Counsel about adverse effects; seek medical attention if any develop. Avoid concomitant intake of high-fat meal. Do not take with grapefruit juice.

**Administration:** Oral route. **Storage:** 20-25°C (68-77°F); excursions permitted to 15-30°C (59-86°F). Protect from moisture. Dispense in tight, light-resistant container.

## SULINDAC RX

sulindac (Various)

**NSAIDs may cause an increased risk of serious cardiovascular thrombotic events, MI, stroke, and serious GI adverse events including bleeding, ulceration, and perforation of the stomach or intestines. Contraindicated for the treatment of perioperative pain in the setting of coronary artery bypass graft (CABG) surgery.**

**OTHER BRAND NAMES:** Clinoril (Merck)

**THERAPEUTIC CLASS:** NSAID

**INDICATIONS:** Acute or long-term use for osteoarthritis (OA), rheumatoid arthritis (RA), ankylosing spondylitis (AS), acute painful shoulder, and acute gouty arthritis.

**DOSAGE:** *Adults:* OA/RA/AS: Initial: 150mg bid. Titrate: May increase or reduce dose depending on clinical response. Acute Painful Shoulder/Acute Gouty Arthritis: 200mg bid for 7-14 days. Max: 400mg/day. Take with food.

**HOW SUPPLIED:** Tab: 150mg, 200mg* *scored

**CONTRAINDICATIONS:** ASA or other NSAID allergy that precipitates acute asthmatic attack, urticaria, or rhinitis. Treatment of perioperative pain in the setting of CABG surgery.

**WARNINGS/PRECAUTIONS:** May lead to onset of new HTN or worsening of pre-existing HTN; monitor BP closely. Fluid retention and edema reported; caution with fluid retention or heart failure. Renal papillary necrosis and other renal injury reported after long-term use. Not recommended for use with advanced renal disease; if therapy must be initiated, monitor renal function. Anaphylactoid reactions may occur. May cause serious skin adverse events (eg, exfoliative dermatitis, Stevens-Johnson syndrome, and toxic epidermal necrolysis). Avoid in late pregnancy; may cause premature closure of ductus arteriosis. May cause elevation of LFTs; d/c if abnormal LFTs persist/worsen, liver disease develops, or systemic manifestations occur. Caution in elderly. Anemia may occur; monitor Hgb/Hct with long-term use. May inhibit platelet aggregation and prolong bleeding time; monitor with coagulation disorders. Caution with asthma and avoid with ASA-sensitive asthma. Keep patients well hydrated and caution with renal lithiasis. Pancreatitis reported; if pancreatitis suspected, d/c and do not restart. Adverse eye findings reported. Monitor closely with poor liver function and consider dose reduction. Increased risk of aseptic meningitis in patients with systemic lupus erythematosus (SLE) and mixed connective tissue disease. Risk of GI ulceration, bleeding, and perforation.

S

**ADVERSE REACTIONS:** GI pain, dyspepsia, N/V, diarrhea, constipation, rash, dizziness, headache, tinnitus, edema, MI, stroke, ulceration, GI perforation, and cardiovascular thrombotic events. As with other NSAIDs anaphylactic/anaphylactoid reactions may occur in patients without known prior exposure to this product.

**INTERACTIONS:** Avoid DMSO, ASA, and other NSAIDs. May increase methotrexate and cyclosporine toxicities. Probenecid may increase plasma levels. Diflunisal may decrease plasma levels. May diminish antihypertensive effect of ACE inhibitors and reduce natriuretic effect of diuretics. May elevate plasma lithium levels. Increased risk of GI bleeding with warfarin.

**PREGNANCY:** Category C, not for use in nursing.

**MECHANISM OF ACTION:** NSAID; suspected to inhibit prostaglandin synthetase; exerts anti-inflammatory, analgesic, and antipyretic actions.

**PHARMACOKINETICS: Absorption:** PO administration of variable doses resulted in different parameters. **Distribution:** Penetrates placental and blood brain barrier. Plasma protein binding: Sulindac (93.1%), sulindac sulfone (95.4%), sulindac sulfide (97.9%). **Metabolism:** Via oxidation and reduction.

**Elimination:** Urine (50%), feces 25% (metabolites); $T_{1/2}$ (sulindac, sulindac sulfide)=7.8, 16.4 hrs.

## NURSING CONSIDERATIONS

**Assessment:** Assess LFTs, renal function, CBCs, and coagulation profile. Assess for history of CABG surgery, asthma and allergic reactions to aspirin or other NSAIDs, active ulceration or chronic inflammation of GI tract, CVD (CHF, MI), asthma, pregnancy status, SLE, possible drug interactions.

**Monitoring:** Monitor for hypersensitivity reactions (anaphylaxis), cardiac complications, stroke, GI bleeding, asthma, skin reactions (Stevens-Johnson syndrome, toxic epidermal necrolysis). Monitor BP, LFTs, renal function, CBCs with differential and platelet count, coagulation profile, ophthalmologic studies.

**Patient Counseling:** Counsel about potential side effects (eg, anaphylaxis, edema, jaundice, GI discomfort, MI, stroke); seek medical attention if any develop. Avoid alcohol and smoking during treatment. Take drug as prescribed. Caution women against use in late pregnancy.

**Administration:** Oral route. **Storage:** 15-30°C (59-86°F). Store in air tight container.

# SUPARTZ RX

sodium hyaluronate (Smith & Nephew)

**THERAPEUTIC CLASS:** Hyaluronan

**INDICATIONS:** Treatment of pain in osteoarthritis of the knee in patients who have failed to respond adequately to conservative non-pharmacologic therapy and simple analgesics (eg, APAP).

**DOSAGE:** *Adults:* Administer 2.5mL by intra-articular injection once a week for a total of 5 injections. Some patients may experience benefit with 3 injections given at weekly intervals. Use strict aseptic technique.

**HOW SUPPLIED:** Inj: 2.5mL

**CONTRAINDICATIONS:** Avoid with knee infections or skin diseases in the area of the injection site.

**WARNINGS/PRECAUTIONS:** Avoid disinfectants containing quaternary ammonium salts for skin preparation; hyaluronic acid can precipitate in their presence. Transient pain and/or swelling of the injected joint may occur. Safety and effectiveness in joints other than the knee or concomitantly with other intra-articular injectables have not been established. Caution in patients who are allergic to avian proteins, feathers, and egg products. Avoid any strenuous activities or prolonged (eg, more than 1 hr) weight-bearing activities within 48 hours following the intra-articular injection. Remove any joint effusion before injecting. Safety and effectiveness have not been demonstrated in children.

**ADVERSE REACTIONS:** Arthralgia, arthropathy, arthrosis, arthritis, back pain, pain (non-specific), injection-site reaction, headache, injection-site pain.

**PREGNANCY:** Safety in pregnancy and nursing not known.

**MECHANISM OF ACTION:** Hyaluronan.

## NURSING CONSIDERATIONS

**Assessment:** Assess for skin infections or disease in area of injection site, use of disinfectants containing quaternary ammonium salts, knee joint infections, and pregnancy/nursing status.

**Monitoring:** Monitor for knee joint swelling/effusion and local skin reaction.

**Patient Counseling:** Inform that drug may cause transient pain/swelling at injection site. Avoid strenuous activities or prolonged weight-bearing activities (jogging, tennis) within 48 hrs following injection.

**Administration:** Intra-articular. **Storage:** Below 25°C (77°F). Do not freeze. Shelf life is 42 months.

## SUPRAX RX

cefixime (Lupin)

**THERAPEUTIC CLASS:** Cephalosporin (3rd generation)

**INDICATIONS:** Otitis media, pharyngitis, tonsillitis, acute bronchitis, acute exacerbation of chronic bronchitis, uncomplicated UTIs, and cervical/urethral gonorrhea caused by susceptible strains.

**DOSAGE:** *Adults:* Usual: 400mg qd. Gonorrhea: 400mg single dose. CrCl 21-60mL/min/Hemodialysis: Give 75% of standard dose. CrCl <20mL/min/CAPD: Give 50% of standard dose.
*Pediatrics:* >12 yrs or >50kg: (Tab/Sus) Usual: 400mg qd. ≥6 months: (Sus) 8mg/kg qd or 4mg/kg bid. Treat for at least 10 days with *S.pyogenes*. CrCl 21-60mL/min/Hemodialysis: Give 75% of standard dose. CrCl <20mL/min/CAPD: Give 50% of standard dose.

**HOW SUPPLIED:** Tab: 400mg; Sus: 100mg/5mL [50mL, 75mL, 100mL]

**WARNINGS/PRECAUTIONS:** Caution with PCN or other allergy, GI disease (eg, colitis). Anaphylactic/anaphylactoid reactions, pseudomembranous colitis reported. May cause false (+) direct Coombs test or false (+) reaction for urinary glucose using Benedict's/Fehling's solution or Clinitest.

**ADVERSE REACTIONS:** Diarrhea, abdominal pain, nausea, dyspepsia, flatulence, superinfection.

**INTERACTIONS:** May increase carbamazepine levels. Increased PT with anticoagulants (eg, warfarin).

**PREGNANCY:** Category B, not for use in nursing.

**MECHANISM OF ACTION:** 3rd-generation cephalosporin; inhibits cell-wall synthesis.

**PHARMACOKINETICS: Absorption:** 40-50% absorbed. $C_{max}$=2mcg/mL (200mg tab), 3.7mcg/mL (400mg tab), 3mcg/mL (200mg sus), 4.6mcg/mL (400mg sus); $T_{max}$=2-6 hrs (200mg tab, 400mg tab/sus), 2-5 hrs (200mg sus). **Distribution:** Serum protein binding (65%). **Elimination:** Urine (50% unchanged); $T_{1/2}$=3-4 up to 9 hrs.

### NURSING CONSIDERATIONS

**Assessment:** Assess for previous hypersensitivity to cephalosporins/PCNs or other drugs, renal/hepatic impairment, GI tract disease (eg, colitis), nutritional status, those receiving protracted course of antibiotics or anticoagulants, pregnancy/nursing status, possible drug interactions.

**Monitoring:** Monitor for PT with vitamin K administration as indicated. Monitor for signs/symtoms of anaphylatic/anaphylactoid reactions, pseudomembranous colitis or CDAD, development of drug resistance, superinfection, pancytopenia, agranulocytosis and lab test interference (eg, false (+) reaction of urinary ketones if using nitroprusside, false (+) reaction for urinary glucose if using Clinitest, Benedict's or Fehling's solution, false (+) Coombs' test). Monitor renal function tests, LFTs, LDH, and CBCs.

**Patient Counseling:** Inform that therapy only treats bacterial, not viral, infections. Take exactly as directed; skipping doses or not completing full course may decrease effectiveness and increase resistance. Inform about benefits/risks. D/C and notify physician if diarrhea or allergic reactions occur. Notify if pregnant/nursing.

**Administration:** Oral route. **Storage:** Sus/Tab, 20-25°C (68-77°F). After mixing, store sus at room temperature or under refrigeration for 14 days; keep tightly closed and shake well before use.



## SUSTIVA RX

efavirenz (Bristol-Myers Squibb)

**THERAPEUTIC CLASS:** Non-nucleoside reverse transcriptase inhibitor

**INDICATIONS:** Treatment of HIV-1 infection in combination with other antiretrovirals.

**DOSAGE:** *Adults:* Initial: 600mg PO qd. Take on an empty stomach hs. Concomitant with voriconazole: Reduce to 300mg PO qd (Sustiva) and 400mg q12h (Voriconazole).
*Pediatrics:* ≥3 yrs: 10-<15kg: 200mg PO qd. 15 to <20kg: 250mg PO qd. 20-<25kg: 300mg PO qd. 25-<32.5kg: 350mg PO qd. 32.5-<40kg: 400mg PO qd. ≥40kg: 600mg PO qd. Take on an empty stomach hs.

**HOW SUPPLIED:** Cap: 50mg, 200mg; Tab: 600mg

**CONTRAINDICATIONS:** Concomitant use with bepridil, cisapride, midazolam, pimozide, triazolam, ergot derivatives (eg, dihydroergotamine, ergonovine, ergotamine, methylergonovine), St. John's wort.

**WARNINGS/PRECAUTIONS:** Not for use as monotherapy. Serious psychiatric symptoms (eg, depression, suicidal ideation) reported. CNS adverse events (eg, dizziness, insomnia) are frequent during 1-2 days after initiating therapy and resolve in 2-4 weeks. May impair mental/physical abilities. Avoid pregnancy while on therapy; use of adequate contraceptive measures for 12 weeks after d/c is recommended. Monitor LFTs with known or suspected hepatitis B (HBV) or C (HCV) infection. D/C if severe rash develops. Caution in patients with history of seizures; convulsions have been reported. Increased total cholesterol and TG levels reported; monitor prior to therapy and periodically thereafter. Possible redistribution/accumulation of body fat. Immune reconstitution syndrome reported.

**ADVERSE REACTIONS:** CNS symptoms (eg, dizziness, insomnia, impaired concentration, somnolence, abnormal dreams), psychiatric symptoms (eg, anxiety, nervousness, severe depression), rash, GI effects (eg, N/V, diarrhea, dyspepsia, abdominal pain), increased ALT/AST/GGT/glucose/amylase levels, and decreased neutrophils.

**INTERACTIONS:** See Contraindications. CYP3A4 inducers (eg, phenobarbital, rifampin, rifabutin) may increase clearance resulting in lowered plasma concentration. Decreased levels of amprenavir, atazanavir, indinavir, lopinavir and saquinavir. Concomitant use with ritonavir result in higher frequency of adverse reaction and laboratory abnormalities; monitor LFTs. May affect warfarin levels. Caution when used with anticonvulsants (carbamazepine, phenytoin); monitor anticonvulsant levels. Decreased sertraline, calcium channel blockers (diltiazem, felodipine, nicardipine, nifedipine, and verapamil), atorvastatin, pravastatin, simvastatin and immmunosuppressants (cyclosporine, tacrolimus, sirolimus) levels. Decreased levels of voriconazole, itraconazole, and ketoconazole. Decreased progestin levels (norelgestromin, levonorgestrel). Decreased levels of clarithromycin; consider alternative. May decrease methadone levels; monitor for signs of withdrawal. Additive CNS effects with alcohol or psychoactive drugs. Increased concentrations reported when taken with food, which may lead to increased frequency of adverse reactions. Do not take with combination products that contain efavirenz. See PI for complete information.

**PREGNANCY:** Category D, not for use in nursing.

**MECHANISM OF ACTION:** Non-nucleoside reverse transcriptase inhibitor; mediated predominantly by noncompetitive inhibition of HIV-1 reverse transcriptase.

**PHARMACOKINETICS: Absorption:** $C_{max}$=12.9µM, $T_{max}$=3-5 hrs; AUC=184µM•h. **Distribution:** Plasma protein binding (99.5-99.75%). **Metabolism:** CYP3A, 2B6 (hydroxylation, glucuronidation). **Elimination:** $T_{1/2}$=40-55 hrs (multiple dose), 52-76 hrs (single dose).

## NURSING CONSIDERATIONS

**Assessment:** Assess for history of HBV or HCV infection, injection drug use, seizures, psychiatric illness, hepatic impairment, pregnancy/nursing status, and possible drug interactions. Perform pregnancy test prior to therapy. Obtain baseline ALT, AST, GGT, amylase, glucose levels, cholesterol, TG and neutrophil count.

**Monitoring:** Monitor for psychiatric events (depression, suicidal ideation), CNS symptoms (dizziness, impaired concentration), severe rash, pregnancy,

S

convulsions, and infection. Monitor LFTs and lipid levels periodically. May enroll patients in the Antiretroviral Pregnancy Registry if they become pregnant while on treatment.

**Patient Counseling:** Inform that therapy is not cure for HIV, does not reduce risk of transmission of HIV and that opportunistic infections may develop. Instruct to take every day as prescribed; take on an empty stomach hs to reduce CNS symptoms (eg, dizziness, insomnia, impaired concentration, abnormal dreams) that may occur during 1st weeks of therapy. Instruct to avoid potentially hazardous tasks such as driving or operating machinery. Inform of pregnancy risks; use reliable barrier and oral contraception during therapy; advise to register in the Antiretroviral Pregnancy Registry. Advise that central obesity, dorsocervical fat enlargement, peripheral and facial wasting and breast enlargement may occur. Advise to seek medical attention if symptoms of seizures, rash, serious psychiatric events (severe depression, suicidal ideation, aggressive behavior), severe infection or hypersensitivity reactions occur. Notify physician of any history of mental illness or substance abuse. Instruct that tablets should not be broken.

**Administration:** Oral route. **Storage:** 25°C (77°F); excursions permitted to 15-30°C (59-86°F).

## SUTENT — RX

sunitinib malate (Pfizer)

**THERAPEUTIC CLASS:** Multikinase inhibitor

**INDICATIONS:** Treatment of gastrointestinal stromal tumor (GIST) after disease progression on or intolerance to imatinib mesylate. Treatment of advanced renal cell carcinoma (RCC).

**DOSAGE:** *Adults:* 50mg once daily; 4 weeks on, 2 weeks off. Dose increase/reduction in 12.5mg increments is recommended. Concomitant Strong CYP3A4 Inhibitors: Consider dose reduction to minimum of 37.5mg daily. Concomitant CYP3A4 Inducer: Consider dose increase to maximum of 87.5mg daily.

**HOW SUPPLIED:** Cap: 12.5mg, 25mg, 50mg

**WARNINGS/PRECAUTIONS:** Cases of decreased left ventricular ejection fraction (LVEF) reported. Patients with cardiac risk factors should be carefully monitored for signs and symptoms of CHF; baseline and periodic evaluation of LVEF should be considered. D/C if clinical manifestations of CHF occur. Prolongation of QT interval and torsades de pointes observed; consider monitoring ECG and electrolytes (magnesium, potassium). Cases of hemorrhagic events reported. Serious, sometimes fatal GI complications including GI perforation have occurred with intra-abdominal malignancies. Cases of HTN reported; monitor for HTN and treat as needed with standard antihypertensive therapy. Temporary suspension recommended if severe HTN occurs. Adrenal toxicity reported; monitor for adrenal insufficiency with stress, trauma, or severe infection. Cases of hypothyroidism reported. Monitor CBCs, platelet count, thyroid function, and serum chemistries beginning each treatment cycle. May cause fetal harm; avoid pregnancy.



**ADVERSE REACTIONS:** Fatigue, asthenia, diarrhea, N/V, mucositis/stomatitis, dyspepsia, abdominal pain, HTN, rash, hand-foot syndrome, skin discoloration, altered taste, anorexia, bleeding.

**INTERACTIONS:** Concomitant CYP3A4 inhibitors (eg, ketoconazole) may increase plasma concentrations, as well as grapefruit; consider dose reduction. CYP3A4 inducers (eg, rifampin) may decrease plasma concentrations; consider dose increase. Avoid concurrent St. John's wort; may decrease plasma concentrations unpredictably.

**PREGNANCY:** Category D, not for use in nursing.

**MECHANISM OF ACTION:** Multikinase inhibitor; inhibits multiple receptor tyrosine kinase, implicated in tumor growth, pathologic angiogenesis, and metastatic cancer progression.

**PHARMACOKINETICS: Absorption:** $T_{max}$=6-12 hrs. **Distribution:** $V_d$=2230L; plasma protein binding (95%). **Metabolism:** CYP3A4. **Elimination:** Feces (61%), renal (16%); $T_{1/2}$=40-60 hrs, 80-110 hrs (metabolite).

## NURSING CONSIDERATIONS

**Assessment:** Assess for risk factors or history of CVD (QT prolongation, bradycardia, HTN, MI, CABG), seizures, liver dysfunction, pregnancy status, hypothyroidism and possible drug interactions. Obtain baseline left ventricular ejection fraction (LVEF) (no risk factors: EF), thyroid function, LFTs, BP, CBC with platelet count, chemistries with phosphate, and renal function.

**Monitoring:** Monitor LVEF, ECG, CBC with platelets, chemistries ($Mg^{2+}$, $K^+$, phosphate), thyroid function, and LFTs periodically. Monitor for signs/symptoms of CVD, electrolyte imbalance, hemorrhagic events, hypothyroidism, adrenal insufficiency, reversible posterior leukoencephalopathy syndrome (RPLS), pancreatitis, muscle toxicity, hypersensitivity reactions, renal/hepatic dysfunction.

**Patient Counseling:** Inform of pregnancy risks. Instruct not to take with grapefruit juice or grapefruit. Advise to seek medical attention if symptoms of CVD (eg, QT prolongation, HTN), electrolyte imbalance, hemorrhagic events (eg, GI perforation; black, tarry stools), hypothyroidism, adrenal insufficiency (during stress), RPLS (eg, HTN, headache, AMS, visual loss), pancreatitis, muscle toxicity, hypersensitivity reactions, renal/hepatic dysfunction occur.

**Administration:** Oral route. **Storage:** 25°C (77°F); excursions permitted to 15-30°C (59-86°F).

# SYMBICORT RX

formoterol fumarate dihydrate - budesonide (AstraZeneca)

**Long-acting $\beta_2$-adrenergic agonists (formoterol) may increase the risk of asthma-related death. Symbicort should only be used for patients not adequately controlled on other asthma-controller medications or whose disease severity clearly requires initiation of treatment with two maintenance therapies.**

**THERAPEUTIC CLASS:** Corticosteroid/beta$_2$ agonist

**INDICATIONS:** Long-term maintenance treatment of asthma in patients ≥12 yrs. Maintenance treatment of airflow obstruction in patients with chronic obstructive pulmonary disease (COPD) including chronic bronchitis and emphysema.

**DOSAGE:** *Adults:* Asthma: Initial: Individualize dose based on asthma severity. 2 inh bid of 80/4.5 or 160/4.5. Maint: 2 inh bid of 80/4.5 or 160/4.5. No Current Inhaled Corticosteroid: 2 inh bid of 80/4.5 or 160/4.5 depending on asthma severity. Max: 160/4.5 bid. Patients not responding to the starting dose after 1-2 weeks of therapy with 80/4.5, replace with 160/4.5 for better asthma control. COPD: 2 inh bid of 160/4.5. If asthma or shortness of breath occurs in period between doses, use short-acting beta$_2$-agonist for immediate relief. Rinse mouth after use.
*Pediatrics:* ≥12 yrs: Asthma: Initial: Individualize dose based on asthma severity. 2 inh bid of 80/4.5 or 160/4.5. Maint: 2 inh bid of 80/4.5 or 160/4.5. No Current Inhaled Corticosteroid: 2 inh bid of 80/4.5 or 160/4.5 depending on asthma severity. Max: 160/4.5 bid. Patients not responding to the starting dose after 1-2 weeks of therapy with 80/4.5, replace with 160/4.5 for better asthma control. If asthma occurs in period between doses, use short-acting beta$_2$-agonist for immediate relief. Rinse mouth after use.

**HOW SUPPLIED:** MDI: (Budesonide-Formoterol) 80mcg-4.5mcg/inh, 160mcg-4.5mcg/inh [10.2g]

**CONTRAINDICATIONS:** Primary treatment of status asthmaticus or other acute asthma attacks or COPD requiring intensive measures.

**WARNINGS/PRECAUTIONS:** Not for asthma managed by inhaled CS with occasional use of short-acting beta$_2$-agonists. Do not use in patients with significantly worsening or acutely deteriorating asthma or COPD. Not for acute treatment of symptoms. Monitor for increasing use of inhaled, short-acting $\beta_2$-

agonists. Deaths due to adrenal insufficiency have occurred with transfer from systemic corticosteroids to inhaled corticosteroids. Resume oral corticosteroids during stress or severe asthma attack. Transferring from oral to inhalation therapy may unmask allergic conditions (eg, rhinitis, conjunctivitis, eczema). Observe for adrenal insufficiency, systemic corticosteroid withdrawal effects, and growth suppression (pediatrics). Increased susceptibility to infections. Not for acute bronchospasm. Do not use any additional inhaled long-acting $\beta_2$-agonist for prevention of exercise-induced bronchospasm or the maintenance treatment of asthma. D/C if paradoxical bronchospasm occurs. Immediate hypersensitivity and upper airway symptom reactions reported. Caution with cardiovascular disorder (eg, coronary insufficiency, arrhythmia, HTN), seizures, thyroid and hepatic problems, diabetes, osteoporosis. QTc interval prolongation reported. Glaucoma, increased IOP, and cataracts reported. Caution in patients with active or quiescent TB infection, untreated systemic fungal, bacterial, viral, or parasitic infections, or ocular herpes simplex. Localized infections with *Candida albicans* may occur in mouth and pharynx. Lower respiratory tract infections, including pneumonia, reported in patients with COPD. Reduction in bone mineral density reported; monitor periodically. Eosinophilic conditions and Churg-Strauss syndrome reported. Hypokalemia and hyperglycemia may occur.

**ADVERSE REACTIONS:** Nasopharyngitis, headache, upper respiratory tract infections, sinusitis, back pain, nasal/sinus congestion, oral candidiasis, influenza, rhinitis, pharyngolaryngeal pain, vomiting, and bronchitis.

**INTERACTIONS:** Oral ketoconazole increases plasma levels. CYP3A4 inhibitors (eg, itraconazole, clarithromycin, erythromycin) may inhibit metabolism and increase systemic exposure. Caution with non-$K^+$-sparing diuretics. Extreme caution within 14 days of using MAOIs or TCAs. Avoid with β-blockers.

**PREGNANCY:** Category C, not for use in nursing.

**MECHANISM OF ACTION:** Budesonide: Corticosteroid; shown to have inhibitory effects on multiple cell types (mast cells, eosinophils, neutrophils, macrophages and lymphocytes) and mediators (histamine, eicosanoids, leukotrienes and cytokines) involved in inflammatory and asthmatic response. Formoterol: $\beta_2$-adrenergic agonist; stimulates intracellular adenyl cyclase, which catalyzes conversion of ATP to cAMP, to produce relaxation of bronchial smooth muscle and inhibition of release of mediators of immediate hypersensitivity from cells (especially mast cells).

**PHARMACOKINETICS: Absorption:** (Asthma) Budesonide: Rapid (lungs). $C_{max}$=4.5nmol/L; $T_{max}$=20 min. Formoterol: Rapid (GI). $C_{max}$=136pmol; $T_{max}$=5-10 min. (COPD) Budesonide: Rapid (lungs). $C_{max}$=3.3nmol/L; $T_{max}$=30 min. Formoterol: Rapid (GI). $C_{max}$=167pmol/L; $T_{max}$=15 min. **Distribution:** Budesonide: $V_d$=3L/kg; plasma protein binding (85-90%). Formoterol: Plasma protein binding (RR enantiomer, 46%), (SS enantiomer, 58%). **Metabolism:** Budesonide: Liver (biotransformation) via CYP3A4. Formoterol: Liver (direct glucuronidation and O-demethylation) via CYP2D6, 2C. **Elimination:** Budesonide: $T_{1/2}$=2-3 hrs. Formoterol: Urine (8%).

S

## NURSING CONSIDERATIONS

**Assessment:** Assess if asthma controlled by inhaled corticosteroids and occasional use of short-acting $\beta_2$-agonists. Assess for risk factors for decreased bone mineral content (eg, tobacco use, advanced age, sedentary lifestyle, family history of osteoporosis, drugs that decrease bone mass), CVD (eg, coronary insufficiency, cardiac arrhythmia, HTN), convulsive disorder, thyrotoxicosis, DM, concomitant diseases such as status asthmaticus, active or quiescent pulmonary TB, ocular herpes simplex, untreated systemic fungal, bacterial, parasitic, or viral infections, and possible drug interactions. Obtain baseline bone mineral density and lung function prior to therapy.

**Monitoring:** Monitor bone mineral density and lung function periodically. Perform periodic eye exams. Monitor for localized oral infections with *Candida albicans*, decreased bone mass, upper airway symptoms (eg, laryngeal spasm, irritation, swelling), worsening or acutely deteriorating asthma (increased use of inhaled $\beta_2$-agonist, decreased lung function), asthma instability (serial objective measures of airflow), body height in children, development of glaucoma, increased IOP, posterior subcapsular cataracts, adrenal insufficiency (eg, fatigue, weakness, N/V and hypotension), paradoxical bronchospasm, eosinophilic conditions, pneumonia, and hypersensitivity reactions.

**Patient Counseling:** Avoid spraying in eyes. Advise to rinse mouth after inhalation. Replace mouthpiece cover after each use and clean inhaler every 7 days by wiping mouthpiece with dry cloth. Do not d/c therapy unless directed by physician. Should not be used for sudden symptoms of SOB or acute bronchospasm. Inform may cause reduction in growth rate (pediatric). May unmask allergies (eg, rhinitis, conjunctivitis, eczema). Avoid exposure to chickenpox or measles; seek medical attention if exposed to chickenpox or measles, or if experience worsening of existing TB, infections or ocular herpes simplex, symptoms do not improve or worsen, during periods of stress or severe asthmatic attack, adrenal insufficiency (fatigue, weakness, N/V and hypotension), paradoxical bronchospasm or hypersensitivity reactions.

**Administration:** Oral inhalation. **Storage:** 20-25°C (68-77°F). Store with mouthpiece down. Shake well.

## SYMBYAX RX

fluoxetine HCl - olanzapine (Lilly)

**Antidepressants increased the risk of suicidal thinking and behavior (suicidality) in short-term studies in children, adolescents, and young adults with major depressive disorder (MDD) and other psychiatric disorders. Patients started on antidepressants should be monitored and observed for clinical worsening, suicidality or unusual changes in behavior. Elderly patients with dementia-related psychosis treated with atypical antipsychotic drugs are at an increased risk of death; most appeared to be cardiovascular (eg, heart failure, sudden death) or infectious (eg, pneumonia) in nature. Symbyax is not approved for pediatric use or for the treatment of patients with dementia-related psychosis.**

**THERAPEUTIC CLASS:** Thienobenzodiazepine/selective serotonin reuptake inhibitor

**INDICATIONS:** Acute treatment of depressive episodes associated with bipolar I disorder, and treatment-resistant depression (Major Depressive Disorder [MDD] patients who do not respond to 2 separate trials of different antidepressants of adequate dose and duration in the current episode) in adults.

**DOSAGE:** *Adults:* Depressive Episodes Associated with Bipolar I Disorder/ Treatment Resistant Depression: Initial: 6mg-25mg qd in evening. Range: 6-12mg (olanzapine)-25-50mg (fluoxetine). Adjust dose based on efficacy and tolerability. Max: 18mg-75mg/day. Re-examine the need for continued pharmacotherapy periodically. Hypotension Risk/Hepatic Impairment/Slow Metabolizers/Olanzapine-Sensitive: Initial: 3mg-25mg to 6mg-25mg qd in evening. Titrate: Increase cautiously. Pregnant: Consider using lower dose during third trimester.

**HOW SUPPLIED:** Cap: (Olanzapine-Fluoxetine): 3mg-25mg, 6mg-25mg, 6mg-50mg, 12mg-25mg, 12mg-50mg

**CONTRAINDICATIONS:** During or within 14 days of d/c therapy with a Monoamine Oxidase Inhibitor (MAOI); during or within 5 weeks of d/c of thioridazine use; concomitant pimozide use.

**WARNINGS/PRECAUTIONS:** Neuroleptic malignant syndrome (NMS) reported; d/c if occurs and instill intensive symptomatic treatment and monitoring. May cause hyperglycemia; caution in patients with DM or in patients with borderline increased blood glucose levels; monitor for worsening of glucose control. Obtain FBG levels at beginning of treatment and periodically during treatment. Hyperlipidemia reported; obtain lipid levels at baseline and periodically thereafter. May cause weight gain; perform regular monitoring of weight. Serotonin syndrome or neuroleptic malignant syndrome (NMS)-like reactions reported; d/c and initiate supportive therapy. D/C if unexplained allergic reaction occurs. Tardive dyskinesia, activation of mania/hypomania, hyponatremia, hyperprolactinemia reported. May cause orthostatic hypotension; caution with CVD (eg, history of MI or ischemia, CHF, conduction abnormalities), cerebrovascular disease, or with conditions that would predispose to hypotension (eg, hypovolemia, dehydration). Leukopenia, neutropenia,

S

and agranulocytosis reported; d/c at first sign of clinically significant decline in WBC without causative factor or if severe neutropenia (ANC<1000/mm³) develops. May cause esophageal dysmotility and aspiration. Not approved for use in patients with Alzheimer's disease. Caution in patients with history of seizures or with conditions that potentially lower the seizure threshold. May increase risk of bleeding events. May cause cognitive/motor impairment and disruption of body temperature regulation. Caution in patients with clinically significant prostatic hypertrophy, narrow-angle glaucoma, a history of paralytic ileus or related conditions, hepatic impairment, and elderly. Avoid abrupt withdrawal.

**ADVERSE REACTIONS:** Asthenia, somnolence, weight gain, increased appetite, peripheral edema, tremor, diarrhea, dry mouth, arthralgia, blurred vision, sedation, fatigue, flatulence, lethargy, restlessness, hypersomnia.

**INTERACTIONS:** See Contraindications. Caution with CYP2D6 substrates including antidepressants (eg, TCAs), antipsychotics (eg, phenothiazines and most atypicals), and antiarrhythmics (eg, propafenone, flecainide). Monitor TCA and lithium levels. Caution with CNS-active drugs, hepatotoxic drugs, other olanzapine- or fluoxetine-containing products, and anticholinergic drugs. May potentiate effects of certain antihypertensive agents. May antagonize levodopa, dopamine agonists. May potentiate orthostatic hypotension with benzodiazepines and alcohol. May increase levels of phenytoin, carbamazepine, haloperidol, clozapine. Increased risk of serotonin syndrome or NMS-like reactions with serotonergic drugs (eg, triptans, linezolid, lithium, tramadol, St. John's wort), MAOIs, antipsychotics, other dopamine antagonists. Avoid with other selective serotonin reuptake inhibitors (SSRIs), serotonin-norepinephrine reuptake inhibitors (SNRIs), or tryptophan. Inducers of CYP1A2 or glucuronyl transferase (eg, omeprazole, rifampin) may increase clearance. CYP1A2 inhibitors (eg, fluvoxamine) and CYP2D6 inhibitors (eg, fluoxetine) may decrease clearance. Increased risk of bleeding events with aspirin, nonsteroidal anti-inflammatory drugs (NSAIDs), warfarin, and other anti-coagulants. May cause a shift in plasma concentration with drugs that are tightly bound to protein (eg, warfarin, digoxin) resulting in an adverse effect. Concomitant use with diuretics, may increase the risk of hyponatremia. Rare reports of prolonged seizures with combined electroconvulsive therapy.

**PREGNANCY:** Category C, not for use in nursing.

**MECHANISM OF ACTION:** SSRI/Thienobenzodiazepine; unknown. Proposed that activation of 3 monoaminergic neural systems (serotonin, norepinephrine, and dopamine) is responsible for its enhanced antidepressant effect. Fluoxetine: SSRI; inhibits serotonin transport; weak inhibitor of norepinephrine and dopamine transporters. Olanzapine: Thienobenzodiazepine; psychotropic agent with high affinity binding to $5HT_{2a/2c}$, $5HT_6$, $D_{1-4}$, $H_1$, and adrenergic $(\alpha)_1$-receptors.

S

**PHARMACOKINETICS: Absorption:** Fluoxetine: $C_{max}$=15-55ng/mL, $T_{max}$=6-8 hrs. Olanzepine: Well absorbed; $T_{max}$=approximately 6 hrs. **Distribution:** Found in breast milk. Fluoxetine: Plasma protein binding (94.5%). Olanzepine: $V_d$=1000L; plasma protein binding (93%). **Metabolism:** Fluoxetine: Liver (extensive); CYP2D6 pathway, norfluoxetine (active metabolite). Olanzapine: Extensively metabolized, via glucuronidation and CYP450 mediated oxidation, 10-N-glucuronide and 4'-N-desmethyl olanzapine (major metabolites). **Elimination:** Fluoxetine: Kidneys; (acute administration) $T_{1/2}$=1-3 days; (chronic administration) $T_{1/2}$=4-6 days. Olanzapine: Urine (57%), feces (30%); $T_{1/2}$=21-54 hrs.

## NURSING CONSIDERATIONS

**Assessment:** Asses for major depressive disorder, bipolar mania, DM, bleeding disorders, prostatic hypertrophy, narrow-angle glaucoma, history of paralytic ileus, history of seizures or conditions that could lower the seizure threshold, risk of hypotension, cardio/cerebrovascular disorders, renal/hepatic impairment, pregnancy/nursing status, and for possible drug interactions (eg, MAOIs). Assess for dementia-related psychosis and Alzheimer's disease in the elderly. Obtain baseline lipid panel, CBC and FBG levels.

**Monitoring:** Monitor for signs/symptoms of NMS, serotonin syndrome. hyperglycemia, hyperlipidemia, weight gain, tardive dyskinesia, orthostatic hypotension, leukopenia, neutropenia, agranulocytosis, hyponatremia, abnormal bleeding, dysphagia, hypersensitivity reactions, seizures, body temperature disruption, cognitive and motor impairment, hyperprolactinemia and for abrupt withdrawal symptoms. Perform periodic monitoring of FBG, lipid levels, and weight of patient. Perform frequent monitoring of CBC in patients with a history of clinically significant low WBC or drug-induced leukopenia/neutropenia. In patient with clinically significant neutropenia, monitor for fever or other symptoms or signs of infection. In high-risk patients, monitor closely for a suicide attempt.

**Patient Counseling:** Advise of risk of orthostatic hypotension. Counsel to avoid hazardous tasks (eg, operating machinery/driving), alcohol use, overheating, dehydration. Instruct to notify physician before taking any other drugs, if pregnant, or intend to become pregnant. Instruct to notify physician if rash or hives develop. Counsel to take exactly as prescribed; instruct to continue even if symptoms improve.

**Administration:** Oral route. **Storage:** 25°C (77°F); excursions permitted to 15-30°C (59-86°F). Keep tightly closed; protect from moisture.

## SYMLIN RX

pramlintide acetate (Amylin)

**Use with insulin. Risk of insulin-induced severe hypoglycemia, particularly with type 1 DM. Severe hypoglycemia usually occurs within 3 hrs of injection. Serious injuries may occur if severe hypoglycemia occurs while operating a motor vehicle, heavy machinery, or other high-risk activities. Appropriate patient selection, careful patient instruction, and insulin dose adjustments are necessary to reduce this risk.**

**OTHER BRAND NAMES:** SymlinPen (Amylin)

**THERAPEUTIC CLASS:** Synthetic amylin analog

**INDICATIONS:** Adjunct treatment in patients with type 1 or type 2 DM who use mealtime insulin therapy and who have failed to achieve desired glucose control despite optimal insulin therapy. May be used with or without sulfonylurea and/or metformin in type 2 DM.

**DOSAGE:** *Adults:* Before initiating therapy, reduce insulin dose by 50%. Monitor blood glucose frequently. Adjust insulin dose once target dose of pramlintide is maintained. Type 2 DM: Initial: 60mcg SQ immediately prior to meals. Titrate: 120mcg as tolerated. Type 1 DM: Initial: 15mcg SQ immediately prior to meals. Titrate: Increase by 15mcg increments to 30mcg or 60mcg as tolerated.

**HOW SUPPLIED:** Inj: 600mcg/mL [5mL]; Pen injector: 1000mcg/mL [1.5mL, 2.7mL]

**CONTRAINDICATIONS:** Confirmed diagnosis of gastroparesis; hypoglycemia unawareness.

**WARNINGS/PRECAUTIONS:** Do not mix with insulin; administer as separate injections.

**ADVERSE REACTIONS:** N/V, headache, anorexia, abdominal pain, fatigue, dizziness, coughing, pharyngitis.

**INTERACTIONS:** Do not administer with agents that alter gastrointestinal motility (eg, anticholinergic agents such as atropine), and agents that slow intestinal absorption of nutrients (eg, α-glucosidase inhibitors). Administer analgesics and other oral agents that require rapid onset 1 hr before or 2 hrs after injection.

**PREGNANCY:** Category C, caution in nursing.

**MECHANISM OF ACTION:** Amylinomimetic agent that modulates gastric emptying, prevents postprandial rise in plasma glucagon, and produces satiety, which leads to a decreased caloric intake.

**PHARMACOKINETICS: Absorption:** Absolute bioavailability (30-40%); SQ administration of variable doses resulted in different parameters. **Distribution:** Not extensively bound to blood cells or albumin (40% unbound). **Metabolism:**

Kidneys (primarily). Des-lys pramlintide (primary active metabolite). **Elimination:** $T_{1/2}$=48 min.

## NURSING CONSIDERATIONS

**Assessment:** Assess patient does not have confirmed diagnosis of gastroparesis or hypoglycemia unawareness. Evaluate patient's $HbA_{1c}$, recent blood glucose monitoring data, history of insulin-induced hypoglycemia, current insulin regimen, and body weight. Assess if patient has failed to achieve proper glycemic control despite individualized insulin management. Assess use in patients with visual or dexterity impairment. Assess for possible drug interactions and pregnancy/nursing status.

**Monitoring:** Monitor for signs/symptoms of hypoglycemia (eg, hunger, headache, sweating, tremor) when using in combination with insulin. Monitor proper glucose control through serum blood glucose levels and $HbA_{1c}$ test.

**Patient Counseling:** Instruct to never mix with insulin and not to transfer from pen-injector to syringe. If dose missed, wait until next scheduled dose and administer usual amount. Instruct to administer immediately prior to each major meal ( ≥250 calories or ≥30g of carbohydrates). Instruct that insulin dose adjustments should be made only by healthcare professional. Patients should have fast-acting sugar (eg, hard candy, glucose tablet, juice) at all times. Self-glucose monitoring should be done on a daily basis. Counsel about signs/symptoms of hypoglycemia (eg, hunger, headache, sweating, tremor, irritability). Instruct regarding the critical importance of maintaining proper glucose control, especially when operating heavy machinery (eg, motor vehicles).

**Administration:** SQ injection to abdomen or thigh; administration to the arm is not recommended because of variable absorption. Rotate injection sites and do not use any site for any concomitant insulin injection. Allow to come to room temperature before injecting. **Storage:** Pen injectors and vials not in use: 2-8°C (36-40°F). Do not freeze. Do not use if frozen. Unused drug (opened or unopened) should not be used after expiration date. Pen-injectors and vials in use: After 1st use, refrigerate or keep at a temperature <30°C (86°F). Use within 30 days.

# SYMMETREL — RX

amantadine HCl (Endo)

**THERAPEUTIC CLASS:** Dopamine receptor agonist

**INDICATIONS:** Prophylaxis and treatment of uncomplicated influenza A infections. Treatment of parkinsonism and drug-induced extrapyramidal reactions.

**DOSAGE:** *Adults:* Influenza A Virus Prophylaxis/Treatment: 200mg qd given as a single dose of two 100mg tabs (or 4 tsp of syrup). May give 100mg (or 2 tsp) bid if CNS effects develop. Elderly: ≥65 yrs: 100mg qd. Parkinsonism: Initial: 100mg bid if used alone. Serious Associated Illness/Concomitant High-Dose Antiparkinson Agent: Initial: 100mg qd. Titrate: May increase to 100mg bid after 1 to several weeks. Max: 400mg/day. Drug-Induced Extrapyramidal Reactions: 100mg bid. Titrate: May increase to 300mg/day in divided doses. CrCl 30-50mL/min: 200mg on Day 1, then 100mg qd. CrCl 15-29mL/min: 200mg on Day 1, then 100mg every other day. CrCl <15mL/min/Hemodialysis: 200mg every 7 days.

*Pediatrics:* Influenza A Virus Prophylaxis/Treatment: 9-12 yrs: 100mg (or 2 tsp of syrup) bid. 1-9 yrs: 4.4-8.8mg/kg/day. Max: 150mg/day.

**HOW SUPPLIED:** Syrup: 50mg/5mL; Tab: 100mg

**WARNINGS/PRECAUTIONS:** Deaths reported from overdose. Suicide attempts, neuroleptic malignant syndrome (NMS) reported. May exacerbate mental illness in patients with history of psychotropic disorder or substance abuse. Caution with CHF, peripheral edema, orthostatic hypotension, renal or hepatic dysfunction, recurrent eczematoid rash, uncontrolled psychosis or severe psychoneurosis. Avoid in untreated angle-closure glaucoma. Do not d/c abruptly in Parkinson's disease. May increase seizure activity. Increased risk of melanoma with Parkinson's disease; monitor periodically. May impair mental/physical abilities. Compulsive behaviors (eg, intense urges to gamble, increased sexual urges) reported.

**ADVERSE REACTIONS:** Nausea, dizziness, insomnia, depression, anxiety, hallucinations, confusion, anorexia, dry mouth, constipation, ataxia, livedo reticularis, peripheral edema, orthostatic hypotension, irritability, and headache.

**INTERACTIONS:** Caution with CNS stimulants. Alcohol may potentiate CNS effects (eg, dizziness, confusion, orthostatic hypotension). Anticholinergic agents may potentiate the anticholinergic side effects. Increased tremor in elderly Parkinson's patients with thioridazine. Increased plasma levels with quinine or quinidine, triamterene/hydrochlorothiazide. Avoid use of attenuated influenza vaccine within 2 weeks before or 48 hours after.

**PREGNANCY:** Category C, not for use in nursing.

**MECHANISM OF ACTION:** Antiviral; appears to prevent release of infectious viral nucleic acid into host cell by interfering with function of transmembrane domain of viral M2 protein, preventing virus assembly during replication. Parkinson's disease; may have direct/indirect effect on dopamine neurons and is a weak, noncompetitive NMDA receptor antagonist.

**PHARMACOKINETICS: Absorption**: Well absorbed; (Tab) $C_{max}$=0.51mcg/mL, $T_{max}$=2-4 hrs. (Syrup) $C_{max}$=0.24mcg/mL, $T_{max}$=2-4 hrs. **Distribution:** (IV) $V_d$=3-8L/kg; plasma protein binding (67%); excreted in breast milk. **Metabolism:** N-acetylation; acetylamantadine (metabolite). **Elimination:** Urine; excreted unchanged; $T_{1/2}$=16 hrs.

## NURSING CONSIDERATIONS

**Assessment:** Assess for history of CHF, peripheral edema, epilepsy or other "seizures", recurrent eczematoid rash, psychiatric illness, untreated angle-closure glaucoma, pregnancy/nursing status, possible drug interactions, renal/hepatic impairment, and hypersensitivity.

**Monitoring:** Monitor for signs/symptoms of CHF, peripheral edema, epilepsy or other "seizures", recurrent eczematoid rash, psychiatric illness, untreated angle-closure glaucoma, NMS (eg, fever, muscle rigidity, altered mental status), renal/hepatic impairment, melanoma, compulsive behaviors (eg, pathological gambling, hypersexuality), and hypersensitivity reactions. Monitor lab tests such as CPK, WBC, serum myoglobin, BUN, SrCr, alkaline phosphatase, LDH, bilirubin, GGT, SGOT and SGPT.

**Patient Counseling:** Advise blurry vision and impaired mental acuity may occur. Avoid excessive alcohol use, getting up suddenly from sitting or lying position, and abrupt d/c. Notify physician if no improvement in a few days or appears less effective after a few weeks. Seek medical attention if experience symptoms of CHF (eg, lightheadedness, SOB), peripheral edema, epilepsy or other "seizures", recurrent eczematoid rash, psychiatric illness (eg, suicidal ideation, mood changes), untreated angle-closure glaucoma, hypersensitivity reaction, NMS (eg, fever, muscle rigidity, altered mental status), renal/hepatic impairment. Consult a physician before discontinuing medication. Caution against driving/working where alertness and adequate motor coordination are important. Notify physician if new or increased gambling urges, increased sexual urges or other intense urges occur.

**Administration:** Oral route. Influenza A: Treatment: should be started within 24-48 hrs after onset and after disappearance of signs and symptoms; continue for at least 10 days after known exposure. Prophylaxis: Administer for 2-4 weeks after vaccine is given. If vaccine unavailable, continue for entire duration of exposure in community. **Storage:** 25°C (77°F); excursions permitted to 15-30°C (59-86°F). Dispense in tight container.



# SYNAGIS — RX

palivizumab (MedImmune)

**THERAPEUTIC CLASS:** Monoclonal antibody/RSV F-protein blocker

**INDICATIONS:** Prevention of serious lower respiratory tract disease caused by respiratory syncytial virus (RSV) in pediatrics at high risk of RSV. Safety and efficacy established in infants with bronchopulmonary dysplasia (BPD), infants with history of prematurity (≤35 weeks gestational age), and children with hemodynamically significant congenital heart disease (CHD).

**DOSAGE:** *Pediatrics:* 15mg/kg IM; give 1st dose before start of RSV season (November-April), then monthly throughout season. Give monthly also if develop RSV infection.

**HOW SUPPLIED:** Inj: 50mg [0.5mL], 100mg [1mL]

**WARNINGS/PRECAUTIONS:** Anaphylactoid reactions (eg, cyanosis, dyspnea, respiratory failure) reported. Administer appropriate medications (eg, epinephrine) in the event of anaphylaxis. Caution with thrombocytopenia or any coagulation disorder due to IM injection. Safety and efficacy not demonstrated for treatment of established RSV disease.

**ADVERSE REACTIONS:** Upper respiratory infection, otitis media, rash, cough, diarrhea, vomiting, liver function abnormality, fever, rhinitis, hernia, gastroenteritis, wheezing, anaphylaxis, thrombocytopenia, injection site reactions.

**PREGNANCY:** Category C, safety in nursing not known.

**MECHANISM OF ACTION:** Monoclonal antibody; exhibits neutralizing and fusion-inhibitory activity against RSV.

**PHARMACOKINETICS: Elimination:** $T_{1/2}$=20 days.

## NURSING CONSIDERATIONS

**Assessment:** Assess for thrombocytopenia and coagulation disorders.

**Monitoring:** Monitor for anaphylaxis or acute hypersensitivity reactions and platelet count.

**Patient Counseling:** Advise to seek medical attention if hypersensitivity reactions occur.

**Administration:** IM (anterolateral aspect of thigh). Administer immediately after withdrawal from vial; do not re-enter vial; gluteal muscle should not be used because of risk of damage to sciatic nerve. Do not dilute, shake, or vigorously agitate vial. **Storage:** 2-8°C (35.5-46.4°F). Do not freeze or use beyond expiration date.

# SYNERA RX

tetracaine - lidocaine (Endo)

**THERAPEUTIC CLASS:** Acetamide local anesthetic

**INDICATIONS:** For use on intact skin to provide local dermal analgesia for superficial venous access and superficial dermatological procedures such as excision, electrodessication, and shave biopsy of skin lesions.

S

**DOSAGE:** *Adults:* Venipuncture or IV Cannulation: Apply to intact skin for 20-30 min prior to procedure. Superficial Dermatological Procedures: Apply to intact skin for 30 min prior to procedure.
*Pediatrics:* ≥3 yrs: Venipuncture or IV Cannulation: Apply to intact skin for 20-30 min prior to procedure. Superficial Dermatological Procedure: Apply to intact skin for 30 min prior to procedure.

**HOW SUPPLIED:** Patch: (Lidocaine-Tetracaine) 70mg-70mg

**CONTRAINDICATIONS:** PABA hypersensitivity.

**WARNINGS/PRECAUTIONS:** Serious adverse events may occur in children or pets if ingested. Caution in acutely ill or debilitated. Risk of allergic/anaphylactoid reactions (eg, urticaria, angioedema, bronchospasm, shock). Increased risk of toxicity in severe hepatic disease. Avoid broken or inflamed skin, eye contact, larger area or longer duration than recommended.

**ADVERSE REACTIONS:** Erythema, blanching, edema, urticaria, angioedema, bronchospasm, shock.

**INTERACTIONS:** Additive toxic effect with concomitant Class I antiarrhythmics (eg, tocainide, mexiletine). Consider total amount absorbed from all formulations with other local anesthetics.

**PREGNANCY:** Category B, caution in nursing.

**MECHANISM OF ACTION:** Lidocaine: Amide-type local anesthetic; blocks $Na^+$ channels required for initiation and conduction of neuronal impulses. Tetracaine: Ester-type local anesthetic; blocks $Na^+$ channels required for initiation and conduction of neuronal impulses.

**PHARMACOKINETICS: Absorption:** $C_{max}$=1.7ng/mL (lidocaine), <0.9ng/mL (tetracaine); $T_{max}$=1.7 hrs. (lidocaine). **Distribution:** Lidocaine: $V_d$=0.8-1.3 L/kg; plasma protein binding (75%); crosses placenta. **Metabolism:** Lidocaine: CYP1A2, CYP3A4 (N-deethylation). Monoethylglycinexylidide, glycinexylidide (active metabolites). Tetracaine: Plasma esterases (hydrolysis). **Elimination:** Lidocaine: Urine; $T_{1/2}$=1.8 hrs.

## NURSING CONSIDERATIONS

**Assessment:** Assess for pseudocholinesterase deficiency, possible drug interactions, cardiac and hepatic impairment.

**Monitoring:** Monitor for allergic or anaphylactoid reactions (eg, erythema, blanching, edema), cardiac and hepatic dysfunction.

**Patient Counseling:** Inform that use may lead to diminished or blocked sensation in treated skin. Instruct to wash hands after application; avoid contact with eyes; remove patch before MRI.

**Administration:** Transdermal. **Storage:** 25°C (77°F) excursions permitted to 15-30°C (59-86°F).

# SYNERCID — RX

dalfopristin - quinupristin (Monarch Pharmaceuticals Inc.)

**Synercid is indicated for treatment of patients with serious or life-threatening infections associated with vancomycin-resistant *Enterococcus faecium* (VREF) bacteremia.**

**THERAPEUTIC CLASS:** Streptogramin

**INDICATIONS:** Treatment of serious or life-threatening infections associated with vancomycin-resistant *Enterococcus faecium* (VREF) bacteremia and complicated skin and skin structure infections (cSSSI) caused by *Staphylococcus aureus* (methicillin-susceptible) or *Streptococcus pyogenes*.

**DOSAGE:** *Adults:* VREF: 7.5mg/kg IV q8h. Duration depends on site and severity of infection. cSSSI: 7.5mg/kg IV q12h for at least 7 days. Hepatic Cirrhosis (Child Pugh A or B): May need dose reduction.
*Pediatrics:* ≥16 yrs: VREF: 7.5mg/kg IV q8h. Duration depends on site and severity of infection. cSSSI: 7.5mg/kg IV q12h for at least 7 days. Hepatic Cirrhosis (Child Pugh A or B): May need dose reduction.

**HOW SUPPLIED:** Inj: (Dalfopristin-Quinupristin) 350mg-150mg, 420mg-180mg

**WARNINGS/PRECAUTIONS:** *C. difficile*-associated diarrhea (CDAD) reported. Flush vein with 5% dextrose after infusion to minimize venous irritation; do not flush with saline or heparin. Arthralgia, myalgia, and bilirubin elevation reported. Superinfections may occur.

**ADVERSE REACTIONS:** Infusion-site reactions (eg, inflammation, pain, edema), N/V, diarrhea, rash, hyperbilirubinemia, arthralgia, myalgia.

**INTERACTIONS:** Significant inhibition of CYP3A4; caution with drugs metabolized by this enzyme system (eg, cyclosporine A, tacrolimus, midazolam, nifedipine, verapamil, diltiazem, astemizole, terfenadine, delaviridine, nevirapine, indinavir, ritonavir, vinca alkaloids, docetaxel, paclitaxel, diazepam, HMG-CoA reductase inhibitors, methylprednisolone, carbamazepine, quinidine, lidocaine, disopyramide). Monitor cyclosporine levels. Avoid drugs metabolized by CYP3A4 that prolong QTc interval. May inhibit gut metabolism of digoxin.

**PREGNANCY:** Category B, caution in nursing.

**MECHANISM OF ACTION:** Bacteriostatic agent; acts on bacterial ribosome. Dalfopristin: Inhibits the early phase of protein synthesis. Quinupristin: Inhibits the late phase of protein synthesis.

**PHARMACOKINETICS: Absorption:** Quinupristin: $C_{max}$=3.2mcg/mL, AUC=7.2mcg•hr/mL; Dalfopristin: $C_{max}$=7.96mcg/mL, AUC=10.57mcg•hr/mL. **Distribution:** Quinupristin: $V_d$=0.45L/kg, plasma protein binding (moderate); Dalfopristin: $V_d$=0.24L/kg, plasma protein binding (moderate). **Metabolism:** Quinupristin: 2 conjugated active metabolites (1 with glutathione; 1 with cysteine); Dalfopristin: 1 nonconjugated active metabolite, via hydrolysis. **Elimination:** Urine: 15% (quinupristin), 19% (dalfopristin), feces (75-77%); $T_{1/2}$=0.85 hrs. (quinupristin), 0.7 hrs. (dalfopristin).

## NURSING CONSIDERATIONS

**Assessment:** Assess for hepatic/renal impairment, pregnancy/nursing status, and for possible drug interactions (eg, concurrent administration with cyclosporine).

**Monitoring:** Monitor for C.*difficile*-associated diarrhea (may range from mild diarrhea to fatal colitis), venous irritation, arthralgia/myalgia, development of superinfection or drug resistance, and isolated hyperbilirubinemia. Lab monitoring of LFTs, renal function, glucose, CBCs, and blood chemistry. Monitor plasma level of drugs metabolized by CYP3A4 (eg, cyclosporine); adjust dose if necessary.

**Patient Counseling:** Inform about risks/benefits of therapy. D/C and notify physician if any adverse reactions occur. Notify if pregnant/nursing.

**Administration:** IV route. Infuse over 60 min; inspect for particulate matter or discoloration; flush only with D5W to minimize venous irritation. Do not dilute with saline solution. Refer to the PI for detailed procedure. **Storage:** Before reconstitution, at 2-8°C (36-46°F); diluted solution stable for 5 hrs at room temperature or for 54 hrs if refrigerated at 2-8°C (36-46°F). Do not freeze.

# SYNTHROID RX

levothyroxine sodium (Abbott)

**THERAPEUTIC CLASS:** Thyroid replacement hormone

**INDICATIONS:** Replacement or supplemental therapy in congenital or acquired hypothyroidism. As a pituitary TSH suppressant in the treatment and prevention of euthyroid goiters, including thyroid nodules, lymphocytic thyroiditis, and multinodular goiter. Adjunct to surgery and radioiodine therapy for thyrotropin-dependent well-differentiated thyroid cancer.

**DOSAGE:** *Adults:* Hypothyroidism: Usual: 1.7mcg/kg/day PO. >200mcg/day (seldom). Patients ≥50 yrs/<50 yrs With Cardiac Disease: May start with 25-50mcg/day and gradually increase every 6-8 weeks until euthyroid. Elderly With Cardiac Disease: Initial: 12.5-25mcg qd PO. Titrate: Increase by 12.5-25mcg every 4-6 weeks until euthyroid. Severe Hypothyroidism: Initial: 12.5-25mcg/day. Titrate: Increase by 25mcg/day every 2-4 weeks. Secondary (Pituitary) or Tertiary (Hypothalamic) Hypothyroidism: Titrate: Increase until clincally euthyroid. Give 1/2 of oral dose for IV/IM. Pregnancy: May require increased doses. Subclinical Hypothyroidism: Lower doses required. *Pediatrics:* Hypothyroidism: 0-3 months: 10-15mcg/kg/day. 3-6 months: 8-10mcg/kg/day. 6-12 months: 6-8mcg/kg/day. 1-5 yrs: 5-6mcg/kg/day. 6-12 yrs: 4-5mcg/kg/day. >12 yrs (growth/puberty incomplete): 2-3mcg/kg/day. Growth/Puberty Complete: 1.7mcg/kg/day. Cardiac Risk: Lower starting dose. Infants with Serum $T_4$ <5mcg/dL: Initial: 50mcg/day. Chronic/Severe Hypothyroidism: Children: Initial: 25mcg/day. Titrate: Increase by 25mcg for 2 weeks then every 2-4 weeks until euthyroid. May crush tab and sprinkle over food (applesauce) or mix with 5-10mL water, formula (non-soy), or breast milk.

S

**HOW SUPPLIED:** Tab: 25mcg*, 50mcg*, 75mcg*, 88mcg*, 100mcg*, 112mcg*, 125mcg*, 137mcg*, 150mcg*, 175mcg*, 200mcg*, 300mcg* *scored

**CONTRAINDICATIONS:** Untreated thyrotoxicosis, acute MI, uncorrected adrenal insufficiency.

**WARNINGS/PRECAUTIONS:** Do not use in the treatment of obesity or for weight loss; larger doses in euthyroid patients can cause serious or even life-threatening toxicity. Not for the treatment of infertility unless associated with hypothyroidism. Caution with CV disorders, angina, CAD, HTN, and the elderly. May aggravate DM, diabetes insipidus, or adrenal cortical insufficiency. Myxedema coma may not be treated with oral thyroid hormone products; administer IV products. May lower seizure threshold.

**ADVERSE REACTIONS:** Fatigue, weight loss, headache, hyperactivity, anxiety, tremors, muscle weakness, palpitations, arrhythmias, diarrhea, hair loss, flushing, decreased bone mineral density, craniosynostosis in infants, pseudotumor cerebri in pediatrics (rare), hypersensitivity reactions, seizures (rare).

**INTERACTIONS:** Increased risk of coronary insufficiency with sympathomimetics and CAD. May potentiate oral anticoagulant effects; adjust dose and monitor PT/INR. Lithium blocks release of $T_4$ and $T_3$. Antidiabetic agents may need adjustment. Decreased absorption with cholestyramine resin, colestipol, ferrous sulfate, aluminum hydroxide, sodium polystyrene sulfonate, soybean flour (infant formula), sucralfate. Altered protein binding with clofibrate, estrogens, androgens/anabolic hormones, asparaginase, 5-FU, furosemide, glucocorticoids, meclofenamic acid, mefenamic acid, methadone, perphenazine, phenytoin, phenylbutazone, tamoxifen, salicylates. Altered thyroid hormone or TSH levels with aminoglutethimide, p-aminosalicyclic acid, amiodarone, androgens/anabolic hormones, complex anions (eg, thiocyanate, perchlorate, pertechnetate), antithyroid drugs, β-adrenergic blockers, carbamazepine, chloral hydrate, diazepam, dopamine/dopamine agonists, ethionamide, glucocorticoids, heparin, hepatic enzyme inducers, insulin, iodinated cholestographic agents, iodine-containing compounds, levodopa, lovastatin, lithium, 6-mercaptopurine, metoclopramide, mitotane, nitroprusside, phenobarbital, phenytoin, resorcinol, rifampin, somatostatin analogs, sulfonamides, sulfonylureas, thiazide diuretics. Adrenocorticoid clearance is decreased with hypothyroidism and increased with hyperthyroidism. Cytokines, amiodarone may induce hypo- or hyperthyroidism. Increased risk of arrhythmias with maprotiline. HTN and tachycardia reported with ketamine. Sympathomimetics may increase risk of coronary insufficiency with CAD. Adverse effects of both drugs with TCAs. Decreased clearance of theophylline with hypothyroidism. Impaired β-blocker effects. Decreased digitalis effects. Decreased uptake of iodine-containing radiolabeled ions. Altered levels of theophylline may occur. Use with somatrem/somatropin may accelerate epiphyseal closure. Additive effects of both agents with TCAs. Avoid mixing crushed tabs with foods/formula with large amounts of iron, soybean or fiber.

**PREGNANCY:** Category A, caution in nursing.

**MECHANISM OF ACTION:** Thyroid hormone; not understood, suspected to control DNA transcription and protein synthesis.

**PHARMACOKINETICS: Distribution:** Plasma protein binding (99%); found in breast milk. **Metabolism:** Deiodination and conjugation in the liver (mainly), kidneys, and other tissues. **Elimination:** Urine, feces; (approximately 20% unchanged). ($T_4$) $T_{1/2}$=6-7 days, and ($T_3$) $T_{1/2}$≤2 days.

## NURSING CONSIDERATIONS

**Assessment:** Assess for suppressed TSH level with normal $T_3$ and $T_4$ or overt thyrotoxicosis, hypersensitivity history, CV disease (angina or acute MI), uncorrected adrenal insufficiency, thyroid diseases (nontoxic diffuse or nodular goiter), endocrine disorders (hypothalamic/pituitary hormone deficiencies and/or autoimmune polyglandular disorders), DM, clotting status, upcoming surgery and possible drug and test interactions. Assess infants for associated congenital anomalies.

**Monitoring:** Perform frequent lab tests and clinical evaluation of thyroid functions (TSH and free $T_4$ levels), glucose/lipid metabolism, blood and/or urinary glucose in diabetics, and clotting parameters. Monitor for CV signs (eg, arrhythmia, coronary insufficiency), growth development, bone metabolism, cognitive function, emotional status, GI functions, reproductive functions, partial hair loss in infants, and signs/symptoms of thyrotoxicosis.

**Patient Counseling:** Inform that drug is to be taken for life and not to be taken for treatment of obesity or weight reduction. Take 1 hr before breakfast on empty stomach with full glass of water. Notify if pregnant/nursing or planning to become pregnant. Notify if taking any other drugs. Do not d/c or change dose without consulting physician. Report any signs/symptoms of thyroid toxicity.

**Administration:** Oral route. **Storage:** Store at 25°C (77°F); excursions permitted to 15-30°C (59-86°F). Protect from light and moisture.

## Synvisc

RX

hylan G-F 20 (Wyeth)

**THERAPEUTIC CLASS:** Hylan polymer

**INDICATIONS:** Treatment of osteoarthritis (OA) knee pain inadequately responsive to conservative nonpharmacologic therapy and simple analgesics.

**DOSAGE:** *Adults:* Usual: Intra-articular injection once weekly (one week apart) for total of three injections.

**HOW SUPPLIED:** Inj: 8mg/mL

**CONTRAINDICATIONS:** Knee joint infections, hyaluronan hypersensitivity, skin diseases or infections in injection site area.

**WARNINGS/PRECAUTIONS:** Avoid with skin disinfectants containing quaternary ammonium salts; hyaluronan can precipitate in their presence. Do not inject extra-articularly or into synovial tissue and capsule. Intravascular injections may cause systemic adverse events. Caution with allergies to avian proteins, feathers, and egg products. Avoid with severely inflamed knee joints. Remove synovial fluid or effusion, if present, before injecting. Follow strict aseptic administration. Caution with lymphatic or venous stasis. Avoid strenuous activity or prolonged weight-bearing activities after injection. Packaging contains dry natural rubber latex.

**ADVERSE REACTIONS:** Injection-site pain, knee swelling/effusion, rash, calf cramps, ankle edema, muscle pain.

**INTERACTIONS:** Do not inject anesthetics or other drugs into knee joint during therapy.

**PREGNANCY:** Safety in pregnancy and nursing not known.

**MECHANISM OF ACTION:** Hylan polymer.

### NURSING CONSIDERATIONS

**Assessment:** Assess for knee joint infection, skin disease, or infection in area of injection site, pregnancy status, lymphatic or venous stasis.

**Monitoring:** Monitor for signs/symptoms of allergic reaction (eg, rash, hives, itching, fever), knee joint effusion/swelling, and local skin reactions.

**Patient Counseling:** Inform that use may cause transient pain/swelling of injected joint. Instruct to avoid any strenuous or prolonged weight-bearing activity (eg, jogging, tennis) within 48 hrs of injection. Seek medical attention if symptoms of allergic reaction occur.

**Administration:** Intra-articular. **Storage:** 30°C (86°F). Do not freeze. Protect from light.



## Talacen

CIV

pentazocine HCl - acetaminophen (Sanofi-Aventis)

**THERAPEUTIC CLASS:** Opioid agonist-antagonist analgesic

**INDICATIONS:** Relief of mild to moderate pain.

**DOSAGE:** *Adults:* 1 tab q4h prn. Max: 6 tabs/day. Elderly: Start at lower end of dosing range.

**HOW SUPPLIED:** Tab: (Pentazocine-APAP) 25mg-650mg* *scored

**WARNINGS/PRECAUTIONS:** May elevate CSF pressure. May produce effects that may obscure diagnosis or clinical course of head injuries. Transient hallucinations, disorientation and confusion reported; closely observe and check vital signs. Psychological and physical dependence may occur in patient with a history of drug abuse. Caution in patients with MI who have N/V, respiratory depression, renal/hepatic dysfunction, seizure disorders and in the elderly.

**ADVERSE REACTIONS:** N/V, constipation, abdominal distress, anorexia, diarrhea, dizziness, lightheadedness, hallucinations, sedation, euphoria, headache, confusion, disorientation, sweating, tachycardia.

**INTERACTIONS:** Increased CNS depressant effects with alcohol or other CNS depressants. Withdrawal symptoms with narcotics.

**PREGNANCY:** Category C, caution in nursing.

**MECHANISM OF ACTION:** Pentazocine: Acts as analgesic and sedative. APAP: Acts as analgesic and antipyretic.

**PHARMACOKINETICS: Absorption:** Pentazocine: Well-absorbed; $T_{max}$=1.7 hrs. APAP: Rapid and complete; $T_{max}$=0.5-2.5 hrs. **Distribution:** Pentazocine: Crosses placental barrier. **Metabolism:** Pentazocine: Liver. APAP: Liver via conjugation. **Elimination:** Pentazocine: Renal excretion, $T_{1/2}$=3.6 hrs. APAP: Urine (80% conjugated drug, 3% unchanged); $T_{1/2}$=2.8 hrs.

## NURSING CONSIDERATIONS

**Assessment:** Assess for asthma, presence of head injury, other intracranial lesions, preexisting increase in intracranial pressure, MI, respiratory depression, impaired renal/hepatic function, seizures, pregnancy status, and possible drug interactions.

**Monitoring:** Monitor signs and symptoms of sulfite hypersensitivity, asthma attack, CNS manifestations (eg, hallucinations, disorientation, confusion), respiratory depression, vital signs, drug abuse or dependence.

**Patient Counseling:** Inform that drug may cause sedation, dizziness, and occasional euphoria. Counsel about drug abuse and dependence. Avoid alcohol and do not abruptly d/c drug as there could be withdrawal symptoms. Exercise caution while driving or operating machinery.

**Administration:** Oral route. **Storage:** 25°C (77°F); excursions permitted to 15-30°C (59-86°F).

# TALWIN NX

CIV

pentazocine HCl - naloxone HCl (Sanofi-Aventis)

**For oral use only. Severe, potentially lethal reactions may result from misuse by injection alone, or in combination with other agents.**

**THERAPEUTIC CLASS:** Opioid agonist-antagonist analgesic

**INDICATIONS:** Relief of moderate to severe pain.

**DOSAGE:** *Adults:* Usual: 1 tab q3-4h. May increase to 2 tabs q3-4h. Max: 12 tabs/day.
*Pediatrics:* ≥12 yrs: Usual: 1 tab q3-4h. May increase to 2 tabs q3-4h. Max: 12 tabs/day.

**HOW SUPPLIED:** Tab. (Pentazocine-Naloxone) 50mg 0.5mg* *scored

**WARNINGS/PRECAUTIONS:** Caution with elderly, drug dependence, head injury, increased ICP, certain respiratory conditions, acute CNS manifestations, renal or hepatic dysfunction, biliary surgery, and MI.

**ADVERSE REACTIONS:** Hypotension, tachycardia, hallucinations, dizziness, sedation, euphoria, sweating, N/V, constipation, diarrhea, anorexia, facial edema, dermatitis, visual problems, chills, insomnia, urinary retention, paresthesia.

**INTERACTIONS:** Increased CNS depressant effects with alcohol. Withdrawal symptoms with narcotics.

**PREGNANCY:** Category C, caution in nursing.

**MECHANISM OF ACTION:** Pentazocine: Acts as analgesic and sedative. Naloxone: Acts as antagonist to pentazocine and pure antagonist to narcotic analgesics.

T

**PHARMACOKINETICS: Absorption:** Pentazocine: GI tract (well absorbed), $T_{max}$=1-3 hrs. **Distribution:** Pentazocine: Crosses placenta. **Metabolism:** Pentazocine: Liver. **Elimination:** Pentazocine: Urine; $T_{1/2}$=2-3 hrs.

## NURSING CONSIDERATIONS

**Assessment:** Assess for head injury, MI, respiratory depression, impaired renal/hepatic function, biliary surgery, seizures, pregnancy status, and possible drug interactions.

**Monitoring:** Monitor vital signs, sedation, seizures, respiratory depression, N/V, BP, HR, allergic reactions, leukopenia, drug abuse or dependence.

**Patient Counseling:** Inform that drug may cause sedation, dizziness, and occasional euphoria. Counsel about drug abuse and dependence. Avoid alcohol and do not abruptly d/c drug as there could be withdrawal symptoms. Exercise caution while driving or operating machinery.

**Administration:** Oral route. **Storage:** 25°C (77°F); excursions permitted to 15-30°C (59-86°F).

# TAMBOCOR

RX

flecainide acetate (Graceway)

**THERAPEUTIC CLASS:** Class IC antiarrhythmic

**INDICATIONS:** Prevention of paroxysmal supraventricular tachycardias (PSVT), paroxysmal atrial fibrillation/flutter (PAF) associated with disabling symptoms in patients without structural heart disease. Prevention of documented ventricular arrhythmias such as sustained ventricular tachycardia (VT).

**DOSAGE:** *Adults:* PSVT/PAF: Initial: 50mg q12h. Titrate: May increase by 50mg bid every 4 days. Max: 300mg/day. Sustained VT: Initial: 100mg q12h. Titrate: May increase by 50mg bid every 4 days. Max: 400mg/day. CrCl ≤35mL/min: Initial: 100mg qd or 50mg bid. Reduce dose by 50% with amiodarone. *Pediatrics:* <6 months: Initial: 50mg/m²/day given bid-tid. ≥6 months: Initial: 100mg/m²/day given bid-tid. Max: 200mg/m²/day. Reduce dose by 50% with amiodarone.

**HOW SUPPLIED:** Tab: 50mg, 100mg*, 150mg* *scored

**CONTRAINDICATIONS:** Right bundle branch block associated with left hemiblock (without a pacemaker), pre-existing 2nd- or 3rd-degree AV block, cardiogenic shock.

**WARNINGS/PRECAUTIONS:** Avoid with non-life-threatening ventricular arrhythmias. Increased mortality and non-cardiac arrests reported. Ventricular proarrhythmic effects may occur with atrial fibrillation/flutter. May cause or worsen CHF, arrhythmias. Slows cardiac conduction; dose related increases in PR, QRS, and QT intervals reported. Conduction changes may cause sinus pause, sinus arrest, bradycardia, 2nd- or 3rd-degree AV block. Extreme caution with sick sinus syndrome. May increase endocardial pacing thresholds and suppress ventricular escape with pacemakers. Correct hypokalemia or hyperkalemia before therapy. Monitor with significant hepatic impairment. Initiate treatment of sustained VT in the hospital.



**ADVERSE REACTIONS:** Arrhythmias, hepatic dysfunction, cardiac arrest, CHF, dizziness, visual disturbances, headache, fatigue, N/V, dyspnea.

**INTERACTIONS:** Additive negative inotropic effects with β-blockers (eg, propranolol). Potentiated by cimetidine, amiodarone, CYP2D6 inhibitors (eg, quinidine). Increases digoxin levels. Increased elimination with phenytoin, phenobarbital, carbamazepine. Diltiazem, nifedipine, verapamil, disopyramide not recommended.

**PREGNANCY:** Category C, safety not known in nursing.

**MECHANISM OF ACTION:** Class 1C antiarrhythmic agent with local anesthetic activity; decreases intracardiac conduction in all parts of the heart with greatest effect on His-Purkinje system (H-V conduction).

**PHARMACOKINETICS: Absorption:** Complete. $T_{max}$=3 hrs. **Distribution:** Plasma protein binding (40%). Found in human milk. **Metabolism:** Extensive, via CYP2D6. Meta-O-dealkylated flecainide (active metabolite). **Elimination:** Urine (30% unchanged), feces (5%); $T_{1/2}$=20 hrs, 29 hrs (at birth), 11-12 hrs (3 months), 6 hrs (1 yr), 8 hrs (1-12 yrs), and 11-12 hrs (12-15 yrs).

## NURSING CONSIDERATIONS

**Assessment:** Assess for pre-existing 2nd- or 3rd-degree AV block, right bundle branch block associated with a left hemiblock, implanted pacemaker, cardiogenic shock, MI, asymptomatic non-life threatening ventricular arrhythmia, atrial fibrillation/flutter, cardiomyopathy, pre-existing severe HF or low ejection fraction, sick sinus syndrome, supraventricular tachycardia, hypersensitivity, pregnancy/nursing status, and possible drug interactions. Correct hypokalemia or hyperkalemia prior to therapy.

**Monitoring:** Determine pacing threshold in patients with pacemaker prior to therapy, after 1 week, and at regular intervals thereafter. Periodically monitor plasma levels with renal/hepatic impairment, CHF, and/or those on concurrent amiodarone therapy. Monitor for HR, ECG changes, paradoxical increase in ventricular rate, proarrhythmic effects (new or worsened supraventricular or ventricular arrhythmia), worsening of CHF, effects on cardiac conduction, bradycardia, and hypersensitivity reactions.

**Patient Counseling:** Advise about importance of initiating therapy in hospital with continuous rhythmic monitoring. Inform about risks/benefits and report any adverse reactions to physician.

**Administration:** Oral route. **Storage:** 15-30°C (59-86°F). Store in tight, light-resistant containers.

# TAMIFLU

**RX**

oseltamivir phosphate (Roche Labs)

**THERAPEUTIC CLASS:** Neuraminidase inhibitor

**INDICATIONS:** Treatment of uncomplicated acute illness due to influenza in adults and children ≥1 yr who have been symptomatic for no more than 2 days. Prophylaxis of influenza in adults and children ≥1 yr.

**DOSAGE:** *Adults:* Prophylaxis: Begin within 2 days of exposure to infection. 75mg qd for at least 10 days. CrCl 10-30mL/min: 75mg every other day or 30mg qd. Treatment: Begin therapy within 2 days of symptom onset. 75mg bid for 5 days. CrCl 10-30mL/min: 75mg qd for 5 days.
*Pediatrics:* Prophylaxis: ≥13 yr: Begin within 2 days of exposure to infection. 75mg qd for at least 10 days. ≥1 yr: (Sus) ≤15kg: 30mg qd. >15-23kg: 45mg qd. >23-40kg: 60mg qd. >40kg: 75mg qd. Duration: 10 days. Treatment: ≥13 yrs: Begin therapy within 2 days of symptom onset. 75mg bid for 5 days. ≥1 yr: (Sus) ≤15kg: 30mg bid. >15-23kg: 45mg bid. >23-40kg: 60mg bid. >40kg: 75mg bid. Duration: 5 days.

**HOW SUPPLIED:** Cap: 30mg, 45mg, 75mg; Sus: 300mg/25mL

**WARNINGS/PRECAUTIONS:** Adjust dose in patients with CrCl <30mL/min. Rare cases of anaphylaxis and serious skin reactions (eg, toxic epidermal necrolysis, Stevens-Johnson syndrome, erythema multiforme) reported; d/c and initiate appropriate treatment if an allergic-like reactions occurs or is suspected. Postmarketing neuropsychiatric events (eg, hallucinations, delirium, abnormal behavior) reported; monitor closely for signs of abnormal behavior.

**ADVERSE REACTIONS:** N/V, diarrhea, cough, headache, fatigue, abdominal pain, bronchitis, dizziness, diarrhea, insomnia, vertigo.

**INTERACTIONS:** Avoid administration of attenuated influenza vaccine within 2 weeks before or 48 hours after; may inhibit replication of live vaccine virus. May increase exposure to oseltamavir carboxylate when coadministered with probenecid.

**PREGNANCY:** Category C, caution in nursing.

**MECHANISM OF ACTION:** Neuraminidase inhibitor; inhibits influenza virus neuraminidase, affecting release of viral particles.

**PHARMACOKINETICS: Absorption:** (GI tract). Oseltamivir: $C_{max}$=65.2ng/mL; $AUC_{0-12h}$=112ng•hr/mL. Oseltamivir carboxylate (metabolite); $C_{max}$=348ng/mL; $AUC_{0-12h}$=2719ng•hr/mL. **Distribution:** Oseltamivir carboxylate: (IV): $V_d$=23-26L; plasma protein binding (3%). Oseltamivir: Plasma protein binding (42%). **Metabolism:** Oseltamivir: Hepatic (esterases). Metabolite: (Oseltamivir carboxylate). **Elimination:** Oseltamivir carboxylate: Renal (>99%); feces (<20%); $T_{1/2}$=6-10 hrs.

## NURSING CONSIDERATIONS

**Assessment:** Assess for renal impairment, neuropsychiatric events, hereditary fructose intolerance, pregnancy/nursing status, and possible drug interactions.

**Monitoring:** Monitor for signs/symptoms of neuropsychiatric events (eg, hallucinations, delirium, abnormal behavior), anaphylaxis/serious skin reactions, renal impairment, and fructose intolerance (eg, dyspepsia, diarrhea).

**Patient Counseling:** Instruct to begin treatment as soon as first appearance of flu symptoms. Advise to take missed doses as soon as possible, unless if next scheduled dose is within 2 hrs. Inform that medication is not a substitute for a flu vaccination. May take with/without food. Seek medical attention if symptoms of neuropsychiatric events (eg, hallucinations, delirium, abnormal behavior), anaphylaxis/serious skin reactions, renal impairment, or fructose intolerance (eg, dyspepsia, diarrhea) occur.

**Administration:** Oral route. **Storage:** Powder/Cap: 25°C (77°F); excursions permitted to 15-30°C (59-86°F). Sus: 2-8°C (36-46°F). Do not freeze.

# TAMOXIFEN RX

tamoxifen citrate (Various)

**For women with ductal carcinoma in situ (DCIS) and women at high risk for breast cancer; serious and life-threatening events including uterine malignancies (eg, endometrial adenocarcinoma, uterine sarcoma), stroke, and PE reported with use in the risk-reduction setting. Discuss the potential benefits vs. the potential risks of these serious events with women at high risk of breast cancer and women with DCIS. The benefits of tamoxifen outweigh risks in women already diagnosed with breast cancer.**

**THERAPEUTIC CLASS:** Antiestrogen

**INDICATIONS:** Treatment of metastatic breast cancer in women and men. Treatment of node-positive and axillary node-negative breast cancer in women following mastectomy, axillary dissection, and breast irradiation. To reduce risk of invasive breast cancer in women with DCIS. Reduction of breast cancer incidence in high risk women. Use for up to 5 yrs.

**DOSAGE:** *Adults:* Breast Cancer Treatment: 20-40mg qd. Divide dosages >20mg into AM and PM doses. Breast Cancer Risk Reduction/DCIS: 20mg qd for 5 yrs.

T

**HOW SUPPLIED:** Tab: 10mg, 20mg

**CONTRAINDICATIONS:** Women who require coumarin-type anticoagulant therapy or have a history of DVT, PE.

**WARNINGS/PRECAUTIONS:** Hypercalcemia reported in patients with bone metastases. Increased incidence of uterine malignancies (eg, endometrial carcinoma, uterine sarcoma) and endometrial changes including hyperplasia and polyps with use. Endometriosis, fibroids, ovarian cysts, and menstrual irregularities also reported. Increased incidence of thromboembolic events (eg, DVT, PE). Malignant and non-malignant effects on the liver and ocular disturbances reported. Leukopenia, anemia, thrombocytopenia, neutropenia, pancytopenia reported. Promptly evaluate abnormal vaginal bleeding if receiving or previously received tamoxifen. Patients receiving or who have previously received tamoxifen should have annual gynecological examinations and should promptly notify physician if experience any abnormal gynecological symptoms (eg, menstrual irregularities, abnormal vaginal bleeding, changes in vaginal discharge, pelvic pain or pressure). May cause fetal harm during pregnancy; avoid pregnancy within 2 months of therapy. May cause hyperlipidemia; periodic monitoring of plasma triglycerides and cholesterol may be indicated in patients with pre-existing hyperlipidemias. Does not cause infertility even with menstrual irregularity. Perform periodic CBC, including platelet counts and periodic LFTs.

**ADVERSE REACTIONS:** Hot flashes, vaginal discharge, fatigue/asthenia, mood disturbances, N/V, irregular menses, fluid retention, pain, headache, infection, flu syndrome, weight loss, vasodilatation; (men) loss of libido, impotence.

**INTERACTIONS:** Increases effects of coumarin-type anticoagulant; monitor PT. Increased risk of thromboembolic events with cytotoxic agents. Increased levels with bromocriptine. May decrease letrozole levels. Decreased levels with rifampin and aminoglutethimide. Decreased plasma levels of major metabolite, N-desmethyl tamoxifen with medroxyprogesterone. Avoid administering with anastrozole.

**PREGNANCY:** Category D, not for use in nursing.

**MECHANISM OF ACTION:** Non-steroidal antiestrogen; competes with estrogen for binding sites in target tissues.

**PHARMACOKINETICS: Absorption:** $C_{max}$=40ng/mL; $T_{max}$=5 hrs. N-desmethyl tamoxifen: $C_{max}$=15ng/mL. **Metabolism:** N-desmethyl tamoxifen (major metabolite). **Elimination:** Feces (primary); $T_{1/2}$=5-7 days.

## NURSING CONSIDERATIONS

**Assessment:** Assess for history of DVT and PE, hepatic impairment, hyperlipidemia, pregnancy/nursing status, and for possible drug interactions. Perform baseline breast exam, gynecologic exam; obtain baseline mammogram.

**Monitoring:** Monitor for signs/symptoms of hypercalcemia, uterine malignancies, endometrial changes, thromboembolic events (eg, PE, DVT), ocular disturbances, and for hypersensitivity reactions. Monitor CBCs with platelets and LFTs periodically. Perform breast exam, mammogram, and gynecologic exam routinely. Perform periodic monitoring of plasma triglycerides and cholesterol levels in patients with pre-existing hyperlipidemia.

**Patient Counseling:** Inform of pregnancy risks; advise to use nonhormonal contraception during therapy and for 2 months after d/c. Instruct women who are taking tamoxifen or have taken tamoxifen to seek medical attention if experience symptoms of new breast lumps, vaginal bleeding, gynecological symptoms (eg, menstrual irregularities, pelvic pain or pressure) leg swelling/tenderness, unexplained SOB, or changes in vision.

**Administration:** Oral route. **Storage:** 20-25°C (68-77°F). Dispense in a well-closed, light-resistant container with a child-resistant closure.

# TARCEVA — RX

erlotinib (Genentech/OSI)

**THERAPEUTIC CLASS:** Epidermal growth factor receptor tyrosine kinase inhibitor

**INDICATIONS:** Treatment of locally advanced or metastatic non-small cell lung cancer (NSCLC) after failure of at least one prior chemotherapy regimen. 1st-line treatment of locally advanced, unresectable, or metastatic pancreatic cancer in combination with gemcitabine.

**DOSAGE:** *Adults:* NSCLC: 150mg qd. Pancreatic Cancer: 100mg qd in combination with gemcitabine. Continue until disease progression or unacceptable toxicity. D/C if patient develops interstitial lung disease (ILD), hepatic failure, GI perforation. Interrupt or d/c in patients with dehydration who are at risk for renal failure, severe bullous, blistering or exfoliative skin conditions, and acute/worsening ocular disorders. Severe Diarrhea/Severe Skin Reactions: May require dose reduction or temporary interruption of therapy. When dose reduction is necessary, reduce dose in 50mg decrements. Concomitant Use With Strong CYP3A4 Inhibitors or Inhibitors of Both CYP3A4 and CYP1A2: Reduce dose if severe adverse events occur. Concomitant Use With CYP3A4 Inducers: Consider alternative treatment or increase the dose at 2-week intervals. Max: 450mg. Cigarette smoker: Increase the dose. Max: 300mg. Interrupt or d/c if total bilirubin >3x ULN and/or transaminases are >5x ULN if pretreatment values normal.

**HOW SUPPLIED:** Tab: 25mg, 100mg, 150mg

**WARNINGS/PRECAUTIONS:** Serious interstitial lung disease (ILD)-like events, including fatalities, reported; d/c if ILD diagnosed. Hepatorenal syndrome, acute renal failure, and renal insufficiency reported. If dehydration occurs, interrupt therapy and intensively rehydrate. If patient is at risk of dehydration, periodically monitor renal function and serum electrolytes. Hepatic failure reported; perform periodic LFTs. If LFTs worsen, interrupt dose or reduce dose and monitor frequently. Take extra caution in patients with total bilirubin >3x ULN. Monitor patients with hepatic impairment closely; interrupt or d/c if changes in liver function are severe. GI perforation reported; caution with history of peptic ulceration or diverticular disease. Bullous, blistering, and exfoliative skin conditions reported; interrupt or d/c if symptoms develop. May cause MI/ischemia, cerebrovascular accidents, and microangiopathic hemolytic anemia with thrombocytopenia. Corneal perforation and ulceration reported; interrupt or d/c if ocular disorders worsen or become acute. INR elevations and infrequent bleeding events reported.

**ADVERSE REACTIONS:** Rash, diarrhea, anorexia, fatigue, dyspnea, cough, N/V, infection, stomatitis, pruritus, dry skin, conjunctivitis, keratoconjunctivitis sicca, abdominal pain, decreased weight.

**INTERACTIONS:** Increased concentrations with ketoconazole and other strong CYP3A4 inhibitors including ciprofloxacin, atazanavir, clarithromycin, indinavir, itraconazole, nefazodone, nelfinavir, ritonavir, saquinavir, telithromycin, troleandomycin, voriconazole, and grapefruit or grapefruit juice. CYP3A4 inducers may decrease plasma concentrations; use of CYP3A4 inducers (eg, rifampin, rifabutin, rifapentine, phenytoin, carbamazepine, phenobarbital, St. John's wort) is not recommended unless alternative therapy is unavailable. Cigarette smoking may reduce AUC. May decrease the AUC of CYP3A4 substrate midazolam. Drugs that alter pH of upper GI tract may alter solubility and bioavailability; concomitant use of proton pump inhibitors should be avoided. Monitor for changes in PT or INR if taking warfarin or other coumarin-derivative anticoagulants. Use with anti-angiogenic agents, corticosteroids, NSAIDs, and/or taxane-based chemotherapy may increase risk of GI perforation.

**PREGNANCY:** Category D, not for use in nursing.

**MECHANISM OF ACTION:** Kinase inhibitor; inhibits the intracellular phosphorylation of tyrosine kinase associated with epidermal growth factor receptor (EGFR).

**PHARMACOKINETICS: Absorption**: $T_{max}$=4 hrs. **Distribution:** $V_d$=232L; plasma protein binding (93%). **Metabolism:** CYP3A4 (major); CYP1A2, 1A1 (minor). **Elimination:** Feces (83%), urine (8%); $T_{1/2}$=36.2hrs.

## NURSING CONSIDERATIONS

T

**Assessment:** Assess for lung disease, lung infection, hepatic/renal impairment, dehydration, history of peptic ulceration or diverticular disease, pregnancy/nursing status, and possible drug interactions. Obtain baseline LFTs and renal function. If taking warfarin or other coumarin anticoagulants, obtain baseline PT/INR.

**Monitoring:** Monitor for signs and symptoms of ILD (eg, dyspnea, cough, fever), hepatorenal syndrome, acute renal failure, renal insufficiency, and dehydration. Perform periodic monitoring of renal function and serum electrolytes if there is a risk of dehydration. Monitor for signs and symptoms of hepatotoxicity; perform periodic monitoring of LFTs (transaminases, bilirubin, alkaline phosphatase). Monitor for signs and symptoms of GI perforation, bullous and exfoliative skin disorders, MI/ischemia, cerebrovascular accident, microangiopathic hemolytic anemia with thrombocytopenia, and for corneal perforation and ulceration. If taking concomitant warfarin or coumarin anticoagulants, monitor PT/INR.

**Patient Counseling:** Instruct to seek medical attention if patients notice onset or worsening of skin rash, severe or persistent diarrhea, N/V, anorexia, onset or worsening of SOB, cough, or if eye irritation occurs. Recommend use of sunscreen and avoidance of sun exposure. Advise to stop smoking and to avoid becoming pregnant while on therapy.

**Administration:** Oral route. Take at least 1 hr before or 2 hrs after ingestion of food. **Storage**: 25°C (77°F); excursions permitted to 15-30° (59-86°F).

## TARKA RX

verapamil HCl - trandolapril (Abbott)

**ACE inhibitors can cause death/injury to developing fetus during 2nd and 3rd trimesters. D/C if pregnancy is detected.**

**THERAPEUTIC CLASS:** ACE inhibitor/calcium channel blocker (nondihydropyridine)

**INDICATIONS:** Treatment of hypertension.

**DOSAGE:** *Adults:* Replacement Therapy: 1 tab qd with food.

**HOW SUPPLIED:** Tab: (Trandolapril-Verapamil) 2mg-180mg, 1mg-240mg, 2mg-240mg, 4mg-240mg

**CONTRAINDICATIONS:** Severe left ventricular dysfunction, hypotension, cardiogenic shock, sick sinus syndrome or 2nd- or 3rd-degree AV block (except with functioning ventricular pacemaker), A-Fib/Flutter with an accessory bypass tract, history of ACE inhibitor-associated angioedema.

**WARNINGS/PRECAUTIONS:** Monitor for hypotension with surgery or anesthesia. Risk of hyperkalemia with renal insufficiency, DM. D/C if jaundice develops. Avoid with moderate to severe cardiac failure and ventricular dysfunction if taking a β-blocker. May cause angioedema, cough, fetal/neonatal morbidity and death, hypotension, AV block, anaphylactoid reactions, transient bradycardia, PR-interval prolongation. Monitor LFTs periodically. Reduce dose with severe hepatic dysfunction. Caution with CHF, hypertrophic cardiomyopathy, renal or hepatic dysfunction. Decrease dose in those with decreased neuromuscular transmission. Monitor WBCs with collagen-vascular disease and/or renal disease. Not for initial treatment.

**ADVERSE REACTIONS:** AV block, constipation, cough, dizziness, fatigue, headache, increased hepatic enzymes, chest pain, upper respiratory tract infection/congestion.

**INTERACTIONS:** Additive effects on HR, AV conduction, and contractility with β-blockers. Potentiates other antihypertensives. May increase digoxin, carbamazepine, theophylline, and cyclosporine levels. Avoid disopyramide within 48 hrs before or 24 hrs after verapamil. Additive negative inotropic effects and AV conduction prolongation with flecainide. Avoid quinidine with hypertrophic cardiomyopathy. Monitor lithium. Increased clearance with phenobarbital. Rifampin may reduce oral bioavailability. May potentiate neuromuscular blockers; both agents may need dose reduction. Risk of hyperkalemia with $K^+$-sparing diuretics, $K^+$ supplements. Caution with inhalation anesthetics. Risks of hypotension, bradyarrhythmias, and lactic acidosis with clarithromycin and erythromycin ethylsuccinate. Nitritoid reactions (eg, facial flushing, NV, hypotension) reported rarely with injectable gold.

**PREGNANCY:** Category C (1st trimester) and D (2nd and 3rd trimesters), not for use in nursing.

**MECHANISM OF ACTION:** Trandolapril: ACE inhibitor; inhibition results in decreased plasma angiotensin II, which leads to decreased vasopressor activity and decreased aldosterone secretion. Verapamil: Calcium channel blocker; modulates influx of ionic calcium across the cell membrane of the arterial smooth muscle as well as in conductile and contractile myocardial cells. Decreases systemic vascular resistance, usually without orthostatic decreases in BP or reflex tachycardia.

**PHARMACOKINETICS: Absorption:** Verapamil: Absolute bioavailability (20-35%), $T_{max}$=4-15 hrs. Trandolopril: Absolute bioavailability (approximate 10%), $T_{max}$=0.5-2 hrs. **Distribution:** Verapamil: Plasma protein binding (90%). Trandolapril: Plasma protein binding (80%). **Metabolism:** Verapamil: Liver.

**Elimination:** Verapamil: Urine 70% (metabolite), 3-4% (unchanged), feces 16% (metabolite). Trandolapril: Urine 33% (metabolite), <1% (unchanged), feces 66% (metabolite).

## NURSING CONSIDERATIONS

**Assessment:** Assess for severe left ventricular dysfunction, hypotension, cardiogenic shock, sick sinus syndrome, 2nd- or 3rd-degree AV block, atrial flutter or atrial fibrillation, history of angioedema, heart failure, hypotension, LFTs, renal function, CHF, accessory bypass tract, hypertrophic cardiomyopathy, CBC with platelets and differential, pregnancy status, neuromuscular disorders (Duchenne's), and possible drug interactions.

**Monitoring:** Monitor for angioedema, cough, anaphylactoid reactions, LFTs, renal function, headaches, URI, heart block, chest pains, CBC with platelets and differential count, serum electrolytes.

**Patient Counseling:** Counsel regarding adverse effects (eg, angioedema, neutropenia, jaundice) and instruct to report any signs/symptoms. Inform of risks when taken during pregnancy. Educate about need for periodic follow-ups and blood tests to rule out adverse effects and to monitor therapeutic effects.

**Administration:** Oral route. **Storage:** 15-25°C (59-77°F). Dispense in tightly closed container with safety closure.

# TASMAR — RX

tolcapone (Valeant)

**Risk of fatal, acute fulminant liver failure. Withdraw if patients fail to show benefit within 3 weeks of initiation. D/C if hepatotoxicity develops, and do not consider retreatment. Perform LFTs before therapy, then every 2 weeks for 1st year, every 4 weeks for next 6 months, then every 8 weeks thereafter. Perform LFTs before increase dose to 200mg tid. Avoid with liver disease or if LFTs ≥2x ULN. Caution with severe dyskinesia or dystonia.**

**THERAPEUTIC CLASS:** COMT inhibitor

**INDICATIONS:** Adjunct to levodopa/carbidopa for the treatment of symptoms of idiopathic Parkinson's disease.

**DOSAGE:** *Adults:* Initial: 100mg tid. Use 200mg tid only if clinical benefit is justified. May need to decrease levodopa dose.

**HOW SUPPLIED:** Tab: 100mg, 200mg

**CONTRAINDICATIONS:** Liver disease, patients withdrawn from therapy due to drug-induced hepatocellular injury. History of non-traumatic rhabdomyolysis, hyperpyrexia or confusion related to medication.

**WARNINGS/PRECAUTIONS:** Dyskinesia, hypotension/syncope, rhabdomyolysis, hallucinations, hyperpyrexia, confusion, diarrhea, hematuria, fibrotic complications reported. Avoid with liver dysfunction. Caution with severe renal dysfunction. Closely monitor when d/c therapy. Increased risk of melanoma with Parkinson's disease; monitor periodically.

T

**ADVERSE REACTIONS:** Dyskinesia, dystonia, excessive dreaming, anorexia, muscle cramps, orthostatic complaints, diarrhea, confusion, hallucination, N/V, constipation, fatigue, increased sweating, xerostomia, urine discoloration, hepatotoxicity.

**INTERACTIONS:** α-methyldopa, dobutamine, apomorphine and isoproterenol may need a dose reduction. Avoid non-selective MAOIs (eg, phenelzine, tranylcypromine). May increase risk of orthostatic hypotension and dyskinesia with levodopa. Caution with tolbutamide, desipramine, warfarin.

**PREGNANCY:** Category C, caution in nursing.

**MECHANISM OF ACTION:** Catecol-*O*-methyltransferase inhibitor; suspected to alter the plasma pharmacokinetics of levodopa, leading to more sustained plasma levels of drug.

**PHARMACOKINETICS: Absorption:** (PO) Rapidly absorbed; absolute bioavailability (65%); $T_{max}$=2 hrs; $C_{max}$=3mcg/mL (100mg, 200mg); $C_{max}$=6mcg/mL (100mg, 200mg). **Distribution:** $V_d$=9L; plasma protein binding (>99.9%).

**Metabolism:** Liver (glucuronidation) via CYP450 enzymes 3A4, 2A6. **Elimination:** Urine (60%, 0.5% unchanged), feces (40%); $T_{1/2}$=2-3 hrs.

## NURSING CONSIDERATIONS

**Assessment:** Assess LFTs, renal function test, dyskinesia, psychosis, depression, and cardiovascular complications.

**Monitoring:** LFTs (SGPT/ALT, SGOT/AST), renal function test, hypotension/syncope, diarrhea, dyskinesia, rhabdomyolysis, hematuria, hyperpyrexia, confusion, melanoma, fibrotic complications, hallucinations, and depression.

**Patient Counseling:** Instruct to take as prescribed. Caution while operating machinery/driving. Regular follow-up needed. Avoid alcohol, OTC agents, and CNS depressants. Report adverse effects. Inform signs and symptoms of onset hepatic injury. Advise that hallucinations and nausea may occur. Inform the possibility of increased dyskinesia and dystonia. Notify physician if new or increased gambling urges, sexual urges or other intense urges occur.

**Administration:** Oral route. **Storage:** 20-25°C (68-77°F). Keep in tight container.

# TAXOL — RX

paclitaxel (Bristol-Myers Squibb)

**Administer under supervision of an experienced physician in the use of cancer chemotherapeutic agents. Anaphylaxis, severe hypersensitivity reactions reported. Pretreat with corticosteroids, diphenhydramine, and $H_2$ antagonists. Do not rechallenge if severe hypersensitivity reaction occurs. Not given to patients with solid tumors having baseline neutrophil counts of <1500 cells/mm³ and with AIDS-related Kaposi's sarcoma having baseline neutrophil count of <1000 cells/mm³. Monitor peripheral blood cell counts frequently.**

**THERAPEUTIC CLASS:** Antimicrotubule agent

**INDICATIONS:** First-line (with cisplatin) and subsequent treatment of advanced ovarian carcinoma and non-small cell lung cancer. Adjuvant treatment of node-positive breast cancer administered sequentially to doxorubicin-containing chemotherapy. Treatment of breast cancer after failure of combination chemotherapy for metastatic disease or relapse within 6 months of adjuvant chemotherapy. Second-line treatment of AIDS-related Kaposi's sarcoma. First-line treatment of non-small cell lung cancer in combination with cisplatin in patients who are not candidates for potentially curative surgery and/or radiation therapy.

**DOSAGE:** *Adults:* IV: Ovarian Carcinoma: Previously Untreated: 175mg/m² over 3 hrs or 135mg/m² over 24 hrs q3 weeks followed by cisplatin. Previously Treated: 135mg/m² or 175mg/m² over 3 hrs q3 weeks. Breast Cancer (adjuvant treatment of node positive/failure of initial chemo for metastatic disease or relapse): 175mg/m² over 3 hrs q3 weeks for 4 courses. Non-Small Cell Lung Cancer: 135mg/m² over 24 hrs q3 weeks followed by cisplatin. Kaposi's Sarcoma: 135mg/m² over 3 hrs q3 weeks or 100mg/m² over 3 hrs q2 weeks. Reduce dose of subsequent courses by 20% if neutrophils <500 cells/mm³ for ≥1 week or severe peripheral neuropathy occurs. Refer to PI for dosing in patients with hepatic impairment.

**HOW SUPPLIED:** Inj: 6mg/mL

**CONTRAINDICATIONS:** Hypersensitivity to drugs formulated in Cremophor® EL, solid tumor patients with baseline neutrophils <1500 cells/mm³, or AIDS-related Kaposi's sarcoma patients with baseline neutrophils <1000 cells/mm³.

**WARNINGS/PRECAUTIONS:** Severe conduction abnormalities documented; appropriate therapy should be adminstered and continuous monitoring should be performed during subsequent therapy if develop. Injection-site reactions, peripheral neuropathy reported. Bone marrow suppression is dose dependent and is the dose limiting toxicity. Can cause fetal harm. Hypotension, bradycardia, and HTN may occur during administration. Contains dehydrated alcohol, CNS and other alcohol effects may occur.

T

**ADVERSE REACTIONS:** Neutropenia, leukopenia, thrombocytopenia, anemia, infections, bleeding, bradycardia, hypotension, peripheral neuropathy, myalgia/arthralgia, N/V, diarrhea, mucositis, alopecia, injection-site reactions.

**INTERACTIONS:** Increases doxorubicin levels. Caution with CYP450 2C8 and 3A4 substrates, inducers (eg, rifampicin, carbamazepine, phenytoin, efavirenz, nevirapine)or inhibitors (eg, erythromycin, fluoxetine, gemfibrozil). Myelosuppression more profound with cisplatin.

**PREGNANCY:** Category D, not for use in nursing.

**MECHANISM OF ACTION:** Antimicrotubule; promotes assembly of microtubules from tubulin dimers and stabilizes microtubules by preventing depolymerization inhibiting microtubule network essential for vital interphase and mitotic cellular functions.

**PHARMACOKINETICS: Absorption:** IV administration of multiple doses resulted in different parameters. **Distribution:** $V_d$=227-688L/m²; plasma protein binding (89-98%). **Metabolism:** CYP2C8 (major), CYP3A4 (minor). 6α-hydroxy paclitaxel (metabolite). **Elimination:** Urine (1.3-12.6%), feces.

## NURSING CONSIDERATIONS

**Assessment:** Assess for pregnancy status, possible drug interactions, neutrophil count (>1500 cells/mm³ for solid tumors; >1000 cells/mm³ for Kaposi's sarcoma), hypersensitivity to Cremophor EL, and hepatic impairment.

**Monitoring:** Monitor blood count frequently; vital signs frequently during 1st hr of infusion. Monitor for signs/symptoms of anaphylaxis/hypersensitivity reactions, injection-site reactions, conduction abnormalities, bone marrow suppression, infections, neutropenia, and hepatic dysfunction.

**Patient Counseling:** Inform of pregnancy risks. Advise to seek medical attention if symptoms of infection, anaphylaxis/hypersensitivity reactions (eg, dyspnea, hypotension, angioedema, urticaria), conduction abnormalities, or injection site reactions (eg, erythema, tenderness, swelling, discoloration) occur. Advise to avoid contact of the undiluted concentrate with plasticized polyvinyl chloride (PVC) equipment or devices in preparing solutions.

**Administration:** IV route. **Storage:** 20-25°C (68-77°F). Protect from light.

# TAXOTERE RX

docetaxel (Sanofi-Aventis)

**Increased treatment-related mortality reported with hepatic dysfunction, high-dose therapy, and in non-small cell lung carcinoma previously treated with platinum-based chemotherapy with docetaxel 100mg/m². Avoid if neutrophils <1500 cells/mm³, bilirubin >ULN, or SGOT/SGPT >1.5x ULN with alkaline phosphatase >2.5x ULN. Severe hypersensitivity reactions reported. Severe fluid retention may occur despite dexamethasone.**

**THERAPEUTIC CLASS:** Antimicrotubule agent

T

**INDICATIONS:** Treatment of locally advanced or metastatic breast cancer and non-small cell lung cancer (NSCLC) after failure of prior chemotherapy. In combination with doxorubicin and cyclophosphamide for the adjuvant treatment of operable, node-positive breast cancer. In combination with cisplatin for treatment of unresectable, locally advanced or metastatic NSCLC in those previously untreated with chemotherapy. In combination with prednisone for treatment of androgen independent (hormone refractory) metastatic prostate cancer. In combination with cisplatin and fluorouracil for the treatment of advanced gastric adenocarcinoma, including adenocarcinoma of the gastroesophageal junction, in patients who have not received prior chemotherapy for advanced disease. In combination with cisplatin and fluorouracil for the induction treatment of patients with locally advanced squamous cell carcinoma of the head and neck (SCCHN).

**DOSAGE:** *Adults:* Premedicate with oral corticosteroids. Adjust dose based on febrile neutropenia, neutrophil count, cutaneous reactions, peripheral neuropathy, neurosensory signs/symptoms, or GI toxicities (see PI). Breast Cancer: 60-100mg/m² IV over 1 hr every 3 weeks. Adjuvant Treatment Operable Node-Positive Breast Cancer: 75mg/m² 1 hr after doxorubicin 50mg/m² and cyclophosphamide 500mg/m² every 3 weeks for 6 courses. NSCLC: 75mg/m² IV over 1 hr every 3 weeks. Prostate Cancer: 75mg/m² every 3 weeks over 1 hr with prednisone 5mg bid. Gastric Adenocarcinoma: Premedicate with antiemetics and appropriate hydration. 75mg/m² IV over 1 hr, followed by cisplatin 75mg/m² IV over 1-3 hrs (both on Day 1 only), followed by fluorouracil 750mg/m²/day IV over 24 hrs for 5 days, starting at end of cisplatin infusion. Repeat treatment every 3 weeks. SCCHN: Induction Followed by Radiotherapy: 75mg/m² IV over 1 hr, followed by cisplatin 75mg/m² IV over 1 hr, on Day 1, followed by fluorouracil as a continuous IV infusion at 750mg/m²/day for 5 days. Administer every 3 weeks for 4 cycles. Induction Followed by Chemoradiotherapy: 75mg/m² IV over 1 hr on Day 1, followed by cisplatin 100mg/m² IV over 30 min to 3 hrs, followed by fluorouracil 1000mg/m²/day as a continuous IV infusion from Day 1 to Day 4. Administer every 3 weeks for 3 cycles.

**HOW SUPPLIED:** Inj: 20mg/0.5mL, 80mg/2mL

**CONTRAINDICATIONS:** Neutrophils <1500 cells/mm³, hypersensitivity to polysorbate 80.

**WARNINGS/PRECAUTIONS:** Toxic deaths, febrile neutropenia, neutropenia, localized erythema of extremities with edema and desquamation, severe neurosensory symptoms, severe asthenia, acute myeloid leukemia reported. Monitor for hypersensitivity reactions. Can cause fetal harm. Caution in elderly. Monitor CBC frequently; avoid subsequent cycles until neutrophils recover to >1500 cells/mm³ and platelets recover to >100,000 cells/mm³.

**ADVERSE REACTIONS:** Arthralgia, myalgia, alopecia, stomatitis, N/V, diarrhea, nail changes, cutaneous and neurosensory reactions, fluid retention, hypersensitivity reactions, leukopenia, thrombocytopenia, anemia, neutropenia, fever.

**INTERACTIONS:** Caution with agents that induce, inhibit, or are metabolized by CYP3A4 (eg, ketoconazole, erythromycin, terfenadine, astemizole, cyclosporine) and with protease inhibitors (eg, ritonavir) which are inhibitors and substrates of CYP3A.

**PREGNANCY:** Category D, not for use in nursing.

**MECHANISM OF ACTION:** Antimicrotubule agent; disrupts microtubular network in cells that is essential for mitotic and interphase cellular functions. Binds to free tubulin and promotes assembly of tubulin into stable microtubules while simultaneously inhibiting their disassembly.

**PHARMACOKINETICS: Distribution:** $V_d$=113L; plasma protein binding (94%). **Metabolism:** CYP3A4. **Elimination:** Urine, feces (80%); $T_{1/2}$=11.1 hrs.

## NURSING CONSIDERATIONS

**Assessment:** Assess CBC with platelet count and differential, LFTs, bilirubin levels, non-small cell lung carcinoma, pregnancy status, and possible drug interactions.

**Monitoring:** Monitor LFTs, bilirubin, CBC with platelets and differential count. Monitor for fluid retention, neurosensory symptoms, skin toxicity, and hypersensitivity reactions.

**Patient Counseling:** Counsel about side effects of drug; report signs/symptoms of side effects. Advise about need for routine blood tests and follow ups. Inform physician before taking any other medications. Advise women of childbearing age not to become pregnant when taking this drug.

**Administration:** IV route; infuse over 1 hr. **Storage:** 2-25°C (36-77°F). Protect from bright light.

# TAZICEF RX

ceftazidime (Hospira)

**THERAPEUTIC CLASS:** Cephalosporin (3rd generation)

**INDICATIONS:** Treatment of lower respiratory tract (eg, pneumonia), skin and skin structure (SSSI), bone and joint, gynecologic, intra-abdominal, CNS (eg, meningitis), and urinary tract infections (UTI), bacterial septicemia, and sepsis caused by susceptible strains of microorganisms.

**DOSAGE:** *Adults:* Usual: 1g IV q8-12h. Uncomplicated UTI: 250mg IM/IV q12h. Complicated UTI: 500mg IM/IV q8-12h. Bone and Joint Infections: 2g IV q12h. Uncomplicated Pneumonia/SSSI: 500mg-1g IM/IV q8h. Gynecological/Intra-Abdominal/Meningitis/Severe Life-Threatening Infection: 2g IV q8h. Lung Infection caused by *Pseudomonas* in Cystic Fibrosis (normal renal function): 30-50mg/kg IV q8h. Max: 6g/day. Renal Impairment: CrCl 31-50mL/min: 1g q12h. CrCl 16-30mL/min: 1g q24h. CrCl 6-15mL/min: 500mg q24h. CrCl <5mL/min: 500mg q48h. For severe infections (6g/day), increase renal impairment dose by 50% or increase dosing interval. Apply reduced dosage recommendations after initial 1g LD is given. Hemodialysis: Give 1g LD before and 1g after each hemodialysis period. Intra-Peritoneal Dialysis/Continuous Ambulatory Peritoneal Dialysis: Give 1g LD followed by 500mg q24h, or add to fluid at 250mg/2L.
*Pediatrics:* Neonates (0-4 weeks): 30mg/kg IV q12h. 1 month-12 yrs: 30-50mg/kg IV q8h. Max: 6g/day. Higher doses for patients with cystic fibrosis or when treating meningitis. Renal Impairment: CrCl 31-50mL/min: 1g q12h. CrCl 16-30mL/min: 1g q24h. CrCl 6-15mL/min: 500mg q24h. CrCl <5mL/min: 500mg q48h. Hemodialysis: Give 1g before and 1g after each hemodialysis. For severe infections (6g/day), increase renal impairment dose by 50% or increase dosing interval. Apply reduced dosage recommendations after initial 1g LD is given. Hemodialysis: Give 1g LD before and 1g after each hemodialysis period. Intra-Peritoneal Dialysis/Continuous Ambulatory Peritoneal Dialysis: Give 1g followed by 500mg q24h, or add to fluid at 250mg/2L.

**HOW SUPPLIED:** Inj: 1g, 2g, 6g

**WARNINGS/PRECAUTIONS:** Monitor renal function; potential for nephrotoxicity. May result in overgrowth of nonsusceptible organisms. Possible cross-sensitivity between PCNs, cephalosporins, and other β-lactams. Pseudomembranous colitis reported. Elevated levels with renal insufficiency can lead to seizures, encephalopathy, asterixis, and neuromuscular excitability. Possible decrease in PT; caution with renal or hepatic impairment, poor nutritional state; monitor PT and give vitamin K if needed. Caution with colitis and other GI diseases. Distal necrosis may occur after inadvertent intra-arterial administration. Continue for 2 days after signs/symptoms of infection resolve; may require longer therapy with complicated infections. Caution in elderly.

**ADVERSE REACTIONS:** Phlebitis and inflammation at injection site, pruritus, rash, fever, diarrhea, N/V.

**INTERACTIONS:** Nephrotoxicity reported with aminoglycosides or potent diuretics (eg, furosemide). Avoid with chloramphenicol; may decrease effect of β-lactam antibiotics.

**PREGNANCY:** Category B, caution in nursing.

**MECHANISM OF ACTION:** 3rd-generation cephalosporin; inhibits enzymes responsible for cell-wall synthesis.

T

**PHARMACOKINETICS: Absorption:** $C_{max}$=90mcg/mL (1g IV), 39mcg/mL (1g IM); see PI for detailed info. **Distribution:** Plasma protein binding (<10%); found in breast milk. **Elimination:** Urine (80-90% unchanged); $T_{1/2}$=1.9 hrs (IV).

## NURSING CONSIDERATIONS

**Assessment:** Assess for previous hypersensitivity reaction to cephalosporins/PCNs or other drugs, renal/hepatic impairment, poor nutritional status, patients receiving protracted course of antibiotics, GI disease (particularly colitis), pregnancy/nursing status, and possible drug interactions.

**Monitoring:** Monitor PT; vitamin K administration as indicated. Monitor for signs/symptoms of allergic reactions (eg, Stevens-Johnson syndrome, toxic epidermal necrolysis), pseudomembranous colitis or *C.difficile*-associated diarrhea (may range in severity from mild diarrhea to fatal colitis), development of drug resistance, overgrowth of nonsusceptible organisms, seizures, encephalopathy, asterixis, neuromuscular excitability, distal necrosis in inadvertent intra-atrial injection, and lab test interactions (eg, false (+) urinary glucose test when using Clinitest, Benedict's solution, or Fehling's solution), (+) Coombs' test without hemolysis, LFTs, renal function tests, and CBCs).

**Patient Counseling:** Only treats bacterial, not viral, infections. Take exactly as directed; skipping doses or not completing full course may decrease effectiveness and increase resistance. Inform about risks/benefits. D/C and notify physician if experience allergic reaction or diarrhea. Notify if pregnant/nursing.

**Administration:** IV and IM route. Do not use flexible container in series connections. **Storage**: Dry state 20-25°C (68-77°F), reconstituted solution for 24 hrs at room temperature, or for 7 days at 5°C; stable for 3 months if frozen at -20°C; thawed solution, store for up to 8 hrs at room temperature or for 4 days at 5°C; do not refreeze thawed solution.

# TAZORAC RX

tazarotene (Allergan)

**THERAPEUTIC CLASS:** Retinoid

**INDICATIONS:** (Gel 0.05%, 0.1%) Stable plaque psoriasis of up to 20% body surface area involvement. (Gel 0.1%) Acne vulgaris of mild to moderate severity.

**DOSAGE:** *Adults:* Psoriasis: Start with 0.05% Gel, increase to 0.1% if tolerated. Apply thin film to psoriatic lesions qpm. Acne: Cleanse and dry skin. Apply thin film of 0.1% Gel to acne lesions qpm.
*Pediatrics:* ≥12 yrs: Psoriasis: Start with 0.05% Gel, increase to 0.1% if tolerated. Apply thin film to psoriatic lesions qpm. Acne: Cleanse and dry skin. Apply thin film of 0.1% Gel to acne lesions qpm.

**HOW SUPPLIED:** Gel: 0.05%, 0.1% [30g, 100g]

**CONTRAINDICATIONS:** Women who are or may become pregnant.

**WARNINGS/PRECAUTIONS:** Use adequate birth control measures. Avoid mouth, eyes, eyelids, exposure to sunlight or sunlamps, or eczematous skin. D/C if pruritus, burning, skin redness, or peeling. Weather extremes (eg, wind, cold) may be irritating.

**ADVERSE REACTIONS:** Pruritus, burning/stinging, erythema, worsening of psoriasis, irritation, skin pain, desquamation, dry skin, rash, fissuring, localized edema, skin discoloration.

**INTERACTIONS:** Avoid topical agents that have a strong drying effect. Caution with photosensitizers (eg, thiazides, tetracyclines, fluoroquinolones, phenothiazines, sulfonamides).

**PREGNANCY:** Category X, caution in nursing.

**MECHANISM OF ACTION:** Retinoic acid derivative; binds to all 3 members of the retinoic acid receptor RAR (RARα, RARβ, and $RAR_{gamma)}$. Treatment of psoriasis not established. Suppresses expression of MRP8, a marker of inflammation; induces expression of a gene which may be a growth suppressor in keratinocytes, and may inhibit epidermal hyperproliferation in treated plaques. Treatment of acne not established; may be due to anti-hyperproliferative, normalizing-of-differentiation, and anti-inflammatory actions.

**PHARMACOKINETICS: Absorption:** Percutaneous; $C_{max}$=18.9ng/mL; $AUC_{0-24hr}$=172ng•hr/mL. **Distribution:** Plasma protein binding (>99%). **Metabolism:** Esterase hydrolysis to form tazarotenic acid (active metabolite). **Excretion:** Urine, feces; $T_{1/2}$=18 hrs.

## NURSING CONSIDERATIONS

**Assessment:** Assess that treatment is not for more than 20% of BSA, and not on eczematous skin. Two weeks prior to treatment, assess pregnancy status in females of childbearing potential. Assess that sexually active females are using effective form of contraception during therapy. Initiate therapy in childbearing females during a normal menstrual period. Assess use in pediatric and nursing patients. Assess for possible drug interactions.

**Monitoring:** Monitor for excessive pruritus, burning, skin redness, or peeling.

**Patient Counseling:** Instruct to avoid contact with eyes, eyelids, and mouth; do not cover treated areas with dressings or bandages. Wash hands following administration. Do not take if pregnant, planning to become or suspected to be pregnant. Instruct females to use effective form of contraception while on medication; advise to begin therapy during menstrual period. Avoid exposure to sunlight/sunlamps while on therapy; wear protective clothing and use sunscreen (minimum SPF15) when exposed to sunlight. Avoid using medication on sunburned skin. Exposure to weather extremes (eg, wind, cold) may cause skin irritation. Contact physician if excessive skin irritation develops. If dose is missed, do not make it up; instead, continue with normal dosing schedule.

**Administration:** Topical route. **Storage:** 25°C (77°F). Excursions permitted to 15-30°C (59-86°F). Keep tube tightly closed when not in use.

## TEGRETOL — RX

carbamazepine (Novartis)

**Serious and fatal dermatologic reactions, including toxic epidermal necrolysis (TEN), Stevens-Johnson syndrome (SJS) reported; increased risk with presence of HLA-B*1502 allele; screen prior to initiation of therapy. Aplastic anemia and agranulocytosis reported. Obtain complete pretreatment hematological testing as a baseline. D/C if evidence of bone marrow depression develops.**

**OTHER BRAND NAMES:** Tegretol-XR (Novartis) - Epitol (Teva)

**THERAPEUTIC CLASS:** Carboxamide

**INDICATIONS:** Treatment of partial seizures with complex symptomatology, generalized tonic-clonic seizures, and mixed seizure patterns of these or other partial or generalized seizures. Treatment of pain associated with trigeminal or glossopharyngeal neuralgia.

**DOSAGE:** *Adults:* Epilepsy: Initial: (Immediate- or Extended-Release Tab) 200mg bid or (Sus) 100mg qid. Titrate: (Immediate-Release Tab/Sus) Increase weekly by 200mg/day given tid-qid. (Extended-Release Tab) Increase weekly by 200mg/day given bid. Maint: 800-1200mg/day. Max: 1600mg/day. Trigeminal Neuralgia: Initial (Day 1): (Immediate- or Extended-Release Tab) 100mg bid or (Sus) 50mg qid. Titrate: May increase by 100mg q12h (Tab) or 50mg qid (Sus). Maint: 400-800mg/day. Max: 1200mg/day. Re-evaluate every 3 months.
*Pediatrics:* Epilepsy: >12 yrs: Initial: (Immediate- or Extended-Release Tab) 200mg bid or (Sus) 100mg qid. Titrate: (Immediate-Release Tab/Sus) Increase weekly by 200mg/day given tid-qid. (Extended-Release Tab) Increase weekly by 200mg/day given bid. Maint: 200-1200mg/day. Max: 12-15 yrs: 1000mg/day. Max: >15 yrs: 1200mg/day. 6-12 yrs: Initial: (Immediate- or Extended-Release Tab) 100mg bid or (Sus) 50mg qid. Titrate: (Immediate-Release Tab/Sus) Increase weekly by 100mg/day given tid-qid. (Extended-Release Tab) Increase weekly by 100mg/day given bid. Maint: 400-800mg/day. Max: 1000mg/day. <6 yrs: Initial: (Immediate-Release Tab) 10-20mg/kg/day given bid-tid or (Sus) 10-20mg/kg/day given qid. Titrate: (Immediate-Release Tab/Sus) Increase weekly tid-qid. Max: 35mg/kg/day.

**HOW SUPPLIED:** Sus: 100mg/5mL [450mL]; Tab: (Tegretol, Epitol) 200mg*; Tab, Chewable: 100mg*; Tab, Extended-Release: (Tegretol-XR) 100mg, 200mg, 400mg *scored

**CONTRAINDICATIONS:** History of bone marrow depression, MAOI use within 14 days, hypersensitivity to TCAs (eg, amitriptyline, desipramine, imipramine, protriptyline, nortriptyline). Coadministration with nefazodone.

**WARNINGS/PRECAUTIONS:** Increased risk of suicidal thoughts or behavior reported. May cause fetal harm with pregnancy. Withdraw gradually to minimize potential increase in seizure frequency. Caution in patients with history of cardiac conduction disturbance; cardiac, hepatic, or renal damage; history of adverse hematologic reactions to other drugs; increased IOP; mixed seizure disorder; previously interrupted course of carbamazepine. AV heart block, slight elevations in LFTs, rare cases of liver failure reported. Avoid in hepatic porphyria (eg, acute intermittent porphyria, variegate porphyria, porphyria cutanea tarda); acute attacks reported. May cause activation of latent psychosis and, in the elderly, confusion or agitation. May impair physical/mental abilities. Start on lower doses and increase slowly to avoid side effects. Avoid suspension in patients with fructose intolerance.

**ADVERSE REACTIONS:** Dizziness, drowsiness, unsteadiness, nausea, vomiting, bone marrow depression, multiorgan hypersensitivity, SIADH, CHF, SJS, TEN.

**INTERACTIONS:** See Contraindications. Do not give suspension with other medicinal liquids or diluents. CYP3A4 inhibitors (eg, cimetidine, macrolides, azoles) increase plasma concentration. CYP3A4 inducers (eg, cisplatin, rifampin, theophylline) decrease plasma concentration. Increases plasma levels of clomipramine, phenytoin, and primidone. Decreases levels of CYP3A4 substrates, APAP, alprazolam, clonazepam, clozapine, dicumarol, doxycycline, ethosuximide, haloperidol, lamotrigine, methsuximide, oral contraceptives, phensuximide, phenytoin, theophylline, tiagabine, topiramate, valproate, and warfarin. May render hormonal contraceptives less effective. Increased risk of neurotoxic side effects with lithium. Alteration of thyroid function with other anticonvulsants. Concomitant use with isoniazid increases risk of isoniazid-induced hepatotoxicity. Symptomatic hyponatremia with concomitant diuretics (eg, hydrochlorothiazide, furosemide). Antagonizes effects of nondepolarizing muscle relaxants (eg, pancuronium).

**PREGNANCY:** Category D, not for use in nursing.

**MECHANISM OF ACTION:** Carboxamide; anticonvulsant: reduces polysynaptic response and blocks post-tetanic potentiation. Neuralgia: depresses thalamic potential and bulbar and polysynaptic reflexes.

**PHARMACOKINETICS: Absorption:** $T_{max}$=1.5 hrs (Sus); $T_{max}$=4-5 hrs (Tab); $T_{max}$=3-12 hrs (Tab, extended-release). **Distribution:** Plasma protein binding (76%). Found in placenta and breast milk. **Metabolism:** Liver via CYP3A4 to carbamazepine-10,11-epoxide (active metabolite). **Elimination:** Urine (72%; 3% unchanged), feces (28%); $T_{1/2}$=25-65 hrs (single dose); $T_{1/2}$=12-17 hrs (multiple doses).

## NURSING CONSIDERATIONS

**Assessment:** Assess use with history of bone marrow depression, hepatic porphyria, hypersensitivity to any tricyclic compound, previous adverse hematological and dermatological reactions with other medications, history of mixed seizure disorders, cardiac damage or cardiac conduction disturbances. Assess renal function (complete urinalysis, BUN), CBC (platelets, reticulocytes), serum iron, presence of HLA-B*1502, LFTs; perform eye exam (slit lamp, funduscopy, tonometry) prior to therapy. Assess pregnancy/nursing status.

**Monitoring:** Monitor for hepatic failure, multiorgan hypersensitivity reactions, bone marrow depression, aplastic anemia, agranulocytosis, dermatological reactions (SJS), latent psychosis, and confusion or agitation in elderly patients. Monitor for emergence of suicidal behavior and ideation, signs and symptoms of depression. Monitor LFTs, SrCr, BUN, IOP.

**Patient Counseling:** Counsel about signs/symptoms of hematological, dermatological, and hepatic complications (eg, fever, sore throat, easy bruising, jaundice). May cause drowsiness or dizziness; caution against using heavy machinery/driving. Avoid alcohol or abrupt d/c. Notify physician if worsening of depression, unusual changes in mood or behavior, or suicidal thoughts/behaviors occur. Notify physician if pregnant or intend to become pregnant. Encourage patients to enroll in North American Antiepileptic Drug (NAAED) Pregnancy Registry by calling 888-233-2334 or go to aedpregnancyregistry.org.

**Administration:** Oral route. Oral sus should not be administered with other liquid medications or diluents. Shake sus well before using. Conversion of patients from tab to sus should be done by administering same number of mg/day in smaller, more frequent doses. XR tab must be swallowed whole; do not chew or crush. **Storage:** Sus: Do not store above 30°C (86°F); dispense in tight, light-resistant container. Tab & Tab, chewable: Do not store above 30°C (86°F). Protect from light and moisture; dispense in tight, light-resistant container. Tab, extended-release: 15-30°C (59-86°F). Protect from moisture. Dispense in tight container.

# TEKTURNA RX

aliskiren (Novartis)

**When used in pregnancy, drugs that act directly on the renin-angiotensin system can cause injury and even death to the developing fetus. D/C therapy when pregnancy is detected.**

**THERAPEUTIC CLASS:** Renin inhibitor

**INDICATIONS:** Treatment of hypertension. May be used alone or with other antihypertensives.

**DOSAGE:** *Adults:* Usual: 150mg qd. Titrate: May increase to 300mg/day if needed. High-fat meals decrease absorption.

**HOW SUPPLIED:** Tab: 150mg, 300mg

**WARNINGS/PRECAUTIONS:** Caution with greater than moderate renal dysfunction (SCr >1.7mg/dL [women] or >2mg/dL [men] and/or GFR <30mL/min), history of dialysis, nephrotic syndrome, or renovascular hypertension. May increase serum $K^+$, especially when used in combination with ACE inhibitors in diabetics. Angioedema of face, extremities, lips, tongue, glottis, and/or larynx reported; d/c and monitor until complete resolution of signs and symptoms and do not readminister. Hypotension rarely seen.

**ADVERSE REACTIONS:** Diarrhea, headache, nasopharyngitis, dizziness, fatigue, upper respiratory tract infection, back pain, cough.

**INTERACTIONS:** Coadministration with atorvastatin may increase $C_{max}$ and AUC up to 50% after multiple dosing. Coadministration of irbesartan may reduce $C_{max}$ up to 50% after multiple dosing. Coadministration of ketoconazole 200mg bid may result in an approximate 80% increase in plasma level. Coadministration with furosemide may reduce AUC and $C_{max}$ by 30% and 50%, respectively. Concomitant use with cyclosporine is not recommended. Concomitant use with $K^+$-sparing diuretics, $K^+$ supplements, salt substitutes containing $K^+$, or other drugs that increase $K^+$ levels may lead to increases in serum $K^+$; caution with concomitant use.

**PREGNANCY:** Category C (1st trimester) and D (2nd and 3rd trimesters); not for use in nursing.

**MECHANISM OF ACTION:** Potent renin inhibitor; lowers BP by directly inhibiting renin, decreasing plasma renin activity, and inhibiting conversion of angiotensinogen to angiotensin I.

**PHARMACOKINETICS: Absorption:** Poor, $T_{max}$=1-3 hrs, bioavailability (2.5%). **Metabolism:** via CYP3A4 enzyme. **Elimination:** Urine (25% of absorbed dose as parent drug), accumulation $T_{1/2}$=24 hrs.

## NURSING CONSIDERATIONS

**Assessment:** Assess BP, renal functions, renal artery stenosis, pregnancy status, and for possible drug interactions.

**Monitoring:** Monitor BP, renal functions, serum $K^+$ levels. Monitor for angioedema of head/neck, N/V, diarrhea, inadequate fluid intake, and excessive perspiration.

**Patient Counseling:** Counsel about fetal risks during pregnancy and signs/symptoms of angioedema (eg, laryngeal or tongue edema); advise to seek prompt medical attention if pregnant or signs/symptoms of angioedema develop. Inform about adverse effects (eg, hypotension, hyperkalemia). Instruct patients not to use $K^+$ supplements or salt substitutes containing $K^+$ without consulting their physician. D/C and notify physician if lightheadedness and syncope develop.

**Administration:** Oral route. **Storage:** 25°C (77°F). Excursions permitted to 15-30°C (59-86°F). Protect from moisture. Dispense in tight container.

# TEKTURNA HCT RX

aliskiren - hydrochlorothiazide (Novartis)

**Drugs that act directly on the renin-angiotensin system can cause injury and even death to the developing fetus. D/C therapy when pregnancy is detected.**

**THERAPEUTIC CLASS:** Renin inhibitor/thiazide diuretic

**INDICATIONS:** Treatment of hypertension in patients not controlled on monotherapy and as initial therapy in patients likely to need multiple medications to control BP.

**DOSAGE:** *Adults*: Initial: Not Controlled on Monotherapy/Initial Therapy: 150mg-12.5mg qd. Titrate: May increase to max of 300mg-12.5mg qd if uncontrolled after 2-4 weeks. Replacement Therapy: May substitute for individually titrated components. Max: 300mg-25mg qd.

**HOW SUPPLIED:** Tab: (Aliskiren-HCTZ) 150mg-12.5mg, 150mg-25mg, 300mg-12.5mg, 300mg-25mg

**CONTRAINDICATIONS:** Anuria, sulfonamide hypersensitivity.

**WARNINGS/PRECAUTIONS:** May cause fetal harm during pregnancy. Angioedema of head and neck may occur; d/c therapy and monitor until signs and symptoms resolve. May cause symptomatic hypotension in volume- and/or salt-depleted patients; correct condition prior to therapy. Avoid with severe renal impairment (CrCl <30mL/min). Titrate dose slowly with renal/hepatic impairment; may precipitate azotemia and hepatic coma. Caution with hepatic impairment, or history of allergy or bronchial asthma. May exacerbate or activate systemic lupus erythematosus (SLE). Monitor serum electrolytes periodically to detect possible electrolyte imbalance. Do not use as initial therapy with intravascular volume depletion.

**ADVERSE REACTIONS:** Dizziness, influenza, diarrhea, cough, vertigo, asthenia, arthralgia.

**INTERACTIONS:** (Aliskiren) Ketoconazole, atorvastatin, cyclosporine may increase plasma levels. Avoid concomitant use of cyclosporine. Irbesartan may reduce levels. Co-administration may diminish furosemide levels. (HCTZ) Potentiation of orthostatic hypotension may occur with alcohol, barbiturates, and narcotics. Dosage adjustment of insulin or oral hypoglycemic agents may be required. Potentiate effects of other antihypertensives. Cholestyramine and colestipol resins may impair absorption. Corticosteroids and ACTH deplete electrolytes. May decrease response to pressor amines (eg, norepinephrine). May increase responsiveness to skeletal muscle relaxants (eg, tubocurarine). Increased risk of lithium toxicity; avoid concurrent use. NSAIDs may reduce diuretic effects; monitor closely.

**PREGNANCY:** Category D, not for use in nursing.

**MECHANISM OF ACTION:** Aliskiren: Direct renin inhibitor. HCTZ: Thiazide diuretic, affects renal tubular mechanisms of electrolyte reabsorption, directly increasing excretion of $Na^+$ and $Cl^-$ in approximately equivalent amounts.

**PHARMACOKINETICS: Absorption:** Aliskiren: $T_{max}$=1 hr. HCTZ: $T_{max}$=2.5 hrs. **Distribution:** HCTZ: Crosses the placenta; found in human milk. **Metabolism:** Aliskiren: CYP3A4 enzyme. HCTZ: Not metabolized. **Elimination:** Aliskiren: Urine (25% parent drug). HCTZ: Urine, $T_{1/2}$=5.8-18.9 hrs.

## NURSING CONSIDERATIONS

**Assessment:** Assess for LFTs, renal function, serum electrolytes, anuria, sulfonamide hypersensitivity, renal/hepatic impairment, allergy or bronchial asthma, SLE, pregnancy/nursing status, and possible drug interactions.

**Monitoring:** Monitor for hypersensitivity and anaphylactic reactions, anuria, urticaria, head/neck angioedema. Monitor renal function, LFTs, serum uric acid, and electrolytes.

**Patient Counseling:** Instruct to notify physician or pharmacist if any unusual symptoms develop or if any known symptoms persist or worsen. Counsel about possible fetal/neonatal disease and death if exposed or while on therapy. Discuss other treatment options if planning to become pregnant. Caution that light-headedness may occur, especially during 1st days of therapy. If syncope occurs, d/c until physician consulted. Caution that inadequate fluid intake, excessive perspiration, diarrhea, or vomiting can lead to an excessive fall in BP, with same consequences as lightheadedness and possible syncope. Advise not to use $K^+$ supplements or salt substitutes containing $K^+$ without consulting a physician. Establish routine pattern for taking medication with regard to meals.

**Administration:** Oral route. **Storage**: 25°C (77°F); excursions permitted to 15-30°C (59-86°F). Protect from moisture.

## Temodar — RX

temozolomide (Schering)

**THERAPEUTIC CLASS:** Alkylating agent (imidazotetrazine derivative)

**INDICATIONS:** Treatment of newly diagnosed glioblastoma multiforme (GBM) concomitantly with radiotherapy and as maintenance treatment. Treatment of refractory anaplastic astrocytoma (eg, patients experiencing disease progression on a drug regimen containing nitrosourea and procarbazine).

**DOSAGE:** *Adults:* Adjust according to nadir neutrophil and platelet counts of previous cycle and at time of initiating next cycle. Newly Diagnosed GBM: (IV/PO) 75mg/m² qd for 42 days with focal radiotherapy; dose may continue up to 49 days if absolute neutrophil count ≥1.5 x $10^9$/L, platelet count ≥100 x $10^9$/L, common toxicity criteria (CTC) non-hematological toxicity ≤Grade 1 (except alopecia, N/V) are met. Maint: Cycle 1 (28 days): 150mg/m² qd for 1st 5 days of each 28-day cycle. Cycle 2-6 (28 days): If Cycle 1 toxicity Grade ≤2, ANC ≥1.5 x $10^9$/L and platelets ≥100 x $10^9$/L, increase to 200mg/m²/day for 5 consecutive days per 28-day cycle. Do not increase dose in subsequent cycles if dose not escalated at Cycle 2. If Cycle 1 toxicity Grade 3, ANC <1.0 x $10^9$/L and platelets <50 x $10^9$/L, reduce to 100mg/m²/day for 5 consecutive days per 28-day cycle. D/C if Cycle 1 toxicity Grade 4, dose reduction to <100mg/m²/day is required or if same Grade 3 toxicity recurs after dose reduction. Refractory Anaplastic Astrocytoma: Initial: (IV/PO) 150mg/m² qd for 5 consecutive days per 28-day cycle. If ANC ≥1.5 x $10^9$/L and platelets ≥100 x $10^9$/L for both the nadir and Day 29 (Day 1 of next cycle), may increase to 200mg/m²/day for 5 consecutive days per 28-day cycle. Start next cycle when ANC >1.5 x $10^9$/L and platelets >100 x $10^9$/L . If ANC <1 x $10^9$/L or platelets <50 x $10^9$/L during any cycle, reduce next cycle by 50mg/m² but not below 100mg/m². If ANC 1.0-1.5 x $10^9$/L or platelets 50-100 x $10^9$/L during any cycle, maintain initial dose.

**HOW SUPPLIED:** Cap: 5mg, 20mg, 100mg, 140mg, 180mg, 250mg. Inj: 100mg

**CONTRAINDICATIONS:** Hypersensitivity to DTIC (dacarbazine).

**WARNINGS/PRECAUTIONS:** Before therapy, must have ANC ≥1.5 x $10^9$/L and platelets ≥100 x $10^9$/L. Myelosuppression may occur, including prolonged pancytopenia, may result in aplastic anemia; greater risk of myelosuppression in women and elderly. May cause fetal harm during pregnancy. Cases of myelodysplastic syndrome and secondary malignancies, including myeloid leukemia, have been observed. Do not open capsules. Caution in elderly, or severe renal/hepatic impairment. *Pneumocystis carinii* pneumonia (PCP) prophylaxis required in all patients with newly diagnosed GBM receiving concomitant radiotherapy for 42-day regimen. Increased risk of infusion-related adverse reactions, and suboptimal dosing with shorter or longer infusion time. Allergic reactions reported.

**ADVERSE REACTIONS:** Anorexia, alopecia, fatigue, myelosuppression (eg, thrombocytopenia, neutropenia), N/V, convulsions, headache, fever, constipation, dizziness, diarrhea, abnormal coordination, viral infection.

**INTERACTIONS:** Valproic acid may decrease clearance. Food reduces the rate and extent of absorption; consistency of administration with respect to food is recommended. Monitor all patients, especially those receiving steroids, for the develpment of PCP. Temzolomide may cause aplastic anemia; exposure to concomitant medications associated with aplastic anemia, including carbamazepine, phenytoin, sulfamethoxazole/trimethoprim complicates assessment.

**PREGNANCY:** Category D, not for use in nursing.

**MECHANISM OF ACTION:** Alkylating agent (imidazotetrazine derivative); exerts action by alkylation of DNA. Alkylation occurs mainly at the $O^6$ and $N^7$ positions of guanine.

**PHARMACOKINETICS: Absorption:** (PO) Rapid and complete, $T_{max}$=1 hr (fasting), 2.25 hrs (fed); $C_{max}$ = 7.5mcg/mL (temozolomide), 282ng/mL (active metabolite); AUC=23.4mcg•hr/mL (temozolomide), 864ng•hr/mL. (IV) $C_{max}$= 7.3mcg/mL (temozolomide), 276ng/mL (active metabolite); AUC=24.6mcg•hr/mL (temozolomide), 891ng•hr/mL (active metabolite). **Distribution:** $V_d$=0.4L/kg; plasma protein binding (15%). **Metabolism:** Via spontaneous hydroxylation; 3-methyl-(triazen-1-yl)imidazole-4-carboxamide (major metabolite) **Elimination:** Urine, feces; $T_{1/2}$=1.8 hrs.

## NURSING CONSIDERATIONS

**Assessment:** Assess for CBC with differential and platelet counts, hepatic/renal functions, pregnancy status. Note other diseases/conditions and possible drug interactions.

**Monitoring:** Obtain CBC on Day 22 (21 days after 1st dose) or within 48 hrs of that day, repeat weekly until ANC >1.5 x $10^9$/L and platelets >100 x $10^9$/L. Monitor for lymphopenia, PCP, secondary malignancies, hypersensitivity reactions, convulsions, hemiparesis.

**Patient Counseling:** Counsel about adverse effects (eg, N/V); seek medical attention if any develop. Take as prescribed. Swallow whole; never chew. Instruct not to open capsule. Avoid inhalation or contact with skin or mucous membranes. Regular follow-ups needed. Keep away from children and pets.

**Administration:** Oral and IV route. See PI for reconstitution. Swallow cap whole with water. IV infusion over 90 min. **Storage:** (Cap) 25°C (77°F); excursions permitted to 15-30°C (59-96°F). (IV) Refrigerate at 2-8°C (36-46°F). After reconstitution, store at room temperature (25°C [77°F]). Reconstituted product must be used within 14 hrs.

# TEMOVATE RX

clobetasol propionate (GlaxoSmithKline)

**OTHER BRAND NAMES:** Temovate-E (GlaxoSmithKline) - Temovate Scalp (GlaxoSmithKline)

**THERAPEUTIC CLASS:** Corticosteroid

**INDICATIONS:** Corticosteroid-responsive dermatoses. Temovate-E is also used to treat moderate to severe plaque-type psoriasis.

**DOSAGE:** *Adults:* Apply bid. Max: 50g/week or 50mL/week. Moderate-Severe Psoriasis: (Temovate-E) Apply bid for up to 4 weeks. May use on 5-10% of BSA. Max: 50g/week. Limit treatment to 2 consecutive weeks. Avoid with occlusive dressings.
*Pediatrics:* ≥12 yrs: Apply bid. Max: 50g/week or 50mL/week. Moderate-Severe Psoriasis: ≥16 yrs: (Temovate-E) Apply bid for up to 4 weeks. May use on 5-10% of BSA. Max: 50g/week. Limit treatment to 2 consecutive weeks. Avoid with occlusive dressings.

**HOW SUPPLIED:** (Temovate) Cre, Oint: 0.05% [15g, 30g, 45g, 60g]; Gel: 0.05% [15g, 30g, 60g]; Sol: 0.05% [25mL]; (Temovate-E) Cre: 0.05% [15g, 30g, 60g]; (Temovate Scalp) Sol: 0.05% [25mL, 50mL]

**CONTRAINDICATIONS:** (Scalp Sol) Primary scalp infections.

**WARNINGS/PRECAUTIONS:** Not for use on face, groin, or axillae, or for treatment of rosacea or perioral dermatitis. May produce reversible HPA axis suppression, manifestations of Cushing's syndrome, hyperglycemia, and glucosuria. Use appropriate antifungal or antibacterial agent with dermatological infections; d/c if infection does not clear. Pediatric patients may be more susceptible to systemic toxicity. Avoid eyes. D/C if irritation occurs.

T

**ADVERSE REACTIONS:** Burning, stinging, pruritus, skin atrophy, cracking/fissuring of the skin, erythema, folliculitis, numbness of fingers, telangiectasia, tingling (Sol), folliculitis (Sol).

**PREGNANCY:** Category C, caution in nursing.

**MECHANISM OF ACTION:** Corticosteroid; possesses anti-inflammatory, antipruritic, and vasoconstrictive properties. Anti-inflammatory effects not established. Suspected to act by induction of phospholipase $A_2$ inhibitory proteins, lipocortins. Lipocortins control biosynthesis of potent inflammation mediators (eg, prostaglandins, leukotrienes) by inhibiting release of their common precursor, arachidonic acid.

**PHARMACOKINETICS: Absorption:** Occlusion, inflammation, other disease states may increase absorption. Use of occlusive dressings ≤24 hrs does not increase penetration, use for 96 hrs markedly enhances penetration.

## NURSING CONSIDERATIONS

**Assessment:** Assess medication not for treatment of perioral dermatitis or rosacea. Assess pregnancy/nursing status.

**Monitoring:** Monitor for signs/symptoms of reversible HPA-axis suppression, Cushing's syndrome, hyperglycemia, glucosuria, skin irritation, allergic contact dermatitis (eg, failure to heal), and concomitant skin infections (eg, fungal, bacterial). With large doses or use of occlusive dressings, perform periodic monitoring for HPA-axis suppression using ACTH stimulation, A.M. plasma cortisol, and urinary free cortisol tests. Following d/c, monitor for glucocorticosteroid insufficiencies. In pediatric patients, monitor for systemic toxicity, HPA-axis suppression (linear growth retardation, delayed weight gain), Cushing's syndrome, and intracranial HTN.

**Patient Counseling:** Counsel to use externally and exactly as directed; avoid contact with eyes, face, groin, or axillae. Advise not to bandage, cover, or wrap treated skin area. Contact physician if adverse reactions occur or improvement not seen after 2 weeks of therapy.

**Administration:** Topical route. **Storage:** 15-30°C (59-86°F). Do not refrigerate.

# TENORETIC RX

chlorthalidone - atenolol (AstraZeneca)

**THERAPEUTIC CLASS:** Selective $beta_1$-blocker/monosulfamyl diuretic

**INDICATIONS:** Treatment of hypertension.

**DOSAGE:** *Adults:* Initial: 50mg-25mg tab qd. May increase to 100mg-25mg tab qd. CrCl 15-35mL/min: Max: 50mg atenolol/day. CrCl <15mL/min: Max: 50mg atenolol qod.

**HOW SUPPLIED:** Tab: (Atenolol-Chlorthalidone) 50mg-25mg, 100mg-25mg

**CONTRAINDICATIONS:** Sinus bradycardia, >1st-degree heart block, cardiogenic shock, overt cardiac failure, anuria, sulfonamide hypersensitivity.

T

**WARNINGS/PRECAUTIONS:** Withdrawal before surgery is not recommended. Caution with bronchospastic disease, conduction abnormalities, left ventricular dysfunction. Caution in patients with impaired renal and hepatic function. Can cause heart failure with prolonged use; d/c if cardiac failure continues despite adequate treatment. Caution with DM; may mask tachycardia occuring with hypoglycemia. May mask hypoglycemia or hyperthyroidism symptoms. Latent DM may become manifest. Avoid abrupt d/c; exacerbation of angina and MI reported. Avoid with untreated pheochromocytoma. Possible fetal harm in pregnancy. May aggravate peripheral arterial circulatory disorders. Enhanced effects in postsympathectomy patient. Electrolyte imbalance (eg, hyponatremia, hypochloremic alkalosis, and hypokalemia) and hyperuricemia may develop. Hypercalcemia and hypophosphatemia observed. Acute gout, hepatic coma, and azotemia may be precipitated. Caution in CHF controlled by digitalis and/or diuretics.

**ADVERSE REACTIONS:** Bradycardia, dizziness, fatigue, and nausea.

**INTERACTIONS:** Additive effects with catecholamine-depleting drugs (eg, reserpine), CCBs, amiodarone, and digitalis. Bradycardia and heart block can occur with verapamil or diltiazem. Exacerbates rebound HTN with clonidine withdrawal. Prostaglandin synthase inhibitors (eg, indomethacin) may decrease hypotensive effects. Caution with anesthetic agents. May block epinephrine effects. May decrease arterial response to norepinephrine. May increase risk of lithium toxicity. Possible hypokalemia with corticosteroids or ACTH. May alter insulin requirements. May increase responsiveness to tubocurarine. Class I antiarrhythimic drugs (eg, disopyramide) may have a potentiating effect on atrial conduction time and induce negative inotropic effect.

**PREGNANCY:** Category D, caution in nursing.

**MECHANISM OF ACTION:** Atenolol: Cardioselective β-adrenoreceptor blocking agent; has not been established. Suspected to competitively antagonize catecholamines at peripheral adrenergic neuron sites, leading to decreased cardiac output; a central effect leading to reduced sympathetic outflow to the periphery and suppression of renin activity. Chlorthalidone: Monosulfamyl diuretic; acts on distal convoluted tubule and produces diuresis with increased excretion of $Na^+$ and $Cl^-$.

**PHARMACOKINETICS: Absorption**: (Atenolol): Rapid, incomplete, $T_{max}$=2-4 hrs. **Distribution**: (Atenolol): Plasma protein binding (6-16%). **Elimination:** (Atenolol): Renal excretion; feces (unchanged); $T_{1/2}$=6-7 hrs.

## NURSING CONSIDERATIONS

**Assessment:** Assess for bradycardia, cardiogenic shock, 2nd- and 3rd-degree heart block, overt cardiac failure, impaired renal/hepatic function, bronchospastic disease, PVD, DM, thyrotoxicosis, pheochromocytoma, anuria, hypersensitivity to sulfonamide-derived drugs, serum electrolytes, parathyroid disease, pregnancy status, SLE, and possible drug interactions.

**Monitoring:** Monitor for cardiac failure, HTN, renal function, exacerbation of ischemia following abrupt withdrawal, bronchospastic disease, arrhythmias, CBC with platelets and differential count, hypersensitivity reactions, mesenteric arterial thrombosis, reversible mental depression, hyperuricemia or acute gout, signs/symptoms of electrolyte imbalance, serum glucose, lipid profile, toxic epidermal necrolysis (TEN), impotence, HR, orthostatic hypotension, pancreatitis, LFTs.

**Patient Counseling:** Instruct not to interrupt or d/c therapy without consulting physician. Notify physician if signs/symptoms of impending CHF or unexplained respiratory symptoms develop. Counsel about signs/symptoms of electrolyte imbalance (eg, dry mouth, thirst, weakness, lethargy, drowsiness, restlessness, muscle pains/cramps, muscular fatigue, hypotension, oliguria, tachycardia, N/V), and advise to seek prompt medical attention.

**Administration:** Oral route. **Storage:** 20-25°C (68-77°F).

# TENORMIN — RX

atenolol (AstraZeneca)

T

**THERAPEUTIC CLASS:** Selective $beta_1$-blocker

**INDICATIONS:** Management of hypertension. Long-term management of angina pectoris. Management of hemodynamically stable patients with definite or suspected Acute MI to reduce cardiovascular mortality.

**DOSAGE:** *Adults:* HTN: Initial: 50mg qd. Titrate: May increase after 1-2 weeks. Max: 100mg qd. Angina: Initial: 50mg qd. Titrate: May increase to 100mg after 1 week. Max: 200mg qd. AMI: Initial: 5mg IV over 5 min, repeat 10 min later. If tolerated, give 50mg PO 10 min after the last IV dose, followed by another 50mg PO 12 hrs later. Maint: 100mg qd or 50mg bid for 6-9 days. Renal Impairment/Elderly: HTN: Initial: 25mg qd. HTN/Angina/AMI: Max: CrCl 15-35mL/min: 50mg/day. CrCl <15mL/min: 25mg/day. Hemodialysis: 25-50mg after each dialysis.

**HOW SUPPLIED:** Tab: 25mg, 50mg*, 100mg *scored

**CONTRAINDICATIONS:** Sinus bradycardia, >1st-degree heart block, cardiogenic shock, overt cardiac failure.

**WARNINGS/PRECAUTIONS:** Avoid abrupt d/c of therapy in coronary artery disease. Severe exacerbation of angina and occurrence of MI and ventricular arrhythmias reported in angina patients following abrupt d/c of therapy with β-blockers. When d/c is planned, patients should be monitored and advised to limit activity. Withdrawal before surgery is not recommended. Caution with bronchospastic disease, conduction abnormalities, left ventricular dysfunction, heart failure controlled by digitalis and/or diuretics, renal or hepatic dysfunction. Can cause heart failure with prolonged use, caution with DM. May mask tachycardia occuring with hypoglycemia or hyperthyroidism symptoms. Avoid abrupt d/c. Avoid with untreated pheochromocytoma. Possible fetal harm in pregnancy. May aggravate peripheral arterial circulatory disorders. Caution in elderly.

**ADVERSE REACTIONS:** Bradycardia, hypotension, dizziness, fatigue, nausea, depression, dyspnea, wheezing, tiredness.

**INTERACTIONS:** Additive effects with catecholamine-depleting drugs (eg, reserpine), CCBs, amiodarone, and digitalis. Use with disopyramide may be associated with severe bradycardia, asystole, and heart failure. Bradycardia and heart block can occur with verapamil or diltiazem. Exacerbates rebound HTN with clonidine withdrawal. Prostaglandin synthase inhibitors (eg, indomethacin) may decrease hypotensive effects. Caution with drugs that depress myocardium (eg, anesthesia). May block epinephrine effects. Concomitant use with digitalis glycosides may increase risk of bradycardia. Coadministration of isoproterenol or dobutamine can reverse effects of beta-blockers.

**PREGNANCY:** Category D, caution in nursing.

**MECHANISM OF ACTION:** Cardioselective β-adrenoreceptor blocking agent; has not been established. Suspected to competitively antagonize catecholamines at peripheral adrenergic neuron sites, leading to decreased cardiac output; a central effect leading to reduced sympathetic outflow to the periphery and suppression of renin activity.

**PHARMACOKINETICS: Absorption**: Rapid, incomplete; $T_{max}$ = 2-4 hrs. **Distribution**: Plasma protein binding (6-16%). **Elimination:** Kidneys; urine (50%); $T_{1/2}$=6-7 hrs.

## NURSING CONSIDERATIONS

**Assessment:** Assess for bradycardia, cardiogenic shock, 2nd- and 3rd-degree heart block, overt cardiac failure, impaired renal/hepatic function, bronchospastic disease, PVD, DM, thyrotoxicosis, pregnancy status, pheochromocytoma, and possible drug interactions.

**Monitoring:** Monitor for cardiac failure, HTN, renal function, exacerbation of ischemia following abrupt withdrawal, bronchospastic disease, arrhythmias, CBC with platelets and differential count, hypersensitivity reactions, mesenteric arterial thrombosis, reversible mental depression.

**Patient Counseling:** Instruct not to interrupt or d/c therapy without consulting physician. Notify physician if signs/symptoms of impending CHF or unexplained respiratory symptoms develop. Educate about signs/symptoms of adverse effects.



**Administration:** Oral route. **Storage:** 20-25°C (68-77°F). Dispense in tightly closed, light-resistant containers.

# TERAZOL 3 RX

terconazole (Ortho-McNeil)

**THERAPEUTIC CLASS:** Azole antifungal

**INDICATIONS:** Local treatment of vulvovaginal candidiasis (moniliasis).

**DOSAGE:** *Adults:* Administer 1 full applicator or sup intravaginally qhs for 3 nights.

**HOW SUPPLIED:** Cre: 0.8% [20g]; Sup: 80mg [2.5g] [3[s]]

**WARNINGS/PRECAUTIONS:** D/C and do not retreat if sensitization, irritation, fever, chills, or flu-like symptoms occur. Confirm diagnosis by KOH smears and/or cultures; reconfirm if no response. Base in suppository may interact with certain rubber or latex products (eg, vaginal contraceptive diaphragms); avoid concurrent use.

**ADVERSE REACTIONS:** Sup: Localized burning, pruritus, genital pain, headache. Cre: Dysmenorrhea, headache, pruritus, burning, abdominal pain.

**PREGNANCY:** Category C, not for use in nursing.

**MECHANISM OF ACTION:** Azole antifungal; uncertain. Suspected to exert antifungal activity by disruption of normal fungal cell membrane permeability.

**PHARMACOKINETICS: Absorption:** $C_{max}$=5.9ng/mL, $T_{max}$=6.6 hrs. **Distribution:** Plasma protein binding (94.9%).

## NURSING CONSIDERATIONS

**Assessment:** Assess for proper diagnosis with appropriate microbiologic studies (KOH smears and/or culture). Assess for hypersensitivity and pregnancy/nursing status.

**Monitoring:** Monitor for signs/symtoms of sensitization, irritation, fever, chills, and flu-like symptoms. Monitor for response to treatment; if lack of response, standard KOH smear and cultures should be repeated to confirm diagnosis.

**Patient Counseling:** Counsel to use as prescribed, even if symptoms improve. Instruct to not use suppository concurrently with rubber or latex products (eg, condoms, diaphragms). Instruct to consult physician if partner has penile itching, redness or discomfort. Advise not to use tampons while on medication. Instruct not to douche unless otherwise directed by physician. Advise to notify physician of all medications currently taking.

**Administration:** Intravaginal route. 1) Lie on back, knees drawn up toward chest. 2) Cre: Insert filled applicator into vagina and press plunger to release cre into vagina. Sup: Insert sup into vagina with finger at hs as directed by physician. **Storage:** 15-30°C (59-86°F).

# Terazol 7 RX

terconazole (Ortho-McNeil)

**THERAPEUTIC CLASS:** Azole antifungal

**INDICATIONS:** Local treatment of vulvovaginal candidiasis (moniliasis).

**DOSAGE:** *Adults:* Administer 1 full applicator intravaginally qhs for 7 nights.

**HOW SUPPLIED:** Cre: 0.4% [45g]

**WARNINGS/PRECAUTIONS:** D/C and do not retreat if sensitization, irritation, fever, chills, or flu-like symptoms occur. Confirm diagnosis by KOH smears and/or cultures; reconfirm if no response.

**ADVERSE REACTIONS:** Headache, body pain, burning, itching, irritation.

**PREGNANCY:** Category C, not for use in nursing.

**MECHANISM OF ACTION:** Azole antifungal; uncertain. Suspected to exert antifungal activity by disruption of normal fungal cell membrane permeability

**PHARMACOKINETICS: Absorption:** 5-8% (hysterectomized), 12-16% (non-hysterectomized); $C_{max}$=5.9ng/mL, $T_{max}$=6.6 hrs. **Distribution:** Plasma protein binding (94.9%).

## NURSING CONSIDERATIONS

**Assessment:** Assess for proper diagnosis with appropriate microbiologic studies (KOH smears and/or culture). Assess for hypersensitivity and pregnancy/nursing status.

**Monitoring:** Monitor for signs/symptoms of sensitization, irritation, fever, chills, flu-like symptoms. Monitor for response to treatment; if lack of response, standard KOH smear and cultures should be repeated to confirm diagnosis.

**Patient Counseling:** Counsel to use as prescribed, even if symptoms improve. Instruct to consult physician if partner has penile itching, redness, or discomfort. Advise to not use tampons while on medication. Instruct not to douche unless otherwise directed by physician. Advise to notify physician of all medications currently taking.

**Administration:** Intravaginal route. 1) Lie on back with knees drawn up towards chest. 2) Insert filled applicator into vagina as far as it will comfortably go. 3) Press plunger to release cre into vagina. 4) Apply at bedtime as directed by doctor. **Storage:** 15-30°C (59-86°F).

## TERAZOSIN HCL — RX

terazosin HCl (Various)

**THERAPEUTIC CLASS:** Alpha$_1$-blocker (quinazoline)

**INDICATIONS:** Treatment of hypertension and symptomatic benign prostatic hyperplasia (BPH).

**DOSAGE:** *Adults:* HTN: Initial: 1mg hs, then slowly increase dose. Usual: 1-5mg/day. Max: 20mg/day. If response is substantially diminished at 24 hrs, may increase dose or use bid regimen. BPH: Initial: 1mg qhs. Titrate: Increase stepwise to 2mg, 5mg, or 10mg qd prn. Usual: 10mg/day. May increase to 20mg/day after 4-6 weeks. Max: 20mg/day. If d/c for several days, restart at initial dose.

**HOW SUPPLIED:** Cap: 1mg, 2mg, 5mg, 10mg

**WARNINGS/PRECAUTIONS:** Monitor for orthostatic hypotension and syncope initially, with dose increase, or introduction of additional antihypertensive agent. May impair physical/mental abilities. Rule out prostate cancer. Priapism (rare) reported. Intraoperative floppy iris syndrome observed during cataract surgery. Significant decreases in Hct, Hgb, WBC, total protein and albumin were observed possibly due to hemodilution. Examine patients with BPH prior to initiation of therapy.

**ADVERSE REACTIONS:** Asthenia, postural hypotension, headache, dizziness, dyspnea, nasal congestion/rhinitis, somnolence, blurred vision, palpitations, nausea, peripheral edema, priapism, thrombocytopenia.

**INTERACTIONS:** Caution with other antihypertensive agents (eg, verapamil). Hypotension reported when coadministering with PDE-5 inhibitors. May need dose reduction or retitration of either agent with other antihypertensive agents.

**PREGNANCY:** Category C, caution with nursing.

**MECHANISM OF ACTION:** Alpha$_1$-blocker; (BPH) antagonizes $\alpha_1$-receptors in bladder neck and prostate, relaxing smooth muscle; (HTN) antagonizes $\alpha_1$-receptors decreasing total peripheral vascular resistance, causing decreased BP.

**PHARMACOKINETICS: Absorption:** Complete; $T_{max}$=1 hr. **Distribution:** Plasma protein binding (90-94%). **Elimination:** Feces (20%), urine (10%); $T_{1/2}$=12 hrs.

T

### NURSING CONSIDERATIONS

**Assessment:** Assess for HTN, BPH, pregnancy/nursing status and possible drug interactions. Rule out prostate cancer.

**Monitoring:** Monitor for Hct, Hgb, WBC, total protein/albumin, and BP periodically. Monitor for signs/symptoms of hypotension, priapism.

**Patient Counseling:** Inform of possibility of syncope and orthostatic symptoms, especially at initiation of therapy. Caution against driving or hazardous tasks for 24 hrs after first dose, dosage increase, or when resuming therapy after interruption. Avoid situations where injury could result should syncope occur. Advise to sit or lie down when symptoms of low BP occur. Inform possibility of priapism; advise to seek medical attention if it occurs.

**Administration:** Oral route. **Storage:** 20°-25°C (68°-77°F). Protect from light and moisture.

## TESSALON — RX

benzonatate (Forest)

**THERAPEUTIC CLASS:** Non-narcotic antitussive

**INDICATIONS:** Symptomatic relief of cough.

**DOSAGE:** *Adults:* Usual: 100-200mg tid as needed. Max: 600mg/day. *Pediatrics:* >10 yrs: Usual: 100-200mg tid as needed. Max: 600mg/day.

**HOW SUPPLIED:** Cap: 100mg, 200mg

**WARNINGS/PRECAUTIONS:** Severe hypersensitivity reactions; confusion and hallucinations reported in combination with other prescribed drugs. Swallow capsules without sucking/chewing to avoid local anesthesia adverse effects.

**ADVERSE REACTIONS:** Sedation, headache, dizziness, confusion, hallucinations, constipation, nausea, GI upset, pruritus.

**PREGNANCY:** Category C, caution in nursing.

**MECHANISM OF ACTION:** Non-narcotic/antitussive agent; acts peripherally by anesthetizing stretch receptors located in respiratory passages, lungs, and pleura by dampening their activity, thereby reducing cough reflex at its source.

### NURSING CONSIDERATIONS

**Assessment:** Assess for drug hypersensitivity.

**Monitoring:** Monitor for hypersensitivity (eg, bronchospasm, laryngospasm, cardiovascular collapse), mental confusion, visual hallucinations, overdose signs/symptoms (eg, restlessness, tremors, clonic convulsions followed by profound CNS depression).

**Patient Counseling:** Caution to swallow caps whole; do not chew or dissolve cap in mouth; may lead to temporary anesthesia of the oral mucosa, hypersensitivity reactions, or choking.

**Administration:** Oral route. **Storage:** 25°C (77°F); excursions permitted to 15-30°C (59-86°F).

## TESTIM — CIII

testosterone (Auxilium)

**Virilization reported in children secondarily exposed to testosterone gel. Children should avoid contact with unwashed or unclothed application sites in men using testosterone gel. Healthcare providers should advise patients to strictly adhere to recommended use instructions.**

**THERAPEUTIC CLASS:** Androgen

**INDICATIONS:** Testosterone replacement in males with primary or hypogonadotropic hypogonadism.

**DOSAGE:** *Adults:* ≥18 yrs: Initial: Apply 5g qd, preferably in the am, to clean, dry, intact skin of shoulders and/or upper arms. Allow to dry prior to dressing. Titrate: May increase to 10g qd if response not achieved or serum concentration is below normal range. Do not apply to genitals or abdomen; wash hands after application. To maintain serum testosterone levels, do not wash site of application for at least 2 hrs.

**HOW SUPPLIED:** Gel: 1% [5g (50mg)/tube, 30^s]

**CONTRAINDICATIONS:** Breast or prostate carcinoma in men. Not for use by women. Pregnant and nursing women should avoid skin contact with application sites on men. Hypersensitivity to soy products.

**WARNINGS/PRECAUTIONS:** Caution men treated with androgens/elderly; at increased risk of worsening prostatic hypertrophy/carcinoma. Evaluate for prostate cancer prior to therapy. Risk of virilization in children (eg, enlarged penis/clitoris, pubic hair, increased erection/libido, aggressive behavior, advanced bone age) and women (eg, changes in body hair distribution, significant increase in acne) due to secondary skin exposure from contact with men using testosterone-containing gel products. Strictly adhere patients to use instructions. Risk of edema with pre-existing cardiac, renal, or hepatic disease; d/c if edema occurs, diuretic therapy may be required. Risk of gynecomastia. May potentiate sleep apnea especially with obesity or chronic lung diseases. Advise patients to report persistent penis erections, changes in skin color, ankle swelling, unexplained N/V, or breathing disturbances. Monitor serum testosterone, LFTs, Hgb, Hct, PSA, cholesterol, lipids. Prolonged use associated with serious hepatic effects (peliosis hepatis, hepatic neoplasms, cholestatic hepatitis, jaundice).

**ADVERSE REACTIONS:** Application-site reactions, benign prostatic hyperplasia, decreased DBP, HTN, gynecomastia, headache, Hct/Hgb increases, hot flushes, insomnia, increased lacrimation, mood swings, smell disorder, virilization from secondary exposure.

**INTERACTIONS:** May elevate oxyphenbutazone levels. May decrease blood glucose and insulin requirements. May increase clearance of propranolol. Corticosteroids may enhance edema; caution with cardiac or hepatic disease.

**PREGNANCY:** Category X, not for use in nursing.

**MECHANISM OF ACTION:** Endogenous androgen; responsible for normal growth and development of male sex organs and for maintenance of secondary sex characteristics.

**PHARMACOKINETICS: Absorption:** 10% absorbed systemically. **Distribution:** Sex hormone-binding globulin (SHBG) binding (40%), albumin- and plasma protein-binding (58%), unbound (2%). **Metabolism:** Skin, liver, male urogenital tract via 5α-reductase; estradiol and dihydrotestosterone (metabolites). **Elimination:** Urine (80%), feces (6%); $T_{1/2}$=10-100 min.

## NURSING CONSIDERATIONS

**Assessment:** Assess for hypersensitivity to soy, breast or prostate carcinoma, cardiac or renal/hepatic disease, obesity; chronic lung disease, pregnancy/nursing status of female partner, and possible drug interactions.

**Monitoring:** Periodically monitor Hgb, Hct, LFTs, PSA, cholesterol, and HDL. Obtain serum testosterone levels 14 days after initiation of therapy. Monitor for signs/symptoms of hypersensitivity reactions, edema with/without CHF, gynecomastia, prostatic hyperplasia/carcinoma in geriatrics, and potentiation of sleep apnea.

**Patient Counseling:** Inform of pregnancy risks; avoid contact with application sites in children and women or if pregnant/nursing. If contact occurs, wash area immediately with soap and water. Instruct not to apply to the scrotum, penis, or abdomen. Cover application site with clothing after gel dries; wash application site with soap and water prior to direct skin-to-skin contact. Advise to wash or swim ≥2 hrs after application. Inform to contact physician if changes in body hair distribution, increase in acne, virilization of female partner or child, too frequent or persistent erections, changes in skin color, ankle swelling, unexplained N/V, breathing disturbances, or hypersensitivity reactions occur.

**Administration:** Transdermal. Apply every day at same time to clean, dry skin of shoulder or upper arms. Wash hands thoroughly after application. **Storage:** 25°C (77°F); excursions permitted to 15-30°C (59-86°F).



# TESTRED

**CIII**

methyltestosterone (Valeant)

**THERAPEUTIC CLASS:** Androgen

**INDICATIONS:** Testosterone replacement therapy in males with primary hypogonadism or hypogonadotropic hypogonadism. To stimulate puberty in males with delayed puberty. Secondary treatment of advancing inoperable metastatic (skeletal) breast cancer in females 1-5 yrs postmenopausal.

**DOSAGE:** *Adults:* Dose based on age, sex and diagnosis. Adjust dose according to clinical response and adverse events. Male Replacement Therapy: 10-50mg/day. Breast Carcinoma: 50-200mg/day.
*Pediatrics:* Dose based on age, sex and diagnosis. Adjust dose according to

clinical response and adverse events. Delayed Puberty: Use lower range of 10-50mg/day for 4-6 months. Caution in children.

**HOW SUPPLIED:** Cap: 10mg

**CONTRAINDICATIONS:** Pregnancy. Males with breast or prostate carcinoma.

**WARNINGS/PRECAUTIONS:** D/C if hypercalcemia occurs in breast cancer; monitor calcium levels. Monitor for virilization in females. Risk of compromised stature in children; monitor bone growth every 6 months. Risk of hepatic damage with long-term use. D/C if jaundice, cholestatic hepatitis occur. Risk of edema; caution with pre-existing cardiac, renal or hepatic disease. Caution in the elderly; increased risk of prostatic hypertrophy and prostatic carcinoma. Should not be used for enhancement of athletic performance. Monitor LFTs, Hct, and Hgb periodically.

**ADVERSE REACTIONS:** Amenorrhea, virilization, menstrual irregularities, gynecomastia, excessive frequency/duration of penile erections, male-pattern baldness, increased/decreased libido, oligospermia, hirsutism, acne, fluid and electrolyte disturbances, nausea, hypercholesterolemia, clotting factor suppression, polycythemia, altered LFTs, priapism, anxiety, depression.

**INTERACTIONS:** Potentiates oral anticoagulants and oxyphenbutazone. May decrease blood glucose and insulin requirements in diabetics.

**PREGNANCY:** Category X, not for use in nursing.

**MECHANISM OF ACTION:** Endogenous androgen (derivative of testosterone); responsible for normal growth and development of male sex organs and maintenance of secondary sex characteristics.

**PHARMACOKINETICS: Metabolism:** Gut, liver. **Elimination:** Urine, feces; $T_{1/2}$=10-100 min.

## NURSING CONSIDERATIONS

**Assessment:** Assess for known or suspected carcinoma of prostate or male breast, pregnancy status, pre-existing cardiac or renal/hepatic disease, and possible drug interactions.

**Monitoring:** Periodically monitor urine and serum calcium levels (female breast cancer), LFTs, Hgb and Hct, and bone age of left wrist and hand every 6 months (bone maturation in pediatrics). Monitor for signs/symptoms of hypersensitivity reactions, peliosis hepatis, hepatic dysfunction, prostatic hyperplasia/carcinoma in geriatrics, edema (with or without CHF), hypercalcemia, and virilization of females.

**Patient Counseling:** Inform of pregnancy risks. Instruct to contact physician if any hypersensitivity reactions, N/V, ankle swelling, changes in skin color, symptoms of hepatotoxicity, frequent or persistent erections (males), hoarseness (females), acne, changes in menstrual periods (females), or more facial hair occur.

**Administration:** Oral route. **Storage:** 25°C (77°F); excursions permitted to 15-30°C (59-86°F).

# TETANUS & DIPHTHERIA TOXOIDS ADSORBED RX

diphtheria toxoid - tetanus toxoid (Sanofi Pasteur)

**THERAPEUTIC CLASS:** Toxoid combination

**INDICATIONS:** Active immunization against tetanus and diphtheria (Td).

**DOSAGE:** *Adults:* 0.5mL IM in the vastus lateralis or deltoid. Repeat 4-8 weeks later. Give 3rd dose 6-12 months after 2nd dose. Booster: 0.5mL IM every 10 yrs.

*Pediatrics:* >7 yrs: 0.5mL IM in the vastus lateralis or deltoid. Repeat 4-8 weeks later. Give 3rd dose 6-12 months after 2nd dose. Booster: 0.5mL IM every 10 yrs.

**HOW SUPPLIED:** Inj: 5LFU-2LFU/0.5mL

**CONTRAINDICATIONS:** Neurological or systemic allergic reaction to previous dose. Defer during febrile illness, acute infection, or an outbreak of poliomyelitis. Thimerosal hypersensitivity.

**WARNINGS/PRECAUTIONS:** Suboptimal response may occur in immunocompromised patients. Avoid booster more frequently than every 10 yrs especially with Arthus-type hypersensitivity reactions or temperature >39.4°C after a previous dose of tetanus toxoid. Caution with IM injection in thrombocytopenia or any coagulation disorder. Increased risk of local/systemic reactions to boosters doses. Have epinephrine available.

**ADVERSE REACTIONS:** Injection-site reactions, fever, malaise, hypotension, nausea, arthralgia.

**INTERACTIONS:** Immunosuppressive therapy may reduce response to active immunization. Caution with anticoagulants.

**PREGNANCY:** Category C, safety in nursing not known.

**MECHANISM OF ACTION:** Toxoid combination; activates neutralizing antibodies to diphtheria and tetanus toxins for protection against diphtheria and tetanus.

**PHARMACOKINETICS: Absorption:** Complete.

## NURSING CONSIDERATIONS

**Assessment:** Assess for history of hypersensitivity including thimerosal (mercury derivative), systemic or neurologic reactions following previous dose of vaccine, acute illness, bleeding disorders (eg, hemophilia, thrombocytopenia), anticoagulant therapy, immunosuppressive therapy, and outbreak of poliomyelitis.

**Monitoring:** Monitor for acute anaphylactic reactions, Arthus-type hypersensitivity reactions, injection-site redness, warmth, edema, induration with/without tenderness, urticaria and rash, malaise, transient fever, pain, hypotension, nausea, arthralgia, and neurological complications (eg, cochlear lesion, brachial plexus neuropathies, paralysis of radical nerve, EEG disturbances, encephalopathy).

**Patient Counseling:** Inform of the benefits and risks of immunization and of importance of completing the primary immunization series or receiving recommended booster doses. Does not treat diphtheria or tetanus infections. Instruct to report any severe or unusual adverse reactions (eg, hives, swelling of mouth, difficulty breathing, hypotension, shock).

**Administration:** IM. Inspect for particulate matter and/or discoloration prior to administration. Shake well before withdrawing each dose. Inject IM only in anterolateral aspect of thigh or deltoid muscle of upper arm. **Storage:** 2-8°C (35-46°F). Do not freeze.

# TETANUS TOXOID ADSORBED — RX

tetanus toxoid (Sanofi Pasteur)

**THERAPEUTIC CLASS:** Toxoid

**INDICATIONS:** Active immunization against tetanus.

T

**DOSAGE:** *Adults:* Primary Immunization: 0.5mL IM. Repeat 4-8 weeks later. Give 3rd dose 6-12 months after 2nd dose. Booster: 0.5mL IM every 10 yrs. *Pediatrics:* <1 yr: 3 doses of 0.5mL IM 4 to 8 weeks apart, then 4th dose (0.5mL) 6 to 12 months after the 3rd dose. Last dose before 4 yrs. Give booster of 0.5mL at 4-6 yrs. No booster needed if last primary dose was given after 4 yrs. ≥1 yrs: Primary Immunization: 0.5mL IM. Repeat 4-8 weeks later. Give 3rd dose 6-12 months after 2nd dose. Booster: 0.5mL IM every 10 yrs.

**HOW SUPPLIED:** Inj: 5 LFU/0.5mL

**CONTRAINDICATIONS:** Neurological or systemic allergic reaction to previous dose. Defer during febrile illness, acute infection, or an outbreak of poliomyelitis. Thimerosal hypersensitivity.

**WARNINGS/PRECAUTIONS:** Suboptimal response may occur in immunocompromised patients. Avoid booster more frequently than every 10 yrs especially with Arthus-type hypersensitivity reactions or temperature >103°F after a previous dose of tetanus toxoid. Caution with IM injections in thrombocytopenia or any coagulation disorders. Have epinephrine injection available. Increased incidence of local/systemic reaction to booster doses.

**ADVERSE REACTIONS:** Local erythema, malaise, transient fever, pain, hypotension, nausea, arthralgia.

**INTERACTIONS:** Caution with anticoagulants. Immunosuppressive therapy (eg, radiation, corticosteroids, chemotherapy) may reduce antibody response to vaccine; defer routine vaccination. Separate syringes and sites should be used when Tetanus Immune Globulin (human) and vaccine are given concurrently.

**PREGNANCY:** Category C, safety in nursing not known.

**MECHANISM OF ACTION:** Development of neutralizing antibodies against tetanus toxin.

## NURSING CONSIDERATIONS

**Assessment:** Review current health status, previous sensitivity/immunization events (eg, Guillain-Barre syndrome, convulsions), and possible drug interactions.

**Monitoring:** Monitor adverse events such as severe Arthus-type hypersensitivity reactions; anaphylactic reactions; injection site for hematoma, redness, warmth, edema, induration, and tenderness; urticaria; rash; malaise; fever; pain; hypotension; nausea; arthralgia; Guillain-Barre syndrome; brachial neuritis; EEG disturbances.

**Patient Counseling:** Inform patient and caregiver of potential benefits/risk ratio; report any adverse reactions to physician. Stress importance of completing vaccination series.

**Administration:** IM in the area of the vastus lateralis or deltoid. **Storage**: 2-8°C (36-46°F). Do not freeze.

# Teveten RX

eprosartan mesylate (Abbott)

**Can cause death/injury to developing fetus during 2nd and 3rd trimesters. D/C therapy if pregnancy detected.**

**THERAPEUTIC CLASS:** Angiotensin II receptor antagonist

**INDICATIONS:** Treatment of hypertension, alone or with other antihypertensives (eg, diuretics, calcium channel blockers).

**DOSAGE:** *Adults:* Initial: 600mg qd. Usual: 400-800mg/day, given qd-bid. Max: 800mg/day. Moderate to Severe Renal Impairment: Max: 600mg/day.

**HOW SUPPLIED:** Tab: 400mg, 600mg

**WARNINGS/PRECAUTIONS:** May cause fetal and neonatal injury/death. Correct volume or salt depletion before therapy or monitor closely. Renal function changes may occur; caution with renal artery stenosis, severe CHF. Oliguria, progressive azotemia, and acute renal failure (rare) reported. Risk of hypotension.

**ADVERSE REACTIONS:** Upper respiratory infection, rhinitis, pharyngitis, cough, viral infection, injury, fatigue, abdominal pain, hypertriglyceridemia, arthralgia, depression, urinary tract infection.

**INTERACTIONS:** Risk of hypotension with diuretics.

**PREGNANCY:** Category C (1st trimester) and D (2nd and 3rd trimesters), not for use in nursing.

**MECHANISM OF ACTION:** Angiotensin II receptor antagonist; blocks vasoconstrictor and aldosterone-secreting effects of angiotensin II by selectively blocking binding of angiotensin II to $AT_1$ receptor found in many tissues.

**PHARMACOKINETICS: Absorption:** Absolute bioavailability (approximately 13%); $T_{max}$=1-2 hrs. **Distribution:** $V_d$=308L; plasma protein binding (approximately 98%). **Elimination:** Feces (90%), urine (7%), (600mg); $T_{1/2}$=20 hrs.

T

## NURSING CONSIDERATIONS

**Assessment:** Assess LFTs, renal function, BP, pregnancy/nursing status, and possible drug interactions.

**Monitoring:** Monitor BP, LFTs, renal function, CBC with platelet count and differential, serum $K^+$ levels. Monitor for angina, bradycardia, angioneurotic edema, hypersensitivity reactions, upper respiratory tract infection, constipation, rhinitis, eczema.

**Patient Counseling:** Counsel about signs/symptoms of adverse effects; advise to seek prompt medical attention. Inform about fetal risks if taken during pregnancy. Instruct to take with or without food.

**Administration:** Oral route. **Storage:** 20-25°C (68-77°F).

# TEVETEN HCT RX

eprosartan mesylate - hydrochlorothiazide (Abbott)

**Can cause death/injury to developing fetus during 2nd and 3rd trimesters. D/C therapy if pregnancy detected.**

**THERAPEUTIC CLASS:** Angiotensin II receptor antagonist/thiazide diuretic

**INDICATIONS:** Treatment of hypertension alone or with other antihypertensive (eg, calcium channel blocker).

**DOSAGE:** *Adults:* Usual (Not Volume Depleted): 600mg-12.5mg qd. If BP not controlled on 600mg-12.5mg qd, may increase to 600mg-25mg qd. Replacement Therapy: May substitute for titrated components.

**HOW SUPPLIED:** Tab: (Eprosartan-HCTZ) 600mg-12.5mg, 600mg-25mg

**CONTRAINDICATIONS:** Anuria, hypersensitivity to other sulfonamide-derived drugs.

**WARNINGS/PRECAUTIONS:** May cause fetal and neonatal injury/death. Hypersensitivity reactions reported. Correct volume or salt depletion before therapy or monitor closely. May cause hypotension. Caution with CHF, renal or hepatic dysfunction, and renal artery stenosis. Monitor electrolytes periodically. Hypercalcemia, hypomagnesemia, hyperuricemia, hyperglycemia, hypokalemia, hyponatremia, hypochloremic alkalosis may occur. Enhanced effects in post-sympathectomy patient. Not for initial therapy.

**ADVERSE REACTIONS:** Dizziness, headache, back pain, fatigue, myalgia, upper respiratory tract infection, sinusitis, viral infection.

**INTERACTIONS:** (Eprosartan) Increased risk of hyperkalemia with $K^+$-sparing diuretics, $K^+$ supplements, or $K^+$-containing salt substitutes. (HCTZ) Potentiates orthostatic hypotension with alcohol, barbiturates, and narcotics. May need to adjust dosages of insulin and antidiabetic drugs. Impaired absorption with cholestyramine, colestipol. Corticosteroids and ACTH deplete electrolytes. May decrease response to pressor amines (eg, norepinephrine). Potentiated effect with other antihypertensives. May increase responsiveness to nondepolarizing skeletal muscle relaxants (eg, tubocurarine). Risk of lithium toxicity; avoid use. NSAIDs may decrease diuretic/antihypertensive effects.

**PREGNANCY:** Category C (1st trimester) and D (2nd and 3rd trimesters), not for use in nursing.

**MECHANISM OF ACTION:** Eprosartan: Angiotensin II receptor antagonist; blocks vasoconstrictor and aldosterone-secreting effects of angiotensin II by selectively blocking binding of angiotensin II to $AT_1$ receptor in vascular smooth muscle and adrenal gland. HCTZ: Thiazide diuretic; mechanism not established. Affects renal tubular mechanism of electrolyte reabsorption, directly increasing excretion of $Na^+$ and $Cl^-$.

**PHARMACOKINETICS: Absorption:** Eprosartan: Absolute bioavailability (13%); $T_{max}$=1-2 hrs. **Distribution:** Eprosartan: $V_d$=308L; plasma protein binding (approximately 98%). HCTZ: Crosses placenta; excreted in breast milk. **Elimination:** Eprosartan: Feces (90%), urine (7%); (600mg) $T_{1/2}$=20 hrs. HCTZ: Urine (61% unchanged); $T_{1/2}$=5.6-14.8 hrs.

## NURSING CONSIDERATIONS

**Assessment:** Assess for anuria, hypersensitivity to other sulfonamide-derived drugs, renal/hepatic insufficiency, hypotension, hyperuricemia, electrolyte imbalance, pregnancy/nursing status, and possible drug interactions.

**Monitoring:** Monitor BP, LFTs, renal function, CBC with platelet count and differential, serum electrolytes, hyperuricemia, lipid profile. Monitor for MI, CHF, angioneurotic edema, hypersensitivity reactions, upper respiratory tract infection, diarrhea, sinusitis, pancreatitis, Stevens-Johnson syndrome (SJS), xanthopsia.

**Patient Counseling:** Inform of risks if taken during pregnancy. Advise that inadequate fluid intake, excessive perspiration, diarrhea, or vomiting can lead to excessive fall in BP, leading to lightheadedness or possible syncope. Advise not to use $K^+$ supplements or salt substitutes containing $K^+$ without consulting physician. Inform about signs/symptoms of adverse effects and advise to seek prompt medical attention.

**Administration:** Oral route. **Storage:** 20-25°C (68-77°F).

# THALOMID — RX

thalidomide (Celgene)

**May cause severe, life-threatening birth defects or death to an unborn baby, if taken during pregnancy. Women of childbearing potential should have a pregnancy test within 24 hrs before starting therapy. Once treatment started, pregnancy testing should occur weekly for the first 4 weeks, then pregnancy testing should be repeated at 4 weeks in women with regular menstrual cycles. Pregnancy testing should occur every 2 weeks in women with irregular menstrual cycles; d/c immediately if pregnancy occurs. Two reliable forms of contraception must be used simultaneously unless continuous abstinence from heterosexual sexual contact is the chosen method. Males must use latex condoms during sexual contact with females of childbearing potential. Effective contraception must be used 4 weeks before, during, and 4 weeks after therapy. Only prescribers and pharmacists registered with the *S.T.E.P.S.®* distribution program can prescribe and dispense. Use in multiple myeloma results in an increased risk of venous thromboembolic events (eg, DVT, PE). Seek immediate medical care if develop symptoms of thromboembolism (eg, SOB, chest pain, arm or leg swelling). Immediately report any suspected fetal exposure to the FDA and the manufacturer.**

**THERAPEUTIC CLASS:** Immunomodulatory agent

**INDICATIONS:** Acute treatment of the cutaneous manifestations of moderate to severe erythema nodosum leprosum (ENL). Maintenance therapy for prevention and suppression of the cutaneous manifestations of ENL recurrence. In combination with dexamethasone for the treatment of newly diagnosed multiple myeloma.

**DOSAGE:** *Adults:* Acute ENL: Initial: 100-300mg qd. <50kg: Start at lower end of dosing range. If severe cutaneous ENL reaction or if previously required higher doses, may initiate at higher doses up to 400mg/day. In moderate to severe neuritis associated with a severe ENL reaction, may use with concomitant corticosteroid therapy. Taper steroid when neuritis is ameliorated. Usual duration: 2 weeks, or until signs/symptoms have subsided. Taper Dose: Decrease by 50mg every 2-4 weeks. Maintenance Therapy for Prevention/Suppression of ENL Recurrence: Use minimum dose to control reaction. Taper Dose: Every 3-6 months, attempt to decrease dose by 50mg every 2-4 weeks. Multiple Myeloma: 200mg qd. Give with dexamethasone in 28-day treatment cycles (40mg po on days 1-4, 9-12, and 17-20). Take with water, preferably at hs, and at least 1hr after the evening meal.
*Pediatrics:* ≥12 yrs: Initial: 100-300mg qd. <50kg: Start at lower end of dosing range. If severe cutaneous ENL reaction or if previously required higher doses, may initiate at higher doses up to 400mg/day. In moderate to severe neuritis associated with a severe ENL reaction, may use with concomitant corticosteroid therapy. Taper steroid when neuritis is ameliorated. Usual duration: 2 weeks, or until signs/symptoms have subsided. Taper Dose: Decrease by 50mg every 2-4 weeks. Maintenance Therapy for Prevention/Suppression of ENL Recurrence: Use minimum dose to control reaction. Taper Dose: Every 3-6 months, attempt to decrease dose by 50mg every 2-4 weeks. Multiple

Myeloma: 200mg qd. Give with dexamethasone in 28-day treatment cycles (40mg po on days 1-4, 9-12, and 17-20). Take with water, preferably at hs, and at least 1hr after the evening meal.

**HOW SUPPLIED:** Cap: 50mg, 100mg, 150mg, 200mg

**CONTRAINDICATIONS:** Pregnancy and women of childbearing potential unless alternative therapies are considered inappropriate and if precautions are taken to avoid pregnancy. Sexually mature males unless they comply with the *S.T.E.P.S.®* program and mandatory contraceptive measures.

**WARNINGS/PRECAUTIONS:** Drowsiness and somnolence reported, caution when operating machinery. May cause irreversible peripheral neuropathy; monitor for neuropathy during the first 3 months of therapy and periodically thereafter; d/c immediately if drug-induced neuropathy develops. May cause dizziness and orthostatic hypotension; sit upright for a few minutes prior to standing. If hypersensitivity reaction occurs (eg, erythematous macular rash); d/c drug. Serious dermatological reactions including Stevens-Johnson syndrome and toxic epidermal necrolysis reported. Decreased WBC, including neutropenia reported; do not initiate if absolute neutrophil count $<750/mm^3$. Measure viral load of HIV patients after 1st and 3rd month of therapy and every 3 months thereafter. Bradycardia and seizures, including grand mal convulsions, reported. Not indicated as monotherapy for cutaneous manifestations of moderate/severe ENL in the presence of moderate/severe neuritis.

**ADVERSE REACTIONS:** Drowsiness/somnolence, peripheral neuropathy, dizziness, orthostatic hypotension, neutropenia, increased HIV viral load, rash, constipation, hypocalcemia, thrombosis/embolism, dyspnea.

**INTERACTIONS:** Enhanced sedation with barbiturates, alcohol, chlorpromazine, and reserpine. Caution with drugs associated with peripheral neuropathy. Concomitant use with chemotherapeutic agents such as dexamethasone may increase risk for thromboembolic events (DVT, PE).

**PREGNANCY:** Category X, not for use in nursing.

**MECHANISM OF ACTION:** Immunomodulatory agent; not fully established. Possesses immunomodulatory, anti-inflammatory, and anti-angiogenic properties. Immunologic effects may be caused by suppression of excessive TNF-α production and down-modulation of selected cell surface adhesion molecules involved in leukocyte migration. Also causes suppression of macrophage involvement in prostaglandin synthesis and modulation of interleukin-10 and 12 production by peripheral blood mononuclear cells. In multiple myeloma, increased circulating natural killer cells and plasma levels of interleukin-2 and INF-gamma are also seen.

**PHARMACOKINETICS: Absorption:** Slow; $T_{max}$=2.9-5.7 hrs, variable doses resulted in different parameters. **Distribution:** Plasma protein binding (55-66%); found in semen. **Metabolism:** Non-enzymatic hydrolysis. **Elimination:** Urine (<0.7% unchanged); $T_{1/2}$=5-7 hrs.

## NURSING CONSIDERATIONS

T

**Assessment:** Assess use in those capable of reproduction. Assess that females of child-bearing potential are committed to either abstaining from heterosexual contact or willing to use 2 forms of reliable contraception including 1 highly effective method (eg, IUD, hormonal contraception, tubal ligation, partner's vasectomy) and 1 additional effective method (eg, latex condom, diaphragm, cervical cap) beginning 4 weeks prior to treatment, during treatment, and continuing 4 weeks after treatment. Prior to therapy, assess that males will wear latex condom during any sexual contact with women of childbearing potential, even if they have undergone a vasectomy. Assess pregnancy status 24 hrs prior to therapy. Assess nursing status, absolute neutrophil count (ANC), and for drug interactions.

**Monitoring:** Monitor for signs/symptoms of venous thromboembolic events (eg, SOB, chest pain, arm or leg swelling), drowsiness, somnolence, peripheral neuropathy, dizziness, orthostatic hypotension, neutropenia, hypersensitivity reactions (eg, erythematous macular rash), bradycardia, seizures, serious dermatological reactions (eg, Stevens-Johnson syndrome, toxic epidermal necrolysis). Perform periodic monitoring of WBC count with differential. Perform pregnancy test weekly during first 4 weeks of therapy, then at

4-week intervals (regular menstrual cycle) or every 2 weeks (irregular menstrual cycle). Monitor for missed periods or abnormal menstrual bleeding. In HIV patients, monitor viral load after first and third months of therapy and every 3 months thereafter.

**Patient Counseling:** Instruct females they must use 2 forms of contraception beginning 4 weeks prior to treatment, during treatment, and 4 weeks following end of therapy. Instruct males to use latex condom during any heterosexual contact. Counsel to not extensively handle caps and maintain medication in blister packs until ingestion. Inform that therapy may cause drowsiness and somnolence and impair mental/physical abilities. Instruct to avoid hazardous tasks (eg, operating machinery/driving) and to avoid alcohol or medications which may cause drowsiness. Advise that therapy may cause dizziness; instruct to sit upright for a few minutes prior to standing up from recumbent position. Instruct about signs/symptoms of peripheral neuropathies (eg, numbness, tingling) and thromboembolism (eg, SOB, chest pain, leg or arm swelling). Inform that not allowed to donate blood and males not allowed to donate sperm while on medication.

**Administration:** Oral route. **Storage:** 25°C (77°F); excursions permitted to 15-30°C (59-86°F). Protect from light.

## TIAZAC — RX

diltiazem HCl (Forest)

**OTHER BRAND NAMES:** Taztia XT (Andrx)

**THERAPEUTIC CLASS:** Calcium channel blocker (nondihydropyridine)

**INDICATIONS:** Treatment of hypertension alone or in combination with other antihypertensives. Treatment of chronic stable angina.

**DOSAGE:** *Adults:* HTN: Initial: 120-240mg qd. Titrate: Adjust at 2-week intervals. Usual: 120-540mg qd. Max: 540mg qd. Angina: Initial: 120-180mg qd Titrate: Increase over 7-14 days. Max: 540mg qd.

**HOW SUPPLIED:** Cap, Extended-Release: (Taztia XT, Tiazac) 120mg, 180mg, 240mg, 300mg, 360mg; (Tiazac) 420mg

**CONTRAINDICATIONS:** Sick sinus syndrome and 2nd- or 3rd-degree AV block (except with functioning pacemaker), severe hypotension (<90mmHg systolic), acute myocardial infarction (MI), pulmonary congestion documented by x-ray.

**WARNINGS/PRECAUTIONS:** Caution in renal, hepatic, or ventricular dysfunction. Monitor LFTs and renal function with prolonged use. D/C if persistent dermatologic reactions (eg, skin eruptions progressing to erythema multiforme and/or exfoliative dermatitis) occurs. Symptomatic hypotension may occur. Acute hepatic injury reported.

**ADVERSE REACTIONS:** Headache, peripheral edema, vasodilation, dizziness, dyspepsia, pain, asthenia, dyspnea, bronchitis, AV block, pharyngitis, infection.

**INTERACTIONS:** Increased levels of buspirone, quinidine, carbamazepine, midazolam, triazolam, lovastatin, and propranolol. Increased levels of diltiazem with cimetidine. Monitor digoxin and cyclosporine levels if used concomitantly. Potentiates cardiac contractility, conductivity, and automaticity; and vascular dilation with anesthetics. Additive cardiac conduction effects with digitalis or β-blockers. Avoid rifampin and other CYP3A4 inducers. Potential additive effects with agents known to affect cardiac contractility and/or conduction.

**PREGNANCY:** Category C, not for use in nursing.

**MECHANISM OF ACTION:** Calcium channel blocker; inhibits cellular influx of calcium ions during membrane depolarization of cardiac and vascular smooth muscle.

**PHARMACOKINETICS: Absorption:** Well-absorbed. Absolute bioavailability (~40%). **Distribution:** Plasma protein binding (70-80%), found in breast milk. **Metabolism:** Hepatic; desacetyldiltiazem, desmethyldiltiazem (major metabolites). **Elimination:** Urine, bile; $T_{1/2}$=3-4.5 hrs.

## NURSING CONSIDERATIONS

**Assessment:** Assess for sick sinus syndrome and 2nd- or 3rd-degree AV block without functional ventricular pacemaker, severe hypotension, Acute MI, pulmonary congestion (documented by x-ray), CHF, renal/hepatic function, drug hypersensitivity, and possible drug interactions.

**Monitoring:** Monitor LFTs, renal function, BP, HR. Monitor for angina, heart block, photosensitivity, ECG abnormalities, headache, edema, pain.

**Patient Counseling:** Counsel about signs/symptoms of adverse effects. Instruct to take as prescribed. Educate on need for routine checkup and lab exams.

**Administration:** Oral route. **Storage:** Controlled room temperature, 20-25°C (68-77°F). Avoid excessive humidity.

# TICLOPIDINE — RX

ticlopidine HCl (Various)

**Can cause life-threatening hematological adverse reactions, including neutropenia/agranulocytosis, thrombotic thrombocytopenic purpura (TTP), and aplastic anemia. Monitor for evidence of neutropenia or TTP during first 3 months; d/c if any seen.**

**THERAPEUTIC CLASS:** Platelet aggregation inhibitor

**INDICATIONS:** To reduce risk of thrombotic stroke in stroke patients or those with stroke precursors who are ASA intolerant, allergic, or failed ASA therapy. Adjunct to ASA to reduce incidence of subacute stent thrombosis in patients undergoing successful coronary artery stent implantation.

**DOSAGE:** *Adults:* Take with food. Stroke: 250mg bid. Coronary Artery Stenting: 250mg bid with ASA up to 30 days after stent implant.

**HOW SUPPLIED:** Tab: 250mg

**CONTRAINDICATIONS:** Hematopoietic disorders (eg, neutropenia, thrombocytopenia), history of TTP or aplastic anemia, hemostatic disorders, active pathological bleeding, severe liver impairment.

**WARNINGS/PRECAUTIONS:** Monitor for hematologic toxicity before treatment, then every 2 weeks for 1st 3 months, and 2 weeks after discontinuation. Monitor more frequently if signs of hematological adverse reactions; d/c if neutrophils <1200/mm$^3$, aplastic anemia or TTP occurs. D/C 10-14 days before surgery. Caution in trauma, surgery, bleeding disorders. May need dose adjustment with renal or hepatic impairment. May elevate LFTs, TG, and cholesterol.

**ADVERSE REACTIONS:** Diarrhea, rash, nausea, GI pain, dyspepsia, neutropenia.

**INTERACTIONS:** Adjust dose with drugs metabolized by CYP450 with low therapeutic ratios or with hepatic impairment. Potentiates ASA and NSAIDs effect on platelet aggregation. Antacids reduce plasma levels. Cimetidine reduces clearance. Decreases digoxin plasma levels. Significant decrease of theophylline plasma clearance. Caution with phenytoin, propranolol. D/C anticoagulants or fibrinolytics. Increased bioavailability with food.

**PREGNANCY:** Category B, not for use in nursing.

**MECHANISM OF ACTION:** Platelet aggregation inhibitor; interferes with platelet membrane function by inhibiting ADP-induced platelet fibrinogen binding and subsequent platelet-platelet interactions. Effect on platelet function is irreversible. Responsible for prolonging bleeding time.

**PHARMACOKINETICS: Absorption:** Rapid; $T_{max}$=2 hrs. **Distribution:** Plasma protein binding (98%). **Metabolism:** Liver (extensive). **Elimination:** Urine (60%), feces (23%); $T_{1/2}$=12.6 hrs (single dose), 4-5 days (multiple dose).

## NURSING CONSIDERATIONS

**Assessment:** Assess for presence of hematopoietic disorders (eg, neutropenia, thrombocytopenia), history of TTP, aplastic anemia, presence of hemostatic disorder or active bleeding (eg, bleeding peptic ulcer, intracranial bleeding), severe liver impairment, renal impairment, nursing status, and drug interactions. Obtain baseline CBC including ANC, platelet count, and peripheral smear.

**Monitoring:** Monitor for signs/symptoms of thrombocytopenia, TTP (eg, weakness, petechiae, purpura, dark urine, neurological changes), aplastic anemia, agranulocytosis, pancytopenia, leukemia, liver dysfunction, and serum cholesterol elevations. During first 3 months of therapy, monitor CBC including ANC, platelet count, and peripheral smear every 2 weeks. If therapy d/c before 3 months, monitor for 2 weeks following d/c. If liver dysfunction suspected, perform liver function testing (eg, ALT, AST, GGT).

**Patient Counseling:** Counsel about possible adverse effects (eg, thrombocytopenia, neutropenia). Contact physician immediately if any signs/symptoms of infection or TTP syndrome (eg, fever, weakness, difficulty speaking, seizures, yellowing of skin or eyes, bloody urine, petechiae) develop. Inform that lab testing is required during therapy. Advise it may take longer than usual to stop bleeding while on medication. Instruct to contact physician if any unusual bleeding occurs. Advise to notify all other physicians of medication. Take with food.

**Administration:** Oral route. **Storage:** 15-30°C (59-86°F).

## TIGAN RX

trimethobenzamide HCl (Various)

**THERAPEUTIC CLASS:** Emetic response modifier

**INDICATIONS:** Treatment of postoperative nausea and vomiting and for nausea associated with gastroenteritis.

**DOSAGE:** *Adults:* (Cap) 300mg tid-qid. (Inj) 200mg IM tid-qid. Renal Impairment: Reduce dose or increase dosing interval. Elderly: Start at low end dose.

**HOW SUPPLIED:** Cap: 300mg; Inj: 100mg/mL

**CONTRAINDICATIONS:** Injection in children

**WARNINGS/PRECAUTIONS:** Caution in children; may cause EPS, which may be confused with CNS signs of undiagnosed primary disease (eg, Reye's syndrome) and may unfavorably alter the course of Reye's syndrome due to hepatotoxic potential. May impair physical/mental abilties. Caution with acute febrile illness, encephalitides, gastroenteritis, dehydration, electrolyte imbalance and in elderly; CNS reactions reported. Caution with renal impairment. May produce drowsiness.

**ADVERSE REACTIONS:** Parkinson-like symptoms, hypotension (inj), blood dyscrasias, blurred vision, coma, convulsions, mood depression, diarrhea, disorientation, dizziness, drowsiness, headache, jaundice, muscle cramps, opisthotonos.

**INTERACTIONS:** Caution with CNS agents (eg, phenothiazines, barbiturates, belladonna derivatives) in acute febrile illness, encephalitides, gastroenteritis, dehydration, and electrolyte imbalance. Adverse drug interactions reported with alcohol.

**PREGNANCY:** Safety in pregnancy and nursing not known.

**MECHANISM OF ACTION:** Mechanism not established; thought to involve chemoreceptor trigger zone, an area in medulla oblongata through which emetic impulses are conveyed to vomiting center (direct impulses to vomiting center apparently not similarly inhibited).

**PHARMACOKINETICS: Absorption:** $T_{max}$=30 min (IM 200mg). **Metabolism:** Oxidation, trimethobenzamide N-oxide (major metabolite). **Elimination:** Urine 30-50% (unchanged); $T_{1/2}$=7-9 hrs.

## NURSING CONSIDERATIONS

**Assessment:** Assess for renal/hepatic impairment, Reye's syndrome in children, pregnancy/nursing status, alcohol intake, acute febrile illness, encephalitides, gastroenteritis, dehydration, electrolyte imbalance, appendicitis, toxicity, possible drug interactions.

**Monitoring:** Monitor renal function, for signs of hepatotoxicity, CNS reactions (eg, opisthotonos, convulsions, coma), EPS, and cerebral edema. Reduce dose in elderly and in patients with renal impairment (CrCl: ≤70ml/min/1.73m$^2$).

**Patient Counseling:** Caution against performing hazardous tasks (operating machinery/driving). Notify if pregnant/nursing.

**Administration:** Oral route and IM. **Storage:** 25°C (77°F); excursions permitted to 15-30°C (59-86°F).

## TIKOSYN RX

dofetilide (Pfizer)

**To minimize risk of arrhythmia, place patients initiated or reinitiated on therapy for minimum of 3 days in a facility that can provide CrCl, ECG monitoring, and cardiac resuscitation. Dofetilide is available only to hospitals and prescribers who have received appropriate dofetilide dosing and treatment initiation education.**

**THERAPEUTIC CLASS:** Class III antiarrhythmic

**INDICATIONS:** Conversion to and maintenance of normal sinus rhythm in atrial fibrillation/flutter.

**DOSAGE:** *Adults:* CrCl: >60mL/min: 500mcg bid. CrCl 40-60mL/min: 250mcg bid. CrCl 20 to <40mL/min: 125mcg bid. Determine QTc interval 2-3 hrs after 1st dose and adjust dose if QTc >500msec or if >15% increase from baseline. QTc/Renal Dose Adjustment: Reduce 500mcg bid to 250mcg bid. Reduce 250mcg bid to 125mcg bid. Reduce 125mcg bid to 125mcg qd. D/C any time after 2nd dose if QTc >500msec (550msec with ventricular conduction abnormalities).

**HOW SUPPLIED:** Cap: 125mcg, 250mcg, 500mcg

**CONTRAINDICATIONS:** Long QT syndromes, baseline QT interval or QTc >440msec (500msec with ventricular conduction abnormalities), severe renal impairment (CrCl <20mL/min). Concomitant verapamil, cimetidine, trimethoprim, ketoconazole, and inhibitors of renal cation transport system (eg, megesterol, prochlorperazine).

**WARNINGS/PRECAUTIONS:** Can cause serious ventricular arrhythmia. Calculate CrCl before 1st dose; adjust dose based on CrCl. Caution in severe hepatic impairment. Maintain normal $K^+$ levels.

**ADVERSE REACTIONS:** Headache, chest pain, dizziness, arrhythmia, conduction disturbances, dyspnea, naûsea, insomnia.

**INTERACTIONS:** See Contraindications. Hypokalemia or hypomagnesemia may occur with $K^+$-depleting diuretics. CYP3A4 inhibitors (eg, macrolides, protease inhibitors, grapefruit juice, etc) may potentiate dofetilide. Avoid verapamil, cimetidine, trimethoprim, ketoconazole, and inhibitors of renal cationic secretion. Caution with drugs actively secreted by cationic secretion (eg, amiloride, triamterene, metformin). Not recommended with drugs that prolong the QT interval. Hold Class I and III antiarrhythmics for at least 3 half-lives before initiating dofetilide. Reduce amiodarone to <0.3mcg/mL or withdraw at least 3 months before initiating dofetilide.

**PREGNANCY:** Category C, not for use in nursing.

**MECHANISM OF ACTION:** Class III antiarrhythmic; blocks cardiac ion channel carrying rapid component of delayed rectifier $K^+$ current, $I_{Kr}$.

**PHARMACOKINETICS: Absorption:** Bioavailability (>90%); $T_{max}$=2-3 hrs. **Distribution:** $V_d$=3L/kg; plasma protein binding (60-70%). **Metabolism:** Liver via CYP3A4 though N-dealkylation and N-oxidation pathways. **Elimination:** Urine (80% unchanged), (20% metabolites); $T_{max}$=10 hrs.

## NURSING CONSIDERATIONS

**Assessment:** Assess for congenital or acquired long QT syndrome, ventricular arrhythmia, CHF, recent MI, structural heart disease, atrial flutter/fibrillation, baseline QT interval or QTc ≥440 msec (500 msec), sick sinus syndrome, HB, implanted pacemaker, renal/hepatic impairment, pregnancy/nursing status, and possible drug interactions. Correct $K^+$ levels prior to therapy.

**Monitoring:** Patient should be in a facility for minimum of 3 days where CrCl, continuous ECG monitoring, and cardiac resuscitation are available. Monitor for ventricular arrhythmias (eg, torsade de pointes and polymorphic ventricular tachycardia associated with QT interval prolongation).

**Patient Counseling:** Inform about risks/benefits and need for compliance with prescribed dosing. Periodic monitoring of QTc and renal function required. Notify physician if pregnant/nursing or if taking concurrent administration of any OTC medication. Advise to not double next dose if dose is missed.

**Administration:** Oral route. **Storage:** 15-30°C (59-86°F). Protect from humidity and moisture.

## TIMENTIN RX

ticarcillin disodium - clavulanate potassium (GlaxoSmithKline)

**THERAPEUTIC CLASS:** Broad-spectrum penicillin/beta-lactamase inhibitor

**INDICATIONS:** Treatment of lower respiratory tract, bone and joint, skin and skin structure, urinary tract (UTI), gynecologic, and intra-abdominal infections, and septicemia caused by susceptible strains of microorganisms.

**DOSAGE:** *Adults:* ≥60kg: UTI/Systemic Infection: 3g-100mg (3.1g vial) IV q4-6h. Gynecologic Infections: Moderate: 200mg/kg/day ticarcillin IV given q6h. Severe: 300mg/kg/day ticarcillin IV given q4h. <60kg: Usual: 200-300mg/kg/day ticarcillin IV given q4-6h. Renal Impairment (based on ticarcillin): LD: 3.1g. Maint: CrCl >60mL/min: 3.1g q4h. CrCl 30-60mL/min: 2g IV q4h. CrCl 10-30mL/min: 2g IV q8h. CrCl <10mL/min: 2g IV q12h (2g IV q24h with hepatic dysfunction). Peritoneal Dialysis: 3.1g IV q12h. Hemodialysis: 2g IV q12h, and 3.1g after each dialysis.
*Pediatrics:* ≥3 months: ≥60kg: Mild to Moderate: 3g-100mg (3.1g vial) IV q6h. Severe: 3g-100mg (3.1g vial) IV q4h. <60 kg: Mild to Moderate: 50mg/kg ticarcillin IV q6h. Severe: 50mg/kg ticarcillin IV q4h. Renal Impairment (based on ticarcillin): LD: 3.1g vial. Maint: CrCl >60mL/min: 3.1g q4h. CrCl 30-60mL/min: 2g IV q4h. CrCl 10-30mL/min: 2g IV q8h. CrCl <10mL/min: 2g IV q12h (2g IV q24h with hepatic dysfunction). Peritoneal Dialysis: 3.1g IV q12h. Hemodialysis: 2g IV q12h, and 3.1g after each dialysis.

**HOW SUPPLIED:** Inj: (Ticarcillin-Clavulanate) 3g-100mg, 3g-100mg/100mL, 30g-1g

**WARNINGS/PRECAUTIONS:** Serious, sometimes fatal, hypersensitivity reactions reported with PCN therapy. *Clostridium difficile*-associated diarrhea reported. Prolonged use may result in overgrowth of nonsusceptible organisms. Risk of convulsions with high doses, especially with renal impairment. Monitor renal, hepatic, hematopoietic functions, and serum $K^+$ with prolonged therapy. Caution with fluid and electrolyte imbalance; hypokalemia reported. Clotting time, platelet aggregation, and PT abnormalities may occur especially with renal impairment; d/c therapy. Continue therapy for at least 2 days after signs/symptoms disappear. Caution in elderly patients with impaired renal function.

**ADVERSE REACTIONS:** Hypersensitivity reactions, headache, giddiness, taste/smell disturbances, stomatitis, flatulence, N/V, diarrhea, hematologic disturbances, hepatic/renal function tests abnormalities, local reactions.

**INTERACTIONS:** May inactivate aminoglycoside if mixed together in parenteral solution. Increased serum levels and prolonged half-life with probenecid. May reduce efficacy of combined oral estrogen/progesterone contraceptives.

**PREGNANCY:** Category B, caution in nursing.

**MECHANISM OF ACTION:** Ticarcillin: Broad-spectrum antibiotic with bactericidal activity against many gram-positive and gram-negative aerobic and anerobic bacteria. Clavulanic acid: β-lactam, which possesses ability to inactivate wide range of β-lactamase enzymes.

**PHARMACOKINETICS: Absorption:** Ticarcillin: $C_{max}$=330mcg/mL, AUC=485mcg•hr/mL. Clavulanic acid: $C_{max}$=8mcg/mL, AUC=8.2mcg•hr/mL. **Distribution:** Ticarcillin: Plasma protein binding (45%). Clavulanic acid: Plasma

T

protein binding (25%). **Elimination:** Ticarcillin: Urine (unchanged 60-70%); $T_{1/2}$=1.1 hrs, 4.4 hrs (neonates), 1 hr (infants/ children). Clavulanic acid: Urine (35-45% unchanged); $T_{1/2}$=1.1hrs, 1.9 hrs (neonates), 0.9 hr (infants/children).

## NURSING CONSIDERATIONS

**Assessment:** Assess for previous hypersensitivity reactions to cephalosporins, PCNs, or other allergens, renal/hepatic impairment, presence of fluid/electrolyte imbalance, pregnancy/nursing status, and possible drug interactions.

**Monitoring:** Periodically monitor renal, hepatic, hematopoietic function and serum $K^+$ levels. Monitor for signs/symptoms of anaphylactic/anaphylactoid reactions, CDAD, drug resistance or superinfection, bleeding manifestations, electrolyte abnormalities, lab test interactions (eg, false (+) Coombs' test).

**Patient Counseling:** Inform drug only treats bacterial, not viral, infections. Take as directed; skipping doses or not completing full course may decrease effectiveness and increase resistance. Inform about risks/benefits. D/C and notify physician if allergic reactions or watery/bloody diarrhea (with/without muscle cramps) occur. Notify if pregnant/nursing.

**Administration:** IV infusion (30 min). Do not use flexible container in series connections. **Storage:** 24°C (75°F). Avoid freezing or excessive heat.

# TIMOLOL MALEATE — RX

timolol maleate (Various)

**THERAPEUTIC CLASS:** Nonselective beta-blocker

**INDICATIONS:** Treatment of hypertension. To reduce cardiovascular mortality and risk of reinfarction with previous MI. Migraine prophylaxis.

**DOSAGE:** *Adults:* HTN: Initial: 10mg bid. Maint: 20-40mg/day. Wait at least 7 days between dose increases. Max: 60mg/day given bid. MI: 10mg bid. Migraine: Initial: 10mg bid. Maint: 20mg qd. Max: 30mg/day in divided doses. May decrease to 10mg qd. D/C if inadequate response after 6-8 weeks with max dose.

**HOW SUPPLIED:** Tab: 5mg, 10mg*, 20mg* *scored

**CONTRAINDICATIONS:** Active or history of bronchial asthma, severe COPD, sinus bradycardia, 2nd- and 3rd-degree AV block, overt cardiac failure, cardiogenic shock.

**WARNINGS/PRECAUTIONS:** Caution with well-compensated cardiac failure, DM, mild to moderate COPD, bronchospastic disease, dialysis, hepatic/renal impairment, or cerebrovascular insufficiency. Exacerbation of ischemic heart disease with abrupt cessation. May mask hyperthyroidism or hypoglycemia symptoms. Withdrawal before surgery is controversial. May potentiate weakness with myasthenia gravis. Can cause cardiac failure. Caution and consider monitoring renal function in elderly.

**ADVERSE REACTIONS:** Fatigue, headache, nausea, arrhythmia, pruritus, dizziness, dyspnea, asthenia, bradycardia.

T

**INTERACTIONS:** Possible additive effects and hypotension and/or marked bradycardia with catecholamine-depleting drugs. NSAIDs may reduce antihypertensive effects. Quinidine may potentiate β-blockade. AV conduction time prolonged with digitalis and either diltiazem or verapamil. Hypotension, AV conduction disturbances, left ventricular failure reported with oral calcium antagonists. Caution with IV calcium antagonists, insulin, oral hypoglycemics. Avoid calcium antagonists with cardiac dysfunction. May exacerbate rebound HTN following clonidine withdrawal. May block effects of epinephrine.

**PREGNANCY:** Category C, not for use in nursing.

**MECHANISM OF ACTION:** $\beta_1$ and $\beta_2$ adrenergic receptor blocking agent; reduces cardiac output and plasma renin activity.

**PHARMACOKINETICS: Absorption:** (PO) Completely absorbed (90%); $T_{max}$=2 hrs. **Metabolism:** Partially, by liver. **Excretion:** Kidneys; $T_{1/2}$= 4 hrs.

## NURSING CONSIDERATIONS

**Assessment:** Assess for bradycardia, cardiogenic shock, 2nd- and 3rd-degree heart block, overt cardiac failure, impaired hepatic/renal function, bronchospastic disease, PVD, DM, thyrotoxicosis, valvular heart disease, and possible drug interactions.

**Monitoring:** Monitor for cardiac failure, HTN, renal function, exacerbation of ischemia following abrupt withdrawal, bronchospastic disease, anaphylactoid reactions, hypersensitivity reactions.

**Patient Counseling:** Counsel if signs suggest reduced cerebral blood flow; may need to d/c therapy. Instruct not to interrupt or d/c therapy without consulting physician. Counsel about signs/symptoms of CHF; notify physician if signs/symptoms of impending CHF or unexplained respiratory symptoms occur.

**Administration:** Oral route. **Storage:** 20-25°C (68-77°F); tight, light-resistant container.

# TIMOPTIC — RX

timolol maleate (Aton)

**OTHER BRAND NAMES:** Timoptic in Ocudose (Aton) - Timoptic-XE (Aton)

**THERAPEUTIC CLASS:** Nonselective beta-blocker

**INDICATIONS:** Treatment of elevated IOP in patients with ocular hypertension or open-angle glaucoma.

**DOSAGE:** *Adults:* (Sol) Initial: 1 drop 0.25% bid. May increase to a max of 1 drop 0.5% bid. Maint: If adequate control, may attempt 1 drop 0.25-0.5% qd. (Sol, Gel Forming) Initial: 1 drop 0.25-0.5% qd. Max: 1 drop 0.5% qd. Dose other ophthalmic drugs 10 min prior to gel-forming drops.

**HOW SUPPLIED:** Sol: (Timoptic) 0.25% [5mL], 0.5% [5mL, 10mL]; Sol: (Timoptic Ocudose) 0.25%, 0.5% [0.2mL 60$^s$]; Sol, Gel Forming: (Timoptic-XE) 0.25%, 0.5% [5mL]

**CONTRAINDICATIONS:** Bronchial asthma, history of bronchial asthma, severe COPD, sinus bradycardia, 2nd- or 3rd-degree AV block, overt cardiac failure, cardiogenic shock.

**WARNINGS/PRECAUTIONS:** Severe cardiac and respiratory reactions reported, including death due to bronchospasm in patients with asthma and rarely death associated with cardiac failure reported. Caution with cardiac failure; d/c if cardiac failure develops. May mask symptoms of hypoglycemia or hyperthyroidism; caution with diabetes mellitus (DM) or thyrotoxicosis. Avoid with COPD, bronchospastic disease. Not for use alone in angle-closure glaucoma. May potentiate muscle weakness. Withdrawal before surgery is controversial.

**ADVERSE REACTIONS:** Ocular: burning, stinging, blurred vision, pain, conjunctivitis, discharge, foreign body sensation, itching, tearing. Systemic: headache, dizziness, upper respiratory infections.

**INTERACTIONS:** May potentiate additive effects with systemic/ophthalmic β-blockers and catecholamine-depleting drugs (eg, reserpine). Oral/IV calcium antagonists may cause AV conduction disturbances, left ventricular failure, or hypotension. Digitalis may cause additive effects in prolonging AV conduction time. Potentiated systemic β-blockade reported with concomitant CYP2D6 inhibitors (eg, quinidine, SSRIs). May antagonize epinephrine. May exacerbate rebound hypertension following clonidine withdrawal. Give other ophthalmic drugs 10 min before use.

**PREGNANCY:** Category C, not for use in nursing.

**MECHANISM OF ACTION:** Nonselective β-blocker; reduces elevated and normal IOP.

**PHARMACOKINETICS: Absorption:** $C_{max}$=0.46ng/mL (morning dosing), 0.35ng/mL (afternoon dosing). **Distribution:** Found in breast milk.

## NURSING CONSIDERATIONS

**Assessment:** Assess for history of asthma or COPD, sinus bradycardia, heart block, cardiac failure, DM, pregnancy/nursing status, undergoing major surgery, hyperthyroidism or thyrotoxicosis, cerebrovascular insufficiency, angle-closure glaucoma, myasthenia gravis or myasthenic syndrome, and possible drug interactions.

**Monitoring:** Monitor BP, HR, IOP, for signs/symptoms of anaphylaxis, increasing muscle weakness in susceptible patients, bronchospasm with severe respiratory and cardiac reactions, thyroid storm, masked symptoms of acute hypoglycemia, psychiatric disturbances, and bacterial keratitis.

**Patient Counseling:** Instruct to avoid touching tip of container to eye or surrounding structures. Counsel to seek physician's advice on continued use of product if patient had ocular surgery or develops intercurrent ocular condition (eg, trauma or infection). Remove contact lenses prior to administration and reinsert 15 min following administration.

**Administration:** Ocular route. **Storage:** 15-30°C (59-86°F); avoid freezing/light. Keep out of reach of children.

# TNKase RX

tenecteplase (Genentech)

**THERAPEUTIC CLASS:** Thrombolytic agent

**INDICATIONS:** To reduce mortality with acute myocardial infarction (AMI).

**DOSAGE:** *Adults:* Administer as single IV bolus over 5 seconds. <60kg: 30mg. ≥60 to <70kg: 35mg. ≥70 to <80kg: 40mg. ≥80 to <90kg: 45mg. ≥90kg: 50mg. Max: 50mg/dose.

**HOW SUPPLIED:** Inj: 50mg

**CONTRAINDICATIONS:** Active internal bleeding, history of cerebrovascular accident (CVA), intracranial or intraspinal surgery or trauma within 2 months, intracranial neoplasm, arteriovenous malformation, aneurysm, bleeding diathesis, severe uncontrolled HTN .

**WARNINGS/PRECAUTIONS:** Weigh benefits/risks with recent major surgery, cerebrovascular disease, recent GI or genitourinary (GU) bleeding, recent trauma, HTN (systolic BP ≥180mmHg and/or diastolic BP ≥110mmHg, left heart thrombus, acute pericarditis, subacute bacterial endocarditis, hemostatic defects, severe hepatic dysfunction, pregnancy, diabetic hemorrhagic retinopathy or other hemorrhagic ophthalmic conditions, septic thrombophlebitis or occluded AV cannula at a seriously infected site, elderly, any other bleeding condition that is difficult to manage. Cholesterol embolism and internal/superficial bleeding reported. Arrhythmias may occur with reperfusion. Avoid IM injection, noncompressible arterial puncture, and internal jugular or subclavian venous puncture. Caution with readministration.

**ADVERSE REACTIONS:** Bleeding.

T

**INTERACTIONS:** Increased risk of bleeding with heparin, vitamin K antagonists, and drugs that alter platelet function (eg, ASA, dipyridamole, GP IIb/IIIa inhibitors) before or after therapy. Weigh benefits/risks with oral anticoagulants, GP IIb/IIIa inhibitors.

**PREGNANCY:** Category C, caution in nursing.

**MECHANISM OF ACTION:** Thrombolytic agent; modified form of human tissue plasminogen activator (tPA) that binds to fibrin and converts plasminogen to plasmin.

**PHARMACOKINETICS: Metabolism:** Liver. **Elimination:** $T_{1/2}$=90-130 min.

## NURSING CONSIDERATIONS

**Assessment:** Assess for active internal bleeding, history of CVA, intracranial or intraspinal surgery or trauma within previous 2 months, intracranial neoplasm, arteriovenous malformation, aneurysm, known bleeding diathesis, acute pericarditis, subacute bacterial endocarditis, hemorrhagic ophthalmic conditions (eg, diabetic hemorrhagic retinopathy), severe uncontrolled

HTN, hepatic function, pregnancy/nursing status, advanced age, and drug interactions.

**Monitoring:** Monitor for signs/symptoms of bleeding (internal or superficial), cholesterol embolization (eg, livedo reticularis, "purple toe" syndrome, acute renal failure), arrhythmia, and hypersensitivity reactions (eg, anaphylaxis).

**Patient Counseling:** Counsel about increased risk of bleeding while on therapy. Contact physician if any type of unusual bleeding or hypersensitivity reactions develop. Inform that arterial and venous punctures should be minimized while on therapy. Instruct that if any serious bleeding occurs, concomitant heparin or antiplatelet agents should be discontinued immediately.

**Administration:** IV route. Reconstitute just prior to use. 1) Inject 10mL of SWFI into vial. 2) Do not shake; gently swirl until contents completely dissolved. 3) May be administered as reconstituted solution (5mg/mL). **Storage:** Lyophilized vial: Store at controlled room temperature not exceeding 30°C (86°F), or under refrigeration 2-8°C (36-46°F). Reconstituted: 2-8°C (36-46°F); use within 8 hrs.

# TobraDex RX

tobramycin - dexamethasone (Alcon)

**THERAPEUTIC CLASS:** Aminoglycoside/corticosteroid

**INDICATIONS:** Ocular inflammation associated with infection or risk of infection.

**DOSAGE:** *Adults:* (Sus) 1-2 drops q4-6h. May increase to 1-2 drops q2h for first 24-48 hrs. (Oint) Apply 1/2 inch in conjunctival sac up to tid-qid. Max: 20mL or 8g for initial RX.

*Pediatrics:* ≥2 yrs: (Sus) 1-2 drops q4-6h. May increase to 1-2 drops q2h for first 24-48 hrs. (Oint) Apply 1/2 inch in conjunctival sac up to tid-qid. Max: 20mL or 8g for initial RX.

**HOW SUPPLIED:** Oint: (Tobramycin-Dexamethasone) 0.3-0.1% [3.5g]; Sus: 0.3-0.1% [2.5mL, 5mL, 10mL]

**CONTRAINDICATIONS:** Viral diseases of the cornea and conjunctiva including epithelial herpes simplex keratitis, vaccinia, and varicella. Mycobacterial infection and fungal diseases of the eye.

**WARNINGS/PRECAUTIONS:** Not for injection into the eye. Prolonged use may result in glaucoma, optic nerve damage, visual acuity and fields of vision defects, cataracts, secondary ocular infections (eg, fungal infections).

**ADVERSE REACTIONS:** Conjunctival erythema, hypersensitivity, lid itching and swelling, secondary infection.

**PREGNANCY:** Category C, caution in nursing.

**MECHANISM OF ACTION:** Tobramycin: Aminoglycoside antibiotic; inhibits synthesis of proteins in bacterial cells. Dexamethasone: Corticoid; suppresses inflammatory response and probably delays or slows healing.

## NURSING CONSIDERATIONS

**Assessment:** Assess for dendritic keratitis, vaccinia, varicella, other viral diseases of cornea or conjunctiva, mycobacterial infection, fungal diseases of eye, and possible drug interactions.

**Monitoring:** Routinely monitor IOP. Monitor for signs/symptoms of hypersensitivity reactions, glaucoma, defects in visual acuity and fields of vision, posterior subcapsular cataracts, perforations, and superinfections.

**Patient Counseling:** Instruct not to touch dropper or tube tip to any surface to avoid contaminating contents and not to wear contact lenses during therapy. Advise to seek medical attention if symptoms of glaucoma, defects in vision, perforations, or superinfections occur.

**Administration:** Ocular route. Shake well before use. **Storage:** 8-27°C (46-80°F). Store upright.

## TOBREX RX
tobramycin (Alcon)

**THERAPEUTIC CLASS:** Aminoglycoside

**INDICATIONS:** External infections of the eye and its adnexa.

**DOSAGE:** *Adults:* Mild to Moderate Infection: Apply half-inch oint bid-tid or 1-2 drops q4h. Severe Infection: Apply half-inch oint q3-4h or 2 drops hourly until improvement, reduce frequency prior to discontinuation.

**HOW SUPPLIED:** Oint: 0.3% [3.5g]; Sol: 0.3% [5mL]

**WARNINGS/PRECAUTIONS:** Oint may retard corneal wound healing.

**ADVERSE REACTIONS:** Hypersensitivity, lid itching, swelling, conjunctival erythema, superinfection.

**INTERACTIONS:** Cross-sensitivity to other aminoglycoside antibiotics may occur.

**PREGNANCY:** Category B, not for use in nursing.

**MECHANISM OF ACTION:** Aminoglycoside antibiotic; inhibits synthesis of proteins in bacterial cells.

### NURSING CONSIDERATIONS

**Assessment:** Assess for proper diagnosis of causative organisms. Assess use in pregnancy/nursing.

**Monitoring:** Monitor for sensitivity reactions while on therapy. With prolonged therapy, monitor for overgrowth of nonsusceptible organisms (eg, fungi) and for development of superinfection. Monitor total serum drug concentrations with concomitant systemic aminoglycoside antibiotics.

**Patient Counseling:** Advise not to wear contact lenses if signs/symptoms of ocular infections develop. Instruct to notify physician if any sensitivity reactions occur. To avoid contamination, avoid touching tube or dropper tip to any surface.

**Administration:** Ocular route. Do not inject into eye. **Storage:** 8-27°C (46-80°F).

## TOFRANIL RX
imipramine HCl (Mallinckrodt)

**Antidepressants increased the risk of suicidal thinking and behavior (suicidality) in short-term studies in children, adolescents, and young adults with major depressive disorder (MDD) and other psychiatric disorders. Imipramine HCl is not approved for use in pediatric patients except for patients with nocturnal enuresis.**

**THERAPEUTIC CLASS:** Tricyclic antidepressant

T

**INDICATIONS:** Treatment of depression. Temporary adjunct in childhood enuresis in ≥6 yrs.

**DOSAGE:** *Adults:* Depression: Initial: (Inpatient) 100mg/day in divided doses. Titrate: Increase to 200mg/day; up to 250-300mg/day after 2 weeks if needed. (Outpatient) 75mg/day. Titrate: Increase to 150mg/day. Maint: 50-150mg/day. Max: 200mg/day. Elderly/Adolescents: Initial: 30-40mg/day. Max: 100mg/day.
*Pediatrics:* Depression: Adolescents: Initial: 30-40mg/day. Max: 100mg/day. Enuresis: ≥6 yrs: Initial: 25mg/day 1 hour before bedtime. Titrate: 6-12 yrs: If inadequate response in 1 week, increase to 50mg before bedtime. ≥12 yrs: Increase to 75mg before bedtime after 1 week if needed. Max: 2.5mg/kg/day.

**HOW SUPPLIED:** Tab: 10mg, 25mg, 50mg

**CONTRAINDICATIONS:** Within 14 days of MAOI therapy, or during acute recovery period following MI.

**WARNINGS/PRECAUTIONS:** Caution with elderly, serious depression, CV disease, hyperthyroidism, urinary retention, narrow-angle glaucoma, increased

IOP, seizure disorders, renal and hepatic impairment. May activate psychosis in schizophrenia; reduce dose. Limit electroshock therapy. May alter blood glucose levels. Photosensitivity reported. D/C prior to elective surgery, or with hypomanic or manic episodes. D/C with pathological neutrophil depression.

**ADVERSE REACTIONS:** Orthostatic hypotension, HTN, confusion, hallucinations, numbness, tremors, dry mouth, urticaria, N/V, diarrhea, gynecomastia (male), breast enlargement (female), galactorrhea.

**INTERACTIONS:** See Contraindications. Increased levels with methylphenidate, CYP2D6 inhibitors (eg, quinidine, cimetidine, SSRIs) and enzyme substrates (eg, phenothiazines, other antidepressants, propafenone, flecainide). Wait 5 weeks after d/c SSRIs before initiating TCAs. Decreased levels with enzyme inducers (eg, barbiturates, phenytoin). May block effects of clonidine, guanethidine. Additive effects with anticholinergics, CNS depressants, alcohol. Caution with drugs that lower BP and thyroid drugs. Paralytic ileus with anticholinergics. Avoid preparations that contain a sympathomimetic amine (eg, epinephrine, norepinephrine); may potentiate catecholamine effect.

**PREGNANCY:** Safety in pregnancy not known; not for use in nursing.

**MECHANISM OF ACTION:** Tricyclic antidepressant; mechanism unknown. Suspected to potentiate adrenergic synapses by blocking uptake of norepinephrine at nerve endings.

## NURSING CONSIDERATIONS

**Assessment:** Assess renal/hepatic function, LFTs, ECG, IOP, major depressive disorder, and for seizures. Note other diseases/conditions and drug therapies.

**Monitoring:** Monitor for clinical worsening, suicidality, or unusual changes in behavior, seizures, increased restlessness, agitation, anxiety, insomnia, neuropsychiatric signs/symptoms (eg, delusions, hallucinations, psychosis, concentration disturbances, paranoia, confusion), ECG, CBC with differential and platelets, blood sugar levels.

**Patient Counseling:** Advise families and caregivers of need for close observation of clinical worsening and suicidal risks. Avoid alcohol, sedatives, OTC agents. Caution against operating machinery/driving. Report adverse reactions. Consult physician before taking any other medications. Avoid excessive exposure to sunlight.

**Administration:** Oral route. **Storage:** 20-25°C (68-77°F).

# TOFRANIL-PM — RX

imipramine pamoate (Mallinckrodt)

**Antidepressants increased the risk of suicidal thinking and behavior (suicidality) in short-term studies in children, adolescents, and young adults with major depressive disorder (MDD) and other psychiatric disorders. Imipramine pamoate is not approved for use in pediatric patients.**

**THERAPEUTIC CLASS:** Tricyclic antidepressant

**INDICATIONS:** Treatment of depression.

**DOSAGE:** *Adults:* (Inpatient) Initial: 100-150mg/day. Titrate: May increase to 200mg/day. If there is no response after 2 weeks may increase up to 250-300mg/day. (Outpatient) Initial: 75mg/day. Titrate: May increase to 150mg/day. If necessary dosage may be increased to 200mg/day. (Inpatient/Outpatient) Maint: Following remission, maintain at lowest possible dose. Usual: 75-150mg/day. Elderly/Adolescents: Initiate with Tofranil 25-50mg/day. Switch to Tofranil-PM with doses ≥75mg. Max: 100mg/day.
*Pediatrics:* Adolescents: Initiate with Tofranil 25-50mg/day. Switch to Tofranil-PM with doses ≥75mg. Max: 100mg/day.

**HOW SUPPLIED:** Cap: 75mg, 100mg, 125mg, 150mg

**CONTRAINDICATIONS:** Within 14 days of MAOI therapy or during acute recovery period following MI.

**WARNINGS/PRECAUTIONS:** Caution with elderly, serious depression, CV disease, hyperthyroidism, urinary retention, narrow-angle glaucoma, increased IOP, seizure disorders, renal and hepatic impairment. May activate psychosis in schizophrenia; reduce dose. Limit electroshock therapy. May alter blood glucose levels. Photosensitivity reported. D/C prior to elective surgery, or with hypomanic or manic episodes. D/C with pathological neutrophil depression.

**ADVERSE REACTIONS:** Orthostatic hypotension, HTN, confusion, hallucinations, numbness, tremors, dry mouth, urticaria, N/V, diarrhea, gynecomastia (male), breast enlargement (female), galactorrhea.

**INTERACTIONS:** See Contraindications. Increased levels with methylphenidate, CYP2D6 inhibitors (eg, quinidine, cimetidine, SSRIs) and enzyme substrates (eg, phenothiazines, other antidepressants, propafenone, flecainide). Wait 5 weeks after d/c SSRIs before initiating TCAs. Decreased levels with enzyme inducers (eg, barbiturates, phenytoin). Blocks effects of clonidine, guanethidine. Additive effects with anticholinergics, CNS depressants, alcohol. Caution with drugs that lower BP and thyroid drugs. Paralytic ileus with anticholinergics. Avoid preparations that contain a sympathomimetic amine (eg, epinephrine, norepinephrine); may potentiate catecholamine effect.

**PREGNANCY:** Safety in pregnancy not known; not for use in nursing.

**MECHANISM OF ACTION:** Tricyclic antidepressant; mechanism unknown. Suspected to potentiate adrenergic synapses by blocking uptake of norepinephrine at nerve endings.

## NURSING CONSIDERATIONS

**Assessment:** Assess for family psychiatric history (suicide, depressive disorder). Assess renal function test, LFTs, ECG, IOP, seizures. Note other diseases/conditions and drug therapies.

**Monitoring:** Monitor for clinical worsening, suicidality, unusual changes in behavior, seizures, increased restlessness, agitation, anxiety, insomnia, neuropsychiatric signs/symptoms (eg, delusions, hallucinations, psychosis, concentration disturbance, paranoia, confusion), ECG, CBC with differential and platelets, blood sugar levels.

**Patient Counseling:** Advise families and caregivers of need for close observation of clinical worsening and suicidal risks. Advise to report new or sudden changes in mood, behavior, thoughts or feelings. Avoid alcohol, sedatives, OTC agents. Caution against operating machinery/driving. Report adverse reactions. Consult physician before taking any other medications. Avoid excessive exposure to sunlight.

**Administration:** Oral route. **Storage**: 20-25°C (68-77°F). Dispense in a tight container with child-resistant closure.

# TOLMETIN RX

tolmetin sodium (Various)

**NSAIDs may cause an increased risk of serious cardiovascular thrombotic events, MI, stroke and serious GI adverse events including bleeding, ulceration and perforation of the stomach or intestines. Contraindicated for the treatment of perioperative pain in the setting of coronary artery bypass graft (CABG) surgery.**

T

**THERAPEUTIC CLASS:** NSAID

**INDICATIONS:** Treatment of acute flares and the long-term management of rheumatoid arthritis (RA) and osteoarthritis (OA). Treatment of juvenile rheumatoid arthritis (JRA) in patients ≥2 yrs of age.

**DOSAGE:** *Adults:* OA/RA: Initial: 400mg tid. Usual: 200-600mg tid. Max: 1800mg/day. Take with antacids other than sodium bicarbonate if GI upset occurs.
*Pediatrics:* JRA: ≥2 yrs: Initial: 20mg/kg/day given tid-qid. Usual: 15-30mg/kg/day. Max: 30mg/kg/day. Take with antacids other than sodium bicarbonate if GI upset occurs.

**HOW SUPPLIED:** Cap: (DS) 400mg; Tab: 200mg*, 600mg *scored

**CONTRAINDICATIONS:** ASA or other NSAID allergy that precipitates asthma, rhinitis, urticaria, or allergic-type reactions. Treatment of perioperative pain in the setting of (CABG) surgery.

**WARNINGS/PRECAUTIONS:** May cause new onset HTN or worsening of pre existing HTN; may contribute to increased incidence of cardiovascular events. Fluid edema and retention reported; caution in patients with fluid retention or heart failure. May cause serious GI events (eg, inflammation, bleeding, ulcer, perforation); caution with a prior history of ulcer or GI bleeding, long duration of therapy, smoking, alcohol, old age and poor general health status. Long term use resulted in renal papillary necrosis and other renal injury. Acute interstitial nephritis with hematuria and proteinuria, nephritic syndrome and renal toxicity reported. Caution with impaired renal/liver function, heart failure and elderly; d/c if needed. Avoid with advanced renal disease and in patients with aspirin (ASA) triad. May develop ASA-sensitive asthma; caution with pre-existing asthma. Anaphylactoid reactions may occur. May cause serious skin adverse events such as exfoliative dermatitis, Stevens-Johnson syndrome (SJS), toxic epidermal necrolysis (TEN); inform about signs and symptoms and d/c at first appearance of rash or any other hypersensitivity reactions. Adverse eye findings reported; perform ophthalmic evaluation if with visual disturbances. Elevation of liver enzymes (eg, ALT, AST) may occur. Hepatic reactions (eg, jaundice, fatal fulminant hepatitis, liver necrosis, hepatic failure) reported; d/c if liver disease or systemic manifestations occur. Anemia reported; monitor Hgb, Hct and for signs and symptoms of anemia. May inhibit platelet aggregation and prolong bleeding time (BT); caution if with coagulation disorders. May diminish utility of diagnostic signs in detecting complications of presumed non-infectious, painful conditions. May cause premature closure of ductus arteriosus late in pregnancy. Not for substitute for corticosteroid nor for treatment of corticosteroid insufficiency.

**ADVERSE REACTIONS:** N/V, dyspepsia, abdominal pain, GI distress, diarrhea, flatulence, headache, asthenia, elevated blood pressure, dizziness, edema, weight gain/loss.

**INTERACTIONS:** Increased PT and bleeding with warfarin. May enhance methotrexate toxicity. May diminish the antihypertensive effect of ACE inhibitors. Concomitant administration with ASA not recommended; potential for increased adverse effects. Can reduce the natriuretic effect of furosemide and thiazides. Can produce elevation of plasma lithium levels and reduction in renal lithium clearance. Increase risk of GI bleeding with alcohol, oral corticosteroids or anticoagulants.

**PREGNANCY:** Category C, not for use in nursing.

**MECHANISM OF ACTION:** NSAID; not established. Suspected to inhibit prostaglandin synthetase, lowers plasma level of PGE.

**PHARMACOKINETICS: Absorption:** Rapid; $C_{max}$=40mcg/mL (400 mg); $T_{max}$=30-60 min. **Elimination:** Urine; $T_{1/2}$=5 hrs.

## NURSING CONSIDERATIONS

**Assessment:** Assess for NSAID or ASA allergy (ASA triad), asthma, HTN, risk factors for CV disease, history of ulcer disease or GI bleeding, coagulation disorder, fluid retention, CHF, pregnancy/nursing status, renal/hepatic impairment and possible drug interactions. Obtain baseline BP, hgb and hct.

**Monitoring:** Monitor BP, CBC, hepatic and renal function periodically. Monitor for signs/symptoms of CV events (eg, thrombosis, MI, stroke), HTN, fluid retention, edema, GI events (eg, ulceration, perforation, bleeding), serious skin reactions, anemia, hypersensitivity reactions and renal/hepatic dysfunction. Perform ophthalmic evaluation if visual disturbances develop.

**Patient Counseling:** Discuss risks and benefits of therapy. Instruct to seek medical attention if experience symptoms of CV events (eg, chest pain, SOB, weakness, slurred speech), ulceration or bleeding (eg, epigastric pain, dyspepsia, melena, hematemesis), skin reactions (eg, rash, blisters, fever, itching), anaphylactoid reactions (eg, swelling, difficulty breathing), hepatotoxicity (eg, nausea, fatigue, pruritus, RUQ pain), weight gain or edema. Inform of pregnancy risks.

**Administration:** Oral route. **Storage**: 20-25°C (68-77°F). Dispense in tight, light, resistant container.

# TOPAMAX RX

topiramate (Ortho-McNeil)

**OTHER BRAND NAMES:** Topamax Sprinkle Capsules (Ortho-McNeil)

**THERAPEUTIC CLASS:** Sulfamate-substituted monosaccharide antiepileptic

**INDICATIONS:** Monotherapy in patients ≥10 yrs with partial onset or primary generalized tonic-clonic seizures. Adjunct therapy in patients 2-16 yrs with partial onset seizures, or primary generalized tonic-clonic seizures, and in patients ≥2 yrs with seizures associated with Lennox-Gastaut syndrome. Migraine prophylaxis in adults.

**DOSAGE:** *Adults:* Epilepsy: Monotherapy: Initial: Week 1: 25mg bid. Titrate: Week 2: 50mg bid. Week 3: 75mg bid. Week 4: 100mg bid. Week 5: 150mg bid. Week 6: 200mg bid. Adjunct Therapy: Initial: 25-50mg/day. Titrate: Increase by 25-50mg/week. Usual: Partial: 100-200mg bid. Tonic-Clonic: 200mg bid. Max: 1600mg/day. Migraine Prophylaxis: Initial: Week 1: 25mg qpm. Titrate: Week 2: 25mg bid. Week 3: 25mg qam and 50mg qpm. Week 4: 50mg bid. Usual: 50mg bid. Renal Dysfunction: 50% of usual dose. Swallow caps whole or sprinkle over food.

*Pediatrics:* Seizures: Monotherapy: ≥10 yrs: Initial: Week 1: 25mg bid. Titrate: Week 2: 50mg bid. Week 3: 75mg bid. Week 4: 100mg bid. Week 5: 150mg bid. Week 6: 200mg bid. Adjunct Therapy: ≥17 yrs: Initial: 25-50mg/day. Titrate: Increase by 25-50mg/week. Usual: Partial: 100-200mg bid. Tonic-Clonic: 200mg bid. Max: 1600mg/day. 2-16 yrs: Initial: 1-3mg/kg nightly for 1 week. Titrate: Increase every 1-2 weeks by 1-3mg/kg/day increments. Usual: 5-9mg/kg/day. Swallow caps whole or sprinkle over food.

**HOW SUPPLIED:** Cap, Sprinkle: 15mg, 25mg; Tab: 25mg, 50mg, 100mg, 200mg

**WARNINGS/PRECAUTIONS:** A syndrome consisting of acute myopia associated with secondary angle-closure glaucoma has been reported. Oligohidrosis leading to hyperthermia and infrequently resulting in hospitalization has been reported; majority in pediatric patients. May increase the risk of suicidal thoughts or behavior; monitor for the emergence or worsening of depression, suicidal thoughts or behavior, and/or any unusual changes in mood or behavior. Hyperchloremic, nonanion gap, metabolic acidosis reported; obtain baseline and periodic serum bicarbonate levels. Cognitive-related dysfunction (eg, difficulty with memory, speech and language problems), dose-related psychiatric/behavioral disturbance, somnolence, fatigue were all reported. Avoid abrupt d/c. Sudden unexplained death in epilepsy (SUDEP) reported. Risk of kidney stones; maintain adequate fluid intake. Caution with renal or hepatic dysfunction.

**ADVERSE REACTIONS:** Abnormal vision, anorexia, ataxia, anxiety, depression, diplopia, dizziness, fatigue, weight decrease, memory difficulty, mood problems, paresthesia, psychomotor slowing, somnolence, speech disorders.

**INTERACTIONS:** Decreased levels with phenytoin, carbamazepine, valproic acid, lamotrigine. Increased levels with HCTZ. Increases levels of amitriptyline, lithium, metformin. Decreases levels of valproic acid, oral contraceptives, pioglitazone, risperidone, digoxin. Potential to cause CNS depression and cognitive/neuropsychiatric adverse events with alcohol and other CNS depressants. Caution when used with drugs that predispose patient to heart-related disorder (eg, carbonic anhydrase inhibitors, drugs with anticholinergic effect). May cause hyperammonemia with/without encephalopathy when used with valproic acid. Increased risk of renal-stone formation and worsening of metabolic acidosis when used with other carbonic anhydrase inhibitors.

**PREGNANCY:** Category C, caution in nursing.

**MECHANISM OF ACTION:** Sulfamate-substituted monosaccharide antiepileptic; unknown mechanism. Suspected to block voltage-dependent Na+ channels, augment activity of the neurotransmitter gamma-aminobutyrate at some subtypes of the GABA-A receptor; antagonizes the AMPA/kainate subtype of the glutamate receptor; and inhibits the carbonic anhydrase enzyme, particularly isoenzymes II and IV.

**PHARMACOKINETICS: Absorption:** Rapid; $T_{max}$=2 hrs. **Distribution:** Plasma protein binding (15-41%). **Metabolism:** Metabolized via hydroxylation, hydrolysis, and glucuronidation. **Elimination:** Urine: (70% unchanged); $T_{1/2}$=21 hrs. For pediatric parameters refer to PI.

## NURSING CONSIDERATIONS

**Assessment:** Assess for renal/hepatic impairment, glaucoma, diarrhea, depression/mood disorders, osteoporosis, lung problems, pregnancy/nursing status, high-fat diet, growth problems, inborn error of metabolism, reduced hepatic mitochondrial activity and possible drug interactions. Obtain baseline serum bicarbonate.

**Monitoring:** Monitor for signs/symptoms of acute myopia, secondary angle glaucoma (decreased visual acuity, ocular pain), oligohidrosis, hyperthermia (eg, decreased sweating, increased body temperature), cognitive or neuropsychiatric impairment (eg, psychomotor slowing, speech difficulty, somnolence), kidney stones, renal dysfunction, metabolic acidosis, parasthesias, emergence of suicidal behavior and ideation, depression. Monitor LFTs and serum bicarbonate.

**Patient Counseling:** Inform can take with/without food. Instruct caregivers of pediatric/adolescent patients that medication may cause decreased sweating and increased body temperature. Advise to take proper precautions and maintain adequate hydration to prevent development of kidney stones. Avoid alcohol use, abrupt d/c, and operating machinery/driving when initiating therapy. Instruct to seek immediate medical attention if blurred vision, visual disturbances, or periorbital pain occur. Instruct to increase food intake if weight loss occurs. Inform females medication may decrease efficacy of oral contraceptives. Notify physician if suicidal thoughts and behavior emerge. Instruct to enroll in the NAAED Pregnancy Registry if patient becomes pregnant during therapy. Visit aedpregnancyregistry.com for more information or call 1-888-233-2334.

**Administration:** Oral route. Sprinkle caps may be swallowed whole or administered by carefully opening cap and sprinkling entire contents on small amount (teaspoonful) of food. The drug/food mixture should be swallowed, not chewed. **Storage:** Tab: 15-30°C (59-86°F). Protect form moisture. Cap, Sprinkle: Below 25°C (77°F). Protect from moisture.

# TOPICORT — RX

desoximetasone (Taro)

**OTHER BRAND NAMES:** Topicort LP (Taro)

**THERAPEUTIC CLASS:** Corticosteroid

**INDICATIONS:** Relief of the inflammatory and pruritic manifestations of corticosteroid-responsive dermatoses.

**DOSAGE:** *Adults:* Apply bid to affected area.
*Pediatrics:* (Cre, Gel) Apply bid to affected area. ≥10 yrs: (Oint) Apply bid to affected area.

**HOW SUPPLIED:** Cre: (LP) 0.05% [15g, 60g, 100g], 0.25% [15g, 60g, 100g]; Gel: 0.05% [15g, 60g]; Oint: 0.25% [15g, 60g, 100g]

**WARNINGS/PRECAUTIONS:** May produce reversible hypothalamic-pituitary-adrenal (HPA) axis suppression, manifestations of Cushing's syndrome, hyperglycemia, and glucosuria. If HPA axis suppression noted, d/c or reduce frequency of application or substitute a less potent steroid. Steroid withdrawal may occur upon d/c. Caution when applied to large surface areas or under occlusive dressings. Use appropriate antifungal or antibacterial agent with dermatological infections; d/c if infection does not clear or if irritation occurs. Avoid contact with eyes. Pediatric patients may be more susceptible to systemic toxicity; chronic therapy may interfere with growth and development.

**ADVERSE REACTIONS:** Burning, itching, irritation, dryness, folliculitis, hypertrichosis, acneiform eruptions, hypopigmentation, perioral dermatitis, allergic contact dermatitis, skin maceration, secondary infection, skin atrophy, striae, miliaria.

**PREGNANCY:** Category C, caution in nursing.

**MECHANISM OF ACTION:** Corticosteroid; possesses anti-inflammatory, anti-pruritic, and vasoconstrictive properties. Anti-inflammatory activity not established.

**PHARMACOKINETICS: Absorption:** Percutaneous; occlusion, inflammation, and other disease states may increase absorption. **Metabolism:** Liver. **Excretion:** Urine (major), bile. Cre 0.25% (men): Urine (4.1%), Feces (1.1%); $T_{1/2}$=15-17 hrs.

## NURSING CONSIDERATIONS

**Assessment:** Assess for hypersensitivity, dermatological infection, and pregnancy/nursing status.

**Monitoring:** Monitor for signs/symptoms of reversible HPA-axis suppression, Cushing's syndrome, hyperglycemia, glucosuria, skin irritation, and for dermatological infections (eg, bacterial, fungal). In patients on large doses or using occlusive dressings, monitor for HPA-axis suppression by using urinary free cortisol and ACTH stimulation tests. Following d/c, monitor for signs of steroid withdrawal. In pediatrics, monitor for signs/symptoms of systemic toxicity, HPA-axis suppression (eg, linear growth retardation, delayed weight gain), Cushing's syndrome, and intracranial HTN.

**Patient Counseling:** Instruct to use externally and exactly as directed; avoid contact with eyes. Report local adverse reactions, especially under occlusive dressings. Do not bandage, cover, or wrap treated skin unless directed by physician. Advise caregivers of pediatric patients not to use tight-fitting diapers or plastic pants on treatment area.

**Administration:** Topical. **Storage:** Cre, Gel: 20-25°C (68-77°F). Oint: 15-30°C (59-86°F).

# TOPROL-XL RX

metoprolol succinate (AstraZeneca)

**Following abrupt cessation of therapy, exacerbation of angina pectoris and, in some cases, MI have occurred. When d/c chronically administered metoprolol, particularly in patients with ischemic heart disease, dosage should be gradually reduced over a period of 1-2 weeks and patients monitored carefully. Avoid interruption or d/c of therapy without physician's advice.**

**THERAPEUTIC CLASS:** Selective $beta_1$-blocker

**INDICATIONS:** Treatment of HTN; may be used alone or in combination with other antihypertensive agents. Long term treatment of angina pectoris. Treatment of stable symptomatic (NYHA Class II or III) heart failure (HF) of ischemic, hypertensive, or cardiomyopathic origin.

**DOSAGE:** *Adults:* Individualized. For once-daily administration. HTN: Initial: 25-100mg qd. Titrate: May increase weekly (or longer) intervals until optimum BP reduction is achieved. Max: 400mg/day. Angina: Initial: 100mg qd. Titrate: May increase weekly until optimum clinical response has been obtained or there is pronounced slowing of heart rate. Max: 400mg/day. HF: Initial: (NYHA Class II) 25mg qd for 2 weeks. Severe HF: 12.5mg qd for 2 weeks. Titrate: Double dose every 2 weeks as tolerated. Max: 200mg/day. Monitor during up-titration. Reduce dose if experiencing symptomatic bradycardia. Dose should not be increased until symptoms of worsening HF have been stabilized. Hepatic impairment: May require lower initial dose; gradually increase dosage to optimize therapy. Elderly: Start at low initial dose.
*Pediatrics:* ≥6 yrs: HTN: Initial: 1mg/kg qd up to 50mg/day. Adjust dose according to BP response. Max: 2.0mg/kg qd.

**HOW SUPPLIED:** Tab, Extended-Release: 25mg*, 50mg*, 100mg*, 200mg* *scored

**CONTRAINDICATIONS:** Severe bradycardia, 2nd-or 3rd-degree heart block, cardiogenic shock, sick sinus syndrome (unless a pacemaker is present), decompensated cardiac failure.

**WARNINGS/PRECAUTIONS:** Caution in patients with HF, bronchospastic disease, DM, on chronic beta-blocking therapy undergoing major surgery, with history of severe anaphylactic reactions and hepatic dysfunction. May precipitate or aggravate symptoms of arterial insufficiency in patients with peripheral vascular disease. May mask symptoms of hyperthyroidism and hypoglycemia. Abrupt withdrawal may precipitate thyroid storm. Avoid initiation of high-dose regimen in patients undergoing non-cardiac surgery. Worsening cardiac failure may occur during up titration; lower dose or temporarily d/c. If used in the setting of pheochromocytoma, give in combination with an alpha blocker; may cause paradoxical increase in BP when given alone. Caution in the elderly.

**ADVERSE REACTIONS:** Bradycardia, shortness of breath (SOB), fatigue/tiredness, dizziness, depression, diarrhea, rash.

**INTERACTIONS:** Additive effects with catecholamine-depleting drugs (eg, reserpine, MAOIs). May block epinephrine effects. CYP2D6 inhibitors (eg, quinidine, fluoxetine, paroxetine, propafenone) may increase levels. May exacerbate rebound HTN following clonidine withdrawal. Caution when used with calcium channel blockers of the verapamil and diltiazem type. Concomitant use of digitalis glycosides and β-blockers can increase the risk of bradycardia.

**PREGNANCY:** Category C, caution with nursing.

**MECHANISM OF ACTION:** $\beta_1$-selective adrenergic receptor blocker; not established. Proposed to competitively antagonize catecholamines at peripheral adrenergic-neuronal sites leading to decreased cardiac output, has central effect leading to reduced symptomatic outflow to periphery and suppression of renin activity.

**PHARMACOKINETICS: Absorption:** Rapid and complete. **Distribution:** Plasma protein binding (12%); crosses blood-brain barrier, found in breast milk. **Metabolism:** Metabolized via CYP2D6. **Elimination:** Liver; Urine (<5% unchanged); $T_{1/2}$=3-7 hrs.

## NURSING CONSIDERATIONS

**Assessment:** Assess for bradycardia, heart block, cardiogenic shock, cardiac failure, sick sinus syndrome (without pacemaker), ischemic heart disease, bronchospastic disease, DM, hyperthyroidism, peripheral vascular disease, arterial insufficiency, impaired hepatic function, pheochromocytoma, upcoming surgery, anaphylactic reactions, pregnancy/nursing status, and possible drug interactions.

**Monitoring:** Monitor BP, hepatic function, difficulty of breathing in patients with bronchospastic disease; signs/symptoms of worsening of cardiac failure during up-titration; hypoglycemia in patients with DM; thyroid function in patients with hyperthyroidism; signs/symptoms of arterial insufficiency in patients with PVD.

**Patient Counseling:** Instruct not to interrupt or d/c therapy without consulting physician. Advise to take drug regularly and continuously, as directed, preferably with or immediately following meals. If dose is missed, take only next scheduled dose (without doubling). Avoid engaging in tasks requiring mental alertness (eg, operating machinery/driving). Contact physician if any difficulty in breathing occurs. Inform physician or dentist of medication use before any type of surgery. Advise HF patients to consult physician if they experience signs/symptoms of worsening HF (eg, weight gain, increasing SOB).

**Administration:** Oral route. Tabs are scored and may be divided. Whole or half-tab should be swallowed whole, not chewed or crushed. **Storage:** 25°C (77°F); excursions permitted to 15-30°C (59-86°F).

# TORISEL RX

temsirolimus (Wyeth)

**THERAPEUTIC CLASS:** Kinase inhibitor

**INDICATIONS:** Treatment of advanced renal cell carcinoma.

**DOSAGE:** *Adults:* 25mg IV over 30-60 min once a week. Hold if ANC <1,000/$mm^3$, platelet count <75,000/$mm^3$, or NCI CTCAE grade 3 or greater adverse reactions. Once toxicities resolve to Grade 2 or less, restart with dose reduced by 5mg/week to a dose no lower than 15mg/week. Concomitant Strong CYP3A4 Inhibitors: Consider dose reduction to 12.5mg/week. If strong inhibitor is d/c, allow wash out period of about 1 week before dose adjustment. Concomitant Strong CYP3A4 Inducers: Consider dose increase to 50mg/week. If strong inducer is d/c, return to dose used prior to initiation of strong inducer.

**HOW SUPPLIED:** Inj: 25mg/mL

**WARNINGS/PRECAUTIONS:** Hypersensitivity reactions manifested by anaphylaxis, dyspnea, flushing, and chest pain have been observed; if develop, stop infusion and observe patient for 30-60 mins; give $H_1$ antihistamine before starting infusion. Hyperglycemia, glucose intolerance, and hyperlipemia may occur; monitor glucose and lipid profiles. Infections may result from immunosuppression. Monitor for interstitial lung disease (ILD); if ILD is suspected, d/c and consider use of corticosteroids and/or antibiotics. Increases in serum triglycerides and cholesterol and should be tested before and during therapy. Bowel perforation may occur; monitor closely. Renal failure, sometimes fatal, reported; monitor renal function. May cause abnormal wound healing; caution during perioperative period. Caution with CNS tumors and/or anticoagulant therapy. Avoid live vaccines and close contact with those who have received live vaccines. Monitor CBC weekly and chemistry panel every 2 weeks. May cause fetal harm; avoid pregnancy during, and for 3 months after, therapy.

**ADVERSE REACTIONS:** Rash, asthenia, mucositis, nausea, edema, anorexia, anemia, hyperlipemia (including hypertriglyceridemia), hyperglycemia, elevated alkaline phosphatase, elevated AST, elevated serum creatinine , leukopenia (including lymphopenia), thrombocytopenia, hypophosphatemia.

**INTERACTIONS:** Strong inducers of CYP3A4/5 (eg, dexamethasone, carbamazepine, phenytoin, phenobarbital, rifampin, rifabutin, rifampicin) may decrease levels. Strong CYP3A4 inhibitors (eg, atazanavir, clarithromycin, indinavir, itraconazole, ketoconazole, nefazodone, nelfinavir, ritonavir, saquinavir, telithromycin, voriconazole) may increase levels. If alternative treatment cannot be administered, dose adjustment should be considered. Concomitant use with sunitinib may result in dose-limiting toxicity. Angioneurotic edema-type reactions may occur with concomitant ACE inhibitors.

**PREGNANCY:** Category D, not for use in nursing.

**MECHANISM OF ACTION:** Kinase inhibitor; binds to an intracellular protein (FKBP-12) and the protein-drug complex inhibits activity of mTOR that controls cell division; this results in reduced levels of hypoxia-inducible factors HIF-1 and HIF-2 α, and the vascular endothelial growth factor.

**PHARMACOKINETICS: Absorption:** $C_{max}$=585ng/mL, AUC=1627ng•h/mL. **Distribution:** $V_d$=172L. **Metabolism:** Liver, via CYP3A4; sirolimus (active metabolite). **Elimination:** Urine (4.6%), feces (78%); $T_{1/2}$(temsirolimus, sirolimus)=17.3, 54.6 hrs.

## NURSING CONSIDERATIONS

**Assessment:** Assess renal function, serum glucose, serum cholesterol, CBC, pregnancy/nursing status. Note other diseases/conditions and drug therapies.

**Monitoring:** Monitor for hypersensitivity reactions, blood glucose levels, infections, ILD, increased cholesterol levels, bowel perforation, renal failure, intracerebral bleeding, wound healing complications, CBC, and chemistry panels.

**Patient Counseling:** Counsel about adverse effects and instruct to report if any develop. Advise to use reliable contraception throughout treatment and continue for 3 months after last dose. Avoid use of live vaccines and close

T

contact with those who receive live vaccines while on this drug. Advise to report promptly any new or worsening abdominal pain or bloody stools.

**Administration:** IV route. Infuse over 30-60 min (See PI for preparation details). **Storage:** 2-8°C (36-46°F). Protect from light.

## Toviaz RX

fesoterodine fumarate (Pfizer)

**THERAPEUTIC CLASS:** Muscarinic antagonist

**INDICATIONS:** Treatment of overactive bladder with symptoms of urge urinary incontinence, urgency, and frequency.

**DOSAGE:** *Adults:* Initial: 4mg qd. Titrate: May increase to 8mg based on individual response and tolerability. Severe Renal Insufficiency (CrCl<30mL/min)/ Potent CYP3A4 Inhibitors: Should not exceed 4mg. Swallow whole; do not chew, divide, or crush.

**HOW SUPPLIED:** Tab, Extended Release: 4mg, 8mg

**CONTRAINDICATIONS:** Urinary retention, gastric retention, or uncontrolled narrow-angle glaucoma.

**WARNINGS/PRECAUTIONS:** Caution with bladder outlet obstruction, decreased GI motility, patients treated for narrow-angle glaucoma, and myasthenia gravis. Avoid in severe hepatic dysfunction. May increase HR.

**ADVERSE REACTIONS:** Dry mouth, constipation, urinary tract infection, dry eyes.

**INTERACTIONS:** Combining with other antimuscarinic agents may increase the frequency and/or severity of dry mouth, constipation, urinary retention, and other anticholinergic pharmacologic effects. May potentially alter the absorption of some concomitantly administered drugs due to anticholinergic effects on GI motility. Doses >4mg are not recommended with concomitant administration of potent CYP3A4 inhibitors (eg, ketoconazole, itraconazole, clarithromycin). Caution with dose titration when taking concomitant weak or moderate CYP3A4 inhibitors (eg, erythromycin). Concomitant use with alcohol may enhance the drowsiness effect produced by fesoterodine.

**PREGNANCY:** Category C, not for use in nursing.

**MECHANISM OF ACTION:** Muscarinic receptor antagonist; muscarinic receptors play a role in contractions of urinary bladder smooth muscle and stimulation of salivary secretion. Inhibition of these receptors in the bladder is presumed to be the mechanism by which effects are produced.

**PHARMACOKINETICS: Absorption:** Well absorbed, $T_{max}$=5 hrs. **Distribution:** Plasma protein binding (50%) (active metabolite). **Metabolism:** Liver via hydrolysis to active metabolite; active metabolite via CYP2D6, CYP3A4 (liver); carboxy-N-desisopropyl and N-desisopropyl metabolites. **Excretion:** Urine (70%), feces (7%); (PO): $T_{1/2}$=7 hrs (active metabolite). Refer to PI for pharmacokinetics parameters for extensive and poor CYP2D6 metabolizers.

### NURSING CONSIDERATIONS

**Assessment:** Assess for presence of urinary retention, gastric retention, narrow-angle glaucoma, myasthenia gravis, bladder outlet obstruction, decreased gastric motility (eg, constipation), hepatic/renal impairment, pregnancy/nursing status, HR, and for possible drug interactions.

**Monitoring:** Monitor for dry mouth, constipation, urinary tract infection, blurred vision, and dry eyes and HR.

**Patient Counseling:** Instruct to swallow whole; do not chew, divide, or crush. Counsel about clinically significant adverse effects (eg, constipation and urinary retention). Inform that heat prostration may occur when used in a hot environment. Advise that alcohol may enhance drowsiness effects caused by fesoterodine. Advise to read the patient leaflet before starting treatment.

**Administration:** Oral route. **Storage:** 20-25°C (68-77°F); excursions permitted between 15-30°C (59-86°F). Protect from moisture.

# TRACLEER RX

bosentan (Actelion)

**Potential liver injury; monitor LFTs before therapy, then monthly; avoid use with elevated aminotransferases (>3 x ULN); d/c use when elevated aminotransferases accompanied by clinical symptoms of liver injury. Contraindicated in pregnancy; likely to cause major birth defects if used during pregnancy. Exclude pregnancy before treatment, throughout treatment, and for one month after stopping treatment. Obtain monthly pregnancy tests. Females of childbearing potential must use two reliable methods of contraception unless have had tubal sterilization or Copper T 380A IUD or LNg 20 IUS inserted, in which case, no other contraception is needed. Prescribe through Tracleer Access Program.**

**THERAPEUTIC CLASS:** Endothelin receptor antagonist

**INDICATIONS:** Treatment of pulmonary arterial hypertension (WHO Group 1) in patients with WHO Class II-IV symptoms, to improve exercise ability and decrease the rate of clinical worsening.

**DOSAGE:** *Adults:* Initial: 62.5mg bid. Titrate/Maint: Increase to 125mg bid after 4 weeks. Low Weight (<40kg): Initial/Maint: 62.5mg bid. Adjust if develop LFT Abnormality: >3 to ≤5x ULN: Reconfirm LFTs. Reduce dose to 62.5mg bid or interrupt therapy. Monitor LFTs every 2 weeks. If LFTs return to pre-treatment levels, reintroduce or continue therapy. >5 to ≤8x ULN: Reconfirm LFTs. Stop treatment and monitor LFTs every 2 weeks. If LFTs return to pre-treatment values, may reintroduce therapy. >8x ULN: D/C; do not reintroduce. Coadministration in Patients on Ritonavir: Initial: 62.5mg qd or qod in patients receiving ritonavir for at least 10 days, based on individual tolerability. D/C use at least 36 hrs prior to initiation of ritonavir.
*Pediatrics:* >12 yrs: <40kg: Initial/Maint: 62.5mg bid.

**HOW SUPPLIED:** Tab: 62.5mg, 125mg

**CONTRAINDICATIONS:** Pregnancy, use with cyclosporine A, use with glyburide.

**WARNINGS/PRECAUTIONS:** May decrease Hgb and Hct; monitor Hgb 1 and 3 months after initiation, then every 3 months. Avoid with moderate to severe hepatic impairment, or LFTs >3x ULN. Fluid retention and peripheral edema reported; d/c if necessary. Consider intervention with diuretic, fluid management, or hospitalization for decompensating heart failure. If signs of pulmonary edema occur, possibility of associated pulmonary veno-occlusive disease (PVOD) should be considered; d/c therapy. May decrease sperm count after 3 or 6 months of therapy.

**ADVERSE REACTIONS:** Liver injury, edema, respiratory tract infection, headache, chest pain, syncope, flushing, hypotension, sinusitis, arthralgia, palpitations, anemia, abnormal LFTs.

**INTERACTIONS:** See Contraindications. May decrease levels of estrogens and progestins in hormonal contraceptives; use additional forms of contraception and do not rely on hormonal contraception alone. May decrease plasma concentrations of simvastatin or other statins metabolized by CYP3A (eg, lovastatin, atorvastatin); monitor cholesterol levels. Concomitant use with ritonavir/lopinavir or other ritonavir-containing HIV agents may increase trough concentrations of bosentan; adjust dose of bosentan when initiating ritonavir/lopinavir. May increased bosentan levels with concomitant use of tacrolimus, caution with use. Rifampin may increase trough levels of bosentan after first concomitant dose, but cause a 60% decrease in bosentan levels at steady-state; measure LFTs weekly for first 4 weeks before reverting to normal monitoring. Concomitant use with ketoconazole may increase plasma concentrations of bosentan. Use with CYP2C9 or CYP3A inhibitors may increase plasma concentrations of bosentan. Concomitant administration of both a CYP2C9 inhibitor (eg, fluconazole, amiodarone) and a strong CYP3A inhibitor (eg, ketoconazole, itraconazole) or a moderate CYP3A inhibitor (eg, amprenavir, erythromycin, fluconazole, diltiazem) with bosentan will likely lead to large increases in plasma concentrations of bosentan; coadministration of a CYP2C9 inhibitor plus a strong or moderate CYP3A inhibitor with bosentan is not recommended. May decrease plasma levels of drugs that are metabolized by CYP3A or CYP2C9.

**PREGNANCY:** Category X, not for use in nursing.

**MECHANISM OF ACTION:** Endothelin receptor antagonist; endothelin-1 (ET-1) is a neurohormone, the effects of which are mediated by binding to $ET_A$ and $ET_B$ receptors in the endothelium and vascular smooth muscle. ET-1 levels are elevated in plasma and lung tissue of patients with PAH; bosentan is a specific and competitive antagonist at endothelin receptor types $ET_A$ and $ET_B$ with slightly higher affinity for $ET_A$ receptors than $ET_B$ receptors.

**PHARMACOKINETICS: Absorption:** Absolute bioavailabilty (50%); $T_{max}$=3-5 hrs. **Distribution:** $V_d$=18L; plasma protein binding (>98%). **Metabolism:** Liver (inducer of CYP2C9, CYP3A, and CYP2C19); three metabolites, one of which is active. **Elimination:** Biliary, urine (<3%); $T_{1/2}$=5 hrs.

## NURSING CONSIDERATIONS

**Assessment:** Prior to therapy, assess serum aminotransferase levels and perform pregnancy test. Prior to therapy, assess that female patients of child bearing potential are on two forms of reliable contraception or assess that the female patient has had a tubal sterilization or that a Copper T 380A IUD or LNg 20 IUS is inserted. Assess for chronic heart failure, hepatic impairment, nursing status, and for possible drug interactions.

**Monitoring:** Monitor for signs and symptoms of liver injury (eg, N/V, abdominal pain, jaundice, lethargy, elevations of liver aminotransferases, elevated bilirubin); perform monthly measurements of liver aminotransferase levels; d/c therapy if liver aminotransferase elevations are accompanied by clinical symptoms of liver injury or if increases in bilirubin ≥2 ULN are seen. Perform monthly pregnancy tests in women of childbearing potential. In male patients, monitor for decreased sperm counts. Monitor for signs and symptoms of fluid retention, CHF, pulmonary edema, and PVOD. Monitor for signs and symptoms of decreased Hgb, and Hct; measure Hgb concentrations after 1 and 3 months of therapy and then every 3 months thereafter.

**Patient Counseling:** Counsel that this medication is only prescribed through TRACLEER Access Program. Counsel about benefits/risks of therapy and the importance of monthly lab monitoring and reporting of any adverse reactions. Instruct that medication is likely to cause birth defects and is not to be used during pregnancy. Instruct to notify physician if pregnant/nursing or planning to become pregnant. Advise women of childbearing potential to use two forms contraception during therapy and for one month after discontinuing therapy. Advise women to practice additional methods of contraception and not rely on hormonal contraception alone. Inform females that if had tubal ligation or a Copper T 380A IUD or LNg 20 IUS that can use these forms of contraception alone.

**Administration:** Oral route. **Storage:** 20-25°C (68-77°F); excursions permitted to 15-30°C (59-86°F).

# TRANDATE RX

labetalol HCl (Prometheus)

**THERAPEUTIC CLASS:** Nonselective beta-blocker/$alpha_1$ blocker

**INDICATIONS:** Management of hypertension.

**DOSAGE:** *Adults:* PO: Initial: 100mg bid. Titrate: May increase by 100mg bid every 2-3 days. Maint: 200-400mg bid. Severe HTN: 1200-2400mg/day given bid-tid. Titrate: Do not increase by more than 200mg bid. Elderly: Initial: 100mg bid. Titrate: May increase by 100mg bid. Maint: 100-200mg bid.

**HOW SUPPLIED:** Tab: 100mg*, 200mg*, 300mg* *scored

**CONTRAINDICATIONS:** Bronchial asthma, overt cardiac failure, greater than first degree heart block, cardiogenic shock, severe bradycardia, other conditions associated with hypotension, history of obstructive airway disease.

**WARNINGS/PRECAUTIONS:** Caution with hepatic dysfunction. Avoid abrupt withdrawal; may exacerbate ischemic heart disease. Caution with latent cardiac insufficiency, may exacerbate cardiac failure, reduce sinus HR, and slow AV conduction. Avoid in overt CHF. Avoid with bronchospastic disease.

T

Paradoxical HTN in pheochromocytoma reported. D/C prior to surgery. Caution with DM; may mask symptoms of hypoglycemia.

**ADVERSE REACTIONS:** Dizziness, fatigue, N/V, dyspepsia, paresthesia, nasal stuffiness, ejaculation failure, impotence, edema, dyspnea, headache, vertigo, postural hypotension, increased sweating.

**INTERACTIONS:** Increased tremor with TCAs. Antagonizes effects of β-agonists (bronchodilators). Potentiated by cimetidine; may need to reduce dose. Synergistic effects with halothane. Synergistic antihypertensive effects blunts the reflex tachycardia with nitroglycerin. Caution with calcium antagonists. May need to adjust dose of antidiabetic drugs.

**PREGNANCY:** Category C, caution in nursing.

**MECHANISM OF ACTION:** Selective $\alpha_1$-adrenergic and nonselective β-adrenergic receptor blocking agent.

**PHARMACOKINETICS: Absorption:** Complete; $T_{max}$=1-2 hrs. **Distribution:** Plasma protein binding (50%); crosses placenta. **Metabolism:** Liver (conjugation, glucuronidation). **Elimination:** Feces, urine (55-60%); $T_{1/2}$=6-8 hrs.

## NURSING CONSIDERATIONS

**Assessment:** Assess for bradycardia, heart block, cardiogenic shock, cardiac failure, ischemic heart disease, severe hypotension, bronchospastic disease, DM, pheochromocytoma, anaphylactic reactions, and possible drug interactions.

**Monitoring:** Monitor for cardiac failure, HTN, renal function, exacerbation of ischemia following abrupt withdrawal, bronchospastic disease, arrhythmias, hypersensitivity reactions, CBC with platelets and differential, anaphylactic reactions.

**Patient Counseling:** Instruct not to interrupt or d/c without consulting physician. Instruct to report signs/symptoms of cardiac failure or hepatic dysfunction (eg, pruritus, dark urine, persistent anorexia, jaundice, RUQ tenderness, or unexplained flu-like symptoms). Transient scalp itching may occur, usually when treatment initiated.

**Administration:** Oral route. **Storage:** 2-30°C (36-86°F); protect from moisture.

# TRANSDERM SCOP — RX

scopolamine (Novartis Consumer)

**THERAPEUTIC CLASS:** Anticholinergic

**INDICATIONS:** Prevention of nausea and vomiting associated with motion sickness or recovery from anesthesia and surgery.

**DOSAGE:** *Adults:* Motion Sickness: Apply 1 patch 4 hrs before travel. Replace after 3 days. Post-OP N/V: Apply 1 patch the evening before surgery or 1 hr prior to cesarean section. Keep in place for 24 hrs. Apply patch to a hairless area behind the ear. Do not cut patch in half.

T

**HOW SUPPLIED:** Patch: 0.33mg/24 hrs [4[s]]

**CONTRAINDICATIONS:** Angle-closure (narrow angle) glaucoma, hypersensitivity to belladonna alkaloids.

**WARNINGS/PRECAUTIONS:** Monitor IOP with open-angle glaucoma. Not for use in children. Caution with pyloric obstruction, urinary bladder neck or intestinal obstruction, and in elderly. Increased CNS effects with liver or kidney dysfunction. May aggravate seizures or psychosis. Idiosyncratic reactions reported (rare). Remove patch before MRI.

**ADVERSE REACTIONS:** Dry mouth, drowsiness, blurred vision, dilation of pupils, dizziness, disorientation, confusion.

**INTERACTIONS:** Caution with anticholinergic drugs (eg, other belladonna alkaloids, antihistamines, TCAs, and muscle relaxants). Increased CNS effects with sedatives, tranquilizers, and alcohol. May decrease absorption of oral medications due to delayed gastric emptying or decreased gastric motility.

**PREGNANCY:** Category C, caution in nursing.

**MECHANISM OF ACTION:** Anticholinergic agent; acts as competitive inhibitor at postganglionic muscarinic receptor sites of parasympathetic nervous system and on smooth muscle that responds to acetylcholine but lacks cholinergic innervation. Acts in the CNS by blocking cholinergic transmission from vestibular nuclei to higher centers in the CNS and from reticular formation to the vomiting center.

**PHARMACOKINETICS: Absorption:** Well-absorbed; $C_{max}$=87pg/mL (free), 354pg/mL (total); $T_{max}$=24 hrs. **Distribution:** Crosses placenta and blood brain barrier; plasma protein binding (reversibly bound); found in breast milk. **Metabolism:** Extensively metabolized. **Elimination:** Urine (10%) parent and metabolite, (5%, unchanged); $T_{1/2}$=9.5 hrs.

## NURSING CONSIDERATIONS

**Assessment:** Assess for angle-closure/chronic open-angle glaucoma, pyloric obstruction or urinary bladder neck obstruction, intestinal obstruction, hepatic/renal impairment, pregnancy/nursing status, seizures, psychosis, alcohol intake, and possible drug interactions.

**Monitoring:** Monitor for interference with gastric secretion test, IOP and glaucoma therapy in chronic open-angle glaucoma during patch use, acute toxic psychosis (eg, confusion, agitation, rambling speech, hallucinations, paranoid behaviors, delusions), drowsiness, and disorientation.

**Patient Counseling:** Caution against performing hazardous tasks (eg, operating machinery/driving). Wash hands thoroughly with soap and water immediately after handling patch; remove patch and consult physician if symptoms of acute-angle glaucoma or difficulty in urinating occur. Dispose properly and keep away from children or pets.

**Administration:** Transdermal route; apply on hairless area behind ear. Do not cut patch. **Storage:** 20-25°C (68-77°F).

# TRANXENE T-TAB

**CIV**

clorazepate dipotassium (Ovation)

**THERAPEUTIC CLASS:** Benzodiazepine

**INDICATIONS:** Management of anxiety disorders. Adjunct therapy for partial seizures. Symptomatic relief of acute alcohol withdrawal.

**DOSAGE:** *Adults:* Anxiety: Initial: (Tab) 15mg qhs. Usual: 30mg/day in divided doses. Max: 60mg/day. Elderly/Debilitated: Initial: 7.5-15mg/day. Alcohol Withdrawal: Day 1: (Tab) 30mg, then 30-60mg/day. Day 2: 45-90mg/day. Day 3: 22.5-45mg/day. Day 4: 15-30mg. Give in divided doses. Reduce dose and continue with 7.5-15mg/day; d/c when stable. Max: 90mg/day. Antiepileptic Adjunct: Initial: (Tab) 7.5mg tid. Titrate: Increase by no more than 7.5mg/week. Max: 90mg/day.
*Pediatrics:* >9 yrs: Anxiety: Initial: (Tab) 15mg qhs. Usual: 30mg/day in divided doses. Max: 60mg/day. Antiepileptic Adjunct: >12 yrs: Initial: (Tab) 7.5mg tid. Titrate: Increase by no more than 7.5mg/week. Max: 90mg/day. 9-12 yrs: Initial: 7.5mg bid. Titrate: Increase by no more than 7.5mg/week. Max: 60mg/day.

**HOW SUPPLIED:** Tab: (Tranxene T-Tab) 3.75mg*, 7.5mg*, 15mg* *scored

**CONTRAINDICATIONS:** Acute narrow-angle glaucoma.

**WARNINGS/PRECAUTIONS:** Avoid with depressive neuroses or psychotic reactions. Withdrawal symptoms with abrupt withdrawal; taper gradually. Caution with known drug dependency, renal/hepatic impairment. Suicidal tendencies reported; give lowest effective dose. Monitor LFTs and blood counts periodically with long-term therapy. Use with caution and lowest effective dose in elderly; dose adjustments should be made slowly. Increased risk of suicidal thoughts or behavior reported; monitor for worsening of depression and any unusual changes in mood or behavior. May impair physical/mental abilities.

**ADVERSE REACTIONS:** Drowsiness, dizziness, GI complaints, nervousness, blurred vision, dry mouth, headache, mental confusion, insomnia, skin rashes, fatigue, ataxia, diplopia, depression, tremor.

**INTERACTIONS:** Additive CNS depression with CNS depressants, alcohol. Potentiated by barbiturates, narcotics, phenothiazines, MAOIs, other antidepressants. Increased sedation with hypnotics.

**PREGNANCY:** Safety in pregnancy not known, not for use in nursing.

**MECHANISM OF ACTION:** Benzodiazepine; antianxiety/hypnotic agent which has CNS depressant effect.

**PHARMACOKINETICS: Absorption:** Orally absorbed; completely decarboxylated to nordiazepam. **Distribution:** Plasma protein binding (97-98%). **Metabolism:** Hydroxylation. **Elimination:** Urine (62-67%), feces (15-19%); $T_{1/2}$=40-50 hrs.

## NURSING CONSIDERATIONS

**Assessment:** Assess for acute narrow-angle glaucoma, renal function tests, LFTs, depressive neurosis, psychotic reactions, pregnancy status. Note other diseases/conditions and drug therapies.

**Monitoring:** Monitor hypersensitivity reactions, renal function, LFTs, CBC, psychological dependence, suicidal ideations.

**Patient Counseling:** Avoid alcohol, sedatives. Caution against operating machinery/driving. Counsel about drug abuse/dependence. Report side effects. Encourage patients to enroll in North American Antiepileptic Drug (NAAED) Pregnancy Registry if they become pregnant. To enroll, call the toll free number 1-888-233-2334.

**Administration:** Oral route. **Storage:** 20-25°C (68-77°F). Protect from moisture; keep bottle tightly closed. Dispense in light-resistant container.

# TRASYLOL RX

aprotinin (Bayer Healthcare)

**May cause fatal anaphylactic or anaphylactoid reactions; increased risk if re-exposed to aprotinin-containing products. Weigh benefit against risks in primary CABG surgery if second exposure to aprotinin is required. Administer only in operative settings where cardiopulmonary bypass can be rapidly initiated.**

**THERAPEUTIC CLASS:** Broad-spectrum protease inhibitor

**INDICATIONS:** Prophylactic use to reduce perioperative blood loss and the need for blood transfusion in patients undergoing cardiopulmonary bypass in the course of coronary artery bypass graft (CABG) surgery who are at an increased risk for blood loss and blood transfusion.

**DOSAGE:** *Adults:* IV: Administer through central line. Do not administer other drugs in same line. Test Dose: 1mL 10 min before LD. Regimen A: LD: 200mL IV over 20-30 min. Pump Prime Dose: Add 200mL to recirculating priming fluid. Constant Infusion Dose: 50mL/hr. Regimen B: Give 1/2 doses of regimen A.



**HOW SUPPLIED:** Inj: 10,000 KIU/mL

**CONTRAINDICATIONS:** Exposure to aprotinin within previous 12 months. Obtain full patient medical history as aprotinin may be a component in fibrant sealant products.

**WARNINGS/PRECAUTIONS:** D/C if hypersensitivity reactions occur. Take precautions with re-exposure to aprotinin: have emergency anaphylactic treatment available; give test dose and LD only when conditions for rapid cannulation present; delay aprotinin addition into pump prime solution until after LD safely given. Consider giving $H_1$ and $H_2$ blockers 15 minutes before test dose. Greater risk of hypersensitivity to aprotinin if history of allergic reactions to other agents. Administer test dose 10 minutes before LD. Administer LD in supine position over 20-30 minutes. Rapid IV administration may cause hypotension. May increase risk of renal dysfunction and possibly cause an increased need for dialysis in the perioperative period.

**ADVERSE REACTIONS:** Fever, infection, arrhythmia, hypotension, MI, CHF, pericarditis, peripheral edema, GI effects, confusion, insomnia, lung disorder, pleural effusion, atelectasis, dyspnea, pneumothorax, nausea, abnormal LFTs and renal function, urinary retention.

**INTERACTIONS:** May inhibit effects of fibrinolytic agents. May block acute hypotensive effect of captopril. Concomitant heparin may prolong activated clotting time. Caution with drugs that affect renal function (eg, aminoglycosides).

**PREGNANCY:** Category B, safety in nursing not known.

**MECHANISM OF ACTION:** Broad-spectrum protease inhibitor; modulates systemic inflammatory response (SIR) associated with cardiopulmonary bypass surgery, resulting in decreased need for blood transfusion, reduced bleeding, and decreased mediastinal re-exploration for bleeding. Inhibits multiple mediators (kallikrein, plasmin), pro-inflammatory cytokine release, and maintains glycoprotein homeostasis.

**PHARMACOKINETICS: Elimination:** Urine (25-40%, 2% unchanged).

## NURSING CONSIDERATIONS

**Assessment:** Assess for possible allergic reaction, history of previous (past year) exposure to drug, potential benefits/risks in those who have experienced allergic reaction after previous administration, history of renal impairment and/or drugs that may alter renal function, and possible drug interactions (eg, heparin). Perform heparin titration-protamine titration prior to administration to determine heparin LD.

**Monitoring:** Monitor for signs of fatal hypersensitivity reactions (eg, hypotension, anaphylactic shock with circulatory failure). During surgery, monitor for deep hypothermic circulatory arrest, anticoagulation test. Regular monitoring of SrCr, glucose, LDH, alkaline phosphatase, AST, PTT, celite ACT, and CPK-MB.

**Patient Counseling:** Inform about the benefits/risks of therapy and the need to report adverse reactions.

**Administration:** IV route. **Storage:** 2-25°C (36-77°F). Avoid freezing.

# TRAVATAN — RX

travoprost (Alcon)

**OTHER BRAND NAMES:** Travatan Z (Alcon)

**THERAPEUTIC CLASS:** Prostaglandin analog

**INDICATIONS:** Reduction of elevated intraocular pressure (IOP) in open-angle glaucoma and ocular hypertension if intolerant to or unresponsive to other IOP therapies.

**DOSAGE:** *Adults:* Usual: 1 drop in affected eye(s) qd in pm. Max: Once-daily dosing. Space dosing with other ophthalmic drugs by at least 5 min.

**HOW SUPPLIED:** Sol: (Travatan) 0.004% [2.5mL]; (Travatan Z) 0.004% [2.5mL, 5mL]

**WARNINGS/PRECAUTIONS:** Contains benzalkonium chloride; remove contact lenses prior to administration, may reinsert after 15 min (Travatan). Avoid with active intraocular inflammation. Caution with history of intraocular inflammation (eg, iritis/uveitis), aphakic patients, pseudophakic patients with torn posterior lens capsule, risk of macular edema. Increased ocular pigmentation (iris, eyelid, eyelashes) reported; may be permanent. Other eyelash changes reported. Not for the treatment of angle-closure, inflammatory, or neovascular glaucoma.

**ADVERSE REACTIONS:** Ocular hyperemia/pruritus/discomfort, foreign body sensation, decreased visual acuity, blepharitis, blurred vision, cataracts, dry eye, photophobia, tearing.

**INTERACTIONS:** Space dosing of other ophthalmics by 5 min.

**PREGNANCY:** Category C, caution in nursing.

**MECHANISM OF ACTION:** Selective FP prostanoid receptor agonist; believed to reduce IOP by increasing outflow of aqueous humor.

**PHARMACOKINETICS: Absorption:** $C_{max}$=0.018ng/mL; $T_{max}$=30 min. **Metabolism:** Cornea, via esterases to active free acid and systemically to inactive metabolites via β-oxidation and reduction. **Elimination:** Urine (2%); $T_{1/2}$=45 min.

## NURSING CONSIDERATIONS

**Assessment:** Assess for intraocular inflammation (iritis/uveitis), active macular edema, aphakic/pseudophakic patient with torn posterior lens capsules, angle-closure, inflammatory, or neovascular glaucoma, pregnancy/nursing status, and possible drug interactions.

**Monitoring:** Monitor for increased brown pigmentation of the iris, periorbital tissue, and eyelid tissue; changes in eyelashes (eg, increased length, thickness, or growth; brown pigmentation; change in number of lashes; misdirected growth of lashes); macular edema (cystoid macular edema); bacterial keratitis.

**Patient Counseling:** Inform about risk of brown pigmentation of iris, which may be permanent, and darkening of eyelid skin. Instruct to avoid touching tip of applicator to eye or surrounding areas. Advise to remove contact lenses prior to administration; reinsert 15 min after administration. Administer at least 5 min apart if using >1 topical ophthalmic drug. Consult physician if having ocular surgery or if intercurrent ocular condition (eg, trauma or infection) or ocular reaction occurs.

**Administration:** Ocular route. **Storage:** 2-25°C (36-77°F).

# TRAZODONE — RX

trazodone HCl (Various)

**Antidepressants increased the risk of suicidal thinking and behavior (suicidality) in short-term studies in children and adolescents with major depressive disorder (MDD) and other psychiatric disorders. Trazodone is not approved for use in pediatric patients.**

**THERAPEUTIC CLASS:** Triazolopyridine derivative

**INDICATIONS:** Treatment of depression.

**DOSAGE:** *Adults:* Initial: 150mg/day in divided doses pc. Titrate: May increase by 50mg/day every 3-4 days. Max: (Outpatient) 400mg/day in divided doses, (Inpatient) 600mg/day in divided doses. Maint: Lowest effective level, and may gradually reduce if adequate response is achieved.

**HOW SUPPLIED:** Tab: 50mg*, 100mg*, 150mg*, 300mg*, *scored

**WARNINGS/PRECAUTIONS:** Monitor for clinical worsening and/or suicidal ideation and behavior (suicidality), especially at initiation of therapy or dose changes. Consideration should be given to changing the therapeutic regimen, including possibly d/c medication if depression is persistently worse or if experience emergent suicidality or symptoms that may be precursors to worsening depression or suicidality. Prior to treatment, adequately screen for bipolar disorder; not approved for use in treating bipolar depression. May cause priapism; d/c use if prolonged or inappropriate erections occur. Not recommended for use during the initial recovery phase of myocardial infarction (MI). Cardiac arrhythmias may occur; caution in patients with pre-existing cardiac disease, and monitor closely. Hypotension, including orthostatic hypotension, and syncope reported. D/C therapy prior to elective surgery. Occasional low WBC and low neutrophil count reported. May impair physical/mental abilities.

**ADVERSE REACTIONS:** Dry mouth, edema, constipation, blurred vision, fatigue, nervousness, drowsiness, dizziness, headache, insomnia, N/V, musculoskeletal pain, hypotension, confusion, priapism.

**INTERACTIONS:** CYP3A4 inhibitors (eg, ritonavir, ketoconazole, indinavir, itraconazole, nefazodone) may increase levels; a lower dose of trazodone may be required when used with potent CYP3A4 inhibitors. Carbamazepine decreases levels; monitor to determine if dosage increase of trazodone is required. Increases digoxin and phenytoin serum levels. Caution with MAOIs.

May enhance response to alcohol, barbiturates and other CNS depressants. May affect PT in patients on warfarin. Concomitant use with antihypertensive therapy, may require a dose reduction of the antihypertensive drug. Avoid electroshock therapy. Changes in prothrombin time may occur with warfarin. May interact with general anesthetics.

**PREGNANCY:** Category C, caution in nursing.

**MECHANISM OF ACTION:** Triazolopyridine derivative; suspected to selectively inhibit serotonin uptake by brain synaptosomes and potentiate behavioral changes induced by the serotonin precursor, 5-hydroxytryptophan.

**PHARMACOKINETICS: Absorption:** Well absorbed; $T_{max}$=1 hr (taken on an empty stomach), 2 hrs (taken with food). **Metabolism:** Liver via CYP3A4 to m-chlorophenylpiperazine (active metabolite).

## NURSING CONSIDERATIONS

**Assessment:** Assess for bipolar disorder, cardiac disease or recent MI, pregnancy/nursing status, and for possible drug interactions. Prior to initiating treatment, assess if patient is planning to undergo surgery.

**Monitoring:** Monitor for signs/symptoms of clinical worsening, suicidality, unusual changes in behavior, priapism, cardiac arrhythmias, and for hypotension.

**Patient Counseling:** Inform about the benefits and risks of therapy. Advise patients, families, and caregivers of need to observe for signs/symptoms of clinical worsening and suicidal risks (eg, anxiety, agitation, panic attacks, mania, changes in behavior, suicidal ideation); instruct to contact physician if such symptoms occur. Counsel to avoid alcohol, sedatives, and other CNS depressants. Instruct males to d/c use and contact physician if develop a prolonged or inappropriate penile erection. Inform that may impair the mental and/or physical ability required for performing potentially hazardous tasks (eg, driving). Instruct to take shortly after a meal or light snack.

**Administration:** Oral route. **Storage:** 20-25°C (68-77°F). Protect from temperatures above 40°C (104°F). Dispense in tight, light-resistant container.

## TREANDA — RX

bendamustine HCl (Cephalon)

**THERAPEUTIC CLASS:** Alkylating agent

**INDICATIONS:** Treatment of chronic lymphocytic leukemia (CLL) and non-Hodgkin's lymphoma (NHL) that has progressed during or within six months of treatment with rituximab or a rituximab-containing regimen.

**DOSAGE:** *Adults:* CLL: 100mg/m² IV over 30 min on Days 1 and 2, of a 28-day cycle. Max: 6 cycles. Delay treatment for Grade 4 hematologic toxicity or clinically significant ≥Grade 2 non-hematologic toxicity. ≥Grade 3 Hematologic Toxicity: Reduce dose to 50mg/m² on Days 1 and 2 of each cycle; if ≥Grade 3 toxicity recurs, reduce dose to 25mg/m² on Days 1 and 2. ≥Grade 3 Non-hematologic Toxicity: Reduce dose to 50mg/m² on Days 1 and 2 of each cycle. Consider dose re-escalation in subsequent cycles. NHL: 120mg/m² IV over 60 mins on Days 1 and 2 of a 21-day cycle. Max: 8 cycles. Delay treatment for Grade 4 hematologic toxicity or clinically significant ≥Grade 2 non-hematologic toxicity. Grade 4 Hematologic Toxicity: Reduce dose to 90mg/m² on days 1 and 2 of each cycle; if grade 4 toxicity recurs, reduce dose to 60mg/m² in days 1 and 2 of each cycle. ≥Grade 3 Non-hematologic Toxicity: Reduce dose to 90mg/m² on days 1 and 2 of each cycle; if ≥Grade 3 toxicity recurs, reduce dose to 60mg/m² on days 1 and 2 of each cycle.

**HOW SUPPLIED:** Inj: 100mg

**CONTRAINDICATIONS:** Hypersensitivity to mannitol.

**WARNINGS/PRECAUTIONS:** Myelosuppression reported; monitor leukocytes, platelets, Hgb, and neutrophils closely. Infection, including pneumonia and sepsis, reported. May cause infusion reactions; monitor clinically and consider d/c with Grade 3 or 4 infusion reactions. May cause tumor lysis syndrome; use preventative measures including maintenance of adequate volume status and monitor potassium and uric acid levels. Skin reactions reported; if severe or

T

progressive, withhold or d/c treatment. Pre-malignant and malignant diseases (eg, myelodysplastic syndrome, myeloproliferative disorders, acute myeloid leukemia, and bronchial carcinoma) reported. Caution with mild hepatic impairment or mild/moderate renal impairment. Avoid with moderate/severe hepatic impairment or CrCl <40mL/min.

**ADVERSE REACTIONS:** Neutropenia, thrombocytopenia, anemia, leukopenia, pyrexia, N/V, diarrhea, fatigue, asthenia, chills, hypersensitivity, rash, hyperuricemia, nasopharyngitis.

**INTERACTIONS:** Concomitant CYP1A2 inducers (eg, fluvoxamine, ciprofloxacin) may decrease plasma concentrations and increase plasma concentrations of active metabolites. Concomitant CYP1A2 inhibitors (eg, omeprazole, smoking) may increase plasma concentrations and decrease plasma concentrations of active metabolites. Cases of Stevens-Johnson syndrome (SJS) and toxic epidermal necrolysis (TEN) reported when administered concomitantly with allopurinol and other medications known to cause these syndromes.

**PREGNANCY:** Category D, not for use in nursing.

**MECHANISM OF ACTION:** Bifunctional mechlorethamine derivative: mechanism not established. Dissociates into electrophilic alkyl groups and forms covalent bonds with electron-rich nucleophilic moieties, leading to cell death via several pathways; active against both quiescent and dividing cells.

**PHARMACOKINETICS: Distribution:** Plasma protein binding (94-96%); $V_d$= 25L. **Metabolism:** Metabolized via hydrolysis and CYP1A2; M3, M4 (minor metabolites). **Elimination:** Feces (90%); $T_{1/2}$=40 min (bendamustine 120mg/m$^2$); $T_{1/2}$=3 hrs, 30 min (M3, M4 ).

## NURSING CONSIDERATIONS

**Assessment:** Prior to initiation of therapy, assess for hypersensitivity to mannitol, renal and hepatic impairment, possible drug interactions, and pregnancy/nursing status. Obtain baseline WBC, neutrophil, platelet count, Hgb/Hct, LFTs, CrCl.

**Monitoring:** Monitor CBCs including platelet counts, Hgb/Hct, LFTs, and renal function periodically. Signs and symptoms of hypersensitivity reaction, infusion reaction (eg, flushing, SOB, facial swelling, headache, chills, back pain, tightness in chest/throat), severe myelosuppression (eg, superinfection, neutropenic fever, bleeding, fatigue), impaired hepatic/renal function, N/V, diarrhea, severe or worsening rash or itching.

**Patient Counseling:** Inform of possibility of mild or serious allergic reactions (eg, rash, facial swelling, difficulty breathing during or soon after infusion), decrease in WBCs, platelets, and RBCs. Advise women to avoid becoming pregnant and men to use reliable contraception throughout treatment and for 3 months after d/c therapy. Caution that may cause tiredness; avoid driving any vehicle or operating any dangerous tools or machinery. May cause N/V, diarrhea, and rash. Report pregnancy or any adverse reactions immediately to physician.

**Administration:** IV route. Aseptically reconstitute each 100mg vial with 20mL of SWFI yielding clear, colorless to pale yellow solution with bendamustine HCl concentration of 5mg/mL. Aseptically withdraw volume needed for required dose (based on 5mg/mL concentration) and immediately transfer to a 500mL infusion bag of 0.9% NS or 2.5% Dextrose/0.45% NS. Transfer reconstituted solution to the infusion bag within 30 min. After transferring, thoroughly mix contents of infusion bag. Admixture should be a clear and colorless to slightly yellow solution. **Storage:** 25°C (77°F); excursions permitted up to 30°C (86°F). Protect from light. Once diluted, final admixture is stable for 24 hrs when stored refrigerated (2-8°C or 36-47°F) or for 3 hrs when stored at room temperature (15-30°C or 59-86°F) and room light.



# TRECATOR RX

ethionamide (Wyeth)

**THERAPEUTIC CLASS:** Peptide synthesis inhibitor

**INDICATIONS:** Treatment of active TB in patients with *M.tuberculosis* resistant to isoniazid or rifampin, or where there is intolerance to other drugs.

**DOSAGE:** *Adults:* 15-20mg/kg qd with food. May give in divided doses with poor GI tolerance. Max: 1g/day. Alternate Regimen: Initial: 250mg qd then titrate gradually to optimal doses as tolerated, or 250mg qd for 1-2 days, then 250mg bid for 1-2 days, then 1g/day in 3-4 divided doses. Continue therapy until bacteriological conversion has become permanent and maximal clinical improvement occurs.
*Pediatrics:* ≥12 yrs: 10-20 mg/kg/day in divided doses given bid or tid with food, or 15mg/kg/day as single dose. Continue therapy until bacteriological conversion has become permanent and maximal clinical improvement occurs.

**HOW SUPPLIED:** Tab: 250mg

**CONTRAINDICATIONS:** Severe hepatic impairment.

**WARNINGS/PRECAUTIONS:** Rapid development of resistance if used alone; should be used with at least 1 or 2 other drugs. Perform ophthalmologic exams before and periodically during therapy. Measure serum transaminases prior to initiation and monthly thereafter. Risk of hypoglycemia in diabetics; monitor blood glucose prior to initiation then periodically. Hypothyroidism reported; monitor TFTs.

**ADVERSE REACTIONS:** N/V, diarrhea, abdominal pain, excessive salivation, metallic taste, stomatitis, anorexia, psychotic disturbances, drowsiness, dizziness, hypersensitivity reactions, increase in serum bilirubin, SGOT or SGPT.

**INTERACTIONS:** D/C all antituberculous medication with elevated serum transaminases until resolved; reintroduce sequentially to determine which drug is responsible. May raise isoniazid levels. May potentiate adverse effects of other antituberculous drugs. Convulsions reported with cycloserine. Risk of psychotic reactions with excessive ethanol ingestion. Give with pyridoxine.

**PREGNANCY:** Category C, not for use in nursing.

**MECHANISM OF ACTION:** Peptide synthesis inhibitor; may be bacteriostatic or bactericidal in action.

**PHARMACOKINETICS: Absorption:** Completely absorbed; $C_{max}$=2.16mcg/mL, $T_{max}$=1.02 hrs, AUC=7.67mcg•hr/mL. **Distribution:** $V_d$=93.5L; plasma protein binding (30%); widely distributed into body tissues. **Metabolism:** Liver (extensive). **Elimination:** Urine ≤1%; $T_{1/2}$=1.92 hrs.

## NURSING CONSIDERATIONS

**Assessment:** Assess for severe hepatic impairment, DM, susceptibility test, and possible drug interactions.

**Monitoring:** Monitor for hypersensitivity reactions (eg, rash, photosensitivity), GI (eg, N/V, diarrhea) and psychotic disturbances (eg, mental depression). Determination of serum transaminases (SGOT, SGPT), blood glucose, thyroid function, and eye exams should be done periodically.

**Patient Counseling:** Advise to report vision loss or blurriness, with/without eye pain. Instruct to avoid excessive ethanol ingestion to avoid psychotic reaction. Take as directed; skipping doses or not completing full course may decrease effectiveness and increase resistance.

**Administration:** Oral route. **Storage:** 20-25°C (68-77°F). Dispense in tight container.

# TRELSTAR RX

triptorelin pamoate (Watson)

**OTHER BRAND NAMES:** Trelstar Depot (Watson) - Trelstar LA (Watson)

**THERAPEUTIC CLASS:** Luteinizing hormone-releasing hormone agonist

**INDICATIONS:** Palliative treatment of advanced prostate cancer.

**DOSAGE:** *Adults:* (Depot) 3.75mg IM every month or (LA) 11.25mg IM every 84 days.

**HOW SUPPLIED:** Inj: (Depot) 3.75mg, (LA) 11.25mg

**CONTRAINDICATIONS:** Pregnancy.

**WARNINGS/PRECAUTIONS:** Anaphylactic shock, angioedema, urethral obstruction, spinal cord compression, renal impairment reported. May worsen symptoms during 1st few weeks of treatment. Closely monitor patients with metastatic vertebral lesions and/or urinary tract obstruction during 1st few weeks of therapy. Monitor serum testosterone levels, PSA.

**ADVERSE REACTIONS:** Hot flushes, HTN, headache, skeletal pain, dysuria, leg edema, pain, impotence.

**INTERACTIONS:** Avoid hyperprolactinemic drugs.

**PREGNANCY:** Category X, not for use in nursing.

**MECHANISM OF ACTION:** Luteinizing hormone-releasing hormone agonist; potent inhibitor of gonadotropin secretion.

**PHARMACOKINETICS: Absorption**: (IM) $C_{max}$=28.43, $T_{max}$=1 hr. **Distribution**: $V_d$=30-33L. **Elimination**: Liver and kidneys; $T_{1/2}$=3 hrs.

## NURSING CONSIDERATIONS

**Assessment:** Assess serum testosterone levels, PSA levels, metastatic vertebral lesions, urinary tract obstruction, pregnancy status.

**Monitoring:** Monitor serum levels of testosterone and PSA. Monitor for new onset of symptoms, bone pain, neuropathy, hematuria, spinal cord compression, pituitary apoplexy, hypersensitivity reactions.

**Patient Counseling:** Counsel about side effects; report if any occur. Counsel about potential hazards to fetus if drug used during pregnancy or if pregnancy occurs during therapy.

**Administration:** IM route. Reconstitute with SWFI. Discard if not used immediately after reconstitution. **Storage**: 20-25°C (68-77°F); excursions permitted to 15-30°C (59-86°F).

# TRENTAL RX

pentoxifylline (Sanofi-Aventis)

**THERAPEUTIC CLASS:** Blood viscosity reducer

**INDICATIONS:** Treatment of intermittent claudication due to chronic occlusive arterial disease of the limbs.

**DOSAGE:** *Adults:* 400mg tid with meals for at least 8 weeks. Reduce to 400mg bid if digestive and CNS side effects occur; d/c if side effects persist.

**HOW SUPPLIED:** Tab, Extended-Release: 400mg

**CONTRAINDICATIONS:** Recent cerebral and/or retinal hemorrhage, intolerance to methylxanthines (eg, caffeine, theophylline, theobromine).

**WARNINGS/PRECAUTIONS:** Monitor Hgb and Hct with risk factors complicated by hemorrhage (eg, recent surgery, peptic ulceration, cerebral/retinal bleeding). Occasional reports of angina, hypotension, and arrhythmia in patients with concurrent coronary artery and cerebrovascular diseases.

**ADVERSE REACTIONS:** Bloating, dyspepsia, N/V, dizziness, headache.

**INTERACTIONS:** Increase risk of bleeding with warfarin; monitor PT/INR more frequently. May increase theophylline levels; risk of theophylline toxicity. May increase effect of antihypertensives.

**PREGNANCY:** Category C, not for use in nursing.

**MECHANISM OF ACTION:** Blood viscosity reducer; not established. Increases blood flow to affected microcirculation and enhances tissue oxygenation. Improves erythrocyte flexibility, increases leukocyte deformability, and inhibits neutrophil adhesion and activation.

**PHARMACOKINETICS: Absorption:** $T_{max}$=1 hr. **Distribution:** Found in breast milk. **Metabolism:** 1st pass; metabolites (major): Metabolite 1(1-[5-hydroxyhexyl]-3,7-dimethylxanthine); metabolite V (1-[3-carboxypropyl]-3,7-dimethylxanthine). **Elimination:** Urine (major), feces (<4%); $T_{1/2}$=0.4-0.8 hrs; $T_{1/2}$=0.4-0.8 hrs (metabolites).

T

## NURSING CONSIDERATIONS

**Assessment:** Assess for recent cerebral and/or retinal hemorrhage, hypersensitivity to methylxanthines (eg, caffeine, theophylline, theobromine), nursing/pregnancy status, renal function, and drug interactions.

**Monitoring:** In presence of concurrent coronary artery disease and cerebrovascular disease, monitor for signs/symptoms of angina, arrhythmia, and hypotension. If on concomitant warfarin therapy, perform more frequent monitoring of prothrombin time. If risk for bleeding (eg, recent surgery, peptic ulceration, recent cerebral and/or retinal bleeding), periodically monitor Hgb and/or Hct. Perform periodic monitoring of renal function in the elderly ( ≥65 yrs).

**Patient Counseling:** Inform to take with meals. Instruct to report if any digestive (eg, dyspepsia, nausea) or CNS (eg, headaches) side effects develop; dose adjustment may be needed. Instruct to report any signs/symptoms of angina or hypotension.

**Administration:** Oral administration. **Storage**: 15-30°C (59-86°F). Dispense in well-closed, light-resistant container. Protect blisters from light.

# TRIAZ RX

benzoyl peroxide (Medicis)

**THERAPEUTIC CLASS:** Antibacterial/keratolytic

**INDICATIONS:** Topical treatment of acne vulgaris.

**DOSAGE:** *Adults:* (Cleanser/Foaming Cloths) Wash affected area for 10-20 seconds qd-bid or ud, then rinse and dry. Rinse off sooner or use less often if drying occurs. (Gel/Pads) Apply qd-bid to affected area after washing with mild cleanser.

**HOW SUPPLIED:** Cleanser: 3%, 6%, 9% [170.3g, 340.2g]; Foaming Cloths: 3%, 6% [3.2g]; Gel: 3%, 6%, 9% [42.5g]; Pads: 3%, 6%, 9% [1g]

**WARNINGS/PRECAUTIONS:** For external use only. Avoid contact with eyes, lips, and mucous membranes. Avoid unnecessary sun exposure and use a sunscreen. D/C if severe irritation develops.

**ADVERSE REACTIONS:** Dryness, allergic contact dermatitis.

**PREGNANCY:** Category C, caution in nursing.

**MECHANISM OF ACTION:** Antibacterial/keratolytic; not established. Produces antibacterial activity against *Propionibacterium acnes*. Also found to reduce lipids and free fatty acids, and produce mild desquamation (drying and peeling activity) with simultaneous reduction in comedones and acne lesions.

**PHARMACOKINETICS: Absorption:** Percutaneous. **Metabolism:** Benzoic acid (metabolite). **Elimination:** Urine (benzoate).

## NURSING CONSIDERATIONS

**Assessment:** Assess use in pregnancy/nursing.

**Monitoring:** Monitor for signs/symptoms of severe skin irritation and for allergic contact dermatitis.

**Patient Counseling:** Instruct to avoid contact with eyes, eyelids, lips, and mucous membranes. If accidental contact occurs, rinse area with water. Contact with hair or fabric may result in bleaching and discoloration. If excessive irritation develops, d/c and consult physician. Avoid unnecessary sun exposure; use sunscreen.

**Administration:** Topical route. **Storage:** 15-25°C (59-77°F).

# TRICOR RX

fenofibrate (Abbott)

**THERAPEUTIC CLASS:** Fibric acid derivative

**INDICATIONS:** Treatment of hypertriglyceridemia (Types IV and V) as adjunct to diet. Reduction of elevated total cholesterol, LDL, Apo B, TG, and to increase HDL in primary hypercholesterolemia or mixed dyslipidemia (Types IIa and IIb) as adjunct to diet.

**DOSAGE:** *Adults:* Hypercholesterolemia/Mixed Dyslipidemia: Initial: 145mg qd. Hypertriglyceridemia: Initial: 48-145mg/day. Titrate: Adjust if needed after repeat lipid determinations at 4-8 week intervals. Max: 145mg/day. Renal Dysfunction/Elderly: Initial: 48mg/day. Take without regard to meals.

**HOW SUPPLIED:** Tab: 48mg, 145mg

**CONTRAINDICATIONS:** Pre-existing gallbladder disease, unexplained persistent liver function abnormality, hepatic or severe renal dysfunction (including primary biliary cirrhosis).

**WARNINGS/PRECAUTIONS:** Monitor LFTs regularly; d/c if >3x ULN. May cause cholelithiasis; d/c if gallstones found. D/C if myopathy or marked CPK elevation occurs. Decreased Hgb, Hct, WBCs, thrombocytopenia, and agranulocytosis reported; monitor CBC during first 12 months of therapy. Acute hypersensitivity reactions (rare) and pancreatitis reported. Monitor lipids periodically initially, d/c if inadequate response after 2 months on 145mg/day. Minimize dose in severe renal impairment. Increased rate of pulmonary embolus (PE) and deep vein thrombosis (DVT) reported.

**ADVERSE REACTIONS:** Abdominal pain, back pain, headache, abnormal LFTs, respiratory disorder, increased creatinine phosphokinase, ALT/AST increase.

**INTERACTIONS:** Potentiates coumarin anticoagulants; reduce anticoagulant dose and monitor PT/INR. Avoid HMG-CoA reductase inhibitors unless benefits outweigh risks. Bile acid sequestrants may impede absorption; take at least 1 hr before or 4-6 hrs after the resin. Evaluate benefits/risks with immunosuppressants (eg, cyclosporine) and other nephrotoxic agents.

**PREGNANCY:** Category C, not for use in nursing.

**MECHANISM OF ACTION:** Fibric acid derivative; activates peroxisome proliferator-activated receptor α (PPARα), increasing lipolysis and elimination of triglyceride-rich particles from plasma by activating lipoprotein lipase and reducing production of apoprotein C-III (lipoprotein lipase inhibitor). Activation of PPARα also induces an increase in synthesis of apoproteins A-I, A-II, and HDL-cholesterol.

**PHARMACOKINETICS: Absorption:** Well absorbed; $T_{max}$=6-8 hrs. **Distribution:** Plasma protein binding (99%). **Metabolism:** Hydrolysis, conjugation; fenofibric acid (active metabolite). **Elimination:** Urine (60%), feces (25%); $T_{1/2}$=20 hrs.

## NURSING CONSIDERATIONS

**Assessment:** Assess for hepatic/renal dysfunction, pre-existing gallbladder disease, pregnancy/nursing status, and drug interactions. Obtain baseline lipid levels.

**Monitoring:** Monitor for signs/symptoms of liver dysfunction, cholelithiasis, pancreatitis, hypersensitivity reactions (eg, Stevens-Johnson syndrome [SJS], toxic epidermal necrosis [TEN]), hematological changes (eg, thrombocytopenia, agranulocytosis), myopathies, rhabdomyolysis, PE, DVT, and elevations in SrCr. Periodically monitor liver function (eg, ALT, AST), cholesterol levels, and blood counts. Evaluate CPK levels in patients suspected of having myopathies. Monitor for clinical response; if adequate response not seen after 2 months with maximum dose, d/c therapy.

**Patient Counseling:** Advise to immediately contact physician if unexplained muscle pain, tenderness, or weakness develop, particularly when accompanied by malaise or fever. Recommend appropriate lipid-lowering diet. Instruct to take with/without meals.

**Administration:** Oral route. **Storage:** 25°C (77°F); excursions permitted to 15-30°C (59-86°F). Keep out of reach of children. Protect from moisture.

# TRIGLIDE RX

fenofibrate (Sciele)

**THERAPEUTIC CLASS:** Fibric acid derivative

**INDICATIONS:** Adjunct to diet for treatment of hypertriglyceridemia (Types IV and V). Reduction of LDL-C, Total-C, TG, and Apo B in primary hypercholesterolemia or mixed dyslipidemia (Types IIa and IIb).

**DOSAGE:** *Adults:* Hypercholesterolemia/Mixed Hyperlipidemia: 160mg qd. Hypertriglyceridemia: Initial: 50-160mg/day. Titrate: Adjust if needed after repeat lipid levels at 4-8 week intervals. Max: 160mg/day. Renal Dysfunction/ Elderly: Initial: 50mg/day. Take without regard to meals.

**HOW SUPPLIED:** Tab: 50mg, 160mg

**CONTRAINDICATIONS:** Severe renal dysfunction, hepatic dysfunction (including primary biliary cirrhosis and unexplained persistent liver function abnormality), pre-existing gallbladder disease.

**WARNINGS/PRECAUTIONS:** Monitor LFTs regularly; d/c if >3x ULN. May cause cholelithiasis; d/c if gallstones found. D/C if myopathy or marked CPK elevation occurs. Decreased Hgb, Hct, WBCs, thrombocytopenia, and agranulocytosis reported; monitor CBCs during first 12 months of therapy. Acute hypersensitivity reactions (rare) and pancreatitis reported. Monitor lipids periodically initially; d/c if inadequate response after 2 months on 160mg/day. Minimize dose in severe renal impairment. Caution in elderly.

**ADVERSE REACTIONS:** Abdominal pain, back pain, headache, abnormal LFTs, respiratory disorder, increased creatinine phosphokinase/SGPT/SGOT.

**INTERACTIONS:** May potentiate coumarin anticoagulants; reduce anticoagulant dose and monitor PT/INR. Avoid HMG-CoA reductase inhibitors unless benefits outweigh risks. Bile acid sequestrants may impede absorption; take at least 1 hr before or 4-6 hrs after the resin. Evaluate benefits/risks with immunosuppressants (eg, cyclosporine) and other nephrotoxic agents; use lowest effective dose.

**PREGNANCY:** Category C, not for use in nursing.

**MECHANISM OF ACTION:** Fibric acid derivative; activates peroxisome proliferator-activated receptor alpha (PPARα). Causes an increase in lipolysis and elimination of triglyceride-rich particles from plasma by activating lipoprotein lipase and reducing production of apoprotein C-III. Induces an increase in apoprotein A-I, A-II and HDL cholesterol synthesis. Reduces serum uric acid levels by increasing urinary excretion of uric acid.

**PHARMACOKINETICS: Absorption:** Well absorbed; $T_{max}$=3 hrs. **Distribution:** Plasma protein binding (99%). **Metabolism:** Hydrolysis, conjugation; fenofibric acid (active metabolite). **Elimination:** Urine (60%), feces (25%); $T_{1/2}$=16 hrs.

## NURSING CONSIDERATIONS

**Assessment:** Assess for hepatic/renal dysfunction, primary biliary cirrhosis, unexplained persistent liver function abnormality, persistent elevation of lipid levels, hypothyroidism, pre-existing gallbladder disease, and DM. Assess pregnancy/nursing status and possible drug interactions. Check baseline liver function and lipid levels.

**Monitoring:** Periodically monitor lipid levels, LFTs, CPK, PT, INR, CBC. Monitor for signs of myopathy (eg, unexplained muscle pain, tenderness, or weakness, with fever or malaise), cholelithiasis/cholecystitis, pancreatitis, hepatocellular, chronic active and cholestatic hepatitis, liver cirrhosis, malignancy, and hypersensitivity reaction or severe skin rash

**Patient Counseling:** Advise to immediately contact physician if unexplained muscle pain, tenderness, or weakness with malaise or fever. Recommend appropriate lipid-lowering diet. Instruct drug may be taken with/without food.

**Administration:** Oral route. **Storage:** 20-25°C (68-77°F); excursions permitted between 15-30°C (59-86°F). Protect from light and moisture.

T

# TRILEPTAL RX

oxcarbazepine (Novartis)

**THERAPEUTIC CLASS:** Dibenzazepine

**INDICATIONS:** Monotherapy or adjunctive therapy in the treatment of partial seizures in adults, and as monotherapy in children aged ≥4 yrs with epilepsy and adjunctive therapy in children aged ≥2 yrs with epilepsy.

**DOSAGE:** *Adults:* Monotherapy: Initial: 300mg bid. Titrate: Increase by 300mg/day every 3rd day. Maint: 1200mg/day. Adjunct Therapy: Initial: 300mg bid. Titrate: Increase weekly by a max of 600mg/day. Maint: 1200mg/day. Conversion to Monotherapy: Initial: 300mg bid while reducing other AEDs. Titrate: Increase weekly by a max of 600mg/day. Withdraw other AEDs over 3-6 weeks. Maint: 2400mg/day. Renal Impairment: CrCl <30mL/min: Initial: 300mg qd. Titrate: Increase gradually.
*Pediatrics:* 4-16yrs: Monotherapy: Initial: 4-5mg/kg bid. Titrate: Increase by 5mg/kg/day every 3rd day. Maint (mg/day): Refer to PI for Dosing Chart. Adjunct Therapy: Initial: 4-5mg/kg bid. Max: 600mg/day. Titrate: Increase over 2 weeks. Maint: 20-29kg: 900mg/day. 29.1-39kg: 1200mg/day. >39kg: 1800mg/day. Conversion to Monotherapy: Initial: 4-5mg/kg bid while reducing other AEDs. Titrate: Increase weekly by max of 10mg/kg/day to target dose. Withdraw other AEDs over 3-6 weeks. Renal Impairment: CrCl <30mL/min: Initial: 300mg qd. Titrate: Increase gradually. Pediatrics 2-<4yrs: Adjunct Therapy: Initial: 4-5mg/kg bid. Max: 600mg/day. <20kg: Initial: 8-10mg/kg bid. Max: 60mg/kg/day. Titrate: 2-4 weeks until maximum dose achieved.

**HOW SUPPLIED:** Sus: 300mg/5mL [250mL]. Tab: 150mg*, 300mg*, 600mg* *scored.

**WARNINGS/PRECAUTIONS:** May develop hyponatremia. Cross-sensitivity with carbamazepine. D/C if anaphylaxis and angioedema involving the larynx, glottis, lips and eyelids develop. Serious dermatologic reactions (eg, Stevens-Johnson syndrome [SJS], toxic epidermal necrolysis [TEN]) and multi-organ hypersensitivity reported. Increased risk of suicidal thoughts or behavior; monitor unusual changes in mood and behavior. Withdraw gradually to minimize the potential of increased seizure frequency. Associated with CNS adverse effects (cognitive symptoms, somnolence or fatigue, coordination disturbances). Rare reports of agranulocytosis, aplastic anemia and pancytopenia; d/c if any evidence of hematologic events. Caution in patients with hepatic and/or renal impairment.

**ADVERSE REACTIONS:** Dizziness, somnolence, diplopia, fatigue, N/V, ataxia, abnormal vision, tremor, abnormal gait, dyspepsia, abdominal pain.

**INTERACTIONS:** Additive sedative effect with alcohol. Verapamil, carbamazepine, phenytoin, phenobarbital and valproic acid may decrease levels. Decreased plasma levels of felodipine, oral contraceptives and dihydropyridine calcium antagonists. May induce metabolism of CYP3A4/5 substrates. Increased plasma levels of phenytoin and phenobarbital. Decreased plasma levels of oxcarbazine with AEDs that are CYP450 inducers.

**PREGNANCY:** Category C, not for use in nursing.

**MECHANISM OF ACTION:** Dibenzazepine; mechanism unknown. Oxcarbazepine and 10-monohydroxy metabolite (MHD) suspected to exert antiseizure effects through blockade of voltage-sensitive $Na^+$ channels, resulting in stabilization of hyperexcited neural membranes, inhibition of repetitive neuronal firing, and diminution of propagation of synaptic impulses. Also, increased $K^+$ conductance and modulation of high-voltage activated calcium channels may contribute to anticonvulsant activity.

**PHARMACOKINETICS: Absorption:** Completely absorbed. $T_{max}$=4.5 hrs (Tab), 6 hrs (Sus). **Distribution:** $V_d$=49L (MHD); plasma protein binding (40%) (MHD); found in breast milk. **Metabolism:** Liver; reduced to MHD (active metabolite), then conjugated. **Elimination:** Urine (>95%), feces (<4%); $T_{1/2}$=2 hrs (parent drug), 9 hrs (MHD). Refer to PI for pediatric parameters.

## NURSING CONSIDERATIONS

**Assessment:** Assess hepatic and renal function. Assess history of hypersensitivity reaction to carbamazepine, depression, pregnancy/nursing status and possible drug interactions.

**Monitoring:** Monitor serum $Na^+$ levels with maintenance treatment, particularly with other medications also known to reduce levels. Monitor $T_4$ levels. Monitor for signs/symptoms of hyponatremia, anaphylaxis and angioedema, severe dermatological reactions, cognitive or neuropsychiatric events, multi-organ hypersensitivity, and hematological effects (eg, agranulocytosis, aplastic anemia). Monitor for the emergence or worsening of depression, suicidal thoughts or behavior, and/or any unusual changes in mood or behavior. Monitor for adverse reactions and hypersensitivity reactions.

**Patient Counseling:** Advise to patients, their caregivers and families to be alert for the emergence or worsening of signs/symptoms of depression, any unusual changes in mood or behavior, or the emergence of suicidal thoughts, behavior, or thoughts about self-harm. Advise to immediately report signs/symptoms suggesting angioedema. Instruct to notify physician if fever with other organ system involvement or serious skin reaction develops. Counsel females that efficacy of oral contraceptives may decrease; use another form of contraception. Avoid operating heavy machinery until gauging effects of drug. Instruct to avoid alcohol. Inform medication can be taken with/without food. If pregnant, encourage to enroll in the North American Antiepileptic Drug (NAEED) Pregnancy Registry at 888-233-2334 or aedpregnancyregistry.org.

**Administration:** Oral route. **Storage:** 25°C (77°F); excursions permitted to 15-30°C (59-86°F). Tab: Dispense in tight container. Sus: Use within 7 weeks after opening. Shake well before use.

# TRILIPIX RX

fenofibric acid (Abbott)

**THERAPEUTIC CLASS:** Fibric acid derivative

**INDICATIONS:** Adjunctive therapy to diet to reduce TG in patients with severe hypertriglyceridemia. Adjunctive therapy to diet to reduce elevated LDL-C, Total-C, TG, and Apo B, and to increase HDL-C in patients with primary hyperlipidemia or mixed dyslipidemia. Adjunct to diet in combination with a statin to reduce TG and increase HDL-C in patients with mixed dyslipidemia and coronary heart disease (CHD) or a CHD risk equivalent who are on optimal statin therapy to achieve LDL-C goal.

**DOSAGE:** *Adults:* Severe Hypertriglyceridemia: Individualize dose. Initial: 45-135mg qd. Titrate: May adjust dose if necessary following repeat lipid determinations at 4-8 week intervals. Max: 135mg qd. Primary Hyperlipidemia or Mixed Dyslipidemia: 135mg qd. Coadministered with Statins in Mixed Dyslipidemia: 135mg qd. Mild-to-Moderate Renal Impairment: Initial: 45mg qd. Titrate: May increase dose after evaluation of effects on renal function and lipid levels. Elderly: Base dose selection on renal function. May take with/without meals. May be taken at same time as statin.

**HOW SUPPLIED:** Cap, Delayed-Release: 45mg, 135mg

**CONTRAINDICATIONS:** Severe renal impairment (including dialysis), active liver disease (including primary biliary cirrhosis and unexplained persistent liver function abnormalities), nursing mothers, and pre-existing gallbladder disease.

**WARNINGS/PRECAUTIONS:** Increases risk of myositis/myopathy and rhabdomyolysis reported; d/c therapy if myopathy or marked CPK elevation occurs. Reversible elevations of serum creatinine reported; monitor renal function in patients with renal impairment and patients at risk for renal insufficiency (eg, elderly, diabetes mellitus [DM]). Hepatocellular, chronic active, and cholestatic hepatitis and cirrhosis (rare) reported. Increase in serum transaminases (eg, ALT, AST) reported; monitor liver function, and d/c therapy if enzyme levels >3x ULN. May cause cholelithiasis; d/c if gallstones are found.

Acute hypersensitivity reactions (rare) and pancreatitis reported. Decreased Hgb, Hct, WBCs, rare thrombocytopenia and agranulocytosis reported. May cause venothromboembolic disease (eg, pulmonary embolism (PE), deep vein thrombosis [DVT]). Avoid in severe renal impairment and caution in elderly.

**ADVERSE REACTIONS:** Headache, back pain, nasopharyngitis, nausea, myalgia, diarrhea, upper respiratory tract infection, constipation, dyspepsia, pain, sinusitis, arthralgia, pain in extremity, dizziness.

**INTERACTIONS:** May potentiate anticoagulant effects; caution with oral coumarin anticoagulants and monitor PT/INR. Bile acid resins may impede absorption; take at least 1 hr before or 4-6 hrs after the bile acid resin. Evaluate benefits/risks with immunosuppressants (eg, cyclosporine) and other potentially nephrotoxic agents; use lowest effective dose. Caution with drugs that are substrates for CYP2C8, CYP2C19, CYP2A6, or CYP2C9.

**PREGNANCY:** Category C, not for use in nursing.

**MECHANISM OF ACTION:** Fibric acid derivative; activates peroxisome proliferator-activated receptor α (PPARα). Increase lipolysis and elimination of triglyceride-rich particles from plasma by activating lipoprotein lipase and reducing production of APO C-III (an inhibitor of lipoprotein lipase activity). Decreases in TG levels produces an alteration in size and composition of LDL particles in which they have a greater affinity for cholesterol receptors and are catabolized rapidly. Activation of PPARα also induces an increase in the synthesis of HDL-C and Apo AI and AII.

**PHARMACOKINETICS: Absorption:** Well-absorbed; absolute bioavailability (81%); $T_{max}$=4-5 hrs. **Distribution:** Plasma protein binding (99%). **Metabolism:** Conjugation with glucuronic acid. **Elimination:** Urine; $T_{1/2}$=20 hrs.

## NURSING CONSIDERATIONS

**Assessment:** Assess for severe renal impairment, active liver disease (eg, primary biliary cirrhosis, unexplained liver function abnormality), pre-existing gallbladder disease, pregnancy/nursing status, and for possible drug interactions. Prior to therapy, obtain baseline LFTs, lipid levels, and renal function.

**Monitoring:** Monitor for signs/symptoms of myositis, myopathy, and rhabdomyolysis; measure CPK levels if myopathy is suspected. Monitor for elevations in SrCr, increases in serum transaminase levels, hepatocellular, chronic active, and cholestatic hepatitis, pancreatitis, hypersensitivity reactions (eg, severe skin rashes), hematological changes (eg, agranulocytosis, thrombocytopenia), and for venothromboembolic disease (eg, DVT, PE). Monitor for signs and symptoms of cholelithiasis; if cholelithiasis is suspected, perform gallbladder studies. Monitor renal function in patients with renal impairment and in patients at risk for renal impairment (eg, DM, elderly). Perform periodic monitoring of LFTs and CBC.

**Patient Counseling:** Inform of the potential benefits and risks of therapy. Inform of medications that should be avoided during treatment. Instruct to take once daily, without regard to food. Inform that if on statin therapy, both drugs may be taken at the same time. Advise to follow appropriate lipid-modifying diet during therapy. Instruct to notify physician of all medications, supplements, and herbal preparations taken and any changes in medical conditions. Instruct to notify physician of any muscle pain, tenderness, or weakness; onset of abdominal pain or if any other new symptoms develop.



**Administration:** Oral route. **Storage:** 25°C (77°F); excursions permitted to 15-30°C (59-86°F). Protect from moisture.

# Tri-Luma RX

fluocinolone acetonide - hydroquinone - tretinoin (Galderma)

**THERAPEUTIC CLASS:** Corticosteroid/depigmenting agent/keratolytic

**INDICATIONS:** Short-term treatment of moderate to severe melasma of the face.

**DOSAGE:** *Adults:* Gently wash face and neck with mild cleanser. Apply thin film to hyperpigmented areas of melasma including 1/2 inch of normal skin surrounding lesion, at least 30 min before bedtime.

**HOW SUPPLIED:** Cre: (Fluocinolone-Hydroquinone-Tretinoin) 0.01%-4%-0.05% [30g]

**WARNINGS/PRECAUTIONS:** Contains sodium metabisulfite. D/C if ochronosis, sensitivity, or irritation occurs. Cutaneous hypersensitivity reported. May produce reversible HPA axis suppression, manifestations of Cushing's syndrome, hyperglycemia, and glucosuria. Avoid eyes, nose, angles of mouth, occlusive dressings, or sunlight/UV exposure. Extreme weather (eg, cold, wind) may irritate skin.

**ADVERSE REACTIONS:** Erythema, desquamation, burning, dryness, pruritus, acne, paresthesia, telangiectasia.

**INTERACTIONS:** Avoid medicated/abrasive soaps or cleansers, soaps/cosmetics with drying effects, products with high concentration of alcohol/astringent, and other irritants or keratolytic agents. Caution with other photosensitizers. Use non-hormonal birth control.

**PREGNANCY:** Category C, caution in nursing.

**MECHANISM OF ACTION:** Fluocinolone: Corticosteroid; acts as anti-inflammatory agent. Hydroquinone: Depigmenting agent; interrupts 1 or more steps in tyrosine-tyrosinase pathway in melanin systhesis. Tretinoin: Keratolytic.

**PHARMACOKINETICS: Absorption:** Hydroquinone: $C_{max}$=25.55-86.52ng/mL. Tretinoin: (gp I) $C_{max}$=2.01-5.34ng/mL, (gp II) $C_{max}$=2-4.99ng/mL. **Distribution:** Corticosteroid; (found in breast milk).

## NURSING CONSIDERATIONS

**Assessment:** Assess for drug or sulfite hypersensitivity, pregnancy/nursing status, and for possible drug interactions with photosensitizer drugs.

**Monitoring:** Monitor for allergic-type reactions (eg, anaphylactic symptoms, life-threatening asthmatic attacks), local irritation (eg, reddening, peeling, burning sensation, dryness, pruritus), ochronosis (gradual blue-black darkening of skin), HPA-axis suppression with potential for glucocorticoid insufficiency after withdrawal, manifestations of Cushing's syndrome, hyperglycemia, and glucosuria. Lab monitoring of HPA-axis supression by ACTH or cosyntropin stimulation test, morning plasma cortisol test, urinary free cortisol test.

**Patient Counseling:** Instruct to avoid sunlight, sunlamp, and UV light exposure. Wearing protective clothing and using sunscreen essential during therapy. Avoid contact with eyes, nose, or angles of mouth. Notify physician if pregnant/nursing or planning to become pregnant.

**Administration:** Topical route. **Storage:** 20-25°C (68-77°F). Avoid freezing.

# TRI-NORINYL RX

ethinyl estradiol - norethindrone (Watson)

**THERAPEUTIC CLASS:** Estrogen/progestogen combination

**INDICATIONS:** Prevention of pregnancy.

**DOSAGE:** *Adults:* 1 tab qd for 28 days, then repeat. Start 1st Sunday after menses begin or 1st day of menses.

**HOW SUPPLIED:** Tab: (Ethinyl Estradiol-Norethindrone) 0.035mg-0.5mg, 0.035mg-1mg

**CONTRAINDICATIONS:** Thrombophlebitis, DVT or thromboembolic disorders, pregnancy, cerebrovascular or coronary artery disease, undiagnosed abnormal genital bleeding, cholestatic jaundice of pregnancy or jaundice with prior pill use, hepatic adenomas or carcinomas, breast cancer or other estrogen-dependent neoplasia.

**WARNINGS/PRECAUTIONS:** Cigarette smoking increases risk of serious cardiovascular side effects. This risk increases with age (especially >35 yrs) and heavy smoking. Increased risk of MI, vascular disease, thromboembolism, stroke and gallbladder disease. Retinal thrombosis, hepatic neoplasia, carcinoma of breast and reproductive organs reported. May cause glucose intolerance. May increase BP, elevate LDL levels or cause other lipid changes, fluid retention, breakthrough bleeding, and spotting. May cause or exacerbate migraine. May develop visual changes with contact lens. Increased risk of MI with HTN, hyperlipidemia, obesity, and diabetes. D/C if jaundice, significant depression or ophthalmic irregularities develop. Perform annual physical exam. Use before menarche is not indicated. May affect certain endocrine, LFTs and blood components.

**ADVERSE REACTIONS:** N/V, breakthrough bleeding, spotting, amenorrhea, migraine, depression, vaginal candidiasis, edema, weight changes.

**INTERACTIONS:** Reduced effects, increased breakthrough bleeding, and menstrual irregularities with rifampin, barbiturates, phenylbutazone, phenytoin, and possibly with griseofulvin, ampicillin, and tetracyclines.

**PREGNANCY:** Category X, not for use in nursing.

**MECHANISM OF ACTION:** Combination oral contraceptive; acts by suppressing gonadotropins. Primarily inhibits ovulation. Also causes changes in cervical mucus (increases difficulty of sperm entry into uterus) and endometrium (reduces likelihood of implantation).

## NURSING CONSIDERATIONS

**Assessment:** Assess family history of breast cancer, presence of certain inherited or acquired thrombophilias, HTN, hyperlipidemia, obesity, DM, renal disease, depression, heavy smoking, and potential drug interactions. Conduct personal and family history and complete physical exam.

**Monitoring:** Monitor for MI, thromboembolism, cerebrovascular disease, benign hepatic adenomas, retinal thrombosis, HTN, headache, bleeding irregularities, jaundice, fluid retention, and emotional disorders. Conduct periodic complete physical exam with emphasis on BP, breasts, abdomen, and pelvic organs including cervical cytology and relevant lab tests (eg, TG, prothrombin clotting factors such as VII, VIII, IX, and X, renal/hepatic functions, TBG, sex steroid binding globulins).

**Patient Counseling:** Inform drug does not protect against HIV infection (AIDS) and other STDs. Inform of potential risks/benefits of oral contraceptives. Do not smoke while on treatment. Take 1 pill at same time daily.

**Administration:** Oral route. **Storage:** 15-25°C (59-77°F).

# TRIPEDIA — RX

pertussis vaccine, acellular - diphtheria toxoid - tetanus toxoid (Sanofi Pasteur)

**THERAPEUTIC CLASS:** Vaccine/toxoid combination

**INDICATIONS:** Active immunization against diphtheria, tetanus, and pertussis in pediatrics 6 weeks to 7 yrs of age (prior to 7th birthday). Combined with ActHIB for active immunization in pediatrics 15-18 months previously immunized against diphtheria, tetanus, and pertussis with 3 doses of whole-cell pertussis DTP or acellular pertussis vaccine and 3 or fewer doses of ActHIB® within 1st year of life for prevention of *H. influenzae* type b, diphtheria, tetanus, and pertussis.

**DOSAGE:** *Pediatrics:* ≥6 weeks up to 7 yrs: Primary Series: 3 doses of 0.5mL IM at 4-8 week intervals. 1st dose usually at 2 months, but can give at 6 weeks up to 7th birthday. Booster: 4th dose (0.5mL IM) at 15-20 months, at least 6 months after 3rd dose, 5th dose at 4-6 yrs; prior to school entry. May give to complete 4th or 5th dose of primary series of 3 doses of whole-cell pertussis DTP (4th dose at 15-20 months and 5th dose before school if 4th dose not given on or before 4th birthday). May combine with ActHIB® for 4th dose at 15-18 months.

**HOW SUPPLIED:** Inj: 0.5mL

**CONTRAINDICATIONS:** Hypersensitivity to thimersal and gelatin, immediate anaphylactic reaction associated with previous dose, encephalopathy not due to an identifiable cause within 7 days of prior pertussis immunization. Defer during poliomyelitis outbreak or acute febrile illness.

**WARNINGS/PRECAUTIONS:** Caution if within 48 hrs of previous whole-cell DTP or acellular DTP vaccine, fever ≥105°F not due to another identifiable cause, collapse or shock-like state, or inconsolable crying lasting ≥3 hrs occurs, or if convulsions occur within 3 days. For high seizure risk, give APAP at time of vaccination and q4-6h for 24 hrs. Caution with neurologic or CNS disorders. Avoid with coagulation disorders. Have epinephrine available. Suboptimal response may occur in immunocompromised patients.

**ADVERSE REACTIONS:** Local erythema and swelling, irritability, drowsiness, anorexia, fever.

**INTERACTIONS:** Avoid with anticoagulants. Immunosuppressive therapy (eg, irradiation, antimetabolites, alkylating agents, cytotoxic drugs, corticosteroids) may decrease response. Do not combine through reconstitution with any vaccine for infants <15 months.

**PREGNANCY:** Category C, safety in nursing not known.

**MECHANISM OF ACTION:** Active immunization against diphtheria, tetanus, and pertussis (whooping cough).

## NURSING CONSIDERATIONS

**Assessment:** Review current health status, previous sensitivity/immunization events (eg, fever, shock, persistent crying, convulsions, Guillain-Barre syndrome), and possible drug interactions.

**Monitoring:** Monitor for Arthus-type hypersensitivity reactions, injection-site for erythema, swelling, and tenderness, fever, irritability, drowsiness, anorexia, N/V, high-pitched/persistent crying, and neurological complications.

**Patient Counseling:** Inform of potential benefits/risks; report any adverse reactions to physician. May not offer 100% protection.

**Administration:** IM route. Inject into anterolateral aspect of thigh or deltoid region. **Storage:** 2-8°C (36-46°F). Do not freeze.

# TRIPHASIL RX

ethinyl estradiol - levonorgestrel (Wyeth)

**OTHER BRAND NAMES:** Enpresse (Barr)

**THERAPEUTIC CLASS:** Estrogen/progestogen combination

**INDICATIONS:** Prevention of pregnancy.

**DOSAGE:** *Adults:* 1 tab qd for 28 days, then repeat. Start 1st Sunday after menses begin or 1st day of menses.

**HOW SUPPLIED:** Tab: (Ethinyl Estradiol-Levonorgestrel) 0.03mg-0.05mg, 0.04mg-0.075mg, 0.03mg-0.125mg

**CONTRAINDICATIONS:** Thrombophlebitis, DVT or thromboembolic disorders, pregnancy, cerebrovascular or coronary artery disease, undiagnosed abnormal genital bleeding, cholestatic jaundice of pregnancy or jaundice with prior pill use, hepatic adenomas or carcinomas, breast cancer or other estrogen-dependent neoplasia, thrombogenic valvulopathies, thrombogenic rhythm disorders, diabetes with vascular involvement, uncontrolled HTN, endometrium carcinoma, active liver disease if liver function has not returned to normal.

**WARNINGS/PRECAUTIONS:** Cigarette smoking increases risk of serious cardiovascular side effects; risk increases with age (especially >35 yrs) and heavy smoking. Increased risk of MI, vascular disease, thromboembolism, stroke and gallbladder disease. Retinal thrombosis, hepatic neoplasia, carcinoma of breast and reproductive organs reported. May cause glucose intolerance. May increase BP, elevate LDL levels or cause other lipid changes, fluid retention, breakthrough bleeding, and spotting. May cause or exacerbate migraine. May develop visual changes with contact lens. Diarrhea and vomiting may decrease hormone absorption. Increased risk of MI with HTN, hyperlipidemia, obesity, and diabetes. D/C if jaundice, significant depression or ophthalmic irregularities develop. Perform annual physical exam. Use before menarche is not indicated. May affect certain endocrine, LFTs and blood components.

**ADVERSE REACTIONS:** N/V, breakthrough bleeding, spotting, amenorrhea, migraine, depression, vaginal candidiasis, edema, weight changes.

**INTERACTIONS:** Reduced effects, increased breakthrough bleeding, and menstrual irregularities with rifampin, rifabutin, barbiturates, phenylbutazone, phenytoin, griseofulvin, topiramate, some protease inhibitors, modafinil, ampicillin, other penicillins, tetracyclines and possibly with St. John's wort. Troleadomycin may increase risk of intrahepatic cholestasis. Increased levels with ascorbic acid, APAP, CYP3A4 inhibitors (eg, indinavir, fluconazole, troleandomycin), and atorvastatin. May alter levels of cyclosporine, theophylline, and corticosteroids.

**PREGNANCY:** Category X, not for use in nursing.

**MECHANISM OF ACTION:** Combination oral contraceptive; acts by suppressing gonadotropins. Inhibits ovulation and produces changes in cervical mucus (increasing difficulty of sperm entry into uterus) and endometrium (reducing likelihood of implantation).

**PHARMACOKINETICS: Absorption**: (LNG): Rapid and complete. (50/30mcg LNG/EE single dose): $C_{max}$=1.7ng/mL, $T_{max}$=1.3 hr, AUC=17ng•hr/mL; (EE) Rapid and complete, (50/30mcg LNG/EE single dose): $C_{max}$=141pg/mL, $T_{max}$=1.5 hr, AUC=1126pg•hr/mL. **Distribution**: Found in breast milk, (EE) plasma protein binding (97%). **Metabolism**: (LNG) reduction, hydroxylation, conjugation; (EE) in liver via CYP3A4 through hydroxylation (major), methylation, glucuronidation. **Elimination**: (LNG) Urine (40%-68%), feces (16-48%); $T_{1/2}$=approximately 36 hrs. (EE) Urine, feces; $T_{1/2}$=18 hrs.

## NURSING CONSIDERATIONS

**Assessment:** Assess family history of breast cancer, presence of certain inherited or acquired thrombophilias, HTN, hyperlipidemia, obesity, DM, renal disease, depression, heavy smoking, and potential drug interactions. Conduct personal/family history and complete physical exam.

**Monitoring:** Monitor for MI, thromboembolism, cerebrovascular disease, benign hepatic adenomas, retinal thrombosis, HTN, headache, bleeding irregularites, jaundice, fluid retention, and emotional disorders. Conduct periodic complete physical exam with emphasis on BP, breasts, abdomen, and pelvic organs including cervical cytology and relevant lab tests (eg, TG, prothrombin and clotting factors as VII, VIII, IX, and X, renal/hepatic functions, TBG, sex steroid binding globulins).

**Patient Counseling:** Inform drug does not protect against HIV infection (AIDS) and other STDs. Inform of potential risks/benefits of oral contraceptives. Do not smoke while on treatment. Take 1 pill at same time daily.

**Administration:** Oral route. **Storage**: 20-25°C (68-77°F).

# TRISENOX — RX

arsenic trioxide (Cephalon)

T

**Administer under supervision of a physician experienced in the management of acute leukemia. Acute promyelocytic leukemia (APL) differentiation syndrome reported. Can cause QT interval prolongation and complete AV block. Monitor ECG, serum electrolytes, and creatinine before and during therapy.**

**THERAPEUTIC CLASS:** DNA fragmentation agent

**INDICATIONS:** For induction of remission and consolidation of APL refractory to or relapsed from retinoid and anthracycline chemotherapy, and has t(15;17) translocation or PML/RAR-alpha gene expression.

**DOSAGE:** *Adults:* Induction: 0.15mg/kg IV qd until bone marrow remission. Max: 60 doses. Consolidation: 0.15mg/kg IV qd for 25 doses over 5 weeks. Begin 3-6 weeks after complete induction therapy.
*Pediatrics:* ≥5 yrs: Induction: 0.15mg/kg IV qd until bone marrow remission. Max: 60 doses. Consolidation: 0.15mg/kg IV qd for 25 doses over 5 weeks. Begin 3-6 weeks after complete induction therapy.

**HOW SUPPLIED:** Inj: 1mg/mL

**WARNINGS/PRECAUTIONS:** Hyperleukocytosis, QT interval prolongation, torsade de pointes, and complete AV block reported. Caution with renal failure. Monitor electrolyte, hematologic, and coagulation profiles at least twice weekly, and more frequently in unstable patients during induction. Obtain ECG weekly, and more frequently for unstable patients. May cause fetal harm; avoid pregnancy.

**ADVERSE REACTIONS:** Fatigue, pyrexia, edema, chest pain, injection-site pain, N/V, abdominal pain, constipation, hypokalemia, hypomagnesemia, hyperglycemia, increased ALT, headache, insomnia, dyspnea.

**INTERACTIONS:** Caution with agents that prolong the QT interval (eg, certain antiarrhythmics, thioridazine) or lead to electrolyte abnormalities (eg, diuretics, amphotericin B).

**PREGNANCY:** Category D, not for use in nursing.

**MECHANISM OF ACTION:** DNA fragmentation agent; suspected to cause morphological changes in cells and DNA fragmentation characteristic of apoptosis, and damage or degradation of fushion protein PML/RAR-α.

**PHARMACOKINETICS: Metabolism:** Liver via reduction and methylation. **Elimination:** Urine.

## NURSING CONSIDERATIONS

**Assessment:** Assess renal/hepatic function, ECG, electrolytes, pregnancy status.

**Monitoring:** Monitor CBC with differential and platelet count, coagulation profile, ECG, electrolytes. Monitor for hypersensitivity reactions, APL differentiation syndrome, pyrexia, nausea.

**Patient Counseling:** Counsel about adverse effects; report if any develop. Advise women of childbearing age to avoid becoming pregnant during treatment.

**Administration:** IV route over 1-2 hrs. **Storage:** 25°C (77°F); excursions permitted to 15-30°C (59-86°F). Do not freeze.

# TRIVORA — RX

ethinyl estradiol - levonorgestrel (Watson)

**OTHER BRAND NAMES:** Enpresse (Barr)

**THERAPEUTIC CLASS:** Estrogen/progestogen combination

**INDICATIONS:** Prevention of pregnancy.

**DOSAGE:** *Adults:* 1 tab qd for 28 days, then repeat. Start 1st Sunday after menses begin or 1st day of menses.

**HOW SUPPLIED:** Tab: (Ethinyl Estradiol-Levonorgestrel) 0.03mg-0.05mg, 0.04mg-0.075mg, 0.03mg-0.125mg

**CONTRAINDICATIONS:** Thrombophlebitis, deep vein thrombophlebitis, thromboembolic disorders, pregnancy, cerebrovascular or coronary artery disease, undiagnosed abnormal genital bleeding, cholestatic jaundice of pregnancy or jaundice with prior pill use, hepatic carcinoma, benign liver tumor, breast cancer, endometrial cancer, or other estrogen-dependent neoplasia.

**WARNINGS/PRECAUTIONS:** Cigarette smoking increases risk of serious cardiovascular side effects. This risk increases with age (especially >35 yrs) and heavy smoking. Increased risk of MI, vascular disease, thromboembolism, stroke, and gallbladder disease. Retinal thrombosis, hepatic neoplasia reported. May cause glucose intolerance. May increase BP, elevate LDL levels or cause other lipid changes, fluid retention, breakthrough bleeding, and spotting. May cause or exacerbate migraine. May develop visual changes with contact lens. Morbidity and mortality risk increased with HTN, hyperlipidemia, obesity, and diabetes. D/C if jaundice, significant depression or ophthalmic irregularities develop. Perform annual physical exam. Use before menarche is not indicated. May affect certain endocrine, LFTs, and blood components.

**ADVERSE REACTIONS:** N/V, breakthrough bleeding, spotting, amenorrhea, migraine, depression, vaginal candidiasis, edema, weight changes.

**INTERACTIONS:** Reduced effects, increased breakthrough bleeding, and menstrual irregularities with rifampin, barbiturates, phenylbutazone, phenytoin, and possibly with griseofulvin, ampicillin, and tetracyclines.

**PREGNANCY:** Category X, not for use in nursing.

**MECHANISM OF ACTION:** Combination oral contraceptive; acts by suppressing gonadotropins, primarily inhibits ovulation. Also causes changes in cervical mucus (increasing difficulty of sperm entry into uterus) and endometrium (reducing likelihood of implantation).

**PHARMACOKINETICS: Absorption:** Triphasic pharmacokinetic parameters varied according to variable dosing. Levonorgestrel: Rapidly and completely absorbed. Absolute bioavailability (100%). Ethinyl: Rapid and almost completely absorbed. Absolute bioavailabilty (38-48%). **Distribution:** Found in breast milk. Levonorgestrel: SHBG binding (60%). Ethinyl: Albumin binding (97%). **Metabolism:** Levonorgestrel: Via hydroxylation and conjugation. Ethinyl: Liver via CYP3A4 enzyme through hydroxylation, methylation and glucuronidation. **Elimination:** Levonorgestrel: Urine (40-68%), feces (16-48%); $T_{1/2}$=36 hrs. Ethinyl: Urine, feces; $T_{1/2}$=18 hrs.

## NURSING CONSIDERATIONS

**Assessment:** Assess family history of breast cancer, presence of inherited or acquired thrombophilias, HTN, hyperlipidemia, obesity, DM, renal disease, depression, heavy smoking, and potential drug interactions. Conduct personal/family history and complete physical exam.

**Monitoring:** Monitor for MI, thromboembolism, cerebrovascular disease, benign hepatic adenomas, retinal thrombosis, HTN, headache, bleeding irregularites, jaundice, fluid retention, and emotional disorders. Conduct periodic complete physical exam with emphasis on BP, breasts, abdomen, and pelvic organs, including cervical cytology and relevant lab tests.

**Patient Counseling:** Inform that drug does not protect against HIV infection and other STDs. Counsel on benefits/risks of drug. Advise to avoid smoking while taking medication. Instruct to take 1 pill at same time daily.

**Administration:** Oral route. **Storage:** 20-25°C (68-77°F).

# TRIZIVIR RX

abacavir sulfate - zidovudine - lamivudine (GlaxoSmithKline)

**Fatal hypersensitivity reactions reported; d/c if hypersensitivity reaction suspected and do not restart to avoid more serious symptoms, including hypotension and death. High risk of hypersensitivity reaction to abacavir in patients with HLA-B*5701 allele; screening is recommended prior to therapy. Hematologic toxicities, lactic acidosis, and severe hepatomegaly with steatosis (including fatal cases) reported. Severe exacerbations of hepatitis B in patients coinfected with HIV upon d/c; monitor hepatic function.**

**THERAPEUTIC CLASS:** Nucleoside analog combination

T

**INDICATIONS:** Treatment of HIV-1 infection alone or in combination with other antiretrovirals.

**DOSAGE:** *Adults:* >40kg and CrCl >50mL/min: 1 tab bid.
*Pediatrics:* Adolescents: >40kg and CrCl >50mL/min: 1 tab bid.

**HOW SUPPLIED:** Tab: (Abacavir-Lamivudine-Zidovudine) 300mg-150mg-300mg

**CONTRAINDICATIONS:** Hepatic impairment.

**WARNINGS/PRECAUTIONS:** Caution with bone marrow compromise. Prolonged use associated with myopathy and myositis with pathological changes. Avoid with mild to moderate hepatic impairment or liver cirrhosis, and renal impairment with <50mL/min. Avoid in adolescents <40kg. Recurrent hepatitis upon d/c of lamivudine reported in hepatitis B patients. Lamivudine-resistant hepatitis B virus reported. Immune reconstitution and fat redistribution was reported. Increased risk of CHD (eg, MI). Caution in elderly. See PI for detailed information.

**ADVERSE REACTIONS:** N/V, diarrhea, decreased appetite, insomnia, fever, chills, fatigue, rash, abdominal pain, stomatitis, hyperglycemia, lab abnormalities.

**INTERACTIONS:** Abacavir (ABC): Ethanol decreases elimination. Zidovudine (AZT): Ganciclovir, interferon-α, and other bone marrow suppressants or cytotoxic agents may increase hematologic toxicity. Antagonistic effects with stavudine. Lamivudine (3TC): Increased 3TC exposure with trimethoprim 160mg/sulfamethoxazole 800mg. Avoid zalcitabine. Hepatic decompensation reported in patients on combination antiretroviral therapy for HIV and interferon-α w/ or w/o ribavirin; monitor closely for treatment-associated toxicities. Avoid concomitant use with other fixed-dose combination drugs (eg, 3TC/AZT, ABC/3TC or emtricitabine and tenofovir).

**PREGNANCY:** Category C, not for use in nursing.

**MECHANISM OF ACTION:** Abacavir: Carbocyclic nucleoside analogue; inhibits HIV-1 reverse transcriptase (RT) by competing with natural substrate dGTP and incorporating into viral DNA. Lamivudine/Zidovudine: Nucleoside analogue; inhibits RT via DNA chain termination.

**PHARMACOKINETICS: Absorption:** Abacavir/Lamivudine: Rapid; bioavailability (86%). Zidovudine: Rapid; bioavailability (64%). **Distribution:** Abacavir: $V_d$=0.86L/kg; plasma protein binding (50%). Lamivudine: $V_d$=1.3L/kg; plasma protein binding (low). Zidovudine: $V_d$=1.6L/kg; plasma protein binding (low). **Metabolism:** Abacavir: Hepatic, via alcohol dehydrogenase and glucuronyl transferase. Lamivudine: Metabolite (trans-sulfoxide). Zidovudine: Hepatic, via glucuronyl transferase. Major metabolite: (3'-azido-3'-deoxy-5'-*O*-β-*D*-glucopyranuronosylthymidine (GZDV). **Elimination:** Abacavir: $T_{1/2}$=1.45 hrs. Lamivudine: (IV): Urine (70%); $T_{1/2}$=5-7 hrs. Zidovudine: Urine (14%); (GZDV): Urine (74%); $T_{1/2}$=0.5-3 hrs.

## NURSING CONSIDERATIONS

**Assessment:** Assess for impaired hepatic/renal function, bone marrow suppression, risk factors for lactic acidosis, myopathy, pregnancy/nursing status and possible drug interactions. Assess for HLA-B*5701 allele.

**Monitoring:** Monitor for signs/symptoms of hypersensitivity reactions (eg, fever, rash, N/V, diarrhea, generalized malaise, fatigue, dyspnea, cough), lactic acidosis, myopathy, exacerbations of hepatitis, immune reconstitution syndrome, hepatic dysfunction (eg, decompensation, failure), and fat redistribution. Monitor blood count. Physician should register patients in the hypersensitivity registry if hypersensitivity reactions occur.

**Patient Counseling:** If treatment interrupted, advise not to restart therapy to avoid more severe symptoms (eg, life-threatening hypotension, death). Seek medical attention if symptoms of hypersensitivity reactions (eg, fever, rash, N/V, diarrhea, generalized malaise, fatigue, dyspnea, cough), lactic acidosis, myopathy, exacerbations of hepatitis, immune reconstitution syndrome, hepatic dysfunction (eg, decompensation, failure), and fat redistribution occur. May enroll patients in the Antiretroviral Pregnancy Registry if they become pregnant while on treatment.

**Administration:** Oral route. **Storage:** 25°C (77°F); excursions permitted to 15-30°C (59-86°F).

# TRUSOPT — RX

dorzolamide HCl (Merck)

**THERAPEUTIC CLASS:** Carbonic anhydrase inhibitor

**INDICATIONS:** Treatment of open-angle glaucoma and ocular hypertension.

**DOSAGE:** *Adults:* 1 drop tid. Space dosing of other ophthalmic drugs by 10 min.
*Pediatrics:* 1 drop tid. Space dosing of other ophthalmic drugs by 10 min.

**HOW SUPPLIED:** Sol: 2% [5mL, 10mL]

**WARNINGS/PRECAUTIONS:** Systemically absorbed. Avoid with sulfonamide allergy or severe renal impairment (CrCl <30mL/ min). Caution with hepatic impairment. Not studied in acute angle-closure glaucoma. Local ocular adverse effects (eg, conjunctivitis, lid reactions) reported with chronic use; d/c use and evaluate patient before considering restarting therapy. Bacterial keratitis reported with contaminated containers. Choroidal detachment reported following filtration procedures.

**ADVERSE REACTIONS:** Ocular burning, stinging, discomfort, superficial punctate keratitis, bitter taste, blurred vision, eye redness, tearing, dryness, photophobia, ocular allergic reactions, lid reactions, conjunctivitis.

**INTERACTIONS:** Acid-base disturbances reported with oral carbonic anhydrase inhibitors, caution with high-dose salicylates. Avoid oral carbonic anhydrase inhibitors due to additive effects. Wait 10 min before using another ophthalmic drug.

**PREGNANCY:** Category C, not for use in nursing.

**MECHANISM OF ACTION:** Carbonic anhydrase inhibitor; inhibition of carbonic anhydrase in the ciliary processes of the eye decreases aqueous humor secretion, presumably by slowing the formation of bicarbonate ions with subsequent reduction in sodium and fluid transport. The result is a reduction in intraocular pressure (IOP).

**PHARMACOKINETICS: Distribution:** Plasma protein binding (33%). **Metabolism:** Metabolites: N-desethyl. **Elimination:** Urine (unchanged, metabolite).

## NURSING CONSIDERATIONS

**Assessment:** Assess for sulfonamide hypersensitivity reaction, acute angle-closure glaucoma, renal/hepatic dysfunction, pregnancy/nursing status, and possible drug interactions.

**Monitoring:** Monitor for sulfonamide hypersensitivity reactions (eg, Stevens-Johnson syndrome, toxic epidermal necrolysis, fulminant hepatic necrosis, agranulocytosis, aplastic anemia, blood dyscrasias). If using chronically, monitor for ocular reactions such as conjunctivitis and lid reactions; d/c therapy and evaluate patient if such reactions occur. Monitor for bacterial keratitis if using multiple dose container. Monitor for choroidal detachment following filtration procedures.

**Patient Counseling:** Advise to d/c and notify physician if allergic/ocular reactions occur. Instruct to contact physician if have ocular surgery or develop an intercurrent ocular condition (eg, trauma, infection). Instruct to avoid allowing tip of dispensing container to contact eye or surrounding structures. Inform that if container becomes contaminated, serious damage to the eye and loss of vision may result. Instruct to remove contact lenses and reinsert 15 min after administration. Separate use by 10 min if using >1 topical ophthalmic drug.

**Administration:** Ocular route. **Storage:** 15-30°C (59-86°F); protect from light.

# TRUVADA RX

tenofovir disoproxil fumarate - emtricitabine (Gilead)

T

**Lactic acidosis and severe hepatomegaly with steatosis, including fatal cases, reported with nucleoside analogs alone or with concomitant antiretrovirals. Severe acute exacerbations of hepatitis B (HBV) reported in patients coinfected with HBV and HIV-1 upon d/c of therapy. Monitor hepatic function closely for at least several months in patients who are coinfected with HIV-1 and HBV. If appropriate, initiation of anti-HBV therapy may be warranted.**

**THERAPEUTIC CLASS:** Nucleoside analog combination

**INDICATIONS:** Treatment of HIV-1 infection in combination with other antiretrovirals.

**DOSAGE:** *Adults:* ≥18 years: CrCl ≥50mL/min: 1 tab qd. CrCl 30-49mL/min: 1 tab q48h.

**HOW SUPPLIED:** Tab: (Emtricitabine-Tenofovir Disoproxil Fumarate ) 200mg-300mg

**WARNINGS/PRECAUTIONS:** Obesity and prolonged nucleoside exposure may be risk factors for lactic acidosis and severe hepatomegaly with steatosis.

Caution in patients with risk factors for liver disease. Suspend therapy in any patients who develop clinical or laboratory findings suggestive of lactic acidosis or pronounced hepatotoxicity. Test for HBV infection before initiating therapy; safety and efficacy has not been established with coinfection. Avoid in patients with CrCl <30mL/min or patients requiring hemodialysis. Renal impairment, including cases of acute renal failure and Fanconi syndrome, reported. All patients should have CrCl calculated prior to and during therapy as clinically appropriate. Monitor Sr phosphorus in patients at risk for renal impairment. May decrease bone mineral density; monitor patients with history of pathologic bone fracture or who are at risk for osteopenia. Possible redistribution/accumulation of body fat. Immune reconstitution syndrome reported. Carefully monitor patients utilizing a triple nucleoside-only regimen and consider treatment modification. Caution in elderly.

**ADVERSE REACTIONS:** Diarrhea, nausea, fatigue, sinusitis, upper respiratory tract infections, nasopharyngitis, headache, dizziness, depression, insomnia, rash.

**INTERACTIONS:** May increase levels of didanosine (ddI); caution when coadministering, monitor for ddI-associated adverse effects and d/c if these develop. Atazanavir (ATV) and lopinavir/ritonavir (LPV/r) may increase tenofovir concentrations; monitor for associated adverse effects. ATV without ritonavir should not be coadministered. Coadministration with drugs eliminated by active tubular secretion may increase levels of emtricitabine, tenofovir or the coadministered drug (eg, acyclovir, adefovir dipivoxil, cidofovir, ganciclovir, valacyclovir, valganciclovir). Drugs that decrease renal function may increase concentrations of emtricitabine and/or tenofovir; avoid with concurrent or recent use of a nephrotoxic agent. Do not coadminister with Atripla, Emtriva or Viread and other drugs containing lamivudine. Do not give with adefovir dipivoxil. See PI for complete information.

**PREGNANCY:** Category B, not for use in nursing.

**MECHANISM OF ACTION:** Emtricitabine: Synthetic nucleoside analog of cytidine. Inhibits activity of HIV-1 reverse transcriptase (RT) by competing with natural substrate deoxycytidine 5'-triphosphate and by being incorporated into nascent viral DNA, which results in chain termination. Tenofovir disoproxil: Acyclic nucleoside phosphonate diester analog of adenosine monophosphate. Inhibits activity of HIV-1 RT by competing with the natural substrate deoxyadenosine 5'-triphosphate and after incorporation into DNA, by DNA chain termination.

**PHARMACOKINETICS: Absorption:** Emtricitabine: Rapid. Bioavailability (92%), $C_{max}$=1.8mcg/mL, $T_{max}$=1-2 hrs, AUC=10mcg•h/mL. Tenofovir disoproxil: Bioavailability (25%), $C_{max}$=0.3mcg/mL, $T_{max}$=1 hr, AUC=2.29mcg•h/mL. **Distribution:** Emtricitabine: Plasma protein binding (<4%). Tenofovir disoproxil: Plasma protein binding (<0.7%). **Elimination:** Emtricitabine: Urine (86%); $T_{1/2}$=10 hrs. Tenofovir disoproxil: (IV) Urine (70-80%); $T_{1/2}$=17 hrs.

## NURSING CONSIDERATIONS

**Assessment:** Assess for risk factors for lactic acidosis, liver disease, HBV status, renal impairment, history of pathologic bone fracture or risk of osteopenia, pregnancy/nursing status and for possible drug interactions. Obtain baseline CrCl.

**Monitoring:** Monitor for signs/symptoms of lactic acidosis, hepatomegaly with steatosis, new onset or worsening renal impairment, decreases in bone mineral density, redistribution/accumulation of body fat, and for immune reconstitution syndrome. In patients coinfected with HBV, upon d/c of therapy, monitor hepatic function closely and monitor for signs/symptoms of acute exacerbation of hepatitis B. Monitor CrCl and monitor Sr phosphorus in patients at risk for renal impairment.

**Patient Counseling:** Inform that therapy is not cure for HIV, does not reduce risk of transmission of HIV and that opportunistic infections may develop. Advise of risks and benefits of therapy and counsel to continue to practice safe sex and to use latex or polyurethane condoms. Advise to never reuse or share needles. Inform that it is important to follow regular dosing schedule and to avoid missing doses. Instruct to seek medical attention if symptoms of lactic acidosis, hepatotoxicity, exacerbation of HBV, renal impairment, fat redistribution/accumulation or immune reconstitution syndrome occur.

**Administration:** Oral route. **Storage:** 25°C (77°F), excursions permitted to 15-30°C (59-86°F).

## TUSSIONEX PENNKINETIC 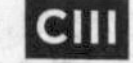

hydrocodone polistirex - chlorpheniramine polistirex (UCB)

**THERAPEUTIC CLASS:** Opioid antitussive/antihistamine

**INDICATIONS:** Relief of cough and upper respiratory symptoms associated with allergy and cold.

**DOSAGE:** *Adults:* ≥12 yrs: 5mL q12h. Max: 10mL/24 hrs.
*Pediatrics:* 6-11 yrs: 2.5mL q12h. Max: 5mL/24 hrs.

**HOW SUPPLIED:** Sus, Extended-Release: (Chlorpheniramine-Hydrocodone) 8mg-10mg/5mL

**CONTRAINDICATIONS:** Should not be used in children less than 6 years of age due to risk of fatal respiratory depression.

**WARNINGS/PRECAUTIONS:** May produce dose-related respiratory depression. Caution with pulmonary disease, post-surgery, head injury, intracranial lesions or pre-existing increase in ICP, narrow-angle glaucoma, asthma, BPH, elderly, debilitated, impaired hepatic/renal functions, hypothyroidosis, Addison's disease or urethral stricture. May mask acute abdominal conditions and the clinical course of head injuries. May cause obstructive bowel disease. Consider risk/benefit ratio in pediatrics, especially with croup. Impairment of mental and physical performance.

**ADVERSE REACTIONS:** Sedation, drowsiness, lethargy, anxiety, dysphoria, euphoria, dizziness, psychotic dependence, rash, pruritus, N/V, ureteral spasm, urinary retention, respiratory depression, dryness of the pharynx, tightness of the chest.

**INTERACTIONS:** Additive CNS depression with narcotics, antipsychotics, antianxiety agents, and alcohol. Increased effect of antidepressant or hydrocodone with MAOIs or TCAs. Concurrent anticholinergics may cause paralytic ileus.

**PREGNANCY:** Category C, not for use in nursing.

**MECHANISM OF ACTION:** Hydrocodone: Opioid antitussive/antihistamine; not established. Suspected to act directly on cough center. Chlorpheniramine: $H_1$-receptor antagonist; possesses anticholinergic and sedative activity. Prevents released histamine from dilating capillaries and causing edema of the respiratory mucosa.

**PHARMACOKINETICS: Absorption:** Hydrocodone: $C_{max}$=22.8ng/mL, $T_{max}$=3.4 hrs. Chlorpheniramine: $C_{max}$=58.4ng/mL, $T_{max}$=6.3 hrs. **Elimination:** Hydrocodone: $T_{1/2}$=4 hrs. Chlorpheniramine: $T_{1/2}$=16 hrs.

### NURSING CONSIDERATIONS

**Assessment:** Assess that patient is ≥6 yrs and females are not nursing. Assess use with pulmonary disease, depressed ventilatory functions, post-op patients, presence of head injury, intracranial lesions, increased intracranial pressure, acute abdominal conditions, elderly/debilitated, severe hepatic/renal impairment, hypothyroidism, Addison's disease, prostatic hypertrophy, urethral stricture, and during pregnancy. Assess for drug interactions.

**Monitoring:** Monitor for signs/symptoms of respiratory depression and development of obstructive bowel disease.

**Patient Counseling:** Inform medication may produce drowsiness and impair mental/physical abilities; use caution when performing hazardous tasks (eg, operating machinery/driving). Instruct not to dilute with fluids or mix with other drugs.

**Administration:** Oral route. Shake well before use. **Storage:** 20-25°C (68-77°F); excursions permitted to 15-30°C (59-86°F). Dispense in a well-closed container.

## TWINJECT RX

epinephrine (Verus)

**THERAPEUTIC CLASS:** Sympathomimetic catecholamine

**INDICATIONS:** Emergency treatment of severe allergic reactions (type 1) including anaphylaxis to insect stings or bites, allergens, foods, drugs, diagnostic testing substances, as well as idiopathic or exercise-induced anaphylaxis.

**DOSAGE:** *Adults:* Administer SQ or IM into thigh. 15-30kg: (Twinject 0.15mg) 0.15mg. May repeat if needed. ≥30kg: (Twinject 0.3mg) 0.3mg. May repeat if needed.

*Pediatrics:* Administer SQ or IM into thigh. 15-30kg: (Twinject 0.15mg) 0.15mg. May repeat if needed. ≥30kg: (Twinject 0.3mg) 0.3mg. May repeat if needed.

**HOW SUPPLIED:** Inj: (Twinject 0.15mg, Twinject 0.3mg) 1mg/mL

**WARNINGS/PRECAUTIONS:** Inject into anterolateral aspect of thigh; avoid injecting into hands, feet, or buttock. Avoid IV use. Contains sodium bisulfite. Caution with cardiac arrhythmias, coronary artery or organic heart disease, or HTN. May precipitate/aggravate angina pectoris or produce ventricular arrhythmias with coronary insufficiency or ischemic heart disease. Light-sensitive; store in tube provided.

**ADVERSE REACTIONS:** Anxiety, apprehensiveness, restlessness, tremor, weakness, dizziness, sweating, palpitations, pallor, N/V, headache, respiratory difficulties, HTN.

**INTERACTIONS:** Monitor for cardiac arrhythmias with cardiac glycosides or diuretics. Effects may be potentiated by TCAs, MAOIs, levothyroxine, and certain antihistamines (notably chlorpheniramine, tripelennamine, diphenhydramine). Cardiostimulating and bronchodilating effects antagonized by β-adrenergic blockers (eg, propranolol). Vasoconstricting and hypertensive effects antagonized by α-adrenergic blockers (eg, phentolamine). Ergot alkaloids and phenothiazines may reverse pressor effects.

**PREGNANCY:** Category C, safety in nursing not known.

**MECHANISM OF ACTION:** Acts on α- and β-adrenergic receptors.

### NURSING CONSIDERATIONS

**Assessment:** Assess for arrhythmias, ischemic/organic heart disease, HTN, DM, hyperthyroidism, pregnancy status, Parkinson's disease, and drug interactions (eg, medications that may sensitize heart to arrhythmia such as digitalis).

**Monitoring:** Monitor BP, HR, blood glucose, signs of cerebral hemorrhage, ventricular arrhythmia, HTN, and anginal pain.

**Patient Counseling:** Inform about side effects of therapy (eg, increased pulse rate, sense of forceful heartbeat, palpitations, throbbing headache, pallor, anxiety, shakiness). Side effects may subside rapidly, especially with rest, quiet, and recumbency but may be severe or persistent with HTN or hyperthyroidism. Never inject into buttocks or by IV route.

**Administration:** IM or SQ route. Inject into anterolateral administration.
**Storage:** 20-25°C (68-77°F); excursions permitted to 15-30°C (59-86°F). Protect from light. Avoid freezing or refrigeration. Discard if discolored.

## TWINRIX RX

hepatitis A vaccine (inactivated) - hepatitis B (recombinant) (GlaxoSmithKline)

**THERAPEUTIC CLASS:** Vaccine

**INDICATIONS:** Active immunization against hepatitis A virus and hepatitis B virus in patients ≥18 yrs of age.

**DOSAGE:** *Adults:* ≥18 yrs: 3-Dose Schedule: 1mL IM in deltoid region at 0, 1, and 6 months. Alternative 4-Dose Schedule: 1 mL IM in deltoid region on Days 0, 7, and 21-30, followed by booster dose at 12 months.

**HOW SUPPLIED:** Inj: (Hepatitis A-Hepatitis B) 720 ELISA U-20mcg/mL

**CONTRAINDICATIONS:** Hypersensitivity to monovalent hepatitis A or B vaccines or any component, including yeast and neomycin.

**WARNINGS/PRECAUTIONS:** Anaphylaxis/anaphylactoid reactions reported; have epinephrine (1:1000) and other appropriate agents available. Hepatitis A and B have long incubation periods, so vaccine may be ineffective with unrecognized hepatitis. May not prevent disease if protective antibody titers are not achieved. Delay vaccine with moderate to severe acute illness. Minor illnesses (eg, mild upper respiratory infection with or without low-grade fever) are not contraindications. Caution with bleeding disorders (eg, hemophilia, thrombocytopenia). Suboptimal response may occur in immunocompromised patients and when administered in gluteal region. Do not give intradermally or IV.

**ADVERSE REACTIONS:** Injection-site reactions (soreness, redness, swelling, induration), respiratory infection, headache, fatigue, diarrhea, nausea, vomiting, fever.

**INTERACTIONS:** Caution with anticoagulants. Immunosuppressive therapy may reduce response.

**PREGNANCY:** Category C, caution in nursing.

**MECHANISM OF ACTION:** Bivalent vaccine; produces immune response against hepatitis A and all known subtypes of hepatitis B virus.

## NURSING CONSIDERATIONS

**Assessment:** Assess current health status (immunosuppression, unrecognized hepatitis A or B infection), medical history, hypersensitivity reactions, adverse reactions related to previous vaccination history, potential benefits/risks, bleeding disorders (eg, hemophilia, thrombocytopenia), pregnancy/nursing status and possible drug interactions.

**Monitoring:** Monitor for possible anaphylaxis/anaphylactoid reactions, injection-site reactions and other possible adverse reactions. Monitor antibody titer.

**Patient Counseling:** Inform about potential benefits/risks. Inform that immunization will not cause hepatitis A or B infection. Report severe or unusual adverse reactions. Encourage to register pregnant women who received vaccination in the pregnancy registry. Counsel on importance of completing vaccination series.

**Administration:** IM route. Inspect for particulate matter, discoloration or cracks on vial/syringe; do not use if present. Shake well before use. **Storage:** 2-8°C (36-46°F). Do not freeze.

# TYGACIL RX

tigecycline (Wyeth)

T

**THERAPEUTIC CLASS:** Glycylcycline

**INDICATIONS:** Treatment of complicated skin and skin structure infections (cSSSI), complicated intra-abdominal infections (cIAI), and community-acquired bacterial pneumonia (CABP) caused by susceptible strains of indicated pathogens in patients ≥18 yrs.

**DOSAGE:** *Adults:* Initial: 100mg IV over 30-60 min then 50mg q12h over 30-60 min for 5-14 days (cSSSI/cIAI) and for 7-14days (CABP). Severe Hepatic Impairment (Child-Pugh C): 100mg IV over 30-60 min then 25mg q12h.

**HOW SUPPLIED:** Inj: 50mg/5mL, 50mg/10mL [vial]

**WARNINGS/PRECAUTIONS:** Anaphylaxis/anaphylactoid reactions reported. Structurally similar to tetracyclines and may have similar adverse effects: photosensitivity, pseudotumor cerebri, pancreatitis, and anti-anabolic action (may lead to increased BUN, azotemia, acidosis, and hyperphosphatemia). Caution with known hypersensitivity to tetracyclines. May cause fetal harm and permanent tooth discoloration (yellow-gray-brown) when administered during tooth development (last half of pregnancy to 8 yrs). *Clostridium difficile*-associated diarrhea reported. Caution when used for cIAI secondary to clinical apparent intestinal perforations. May result in overgrowth of non-susceptible organisms, including fungi; monitor during therapy. Caution with hospital acquired pneumonia, liver associated toxicity, and severe hepatic impairment.

**ADVERSE REACTIONS:** N/V, diarrhea, abdominal pain, infection, fever, headache, HTN, thrombocythemia, anemia, hypoproteinemia, increased liver enzymes, anaphylaxis/anaphylactoid reactions, acute pancreatitis, hyperbilirubinemia, hepatic cholestasis, and jaundice.

**INTERACTIONS:** Decreased effectiveness of oral contraceptives. Monitor PT with warfarin.

**PREGNANCY:** Category D, caution in nursing.

**MECHANISM OF ACTION:** Glycylcycline; inhibits protein translation in bacteria by binding to the 30S ribosomal subunit and blocking entry of amino-acyl tRNA molecules into A site of the ribosome.

**PHARMACOKINETICS: Absorption:** IV infusion of variable doses resulted in different parameters. **Distribution:** $V_d$=7-9L/kg; plasma protein binding (71-89%). **Metabolism:** Liver. **Elimination:** Bile (primary), urine; $T_{1/2}$(100mg)=27.1 hrs.

## NURSING CONSIDERATIONS

**Assessment:** Assess for known hypersensitivity to tetracycline antibiotics, complicated intra-abdominal infections secondary to clinically apparent intestinal perforation. Document indications for therapy, culture and susceptibility testing, and possible drug interactions.

**Monitoring:** Monitor for signs/symptoms of hypersensitivity reactions (eg, anaphylaxis), PT, pancreatitis, photosensitivity, superinfection, *C. difficile*-associated diarrhea, vaginal candidiasis, benign intracranial HTN, LFTs, renal function, HTN, CBC with platelets and differential, hyperglycemia, hepatic impairment.

**Patient Counseling:** Inform of pregnancy risks (eg, fetal harm, discoloration of teeth) and photosensitivity reactions. Inform that therapy treats bacterial, not viral, infections. Take as directed; skipping doses or not completing full course of therapy may decrease effectiveness and increase resistance. May experience diarrhea; notify physician if watery/bloody stools, hypersensitivity reactions, superinfection, or photosensitivity develops.

**Administration:** IV route. Reconstituted solution should be yellow to orange in color; if not, discard solution. **Storage:** Room temperature for up to 24 hrs (reconstituted). Store refrigerated 2-8°C (36-46°F) up to 48 hrs following immediate transfer of reconstituted solution into IV bag.

# TYKERB RX

lapatinib (GlaxoSmithKline)

**Hepatotoxicity reported. Hepatotoxicity may be severe and deaths have been reported.**

**THERAPEUTIC CLASS:** Kinase inhibitor

**INDICATIONS:** Treatment of advanced or metastatic breast cancer, in combination with capecitabine, whose tumors overexpress HER2 and who received prior therapy including an anthracycline, a taxane, and trastuzumab. In combination with letrozole for the treatment of postmenopausal women with hormone receptor positive metastatic breast cancer that overexpresses the HER2 receptor, for whom hormonal therapy is indicated.

**DOSAGE:** *Adults:* HER2 Positive Metastatic Breast Cancer: Usual: 1250mg qd on Days 1-21 continuously with capecitabine 2000mg/m²/day (2 doses 12 hrs apart) on Days 1-14 in a repeating 21-day cycle. Do not double the dose the next day, if a day's dose is missed. Continue treatment until disease progressess or unacceptable toxicity occurs. Take capecitabine with food or within 30 min after food. Hormone Receptor Positive, HER2 Positive Metastatic Breast Cancer: Usual: 1500mg qd continuously with letrozole 2.5mg qd. Dividing daily dosing not recommended. ≥Grade 2 Left Ventricular Ejection Fraction (LVEF): D/C dose. If LVEF recovers to normal and asymptomatic after 2 weeks, restart at 1000mg/day with capecitabine and 1250mg/day with letrozole. Hepatic Impairment (Child-Pugh Class C): Reduce dose from 1250mg/day to 750mg/day (HER2 positive metastatic breast cancer) or from 1500mg/day to 1000mg/day (hormone receptor positive, HER2 positive breast cancer). Concomitant Strong CYP3A4 Inhibitors: Reduce dose to 500mg/day. Concomitant Strong CYP3A4 Inducers: Titrate gradually from 1250mg/day up to 4500mg/day (HER2 positive metastatic breast cancer) and 1500mg/day up to 5500mg/day (hormone receptor positive, HER2 positive breast cancer) based on tolerability. ≥Grade 2 NCI CTCAE Toxicity: D/C or interrupt dose and restart with 1250mg/day when toxicity <Grade 1. Restart at 1000mg/day (with capecitabine) or 1250mg/day (with letrozole) if toxicity recurs. Take at least 1 hr before or after a meal.

**HOW SUPPLIED:** Tab: 250mg

**WARNINGS/PRECAUTIONS:** Decreased LVEF reported; confirm normal LVEF prior to therapy and evaluate during treatment. Caution in patients with conditions that may impair left ventricular function. Monitor LFTs prior to initiation of treatment, every 4-6 weeks during therapy, and as clinically indicated. Reduce dose with severe pre-existing hepatic impairment. Diarrhea including severe diarrhea reported; manage with antidiarrheals, replace electrolytes/fluids, and consider interrupting or d/c therapy if severe diarrhea occurs. QT prolongation observed. Caution with hypokalemia/hypomagnesemia, and congenital long QT syndrome; correct hypokalemia/hypomagnesemia prior to administration. Associated with interstitial lung disease and pneumonitis in monotherapy or in combination with other chemotherapies; d/c if pulmonary symptoms indicative of interstitial lung disease/pneumonitis ≥Grade 3 is experienced. May cause fetal harm.

**ADVERSE REACTIONS:** Diarrhea, N/V, stomatitis, dyspepsia, palmar-plantar erythrodysesthesia, rash, dry skin, mucosal inflammation, pain in extremity, back pain, dyspnea, insomnia, fatigue, anorexia, asthenia.

**INTERACTIONS:** Caution with CYP3A4 or CYP2C8 substrates; consider dose reduction. Avoid with strong CYP3A4 inhibitors (eg, ketoconazole, itraconazole, clarithromycin, atazanavir, indinavir, nefazodone, nelfinavir, ritonavir, saquinavir, telithromycin, voriconazole) and inducers (eg, dexamethasone, phenytoin, carbmazepine, rifampin, rifabutin, rifapentin, phenobarbital, St. John's wort); if unavoidable, consider dose reduction with concomitant CYP3A4 inhibitors, and gradual dose increase with concomitant CYP3A4 inducers. May increase plasma concentrations with grapefruit; avoid coadministration. Caution with concomitant use of anti-arrhythmic medications or medications which lead to QT prolongation and with cumulative high-dose anthracycline therapy. May increase concentrations with P-glycoprotein inhibitors. May increase concentrations of P-glycoprotein substrates and paclitaxel.

**PREGNANCY:** Category D, not for use in nursing.

**MECHANISM OF ACTION:** Kinase inhibitor; inhibits intracellular tyrosine kinase domains of both Epidermal Growth Factor Receptor (EGFR) and Human Epidermal Receptor Type 2 (HER2) receptors.

**PHARMACOKINETICS: Absorption**: Incomplete and variable. $C_{max}$=2.43mcg/mL, $T_{max}$=4 hrs, AUC=36.2mcg•hr/mL. **Distribution**: Plasma protein binding (>99%). **Metabolism**: CYP3A4, CYP3A5. **Elimination**: Feces (27%), urine (<2%); $T_{1/2}$(single dose, repeated dose)=14.2 hrs, 24 hrs.

T

## NURSING CONSIDERATIONS

**Assessment:** Assess for severe hepatic impairment, decreased LVEF or conditions which may impair left ventricular function, QT prolongation, hypokalemia, hypomagnesemia, pregnancy/nursing status, and for possible drug interactions. Obtain baseline LVEF, LFTs, serum $K^+$, and magnesium levels.

**Monitoring:** Monitor for signs/symptoms of hepatotoxicity, diarrhea, interstital lung disease, hypokalemia, hypomagnesemia, and for QT prolongation. Monitor LVEF. Monitor LFTs (transaminases, bilirubin, and alkaline phosphatase) every 4-6 weeks during therapy and as clinically indicated.

**Patient Counseling:** Advise to notify physician if SOB, palpitations, fatigue, persistent cough, or diarrhea occurs. Advise to report use of any Rx/OTC drugs or herbal products. Inform to avoid grapefruit products. Instruct to take at least 1 hr before or 1 hr after a meal; take capecitabine with food or within 30 min after food. Instruct to take once daily and inform that dividing daily dose is not recommended.

**Administration:** Oral route. **Storage**: 25°C (77°F); excursions permitted to 15-30°C (59-86°F).

## TYLENOL WITH CODEINE

CIII

codeine phosphate - acetaminophen (Ortho-McNeil)

**THERAPEUTIC CLASS:** Opioid analgesic

**INDICATIONS:** Relief of mild to moderately severe pain.

**DOSAGE:** *Adults:* (Sol) Usual: 15mL PO q4h prn. (Tab) Usual: 15-60mg codeine/dose, 300-1000mg APAP/dose up to q4h prn. Adjust according to severity of pain and response of the patient. Max: 360mg codeine/day, 4g APAP/day.
*Pediatrics:* (Sol) Usual: 0.5mg/kg/dose. 7-12 yrs: 10mL PO tid-qid. 3-6 yrs: 5mL PO tid-qid. Adjust according to severity of pain and response of the patient.

**HOW SUPPLIED:** (APAP-Codeine) Elix/Sol (generic): (CV) 120mg-12mg/5mL; Tab: (#3, CIII) 300mg-30mg, (#4, CIII) 300mg-60mg

**WARNINGS/PRECAUTIONS:** Respiratory depressant effects may be exacerbated with head injury or increased ICP. May obscure head injuries, acute abdominal conditions. Potential for physical dependence and tolerance. Caution in the elderly, debilitated, severe hepatic or renal dysfunction, hypothyroidism, Addison's disease, prostatic hypertrophy, or urethral stricture. Tab contains sodium metabisulfite; may cause allergic-type reactions including anaphylactic symptoms and life-threatening or less severe asthmatic episodes in certain susceptible patients. Extreme sleepiness, confusion or shallow breathing may occur with ultra-rapid metabolizers of codeine; choose the lowest effective dose for the shortest period of time.

**ADVERSE REACTIONS:** Drowsiness, lightheadedness, dizziness, sedation, SOB, N/V.

**INTERACTIONS:** May enhance the effects of other narcotic analgesics, alcohol, general anesthetics, tranquilizers (eg, chlordiazepoxide), sedative-hypnotics, or other CNS depressants causing increased CNS depression.

**PREGNANCY:** Category C, not for use in nursing.

**MECHANISM OF ACTION:** Codeine: Opiate analgesic and antitussive; produces centrally acting analgesic effects. APAP: Non-opiate, non-salicylate analgesic and antipyretic; produces peripherally acting analgesic effects.

**PHARMACOKINETICS: Absorption:** Rapid; $T_{max}$=2 hrs. **Distribution:** Codeine: Rapid; to liver, spleen and kidneys. Crosses blood-brain barrier; found in fetal tissue and breast milk. APAP: Found in breast milk. **Metabolism:** APAP: Liver (conjugation). **Elimination:** Codeine: Urine (90%, parent and metabolites); $T_{1/2}$=2.9 hrs. APAP: Urine (85%); $T_{1/2}$=1.25-3 hrs.

### NURSING CONSIDERATIONS

**Assessment:** Assess for head injury or other intracranial lesions, presence of increased ICP, acute abdominal conditions, asthma, hypersensitivity to sulfite and other ingredients of the formulation, presence of renal/hepatic impairment, hypothyroidism, urethral stricture, Addison's disease, prostatic hypertrophy, pregnancy/nursing status, and possible drug interactions.

**Monitoring:** Monitor for signs/symptoms of respiratory depression, elevations in CSF pressure, drowsiness, allergic type reactions (eg, anaphylaxis), elevations in serum amylase levels, medication abuse, and medication dependence. Monitor hepatic/renal function with severe hepatic/renal disease.

**Patient Counseling:** Inform that drug may be habit-forming; take only for as long as prescribed, in amounts prescribed, and no more frequently than prescribed. Caution to avoid performing hazardous tasks (eg, operating machinery/driving) while on therapy. Counsel to avoid alcohol and other CNS depressants during therapy. Counsel about possible adverse events if used during pregnancy/nursing.

**Administration:** Oral route. **Storage:** (Sol) 15-30°C (59-86°F); (Tab) 20-25°C (68-77°F). Do not refrigerate. Dispense in tight, light-resistant container.

## TYLOX CII

oxycodone HCl - acetaminophen (Ortho-Mcneil/Janssen)

**OTHER BRAND NAMES:** Roxilox (Roxane)

**THERAPEUTIC CLASS:** Opioid analgesic

**INDICATIONS:** Relief of moderate to moderately severe pain.

**DOSAGE:** *Adults:* Usual: 1 cap q6h prn. Dosage should be adjusted according to the severity of pain and patient's response.

**HOW SUPPLIED:** Cap: (Oxycodone-APAP) 5mg-500mg

**WARNINGS/PRECAUTIONS:** Contains sulfites; may cause allergic-type reactions including anaphylactic symptoms and life-threatening or less severe asthmatic episodes. Sulfite sensitivity is seen more frequently in asthmatic people. Can produce drug dependence; has the potential for being abused. Psychic dependence, physical dependence and tolerance may develop; caution should be exercised. May increase respiratory depressant effects and CSF pressure in presence of head injury. May obscure the diagnosis or clinical course when have acute abdominal conditions. Caution in elderly, debilitated, severe hepatic or renal dysfunction, hypothyroidism, Addison's disease, prostatic hypertrophy, or urethral stricture. Inappropriate for intractable/severe pain. May result in some degree of respiratory depression in the newborn and mother.

**ADVERSE REACTIONS:** Lightheadedness, dizziness, sedation, N/V, allergic reactions, euphoria, dysphoria, constipation, skin rashes, pruritus.

**INTERACTIONS:** Additive CNS depression with alcohol, tranquilizers, sedative-hypnotics, narcotic analgesics, general anesthetics, phenothiazines, antipsychotics, antianxiety agents, other CNS depressants. May produce paralytic ileus with anticholinergics.

**PREGNANCY:** Category C, caution in nursing.

**MECHANISM OF ACTION:** Oxycodone: Narcotic analgesic. Produces similiar action to morphine, prominently in CNS and smooth muscle organs. Produces analgesia and sedative effects. APAP: Nonopiate, nonsalicylate analgesic and antipyretic.

### NURSING CONSIDERATIONS

**Assessment:** Assess for sulfite sensitivity, history of asthma, presence of head injury or other intracranial lesions, acute abdominal conditions, age, presence of debilitation, hepatic/renal impairment, hypothyroidism, Addison's disease, prostatic hypertrophy or urethral stricture, pregnancy/nursing status, and possible drug interactions.



**Monitoring:** Monitor for signs/symptoms of hypersensitivity reactions (eg, anaphylaxis), asthmatic episodes, sulfite sensitivity, respiratory depression, elevations in CSF pressure, respiratory depression, drug dependence, tolerance and drug abuse.

**Patient Counseling:** Instruct to report any adverse reactions (eg, allergic reactions, respiratory depression). May impair mental/physical abilities required for the performance of potentially hazardous tasks (eg, operating machinery/driving); caution patient accordingly. May produce dependence and has potential for abuse.

**Administration:** Oral route. **Storage:** 15-30°C (59-86°F). Protect from moisture. Dispense in tight, light-resistant container.

# TYSABRI RX

natalizumab (Elan)

**Increases risk of progressive multifocal leukoencephalopathy (PML). Because of risk of PML, natalizumab is available only through a special restricted distribution program called the TOUCH™ Prescribing Program. Administer only to patients who are enrolled in and meet all conditions of the TOUCH™ Prescribing Program. Monitor patients for any new signs or symptoms that may be suggestive of PML. Dosing should be withheld immediately at the first sign or symptom suggestive of PML.**

**THERAPEUTIC CLASS:** Monoclonal antibody/VCAM-1 blocker

**INDICATIONS:** Treatment of patients with relapsing forms of multiple sclerosis (MS) to delay the accumulation of physical disability and reduce the frequency of clinical exacerbations. Treatment for inducing and maintaining clinical response and remission in adult patients with moderately to severely active Crohn's disease (CD) with evidence of inflammation who have had an inadequate response to, or are unable to tolerate, conventional CD therapies and TNF-α inhibitors.

**DOSAGE:** *Adults:* MS/CD: 300mg IV infusion over 1 hr every 4 weeks. (CD) D/C therapy if no therapeutic benefit by 12 weeks, if patient cannot be tapered off corticosteroids within 6 months, or in patients who require additional steroid use that exceeds 3 months within a calendar year to control their CD.

**HOW SUPPLIED:** Inj: 300mg/15mL

**CONTRAINDICATIONS:** Progressive multifocal leukoencephalopathy (PML).

**WARNINGS/PRECAUTIONS:** Possible hypersensitivity reactions, including anaphylaxis; d/c and do not re-treat. Liver injury reported. D/C if evidence of jaundice or abnormal LFT. Induces increases in circulating lymphocytes, monocytes, eosinophils, basophils, and nucleated RBCs. Additional cases of PML reported in patients with MS who are not receiving concomitant immunomodulatory therapy. Avoid in patients treated with chronic immunosuppressants or immunomodulatory therapy, or serious medical conditions resulting in significantly compromised immune system function. Immune reconstitution inflammatory syndrome (IRIS) reported with PML. May increase risk for infections.

**ADVERSE REACTIONS:** Headache, fatigue, urinary tract infection (UTI), depression, lower/upper respiratory tract infection, arthralgia, abdominal discomfort, rash, gastroenteritis, vaginitis, urinary urgency/frequency, irregular menstruation/dysmenorrhea, dermatitis, abnormal LFTs.

**INTERACTIONS:** Avoid with concomitant immunosuppressants (eg, 6-mercaptopurine, azathioprine, cyclosporine, or methotrexate) or inhibitors of TNF-α. Taper corticosteroids in CD patients before starting therapy. Concurrent use with antineoplastic, immunosuppressive, or immunomodulating agents may further increase risk of infections, including PML and other opportunistic infections.

**PREGNANCY:** Category C, not for use in nursing.

**MECHANISM OF ACTION:** Recombinant humanized IgG4k monoclonal antibody; not established. Binds to α4-subunit of α4β1 and α4β7 integrins expressed on surface of all leukocytes except neutrophils. Inhibits α4-mediated adhesion of leukocytes to their counter-receptor(s).

**PHARMACOKINETICS: Absorption:** (MS) $C_{max}$=110mcg/mL, $T_{max}$= 24 weeks; (CD) $C_{max}$=101mcg/mL, $T_{max}$= 16-24 weeks. **Distribution:** (MS) $V_d$=5.7L; (CD) $V_d$=5.2L. **Elimination:** (MS) $T_{1/2}$=11 days; (CD) $T_{1/2}$=10 days.

## NURSING CONSIDERATIONS

**Assessment:** Assess for risk of PML, history of chronic immunosuppressant or immunomodulatory therapy and immunocompromised status, drug hypersensitivity, and drug interactions. Perform MRI prior to initiating therapy in MS. Obtain baseline MRI in patients with CD.

**Monitoring:** Monitor for PML (eg, progressive weakness on one side of body, clumsiness, vision problems, changes in thinking, memory, and orientation leading to confusion and personality changes); a gadolinium-enhanced MRI scan of brain and CSF analysis for JC viral DNA recommended for diagnosis. Monitor for anaphylactic reactions, infections (eg, pneumonia, UTI), opportunistic infections, hepatotoxicity, and development of IRIS. Antibody testing recommended if presence of persistent antibodies suspected. Monitor CBC, LFTs, and bilirubin.

**Patient Counseling:** Inform about TOUCH™ Prescribing Program. Educate on risks/benefits. Instruct to report signs of infections, hypersensitivity reactions, liver toxicity. Counsel on importance of follow-up schedule (3 and 6 months after 1st infusion, then every 6 months). Instruct to contact their physician if symptoms suggestive of PML develop.

**Administration:** IV infusion. Refer to PI for dilution/administration instructions. **Storage:** 2-8°C (36-46°F). Administer within 8 hrs of preparation. Do not shake or freeze. Protect from light.

## Tyvaso RX

treprostinil (United Therapeutics)

**THERAPEUTIC CLASS:** Pulmonary and systemic vasodilator

**INDICATIONS:** Treatment of pulmonary arterial hypertension (PAH) in WHO Group I and NYHA Class III symptoms. To increase walk distance.

**DOSAGE:** *Adults:* Initial: 3 breaths (18mcg of treprostinil) qid. Reduce 1-2 breaths if not tolerated and subsequently increase to 3 breaths, as tolerated. Maint: increased by an additional 3 breaths at 1-2 week intervals, if tolerated. Usual max: 9 breaths (54mcg of treprostinil) qid.

**HOW SUPPLIED:** Sol: 0.6mg/mL [2.9mL]

**WARNINGS/PRECAUTIONS:** Caution use with underlying lung disease (eg, asthma, chronic obstructive pulmonary disease) and pulmonary infections; monitor carefully to detect worsening of lung disease and loss of drug effect. May produce symptomatic hypotension. Caution with hepatic or renal impairment. Increase risk of bleeding. Caution in elderly.

**ADVERSE REACTIONS:** Symptomatic hypotension, bleeding, cough, headache, throat irritation, nausea, flushing, syncope.

**PREGNANCY:** Category B, caution in nursing

**MECHANISM OF ACTION:** Prostacyclin analogue: pulmonary and systemic vasodilator; causes direct vasodilation of pulmonary and systemic arterial vascular beds. Inhibits platelet aggregation.

**PHARMACOKINETICS: Absorption:** $C_{max}$=0.91-1.32mg/mL, $T_{max}$=0.12-0.25 hrs, AUC=0.81-0.97mg/mL/hr. Absolute bioavailability: 18mcg (64%), 36mcg (72%). **Distribution:** plasma protein binding (91%)

### NURSING CONSIDERATIONS

T

**Assessment:** Assess for underlying lung disease or infections, hepatic/renal impairment, pregnancy/nursing status, possible drug interactions.

**Monitoring:** Monitor LFTs, renal function tests, bleeding time, blood pressure. Monitor for worsening of symptoms, and hypersensitivity reactions.

**Patient Counseling:** Counsel for proper administration process including dosing, set-up, operation, cleaning, and maintenance according to the instruction for use. Advise to avoid potential interruptions in drug delivery. Therapy should be resumed as soon as possible if treatment session is missed or interrupted. Advise to immediately rinse with water if in contact with skin or eyes. Notify healthcare professional if worsening of symptoms, hypotensive symptoms, bleeding or hypersensitivity reactions are experienced.

**Administration:** Oral route. If opened or transferred in a device, it should remain for no >1 day. Use within 7 days if foil pack is opened. **Storage:** 25°C (77°F); excursions permitted to 15-30°C (59-86°F). Protect from light

# TYZEKA RX

telbivudine (Novartis)

**Lactic acidosis and severe hepatomegaly with steatosis reported. D/C may result in severe acute exacerbations of hepatitis; monitor hepatic function closely for at least several months following d/c of therapy.**

**THERAPEUTIC CLASS:** Nucleoside analogue

**INDICATIONS:** Treatment of chronic hepatitis B.

**DOSAGE:** *Adults:* Usual: 600mg or 30mL qd. Dose Adjustment: CrCl ≥50mL/min: 600mg q24h or 30mL qd. CrCl 30-49mL/min: 600mg q48h or 20mL qd. CrCl <30mL/min (not requiring dialysis): 600mg q72h or 10mL qd. ESRD: 600mg q96h.
*Pediatrics:* ≥16 yrs: Usual: 600mg or 30mL qd. Dose Adjustment: CrCl ≥50mL/min: 600mg q24h or 30mL qd. CrCl 30-49mL/min: 600mg q48h or 20mL qd. CrCl <30mL/min (not requiring dialysis): 600mg q72h. ESRD: 600mg q96h.

**HOW SUPPLIED:** Tab: 600mg; Sol: 100mg/5mL(300mL)

**WARNINGS/PRECAUTIONS:** Myopathy/myositis, rhabdomyolysis and uncomplicated myalgia reported; interrupt therapy if myopathy suspected and d/c if myopathy diagnosed. Peripheral neuropathy reported; d/c if peripheral neuropathy confirmed. Caution in elderly. Oral solution contains sodium and should be used cautiously in patients with sodium-restricted diet.

**ADVERSE REACTIONS:** Abdominal distention and pain, arthralgia, back pain, cough, diarrhea, dizziness, dyspepsia, elevated ALT and blood creatinine kinase levels, fatigue, headache, maculopathy, myalgia, myopathy, nausea, pain, sore throat.

**INTERACTIONS:** Drugs that alter renal function may alter plasma concentrations of telbivudine. Risk of peripheral neuropathy reported with pegylated interferon alfa-2a and other interferons.

**PREGNANCY:** Category B, not for use in nursing.

**MECHANISM OF ACTION:** Thymidine nucleoside analogue; inhibits HBV DNA polymerase by competing with thymidine 5'-triphosphate and inhibits viral replication by incorporating into viral DNA causing DNA chain termination.

**PHARMACOKINETICS: Absorption:** $C_{max}$=3.69mcg/mL, $T_{max}$=2 hrs, AUC=26.1mcg•h/mL. **Distribution:** Plasma protein binding (3.3%). **Elimination:** Urine; $T_{1/2}$=40-49 hrs.

## NURSING CONSIDERATIONS

**Assessment:** Assess for renal/hepatic impairment, pregnancy/nursing status, and possible drug interactions. Check if patient on low-sodium diet.

**Monitoring:** Monitor LFTs periodically and for several months after d/c. Monitor for signs/symptoms of exacerbation of unexplained muscle pain, tenderness, weakness, HBV after d/c, hepatotoxicity, hypersensitivity reactions, and myopathy.

**Patient Counseling:** Inform of possibility of liver disease deterioration; not shown to reduce risk of HBV transmission to others through sexual contact or blood contamination. Advise not to change dose or d/c without consultation. If dose missed, instruct to take as soon as remembered and next dose at regular time. If almost time for next dose, skip missed dose (do not take 2 doses at same time). Advise to seek medical attention if symptoms of exacerbation, hepatotoxicity, hypersensitivity reactions, or myopathy (eg, myalgia, muscle tenderness, weakness) occur. Advise to register in the antiretroviral Pregnancy Registry (1-800-258-4263) if patient becomes pregnant while on medication. Inform that oral solution contains sodium; seek medical advice before use in patients with a low-sodium diet requirement.

**Administration:** Oral route. **Storage:** (Tab/Sol) 25°C (77°F); excursions permitted to 15-30°C (59-86°F). Avoid storage in damp places (eg, bathroom medicine cabinet or kitchen sink). (Sol) Use within two months after opening. Do not freeze.

T

## Uloric

**RX**

febuxostat (Takeda)

**THERAPEUTIC CLASS:** Xanthine oxidase inhibitor

**INDICATIONS:** Chronic management of hyperuricemia in patients w/ gout.

**DOSAGE:** *Adults:* Initial: 40mg qd. Range: 40-80mg qd. Serum Uric Acid (sUA) >6mg/dL After 2 Weeks at 40mg: 80mg qd.

**HOW SUPPLIED:** Tab: 40mg, 80mg

**CONTRAINDICATIONS:** Patients treated with azathioprine, mercaptopurine, or theophylline.

**WARNINGS/PRECAUTIONS:** May increase risk of gout flares; prophylactic treatment with NSAIDs or colchicine is recommended. Higher rate of CV thromboembolic events (eg, CV deaths, non-fatal MI, non-fatal strokes) vs. allopurinol reported; monitor for signs and symptoms of MI and stroke. Elevated serum transaminase levels observed; monitor LFTs periodically. Caution with severe hepatic impairment. Avoid with asymptomatic or secondary hyperuricemia (eg, malignant disease, Lesch-Nyhan syndrome).

**ADVERSE REACTIONS:** Liver function abnormalities, nausea, arthralgia, rash.

**INTERACTIONS:** See Contraindications. Concomitant use with xanthine oxidase substrates may increase plasma concentrations of these drugs, resulting in severe toxicity.

**PREGNANCY:** Category C, caution in nursing.

**MECHANISM OF ACTION:** Xanthine oxidase inhibitor; achieves therapeutic effect by decreasing serum uric acid.

**PHARMACOKINETICS: Absorption:** (40mg) $C_{max}$ = 1.6mcg/mL. (80mg) $C_{max}$ = 2.6mcg/mL. $T_{max}$=1-1.5 hrs. **Distribution:** $V_d$=50L; plasma protein binding (99.2%). **Metabolism:** Conjugation via uridine diphosphate glucuronosyltransferase (UGT), and oxidation via CYP450 enzymes. **Elimination:** Hepatic and renal pathways; Urine (49%), feces (45%); $T_{1/2}$=5-8 hrs.

### NURSING CONSIDERATIONS

**Assessment:** Assess for treatment with azathioprine, mercaptopurine, or theophylline, secondary/asymptomatic hyperuricemia, hepatic/renal impairment, possible drug interactions, and pregnancy/nursing status. Assess for sUA, LFTs, and ECG.

**Monitoring:** Monitor for sUA levels, LFTs, QTc interval, MI, and stroke.

**Patient Counseling:** May take without regard to food or antacid use. Counsel about potential benefits and risks. Inform that gout flares, elevated liver enzymes, and adverse CV events may occur. Counsel about concomitant prophylaxis with NSAIDs or colchicine for gout flares. Instruct to notify physician if rash, chest pain, SOB, or neurologic symptoms occur. Advise to inform physician of any other medications currently taking, including OTC drugs.

**Administration:** Oral route. **Storage:** Store at 25°C (77°F); excursions permitted to 15°-30°C (59°-86°F). Protect from light.



## Ultiva

**CII**

remifentanil HCl (Abbott)

**THERAPEUTIC CLASS:** Opioid analgesic

**INDICATIONS:** As an analgesic agent for use during the induction and maintenance of general anesthesia. For continuation as an analgesic into the immediate postoperative period in adults under the direct supervision of an anesthesia practitioner in a postoperative anesthesia care unit or intensive care setting. As an analgesic component of monitored anesthesia care in adults.

**DOSAGE:** *Adults:* Continuous IV Infusion: Induction: 0.5-1mcg/kg/min. Maint: 0.4mcg/kg with nitrous oxide 66%; 0.25mcg/kg with isoflurane (0.4-1.25 MAC); 0.25 with propofol (100-200mcg/kg/min). Post-Op Continuation:

0.1mcg/kg/min. CABG: Induction/Maint/Continuation: 1mcg/kg/min. Elderly (>65 yrs): Use 50% of adult dose. Titrate carefully.
*Pediatrics:* Anesthesia Maint: Continuous IV Infusion: 1-12 yrs: 0.25mcg/kg/min with halothane (0.3-1.5 MAC), sevoflurane (0.3-1.5 MAC, or isoflurane (0.4-1.5 MAC). Range: 0.05-1.3mcg/kg/min. Birth-2 months: 0.4mcg/kg/min. Range: 0.4-1mcg/kg/min.

**HOW SUPPLIED:** Inj: 1mg, 2mg, 5mg

**CONTRAINDICATIONS:** Epidural or intrathecal administration, hypersensitivity to fentanyl analogs.

**WARNINGS/PRECAUTIONS:** Administer only with infusion device. IV bolus administration should be used only during the maintenance of general anesthesia. Interruption of infusion will result in rapid offset of effect. Use associated with apnea and respiratory depression. Not for use in diagnostic or therapeutic procedures outside the monitored anesthesia care setting. Resuscitative and intubation equipment, oxygen, and opioid antagonist must be readily available. May cause skeletal muscle rigidity and is related to the dose and speed of administration. Do not administer into the same IV tubing with blood due to potential inactivation by nonspecific esterases in blood products. Continuously monitor vital signs and oxygenation. Bradycardia, hypotension, intraoperative awareness reported. Not recommended as sole agent for induction of anesthesia.

**ADVERSE REACTIONS:** N/V, hypotension, muscle rigidity, bradycardia, shivering, fever, dizziness, visual disturbances, respiratory depression, apnea.

**INTERACTIONS:** Synergism with thiopental, propofol, isoflurane, midazolam; reduce doses of these drugs by up to 75%.

**PREGNANCY:** Category C, caution in nursing.

**MECHANISM OF ACTION:** Opioid analgesic.

**PHARMACOKINETICS: Distribution**: $V_d$=100mL/kg, 350mL/kg (initial, steady-state), plasma protein binding (70%). **Metabolism**: Hydrolysis via nonspecific blood and tissue esterases to carboxylic acid metabolite. **Elimination**: $T_{1/2}$=10-20 min.

## NURSING CONSIDERATIONS

**Assessment:** Assess for pulmonary disease, decreased respiratory reserve, and possible drug interactions.

**Monitoring:** Monitor for cardiovascular depression (eg, bradycardia, hypotension), respiratory depression, muscle rigidity of neck and extremities, N/V, chills, arrhythmias, chest wall rigidity. Monitor vital signs routinely. Appropriate post-op monitoring should ensure adequate spontaneous breathing established and maintained prior to discharge.

**Patient Counseling:** Advise to use caution while performing potentially hazardous tasks (eg, operating machinery/driving). Counsel about side effects of drug and abuse potential.

**Administration:** IV infusion. Continuous infusions should only be administered using an infusion device. **Storage**: 2-25°C (36-77°F).

# ULTRACET — RX

tramadol HCl - acetaminophen (Ortho-McNeil)

U

**THERAPEUTIC CLASS:** Analgesic combination

**INDICATIONS:** Short-term (≤5 days) management of acute pain.

**DOSAGE:** *Adults:* 2 tabs q4-6h prn for 5 days or less. Max: 8 tabs/24 hrs. CrCl <30mL/min: Max: 2 tabs q12h. Elderly: Start at lower end of dosing range.

**HOW SUPPLIED:** Tab: (Tramadol-APAP) 37.5mg-325mg

**CONTRAINDICATIONS:** Acute intoxication with any of the following: alcohol, hypnotics, narcotics, centrally acting analgesics, opioids, or psychotropic drugs.

**WARNINGS/PRECAUTIONS:** Increased risk of convulsion in patients with history of seizures and epilepsy. Avoid use with suicidal, depressed or addiction-prone patients. Seizures and anaphylactic reactions reported. May complicate clinical assessment with acute abdominal conditions. Caution with risk of respiratory depression, increased intracranial pressure (ICP), or head injury. May impair mental or physical abilities. Avoid abrupt withdrawal and overdosage. Caution in elderly. Avoid use in opioid-dependent patients and with hepatic impairment.

**ADVERSE REACTIONS:** Constipation, diarrhea, nausea, somnolence, anorexia, increased sweating, dizziness.

**INTERACTIONS:** See Contraindications. Caution and reduce dose with CNS depressants (eg, alcohol, opioids, anesthetics, phenothiazines, tranquilizers, narcotics, sedative hypnotics, muscle relaxants); may increase risk of CNS and respiratory depression. May reduce analgesic effects with carbamazepine; not recommended. Possible digoxin toxicity and altered warfarin effects; monitor PT periodically. CYP2D6 inhibitors (eg, fluoxetine, paroxetine, amitriptyline) may inhibit metabolism of tramadol. CYP3A4 inhibitors (eg, ketoconazole, erythromycin) and CYP3A4 inducers (eg, rifampin, St. John's wort) may alter tramadol exposure. May potentiate seizure risk with MAOIs, SSRIs, naloxone (with overdose), TCAs, tricyclics (eg, cyclobenzaprine, promethazine), neuroleptics, other opioids, and drugs that lower seizure threshold. May cause serotonin syndrome with serotonergic agents (eg, SSRIs, SNRIs, TCAs, MAOIs, triptans) and drugs that impair metabolism of tramadol (CYP2D6, 3A4 inhibitors). Avoid alcohol and other tramadol- or APAP-containing products.

**PREGNANCY:** Category C, not for use in nursing.

**MECHANISM OF ACTION:** Tramadol: Centrally acting synthetic opioid analgesic; mechanism not fully understood. Binds to μ-opioid receptors and inhibits reuptake of norepinephrine and serotonin. APAP: Nonopiate, nonsalicylate analgesic.

**PHARMACOKINETICS: Absorption:** Tramadol: Bioavailability (75%), $T_{max}$=2 hrs, 3 hrs (M1). APAP: Small intestines; $T_{max}$=1 hr. **Distribution:** (IV) Tramadol: $V_d$=2.6L/kg (male), 2.9L/kg (female); found in breast milk (0.1%); plasma protein binding (20%). APAP: $V_d$=0.9L/kg; plasma protein binding (20%). **Metabolism:** Tramadol: CYP2D6, 3A4 (N- and O-demethylation, glucuronidation, or sulfation); M1 (active metabolite). APAP: CYP2E1, 1A2, 3A4 (glucuronidation, sulfation, oxidation). **Elimination:** Tramadol: $T_{1/2}$=5-6 hrs, 7 hrs (M1); urine (30%, unchanged), (60%, metabolites). APAP: $T_{1/2}$=2-3 hrs; urine (<9%, unchanged).

## NURSING CONSIDERATIONS

**Assessment:** Assess for acute intoxication, CNS/respiratory depression, seizures, serotonin syndrome, head trauma, metabolic disorders, CNS infection, acute abdominal conditions, increased ICP, drug abuse, opioid dependence, renal/hepatic impairment, pregnancy/nursing status, and possible drug interactions.

**Monitoring:** Monitor for signs/symptoms of seizures, serotonin syndrome, respiratory depression, withdrawal symptoms, hepatotoxicity, and hypersensitivity reactions.



**Patient Counseling:** Inform that drug may cause seizures and/or serotonin syndrome with concomitant use of serotonergic agents. Caution when taking tranquilizers, hypnotics, or other opiate-containing analgesics. Caution when driving and operating machinery. Instruct to avoid alcohol. Advise to seek medical attention if experience symptoms of seizures, respiratory depression, hypersensitivity reactions, hepatotoxicity, or withdrawal symptoms (eg, anxiety, sweating, insomnia, rigors). Warn not to exceed the recommended dose. Instruct to inform physician if pregnant or are trying to become pregnant.

**Administration:** Oral route. **Storage:** 25°C (77°F); excursions permitted to 15-30°C (59-86°F).

# Ultram RX

tramadol HCl (Ortho-McNeil)

**OTHER BRAND NAMES:** Ultram ER (PRICARA)

**THERAPEUTIC CLASS:** Central acting analgesic

**INDICATIONS:** Management of moderate to moderately severe pain.

**DOSAGE:** *Adults:* ≥17 yrs: (Tab) Initial: 25mg qam. Titrate: Increase by 25mg every 3 days to 25mg qid, then increase by 50mg every 3 days to 50mg qid. Usual: 50-100mg q4-6h as needed. Max: 400mg/day. Individualize dose. CrCl <30mL/min: Dose q12h. Max: 200mg/day. Cirrhosis: 50mg q12h. Elderly: Start at low end of dosing range. >75 yrs: Max: 300mg/day. ≥18 yrs: (Tab, ER) Initial: 100mg qd. Titrate: Increase by 100mg every 5 days. Max: 300mg/day. Elderly: Start at low end of dosing range.

**HOW SUPPLIED:** Tab: 50mg*; Tab, Extended-Release: 100mg, 200mg, 300mg *scored

**CONTRAINDICATIONS:** Any situation where opiods are contraindicated including acute intoxication with any of the following: alcohol, hypnotics, narcotics, centrally acting analgesics, opioids or psychotropic drugs.

**WARNINGS/PRECAUTIONS:** Seizures and anaphylactoid reactions reported. Do not prescribe for suicidal or addiction-prone patients. Caution with patients at risk for respiratory depression, with increased intracranial pressure (ICP), or head trauma. May complicate clinical assessment of acute abdominal conditions. Do not d/c abruptly. Adjust dose with renal/hepatic impairment and patients older than 75 yrs of age. Development of serotonin syndrome including mental status changes, autonomic instability, neuromuscular aberrations, and GI symptoms reported. May impair physical or mental abilities.

**ADVERSE REACTIONS:** Dizziness, N/V, constipation, headache, somnolence, sweating, asthenia, dyspepsia, dry mouth, diarrhea, CNS stimulation, pruritus.

**INTERACTIONS:** See Contraindications. Caution and reduce dose with CNS depressants (eg, alcohol, opioids, anesthetics, phenothiazines, tranquilizers, sedatives, hypnotics). Avoid with carbamazepine. Possible digoxin toxicity and altered warfarin effects. Increased risk of adverse events with CYP2D6 inhibitors (eg, quinidine, fluoxetine, paroxetine, amtriptyline), CYP3A4 inhibitors (eg, ketoconazole, erythromycin), TCAs and other tricyclic compounds (eg, cyclobenzaprine, promethazine, etc), other opioids, neuroleptics, and drugs that reduce seizure threshold. Caution with SSRIs, MAOIs, triptans, linezolid, lithium, or St. John's wort; increased risk of serotonin syndrome. Increased levels with quinidine.

**PREGNANCY:** Category C, not for use in nursing.

**MECHANISM OF ACTION:** Centrally acting synthetic opioid analgesic; not established. Binding of parent and M1 metabolite to μ-opioid receptors and weak inhibition reuptake of norepinephrine and serotonin.

**PHARMACOKINETICS: Absorption:** (100mg) Bioavailability (75%); $T_{max}$=2 hrs (drug), 3 hrs (M1). **Distribution:** $V_d$=2.6L/kg (male), 2.9L/kg (female); plasma protein binding (20%). **Metabolism:** Liver (extensive); through N-and O-demethylation and glucuronidation or sulfation pathways via CYP3A4, 2D6. M1 (active metabolite). **Elimination:** Urine: (30% unchanged), (60% as metabolite); $T_{1/2}$=6.3 hrs (drug), 7.4 hrs (M1).

## NURSING CONSIDERATIONS

**Assessment:** Assess for acute intoxication with alcohol, hypnotics, centrally acting analgesics, opioids, or psychotropic drugs. Assess for epilepsy, risk for seizure (eg, head trauma, metabolic disorders, alcohol and drug withdrawal, CNS infections), risk for respiratory depression, increased ICP, renal/hepatic impairment, pregnancy/nursing status, and possible drug interactions.

**Monitoring:** Monitor for anaphylactoid reactions (eg, pruritus, hives, bronchospasm, angioedema, toxic epidermal necrolysis and Stevens-Jonhson syndrome), respiratory/CNS depression, physical dependence/abuse, seizures, serotonin syndrome, withdrawal symptoms with abrupt d/c (eg, anxiety, sweating, insomnia, rigors, upper respiratory symptoms, diarrhea, piloerection and rarely, hallucinations).

**Patient Counseling:** Advise to use caution while performing hazardous tasks (operating machinery/driving). Do not take with alcohol, tranquilizers, or hypnotics. Notify physician if pregnant/nursing or planning to become pregnant.

**Administration:** Oral route. **Storage:** 25°C (77°F); excursions permitted to 15-30°C (59-86°F).

## ULTRAVATE **RX**

halobetasol propionate (Ranbaxy)

**THERAPEUTIC CLASS:** Corticosteroid

**INDICATIONS:** Relief of the inflammatory and pruritic manifestations of corticosteroid-responsive dermatoses.

**DOSAGE:** *Adults:* Apply qd-bid. Rub in gently and completely. Max: 50g/week.Limit treatment to 2 weeks.
*Pediatrics:* ≥12 yrs: Apply qd-bid. Rub in gently. Max: 50g/week.Limit treatment to 2 weeks.

**HOW SUPPLIED:** Cre, Oint: 0.05% [15g, 50g]

**WARNINGS/PRECAUTIONS:** Avoid face, groin, or axillae. Not for treatment of rosacea or perioral dermatitis. May produce reversible HPA axis suppression, manifestations of Cushing's syndrome, hyperglycemia, and glucosuria. Caution when applied to large surface areas or under occlusive dressings. Withdraw, reduce frequency or substitute to a less potent steroid if adrenal suppression noted. Use appropriate antifungal or antibacterial agent with dermatological infections; d/c until infection controlled. Pediatrics may be more susceptible to systemic toxicity. Striae, HPA axis suppression (low plasma cortisol, no response to ACTH stimulation), Cushing's syndrome, linear growth retardation, delayed weight gain and intracranial HTN (bulging fontanelles, headache, bilateral papilledema) reported in pediatrics. Not recommended in pediatrics <12 yrs. Avoid eyes. D/C if irritation occurs and institute appropriate therapy. Re-assess if no improvement after 2 weeks. D/C when control is acheived.

**ADVERSE REACTIONS:** Stinging, burning, itching, pustulation, erythema, skin atrophy, leukoderma, acne, secondary infection, urticaria, dry skin, miliaria, paresthesia, rash.

**PREGNANCY:** Category C, caution in nursing.

**MECHANISM OF ACTION:** Corticosteroid; possesses anti-inflammatory, antipruritic, and vasoconstrictive properties. Anti-inflammatory activity not established; suspected to act by induction of phospholipase $A_2$ inhibitory proteins called lipocortins. Lipocortins control biosynthesis of potent inflammation mediators (eg, prostaglandins, leukotrienes) by inhibiting release of their common precursor, arachidonic acid.

**PHARMACOKINETICS: Absorption:** Percutaneous; occlusion, inflammation and other disease states may increase absorption. **Distribution:** Systemically administered corticosteroids appear in breast milk.

U

### NURSING CONSIDERATIONS

**Assessment:** Assess for hypersensitivity, pregnancy/nursing status and for presence of concomitant skin infections. Assess that treatment is not for rosacea or perioral dermatitis.

**Monitoring:** Monitor for signs/symptoms of reversible HPA-axis suppression, Cushing's syndrome, hyperglycemia, glucosuria, treatment-site irritation, allergic contact dermatitis (eg, failure to heal), dermatological infections (eg, bacterial, fungal) and for hypersensitivity reactions. Monitor for glucocorticosteroid insufficiencies and treat appropriately. If applying to large area or to areas under occlusion, perform periodic monitoring for HPA-axis suppression using ACTH stimulation, AM plasma cortisol and urinary free cortisol tests. In pediatric patients, monitor for signs/symptoms of systemic toxicity, HPA-axis suppression (linear growth retardation, delayed weight gain), Cushing's syndrome and intracranial HTN. Monitor for signs of clinical improvement; if no improvement within 2 weeks, reassess diagnosis.

**Patient Counseling:** Instruct to use externally and as directed; avoid contact with eyes, use on face, groin or axillae. Counsel not to bandage or wrap treatment area so as to be occlusive unless directed by physician. Instruct to report signs of local adverse reactions (eg, irritation).

**Administration:** Topical route. **Storage**: 15-30°C (59-86°F).

## UNASYN RX

ampicillin sodium - sulbactam sodium (Pfizer)

**THERAPEUTIC CLASS:** Semisynthetic penicillin/beta-lactamase inhibitor

**INDICATIONS:** Treatment of skin and skin structure (SSSI), intra-abdominal, and gynecological infections caused by susceptible microorganisms.

**DOSAGE:** *Adults:* 1.5-3g (ampicillin+sulbactam) IM/IV q6h. Max: 4g sulbactam/day. Renal Impairment: CrCl ≥30mL/min: 1.5-3g q6-8h. CrCl 15-29mL/min: 1.5-3g q12h. CrCl 5-14mL/min: 1.5-3g q24h.
*Pediatrics:* ≥1 yr: 300mg/kg/day (ampicillin+sulbactam) IV in equally divided doses q6h. Max: 4g sulbactam/day. ≥40kg: Dose according to adult recommendations.

**HOW SUPPLIED:** Inj: (Ampicillin-Sulbactam) 1g-0.5g, 2g-1g, 10g-5g

**WARNINGS/PRECAUTIONS:** Serious, sometimes fatal, hypersensitivity reactions reported with PCN therapy; d/c use and initiate appropriate therapy. *Clostridium difficile*-associated diarrhea (CDAD) reported; if suspected or confirmed d/c ongoing antibiotics not for *C.difficile*. Increased risk of skin rash with mononucleosis; use alternate agent. Possible superinfections with mycotic or bacterial pathogens; d/c therapy if superinfection occurs. Use in the absence a proven or strongly suspected bacterial infection or a prophylactic indication is unlikely to provide benefit and increases the risk of drug resistant bacteria. False positive reactions may occur when using Benedict's or Fehling solution for urinary glucose test. Decreases in total conjugated estriol, estriol-glucoronide, conjugated estrone, and estradiol reported in pregnant women.

**ADVERSE REACTIONS:** Injection-site pain, thrombophlebitis, diarrhea.

**INTERACTIONS:** Probenecid may increase and prolong blood levels and decreases renal tubular secretion. Increased incidence of rash with allopurinol. Do not reconstitute with aminoglycosides; ampicillin component may inactivate aminoglycosides.

**PREGNANCY:** Category B, caution in nursing.

**MECHANISM OF ACTION:** Ampicillin: Semi-synthetic penicillin; acts through inhibition of cell wall mucopeptide biosynthesis. Has a broad spectrum of bactericidal activity against many gram-positive and gram-negative aerobic and anaerobic bacteria. Sulbactam: beta-lactamase inhibitor: provides good inhibitory activity against clinically important plasmid mediated β-lactamases most frequently responsible for transferred drug resistance.

**PHARMACOKINETICS: Absorption**: IV/IM administration of variable doses resulted in different parameters. **Distribution**: Plasma protein binding (28% ampicillin), (38% sulbactam); found in breast milk. **Elimination:** Urine (75-85% unchanged); $T_{1/2}$=1 hr.

U

### NURSING CONSIDERATIONS

**Assessment:** Assess for history of hypersensitivity to cephalosporins/PCNs or other allergens, nursing status, mononucleosis, renal impairment, and for possible drug interactions. Document indications for therapy, culture, and susceptibility testing.

**Monitoring:** Monitor for signs/symptoms of hypersensitivity reactions (eg, anaphylaxis), CDAD, superinfection, gastrointestinal changes, hematological changes (eg, agranulocytosis), and for changes in hepatic/renal function. Monitor for changes in estrogen levels in pregnant women and for false positive reactions when testing for glucose in urine if using Clinitest, Benedict's Solution, or Fehling's Solution.

**Patient Counseling:** Inform that drug only treats bacterial, not viral infections. Instruct to take as directed; skipping doses or not completing full course may decrease effectiveness and increase resistance. Counsel that may experience diarrhea. Instruct to contact physician if GI symptoms including watery/bloody stools develop or if allergic reaction develops.

**Administration:** IV/IM route. IV: Refer to PI for reconstitution instructions. IM: Reconstitute with sterile water for injection (SWFI) or lidocaine 0.5% or 2%. For 1.5g vial, add 3.2mL diluent; withdrawal volume is 4mL. For 3g vial, add 6.4mL diluent; withdrawal volume is 8mL. **Storage:** Prior to reconstitution: 30°C(86°F). IV Reconstituted Solution: Refer to PI for storage requirements. IM Reconstituted Solution: Use only freshly prepared solutions and administer within 1 hr after preparation.

## UNIPHYL RX

theophylline (Purdue Pharmaceutical)

**THERAPEUTIC CLASS:** Xanthine bronchodilator

**INDICATIONS:** Treatment of the symptoms and reversible airflow obstruction associated with chronic asthma and other chronic lung disease (eg, emphysema, chronic bronchitis).

**DOSAGE:** *Adults:* Initial: 300-400mg qd for 3 days with meals. Titrate: Increase to 400-600mg qd. After 3 days and if needed/tolerated, increase dose according to blood levels. Tab may be split in half; do not chew or crush. Renal Dysfunction/Elderly (>60 yrs): Max: 400mg/day. Conversion from Immediate-Release Theophylline: Give same daily dose as once daily. *Pediatrics:* 12-15 yrs: (<45kg): Initial: 12-14mg/kg/day up to 300mg qd for 3 days with meals. Titrate: Increase to 16mg/kg/day up to 400mg qd. After 3 days if needed/tolerated increase to 20mg/kg/day up to 600mg qd. (>45kg): Follow adult dose schedule. Tab may be split in half; do not chew or crush. Conversion from Immediate-Release Theophylline: ≥12 yrs: Give same daily dose as once daily. Renal Dysfunction: Max: 400mg qd.

**HOW SUPPLIED:** Tab, Extended-Release: 400mg, 600mg

**WARNINGS/PRECAUTIONS:** Extreme caution in peptic ulcer disease, seizure disorders, and/or cardiac arrhythmias (except bradycardia). Caution in neonates, children <1 yr, and the elderly. Caution in pulmonary edema, CHF, fever ≥102°F for 24 hrs, cor pulmonale, hypothyroidism, liver disease, reduced renal function, sepsis, shock, and HTN. If toxicity develops (eg, repetitive vomiting), monitor serum levels and adjust dosage.

**ADVERSE REACTIONS:** Vomiting, headache, insomnia, diarrhea, restlessness, tremors, hematemesis, hypokalemia, hyperglycemia, tachycardia, hypotension/shock, nervousness, disorientation, arrhythmias, seizures.

**INTERACTIONS:** Diminished effects with charcoal-broiled food, phenytoin, carbamazepine, phenobarbital, hydantoins, rifampin, ritonavir, aminoglutethimide, barbiturates, ketoconazole, sulfinpyrazone, INH, loop diuretics, sympathomimetics, high protein/low carbohydrate diet, alcohol, St. John's wort. Potentiated by propranolol, allopurinol, erythromycin, troleandomycin, ciprofloxacin, quinolone antibiotics, oral contraceptives, CCBs, corticosteroids, disulfiram, ephedrine, influenza virus vaccine, interferon, macrolides, mexiletine, thiabendazole, thyroid hormones, carbamazepine, loop diuretics, high carbohydrate/low protein diet and parenteral nutrition.

**PREGNANCY:** Category C, caution in nursing.

**MECHANISM OF ACTION:** Methylxanthine; acts via smooth muscle relaxation and suppression of airway response to stimuli. Bronchodilatation suggested to be mediated by inhibiting isozymes of phosphodiesterase. Also increases the force of contraction of diaphragmatic muscles due to enhancement of calcium uptake through adenosine-mediated channel.

**PHARMACOKINETICS: Absorption:** Rapid, complete; (800 qam, fed) $C_{max}$=12.1mcg/mL, $C_{min}$=4.5mcg/mL, $T_{max}$=8.8 hrs, AUC=203mcg•hr/

mL. (600 qd, fed) $C_{max}$=12.91mcg/mL, $C_{min}$=5.52mcg/mL, $T_{max}$=8.62 hrs, AUC=209mcg•hr/mL. Bioavailability Ratio 600/400: 98.8%. **Distribution:** $V_d$= 0.45L/kg; plasma protein binding (40%). **Metabolism:** Extensive; CYP1A2, 2E1, 3A3; Caffeine and 3-methylxanthine (active metabolites). **Elimination:** Urine (10% unchanged), $T_{1/2}$=8 hrs.

## NURSING CONSIDERATIONS

**Assessment:** Assess risk of exacerbation of concurrent conditions (eg, active PUD, seizure disorder, cardiac arrhythmias). Assess use with neonates, children <1 yr, elderly, pulmonary edema, CHF, fever ≥102°F for 24 hrs, cor pulmonale, hypothyroidism, liver disease (eg, cirrhosis, acute hepatitis), reduced renal function, sepsis, shock, and HTN. Assess known hypersensitivity, renal/hepatic functions, and possible drug interactions.

**Monitoring:** Carefully monitor serum drug levels (target unbound concentration: 6-12mcg/mL) for dose adjustments, drug toxicity, worsening of chronic illness, hepatic dysfunction. Monitor plasma glucose, uric acid, free fatty acids, cholesterol, HDL, LDL, LFTs, and urine free cortisol excretion. If toxicity develops (eg, repetitive vomiting), adjust dosage based on serum levels.

**Patient Counseling:** Instruct to seek medical attention if N/V, persistent headache, insomnia, or rapid heartbeat occur. Counsel not to take St. John's wort concurrently; may result in decreased drug levels. Inform to take once daily in morning or evening. Advise to consistently take with/without food, do not chew or crush, and inform physician if new illness (especially if accompanied with persistent fever) or worsening of chronic illness occurs. Advise to inform all physicians of theophylline use especially if medication is being added or removed from treatment.

**Administration:** Oral route. **Storage:** 25°C (77°F); excursions permitted to 15-30°C (59-86°F).

# UNIRETIC RX

moexipril HCl - hydrochlorothiazide (Schwarz)

**ACE inhibitors can cause death/injury to developing fetus during 2nd and 3rd trimesters. D/C if pregnancy detected.**

**THERAPEUTIC CLASS:** ACE inhibitor/thiazide diuretic

**INDICATIONS:** Treatment of hypertension. Not for initial therapy.

**DOSAGE:** *Adults:* Initial (if not controlled on moexipril/HCTZ monotherapy): Switch to 7.5mg-12.5mg tab, 15mg-12.5mg tab, or 15mg-25mg tab qd. Titrate: Based on clinical response. May increase after 2-3 weeks. Initial (if controlled on 25mg HCTZ/day with hypokalemia): 3.75mg-6.25mg (1/2 of 7.5mg-12.5mg tab). If excessive reduction with 7.5mg-12.5mg tab, may switch to 3.75mg-6.25mg. Replacement Therapy: Substitute combination for titrated components. Take 1 hr before meals.

**HOW SUPPLIED:** Tab: (Moexipril-HCTZ) 7.5mg-12.5mg*, 15mg-12.5mg*, 15mg-25mg* *scored

**CONTRAINDICATIONS:** History of ACE inhibitor-associated angioedema, anuria, sulfonamide hypersensitivity.

**WARNINGS/PRECAUTIONS:** Angioedema involving the face, extremities, lips, tongue, glottis, and/or larynx reported; d/c if it occurs as it may be fatal due to airway obstruction. Intestinal angioedema reported. Can cause symptomatic hypotension; caution in patients with ischemic heart disease, aortic stenosis, cerebrovascular disease. Caution in patients with severe renal disease; may precipitate azotemia. Monitor WBCs in renal and collagen vascular disease. Fetal/neonatal morbidity and death reported. Risk of hyperkalemia with DM, renal dysfunction. Persistent nonproductive cough reported. Anaphylactoid reactions reported. Rarely, associated with syndrome that starts with cholestatic jaundice and progresses to fulminant necrosis and sometimes death; d/c if jaundice or marked elevations of hepatic enzymes. Caution in patients with hepatic impairment or progressive liver disease. May exacerbate or activate SLE. May cause electrolyte imbalance (hyperkalemia, hypokalemia, hyponatremia, hypochloremic alkalosis, hypomagnesemia, hypercalcemia); monitor electrolytes. May reduce glucose tolerance and increase cholesterol, TG.

**ADVERSE REACTIONS:** Cough.

**INTERACTIONS:** Increase risk of hyperkalemia with $K^+$-sparing diuretics, $K^+$ supplements, or $K^+$-containing salt substitutes. Potentiates orthostatic hypotension with alcohol, barbiturates, and narcotics. Adjust antidiabetic drugs. Reduced absorption with cholestyramine, colestipol. Corticosteroids, ACTH deplete electrolytes. May decrease response to pressor amines. Potentiates other antihypertensives. May increase responsiveness to skeletal muscle relaxants. Risk of lithium toxicity. NSAIDs reduce effects. Increased absorption of HCTZ with guanabenz and propantheline. Nitritoid reactions have been reported rarely with injectable gold (sodium aurothiomalate).

**PREGNANCY:** Category C (1st trimester) and D (2nd and 3rd trimesters), not for use in nursing.

**MECHANISM OF ACTION:** Moexipril: ACE inhibitor; inhibition results in decreased plasma angiotensin II, leading to decreased vasopressor activity and decreased aldosterone secretion. HCTZ: Thiazide diuretic; affects renal tubular mechanism of electrolyte reabsorption, directly increasing excretion of $Na^+$ and $Cl^-$.

**PHARMACOKINETICS: Absorption:** Moexipril-HCTZ: $T_{max}$=0.8 hrs. Moexipril: Incomplete; bioavailability (13%), $T_{max}$= 1.5 hrs. **Distribution:** Moexiprilat: $V_d$=2.8L/kg; plasma protein binding (50%). HCTZ: $V_d$=1.5-4.2L/kg; crosses the placenta; found in breast milk; plasma protein binding (21-24%). **Metabolism:** Moexiprilat (active metabolite). **Elimination**: Urine (7% moexiprilat, 1% moexpril, 5% other metabolites), feces (52% moexiprilat, 1% moexipril); $T_{1/2}$=2-9 hrs (Moexiprilat). HCTZ: Renal excretion; $T_{1/2}$=5.6-14.8 hrs.

## NURSING CONSIDERATIONS

**Assessment:** Assess BP, history of angioedema, collagen-vascular disease, hepatic/renal function, CHF, renal artery stenosis, SLE, serum electrolytes, pregnancy status, history of allergy to sulfonamides, bronchial asthma, parathyroid disorders, and possible drug interactions. Obtain baseline electrolytes ($K^+$, Na, Cl, Mg), blood glucose, cholesterol, TG and uric acid.

**Monitoring:** Monitor for signs of angioedema (face, extremities, lips, glottis, and/or larynx), hypotension, infections, electrolyte imbalance (hyperkalemia, hypokalemia, hyponatremia, hypochloremic alkalosis, hypomagnesemia, hypercalcemia). Monitor BP, WBC counts, electrolytes ($K^+$, Na, Cl, Mg), blood glucose, cholesterol, TG and uric acid.

**Patient Counseling:** Inform about fetal risks if taken during pregnancy. Caution that inadequate fluid intake, excessive perspiration, diarrhea, or vomiting can lead to excessive fall in BP. Advise patient that lightheadedness and possible syncope may occur, especially during first few days of therapy. Advise not to use $K^+$ supplements or salt substitutes containing $K^+$ without consulting physician. Counsel about signs/symptoms of neutropenia (eg, infections, sore throat, fever), angioedema, electrolyte imbalance (eg, thirst, weakness, lethargy), and other adverse effects; advise to seek prompt medical attention if any occur. Instruct to take medication 1 hr before meals.

U

**Administration:** Oral route. **Storage:** 20-25°C (68-77°F). Protect from excessive moisture.

# UNITHROID RX

levothyroxine sodium (Lannett)

**THERAPEUTIC CLASS:** Thyroid replacement hormone

**INDICATIONS:** Hypothyroidism. As a pituitary TSH suppressant in the treatment and prevention of euthyroid goiters, including thyroid nodules, lymphocytic thyroiditis, and multinodular goiter. Adjunct to surgery and radioiodine therapy for thyrotropin-dependent well-differentiated thyroid cancer.

**DOSAGE:** *Adults:* Take in AM at least 1/2-1 hr before food. Hypothyroid: Usual: 1.7mcg/kg/day. >200mcg/day (seldom). >50 yrs/<50 yrs with Cardiac Disease: Initial: 25-50mcg/day. Titrate: Increase by 12.5-25mcg/day every 6-8 weeks until euthyroid. Elderly with Cardiac Disease: Initial: 12.5-25mcg/day. Titrate: Increase by 12.5-25mcg/day every 4-6 weeks until euthyroid. Severe Hypothyroidism: Initial: 12.5-25mcg/day. Titrate: Increase by 25mcg/day every 2-4 weeks until euthyroid. Pregnancy: May increase dose requirements. Subclinical Hypothyroidism: Lower doses required. *Pediatrics:* Take in AM at least 1/2-1 hr before food. Hypothyroidism: 0-3 months: 10-15mcg/kg/day. 3-6 months: 8-10mcg/kg/day. 6-12 months: 6-8mcg/kg/day. 1-5 yrs: 5-6mcg/kg/day. 6-12 yrs: 4-5mcg/kg/day. >12 yrs: 2-3mcg/kg/day. Growth/Puberty Complete: 1.7mcg/kg/day. Cardiac Risk: Initial: Use lower dose. Titrate: Increase dose every 4-6 weeks until euthyroid. Infants with Serum $T_4$ <5mcg/dL: Initial: 50mcg/day. Chronic/Severe Hypothyroidism: Children: Initial: 25mcg/day. Titrate: Increase by 25mcg/day every 2-4 weeks until desired effect. Minimize Hyperactivity in Older Children: Initial: Give 1/4 of full replacement dose. Titrate: Increase by same amount weekly until full dose achieved. May crush tab and mix with 5-10mL water.

**HOW SUPPLIED:** Tab: 25mcg*, 50mcg*, 75mcg*, 88mcg*, 100mcg*, 112mcg*, 125mcg*, 150mcg*, 175mcg*, 200mcg*, 300mcg* *scored

**CONTRAINDICATIONS:** Untreated thyrotoxicosis, acute MI, uncorrected adrenal insufficiency.

**WARNINGS/PRECAUTIONS:** Do not use in the treatment of obesity; larger doses in euthyroid patients can cause serious or even life threatening toxicity. Caution with cardiovascular disease, CAD, adrenal insufficiency, autonomous thyroid tissue, hypothalamic/pituitary hormone deficiencies, and the elderly with risk of occult cardiac disease. Carefully titrate dose to avoid over or under treatment. Decreased bone mineral density with long term use. With adrenal insufficiency supplement with glucocorticoids before therapy.

**INTERACTIONS:** Sympathomimetics may increase risk of coronary insufficiency with CAD. Upward dose adjustments needed for insulin and oral hypoglycemic agents. Decreased absorption with soybean flour (infant formula), cotton seed meal, walnuts, and fiber. May potentiate oral anticoagulant effects; adjust dose and monitor PT/INR. May decrease levels and effects of digitalis glycosides. Cholestyramine, colestipol, ferrous sulfate, aluminum hydroxide, sodium polystyrene, soybean flour, sucralfate may decrease absorption. Reduced TSH secretion with dopamine/dopamine agonists, glucocorticoids, octreotide. Decreased thyroid hormone secretion with aminoglutethimide, amiodarone, iodine (including iodine-containing radiographic contrast agents), lithium, methimazole, PTU, sulfonamides, tolbutamide. Increased thyroid hormone secretion with amiodarone, iodide (including iodine-containing radiographic contrast agents). Decreased $T_4$ absorption with antacids (aluminum & magnesium hydroxides), simethicone, bile acid sequestrants (cholestyramine, colestipol), calcium carbonate, cation exchange resins (eg, Kayexalate), ferrous sulfate, sucralfate. Increased serum TBG concentration with clofibrate, estrogens, heroin/methadone, 5-FU, mitotane, tamoxifen. Decreased serum TBG concentration with androgens/anabolic steroids, asparaginase, glucocorticoids, nicotinic acid (slow-release). Protein-binding site displacement with furosemide, heparin, hydantoins, NSAIDs, salicylates. Increased hepatic metabolism with carbamazepine, hydantoins, phenobarbital, rifampin. Decreased conversion of $T_4$ to $T_3$ levels with amiodarone, β-adrenergic antagonists (propranolol >160mg/day), glucocorticoids (dexamethasone >4mg/day), PTU. Additive effects of both agents with antidepressants. Interferon-(alpha) may cause development of antithyroid microsomal antibodies causing transient hypothyroidism, hyperthyroidism, or both. Interleukin-2 has been associated with transient painless thyroiditis. Excessive use with growth hormones may accelerate epiphyseal closure. Ketamine use may produce marked HTN and tachycardia. May reduce uptake of iodine-containing radiographic contrast agents. Altered levels of thyroid hormone and/or TSH level with choral hydrate, diazepam, ethionamide, lovastatin, metoclopramide, 6-mercaptopurine, nitroprusside, para-aminosalicylate sodium, perphenazine, resorcinol (excessive topical use), thiazide diuretics.

**PREGNANCY:** Category A, caution in nursing.

U

**MECHANISM OF ACTION:** Thyroid hormone; not understood, suspected to control DNA transcription and protein synthesis.

**PHARMACOKINETICS: Distribution:** Plasma protein binding (99%), found in breast milk. **Metabolism:** Liver via sequential deiodination (major pathway), conjugation in liver (mainly), kidneys, other tissues. **Elimination:** Urine, feces (20% unchanged); ($T_4$) $T_{1/2}$=6-7 days, ($T_3$) $T_{1/2}$≤2days.

## NURSING CONSIDERATIONS

**Assessment:** Assess for suppressed serum TSH with normal $T_3$ and $T_4$ levels, overt thyrotoxicosis, thyroid diseases (eg, nontoxic diffuse or nodular goiter), endocrine disorders (eg, hypothalmic/pituitary hormone deficiencies, autoimmune polyglandular disorders), infants for congenital anomalies, cardiovascular diseases (eg, angina pectoris, acute MI), DM, hypersensitivity history, clotting status, upcoming surgery, and for possible drug and test interactions.

**Monitoring:** Perform frequent lab tests and clinical evaluations of thyroid functions (TSH and free $T_4$ levels, lipid metabolism, blood/urinary glucose in DM, clotting parameters). Monitor cardiovascular signs (eg, arrhythmias, coronary insufficiency), growth/development, bone metabolism, cognitive function, emotional status, GI functions, reproductive functions, partial hair loss in infants, and signs/symptoms of thyroid toxicity.

**Patient Counseling:** Inform that drug is to be taken for life and not for treatment of obesity or weight loss. Take on empty stomach, 1 hr before breakfast with full glass of water. Notify physician if pregnant/nursing or planning to become pregnant. Notify if taking any other drugs. Do not d/c or change dosage unless directed by physician. Report any signs/symptoms of thyroid toxicity to physician.

**Administration:** Oral route. **Storage**: 20-25°C (68-77°F); excursions permitted to 15-30°C (59-86°F).

# UNIVASC **RX**

moexipril HCl (Schwarz)

**ACE inhibitors can cause death/injury to developing fetus during 2nd and 3rd trimesters. D/C if pregnancy detected.**

**THERAPEUTIC CLASS:** ACE inhibitor

**INDICATIONS:** Treatment of hypertension alone or in combination with thiazide diuretics.

**DOSAGE:** *Adults:* D/C diuretic 2-3 days prior to therapy if possible. Take 1 hr before meals. Initial: 7.5mg qd, 3.75mg with concomitant diuretic therapy. Maint: 7.5-30mg/day given qd-bid. Resume diuretic if BP not controlled. Max: 60mg/day. CrCl ≤40mL/min: Initial: 3.75mg qd. Max: 15mg/day. Elderly: Start at lower end of dosing range.

**HOW SUPPLIED:** Tab: 7.5mg*, 15mg* *scored

**CONTRAINDICATIONS:** History of ACE inhibitor-associated angioedema.

U

**WARNINGS/PRECAUTIONS:** Angioedema involving the face, extremities, lips, tongue, glottis, and/or larynx reported; d/c if it occur. Angioedema associated with involvement of tongue, glottis, or larynx, may be fatal due to airway obstruction. Can cause symptomatic hypotension; caution in patients with ischemic heart disease, aortic stenosis, cerebrovascular disease. Monitor WBCs in renal and collagen vascular disease. Fetal and neonatal injury and death reported. Rarely, associated with syndrome that starts with cholestatic jaundice and progresses to fulminant necrosis and sometimes death; d/c if experience jaundice or marked elevations of hepatic enzymes. Caution in patients with impaired renal function, CHF, and renal artery stenosis. Risk of hyperkalemia with DM, renal dysfunction. Persistent nonproductive cough reported. Minor increases in BUN or SrCr reported.

**ADVERSE REACTIONS:** Cough, dizziness, diarrhea, flu syndrome.

**INTERACTIONS:** May increase lithium levels. Hypotension risk with diuretics. Increased risk of hyperkalemia with $K^+$-sparing diuretics, $K^+$-containing salt substitutes, or $K^+$ supplements. Nitritoid reactions reported rarely with injectable gold (sodium aurothiomalate).

**PREGNANCY:** Category C (1st trimester) and D (2nd and 3rd trimesters), caution in nursing.

**MECHANISM OF ACTION:** ACE inhibitor; inhibition results in decreased plasma angiotensin II, which leads to decreased vasopressor activity, increased plasma renin activity, and decreased aldosterone secretion.

**PHARMACOKINETICS: Absorption:** Incomplete; bioavailability (13%). **Distribution:** $V_d$=183L; plasma protein binding (50%). **Metabolism:** Moexiprilat (active metabolite). **Elimination:** Urine (7% moexiprilat, 1% moexipril, 5% other metabolites), feces (52% moexiprilat, 1% moexipril); $T_{1/2}$=2-9 hrs.

## NURSING CONSIDERATIONS

**Assessment:** Assess for history of angioedema, BP, LFTs, renal function, CHF, renal artery stenosis, pregnancy status, and possible drug interactions. Obtain baseline serum $K^+$, $Na^+$, WBC count, LFTs, serum creatinine, BUN, uric acid.

**Monitoring:** Monitor BP, LFTs, renal function, WBC, BUN, SrCr, serum electrolytes, and serum $K^+$ levels. Monitor for MI, CHF, head/neck and intestinal angioedema, anaphylactoid reactions, hepatic failure, hypersensitivity reactions, cough, N/V, dizziness, oliguria and azotemia.

**Patient Counseling:** Counsel about fetal risks during pregnancy and signs/symptoms of angioedema (eg, laryngeal/tongue edema, abdominal pain); advise to seek prompt medical attention if symptoms develop. Inform about adverse effects (eg, anaphylaxis, cough, hypotension, hyperkalemia, neutropenia). Inform about need for periodic monitoring of electrolytes and blood counts. Caution that inadequate fluid intake, excessive perspiration, diarrhea, vomiting may lead to excessive fall in BP, resulting in lightheadedness and possible syncope. Advise not to use $K^+$ supplements or salt substitutes. Instruct to take 1 hr before meals.

**Administration:** Oral route. **Storage:** Room temperature; protect from excessive moisture.

# UROXATRAL **RX**

alfuzosin HCl (Sanofi-Aventis)

**THERAPEUTIC CLASS:** $Alpha_1$-antagonist

**INDICATIONS:** Treatment of signs and symptoms of benign prostatic hyperplasia (BPH).

**DOSAGE:** *Adults:* 10mg qd, taken immediately after same meal, each day.

**HOW SUPPLIED:** Tab, Extended-Release: 10mg

**CONTRAINDICATIONS:** Moderate or severe hepatic insufficiency (Child-Pugh B and C). Concomitant potent CYP3A4 inhibitors (eg, ketoconazole, itraconazole, ritonavir).

**WARNINGS/PRECAUTIONS:** Increased risk of hypotension/postural hypotension and syncope; monitor for any occurrences within a few hours of administration. Rule out prostatic cancer prior to therapy. D/C with new or worsening angina. Caution with severe renal impairment. Caution in patients with congenital or acquired QT prolongation. Intraoperative Floppy Iris syndrome (IFIS) observed in some patients during cataract surgery.

**ADVERSE REACTIONS:** Angina pectoris, postural/orthostatic hypotension, syncope, QT prolongation, IFIS, dizziness, upper respiratory tract infection, headache, fatigue, abdominal pain, dyspepsia, constipation, nausea, impotence, bronchitis.

**INTERACTIONS:** See Contraindications. Avoid use with other α-blockers. Increased levels with cimetidine, diltiazem, atenolol. Increased risk of hypotension/postural hypotension and syncope with nitrates and other antihypertensives. Caution with medications that prolong the QT interval.

**PREGNANCY:** Category B, safety not known in nursing.

**MECHANISM OF ACTION:** $\alpha_1$-antagonist; inhibits adrenoreceptors in lower urinary tract causing smooth muscle in bladder neck and prostate to relax, which results in improved urine flow and decreased symptoms of BPH.

**PHARMACOKINETICS: Absorption:** Absolute bioavailability (49%); $C_{max}$=13.6ng/mL; $T_{max}$=8 hrs; AUC=194ng•hr/mL. **Distribution:** $V_d$=3.2L/kg; plasma protein binding (82-90%). **Metabolism:** Liver via CYP3A4 (oxidation, O-demethylation, N-dealkylation). **Elimination:** Feces (69%), urine (24%, 11% unchanged); $T_{1/2}$=10 hrs.

## NURSING CONSIDERATIONS

**Assessment:** Assess for BPH, prostatic cancer, symptomatic hypotension, history of QT prolongation, hepatic/renal impairment, hypersensitivity, and possible drug interactions.

**Monitoring:** Monitor for postural hypotension (syncope), hypersensitivity reactions, IFIS, QT prolongation, hepatic/renal dysfunction. Monitor for adverse reactions.

**Patient Counseling:** Advise that postural hypotension may occur during the first few hours of administration and avoid situations where injury could result in case syncope occurs. Dizziness may occur. Advise to use caution while driving, operating machinery, or performing any other hazardous tasks. Notify ophthalmologist about drug use/history prior to ophthalmological procedures including cataract surgery. Advise to take with food, with the same meal each day, and not to crush or chew. Notify physician if symptoms of postural hypotension, cardiovascular effects, hypersensitivity, or hepatic/renal dysfunction occur.

**Administration:** Oral route. **Storage:** 25°C (77°F); excursions permitted to 15-30°C (59-86°F). Protect from light and moisture.

# VAGIFEM

RX

estradiol (Novo Nordisk)

**Estrogens increase the risk of endometrial cancer. Perform adequate diagnostic measures including directed or random endometrial sampling when indicated, to rule out malignancy in postmenopausal women with undiagnosed persistent or recurring abnormal genital bleeding. Do not use as monotherapy or concomitant with progestin for the prevention of cardiovascular (CV) disease or probable dementia. Increased risk of stroke, deep vein thrombosis (DVT), pulmonary embolism, myocardial infarction (MI), and invasive breast cancer in postmenopausal women. Should be prescribed at lowest effective doses and for shortest duration consistent with treatment goals and risks for individual women.**

**THERAPEUTIC CLASS:** Estrogen

**INDICATIONS:** Treatment of atrophic vaginitis due to menopause.

**DOSAGE:** *Adults:* Initial: Insert 1 tab vaginally qd for 2 weeks. Maint: Insert 1 tab twice weekly. Generally, women should be started at the 10mcg dosage strength.

**HOW SUPPLIED:** Tab, Vaginal: 10mcg, 25mcg

**CONTRAINDICATIONS:** Breast carcinoma or other estrogen-dependent neoplasia, abnormal genital bleeding, pregnancy, active DVT, pulmonary embolism, arterial thromboembolic disease (eg, stroke, MI) or history of these conditions, and liver dysfunction or disease.

V

**WARNINGS/PRECAUTIONS:** Risk of gallbladder disease, thromboembolism, thrombotic disease, retinal vascular disease. May elevate BP, thyroid binding globulin levels, and plasma TG leading to pancreatitis. Monitor for hypercalcemia in breast cancer and bone metastases. Caution in asthma, epilepsy, migraine, porphyria, systemic lupus erythematosus, DM, hepatic hemangiomas, cardiac or renal dysfunction due to fluid retention, liver dysfunction and metabolic bone disease associated with hypercalcemia. Few cases of local abrasion and malignant transformation of residual endometrial implants reported. Caution in young patients. For vaginal administration only.

**ADVERSE REACTIONS:** Headache, abdominal pain, respiratory infection, genital moniliasis, back pain, diarrhea, vulvovaginal mycotic infection, vulvovaginal pruritis.

**INTERACTIONS:** Reduced plasma concentration resulting in decrease in therapeutic effects and/or changes in uterine bleeding profile with CYP3A4 inducers (eg, St. Johns wort, phenobarbital, carbamazepine, rifampin). Increases plasma concentrations, which may result in side effects with CYP3A4 inhibitors (eg, erythromycin, clarithromycin, ketoconazole, itraconazole, ritonavir, and grapefruit juice).

**PREGNANCY:** Not safe in pregnancy. Caution in nursing.

**MECHANISM OF ACTION:** Estrogen (estradiol); acts through binding to nuclear receptors in estrogen-responsive tissues. Reduce elevated levels of gonodotropins, luteinizing hormone (LH), and follicle-stimulating hormone (FSH) seen in postmenopausal women through a negative feedback mechanism.

**PHARMACOKINETICS: Absorption:** Well absorbed. **Metabolism:** Liver; estrone, estriol (metabolites). **Elimination:** Urine.

## NURSING CONSIDERATIONS

**Assessment:** Assess for abnormal genital bleeding, strong family history of breast cancer, abnormal mammograms, known/suspected breast or estrogen-dependent neoplasia, thromboembolic disorders, DM, atrophic vaginal mucosa, porphyria, asthma, epilepsy, migraine, vaginal infections, fibrocystic disease, cardiac, hepatic/renal impairment, pregnancy status, and possible drug interactions. Perform exam of breast, and pelvic organs; obtain BP, serum TG, and calcium levels.

**Monitoring:** Monitor BP, serum TG, and calcium levels periodically; perform exams routinely. Monitor for abnormal vaginal bleeding, gallbladder disease, HTN, hyperglycemia, fluid retention, trauma from applicator, hypercalcemia, hepatic dysfunction, and hypersensitivity reactions.

**Patient Counseling:** Advise to seek medical attention for symptoms of abnormal vaginal bleeding, gallbladder disease, abdominal pain/tenderness, HTN, hyperglycemia, fluid retention, trauma from applicator, hypercalcemia, hepatic dysfunction (eg, jaundice), or hypersensitivity reactions. Instruct to insert applicator carefully if atrophic vaginal mucosa present.

**Administration:** Intravaginal route. **Storage:** 25°C (77°F); excursions permitted to 15-30°C (59-86°F). Do not refrigerate

# VALCYTE — RX

valganciclovir HCl (Roche Labs)

**Granulocytopenia, anemia, and thrombocytopenia reported. Carcinogenic, teratogenic, and may cause aspermatogenesis based on animal studies.**

**THERAPEUTIC CLASS:** Synthetic guanine derivative nucleoside analogue

**INDICATIONS:** Treatment of cytomegalovirus (CMV) retinitis in AIDS patients. Prevention of CMV disease in kidney and heart transplant patients (age ≥4 months) and adult kidney-pancreas transplant patients at high risk (donor CMV seropositive/recipient CMV seronegative).

**DOSAGE:** *Adults:* Treatment of CMV Retinitis: Initial: 900mg bid for 21 days. Maint: 900mg qd. Prevention of CMV Disease: 900mg qd starting within 10 days of transplantation until 100 days post-transplantation. Renal Impairment (CrCl 40-59mL/min): Initial: 450mg bid. Maint: 450mg qd. CrCl 25-39mL/min: Initial: 450mg qd. Maint: 450mg q2d. CrCl 10-24mL/min: Initial: 450mg q2d. Maint: 450mg biw. Take with food.
*Pediatrics*: 4 months-16 yrs: Prevention of CMV Disease: Recommended once-daily dose starting within 10 days of transplantation until 100 days post-transplantation is based on body surface area (BSA) and creatinine clearance (CrCl) derived from modified Schwartz formula. Refer to PI for dose calculations.

**HOW SUPPLIED:** Tab: 450mg; Sol: 50mg/mL

**WARNINGS/PRECAUTIONS:** Severe leukopenia, neutropenia, anemia, thrombocytopenia, pancytopenia, bone marrow aplasia, and aplastic anemia observed. Avoid if the neutrophils <500cells/μL, platelet count <25,000/μL, or Hgb <8g/dL. Acute renal failure may occur; caution in the elderly and adjust dose in renal impairment. May cause temporary or permanent inhibition of spermatogenesis.

**ADVERSE REACTIONS:** Diarrhea, N/V, graft rejection, abdominal pain, pyrexia, headache, neutropenia, thrombocytopenia, anemia, cough, HTN, constipation.

**INTERACTIONS:** Greater risk for neutropenia and anemia with zidovudine. Monitor for toxicity with probenecid. Increased levels of metabolites of both drugs with mycophenolate mofetil. Caution with myelosuppressive drugs or irradiation. Increased risk of didanosine toxicity. Acute renal failure may occur in patients receiving nephrotoxic drugs; caution with use.

**PREGNANCY:** Category C, not for use in nursing.

**MECHANISM OF ACTION:** Guanine derivative; inhibits viral DNA synthesis, resulting in inhibition of human CMV replication.

**PHARMACOKINETICS: Absorption:** Absolute bioavailability (59.4%, Adult) (60%, Pediatrics); $C_{max}$=5.61mcg/mL; $T_{max}$=1-3 hrs; AUC=29.1mcg•h/mL (Tab), 23.6mcg•h/L (Sol). **Distribution:** (Ganciclovir) $V_d$=0.703L/kg; plasma protein binding (1-2%). **Metabolism:** Intestinal wall, liver (hydrolysis). **Elimination:** Renal; $T_{1/2}$=4.08 hrs.

## NURSING CONSIDERATIONS

**Assessment:** Assess for renal impairment, pre-existing cytopenia, pregnancy/nursing status, prior/current irradiation, and possible drug interactions. Obtain baseline neutrophil ( ≥500cells/μL), platelet ( ≥25000/μL), and Hgb ( ≥8g/dL) count.

**Monitoring:** Monitor CBC, differential, and platelet count, and renal function (SrCr) frequently. Perform ophthalmologic exams every 4-6 weeks during therapy. Monitor for signs/symptoms of drug toxicity (eg, granulocytopenia, anemia, thrombocytopenia), infertility, renal dysfunction, and hypersensitivity reactions.

**Patient Counseling:** Counsel to avoid direct contact of broken or crushed tab and oral solution with skin or mucous membranes; if contact occurs, wash thoroughly with soap and water. Advise to use effective contraception due to pregnancy risks. Strict adherence to dosage recommendations is essential to avoid overdose. Do not substitute for ganciclovir caps on 1:1 basis. Inform of major toxicities (eg, anemia, granulocytopenia, thrombocytopenia). Notify physician if convulsions, sedation, dizziness, ataxia, and/or confusion occur as these may affect physical/mental abilities.

**Administration:** Oral route. Take with food; do not break or crush. **Storage:** Tab/dry powder: 25°C (77°F); excursions permitted to 15-30°C (59-86°F). Reconstituted sol: 2-8°C (36-46°F) for no longer 49 days. Do not freeze.

# VALIUM

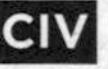


diazepam (Roche Labs)



**THERAPEUTIC CLASS:** Benzodiazepine

**INDICATIONS:** Management of anxiety disorders and short-term relief of anxiety symptoms. Symptomatic relief of acute alcohol withdrawal. Adjunct therapy in skeletal muscle spasm and convulsive disorders.

**DOSAGE:** *Adults:* Individualize dose. Anxiety Disorders/Anxiety Symptoms: 2-10mg bid-qid. Acute Alcohol Withdrawal: 10mg tid-qid for 24 hrs. Reduce to 5mg tid-qid prn. Skeletal Muscle Spasm: 2-10mg tid-qid. Convulsive Disorders: 2-10mg bid-qid. Elderly/Debilitated: 2-2.5mg qd-bid initially. May increase gradually prn and tolerated.
*Pediatrics:* ≥6 months: 1-2.5mg tid-qid initially. May increase gradually prn if tolerated.

**HOW SUPPLIED:** Tab: 2mg*, 5mg*, 10mg* *scored

**CONTRAINDICATIONS:** Acute narrow-angle glaucoma, patients <6 months, myasthenia gravis, severe respiratory insufficiency, severe hepatic insufficiency, sleep apnea syndrome.

**WARNINGS/PRECAUTIONS:** Not recommended in treatment of psychotic patients. Avoid simultaneous ingestion of alcohol and other CNS depressants during therapy. Temporarily increases frequency and severity of seizures during abrupt withdrawal. May produce irregularities in fetal heart rate and hypotonia, poor sucking, hypothermia, and moderate respiratory depression in neonates. Psychiatric and paradoxical reactions may occur. Lower dose with chronic respiratory insufficiency; smallest effective amount recommended in debilitated patients. Caution with history of alcohol and drug abuse. Prolonged use may result in loss of response to the effects of benzodiazepines.

**ADVERSE REACTIONS:** Drowsiness, fatigue, muscle weakness, ataxia, confusion, vertigo, constipation, blurred vision, dizziness, hypotension, stimulation, agitation, incontinence, skin reactions, hypersalivation.

**INTERACTIONS:** Mutually potentiates effects with phenothiazines, antipsychotics, anxiolytics/sedatives, hypnotics, anticonvulsants, narcotic analgesics, anesthetics, sedative antihistamines, narcotics, barbiturates, MAOIs, and other antidepressants. Alcohol enhances sedative effects. Increased and prolonged sedation with cimetidine, ketoconazole, fluvoxamine, fluoxetine, and omeprazole. Diazepam decreases metabolic elimination of phenytoin.

**PREGNANCY:** Category D, not for use in nursing.

**MECHANISM OF ACTION:** Benzodiazepine; exerts anxiolytic, sedative, muscle-relaxant, anticonvulsant, and amnestic effect. Facilitates GABA, an inhibitory neurotransmitter in CNS.

**PHARMACOKINETICS: Absorption:** $T_{max}$=1-1.5 hrs. **Distribution:** $V_d$=0.8-1.0 L/kg, plasma protein binding (98%), crosses blood-brain and placental barrier, appears in breast milk. **Metabolism:** Via N-desmethylation, hydroxylation, glucuronidation to N-desmethyldiazepam, temazepam, oxazepam by CYP3A4, CYP2C19 enzymes. **Elimination:** Urine; $T_{1/2}$=48 hrs, $T_{1/2}$(N-desmethyldiazepam)=100 hrs.

## NURSING CONSIDERATIONS

**Assessment:** Assess for anxiety disorders/symptoms, acute alcohol withdrawal, skeletal muscle spasm, convulsive disorders, acute narrow-angle glaucoma, myasthenia gravis, severe respiratory/hepatic insufficiency, sleep apnea syndrome, history of alcohol or drug abuse, pregnancy/nursing status, and possible drug interactions.

**Monitoring:** Monitor for hypersensitivity reactions, rebound or withdrawal symptoms, seizures, HR, and respiratory depression.

**Patient Counseling:** Advise to consult physician before increasing dose or abruptly d/c the drug. Advise against simultaneous ingestion of alcohol and other CNS depressants during therapy. Caution against engaging in hazardous occupations requiring complete mental alertness, such as operating machinery or driving a motor vehicle.

**Administration:** Oral route. **Storage:** 15-30°C (59-86°F). Dispense in tight, light-resistant containers.

# VALSTAR — RX

valrubicin (Endo)

**THERAPEUTIC CLASS:** Anthracycline

**INDICATIONS:** Intravesical therapy of BCG-refractoray carcinoma *in-situ* (CIS) of the urinary bladder in patients for whom immediate cystectomy would be associated with unacceptable morbidity or mortality.

**DOSAGE:** *Adults:* 800mg intravesically once weekly for 6 weeks. Delay administration for at least 2 weeks after transurethral resection and/or fulguration.

**HOW SUPPLIED:** Inj: 40mg/mL

**CONTRAINDICATIONS:** Concurrent UTI, small bladder capacity (unable to tolerate a 75mL instillation). Hypersensitivity to anthracyclines or Cremophor® EL (polyoxyethyleneglycol triricinoleate).

**WARNINGS/PRECAUTIONS:** Avoid in patients with a perforated bladder or to those in whom the integrity of the bladder mucosa has been compromised. Caution with severe irritable bladder symptoms. Bladder spasm and spontaneous discharge of the intravesical instillate may occur; clamping of urinary catheter is not advised and, if performed, should be executed under medical supervision and with caution.

**ADVERSE REACTIONS:** Local bladder symptoms: urinary frequency, dysuria, urinary urgency, bladder spasm, hematuria, bladder pain, urinary incontinence, cystitis, nocturia, local burning symptoms, urethral pain. Systemic symptoms: UTI, nausea, abdominal pain.

**PREGNANCY:** Category C, not for use in nursing.

## VALTREX — RX

valacyclovir HCl (GlaxoSmithKline)

**THERAPEUTIC CLASS:** Nucleoside analogue

**INDICATIONS:** Treatment of herpes labialis (cold sores) in patients ≥12 yrs. Treatment of herpes zoster (shingles) in immunocompetent adults. Treatment of initial and recurrent episodes of genital herpes in immunocompetent adults, chronic suppressive therapy of recurrent episodes of genital herpes in immunocompetent and in HIV-infected adults, and reduction of transmission of genital herpes in immunocompetent adults. Treatment of chickenpox in immunocompetent patients 2 to <18 yrs.

**DOSAGE:** *Adults:* Herpes Zoster: 1g tid for 7 days. Start within 48 hrs after onset of rash. CrCl 30-49mL/min: 1g q12h. CrCl 10-29mL/min: 1g q24h. CrCl <10mL/min: 500mg q24h. Genital Herpes: Initial Episode: 1g bid for 10 days. Start within 48 hrs after onset of symptoms. CrCl 10-29mL/min: 1g q24h. CrCl <10mL/min: 500mg q24h. Recurrent Episodes: Treatment: 500mg bid for 3 days. Start at 1st sign/symptom of episode. CrCl ≤10-29mL/min: 500mg q24h. Suppressive Therapy w/ Normal Immune Function: 1g qd. CrCl ≤10-29mL/min: 500mg q24h. Alternative: (≤9 episodes/yr) 500mg qd. CrCl ≤10-29mL/min: 500mg q48h. Suppressive Therapy with HIV and CD4 ≥100 cells/mm$^3$: 500mg q12h. CrCl ≤10-29mL/min: 500mg q24h. Reduction of Transmission of Genital Herpes (≤9 episodes/yr): 500mg qd for the source partner. Herpes Labialis: 2g q12h for 1 day. Start at earliest symptom of cold sore. CrCl 30-49mL/min: 1g q12h. CrCl 10-29mL/min: 500mg q12h. CrCl <10mL/min: 500mg single dose. Do not exceed 1 day of treatment. *Pediatrics:* Herpes Labialis: ≥12 yrs: 2g q12h for 1 day. Start at earliest symptom of cold sore. Chickenpox: 2 to <18 yrs: 20mg/kg tid for 5 days. Max: 1g tid. Initiate at the earliest sign/symptom of chickenpox.

**HOW SUPPLIED:** Tab: 500mg, 1g* *partially scored

**WARNINGS/PRECAUTIONS:** Thrombotic thrombocytopenic purpura/hemolytic uremic syndrome (TTP/HUS) reported with advanced HIV disease, allogeneic bone marrow transplants, and in renal transplant patients. Cases of acute renal failure reported in elderly patients with or without reduced renal function, in patients with underlying renal disease who receive higher than recommended doses of valacyclovir for their level of renal function, and in patients without adequate hydration; reduce dose with renal dysfunction and maintain adequate hydration. Caution in elderly. CNS adverse reactions (eg, agitation, hallucinations, confusion, delirium, seizures, encephalopathy) are more likely in elderly but are also reported in adult and pediatric patients with or without reduced renal function and in patients with underlying renal disease; d/c if these occur.

**ADVERSE REACTIONS:** Headache, N/V, abdominal pain, dysmenorrhea, arthralgia, nasopharyngitis, fatigue, rash, upper respiratory tract infections, pyrexia, decreased neutrophil counts, diarrhea, elevated ALT/AST.

**INTERACTIONS:** Caution with other potentially nephrotoxic drugs.

**PREGNANCY:** Category B, caution in nursing.

**MECHANISM OF ACTION:** Nucleoside analogue; converted to acyclovir which inhibits replication of herpes viral DNA by competitively inhibiting viral DNA polymerase, incorporating and terminating growing viral DNA chain, and inactivating viral DNA polymerase.

**PHARMACOKINETICS: Absorption:** Rapid (GI tract); Acyclovir absolute bioavailability (54.5%). Oral administration of variable doses resulted in different parameters. **Distribution:** Valacyclovir: Plasma protein binding (13.5-17.9%). Acyclovir: Plasma protein binding (9-33%). Found in breast milk. **Metabolism:** Hepatic/Intestinal (1st pass) to acyclovir and L-valine. **Elimination:** Urine (46%), feces (47%); $T_{1/2}$=2.5-3.3 hrs.

## NURSING CONSIDERATIONS

**Assessment:** Assess for renal impairment, age of patient, pregnancy/nursing status, hydration status, and for possible drug interactions. Assess for presence of advanced HIV disease, an allogeneic bone transplant, and for the presence of a renal transplant.

**Monitoring:** Monitor for signs/symptoms of renal toxicity. Monitor for signs/symptoms of TTP/HUS in patients with advanced HIV disease, allogeneic bone marrow transplant patients, and in patients who are renal transplant recipients. Monitor for CNS effects such as agitation, hallucinations, confusion, delirium, seizures and encephalopathy.

**Patient Counseling:** Advise to maintain adequate hydration. Inform that product is not a cure for cold sores or genital herpes. In patients with genital herpes, instruct to avoid contact with lesions or sexual intercourse when lesions and/or symptoms are present to avoid infecting partner(s); use safe sex practice in combination with suppressive therapy. In patients with cold sores, instruct to initiate treatment at earliest symptom of a cold sore (eg, tingling, itching, burning); treatment should not exceed 1 day (2 doses) and that doses should be taken 12 hrs apart. In patients with herpes zoster, advise to initiate treatment as soon as possible after diagnosis. In patients with chicken pox, advise to initiate treatment at the earliest sign or symptom of chickenpox.

**Administration:** Oral route. **Storage:** 15-25°C (59-77°F). Dispense in well-closed container.

# VALTROPIN — RX

somatropin (LG Life)

**THERAPEUTIC CLASS:** Human growth hormone

**INDICATIONS:** Treatment of pediatric patients who have growth failure due to inadequate secretion of endogenous growth hormone. Treatment of growth failure associated with Turner syndrome in pediatric patients who have open epiphyses. Long-term replacement therapy in adults with growth hormone deficiency (GHD) of either adult or childhood onset etiology.

**DOSAGE:** *Adults:* Individualize dose. Initial: 0.33mg/day SQ 6 days a week. Dosage may be increased to individual patient requirement to maximum of 0.66mg/day after 4 weeks. Alternative Dosing: 0.2mg/day (Range: 0.15-0.3mg/day). May increase gradually every 1-2 months by 0.1-0.2mg/day based on individual patient requirements.

*Pediatrics:* Individualize dose. Divide weekly dose into equal amounts given either daily or 6 days a week by SQ injection. GHD: 0.17-0.3mg/kg of body weight/week. Turner Syndrome: Up to 0.375mg/kg of body weight/week.

**HOW SUPPLIED:** Inj: 5mg

**CONTRAINDICATIONS:** Pediatrics with closed epiphyses. Active proliferative and severe non-proliferative diabetic retinopathy. Presence of active malignancy. Acute critical illness due to complications following open heart surgery, abdominal surgery, or multiple accidental trauma, or those with acute respiratory failure. Patients with Prader-Willi syndrome who are severely obese or have severe respiratory impairment.

**WARNINGS/PRECAUTIONS:** Known sensitivity to supplied diluent (metacresol). Caution in pediatric pateints with Prader-Willi syndrome with 1 or more risk factors (severe obesity, history of upper airway destruction or sleep apnea, or unidentified respiratory infection). May decrease insulin sensitivity. Patients with GHD secondary to intracranial lesion should be monitored closely for progression or recurrence of underlying disease process. Intracranial HTN reported. Monitor closely with DM, glucose intolerance, hypopituitarism. Funduscopic exam recommended at initiation and periodically during course of therapy. Monitor carefully for any malignant transformation of skin lesions.

**ADVERSE REACTIONS:** Headache, pyrexia, cough, respiratory tract infection, diarrhea, vomiting, pharyngitis.

**INTERACTIONS:** Growth-promoting effects may be inhibited by glucocorticoids. May alter clearance of compounds metabolized by CP450 liver enzymes (eg, corticosteroids, sex steroids, anticonvulsants, cyclosporine); monitor closely. May need insulin adjustment.

**PREGNANCY:** Category B, caution in nursing.

**MECHANISM OF ACTION:** Human growth hormone; stimulates linear growth synthesis, metabolizes lipids, reduces body fat stores by increasing cellular protein, and increases plasma fatty acids.

**PHARMACOKINETICS: Absorption:** $C_{max}$=43.97ng/mL, $T_{max}$=4 hrs, AUC=369.9ng•hr/mL. **Metabolism:** Liver, kidneys (protein catabolism). **Elimination:** $T_{1/2}$=3.03 hrs.

## NURSING CONSIDERATIONS

**Assessment:** Assess for hypersensitivity to benzyl alcohol, closed epiphyses (pediatric), proliferative diabetic retinopathy, active malignancy, acute critical illness (complications of surgery, multiple accidental trauma, or acute respiratory failure), pre-existing type 1 or type 2 DM or impaired glucose tolerance, history of scoliosis, pre-existing papilledema, hypothyroidism, diagnostic imaging (pituitary or intracranial tumor), hypopituitarism, and possible drug interactions. Obtain baseline funduscopic exam. Prader-Willi syndrome: Evaluate for signs of upper airway obstruction or sleep apnea before initiation. Turner syndrome: Evaluate for otitis media or other ear disorders, and CV disorders before initiation.

**Monitoring:** Monitor fasting blood glucose and thyroid function tests periodically, periodic fundoscopic exam, weight control (Prader-Willi syndrome), signs/symptoms of malignant transformation of skin lesions, intracranial HTN, slipped capital femoral epiphysis (eg, onset of limp, hip or knee pain), hypersensitivity/allergic reactions, respiratory infections (Prader-Willi syndrome), otitis media or ear disorders, CV disorders and progression of scoliosis.

**Patient Counseling:** Instruct thoroughly as to proper usage, proper disposal, caution against any reuse of needles and syringes. Seek medical attention if signs/symptoms of slipped capital femoral epiphysis (eg, onset of limp, hip or knee pain), hypersensitivity/allergic reactions, respiratory infections (Prader-Willi syndrome), otitis media or CV disorders or progression of scoliosis occur.

**Administration:** SQ route (thighs). **Storage:** Before reconstitution: 2-8°C (36-46°F). Do not freeze. After reconstitution: 2-8°C (36-46°F) for up to 21 days. Do not freeze.



# VALTURNA RX

aliskiren - valsartan (Novartis)

**When used in pregnancy, drugs that act directly on the renin-angiotensin system can cause injury and death to the developing fetus. D/C immediately if pregnancy is detected.**

**THERAPEUTIC CLASS:** Renin inhibitor/angiotensin II receptor antagonist

**INDICATIONS:** Treatment of hypertension. May be used as an add-on therapy in patients whose BP is not adequately controlled alone. May be substituted for titrated components. May be used as initial therapy in patients who are likely to need multiple drugs to achieve BP goals.

**DOSAGE:** *Adults:* Usual: 150-160mg or 300-320mg qd. Initial: 150-160mg qd. Titrate: May increase up to 300-320mg if BP remains uncontrolled after 2-4 weeks. Max: 300-320mg/day.

**HOW SUPPLIED:** Tab: (Aliskiren-Valsartan) 150mg-160mg, 300mg-320mg

**WARNINGS/PRECAUTIONS:** Angioedema of the face, extremities, lips, tongue, lips glottis and/or larynx reported. D/C immediately if angioedema develops; do not readminister. Hypotension seen rarely; correct volume or salt depletion prior to administration in patients on high-dose diuretics to avoid symptomatic hypotension. Caution when initiating therapy in heart failure or post-MI patients. Caution with hepatic dysfunction including biliary obstructive disorders. Changes in renal function may occur; caution with renal artery stenosis, severe CHF. Minor and transient increases in BUN, SrCr, and $K^+$ may occur in patients with CHF and pre-existing renal impairment; consider dose reduction or d/c completely. Periodic determinations of serum electrolyte imbalances recommended.

**ADVERSE REACTIONS:** Fatigue, nasopharyngitis, diarrhea, upper respiratory tract infection, urinary tract infection, influenza, vertigo, hyperkalemia.

**INTERACTIONS:** Coadministration with atorvastatin and ketoconazole may increase aliskiren plasma levels. Coadministration with irbesartran and furosemide may reduce aliskiren plasma levels. Avoid with cyclosporine. Coadministration of inhibitors of the hepatic uptake transporter OATP1B1 (eg, rifampin, cyclosporine) or the hepatic efflux transporter MRP2 (eg, ritonavir) may increase systemic exposure to valsartan. Concomitant use with $K^+$-sparing diuretics, $K^+$ supplements, salt substitutes containing $K^+$ or other drugs that increase $K^+$ levels may lead to increase in serum $K^+$ levels, and increase SrCr in heart failure patients; caution when coadministering.

**PREGNANCY:** Category D, not for use in nursing.

**MECHANISM OF ACTION:** Aliskiren: Renin inhibitor; lowers BP by directly inhibiting renin, decreasing plasma renin activity, and inhibiting conversion of angiotensinogen to angiotensin I. Valsartan: Angiotensin II receptor antagonist; blocks vasoconstrictor and aldosterone-ecreting effects of angiotensin II by selectively blocking the binding of angiotensin II to the $AT_1$ receptor.

**PHARMACOKINETICS: Absorption:** Aliskiren: $T_{max}$ =1 hr. Valsartan: $T_{max}$=3 hrs. **Distribution:** Valsartan: (IV) $V_d$=17L; plasma protein binding (95%). **Metabolism:** Aliskiren: via CYP3A4 enzyme. Valsartan: Valeryl 4-hydroxy valsartan (primary metabolite). **Elimination:** Valsartan: Feces (83%), urine (13%); $T_{1/2}$=6 hrs.

## NURSING CONSIDERATIONS

**Assessment:** Assess BP, renal function, renal artery stenosis, renal/hepatic impairment, history of dialysis, nephrotic syndrome, heart failure, post-MI status, pregnancy/nursing status, and possible drug interactions.

**Monitoring:** Monitor BP, renal function including BUN, SrCr, and $K^+$levels, serum electrolytes, and signs/symptoms of hypotension or angioedema of head/neck.

**Patient Counseling:** Counsel about fetal risks during pregnancy and signs/symptoms of angioedema (eg, laryngeal or tongue edema); advise to seek prompt medication if any develop. Inform about adverse effects (eg, hypotension, hyperkalemia). Inform about need for periodic monitoring of electrolytes. Caution that lightheadness may occur especially during the first days of therapy, and should be reported immediately to physician; d/c if syncope occurs. Advise to avoid taking potassium supplements or salt substitutes containing potassium without consulting a physician.

**Administration:** Oral route. **Storage:** 25°C (77°F). Excursion permitted to 15-30°C (59-86°F). Protect from moisture. Dispense in tight container.

# VANCOCIN ORAL — RX

vancomycin HCl (Viro Pharma)

**THERAPEUTIC CLASS:** Tricyclic glycopeptide antibiotic

**INDICATIONS:** Treatment of enterocolitis caused by *Staphylococcus aureus* and antibiotic-associated pseudomembranous colitis caused by *Clostridium difficile*.

**DOSAGE:** *Adults:* 500mg-2g/day given tid-qid for 7-10 days. Elderly: Start at lower end of dosing range.
*Pediatrics:* 40mg/kg/day given tid-qid for 7-10 days. Max: 2g/day.

**HOW SUPPLIED:** Cap: 125mg, 250mg

**WARNINGS/PRECAUTIONS:** Use in the absence of a proven or strongly suspected bacterial infection or a prophylactic indication is unlikely to provide benefit and increases the risk of drug-resistant bacteria. Monitoring serum concentrations may be appropriate in some instances (eg, renal insufficiency and/or colitis). Not effective for other types of infection. Caution with inflammatory disorders of intestinal mucosa, renal impairment; may have increased systemic absorption and may be at risk for development of adverse reactions associated with parenteral administration of vancomycin. Ototoxicity reported; caution in patients with underlying hearing loss; consider performing serial tests of auditory function during use to minimize ototoxicity risk. Monitor renal function in patients with underlying renal dysfunction. May cause overgrowth of nonsusceptible organisms; take appropriate measures if superinfection develops. Caution in elderly.

**ADVERSE REACTIONS:** Nephrotoxicity, ototoxicity, reversible neutropenia, anaphylactoid reactions (hypotension, wheezing, "Red Man syndrome," pruritus)

**INTERACTIONS:** Monitor renal function with aminoglycosides. Increased risk of ototoxicity when used concurrently with other ototoxic agents (eg, aminoglycosides).

**PREGNANCY:** Category B, caution in nursing.

**MECHANISM OF ACTION:** Tricyclic glycopeptide antibiotic; inhibits cell-wall biosynthesis. Also alters bacterial cell membrane permeabilty and RNA synthesis.

**PHARMACOKINETICS: Absorption:** Poor. **Elimination:** Urine, feces.

## NURSING CONSIDERATIONS

**Assessment:** Assess for inflammatory intestinal disorders, renal dysfunction, hearing disturbances, pregnancy/nursing status, and for possible drug interactions. Document indications for therapy, culture, and susceptibility testing.

**Monitoring:** Monitor signs/symptoms of ototoxicity, superinfection, and for anaphylactoid reactions. Monitor drug levels when appropriate (eg, renal insufficiency and/or colitis). Monitor renal function in patients with underlying renal dysfunction.

**Patient Counseling:** Inform that therapy treats bacterial, not viral infections. Instruct to take as directed; inform that skipping doses or not completing full course may decrease effectiveness and increase resistance.

**Administration:** Oral route. **Storage:** 59-86°F (15-30°C).

# VANCOMYCIN INJECTION RX

vancomycin HCl (Various)

V

**THERAPEUTIC CLASS:** Tricyclic glycopeptide antibiotic

**INDICATIONS:** Treatment of serious or severe infections caused by susceptible strains of methicillin-resistant (β-lactam resistant) staphylococci. Indicated for penicillin-allergic patients who cannot receive or have failed to respond to other drugs, and for infections caused by vancomycin-susceptible organisms that are resistant to other antimicrobials. Indicated for initial therapy when methicillin-resistant staphylococci are suspected. Effective in the treatment of staphylococcal endocarditis, other infections due to staphylococci, including septicemia, bone infections, lower respiratory tract infections, and skin and skin-structure infections. Effective alone or in combination with an aminoglycoside for endocarditis caused by *S.viridans* or *S.bovis*. Effective only in combination with an aminoglycoside for endocarditis caused by enterococci (eg, *E.faecalis*). Effective for treatment of diphtheroid endocarditis. Successfully used in combination with either rifampin, an aminoglycoside, or both in early-onset prosthetic valve endocarditis caused by *S.epidermidis* or diphtheroids. Parenteral form may be administered orally for treatment of antibiotic-associated pseudomembranous colitis produced by *C.difficile* and for staphylococcal enterocolitis.

**DOSAGE:** *Adults*: Usual: 500mg IV q6h or 1g IV q12h. Administer at no more than 10mg/min or over at least 60 min, whichever is longer. Renal Impairment: Initial: Not <15mg/kg. Dosage per day in mg is about 15x the GFR in mL/min (refer to dosage table in PI). Elderly: Require greater dose reductions than expected. Functionally Anephric Patients: Initial: 15mg/kg, then 1.9mg/kg/24 hrs. Marked Renal Impairment: 250-1000mg once every several days. Anuria: 1000mg every 7-10 days. For PO Administration: 500-2000mg/day in 3-4 divided doses for 7-10 days. Max: 2000mg/day. May dilute in 1oz of water. May also be administered via NG tube.

*Pediatrics*: Usual: 10mg/kg IV q6h. Infants/Neonates: Initial: 15mg/kg, then 10mg/kg q12h for neonates in 1st week of life and q8h thereafter until 1 month of age. Administer over at least 60 min. Renal Impairment: Initial: Not <15mg/kg. Dosage per day in mg is about 15x the GFR in mL/min (refer to table in PI). Premature Infants: Requires longer dosing intervals. ADD-Vantage vials should not be used in neonates, infants, and pediatrics who require doses <500mg. For PO Administration: 40mg/kg/day in 3-4 divided doses for 7-10 days. Max: 2000mg/day. May dilute in 1oz of water. May also be administered via NG tube.

**HOW SUPPLIED:** Inj: 500mg, 1g

**WARNINGS/PRECAUTIONS:** Not effective by the oral route for other types of infections. Rapid bolus administration may cause hypotension and cardiac arrest (rare); administer in diluted solution over a period not <60 min. Ototoxicity reported; caution if with underlying hearing loss. Caution with renal insufficiency and adjust dose with renal dysfunction. Pseudomembranous colitis reported. Prolonged use may result in overgrowth of nonsusceptible organisms. Reversible neutropenia reported; monitor leukocyte count periodically. Administer via IV route. Thrombophlebitis may occur; infuse slowly and rotate injection sites. Safety and efficacy of administration via the intraperitoneal and intrathecal (intralumbar and intraventricular) routes has not been established. Administration via intraperitoneal route during continuous ambulatory peritoneal dialysis (CAPD) has resulted in a syndrome of chemical peritonitis. Caution in elderly.

**ADVERSE REACTIONS:** Infusion-related events, hypotension, wheezing, pruritus, chest and back muscle spasm or pain, dyspnea, urticaria, nephrotoxicity, pseudomembranous colitis, ototoxicity, neutropenia, phlebitis.

**INTERACTIONS:** Concomitant use of anesthetic agents associated with erythema, histamine-like flushing, and anaphylactoid reactions. Concurrent and/or sequential systemic or topical use of other potentially neurotoxic and/or nephrotoxic drugs (eg, amphotericin B, aminoglycosides, bacitracin, polymyxin B, colistin, viomycin, cisplatin) requires careful monitoring. Increased risk of ototoxicity with concomitant ototoxic agents (eg, aminoglycoside). Periodic leukocyte count monitoring with drugs that may cause neutropenia. Serial monitoring of renal function and particular care following appropriate dosing to minimize risk of nephrotoxicity with concomitant aminoglycoside.

**PREGNANCY:** Category C, not for use in nursing.

**MECHANISM OF ACTION:** Tricyclic glycopeptide antibiotic; inhibits cell-wall biosynthesis, alters bacterial cell membrane permeability and RNA synthesis.

**PHARMACOKINETICS: Absorption:** (1g at 2 hrs) $C_{max}$ =23mcg/mL; (500mg at 2 hrs) $C_{max}$=19mcg/mL. **Distribution:** Serum protein binding (55%). **Elimination:** Urine (75%); $T_{1/2}$=4-6 hrs.

## NURSING CONSIDERATIONS

**Assessment:** Assess for renal function, underlying hearing loss, ototoxicity, pregnancy/nursing status and possible drug interactions. Perform culture and susceptibility testing.

**Monitoring:** Monitor for hypersensitivity reactions (eg, Stevens-Johnson syndrome, vasculitis), infusion reactions (eg, hypotension, arrhythmias, "Red Neck"), thrombophlebitis, ototoxicity, renal function, diarrhea, pseudomembranous colitis, neutropenia, superinfection, and chemical peritonitis (intraperitoneal route). Monitor leukocyte count periodically.

**Patient Counseling:** Inform that drug treats bacterial, not viral, infections. Take as directed; skipping doses or not completing full course may decrease effectiveness and increase bacterial resistance. Inform that may experience diarrhea; notify physician if watery/bloody stools, hypersensitivity reactions, or superinfection develops.

**Administration:** IV, Oral route. Refer to PI for preparation for IV use. Intermittent infusion recommended. Physically incompatible with β-lactam antibiotics. Diluted sol may be given via NGT. (PO) Common flavoring syrup may be added to improve taste. **Storage:** 20-25°C (68-77°F). After reconstitution: may refrigerate for 14 days. After further dilution: may refrigerate for 14 days or 96 hrs depending on diluent used (refer to PI).

## VANOS — RX
fluocinonide (Medicis)

**THERAPEUTIC CLASS:** Corticosteroid

**INDICATIONS:** To relieve inflammatory and pruritic manifestations of corticosteroid-responsive dermatoses in patients ≥12 yrs.

**DOSAGE:** *Adults:* Psoriasis/Corticosteroid Responsive Dermatoses: Apply thin layer to affected areas qd-bid. Atopic Dermatitis: Apply thin layer to affected areas qd. Max: 60g/week. Do not exceed 2 weeks.
*Pediatrics:* ≥12 yrs: Psoriasis/Corticosteroid Responsive Dermatoses: Apply thin layer to affected areas qd-bid. Atopic Dermatitis: Apply thin layer to affected areas qd. Max: 60g/week. Do not exceed 2 weeks.

**HOW SUPPLIED:** Cre: 0.1% [30g, 60g, 120g]

**WARNINGS/PRECAUTIONS:** May produce reversible hypothalamic-pituitary-adrenal (HPA) axis suppression, manifestations of Cushing's syndrome, hyperglycemia, and glucosuria; pediatric patients are at greater risk. Caution when applied to large surface areas or under occlusive dressings; evaluate periodically for HPA suppression. Do not use for more than 2 weeks at a time and apply on small areas when HPA suppression develops. Use appropriate antifungal or antibacterial agent with dermatological infections. D/C if infection does not clear or irritation develops. Not recommended for treatment of rosacea or perioral dematitis. Do not use on face, groin, or underarms. Caution in elderly. D/C therapy when control is achieved.

**ADVERSE REACTIONS:** Headache, application-site burning, nasopharyngitis, nasal congestion, unspecified application-site reaction.

**PREGNANCY:** Category C, not for use in nursing.

**MECHANISM OF ACTION:** Synthetic corticosteroid; possesses anti-inflammatory, antipruritic, and vasoconstrictive properties. Anti-inflammatory activity not established; suspected to act by induction of phospholipase $A_2$ inhibitory proteins, lipocortins. Lipocortins control biosynthesis of potent inflammation mediators (eg, prostaglandins, leukotrienes) by inhibiting release of their common precursor, arachidonic acid.



### NURSING CONSIDERATIONS

**Assessment:** Assess for serum cortisol level, HPA suppression, rosacea or perioral dermatitis, pregnancy/nursing status. Obtain cosyntropin (ACTH) stimulation result.

**Monitoring:** Monitor for signs/symptoms of reversible HPA-axis suppression, Cushing's syndrome, hyperglycemia, glucosuria, skin irritation, allergic contact dermatitis (eg, failure to heal), and for development of concomitant skin infections (eg, bacterial, fungal). With large doses or use of occlusive dressings, monitor for HPA-axis suppression using cosyntropin ($ACTH_{1-24}$) stimulation test. Following withdrawal of therapy, monitor for glucocorticosteroid insufficiency. In pediatric patients, monitor for systemic toxicity, HPA-axis suppression (linear growth retardation, delayed weight gain), Cushing's syndrome, and intracranial HTN.

**Patient Counseling:** Counsel to use externally and exactly as directed; avoid contact with eyes, face, groin, and underarms. Instruct not to cover, wrap, or bandage treatment areas unless directed by physician. Inform not to use more than 60 g per week. Wash hands following application. Contact physician if adverse reactions (eg, burning, itching, irritation) occur or no clinical improvement after 2 weeks. Contact physician before using other corticosteroid-containing products. Notify physician if planning surgery during therapy.

**Administration:** Topical route. **Storage:** 15-30°C (59-86°F).

## VANTAS — RX

histrelin acetate (Indevus)

**THERAPEUTIC CLASS:** Luteinizing hormone-releasing hormone agonist

**INDICATIONS:** Palliative treatment of advanced prostate cancer.

**DOSAGE:** *Adults:* 50mg every 12 months. Inject SQ into inner aspect of the upper arm. Refrain from wetting the inserted arm for 24 hrs. Refrain from heavy lifting or strenuous exercise of the inserted arm for 7 days after implant insertion. Must remove after 12 months of therapy.

**HOW SUPPLIED:** Implant: 50mg

**CONTRAINDICATIONS:** Women and pediatric patients.

**WARNINGS/PRECAUTIONS:** Transient increase in serum testosterone and worsening of symptoms of prostate cancer with initial therapy. Urethral obstruction and spinal cord compression reported. Anaphylactic reactions may occur.

**ADVERSE REACTIONS:** Hot flashes, fatigue, implant site reaction, testicular atrophy, renal impairment, gynecomastia, constipation, erectile dysfunction.

**PREGNANCY:** Category X, not for use in nursing.

**MECHANISM OF ACTION:** LH-RH agonist; acts as potent inhibitor of gonadotropin secretion, desensitizes responsiveness of pituitary gonadotropin, causing reduction in testicular steroidogenesis.

**PHARMACOKINETICS: Absorption:** $C_{max}$=1.1ng/mL; $T_{max}$=12 hrs. **Distribution:** $V_d$=58.4L. **Elimination:** $T_{1/2}$=3.92 hrs.

## NURSING CONSIDERATIONS

**Assessment:** Assess pregnancy status, for metastatic vertebral lesions, urinary tract obstruction, and possible drug interactions. Obtain baseline serum testosterone and PSA levels.

**Monitoring:** Periodically monitor serum testosterone and PSA levels. Monitor for signs/symptoms of anaphylactoid reactions, transient worsening of symptoms, and implant-site reaction.

**Patient Counseling:** Instruct to refrain from wetting arm for 24 hrs and from heavy lifting or strenuous exertion for 7 days after implant insertion. Monitor for signs/symptoms of anaphylactoid reactions, transient worsening of symptoms, and implant-site reaction.

**Administration:** Dermal implant. Inserting implant: 1) Clean and anesthesize area; make 2-3mm incision SQ and perpendicular to shoulder. 2) Grasp tool by handle; insert tip into incision with bevel up and advance along track to inscribed line on cannula. 3) Hold tool in place; move thumb to green retraction button; press down to release lock; draw button back towards handle until it stops. Withdraw tool from incision. Check implant by palpation. **Storage:** Refrigerate; 2-8°C (36-46°F). Protect from light. Do not freeze.

# VANTIN RX

cefpodoxime proxetil (Pharmacia & Upjohn)

**THERAPEUTIC CLASS:** Cephalosporin (3rd generation)

**INDICATIONS:** Treatment of mild to moderate infections (acute otitis media, pharyngitis/tonsillitis, community-acquired pneumonia [CAP], acute bacterial exacerbation of chronic bronchitis [ABECB], acute uncomplicated urethral and cervical gonorrhea, acute uncomplicated anorectal infections in women, uncomplicated skin and skin structure infections [SSSI], acute maxillary sinusitis, and uncomplicated urinary tract infections [cystitis]) caused by susceptible strains of microorganisms.

**DOSAGE:** *Adults:* Pharyngitis/Tonsillitis: 100mg q12h for 5-10 days. CAP: 200mg q12h for 14 days. ABECB: 200mg q12h for 10 days. Uncomplicated Gonorrhea (Men/Women)/Rectal Gonococcal Infections (Women): 200mg single dose. SSSI: 400mg q12h for 7-14 days. Sinusitis: 200mg q12h for 10 days. Cystitis: 100mg q12h for 7 days. CrCl <30mL/min: Increase interval to q24h. Hemodialysis: Dose 3 times weekly after dialysis. Take with food. *Pediatrics:* ≥12 yrs: (Susp/Tabs): Pharyngitis/Tonsillitis: 100mg q12h for 5-10 days. CAP: 200mg q12h for 14 days. Uncomplicated Gonorrhea (Men/Women)/Rectal Gonococcal Infections (Women): 200mg single dose. SSSI: 400mg q12h for 7-14 days. Sinusitis: 200mg q12h for 10 days. Cystitis: 100mg q12h for 7 days. (Tabs) ABECB: 200mg q12h for 10 days. 2 months to 12 yrs: (Susp): Otitis media: 5mg/kg (max 200mg/dose) q12h for 5 days. Pharyngitis/Tonsillitis: 5mg/kg/dose (max 100mg/dose) q12h for 5-10 days. Sinusitis: 5mg/kg (max 200mg/dose) for 10 days. CrCl <30mL/min: Increase interval to q24h. Hemodialysis: Dose 3 times weekly after dialysis. Take with food.

**HOW SUPPLIED:** Sus: (Generic) 50mg/5mL, 100mg/5mL; Tab: 100mg, 200mg

**WARNINGS/PRECAUTIONS:** Cross-sensitivity to PCNs and other cephalosporins may occur. *Clostridium difficile*-associated diarrhea reported. Positive direct Coombs' tests reported. Caution with renal impairment; dose reduction may be needed. May result in overgrowth of nonsusceptible organisms with prolonged use.

**ADVERSE REACTIONS:** Diarrhea, nausea.

**INTERACTIONS:** Decreased plasma levels and absorption with antacids and $H_2$-blockers. Delayed peak plasma levels with oral anticholinergics. Probenecid inhibits renal excretion. Closely monitor renal function with nephrotoxic agents. Caution with potent diuretics.

**PREGNANCY:** Category B, not for use in nursing.

**MECHANISM OF ACTION:** Cephalosporin; inhibits cell-wall synthesis.

**PHARMACOKINETICS: Absorption**: $C_{max}$(100mg)=1.4mcg/mL, (200mg)=2.3mcg/mL, (400mg)=3.9mcg/mL; $T_{max}$=2-3 hrs. **Distribution:** Plasma protein binding (21-29%), found in breast milk. **Metabolism:** Via desterification; cefpodoxime (active metabolite). **Elimination**: Urine; $T_{1/2}$= 2.09-2.84 hrs.

## NURSING CONSIDERATIONS

**Assessment:** Assess for history of hypersensitivity to cephalosporins/PCNs, pregnancy status, possible drug interactions, renal impairment. Document indications for therapy, culture, and susceptibility testing.

V

**Monitoring:** Monitor for signs/symptoms of hypersensitivity reactions (anaphylaxis, Stevens-Johnsons syndrome), *C.difficile*-associated diarrhea, seizures, LFTs, CBC with platelets and differential, renal function, PT, LDH, superinfections.

**Patient Counseling:** Inform that drug only treats bacterial, not viral, infections. Instruct to take as directed; skipping doses or not completing full course may decrease effectiveness and increase resistance. Inform may experience diarrhea; contact physician if watery/bloody stools occur.

**Administration:** Oral route. **Storage:** 20°-25°C (68°-77°F). Protect from excessive moisture.

## Vaqta RX
hepatitis B immune globulin (Merck)

**THERAPEUTIC CLASS:** Vaccine

**INDICATIONS:** Active immunization against hepatitis A virus. Give primary immunization at least 2 weeks before expected exposure.

**DOSAGE:** *Adults:* ≥19 yrs: 1mL (50 U) IM followed by a booster of 1mL (50 U) 6-18 months later.
*Pediatrics:* 1-18 yrs: 0.5mL (25 U) IM followed by a booster of 0.5mL (25 U) 6-18 months later.

**HOW SUPPLIED:** Inj: 25 U/0.5mL, 50 U/mL

**WARNINGS/PRECAUTIONS:** Have epinephrine (1:1000) available. May not prevent hepatitis A with unrecognized infection. Caution with bleeding disorders (eg, hemophilia or thrombocytopenia or patients on anticoagulant therapy). Defer use with acute infection or febrile illness. Suboptimal response may occur in immunocompromised patients.

**ADVERSE REACTIONS:** Injection-site pain, tenderness, erythema, swelling, warmth, fever.

**INTERACTIONS:** Immunosuppressive therapy may reduce response to active immunization.

**PREGNANCY:** Category C, caution in nursing.

**MECHANISM OF ACTION:** Vaccine; produces an antibody response against hepatitis A virus.

### NURSING CONSIDERATIONS

**Assessment:** Assess for immune status, vaccination history, bleeding disorders (eg, hemophilia, thrombocytopenia), acute infection or febrile illness, pregnancy/nursing status, and possible drug interactions (eg, anticoagulants).

**Monitoring:** Monitor for signs/symptoms of hypersensitivity reactions (eg, anaphylaxis), injection-site reactions, or hematoma, immune response, fever, elevated LFTs, eosinophilia, and increased urine protein.

**Patient Counseling:** Inform of potential risks/benefits; report any adverse reactions to physician. Primary immunization should be given 2 weeks prior to expected exposure to hepatitis A virus.

**Administration:** IM route; inject preferably into deltoid muscle. Do not inject intravascularly, intradermally, or SQ. **Storage:** 2-8°C (36-46°F). Do not freeze.

## Varivax RX
varicella virus vaccine live (Merck)

**THERAPEUTIC CLASS:** Vaccine

**INDICATIONS:** Vaccination against varicella.

**DOSAGE:** *Adults:* 0.5mL SQ at elected date, repeat 4-8 weeks later.
*Pediatrics:* 12 months-12 yrs: 0.5mL SQ. If a second dose is given; administer a minimum of 3 months later. ≥13 yrs: 0.5mL SQ at elected date, repeat 4-8 weeks later.

**HOW SUPPLIED:** Inj: 1350PFU/0.5mL

**CONTRAINDICATIONS:** Pregnancy (avoid pregnancy for 3 months after vaccine); gelatin hypersensitivity; anaphylactoid reactions to neomycin, blood dyscrasias, leukemia, lymphomas, malignant neoplasms affecting bone marrow or lymphatic system, febrile respiratory illness or other active febrile infection, active untreated TB, immunosuppressive therapy, immunosuppressant doses of corticosteroids, immunodeficiency states and family history of congenital or hereditary immunodeficiency.

**WARNINGS/PRECAUTIONS:** Children and adolescents with ALL in remission can receive the vaccine under an investigational protocol. Defer vaccine for at least 5 months after blood or plasma transfusions, or administration of immune globulin or varicella zoster immune globulin. Defer vaccine with family history of congenital, hereditary immunodeficiency until immune system evaluated. Rarely, vaccine virus transmission through varicella-like rash can occur; avoid close association with susceptible high-risk individuals for up to six weeks (eg, immunocompromised patients, pregnant women without history of chickenpox, newborns of mothers without documented history of chickenpox). Have epinephrine available. Do not inject into a blood vessel.

**ADVERSE REACTIONS:** Fever, local reactions, pain, varicella-like rashes.

**INTERACTIONS:** Avoid immune globulins for 2 months after vaccination. Avoid salicylates for 6 weeks after vaccination. Contraindicated with immunosuppressive therapy or immunosuppressant doses of corticosteroids.

**PREGNANCY:** Category C, caution in nursing.

**MECHANISM OF ACTION:** Vaccine; cell-mediated immune response stimulation against varicella zoster virus (VZV) infection.

## NURSING CONSIDERATIONS

**Assessment:** Assess for immunity, health status, blood dyscrasias, immunization/family history, and possible drug interactions.

**Monitoring:** Monitor for signs/symptoms of allergic reactions, injection-site reactions (eg, pain, swelling, rash, hematoma, pruritus), fever, URI, irritability, diarrhea, anorexia, N/V, headache, and thrombocytopenia.

**Patient Counseling:** Inform of potential benefits/risks; report adverse reactions to physician. May not offer 100% protection.

**Administration:** SQ route; inject into outer aspect of deltoid region. **Storage:** Frozen at -15°C (+5°F) or colder; diluent stored at room temperature or refrigerated.

# VASERETIC RX

enalapril maleate - hydrochlorothiazide (Merck)

**ACE inhibitors can cause death/injury to developing fetus during 2nd and 3rd trimesters. D/C therapy if pregnancy detected.**

**THERAPEUTIC CLASS:** ACE inhibitor/thiazide diuretic

**INDICATIONS:** Treatment of hypertension. Not indicated for initial treatment.

**DOSAGE:** *Adults:* If BP is not controlled on either enalapril or HCTZ monotherapy may give 5mg-12.5mg or 10mg-25mg qd. Titrate: Dose titration must be guided by clinical effect; at 2-3 week intervals. Max: 20mg-50mg qd. Renal impairment: Not recommended. Replacement Therapy: Substitute combination for titrated components. Elderly: Start at lower end of dosing range.

**HOW SUPPLIED:** Tab: (Enalapril-HCTZ) 5mg-12.5mg, 10mg-25mg

**CONTRAINDICATIONS:** History of ACE inhibitor-associated angioedema and hereditary or idiopathic angioedema. Anuria, sulfonamide hypersensitivity.

**WARNINGS/PRECAUTIONS:** D/C if angioedema, jaundice, or if marked LFT elevation occurs. Risk of hyperkalemia with DM, renal dysfunction. Persistent nonproductive cough reported. Monitor WBCs in renal and collagen vascular disease. Anaphylactoid reactions reported. Fetal/neonatal morbidity and death reported. Monitor for hypotension in high-risk patients (heart failure, surgery/anesthesia, hyponatremia, severe volume/salt depletion, etc.). Caution with CHF, renal or hepatic dysfunction, obstruction to left ventricle outflow tract, elderly, renal artery stenosis. More reports of angioedema in blacks than nonblacks. May exacerbate or activate systemic lupus erythematosus (SLE). Monitor serum electrolytes. Avoid if CrCl≤30mL/min/1.73m². May increase cholesterol, TG, uric acid levels, and blood glucose. Intestinal angioedema reported. Oliguria, progressive azotemia, acute renal failure, and death (rare) may occur in patients with CHF. Not for initial therapy. Caution with severe renal disease, impaired hepatic function, and progressive liver disease. Hypokalemia may occur and cause cardiac arrhythmia and may sensitize or exaggerate the response of the heart to toxic effects of digitalis (eg, increased ventricular irritability). Hyponatremia (including dilutional hyponatremia in edematous patients in hot weather), hypochloremic alkalosis, hyperuricemia (or frank gout), hyperglycemia, hypomagnesemia and hypocalcemia may occur. Enhanced effects in the postsympathectomy patient.

**ADVERSE REACTIONS:** Dizziness, cough, fatigue, and headache.

**INTERACTIONS:** Increased risk of hyperkalemia with $K^+$-sparing diuretics, $K^+$ supplements, or $K^+$-containing salt substitutes. Potentiates orthostatic hypotension with alcohol, barbiturates, and narcotics. Adjust insulin and antidiabetic drugs. Impaired absorption with cholestyramine, colestipol. Corticosteroids and ACTH deplete electrolytes. May decrease response to pressor amines. Potentiates other antihypertensives that cause renin release (eg, diuretics). May increase responsiveness to skeletal muscle relaxants, nondepolarizing (eg, tubocurarine). Risk of lithium toxicity. NSAIDs may reduce antihypertensive effect and worsen renal dysfunction. Concomitant use of diuretic may increase blood urea and serum creatinine with HTN or CHF.

**PREGNANCY:** Category C (1st trimester) and D (2nd and 3rd trimesters); not for use in nursing.

**MECHANISM OF ACTION:** Enalapril: ACE inhibitor; inhibition results in decreased plasma angiotensin II, which leads to decreased vasopressor activity and decreased aldosterone secretion. HCTZ: Thiazide diuretic; affects renal tubular mechanism of electrolyte reabsorption, directly increasing excretion of $Na^+$ and chloride.

**PHARMACOKINETICS: Absorption:** (60%); $T_{max}$ (enalapril, enalaprilat)=1, 3-4 hrs. **Distribution:** Found in breast milk. HCTZ: Crosses placental barrier. **Metabolism:** Via hydrolysis; Enalaprilat (metabolite). **Elimination:** Enalapril: Urine, feces (94%); $T_{1/2}$ (enalaprilat)=11 hrs. HCTZ: Kidneys; $T_{1/2}$=5.6-14.8 hrs.

## NURSING CONSIDERATIONS

**Assessment:** Assess BP, LFTs, renal function, CVD (eg, cardiomyopathy, aortic stenosis), renal artery stenosis, SLE, serum electrolytes, pregnancy status, history of allergy to sulfonamides, bronchial asthma, parathyroid disorders, and for possible drug interactions.

**Monitoring:** Monitor BP, LFTs, renal function, CBC with platelet count and differential, serum electrolytes. Monitor for MI, CHF, angioedema (head, neck, intestinal), anaphylactoid reactions, hepatic failure, hyperuricemia, hyperglycemia, hypersensitivity reactions, cough, N/V, dizziness.

**Patient Counseling:** Inform about fetal risks if taken during pregnancy. Caution that inadequate fluid intake, excessive perspiration, diarrhea, or vomiting may lead to excessive fall in BP, resulting in lightheadedness and possible syncope. Advise not to use $K^+$ supplements or salt substitutes containing $K^+$ without consulting physician. Counsel about signs/symptoms of neutropenia (eg, fever, sore throat, infection), angioedema, electrolyte imbalance (eg, thirst, weakness, lethargy) and other adverse effects; advise to seek prompt medical attention if any occur.

**Administration:** Oral route. Not recommended in patients with severe renal impairment. **Storage:** Below 30°C(86°F); avoid temperature above 50°C(122°F). Keep container tightly closed. Protect from moisture.

# VASOTEC — RX

enalapril maleate (Merck)

**ACE inhibitors can cause death/injury to developing fetus during 2nd and 3rd trimesters. D/C therapy if pregnancy detected.**

**THERAPEUTIC CLASS:** ACE inhibitor

**INDICATIONS:** Treatment of hypertension, alone or with other antihypertensive agents (thiazide diuretics). Treatment of symptomatic chronic heart failure (CHF) usually in combination with diuretics and digitalis. To decrease overt heart failure development and hospitalization in stable asymptomatic left ventricular dysfunction.

**DOSAGE:** *Adults:* HTN: If possible, d/c diuretic 2-3 days prior to therapy. Initial: 5mg qd, 2.5mg qd with concomitant diuretic. Usual: 10-40mg given qd or bid. Resume diuretic if BP not controlled. CrCl>80mL/min: Initial: 5mg qd. CrCl≤80>30mL/min: Initial: 5mg. CrCl ≤30mL/min: Initial: 2.5mg qd. Dialysis: Initial: 2.5mg qd on dialysis days. Max: 40mg qd. Heart Failure: Initial: 2.5mg qd. Usual: 2.5-20mg given bid. Max: 40mg qd. Asymptomatic Left Ventricular Dysfunction: Initial: 2.5mg bid. Titrate: Increase to 20mg qd. Hyponatremia or SrCr 1.6mg/dL with Heart Failure: Initial: 2.5mg qd. Titrate: Increase to 2.5mg bid, then 5mg bid. Max: 40mg qd.
*Pediatrics:* HTN: Initial: 0.08mg/kg (up to 5mg) qd. Titrate: Adjust according to response. Max: 0.58mg/kg/dose (or 40mg/dose). Avoid if GFR <30mL/min/1.73m$^2$.

**HOW SUPPLIED:** Tab: 2.5mg*, 5mg*, 10mg,* 20mg* *scored

**CONTRAINDICATIONS:** History of ACE inhibitor-associated angioedema and hereditary or idiopathic angioedema.

**WARNINGS/PRECAUTIONS:** D/C if angioedema, jaundice, or if marked LFT elevation occurs. Risk of hyperkalemia with DM, renal dysfunction. Persistent nonproductive cough reported. Monitor WBCs in renal or collagen vascular disease. Anaphylactoid reactions reported. Fetal/neonatal morbidity and death reported. Monitor for hypotension in high-risk patients (heart failure, surgery/anesthesia, hyponatremia, high-dose diuretic therapy, severe volume and/or salt depletion, etc). Caution with CHF, obstruction to left ventricle outflow tract, renal dysfunction, and renal artery stenosis. Less effective on BP in blacks and more reports of angioedema than nonblacks. Intestinal angioedema reported. Oliguria, progressive azotemia, acute renal failure, and death (rare) may occur in patients at high risk for hypotension.

**ADVERSE REACTIONS:** Fatigue, headache, dizziness, hypotension.

**INTERACTIONS:** May increase lithium levels. Hypotension risk with diuretics. May further decrease renal dysfunction with NSAIDs. Increased risk of hyperkalemia with $K^+$-sparing diuretics, $K^+$-containing salt substitutes, or $K^+$ supplements. Augmented effect by antihypertensives that cause renin release (eg, thiazides). NSAIDs may diminish antihypertensive effect. Nitritoid reactions (eg, facial flushing, N/V, hypotension) reported rarely with injectable gold. Concomitant use of diuretic may increase blood urea and serum creatinine with HTN or CHF.

**PREGNANCY:** Category C (1st trimester) and D (2nd and 3rd trimesters), not for use in nursing.

**MECHANISM OF ACTION:** ACE inhibitor; inhibition results in decreased plasma angiotensin II, which leads to decreased vasopressor activity and decreased aldosterone secretion.

**PHARMACOKINETICS: Absorption:** $T_{max}$=1, 3-4 hrs (enalapril, enalaprilat). **Metabolism:** Via hydrolysis, enalaprilat (metabolite). **Elimination:** Urine,/feces (94%); $T_{1/2}$=11 hrs (enalaprilat).

## NURSING CONSIDERATIONS

**Assessment:** Assess BP, LFTs, renal function, CHF, renal artery stenosis, pregnancy status, history of angioedema, and possible drug interactions.

**Monitoring:** Monitor BP, LFTs, renal function, CBC with platelet count and differential, serum $K^+$ levels. Monitor for MI, CHF, angioedema (head, neck, intestinal), anaphylactoid reactions, hepatic failure, hypersensitivity reactions, cough, N/V, dizziness.

**Patient Counseling:** Counsel about fetal risks during pregnancy and signs/symptoms of angioedema (eg, laryngeal/tongue edema, abdominal pain); advise to seek prompt medical attention if symptoms develop. Inform about adverse effects (eg, anaphylaxis, cough, hypotension, hyperkalemia). Infants with histories of *in utero* exposure should be closely observed for hypotension, oliguria, hyperkalemia. Inform about need for periodic monitoring of electrolytes and blood counts. Caution that inadequate fluid intake, excessive perspiration, diarrhea, vomiting may lead to excessive fall in BP, which can result in lightheadedness or possible syncope. Advise not to use $K^+$ supplements or salt substitutes containing $K^+$ without consulting physician. Advise patient to report any signs of infection.

**Administration:** Oral route. See PI for preparation of suspension. **Storage:** (Cap) 25°C (77°F); excursions permitted to 15-30°C (59-86°F). Protect from moisture. Dispense in tight container. (Sus) Refrigerate at 2-8°C (36-46°F) and can be stored for up to 30 days. Shake the suspension before each use.

## VASOTEC I.V. RX

enalaprilat (Merck)

**ACE inhibitors can cause death/injury to developing fetus during 2nd and 3rd trimesters. Stop therapy if pregnancy detected.**

**THERAPEUTIC CLASS:** ACE inhibitor

**INDICATIONS:** Treatment of hypertension when oral therapy is not practical.

**DOSAGE:** *Adults:* Administer IV over 5 min. Usual: 1.25mg q6h for no longer than 48 hrs. Max: 20mg/day. Concomitant Diuretic/CrCl ≤30mL/min: Initial: 0.625mg, may repeat after 1 hr. Maint: 1.25mg q6h. Risk of Excessive Hypotension: Initial: 0.625mg over 5 min to 1 hr. PO/IV Conversion: Give 5mg/day PO for 1.25mg IV q6h and 2.5mg/day PO for 0.625mg q6h IV.

**HOW SUPPLIED:** Inj: 1.25mg/mL

**CONTRAINDICATIONS:** History of ACE inhibitor associated angioedema and hereditary or idiopathic angioedema.

**WARNINGS/PRECAUTIONS:** D/C if angioedema, jaundice, or if marked LFT elevation occurs. Risk of hyperkalemia with DM, renal dysfunction. Persistent nonproductive cough reported. Monitor WBCs in renal or collagen vascular disease. Anaphylactoid reactions reported. Fetal/neonatal morbidity and death reported. Monitor for hypotension in high risk patients (heart failure, surgery/anesthesia, hyponatremia, high dose diuretic therapy, severe volume and/or salt depletion, etc). Caution with CHF, obstruction to left ventricle outflow tract, renal dysfunction, and renal artery stenosis. Less effective on BP in blacks and more reports of angioedema than nonblacks.

**ADVERSE REACTIONS:** Hypotension, headache, angioedema, myocardial infarction, fatigue, dizziness, fever, rash, constipation, cough.

**INTERACTIONS:** May increase lithium levels. Hypotension risk with diuretics. May further decrease renal dysfunction with NSAIDs. Increase risk of hyperkalemia with $K^+$-sparing diuretics, $K^+$-containing salt substitutes or $K^+$ supplements. Augmented effect by antihypertensives that cause renin release (eg, thiazides). NSAIDs may diminish antihypertensive effect.

**PREGNANCY:** Category C (1st trimester) and D (2nd and 3rd trimesters), not for use in nursing.

**MECHANISM OF ACTION:** ACE inhibitor; inhibition results in decreased plasma angiotensin II, which leads to decreased vasopressor activity and decreased aldosterone secretion.

**PHARMACOKINETICS: Absorption:** (PO) Poorly absorbed. **Elimination:** Urine (90% unchanged ); $T_{1/2}$=11 hrs.

### NURSING CONSIDERATIONS

**Assessment:** Assess BP, LFTs, renal function, CVD (eg, aortic stenosis, cardiomyopathy), renal artery stenosis, pregnancy status, and possible drug interactions.

**Monitoring:** Monitor BP, LFTs, renal function, CBC with platelet count and differential, serum $K^+$ levels. Monitor for MI, CHF, angioedema (head, neck, intestinal), anaphylactoid reactions, hepatic failure, hypersensitivity reactions, cough, NV, dizziness.

**Patient Counseling:** Counsel about fetal risks during pregnancy and signs/symptoms of angioedema (eg, laryngeal/tongue edema, abdominal pain); seek prompt medical attention if any develop. Inform about adverse effects (eg, anaphylaxis, cough, hypotension, hyperkalemia, neutropenia). Infants with histories of *in utero* exposure should be closely observed for hypotension, oliguria, hyperkalemia. Inform about need for periodic monitoring of electrolytes and blood counts. Advise not to use $K^+$ supplements or salt substitutes containing $K^+$ without consulting physician.

**Administration:** IV route; inject over 5 min. **Storage:** Store below 30°C (86°F).

## VECTIBIX RX

panitumumab (Amgen)

**Dermatologic toxicities and severe infusion reactions reported.**

**THERAPEUTIC CLASS:** Monoclonal antibody/EGFR-blocker

**INDICATIONS:** Treatment as a single agent of epidermal growth factor receptor (EGFR)-expressing, metastatic colorectal carcinoma with disease progression on or following fluoropyrimidine-, oxaliplatin-, and irinotecan-containing chemotherapy regimens.

**DOSAGE:** *Adults:* 6mg/kg IV infusion over 60 min q14 days. Infuse doses >1000mg over 90 min. Reduce infusion rate by 50% with mild or moderate (Grade 1 or 2) infusion reaction for duration of that infusion. Immediately and permanently d/c infusion with severe (Grade 3 or 4) infusion reactions. Withhold for dermatologic toxicities that are ≥Grade 3 or considered intolerable. If toxicity does not improve to ≤Grade 2 within 1 month, permanently d/c. If dermatologic toxicity improves to ≤Grade 2 and symptoms improve after withholding no more than 2 doses, treatment may be resumed at 50% of original dose. If toxicities recur, permanently d/c. If toxicities do not recur, subsequent doses may be increased by increments of 25% of original dose until recommended dose of 6mg/kg is reached.

**HOW SUPPLIED:** Inj: 20mg/mL [5mL, 10mL, 20mL]

**WARNINGS/PRECAUTIONS:** D/C if severe dermatologic toxicities and infusion reactions occur. Pulmonary fibrosis reported; d/c therapy in patients developing interstitial lung disease, pneumonitis, or lung infiltrates. Hypomagnesemia and hypocalcemia may occur; monitor periodically during and for 8 weeks after completion of therapy and institute appropriate treatment such as oral or IV electrolyte repletion. Exacerbation of dermatologic toxicity upon sun exposure; wear sunscreen, hats and limit exposure while on therapy. EGFR protein expression is necessary for appropriate selection of patients. Refer to PI for FDA-approved test kits.

**ADVERSE REACTIONS:** Skin toxicities (eg, erythema, dermatitis acneiform, pruritus, exfoliation, rash, fissures), hypomagnesemia, paronychia, fatigue, abdominal pain, N/V, diarrhea, constipation.

**INTERACTIONS:** Avoid use in combination with chemotherapy.

**PREGNANCY:** Category C, not for use in nursing.

**MECHANISM OF ACTION:** IgG2 kappa monoclonal antibody; binds specifically to EGFR on both normal and tumor cells, and competitively inhibits binding of ligands for EGFR.

**PHARMACOKINETICS: Absorption:** $C_{max}$=213mcg/mL, AUC=1306mcg•day/mL. **Elimination:** $T_{1/2}$=7.5 days.

### NURSING CONSIDERATIONS

V

**Assessment:** Assess electrolyte baseline levels, EGFR protein expression, pulmonary disease, and pregnancy/nursing status.

**Monitoring:** Monitor electrolytes periodically during, and for 8 weeks after, therapy. Monitor for signs/symptoms of dermatologic toxicities (eg, dermatitis acneiform, pruritus, erythema, rash, skin exfoliation, paronychia, dry skin, skin fissures), severe infusion reactions (eg, anaphylactic reactions, bronchospasm, fever, chills, hypotension), angioedema, and pulmonary fibrosis.

**Patient Counseling:** Advise to report skin/ocular changes and dyspnea. Instruct to wear sunscreen, hats and limit sun exposure to prevent exacerbation of skin reactions. Instruct to d/c nursing during and 2 months after therapy. Advise to report severe cases of diarrhea and dehydration.

**Administration:** IV infusion; do not administer as bolus or push. Administer through IV pump using low-protein binding 0.2µm or 0.22µm in-line filter.
**Storage:** 2-8°C (36-46°F). Protect from sunlight. (Diluted): Room temperature; use within 6 hrs, or at 2-8°C (36-46°F); stable for 24 hrs. Do not freeze.

## VELCADE

**RX**

bortezomib (Millennium)

**THERAPEUTIC CLASS:** Proteasome inhibitor

**INDICATIONS:** Treatment of multiple myeloma and mantle cell lymphoma in patients who have received at least 1 prior therapy.

**DOSAGE:** *Adults:* Previously Untreated Multiple Myeloma: Initial: 1.3mg/m²/dose IV bolus (3-5 sec) in combination with oral melphalan and oral prednisone for nine 6-week cycles. In Cycles 1-4 administer twice weekly (Days 1, 4, 8, 11, 22, 25, 29, and 32). In Cycles 5-9 administer once weekly (Days 1, 8, 22, and 29). At least 72 hrs should elapse between consecutive doses. Relapsed Multiple Myeloma/ Mantle Cell Lymphoma: 1.3mg/m²/dose IV bolus (3-5 sec) twice weekly for 2 weeks (Days 1, 4, 8, 11); followed by 10-day rest period (Days 12-21). For extended therapy of more than 8 cycles, administer on standard schedule or on a maintenance schedule of once weekly for 4 weeks (Days 1, 8, 15, 22). At least 72 hrs should elapse between consecutive doses. Moderate/Severe Hepatic Impairment: Initial: 0.7mg/m² during 1st cycle. Titrate: May increase to 1.0mg/m² or further dose reduction to 0.5mg/m² may be considered based on patient tolerance. Please refer to PI on dose modification guidelines for grade 3/4 hematological toxicity and for peripheral neuropathy.

**HOW SUPPLIED:** Inj: 3.5mg

**CONTRAINDICATIONS:** Hypersensitivity to boron or mannitol.

**WARNINGS/PRECAUTIONS:** Avoid pregnancy. May cause or worsen peripheral neuropathy; change dose or schedule if occurs. Thrombocytopenia and neutropenia reported; monitor CBC and platelets frequently. May cause orthostatic/postural hypotension; caution with history of syncope or dehydration. May cause acute development or exacerbation of CHF and/or new onset of decreased left ventricular ejection fraction. Reports of acute diffuse infiltrative pulmonary disease of unknown etiology (eg, pneumonitis, interstitial pneumonia, lung infiltration and ARDS). May cause nausea, diarrhea, constipation, and vomiting; use of antiemetic and antidiarrheal medications may be necessary. Rare reports of reversible posterior leukoencephalopathy syndrome. May cause tumor lysis syndrome. Acute liver failure reported. Caution in patients with moderate to severe hepatic failure; lower starting dose recommended. Patients on oral antidiabetic agents may require close monitoring of blood glucose levels. Should be administered after dialysis procedure.

**ADVERSE REACTIONS:** Thrombocytopenia, N/V, peripheral neuropathy, diarrhea, anemia, constipation, pyrexia, asthenia, appetite decreased, paresthesia, headache, cough, edema, dyspnea.

**INTERACTIONS:** Increased exposure with ketoconazole and melphalan-prednisone. Caution with concomitant use of medications that cause hypotension. Oral antidiabetic agents may require dosage adjustment. Caution with CYP3A4 inducers and inhibitors; monitor for toxicities or reduced efficacy.

**PREGNANCY:** Category D, not for use in nursing.

**MECHANISM OF ACTION:** Proteasome inhibitor; inhibits chymotrypsin-like activity of 26s proteosome cell.

**PHARMACOKINETICS: Absorption:** (1st dose: 1mg/m²; 1.3mg/m²) $C_{max}$=57ng/mL, 112ng/mL; (Twice weekly: 1mg/m²; 1.3mg/m²) $C_{max}$=67-106ng/mL, 89-120ng/mL. **Distribution:** $V_d$=498-1884L/m²; plasma protein binding (83%). **Metabolism:** Oxidation via CYP3A4, 2C19, 1A2; 2D6, 2C9 (minor). Deboronation (major). **Elimination:** (1mg/m²; 1.3mg/m²) $T_{1/2}$=40-193 hrs, 76-108 hrs.

V

## NURSING CONSIDERATIONS

**Assessment:** Assess for peripheral neuropathy, hypersensitivity to boron or mannitol, syncope, dehydration, risk factors for or existing heart disease (eg, CHF, hypotension, HTN), DM, hepatic dysfunction, pregnancy status, and possible drug interactions. Obtain baseline CBC, LFTs, BP.

**Monitoring:** Monitor CBC, blood glucose, and LFTs periodically. Monitor for signs/symptoms of dehydration, hypoglycemia, hyperglycemia, new/worsening neuropathy, cardiopulmonary symptoms, reversible posterior leukoencephalopathy syndrome (RPLS), tumor lysis syndrome, and hypersensitivity reactions.

**Patient Counseling:** Advise not to drive or operate heavy machinery. Take appropriate measures to avoid dehydration. Seek medical advice if symptoms of dizziness, light headedness and fainting spells are experienced. Use effective measures to prevent pregnancy. Instruct to inform physician immediately if become pregnant. Advise not to take this medication during pregnancy or while breastfeeding. Consult a physician about any other medications they are currently taking. Check blood sugar frequently if taking oral antidiabetic medication. Instruct to seek medical attention if symptoms of new/worsening peripheral neuropathy (eg, burning, paresthesia, weakness), rash, shortness of breath, cough, swelling of the feet, ankles, or legs, convulsion, persistent headache, reduced eyesight, an increase in BP or blurred vision develops.

**Administration:** IV route. Refer to PI for reconstitution procedure. Should be administered within 8 hrs after reconstitution. **Storage:** 25°C (77°F); excursions permitted to 15-30°C (59-86°F). Protect from light. Reconstituted: 25°C (77°F); stable for 8 hrs.

# VENTAVIS — RX

iloprost (Actelion)

**THERAPEUTIC CLASS:** Systemic and pulmonary arterial vascular bed dilator

**INDICATIONS:** Treatment of pulmonary arterial hypertension (WHO Group I) in patients with NYHA Class III or IV symptoms.

**DOSAGE:** *Adults:* Administer via I-neb™ or Prodose™ AAD® systems. Initial: 2.5mcg. Titrate: May increase to 5mcg and maintain if well tolerated; otherwise maintain at 2.5mcg. Maint: 2.5-5mcg taken 6 to 9 times per day, no more than once q2h. Max: 45mcg/day. Elderly: Start at lower end of dosing range.

**HOW SUPPLIED:** Sol, Inhalation: 10mcg/mL [1mL], 20mcg/mL [1mL]

**WARNINGS/PRECAUTIONS:** Risk of syncope and hypotension; exertional syncope may signify insufficient therapy. Avoid with systolic BP <85mmHg. D/C if signs of pulmonary edema occur. Administer only via I-neb™ or Prodose™ AAD® systems. Direct mixing of iloprost with other medications in the I-neb™ or Prodose AAD® systems has not been evaluated. Should not come in contact with the skin or eyes and oral ingestion should be avoided. May induce bronchospasm. Use has not been evaluated in patients with COPD, severe asthma, or with acute pulmonary infections; such patients should be carefully monitored during therapy. Caution in patients with at least Child Pugh Class B hepatic impairment, patients on dialysis, and in elderly patients.

**ADVERSE REACTIONS:** Vasodilation, increased cough, headache, trismus, insomnia, N/V, hypotension, flu syndrome, back pain, syncope, palpitations, tongue pain, increased GGT, increase alkaline phosphotase.

**INTERACTIONS:** May increase hypotensive effect of vasodilators and antihypertensive agents. Increased risk of bleeding with anticoagulants. Caution with concomitant use of drugs that may increase the risk of syncope.

**PREGNANCY:** Category C, not for use in nursing.

**MECHANISM OF ACTION:** Synthetic analogue of prostacyclin $PGI_2$; dilates systemic and pulmonary arterial vascular beds. Affects platelet aggregation.

**PHARMACOKINETICS: Absorption:** $C_{max}$=150pg/mL. **Distribution:** (IV) $V_d$=0.7-0.08L/kg; plasma protein binding (60%). **Metabolism:** via β-oxidation.

Tetranor-iloprost (main metabolite). **Elimination:** Urine (68%), feces (12%); $T_{1/2}$=20-30 min.

## NURSING CONSIDERATIONS

**Assessment:** Assess for renal/hepatic impairment, hypotension, COPD, severe asthma, acute pulmonary infections, pregnancy/nursing status, and for possible drug interactions. Assess for risk of syncope.

**Monitoring:** Monitor for signs and symptoms of syncope and for pulmonary edema (may be a sign of pulmonary venous HTN). Monitor vital signs. Monitor for signs/symptoms of bronchospasm, especially in patients with COPD, severe asthma, and in patients with acute pulmonary infections.

**Patient Counseling:** Counsel to use drug as prescribed with either I-neb™ or Prodose™ AAD® Systems. Instruct on proper administration techniques, including dosing frequency, amp dispensing, and equipment cleaning. Advise that a drop in BP during therapy is possible and may become dizzy or faint; advise to stand up slowly when getting out of a chair or bed. Consult a physician if fainting gets worse. Inform that medication should be inhaled at intervals of not less than 2 hours and that acute benefits of therapy may not last 2 hours; advise that may want to adjust times of administration to cover planned activities.

**Administration:** Inhalation route. **Storage:** 20-25°C (68-77°F); excursions permitted to 15-30°C (59-86°F).

# VENTOLIN HFA — RX

albuterol sulfate (GlaxoSmithKline)

**THERAPEUTIC CLASS:** $Beta_2$-agonist

**INDICATIONS:** Treatment or prevention of bronchospasm in patients with reversible obstructive airway disease. Prevention of exercise-induced bronchospasm (EIB).

**DOSAGE:** *Adults:* Bronchospasm: 2 inh q4-6h or 1 inh q4h. EIB: 2 inh 15-30 min before exercise. Elderly: Start at lower end of dosing range.
*Pediatrics:* ≥4 yrs: Bronchospasm: 2 inh q4-6h or 1 inh q4h. EIB: 2 inh 15-30 min before exercise.

**HOW SUPPLIED:** MDI: 90mcg/inh [8g, 18g]

**WARNINGS/PRECAUTIONS:** D/C if paradoxical bronchospasm or CV events occur. Avoid excessive use; may be marker of destabilization of asthma and require reevaluation of the patient. Caution with convulsive disorders, coronary insufficiency, arrhythmias, HTN, diabetes mellitus (DM), hyperthyroidism, sensitivity to sympathomimetics. Hypersensitivity reactions may occur. Fatalities reported with excessive use. May need concomitant corticosteroids. May produce significant hypokalemia. Caution in elderly.

**ADVERSE REACTIONS:** Throat irritation, viral respiratory infections, upper respiratory inflammation, cough, musculoskeletal pain, parodoxical bronchospasm, hoarseness, arrhythmias, hypersensitivity reactions, hypokalemia, hypertension, peripheral vasodilation, angina, tremor.

**INTERACTIONS:** Avoid other short-acting sympathomimetic bronchodilators; caution with oral sympathomimetics. Extreme caution with MAOIs, TCAs during or within 2 weeks of d/c. β-blockers may block pulmonary effects and cause severe bronchospasm. Decreases digoxin levels. ECG changes and/or hypokalemia caused by non-$K^+$-sparing diuretics (eg, loop or thiazide diuretics) may be worsened.

**PREGNANCY:** Category C, caution in nursing.

**MECHANISM OF ACTION:** $\beta_2$-adrenergic agonist; activates $\beta_2$-adrenergic receptors on airway smooth muscle leading to the activation of adenylcyclase and to an increase in the intracellular concentration of cAMP. This increase of cAMP leads to the activation of protein kinase A, which inhibits the phosphorylation of myosin and lowers intracellular ionic calcium concentrations, resulting in relaxation of the smooth muscles of all airways, from the trachea to the terminal bronchioles. Albuterol acts as a functional antagonist to relax the airway irrespective of the spasmogen involved, thus protecting against all bronchoconstrictor challenges. Increased cAMP concentrations are also associated with the inhibition of release of mediators from mast cells in the airway.

**PHARMACOKINETICS: Absorption:** $C_{max}$=3ng/mL; $T_{max}$=0.42 hrs. **Elimination:** $T_{1/2}$=4.6 hrs.

## NURSING CONSIDERATIONS

**Assessment:** Assess renal/hepatic function, history of hypersensitivity to drug, CVD (eg, coronary insufficiency, HTN, cardiac arrhythmias), convulsive disorders, hyperthyroidism, DM and ketoacidosis, pregnancy/nursing status, and possible drug interactions. Assess use in patients unusually responsive to sympathomimetic amines.

**Monitoring:** Monitor for possible paradoxical bronchospasm, deterioration of asthma, CV effects, hypokalemia, immediate hypersensitivity reactions and common adverse effects (eg, palpitation, rapid heart rate, tremor and nervousness. Monitor BP, HR, ECG changes and blood glucose.

**Patient Counseling:** Advise to seek medical attention if treatment becomes less effective for symptomatic relief, symptoms become worse, or usage becomes more frequent than usual. Inform to take as directed and to report lack of response or adverse side effects. Instruct how to properly prime, clean and use inhaler. Advise to prime inhaler before using for first time or if inhaler has not been used for 2 weeks, or if it has been dropped by releasing 4 test sprays into air, away from face; shake well before each spray. Counsel to clean inhaler at least once a week, wash the actuator with warm water and let it air-dry completely. Use only with actuator supplied with product. Advise to refill prescription when the counter reads 020 or discard when the counter reads 000 or if it is 12 months after removal from the moisture-protective foil pouch, whichever comes first. Advise to never immerse the canister in water to determine the amount of drug remaining in the canister. Advise to avoid spraying in eyes and shake well before each spray.

**Administration:** Oral inhalation route. **Storage:** 15-25°C (59-77°F). Keep out of the reach of children. Do not puncture. Do not use or store near heat or open flame. Exposure to temperatures above 120°F may cause bursting. Store inhaler with mouthpiece down.

# VERAMYST RX

fluticasone furoate (GlaxoSmithKline)

**THERAPEUTIC CLASS:** Corticosteroid

**INDICATIONS:** Treatment of the symptoms of seasonal and perennial allergic rhinitis in patients ≥2 yrs.

**DOSAGE:** *Adults:* Initial: 2 sprays per nostril qd. Maint: 1 spray per nostril qd. Elderly: Start at the low end of dosing range.
*Pediatrics:* ≥12 yrs: Initial: 2 sprays per nostril qd. Maint: 1 spray per nostril qd. 2-11 yrs: Initial: 1 spray per nostril qd. Titrate: If inadequate response, may increase to 2 sprays per nostril qd.

**HOW SUPPLIED:** Spray: 27.5mcg/spray [10g]

**WARNINGS/PRECAUTIONS:** Excessive use may cause hypercorticism and adrenal suppression. Risk of adrenal insufficiency and withdrawal symptoms when replacing systemic corticosteroids with topical corticosteroids. Caution with active or quiescent TB, ocular herpes simplex, or untreated bacterial, fungal, and systemic viral infections. Risk for more severe/fatal course of infections (eg, chickenpox, measles); avoid exposure in patients who have not had disease or have not been properly immunized. Epistaxis and nasal ulcerations may occur. *Candida* infection of nose reported. Avoid with recent nasal trauma, ulcers, or surgery. May result in glaucoma and cataracts. Hypersensitivity reactions, including anaphylaxis, angioedema, rash and urticaria may occur. Potential for reduced growth velocity in pediatrics. Caution in elderly.

**ADVERSE REACTIONS:** Headache, epistaxis, nasopharyngitis, pyrexia, pharynolaryngeal pain, cough.

**INTERACTIONS:** Ketoconazole or other potent CYP3A4 inhibitors may increase serum fluticasone levels; co-administer with caution. Increased levels with ritonavir; avoid coadministering.

**PREGNANCY:** Category C, caution in nursing.

**MECHANISM OF ACTION:** Corticosteroid; mechanism not established. May activate glucocorticoid response element, inhibits pro-inflammatory transcription factors such as NFkB, and inhibition of antigen-induced lung eosinophilia (animal studies).

**PHARMACOKINETICS: Absorption:** Incomplete absorption, absolute bioavailability (0.5%). **Distribution:** $V_d$=608L. Plasma protein binding (>99%). **Metabolism:** Hepatic via hydrolysis; CYP3A4. **Elimination:** Feces.

## NURSING CONSIDERATIONS

**Assessment:** Assess for active or quiescent TB, untreated localized or systemic fungal/bacterial infection, systemic viral infection, ocular herpes simplex, history of glaucoma or cataracts, history of nasal polyps, recent nasal septal ulcers, nasal surgery/trauma, glaucoma, concomitant use with other inhaled or systemic corticosteroids, hepatic function, pregnancy/nursing status, and possible drug interactions.

**Monitoring:** Monitor for acute adrenal insufficiency, hypercorticism, HPA-axis suppression, chickenpox, measles, nasal or pharyngeal *Candida* infections, epistaxis, nasal ulceration, nasal septal perforation, hypoadrenalism (in infant born to mother who received corticosteroids during pregnancy), suppression of growth velocity in children, vision changes, increased IOP.

**Patient Counseling:** Counsel to take as directed. Avoid exposure to chickenpox and measles; consult physician immediately if exposed, if symptoms worsen, or if adverse reactions (eg, epistaxis, nasal ulceration, nasal/pharyngeal *Candida* infection, vision changes, nasal perforation and impaired wound healing) occur. Avoid spraying into eyes.

**Administration:** Intranasal route. If not used >30 days, or cap left off >5 days, prime pump until fine mist appears. Shake well before each use. **Storage:** 15-30°C (59-86°F). Store device in upright position with cap in place. Do not freeze or refrigerate.

# VERELAN — RX

verapamil HCl (UCB)

**THERAPEUTIC CLASS:** Calcium channel blocker (nondihydropyridine)

**INDICATIONS:** Management of hypertension.

**DOSAGE:** *Adults:* Usual: 240mg qam. Titrate: May increase by 120mg qam. Max: 480mg qam. Elderly/Small People: Initial: 120mg qam. Titrate: May increase to 180mg qam, then 240mg qam, then 360mg qam, then 480mg qam. May sprinkle on applesauce; do not crush or chew.

**HOW SUPPLIED:** Cap, Extended-Release: 120mg, 180mg, 240mg, 360mg

**CONTRAINDICATIONS:** Severe ventricular dysfunction, hypotension, cardiogenic shock, sick sinus syndrome or 2nd- or 3rd-degree AV block (except with functioning ventricular pacemaker), A-Fib/Flutter with an accessory bypass tract.

**WARNINGS/PRECAUTIONS:** Avoid with moderate to severe cardiac failure, and ventricular dysfunction if taking a β-blocker. May cause hypotension, AV block, transient bradycardia, PR interval prolongation. Monitor LFTs periodically; hepatocellular injury reported. Give 30% of normal dose with severe hepatic dysfunction. Caution with hypertrophic cardiomyopathy, renal or hepatic dysfunction. Decrease dose in those with decreased neuromuscular transmission.

**ADVERSE REACTIONS:** Constipation, dizziness, nausea, hypotension, headache, peripheral edema, infection, flu syndrome, fatigue, bradycardia, AV block.

**INTERACTIONS:** Additive negative effects on HR, AV conduction, and contractility with β-blockers. Potentiates other antihypertensives. May increase digoxin, carbamazepine, theophylline, cyclosporine, and alcohol levels. Avoid disopyramide within 48 hrs before or 24 hrs after verapamil. Additive negative inotropic effects and AV conduction prolongation with flecainide. Avoid quinidine with hypertrophic cardiomyopathy. Monitor lithium levels. Increased clearance with phenobarbital. Rifampin may reduce oral bioavailability. May potentiate neuromuscular blockers; both agents may need dose reduction. Caution with inhalation anesthetics. Increased bleeding time with ASA. Increased efficacy of doxorubicin. Reduced absorption with COPP and VAC cytotoxic drug regimens. May decrease clearance of paclitaxel. CYP3A4 inhibitors (eg, erythromycin, ritonavir) or grapefruit juice may increase levels. CYP3A4 inducers (eg, rifampin) may lower levels.

**PREGNANCY:** Category C, not for use in nursing.

## NURSING CONSIDERATIONS

**Assessment:** Assess for left ventricular dysfunction, hypotension, sick sinus syndrome, 2nd- or 3rd-degree AV block, atrial flutter, accessory bypass tract, CHF, LFTs, cardiomyopathy, attenuated neuromuscular transmission, renal impairment, and possible drug interactions.

**Monitoring:** Monitor for hypotension, CHF, arrhythmias, heart block, LFTs, constipation, headache, dizziness.

**Patient Counseling:** Counsel about adverse effects. Instruct to take as prescribed. Advise to swallow cap whole; do not crush or chew. May administer by opening and sprinkling pellets on spoonful of applesauce (should not be hot), and swallow immediately without chewing with a glass of cool water. Subdividing contents of capsule not recommended.

# VERELAN PM — RX

verapamil HCl (Schwarz Pharma)

**THERAPEUTIC CLASS:** Calcium channel blocker (nondihydropyridine)

**INDICATIONS:** Management of essential hypertension.

**DOSAGE:** *Adults:* Individualize dose. Usual: 200mg qhs. Titrate: May increase to 300mg qhs, then 400mg qhs. Renal or Hepatic Dysfunction/Elderly/Low-Weight Patients: Initial: 100mg qhs. Titrate: May increase dose based on therapeutic efficacy and safety evaluated 24 hrs after initial dosing. May sprinkle on applesauce; do not crush or chew.

**HOW SUPPLIED:** Cap, Extended-Release: 100mg, 200mg, 300mg

**CONTRAINDICATIONS:** Severe left ventricular dysfunction, hypotension (SBP <90mmHg) or cardiogenic shock, sick sinus syndrome or 2nd- or 3rd-degree AV block (except in patients with a functioning ventricular pacemaker), A-fib/A-flutter and an accessory bypass tract (eg, Wolff-Parkinson-White, Lown-Ganong-Levine syndromes).

**WARNINGS/PRECAUTIONS:** Congestive heart failure or pulmonary edema may develop. Hypotension/dizziness may occur. Elevated transaminases have occurred; monitor liver function. Ventricular fibrillation has occurred in patients with A-fib or A-flutter or atrial fibrillation and an accessory bypass tract. Reduce dose or d/c therapy if marked first-degree AV block or progression to second- or third-degree AV block occurs. Sinus bradycardia, pulmonary edema, severe hypotension, second-degree AV block, sinus arrest and death occurred in patients with hypertrophic cardiomyopathy.

V

**ADVERSE REACTIONS:** Headache, infection, constipation, flu syndrome, peripheral edema, dizziness, pharyngitis, sinusitis.

**INTERACTIONS:** Additive negative effects on HR, AV conduction, and contractility with β-blockers. Additive effects with other antihypertensives. May increase digoxin, metoprolol, propranolol, quinidine, carbamazepine, theophylline, cyclosporine, doxorubucin and alcohol levels. May alter levels of atenolol. Sinus bradycardia resulting in hospitalization and pacemaker insertion has been reported in association with the use of clonidine; monitor heart rate. Hypotension and bradyarrhythmias have been observed in patients receiving concurrent telethromycin, an antibiotic in the ketolide class of antibiotics. Avoid disopyramide within 48 hrs before or 24 hrs after verapamil. Additive negative inotropic effects and AV conduction prolongation with flecainide. Avoid quinidine with hypertrophic cardiomyopathy. May increase sensitivity to neurotoxic effects of lithium with or without an increase in serum lithium levels. Increased clearance with phenobarbital. Cimetidine may reduce the levels of verapamil. Rifampin may reduce oral bioavailability. May potentiate neuromuscular blockers (eg, vecuronium); both agents may need dose reduction. Caution with inhalation anesthetics. Increased bleeding time with ASA. Reduced absorption with COPP and VAC cytotoxic drug regimens. May decrease clearance of paclitaxel. CYP3A4 inhibitors (eg, erythromycin, ritonavir) or grapefruit juice may increase levels. CYP3A4 inducers (eg, rifampin) may decrease levels.

**PREGNANCY:** Category C, safety not known in nursing.

**MECHANISM OF ACTION:** Calcium channel blocker (non-dihydropyridine); inhibits transmembrane influx of ionic calcium into arterial smooth muscle as well as in conductile and contractile myocardial cells without altering serum calcium concentrations.

**PHARMACOKINETICS: Absorption:** Absolute bioavailability (33-65% R-enantiomer), (13-34% S-enantiomer); $C_{max}$=77.8ng/mL (R), 16.8ng/mL (S); $AUC_{0-24}$=1037ng•h/mL (R), 195ng•h/mL (S); $T_{max}$=11 hrs. **Distribution:** Plasma protein binding (94% R), (88% S); α-1-acid glycoprotein binding (92% R), (86% S); crosses placenta and excreted in breast milk. **Metabolism:** Liver via CYP450; O-demethylation and N-dealkylation; norverapamil (active metabolite). **Elimination:** Urine (70% metabolites, 4% unchanged), feces (16% metabolites).

## NURSING CONSIDERATIONS

**Assessment:** Assess for left ventricular dysfunction, hypotension, cardiogenic shock, sick sinus syndrome, 2nd- or 3rd-degree AV block, A-fib/A-flutter, accessory bypass tract, CHF, LFTs, hypertrophic cardiomyopathy, attenuated neuromuscular transmission, impaired renal function, pregnancy/nursing status, and possible drug interactions.

**Monitoring:** Monitor for hypotension, CHF, arrhythmias, AV block, angina pectoris, MI, ECG, LFTs, constipation, headache, dizziness, and infections.

**Patient Counseling:** Advise to immediately seek medical help if a drop in BP, chest pain, headache, dizziness, N/V, or edema develops. Instruct to take as prescribed. Swallow capsule whole; do not crush or chew. May administer by opening and sprinkling pellets on spoonful of applesauce (should not be hot), and swallow immediately, without chewing, with a glass of cool water. Instruct to use any pellet/applesauce mixture immediately.

**Administration:** Oral route. **Storage:** 25°C (77°F); excursions permitted to 15-30°C (59-86°F). Protect from moisture. Dispense in tight, light-resistant container.

# VESIcare — RX

solifenacin succinate (Astellas/GlaxoSmithKline)

**THERAPEUTIC CLASS:** Muscarinic antagonist

**INDICATIONS:** Treatment of overactive bladder with symptoms of urge urinary incontinence, urgency, and urinary frequency.

**DOSAGE:** *Adults:* Usual: 5mg qd. Max: 10mg qd. Renal Impairment (CrCl <30mL/min)/Moderate Hepatic Impairment (Child-Pugh B)/Potent CYP3A4 Inhibitors: Max: 5mg qd.

**HOW SUPPLIED:** Tab: 5mg, 10mg

**CONTRAINDICATIONS:** Urinary retention, gastric retention, uncontrolled narrow-angle glaucoma.

**WARNINGS/PRECAUTIONS:** Caution with bladder outflow obstruction, GI obstructive disorders, decreased GI motility, and narrow-angle glaucoma.

Caution with renal and hepatic impairment. Avoid with severe hepatic impairment (Child-Pugh C).

**ADVERSE REACTIONS:** Dry mouth, constipation, nausea, dyspepsia, UTI, blurred vision.

**INTERACTIONS:** Do not exceed 5mg daily dose when administered with therapeutic doses of ketoconazole or other potent CYP3A4 inhibitors.

**PREGNANCY:** Category C, not for use in nursing.

**MECHANISM OF ACTION:** Muscarinic receptor antagonist; inhibits muscarinic receptors, resulting in decreased urinary smooth muscle contraction and salivary secretion.

**PHARMACOKINETICS: Absorption:** Absolute bioavailabilty (90%); $T_{max}$=3-8 hrs. **Distribution:** $V_d$=600L; plasma protein binding (98%). **Metabolism:** Liver (extensive) via CYP3A4 (N-oxidation; 4R-hydroxylation), 4R-hydroxy solifenacin (active metabolite). **Elimination:** Urine (<15%), feces; $T_{1/2}$=45-68 hrs.

## NURSING CONSIDERATIONS

**Assessment:** Assess for bladder outflow obstruction (eg, urinary retention), gastric retention, narrow-angle glaucoma, decreased GI motility, renal/hepatic impairment, pregnancy/nursing status, and possible drug interactions. Assess EKG, renal function, LFTs.

**Monitoring:** Monitor for signs/symptoms of urinary retention, gastric retention, blurred vision, hypersensitivity reaction, renal/hepatic impairment. Monitor for EKG changes (eg, QT prolongation).

**Patient Counseling:** Inform that therapy associated with constipation and blurred vision. Caution against potentially dangerous activities. Advise to seek medical attention if symptoms of severe abdominal pain, constipation (>3 days), blurred vision, heat prostration (eg, decreased sweating), or hypersensitivity reactions occur.

**Administration:** Oral route. **Storage:** 25°C (77°F); excursions permitted to 15-30°C (59-86°F).

# VFEND RX

voriconazole (Pfizer)

**THERAPEUTIC CLASS:** Azole antifungal

**INDICATIONS:** Treatment of invasive aspergillosis, esophageal candidiasis. Treatment of candidemia in nonneutropenic patients and the following *Candida* infections: disseminated infections in skin and infections in abdomen, kidney, bladder wall, and wounds. Treatment of serious fungal infections caused by *Scedosporium apiospermum* and *Fusarium* spp. including *Fusarium solani* in patients intolerant of, or refractory to, other therapy.

**DOSAGE:** *Adults:* (Inj) LD: 6mg/kg IV q12h x 2 doses. Maint: 4mg/kg IV q12h. Switch to PO when appropriate. (PO) Maint: ≥40kg: 200mg q12h; 300mg q12h if inadequate response. <40kg: 100mg q12h; 150 mg q12h if inadequate response. Esophageal Candidiasis: (PO) ≥40kg: 200mg q12h. <40kg: 100mg q12h. Treat for minimum of 14 days and at least 7 days following resolution of symptoms. Intolerant: (Inj/PO) Maint: IV: 3mg/kg q12h. PO: Reduce by 50mg steps to minimum of 200mg q12h for >40kg or 100mg q12h for <40kg. Concomitant Phenytoin: Maint: IV: 5mg/kg q12h. PO: ≥40kg: 400mg q12h. <40kg: 200mg q12h. Concomitant Efavirenz: Maint: 400mg q12h and efavirenz should be decreased to 300mg q24h. Mild to Moderate Hepatic Cirrhosis: Maint: 1/2 of maint dose. CrCl <50mL/min: Use PO. Give PO 1 hr before or 1 hr after a meal. Base duration on severity of underlying disease, recovery from immunosuppression, and clinical response.

**HOW SUPPLIED:** Inj: 200mg; Sus: 40mg/mL; Tab: 50mg, 200mg

**CONTRAINDICATIONS:** Concomitant CYP3A4 substrates (terfenadine, astemizole, cisapride, pimozide, quinidine), sirolimus, rifampin, carbamazepine, long-acting barbiturates, high-dose ritonavir (400mg q12h), low-dose ritonavir (100mg q12h; assess benefit/risk), rifabutin, ergot alkaloids, St. John's wort.

**WARNINGS/PRECAUTIONS:** Monitor visual function with treatment >28 days. Hepatic reactions (clinical hepatitis, cholestasis, fulminant hepatic failure) reported; monitor LFTs at initiation and during therapy. D/C if liver dysfunction occurs. Tabs contain lactose; avoid with galactose intolerance, Lapp lactase deficiency, or glucose-galactose malabsorption. Anaphylactoid-type reactions reported with infusion. Avoid strong, direct sunlight. Monitor renal function. May prolong QT interval; caution with proarrhythmic conditions. Correct electrolyte disturbances before starting therapy. If rash develops, monitor closely and consider discontinuation of voriconazole.

**ADVERSE REACTIONS:** Visual disturbances, fever, chills, rash, headache, N/V, sepsis, peripheral edema, abdominal pain, respiratory disorder, increased LFTs and alkaline phosphatase.

**INTERACTIONS:** See Contraindications. Avoid with low-dose ritonavir (100mg q12h). Efavirenz reduces levels. May increase levels of CYP3A4 inhibitors; monitor for adverse events and toxicity with HIV protease inhibitors, NNRTIs, benzodiazepines, HMG-CoA reductase inhibitors, dihydropyridine CCBs, and vinca alkaloids. May increase levels of CYP2C9 inhibitors; monitor phenytoin, warfarin, hypoglycemics, tacrolimus (reduce tacrolimus to 1/3 of initial dose), and cyclosporine (reduce cyclosporine to 1/2 of initial dose). Omeprazole is CYP2C19/3A4 inhibitor; reduce omeprazole by 1/2 if voriconazole ≥40mg. Proton pump inhibitors that are CYP2C19 substrates may increase levels. Phenytoin may decrease levels. Oral contraceptives containing ethinyl estradiol and norethindrone may increase levels. May increase levels of oral contraceptives containing ethinyl estradiol and norethindrone. May increase levels of methadone; may prolong QT interval; dose reduction may be needed. Do not infuse into same line or cannula with other drug infusions or parenteral nutrition. Do not infuse simultaneously with blood products or electrolyte supplements.

**PREGNANCY:** Category D, not for use in nursing.

**MECHANISM OF ACTION:** Triazole antifungal agent; inhibits fungal CYP450 mediated 14α-lanosterol demethylation, an essential step in fungal ergosterol biosynthesis. Accumulation of 14-α methyl-sterols correlates with subsequent loss of ergosterol in fungal cell wall and may be responsible for antifungal activity of vorconizole.

**PHARMACOKINETICS: Absorption:** Administration of different doses led to varying parameters. $T_{max}$=1-2 hrs. **Distribution:** $V_d$=4.6L/kg; plasma protein binding (58%). **Metabolism:** Hepatic, via CYP2C19, CYP2C9, CYP3A4; N-oxide (major metabolite). **Elimination:** <2% excreted unchanged in urine.

## NURSING CONSIDERATIONS

**Assessment:** Obtain fungal cultures prior to therapy to properly identify causative organisms. Assess for possible drug interactions. Assess pregnancy status, renal (SrCr) and hepatic function (LFTs, bilirubin), serum electrolytes ($K^+$, Mg, Ca), and correct deficiencies. Assess use with proarrhythmic conditions. Give oral formulation to patients with CrCl<50mL/min unless benefits of IV use outweigh risks. Assess with known hypersensitivity to drug or excipient, history of cardiotoxic chemotherapy, cardiomyopathy, hypokalemia, concomitant medications, arrhythmias, hepatic insufficiency (CrCl 50mL/min), and renal insufficiency.

**Monitoring:** Monitor visual acuity, visual field, and color perception with therapy for longer than 28 days. Monitor for infusion-related reactions, hepatotoxicity, arrhythmias, QT prolongation, acute renal failure, and dermatological reactions (eg, Stevens-Johnson syndrome). Monitor for drug toxicity with hepatic insufficiencies. Monitor renal function (SrCr) and hepatic function (LFTs, bilirubin) during therapy.

**Patient Counseling:** Counsel to take tabs or oral sus at least 1 hr before or after a meal. Avoid driving at night; drug may affect vision. Counsel to avoid hazardous tasks if visual changes occur and avoid direct sunlight. Oral sus contains sucrose and is not recommended with rare problems of fructose intolerance, sucrase-isomalate deficiency, or glucose-galactose malabsorption. Counsel females to use proper contraception during therapy.

**Administration:** Oral and IV route. IV: Do not infuse concomitantly into same line or cannula with other drug infusions, including parenteral nutrition. Reconstitute. 1) Add 19mL of SWFI to vial for a concentration of 10mg/mL. 2) Further dilute so final concentration is ≤5mg/mL. Infusion should be administered at maximum rate of 3/mg/kg/hr over 1 hr. Refer to prescribing guidelines. Oral Sus: Reconstitute: 1) Add 46mL of water to bottle and shake. **Storage:** IV: (unreconstituted) 15-30°C (59-86°F). Tab: 15-30°C (59-86°F). Oral Sus: (reconstituted) 15-30°C (59-86°F) for 14 days; (refrigerate before reconstitution) 2-8°C (36-46°F).

## VIADUR — RX

leuprolide acetate (Bayer Healthcare)

**THERAPEUTIC CLASS:** Synthetic gonadotropin releasing hormone analog

**INDICATIONS:** Palliative treatment of advanced prostate cancer.

**DOSAGE:** *Adults:* Insert 1 implant SQ in upper arm every 12 months.

**HOW SUPPLIED:** Implant: 65mg

**CONTRAINDICATIONS:** Women, pregnancy, pediatrics.

**WARNINGS/PRECAUTIONS:** Transient worsening of symptoms may occur during 1st few weeks of therapy. Closely monitor patients with metastatic vertebral lesions and/or urinary tract obstruction during 1st few weeks of therapy. Monitor serum testosterone, PSA. Ureteral obstruction and spinal cord decompression reported.

**ADVERSE REACTIONS:** Headache, asthenia, hot flashes, ecchymosis, peripheral edema, depression, sweating, gynecomastia, nocturia, testis atrophy, breast pain, urinary retention/frequency, local bruising/burning.

**PREGNANCY:** Category X, safety in nursing not known.

**MECHANISM OF ACTION:** LH-RH agonist; acts as a potent inhibitor of gonadotropin secretion resulting in suppression of testicular and ovarian steroidogenesis.

**PHARMACOKINETICS: Absorption:** $C_{max}$=16.9ng/mL; $T_{max}$=4 hrs. **Distribution:** $V_d$=27L; plasma protein binding (43-49%). **Metabolism:** (Major metabolite): M-I. **Elimination:** $T_{1/2}$=3 hrs.

### NURSING CONSIDERATIONS

**Assessment:** Assess pregnancy status, metastatic vertebral lesions, urinary tract obstruction, and possible drug interactions. Obtain baseline serum testosterone and PSA levels.

**Monitoring:** Periodically monitor serum testosterone and PSA levels and for signs/symptoms of anaphylactoid reactions, transient worsening of symptoms, and insertion-site reaction.

**Patient Counseling:** Inform to keep site clean and dry for 24 hrs; do not bathe or swim for 24 hrs. Avoid heavy lifting and physical activity for 48 hrs. Avoid bumping site for few days. After healed, should be able to go back to normal activities. Inform of pregnancy risks. Advise to seek medical attention if symptoms of hot flushes, transient worsening of symptoms (eg, bone pain, increased difficulty in urinating, onset or aggravation of nerve symptoms), insertion-site reaction (eg, unusual bleeding, redness, pain, weakness, numbness), or anaphylactoid reaction occurs.



**Administration:** Dermal implant. Inserting implant: 1) After cleansing and anesthetizing area, make 5mm incision just through dermis in groove between biceps and triceps. 2) Grasp handle and extend index finger to rest on back of actuator. Insert cannula tip into incision with level up and advance into intended track. Advance to depth indicator on cannula. 3) Hold handle in place; using index finger slide actuator back until stops. Do not pull back on handle. Withdraw implanter from incision. Check implant by palpation. **Storage:** 25°C (77°F); excursions permitted to 15-30°C (59-86°F).

# VIAGRA RX

## sildenafil citrate (Pfizer)

**THERAPEUTIC CLASS:** Phosphodiesterase type 5 inhibitor

**INDICATIONS:** Treatment of erectile dysfunction (ED).

**DOSAGE:** *Adults:* Usual: 50mg 1 hr (recommended) or 0.5-4 hrs prior to sexual activity qd. Titrate: May decrease to 25mg qd or increase to 100mg qd based on effectiveness and toleration. Max: 100mg qd. Elderly/Hepatic Impairment/CrCl <30mL/min/Concomitant CYP450 3A4 Inhibitors (eg, ketoconazole, itraconazole, erythromycin, saquinavir): Initial: 25mg qd. Concomitant Ritonavir: Max: 25mg q48h. Concomitant α-blocker: Patient should be on stable α-blocker therapy. Initiate sildenafil at lowest dose.

**HOW SUPPLIED:** Tab: 25mg, 50mg, 100mg

**CONTRAINDICATIONS:** Organic nitrates taken regularly and/or intermittently.

**WARNINGS/PRECAUTIONS:** Caution with MI, stroke or life-threatening arrhythmia within last 6 months; with resting hypotension (BP<90/50) or HTN (BP>170/110); unstable angina due to cardiac failure or CAD; anatomical penile deformation; predisposition to priapism; and retinitis pigmentosa. Avoid in men where sexual activity is inadvisable due to underlying CV status. Decrease in supine BP reported. Rare reports of non-arteritic anterior ischemic optic neuropathy (NAION) with PDE5 inhibitors. Cases of sudden decrease or loss of hearing reported. D/C if experienced these symptoms. Not indicated for use in newborns, children, and women.

**ADVERSE REACTIONS:** Headache, flushing, dyspepsia, nasal congestion, UTI, abnormal vision (eg, color tinge, increased light sensitivity, blurred vision), diarrhea, cardiovascular events, sudden decrease or loss of hearing.

**INTERACTIONS:** See Contraindications. Increased levels with CYP3A4 inhibitors (eg, cimetidine, ketoconazole, itraconazole, erythromycin) and protease inhibitors (eg, ritonavir, saquinavir). CYP2C9 inhibitors may decrease sildenafil clearance. CYP3A4 inducers (eg, rifampin) and CYP2C9 may decrease levels. Potentiates hypotensive effects of nitrates. Additional supine BP reduction with amlodipine reported. Simultaneous administration with α-blockers may lead to symptomatic hypotension. Avoid with other ED treatments. Loop and potassium sparing diuretics and non selective β-blockers increase AUC of active metabolite, N-desmethyl sildenafil.

**PREGNANCY:** Category B.

**MECHANISM OF ACTION:** Phosphodiesterase type 5 inhibitor; enhances effect of nitric oxide by inhibiting phosphodiesterase type 5, which is responsible for the degradation of cGMP in corpus cavernosum resulting in smooth muscle relaxation and inflow of blood to corpus cavernosum.

**PHARMACOKINETICS: Absorption:** Rapid; absolute bioavailability (41%). Fasted state: $T_{max}$=120min. Fed state: $T_{max}$=60min. **Distribution:** $V_d$=105L; plasma protein binding (96%). **Metabolism:** Liver, via CYP450 3A4 (major), 2C9 (minor); N-desmethyl sildenafil (major metabolite). **Elimination:** Feces (80% metabolites), urine (13%); $T_{1/2}$=4 hrs.

## NURSING CONSIDERATIONS

**Assessment:** Assess for CVD, retinitis pigmentosa, bleeding disorders, active peptic ulceration, anatomical deformation of penis, renal/hepatic impairment, potential underlying causes of ED and for possible drug interactions.

**Monitoring:** Monitor potential for cardiac risk due to sexual activity, postural hypotension, color vision changes, hypersensitivity reactions, stomach ulcers. Monitor therapeutic effect when used in combination with other drugs.

**Patient Counseling:** Instruct to seek medical assistance if erection persists >4 hrs. Inform of potential BP-lowering effect with α-blockers and antihypertensive drugs, and potential cardiac risk of sexual activity in patients with preexisting cardiovascular risk factors. Counsel about protective measures necessary to guard against STDs, including HIV. D/C and inform physician if sudden loss of vision, color vision, or hearing occur. Counsel to take tab 1 hr before intercourse.

**Administration:** Oral route. **Storage:** 25°C (77°F); excursions permitted to 15-30°C (59-86°F).

## VIBRAMYCIN RX

doxycycline hyclate (Pfizer)

**OTHER BRAND NAMES:** Vibra-Tabs (Pfizer)

**THERAPEUTIC CLASS:** Tetracycline derivative

**INDICATIONS:** Treatment of the following infections caused by susceptible microorganisms: Rocky Mountain spotted fever; typhus fever and the typhus group; Q fever; rickettsialpox; tick fevers; respiratory tract infections; lymphogranuloma venereum; psittacosis (ornithosis); trachoma; inclusion conjunctivitis; uncomplicated urethral, endocervical, or rectal infections; nongonococcal urethritis; relapsing fever; chancroid; plague; tularemia; cholera; *Campylobacter fetus* infections; brucellosis; bartonellosis; granuloma inguinale; respiratory tract and urinary tract infections; anthrax. Treatment of infections caused by *Escherichia coli*, *Enterobacter aerogenes*, *Shigella* species, *Acinetobacter* species. When penicillin is contraindicated, treatment of the following infections caused by susceptible microorganisms: uncomplicated gonorrhea, syphilis, yaws, listeriosis, Vincent's infection, actinomycosis, infections caused by *Clostridium* species. Adjunct in acute intestinal amebiasis and severe acne. Prophylaxis of malaria.

**DOSAGE:** *Adults:* Usual: 100mg q12h on Day 1, then 100mg qd or 50mg q12h. Severe Infection: 100mg q12h. Treat for 10 days with strep infection. Uncomplicated Gonococcal Infection (Except Anorectal in Men): 100mg bid for 7 days or 300mg followed by 300mg in 1 hr. Uncomplicated Urethral/Endocervical/Rectal Infection and Nongonococcal Urethritis: 100mg bid for 7 days. Syphilis: 100mg bid for 2 weeks. Syphilis for >1 yr: 100mg bid for 4 weeks. Acute Epididymo-orchitis: 100mg bid for at least 10 days. Inhalation Anthrax (Post-Exposure): 100mg bid for 60 days. Malaria Prophylaxis: 100mg qd. Begin 1-2 days before travel and continue for 4 weeks after leaving malarious area.

*Pediatrics:* >8 yrs: ≤100 lbs: 1mg/lb bid on Day 1, then 1mg/lb qd or 0.5mg/lb bid. Severe Infections: Maint: 2mg/lb. >100 lbs: Usual: 100mg q12h on Day 1, then 100mg qd or 50mg q12h. Severe Infection: 100mg q12h. Treat for 10 days with strep infection. Inhalation Anthrax (Post-Exposure): <100 lbs: 1mg/lb bid for 60 days. ≥100 lbs: 100mg bid for 60 days. Malaria Prophylaxis: >8 yrs: 2mg/kg qd. Max: 100mg/day. Begin 1-2 days before travel and continue for 4 weeks after leaving malarious area.

**HOW SUPPLIED:** Cap: (Doxycycline Hyclate) 50mg, 100mg; Syrup: (Doxycycline Calcium) 50mg/5mL; Sus: (Doxycycline Monohydrate) 25mg/5mL [60mL]; Tab: (Vibra-Tabs) 100mg

**WARNINGS/PRECAUTIONS:** May cause fetal harm with pregnancy. Permanent tooth discoloration during tooth development (last half of pregnancy, infancy, and children <8 yrs) reported. *Clostridium difficile*-associated diarrhea reported. May increase BUN. Photosensitivity, enamel hypoplasia reported. Superinfection with prolonged use. Syrup contains sodium metabisulfite. Bulging fontanels in infants and benign intracranial HTN in adults reported. Monitor renal/hepatic and hematopoietic function with long-term use. Take adequate fluids with caps or tabs to reduce esophageal irritation. Take with food or milk if GI irritation occurs.

**ADVERSE REACTIONS:** GI effects (eg, anorexia, nausea, vomiting, diarrhea), photosensitivity, increased BUN, hypersensitivity reactions, hemolytic anemia, thrombocytopenia, neutropenia, eosinophilia.

**INTERACTIONS:** May decrease PT, adjust anticoagulants. May interfere with bactericidal agents (eg, penicillin). May decrease effects of oral contraceptives. Aluminum-, calcium-, iron-, and magnesium-containing products and bismuth subsalicylate impair absorption. Decreased half-life with barbiturates, carbamazepine, and phenytoin. Fatal renal toxicity with methoxyflurane.

**PREGNANCY:** Category D, not for use in nursing.

**MECHANISM OF ACTION:** Tetracycline derivative; thought to inhibit protein synthesis.

**PHARMACOKINETICS: Absorption:** (PO) completely absorbed, $C_{max}$=2.6 mcg/mL, $T_{max}$=2 hrs. **Distribution:** Crosses placenta. **Elimination:** Urine, feces.

## NURSING CONSIDERATIONS

**Assessment:** Assess for pregnancy status, possible drug interactions, and renal impairment. Document indications for therapy, culture, and susceptibility testing. Perform incision and drainage in conjunction with antibiotic therapy when indicated.

**Monitoring:** Monitor for signs/symptoms of hypersensitivity reactions, photosensitivity, superinfection, *C. difficile*-associated diarrhea, vaginal candidiasis, benign intracranial HTN, LFTs, renal function. In venereal disease with coexistent syphilis, conduct dark field exam before treatment and monthly for 4 months.

**Patient Counseling:** Inform of pregnancy risks and photosensitivity reactions (d/c at 1st sign of skin erythema). Advise to avoid excessive sunlight and UV light and wear sunscreen/sunblock. Instruct to drink fluids liberally to reduce risk of esophageal irritation or ulceration. Inform that therapy only treats bacterial, not viral, infections. Take as directed; skipping doses or not completing full course may decrease effectiveness and increase resistance. Inform may experience diarrhea; notify physician if watery/bloody stools, hypersensitivity reactions, superinfections, photosensitivity, or benign intracranial HTN occur. Advise to avoid foods with calcium. Advise patients on malaria prophylaxis to begin therapy 2 days before travel, continue while in malarious area, and continue for 4 weeks after returning from area. Therapy should not exceed 4 months.

**Administration:** Oral route. **Storage:** Below 30°C (86°F); dispense in tight, light-resistant container.

# VICODIN

**CIII**

hydrocodone bitartrate - acetaminophen (Abbott)

**OTHER BRAND NAMES:** Vicodin ES (Abbott) - Vicodin HP (Abbott)

**THERAPEUTIC CLASS:** Opioid analgesic

**INDICATIONS:** Relief of moderate to moderately severe pain.

**DOSAGE:** *Adults:* Usual: Vicodin: 1-2 tabs q4-6h prn. Max: 8 tabs/day. Vicodin HP: 1 tab q4-6h prn. Max: 6 tabs/day. Vicodin ES: 1 tab q4-6h prn. Max: 5 tabs/day.

**HOW SUPPLIED:** (Hydrocodone-APAP) Tab: Vicodin: 5mg-500mg*; Vicodin HP: 10mg-660mg*; Vicodin ES: 7.5mg-750mg* *scored

**WARNINGS/PRECAUTIONS:** Caution in elderly, debilitated, severe hepatic or renal dysfunction, hypothyroidism, Addison's disease, prostatic hypertrophy, urethral stricture, pulmonary disease and postoperative use. May obscure acute abdominal conditions or head injuries. May produce dose-related respiratory depression. Monitor for tolerance. Suppresses cough reflex.

**ADVERSE REACTIONS:** Lightheadedness, dizziness, sedation, NV, constipation, rash, respiratory depression.

**INTERACTIONS:** Additive CNS depression with other narcotic analgesics, antihistamines, antipsychotics, antianxiety agents, alcohol and other CNS depressants. Increased effect of antidepressant or hydrocodone with MAOIs or TCAs.

**PREGNANCY:** Category C, not for use in nursing.

**MECHANISM OF ACTION:** Hydrocodone: Opioid analgesic; precise mechanism not known. Suspected to relate to existence of opiate receptors in CNS. APAP: Nonopiate, nonsalicylate analgesic and antipyretic. Analgesic action involves peripheral influences; specific mechanism not established. Antipyretic activity mediated through hypothalmic heat-regulating centers. Inhibits prostaglandin synthetase.

**PHARMACOKINETICS: Absorption:** Hydrocodone: $C_{max}$=23.6ng/mL; $T_{max}$=1.3 hrs. APAP: Rapidly absorbed. **Distribution:** APAP: Found in breast milk. **Metabolism:** Hydrocodone: O-demethylation, N-demethylation and 6-keto reduction. APAP: Liver (conjugation). **Elimination:** Hydrocodone: $T_{1/2}$=3.8 hrs. APAP: Urine (85%) (parent compound and metabolites); $T_{1/2}$=1.25-3 hrs.

## NURSING CONSIDERATIONS

**Assessment:** Assess for hypersensitivity to other opioids, head injury or other intracranial lesions, elevated ICP, acute abdominal conditions, pulmonary disease, presence of debilitation (eg, elderly), hepatic/renal impairment, hypothyroidism, Addison's disease, prostatic hypertrophy or urethral stricture, nursing/pregnancy status, potential for misuse or abuse, and possible drug interactions.

**Monitoring:** Monitor for signs/symptoms of respiratory depression, elevations in CSF pressure, drug abuse, and drug dependence. In presence of severe hepatic/renal disease, monitor serial liver and/or renal function tests.

**Patient Counseling:** Caution that may impair mental/physical abilities required for performance of potentially hazardous tasks (eg, operating machinery). Avoid alcohol and other CNS depressants. Advise that drug may be habit forming; should only take for as long as prescribed, in amounts prescribed, and no more frequently than prescribed.

**Administration:** Oral route. **Storage:** 25°C (77°F); excursions permitted to 15-30°C (59-86°F). Dispense in tight, light-resistant container.

# VICOPROFEN CIII

hydrocodone bitartrate - ibuprofen (Abbott)

**OTHER BRAND NAMES:** Reprexain (Centrix)

**THERAPEUTIC CLASS:** Opioid analgesic

**INDICATIONS:** Short-term (generally <10 days) management of acute pain.

**DOSAGE:** *Adults:* Usual: 1 tab q4-6h prn. Max: 5 tabs/day. Elderly: Use lowest dose or longest interval.
*Pediatrics:* ≥16 yrs: Usual: 1 tab q4-6h prn. Max: 5 tabs/day.

**HOW SUPPLIED:** (Hydrocodone-Ibuprofen) Tab: (Vicoprofen) 7.5mg-200mg; (Reprexain) 5mg-200mg, 7.5mg-200mg *scored

**CONTRAINDICATIONS:** ASA or other NSAID allergy that precipitates asthma, urticaria, or other allergic reaction.

**WARNINGS/PRECAUTIONS:** May produce dose-related respiratory depression. May obscure acute abdominal conditions or head injuries. Avoid with ASA triad, late pregnancy, advanced renal disease, ASA-sensitive asthma. Caution in elderly, debilitated, dehydration, renal disease, intrinsic coagulation defects, severe hepatic dysfunction, asthma, hypothyroidism, Addison's disease, prostatic hypertrophy, urethral stricture, heart failure, HTN, ulcer disease, pulmonary disease, postoperative use. May be habit-forming. Suppresses cough reflex. Risk of GI ulceration, bleeding, perforation. Anemia, fluid retention, edema, severe hepatic reactions reported. Possible risk of aseptic meningitis, especially in SLE patients. Increased risk of serious cardiovascular thrombotic events, MI and stroke. Fluid retention and edema observed. Skin reactions (eg, exfoliative dermatitis, TEN, SJS) can occur.



**ADVERSE REACTIONS:** Headache, somnolence, dizziness, constipation, dyspepsia, N/V, infection, edema, nervousness, anxiety, pruritus, diarrhea, asthenia, abdominal pain, insomnia, dry mouth, sweating.

**INTERACTIONS:** Additive CNS depression with other narcotics, antihistamines, antipsychotics, antianxiety agents, alcohol, CNS depressants. Increased effect of antidepressant or hydrocodone with MAOIs or TCAs. May produce paralytic ileus with anticholinergics. May decrease effects of furosemide and thiazide diuretics, ACE-inhibitors. Avoid ASA. Risk of serious GI bleeding with warfarin. May enhance methotrexate toxicity. Monitor for lithium toxicity.

**PREGNANCY:** Category C, not for use in nursing.

**MECHANISM OF ACTION:** Hydrocodone: Opioid analgesic and antitussive. Not known; suspected to be related to existence of opiate receptors in CNS. Produces actions similiar to codeine; most occur in CNS and smooth muscle. Ibuprofen: Non-steroidal anti-inflammatory agent. Not established; suspected to inhibit cyclooxygenase activity and prostaglandin synthesis. Peripherally acting analgesic; has no known effects on opiate receptors. Possesses anti-pyretic activity.

**PHARMACOKINETICS: Absorption:** Hydrocodone: $C_{max}$=27ng/mL; $T_{max}$=1.7 hrs. Ibuprofen: $C_{max}$=30mcg/mL; $T_{max}$=1.8 hrs. **Distribution:** Ibuprofen: Plasma protein binding (99%). **Metabolism:** Hydrocodone: CYP2D6, via O-demethylation to hydromorphone (active metabolite); CYP3A4 via N-demethylation; 6-keto reduction. Ibuprofen: Interconversion from R-isomer to S-isomer; (+)-2-4'-(2-hydroxy-2-methyl-propyl) phenyl propionic acid and (+)-2-4-(2-carboxypropyl) phenyl propionic acid (primary metabolites). **Elimination:** Hydrocodone: Urine (primary); $T_{1/2}$=4.5 hrs. Ibuprofen: Urine (50-60% metabolites, 15% unchanged, conjugate), $T_{1/2}$=2.2 hrs.

## NURSING CONSIDERATIONS

**Assessment:** Assess for hypersenstivity to other opioids, previous reaction to ASA or NSAIDs (eg, asthma, urticaria), type of pain (eg, CABG surgery), cardiovascular disease, HTN, heart failure, fluid retention, drug abuse potential, head injury, intracranial lesions, presence of increased ICP, acute abdominal conditions, history of peptic ulcers and/or GI bleeding, impaired renal/hepatic function, presence of debilitation (eg, elderly), hypothyroidism, Addison's disease, prostatic hypertrophy or urethral stricture, pulmonary disease (eg, asthma), SLE, pregnancy/nursing status, and possible drug interactions. Obtain baseline BP.

**Monitoring:** Monitor for signs/symptoms of cardiovascular thrombotic events, MI, stroke, HTN, fluid retention and edema, drug abuse and dependence, respiratory depression, elevations in CSF pressure, GI effects (eg, inflammation, bleeding, ulceration, perforation of stomach, small intestine, or large intestine), renal effects (eg, renal papillary necrosis), anaphylactoid reactions, skin reactions (eg, exfoliative dermatitis, Stevens-Johnson syndrome, toxic epidermal necrolysis), hepatic effects (eg, elevations in hepatic enzymes, jaundice, liver necrosis), hematological effects (eg, anemia), bronchospasm, and aseptic meningitis. If signs/symptoms of anemia develop, evaluate Hgb or Hct. Monitor BP while on therapy. If on long-term therapy, perform periodic monitoring of CBC and chemistry profile.

**Patient Counseling:** Inform drug cannot be substitute for corticosteroids or treat corticosteroid insufficiency. Caution that may impair mental and/or physical abilities required to perform potentially hazardous tasks (eg, operating machinery/driving). Avoid alcohol and other CNS depressants while on therapy. Advise drug may be habit forming; only take for as long as prescribed, and no more frequently than prescribed. Inform to contact physician if cardiovascular events (eg, CP, SOB, slurring of speech), GI effects (eg, ulcers, bleeding), edema, or weight gain occur. Immediately stop therapy and contact physician if signs/symptoms of skin reactions or hepatotoxicity (eg, nausea, fatigue, jaundice) develop. Seek immediate medical attention if any anaphylactoid reactions (eg, difficulty breathing, facial swelling) develop. Report any signs of blurred vision or other eye symptoms.

**Administration:** Oral route. **Storage:** 25°C (77°F); excursions permitted to 15-30°C (59-86°F). Dispense in a tight, light-resistant container.

# VICTOZA RX

## liraglutide (Novo Nordisk)

**Liraglutide causes dose-dependent and treatment duration-dependent thyroid C-cell tumors at clinically relevant exposure in animal studies. It is unknown whether it causes thyroid C-cell tumors, including medullary thyroid carcinoma (MTC), in humans, as human relevance could not be ruled out by clinical or nonclinical studies. It is contraindicated in patients with a personal or family history of MTC and in patients with multiple endocrine neoplasia syndrome type 2 (MEN 2). It is unknown whether monitoring with serum calcitonin or thyroid ultrasound will mitigate human risk of thyroid C-cell tumors. Patients should be counseled regarding the risks and symptoms of thyroid tumors.**

**THERAPEUTIC CLASS:** Incretin mimetic

**INDICATIONS:** Adjunct to diet and exercise to improve glycemic control in adults with type 2 diabetes mellitus (DM).

**DOSAGE:** *Adults:* Initial: 0.6mg qd SQ (abdomen, thigh, or upper arm) for 1 week. Titrate: Increase to 1.2mg after 1 week, then to 1.8mg if acceptable glycemic control not achieved.

**HOW SUPPLIED:** Inj: 0.6mg, 1.2mg, 1.8mg (6mg/mL, 3mL)

**CONTRAINDICATIONS:** MEN 2; personal or family history of MTC.

**WARNINGS/PRECAUTIONS:** Not recommended as first-line therapy for patients who have inadequate glycemic control on diet and exercise. Not a substitute for insulin therapy, and should not be used in type 1 DM or treatment of diabetic ketoacidosis. Not been studied in patients with history of pancreatitis; caution with history of pancreatitis. Refer patient to an endocrinologist if thyroid nodule and/or elevated calcitonin level are detected. Pancreatitis reported; observe for signs and symptoms after initiation and dose increases; d/c if suspected and do not restart if confirmed. Caution with renal/hepatic impairment. Slows gastric emptying.

**ADVERSE REACTIONS:** N/V, diarrhea, constipation, upper respiratory tract infection, headache, influenza, urinary tract infection, dizziness, sinusitis, nasopharyngitis, back pain, HTN.

**INTERACTIONS:** Sulfonylureas or other insulin secretagogues may increase the risk of hypoglycemia. May cause delay in gastric emptying; use caution with concomitantly administered oral medications. Interferes with absorption of digoxin, lisinopril, atorvastatin, acetaminophen, griseofulvin, ethinylestradiol and levonorgestrel.

**PREGNANCY:** Category C, not for use in nursing

**MECHANISM OF ACTION:** Human glucagon-like peptide-1 (GLP-1) receptor agonist; increases intracellular cyclic AMP (cAMP) leading to insulin release in presence of elevated glucose concentrations. Also decreases glucagon secretion in a glucose-dependent manner and delays gastric emptying.

**PHARMACOKINETICS: Absorption:** Absolute bioavailability is 55%; $T_{max}$=8-12 hrs; (0.6mg) $C_{max}$=35ng/mL, AUC= 960ng•h/mL. **Distribution:** Plasma protein binding (>98%); $V_d$=13L. **Metabolism:** Endogenously metabolized. **Elimination:** Urine (6%); feces (5%); $T_{1/2}$=13 hrs.

## NURSING CONSIDERATIONS

V

**Assessment:** Assess for history of pancreatitis, MTC and MEN 2, pregnancy/nursing status, and possible drug interactions. Check blood glucose and $HbA_{1c}$ levels.

**Monitoring:** Monitor for signs and symptoms of thyroid tumor (eg, a lump in the neck, hoarseness, dysphagia, or dyspnea), pancreatitis (eg, persistent abdominal pain, sometimes radiating to the back and which may or may not be accompanied by vomiting), MTC, hypoglycemia. Monitor blood glucose and $HbA_{1c}$ levels.

**Patient Counseling:** Advise to contact physician if signs and symptoms of pancreatitis and thyroid C-cell tumors noted. Inform not to share pen to prevent transmission of infection. Counsel regarding potential risk and benefits of treatment, and alternative modes of therapy, importance of adherence to dietary instructions, regular physical activity, and periodic blood glucose monitoring and $HbA_{1c}$ testing.

**Administration:** SQ route. Inspect solution before administration; it should be clear, colorless, and with no particles. **Storage:** 2-8°C (36-46°F). Do not freeze. After the initial use, store at room temperature, 15-30°C (59-86°F), or refrigerate at 2-8°C (36-46°F) for up to 30 days.

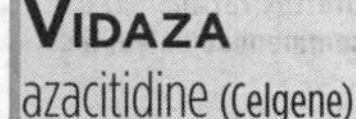

## VIDAZA — RX

azacitidine (Celgene)

**THERAPEUTIC CLASS:** Pyrimidine nucleoside analog

**INDICATIONS:** Treatment of myelodysplastic syndrome subtypes: refractory anemia (RA) or refractory anemia with ringed sideroblasts (if accompanied by neutropenia or thrombocytopenia or requiring transfusions), refractory anemia with excess blasts (RAEB), refractory anemia with excess blasts in transformation (RAEB-T), and chronic myelomonocytic leukemia (CMMoL).

**DOSAGE:** *Adults:* Initial: 75mg/m² SQ or IV daily for 7 days. Repeat cycle every 4 weeks. May increase to 100mg/m² after 2 cycles if no beneficial effect and no toxicity other than N/V. Treat for a minimum of 4-6 cycles. Premedicate for N/V. If administer IV, administer over 10-40 min. Adjust dose based on hematology lab values, renal function, and serum electrolytes; refer to PI for further detail.

**HOW SUPPLIED:** Inj: 100mg

**CONTRAINDICATIONS:** Advanced malignant hepatic tumors and hypersensitivity to mannitol.

**WARNINGS/PRECAUTIONS:** Anemia, neutropenia and thrombocytopenia may occur; monitor CBC periodically (at minimum, before each cycle). Potentially hepatotoxic in patients with severe pre-existing hepatic impairment; caution with liver disease. Renal abnormalities reported; reduce dose or hold for unexplained reductions in serum bicarbonate <20mEq/L or elevations of BUN or SrCr occur. Monitor for toxicity with renal impairment. Obtain liver chemistries and SrCr prior to initiation of therapy. May cause fetal harm; avoid pregnancy in women of childbearing potential. Men should not father a child while receiving treatment.

**ADVERSE REACTIONS:** (SQ) N/V, anemia, thrombocytopenia, pyrexia, leukopenia, diarrhea, fatigue, injection-site erythema, constipation, neutropenia, ecchymosis, cough, dyspnea, weakness. (IV) Petechiae, rigors, weakness, hypokalemia.

**PREGNANCY:** Category D, not for use in nursing.

**MECHANISM OF ACTION:** Pyrimidine nucleoside analogue; believed to exert its antineoplastic effects by causing hypomethylation of DNA and direct cytotoxicity on abnormal hematopoietic cells in the bone marrow.

**PHARMACOKINETICS: Absorption:** (SQ) Rapid; Bioavailability (89%). $C_{max}$=750ng/mL; $T_{max}$=0.5 hr. **Distribution:** (IV) $V_d$=76L. **Elimination:** (SQ) $T_{1/2}$=41 min.

## NURSING CONSIDERATIONS

**Assessment:** Assess for hypersensitivity to mannitol, advanced malignant hepatic tumors, renal/hepatic impairment, pregnancy/nursing status, and for possible drug interactions. Obtain baseline CBC, LFTs, and SrCr.

**Monitoring:** Monitor for signs/symptoms of renal/hepatic dysfunction, anemia, neutropenia, and for thrombocytopenia. Perform periodic monitoring of CBC, liver chemistries, and SrCr.

**Patient Counseling:** Instruct to notify physician of any underlying liver or renal disease. Inform of pregnancy risks; advise women to avoid pregnancy and men not to father children while on therapy.

**Administration:** IV/SQ route. **Storage:** 25°C (77°F); excursions permitted to 15-30°C (59-86°F). Reconstituted: Vials: Stable for 1 hr at 25°C (77°F); stable for 8 hrs at 2-8°C (36-46°F).

# VIDEX RX

didanosine (Bristol-Myers Squibb)

**Fatal and nonfatal pancreatitis reported when used alone or part of a combination regimen. Lactic acidosis and severe hepatomegaly with steatosis, including fatal cases, reported with nucleoside analogs alone or in combination. Fatal lactic acidosis reported in pregnant women who received the combination of stavudine and didanosine with other antiretroviral agents. Use with caution in pregnancy when coadministered with stavudine and is recommended only if the potential benefit clearly outweighs the risk.**

**OTHER BRAND NAMES:** Videx EC (Bristol-Myers Squibb)

**THERAPEUTIC CLASS:** Nucleoside analogue

**INDICATIONS:** Treatment of HIV-1 infection in combination with other antiretrovirals.

**DOSAGE:** *Adults:* ≥18yrs: ≥60kg: (Cap) 400mg qd; (Sol) 200mg bid or 400mg qd. 25-<60kg: (Cap) 250mg qd; (Sol) 125mg bid or 250mg qd. 20-<25kg: (Cap) 200mg qd. CrCl ≥60mL/min: ≥60kg: (Cap) 400mg qd; (Sol) 400mg qd or 200mg bid. <60kg: (Cap) 250mg qd; (Sol) 250mg qd or 125mg bid. CrCl 30-59mL/min: ≥60kg: (Cap) 200mg qd; (Sol) 200mg qd or 100mg bid. <60kg: (Cap) 125mg qd; (Sol) 150mg qd or 75mg bid. CrCl 10-29mL/min: ≥60kg: (Cap) 125mg qd; (Sol) 150mg qd. <60kg: (Cap) 125mg qd; (Sol) 100mg qd. CrCl <10mL/min: ≥60kg: (Cap) 125mg qd; (Sol) 100mg qd. <60kg: (Sol) 75mg qd. Continous Ambulatory Peritoneal Dialysis/Hemodialysis: CrCl <10mL/min: ≥60kg: (Cap) 125mg qd; (Sol) 100mg qd. <60kg: (Sol) 75mg qd. Concomitant Therapy with Tenofovir Disoproxil Fumarate: CrCl ≥60mL/min: ≥60kg: 250mg qd; <60kg: 200mg qd. (Cap) Take on empty stomach; swallow caps whole. (Sol) Take on empty stomach, at least 30 min ac or 2 hrs pc.

*Pediatrics:* (Cap) 6-17 yrs: 20-<25kg: 200mg qd. 25-<60kg: 250mg qd. ≥60kg: 400mg qd. (Sol) 2 weeks-8 months: 100mg/m$^2$ bid. >8 months: 120mg/m$^2$ bid. Do not exceed adult dosing recommendations. Renal Impairment: CrCl ≥60mL/min: ≥60kg: (Cap) 400mg qd; (Sol) 400mg qd or 200mg bid. <60kg: (Cap) 250mg qd; (Sol) 250mg qd or 125mg bid. CrCl 30-59mL/min: ≥60kg: (Cap) 200mg qd; (Sol) 200mg qd or 100mg bid. <60kg: (Cap) 125mg qd; (Sol) 150mg qd or 75mg bid. CrCl 10-29mL/min: ≥60kg: (Cap) 125mg qd; (Sol) 150mg qd. <60kg: (Cap) 125mg qd; (Sol) 100mg qd. CrCl <10mL/min: ≥60kg: (Cap) 125mg qd; (Sol) 100mg qd. <60kg: (Sol) 75mg qd. (Cap) Take on empty stomach; swallow caps whole. (Sol) Take on empty stomach, at least 30 min ac or 2 hrs pc.

**HOW SUPPLIED:** Sol: 2g, 4g; Cap, Delayed-Release: (Videx EC) 125mg, 200mg, 250mg, 400mg

**CONTRAINDICATIONS:** Concomitant use with allopurinol and ribavirin.

**WARNINGS/PRECAUTIONS:** Risk of toxicity with CrCl <60mL/min; reduce dose. Retinal changes and optic neuritis reported; perform periodic retinal exams. D/C with peripheral neuropathy and evidence of non-cirrhotic portal hypertension. Caution with hepatic dysfunction. May cause redistribution/accumulation of fat including central obesity, dorsocervical fat enlargement, peripheral wasting, facial wasting, breast enlargement, and "cushingoid appearance". Immune reconstitution syndrome has been reported in patients treated with combination antiretroviral therapy.



**ADVERSE REACTIONS:** Pancreatitis, lactic acidosis, hepatomegaly with steatosis, visual changes, diarrhea, neuropathy, abdominal pain, headache, N/V, rash, elevated LFTs.

**INTERACTIONS:** (Sol, Caps) See Contraindications. Extreme caution with drugs that may cause pancreatitis. Increased risk of peripheral neuropathy with neurotoxic agents (eg, stavudine). Use with ciprofloxacin may decrease the AUC and $C_{max}$ of didanosine (ddI). Concomitant use with ganciclovir may increase ddI levels; use with caution and monitor for ddI toxicity. Use with ketoconazole may decrease the $C_{max}$ of ddI. Use with methadone may decrease ddI concentrations; do not use concomitantly with ddI pediatric powder; if necessary use ddI delayed-release capsules and monitor clinical response.

Administer nelfinavir 1 hr after ddI. Administration of indinavir 1 hr before ddI, may decrease the AUC and $C_{max}$ of ddI. Use with tenofovir disoproxil fumarate may increase ddI concentrations; reduce dose of ddI and monitor for ddI toxicities and clinical response. Use of ddI in combination with stavudine, with or without hydroxyurea, may increase the risk for pancreatitis and hepatotoxicity (which may be fatal) and severe peripheral neuropathy; avoid ddI and hydroxyurea with or without stavudine. Use with loperamide may decrease the $C_{max}$ of ddI. Concurrent use with metoclopramide may increase the $C_{max}$ of ddI. Administration of ranitidine 2 hrs before ddI, may increase the AUC and $C_{max}$ of ddI and decrease the AUC of ranitidine. Use with rifabutin may increase the AUC and $C_{max}$ of ddI. Use with ritonavir may decrease the AUC and $C_{max}$ of ddI. Concomitant use with trimethoprim may increase the $C_{max}$ of ddI, increase the AUC of trimethoprim, and decrease the $C_{max}$ of trimethoprim. (Sol) Aluminum- and magnesium-containing antacids may potentiate adverse events. Administer ketoconazole or itraconazole at least two hrs before ddI. May decrease quinolone antibiotic concentrations; administer ddI at least 2 hrs after or 6 hrs before ciprofloxacin. May decrease delavirdine concentrations; administer ddI 1 hr after delavirdine. Administer ddI at least 1 hr after indinavir. May decrease tetracycline antibiotic concentrations.

**PREGNANCY:** Category B, not for use in nursing.

**MECHANISM OF ACTION:** Synthetic purine nucleoside analogue; inhibits activity of HIV-1 reverse transcriptase both by competing with natural substrate deoxyadenosine 5'-triphosphate and by incorporation into viral DNA, causing termination of viral DNA chain elongation.

**PHARMACOKINETICS: Absorption:** Rapid. $T_{max}$=0.25-1.5 hrs. **Distribution:** Plasma protein bound (<5%). (Sol) $V_d$= (Adults) 43.70L/m²; (Pediatrics, 8 months-19 yrs) 28L/m². (Cap) $V_d$= (Adults, ≥60 kg) 308.3L; (Pediatrics, 20-<25kg) 98.1L; (Pediatrics, 25-<60kg) 154.7L; (Pediatrics, ≥60kg) 363L; (Cap) AUC= (Adults, ≥60kg) 2.65mg•h/L; (Pediatrics, 20-<25kg) 2.38mg•h/L; (Pediatrics, 25-<60kg) 2.36mg•h/L; (Pediatrics, ≥60kg) 2.25mg•h/L. **Elimination:** (Sol) $T_{1/2}$= (Adults) 1.5 hrs; (Pediatrics, 8 months-19 yrs) 0.8 hrs; (Pediatrics, 2 weeks-4 months) 1.2 hrs. (Cap) $T_{1/2}$= (Adults) 1.19 hrs; (Pediatrics, 20-<25kg) 0.75 hrs; (Pediatrics, 25-<60kg) 0.92 hrs; (Pediatrics, ≥60kg) 1.26 hrs.

## NURSING CONSIDERATIONS

**Assessment:** Assess for pre-existing liver dysfunction, renal impairment, pregnancy/nursing status, for possible drug interactions.

**Monitoring:** Monitor for signs/symptoms of pancreatitis, lactic acidosis, hepatomegaly with steatosis, peripheral neuropathy, portal hypertension, retinal changes, optic neuritis, immune reconstitution syndrome, and for fat redistribution. Closely monitor renal/hepatic function. Perform periodic retinal exams.

**Patient Counseling:** Inform about possible serious toxicity of pancreatitis and about signs/symptoms of lactic acidosis, hepatotoxicity including fatal hepatic events, and peripheral neuropathy. Inform about retinal changes/optic neuritis and non-cirrhotic portal hypertension, including cases leading to liver transplant or death. Caution about use of medications or other substances, including alcohol. Instruct to notify physician if changes in visual acuity occur. Inform about fat redistribution effect. Inform that medication does not cure HIV and may continue to develop opportunistic infections and other complications of HIV. Advise HIV-infected females they should avoid nursing to reduce the risk of transmission. Advise to take on empty stomach, at least 30 min ac or 2 hrs pc. Instruct to swallow capsule whole and not to open. Instruct to not miss a dose but if they do, take medication immediately. Advise to continue to practice safe sex and take precautions to prevent from coming in contact with infected blood and other body fluids. Instruct to contact poison control center or emergency room right away in case of overdose.

**Administration:** Oral route. Cap: Take on empty stomach; swallow caps whole. Pediatric Powder for Oral Sol: 1) Reconstitute dry powder with purified water, USP, to initial concentration of 20mg/mL. 2) Immediately mix resulting sol with antacids to final concentration of 10mg/mL. Sol: Take on empty stomach, at least 30 min ac or 2 hrs pc. **Storage:** Cap: 25°C (77°F); excursions permitted

15-30°C (59-86°F). Store in tightly closed container. Powder: 15-30°C (59-86°F). Admixture: May be stored up to 30 days in refrigerator at 2-8°C (36-46°F). Discard unused medication after 30 days.

## VIGAMOX **RX**
moxifloxacin HCl (Alcon)

**THERAPEUTIC CLASS:** Fluoroquinolone

**INDICATIONS:** Treatment of bacterial conjunctivitis.

**DOSAGE:** *Adults:* 1 drop tid for 7 days.
*Pediatrics:* ≥1 yr: 1 drop tid for 7 days.

**HOW SUPPLIED:** Sol: 0.5% [3mL]

**WARNINGS/PRECAUTIONS:** Not for injection. Do not inject subconjunctivally or into the anterior chamber of the eye. Superinfection may result with prolonged use. Fatal hypersensitivity reactions reported after first dose of systemic quinolone therapy. Avoid contact lenses when symptoms are present.

**ADVERSE REACTIONS:** Conjunctivitis, decreased visual acuity, dry eye, keratitis, ocular discomfort/hyperemia, ocular pain/pruritus, subconjunctival hemorrhage, tearing.

**PREGNANCY:** Category C, caution in nursing.

**MECHANISM OF ACTION:** Fluoroquinolone antibiotic; inhibits topoisomerase II (DNA gyrase) and topoisomerase IV. DNA gyrase is essential enzyme involved in replication, transcription, and repair of bacterial DNA. Topoisomerase IV is enzyme known to play key role in partitioning of chromosomal DNA during bacterial cell division.

**PHARMACOKINETICS: Absorption:** $C_{max}$=2.7ng/mL; AUC=45ng•hr/mL.
**Distribution:** Presumed to be excreted in breast milk.

### NURSING CONSIDERATIONS

**Assessment:** Assess for proper diagnosis of causative organisms (eg, slit lamp biomicroscopy, fluorescein staining). Assess for allergies to other quinolones. Assess use in pregnant/nursing females.

**Monitoring:** Monitor for signs/symptoms of hypersensitivity or anaphylactic reactions (eg, cardiovascular collapse, angioedema, airway obstruction, dyspnea, urticaria). With prolonged therapy, monitor for overgrowth of nonsusceptible organisms (eg, fungi) and for development of superinfection.

**Patient Counseling:** Instruct to avoid contaminating applicator tip with material from eye, fingers, or other sources. Instruct to d/c medication and contact physician if rash or allergic reaction occurs. Advise with bacterial conjunctivitis not to wear contact lenses.

**Administration:** Ocular route. Do not inject into eye. **Storage:** Store at 2-25°C (36-77°F).

## VIMPAT **CV**
lacosamide (UCB)



**THERAPEUTIC CLASS:** Sodium channel inactivator

**INDICATIONS:** (Tab) Adjunctive therapy for the treatment of partial-onset seizures in patients ≥17 yrs with epilepsy. (Inj) IV use indicated when oral administration temporarily not feasible.

**DOSAGE:** *Adults:* Partial-Onset Seizures: (PO/Inj) Initial: 50mg bid (100mg/day). Titrate: May increase, at weekly intervals by 100mg/day given as two divided doses. Maint: 200-400mg/day based on response and tolerability. Mild/Moderate Hepatic Impairment/End-Stage Renal Disease (ESRD)/CrCl ≤30mL/min: Max: 300mg/day. Switching from Oral to IV Dosing: Initial total daily IV dosage should be equivalent to total daily dosage and frequency of PO dosing and infused over 30-60 min. Switching from IV to Oral Dosing: Oral administration may be given at equivalent daily dosage and frequency of

IV treatment. May be taken with/without food.
*Pediatrics:* ≥17 yrs: Partial-Onset Seizures: (PO/Inj) Initial: 50mg bid (100mg/day). Titrate: May increase at weekly intervals by 100mg/day given as two divided doses. Maint: 200-400mg/day based on response and tolerability. Mild/Moderate Hepatic Impairment/End-Stage Renal Disease/ CrCl ≤30mL/min: Max: 300mg/day. Switching from Oral to IV Dosing: Initial total daily IV dosage should be equivalent to total daily dosage and frequency of PO dosing and infused over 30-60 min. Switching from IV to Oral Dosing: Oral administration may be given at equivalent daily dosage and frequency of IV treatment. May be taken with/without food.

**HOW SUPPLIED:** Tab, Delayed Release: 50mg, 100mg, 150mg, 200mg. Inj: 200mg/20mL

**WARNINGS/PRECAUTIONS:** May increase risk of suicidal behavior and ideation; monitor emergence or worsening of depression, suicidal thoughts/ behavior and changes in mood/behavior. May cause dizziness and ataxia; may impair physical/mental abilities. Prolongations in PR interval reported. Caution with known conduction abnormalities (eg, AV block, sick sinus syndrome without pacemaker) or severe cardiac disease (eg, myocardial ischemia, heart failure). May predispose to atrial arrhythmias especially in patients with diabetic neuropathy and/or cardiovascular disease (CVD). Syncope or loss of consciousness reported in patients with diabetic neuropathy. Withdraw gradually over minimum of 1 week to minimize potential of increased seizure frequency in patients with seizure disorders. Multi-organ hypersensitivity reactions (Drug Reaction with Eosinophilia and Systemic Symptoms [DRESS]) may occur; d/c if suspected. Caution in elderly. Avoid use with severe hepatic impairment. Monitor closely during dose titration with co-existing hepatic or renal impairment; abnormalities in LFTs reported.

**ADVERSE REACTIONS:** Dizziness, headache, N/V, fatigue, diplopia, vertigo, somnolence, ataxia, tremor, memory impairment, nystagmus, balance disorder, diarrhea, contusion.

**INTERACTIONS:** Caution with drugs known to induce PR interval prolongation. Small decreases in concentrations with carbamazepine, phenobarbital or phenytoin. Possibility of pharmacodynamic interactions with drugs that affect the heart conduction system. Potential to inhibit CYP2C19. Abnormality in LFTs with concomitant anti-epileptic drugs.

**PREGNANCY:** Category C, not for use in nursing.

**MECHANISM OF ACTION:** Not established; selectively enhances slow inactivation of voltage-gated sodium channels, resulting in stabilization of hyperexcitable neuronal membranes and inhibition of repetitive neuronal firing (in vitro studies).

**PHARMACOKINETICS: Absorption:** Complete; Absolute Bioavailability (100%); (Tab) $T_{max}$=1-4 hrs. **Distribution:** $V_d$=0.6L/kg; plasma protein binding (<15%). **Metabolism:** CYP2C19; O-desmethyl-lacosamide (major metabolite). **Elimination:** Urine (95%), feces (<0.5%); $T_{1/2}$=13 hrs.

## NURSING CONSIDERATIONS

**Assessment:** Assess hepatic/renal function. Assess history of depression, conduction problems and/or cardiovascular disease, diabetic neuropathy, pregnancy/nursing status, and possible drug interactions. Obtain baseline LFTs, and ECG.

**Monitoring:** Monitor renal/hepatic function, ECG abnormalities, emergence or worsening of depression, suicidal thoughts or behavior and/or any unusual changes in mood or behavior and DRESS. Monitor if pregnant or intend to get pregnant.

**Patient Counseling:** Instruct to take only as prescribed with or without food. Counsel about high risk of suicidal thoughts and behavior. Carefully monitor emergence or worsening symptoms of depression, unusual changes in behavior or mood, suicidal thoughts, behavior or self-harm. Counsel about dizziness, blurred vision and somnolence. Advise not to drive, operate complex machinery or engage in other hazardous activities until effects of drug are known. Counsel that electrocardiographic changes may predispose to irregular HR and syncope. Inform about DRESS and to d/c therapy immediately if it occurs. May cause hypersensitivity reactions affecting multiple organs such as liver and kidney; d/c if suspected. Instruct to seek consultation if symptoms of liver toxicity (eg, fatigue, jaundice, dark urine) occur. Notify physician if pregnant or intend to get pregnant; encourage to enroll in the North American Antiepileptic Drug Pregnancy Registry.

**Administration:** Oral/IV route. **Storage:** Store at 20-25°C (68-77°F); excursions permitted between 15-30°C (59-86°F).

## VINBLASTINE RX

vinblastine sulfate (Various)

**For IV use only; fatal if given intrathecally. Considerable irritation if leakage occurs into surrounding tissue. If this occurs, d/c and restart in another vein. Heat and hyaluronidase minimize discomfort and cellulitis.**

**THERAPEUTIC CLASS:** Vinca alkaloid

**INDICATIONS:** Palliative treatment of generalized Hodgkin's disease (Stages III and IV), lymphocytic lymphoma, histiocytic lymphoma, advanced mycosis fungoides, advanced testis carcinoma, Kaposi's sarcoma, Letterer-Siwe disease, and resistant choriocarcinoma and unresponsive breast carcinoma.

**DOSAGE:** *Adults:* Dose at intervals of ≤7 days. 1st Dose: 3.7mg/m². 2nd Dose: 5.5mg/m². 3rd Dose: 7.4mg/m². 4th Dose: 9.25mg/m². 5th Dose: 11.1mg/m². Max: 18.5mg/m². Do not increase dose after that dose which reduces WBC to 3000 cells/mm³. Maint: Use dose of 1 increment smaller than this dose at weekly intervals. Reduce to 50% dose if direct serum bilirubin >3mg/100mL. Only dose if WBC ≥4000 cells/mm³.

*Pediatrics:* Letterer-Siwe Disease as Single Agent: Initial: 6.5mg/m². Hodgkin's Disease in Combination Therapy: Initial: 6mg/m². Testicular Germ Cell Carcinoma in Combination Therapy: Initial: 3mg/m².

**HOW SUPPLIED:** Inj: 1mg/mL [10mL]

**CONTRAINDICATIONS:** Significant granulocytopenia (unless result of disease being treated), bacterial infections.

**WARNINGS/PRECAUTIONS:** Avoid pregnancy. Acute shortness of breath, severe bronchospasm, aspermia, stomatitis, neurologic toxicity reported. Increased toxicity with hepatic insufficiency. Monitor for infection with WBC <2000 cells/mm³. Avoid with malignant-cell infiltration of bone marrow, or in older persons with cachexia or ulcerated skin. Small daily amounts for long periods is not advised. Avoid eye contamination. Monitor WBCs. May cause fetal harm during pregnancy. Caution with ischemic cardiac disease.

**ADVERSE REACTIONS:** Leukopenia (granulocytopenia), anemia, thrombocytopenia, alopecia, constipation, anorexia, N/V, abdominal pain, diarrhea, HTN, paresthesis.

**INTERACTIONS:** May increase phenytoin metabolism/elimination, or decrease phenytoin absorption. Caution with CYP3A inhibitors (eg, erythromycin, doxorubicin, etoposide), or with hepatic dysfunction; may cause earlier onset and/or an increased severity of side effects. Increased risk of acute shortness of breath and severe bronchospasm with mitomycin-C.

**PREGNANCY:** Category D, not for use in nursing.

**MECHANISM OF ACTION:** Vinca alkaloid; inhibits microtubule formation in mitotic spindle, resulting in cell division arrest.

**PHARMACOKINETICS: Metabolism:** CYP3A. **Elimination:** $T_{1/2}$=24.8 hrs.

### NURSING CONSIDERATIONS

**Assessment:** Assess for hepatic dysfunction, granulocytopenia, bacterial infection, ischemic heart disease, pulmonary dysfunction, malignant-cell infiltration of bone marrow, elderly with cachexia or ulcerated area of skin, pregnancy status, and possible drug interactions.

**Monitoring:** Monitor CBC and LFTs periodically and for signs/symptoms of leukopenia (infection), extravasation, hepatic dysfunction, and hypersensitivity reactions.

**Patient Counseling:** Instruct to avoid pregnancy during therapy. Inform that alopecia, jaw pain, and pain in organs containing tumor tissue may occur during treatment. Avoid contact with eyes; if contamination occurs, wash immediately and thoroughly. Advise to seek medical attention if symptoms of sore throat, fever, chills, or sore mouth occur.

**Administration:** IV route. **Storage:** 2-8°C (36-46°F).

## VINCRISTINE RX

vincristine sulfate (Various)

**Properly position IV needle or catheter before injection; considerable irritation with extravasation. If extravasation occurs, d/c immediately, and any remaining portion of the dose introduced into another vein. Use hyaluronidase and heat to minimize discomfort and cellulitis with extravasation. Fatal with intrathecal use. For IV use only.**

**THERAPEUTIC CLASS:** Vinca alkaloid

**INDICATIONS:** For treatment of acute leukemia. As an adjunct in the treatment of Hodgkin's disease, non-Hodgkin's malignant lymphomas (lymphocytic, mixed cell, histiocytic, undifferentiated, nodular and diffuse types), rhabdomyosarcoma, neuroblastoma, and Wilms' tumor.

**DOSAGE:** *Adults:* Usual: 1.4mg/m² IV at weekly intervals. Bilirubin >3mg/dL: 50% dose reduction. If given together with L-asparaginase, give 12-24 hrs before the enzyme.
*Pediatrics:* Usual: 1.5-2mg/m² IV at weekly intervals. ≤10kg: Initial: 0.05mg/kg IV once weekly. Bilirubin >3mg/dL: 50% dose reduction. If given together with L-asparaginase, give 12-24 hrs before the enzyme.

**HOW SUPPLIED:** Inj: 1mg/mL, 2mg/2mL

**CONTRAINDICATIONS:** Demyelinating form of Charcot-Marie-Tooth syndrome.

**WARNINGS/PRECAUTIONS:** Acute uric acid nephropathy may occur. May require additional agents with CNS leukemia. Neurotoxicity is dose-limiting toxicity. Perform CBC before each dose. Determine serum uric acid levels frequently during 1st 3-4 weeks. Acute shortness of breath, severe bronchospasm reported. Monitor with pre-existing neuromuscular disease. Avoid eye contamination. May cause fetal harm during pregnancy.

**ADVERSE REACTIONS:** Alopecia, abdominal cramps, weight loss, nausea, vomiting, diarrhea, constipation, paralytic ileus, HTN, hypotension, polyuria, dysuria, urinary retention, sensory impairment, paresthesia.

**INTERACTIONS:** Reduced levels of phenytoin and increased seizures reported. Increased risk of acute shortness of breath and severe bronchospasm with mitomycin-C. Monitor with other neurotoxic agents. Discontinue drugs known to cause urinary retention for 1st few days after administration. Give 12-24 hrs before L-asparaginase therapy to minimize toxicity. Do not give with radiation therapy through ports that include the liver. Do not dilute in solutions that raise or lower the pH outside the range of 3.5-5.5. Inhibition of metabolism and increased severity of neuromuscular side effects with itraconazole. Caution with drugs known to be ototoxic such as platinum-containing oncolytics.

**PREGNANCY:** Category D, not for use in nursing.

**MECHANISM OF ACTION:** Antineoplastic agent; inhibits microtubule formation in mitotic spindle, resulting in cell division arrest at metaphase stage.

**PHARMACOKINETICS: Metabolism:** Liver, via CYP450 isoenzyme 3A **Elimination:** Feces (80%), urine (10-20%); $T_{1/2}$=85 hrs.

## NURSING CONSIDERATIONS

**Assessment:** Assess for hepatic dysfunction, presence of leukopenia or complicating infection, demyelinating form of Charcot-Marie-Tooth syndrome, pregnancy/nursing status, and possible drug interactions.

**Monitoring:** Monitor for acute uric acid nephropathy, acute SOB, and severe bronchospasm. Monitor bone marrow function and CBC (WBC, platelet).

Acute elevation of serum uric acid may occur, thus such levels should be determined frequently during first 3-4 weeks of treatment.

**Patient Counseling:** Avoid contamination of eye with concentrated drug. If accidental contamination occurs, severe irritation (or if drug was delivered under pressure, even corneal ulceration) may result. Wash eye immediately and thoroughly.

**Administration:** IV route. **Storage:** 2-8°C (36-46°F). Protect from light.

## Viracept RX

nelfinavir mesylate (Pfizer)

**THERAPEUTIC CLASS:** Protease inhibitor

**INDICATIONS:** Treatment of HIV infection in combination with other antiretrovirals.

**DOSAGE:** *Adults:* 1250mg bid or 750mg tid. Take with meal. May dissolve whole tab in small amount of water. Once dissolved, mix cloudy liquid well and consume immediately. Rinse glass with water and swallow rinse to ensure that entire dose is consumed.
*Pediatrics:* 2-13 yrs: 45-55mg/kg bid or 25-35mg/kg tid. Take with meal. May mix powder with small amount of water, milk, formula, soy formula, soy milk, or dietary supplements; once mixed entire contents must be consumed in order to obtain the full dose. If mixture is not consumed immediately, must be stored under refrigeration for not more than 6 hrs. Acidic food or juice are not recommended to be used in combination (eg, orange juice, apple juice, applesauce). Do not reconstitute powder with water in its original container. Refer to PI for further dosing guidelines.

**HOW SUPPLIED:** Sus: (powder) 50mg/g [144g]; Tab: 250mg, 625mg

**CONTRAINDICATIONS:** Concomitant use with amiodarone, quinidine, dihydroergotamine, ergonovine, ergotamine, methylergonovine, pimozide, midazolam, triazolam.

**WARNINGS/PRECAUTIONS:** Powder contains phenylalanine. New-onset diabetes mellitus (DM), exacerbation of DM, and hyperglycemia reported. Register pregnant patients. Avoid use in patients with moderate or severe hepatic impairment. HIV cross-resistance reported. Increased bleeding reported in patients with hemophilia A and B (eg, hematomas, hemarthrosis). Possible fat redistribution/accumulation of body fat and immune reconstitution syndrome reported.

**ADVERSE REACTIONS:** Diarrhea, N/V, flatulence, rash, redistribution of body fat, jaundice, allergic reactions, bilirubinemia, hyperglycemia, metabolic acidosis, anemia, anxiety, rhinitis, pruritus.

**INTERACTIONS:** See Contraindications. CYP3A or CYP2C19 inducers (eg, rifampin) may decrease plasma levels and reduce therapeutic effect. Use with rifampin may lead to loss of virologic response and possible resistance to nelfinavir or other coadministered antiretroviral agents. CYP3A or CYP2C19 inhibitors may increase plasma levels. Avoid lovastatin or simvastatin; caution with other HMG-CoA reductase inhibitors that are metabolized by CYP3A. Reduce dose of rifubatin to 50% of the usual dose when coadministering. May increase sildenafil or other PDE5 inhibitor levels and adverse effects. Avoid St. John's wort; may decrease levels of nelfinavir. May increase levels of drugs metabolized by CYP3A (eg, dihydropyridine CCBs, immunosuppressants, etc). Caution with drugs that are metabolized by CYP3A and that prolong the QT interval. Use alternative or additional contraception with oral contraceptives. May increase levels of cyclosporine, tacrolimus, sirolimus, atorvastatin, rosuvastatin, fluticasone, azithromycin, trazadone. Carbamazepine, phenobarbital may decrease levels of nelfinavir. May decrease levels of phenytoin, methadone. Give didanosine 1 hr before or 2 hrs after nelfinavir. Concomitant use with indinavir may increase nelfinavir and indinavir concentrations. Concomitant use with ritonavir may increase nelfinavir concentrations. Concomitant use with saquinavir may increase saquinavir levels. Concomitant use with delavirdine may increase nelfinavir levels, decrease delavirdine levels and decrease nelfinavir $C_{min}$. Coadministration with amprenavir may decrease

$C_{max}$ of amprenavir and increase the $C_{min}$ of amprenavir. Omeprazole decreases levels of nelfinavir; concomitant use with proton pump inhibitors may lead to loss of virologic response and development of resistance.

**PREGNANCY:** Category B, not for use in nursing.

**MECHANISM OF ACTION:** HIV-1 protease inhibitor; prevents cleavage of Gag and Gag-Pol polyprotein resulting in production of immature, noninfectious virus.

**PHARMACOKINETICS: Absorption:** (1250mg bid) $C_{max}$=4mg/L; AUC=52.8mg•h/L. (750mg tid) $C_{max}$=3mg/L; AUC=43.6mg•h/L. **Distribution:** $V_d$=2-7L/kg; plasma protein binding (>98%). **Metabolism:** Liver via CYP3A, 2C19 (oxidation). **Elimination:** Feces (78%, metabolites), (22%, unchanged), urine (1-2%); $T_{1/2}$=3.5-5 hrs.

## NURSING CONSIDERATIONS

**Assessment:** Assess for hepatic impairment, DM, hemophilia, pregnancy/nursing status, and for possible drug interactions. Assess for phenylketonuria if planning to use oral powder formulation.

**Monitoring:** Monitor for signs/symptoms of hypersensitivity reactions, new onset or exacerbation of DM and hyperglycemia, immune reconstitution syndrome, fat redistribution/accumulation, and hepatic dysfunction. In patients with hemophilia, monitor for signs/symptoms of increased bleeding (eg, hematomas, hemarthrosis). May enroll patients in the Antiretroviral Pregnancy Registry if they become pregnant while on treatment.

**Patient Counseling:** Inform that therapy does not cure HIV; may continue to acquire illnesses including opportunistic infections. Inform that therapy does not reduce risk of transmitting HIV. Instruct to take every day with meals. Counsel to not alter dose or d/c therapy without consulting physician. Advise if dose is missed, take as soon as possible and then return to normal dosing schedule. However, inform that if a dose is skipped, do not double the next dose. Instruct to report all prescription, nonprescription, and herbal products currently taking to physician. Inform that if taking oral contraceptives, alternate or additional contraceptive measures should be used during therapy. Instruct to seek medical attention if symptoms of hypersensitivity reactions, infections, or fat redistribution/accumulation occur.

**Administration:** Oral route. **Storage:** Tab/Oral Powder: 15-30°C (59-86°F). Keep container tightly closed.

# VIRAMUNE — RX

nevirapine (Boehringer Ingelheim)

**Severe, life-threatening, in some cases fatal, hepatotoxicity and skin reactions (eg, Stevens-Johnson syndrome, toxic epidermal necrolysis, hypersensitivity) reported. Women, including pregnant women, and/or patients with higher CD4 counts are at higher risk of hepatotoxicity. Seek medical evaluation and d/c if signs or symptoms of hepatitis, skin or hypersensitivity reactions develop. Monitoring during the first 18 weeks of therapy is essential; extra vigilance is warranted during the first 6 weeks of therapy.**

**THERAPEUTIC CLASS:** Non-nucleoside reverse transcriptase inhibitor

**INDICATIONS:** Treatment of HIV-1 infection in combination with other antiretrovirals.

**DOSAGE:** *Adults:* 200mg qd for 14 days (lead-in period), then 200mg bid. If severe rash occurs, d/c therapy. If mild-to-moderate rash occurs during 14-day lead-in period, do not increase dose until rash resolves. If dosing interrupted for >7 days, restart 14-day lead-in dosing. Additional 200mg dose following each dialysis treatment for patients requiring dialysis.
*Pediatrics:* ≥15 days:150mg/m$^2$ qd for 14 days, followed by 150mg/m$^2$ bid. Max: 400mg/day. If severe rash occurs, d/c therapy. If mild-to-moderate rash occurs during 14-day lead-in period, do not increase dose until rash resolves. If dosing interrupted for >7 days, restart lead-in dosing. Additional 200mg dose following each dialysis treatment for patients requiring dialysis. Refer to PI for dose calculation based on BSA.

**HOW SUPPLIED:** Sus: 50mg/5mL [240mL]; Tab: 200mg

**CONTRAINDICATIONS:** Moderate or severe (Child-Pugh Class B or C) hepatic impairment.

**WARNINGS/PRECAUTIONS:** May cause rhabdomyolysis in patients with skin or liver reactions. D/C permanently if clinical hepatitis or transaminase elevations accompanied with rash or other systemic symptoms occur; do not restart therapy after recovery. Do not use as single agent to treat HIV or add on as a sole agent to a failing regimen. Immune reconstitution syndrome reported. Possible fat redistribution/accumulation. Caution in elderly.

**ADVERSE REACTIONS:** Hepatitis, hepatic failure, Stevens-Johnson syndrome, toxic epidermal necrolysis, neutropenia, anemia, hepatotoxicity, rash, asymptomatic transaminase elevations, liver enzyme abnormalities.

**INTERACTIONS:** Avoid use of prednisone for prevention of therapy-associated rash. Decreased levels of clarithromycin; consider alternative. Decreased levels of efavirenz, indinavir, nelfinavir, saquinavir. May decrease effectiveness of oral contraceptives and other hormonal contraceptives; use alternate or additional method of contraception. Increased levels with fluconazole. Avoid with ketoconazole, St. John's wort, rifampin. Decreased levels of lopinavir; adjust lopinavir/ritonavir doses. May decrease levels of methadone; monitor for signs of withdrawal. Increased levels of rifabutin. Possible decreased levels with antiarrhythmics (eg, amiodarone, disopyramide, lidocaine), anticonvulsants (eg, carbamazepine, clonazepam, ethosuximide), itraconazole, CCBs (eg, diltiazem, nifedipine, verapamil), cyclophosphamide, ergotamine, immunosuppressants (eg, cyclosporine, tacrolimus, sirolimus), cisapride, fentanyl. Monitor with warfarin.

**PREGNANCY:** Category B, not for use in nursing.

**MECHANISM OF ACTION:** Non-nucleoside reverse transcriptase inhibitor; binds directly to reverse transcriptase and blocks RNA-dependent DNA polymerase activities by causing disruption of the enzyme's catalytic site.

**PHARMACOKINETICS: Absorption:** Absolute bioavailability: 93% (tab), 91% (sol); $C_{max}$=2 mcg/mL; $T_{max}$=4 hrs. **Distribution:** $V_d$=1.21L/Kg; plasma protein binding (60%); readily crosses placenta; found in breast milk. **Metabolism:** Liver; oxidative metabolism, via CYP3A4 and CYP2B6 (extensively); glucuronidated metabolites. **Elimination:** Urine (<3% excreted as parent drug); $T_{1/2}$=45 hrs.

## NURSING CONSIDERATIONS

**Assessment:** Assess for CD4, LFTs, renal or cardiac function, concomitant disease or other drug therapy, moderate or severe hepatic impairment, pregnancy/nursing, possible drug interactions.

**Monitoring:** Monitor for hepatotoxicity, rhabdomyolysis, and skin reactions (eg, Steven-Johnson syndrome, toxic epidermal necrolysis) during therapy. Perform LFTs prior to dose escalation and 2 weeks following dose escalation. Monitor patients on methadone for evidence of narcotic withdrawal. May enroll patients in the Antiretroviral Pregnancy Registry if they become pregnant while on medication.

**Patient Counseling:** Counsel about signs/symptoms of hepatotoxicity. Notify physician immediately if any rash or skin reactions develop. Inform may experience redistribution or accumulation of fat tissue during medication. Counsel that drug does not cure HIV and may continue to develop opportunistic infections and other complications of HIV. Instruct females to avoid nursing to reduce risk transmission. Inform females that oral contraceptives and other hormonal methods of birth control should not be used as sole method of birth control since drug may lower plasma levels of those medications.

**Administration:** Oral route. **Storage:** 25°C (77°F); excursions permitted to 15-30°C (59-86°F).

## VIRAZOLE RX

ribavirin (Valeant)

**Sudden deterioration of respiratory function associated with initiation in infants. Monitor respiratory function carefully. Not for use in adults. Use with mechanical ventilator assistance with staff familiar with mode of administration and specific type of ventilator.**

**THERAPEUTIC CLASS:** Nucleoside analogue

**INDICATIONS:** Treatment of hospitalized infants and young children with severe lower respiratory tract infections due to respiratory syncytial virus.

**DOSAGE:** *Pediatrics:* Continuous aerosol administration of 20mg/mL in the drug reservoir of the SPAG-2 unit for 12-18 hrs/day for 3-7 days.

**HOW SUPPLIED:** Sol, Inhalation: 6g

**CONTRAINDICATIONS:** Women who are or may become pregnant during exposure to drug.

**WARNINGS/PRECAUTIONS:** Monitor respiratory function and fluid status according to SPAG-2 manual. Accumulation of drug precipitate can result in mechanical ventilator dysfunction and associated increased pulmonary pressures.

**ADVERSE REACTIONS:** Worsening of respiratory status, bronchospasm, pulmonary edema, hypoventilation, cyanosis, dyspnea, bacterial pneumonia, pneumothorax, apnea, atelectasis, ventilator dependence, cardiac arrest, hypotension, bradycardia.

**INTERACTIONS:** Digoxin toxicity reported.

**PREGNANCY:** Category X, safety in nursing not known.

**MECHANISM OF ACTION:** Nucleoside analogue; mechanism unknown. Suspected to be analogue of guanosine or xanthosine.

**PHARMACOKINETICS: Elimination:** $T_{1/2}$=9.5 hrs.

### NURSING CONSIDERATIONS

**Assessment:** Assess for pregnancy status and possible drug interactions.

**Monitoring:** Monitor respiratory function and fluid status periodically.

**Administration:** Inhalation route. **Storage:** 25°C (77°F); excursions permitted to 15-30°C (59-86°F). Reconstituted: 20-30°C (68-86°F); stable for 24 hrs.

## VIREAD RX

tenofovir disoproxil fumarate (Gilead)

**Lactic acidosis and severe hepatomegaly with steatosis, including fatal cases, reported with nucleoside analogs alone or with concomitant antiretrovirals. Severe acute exacerbations of hepatitis B virus (HBV) have been reported in patients coinfected with HIV and HBV and who have discontinued Viread. Monitor hepatic function closely for at least several months in patients who d/c anti HBV therapy. If appropriate, resumption of anti-HBV therapy may be warranted.**

**THERAPEUTIC CLASS:** Nucleotide analog reverse transcriptase inhibitor

**INDICATIONS:** Treatment of HIV-1 infection in combination with other antiretrovirals and for chronic HBV in adults.

**DOSAGE:** *Adults:* 300mg qd without regard to food. Renal Impairment: CrCl 30-49mL/min: 300mg q48 hr. CrCl 10-29mL/min: 300mg q72-96 hrs. Hemodialysis: 300mg every 7 days or after a total of approximately 12 hrs of dialysis.

**HOW SUPPLIED:** Tab: 300mg

**WARNINGS/PRECAUTIONS:** Obesity and prolonged nucleoside exposure may be risk factors for lactic acidosis and severe hepatomegaly with steatosis. Caution if risk factors for hepatic disease present. Renal impairment, including cases of acute renal failure and Fanconi syndrome, reported. All patients should have CrCl calculated prior to and during therapy as clinically appropriate. Dose adjust and monitor renal function when CrCl <50mL/min. Monitor

V

serum phosphorous levels in patients at risk for or with history of renal dysfunction. Should only be used in HIV-1 and HBV coinfected patients as part of an appropriate antiretroviral combination regimen. HIV-1 antibody testing should be offered to all HBV-infected patients prior to therapy. Testing for chronic HBV infection recommended prior to therapy in HIV-1 patients. Bone mineral density (BMD) monitoring should be considered for HIV patients at risk for osteopenia. Cases of osteomalacia reported. Possible fat redistribution/accumulation including central obesity, dorsocervical fat enlargement, peripheral wasting, facial wasting, breast enlargement, and "cushingoid appearance" may develop. Immune reconstitution syndrome observed in HIV-infected patients. Early virological failure and high rates of resistance substitutions reported with certain regimens that only contain three nucleoside reverse transcriptase inhibitors (NRTIs); triple nucleoside regimens should be used with caution and patients carefully monitored and considered for treatment modification.

**ADVERSE REACTIONS:** Lactic acidosis, hepatomegaly with steatosis, acute exacerbations of hepatitis, N/V, diarrhea, depression, asthenia, headache, pain, rash, elevated cholesterol levels, elevated creatine kinase, elevated serum amylase, increased AST/ALT, hematuria.

**INTERACTIONS:** Increases levels of didanosine, use caution when coadministered and monitor for didanosine-associated adverse events. Concomitant use with atazanavir may increase tenofovir (TDF) levels and decrease atazanavir levels; monitor for TDF-associated adverse reactions and d/c if adverse reactions develop. Levels of renally eliminated drugs (eg, cidofovir, acyclovir, valacyclovir, ganciclovir, valganciclovir) may increase, along with TDF. Lopinavir/ritonavir, and drugs that decrease renal function may increase levels. Concomitant use with indinavir, may decrease indinavir levels and increase TDF levels. Concomitant use with saquinavir/ritonavir may increase increase saquinavir levels and increase the $C_{min}$ of ritonavir and TDF. Concomitant use with tacrolimus may increase levels. Concomitant use with emtricitabine, may increase the $C_{min}$ of emtricitabine. Concomitant use with entecavir may increase the AUC of entecavir. May decrease lamivudine plasma levels. Avoid with concurrent or recent use of nephrotoxic agents. Do not use in combination with other TDF containing products and do not administer in combination with adefovir.

**PREGNANCY:** Category B, not for use in nursing.

**MECHANISM OF ACTION:** Nucleotide analog reverse transcriptase inhibitor; inhibits activity of HIV-1 reverse transcriptase and HBV polymerase by competing with natural substrate deoxyadenosine 5'-triphosphate and, after incorporation into DNA, by DNA termination.

**PHARMACOKINETICS: Absorption:** $C_{max}$=0.30mcg/mL; $T_{max}$=1.0 hr; AUC=2.29mcg•hr/mL. **Distribution:** Serum protein bound (7.2%), human plasma bound (<0.7%); $V_d$=1.3L/kg (1mg/kg IV dose); $V_d$=1.2L/kg (3mg/kg IV dose). **Elimination:** Urine (70-80% unchanged); $T_{1/2}$=17 hrs.

## NURSING CONSIDERATIONS

**Assessment:** Assess for renal impairment, risk factors for liver disease, obesity, pregnancy/nursing status, and for possible drug interactions. Prior to therapy, assess CrCl in all patients. In HBV-infected patients, perform HIV-1 antibody testing. In HIV-1 patients, perform testing for presence of chronic hepatitis B.



**Monitoring:** Monitor for signs/symptoms of lactic acidosis, severe hepatomegaly with steatosis, fat accumulation/redistribution, new onset or worsening renal impairment, immune reconstitution syndrome, and for osteomalacia. Upon d/c of tenofovir in patients with HBV, monitor with clinical and laboratory followup for acute exacerbations of hepatitis. Monitor BMD in patients who have a history of pathologic bone fracture or are at risk for osteopenia. Monitor CrCl in all patients and monitor serum phosphorus levels in patients with at risk for renal impairment. Monitor renal function in all patients with CrCl <50mL/min.

**Patient Counseling:** Inform that medication is not a cure for HIV-1 infection and may continue to experience illness associated with HIV-1 infection, including opportunistic infections. Counsel that medication has not been shown to reduce the risk of transmission of HIV-1 or HBV to others through sexual contact or blood contamination; advise to continue to practice safe sex and to use latex or polyurethane condoms. Advise to never re-use or share needles. Inform that tablets are for oral ingestion only. Advise not to d/c without informing their physician. Counsel about the importance of adherence to regimen and avoid missing doses. Inform of medications that that may interact and adverse effects that might occur during therapy.

**Administration:** Oral route. **Storage:** 25°C (77°F); excursions permitted to 15-30°C (59-86°F).

## VIROPTIC — RX

trifluridine (Monarch Pharmaceuticals Inc.)

**THERAPEUTIC CLASS:** Fluorinated pyrimidine nucleoside antiviral

**INDICATIONS:** Treatment of primary keratoconjunctivitis and recurrent epithelial keratitis due to herpes simplex virus, types 1 and 2.

**DOSAGE:** *Adults:* 1 drop into cornea of the affected eye q2h while awake until corneal ulcer has completely re-epithelialized. Max: 9 drops/day. Following Re-epithelialization: 1 drop q4h while awake for 7 days; minimum of 5 drops/day. If no improvement after 7 days or if complete re-epithelialization has not occurred after 14 days, consider other forms of therapy. Avoid using >21 days.
*Pediatrics:* ≥6 yrs: 1 drop into cornea of the affected eye q2h while awake until corneal ulcer has completely re-epithelialized. Max: 9 drops/day. Following Re-epithelialization: 1 drop q4h while awake for 7 days; minimum of 5 drops/day. If no improvement after 7 days or if complete re-epithelialization has not occurred after 14 days, consider other forms of therapy. Avoid using >21 days.

**HOW SUPPLIED:** Sol: 1% [7.5mL]

**WARNINGS/PRECAUTIONS:** Only use with a clinical diagnosis of herpetic keratitis. May cause transient, mild local irritation of the conjunctiva and cornea when instilled. Possibility of development of viral resistance.

**ADVERSE REACTIONS:** Burning, stinging, palpebral edema, superficial punctate keratopathy, epithelial keratopathy, hypersensitivity reaction, stromal edema, irritation, keratitis sicca, hyperemia, IOP.

**PREGNANCY:** Category C, not for use in nursing.

**MECHANISM OF ACTION:** Fluorinated pyrimidine nucleoside antiviral; unknown, suspected to interfere with DNA synthesis.

**PHARMACOKINETICS: Absorption:** Intraocular penetration; decreased corneal integrity or stromal/uveal inflammation may enhance penetration into the aqueous humor.

### NURSING CONSIDERATIONS

**Assessment:** Assess for clinical diagnosis of herpetic keratitis and for pregnancy/nursing status.

**Monitoring:** Monitor for clinical signs of improvement after 7 days of therapy and complete re-epithelialization after 14 days of therapy. Monitor for signs/symptoms of mild local irritation of conjunctiva and cornea. Monitor for possible viral resistance and hypersensitivity reactions.

**Patient Counseling:** Advise that recommended dosage and frequency of administration should not be exceeded. Inform that continuous administration for periods exceeding 21 days should be avoided because of potential for ocular toxicity. Instruct to report any adverse reactions that develop.

**Administration:** Ocular route. **Storage:** Store under refrigeration 2-8°C (36-46°F).

# VISICOL

RX

sodium phosphate (Salix)

**Serious acute phosphate nephropathy (rare) reported. Some cases resulted in permanent renal impairment requiring long-term dialysis. Increased risk of acute phosphate nephropathy may occur with increased age, hypovolemia, increased bowel transit time (eg, bowel obstruction), active colitis or baseline kidney disease and using medicines that affect renal perfusion or function (eg, diuretics, ACE inhibitors, ARBs, and possibly NSAIDs). Use the recommended dose and dosing regimen (pm/am split dose).**

**THERAPEUTIC CLASS:** Bowel cleanser

**INDICATIONS:** For cleansing the colon in preparation for colonoscopy in adults ≥18 yrs.

**DOSAGE:** *Adults:* ≥18 yrs: Adequately hydrate before, during, and after use. Evening Before Colonoscopy Procedure: 3 tabs with 8 oz clear liquids every 15 min for total of 20 tabs (last dose is 2 tabs). Day of Colonoscopy Procedure: Repeat dosing on day of exam 3-5 hrs before procedure. May re-treat after 7 days.

**HOW SUPPLIED:** Tab: (Sodium Phosphate Monobasic Monohydrate-Sodium Phosphate Dibasic Anhydrous) 1.102g-0.398g

**CONTRAINDICATIONS:** Patients with biopsy-proven acute phosphate nephropathy.

**WARNINGS/PRECAUTIONS:** Fatalities reported due to significant fluid shift, severe electrolyte imbalances and arrhythmias with administration of sodium phosphate products. Caution with severe renal insufficiency (CrCl <30 mL/min), CHF, ascites, unstable angina, acute bowel obstruction, bowel perforation, toxic megacolon, gastric retention, ileus, pseudo-obstruction of the bowel, severe chronic constipation, acute colitis, gastric bypass, stapling surgery or hypomotility syndrome. Caution with impaired renal function, history of acute phosphate nephropathy, known or suspected electrolyte disturbances (eg, dehydration). Correct electrolyte disturbance before use. Reports of generalized tonic-clonic seizures and/or loss of consciousness in patients with no prior history of seizures. Caution in patients with history of seizures and in patients at high risk of seizure (eg, withdrawing from alcohol or benzodiazepines, known or suspected hyponatremia). Caution in patients with higher risk of arrhythmias (eg, history of cardiomyopathy, prolonged QT interval, uncontrolled arrhythmias, recent MI). Pre-dose and post-colonoscopy ECGs should be done in patients with high risk of serious, cardiac arrhythmias. May induce colonic mucosal aphthous ulcerations and exacerbate IBD. Difficulty of swallowing may occur in patients with a history of difficulties or anatomic narrowing of the esophagus (eg, stricture). Caution with recent cardiac surgery (eg, coronary artery bypass graft surgery). Caution in elderly.

**ADVERSE REACTIONS:** N/V, abdominal bloating, abdominal pain, hyperphosphatemia, hypocalcemia, hypokalemia and acute phosphate nephropathy (rare).

**INTERACTIONS:** See Black Box Warning. May reduce absorption of other drugs. Caution with agents that prolong QT interval or affect electrolyte levels. Avoid use of additional purgative or laxative (eg, other sodium phosphate-containing products) agents. Caution with concomitant use of medications lowering seizure threshold (eg, TCAs).

V

**PREGNANCY:** Category C, safety not known in nursing.

**MECHANISM OF ACTION:** Osmotic laxative; causes large amounts of water to be drawn into colon, promoting colon evacuation.

## NURSING CONSIDERATIONS

**Assessment:** Assess for acute phosphate nephropathy, known hypersensitivity to sodium phosphates, cardiac arrhythmias, severe electrolyte abnormalities, severe renal insufficiency, CHF, unstable angina, bowel obstruction, bowel perforation, gastric retention, severe chronic constipation, acute colitis, history of seizures, pregnancy status and possible drug interactions. Perform baseline ECG, phosphate, calcium, $K^+$, $Na^+$, creatinine and BUN levels.

**Monitoring:** Monitor CrCl, ECG, phosphate, calcium, $K^+$, $Na^+$, creatinine and BUN levels post-colonoscopy. Watch out for vomiting, arrhythmias and seizures.

**Patient Counseling:** Discuss the benefits and risks of therapy. Inform healthcare provider of any concomitant medical condition or medication being taken. Instruct to follow the dose and dosing regimen. Drink 8 oz clear liquid with each 3-tab dose. Ingest total of 3.6 quarts clear liquid. Do not use within 7 days of previous administration. Do not take additional laxatives or purgatives.

**Administration:** Oral route. **Storage:** 25°C (77°F); excursions permitted to 15-30°C (59-86°F). Discard any unused portion.

## VISTIDE RX

cidofovir (Gilead)

**Renal impairment is a major toxicity; prehydrate with IV normal saline (NS) and administer probenecid with each dose. Monitor serum creatinine (SrCr) and urine protein within 48 hrs prior to each dose. Modify dose with renal function changes. Contraindicated with nephrotoxic agents. Neutropenia reported; monitor neutrophils. Carcinogenic, teratogenic, and hypospermatic in animal studies.**

**THERAPEUTIC CLASS:** Viral DNA synthesis inhibitor

**INDICATIONS:** Treatment of cytomegalovirus (CMV) retinitis in AIDS patients.

**DOSAGE:** *Adults:* IV: Induction: 5mg/kg once weekly for 2 weeks. Maint: 5mg/kg once every 2 weeks. Reduce maint from 5mg/kg to 3mg/kg for an increase in SrCr of 0.3-0.4mg/dL above baseline. D/C with increase in SrCr ≥0.5mg/dL above baseline or ≥3+ proteinuria. Administer probenecid 2g PO 3 hrs before cidofovir, then 1g at 2 hrs and 8 hrs after completion of cidofovir infusion. Administer at least 1L 0.9% NS immediately before infusion. If tolerated, give 2nd liter at start of or immediately after infusion.

**HOW SUPPLIED:** Inj: 75mg/mL

**CONTRAINDICATIONS:** SrCr >1.5mg/dL, CrCl ≤55mL/min, or urine protein ≥100mg/dL ( ≥2+ proteinuria) with therapy initiation. Nephrotoxic agents (d/c at least 7 days before therapy), severe hypersensitivity to probenecid or other sulfa-containing agents, direct intraocular use.

**WARNINGS/PRECAUTIONS:** Dose-dependent nephrotoxicity. Monitor IOP, visual acuity, ocular symptoms, uveitis/iritis, and renal function periodically. Monitor WBC with differential before each dose. Avoid during pregnancy. Adequate contraception for both sexes during and following treatment is advised. May cause male infertility. Potentially carcinogenic.

**ADVERSE REACTIONS:** N/V, neutropenia, proteinuria, decreased IOP/ocular hypotony, anterior uveitis/iritis, metabolic acidosis, nephrotoxicity, pneumonia, dyspnea, infection, fever, creatinine ≥2mg/dL, decreased sodium bicarbonate.

**INTERACTIONS:** Avoid nephrotoxic agents (aminoglyosides, amphotericin B, foscarnet, IV pentamidine, vancomycin, and NSAIDs); d/c nephrotoxic agents at least 7 days before therapy. Temporarily d/c zidovudine or decrease zidovudine by 50% with probenecid.

**PREGNANCY:** Category C, not for use in nursing.

**MECHANISM OF ACTION:** Viral DNA synthesis inhibitor; suppresses CMV replication by selective inhibition of viral DNA synthesis.

**PHARMACOKINETICS: Administration:** Variable doses resulted in altered parameters. **Absorption:** 5mg/kg: AUC=28.3 mcg•mL/hr (without probenecid), AUC=40.8 mcg•mL/hr (with probenecid); $C_{max}$=11.5mcg/mL (without probenecid), $C_{max}$=19.6mcg/mL (with probenecid); 3mg/kg: AUC=20.0mcg•mL/hr (without probenecid), AUC=25.7 mcg•mL/hr (with probenecid); $C_{max}$=7.3 mcg/mL (without probenecid), $C_{max}$=9.8 mcg/mL (with probenecid). **Distribution:** $V_d$=537mL/kg (without probenecid), $V_d$= 410mL/kg (with probenecid); Plasma protein binding (≤6%). **Elimination:** 80-100% excreted unchanged in urine.

## NURSING CONSIDERATIONS

**Assessment:** Assess renal function prior to therapy.

**Monitoring:** Monitor renal function, SrCr, urine protein, WBC, neutrophils, serum bicarbonate, IOP, and visual acuity. Monitor for signs/symptoms of nephrotoxicity, metabolic acidosis, uveitis, or iritis. Monitor for allergic reactions when using in combination with probenecid.

**Patient Counseling:** Counsel to take full course of probenecid with drug. If nausea develops, take with food. Inform drug does not cure CMV retinitis; may continue to experience progression of retinitis during, and following, treatment. Advise for regular follow-up ophthalmologic exams. Advise females to use proper contraception while on medication and to continue using contraception for at least 1 month following therapy. Counsel males to use proper contraception while on medication and for 3 months following therapy. Advise drug is not for direct intraocular injection.

**Administration:** IV route. 1) Inspect for particulate matter and discoloration. 2) Add appropriate volume to 100mL 0.9% NS. 3) Infuse over 1 hr at constant rate. 4) Probenecid and IV saline prehydration must be administered with each infusion. **Storage:** Vial: 20-25°C (68-77°F). Admixture: Under refrigeration, 2-8°C, for no more than 24 hrs. If refrigerated, allow admixture to reach room temperature prior to use.

# VISUDYNE — RX

verteporfin (Novartis Ophthalmics)

**THERAPEUTIC CLASS:** Photosensitizing agent

**INDICATIONS:** Treatment of age-related macular degeneration with subfoveal choroidal neovascularization.

**DOSAGE:** *Adults:* 6mg/m² IV over 10 min at 3mL/min. Photoactivation with laser light therapy with nonthermal diode laser 15 min after start IV infusion. Re-evaluate every 3 months and repeat if choroidal neovascular leakage detected on fluorescein angiography.

**HOW SUPPLIED:** Inj: 15mg

**CONTRAINDICATIONS:** Porphyria.

**WARNINGS/PRECAUTIONS:** Avoid direct sunlight or bright indoor light for 5 days. Avoid extravasation. If extravasation occurs, protect area from direct light until swelling and discoloration fade. Protect from intense light if surgery within 48 hrs after therapy. Do not retreat if severe vision decrease of 4 lines or more occurs within 1 week after therapy. Only use compatible lasers. Caution with moderate to severe hepatic dysfunction. Reduced effects with increasing age.

**ADVERSE REACTIONS:** Headache, injection-site reactions, visual disturbances, asthenia, HTN, eczema, constipation, nausea, anemia, arthralgia, vertigo, pharyngitis.

**INTERACTIONS:** CCBs, polymyxin B, and radiation therapy may enhance rate of uptake by vascular endothelium. Increased photosensitivity with tetracyclines, sulfonamides, phenothiazines, sulfonylureas, thiazide diuretics, and griseofulvin. Decreased effects with dimethyl sulfoxide, β-carotene, ethanol, formate, mannitol, and drugs that decrease clotting, vasoconstriction, or platelet aggregation (eg, thromboxane $A_2$ inhibitors).



**PREGNANCY:** Pregnancy C, not for use in nursing.

**MECHANISM OF ACTION:** Photosensitizing agent; transported into plasma by lipoproteins. Activated by light in presence of oxygen; light activation causes local damage to neovascular endothelium, subsequently leading to vessel occlusion. Damaged endothelium releases procoagulant and vasoactive factors through lipo-oxygenase and cyclo-oxygenase pathways, resulting in platelet aggregation, fibrin clot formation, and vasoconstriction.

**PHARMACOKINETICS: Absorption:** Dose proportional. **Distribution:** Found in breast milk. **Metabolism:** Liver and plasma esterases; diacid metabolite. **Elimination:** Feces (major), urine (≤0.01%); $T_{1/2}$=5-6 hrs.

## NURSING CONSIDERATIONS

**Assessment:** Assess patient does not have porphyria and that females are not nursing. Assess use in pregnancy, with severe hepatic impairment, or biliary obstruction. Assess for drug interactions.

**Monitoring:** Monitor for signs/symptoms of extravasation or injection site reactions, severe decreases in vision, severe CP, vasovagal and hypersensitivity reactions (eg, syncope, rash, dyspnea, flushing, changes in BP and HR). Monitor that IV line is free-flowing.

**Patient Counseling:** Instruct to avoid exposure of unprotected skin, eyes, or other body organs to direct sunlight, bright light (eg, tanning salon, bright halogen lighting, high powered lighting), or light-emitting medical devices (eg, pulse oximeters) for 5 days following therapy. Instruct to protect eyes and skin if going outdoors during first 5 days following treatment. Instruct to avoid staying in dark when indoors; skin should be exposed to ambient indoor lighting. Darkness inactivates drug in skin through process called photobleaching. Inform that visual changes may occur; avoid using machinery/driving until symptoms have subsided.

**Administration:** IV route. Reconstitute. 1) Use 7mL SWFI to provide 7.5mL containing 2mg/mL; do not use NS or other parenteral solutions. Do not mix in same sol with other drugs. 2) Dilute using D5W to total infusion volume of 30mL. **Storage:** 20-25°C (68-77°F). Following dilution, protect from light and use within maximum of 4 hrs.

# VITRASERT — RX

ganciclovir (Bausch & Lomb)

**THERAPEUTIC CLASS:** Nucleoside analogue

**INDICATIONS:** Treatment of cytomegalovirus (CMV) retinitis in AIDS patients.

**DOSAGE:** *Adults:* Each implant releases 4.5mg over 5-8 months. Remove and replace when evidence of retinitis progression.
*Pediatrics:* ≥9 yrs: Each implant releases 4.5mg over 5-8 months. Remove and replace when evidence of retinitis progression.

**HOW SUPPLIED:** Implant: 4.5mg

**CONTRAINDICATIONS:** Hypersensitivity to acyclovir, patients with contraindication for intraocular surgery (eg, external infection, severe thrombocytopenia).

**WARNINGS/PRECAUTIONS:** For intravitreal implantation only. Monitor for extraocular CMV disease. Implant does not treat systemic CMV. Complications from surgery include vitreous loss or hemorrhage, cataract formation, retinal detachment, uveitis, endophthalmitis, decrease in visual acuity. Immediate decrease in visual acuity will last 2-4 weeks postop. Maintain sterility of the surgical field, implant. Handle implant by suture tab to avoid damage to polymer coating. Handling and disposal of the implant should follow guidelines for antineoplastics.

**ADVERSE REACTIONS:** Visual acuity loss, vitreous hemorrhage, retinal detachments, cataract formation/lens opacities, macular abnormalities, IOP spikes, optic disk/nerve changes, uveitis, hyphemas.

**PREGNANCY:** Category C, not for use in nursing.

**MECHANISM OF ACTION:** Nucleoside analogue antiviral; inhibits replication of herpes viruses.

## NURSING CONSIDERATIONS

**Assessment:** Assess for proper diagnosis of CMV retinitis (eg, indirect opthalmoscopy). Assess patient does not have contraindications for intraocular surgery (eg, external infection, severe thrombocytopenia) and does not have allergy to acyclovir. Assess use in pregnancy/nursing.

**Monitoring:** Monitor for extraocular CMV disease and infections (eg, pneumonitis, colitis), vitreous loss or hemorrhage, cataract formation, retinal detachment, uvelitis, intraocular infection, and decrease in visual acuity.

V

**Patient Counseling:** Advise that implant is not a cure for CMV retinitis; some patients may continue to experience progression of retinitis. Counsel about potential complications following intraocular surgery (eg, intraocular infection, retina detachment, formation of cataracts). Inform patient will experience immediate and temporary decrease in visual acuity for 2-4 weeks after surgery and will require follow-up ophthalmological exams at regular intervals following surgery. Inform medication may cause infertility and may be carcinogenic.

**Administration:** Ocular implant. **Storage:** 15-30°C (59-86°F). Protect from freezing, excessive heat, and light.

## VIVELLE RX

estradiol (Novartis)

**Estrogens increase risk of endometrial cancer in postmenopausal women. Estrogens, with or without progestins, should not be used for the prevention of cardiovascular disease. Increased risks of MI, stroke, invasive breast cancer, PE, and DVT in postmenopausal women (50-79 yrs of age) reported. Increased risk of developing probable dementia in postmenopausal women ≥65 yrs of age reported.**

**OTHER BRAND NAMES:** Vivelle-Dot (Novartis)

**THERAPEUTIC CLASS:** Estrogen

**INDICATIONS:** Treatment of moderate to severe vasomotor symptoms and/or vulvar/vaginal atrophy associated with menopause. Treatment of hypoestrogenism due to hypogonadism, castration, or primary ovarian failure. Prevention of postmenopausal osteoporosis.

**DOSAGE:** *Adults:* Vasomotor Symptoms/Vulvar/Vaginal Atrophy: Initial: 0.0375mg/day twice weekly. Titrate: Adjust after at least 1 month. D/C or taper at 3-6 month intervals. Wait 1 week after withdrawal of oral therapy before initiating therapy. Osteoporosis Prevention: Minimum Effective Dose: 0.025mg/day twice weekly. Apply to clean, dry area of the trunk; avoid breasts and waistline. Rotate sites; allow 1 week between same site. Without intact uterus, may give continuously; with intact uterus, may give cyclically (3 weeks on, 1 week off) with a progestin.

**HOW SUPPLIED:** Patch: (Vivelle) 0.05mg/day, 0.1mg/day [8[s], 48[s]]; (Vivelle-Dot) 0.025mg/day, 0.0375mg/day, 0.05mg/day, 0.075mg/day, 0.1mg/day [8[s], 24[s]]

**CONTRAINDICATIONS:** Pregnancy, undiagnosed abnormal genital bleeding, breast cancer, estrogen dependent neoplasia, DVT/PE, active or recent (eg, within past year) arterial thromboembolic disease (eg, stroke, MI), liver dysfunction or disease.

**WARNINGS/PRECAUTIONS:** May increase risk of cardiovascular events (eg, MI, stroke), venous thrombosis, and PE; d/c immediately if any of these events occur or are suspected. May increase risk of breast/endometrial cancer and gallbladder disease. May lead to severe hypercalcemia with breast cancer and bone metastases; monitor and d/c if hypercalcemia occurs. Retinal vascular thrombosis reported; monitor and d/c if papilledema or retinal vascular lesions occur. Consider addition of a progestin if no hysterectomy. May elevate BP; monitor at regular intervals. May cause elevations of plasma triglycerides with pre-existing hypertriglyceridemia. Caution with history of cholestatic jaundice associated with past estrogen use or with pregnancy; d/c with recurrence. May lead to increased thyroid-binding globulin levels; monitor thyroid function. May cause fluid retention; caution with cardiac/renal dysfunction. Caution with severe hypocalcemia. May increase risk of ovarian cancer. May exacerbate endometriosis, asthma, DM, epilepsy, migraine, porphyria, SLE, and hepatic hemangiomas; use with caution.

**ADVERSE REACTIONS:** Altered vaginal bleeding, vaginal candidiasis, breast tenderness/enlargement, N/V, melasma, headache, weight changes, edema, altered libido.

**INTERACTIONS:** CYP3A4 inducers (eg, St. John's wort, phenobarbital, carbamazepine, rifampin) may decrease levels which may decrease therapeutic

V

effects and/or change uterine bleeding profile. CYP3A4 inhibitors (eg, erythromycin, clarithromycin, ketoconazole, itraconazole, ritonavir, grapefruit juice) may increase levels which may result in side effects.

**PREGNANCY:** Contraindicated in pregnancy, caution in nursing.

**MECHANISM OF ACTION:** Estrogen; responsible for development and maintenance of female reproductive system, and secondary sexual characteristics by modulating pituitary secretion of gonadotropins, LH and FSH.

**PHARMACOKINETICS: Absorption**: Transdermal administration of variable doses resulted in different parameters. **Metabolism**: Liver, estrone (metabolite), estriol (major urinary metabolite). **Elimination**: Urine; $T_{1/2}$=4.4 hrs, 5.9-7.7 hrs (Dot).

## NURSING CONSIDERATIONS

**Assessment:** Assess for abnormal bleeding, breast or estrogen-dependent neoplasia, CAD, asthma, endometriosis, DM, epilepsy, migraine, porphyrias, SLE, hypothyroidism, pregnancy status, thromboembolic disease, hypocalcemia, and hepatic impairment.

**Monitoring:** Monitor BP regularly; TFTs periodically. Breast exam by physician yearly and self-exam monthly; mammogram as required. Monitor for signs/symptoms of dementia, gallbladder disease, hypercalcemia, CV events (eg, MI, stroke), abnormal vaginal bleeding, thromboembolic disorders, fluid retention, visual abnormalities, hypersensitivity reactions, hepatic dysfunction, exacerbation of asthma, DM, epilepsy, SLE, migraines, and porphyria.

**Patient Counseling:** Inform of pregnancy risks. Advise to seek medical attention if symptoms of hepatic dysfunction (eg, jaundice), hypercalcemia, visual abnormalities (eg, partial/complete loss of vision, diplopia), migraines, abnormal vaginal bleeding, hypersensitivity reactions, HTN, thromboembolic disorders, fluid retention, exacerbation of diseases, CV events, or dementia occur.

**Administration:** Transdermal route. Apply immediately after removed from pouch. **Storage**: Below 30°C (86°F). Dot: 25°C (77°F).

# VIVITROL — RX

naltrexone (Alkermes)

**THERAPEUTIC CLASS:** Opioid antagonist

**INDICATIONS:** Treatment of alcohol dependence in patients who are able to abstain from alcohol in an outpatient setting prior to initiation of therapy.

**DOSAGE:** *Adults:* Administer 380mg IM gluteal inj every 4 weeks or once a month, alternating buttocks.

**HOW SUPPLIED:** Inj, Extended-Release: 380mg

**CONTRAINDICATIONS:** Acute hepatitis or liver failure, concomitant opioid analgesics, physiologic opioid dependence, acute opiate withdrawal, positive urine screen for opioids or failed naloxone challenge test.

**WARNINGS/PRECAUTIONS:** Hepatotoxicity with excessive doses; does not appear to be heptatotoxic at recommended doses. Eosinophilic pneumonia reported. Only treat patients opioid-free for 7-10 days. Perform naloxone challenge test if risk of precipitating withdrawal. Not indicated for opioid blockade or the treatment of opiate dependence. Attempting to overcome the opiate blockade using opioids is very dangerous. More sensitive to lower doses of opioids after naltrexone is d/c. In emergency situation, suggested plan for pain management is regional analgesia, conscious sedation with a benzodiazepine, or use of non-opioid analgesics or general anesthesia. Monitor for development of depression or suicidal thinking. Caution in renal or hepatic impairment. Administration will not eliminate or diminish alcohol withdrawal symptoms. Injection-site reactions reported; inadvertent SQ injection may increase likelihood of severe injection-site reactions. As with any intramuscular injection, caution with thrombocytopenia or any coagulation disorder (eg, hemophilia, severe hepatic failure).

**ADVERSE REACTIONS:** N/V, diarrhea, abdominal pain, upper respiratory tract infection, pharyngitis, insomnia, anxiety, depression, injection-site reactions, arthralgia, muscle cramps, dizziness, syncope, appetite disorder.

**INTERACTIONS:** See Contraindications. May antagonize effects of opioid-containing medicines (eg, cough and cold remedies, antidiarrheals, opioid analgesics).

**PREGNANCY:** Category C, not for use in nursing.

**MECHANISM OF ACTION:** Opioid antagonist; blocks the effects of opioids by competitive binding at opioid receptors.

**PHARMACOKINETICS: Absorption:** $T_{max}$=2 hrs. **Distribution:** Plasma protein binding (21%); found in breast milk. **Metabolism:** Extensive, via dihydrodiol dehydrogenase, 6β-naltrexol (primary metabolite). **Elimination:** Urine; $T_{1/2}$=5-10 days.

## NURSING CONSIDERATIONS

**Assessment:** Assess opioid use or dependence, acute opiate withdrawal, hepatic failure or hepatitis, renal impairment, pre-existing subclinical abstinence syndrome, hypersensitivity, pregnancy/nursing status, alcohol intake, and for possible drug interactions. Assess patient's body habitus, to assure the needle length is adequate.

**Monitoring:** Monitor for injection-site reactions, signs/symptoms of hepatotoxicity, respiratory arrest, eosinophilic pneumonia, suicidal ideation attempt, acute abstinence syndrome, and hypersensitivity reactions. Monitor CBC, LFTs, and CPK.

**Patient Counseling:** Alert families and caregivers to monitor for emergence of symptoms of depression or suicidality. Advise to carry documentation to alert medical personnel to therapy. Advise that concomitant large doses of heroin, or other opioids, may lead to serious injury, coma, or death; reduced sensitivity to lower doses of opioids. Notify if pregnant/nursing or planning to become pregnant. Inform that injection-site reactions may occur and to seek medical attention for worsening skin reactions. Inform that can cause liver injury and allergic pneumonia. Advise to notify physician if signs/symptoms of liver injury or pneumonia develop. Counsel that therapy treats alcohol dependence only when used as part of treatment program. Caution in engaging in hazardous activities (eg, operating machinery or vehicles). Instruct to receive the next dose as soon as possible if a dose is missed.

**Administration:** IM route; gluteal region. Must be administrated by healthcare professional. Not for IV/SQ use. **Storage:** 2-8°C (36-46°F). Do not freeze. Can be stored at <25°C (77°F) for <7 days prior administration.

# VOLTAREN GEL — RX

diclofenac sodium (Novartis Consumer)

**NSAIDs may cause an increased risk of serious cardiovascular thrombotic events, MI, stroke and serious GI adverse events including bleeding, ulceration, and perforation of the stomach or intestines. Contraindicated for the treatment of perioperative pain in the setting of coronary artery bypass graft (CABG) surgery.**

V

**THERAPEUTIC CLASS:** NSAID

**INDICATIONS:** Relief of the pain of osteoarthritis of joints amenable to topical treatment, such as knees and hands.

**DOSAGE:** *Adults:* Measure onto enclosed dosing card to appropriate 2g or 4g line. Lower Extremities: Apply 4g to affected foot, knee, or ankle qid. Max: 16g/day to any single joint. Upper Extremities: Apply 2g to affected hand, elbow, or wrist qid. Max: 8g/day to any single joint. Total dose should not exceed 32g/day over all affected joints. Avoid showering or bathing for at least 1 hour after application. Avoid open wounds, eyes, mucous membranes, external heat, and/or occlusive dressings. Avoid wearing clothing or gloves for at least 10 min after application.

**HOW SUPPLIED:** Gel: 1%

**CONTRAINDICATIONS:** ASA or other NSAID allergy that precipitates asthma, urticaria, or allergic-type reactions. Treatment of perioperative pain in the setting of CABG surgery.

**WARNINGS/PRECAUTIONS:** Not evaluated for use on spine, hip, or shoulder. May lead to onset of new HTN or worsening of pre-existing HTN; monitor BP closely. Fluid retention and edema reported; caution with fluid retention or heart failure. Renal papillary necrosis and other renal injury reported after long-term use. Not recommended for use with advanced renal disease; if therapy must be initiated, monitor renal function. Anaphylactoid reactions may occur. May cause serious skin adverse events (eg, exfoliative dermatitis, Stevens-Johnson syndrome [SJS], and toxic epidermal necrolysis [TEN]). Avoid in late pregnancy; may cause premature closure of ductus arteriosus. May cause elevations of LFTs; d/c if liver disease develops or systemic manifestations occur. To minimize the potential for adverse liver-related events, use the lowest effective dose for the shortest duration possible. Caution in elderly. Anemia may occur; with long-term use, monitor Hgb/Hct if signs or symptoms of anemia develop. May inhibit platelet aggregation and prolong bleeding time; monitor with coagulation disorders. Caution with asthma and avoid with ASA-sensitive asthma. Patients should minimize or avoid exposure to natural or artificial sunlight on treated areas. Caution in patients with prior history of ulcer or GI bleeding; monitor for signs or symptoms of GI bleeding. May diminish utility of diagnostic signs (eg, inflammation, fever) in detecting infectious complications of presumed noninfectious, painful conditions.

**ADVERSE REACTIONS:** Application-site reactions, dermatitis.

**INTERACTIONS:** See Contraindications. May enhance methotrexate toxicity and cyclosporine nephrotoxicity; caution when coadministering. May diminish antihypertensive effect of ACE-inhibitors. May reduce natriuretic effect of furosemide and thiazides; monitor for renal failure. May increase lithium levels; monitor for toxicity. Synergistic effects on GI bleeding with anticoagulants (eg, warfarin). Avoid concomitant use with other topical products, including topical medications, sunscreens, lotions, moisturizers, and cosmetics, on the same skin site; may alter tolerability and absorption. Coadministration with oral NSAIDs or ASA may result in increased adverse NSAID effects. Caution with concomitant hepatotoxic drugs (eg, antibiotics, anti-epileptics).

**PREGNANCY:** Category C, not for use in nursing.

**MECHANISM OF ACTION:** NSAID; inhibits cyclooxygenase, resulting in reduced formation of prostaglandins, thromboxanes, and prostacylin.

**PHARMACOKINETICS: Absorption:** (4g) $C_{max}$=15ng/mL; $T_{max}$=14 hrs; AUC=233ng•h/mL. (12g)$C_{max}$=53.8ng/mL; $T_{max}$=10 hrs; AUC=807ng•h/mL.

## NURSING CONSIDERATIONS

**Assessment:** Assess for hypersensitivity to ASA or NSAIDs, history of ulcer or GI bleeding, HTN, fluid retention, CHF, asthma, CV disease (or risk factors), renal/hepatic impairment, pregnancy/nursing status and possible drug interactions. Obtain baseline BP.

**Monitoring:** Monitor BP, LFTs, and renal function periodically. Monitor for signs/symptoms of CV events, GI events (eg, ulcerations, bleeding), hepatotoxicity, renal dysfunction, HTN, skin reactions, anemia, blood loss and hypersensitivity reactions.

**Patient Counseling:** Instruct to avoid contact with eyes and mucous membranes; if contact occurs, wash with water or saline and if irritation persists for >1 hr call physician. Advise to minimize sun exposure. Inform to avoid late in pregnancy. Seek medical attention for symptoms of cardiovascular events (eg, chest pain, SOB, weakness, slurring of speech), GI events (eg, epigastric pain, dyspepsia, melena, hematemesis), hepatotoxicity (eg, RUQ pain, pruritus, fatigue), unexplained weight gain or edema, skin reactions (eg, rash, blisters, fever, SJS, TEN, exfoliative dermatitis) or hypersensitivity reactions (eg, difficulty breathing, swelling of face/throat); d/c at first appearance of rash/hypersensitivity reactions.

**Administration:** Topical route. **Storage:** 25°C (77°F), excursions permitted to 15-30°C (59-86°F). Avoid freezing.

# VOLTAREN OPHTHALMIC RX

diclofenac sodium (Novartis Ophthalmics)

**THERAPEUTIC CLASS:** NSAID

**INDICATIONS:** Treatment of postoperative inflammation following cataract surgery. Temporary relief of pain and photophobia in corneal refractive surgery.

**DOSAGE:** *Adults:* Cataract Surgery: 1 drop qid, start 24 hrs after surgery and continue for 2 weeks. Corneal Refractive Surgery: 1-2 drops within 1 hr prior to, and within 15 min after surgery. Continue qid for up to 3 days.

**HOW SUPPLIED:** Sol: 0.1% [2.5mL, 5mL]

**WARNINGS/PRECAUTIONS:** May delay wound healing. Caution with bleeding tendencies. Monitor for 1 yr after use in corneal refractive procedures. May increase bleeding of ocular tissues. No significant increase in tumor incidence. No differences in safety and effectiveness observed between elderly and younger adult patients.

**ADVERSE REACTIONS:** Transient burning/stinging, keratitis, elevated IOP, lacrimation, abnormal vision, conjunctivitis, eyelid swelling, discharge, iritis, itching.

**INTERACTIONS:** Caution with agents that prolong bleeding time (eg, NSAIDs). Potential for cross-sensitivity to acetylsalicylic acid, phenylacetic acid derivatives, and other NSAIDs.

**PREGNANCY:** Category C, safety in nursing not known.

**MECHANISM OF ACTION:** NSAID; anti-inflammatory and analgesic that inhibits the enzyme cyclo-oxygenase, which is essential for biosynthesis of prostaglandins.

**PHARMACOKINETICS: Absorption:** $C_{max}$<10ng/mL; $T_{max}$=4 hrs.

## NURSING CONSIDERATIONS

**Assessment:** Assess for hypersensitivity or cross-sensitivity with some drugs (eg, ASA), history of complicated or repeated ocular surgeries, corneal denervation, corneal epithelial defects, DM, ocular surface diseases (eg, dry eye syndrome), RA, bleeding tendencies, and history of concomitant use of medications that may prolong bleeding time or delay wound healing.

**Monitoring:** Monitor for corneal thinning, erosion, ulceration, or perforation and for hypersensitivity reactions, wound healing problems, keratitis, increased bleeding time, bleeding of ocular tissues (hyphemas) in conjunction with ocular surgery, and increased IOP after cataract surgery.

**Patient Counseling:** Instruct not to administer while wearing contact lenses.

**Administration:** Ocular route. **Storage:** 15-25°C (59-77°F).

# VOLTAREN-XR RX

diclofenac sodium (Novartis)

**NSAIDs may cause an increased risk of serious cardiovascular thrombotic events, MI, stroke and serious GI adverse events including bleeding, ulceration, and perforation of the stomach or intestines. Contraindicated for the treatment of perioperative pain in the setting of coronary artery bypass graft (CABG) surgery.**

V

**OTHER BRAND NAMES:** Voltaren (Novartis)

**THERAPEUTIC CLASS:** NSAID

**INDICATIONS:** (Voltaren) Relief of signs and symptoms of osteoarthritis (OA), rheumatoid arthritis (RA), and ankylosing spondylitis (AS). (Voltaren-XR) Relief of signs and symptoms of OA and RA.

**DOSAGE:** *Adults:* (Voltaren) OA: 50mg bid-tid or 75mg bid. Max: 150mg/day. RA: 50mg tid-qid or 75mg bid. Max: 200mg/day. AS: 25mg qid and 25mg qhs prn. Max: 125mg/day. (Voltaren-XR) OA: 100mg qd. RA: 100mg qd-bid.

**HOW SUPPLIED:** Tab, Delayed-Release: (Voltaren) 75mg; (Generic) 25mg, 50mg, 75mg; Tab, Extended-Release: (Voltaren-XR) 100mg

**CONTRAINDICATIONS:** ASA or other NSAID allergy that precipitates asthma, urticaria, or allergic-type reactions. Treatment of perioperative pain in the setting of CABG surgery.

**WARNINGS/PRECAUTIONS:** Cannot replace corticosteroid or to treat corticosteroid insufficiency. May lead to onset of new HTN or worsening of preexisting HTN; monitor BP closely. Fluid retention and edema reported; caution with fluid retention or heart failure. Caution with considerable dehydration. Renal papillary necrosis and other renal injury reported after long-term use. Not recommended for use with advanced renal disease; if therapy must be initiated, monitor renal function. Anaphylactoid reactions may occur. May cause serious skin adverse events (eg, exfoliative dermatitis, Stevens-Johnson syndrome, and toxic epidermal necrolysis). Avoid in late pregnancy; may cause premature closure of ductus arteriosus. May cause elevations of LFTs; d/c if liver disease develops or systemic manifestations occur. Caution in elderly. Anemia may occur; with long-term use, monitor Hgb/Hct if signs or symptoms of anemia develop. May inhibit platelet aggregation and prolong bleeding time; monitor with coagulation disorders. Caution with asthma and avoid with ASA-sensitive asthma. Risk of GI ulceration, bleeding, and perforation.

**ADVERSE REACTIONS:** Abdominal pain, constipation, diarrhea, dyspepsia, flatulence, gross bleeding/perforation, heartburn, N/V, GI ulcers (gastric/duodenal), renal function abnormalities, anemia, dizziness, edema, elevated liver enzymes, headaches, increased bleeding time, pruritus, rashes, and tinnitus.

**INTERACTIONS:** Avoid with other diclofenac products. Increased adverse effects with ASA; avoid use. May enhance methotrexate toxicity; caution when coadministering. May increase nephrotoxicity of cyclosporine; caution when coadministering. May diminish antihypertensive effect of ACE-inhibitors. May reduce natriuretic effect of furosemide and thiazides; monitor for renal failure. May increase lithium levels; monitor for toxicity. Synergistic effects on GI bleeding with warfarin.

**PREGNANCY:** Category C, not for use in nursing.

**MECHANISM OF ACTION:** NSAID; not known, suspected to inhibit prostaglandin synthetase.

**PHARMACOKINETICS: Absorption:** Absolute bioavailability (55%); $T_{max}$=5.3 hrs. **Distribution:** $V_d$=1.4L/kg; plasma protein binding (99%). **Metabolism:** Liver (glucuronidation and sulfation). **Elimination:** Urine (65%), bile (35%); $T_{1/2}$=2.3 hrs.

## NURSING CONSIDERATIONS

**Assessment:** Assess for history of asthma, cardiovascular thrombotic events, CABG surgery, stroke, MI, CVD (eg, pre-existing HTN, CHF) or risk factors, fluid retention, edema, pregnancy status, GI events (eg, bleeding, ulceration, perforation) or risk factors, possible drug interactions, renal/hepatic impairment.

**Monitoring:** Monitor BP, CBC, LFTs, renal function, and chemistries periodically. Monitor for signs/symptoms of GI events (eg, bleeding, ulceration, perforation), cardiovascular thrombotic events, CHF, HTN, salt depletion, allergic reactions (eg, rash, eosinophilia), renal/liver dysfunction.

**Patient Counseling:** Advise to seek medical attention if symptoms of hepatotoxicity (eg, nausea, fatigue, pruritus), anaphylactic reactions (eg, difficulty breathing, swelling of face/throat), hypersensitivity reactions (eg, rash), cardiovascular events (eg, chest pain, SOB, weakness, slurring of speech), GI ulceration or bleeding (eg, epigastric pain, dyspepsia, melena, hematemesis), weight gain, or edema occur. Inform of pregnancy risks.

**Administration:** Oral route. **Storage:** Below 30°C (86°F). Protect from moisture.

V

## VoSpire ER

RX

albuterol sulfate (Dava)

**THERAPEUTIC CLASS:** $Beta_2$-agonist

**INDICATIONS:** Treatment of bronchospasm in reversible obstructive airway disease.

**DOSAGE:** *Adults:* Usual: 4-8mg q12h. Low Body Weight: Initial: 4mg q12h. Titrate: May increase to 8mg q12h. Max: 32mg/day in divided doses. Swallow whole with liquids; do not chew or crush.
*Pediatrics:* >12 yrs: Usual: 4-8mg q12h. Low Body Weight: Initial: 4mg q12h. Titrate: May increase to 8mg q12h. Max: 32mg/day in divided doses. 6-12 yrs: Usual: 4mg q12h. Max: 24mg/day in divided doses. Swallow whole with liquids; do not chew or crush.

**HOW SUPPLIED:** Tab, Extended-Release: 4mg, 8mg

**WARNINGS/PRECAUTIONS:** Hypersensitivity reactions reported. Caution with cardiovascular disorders, especially coronary insufficiency, arrhythmias and HTN. Increased doses may signify need for concomitant corticosteroids. Can produce paradoxical bronchospasm. Caution with DM, hyperthyroidism, seizures. May produce transient hypokalemia. Erythema multiforme and Stevens-Johnson syndrome (rare) reported in children.

**ADVERSE REACTIONS:** Tremor, headache, nervousness, tachycardia, palpitations, N/V, muscle cramps.

**INTERACTIONS:** Avoid oral sympathomimetic agents. Extreme caution within 14 days of MAOI or TCA therapy. Monitor digoxin. May worsen ECG changes and/or hypokalemia with non-$K^+$-sparing diuretics. Antagonized by β-blockers.

**PREGNANCY:** Category C, not for use in nursing.

**MECHANISM OF ACTION:** $\beta_2$-adrenergic bronchodilator; stimulates adenyl cylase, enzyme that catalyzes formation of cAMP from ATP. Increased cAMP levels associated with relaxation of bronchial smooth muscle and inhibition of release of mediators of immediate hypersensitivity.

**PHARMACOKINETICS: Absorption:** $C_{max}$=13.7ng/mL; $T_{max}$=6 hrs; AUC=134ng•hr/mL. **Elimination:** $T_{1/2}$=9.3 hrs.

### NURSING CONSIDERATIONS

**Assessment:** Assess for renal/hepatic functions, history of hypersensitivity to drug, cardiovascular disorder (coronary insufficiency, HTN, cardiac arrhythmias), convulsive disorders, hyperthyroidism, DM and ketoacidosis, and possible drug interactions.

**Monitoring:** Monitor for possible paradoxical bronchospasm, asthma deterioration, cardiovascular effects, immediate hypersensitivity reactions, CBC with differential count, ketoacidosis, hypokalemia, serum glucose concentrations, tremors.

**Patient Counseling:** Instruct to swallow tablet; do not chew or crush. Report lack of response or adverse effects.

**Administration:** Oral route. **Storage:** Store at 20-25°C (68-77°F). Dispense in well-closed, light-resistant container.



## Vytorin

RX

simvastatin - ezetimibe (Merck/Schering-Plough)

**THERAPEUTIC CLASS:** Cholesterol absorption inhibitor/HMG-CoA reductase inhibitor

**INDICATIONS:** When treatment with both components is appropriate, used as an adjunct to diet for the reduction of elevated total-C, LDL-C, Apo B, TG, non-HDL-C, and to increase HDL-C in primary hyperlipidemia (heterozygous familial and non-familial) or mixed hyperlipidemia. For the reduction of elevated total-C, LDL-C in homozygous familial hypercholesterolemia, as an adjunct to other lipid-lowering treatments or if such treatments are unavailable.

**DOSAGE:** *Adults:* Take qpm, with or without food. Initial: 10mg-20mg qd. Less Aggressive LDL-C Reductions: Initial: 10mg-10mg qd. LDL-C Reduction >55%: Initial: 10mg-40mg qd. Titrate: Adjust at ≥2 weeks. Homozygous Familial Hypercholesterolemia: 10mg-40mg or 10mg-80mg qd in pm. Severe Renal Insufficiency: Avoid unless tolerant of ≥5mg of simvastatin; monitor closely. Concomitant Bile Acid Sequestrant: Take either ≥2 hrs before or ≥4 hrs after bile acid sequestrant. Concomitant Cyclosporine/Danazol: Avoid unless tolerant of ≥5mg of simvastatin. Max: 10mg-10mg/day. Concomitant Amiodarone/Verapamil: Max: 10mg-20mg/day.

**HOW SUPPLIED:** Tab: (Ezetimibe-Simvastatin) 10mg-10mg, 10mg-20mg, 10mg-40mg, 10mg-80mg

**CONTRAINDICATIONS:** Active liver disease, unexplained persistent elevations in hepatic transaminase, pregnancy, lactation.

**WARNINGS/PRECAUTIONS:** Rhabdomyolysis (rare), myopathy reported. Predisposing risk factors for myopathy include advanced age ( ≥65 yrs), uncontrolled hypothyroidism, and renal impairment. D/C therapy if myopathy is suspected or diagnosed, if AST or ALT ≥3x ULN persists, a few days prior to major surgery, or when any major medical or surgical condition supervenes. Monitor LFTs prior to therapy and thereafter when clinically indicated. With 10mg-80mg dose, monitor LFTs prior to titration, 3 months after titration, and periodically thereafter for 1st yr. Caution with heavy alcohol use, severe renal insufficiency, or history of hepatic disease. Avoid use in moderate or severe hepatic insufficiency. Caution in elderly and in severe renal impairment. Females with child-bearing potential should use effective contraception. D/C if pregnancy occurs.

**ADVERSE REACTIONS:** Myopathy/rhabdomyolysis, liver enzyme abnormalities (eg, transaminase elevations), headache, upper respiratory tract infection, myalgia, diarrhea, pain in extremity.

**INTERACTIONS:** Use with CYP3A4 inhibitors may increase simvastatin levels and increase risk for myopathy and rhabdomyolysis. Avoid use with the following CYP3A4 inhibitors: antifungal azoles (eg, itraconazole, ketoconazole), erythromycin, clarithromycin, telithromycin, HIV protease inhibitors, nefazodone, grapefruit juice [>1 quart/day], and other strong CYP3A4 inhibitors. Increased risk for myopathy/rhabdomyolysis with fibrates (eg, gemfibrozil), niacin, amiodarone, verapamil, cyclosporine, danazol. Avoid use with fibrates. Monitor cyclosporine levels. Dose should not exceed 10mg-10mg daily with gemfibrozil, cyclosporine, or danazol. Dose should not exceed 10mg-20mg daily with amiodarone or verapamil. Caution with ≥1g/day of niacin. Reduced ezetimibe levels with cholestyramine; incremental LDL-C reduction with concomitant use may be reduced. May increase plasma digoxin concentrations. Simvastatin may potentiate effect of coumarin anticoagulants; monitor PT levels. Use with cimetidine may increase ezetimibe levels. Use with aluminum and magnesium hydroxide antacids may decrease ezetimibe levels. Lovastatin and ezetimibe levels may be increased when used concomitantly. Use with pravastatin may increase ezetimibe levels and decrease pravastatin levels. Use with atorvastatin may affect ezetimibe and atorvastatin levels. Use with rosuvastatin may increase ezetimibe and rosuvastatin levels. Concomitant use with fluvastatin may affect ezetimibe levels and fluvastatin levels. Use with glipizide may affect ezetimibe and glipizide levels. May decrease ethinyl estradiol & levonorgestrel levels.

**PREGNANCY:** Category X, not for use in nursing.

**MECHANISM OF ACTION:** Ezetimibe: Cholesterol absorption inhibitor. Reduces blood cholesterol by inhibiting absorption of cholesterol by small intestine. Molecular target is sterol transporter, Niemann-Pick C1-Like 1 (NPC1L1), which is involved in intestinal uptake of cholesterol and phytosterols. Simvastatin: HMG-CoA reductase inhibitor. Inhibits conversion of HMG-CoA to mevalonate. Also reduces VLDL, TG, and increases HDL-C.

**PHARMACOKINETICS: Distribution:** Ezetimibe: Plasma protein binding (>90%). Simvastatin: Plasma protein binding (95%); crosses blood-brain barrier. **Metabolism:** Ezetimibe: Small intestine, liver via glucuronide conjugation, ezetimibe-glucuronide (active metabolite). Simvastatin: Hydrolysis; β-hydroxyacid; 6'-hydroxy; 6'hydroxymethyl, and 6'-exomethylene (major active metabolites). **Elimination:** Ezetimibe: Feces (78%), urine (11%). Simvastatin: Feces (60%), urine (13%).

## NURSING CONSIDERATIONS

**Assessment:** Assess for active liver disease or unexplained persistent elevations in hepatic transaminases, pregnancy/nursing status, risk factors for developing myopathy (eg, advanced age, uncontrolled hypothyroidism, renal impairment), severe renal impairment, and for possible drug interactions. Assess use in patients who consume substantial quantities of alcohol and/or have a past history of liver disease. Obtain baseline lipid profile (total-C, LDL-C, HDL-C, TG) and liver function (eg, AST, ALT) parameters.

**Monitoring:** Monitor for signs/symptoms of myopathy (unexplained muscle pain, tenderness, weakness), rhabdomyolysis, and for liver dysfunction. Perform periodic monitoring of CK levels, LFTs, and lipid profile.

**Patient Counseling:** Recommend cholesterol-lowering diet while taking drug. Instruct to take in evening, with/without food. Advise to contact physician immediately if unexplained muscle pain, tenderness, or weakness develops. Advise about possible drug interactions and interaction with grapefruit juice. Advise to d/c therapy if pregnant or planning to become pregnant. Females with child-bearing potential should use effective contraception. Counsel not to use if breast-feeding.

**Administration:** Oral route. **Storage:** 20-25°C (68-77°F). Keep container tightly closed.

# VYVANSE

**CII**

lisdexamfetamine dimesylate (Shire)

**High abuse potential; prolonged periods of administration may lead to dependence. Misuse of amphetamine may cause sudden death and serious cardiovascular events.**

**THERAPEUTIC CLASS:** Sympathomimetic amine

**INDICATIONS:** Treatment of ADHD.

**DOSAGE:** *Adults:* Individualize dose. Usual: 30mg qam. Titrate: If needed, may increase in increments of 10mg or 20mg at weekly intervals. Max: 70mg/day. Swallow caps or dissolve contents in glass of water; do not store once dissolved. Re-evaluate periodically.
*Pediatrics:* 6-12 yrs: Individualize dose. Usual: 30mg qam. Titrate: If needed, may increase in increments of 10mg or 20mg at weekly intervals. Max: 70mg/day. Swallow caps or dissolve contents in glass of water; do not store once dissolved. Re-evaluate periodically.

**HOW SUPPLIED:** Cap: 20mg, 30mg, 40mg, 50mg, 60mg, 70mg

**CONTRAINDICATIONS:** Advanced arteriosclerosis, symptomatic CVD, moderate to severe HTN, hyperthyroidism, glaucoma, agitated states, history of drug abuse, during or within 14 days of MAOI use.

**WARNINGS/PRECAUTIONS:** May exacerbate symptoms of behavior disturbance and thought disorder in psychotic patients. Caution when using stimulants to treat patients with comorbid bipolar disorder because of concern for possible induction of mixed/manic episodes in such patients. Stimulants at usual doses can cause treatment emergent psychotic or manic symptoms (eg, hallucinations, delusional thinking, mania) in children and adolescents without prior history of psychotic illness. Aggressive behavior or hostility reported in clinical trials and postmarketing experience of some medications indicated for the treatment of ADHD. Monitor growth in children. May lower convulsive threshold; d/c in presence of seizure. Visual disturbances reported with stimulant treatment. May exacerbate Tourette's syndrome and phonic or motor tics. Caution with HTN and monitor BP. Sudden death reported in children or adults with structural cardiac abnormalities.

**ADVERSE REACTIONS:** Ventricular hypertrophy, tics, N/V, psychomotor hyperactivity, insomnia, rash, upper abdominal pain, decreased appetite, dizziness, dry mouth, irritability, weight loss, headache, affect lability, seizure, visual disturbances.

**INTERACTIONS:** Urinary acidifying agents (eg, ammonium chloride, sodium acid phosphate) and methenamine decrease efficacy. Inhibits adrenergic blockers, antihistamines, and antihypertensives (veratrum alkaloids). Potentiated effects of both agents with TCAs. Urinary alkalinizing agents (eg, acetazolamide and some thiazides), MAOIs, and furazolidone may increase levels. MAOIs and furazolidone metabolites may cause hypertensive crisis. Antagonized by chlorpromazine, haloperidol, and lithium carbonate. May delay absorption of ethosuximide, phenobarbital, and phenytoin. Potentiates meperidine, norepinephrine, phenobarbital, and phenytoin. Potentiated by propoxyphene overdose; fatal convulsions may occur.

**PREGNANCY:** Category C, not for use in nursing.

**MECHANISM OF ACTION:** Dextroamphetamine; blocks reuptake of norepinephrine and dopamine into presynaptic neuron and increases release of these monoamines into extraneuronal space.

**PHARMACOKINETICS: Absorption:** Rapidly absorbed; $T_{max}$=1 hr. **Metabolism:** 1st-pass intestinal and/or hepatic metabolism to dextroamphetamine and L-lysine. **Elimination:** Urine, feces; $T_{1/2}$=1hr.

## NURSING CONSIDERATIONS

**Assessment:** Assess for agitation, glaucoma, tics, cardiovascular conditions (eg, severe HTN, angina pectoris, cardiac structural abnormalities, arrhythmias, HF, recent MI), hyperthyroidism or thyrotoxicosis, bipolar disorder, psychosis. Assess for family history of Tourette's syndrome and history of drug dependence or alcoholism. Assess pregnancy/nursing status and for possible drug interactions.

**Monitoring:** Monitor HR, BP, cardiovascular abnormalities, exacerbation of behavioral disturbances and thought disorders, bipolar disorder, aggression, seizures, visual disturbances, impotence, and changes in libido. Monitor growth in children.

**Patient Counseling:** Inform about risks of treatment, appropriate use, and drug abuse/dependence. Advise about serious cardiovascular risks including sudden death, myocardial infarction, stroke and hypotension. Advise to notify physician if pregnant or intend to become pregnant. Advise not to breastfeed. Use caution while operating machinery/driving. Avoid afternoon dose to reduce potential insomnia. May be taken with/without food.

**Administration:** Oral route. **Storage:** Store at 25°C (77°F); excursions permitted to 15-30°C (59-86°F).

# WELCHOL — RX

colesevelam HCl (Daiichi Sankyo)

**THERAPEUTIC CLASS:** Bile acid sequestrant

**INDICATIONS:** Adjunct to diet and exercise to reduce elevated LDL-C in adults with primary hyperlipidemia (Fredrickson Type IIa) as monotherapy or with an HMG-CoA reductase inhibitor and to reduce LDL-C levels in boys and postmenarchal girls 10-17 yrs old with heterozygous familial hypercholesterolemia as monotherapy or in combination with statin after failing an adequate trial of diet therapy. Adjunct to diet and exercise to improve glycemic control in adults with type 2 diabetes mellitus (DM).

**DOSAGE:** *Adults:* Hyperlipidemia/Type 2 DM: 3 tabs bid or 6 tabs qd. Sus: 3.75g qd or 1.875g bid in 4-8oz of water. Stir well and drink. Take with meals. Avoid taking in dry form.

*Pediatrics:* 10-17 yrs: Sus: 3.75g qd or 1.875g bid. Add 4-8oz of water. Stir well and drink. Take with meals. Avoid taking in dry form.

**HOW SUPPLIED:** Sus: 3.75g, 1.875g [pkt]; Tab: 625mg

**CONTRAINDICATIONS:** History of bowel obstruction, history of hypertriglyceridemia-induced pancreatitis, serum TG concentrations >500mg/dL.

**WARNINGS/PRECAUTIONS:** Increases serum TG concentrations; causes acute pancreatitis. Monitor lipids, including TG and non-HDL-cholesterol levels prior to initiation of treatment and periodically thereafter. Caution in TG levels >300mg/dL, dysphagia or swallowing disorders, gastroparesis, GI motility disorders, major GI tract surgery, bowel obstruction, and those susceptible to vitamin K or fat-soluble vitamin deficiencies. Coadministered drugs with/without known interaction especially those with narrow therapeutic index should be given at least 4 hrs prior to treatment; monitor drug levels. Not for use in treatment of type 1 DM or for diabetic ketoacidosis. Has not been studied in type 2 DM as monotherapy or in combination with dipeptidyl peptidase 4 inhibitor and thiazolidinediones. Not studied in Friedrickson Type I, III, IV or V dyslipidemias. Not studied in children <10 yrs or in pre-menarchal girls. (Sus) Contains phenylalanine.

**ADVERSE REACTIONS:** Asthenia, constipation, dyspepsia, nausea, hypoglycemia, rhinitis, fatigue, flu syndrome, nasopharyngitis, headache.

**INTERACTIONS:** May increase TG levels when used with insulin or sulfonylureas. May decrease level of glyburide, levothyroxine, and oral contraceptives containing ethinyl estradiol and norethindrone. Concomitant use with warfarin decreases INR; monitor INR. May elevate TSH in patients receiving thyroid hormone replacement therapy. May decrease phenytoin levels.

**PREGNANCY:** Category B, caution in nursing.

**MECHANISM OF ACTION:** Bile acid sequestrant; non-absorbed, lipid-lowering polymer that binds bile acids in intestine, impeding their reabsorption. Consequently, compensatory effects lead to increased LDL-C clearance from blood, resulting in decreased serum LDL-C levels.

**PHARMACOKINETICS: Absorption:** Not hydrolyzed by digestive enzymes and not absorbed. **Distribution:** Limited to GI tract. **Metabolism:** Not metabolized systemically. **Excretion:** Urine.

## NURSING CONSIDERATIONS

**Assessment:** Prior to initiation, assess history of bowel obstruction, gastroparesis, other GI motility disorder, or hypertriglyceridemia-induced pancreatitis; serum TG concentrations >500mg/dL; susceptibility to deficiencies of Vitamin K or other fat soluble vitamins; dysphagia or swallowing disorders; possible drug interactions. Obtain baseline lipid parameters (eg, TG, non-HDL-C).

**Monitoring:** Monitor signs/symptoms of increased TG levels (eg, hypertriglyceridemia-induced pancreatitis), hypoglycemia, vitamin K or fat-soluble vitamin deficiencies, dysphagia, or esophageal obstruction. Periodically monitor lipid profile (eg, TG, non-HDL-C), $HbA_{1c}$, and coadministered drug levels.

**Patient Counseling:** Instruct to take with meal/liquid and consume diet that promotes bowel regularity; take drugs that may interact (eg, glyburide, levothyroxine, oral contraceptives) ≥4 hrs prior. Instruct to promptly d/c and seek medical attention if severe abdominal pain or constipation occurs. Inform that dysphagia or esophageal obstruction may occur because of tab size; caution with swallowing disorders. (Sus) Instruct to mix with water before ingesting.

**Administration:** Oral route. **Storage:** (Tab/Sus) 25°C (77°F); excursions permitted to 15-30°C (59-86°F). Brief exposure to 40°C does not affect the product. Protect from moisture.

# WELLBUTRIN SR

**RX**

bupropion HCl (GlaxoSmithKline)

**Antidepressants increased the risk of suicidal thinking and behavior (suicidality) in short-term studies in children, adolescents, and young adults with major depressive disorder (MDD) and other psychiatric disorders. Bupropion is not approved for use in pediatric patients. Wellbutrin, Wellbutrin SR, and Wellbutrin XL are not approved for smoking cessation treatment but bupropion under the name Zyban is approved for this use. Serious neuropsychiatric events including suicidal ideation, suicide attempt, and completed suicide reported in patients taking bupropion for smoking cessation. Monitor appropriately and observe closely for clinical worsening, suicidality, or unusual changes in behavior and for neuropsychiatric symptoms (eg, behavioral changes, hostility, agitation, depressed mood, and suicide-related events) or worsening of pre-existing psychiatric illness. D/C if psychiatric symptoms observed.**

**OTHER BRAND NAMES:** Wellbutrin (GlaxoSmithKline)

**THERAPEUTIC CLASS:** Aminoketone

**INDICATIONS:** Treatment of MDD.

**DOSAGE:** *Adults:* ≥18 yrs: (Tab, Sustained-Release) Initial: 150mg qd, may increase to 150mg bid after 3 days. Usual: 150mg bid. Max: 200mg bid. Separate doses by at least 8 hrs. Severe Hepatic Cirrhosis: 100mg/day or 150mg qod. Mild-Moderate Hepatic Cirrhosis/Renal Impairment: Consider reduced frequency and/or dose. (Tab) Initial: 100mg bid, may increase to 100mg tid after 3 days. Usual: 100mg tid. Max: 450mg/day, given in divided doses of not more than 150mg each. Severe Hepatic Cirrhosis: Max: 75mg qd. Mild-Moderate Hepatic Cirrhosis/Renal Impairment: Consider reduced frequency and/or dose.

**HOW SUPPLIED:** Tab: 75mg, 100mg; Tab, Sustained-Release: 100mg, 150mg, 200mg

**CONTRAINDICATIONS:** Seizure disorder, bulimia or anorexia nervosa, use of MAOIs or within 14 days of use, other forms of bupropion, abrupt d/c of alcohol or sedatives.

**WARNINGS/PRECAUTIONS:** Dose-related risk of seizures. D/C and do not restart if seizure occurs. Extreme caution with history of seizure, cranial trauma, CNS tumor, severe hepatic cirrhosis. Screen for bipolar disorder. May precipitate manic episodes in bipolar disorder patients. Agitation, anxiety, insomnia, psychosis, confusion and other neuropsychiatric signs reported. Caution with recent MI, unstable heart disease, renal impairment, and hepatic impairment. Altered appetite/weight, allergic reactions, HTN reported. Potential for hepatotoxicity. Monitor for clinical worsening and/or suicidality, especially at initiation of therapy or dose changes.

**ADVERSE REACTIONS:** Dry mouth, excessive sweating, headache/migraine, insomnia, tremor, agitation, weight loss, N/V, constipation, dizziness, sedation, blurred vision, decreased libido, pharyngitis.

**INTERACTIONS:** See Contraindications. Extreme caution with drugs that lower seizure threshold (eg, antidepressants, antipsychotics, theophylline, systemic steroids). Increased seizure risk with opioids, cocaine, or stimulant addiction, use of OTC stimulants or anorectics, oral hypoglycemics, insulin, excessive use or abrupt d/c of alcohol or sedatives (including benzodiazepines). Caution with levodopa and amantadine. Caution with drugs that are metabolized by CYP2D6 (eg, SSRIs, TCAs, antipsychotics, β-blockers, type 1C antiarrhythmics); use low initial dose and gradually titrate. Monitor HTN with nicotine replacement. Caution with CYP2B6 substrates or inhibitors (eg, orphenadrine, cyclophosphamide, thiotepa). Carbamazepine, phenytoin, and phenobarbital may induce metabolism of bupropion. Caution with concomitant use of cimetidine. Minimize or avoid alcohol. Hemorrhagic or thrombotic complications reported with warfarin.

**PREGNANCY:** Category C, not for use in nursing.

**MECHANISM OF ACTION:** Aminoketone antidepressant; unknown. Suspected to inhibit neuronal uptake of norepinephrine and dopamine.

**PHARMACOKINETICS: Absorption**: $T_{max}$=3 hrs (bupropion, sustained-release). **Distribution**: Plasma protein binding (84%); found in breast milk. **Metabolism**:

W

Extensive. Hydroxylation, hydroxybupropion (active metabolite)(CYP2B6); Reduction of carbonyl group, threohydrobupropion (active metabolite), erythrohydrobupropion (active metabolite). **Elimination**: Urine (87%), feces (10%), (0.5% unchanged); $T_{1/2}$=21 hrs, 20 hrs, 33 hrs, 37 hrs (bupropion, hydroxybupropion, erythrohydrobupropion, threohydrobupropion, respectively).

## NURSING CONSIDERATIONS

**Assessment:** Assess for seizure disorder, presence of increased seizure risk (eg, head trauma, excessive use of alcohol or sedatives, addiction to opiates, cocaine, or stimulants, use of OTC stimulants and anorectics, use of insulin or oral hypoglycemics), pre-existing psychiatric illness, bulimia/anorexia nervosa, renal/hepatic impairment, pregnancy/nursing status, and possible drug interactions. Note other diseases/conditions.

**Monitoring:** Monitor for clinical worsening, suicidality, or unusual changes in behavior, seizures, increased restlessness, agitation, anxiety, insomnia, neuropsychiatric signs/symptoms (eg, delusions, hallucinations, psychosis, concentration disturbance, paranoia, confusion), changes in weight or appetite, anaphylactoid/anaphylactic reactions (eg, pruritus, urticaria, angioedema, dyspnea), delayed hypersensitivity reactions (eg, arthralgia, myalgia, fever with rash), and HTN.

**Patient Counseling:** Advise patients and caregivers of need for close observation for clinical worsening and/or suicidal risks. Instruct to discontinue and not restart if experience a seizure while on therapy. Inform that excessive use or abrupt discontinuation of alcohol or sedatives may alter seizure threshold. Advise to minimize or avoid alcohol use. Inform that may impair the ability to perform tasks requiring judgment or motor or cognitive skills; use caution while operating hazardous machinery/driving. Instruct to report to physician all prescription or OTC medications taking. Advise to contact physician if become pregnant or planning to become pregnant during therapy.

**Administration:** Oral route. **Storage:** Tab: 15-25°C (59-77°F); protect from light and moisture. SR Tab: 20-25°C (68-77°F); dispense in a tight, light-resistant container.

# WELLBUTRIN XL — RX

bupropion HCl (GlaxoSmithKline)

**Antidepressants increased the risk of suicidal thinking and behavior (suicidality) in short-term studies in children, adolescents, and young adults with major depressive disorder (MDD) and other psychiatric disorders. Bupropion is not approved for use in pediatric patients. Wellbutrin, Wellbutrin SR, and Wellbutrin XL are not approved for smoking cessation treatment but bupropion under the name Zyban is approved for this use. Serious neuropsychiatric events including suicidal ideation, suicide attempt, and completed suicide reported in patients taking bupropion for smoking cessation. Monitor appropriately and observe closely for clinical worsening, suicidality, or unusual changes in behavior and for neuropsychiatric symptoms (eg, behavioral changes, hostility, agitation, depressed mood, and suicide-related events) or worsening of pre-existing psychiatric illness. D/C if psychiatric symptoms observed.**

**THERAPEUTIC CLASS:** Aminoketone

**INDICATIONS:** Treatment of MDD and prevention of seasonal major depressive episodes in patients diagnosed with seasonal affective disorder (SAD).

**DOSAGE:** *Adults:* ≥18 yrs: Give in AM. Swallow whole. MDD: Initial: 150mg qd. May increase to 300mg qd on Day 4. There should be an interval of at least 24 hours between successive doses. Usual: 300mg qd. Max: 450mg qd. SAD: The timing of initiation and duration of treatment should be individualized based on the patient's historical pattern of SAD episodes. Start in autumn; stop in early spring. Initial: 150mg qd. May increase to 300mg after 1 week. If the 300mg dose is not adequately tolerated, the dose can be reduced to 150 mg/day. Usual/Max: 300mg qd. Taper dose to 150mg for 2 weeks prior to d/c. Mild-Moderate Hepatic Cirrhosis/Renal Impairment: Reduce frequency and/or dose. Severe Hepatic Cirrhosis: Max: 150mg every other day. Switching from Wellbutrin Tablet/Wellbutrin SR: Give the same total daily dose when possible.

**HOW SUPPLIED:** Tab, Extended-Release: 150mg, 300mg

**CONTRAINDICATIONS:** Seizure disorder, bulimia or anorexia nervosa, within 14 days of MAOIs, other forms of bupropion, abrupt d/c of alcohol or sedatives.

**WARNINGS/PRECAUTIONS:** Dose-related risk of seizures. D/C and do not restart if seizure occurs. Risk of seizure may be minimized if daily dose does not exceed 450mg and if the rate of incrementation of dose is gradual. Extreme caution with history of seizures, cranial trauma, CNS tumor, severe hepatic cirrhosis. Screen for bipolar disorder. May precipitate mixed/manic episode in bipolar disorder patients. Agitation, increased restlessness, anxiety, insomnia, psychosis, confusion and other neuropsychiatric signs reported. Caution with recent MI, unstable heart disease, renal/hepatic impairment. Altered appetite/weight, allergic reactions, HTN reported. Monitor for clinical worsening and/or suicidality, especially at initiation of therapy or dose changes.

**ADVERSE REACTIONS:** Headache, dry mouth, nausea, insomnia, dizziness, nasopharyngitis, flatulence, tremor, URI, sinusitis, cough, myalgia, anxiety, constipation, decreased appetite.

**INTERACTIONS:** See Contraindications. Extreme caution with drugs that lower seizure threshold (eg, antidepressants, antipsychotics, theophylline, systemic steroids). Increased seizure risk with opioid, cocaine, or stimulant addiction, OTC stimulants or anorectics; oral hypoglycemics; insulin; excessive use or abrupt d/c of alcohol or sedatives. Caution with levodopa, amantadine, and drugs that are metabolized by CYP2D6 (eg, SSRIs, TCAs, antipsychotics, β-blockers, type 1C antiarrhythmics); use low initial dose and gradually titrate. Monitor HTN with transdermal nicotine. Caution with CYP2B6 substrates or inhibitors (eg, orphenadrine, cyclophosphamide, thiotepa). Carbamazepine, phenytoin, cimetidine, and phenobarbital may induce metabolism of bupropion. *In vitro* studies suggest that paroxetine, sertraline, norfluoxetine, fluvoxamine, nelfinavir, ritonavir, and efavirenz inhibit the hydroxylation of bupropion

**PREGNANCY:** Category C, not for use in nursing.

**MECHANISM OF ACTION:** Aminoketone antidepressant; suspected to inhibit neuronal uptake of norepinephrine and dopamine.

**PHARMACOKINETICS: Absorption**: $T_{max}$=5 hrs. **Distribution**: Plasma protein binding (84%); found in breast milk. **Metabolism**: Extensive to hydroxybupropion (CYP2B6) via hydroxylation; threohydrobupropion, eythrohydrobupropion via reduction of carbonyl group. **Elimination**: Urine (87%), feces (10%), (0.5% unchanged); $T_{1/2}$=21 hrs, 20 hrs, 33 hrs, 37 hrs (bupropion, hydroxybupropion, erythrohydrobupropion, threohydrobupropion respectively).

## NURSING CONSIDERATIONS

**Assessment:** Assess for history of seizures, bulimia/anorexia nervosa, LFTs, renal function tests, DM, head trauma, use of alcohol, opiate sedatives, history of MI or unstable heart disease, psychosis, mixed/manic episodes, hypersensitivity, pregnancy/nursing status. Note other diseases/conditions and drug therapies, especially other bupropion products.

**Monitoring:** Monitor for clinical worsening, suicidality, unusual changes in behavior, seizures, increased restlessness, agitation, anxiety, insomnia, neuropsychiatric signs/symptoms (eg, delusions, hallucinations, psychosis, concentration disturbances, paranoia, confusion), weight loss, loss of appetite, arthralgia, myalgia, HTN, and fever with rash.

**Patient Counseling:** Advise families and caregivers of need for close observation of clinical worsening and suicidal risks. Avoid alcohol, sedatives, OTC drugs. Exercise caution while operating machinery/driving. Report adverse reactions and consult physician before taking any other medications or plan to become pregnant. Advise to swallow tablets whole; do not chew, divide, or crush. D/C and do not restart if experience seizure while on treatment.

**Administration:** Oral route. Swallow whole; do not chew, divide or crush tablets. **Storage**: 25°C (77°F); excursions permitted to 15-30°C (59-86°F).

## WESTCORT RX
hydrocortisone valerate (Ranbaxy)

**THERAPEUTIC CLASS:** Corticosteroid

**INDICATIONS:** Relief of inflammatory and pruritic manifestations of corticosteroid-responsive dermatoses.

**DOSAGE:** *Adults:* Apply bid-tid.

**HOW SUPPLIED:** Cre, Oint: 0.2% [15g, 45g, 60g]

**WARNINGS/PRECAUTIONS:** May produce reversible HPA axis suppression, manifestations of Cushing's syndrome, hyperglycemia, and glucosuria. Caution when applied to large surface areas or under occlusive dressings. Use appropriate antifungal or antibacterial agent with dermatological infections; d/c if infection does not clear. Pediatric patients may be more susceptible to systemic toxicity. Avoid contact with eyes or use on face, underarms, or groin area. D/C if irritation occurs.

**ADVERSE REACTIONS:** Burning, itching, dryness, irritation, folliculitis, hypertrichosis, acneiform eruptions, hypopigmentation, allergic contact dermatitis, skin maceration, secondary infection, skin atrophy, striae, miliaria.

**PREGNANCY:** Category C, caution in nursing.

**MECHANISM OF ACTION:** Corticosteroid; possesses anti-inflammatory, antipruritic, and vasoconstrictive properties. Anti-inflammatory effects not established; suspected to act by induction of phospholipase $A_2$ inhibitory proteins, lipocortins. Lipocortins control biosynthesis of potent inflammation mediators (eg, prostaglandins, leukotrienes) by inhibiting release of their common precursor, arachidonic acid.

**PHARMACOKINETICS: Absorption:** Percutaneous; inflammation and other disease states may increase absorption. Use of occlusive dressings for ≤24 hrs not shown to increase penetration; use for ≥96 hrs markedly enhances penetration. **Distribution:** Systemically administered corticosteroids found in breast milk.

### NURSING CONSIDERATIONS

**Assessment:** Assess use in pregnant/nursing patients.

**Monitoring:** Monitor for signs/symptoms of reversible HPA-axis suppression, Cushing's syndrome, hyperglycemia, glucosuria, skin irritation, allergic contact dermatitis (eg, failure to heal), and concomitant skin infections (eg, bacterial, fungal). If large doses or using occlusive dressings, monitor for HPA-axis suppression using ACTH stimulation test, AM plasma cortisol test, and urinary free cortisol test. Monitor for glucocorticosteroid insufficiencies following d/c of therapy. In pediatric patients, monitor for signs/symptoms of systemic toxicity, HPA-axis suppression (linear growth retardation, delayed weight gain), Cushing's syndrome, and intracranial HTN.

**Patient Counseling:** Instruct to use externally and exactly as directed; avoid contact with eyes or using on face, underarms, or groin areas. Instruct not to bandage or wrap treatment areas unless directed by physician. Contact physician if adverse reactions or if no clinical improvement within 2 weeks. Instruct parents of pediatric patients not to apply medication to diaper areas.

**Administration:** Topical route. **Storage:** 20-25°C (68-77°F); excursions permitted to 15-30°C.



## XALATAN RX
latanoprost (Pharmacia & Upjohn)

**THERAPEUTIC CLASS:** Prostaglandin analog

**INDICATIONS:** Reduction of elevated intraocular pressure (IOP) in open-angle glaucoma or ocular hypertension.

**DOSAGE:** *Adults:* Usual: 1 drop in affected eye(s) qd in pm. Max: Once-daily dosing. Space dosing with other ophthalmic drugs by at least 5 min.

**HOW SUPPLIED:** Sol: 0.005% [2.5mL]

**WARNINGS/PRECAUTIONS:** Changes to pigmented tissues, including increased pigmentation of iris (may be permanent), eyelids and eyelashes (may be reversible), and growth of eyelashes. Macular edema reported. May change eye color. Caution with history of intraocular inflammation, aphakic patients, pseudophakic patients with a torn posterior lens capsule, patients at risk of macular edema. Avoid with active intraocular inflammation. Remove contact lenses prior to use and reinsert 15 min after administration.

**ADVERSE REACTIONS:** Eyelash changes (increased length, thickness, pigmentation, number of lashes), eyelid skin darkening, intraocular inflammation, iris pigmentation changes, macular edema.

**INTERACTIONS:** Administer at least 5 min apart from other topical ophthalmic agents.

**PREGNANCY:** Category C, caution in nursing.

**MECHANISM OF ACTION:** Prostanoid selective FP receptor agonist; believed to reduce IOP by increasing outflow of aqueous humor.

**PHARMACOKINETICS: Absorption:** $C_{max}$=2 hrs. **Distribution:** $V_d$=0.16L/kg. **Metabolism:** Cornea, via esterases to active free acid; Liver, via fatty acid β-oxidation to 1,2-dinor and 1,2,3,4-tetranor (metabolites). **Elimination:** Urine (88-98%); $T_{1/2}$=17 min.

## NURSING CONSIDERATIONS

**Assessment:** Assess for intraocular inflammation (iritis/uveitis), active or high risk for macular edema, aphakic/pseudophakic patient with torn posterior lens capsules, angle-closure inflammatory or neovascular glaucoma, pregnancy/nursing status, and possible drug interactions.

**Monitoring:** Monitor for increased brown pigmentation of iris, periorbital tissue, and eyelid tissue; changes in eyelashes (eg, increased length, thickness, or growth; brown pigmentation; change in number of lashes; misdirected growth of lashes); macular edema (cystoid macular edema); bacterial keratitis.

**Patient Counseling:** Inform about risk of brown pigmentation of iris, which may be permanent; darkening of eyelid skin; eyelashes and vellus hair changes. Instruct to avoid touching tip of applicator to eye or surrounding areas. Advise to remove contact lenses prior to administration; reinsert 15 min after administration. Administer at least 5 min apart if using >1 topical ophthalmic drug. Consult physician if having ocular surgery, if intercurrent ocular condition (eg, trauma or infection) develops, or if ocular reaction occurs.

**Administration:** Ocular route. **Storage:** 2-8°C (36-46°F); may store opened bottle for 6 weeks at room temperature.

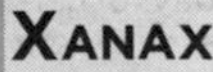

# Xanax

**CIV**

alprazolam (Pharmacia & Upjohn)

**THERAPEUTIC CLASS:** Benzodiazepine

**INDICATIONS:** Anxiety disorders and short-term relief of anxiety symptoms. Panic disorder with or without agoraphobia.

**DOSAGE:** *Adults:* Anxiety: Initial: 0.25-0.5mg tid. Titrate: May increase every 3-4 days. Max: 4mg/day. Elderly/Advanced Liver Disease/Debilitated: Initial: 0.25mg bid-tid. Titrate: Increase gradually as tolerated. Panic Disorder: Initial: 0.5mg tid. Titrate: Increase by no more than 1mg/day every 3-4 days; slower titration if ≥4mg/day. Usual: 1-10mg/day. Decrease dose slowly (no more than 0.5mg every 3 days).

**HOW SUPPLIED:** Tab: 0.25mg*, 0.5mg*, 1mg*, 2mg* *scored

**CONTRAINDICATIONS:** Acute narrow-angle glaucoma, untreated open angle-glaucoma, concomitant ketoconazole or itraconazole.

**WARNINGS/PRECAUTIONS:** Risk of dependence. Withdrawal symptoms, including seizures, reported with dose reduction or abrupt d/c; avoid abrupt withdrawal. Caution with impaired renal, hepatic, or pulmonary function, severe depression, obesity, elderly, and debilitated. May cause fetal harm. Hypomania/mania reported with depression. Weak uricosuric effect. Periodically reassess usefulness.

**ADVERSE REACTIONS:** Drowsiness, lightheadedness, depression, headache, confusion, insomnia, dry mouth, constipation, diarrhea, N/V, tachycardia/palpitations, blurred vision, nasal congestion.

**INTERACTIONS:** See Contraindications. Increases plasma levels of imipramine, desipramine. Additive CNS depressant effects with psychotropics, anticonvulsants, antihistamines, ethanol. Potentiated by fluoxetine, fluvoxamine, nefazodone, cimetidine, oral contraceptives. Propoxyphene decreases plasma levels. Caution with diltiazem, isoniazid, macrolides, grapefruit juice, sertraline, paroxetine, ergotamine, cyclosporine, amiodarone, nicardipine, nifedipine and other CYP3A inhibitors. Avoid azole antifungals.

**PREGNANCY:** Category D, not for use in nursing.

**MECHANISM OF ACTION:** Benzodiazepine; mechanism unknown, suspected to bind at stereo specific receptors at several sites within the CNS.

**PHARMACOKINETICS: Absorption:** (PO) Readily absorbed; $T_{max}$=1-2 hrs; $C_{max}$(0.5-3mg)=8-37ng/mL. **Distribution:** Plasma protein binding (80%). **Metabolism:** Liver via CYP3A4; 4-hydroxyalprazolam and α-hydroxyalprazolam (metabolites). **Elimination:** Urine; $T_{1/2}$=11.2 hrs.

## NURSING CONSIDERATIONS

**Assessment:** Assess for acute narrow-angle glaucoma, renal/hepatic/pulmonary function, pregnancy status. Note other diseases/conditions and drug therapies.

**Monitoring:** Monitor hypersensitivity reactions, rebound/withdrawal symptoms (eg, seizures), renal function, LFTs, pulmonary function tests, HR, insomnia.

**Patient Counseling:** Avoid alcohol, sedatives, smoking. Caution while operating machinery/driving. Take as directed. Counsel about drug abuse/dependence, potential side effects, advise to report if any occur.

**Administration:** Oral route. **Storage:** 20-25°C (68-77°F).

# Xanax XR

CIV

alprazolam (Pharmacia & Upjohn)

**THERAPEUTIC CLASS:** Benzodiazepine

**INDICATIONS:** Panic disorder with or without agoraphobia.

**DOSAGE:** *Adults:* ≥18 yrs: Initial: 0.5-1mg qd, preferably in the am. Titrate: Increase by no more than 1mg/day every 3-4 days. Maint: 1-10mg/day. Usual: 3-6mg/day. Decrease dose slowly (no more than 0.5mg every 3 days). Elderly/Advanced Liver Disease/Debilitated: Initial: 0.5mg qd.

**HOW SUPPLIED:** Tab, Extended-Release: 0.5mg, 1mg, 2mg, 3mg

**CONTRAINDICATIONS:** Acute narrow-angle glaucoma, untreated open-angle glaucoma, concomitant ketoconazole or itraconazole.

**WARNINGS/PRECAUTIONS:** Risk of dependence. Withdrawal symptoms, including seizures, reported with dose reduction or abrupt d/c; avoid abrupt withdrawal. Caution with impaired renal, hepatic, or pulmonary function, severe depression, obesity, elderly, and debilitated. May cause fetal harm. Hypomania/mania reported with depression. Weak uricosuric effect. Periodically reassess usefulness.

**ADVERSE REACTIONS:** Sedation, somnolence, memory impairment, dysarthria, abnormal coordination, fatigue, depression, constipation, mental impairment, ataxia, dry mouth, decreased libido, increased/decreased appetite.



**INTERACTIONS:** See Contraindications. Increases plasma levels of imipramine, desipramine. Additive CNS depressant effects with psychotropics, anticonvulsants, antihistamines, ethanol. Potentiated by fluoxetine, fluvoxamine, nefazodone, cimetidine, oral contraceptives. Decreased levels with CYP3A inducers (eg, carbamazepine) or propoxyphene. Caution with diltiazem, isoniazid, macrolides, grapefruit juice, sertraline, paroxetine, ergotamine, cyclosporine, amiodarone, nicardipine, nifedipine and other CYP3A inhibitors. Avoid azole antifungals.

**PREGNANCY:** Category D, not for use in nursing.

**MECHANISM OF ACTION:** Benzodiazepine; mechanism unknown, suspected to bind at stereo specific receptors at several sites within the CNS.

**PHARMACOKINETICS: Absorption:** Readily absorbed; absolute bioavailability (90%); $C_{max}$(0.5-3mg)=8-37ng/mL; $T_{max}$=1-2 hrs. **Distribution:** Plasma protein binding (80%). **Metabolism:** Liver, via CYP3A4; 4-hydroxyalprazolam and α-hydroxyalprazolam (metabolites). **Elimination:** Urine (unchanged and metabolites); $T_{1/2}$=10.7-15.58 hrs.

## NURSING CONSIDERATIONS

**Assessment:** Assess for acute narrow-angle glaucoma, seizures, renal/hepatic/pulmonary function, and pregnancy status. Note other diseases/conditions and drug therapies.

**Monitoring:** Monitor for hypersensitivity reactions, rebound or withdrawal symptoms, seizures, LFTs, renal/pulmonary function tests, HR, insomnia.

**Patient Counseling:** Instruct to avoid alcohol, sedatives, smoking. Caution while operating machinery/driving. Take as directed. Counsel about drug abuse/dependence, side effects, and advise to report if any signs/symptoms occur. Advise to take in the AM; do not crush or chew tabs.

**Administration:** Oral route. **Storage:** 25°C (77°F); excursions permitted to 15-30°C (59-86°F).

# XELODA RX

capecitabine (Roche Labs)

**Altered coagulation parameters and/or bleeding, including death, reported with concomitant coumarin-derivative anticoagulants (eg, warfarin, phenprocoumon). Monitor PT and INR frequently to adjust anticoagulant dose; post-marketing reports have shown clinically significant increases in PT and INR in patients who were stabilized on anticoagulants at start of therapy.**

**THERAPEUTIC CLASS:** Fluoropyrimidine carbamate

**INDICATIONS:** First-line treatment of metastatic colorectal carcinoma when fluoropyrimidine therapy alone is preferred. Adjuvant treatment in patients with Dukes' C colon cancer who have undergone complete resection of the primary tumor when treatment with fluoropyrimidine therapy alone is preferred. Treatment of metastatic breast cancer in combination with docetaxel after failure of prior anthracycline-containing chemotherapy. Treatment of metastatic breast cancer in patients resistant to paclitaxel and anthracycline-containing chemotherapy or resistant to paclitaxel and for whom further anthracycline therapy is not indicated.

**DOSAGE:** *Adults:* Take with water within 30 min after meals, morning and evening. Usual/Concomitantly w/ docetaxel: 1250mg/m² bid for 2 weeks, then 1 week off (rest period). Give as 3-week cycles. For adjuvant treatment of Dukes' C colon cancer give as 3-week cycles for a total of 8 cycles (24 weeks). CrCl 30-50mL/min: Reduce to 75% of starting dose. Interrupt and/or reduce dose if toxicity occurs. Readjust according to adverse effects (see PI for details).

**HOW SUPPLIED:** Tab: 150mg, 500mg

**CONTRAINDICATIONS:** Hypersensitivity to 5-FU. Dihydropyrimidine dehydrogenase (DPD) deficiency. Severe renal impairment (CrCl <30mL/min).

**WARNINGS/PRECAUTIONS:** Reduce dose with moderate renal dysfunction. Carefully monitor for adverse events with mild to moderate renal dysfunction. Carefully monitor fluid/electrolyte balance with severe diarrhea; if grade 2/3/4 diarrhea occurs, d/c until diarrhea resolves or decreases in intensity. May need dose reduction if grade 2 diarrhea reoccurs or if grade 3/4 diarrhea occurs. Necrotizing enterocolitis reported. Patients ≥80 yrs may experience greater incidence of grade 3/4 adverse events. May cause fetal harm in pregnancy. Monitor for hand-and-foot syndrome; d/c if grade 2/3 symptoms occur and may restart if symptoms resolve or decrease in intensity. Cardiotoxicity reported; more common with history of coronary artery disease (CAD). Carefully monitor with mild to moderate hepatic dysfunction due to hepatic metastases. Hyperbilirubinemia, neutropenia, thrombocytopenia, and decrease in hemoglobin reported. Rarely, severe toxicity associated with 5-FU has been attributed to DPD deficiency.

**ADVERSE REACTIONS:** Diarrhea, hand-and-foot syndrome, pyrexia, anemia, N/V, fatigue/weakness, dermatitis, thrombocytopenia, constipation, taste disturbance, stomatitis, alopecia, abdominal pain, decreased appetite, leukopenia.

**INTERACTIONS:** May increase phenytoin levels; reduce phenytoin dose and monitor carefully. Leucovorin may increase levels and toxicity of 5-FU. Altered coagulation parameters and/or bleeding reported with anticoagulants (eg, coumarin, phenprocoumon); monitor PT/INR frequently and for up to 1 month after stopping therapy. Caution with CYP2C9 substrates. Aluminum and magnesium antacids may increase levels.

**PREGNANCY:** Category D, not for use in nursing.

**MECHANISM OF ACTION:** Fluoropyrimidine carbamate; binds to thymidylate synthetase forming covalently bound ternary complex that inhibits formation of thymidylate from 2'-deoxyuridylate, inhibits DNA synthesis, and interferes with RNA processing and protein synthesis. Prodrug of 5-FU.

**PHARMACOKINETICS: Absorption:** $T_{max}$=1.5 hrs. **Distribution:** Plasma protein binding (<60%). **Metabolism:** Extensive enzymatic conversion to 5-FU; hydrogenated to less toxic metabolite via dihydropyrimidine dehydrogenase. 5-FU (metabolite), α-fluoro-β-alanine (major metabolite). **Elimination:** Urine 95.5% (3% unchanged), feces 2.6%; $T_{1/2}$=0.75 hr.

## NURSING CONSIDERATIONS

**Assessment:** Assess for hypersensitivity to 5-FU, DPD deficiency, renal/hepatic impairment, history of CAD, and possible drug interactions. Assess pregnancy/nursing status.

**Monitoring:** Monitor LFTs, CBC, and renal function periodically. Monitor for signs/symptoms of renal/hepatic impairment, fever ( ≥100.5°F), infections, and hypersensitivity reactions. Monitor for diarrhea, N/V, and hand-and-foot syndrome toxicity with severity of grade 2 and up.

**Patient Counseling:** Inform of pregnancy risks; avoid pregnancy during therapy. Advise to seek medical attention if fever ( ≥100.5°F), infections, or hypersensitivity reactions occur. Advise patients to stop therapy immediately if grade 2 level toxicities are experienced and to seek medical attention for symptomatic treatment. Toxicities to be aware of include diarrhea (increase of 4-6 stools/day or nocturnal stools), N/V (food intake significantly decreased and 2-5 episodes/day), hand-and-foot syndrome (painful erythema and swelling of hands and/or feet affecting daily activities), and stomatitis (painful erythema, edema, or ulcers of mouth or tongue, but able to eat).

**Administration:** Oral route. **Storage:** 25°C (77°F); excursions permitted to 15-30°C (59-86°F).

# XENICAL RX

orlistat (Roche Labs)

**THERAPEUTIC CLASS:** Lipase inhibitor

**INDICATIONS:** For weight loss and weight maintenance and to reduce risk of weight regain after weight loss in obese patients with initial BMI ≥30kg/m² or ≥27kg/m² in presence of other risk factors.



**DOSAGE:** *Adults:* 120mg tid with each main meal containing fat. Take during or up to 1 hr after meals. Use with reduced-calorie diet with about 30% of calories from fat. Omit dose if meal is missed or contains no fat. Separate multivitamin (containing fat-soluble vitamins) by at least 2 hrs, separate by 4 hrs if taking levothyroxine concomitantly.

*Pediatrics:* ≥12 yrs: 120mg tid with each main meal containing fat. Take during or up to 1 hr after meals. Use with reduced-calorie diet with about 30% of calories from fat. Omit dose if meal is missed or contains no fat. Separate multivitamin (containing fat-soluble vitamins) by at least 2 hrs, separate by 4 hrs if taking levothyroxine concomitantly.

**HOW SUPPLIED:** Cap: 120mg

**CONTRAINDICATIONS:** Chronic malabsorption syndrome, cholestasis.

**WARNINGS/PRECAUTIONS:** Exclude organic causes of obesity (eg, hypothyroidism). Caution with history of hyperoxaluria or calcium oxalate nephrolithiasis. GI effects may increase with a high-fat diet (>30%). Weight loss may improve metabolic control; monitor dosage of antidiabetic agents. Increased risk of cholelithiasis due to substantial weight loss.

**ADVERSE REACTIONS:** Oily spotting, flatus with discharge, fecal urgency, fatty/oily stool, oily evacuation, increased defecation, fecal incontinence, and hypothyroidism.

**INTERACTIONS:** Monitor warfarin and cyclosporine (separate cyclosporine dose by 2 hrs). May decrease absorption of fat-soluble vitamins and β-carotene; supplement with fat-soluble multivitamin. Risk of hypothyroidism with levothyroxine; monitor changes in thyroid function.

**PREGNANCY:** Category B, not for use in nursing.

**MECHANISM OF ACTION:** Lipase inhibitor; inhibits absorption of dietary fats. Acts in lumen of stomach and small intestine by forming covalent bond with active serine residue site of gastric and pancreatic lipases, inactivating enzymes making them unavailable to hydrolyze dietary fats.

**PHARMACOKINETICS: Absorption:** $T_{max}$=8 hrs; $C_{max}$=<5ng/mL. **Distribution:** Plasma protein binding (>99%). **Metabolism:** GI wall; $M_1$ and $M_2$ (metabolites). **Elimination:** Feces (83%, unchanged); $T_{1/2}$=1-2 hrs.

## NURSING CONSIDERATIONS

**Assessment:** Assess for chronic malabsorption syndrome, cholestasis, hypothyroidism, calcium oxalate nephrolithiasis, hyperoxaluria, anorexia nervosa, bulimia, nursing status, and possible drug interactions.

**Monitoring:** Monitor urinary oxalate levels, coagulation parameters, changes in thyroid function, and signs/symptoms of hypersensitivity reactions.

**Patient Counseling:** Inform that GI events may increase when taken with high-fat diet. Advise that daily intake of fat, carbohydrates, and protein should be distributed for 3 main meals. Encourage patients to take multivitamin supplement containing fat-soluble vitamins.

**Administration:** Oral route. **Storage:** 25°C (77°F); excursions permitted to 15-30°C (59-86°F).

# XIBROM — RX

bromfenac (Ista)

**THERAPEUTIC CLASS:** NSAID

**INDICATIONS:** Treatment of postoperative inflammation after cataract extraction.

**DOSAGE:** *Adults:* 1 drop bid in affected eye(s), start 24 hrs post-op and continue for 2 weeks.

**HOW SUPPLIED:** Sol: 0.09% [5mL]

**WARNINGS/PRECAUTIONS:** Contains sodium sulfite; may cause allergic-type reactions including anaphylactic symptoms and life-threatening or less severe asthmatic episodes. Potential cross-sensitivity to acetylsalicylic acid, phenylacetic acid derivatives, and other NSAIDs. May cause increased bleeding of ocular tissues; slow or delay healing; keratitis. Continued use may lead to sight-threatening epithelial breakdown, corneal thinning, corneal erosion, corneal ulceration, corneal perforation; d/c if this occurs. Caution in complicated ocular surgeries, corneal denervation, corneal epithelial defects, diabetes mellitus (DM), ocular surface diseases (eg, dry eye syndrome), rheumatoid arthritis (RA), repeat ocular surgeries within a short period of time, bleeding tendencies, or receiving other medication which may prolong bleeding time.

**ADVERSE REACTIONS:** Abnormal sensation in eye, conjunctival hyperemia, eye irritation (burning/stinging), eye pain, eye pruritus, eye redness, headache, iritis.

**INTERACTIONS:** Concomitant use of topical NSAIDs and topical steroids may increase potential for healing problems. Caution with other medications which may prolong bleeding time.

**PREGNANCY:** Category C, caution in nursing.

**MECHANISM OF ACTION:** NSAID; thought to block prostaglandin synthesis by inhibiting cyclooxygenase 1 and 2.

## NURSING CONSIDERATIONS

**Assessment:** Assess for hypersensitivity reactions (eg, sulfite) or cross-sensitivity (eg, ASA), history of complicated or repeated ocular surgeries, corneal denervation, corneal epithelial defects, DM, ocular surface diseases (eg, dry eye syndrome), RA, bleeding tendencies, and concomitant medications that may prolong bleeding time or delay wound-healing.

**Monitoring:** Monitor for anaphylactic symptoms, severe asthma attacks, wound-healing problems, keratitis, corneal thinning, corneal erosion/ulceration/perforation, increased bleeding time, and bleeding of ocular tissues (hyphemas) in conjunction with ocular surgery.

**Patient Counseling:** Advise not to wear contact lenses during therapy.

**Administration:** Ocular route. **Storage:** Store at 15-25°C (59-77°F).

# XIFAXAN RX

rifaximin (Salix)

**THERAPEUTIC CLASS:** Semisynthetic rifampin analog

**INDICATIONS:** Traveler's diarrhea caused by noninvasive strains of *E.coli*

**DOSAGE:** *Adults:* 1 tab tid for 3 days.
*Pediatrics:* ≥12 yrs: 1 tab tid for 3 days.

**HOW SUPPLIED:** Tab: 200mg

**WARNINGS/PRECAUTIONS:** Avoid in diarrhea complicated by fever or blood in the stool or diarrhea due to pathogens other than *E.coli*. D/C if diarrhea symptoms worsen or persist >24-48 hrs; consider alternative antibiotic therapy. Pseudomembranous colitis reported.

**ADVERSE REACTIONS:** Flatulence, headache, abdominal pain, rectal tenesmus, defecation urgency, nausea, constipation, pyrexia.

**PREGNANCY:** Category C; not for use in nursing.

**MECHANISM OF ACTION:** Antibacterial agent; binds to β-subunit of bacterial DNA-dependent RNA polymerase, resulting in inhibition of bacterial RNA synthesis.

**PHARMACOKINETICS: Absorption:** $C_{max}$=4.3ng/mL; $T_{max}$=1.25 hrs. **Metabolism:** CYP3A4. **Elimination:** Feces (97%), urine (0.32%).

## NURSING CONSIDERATIONS

**Assessment:** Assess for pregnancy status, diarrhea complicated by fever or blood in stool, diarrhea by pathogens other than *Escherichia coli* (eg, *Campylobacter jejuni, Shigella* spp. *Salmonella* spp).

**Monitoring:** Monitor for pseudomembranous colitis, antibiotic-associated colitis, worsening of symptoms, superinfection, pyrexia. Monitor CBC.

**Patient Counseling:** Inform to take with/without food. D/C and seek medical attention for persistent diarrhea (>24-48 hrs), blood in stools.

**Administration:** Oral route. **Storage:** 20-25°C (68-77°F); excursions permitted to 15-30°C (59-86°F).

# XIGRIS RX

## drotrecogin alfa (Lilly)

**THERAPEUTIC CLASS:** Activated protein C

**INDICATIONS:** For reduction of mortality in adult patients with severe sepsis (sepsis associated with acute organ dysfunction) at a high risk of death (eg, as determined by APACHE II score ≥25).

**DOSAGE:** *Adults:* Infuse at 24mcg/kg/hr IV for 96 hrs (based on actual body weight). Dose adjustment, dose escalation or bolus doses are not recommended. If infusion interrupted, restart at same rate.

**HOW SUPPLIED:** Inj: 5mg, 20mg

**CONTRAINDICATIONS:** Clinical conditions where bleeding could lead to significant morbidity or death, namely: active internal bleeding, hemorrhagic stroke within 3 months, intracranial or intraspinal surgery or severe head trauma within 2 months, trauma with an increased risk of life-threatening bleeding, presence of an epidural catheter, and intracranial neoplasm or mass lesion or evidence of cerebral herniation.

**WARNINGS/PRECAUTIONS:** Not indicated for adult patients with severe sepsis and lower risk of death, and pediatric patients. May not be indicated in patients with single organ dysfunction and recent surgery. Carefully evaluate and anticipate the benefits against potential risks of therapy. Increased risk of bleeding with therapy in patients with platelets <30,000 x $10^6$/L (even if count is increased by transfusions), PT/INR >3.0, GI bleed within 6 weeks, ischemic stroke within 3 months, intracranial arteriovenous malformation or aneurysm, known bleeding diathesis, chronic severe hepatic disease, and conditions where bleeding is a significant hazard or difficult to manage due to location. If bleeding occurs, stop infusion. D/C 2 hrs before invasive surgical procedures or procedures with risk of bleeding. Restart 12 hrs after surgery and major invasive procedures. Arterial and central venous puncture should be minimized. Avoid noncompressible puncture sites. Prolongs activated partial thromboplastin time (APTT). Monitor coagulopathy with prothrombin time (PTT).

**ADVERSE REACTIONS:** Bleeding, GI bleeding, intrathoracic bleeding, retroperitoneal bleeding, immunogenicity.

**INTERACTIONS:** Caution with drugs that affect hemostasis; increased risk of bleed with therapeutic heparin, thrombolytic therapy within 3 days, and oral anticoagulants, ASA >650mg per day, platelet inhibitors or glycoprotein IIb/IIIa inhibitors within 7 days.

**PREGNANCY:** Category C, not for use in nursing.

**MECHANISM OF ACTION:** Activated protein C; exerts antithrombotic effect by inhibiting Factors Va and VIIIa.

**PHARMACOKINETICS: Absorption:** $C_{max}$=45ng/mL; $T_{max}$=2 hrs.

## NURSING CONSIDERATIONS

**Assessment:** Assess for active internal bleeding, recent (within 3 months) hemorrhagic stroke, recent (within 2 months) intracranial or intraspinal surgery, severe head trauma, trauma with increased risk of life-threatening bleeding, presence of epidural catheter, intracranial neoplasm or mass lesion or evidence of cerebral herniation, platelet count, bleeding diathesis, LFTs, GI bleeding, recent administration of heparin, ASA, thrombolytic therapy, oral anticoagulants. Assess for possible drug interactions.

**Monitoring:** Monitor for hypersensitivity reactions and active bleeding. Monitor PTT, and platelet count.

**Patient Counseling:** Advise to report any side effects. Counsel about the potential risk and benefits associated with therapy.

**Administration:** IV route. Administer via dedicated IV line or lumen of a multilumen venous catheter; compatible with 0.9% sodium chloride injection, lactated Ringer's injection, dextrose injection, and dextrose sodium chloride injection. Refer PI for preparation of concentrated solution, dilution and administration of IV infusion pump and syringe pump. **Storage:** Do not freeze.

Protect from light. Lyophilized Powder: Refrigerate at 2-8°C (36-46°F). Reconstituted Solution: Prepare IV solution immediately after reconstitution; may keep at room temperature 20-25°C (68-77°F) but use within 3 hrs. Infusion solution with an infusion bag or syringe pump: IV solution should be used at controlled room temperature 20-25°C (68-77°F) within 12 hrs. May refrigerate at 2-8°C (36-46°F) up to 12 hrs. If prepared solution is refrigerated prior to administration, may use within 24 hours (maximum time limit).

## XOLAIR RX

omalizumab (Genentech/Novartis)

**Anaphylaxis, presenting as bronchospasm, hypotension, syncope, urticaria, and/or angioedema of the throat or tongue has been reported. Monitor patients closely for an appropriate time period after administration.**

**THERAPEUTIC CLASS:** Monoclonal antibody/IgE-blocker

**INDICATIONS:** For adults and adolescents ( ≥12 yrs) with moderate-severe persistent asthma in those who have a positive skin test or *in vitro* reactivity to a perennial aeroallergen and whose symptoms are inadequately controlled with inhaled corticosteroids.

**DOSAGE:** *Adults:* 150-375mg SQ every 2 or 4 weeks based on body weight and pretreatment serum total IgE level. Max: 150mg/site. 30-90kg & IgE ≥30-100 IU/mL: 150mg every 4 weeks. >90-150kg & IgE ≥30-100 IU/mL OR 30-90kg & IgE >100-200 IU/mL OR 30-60kg & IgE >200-300 IU/mL: 300mg every 4 weeks. >90-150kg & IgE >100-200 IU/mL OR >60-90kg & IgE >200-300 IU/mL OR 30-70kg & IgE >300-400 IU/mL: 225mg every 2 weeks. >90-150kg & IgE >200-300 IU/mL OR >70-90kg & IgE >300-400 IU/mL OR 30-70kg & IgE >400-500 IU/mL OR 30-60kg & IgE >500-600 IU/mL: 300mg every 2 weeks. >70-90kg & IgE >400-500 IU/mL OR >60-70kg & IgE >500-600 IU/mL OR 30-60kg & IgE >600-700 IU/mL: 375mg every 2 weeks.

*Pediatrics:* ≥12 yrs: 150-375mg SQ every 2 or 4 weeks based on body weight and pretreatment serum total IgE level. Max: 150mg/site. 30-90kg & IgE ≥30-100 IU/mL: 150mg every 4 weeks. >90-150kg & IgE ≥30-100 IU/mL OR 30-90kg & IgE >100-200 IU/mL OR 30-60kg & IgE >200-300 IU/mL: 300mg every 4 weeks. >90-150kg & IgE >100-200 IU/mL OR >60-90kg & IgE >200-300 IU/mL OR 30-70kg & IgE >300-400 IU/mL: 225mg every 2 weeks. >90-150kg and IgE >200-300 IU/mL OR >70-90kg & IgE >300-400 IU/mL OR 30-70kg & IgE >400-500 IU/mL OR 30-60kg & IgE >500-600 IU/mL: 300mg every 2 weeks. >70-90kg & IgE >400-500 IU/mL OR >60-70kg & IgE >500-600 IU/mL OR 30-60kg & IgE >600-700 IU/mL: 375mg q2 weeks.

**HOW SUPPLIED:** Inj: 150mg [5mL]

**WARNINGS/PRECAUTIONS:** Malignant neoplasms reported. Not for use in treatment of acute bronchospasm or status asthmaticus. Systemic or inhaled corticosteroids should not be abruptly d/c when initiating therapy. Rarely, serious systemic eosinophilia reported with clinical features of vasculitis consistent with Churg-Strauss syndrome. Geohelminth (roundworm, hookworm, whipworm, threadworm) infections reported in patients with risk factors.

**ADVERSE REACTIONS:** Anaphylaxis, malignancies, injection-site reactions, viral infections, upper respiratory infection, sinusitis, headache, pharyngitis, pain, arthralgia, eosinophilic conditions, severe thrombocytopenia, hair loss.

**PREGNANCY:** Category B, caution in nursing.

**MECHANISM OF ACTION:** Monoclonal antibody/IgE blocker; inhibits binding of IgE to high-affinity IgE receptor on surface of mast cells and basophils and limits degree of release of mediators of allergic response.

X

**PHARMACOKINETICS: Absorption:** (SQ) Absolute bioavailability (62%); $T_{max}$=7-8 days. **Distribution:** $V_d$=78mL/kg; crosses placental barrier. **Elimination:** $T_{1/2}$=26 days.

## NURSING CONSIDERATIONS

**Assessment:** Assess for acute asthma, malignancies, IgE levels, hypersensitivity to drug, and pregnancy/nursing status.

**Monitoring:** Monitor IgE levels, hypersensitivity reactions, injection-site reactions, viral infections, sinusitis, pharyngitis, headaches, malignancies, upper respiratory tract infections. Identify and monitor patients at risk for geohelminth infections (roundworm, hookworm, whipworm, threadworm).

**Patient Counseling:** Advise of the risk of life-threatening anaphylaxis; inform signs/symptoms. Notify physician immediately if signs/symptoms occur and report any adverse reactions. Take as directed. Decreases in corticosteroid therapy should be gradual and under medical supervision.

**Administration:** SQ route. See PI for proper reconstitution. **Storage:** 2-8°C (36-46°F). Reconstituted vial may be stored at 2-8°C (36-46°F) for up to 8 hrs or 4 hrs at room temperature. Protect reconstituted vial from direct sunlight.

## XOPENEX RX

levalbuterol HCl (Sepracor)

**THERAPEUTIC CLASS:** $Beta_2$-agonist

**INDICATIONS:** Prevention and treatment of bronchospasm with reversible obstructive airway disease.

**DOSAGE:** *Adults:* Initial: 0.63mg tid, q6-8h. Severe Asthma: 1.25mg tid, q6-8h. Administer by nebulizer.
*Pediatrics:* ≥12 yrs: Initial: 0.63mg tid, q6-8h. Severe Asthma: 1.25mg tid, q6-8h. 6-11 yrs: 0.31mg tid. Max: 0.63mg tid. Administer by nebulizer.

**HOW SUPPLIED:** Sol, Inhalation: 0.31mg/3mL, 0.63mg/3mL, 1.25mg/3mL [3mL, 24$^s$]

**WARNINGS/PRECAUTIONS:** Hypersensitivity reactions reported. D/C immediately if paradoxical bronchospasm occurs. May produce ECG changes; caution with cardiovascular disorders, coronary insufficiency, arrhythmias, and HTN. Caution with convulsive disorders, hyperthyroidism, and diabetes. May produce transient hypokalemia.

**ADVERSE REACTIONS:** Tachycardia, migraine, dyspepsia, leg cramps, nervousness, dizziness, tremor, rhinitis, increased cough, chest pain, HTN, hypotension, diarrhea, dry mouth, anxiety, insomnia, paresthesia, wheezing.

**INTERACTIONS:** Avoid other sympathomimetic agents. Extreme caution with MAOIs and TCAs. Monitor digoxin. ECG changes and/or hypokalemia with non-$K^+$-sparing diuretics. Antagonized by β-blockers.

**PREGNANCY:** Category C, not for use in nursing.

**MECHANISM OF ACTION:** $\beta_2$-adrenergic bronchodilator; stimulates adenyl cylase, the enzyme that catalyzes formation of cAMP from ATP. Increased cAMP levels associated with relaxation of bronchial smooth muscle and inhibition of release of mediators of immediate hypersensitivity.

**PHARMACOKINETICS: Absorption:** $C_{max}$(1.25, 5mg)=1.1, 4.5ng/ml; $T_{max}$(1.25, 5mg)=0.2, 0.2 hrs. **Metabolism:** GI tract by SULT1A3. **Elimination:** Renal (80-100%), urine (25-46% unchanged), feces (≤20%); $T_{1/2}$(1.25, 5mg)=3.3, 4 hrs.

### NURSING CONSIDERATIONS

**Assessment:** Assess for convulsive disorders, hyperthyroidism, DM, CVD, renal/hepatic impairment, and possible drug interactions.

**Monitoring:** Monitor cardiovascular effects (eg, HR, BP, arrhythmias), paradoxical bronchospasm, hypersensitivity reactions, deterioration of asthma, tremors.

**Patient Counseling:** Take as directed. Report lack of response or any adverse side effects.

**Administration:** Inhalation route. 1) Open unit dose vial and squeeze contents into nebulizer reservoir. 2) Connect nebulizer to compressor and nebulizer reservoir to mouthpiece or face mask. 3) Breathe as calmly and deeply as possible until no more mist is formed. 4) Clean nebulizer. **Storage:** 20-25°C (68-77°F). Protect from light and excessive heat.

## XOPENEX HFA RX

levalbuterol tartrate (Sepracor)

**THERAPEUTIC CLASS:** $Beta_2$-agonist

**INDICATIONS:** Prevention and treatment of bronchospasm with reversible obstructive airway disease.

**DOSAGE:** *Adults:* 2 inh (90mcg) q4-6h or 1 inh (45mcg) q4h may be sufficient. *Pediatrics:* ≥4 yrs: 2 inh (90mcg) q4-6h or 1 inh (45mcg) q4h may be sufficient.

**HOW SUPPLIED:** MDI: 45mcg/inh [15g]

**WARNINGS/PRECAUTIONS:** D/C immediately if paradoxical bronchospasm occurs. May produce ECG changes; caution with cardiovascular disorders, coronary insufficiency, arrhythmias, and HTN. Caution with convulsive disorders, hyperthyroidism, and diabetes. May produce transient hypokalemia.

**ADVERSE REACTIONS:** Asthma, pharyngitis, rhinitis, pain, vomiting.

**INTERACTIONS:** Avoid other sympathomimetic agents. Extreme caution with MAOIs and TCAs. Monitor digoxin. ECG changes and/or hypokalemia with non-$K^+$-sparing diuretics. Antagonized by β-blockers.

**PREGNANCY:** Category C, not for use in nursing.

**MECHANISM OF ACTION:** $\beta_2$-adrenergic bronchodilator; stimulates adenyl cylase, the enzyme that catalyzes formation of cAMP from ATP. Increased cAMP levels associated with relaxation of bronchial smooth muscle and inhibition of release of mediators of immediate hypersensitivity.

**PHARMACOKINETICS: Absorption:** $C_{max}$=0.199ng/mL ( ≥12 yrs), 0.163ng/mL (4-11 yrs); $T_{max}$=0.54 hrs ( ≥12 yrs), 0.76 hrs (4-11 yrs); AUC=0.695ng•hr/mL ( ≥12 yrs), 0.579ng•hr/mL (4-11 yrs). **Metabolism:** GI tract by SULT1A3. **Elimination:** Renal (80-100%), urine (25-46% unchanged), feces (≤20%).

### NURSING CONSIDERATIONS

**Assessment:** Assess for convulsive disorders, hyperthyroidism, DM and ketoacidosis, CVD (eg, coronary insufficiency, HTN, cardiac arrhythmias), renal/hepatic impairment, history of hypersensitivity to drug, and possible drug interactions.

**Monitoring:** Monitor cardiovascular effects (eg, BP, HR, arrhythmias), for possible paradoxical bronchospasm, asthma deterioration, tremors, and immediate hypersensitivity reactions.

**Patient Counseling:** Instruct to shake inhaler well before using. If first time or inhaler not used >3 days, release 4 test sprays into air, away from face. Keep plastic actuator clean to prevent build-up and blockage. Wash actuator by running warm water through top and bottom for 30 seconds at least once a week. Shake to remove excess water and air-dry thoroughly. Avoid spraying in eyes.

**Administration:** Oral inhalation. 1) Shake and test spray into air 4 times. 2) Shake inhaler well. 3) Breathe out through mouth. 4) Breathe in through mouth and at same time spray product into mouth. 5) Hold breath for 10 seconds and remove mouthpiece. 6) Wait for 1 min before next spray. 7) Replace cap and keep mouthpiece clean. 8) Discard after 200 sprays. **Storage:** 20-25°C (68-77°F). Protect from freezing and direct sunlight.

## XYLOCAINE INJECTION RX

lidocaine HCl (APP Pharmaceuticals)



**OTHER BRAND NAMES:** Xylocaine-MPF (Abraxis)

**THERAPEUTIC CLASS:** Local anesthetic

**INDICATIONS:** For production of local or regional anesthesia by infiltration techniques such as percutaneous injection and IV regional anesthesia by peripheral nerve block techniques such as brachial plexus and intercostal and by central neural techniques such as lumbar and caudal epidural blocks.

**DOSAGE:** *Adults:* Dosage varies depending on procedure, depth, and duration of anesthesia, degree of muscular relaxation, and patient physical condition. Max: 4.5mg/kg or total dose of 300mg. Epidural/Caudal Anesthesia: Max: Intervals not less than 90 min. Paracervical Block: Max: 200mg/90 min. Regional Anesthesia: IV: Max: 4mg/kg. Children/Elderly/Debilitated/Cardiac or Liver Disease: Reduce dose.
*Pediatrics:* >3 yrs: Max: 1.5-2mg/lb. Regional Anesthesia: IV: Max: 3mg/kg.

**HOW SUPPLIED:** Inj: 0.5%, 1%, 2%; (MPF) 0.5%, 1%, 1.5%, 2%

**WARNINGS/PRECAUTIONS:** Acidosis, cardiac arrest, death reported from delay in toxicity management. Local anesthetic solutions containing antimicrobial preservatives should not be used for epidural or spinal anesthesia. Use lowest effective dose. During epidural anesthesia, administer initial test dose and monitor for CNS and cardiovascular toxicity as well as for signs of unintended intrathecal administration. Reduce dose with debilitated, elderly, acutely ill, and children. Extreme caution when using lumbar and caudal epidural anesthesia with existing neurological disease, spinal deformities, septicemia, and severe HTN. Monitor cardiovascular and respiratory vital signs and state of consciousness after each injection. Caution with hepatic disease, cardiovascular disorders. Monitor circulation and respiration with injections into head and neck area.

**ADVERSE REACTIONS:** Lightheadedness, nervousness, euphoria, confusion, dizziness, drowsiness, tinnitus, blurred vision, vomiting, heat/cold sensations, twitching, tremors, convulsions, respiratory depression, bradycardia, hypotension, urticaria, edema, anaphylactoid reactions.

**PREGNANCY:** Category B, caution in nursing.

**MECHANISM OF ACTION:** Anesthetic; stabilizes neuronal membrane by inhibiting ionic fluxes required for initiation and conduction of impulses, thereby effecting local anesthetic action.

**PHARMACOKINETICS: Absorption:** Complete. **Distribution:** Crosses blood-brain and placental barriers. **Metabolism:** Liver (rapid), oxidative N-alkylation (major pathway), yields monoethylglycinexylidide and glycinexylidide (metabolites). **Elimination:** Urine, (90% metabolites), (≤10% unchanged); $T_{1/2}$=1.5-2.0 hrs.

## NURSING CONSIDERATIONS

**Assessment:** Assess for drug hypersensitivity, hepatic functions, pregnancy/nursing status, shock, heart block, and possible drug/test interactions.

**Monitoring:** Monitor for allergic-type reactions, cardiac/respiratory vital signs (eg, adequacy of ventilation, tachypnia, tachycardia, labile BP), state of consciousness, signs of CNS toxicity (restlessness, anxiety, tinnitus, dizziness, blurred vision, tremors, depression, drowsiness), confusion, convulsions, and increased creatine phosphokinase levels after IM injection, which interacts with diagnosis of MI.

**Patient Counseling:** Counsel about possibilty of temporary loss of sensation and muscle function following injection; avoid inadvertent trauma until normal functions return. Consult physician/dentist if anesthesia persists or rash occurs.

**Administration:** IM/IV routes. **Storage:** 25°C (77°F).

# XYLOCAINE JELLY — RX

lidocaine HCl (AstraZeneca)

**THERAPEUTIC CLASS:** Acetamide local anesthetic

**INDICATIONS:** Prevention and control of pain in procedures involving the male and female urethra. Topical treatment of painful urethritis. Anesthetic lubricant for endotracheal intubation.

**DOSAGE:** *Adults:* Max: 600mg/12 hrs. Surface Anesthesia of Male Urethra: Instill about 15mL (300mg). Instill an additional dose of not more than 15mL if needed. Prior to Sounding or Cystoscopy: A total dose of 30mL (600mg) is usually required. Prior to Catheterization: 5-10mL usually adequate. Surface Anesthesia of Female Urethra: Instill 3-5mL. Elderly/Debilitated: Reduce dose. *Pediatrics:* Determine dose by age and weight. Max: 4.5mg/kg.

**HOW SUPPLIED:** Jelly: 2% [Tube: 5mL, 30mL; Syringe: 10mL, 20mL]

**WARNINGS/PRECAUTIONS:** Avoid excessive dosage or frequent administration; may result in serious adverse effects requiring resuscitative measures. Caution with heart block and severe shock. Extreme caution if mucosa traumatized or sepsis is present in the area of application; risk of rapid systemic absorption.

**ADVERSE REACTIONS:** Lightheadedness, nervousness, confusion, euphoria, dizziness, drowsiness, blurred vision, tremors, convulsions, respiratory depression, bradycardia, hypotension, urticaria, edema, anaphylactoid reactions.

**PREGNANCY:** Category B, caution in nursing.

**MECHANISM OF ACTION:** Local anesthetic; stabilizes neuronal membrane by initiating ionic fluxes required for initiation and conduction of impulses.

**PHARMACOKINETICS: Absorption:** Rapid. **Metabolism:** Biotransformation. **Distribution:** Plasma protein binding (60-80%); crosses placenta. **Elimination:** Urine; $T_{1/2}$=1.5-2 hrs.

## NURSING CONSIDERATIONS

**Assessment:** Assess for acidosis, severe shock, heart block, possible drug interactions, renal/hepatic impairment.

**Monitoring:** Monitor for signs/symptoms of hypersensitivity reactions, malignant hyperthermia, renal/hepatic dysfunction.

**Patient Counseling:** Instruct not to ingest food or drink within 60 min of using local anesthetics in mouth or throat area. Numbness of tongue or buccal mucosa may enhance danger of unintentional biting trauma. Inform to strictly adhere to dosing instructions and keep out of reach of children. Instruct to notify physician if pregnant/nursing or planning to become pregnant.

**Administration:** Topical route. **Storage:** 20-25°C (68-77°F).

# Xylocaine Viscous RX

lidocaine HCl (AstraZeneca)

**THERAPEUTIC CLASS:** Acetamide local anesthetic

**INDICATIONS:** Production of topical anesthesia of irritated or inflamed mucous membranes of the mouth and pharynx. Also useful for reducing gagging during the taking of X-ray pictures and dental impressions.

**DOSAGE:** *Adults:* Irritated/Inflamed Mucous Membranes: Usual: 15mL undiluted. (Mouth) Swish and spit out. (Pharynx) Gargle and may swallow. Do not administer in <3 hr intervals. Max: 8 doses/24hr; (Single Dose) 4.5mg/kg and should not in any case exceed a total of 300mg.
*Pediatrics:* >3 yrs: Max: Determine by age and weight. Infants - <3 yrs: Apply 1/4 tsp should be applied with cotton-tipped applicator to immediate area. Do not administer in <3 hour intervals. Max: 4 doses/24hr.

**HOW SUPPLIED:** Sol: 2% [100mL, 450mL]

**WARNINGS/PRECAUTIONS:** Excessive dosage or too frequent administration may result in high plasma levels and serious adverse effects requiring resuscitative measures. Use lowest effective dose. Tolerance varies with the status of the patient. Extreme caution if mucosa in the treatment area has been severely traumatized; risk of rapid systemic absorption. Elderly, debilitated, acutely ill, and children should be given reduced doses commensurate with their age, weight, and physical condition. Caution with severe shock or heart block, and in patients with known drug sensitivities. Overdose reported in pediatrics due to inappropriate dosing. Acidosis affects the CNS levels of lidocaine required to produce overt systemic effects.

**ADVERSE REACTIONS:** Lightheadedness, nervousness, confusion, euphoria, dizziness, drowsiness, blurred vision, tremors, convulsions, respiratory depression, bradycardia, hypotension, urticaria, edema, anaphylactoid reactions.

**INTERACTIONS:** Use of CNS stimulants and depressants affects the CNS levels of lidocaine required to produce overt systemic effects.

**PREGNANCY:** Category B, caution in nursing.

**MECHANISM OF ACTION:** Local anesthetic; stabilizes the neuronal membrane by inhibiting the ionic fluxes required for the initiation and conduction of impulses, thereby effecting local anesthetic action.

**PHARMACOKINETICS: Absorption:** Rate and extent of absorption is dependent on the concentration and total dose administered, the specific site of application, and duration of exposure. Well-absorbed from the GI tract. **Distribution:** Crosses blood-brain and placental barriers; plasma protein binding (60-80%). **Metabolism:** Liver (rapid), oxidative N-dealkylation, ring hydroxylation, cleavage of amide linkage, conjugation; monoethylglycinexylidide and glycinexylidide (metabolites). **Elimination:** Urine; $T_{1/2}$=1.5-2 hrs.

## NURSING CONSIDERATIONS

**Assessment:** Assess for traumatized mucosa in the area of application, acidosis, renal/hepatic dysfunction, debilitation or acute illness, severe shock or heart block, known drug sensitivities, pregnancy/nursing status, and for possible drug interactions.

**Monitoring:** Monitor for signs/symptoms of CNS manifestations (eg, lightheadedness, nervousness, euphoria, confusion, dizziness, tremors, convulsions, unconsciousness, respiratory depression), cardiovascular manifestations (eg, bradycardia, hypotension, cardiovascular collapse), and for allergic reactions (eg, urticaria, edema, anaphylactoid reactions).

**Patient Counseling:** Inform that when topical anesthetics are used in the mouth or throat, that swallowing may be impaired and consequently the danger of aspiration may be enhanced; instruct not to ingest food or drink within 60 min of using local anesthetics in mouth or throat area. Advise that numbness of tongue or buccal mucosa may enhance danger of unintentional biting trauma. Counsel to strictly adhere to dosing instructions and keep out of reach of children.

**Administration:** Topical route. **Storage**: 15-30°C (59-86°F).

# XYZAL — RX

levocetirizine dihydrochloride (Sanofi-Aventis/UCB)

**THERAPEUTIC CLASS:** $H_1$-antagonist

**INDICATIONS:** Relief of symptoms associated with allergic rhinitis: seasonal (for adults and children ≥2 yrs) and perennial (for adults and children ≥6 months of age). Treatment of uncomplicated skin manifestations of chronic idiopathic urticaria in adults and children ≥6 months of age.

**DOSAGE:** *Adults:* 5mg (1 tab or 2 tsp [10mL] oral solution) qd in evening. Mild Renal Impairment: CrCl=50-80mL/min: 2.5mg qd. Moderate Renal Impairment: CrCl=30-50mL/min: 2.5mg qod. Severe Renal Impairment: CrCl=10-30mL/min: 2.5mg biw (administered q3-4d). Adjust dose with decreased renal function. Elderly: Start at lower end of dosing range.
*Pediatrics:* ≥12 yrs: 5mg (1 tab or 2tsp [10mL] oral solution) qd in evening. Mild Renal Impairment: CrCl=50-80mL/min: 2.5mg qd. Moderate Renal Impairment: CrCl=30-50mL/min: 2.5mg qod. Severe Renal Impairment: CrCl=10-30mL/min: 2.5mg biw (administer q3-4d). Adjust dose with decreased renal function. 6-11 yrs: 2.5mg (1/2 tab or 1 tsp [5mL] oral solution) qd in evening. 6 months-5 yrs: 1.25mg (1/2 tsp [2.5mL] oral solution) qd in evening.

**HOW SUPPLIED:** Sol: 2.5mg/5mL; Tab: 5mg* *scored

**CONTRAINDICATIONS:** End stage renal disease (CrCl <10mL/min) or hemodialysis. Pediatrics 6-11 yrs with renal impairment.

**WARNINGS/PRECAUTIONS:** Somnolence, fatigue, and asthenia reported. May impair mental/physical abilities. Transient elevations of bilirubin and transaminases reported. Caution in the elderly. Reduce dose in patient with renal impairment.

**ADVERSE REACTIONS:** Somnolence, fatigue, dry mouth, diarrhea, nasopharyngitis, constipation, cough, pyrexia, vomiting, pharyngitis, otitis media, angioneurotic edema, convulsion, aggression, agitation.

**INTERACTIONS:** Avoid alcohol and CNS depressants. Possible decreased clearance with large doses of theophylline. Increase plasma concentration with ritonavir.

**PREGNANCY:** Category B, not for use in nursing.

**MECHANISM OF ACTION:** $H_1$-Antagonist; antihistamine that selectively inhibits $H_1$-receptor.

**PHARMACOKINETICS: Absorption:** Rapid, extensive; $C_{max}$=270ng/mL (single dose), 308ng/mL (multiple doses); $T_{max}$=0.9 hrs(fasted), 3.15 hrs (fed). **Distribution:** $V_d$=0.4L/kg; plasma protein binding (91-92%). **Metabolism**: <14% metabolized through aromatic oxidation (via CYP 450 system), N and O- dealkylation (via CYP3A4) and taurine conjugation pathways. **Elimination:** Urine (85.4%), feces (12.9%); $T_{1/2}$=8-9 hrs.

## NURSING CONSIDERATIONS

**Assessment:** Assess for renal impairment, ESRD or hemodialysis, nursing status, alcohol consumption, and possible drug interactions (eg, CNS depressants).

**Monitoring:** Monitor for allergic reactions and adverse events. Check renal function in elderly/renal impairment and LFTs.

**Patient Counseling:** Caution against performing hazardous tasks requiring mental alertness and motor coordination (eg, operating machinery, driving). Advise against concurrent use of alcohol or other CNS depressants since additional reduction in mental alertness may occur. Notify physician if nursing.

**Administration:** Oral route. **Storage:** 20-25°C (68-77°F), excursions permitted to 15-30°C (59-86°F).

# YASMIN RX

drospirenone - ethinyl estradiol (Bayer Healthcare)

**THERAPEUTIC CLASS:** Estrogen/progestogen combination

**INDICATIONS:** Prevention of pregnancy.

**DOSAGE:** *Adults:* 1 tab qd for 28 days, then repeat. Start 1st Sunday after menses begin or 1st day of menses.

**HOW SUPPLIED:** Tab: (Ethinyl Estradiol-Drospirenone) 0.03mg-3mg

**CONTRAINDICATIONS:** Renal or adrenal insufficiency, hepatic dysfunction, thrombophlebitis, thromboembolic disorders, history of deep vein thrombophlebitis or thromboembolic disorders, cerebrovascular or coronary artery disease (CAD), valvular heart disease with thrombogenic complications, severe hypertension (HTN), diabetes with vascular involvement, headaches with focal neurological symptoms, breast carcinoma, endometrial carcinoma, estrogen-dependent neoplasia, undiagnosed abnormal genital bleeding, cholestatic jaundice of pregnancy or jaundice with prior pill use, liver tumor (benign or malignant) or active liver disease, pregnancy, heavy smoking ( ≥15 cigarettes daily) and >35 yrs.

**WARNINGS/PRECAUTIONS:** Cigarette smoking increases risk of serious CV side effects; risk increases with age (especially >35 yrs) and heavy smoking. Risk of hyperkalemia in high-risk patients; avoid use in patients predisposed to hyperkalemia (eg, renal insufficiency, hepatic dysfunction, adrenal insufficiency). Monitor $K^+$ levels during first cycle with conditions predisposing to hyperkalemia. Increased risk of MI, vascular disease, thromboembolism, stroke, hepatic neoplasia, and gallbladder disease. Retinal thrombosis reported; d/c use if unexplained partial or complete loss of vision occurs, onset of proptosis or diplopia, papilledema, or retinal vascular lesions develop. May increase the risk of breast cancer and cervical intraepithelial neoplasia. May elevate LDL levels or cause other lipid changes. May cause glucose intolerance, fluid retention, breakthrough bleeding, and spotting. May increase BP; d/c if significant elevations in BP occur. May cause or exacerbate migraine headaches. May develop visual changes with contact lens. Increased risk of morbidity and mortality with HTN, hyperlipidemia, obesity, and DM. D/C if jaundice or if significant depression develops. Perform annual physical exam. Use before menarche is not indicated. Does not protect against against HIV infection (AIDS) and other sexually transmitted diseases. May affect certain endocrine, LFTs, and blood components in laboratory tests.

**ADVERSE REACTIONS:** N/V, breakthrough bleeding, spotting, amenorrhea, migraine, depression, vaginal candidiasis, edema, weight changes, breast changes.

**INTERACTIONS:** Concomitant use with rifampin may reduce contraceptive effectiveness and increase menstrual irregularities. Use with anticonvulsants (eg, phenobarbital, phenytoin, carbamazepine) may reduce contraceptive effectiveness. Pregnancy reported with antimicrobials (eg, ampicillin, tetracycline, griseofulvin). St. John's wort may reduce contraceptive effectiveness and cause breakthrough bleeding. Concomitant use with phenylbutazone may decrease contraceptive effectiveness and cause menstrual irregularities. Increased levels with atorvastatin, ascorbic acid and APAP. Risk of hyperkalemia with ACE inhibitors, angiotensin-II receptor antagonists, $K^+$-sparing diuretics, heparin, aldosterone antagonists, and NSAIDs; monitor $K^+$ levels during 1st cycle. May increase levels of cyclosporine, prednisolone, and theophylline. May decrease APAP levels and increase clearance of temazepam, salicylic acid, morphine, and clofibric acid.

**PREGNANCY:** Category X, not for use in nursing.

**MECHANISM OF ACTION:** Estrogen/progestogen oral contraceptive; acts by suppressing gonadotropins. Inhibits ovulation and produces changes in cervical mucus (increasing difficulty of sperm entry into uterus) and endometrium (reducing likelihood of implantation).

**PHARMACOKINETICS: Absorption:** Drospirenone (DRSP): Absolute bioavailability (76%); (Cycle 13/Day 21) $C_{max}$=78.7ng/mL; $T_{max}$=1.6 hrs; AUC=968ng•h/mL. Ethinyl estradiol (EE): Absolute bioavailability (40%); (Cycle 13/Day 21) $C_{max}$=90.5pg/mL; $T_{max}$=1.6 hrs; AUC=469.5pg•h/mL. **Distribution:** Found in breast milk; DRSP: $V_d$=4L/kg; serum protein binding (97%). EE: $V_d$=4-5L/kg; serum albumin binding (98.5%). **Metabolism:** DRSP: Liver, via CYP3A4 (minor). EE: Hydroxylation (via CYP3A4), conjugation (glucuronidation and sulfation). **Elimination:** DRSP: Urine, feces; $T_{1/2}$=30 hrs. EE: Urine, feces; $T_{1/2}$=24 hrs.

## NURSING CONSIDERATIONS

**Assessment:** Assess for current or history of thrombophlebitis or thromboembolic disorders, cerebrovascular disorders, CAD, valvular heart disease with thrombogenic complications, renal insufficiency, hepatic dysfunction or active liver disease, adrenal insufficiency, headaches with focal neurological symptoms, severe HTN, DM with vascular involvement, known or suspected carcinoma of the breast, carcinoma of endometrium or other known/suspected estrogen-dependent neoplasia, abnormal genital bleeding, cholestatic jaundice of pregnancy or jaundice with prior pill use, liver tumor (benign or malignant), heavy smoking, mental depression, pregnancy/nursing status, and for possible drug interactions. Assess use in patients with HTN, DM, hyperlipidemias, and obesity.

**Monitoring:** Monitor for signs/ symptoms of MI, thromboembolism, cerebrovascular disease, carcinoma of the breast, cervical intraepithelial neoplasia, hepatic neoplasia, onset or exacerbation of a migraine headache, gallbladder disease, ocular lesions, hyperlipidemia, HTN, bleeding irregularites, jaundice, and for fluid retention. Monitor for signs of worsening depression in patients with a history of depression. Monitor lipid levels in patients with a history of hyperlipidemia. Monitor blood glucose levels in patients with DM. Monitor BP in patients with HTN. Perform annual history and physicial exam. Monitor $K^+$ levels in patients at risk for hyperkalemia. Refer patients with contact lenses to an ophthalmologist if visual changes or changes in contact lens tolerance occur.

**Patient Counseling:** Inform that drug does not protect against HIV infection (AIDS) and other STDs. Inform of potential risks/benefits of oral contraceptives. Counsel not to smoke while on treatment. Instruct to take 1 pill at same time daily. Inform that if dose missed, take as soon as possible; take next dose regularly scheduled time. Inform may have spotting, light bleeding or nausea during first 1-3 packs of pills; advise not to d/c medication and if symptoms persist, notify physician.

**Administration:** Oral route. **Storage:** 25°C (77°F); excursions permitted to 15-30° (59-86°F).

## YAZ RX

drospirenone - ethinyl estradiol (Bayer Healthcare)

**THERAPEUTIC CLASS:** Estrogen/progestogen combination

**INDICATIONS:** Prevention of pregnancy. Treatment of symptoms of premenstrual dysphoric disorder (PMDD). Treatment of moderate acne vulgaris in women ≥14 yrs.

**DOSAGE:** *Adults:* 1 tab qd for 28 days (24 active plus 4 inert pills), then repeat. Start 1st Sunday after menses begin or 1st day of menses.
*Pediatrics:* ≥14 yrs: Acne: 1 tab qd for 28 days (24 active plus 4 inert pills), then repeat. Start 1st Sunday after menses begin or 1st day of menses.

**HOW SUPPLIED:** Tab: (Ethinyl Estradiol-Drospirenone) 0.02mg-3mg

**CONTRAINDICATIONS:** Renal or adrenal insufficiency, hepatic dysfunction, thrombophlebitis, thromboembolic disorders, history of deep vein thrombophlebitis, valvular heart disease with thrombogenic complications, severe HTN, DM with vascular involvement, headaches with focal neurological symptoms, major surgery with prolonged immobilization, cerebrovascular or CAD, breast carcinoma, endometrial carcinoma, estrogen-dependent neoplasia, undiagnosed abnormal genital bleeding, cholestatic jaundice of pregnancy or jaundice with prior pill use, liver tumor, active liver disease, pregnancy, heavy smoking (>15 cigarettes daily) and >35 yrs.

**WARNINGS/PRECAUTIONS:** Cigarette smoking increases risk of serious CV side effects. Risk increases with age (especially >35 yrs) and with heavy smoking. Increased risk of MI, thromboembolism, thrombotic disease, cerebrovascular events, and gallbladder disease. Monitor $K^+$ levels during first cycle with conditions predisposing to hyperkalemia. Retinal thrombosis, hepatic neoplasia, carcinoma of breast and reproductive organs reported. May cause glucose intolerance. May increase BP, elevate LDL levels or cause other lipid changes, fluid retention, breakthrough bleeding and spotting. May cause or exacerbate migraine. May develop visual changes with contact lens. Increased risk of MI with HTN, hyperlipidemia, obesity and DM. D/C if jaundice, significant depression or ophthalmic irregularities develop. Use before menarche is not indicated.

**ADVERSE REACTIONS:** N/V, breakthrough bleeding, spotting, amenorrhea, migraine, mental depression, vaginal candidiasis, edema, weight changes, depression, decrease in serum folate levels, aggravation of varicose veins, uriticaria, angioedema, severe reactions with respiratory and circulatory symptoms, dysmenorrhea.

**INTERACTIONS:** Reduced effects, increased breakthrough bleeding, and menstrual irregularities with rifampin, phenobarbital, phenytoin, carbamazepine, possibly with griseofulvin, ampicillin, tetracycline, St. John's wort, and phenylbutazone. Increased levels with atorvastatin, ascorbic acid and APAP. Risk of hyperkalemia with ACE inhibitors, angiotensin-II receptor antagonists, potassium-sparing diuretics, heparin, aldosterone antagonists, and NSAIDs; monitor $K^+$ levels during 1st cycle. Increased levels of cyclosporine, prednisolone, and theophylline. May decrease APAP levels and increase clearance of temazepam, salicylic acid, morphine, and clofibric acid.

**PREGNANCY:** Category X, not for use in nursing.

**MECHANISM OF ACTION:** Estrogen/progestogen oral contraceptive; acts by suppressing gonadotropins, inhibiting ovulation. Also causes changes in cervical mucus (increases difficulty of sperm entry into uterus) and endometrium (reduces likelihood of implantation).

**PHARMACOKINETICS: Absorption:** Drospirenone (DRSP): Absolute bioavailability (76%); (Cycle 1/Day 21) $C_{max}$=70.3ng/mL; $T_{max}$=1.5 hrs; AUC=763ng•h/mL. Ethinyl estradiol (EE): Absolute bioavailability (40%); (Cycle 1/Day 21) $C_{max}$=45.1pg/mL; $T_{max}$=1.5 hrs; AUC=220pg•h/mL. **Distribution:** DRSP: $V_d$=4L/kg; serum protein binding (97%). EE: $V_d$=4-5L/kg; serum albumin binding (98.5%). **Metabolism:** DRSP: Liver, via CYP3A4 (minor). EE: Hydroxylation (via CYP3A4), conjugation (glucuronidation and sulfation). **Elimination:** DRSP: Urine, feces; $T_{1/2}$=30 hrs. EE: Urine, feces; $T_{1/2}$=24 hrs.

## NURSING CONSIDERATIONS

**Assessment:** Assess family history of breast cancer, presence of inherited or acquired thrombophilias, HTN, hyperlipidemias, obesity, DM, renal disease, depression, heavy smoking, and potential drug interactions. Assess personal/family history; complete physical exam.

**Monitoring:** Monitor for MI, thromboembolism, cerebrovascular disease, benign hepatic adenomas, retinal thrombosis, HTN, headache, bleeding irregularites, jaundice, fluid retention, and emotional disorders. Conduct periodic complete physical exam with emphasis on BP, breasts, abdomen, and pelvic organs including cervical cytology and relevant lab tests (eg, $K^+$ levels, prothrombin time, clotting factors VII, VIII, IX, X, cholesterol, TG, serum folate, TBG, glucose tolerance).

**Patient Counseling:** Inform that drug does not protect against HIV infection (AIDS) and other STDs. Inform of potential risks/benefits of oral contraceptives. Counsel not to smoke while on treatment. Take 1 pill at same time daily. Notify physician if nursing or need more information about therapy.

**Administration:** Oral route. **Storage:** 25°C (77°F); excursions permitted to 15-30°C (59-86°F).

# ZANAFLEX — RX

tizanidine HCl (Acorda)

**THERAPEUTIC CLASS:** Centrally acting alpha$_2$-adrenergic agonist

**INDICATIONS:** Short-term treatment of spasticity.

**DOSAGE:** *Adults:* Initial: 4mg single dose q6-8h. Titrate: Increase by 2-4mg. Usual: 8mg single dose q6-8h. Max: 3 doses/24h or 36mg/day.

**HOW SUPPLIED:** Cap: 2mg, 4mg, 6mg; Tab: 2mg*, 4mg* *scored

**CONTRAINDICATIONS:** Concomitant use with fluvoxamine, ciprofloxacin or potent inhibitors of CYP1A2.

**WARNINGS/PRECAUTIONS:** May prolong QT interval. May cause liver damage; monitor baseline LFTs and at 1, 3, and 6 months. Retinal degeneration and corneal opacities reported. Caution with renal impairment or elderly. May cause hypotension, caution with antihypertensives; avoid ciprofloxacin and fluvoxamine. Use with extreme caution in patients with hepatic impairment. May cause sedation and hallucinations. Avoid concomitant use with oral contraceptives. When discontinuing, taper dose to avoid withdrawal and rebound HTN, tachycardia, and hypertonia.

**ADVERSE REACTIONS:** Dry mouth, somnolence, asthenia, dizziness, UTI, urinary frequency, flu-like syndrome, rhinitis.

**INTERACTIONS:** See Contraindications. Potentiated depressant effect with alcohol. Potentiated by oral contraceptives. Avoid α-adrenergic agonists. Avoid with CYP1A2 inhibitors.

**PREGNANCY:** Category C, caution in nursing.

**MECHANISM OF ACTION:** Centrally acting $\alpha_2$-adrenergic agonist: reduces spasticity by increasing presynaptic inhibition of motor neurons.

**PHARMACOKINETICS: Absorption:** Complete; (Fasting) $T_{max}$=1 hr. (Fed) Absolute bioavailability (40%); $C_{max}$ increased by 30%; $T_{max}$=1.25 hrs. **Distribution:** $V_d$=2.4L/kg; plasma protein binding (30%); excreted in breast milk. **Metabolism:** CYP1A2. **Elimination:** Urine (60%), feces (20%); $T_{1/2}$=2.5 hrs.

## NURSING CONSIDERATIONS

**Assessment:** Assess for hypersensitivity, hypotension, hepatic/renal dysfunction, corneal opacities, retinal degeneration, CVD, QT prolongation, pregnancy/nursing status, and possible drug interactions. Obtain baseline LFTs.

**Monitoring:** Monitor for hypotension, bradycardia, lightheadedness/dizziness, syncope, hepatic impairment, sedation, hallucinosis/psychotic-like symptoms, corneal opacities, retinal degeneration, dry mouth, somnolonce, asthenia, and withdrawal symptoms (eg, rebound HTN, tachycardia, hypertonia). Evaluate LFTs at 1, 3, and 6 months, BP, HR, ECG.

**Patient Counseling:** Counsel to take exactly as directed, not to increase dose unless directed by physician, and about possibility of orthostatic hypotension. Caution against performing hazardous tasks (eg, operating machinery/driving). To avoid withdrawal symptoms, do not suddenly d/c therapy. Avoid alcohol and CNS depressants. Advise that food changes absorption; may lead to potentiation in efficacy and adverse effects. Instruct to inform physician if taking oral contraceptives, fluvoxamine, ciprofloxacin, or if pregnant/nursing.

**Administration:** Oral route. **Storage:** 25°C (77°F); excursions permitted to 15-30°C (59-86°F). Dispense in tight, child-resistant container.

# ZANTAC — RX

ranitidine HCl (GlaxoSmithKline)

**THERAPEUTIC CLASS:** $H_2$-blocker

**INDICATIONS:** (PO) Short-term treatment of active duodenal (DU) and benign gastric ulcers (GU). Maintenance therapy for duodenal and gastric ulcers. Treatment of pathological hypersecretory conditions (eg, Zollinger-Ellison) and GERD. Treatment and maintenance of erosive esophagitis. (Inj) Hospitalized patients with pathological hypersecretory conditions or intractable duodenal ulcer. Short-term alternate to oral therapy.

**DOSAGE:** *Adults:* (PO) DU/GU: 150mg bid or (DU) 300mg after evening meal or qhs. Maint: 150mg qhs. GERD: 150mg bid. Erosive Esophagitis: 150mg qid. Maint: 150mg bid. Hypersecretory Conditions: 150mg bid. May give up to 6g/day with severe disease. Do not chew. Swallow whole or dissolve in tongue. (Inj) Usual: 50mg IV/IM q6-8 hrs or 6.25mg/hr continuous IV. Max: 400mg/day. Zollinger Ellison: Initial: 1mg/kg/hr. Titrate: May increase after 4 hrs by 0.5mg/kg/hr increments. Max: 2.5mg/kg/hr or 220mg/hr. CrCl <50mL/min: 50mg IV q18-24 hrs or 150mg PO q24h. Give more frequent (q12h) if necessary. Hemodialysis: Give dose at the end of treatment.
*Pediatrics:* 1 month-16 yrs: (PO) DU/GU: 2-4mg/kg bid. Max: 300mg/day. Maint: 2-4mg/kg qd. Max: 150mg/day. GERD/Erosive Esophagitis: 2.5-5mg/kg bid. (Inj) DU: 2-4mg/kg/day IV given q6-8 hrs. Max: 50mg q6-8 hrs. CrCl <50mL/min: 50mg IV q18-24 hrs or 150mg PO q24h. Give more frequent (q12h) if necessary.

**HOW SUPPLIED:** Inj: 25mg/mL, 50mg/50mL (premixed); Syrup: 15mg/mL; Tab: 150mg, 300mg; Tab, Effervescent: 25mg.

**WARNINGS/PRECAUTIONS:** Do not exceed recommended infusion rates; bradycardia reported with rapid infusion. Caution with liver and renal dysfunction. SGPT elevations reported; monitor SGPT if on IV therapy for ≥5 days at dose >100mg qid. Avoid use with history of acute porphyria. Symptomatic response does not preclude the presence of gastric malignancy. May cause false (+) urine protein test. Caution in elderly. (PO) Granules and effervescent tablets contain phenylalanine.

**ADVERSE REACTIONS:** Headache, constipation, diarrhea, N/V, abdominal discomfort, hepatitis, blood dyscrasias, rash, injection-site reactions (IV/IM).

**INTERACTIONS:** Increases plasma levels of triazolam, midazolam, glipizide, and procainamide. Decreases plasma levels of ketoconazole, atazanavir, delaviridine, and gefitinib. Altered anticoagulant effects with warfarin. Avoid chronic use with delavirdine. Monitor for prolonged sedation with midazolam. Caution with gefitinib and atazanavir. (PO) Propantheline delays and increases peak blood levels of ranitidine. High-potency antacid in fasting subjects decreases absorption of ranitidine.

**PREGNANCY:** Category B, caution with nursing.

**MECHANISM OF ACTION:** $H_2$-blocker; competitive, reversible inhibitor of histamine at histamine $H_2$-receptors, including those found on gastric cells.

**PHARMACOKINETICS: Absorption:** (PO, 150mg) $C_{max}$=440-545ng/mL, $T_{max}$=2-3 hrs; Absolute bioavailability=50%. (IM) Rapid; $C_{max}$=576ng/mL, $T_{max}$=15 min; Absolute bioavailability (90%-100%) IM. **Distribution**: $V_d$=1.4L/kg; plasma protein binding (15%); found in breast milk. **Metabolism**: Liver, N-oxide (principal metabolite). **Elimination**: Urine: (PO) 30% unchanged; (IV) 70% unchanged; (PO) $T_{1/2}$=2.5-3 hrs, (IV) $T_{1/2}$=2-2.5 hrs. Refer to PI for pediatric parameters.

## NURSING CONSIDERATIONS

**Assessment:** Assess for renal/hepatic dysfunction, gastric malignancy, history of acute porphyria, pregnancy/nursing status, and possible drug interactions.

**Monitoring:** Monitor for signs/symptoms of hepatic effects (eg, elevations in SGPT values), CV effects, headache, GI effects (eg, constipation, diarrhea), and prolonged sedation. In patients receiving IV formulation at dosages ≥100mg qid for ≥5 days, monitor SGPT daily from Day 5 to the conclusion of IV therapy.

**Patient Counseling:** Antacids may be given as pain relief for GI symptoms. If taking efferdose tab formulation, do not chew tab, swallow whole, or dissolve on tongue; should be completely dissolved in ≥5mL of water before administration; may be given by medicine dropper or oral syringe. Notify physician if any adverse events develop.

**Administration:** Oral/IM/IV routes. **Storage:** Tab: 15-30°C (59-86°F) in dry place. Protect from light. Replace cap securely after each use. Efferdose Tab: 2-30°C (36-86°F). Syrup: 4-25°C (39-77°F). Dispense in tight, light resistant containers. Inj: 4-25°C (39-77°F); excursions permitted to 30°C (86°F). Protect from light. Premixed Inj: 2-25°C (36-77°F). Protect from light.

# ZARONTIN — RX

ethosuximide (Parke-Davis)

**THERAPEUTIC CLASS:** Succinimide

**INDICATIONS:** Control of absence (petit mal) epilepsy.

**DOSAGE:** *Adults:* Initial: 500mg qd. Titrate: May increase daily dose by 250mg every 4-7 days. Max: 1.5g/day.
*Pediatrics:* Initial: 3-6 yrs: 250mg qd. ≥6 yrs: 500mg qd. Titrate: May increase daily dose by 250mg every 4-7 days. Usual: 20mg/kg/day. Max: 1.5g/day.

**HOW SUPPLIED:** Cap: 250mg; Syrup: 250mg/5mL

**WARNINGS/PRECAUTIONS:** Extreme caution in liver and renal dysfunction. Monitor blood counts, liver and renal function periodically. SLE, blood dyscrasias reported. Adjust dose slowly and avoid abrupt withdrawal. May increase grand mal seizures in mixed types of epilepsy when used alone. May impair mental/physical abilities. Cases of birth defects reported. Increased risk of suicidal thoughts or behavior reported; monitor for worsening of depression and any unusual changes in mood or behavior.

**ADVERSE REACTIONS:** Anorexia, N/V, abdominal pain, leukopenia, drowsiness, headache, urticaria, SLE, myopia, vaginal bleeding, diarrhea, euphoria, hirsutism, hematuria, pancytopenia.

**INTERACTIONS:** May increase phenytoin levels. Valproic acid may alter levels.

**PREGNANCY:** Safety not known in pregnancy or nursing.

**MECHANISM OF ACTION:** Succinimide; suppresses paroxysmal three cycles per second spike and wave activity associated with lapses of consciousness, which is common in absence (petit mal) seizures. Frequency of attacks is reduced through depression of motor cortex and elevation of the CNS threshold to convulsive stimuli.

**PHARMACOKINETICS: Distribution:** Crosses placenta, found in breast milk.

## NURSING CONSIDERATIONS

**Assessment:** Assess renal/hepatic function prior to therapy. Assess for pregnancy/nursing status and for possible drug interactions. Obtain baseline CBC.

**Monitoring:** Monitor for blood dyscrasias and signs/symptoms of SLE. Monitor for occurrence of grand mal seizures in patients with mixed types of epilepsy who are on monotherapy. Monitor CBC, LFTs, urinalysis, signs/symptoms of infection (eg, sore throat, fever), and hypersensitivity reactions.

**Patient Counseling:** Advise to contact physician if any signs/symptoms of infection develop. Counsel not to abruptly d/c therapy. Inform that therapy may impair mental/physical abilities; avoid activities requiring alertness (eg, operating vehicles). Monitor for worsening of depression and any unusual changes in mood or behavior. Encourage patients to enroll in NAAED Pregnancy Registry if they become pregnant. To enroll, call 888-233-2334 or go to aedpregnancyregistry.org.

**Administration:** Oral. **Storage:** (Oral Sol) 20-25°C (68-77°F). Preserve in tight containers. Protect from freezing and light. (Caps) 25°C (77°F); excursions permitted to 15-30°C (59-86°F).

# ZAROXOLYN RX

metolazone (Celltech)

**Do not interchange rapid and complete bioavailability metolazone formulations for other slow and incomplete bioavailability metolazone formulations; they are not therapeutically equivalent.**

**THERAPEUTIC CLASS:** Quinazoline diuretic

**INDICATIONS:** Treatment of hypertension and of salt and water retention in edema accompanying CHF or renal disease.

**DOSAGE:** *Adults:* Edema: 5-20mg qd. HTN: 2.5-5mg qd. Elderly: Start at low end of dosing range.

**HOW SUPPLIED:** Tab: 2.5mg, 5mg, 10mg

**CONTRAINDICATIONS:** Anuria, hepatic coma or precoma.

**WARNINGS/PRECAUTIONS:** Risk of hypokalemia, orthostatic hypotension, hypercalcemia, hyperuricemia, azotemia, and rapid-onset hyponatremia. Cross-allergy with sulfonamide-derived drugs, thiazides, or quinethazone. Sensitivity reactions may occur with 1st dose. Monitor electrolytes. May cause hyperglycemia and glycosuria in diabetics. Caution in elderly or severe renal impairment. May exacerbate or activate SLE.

**ADVERSE REACTIONS:** Chest pain/discomfort, orthostatic hypotension, syncope, neuropathy, necrotizing angiitis, hepatitis, jaundice, pancreatitis, blood dyscrasias, joint pain.

**INTERACTIONS:** Furosemide and other loop diuretics prolong fluid and electrolyte loss. Adjust dose of other antihypertensives. Potentiates hypotensive effects of alcohol, barbiturates, and narcotics. Lithium, digitalis toxicity. Corticosteroids and ACTH increase hypokalemia and salt and water retention. Enhanced neuromuscular blocking effects of curariform drugs. Salicylates and NSAIDs decrease effects. Decreased arterial response to norepinephrine. Decrease in methenamine efficacy. Adjust anticoagulants, antidiabetics.

**PREGNANCY:** Category B, not for use in nursing.

**MECHANISM OF ACTION:** Quinazoline diuretic; acts primarily to inhibit $Na^+$ reabsorption at cortical diluting site and, to a lesser extent, in proximal convoluted tubule.

**PHARMACOKINETICS: Absorption:** $T_{max}$=8 hrs. **Elimination:** Urine (unchanged).

## NURSING CONSIDERATIONS

**Assessment:** Assess for anuria, SLE, DM, sulfonamide hypersensitivity, history of allergy or bronchial asthma, hepatic/renal impairment, possible drug interactions.

**Monitoring:** Monitor serum electrolytes periodically. Monitor for signs/symptoms of electrolyte imbalance, exacerbation or activation of SLE, hyperglycemia, hyperuricemia or precipitation of gout, hypersensitivity reactions (eg, angioedema, bronchospasm, toxic epidermal necrolysis, Stevens-Johnson syndrome), orthostatic hypotension, renal/hepatic dysfunction.

**Patient Counseling:** Counsel to take medication as directed and promptly report adverse reactions. Advise not to interchange formulations. Instruct to seek medical attention if symptoms of electrolyte imbalance (eg, dry mouth, thirst, weakness) or hypersensitivity reactions occur.

**Administration:** Oral route. **Storage:** 25°C (77°F); excursions permitted to 15-30°C (59-86°F). Protect from light.

# ZEBETA RX

bisoprolol fumarate (Duramed)

**THERAPEUTIC CLASS:** Selective $beta_1$-blocker

**INDICATIONS:** Management of hypertension alone or in combination with other antihypertensive agents.

**DOSAGE:** *Adults:* Individualize dosing. Initial: 5mg qd. Titrate: May increase to 10mg and then, if necessary, to 20mg/day if antihypertensive effect is inadequate. Max: 20mg/day. Bronchospastic Disease: Initial: 2.5mg qd. Hepatic/Renal Dysfunction (CrCl <40mL/min): Initial: 2.5mg qd; caution with dose titration.

**HOW SUPPLIED:** Tab: 5mg*, 10mg *scored

**CONTRAINDICATIONS:** Cardiogenic shock, overt cardiac failure, 2nd- or 3rd-degree AV block, marked sinus bradycardia.

**WARNINGS/PRECAUTIONS:** Avoid abrupt withdrawal. May mask manifestations of hypoglycemia or clinical signs of hyperthyroidism. Avoid with overt congestive heart failure. Caution with compensated cardiac failure, diabetes mellitus (DM), bronchospastic disease, hepatic/renal impairment, or peripheral vascular disease (PVD). May precipitate cardiac failure and symptoms of arterial insufficiency in patients with PVD. Caution with history of severe anaphylactic reaction to a variety of allergens; reactivity may increase with repeated challenge.

**ADVERSE REACTIONS:** Headache, URI, cough, rhinitis, peripheral edema, dizziness.

**INTERACTIONS:** Patients with a history of severe anaphylactic reaction to a variety of allergens taking β-blockers may be unresponsive to usual doses of epinephrine. Caution with clonidine withdrawal; d/c bisoprolol several days before clonidine. Excessive reduction of sympathetic activity with catecholamine-depleting drugs (eg, reserpine, guanethidine); monitor closely. Avoid other β-blockers. Caution with myocardial depressants or inhibitors of AV conduction such as calcium antagonists (eg, verapamil, diltiazem), antiarrhythmics (eg, disopyramide), and anesthetics that depress myocardial function. Caution with digitalis glycosides; both agents slow AV conduction and decrease HR. Rifampin increases clearance. Caution with antidiabetic agents.

**PREGNANCY:** Category C, caution in nursing.

**MECHANISM OF ACTION:** $\beta_1$-selective adrenoreceptor blocking agent; not established. May decrease cardiac output, inhibit renin release in the kidneys, and diminution of tonic sympathetic outflow from the vasomotor centers in the brain.

**PHARMACOKINETICS: Absorption:** (10mg) Absolute bioavailability 80%; $C_{max}$= (5mg) 16ng/mL, (20mg) 70ng/mL; (5-20mg) $T_{max}$=2-4 hrs. **Distribution:** Plasma protein binding (30%). **Metabolism:** CYP2D6. **Elimination:** Urine (50%, unchanged), feces (<2%); $T_{1/2}$=9-12 hrs.

## NURSING CONSIDERATIONS

**Assessment:** Assess for bradycardia, cardiogenic shock, 2nd- and 3rd-degree heart block, overt cardiac failure, renal/hepatic impairment, bronchospastic disease, PVD, DM, hyperthyroidism, severe anaphylactic reactions, pregnancy/nursing status, and possible drug interactions.

**Monitoring:** Monitor for cardiac failure, renal/hepatic function, hypersensitivity reactions, symptoms of arterial insufficiency in patients with PVD and hypoglycemia. Monitor for exacerbation of angina pectoris, MI and ventricular arrhythmia in patients with coronary artery disease, symptoms of hyperthyroidism or thyroid storm following abrupt withdrawal. Monitor HR, ECG, CBC with platelet and differential count.

**Patient Counseling:** Instruct not to interrupt or d/c therapy without consulting physician. Notify physician if difficulty in breathing, signs/symptoms of CHF or excessive bradycardia develop. Educate about signs/symptoms of drug's potential adverse effects. Advise to exercise caution while driving, operating machinery or other tasks requiring alertness.

**Administration:** Oral route. **Storage**: 20-25°C (68-77°F). Protect from moisture. Dispense in tight container.

# ZEGERID RX

## sodium bicarbonate - omeprazole (Santarus)

**THERAPEUTIC CLASS:** Proton pump inhibitor

**INDICATIONS:** (Cap, Powder, Tab) Short-term treatment of erosive esophagitis diagnosed by endoscopy, active duodenal ulcer, and active benign gastric ulcer. Treatment of heartburn and other symptoms associated with GERD. Maintain healing of erosive esophagitis. (Powder, 40mg-1680mg) Reduction of risk of upper GI bleeding in critically ill patients.

**DOSAGE:** *Adults:* Cap/Powder/Tab: Duodenal Ulcer: 20mg qd for 4-8 weeks. Gastric Ulcer: 40mg qd for 4-8 weeks. GERD: 20mg qd for up to 4 weeks without esophageal lesions and for 4-8 weeks with erosive esophagitis. Maintenance of Healing Erosive Esophagitis: 20mg qd. Powder (40mg-1680mg): Risk Reduction of Upper GI Bleeding in Critically Ill Patients: Initial: 40mg, followed by 40mg after 6-8 hrs. Maint: 40mg qd for 14 days. Take 1 hr before a meal. Add pkt contents to 2 tablespoons of water; do not use other liquids or foods. Stir powder well and drink immediately. Swallow caps whole with water.

**HOW SUPPLIED:** (Omeprazole-Sodium Bicarbonate) Cap: 20mg-1100mg, 40mg-1100mg; Powder: 20mg-1680mg/pkt [30s], 40mg-1680mg/pkt [30s]; (Omeprazole-Sodium Bicarbonate-Magnesium Hydroxide) Tab, Chewable: 20mg-600mg-700mg, 40mg-600mg-700mg

**WARNINGS/PRECAUTIONS:** Atrophic gastritis reported with long-term use. Symptomatic response does not preclude the presence of gastric malignancy. Due to sodium bicarbonate content, avoid with metabolic alkalosis, hypocalcemia and use caution with a sodium-restricted diet, Bartter's syndrome, hypokalemia, respiratory alkalosis. Long-term use of bicarbonate with calcium or milk may cause milk-alkali syndrome.(Tab) Magnesium content may increase hypermagnesemia and magnesium toxicity in neonates, elderly and in patients with renal impairment/renal disease.

**ADVERSE REACTIONS:** Abdominal pain, headache, nausea, vomiting.

**INTERACTIONS:** May prolong elimination of diazepam, warfarin, phenytoin, and drugs metabolized by oxidation. May increase PT and INR if given concomitantly with warfarin. May alter absorption of pH-dependent drugs (eg, ketoconazole, ampicillin esters, and iron salts). Monitor when given with drugs metabolized by CYP450 (eg, cyclosporine, disulfiram, benzodiazepines).

Clarithromycin may increase levels. May increase levels of tacrolimus, clarithromycin. May reduce levels of atazanavir.

**PREGNANCY:** Category C, not for use in nursing.

**MECHANISM OF ACTION:** Omeprazole: Proton-pump inhibitor; suppresses gastric acid secretion by specific inhibition of the ($H^+/K^+$)-ATPase enzyme at secretory surface of gastric parietal cell. Sodium Bicarbonate: Acts as antacid.

**PHARMACOKINETICS: Absorption:** Omeprazole: Rapid absorption; $T_{max}$=30 min; (Sus) Absolute bioavailability (30-40%); $C_{max}$=1954ng/mL. (Cap) $C_{max}$=1526ng/mL. **Distribution:** Omeprazole: Plasma protein binding (95%); found in breast milk. **Metabolism:** Omeprazole: Hydroxyomeprazole and corresponding carboxylic acid (metabolites). **Elimination:** Omeprazole: Urine (77% as metabolites), feces; $T_{1/2}$=1 hr.

## NURSING CONSIDERATIONS

**Assessment:** Assess for hepatic impairment, gastric malignancy, $Na^+$-restricted diet, metabolic alkalosis, respiratory alkalosis, problems with acid-base balance, hypocalcemia, Bartter's syndrome, hypokalemia, pregnancy/nursing status, and possible drug interactions. Assess dosing in Asian patients.

**Monitoring:** Monitor for signs/symptoms of atrophic gastritis. Monitor for milk-alkali syndrome in presence of long-term use of bicarbonate with calcium or milk.

**Patient Counseling:** Counsel to take on empty stomach at least 1 hr before meals. If taking cap, swallow whole, do not open cap and sprinkle contents on food. For sus, empty packet contents into small cup containing 1-2 tbl of water; do not use other liquids or foods; stir well and drink immediately; refill cup with water and drink. Notify physician of adverse events (eg, GI effects).

**Administration:** Oral route. **Storage:** 25°C (77°F); excursions permitted to 15-30°C (59-86°F).

# ZEGERID OTC — OTC

sodium bicarbonate - omeprazole (Schering-Plough)

**THERAPEUTIC CLASS:** Proton pump inhibitor

**INDICATIONS:** Treatment of frequent heartburn ( ≥2 days per week).

**DOSAGE: Adults:** 1 cap qd for 14 days. Take with water 1 hr before breakfast. May repeat q4months.

**HOW SUPPLIED:** Cap: (Omeprazole-Sodium Bicarbonate) 20mg-1100mg

**WARNINGS/PRECAUTIONS:** Not for immediate relief of heartburn. D/C if heartburn continues or worsens, or if need to take for more than 14 days. Avoid use if having trouble/pain swallowing food, vomiting with blood or if have bloody/black stools.

**INTERACTIONS:** Caution with warfarin, diazepam, digoxin, antifungals, tacrolimus and antiretroviral agents.

**PREGNANCY:** Safety in pregnancy and nursing not known.

## NURSING CONSIDERATIONS

**Assessment:** Assess for proper diagnosis, difficulty/pain in swallowing, vomiting with blood, bloody/black stools, hypersensitivity reactions, pregnancy/nursing status and possible drug interactions.

**Monitoring:** Monitor for continuing/worsening of heartburn and allergic/hypersensitivity reactions.

**Patient Counseling:** Instruct to take 1 hr before breakfast; do not chew, crush, open and sprinkle on food. Advise not to take for more than 14 days or more often than every 4 months unless directed by a doctor. Advise to consult a physician if heartburn >3 months or continuing/worsening, experiencing lightheadedness, sweating, dizziness, chest/shoulder pain with shortness of breath, pain radiating to the arms, neck or shoulder, frequent chest pain/

wheezing, unexplained weight loss, nausea, vomiting, stomach pain and if on sodium restricted diet. Advise to inform any other medications being taken.

**Administration:** Oral route. Do not chew, crush or open capsule. **Storage:** 20-25°C (68-77°F). Tamper-evident. Keep out of high heat and humidity. Protect from moisture.

## ZELAPAR RX

selegiline HCl (Valeant)

**THERAPEUTIC CLASS:** Monoamine oxidase inhibitor (Type B)

**INDICATIONS:** Adjunct in the management of Parkinson's disease in patients exhibiting a deteriorated response to levodopa/carbidopa therapy.

**DOSAGE:** *Adults:* 1.25mg qd for 6 weeks. Titrate: After 6 weeks, may increase to 2.5mg if desired benefit not achieved. Max: 2.5mg/day.

**HOW SUPPLIED:** Tab, Orally Disintegrating: 1.25mg

**CONTRAINDICATIONS:** Concomitant meperidine, tramadol, methadone, propoxyphene dextromethorphan, and other MAOIs.

**WARNINGS/PRECAUTIONS:** Do not exceed 2.5mg/day; risk of non-selective MAO inhibition. Greater risk of orthostatic hypotension and dizziness in geriatric patients. Decrease levodopa/carbidopa to prevent exacerbation of levodopa side effects (eg, preexisting dyskinesias). Melanoma reported; perform periodic dermatologic screening. May increase frequency of mild oropharyngeal abnormality. Caution with renal or hepatic impairment. Neuroleptic malignant syndrome reported in association with rapid dose reduction, withdrawal of, or changes in antiparkinsonian therapy. Compulsive behaviors (eg, intense urges to gamble, increased sexual urges) reported.

**ADVERSE REACTIONS:** Nausea, dizziness, pain, headache, insomnia, rhinitis, skin disorders, dyskinesia, backache, dyspepsia, stomatitis, constipation, hallucinations, pharyngitis, rash.

**INTERACTIONS:** See Contraindications. Serious, sometimes fatal, reactions have been precipitated with meperidine, tramadol, methadone, and propoxyphene; avoid concomitant use. Episodes of psychosis or bizarre behavior reported with dextromethorphan; avoid concomitant use. Severe toxicity reported with SSRIs or TCAs; avoid concurrent use and allow 2 weeks between d/c of selegiline and initiation of TCAs or SSRIs. Allow 5 weeks for fluoxetine due to a longer half-life. Caution with sympathomimetics and CYP3A4 inducers (eg, phenytoin, carbamazepine, nafcillin, phenobarbital, and rifampin).

**PREGNANCY:** Category C, not for use in nursing.

**MECHANISM OF ACTION:** Irreversible MAO inhibitor; blocks catabolism of dopamine and increases net amount of dopamine available.

**PHARMACOKINETICS: Absorption**: $C_{max}$(1.25mg, 2.5mg, 5mg)=3.34, 4.47, 1.12ng/mL. $T_{max}$(1.25mg, 2.5mg, 5mg)=10-15 min, 10-15 min, 40-90 min. **Distribution:** Plasma protein binding (85%). **Metabolism:** Liver (1st-pass metabolism). **Elimination:** Urine; $T_{1/2}$=10 hrs (steady state).

### NURSING CONSIDERATIONS

**Assessment:** Assess renal function, LFTs, dyskinesia, phenylalanine levels, BP, melanomas, pregnancy/nursing status, and possible drug interactions.

**Monitoring:** Monitor LFTs, renal function, BP, exacerbation of pre-existing dyskinesia, melanomas, hyperpyrexia, hallucinations, compulsive behaviors (eg, pathological gambling, hypersexuality).

**Patient Counseling:** Should be taken every morning before breakfast without liquid. Do not remove blister from outer pouch until just prior to dosing. Report any side effects. Notify physician if new or increased gambling urges, sexual urges, or other urges occur.

**Administration:** Oral route; dissolve on tongue. **Storage:** 25°C (77°F); excursions permitted to 15-30°C (59-86°F). Use within 3 months after opening.

# ZEMPLAR IV RX

paricalcitol (Abbott)

**THERAPEUTIC CLASS:** Vitamin D analog

**INDICATIONS:** Prevention and treatment of secondary hyperparathyroidism associated with chronic kidney disease Stage 5.

**DOSAGE:** *Adults:* Initial: 0.04-0.1mcg/kg bolus no more frequently than every other day during dialysis. Titrate: May increase by 2-4mcg at 2-to 4-week intervals. Monitor serum Ca and phosphorus more frequently during dose adjustments. Reduce or interrupt dose if elevated Ca level or Ca x P product >75; may reinitiate at lower dose once normalized. May need dose reduction as PTH levels decrease (see PI).
*Pediatrics:* ≥5 yrs: (Inj) Initial: 0.04-0.1mcg/kg bolus no more frequently than every other day during dialysis. Titrate: May increase by 2-4mcg at 2-to 4-week intervals. Monitor serum Ca and phosphorus more frequently during dose adjustments. Reduce or interrupt dose if elevated Ca level or Ca x P product >75; may reinitiate at lower dose once normalized. May need dose reduction as PTH levels decrease (see PI).

**HOW SUPPLIED:** Inj: 2mcg/mL, 5mcg/mL

**CONTRAINDICATIONS:** Vitamin D toxicity, hypercalcemia.

**WARNINGS/PRECAUTIONS:** May cause hypercalcemia with acute overdose. Monitor serum Ca and phosphorus levels during dose adjustment. If clinically significant hypercalcemia develops, reduce or interrupt dose. May increase risk of hypercalcemia, elevated Ca x P product, and metastatic calcification with chronic administration. Adynamic bone lesions may develop if PTH levels are suppressed to abnormal levels.

**ADVERSE REACTIONS:** N/V, GI bleeding, edema, light-headedness, pneumonia, sepsis, flu, fever, chills, palpitations.

**INTERACTIONS:** Digitalis toxicity potentiated by hypercalcemia. Avoid excessive use of aluminum-containing compounds. Avoid use with phosphate or vitamin D-related compounds. Caution with ketoconazole and other strong CYP450 3A inhibitors (eg, atazanavir, clarithromycin, indinavir, itraconazole, nefazodone, nelfinavir, ritonavir, saquinavir, telithromycin, voriconazole).

**PREGNANCY:** Category C, not for use in nursing.

**MECHANISM OF ACTION:** Synthetic vitamin D analog; binds to vitamin D receptor, which results in selective activation of vitamin D pathways. Shown to reduce parathyroid hormone levels by inhibiting PTH synthesis and secretion.

**PHARMACOKINETICS: Absorption:** $C_{max}$=1.680ng/mL (hemodialysis), 1.832ng/mL (peritoneal dialysis); AUC=14.51ng•h/mL (hemodialysis), 16.01ng•h/mL (peritoneal dialysis). **Distribution:** $V_d$=23.8L (healthy), 31L (hemodialysis), and 35L (peritoneal dialysis); plasma protein binding ( ≥99.8%). **Metabolism:** Hepatic, via hydroxylation and glucuronidation; CYP24, CYP3A4, UGT1A4. **Elimination:** Hepatobiliary excretion (primary), urine (19%), feces (63%); $T_{1/2}$=5-7 hrs (healthy), 13.9 hrs (hemodialysis), 15.4 hrs (peritoneal dialysis).

## NURSING CONSIDERATIONS

**Assessment:** Assess for vitamin D toxicity and hypercalcemia prior to therapy. Assess pregnancy/nursing status and for possible drug interactions.

**Monitoring:** Monitor for signs/symptoms of hypercalcemia, hyperphosphatemia, and metastatic calcification. If hypercalcemia develops, monitor for fluid and electrolyte imbalances, ECG abnormalities, and serum Ca levels; monitor serum Ca levels frequently until levels normalized. Monitor for adynamic bone lesions with suppressed PTH levels. Monitor Ca and phosphorus levels twice weekly when initiating therapy. Once dosage established, monitor serum Ca and phosphorus monthly. Monitor serum/plasma PTH levels every 3 months.

**Patient Counseling:** Inform of importance of adherence to dietary regimen of Ca supplementation and phosphorus restriction. Instruct to avoid excessive use of aluminum containing compounds. Counsel about signs/symptoms of

Z

hypercalcemia. Advise to avoid taking phosphate- or vitamin D-containing compounds.

**Administration:** IV route. **Storage:** 25°C (77°F); excursions permitted to 15-30°C (59-86°F).

## ZEMPLAR ORAL RX

paricalcitol (Abbott)

**THERAPEUTIC CLASS:** Vitamin D analog

**INDICATIONS:** Prevention and treatment of secondary hyperparathyroidism associated with Stage 3 and 4 chronic kidney disease (CKD), and CKD Stage 5 on hemodialysis or peritoneal dialysis.

**DOSAGE:** *Adults:* CKD Stage 3 and 4: Initial: Baseline iPTH Level ≤500pg/mL: 1mcg qd or 2mcg tiw. Baseline iPTH Level >500pg/mL: 2mcg qd or 4mcg tiw. May need dose adjustment based on iPTH level relative to baseline (see PI). CKD Stage 5: Initial: Baseline iPTH level (pg/mL)/80. May need to decrease dose by 2-4mcg lower than the calculated baseline iPTH level/80 if serum calcium levels are elevated.

**HOW SUPPLIED:** Cap: 1mcg, 2mcg, 4mcg

**CONTRAINDICATIONS:** Vitamin D toxicity, hypercalcemia.

**WARNINGS/PRECAUTIONS:** May cause over suppression of PTH, hypercalcemia, hypercalciuria, hyperphosphatemia, and adynamic bone disease. Overdose may cause progressive hypercalcemia.

**ADVERSE REACTIONS:** Pain, allergic reactions, headache, infection, hypotension, HTN, diarrhea, N/V, constipation, edema, arthritis, dizziness, vertigo, rhinitis, rash.

**INTERACTIONS:** Digitalis toxicity potentiated by hypercalcemia. Caution with strong CYP3A inhibitors (eg, ketoconazole, atazanavir, clarithromycin, indinavir, itraconazole, nefazodone, nelfinavir, ritonavir, saquinavir, telithromycin, voriconazole). Drugs that may impair intestinal absorption of fat-soluble vitamins (eg, cholestyramine) may intefere with absorption.

**PREGNANCY:** Category C, not for use in nursing.

**MECHANISM OF ACTION:** Synthetic vitamin D analog; binds to vitamin D receptor (VDR), which results in selective activation of vitamin D pathways. Shown to reduce parathyroid hormone levels by inhibiting PTH synthesis and secretion.

**PHARMACOKINETICS: Absorption:** Well absorbed; absolute bioavailability (72%); $C_{max}$=0.630ng/mL; $T_{max}$=3 hrs; AUC=5.25ng•h/mL. **Distribution:** $V_d$=34L (healthy); 44-46L (CKD stage 3 and 4); plasma protein binding ( ≥99.8%). **Metabolism:** Hepatic, via hydroxylation and glucuronidation; extensively metabolized by CYP24, as well as CYP3A4, UGT1A4. 24(R)-hydroxy paracalcitol (minor metabolite). **Elimination:** Hepatobiliary excretion (primary); urine (18%), feces (70%); $T_{1/2}$=17 hrs (CKD Stage 3), 20 hrs (CKD Stage 4).

### NURSING CONSIDERATIONS

**Assessment:** Assess for vitamin D toxicity or hypercalcemia prior to therapy. Assess for pregnancy/nursing status, possible drug interactions (digitalis compounds).

**Monitoring:** Monitor for signs/symptoms of hypercalcemia (eg, cardiac arrhythmias, seizures, vascular calcification, soft tissue calcification). Monitor for PTH suppression, hypercalciuria, hyperphosphatemia and adynamic bone disease. Monitor serum calcium, serum phosphorus, and serum/plasma PTH every 2 weeks for 3 months after initiation of therapy or following dosage adjustment. Levels should then be assessed monthly for 3 months, and then every 3 months thereafter.

**Patient Counseling:** Inform about compliance with dosage instructions, proper diet, phosphorus restrictions, and avoidance of unapproved OTC drugs. Advise about signs/symptoms of hypercalcemia. Instruct to avoid use of aluminum-containing compounds and pharmacological doses of vitamin D and its derivatives while on therapy. Inform medication may be taken without regard to food.

**Administration:** Oral route. **Storage:** 25°C (77°F); excursions permitted to 15-30°C (59-86°F).

## ZENAPAX RX

daclizumab (Roche Labs)

**Should only be prescribed by physicians experienced in immunosuppressive therapy and management of organ transplant patients. Physician should have complete information requisite for the follow-up of the patient. Only healthcare personnel trained in the administration of the drug who have available adequate laboratory and supportive medical resources should administer.**

**THERAPEUTIC CLASS:** Interleukin-2 receptor antagonist

**INDICATIONS:** For prophylaxis of acute organ rejection in renal transplants, in combination with cyclosporine and corticosteroids.

**DOSAGE:** *Adults:* 1mg/kg IV over 15 min for 5 doses. Administer 1st dose no more than 24 hrs prior to transplant and remaining 4 doses at 14-day intervals. *Pediatrics:* ≥11 months: 1mg/kg IV over 15 min for 5 doses. Administer 1st dose no more than 24 hrs prior to transplant and remaining 4 doses at 14-day intervals.

**HOW SUPPLIED:** Inj: 25mg/5mL

**WARNINGS/PRECAUTIONS:** May be associated with increased risk in mortality, lymphoproliferative disorder, and opportunistic infections; monitor accordingly. Hypersensitivity reactions including anaphylaxis reported on initial and re-exposure. Postmarketing reports of cytokine release syndrome. D/C if severe hypersensitivity reaction occurs. Caution in elderly. Re-administration after initial course of therapy has not been studied in humans.

**ADVERSE REACTIONS:** GI disorders, constipation, N/V, diarrhea, abdominal pain, pyrosis, dyspepsia, abdominal distention, epigastric pain, edema extremities, edema, tremor, headache, dizziness, oliguria.

**INTERACTIONS:** Immunosuppressive regimens including cyclosporine, mycophenolate mofetil, and corticosteroids are associated with an increase in mortality, particularly in patients receiving anti-lymphocyte antibody therapy and who develop severe infections. Very limited experience exists with tacrolimus, muromonab-CD3, antithymocyte globulin, and anti-lymphocyte globulin.

**PREGNANCY:** Category C, not for use in nursing.

**MECHANISM OF ACTION:** IL-2 receptor antagonist; binds with high affinity to the Tac subunit of the high affinity IL-2 receptor complex and inhibits IL-2 binding.

**PHARMACOKINETICS: Absorption:** $C_{max}$=21mcg/mL (adult); 16mcg/mL (pediatric). **Elimination:** $T_{1/2}$=20 days (adult), 13 days (pediatric).

### NURSING CONSIDERATIONS

**Assessment:** Assess for drug hypersensitivity, DM, pregnancy status, and possible drug interactions.

**Monitoring:** Monitor for hypersensitivity reactions, including hypotension, bronchospasm, wheezing, laryngeal edema, pulmonary edema, cyanosis, hypoxia, respiratory arrest, cardiac arrhythmia, cardiac arrest, peripheral edema, loss of consciousness, fever, rash, urticaria, diaphoresis, pruritus, injection-site reactions, lymphoproliferative disorders, infectious episodes (eg, viral and fungal infections, bacteremia, and septicemia), pneumonia, and opportunistic infections (eg, CMV, cellulitis, and wound infection). Monitor fasting blood glucose.

**Patient Counseling:** Inform about potential risks/benefits. Instruct not to take while pregnant/nursing.

**Administration:** IV route. Not for direct injection; dilute with 50mL of 0.9% NaCl solution and administer via central or peripheral vein for 15 mins. When mixing, invert the bag without shaking. **Storage:** 2-8°C (36-46°F).

Do not shake or freeze. Protect diluted solution against direct light. Diluted medication is stable for 24 hrs at 4°C or for 4 hrs at room temp.

## ZENPEP RX

protease - amylase - lipase (Eurand Pharmaceuticals, Inc.)

**THERAPEUTIC CLASS:** Pancreatic enzyme supplement

**INDICATIONS:** Treatment of exocrine pancreatic insufficiency due to cystic fibrosis or other conditions.

**DOSAGE:** *Adults:* Individualize dose. Initial: 500 U lipase/kg/meal. Titrate: May increase dose based on clinical symptoms, degree of steatorrhea present, and fat content of diet. Max: 2500 U lipase/kg/meal. Swallow whole; do not crush or chew.
*Pediatrics:* Individualize dose. ≥4 yrs: Initial: 500 U lipase/kg/meal. Titrate: May increase dose based on clinical symptoms, degree of steatorrhea present, and fat content of diet. Max: 2500 U lipase/kg/meal. >12 mos-<4 yrs: Initial: 1000 U lipase/kg/meal. Titrate: May increase dose based on clinical symptoms, degree of steatorrhea present, and fat content of diet. Max: 2500 U lipase/kg/meal. Infants-≤12 mos: 2000-4000 lipase units/120 mL of formula or per breastfeeding.

**HOW SUPPLIED:** Cap, Delayed-Release (Amylase-Lipase-Protease) (Eurand 5) 27,000 U-5,000 U-17,000 U, (Eurand 10) 55,000 U-10,000 U-34,000 U, (Eurand 15) 82,000 U-15,000 U-51,000 U, (Eurand 20) 109,000 U-20,000 U-68,000 U

**WARNINGS/PRECAUTIONS:** Fibrosing colonopathy reported; patients with fibrosing colonopathy should be closely monitored because some patients may be at risk of progressing to stricture formation. Caution in doses >2500 U lipase/kg/meal. May irritate oral mucosa; care should be taken to ensure that no drug is retained in the mouth. Do not crush, chew, or mix in foods with a pH >4.5. If unable to swallow, carefully open and add contents to a small amount of acidic food with a pH of 4.5 or less (eg, applesauce); swallow food mixture immediately and follow with water or juice to ensure complete ingestion. Caution with gout, renal impairment, or hyperuricemia. May increase serum uric acid levels. Risk for transmission of viral disease, including diseases caused by novel or unidentified viruses. Caution with a known allergy to porcine protein. Allergic reactions may occur. Do not interchange with any other pancrealipase products. Not recommended to mix directly with milk formula or breast milk.

**ADVERSE REACTIONS:** Abdominal pain, flatulence, headache, cough, weight loss, early satiety, contusion, steatorrhea, diarrhea, constipation, nausea, skin disorders (eg, pruritus, urticaria, rash).

**PREGNANCY:** Category C, caution in nursing.

**MECHANISM OF ACTION:** Pancreatic enzyme; catalyzes the hydrolysis of fats to monoglycerol, glycerol and fatty acids, protein into peptides and amino acids, and starch into dextrins and short chain sugars, acting like digestive enzymes physiologically secreted by the pancreas.

### NURSING CONSIDERATIONS

**Assessment:** Assess for gout, renal impairment, hyperuricemia, known allergy to porcine proteins, and pregnancy/nursing status.

**Monitoring:** Monitor for signs/symptoms of fibrosing colonopathy, oral mucosa irritation, hyperuricemia, viral diseases, and for allergic reactions.

**Patient Counseling:** Instruct to take medication as prescribed. Inform that if dose is missed, the next dose should be taken with the next meal or snack as directed; instruct not to take a double dose. Instruct to take with food. Advise to swallow cap whole; do not crush, chew, or mix directly with formula or breast milk. Inform that cap should be swallowed with adequate amount of liquid. Inform that if cannot swallow intact cap, cap may be opened carefully and the contents may be added or sprinkled onto a small amount of acidic soft food (pH <4.5) such as applesauce. Inform care should be taken to ensure that no drug is retained in the mouth to avoid oral mucosa irritation. Advise to notify physician if pregnant or thinking of becoming pregnant during treatment. Instruct to immediately contact physician if an allergic reaction develops.

**Administration:** Oral route. Administer to infants immediately prior to each feeding; contents may be administered directly to the mouth or with a small amount of applesauce or other acidic food with a pH of 4.5 or less; avoid mixing contents of cap directly into formula or breast milk; administration should be followed by breast milk or formula. **Storage:** 20-25°C (68-77°F); excursions permitted to 15-40°C (59-104°F). Keep tightly closed. Protect from moisture.

## ZERIT RX

stavudine (Bristol-Myers Squibb)

**Lactic acidosis and severe hepatomegaly with steatosis, including fatal cases, reported with nucleoside analogs alone or in combination. Fatal lactic acidosis reported in pregnant women who received the combination of stavudine and didanosine with other antiretroviral agents. Use with caution in pregnancy when coadministered with didanosine. Fatal and nonfatal pancreatitis reported when part of a combination regimen that included didanosine.**

**THERAPEUTIC CLASS:** Synthetic thymidine nucleoside analogue

**INDICATIONS:** Treatment of HIV-1 infection in combination with other antiretrovirals.

**DOSAGE:** *Adults:* ≥60kg: 40mg q12h. <60kg: 30mg q12h. Interrupt therapy if symptoms of peripheral neuropathy develop; resume at 1/2 dose when neuropathy resolves. D/C permanently if neuropathy recurs after resumption. CrCl 26-50mL/min: ≥60kg: 20mg q12h. <60kg: 15mg q12h. CrCl 10-25mL/min/ Hemodialysis: ≥60kg: 20mg q24h. <60kg: 15mg q24h. May be taken with or without food.

*Pediatrics:* ≥14 days old and <30kg: 1mg/kg q12h. ≥30-<60kg: 30mg q12h. ≥60kg: 40mg q12h. Birth-13 days old: 0.5mg/kg q12h. Interrupt therapy if symptoms of peripheral neuropathy develop; resume with 1/2 dose when neuropathy resolves. D/C permanently if neuropathy recurs after resumption. Renal Impairment: Reduce dose and/or increase interval between doses. May be taken with or without food.

**HOW SUPPLIED:** Cap: 15mg, 20mg, 30mg, 40mg; Sol: 1mg/mL [200mL]

**WARNINGS/PRECAUTIONS:** Patients with pre-existing liver dysfunction, including chronic active hepatitis, have an increased frequency of liver function abnormalities (eg, severe and fatal hepatic adverse events); monitor accordingly and d/c if evidence of worsening liver disease. Suspend therapy in patients who develop clinical or laboratory findings suggestive of symptomatic hyperlactatemia, lactic acidosis or pronounced hepatotoxicity. Caution in patients with risk factors for liver disease. Motor weakness, peripheral neuropathy, redistribution/accumulation of body fat and immune reconstitution syndrome reported.

**ADVERSE REACTIONS:** Peripheral neuropathy, rash, headache, diarrhea, N/V, pancreatitis, lactic acidosis, increased AST/ALT, increased GGT, increased amylase, increased lipase, increased bilirubin.

**INTERACTIONS:** See Black Box Warning. Avoid with zidovudine. Increased risk of pancreatitis, peripheral neuropathy and hepatotoxicity, which may be fatal, may occur when concomitantly used in combination with didanosine with or without hydroxyurea; avoid concomitant use. Fatal hepatic decompensation may occur in HIV/HCV coinfected patients with concomitant use of interferon/ribavirin; monitor for clinical toxicities. Caution with concomitant use of doxorubicin or ribavirin. Incidence of peripheral neuropathy may occur more frequently if receiving other drugs that have been associated with neuropathy.

**PREGNANCY:** Category C, not for use in nursing.

**MECHANISM OF ACTION:** Thymidine nucleoside analogue; inhibits activity of HIV-1 reverse transcriptase by competing with natural substrate thymidine triphosphate and by causing DNA chain termination following incorporation into viral DNA. Inhibits cellular DNA polymerases β and gamma and markedly reduces synthesis of mitochondrial DNA.

**PHARMACOKINETICS: Absorption**: Rapid; $C_{max}$=536ng/mL; $T_{max}$=1 hr; AUC=2568ng•hr/mL. **Distribution**: $V_d$=46L (adults); $V_d$=0.73L/kg (age 5 weeks to 15 yrs). **Metabolism:** Oxidized stavudine, glucuronide conjugates and N-acetylcysteine conjugate (minor metabolites). **Elimination**: Renal (40% unchanged); $T_{1/2}$=2.3 hrs.

## NURSING CONSIDERATIONS

**Assessment:** Assess for liver dysfunction including chronic active hepatitis, renal impairment, pregnancy/nursing status and for possible drug interactions.

**Monitoring:** Monitor for signs/symptoms of lactic acidosis, severe hepatomegaly with steatosis, pancreatitis, immune reconstitution syndrome, motor weakness, peripheral neuropathy, redistribution/accumulation of body fat and for evidence of worsening liver disease. Monitor LFTs and renal function. Enroll patients in the Antiretroviral Pregnancy Registry if they become pregnant while on therapy.

**Patient Counseling:** Inform that therapy is not cure for HIV, does not reduce risk of transmission of HIV and that opportunistic infections may develop. Instruct to seek medical attention if symptoms of hyperlactatemia or lactic acidosis syndrome (eg, unexplained weight loss, abdominal discomfort, N/V, fatigue, dyspnea) occur. Inform that may develop peripheral neuropathy while on therapy; instruct to contact physician if symptoms of numbness, tingling or pain in the hands or feet occur. Counsel that redistribution/accumulation of fat tissue may occur. Advise patients and caregivers of the importance of adherence to an antiretroviral regimen. Inform about the higher incidence of adverse events when used in combination with agents with similar toxicities.

**Administration:** Oral route. Refer to PI for preparation of oral solution. **Storage**: 25°C (77°F); excursions permitted to 15-30°C (59-86°F); keep in a tightly closed container. Sol: Protect from excessive moisture. After reconstitution, refrigerate at 2-8°C (36-46°F). Discard any unused portion after 30 days.

# ZESTORETIC — RX

lisinopril - hydrochlorothiazide (AstraZeneca)

**ACE inhibitors can cause injury/death to developing fetus during 2nd and 3rd trimesters. D/C if pregnancy is detected.**

**THERAPEUTIC CLASS:** ACE inhibitor/thiazide diuretic

**INDICATIONS:** Treatment of hypertension. Not for initial therapy.

**DOSAGE:** *Adults:* Initial (If Not Controlled with Either Lisinopril or HCTZ Monotherapy): 10mg-12.5mg tab or 20mg-12.5mg tab qd depending on current monotherapy dose. Titrate: May increase after 2-3 weeks. Initial (If Controlled on 25mg HCTZ/day with Hypokalemia): 10mg-12.5mg tab. Replacement Therapy: Substitute combination for titrated components.

**HOW SUPPLIED:** Tab: (HCTZ-Lisinopril) 12.5mg-10mg, 12.5-20mg, 25-20mg

**CONTRAINDICATIONS:** History of ACE inhibitor-associated angioedema, hereditary or idiopathic angioedema, anuria, sulfonamide hypersensitivity.

**WARNINGS/PRECAUTIONS:** D/C if angioedema, jaundice, or marked LFT elevation occur. Anaphylactoid reactions during membrane exposure, angioedema of head and neck (rarely fatal), and intestinal angioedema reported; more reports of angioedema in blacks. Sensitivity reactions with/without history of allergy or bronchial asthma may occur. Association with syndrome of cholestatic jaundice progressing to fulminant necrotic hepatitis and death reported. Risk of hyperkalemia with DM, renal dysfunction. Persistent nonproductive cough may occur. Monitor WBCs in renal and collagen vascular disease. Caution with CHF, aortic stenosis/hypertrophic cardiomyopathy, renal/hepatic dysfunction, renal artery stenosis and left ventricular outflow obstruction.

Monitor for hypotension in high-risk patients (eg, surgery/anesthesia, volume/salt depletion). May precipitate azotemia in renal disease. Sensitivity reactions with/without history of allergy or bronchial asthma may occur. May exacerbate or activate systemic lupus erythematosus (SLE). Monitor electrolytes. Dilutional hyponatremia in edematous patients, hypokalemia with severe cirrhosis or prolonged treatment, hypercalcemia, hypomagnesemia, hyperuricemia or frank gout may occur. Avoid if CrCl ≤30mL/min/1.7m². May increase cholesterol and TG. Latent DM may manifest with therapy. Syncope reported.

**ADVERSE REACTIONS:** Dizziness, headache, cough, fatigue, orthostatic effects, angiodema/anaphylactoid reactions.

**INTERACTIONS:** Lisinopril: May increase lithium levels. Hypotension risk with diuretics. Concomitant use with antidiabetic medications may increase risk of hypoglycemia. Coadministration with NSAIDs in patients with compromised renal function may cause further deterioration. Increased risk of hyperkalemia with $K^+$-sparing diuretics, $K^+$-containing salt substitutes, or $K^+$ supplements. Indomethacin may reduce effects. Nitritoid reactions with gold. HCTZ: Potentiates orthostatic hypotension with alcohol, barbiturates, and narcotics. Dose adjustment may be required with antidiabetics. Reduced absorption with cholestyramine, colestipol. Corticosteroids and ACTH may deplete electrolytes. May decrease response to pressor amines. Potentiates other antihypertensives. May increase responsiveness to skeletal muscle relaxants. Risk of lithium toxicity. NSAIDs may worsen renal dysfunction and reduce diuretic, natriuretic, and antihypertensive effects.

**PREGNANCY:** Category C (1st trimester) and D (2nd and 3rd trimesters), not for use in nursing.

**MECHANISM OF ACTION:** Lisinopril: ACE inhibitor; inhibition results in decreased plasma angiotensin II, which leads to decreased vasopressor activity and aldosterone secretion. HCTZ: Thiazide diuretic; affects renal tubular mechanism of electrolyte reabsorption, directly increasing excretion of $Na^+$ and $Cl^-$.

**PHARMACOKINETICS: Absorption:** Lisinopril: $T_{max}$=7 hrs. **Distribution:** HCTZ: Crosses placenta. **Elimination:** Lisinopril: Urine (unchanged); $T_{1/2}$=12 hrs. HCTZ: Kidneys; $T_{1/2}$=5.6-14.8 hrs.

## NURSING CONSIDERATIONS

**Assessment:** Assess BP, LFTs, renal function, CVD (eg, cardiomyopathy, aortic stenosis), renal artery stenosis, SLE, serum electrolytes, history of angioedema and allergy to sulfonamides, bronchial asthma, parathyroid disorders. Assess pregnancy/nursing status and for possible drug interactions.

**Monitoring:** Monitor BP, LFTs, renal function, CBC with platelet count and differential, serum electrolytes. Monitor for MI, CHF, angioedema (head/neck, intestinal), anaphylactoid reactions, hepatic failure, hyperuricemia, hyperglycemia, hypersensitivity reactions, cough, N/V, dizziness, mood alterations.

**Patient Counseling:** Inform about fetal risks if taken during pregnancy. Advise to report if pregnant. Advise to watch for signs and symptoms of angioedema (eg, swelling of face, extremities, eyes, lips, SOB). Caution that inadequate fluid intake, excessive perspiration, diarrhea, and vomiting may lead to excessive fall in BP, resulting in lightheadedness or possible syncope. Advise not to use $K^+$ supplements or salt substitutes containing $K^+$ without consulting physician. Inform about need for periodic monitoring of electrolytes and blood counts. Counsel about signs/symptoms of neutropenia (eg, infection, sore throat, fever), angioedema, electrolyte imbalance (eg, thirst, weakness, lethargy), and other potential adverse effects; seek prompt medical attention if any occur.

**Administration:** Oral route. **Storage:** 20-25°C (68-77°F). Protect from excessive light and humidity.

# ZESTRIL

RX

lisinopril (AstraZeneca)

**ACE inhibitors can cause injury/death to developing fetus during 2nd and 3rd trimesters. D/C if pregnancy is detected.**

**THERAPEUTIC CLASS:** ACE inhibitor

**INDICATIONS:** Treatment of HTN. Adjunct therapy in heart failure if inadequately controlled by diuretics and digitalis. Adjunct therapy in stable patients within 24 hrs of AMI to improve survival.

**DOSAGE:** *Adults:* HTN: Initial: 10mg qd. Adjust dose according to BP response. Usual: 20-40mg qd. Max: 80mg/day. May add a low-dose diuretic if BP not controlled. Diuretic-Treated Patients: D/C diuretic 2-3 days prior to therapy to reduce hypotension. Adjust dose according to BP response. If diuretic cannot be d/c; give initial dose of 5mg under medical supervision for at least 2 hrs and BP stabilized for 1 hr. CrCl 10-30mL/min: Initial: 5mg/day. CrCl <10mL/min: Initial: 2.5mg/day. Titrate up until BP is controlled. Max: 40mg/day. Heart Failure: Initial: 5mg qd. Usual: 5-40mg qd. May increase by 10mg every 2 weeks. Max: 40mg/day. Heart failure/Hyponatremia or CrCl ≤30mL/min or SrCr >3mg/dL: Initial: 2.5mg qd under close medical supervision. AMI: Initial: 5mg within 24 hrs, then 5mg after 24 hrs, then 10mg after 48 hrs, then 10mg qd. Patients with low SBP (≤120mmHg) when treatment is started or during the 1st 3 days after the infact should be given 2.5mg PO. Maintenance dose of 5mg qd may be given with temporary reductions to 2.5mg prn if prolonged hypotension (SBP≤100mmHg) occurs. D/C with prolonged hypotension (SBP<90mmHg for more than 1 hr). Dose Adjustment with MI with Renal Impairment: Initiate treatment with caution. Elderly: Caution with dose adjustment.

*Pediatrics:* ≥6 yrs: HTN: Initial: 0.07mg/kg qd up to 5mg total. Adjust dose according to response. Max: 0.61mg/kg or 40mg.

**HOW SUPPLIED:** Tab: 2.5mg, 5mg*, 10mg, 20mg, 30mg, 40mg *scored

**CONTRAINDICATIONS:** History of ACE inhibitor-associated angioedema, hereditary or idiopathic angioedema.

**WARNINGS/PRECAUTIONS:** Anaphylactoid reactions during membrane exposure, and angioedema of the head and neck (rarely with fatalities) and of the intestines reported. Rate of angioedema higher in blacks. Rarely, syndrome of cholestatic jaundice progressing to fulminant necrotic hepatitis and death reported. D/C if angioedema, jaundice, or marked LFT elevation occur. Risk of hyperkalemia, hypoglycemia with DM, renal dysfunction. Persistent nonproductive cough reported; resolves upon d/c. Monitor WBCs in renal and collagen vascular disease; agranulocytosis and bone marrow depression may occur. Monitor for hypotension in high-risk patients (heart failure with SBP <100mmHg, surgery/anesthesia, hyponatremia, high-dose diuretic therapy, severe volume, and/or salt depletion, etc.). Caution with CHF, aortic stenosis/hypertrophic cardiomyopathy, renal dysfunction, and renal artery stenosis. Less effective on BP in blacks. Not recommended in pediatric patients with GFR <30mL/min/1.73min².

**ADVERSE REACTIONS:** Chest pain, cough, diarrhea, dizziness, headache, hyperkalemia, hypotension, syncope, angioedema, increased creatinine and non-protein nitrogen.

**INTERACTIONS:** May increase lithium levels. Hypotension risk with diuretics. Concomitant use with antidiabetic medications may increase risk of hypoglycemia. Coadministration with NSAIDs in patients with compromised renal function may cause further deterioration. Increased risk of hyperkalemia with $K^+$-sparing diuretics, $K^+$-containing salt substitutes, or $K^+$ supplements. Indomethacin may reduce effects. Nitritoid reactions with gold.

**PREGNANCY:** Category C (1st trimester) and D (2nd and 3rd trimesters), not for use in nursing.

**MECHANISM OF ACTION:** ACE inhibitor; inhibition results in decreased plasma angiotensin II, which leads to decreased vasopressor activity and aldosterone secretion.

**PHARMACOKINETICS: Absorption:** $T_{max}$=7 hrs. **Elimination:** Urine (unchanged); $T_{1/2}$=12 hrs.

## NURSING CONSIDERATIONS

**Assessment:** Assess BP, LFTs, renal function, CVD (eg, aortic stenosis, cardiomyopathy), renal artery stenosis, pregnancy/nursing status, and for possible drug interactions.

**Monitoring:** Monitor BP, LFTs, renal function, CBC with platelet count and differential, serum $K^+$ levels. Monitor for MI, CHF, angioedema (head, neck, intestinal), anaphylactoid reactions, hepatic failure, hypoglycemia, hypersensitivity reactions, cough, N/V, dizziness, mood alterations.

**Patient Counseling:** Inform about fetal risks during pregnancy. Advise to report if pregnant. Advise to watch for signs/symptoms of angioedema (laryngeal/tongue edema, abdominal pain); seek prompt medical attention if symptoms develop. Inform about potential adverse effects (eg, anaphylaxis, cough, hypotension, hyperkalemia, diarrhea, dizziness, headaches, mood alterations). Report any indication of infection (eg, sore throat, fever) which may be a sign of leukopenia/neutropenia. Inform about need for periodic monitoring of electrolytes and blood counts. Caution that inadequate fluid intake, excessive perspiration, diarrhea, vomiting may lead to excessive fall in BP, which can result in lightheadedness or possible syncope. Advise not to use $K^+$ supplements or salt substitutes containing $K^+$ without consulting physician. Advise to report if pregnant.

**Administration:** Oral route. **Storage:** 20-25°C (68-77°F). Protect from moisture, freezing, and excessive heat.

# ZETIA RX

ezetimibe (Merck/Schering-Plough)

**THERAPEUTIC CLASS:** Cholesterol absorption inhibitor

**INDICATIONS:** Adjunct to diet, as monotherapy or with concomitant HMG-CoA reductase inhibitors, to reduce total cholesterol (total-C), low-density lipoprotein cholesterol (LDL-C), and apolipoprotein B (Apo B) levels in primary (heterozygous familial and nonfamilial) hyperlipidemia. Adjunct to diet, with concomitant fenofibrate, to reduce elevated total-C, LDL-C, Apo B, and non-high-density lipoprotein cholesterol (non-HDL-C) in adults with mixed hyperlipidemia. Adjunct to other lipid-lowering treatments or if such treatments are unavailable, with concomitant atorvastatin or simvastatin, to reduce total-C and LDL-C in homozygous familial hypercholesterolemia (HoFH). Adjunct to diet, to reduce sitosterol and campesterol levels in homozygous familial sitosterolemia.

**DOSAGE:** *Adults:* 10mg qd. May give with HMG-CoA reductase inhibitor (with primary hypercholesterolemia) or fenofibrate (with mixed hyperlipidemia) for incremental effect. Concomitant Bile Acid Sequestrant: Give either ≥2 hrs before or ≥4 hrs after bile acid sequestrant.

**HOW SUPPLIED:** Tab: 10mg

**CONTRAINDICATIONS:** When used with a statin, ezetimibe is contraindicated in pregnancy, nursing, and in patients with active liver disease or unexplained persistent elevations in hepatic transaminase levels.

**WARNINGS/PRECAUTIONS:** Concurrent statin therapy may lead to transaminase elevations; monitor LFTs. May increase risk of rhabdomyolysis/myopathy especially during concomitant use with fibrate or statin therapy; d/c use of ezetimibe, fibrate, or statin if myopathy is suspected. Not recommended with moderate or severe hepatic insufficiency.

**ADVERSE REACTIONS:** Upper respiratory tract infection, nasopharyngitis, arthralgia, diarrhea, myalgia, sinusitis, pain in extremities, liver enzyme abnormalities, rhabdomyolysis/myopathy.

**INTERACTIONS:** See Contraindications. Monitor cyclosporine levels during concomitant use; may increase exposure to both drugs. Use with fenofibrate may increase fenofibrate and ezetimibe levels; concomitant use with fenofibrate may cause cholelithiasis requiring gallbladder studies and alternate lipid-lowering therapy. Use with gemfibrozil may increase levels of ezetimibe and may decrease gemfibrozil levels; fibrates may increase cholesterol excretion in the bile, leading to cholelithiasis; co-administration of ezetimibe with fibrates other than fenofibrate is not recommended. Use with cholestyramine may decrease ezetimibe concentrations; incremental LDL-C reduction may be reduced by this interaction. Monitor INR when administered with warfarin. Use with aluminum and magnesium hydroxide may lead to a decrease in ezetimibe concentrations. Use with cimetidine may increase ezetimibe concentrations. Use with glipizide may cause an increase in AUC of ezetimibe, a decrease in $C_{max}$ of ezetimibe, and a decrease in glipizide concentrations. Use with digoxin may lead to an increase in AUC of digoxin and a decrease in $C_{max}$ of digoxin. Use with ethinyl estradiol and levonorgestrel may lead to a decrease in $C_{max}$ of ethinyl estradiol and levonorgestrel. Use with lovastatin may lead to an increase in ezetimibe and lovastatin concentrations. Concomitant use with pravastatin may lead to an increase in ezetimibe and a decrease in pravastatin concentrations. Use with atorvastatin may lead to a decrease in the AUC of atorvastatin, an increase in the $C_{max}$ of atorvastatin, a decrease in the AUC of ezetimibe, and an increase in the $C_{max}$ of ezetimibe. Use with rosuvastatin may lead to a increase in ezetimibe and rosuvastatin concentrations. Use with fluvastatin may lead to a decrease in AUC of ezetimibe, an increase in $C_{max}$ of ezetimibe, and a decrease in fluvastatin concentrations.

**PREGNANCY:** Category C, caution in nursing.

**MECHANISM OF ACTION:** Cholesterol absorption inhibitor; inhibits absorption of cholesterol by small intestine. Targets the sterol transporter, Neimann-Pick C1-like 1 (NPC1L1), which is involved in intestinal uptake of cholesterol and phytosterols; inhibited uptake leads to decrease in delivery of intestinal cholesterol to the liver, causing reduction of hepatic cholesterol stores and increase in clearance of cholesterol from the blood. Mechanism is complementary to that of statins and of fenofibrate.

**PHARMACOKINETICS: Absorption:** Ezetimibe: $C_{max}$=3.4-5.5ng/mL; $T_{max}$=4-12 hrs. Ezetimibe-glucuronide (active metabolite) $C_{max}$=45-71ng/mL; $T_{max}$=1-2 hrs. **Distribution:** Plasma protein binding (>90%). **Metabolism:** Small intestine, liver via glucuronide conjugation; Ezetimibe-glucuronide (major active metabolite). **Elimination:** Feces (78%), urine (11%); $T_{1/2}$=22 hrs.

## NURSING CONSIDERATIONS

**Assessment:** Assess for presence of hepatic impairment, pregnancy/nursing status, and for possible drug interactions. If using in combination with statin therapy, assess for risk factors for skeletal muscle toxicity (eg, use with higher doses of statins, advanced age, hypothyroidism, renal impairment, concomitant drug use). Obtain baseline lipid profile (total-C, LDL-C, HDL-C, TG). If using in combination with statin therapy, obtain baseline LFTs.

**Monitoring:** Monitor for signs/symptoms of elevated liver enzymes, myopathy, and rhabdomyolysis. Periodically monitor LFTs if during concomitant therapy with a HMG-CoA reductase inhibitor. Monitor lipid profile while on therapy.

**Patient Counseling:** Recommend standard cholesterol-lowering diet before and during treatment. Advise drug may be taken with/without food. Counsel about risk of myopathy and instruct to contact physician promptly if any unexplained muscle pain, tenderness, or weakness occur. Counsel to undergo LFTs when drug is added to statin therapy. Inform that if using ezetimibe in combination with statin therapy that should use an effective method of birth control or stop treatment if trying to conceive due to the potential risk to the fetus. Advise not to breastfeed if using ezetimibe with statin therapy. Instruct that, if on concomitant therapy with bile acid sequestrant, dosing of drug should occur either ≥2 hrs before or ≥4 hrs after administration of the bile acid sequestrant.

**Administration:** Oral route. **Storage:** 25°C (77°F); excursions permitted to 15-30°C (59-86°F). Protect from moisture.

# ZEVALIN RX

ibritumomab tiuxetan (Spectrum)

**D/C if severe infusion reactions occur, fatalities reported. Severe and prolonged cytopenias reported; avoid if ≥25% lymphoma marrow involvement and/or impaired bone marrow reserve. Severe, some fatal, cutaneous and mucocutaneous reactions reported. Do not exceed the maximum dose and do not admnister to patients with altered biodistribution.**

**THERAPEUTIC CLASS:** Monoclonal antibody

**INDICATIONS:** Treatment of relapsed or refractory low-grade or follicular B-cell non-Hodgkin's lymphoma (NHL) and previously untreated follicular NHL in patients who achieve partial or complete response to first-line chemotherapy.

**DOSAGE:** *Adults:* Day 1: Rituximab 250mg/m² IV single infusion. Within 4 hrs, give 5mCi of In-111 ibritumomab IV. Assess biodistribution scan at 48-72 hrs after In-111 and may be optional at other points. If biodistribution acceptable, Day 7-9: Rituximab 250mg/m² IV. Within 4 hrs, give Y-90 Ibritumomab 0.4mCi/kg (or 0.3mCi/kg if platelets 100,000-149,000 cells/mm³). Max: Y-90 ibritumomab 32mCi.

**HOW SUPPLIED:** Inj: 3.2mg/2mL

**WARNINGS/PRECAUTIONS:** To be used with rituximab. Leukemia and mylodysplastic syndrome reported. May cause fetal harm. Single-course treatment only. Monitor closely for evidence of extravasation; d/c infusion if with signs or symptoms of extravasation and restart in another limb. Monitor CBC and platelets weekly until levels recover. Minimize radiation exposure to patients. Contains albumin; remote risk of transmission of viral disease and CJD.

**ADVERSE REACTIONS:** Cytopenias (eg, neutropenia, thrombocytopenia, anemia), fatigue, abdominal pain, nausea, nasopharyngitis, asthenia, diarrhea, cough, pyrexia, myalgia, anorexia, night sweats and influenza-like illness.

**INTERACTIONS:** Avoid with live vaccines.

**PREGNANCY:** Category D, not for use in nursing.

**MECHANISM OF ACTION:** Monoclonal antibody; binds specifically to CD20 antigen, which is expressed on pre-B and mature B lymphocytes, and on B-cell non-Hodgkin's lymphomas.

**PHARMACOKINETICS: Elimination:** Urine (7.5%); $T_{1/2}$=30 hrs.

## NURSING CONSIDERATIONS

**Assessment:** Assess for hypersensitivity, infusion reactions, cytopenia, hemorrhage, severe infections, erythema multiforme, Stevens-Johnson syndrome, lymphoma marrow involvement and/or impaired bone marrow reserves, history of failed stem cell collection, altered biodistribution, and pregnancy status.

**Monitoring:** Monitor for infusion reactions (eg, urticaria, hypotension, angioedema, hypoxia, bronchospasm, pulmonary infiltrates, acute respiratory distress, MI, ventricular filtration, cardiogenic shock), thrombocytopenia, neutropenia, hemorrhage, cerebral hemorrhage, severe infections, Stevens-Johnson syndrome, exfoliative dermatitis, toxic epidermal necrolysis, leukemia, myelodysplastic syndrome, pregnancy, extravasation during drug infusion, radiation exposure, viral diseases (Creutzfeldt-Jakob disease), and lab tests (eg, CBC, platelets).

**Patient Counseling:** Counsel about risk of allergic or serious hypersensitivity, to avoid pregnancy/nursing, and use of effective contraceptives in females of childbearing potential. Advise to immediately seek medical intervention if bleeding, easy bruising, painful sores, ulcers, blisters or peeling skin, hives, swelling, dizziness, blurred vision, drowsiness, headache, cough, wheezing, difficulty breathing, weakness, fatigue, or infection occur. Caution against immunization with live vaccines.

**Administration:** IV route. Refer to PI for specific instructions. **Storage:** 2-8°C (36-46°F). Do not freeze.

# ZIAC RX

## bisoprolol fumarate - hydrochlorothiazide (Duramed)

**THERAPEUTIC CLASS:** Selective $beta_1$-blocker/thiazide diuretic

**INDICATIONS:** Management of hypertension.

**DOSAGE:** *Adults:* Initial: 2.5mg-6.25mg qd. Maint: May increase every 14 days. Max: 20mg-12.5mg/day. Replacement therapy: Substitute for titrated individual components. Renal/Hepatic Dysfunction: Caution in dosing/titrating. Cessation of therapy: Withdraw gradually over 2 weeks.

**HOW SUPPLIED:** Tab: (Bisoprolol-HCTZ) 2.5mg-6.25mg, 5mg-6.25mg, 10mg-6.25mg

**CONTRAINDICATIONS:** Cardiogenic shock, overt cardiac failure, 2nd- or 3rd-degree AV block, marked sinus bradycardia, anuria, sulfonamide hypersensitivity.

**WARNINGS/PRECAUTIONS:** Caution with compensated cardiac failure, diabetes mellitus (DM), bronchospastic disease, hepatic/renal impairment, or peripheral vascular disease (PVD). Avoid abrupt withdrawal; exacerbation of angina pectoris, myocardial infarctions, and ventricular arrhythmias observed. Monitor for fluid/electrolyte imbalance; hypokalemia, hypercalcemia, hypophosphatemia reported. May activate/exacerbate systemic lupus erythematosus (SLE). Enhanced effects in post-sympathectomy patients. May mask hyperthyroidism or hypoglycemia symptoms. May precipitate hyperuricemia, acute gout, cardiac failure. May impair physical/mental abilities.

**ADVERSE REACTIONS:** Diarrhea, headache, dizziness, fatigue.

**INTERACTIONS:** Alcohol, barbiturates, or narcotics may potentiate orthostatic hypotension. Adjust dose of antidiabetic drugs. Potentiates other antihypertensives. Avoid other β-blockers. Impaired absorption with cholestyramine, colestipol. Corticosteroids, ACTH intensify electrolyte depletion. May decrease response to pressor amines. May increase response to nondepolarizing muscle relaxants. Risk of lithium toxicity. NSAIDs may reduce effects. May block epinephrine effects. Excessive reduction of sympathetic activity with catecholamine-depleting drugs. Caution with clonidine withdrawal. Increased clearance with rifampin. Caution with CCBs, myocardial depressants, anesthesia, and antiarrhythmics. Digitalis glycosides and β-blockers slow atrioventricular conduction and decrease HR; concomitant use can increase the risk of bradycardia.

**PREGNANCY:** Category C, not for use in nursing.

**MECHANISM OF ACTION:** Bisoprolol: $\beta_1$-selective, cardioselective, adrenoreceptor-blocking agent; decreases HR, increases sinus node recovery time, prolongs AV-node refractory periods, and prolongs AV-nodal conduction with rapid atrial stimulation. HCTZ: Thiazide diuretic; affects renal tubular mechanisms of electrolyte reabsorption and increases excretion of $Na^+$ and $Cl^-$.

**PHARMACOKINETICS: Absorption:** Bisoprolol: Absolute bioavailability (80%); (2.5mg) $C_{max}$=9ng/mL, $T_{max}$=3 hrs. HCTZ: Well-absorbed; $C_{max}$=30ng/mL, $T_{max}$=2.5 hrs. **Distribution**: Bisoprolol: Plasma protein binding (30%). HCTZ: Plasma protein binding (40-68%). **Elimination:** Bisoprolol: $T_{1/2}$=7-15 hrs; urine (55% unchanged). HCTZ: $T_{1/2}$=4-10 hrs; urine (60% unchanged).

## NURSING CONSIDERATIONS

**Assessment:** Assess for bradycardia, cardiogenic shock, 2nd- or 3rd-degree heart block, overt cardiac failure, impaired renal/hepatic function, bronchospastic disease, PVD, DM, thyrotoxicosis, anuria, sulfonamide hypersensitivity, history of allergy or bronchial asthma, parathyroid disease, possible drug interactions.

**Monitoring:** Monitor for cardiac failure, exacerbation of ischemia following abrupt withdrawal, bronchospastic disease, arrhythmias, WBC and platelet count, hypersensitivity reactions and reversible mental depression. Serum electrolytes should be checked periodically. Monitor for signs/symptoms of electrolyte imbalance, hyperglycemia, hyperuricemia or precipitation of gout, hypersensitivity reactions, and renal/hepatic dysfunction.

**Patient Counseling:** Instruct not to interrupt or d/c therapy without consulting a physician. Notify healthcare provider if signs/symptoms of impending CHF or unexplained respiratory symptoms develop. Advise to exercise caution while operating machinery/driving. Advise to seek medical attention if symptoms of electrolyte imbalance (eg, dry mouth, thirst, weakness) or hypersensitivity/photosensitivity reactions occur. Inform diabetics that drug may mask symptoms of hypoglycemia.

**Administration:** Oral route. **Storage**: 20-25°C (68-77°F).

## Ziagen

RX

abacavir sulfate (GlaxoSmithKline)

**Fatal hypersensitivity reactions reported; d/c if hypersensitivity reaction suspected and do not restart to avoid more serious symptoms, including hypotension and death. High risk of hypersensitivity reaction to abacavir in patients with HLA-B*5701 allele; screening is recommended prior to therapy. Lactic acidosis and severe hepatomegaly with steatosis (including fatal cases) reported.**

**THERAPEUTIC CLASS:** Synthetic carbocyclic nucleoside analogue

**INDICATIONS:** Treatment of HIV-1 infection in combination with other antiretrovirals.

**DOSAGE:** *Adults:* 300mg bid or 600mg qd. Mild Hepatic Impairment (Child-Pugh: 5-6): 200mg bid.
*Pediatrics:* Oral Sol: ≥3 months: 8mg/kg bid. Max: 300mg bid. Tab: 14-21 kg: 150mg (1/2 tab) bid. >21-<30 kg: 150mg (1/2 tab) in AM, 300mg (1 tab) in PM. ≥30 kg: 300mg (1 tab) bid. Max: 600mg/day.

**HOW SUPPLIED:** Sol: 20mg/mL [240mL]; Tab: 300mg* *scored

**CONTRAINDICATIONS:** Moderate or severe hepatic impairment.

**WARNINGS/PRECAUTIONS:** Caution in patients with known risk factors for liver disease. Suspend therapy in any patient who develops clinical or laboratory findings suggestive of lactic acidosis or pronounced hepatotoxicity. Immune reconstitution syndrome reported. Redistribution/accumulation of body fat including central obesity, dorsocervical fat enlargement, peripheral wasting, facial wasting, breast enlargement, and "cushingoid appearance" reported. Increased risk of MI; caution in patients with underlying risk factors for coronary heart disease (eg, hyperlipidemia, HTN, DM, smoking). Caution in elderly.

**ADVERSE REACTIONS:** Headache/migraine, malaise/fatigue, nausea, dream/sleep disorders, hypersensitivity, diarrhea, rashes, GI disturbances, depressive disorders, dizziness, musculoskeletal pain, fever/chills, elevated CPK, elevated ALT/AST, hypertriglyceridemia.

**INTERACTIONS:** Concomitant use with ethanol may decrease the elimination of abacavir and increase overall exposure. Concomitant use with methadone may increase the clearance of methadone and may require an increased dose of methadone.

**PREGNANCY:** Category C, not for use in nursing.

**MECHANISM OF ACTION:** Carbocyclic nucleoside analogue; inhibits HIV-1 reverse transcriptase (RT) by competing with natural substrate dGTP and its incorporation into viral DNA.

**PHARMACOKINETICS: Absorption:** Rapid; absolute bioavailabilty (83%). (300 mg bid) $C_{max}$= 3mcg/mL, $AUC_{0\text{-}12h}$=6.02mcg•hr/mL. (600 mg qd) $C_{max}$= 4.26mcg/mL, AUC=11.95mcg•hr/mL. **Distribution:** (IV) $V_d$=0.86L/kg; plasma protein binding (50%). **Metabolism:** Via alcohol dehydrogenase and glucuronyl transferase. **Elimination:** Urine (1.2%, abacavir), (30%, 5'-carboxylic acid metabolite), (36%, 5'glucuronide metabolite), (15% unidentified minor metabolites); $T_{1/2}$=1.54 hrs (single dose).

## NURSING CONSIDERATIONS

**Assessment:** Assess for moderate or severe hepatic impairment, risk factors for coronary heart disease (eg, HTN, hyperlipidemia, DM, smoking),

Z

pregnancy/nursing status, and for possible drug interactions. Assess for HLA-B*5701 allele prior to initiation of therapy and prior to reinitiation of therapy.

**Monitoring:** Monitor for signs/symptoms of hypersensitivity (eg, fever, rash, N/V, diarrhea, generalized malaise, fatigue, dyspnea, cough), immune reconstitution syndrome, fat redistribution/accumulation, lactic acidosis, and for hepatomegaly with steatosis. Monitor CPK, ALT/AST, and triglycerides. May enroll patients in the Antiretroviral Pregnancy Registry if they become pregnant while on treatment.

**Patient Counseling:** Inform that therapy is not cure for HIV, does not reduce risk of transmission of HIV and that opportunistic infections may develop. Inform if treatment is interrupted, do not restart or replace with any drug containing abacavir without medical consultation. Instruct to seek medical attention if experience symptoms of hypersensitivity (eg, fever, rash, N/V, diarrhea, generalized malaise, fatigue, dyspnea, cough), lactic acidosis, hepatomegaly, immune reconstitution syndrome, or fat redistribution/accumulation.

**Administration:** Oral route. **Storage**: 20-25°C (68-77°F). Sol: Do not freeze. May be refrigerated.

## ZIANA RX

clindamycin phosphate - tretinoin (Medicis)

**THERAPEUTIC CLASS:** Lincosamide derivative/retinoid

**INDICATIONS:** Topical treatment of acne vulgaris in patients ≥12 yrs.

**DOSAGE:** *Adults:* Apply at hs a pea-sized amount of medication onto one fingertip, dot onto the chin, cheeks, nose, and forehead, then gently rub over entire face.

*Pediatrics:* ≥12 yrs: Apply at hs a pea-sized amount of medication onto one fingertip, dot onto the chin, cheeks, nose, and forehead, then gently rub over entire face.

**HOW SUPPLIED:** Gel: (Clindamycin-Tretinoin) 1.2%-0.025% [2g, 30g, 60g]

**CONTRAINDICATIONS:** Regional enteritis, ulcerative colitis, or history of antibiotic-associated colitis.

**WARNINGS/PRECAUTIONS:** May cause severe colitis; d/c if significant diarrhea occurs. Avoid exposure to sunlight and sunlamps; wear sunscreen and protective apparel daily. Avoid eyes, mouth, angles of nose, or mucous membranes. Not for oral, ophthalmic, or intravaginal use.

**ADVERSE REACTIONS:** Nasopharyngitis, erythema, scaling, itching, burning, gastrointestinal symptoms.

**INTERACTIONS:** Caution with concomitant topical medications, medicated/abrasive soaps and cleansers, soaps/cosmetics with strong drying effect, products with high concentrations of alcohol, astringents, spices, or lime. Avoid with erythromycin-containing products. Caution with neuromuscular blocking agents. Antiperistaltic agents (eg, opiates, diphenoxylate with atropine) may prolong and/or worsen severe colitis.

**PREGNANCY:** Category C, not for use in nursing.

**MECHANISM OF ACTION:** Clindamycin: Lincosamide antibiotic; binds to 50S ribosomal subunits of susceptible bacteria and prevents elongation of peptide chains by interfering with peptidyl transfer, thereby suppressing bacterial protein synthesis. Found to have activity against *P. acnes*. Tretinoin: Retinoid; not established. Suspected to decrease cohesiveness of follicular epithelial cells with decreased microcomedo formation. Also responsible for stimulating miotic activity and increasing turnover of follicular epithelial cells, causing extrusion of comedones.

**PHARMACOKINETICS: Absorption:** Tretinoin: Percutaneous (minimal). **Distribution:** Orally and parenterally administered clindamycin found in breast milk. **Metabolism:** Tretinoin: 13-cis-retinoic acid and 4-oxo-13-cis-retinoic acid (metabolites).

## NURSING CONSIDERATIONS

**Assessment:** Assess for regional enteritis, ulcerative colitis, or history of antibiotic-associated colitis. Assess use in pregnancy/nursing and for possible drug interactions.

**Monitoring:** Monitor for signs/symptoms of diarrhea, bloody diarrhea, and colitis (including pseudomembranous colitis). Perform stool cultures to identify *Clostridium difficile* and stool assay to identify *C.difficile* toxin. Monitor for signs/symptoms of skin irritation (eg, erythema, scaling, burning, stinging).

**Patient Counseling:** Instruct to wash face gently with mild soap and warm water at bedtime before applying. Advise not to use excessive amount; may cause skin irritation. Avoid washing face more than 2-3 times a day; may worsen acne. Advise to avoid exposure to sunlight/sunlamps; use sunscreen and protective clothing outdoors. Inform that weather extremes, such as wind or cold, may irritate skin during therapy.

**Administration:** Topical route. **Storage:** Store at room temperature, 15-30°C (59-86°F). Do not freeze. Keep away from heat and light.

# ZINACEF RX

cefuroxime (GlaxoSmithKline)

**THERAPEUTIC CLASS:** Cephalosporin (2nd generation)

**INDICATIONS:** Treatment of septicemia; meningitis; gonorrhea; lower respiratory tract, urinary tract, skin and skin structure (SSSI), and bone and joint infections caused by susceptible strains of microorganisms. For preoperative and perioperative surgical prophylaxis.

**DOSAGE:** *Adults:* Usual: 750mg-1.5g q8h for 5-10 days. Uncomplicated Pneumonia and UTI/SSSI/Disseminated Gonococcal Infections: 750mg q8h. Severe/Complicated Infections: 1.5g q8h. Bone and Joint Infections: 1.5g q8h. Life-Threatening Infections/Infections With Susceptible Organisms: 1.5g q6h. Meningitis: Max: 3g q8h. Uncomplicated Gonococcal Infection: 1.5g IM single dose at 2 different sites with 1g PO probenecid. Surgical Prophylaxis: 1.5g IV 0.5-1 hr before incision, then 750mg IM/IV q8h with prolonged procedure. Open Heart Surgery (Perioperative): 1.5g IV at induction of anesthesia and q12h thereafter, for total of 6g. Renal Impairment: CrCl 10-20mL/min: 750mg q12h. CrCl <10mL/min: 750mg q24h. Hemodialysis: Give further dose at end of dialysis.

*Pediatrics:* >3 months: Usual: 50-100mg/kg/day in divided doses q6-8h. Severe Infections: 100mg/kg/day (not to exceed max adult dose). Bone and Joint Infections: 150mg/kg/day in divided doses q8h (not to exceed max adult dose). Meningitis: 200-240mg/kg/day IV in divided doses q6-8h. Renal Insufficiency: Modify dosing frequency consistent with adult recommendations.

**HOW SUPPLIED:** Inj: 750mg, 1.5g, 7.5g, 750mg/50mL, 1.5g/50mL.

**WARNINGS/PRECAUTIONS:** Caution with use in penicillin-sensitive patients or patients who have demonstrated some form of allergy, particularly drugs. D/C use if an allergic reaction occurs. *Clostridium difficile*-associated diarrhea (CDAD) reported, ranging in severity from mild diarrhea to fatal colitis. Monitor renal function. Prolonged use may result in overgrowth of nonsusceptible organisms; take appropriate measures if superinfection develops. Caution with history of GI disease, particularly colitis. Hearing loss reported in peds being treated for meningitis. Risk of decreased prothrombin activity with renal or hepatic impairment, poor nutritional state, or protracted course of therapy. Use in the absence of a proven or strongly suspected bacterial infection or a prophylactic indication is unlikely to provide benefit and increases the risk of the development of drug-resistant bacteria. False (+) urine glucose with copper reduction tests and false (-) with ferricyanide test.

**ADVERSE REACTIONS:** Thrombophlebitis, GI symptoms, decreased Hgb and Hct, eosinophilia. Transient rise in SGOT, SGPT, alkaline phosphatase, bilirubin, and LDH.

**INTERACTIONS:** Possible nephrotoxicity with concomitant administration of aminoglycosides. Caution with potent diuretics; may adversely affect renal function. May decrease prothrombin activity; caution with anticoagulants. May affect the gut flora, leading to lower estrogen reabsorption and reduced efficacy of combined estrogen/progesterone oral contraceptives. Concomitant oral administration of probenecid with cefuroxime may increase peak serum levels and the serum-half life.

**PREGNANCY:** Category B, caution in nursing.

**MECHANISM OF ACTION:** 2nd-generation cephalosporin; inhibits cell-wall synthesis.

**PHARMACOKINETICS: Absorption**: $C_{max}$(750mg IM, IV)=27mcg/mL, 50mcg/mL; $T_{max}$(750mg IM, IV)=45 min, 15 min. **Distribution:** Plasma protein binding (50%); found in breast milk. **Elimination**: Urine; $T_{1/2}$=80 min.

## NURSING CONSIDERATIONS

**Assessment:** Assess for presence of allergies including allergy to penicillin, renal/hepatic impairment, nutritional status, history of GI disease (eg, colitis), pregnancy/nursing status, and for possible drug interactions. Document indications for therapy, culture, and susceptibility testing.

**Monitoring:** Monitor for signs/symptoms of an allergic reaction, CDAD, and for overgrowth of nonsusceptible organisms. In pediatric patients with meningitis, monitor for hearing loss. Monitor renal function and PT.

**Patient Counseling:** Inform therapy only treats bacterial, not viral, infections. Instruct to take as directed. Advise that skipping doses or not completing full course may decrease effectiveness and increase resistance. Inform that may experience diarrhea. Instruct to notify physician if watery/bloody stools, superinfections, or an allergic reaction develops.

**Administration:** IV/IM routes. Refer to PI for administration procedures.
**Storage:** (Dry State) 15-30°C (59-86°F). Protect from light. (Frozen Premixed Solution) Should not be stored above -20°C.

# ZINECARD RX

dexrazoxane (Pharmacia & Upjohn)

**THERAPEUTIC CLASS:** EDTA derivative

**INDICATIONS:** To reduce the incidence and severity of cardiomyopathy associated with doxorubicin in women with metastatic breast cancer who received a cumulative doxorubicin dose of 300mg/m² and who will continue doxorubicin therapy.

**DOSAGE:** *Adults:* IV: 10:1 ratio of dexrazoxane:doxorubicin (eg, 500mg/m² dexrazoxane:50mg/m² doxorubicin). Hepatic Impairment: Reduce dose proportionally. Give by slow IV push or rapid IV infusion. Give doxorubicin within 30 min after start of infusion.

**HOW SUPPLIED:** Inj: 250mg, 500mg

**CONTRAINDICATIONS:** Chemotherapy regimens not containing an anthracycline.

**WARNINGS/PRECAUTIONS:** Not for use with initiation of doxorubicin therapy. Monitor cardiac function. May cause secondary malignancies. Obtain frequent CBCs. Caution with moderate or severe renal insufficiency; reduce dose by 50% if CrCl <40mL/min.

**ADVERSE REACTIONS:** Alopecia, nausea, vomiting, fatigue, malaise, anorexia, stomatitis, fever, infection, diarrhea, pain on injection, sepsis, neurotoxicity, streaking/erythema.

**INTERACTIONS:** Avoid use during the initiation of FAC (fluorouracil, doxorubicin, cyclophosphamide) therapy. Additive myelosuppression with other chemotherapies.

**PREGNANCY:** Category C, not for use in nursing.

Z

**MECHANISM OF ACTION:** EDTA derivative; suspected to interfere with iron-mediated free radical generation.

**PHARMACOKINETICS: Absorption:** $C_{max}$(500mg/m²)=36.5mcg/ml. **Distribution**: $V_d$=25L/m². **Elimination:** Urine (42%).

## NURSING CONSIDERATIONS

**Assessment:** Assess renal/hepatic function, CBC with differential and platelet count, LVEF, pregnancy status, and for possible drug interactions. Should not be used with chemotherapy regimens that do not contain an anthracycline.

**Monitoring:** Monitor for myelosuppression, abnormalities in hepatic/renal function, neurotoxicity, infections, stomatitis, diarrhea, LVEF.

**Patient Counseling:** Instruct to avoid nursing during therapy. Discuss signs/symptoms of adverse side effects and advise to report any if they develop.

**Administration:** IV route. Refer to PI for details. **Storage:** 25°C (77°F); excursions permitted to 15-30°C (59-86°F). Reconstituted solutions stable for 6 hrs at room temperature or 2-8°C (36-46°F). Discard unused solutions.

# ZIPSOR RX

diclofenac potassium (Xanodyne)

**NSAIDs may cause an increased risk of serious cardiovascular thrombotic events, MI, stroke, and serious GI adverse events including bleeding, ulceration, and perforation of the stomach or intestines. Contraindicated for the treatment of perioperative pain in the setting of coronary artery bypass graft (CABG) surgery.**

**THERAPEUTIC CLASS:** NSAID

**INDICATIONS:** Relief of mild to moderate acute pain in adults ≥18 yrs.

**DOSAGE:** *Adults:* ≥18 yrs: 25mg qid. Elderly: Start at low end of dosing range.

**HOW SUPPLIED:** Cap: 25mg

**CONTRAINDICATIONS:** Asthma, urticaria, or allergic reactions after taking aspirin or other NSAIDs. Hypersensitivity to bovine protein. Treatment of perioperative pain in the setting of CABG surgery.

**WARNINGS/PRECAUTIONS:** May lead to onset of new HTN or worsening of pre-existing HTN; monitor BP closely. Fluid retention and edema reported; caution with fluid retention or heart failure. Caution in patients with considerable dehydration. Renal papillary necrosis and other renal injury reported after long-term use. Not recommended for use with advanced renal disease. If therapy must be initiated, monitor renal function. Anaphylactoid reactions may occur. Contraindicated in aspirin-triad patients. May cause serious skin adverse events (eg, exfoliative dermatitis, Stevens-Johnson syndrome, and toxic epidermal necrolysis). Avoid in late pregnancy; may cause premature closure of ductus arteriosus. May cause elevations of LFTs; d/c if liver disease develops or systemic manifestations occur. Caution in elderly. Anemia may occur; with long-term use, monitor Hgb/Hct if signs or symptoms of anemia develop. May inhibit platelet aggregation and prolong bleeding time; monitor with coagulation disorders. Caution with asthma and avoid with ASA-sensitive asthma. May mask symptoms of infection (eg, fever, inflammation). Caution in patients with history of ulcer disease or GI bleeding, or with risk factors (eg, concomitant oral corticosteroids or anticoagulants, smoking, alcohol). Not a substitute for corticosteroids or to treat corticosteroid insufficiency.

**ADVERSE REACTIONS:** Abdominal pain, constipation, diarrhea, dyspepsia, N/V, dizziness, headache, somnolence, pruritus, increased sweating.

**INTERACTIONS:** Avoid use with other diclofenac products. Increased adverse effects with ASA. May impair therapeutic response to ACE inhibitors, thiazides or loop diuretics; monitor for renal failure. Avoid acetaminophen unless prescribed. Synergistic effects on GI bleeding with warfarin. May increase lithium levels; monitor for toxicity. May enhance methotrexate toxicity; caution when coadministering. May increase nephrotoxicity of cyclosporine; caution when coadministering. Caution with coadministration of other drugs that are substrates or inhibitors of CYP2C9.

**PREGNANCY:** Category C <30 weeks gestation, Category D after 30 weeks. Not for use in nursing.

**MECHANISM OF ACTION:** NSAID (benzeneacetic acid derivative); suspected to inhibit prostaglandin synthetase, exerts anti-inflammatory, analgesic, and antipyretic actions.

**PHARMACOKINETICS: Absorption:** Mean absolute bioavailability (50%), $C_{max}$=1087ng/mL, AUC=597ng•h/mL, $T_{max}$=0.5 hr. **Distribution:** $V_d$=1.3L/kg; serum protein binding (>99%). **Metabolism:** Metabolites: 4'-hydroxy-, 5-hydroxy-, 3'-hydroxy-, 4',5-dihydroxy- and 3'-hydroxy-4'-methoxy diclofenac. **Elimination:** Urine (65%), bile (35%); $T_{1/2}$= approximately 1 hr.

## NURSING CONSIDERATIONS

**Assessment:** Assess LFTs, renal function, CBC and coagulation profile. Assess for history of CABG surgery, asthma and allergic reactions to ASA or other NSAIDS, active ulceration, bleeding or chronic inflammation of GI tract, CVD, pregnancy/nursing status, and possible drug interactions. Note other diseases/conditions and drug therapies. Elderly or debilitated patients may be at greater risk for GI events.

**Monitoring:** Monitor for hypersensitivity reactions, cardiac complications, stroke, GI bleeding, asthma, skin side effects. Monitor BP, LFTs, renal function, CBC with differential and platelet count, coagulation profile (especially if on anticoagulation therapy), hyperglycemia.

**Patient Counseling:** Counsel about potential cardiovascular, GI, hepatotoxic and dermatological events, as well as possible weight gain/edema. Take as prescribed. Caution women against using late in pregnancy.

**Administration:** Oral route. **Storage:** 25°C (77°F); excursions permitted to 15-30°C (59-86°F). Protect from moisture. Dispense in tight container.

# ZITHROMAX — RX

azithromycin (Pfizer)

**THERAPEUTIC CLASS:** Macrolide

**INDICATIONS:** Treatment of the following infections caused by susceptible microorganisms: (PO) Acute bacterial exacerbations of COPD, acute bacterial sinusitis (ABS), community-acquired pneumonia (CAP), pharyngitis/tonsillitis, uncomplicated skin and skin structure infections (SSSI), urethritis/cervicitis, genital ulcer disease (men) in adults, acute otitis media. Prevention of disseminated *Mycobacterium avium* complex (MAC) disease alone, or in combination with rifabutin, in persons with advanced HIV infection. Treatment of disseminated MAC disease in combination with ethambutol in persons with advanced HIV infection. (IV) CAP and pelvic inflammatory disease (PID).

**DOSAGE:** *Adults:* PO: CAP/Pharyngitis/Tonsillitis (2nd-line therapy)/SSSI: 500mg on Day 1, then 250mg qd on Days 2-5. COPD: 500mg qd for 3 days or 500mg on Day 1, then 250mg qd on Days 2-5. ABS: 500mg qd for 3 days. Genital Ulcer Disease and Nongonococcal Urethritis/Cervicitis: 1g single dose. Gonococcal Urethritis/Cervicitis: 2g single dose. Prevention of Disseminated MAC Infections: 1200mg once weekly. May be combined with rifabutin. Treatment of Disseminated MAC Infections: 600mg qd in combination with ethambutol at 15mg/kg qd. IV: CAP: 500mg qd for at least 2 days, then 500mg PO qd to complete 7-10-day course. PID: 500mg qd for 1-2 days, then 250mg PO qd to complete 7- day course of therapy.

*Pediatrics:* Sus: Otitis Media: ≥6 months: 30mg/kg single dose; 10mg/kg qd for 3 days; or 10mg/kg qd on Day 1, then 5mg/kg qd on Days 2-5. CAP: ≥ 6 months:10 mg/kg on Day 1, then 5mg/kg on Days 2-5. ABS: ≥6 months: 10mg/kg qd for 3 days. Pharyngitis/Tonsillitis: ≥2 yrs: 12mg/kg qd for 5 days.

**HOW SUPPLIED:** Inj: 500mg; Sus: 100mg/5mL [15mL], 200mg/5mL [15mL, 22.5mL, 30mL]; 1g. Tab: 250mg [Z-PAK, 6 tabs], 500mg [TRI-PAK, 3 tabs], 600mg

**WARNINGS/PRECAUTIONS:** (Inj, PO) Serious allergic reactions reported including angioedema, anaphylaxis, dermatologic reactions including Stevens-Johnson syndrome and toxic epidermal necrolysis rarely reported. D/C if allergic reaction occurs. Hypersensitivity reactions may recur after initial successful symptomatic treatment. *Clostridium difficile*-associated diarrhea (CDAD) reported. Myasthenia gravis exacerbation and new onset of myasthenic syndrome reported. Prescribing in absence of a proven or strongly suspected bacterial infection or prophylactic indication is unlikely to provide benefit and increases the risk of drug-resistant bacteria. May increase risk of developing a cardiac arrhythmia and torsades de pointes. Caution in patients at increased risk for prolonged cardiac repolarization. Caution in patients with hepatic impairment and in patients with GFR<10mL/min. Should not be relied on to treat gonorrhea or syphilis. All patients with sexually transmitted urethritis or cervicitis should have a serologic test for syphilis and appropriate cultures for gonorrhea performed at the time of diagnosis. In all patients, perform appropriate culture and susceptibility tests prior to treatment. (PO): Should not be used in patients with pneumonia who are judged to be inappropriate for PO therapy because of moderate to severe illness or risk factors such as nosocomial acquired infections, known or suspected bacteremia, patients requiring hospitalization, elderly or debilititated patients, or in patients with significant underlying health problems that may compromise their ability to respond to their illness (including immunodeficiency or functional asplenia). (Inj): Local IV-site reactions reported.

**ADVERSE REACTIONS:** Diarrhea/loose stools, N/V, abdominal pain.

**INTERACTIONS:** Monitor terfenadine, cyclosporine, hexobarbital, phenytoin levels when coadministered. May increase digoxin levels. May potentiate effects of oral anticoagulants; monitor for prothrombin time. May increase serum concentrations with nelfinavir. May produce modest effect on pharmacokinetics of atorvastatin, carbamazepine, cetirizine, didanosine, efavirenz, fluconazole, indinavir, midazolam, rifabutin, sildenafil, theophylline (PO and IV), triazolam, trimethoprim/sulfamethoxazole, and zidovudine. Coadministration with efavirenz or fluconazole may have a modest effect on pharmacokinetics of azithromycin. Aluminum- and magnesium-containing antacids may reduce PO levels. Acute ergot toxicity may occur with ergotamine or dihydroergotamine.

**PREGNANCY:** Category B, caution in nursing.

**MECHANISM OF ACTION:** Macrolide; inhibits protein synthesis by binding 50S ribosomal subunits of susceptible organisms, and thus interfering with microbial protein synthesis.

**PHARMACOKINETICS: Absorption:** Administration of variable doses resulted in different parameters. **Distribution:** Plasma protein binding (7-51%); $V_d$=31.1L/kg. **Elimination:** Biliary (major), urine (6%, unchanged); $T_{1/2}$=68 hrs.

## NURSING CONSIDERATIONS

**Assessment:** Assess for liver/renal dysfunction, pregnancy/nursing status, myasthenia gravis, and for possible drug interactions. Assess use in patients at risk for prolonged cardiac repolarization. In patients with sexually transmitted urethritis or cervicitis, perform serologic test for syphilis and perform appropriate cultures for gonorrhea at the time of diagnosis. In all patients, perform appropriate culture and susceptibility tests prior to treatment. In patients planning to use oral therapy for the treatment of pneumonia, assess that oral therapy is appropriate.

**Monitoring:** Monitor for signs/symptoms of allergic reactions (eg, angioedema, Stevens-Johnson syndrome), CDAD, arrhythmias, torsades de pointes, and for new onset of myasthenic syndrome or exacerbation of myasthenia gravis. Monitor PT with oral anticoagulants.

**Patient Counseling:** Caution not to take aluminum- or magnesium-containing antacids. Inform that therapy treats bacterial, not viral, infections. Instruct to take as directed; skipping doses or not completing full course may decrease effectiveness and increase resistance. Inform that may experience diarrhea; notify physician if watery/bloody stools, superinfection, or hypersensitivity reactions occur.

**Administration:** Oral/IV routes. IV: Refer to PI for reconstitution instructions. **Storage:** (Tab) Store at 15-30°C (59-86°F). (Sus) Store dry powder below 30°C (86°F); reconstituted sus between 5-30°C (41-86°F). Reconstituted Inj:

Stable for 24 hrs at or below room temperature (30°C or 86°F) or for 7 days if stored under refrigeration (5°C or 41°F).

## ZMAX RX

azithromycin (Pfizer)

**THERAPEUTIC CLASS:** Macrolide

**INDICATIONS:** Treatment of community-acquired pneumonia in adults and children >6 months and mild-to-moderate acute bacterial sinusitis in adults caused by susceptible bacteria.

**DOSAGE:** *Adults:* 2g single dose. Take on empty stomach (1 hr before or 2 hrs after a meal).
*Pediatrics:* ≥6 months: 60mg/kg single dose. Take on empty stomach (1 hr before or 2 hrs after a meal). Max: 2g single dose. Patients weighing >34kg should receive adult dose. See PI for specific pediatric dosage info.

**HOW SUPPLIED:** Sus, Extended-Release: 2g (27mg/mL)

**CONTRAINDICATIONS:** Hypersensitivity to macrolide or ketolide antibiotics.

**WARNINGS/PRECAUTIONS:** Rare reports of angioedema, anaphylaxis, and dermatologic reactions including Stevens-Johnson syndrome and toxic epidermal necrolysis. D/C if allergic reaction occurs. Hypersensitivity reactions may recur after initial successful symptomatic treatment. *Clostridium difficile*-associated diarrhea reported. Caution with renal/hepatic dysfunction and patients with increased risk for prolonged cardiac repolarization. Exacerbation and new onset of symptoms of myasthenia gravis reported.

**ADVERSE REACTIONS:** Diarrhea/loose stools, N/V, abdominal pain, headache, and taste/smell perversion.

**INTERACTIONS:** Monitor for azithromycin side effects (eg, liver enzyme abnormalities, hearing impairment) with nelfinavir. Monitor cyclosporine, hexobarbital, phenytoin, warfarin concentrations. May increase digoxin levels. Acute ergot toxicity may occur with ergotamine or dihydroergotamine.

**PREGNANCY:** Category B, caution in nursing.

**MECHANISM OF ACTION:** Macrolide antibiotic; inhibits protein synthesis by binding 50S ribosomal subunits of susceptible organisms.

**PHARMACOKINETICS: Absorption:** Oral administration of variable doses resulted in different parameters. **Distribution:** $V_d$=31.1L/kg; plasma protein binding (7-51%). **Elimination:** Bile (major route), urine; $T_{1/2}$=59 hrs.

### NURSING CONSIDERATIONS

**Assessment:** Assess LFTs, prolonged QT interval, and possible drug interactions. Document indications for therapy, culture and susceptibility testing.

**Monitoring:** Monitor for signs/symptoms of hypersensitivity reactions (eg, angioedema, Stevens-Johnson syndrome), *C.difficile*-associated diarrhea, neutropenia, arrhythmia, jaundice, LFTs, hearing loss, seizures, and myasthenia gravis.

**Patient Counseling:** Inform to take on empty stomach. Instruct to immediately report any signs of allergic reaction. Contact physician if vomiting occurs within 1st hr. Advise to keep bottle tightly closed, use within 12 hrs of reconstitution, shake well before use, and to consume entire contents of bottle. Instruct that drug may be taken without regard to magnesium- or aluminum-containing antacids. Inform that therapy treats bacterial, not viral, infections. Take as directed; skipping doses or not completing full course may decrease effectiveness and increase resistance. Inform may experience diarrhea; notify physician if watery/bloody stools, superinfection, or hypersensitivity reactions occur.

**Administration:** Oral route. Reconstitute with 60mL water. Shake well.
**Storage:** Store dry powder at or below 30°C (86°F). Reconstituted sus should be consumed within 12 hrs and stored at 25°C (77°F); excursions permitted to 15-30°C (59-86°F). Do not refrigerate or freeze.

# Zocor RX

simvastatin (Merck)

**THERAPEUTIC CLASS:** HMG-CoA reductase inhibitor

**INDICATIONS:** May initiate with diet in patients with, or at high-risk for, coronary heart disease (CHD). In high risk patients with CHD, diabetes, peripheral vessel disease, history of stroke or other cerebrovascular disease, to reduce risk of total mortality by reducing CHD deaths, risk of non-fatal MI and stroke, need for revascularization procedures. To reduce elevated total-C, LDL-C, Apo B, TG, and increase HDL-C in primary hypercholesterolemia (heterozygous familial and nonfamilial) and mixed dyslipidemia (Types IIa and IIb). To treat hypertriglyceridemia (Type IV) and primary dysbetalipoproteinemia (Type III). To reduce total-C, LDL-C in homozygous familial hypercholesterolemia as adjunct to other lipid-lowering agents or if such treatments are unavailable. To reduce total-C, LDL-C, Apo B in adolescents 10-17 yrs old, at least 1 yr postmenarche, with heterozygous familial hypercholesterolemia. To reduce elevated LDL-C, TG in Type IIb hyperlipidemia.

**DOSAGE:** *Adults:* Initial: 20-40mg qpm. Usual: 5-80mg/day. Titrate: Adjust at ≥4-week intervals. High Risk for CHD Events: Initial: 40mg/day. Homozygous Familial Hypercholesterolemia: 40mg qpm or 80mg/day given as 20mg bid plus 40mg qpm. Concomitant Cyclosporine: Initial: 5mg/day. Max: 10mg/day. Concomitant Gemfibrozil (try to avoid): Max: 10mg/day. Concomitant Amiodarone/Verapamil: Max: 20mg/day. Severe Renal Insufficiency: 5mg/day; monitor closely.
*Pediatrics:* Heterozygous Familial Hypercholesterolemia: 10-17 yrs (at least 1 yr postmenarchal): Initial: 10mg qpm. Usual: 10-40mg/day. Titrate: Adjust at ≥4-week intervals. Max: 40mg/day.

**HOW SUPPLIED:** Tab: 5mg, 10mg, 20mg, 40mg, 80mg

**CONTRAINDICATIONS:** Active liver disease, unexplained persistent elevations of serum transaminases, pregnancy, nursing mothers.

**WARNINGS/PRECAUTIONS:** Caution with heavy alcohol use, severe renal insufficiency or history of hepatic disease. Monitor LFTs prior to therapy, periodically thereafter for 1st yr, or until 1 yr after last dose elevation (additional test at 3 months for 80mg dose). D/C if AST or ALT ≥3x ULN persists, if myopathy is suspected or diagnosed, a few days prior to major surgery. Rhabdomyolysis (rare), myopathy reported.

**ADVERSE REACTIONS:** Abdominal pain, headache, CK and transaminase elevations, constipation, upper respiratory infection, hepatic failure.

**INTERACTIONS:** Avoid use with concomitant itraconazole, ketoconazole, erythromycin, clarithromycin, telithromycin, HIV protease inhibitors, nefazodone, grapefruit juice (>1 quart/day); increased risk of myopathy/rhabdomyolysis. Max 10mg/day with gemfibrozil, cyclosporine, danazol. Max 20mg/day with amiodarone, verapamil. Caution with other fibrates, ≥1g/day of niacin. Monitor digoxin, warfarin.

**PREGNANCY:** Category X, not for use in nursing.

**MECHANISM OF ACTION:** HMG-CoA reductase inhibitor; lipid-lowering agent.

**PHARMACOKINETICS: Absorption:** $T_{max}$=1.3-2.4 hrs. **Distribution:** Plasma protein binding (95%); crosses blood-brain barrier. **Metabolism:** Liver (1st pass); β-hydroxyacid; 6'hydroxy. 6'-hydroxymethyl, 6'-exomethylene (active metabolites). **Elimination:** Feces (60%), urine (13%).

## NURSING CONSIDERATIONS

**Assessment:** Assess for secondary causes of hypercholesterolemia (eg, hypothyroidism, nephrotic syndrome, dysproteinemias, obstructive liver disease, other drug therapy, alcoholism), active liver disease or unexplained elevations in serum transaminases, renal insufficiencies, pregnancy/nursing status. Obtain baseline lipid profile (total-C, HDL-C, TG) and LFTs. Assess for drug interactions.

**Monitoring:** Monitor for signs/symptoms of myopathy (eg, muscle pain, tenderness, weakness), rhabdomyolysis, liver dysfunction, and CNS toxicity (eg, optic nerve degeneration, CNS vascular lesions). Periodically monitor lipid levels (LDL-C), creatine kinase levels (CK), and LFTs. Patients titrated to 80mg dose should have LFTs evaluated prior to titration, 3 months after titration, and periodically thereafter.

**Patient Counseling:** Recommend standard cholesterol-lowering diet. Counsel to contact physician immediately if unexplained muscle pain, tenderness, or weakness occurs. Advise about possible drug interactions and interaction with grapefruit juice. Notify all physicians of all concurrently taken medications. Counsel about risks during pregnancy/nursing.

**Administration:** Oral route. **Storage:** 5-30°C (41-86°F).

## ZOFRAN RX

ondansetron (GlaxoSmithKline)

**THERAPEUTIC CLASS:** 5-$HT_3$ receptor antagonist

**INDICATIONS:** (Inj) Prevention of nausea and vomiting (N/V) associated with initial and repeat courses of emetogenic cancer chemotherapy, including high-dose cisplatin. Prevention of postoperative nausea and/or vomiting (PONV). (Sol/Tab) Prevention of N/V associated with: highly emetogenic cancer chemotherapy, including cisplatin ≥50mg/m²; initial and repeat courses of moderately emetogenic cancer chemotherapy; and radiotherapy in patients receiving either total body irradiation, single high-dose fraction to the abdomen, or daily fractions to the abdomen. Prevention of postoperative nausea and/or vomiting.

**DOSAGE:** *Adults:* Prevention of Chemotherapy-Induced N/V: (Inj) 32mg single IV dose or three 0.15mg/kg IV doses, 1st dose 30 min before chemotherapy, then 4 and 8 hrs after 1st dose. Prevention of N/V Associated With Highly Emetogenic Cancer Chemotherapy: (Tab) 24mg (given as three 8mg tab) 30 min before chemotherapy. Prevention of N/V Associated With Moderately Emetogenic Cancer Chemotherapy: (Sol/Tab) 8mg bid, 1st dose 30 min before chemotherapy, then 8 hrs later, then bid for 1-2 days after completion of chemotherapy. Prevention of PONV: (Inj) 4mg IM/IV immediately before anesthesia or post-op if nausea or vomiting occurs. (Sol/Tab) 16mg 1 hr before anesthesia. Prevention of N/V Associated with Radiation Therapy: (Sol/Tab) Usual: 8mg tid. Total Body Irradiation: 8mg 1-2 hrs before each fraction of radiotherapy administered each day. Single High-Dose Therapy Fraction Radiotherapy to Abdomen: 8mg 1-2 hrs before therapy then q8h after 1st dose for 1-2 days after completion of therapy. Daily Fractionated Radiotherapy Therapy to Abdomen: 8mg 1-2 hrs before therapy then q8h after 1st dose for each day radiotherapy is given. Severe Hepatic Dysfunction (Child-Pugh ≥10): Max: 8mg/day IV single dose infused over 15 min, start 30 min before chemotherapy or 8mg/day PO.

*Pediatrics:* Prevention of Chemotherapy-Induced N/V: (Inj) 6 months-18 yrs: Three 0.15mg/kg doses, 1st dose 30 min before chemotherapy, then 4 and 8 hrs after the 1st dose. (Sol/Tab) Prevention of N/V Associated With Moderately Emetogenic Cancer Chemotherapy: ≥12 yrs: 8mg bid, 1st dose 30 min before chemotherapy, then 8mg 8 hrs later, then bid for 1-2 days after completion of chemotherapy. 4-11 yrs: 4mg tid, 1st dose 30 min before chemotherapy, then 4 and 8 hrs after 1st dose, then tid for 1-2 days after completion of chemotherapy. Prevention of PONV: (Inj) 1 month-12 yrs: ≤40kg: 0.1mg/kg IV single dose. >40kg: 4mg IV single dose. Severe Hepatic Dysfunction (Child Pugh ≥10): Max: 8mg/day IV single dose infused over 15 min, start 30 min before chemotherapy or 8mg/day PO.

**HOW SUPPLIED:** Inj: 2mg/mL, 32mg/50mL; Sol: 4mg/5mL [50mL]; Tab: 4mg, 8mg; Tab, Disintegrating: 4mg, 8mg

**WARNINGS/PRECAUTIONS:** Hypersensitivity reactions reported in those hypersensitive to other 5-$HT_3$ receptor antagonists. Do not use instead of nasogastric suction. May mask progressive ileus or gastric distension. Rarely and predominantly with IV administration, transient ECG changes including QT interval prolongation reported. Orally disintegrating tabs contain phenylalanine; caution in phenylketonurics.

**ADVERSE REACTIONS:** Headache, diarrhea, dizziness, drowsiness/sedation, bradycardia, constipation, LFT abnormalities, wound problem, hypoxia, pyrexia, gynecological disorder, anxiety/agitation.

**INTERACTIONS:** Ondansetron is metabolized by CYP450 enzymes (CYP3A4, CYP2D6, CYP1A2); inducers or inhibitors of these enzymes may change the clearance and half-life of ondansetron. Concomitant use with tramadol may be associated with an increase in patient-controlled administration of tramadol.

**PREGNANCY:** Category B, caution in nursing.

**MECHANISM OF ACTION:** Serotonin 5-$HT_3$ receptor blocker; not established. Blocks 5-$HT_3$ receptors from serotonin, which may stimulate vagal afferents through 5-$HT_3$ receptors, which initiate vomiting reflex.

**PHARMACOKINETICS: Absorption:** IV and oral administration to various age groups resulted in different parameters. PO: Well absorbed from GI tract. **Distribution:** Plasma protein binding (70-76%). **Metabolism:** Hydroxylation, conjugation. **Elimination:** Urine.

## NURSING CONSIDERATIONS

**Assessment:** Assess for hepatic impairment, pregnancy/nursing status, and for possible drug interactions. If planning to use orally disintegrating tablet formulation, assess for phenylketonuria.

**Monitoring:** Monitor signs/symptoms of ECG changes and for hypersensitivity reactions. In patients who recently underwent abdominal surgery or in patients with chemotherapy-induced n/v, monitor for masking of signs of a progressive ileus and/or gastric distension.

**Patient Counseling:** Instruct not to remove disintegrating tab from blister until just prior to dosing; do not push through foil. Remove gently and immediately place on tongue to dissolve and swallow; liquid not necessary. Inform that disintegrating tab contains phenylalanine. Advise to seek medical attention if symptoms of hypersensitivity reactions, progressive ileus, or gastric distention occur.

**Administration:** IM/IV/Oral routes. Inj: Refer to prescribing information for reconstitution guidelines. **Storage:** Inj/Tab: 2-30°C (36-86°F). Protect from light. Inj: Avoid excessive heat. Sol: 15-30°C (59-86°F). Protect from light; store upright.

# ZOLADEX 1-MONTH — RX

goserelin acetate (AstraZeneca)

**THERAPEUTIC CLASS:** Synthetic gonadotropin releasing hormone analog

**INDICATIONS:** Palliative treatment of advanced prostatic carcinoma, and advanced breast cancer in pre-and peri-menopausal women. Adjunct to and during radiotherapy, and in combination with flutamide, for management of locally confined Stage T2b-T4 (Stage B2-C) prostatic carcinoma. Management of endometriosis, including pain relief and reduction of endometriotic lesions. Use as an endometrial thinning agent prior to ablation for dysfunctional uterine bleeding.

**DOSAGE:** *Adults:* Inject SQ into anterior abdominal wall below navel line. Advanced Prostatic Carcinoma/Breast Cancer: 3.6mg every 28 days. Stage B2-C Prostatic Carcinoma: 3.6mg starting 8 weeks before radiotherapy, then 10.8mg formulation 28 days after 1st injection, or 3.6mg at 28-day intervals for 4 doses (2 before and 2 during radiotherapy). Endometriosis: 3.6mg every 28 days for up to 6 months. Endometrial Thinning: 3.6mg then surgery 4 weeks later, or 2 doses of 3.6mg (given 4 weeks apart) followed by surgery 2-4 weeks after 2nd dose.

**HOW SUPPLIED:** Implant: 3.6mg

**CONTRAINDICATIONS:** Pregnancy.

**WARNINGS/PRECAUTIONS:** Exclude pregnancy before initiating therapy; may cause fetal harm. Premenopausal women should use nonhormonal contraception during therapy and for 12 weeks post-therapy. Transient worsening of symptoms (or emergence of additional signs/symptoms) of prostate/breast cancer may occur during initial therapy; causes transient increases in testosterone levels (in men) and estrogen levels (in women). Ureteral obstruction and spinal cord compression reported in patients with prostate cancer. Temporary increases in bone pain may occur. May cause hyperglycemia; monitor blood glucose levels. Hypercalcemia reported in prostate/breast cancer patients with bone metastases. May increase cervical resistance. Hypersensitivity, antibody formation, and acute anaphylactic reactions may occur.

**ADVERSE REACTIONS:** Hot flashes/flushes, sexual dysfunction, decreased erections, seborrhea, peripheral edema, breast enlargement/atrophy, pain, vaginitis, emotional lability, decreased libido, sweating, depression, headache, acne, changes in bone mineral density (BMD).

**INTERACTIONS:** Ovarian hyperstimulation syndrome reported when used concomitantly with other gonadotropins.

**PREGNANCY:** Category X (endometriosis and endometrial thinning), Category D (breast cancer), not for use in nursing.

**MECHANISM OF ACTION:** Synthetic decapeptide analog of GnRH; acts as potent inhibitor of pituitary gonadotropin secretion. In males, causes initial increase in serum LH and FSH levels, causing subsequent increases in serum testosterone levels; chronic administration suppresses pituitary gonadotropins causing fall in testosterone levels to post-castration levels. In females, chronic exposure causes decrease in serum estradiol levels consistent with postmenopausal state, leading to reduction of ovarian size and function, reduction in size of uterus and mammary gland, and regression of sex hormone-responsive tumors.

**PHARMACOKINETICS: Absorption:** $C_{max}$=2.84ng/mL (male), 1.46ng/mL (female); $T_{max}$=12-15 days (male), 8-22 days (female); AUC=27.8ng•d/mL (male), 18.5ng•d/mL (female). **Distribution:** $V_d$=44.1L (male), 20.3L (female); plasma protein binding (27.3%). **Metabolism:** Liver; hydrolysis; 1-7 fragment (major circulating component). **Elimination:** Urine: 90% (20% unchanged); clearance greater in females.

## NURSING CONSIDERATIONS

**Assessment:** Assess for endometriosis, serum testosterone levels, PSA, psychotic disorders. Assess for ureteral obstruction and spinal cord compression prior to initiation of treatment. Note other diseases/conditions and drug therapies. Assess pregnancy/nursing status.

**Monitoring:** Monitor for ureteral obstruction, spinal cord compression, renal impairment, hypersensitivity reactions, pituitary apoplexy, sexual dysfunction. Monitor BMD, serum cholesterol levels, and blood glucose levels.

**Patient Counseling:** Counsel about potential side effects (regular menstrual bleeding, allergic reactions, hypoestrogenism, reduction in BMD, and amenorrhea); seek medical attention if any occur. Inform that diabetes/loss of glycemic control has been reported. Advise against pregnancy and/or breastfeeding; instruct to d/c use if pregnancy occurs during treatment for endometriosis/endometrial thinning. Counsel to not initiate treatment with abnormal vaginal bleeding or known allergy. Advise to not use for periods >6 months.

**Administration:** SQ route. Inject into anterior abdominal wall below navel line. See PI for extensive details of administration. **Storage:** Room temperature; do not exceed 25°C (77°F).

# Zoladex 3-Month RX

goserelin acetate (AstraZeneca)

**THERAPEUTIC CLASS:** Synthetic gonadotropin releasing hormone analog

**INDICATIONS:** Palliative treatment of advanced prostate cancer. Adjunct to radiotherapy and flutamide for management of locally confined Stage T2b-T4 (Stage B2-C) prostate cancer.

**DOSAGE:** *Adults:* Inject SQ into anterior abdominal wall below navel line. Advanced Prostate Cancer: 10.8mg every 12 weeks. Stage B2-C Prostate Cancer: 3.6mg depot formulation 8 weeks before radiotherapy then 10.8mg 28 days after 1st injection.

**HOW SUPPLIED:** Implant: 10.8mg

**CONTRAINDICATIONS:** Pregnancy, 10.8mg implant is not indicated in women.

**WARNINGS/PRECAUTIONS:** Worsening of symptoms of prostate cancer with initial therapy. Ureteral obstruction and spinal cord compression reported. Temporary increase in bone pain may occur. Hypersensitivity, antibody formation, and acute anaphylactic reactions may occur.

**ADVERSE REACTIONS:** Hot flashes, sexual dysfunction, decreased erections, osteoporosis, pain, asthenia, gynecomastia.

**PREGNANCY:** Category X, not for use in nursing.

**MECHANISM OF ACTION:** Synthetic analog of luteinizing hormone-releasing hormone (LHRH); acts as potent inhibitor of pituitary gonadotropin secretion. In males, causes initial increase in serum LH and FSH levels, causing increase in testosterone. In females, causes decrease in serum estradiol levels consistent with postmenopausal state, reduction of ovarian size and function, reduction in size of uterus and mammary gland, and regression of sex hormone-responsive tumors.

**PHARMACOKINETICS: Absorption:** $C_{max}$=8.85ng/mL; $T_{max}$=1.8 hrs. **Distribution:** $V_d$=44.1 L; plasma protein binding (27%). **Metabolism:** Hydrolysis of C-terminal amino acids. **Elimination:** Urine (90%, 20% unchanged); $T_{1/2}$=4.16 hrs.

## NURSING CONSIDERATIONS

**Assessment:** Assess serum testosterone levels, PSA, DM, CVD. Note other diseases/conditions and drug therapies.

**Monitoring:** Monitor for ureteral obstruction, spinal cord compression, renal impairment, BMD, hypersensitivity reactions, pituitary apoplexy, sexual dysfunction, serum cholesterol levels, CVD, CBC.

**Patient Counseling:** Counsel about potential side effects; seek medical attention if any occur.

**Administration:** SQ route. Inject into anterior abdominal wall below navel line. **Storage:** Room temperature; do not exceed 25°C (77°F).

# ZOLINZA RX

vorinostat (Merck)

**THERAPEUTIC CLASS:** Histone deacetylase inhibitor

**INDICATIONS:** Treatment of cutaneous manifestations in patients with cutaneous T-cell lymphoma who have progressive, persistent, or recurrent disease on or following 2 systemic therapies.

**DOSAGE:** *Adults.* 400mg PO qd with food. Intolerant to Therapy: May reduce dose to 300mg PO qd with food. If necessary, may further reduce dose to 300mg PO qd with food for 5 consecutive days each week. Do not open or crush.

**HOW SUPPLIED:** Cap: 100mg

**WARNINGS/PRECAUTIONS:** Pulmonary embolism and deep vein thrombosis (DVT) reported; monitor for signs and symptoms. Dose-related thrombocytopenia and anemia may occur; consider dose modification or d/c of therapy if platelet counts and/or Hgb are reduced during treatment. GI disturbances (eg, N/V, diarrhea) reported; pre-existing N/V and diarrhea should be adequately controlled before beginning therapy. Hyperglycemia observed; monitor glucose levels. Monitor CBC and chemistry tests including electrolytes (including potassium, magnesium, calcium), glucose, and SrCr every 2 weeks during first 2 months of therapy and monthly thereafter; correct hypokalemia or hypomagnesemia prior to therapy. May cause fetal harm. Caution with renal/hepatic impairment.

**ADVERSE REACTIONS:** Diarrhea, fatigue, N/V, thrombocytopenia, anorexia, dysgeusia, decreased weight, muscle spasms, alopecia, dry mouth, increased SrCr, chills, constipation, dizziness.

**INTERACTIONS:** Prolongation of PT and INR observed with coumarin-derivative anticoagulants; monitor closely. Severe thrombocytopenia and GI bleeding reported with concomitant use of other histone deacetylase inhibitors (eg, valproic acid); monitor platelet count every 2 weeks for the first 2 months of therapy.

**PREGNANCY:** Category D, not for use in nursing.

**MECHANISM OF ACTION:** Histone deacetylase inhibitor; inhibits activity of histone deacetylases (HDAC) allowing for accumulation of acetyl groups on the histone lysine residues, resulting in open chromatin structure and transcriptional activation.

**PHARMACOKINETICS: Absorption:** Fasted: $C_{max}$=1.2µM, $T_{max}$=1.5 hrs, AUC=4.2µM•hr. Fed: $C_{max}$=1.2µM, $T_{max}$=4 hrs, AUC=6.0µM•hr. **Distribution:** Plasma protein binding (71%). **Metabolism:** Liver, via glucuronidation, hydrolysis and β-oxidation. **Elimination:** Urine (<1% unchanged); $T_{1/2}$=2 hrs.

## NURSING CONSIDERATIONS

**Assessment:** Assess for renal/hepatic impairment, history of thromboembolic events, GI disturbances (eg, N/V, diarrhea), diabetes, hypokalemia, hypomagnesemia, fluid imbalance, pregnancy/nursing status, and for possible drug interactions.

**Monitoring:** Monitor for signs/symptoms of pulmonary embolism, DVT, thrombocytopenia, anemia, GI disturbances (eg, N/V, diarrhea), and hyperglycemia. Monitor blood cell counts and chemistry tests, including electrolytes (including potassium, magnesium, calcium), glucose, and SrCr every 2 weeks for first 2 months.

**Patient Counseling:** Counsel to take with food, not to open or crush, and to drink at least 2L of fluid per day to prevent dehydration. Instruct to contact physician if excessive vomiting or diarrhea occur, if signs of DVT develop, or if unusual bleeding develops.

**Administration:** Oral route. **Storage:** 20-25°C (68-77°F); excursions permitted between 15-30°C (59-86°F).

# ZOLOFT — RX

sertraline HCl (Pfizer)

**Antidepressants increased the risk of suicidal thinking and behavior (suicidality) in short-term studies in children, adolescents, and young adults with major depressive disorder (MDD) and other psychiatric disorders. Sertraline HCl is not approved for use in pediatric patients except for patients with obsessive compulsive disorder (OCD).**

**THERAPEUTIC CLASS:** Selective serotonin reuptake inhibitor

**INDICATIONS:** Treatment of major depressive disorder (MDD), social anxiety disorder (SAD), obsessive compulsive disorder (OCD), panic disorder with or without agoraphobia, premenstrual dysphoric disorder (PMDD) and post-traumatic stress disorder (PTSD).

**DOSAGE:** *Adults:* MDD/OCD: 50mg qd. Titrate: Adjust dose at 1-week intervals. Max: 200mg/day. Panic Disorder/PTSD/SAD: Initial: 25mg qd. Titrate: Increase to 50mg qd after 1 week. Adjust dose at 1 week intervals. Max: 200mg/day. PMDD: Initial: 50mg qd continuous or limited to luteal phase of cycle. Titrate: Increase 50mg/cycle if needed up to 150mg/day for continuous or 100mg/day for luteal phase dosing. If 100mg/day is established for luteal phase dosing, a 50mg/day titration step for 3 days should take place at the beginning of each luteal phase dosing period. Hepatic Impairment: Use lower or less frequent doses. Dilute sol with 4oz water, ginger ale, lemon/lime soda, lemonade or orange juice. Take immediately after mixing.
*Pediatrics:* OCD: Initial: 6-12 yrs: 25mg qd. 13-17 yrs: 50mg qd. Titrate: Adjust dose at 1 week intervals. Max: 200mg/day. Hepatic Impairment: Use lower or

less frequent doses. Dilute sol with 4oz water, gingerale, lemon/lime soda, lemonade or orange juice. Take immediately after mixing.

**HOW SUPPLIED:** Sol: 20mg/mL [60mL]; Tab: 25mg*, 50mg*, 100mg* *scored

**CONTRAINDICATIONS:** Concomitant use of MAOIs or pimozide. Concomitant disulfiram with solution.

**WARNINGS/PRECAUTIONS:** Avoid abrupt withdrawal. May increase risk of bleeding events. Activation of mania/hypomania, SIADH, hyponatremia, altered platelet function reported. Caution with diseases or conditions that could affect hemodynamic responses or metabolism, seizure disorder, suicidal tendencies. Decreased appetite and weight loss reported. Caution in third trimester of pregnancy due to risk of serious neonatal complications. Serotonin syndrome and neuroleptic malignant syndrome (NMS)-like reactions reported. Monitor for clinical worsening and/or suicidality, especially at initiation of therapy or dose changes.

**ADVERSE REACTIONS:** Ejaculation failure, dry mouth, increased sweating, somnolence, tremor, anorexia, dizziness, headache, diarrhea, dyspepsia, N/V, agitation, insomnia, nervousness, abnormal vision.

**INTERACTIONS:** See Contraindications. Avoid alcohol, tryptophan, other SNRIs, and SSRIs. Caution with other centrally acting drugs, TCAs. May shift concentrations with plasma-bound drugs (eg, warfarin, digitoxin). May alter warfarin effects. Increased levels with cimetidine. Decreases clearance of tolbutamide. Rare reports of weakness, hyperreflexia, incoordination with an SSRI and sumatriptan. May potentiate drugs metabolized by CYP2D6 (eg, TCAs, Type 1C antiarrhythmics). Monitor lithium. Caution with OTC products. May induce metabolism of cisapride. Increased risk of bleeding with NSAIDs, ASA, warfarin. Concomitant use of serotonergic drugs and drugs that impair metabolism of serotonin may cause serotonin syndrome. Caution with other agents that may affect serotonergic neurotransmitter systems (eg, triptans, linezolid, tramadol, or St. John's wort).

**PREGNANCY:** Category C, caution in nursing.

**MECHANISM OF ACTION:** SSRI; inhibits CNS neuronal uptake of serotonin.

**PHARMACOKINETICS: Absorption:** $T_{max}$ =4.5-8.4 hrs. **Distribution:** Plasma protein binding (98%). **Metabolism:** Liver (extensive). **Elimination:** Feces (12-14% unchanged), urine (minor); $T_{1/2}$=26 hrs.

## NURSING CONSIDERATIONS

**Assessment:** Assess for risk of bipolar disorder, history of seizures, disease/condition that alters metabolism or hemodynamic response, hepatic/renal impairment, MAOI, thioridazine, or pimozide therapy, renal/hepatic impairment, pregnancy/nursing status, and possible drug interactions.

**Monitoring:** Monitor for worsening of depression, emergence of suicidal ideation and behavior (suicidality), or unusual changes in behavior. Monitor for possible serotonin syndrome and hyponatremia (eg, headache, difficulty concentrating, memory impairment, confusion, weakness, and unsteadiness, which may lead to falls), and NMS-like reactions. Monitor platelets, body weight, $Na^+$, and uric acid.

**Patient Counseling:** Advise to avoid alcohol. Seek medical attention for symptoms of serotonin syndrome (mental status changes, tachycardia, hyperthermia, N/V, diarrhea, incoordination), abnormal bleeding (eg, NSAIDs or ASA), hyponatremia, activation of mania, seizures, clinical worsening (suicidal ideation, unusual changes in behavior) and discontinuation symptoms (irritability, agitation, dizziness, anxiety, headache, insomnia). May cause motor/mental skills impairment; use caution when operating machinery/driving. May notice improvement in 1-4 weeks; continue therapy as directed. Notify physician if pregnant/intend to become pregnant, or breastfeeding. Counsel about benefits and risks of therapy. Inform physician if taking, or plan to take any over-the-counter prescriptions.

**Administration:** Oral route. Mix sol with 4oz water, ginger ale, lemon/lime soda, lemonade, or orange juice. Do not mix with anything other than liquids listed. Dose should be taken immediately after mixing. **Storage:** 25°C (77°F); excursions permitted to 15-30°C (59-86°F).

## ZOLPIMIST

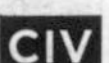

zolpidem tartrate (NovaDel Pharma)

**THERAPEUTIC CLASS:** Imidazopyridine hypnotic

**INDICATIONS:** Short-term treatment of insomnia characterized by difficulties with sleep initiation.

**DOSAGE:** *Adults:* Individualize dose. 10mg qhs. Max: 10mg/day. Elderly/Debilitated/Hepatic Insufficiency: 5mg qhs.

**HOW SUPPLIED:** Spray: 5mg/spray [8.2g]

**WARNINGS/PRECAUTIONS:** Evaluate for primary psychiatric and/or medical illness if insomnia fails to remit after 7-10 days of treatment. Severe anaphylactic and anaphylactoid reactions reported. Visual/auditory hallucinations, complex behavior (eg, sleep-driving), abnormal thinking and behavior changes reported. Worsening of depression, including suicidal thoughts and actions have been reported in depressed patients. Caution with conditions that could affect metabolism or hemodynamic responses, sleep apnea syndrome, myasthenia gravis, and worsening depression. Signs and symptoms of withdrawal reported with abrupt d/c of sedative/hypnotics. Monitor elderly and debilitated patients for impaired motor and/or cognitive performance.

**ADVERSE REACTIONS:** Drowsiness, dizziness, headache, N/V, diarrhea.

**INTERACTIONS:** CNS-active drugs may potentially enhance effects; downward dose adjustment may be necessary. Additive effects seen with alcohol use. Decreased alertness observed with combination use of imipramine/chlorpromazine. Ketoconazole may enhance sedative effects; consider lowering dose when given with ketoconazole.

**PREGNANCY:** Category C, safety not known in nursing.

**MECHANISM OF ACTION:** Imidazopyridine, non-benzodiazepine hypnotic; interacts with a GABA-BZ receptor complex and preferentially binds to the $BZ_1$ receptor subtype at the $\alpha_1/\alpha_5$ subunits.

**PHARMACOKINETICS: Absorption:** Rapid; (5mg) $C_{max}$=114ng/mL, (10mg) $C_{max}$=210ng/mL; $T_{max}$=0.9 hrs. **Distribution:** Plasma protein binding (92.5%). **Elimination:** Renal; (5mg) $T_{1/2}$=2.7 hrs, (10mg) $T_{1/2}$= 3.

### NURSING CONSIDERATIONS

**Assessment:** Assess for primary psychiatric and/or medical illness, pre-existing respiratory impairment (eg, sleep apnea syndrome), myasthenia gravis, hypersensitivity reactions, hepatic impairment, possible drug interactions, history of alcohol abuse, and pregnancy/nursing status.

**Monitoring:** Monitor for anaphylactic/anaphylactoid reactions, abnormal thinking, behavioral changes, complex behavior (eg, sleep-driving, hallucinations). Monitor patients with hepatic impairment, and those on long-term treatment for drug abuse/dependence.

**Patient Counseling:** Instruct not to take with or immediately after meals. Counsel to take just before bedtime (prior to a full 7-8 hrs of sleep) without food and do not take with alcohol. Caution against hazardous tasks (eg, driving/operating machines). Inform about risks/benefits of use.

**Administration:** Oral route. **Storage:** Store upright at 25°C (77°F); with excursions permitted to 15-30°C (59-86°F). Do not freeze. Avoid prolonged exposure to heat.

## ZOMETA

RX

zoledronic acid (Novartis)

**THERAPEUTIC CLASS:** Bisphosphonate

**INDICATIONS:** Treatment of hypercalcemia of malignancy. Treatment of multiple myeloma and bone metastases from solid tumors, in conjunction with antineoplastic therapy.

**DOSAGE:** *Adults:* Hypercalcemia of Malignancy: Max: 4mg IV over no less than 15 min. Retreatment (if necessary): Wait at least 7 days from initial dose. Multiple Myeloma/Bone Metastases: 4mg IV over 15 min every 3-4 weeks. CrCl >60mL/min: 4mg; CrCl 50-60mL/min: 3.5mg; CrCl 40-49mL/min: 3.3mg; CrCl 30-39mL/min: 3mg. Measure SrCr prior to each dose. Withhold dose with renal deterioration; resume when SrCr returns to within 10% of baseline. Take with oral calcium 500mg/day and vitamin D 400 IU/day.

**HOW SUPPLIED:** Inj: 4mg/5mL

**WARNINGS/PRECAUTIONS:** Caution with hepatic insufficiency, ASA-sensitive asthma, and the elderly. Risk of renal toxicity/failure. In severe renal impairment, avoid with bone metastases and use caution with hypercalcemia of malignancy. Rehydrate before use with hypercalcemia of malignancy. Monitor SrCr before each dose, and serum calcium, electrolytes, phosphate, magnesium, and Hct/Hgb regularly. May cause fetal harm during pregnancy. Osteonecrosis of the jaw reported in cancer patients treated with bisphosphonates; avoid invasive dental procedures during therapy. Severe and occasionally incapacitating bone, joint, and/or muscle pain reported; d/c if severe symptoms develop. Bronchoconstriction in aspirin-sensitive patients reported. Hypersensitivity reactions reported.

**ADVERSE REACTIONS:** Fever, chills, bone pain, arthralgia, myalgia, N/V, diarrhea, constipation, injection-site reactions, hypophosphatemia, anorexia, anemia, insomnia, anxiety, dyspnea, fatigue.

**INTERACTIONS:** Additive effect/risk of hypocalcemia with aminoglycosides and loop diuretics. Caution with other nephrotoxic drugs. Increased risk of renal dysfunction with thalidomide in multiple myeloma patients.

**PREGNANCY:** Category D, not for use in nursing.

**MECHANISM OF ACTION:** Bisphosphonate; inhibits bone resorption through osteoclastic activity and induces osteoclast apoptosis. Also blocks osteoclastic resorption of mineralized bone and cartilage through binding to bone.

**PHARMACOKINETICS: Absorption:** IV administration of different doses resulted in different parameters. **Distribution:** Plasma protein binding: 28-53%. **Elimination:** Urine (39%); $T_{1/2}$=146 hrs.

## NURSING CONSIDERATIONS

**Assessment:** Assess hydration status, serum levels of calcium, phosphate, magnesium, SrCr, renal function, LFTs, asthma, pregnancy status, and for possible drug interactions.

**Monitoring:** Monitor serum levels of calcium, phosphate, magnesium, SrCr, renal function, LFTs. Monitor adverse events (eg, osteonecrosis of jaw, musculoskeletal pain, bronchoconstriction, fever, nausea, constipation, anemia, and dyspnea) and hypersensitivity reactions.

**Patient Counseling:** Advise to take oral calcium supplement of 500mg and multiple vitamin containing 400IU vitamin D daily in patients with multiple myeloma or bone metastasis of solid tumor. Cancer patients should maintain good oral hygiene, have dental exam with preventive dentistry prior to therapy with bisphosphonates, and avoid invasive dental procedures. Inform about importance of blood tests. Advise to avoid pregnancy during course of therapy.

**Administration:** IV route. Single doses should not exceed 4mg and duration of infusion should not be less than 15 min. **Storage:** 25°C (77°F); excursions permitted to 15-30°C (59-86°F).

# Zomig — RX

zolmitriptan (AstraZeneca)

**OTHER BRAND NAMES:** Zomig-ZMT (AstraZeneca) - Zomig Nasal Spray (AstraZeneca)

**THERAPEUTIC CLASS:** 5-$HT_{1B/1D}$ agonist

**INDICATIONS:** Acute treatment of migraine attacks with or without aura.

**DOSAGE:** *Adults:* ≥18 yrs: (Spray) 5mg single dose; may repeat once after 2 hrs. Max: 10mg/24 hrs. Safety of treating >4 headaches/30 days unknown. (Tab) Initial: 2.5mg or lower (2.5mg tab may be broken in 1/2); may repeat after 2 hrs. Max: 10mg/24 hrs. Safety of treating >3 headaches/30 days unknown. (ZMT) 2.5mg single dose; may repeat after 2 hrs. Max: 10mg/24 hrs. Dissolve on tongue without water. Safety of treating >3 headaches/30 days unknown. Hepatic Impairment: Use low dose and monitor blood pressure.

**HOW SUPPLIED:** Nasal Spray: 5mg [0.1mL, 6[s]]; Tab: 2.5mg*, 5mg; Tab, Disintegrating: (ZMT) 2.5mg, 5mg *scored

**CONTRAINDICATIONS:** Ischemic heart disease, coronary artery vasospasm (eg, Prinzmetal's angina), uncontrolled HTN, cerebrovascular syndromes, other significant cardiovascular disease, hemiplegic or basilar migraine, MAOI use during or within 14 days, other 5-$HT_1$ agonist or ergot-type agent (eg, dihydroergotamine, methysergide) use within 24 hrs.

**WARNINGS/PRECAUTIONS:** Confirm migraine diagnosis. Supervise 1st dose and monitor cardiac function in those at risk of CAD (eg, HTN, hypercholesterolemia, smoker, obesity, diabetes, CAD family history, postmenopausal women, males >40 yrs). Serious adverse cardiac events, cerebrovascular events, vasospastic reactions reported with 5-$HT_1$ agonists. Disintegrating tabs contain phenylalanine. Caution with hepatic dysfunction. Reconsider diagnosis before 2nd dose, if no response seen after 1st dose. Serotonin syndrome symptoms (eg, mental status changes, autonomic instability, neuromuscular aberrations, and GI symptoms) reported. Avoid in patients with symptomatic Wolff-Parkinson-White syndrome or arrhythmias associated with other cardiac accessory conduction pathway disorders.

**ADVERSE REACTIONS:** Paresthesia, hyperesthesia, paresthesia, asthenia, warm/cold sensation, neck/throat/jaw pain, dry mouth, nausea, dizziness, somnolence, unusual taste (nasal spray).

**INTERACTIONS:** Ergot-containing agents may prolong vasospastic reactions. Avoid MAOIs during or within 14 days of therapy. Serotonin syndrome reported with combined use of an SSRI or SNRI. Half-life and AUC doubled with cimetidine. Avoid 5-$HT_{1B/1D}$ agonists within 24 hrs.

**PREGNANCY:** Category C, caution in nursing.

**MECHANISM OF ACTION:** 5-$HT_{1D/1B}$ agonist; binds with high affinity to 5-$HT_{1D/1B}$ receptors on intracranial vessels (including arteriovenous anastomoses) and sensory nerves of trigeminal system, which results in cranial vessel constriction and inhibition of pro-inflammatory neuropeptide release.

**PHARMACOKINETICS: Absorption:** Well-absorbed; absolute bioavailability (40%); $T_{max}$=3 hrs (ODT/Nasal Spray), 1.5 hrs (Tab). **Distribution:** (Oral) $V_d$=7L/kg, (Nasal Spray) $V_d$=8.4L/kg. Plasma protein binding (25% ). **Metabolism:** N-desmethyl (active metabolite). **Elimination:** Urine (65%, 8% unchanged), feces (30% Oral); $T_{1/2}$=3 hrs (Nasal Spray).

## NURSING CONSIDERATIONS

**Assessment:** Confirm diagnosis of migraine before therapy. Assess for ischemic heart disease (eg, angina pectoris, Prinzmetal's variant angina, MI or documented silent MI), HTN, hemiplegic or basilar migraine, presence of risk factors (eg, hypercholesterolemia, smoking, obesity, DM, strong family history of CAD, female with surgical or physiological menopause, or male >40 yrs), ECG changes, hepatic/renal impairment, pregnancy/nursing status, and possible drug interactions.

**Monitoring:** Administration of 1st dose should be in physician's office or medically staffed and equipped facility as cardiac ischemia may occur in absence of clinical symptoms. ECG should be obtained immediately after administration in those with risk factors. Monitor for signs/symptoms of cardiac events (eg, coronary vasospasm, acute MI, arrhythmia, ECG changes, follow-up coronary angiography), cerebrovascular events (eg, hemorrhage, stroke, TIAs), peripheral vascular ischemia, colonic ischemia with bloody diarrhea and abdominal pain, serotonin syndrome (eg, mental status changes, autonomic instability, neuromuscular aberrations and/or GI symptoms), ophthalmic effects, and increased BP.

**Patient Counseling:** Inform about risk of serotonin syndrome, especially if taken with SSRIs or SNRIs. Advise to notify physician if pregnant/nursing or planning to become pregnant. Counsel on proper administration technique for nasal spray.

**Administration:** Oral/Nasal routes. ODT: Immediately prior to dosing, remove blister from outer pouch with dry hands. Dissolve on tongue and swallow.
**Storage:** 20-25°C (68-77°F).

## ZONEGRAN — RX

zonisamide (Eisai)

**THERAPEUTIC CLASS:** Sulfonamide anticonvulsant

**INDICATIONS:** Adjunctive therapy in the treatment of partial seizures in adults.

**DOSAGE:** *Adults:* Initial: 100mg qd for 2 weeks. Titrate: May increase to 200mg/day for at least 2 weeks. May then increase to 300mg/day, then to 400mg/day for at least 2-week intervals. Max: 400mg/day. Elderly: Start at low end of dosing range.
*Pediatrics:* ≥16 yrs: Initial: 100mg qd for 2 weeks. Titrate: May increase to 200mg/day for at least 2 weeks. May then increase to 300mg/day, then to 400mg/day for at least 2-week intervals. Max: 400mg/day.

**HOW SUPPLIED:** Cap: 25mg, 100mg

**CONTRAINDICATIONS:** Hypersensitivity to sulfonamides.

**WARNINGS/PRECAUTIONS:** Fatal sulfonamide hypersensitivity reactions (eg, Stevens-Johnson syndrome [SJS], toxic epidermal necrolysis [TEN], fulminant hepatic necrosis, blood dyscrasias) reported; d/c if with unexplained rash. Increased risk of suicidal thoughts or behavior reported; monitor for worsening of depression and any unusual changes in mood or behavior. Increased risk of oligohidrosis and hyperthermia in pediatrics; monitor for decreased sweating and increased body temperature. Avoid abrupt withdrawal, may precipitate increased seizure frequency or status epilecticus. Advise females to use contraceptives to prevent pregnancy; should only be used in pregnancy if potential benefit justifies the potential risk to fetus. May cause cognitive/neuropsychiatric adverse events. May impair physical/mental abilities. Caution with renal/hepatic impairment. Increased SrCr and BUN, kidney stones reported during therapy; d/c if acute renal failure or if a sustained increase in BUN or SrCr develops. Status epilepticus reported. Caution in elderly.

**ADVERSE REACTIONS:** Headache, abdominal pain, anorexia, N/V, dizziness, ataxia, confusion, difficulty concentrating, memory difficulties, agitation/irritability, insomnia, somnolence, fatigue, speech abnormalities, diplopia.

**INTERACTIONS:** Liver enzyme inducers increase metabolism and clearance and decrease half-life of zonisamide. Concomitant administration of phenytoin and carbamazepine increases zonisamide plasma clearance and decreases the half-life of zonisamide. Concomitant use with phenobarbital or valproate decreases the half-life of zonisamide. Caution with drugs that predispose patients to heat-related disorders (eg, carbonic anhydrase inhibitors, anticholinergic drugs). Drugs that induce or inhibit CYP3A4 may alter zonisamide serum concentrations.

**PREGNANCY:** Category C, not for use in nursing.

**MECHANISM OF ACTION:** Sulfonamide; mechanism unknown. Found to block $Na^+$ channels and reduce voltage-dependent, transient inward currents (T-type $Ca^{2+}$ currents), which then stabilize neuronal membranes and suppress neuronal hypersynchronization. Facilitates both dopaminergic and serotonergic neurotransmission.

**PHARMACOKINETICS: Absorption:** $C_{max}$=2-5mcg/mL; $T_{max}$ =2 to 6 hrs. **Distribution:** $V_d$=1.45L/kg; plasma protein binding (40%). **Metabolism:** Liver, via acetylation and reduction by CYP3A4; N-acetyl zonisamide, 2-sulfamoylacetyl phenol (metabolites). **Elimination**: Urine (62%), feces (3%); $T_{1/2}$=63 hrs.

## NURSING CONSIDERATIONS

**Assessment:** Assess renal/hepatic function, drug allergy to sulfonamides, history of depression, suicidal thoughts or behavior, pregnancy/nursing status, and possible drug interactions. Obtain baseline CBC, renal function (SrCr, BUN).

**Monitoring:** Monitor for signs/symptoms of sulfonamide reactions (eg, SJS, TEN, fulminant hepatic necrosis, agranulocytosis, aplastic anemia, other blood dyscrasias), oligohidrosis, hyperthermia, emergence or worsening of depression, suicidal thoughts or behavior, cognitive or other neuropsychiatric disorders (eg, psychosis, psychomotor slowing, somnolence), kidney stones, and status epilepticus. If abruptly withdraw from therapy, monitor for increased seizure frequency. Monitor renal function (SrCr, BUN); d/c if develop acute renal failure or sustained increases in BUN and SrCr. Monitor for severe muscle pain and/or weakness.

**Patient Counseling:** Inform that may produce drowsiness; do not drive or operate complex machinery until accustomed to effects of medication. Instruct to contact physician if skin rash develops or seizures worsen. Contact physician if develop signs or symptoms that could indicate a kidney stone (eg, sudden back pain, abdominal pain, blood in urine); inform that increasing fluid intake and urine output may decrease risk of kidney stones. Instruct to contact physician if a child has been taking zonisamide and is not sweating as usual with or without a fever. Notify physician if develop any signs or symptoms of hematological complications (eg, fever, sore throat, easy bruising). Zonisamide may increase the risk of suicidal thoughts and behavior; contact physician if develop emergence or worsening symptoms of depression, changes in mood or behavior, or the emergence of suicidal thoughts or behavior. Instruct to contact physician if severe muscle pain or weakness. develop. Inform females to use proper contraception while on therapy; contact physician if become pregnant, plan to become pregnant, or are breastfeeding during therapy. Advise to enroll in NAAED Pregnancy Registry at aedpregnancyregistry.org or by calling 888-233-2334.

**Administration:** Oral route. Caps should be swallowed whole. **Storage:** 25°C (77°F); excursions permitted to 15-30°C (59-86°F). Store in dry place and protected from light.

# ZORBTIVE RX

somatropin (EMD Serono)

**THERAPEUTIC CLASS:** Human growth hormone

**INDICATIONS:** Treatment of short bowel syndrome in patients receiving specialized nutritional support.

**DOSAGE:** *Adults:* 0.1mg/kg qd SC for 4 weeks. Max: 8mg qd. Rotate injection site.

**HOW SUPPLIED:** Inj: 8.8mg

**CONTRAINDICATIONS:** Acute critical illness due to complications following open heart or abdominal surgery, multiple accidental trauma, or acute respiratory failure; active neoplasia (either newly diagnosed or recurrent); benzyl alcohol sensitivity.

**WARNINGS/PRECAUTIONS:** Associated with acute pancreatitis. New onset impaired glucose intolerance, new onset type 2 DM, exacerbation of preexisting DM, ketoacidosis, diabetic coma reported; closely monitor with risk factors for glucose intolerance. Perform funduscopic evaluations periodically. Increased tissue turgor, musculoskeletal discomfort, and carpal tunnel syndrome may occur.

**ADVERSE REACTIONS:** Peripheral/facial edema, chest/back pain, fever, flu-like disorder, malaise, flatulence, abdominal pain, N/V, viral infection, dizziness, headache, rash.

**PREGNANCY:** Category B, caution in nursing.

**MECHANISM OF ACTION:** Human growth hormone; anabolic and anticatabolic agent, exerts influence by interacting with specific receptors. On gut, actions may be direct or mediated via local or systemic production of IGF-1; also enhances transmucosal transport of water, electrolytes, and nutrients.

**PHARMACOKINETICS: Absorption:** (SQ) Absolute bioavailability (70-90%). **Distribution:** $V_d$=12.0L. **Metabolism:** Liver, kidneys. **Elimination:** Urine; (SQ) $T_{1/2}$=3.94 hrs. (IV) $T_{1/2}$=0.58 hrs.

## NURSING CONSIDERATIONS

**Assessment:** Assess for acute critical illness (eg, complications after open heart or abdominal surgery, multiple accidental trauma, acute respiratory failure), active malignancy, hypersensitivity to benzyl alcohol, and possible drug interactions. Perform baseline fundoscopic exam.

**Monitoring:** Perform fundoscopic exam periodically. Monitor for signs/symptoms of impaired glucose intolerance, new onset type 2 DM, exacerbation of pre-existing DM, diabetic ketoacidosis, diabetic coma, carpal tunnel syndrome, acute pancreatitis, tissue atrophy at injection site, increased tissue turgor (swelling), musculoskeletal discomfort (eg, pain, swelling, stiffness), and hypersensitivity/allergic reactions.

**Patient Counseling:** Instruct thoroughly as to proper usage and disposal; caution against any reuse of needles or syringes. Advise to seek medical attention if symptoms of impaired glucose intolerance, new onset type 2 DM, exacerbation of pre-existing DM, diabetic ketoacidosis, diabetic coma, carpal tunnel syndrome, acute pancreatitis, tissue atrophy at injection site, increased tissue turgor (swelling), musculoskeletal discomfort (pain, swelling, stiffness), or hypersensitivity/allergic reactions occur.

**Administration:** SQ route. **Storage:** (Before reconstitution): 15-30°C (59-86°F). (After reconstitution): Refrigerate; 2-8°C (36-46°F) for up to 14 days. Avoid freezing.

# ZOSTAVAX — RX

zoster vaccine live (Merck)

**THERAPEUTIC CLASS:** Vaccine

**INDICATIONS:** Prevention of herpes zoster in individuals ≥60.

**DOSAGE:** *Adults:* ≥60 yrs: Inject SQ immediately after reconstitution with supplied diluent.

**HOW SUPPLIED:** Inj: 19,400 PFU/0.65mL

**CONTRAINDICATIONS:** Anaphylactic/anaphylactoid reactions to gelatin or neomycin. Primary or acquired immunodeficiency states (eg, leukemia); lymphomas or other malignant neoplasms affecting the bone marrow or lymphatic system; AIDS or other clinical manifestations HIV infections. Immunosuppressive therapy, including high-dose corticosteroids. Active untreated tuberculosis. Pregnancy.

**WARNINGS/PRECAUTIONS:** More extensive vaccine-associated rash or disseminated disease with immunosuppression. Anaphylactic/anaphylactoid reaction may occur. Deferral of vaccination should be considered in acute illness. Not indicated for prevention of primary varicella infection. Have epinephrine (1:1000) available.

**ADVERSE REACTIONS:** Erythema, pain, tenderness, swelling, pruritus.

**INTERACTIONS:** See Contraindications.

**PREGNANCY:** Category C, caution in nursing.

**MECHANISM OF ACTION:** Vaccine; stimulates immune system to produce antibodies that may protect against herpes zoster infection (shingles).

## NURSING CONSIDERATIONS

**Assessment:** Assess current health status and previous vaccination history.

**Monitoring:** Monitor for hypersensitivity reactions, injection-site reactions (eg, hematoma, pain, swelling, erythema, pruritus), and headache.

**Patient Counseling:** Inform of potential benefits/risks; report any adverse reactions to physician. Inform may not provide protection in all vaccine recipients.

**Administration:** SQ route. Inject into deltoid region of upper arm. **Storage:** Frozen at average temperature of 15°C (+5°F) or colder; diluent stored at room temperature 20-25°C (68-77°F) or refrigerated 2-8°C (36-46°F).

## Zosyn RX

tazobactam sodium - piperacillin sodium (Wyeth)

**THERAPEUTIC CLASS:** Broad-spectrum penicillin/beta-lactamase inhibitor

**INDICATIONS:** Treatment of appendicitis, peritonitis, uncomplicated/complicated skin and skin structure infections, postpartum endometritis, pelvic inflammatory disease, moderate severity of community-acquired pneumonia (CAP), and moderate to severe nosocomial pneumonia caused by susceptible strains of microorganisms.

**DOSAGE:** *Adults:* Usual: 3.375g q6h for 7-10 days. CrCl 20-40mL: 2.25g q6h. CrCl <20mL/min: 2.25g q8h. Hemodialysis/CAPD: 2.25g q12h. Give 1 additional 0.75g dose after each dialysis period. Nosocomial Pneumonia: 4.5g q6h for 7-14 days plus aminoglycoside. CrCl 20-40mL/min: 3.375g q6h. CrCl <20mL/min: 2.25g q6h. Hemodialysis/CAPD: 2.25g q8h. Give 1 additional 0.75g dose after each dialysis period. Elderly: Start at low end of dosing range. *Pediatrics:* Appendicitis/Peritonitis: ≤40kg: ≥9 months: 100mg piperacillin-12.5mg tazobactam/kg q8h. 2-9 months: 80mg piperacillin-10mg tazobactam/kg q8h. >40kg: Use adult dose.

**HOW SUPPLIED:** Inj: (Piperacillin-Tazobactam) 2g-0.25g, 3g-0.375g, 4g-0.5g, 2g-0.25g/50mL, 3g-0.375g/50mL, 4g-0.5g/100mL, 36g-4.5g.

**CONTRAINDICATIONS:** History of allergic reactions to cephalosporins.

**WARNINGS/PRECAUTIONS:** Serious, fatal hypersensitivity reactions reported; hypersensitivity reaction more likely to occur with history of PCN allergy or history of sensitivity to multiple allergens. *Clostridium difficile*-associated diarrhea (CDAD ) reported. D/C if bleeding manifestations occur. Emergence of treatment resistant organisms may develop; take appropriate measures if superinfection develops. May experience neuromuscular excitability or convulsions with higher doses. Contains 2.79mEq (64 mg) of $Na^+$ per gram of piperacillin; caution with restricted salt intake. Increased incidence of rash and fever in cystic fibrosis. Monitor electrolytes periodically with low $K^+$ reserves. Therapy may lead to emergence of resistant organisms that can cause superinfections. Caution with renal impairment (CrCl <40mL/min). Caution in elderly.

**ADVERSE REACTIONS:** Diarrhea, headache, constipation, N/V, insomnia, rash, dyspepsia, pruritus.

**INTERACTIONS:** Probenecid prolongs half-life. Monitor coagulation parameters with high doses of heparin, oral anticoagulants, or other drugs which may affect blood coagulation system or thrombocyte function. (Piperacillin) May prolong neuromuscular blockade of vecuronium or any non-depolarizing muscle relaxant. (Tazobactam) May inactivate aminoglycosides if mixed together.

**PREGNANCY:** Category B, caution in nursing.

**MECHANISM OF ACTION:** Piperacillin: Broad-spectrum penicillin; exerts bactericidal activity by inhibiting septum formation and cell-wall synthesis of susceptible bacteria. Tazobactam: β-lactamase enzyme inhibitor.

**PHARMACOKINETICS: Absorption:** Piperacillin (2.25g, 3.375g, 4.5g): $C_{max}$=134mcg/mL, 242mcg/mL, 298mcg/mL. Tazobactam (2.25g, 3.375g, 4.5g): $C_{max}$= 15mcg/mL, 24mcg/mL, 34mcg/mL. **Distribution:** Plasma protein binding (30%); wide distribution into tissues and bodily fluids; crosses placental barrier. Piperacillin: $V_d$=0.243L/kg, found in breast milk. **Elimination:** Kidneys; $T_{1/2}$=0.7-1.2 hrs. Piperacillin: Urine (68% unchanged). Tazobactam: Urine (80% unchanged, 20% as single metabolite).

## NURSING CONSIDERATIONS

**Assessment:** Assess for previous hypersensitivity reaction to cephalosporins, PCNs or other allergens, renal/hepatic impairment, hypokalemia, pregnancy/nursing status, and for possible drug interactions.

**Monitoring:** Periodically monitor renal/hepatic function, hematopoietic function, and serum $K^+$ levels. Monitor for signs/symptoms of anaphylactic/anaphylactoid reactions, CDAD, drug resistance or superinfection, bleeding manifestations, and electrolyte abnormalities.

**Patient Counseling:** Advise of risks/benefits of therapy. Inform drug only treats bacterial, not viral, infections. Instruct to take as directed; advise that skipping doses or not completing full course may decrease effectiveness and increase resistance. Advise to d/c and notify physician if allergic reaction or watery/bloody diarrhea (with or without muscle cramps) occur. Instruct to notify physician if pregnant/nursing.

**Administration:** IV route. Administer as infusion over 30 min. **Storage:** 20-25°C (68-77°F); discard any unused portion of reconstituted solution after 24 hrs if at room temperature at 20-25°C (68-77°F) after 48 hrs if refrigerated at 2-8°C (36-46°).

# Zovirax Cream RX

acyclovir (Biovail)

**THERAPEUTIC CLASS:** Nucleoside analogue

**INDICATIONS:** Treatment of recurrent herpes labialis (cold sores).

**DOSAGE:** *Adults:* Apply 5x/day for 4 days. Initiate with 1st sign/symptom. *Pediatrics:* ≥12 yrs: Apply 5x/day for 4 days. Initiate with 1st sign/symptom.

**HOW SUPPLIED:** Cre: 5% [2g, 5g]

**WARNINGS/PRECAUTIONS:** Cutaneous use only; not for use in the eye, mouth or nose.

**ADVERSE REACTIONS:** Dry lips, desquamation, dryness of skin, cracked lips, burning skin, pruritus, flakiness of skin, stinging on skin.

**PREGNANCY:** Category B, caution in nursing.

**MECHANISM OF ACTION:** Synthetic purine nucleoside analogue; possesses inhibitory activity against herpes simplex virus types 1 and 2, and varicella-zoster virus. Stops replication of herpes viral DNA by competitive inhibition of viral DNA polymerase, incorporation into and termination of growing viral DNA chain, and inactivation of viral DNA polymerase.

**PHARMACOKINETICS: Absorption:** Minimal systemic absorption.

## NURSING CONSIDERATIONS

**Assessment:** Assess nursing and immunocompromised status.

**Monitoring:** Monitor for signs/symptoms of irritation and contact sensitization.

**Patient Counseling:** Inform that medication is for treatment of cold sores. Instruct that medication for external use only; avoid application to eyes, inside mouth or nose, or unaffected skin areas. Inform that drug not for treatment of genital herpes and not a cure for cold sores. Instruct to use at first sign of cold sore (eg, tingling, redness, bump, or itch). Counsel to wash hands prior to and following administration, apply to clean/dry skin, and do not cover cold sores with bandages or dressings unless directed by physician. Advise to avoid applying another type of skin product (eg, cosmetics, sunscreen, lip balms) or medication to cold sore area during therapy, unless directed by physician. Instruct not to bathe, shower, or swim immediately after application.

**Administration:** Topical route. **Storage:** 25°C (77°F); excursions permitted to 15-30°C (59-86°F).

# ZOVIRAX INJECTION RX

acyclovir sodium (GlaxoSmithKline)

**THERAPEUTIC CLASS:** Nucleoside analogue

**INDICATIONS:** Treatment of neonatal herpes simplex infections and herpes simplex encephalitis. Treatment of varicella-zoster (shingles), initial and recurrent mucosal and cutaneous herpes simplex in immunocompromised patients. Treatment of severe initial clinical episodes of herpes genitalis in immunocompetent patients.

**DOSAGE:** *Adults:* Initiate with 1st sign/symptom. Max: 20mg/kg q8h for any patient. Mucosal/Cutaneous Herpes Simplex Infections: 5mg/kg q8h for 7 days. Herpes Genitalis: 5mg/kg q8h for 5 days. Herpes Simplex Encephalitis: 10mg/kg q8h for 10 days. Varicella Zoster: 10mg/kg q8h for 7 days. Obese Patients: Dose according to IBW. CrCl 25-50mL/min: Give 100% of recommended dose q12h. CrCl 10-25: Give 100% of recommended dose q24h. CrCl 0-10mL/min: Give 50% of recommended dose q24h. Elderly: Reduce dose and monitor renal function.
*Pediatrics:* Initiate with 1st sign/symptom. Max: 20mg/kg q8h for any patient. Mucosal/Cutaneous Herpes Simplex: ≥12 yrs: 5mg/kg q8h for 7 days. <12 yrs: 10mg/kg q8h for 7 days. Herpes Genitalis: ≥12 yrs: 5mg/kg q8h for 5 days. Herpes Simplex Encephalitis: ≥12 yrs: 10mg/kg q8h for 10 days. 3 months-12 yrs: 20mg/kg q8h for 10 days. Neonatal Herpes Simplex: Birth-3 months: 10mg/kg q8h for 10 days. Varicella Zoster: ≥12 yrs: 10mg/kg q8h for 7 days. <12 yrs: 20mg/kg q8h for 7 days. Obese Patients: Dose according to IBW. CrCl 25-50mL/min: Give 100% of recommended dose q12h. CrCl 10-25: Give 100% of recommended dose q24h. CrCl 0-10mL/min: Give 50% of recommended dose q24h.

**HOW SUPPLIED:** Inj: 500mg, 1000mg

**CONTRAINDICATIONS:** Hypersensitivity to valacyclovir.

**WARNINGS/PRECAUTIONS:** Do not administer topically, IM, PO, SQ, or in the eye. Adjust dose in renal impairment and the elderly. Renal failure and death reported. Thrombotic thrombocytopenic purpura/hemolytic uremic syndrome in immunocompromised patients reported. Patient must be adequately hydrated. Caution with underlying neurologic abnormalities, electrolyte abnormalities, significant hypoxia, and serious renal or hepatic abnormalities. Infusion must not be given over <1 hr.

**ADVERSE REACTIONS:** Injection-site inflammation, phlebitis, transient serum creatinine and BUN elevations, N/V.

**INTERACTIONS:** Increased serum levels with probenecid. Avoid with nephrotoxic drugs.

**PREGNANCY:** Category B, caution in nursing.

**MECHANISM OF ACTION:** Synthetic purine nucleoside analogue; possesses inhibitory activity against herpes simplex virus types 1 and 2, and varicella-zoster virus. Stops replication of herpes viral DNA by competitive inhibition of viral DNA polymerase, incorporation into and termination of growing viral DNA chain, and inactivation of viral DNA polymerase.

**PHARMACOKINETICS: Absorption:** $C_{max}$=9.8mcg/mL (5mg/kg), 22.9mcg/mL (10mg/kg). **Distribution:** Plasma protein binding (9-33%); found in breast milk. **Metabolism:** 9-carboxymethoxymethylguanine (major metabolite). **Elimination:** Urine (62-91% unchanged) (14.1% metabolite). Refer to PI for detailed info regarding renal function and pediatrics.

## NURSING CONSIDERATIONS

**Assessment:** Assess for immunosuppression, renal/hepatic disease, electrolyte abnormalities, significant hypoxia, pregnancy/nursing status, hydration status, possible drug interactions.

**Monitoring:** Monitor signs/symptoms of renal failure, thrombocytopenic purpura/hemolytic uremic syndrome, encephalopathic changes (eg, lethargy, obtundation, tremors, confusion, hallucinations, agitation, seizures, or coma). Monitor renal function (CrCl), LFTs, and CBC.

**Patient Counseling:** Notify physician if pregnant/nursing. Inform about potential risks of therapy and advise to report any adverse reactions.

**Administration:** IV route. Infuse over period of ≥ 1 hr to reduce risk of renal tubular damage, with adequate hydration. Not for topical, IM, oral, ocular, or SQ use. **Storage:** 15-25°C (59-77°F).

## Zovirax Ointment RX

acyclovir (Biovail)

**THERAPEUTIC CLASS:** Nucleoside analogue

**INDICATIONS:** Management of initial genital herpes and in limited non-life-threatening mucocutaneous herpes simplex infections in immunocompromised patients.

**DOSAGE:** *Adults:* Apply to all lesions q3h, 6x/day for 7 days. Apply with finger cot or rubber glove to prevent autoinoculation and transmission. Initiate with 1st sign/symptom.

**HOW SUPPLIED:** Oint: 5% [15g]

**WARNINGS/PRECAUTIONS:** Not for use for the prevention of recurrent HSV infections. Cutaneous use only; avoid eyes.

**ADVERSE REACTIONS:** Pain with application, transient burning and stinging, pruritus.

**PREGNANCY:** Category B, not for use in nursing.

**MECHANISM OF ACTION:** Synthetic purine nucleoside analogue; possesses inhibitory activity against herpes simplex virus types 1 and 2, and varicella-zoster virus. Stops replication of herpes viral DNA by competitive inhibition of viral DNA polymerase, incorporation into and termination of growing viral DNA chain, and inactivation of viral DNA polymerase.

**PHARMACOKINETICS: Absorption:** Minimal systemic absorption.

### NURSING CONSIDERATIONS

**Assessment:** Assess for active signs/symptoms of herpes simplex virus. Assess nursing status.

**Monitoring:** Monitor for signs/symptoms of mild pain (eg, transient burning, stinging) and for pruritus at treatment site.

**Patient Counseling:** Counsel that ointment is for cutaneous administration only; should not be used in eyes. Advise to initiate as soon as possible following onset of signs/symptoms; not to use in absence of signs/symptoms. Counsel to use finger cot or rubber glove when applying to prevent autoinoculation of other body sites and transmission of infection to others.

**Administration:** Topical route. **Storage:** 15-25°C (59-77°F); store in dry place.

## Zovirax Oral RX

acyclovir (GlaxoSmithKline)

**THERAPEUTIC CLASS:** Nucleoside analogue

**INDICATIONS:** Acute treatment of herpes zoster (shingles). Treatment of initial and recurrent episodes of genital herpes. Treatment of chickenpox (varicella).

**DOSAGE:** *Adults:* Herpes Zoster: 800mg q4h, 5x/day for 7-10 days. Start within 72 hrs after onset of rash. Genital Herpes: Initial: 200mg q4h, 5x/day for 10 days. Chronic Therapy: 400mg bid or 200mg 3-5x/day up to 12 months, then re-evaluate. Intermittent Therapy: 200mg q4h, 5x/day for 5 days. Start with 1st sign/symptom of recurrence. Chickenpox: 800mg qid for 5 days. CrCl 10-25mL/min: For a dose of 800mg q4h, give 800mg q8h. CrCl 0-10mL/min: For a dose of 200mg q4h, give 200mg q12h. For a dose of 400mg q12h, give 200mg q12h. For a dose of 800mg q4h, give 800mg q12h. Elderly: Reduce dose.

*Pediatrics:* ≥2 yrs: ≤40kg: Chickenpox: 20mg/kg qid for 5 days. >40kg: 800mg qid for 5 days.

**HOW SUPPLIED:** Cap: 200mg; Sus: 200mg/5mL; Tab: 400mg, 800mg

**CONTRAINDICATIONS:** Hypersensitivity to valacyclovir.

**WARNINGS/PRECAUTIONS:** Adjust dose in renal impairment, elderly. Renal failure and death reported. Thrombotic thrombocytopenic purpura/hemolytic uremic syndrome in immunocompromised patients reported.

**ADVERSE REACTIONS:** Nausea, diarrhea, headache, malaise, and renal dysfunction, seizures, tremors, anemia, leukopenia, elevated LFTs.

**INTERACTIONS:** Probenecid increased levels of IV formulation. Caution with potentially nephrotoxic agents.

**PREGNANCY:** Category B, caution in nursing.

**MECHANISM OF ACTION:** Synthetic purine nucleoside analogue; possesses inhibitory activity against herpes simplex virus types 1 and 2, and varicella-zoster virus. Stops replication of herpes viral DNA by competitive inhibition of viral DNA polymerase, incorporation into and termination of growing viral DNA chain, and inactivation of viral DNA polymerase.

**PHARMACOKINETICS: Absorption:** Absolute bioavailability (10-20%). Oral administration of variable doses resulted in different parameters. **Distribution:** Plasma protein binding (9-33%). **Elimination:** $T_{1/2}$=2.5-3.3 hrs.

## NURSING CONSIDERATIONS

**Assessment:** Assess if immunocompromised (eg, transplant, advanced HIV, AIDS), renal impairment, and possible drug interactions.

**Monitoring:** Monitor for signs/symptoms of thrombotic thrombocytopenic purpura/hemolytic syndrome. Check renal function, LFTs, BUN, and SrCr.

**Patient Counseling:** Inform may be taken with/without food and to maintain adequate hydration. Advise to avoid contact when lesions or symptoms are present to avoid infecting partners. Advise to use safe sex practice in combination with suppressive therapy. Instruct to initiate treatment at earliest symptom of cold sores (eg, tingling, itching, burning).

**Administration:** Oral route. **Storage:** 15-25°C (59-77°F); protect from moisture.

# Zyban RX

bupropion HCl (GlaxoSmithKline)

**Serious neuropsychiatric events including depression, suicidal ideation, suicide attempt, and completed suicide have been reported. Some cases may be complicated by nicotine withdrawal symptoms. Advise patients and caregivers that patient should stop taking bupropion and contact a healthcare provider immediately if agitation, hostility, depressed mood, changes in thinking or behavior, suicidal ideation, or suicidal behavior occur. The risks of bupropion should be weighed against the benefits of its use. Although Zyban is not indicated for the treatment of depression, it contains the same active ingredient found in antidepressant medications. Antidepressants increase the risk of suicidal thinking and behavior in children, adolescents, and young adults with major depressive disorder (MDD) and other psychiatric disorders. Bupropion is not approved for use in pediatric patients.**

**THERAPEUTIC CLASS:** Aminoketone

**INDICATIONS:** Aid to smoking cessation treatment.

**DOSAGE:** *Adults:* Initial: 150mg qd for 3 days. Usual: 150mg bid. Max: 300mg/day. Separate doses by at least 8 hrs. Initiate treatment while patient is still smoking. Patients should set a "target quit date" within the first 2 weeks. Treat for 7 to 12 weeks; d/c at 7 weeks if no progress seen. Renal Dysfunction: Reduce frequency of dosing. Severe Hepatic Cirrhosis: 150mg qod. Swallow whole, do not crush, chew, or divide.

**HOW SUPPLIED:** Tab, Sustained-Release: 150mg

**CONTRAINDICATIONS:** Seizure disorder, bulimia or anorexia nervosa, use of MAOIs or within 14 days of use, other forms of bupropion, abrupt d/c of alcohol or sedatives (including benzodiazepines).

**WARNINGS/PRECAUTIONS:** Patients with major depressive disorder (MDD) may experience worsening of depression and/or emergence of suicidal ideation and behavior (suicidality) or unusual changes in behavior; monitor appropriately especially during the initial few months of a course of drug therapy, or during dosing changes. Screen for bipolar disorder; may precipitate a mixed/manic episode. Dose-dependent risk of seizures; do not prescribe doses over 300mg/day for smoking cessation. D/C bupropion use and do not restart if seizure occurs. Extreme caution with history of seizure, cranial trauma, or other predisposition toward seizures, and in patients with severe hepatic cirrhosis. Potential for hepatotoxicity. Allergic reactions (eg, anaphylactoid/anaphylactic) and HTN reported. Insomnia, neuropsychiatric symptoms (eg, mood changes, psychosis, hallucinations, paranoia, delusions, hostility, agitation) reported. May activate latent psychosis. Caution in use with hepatic impairment, recent history of myocardial infarction (MI), unstable heart disease, and renal impairment.

**ADVERSE REACTIONS:** Serious neuropsychiatric events (including depression, suicidal ideation, suicide attempt, completed suicide), insomnia, dry mouth, dizziness, disturbed concentration, dream abnormality, rhinitis, rash, pruritus, nausea, diarrhea, anorexia, constipation, arthralgia.

**INTERACTIONS:** See Contraindications. Extreme caution with drugs that lower seizure threshold (eg, antidepressants, antipsychotics, theophylline, systemic steroids). Increased seizure risk with opioid, cocaine, or stimulant addiction, use of OTC stimulants or anorectics, oral hypoglycemics or insulin, excessive use or abrupt d/c of alcohol or sedatives (including benzodiazepines). Caution with levodopa and amantadine. Caution with drugs that are metabolized by CYP2D6 (eg, SSRIs, TCAs, antipsychotics, β-blockers, type 1C antiarrhythmics); use low initial dose and gradually titrate. Monitor HTN with nicotine replacement. Caution with CYP2B6 substrates or inhibitors (eg, orphenadrine, thiotepa, cyclophosphamide). Carbamazepine, phenytoin, and phenobarbital may induce metabolism of bupropion. Cimetidine may inhibit the metabolism of bupropion. Minimize or avoid alcohol. Hemorrhagic or thrombotic complications were observed when bupropion was coadministered with warfarin.

**PREGNANCY:** Pregnancy C, not for use in nursing.

**MECHANISM OF ACTION:** Aminoketone: unknown; suspected to inhibit neuronal uptake of norepinephrine and dopamine.

**PHARMACOKINETICS: Absorption:** $C_{max}$=136ng/mL; $T_{max}$=3 hrs. **Distribution:** $V_d$=1,950L; plasma protein binding (84%); found in breast milk. **Metabolism:** Extensive, through hydroxylation and reduction pathways. Hydroxybupropion, threohydrobupropion, and erythrohydrobupropion (active metabolites). **Elimination:** Urine; $T_{1/2}$=21 hrs, 20 hrs, 37 hrs, 33 hrs (bupropion, hydroxybupropion, threohydrobupropion, erythrohydrobupropion, repectively).

## NURSING CONSIDERATIONS

**Assessment:** Assess for hepatic/renal dysfunction, seizure disorder, risk of seizure development (eg, cranial trauma, excessive use of alcohol or sedatives, addiction to opiates, cocaine, stimulants, use of insulin or oral hypoglycemics), presence or history of bulimia or anorexia nervosa, MDD, bipolar disorder, recent MI, presence of unstable heart disease, pregnancy/nursing status, and possible drug interactions. Detailed psychiatric history (eg, family history of suicide, bipolar disorder, depression) should be taken.

**Monitoring:** Monitor signs and symptoms of neuropsychiatric events (eg, depression, suicidal ideation, mood changes, psychosis, hallucinations, paranoia), hepatotoxicity, allergic reactions (eg, anaphylactoid/anaphylactic reactions), insomnia, activation of psychosis and/or mania, HTN, and seizures.

**Patient Counseling:** Advise patients and caregivers to discontinue therapy and notify physician if agitation, hostility, depressed mood, changes in thinking or behavior, or if suicidal ideation or suicidal behavior occur. Inform patient to notify physician if pregnant/nursing. Instruct to swallow whole and not to crush or chew the tablet. Instruct to read medication guide and discuss with physician.

**Administration:** Oral route. **Storage:** 20-25°C (68-77°F); dispense in a tight closed, light-resistant container.

## ZYDONE CIII

hydrocodone bitartrate - acetaminophen (Endo)

**THERAPEUTIC CLASS:** Opioid analgesic

**INDICATIONS:** Relief of moderate to moderately severe pain.

**DOSAGE:** *Adults:* (5/400): 1-2 tabs q4-6h prn. Max: 8 tabs/day. (7.5/400, 10/400): 1 tab q4-6h prn. Max: 6 tabs/day.

**HOW SUPPLIED:** Tab: (Hydrocodone-APAP) 5mg-400mg, 7.5mg-400mg, 10mg-400mg

**WARNINGS/PRECAUTIONS:** May produce dose-related respiratory depression. May obscure diagnosis of acute abdominal conditions or head injuries. Caution in elderly, debilitated, severe hepatic or renal dysfunction, hypothyroidism, Addison's disease, prostatic hypertrophy, urethral stricture, pulmonary disease, and postoperative use. May be habit-forming. May impair mental/physical abilities. Suppresses cough reflex.

**ADVERSE REACTIONS:** Lightheadedness, dizziness, sedation, N/V.

**INTERACTIONS:** Additive CNS depression with opioids, antihistamines, antipsychotics, antianxiety agents, or other CNS depressants (including alcohol). Increased effect of antidepressant or hydrocodone with MAOIs or TCAs.

**PREGNANCY:** Category C, not for use in nursing.

**MECHANISM OF ACTION:** Hydrocodone: Opioid analgesic and antitussive; not established. Possibly related to existence of opiate receptors in CNS. Most actions involve CNS and smooth muscle. APAP: Nonopiate, nonsalicylate analgesic and antipyretic. Mechanism of analgesic effect not established; involves peripheral influences. Antipyretic activity mediated through hypothalamic heat-regulating centers. Inhibits prostaglandin synthetase.

**PHARMACOKINETICS: Absorption:** Hydrocodone: $C_{max}$=23.6ng/mL; $T_{max}$=1.3 hrs. APAP: Rapidly absorbed. **Distribution:** APAP: Found in breast milk. **Metabolism:** Hydrocodone: O-demethylation, N-demethylation and 6-keto reduction. APAP: Liver (conjugation). **Elimination:** Hydrocodone: $T_{1/2}$=3.8 hrs. APAP: Urine (85%); $T_{1/2}$=1.25-3 hrs.

### NURSING CONSIDERATIONS

**Assessment:** Assess for hypersensitivity to other opioids, head injury or other intracranial lesions, presence of increased ICP, acute abdominal conditions, presence of debilitation (eg, elderly), hepatic/renal impairment, hypothyroidism, Addison's disease, prostatic hypertrophy or urethral stricture, pulmonary disease, pregnancy/nursing status, and possible drug interactions.

**Monitoring:** Monitor for signs/symptoms of respiratory depression, elevations in CSF pressure, hepatic/renal dysfunction, drug abuse and dependence.

**Patient Counseling:** Inform that drug may impair mental/physical abilities required for performing potentially hazardous tasks (eg, operating machinery/driving). Advise to avoid alcohol and other CNS depressants. Counsel drug may be habit forming; take only as long as prescribed, in amounts prescribed, and no more frequently than prescribed.

**Administration:** Oral route. **Storage:** 25°C (77°F); excursions permitted to 15-30°C (59-86°F). Dispense in a tight, light-resistant container with child-resistant closure.

## ZYFLO CR RX

zileuton (Cornerstone)

**THERAPEUTIC CLASS:** Leukotriene inhibitor

**INDICATIONS:** Prophylaxis and chronic treatment of asthma in adults and children ≥12 yrs.

**DOSAGE:** *Adults:* 1200mg bid within 1 hr after am and pm meals. Max: 2400mg/day. If a dose is missed, take the next dose at the scheduled time and do not double the dose. Do not chew, cut, or crush.
*Pediatrics:* ≥12 yrs: 1200mg bid within 1 hr after am and pm meals. Max: 2400mg/day. If a dose is missed, take the next dose at the scheduled time and not double the dose. Do not chew, cut, or crush.

**HOW SUPPLIED:** Tab: Extended-Release: 600mg* *scored

**CONTRAINDICATIONS:** Active liver disease or persistent transaminase elevations ( ≥3x ULN).

**WARNINGS/PRECAUTIONS:** Not for treatment of acute attacks. Elevations of one or more liver function enzymes and bilirubin may occur; evaluate and monitor periodically. D/C if signs of liver disease occur. Neuropsychiatric events including sleep disorders and behavior changes reported; evaluate risks and benefits of continuing treatment.

**ADVERSE REACTIONS:** Headache, elevation of hepatic function enzyme (ALT) and bilirubin, nausea, myalgia, upper respiratory tract infection, sinusitis, pharyngolaryngeal pain, neuropsychiatric events.

**INTERACTIONS:** Monitor drugs metabolized by CYP3A4. Increases theophylline levels; reduce theophylline by 50% and monitor levels. May increase propranolol levels when coadministering; monitor closely and reduce dose if necessary. May decrease warfarin clearance; monitor prothrombin time, or other coagulation tests.

**PREGNANCY:** Category C, not for use in nursing.

**MECHANISM OF ACTION:** Leukotriene inhibitor; anti-asthmatic agent, inhibits leukotriene ($LTB_4$, $LTC_4$, $LTD_4$, and $LTE_4$) formation by inhibiting the enzyme 5-lipoxygenase.

**PHARMACOKINETICS: Absorption:** $T_{max}$=4.3 hrs. **Distribution:** $V_d$=1.2L/kg; plasma protein binding (93%). **Metabolism:** Liver, via oxidation by CYP1A2, CYP2C9, CYP3A4; glucuronidation. **Elimination:** Urine, feces; $T_{1/2}$=3.2 hrs.

## NURSING CONSIDERATIONS

**Assessment:** Assess LFTs and evaluate for hepatic impairment, acute asthma, status asthmaticus, pregnancy/nursing status, neuropsychiatric events, alcoholism, allergic reactions, and possible drug interactions.

**Monitoring:** Monitor LFTs such as hepatic enzymes, bilirubin. Monitor for hypersensitivity reactions, sinusitis, pharyngolaryngeal pain, and neuropsychiatric events (eg, sleep disorders, behavior changes). Monitor concomitant use of propranolol closely; reduce dose if necessary.

**Patient Counseling:** Inform that drug is indicated for chronic treatment of asthma and not indicated for used to treat acute epsiodes of asthma; take regularly as prescribed one hour after am and pm meals. Advise not to reduce dose or d/c other anti-asthma medications unless instructed. If a dose is missed, take the next dose at the scheduled time and do not double the dose. Instruct to notify healthcare provider if signs/symptoms of liver dysfunction (eg, right upper quadrant pain, nausea, fatigue, lethargy, pruritus, jaundice, "flu-like" symptoms) or neuropsychiatric events (eg, sleep disorder, behavior changes) occur. Consult physician before starting or stopping any prescription or non-prescription medications. Counsel about possibilities of liver damage and need for liver enzyme monitoring on regular basis. Avoid alcohol.

**Administration:** Oral route. **Storage:** 20-25°C (68-77°F); excursions permitted to 15-30°C (59-86°F). Protect from light and replace cap after use.

# ZYLET RX

loteprednol etabonate - tobramycin (Bausch & Lomb)

**THERAPEUTIC CLASS:** Aminoglycoside/corticosteroid

**INDICATIONS:** Treatment of steroid-responsive inflammatory ocular conditions for which a corticosteroid is indicated and where superficial bacterial ocular infection or a risk of bacterial ocular infection exists.

**DOSAGE:** *Adults:* Initial: 1-2 drops q4-6h. May increase to 1-2 drops q1-2h for first 24-48 hrs. Max: 20mL for initial Rx.

**HOW SUPPLIED:** Sus: 2.5mL, 5mL, 10mL

**CONTRAINDICATIONS:** Viral diseases of the cornea and conjunctiva including epithelial herpes simplex keratitis (dendritic keratitis), vaccinia, and varicella, and also in mycobacterial infection of the eye and fungal diseases of ocular structures.

**WARNINGS/PRECAUTIONS:** Not for injection into the eye. Prolonged use may result in glaucoma, optic nerve damage, visual acuity and fields of vision defects, cataracts, secondary ocular infections. May exacerbate the severity of many viral infections of the eye (including herpes simplex). May delay healing and increase incidence of bleb formation after cataract surgery.

**ADVERSE REACTIONS:** Injection and superficial punctate keratitis, increased IOP, burning, stinging, headache, secondary infection, vision disorders, discharge, itching, lacrimation disorder, photophobia, corneal deposits, ocular discomfort, eyelid disorder.

**PREGNANCY:** Category C, caution in nursing.

**MECHANISM OF ACTION:** Loteprednol: Corticosteroid; not understood. Thought to act by induction of phospholipase $A_2$ inhibitory proteins, lipocortins. Tobramycin: Aminoglycoside antibiotic; inhibits synthesis of proteins in bacterial cells.

## NURSING CONSIDERATIONS

**Assessment:** Assess for viral disease of cornea and conjunctiva (eg, dendritic keratitis, vaccinia, varicella), mycobacterial infection of eye, fungal disease of eye, glaucoma, and possible drug interactions.

**Monitoring:** Routinely monitor IOP (use >10 days). Monitor for signs/symptoms of hypersensitivity reactions, glaucoma, defects in visual acuity and fields of vision, posterior subcapsular cataracts, perforations, and superinfections.

**Patient Counseling:** Instruct not to touch dropper tip to any surface to avoid contamination and not to wear contact lenses during therapy. Advise to seek medical attention if pain develops, if itching/inflammation becomes aggravated, or if hypersensitivity reactions, defects in vision, glaucoma, perforations, or superinfections occur.

**Administration:** Ocular route. **Storage:** 15-25°C (59-77°F). Protect from freezing; store upright.

# ZYLOPRIM RX

allopurinol (Prometheus)

**THERAPEUTIC CLASS:** Xanthine oxidase inhibitor

**INDICATIONS:** Management of symptoms of primary and secondary gout (acute attacks, tophi, joint destruction, uric acid lithiasis, and/or nephropathy). Management of hyperuricosuria and hyperuricemia in patients with leukemia, lymphoma and malignancies due to chemotherapy. Management of recurrent calcium oxalate calculi in those with hyperuricosuria (uric acid excretion >800mg/day in males and >750mg/day in females).

**DOSAGE:** *Adults:* Individualize dose. Reduction of Flare-Up of Acute Gouty Attacks: Initial: 100mg/day. Titrate: Increase by 100mg/week until serum uric acid level is ≤6mg/dL. Mild Gout: Usual: 200-300mg/day. Moderately Severe Tophaceous Gout: Usual: 400-600mg/day. Max: 800mg/day. Concomitant Colchicine/Anti-Inflammtatory Agents: While adjusting dose of allopurinol, continue therapy until serum uric acid normal and no acute gouty attacks for months. Transfer from a Uricosuric Agent: Gradually reduce dose of uricosuric agent over several weeks while gradually increasing allopurinol to the required dose. Recurrent Calcium Oxalate Stones: Usual: 200-300mg/day in divided doses or as single equivalent. Prevention of Uric Acid Nephropathy with Chemotherapy: Usual: 600-800mg/day for 2-3 days with high fluid intake. CrCl 10-20mL/min: 200mg/day. CrCl <10mL/min: Max: 100mg/day.

CrCl <3mL/min: Also increase dosing intervals. Take after meals. Divide dose if >300mg.
*Pediatrics:* Hyperuricemia with Malignancies: 6-10 yrs: 300mg/day. <6 yrs: 150mg/day. Evaluate response after 48 hrs. Take after meals.

**HOW SUPPLIED:** Tab: 100mg*, 300mg* *scored

**WARNINGS/PRECAUTIONS:** Not for treatment of asymptomatic hyperuricemia. D/C at first appearance of skin rash or other signs of allergic reaction. Severe hypersensitivity reactions, hepatotoxicity, and bone marrow depression reported. Monitor LFTs during early stages of therapy with liver disease. Caution with activities that require alertness. Caution with renal impairment. Renal failure reported with hyperuricemia secondary to neoplastic diseases; caution with multiple myeloma and congestive myocardial disease. Fluid intake should yield ≥2L of urinary output/day. Maintain neutral or slightly alkaline urine. Acute gouty attacks increase during early stages of therapy; give colchicine or anti-inflammatory agents.

**ADVERSE REACTIONS:** Acute gout attacks, rash, diarrhea, SGOT/SGPT increase, alkaline phosphatase increase, nausea.

**INTERACTIONS:** Increased toxicity with thiazide diuretics; monitor renal function. Reduce mercaptopurine or azathioprine to 1/3 or 1/4 of usual dose with concomitant use. Prolongs half-life of dicumarol and chlorpropamide. May increase cyclosporine levels. Decreased effects with uricosuric agents. Increased skin rash with ampicillin and amoxicillin. Enhanced bone marrow suppression by cyclophosphamide and other cytotoxic agents among patients with neoplastic disease, except leukemia. Caution with sulfinpyrazone.

**PREGNANCY:** Category C, caution in nursing.

**MECHANISM OF ACTION:** Xanthine oxidase inhibitor; acts on purine catabolism; reduces production of uric acid by inhibiting biochemical reactions immediately preceding its formation.

**PHARMACOKINETICS: Absorption:** $C_{max}$=3mcg/mL, $T_{max}$=1.5 hrs. Oxipurinol: $C_{max}$=6.5mcg/mL, $T_{max}$=4.5 hrs. **Metabolism:** Oxidation to oxipurinol (metabolite). **Elimination:** Kidneys, feces (20%); $T_{1/2}$=1-2 hrs. Oxipurinol: $T_{1/2}$=15 hrs.

## NURSING CONSIDERATIONS

**Assessment:** Assess for HTN, DM, multiple myeloma, congestive myocardial diseases, pre-existing hepatic/renal disease, pregnancy/nursing status and possible drug interactions.

**Monitoring:** Monitor LFTs, serum uric acid, and renal function periodically. Monitor for signs/symptoms of hepatotoxicity, hypersensitivity/allergic reaction, bone marrow depression, and renal dysfunction.

**Patient Counseling:** Inform that full benefit will not be seen until after 2-6 weeks of therapy. Increase fluid intake during therapy to prevent renal stones. Instruct to take after meals to minimize gastric irritation. Caution that drowsiness may occur and physical/mental abilities may be impaired. Caution about possible drug interactions. Advise to seek medical attention immediately at 1st sign of allergic reaction (skin rash), painful urination, blood in urine, irritation of eyes, swelling of lips/mouth, or hepatotoxicity (anorexia, weight loss, pruritus).

**Administration:** Oral route. **Storage:** 15-25°C (59-77°F); store in dry place and protect from light.

# Zymar — RX

gatifloxacin (Allergan)

**THERAPEUTIC CLASS:** Fluoroquinolone

**INDICATIONS:** Treatment of bacterial conjunctivitis.

**DOSAGE:** *Adults:* 1 drop q2h while awake, up to 8x/day for 2 days; then 1 drop up to qid while awake for 5 days.
*Pediatrics:* ≥1 yr: 1 drop q2h while awake, up to 8x/day for 2 days; then 1 drop up to qid while awake for 5 days.

**HOW SUPPLIED:** Sol: 0.3% [5mL]

**WARNINGS/PRECAUTIONS:** Not for injection. Do not inject subconjunctivally or into the anterior chamber of the eye. Superinfection may result with prolonged use. Fatal hypersensitivity reactions reported after 1st dose of systemic quinolone therapy. Avoid contact lenses when symptoms are present.

**ADVERSE REACTIONS:** Conjunctival irritation, increased lacrimation, keratitis, papillary conjunctivitis, chemosis, conjunctival hemorrhage, dry eye, eye discharge/irritation/pain, red eye, eyelid edema, headache, reduced visual acuity, taste disturbance.

**INTERACTIONS:** Systemic quinolone therapy may increase theophylline levels, interfere with caffeine metabolism, enhance warfarin effects, and elevate SrCr with cyclosporine.

**PREGNANCY:** Category C, caution in nursing.

**MECHANISM OF ACTION:** Fluoroquinolone antibiotic; inhibits topoisomerase II (DNA gyrase) and topoisomerase IV. DNA gyrase is essential enzyme involved in replication, transcription, and repair of bacterial DNA. Topoisomerase IV is enzyme known to play key role in partitioning of chromosomal DNA during bacterial cell division.

## NURSING CONSIDERATIONS

**Assessment:** Assess for proper diagnosis of causative organisms (eg, slit lamp biomicroscopy, fluorescein staining). Assess for hypersensitivity to other quinolones, possible drug interactions, and use in pregnancy/nursing.

**Monitoring:** Monitor for signs/symptoms of hypersensitivity or anaphylactic reactions (eg, cardiovascular collapse, loss of consciousness, angioedema). Monitor for overgrowth of nonsusceptible organisms (eg, fungi) with prolonged therapy.

**Patient Counseling:** Advise to avoid contaminating applicator tip with material from eye, fingers, or other sources. Instruct to d/c therapy and contact physician at first sign of rash or allergic reaction. Advise not to wear contact lenses if there are signs/symptoms of bacterial conjunctivitis.

**Administration:** Ocular route. Do not inject into eye. **Storage:** Store at 15-25°C (59-77°F). Protect from freezing.

# ZYPREXA — RX

olanzapine (Lilly)

**Elderly patients with dementia-related psychosis treated with antipsychotic drugs are at an increased risk of death. Most deaths reported appeared to be cardiovascular (eg, heart failure, sudden death) or infectious (eg, pneumonia) in nature. Olanzapine is not approved for the treatment of patients with dementia-related psychosis.**

**OTHER BRAND NAMES:** Zyprexa Zydis (Lilly) - Zyprexa IntraMuscular (Lilly)

**THERAPEUTIC CLASS:** Thienobenzodiazepine

**INDICATIONS:** (PO) Treatment of schizophrenia in adults and adolescent patients (ages 13-17 yrs). Acute treatment of manic or mixed episodes associated with bipolar I disorder and maintenance treatment of bipolar I disorder in adults and adolescent patients (ages 13-17 yrs). Adjunct to lithium or valproate for the treatment of manic episodes or mixed episodes associated with bipolar I disorder in adults. In combination with fluoxetine for the treatment of depressive episodes associated with bipolar I disorder and for treatment of treatment-resistant depression. (Inj) Treatment of acute agitation associated with schizophrenia and bipolar I mania.

**DOSAGE:** *Adults:* (PO) Schizophrenia: Initial/Usual: 5-10mg qd. Target dose: 10mg/day. Titrate: Adjust by 5mg daily at weekly intervals. Max: 20mg/day. Debilitated/Hypotension Risk/Slow Metabolizers/Sensitivity to Olanzapine Effects: Initial: 5mg qd. Titrate: Increase cautiously. Maint: 10-20mg/day. Periodically reevaluate. Bipolar I Disorder (Manic or Mixed Episodes): Initial: 10-15mg qd. Titrate: May increase/decrease dose by 5mg daily at intervals of not less than 24 hrs. Maint: 5-20mg/day. Periodically reevaluate. Max:

20mg/day. With Lithium or Valproate: Initial/Usual: 10mg qd. Max: 20mg/day. Concomitant Use with Fluoxetine: Depressive Episodes Associated with Bipolar I Disorder/Resistant Depression: Initial: 5mg with 20mg fluoxetine qd in the evening. Titrate: Adjust dose based on efficacy and tolerability. Usual: 5-12.5mg with 20-50mg fluoxetine (depressive episodes associated with Bipolar I disorder) or 5-20mg with 20-50mg fluoxetine (resistant depression). Max: 18mg plus fluoxetine 75mg. Hypotension Risk/Hepatic Impairment/Slow Metabolizers/Sensitivity to Olanzapine Effects: Initial: 2.5-5mg plus fluoxetine 20mg qd. Titrate: Increase cautiously. (IM) Agitation: Initial: 10mg IM. Usual: 2.5-10mg IM. Assess for orthostatic hypotension prior to subsequent dosing. Max: 3 doses of 10mg IM q 2-4h. Elderly: 5mg IM. Debilitated/Hypotension Risk/Sensitivity to Olanzapine Effects: 2.5mg IM. May initiate PO therapy when clinically appropriate.

*Pediatrics:* 13-17 yrs: (PO) Schizophrenia/ Bipolar I Disorder (Manic or Mixed Episodes): Initial: 2.5-5mg qd. Target dose: 10mg/day. Titrate: Adjust by dose increments/decrements of 2.5-5mg. Max: 20mg/day. Periodically reassess to determine the need for maintenance treatment. Use lowest dose to maintain remission.

**HOW SUPPLIED:** Inj: 10mg; Tab: 2.5mg, 5mg, 7.5mg, 10mg, 15mg, 20mg; Tab, Disintegrating: (Zydis) 5mg, 10mg, 15mg, 20mg

**WARNINGS/PRECAUTIONS:** May cause hyperglycemia; caution in patients with DM or in patients with borderline increased blood glucose levels; monitor for worsening of glucose control. Obtain FBG levels at beginning of treatment and periodically during treament. Supervise suicidal patients at risk . Neuroleptic malignant syndrome (NMS) reported; d/c if occurs and instill intensive symptomatic treatment and monitoring. Tardive dyskinesia reported; d/c if signs/symptoms develop. Hyperlipidemia reported; obtain lipid levels at baseline and periodically thereafter. May cause weight gain; perform regular monitoring of weight. May cause orthostatic hypotension; caution with CVD (eg, history of MI or ischemia, CHF, conduction abnormalities), cerebrovascular disease and conditions that would predispose to hypotension (eg, hypovolemia, dehydration). May cause esophageal dysmotility and aspiration. Not approved for use in patients with Alzheimer's disease. Seizures reported; caution in patients with history of seizures or with conditions that potentially lower the seizure threshold. Leukopenia, neutropenia, and agranulocytosis reported; d/c in first sign of clinically significant decline in WBC without causative factor or if severe neutropenia (ANC<1000/mm$^3$) develops. May cause cognitive and motor impairment. Hyperprolactinemia reported. May cause disruption of body temperature regulation. Caution in patients with clinically significant prostatic hypertrophy, narrow-angle glaucoma, a history of paralytic ileus or related conditions, hepatic impairment, and elderly.

**ADVERSE REACTIONS:** Postural hypotension, constipation, dry mouth, weight gain, somnolence, dizziness, personality disorder, akathisia, asthenia, dyspepsia, tremor, increased appetite, abdominal pain, headache, insomnia.

**INTERACTIONS:** May potentiate orthostatic hypotension with diazepam and alcohol. May potentiate effects of certain antihypertensive agents. Decreased levels with activated charcoal. Increased clearance with carbamazepine (CYP1A2 inducer). Caution with other CNS-acting drugs and alcohol. May antagonize levodopa, dopamine agonists. Inducers of CYP1A2 or glucuronyl transferase (eg, omeprazole, rifampin) may increase clearance. CYP1A2 inhibitors (eg, fluvoxamine) and CYP2D6 inhibitors (eg, fluoxetine) may decrease clearance. Caution with concomitant use of drugs whose effects can induce hypotension, bradycardia, respiratory or CNS depression. Concomitant administration of IM olanzapine and parenteral benzodiazepines is not recommended. Coadministration of IM lorazepam with IM olanzapine may increase the incidence of somnolence. Caution in patients receiving concomitant therapy with potentially hepatotoxic drugs. Caution with anticholinergic drugs; olanzapine disrupts body's ability to reduce core body temperature.

**PREGNANCY:** Category C, not for use in nursing.

**MECHANISM OF ACTION:** Thienobenzodiazepine; not established. Proposed that mechanism of action for the treatment of schizophrenia is mediated through a combination of dopamine and serotonin type 2 ($5HT_2$) antagonism.

**PHARMACOKINETICS: Absorption:** (PO) Well-absorbed, $T_{max}$=6 hrs; (IM) Rapid, $T_{max}$=15-45 min. **Distribution:** Found in breast milk. (PO) $V_d$=1000L; plasma protein binding (93%). **Metabolism**: (PO) Via CYP450 mediated oxidation and direct glucuronidation; 10-N-glucuronide, 4'-N-desmethyl olanzapine (major metabolites). **Elimination:** (PO) Urine (57%, 7% unchanged), feces (30%); $T_{1/2}$=21-54 hrs.

## NURSING CONSIDERATIONS

**Assessment:** Assess for DM, CV disease, cerebrovascular disease, risk of hypotension, history of seizures or conditions that could lower the seizure threshold, prostatic hypertrophy, narrow-angle glaucoma, history of paralytic ileus, hepatic impairment, pregnancy/nursing status, and for possible drug interactions. Assess for dementia-related psychosis and Alzheimer's disease in the elderly. Obtain baseline lipid panel, CBC and FBG levels.

**Monitoring:** Monitor for signs/symptoms of NMS, hyperglycemia, hyperlipidemia, weight gain, tardive dyskinesia, orthostatic hypotension, leukopenia, neutropenia, agranulocytosis, dysphagia, seizures, body temperature disruption, cognitive and motor impairment, and for hyperprolactinemia. Perform periodic monitoring of FBG, lipid levels, and weight of patient. Perform frequent monitoring of CBC in patients with a history of clinically significant low WBC or drug-induced leukopenia/neutropenia. In patient with clinically significant neutropenia, monitor for fever or other symptoms or signs of infection. In high-risk patients, monitor closely for a suicide attempt.

**Patient Counseling:** Advise of benefits/risks of therapy. Counsel about signs and symptoms of NMS. Inform of potential risk of hyperglycemia-related adverse events. Advise that medication may cause hyperlipidemia and weight gain. Counsel that medication may cause orthostatic hypotension; instruct to contact physician if dizziness, fast or slow heart beat, or if fainting occurs. Advise that medication may impair judgment, thinking, or motor skills; instruct to use caution when operating hazardous machinery. Counsel to avoid overheating and dehydration. Advise to avoid alcohol. Inform that olanzapine orally disintegrating tablets contain phenylalanine. Instruct to notify physician if taking, planning to take, or have stopped taking any prescription or OTC products, including herbal supplements. Counsel to notify physician if pregnant or planning to become pregnant during treatment. Advise to avoid breastfeeding during therapy.

**Administration:** Oral/IM routes. (IM) Do not administer IV or SQ. Inject slowly, deep into the muscle mass. Should not be combined in a syringe with diazepam, lorazepam, or haloperidol. See PI for proper reconstitution procedures.
**Storage:** Tab; Tab, Disintegrating; Inj vial (before reconstitution): 20-25°C (68-77°F); excursions permitted between 15°-30°C (59°-86°F). Reconstituted Inj: May be stored at 20-25°C (68-77°F) for up to 1 hr; excursions permitted between 15°-30°C (59°-86°F). Tab; Tab, Disintegrating: Protect from light and moisture. Inj: Protect from light and do not freeze.

# ZYPREXA RELPREVV RX

olanzapine (Lilly)

**Elderly patients with dementia-related psychosis treated with antipsychotic drugs are at an increased risk of death; most appeared to be cardiovascular (eg, heart failure, sudden death) or infectious (eg, pneumonia) in nature. Olanzapine is not approved for the treatment of patients with dementia-related psychosis. Post-injection delirium and sedation reported. Must be administered in a registered healthcare facility with ready access to emergency response services. After each injection, patient must be observed for 3 hrs. Available only through a restricted distribution program called Zyprexa Relprevv Patient Care Program and requires prescriber, healthcare facility, patient, and pharmacy enrollment.**

**THERAPEUTIC CLASS:** Thienobenzodiazepine

**INDICATIONS:** Treatment of schizophrenia.

**DOSAGE:** *Adults:* IM: Establish tolerability with oral olanzapine prior to initiating treatment. Administered by a healthcare professional every 2-4 weeks. Usual: 150-300mg/2 weeks or 405mg/4 weeks. Debilitated/ Hypotension

Risk/Slower Metabolism to Olanzapine/Pharmacodynamic Sensitivity to Olanzapine: 150mg/4 weeks. Max: 405mg q4 weeks or 300mg q2 weeks. Refer to PI for recommended dosing based on corresponding oral olanzapine doses. Reassess periodically to determine the need for continued treatment. IM injection only.

**HOW SUPPLIED:** Inj, Extended-release: 210mg, 300mg, 405mg

**WARNINGS/PRECAUTIONS:** May cause hyperglycemia; caution in patients with DM or borderline increased blood glucose levels; monitor for worsening of glucose control. Obtain FBG levels at beginning of treatment and periodically during treatment. Supervise suicidal patients at high risk. Neuroleptic malignant syndrome (NMS) reported; d/c if occurs and instill symptomatic treatment and monitoring. May cause tardive dyskinesia; d/c if signs/symptoms develop. May induce orthostatic hypotension; caution with known CVD (eg, history of MI or ischemia, heart failure, conduction abnormalities), cerebrovascular disease, and conditions that would predispose to hypotension (eg, hypovolemia, dehydration). May cause esophageal dysmotility and aspiration. Not approved for use in patients with Alzheimer's disease. Seizures reported; caution with history of seizures or with conditions that potentially lower the seizure threshold. Leukopenia, neutropenia, and agranulocytosis reported; d/c in first sign of clinically significant decline in WBC without causative factor or severe neutropenia (ANC<1000/$mm^3$). Hyperlipidemia reported; obtain lipid levels at baseline and periodically thereafter. May cause weight gain; perform regular monitoring of weight. May cause cognitive and motor impairment. Hyperprolactinemia reported. May cause disruption of body temperature regulation. Caution in patients with clinically significant prostatic hypertrophy, narrow-angle glaucoma, history of paralytic ileus or related conditions, hepatic impairment, and in the elderly.

**ADVERSE REACTIONS:** Headache, sedation, weight gain, cough, diarrhea, back pain, N/V, somnolence, dry mouth, nasopharyngitis, increased appetite, arthralgia, toothache.

**INTERACTIONS:** May potentiate orthostatic hypotension with diazepam and alcohol. May potentiate the effects of certain antihypertensive agents. Increased clearance with carbamazepine (CYP1A2 inducer). May antagonize levodopa, dopamine agonists. Caution with other CNS-acting drugs and alcohol. Inducers of CYP1A2 or glucuronyl transferase (eg, omeprazole, rifampin) may increase clearance. CYP1A2 inhibitors (eg, fluvoxamine) and CYP2D6 inhibitors (eg, fluoxetine) may decrease clearance. Caution with concomitant use of drugs whose effects that can induce hypotension, bradycardia, respiratory or CNS depression. Coadministration with lorazepam may increase the incidence of somnolence. Caution in patients receiving concomitant therapy with potentially hepatotoxic drugs. Caution with anticholinergic drugs; olanzapine disrupts body's ability to reduce core body temperature.

**PREGNANCY:** Category C, not for use in nursing.

**MECHANISM OF ACTION:** Thienobenzodiazepine; not established. Proposed that mechanism of action for the treatment of schizophrenia is mediated through a combination of dopamine and serotonin type 2 ($5HT_2$) antagonism.

**PHARMACOKINETICS: Absorption:** (IM) Rapid. $T_{max}$: 15-45 mins. **Distribution:** Found in breast milk. $V_d$=1000L; plasma protein binding (93%). **Metabolism**: (PO) Via CYP450 mediated oxidation and direct glucuronidation; 10-N-glucuronide, 4'-N-desmethyl olanzapine (major metabolites). **Elimination:** (PO) Urine (57%, 7% unchanged), feces (30%), $T_{1/2}$ =30 days.

## NURSING CONSIDERATIONS

**Assessment:** Assess for DM, hyperlipidemia, CV disease, cerebrovascular disease, risk of hypotension, history of seizures or conditions that could lower the seizure threshold, prostatic hypertrophy, narrow-angle glaucoma, history of paralytic ileus or related conditions, hepatic impairment, pregnancy/nursing status, and for possible drug interactions. Assess for dementia-related psychosis and Alzheimer's disease in elderly. Obtain baseline lipid panel, CBC and FBG levels.

**Monitoring:** Monitor for sedation and/or delirium for at least 3 hrs post-injection. Monitor for signs/symptoms of NMS, hyperglycemia, hyperlipidemia,

Z

weight gain, tardive dyskinesia, orthostatic hypotension, leukopenia, neutropenia, agranulocytosis, dysphagia, seizures, cognitive and motor impairment, body temperature disruption, and for hyperprolactinemia. Perform periodic monitoring of FBG, lipid levels, and weight of patient. Perform frequent monitoring of CBC in patients with a history of clinically significant low WBC or drug-induced leukopenia/neutropenia. In patients with clinically significant neutropenia, monitor for fever or other symptoms or signs of infection. In high-risk patients, monitor closely for a suicide attempt.

**Patient Counseling:** Advise to call physician if not improving or have concerns. Inform about potential risks and benefits associated with treatment. Advise of risk of developing delrium and sedation following administration of the medication. Inform that drug is not approved for elderly with dementia-related psychosis. Counsel about the signs/symptoms of NMS (eg, hyperpyrexia, muscle rigidity, altered mental status, autonomic instability) and instruct to contact physician if they develop. Advise of the potential risk of hyperglycemia-related adverse reactions and orthostatic hypotension. Counsel about hyperlipidemia and weight gain. Inform that medication may impair judgment, thinking, or motor skills. Instruct to avoid alcohol. Advise to notify physician if planning to take or have stopped taking any prescription or over the counter drugs, including herbal supplements. Instruct to notify physician if become pregnant or are breastfeeding.

**Administration:** IM route. Do not administer IV or SQ. Do not massage injection site. See PI for proper reconstitution technique. **Storage:** Room temperature not to exceed 30°C (86°F). Reconstituted solution may be held at room temperature for 24 hrs.

## ZYRTEC-D OTC

pseudoephedrine HCl - cetirizine HCl (McNeil Consumer)

**THERAPEUTIC CLASS:** Antihistamine/decongestant

**INDICATIONS:** Relief of nasal and non-nasal symptoms associated with seasonal or perennial allergic rhinitis in patients ≥12 yrs.

**DOSAGE:** *Adults:* 1 tab bid. Hepatic Impairment/Renal Dysfunction (CrCl <31mL/min): 1 tab qd. Swallow whole.
*Pediatrics:* ≥12 yrs: 1 tab bid. Hepatic Impairment/Renal Dysfunction (CrCl <31mL/min): 1 tab qd. Swallow tabs whole.

**HOW SUPPLIED:** Tab, Extended-Release: (Cetirizine-Pseudoephedrine) 5mg-120mg

**CONTRAINDICATIONS:** Narrow-angle glaucoma, urinary retention, MAOIs during or within 14 days of use, severe HTN, severe CAD, hypersensitivity to adrenergics.

**WARNINGS/PRECAUTIONS:** Caution with HTN, DM, ischemic heart disease, increased IOP, hyperthyroidism, renal impairment, or prostatic hypertrophy. May produce CNS stimulation with convulsions or cardiovascular collapse. May impair mental/physical abilities. The elderly are more likely to have adverse reactions.

**ADVERSE REACTIONS:** Insomnia, dry mouth, fatigue, somnolence.

**INTERACTIONS:** See Contraindications. Avoid alcohol or other CNS depressants due to additional reduction in alertness and CNS impairment. May reduce antihypertensive effects of antihypertensive drugs that interfere with sympathetic activity (eg, methyldopa, mecamylamine, reserpine). Caution with sympathomimetic amines; combined effects on the cardiovascular system may be harmful. Theophylline may decrease clearance of cetirizine; larger doses may have greater effect. Increased ectopic pacemaker may occur when pseudoephedrine is used concomitantly with digitalis.

**PREGNANCY:** Category C, not for use in nursing.

**MECHANISM OF ACTION:** Cetirizine: Antihistamine/decongestant; selectively inhibits $H_1$-receptors. Pseudoephedrine: Orally active sympathomimetic amine; exerts a decongestant effect on the nasal mucosa.

**PHARMACOKINETICS: Absorption:** Cetirizine: $C_{max}$=114ng/mL (single dose), 178ng/mL (multiple doses); $T_{max}$=2.2 hrs. Pseudoephedrine: $C_{max}$=309ng/mL, 526ng/mL (multiple doses); $T_{max}$=4.4 hrs. **Distribution:** Found in breast milk. Cetirizine: Plasma protein binding (93%). Pseudoephedrine: $V_d$=2.6-3.3L/kg. **Metabolism:** Cetirizine: Oxidative-O-dealkylation. Pseudoephedrine: N-demethylation; (1%-7%) metabolized to norpseudoephedrine. **Elimination:** Cetirizine: Urine (70%), feces (10%); $T_{1/2}$=7.9 hrs. Pseudoephedrine: $T_{1/2}$=6 hrs.

## NURSING CONSIDERATIONS

**Assessment:** Assess for narrow-angle glaucoma, urinary retention, current or recent use (within 14 days) of MAO inhibitors, severe HTN, and CAD. Assess use in pregnant/nursing females, patients with idiosyncratic reactions to adrenergic agents or other drugs with similiar structures, patients with HTN, DM, ischemic heart disease, increased IOP, hyperthyroidism, renal impairment, prostatic hypertrophy, and in elderly patients. Assess for possible drug interactions.

**Monitoring:** Monitor for manifestations of idiosyncratic reactions to adrenergic agents (eg, insomnia, dizziness, weakness, tremor, or arrhythmia).

**Patient Counseling:** Inform drug may cause somnolence and decreased alertness; caution when operating machinery/driving. Advise to avoid concurrent use with alcohol or other CNS depressants. Instruct to swallow whole, do not chew or break. May be given with/without food.

**Administration:** Oral route. **Storage:** 20-25°C (68-77°F); excursions permitted to 15-30°C (59-86°F).

# ZYVOX RX

linezolid (Pharmacia & Upjohn)

**THERAPEUTIC CLASS:** Oxazolidinone class antibacterial

**INDICATIONS:** Treatment of vancomycin-resistant *Enterococcus faecium* (VRE) infections, nosocomial pneumonia caused by *Staphylococcus aureus* (methicillin-susceptible and -resistant strains) or *Streptococcus pneumoniae* (including multi drug-resistant strains [MDRSP]), complicated skin and skin structure infections (SSSI) including diabetic foot infections without concomitant osteomyelitis caused by *Staphylococcus aureus* (methicillin-susceptible and -resistant strains), *Streptococcus pyogenes*, or *Streptococcus agalactiae*, uncomplicated SSSI caused by *Staphylococcus aureus* (methicillin-susceptible only) or *Streptococcus pyogenes*, community-acquired pneumonia (CAP) caused by *Streptococcus pneumoniae* (MDRSP), including concurrent bacteremia, or *Staphylococcus aureus* (methicillin-susceptible strains only).

**DOSAGE:** *Adults:* Complicated SSSI/CAP/Nosocomial Pneumonia: 600mg IV/PO q12h for 10-14 days. Vancomycin-resistant *Enterococcus faecium* infections (VRE): 600mg IV/PO q12h for 14-28 days. Uncomplicated SSSI: 400mg PO q12h for 10-14 days. Methicillin-Resistant *Staphylococcus Aureus* (MRSA) infection: 600mg PO q12h.

*Pediatrics:* Complicated SSSI/CAP/Nosocomial Pneumonia: Treat for 10-14 days. ≥12 yrs: 600mg IV/PO q12h. Birth-11 yrs: 10mg/kg IV/PO q8h. VRE: Treat for 14-28 days: ≥12 yrs: 600mg IV/PO q12h; Birth-11 yrs: 10mg/kg IV/PO q8h. Uncomplicated SSSI: Treat for 10-14 days: ≥12 yrs: 600mg PO q12h; 5-11 yrs: 10mg/kg PO q12h; <5 yrs: 10mg/kg PO q8h. Neonates <7 days: Initiate with dosing regimen of 10mg/kg q12h; may increase to 10mg/kg q8h if suboptimal response. All neonatal patients should receive 10mg/kg q8h by 7 days of life.

**HOW SUPPLIED:** Inj: 2mg/mL [100mL, 200mL, 300mL]; Sus: 100mg/5mL [240mL]; Tab: 600mg

**CONTRAINDICATIONS:** Uncontrolled HTN, pheochromocytoma, thyrotoxicosis, carcinoid syndrome, and patients taking any of the following types of medication: MAOIs (within two weeks), directly and indirectly acting sympathomimetic agents (eg, pseudoephedrine), vasopressive agents (eg, epinephrine, norepinephrine), dopaminergic agents (eg, dopamine, dobutamine), SSRIs, TCAs, serotonin 5-$HT_1$ receptor agonists (triptans), meperidine or buspirone.

**WARNINGS/PRECAUTIONS:** Myelosuppression, including anemia, thrombocytopenia, pancytopenia, and leukopenia reported; monitor CBC weekly; d/c if myelosuppression develop or worsens. *Clostridium difficile*-associated diarrhea reported. Peripheral and optic neuropathy reported; monitor visual function if for extended treatment periods ( ≥3 months). Lactic acidosis and convulsions reported. May promote overgrowth of nonsusceptible organisms. Not approved for treatment of catheter-related bloodstream infections, catheter-site infections, or Gram-negative infections. Oral sus contains phenylalanine.

**ADVERSE REACTIONS:** Diarrhea, headache, N/V.

**INTERACTIONS:** See Contraindications. Potential interaction with adrenergic and serotonergic agents. May enhance pressor response to sympathomimetics, vasopressors, and dopaminergic agents; caution with dopamine, epinephrine, pseudoephedrine, and phenylpropanolamine. Serotonin syndrome may occur with concomitant serotonergic agents, including antidepressants such as SSRIs. Avoid large quantities of tyramine-containing foods or beverages. Reduced plasma concentration with rifampin.

**PREGNANCY:** Category C, caution in nursing.

**MECHANISM OF ACTION:** Oxazolidinone antibacterial; inhibits bacterial protein synthesis; binds to a site on the bacterial 23S ribosomal RNA of the 50S subunit and prevents formation of functional 70S initiation complex, which is an essential component of the bacterial translation process.

**PHARMACOKINETICS: Absorption:** Rapid/extensive; absolute bioavailability (100%); $T_{max}$=1-2 hrs. **Distribution:** $V_d$=40-50L; plasma protein binding (31%); distributes to well-perfused tissues. **Metabolism:** Via oxidation; aminoethoxyacetic acid (A), hydroxyethyl glycine (B) (inactive metabolites). **Elimination:** Urine (30% as parent drug, 40% as B, 10% as A), feces (6% as B, 3% as A).

## NURSING CONSIDERATIONS

**Assessment:** Assess for pre-existing myelosuppression (including anemia, leukopenia, pancytopenia, thrombocytopenia), concomitant drugs that produce myelosuppression, presence of chronic infections, previous or concomitant antibiotic therapy, catheter-related bloodstream infections or catheter-site infections, pregnancy/nursing status, uncontrolled HTN, carcinoid syndrome, pheochromocytoma, untreated hyperthyroidism, phenylketonuria, renal/hepatic impairment, and possible drug interactions (eg, SSRIs).

**Monitoring:** Perform weekly monitoring of CBC. Monitor for signs/symptoms of myelosuppresion (eg, anemia, leukopenia, pancytopenia, thrombocytopenia), pseudomembranous colitis or *C.difficile*-associated diarrhea (may range from mild diarrhea to fatal colitis), lactic acidosis with repeated N/V, convulsions, development of drug resistance or superinfection, serotonin syndrome (eg, cognitive dysfunction, hyperpyrexia, hyperreflexia, incoordination), blurred vision, optic/peripheral neuropathy. Monitor visual function with long-term therapy or if new visual symptoms occur.

**Patient Counseling:** Instruct to notify if pregnant/nursing, have HTN or history of seizures, or if taking cold remedies, decongestants or SSRIs. Inform about risks/benefits of therapy. D/C and notify physician if visual changes or other side effects occur. Inform that drug treats bacterial, not viral, infections. Instruct to take drug exactly as directed to prevent drug resistance and maintain effectiveness. Caution to avoid large quantities of food or beverages with high tyramine content.

**Administration:** IV/Oral routes. **Storage:** 25°C (77°F); excursions permitted to 15-30°C (59-86°F); store in tightly closed bottles. Protect from light. Protect infusion bags from freezing.

# Appendix: Reference Tables

# Abbreviations, Acronyms, and Symbols

| ABBREVIATIONS | DESCRIPTIONS |
|---|---|
| - (eg, 6-8) | to (eg, 6 to 8) |
| / | per |
| < | less than |
| > | greater than |
| ≤ | less than or equal to |
| ≥ | greater than or equal to |
| α | alpha |
| β | beta |
| 5-FU | 5-fluorouracil |
| 5-HT | 5-hydroxytryptamine (serotonin) |
| ABECB | acute bacterial exacerbation of chronic bronchitis |
| aa | of each |
| ACTH | adrenocorticotrophic hormone |
| ad | right ear |
| ADHD | attention-deficit/hyperactivity disorder |
| A-fib | atrial fibrillation |
| A-flutter | atrial flutter |
| AIDS | acquired immunodeficiency syndrome |
| ALT | alanine transaminase (SGPT) |
| am or AM | morning |
| AMI | acute myocardial infarction |
| ANA | antinuclear antibodies |
| ANC | absolute neutrophil count |
| APAP | acetaminophen |
| as | left ear |
| ASA | aspirin |
| AST | aspartate transaminase (SGOT) |
| au | each ear |
| AUC | area under the curve |
| AV | atrioventricular |
| bid | twice daily |
| BMI | body mass index |
| BP | blood pressure |
| BPH | benign prostatic hypertrophy |
| BSA | body surface area |
| BUN | blood urea nitrogen |
| CABG | coronary artery bypass graft |
| CAD | coronary artery disease |
| Cap | capsule or gelcap |
| CAP | community-acquired pneumonia |
| CBC | complete blood count |
| CF | cystic fibrosis |
| CHF | congestive heart failure |
| cm | centimeter |
| CMV | cytomegalovirus |
| $C_{max}$ | peak plasma concentration |
| CNS | central nervous system |
| COPD | chronic obstructive pulmonary disease |
| CrCl | creatinine clearance |
| Cre | cream |
| CRF | chronic renal failure |

(Continued)

| ABBREVIATIONS | DESCRIPTIONS |
|---|---|
| CSF | cerebrospinal fluid |
| CVA | cerebrovascular accident |
| CVD | cardiovascular disease |
| CYP450 | cytochrome P450 |
| d/c or D/C | discontinue |
| DHEA | dehydroepiandrosterone |
| DM | diabetes mellitus |
| DVT | deep vein thrombosis |
| ECG | electrocardiogram |
| EEG | electroencephalogram |
| eg | for example |
| EPS | extrapyramidal symptom |
| ESRD | end-stage renal disease |
| FPG | fasting plasma glucose |
| FSH | follicle-stimulating hormone |
| g | gram |
| GABA | gamma-aminobutyric acid |
| GAD | general anxiety disorder |
| GERD | gastroesophageal reflux disease |
| GFR | glomerular filtration rate |
| GI | gastrointestinal |
| GnRH | gonadotropin-releasing hormone |
| GVHD | graft versus host disease |
| HCG | human chorionic gonadotropin |
| Hct | hematocrit |
| HCTZ | hydrochlorothiazide |
| HDL | high-density lipoprotein |
| Hgb | hemoglobin |
| HIV | human immunodeficiency virus |
| HMG-CoA | 3-hydroxy-3-methylglutaryl-coenzyme A |
| HR | heart rate |
| hr or hrs | hour or hours |
| hs | bedtime |
| HSV | herpes simplex virus |
| HTN | hypertension |
| IBD | inflammatory bowel disease |
| IBS | irritable bowel syndrome |
| ICH | intracranial hemorrhage |
| ICP | intracranial pressure |
| IM | intramuscular |
| INH | isoniazid |
| Inj | injection |
| INR | international normalized ratio |
| IOP | intraocular pressure |
| IU | international units |
| IV | intravenous/intravenously |
| $K^+$ | potassium |
| kg | kilogram |
| KIU | kallikrein inhibitor unit |
| L | liter |
| lbs | pounds |
| LD | loading dose |
| LDL | low-density lipoprotein |
| LFT | liver function test |

*(Continued)*

| ABBREVIATIONS | DESCRIPTIONS |
|---|---|
| LH | luteinizing hormone |
| LHRH | luteinizing-hormone releasing hormone |
| Lot | lotion |
| Loz | lozenge |
| LVH | left ventricular hypertrophy |
| M | molar |
| MAC | mycobacterium avium complex |
| Maint | maintenance |
| MAOI | monoamine oxidase inhibitor |
| Max | maximum |
| mcg | microgram |
| mEq | milli-equivalent |
| mg | milligram |
| MI | myocardial infarction |
| min | minute (usually as mL/min) |
| mL | milliliter |
| mm | millimeter |
| mM | millimolar |
| MRI | magnetic resonance imaging |
| MS | multiple sclerosis |
| msec | millisecond |
| MTX | methotrexate |
| Na | sodium |
| NaCl | sodium chloride |
| NG | nasogastric |
| NKA | no known allergies |
| NMS | neuroleptic malignant syndrome |
| NPO | nothing by mouth |
| NSAID | nonsteroidal anti-inflammatory drug |
| NV or N/V | nausea and vomiting |
| OA | osteoarthritis |
| OCD | obsessive-compulsive disorder |
| od | right eye |
| Oint | ointment |
| os | left eye |
| ou | each eye |
| PAT | paroxysmal atrial tachycardia |
| pc | after meals |
| PCN | penicillin |
| PCP | *Pneumocystis carinii* pneumonia |
| PD | Parkinson's disease |
| PID | pelvic inflammatory disease |
| pkt, pkts | packet, packets |
| pm | evening |
| po or PO | orally |
| PONV | postoperative nausea and vomiting |
| pr | rectally |
| prn | as needed |
| PSA | prostate-specific antigen |
| PSVT | paroxysmal supraventricular tachycardia |
| PT | prothrombin time |
| PTSD | post-traumatic stress disorder |
| PTT | partial thromboplastin time |
| PTU | propylthiouracil |

*(Continued)*

| ABBREVIATIONS | DESCRIPTIONS |
|---|---|
| PUD | peptic ulcer disease |
| PVD | peripheral vascular disease |
| q4h, q6h, q8h, etc. | every four hours, every six hours, every eight hours, etc. |
| qd | once daily |
| qh | every hour |
| qid | four times daily |
| qod | every other day |
| qs | a sufficient quantity |
| qs ad | a sufficient quantity up to |
| RA | rheumatoid arthritis |
| RBC | red blood cells |
| RDS | respiratory distress syndrome |
| REM | rapid eye movement |
| SAH | subarachnoid hemorrhage |
| SBP | systolic blood pressure |
| sec | second(s) |
| SGOT | serum glutamic-oxaloacetic transaminase (AST) |
| SGPT | serum glutamic-pyruvic transaminase (ALT) |
| SIADH | syndrome of inappropriate antidiuretic hormone secretion |
| SLE | systemic lupus erythematosus |
| SOB | shortness of breath |
| Sol | solution |
| SQ, SC | subcutaneous |
| SrCr | serum creatinine |
| SSRI | selective serotonin reuptake inhibitor |
| SSSI | skin and skin structure infection |
| STD | sexually transmitted disease |
| Sup | suppository |
| Sus | suspension |
| SVT | supraventricular tachycardia |
| $T_{1/2}$ | half-life |
| Tab | tablet or caplet |
| Tab, SL | sublingual tablet |
| TB | tuberculosis |
| TBG | thyroxine binding globulin |
| tbl or tbsp | tablespoon |
| TCA | tricyclic antidepressant |
| TD | tardive dyskinesia |
| TFT | thyroid function test |
| TG | triglyceride |
| tid | three times daily |
| $T_{max}$ | time to maximum concentration |
| TNF | tumor necrosis factor |
| TPN | total parenteral nutrition |
| TSH | thyroid stimulating hormone |
| tsp | teaspoonful |
| TTP | thrombotic thrombocytopenic purpura |

*(Continued)*

| ABBREVIATIONS | DESCRIPTIONS |
|---|---|
| U | unit |
| ud | as directed |
| ULN | upper limit of normal |
| URTI/URI | upper respiratory tract infection |
| UTI | urinary tract infection |
| UV | ultraviolet |
| WBC | white blood cell count |
| Vd | volume of distribution |
| VTE | venous thromboembolism |
| X | times (eg, >2X ULN) |
| yr or yrs | year or years |

# CALCULATIONS AND FORMULAS

## WEIGHTS AND MEASURES

| METRIC MEASURES | |
|---|---|
| 1 kilogram (kg) | 1000 g |
| 1 gram (g) | 1000 mg |
| 1 milligram (mg) | 0.001 g |
| 1 microgram (mcg or µg) | 0.001 mg; 1 x $10^{-6}$ g |
| 1 liter (L) | 1000 mL |
| 1 milliliter (mL) | 0.001 L; 1 cc (cubic centimeter) |
| **APOTHECARY MEASURES (AP)** | |
| 1 scruple | 20 grains (gr) |
| 1 drachm | 3 scruples; 60 gr |
| 1 ounce (oz) | 8 drachms; 24 scruples; 480 gr |
| 1 pound (lb) | 12 oz; 96 drachms; 288 scruples; 5760 gr |
| **U.S. FLUID MEASURES** | |
| 1 fluidrachm | 60 minim |
| 1 fluid ounce | 8 fluidrachm; 480 minim |
| 1 pint (pt) | 16 fl oz; 7680 minim |
| 1 quart (qt) | 2 pt; 32 fl oz |
| 1 gallon (gal) | 4 qt; 128 fl oz |
| **AVOIRDUPOIS WEIGHT (AV)** | |
| 1 ounce | 437.5 gr |
| 1 pound | 16 oz |
| **CONVERSION FACTORS** | |
| 1 gram | 15.4 gr |
| 1 grain | 64.8 mg |
| 1 ounce (Av) | 28.35 g; 437.5 gr |
| 1 ounce (Ap) | 31.1 g; 480 gr |
| 1 pound (Av) | 453.6 g; 2.68 lb (Ap); 2.20 lb (Av) |
| 1 fluid ounce | 29.57 mL |
| 1 fluidrachm | 3.697 mL |
| 1 minim | 0.06 mL |
| **COMMON MEASURES** | |
| 1 teaspoonful | 5 mL; 1/6 fl oz |
| 1 tablespoonful | 15 mL; 1/2 fl oz |
| 1 wineglassful | 60 mL; 2 fl oz |
| 1 teacupful | 120 mL; 4 fl oz |
| 1 gallon | 3800 mL; 128 fl oz |
| 1 quart | 960 mL; 32 fl oz |
| 1 pint | 480 mL; 16 fl oz (exactly 473.2 mL) |
| 8 fluid ounces | 240 mL |
| 4 fluid ounces | 120 mL |
| 2.2 lb | 1 kg |

## DOSE EQUIVALENTS

| WEIGHT (METRIC) | WEIGHT (APOTHECARY) |
|---|---|
| 30 g | 1 ounce |
| 15 g | 4 drams |
| 10 g | 2 1/2 drams |
| 7.5 g | 2 drams |
| 6 g | 90 grains |
| 5 g | 75 grains |
| 4 g | 60 grains; 1 dram |
| 3 g | 45 grains |
| 2 g | 30 grains; 1/2 dram |
| 1.5 g | 22 grains |
| 1 g | 15 grains |
| 750 mg | 12 grains |
| 600 mg | 10 grains |
| 500 mg | 7 1/2 grains |
| 400 mg | 6 grains |
| 300 mg | 5 grains |
| 250 mg | 4 grains |

*(Continued)*

## DOSE EQUIVALENTS *(Continued)*

| WEIGHT (METRIC) | WEIGHT (APOTHECARY) |
|---|---|
| 200 mg | 3 grains |
| 150 mg | 2 1/2 grains |
| 125 mg | 2 grains |
| 100 mg | 1 1/2 grains |
| 75 mg | 1 1/4 grains |
| 60 mg | 1 grain |
| 50 mg | 3/4 grain |
| 40 mg | 2/3 grain |
| 30 mg | 3/8 grain |
| 25 mg | 3/8 grain |
| 20 mg | 1/3 grain |
| 15 mg | 1/5 grain |
| 12 mg | 1/5 grain |
| 10 mg | 1/6 grain |
| 8 mg | 1/8 grain |
| 6 mg | 1/10 grain |
| 5 mg | 1/12 grain |
| 4 mg | 1/15 grain |
| 3 mg | 1/20 grain |
| 2 mg | 1/30 grain |
| 1.5 mg | 1/40 grain |
| 1.2 mg | 1/50 grain |
| 1 mg | 1/60 grain |

| LIQUID MEASURES (METRIC) | LIQUID MEASURES (APOTHECARY) |
|---|---|
| 1000 mL | 1 quart |
| 750 mL | 1 1/2 pints |
| 500 mL | 1 pint |
| 230 mL | 8 fluid ounces |
| 200 mL | 7 fluid ounces |
| 100 mL | 3 1/2 fluid ounces |
| 50 mL | 1 3/4 fluid ounces |
| 30 mL | 1 fluid ounces |
| 15 mL | 4 fluid drams |
| 10 mL | 2 1/2 fluid drams |
| 8 mL | 2 fluid drams |
| 5 mL | 1 1/4 fluid drams |
| 4 mL | 1 fluid dram |
| 3 mL | 45 minims |
| 2 mL | 30 minims |
| 1 mL | 15 minims |
| 0.75 mL | 12 minims |
| 0.6 mL | 10 minims |
| 0.5 mL | 8 minims |
| 0.3 mL | 5 minims |
| 0.25 mL | 4 minims |
| 0.2 mL | 3 minims |
| 0.1 mL | 1 1/2 minims |
| 0.06 mL | 1 minim |
| 0.05 mL | 3/4 minim |
| 0.03 mL | 1/2 minim |

## MILLIEQUIVALENT (mEq) AND MILLIMOLE (mmol)

### CALCULATIONS

$$\text{moles} = \frac{\text{weight of a substance (grams)}}{\text{molecular weight of that substance (grams)}} \quad \textbf{OR} \quad = \frac{\text{equivalent}}{\text{valence of ion}}$$

$$\text{millimoles} = \frac{\text{weight of a substance (milligrams)}}{\text{molecular weight of that substance (milligrams)}} \quad \textbf{OR} \quad = \frac{\text{milliequivalents}}{\text{valence of ion}} \quad \textbf{OR} \quad = \text{moles} \times 1000$$

$$\text{equivalents} = \text{moles} \times \text{valence of ion}$$

$$\text{milliequivalents} = \text{millimoles} \times \text{valence of ion} \quad \textbf{OR} \quad = \text{equivalents} \times 1000$$

*(Continued)*

## CONVERSIONS

| | |
|---|---|
| mg/100mL to mEq/L | mEq/L = $\frac{(\text{mg/100mL}) \times 10 \times \text{valence}}{\text{atomic weight}}$ |
| mEq/L to mg/100mL | mg/100mL = $\frac{(\text{mEq/L}) \times \text{atomic weight}}{10 \times \text{valence}}$ |
| mEq/L to volume percent of a gas | volume % = $\frac{(\text{mEq/L}) \times 22.4}{10}$ |

# ACID-BASE ASSESSMENT

## DEFINITIONS

| | |
|---|---|
| $PIO_2$ | Oxygen partial pressure of inspired gas (mmHg); 150 mmHg in room air at sea level |
| $FiO_2$ | Fractional pressure of oxygen in inspired gas (0.21 in room air) |
| $PAO_2$ | Alveolar oxygen partial pressure |
| $PACO_2$ | Alveolar carbon dioxide partial pressure |
| $PaO_2$ | Arterial oxygen partial pressure |
| $PaCO_2$ | Arterial carbon dioxide partial pressure |
| R | Respiratory exchange quotient (typically 0.8, increases with high carbohydrate diet, decreases with high fat diet) |

## HENDERSON-HASSELBALCH EQUATION

$pH = 6.1 + \log [HCO_3^- / (0.03)(pCO_2)]$

## ALVEOLAR GAS EQUATION

$PIO_2 = FiO_2 \times$ (total atmospheric pressure - vapor pressure of $H_2O$ at 37°C)
$= FiO_2 \times (760 \text{ mmHg} - 47 \text{ mmHg})$

$PaO_2 = PIO_2 - PaCO_2/R$

## ALVEOLAR/ARTERIAL OXYGEN GRADIENT

$PAO_2 - PaO_2$

# ACID-BASE DISORDERS

| Disorder | pH | $HCO_3^-$ | $PCO_2$ | Compensation |
|---|---|---|---|---|
| Metabolic acidosis | < 7.35 | Primary decrease | Compensatory decrease | 1.2-mmHg decrease in $PCO_2$ for every 1-mmol/L decrease in $HCO_3^-$ **or** $PCO_2 = (1.5 \times HCO_3^-) + 8 (\pm 2)$ **or** $PCO_2 = HCO_3^- + 15$ **or** $PCO_2$ = last 2 digits of pH x 100 |
| Metabolic alkalosis | > 7.45 | Primary increase | Compensatory increase | 0.6-0.75 mmHg increase in $PCO_2$ for every 1-mmol/L increase in $HCO_3^-$. $PCO_2$ should not rise above 60 mm Hg in compensation. |
| Respiratory acidosis | < 7.35 | Compensatory increase | Primary increase | ***Acute:*** 1-2 mmol decrease in $HCO_3^-$. for every 10-mmHg decrease in $PCO_2$. ***Chronic:*** 3-4 mmol increase in $HCO_3^-$. for every 10-mmHg increase in $PCO_2$. |
| Respiratory alkalosis | > 7.45 | Compensatory decrease | Primary decrease | ***Acute:*** 1-2 mmol increase in $HCO_3^-$. for every 10-mmHg increase in $PCO_2$. ***Chronic:*** 4-5 mmol decrease in $HCO_3^-$. for every 10-mmHg decrease in $PCO_2$. |

## ACID-BASE EQUATION

$H^+$ (in mEq/L) = $(24 \times PaCO_2)$ divided by $HCO_3^-$

*(Continued)*

# OTHER CALCULATIONS

## ANION GAP

Anion gap = $Na^+$ - ($Cl^-$ + $HCO_3^-$ measured)

## AA GRADIENT

Aa gradient [(713) ($FiO_2$ - ($PaCO_2$ divided by 0.8))] - $PaO_2$

## OSMOLALITY

**Definition:**
Osmolality is a measure of the total number of particles in a solution.

U.S. units (sodium as mEq/L, BUN (blood urea nitrogen) and glucose as (mg/dL)
Plasma osmolality (mOsm/kg) = 2([$Na^+$] + [$K^+$]) + ([BUN]/2.8) + ([glucose]/18)

SI units (all variables in mmol/L):
Plasma osmolality (mOsm/kg) = 2[$Na^+$] + [urea] + [glucose]
Normal range plasma osmolality: 280 - 303 mOsm/kg

**Corrected Sodium**
Corrected Na+ = measured $Na^+$ + [1.5 x (glucose - 150 divided by 100)]*
*Do not correct for glucose <150.

**Total Serum Calcium Corrected for Albumin Level**
[(Normal albumin - patient's albumin) x 0.8] + patient's measured total calcium

**Water Deficit**
Water deficit = 0.6 x body weight [1 - (140 divided by $Na^+$)]*
*Body weight is estimated weight in kg; $Na^+$ is serum or plasma sodium.

**Bicarbonate Deficit**
$HCO_3^-$ deficit = [0.4 x weight (kg)] x ($HCO_3^-$ desired - $HCO_3^-$ measured)

## CHILD-PUGH SCORE

The Child-Pugh classification is used to assess the prognosis of chronic liver disease, mainly cirrhosis. Child-Pugh is also used to determine the required strength of treatment and the necessity of liver transplantation.

Score:
The score employs five clinical measures of liver disease. Each measure is scored 1-3, with 3 indicating the most severe derangement.

| Measure | 1 point | 2 points | 3 points | Units |
|---|---|---|---|---|
| Bilirubin (total)* | <34 (<2) | 34-50 (2-3) | >50 (>3) | mol/L (mg/dL) |
| Serum albumin | >35 | 28-35 | <28 | mg/L |
| INR** | <1.7 | 1.71-2.20 | > 2.20 | no unit |
| Ascites | None | Suppressed with medication | Refractory | no unit |
| Hepatic encephalopathy | None | Grade I-II (or suppressed with medication) | Grade III-IV (or refractory) | no unit |

* In primary sclerosing cholangitis and primary biliary cirrhosis, the bilirubin references are changed to reflect the fact that these diseases feature high conjugated bilirubin levels. The upper limit for 1 point is 68 mol/L (4 mg/dL) and the upper limit for 2 points is 170 mol/L (10 mg/dL).

** Some older reference works substitute PT prolongation for INR.

Interpretation:
Chronic liver disease is classified into Child-Pugh class A to C, employing the added score from above.

| Points | Class | One year survival | Two year survival |
|---|---|---|---|
| 5-6 | A | 100% | 85% |
| 7-9 | B | 81% | 57% |
| 10-15 | C | 45% | 35% |

## CREATININE CLEARANCE

Clinically, creatinine clearance is a useful measure for estimating the glomerular filtration rate (GFR) of the kidneys.

| Factors | Abbreviations |
|---|---|
| Creatinine clearance | $Cl_{Cr}$ |
| Plasma creatinine concentration | $P_{Cr}$ |
| Serum creatinine concentration | $S_{Cr}$ |
| Urine creatinine concentration | $U_{Cr}$ |
| Urine flow rate | V |
| Plasma creatinine concentration | $P_{Cr}$ |

*(Continued)*

## CREATININE CLEARANCE *(Continued)*

**Calculations:**

$$Cl_{Cr} = \frac{U_{Cr} \times V}{P_{Cr}}$$

**Example:**

Patient with $P_{Cr}$ 1 mg/dL, $U_{Cr}$ 60 mg/dL, and V of 0.5 dL/hr.

$$Cl_{Cr} = \frac{60\ \text{mg/dL} \times 0.5\ \text{dL/hr}}{1\ \text{mg/dL}} = 30\ \text{dL/hr}$$

**Cockcroft-Gault formula:** Estimates creatinine clearance (mL/min).

**Male:**

$$Cl_{Cr} = \frac{(140 - \text{age}) \times \text{mass (kg)}}{72 \times S_{Cr}\ \text{(mg/dL)}}$$

**Example:**

Male patient, 67 years of age, weight 75 kg, and $S_{Cr}$ 1 mg/dL.

$$Cl_{Cr} = \frac{(140 - 67) \times 75}{72 \times 1} = 76\ \text{mL/min}$$

**Female:**

$$Cl_{Cr} = \frac{(140 - \text{age}) \times \text{mass (kg)} \times 0.85}{72 \times S_{Cr}\ \text{(mg/dL)}}$$

**Example:**

Female patient, 67 years of age, weight 75 kg, and $S_{Cr}$ 1 mg/dL.

$$Cl_{Cr} = \frac{(140 - 67) \times 75}{72 \times 1} \times 0.85 = 64.6\ \text{mL/min}$$

Note: Using actual body weight (ABW) in obese patients can significantly overestimate creatinine clearance. Adjusted ideal body weight (IBW) can provide a more approximate estimate. Adjusted IBW = IBW + 0.4 (ABW - IBW).

## BASAL ENERGY EXPENDITURE (BEE)

Basal energy expenditure: the amount of energy required to maintain the body's normal metabolic activity (eg, respiration, maintenance of body temperature, etc).

H = height (cm), W = weight (kg), A = age (years)

**Male:**

BEE = 66.67 + 13.75W + 5H - 6.76A

**Female:**

BEE = 665.1 + 9.56W +1.85H -4.68A

## BODY MASS INDEX (BMI)

$$BMI = \frac{\text{weight (kg)}}{[\text{height (m)}]^2}$$

## BODY SURFACE AREA (BSA)

$$BSA\ (m^2) = \sqrt{\frac{\text{height (in)} \times \text{weight (lb)}}{3131}}$$

**OR**

$$BSA\ (m^2) = \sqrt{\frac{\text{height (cm)} \times \text{weight (kg)}}{3600}}$$

## IDEAL BODY WEIGHT (IBW)

Adults (18 years and older; IBW is in kg):

IBW (male) = 50 + (2.3 x height [inches] over 5 feet)
IBW (female) = 45.5 + (2.3 x height [inches] over 5 feet)

Children (IBW is in kg; height is in cm):

1-18 years of age:

$$IBW = \frac{(\text{height}^2 \times 1.65)}{100}$$

5 feet and taller:

IBW (male) = 39 + (2.27 x height [inches] over 5 feet)
IBW (female) = 42.2 + (2.27 x height [inches] over 5 feet)

*(Continued)*

## POUNDS/KILOGRAM CONVERSION

| 1 pound = 0.45359 kilogram | | | | 1 kilogram = 2.2 pounds | | | |
|---|---|---|---|---|---|---|---|
| lb | kg | lb | kg | lb | kg | lb | kg |
| 1 | 0.45 | 105 | 47.63 | 210 | 95.25 | 315 | 142.88 |
| 5 | 2.27 | 110 | 49.89 | 215 | 97.52 | 320 | 145.15 |
| 10 | 4.54 | 115 | 52.16 | 220 | 99.79 | 325 | 147.42 |
| 15 | 6.80 | 120 | 54.43 | 225 | 102.06 | 330 | 149.68 |
| 20 | 9.07 | 125 | 56.70 | 230 | 104.33 | 335 | 151.95 |
| 25 | 11.34 | 130 | 58.97 | 235 | 106.59 | 340 | 154.22 |
| 30 | 13.61 | 135 | 61.23 | 240 | 108.86 | 345 | 156.49 |
| 35 | 15.88 | 140 | 63.50 | 245 | 111.13 | 350 | 158.76 |
| 40 | 18.14 | 145 | 65.77 | 250 | 113.40 | 355 | 161.02 |
| 45 | 20.41 | 150 | 68.04 | 255 | 115.67 | 360 | 163.29 |
| 50 | 22.68 | 155 | 70.31 | 260 | 117.93 | 365 | 165.56 |
| 55 | 24.95 | 160 | 72.57 | 265 | 120.20 | 370 | 167.83 |
| 60 | 27.22 | 165 | 74.84 | 270 | 122.47 | 375 | 170.10 |
| 65 | 29.48 | 170 | 77.11 | 275 | 124.74 | 380 | 172.36 |
| 70 | 31.75 | 175 | 79.38 | 280 | 127.01 | 385 | 174.63 |
| 75 | 34.02 | 180 | 81.65 | 285 | 129.27 | 390 | 176.90 |
| 80 | 36.29 | 185 | 83.91 | 290 | 131.54 | 395 | 179.17 |
| 85 | 38.56 | 190 | 86.18 | 295 | 133.81 | 400 | 181.44 |
| 90 | 40.82 | 195 | 88.45 | 300 | 136.08 | 405 | 183.70 |
| 95 | 43.09 | 200 | 90.72 | 305 | 138.34 | 410 | 185.97 |
| 100 | 45.36 | 205 | 92.99 | 310 | 140.61 | 415 | 188.24 |

## TEMPERATURE CONVERSION

| Fahrenheit to Celsius = (°F - 32) x 5/9 = °C | | | | Celsius to Fahrenheit = (°C x 9/5) + 32 = °F | | | |
|---|---|---|---|---|---|---|---|
| °F | °C | °F | °C | °C | °F | °C | °F |
| 0.0 | -17.8 | 92.0 | 33.3 | 0.0 | 32.0 | 49.0 | 120.2 |
| 5.0 | -15.0 | 93.0 | 33.9 | 5.0 | 41.0 | 50.0 | 122.0 |
| 10.0 | -12.2 | 94.0 | 34.4 | 10.0 | 50.0 | 51.0 | 123.8 |
| 15.0 | -9.4 | 95.0 | 35.0 | 15.0 | 59.0 | 52.0 | 125.6 |
| 20.0 | -6.7 | 96.0 | 35.6 | 20.0 | 68.0 | 53.0 | 127.4 |
| 25.0 | -3.9 | 97.0 | 36.1 | 25.0 | 77.0 | 54.0 | 129.2 |
| 30.0 | -1.1 | 98.0 | 36.7 | 30.0 | 86.0 | 55.0 | 131.0 |
| 35.0 | 1.7 | 98.6 | 37.0 | 35.0 | 95.0 | 56.0 | 132.8 |
| 40.0 | 4.4 | 99.0 | 37.2 | 36.0 | 96.8 | 57.0 | 134.6 |
| 45.0 | 7.2 | 100.0 | 37.8 | 37.0 | 98.6 | 58.0 | 136.4 |
| 50.0 | 10.0 | 101.0 | 38.3 | 38.0 | 100.4 | 59.0 | 138.2 |
| 55.0 | 12.8 | 102.0 | 38.9 | 39.0 | 102.2 | 60.0 | 140.0 |
| 60.0 | 15.6 | 103.0 | 39.4 | 40.0 | 104.0 | 65.0 | 149.0 |
| 65.0 | 18.3 | 104.0 | 40.0 | 41.0 | 105.8 | 70.0 | 158.0 |
| 70.0 | 21.1 | 105.0 | 40.6 | 42.0 | 107.6 | 75.0 | 167.0 |
| 75.0 | 23.9 | 106.0 | 41.1 | 43.0 | 109.4 | 80.0 | 176.0 |
| 80.0 | 26.7 | 107.0 | 41.7 | 44.0 | 111.2 | 85.0 | 185.0 |
| 85.0 | 29.4 | 108.0 | 42.2 | 45.0 | 113.0 | 90.0 | 194.0 |
| 90.0 | 32.2 | 109.0 | 42.8 | 46.0 | 114.8 | 95.0 | 203.0 |
| 91.0 | 32.8 | 110.0 | 43.3 | 47.0 | 116.6 | 100.0 | 212.0 |
| | | | | 48.0 | 118.4 | 105.0 | 221.0 |

*(Continued)*

## PEDIATRIC DOSAGE ESTIMATION FORMULAS

The following formulas can be used to estimate the approximate pediatric dosage of a medication. These formulas are based on the adult dose and either the child's age or weight. These formulas should be used with caution as the response to any drug is not always directly proportional to the age or weight of the child relative to the usual adult dose. Dosage will also vary based on the formula used. Care should be taken when using any of these methods to calculate the child's dosage. Some products have FDA-approved pediatric indications and dosages; always refer to the full prescribing information first before calculating a pediatric dosage.

### BASED ON WEIGHT

**Augsberger's Rule:**

$$\frac{[(1.5 \times \text{weight [kg]}) + 10]}{100} \times \text{adult dose} = \text{approximate child's dose}$$

**Example:** If the child's weight is 15 kg (33 lb) and the adult dose is 50 mg then the child's dose is 16.25 mg.

$$\frac{[(1.5 \times 15 \text{ kg}) + 10]}{100} \times 50 \text{ mg} = 0.325 \times 50 \text{ mg} = 16.25 \text{ mg}$$

**Clark's Rule:**

(weight [lb]/150) x adult dose = approximate child's dose

**Example:** If the child's weight is 15 kg (33 lb) and the adult dose is 50 mg then the child's dose is 11 mg.

(33/150) x 50 mg = 0.22 x 50 mg = 11 mg

### BASED ON AGE

**Augsberger's Rule:**

$$\frac{[(4 \times \text{age [years]}) + 20]}{100} \times \text{adult dose} = \text{approximate child's dose}$$

**Example:** If the child's age is 8 years and the adult dose is 50 mg then the child's dose is 26 mg.
[(4 x 8) + 20)/100] x 50 mg = 0.52 X 50 mg = 26 mg

**Dilling's Rule:**

(age [years]/20) x adult dose = approximate child's dose

**Example:** If the child's age is 8 years and the adult dose is 50 mg then the child's dose is 20 mg.
(8/20) x 50 mg = 0.40 x 50 mg = 20 mg

**Cowling's Rule:**

$$\frac{[\text{age at next birthday (years)}]}{24} \times \text{adult dose} = \text{approximate child's dose}$$

**Example:** If the child is going to turn 8 years old in a few months and the adult dose is 50 mg then the child's dose is 16.7 mg. (8/24) x 50 mg = 0.33 x 50 mg = 16.7 mg

**Younge's Rule:**

$$\frac{[\text{age (years)}]}{\text{age} + 12} \times \text{adult dose} = \text{approximate child's dose}$$

**Example:** If the child's age is 8 years and the adult dose is 50 mg then the child's dose is 20 mg.
[8/(8+12)] x 50 mg = 0.4 x 50 mg = 20 mg

**Fried's Rule** (younger than 1 year):

$$\frac{[\text{age (months)}]}{150} \times \text{adult dose} = \text{approximate infant's dose}$$

**Example:** If the child's age is 10 months and the adult dose is 50 mg then the child's dose is 3.33 mg.
(10/150) x 50 mg = 0.067 x 50 mg = 3.33 mg

# TABLES FOR PHARMACY CALCULATIONS

## WEIGHTS AND MEASURES

### Metric Measure

*Weight*

| | | |
|---|---|---|
| 1 kilogram (kg) | = | 1,000 g |
| 1 gram (g) | = | 1,000 mg |
| 1 milligram (mg) | = | 0.001 g |
| 1 microgram (mcg) | = | 0.001 mg |
| 1 gamma | = | 1 mcg |

*Liquid*

| | | |
|---|---|---|
| 1 liter (L) | = | 1,000 mL |
| 1 milliliter (mL) | = | 1 cc (cubic centimeter) |

### Apothecary (Ap)

*Weight*

| | | |
|---|---|---|
| 1 scruple | = | 20 grains (gr) |
| 1 drachm | = | 3 scruples |
| | = | 60 gr |
| 1 ounce (oz) | = | 8 drachms |
| | = | 24 scruples |
| | = | 480 gr |
| 1 pound (lb) | = | 12 oz |
| | = | 96 drachms |
| | = | 288 scruples |
| | = | 5,760 gr |

### U.S. Fluid Measure

| | | |
|---|---|---|
| 1 fluidrachm | = | 60 minim (min) |
| 1 fluid ounce | = | 8 fld drachm |
| | = | 480 min |
| 1 pint (pt) | = | 16 fl oz |
| | = | 7,680 min |
| 1 quart (qt) | = | 2 pt |
| | = | 32 fl oz |
| 1 gallon (gal) | = | 4 qts |
| | = | 128 fl oz |

### Avoirdupois (Av)

*Weight*

| | | |
|---|---|---|
| 1 ounce | = | 437.5 gr |
| 1 pound | = | 16 oz |

### Conversion Factors

| | | |
|---|---|---|
| 1 gram | = | 15.4 gr |
| 1 grain | = | 64.8 mg |
| 1 ounce (Av) | = | 28.35 g |
| | = | 437.5 gr |
| 1 ounce (Ap) | = | 31.1 g |
| | = | 480 gr |
| 1 pound (Av) | = | 453.6 g |
| 1 kilogram | = | 2.68 pounds Ap |
| | = | 2.20 lbs Av |
| 1 fluid ounce | = | 29.57 mL |
| 1 fluidrachm | = | 3.697 mL |
| 1 minim | = | 0.06 mL |

### Converting °F to °C

For °F to °C, the formula is:

$°C = \frac{5}{9}(°F - 32)$

For °C to °F, the formula is:

$°F = (\frac{9}{5} \times °C) + 32$

### Common Measures

| | | |
|---|---|---|
| 1 teaspoonful | = | 5 mL |
| | = | 1/6 fl oz |
| 1 tablespoonful | = | 15 mL |
| | = | 1/2 fl oz |
| 1 wineglassful | = | 60 mL |
| | = | 2 fl oz |
| 1 teacupful | = | 120 mL |
| | = | 4 fl oz |

## TABLE OF SATURATED SOLUTIONS

This table shows the quantity of the substance and milliliters (mL) of water for 100 mL of a saturated solution at about 25° C.

| Substance | Gram | mL Water |
|---|---|---|
| Alum | 13.00 | 92.0 |
| Ammonium Carbonate | 22.00 | 88.0 |
| Ammonium Chloride | 28.30 | 79.3 |
| Ammonium Nitrate | 90.20 | 41.8 |
| Ammonium Sulfate | 53.10 | 71.7 |
| Borax | 5.90 | 98.0 |
| Boric Acid | 5.10 | 97.0 |
| Calcium Lactate | 5.00 | 96.0 |
| Chloral Hydrate | 120.00 | 31.0 |
| Citric Acid | 88.60 | 42.7 |
| Copper Sulfate | 22.30 | 98.7 |
| Dextrose | 59.00 | 60.0 |
| Ferric Chloride | 125.00 | 29.0 |
| Ferrous Sulfate | 52.80 | 72.7 |
| Lactose | 17.00 | 90.0 |
| Lead Acetate | 55.00 | 79.0 |
| Lithium Chloride | 59.50 | 70.2 |
| Lithium Sulfate | 33.00 | 88.5 |
| Magnesium Sulfate | 72.00 | 58.5 |
| Manganese Chloride | 90.00 | 54.0 |
| Mercuric Chloride | 6.96 | 98.5 |
| Methylene Blue | 4.30 | 97.0 |
| Oxalic Acid | 10.30 | 94.2 |
| Potassium Bromide | 56.00 | 82.0 |
| Potassium Carbonate | 82.20 | 73.5 |
| Potassium Chloride | 8.41 | 96.6 |
| Potassium Citrate | 92.00 | 56.5 |
| Potassium Iodide | 103.20 | 69.1 |
| Potassium Nitrate | 33.40 | 86.0 |
| Potassium Permanganate | 7.43 | 97.3 |
| Resorcinol | 67.20 | 47.2 |
| Rochelle Salt | 51.90 | 78.8 |
| Silver Nitrate | 164.00 | 65.5 |
| Sodium Acetate | 65.00 | 53.0 |
| Sodium Benzoate | 41.50 | 73.9 |
| Sodium Bicarbonate | 8.80 | 97.6 |
| Sodium Bromide | 73.00 | 78.0 |
| Sodium Carbonate | 27.50 | 96.0 |
| Sodium Chloride | 31.50 | 88.1 |
| Sodium Citrate | 55.50 | 72.5 |
| Sodium Iodide | 124.30 | 67.7 |
| Sodium Nitrate | 62.30 | 73.8 |
| Sodium Salicylate | 67.00 | 58.0 |
| Sodium Sulfate | 33.30 | 87.0 |
| Sodium Thiocyanate | 87.00 | 51.0 |
| Sodium Thiosulfate | 93.00 | 46.0 |
| Tartaric Acid | 76.90 | 54.7 |
| Urea | 62.00 | 53.5 |
| Zinc Sulfate | 93.00 | 56.0 |

## DOSE EQUIVALENTS

These approximate dose equivalents have been adopted by U.S.P. XXII, N.F. XVII. They are approved by the Food and Drug Administration.

When converting specific quantities or a prescription that requires compounding, or when converting a pharmaceutical formula from one system of weights or measures to the other, the following must be used.

### Weight

| Metric | Apothecary |
|---|---|
| 030 g | 1 ounce |
| 015 g | 4 drachms |
| 010 g | 2 1/2 drachms |
| 07.5 g | 2 drachms |
| 006 g | 90 grains |
| 005 g | 75 grains |
| 004 g | 60 grains (1 drachm) |
| 003 g | 45 grains |
| 002 g | 30 grains (1/2 drachm) |
| 01.5 g | 22 grains |
| 001 g | 15 grains |
| 750 mg | 12 grains |
| 600 mg | 10 grains |
| 500 mg | 7 1/2 grains |
| 400 mg | 6 grains |
| 300 mg | 5 grains |
| 250 mg | 4 grains |
| 200 mg | 3 grains |
| 150 mg | 2 1/2 grains |
| 125 mg | 2 grains |
| 100 mg | 1 1/2 grains |
| 75 mg | 1 1/4 grains |
| 60 mg | 1 grain |
| 50 mg | 3/4 grain |
| 40 mg | 2/3 grain |
| 30 mg | 1/2 grain |
| 25 mg | 3/8 grain |
| 20 mg | 1/3 grain |
| 15 mg | 1/4 grain |
| 12 mg | 1/5 grain |
| 10 mg | 1/6 grain |
| 08 mg | 1/8 grain |
| 06 mg | 1/10 grain |
| 05 mg | 1/12 grain |
| 04 mg | 1/15 grain |
| 03 mg | 1/20 grain |
| 02 mg | 1/30 grain |
| 1.5 mg | 1/40 grain |
| 1.2 mg | 1/50 grain |
| 01 mg | 1/60 grain |

*(Continued)*

**Liquid Measure**

| Metric | Apothecary |
|---|---|
| 1000 mL | 1 quart |
| 0750 mL | 1½ pints |
| 0500 mL | 1 pint |
| 0250 mL | 8 fluid ounces |
| 0200 mL | 7 fluid ounces |
| 0100 mL | 3½ fluid ounces |
| 0050 mL | 1¾ fluid ounces |
| 0030 mL | 1 fluid ounce |
| 0015 mL | 4 fluidrachms |
| 0010 mL | 2½ fluidrachms |
| 0008 mL | 2 fluidrachms |
| 0005 mL | 1¼ fluidrachms |
| 0004 mL | 1 fluidrachm |
| 0003 mL | 45 minims |
| 0002 mL | 30 minims |
| 0001 mL | 15 minims |
| 0.75 mL | 12 minims |
| 00.6 mL | 10 minims |
| 00.5 mL | 8 minims |
| 00.3 mL | 5 minims |
| 0.25 mL | 4 minims |
| 00.2 mL | 3 minims |
| 00.1 mL | 1½ minims |
| 0.06 mL | 1 minim |
| 0.05 mL | ¾ minim |
| 0.03 mL | ½ minim |

# Poison Control Centers

The American Association of Poison Control Centers (AAPCC) uses a single, nationwide emergency number to automatically link callers with their regional poison center. This toll-free number, **800-222-1222**, also works for **teletype lines (TTY)** for the hearing-impaired and **telecommunication devices (TTD)** for individuals who are deaf. However, a few local poison centers and the ASPCA/Animal Poison Control Center are not part of this nationwide system and continue to use separate numbers.

Most of the centers listed below are accredited by the AAPCC. **Certified centers are marked by an asterisk after the name.** Each has to meet certain criteria. It must, for example, serve a large geographic area; it must be open 24 hours a day and provide direct-dial or toll-free access; it must be supervised by a medical director; and it must have registered pharmacists or nurses available to answer questions from the public.

Within each state, centers are listed alphabetically by city. Some state poison centers also list their original emergency numbers (including TTY/TDD) that only work within that state. For these listings, callers may use either the state number or the nationwide 800 number.

## ALABAMA

### BIRMINGHAM

**Regional Poison Control Center (*)**
**Children's Hospital of Alabama**

1600 7th Ave. South
Birmingham, AL 35233
Business: 205-939-6334
**Emergency:** 800-222-1222
www.chsys.org

### TUSCALOOSA

**Alabama Poison Center (*)**

2503 Phoenix Dr.
Tuscaloosa, AL 35405
Business: 800-462-0609
**Emergency:** 800-222-1222
800-462-0800 (AL)
www.alapoisoncenter.org

## ALASKA

### JUNEAU

**Alaska Poison Control System**
**Section of Injury Prevention and EMS**

410 Willoughby Ave., Room 103
Box 110616
Juneau, AK 99811-0616
Business: 907-465-3027
**Emergency:** 800-222-1222
www.chems.alaska.gov

### (PORTLAND, OR)

**Oregon Poison Center (*)**
**Oregon Health and Science University**

3181 SW Sam Jackson Park Rd.
CB550
Portland, OR 97239
Business: 503-494-8600
**Emergency:** 800-222-1222
www.oregonpoison.com

## ARIZONA

### PHOENIX

**Banner Poison Control Center (*)**
**Banner Good Samaritan Medical Center**

1111 E. McDowell
Phoenix, AZ 85006
Business: 602-495-4884
**Emergency:** 800-222-1222
www.bannerpoisoncontrol.com

### TUCSON

**Arizona Poison and Drug Information Center (*)**
**Arizona Health Sciences Center**

1295 N. Martin Ave., Room B308
Tucson, AZ 85721
Business: 520-626-7899
**Emergency:** 800-222-1222
www.pharmacy.arizona.edu/outreach/poison

## ARKANSAS

### LITTLE ROCK

**Arkansas Poison and Drug Information Center (*)**
**College of Pharmacy - UAMS**

4301 West Markham St.
Mail Slot 522-2
Little Rock, AR 72205
Business: 501-686-6161
**Emergency:** 800-222-1222
800-376-4766 (AR)
TDD/TTY: 800-641-3805

## ASPCA/Animal Poison Control Center

1717 South Philo Rd.
Suite 36
Urbana, IL 61802
Business: 217-337-5030
**Emergency:** 888-426-4435
800-548-2423
www.aspca.org/apcc

## CALIFORNIA

### FRESNO/MADERA

**California Poison Control System-Fresno/Madera Div. (*)**
**Children's Hospital Central California**

9300 Valley Children's Place, MB 15
Madera, CA 93638-8762
Business: 559-622-2300
**Emergency:** 800-222-1222
800-876-4766 (CA)
TDD/TTY: 800-972-3323
www.calpoison.org

### SACRAMENTO

**California Poison Control System-Sacramento Div. (*)**
**UC Davis Medical Center**

2315 Stockton Blvd.
Sacramento, CA 95817
Business: 916-227-1400
**Emergency:** 800-222-1222
800-876-4766 (CA)
TDD/TTY: 800-972-3323
www.calpoison.org

### SAN DIEGO

**California Poison Control System-San Diego Div. (*)**
**UC San Diego Medical Center**

200 West Arbor Dr.
San Diego, CA 92103-8925
Business: 858-715-6300
**Emergency:** 800-222-1222
800-876-4766 (CA)
TDD/TTY: 800-972-3323
www.calpoison.org

### SAN FRANCISCO

**California Poison Control System-San Francisco Div. (*)**
**University of California San Francisco**

Box 1369
San Francisco, CA 94143-1369
Business: 415-502-6000
**Emergency:** 800-222-1222
800-876-4766 (CA)
TDD/TTY: 800-972-3323
www.calpoison.org

## COLORADO

### DENVER

**Rocky Mountain Poison and Drug Center (*)**

777 Bannock St., Mail Code 0180
Denver, CO 80204
Business: 303-739-1100
**Emergency**: 800-222-1222
TDD/TTY: 303-739-1127 (CO)
www.RMPDC.org

## CONNECTICUT

### FARMINGTON

**Connecticut Poison Control Center (*)**
**University of Connecticut Health Center**

263 Farmington Ave.
Farmington, CT 06030-5365
Business: 860-679-4540
**Emergency**: 800-222-1222
TDD/TTY: 866-218-5372
http://poisoncontrol.uchc.edu

## DELAWARE

### (PHILADELPHIA, PA)

**The Poison Control Center (*)**
**Children's Hospital of Philadelphia**

34th St. & Civic Center Blvd.
Philadelphia, PA 19104-4399
Business: 215-590-2003
**Emergency**: 800-222-1222
TDD/TTY: 215-590-8789
www.poisoncontrol.chop.edu

## DISTRICT OF COLUMBIA

### WASHINGTON, DC

**National Capital Poison Center (*)**

3201 New Mexico Ave., NW
Suite 310
Washington, DC 20016
Business: 202-362-3867
**Emergency**: 800-222-1222
www.poison.org

## FLORIDA

### JACKSONVILLE

**Florida Poison Information Center-Jacksonville (*)**

655 West 8th St.
Box C23
Jacksonville, FL 32209
Business: 904-244-4465
**Emergency**: 800-222-1222
http://fpicjax.org

### MIAMI

**Florida Poison Information Center (*)**
**University of Miami, Dept. of Pediatrics**

P.O. Box 016960 (R-131)
Miami, FL 33101
Business: 305-585-5250
**Emergency**: 800-222-1222
www.med.miami.edu/poisoncontrol

### TAMPA

**Florida Poison Information Center (*)**
**Tampa General Hospital**

P.O. Box 1289
Tampa, FL 33601-1289
Business: 813-844-7044
**Emergency**: 800-222-1222
www.poisoncentertampa.org

## GEORGIA

### ATLANTA

**Georgia Poison Center (*)**
**Hughes Spalding Children's Hospital, Grady Health System**

80 Jesse Hill Jr. Dr., SE
P.O. Box 26066
Atlanta, GA 30303-3050
Business: 404-616-9237
**Emergency**: 800-222-1222
(Atlanta) 404-616-9000
TDD: 404-616-9287
www.georgiapoisoncenter.org

## HAWAII

### (DENVER, CO)

**Rocky Mountain Poison and Drug Center (*)**

777 Bannock St., Mail Code 0180
Denver, CO 80204
Business: 303-739-1100
**Emergency**: 800-222-1222
TDD/TTY: 303-739-1127 (CO)
www.RMPDC.org

## IDAHO

### (Denver, CO)

**Rocky Mountain Poison and Drug Center (*)**

777 Bannock St., Mail Code 0180
Denver, CO 80204
Business: 303-739-1100
**Emergency**: 800-222-1222
TDD/TTY: 303-739-1127 (CO)
www.RMPDC.org

## ILLINOIS

### CHICAGO

**Illinois Poison Center (*)**

222 South Riverside Plaza
Suite 1900
Chicago, IL 60606
Business: 312-906-6136
**Emergency**: 800-222-1222
TDD/TTY: 312-906-6185
www.mchc.org/ipc

## INDIANA

### INDIANAPOLIS

**Indiana Poison Control Center (*)**
**Methodist Hospital, Clarian Health Partners**

I-65 at 21st St.
P.O. Box 1367
Indianapolis, IN 46206-1367
Business: 317-962-2335
**Emergency**: 800-222-1222
800-382-9097
317-962-2323
(Indianapolis)
www.clarian.org/poisoncontrol

## IOWA

### SIOUX CITY

**Iowa Statewide Poison Control Center (*)**
**Iowa Health System and the University of Iowa Hospitals and Clinics**

401 Douglas St., Suite 402
Sioux City, IA 51101
Business: 712-279-3710
**Emergency**: 800-222-1222
712-277-2222 (IA)
www.iowapoison.org

## KANSAS

### KANSAS CITY

**University of Kansas Poison Control Hospital Center**

3901 Rainbow Blvd.
Delp - Room 4043
Kansas City, KS 66160-7231
Business: 913-588-6638
**Emergency**: 800-222-1222
800-332-6633 (KS)
www.kumed.com/poison

## KENTUCKY

### LOUISVILLE

**Kentucky Regional Poison Center (*)**
**Medical Towers South**

234 E Gray St, Suite 847
Louisville, KY 40202
Business: 502-629-7264
**Emergency:** 800-222-1222
www.krpc.com

## LOUISIANA

### SHREVEPORT

**Louisiana Poison Center (*)**
**LSUHSC - Shreveport**
**Dept. of Emergency Medicine**
**Section of Clinical Toxology**

1455 Wilkinson St
Shreveport, LA 71130
Business: 318-813-3314
**Emergency:** 800-222-1222

## MAINE

### PORTLAND

**Northern New England Poison Center (*)**

22 Bramhall St.
Portland, ME 04102
Business: 207-662-7042
**Emergency:** 800-222-1222
800-442-6035
207-871-2879 (ME)
TDD/TTY: 207-662-2879 (ME)
www.nnepc.org

## MARYLAND

### BALTIMORE

**Maryland Poison Center (*)**
**University of Maryland at Baltimore**
**School of Pharmacy**

220 Arch St.
Office Level 01
Baltimore, MD 21201
Business: 410-706-7604
**Emergency:** 800-222-1222
TDD: 410-528-7530
www.mdpoison.com

### (WASHINGTON, DC)

**National Capital Poison Center (*)**

3201 New Mexico Ave., NW
Suite 310
Washington, DC 20016
Business: 202-362-3867
**Emergency:** 800-222-1222
www.poison.org

## MASSACHUSETTS

### BOSTON

**Regional Center for Poison Control and Prevention (*)**
**(Serving Massachusetts and Rhode Island)**

300 Longwood Ave.
Boston, MA 02115
Business: 617-355-6609
**Emergency:** 800-222-1222
TDD/TTY: 888-244-5313
www.maripoisoncenter.com

## MICHIGAN

### DETROIT

**Regional Poison Control Center (*)**
**Children's Hospital of Michigan**

4160 John R. Harper Professional Office Bldg.
Suite 616
Detroit, MI 48201
Business: 313-745-5335
**Emergency:** 800-222-1222
www.mitoxic.org/pcc

## MINNESOTA

### MINNEAPOLIS

**Hennepin Regional Poison Center (*)**
**Hennepin County Medical Center**

701 Park Ave.
Mail Code RL
Minneapolis, MN 55415
Business: 612-873-3144
**Emergency:** 800-222-1222
www.mnpoison.org

## MISSISSIPPI

### JACKSON

**Mississippi Regional Poison Control Center**
**University of Mississippi Medical Center**

2500 North State St.
Jackson, MS 39216
Business: 601-984-1680
**Emergency:** 800-222-1222
http://poisoncontrol.umc.edu

## MISSOURI

### ST. LOUIS

**Missouri Regional Poison Center (*)**

7980 Clayton Rd. Suite 200
St. Louis, MO 63117
Business: 314-772-8300
**Emergency:** 800-222-1222
www.cardinalglennon.com

## MONTANA

### (DENVER, CO)

**Rocky Mountain Poison and Drug Center (*)**

777 Bannock St., Mail Code 0180
Denver, CO 80204
Business: 303-739-1100
**Emergency:** 800-222-1222
TDD/TTY: 303-739-1127 (CO)
www.RMPDC.org

## NEBRASKA

### OMAHA

**Nebraska Regional Poison Center (*)**

8401 W. Dodge Rd., Suite 115
Omaha, NE 68114
Business: 402-390-5555
**Emergency:** 800-222-1222
www.nebraskapoison.com

## NEVADA

### (DENVER, CO)

**Rocky Mountain Poison and Drug Center (*)**

777 Bannock St., Mail Code 0180
Denver, CO 80204
Business: 303-739-1100
**Emergency:** 800-222-1222
TDD/TTY: 303-739-1127 (CO)
www.RMPDC.org

## NEW HAMPSHIRE

### (PORTLAND, ME)

**Northern New England Poison Center**
**Maine Medical Center**

22 Bramhall St.
Portland, ME 04102
Business: 207-662-0111
**Emergency:** 800-222-1222
www.nnepc.org

## NEW JERSEY

### NEWARK

**New Jersey Poison Information and Education System (*)**
**UMDNJ**

140 Bergen St. PO Box 1709
Newark, NJ 07101
Business: 973-972-9280
**Emergency**: 800-222-1222
TDD/TTY: 973-926-8008
www.njpies.org

## NEW MEXICO

### ALBUQUERQUE

**New Mexico Poison and Drug Information Center (*)**

MSC09/5080
1 University of New Mexico
Albuquerque, NM 87131-0001
Business: 505-272-4261
**Emergency**: 800-222-1222
http://hsc.unm.edu/pharmacy/poison

## NEW YORK

### MINEOLA

**Long Island Regional Poison and Drug Information Center (*)**
**Winthrop University Hospital**

259 First St.
Mineola, NY 11501
Business: 516-663-4574
**Emergency**: 800-222-1222
www.lirpdic.org

### NEW YORK CITY

**New York City Poison Control Center (*)**
**NYC Bureau of Public Health**

455 First Ave., Room 123, Box 81
New York, NY 10016
Business: 212-447-8152
**Emergency**: 800-222-1222
(English) 212-340-4494
212-POISONS
(212-764-7667)
**Emergency**: 212-venenos
(Spanish) (212-836-3667)
TDD: 212-689-9014
www.nyc.gov/html/doh/html/poison/poison.shtml

### ROCHESTER

**The Ruth A. Lawrence Regional Poison and Drug Information Center (*)**
**University of Rochester Medical Center**

601 Elmwood Ave.
Box 321
Rochester, NY 14642
Business: 585-273-4155
**Emergency**: 800-222-1222
TTY: 585-273-3854
www.fingerlakespoison.org

### SYRACUSE

**Upstate New York Poison Center (*)**
**SUNY Upstate Medical University**

750 East Adams St.
Syracuse, NY 13210
Business: 315-464-7078
**Emergency**: 800-222-1222
TTY: 315-464-5424
www.upstatepoison.org

## NORTH CAROLINA

### CHARLOTTE

**Carolinas Poison Center (*)**
**Carolinas Medical Center**

PO Box 32861
Charlotte, NC 28232-2861
Business: 704-512-3795
**Emergency**: 800-222-1222
www.ncpoisoncenter.org

## NORTH DAKOTA

### (MINNEAPOLIS, MN)

**Hennepin Regional Poison Center (*)**
**Hennepin County Medical Center**

701 Park Ave., Mail Code RL
Minneapolis, MN 55415
Business: 612-873-3144
**Emergency**: 800-222-1222
www.mnpoison.org

## OHIO

### CINCINNATI

**Cincinnati Drug and Poison Information Center (*)**

3333 Burnet Ave., MLC 9004
Cincinnati, OH 45229
Business: 513-636-5063
**Emergency**: 800-222-1222
www.cincinnatichildrens.org/dpic

### CLEVELAND

**Northern Ohio Poison Center**
**Rainbow Babies and Children's Hospital**

11100 Euclid Ave.
B261 MP 6007
Cleveland, OH 44106-6010
Business: 216-844-1573
**Emergency**: 800-222-1222
www.uhhospitals.org/rainbowchildren/tabid/195/Default.aspx

### COLUMBUS

**Central Ohio Poison Center (*)**

700 Children's Dr.
Columbus, OH 43205
Business: 614-355-0435
**Emergency**: 800-222-1222
TTY: 866-688-0088
www.bepoisonsmart.com

## OKLAHOMA

### OKLAHOMA CITY

**Oklahoma Poison Control Center (*)**
**OU Health Sciences Center**

940 Northeast 13th St.
Room 3N3510
Oklahoma City, OK 73104
Business: 405-271-5062
**Emergency**: 800-222-1222
www.oklahomapoison.org

## OREGON

### PORTLAND

**Oregon Poison Center (*)**
**Oregon Health and Science University**

3181 S.W. Sam Jackson Park Rd.
CB550
Portland, OR 97239
Business: 503-494-8600
**Emergency**: 800-222-1222
www.ohsu.edu/poison

## PENNSYLVANIA

### PHILADELPHIA

**The Poison Control Center (*)**
**Children's Hospital of Philadelphia**

34th Street & Civic Center Blvd.
Philadelphia, PA 19104
Business: 215-590-2003
**Emergency**: 800-222-1222
215-386-2100 (PA)
TDD/TTY: 215-590-8789
www.poisoncontrol.chop.edu

### PITTSBURGH

**Pittsburgh Poison Center (*)**
**University of Pittsburgh**

200 Lothrop Street
Pittsburgh, PA 15213
Business: 412-390-3300
**Emergency**: 800-222-1222
412-681-6669
www.upmc.com/services/poisoncenter

## RHODE ISLAND

### (BOSTON, MA)

**Regional Center for Poison Control and Prevention (*)**
**(Serving Massachusetts and Rhode Island)**

300 Longwood Ave.
Boston, MA 02115
Business: 617-355-6609
**Emergency**: 800-222-1222
TDD/TTY: 888-244-5313
www.maripoisoncenter.com

## SOUTH CAROLINA

### COLUMBIA

**Palmetto Poison Center (*)**
**South Carolina College of Pharmacy**
**University of South Carolina**

Columbia, SC 29208
Business: 803-777-7909
**Emergency**: 800-222-1222
http://poison.sc.edu

## SOUTH DAKOTA

### (MINNEAPOLIS, MN)

**Hennepin Regional Poison Center (*)**
**Hennepin County Medical Center**

701 Park Ave., Mail Code RL
Minneapolis, MN 55415
Business: 612-873-3144
**Emergency**: 800-222-1222
www.mnpoison.org

## TENNESSEE

### NASHVILLE

**Tennessee Poison Center (*)**

1161 21st Ave. South
501 Oxford House
Nashville, TN 37232-4632
Business: 615-936-0760
**Emergency**: 800-222-1222
www.tnpoisoncenter.org

## TEXAS

### AMARILLO

**Texas Panhandle Poison Center (*)**

1501 S. Coulter Dr.
Amarillo, TX 79106
Business: 806-354-1630
**Emergency**: 800-222-1222
www.poisoncontrol.org

### DALLAS

**North Texas Poison Center (*)**
**Texas Poison Center Network**
**Parkland Memorial Hospital**

5201 Harry Hines Blvd.
Dallas, TX 75235
Business: 214-589-0911
**Emergency**: 800-222-1222
www.poisoncontrol.org

### EL PASO

**West Texas Regional Poison Center (*)**
**At University Medical Center of El Paso**

4815 Alameda Ave.
El Paso, TX 79905
Business 915-534-3800
**Emergency**: 800-222-1222
www.poisoncontrol.org

### GALVESTON

**Southeast Texas Poison Center (*)**
**The University of Texas Medical Branch**

3.112 Trauma Center
Galveston, TX 77555-1175
Business: 409-772-3332
**Emergency**: 800-222-1222
www.utmb.edu/setpc

### SAN ANTONIO

**South Texas Poison Center (*)**
**The University of Texas Health Science Center–San Antonio**
**Dept. of Surgery**

7703 Floyd Curl Dr., MSC 7849
San Antonio, TX 78229-3900
Business: 210-567-5762
**Emergency**: 800-222-1222
www.texaspoison.com

### TEMPLE

**Central Texas Poison Center (*)**
**Scott & White Memorial Hospital**

2401 South 31st St.
Temple, TX 76508
Business: 254-724-7405
**Emergency**: 800-222-1222
http://www.sw.org/web/patientsAndVisitors/iwcontent/public/poison/en_us/html/poison.jsp

## UTAH

### SALT LAKE CITY

**Utah Poison Control Center (*)**
**University of Utah**

585 Komas Dr. Suite #200
Salt Lake City, UT 84108-1234
Business: 801-587-0600
**Emergency**: 800-222-1222
http://uuhsc.utah.edu/poison

## VERMONT

### (PORTLAND, ME)

**Northern New England Poison Center (*)**
**Maine Medical Center**

22 Bramhall St.
Portland, ME 04102
Business: 207-662-0111
**Emergency**: 800-222-1222
www.nnepc.org

## VIRGINIA

### CHARLOTTESVILLE

**Blue Ridge Poison Center (*)**
**Jefferson Park Place**

1222 Jefferson Park Ave.
Charlottesville, VA 22908-0774
Business: 434-924-0347
**Emergency**: 800-222-1222
www.healthsystem.virginia.edu/brpc

### RICHMOND

**Virginia Poison Center (*)**
**Medical College of Virginia Hospitals**
**Virginia Commonwealth University Health System**

P.O. Box 980522
Richmond, VA 23298-0522
Business: 804-828-4780
**Emergency**: 800-222-1222
www.poison.vcu.edu

## WASHINGTON

### SEATTLE

**Washington Poison Center (*)**

155 NE 100th St.
Seattle, WA 98125-8007
Business: 206-517-2350
**Emergency**: 800-222-1222
www.wapc.org

## WEST VIRGINIA

### CHARLESTON

**West Virginia Poison Center (*)**
**WVU Charleston Division**

3110 MacCorkle Ave. SE
Charleston, WV 25314
Business: 304-347-1212
**Emergency**: 800-222-1222
www.wvpoisoncenter.org

## WISCONSIN

### MILWAUKEE

**Wisconsin Poison Center**

Mail Station 660
P.O. Box 1997
Milwaukee, WI 53201-1997
Business: 414-266-6973
**Emergency**: 800-222-1222
www.wisconsinpoison.org

## WYOMING

### (OMAHA, NE)

**Nebraska Regional Poison Center (*)**

8401 W. Dodge St., Suite 115
Omaha, NE 68114
Business: 402-390-5555
**Emergency**: 800-222-1222
www.nebraskapoison.com

# CERTIFICATION PROGRAMS FOR NURSES

| Organization | Website |
|---|---|
| **American Nurses Credentialing Center (ANCC)**<br>• Acute Care Nurse Practitioner<br>• Adult Health Clinical Nurse Specialist (formerly Med-Surg)<br>• Adult Nurse Practitioner<br>• Adult Psychiatric & Mental Health Clinical Nurse Specialist<br>• Adult Psychiatric & Mental Health Nurse Practitioner<br>• Ambulatory Care Nurse<br>• Cardiac Rehabilitation Nurse<br>• Cardiac Vascular Nurse<br>• Case Management Nurse<br>• Child/Adolescent Psychiatric & Mental Health Clinical Nurse Specialist<br>• College Health Nurse<br>• Community Health Nurse<br>• Diabetes Management, Advanced<br>• Family Nurse Practitioner<br>• Family Psychiatric & Mental Health Nurse Practitioner<br>• General Nursing Practice<br>• Gerontological Clinical Nurse Specialist<br>• Gerontological Nurse<br>• Gerontological Nurse Practitioner<br>• High-Risk Perinatal Nurse<br>• Home Health Clinical Nurse Specialist<br>• Home Health Nurse<br>• Informatics Nurse<br>• Maternal-Child Nurse<br>• Medical-Surgical Nurse<br>• Nurse Executive (*formerly Nursing Administration*)<br>• Nurse Executive, Advanced (*formerly Nursing Administration, Advanced*)<br>• Nursing Professional Development<br>• Pain Management<br>• Pediatric Clinical Nurse Specialist<br>• Pediatric Nurse<br>• Pediatric Nurse Practitioner<br>• Perinatal Nurse<br>• Psychiatric and Mental Health Nurse<br>• Public/Community Health Clinical Nurse Specialist<br>• Public Health Nurse, Advanced<br>• School Nurse<br>• School Nurse Practitioner | **nursecredentialing.org** |
| **American Academy of Medical Esthetic Professionals (AAMEP)**<br>• Medical Esthetics-Certified (ME-C) | **www.amen-usa.org** |
| **Association for the Advancement of Medical Instrumentation (AAMI)**<br>• Biomedical Equipment Technicians (CBET)<br>• Radiology Equipment Specialists (CRES)<br>• Clinical Laboratory Equipment Specialists (CLES) | **www.aami.org** |
| **American Society of Ophthalmic Registered Nurses (ASORN)**<br>• Ophthalmic Registered Nurses (CORN) | **webeye.ophth.uiowa.edu/asorn** |
| **American Board of Certification for Gastroenterology Nurses (ABCGN)**<br>• Certified Gastroenterology Registered Nurses (CGRN) | **www.abcgn.org** |
| **National Council of State Boards of Nursing (NCSBN)**<br>• Nurse Practitioner Certification<br>• Nurse Licensure Compact (NLC) | **www.ncsbn.org** |
| **National Certification Board for Diabetes Educators (NCBDE)**<br>• Certified Diabetes Educator | **www.ncbde.org** |
| **Board of Certification for Emergency Nursing (BCEN)**<br>• Certified Emergency Nursing (CEN)<br>• Certified Flight Registered Nurse (CFRN) | **www.ena.org/bcen** |
| **HIV/AIDS Nursing Certification Board (HANCB)**<br>• HIV/AIDS Nursing | **www.hancb.org** |
| **Certification Board of Infection Control & Epidemiology (CBIC)**<br>• Infectious Disease Nursing | **www.cbic.org** |

## Certification Programs for Nurses

| Organization | Website |
|---|---|
| **Infusion Nurses Society (INS)**<br>• Infusion Nursing | **www.ins1.org** |
| **National Certification Corporation (NCC)**<br>• Inpatient OB/GYN (INPT)<br>• Maternal Newborn (MN)<br>• Low Risk Neonatal (LRN)<br>• Neonatal Intensive Care (NIC) | **www.nccwebsite.org** |
| **Oncology Nursing Certification Corporation**<br>• Oncology Certified Nurse (OCN®)<br>• Certified Pediatric Oncology Nurse (CPON®)<br>• Advanced Oncology Certified Nurse Practitioner (AOCNP®)<br>• Advanced Oncology Certified Clinical Nurse Specialists (AOCNS®) | **www.oncc.org** |
| **American Academy of Pain Management (AAPM)**<br>• Credentialed Pain Practitioner (CPP) | **www.aapainmanage.org** |
| **Competency & Credentialing Institute (CCI)**<br>• Perioperative Nursing (CNOR & CRNFA) | **www.cc-institute.org** |
| **American Society of Plastic Surgical Nurses (ASPSN)**<br>• Certified Plastic Surgical Nurse (CPSN) | **www.aspsn.org** |
| **American Board of Perianesthesia Nursing Certification (ABPANC)**<br>• Certified Post Anesthesia Nurse (CPAN®)<br>• Certified Ambulatory Perianesthesia Nurse (CAPA®) | **www.cpancapa.org** |
| **National Board for Certification of School Nurses (NCSN)**<br>• School Nursing (NBCSN) | **www.nbcsn.com** |
| **Genetic Nursing Credentialing Commission (GNCC)**<br>• Advanced Practice Nurse in Genetics (APNG)<br>• Genetics Clinical Nurse (GCN) | **www.geneticnurse.org** |
| **Center for Nursing Education and Testing (C-NET®)**<br>• Certified Board for Urology Nurses & Associates (CBUNA)<br>• Dermatology Nurses Certification Board (DNCB)<br>• Certified Medical-Surgical Nurse (CMSRN)<br>• Certified Nephrology Nurse (CNN)<br>• Certified Nephrology Nurse – Nurse Practitioner (CNN-NP)<br>• Plastic Surgical Nursing Certification Board (PSNCB)<br>• Radiological Nurse (RNC) | **www.cnetnurse.com** |
| **Prepared Childbirth Educators, Inc.**<br>• Certified Breastfeeding Counselor (CBC)<br>• Certified Childbirth Educator (CCE)<br>• Certified Labor Support Specialist (CLSS)<br>• Certified Prenatal/Postnatal Fitness Instructor<br>• Certified Infant Massage Instructor/Educator | **www.childbirtheducation.org** |
| **American Association of Nurse Anesthetists**<br>• Certified Registered Nurse Anesthetist (CRNA) | **www.aana.com** |

# PROFESSIONAL ASSOCIATIONS FOR NURSES

## COMMUNITY HEALTH

**American Academy of Ambulatory Care Nursing**
East Holly Ave.
Box 56
Pitman, NJ 08071-0056
800-262-6877
www.aaacn.org

**American Public Health Association**
800 I St., NW
Washington, DC 20001-3710
202-777-2742
www.apha.org

## CRITICAL CARE

**American Association of Critical-Care Nurses**
101 Columbia
Aliso Viejo, CA 92656-4109
800-899-2226
www.aacn.org

**Northeast Pediatric Cardiology Nurses Association**
www.npcna.org

**Society of Critical Care Medicine**
500 Midway Dr.
Mount Prospect, IL 60056
847-827-6869
www.sccm.org

## EMERGENCY NURSING

**Air & Surface Transport Nurses Association**
7995 East Prentice Ave., Suite 100
Greenwood Village, CO 80111
800-897-6362
www.astna.org

**Emergency Nurses Association**
915 Lee St.
Des Plaines, IL 60016-6569
800-900-9659
www.ena.org

## GERIATRICS

**American Geriatrics Society**
The Empire State Building
350 Fifth Ave., Suite 801
New York, NY 10118
212-308-1414
www.americangeriatrics.org

**Gerontological Advanced Practice Nurses Association**
7794 Grow Dr.
Pensacola, FL 32514
866-355-1392
www.ncgnp.org

**Gerontological Society of America**
1220 L St. NW, Suite 901
Washington, DC 20005
202-842-1275
www.geron.org

## MIDWIFERY

**American College of Nurse-Midwives**
8403 Colesville Rd., Suite 1550
Silver Spring, MD 20910
240-485-1800
www.acnm.org

## NEONATAL

**Association of Women's Health, Obstetric & Neonatal Nurses**
2000 L St., NW, Suite 740
Washington, DC 20036
800-673-8499
www.awhonn.org

**National Association of Neonatal Nurses**
4700 W. Lake Ave.
Glenview, IL 60025-1468
800-451-3795
www.nann.org

## NEPHROLOGY

**American Nephrology Nurses' Association**
East Holly Ave.
Box 56
Pitman, NJ 08071-0056
888-600-2662
www.annanurse.org

**National Kidney Foundation**
30 East 33rd St.
New York, NY 10016
800-622-9010
www.kidney.org

## NEUROSCIENCE

**American Association of Neuroscience Nurses**
4700 West Lake Ave.
Glenview, IL 60025
888-557-2266
www.aann.org

**American Association of Spinal Cord Injury Professionals**
801 18th St., NW
Washington, DC 20006
202-416-7704
www.aascin.org

## ONCOLOGY

**Association of Pediatric Hematology/Oncology Nurses**
4700 West Lake Ave.
Glenview, IL 60025-1485
847-375-4724
www.apon.org

**Oncology Nursing Society**
125 Enterprise Dr.
Pittsburgh, PA 15275
866-257-4667
www.ons.org

## PALLIATIVE CARE

**Hospice and Palliative Nurses Association**
One Penn Center West, Suite 229
Pittsburgh, PA 15276-0100
412-787-9301
www.hpna.org

## PEDIATRICS

**Pediatric Nursing Certification Board**
800 South Frederick Ave.
Suite 204
Gaithersburg, MD 20877-4152
888-641-2767
www.pncb.org

## PREOPERATIVE & PERIOPERATIVE

**American Association of Nurse Anesthetists**
222 South Prospect Ave.
Park Ridge, IL 60068
Phone: 847-692-7050
Fax: 847-692-6968
www.aana.com

**American Society of PeriAnesthesia Nurses**
90 Frontage Rd
Cherry Hill, NJ 08034-1424
877-737-9696
www.aspan.org

**American Society of Plastic Surgical Nurses**
7794 Grow Dr.
Pensacola, FL 32514
800-272-0136
www.aspsn.org

**Association of Perioperative Registered Nurses (AORN)**
2170 South Parker Rd., Suite 400
Denver, CO 80231
800-755-2676
www.aorn.org

## PSYCHIATRIC

**American Psychiatric Nurses Association**
1555 Wilson Blvd., Suite 530
Arlington, VA 22209
866-243-2443
www.apna.org

## REHABILITATION

**Association of Rehabilitation Nurses**
4700 West Lake Ave.
Glenview, IL 60025
800-229-7530
www.rehabnurse.org

## SCHOOL NURSING

**American School Health Association**
7263 State Route 43
PO Box 708
Kent, OH 44240
330-678-1601
www.ashaweb.org

**National Association of School Nurses**
8484 Georgia Ave., Suite 420
Silver Spring, MD 20910
866-627-6767
www.nasn.org

## STATE ASSOCIATIONS/ ANESTHETISTS

**California Association of Nurse Anesthetists**
PO Box 1426
Boyes Hot Springs, CA 95416
206-984-1624
www.canainc.org

**Connecticut Association of Nurse Anesthetists**
377 Research Parkway
Suite 2D
Meriden, CT 06450
203-238-1207
www.ctana.com

**New York State Association of Nurse Anesthetists**
1450 Western Ave., Suite 101
Albany, NY 12203
518-861-8876
www.nysana.com

**Pennsylvania Association of Nurse Anesthetists**
234 North Third St.
Harrisburg, PA 17101
800-495-7262
www.pana.org

**Texas Association of Nurse Anesthetists**
PO Box 40775
Austin, TX 78704
512-495-9004
www.txana.org

## STUDENT NURSING

**National Student Nurses' Association**
45 Main St., Suite 606
Brooklyn, NY 11201
718-210-0705
www.nsna.org

## WOUND CARE

**Wound, Ostomy and Continence Nurses Society**
15000 Commerce Parkway, Suite C
Mt. Laurel, NJ 08054
888-224-9626
www.wocn.org

# Nurse Practitioner Programs by State

## ALABAMA

University of Alabama–Huntsville
College of Nursing
Nursing Building, Room 207
301 Sparkman Dr.
Huntsville, AL 35899
256-824-6345
onlinenurse.nb.uah.edu

## ARIZONA

Arizona State University
College of Nursing & Health Innovation
500 N. 3rd St.
Phoenix, AZ 85004
602-496-2264
nursingandhealth.asu.edu

University of Arizona
College of Nursing
1305 N. Martin St.
PO Box 210203
Tucson, AZ 85721
520-626-6154
www.nursing.arizona.edu

## CALIFORNIA

Azusa Pacific University
School of Nursing
PO Box 7000
Azusa, CA 91702-7000
626-815-5386
www.apu.edu/nursing

California State University–Bakersfield
Dept. of Nursing, 29 RNC
9001 Stockdale Hwy.
Bakersfield, CA 93311
661-654-3110
www.csub.edu/nursing

California State University–Fresno
Dept. of Nursing
College of Health & Human Services
2345 E. San Ramon
M/S MH26
Fresno, CA 93740
559-278-4004
www.csufresno.edu/chhs

California State University–Long Beach
Dept. of Nursing
College of Health & Human Services
1250 Bellflower Blvd.
Long Beach, CA 90840
562-985-4194
www.csulb.edu/colleges/chhs

Loma Linda University
School of Nursing, West Hall
Loma Linda, CA 92350
800-422-4558
www.llu.edu/llu/nursing

UCLA School of Nursing
Factor Building
700 Tiverton Ave.
Los Angeles, CA 90095
310-825-7181
www.nursing.ucla.edu

University of California–San Francisco
School of Nursing
2 Koret Way, #N-319X
UCSF Box 0602
San Francisco, CA 94143-0602
415-476-9710
www.nurseweb.ucsf.edu

University of San Diego
Hahn School of Nursing & Health Science
5998 Alcala Park
San Diego, CA 92110
619-260-4600
www.sandiego.edu

University of San Francisco
School of Nursing
2130 Fulton St.
San Francisco, CA 94117-1080
415-422-6681
www.usfca.edu/nursing

## COLORADO

Regis University
Rueckert-Hartman College for Health Professions
3333 Regis Blvd.
Mail Code G-9
Denver, CO 80221-1099
303-458-4126
www.regis.edu

University of Colorado–Denver
College of Nursing
Campus Box C288
Education 2 North
13120 E. 19th Ave.
Aurora, CO 80045
303-724-1812
www.nursing.ucdenver.edu

## CONNECTICUT

Quinnipiac University
Dept. of Nursing
275 Mount Carmel Ave.
Hamden, CT 06518-1908
203-582-5397
www.quinnipiac.edu

Saint Joseph College
Div. of Nursing
1678 Asylum Ave.
West Hartford, CT 06117
860-231-5211
www.sjc.edu

Yale University
School of Nursing
100 Church St. South
PO Box 9740
New Haven, CT 06536-0740
203-785-2389
www.nursing.yale.edu

## DELAWARE

University of Delaware
College of Health Sciences
School of Nursing
McDowell Hall
25 N. College
Newark, DE 19716
302-831-1253
www.udel.edu/nursing

## DISTRICT OF COLUMBIA

Catholic University of America
School of Nursing
125 Gowan Hall
620 Michigan Ave., NE
Washington, DC 20064
202-319-5400
nursing.cua.edu

Georgetown University
School of Nursing & Health Studies
3700 Reservoir Rd., NW
PO Box 571107
Washington, DC 20057-1107
202-687-4647
snhs.georgetown.edu

## FLORIDA

Barry University
School of Nursing
11300 NE Second Ave.
Miami Shores, FL 33161-6695
305-899-3800
www.barry.edu

Florida State University
College of Nursing
98 Varsity Way
PO Box 3064310
Tallahassee, FL 32306
850-644-3296
www.nursing.fsu.edu

University of Florida
College of Nursing
PO Box 100197
Gainesville, FL 32610-0197
352-273-6001
www.con.ufl.edu

University of Miami
School of Nursing & Health Studies
PO Box 248153
Coral Gables, FL 33124
305-284-3666
www.miami.edu/sonhs

## GEORGIA

Emory University
School of Nursing
1520 Clifton Rd., NE
Atlanta, GA 30322-4207
404-727-7980
www.nursing.emory.edu

Georgia State University
School of Nursing
PO Box 4019
Atlanta, GA 30303
404-413-1200
www.chhs.gsu.edu/nursing

## HAWAII

Hawaii Pacific University
School of Nursing
45-045 Kamehameha Hwy.
Kaneohe, HI 96744-5297
808-236-3552
www.hpu.edu

## IDAHO

Boise State University
Dept. of Nursing
1910 University Dr.
Boise, ID 83725-1840
208-426-4143
www.nursing.boisestate.edu

Idaho State University
School of Nursing
650 Memorial Dr.
Building 66, Room 329
Pocatello, ID 83209
208-282-2132
www.isu.edu/nursing

## ILLINOIS

DePaul University
Dept. of Nursing
990 West Fullerton Pkwy.
Chicago, IL 60614
773-325-7280
www.depaul.edu

North Park University
School of Nursing
3225 West Foster Ave.
Chicago, IL 60625-4895
773-244-5680
www.northpark.edu

Southern Illinois
University–Edwardsville
School of Nursing, Alumni Hall
Room 2117
PO Box 1066
Edwardsville, IL 62026
800-234-4844
www.siue.edu/nursing

University of Illinois–Chicago
College of Nursing
845 South Damen Ave., MC 802
Chicago, IL 60612
312-996-7800
www.uic.edu/nursing

## INDIANA

Indiana Wesleyan University–Marion
School of Nursing
4201 S. Washington St.
Marion, IN 46953
800-332-6901
www.indwes.edu/nursing

Purdue University
School of Nursing
502 N. University St.
West Lafayette, IN 47907-2069
765-494-4004
www.nursing.purdue.edu

## KENTUCKY

University of Kentucky
College of Nursing
315 College of Nursing Building
Lexington, KY 40536-0232
859-323-5108
www.mc.uky.edu/nursing

## LOUISIANA

Louisiana State University
School of Nursing
1900 Gravier St., 4th Floor
New Orleans, LA 70112
504-568-4106
www.nursing.lsuhsc.edu

## MARYLAND

Johns Hopkins University
School of Nursing
525 N. Wolfe St.
Baltimore, MD 21205
410-955-7548
www.son.jhmi.edu

## MASSACHUSETTS

Northeastern University
College of Health Sciences
School of Nursing
102 Robinson Hall
Boston, MA 02115
617-373-3649
www.neu.edu

University of
Massachusetts–Dartmouth
College of Nursing
285 Old Westport Rd.
North Dartmouth, MA 02747
508-999-8586
www.umassd.edu/nursing

University of
Massachusetts–Worcester
Graduate School of Nursing
55 Lake Ave. North
Worcester, MA 01655
508-856-5801
www.umassmed.edu

## MICHIGAN

Michigan State University
College of Nursing
A117 Life Sciences Building
East Lansing, MI 48824-1317
800-605-6424
www.nursing.msu.edu

University of Michigan
School of Nursing Building
400 North Ingalls
Ann Arbor, MI 48109-5482
734-763-5985
www.nursing.umich.edu

University of Michigan–Flint
School of Health Professions &
Studies
2180 William S. White Building
303 East Kearsley St.
Flint, MI 48502
810-237-6503
www.umflint.edu

## MINNESOTA

University of Minnesota
School of Nursing
5-140 Weaver-Densford Hall
308 Harvard St., SE
Minneapolis, MN 55455
612-624-9600
www.nursing.umn.edu

## MISSOURI

Missouri State University
Dept. of Nursing
Professional Building, Suite 300
901 S. National Ave.
Springfield, MO 65897
417-836-5310
www.missouristate.edu

Saint Louis University
School of Nursing
3525 Caroline St.
St. Louis, MO 63104
314-977-8995
www.slu.edu

University of Missouri–Kansas City
School of Nursing
Health Sciences Building
2464 Charlotte
Kansas City, MO 64108
816-235-1700
www.nursing.umkc.edu

## NEBRASKA

Creighton University
School of Nursing
2500 California Plaza
Omaha, NE 68178
800-544-5071
www.creighton.edu

## NEW JERSEY

The College of New Jersey
Dept. of Nursing
Paul Loser Hall 206
PO Box 7718
Ewing, NJ 08628-0718
609-771-2591
www.tcnj.edu

Felician College
Div. of Health Sciences
262 South Main St.
Lodi, NJ 07644
201-559-6000
www.felician.edu

Monmouth University
School of Nursing & Health Studies
400 Cedar Ave.
West Long Branch, NJ 07764-1898
732-571-3443
www.monmouth.edu

Ramapo College of New Jersey
Nursing Programs at Ramapo
School of Theoretical & Applied Science
505 Ramapo Valley Rd.
Mahwah, NJ 07430
201-684-7737
www.ramapo.edu

Rutgers College of Nursing
Ackerson Hall, Rm. 102
108 University Ave.
Newark, NJ 07102
973-353-1157
www.nursingrutgers.edu

## NEW MEXICO

New Mexico State University
School of Nursing
MSC 3185
PO Box 30001
Las Cruces, NM 88003-8001
575-646-3812
www.nmsu.edu/~nursing

University of New Mexico
College of Nursing
MSC09 5350
Albuquerque, NM 87131-0001
505-272-4223
hsc.unm.edu/consg

## NEW YORK

Adelphi University
School of Nursing
One South Ave.
Garden City, NY 11530-0701
516-877-4540
www.nursing.adelphi.edu

Binghamton University–SUNY
Decker School of Nursing
PO Box 6000
Binghamton, NY 13902-6000
607-777-4954
www.binghamton.edu

College of Mount Saint Vincent
Dept. of Nursing
6301 Riverdale Ave.
Riverdale, NY 10471
718-405-3365
www.mountsaintvincent.edu

Columbia University
School of Nursing
630 West 168th St.
PO Box 6
New York, NY 10032
212-305-5756
www.columbia.edu

D'Youville College
Nursing Department
320 Porter Ave.
Buffalo, NY 14201-9985
716-829-7613
www.dyc.edu

Long Island University–Brooklyn
School of Nursing
1 University Plaza
Brooklyn, NY 11201-8423
(718) 488-1508
www.liu.edu

Long Island University–Brookville
C.W. Post Campus
Dept. of Nursing
720 Northern Blvd.
Brookville, NY 11548
516-299-2485
www.liu.edu

New York University
College of Nursing
726 Broadway, 10th Fl.
New York, NY 10003
212-998-5300
www.nyu.edu/nursing

Pace University
Lienhard School of Nursing
41 Park Row, Room 300
New York, NY 10038
914-773-3552
www.pace.edu

SUNY Institute of Technology
School of Nursing & Health Systems
PO Box 3050
Utica, NY 13504
315-792-7295
www.sunyit.edu

University at Buffalo
School of Nursing
Wende Hall
3435 Main St.
Buffalo, NY 14214
716-829-2533
www.nursing.buffalo.edu

University of Rochester
School of Nursing
601 Elmwood Ave.
Rochester, NY 14642
585-273-2375
www.son.rochester.edu

## NORTH CAROLINA

University of North Carolina–Chapel Hill
School of Nursing
301 Carrington Hall, CB# 7460
Chapel Hill, NC 27599-7460
919-966-3638
www.nursing.ce.unc.edu

University of North Carolina–Charlotte
School of Nursing
9201 University City Blvd.
Charlotte, NC 28223-0001
704-687-7952
www.nursing.uncc.edu

## OHIO

Case Western Reserve University
School of Nursing
10900 Euclid Ave.
Cleveland, OH 44106
216-368-2529
www.fpb.case.edu

Kent State University
College of Nursing
113 H Henderson Hall
Kent, OH 44242
330-672-7930
www.kent.edu/nursing

Ohio State University
College of Nursing
Newton Hall
1585 Neil Ave.
Columbus, OH 43210
614-292-8900
www.con.ohio-state.edu

University of Akron
College of Nursing
Mary Gladwin Hall
209 Carroll St.
Akron, OH 44325-3701
330-972-7551
www.uakron.edu/nursing

University of Toledo
College of Nursing
2801 W. Bancroft
Toledo, OH 43606-3390
800-586-5336
www.utoledo.edu

## OKLAHOMA

University of Oklahoma
College of Nursing
PO Box 26901
1100 N. Stonewall Ave.
Oklahoma City, OK 73117
877-367-6876
www.nursing.ouhsc.edu

## OREGON

Oregon Health & Science University
School of Nursing
3455 SW US Veterans Hospital Rd.
Portland, OR 97239
866-223-1811
www.ohsu.edu/nursing

University of Portland
School of Nursing
5000 North Willamette Blvd.
Portland, OR 97203-5798
503-943-7211
www.nursing.up.edu

## PENNSYLVANIA

Bloomsburg University
Dept. of Nursing
3121 McCormick Center for Human Services
400 E. Second St.
Bloomsburg, PA 17815
570-389-4615
www.bloomu.edu

Drexel University
College of Nursing & Health Professions
Bellet Building
1505 Race St., Ms 501
Philadelphia, PA 19102
215-895-2000
www.drexel.edu

Millersville University
Dept. of Nursing
127 Caputo Hall
PO Box 1002
1 South George St.
Millersville, PA 17551
717-872-3410
www.millersville.edu

Pennsylvania State University
School of Nursing Graduate Programs
201 Health & Human Development East
University Park, PA 16802
814-863-0245
www.psu.edu

Temple University
College of Health Professions–Nursing Dept.
3307 N. Broad St.
Philadelphia, PA 19140
215-707-4686
www.temple.edu

University of Pennsylvania
School of Nursing
Claire M. Fagin Hall
418 Curie Blvd.
Philadelphia, PA 19104-4217
215-898-8281
www.nursing.upenn.edu

University of Pittsburgh
School of Nursing
3500 Victoria St.
Victoria Building
Pittsburgh, PA 15261
412-624-4586
www.nursing.pitt.edu

Villanova University
College of Nursing
800 Lancaster Ave.
Villanova, PA 19085-1690
610-519-4933
www.villanova.edu/nursing

## TENNESSEE

Belmont University
School of Nursing
1900 Belmont Blvd
Nashville, TN 37212-3757
615-460-6781
www.belmont.edu

East Tennessee State University
College of Nursing
310 Roy S. Nicks Hall
PO Box 70617
Johnson City, TN 37614-0617
423-439-7199
www.etsu.edu/nursing

Union University
School of Nursing
Nursing Admissions Coordinator
1050 Union University Dr.
Jackson, TN 38305
731-661-5538
www.uu.edu

University of Tennessee–Memphis
College of Nursing
877 Madison Ave.
Memphis, TN 38163
800-733-2498
www.uthsc.edu/nursing

Vanderbilt University
School of Nursing
Godchaux Hall 207
461 21st Ave. South
Nashville, TN 37240
888-333-9192
www.nursing.vanderbilt.edu

## TEXAS

Texas A&M University–Corpus Christi
College of Nursing & Health Sciences
6300 Ocean Dr.
Corpus Christi, TX 78412
361-825-2648
www.tamucc.edu

University of Texas–Austin
School of Nursing, D0100
1700 Red River St.
Austin, TX 78701
512-471-7311
www.utexas.edu/nursing

## VIRGINIA

Marymount University
School of Health Professions
Dept. of Nursing
2807 North Glebe Rd.
Arlington, VA 22207
703-284-1580
www.marymount.edu

Shenandoah University
Div. of Nursing
1775 N. Sector Ct.
Winchester, VA 22601
540-678-4374
www.su.edu/nursing

University of Virginia
School of Nursing
McLeod Hall
PO Box 800782
Charlottesville, VA 22908-3388
434-924-0063
www.nursing.virginia.edu

Virginia Commonwealth University
School of Nursing
PO Box 980567
1100 E. Leigh St.
Richmond, VA 23298
800-828-9451
www.nursing.vcu.edu

## WASHINGTON

Gonzaga University
Dept. of Nursing
502 E. Boone Ave.
Spokane, WA 99258-0102
509-313-3569
www.gonzaga.edu

Pacific Lutheran University
School of Nursing
Ramstad Building #214
Tacoma, WA 98447
253-535-7672
www.plu.edu

Seattle University
College of Nursing
901 12th Ave.
PO Box 222000
Seattle, WA 98122
206-296-5660
www.seattleu.edu

University of Washington
School of Nursing
PO Box 357260
Seattle, WA 98195
206-543-8736
www.son.washington.edu

Washington State University
Intercollegiate College of Nursing
PO Box 1495
Spokane, WA 99210-1495
509-324-7360
www.nursing.wsu.edu

## WISCONSIN

University of Wisconsin–Milwaukee
College of Nursing
1921 E. Hartford Ave.
PO Box 413
Milwaukee, WI 53201
414-229-4801
www.uwm.edu

## WYOMING

University of Wyoming
School of Nursing
Dept. 3065
1000 E. University Ave.
Laramie, WY 82071
307-766-4312
www.uwyo.edu

# PROFESSIONAL ASSOCIATIONS FOR NPs

## NATIONAL ASSOCIATIONS

**American Academy of Nurse Practitioners**
PO Box 12846
Austin, TX 78711
512-442-4262
www.aanp.org

**Gerontological Advanced Practice Nurses Association**
7794 Grow Dr.
Pensacola, FL 32514
866-355-1392
www.gapna.org

**National Association of Pediatric Nurse Practitioners**
20 Brace Rd., Suite 200
Cherry Hill, NJ 08034-2634
856-857-9700
www.napnap.org

**Nurse Practitioner Wellness Alliance**
2813 East Main Ave.
Puyallup, WA 98372
253-445-8943
www.npwellnessalliance.com

**Nurse Practitioners in Women's Health**
505 C St., NE
Washington, DC 20002
202-543-9693
www.npwh.org

## STATE ASSOCIATIONS

**ALABAMA**
North Alabama Nurse Practitioner Association
PO Box 14055
Huntsville, AL 35815
www.enpnetwork.com

**ALASKA**
Alaska Nurse Practitioner Association
3701 E. Tudor Rd., Suite #208
Anchorage, AK 99507
907-222-6847
www.alaskanp.org

**ARIZONA**
Arizona Nurse Practitioner Council
1850 E. Southern Ave., Suite 1
Tempe, AZ 85282
480-831-0404
www.arizonanp.com

**ARKANSAS**
Arkansas Nurses Association
1123 South University, Suite 1015
Little Rock, AR 72204
501-244-2363
www.arna.org

**CALIFORNIA**
California Association for Nurse Practitioners
One Capitol Mall, Suite 320
Sacramento, CA 95814
916-441-1361
www.canpweb.org

**COLORADO**
Colorado Society of Advanced Practice Nurses
PO Box 100158
Denver, CO 80250-0158
303-757-7483
www.csapn.org

**CONNECTICUT**
Connecticut Advanced Practice Registered Nurse Society
2842 Main St., PO Box 323
Glastonbury, CT 06033
www.ctaprns.org

**DELAWARE**
Delaware Nurses Association
5586 Kirkwood Hwy.
Wilmington, DE 19808
800-381-0939
www.denurses.org

**DISTRICT OF COLUMBIA**
Nurse Practitioner Association of DC
PO Box 77424
Washington, DC 20013-7424
www.npadc.org

**FLORIDA**
Florida Nurses Association
PO Box 536985
Orlando, FL 32803
407-896-3261
www.floridanurse.org

Florida Nurse Practitioner Network
PO Box 25422
Tampa, FL 33622
866-535-3676
www.fnpn.org

**GEORGIA**
Nurse Practitioner Council of Coastal Georgia
PO Box 14046
Savannah, GA 31416
912-351-7800
www.npcouncilofcoastalga.org

**IDAHO**
Nurse Practitioners of Idaho
5120 W Overland Rd #218
Boise, ID 83705
208-914-0138
www.npidaho.org

**ILLINOIS**
Illinois Nurses Association
105 W. Adams St., Suite 2101
Chicago, IL 60603
312-419-2900
www.illinoisnurses.com

**INDIANA**
Coalition of Advanced Practice Nurses of Indiana
PO Box 10239
Fort Wayne, IN 46851
www.capni.org

**IOWA**
Iowa Nurse Practitioner Society
Hoskins Geriatrics, PC
www.iowanpsociety.org

**KENTUCKY**
Kentucky Coalition of Nurse Practitioners and Nurse Midwives
1017 Ash St.
Louisville, KY 40217
502-333-0076
www.kcnpnm.org

**LOUISIANA**
Louisiana Association of Nurse Practitioners
5713 Superior Dr., Suite A5
Baton Rouge, LA 70816
225-293-7950
www.lanp.org

**MAINE**
Maine Nurse Practitioner Association
11 Columbia St.
Augusta, ME 04330
207-621-0313
www.mnpa.us

**MARYLAND**
Nurse Practitioner Association of Maryland
PO Box 540
Ellicott City, MD 21041-0540
888-405-NPAM
www.npamonline.org

**MASSACHUSETTS**
Massachusetts Coalition of Nurse Practitioners
PO Box 1153
Littleton, MA 01460
781-575-1565
www.mcnpweb.org

**MICHIGAN**
Michigan Council of Nurse Practitioners
PO Box 87934
Canton, MI 48187
734-432-9881
www.micnp.org

**MINNESOTA**
Association of Southeast Minnesota Nurse Practitioners
www.asmnp.org

**MISSISSIPPI**
Mississippi Nurses Association
31 Woodgreen Pl.
Madison, MS 39110
601-898-0670
www.msnurses.org

**MISSOURI**
Missouri Nurses Association
PO Box 105228
1904 Bubba Lane
Jefferson City, MO 65110
573-636-4623
www.missourinurses.org

**MONTANA**
Montana Nurses Association
20 Old Montana State Highway
Clancy, MT 59634
406-442-6710
www.mtnurses.org

**NEVADA**
Nevada Nurses Association
PO Box 34660
Reno, NV 89533
775-747-2333
www.nvnurses.org

**NEW HAMPSHIRE**
New Hampshire Nurse Practitioner Association
603-648-2233
www.npweb.org

**NEW JERSEY**
New Jersey State Nurses Association
1479 Pennington Rd.
Trenton, NJ 08618
www.njsna.org

**NEW MEXICO**
New Mexico Nurse Practitioner Council
PO Box 40682
Albuquerque, NM 87196-0682
505-414-8449
www.nmnpc.org

**NEW YORK**
Nurse Practitioner Association New York State
12 Corporate Dr.
Clifton Park, NY 12065
518-348-0719
www.thenpa.org

**NORTH CAROLINA**
North Carolina Nurses Association
PO Box 12025
Raleigh, NC 27605
800-626-2153
www.ncnurses.org

**OHIO**
Ohio Association of Advanced Practice Nurses
5818 Wilmington Pike #300
Dayton, OH 45459
866-668-3839
www.oaapn.org

**OKLAHOMA**
Oklahoma Nurse Practitioners Association
337 NE 4th
Oklahoma City, OK 73104
405-445-4874
www.npofoklahoma.com

**OREGON**
Nurse Practitioners of Oregon
18765 SW Boones Ferry Rd
Suite 200
Tualatin, OR 97062
503-293-0011
www.nursepractitionersoforegon.org

**PENNSYLVANIA**
Pennsylvania Coalition of Nurse Practitioners
PO Box 545
Mechanicsburg, PA 17055
717-766-4458
www.pacnp.org

**SOUTH DAKOTA**
Nurse Practitioner Association of South Dakota
PO Box 2822
Rapid City, SD 57709
www.npasd.org

**TENNESSEE**
Tennessee Nurses Association
545 Mainstream Dr., Suite 405
Nashville, TN 37228-1296
615-254-0350
www.tnaonline.org

**TEXAS**
Texas Nurse Practitioners
4425 S. Mopac Expswy
Building 111, Suite 405
Austin, TX 78735
512-291-6225
www.texasnp.org

**UTAH**
Utah Nurse Practitioners
www.utahnp.org

**VERMONT**
Vermont Nurse Practitioners Association
PO Box 64773
Burlington, VT 05406
www.vtnpa.org

**VIRGINIA**
Virginia Council of Nurse Practitioners
2209 Dickens Rd.
Richmond, VA 23230-2005
804-565-6360
www.vcnp.net

**WASHINGTON**
ARNPs United of Washington State
10024 SE 240th St., Suite 102
Kent, WA 98031
253-480-1035
www.auws.org

**WEST VIRGINIA**
West Virginia Nurses Association
405 Capitol St.,
Suite 600
Charleston, WV 25301
304-342-1169
www.wvnurses.org

**WISCONSIN**
Wisconsin Nurses Association
6117 Monona Dr., #1
Monona, WI 53716
608-221-0383
www.wisconsinnurses.org

# ANTIPYRETIC PRODUCTS

| BRAND | INGREDIENT/STRENGTH | DOSE |
|---|---|---|
| **ACETAMINOPHEN** | | |
| Anacin Extra Strength Aspirin Free Tablets | Acetaminophen 500mg | **Adults & Peds ≥12 yrs:** 2 tabs q6h. **Max:** 8 tabs q24h. |
| FeverAll Childrens' Suppositories | Acetaminophen 120mg | **Peds 3-6 yrs:** 1 supp. q4-6h. **Max:** 6 supp. q24h. |
| FeverAll Infants' Suppositories | Acetaminophen 80mg | **Peds 3-11 months:** 1 supp. q6h. **12-36 months:** 1 supp. q4h. **Max:** 6 supp. q24h. |
| FeverAll Jr. Strength Suppositories | Acetaminophen 325mg | **Peds 6-12 yrs:** 1 supp. q4-6h. **Max:** 6 supp. q24h. |
| Tylenol 8 Hour Caplets | Acetaminophen 650mg | **Adults & Peds ≥12 yrs:** 2 tabs q8h prn. **Max:** 6 tabs q24h. |
| Tylenol Arthritis Caplets | Acetaminophen 650mg | **Adults:** 2 tabs q8h prn. **Max:** 6 tabs q24h. |
| Tylenol Arthritis Gelcaps | Acetaminophen 650mg | **Adults:** 2 tabs q8h prn. **Max:** 6 tabs q24h. |
| Tylenol Arthritis Geltabs | Acetaminophen 650mg | **Adults:** 2 tabs q8h prn. **Max:** 6 tabs q24h. |
| Tylenol Children's Meltaways Tablets | Acetaminophen 80mg | **Peds 2-3 yrs (24-35 lbs):** 2 tabs. **4-5 yrs (36-47 lbs):** 3 tabs. **6-8 yrs (48-59 lbs):** 4 tabs. **9-10 yrs (60-71 lbs):** 5 tabs. **11 yrs (72-95 lbs):** 6 tabs. May repeat q4h. **Max:** 5 doses q24h. |
| Tylenol Children's Suspension | Acetaminophen 160mg/5mL | **Peds 2-3 yrs (24-35 lbs):** 1 tsp (5mL). **4-5 yrs (36-47 lbs):** 1.5 tsp (7.5mL). **6-8 yrs (48-59 lbs):** 2 tsp (10mL). **9-10 yrs (60-71 lbs):** 2.5 tsp (12.5mL). **11 yrs (72-95 lbs):** 3 tsp (15mL). May repeat q4h. **Max:** 5 doses q24h. |
| Tylenol Extra Strength Caplets | Acetaminophen 500mg | **Adults & Peds ≥12 yrs:** 2 tabs q4-6h prn. **Max:** 8 tabs q24h. |
| Tylenol Extra Strength Cool Caplets | Acetaminophen 500mg | **Adults & Peds ≥12 yrs:** 2 tabs q4-6h prn. **Max:** 8 tabs q24h. |
| Tylenol Extra Strength EZ Tablets | Acetaminophen 500mg | **Adults & Peds ≥12 yrs:** 2 tabs q4-6h prn. **Max:** 8 tabs q24h. |
| Tylenol Extra Strength Rapid Blast Liquid | Acetaminophen 1000mg/30mL | **Adults & Peds ≥12 yrs:** 2 tbl (30mL) q4-6h prn. **Max:** 8 tbl (120mL) q24h. |
| Tylenol Extra Strength Rapid Release Gelcaps | Acetaminophen 500mg | **Adults & Peds ≥12 yrs:** 2 caps q4-6h prn. **Max:** 8 caps q24h. |
| Tylenol Infants' Drops | Acetaminophen 80mg/0.8mL | **Peds 2-3 yrs (24-35 lbs):** 1.6 mL q4h prn. **Max:** 5 doses (8mL) q24h. |
| Tylenol Junior Meltaways Tablets | Acetaminophen 160mg | **Peds 6-8 yrs (48-59 lbs):** 2 tabs. **9-10 yrs (60-71 lbs):** 2.5 tabs. **11 yrs (72-95 lbs):** 3 tabs. **12 yrs (≥96 lbs):** 4 tabs. May repeat q4h. **Max:** 5 doses q24h. |
| Tylenol Regular Strength Tablets | Acetaminophen 325mg | **Adults & Peds ≥12 yrs:** 2 tabs q4-6h prn. **Max:** 12 tabs q24h. **Peds 6-11 yrs:** 1 tab q4-6h. **Max:** 5 tabs q24h. |

*(Continued)*

| BRAND | INGREDIENT/STRENGTH | DOSE |
|---|---|---|
| **NONSTEROIDAL ANTI-INFLAMMATORY DRUGS (NSAIDs)** | | |
| Advil Caplets | Ibuprofen 200mg | **Adults & Peds ≥12 yrs:** 1-2 tabs q4-6h. **Max:** 6 tabs q24h. |
| Advil Children's Suspension | Ibuprofen 100mg/5mL | **Peds 2-3 yrs (24-35 lbs):** 1 tsp (5mL). **4-5 yrs (36-47 lbs):** 1.5 tsp (7.5mL). **6-8 yrs (48-59 lbs):** 2 tsp (10mL). **9-10 yrs (60-71 lbs):** 2.5 tsp (12.5mL). **11 yrs (72-95 lbs):** 3 tsp (15mL). May repeat q6-8h. **Max:** 4 doses q24h. |
| Advil Gel Caplets | Ibuprofen 200mg | **Adults & Peds ≥12 yrs:** 1-2 tabs q4-6h. **Max:** 6 tabs q24h. |
| Advil Infants' Concentrated Drops | Ibuprofen 50mg/1.25mL | **Peds 6-11 months (12-17 lbs):** 1.25mL. **12-23 months (18-23 lbs):** 1.875mL. May repeat q6-8h. **Max:** 4 doses q24h. |
| Advil Liqui-Gels | Ibuprofen 200mg | **Adults & Peds ≥12 yrs:** 1-2 caps q4-6h. **Max:** 6 caps q24h. |
| Advil Tablets | Ibuprofen 200mg | **Adults & Peds ≥12 yrs:** 1-2 tabs q4-6h. **Max:** 6 tabs q24h. |
| Aleve Caplets | Naproxen Sodium 220mg | **Adults & Peds ≥12 yrs:** 1 tab q8-12h. May take 1 additional tab within 1 hour of first dose. **Max:** 2 tabs q8-12h or 3 tabs q24h. |
| Aleve Liquid Gels | Naproxen Sodium 220mg | **Adults & Peds ≥12 yrs:** 1 cap q8-12h. May take 1 additional cap within 1 hour of first dose. **Max:** 2 caps q8-12h or 3 caps q24h. |
| Aleve Smooth Gels | Naproxen Sodium 220mg | **Adults & Peds ≥12 yrs:** 1 cap q8-12h. May take 1 additional cap within 1 hour of first dose. **Max:** 2 caps q8-12h or 3 caps q24h. |
| Aleve Tablets | Naproxen Sodium 220mg | **Adults & Peds ≥12 yrs:** 1 tab q8-12h. May take 1 additional tab within 1 hour of first dose. **Max:** 2 tabs q8-12h or 3 tabs q24h. |
| Motrin Children's Suspension | Ibuprofen 100mg/5mL | **Peds 2-3 yrs (24-35 lbs):** 1 tsp (5mL). **4-5 yrs (36-47 lbs):** 1.5 tsp (7.5mL). **6-8 yrs (48-59 lbs):** 2 tsp (10mL). **9-10 yrs (60-71 lbs):** 2.5 tsp (12.5mL). **11 yrs (72-95 lbs):** 3 tsp (15mL). May repeat q6-8h. **Max:** 4 doses q24h. |
| Motrin IB Caplets | Ibuprofen 200mg | **Adults & Peds ≥12 yrs:** 1-2 tabs q4-6h. **Max:** 6 tabs q24h. |
| Motrin IB Tablets | Ibuprofen 200mg | **Adults & Peds ≥12 yrs:** 1-2 tabs q4-6h. **Max:** 6 tabs q24h. |
| Motrin Infants' Drops | Ibuprofen 50mg/1.25mL | **Peds 6-11 months (12-17 lbs):** 1.25mL. **12-23 months (18-23 lbs):** 1.875mL. May repeat q6-8h. **Max:** 4 doses q24h. |
| Motrin Junior Strength Caplets | Ibuprofen 100mg | **Peds 6-8 yrs (48-59 lbs):** 2 tabs. **9-10 yrs (60-71 lbs):** 2.5 tabs. **11 yrs (72-95 lbs):** 3 tabs. May repeat q6-8h. **Max:** 4 doses q24h. |

*(Continued)*

| BRAND | INGREDIENT/STRENGTH | DOSE |
|---|---|---|
| **NONSTEROIDAL ANTI-INFLAMMATORY DRUGS (NSAIDs)** *(Continued)* | | |
| Motrin Junior Strength Chewable Tablets | Ibuprofen 100mg | **Peds 2-3 yrs (24-35 lbs):** 1 tab. **4-5 yrs (36-47 lbs):** 1.5 tabs. **6-8 yrs (48-59 lbs):** 2 tabs. **9-10 yrs (60-71 lbs):** 2.5 tabs. **11 yrs (72-95 lbs):** 3 tabs. May repeat q6-8h. **Max:** 4 doses q24h. |
| **SALICYLATES** | | |
| Bayer Aspirin Extra Strength Caplets | Aspirin 500mg | **Adults & Peds ≥12 yrs:** 1-2 tabs q4-6h. **Max:** 8 tabs q24h. |
| Bayer Aspirin Safety Coated Caplets | Aspirin 325mg | **Adults & Peds ≥12 yrs:** 1-2 tabs q4h. **Max:** 12 tabs q24h. |
| Bayer Genuine Aspirin Tablets | Aspirin 325mg | **Adults & Peds ≥12 yrs:** 1-2 tabs q4h or 3 tabs q6h. **Max:** 12 tabs q24h. |
| Bayer Low-Dose Aspirin Chewable Tablets | Aspirin 81mg | **Adults & Peds ≥12 yrs:** 4-8 tabs q4h. **Max:** 48 tabs q24h. |
| Bayer Low-Dose Aspirin Safety Coated Tablets | Aspirin 81mg | **Adults & Peds ≥12 yrs:** 4-8 tabs q4h. **Max:** 48 tabs q24h. |
| Ecotrin Low Strength Tablets | Aspirin 81mg | **Adults:** 4-8 tabs q4h. **Max:** 48 tabs q24h. |
| Ecotrin Regular Strength Tablets | Aspirin 325mg | **Adults & Peds ≥12 yrs:** 1-2 tabs q4h. **Max:** 12 tabs q24h. |
| Halfprin 162mg Tablets | Aspirin 162mg | **Adults & Peds ≥12 yrs:** 2-4 tabs q4h. **Max:** 24 tabs q24h. |
| Halfprin 81mg Tablets | Aspirin 81mg | **Adults & Peds ≥12 yrs:** 4-8 tabs q4h. **Max:** 48 tabs q24h. |
| St. Joseph Aspirin Chewable Tablets | Aspirin 81mg | **Adults & Peds ≥12 yrs:** 4-8 tabs q4h. **Max:** 48 tabs q24h. |
| St. Joseph Enteric Safety-Coated Tablets | Aspirin 81mg | **Adults & Peds ≥12 yrs:** 4-8 tabs q4h. **Max:** 48 tabs q24h. |
| **SALICYLATES, BUFFERED** | | |
| Bayer Extra Strength Plus Caplets | Aspirin 500mg Buffered with Calcium Carbonate | **Adults & Peds ≥12 yrs:** 1-2 tabs q4-6h. **Max:** 8 tabs q24h. |
| Bayer Women's Low Dose Aspirin Caplets | Aspirin 81mg Buffered with Calcium Carbonate 777mg | **Adults & Peds ≥12 yrs:** 4-8 tabs q4h. **Max:** 10 tabs q24h. |
| Bufferin Extra Strength Tablets | Aspirin 500mg Buffered with Calcium Carbonate/Magnesium Oxide/Magnesium Carbonate | **Adults & Peds ≥12 yrs:** 2 tabs q6h. **Max:** 8 tabs q24h. |
| Bufferin Tablets | Aspirin 325mg Buffered with Benzoic Acid/Citric Acid | **Adults & Peds ≥12 yrs:** 2 tabs q4h. **Max:** 12 tabs q24h. |

# HEADACHE/MIGRAINE PRODUCTS

| BRAND | INGREDIENT/STRENGTH | DOSE |
|---|---|---|
| **ACETAMINOPHEN** | | |
| Anacin Extra Strength Aspirin Free Tablets | Acetaminophen 500mg | **Adults & Peds ≥12 yrs:** 2 tabs q6h. **Max:** 8 tabs q24h. |
| Tylenol 8 Hour Caplets | Acetaminophen 650mg | **Adults & Peds ≥12 yrs:** 2 tabs q8h prn. **Max:** 6 tabs q24h. |
| Tylenol Arthritis Caplets | Acetaminophen 650mg | **Adults:** 2 tabs q8h prn. **Max:** 6 tabs q24h. |
| Tylenol Arthritis Gelcaps | Acetaminophen 650mg | **Adults:** 2 tabs q8h prn. **Max:** 6 tabs q24h. |
| Tylenol Arthritis Geltabs | Acetaminophen 650mg | **Adults:** 2 tabs q8h prn. **Max:** 6 tabs q24h. |
| Tylenol Children's Meltaways Tablets | Acetaminophen 80mg | **Peds 2-3 yrs (24-35 lbs):** 2 tabs. **4-5 yrs (36-47 lbs):** 3 tabs. **6-8 yrs (48-59 lbs):** 4 tabs. **9-10 yrs (60-71 lbs):** 5 tabs. **11 yrs (72-95 lbs):** 6 tabs. May repeat q4h. **Max:** 5 doses q24h. |
| Tylenol Children's Suspension | Acetaminophen 160mg/5mL | **Peds 2-3 yrs (24-35 lbs):** 1 tsp (5mL). **4-5 yrs (36-47 lbs):** 1.5 tsp (7.5mL). **6-8 yrs (48-59 lbs):** 2 tsp (10mL). **9-10 yrs (60-71 lbs):** 2.5 tsp (12.5mL). **11 yrs (72-95 lbs):** 3 tsp (15mL). May repeat q4h. **Max:** 5 doses q24h. |
| Tylenol Extra Strength Caplets | Acetaminophen 500mg | **Adults & Peds ≥12 yrs:** 2 tabs q4-6h prn. **Max:** 8 tabs q24h. |
| Tylenol Extra Strength Cool Caplets | Acetaminophen 500mg | **Adults & Peds ≥12 yrs:** 2 tabs q4-6h prn. **Max:** 8 tabs q24h. |
| Tylenol Extra Strength Rapid Release Gelcaps | Acetaminophen 500mg | **Adults & Peds ≥12 yrs:** 2 caps q4-6h prn. **Max:** 8 caps q24h. |
| Tylenol Extra Strength Rapid Blast Liquid | Acetaminophen 1000mg/30mL | **Adults & Peds ≥12 yrs:** 2 tbl (30mL) q4-6h prn. **Max:** 8 tbl (120mL) q24h. |
| Tylenol Extra Strength EZ Tabs | Acetaminophen 500mg | **Adults & Peds ≥12 yrs:** 2 tabs q4-6h prn. **Max:** 8 tabs q24h. |
| Tylenol Infants' Drops | Acetaminophen 80mg/0.8mL | **Peds 2-3 yrs (24-35 lbs):** 1.6 mL q4h prn. **Max:** 5 doses (8mL) q24h. |
| Tylenol Junior Meltaways Tablets | Acetaminophen 160mg | **Peds 6-8 yrs (48-59 lbs):** 2 tabs. **9-10 yrs (60-71 lbs):** 2.5 tabs. **11 yrs (72-95 lbs):** 3 tabs. **12 yrs (≥96 lbs):** 4 tabs. May repeat q4h. **Max:** 5 doses q24h. |
| Tylenol Regular Strength Tablets | Acetaminophen 325mg | **Adults & Peds ≥12 yrs:** 2 tabs q4-6h prn. **Max:** 12 tabs q24h. **Peds 6-11 yrs:** 1 tab q4-6h. **Max:** 5 tabs q24h. |
| **ACETAMINOPHEN COMBINATIONS** | | |
| Anacin Advanced Headache Tablets | Acetaminophen/Aspirin/Caffeine 250mg-250mg-65mg | **Adults & Peds ≥12 yrs:** 2 tabs q6h. **Max:** 8 tabs q24h. |
| Excedrin Back & Body Caplets | Acetaminophen/Aspirin Buffered 250mg-250mg | **Adults & Peds ≥12 yrs:** 2 tabs q6h. **Max:** 8 tabs q24h. |
| Excedrin Extra Strength Caplets | Acetaminophen/Aspirin/Caffeine 250mg-250mg-65mg | **Adults & Peds ≥12 yrs:** 2 tabs q6h. **Max:** 8 tabs q24h. |
| Excedrin Extra Strength Express Gels | Acetaminophen/Aspirin/Caffeine 250mg-250mg-65mg | **Adults & Peds ≥12 yrs:** 2 caps q6h. **Max:** 8 caps q24h. |
| Excedrin Extra Strength Geltabs | Acetaminophen/Aspirin/Caffeine 250mg-250mg-65mg | **Adults & Peds ≥12 yrs:** 2 tabs q6h. **Max:** 8 tabs q24h. |
| Excedrin Extra Strength Tablets | Acetaminophen/Aspirin/Caffeine 250mg-250mg-65mg | **Adults & Peds ≥12 yrs:** 2 tabs q6h. **Max:** 8 tabs q24h. |

*(Continued)*

| BRAND | INGREDIENT/STRENGTH | DOSE |
|---|---|---|
| **ACETAMINOPHEN COMBINATIONS** *(Continued)* | | |
| Excedrin Migraine Caplets | Acetaminophen/Aspirin/Caffeine 250mg-250mg-65mg | **Adults:** 2 tabs. **Max:** 2 tabs q24h. |
| Excedrin Migraine Geltabs | Acetaminophen/Aspirin/Caffeine 250mg-250mg-65mg | **Adults:** 2 tabs. **Max:** 2 tabs q24h. |
| Excedrin Migraine Tablets | Acetaminophen/Aspirin/Caffeine 250mg-250mg-65mg | **Adults:** 2 tabs. **Max:** 2 tabs q24h. |
| Excedrin Sinus Headache Caplets | Acetaminophen/Phenylephrine HCl 325mg-5mg | **Adults & Peds ≥12 yrs:** 2 tabs q4h. **Max:** 12 tabs q24h. |
| Excedrin Tension Headache Caplets | Acetaminophen/Caffeine 500mg-65mg | **Adults & Peds ≥12 yrs:** 2 tabs q6h. **Max:** 8 tabs q24h. |
| Excedrin Tension Headache Express Gels | Acetaminophen/Caffeine 500mg-65mg | **Adults & Peds ≥12 yrs:** 2 caps q6h. **Max:** 8 caps q24h. |
| Excedrin Tension Headache Geltabs | Acetaminophen/Caffeine 500mg-65mg | **Adults & Peds ≥12 yrs:** 2 tabs q6h. **Max:** 8 tabs q24h. |
| Goody's Body Pain Powder | Acetaminophen/Aspirin 325mg-500mg | **Adults & Peds ≥12 yrs:** 1 powder q4-6h. **Max:** 4 powders q24h. |
| Goody's Cool Orange | Acetaminophen/Aspirin/Caffeine 325mg-500mg-65mg | **Adults & Peds ≥12 yrs:** 1 powder q6h. **Max:** 4 powders q24h. |
| Goody's Extra Strength Headache Powders | Acetaminophen/Aspirin/Caffeine 260mg-520mg-32.5mg | **Adults & Peds ≥12 yrs:** 1 powder q4-6h. **Max:** 4 powders q24h. |
| Sudafed PE Sinus Headache | Acetaminophen/Phenylephrine HCl 325mg-5mg | **Adults & Peds ≥12 yrs:** 2 tabs q4h. **Max:** 12 tabs q24h. |
| Tylenol Sinus Congestion and Pain Daytime Cool Burst Caplets | Acetaminophen/Phenylephrine HCl 325mg-5mg | **Adults & Peds ≥12 yrs:** 2 tabs q4h. **Max:** 12 tabs q24h. |
| Tylenol Sinus Congestion & Pain Daytime Rapid Release Gelcaps | Acetaminophen/Phenylephrine HCl 325mg-5mg | **Adults & Peds ≥12 yrs:** 2 caps q4h. **Max:** 12 caps q24h. |
| Vanquish Caplets | Acetaminophen/Aspirin/Caffeine 194mg-227mg-33mg | **Adults & Peds ≥12 yrs:** 2 tabs q6h. **Max:** 8 tabs q24h. |
| **ACETAMINOPHEN/SLEEP AIDS** | | |
| Excedrin PM Caplets | Acetaminophen/Diphenhydramine Citrate 500mg-38mg | **Adults & Peds ≥12 yrs:** 2 tabs qhs. **Max:** 2 tabs q24h. |
| Excedrin PM Expess Gels | Acetaminophen/Diphenhydramine Citrate 500mg-38mg | **Adults & Peds ≥12 yrs:** 2 tabs qhs. **Max:** 2 tabs q24h. |
| Excedrin PM Tablets | Acetaminophen/Diphenhydramine Citrate 500mg-38mg | **Adults & Peds ≥12 yrs:** 2 tabs qhs. **Max:** 2 tabs q24h. |
| Goody's PM Powder | Acetaminophen/Diphenhydramine 1000mg-76mg/dose | **Adults & Peds ≥12 yrs:** 1 packet (2 powders) qhs. |
| Tylenol PM Caplets | Acetaminophen/Diphenhydramine 500mg-25mg | **Adults & Peds ≥12 yrs:** 2 tabs qhs. **Max:** 2 tabs q24h. |
| Tylenol PM Geltabs | Acetaminophen/Diphenhydramine 500mg-25mg | **Adults & Peds ≥12 yrs:** 2 tabs qhs. **Max:** 2 tabs q24h. |
| Tylenol PM Rapid Release Gels | Acetaminophen/Diphenhydramine 500mg-25mg | **Adults & Peds ≥12 yrs:** 2 caps qhs. **Max:** 2 caps q24h. |
| Tylenol PM Vanilla Liquid | Acetaminophen/Diphenhydramine 1000mg-50mg/30mL | **Adults & Peds ≥12 yrs:** 2 tbl (30mL) qhs. **Max:** 2 tbl (30mL) q24h. |
| Tylenol Sinus Congestion and Pain Nighttime | Acetaminophen/Chlorpheniramine/ Phenylephrine HCl 325mg-2mg-5mg | **Adults & Peds ≥12 yrs:** 2 caps q4h. **Max:** 12 caps q24h. |
| **NONSTEROIDAL ANTI-INFLAMMATORY DRUGS (NSAIDS)** | | |
| Advil Caplets | Ibuprofen 200mg | **Adults & Peds ≥12 yrs:** 1-2 tabs q4-6h. **Max:** 6 tabs q24h. |
| Advil Children's Suspension | Ibuprofen 100mg/5mL | **Peds 2-3 yrs (24-35 lbs):** 1 tsp (5mL). **4-5 yrs (36-47 lbs):** 1.5 tsp (7.5mL). **6-8 yrs (48-59 lbs):** 2 tsp (10mL). **9-10 yrs (60-71 lbs):** 2.5 tsp (12.5mL). **11 yrs (72-95 lbs):** 3 tsp (15mL). May repeat q6-8h. **Max:** 4 doses q24h. |

*(Continued)*

| BRAND | INGREDIENT/STRENGTH | DOSE |
|---|---|---|
| **NONSTEROIDAL ANTI-INFLAMMATORY DRUGS (NSAIDS)** *(Continued)* | | |
| Advil Gel Caplets | Ibuprofen 200mg | **Adults & Peds ≥12 yrs:** 1-2 tabs q4-6h. **Max:** 6 tabs q24h. |
| Advil Infants' Concentrated Drops | Ibuprofen 50mg/1.25mL | **Peds 6-11 months (12-17 lbs):** 1.25mL. **12-23 months (18-23 lbs):** 1.875mL. May repeat q6-8h. **Max:** 4 doses q24h. |
| Advil Liqui-Gels | Ibuprofen 200mg | **Adults & Peds ≥12 yrs:** 1-2 caps q4-6h. **Max:** 6 caps q24h. |
| Advil Migraine Capsules | Ibuprofen 200mg | **Adults:** 2 caps prn. **Max:** 2 caps q24h. |
| Advil Tablets | Ibuprofen 200mg | **Adults & Peds ≥12 yrs:** 1-2 tabs q4-6h. **Max:** 6 tabs q24h. |
| Aleve Caplets | Naproxen Sodium 220mg | **Adults & Peds ≥12 yrs:** 1 tab q8-12h. May take 1 additional tab within 1 hour of first dose. **Max:** 2 tabs q8-12h or 3 tabs q24h. |
| Aleve Liquid Gels | Naproxen Sodium 220mg | **Adults & Peds ≥12 yrs:** 1 cap q8-12h. May take 1 additional cap within 1 hr of first dose. **Max:** 2 caps q8-12hr or 3 caps q24h. |
| Aleve Smooth Gels | Naproxen Sodium 220mg | **Adults & Peds ≥12 yrs:** 1 cap q8-12h. May take 1 additional cap within 1 hour of first dose. **Max:** 2 caps q8-12h or 3 caps q24h. |
| Aleve Tablets | Naproxen Sodium 220mg | **Adults & Peds ≥12 yrs:** 1 tab q8-12h. May take 1 additional tab within 1 hour of first dose. **Max:** 2 tabs q8-12h or 3 tabs q24h. |
| Motrin Children's Suspension | Ibuprofen 100mg/5mL | **Peds 2-3 yrs (24-35 lbs):** 1 tsp (5mL). **4-5 yrs (36-47 lbs):** 1.5 tsp (7.5mL). **6-8 yrs (48-59 lbs):** 2 tsp (10mL). **9-10 yrs (60-71 lbs):** 2.5 tsp (12.5mL). **11 yrs (72-95 lbs):** 3 tsp (15mL). May repeat q6-8h. **Max:** 4 doses q24h. |
| Motrin IB Caplets | Ibuprofen 200mg | **Adults & Peds ≥12 yrs:** 1-2 tabs q4-6h. **Max:** 6 tabs q24h. |
| Motrin IB Tablets | Ibuprofen 200mg | **Adults & Peds ≥12 yrs:** 1-2 tabs q4-6h. **Max:** 6 tabs q24h. |
| Motrin Infants' Drops | Ibuprofen 50mg/1.25mL | **Peds 6-11 months (12-17 lbs):** 1.25mL. **12-23 months (18-23 lbs):** 1.875mL. May repeat q6-8h. **Max:** 4 doses q24h. |
| Motrin Junior Strength Caplets | Ibuprofen 100mg | **Peds 6-8 yrs (48-59 lbs):** 2 tabs. **9-10 yrs (60-71 lbs):** 2.5 tabs. **11 yrs (72-95 lbs):** 3 tabs. May repeat q6-8h. **Max:** 4 doses q24h. |
| Motrin Junior Strength Chewable Tablets | Ibuprofen 100mg | **Peds 2-3 yrs (24-35 lbs):** 1 tab. **4-5 yrs (36-47 lbs):** 1.5 tabs. **6-8 yrs (48-59 lbs):** 2 tabs. **9-10 yrs (60-71 lbs):** 2.5 tabs. **11 yrs (72-95 lbs):** 3 tabs. May repeat q6-8h. **Max:** 4 doses q24h. |
| **NSAID COMBINATIONS** | | |
| Advil Allergy Sinus Caplets | Ibuprofen/Chlorpheniramine/Pseudoephedrine HCl 200mg-2mg-30mg | **Adults & Peds ≥12 yrs:** 1 tab q4-6h. **Max:** 6 tabs q24h. |

*(Continued)*

| BRAND | INGREDIENT/STRENGTH | DOSE |
|---|---|---|
| **NSAID COMBINATIONS** *(Continued)* | | |
| Advil Cold & Sinus Caplets | Ibuprofen/Pseudoephedrine HCl 200mg-30mg | **Adults & Peds ≥12 yrs:** 1-2 tabs q4-6h. **Max:** 6 tabs q24h. |
| Advil Cold & Sinus Liqui-Gels | Ibuprofen/Pseudoephedrine HCl 200mg-30mg | **Adults & Peds ≥12 yrs:** 1-2 caps q4-6h. **Max:** 6 caps q24h. |
| Aleve-D Sinus & Cold | Naproxen Sodium/Pseudoephedrine HCl 220mg-120mg | **Adults & Peds ≥12 yrs:** 1 tab q12h. **Max:** 2 tabs q24h. |
| Sudafed Sinus & Pain 12-Hour Caplets | Naproxen Sodium/Pseudoephedrine HCl 220mg-120mg | **Adults & Peds ≥12 yrs:** 1 tab q12h. **Max:** 2 tabs q24h. |
| **NSAID SLEEP AIDS** | | |
| Advil PM Caplets | Ibuprofen/Diphenhydramine Citrate 200mg-38mg | **Adults & Peds ≥12 yrs:** 2 tabs qhs. **Max:** 2 tabs q24h. |
| Advil PM Liqui-Gels | Ibuprofen/Diphenhydramine HCl 200mg-25mg | **Adults & Peds ≥12 yrs:** 2 caps qhs. **Max:** 2 caps q24h. |
| Motrin PM Caplets | Ibuprofen/Diphenhydramine Citrate 200mg-38mg | **Adults & Peds ≥12 yrs:** 2 tabs qhs. **Max:** 2 tabs q24h. |
| **SALICYLATES** | | |
| Bayer Aspirin Extra Strength Caplets | Aspirin 500mg | **Adults & Peds ≥12 yrs:** 1-2 tabs q4-6h. **Max:** 8 tabs q24h. |
| Bayer Aspirin Safety Coated Caplets | Aspirin 325mg | **Adults & Peds ≥12 yrs:** 1-2 tabs q4h. **Max:** 12 tabs q24h. |
| Bayer Genuine Aspirin Tablets | Aspirin 325mg | **Adults & Peds ≥12 yrs:** 1-2 tabs q4h or 3 tabs q6h. **Max:** 12 tabs q24h. |
| Bayer Low-Dose Aspirin Chewable Tablets | Aspirin 81mg | **Adults & Peds ≥12 yrs:** 4-8 tabs q4h. **Max:** 48 tabs q24h. |
| Bayer Low-Dose Aspirin Safety Coated Tablets | Aspirin 81mg | **Adults & Peds ≥12 yrs:** 4-8 tabs q4h. **Max:** 48 tabs q24h. |
| Doan's Extra Strength Caplets | Magnesium Salicylate Tetrahydrate 580mg | **Adults & Peds ≥12 yrs:** 2 tabs q6h. **Max:** 8 tabs q24h. |
| Ecotrin Low Strength Tablets | Aspirin 81mg | **Adults:** 4-8 tabs q4h. **Max:** 48 tabs q24h. |
| Ecotrin Regular Strength Tablets | Aspirin 325mg | **Adults & Peds ≥12 yrs:** 1-2 tabs q4h. **Max:** 12 tabs q24h. |
| Halfprin 162mg Tablets | Aspirin 162mg | **Adults & Peds ≥12 yrs:** 2-4 tabs q4h. **Max:** 24 tabs q24h. |
| Halfprin 81mg Tablets | Aspirin 81mg | **Adults & Peds ≥12 yrs:** 4-8 tabs q4h. **Max:** 48 tabs q24h. |
| St. Joseph Aspirin Chewable Tablets | Aspirin 81mg | **Adults & Peds ≥12 yrs:** 4-8 tabs q4h. **Max:** 48 tabs q24h. |
| St. Joseph Enteric Safety-Coated Tablets | Aspirin 81mg | **Adults & Peds ≥12 yrs:** 4-8 tabs q4h. **Max:** 48 tabs q24h. |
| **SALICYLATES, BUFFERED** | | |
| Alka-Seltzer Extra Strength Effervescent Tablets | Aspirin/Citric Acid/Sodium Bicarbonate 500mg-1000mg-1985mg | **Adults & Peds ≥12 yrs:** 2 tabs q6h. **Max:** 7 tabs q24h. **≥60 yrs: Max:** 3 tabs q24h. |
| Alka-Seltzer Lemon-Lime Tablets | Aspirin/Citric Acid/Sodium Bicarbonate 325mg-1000mg-1700mg | **Adults & Peds ≥12 yrs:** 2 tabs q4h. **Max:** 8 tabs q24h. **≥60 yrs: Max:** 4 tabs q24h. |
| Alka-Seltzer Original Effervescent Tablets | Aspirin/Citric Acid/Sodium Bicarbonate 325mg-1000mg-1916mg | **Adults & Peds ≥12 yrs:** 2 tabs q4h. **Max:** 8 tabs q24h. **≥60 yrs: Max:** 4 tabs q24h. |
| Ascriptin Maximum Strength Tablets | Aspirin Buffered with Maalox/Calcium Carbonate 500mg | **Adults & Peds ≥12 yrs:** 2 tabs q4h. **Max:** 8 tabs q24h. |
| Ascriptin Regular Strength Tablets | Aspirin 325mg Buffered with Maalox/ Calcium Carbonate | **Adults & Peds ≥12 yrs:** 2 tabs q4h. **Max:** 12 tabs q24h. |
| Bayer Extra Strength Plus Caplets | Aspirin 500mg Buffered with Calcium Carbonate | **Adults & Peds ≥12 yrs:** 1-2 tabs q4-6h. **Max:** 8 tabs q24h. |

*(Continued)*

| BRAND | INGREDIENT/STRENGTH | DOSE |
|---|---|---|
| **SALICYLATES, BUFFERED** *(Continued)* | | |
| Bayer Women's Low Dose Aspirin Caplets | Aspirin 81mg Buffered with Calcium Carbonate 777mg | **Adults & Peds ≥12 yrs:** 4-8 tabs q4h. **Max:** 10 tabs q24h. |
| Bufferin Extra Strength Tablets | Aspirin 500mg Buffered with Calcium Carbonate/Magnesium Oxide/ Magnesium Carbonate | **Adults & Peds ≥12 yrs:** 2 tabs q6h. **Max:** 8 tabs q24h. |
| Bufferin Tablets | Aspirin 325mg Buffered with Benzoic Acid/ Citric Acid | **Adults & Peds ≥12 yrs:** 2 tabs q4h. **Max:** 12 tabs q24h. |
| Alka-Seltzer Wake-Up Call! | Aspirin/Caffeine 500mg-65mg | **Adults & Peds ≥12 yrs:** 2 tabs q6h. **Max:** 8 tabs q24h. **≥60 yrs: Max:** 4 tabs q24h. |
| Anacin Max Strength Tablets | Aspirin/Caffeine 500mg-32mg | **Adults & Peds ≥12 yrs:** 2 tabs q6h. **Max:** 8 tabs q24h. |
| Anacin Regular Strength Caplets | Aspirin/Caffeine 400mg-32mg | **Adults & Peds ≥12 yrs:** 2 tabs q6h. **Max:** 8 tabs q24h. |
| Anacin Tablets | Aspirin/Caffeine 400mg-32mg | **Adults & Peds ≥12 yrs:** 2 tabs q6h. **Max:** 8 tabs q24h. |
| Bayer Back & Body Pain Caplets | Aspirin/Caffeine 500mg-32.5mg | **Adults & Peds ≥12 yrs:** 2 tabs q6h. **Max:** 8 tabs q24h. |
| Bayer Quick Release Crystals | Aspirin/Caffeine 850mg-65mg | **Adults & Peds ≥12 yrs:** 1 powder pouch q6h. **Max:** 4 powder pouches q24h. |
| BC Arthritis Strength Powders | Aspirin/Caffeine/Salicylamide 742mg-38mg-222mg | **Adults & Peds ≥12 yrs:** 1 powder q3-4h. **Max:** 4 powders q24h. |
| BC Original Formula Powders | Aspirin/Caffeine/Salicylamide 650mg-33.3mg-195mg | **Adults & Peds ≥12 yrs:** 1 powder q3-4h. **Max:** 4 powders q24h. |
| **SALICYLATES/SLEEP AIDS** | | |
| Alka-Seltzer PM Effervescent Tablets | Aspirin/Diphenhydramine Citrate 325mg-38mg | **Adults & Peds ≥12 yrs:** 2 tabs qhs. **Max:** 2 tabs q24h. |
| Bayer PM Caplets | Aspirin/Diphenhydramine Citrate 500mg-38.3mg | **Adults & Peds ≥12 yrs:** 2 tabs qhs. |
| Doan's Extra Strength PM Caplets | Magnesium Salicylate Tetrahydrate/Diphenhydramine 580mg-25mg | **Adults & Peds ≥12 yrs:** 2 tabs qhs. |

# INSOMNIA PRODUCTS

| BRAND | INGREDIENT/STRENGTH | DOSE |
|---|---|---|
| **DIPHENHYDRAMINE** | | |
| Nytol Quick Caps Caplets | Diphenhydramine 25mg | **Adults & Peds ≥12 yrs:** 2 tabs qhs. |
| Simply Sleep Nighttime Sleep Aid Caplets | Diphenhydramine 25mg | **Adults & Peds ≥12 yrs:** 2 tabs qhs. |
| Sominex Original Formula | Diphenhydramine 25mg | **Adults & Peds ≥12 yrs:** 2 tabs qhs. |
| Sominex Maximum Strength Formula | Diphenhydramine 50mg | **Adults & Peds ≥12 yrs:** 1 tab qhs. |
| Unisom Nighttime Sleep-Aid Sleep Gels | Diphenhydramine 50mg | **Adults & Peds ≥12 yrs:** 1 cap qhs. |
| Unisom Sleep Melts | Diphenhydramine 25mg | **Adults & Peds ≥12 yrs:** 2 tabs qhs. |
| **DIPHENHYDRAMINE COMBINATION** | | |
| Alka-Seltzer PM | Aspirin/Diphenhydramine Citrate 325mg-38mg | **Adults & Peds ≥12 yrs:** 2 tabs qhs. |
| Bayer PM Relief Caplets | Aspirin/Diphenhydramine Citrate 500mg-38.3mg | **Adults & Peds ≥12 yrs:** 2 tabs qhs. |
| Doan's Extra Strength PM Caplets | Magnesium Salicylate Tetrahydrate/ Diphenhydramine 580mg-25mg | **Adults & Peds ≥12 yrs:** 2 tabs qhs. |
| Excedrin PM Caplets | Acetaminophen/Diphenhydramine Citrate 500mg-38mg | **Adults & Peds ≥12 yrs:** 2 tabs qhs. |
| Excedrin PM Tablets | Acetaminophen/Diphenhydramine Citrate 500mg-38mg | **Adults & Peds ≥12 yrs:** 2 tabs qhs. |
| Goody's PM Powder | Acetaminophen/Diphenhydramine Citrate 1000mg-76mg/dose | **Adults & Peds ≥12 yrs:** 1 packet (2 powders) qhs. |
| Tylenol PM Caplets | Acetaminophen/Diphenhydramine HCl 500mg-25mg | **Adults & Peds ≥12 yrs:** 2 tabs qhs. |
| Tylenol PM Rapid Release Gelcaps | Acetaminophen/Diphenhydramine HCl 500mg-25mg | **Adults & Peds ≥12 yrs:** 2 caps qhs. |
| Tylenol PM Geltabs | Acetaminophen/Diphenhydramine HCl 500mg-25mg | **Adults & Peds ≥12 yrs:** 2 tabs qhs. |
| Tylenol PM Liquid | Acetaminophen/Diphenhydramine HCl 1000mg-50mg/30mL | **Adults & Peds ≥12 yrs:** 2 tbl (30mL) qhs. **Max:** 2 tbl (30mL) q24h. |
| **DOXYLAMINE** | | |
| Unisom Nighttime Sleep-Aid Sleep Tabs | Doxylamine Succinate 25mg | **Adults & Peds ≥12 yrs:** 1 tab 30 min before hs. |

# SMOKING CESSATION PRODUCTS

| BRAND | INGREDIENT/STRENGTH | DOSE |
|---|---|---|
| Commit Stop Smoking 2mg Lozenges | Nicotine Polacrilex 2mg | **Adults:** If smoking first cigarette >30 minutes after waking up use 2mg lozenge. **Weeks 1 to 6:** 1 lozenge q1-2h. **Weeks 7 to 9:** 1 lozenge q2-4h. **Weeks 10 to 12:** 1 lozenge q4-8h. **Max:** 5 lozenges/6 hours; 20 lozenges/day. Stop using at the end of 12 weeks. |
| Commit Stop Smoking 4mg Lozenges | Nicotine Polacrilex 4mg | **Adults:** If smoking first cigarette within 30 minutes after waking up use 4mg lozenge. **Weeks 1 to 6:** 1 lozenge q1-2h. **Weeks 7 to 9:** 1 lozenge q2-4h. **Weeks 10 to 12:** 1 lozenge q4-8h. **Max:** 5 lozenges/6 hours; 20 lozenges/day. Stop using at the end of 12 weeks. |
| NicoDerm CQ Step 1 Clear Patch | Nicotine 21mg | **Adults:** If smoking >10 cigarettes/day. **Weeks 1 to 6:** Apply one 21mg patch/ day. **Weeks 7 to 8:** Apply one 14mg patch/day. **Weeks 9 to 10:** Apply one 7mg patch/day. |
| NicoDerm CQ Step 2 Clear Patch | Nicotine 14mg | **Adults:** If smoking >10 cigarettes/day. **Weeks 1 to 6:** Apply one 21mg patch/day. **Weeks 7 to 8:** Apply one 14mg patch/day. **Weeks 9 to 10:** Apply one 7mg patch/day. If smoking <10 cigarettes/day. **Weeks 1 to 6:** Apply one 14mg patch/day. **Weeks 7 to 8:** Apply one 7mg patch/day. |
| NicoDerm CQ Step 3 Clear Patch | Nicotine 7mg | **Adults:** Apply 1 patch qd Weeks 9 to 10 if smoking >10 cigarettes/day or Weeks 7 to 8 if smoking <10 cigarettes/day. |
| Nicorette 2mg | Nicotine Polacrilex 2mg | **Adults:** If smoking <25 cigarettes/day use 2mg gum. **Weeks 1 to 6:** 1 piece q1-2h. **Weeks 7 to 9:** 1 piece q2-4h. **Weeks 10 to 12:** 1 piece q4-8h. **Max:** 24 pieces/day. |
| Nicorette 4mg | Nicotine Polacrilex 4mg | **Adults:** If smoking ≥25 cigarettes/day use 4mg gum. **Weeks 1 to 6:** 1 piece q1-2h. **Weeks 7 to 9:** 1 piece q2-4h. **Weeks 10 to 12:** 1 piece q4-8h. **Max:** 24 pieces/day. |
| Habitrol Nicotine Transdermal System Patch Step 1 | Nicotine 21mg/24hr | **Adults:** If smoking >10 cigarettes/day. **Weeks 1 to 4:** Apply one 21mg patch/ day. **Weeks 5 to 6:** Apply one 14mg patch/day. **Weeks 7 to 8:** Apply one 7mg patch/day. |
| Habitrol Nicotine Transdermal System Patch Step 2 | Nicotine 14mg/24hr | **Adults:** If smoking >10 cigarettes/day. **Weeks 1 to 4:** Apply one 21mg patch/ day. **Weeks 5 to 6:** Apply one 14mg patch/day. **Weeks 7 to 8:** Apply one 7mg patch/day. If smoking <10 cigarettes/day. **Weeks 1 to 6:** Apply one 14 mg patch/day. **Weeks 7 to 8:** Apply one 7mg patch/day. |
| Habitrol Nicotine Transdermal System Patch Step 3 | Nicotine 7mg/24hr | **Adults:** If smoking >10 cigarettes/day. **Weeks 1 to 4:** Apply one 21mg patch/ day. **Weeks 5 to 6:** Apply one 14mg patch/day. **Weeks 7 to 8:** Apply one 7mg patch/day. If smoking <10 cigarettes/day. **Weeks 1 to 6:** Apply one 14mg patch/ day. **Weeks 7 to 8:** Apply one 7mg patch/day. |

# WEIGHT MANAGEMENT PRODUCTS

| BRAND | DOSE |
|---|---|
| Alli Weight-Loss Aid | **Adults:** 1 cap with each fat-containing meal. **Max:** 3 caps per day. |
| Applied Nutrition 10-Day Hoodia Diet Capsules | **Adults:** Take 1-2 caps with meals tid. |
| Applied Nutrition Carb Blocker | **Adults:** Take 2 caps with meals bid. |
| Applied Nutrition Green Tea Fat Burner | **Adults:** Take 2 caps with meals bid. |
| Applied Nutrition Green Tea Triple Fat Burner | **Adults:** Take 2 caps with meals bid. |
| Applied Nutrition Natural Fat Burner Capsules | **Adults:** Take 2 caps with meals bid. |
| Applied Nutrition Oolong Tea Diet | **Adults:** Take 1 cap with meals tid. |
| Applied Nutrition Resveratol Rapid Calorie Burn | **Adults:** Take 2 tabs qam and 2 tabs qpm. |
| Aqua-Ban Maximum Strength Diuretic Tablets | **Adults:** Take 1 tab qid. **Max:** 4 tabs q24h. |
| BioMD Nutraceuticals Metabolism T3 Capsules | **Adults:** Take 2 caps with meals bid-tid. **Max:** 6 caps q24h. |
| Biotest Hot-Rox Capsules | **Adults:** Take 1-2 caps bid. **Max:** 6 caps q24h. |
| Carb Cutter Original Formula Tablets | **Adults:** Take 1-2 tabs with meals bid. |
| Carb Cutter Phase 2 Starch Neutralizer Tablets | **Adults:** Take 1-2 tabs with meals bid. |
| Dexatrim Max | **Adults:** Take 1-2 caps with water, one in AM and one in afternoon. **Max:** 2 caps q24h. |
| Dexatrim Max Slim Packs | **Adults:** Dissolve 1 packet in 16.9 ounces of water. **Max:** 6 packs q24h. |
| Dexatrim Natural Extra Energy Formula Caplets | **Adults:** Take 1 tab with meals tid. **Max:** 3 tabs q24h. |
| Dexatrim Natural Green Tea Formula Caplets | **Adults:** Take 1 tab with meals tid. **Max:** 3 tabs q24h. |
| Dexatrim Max Complex 7 | **Adults:** Take 2 caps qam. Second serving mid-afternoon. **Max:** 4 caps q24h. |
| EAS CLA Capsules | **Adults:** Take 2 caps with meals tid. |
| Estrin-D Capsules | **Adults:** Take 2 caps 30 min before meals. **Max:** 6 caps q24h. |
| Isatori Flash Point Sublingual Fat Burner | **Adults:** Dissolve 1 tab in mouth bid. **Max:** 10 tabs q24h. |
| Isatori Lean System 7 Advanced Metabolic Support Formula | **Adults:** Take 2 caps 30 min before meals bid-tid. **Max:** 6 caps q24h. |
| Isatori MX-LS7 Maximum Strength Lean System 7 | **Adults:** Take 3 caps 30 min before meals bid. **Max:** 4 caps q4h. |
| Metabolife Break Through | **Adults:** Take 2 tabs 1 hr before meals tid, at least 3-4 hrs apart. **Max:** 6 tabs q24h. |
| Metabolife Extreme Energy | **Adults:** Take 1-2 tabs tid at least 3-4 hrs apart. **Max:** 4 tabs q8h. |
| Metabolife Ultra Caplets | **Adults:** Take 2 tabs tid 30-60 min before meals, at least 3-4 hrs apart. **Max:** 6 tabs q24h. |
| Metabolife Caffeine Free Caplets | **Adults:** Take 2 tabs tid 30-60 min before meals, at least 3-4 hrs apart. **Max:** 6 tabs q24h. |
| Metabolife Green Tea | **Adults:** Take 2 tabs tid 30-60 min before meals, at least 3-4 hrs apart. **Max:** 6 tabs q24h. |
| MHP TakeOff, Hi-Energy Fat Burner Capsules | **Adults:** Take 2 caps qd or bid. |
| Natrol Carb Intercept with Phase 2 Starch Neutralizer Capsules | **Adults:** Take 2 caps before carbohydrate-containing meals. |
| Natrol Green Tea 500mg Capsules | **Adults:** Take 1 cap with meals qd. |
| Natural Balance Fat Magnet Capsules | **Adults:** Take 2 caps with meals bid. |
| Nature Made Chromium Picolinate, Extra Strength | **Adults:** Take 1 tab qd. |
| Nature's Bounty Super Green Tea Diet Capsules | **Adults:** Take 1 cap bid. **Max:** 2 caps q24h. |
| Nature's Bounty Xtreme Lean Zn-3 Ephedra Free Capsules | **Adults:** Take 2 caps bid. **Max:** 4 caps q24h. |
| Nunaturals LevelRight for Blood Sugar Management Capsules | **Adults:** Take 1 cap with meals tid. |
| One-A-Day Weight Smart Dietary Supplement Tablets | **Adults:** Take 1 tab with meals qd. |
| Prolab Enhanced CLA | **Adults:** Take 3 caps with meals qd. |

*(Continued)*

| BRAND | DOSE |
|---|---|
| Stacker 2 Ephedra Free Capsules | **Adults:** Take 1 cap after meals. **Max:** 3 caps q24h. |
| Stacker 3 Ephedra Free Formula with Chitosan Capsules | **Adults:** Take 1 cap after meals. **Max:** 3 caps q24h. |
| Stacker 3 XPLC Extreme Performance Formula Ephedra Free | **Adults:** Take 1 cap after meals. **Max:** 3 caps q24h. |
| Tetrazene ES-50 Ultra High-Energy Weight Loss Catalyst Capsules | **Adults:** Take 2 caps with meals tid. **Max:** 6 caps q24h. |
| Tetrazene KGM-90 Rapid Weight Loss Catalyst Capsules | **Adults:** Take 2 caps with meals tid. **Max:** 6 caps q24h. |
| Twinlab CLA Fuel | **Adults:** Take 1 cap tid. |
| Twinlab GTF Chromium | **Adults:** Take 1 tab qd. |
| Twinlab Mega L-Carnitine | **Adults:** Take 1 tab daily on an empty stomach. |
| Twinlab Metabolift, Ephedra Free Formula Capsules | **Adults:** Take 2 caps before each meal. **Max:** 6 caps q24h. |
| Twinlab Ripped Fuel 5X | **Adults:** Take 1 tab before meals bid. |
| Twinlab Ripped Fuel Ephedra Free | **Adults:** Take 2 caps before each meal. **Max:** 6 caps q24h. |
| Twinlab Ripped Fuel Extreme | **Adults:** Take 2 caps bid. |
| Twinlab Ripped Fuel Xtendr | **Adults:** Take 2 tabs 30 min before meals. **Max:** 6 tabs q24h. |
| Twinlab 7-Keto Fuel | **Adults:** Take 2-4 caps daily. |
| Ultra Diet Pep Tablets | **Adults:** Take 1 tab with meals bid. |
| XtremeLean Advanced Formula, Ephedra Free Capsules | **Adults:** Take 2 caps before meals bid. |
| Zantrex 3, Ephedrine Free | **Adults:** Take 2 caps with meals qd. **Max:** 6 caps q24h. |
| Zantrex 3 High Energy Fat Burner | **Adults:** Take 2 caps qam and 2 caps with main meal. **Max:** 4 caps q24h. |
| Zantrex 3 Power Crystals | **Adults:** Add 1 packet to 16 oz of water. **Max:** 3 packets q24h. |

# ANTIFUNGAL PRODUCTS

| BRAND | INGREDIENT/STRENGTH | DOSE |
|---|---|---|
| **BUTENAFINE** | | |
| Lotrimin Ultra Athlete's Foot Cream | Butenafine HCl 1% | **Adults & Peds ≥12 yrs:** Athlete's Foot: Apply bid for 1 week or qd for 4 weeks. Jock Itch/Ringworm: Apply qd for 2 weeks. |
| Lotrimin Ultra Jock Itch Cream | Butenafine HCl 1% | **Adults & Peds ≥12 yrs:** Apply qd for 2 weeks. |
| **CLOTRIMAZOLE** | | |
| Clearly Confident Triple Action Treatment | Clotrimazole 1% | **Adults & Peds ≥2 yrs:** Apply bid for 4 weeks. |
| Desenex Antifungal Cream | Clotrimazole 1% | **Adults & Peds ≥2 yrs:** Athlete's Foot/Ringworm: Apply bid for 4 weeks. Jock Itch: Apply bid for 2 weeks. |
| FungiCure Anti-Fungal Liquid Manicure/Pedicure Formula | Clotrimazole 1% | **Adults & Peds ≥2 yrs:** Apply bid for 4 weeks. |
| FungiCure Anti-Fungal Liquid Pump Spray | Clotrimazole 1% | **Adults & Peds ≥2 yrs:** Athlete's Foot/Ringworm: Apply bid for 4 weeks. Jock Itch: Apply bid for 2 weeks. |
| FungiCure Intensive Anti-Fungal Treatment | Clotrimazole 1% | **Adults & Peds ≥2 yrs:** Athlete's Foot/Ringworm: Apply bid for 4 weeks. Jock Itch: Apply bid for 2 weeks. |
| Lotrimin AF Athlete's Foot Cream | Clotrimazole 1% | **Adults & Peds ≥2 yrs:** Athlete's Foot/Ringworm: Apply bid for 4 weeks. Jock Itch: Apply bid for 2 weeks. |
| Lotrimin AF For Her Athlete's Foot Cream | Clotrimazole 1% | **Adults & Peds ≥2 yrs:** Apply bid for 4 weeks. |
| Lotrimin AF Jock Itch Cream | Clotrimazole 1% | **Adults & Peds ≥2 yrs:** Apply bid for 2 weeks. |
| Lotrimin AF Ringworm Cream | Clotrimazole 1% | **Adults & Peds ≥2 yrs:** Apply bid for 4 weeks. |
| **MICONAZOLE** | | |
| Desenex Antifungal Liquid Spray | Miconazole Nitrate 2% | **Adults & Peds ≥2 yrs:** Apply bid for 4 weeks. |
| Desenex Antifungal Powder | Miconazole Nitrate 2% | **Adults & Peds ≥2 yrs:** Athlete's Foot/Ringworm: Apply bid for 4 weeks. Jock Itch: Apply bid for 2 weeks. |
| Desenex Antifungal Spray Powder | Miconazole Nitrate 2% | **Adults & Peds ≥2 yrs:** Apply bid for 4 weeks. |
| Desenex Jock Itch Spray | Miconazole Nitrate 2% | **Adults & Peds ≥2 yrs:** Apply bid for 2 weeks. |
| Lotrimin AF Athlete's Foot Deodorant Powder Spray | Miconazole Nitrate 2% | **Adults & Peds ≥2 yrs:** Athlete's Foot/Ringworm: Apply bid for 4 weeks. Jock Itch: Apply bid for 2 weeks. |
| Lotrimin AF Athlete's Foot Liquid Spray | Miconazole Nitrate 2% | **Adults & Peds ≥2 yrs:** Athlete's Foot/Ringworm: Apply bid for 4 weeks. Jock Itch: Apply bid for 2 weeks. |
| Lotrimin AF Athlete's Foot Powder | Miconazole Nitrate 2% | **Adults & Peds ≥2 yrs:** Athlete's Foot/Ringworm: Apply bid for 4 weeks. Jock Itch: Apply bid for 2 weeks. |

*(Continued)*

| BRAND | INGREDIENT/STRENGTH | DOSE |
|---|---|---|
| **MICONAZOLE** *(Continued)* | | |
| Lotrimin AF Athlete's Foot Powder Spray | Miconazole Nitrate 2% | **Adults & Peds ≥2 yrs:** Athlete's Foot/Ringworm: Apply bid for 4 weeks. Jock Itch: Apply bid for 2 weeks. |
| Lotrimin AF Jock Itch Powder Spray | Miconazole Nitrate 2% | **Adults & Peds ≥2 yrs:** Apply bid for 2 weeks. |
| Micatin Cream | Miconazole Nitrate 2% | **Adults & Peds ≥2 yrs:** Athlete's Foot/Ringworm: Apply bid for 4 weeks. Jock Itch: Apply bid for 2 weeks. |
| Miranel AF Antifungal Treatment | Miconazole Nitrate 2% | **Adults & Peds ≥12 yrs:** Apply bid for 4 weeks. |
| Ting Spray Powder | Miconazole Nitrate 2% | **Adults & Peds ≥2 yrs:** Athlete's Foot/Ringworm: Apply bid for 4 weeks. Jock Itch: Apply bid for 2 weeks. |
| Zeasorb-AF Antifungal Drying Gel | Miconazole Nitrate 2% | **Adults & Peds ≥2 yrs:** Athlete's Foot/Ringworm: Apply bid for 4 weeks. Jock Itch: Apply bid for 2 weeks. |
| Zeasorb-AF Super Absorbent Antifungal Powder | Miconazole Nitrate 2% | **Adults & Peds ≥2 yrs:** Athlete's Foot/Ringworm: Apply bid for 4 weeks. Jock Itch: Apply bid for 2 weeks. |
| **TERBINAFINE** | | |
| Lamisil AT Antifungal Continuous Spray, Athlete's Foot | Terbinafine HCl 1% | **Adults & Peds ≥12 yrs:** Athlete's Foot (between toes): Apply bid for 1 week. Jock Itch/Ringworm: Apply qd for 1 week. |
| Lamisil AT Antifungal Continuous Spray, Jock Itch | Terbinafine HCl 1% | **Adults & Peds ≥12 yrs:** Apply qd for 1 week. |
| Lamisil AT Antifungal Spray Pump | Terbinafine HCl 1% | **Adults & Peds ≥12 yrs:** Athlete's Foot (between toes): Apply bid for 1 week. Jock Itch/Ringworm: Apply qd for 1 week. |
| Lamisil AT Athlete's Foot Treatment Cream | Terbinafine HCl 1% | **Adults & Peds ≥12 yrs:** Athlete's Foot (between toes): Apply bid for 1 week. Athlete's Foot (on side or bottom of foot): Apply bid for 2 weeks. Jock Itch/ Ringworm: Apply qd for 1 week. |
| Lamisil AT Athlete's Foot Treatment Gel | Terbinafine HCl 1% | **Adults & Peds ≥12 yrs:** Athlete's Foot (between toes): Apply qhs for 1 week. Jock Itch/Ringworm: Apply qd for 1 week |
| Lamisil AT for Women Antifungal Cream | Terbinafine HCl 1% | **Adults & Peds ≥12 yrs:** Apply bid for 2 weeks. |
| **TOLNAFTATE** | | |
| Flexitol Medicated Foot Cream | Tolnaftate 1% | **Adults & Peds ≥2 yrs:** Apply bid for 4 weeks. |
| FungiCure Anti-Fungal Gel | Tolnaftate 1% | **Adults & Peds ≥2 yrs:** Athlete's Foot/Ringworm: Apply bid for 4 weeks. Jock Itch: Apply bid for 2 weeks. |
| Lamisil AF Defense Antifungal Cream to Powder | Tolnaftate 1% | **Adults & Peds ≥2 yrs:** Athlete's Foot: Apply bid for 4 weeks. Prevention: Apply qd-bid. |
| Lamisil AF Defense Antifungal Shake Powder | Tolnaftate 1% | **Adults & Peds ≥2 yrs:** Athlete's Foot: Apply bid for 4 weeks. Prevention: Apply qd-bid. |
| Lamisil AF Defense Spray Powder | Tolnaftate 1% | **Adults & Peds ≥2 yrs:** Athlete's Foot: Apply bid for 4 weeks. Prevention: Apply qd-bid. |

| BRAND | INGREDIENT/STRENGTH | DOSE |
|---|---|---|
| **TOLNAFTATE** *(Continued)* | | |
| Tinactin Athlete's Foot Cream | Tolnaftate 1% | **Adults & Peds ≥2 yrs:** Apply bid for 4 weeks. |
| Tinactin Deodorant Powder Spray | Tolnaftate 1% | **Adults & Peds ≥2 yrs:** Athlete's Foot: Apply bid for 4 weeks. Prevention: Apply qd-bid. |
| Tinactin Jock Itch Cream | Tolnaftate 1% | **Adults & Peds ≥2 yrs:** Apply bid for 2 weeks. |
| Tinactin Jock Itch Powder Spray | Tolnaftate 1% | **Adults & Peds ≥2 yrs:** Apply bid for 2 weeks. |
| Tinactin Liquid Spray | Tolnaftate 1% | **Adults & Peds ≥2 yrs:** Athlete's Foot: Apply bid for 4 weeks. Prevention: Apply qd-bid. |
| Tinactin Powder Spray | Tolnaftate 1% | **Adults & Peds ≥2 yrs:** Athlete's Foot: Apply bid for 4 weeks. Prevention: Apply qd-bid. |
| Tinactin Pump Spray | Tolnaftate 1% | **Adults & Peds ≥2 yrs:** Athlete's Foot: Apply bid for 4 weeks. Prevention: Apply qd-bid. |
| Tinactin Super Absorbent Powder | Tolnaftate 1% | **Adults & Peds ≥2 yrs:** Athlete's Foot: Apply bid for 4 weeks. Prevention: Apply qd-bid. |
| Ting Antifungal Cream | Tolnaftate 1% | **Adults & Peds ≥2 yrs:** Athlete's Foot/Ringworm: Apply bid for 4 weeks. Jock Itch: Apply bid for 2 weeks. |
| Ting Spray Liquid | Tolnaftate 1% | **Adults & Peds ≥2 yrs:** Apply bid for 4 weeks. |
| **UNDECYLENIC ACID** | | |
| DiabetiDerm Toenail & Foot Fungus Antifungal Cream | Undecylenic Acid 10% | **Adults & Peds ≥2 yrs:** Athlete's Foot/Ringworm: Apply bid for 4 weeks. Jock Itch: Apply bid for 2 weeks. |
| Flexitol Anti-Fungal Liquid | Undecylenic Acid 25% | **Adults & Peds ≥2 yrs:** Apply bid. |
| Fungi Nail Anti-Fungal Solution | Undecylenic Acid 25% | **Adults & Peds ≥2 yrs:** Apply bid. |
| Fungi Nail Anti-Fungal Pen | Undecylenic Acid 25% | **Adults & Peds ≥2 yrs:** Apply bid. |
| FungiCure Extra Strength Anti-Fungal Liquid | Undecylenic Acid 12.5% | **Adults & Peds ≥2 yrs:** Apply bid for 4 weeks. |
| FungiCure Maximum Strength Anti-Fungal Liquid | Undecylenic Acid 25% | **Adults & Peds ≥2 yrs:** Apply bid for 4 weeks. |
| FungiCure Professional Formula Anti-Fungal Liquid | Undecylenic Acid 15% | **Adults & Peds ≥2 yrs:** Apply bid for 4 weeks. |
| Tineacide Antifungal Cream | Undecylenic Acid 10% | **Adults & Peds ≥12 yrs:** Athlete's Foot (between toes): Apply bid for 4 weeks. Jock Itch/Ringworm: Apply bid for 2 weeks. |

# CONTACT DERMATITIS PRODUCTS

| BRAND | INGREDIENT/STRENGTH | DOSE |
|---|---|---|
| **ANTIHISTAMINE** | | |
| Benadryl Itch Stopping Extra Strength Gel | Diphenhydramine HCl 2% | **Adults & Peds ≥2 yrs:** Apply to affected area tid-qid. |
| **ANTIHISTAMINE COMBINATION** | | |
| Benadryl Extra Strength Itch Stopping Cream | Diphenhydramine HCl/Zinc Acetate 2%-0.1% | **Adults & Peds ≥2 yrs:** Apply to affected area tid-qid. |
| Benadryl Extra Strength Spray | Diphenhydramine HCl/Zinc Acetate 2%-0.1% | **Adults & Peds ≥2 yrs:** Apply to affected area tid-qid. |
| Benadryl Extra Strength Itch Relief Stick | Diphenhydramine HCl/Zinc Acetate 2%-0.1% | **Adults & Peds ≥2 yrs:** Apply to affected area tid-qid. |
| Benadryl Original Strength Itch Stopping Cream | Diphenhydramine HCl/Zinc Acetate 1%-0.1% | **Adults & Peds ≥2 yrs:** Apply to affected area tid-qid. |
| CalaGel Anti-Itch Gel | Diphenhydramine HCl/Zinc Acetate/ Benzenthonium Chloride 2%-0.215%-0.15% | **Adults & Peds ≥2 yrs:** Apply to affected area no more than tid. |
| Ivarest Double Relief Formula | Diphenhydramine HCl/Benzyl Alcohol/ Calamine 2%-10.5%-14% | **Adults & Peds ≥2 yrs:** Apply to affected area tid-qid. |
| **ASTRINGENT** | | |
| Domeboro Astringent Solution Powder Packets | Aluminum Acetate (combination of Calcium Acetate 893mg and Aluminum Sulfate 1191mg) | **Adults & Peds:** Dissolve 1-3 pkts and apply to affected area for 15-30 min tid. |
| Ivy-Dry Super with Zytrel | Zinc Acetate/Benzyl Alcohol/Camphor/ Menthol 2%-10%-0.5%-0.25% | **Adults & Peds ≥6 yrs:** Apply to affected area tid. |
| Ivy-Dry Anti-Itch Cream with Zytrel | Zinc Acetate/Camphor/Menthol 2%-0.6%-0.4% | **Adults & Peds ≥6 yrs:** Apply to affected area tid. |
| Ivy-Dry Cream with Zytrel | Zinc Acetate/Camphor/Menthol 2%-0.6%-0.4% | **Adults & Peds ≥6 yrs:** Apply to affected area tid. |
| Ivy-Dry Kids with Zytrel | Zinc Acetate 2% | **Adults & Peds ≥2 yrs:** Apply to affected area tid. |
| **ASTRINGENT COMBINATION** | | |
| Aveeno Calamine and Pramoxine HCl Anti-Itch Cream | Calamine/Camphor/Pramoxine HCl 3%-0.5%-1% | **Adults & Peds ≥2 yrs:** Apply to affected area tid-qid. |
| Aveeno Anti-Itch Concentrated Lotion | Calamine/Camphor/Pramoxine HCl 3%-0.47%-1% | **Adults & Peds ≥2 yrs:** Apply to affected area qid. |
| Caladryl Clear Anti-Itch Lotion | Zinc Acetate/Pramoxine HCl 0.1%-1% | **Adults & Peds ≥2 yrs:** Apply to affected area tid-qid. |
| Caladryl Anti-Itch Lotion | Calamine/Pramoxine HCl 8%-1% | **Adults & Peds ≥2 yrs:** Apply to affected area tid-qid. |
| Calamine Lotion (generic) | Calamine/Zinc Oxide 8%-8% | **Adults & Peds:** Apply to affected area prn. |
| Cortaid Poison Ivy Care Treatment Kit | (Scrub) Water, polyethylene, laureth-4, sodium lauryl sarcosinate, glycol distearate, acrylates/ C10-30, alkyl acrylate crosspolymer, coco-glucoside, sodium hydroxide, microcrystalline wax, tetrasodium EDTA, glyceryl oleate, glyceryl stearate, quaternium-15, chromium hydroxide green, tocopherol (Spray) Zinc Acetate/Pramoxine 0.12%-1% | **Adults & Peds:** (Scrub) Apply quarter-sized amount into hand and rub onto affected area for 30 seconds. Rinse area thoroughly and pat dry. (Spray) Apply to affected area tid-qid. |
| **CLEANSER** | | |
| Cortaid Poison Ivy Care Toxin Removal Cloths | Water, laureth-4, sodium lauryl sarcosinate, glycerin, DMDM, hydantoin, methylparaben, tetrasodium EDTA, *Aloe barbadensis* leaf extract, citric acid | **Adults & Peds:** Wipe affected area at least 15 seconds. Rinse or wipe dry. |
| Ivarest Poison Ivy Cleansing Foam | Menthol 1% | **Adults & Peds ≥2 yrs:** Gently rub into affected area and rinse under running water. |
| Ivy-Dry Scrub with Zytrel | Polyethylene, sodium laureth sulfate, zinc actate, panthenol, PEG-14M, nonoxynol-9, zinc gluconate, zinc acetate, glycerin, tocopheryl acetate, C12-15 pareth-9, *Aloe barbadensis* extract, carbomer, allantoin, sodium hydroxide | **Adults & Peds:** Gently rub into affected area for at least 30 seconds; rinse. |

*(Continued)*

| BRAND | INGREDIENT/STRENGTH | DOSE |
|---|---|---|
| **CORTICOSTEROID** | | |
| Aveeno 1% Hydrocortisone Anti-Itch Cream | Hydrocortisone 1% | **Adults & Peds ≥2 yrs:** Apply to affected area tid-qid. |
| Cortaid Advanced 12-Hour Anti-Itch Cream | Hydrocortisone 1% | **Adults & Peds ≥2 yrs:** Apply to affected area tid-qid. |
| Cortaid Intensive Therapy Cooling Spray | Hydrocortisone 1% | **Adults & Peds ≥2 yrs:** Apply to affected area tid-qid. |
| Cortaid Intensive Therapy Moisturizing Cream | Hydrocortisone 1% | **Adults & Peds ≥2 yrs:** Apply to affected area tid-qid. |
| Cortaid Maximum Strength Cream | Hydrocortisone 1% | **Adults & Peds ≥2 yrs:** Apply to affected area tid-qid. |
| Cortaid Maximum Strength Ointment | Hydrocortisone 1% | **Adults & Peds ≥2 yrs:** Apply to affected area tid-qid. |
| Cortizone-10 Easy Relief Applicator | Hydrocortisone 1% | **Adults & Peds ≥2 yrs:** Apply to affected area tid-qid. |
| Cortizone-10 Cooling Relief Gel | Hydrocortisone 1% | **Adults & Peds ≥2 yrs:** Apply to affected area tid-qid. |
| Cortizone-10 Creme | Hydrocortisone 1% | **Adults & Peds ≥2 yrs:** Apply to affected area tid-qid. |
| Cortizone-10 Ointment | Hydrocortisone 1% | **Adults & Peds ≥2 yrs:** Apply to affected area tid-qid. |
| Cortizone-10 Creme Plus | Hydrocortisone 1% | **Adults & Peds ≥2 yrs:** Apply to affected area tid-qid. |
| Cortizone-10 Intensive Healing Formula | Hydrocortisone 1% | **Adults & Peds ≥2 yrs:** Apply to affected area tid-qid. |
| Corticool 1% Hydrocortisone Anti-Itch Gel | Hydrocortisone 1% | **Adults & Peds ≥2 yrs:** Apply to affected area tid-qid. |
| **COUNTERIRRITANT** | | |
| Gold Bond Quick Spray | Menthol/Benzethonium Chloride 1%-0.13% | **Adults & Peds ≥2 yrs:** Apply to affected area tid-qid. |
| Gold Bond Medicated Maximum Strength Anti-Itch Cream | Menthol/Pramoxine HCl 1%-1% | **Adults & Peds ≥2 yrs:** Apply to affected area tid-qid. |
| Ivy Block Lotion | Bentoquatam 5% | **Adults & Peds ≥6 yrs:** Apply 15 minutes before exposure risk and q4h for continued protection. |
| **LOCAL ANESTHETIC** | | |
| Solarcaine Aloe Extra Burn Relief Gel | Lidocaine HCl 0.5% | **Adults & Peds ≥2 yrs:** Apply to affected area tid-qid. |
| Solarcaine Aloe Extra Burn Relief Spray | Lidocaine HCl 0.5% | **Adults & Peds ≥2 yrs:** Apply to affected area tid-qid. |
| Solarcaine First Aid Medicated Spray | Benzocaine/Triclosan 20%-0.13% | **Adults & Peds ≥2 yrs:** Apply to affected area qd-tid. |
| **LOCAL ANESTHETIC COMBINATION** | | |
| Bactine Pain Relieving Cleansing Spray | Lidocaine/Benzalkonium Chloride 2.5%-0.13% | **Adults & Peds ≥2 yrs:** Apply to affected area qd-tid. |
| Bactine Original First Aid Liquid | Lidocaine HCl/Benzalkonium Chloride 2.5%-0.13% | **Adults & Peds ≥2 yrs:** Apply to affected area qd-tid. |
| Lanacane Maximum Strength Cream | Benzocaine/Benzethonium Chloride 20%-0.2% | **Adults & Peds ≥2 yrs:** Apply to affected area qd-tid. |
| Lanacane Antibacterial First Aid Spray | Benzocaine/Benzethonium Chloride 20%-0.2% | **Adults & Peds ≥2 yrs:** Apply to affected area qd-tid. |
| Lanacane Original Strength Cream | Benzocaine/Benzethonium Chloride 6%-0.2% | **Adults & Peds ≥2 yrs:** Apply to affected area qd-tid. |

*(Continued)*

| BRAND | INGREDIENT/STRENGTH | DOSE |
|---|---|---|
| **SKIN PROTECTANT** | | |
| Aveeno Skin Relief Moisturizing Cream | Dimethicone 2.5% | **Adults & Peds ≥2 yrs:** Apply to affected area prn. |
| Aveeno Skin Relief Moisturizing Lotion | Dimethicone 1.3% | **Adults & Peds:** Apply to affected area prn. |
| Vaseline Intensive Rescue Clinical Therapy Lotion | Dimethicone 1% | **Adults & Peds:** Apply to affected area prn. |
| **SKIN PROTECTANT COMBINATION** | | |
| Gold Bond Extra Strength Medicated Body Lotion | Dimethicone/Menthol 5%-0.5% | **Adults & Peds:** Apply to affected area tid-qid. |
| Gold Bond Medicated Body Lotion | Dimethicone/Menthol 5%-0.15% | **Adults & Peds:** Apply to affected area prn. |
| Gold Bond Medicated Powder | Zinc Oxide/Menthol 1%-0.15% | **Adults & Peds ≥2 yrs:** Apply to affected area tid-qid. |
| Gold Bond Extra Strength Medicated Powder | Zinc Oxide/Menthol 5%-0.8% | **Adults & Peds ≥2 yrs:** Apply to affected area tid-qid. |

# DIAPER RASH PRODUCTS

| BRAND | INGREDIENT/STRENGTH | DOSE |
|---|---|---|
| **WHITE PETROLATUM** | | |
| Balmex Multi-Purpose Healing Ointment | White Petrolatum 51.1% | **Peds:** Apply prn. |
| Desitin Multi-Purpose Skin Protectant and Diaper Rash Ointment | White Petrolatum 60.4% | **Peds:** Apply prn. |
| Vaseline Baby, Baby Fresh Scent | White Petrolatum 100% | **Peds:** Apply prn. |
| Vaseline Petroleum Jelly | White Petrolatum 100% | **Peds:** Apply prn. |
| **ZINC OXIDE** | | |
| Aveeno Baby Soothing Relief Diaper Rash Cream | Zinc Oxide 13% | **Peds:** Apply prn. |
| Balmex Diaper Rash Cream with ActivGuard | Zinc Oxide 11.3% | **Peds:** Apply prn. |
| Balmex Prevention Baby Powder with ActivGuard | Zinc Oxide 11.3% | **Adults & Peds ≥2 yrs:** Apply tid-qid. **Peds <2 yrs:** Apply prn. |
| Boudreaux's Butt Paste, Diaper Rash Ointment | Zinc Oxide 16% | **Peds:** Apply prn. |
| California Baby Calming Diaper Rash Cream | Zinc Oxide 12% | **Peds:** Apply prn. |
| Canus Li'l Goat's Milk Ointment | Zinc Oxide 40% | **Peds:** Apply prn. |
| Desitin Rapid Relief Cream | Zinc Oxide 13% | **Peds:** Apply prn. |
| Desitin Maximum Strength Original Paste | Zinc Oxide 40% | **Peds:** Apply prn. |
| Johnson's Baby Powder Medicated with Aloe & Vitamin E Medicated | Zinc Oxide 10% | **Peds:** Apply prn. |
| Mustela Bebe Vitamin Barrier Cream | Zinc Oxide 10% | **Peds:** Apply prn. |
| Triple Paste Medicated Ointment | Zinc Oxide 12.8% | **Peds:** Apply prn. |
| **COMBINATION PRODUCTS** | | |
| A+D Original Ointment | Petrolatum/Lanolin 53.4%-15.5% | **Peds:** Apply prn. |
| A+D Zinc Oxide Cream | Dimethicone/Zinc Oxide 1%-10% | **Peds:** Apply prn. |
| Lansinoh Diaper Rash Ointment | Dimethicone/USP Modified Lanolin/ Zinc Oxide 5.0%-15.5%-5.5% | **Peds:** Apply prn. |

# PSORIASIS PRODUCTS

| BRAND | INGREDIENT/STRENGTH | DOSE |
|---|---|---|
| **COAL TAR** | | |
| DHS Tar Gel Shampoo | Coal Tar 0.5% | Use at least biw. |
| DHS Tar Shampoo | Coal Tar 0.5% | Use at least biw. |
| Ionil Plus Shampoo | Coal Tar 2% | Use at least biw. |
| Ionil-T Plus Shampoo | Coal Tar 2% | Use at least biw. |
| Ionil-T Shampoo | Coal Tar 2% | Use at least biw. |
| MG217 Medicated Tar Lotion | Coal Tar 1% | Apply to affected area qd-qid. |
| MG217 Medicated Tar Ointment | Coal Tar 2% | Apply to affected area qd-qid. |
| MG217 Medicated Tar Shampoo | Coal Tar 3% | Use at least biw. |
| Neutrogena T/Gel Shampoo Extra Strength | Coal Tar 1% | Use at least biw. |
| Neutrogena T/Gel Shampoo Original Formula | Coal Tar 0.5% | Use at least biw. |
| Neutrogena T/Gel Shampoo Stubborn Itch Control | Coal Tar 0.5% | Use at least biw. |
| Psoriasin Gel | Coal Tar 1.25% | **Adults:** Apply to affected area qd-qid. |
| Psoriasin Liquid For Skin & Scalp | Coal Tar 0.66% | **Adults:** Apply to affected area qd-qid. |
| Psoriasin Ointment | Coal Tar 2% | **Adults:** Apply to affected area qd-qid. |
| **CORTICOSTEROID** | | |
| Aveeno 1% Hydrocortisone Anti-Itch Cream | Hydrocortisone 1% | **Adults & Peds ≥2 yrs:** Apply to affected area tid-qid. |
| Cortaid Advanced 12-Hour Anti-Itch Cream | Hydrocortisone 1% | **Adults & Peds ≥2 yrs:** Apply to affected area tid-qid. |
| Cortaid Intensive Therapy Cooling Spray | Hydrocortisone 1% | **Adults & Peds ≥2 yrs:** Apply to affected area tid-qid. |
| Cortaid Intensive Therapy Moisturizing Cream | Hydrocortisone 1% | **Adults & Peds ≥2 yrs:** Apply to affected area tid-qid. |
| Cortaid Maximum Strength Cream | Hydrocortisone 1% | **Adults & Peds ≥2 yrs:** Apply to affected area tid-qid. |
| Cortaid Maximum Strength Ointment | Hydrocortisone 1% | **Adults & Peds ≥2 yrs:** Apply to affected area tid-qid. |
| Corticool 1% Hydrocortisone Anti-Itch Gel | Hydrocortisone 1% | **Adults & Peds ≥2 yrs:** Apply to affected area tid-qid. |
| Cortizone-10 Cooling Relief Gel | Hydrocortisone 1% | **Adults & Peds ≥2 yrs:** Apply to affected area tid-qid. |
| Cortizone-10 Creme | Hydrocortisone 1% | **Adults & Peds ≥2 yrs:** Apply to affected area tid-qid. |
| Cortizone-10 Creme Plus | Hydrocortisone 1% | **Adults & Peds ≥2 yrs:** Apply to affected area tid-qid. |
| Cortizone-10 Ointment | Hydrocortisone 1% | **Adults & Peds ≥2 yrs:** Apply to affected area tid-qid. |
| Cortizone-10 Easy Relief Applicator | Hydrocortisone 1% | **Adults & Peds ≥2 yrs:** Apply to affected area tid-qid. |
| Cortizone-10 Intensive Healing Formula | Hydrocortisone 1% | **Adults & Peds ≥2 yrs:** Apply to affected area tid-qid. |
| **SALICYLIC ACID** | | |
| Dermarest Psoriasis Medicated Moisturizer | Salicylic Acid 2% | **Adults & Peds:** Apply to affected area qd-qid. |
| Dermarest Psoriasis Medicated Overnight Treatment | Salicylic Acid 3% | **Adults & Peds:** Apply to affected area qhs. **Max:** qid. |
| Dermarest Psoriasis Medicated Scalp Treatment | Salicylic Acid 3% | **Adults & Peds:** Apply to affected area qd-qid. |
| Dermarest Psoriasis Medicated Shampoo Plus Conditioner | Salicylic Acid 3% | **Adults & Peds:** Use at least biw. |
| Dermarest Psoriasis Medicated Skin Treatment | Salicylic Acid 3% | **Adults & Peds:** Apply to affected area qd-qid. |

*(Continued)*

| BRAND | INGREDIENT/STRENGTH | DOSE |
|---|---|---|
| **SALICYLIC ACID** *(Continued)* | | |
| DHS Sal Shampoo | Salicylic Acid 3% | **Adults & Peds:** Use at least biw. |
| MG217 Sal-Acid Ointment | Salicylic Acid 3% | **Adults & Peds:** Apply to affected area qd-qid. |
| Neutrogena T/Gel Therapeutic Conditioner | Salicylic Acid 2% | **Adults & Peds:** Use at least biw. |
| Neutrogena T/Sal Therapeutic Shampoo | Salicylic Acid 3% | **Adults & Peds:** Use at least tiw. |
| Psoriasin Therapeutic Shampoo and Body Wash | Salicylic Acid 3% | **Adults & Peds:** Use at least biw. |

# WOUND CARE PRODUCTS

| BRAND | INGREDIENT/STRENGTH | DOSE |
|---|---|---|
| **NEOMYCIN/POLYMYXIN B/BACITRACIN COMBINATIONS** | | |
| Bacitracin Ointment | Bacitracin 500 U | **Adults & Peds:** Apply to affected area qd-tid. |
| Neosporin First Aid Antibiotic Ointment | Neomycin/polymyxin B/bacitracin 3.5mg-5,000 U-400 U | **Adults & Peds:** Apply to affected area qd-tid. |
| Neosporin Neo To Go! Single Use Packets | Neomycin/polymyxin B/bacitracin 3.5mg-5,000 U-400 U | **Adults & Peds:** Apply to affected area qd-tid. |
| Neosporin Plus Pain Relief Cream | Neomycin/polymyxin B/pramoxine HCl 3.5mg-10,000 U-10mg | **Adults & Peds ≥2 yrs:** Apply to affected area qd-tid. |
| Neosporin Plus Pain Relief Ointment | Neomycin/polymyxin B/bacitracin/pramoxine HCl 3.5mg-10,000 U-400 U-10mg | **Adults & Peds ≥2 yrs:** Apply to affected area qd-tid. |
| Polysporin First Aid Antibiotic Ointment | Polymyxin B/bacitracin 10,000 U-500 U | **Adults & Peds:** Apply to affected area qd-tid. |
| Polysporin First Aid Antibiotic Powder | Polymyxin B/bacitracin 10,000 U-500 U | **Adults & Peds:** Apply to affected area qd-tid. |
| **BENZALKONIUM CHLORIDE COMBINATIONS** | | |
| Bactine Original First Aid Liquid | Benzalkonium chloride/lidocaine HCl 0.13%-2.5% | **Adults & Peds ≥2 yrs:** Use to clean affected area qd-tid. |
| Bactine Pain Relieving Cleansing Spray | Benzalkonium chloride/lidocaine HCl 0.13%-2.5% | **Adults & Peds ≥2 yrs:** Use to clean affected area qd-tid. |
| Band-Aid Hurt Free Antiseptic Wash | Benzalkonium chloride/lidocaine HCl 0.13%-2% | **Adults & Peds ≥2 yrs:** Use to clean affected area qd-tid. |
| Neosporin Neo To Go! First Aid Antiseptic/Pain Relieving Spray | Benzalkonium chloride/pramoxine HCl 0.13%-1% | **Adults & Peds ≥2 yrs:** Use to clean affected area qd-tid. |
| **BENZETHONIUM CHLORIDE COMBINATIONS** | | |
| Gold Bond Quick Spray | Benzethonium chloride/menthol 0.13%-1% | **Adults & Peds ≥2 yrs:** Apply to affected area qd-tid. |
| Lanacane Anti-Bacterial First Aid Spray | Benzethonium chloride/benzocaine 0.2%-20% | **Adults & Peds ≥2 yrs:** Apply to affected area qd-tid. |
| Lanacane Maximum Strength Pain & Intense Itch Anti-Itch Cream | Benzethonium chloride/benzocaine 0.2%-20% | **Adults & Peds ≥2 yrs:** Apply to affected area qd-tid. |
| Lanacane Original Strength Itch & Irritation Anti-Itch Cream | Benzethonium chloride/benzocaine 0.2%-6% | **Adults & Peds ≥2 yrs:** Apply to affected area qd-tid. |
| **CHLORHEXIDINE GLUCONATE** | | |
| Hibiclens | Chlorhexidine gluconate 4% | **Adults:** Apply sparingly to affected area and wash. |
| Hibistat | Chlorhexidine gluconate/isopropyl alcohol 0.5%-70% | **Adults:** Rub vigorously with the towelette for about 15 seconds. |
| **IODINE** | | |
| Betadine Skin Cleanser | Povidone-iodine 7.5% | **Adults & Peds:** Apply to affected area, wash vigorously for 15 seconds, rinse and dry. |
| Betadine Solution | Povidone-iodine 10% | **Adults & Peds:** Apply to affected area qd-tid. |
| **MISCELLANEOUS** | | |
| Aquaphor Healing Ointment | Petrolatum (41%), mineral oil, ceresin, lanolin alcohol, panthenol, glycerin, bisabolol | **Adults & Peds:** Apply to affected area prn. |
| Wound Wash Saline | Sterile 0.9% sodium chloride solution | **Adults & Peds:** Use to clean affected area prn. |

# ANTACID AND HEARTBURN PRODUCTS

| BRAND | INGREDIENT/STRENGTH | DOSE |
|---|---|---|
| **ANTACID** | | |
| Alka-Seltzer Gold Tablets | Citric Acid/Potassium Bicarbonate/ Sodium Bicarbonate 1000mg-344mg-1050mg | **Adults ≥60 yrs:** 2 tabs q4h prn. **Max:** 6 tabs q24h. **Adults & Peds ≥12 yrs:** 2 tabs q4h prn. **Max:** 8 tabs q24h. **Peds ≤12 yrs:** 1 tab q4h prn. **Max:** 4 tabs q24h. |
| Alka-Seltzer Heartburn Relief Tablets | Citric Acid/Sodium Bicarbonate 1000mg-1940mg | **Adults ≥60 yrs:** 2 tabs q4h prn. **Max:** 4 tabs q24h. **Adults & Peds ≥12 yrs:** 2 tabs q4h prn. **Max:** 8 tabs q24h. |
| Alka-Seltzer Lemon Lime Tablets | Aspirin/Citric Acid/Sodium Bicarbonate 325mg-1000mg-1700mg | **Adults ≥60 yrs:** 2 tabs q4h prn. **Max:** 4 tabs q24h. **Adults & Peds ≥12 yrs:** 2 tabs q4h prn. **Max:** 8 tabs q24h. |
| Alka-Seltzer Tablets, Extra-Strength | Aspirin/Citric Acid/Sodium Bicarbonate 500mg-1000mg-1985mg | **Adults ≥60 yrs:** 2 tabs q6h prn. **Max:** 3 tabs q24h. **Adults & Peds ≥12 yrs:** 2 tabs q6h prn. **Max:** 7 tabs q24h. |
| Alka-Seltzer Tablets, Original | Aspirin/Citric Acid/Sodium Bicarbonate 325mg-1000mg-1916mg | **Adults ≥60 yrs:** 2 tabs q4h prn. **Max:** 4 tabs q24h. **Adults & Peds ≥12 yrs:** 2 tabs q4h prn. **Max:** 8 tabs q24h. |
| Brioschi Powder | Sodium Bicarbonate/Tartaric Acid 2.69g-2.43g/dose | **Adults & Peds ≥12 yrs:** 1 capful (6g) dissolved in 4-6 oz water q1h. **Max:** 6 doses q24h. **Adults ≥60 yrs:** 1 capful (6g) dissolved in 4-6 oz water q1h. **Max:** 3 doses q24h. |
| Gaviscon Extra Strength Liquid | Aluminum Hydroxide/Magnesium Carbonate 254mg-237.5mg/5mL | **Adults:** 2-4 tsp (10-20mL) qid. |
| Gaviscon Extra Strength Tablets | Aluminum Hydroxide/Magnesium Carbonate 160mg-105mg | **Adults:** 2-4 tabs qid. **Max:** 16 doses q24h. |
| Gaviscon Regular Strength Liquid | Aluminum Hydroxide/Magnesium Carbonate 95mg-358mg/15mL | **Adults:** 1-2 tbl (15-30mL) qid. **Max:** 8 tbl q24h. |
| Gaviscon Regular Strength Tablets | Aluminum Hydroxide/Magnesium Trisilicate 80mg-14.2mg | **Adults:** 2-4 tabs qid. **Max:** 16 tabs q24h. |
| Maalox Children's Relief Chewables | Calcium Carbonate 400mg | **Peds 6-11 yrs (48-95 lbs):** 2 tabs prn. **Max:** 6 tabs q24h. **Peds 2-5 yrs (24-47 lbs):** 1 tab prn. **Max:** 3 tabs q24h. |
| Maalox Regular Strength Chewable Tablets | Calcium Carbonate 600mg | **Adults:** 1-2 tabs prn. **Max:** 12 tabs q24h. |
| Mylanta, Children's | Calcium Carbonate 400mg | **Peds 6-11 yrs (48-95 lbs):** Take 2 tabs prn. **Max:** 6 tabs q24h. **Peds 2-5 yrs (24-47 lbs):** Take 1 tab prn. **Max:** 3 tabs q24h. |
| Mylanta Supreme Antacid Liquid | Calcium Carbonate/Magnesium Hydroxide 400mg-135mg/5mL | **Adults:** 2-4 tsp (10-20mL) qid (between meals & hs). **Max:** 18 tsp (90mL) q24h. |
| Mylanta Ultimate Strength Chewable Tablets | Calcium Carbonate/Magnesium Hydroxide 700mg-300mg | **Adults:** 2-4 tabs qid (between meals & hs). **Max:** 10 tabs q24h for ≤2 weeks. |
| Mylanta Ultimate Strength Liquid | Aluminum Hydroxide/Magnesium Hydroxide 500mg-500mg/5mL | **Adults & Peds ≥12 yrs:** 2-4 tsp (10-20mL) qid (between meals & hs). **Max:** 9 tsp (45mL) q24h for ≤2 weeks. |
| Pepto Bismol Children's Pepto Chewable Tablets | Calcium Carbonate 400mg | **Peds 6-11 yrs (48-95 lbs):** Take 2 tabs prn. **Max:** 6 tabs q24h. **Peds 2-5 yrs (24-47 lbs):** Take 1 tab prn. **Max:** 3 tabs q24h. |
| Rolaids Extra Strength Softchews | Calcium Carbonate 1177mg | **Adults:** 2-3 chews q1h prn. **Max:** 6 chews q24h. |
| Rolaids Extra Strength Tablets | Calcium Carbonate/Magnesium Hydroxide 675mg-135mg | **Adults:** 2-4 tabs q1h prn. **Max:** 10 tabs q24h. |

*(Continued)*

| BRAND | INGREDIENT/STRENGTH | DOSE |
|---|---|---|
| **ANTACID** *(Continued)* | | |
| Rolaids Tablets | Calcium Carbonate/Magnesium Hydroxide 550mg-110mg | **Adults:** 2-4 tabs q1h prn. **Max:** 12 tabs q24h. |
| Titralac Chewable Tablets | Calcium Carbonate 420mg | **Adults:** 2 tabs q2-3h prn. **Max:** 19 tabs q24h. |
| Tums Chewable Tablets | Calcium Carbonate 500mg | **Adults:** 2-4 tabs prn. **Max:** 15 tabs q24h. |
| Tums E-X 750 Chewable Tablets | Calcium Carbonate 750mg | **Adults:** 2-4 tabs prn. **Max:** 10 tabs q24h. |
| Tums E-X 750 Sugar Free Chewable Tablets | Calcium Carbonate 750mg | **Adults:** 2-4 tabs prn. **Max:** 9 tabs q24h. |
| Tums Kids Chewable Tablets | Calcium Carbonate 750mg | **Peds >4 yrs (>49 lbs):** Take 1 tab tid. **Max:** 4 tabs q24h. **Peds 2-4 yrs (24-47 lbs):** Take ½-1 tab bid. **Max:** 2 tabs q24h. |
| Tums Quik Pak Instant Dissolve Powder | Calcium Carbonate 1000mg | **Adults:** Pour 1 packet onto tongue and allow powder to dissolve. **Max:** 7 packets q24h. |
| Tums Smoothies Tablets | Calcium Carbonate 750mg | **Adults:** 2-4 tabs prn. **Max:** 10 tabs q24h. |
| Tums Ultra 1000 Chewable Tablets | Calcium Carbonate 1000mg | **Adults:** 2-3 tabs prn. **Max:** 7 tabs q24h for ≤2 weeks. |
| **ANTACID/ANTIFLATULANT** | | |
| Gelusil Chewable Tablets | Aluminum Hydroxide/Magnesium Hydroxide/Simethicone 200mg-200mg-25mg | **Adults:** 2-4 tabs q1h prn. **Max:** 12 tabs q24h. |
| Maalox Advanced Maximum Strength Chewable Tablets | Calcium Carbonate/Simethicone 1000mg-60mg | **Adults & Peds ≥12 yrs:** 1-2 tabs prn. **Max:** 8 tabs q24h. |
| Maalox Advanced Maximum Strength Liquid | Aluminum Hydroxide/Magnesium Hydroxide/Simethicone 400mg-400mg-40mg/5mL | **Adults & Peds ≥12 yrs:** 2-4 tsp (10-20mL) bid. **Max:** 8 tsp (40mL) q24h. |
| Maalox Advanced Regular Strength Liquid | Aluminum Hydroxide/Magnesium Hydroxide/Simethicone 200mg-200mg-20mg/5mL | **Adults & Peds ≥12 yrs:** 2-4 tsp (10-20mL) qid. **Max:** 16 tsp (80mL) q24h. |
| Maalox Junior Relief Chewables | Calcium Carbonate/Simethicone 400mg-24mg | **Peds 6–11 yrs:** 2 tabs prn. **Max:** 6 tabs q24h. |
| Mylanta Maximum Strength Liquid | Aluminum Hydroxide/Magnesium Hydroxide/Simethicone 400mg-400mg-40mg/5mL | **Adults & Peds ≥12 yrs:** 2-4 tsp (between meals and hs) (10-20mL) qid. **Max:** 12 tsp (60mL) q24h. |
| Mylanta Regular Strength Liquid | Aluminum Hydroxide/Magnesium Hydroxide/Simethicone 200mg-200mg-20mg/5mL | **Adults & Peds ≥12 yrs:** 2-4 tsp (between meals and hs) (10-20mL) qid. **Max:** 24 tsp (120mL) q24h. |
| Rolaids Extra Strength Plus Gas Soft Chews | Calcium Carbonate/Simethicone 1177mg-80mg | **Adults:** 2-3 chews q1h prn. **Max:** 6 chews q24h. |
| Rolaids Multi-Symptom Chewable Tablets | Calcium Carbonate/Magnesium Hydroxide/Simethicone 675mg-135mg-60mg | **Adults:** 2-4 tabs q1h prn. **Max:** 8 tabs q24h. |
| Titralac Plus Chewable Tablets | Calcium Carbonate/Simethicone 420mg-21mg | **Adults:** 2 tabs q2-3h prn. **Max:** 19 tabs q24h. |
| **BISMUTH SUBSALICYLATE** | | |
| Maalox Total Relief Maximum Strength Liquid | Bismuth Subsalicylate 525mg/15mL | **Adults & Peds ≥12 yrs:** 2 tbl (30mL) q1h prn. **Max:** 8 tbl (120mL) q24h. |
| Pepto Bismol Caplets | Bismuth Subsalicylate 262mg | **Adults & Peds ≥12 yrs:** 2 tabs q1/2-1h prn. **Max:** 8 doses q24h. |

*(Continued)*

| BRAND | INGREDIENT/STRENGTH | DOSE |
|---|---|---|
| **BISMUTH SUBSALICYLATE** *(Continued)* | | |
| Pepto Bismol Chewable Tablets | Bismuth Subsalicylate 262mg | **Adults & Peds ≥12 yrs:** 2 tabs q1/2-1h prn. **Max:** 8 doses q24h. |
| Pepto Bismol Liquid | Bismuth Subsalicylate 262mg/15mL | **Adults & Peds ≥12 yrs:** 2 tbl (30mL) q1/2-1h prn. **Max:** 8 doses (240mL) q24h. |
| Pepto Bismol Liquid Max | Bismuth Subsalicylate 525mg/15mL | **Adults & Peds ≥12 yrs:** 2 tbl (30mL) q1h prn. **Max:** 4 doses (120mL) q24h. |
| **$H_2$-RECEPTOR ANTAGONIST** | | |
| Axid AR | Nizatidine 75mg | **Adults & Peds ≥12 yrs:** 1 tab qd. **Max:** 2 tabs q24h. |
| Pepcid AC Gelcaps | Famotidine 10mg | **Adults & Peds ≥12 yrs:** 1 cap qd. **Max:** 2 caps q24h. |
| Pepcid AC Maximum Strength EZ Chews | Famotidine 20mg | **Adults & Peds ≥12 yrs:** 1 tab qd. **Max:** 2 tabs q24h. |
| Pepcid AC Maximum Strength Tablets | Famotidine 20mg | **Adults & Peds ≥12 yrs:** 1 tab qd. **Max:** 2 tabs q24h. |
| Pepcid AC Tablets | Famotidine 10mg | **Adults & Peds ≥12 yrs:** 1 tab qd. **Max:** 2 tabs q24h. |
| Tagamet HB Tablets | Cimetidine 200mg | **Adults & Peds ≥12 yrs:** 1 tab qd. **Max:** 2 tabs q24h. |
| Zantac 75 Tablets | Ranitidine 75mg | **Adults & Peds ≥12 yrs:** 1 tab qd. **Max:** 2 tabs q24h. |
| Zantac 150 Tablets | Ranitidine 150mg | **Adults & Peds ≥12 yrs:** 1 tab qd. **Max:** 2 tabs q24h. |
| **$H_2$-RECEPTOR ANTAGONIST/ANTACID** | | |
| Pepcid Complete Chewable Tablets | Famotidine/Calcium Carbonate/ Magnesium Hydroxide 10mg-800mg-165mg | **Adults & Peds ≥12 yrs:** 1 tab qd. **Max:** 2 tabs q24h. |
| Tums Dual Action | Famotidine/Calcium Carbonate/ Magnesium Hydroxide 10mg-800mg-165mg | **Adults & Peds ≥12 yrs:** 1 tab qd. **Max:** 2 tabs q24h. |
| **PROTON PUMP INHIBITOR** | | |
| Prevacid 24HR | Lansoprazole 15mg | **Adults:** 1 cap qd x 14 days. May repeat 14-day course q4 months. |
| Prilosec OTC Tablets | Omeprazole 20mg | **Adults:** 1 tab qd x 14 days. May repeat 14-day course q4 months. |
| Zegerid OTC | Omeprazole/Sodium bicarbonate 20mg-1100mg | **Adults:** 1 cap qd x 14 days. May repeat 14-day course q4 months. |

# ANTIDIARRHEAL PRODUCTS

| BRAND | INGREDIENT/STRENGTH | DOSE |
|---|---|---|
| **ABSORBENT AGENTS** | | |
| Equalactin Chewable Tablets | Calcium Polycarbophil 625mg | **Adults & Peds ≥12 yrs:** 2 tabs/dose. **Max:** 8 tabs q24h. **Peds 6-12 yrs:** 1 tab/dose. **Max:** 4 tabs q24h. **Peds 2 to ≤6 yrs:** 1 tab/dose. **Max:** 2 tabs q24h. |
| Fibercon Caplets | Calcium Polycarbophil 625mg | **Adults & Peds ≥12 yrs:** 2 tabs qd. **Max:** 8 tabs q24h. |
| Konsyl Fiber Caplets | Calcium Polycarbophil 625mg | **Adults & Peds ≥12 yrs:** 2 tabs qd-qid. **Peds 6-12 yrs:** 1 tab qd-tid. **Max:** 8 tabs q24h. |
| **ANTIPERISTALTIC AGENTS** | | |
| Imodium A-D Caplets | Loperamide HCl 2mg | **Adults & Peds ≥12 yrs:** 2 tabs after first loose stool; 1 tab after each subsequent loose stool. **Max:** 4 tabs q24h. **Peds 9-11 yrs (60-95 lbs):** 1 tab after first loose stool; ½ tab after each subsequent loose stool. **Max:** 3 tabs q24h. **Peds 6-8 yrs (48-59 lbs):** 1 tab after first loose stool; ½ tab after each subsequent loose stool. **Max:** 2 tabs q24h. |
| Imodium A-D E-Z Chews | Loperamide HCl 2mg | **Adults & Peds ≥12 yrs:** 2 tabs after first loose stool; 1 tab after each subsequent loose stool. **Max:** 4 tabs q24h. **Peds 9-11 yrs (60-95 lbs):** 1 tab after first loose stool; ½ tab after each subsequent loose stool. **Max:** 3 tabs q24h. **Peds 6-8 yrs (48-59 lbs):** 1 tab after first loose stool; ½ tab after each subsequent loose stool. **Max:** 2 tabs q24h. |
| Imodium A-D Liquid | Loperamide HCl 1mg/7.5mL | **Adults & Peds ≥12 yrs:** 4 tsp (20mL) after first loose stool; 2 tsp (10mL) after each subsequent loose stool. **Max:** 8 tsp (40mL) q24h. **Peds 9-11 yrs (60-95 lbs):** 2 tsp (10mL) after the first loose stool; 1 tsp (5mL) after each subsequent loose stool. **Max:** 6 tsp (30mL) q24h. **Peds 6-8 yrs (48-59 lbs):** 2 tsp (10mL) after the first loose stool; 1 tsp (5mL) after each subsequent loose stool. **Max:** 4 tsp (20mL) q24h. |
| Imodium A-D Liquid For Use In Children (Mint Flavor) | Loperamide HCl 1mg/7.5mL | **Adults & Peds ≥12 yrs:** 6 tsp (30mL) after first loose stool; 3 tsp (15mL) after each subsequent loose stool. **Max:** 12 tsp (60mL) q24h. **Peds 9-11 yrs (60-95 lbs):** 3 tsp (15mL) after the first loose stool; 1½ tsp (7.5mL) after each subsequent loose stool. **Max:** 9 tsp (45mL) q24h. **Peds 6-8 yrs (48-59 lbs):** 3 tsp (15mL) after first loose stool; 1½ tsp (7.5mL) after each subsequent loose stool. **Max:** 6 tsp (30mL) q24h. |

*(Continued)*

| BRAND | INGREDIENT/STRENGTH | DOSE |
|---|---|---|
| **ANTIPERISTALTIC/ANTIFLATULENT AGENTS** | | |
| Imodium Multi-Symptom Relief Caplets | Loperamide HCl/Simethicone 2mg-125mg | **Adults & Peds ≥12 yrs:** 2 tabs after first loose stool; 1 tab after each subsequent loose stool. **Max:** 4 tabs q24h. **Peds 9-11 yrs (60-95 lbs):** 1 tab after first loose stool; ½ tab after each subsequent loose stool. **Max:** 3 tabs q24h. **6-8 yrs (48-59 lbs):** 1 tab after first loose stool; ½ tab after each subsequent loose stool. **Max:** 2 tabs q24h. |
| Imodium Multi-Symptom Relief Chewable Tablets | Loperamide HCl/Simethicone 2mg-125mg | **Adults & Peds ≥12 yrs:** 2 tabs with 4-8 oz water after first loose stool; 1 tab with 4-8 oz water after each subsequent loose stool. **Max:** 4 tabs q24h. **Peds 9-11 yrs (60-95 lbs):** 1 tab with 4-8 oz water after first loose stool; ½ tab after each subsequent loose stool. **Max:** 3 tabs q24h. **Peds 6-8 yrs (48-59 lbs):** 1 tab with 4-8 oz water after first loose stool; ½ tab with 4-8 oz water after each subsequent loose stool. **Max:** 2 tabs q24h. |
| **BISMUTH SUBSALICYLATE** | | |
| Kaopectate Extra Strength Liquid | Bismuth Subsalicylate 525mg/15mL | **Adults & Peds ≥12 yrs:** 2 tbl (30mL) q1h prn. **Max:** 4 doses (8 tbl) q24h. |
| Kaopectate Liquid | Bismuth Subsalicylate 262mg/15mL | **Adults & Peds ≥12 yrs:** 2 tbl (30mL) q½-1h prn. **Max:** 8 doses (16 tbl) q24h. |
| Maalox Total Relief Liquid | Bismuth Subsalicylate 525mg/15mL | **Adults & Peds ≥12 yrs:** 2 tbl (30mL) q1h prn. **Max:** 4 doses (8 tbl) q24h. |
| Pepto Bismol Caplets | Bismuth Subsalicylate 262mg | **Adults & Peds ≥12 yrs:** 2 tabs q½-1h. **Max:** 8 doses (16 tabs) q24h. |
| Pepto Bismol Chewable Tablets | Bismuth Subsalicylate 262mg | **Adults & Peds ≥12 yrs:** 2 tabs q½-1h. **Max:** 8 doses (16 tabs) q24h. |
| Pepto Bismol Liquid | Bismuth Subsalicylate 262mg/15mL | **Adults & Peds ≥12 yrs:** 2 tbl (30mL) q½-1h prn. **Max:** 8 doses (16 tbl) q24h. |
| Pepto Bismol Liquid Max | Bismuth Subsalicylate 525mg/15mL | **Adults & Peds ≥12 yrs:** 2 tbl (30mL) q1h prn. **Max:** 4 doses (8 tbl) q24h. |

# ANTIFLATULANT PRODUCTS

| BRAND | INGREDIENT/STRENGTH | DOSE |
|---|---|---|
| **ALPHA-GALACTOSIDASE** | | |
| Beano Food Enzyme Dietary Supplement Drops | Alpha-Galactosidase Enzyme 150 GalU (per 5 drops) | **Adults:** Add 5 drops to first bite of food serving. |
| Beano Food Enzyme Dietary Supplement Tablets | Alpha-Galactosidase Enzyme 150 GalU | **Adults:** Take 3 tabs before meals. |
| **ANTACID/ANTIFLATULANT** | | |
| Gas-X Extra Strength with Maalox Chewable Tablets | Calcium Carbonate/Simethicone 500mg-125mg | **Adults:** Chew 1-2 tabs prn. **Max:** 4 tabs q24h. |
| Gelusil Chewable Tablets | Aluminum Hydroxide/Magnesium Hydroxide/Simethicone 200mg-200mg-25mg | **Adults:** Chew 2-4 tabs q1h prn. **Max:** 12 tabs q24h. |
| Maalox Advanced Maximum Strength Liquid | Aluminum Hydroxide/Magnesium Hydroxide/Simethicone 400mg-400mg-40mg/5mL | **Adults & Peds ≥12 yrs:** 2-4 tsp (10-20mL) bid. **Max:** 8 tsp (40mL) q24h. |
| Maalox Advanced Maximum Strength Chewable Tablets | Calcium Carbonate/Simethicone 1000mg-60mg | **Adults & Peds ≥12 yrs:** Chew 1-2 tabs prn. **Max:** 8 tabs q24h. |
| Maalox Advanced Regular Strength Liquid | Aluminum Hydroxide/Magnesium Hydroxide/Simethicone 200mg-200mg-20mg/5mL | **Adults & Peds ≥12 yrs:** 2-4 tsp (10-20mL) qid. **Max:** 16 tsp (80mL) q24h. |
| Mylanta Maximum Strength Liquid | Aluminum Hydroxide/Magnesium Hydroxide/Simethicone 400mg-400mg-40mg/5mL | **Adults & Peds ≥12 yrs:** 2-4 tsp (10-20mL) between meals & hs. **Max:** 12 tsp (60mL) q24h. |
| Mylanta Regular Strength Liquid | Aluminum Hydroxide/Magnesium Hydroxide/Simethicone 200mg-200mg-20mg/5mL | **Adults & Peds ≥12 yrs:** 2-4 tsp (10-20mL) between meals & hs. **Max:** 24 tsp (120mL) q24h. |
| Rolaids Antacid & Antigas Soft Chews | Calcium Carbonate/Simethicone 1177mg-80mg | **Adults:** 2-3 chews hourly prn. **Max:** 6 chews q24h. |
| Rolaids Multi-Symptom Tablets | Calcium Carbonate/Magnesium Hydroxide/Simethicone 675mg-135mg-60mg | **Adults:** Chew 2-4 tabs hourly prn. **Max:** 8 tabs q24h. |
| Titralac Plus Chewable Tablets | Calcium Carbonate/Simethicone 420mg-21mg | **Adults:** Chew 2 tabs q2-3h prn. **Max:** 19 tabs q24h. |
| **SIMETHICONE** | | |
| GasAid Maximum Strength Anti-Gas Softgels | Simethicone 125mg | **Adults & Peds ≥12 yrs:** Take 1-2 caps prn and qhs. **Max:** 4 caps q24h. |
| Baby Gas-X Infant Drops | Simethicone 20mg/0.3mL | **Peds ≥2 yrs (≥24 lbs):** 0.6mL prn after meals and qhs. **Peds <2 yrs (<24 lbs):** 0.3mL prn after meals and qhs. **Max:** 6 doses q24h. |
| Gas-X Children's Thin Strips | Simethicone 40mg | **Peds 2-12 yrs:** 1 strip prn after meals and qhs. **Max:** 6 strips q24h. |
| Gas-X Thin Strips | Simethicone 62.5mg | **Adults:** Allow 2-4 strips to dissolve prn after meals and qhs. **Max:** 8 strips q24h. |
| Gas-X Antigas Chewable Tablets | Simethicone 80mg | **Adults:** Chew 1-2 tabs prn after meals and qhs. **Max:** 6 tabs q24h. |
| Gas-X Extra Strength Antigas Softgels | Simethicone 125mg | **Adults:** Take 1-2 caps prn after meals and qhs. **Max:** 4 caps q24h. |
| Gas-X Extra Strength Chewable Tablets | Simethicone 125mg | **Adults:** Chew 1-2 tabs prn after meals and qhs. **Max:** 4 tabs q24h. |

*(Continued)*

| BRAND | INGREDIENT/STRENGTH | DOSE |
|---|---|---|
| **SIMETHICONE** *(Continued)* | | |
| Gas-X Ultra Strength Softgels | Simethicone 180mg | **Adults:** Take 1-2 caps prn after meals and qhs. **Max:** 2 caps q24h. |
| Little Tummys Gas Relief Drops | Simethicone 20mg/0.3mL | **Peds ≥2 yrs (≥24 lbs):** 0.6mL prn (after meals & hs). **Peds <2 yrs (<24 lbs):** 0.3mL prn (after meals & hs). **Max:** 12 doses q24h. |
| Mylanta Gas Maximum Strength Softgels | Simethicone 125mg | **Adults:** Take 1-2 caps (after meals & hs). **Max:** 4 caps q24h. |
| Mylanta Gas Maximum Strength Chewable Tablets | Simethicone 125mg | **Adults:** Chew 1-2 tabs (after meals & hs). **Max:** 4 tabs q24h. |
| Mylicon Infants' Gas Relief Drops | Simethicone 20mg/0.3mL | **Peds ≥2 yrs (≥24 lbs):** 0.6mL (after meals & hs). **Peds <2 yrs (<24 lbs):** 0.3mL (after meals & hs). **Max:** 12 doses q24h. |

# LAXATIVE PRODUCTS

| BRAND | INGREDIENT/STRENGTH | DOSE |
|---|---|---|
| **BULK-FORMING** | | |
| Citrucel Caplets | Methylcellulose 500mg | **Adults & Peds ≥12 yrs:** 2 tabs qd prn. **Max:** 12 tabs q24h. **Peds 6-11 yrs:** 1 tab qd prn. **Max:** 6 tabs q24h. |
| Citrucel Powder | Methylcellulose 2g/tbl | **Adults & Peds ≥12 yrs:** 1 tbl (11.5g) qd-tid. **Peds 6-11 yrs:** ½ tbl (5.75g) qd. |
| Equalactin Chewable Tablets | Calcium Polycarbophil 625mg | **Adults & Peds ≥12 yrs:** 2 tabs qd. **Max:** 8 tabs q24h. **Peds 6-11 yrs:** 1 tab qd. **Max:** 4 tabs q24h. **Peds 2-5 yrs:** 1 tab qd. **Max:** 2 tabs q24h. |
| Fibercon Caplets | Calcium Polycarbophil 625mg | **Adults & Peds ≥12 yrs:** 2 tabs qd. **Max:** 8 tabs qd. |
| Konsyl Easy Mix Powder | Psyllium 4.3g/tsp | **Adults & Peds ≥12 yrs:** 1 tsp qd-tid. **Peds 6-11 yrs:** ½ tsp qd-tid. |
| Konsyl Fiber Caplets | Calcium Polycarbophil 625mg | **Adults:** 2 tabs qd-qid. **Max:** 8 tabs q24h. **Peds 6-12 yrs:** 1 tab qd-tid. **Max:** 3 tabs q24h. |
| Konsyl Orange Powder | Psyllium 3.4g/tbl | **Adults & Peds ≥12 yrs:** 1 tbl qd-tid. **Peds 6-11 yrs:** ½ tbl qd-tid. |
| Konsyl Original Powder | Psyllium 6g/tsp | **Adults & Peds ≥12 yrs:** 1 tsp qd-tid. **Peds 6-11 yrs:** ½ tsp qd-tid. |
| Konsyl-D Powder | Psyllium 3.4g/tsp | **Adults & Peds ≥12 yrs:** 1 tsp qd-tid. **Peds 6-11 yrs:** ½ tsp qd-tid. |
| Metamucil Capsules | Psyllium 0.52g | **Adults & Peds ≥12 yrs:** 5 caps qd-tid. |
| Metamucil Original Texture Powder (multi-flavor) | Psyllium 3.4g/tbl | **Adults & Peds ≥12 yrs:** 1 tbl up to tid. **Peds 6-11 yrs:** ½ tbl up to tid. |
| Metamucil Smooth Texture Powder (multi-flavor) | Psyllium 3.4g/tbl | **Adults & Peds ≥12 yrs:** 1 tbl up to tid. **Peds 6-11 yrs:** ½ tbl up to tid. |
| Metamucil Wafers | Psyllium 3.4g/dose | **Adults & Peds ≥12 yrs:** 2 wafers qd-tid. **Peds 6-11 yrs:** 1 wafer qd-tid. |
| **HYPEROSMOTICS** | | |
| Colace Glycerin Suppositories for Adults and Children | Glycerin 2.1g | **Adults & Peds ≥6 yrs:** 1 supp. **Max:** 1 supp. q24h. |
| Colace Glycerin Suppositories for Infants and Children | Glycerin 1.2g | **Peds 2-5 yrs:** 1 supp. **Max:** 1 supp. q24h. |
| Dulcolax Balance | Polyethylene Glycol 3350, 17g | **Adults & Peds ≥17 yrs:** 1 capful (17g) qd. **Max:** 7 days. |
| Fleet Glycerin Suppositories | Glycerin 2g | **Adults & Peds ≥6 yrs:** 1 supp. ud. |
| Fleet Liquid Glycerin Suppositories | Glycerin 5.6g | **Adults & Peds ≥6 yrs:** 1 supp. ud. |
| Fleet Mineral Oil Enema | Mineral Oil 118mL | **Adults & Peds ≥12 yrs:** 1 bottle (118mL). **Peds 2-11 yrs:** ½ bottle (59mL). |
| Fleet Pedia-Lax Glycerin Suppositories | Glycerin 1g | **Peds 2-6 yrs:** 1 supp. ud. |
| Fleet Pedia-Lax Liquid Glycerin Suppositories | Glycerin 2.3g | **Peds 2-6 yrs:** 1 supp. ud. |

*(Continued)*

| BRAND | INGREDIENT/STRENGTH | DOSE |
|---|---|---|
| **SALINES** | | |
| Fleet Enema | Monobasic Sodium Phosphate/Dibasic Sodium Phosphate 19g-7g/118mL | **Adults & Peds ≥12 yrs:** 1 bottle (118mL). |
| Fleet Enema Extra | Monobasic Sodium Phosphate/Dibasic Sodium Phosphate 19g-7g/197mL | **Adults & Peds ≥12 yrs:** 1 bottle (197mL). |
| Fleet Pedia-Lax Chewable Tablets | Magnesium Hydroxide 400mg | **Peds 6-<12 yrs:** 3-6 tabs qd. **Max:** 6 tabs q24h. **Peds 2-<6 yrs:** 1-3 tabs qd. **Max:** 3 tabs q24h. |
| Fleet Pedia-Lax Enema | Monobasic Sodium Phosphate/Dibasic Sodium Phosphate 9.5g-3.5g/59mL | **Peds 5-11 yrs:** 1 bottle (59mL). **Peds 2-<5 yrs:** ½ bottle (29.5mL). |
| Magnesium Citrate Solution | Magnesium Citrate 1.75g/30mL | **Adults & Peds ≥12 yrs:** 300mL. **Peds 6-<12 yrs:** 90-210mL. **Peds 2-<6 yrs:** 60mL. |
| Little Phillips' Milk of Magnesia Safe and Gentle | Magnesium Hydroxide 800mg/5mL | **Adults & Peds ≥12 yrs:** 3-6 tsp qd. **Peds 6-11 yrs:** 1.5-3 tsp qd. **Peds 2-5 yrs:** 1/2-1.5 tsp qd. |
| Phillips' Antacid/Laxative Chewable Tablets | Magnesium Hydroxide 311mg | **Adults & Peds ≥12 yrs:** 8 tabs qd. **Peds 6-11 yrs:** 4 tabs qd. **Peds 3-5 yrs:** 2 tabs qd. |
| Phillips' Cramp-Free Laxative Caplets | Magnesium 500mg | **Adults & Peds ≥12 yrs:** Take 2-4 tabs qd. **Max:** 4 tabs q24h. |
| Phillips' Milk of Magnesia Concentrated Liquid | Magnesium Hydroxide 800mg/5mL | **Adults & Peds ≥12 yrs:** 1-2 tbl qd. **Peds 6-11 yrs:** ½-1 tbl qd. |
| Phillips' Milk of Magnesia Liquid | Magnesium Hydroxide 400mg/5mL | **Adults & Peds ≥12 yrs:** 2-4 tbl qd. **Peds 6-11 yrs:** 1-2 tbl qd. |
| **SALINE COMBINATION** | | |
| Phillips' M-O Liquid | Magnesium Hydroxide/Mineral Oil 300mg-1.25mL/5mL | **Adults & Peds ≥12 yrs:** 3-4 tbl qd. **Peds 6-11 yrs:** 4-6 tsp qd. |
| **STIMULANTS** | | |
| Alophen Enteric Coated Stimulant Laxative Pills | Bisacodyl 5mg | **Adults & Peds ≥12 yrs:** Take 1-3 tabs qd. **Peds 6-11 yrs:** Take 1 tab qd. |
| Carter's Laxative, Sodium Free Pills | Bisacodyl 5mg | **Adults & Peds ≥12 yrs:** Take 1-3 tabs (usually 2 tabs) qd. **Peds 6-<12 yrs:** Take 1 tab qd. |
| Castor Oil | Castor Oil | **Adults & Peds ≥12 yrs:** 15-60mL. **Peds 2-<12 yrs:** 5-15mL. |
| Dulcolax Suppository | Bisacodyl 10mg | **Adults & Peds ≥12 yrs:** 1 supp. qd. **Peds 6-<12 yrs:** ½ supp. qd. |
| Dulcolax Tablets | Bisacodyl 5mg | **Adults & Peds ≥12 yrs:** 1-3 tabs qd. **Peds 6-<12 yrs:** 1 tab qd. |
| Ex-Lax Maximum Strength Tablets | Sennosides 25mg | **Adults & Peds ≥12 yrs:** 2 tabs qd-bid. **Peds 6-<12 yrs:** 1 tab qd-bid. |
| Ex-Lax Tablets | Sennosides 15mg | **Adults & Peds ≥12 yrs:** 2 tabs qd-bid. **Peds 6-<12 yrs:** 1 tab qd-bid. |
| Ex-Lax Ultra Stimulant Laxative Tablets | Bisacodyl 5mg | **Adults & Peds ≥12 yrs:** 1-3 tabs qd. **Peds 6-<12 yrs:** 1 tab qd-bid. |
| Fleet Bisacodyl Enema | Bisacodyl 10mg/30mL | **Adults & Peds ≥12 yrs:** 1 bottle (30mL). |
| Fleet Bisacodyl Suppositories | Bisacodyl 10mg | **Adults & Peds ≥12 yrs:** 1 supp. qd. **Peds 6-<12 yrs:** ½ supp. qd. |

*(Continued)*

| BRAND | INGREDIENT/STRENGTH | DOSE |
|---|---|---|
| **STIMULANTS** *(Continued)* | | |
| Fleet Pedia-Lax Quick Dissolve Strips | Sennosides 8.6mg | **Peds 6-<12 yrs:** 2 strips. **Max:** 4 strips q24h. **Peds 2-<6 yrs:** 1 strip. **Max:** 2 strips q24h. |
| Fleet Stimulant Laxative Tablets | Bisacodyl 5mg | **Adults & Peds ≥12 yrs:** 1-3 tabs qd. **Peds 6-<12 yrs:** 1 tab qd. |
| Perdiem Overnight Relief Tablets | Sennosides 15mg | **Adults & Peds ≥12 yrs:** 2 tabs qd-bid. **Peds 6-<12 yrs:** 1 tab qd-bid. |
| Senokot Tablets | Sennosides 8.6mg | **Adults & Peds ≥12 yrs:** 2 tabs qd. **Max:** 4 tabs bid. **Peds 6-<12 yrs:** 1 tab qd. **Max:** 2 tabs bid. **Peds 2-<6 yrs:** ½ tab qd. **Max:** 1 tab bid. |
| SenokotXTRA Tablets | Sennosides 17.2mg | **Adults & Peds ≥6 yrs:** Starting dose 1 tab qd. **Max:** 2 tabs bid. **Peds 2-<6 yrs:** ½ tab qd. **Max:** 1 tab bid. |
| **STIMULANT COMBINATIONS** | | |
| Konsyl Senna Prompt | Psyllium/Sennosides 500mg-9mg | **Adults & Peds ≥12 yrs:** 1-5 caps qd-bid. |
| Peri-Colace Tablets | Sennosides/Docusate 8.6mg-50mg | **Adults & Peds ≥12 yrs:** 2-4 tabs qd. **Peds 6-<12 yrs:** 1-2 tabs qd. **Peds 2-5 yrs:** 1 tab qd. |
| Senokot S Tablets | Sennosides/Docusate 8.6mg-50mg | **Adults ≥12 yrs:** 2 tabs qd. **Max:** 4 tabs bid. **Peds 6-<12 yrs:** 1 tab qd. **Max:** 2 tabs bid. **Peds 2-<6 yrs:** ½ tab qd. **Max:** 1 tab bid. |
| **SURFACTANTS (STOOL SOFTENERS)** | | |
| Colace Capsules | Docusate Sodium 100mg | **Adults & Peds ≥12 yrs:** 1-3 caps qd. **Peds 2-<12 yrs:** 1 cap qd. |
| Colace Capsules | Docusate Sodium 50mg | **Adults & Peds ≥12 yrs:** 1-6 caps qd. **Peds 2-<12 yrs:** 1-3 caps qd. |
| Colace Liquid | Docusate Sodium 10mg/mL | **Adults & Peds ≥12 yrs:** 5-15mL qd-bid. **Peds 2-<12 yrs:** 5-15mL qd. |
| Colace Syrup | Docusate Sodium 60mg/15mL | **Adults & Peds ≥12 yrs:** 1-6 tbl qd. **Peds 2-<12 yrs:** 1-2½ tbl qd. |
| Docusol Constipation Relief, Mini Enemas | Docusate Sodium 283mg | **Adults & Peds ≥12 yrs:** Take 1-3 units qd. **Peds 6-12 yrs:** Take 1 unit qd. |
| Dulcolax Stool Softener Capsules | Docusate Sodium 100mg | **Adults & Peds ≥12 yrs:** 1-3 caps qd. **Peds 2-<12 yrs:** 1 cap qd. |
| Fleet Pedia-Lax Liquid Stool Softener | Docusate 50mg/15mL | **Peds 2-12 yrs:** 1-3 tbl qd. **Max:** 3 tbl q24h. |
| Fleet Sof-Lax | Docusate 100mg | **Adults & Peds ≥12 yrs:** 1-3 caps qd. **Peds 2-<12 yrs:** 1 cap qd. |
| Kaopectate Liqui-Gels | Docusate Calcium 240mg | **Adults & Peds ≥12 yrs:** 1 cap qd until normal bowel movement. |
| Phillips' Stool Softener Capsules | Docusate Sodium 100mg | **Adults & Peds ≥12 yrs:** 1-3 caps qd. **Peds 6-<12 yrs:** 1 cap qd. |

# ALLERGIC RHINITIS PRODUCTS

| BRAND | INGREDIENT/STRENGTH | DOSE |
|---|---|---|
| **ANTIHISTAMINE** | | |
| Alavert Quick Dissolving Tablets | Loratadine 10mg | **Adults & Peds ≥6 yrs:** 1 tab qd. **Max:** 1 tab q24h. |
| Alavert For Kids 6+ | Loratadine 10mg | **Adults & Peds ≥6 yrs:** 1 tab qd. **Max:** 1 tab q24h. |
| Alavert Tablets | Loratadine 10mg | **Adults & Peds ≥6 yrs:** 1 tab qd. **Max:** 1 tab q24h. |
| Benadryl Allergy Quick Dissolve Strips | Diphenhydramine HCl 25mg | **Adults & Peds ≥12 yrs:** Dissolve 1-2 strips on tongue q4-6h. **Peds 6-<12 yrs:** Dissolve 1 strip on tongue q4-6h. **Max:** 6 doses q24h. |
| Benadryl Allergy Kapgels | Diphenhydramine HCl 25mg | **Adults & Peds ≥12 yrs: 1-2 caps** q4-6h. **Peds 6-<12 yrs:** 1 cap q4-6h. **Max:** 6 doses q24h. |
| Benadryl Allergy Ultratab Tablets | Diphenhydramine HCl 25mg | **Adults & Peds ≥12 yrs:** 1-2 tabs q4-6h. **Peds 6-<12 yrs:** 1 tab q4-6h. **Max:** 6 doses q24h. |
| Benadryl Dye-Free Allergy Liqui-Gels | Diphenhydramine HCl 25mg | **Adults & Peds ≥12 yrs:** 1-2 caps q4-6h. **Peds 6-<12 yrs:** 1 cap q4-6h. **Max:** 6 doses q24h. |
| Children's Benadryl Allergy Fastmelt Tablets | Diphenhydramine HCl 12.5mg | **Adults & Peds ≥12 yrs:** 2-4 tabs q4-6h. **Peds 6-<12 yrs:** 1-2 tabs q4-6h. **Max:** 6 doses q24h. |
| Children's Benadryl Perfect Measure Pre-Filled Single Use Spoons | Diphenhydramine HCl 12.5mg/5mL | **Adults & Peds ≥12 yrs:** 2-4 pre-filled spoons (10-20mL) q4-6h. **Peds 6-<12 yrs:** 1-2 pre-filled spoons (5-10mL) q4-6h. **Max:** 6 doses q24h. |
| Children's Benadryl Allergy Liquid | Diphenhydramine HCl 12.5mg/5mL | **Peds 6-<12 yrs:** 1-2 tsp (5-10mL) q4-6h. **Max:** 6 doses q24h. |
| Children's Benadryl Dye-Free Allergy Liquid | Diphenhydramine HCl 12.5mg/5mL | **Peds 6-<12 yrs:** 1-2 tsp (5-10mL) q4-6h. **Max:** 6 doses q24h. |
| Claritin Tablets | Loratadine 10mg | **Adults & Peds ≥6 yrs:** 1 tab qd. **Max:** 1 tab q24h. |
| Claritin Liqui-Gels | Loratadine 10mg | **Adults & Peds ≥6 yrs:** 1 tab qd. **Max:** 1 tab q24h. |
| Claritin RediTabs 24-Hour | Loratadine 10mg | **Adults & Peds ≥6 yrs:** 1 tab qd. **Max:** 1 tab q24h. |
| Claritin 12-Hour RediTabs | Loratadine 5mg | **Adults & Peds ≥6 yrs:** 1 tab q12h. **Max:** 2 tabs q24h. |
| Claritin 24-Hour RediTabs For Kids | Loratadine 10mg | **Adults & Peds ≥6 yrs:** 1 tab qd. **Max:** 1 tab q24h. |
| Claritin 12-Hour RediTabs For Kids | Loratadine 5mg | **Adults & Peds ≥6 yrs:** 1 tab q12h. **Max:** 2 tabs q24h. |
| Children's Claritin Chewables | Loratadine 5mg | **Adults & Peds ≥6 yrs:** 2 tabs qd. **Max:** 2 tabs q24h. **Peds 2-<6 yrs:** 1 tab qd. **Max:** 1 tab q24h. |
| Children's Claritin Syrup | Loratadine 5mg/5mL | **Adults & Peds ≥6 yrs:** 2 tsp (10mL) qd. **Max:** 2 tsp q24h. **Peds 2-<6 yrs:** 1 tsp (5mL) qd. **Max:** 1 tsp q24h. |
| Zyrtec Tablets | Cetirizine HCl 10mg | **Adults & Peds 6-<65 yrs:** 1 tab qd. **Max:** 1 tab q24h. |
| Children's Zyrtec Chewable 5mg | Cetirizine HCl 5mg | **Adults & Peds 6-<65 yrs:** 1-2 tabs qd. **Max:** 2 tabs q24h. **Adults ≥65 yrs:** 1 tab qd. **Max:** 1 tab q24h. |

*(Continued)*

| BRAND | INGREDIENT/STRENGTH | DOSE |
|---|---|---|
| **ANTIHISTAMINE** *(Continued)* | | |
| Children's Zyrtec Chewable 10mg | Cetirizine HCl 10mg | **Adults & Peds 6-<65 yrs:** 1 tab qd. **Max:** 1 tab q24h. |
| Children's Zyrtec Perfect Measure | Cetirizine HCl 5mg/5mL | **Adults & Peds 6-<65 yrs:** 1-2 prefilled spoons (5-10mL) qd. **Max:** 2 prefilled spoons q24h. **Adults ≥65 yrs:** 1 prefilled spoon (5mL) qd. **Max:** 1 prefilled spoon q24h. |
| Children's Zyrtec Allergy Syrup | Cetirizine HCl 5mg/5mL | **Adults & Peds 6-<65 yrs:** 1-2 tsp (5-10mL) qd. **Max:** 2 tsp q24h. **Adults ≥65 yrs:** 1 tsp qd. **Max:** 1 tsp q24h. **Peds 2-<6 yrs:** ½-1 tsp (2.5-5mL) qd or ½ tsp q12h. **Max:** 1 tsp q24h. |
| **ANTIHISTAMINE COMBINATIONS** | | |
| Advil Allergy Sinus Caplets | Chlorpheniramine Maleate/ Ibuprofen/Pseudoephedrine HCl 2mg-200mg-30mg | **Adults & Peds ≥12 yrs:** 1 tab q4-6h. **Max:** 6 tabs q24h. |
| Alavert Allergy & Sinus D-12 | Loratadine/Pseudoephedrine Sulfate 5mg-120mg | **Adults & Peds ≥12 yrs:** 1 tab q12h. **Max:** 2 tabs q24h. |
| Allerest PE | Chlorpheniramine Maleate/ Phenylephrine HCl 4mg-10mg | **Adults & Peds ≥12 yrs:** 1 tab q4h. **Peds 6-<12 yrs:** ½ tab q4h **Max:** 6 doses q24h. |
| Benadryl-D Allergy Plus Sinus | Diphenhydramine HCl/ Phenylephrine HCl 25mg-10mg | **Adults & Peds ≥12 yrs:** 1 tab q4h. **Max:** 6 tabs q24h. |
| Benadryl Severe Allergy Plus Sinus Headache Caplets | Diphenhydramine HCl/ Acetaminophen/Phenylephrine HCl 25mg-325mg-5mg | **Adults & Peds ≥12 yrs:** 2 tabs q4h. **Max:** 12 tabs q24h. |
| Benadryl Severe Allergy Plus Sinus Headache Kapgels | Diphenhydramine HCl/ Acetaminophen/Phenylephrine HCl 12.5mg-325mg-5mg | **Adults & Peds ≥12 yrs:** 2 caps q4h. **Max:** 12 caps q24h. |
| Benadryl Severe Allergy Plus Cold Kapgels | Diphenhydramine HCl/ Acetaminophen/Phenylephrine HCl 12.5mg-325mg-5mg | **Adults & Peds ≥12 yrs:** 2 caps q4h. **Max:** 12 caps q24h. |
| Children's Benadryl-D Allergy & Sinus Liquid | Diphenhydramine HCl/ Phenylephrine HCl 12.5mg-5mg/5mL | **Adults & Peds ≥12 yrs:** 2 tsp (10mL) q4h. **Peds 6-<12 yrs:** 1 tsp (5mL) q4h. **Max:** 6 doses q24h. |
| Claritin-D 12 Hour | Loratadine/Pseudoephedrine Sulfate 5mg-120mg | **Adults & Peds ≥12 yrs:** 1 tab q12h. **Max:** 2 tabs q24h. |
| Claritin-D 24 Hour | Loratadine/Pseudoephedrine Sulfate 10mg-240mg | **Adults & Peds ≥12 yrs:** 1 tab qd. **Max:** 1 tab q24h. |
| Children's Dimetapp Cold & Allergy Chewable Tablets | Brompheniramine Maleate/ Phenylephrine HCl 1mg-2.5mg | **Peds 6-<12 yrs:** 2 tabs q4h. **Max:** 6 doses q24h. |
| Children's Dimetapp Cold & Allergy Syrup | Brompheniramine Maleate/ Phenylephrine HCl 1mg-2.5mg/5mL | **Adults & Peds ≥12 yrs:** 4 tsp (20mL) q4h. **Peds 6-<12 yrs:** 2 tsp (10mL) q4h. **Max:** 6 doses q24h. |
| Sudafed PE Maximum Sinus & Allergy Tablets | Chlorpheniramine Maleate/ Phenylephrine HCl 4mg-10mg | **Adults & Peds ≥12 yrs:** 1 tab q4h. **Max:** 6 tabs q24h. |
| Tylenol Sinus Congestion and Pain Nighttime | Chlorpheniramine Maleate/ Acetaminophen/Phenylephrine HCl 2mg-325mg-5mg | **Adults & Peds ≥12 yrs:** 2 tabs q4h. **Max:** 12 tabs q24h. |
| Tylenol Allergy Multi-Symptom | Chlorpheniramine Maleate/ Acetaminophen/Phenylephrine HCl 2mg-325mg-5mg | **Adults & Peds ≥12 yrs:** 2 tabs q4h. **Max:** 12 tabs q24h. |
| Tylenol Allergy Multi-Symptom Nighttime | Diphenhydramine HCl/ Acetaminophen/Phenylephrine HCl 25mg-325mg-5mg | **Adults & Peds ≥12 yrs:** 2 tabs q4h. **Max:** 12 tabs q24h. |

*(Continued)*

| BRAND | INGREDIENT/STRENGTH | DOSE |
|---|---|---|
| **ANTIHISTAMINE COMBINATIONS** *(Continued)* | | |
| Tylenol Severe Allergy | Diphenhydramine HCl/ Acetaminophen 12.5mg-500mg | **Adults & Peds ≥12 yrs:** 2 tabs q4-6h. **Max:** 8 tabs q24h. |
| Zyrtec-D Tablets | Cetirizine HCl/ Pseudoephedrine HCl 5mg-120mg | **Adults & Peds 12-<65 yrs:** 1 tab q12h. **Max:** 2 tabs q24h. |
| **TOPICAL NASAL DECONGESTANTS** | | |
| 4-Way Fast Acting Nasal Decongestant Spray | Phenylephrine HCl 1% | **Adults & Peds ≥12 yrs:** Instill 2-3 sprays per nostril q4h. |
| 4-Way Mentholated Nasal Decongestant Spray | Phenylephrine HCl 1% | **Adults & Peds ≥12 yrs:** Instill 2-3 sprays per nostril q4h. |
| Afrin Original 12 Hour Pump Mist | Oxymetazoline HCl 0.05% | **Adults & Peds ≥6 yrs:** Instill 2-3 sprays per nostril q10-12h. **Max:** 2 doses q24h. |
| Afrin Extra Moisturizing 12 Hour Pump Mist | Oxymetazoline HCl 0.05% | **Adults & Peds ≥6 yrs:** Instill 2-3 sprays per nostril q10-12h. **Max:** 2 doses q24h. |
| Afrin All Night 12 Hour Pump Mist | Oxymetazoline HCl 0.05% | **Adults & Peds ≥6 yrs:** Instill 2-3 sprays per nostril q10-12h. **Max:** 2 doses q24h. |
| Afrin Sinus 12 Hour Pump Mist | Oxymetazoline HCl 0.05% | **Adults & Peds ≥6 yrs:** Instill 2-3 sprays per nostril q10-12h. **Max:** 2 doses q24h. |
| Afrin Severe Congestion 12 Hour Pump Mist | Oxymetazoline HCl 0.05% | **Adults & Peds ≥6 yrs:** Instill 2-3 sprays per nostril q10-12h. **Max:** 2 doses q24h. |
| Benzedrex Inhaler | Propylhexedrine 250mg | **Adults & Peds ≥6 yrs:** Inhale 2 sprays per nostril q2h. |
| Dristan 12-hr Nasal Spray | Oxymetazoline HCl 0.05% | **Adults & Peds ≥12 yrs:** Instill 2-3 sprays per nostril q10-12h. **Max:** 2 doses q24h. |
| Little Noses Decongestant Nose Drops | Phenylephrine HCl 0.125% | **Peds 2-<6 yrs:** Instill 2-3 sprays per nostril q4h. **Max:** 2 doses q24h. |
| Mucinex Moisture Smart Nasal Spray | Oxymetazoline HCl 0.05% | **Adults & Peds ≥6 yrs:** Instill 2-3 sprays per nostril q10-12h. **Max:** 2 doses q24h. |
| Mucinex Full Force Nasal Spray | Oxymetazoline HCl 0.05% | **Adults & Peds ≥6 yrs:** Instill 2-3 sprays per nostril q10-12h. **Max:** 2 doses q24h. |
| Neo-Synephrine Regular Strength Nasal Spray | Phenylephrine HCl 0.5% | **Adults & Peds ≥12 yrs:** Instill 2-3 sprays per nostril q4h. |
| Neo-Synephrine Extra Strength Nasal Spray | Phenylephrine HCl 1% | **Adults & Peds ≥12 yrs:** Instill 2-3 sprays per nostril q4h. |
| Neo-Synephrine Nighttime Nasal Spray | Oxymetazoline HCl 0.05% | **Adults & Peds ≥≥6 yrs:** Instill 2-3 sprays per nostril q10-12h. **Max:** 2 doses q24h. |
| Nostrilla Fast Relief | Oxymetazoline HCl 0.05% | **Adults & Peds ≥6 yrs:** Instill 2-3 sprays per nostril q10-12h. **Max:** 2 doses q24h. |
| Nostrilla Complete Congestion Relief | Oxymetazoline HCl 0.05% | **Adults & Peds ≥6 yrs:** Instill 2-3 sprays per nostril q10-12h. **Max:** 2 doses q24h. |
| Privine Nasal Drops | Naphazoline HCl 0.05% | **Adults & Peds ≥12 yrs:** Instill 1-2 sprays per nostril q6h. |
| Privine Nasal Spray | Naphazoline HCl 0.05% | **Adults & Peds ≥12 yrs:** Instill 1-2 sprays per nostril q6h. |
| Sudafed OM Sinus Congestion Spray | Oxymetazoline HCl 0.05% | **Adults & Peds ≥6 yrs:** Instill 2-3 sprays per nostril q10-12h. **Max:** 2 doses q24h. |

*(Continued)*

| BRAND | INGREDIENT/STRENGTH | DOSE |
|---|---|---|
| **TOPICAL NASAL DECONGESTANTS** *(Continued)* | | |
| Sudafed OM Sinus Cold Spray | Oxymetazoline HCl 0.05% | **Adults & Peds ≥6 yrs:** Instill 2-3 sprays per nostril q10-12h. **Max:** 2 doses q24h. |
| Vicks Sinex VapoSpray 12-Hour Decongestant UltraFine Mist | Oxymetazoline HCl 0.05% | **Adults & Peds ≥6 yrs:** Instill 2-3 sprays per nostril q10-12h. **Max:** 2 doses q24h. |
| Vicks Sinex VapoSpray 12-Hour Decongestant Nasal Spray | Oxymetazoline HCl 0.05% | **Adults & Peds ≥6 yrs:** Instill 2-3 sprays per nostril q10-12h. **Max:** 2 doses q24h. |
| Vicks Sinex VapoSpray 4-Hour | Phenylephrine HCl 0.5% | **Adults & Peds ≥12 yrs:** Instill 2-3 sprays per nostril q4h. |
| Vicks VapoInhaler | Levmetamfetamine 50mg | **Adults & Peds ≥12 yrs:** Inhale 2 sprays per nostril q2h. **Peds 6-<12 yrs:** Inhale 1 spray per nostril q2h. |
| Zicam Extreme Congestion Relief Nasal Gel | Oxymetazoline HCl 0.05% | **Adults & Peds ≥6 yrs:** Instill 2-3 sprays per nostril q10-12h. **Max:** 2 doses q24h. |
| Zicam Intense Sinus Relief Nasal Gel | Oxymetazoline HCl 0.05% | **Adults & Peds ≥6 yrs:** Instill 2-3 sprays per nostril q10-12h. **Max:** 2 doses q24h. |
| **TOPICAL NASAL MOISTURIZERS** | | |
| 4-Way Saline Moisturizing Mist | Water, Boric Acid, Glycerin, Sodium Chloride, Sodium Borate, Eucalyptol, Menthol, Polysorbate 80, Benzalkonium Chloride | **Adults & Peds ≥2 yrs:** Instill 2-3 sprays per nostril prn. |
| Afrin PureSea Medium Stream | Sea Water | **Adults & Peds ≥2 yrs:** Use to rinse nostrils qid. |
| Afrin PureSea Gentle Mist | Sea Water | **Adults & Peds ≥2 yrs:** Use to rinse nostrils qid. |
| Afrin PureSea Ultra-Gentle Mist | Sea Water | **Peds ≥6 mos:** Use to rinse nostrils qid. |
| Ayr Saline Nasal Mist | Sodium Chloride 0.65% | **Adults & Peds:** Instill 1 spray per nostril prn. |
| Ayr Saline Nasal Drops | Sodium Chloride 0.65% | **Adults & Peds:** Instill 2-6 drops per nostril prn |
| Ayr Allergy & Sinus Hypertonic Saline Nasal Mist | Sodium Chloride 2.65% | **Adults & Peds:** Instill 2 sprays per nostril bid-tid |
| Baby Ayr Saline Nose Spray/Drops | Sodium Chloride 0.65% | **Peds:** Instill 2-6 drops per nostril. |
| Ayr Saline Nasal Gel No-Drip Sinus Spray | Water, Sodium Carbomethyl Starch, Propylene Glycol, Glycerin, *Aloe Barbadensis* Leaf Juice (Aloe Vera), Sodium Chloride, Cetylpyridinium Chloride, Citric Acid, Disodium EDTA, *Glycine Soja* (Soybean) Oil, Tocopheryl Acetate, Benzyl Alcohol, Benzalkonium Chloride, *Geranium Maculatum* Oil | **Adults & Peds:** Instill 1 spray per nostril. |
| Ayr Saline Nasal Gel | Water, Methyl Gluceth-10, Propylene Glycol, Glycerin, Glyceryl Polymethacrylate, Triethanolamine, *Aloe Barbadensis* Leaf Juice (Aloe Vera Gel), PEG/PPG-18/18 Dimethicone, Carbomer, Poloxamer 184, Sodium Chloride, Xanthan Gum, Diazolidinyl Urea, Methylparaben, Propylparaben, *Glycine Soja* (Soybean) Oil, *Geranium Maculatum* Oil, Tocopheryl Acetate, Blue 1 | **Adults & Peds:** Apply around nostrils and under nose prn. |

*(Continued)*

| BRAND | INGREDIENT/STRENGTH | DOSE |
|---|---|---|
| **TOPICAL NASAL MOISTURIZERS** *(Continued)* | | |
| Ayr Saline Nasal Gel Swabs | Water, Methyl Gluceth-10, Propylene Glycol, Glycerin, Glyceryl Polymethacrylate, Triethanolamine, *Aloe Barbadensis* Leaf Juice (Aloe Vera Gel), PEG/PPG-18/18 Dimethicone, Carbomer, Poloxamer 184, Sodium Chloride, Xanthan Gum, Diazolidinyl Urea, Methylparaben, Propylparaben, *Glycine Soja* (Soybean) Oil, *Geranium Maculatum* Oil, Tocopheryl Acetate, Blue 1 | **Adults & Peds:** Apply around nostrils and under nose prn. |
| Little Noses Saline Spray/Drops | Sodium Chloride 0.65% | **Adults & Peds:** Instill 2-6 drops/sprays per nostril prn. |
| Little Noses Sterile Saline Nasal Mist | Sodium Chloride 0.9% | **Adults & Peds:** Instill 1-3 short sprays per nostril prn. |
| Nostrilla Conditioning Double-Moisture | Benzalkonium Chloride Solution, Carboxymethylcellulose Sodium, Eucalyptol, Glycine, Hyaluronic Acid Sodium, Polyethylene Glycol, Povidone, Propylene Glycol, Sodium Chloride (as 1.9% saline solution), Spearmint Oil, Wintergreen Oil, Water | **Adults & Peds:** Instill 1-2 sprays per nostril bid. |
| Ocean Gel Ultra Moisturizing Gel | Purified water, Glycerin, Carbomer 940, Trolamine, Hyaluranon, Methlyparaben, Propylparaben | **Adults & Peds:** Apply around nostrils and under nose prn. |
| Ocean Sinus Irrigation | Purified Water, Glycerin, Sodium Chloride, Monobasic Sodium Phosphate, Dibasic Sodium Phosphate, Potassium Chloride, Calcium Chloride, Magnesium Chloride | **Adults & Peds:** Attach white actuator and spray into each nostril prn. |
| Ocean Ultra Sterile Saline Mist | Purified Water, Glycerin, Sodium Chloride, Monobasic Sodium Phosphate, Sodium Hyaluronan, Dibasic Sodium Phosphate, Potassium Chloride, Calcium Chloride, Magnesium Chloride | **Adults & Peds:** Spray into each nostril prn. |
| Ocean for Kids Premium Saline Nasal Spray | Sodium Chloride 0.65%, Purified Water, Glycerin, Sodium Phosphate Monobasic, Sodium EDTA, Benzalkonium Chloride | **Peds:** Instill 2 sprays per nostril prn. |
| Ocean Premium Saline Nasal Spray | Sodium Chloride 0.65% | **Adults & Peds:** Instill 2 sprays per nostril prn. |
| Simply Saline Nasal Mist | Sodium Chloride 0.9% | **Adults & Peds:** Spray into each nostril prn. |
| Baby Simply Saline Sterile Saline Mist | Sodium Chloride 0.9% | **Peds:** Spray into each nostril prn. |
| Simply Saline Nasal Moist Gel | Propylene Glycol, Hydroxyethylcellulose, Aloe Vera, Sodium Chloride, Allantoin, Methylparaben, Propylparaben, Purified Water | **Adults & Peds:**: Apply around nostrils and under nose prn. |

*(Continued)*

| BRAND | INGREDIENT/STRENGTH | DOSE |
|---|---|---|
| **MISCELLANEOUS** | | |
| NasalCrom Nasal Spray | Cromolyn Sodium 5.2 mg | **Adults & Peds ≥2 yrs:** Instill 1 spray per nostril q4-6h. **Max:** 6 doses q24h. |
| Similasan Hay Fever Relief Nasal Spray | *Cardiospermum* 6X, *Galphimia glauca* 6X, *Luffa operculata* 6X, *Sabadilla* 6X | **Adults & Peds:** Instill 1-3 sprays per nostril prn. |
| SinoFresh Nasal & Sinus Care | *Eucalyptus Globulus* 20x, *Kalium Bichromicum* 30x | **Adults:** Instill 1-2 sprays per nostril every morning and evening. Gently sniff to distribute solution. Blow nose to clear it of loosened debris and mucus. Re-apply 1 spray to each nostril. |
| Zicam Allergy Relief Nasal Gel | *Luffa Operculata* (4x, 12x, 30x), *Galphimia Glauca* (12x, 30x), *Histaminum Hydrochloricum* (12x, 30x, 200x), *Sulphur* (12x, 30x, 200x) | **Adults & Peds ≥6 yrs:** Instill 1 spray per nostril q4h. |
| Zicam Allergy Relief Gel Swabs | *Galphimia Glauca* (12x, 30x), *Histaminum Hydrochloricum* (12x, 30x, 200x), *Luffa Operculata* (4x, 12x, 30x), *Sulphur* (12x, 30x, 200x) | **Adults & Peds ≥6 yrs:** Apply medication just inside first nostril. Remove swab and press lightly on the outside of first nostril for 5 sec. Re-dip swab in tube and repeat with 2nd nostril. |

# IS IT A COLD, THE FLU, OR AN ALLERGY?

| | COLD | FLU | AIRBORNE ALLERGY |
|---|---|---|---|
| **SYMPTOMS** | | | |
| Chest discomfort | Mild to moderate | Common; can become severe | Sometimes |
| Cough | Common (hacking cough) | Sometimes | Sometimes |
| Duration | 3-14 days | Days to weeks | Weeks (eg, 6 weeks for ragweed or grass pollen seasons) |
| Extreme exhaustion | Never | Early and prominent | Never |
| Fatigue, weakness | Sometimes | Can last up to 2-3 weeks | Sometimes |
| Fever | Rare | Characteristic, high (100-102°F); lasts 3-4 days | Never |
| General aches, pains | Slight | Usual; often severe | Never |
| Headache | Rare | Common | Sometimes |
| Itchy eyes | Rare or never | Rare or never | Common |
| Runny nose | Common | | Common |
| Sneezing | Usual | Sometimes | Usual |
| Sore throat | Common | Sometimes | Sometimes |
| Stuffy nose | Common | Sometimes | Common |
| **TREATMENT*** | | | |
| | Antihistamines | Amantadine | Antihistamines |
| | Decongestants | Rimantadine | Nasal steroids |
| | Nonsteroidal anti-inflammatories | Oseltamivir | Decongestants |
| | | Zanamivir | |
| **PREVENTION** | | | |
| | Wash your hands often; avoid close contact with anyone with a cold | Annual vaccination<br>Amantadine<br>Rimantadine<br>Oseltamivir | Avoid allergens such as pollen, house flies, dust mites, mold, pet dander, cockroaches |
| **COMPLICATIONS** | | | |
| | Sinus infection | Bronchitis | Sinus infections |
| | Middle ear infection | Pneumonia | Asthma |
| | Asthma | Can be life-threatening | |

Adapted from the National Institute of Allergy and Infectious Diseases, November 2008.

*Used only for temporary relief of cold symptoms.

# Cough-Cold-Flu Products

| BRAND NAME | ANALGESIC | ANTIHISTAMINE | DECONGESTANT | COUGH SUPPRESSANT | EXPECTORANT | DOSE |
|---|---|---|---|---|---|---|
| **ANTIHISTAMINE + DECONGESTANT** | | | | | | |
| Actifed Cold & Allergy Tablets | | Chlorpheniramine Maleate 4mg | Phenylephrine HCl 10mg | | | **Adults & Peds ≥12 yrs:** 1 tab q4h. **Max:** 6 tabs q24h. |
| Benadryl-D Allergy Plus Sinus | | Diphenhydramine HCl 25mg | Phenylephrine HCl 10mg | | | **Adults & Peds ≥12 yrs:** 1 tab q4h. **Max:** 6 tabs q24h. |
| Children's Benadryl-D Allergy & Sinus Liquid | | Diphenhydramine HCl 12.5mg/5mL | Phenylephrine HCl 5mg/5mL | | | **Adults ≥12 yrs:** 2 tsp (10mL) q4h. **Peds 6-<12 yrs:** 1 tsp (5mL) q4h. **Max:** 6 doses q24h. |
| Children's Dimetapp Cold & Allergy Chewable Tablets | | Brompheniramine Maleate 1mg | Phenylephrine HCl 2.5mg | | | **Peds 6-<12 yrs:** 2 tabs q4h. **Max:** 6 doses q24h. |
| Children's Dimetapp Cold & Allergy Syrup | | Brompheniramine Maleate 1mg/5mL | Phenylephrine HCl 2.5mg/5mL | | | **Adults & Peds ≥12 yrs:** 4 tsp (20mL) q4h. **Peds 6-<12 yrs:** 2 tsp (10mL) q4h. **Max:** 6 doses q24h. |
| Children's Dimetapp Nighttime Cold & Congestion Liquid | | Diphenhydramine HCl 6.25mg/5mL | Phenylephrine HCl 2.5mg/5mL | | | **Adults & Peds ≥12 yrs:** 4 tsp (20mL) q4h. **Peds 6-<12 yrs:** 2 tsp (10mL) q4h. **Max:** 6 doses q24h. |
| Pediacare Children's Allergy & Cold | | Diphenhydramine HCl 12.5mg/5mL | Phenylephrine HCl 5mg/5mL | | | **Peds 6-11 yrs:** 1 tsp (5mL) q4h. **Max:** 6 doses q24h. |
| Robitussin Night Time Cough & Cold | | Diphenhydramine HCl 6.25mg/5mL | Phenylephrine HCl 2.5mg/5mL | | | **Adults & Peds ≥12 yrs:** 4 tsp (20mL) q4h. **Max:** 6 doses q24h. |
| Sudafed PE Maximum Strength Sinus & Allergy Tablets | | Chlorpheniramine Maleate 4mg | Phenylephrine HCl 10mg | | | **Adults & Peds ≥12 yrs:** 1 tab q4h. **Max:** 6 tabs q24h. |
| Sudafed PE Nighttime Nasal Decongestant | | Diphenhydramine HCl 25mg | Phenylephrine HCl 10mg | | | **Adults & Peds ≥12 yrs:** 1 tab q4h. **Max:** 6 tabs q24h. |
| Night Time Triaminic Thin Strips Cold & Cough | | Diphenhydramine HCl 12.5mg/strip | Phenylephrine HCl 5mg/strip | | | **Peds 6-12 yrs:** 1 strip q4h. **Max:** 6 strips q24h. |
| Triaminic Night Time Cold & Cough | | Diphenhydramine HCl 6.25mg/5mL | Phenylephrine HCl 2.5mg/5mL | | | **Peds 6-<12 yrs:** 2 tsp (10mL) q4h. **Max:** 6 doses q24h. |
| Triaminic Syrup Cold & Allergy | | Chlorpheniramine Maleate 1mg/5mL | Phenylephrine HCl 2.5mg/5mL | | | **Peds 6-<12 yrs:** 2 tsp (10mL) q4h. **Max:** 6 doses q24h. |

| BRAND NAME | ANALGESIC | ANTIHISTAMINE | DECONGESTANT | COUGH SUPPRESSANT | EXPECTORANT | DOSE |
|---|---|---|---|---|---|---|
| **ANTIHISTAMINE + DECONGESTANT + ANALGESIC** | | | | | | |
| Advil Allergy Sinus Caplets | Ibuprofen 200mg | Chlorpheniramine Maleate 2mg | Pseudoephedrine HCl 30mg | | | **Adults & Peds ≥12 yrs:** 1 tab q4-6h. **Max:** 6 tabs q24h. |
| Alka-Seltzer Plus Cold Formula Effervescent Tablets | Aspirin 325mg | Chlorpheniramine Maleate 2mg | Phenylephrine Bitartrate 7.8mg | | | **Adults & Peds ≥12 yrs:** 2 tabs q4h. **Max:** 8 tabs q24h. |
| Alka-Seltzer Plus Fast Crystal Packs | Acetaminophen 650mg/packet | Chlorpheniramine Maleate 2mg/packet | Phenylephrine HCl 10mg/packet | | | **Adults & Peds ≥12 yrs:** 1 packet q4h. **Max:** 6 packets q24h. |
| Benadryl Severe Allergy Plus Cold Kapgels | Acetaminophen 325mg | Diphenhydramine HCl 12.5mg | Phenylephrine HCl 5mg | | | **Adults & Peds ≥12 yrs:** 2 caps q4h. **Max:** 12 caps q24h. |
| Benadryl Severe Allergy Plus Sinus Headache Caplets | Acetaminophen 325mg | Diphenhydramine HCl 25mg | Phenylephrine HCl 5mg | | | **Adults & Peds ≥12 yrs:** 2 tabs q4h. **Max:** 12 tabs q24h. |
| Benadryl Severe Allergy Plus Sinus Headache Kapgels | Acetaminophen 325mg | Diphenhydramine HCl 12.5mg | Phenylephrine HCl 5mg | | | **Adults & Peds ≥12 yrs:** 2 caps q4h. **Max:** 12 caps q24h. |
| Comtrex Day & Night Flu Therapy Caplets | Acetaminophen 325mg | Chlorpheniramine Maleate 2mg | Phenylephrine HCl 5mg | | | **Adults & Peds ≥12 yrs:** 2 tabs q4h. **Max:** 12 tabs q24h. |
| Comtrex Severe Cold & Sinus Caplets | Acetaminophen 325mg | Chlorpheniramine Maleate 2mg | Phenylephrine HCl 5mg | | | **Adults & Peds ≥12 yrs:** 2 tabs q4h. **Max:** 12 tabs q24h. |
| Contac Cold Plus Flu Maximum Strength Caplets | Acetaminophen 500mg | Chlorpheniramine Maleate 2mg | Phenylephrine HCl 5mg | | | **Adults & Peds ≥12 yrs:** 2 tabs q4-6h. **Max:** 8 tabs q24h. |
| Dristan Cold Multi-Symptom Formula Tablets | Acetaminophen 325mg | Chlorpheniramine Maleate 2mg | Phenylephrine HCl 5mg | | | **Adults & Peds ≥12 yrs:** 2 tabs q4h. **Max:** 12 tabs q24h. |
| Sudafed PE Nighttime Cold Caplets | Acetaminophen 325mg | Diphenhydramine HCl 25mg | Phenylephrine HCl 5mg | | | **Adults & Peds ≥12 yrs:** 2 tabs q4h. **Max:** 12 tabs q24h. |
| Sudafed PE Severe Cold Formula Caplets | Acetaminophen 325mg | Diphenhydramine HCl 12.5mg | Phenylephrine HCl 5mg | | | **Adults & Peds ≥12 yrs:** 2 tabs q4h. **Max:** 12 tabs q24h. **Peds 6-<12 yrs:** 1 tab q4h. **Max:** 5 tabs q24h. |
| Theraflu Cold & Sore Throat Hot Liquid | Acetaminophen 325mg/packet | Pheniramine Maleate 20mg/packet | Phenylephrine HCl 10mg/packet | | | **Adults & Peds ≥12 yrs:** 1 pkt q4h. **Max:** 6 pkts q24h. |
| Theraflu Nighttime Severe Cold & Cough Hot Liquid | Acetaminophen 650mg/packet | Diphenhydramine HCl 25mg/packet | Phenylephrine HCl 10mg/packet | | | **Adults & Peds ≥12 yrs:** 1 pkt q4h. **Max:** 6 pkts q24h. |
| Theraflu Sugar Free Nighttime Severe Cold & Cough Hot Liquid | Acetaminophen 650mg/packet | Diphenhydramine HCl 25mg/packet | Phenylephrine HCl 10mg/packet | | | **Adults & Peds ≥12 yrs:** 1 pkt q4h. **Max:** 6 pkts q24h. |

*(Continued)*

| BRAND NAME | ANALGESIC | ANTIHISTAMINE | DECONGESTANT | COUGH SUPPRESSANT | EXPECTORANT | DOSE |
|---|---|---|---|---|---|---|
| **ANTIHISTAMINE + DECONGESTANT + ANALGESIC** *(Continued)* | | | | | | |
| Theraflu Flu & Sore Throat Hot Liquid | Acetaminophen 650mg/packet | Pheniramine Maleate 20mg/packet | Phenylephrine HCl 10mg/packet | | | **Adults & Peds ≥12 yrs:** 1 pkt q4h. **Max:** 6 pkts q24h. |
| Theraflu Warming Relief Nighttime Severe Cough & Cold | Acetaminophen 325mg/15mL | Diphenhydramine HCl 12.5mg/15mL | Phenylephrine HCl 5mg/15mL | | | **Adults & Peds ≥12 yrs:** 2 tbl (30mL) q4h. **Max:** 6 doses (12 tbl or 180 mL) q24h. |
| Theraflu Warming Relief Flu & Sore Throat | Acetaminophen 325mg/15mL | Diphenhydramine HCl 12.5mg/15mL | Phenylephrine HCl 5mg/15mL | | | **Adults & Peds ≥12 yrs:** 2 tbl (30mL) q4h. **Max:** 6 doses (12 tbl or 180mL) q24h. |
| Children's Tylenol Plus Cold | Acetaminophen 160mg/5mL | Chlorpheniramine Maleate 1mg/5mL | Phenylephrine HCl 2.5mg/5mL | | | **Peds 6-11 yrs (48-95 lbs):** 2 tsp (10mL) q4h. **Max:** 5 doses q24h. |
| Children's Tylenol Plus Cold and Allergy | Acetaminophen 160mg/5mL | Diphenhydramine HCl 12.5mg/5mL | Phenylephrine HCl 2.5mg/5mL | | | **Peds 6-11 yrs (48-95 lbs):** 2 tsp (10mL) q4h. **Max:** 5 doses q24h. |
| Tylenol Allergy Multi-Symptom | Acetaminophen 325mg | Chlorpheniramine Maleate 2mg | Phenylephrine HCl 5mg | | | **Adults & Peds ≥12 yrs:** 2 tabs q4h. **Max:** 12 tabs q24h. |
| Tylenol Allergy Multi-Symptom Nighttime | Acetaminophen 325mg | Diphenhydramine HCl 25mg | Phenylephrine HCl 5mg | | | **Adults & Peds ≥12 yrs:** 2 tabs q4h. **Max:** 12 tabs q24h. |
| Tylenol Sinus Congestion & Pain Nighttime | Acetaminophen 325mg | Chlorpheniramine Maleate 2mg | Phenylephrine HCl 5mg | | | **Adults & Peds ≥12 yrs:** 2 tabs q4h. **Max:** 12 tabs q24h. |
| Vicks NyQuil Sinus LiquiCaps | Acetaminophen 325mg | Doxylamine Succinate 6.25mg | Phenylephrine HCl 5mg | | | **Adults & Peds ≥12 yrs:** 2 caps q4h. **Max:** 4 doses q24h. |
| **COUGH SUPPRESSANT** | | | | | | |
| Children's Delsym Cough Medicine | | | | Dextromethorphan HBr 30mg/5mL | | **Adults & Peds ≥12 yrs:** 2 tsp (10mL) q12h. **Max:** 4 tsp (20mL) q24h. **Peds 6-<12 yrs:** 1 tsp (5mL) q12h. **Max:** 2 tsp (10mL) q24h. **Peds 4-<6 yrs:** 1/2 tsp (2.5mL) q12h. **Max:** 1 tsp (5mL) q24h. |
| Delsym Cough Medicine | | | | Dextromethorphan HBr 30mg/5mL | | **Adults & Peds ≥12 yrs:** 2 tsp (10mL) q12h. **Max:** 4 tsp (20mL) q24h. **Peds 6-<12 yrs:** 1 tsp (5mL) q12h. **Max:** 2 tsp (10mL) q24h. **Peds 4-<6 yrs:** 1/2 tsp (2.5mL) q12h. **Max:** 1 tsp (5mL) q24h. |

| BRAND NAME | ANALGESIC | ANTIHISTAMINE | DECONGESTANT | COUGH SUPPRESSANT | EXPECTORANT | DOSE |
|---|---|---|---|---|---|---|
| PediaCare Children's Long-Acting Cough | | | | Dextromethorphan HBr 7.5mg/5mL | | **Peds 6-11 yrs:** 2 tsp (10mL) q6-8h. **Peds 4-5 yrs:** 1 tsp (5mL) q6-8h. **Max:** 4 doses q24h. |
| Children's Robitussin Cough Long-Acting | | | | Dextromethorphan HBr 7.5mg/5mL | | **Adults & Peds ≥12 yrs:** 4 tsp (20mL) q6-8h. **Peds 6-<12 yrs:** 2 tsp (10mL) q6-8h. **Peds 4-<6 yrs:** 1 tsp (5mL) q6-8h. **Max:** 4 doses q24h. |
| Robitussin Cough Long-Acting | | | | Dextromethorphan HBr 15mg/5mL | | **Adults & Peds ≥12 yrs:** 2 tsp (10mL) q6-8h. **Max:** 4 doses q24h. |
| Robitussin CoughGels | | | | Dextromethorphan HBr 15mg | | **Adults & Peds ≥12 yrs:** 2 caps q6-8h. **Max:** 8 caps q24h. |
| Triaminic Long-Acting Cough | | | | Dextromethorphan HBr 7.5mg/5mL | | **Peds 6-<12 yrs:** 2 tsp (10mL) q6-8h. **Peds 4-<6 yrs:** 1 tsp (5mL) q6-8h. **Max:** 4 doses q24h. |
| Triaminic Thin Strips Long-Acting Cough | | | | Dextromethorphan HBr 7.5mg/strip | | **Peds 6-<12 yrs:** 2 strips q6-8h. **Peds 4-<6 yrs:** 1 strip q6-8h. **Max:** 4 doses q24h. |
| Vicks DayQuil Cough | | | | Dextromethorphan HBr 15mg/15mL | | **Adults & Peds ≥12 yrs:** 2 tbl (30mL) q6-8h. **Peds 6-12 yrs:** 1 tbl (15mL) q6-8h. **Max:** 4 doses q24h. |
| Vicks Formula 44 Custom Care Dry Cough Suppressant | | | | Dextromethorphan HBr 30mg/15mL | | **Adults & Peds ≥12 yrs:** 1 tbl (15mL) q6-8h. **Peds 6-<12 yrs:** 1½ tsp (7.5mL) q6-8h. **Max:** 4 doses q24h. |
| Vicks BabyRub | | | | Petrolatum, fragrance, aloe extract, eucalyptus oil, lavender oil, rosemary oil | | **Peds:** Gently massage on the chest, neck, and back to help soothe and comfort. |
| Vicks VapoRub Topical Cream | | | | Camphor 5.2%, Menthol 2.8%, Eucalyptus 1.2% | | **Adults & Peds ≥2 yrs:** Apply to chest and throat. **Max:** tid per 24h. |
| Vicks VapoRub Topical Ointment | | | | Camphor 4.8%, Menthol 2.6%, Eucalyptus 1.2% | | **Adults & Peds ≥2 yrs:** Apply to chest and throat. **Max:** tid per 24h. |

*(Continued)*

| BRAND NAME | ANALGESIC | ANTIHISTAMINE | DECONGESTANT | COUGH SUPPRESSANT | EXPECTORANT | DOSE |
|---|---|---|---|---|---|---|
| **COUGH SUPPRESSANT** *(Continued)* | | | | | | |
| Vicks VapoSteam | | | | Camphor 6.2% | | **Adults & Peds ≥2 yrs:** 1 tbl/quart q8h or 1½ tsp/pint q8h (for use in a hot steam vaporizer). **Max:** tid per 24h. |
| **COUGH SUPPRESSANT + ANTIHISTAMINE** | | | | | | |
| Coricidin HBP Cough & Cold | | Chlorpheniramine Maleate 4mg | | Dextromethorphan HBr 30mg | | **Adults & Peds ≥12 yrs:** 1 tab q6h. **Max:** 4 tabs q24h. |
| Children's Dimetapp Long-Acting Cough Plus Cold | | Chlorpheniramine Maleate 1mg/5mL | | Dextromethorphan HBr 7.5mg/5mL | | **Adults & Peds ≥12 yrs:** 4 tsp (20mL) q6h. **6-<12 yrs:** 2 tsp (10mL) q6h. **Max:** 4 doses q24h. |
| Children's Robitussin Cough & Cold Long-Acting | | Chlorpheniramine Maleate 1mg/5mL | | Dextromethorphan HBr 7.5mg/5mL | | **Adults & Peds ≥12 yrs:** 4 tsp (20mL) q6h. **Peds 6-<12 yrs:** 2 tsp (10mL) q6h. **Max:** 4 doses q24h. |
| Robitussin Cough & Cold Long-Acting | | Chlorpheniramine Maleate 2mg/5mL | | Dextromethorphan HBr 15mg/5mL | | **Adults & Peds ≥12 yrs:** 2 tsp (10mL) q6h. **Max:** 4 doses q24h. |
| Triaminic Softchews Cough and Runny Nose | | Chlorpheniramine Maleate 1mg | | Dextromethorphan HBr 5mg | | **Peds 6-<12 yrs:** 2 tabs q4-6h. **Max:** 5 doses q24h. |
| Pediatric Vicks Formula 44m Cough & Cold Relief | | Chlorpheniramine Maleate 2mg/15mL | | Dextromethorphan HBr 15mg/15mL | | **Adults & Peds ≥12 yrs:** 2 tbl (30mL) q6h. **Peds 6-<12 yrs:** 1 tbl (15mL) q6h. **Max:** 4 doses q24h. |
| Vicks Children's NyQuil | | Chlorpheniramine Maleate 2mg/15mL | | Dextromethorphan HBr 15mg/15mL | | **Adults & Peds ≥12 yrs:** 2 tbl (30mL) q6h. **Peds 6-11 yrs:** 1 tbl (15mL) q6h. **Max:** 4 doses q24h. |
| Vicks NyQuil Cough | | Doxylamine Succinate 6.25mg/15mL | | Dextromethorphan HBr 15mg/15mL | | **Adults & Peds ≥12 yrs:** 2 tbl (30mL) q6h. **Max:** 4 doses q24h. |
| **COUGH SUPPRESSANT + ANALGESIC** | | | | | | |
| Triaminic Cough & Sore Throat | Acetaminophen 160mg/5mL | | | Dextromethorphan HBr 5mg/5mL | | **Peds 6-<12 yrs:** 2 tsp (10mL) q4h. **Peds 4-<6 yrs:** 1 tsp (5mL) q4h. **Max:** 5 doses q24h. |
| Triaminic Softchews Cough & Sore Throat | Acetaminophen 160mg | | | Dextromethorphan HBr 5mg | | **Peds 6-<12 yrs:** 2 tabs q4h. **Peds 4-<6 yrs:** 1 tab q4h. **Max:** 5 doses q24h. |

| BRAND NAME | ANALGESIC | ANTIHISTAMINE | DECONGESTANT | COUGH SUPPRESSANT | EXPECTORANT | DOSE |
|---|---|---|---|---|---|---|
| Children's Tylenol Plus Cough and Sore Throat | Acetaminophen 160mg/5mL | | | Dextromethorphan HBr 5mg/5mL | | **Peds 6-11 yrs (48-95 lbs):** 2 tsp (10mL) q4h. **Peds 4-5 yrs (36-47 lbs):** 1 tsp (5mL) q4h. **Max:** 5 doses q24h. |
| Tylenol Cough & Sore Throat Daytime | Acetaminophen 1000mg/30mL | | | Dextromethorphan HBr 30mg/30mL | | **Adults & Peds ≥12 yrs:** 2 tbl (30mL) q6h. **Max:** 8 tbl q24h. |
| **COUGH SUPPRESSANT + ANTIHISTAMINE + ANALGESIC** | | | | | | |
| Alka-Seltzer Plus Flu Formula Effervescent Tablets | Aspirin 500mg | Chlorpheniramine Maleate 2mg | | Dextromethorphan HBr 15mg | | **Adults & Peds ≥12 yrs:** 2 tabs q6h. **Max:** 8 tabs q24h. |
| Coricidin HBP Day & Night Multi-Symptom Cold | Acetaminophen 500mg (nighttime dose only) | Chlorpheniramine Maleate 2mg (nighttime dose only) | | Dextromethorphan HBr 10mg (daytime dose), 15mg (nighttime dose) | Guaifenesin 200mg (daytime dose only) | **Adults & Peds ≥12 yrs:** 2 tabs hs and q6h prn. **Max:** 4 tablets q12h. |
| Coricidin HBP Maximum Strength Flu | Acetaminophen 500mg | Chlorpheniramine Maleate 2mg | | Dextromethorphan HBr 15mg | | **Adults & Peds ≥12 yrs:** 2 tabs q6h. **Max:** 8 tabs q24h. |
| Coricidin HBP Nighttime Multi-Symptom Cold Relief Liquid | Acetaminophen 500mg/15mL | Doxylamine 6.25mg/15mL | | Dextromethorphan HBr 15mg/15mL | | **Adults & Peds ≥12 yrs:** 2 tbl (30mL) q6h. **Max:** 4 doses q24h. |
| Triaminic Multisymptom Fever | Acetaminophen 160mg/5mL | Chlorpheniramine Maleate 1mg/5mL | | Dextromethorphan HBr 7.5mg/5mL | | **Peds 6-<12 yrs:** 2 tsp (10mL) q6h. **Max:** 4 doses q24h. |
| Children's Tylenol Plus Cough & Runny Nose | Acetaminophen 160mg/5mL | Chlorpheniramine Maleate 1mg/5mL | | Dextromethorphan HBr 5mg/5mL | | **Peds 6-11 yrs (48-95 lbs):** 2 tsp (10mL) q4h. **Max:** 5 doses q24h. |
| Tylenol Cough & Sore Throat Nighttime | Acetaminophen 500mg/15mL | Doxylamine 6.25mg/15mL | | Dextromethorphan HBr 15mg/15mL | | **Adults & Peds ≥12 yrs:** 2 tbl (30mL) q6h. **Max:** 8 tbl (120mL) q24h. |
| Vicks Formula 44 Custom Care Cough & Cold PM | Acetaminophen 650mg/15mL | Chlorpheniramine Maleate 4mg/15mL | | Dextromethorphan HBr 30mg/15mL | | **Adults & Peds ≥12 yrs:** 1 tbl q6h. **Max:** 4 doses q24h. |
| Vicks NyQuil Cold & Flu Relief Liquid | Acetaminophen 500mg/15mL | Doxylamine Succinate 6.25mg/15mL | | Dextromethorphan HBr 15mg/15mL | | **Adults & Peds ≥12 yrs:** 2 tbl (30mL) q6h. **Max:** 4 doses q24h. |
| Vicks NyQuil Cold & Flu Relief LiquiCaps | Acetaminophen 325mg | Doxylamine Succinate 6.25mg | | Dextromethorphan HBr 15mg | | **Adults & Peds ≥12 yrs:** 2 caps q6h. **Max:** 4 doses q24h. |

*(Continued)*

| BRAND NAME | ANALGESIC | ANTIHISTAMINE | DECONGESTANT | COUGH SUPPRESSANT | EXPECTORANT | DOSE |
|---|---|---|---|---|---|---|
| **COUGH SUPPRESSANT + ANTIHISTAMINE + ANALGESIC** *(Continued)* | | | | | | |
| Vicks NyQuil Cold & Flu Symptom Relief Plus Vitamin C | Acetaminophen 325mg | Doxylamine Succinate 6.25mg | | Dextromethorphan HBr 15mg | | **Adults & Peds ≥12 yrs:** 2 caps q6h. **Max:** 4 doses q24h. |
| Vicks NyQuil Less Drowsy Cold & Flu Relief Liquid | Acetaminophen 325mg/15mL | Chlorpheniramine Maleate 2mg/15mL | | Dextromethorphan HBr 15mg/15mL | | **Adults & Peds ≥12 yrs:** 2 tbl (30mL) q6h. **Max:** 4 doses q24h. |
| **COUGH SUPPRESSANT + ANTIHISTAMINE + ANALGESIC + DECONGESTANT** | | | | | | |
| Alka-Seltzer Plus Cold & Cough Formula Effervescent Tablets | Aspirin 325mg | Chlorpheniramine Maleate 2mg | Phenylephrine Bitartrate 7.8mg | Dextromethorphan HBr 10mg | | **Adults & Peds ≥12 yrs:** 2 tabs q4h. **Max:** 8 tabs q24h. |
| Alka-Seltzer Plus Cold & Cough Formula Liquid Gels | Acetaminophen 325mg | Chlorpheniramine Maleate 2mg | Phenylephrine HCl 5mg | Dextromethorphan HBr 10mg | | **Adults & Peds ≥12 yrs:** 2 caps q4h. **Max:** 12 caps q24h. |
| Alka-Seltzer Plus Night Cold Formula Effervescent Tablets | Aspirin 500mg | Doxylamine 6.25mg | Phenylephrine Bitartrate 7.8mg | Dextromethorphan HBr 10mg | | **Adults & Peds ≥12 yrs:** 2 tabs q4-6h. **Max:** 8 tabs q24h. |
| Alka-Seltzer Plus Night Cold Formula Liquid Gels | Acetaminophen 325mg | Doxylamine 6.25mg | Phenylephrine HCl 5mg | Dextromethorphan HBr 10mg | | **Adults & Peds ≥12 yrs:** 2 caps q4h. **Max:** 12 caps q24h. |
| Comtrex Nighttime Cough & Cold Caplets | Acetaminophen 325mg | Chlorpheniramine Maleate 2mg | Phenylephrine HCl 5mg | Dextromethorphan HBr 10mg | | **Adults & Peds ≥12 yrs:** 2 tabs q4h. **Max:** 12 tabs q24h. |
| Robitussin Night Time Cough, Cold & Flu | Acetaminophen 160mg/5mL | Chlorpheniramine Maleate 1mg/5mL | Phenylephrine HCl 2.5mg/5mL | Dextromethorphan HBr 5mg/5mL | | **Adults & Peds ≥12 yrs:** 4 tsp (20mL) q4h. **Max:** 6 doses q24h. |
| Theraflu Nighttime Severe Cold & Cough Caplets | Acetaminophen 325mg | Chlorpheniramine Maleate 2mg | Phenylephrine HCl 5mg | Dextromethorphan HBr 10mg | | **Adults & Peds ≥12 yrs:** 2 tabs q4h. **Max:** 12 tabs q24h. |
| Children's Tylenol Plus Flu | Acetaminophen 160mg/5mL | Chlorpheniramine Maleate 1mg/5mL | Phenylephrine HCl 2.5mg/5mL | Dextromethorphan HBr 5mg/5mL | | **Peds 6-11 yrs (48-95 lbs):** 2 tsp (10mL) q4h. **Max:** 5 doses q24h. |
| Children's Tylenol Plus Multi-Symptom Cold | Acetaminophen 160mg/5mL | Chlorpheniramine Maleate 1mg/5mL | Phenylephrine HCl 2.5mg/5mL | Dextromethorphan HBr 5mg/5mL | | **Peds 6-11 yrs (48-95 lbs):** 2 tsp (10mL) q4h. **Max:** 5 doses q24h. |
| Tylenol Cold Head Congestion Nighttime | Acetaminophen 325mg | Chlorpheniramine Maleate 2mg | Phenylephrine HCl 5mg | Dextromethorphan HBr 10mg | | **Adults & Peds ≥12 yrs:** 2 tabs q4h. **Max:** 12 tabs q24h. |
| Tylenol Cold Multi-Symptom Nighttime Gelcaps | Acetaminophen 325mg | Chlorpheniramine Maleate 2mg | Phenylephrine HCl 5mg | Dextromethorphan HBr 10mg | | **Adults & Peds ≥12 yrs:** 2 tabs q4h. **Max:** 12 tabs q24h. |
| Tylenol Cold Multi-Symptom Nighttime Liquid | Acetaminophen 325mg/15mL | Doxylamine 6.25mg/30mL | Phenylephrine HCl 5mg/15mL | Dextromethorphan HBr 10mg/15mL | | **Adults & Peds ≥12 yrs:** 2 tbl (30mL) q4h. **Max:** 12 tbl (180mL) q24h. |
| Vicks NyQuil D | Acetaminophen 500mg/15mL | Doxylamine 6.25mg/15mL | Pseudoephedrine HCl 30mg/15mL | Dextromethorphan HBr 15mg/15mL | | **Adults & Peds ≥12 yrs:** 2 tbl (30mL) q6h. **Max:** 4 doses q24h. |

| BRAND NAME | ANALGESIC | ANTIHISTAMINE | DECONGESTANT | COUGH SUPPRESSANT | EXPECTORANT | DOSE |
|---|---|---|---|---|---|---|
| **COUGH SUPPRESSANT + ANTIHISTAMINE + DECONGESTANT** | | | | | | |
| Children's Dimetapp Cold & Cough | | Brompheniramine Maleate 1mg/5mL | Phenylephrine HCl 2.5mg/5mL | Dextromethorphan HBr 5mg/5mL | | **Adults & Peds ≥12 yrs:** 4 tsp (20mL) q4h. **Peds 6-<12 yrs:** 2 tsp (10mL) q4h. **Max:** 6 doses q24h. |
| Theraflu Cold & Cough Hot Liquid | | Pheniramine Maleate 20mg/packet | Phenylephrine HCl 10mg/packet | Dextromethorphan HBr 20mg/packet | | **Adults & Peds ≥12 yrs:** 1 pkt q4h. **Max:** 6 pkts q24h. |
| Triaminic-D Multi-Symptom Cold | | Chlorpheniramine Maleate 1mg/5mL | Pseudoephedrine HCl 15mg/5mL | Dextromethorphan HBr 7.5mg/5mL | | **Peds 6-<12 yrs:** 2 tsp q6h. **Max:** 4 doses q24h. |
| **COUGH SUPPRESSANT + DECONGESTANT** | | | | | | |
| PediaCare Children's Multi-Symptom Cold | | | Phenylephrine HCl 2.5mg/5mL | Dextromethorphan HBr 5mg/5mL | | **Peds 6-11 yrs:** 2 tsp (10mL) q4h. **Peds 4-5 yrs:** 1 tsp (5mL) q4h. **Max:** 6 doses q24h. |
| Children's Sudafed PE Cold & Cough Liquid | | | Phenylephrine HCl 2.5mg/5mL | Dextromethorphan HBr 5mg/5mL | | **Peds 6-11 yrs:** 2 tsp (10mL) q4h. **Peds 4-5 yrs:** 1 tsp (5mL) q4h. **Max:** 6 doses q24h. |
| Day Time Triaminic Thin Strips Cold & Cough | | | Phenylephrine HCl 2.5mg/strip | Dextromethorphan HBr 5mg/strip | | **Peds 6-<12 yrs:** 2 strips q4h. **Peds 4-<6 yrs:** 1 strip q4h. **Max:** 6 doses q24h. |
| Triaminic Day Time Cold & Cough | | | Phenylephrine HCl 2.5mg/5mL | Dextromethorphan HBr 5mg/5mL | | **Peds 6-<12 yrs:** 2 tsp (10mL) q4h. **Peds 4-<6 yrs:** 1 tsp (5mL) q4h. **Max:** 6 doses q24h. |
| Vicks Formula 44 Custom Care Congestion | | | Phenylephrine HCl 10mg/15mL | Dextromethorphan HBr 20mg/15mL | | **Adults & Peds ≥12 yrs:** 1 tbl (15mL) q4h. **Peds 6-<12 yrs:** 1½ tsp (7.5mL) q4h. **Max:** 6 doses q24h. |
| **COUGH SUPPRESSANT + DECONGESTANT + ANALGESIC** | | | | | | |
| Alka-Seltzer Plus Day Non-Drowsy Cold Formula Liquid Gels | Acetaminophen 325mg | | Phenylephrine HCl 5mg | Dextromethorphan HBr 10mg | | **Adults & Peds ≥12 yrs:** 2 caps q4h. **Max:** 12 caps q24h. |
| Alka-Seltzer Plus Day & Night Cold Formula Liquid Gels | Acetaminophen 325mg | Doxylamine 6.25mg (nighttime dose only) | Phenylephrine HCl 5mg | Dextromethorphan HBr 10mg | | **Adults & Peds ≥12 yrs:** 2 caps q4h. **Max:** 12 caps q24h. |
| Alka-Seltzer Plus Day & Night Cold Formula Effervescent Tablets | Aspirin 325mg | Doxylamine 6.25mg (nighttime dose only) | Phenylephrine Bitartrate 7.8mg | Dextromethorphan HBr 10mg | | **Adults & Peds ≥12 yrs:** 2 tabs q4h. **Max:** 8 tabs q24h. |
| Comtrex Non-Drowsy Day Cold & Cough Caplets | Acetaminophen 325mg | | Phenylephrine HCl 5mg | Dextromethorphan HBr 10mg | | **Adults & Peds ≥12 yrs:** 2 tabs q4h. **Max:** 12 tabs q24h. |

*(Continued)*

| BRAND NAME | ANALGESIC | ANTIHISTAMINE | DECONGESTANT | COUGH SUPPRESSANT | EXPECTORANT | DOSE |
|---|---|---|---|---|---|---|
| **COUGH SUPPRESSANT + DECONGESTANT + ANALGESIC** *(Continued)* | | | | | | |
| Theraflu Daytime Severe Cold & Cough Caplets | Acetaminophen 325mg | | Phenylephrine HCl 5mg | Dextromethorphan HBr 10mg | | **Adults & Peds ≥12 yrs:** 2 tabs q4h. **Max:** 12 tabs q24h. |
| Theraflu Daytime Severe Cold & Cough Hot Liquid | Acetaminophen 650mg/packet | | Phenylephrine HCl 10mg/packet | Dextromethorphan HBr 20mg/packet | | **Adults & Peds ≥12 yrs:** 1 pkt q4h. **Max:** 6 pkts q24h. |
| Theraflu Warming Relief Daytime Severe Cough & Cold | Acetaminophen 325mg/15mL | | Phenylephrine HCl 5mg/15mL | Dextromethorphan HBr 10mg/15mL | | **Adults & Peds ≥12 yrs:** 2 tbl (30mL) q4h. **Max:** 6 doses q24h. |
| Children's Tylenol Plus Cold & Cough | Acetaminophen 160mg/5mL | | Phenylephrine HCl 2.5mg/5mL | Dextromethorphan HBr 5mg/5mL | | **Peds 6-11 yrs (48-95 lbs):** 2 tsp (10mL) q4h. **Peds 4-5 yrs (36-47 lbs):** 1 tsp (5mL) q4h. **Max:** 5 doses q24h. |
| Tylenol Cold Head Congestion Daytime | Acetaminophen 325mg | | Phenylephrine HCl 5mg | Dextromethorphan HBr 10mg | | **Adults & Peds ≥12 yrs:** 2 caps q4h. **Max:** 12 caps q24h. |
| Tylenol Cold Multi-Symptom Daytime Gelcaps/Caplets | Acetaminophen 325mg | | Phenylephrine HCl 5mg | Dextromethorphan HBr 10mg | | **Adults & Peds ≥12 yrs:** 2 caps q4h. **Max:** 12 caps q24h. |
| Tylenol Cold Multi-Symptom Daytime Liquid | Acetaminophen 325mg/15mL | | Phenylephrine HCl 5mg/15mL | Dextromethorphan HBr 10mg/15mL | | **Adults & Peds ≥12 yrs:** 2 tbl (30mL) q4h. **Max:** 12 tbl (180mL) q24h. |
| Vicks DayQuil Cold & Flu Relief LiquiCaps | Acetaminophen 325mg | | Phenylephrine HCl 5mg | Dextromethorphan HBr 10mg | | **Adults & Peds ≥12 yrs:** 2 doses q4h. **Max:** 6 doses q24h. |
| Vicks DayQuil Cold & Flu Relief Liquid | Acetaminophen 325mg/15mL | | Phenylephrine HCl 5mg/15mL | Dextromethorphan HBr 10mg/15mL | | **Adults & Peds ≥12 yrs:** 2 tbl (30 mL) q4h. **Max:** 6 doses q24h. **Peds 6-<12 yrs:** 1 tbl (15mL) q4h. **Max:** 5 doses q24h. |
| Vicks DayQuil Cold & Flu Symptom Relief Plus Vitamin C | Acetaminophen 325mg | | Phenylephrine HCl 5mg | Dextromethorphan HBr 15mg | | **Adults & Peds ≥12 yrs:** 2 caps q4h. **Max:** 6 doses q24h. |
| **COUGH SUPPRESSANT + DECONGESTANT + EXPECTORANT** | | | | | | |
| Children's Robitussin Cough & Cold CF | | | Phenylephrine HCl 2.5mg/5mL | Dextromethorphan HBr 5mg/5mL | Guaifenesin 50mg/5mL | **Adults & Peds ≥12 yrs:** 4 tsp (20mL) q4h. **Peds 6-<12 yrs:** 2 tsp (10mL) q4h. **Peds 4-<6 yrs:** 1 tsp (5mL) q4h. **Max:** 6 doses q24h. |
| Robitussin Cough & Cold CF | | | Phenylephrine HCl 5mg/5mL | Dextromethorphan HBr 10mg/5mL | Guaifenesin 100mg/5mL | **Adults & Peds ≥12 yrs:** 2 tsp (10mL) q4h. **Max:** 6 doses q24h. |
| Robitussin Cough & Cold D | | | Pseudoephedrine HCl 30mg/5mL | Dextromethorphan HBr 15mg/5mL | Guaifenesin 200mg/5mL | **Adults & Peds ≥12 yrs:** 2 tsp (10mL) q4h. **Max:** 4 doses q24h. |
| Robitussin To Go Cough & Cold CF | | | Phenylephrine HCl 10mg/10mL | Dextromethorphan HBr 20mg/10mL | Guaifenesin 200mg/10mL | **Adults & Peds ≥12 yrs:** 1 pre-filled spoon (10 mL) q4h. **Max:** 6 doses q24h. |

| BRAND NAME | ANALGESIC | ANTIHISTAMINE | DECONGESTANT | COUGH SUPPRESSANT | EXPECTORANT | DOSE |
|---|---|---|---|---|---|---|
| **COUGH SUPPRESSANT + DECONGESTANT + EXPECTORANT + ANALGESIC** | | | | | | |
| Sudafed PE Cold & Cough Caplets | Acetaminophen 325mg | | Phenylephrine HCl 5mg | Dextromethorphan HBr 10mg | Guaifenesin 100mg | **Adults & Peds ≥12 yrs:** 2 tabs q4h. **Max:** 12 tabs q24h. |
| Tylenol Cold Multi-Symptom Severe Caplets | Acetaminophen 325mg | | Phenylephrine HCl 5mg | Dextromethorphan HBr 10mg | Guaifenesin 200mg | **Adults & Peds ≥12 yrs:** 2 tabs q4h. **Max:** 12 tabs q24h. |
| Tylenol Cold Multi-Symptom Severe Liquid | Acetaminophen 325mg/15mL | | Phenylephrine HCl 5mg/15mL | Dextromethorphan HBr 10mg/15mL | Guaifenesin 200mg/15mL | **Adults & Peds ≥12 yrs:** 2 tbl (30mL) q4h. **Max:** 12 tbl (180mL) q24h. |
| Tylenol Cold Severe Congestion Daytime | Acetaminophen 325mg | | Phenylephrine HCl 30mg | Dextromethorphan HBr 15mg | Guaifenesin 200mg | **Adults & Peds ≥12 yrs:** 2 tabs q6h. **Max:** 8 tabs q24h. |
| Tylenol Cold Severe Head Congestion | Acetaminophen 325mg | | Phenylephrine HCl 5mg | Dextromethorphan HBr 10mg | Guaifenesin 200mg | **Adults & Peds ≥12 yrs:** 2 tabs q4h. **Max:** 12 tabs q24h. |
| Tylenol Cough & Severe Congestion Daytime | Acetaminophen 325mg/15mL | | Phenylephrine HCl 5mg/15mL | Dextromethorphan HBr 10mg/15mL | Guaifenesin 200mg/15mL | **Adults & Peds ≥12 yrs:** 2 tbl (30mL) q4h. **Max:** 12 tbl (180mL) q24h. |
| **COUGH SUPPRESSANT + EXPECTORANT** | | | | | | |
| Alka-Seltzer Plus Mucus & Congestion Effervescent Tablets | | | | Dextromethorphan HBr 10mg | Guaifenesin 200mg | **Adults & Peds ≥12 yrs:** 2 tabs q4h. **Max:** 8 tabs q24h. |
| Alka-Seltzer Plus Mucus & Congestion Liquid Gels | | | | Dextromethorphan HBr 10mg | Guaifenesin 200mg | **Adults & Peds ≥12 yrs:** 2 caps q4h. **Max:** 12 caps q24h. |
| Coricidin HBP Chest Congestion & Cough | | | | Dextromethorphan HBr 10mg | Guaifenesin 200mg | **Adults & Peds ≥12 yrs:** 1-2 caps q4h. **Max:** 12 caps q24h. |
| Maximum Strength Mucinex DM | | | | Dextromethorphan HBr 60mg | Guaifenesin 1200mg | **Adults & Peds ≥12 yrs:** 1 tab q12h. **Max:** 2 tabs q24h. |
| Mucinex Cough Liquid (Cherry Flavor) | | | | Dextromethorphan HBr 5mg/5mL | Guaifenesin 100mg/5mL | **Peds 6-<12 yrs:** 1-2 tsp (5-10mL) q4h. **Peds 4-<6yrs:** ½-1 tsp (2.5-5mL) q4h. **Max:** 6 doses q24h. |
| Mucinex Cough Mini-Melts (Orange Crème Flavor) | | | | Dextromethorphan HBr 5mg | Guaifenesin 100mg | **Adults & Peds ≥12 yrs:** 2-4 pkts q4h. **Peds 6-<12 yrs:** 1-2 pkts q4h. **Peds 4-<6yrs:** 1 pkt q4h. **Max:** 6 doses q24h. |
| Mucinex DM | | | | Dextromethorphan HBr 30mg | Guaifenesin 600mg | **Adults & Peds ≥12 yrs:** 1-2 tabs q12h. **Max:** 4 tabs q24h. |
| Robitussin Cough & Chest Congestion DM Max | | | | Dextromethorphan HBr 10mg/5mL | Guaifenesin 200mg/5mL | **Adults & Peds ≥12 yrs:** 2 tsp (10mL) q4h. **Max:** 6 doses q24h. |

*(Continued)*

| BRAND NAME | ANALGESIC | ANTIHISTAMINE | DECONGESTANT | COUGH SUPPRESSANT | EXPECTORANT | DOSE |
|---|---|---|---|---|---|---|
| **COUGH SUPPRESSANT + EXPECTORANT** *(Continued)* | | | | | | |
| Robitussin Cough & Chest Congestion DM | | | | Dextromethorphan HBr 10mg/5mL | Guaifenesin 100mg/5mL | **Adults & Peds ≥12 yrs:** 2 tsp (10mL) q4h. **Max:** 6 doses q24h. |
| Robitussin Cough & Chest Congestion Sugar-Free DM | | | | Dextromethorphan HBr 10mg/5mL | Guaifenesin 100mg/5mL | **Adults & Peds ≥12 yrs:** 2 tsp (10mL) q4h. **Max:** 6 doses q24h. |
| Robitussin To Go Cough & Chest Congestion DM | | | | Dextromethorphan HBr 20mg/10mL | Guaifenesin 200mg/10mL | **Adults & Peds ≥12 yrs:** 1 pre-filled spoon (10mL) q4h. **Max:** 6 doses q24h. |
| Pediatric Vicks Formula 44e Cough & Chest Congestion Relief | | | | Dextromethorphan HBr 10mg/15mL | Guaifenesin 100mg/15mL | **Adults & Peds ≥12 yrs:** 2 tbl (30 mL) q4h. **Peds 6-<12 yrs:** 1 tbl (15 mL) q4h. **Peds 4-<6 yrs:** ½ tbl (7.5 mL) q4h. **Max:** 6 doses q24h. |
| Vicks DayQuil Mucus Control DM | | | | Dextromethorphan HBr 10mg/15mL | Guaifenesin 200mg/15mL | **Adults & Peds ≥12 yrs:** 2 tbl (30mL) q4h. **Peds 6-12 yrs:** 1 tbl (15mL) q4h. **Max:** 6 doses q24h. |
| Vicks Formula 44 Custom Care Chesty Cough | | | | Dextromethorphan HBr 20mg/15mL | Guaifenesin 200mg/15mL | **Adults & Peds ≥12 yrs:** 1 tbl (15mL) q4h. **Peds 6-<12 yrs:** 1½ tsp (7.5mL) q4h. **Max:** 6 doses q24h. |
| **DECONGESTANT** | | | | | | |
| Contac-D Cold Decongestant Tablets | | | Phenylephrine HCl 10mg | | | **Adults & Peds ≥12 yrs:** 1 tab q4h. **Max:** 6 tabs q24h. |
| Mucinex Moisture Smart Nasal Spray | | | Oxymetazoline HCl 0.05% | | | **Adults & Peds ≥12 yrs:** 2-3 sprays in each nostril q10-12h. **Max:** 2 doses q24h. |
| Mucinex Full Force Nasal Spray | | | Oxymetazoline HCl 0.05% | | | **Adults & Peds ≥12 yrs:** 2-3 sprays in each nostril q10-12h. **Max:** 2 doses q24h. |
| PediaCare Children's Decongestant | | | Phenylephrine HCl 2.5mg/5mL | | | **Peds 6-11 yrs:** 2 tsp (10mL) q4h. **Peds 4-5 yrs:** 1 tsp (5mL) q4h. **Max:** 6 doses q24h. |
| Children's Sudafed Nasal Decongestant Liquid | | | Pseudoephedrine HCl 15mg/5mL | | | **Peds 6-11 yrs:** 2 tsp (10mL) q4-6h. **Peds 4-5 yrs:** 1 tsp (5mL) q4-6h. **Max:** 4 doses q24h. |

| BRAND NAME | ANALGESIC | ANTIHISTAMINE | DECONGESTANT | COUGH SUPPRESSANT | EXPECTORANT | DOSE |
|---|---|---|---|---|---|---|
| Children's Sudafed PE Nasal Decongestant Liquid | | | Phenylephrine HCl 2.5mg/5mL | | | **Peds 6-11 yrs:** 2 tsp (10mL) q4h. **Peds 4-5 yrs:** 1 tsp (5mL) q4h. **Max:** 6 doses q24h. |
| Sudafed 12-Hour Tablets | | | Pseudoephedrine HCl 120mg | | | **Adults & Peds ≥12 yrs:** 1 tab q12h. **Max:** 2 tabs q24h. |
| Sudafed 24-Hour Tablets | | | Pseudoephedrine HCl 240mg | | | **Adults & Peds ≥12 yrs:** 1 tab q24h. **Max:** 1 tab q24h. |
| Sudafed Nasal Decongestant Tablets | | | Pseudoephedrine HCl 30mg | | | **Adults ≥12 yrs:** 2 tabs q4-6h. **Max:** 8 tabs q24h. **Peds 6-12 yrs:** 1 tab q4-6h. **Max:** 4 tabs q24h. |
| Sudafed OM Sinus Cold Spray | | | Oxymetazoline HCl 0.05% | | | **Adults & Peds ≥6 yrs:** 2-3 sprays in each nostril q10-12h. **Max:** 2 doses q24h. |
| Sudafed OM Sinus Congestion Spray | | | Oxymetazoline HCl 0.05% | | | **Adults & Peds ≥6 yrs:** 2-3 sprays in each nostril q10-12h. **Max:** 2 doses q24h. |
| Sudafed PE Nasal Decongestant Tablets | | | Phenylephrine HCl 10mg | | | **Adults & Peds ≥12 yrs:** 1 tab q4h. **Max:** 6 tabs q24h. |
| Triaminic Thin Strips Cold with Stuffy Nose | | | Phenylephrine HCl 2.5mg/strip | | | **Peds 6-<12 yrs:** 2 strips q4h. **Peds 4-<6 yrs:** 1 strip q4h. **Max:** 6 doses q24h. |
| Triaminic Decongestant Spray Nasal & Sinus Congestion | | | Xylometazoline HCl 0.05% | | | **Peds 2-<12 yrs:** 1-2 sprays in each nostril q8-10h. **Max:** 3 doses q24h. |
| Vicks Sinex VapoSpray 4-Hour | | | Phenylephrine HCl 0.5% | | | **Adults & Peds ≥12 yrs:** Instill 2-3 sprays per nostril q4h. |
| Vicks Sinex VapoSpray 12-Hour Decongestant Nasal Spray | | | Oxymetazoline HCl 0.05% | | | **Adults & Peds ≥6 yrs:**. Instill 2-3 sprays per nostril q10-12h. **Max:** 2 doses q24h. |
| Vicks Sinex VapoSpray 12-Hour Decongestant UltraFine Mist | | | Oxymetazoline HCl 0.05% | | | **Adults & Peds ≥6 yrs:** Instill 2-3 sprays per nostril q10-12h. **Max:** 2 doses q24h. |
| Vicks VapoInhaler | | | Levmetamfetamine 50mg | | | **Adults & Peds ≥12 yrs:** 2 inhalations q2h. **Max:** 24 inhalations q24h. **Peds 6-<12 yrs:** 1 inhalation q2h. |

*(Continued)*

| BRAND NAME | ANALGESIC | ANTIHISTAMINE | DECONGESTANT | COUGH SUPPRESSANT | EXPECTORANT | DOSE |
|---|---|---|---|---|---|---|
| **DECONGESTANT + ANALGESIC** | | | | | | |
| Children's Advil Cold Suspension | Ibuprofen 100mg/5mL | | Pseudoephedrine HCl 15mg/5mL | | | **Peds 6-11 yrs (48-95 lbs):** 2 tsp (10mL) q6h. **2-5 yrs (24-47 lbs):** 1 tsp (5mL) q6h. **Max:** 4 doses q24h. |
| Advil Cold & Sinus Caplets/Liqui-Gels | Ibuprofen 200mg | | Pseudoephedrine HCl 30mg | | | **Adults & Peds ≥12 yrs:** 1-2 caps q4-6h. **Max:** 6 caps q24h. |
| Alka-Seltzer Plus Sinus Formula Effervescent Tablets | Aspirin 325mg | | Phenylephrine Bitartrate 7.8mg | | | **Adults & Peds ≥12 yrs:** 2 tabs q4h. **Max:** 8 tabs q24h. |
| Contac Cold & Flu Day & Night Caplets | Acetaminophen 500mg | Chlorpheniramine Maleate 2mg (nighttime dose only) | Phenylephrine HCl 5mg | | | **Adults & Peds ≥12 yrs:** 2 tabs q4-6h. **Max:** 8 tabs q24h. |
| Contac Cold Plus Flu Non-Drowsy Maximum Strength Caplets | Acetaminophen 500mg | | Phenylephrine HCl 5mg | | | **Adults & Peds ≥12 yrs:** 2 tabs q4-6h. **Max:** 8 tabs q24h. |
| Children's Motrin Cold | Ibuprofen 100mg/5mL | | Pseudoephedrine HCl 15mg/5mL | | | **Peds 6-11 yrs (48-95 lbs):** 2 tsp (10mL) q6h. **2-5 yrs (24-47 lbs):** 1 tsp (5mL) q6h. **Max:** 4 doses q24h. |
| Sinutab Sinus Caplets | Acetaminophen 325mg | | Phenylephrine HCl 5mg | | | **Adults & Peds ≥12 yrs:** 2 tabs q4h. **Max:** 12 tabs q24h. |
| Sudafed PE Sinus Headache Caplets | Acetaminophen 325mg | | Phenylephrine HCl 5mg | | | **Adults & Peds ≥12 yrs:** 2 tabs q4h. **Max:** 12 tabs q24h. |
| Sudafed Sinus Pain 12 Hour Caplets | Naproxen Sodium 220mg | | Pseudoephedrine HCl 120mg | | | **Adults & Peds ≥12 yrs:** 1 tab q12h. **Max:** 2 tabs q24h. |
| Children's Tylenol Plus Cold & Stuffy Nose | Acetaminophen 160mg/5mL | | Phenylephrine HCl 2.5mg/5mL | | | **Peds 6-11 yrs (48-95 lbs):** 2 tsp (10mL) q4h. **Peds 4-5 yrs (36-47 lbs):** 1 tsp (5mL) q4h. **Max:** 5 doses q24h. |
| Tylenol Sinus Congestion & Pain Daytime | Acetaminophen 325mg | | Phenylephrine HCl 5mg | | | **Adults & Peds ≥12 yrs:** 2 caps q4h. **Max:** 12 caps q24h. |
| Vicks DayQuil Sinus Liquicaps | Acetaminophen 325mg | | Phenylephrine HCl 5mg | | | **Adults & Peds ≥12 yrs:** 2 caps q4h. **Max:** 12 caps q24h. |
| **DECONGESTANT + EXPECTORANT** | | | | | | |
| Maximum Strength Mucinex D | | | Pseudoephedrine HCl 120mg | | Guaifenesin 1200mg | **Adults & Peds ≥12 yrs:** 1 tab q12h. **Max:** 2 tabs q24h. |
| Mucinex Cold Liquid (Mixed Berry Flavor) | | | Phenylephrine HCl 2.5mg/5mL | | Guaifenesin 100mg/5mL | **Peds 6-<12 yrs:** 2 tsp (10mL) q4h. **Peds 4-<6 yrs:** 1 tsp (5mL) q4h. **Max:** 6 doses q24h. |

| BRAND NAME | ANALGESIC | ANTIHISTAMINE | DECONGESTANT | COUGH SUPPRESSANT | EXPECTORANT | DOSE |
|---|---|---|---|---|---|---|
| Mucinex D | | | Pseudoephedrine HCl 60mg | | Guaifenesin 600mg | **Adults & Peds ≥12 yrs:** 2 tabs q12h. **Max:** 4 tabs q24h. |
| Sudafed PE Non-Drying Sinus Caplets | | | Phenylephrine HCl 5mg | | Guaifenesin 200mg | **Adults & Peds ≥12 yrs:** 2 tabs q4h. **Max:** 12 tabs q24h. |
| Triaminic Chest & Nasal Congestion | | | Phenylephrine HCl 2.5mg/5mL | | Guaifenesin 50mg/5mL | **Peds 6-<12 yrs:** 2 tsp (10mL) q4h. **Peds 4-<6 yrs:** 1 tsp (5mL) q4h. **Max:** 6 doses q24h. |
| **DECONGESTANT + EXPECTORANT + ANALGESIC** | | | | | | |
| Sudafed PE Triple Action Caplets | Acetaminophen 325mg | | Phenylephrine HCl 5mg | | Guaifenesin 200mg | **Adults & Peds ≥12 yrs:** 2 tabs q4h. **Max:** 12 tabs q24h. |
| Sudafed Triple Action Caplets | Acetaminophen 325mg | | Pseudoephedrine HCl 30mg | | Guaifenesin 200mg | **Adults & Peds ≥12 yrs:** 2 tabs q4-6h. **Max:** 8 tabs q24h. |
| Theraflu Warming Relief Cold & Chest Congestion | Acetaminophen 325mg/15mL | | Phenylephrine HCl 5mg/15mL | | Guaifenesin 200mg/15mL | **Adults & Peds ≥12 yrs:** 2 tbl (30mL) q4h. **Max:** 6 doses q24h. |
| Tylenol Sinus Severe Congestion & Pain | Acetaminophen 325mg | | Phenylephrine HCl 5mg | | Guaifenesin 200mg | **Adults & Peds ≥12 yrs:** 2 tabs q4h. **Max:** 12 tabs q24h. |
| Tylenol Sinus Severe Congestion Daytime | Acetaminophen 325mg | | Pseudoephedrine HCl 30mg | | Guaifenesin 200mg | **Adults & Peds ≥12 yrs:** 2 tabs q4-6h. **Max:** 8 tabs q24h. |
| **EXPECTORANT** | | | | | | |
| Maximum Strength Mucinex | | | | | Guaifenesin 1200mg | **Adults & Peds ≥12 yrs:** 1 tab q12h. **Max:** 2 tabs q24h. |
| Mucinex | | | | | Guaifenesin 600mg | **Adults & Peds ≥12 yrs:** 1-2 tabs q12h. **Max:** 4 tabs q24h. |
| Mucinex Liquid (Grape Flavor) | | | | | Guaifenesin 100mg | **Peds 6-<12 yrs:** 1-2 tsp (5-10mL) q4h. **Peds 4-<6 yrs:** ½-1 tsp (2.5-5mL) q4h. **Max:** 6 doses q24h. |
| Mucinex Mini-Melts (Bubble Gum Flavor) | | | | | Guaifenesin 100mg | **Adults & Peds ≥12 yrs:** 2-4 pkts q4h. **Peds 6-<12 yrs:** 1-2 pkts q4h. **Peds 4-<6 yrs:** 1 pkt q4h. **Max:** 6 doses q24h. |
| Mucinex Mini-Melts (Grape Flavor) | | | | | Guaifenesin 50mg | **Peds 6-<12 yrs:** 2-4 pkts q4h. **Peds 4-<6 yrs:** 1-2 pkts q4h. **Max:** 6 doses q24h. |

(Continued)

| BRAND NAME | ANALGESIC | ANTIHISTAMINE | DECONGESTANT | COUGH SUPPRESSANT | EXPECTORANT | DOSE |
|---|---|---|---|---|---|---|
| **EXPECTORANT** *(Continued)* | | | | | | |
| Robitussin Chest Congestion | | | | | Guaifenesin 100mg/5mL | **Adults & Peds ≥12 yrs:** 2-4 tsp (10-20mL) q4h. **Max:** 6 doses q24h. |
| Vicks DayQuil Mucus Control Liquid | | | | | Guaifenesin 200mg | **Adults & Peds ≥12 yrs:** 2 tbl (30mL) q4h. **Peds 6-<12 yrs:** 1 tbl (15mL) q4h. **Max:** 6 doses q24h. |
| **EXPECTORANT + ANALGESIC** | | | | | | |
| Comtrex Day & Night Cold & Cough Caplets | Acetaminophen 325mg | | | | Guaifenesin 200mg | **Adults & Peds ≥12 yrs:** 2 tabs q6h. **Max:** 4 tabs q24h. |
| Comtrex Deep Chest Cold Caplets | Acetaminophen 325mg | | | | Guaifenesin 200mg | **Adults & Peds ≥12 yrs:** 2 tabs q4h. **Max:** 12 tabs q24h. |
| Theraflu Flu & Chest Congestion Hot Liquid | Acetaminophen 1000mg/packet | | | | Guaifenesin 400mg/packet | **Adults & Peds ≥12 yrs:** 1 pkt q6h. **Max:** 4 pkts q24h. |
| **ANTIHISTAMINE + ANALGESIC** | | | | | | |
| Advil PM Caplets/Liqui-Gels | Ibuprofen 200mg | Diphenhydramine Citrate 38mg | | | | **Adults & Peds ≥12 yrs:** 2 caps hs. **Max:** 2 caps q24h. |
| Coricidin HBP Cold & Flu | Acetaminophen 325mg | Chlorpheniramine Maleate 2mg | | | | **Adults & Peds ≥12 yrs:** 2 tabs q4-6h. **Max:** 12 tabs q24h. **Peds 6-<12 yrs:** 1 tab q4-6h. **Max:** 5 tabs q24h. |
| Motrin PM | Ibuprofen 200mg | Diphenhydramine Citrate 38mg | | | | **Adults & Peds ≥12 yrs:** 2 tabs hs. **Max:** 2 tabs q24h. |
| Tylenol Severe Allergy | Acetaminophen 500mg | Diphenhydramine HCl 12.5mg | | | | **Adults & Peds ≥12 yrs:** 2 tabs q4–6h. **Max:** 8 tabs q24h. |

# ANALGESIC PRODUCTS

| BRAND | INGREDIENT/STRENGTH | DOSE |
|---|---|---|
| **ACETAMINOPHEN** | | |
| Anacin Extra Strength Aspirin Free Tablets | Acetaminophen 500mg | **Adults & Peds ≥12 yrs:** 2 tabs q6h. **Max:** 8 tabs q24h. |
| FeverAll Childrens' Suppositories | Acetaminophen 120mg | **Peds 3-6 yrs:** 1 supp. q4-6h. **Max:** 6 supp. q24h. |
| FeverAll Infants' Suppositories | Acetaminophen 80mg | **Peds 3-11 months:** 1 supp. q6h. **12-36 months:** 1 supp. q4h. **Max:** 6 supp. q24h. |
| FeverAll Jr. Strength Suppositories | Acetaminophen 325mg | **Peds 6-12 yrs:** 1 supp. q4-6h. **Max:** 6 supp. q24h. |
| Tylenol 8 Hour Caplets | Acetaminophen 650mg | **Adults & Peds ≥12 yrs:** 2 tabs q8h prn. **Max:** 6 tabs q24h. |
| Tylenol Arthritis Caplets | Acetaminophen 650mg | **Adults:** 2 tabs q8h prn. **Max:** 6 tabs q24h. |
| Tylenol Arthritis Gelcaps | Acetaminophen 650mg | **Adults:** 2 tabs q8h prn. **Max:** 6 tabs q24h. |
| Tylenol Arthritis Geltabs | Acetaminophen 650mg | **Adults:** 2 tabs q8h prn. **Max:** 6 tabs q24h. |
| Tylenol Children's Meltaways Tablets | Acetaminophen 80mg | **Peds 2-3 yrs (24-35 lbs):** 2 tabs. **4-5 yrs (36-47 lbs):** 3 tabs. **6-8 yrs (48-59 lbs):** 4 tabs. **9-10 yrs (60-71 lbs):** 5 tabs. **11 yrs (72-95 lbs):** 6 tabs. May repeat q4h. **Max:** 5 doses q24h. |
| Tylenol Children's Suspension | Acetaminophen 160mg/5mL | **Peds 2-3 yrs (24-35 lbs):** 1 tsp (5mL). **4-5 yrs (36-47 lbs):** 1.5 tsp (7.5mL). **6-8 yrs (48-59 lbs):** 2 tsp (10mL). **9-10 yrs (60-71 lbs):** 2.5 tsp (12.5mL). **11 yrs (72-95 lbs):** 3 tsp (15mL). May repeat q4h. **Max:** 5 doses q24h. |
| Tylenol Extra Strength Caplets | Acetaminophen 500mg | **Adults & Peds ≥12 yrs:** 2 tabs q4-6h prn. **Max:** 8 tabs q24h. |
| Tylenol Extra Strength Cool Caplets | Acetaminophen 500mg | **Adults & Peds ≥12 yrs:** 2 tabs q4-6h prn. **Max:** 8 tabs q24h. |
| Tylenol Extra Strength Rapid Release Gelcaps | Acetaminophen 500mg | **Adults & Peds ≥12 yrs:** 2 caps q4-6h prn. **Max:** 8 caps q24h. |
| Tylenol Extra Strength Rapid Blast Liquid | Acetaminophen 1000mg/30mL | **Adults & Peds ≥12 yrs:** 2 tbl (30mL) q4-6h prn. **Max:** 8 tbl (120mL) q24h. |
| Tylenol Extra Strength EZ Tablets | Acetaminophen 500mg | **Adults & Peds ≥12 yrs:** 2 tabs q4-6h prn. **Max:** 8 tabs q24h. |
| Tylenol Infants' Drops | Acetaminophen 80mg/0.8mL | **Peds 2-3 yrs (24-35 lbs):** 1.6 mL q4h prn. **Max:** 5 doses (8mL) q24h. |
| Tylenol Junior Meltaways Tablets | Acetaminophen 160mg | **Peds 6-8 yrs (48-59 lbs):** 2 tabs. **9-10 yrs (60-71 lbs):** 2.5 tabs. **11 yrs (72-95 lbs):** 3 tabs. **12 yrs (≥96 lbs):** 4 tabs. May repeat q4h. **Max:** 5 doses q24h. |
| Tylenol Regular Strength Tablets | Acetaminophen 325mg | **Adults & Peds ≥12 yrs:** 2 tabs q4-6h prn. **Max:** 12 tabs q24h. **Peds 6-11 yrs:** 1 tab q4-6h. **Max:** 5 tabs q24h. |
| **ACETAMINOPHEN COMBINATIONS** | | |
| Anacin Advanced Headache Tablets | Acetaminophen/Aspirin/Caffeine 250mg-250mg-65mg | **Adults & Peds ≥12 yrs:** 2 tabs q6h. **Max:** 8 tabs q24h. |
| Excedrin Back & Body Caplets | Acetaminophen/Aspirin Buffered 250mg-250mg | **Adults & Peds ≥12 yrs:** 2 tabs q6h. **Max:** 8 tabs q24h. |
| Excedrin Extra Strength Caplets | Acetaminophen/Aspirin/Caffeine 250mg-250mg-65mg | **Adults & Peds ≥12 yrs:** 2 tabs q6h. **Max:** 8 tabs q24h. |

*(Continued)*

| BRAND | INGREDIENT/STRENGTH | DOSE |
|---|---|---|
| **ACETAMINOPHEN COMBINATIONS** *(Continued)* | | |
| Excedrin Extra Strength Geltabs | Acetaminophen/Aspirin/Caffeine 250mg-250mg-65mg | **Adults & Peds ≥12 yrs:** 2 tabs q6h. **Max:** 8 tabs q24h. |
| Excedrin Extra Strength Express Gels | Acetaminophen/Aspirin/Caffeine 250mg-250mg-65mg | **Adults & Peds ≥12 yrs:** 2 tabs q6h. **Max:** 8 tabs q24h. |
| Excedrin Extra Strength Tablets | Acetaminophen/Aspirin/Caffeine 250mg-250mg-65mg | **Adults & Peds ≥12 yrs:** 2 tabs q6h. **Max:** 8 tabs q24h. |
| Excedrin Menstrual Complete Express Gels | Acetaminophen/Aspirin/Caffeine 250mg-250mg-65mg | **Adults & Peds ≥12 yrs:** 2 tabs q6h. **Max:** 8 tabs q24h. |
| Excedrin Migraine Caplets | Acetaminophen/Aspirin/Caffeine 250mg-250mg-65mg | **Adults:** 2 tabs prn. **Max:** 2 tabs q24h. |
| Excedrin Migraine Geltabs | Acetaminophen/Aspirin/Caffeine 250mg-250mg-65mg | **Adults:** 2 tabs prn. **Max:** 2 tabs q24h. |
| Excedrin Migraine Tablets | Acetaminophen/Aspirin/Caffeine 250mg-250mg-65mg | **Adults:** 2 tabs prn. **Max:** 2 tabs q24h. |
| Excedrin Sinus Headache Caplets | Acetaminophen/Phenylephrine HCl 325mg-5mg | **Adults & Peds ≥12 yrs:** 2 tabs q4h. **Max:** 12 tabs q24h. |
| Excedrin Tension Headache Caplets | Acetaminophen/Caffeine 500mg-65mg | **Adults & Peds ≥12 yrs:** 2 tabs q6h. **Max:** 8 tabs q24h. |
| Excedrin Tension Headache Express Gels | Acetaminophen/Caffeine 500mg-65mg | **Adults & Peds ≥12 yrs:** 2 caps q6h. **Max:** 8 caps q24h. |
| Excedrin Tension Headache Geltabs | Acetaminophen/Caffeine 500mg-65mg | **Adults & Peds ≥12 yrs:** 2 tabs q6h. **Max:** 8 tabs q24h. |
| Goody's Body Pain Powder | Acetaminophen/Aspirin 325mg-500mg | **Adults & Peds ≥12 yrs:** 1 powder q4-6h. **Max:** 4 powders q24h. |
| Goody's Cool Orange | Acetaminophen/Aspirin/Caffeine 325mg-500mg-65mg | **Adults & Peds ≥12 yrs:** 1 powder q6h. **Max:** 4 powders q24h. |
| Goody's Extra Strength Headache Powder | Acetaminophen/Aspirin/Caffeine 260mg-520mg-32.5mg | **Adults & Peds ≥12 yrs:** 1 powder q4-6h. **Max:** 4 powders q24h. |
| Midol Menstrual Complete Caplets | Acetaminophen/Caffeine/Pyrilamine Maleate 500mg-60mg-15mg | **Adults & Peds ≥12 yrs:** 2 tabs q6h. **Max:** 8 tabs q24h. |
| Midol Menstrual Complete Gelcaps | Acetaminophen/Caffeine/Pyrilamine Maleate 500mg-60mg-15mg | **Adults & Peds ≥12 yrs:** 2 caps q6h. **Max:** 8 caps q24h. |
| Midol Teen Formula Caplets | Acetaminophen/Pamabrom 500mg-25mg | **Adults & Peds ≥12 yrs:** 2 tabs q6h. **Max:** 8 tabs q24h. |
| Pamprin Cramp Caplets | Acetaminophen/Magnesium Salicylate/ Pamabrom 250mg-250mg-25mg | **Adults & Peds ≥12 yrs:** 2 tabs q4-6h. **Max:** 8 tabs q24h. |
| Pamprin Max Caplets | Acetaminophen/Aspirin/Caffeine 250mg-250mg-65mg | **Adults & Peds ≥12 yrs:** 2 tabs q4-6h. **Max:** 8 tabs q24h. |
| Pamprin Multi-Symptom Caplets | Acetaminophen/Pamabrom/Pyrilamine 500mg-25mg-15mg | **Adults & Peds ≥12 yrs:** 2 tabs q4-6h. **Max:** 8 tabs q24h. |
| Premsyn PMS Caplets | Acetaminophen/Pamabrom/Pyrilamine 500mg-25mg-15mg | **Adults & Peds ≥12 yrs:** 2 tabs q4-6h. **Max:** 8 tabs q24h. |
| Vanquish Caplets | Acetaminophen/Aspirin/Caffeine 194mg-227mg-33mg | **Adults & Peds ≥12 yrs:** 2 tabs q6h. **Max:** 8 tabs q24h. |
| **ACETAMINOPHEN/SLEEP AIDS** | | |
| Excedrin PM Caplets | Acetaminophen/Diphenhydramine Citrate 500mg-38mg | **Adults & Peds ≥12 yrs:** 2 tabs qhs. **Max:** 2 tabs q24h. |
| Excedrin PM Express Gels | Acetaminophen/Diphenhydramine Citrate 500mg-38mg | **Adults & Peds ≥12 yrs:** 2 tabs qhs. **Max:** 2 tabs q24h. |
| Excedrin PM Tablets | Acetaminophen/Diphenhydramine Citrate 500mg-38mg | **Adults & Peds ≥12 yrs:** 2 tabs qhs. **Max:** 2 tabs q24h. |
| Goody's PM Powder | Acetaminophen/Diphenhydramine 1000mg-76mg/dose | **Adults & Peds ≥12 yrs:** 1 packet (2 powders) qhs. |
| Tylenol PM Caplets | Acetaminophen/Diphenhydramine 500mg-25mg | **Adults & Peds ≥12 yrs:** 2 tabs qhs. **Max:** 2 tabs q24h. |
| Tylenol PM Rapid Release Gels | Acetaminophen/Diphenhydramine 500mg-25mg | **Adults & Peds ≥12 yrs:** 2 caps qhs. **Max:** 2 caps q24h. |

*(Continued)*

| BRAND | INGREDIENT/STRENGTH | DOSE |
|---|---|---|
| **ACETAMINOPHEN/SLEEP AIDS** *(Continued)* | | |
| Tylenol PM Geltabs | Acetaminophen/Diphenhydramine 500mg-25mg | **Adults & Peds ≥12 yrs:** 2 tabs qhs. **Max:** 2 tabs q24h. |
| Tylenol PM Vanilla Liquid | Acetaminophen/Diphenhydramine 1000mg-50mg/30mL | **Adults & Peds ≥12 yrs:** 2 tbl (30mL) qhs. **Max:** 2 tbl (30mL) q24h. |
| **NSAIDs** | | |
| Advil Caplets | Ibuprofen 200mg | **Adults & Peds ≥12 yrs:** 1-2 tabs q4-6h. **Max:** 6 tabs q24h. |
| Advil Children's Suspension | Ibuprofen 100mg/5mL | **Peds 2-3 yrs (24-35 lbs):** 1 tsp (5mL). **4-5 yrs (36-47 lbs):** 1.5 tsp (7.5mL). **6-8 yrs (48-59 lbs):** 2 tsp (10mL). **9-10 yrs (60-71 lbs):** 2.5 tsp (12.5mL). **11 yrs (72-95 lbs):** 3 tsp (15mL). May repeat q6-8h. **Max:** 4 doses q24h. |
| Advil Gel Caplets | Ibuprofen 200mg | **Adults & Peds ≥12 yrs:** 1-2 tabs q4-6h. **Max:** 6 tabs q24h. |
| Advil Infants' Concentrated Drops | Ibuprofen 50mg/1.25mL | **Peds 6-11 months (12-17 lbs):** 1.25mL. **12-23 months (18-23 lbs):** 1.875mL. May repeat q6-8h. **Max:** 4 doses q24h. |
| Advil Liqui-Gels | Ibuprofen 200mg | **Adults & Peds ≥12 yrs:** 1-2 caps q4-6h. **Max:** 6 caps q24h. |
| Advil Migraine Capsules | Ibuprofen 200mg | **Adults:** 2 caps prn. **Max:** 2 caps q24h. |
| Advil Tablets | Ibuprofen 200mg | **Adults & Peds ≥12 yrs:** 1-2 tabs q4-6h. **Max:** 6 tabs q24h. |
| Aleve Caplets | Naproxen Sodium 220mg | **Adults & Peds ≥12 yrs:** 1 tab q8-12h. May take 1 additional tab within 1h of first dose. **Max:** 2 tabs q8-12h or 3 tabs q24h. |
| Aleve Liquid Gels | Naproxen Sodium 220mg | **Adults & Peds ≥12 yrs:** 1 cap q8-12h. May take 1 additional cap within 1 hour of first dose. **Max:** 2 caps q8-12h or 3 caps q24h. |
| Aleve Smooth Gels | Naproxen Sodium 220mg | **Adults & Peds ≥12 yrs:** 1 cap q8-12h. May take 1 additional cap within 1 hour of first dose. **Max:** 2 caps q8-12h or 3 caps q24h. |
| Aleve Tablets | Naproxen Sodium 220mg | **Adults & Peds ≥12 yrs:** 1 tab q8-12h. May take 1 additional tab within 1 hour of first dose. **Max:** 2 tabs q8-12h or 3 tabs q24h. |
| Midol Liquid Gels | Ibuprofen 200mg | **Adults & Peds ≥12 yrs:** 1-2 caps q4-6h. **Max:** 6 caps q24h. |
| Midol Extended Relief Caplets | Naproxen Sodium 220mg | **Adults & Peds ≥12 yrs:** 1-2 tabs q8-12h. **Max:** 2 tabs q8-12h or 3 tabs q24h. |
| Motrin Children's Suspension | Ibuprofen 100mg/5mL | **Peds 2-3 yrs (24-35 lbs):** 1 tsp (5mL). **4-5 yrs (36-47 lbs):** 1.5 tsp (7.5mL). **6-8 yrs (48-59 lbs):** 2 tsp (10mL). **9-10 yrs (60-71 lbs):** 2.5 tsp (12.5mL). **11 yrs (72-95 lbs):** 3 tsp (15mL). May repeat q6-8h. **Max:** 4 doses q24h. |
| Motrin IB Caplets | Ibuprofen 200mg | **Adults & Peds ≥12 yrs:** 1-2 tabs q4-6h. **Max:** 6 tabs q24h. |
| Motrin IB Tablets | Ibuprofen 200mg | **Adults & Peds ≥12 yrs:** 1-2 tabs q4-6h. **Max:** 6 tabs q24h. |

*(Continued)*

| BRAND | INGREDIENT/STRENGTH | DOSE |
|---|---|---|
| **NSAIDs** *(Continued)* | | |
| Motrin Infants' Drops | Ibuprofen 50mg/1.25mL | **Peds 6-11 months (12-17 lbs):** 1.25mL. **12-23 months (18-23 lbs):** 1.875mL. May repeat q6-8h. **Max:** 4 doses q24h. |
| Motrin Junior Strength Caplets | Ibuprofen 100mg | **Peds 6-8 yrs (48-59 lbs):** 2 tabs. **9-10 yrs (60-71 lbs):** 2.5 tabs. **11 yrs (72-95 lbs):** 3 tabs. May repeat q6-8h. **Max:** 4 doses q24h. |
| Motrin Junior Strength Chewable Tablets | Ibuprofen 100mg | **Peds 2-3 yrs (24-35 lbs):** 1 tab. **4-5 yrs (36-47 lbs):** 1.5 tabs. **6-8 yrs (48-59 lbs):** 2 tabs. **9-10 yrs (60-71 lbs):** 2.5 tabs. **11 yrs (72-95 lbs):** 3 tabs. May repeat q6-8h. **Max:** 4 doses q24h. |
| Pamprin All Day Caplets | Naproxen Sodium 220mg | **Adults & Peds ≥12 yrs:** 1-2 tabs q8-12h. **Max:** 2 tabs q8-12h or 3 tabs q24h. |
| **NSAID SLEEP AIDS** | | |
| Advil PM Caplets | Ibuprofen/Diphenhydramine Citrate 200mg-38mg | **Adults & Peds ≥12 yrs:** 2 tabs qhs. **Max:** 2 tabs q24h. |
| Advil PM Liqui-Gels | Ibuprofen/Diphenhydramine 200mg-25mg | **Adults & Peds ≥12 yrs:** 2 caps qhs. **Max:** 2 caps q24h. |
| Motrin PM Caplets | Ibuprofen/Diphenhydramine Citrate 200mg-38mg | **Adults & Peds ≥12 yrs:** 2 tabs qhs. **Max:** 2 tabs q24h. |
| **SALICYLATES** | | |
| Bayer Aspirin Extra Strength Caplets | Aspirin 500mg | **Adults & Peds ≥12 yrs:** 1-2 tabs q4-6h. **Max:** 8 tabs q24h. |
| Bayer Aspirin Safety Coated Caplets | Aspirin 325mg | **Adults & Peds ≥12 yrs:** 1-2 tabs q4h. **Max:** 12 tabs q24h. |
| Bayer Low Dose Aspirin Chewable Tablets | Aspirin 81mg | **Adults & Peds ≥12 yrs:** 4-8 tabs q4h. **Max:** 48 tabs q24h. |
| Bayer Low Dose Aspirin Safety Coated Tablets | Aspirin 81mg | **Adults & Peds ≥12 yrs:** 4-8 tabs q4h. **Max:** 48 tabs q24h. |
| Bayer Genuine Aspirin Tablets | Aspirin 325mg | **Adults & Peds ≥12 yrs:** 1-2 tabs q4h or 3 tabs q6h. **Max:** 12 tabs q24h. |
| Doan's Extra Strength Caplets | Magnesium Salicylate Tetrahydrate 580mg | **Adults & Peds ≥12 yrs:** 2 tabs q6h. **Max:** 8 tabs q24h. |
| Ecotrin Low Strength Tablets | Aspirin 81mg | **Adults:** 4-8 tabs q4h. **Max:** 48 tabs q24h. |
| Ecotrin Regular Strength Tablets | Aspirin 325mg | **Adults & Peds ≥12 yrs:** 1-2 tabs q4h. **Max:** 12 tabs q24h. |
| Halfprin 162mg Tablets | Aspirin 162mg | **Adults & Peds ≥12 yrs:** 2-4 tabs q4h. **Max:** 24 tabs q24h. |
| Halfprin 81mg Tablets | Aspirin 81mg | **Adults & Peds ≥12 yrs:** 4-8 tabs q4h. **Max:** 48 tabs q24h. |
| St. Joseph Chewable Aspirin Tablets | Aspirin 81mg | **Adults & Peds ≥12 yrs:** 4-8 tabs q4h. **Max:** 48 tabs q24h. |
| St. Joseph Enteric Safety-Coated Tablets | Aspirin 81mg | **Adults & Peds ≥12 yrs:** 4-8 tabs q4h. **Max:** 48 tabs q24h. |
| **SALICYLATES, BUFFERED** | | |
| Alka-Seltzer Lemon-Lime Tablets | Aspirin/Citric Acid/Sodium Bicarbonate 325mg-1000mg-1700mg | **Adults & Peds ≥12 yrs:** 2 tabs q4h. **Max:** 8 tabs q24h. **≥60 yrs: Max:** 4 tabs q24h. |
| Alka-Seltzer Original Effervescent Tablets | Aspirin/Citric Acid/Sodium Bicarbonate 325mg-1000mg-1916mg | **Adults & Peds ≥12 yrs:** 2 tabs q4h. **Max:** 8 tabs q24h. **≥60 yrs: Max:** 4 tabs q24h. |
| Alka-Seltzer Extra Strength Effervescent Tablets | Aspirin/Citric Acid/Sodium Bicarbonate 500mg-1000mg-1985mg | **Adults & Peds ≥12 yrs:** 2 tabs q6h. **Max:** 7 tabs q24h. **≥60 yrs: Max:** 3 tabs q24h. |

*(Continued)*

| BRAND | INGREDIENT/STRENGTH | DOSE |
|---|---|---|
| **SALICYLATES, BUFFERED** *(Continued)* | | |
| Ascriptin Maximum Strength Tablets | Aspirin 500mg Buffered with Aluminum Hydroxide/Calcium Carbonate/Magnesium Hydroxide | **Adults:** 2 tabs q6h. **Max:** 8 tabs q24h. |
| Ascriptin Regular Strength Tablets | Aspirin 325mg Buffered with Aluminum Hydroxide/Calcium Carbonate/Magnesium Hydroxide | **Adults:** 2 tabs q4h. **Max:** 12 tabs q24h. |
| Bayer Extra Strength Plus Caplets | Aspirin 500mg Buffered with Calcium Carbonate | **Adults & Peds ≥12 yrs:** 1-2 tabs q4-6h. **Max:** 8 tabs q24h. |
| Bayer Women's Low Dose Aspirin Caplets | Aspirin 81mg Buffered with Calcium Carbonate 777mg | **Adults & Peds ≥12 yrs:** 4-8 tabs q4h. **Max:** 10 tabs q24h. |
| Bufferin Extra Strength Tablets | Aspirin 500mg Buffered with Calcium Carbonate/Magnesium Oxide/Magnesium Carbonate | **Adults & Peds ≥12 yrs:** 2 tabs q6h. **Max:** 8 tabs q24h. |
| Bufferin Tablets | Aspirin 325mg Buffered with Benzoic Acid/Citric Acid | **Adults & Peds ≥12 yrs:** 2 tabs q4h. **Max:** 12 tabs q24h. |
| **SALICYLATE COMBINATIONS** | | |
| Alka-Seltzer Wake-Up Call | Aspirin/Caffeine 500mg-65mg | **Adults & Peds ≥12 yrs:** 2 tabs q6h. **Max:** 8 tabs q24h. **≥60 yrs: Max:** 4 tabs q24h. |
| Anacin Max Strength Tablets | Aspirin/Caffeine 500mg-32mg | **Adults & Peds ≥12 yrs:** 2 tabs q6h. **Max:** 8 tabs q24h. |
| Anacin Regular Strength Caplets | Aspirin/Caffeine 400mg-32mg | **Adults & Peds ≥12 yrs:** 2 tabs q6h. **Max:** 8 tabs q24h. |
| Anacin Tablets | Aspirin/Caffeine 400mg-32mg | **Adults & Peds ≥12 yrs:** 2 tabs q6h. **Max:** 8 tabs q24h. |
| Bayer Back & Body Pain Caplets | Aspirin/Caffeine 500mg-32.5mg | **Adults & Peds ≥12 yrs:** 2 tabs q6h. **Max:** 8 tabs q24h. |
| Bayer Quick Release Crystals | Aspirin/Caffeine 850mg-65mg | **Adults & Peds ≥12 yrs:** 1 powder pouch q6h. **Max:** 4 powder pouches q24h. |
| BC Arthritis Strength Powders | Aspirin/Caffeine/Salicylamide 742mg-38mg-222mg | **Adults & Peds ≥12 yrs:** 1 powder q3-4h. **Max:** 4 powders q24h. |
| BC Original Formula Powders | Aspirin/Caffeine/Salicylamide 650mg-33.3mg-195mg | **Adults & Peds ≥12 yrs:** 1 powder q3-4h. **Max:** 4 powders q24h. |
| **SALICYLATE/SLEEP AID** | | |
| Alka-Seltzer PM Effervescent Tablets | Aspirin/Diphenhydramine Citrate 325mg-38mg | **Adults & Peds ≥12 yrs:** 2 tabs qhs. **Max:** 2 tabs q24h. |
| Bayer PM Caplets | Aspirin/Diphenhydramine Citrate 500mg-38.3mg | **Adults & Peds ≥12 yrs:** 2 tabs qhs. |
| Doan's Extra Strength PM Caplets | Magnesium Salicylate Tetrahydrate/Diphenhydramine 580mg-25mg | **Adults & Peds ≥12 yrs:** 2 tabs qhs. |

# ACE INHIBITORS

| DRUG (BRAND) | PEAK PLASMA LEVEL | FOOD EFFECT ON AMOUNT ABSORBED | HYPERTENSION DOSING* | HEART FAILURE DOSING | RENAL DOSE ADJUSTMENT |
|---|---|---|---|---|---|
| **Benazepril** (Lotensin) | 1-2 hrs (fasting); 2-4 hrs (non-fasting**) | None | **Initial:** 10mg qd. **Usual:** 20-40mg/day given qd-bid. **Max:** 80mg/day. | Not FDA approved. | CrCl<30mL/min/1.73m$^2$: **Initial:** 5mg qd. **Max:** 40mg/day. |
| **Captopril** (Capoten) | 1 hr | Reduced*** | **Initial:** 25mg bid-tid. **Usual:** 25-150mg bid-tid. **Max:** 450mg/day. | **Initial:** 25mg tid. **Usual:** 50-100mg tid. **Max:** 450mg/day. | **Significant Renal Dysfunction:** Lower initial dose and titrate slowly. |
| **Enalapril** (Vasotec) | 3-4 hrs** | None | **Initial:** 5mg qd. **Usual:** 10-40mg/day given qd-bid. **Max:** 40mg/day.† | **Initial:** 2.5mg qd. **Usual:** 2.5-20mg given bid. **Max:** 40mg/day. | **HTN:** CrCl ≤30mL/min: **Initial:** 2.5mg/day. **Max:** 40mg/day. **Dialysis:** 2.5mg/day on dialysis day. **HF:** SCr 1.6mg/dL: **Initial:** 2.5mg qd. **Max:** 40mg/day. |
| **Fosinopril** (Monopril) | 3 hrs** | None | **Initial:** 10mg qd. **Usual:** 20-40mg/day. **Max:** 80mg/day.† | **Initial:** 10mg qd. **Usual:** 20-40mg qd. **Max:** 40mg/day. | **HTN:** No dosage adjustment needed. **HF:** Moderate to severe renal failure/vigorous diuresis: initial: 5mg qd. |
| **Lisinopril** (Prinivil, Zestril) | 7 hrs | None | **Initial:** 10mg qd. **Usual:** 20-40mg qd. **Max:** 80mg/day.† | (Prinivil) **Initial:** 5mg qd. **Usual:** 5-20mg qd. (Zestril) **Initial:** 5mg qd. **Usual:** 5-40mg qd. **Max:** 40mg/day. | **HTN:** CrCl 10-30mL/min: **Initial:** 5mg qd. **Max:** 40mg/day. CrCl <10mL/min: **Initial:** 2.5mg qd. **Max:** 40mg/day. **HF:** CrCl ≤30mL/min: **Initial:** 2.5mg qd. |
| **Moexipril** (Univasc) | 1.5 hrs** | Reduced*** | **Initial:** 7.5mg qd. **Usual:** 7.5-30mg/day given qd-bid. **Max:** 60mg/day. | Not FDA approved. | CrCl ≤40mL/min/1.73m$^2$: **Initial:** 3.75mg qd. **Max:** 15mg/day. |
| **Perindopril** (Aceon) | 3-7 hrs** | None | **Initial:** 4mg qd. **Usual:** 4-8mg/day qd. **Max:** 16mg/day. | Not FDA approved. | CrCl >30mL/min: **Initial:** 2mg qd. **Max:** 8mg/day. |
| **Quinapril** (Accupril) | 2 hrs** | Reduced (after high-fat meals) | **Initial:** 10-20mg qd. **Usual:** 20-80mg/day given qd-bid. | **Initial:** 5mg bid. **Usual:** 10-20mg bid. | CrCl 30-60mL/min: **Initial:** 5mg/day. CrCl 10-30mL/min: **Initial:** 2.5mg/day. |
| **Ramipril** (Altace) | 2-4 hrs** | None | **Initial:** 2.5mg qd. **Usual:** 2.5-20mg/day given qd-bid. | **Post MI:** **Initial:** 2.5mg bid; 1.25mg bid if hypotensive. Titrate to 5mg bid. | **HTN:** **Initial:** 1.25mg qd. **Max:** 5mg/day. **Post MI:** **Initial:** 1.25mg/day. **Max:** 2.5mg/bid. |
| **Trandolapril** (Mavik) | 4-10 hrs** | None | **Initial:** 1mg qd in non-black patients. 2mg qd in black patients. **Usual:** 2-4mg/day. **Max:** 8mg/day. | **Post MI:** **Initial:** 1mg qd. Titrate to 4mg qd if tolerated. | CrCl <30mL/min: **Initial:** 0.5mg qd. Titrate slowly. |

* Note: Dosages may need to be adjusted when used in combination with other antihypertensives (ie, diuretics). Monitor patient closely. For more information, refer to monograph listings or drug's FDA-approved labeling.
** Peak effect of active metabolite.
*** Administer 1 hour before meals.
† Refer to monograph for pediatric dosing.

# ANTIARRHYTHMIC AGENTS

| DRUG (BRAND) | HOW SUPPLIED | INDICATION | DOSAGE | HEPATIC/RENAL DOSE ADJUSTMENT* |
|---|---|---|---|---|
| **Class IA Antiarrhythmics** | | | | |
| **Disopyramide** (Norpace, Norpace CR) | Cap: (Norpace) 100mg, 150mg; Cap, Extended-Release: (Norpace CR) 100mg, 150mg | Treatment of documented life-threatening ventricular arrhythmias. | **Adults:** Usual: 400-800mg/day in divided dose. Recommended: 150mg q6h immediate-release (IR) or 300mg q12h extended-release (CR). Adjust dose with anticholinergic effects. Rapid Control of Ventricular Arrhythmia: LD: 300mg IR (200mg if <110lbs). Follow with maint dose. Cardiomyopathy/Cardiac Decompensation: Initial: 100mg q6-8h IR. Adjust gradually. See labeling if no response or toxicity occurs. Elderly: Start at low end of dosing range. **Pediatrics:** <1 yr: 10-30mg/kg/day. 1-4 yrs: 10-20mg/kg/day. 4-12 yrs: 10-15mg/kg/day. 12-18 yrs: 6-15mg/kg/day. Give in equally divided doses q6h. Hospitalize patient during initial therapy. Start dose titration at lower end of range. | Weight <110lbs/Moderate Hepatic or Renal Insufficiency (CrCl >40mL/min): 100mg q6h IR or 200mg q12h CR. Severe Renal Insufficiency (with or without initial 150mg LD): CrCl 30-40mL/min: 100mg q8h IR. CrCl 30-15mL/min: 100mg q12h IR. CrCl <15mL/min: 100mg q24h IR. |
| **Quinidine Gluconate** | Tab, Extended-Release: 324mg; Inj: 80mg/mL | Conversion of symptomatic atrial fibrillation/flutter (A-Fib/Flutter) to normal sinus rhythm, and suppression of ventricular arrhythmias. Tab: reduction of relapse frequency into A-Fib/Flutter. | **Adults:** A-Fib/Flutter Conversion: Initial: 2 tabs q8h. Titrate: Increase cautiously if no effect after 3-4 doses. Alternate Regimen: 1 tab q8h for 2 days, then 2 tabs q12h for 2 days, then 2 tabs q8h up to 4 days. A-Fib/Flutter Relapse Reduction: 1 tab q8-12h. Titrate: Increase cautiously if needed. Ventricular Arrhythmia: Dosing regimens not adequately studied. May break tab in half. Do not chew or crush. IV: A-Fib/Flutter and Ventricular Arrhythmia: 0.25mg/kg/min. Max: 5-10mg/kg. Consider alternate therapy if conversion to sinus rhythm not achieved. Elderly: Start at low end of dosing range. | Renal/Hepatic Impairment or CHF: Reduce dose. |
| **Quinidine Sulfate** | Tab: 200mg, 300mg; 300mg ER | Conversion of symptomatic A-fib/flutter to normal sinus rhythm, reduction of relapse frequency into A-fib/flutter, and suppression of ventricular arrhythmias. | **Adults:** A-Fib/Flutter Conversion: Initial: 400mg q6h. Titrate: Increase cautiously if no effect after 4-5 doses. (ER): 300mg q8-12h. Titrate: Increase dose cautiously. A-Fib/Flutter Relapse Reduction: 200mg q6h. (ER): 300mg q8-12h. Titrate: Increase cautiously if needed. Ventricular Arrhythmia: Dosing regimens not adequately studied. | Renal or hepatic impairment: Reduce dose. |

| DRUG (BRAND) | HOW SUPPLIED | INDICATION | DOSAGE | HEPATIC/RENAL DOSE ADJUSTMENT* |
|---|---|---|---|---|
| **Class IB Antiarrhythmics** | | | | |
| **Mexiletine** | Cap: 150mg, 200mg, 250mg | Treatment of life-threatening ventricular arrhythmias. | **Adults:** Initial: 200mg q8h when rapid control is not essential. Titrate: Adjust by 50-100mg, not less than every 2-3 days. Usual: 200-300mg q8h. Max: 1200mg/day. If control with ≤300mg q8h, then may divide daily dose and give q12h. Max: 450mg q12h. For Rapid Control: LD: 400mg, then 200mg in 8 hrs. Transfer from Class I Oral Agents: Initial: 200mg and titrate as above, 6-12 hrs after last quinidine sulfate or disopyramide dose, 3-6 hrs after last procainamide dose, or 8-12 hrs after last tocainide dose. Take with food or antacid. | Severe Hepatic Disease: May need lower dose. |
| **Class IC Antiarrhythmics** | | | | |
| **Flecainide** (Tambocor) | Tab: 50mg, 100mg*, 150mg* *scored | Prevention of paroxysmal supraventricular tachycardias (PSVT), paroxysmal atrial fibrillation/flutter (PAF) associated with disabling symptoms in patients without structural heart disease. Prevention of life-threatening ventricular arrhythmias (VT). | **Adults:** PSVT/PAF: Initial: 50mg q12h. Titrate: May increase by 50mg bid every 4 days. Max: 300mg/day. Sustained VT: Initial: 100mg q12h. Titrate: May increase by 50mg bid every 4 days. Max: 400mg/day. Reduce dose by 50% with amiodarone. **Pediatrics:** <6 months: Initial: $50mg/m^2$/day given bid-tid. ≥6 months: Initial: $100mg/m^2$/day given bid-tid. Max: $200mg/m^2$/day. Reduce dose by 50% with amiodarone. | CrCl ≤35mL/min: Initial: 100mg qd or 50mg bid. |
| **Propafenone** (Rythmol, Rythmol SR) | Tab: 150mg*, 225mg*, 300mg*; *scored SR: 225mg, 325mg, 425mg | To prolong the time to recurrence of paroxysmal atrial fibrillation/flutter (PAF) and paroxysmal supraventricular tachycardia (PSVT) associated with disabling symptoms in patients without structural heart disease. Treatment of life-threatening documented ventricular arrhythmias. | **Adults:** Initial: 150mg q8h. Titrate: May increase at minimum 3-4 day intervals to 225mg q8h, then to 300mg q8h if needed. Max: 900mg/day. Elderly/Marked Myocardial Damage: Increase more gradually during initial phase. **SR: Adults:** Initial: 225mg q12h. Titrate: May increase at minimum 5-day intervals to 325mg q12h, then to 425mg q12h if needed. QRS Widening/ 2nd- or 3rd-degree AV Block: Reduce dose. | Hepatic Dysfunction: Give 20-30% of normal dosage. (SR) Hepatic Impairment: Reduce dose. |
| **Class II Antiarrhythmics (Beta-Blockers)** | | | | |
| **Acebutolol** (Sectral) | Cap: 200mg, 400mg | Management of hypertension and ventricular arrhythmias. | **Adults:** Ventricular Arrhythmia: Initial: 200mg bid. Maint: Increase gradually to 600-1200mg/day. Elderly: Lower daily doses. Max: 800mg/day. | CrCl <50mL/min: Decrease daily dose by 50%. CrCl <25mL/min: Decrease daily dose by 75%. |

*(Continued)*

| DRUG (BRAND) | HOW SUPPLIED | INDICATION | DOSAGE | HEPATIC/RENAL DOSE ADJUSTMENT* |
|---|---|---|---|---|
| **Class II Antiarrhythmics (Beta-Blockers)** *(Continued)* | | | | |
| **Esmolol** (Brevibloc) | Inj: 10mg/mL [10mL, 250mL], 20mg/mL [5mL, 100mL] | For rapid control of ventricular rate in atrial fibrillation or atrial flutter in perioperative, postoperative, or other emergent circumstances. For non-compensatory sinus tachycardia. | **Adults:** Supraventricular Tachycardia: Titrate dose based on ventricular rate. Load: 0.5mg/kg over 1 min. Maint: 0.05mg/kg/min for next 4 min. May continue at 0.05mg/kg/min at intervals of 4 min or increase stepwise to max 0.2mg/kg/min. Rapid slowing of ventricular response: Repeat 0.5mg/kg load over 1 min, then 0.1mg/kg/min for 4 min. If needed, another (final) load of 0.5mg/kg over 1 min, then 0.15mg/kg/min for 4 min up to 0.2mg/kg/min. May continue infusions for 24 hrs. Intraoperative/Postoperative Tachycardia: Immediate Control: Initial: 80mg bolus over 30 sec. Maint: 0.15mg/kg/min. May titrate up to 0.3mg/kg/min. Gradual Control: Initial: 0.5mg/kg over 1 min. Maint: 0.05mg/kg/min for 4 min. Then, if needed, may repeat load and increase to 0.1mg/kg/min. | |
| **Propranolol** (Inderal) | Inj: 1mg/mL; Tab: 10mg*, 20mg*, 40mg*, 60mg*, 80mg* *scored | (Inj) For cardiac arrhythmias (supraventricular, ventricular tachycardia, tachyarrhythmia of digitalis intoxication, resistant tachyarrhythmia). (Tab) To control ventricular rate in patients with atrial fibrillation and a rapid ventricular response. | **Adults:** (Inj) 1-3mg IV at 1 mg/min. May give 2nd dose after 2 min, subsequent doses q4h prn. A Fib: 10-30mg PO tid-qid ac and hs. | Hepatic insufficiency: May need to lower dose. |
| **Sotalol** (Betapace) | Tab: 80mg*, 120mg*, 160mg* *scored | Treatment of documented life threatening ventricular arrhythmias. | **Adults:** Initial: 80mg bid. Titrate: Increase to 120-160mg bid if needed. Allow 3 days between dose increments. Usual: 160-320mg/day given bid-tid. Refractory Patients: 480-640mg/day. **Pediatrics:** ≥2 yrs: Initial: 30mg/m² tid. Titrate: Wait at least 36 hrs between dose increases. Guide dose by response, HR, and QTc. Max: 60mg/m². <2 yrs: See dosing chart in PI. Reduce dose or d/c if QTc >550msec. | **Adults:** CrCl 30-59mL/min: Dose q24h. CrCl 10-29mL/min: Dose q36-48h. CrCl <10mL/min: Individualize dose. May increase dose with renal impairment after at least 5-6 doses at appropriate intervals. **Pediatrics:** Renal Impairment: Reduce dose or increase interval. |

| DRUG (BRAND) | HOW SUPPLIED | INDICATION | DOSAGE | HEPATIC/RENAL DOSE ADJUSTMENT* |
|---|---|---|---|---|
| **Class II Antiarrhythmics (Beta-Blockers)** *(Continued)* | | | | |
| **Sotalol** (Betapace AF) | Tab: 80mg*, 120mg*, 160mg* *scored | Maintenance of normal sinus rhythm with symptomatic atrial fibrillation/atrial flutter (AFIB/AFL) in patients who are currently in sinus rhythm. | **Adults:** Initiate with continuous ECG monitoring. Give dose qd for CrCl 40-60mL/min and bid for CrCl >60mL/min. Initial: 80mg. Monitor QT 2-4 hrs after each dose. Reduce dose or d/c if QT ≥500msec. If QT <500msec after 3 days (after 5th or 6th dose if receiving qd dosing), discharge on current treatment. Alternately, may increase dose to 120mg during hospitalization, and follow for 3 days with bid dose and for 5 or 6 doses if receiving qd dose. Max: 160mg qd or bid depending on CrCl. **Pediatrics:** ≥2 yrs: Initial: 30mg/m$^2$ tid. Titrate: Wait at least 36 hrs between dose increases. Guide dose by response, heart rate and QTc. Max: 60mg/m$^2$. <2 yrs: See dosing chart in PI. Reduce dose or d/c if QTc >550msec. | Renal Impairment: Reduce dose or increase interval. |
| **Class III Antiarrhythmics** | | | | |
| **Amiodarone** (Cordarone, Nexterone, Pacerone) | Tab: 100mg, 200mg*, 400mg* *scored; Inj: 50mg/mL [3mL] | Treatment of documented, life-threatening recurrent ventricular fibrillation and recurrent hemodynamically unstable ventricular tachycardia. | **Adults:** Give LD in hospital. LD: 800-1600mg/day in divided doses for 1-3 weeks. After control is achieved, then 600-800mg/day for 1 month. Maint: 400mg/day; up to 600mg/day if needed. Use lowest effective dose. Take with meals. Elderly: Start at low end of dosing range. IV: Adults: LD: 150mg over 1st 10 min (15mg/min), then 360mg over next 6 hrs (1mg/min), then 540mg over remaining 18 hrs (0.5mg/min). Maint: 0.5mg/min for 2-3 weeks. Breakthrough Ventricular Tachycardia/Ventricular Fibrillation: 150mg supplement IV over 10 min. Increase rate to achieve suppression. Elderly: Start at low end of dosing range. Administer infusions >2 hrs in a glass or polyolefin bottle containing D5W. Amiodarone leaches out plasticizers (eg, DEHP from IV tubing) especially at higher infusion concentrations, and lower flow rates. | |

(Continued)

| DRUG (BRAND) | HOW SUPPLIED | INDICATION | DOSAGE | HEPATIC/RENAL DOSE ADJUSTMENT* |
|---|---|---|---|---|
| **Class III Antiarrhythmics** *(Continued)* | | | | |
| **Dofetilide** (Tikosyn) | Cap: 125mcg, 250mcg, 500mcg | Conversion to and maintenance of normal sinus rhythm in atrial fibrillation/flutter. | **Adults:** Individualize dose based on CrCl and QTc. Use QT interval if HR <60 beats/min. Initiate with continuous ECG monitoring. Determine QTc interval 2-3 hrs after 1st dose and adjust dose if QTc >500msec or if >15% increase from baseline. QTc Adjustment: Reduce 500mcg bid to 250mcg bid. Reduce 250mcg bid to 125mcg bid. Reduce 125mcg bid to 125mcg qd. D/C anytime after 2nd dose if QTc >500 msec (550msec with ventricular conduction abnormalities). | CrCl: >60mL/min: 500mcg bid. CrCl 40-60mL/min: 250mcg bid. CrCl 20 to <40mL/min: 125mcg bid. CrCl <20mL/min: do not use. Monitor ECG. |
| **Ibutilide** (Corvert) | Inj: 0.1mg/mL | For rapid conversion of atrial fibrillation or flutter (A-Fib/Flutter) of recent onset to sinus rhythm. | **Adults:** ≥60kg: 1mg over 10 min. <60 kg: 0.01mg/kg over 10 min. If arrhythmia still present within 10 min after the end of the initial infusion, repeat infusion 10 min after completion of 1st infusion. Continuous ECG monitoring for 4 hrs after infusion or until QTc returns to baseline. | |
| **Class IV Antiarrhythmics (Calcium Channel Blockers)** | | | | |
| **Diltiazem Injection** | Inj: 5mg/mL | Temporary control of rapid ventricular rate in atrial fibrillation/flutter (A-Fib/Flutter). Rapid conversion of paroxysmal supraventricular tachycardia (PSVT) to sinus rhythm. | **Adults:** Bolus: (Injection/Lyo-Ject) 0.25mg/kg IV over 2 minutes. If no response after 15 minutes, may give 2nd dose of 0.35mg/kg over 2 minutes. Continuous Infusion: (Injection/Lyo-Ject/Monovial) 0.25-0.35mg/kg IV bolus, then 10mg/hr. Titrate: Increase by 5mg/hr. Max: 15mg/hr and duration up to 24 hrs. | |
| **Verapamil** (Calan) | Tab: 40mg, 80mg*, 120mg* *scored<br>Inj: 2.5mg/mL<br>(available in generic) | (Tab): With digitalis, for control of ventricular rate at rest and during stress in patients with chronic atrial flutter and/or atrial fibrillation and prophylaxis of repetitive PSVT.<br>(Inj): Rapid conversion of PSVT to sinus rhythm, including those associated with accessory bypass tracts and temporary control of rapid ventricular rate in A-fib/flutter except when associated with accessory bypass tracts. | **Adults:** A-Fib (Digitalized): Usual: 240-320mg/day PO given tid-qid. PSVT Prophylaxis (Non-Digitalized): 240-480mg/day PO given tid-qid. Max: 480mg/day. **(Inj): Adults:** Initial: 5-10mg IV bolus over 2 min. If 1st dose not adequate, repeat 10mg over 2 min 30 min after first dose. Elderly: Administer dose over at least 3 min. **Pediatrics:** Continuously monitor ECG. **<1 yr:** 0.1-0.2mg/kg IV bolus over 2 min. If 1st dose not adequate, repeat 0.1-0.2mg/kg over 2 min 30 min after 1st dose. **1-15 yrs:** 0.1-0.3 mg/kg IV bolus over 2 min. Max: 5mg. If 1st dose not adequate, repeat 0.1-0.3mg/kg over 2 min 30 min after 1st dose. Max: 10mg single dose. | Severe hepatic dysfunction: (Tab) Give 30% of normal dose. |

| DRUG (BRAND) | HOW SUPPLIED | INDICATION | DOSAGE | HEPATIC/RENAL DOSE ADJUSTMENT* |
|---|---|---|---|---|
| **Class V Antiarrhythmics** | | | | |
| **Adenosine** (Adenocard) | Inj: 3mg/mL [2mL, 4mL] | Conversion of paroxysmal supraventricular tachycardia (including Wolff-Parkinson-White syndrome) to sinus rhythm (SR). | **Adults:** 6mg rapid IV bolus infusion over 1-2 seconds. If not converted to SR within 1-2 min, give 12mg rapid IV bolus; may give 2nd 12mg dose if needed. Max: 12mg/dose. **Pediatrics:** <50kg: 0.05-0.1mg/kg rapid IV bolus. If not converted to SR within 1-2 min, give additional bolus doses incrementally increasing amount by 0.05-0.1mg/kg. Follow each bolus with a saline flush. Continue process until SR or a maximum single dose of 0.3mg/kg is used. ≥50kg: 6mg rapid IV bolus infusion over 1-2 sec. If not converted to SR within 1-2 min, give 12mg rapid IV bolus; may give 2nd 12mg dose if needed. Max: 12mg/dose. | |
| **Digoxin** (Lanoxin) | Inj: (Pediatric Inj) 0.1mg/mL, 0.25mg/mL; Sol: (Pediatric Sol) 0.05mg/mL [60mL]; Tab: 0.125mg*, 0.25mg* *scored | Treatment of mild to moderate heart failure and to control ventricular response rate with chronic atrial fibrillation. | **Adults:** Rapid Digitalization: LD: (Inj) 0.4-0.6mg IV single dose or (Tab) 0.5-0.75mg PO, may give additional (Inj) 0.1-0.3mg or (Tab) 0.125-0.375mg at 6-8 hr intervals until clinical effect. Maint: (Tab) 0.125-0.5mg qd. A-Fib: Titrate to minimum effective dose for desired response. **Pediatrics:** See PI for full pediatric dosing information. | Elderly (>70 yrs)/Renal Dysfunction: Initial: 0.125mg qd. Marked Renal Dysfunction: Initial: 0.0625mg qd. Titrate: Increase every 2 weeks based on response. |

# ARBs* AND COMBINATIONS

| DRUG | BRAND | USUAL HTN† DOSAGE RANGE | HOW SUPPLIED |
|---|---|---|---|
| **ANGIOTENSIN II RECEPTOR BLOCKERS** | | | |
| Candesartan | Atacand | 8–32mg/day. | **Tab:** 4mg, 8mg, 16mg, 32mg |
| Eprosartan | Teveten | 400–800mg/day. | **Tab:** 400mg, 600mg |
| Irbesartan | Avapro | 150–300mg/day. | **Tab:** 75mg, 150mg, 300mg |
| Losartan | Cozaar | 25–100mg/day. | **Tab:** 25mg, 50mg, 100mg |
| Olmesartan | Benicar | 20–40mg/day.‡ | **Tab:** 5mg, 20mg, 40mg |
| Telmisartan | Micardis | 20–80mg/day. | **Tab:** 20mg, 40mg, 80mg |
| Valsartan | Diovan | 80–320mg/day.‡ | **Tab:** 40mg, 80mg, 160mg, 320mg |
| **COMBINATIONS** | | | |
| Candesartan-Hydrochlorothiazide | Atacand HCT | 16/12.5–32/25mg/day. | **Tab:** 16mg-12.5mg, 32mg-12.5mg, 32mg-25mg |
| Eprosartan-Hydrochlorothiazide | Teveten HCT | 600/12.5–600/25mg/day. | **Tab:** 600mg-12.5mg, 600mg-25mg |
| Irbesartan-Hydrochlorothiazide | Avalide | 150/12.5–300/25mg/day. | **Tab:** 150mg-12.5mg, 300mg-12.5mg, 300mg-25mg |
| Losartan-Hydrochlorothiazide | Hyzaar | 50/12.5–100/25mg/day. | **Tab:** 50mg-12.5mg, 100mg-12.5mg, 100mg-25mg |
| Olmesartan-Amlodipine | Azor | 20/5-40/10mg/day. | **Tab:** 20mg-5mg, 20mg-10mg, 40mg-5mg, 40mg-10mg |
| Olmesartan-Hydrochlorothiazide | Benicar HCT | 20/12.5–40/25mg/day. | **Tab:** 20mg-12.5mg, 40mg-12.5mg, 40mg-25mg |
| Telmisartan-Amlodipine | Twynsta | 40/5-80/10mg/day. | **Tab:** 40mg-5mg, 40mg-10mg, 80mg-5mg, 80mg-10mg |
| Telmisartan-Hydrochlorothiazide | Micardis HCT | 40/12.5–160/25mg/day. | **Tab:** 40mg-12.5mg, 80mg-12.5mg, 80mg-25mg |
| Valsartan-Amlodipine | Exforge | 160/5-320/10mg/day. | **Tab:** 160mg-5mg, 160mg-10mg, 320mg-5mg, 320mg-10mg |
| Valsartan-Amlodipine-Hydrochlorothiazide | Exforge HCT | Individualize dose up to 320/10/25mg/day.§ | **Tab:** 160mg-5mg-12.5mg, 160mg-5mg-25mg, 160mg-10mg-12.5mg, 160mg-10mg-25mg, 320mg-10mg-25mg |
| Valsartan-Hydrochlorothiazide | Diovan HCT | 160/12.5–320/25mg/day. | **Tab:** 80mg-12.5mg, 160mg-12.5mg, 160mg-25mg, 320mg-12.5mg, 320mg-25mg |

*ARBs: Angiotensin II receptor blockers.

†HTN: Hypertension.

‡Refer to monograph for pediatric dosing.

§Exforge HCT is not indicated for initial therapy of hypertension. May be used for patients not adequately controlled on any two of the following antihypernsive classes: calcium channel blockers, angiotensin receptor blockers, and diuretics.

Adopted from the Seventh Report of the Joint National Committee on Prevention, Detection, Evaluation, and Treatment of High Blood Pressure (JNC 7); http://www.nhlbi.nih.gov/guidelines/hypertension/jnc7full.htm.

# BETA-BLOCKERS

| DRUG | BRAND | HOW SUPPLIED | HYPERTENSION DOSING | ANGINA DOSING | POST-MI DOSING |
|---|---|---|---|---|---|
| **NONSELECTIVE BETA-BLOCKERS** | | | | | |
| Nadolol | Corgard | **Tab:** 20mg, 40mg, 80mg | **Initial:** 40mg qd. **Usual:** 40mg–80mg qd. **Max:** 320mg/day. | **Initial:** 40mg qd. **Usual:** 40mg–80mg qd. **Max:** 240mg/day. | Not FDA approved |
| Penbutolol sulfate | Levatol | **Tab:** 20mg | **Initial** and **Usual:** 20mg qd. | Not FDA approved | Not FDA approved |
| Pindolol | Visken | **Tab:** 5mg, 10mg | **Initial:** 5mg bid. **Max:** 60mg/day. | Not FDA approved | Not FDA approved |
| Propranolol HCl | Inderal | **Tab:** 10mg, 20mg, 40mg, 60mg, 80mg | **Initial:** 40mg bid. **Usual:** 120mg–240mg/day. **Max:** 640mg/day. | **Usual:** 80mg–320mg/day. | **Initial:** 40mg bid. **Usual:** 180mg–240mg/day. **Max:** 240mg/day. |
| | Inderal LA | **Cap, LA:** 60mg, 80mg, 120mg, 160mg | **Initial:** 80mg qd. **Usual:** 120mg–160mg qd. **Max:** 640mg/day. | **Initial:** 80mg qd. **Usual:** 160mg qd. **Max:** 320mg. | Not FDA approved |
| | Innopran XL | **Cap, ER:** 80mg, 120mg | **Initial:** 80mg qhs. **Max:** 120mg qhs. | Not FDA approved | Not FDA approved |
| Timolol maleate | Various generics | **Tab:** 5mg, 10mg 20mg | **Initial:** 10mg bid. **Usual:** 20mg–40mg/day. **Max:** 60mg/day. | Not FDA approved | **Usual:** 10mg bid (post acute MI). |
| **SELECTIVE BETA$_1$-BLOCKERS** | | | | | |
| Acebutolol | Sectral | **Cap:** 200mg, 400mg | **Initial:** 400mg qd or bid. **Usual:** 400mg–800mg/day. **Max:** 1200mg/day. | Not FDA approved | Not FDA approved |
| Atenolol | Tenormin | **Tab:** 25mg, 50mg, 100mg | **Initial:** 50mg qd. **Max:** 100mg qd. | **Initial:** 50mg qd. **Usual:** 100mg qd. **Max:** 200mg qd. | **Usual:** 50mg bid or 100mg qd for 6–9 days post MI. |
| Betaxolol HCl | Kerlone | **Tab:** 10mg, 20mg | **Initial:** 10mg qd. **Max:** 40mg qd. | Not FDA approved | Not FDA approved |
| Bisoprolol fumarate | Zebeta | **Tab:** 5mg, 10mg | **Initial:** 2.5mg–5mg qd. **Usual:** 2.5mg–20mg qd. **Max:** 20mg qd. | Not FDA approved | Not FDA approved |
| Esmolol | Brevibloc | **Inj:** 10mg/mL [10mL, 250mL], 20mg/mL [5mL, 100mL], 250mg/mL concentrate | **Immediate Control: Initial:** 80mg bolus over 30 sec. **Maint:** 0.15mg/kg/min. May titrate up to 0.3mg/kg/min. **Gradual Control: Initial:** 0.5mg/kg over 1 min. **Maint:** 0.05mg/kg/min for 4 min. If needed, may repeat loading dose. **Maint:** follow and increase to 0.1mg/kg/min.** | Not FDA approved | Not FDA approved |
| Metoprolol succinate | Toprol-XL† | **Tab, XL:** 25mg, 50mg, 100mg, 200mg | **Initial:** 25mg–100mg qd. **Max:** 400mg/day. | **Initial:** 100mg qd. **Max:** 400mg/day. | Not FDA approved |

*(Continued)*

| DRUG | BRAND | HOW SUPPLIED | HYPERTENSION DOSING | ANGINA DOSING | POST-MI DOSING |
|---|---|---|---|---|---|
| **SELECTIVE BETA$_1$-BLOCKERS** *(Continued)* | | | | | |
| Metoprolol tartrate | Lopressor | **Tab:** 50mg, 100mg | **Initial:** 100mg qd or in divided doses. **Usual:** 100mg–450mg/day. **Max:** 450mg/day. | **Initial:** 50mg bid. **Usual:** 100mg–400mg/day. **Max:** 400mg/day. | **Usual:** 100mg bid for at least 3 months. |
| | Various generics | **Tab:** 25mg, 50mg 100mg | **Initial:** 100mg qd or in divided doses. **Usual:** 100mg–450mg/day. **Max:** 450mg/day. | **Initial:** 50mg bid. **Usual:** 100mg–400mg/day. **Max:** 400mg/day. | **Usual:** 100mg bid for at least 3 months. |
| Nebivolol | Bystolic | **Tab:** 2.5mg, 5mg 10mg, 20mg | **Initial:** 5mg qd. Titrate: May increase dose if needed at 2-week intervals. **Max:** 40mg. **Hepatic impairment/ CrCl <30mL/min:** 2.5mg qd. | Not FDA approved | Not FDA approved |
| **MIXED ALPHA- AND BETA-BLOCKERS** | | | | | |
| Carvedilol | Coreg† | **Tab:** 3.125mg, 6.25mg, 12.5mg, 25mg | **Initial:** 6.25mg bid. **Max:** 25mg bid. | Not FDA approved | Left Ventricular Dysfunction post MI: **Initial:** 6.25mg bid, then increase to 12.5mg bid after 3-10 days. **Usual Target:** 25mg bid. |
| | Coreg CR† | **Tab, CR:** 10mg, 20mg, 40mg, 80mg | **Initial:** 20mg qd. **Max:** 80mg/day. | Not FDA approved | Left Ventricular Dysfunction post MI: **Initial:** 10mg–20mg qd. **Usual:** 80mg qd. |
| Labetalol HCl | Trandate | **Tab:** 100mg, 200mg, 300mg | **Initial:** 100mg bid. **Usual:** 200mg–400mg bid. | Not FDA approved | Not FDA approved |
| **COMBINATIONS** | | | | | |
| Atenolol/ Chlorthalidone | Tenoretic | **Tab:** 50mg/25mg, 100mg/25mg | **Initial:** 50mg/25mg qd. **Max:** 100mg/ 25mg/day. | Not FDA approved | Not FDA approved |
| Nadolol/ Bendroflumethiazide | Corzide | **Tab:** 40mg/5mg, 80mg/5mg | **Initial:** 40mg/5mg qd. **Max:** 80mg/ 5mg/day. | Not FDA approved | Not FDA approved |
| Bisoprolol/ fumarate/ HCTZ* | Ziac | **Tab:** 2.5mg/ 6.25mg, 5mg/ 6.25mg, 10mg/ 6.25mg | **Initial:** 2.5mg/ 6.25mg qd. **Max:** 20mg/12.5mg/day. | Not FDA approved | Not FDA approved |

*(Continued)*

| DRUG | BRAND | HOW SUPPLIED | HYPERTENSION DOSING | ANGINA DOSING | POST-MI DOSING |
|---|---|---|---|---|---|
| **COMBINATIONS** *(Continued)* | | | | | |
| Metoprolol tartrate/ HCTZ* | Lopressor HCT | **Tab:** 50mg/25mg, 100mg/25mg, 100mg/50mg | Individualize dose. **Lopressor usual initial:** 100mg/day qd or divided. **Lopressor max:** 450mg/day. **HCTZ usual:** 12.5mg-50mg/day. HCTZ dose >50mg/day not recommended. | Not FDA approved | Not FDA approved |
| Propranolol/ HCTZ* | Inderide | **Tab:** 40mg/25mg, 80mg/25mg | Individualize dose. **Propranolol alone initial:** 80mg/day. **Usual:** 160mg-480mg/day. **HCTZ alone usual:** 12.5-50mg/day. **Inderide max dose:** 160mg/50mg. | Not FDA approved | Not FDA approved |

*Hydrochlorothiazide.

**Brevibloc is used for the treatment of tachycardia and hypertension that occur during induction and tracheal intubation, during surgery, on emergence from anesthesia, and in the postoperative period.

†For additional indications, refer to FDA-approved labeling.

Note: Sotalol (Betapace) is indicated for ventricular arrhythmias. Refer to FDA-approved labeling for dosing and additional information.

**Source:** FDA-approved labeling.

# CALCIUM CHANNEL BLOCKERS

| DRUG | BRAND | HOW SUPPLIED | HYPERTENSION DOSING* | ANGINA DOSING* |
|---|---|---|---|---|
| **DIHYDROPYRIDINES** | | | | |
| **Amlodipine besylate** | Norvasc | **Tab:** 2.5mg, 5mg, 10mg | **Initial:** 5mg qd. **Max:** 10mg qd. | **Initial/Usual:** 10mg qd. |
| **Felodipine** | Plendil | **Tab, ER:** 2.5mg, 5mg, 10mg | **Initial:** 5mg qd. **Usual:** 2.5-10mg qd. | Not FDA approved |
| **Isradipine** | DynaCirc CR, Generic | **Tab, CR:** 5mg, 10mg **Cap:** 2.5mg, 5mg | **Initial:** Cap: 2.5mg bid or (CR): 5mg qd. **Max:** 20mg/day. | Not FDA approved |
| **Nicardipine HCl** | Cardene | **Cap:** 20mg, 30mg | **Initial:** 20mg tid. **Usual:** 20-40mg tid. | **Initial:** 20mg tid. **Usual:** 20-40mg tid. |
| | Cardene SR | **Cap, ER:** 30mg, 45mg, 60mg | **Initial:** 30mg bid. **Usual:** 30-60mg bid. | Not FDA approved |
| **Nifedipine** | Adalat CC | **Tab, ER:** 30mg, 60mg, 90mg | **Initial:** 30mg qd. **Usual:** 30-60mg qd. **Max:** 90mg/day. | Not FDA approved |
| | Afeditab CR | **Tab, ER:** 30mg, 60mg | **Initial:** 30mg qd. **Usual:** 30-60mg qd. **Max:** 90mg/day. | Not FDA approved |
| | Procardia | **Cap:** 10mg, 20mg | Not FDA approved | **Initial:** 10mg tid. **Usual:** 10-20mg tid. **Max:** 180mg/day. |
| | Procardia XL | **Tab, ER:** 30mg, 60mg, 90mg | **Initial:** 30-60mg qd. **Max:** 120mg/day. | **Initial:** 30-60mg qd. **Max:** 90-120mg/day. |
| **Nisoldipine** | Generic | **Tab, ER:** 20mg, 30mg, 40mg | **Initial:** 20mg qd. **Usual:** 20-40mg qd. **Max:** 60mg/day. | Not FDA approved |
| | Sular | **Tab, ER:** 8.5mg, 17mg, 25.5mg, 34mg | **Initial:** 17mg qd. **Usual:** 17-34mg qd. **Max:** 34mg/day. | Not FDA approved |
| **NON-DIHYDROPYRIDINES** | | | | |
| **Diltiazem HCl** | Cardizem | **Tab:** 30mg, 60mg, 90mg, 120mg | Not FDA approved | **Initial:** 30mg qid. **Usual:** 180-360mg/day. |
| | Cardizem CD, Cartia XT | **Cap, ER:** 120mg, 180mg, 240mg, 300mg, (Cardizem CD) 360mg | **Initial:** 180-240mg qd. **Usual:** 240-360mg qd. **Max:** 480mg qd. | **Initial:** 120-180mg qd. **Max:** 480mg/day. |
| | Cardizem LA | **Tab, ER:** 120mg, 180mg, 240mg, 300mg, 360mg, 420mg | **Initial:** 180-240mg qd. **Max:** 540mg/day. | **Initial:** 180 qd. **Max:** 360mg/day. |
| | Dilacor XR | **Cap, ER:** 120mg, 180mg, 240mg | **Initial:** 180-240mg qd. **Usual:** 180-480mg qd. **Max:** 540mg qd. | **Initial:** 120mg qd. **Max:** 480mg/day. |
| | Dilt-CD | **Cap, ER:** 120mg 180mg, 240mg, 300mg | **Initial:** 180-240mg qd. **Usual:** 240-360mg qd. **Max:** 540mg/day. | **Initial:** 120-180mg qd. **Max:** 540mg/day. |
| | Diltzac | **Cap, ER:** 120mg, 180mg, 240mg, 300mg, 360mg | **Initial:** 120-240mg qd. **Usual:** 120-540mg qd. **Max:** 540mg/day. | **Initial:** 120-180mg qd. **Max:** 540mg/day. |
| | Tiazac, Taztia XT | **Cap, ER:** 120mg, 180mg, 240mg, 300mg, 360mg, (Tiazac) 420mg | **Initial:** 120-240mg qd. **Usual:** 120-540mg qd. **Max:** 540mg qd. | **Initial:** 120-180mg qd. **Max:** 540mg/day. |

*(Continued)*

| DRUG | BRAND | HOW SUPPLIED | HYPERTENSION DOSING* | ANGINA DOSING* |
|---|---|---|---|---|
| **NON-DIHYDROPYRIDINES** *(Continued)* | | | | |
| **Verapamil HCl** | Calan** | **Tab:** 40mg, 80mg, 120mg | **Initial:** 80mg tid. **Usual:** 360-480mg/day. | **Usual:** 80-120mg tid. **Max:** 480mg/day. |
| | Calan SR | **Cap, ER:** 120mg, 180mg, 240mg | **Initial:** 180mg qam. **Max:** 480mg/day. | Not FDA approved |
| | Covera HS | **Tab, ER:** 180mg, 240mg | **Initial:** 180mg qhs. **Max:** 480mg qhs. | **Initial:** 180mg qhs. **Max:** 480mg qhs. |
| | Isoptin SR | **Tab, ER:** 120mg, 180mg, 240mg | **Initial:** 180mg qam. **Max:** 480mg/day. | Not FDA approved |
| | Verelan | **Cap, ER:** 120mg, 180mg, 240mg, 360mg | **Usual:** 240mg qam. **Max:** 480mg/day. | Not FDA approved |
| | Verelan PM | **Cap, ER:** 100mg, 200mg, 300mg | **Usual:** 200mg qhs. **Max:** 400mg qhs. | Not FDA approved |

* NOTE: Adult dosing shown is for monotherapy. Dosage needs to be adjusted by titration to individual patient needs. Dosages may need to be reduced in the elderly, or with renal/hepatic impairment. When used in combination with other antihypertensives the dosage of the calcium channel blocker or the concomitant antihypertensives may need to be adjusted due to possible additive effect. Monitor patient closely. For more information refer to monograph listings or drug's FDA-approved labeling.

** For additional indications refer to monograph listings or drug's FDA-approved labeling.

# CHOLESTEROL-LOWERING AGENTS

| BRAND (GENERIC) | HOW SUPPLIED (MG)* | USUAL DOSAGE RANGE** | T-CHOL (% DECREASE) | LDL (% DECREASE) | HDL (% INCREASE) | TG (% DECREASE) |
|---|---|---|---|---|---|---|
| **HMG-CoA REDUCTASE INHIBITORS (STATINS)** | | | | | | |
| Altoprev (Lovastatin) | **Tab, ER:** 20, 40, 60 | 20-60mg/day | 20.9 to 29.2 | 29.6 to 40.8 | 11.6 to 13.1 | 9.9 to 25.1 |
| Crestor (Rosuvastatin) | **Tabs:** 5, 10, 20, 40 | 5-40mg/day | 33 to 46 | 45 to 63 | 8 to 14 | 10 to 35 |
| Lescol (Fluvastatin) | **Tabs:** 20, 40 | 20-80mg/day | 17 to 27 | 22 to 36 | 3 to 6 | 12 to 18 |
| Lescol XL (Fluvastatin) | **Tabs, ER:** 80 | 80mg/day | 25 | 35 | 7 | 19 |
| Lipitor (Atorvastatin) | **Tabs:** 10, 20, 40 80 | 10-80mg/day | 29 to 45 | 39 to 60 | 5 to 9 | 19 to 37 |
| Mevacor (Lovastatin) | **Tabs:** 10, 20, 40 | 10-80mg/day given qd or bid | 17 to 29 | 24 to 40 | 6.6 to 9.5 | 10 to 19 |
| Pravachol (Pravastatin) | **Tabs:** 10, 20, 40, 80 | 40-80mg/day qd; renal/hepatic dysfunction: 10mg qd | 16 to 27 | 22 to 37 | 2 to 12 | 11 to 24 |
| Zocor (Simvastatin) | **Tabs:** 5, 10, 20, 40, 80 | 5-80mg/day | 19 to 36 | 26 to 47 | 8 to 16 | 12 to 33 |
| **FIBRATES** | | | | | | |
| Antara (Fenofibrate) | **Caps:** 43, 130 | 43-130mg/day | 18.7 | 20.6 | 11 | 28.9 |
| Fenoglide (Fenofibrate) | **Tabs:** 40, 120 | 40-120mg/day | 16.8 to 22.4 | 20.1 to 31.4 | 9.8 to 14.6 | 23.5 to 35.9 |
| Fibricor (Fenofibric acid) | **Tabs:** 35, 105 | 35-105mg/day | 16.8 to 22.4 | 20.1 to 31.4 | 9.8 to 14.6 | 23.5 to 35.9 |
| Lipofen (Fenofibrate) | **Caps:** 50, 150 | 50-150mg/day | 9.1 to 13.8 | 14.5 to +45.0 | 19.6 to 22.9 | 46.2 to 54.5 |
| Lofibra (Fenofibrate) | **Tabs:** 54, 160; **Caps:** 67, 134, 200 | 54-160mg/day, 67-200mg/day | 18.7 | 20.6 | 11 | 28.9 |
| Lopid (Gemfibrozil) | **Tab:** 600 | 1200mg/day in divided doses | n/a | 4.1 | 12.6 | Not specified-but decrease |
| Tricor (Fenofibrate) | **Tab:** 48, 145 | 48-145mg/day | 18.7 | 20.6 | 11 | 28.9 |
| Triglide (Fenofibrate) | **Tabs:** 50, 160 | 50-160mg/day | 18.7 | 20.6 | 11 | 28.9 |
| Trilipix (Fenofibric acid) | **Caps, Delayed-Release:** 45, 135 | 45-135mg/day | 12.4 | 5.1 | 16.3 | 31 |
| **BILE-ACID SEQUESTRANTS** | | | | | | |
| Colestid (Colestipol) | **Granules:** 5g/pkt or scoop; **Tab:** 1000 | **Granules:** 1-6 pkts or scoopfuls/day given qd or in divided doses; **Tab:** 2-16g/day given qd or in divided doses | Not specified | Not specified | Not specified | Not specified |
| Questran, Questran Light (Cholestyramine) | **Granules:** 4g/pkt or scoop | 2-4 packets or scoopfuls daily (8-16 g) divided into two doses | 7.2 | 10.4 | n/a | n/a |
| Welchol (Colesevelam HCl) | **Tabs:** 625 **Sus:** 3.75g, 1.875g [pkt] | 3750mg/day given qd or bid | 7 | 15 | 3 | 10 |
| **CHOLESTEROL ABSORPTION INHIBITOR** | | | | | | |
| Zetia (Ezetimibe) | **Tab:** 10 | 10mg qd | 13 | 18 | 1 | 8 |

*(Continued)*

| BRAND (GENERIC) | HOW SUPPLIED (MG)* | USUAL DOSAGE RANGE** | T-CHOL (% DECREASE) | LDL (% DECREASE) | HDL (% INCREASE) | TG (% DECREASE) |
|---|---|---|---|---|---|---|
| **NICOTINIC ACID DERIVATIVE** | | | | | | |
| Niaspan (Niacin, Extended-Release) | **Tabs, ER:** 500, 750, 1000 | 1-2g qhs | 3 to 10 | 5 to 14 | 18 to 22 | 13 to 28 |
| **LIPID-REGULATING AGENT** | | | | | | |
| Lovaza (Omega-3-Acid Ethyl Esters) | **Cap:** 1000 | 4g/day given qd or bid | 9.7 | +44.5 | 9.1 | 44.9 |
| **COMBINATIONS** | | | | | | |
| Advicor (Niacin ER/ Lovastatin) | **Tabs:** 500/20, 750/20, 1000/20, 1000/40 | 500/20mg to 2000mg/40mg | Not specified | 30 to 42 | 20 to 30 | 32 to 44 |
| Caduet (Amlodipine/ Atorvastatin) | **Tabs:** 2.5/10, 2.5/20, 2.5/40, 5/10, 5/20, 5/40, 5/80, 10/10, 10/20, 10/40, 10/80 | 5/10mg to 10/80mg | n/a | n/a | n/a | n/a |
| Simcor (Niacin ER/ Simvastatin) | **Tabs:** 500/20, 750/20, 1000/20 | 500mg/20mg to 2000mg/40mg | 8.8 to 11.1 | 11.9 to 14.3 | 20.7 to 29 | 26.5 to 38.0 |
| Vytorin (Ezetimibe/ Simvastatin) | **Tabs:** 10/10, 10/20, 10/40, 10/80 | 10/10 to 10/80mg/day | 31 to 43 | 45 to 60 | 6 to 10 | 23 to 31 |

* Unless otherwise indicated.

** NOTE: Dosage shown is for adults and may need to be adjusted to individual patient needs. For pediatric dosing and additional information please refer to the individual monograph listing or the drug's FDA-approved labeling. According to NCEP-ATP III guidelines, lipid-altering agents should be used in addition to a diet restricted in saturated fat and cholesterol only when the response to diet and other nonpharmacological measures has been inadequate.

**Abbreviation:** ER: Extended-Release.

**Major Contraindications** (refer to PI for a complete list of warnings and precautions)

Statins: Active liver disease or unexplained persistent elevations of hepatic transaminase levels; pregnancy; nursing mothers.

Fibrates: Hepatic or severe renal dysfunction, including primary biliary cirrhosis; pre-existing gallbladder disease; combination therapy with repaglinide; nursing mothers.

Bile-acid sequestrants: History of bowel obstruction; serum triglycerides >500 mg/dL; history of hypertriglyceridemia-induced pancreatitis.

Cholesterol absorption inhibitor: Statin contraindications apply when used with a statin; active liver disease or unexplained persistent elevations in hepatic transaminase levels; pregnancy; nursing mothers.

Nicotinic acid derivative: Active liver disease or unexplained persistent elevations in hepatic transaminases; active peptic ulcer disease; arterial bleeding.

Combinations: Refer to individual therapeutic class contraindications.

# COAGULATION MODIFIERS

| DRUG (BRAND) | HOW SUPPLIED | INDICATIONS | DOSAGE | HEPATIC/RENAL IMPAIRMENT |
|---|---|---|---|---|
| **THROMBOLYTICS** | | | | |
| **Alteplase** (Activase) | Inj: 50mg, 100mg | To improve ventricular function, reduce incidence of congestive heart failure, and reduce mortality with acute myocardial infarction (AMI). Management of acute ischemic stroke and acute massive pulmonary embolism (PE). | AMI: Accelerated Infusion: >67kg: 15mg IV bolus, then 50mg over next 30 min, and then 35mg over next 60 min. ≤67kg: 15mg IV bolus, then 0.75mg/kg (max 50mg) over next 30 min, then 0.5mg/kg (max 35mg) over next 60 min. Max: 100mg total dose. 3-Hr Infusion: ≥65kg: 60mg in 1st hr (give 6-10mg as IV bolus), then 20mg over 2nd hr, then 20mg over 3rd hr. <65kg: 1.25mg/kg over 3 hrs as described above. Stroke: 0.9mg/kg IV over 1 hr (max 90mg total dose). Administer 10% of total dose as IV bolus over 1 min. PE: 100mg IV over 2 hrs. Start heparin at end or immediately after infusion when PTT or PT ≤2× normal. | |
| **Reteplase** (Retavase) | Inj: 10.4 U | To improve ventricular function following acute myocardial infarction (AMI), reduce the incidence of congestive heart failure (CHF) and reduce the mortality associated with AMI. | 10 U IV over 2 min. Repeat in 30 min. | |
| **Tenecteplase** (TNKase) | Inj: 50mg | To reduce mortality with AMI. | Administer as single IV bolus over 5 seconds. <60kg: 30mg. 60 to <70kg: 35mg. 70 to <80kg: 40mg. 80 to <90kg: 45mg. ≥90kg: 50mg. Max: 50mg/dose. | |
| **Urokinase** (Kinlytic) | Inj: 250,000 IU | Lysis of acute massive pulmonary emboli (PE) and PE accompanied by unstable hemodynamics. | LD: 4400 IU/kg IV at 90mL/hr over 10 min. Maint: 4400 IU/kg/hr IV at 15mL/hr for 12 hrs. Flush line after each cycle. For IV use only. | |
| **PLATELET AGGREGATION INHIBITORS** | | | | |
| **Abciximab** (Reopro) | Inj: 2mg/mL | Adjunct to percutaneous coronary intervention (PCI) for prevention of cardiac ischemic complications in patients undergoing PCI or with unstable angina unresponsive to conventional therapy when PCI is planned within 24 hrs. Intended for use with aspirin and heparin. | PCI: 0.25mg/kg IV bolus given 10-60 min before start PCI, followed by 0.125mcg/kg/min IV infusion (Max: 10mcg/min) for 12 hrs. Unstable Angina: 0.25mg/kg IV bolus followed by 10mcg/min infusion for 18-24 hrs, concluding 1 hr after PCI. | |

(Continued)

| DRUG (BRAND) | HOW SUPPLIED | INDICATIONS | DOSAGE | HEPATIC/RENAL IMPAIRMENT |
|---|---|---|---|---|
| **PLATELET AGGREGATION INHIBITORS** *(Continued)* | | | | |
| **Anagrelide** (Agrylin) | Cap: 0.5mg | Treatment of thrombocythemia secondary to myeloproliferative disorders, to reduce the elevated platelet count and the risk of thrombosis and to ameliorate associated symptoms including thrombo-hemorrhagic events. | Initial: 0.5mg qid or 1mg bid for at least 1 week. Titrate: Increase by no more than 0.5mg/day per week. Max: 10mg/day or 2.5mg/dose. Adjust lowest effective dose to reduce and maintain platelets <600,000/mcL. Monitor platelets every 2 days during first week, then weekly thereafter until reach maintenance dose. **Pediatrics:** Initial: 0.5mg qd. Titrate: Increase by no more than 0.5mg/day per week. Max:10mg/day or 2.5mg/dose. Adjust to lowest effective dose to reduce and maintain platelets <600,000/mcL. Monitor platelets every 2 days during first week, then weekly thereafter until reach maintenance dose. | Moderate Hepatic Impairment: Initial: 0.5mg qd for at least 1 week. Titrate: Increase by no more than 0.5mg/day per week. Max: 10mg/day or 2.5mg/dose. |
| **Aspirin** (Halfprin) | Tab, Delayed-Release: 81mg, 162mg | To reduce the risk of vascular mortality and fatal and nonfatal cardiovascular and cerebrovascular events in patients with a suspected acute MI. | 162mg as soon as MI suspected; continue qd for 30 days. May need to continue as prophylaxis for recurrent MI. Crush, chew, or suck the 1st dose. | |
| **Cilostazol** (Pletal) | Tab: 50mg, 100mg | Reduction of symptoms with intermittent claudication. | 100mg bid, ½ hr before or 2 hrs after breakfast and dinner. Concomitant CYP3A4 and CYP2C19 Inhibitors: Consider 50mg bid. | |
| **Clopidogrel** (Plavix) | Tab: 75mg, 300mg | For reduction of thrombotic events in those with recent stroke or MI, established peripheral arterial disease (PAD); or with non-ST-segment elevation acute coronary syndrome (unstable angina/non-Q-wave MI); and patients with ST-segment elevation acute myocardial infarction (STEMI). | MI/Stroke/PAD: 75mg qd. Acute Coronary Syndrome: Take with 75-325mg ASA qd. LD: 300mg. Maint: 75mg qd. STEMI: 75mg, with 75-325mg ASA, qd with or without LD. | |
| **Dipyridamole** (Persantine) | Tab: 25mg, 50mg, 75mg | Adjunct to coumarin anticoagulants for prevention of postoperative thromboembolic complications of cardiac valve replacement. | 75-100mg qid. | |
| **Dipyridamole and aspirin** (Aggrenox) | Cap: (Dipyridamole Extended-Release/ ASA) 200mg-25mg | Reduce risk of stroke in patients with transient brain ischemia or complete ischemic stroke due to thrombosis. | 1 cap bid (am and pm). | |
| **Eptifibatide** (Integrilin) | Sol: 0.75mg/mL, 2mg/mL | Treatment of acute coronary syndrome (ACS) in patients being medically managed or undergoing percutaneous coronary intervention (PCI) including intracoronary stenting. | ACS: 180mcg/kg IV bolus, then 2mcg/kg/min IV infusion until discharge, initiation of CABG, or up to 72 hrs. If undergoing PCI, continue until discharge or 18-24 hrs post-PCI. PCI: 180mcg/kg IV bolus immediately before PCI, then 2mcg/kg/min IV infusion. Give 2nd bolus of 180mcg/kg 10 min after 1st bolus. Continue until discharge or 18-24 hrs post-PCI. See PI for concomitant ASA and heparin doses. | ACS: CrCl <50mL/min: 180mcg/kg IV bolus, then 1mcg/kg/min IV infusion. PCI: CrCl <50mL/min: 180mcg/kg IV bolus immediately before PCI, then 1mcg/kg/min IV infusion. Give 2nd bolus of 180mcg/kg 10 min after 1st bolus. |

| DRUG (BRAND) | HOW SUPPLIED | INDICATIONS | DOSAGE | HEPATIC/RENAL IMPAIRMENT |
|---|---|---|---|---|
| **PLATELET AGGREGATION INHIBITORS** *(Continued)* | | | | |
| **Prasugrel** (Effient) | Tab: 5mg, 10mg | Reduction of thrombotic CV events (eg, stent thrombosis) in patients with ACS (eg, unstable angina, non ST-elevation MI, ST-elevation MI) who are to be managed with percutaneous coronary intervention (PCI). | Adults: LD: 60mg PO single dose. Maint: 10mg qd. ≤60 kg: Reduce to 5mg qd. Should be taken with ASA 75mg-325mg qd. | |
| **Ticlopidine** | Tab: 250mg | To reduce risk of thrombotic stroke in stroke patients or those with stroke precursors who are ASA intolerant, allergic, or failed ASA therapy. Adjunct to ASA to reduce incidence of subacute stent thrombosis in patients undergoing successful coronary artery stent implantation. | Take with food. Stroke: 250mg bid. Coronary Artery Stenting: 250mg bid with ASA for up to 30 days after stent implant. | |
| **Tirofiban** (Aggrastat) | Inj: 0.05mg/mL | In combination with heparin, for treatment of acute coronary syndrome, in patients being medically managed or undergoing PTCA or atherectomy. | Initial: 0.4mcg/kg/min IV for 30 min. Maint: 0.1mcg/kg/min IV. Continue through angiography and for 12-24 hrs after angioplasty or atherectomy. | CrCl <30mL/min: Administer half of the usual rate of infusion. |
| **COAGULATION FACTOR INHIBITORS** | | | | |
| **Dalteparin** (Fragmin) | Inj: (Syringe) 2,500 IU/0.2mL, 5,000 IU/0.2mL, 7,500 IU/0.3mL, 10,000 IU/0.4mL, 10,000 IU/1mL, 12,500 IU/0.5mL, 15,000 IU/0.6mL, 18,000 IU/0.72mL; (MDV) 25,000 IU/mL [3.8mL], 10,000 IU/mL [9.5mL] | Prevention of ischemic complications in unstable angina and non-Q-wave MI with concurrent ASA therapy. Prophylaxis of DVT in hip replacement surgery, abdominal surgery in patients who are at high risk for thromboembolic complications, and for those at risk for thromboembolic complications due to severely restricted mobility during acute illness. Extended treatment of symptomatic VTE (proximal DVT and/or PE), to reduce the recurrence of VTE in patients with cancer. | Administer SQ. Unstable Angina/Non-Q-Wave MI: 120 IU/kg up to 10,000 IU q12h with ASA (75-165mg/day) for 5-8 days. Hip Surgery: Pre-Op Start: Initial (if start 2 hrs pre-op): 2500 IU within 2 hrs pre-op, then 2500 IU 4-8 hrs post-op. Initial (if start 10-14 hrs pre-op): 5000 IU 10-14 hrs pre-op, then 5000 IU 4-8 hrs post-op. Maint (for either initial dose): 5000 IU SQ qd for 5-10 days post-op (up to 14 days). Post-Op Start: 2500 IU 4-8 hrs post-op. Maint: 5000 IU qd. Abdominal Surgery: 2500 IU 1-2 hrs pre-op. Maint: 2500 IU qd for 5-10 days post-op. Abdominal Surgery with High Risk: 5000 IU evening before surgery. Maint: 5000 IU qd for 5-10 days post-op. Abdominal Surgery with Malignancy: Initial: 2500 IU 1-2 hrs pre-op, then 2500 IU 12 hrs later. Maint: 5000 IU qd for 5-10 days post-op. Severely Restricted Mobility During Acute Illness: 5000 IU qd for 12-14 days. Symptomatic VTE in Cancer Patients: 200 IU/kg qd for first 30 days, then 150 IU/kg qd for months 2-6. Max: 18,000 IU/day. Platelet Count 50,000-100,000/$mm^3$: Reduce dose by 2500 IU until platelet count ≥100,000/$mm^3$. Platelet Count <50,000/$mm^3$: D/C therapy until platelet count >50,000/$mm^3$. | Renal Impairment (CrCl <30mL/min): Monitor anti-Xa levels to determine appropriate dose. |

*(Continued)*

| DRUG (BRAND) | HOW SUPPLIED | INDICATIONS | DOSAGE | HEPATIC/RENAL IMPAIRMENT |
|---|---|---|---|---|
| **COAGULATION FACTOR INHIBITORS** *(Continued)* | | | | |
| **Enoxaparin** (Lovenox) | Inj: (MDV) 300mg/3mL; (Syringe) 30mg/0.3mL, 40mg/0.4mL, 60mg/0.6mL, 80mg/0.8mL, 100mg/mL, 120mg/0.8mL, 150mg/mL | Prevention of DVT in hip or knee replacement surgery, abdominal surgery, or with severely restricted mobility during acute illness. With concomitant warfarin, inpatient treatment of acute DVT with or without PE and outpatient treatment of DVT without PE. Prevention of ischemic complications in unstable angina and non-Q-wave MI with concurrent ASA therapy. Treatment of acute ST-segment elevation MI (STEMI) in patients receiving thrombolysis and being managed medically or with percutaneous coronary intervention (PCI). | Hip/Knee Surgery: 30mg SQ q12h, starting 12-24 hrs post-op, for 7-10 days (up to 14 days) or 40mg SQ qd, starting 12 hrs pre-op for hip surgery for 3 weeks. Abdominal Surgery: 40mg SQ qd, starting 2 hrs pre-op, for 7-10 days (up to12 days). DVT with or without PE treatment: (inpatient/outpatient) 1mg/kg SQ q12h or (inpatient) 1.5mg/kg SQ qd with warfarin (start within 72 hrs) for 7 days (up to 17 days). Acute Illness: 40mg SQ qd for 6-11 days (up to 14 days). Unstable Angina/Non-Q-Wave MI: 1mg/kg SQ q12h with 100-325mg/day of ASA for 2-8 days (up to 12.5 days). Acute STEMI (<75 yrs): 30mg single IV bolus plus a 1mg/kg SQ dose followed by 1mg/kg SQ q12h with ASA. Max: 100mg for 1st 2 doses only. Acute STEMI (≥75 yrs): 0.75mg/kg SQ q12h (no initial bolus) with ASA. Max: 75mg for 1st 2 doses only. When given with thrombolytic, give enoxaparin dose between 15 min before and 30 min after start of fibrinolytic therapy. With PCI, if last enoxaparin SQ dose was given >8 hrs before balloon inflation, an IV bolus of 0.3mg/kg of enoxaparin should be given. | CrCl <30mL/min: Surgery/Acute Illness: 30mg SQ qd. DVT with or without PE treatment (inpatient/outpatient)/Unstable Angina/Non-Q-Wave MI: 1mg/kg SQ qd. Acute STEMI: <75 yrs: 30mg single IV bolus plus a 1mg/kg SQ dose followed by 1mg/kg SQ qd. ≥75 yrs: 1mg/kg SQ qd (no initial bolus) |
| **Fondaparinux** (Arixtra) | Inj: (Syringe) 2.5mg/0.5mL, 5mg/0.4mL, 7.5mg/0.6mL, 10mg/0.8mL | Prophylaxis of DVT in patients undergoing hip fracture surgery, including extended prophylaxis; hip replacement surgery; knee replacement surgery; abdominal surgery who are at risk of thromboembolic complications. With concomitant warfarin, treatment of acute PE when initial therapy is administered in hospital and acute DVT. | DVT Prophylaxis: 2.5mg SQ qd, starting 6-8 hrs post-op for 5-9 days (up to 11 days). Hip Fracture Surgery: Extended prophylaxis up to 24 additional days is recommended. DVT/PE Treatment: <50kg: 5mg SQ qd. 50-100kg: 7.5mg SQ qd. >100kg: 10mg SQ qd. Add concomitant warfarin ASAP (usually within 72 hrs) and continue for 5-9 days (up to 26 days) until INR=2-3. | CrCl <30mL/min: Avoid use. |
| **Heparin** | Inj: 1,000 U/mL, 5000 U/mL, 10,000 U/mL | Prophylaxis and treatment of venous thrombosis and its extension, PE in atrial fibrillation, and peripheral arterial embolism. Prevention of post-operative DVT and PE. Diagnosis and treatment of acute and chronic consumptive coagulopathies, for prevention of clotting in arterial and cardiac surgery. | Based on 68kg: Initial: 5000 U IV, then 10,000-20,000 U SQ. Maint: 8000-10,000 U SQ q8h or 15,000-20,000 U SQ q12h. Intermittent IV Injection: Initial: 10,000 U. Maint: 5000-10,000 U q4-6h. Continuous IV Infusion:Initial: 5000U. Maint: 20,000-40,000 U/24 hrs. Adjust to coagulation test results. See PI for details in specific disease states. Pediatrics: Initial: 50 U/kg IV drip. Maint: 100 U/kg IV drip q4h or 20,000 U/$m^2$/24 hrs continuously. | |

| DRUG (BRAND) | HOW SUPPLIED | INDICATIONS | DOSAGE | HEPATIC/RENAL IMPAIRMENT |
|---|---|---|---|---|
| **COAGULATION FACTOR INHIBITORS** *(Continued)* | | | | |
| **Tinzaparin** (Innohep) | Inj: 20,000 anti-Xa IU/mL | Treatment of acute symptomatic DVT with or without PE with concomitant warfarin. | 175 anti-Xa IU/kg SQ qd for at least 6 days and until anticoagulated with warfarin (INR is at least 2.0 for 2 consecutive days). Begin warfarin within 1-3 days of therapy. | |
| **Warfarin** (Coumadin, Jantoven) | Inj: (Coumadin) 5mg; Tab: (Coumadin, Jantoven) 1mg*, 2mg*, 2.5mg*, 3mg*, 4mg*, 5mg*, 6mg*, 7.5mg*, 10mg* *scored | Prophylaxis and treatment of venous thrombosis, PE, and thromboembolic disorders associated with atrial fibrillation and/or cardiac valve replacement. To reduce risk of death, recurrent MI, and thromboembolic events after MI. | ≥18 yrs: Adjust dose based on PT/INR. Give IV as alternate to PO. Initial: 2-5mg qd. Usual: 2-10mg qd. Venous Thromboembolism (including pulmonary embolism): INR 2-3. Atrial Fibrillation: INR 2-3. Post-MI: Initiate 2-4 weeks post-infarct and maintain INR 2.5-3.5. Mechanical/Bioprosthetic Heart Valve: INR 2-3 for 12 weeks after valve insertion, then INR 2.5-3.5 long term. | |
| **THROMBIN INHIBITORS** | | | | |
| **Argatroban** | Inj: 100mg/mL | Prophylaxis or treatment of thrombosis in heparin-induced thrombocytopenia (HIT). As an anticoagulant in patients with or at risk for HIT undergoing percutaneous coronary intervention (PCI). | Thrombosis: D/C heparin and obtain baseline aPTT. Initial: 2mcg/kg/min IV. Check aPTT after 2 hrs. Titrate: Increase dose until aPTT is 1.5-3× the initial baseline. Max: 10mcg/kg/min. PCI: Initial: 350mcg/kg bolus with 25mcg/kg/min IV. Check activated clotting time (ACT) 5-10 min after bolus. Proceed with PCI if ACT >300 seconds. See PI for detailed information for dose adjustment. | Thrombosis: Moderate Hepatic Impairment: Initial: 0.5mcg/kg/min |
| **Bivalirudin** (Angiomax) | Inj: 250mg | Adjunct to aspirin for anticoagulation in patients with unstable angina undergoing percutaneous transluminal coronary angioplasty (PTCA) or percutaneous coronary intervention (PCI). Patients with, or at risk of, HIT/HITTS undergoing PCI. | Initial: 0.75mg/kg IV bolus, then 1.75mg/kg/hr for duration of PCI procedure. Additional bolus of 0.3mg/kg can be given if needed based on ACT. Continuation of infusion for up to 4 hrs post-procedure is optional. After 4 hrs, if needed, an additional 0.2mg/kg/hr IV for up to 20 hrs may be initiated. | Renal Impairment: CrCl <30mL/min: 1mg/kg/hr infusion. Hemodialysis: 0.25mg/kg/hr infusion. Reduction in bolus dose not necessary; monitor anticoagulation. |
| **Lepirudin** (Refludan) | Inj: 50mg | Anticoagulant for heparin-induced thrombocytopenia (HIT) and associated thromboembolic disease. | LD: 0.4mg/kg (max 44mg) IV over 15-20 seconds. Initial: 0.15mg/kg/hr (max 16.5mg/hr) continuous infusion for 2-10 days. Adjust dose based on aPTT. Concomitant Thrombolytic Therapy: LD: 0.2mg/kg. Initial: 0.1mg/kg/hr. See PI for monitoring and adjusting therapy details. | Renal Impairment: LD: 0.2mg/kg. Initial: CrCl 45-60 mL/min: 0.075mg/kg/hr. CrCl 30-44mL/min: 0.045mg/kg/hr. CrCl 15-29 mL/min: 0.0225mg/kg/hr. CrCl <15mL/min/Hemodialysis: Avoid or stop infusion. |

*(Continued)*

| DRUG (BRAND) | HOW SUPPLIED | INDICATIONS | DOSAGE | HEPATIC/RENAL IMPAIRMENT |
|---|---|---|---|---|
| **MISCELLANEOUS** | | | | |
| **Aminocaproic Acid** (Amicar) | Inj: 250mg/mL [20mL]; Syrup: 1.25g/5mL; Tab: 500mg*, 1,000mg* *scored | To enhance hemostasis when fibrinolysis contributes to bleeding. | IV: 16-20mL (4-5g) in 250mL diluent during 1st hr, then 4mL/hr (1g) in 50mL of diluent. PO: 5g during 1st hr, then 5mL (syr) or 1g (tabs) per hr. Continue IV/PO therapy for 8 hrs or until bleeding is controlled. | |
| **Pentoxifylline** (Trental) | Tab, Extended-Release: 400mg | Treatment of intermittent claudication due to chronic occlusive arterial disease of the limbs. | 400mg tid with meals for at least 8 weeks. Reduce to 400mg bid if digestive and CNS side effects occur; d/c if side effects persist. | |
| **Phytonadione** (Mephyton) | Tab: 5mg* *scored; Inj: 1mg/0.5 mL | For coagulation disorders caused by vitamin K deficiency or interference with vitamin K activity, including anticoagulant-induced prothrombin deficiency caused by coumarin or indanedione derivatives; and hypoprothrombinemia secondary to antibacterials, salicylates, obstructive jaundice, or biliary fistulas. | (Tab): Anticoagulant-Induced Prothrombin Deficiency: Initial: 2.5-10mg up to 25mg (rarely 50mg). May repeat if PT is still elevated 12-48 hrs after initial dose. Hypoprothrombinemia Due to Other Causes: 2.5-25mg or more (rarely up to 50mg). Give bile salts when endogenous bile supply to GIT is deficient. **Adults (IV):** Administer SQ when possible. Anticoagulant-Induced PT Deficiency: Initial: 2.5-10mg up to 25mg (rarely 50mg). May repeat if PT is still elevated 6-8 hrs after initial dose. Hypoprothrombinemia Due to Other Causes: 2.5-25mg or more (rarely up to 50mg); route depends on severity of condition and response. **Pediatrics** (IV): Prophylaxis of Hemorrhagic Disease in Newborn: 0.5-1mg IM within 1 hr of birth. Treatment of Hemorrhagic Disease in Newborn: 1mg SQ/IM (may need higher dose if mother has received oral anticoagulants). | |
| **Thrombin** (Recombinant, Recothrom) | Powder: 5,000 IU, 20,000 IU | Aid to hemostasis whenever oozing blood and minor bleeding from capillaries and small venules is accessible and control of bleeding by standard surgical techniques is ineffective or impractical. May be used in conjunction with an absorbable gelatin sponge, USP. | Apply directly on the surface of bleeding tissue or in conjunction with absorbable gelatin sponge. Required amount depends upon the tissue area to be treated. Reconstitute with sterile isotonic saline at a recommended concentration of 1000 IU/mL. | |
| **Topical Thrombin** (Thrombi-Gel, Thrombi-Pad, Thrombin-JMI) | Powder: 5,000 IU, 20,000 IU; Kit: Powder: 20,000 IU [Spray; Syringe Spray] | An aid to hemostasis whenever oozing blood and minor bleeding from capillaries and small venules is accessible. In various types of surgery, may be used in conjuction with an absorbable gelatin sponge, USP for hemostasis. | Spray topically on surface of bleeding tissue. Reconstitute with sterile isotonic saline at a recommended concentration of 1,000-2,000 IU/mL. Profuse Bleeding: Use 1,000 IU/mL. General use (eg, plastic surgery, dental extractions, skin grafting): 100 IU/mL. Intermediate strengths may be prepared by diluting in appropriate isotonic saline volume if needed. Oozing surfaces: Use dry form. May be used with FlowSeal™ NT. | |

# DIURETICS

| DRUG | BRAND | USUAL HYPERTENSION DOSAGE RANGE | HOW SUPPLIED |
|---|---|---|---|
| **ALDOSTERONE-RECEPTOR BLOCKERS** | | | |
| Eplerenone | Inspra | 50mg qd or bid. | **Tab:** 25mg, 50mg |
| Spironolactone | Aldactone | 50mg–100mg/day. | **Tab:** 25mg, 50mg, 100mg |
| **LOOP DIURETICS** | | | |
| Bumetanide | — | 0.5mg–2mg qd. | **Tab:** 0.5mg, 1mg, 2mg |
| Furosemide | Lasix | 40mg bid.† | **Tab:** 20mg, 40mg, 80mg |
| Torsemide | Demadex | 5mg–10mg qd. | **Tab:** 5mg, 10mg, 20mg, 100mg |
| **POTASSIUM-SPARING DIURETICS** | | | |
| Amiloride | Midamor | 5mg–10mg qd. | **Tab:** 5mg |
| Triamterene | Dyrenium | 100mg bid pc. | **Cap:** 50mg, 100mg |
| **THIAZIDE DIURETICS** | | | |
| Chlorothiazide | Diuril | **Sus:** 0.5–1g/day.† | **Sus:** 250mg/5mL |
| | Various generics | **Tab:** 0.5g–1g/day.† | **Tab:** 250mg, 500mg |
| Chlorthalidone | Thalitone | 15mg–50mg qd. | **Tab:** 15mg |
| | Various generics | 25mg–100mg qd. | **Tab:** 25mg, 50mg |
| Hydrochlorothiazide | Microzide | 12.5mg–50mg qd. | **Cap:** 12.5mg |
| | Various generics | 25mg–50mg qd.† | **Cap:** 12.5mg; **Tab:** 12.5mg, 25mg, 50mg |
| Indapamide | Various generics | 1.25mg–5mg qd. | **Tab:** 1.25mg, 2.5mg |
| **QUINAZOLINE DIURETIC** | | | |
| Metolazone | Zaroxolyn | 2.5mg–5mg qd. | **Tab:** 2.5mg, 5mg, 10mg |
| **COMBINATION DIURETICS*** | | | |
| Amiloride-Hydrochlorothiazide | Various generics | 1-2 tabs qd (5/50mg–10/100mg/day). | **Tab:** 5/50mg |
| Spironolactone-Hydrochlorothiazide | Aldactazide | 50/50mg–100/100mg/day. | **Tab:** 25/25mg, 50/50mg |
| Triamterene-Hydrochlorothiazide | Dyazide, Maxzide | 37.5/25mg–75/50mg/day. | **Cap:** 37.5/25mg<br>**Tab:** 37.5/25mg, 75/50mg |

* Fixed combination drugs are indicated for the treatment of hypertension in patients who develop hypokalemia on hydrochlorothiazide alone.

† Pediatric dosing available.

# ACNE MANAGEMENT: SYSTEMIC THERAPIES

| DRUG (BRAND) | HOW SUPPLIED | DOSAGE | SIDE EFFECTS |
|---|---|---|---|
| **ANTIBIOTICS** | | | |
| **Doxycycline hyclate** (Adoxa, Doryx, Vibramycin) | Adoxa: 75mg, 100mg, 150mg<br>Doryx: (Tab, Delayed-Release) 75mg, 100mg, 150mg<br>Vibramycin: (Cap) 50mg, 100mg | 100mg q12h on 1st day, followed by 100mg qd. | Anorexia, nausea, vomiting, diarrhea, dysphagia, enterocolitis, rash, exfoliative dermatitis, renal toxicity, hypersensitivity reactions, blood dyscrasias, tooth discoloration, photosensitivity |
| **Doxycycline monohydrate** (Monodox) | Cap: 50mg, 75 mg, 100mg | 100mg q12h or 50mg q6h for 1 day, then 100mg/day. | GI effects, photosensitivity, rash, blood dyscrasias, hypersensitivity reactions, tooth discoloration |
| **Doxycycline, USP** (Oracea) | Cap: 40mg | 40mg qd am. | Anorexia, nausea, sinusitis, diarrhea, abdominal pain |
| **Minocycline HCl** (Dynacin, Minocin) | Dynacin: Tab: 50mg, 75mg, 100mg<br>Minocin: Cap: 50mg, 100mg | 200mg initially, then 100mg q12h; alternative is 100-200mg initially, then 50mg qid. | Anorexia, nausea, vomiting, diarrhea, dysphagia, enterocolitis, pancreatitis, increased LFTs, hepatitis, liver failure, renal toxicity, rash, exfoliative dermatitis, Stevens-Johnson syndrome, skin and mucous membrane pigmentation, blood dyscrasias, headache, tooth discoloration, photosensitivity, intracranial HTN |
| **Minocycline HCl** (Solodyn) | Tab, Extended-Release: 45mg, 65mg, 90mg, 115mg, 135mg | 1mg/kg qd for 12 weeks. | Headache, fatigue, dizziness, pruritus, malaise, mood alteration, Stevens-Johnson syndrome, photosensitivity, tooth discoloration |
| **Tetracycline HCl** (Sumycin) | Sus: 125mg/5mL;<br>Tab: 250mg, 500mg | Mild-Moderate: 250mg qid or 500mg bid. Severe: 500mg qid. Severe Acne: Initial: 1g/day in divided doses. Maint: After improvement, 125-500mg/day. | GI effects, photosensitivity, increased BUN, hypersensitivity reactions, blood dyscrasias, dizziness, headache, tooth discoloration |
| **ORAL CONTRACEPTIVES** | | | |
| **Ethinyl Estradiol and Drospirenone** (YAZ) | Tab: (Ethinyl Estradiol-Drospirenone) 0.02mg-3mg | 1 tab qd for 28 days, then repeat. Start on first Sunday of menses or begin 1st day of menses. | Nausea, vomiting, breakthrough bleeding, spotting, amenorrhea, migraine, vaginal candidiasis, edema, weight changes, depression, urticaria, angioedema, circulatory symptoms, dysmenorrhea |
| **Ethinyl Estradiol and Norgestimate** (Ortho Tri-Cyclen) | Tab: (Ethinyl Estradiol-Norgestimate) 0.035mg-0.18mg, 0.035mg-0.215mg, 0.035mg-0.25mg | 1 tab qd for 28 days, then repeat. Start on first Sunday of menses or begin 1st day of menses. | Nausea, vomiting, breakthrough bleeding, spotting, amenorrhea, migraine, depression, vaginal candidiasis, edema, weight changes |
| **Ethinyl Estradiol and Norethindrone** (Estrostep Fe) | Tab: (Ethinyl Estradiol-Norethindrone) 0.035mg-1mg, 0.030mg-1mg, 0.020mg-1mg and 75mg ferrous fumarate | 1 tab qd for 28 days, then repeat. Start on first Sunday of menses or begin 1st day of menses. | Nausea, vomiting, breakthrough bleeding, spotting, amenorrhea, migraine, depression, vaginal candidiasis, edema, weight changes |

*(Continued)*

| DRUG (BRAND) | HOW SUPPLIED | DOSAGE | SIDE EFFECTS |
|---|---|---|---|
| **RETINOID** | | | |
| **Isotretinoin** (Amnesteem, Claravis, Sotret) | Amnesteem, Claravis: (Cap) 10mg, 20mg, 40mg<br>Sotret: (Cap) 10mg, 20mg, 30mg, 40mg | 0.5-1mg/kg/day given bid for 15-20 weeks. | Cheilitis, dry skin and mucous membranes, conjunctivitis, blood dyscrasias, epistaxis, decreased HDL, elevated cholesterol and TG, elevated blood sugar, arthralgias, back pain, hearing/vision impairment, rash, photosensitivity reactions, psychiatric disorders |

**Source:** FDA-approved product labeling.

# ACNE MANAGEMENT: TOPICAL THERAPIES

| DRUG (BRAND) | HOW SUPPLIED | DOSAGE | SIDE EFFECTS |
|---|---|---|---|
| **ANTIBACTERIAL/KERATOLYTIC AGENTS & COMBINATIONS** | | | |
| **Adapalene/Benzoyl peroxide** (Epiduo) | (Gel) 0.1%-2.5% [45g] | Apply qd. | Erythema, dry skin, scaling, dryness, skin irritation |
| **Benzoyl peroxide** (Benzac AC, Benzagel, Triaz) | Benzac AC: (Gel) 5%, 10% [60g], (Wash) 10% [60g]; Benzagel: (Gel) 5%, 10% [42.5g], (Wash) 10% [60g]; Triaz: (Gel) 3%, 6%, 9% [42.5g], (Cleanser) 3%, 6%, 9% [170.3g, 340.2g], (Pads) 3%, 6%, 9% [30g, 60g] | (Benzac) Apply qd-bid. (Benzagel) Apply wash qd-bid; apply gel qd initially or qhs for light skin. (Triaz) Apply gel/wash qd-bid. | Erythema, peeling, contact dermatitis, dryness, irritation |
| (Brevoxyl, Zoderm) | Brevoxyl: (Gel) 4%, 8% [42.5g], (Lot, Creamy Wash) 4%, 8% [170g]; Zoderm: (Cleanser) 4.5%, 6.5%, 8.5% [400mL], (Cre/Gel) 4.5%, 6.5%, 8.5% [125mL] | (Brevoxyl) Apply gel qd-bid; apply lotion qd for first week then bid as tolerated. (Zoderm) Apply qd-bid. | Erythema, peeling, contact dermatitis, dryness |
| **Benzoyl peroxide/ Erythromycin** (Benzamycin) | Gel: 5%-3% [23.3g, 46.6g, $60^{s}$] | Apply bid. | Dryness, urticaria, skin irritation, skin discoloration, oiliness |
| **Clindamycin/ Benzoyl peroxide** (Acanya, Benzaclin, Duac) | Acanya: (Gel): 1.2%-2.5% [50g] Benzaclin: (Gel) 1%-5% [25g, 50g]; Duac: (Gel) 1%-5% [45g] | (Acanya) Apply qd. (Benzaclin) Apply bid. (Duac) Apply once in the evening. | Dry skin, erythema, peeling, and burning |
| **ANTIBIOTICS & COMBINATIONS** | | | |
| **Azelaic acid** (Azelex) | (Cre) 20% [30g, 50g] | Apply bid. | Dryness, scaling, erythema, burning, irritation, pruritus; rarely, hypopigmentation |
| **Azelaic acid** (Finacea) | (Gel) 15% [30g, 50g] | Apply bid. | Burning, stinging, tingling, pruritus, scaling, dry skin |
| **Adapalene** (Differin) | (Cre) 0.1% [45g]; (Gel) 0.1%, 0.3% [45g] | Apply hs. | Erythema, scaling, dryness, pruritus, burning, sunburn, acne flares |
| **Clindamycin** (Cleocin T, Clinda-derm, Clindagel, Clindets, Evoclin Foam) | Cleocin T: (Gel) 1% [30g, 60g], (Lot) 1% [60mL], (Sol) 1% [30mL, 60mL], (Swab, Pledgets) 1% [$60^{s}$]; Clinda-derm: (Sol): 1% [60mL]; Clindagel: 1% [40mL, 75mL]; Clindets: (Swab) 1% [$60^{s}$]; Evoclin: (Foam) 1% [50g, 100g] | (Cleocin T) Apply bid. (Clinda-derm) Apply bid. (Clindagel) Apply qd. (Clindets) Apply bid. (Evoclin Foam) Apply qd. | Local irritation, stains clothing |
| **Clindamycin/ Tretinoin** (Ziana) | Gel: 1.2%-0.025% [30g, 60g] | Apply qd at bedtime. | Nasopharyngitis, erythema, scaling, itching, burning |
| **Erythromycin** (Erygel, EryPads) | Erygel: 2% [30g, 60g]; EryPads: 2% [60g] | (Erygel) Apply qd-bid. (EryPads) Apply bid. | Local irritation, stains clothing, peeling, dryness, itching, erythema, oiliness |
| **Sulfacetamide** (Klaron, Ovace Wash, Rosula NS) | Lot: 10% [118mL]; Ovace: (Lot) 10% [360mL]; Rosula NS: (Pads) 10% [$30^{s}$] | Apply bid. | Itching, erythema, edema |

*(Continued)*

| DRUG (BRAND) | HOW SUPPLIED | DOSAGE | SIDE EFFECTS |
|---|---|---|---|
| **ANTIBIOTICS & COMBINATIONS** *(Continued)* | | | |
| **Sulfacetamide/ Sulfur** (Clenia, Plexion, Rosula) | Clenia: (Cleanser) 10%-5% [170g, 340g], Cre: 10%-5% [28g]; Plexion: (Cleanser) 10%-5% [170.3g, 340.2g]; Rosula: (Cleanser) 10%-5% [355mL], Gel 10%-5% [45mL] | (Clenia) Apply wash qd-bid; apply cream qd-tid. (Plexion) Apply qd-bid. (Rosula) Apply cleanser qd-bid; apply gel qd-tid. | Local irritation |
| (Plexion SCT, Rosac) | Plexion SCT: (Cre) 10%-5% [4oz] Rosac: (Cre) 10%-5% [45g] | (Rosac) Apply qd-tid. (Plexion SCT) Apply qd. | Local irritation |
| (Plexion TS, Sulfacet-R) | Plexion TS: (Lot) 10%-5% [30g]; Sulfacet-R: (Lot) 10%-5% [25g] | Apply qd-tid. | Local irritation |
| **Tazarotene** (Avage, Tazorac) | Avage: (Cre) 0.1% [30g]; Tazorac: (Cre) 0.05%, 0.1% [30g, 60g]; (Gel) 0.05%, 0.1% [30g, 100g] | Apply hs. | Pruritus, burning/stinging, erythema, irritation, skin pain, desquamation, dry skin, rash |
| **Tretinoin** (Atralin, Avita, Retin-A) | Atralin: (Gel) 0.05% [45g] Avita: (Cre, Gel) 0.025% [20g, 45g] Retin-A: (Cre) 0.025%, 0.05%, 0.1% [20g, 45g]; (Gel) 0.01%, 0.025% [15g, 45g]; (Sol) 0.05% [28mL] | Apply hs. | Local skin reactions (red, edematous, blistered, crusted), photosensitivity, temporary skin pigmentation changes |
| **Tretinoin microsphere** (Retin-A-Micro) | (Gel) 0.04%, 0.1% [20g, 45g] | Apply hs. | |

**Source:** FDA-approved product labeling.

# PSORIASIS MANAGEMENT: SYSTEMIC THERAPIES

| DRUG (BRAND) | HOW SUPPLIED | DOSAGE | SIDE EFFECTS |
|---|---|---|---|
| **ANTIMETABOLITE** | | | |
| **Methotrexate** | **Inj:** 25mg/mL; **Tab:** 2.5mg | **Initial:** 10-25mg weekly until response or use divided oral dose schedule, 2.5mg at 12-hr intervals for 3 doses. **Titrate:** Increase gradually until optimal response. **Maint:** Reduce to lowest effective dose. **Max:** 30mg/wk. | Ulcerative stomatitis, leukopenia, nausea, abdominal distress, malaise, fatigue, chills, fever, dizziness, decreased resistance to infection |
| **IMMUNOSUPPRESSIVES** | | | |
| **Alefacept** (Amevive) | **Inj:** (IM) 15mg | 15mg IM once wkly for 12 wks. May repeat cycle 12 wks after first cycle complete. Adjust dose, D/C, based on CD4+ T-lymphocyte counts. | Lymphopenia, injection-site reactions, influenza-like symptoms, pruritus, hypersensitivity reactions |
| **Cyclosporine** (Gengraf, Neoral) | (Gengraf, Neoral) **Cap:** 25mg, 100mg; **Sol:** 100mg/mL [50mL] | Gengraf: **Initial:** 2.5mg/kg/day for 4 weeks. Titrate: May increase by 0.5mg/kg/day every 2 weeks. **Max:** 4mg/kg/day. Neoral: **Initial:** 1.25mg/kg bid for 4 wks. **Titrate:** May increase by 0.5mg/kg/day every 2 weeks. **Max:** 4mg/kg/day. | Infection, renal dysfunction, HTN, malignancy risk w/certain psoriasis therapies, hirsutism, muscle cramps, acne, tremor, headache, gingival hyperplasia, diarrhea, nausea, vomiting |
| **MONOCLONAL ANTIBODY** | | | |
| **Ustekinumab** (Stelara) | **Inj:** 45mg/0.5mL, 90mg/1mL | ≤100kg: **Initial:** 45mg SQ and 4 weeks later, followed by 45mg q12 weeks. >100kg: **Initial:** 90mg SQ and 4 weeks later, followed by 90mg q12 weeks. | Infection, malignancies, RPLS, nasopharyngitis, upper respiratory infection, headache, fatigue. |
| **MONOCLONAL ANTIBODIES/TNF BLOCKERS** | | | |
| **Adalimumab** (Humira) | **Inj:** 20mg/0.4mL, 40mg/0.8mL | **Initial:** 80mg. **Maint:** 40mg every other week starting 1 week after initial dose. | URI, injection-site pain/reactions, headache, rash, sinusitis, nausea, UTI, flu syndrome, abdominal pain, hyperlipidemia, hypercholesterolemia, back pain, hematuria, HTN, immunogenicity |
| **Infliximab** (Remicade) | **Inj:** 100mg | 5mg/kg IV infusion; repeat at 2 and 6 weeks. **Maint:** 5mg/kg every 8 weeks. | Infusion reactions, nausea, infections, URI, pruritus, headache, sore throat, potential risk of reactivating TB, hepatotoxicity |
| **PSORALENS** | | | |
| **Methoxsalen*** (8-Mop, Oxsoralen-Ultra) | **Cap:** 10mg | Take with food or milk. **Initial:** <30kg: 10mg. 30-50kg: 20mg. 51-65kg: 30mg. 66-80kg: 40mg. 81-90kg: 50mg. 91-115kg: 60mg. >115kg: 70mg. Take 2 hrs before UVA exposure. **Titrate:** May increase by 10mg after 15th treatment under certain conditions. **Max:** Do not treat more often than qod. | Nausea, nervousness, insomnia, depression, pruritus, erythema |
| **RETINOID** | | | |
| **Acitretin** (Soriatane) | **Cap:** 10mg, 25mg | **Initial:** 25-50mg qd w/food. Individualize dose. **Maint:** 25-50mg qd. Terminate therapy when lesions resolve. May treat relapses. | Ophthalmologic effects, cheilitis, rhinitis, dry mouth, epistaxis, alopecia, dry skin, rash, skin peeling, nail disorder, pruritus, paresthesia, paronychia, skin atrophy, sticky skin, xerophthalmia, arthralgia |

*(Continued)*

| DRUG (BRAND) | HOW SUPPLIED | DOSAGE | SIDE EFFECTS |
|---|---|---|---|
| **TNF-BLOCKING AGENT** | | | |
| **Etanercept** (Enbrel) | **Inj:** 25mg [vial], 25mg/0.5mL [syringe] 50mg/mL [syringe] | **Initial:** 50mg SQ twice weekly given 3 or 4 days apart for 3 months. May begin with 25-50mg/wk. **Maint:** 50mg/wk. | Injection-site reactions, infections, headache |

* Oxsoralen-Ultra and 8-MOP are not interchangeable due to significantly greater bioavailability and earlier photosensitization onset time of Oxsoralen-Ultra.

**Sources:** FDA-approved product labeling.

# Psoriasis Management: Topical Therapies

| DRUG (BRAND) | HOW SUPPLIED | DOSAGE | SIDE EFFECTS |
|---|---|---|---|
| **TOPICAL IMMUNOSUPPRESSANT** | | | |
| **Pimecrolimus** (Elidel) | Cre: 1% [30g, 60g, 100g] | Apply bid. | Stinging, soreness, burning, headache, nasopharyngitis, pyrexia, influenza, bacterial and viral skin infections. |
| **TOPICAL STEROIDS** | | | |
| **Betamethasone** (Luxiq) | Foam: 0.12% [50g, 100g, 150g] | Apply bid. | Burning, itching, stinging, pruritus, paresthesia, acne, alopecia, conjunctivitis |
| **Clobetasol** (Temovate, Temovate-E, Clobex, Embeline E, Olux, Olux-E) | (Temovate) Cre, Oint: 0.05% [15g, 30g, 60g]; Gel: 0.05% [15g, 30g, 60g]; Sol: 0.05% [25mL, 50mL]; (Temovate-E) Cre: 0.05% [15g, 30g, 60g]; (Clobex) Lot: 0.05% [30mL, 59mL, 118mL]; Shampoo: 0.05% [118mL]; Spray: 0.05% [2oz, 4.25oz]; (Embeline E) Cre: 0.05% [15g, 30g,60g]; (Olux) Foam: 0.05% [50g, 100g] (Olux-E) Foam: 0.05% [50g, 100g] | Apply bid. | Hypopigmentation, tachyphylaxis, striae, skin atrophy. Other common side effects: burning, stinging, pruritus, erythema, folliculitis, cracking/ fissures of the skin, numbness in fingers, tenderness |
| **Fluocinolone** | Cre: 0.01%, 0.025% [15g, 60g]; Oint: 0.025% [15g, 30g, 60g]; Sol: 0.01% [20mL, 60mL] | Apply bid-qid. | Dryness, folliculitis, acne, skin atrophy, burning, itching, irritation |
| **Fluocinonide** (Vanos) | (Generic) Cre: 0.05% [15g, 30g, 60g,120g] Cre (Emulsified base): 0.05% [15g, 30g, 60g, 120g] Gel, Oint: 0.05% [15g, 30g, 60g] Sol: 0.05% [20mL, 60mL] (Vanos) Cre: 0.1% [30mg, 60mg, 120mg] | (Generic) Apply bid-qid. (Vanos) Apply qd-bid. | Burning, itching, irritation, dryness, folliculitis, acne, hypopigmentation, skin atrophy |
| **Halcinonide** (Halog) | (Halog) Cre, Oint: 0.1% [15g, 30g, 60g] | Apply bid-tid. | Burning, itching, irritation, dryness, folliculitis, hypopigmentation, contact dermatitis, skin maceration |
| **Hydrocortisone** (Hytone, Locoid, Locoid Lipocream, Pandel, Westcort) | (Hytone 1%, 2.5%) Cre: [1oz, 2oz] Lot: [2oz] (Locoid 0.1%) Lot: [2oz] Oint: [15g, 45g] Cre: [15g, 45g] (Locoid Lipocream) Cre: [15g, 45g, 60g] Sol: [20mL, 60mL] (Pandel) Cre: 0.1% [15g, 45g, 80g]; (Westcort) Oint: 0.2% [15g, 45g, 60g] | (Hytone) bid-qid; (Locoid) Lot: bid; Oint, Cre, Sol: bid-tid. (Locoid Lipocream) Apply bid-tid. (Pandel) Apply qd-bid. (Westcort) Apply bid-tid. | Burning, stinging, moderate paresthesia, itching, dryness, folliculitis, hypopigmentation, skin atrophy |
| **Hydrocortisone/ Pramoxine** (Epifoam, Novacort, Pramosone) | (Epifoam) Foam: (Hydrocortisone-Pramoxine) 1%-1% [10g]; (Novacort) Gel: 2%-1% [29g]; (Pramosone) Cre: 1%-1%, 1%-2.5% Lot: 1%-1% [60mL, 120mL, 240mL], 1%-2.5% [60mL, 120mL]; Oint: 1%-1%, 1%-2.5% [30mL] | Apply tid-qid. | Burning, itching, irritation, dryness, folliculitis, hypopigmentation, maceration, skin atrophy |
| **Mometasone** (Elocon) | Cre, Oint: 0.1% [15g, 45g]; Lot: 0.1% [30mL, 60mL] | Apply qd. | Burning, pruritus, skin atrophy, rosacea, acneiform reaction, tingling, stinging, furunculosis, folliculitis |

*(Continued)*

| DRUG (BRAND) | HOW SUPPLIED | DOSAGE | SIDE EFFECTS |
|---|---|---|---|
| **TOPICAL STEROIDS** *(Continued)* | | | |
| **Prednicarbate** (Dermatop) | Cre, Oint: 0.1% [15g, 60g] | Apply bid. | Burning, itching, irritation, dryness, folliculitis, hypertrichosis, acneiform eruptions, hypopigmentation |
| **Triamcinolone** (Kenalog) | (Kenalog) Cre: 0.1% [15g, 60g, 80g], 0.5% [20g]; Lot: 0.025%, 0.1% [60mL]; 0.1%: [15g, 60g]; Spray: 0.147mg/g [63g] | (Kenalog) Cre, Lot, Oint: Apply 0.025% bid-qid. Apply 0.1% or 0.5% bid-tid. Spray: Apply tid-qid. | Burning, itching, irrita-, tion, dryness, folliculitis, hypopigmentation, allergic contact dermatitis |
| **Tazarotene** (Avage, Tazorac) | (Avage) Cre: 0.1% [30g] (Tazorac) Cre: 0.05%, 0.1% [30g, 60g]; Gel: 0.05%, 0.1% [30g, 100g] | Apply hs. | Pruritus, erythema, irritation, dry skin, rash, skin discoloration |
| **VITAMIN D DERIVATIVES & COMBINATIONS** | | | |
| **Calcitriol** (Vectical) | Oint: 3mcg/g [5g, 100g] | Apply to affected area(s) bid, am and pm. | Laboratory test abnormality, urine abnormality, psoriasis, hypercalciuria, pruritus. |
| **Calcipotriene** (Dovonex, Dovonex Scalp) | (Dovonex) Cre, 0.005% [60g, 120g]; (Dovonex Scalp) Sol: 0.005% [60mL] | Apply bid. | Skin irritation, pruritus, burning, hypercalcemia |
| **Calcipotriene/ betamethasone** (Taclonex, Taclonex Scalp) | Oint: (Calcipotriene-Betamethasone) 0.005%-0.064% [60g, 100g] Scalp Sus: [60g] | Apply qd up to 4 weeks. | Pruritus, headache |
| **MISCELLANEOUS AGENTS** | | | |
| **Anthralin** (Anthra-Derm, Zithranol-RR) | Cre: 1% [50g] (Zithranol-RR) Cre: 1.2% [45g] | Apply qd-bid. (Zithranol-RR) Apply qd. | Skin irritation, erythema, staining (skin and clothing), odor |
| **Coal Tar** (Zetar) | Sol 10%: 2% [3.8oz] | Apply hs. | Skin irritation, folliculitis, odor, staining of clothing |
| **Urea** (Carmol 40) | Cre: 40% [28.35g, 85g, 198.6g]; Gel: 40% [15mL]; Lot: 40% [236.6 mL] | Apply bid. | Transient stinging, burning, itching, irritation |

**Sources:**
FDA-approved drug labeling.
Luba KM, Stulberg DL. Chronic plaque psoriasis. *Am Fam Physician.* 2006 Feb 15;73(4):636-44. Review.

# Topical Corticosteroids

| STEROID | DOSAGE FORM(S) | STRENGTH (%) | POTENCY | FREQUENCY |
|---|---|---|---|---|
| Alclometasone Dipropionate (Aclovate) | Cre, Oint | 0.05 | Low-Med | bid/tid |
| Augmented Betamethasone Dipropionate (Diprolene, Diprolene AF) | Oint | 0.05 | Very High | qd/bid |
| | Cre, Lot | 0.05 | High | qd/bid |
| Betamethasone Dipropionate | Cre, Lot, Oint | 0.05 | High | qd/bid |
| Betamethasone Valerate (Luxiq) | Foam | 0.12 | Medium | bid |
| Clobetasol Propionate (Clobevate, Clobex, Cormax, Embeline E, Olux, Olux E, Temovate, Temovate-E) | Cre, Foam (Olux) | 0.05 | Very High | bid |
| | Cream (Embeline E), Foam, Gel (Clobevate), Lotion (Clobex), Oint, Shampoo (Clobex), Sol | 0.05 | Very High | qd (shampoo) |
| Clocortolone Pivalate (Cloderm) | Cre | 0.1 | Med | tid |
| Desonide (Desonate, DesOwen, Verdeso) | Cre, Foam, Gel (Desonate), Lot, Oint | 0.05 | Low-Med | bid/tid |
| Desoximetasone (Topicort, Topicort LP) | Cre | 0.05 | Medium | bid |
| | Cre, Oint | 0.25 | High | bid |
| | Gel | 0.05 | High | bid |
| Diflorasone Diacetate (Psorcon) | Cre (Psorcon), Oint | 0.05 | High | bid |
| Fluocinolone Acetonide (Capex, Derma-Smoothe/FS) | Cre, Oint | 0.025 | Medium | tid/qid |
| | Cre, Sol | 0.01 | Medium | tid/qid |
| | Oil (Derma-Smoothe/FS) | 0.01 | Low-Med | qd hs |
| | Shampoo (Capex) | 0.01 | Low-Med | qd |
| Fluocinonide (Vanos) | Cre, Gel, Oint, Sol | 0.05 | High | bid/qid |
| | Cre (Vanos) | 0.1 | Very High | qd/bid |
| Flurandrenolide (Cordran, Cordran SP) | Cre, Oint | 0.025 | Medium | bid/tid |
| | Cre, Lot, Oint | 0.05 | Medium | bid/tid |
| | Tape | 4mcg/cm$^2$ | Medium | qd/bid |
| Fluticasone Propionate (Cutivate) | Cre, Lot | 0.05 | Medium | qd/bid |
| | Oint | 0.005 | Medium | bid |
| Halcinonide (Halog) | Cre, Oint | 0.1 | High | bid/tid |
| Halobetasol Propionate (Ultravate, Ultravate PAC) | Cre, Oint | 0.05 | Very High | qd/bid |
| Hydrocortisone (Anusol HC, Hytone, Proctocort) | Cre, Lot | 1 | Low | tid/qid |
| | Cre, Lot, Oint | 2.5 | Low | bid/qid |
| Hydrocortisone Butyrate (Locoid, Locoid Lipo Cream) | Cre, Lot, Oint, Sol | 0.1 | Medium | bid/tid |
| Hydrocortisone Probutate (Pandel) | Cre | 0.1 | Medium | qd/bid |
| Hydrocortisone Valerate (Westcort) | Cre, Oint | 0.2 | Medium | bid/tid |
| Mometasone Furoate (Elocon) | Cre, Lot, Oint | 0.1 | Medium | qd |
| Prednicarbate (Dermatop) | Cre, Oint | 0.1 | Medium | bid |
| Triamcinolone Acetonide (Kenalog, Triderm) | Cre, Lot, Oint | 0.025 | Medium | bid/qid |
| | Cre, Lot, Oint | 0.1 | Medium | bid/tid |
| | Cre, Oint | 0.5 | High | bid/tid |
| | Spray | 0.147 | Medium | bid/qid |

# INSULIN FORMULATIONS

| TYPE OF INSULIN | BRAND | ONSET* (hrs) | PEAK* (hrs) | DURATION* (hrs) |
|---|---|---|---|---|
| **Rapid-acting** | | | | |
| Insulin Glulisine | Apidra | – | 0.5 to 1.7 | 1 to 3 |
| Insulin Lispro | Humalog | <0.25 | 0.5 to 1.5 | 3 to 5 |
| Insulin Aspart | Novolog | <0.25 | 0.5 to 1 | 3 to 5 |
| **Short-acting** | | | | |
| Regular Insulin | Humulin R† | 0.5 to 1 | 2 to 4 | 4 to 12 |
| | Novolin R | 0.5 | 2.5 to 5 | 8 |
| **Intermediate-acting** | | | | |
| NPH (Isophane) | Humulin N | 1 to 3 | 6 to 12 | 18 to 24 |
| | Novolin N | 1.5 | 4 to 12 | 24 |
| **Long-acting** | | | | |
| Insulin glargine | Lantus | 1 | Flat | 24 |
| Insulin detemir | Levemir | – | 6 to 8 | 24 |
| **Combinations** | | | | |
| Isophane insulin suspension (70%)/ regular insulin (30%) | Humulin 70/30 | 0.5 to 1 | 4 to 6 | 24 |
| | Novolin 70/30 | 0.5 | 2 to 12 | 24 |
| Isophane insulin suspension (50%)/ regular insulin (50%) | Humulin 50/50 | 0.5 to 1 | 3 to 5 | 24 |
| Insulin aspart protamine (70%)/ insulin aspart (30%) | Novolog Mix 70/30 | ≤0.25 | 1 to 4 | 24 |
| Insulin lispro protamine (50%)/ insulin lispro (50%) | Humalog Mix 50/50 | ≤0.25 | 0.75 to 2 | 24 |
| Insulin lispro protamine (75%)/ insulin lispro (25%) | Humalog Mix 75/25 | ≤0.25 | 0.5 to 4 | 24 |

*Approximate parameters following SC injection of an average patient dose; insulin concentration: 100 U/mL.

†Also available as 500 U/mL for insulin-resistant patients (rapid onset; up to 24-hr duration).

# ORAL ANTIDIABETIC AGENTS

| DRUG | HOW SUPPLIED | INITIAL* & (MAX) DOSE | USUAL DOSE RANGE* |
|---|---|---|---|
| **BIGUANIDES** | | | |
| **Metformin HCl** | | | |
| Fortamet | **Tab: ER:** 500mg, 1000mg | 1000mg qd with evening meal (2500mg/day). | 500-2500mg qd. |
| Glumetza | **Tab: ER:** 500mg, 1000mg | 1000mg qd with evening meal (2000mg/day). | 1500mg-2000mg/day. |
| Glucophage, Riomet | **Tab:** 500mg, 850mg, 1000mg **Sol:** 500mg/5mL | 500mg bid or 850mg qd with meals (2550mg/day). | 850mg-2000mg/day qd or divided doses. |
| Glucophage XR | **Tab: ER:** 500mg, 750mg | 500mg qd with evening meal (2000mg/day). | 500-2000mg/day qd or divided doses. |
| **BILE-ACID SEQUESTRANT** | | | |
| **Colesevelam HCl** Welchol | **Tab:** 625mg **Sus:** 3.75g, 1.875g [pkt] | 1875mg bid or 3750mg qd (3750mg/day). | 3750mg qd. |
| **DIPEPTIDYL PEPTIDASE-4 INHIBITOR** | | | |
| **Saxagliptin** Onglyza | **Tab:** 2.5mg, 5mg | 2.5-5mg qd. | 2.5-5mg qd. |
| **Sitagliptin** Januvia | **Tab:** 25mg, 50mg, 100mg | 100mg qd. | 100mg qd. |
| **GLUCOSIDASE INHIBITORS** | | | |
| **Acarbose** Precose | **Tab:** 25mg, 50mg, 100mg | 25mg tid at start of each meal ($\leq$60kg: 50mg tid, $>$60kg: 100mg tid). | 25-100mg tid. |
| **Miglitol** Glyset | **Tab:** 25mg, 50mg, 100mg | 25mg tid at start of each meal (300mg/day). | 50-100mg tid. |
| **MEGLITINIDES** | | | |
| **Nateglinide** Starlix | **Tab:** 60mg, 120mg | 120mg tid before meals (360mg/day). | 120mg tid. |
| **Repaglinide** Prandin | **Tab:** 0.5mg, 1mg, 2mg | 0.5-2mg with each meal (16mg/day). | 0.5-4mg with each meal. |
| **SULFONYLUREAS** | | | |
| **Chlorpropamide** | **Tab:** 100mg, 250mg | Initial: 250mg daily. Elderly: 100-125mg/day. (750mg/day). | $<$100-500mg daily. Most patients controlled with 250mg daily. |
| **Glimepiride** Amaryl | **Tab:** 1mg, 2mg, 4mg | 1-2mg qd w/breakfast or first main meal (8mg/day). | 1-4mg qd. |
| **Glipizide** | | | |
| Glucotrol | **Tab:** 5mg, 10mg | 5mg qd before breakfast (40mg/day). | 5-40mg qd or divided if $>$15mg/day. |
| Glucotrol XL | **Tab, ER:** 2.5mg, 5mg, 10mg | 5mg qd w/breakfast (20mg/day). | 5-10mg qd. |
| **Glyburide** Diabeta | **Tab:** 1.25mg, 2.5mg, 5mg | 2.5-5mg qd w/breakfast or first main meal (20mg/day). | 1.25-20mg qd or divided doses. |
| **Glyburide Micronized** Glynase PresTab | **Tab:** 1.5mg, 3mg, 6mg | 1.5-3mg qd w/breakfast or first main meal (12mg/day). | 0.75-12mg qd or divided doses. |

*(Continued)*

| DRUG | HOW SUPPLIED | INITIAL* & (MAX) DOSE | USUAL DOSE RANGE* |
|---|---|---|---|
| **SULFONYLUREAS** *(Continued)* | | | |
| **Tolazamide** | **Tab:** 100mg, 250mg, 500mg | 100-250mg qd with breakfast or first main meal (1000mg/day). | 100-1000mg qd or divided if >500mg/day. |
| **Tolbutamide** | **Tab:** 500mg | 1000-2000mg qd or divided doses (3000mg/day). | 250-3000mg/day qd or divided doses. |
| **THIAZOLIDINEDIONES** | | | |
| **Pioglitazone HCl** Actos | **Tab:** 15mg, 30mg, 45mg | 15-30mg qd (45mg/day). | 15-30mg qd. |
| **Rosiglitazone maleate** Avandia | **Tab:** 2mg, 4mg, 8mg | 2mg bid or 4mg qd (8mg/day). | 4mg bid or 8mg qd. |
| **COMBINATIONS** | | | |
| **Glipizide/ Metformin HCl** Metaglip | **Tab:** 2.5mg/250mg, 2.5mg/500mg, 5mg/500mg | 2.5mg/250mg qd w/meals or 2.5mg/500mg bid (20mg/2g/day). | 2.5mg/250mg qd-2.5mg/500mg bid. |
| **Glyburide/ Metformin HCl** Glucovance | **Tab:** 1.25mg/250mg, 2.5mg/500mg, 5mg/500mg | 1.25mg/250mg qd or bid with meals (20mg/2g/day). | 1.25mg/250mg qd-5mg/500mg bid. |
| **Pioglitazone/ Glimepiride** Duetact | **Tab:** 30mg/2mg, 30mg/4mg | 30mg/2mg qd or 30mg/4mg qd Do not give more than once daily at any of the tablet strengths. | 1 tab qd. |
| **Pioglitazone/ Metformin HCl** Actoplus Met | **Tab:** 15mg/500mg, 15mg/850mg | 15mg/500mg or 15mg/850mg qd-bid (45mg/2550mg/day). | 1 tab qd-bid. |
| Actoplus Met XR | **Tab: ER:** 15mg/1000mg, 30mg/1000mg | 15mg/1000mg or 30mg/1000mg qd with evening meal (45mg/2000mg/day). | 1 tab qd. |
| **Repaglinide/ Metformin HCl** PrandiMet | **Tab:** 1mg/500mg, 2mg/500mg | 1mg/500mg bid-tid before meals or 2mg/500mg bid-tid before meals (10mg/2500/day). | 1 tab bid-tid. |
| **Rosiglitazone/ Glimepiride** Avandaryl | **Tab:** 4mg/1mg, 4mg/2mg, 4mg/4mg, 8mg/2mg, 8mg/4mg | 4mg/1mg qd or 4mg/2mg qd w/first meal (8mg/4mg/day). | 1 tab am. |
| **Rosiglitazone/ Metformin HCl** Avandamet | **Tab:** 2mg/500mg, 4mg/500mg, 2mg/1g, 4mg/1g | 2mg/500mg qd-bid w/meals (8mg/2g/day). | 1 tab bid. |
| **Sitagliptin/ Metformin** Janumet | **Tab:** 50mg/500mg, 50mg/1000mg | 50mg/500mg or 50mg/1000mg bid w/meals (100mg/2g/day). | 1 tab bid. |

*NOTE: Usual dose ranges are derived from the drug's FDA-approved labeling. There is no fixed dosage regimen for the management of diabetes mellitus with any hypoglycemic agent. The initial and maintenance dosing should be conservative, depending on the patient's individual needs, especially in elderly, debilitated or malnourished patients, and with impaired renal or hepatic function. Management of type 2 diabetes should include blood glucose and HbA1c monitoring, nutritional counseling, exercise, and weight reduction as needed. For more detailed information refer to the individual monograph listings or the drug's FDA-approved labeling.

# ANTIEMETICS

| DRUG (BRAND) | INDICATIONS | HOW SUPPLIED | ADULT DOSING | PEDIATRIC DOSING |
|---|---|---|---|---|
| **Anticholinergic Agent** | | | | |
| **Scopolamine** (Transderm Scop) | Prevention of nausea and vomiting associated with motion sickness or recovery from anesthesia and surgery. | Patch: 1mg/72 hrs [4[s]] | Apply 1 patch the evening before surgery or 1 hr prior to cesarean section. Keep in place for 24 hrs. Apply patch to a hairless area behind the ear at least 4 hrs before needed. Do not cut patch in half. | |
| **Antihistamines** | | | | |
| **Dimenhydrinate** (Dramamine Original Formula) | Prevention and treatment of nausea, vomiting, or vertigo caused by motion sickness. | Inj: 50mg/mL | (Inj) 50mg q4h, may increase to 100mg q4h if drowsiness is desirable. For IV administration, dilute each mL of solution in 10mL of 0.9% sodium chloride and inject over 2 minutes. IM injection is administered undiluted. | (IM) 1.25mg/kg or 37.5mg/m$^2$ body surface area qid. Max: 300mg/day. |
| **Meclizine HCl** (Antivert) | Management of nausea, vomiting and dizziness associated with motion sickness. Management of vertigo associated with diseases affecting the vestibular system. | Tab: 12.5mg, 25mg, 50mg* *scored | 25-50mg 1 hr prior to trip/departure, repeat q24h prn. | **≥12 yrs:** Motion Sickness: 25-50mg 1 hr prior to trip/departure, repeat q24h prn. Vertigo: 25-100mg/day in divided doses. |
| **Promethazine HCl** (Phenergan) | Prevention and control of nausea and vomiting in surgery. Active and prophylactic treatment of motion sickness. Postoperative antiemetic therapy. | Liq: 6.25/5mL [473mL, 118mL]; Sup: 12.5mg, 25mg, 50mg; Tab: 12.5mg, 25mg, 50mg* *scored Inj: 25mg/mL, 50mg/mL | Nausea/Vomiting: 12.5-25mg q4h; Motion Sickness: 25mg bid 0.5-1h prior to trip/departure. | **≥2 yrs:** Motion Sickness: 12.5-25mg bid. Nausea/Vomiting: 12.5-25mg may be repeated at 4-6h intervals. Dose should not exceed half of adult dose. Premedication: Usual: 0.5mg/lb. Do not give IV administration >25mg/mL and at a rate >25mg/min. |
| **Cannabinoids** | | | | |
| **Dronabinol** (Marinol) | Treatment of nausea and vomiting associated with chemotherapy when conventional treatment has failed. | Cap: 2.5mg, 5mg, 10mg | Initial: 5mg/m$^2$ given 1-3 hrs before chemotherapy, then q2-4h after chemotherapy, up to 4-6 doses/day. Titrate: May increase by 2.5mg/m$^2$ increments. Max: 15mg/m$^2$/dose. | |
| **Nabilone** (Cesamet) | Treatment of the nausea and vomiting associated with chemotherapy when conventional treatment has failed. | Cap: 1mg | Initial: 1 or 2mg bid; given 1-3 hrs before chemotherapy. A dose of 1 or 2mg the night before may be useful. Max: 6mg/day given in divided doses tid. | |

(Continued)

| DRUG (BRAND) | INDICATIONS | HOW SUPPLIED | ADULT DOSING | PEDIATRIC DOSING |
|---|---|---|---|---|
| **5-HT3 Antagonists** | | | | |
| **Dolasetron mesylate** (Anzemet) | (Inj) Prevention of nausea/vomiting associated with emetogenic cancer chemotherapy including high-dose cisplatin. Prevention and treatment of post-op nausea/vomiting (PONV). (Tab) Prevention of nausea/vomiting associated with moderately emetogenic cancer chemotherapy and prevention of PONV. | Inj: 20mg/mL; Tab: 50mg, 100mg | (Inj) Prevention of Chemotherapy-Induced Nausea/Vomiting (CINV): 1.8mg/kg IV single dose or 100mg IV 30 min before chemotherapy. Prevention/Treatment of PONV: 12.5mg IV single dose 15 min before cessation of anesthesia or as soon as nausea/vomiting presents. (Tab) Prevention of CINV: 100mg PO within 1 hr before chemotherapy. Prevention of PONV: 100mg PO within 2 hrs before surgery. | **2-16 yrs:** (Inj) Prevention of CINV: 1.8mg/kg IV single dose 30 min before chemotherapy. Max: 100mg. May mix inj in apple or grape juice and take orally within 1 hr before chemotherapy. Prevention/Treatment of PONV: 0.35mg/kg IV single dose 15 min before cessation of anesthesia or as soon as nausea/vomiting presents. Max: 12.5mg single dose. May mix 1.2mg/kg inj in apple or grape juice and take orally within 2 hrs before surgery. Max: 100mg/dose. (Tab) Prevention of CINV: 1.8mg/kg PO within 1 hr before chemotherapy. Max: 100mg. Prevention of PONV: 1.2mg/kg PO within 2 hrs before surgery. Max: 100mg. |
| **Granisetron hydrochloride** (Kytril) | (Inj, Sol, Tab) Prevention of nausea and vomiting associated with chemotherapy including high-dose cisplatin. (Sol, Tab) Prevention of nausea and vomiting associated with radiation. (Inj) Prevention and treatment of post-op nausea and vomiting (PONV). | Inj: 0.1mg/mL, 1mg/mL; Sol: 2mg/10mL [30mL]; Tab: 1mg | (Sol/Tab) Prevention of Chemotherapy-Induced Nausea/Vomiting (CINV): 2mg qd up to 1 hr before chemotherapy or 1mg bid (up to 1 hr before chemotherapy and 12 hrs later). (Inj) 10mcg/kg within 30 min before chemotherapy. Prevention with Radiation: (Sol/Tab) 2mg within 1 hr of radiation. Prevention and treatment of PONV: (Inj) Administer 1mg over 30 sec before induction of anesthesia or immediately before anesthesia reversal. | **2-16 yrs:** Prevention of CINV: 10mcg/kg IV within 30 min before chemotherapy. |
| **Granisetron transdermal system** (Sancuso) | Prevention of nausea and vomiting in patients receiving moderately and/or highly emetogenic chemotherapy regimens of up to 5 consecutive days duration. | Patch: 3.1mg/24hrs [1[s]] | Apply patch to upper outer arm 24 hrs prior to chemotherapy. The patch may be applied up to a maximum of 48 hrs before chemotherapy. | |

| DRUG (BRAND) | INDICATIONS | HOW SUPPLIED | ADULT DOSING | PEDIATRIC DOSING |
|---|---|---|---|---|
| **5-$HT_3$ Antagonists** *(Continued)* | | | | |
| **Ondansetron hydrochloride** (Zofran) | (Inj) Prevention of nausea and vomiting associated with initial and repeat courses of emetogenic cancer chemotherapy, including high-dose cisplatin. Prevention of post-op nausea and/or vomiting (PONV). (Sol/Tab) Prevention of nausea and vomiting associated with: highly emetogenic cancer chemotherapy, including cisplatin ≥50mg/m²; initial and repeat courses of moderately emetogenic cancer of moderately emetogenic cancer chemotherapy; and radiotherapy in patients receiving either total body irradiation, single high-dose fraction to the abdomen, or daily fractions to the abdomen. Prevention of PONV. | Inj: 2mg/mL;<br>Sol: 4mg/5mL [50mL];<br>Tab: 4mg, 8mg;<br>Tab, Disintegrating: 4mg, 8mg | Prevention of Chemotherapy-Induced Nausea/Vomiting (CINV): (Inj) 32mg single dose over 15 min or three 0.15mg/kg doses, 1st dose 30 min before chemotherapy, then 4 and 8 hrs after 1st dose. Prevention of CINV, Highly Emetogenic Therapy: (Tab) 24mg given as three 8mg tablets administered 30 min before chemotherapy. Prevention of CINV, Moderately Emetogenic Therapy: (Sol/Tab) 8mg bid, 1st dose 30 min before chemotherapy, then 8 hrs later, then bid for 1-2 days after chemotherapy. Prevention of PONV: (Inj) 4mg IM/IV immediately before anesthesia or post-op after surgery if nausea or vomiting occurs. (Sol/Tab) 16mg 1 hr before anesthesia. Prevention of Nausea/Vomiting Associated with Radiation Therapy: (Sol/Tab) Usual: 8mg tid. Total Body Irradiation: before therapy daily. Single 8mg 1-2 hrs High-Dose Therapy To Abdomen: 8mg 1-2 hrs before therapy then q8h after 1st dose for 1-2 days after completion of therapy. Daily Fractionated Therapy To Abdomen: 8mg 1-2 hrs before therapy then q8h after 1st dose.<br>Severe Hepatic Dysfunction (Child-Pugh ≥10): Max: 8mg/day IV single dose infused over 15 min, start 30 min before chemotherapy or 8mg/day PO. | Prevention of CINV: (Inj) **6 months-18 yrs:** Three 0.15mg/kg doses, 1st dose 30 min before chemotherapy, then 4 and 8 hrs after the 1st dose. (Sol/Tab) Prevention of CINV, Moderately Emetogenic Therapy: ≥**12 yrs:** 8mg bid, 1st dose 30 min before chemotherapy, then 8mg 8 hrs later, then bid for 1-2 days. **4-11 yrs:** 4mg tid, 1st dose 30 min before chemotherapy, then 4 and 8 hrs after 1st dose, then tid for 1-2 days. Prevention of PONV: (Inj) >**12 yrs:** 4mg IM/IV immediately before anesthesia or post-op after surgery if nausea or vomiting occurs. **1 month-12 yrs**: ≤40kg: 0.1mg/kg single dose. >40kg: 4mg single dose. Severe Hepatic Dysfunction: Max: 8mg/day IV single dose infused over 15 min, start 30 min before chemotherapy or 8mg/day PO. |
| **Palonosetron hydrochloride** (Aloxi) | (Inj) Prevention of acute and delayed nausea and vomiting associated with initial and repeat courses of moderately emetogenic cancer chemotherapy and prevention of acute N/V associated with initial and repeat courses of highly emetogenic cancer chemotherapy. Prevention of post-op nausea and vomiting (PONV) for up to 24 hrs following surgery. | Inj: 0.25mg/5mL, 0.075mg/1.5mL | Chemo-Induced N/V: 0.25mg IV single dose 30 min before start of chemotherapy. Repeated dosing within a 7-day interval not recommended. PONV: 0.075mg IV single dose 10 sec before induction of anesthesia. | |

*(Continued)*

| DRUG (BRAND) | INDICATIONS | HOW SUPPLIED | ADULT DOSING | PEDIATRIC DOSING |
|---|---|---|---|---|
| **Miscellaneous** | | | | |
| **Droperidol** (Inapsine) | To reduce incidence of nausea and vomiting associated with surgical and diagnostic procedures. | Inj: 2.5mg/mL | Initial (Max): 2.5mg IM/IV. May give additional 1.25mg cautiously to achieve desired effect. Lower initial doses in elderly, debilitated, poor-risk patients. | **2-12 yrs:** Initial (Max): 0.1 mg/kg IM/IV. May give additional dose cautiously. Lower initial doses in debilitated, poor-risk patients. |
| **Metoclopramide** (Reglan) | (Inj) Prevention of post-op or chemo-induced nausea/vomiting. | Inj: 5mg/mL | Antiemetic: (Postoperative) 10-20mg IM near end of surgery. (Chemotherapy-Induced) 1-2mg/kg 30 min before chemotherapy then q2h for two doses, then q3h for three doses. Give 2mg/kg for highly emetogenic drugs for initial 2 doses. For CrCl <40mL/min: Give approx. half the recommended dosage. | |
| **Trimethobenzamide hydrochloride** (Tigan) | Treatment of postoperative nausea and vomiting and for nausea associated with gastroenteritis. | Cap: 300mg; Inj: 100mg/mL | (Cap) 300mg tid-qid. (Inj) 200mg IM tid-qid. | |
| **Phenothiazine Derivative** | | | | |
| **Prochlorperazine** (Compazine) | Control of severe nausea and vomiting. | Inj: (Edisylate) 5mg/mL; Supp: 2.5mg, 5mg, 25mg; Tab: (Maleate) 5mg, 10mg; Cap: (Maleate) 10mg, 15mg; Syr: 5mg/5ml | Nausea/Vomiting: (Tab) Usual: 5-10mg tid-qid. Max: 40mg/day. (Cap) 15mg qam or 10mg q12h. Max: 40mg/day. (Supp) 25mg bid. (IM) 5-10mg IM q3-4h prn. Max: 40mg/day. (IV) 2.5-10mg IV (not bolus). Max: 10mg single dose and 40mg/day. Nausea/Vomiting with Surgery: 5-10mg IM 1-2 hrs or 5-10mg IV 15-30 min before anesthesia, or during or after surgery; repeat once if needed. | Nausea/Vomiting: >**2 yrs** and >20 lbs: (PO/PR) 20-29 lbs: Usual: 2.5mg qd-bid. Max: 7.5mg/day. 30-39 lbs: 2.5mg bid-tid. Max: 10mg/day. 40-85 lbs: 2.5mg tid or 5mg bid. Max: 15mg/day. (IM) 0.06mg/lb, usually single dose for control. |

| DRUG (BRAND) | INDICATIONS | HOW SUPPLIED | ADULT DOSING | PEDIATRIC DOSING |
|---|---|---|---|---|
| **Substance P/Neurokinin 1 Receptor Antagonists** | | | | |
| **Aprepitant** (Emend) | In combination with other antiemetics for prevention of acute and delayed nausea and vomiting associated with initial and repeat courses of highly emetogenic cancer chemotherapy (eg, high-dose cisplatin) and for moderately emetogenic cancer chemotherapy. For the prevention of post-op nausea and vomiting (PONV). | Cap: 40mg, 80mg, 125mg; Tri-Pak: (one 125mg & two 80mg caps) | Prevention of Chemotherapy-Induced Nausea/Vomiting: Day 1: 125mg 1 hr prior to chemotherapy. Days 2 and 3: 80mg qam. Regimen should include a corticosteroid and a 5-$HT_3$ antagonist. Prevention of PONV: 40mg within 3 hrs prior to induction of anesthesia. | |
| **Fosaprepitant Dimeglumine** (Emend for injection) | In combination with other antiemetics for prevention of acute and delayed nausea and vomiting associated with initial and repeat courses of highly emetogenic cancer chemotherapy (eg, high-dose cisplatin) and for moderately emetogenic cancer chemotherapy. | Powder (Vial): 115mg/10mL [10mL] | 115mg IV over 15 min or 125mg PO 30 min prior to chemotherapy on day 1, 80mg PO days 2 and 3 only of a 3-day regimen, in addition to corticosteroid and 5-$HT_3$ antagonist. | |

# $H_2$ ANTAGONISTS AND PPIs COMPARISON[§]

| | | | INDICATIONS | | | | | | |
|---|---|---|---|---|---|---|---|---|---|
| | DRUG | HOW SUPPLIED | Heart-burn | PUD | GERD | Zollinger-Ellison | *H.pylori* | NSAID† Induced | Upper GI‡ Bleeding |
| $H_2$ ANTAGONISTS | **CIMETIDINE** | | | | | | | | |
| | Tagamet | **Inj:** 300mg/50mL** **Sol:** 300mg/5mL** **Tab:** 200mg, 300mg, 400mg, 800mg | | X | X | X | | | X |
| | **FAMOTIDINE** | | | | | | | | |
| | Pepcid | **Inj:** 0.4mg/mL, 10mg/mL **Sus:** 40mg/5mL; **Tab:** 20mg, 40mg | | X | X | X | | | |
| | **NIZATIDINE** | | | | | | | | |
| | Axid | **Cap:** 150mg, 300mg **Sol:** 15mg/mL | | X | X | | | | |
| | **RANITIDINE** | | | | | | | | |
| | Zantac | **Inj:** 1mg/mL, 25mg/mL **Syrup:** 15mg/mL **Tab:** 150mg, 300mg **Tab, Effervescent:** 25mg | | X | X | X | | | |
| PROTON PUMP INHIBITORS | **DEXLANSOPRAZOLE** | | | | | | | | |
| | Dexilant (formerly known as Kapidex) | **Cap, DR:** 30mg, 60mg | X | | X | | | | |
| | **ESOMEPRAZOLE** | | | | | | | | |
| | Nexium | **Cap, DR:** 20mg, 40mg; **Inj:** 20mg, 40mg **Sus, DR:** 10mg, 20mg, 40mg (granules/packet) | X | X | X | X | X | X | |
| | **LANSOPRAZOLE** | | | | | | | | |
| | Prevacid | **Cap, DR:** 15mg, 30mg; **Inj:** 30mg **Sus:** 15mg/packet, 30mg/packet **Tab, Disintegrating:** 15mg, 30mg | X | X | X | X | X | X | |
| | Prevpac | **Cap:** (Amoxicillin) 500mg **Tab:** (Clarithromycin) 500mg **Cap, DR:** (Lansoprazole) 30mg | | | | | X | | |
| | Prevacid NapraPAC | **Cap, DR:** (Naproxen Lansoprazole): 500mg-15mg | | | | | | X | |
| | **OMEPRAZOLE** | | | | | | | | |
| | Prilosec | **Cap, DR:** 10mg, 20mg, 40mg; **Sus, DR:** 2.5mg, 10mg (granules/packet) | | X | X | X | X | | |
| | Zegerid | (Omeprazole-Sodium Bicarbonate); **Cap:** 20mg-1100mg, 40mg-1100mg; **Pow:** 20mg-1680mg/packet, 40mg-1680mg/packet **Tab, Chewable:** (Omeprazole-Sodium Bicarbonate-Magnesium Hydroxide) 20mg-600mg-700mg, 40mg-600mg-700mg | X | X | X | | | | X |
| | **PANTOPRAZOLE** | | | | | | | | |
| | Protonix | **Inj:** 40mg; **Tab, DR:** 20mg, 40mg **Sus, DR:** 40mg (granules/packet) | X | | X | X | | | |
| | **RABEPRAZOLE** | | | | | | | | |
| | Aciphex | **Tab, DR:** 20mg | | X | X | X | X | | |

DR=Delayed-Release *Product available generically only. †Prevention of NSAID-induced gastric ulcers.

‡Prevention of upper GI bleeding in critically ill patients.

§Rx products only. For OTC products, refer to Antacid and Heartburn Products on page A63.

# ANTIBIOTIC SENSITIVITY – AMINOGLYCOSIDES*

| ORGANISMS | Amikacin | Gentamicin | Kanamycin | Neomycin | Streptomycin | Tobramycin | |
|---|---|---|---|---|---|---|---|
| **ANAEROBES** | | | | | | | |
| *Actinomyces* | | | | | | | |
| *Bacillus anthracis* | | | | | | | |
| *Bacteroides fragilis* | | | | | | | |
| *Clostridium difficile* | | | | | | | |
| *Clostridium species* | | | | | | | |
| **GRAM-NEGATIVE AEROBES** | | | | | | | |
| *Acinetobacter baumannii* | ✓ | | ✓ | | | | |
| *Aeromonas hydrophila* | | | | | | | |
| *Bartonella henselae* | | | | | | | |
| *Bordetella species* | | | | | | | |
| *Brucella* | | | | | ✓ | | |
| *Burkholderia cepacia* | | | | | | | |
| *Calymmatobacterium granulomatis* | | | | | ✓ | | |
| *Campylobacter jejuni* | | | | | | | |
| *Citrobacter species* | ✓ | ✓ | ✓ | | | ✓ | |
| *Coxiella burnetti* | | | | | | | |
| *Enterobacter species* | ✓ | ✓ | ✓ | ✓ | | ✓ | |

*These are generalizations. There are major differences among countries, areas, and hospitals depending on antibiotic usage patterns. The organisms checked for each antibiotic are not all-inclusive; only the major organisms are listed.
Blank = no or insufficient activity, or unknown.

| ORGANISMS | Amikacin | Gentamicin | Kanamycin | Neomycin | Streptomycin | Tobramycin | |
|---|---|---|---|---|---|---|---|
| **GRAM-NEGATIVE AEROBES** *(Continued)* | | | | | | | |
| *Escherichia coli* | ✓ | ✓ | ✓ | ✓ | ✓ | ✓ | |
| *Francisella tularensis* | | | | | ✓ | | |
| *Haemophilus ducreyi* | | | | | ✓ | | |
| *Haemophilus influenzae* | | | ✓ | | ✓ | | |
| *Klebsiella species* | ✓ | ✓ | ✓ | ✓ | ✓ | ✓ | |
| *Legionella species* | | | | | | | |
| *Moraxella catarrhalis* | | | | | | | |
| *Morganella morganii* | | | | | | ✓ | |
| *Neisseria gonorrhoeae* | | ✓ | ✓ | | | | |
| *Neisseria meningitidis* | | | | | | | |
| *Pasteurella multocida* | | | | | | | |
| *Pasteurella pestis* | | | | | ✓ | | |
| *Proteus mirabilis* | ✓ | ✓ | ✓ | | ✓ | ✓ | |
| *Proteus vulgaris* | ✓ | ✓ | ✓ | | ✓ | ✓ | |
| *Providencia stuartii* | ✓ | ✓ | ✓ | | | ✓ | |
| *Pseudomonas aeruginosa* | ✓ | ✓ | | | | ✓ | |
| *Rickettsia species* | | | | | | | |
| *Salmonella species* | | ✓ | ✓ | | | | |
| *Serratia species* | ✓ | ✓ | ✓ | | | ✓ | |

*These are generalizations. There are major differences among countries, areas, and hospitals depending on antibiotic usage patterns. The organisms checked for each antibiotic are not all-inclusive; only the major organisms are listed.
Blank = no or insufficient activity, or unknown.

**AMINOGLYCOSIDES (CONTINUED)**

| ORGANISMS | Amikacin | Gentamic | Kanamycin | Neomycin | Streptomycin | Tobramyc | |
|---|---|---|---|---|---|---|---|
| **GRAM-NEGATIVE AEROBES** *(Continued)* | | | | | | | |
| *Shigella species* | | ✓ | ✓ | | | | |
| *Stenotrophomonas maltophilia* | | | | | | | |
| *Vibrio vulnificus* | | | | | | | |
| *Yersinia enterocolitica* | | | | | | | |
| *Yersinia pestis* | | | | | | | |
| **GRAM-POSITIVE AEROBES** | | | | | | | |
| *Enterococcus faecalis* | | | | | ✓ | | |
| *Enterococcus faecium* | | | | | | | |
| *Enterococcus faecium (VRE)* | | | | | | | |
| *Listeria monocytogenes* | | | | | | | |
| *Nocardia* | | | | | | | |
| *Staphylococcus aureus (MSSA)* | | ✓ | ✓ | | | ✓ | |
| *Staphylococcus aureus (MRSA)* | | | ✓ | | | | |
| *Staphylococcus epidermidis* | | ✓ | ✓ | | | | |
| *Staphylococcus epidermidis (MRSE)* | | | | | | | |
| *Streptococcus pneumoniae*† | | ✓ | | | | | |

*These are generalizations. There are major differences among countries, areas, and hospitals depending on antibiotic usage patterns. The organisms checked for each antibiotic are not all-inclusive; only the major organisms are listed.

Blank = no or insufficient activity, or unknown.

† Penicillin sensitive; MIC ≤1.0 mcg/mL.

| ORGANISMS | Amikacin | Gentamicin | Kanamycin | Neomycin | Streptomycin | Tobramycin | |
|---|---|---|---|---|---|---|---|
| **GRAM-POSITIVE AEROBES** *(Continued)* | | | | | | | |
| *Streptococcus pneumoniae*§§ | | ✓ | | | | | |
| *Streptococcus (Group A,B,C,F,G)* | | ✓ | | | | | |
| *Streptococcus species* | | ✓ | ✓ | | | | |
| **MISCELLANEOUS** | | | | | | | |
| *Chlamydia pneumoniae* | | | | | | | |
| *Chlamydia trachomatis* | | | | | | | |
| *Ehrlichia/Anaplasma species* | | | | | | | |
| **MYCOBACTERIA** | | | | | | | |
| *Mycobacterium avium (MAI) (non-HIV)* | | | | | | | |
| *Mycobacterium tuberculosis* | | | | | ✓ | | |
| *Mycoplasma pneumoniae* | | | | | | | |
| **SPIROCHETES** | | | | | | | |
| *Leptospira interrogans* | | | | | | | |
| *Treponema pallidum (syphilis)* | | | | | | | |

*These are generalizations. There are major differences among countries, areas, and hospitals depending on antibiotic usage patterns. The organisms checked for each antibiotic are not all-inclusive; only the major organisms are listed.

Blank = no or insufficient activity, or unknown.

§§ Penicillin resistant; MIC ≥2.0 mcg/mL.

# ANTIBIOTIC SENSITIVITY – CARBAPENEMS/MONOBACTAMS*

| ORGANISMS | Aztreonam | Doripenem | Ertapenem | Imipenem/Cilastatin | Meropenem |
|---|---|---|---|---|---|
| **ANAEROBES** | | | | | |
| *Actinomyces* | | | | | |
| *Bacillus anthracis* | | | | ✓ | |
| *Bacteroides fragilis* | | ✓ | ✓ | ✓ | ✓ |
| *Bacteroides species* | | ✓ | ✓ | ✓ | ✓ |
| *Clostridium difficile* | | | ✓ | ✓ | ✓ |
| *Clostridium species* | | | ✓ | ✓ | ✓ |
| **GRAM-NEGATIVE AEROBES** | | | | | |
| *Acinetobacter baumannii* | | ✓ | | ✓ | ✓ |
| *Aeromonas hydrophila* | ✓ | | | ✓ | ✓ |
| *Bartonella henselae* | | | | | |
| *Bordetella species* | | | | | |
| *Burkholderia cepacia* | | | | | |
| *Campylobacter jejuni* | | | | | ✓ |
| *Citrobacter species* | ✓ | ✓ | ✓ | ✓ | ✓ |
| *Coxiella burnetti* | | | | | |
| *Enterobacter species* | ✓ | ✓ | ✓ | ✓ | ✓ |
| *Escherichia coli* | ✓ | ✓ | ✓ | ✓ | ✓ |

*These are generalizations. There are major differences among countries, areas, and hospitals depending on antibiotic usage patterns. The organisms checked for each antibiotic are not all-inclusive; only the major organisms are listed.

Blank = no or insufficient activity, or unknown.

| ORGANISMS | Aztreonam | Doripenem | Ertapenem | Imipenem/Cilastatin | Meropenem | |
|---|---|---|---|---|---|---|
| **GRAM-NEGATIVE AEROBES** *(Continued)* | | | | | | |
| *Francisella tularensis* | | | | | | |
| *Haemophilus influenzae* | ✓ | | ✓ | ✓ | ✓ | |
| *Klebsiella species* | ✓ | ✓ | ✓ | ✓ | ✓ | |
| *Legionella species* | | | | | | |
| *Moraxella catarrhalis* | | | ✓ | | ✓ | |
| *Morganella morganii* | ✓ | ✓ | ✓ | ✓ | ✓ | |
| *Neisseria gonorrhoeae* | ✓ | | | ✓ | | |
| *Neisseria meningitidis* | ✓ | | | | ✓ | |
| *Pasteurella multocida* | ✓ | | | ✓ | ✓ | |
| *Proteus mirabilis* | ✓ | ✓ | ✓ | ✓ | ✓ | |
| *Proteus vulgaris* | ✓ | | | ✓ | ✓ | |
| *Providencia stuartii* | ✓ | | ✓ | ✓ | | |
| *Pseudomonas aeruginosa* | ✓ | ✓ | | ✓ | ✓ | |
| *Rickettsia species* | | | | | | |
| *Salmonella species* | | | | | ✓ | |
| *Serratia species* | ✓ | ✓ | ✓ | ✓ | ✓ | |
| *Shigella species* | | | | | ✓ | |
| *Stenotrophomonas maltophilia* | | | | | | |

*These are generalizations. There are major differences among countries, areas, and hospitals depending on antibiotic usage patterns. The organisms checked for each antibiotic are not all-inclusive; only the major organisms are listed.

Blank = no or insufficient activity, or unknown.

**CARBAPENEMS/MONOBACTAMS (CONTINUED)**

| ORGANISMS | Aztreonam | Doripenem | Ertapenem | Imipenem/Cilastatin | Meropenem |
|---|---|---|---|---|---|
| **GRAM-NEGATIVE AEROBES** *(Continued)* | | | | | |
| *Vibrio vulnificus* | | | | | |
| *Yersinia enterocolitica* | ✓ | | | | ✓ |
| *Yersinia pestis* | | | | | |
| **GRAM-POSITIVE AEROBES** | | | | | |
| *Enterococcus faecalis* | | | | ✓ | ✓ |
| *Enterococcus faecium* | | | | | |
| *Enterococcus faecium (VRE)* | | | | | |
| *Listeria monocytogenes* | | | | ✓ | ✓ |
| *Nocardia* | | | | ✓ | |
| *Staphylococcus aureus (MSSA)* | | ✓ | ✓ | ✓ | ✓ |
| *Staphylococcus aureus (MRSA)* | | | | | |
| *Staphylococcus epidermidis* | | | ✓ | ✓ | ✓ |
| *Staphylococcus epidermidis (MRSE)* | | | | | |
| *Streptococcus pneumoniae†* | | | ✓ | ✓ | ✓ |
| *Streptococcus pneumoniae§§* | | | | | |

*These are generalizations. There are major differences among countries, areas, and hospitals depending on antibiotic usage patterns. The organisms checked for each antibiotic are not all-inclusive; only the major organisms are listed.

Blank = no or insufficient activity, or unknown.

† Penicillin sensitive; MIC ≤1.0 mcg/mL. §§ Penicillin resistant; MIC ≥2.0 mcg/mL.

| ORGANISMS | ztreonam | Doripenem | Ertapenem | Imipenem/Cilastati | eropenem | |
|---|---|---|---|---|---|---|
| **GRAM-POSITIVE AEROBES** *(Continued)* | | | | | | |
| *Streptococcus (Group A,B,C,F,G)* | | ✓ | ✓ | ✓ | ✓ | |
| *Streptococcus species* | | ✓ | ✓ | ✓ | ✓ | |
| **MISCELLANEOUS** | | | | | | |
| *Chlamydia pneumoniae* | | | | | | |
| *Chlamydia trachomatis* | | | | | | |
| *Ehrlichia/Anaplasma species* | | | | | | |
| **MYCOBACTERIA** | | | | | | |
| *Mycobacterium avium (MAI) (non-HIV)* | | | | | | |
| *Mycoplasma pneumoniae* | | | | | | |
| **SPIROCHETES** | | | | | | |
| *Leptospira interrogans* | | | | | | |
| *Treponema pallidum (syphilis)* | | | | | | |

*These are generalizations. There are major differences among countries, areas, and hospitals depending on antibiotic usage patterns. The organisms checked for each antibiotic are not all-inclusive; only the major organisms are listed.
Blank = no or insufficient activity, or unknown.

# ANTIBIOTIC SENSITIVITY – CEPHALOSPORINS*

| ORGANISMS | Cefaclor | Cefadroxil | Cefazolin | Cefdinir | Cefepime | Cefixime | Cefotaxime | Cefoxitin | Cefpodoxime Proxetil | Cefprozil | Ceftazidime | Ceftibuten | Ceftizoxime | Ceftriaxone | Cefuroxime Axetil | Cephalexin |
|---|---|---|---|---|---|---|---|---|---|---|---|---|---|---|---|---|
| **ANAEROBES** | | | | | | | | | | | | | | | | |
| *Actinomyces* | | | | | | | | | | | | | | | | |
| *Bacillus anthracis* | | | | | | | | | | | | | | | | |
| *Bacteroides fragilis* | | | | | | | | ✓ | | | | | | ✓ | | |
| *Bacteroides species* | ✓ | | | | | | ✓ | ✓ | | | | | ✓ | | | |
| *Clostridium difficile* | | | | | | | | | | ✓ | | | | | | |
| *Clostridium species* | | | | | | | ✓ | ✓ | | ✓ | ✓ | | | ✓ | | |
| **GRAM-NEGATIVE AEROBES** | | | | | | | | | | | | | | | | |
| *Acinetobacter baumannii* | | | | | ✓ | | ✓ | | | | ✓ | | | ✓ | | |
| *Aeromonas hydrophila* | | | | | | | | | | | | | ✓ | | | |
| *Bartonella henselae* | | | | | | | | | | | | | | | | |
| *Bordetella species* | | | | | | | | | | | | | | | | |
| *Burkholderia cepacia* | | | | | | | | | | | | | | | | |
| *Campylobacter jejuni* | | | | | | | | | | | | | | | | |
| *Citrobacter species* | ✓ | | | ✓ | ✓ | ✓ | ✓ | | ✓ | ✓ | ✓ | | ✓ | ✓ | ✓ | |
| *Coxiella burnetti* | | | | | | | | | | | | | | | | |
| *Enterobacter species* | | | | | ✓ | | ✓ | | | | ✓ | | ✓ | ✓ | | |
| *Escherichia coli* | ✓ | ✓ | ✓ | ✓ | ✓ | ✓ | ✓ | ✓ | ✓ | ✓ | ✓ | | ✓ | ✓ | ✓ | ✓ |

*These are generalizations. There are major differences among countries, areas, and hospitals depending on antibiotic usage patterns. **The organisms checked for each antibiotic are not all-inclusive; only the major organisms are listed.**

Blank = no or insufficient activity, or unknown.

| ORGANISMS | Cefaclor | Cefadroxil | Cefazolin | Cefdinir | Cefepime | Cefixime | Cefotaxime | Cefoxitin | Cefpod Proxeti | Cefprozil | Ceftazidime | Ceftibuten | Ceftizoxime | Ceftriaxone | Cefu Axeti | Cephalexin |
|---|---|---|---|---|---|---|---|---|---|---|---|---|---|---|---|---|
| **GRAM-NEGATIVE AEROBES** *(Continued)* | | | | | | | | | | | | | | | | |
| *Francisella tularensis* | | | | | | | | | | | | | | | | |
| *Haemophilus influenzae* | ✓ | | | ✓ | ✓ | ✓ | ✓ | ✓ | ✓ | ✓ | ✓ | ✓ | ✓ | ✓ | ✓ | ✓ |
| *Klebsiella species* | ✓ | ✓ | | ✓ | ✓ | ✓ | ✓ | ✓ | ✓ | ✓ | ✓ | | ✓ | ✓ | ✓ | ✓ |
| *Legionella species* | | | | | | | | | | | | | | | | |
| *Moraxella catarrhalis* | ✓ | ✓ | | ✓ | ✓ | ✓ | | | ✓ | ✓ | | ✓ | ✓ | ✓ | ✓ | ✓ |
| *Morganella morganii* | | | | | ✓ | | ✓ | ✓ | | | ✓ | | ✓ | ✓ | ✓ | |
| *Neisseria gonorrhoeae* | ✓ | | | | | ✓ | ✓ | ✓ | ✓ | ✓ | ✓ | | ✓ | ✓ | ✓ | |
| *Neisseria meningitidis* | | | | | | | ✓ | | | | ✓ | | ✓ | ✓ | | |
| *Pasteurella multocida* | | | | | | ✓ | | | | | ✓ | | | | | |
| *Proteus mirabilis* | ✓ | ✓ | ✓ | ✓ | ✓ | ✓ | ✓ | ✓ | ✓ | ✓ | ✓ | | ✓ | ✓ | ✓ | ✓ |
| *Proteus vulgaris* | | | | | ✓ | ✓ | ✓ | ✓ | ✓ | | ✓ | | ✓ | ✓ | | |
| *Providencia stuartii* | | | | | ✓ | ✓ | ✓ | ✓ | ✓ | | ✓ | | ✓ | ✓ | | |
| *Pseudomonas aeruginosa* | | | | | ✓ | | ✓ | | | | ✓ | | ✓ | | | |
| *Rickettsia species* | | | | | | | | | | | | | | | | |
| *Salmonella species* | | | | | | ✓ | ✓ | | | ✓ | ✓ | | | ✓ | | |
| *Serratia species* | | | | | ✓ | ✓ | ✓ | | | | ✓ | | ✓ | ✓ | | |

*These are generalizations. There are major differences among countries, areas, and hospitals depending on antibiotic usage patterns. The organisms checked for each antibiotic are not all-inclusive; only the major organisms are listed.

Blank = no or insufficient activity, or unknown.

**CEPHALOSPORINS (CONTINUED)**

| ORGANISMS | Cefaclor | Cefadroxil | Cefazolin | Cefdinir | Cefepime | Cefixime | Cefotaxime | Cefoxitin | Cefpodoxime Proxetil | Cefprozil | Ceftazidime | Ceftibuten | Ceftizoxime | Ceftriaxone | Cefuroxime Axetil | Cephalexin |
|---|---|---|---|---|---|---|---|---|---|---|---|---|---|---|---|---|
| **GRAM-NEGATIVE AEROBES** *(Continued)* | | | | | | | | | | | | | | | | |
| *Shigella species* | | | | | | ✓ | ✓ | | | ✓ | ✓ | | | ✓ | | |
| *Stenotrophomonas maltophilia* | | | | | | | | | | | | | | | | |
| *Vibrio vulnificus* | | | | | | | | | | ✓ | | | | | | |
| *Yersinia enterocolitica* | | | | | | | | | | | ✓ | | | | | |
| *Yersinia pestis* | | | | | | | | | | | | | | | | |
| **GRAM-POSITIVE AEROBES** | | | | | | | | | | | | | | | | |
| *Enterococcus faecalis* | | | | | | | ✓ | | | ✓ | | | | | | |
| *Enterococcus faecium* | | | | | | | ✓ | | | | | | | | | |
| *Enterococcus faecium (VRE)* | | | | | | | ✓ | | | | | | | | | |
| *Listeria monocytogenes* | | | | | | | | | | ✓ | | | | | | |
| *Nocardia* | | | | | | | | | | | | | | | | |
| *Staphylococcus aureus (MSSA)* | ✓ | ✓ | ✓ | ✓ | ✓ | | ✓ | ✓ | ✓ | ✓ | ✓ | | ✓ | ✓ | ✓ | ✓ |
| *Staphylococcus aureus (MRSA)* | | | | | | | | | | | | | | | | |

*These are generalizations. There are major differences among countries, areas, and hospitals depending on antibiotic usage patterns. The organisms checked for each antibiotic are not all-inclusive; only the major organisms are listed.

Blank = no or insufficient activity, or unknown.

| ORGANISMS | Cefaclor | Cefadroxil | Cefazolin | Cefdinir | Cefepime | Cefixime | Cefotaxime | Cefoxitin | Cefpodoxime Proxetil | Cefprozil | Ceftazidime | Ceftibuten | Ceftizoxime | Ceftriaxone | Cefuroxime Axetil | Cephalexin |
|---|---|---|---|---|---|---|---|---|---|---|---|---|---|---|---|---|
| **GRAM-POSITIVE AEROBES** *(Continued)* | | | | | | | | | | | | | | | | |
| *Staphylococcus epidermidis* | | ✓ | ✓ | ✓ | ✓ | | ✓ | ✓ | | ✓ | | | ✓ | ✓ | ✓ | ✓ |
| *Staphylococcus epidermidis (MRSE)* | | | | | | | | | | | | | | | | |
| *Streptococcus pneumoniae†* | ✓ | ✓ | ✓ | ✓ | ✓ | ✓ | ✓ | ✓ | ✓ | ✓ | ✓ | ✓ | ✓ | ✓ | ✓ | ✓ |
| *Streptococcus pneumoniae§§* | | | | | ✓ | | ✓ | | ✓ | | | | ✓ | ✓ | | |
| *Streptococcus (Group A,B,C,F,G)* | ✓ | ✓ | ✓ | ✓ | ✓ | ✓ | ✓ | ✓ | ✓ | ✓ | ✓ | ✓ | ✓ | ✓ | ✓ | ✓ |
| *Streptococcus species* | ✓ | ✓ | ✓ | ✓ | ✓ | | ✓ | ✓ | ✓ | ✓ | ✓ | ✓ | ✓ | ✓ | ✓ | ✓ |
| **MISCELLANEOUS** | | | | | | | | | | | | | | | | |
| *Chlamydia pneumoniae* | | | | | | | | | | | | | | | | |
| *Chlamydia trachomatis* | | | | | | | | | | | | | | | | |
| *Ehrlichia/Anaplasma species* | | | | | | | | | | | | | | | | |
| **MYCOBACTERIA** | | | | | | | | | | | | | | | | |
| *Mycobacterium avium (MAI) (non-HIV)* | | | | | | | | | | | | | | | | |

*These are generalizations. There are major differences among countries, areas, and hospitals depending on antibiotic usage patterns. The organisms checked for each antibiotic are not all-inclusive; only the major organisms are listed.

Blank = no or insufficient activity, or unknown.

† Penicillin sensitive; MIC ≤1.0 mcg/mL. §§ Penicillin resistant; MIC ≥2.0 mcg/mL.

**CEPHALOSPORINS (CONTINUED)**

| ORGANISMS | Cefaclor | Cefadroxil | Cefazolin | Cefdinir | Cefepime | Cefixime | Cefotaxime | Cefoxitin | Cefpodoxime Proxetil | Cefprozil | Ceftazidime | Ceftibuten | Ceftizoxime | Ceftriaxone | Cefuroxime axetil | Cephalexin |
|---|---|---|---|---|---|---|---|---|---|---|---|---|---|---|---|---|
| **MYCOBACTERIA** *(Continued)* | | | | | | | | | | | | | | | | |
| *Mycoplasma pneumoniae* | | | | | | | | | | | | | | | | |
| **SPIROCHETES** | | | | | | | | | | | | | | | | |
| *Leptospira interrogans* | | | | | | | | | | | | | | | | |
| *Treponema pallidum (syphilis)* | | | | | | | | | | | | | | | | |

*These are generalizations. There are major differences among countries, areas, and hospitals depending on antibiotic usage patterns. The organisms checked for each antibiotic are not all-inclusive; only the major organisms are listed.

Blank = no or insufficient activity, or unknown.

# Antibiotic Sensitivity – Fluoroquinolones*

| ORGANISMS | Ciprofloxacin | Gemifloxacin | Levofloxacin | Moxifloxacin | Norfloxacin | Ofloxacin |
|---|---|---|---|---|---|---|
| **ANAEROBES** | | | | | | |
| *Actinomyces* | | | | | | |
| *Bacillus anthracis* | ✓ | | | | | |
| *Bacteroides fragilis* | | | | ✓ | | |
| *Clostridium difficile* | | | | | | |
| *Clostridium species* | | | ✓ | ✓ | | |
| **GRAM-NEGATIVE AEROBES** | | | | | | |
| *Acinetobacter baumannii* | | | ✓ | | ✓ | |
| *Aeromonas hydrophila* | ✓ | | | | | |
| *Bartonella henselae* | | | | | | |
| *Bordetella species* | | | ✓ | | | |
| *Burkholderia cepacia* | | | | | | |
| *Campylobacter jejuni* | ✓ | | | | | |
| *Citrobacter species* | ✓ | | ✓ | ✓ | ✓ | ✓ |
| *Coxiella burnetti* | | | | | | |
| *Enterobacter species* | ✓ | | ✓ | ✓ | ✓ | ✓ |
| *Escherichia coli* | ✓ | | ✓ | ✓ | ✓ | ✓ |

*These are generalizations. There are major differences among countries, areas, and hospitals depending on antibiotic usage patterns. The organisms checked for each antibiotic are not all-inclusive; only the major organisms are listed.

Blank = no or insufficient activity, or unknown.

**FLUOROQUINOLONES (CONTINUED)**

| ORGANISMS | Ciprofloxacin | Gemifloxacin | Levofloxacin | Moxifloxacin | Norfloxacin | Ofloxacin |
|---|---|---|---|---|---|---|
| **GRAM-NEGATIVE AEROBES** *(Continued)* | | | | | | |
| *Francisella tularensis* | | | | | | |
| *Haemophilus influenzae* | | ✓ | ✓ | ✓ | | ✓ |
| *Klebsiella species* | ✓ | ✓ | ✓ | ✓ | ✓ | ✓ |
| *Legionella species* | ✓ | ✓ | ✓ | ✓ | | |
| *Moraxella catarrhalis* | ✓ | ✓ | ✓ | ✓ | | ✓ |
| *Morganella morganii* | ✓ | | ✓ | | ✓ | ✓ |
| *Neisseria gonorrhoeae* | ✓ | | | | ✓ | ✓ |
| *Neisseria meningitidis* | | | | | | |
| *Pasteurella multocida* | | | | | | |
| *Proteus mirabilis* | ✓ | | ✓ | ✓ | ✓ | ✓ |
| *Proteus vulgaris* | ✓ | ✓ | ✓ | | ✓ | |
| *Providencia stuartii* | ✓ | | ✓ | | ✓ | |
| *Pseudomonas aeruginosa* | ✓ | | ✓ | | ✓ | ✓ |
| *Rickettsia species* | | | | | | |
| *Salmonella species* | ✓ | | | | | |
| *Serratia species* | ✓ | | ✓ | | ✓ | ✓ |
| *Shigella species* | ✓ | | | | | ✓ |
| *Stenotrophomonas maltophilia* | | | | | | |

*These are generalizations. There are major differences among countries, areas, and hospitals depending on antibiotic usage patterns. The organisms checked for each antibiotic are not all-inclusive; only the major organisms are listed.

Blank = no or insufficient activity, or unknown.

| ORGANISMS | Ciprofloxa | Gemifloxacin | Levofloxacin | Moxifloxacin | Norfloxaci | Ofloxacin | |
|---|---|---|---|---|---|---|---|
| **GRAM-NEGATIVE AEROBES** *(Continued)* | | | | | | | |
| *Vibrio vulnificus* | ✓ | | | | | | |
| *Yersinia enterocolitica* | ✓ | | | | | | |
| *Yersinia pestis* | | | | | | | |
| **GRAM-POSITIVE AEROBES** | | | | | | | |
| *Enterococcus faecalis* | ✓ | | ✓ | ✓ | ✓ | ✓ | |
| *Enterococcus faecium* | | | | | | | |
| *Enterococcus faecium (VRE)* | | | | | | | |
| *Listeria monocytogenes* | | | | | | ✓ | |
| *Nocardia* | | | | | | | |
| *Staphylococcus aureus (MSSA)* | ✓ | ✓ | ✓ | ✓ | ✓ | ✓ | |
| *Staphylococcus aureus (MRSA)* | | | | | | | |
| *Staphylococcus epidermidis* | ✓ | | ✓ | ✓ | ✓ | ✓ | |
| *Staphylococcus epidermidis (MRSE)* | | | | | | | |
| *Streptococcus pneumoniae†* | ✓ | ✓ | ✓ | ✓ | | ✓ | |
| *Streptococcus pneumoniae§§* | ✓ | ✓ | ✓ | ✓ | | ✓ | |

*These are generalizations. There are major differences among countries, areas, and hospitals depending on antibiotic usage patterns. The organisms checked for each antibiotic are not all-inclusive; only the major organisms are listed.

Blank = no or insufficient activity, or unknown.

† Penicillin sensitive; MIC ≤1.0 mcg/mL. §§ Penicillin resistant; MIC ≥2.0 mcg/mL.

**FLUOROQUINOLONES (CONTINUED)**

| ORGANISMS | Ciprofloxac | Gemifloxacin | Levofloxacin | Moxifloxacin | Norfloxacin | Ofloxacin | |
|---|---|---|---|---|---|---|---|
| **GRAM-POSITIVE AEROBES** *(Continued)* | | | | | | | |
| *Streptococcus (Group A,B,C,F,G)* | ✓ | ✓ | ✓ | ✓ | | ✓ | |
| *Streptococcus species* | ✓ | ✓ | ✓ | ✓ | ✓ | ✓ | |
| **MISCELLANEOUS** | | | | | | | |
| *Chlamydia pneumoniae* | | ✓ | ✓ | ✓ | | | |
| *Chlamydia trachomatis* | | | | | | ✓ | |
| *Ehrlichia/Anaplasma species* | | | | | | | |
| **MYCOBACTERIA** | | | | | | | |
| *Mycobacterium avium (MAI) (non-HIV)* | | | | | | | |
| *Mycoplasma pneumoniae* | | ✓ | ✓ | ✓ | | | |
| **SPIROCHETES** | | | | | | | |
| *Leptospira interrogans* | | | | | | | |
| *Treponema pallidum (syphilis)* | | | | | | | |

*These are generalizations. There are major differences among countries, areas, and hospitals depending on antibiotic usage patterns. The organisms checked for each antibiotic are not all-inclusive; only the major organisms are listed. Blank = no or insufficient activity, or unknown.

# ANTIBIOTIC SENSITIVITY – MACROLIDES & CLINDAMYCIN*

| ORGANISMS | Azit | Clarithromycin | Clindamycin | Erythromycin | elithromycin | |
|---|---|---|---|---|---|---|
| **ANAEROBES** | | | | | | |
| *Actinomyces* | | | | | | |
| *Bacillus anthracis* | | | | | | |
| *Bacteroides fragilis* | | | | | | |
| *Clostridium difficile* | | | | | | |
| *Clostridium species* | | ✓ | ✓ | | | |
| **GRAM-NEGATIVE AEROBES** | | | | | | |
| *Acinetobacter baumannii* | | | | | | |
| *Aeromonas hydrophila* | | | | | | |
| *Bartonella henselae* | | | | | | |
| *Bordetella species* | ✓ | ✓ | | ✓ | | |
| *Burkholderia cepacia* | | | | | | |
| *Campylobacter jejuni* | | | | | | |
| *Citrobacter species* | | | | | | |
| *Coxiella burnetti* | | | | | | |
| *Enterobacter species* | | | | | | |
| *Escherichia coli* | | | | | | |

*These are generalizations. There are major differences among countries, areas, and hospitals depending on antibiotic usage patterns. The organisms checked for each antibiotic are not all-inclusive; only the major organisms are listed.
Blank = no or insufficient activity, or unknown.

**MACROLIDES & CLINDAMYCIN (CONTINUED)**

| ORGANISMS | Azithromyc | Clarithromyc | Clindamycin | Erythromycin | Telithromyc |
|---|---|---|---|---|---|
| **GRAM-NEGATIVE AEROBES** *(Continued)* | | | | | |
| *Francisella tularensis* | | | | | |
| *Haemophilus influenzae* | ✓ | ✓ | | | ✓ |
| *Klebsiella species* | | | | | |
| *Legionella species* | ✓ | ✓ | | ✓ | ✓ |
| *Moraxella catarrhalis* | ✓ | ✓ | | ✓ | ✓ |
| *Morganella morganii* | | | | | |
| *Neisseria gonorrhoeae* | ✓ | | | ✓ | |
| *Neisseria meningitidis* | | | | | |
| *Pasteurella multocida* | | ✓ | | | |
| *Proteus mirabilis* | | | | | |
| *Proteus vulgaris* | | | | | |
| *Providencia stuartii* | | | | | |
| *Pseudomonas aeruginosa* | | | | | |
| *Rickettsia species* | | | | | |
| *Salmonella species* | | | | | |
| *Serratia species* | | | | | |
| *Shigella species* | | | | | |
| *Stenotrophomonas maltophilia* | | | | | |

*These are generalizations. There are major differences among countries, areas, and hospitals depending on antibiotic usage patterns. The organisms checked for each antibiotic are not all-inclusive; only the major organisms are listed.

Blank = no or insufficient activity, or unknown.

| ORGANISMS | Azithromycin | Clarithromycin | Clindamycin | Erythromycin | Telithromycin | |
|---|---|---|---|---|---|---|
| **GRAM-NEGATIVE AEROBES** *(Continued)* | | | | | | |
| *Vibrio vulnificus* | | | | | | |
| *Yersinia enterocolitica* | | | | | | |
| *Yersinia pestis* | | | | | | |
| **GRAM-POSITIVE AEROBES** | | | | | | |
| *Enterococcus faecalis* | | | | | | |
| *Enterococcus faecium* | | | | | | |
| *Enterococcus faecium (VRE)* | | | | | | |
| *Listeria monocytogenes* | | | | ✓ | | |
| *Nocardia* | | | | | | |
| *Staphylococcus aureus (MSSA)* | ✓ | ✓ | ✓ | ✓ | ✓ | |
| *Staphylococcus aureus (MRSA)* | | | | | | |
| *Staphylococcus epidermidis* | | | ✓ | | | |
| *Staphylococcus epidermidis (MRSE)* | | | | | | |
| *Streptococcus pneumoniae†* | | ✓ | ✓ | ✓ | ✓ | |
| *Streptococcus pneumoniae§§* | ✓ | | | | ✓ | |

*These are generalizations. There are major differences among countries, areas, and hospitals depending on antibiotic usage patterns. The organisms checked for each antibiotic are not all-inclusive; only the major organisms are listed.

Blank = no or insufficient activity, or unknown.

† Penicillin sensitive; MIC ≤1.0 mcg/mL. §§ Penicillin resistant; MIC ≥2.0 mcg/mL.

## MACROLIDES & CLINDAMYCIN (CONTINUED)

| ORGANISMS | Azithromyc | Clarithromycin | Clindamycin | Erythromycin | Telithromyc | |
|---|---|---|---|---|---|---|
| **GRAM-POSITIVE AEROBES** *(Continued)* | | | | | | |
| *Streptococcus (Group A,B,C,F,G)* | ✓ | ✓ | ✓ | ✓ | ✓ | |
| *Streptococcus species* | ✓ | ✓ | ✓ | ✓ | ✓ | |
| **MISCELLANEOUS** | | | | | | |
| *Chlamydia pneumoniae* | ✓ | ✓ | | | ✓ | |
| *Chlamydia trachomatis* | ✓ | | | ✓ | | |
| *Ehrlichia/Anaplasma species* | | | | | | |
| **MYCOBACTERIA** | | | | | | |
| *Mycobacterium avium (MAI) (non-HIV)* | | ✓ | | | ✓ | |
| *Mycobacterium avium complex (MAC)* | | ✓ | | | | |
| *Mycoplasma pneumoniae* | ✓ | ✓ | | ✓ | ✓ | |
| **SPIROCHETES** | | | | | | |
| *Leptospira interrogans* | | | | | | |
| *Treponema pallidum (syphilis)* | | | | ✓ | | |

*These are generalizations. There are major differences among countries, areas, and hospitals depending on antibiotic usage patterns. The organisms checked for each antibiotic are not all-inclusive; only the major organisms are listed.

Blank = no or insufficient activity, or unknown.

# ANTIBIOTIC SENSITIVITY – PENICILLINS*

| ORGANISMS | Amoxicillin | Amoxicillin + Clavulanate | Ampicillin | Ampicillin + Sulbactam | Dicloxacillin | Nafcillin/ Oxacillin | Penicillin | Piperacillin | Piperacillin + Tazobactam | Ticarcillin + Clavulanic Acid |
|---|---|---|---|---|---|---|---|---|---|---|
| **ANAEROBES** | | | | | | | | | | |
| *Actinomyces* | | | | | | | ✓ | ✓ | | |
| *Bacillus anthracis* | | | ✓ | | | | ✓ | | | |
| *Bacteroides fragilis* | | ✓ | | ✓ | | | | ✓ | ✓ | ✓ |
| *Clostridium difficile* | | | | | | | | | | ✓ |
| *Clostridium species* | | | ✓ | ✓ | | | ✓ | ✓ | ✓ | ✓ |
| **GRAM-NEGATIVE AEROBES** | | | | | | | | | | |
| *Acinetobacter baumannii* | | | | | | | | ✓ | ✓ | ✓ |
| *Aeromonas hydrophila* | | | | | | | | | | |
| *Bartonella henselae* | | | | | | | | | | |
| *Bordetella species* | | | | | | | | | | |
| *Burkholderia cepacia* | | | | | | | | | | |
| *Campylobacter jejuni* | | | | | | | | | | |
| *Citrobacter species* | | | | | | | | ✓ | ✓ | ✓ |
| *Coxiella burnetti* | | | | | | | | | | |
| *Enterobacter species* | | ✓ | | ✓ | | | | ✓ | ✓ | ✓ |
| *Escherichia coli* | ✓ | ✓ | ✓ | ✓ | | | | ✓ | ✓ | ✓ |

*These are generalizations. There are major differences among countries, areas, and hospitals depending on antibiotic usage patterns. The organisms checked for each antibiotic are not all-inclusive; only the major organisms are listed.
Blank = no or insufficient activity, or unknown.

**PENICILLINS (CONTINUED)**

| ORGANISMS | Amoxicillin | Amoxicillin + Clavulanate | Ampicillin | Ampicillin + Sulbactam | Dicloxacillin | Nafcillin/ Oxacillin | Penicillin | Piperacillin | Piperacillin + Tazobactam | Ticarcillin + Clavulanic Acid |
|---|---|---|---|---|---|---|---|---|---|---|
| **GRAM-NEGATIVE AEROBES** *(Continued)* | | | | | | | | | | |
| *Francisella tularensis* | | | | | | | | | | |
| *Haemophilus influenzae* | ✓ | ✓ | ✓ | ✓ | | | | ✓ | ✓ | ✓ |
| *Helicobacter pylori* | ✓ | | | | | | | | | |
| *Klebsiella species* | | ✓ | | ✓ | | | | ✓ | ✓ | |
| *Legionella species* | | | | | | | | | | |
| *Moraxella catarrhalis* | | ✓ | | ✓ | | | | | ✓ | ✓ |
| *Morganella morganii* | | | | ✓ | | | | ✓ | ✓ | ✓ |
| *Neisseria gonorrhoeae* | ✓ | ✓ | ✓ | ✓ | | | ✓ | ✓ | ✓ | ✓ |
| *Neisseria meningitidis* | | | ✓ | | | | ✓ | | | |
| *Pasteurella multocida* | | | | | | | ✓ | | | ✓ |
| *Proteus mirabilis* | ✓ | ✓ | ✓ | ✓ | | | | ✓ | ✓ | ✓ |
| *Proteus vulgaris* | | | | ✓ | | | | ✓ | ✓ | ✓ |
| *Providencia stuartii* | | | | ✓ | | | | | | ✓ |
| *Pseudomonas aeruginosa* | | | | | | | | ✓ | ✓ | ✓ |
| *Rickettsia species* | | | | | | | | | | |
| *Salmonella species* | | | ✓ | | | | | | ✓ | |
| *Serratia species* | | | | | | | | ✓ | ✓ | ✓ |
| *Shigella species* | | | ✓ | | | | | | | |

*These are generalizations. There are major differences among countries, areas, and hospitals depending on antibiotic usage patterns. The organisms checked for each antibiotic are not all-inclusive; only the major organisms are listed.
Blank = no or insufficient activity, or unknown.

| ORGANISMS | Amoxicillin | Amoxicillin + Clavulanate | Ampicillin | Ampicillin + Sulbactam | Dicloxacillin | Nafcillin/ Oxacillin | Penicillin | Piperacillin | Piperacillin + Tazobactam | Ticarcillin + Clavulanic Acid |
|---|---|---|---|---|---|---|---|---|---|---|
| **GRAM-NEGATIVE AEROBES** *(Continued)* | | | | | | | | | | |
| *Stenotrophomonas maltophilia* | | | | | | | | ✓ | | ✓ |
| *Vibrio vulnificus* | | | | | | | | | | |
| *Yersinia enterocolitica* | | | | | | | | ✓ | | |
| *Yersinia pestis* | | | | | | | | | | |
| **GRAM-POSITIVE AEROBES** | | | | | | | | | | |
| *Corynebacterium diphtheriae* | | | | | | | ✓ | | | |
| *Enterococcus faecalis* | ✓ | ✓ | ✓ | ✓ | | | | ✓ | ✓ | |
| *Enterococcus faecium* | | | | | | | | ✓ | | |
| *Enterococcus faecium (VRE)* | | | | | | | | | | |
| *Listeria monocytogenes* | | | ✓ | | | | ✓ | | | |
| *Nocardia* | | | | | | | | | | |
| *Staphylococcus aureus (MSSA)* | ✓ | ✓ | ✓ | ✓ | ✓ | ✓ | ✓ | | ✓ | ✓ |
| *Staphylococcus aureus (MRSA)* | | | | | | | | | | |
| *Staphylococcus epidermidis* | ✓ | ✓ | ✓ | ✓ | ✓ | | | | ✓ | ✓ |
| *Staphylococcus epidermidis (MRSE)* | | | | | | | | | | |
| *Streptococcus pneumoniae†* | ✓ | ✓ | ✓ | ✓ | | | ✓ | ✓ | ✓ | ✓ |
| *Streptococcus pneumoniae§§* | ✓ | ✓ | ✓ | ✓ | | | | | | ✓ |

*These are generalizations. There are major differences among countries, areas, and hospitals depending on antibiotic usage patterns. The organisms checked for each antibiotic are not all-inclusive; only the major organisms are listed.

Blank = no or insufficient activity, or unknown.

† Penicillin sensitive; MIC ≤1.0 mcg/mL. §§ Penicillin resistant; MIC ≥2.0 mcg/mL.

**PENICILLINS (CONTINUED)**

| ORGANISMS | Amoxicillin | Amoxicillin + Clavulanate | Ampicillin | Am Sul | Dicloxacillin | Nafcillin/ Oxacillin | Penicillin | Piperacillin | peracillin + zobactam | Ticarcillin + C anic Acid |
|---|---|---|---|---|---|---|---|---|---|---|
| **GRAM-POSITIVE AEROBES** *(Continued)* | | | | | | | | | | |
| *Streptococcus (Group A,B,C,F,G)* | ✓ | ✓ | ✓ | ✓ | | | ✓ | ✓ | ✓ | ✓ |
| *Streptococcus species* | ✓ | ✓ | ✓ | ✓ | | | ✓ | ✓ | ✓ | ✓ |
| **MISCELLANEOUS** | | | | | | | | | | |
| *Chlamydia pneumoniae* | | | | | | | | | | |
| *Chlamydia trachomatis* | | | | | | | | | | |
| *Ehrlichia/Anaplasma species* | | | | | | | | | | |
| **MYCOBACTERIA** | | | | | | | | | | |
| *Mycobacterium avium (MAI) (non-HIV)* | | | | | | | | | | |
| *Mycoplasma pneumoniae* | | | | | | | | | | |
| **SPIROCHETES** | | | | | | | | | | |
| *Leptospira interrogans* | | | | | | | | | | |
| *Treponema pallidum (syphilis)* | | | | | | | ✓ | | | |

*These are generalizations. There are major differences among countries, areas, and hospitals depending on antibiotic usage patterns. The organisms checked for each antibiotic are not all-inclusive; only the major organisms are listed.

Blank = no or insufficient activity, or unknown.

## ANTIBIOTIC SENSITIVITY – SULFONAMIDES*

| ORGANISMS | Trimethoprim + Sulfamethoxazole |
|---|---|
| **ANAEROBES** | |
| *Actinomyces* | |
| *Bacillus anthracis* | |
| *Bacteroides fragilis* | |
| *Clostridium difficile* | |
| *Clostridium species* | |
| **GRAM-NEGATIVE AEROBES** | |
| *Acinetobacter baumannii* | |
| *Aeromonas hydrophila* | |
| *Bartonella henselae* | |
| *Bordetella species* | |
| *Burkholderia cepacia* | |
| *Campylobacter jejuni* | |
| *Citrobacter species* | |
| *Coxiella burnetti* | |
| *Enterobacter species* | ✓ |

## ANTIBIOTIC SENSITIVITY – TETRACYCLINES*

| ORGANISMS | Doxycycline | Minocycline | Tetracycline | |
|---|---|---|---|---|
| **ANAEROBES** | | | | |
| *Actinomyces* | ✓ | ✓ | ✓ | |
| *Bacillus anthracis* | ✓ | ✓ | ✓ | |
| *Bacteroides fragilis* | ✓ | | ✓ | |
| *Clostridium difficile* | | | | |
| *Clostridium species* | ✓ | ✓ | ✓ | |
| **GRAM-NEGATIVE AEROBES** | | | | |
| *Acinetobacter baumannii* | ✓ | ✓ | ✓ | |
| *Aeromonas hydrophila* | | | | |
| *Bartonella henselae* | | | | |
| *Bordetella species* | | | | |
| *Burkholderia cepacia* | | | | |
| *Campylobacter jejuni* | | | | |
| *Citrobacter species* | | | | |
| *Coxiella burnetti* | | | | |
| *Enterobacter species* | ✓ | | | |

*These are generalizations. There are major differences among countries, areas, and hospitals depending on antibiotic usage patterns. The organisms checked for each antibiotic are not all-inclusive; only the major organisms are listed.

Blank = no or insufficient activity, or unknown.

**SULFONAMIDES (CONTINUED)**

| ORGANISMS | Trimethopr Sulfamethoxazo |
|---|---|
| **GRAM-NEGATIVE AEROBES** *(Continued)* | |
| *Escherichia coli* | ✓ |
| *Francisella tularensis* | |
| *Haemophilus influenzae* | ✓ |
| *Klebsiella species* | ✓ |
| *Legionella species* | |
| *Moraxella catarrhalis* | ✓ |
| *Morganella morganii* | ✓ |
| *Neisseria gonorrhoeae* | |
| *Neisseria meningitidis* | |
| *Pasteurella multocida* | |
| *Proteus mirabilis* | ✓ |
| *Proteus vulgaris* | ✓ |
| *Providencia stuartii* | |
| *Pseudomonas aeruginosa* | |
| *Rickettsia species* | |
| *Salmonella species* | |
| *Serratia species* | |

**TETRACYCLINES (CONTINUED)**

| ORGANISMS | Doxycyc | Minocycl | Tetracycline | |
|---|---|---|---|---|
| **GRAM-NEGATIVE AEROBES** *(Continued)* | | | | |
| *Escherichia coli* | ✓ | ✓ | ✓ | |
| *Francisella tularensis* | ✓ | ✓ | ✓ | |
| *Haemophilus influenzae* | ✓ | ✓ | ✓ | |
| *Klebsiella species* | ✓ | ✓ | ✓ | |
| *Legionella species* | | | | |
| *Moraxella catarrhalis* | | | | |
| *Morganella morganii* | | | | |
| *Neisseria gonorrhoeae* | ✓ | ✓ | ✓ | |
| *Neisseria meningitidis* | | ✓ | | |
| *Pasteurella multocida* | | | | |
| *Proteus mirabilis* | | | | |
| *Proteus vulgaris* | | | | |
| *Providencia stuartii* | | | | |
| *Pseudomonas aeruginosa* | | | | |
| *Rickettsia species* | ✓ | ✓ | ✓ | |
| *Salmonella species* | | | | |
| *Serratia species* | | | | |

*These are generalizations. There are major differences among countries, areas, and hospitals depending on antibiotic usage patterns. The organisms checked for each antibiotic are not all-inclusive; only the major organisms are listed.
Blank = no or insufficient activity, or unknown.

| ORGANISMS | Trimethoprim + Sulfamethoxazole |
|---|---|
| **GRAM-NEGATIVE AEROBES** *(Continued)* | |
| *Shigella species* | ✓ |
| *Stenotrophomonas maltophilia* | |
| *Vibrio vulnificus* | |
| *Yersinia enterocolitica* | |
| *Yersinia pestis* | |
| **GRAM-POSITIVE AEROBES** | |
| *Enterococcus faecalis* | |
| *Enterococcus faecium* | |
| *Enterococcus faecium (VRE)* | |
| *Listeria monocytogenes* | |
| *Nocardia* | |
| *Staphylococcus aureus (MSSA)* | |
| *Staphylococcus aureus (MRSA)* | |
| *Staphylococcus epidermidis* | |
| *Staphylococcus epidermidis (MRSE)* | |
| *Streptococcus pneumoniae†* | ✓ |

| ORGANISMS | Doxycycline | Minocycline | Tetracycline | |
|---|---|---|---|---|
| **GRAM-NEGATIVE AEROBES** *(Continued)* | | | | |
| *Shigella species* | ✓ | ✓ | ✓ | |
| *Stenotrophomonas maltophilia* | | | | |
| *Vibrio vulnificus* | | | | |
| *Yersinia enterocolitica* | | | | |
| *Yersinia pestis* | ✓ | ✓ | ✓ | |
| **GRAM-POSITIVE AEROBES** | | | | |
| *Enterococcus faecalis* | ✓ | | ✓ | |
| *Enterococcus faecium* | ✓ | | ✓ | |
| *Enterococcus faecium (VRE)* | | | | |
| *Listeria monocytogenes* | ✓ | ✓ | ✓ | |
| *Nocardia* | | | | |
| *Staphylococcus aureus (MSSA)* | | ✓ | | |
| *Staphylococcus aureus (MRSA)* | | | | |
| *Staphylococcus epidermidis* | | | | |
| *Staphylococcus epidermidis (MRSE)* | | | | |
| *Streptococcus pneumoniae†* | ✓ | ✓ | ✓ | |

*These are generalizations. There are major differences among countries, areas, and hospitals depending on antibiotic usage patterns. The organisms checked for each antibiotic are not all-inclusive; only the major organisms are listed.

Blank = no or insufficient activity, or unknown.

† Penicillin sensitive; MIC ≤1.0 mcg/mL.

## SULFONAMIDES (CONTINUED)

| ORGANISMS | Trimethoprim + Sulfamethoxazole |
|---|---|
| **GRAM-POSITIVE AEROBES** *(Continued)* | |
| *Streptococcus pneumoniae§§* | |
| *Streptococcus (Group A,B,C,F,G)* | |
| *Streptococcus species* | |
| **MISCELLANEOUS** | |
| *Chlamydia pneumoniae* | |
| *Chlamydia trachomatis* | |
| *Ehrlichia/Anaplasma species* | |
| **MYCOBACTERIA** | |
| *Mycobacterium avium (MAI) (non-HIV)* | |
| *Mycoplasma pneumoniae* | |
| **SPIROCHETES** | |
| *Leptospira interrogans* | |
| *Treponema pallidum (syphilis)* | |

## TETRACYCLINES (CONTINUED)

| ORGANISMS | Doxycycline | Minocycline | Tetracycline | |
|---|---|---|---|---|
| **GRAM-POSITIVE AEROBES** *(Continued)* | | | | |
| *Streptococcus pneumoniae§§* | | | | |
| *Streptococcus (Group A,B,C,F,G)* | | | | |
| *Streptococcus species* | ✓ | ✓ | ✓ | |
| **MISCELLANEOUS** | | | | |
| *Chlamydia pneumoniae* | | | | |
| *Chlamydia trachomatis* | ✓ | ✓ | ✓ | |
| *Ehrlichia/Anaplasma species* | | | | |
| **MYCOBACTERIA** | | | | |
| *Mycobacterium avium (MAI) (non-HIV)* | | | | |
| Mycoplasma pneumoniae | ✓ | ✓ | ✓ | |
| **SPIROCHETES** | | | | |
| *Leptospira interrogans* | | | | |
| *Treponema pallidum (syphilis)* | ✓ | ✓ | ✓ | |

*These are generalizations. There are major differences among countries, areas, and hospitals depending on antibiotic usage patterns. The organisms checked for each antibiotic are not all-inclusive; only the major organisms are listed.

Blank = no or insufficient activity, or unknown.

§§ Penicillin resistant; MIC ≥2.0 mcg/mL.

# ANTIBIOTIC SENSITIVITY – MISCELLANEOUS*

| ORGANISMS | Chloramphenicol | Colistimethate | Daptomycin | Fosfomycin | Linezolid | Metronidazole | Nitrofurantoin | Quinupristin + Dalfopristin | Rifampin | Vancomycin |
|---|---|---|---|---|---|---|---|---|---|---|
| **ANAEROBES** | | | | | | | | | | |
| *Actinomyces* | | | | | | | | ✓ | | ✓ |
| *Bacillus anthracis* | | | | | | | | | | ✓ |
| *Bacteroides fragilis* | | | | | | ✓ | | ✓ | | |
| *Clostridium difficile* | | | | | | ✓ | | | | ✓ |
| *Clostridium species* | | | | | | ✓ | | ✓ | | ✓ |
| **GRAM-NEGATIVE AEROBES** | | | | | | | | | | |
| *Aeromonas hydrophila* | | | | | | | | | | |
| *Bartonella henselae* | | | | | | | | | | |
| *Bordetella species* | | | | | | | | | | |
| *Burkholderia cepacia* | | | | | | | | | | |
| *Campylobacter jejuni* | | | | | | | | | | |
| *Citrobacter species* | | | | ✓ | | | ✓ | | | |
| *Coxiella burnetti* | | | | | | | | | | |
| *Enterobacter species* | | ✓ | | ✓ | | | ✓ | | | |
| *Escherichia coli* | ✓ | ✓ | | ✓ | | | ✓ | | ✓ | |
| *Francisella tularensis* | | | | | | | | | | |

*These are generalizations. There are major differences among countries, areas, and hospitals depending on antibiotic usage patterns. The organisms checked for each antibiotic are not all-inclusive; only the major organisms are listed. Blank = no or insufficient activity, or unknown.

**MISCELLANEOUS (CONTINUED)**

| ORGANISMS | Chloramphenicol | Colistimethate | Daptomycin | Fosfomycin | Linezolid | Metronidazole | Nitrofurantoin | Quinupristin + Dalfopristin | Rifampin | Vancomycin |
|---|---|---|---|---|---|---|---|---|---|---|
| **GRAM-NEGATIVE AEROBES** *(Continued)* | | | | | | | | | | |
| *Haemophilus influenzae* | ✓ | | | | | | | | ✓ | |
| *Klebsiella species* | ✓ | ✓ | | ✓ | | | ✓ | | | |
| *Legionella species* | | | | | | | | | | |
| *Moraxella catarrhalis* | | | | | | | | | | |
| *Morganella morganii* | | | | | | | | | | |
| *Neisseria gonorrhoeae* | | | | | | | | | | |
| *Neisseria meningitidis* | | | | | | | | | ✓ | |
| *Pasteurella multocida* | | | | | ✓ | | | | | |
| *Proteus mirabilis* | ✓ | | | ✓ | | | | | | |
| *Proteus vulgaris* | ✓ | | | ✓ | | | | | | |
| *Providencia stuartii* | | | | | | | | | | |
| *Pseudomonas aeruginosa* | ✓ | ✓ | | | | | | | | |
| *Rickettsia species* | | | | | | | | | | |
| *Salmonella species* | | | | | | | | | | |
| *Serratia species* | | | | ✓ | | | | | | |
| *Shigella species* | | | | | | | | | | |
| *Stenotrophomonas maltophilia* | | | | | | | | | | |

*These are generalizations. There are major differences among countries, areas, and hospitals depending on antibiotic usage patterns. The organisms checked for each antibiotic are not all-inclusive; only the major organisms are listed.
Blank = no or insufficient activity, or unknown.

| ORGANISMS | Chloramphenicol | Colistimethate | Daptomycin | Fosfomycin | Linezolid | Metronidazole | Nitrofurantoin | Quinupristin + Dalfopristin | Rifampin | Vancomycin |
|---|---|---|---|---|---|---|---|---|---|---|
| **GRAM-NEGATIVE AEROBES** *(Continued)* | | | | | | | | | | |
| *Vibrio vulnificus* | | | | | | | | | | |
| *Yersinia enterocolitica* | | | | | | | | | | |
| *Yersinia pestis* | | | | | | | | | | |
| **GRAM-POSITIVE AEROBES** | | | | | | | | | | |
| *Enterococcus faecalis* | | | ✓ | ✓ | ✓ | | ✓ | | ✓ | ✓ |
| *Enterococcus faecium* | | | ✓ | ✓ | ✓ | | ✓ | ✓ | | ✓ |
| *Enterococcus faecium (VRE)* | | | ✓ | | ✓ | | | ✓ | | |
| *Listeria monocytogenes* | | | | | | | | | | ✓ |
| *Nocardia* | | | | | | | | | | |
| *Staphylococcus aureus (MSSA)* | ✓ | | ✓ | | ✓ | | ✓ | ✓ | ✓ | ✓ |
| *Staphylococcus aureus (MRSA)* | | | ✓ | | ✓ | | | ✓ | ✓ | ✓ |
| *Staphylococcus epidermidis* | | | ✓ | | ✓ | | ✓ | ✓ | ✓ | ✓ |
| *Staphylococcus epidermidis (MRSE)* | | | ✓ | | ✓ | | | ✓ | | ✓ |
| *Streptococcus pneumoniae†* | | | ✓ | | ✓ | | | | | ✓ |
| *Streptococcus pneumoniae§§* | | | | | ✓ | | | | | ✓ |

*These are generalizations. There are major differences among countries, areas, and hospitals depending on antibiotic usage patterns. The organisms checked for each antibiotic are not all-inclusive; only the major organisms are listed.
Blank = no or insufficient activity, or unknown.
† Penicillin sensitive; MIC ≤1.0 mcg/mL. §§ Penicillin resistant; MIC ≥2.0 mcg/mL.

## MISCELLANEOUS (CONTINUED)

| ORGANISMS | Chloramphenicol | Colistimethate | Daptomycin | Fosfomycin | Linezolid | Metronidazole | Nitrofurantoin | Quinupristin + Dalfopristin | Rifampin | Vancomycin |
|---|---|---|---|---|---|---|---|---|---|---|
| **GRAM-POSITIVE AEROBES** *(Continued)* | | | | | | | | | | |
| *Streptococcus (Group A,B,C,F,G)* | | | ✓ | | ✓ | | | ✓ | | ✓ |
| *Streptococcus species* | | | ✓ | | ✓ | | | ✓ | | ✓ |
| **MISCELLANEOUS** | | | | | | | | | | |
| *Chlamydia pneumoniae* | | | | | | | | | | |
| *Chlamydia trachomatis* | | | | | | | | | | |
| *Ehrlichia/Anaplasma species* | | | | | | | | | | |
| **MYCOBACTERIA** | | | | | | | | | | |
| *Mycobacterium avium (MAI) (non-HIV)* | | | | | | | | | | |
| *Mycoplasma pneumoniae* | | | | | | | | | | |
| **SPIROCHETES** | | | | | | | | | | |
| *Leptospira interrogans* | | | | | | | | | | |
| *Treponema pallidum (syphilis)* | | | | | | | | | | |

*These are generalizations. There are major differences among countries, areas, and hospitals depending on antibiotic usage patterns. The organisms checked for each antibiotic are not all-inclusive; only the major organisms are listed.

Blank = no or insufficient activity, or unknown.

# Drug Treatments for Common STDs*

| DISEASE | DRUG | RECOMMENDED DOSAGE |
|---|---|---|
| **Bacterial Vaginosis** | | |
| Nonpregnant Women | Metronidazole (Flagyl) *or* | 500mg PO bid x 7d. |
| | Clindamycin cream (Cleocin) *or* | 2%, 1 full applicator intravaginally qhs x 7d. |
| | Metronidazole gel (MetroGel) | 0.75%, 1 full applicator intravaginally qd x 5d. |
| *Alternative Regimens* (Nonpregnant Women) | Clindamycin *or*<br>Clindamycin ovules | 300mg PO bid x 7d.<br>100mg intravaginally qhs x 3d. |
| Pregnant Women | Metronidazole *or* | 250mg PO tid x 7d (metronidazole) or<br>500mg PO bid x 7d. |
| | Clindamycin | 300mg PO bid x 7d (clindamycin). |
| **Chancroid** | Azithromycin (Zithromax) *or* | 1g PO single dose. |
| | Ceftriaxone (Rocephin) *or* | 250mg IM single dose. |
| | Ciprofloxacin (Cipro) *or* | 500mg PO bid x 3d. |
| | Erythromycin base | 500mg PO tid x 7d. |
| **Chlamydial Infection** | | |
| Nonpregnant Women | Azithromycin (Zithromax) *or* | 1g PO single dose. |
| | Doxycycline (Vibramycin) | 100mg PO bid x 7d. |
| *Alternative Regimens* (Nonpregnant/pregnant) | Erythromycin base or | 500mg PO qid x 7d or<br>250mg PO qid x 14d (pregnancy). |
| | Erythromycin Ethylsuccinate or | 800mg PO qid x 7d or<br>400mg PO qid x 14d (pregnancy). |
| | Ofloxacin (Floxin) *or* | 300mg PO bid x 7d (nonpregnant). |
| | Levofloxacin (Levaquin) | 500mg PO qd x 7d (nonpregnant). |
| Pregnant Women | Azithromycin (Zithromax) *or* | 1g PO single dose. |
| | Amoxicillin | 500mg PO tid x 7d. |
| **Epididymitis** | | |
| Gonococcal or Chlamydial Infection | Ceftriaxone (Rocephin) *plus*<br>Doxycycline (Vibramycin) | 250mg IM single dose.<br>100mg PO bid x 10d. |
| Enteric organisms, negative gonococcal culture, or nucleic acid amplification test | Ofloxacin (Floxin) *or*<br>Levofloxacin (Levaquin) | 300mg PO bid x 10d.<br>500mg PO qd x 10d. |
| **Granuloma Inguinale** | Doxycycline (Vibramycin) | 100mg PO bid for at least 3 weeks. |
| *Alternative Regimens* | Ciprofloxacin (Cipro) *or* | 750mg PO bid for at least 3 weeks. |
| | Erythromycin base (during pregnancy) *or* | 500mg PO qid for at least 3 weeks. |
| | Azithromycin (Zithromax) | 1g PO once weekly for at least 3 weeks. |
| | Trimethoprim/Sulfamethoxazole (Bactrim, Septra) | 1 tab (DS) PO bid for at least 3 weeks. |
| | plus (if no improvement w/in first few days)<br>Aminoglycoside (ie, gentamicin) | 1mg/kg IV q8h for at least 3 weeks. |
| **Herpes Simplex Virus (HSV)** | | |
| First Episode | Acyclovir (Zovirax) *or* | 400mg PO tid x 7-10d or 200mg PO 5x/d x 7-10d. |
| | Famciclovir (Famvir) *or* | 250mg PO tid x 7-10d. |
| | Valacyclovir (Valtrex) | 1g PO bid x 7-10d. |
| Recurrent Episodes | Acyclovir *or* | 400mg PO tid x 5d or 800mg PO bid x 5d or 800mg PO tid x 2d. |
| | Famciclovir *or* | 1g bid x 1d or 125mg PO bid x 5d or |
| | Valacyclovir | 500mg PO bid x 3d or<br>1g PO qd x 5d. |
| Daily Suppressive Therapy | Acyclovir *or* | 400mg PO bid. |
| | Famciclovir *or* | 250mg PO bid. |
| | Valacyclovir | 500mg PO qd (<10 episodes/yr) or<br>1g PO qd. |

*(Continued)*

| DISEASE | DRUG | RECOMMENDED DOSAGE |
|---|---|---|
| **Human Papillomavirus (HPV) Infection** | | |
| External Genital Area | Podofilox (Condylox) *or* | 0.5% sol or gel (patient-applied) bid x 3d, wait 4d, repeat as necessary x 4 cycles. Limit application to 0.5mL/day and to <10cm² wart area. |
| | Imiquimod (Aldara) | 5% cre (patient-applied) tiw at bedtime up to 16 wks. |
| | Cryotherapy *or* | Physician-applied every 1-2 wks. |
| | Podophyllum resin | 10-25% (physician-applied) qwk if necessary. Limit application to 0.5mL/day and to <10cm² wart area. Do not apply to area with open lesions or wounds. |
| | Trichloroacetic acid *or* | 80-90% (physician-applied) qwk if necessary. |
| | Bichloroacetic acid *or* | 80-90% (physician-applied) qwk if necessary. |
| | Surgical removal | |
| *Alternative Regimens* | Intralesional interferon *or* laser surgery | |
| Vaginal warts | Cryotherapy *or* | With liquid nitrogen. |
| | Trichloroacetic acid *or* | 80-90% (physician-applied) qwk if necessary. |
| | Bichloroacetic acid | 80-90% (physician-applied) qwk if necessary. |
| Urethral Meatus warts | Cryotherapy *or* | With liquid nitrogen. |
| | Podophyllum | 10-25% (physician-applied) qwk if necessary. |
| Anal warts | Cryotherapy | With liquid nitrogen. |
| | Trichloroacetic acid *or* | 80-90% (physician-applied) qwk if necessary. |
| | Bichloroacetic acid *or* | 80-90% (physician-applied) qwk if necessary. |
| | Surgical removal | |
| **Lymphogranuloma Venereum** | Doxycycline (Vibramycin) | 100mg PO bid x 21d. |
| *Alternative Regimen* (including pregnancy) | Erythromycin base | 500mg PO qid x 21d. |
| **Nongonococcal Urethritis** | Azithromycin (Zithromax) *or* | 1g PO single dose. |
| | Doxycycline (Vibramycin) | 100mg PO bid x 7d. |
| *Alternative Regimens* | Erythromycin base or | 500mg PO qid x 7d. |
| | Erythromycin ethylsuccinate *or* | 800mg PO qid x 7d. |
| | Ofloxacin (Floxin) *or* | 300mg PO bid x 7d. |
| | Levofloxacin (Levaquin) | 500mg PO qd x 7d. |
| Recurrent and Persistent Urethritis | Metronidazole *or* | 2g PO single dose. |
| | Tinidazole *plus* | 2g PO single dose. |
| | Azithromycin | 1g PO single dose (if not used for initial episodes). |
| **Pediculosis Pubis** | Permethrin cream (NIX) | 1% cre: Apply to affected area & wash off after 10 min. |
| | Pyrethrins with piperonyl butoxide (compounded by pharmacist) | Apply to affected area and wash off after 10 min. |
| *Alternative Regimens* | Malathion | 0.5% lotion: Apply for 8-12 hours and wash off. |
| | Ivermectin | 250μg/kg repeat in 2 weeks. |
| **Pelvic Inflammatory Disease** | | |
| Parenteral Regimen A | Cefotetan (Cefotan) *or* | 2g IV q12h. |
| | Cefoxitin (Mefoxin) *plus* | 2g IV q6h. |
| | Doxycycline (Vibramycin) | 100mg IV q12h. |
| Parenteral Regimen B | Clindamycin (Cleocin) *plus* | 900mg IV q8h. |
| | Gentamicin | LD: 2mg/kg IM/IV. MD: 1.5mg/kg IM/IV q8h (may substitute single daily dosing). |
| *Alternative Regimen* | Ampicillin/Sulbactam *plus* | 3g IV q6h. |
| | Doxycycline | 100mg PO/IV q12h. |
| Oral Regimen | Ceftriaxone (Rocephin) *plus* | 250mg IM single dose. |
| | Doxycycline w/ or w/o | 100mg PO bid x 14d. |
| | Metronidazole | 500mg PO bid x 14d. |
| | or | |
| | Cefoxitin *plus* | 2g IM single dose with probenecid 1g PO single dose. |
| | Doxycycline w/ or w/o | 100mg PO bid x 14d. |
| | Metronidazole | 500mg PO bid x 14d. |
| | or | |
| | 3rd Gen Cephalosporin *plus* | Given IV/IM |
| | Doxycycline w/ or w/o | 100mg PO bid x 14d. |
| | Metronidazole | 500mg PO bid x 14d. |
| *Alternative Oral Regimen (Use only if negative NAAT test or negative gonococcal culture)* | Levofloxacin *or* | 500mg PO qd x 14d. |
| | Ofloxacin w/ or w/o | 400mg PO bid x 14d. |
| | Metronidazole | 500mg PO bid x 14d. |

*(Continued)*

| DISEASE | DRUG | RECOMMENDED DOSAGE |
|---|---|---|
| **Proctitis, Proctocolitis & Enteritis** | Ceftriaxone (Rocephin) *plus*<br>Doxycycline (Vibramycin) | 125mg IM single dose.<br>100mg PO bid x 7d. |
| **Scabies** | Permethrin cream (Elimite)<br><br>or<br>Ivermectin | 5% cre: Apply to body from the neck down & wash off after 8-14h; re-evaluate in 1 week.<br>200mcg/kg PO; repeat in 2 weeks. |
| *Alternative Regimens* | Lindane (Kwell) | 1% lot or cre: Apply 1oz lotion or 30g cream to body from the neck down & wash off after 8h; re-evaluate in 1 wk (not recommended in pregnancy, lactating women or children <2 yrs). |
| **Syphilis** | | |
| Primary & Secondary Disease | Benzathine Penicillin G | **Adults:** 2.4 MU IM single dose.<br>**Pediatrics:** 50,000 U/kg IM single dose.<br>**Max:** 2.4 MU/dose. |
| Penicillin Allergy | Doxycycline (Vibramycin) *or*<br>Tetracycline | 100mg PO bid x 14d.<br>500mg PO qid x 14d. |
| Early Latent Disease | Benzathine Penicillin G | **Adults:** 2.4 MU IM single dose.<br>**Pediatrics:** 50,000 U/kg IM single dose.<br>**Max:** 2.4 MU/dose. |
| Late Latent, Unknown Duration | Benzathine Penicillin G | **Adults:** 2.4 MU IM qwk x 3 doses.<br>**Pediatrics:** 50,000 U/kg IM qwk x 3 doses.<br>**Max:** 2.4 MU/dose. |
| Tertiary Disease | Benzathine Penicillin G | 2.4 MU IM qwk x 3 doses. |
| Neurosyphilis | Aqueous Crystalline Penicillin G | 3-4 MU IV q4h or continuous infusion x 10-14d. |
| *Alternative Regimen* | Procaine Penicillin *plus*<br>Probenecid | 2.4 MU IM qd x 10-14d.<br>500mg PO qid x 10-14d. |
| **Trichomoniasis** | Metronidazole (Flagyl)<br>Tinidazole (Tindamax) | 2g PO single dose.<br>2g PO single dose. |
| *Alternative Regimen* | Metronidazole | 500mg PO bid x 7d. |
| Pregnant Women | Metronidazole (CI in 1st trimester) | 2g PO single dose. |
| **Uncomplicated Gonococcal Infections** | | |
| Cervix, Urethra, and Rectum<br>*Recommended Regimens* | Ceftriaxone or<br>Cefixime Plus | 125mg IM single dose.<br>400mg PO single dose.<br>or 400mg by susp 200mg/5mL. |
| | *If Chlamydial infection is not ruled out:*<br>Azithromycin (Zithromax) *or*<br>Doxycycline (Vibramycin) | <br>1g PO single dose.<br>100mg PO bid x 7d. |
| *Alternative Regimens* | Spectinomycin or<br>*Cephalosporin regimens:*<br>Ceftizoxime *or*<br>Cefotaxime *or*<br>Cefoxitin plus | 2g IM single dose.<br><br>500mg IM single dose.<br>500mg IM single dose.<br>2g IM. |
| | Probenecid | 1g PO. |
| Pharynx<br>*Recommended Regimens* | Ceftriaxone<br>*plus*<br>*If Chlamydial infection is not ruled out:*<br>Azithromycin (Zithromax) or<br>Doxycycline (Vibramycin) | 125mg IM single dose.<br><br><br>1g PO single dose.<br>100mg PO bid x 7d. |

*(Continued)*

| DISEASE | DRUG | RECOMMENDED DOSAGE |
|---|---|---|
| **Vulvovaginal Candidiasis** | | |
| Intravaginal Agents | Butoconazole *or* | 2% cre, 5g intravaginally x 3d (sustained release) |
| | Butoconazole *or* | 2% cre, 5g intravaginally single dose. |
| | Clotrimazole *or* | 1% cre, 5g intravaginally x 7-14d. |
| | Clotrimazole *or* | 100mg vaginal tab qd x 7 days or 2 tabs qd x 3d. |
| | Miconazole *or* | 2% cre, 5g intravaginally qd x 7d. |
| | Miconazole *or* | 200mg vaginal supp qd x 3d. |
| | Miconazole *or* | 100mg vaginal supp qd x 7d. |
| | Miconazole | 1200mg vaginal supp single dose. |
| | Nystatin *or* | 100,000-U vaginal tab qd x 14d. |
| | Tioconazole *or* | 6.5% oint, 5g intravaginally single dose. |
| | Terconazole *or* | 0.4% cre, 5g intravaginally x 7d. |
| | Terconazole *or* | 0.8% cre, 5g intravaginally x 3d. |
| | Terconazole | 80mg vaginal supp qd x 3d. |
| Oral Agent | Fluconazole | 150mg tab PO single dose. |

*Adapted from: Centers for Disease Control and Prevention. Sexually Transmitted Diseases Treatment Guidelines 2006. MMWR 2002; 51 (No. RR-6): 1-77.

# HIV/AIDS PHARMACOTHERAPY

| DRUG | BRAND | HOW SUPPLIED | USUAL DOSE | FOOD EFFECT |
|---|---|---|---|---|
| **CCR5 ANTAGONIST** | | | | |
| Maraviroc (MVC) | Selzentry | **Tab:** 150mg, 300mg | **Adults >16 yrs:** Give in combination with other antiretroviral medications. With Strong CYP3A Inhibitors (with or without CYP3A inducers) Including PIs (excepts tipranavir/ritonavir), Delavirdine: 150mg bid. With NRTIs, Tipranavir/Ritonavir, Nevirapine, Other Drugs That Are Not Strong CYP3A Inhibitors/Inducers: 300mg bid. With CYP3A Inducers (without strong CYP3A inhibitor): 600mg bid. | Take without regard to meals. |
| **HIV INTEGRASE STRAND TRANSFER INHIBITOR** | | | | |
| Raltegravir | Isentress | **Tab:** 400mg | **Adults:** 400mg bid. | Take without regard to meals. |
| **NUCLEOSIDE REVERSE TRANSCRIPTASE INHIBITORS (NRTIs)** | | | | |
| Abacavir (ABC) | Ziagen | **Sol:** 20mg/mL [240mL]; **Tab:** 300mg | **Adults >16 yrs:** 300mg bid or 600 mg qd. **Pediatrics 3 months-16 yrs:** 8mg/kg bid. **Max:** 300mg bid. | Take without regard to meals. |
| Didanosine (ddI) | Videx Powder for Oral Sol; Videx EC | **Powder for Sol:** 10mg/mL [2g, 4g]; **Cap, Delayed Release:** (Videx EC) 125mg, 200mg, 250mg, 400mg | **Adults ≥60kg: (Cap)** 400mg qd; **(Sol)** 200mg bid or 400mg qd. **<60kg: (Sol)** 125mg bid. or 250mg qd. 25-60 kg; **(Cap)** 250mg qd. 20-25 kg: **(Cap)** 200mg qd. **Pediatrics 2 weeks-8 months: (Sol)** 100$mg/m^2$ bid. **>8 months:** 120$mg/m^2$ bid. | Take on empty stomach at least 30 minutes before or 2 hrs after meals. Swallow caps whole. |
| Emtricitabine (FTC) | Emtriva | **Cap:** 200mg; **Sol:** 10mg/mL [170mL] | **Adults ≥18 yrs: Cap:** 200 mg qd. **Sol:** 240mg (24mL) qd. **Pediatrics 0-3 mos:** 3mg/kg qd. **3 mos-17 yrs: Cap: >33kg:** 200mg qd. **Sol:** 6mg/kg qd. **Max:** 240mg (24mL). | Take without regard to meals. |
| Lamivudine | Epivir | **Sol:** 10mg/mL [240mL]; **Tab:** 150mg, 300mg | **Adults:** 150mg bid or 300mg qd. **Pediatrics 3 months-16 yrs:** 4mg/kg bid. **Max:** 150mg bid. | Take without regard to meals. |
| Stavudine (d4T) | Zerit | **Cap:** 15mg, 20mg, 30mg, 40mg; **Sol:** 1mg/mL [200mL] | **Adults ≥60kg:** 40mg q12h. **<60kg:** 30mg q12h. **Pediatrics ≥60kg:** 40mg q12h. **30-59 kg:** 30mg q12h. **≥14 days and <30kg:** 1mg/kg q12h. **Birth-13 days:** 0.5mg/kg q12h. | Take without regard to meals. |
| Tenofovir Disoproxil Fumarate (TDF) | Viread | **Tab:** 300mg | **Adults:** 300mg once daily. | Take without regard to meals. |
| Zidovudine (AZT, ZDV) | Retrovir | **Cap:** 100mg; **Inj:** 10mg/mL; **Syrup:** 50mg/5mL [240mL]; **Tab:** 300mg | **Adults: (Cap, Tab)** 600mg/day in divided doses (300mg bid or 200mg tid). (Inj) 1mg/kg IV over 1 hr 5-6 times/day. **Pediatrics 6 weeks-12 yrs:** 160$mg/m^2$ PO q8h. **Max:** 200mg PO q8h. | Take without regard to meals. |

*(Continued)*

| DRUG | BRAND | HOW SUPPLIED | USUAL DOSE | FOOD EFFECT |
|---|---|---|---|---|
| **NON-NUCLEOSIDE REVERSE TRANSCRIPTASE INHIBITORS (NNRTIs)** | | | | |
| Delavirdine (DLV) | Rescriptor | **Tab:** 100mg, 200mg | **Adults: Usual:** 400mg tid. **Pediatrics ≥16 yrs: Usual:** 400mg tid. | Take without regard to meals. |
| Efavirenz (EFV) | Sustiva | **Cap:** 50mg, 200mg; **Tab:** 600mg | **Adults Initial:** 600mg qd at bedtime. **Pediatrics ≥3 yrs: 10 to <15kg:** 200mg qd. **15 to <20kg:** 250mg qd. **20 to <25kg:** 300mg qd. **25 to <32.5kg:** 350mg qd. **32.5 to <40kg:** 400mg qd. **≥40kg:** 600mg qd at bedtime. | Take on an empty stomach. |
| Etravirine (ETR) | Intelence | **Tab:** 100mg | **Adults:** 200mg bid. | Take with meals. |
| Nevirapine (NVP) | Viramune | **Sus:** 50mg/5mL [240mL]; **Tab:** 200mg* *scored | **Adults ≥16 yrs:** 200mg qd for 14 days (lead-in period), then 200mg bid. **Pediatrics >15 days:** 150mg/m$^2$ qd for 14 days, then 150mg/m$^2$ bid. **Max:** 400mg/day. | Take without regard to meals. |
| **PROTEASE INHIBITORS (PIs)** | | | | |
| Atazanavir (ATV) | Reyataz | **Cap:** 100mg, 150mg, 200mg, 300mg | **Adults:** Therapy-naive: 400mg qd. Therapy Experienced: (ATV 300mg + RTV 100mg) qd. | Take with food; avoid taking with antacids. |
| Darunavir (DRV) | Prezista | **Tab:** 75mg, 150mg, 300mg, 400mg, 600mg | **Adults:** Therapy-naïve: (DRV 800mg + RTV 100mg) qd. Therapy-experienced: (DRV 600mg + RTV 100mg) bid. **Pediatrics:** (6 to <18 yrs): ≥40kg: (DRV 600mg + RTV 100mg) bid. ≥30- <40kg: (DRV 450mg + RTV 60mg) bid. ≥20-<30kg: (DRV 375mg + RTV 50mg) bid. **Max:** (DRV 600mg + RTV 100mg) bid. | Take with food. |
| Fosamprenavir (fAPV) | Lexiva | **Tab:** 700mg **Sus:** 50mg/mL [225mL] | **Adults:** Therapy-naïve: fAPV 1,400mg bid OR fAPV 1400mg qd + RTV 200mg qd OR fAPV 1400mg qd + RTV 100mg qd OR fAPV 700mg bid + RTV 100mg bid. PI-experienced: fAPV 700mg bid + RTV 100mg bid. **Pediatrics:** (Sus): Therapy-naïve: (2-5 yrs) fAPV 30mg/kg bid **Max:** fAPV 1,400mg bid. (≥6 yrs): fAPV 30mg/kg bid **Max:** fAPV 1,400mg bid. OR fAPV 18mg/kg bid + RTV 3mg/kg bid **Max:** fAPV 700mg bid + RTV 100mg bid. Therapy-experienced: (≥6 yrs) fAPV 18mg/kg bid + RTV 3mg/kg bid **Max:** fAPV 700mg bid + RTV 100mg bid. | **Tab:** Take with or w/o food. **Sus: Adults:** Take w/o food. **Pediatrics:** Take with food. |

*(Continued)*

| DRUG | BRAND | HOW SUPPLIED | USUAL DOSE | FOOD EFFECT |
|---|---|---|---|---|
| **PROTEASE INHIBITORS (PIs)** *(Continued)* | | | | |
| Indinavir (IDV) | Crixivan | **Cap:** 100mg, 200mg, 400mg | **Adults:** 800mg q8h RTV Boost: (IDV 800mg + RTV 100 or 200mg) q12h. | Take 1 hr before or 2 hr after meals; may take with skim milk or low-fat meal. |
| Nelfinavir (NFV) | Viracept | **Sus:** (powder) 50mg/g [144g] **Tab:** 250mg, 625mg | **Adults:** 1250mg bid or 750mg tid. **Pediatrics 2-13 yrs:** 45-55mg/kg bid; 25-35mg/kg tid. **Max:** 2500mg/day. | Take with meals. |
| Ritonavir (RTV) | Norvir | **Cap:** 100mg **Sol:** 80mg/mL [240mL] | **Adults: Initial:** 300mg bid. **Titrate:** Increase every 2-3 days by 100mg bid. **Maint:** 600mg bid. **Pediatrics >1 month: Initial:** $250mg/m^2$ po bid. **Titrate:** Increase by $50mg/m^2$ every 2-3 days. **Maint:** 350-$400mg/m^2$ po bid or highest tolerated dose. **Max:** 600mg bid. | Take with food, may improve tolerability. |
| Saquinavir (SQV) | Invirase | **Cap:** 200mg **Tab:** 500mg | **Adults/Pediatrics >16 yrs:** 1000mg bid with RTV 100mg bid OR 1000mg bid with LPV/RTV 400/100mg bid (no additional RTV). | Take within 2 hrs after a meal when taken with RTV. |
| Tipranavir (TPV) | Aptivus | **Cap:** 250mg **Sol:** 100mg/mL | **Adults:** (500mg + RTV 200mg) bid. **Pediatrics:** (≥2 yrs) 14mg/kg + RTV 6mg/kg (or $375mg/m^2$ + RTV 150 $mg/m^2$) bid. **Max:** (500mg + RTV 200mg) bid. | Take with or w/o food. |
| **FUSION INHIBITOR** | | | | |
| Enfuvirtide (T20) | Fuzeon | **Inj:** 90mg/mL [60[s]] | **Adults:** 90mg SQ bid. **Pediatrics 6-16 yrs:** 2mg/kg SQ bid. **Max:** 90mg bid. 11-15.5kg: 27mg bid. 15.6-20.0kg: 36mg bid. 20.1-24.5kg: 45mg bid. 24.6-29.0kg: 54mg bid. 29.1-33.5kg: 63mg bid. 33.6-38.0kg: 72mg bid. 38.1-42.5kg: 81mg bid. ≥42.6kg: 90mg bid. | |
| **COMBINATIONS** | | | | |
| EFV/FTC/TDF | Atripla | **Tab:** (Efavirenz-Emtricitabine-Tenofovir DF) 600mg-200mg-300mg | **Adults ≥18 yrs:** 1 tab qd, preferably at bedtime. | Take on empty stomach. |
| 3TC/ZDV | Combivir | **Tab:** (Lamivudine-Zidovudine) 150mg-300mg | **Adults/Pediatrics:** (≥30kg) 1 tab bid. Do not give if CrCl <50mL/min or if <30kg weight. | Take without regard to meals. |
| ABC/3TC | Epzicom | **Tab:** (Abacavir Sulfate-Lamivudine) 600mg-300mg | **Adults ≥18 yrs:** CrCl >50 mL/min: 1 tab qd. Do not give if CrCl <50mL/min. | Take without regard to meals. |

*(Continued)*

| DRUG | BRAND | HOW SUPPLIED | USUAL DOSE | FOOD EFFECT |
|---|---|---|---|---|
| **COMBINATIONS** *(Continued)* | | | | |
| LPV/RTV | Kaletra | **Cap:** (LPV-RTV) 133.3mg-33.3mg **Tab:** (LPV-RTV) 200mg-50mg; 100mg-25mg; **Sol:** (LPV-RTV) 80mg-20mg/mL [160mL] | **Adults:** Therapy-naive: 400/100mg bid or 800/200mg qd. Therapy-experienced: 400/100mg bid. **Pediatrics: Sol:** (14 days-6 months) LPV/RTV 16/4 mg/kg or 300/75 mg/m$^2$ bid. (6 months-18 yrs) LPV/RTV 230/57.5 mg/m$^2$ bid or weight-based (<15kg) 12/3 mg/kg bid (≥15-40kg) 10/2.5 mg/kg bid. | **Tab:** Take without regard to meals. **Cap/Sol:** Take with meals. |
| ABC/ZDV/3TC | Trizivir | **Tab:** (Abacavir-Lamivudine-Zidovudine) 300mg-150mg-300mg | **Adults/Adolescents:** >40kg and CrCl >50mL/min: 1 tab bid. | Take without regard to meals. |
| FTC/TDF | Truvada | **Tab:** (Emtricitabine-Tenofovir Disoproxil Fumarate) 200mg-300mg | **Adults ≥18 yrs:** CrCl ≥50mL/min: 1 tab qd. CrCl 30-49mL/min: 1 tab q48h. | Take without regard to meals. |
| Sources: FDA Approved Labeling; Guidelines for the Use of Antiretroviral Agents in HIV-1-Infected Adults and Adolescents - December 1, 2009. | | | | |

# HIV/AIDS COMPLICATIONS THERAPY

| DISEASE-RELATED COMPLICATION | GENERIC (BRAND) | RECOMMENDED DOSAGE |
|---|---|---|
| **ASPERGILLOSIS, INVASIVE** | | |
| Recommended Treatment Regimen | Voriconazole (VFEND)* | **Adults: LD:** 6mg/kg q12h for 1st 24 hrs. **MD:** (IV) 4mg/kg q12h or (PO) ≥40kg: 200mg q12h. <40kg: 100mg q12h. Continue treatment until at least 7 days following resolution of symptoms. |
| Alternative Treatment Regimen | Amphotericin B (AmBisome) | **Adults/Pediatrics:** 3-5mg/kg/day IV controlled infusion over 1-2 hrs. |
| | Amphotericin B lipid-formulation | **Adults/Pediatrics:** 5mg/kg at 2.5mg/kg/hr. |
| | Caspofungin (Cancidas) | **Adults: LD:** 70mg slow IV infusion over 1 hr on Day 1. **MD:** 50mg IV qd. **Pediatrics:** (3 months-17 yrs). **LD:** 70mg/m$^2$ slow IV infusion over 1 hr on Day 1. **MD:** 50mg/m$^2$ qd. **Max:** LD and MD should not exceed 70mg. |
| | Posaconazole (Noxafil) | **Adults/Pediatrics ≥13 yrs:** 400mg PO bid. Duration of treatment based on neutropenia/immunosuppression. |
| **CANDIDIASIS** | | |
| Prevention/Treatment | Amphotericin B (AmBisome) | **Adults/Pediatrics:** 3-5mg/kg/day IV controlled infusion over 1-2 hrs. |
| | Amphotericin B lipid-formulation | **Adults/Pediatrics:** 5mg/kg at 2.5mg/kg/hr. |
| | Anidulafungin (Eraxis) | **Esophageal: Adults:** 100mg IV x 1, then 50mg IV qd x 14-21 days. |
| | Caspofungin (Cancidas) | **Adults: LD:** 70mg slow IV infusion over 1 hr on Day 1. **MD:** 50mg IV qd. **Esophageal:** 50mg/day slow IV infusion over 1 hr. |
| | Fluconazole (Diflucan)† | **Oropharngeal: Adults:** 200mg PO Day 1, then 100mg qd q 2 weeks. **Pediatrics:** 6mg/kg Day 1, then 3mg/kg qd q 2 weeks. **Esophageal: Adults:** 200mg Day 1, then 100mg qd. Continue until 2 weeks after resolution of symptoms. Max: 400mg/day. **Pediatrics:** 6mg/kg Day 1, then 3mg/kg qd for a minimum of 3 weeks and for at least 2 weeks following resolution of symptoms. Max: 12mg/kg/day. |
| | Itraconazole (Sporanox) | **Oropharngeal: Adults:** Swish and swallow 200mg (20mL) oral solution qd x 1-2 weeks. **Esophageal: Adults:** 200mg qd x 14-21 days. |
| | Micafungin (Mycamine) | **Esophageal: Adults:** 150mg IV qd x 14-21 days. |
| | Posaconazole (Noxafil) | **Oropharngeal: ≥13 yrs:** 100mg bid Day 1, then 100mg qd x 13d. **Refractory to fluconazole:** 400mg bid. Duration of therapy individualized. |
| | Voriconazole (VFEND)* | **Esophageal: Adults:** ≥40kg: 200mg PO q12h. <40kg: 100mg PO q12h. Continue treatment until at least 7 days following resolution of symptoms. |
| **CMV RETINITIS** | | |
| Treatment | Cidofovir (Vistide)† | **Adults:** Induction: 5mg/kg IV infusion over 1 hr q week x 2 weeks. Maint: 5mg/kg IV over 1 hr q 2 weeks. |
| | Foscarnet (Foscavir) | **Adults:** Induction: 90mg/kg over 1.5-2 hrs IV infusion q12h or 60mg/kg 1 hr IV infusion q8h x 2-3 weeks. **Maint:** 90-120mg/kg/day IV over 2 hrs. |
| | Ganciclovir (Cytovene)† | **Adults:** Induction: 5mg/kg IV over 1hr q12h x 14-21days. Maint: 5mg/kg IV over 1 hr qd x 7 days/week or 6mg/kg IV qd x 5 days/week. |
| | Ganciclovir (Vitrasert) | **Adults/Pediatrics ≥9 yrs:** One implant q 5-8 months. |
| | Valganciclovir (Valcyte) | **Adults:** Induction: 900mg PO bid x 21 days w/ food. Maint: 900mg PO qd w/ food. |

*(Continued)*

| DISEASE-RELATED COMPLICATION | GENERIC (BRAND) | RECOMMENDED DOSAGE |
|---|---|---|
| **CRYPTOCOCCAL MENINGITIS** | | |
| Treatment | Amphotericin B (AmBisome) | **Adults:** 6mg/kg/day IV over 1-2 hrs. |
| | Fluconazole (Diflucan) | **Adults:** 400mg on Day 1, then 200-400mg qd x 10-12 weeks. Relapse: 200mg qd. **Pediatrics:** 12mg/kg on Day 1, then 6-12mg/kg qd x 10-12 weeks. Relapse: 6mg/kg qd. |
| **HSV** | | |
| Recommended Regimen for Daily Suppressive Therapy | Acyclovir *or*<br>Famciclovir (Famvir) *or*<br>Valacyclovir | 400-800mg PO bid-tid.<br>500mg PO bid.<br>1000mg PO bid. |
| Recommended Regimen for Episodic Infection | Acyclovir *or*<br>Famiciclovir† *or*<br>Valacyclovir | 400mg PO tid x 5-10 days.<br>500mg PO bid x 5-10 days.<br>1g PO bid x 5-10 days. |
| **KAPOSI'S SARCOMA** | | |
| Treatment | Alitretinoin (Panretin) | **0.1% gel: Adults: Initial:** Apply bid to lesions. Can increase to tid-qid based on individual lesion tolerance. |
| | Daunorubicin (DaunoXome) | **Adults:** 40mg/m$^2$ IV over 60 min q 2 weeks. |
| | Doxorubicin (Doxil) | **Adults:** 20mg/m$^2$ IV q 3 weeks. Initial rate: 1mg/min. May be increased to administer over 1 hr if tolerated. |
| | Interferon alfa-2b (INTRON A) | **Adults:** 30 MIU/m$^2$/dose SQ/IM tiw until max response achieved after 16 weeks. Must use Powder for Injection/Reconstitution only. Solution for Injection in vials or Multidose Pens should not be used. |
| | Paclitaxel (Taxol) | **Adults:** 135mg/m$^2$ IV over 3 hrs q 3 weeks or 100mg/m2 IV over 3 hrs q 2 weeks. Dose Intensity: 45-50mg/m$^2$/week. |
| **MAC** | | |
| Prevention/Treatment | Azithromycin (Zithromax) | **Adults:** Prevention: 1200mg once weekly. Treatment: 600mg qd with ethambutol 15mg/kg/day. |
| Prevention/Treatment | Clarithromycin (Biaxin) | **Adults:** 500mg PO bid. **Pediatrics:** 7.5mg/kg bid up to 500mg bid. |
| Prevention | Rifabutin (Mycobutin)† | **Adults:** 300mg PO qd. N/V/GI upset: 150mg bid w/ food. |
| **PCP** | | |
| Prevention/Treatment | Atovaquone (Mepron) | **Adults/Pediatrics ≥13 yrs:** 1500mg PO qd w/ meals. **Adults/Pediatrics ≥13 yrs (mild-moderate PCP):** 750mg PO bid w/ meals x 21 days. |
| | TMP/SMX (Bactrim) | **Adults/Pediatrics:** Treatment: 15-20mg/kg/day TMP and 75-100mg/kg/day SMX in divided doses q6h x 14-21days. |
| | TMP/SMX DS (Bactrim DS) | **Adults:** Prevention: 1 DS tab (160/800mg) qd. **Pediatrics:** Prevention: 150mg/m$^2$/day TMP with 750mg/m$^2$/day SMX PO bid in equally divided doses on 3 consecutive days/week. |
| **VISCERAL LEISHMANIASIS** | | |
| Treatment | Amphotericin B (AmBisome) | **Adults:** Immunocompetent: 3mg/kg/day IV Days 1-5, then on Days 14 and 21. Immunocompromised: 4mg/kg/day IV Days 1-5, then on Days 10, 17, 24, 31, and 38. |
| **WEIGHT LOSS** | | |
| Anorexia | Dronabinol (Marinol) | **Adults:** 2.5mg qhs or bid ac. **Max:** 20mg/day in divided doses. |
| Anorexia, cachexia, unexplained weight loss | Megesterol (Megace) | **Adults:** Initial: 800mg/d. **Usual:** 400-800mg/day. |
| Cachexia/Wasting | Somatropin (Serostim) | **Adults:** >55kg: 6mg SQ qhs. 45-55kg: 5mg SQ qhs. 35-45kg: 4mg SQ qhs. <35kg: 0.1mg/kg SQ qhs. **Max:** 6mg/day. |

Abbreviations: CMV=cytomegalovirus; HSV=herpes simplex virus; MAC=*Mycobacterium avium* complex; PCP=*Pneumocystis carinii* pneumonia.

*Use cautiously in patients on protease inhibitors and efavirenz.

†For dosing in special populations, see the complete prescribing information.

Sources: Prescribing information; Guidelines for prevention and treatment of opportunistic infections in HIV-infected adults and adolescents. MMWR; Vol 58, No. RR-4. April 10, 2009.

# MANAGEMENT OF HEPATITIS B AND HEPATITIS C

| BRAND NAME (GENERIC) | HOW SUPPLIED | ADULTS | COMMENTS |
|---|---|---|---|
| **HEPATITIS B** | | | |
| **Acyclic Nucleotide Analog** | | | |
| **Hepsera** (Adefovir dipivoxil) | **Tab:** 10mg | **Adults:** 10mg QD PO without regard to food. **Pediatrics ≥12 yrs:** 10mg QD PO without regard to food. | Renal Impairment: CrCl 30-49mL/min: 10mg q48h. CrCl 10-29mL/min: 10mg q72h. Hemodialysis Patients: 10mg every 7 days following dialysis. |
| **Biological Response Modifier** | | | |
| **Intron-A** (Interferon alfa-2b, recombinant) | **Inj:** 10 MIU, 18 MIU, 50 MIU, 3 MIU/0.2mL, 5 MIU/0.2mL, 10 MIU/0.2mL, 3MIU/0.5mL, 5MIU/0.5mL | **Adults ≥18 yrs:** IM/SQ: 5 MIU qd or 10 MIU IM/SQ 3x/week for 16 weeks. **Pediatrics 1-17yrs:** 3 MIU/$m^2$ SQ 3x/week for 1 week, then 6 MIU/$m^2$ 3x/week (max 10 MIU TIW) for total therapy of 16-24 weeks. | Adjust dose according to severe adverse reactions and laboratory abnormalities (See PI for more information). Reduce dose by 50% or stop therapy with severe reactions. Adjust based on WBC, granulocyte, and/or platelet counts. |
| **Guanosine Nucleoside Analogue** | | | |
| **Baraclude** (Entecavir) | **Sol:** 0.05mg/mL; **Tab:** 0.5mg, 1mg | **Adults/Pediatrics >16 yrs:** Nucleoside-Treatment-Naive: 0.5mg qd. CrCl 30 to <50mL/min: 0.25mg qd or 0.5mg q48h. CrCl 10 to <30mL/min: 0.15mg qd or 0.5mg q72h. CrCl <10mL/min: 0.05mg qd or 0.5mg q7 days. Receiving Lamivudine or Known Lamivudine Resistance Mutation: 1mg qd. CrCl 30 to <50mL/min: 0.5mg qd or 1mg q48h. CrCl 10 to <30mL/min: 0.3mg qd or 1mg q72h. CrCl <10mL/min: 0.1mg qd or 1mg q7 days. | Take on empty stomach. |
| **Immune Globulin** | | | |
| **Nabi-HB** (Hepatitis B immune globulin, human) | **Inj:** >312 IU/1mL | **Adults:** 0.06mL/kg IM and should begin the hepatitis B vaccine series. | See PI for special populations. |
| **Nucleoside Analogues** | | | |
| **Epivir-HBV** (Lamivudine) | **Sol:** 5mg/mL [240mL]; **Tab:** 100mg | **Adults:** 100mg qd. CrCl 30-49mL/min: 100mg Day 1, then 50mg qd. CrCl: 15-29mL/min: 100mg Day 1, then 25mg qd. CrCl 5-14mL/min: 35mg Day 1, then 15mg qd. CrCl <5mL/min: 35mg Day 1, then 10mg qd. **Pediatrics 2-17 yrs:** 3mg/kg qd. Max: 100mg/day. | |

(Continued)

| BRAND NAME (GENERIC) | HOW SUPPLIED | ADULTS | COMMENTS |
|---|---|---|---|
| **Nucleoside Analogues** *(Continued)* | | | |
| **Tyzeka**<br>(Telbivudine) | **Tab:** 600mg; **Sol:** 100mg/5mL | **Adults/Pediatrics ≥16 yrs: Tab:** CrCl ≥50mL/min: 600mg qd. CrCl 30-49mL/min: 600mg every 48 hrs. CrCl <30mL/min (not requiring dialysis): 600mg every 72 hrs. ESRD: 600mg every 96 hrs. **Sol:** CrCL ≥50mL/min: 30mL qd. CrCl 30-49mL/min: 20mL qd. CrCl <30mL/min: 10mL qd. | Take with or without food. |
| **Viread**<br>(Tenofovir disoproxil fumarate) | **Tab:** 300mg | **Adults:** 300mg qd without regard to food. Renal Impairment: CrCl 30-49mL/min: 300mg q48 hrs. CrCl 10-29mL/min: 300mg q72-96 hrs. | Hemodialysis: 300mg every 7 days after total of approx. 12 hrs of dialysis. |
| **Pegylated Virus Proliferation Inhibitor** | | | |
| **Pegasys**<br>(Peginterferon alfa-2a) | **Inj:** Prefilled syringe: 180mcg/0.5mL; **Single Dose Vial:** 180mcg/mL | **Monotherapy:** 180mcg SQ in abdomen or thigh once weekly for 48 wks. | Adjust dose based on hematological parameters and depression severity (see PI for dose modifications). |
| **Vaccines** | | | |
| **Engerix-B**<br>(Hepatitis B vaccine [recombinant]) | **Inj:** 10mcg/0.5mL, 20mcg/mL | **Adults >19 yrs:** 20mcg/1mL IM in deltoid region at 0, 1, 6 months. Hemodialysis: 40mcg/2mL IM at 0, 1, 2, 6 months. Booster: 20mcg IM. Hemodialysis Booster: 40mcg IM. May give SQ with risk of hemorrhage. **Pediatrics ≤19 yrs:** 10mcg/0.5mL IM at 0, 1, 6 months. Booster: ≤10 yrs: 10mcg IM. 11-19 yrs: 20mcg IM. | See PI for special populations. May give SQ with risk of hemorrhage. |
| **Recombivax HB, Recombivax HB Adult, Recombivax HB Dialysis, Recombivax HB Pediatric/Adolescent**<br>(Hepatitis B vaccine [recombinant]) | **Inj:** Pediatric/Adolescent Formulation Preservative-Free: 5mcg/0.5mL, Adult Formulation Preservative-Free: 10mcg/1mL, Dialysis Formulation Preservative-Free: 40mcg/1mL | **Adults:** IM into deltoid muscle. If at risk of hemorrhage with IM injection, give SQ. ≥20 years (Adult Formulation): 10mcg at 0, 1, 6 months. Predialysis/Dialysis (Dialysis Formulation): 40mcg at 0, 1, 6 months; consider booster dose or revaccination if anti-HBs level <l0mIU/mL 1 to 2 months after the 3rd dose. **Pediatrics:** IM injection into anterolateral thigh in infants and young children. Give SQ if risk of hemorrhage following IM injection. 0-19 years (Pediatric/Adolescent Formulation): 5mcg at 0, 1, 6 months. 11-15 years (Adult Formulation): 10mcg as first dose, then 10mcg 4-6 months later. | |

| BRAND NAME (GENERIC) | HOW SUPPLIED | ADULTS | COMMENTS |
|---|---|---|---|
| **Combination Vaccines** | | | |
| **Comvax**<br>(*Haemophilus* B conjugate [Meningococcal protein conjugate] and Hepatitis B [recombinant] vaccine) | **Inj:** 7.5mcg PRP polysaccaride conjugated to about 125mcg OMPC and 5 mcg HBsAg [0.5mL] | **Pediatrics ≥6 weeks:** 0.5mL IM at 2, 4, and 12-15 months of age. If schedule cannot be followed, wait at least 6 wks between 1st 2 doses. The 2nd and 3rd dose should be close to 8-11 months apart. | See PI for special populations. |
| **Pediarix**<br>(Diphtheria and tetanus toxoids and acellular pertussis adsorbed, Hepatitis B [recombinant] and Inactivated poliovirus vaccine combined) | **Inj:** 0.5mL | **Pediatrics ≥6 weeks to <7 yrs:** 3 doses of 0.5mL IM at 6-8 wk intervals. Start at 2 months old or as early as 6 wks old if necessary. | Preferred site is anterolateral aspect of the thigh for children <1yr. In older children, deltoid muscle. May use to complete primary series in infants who have received 1 or 2 doses of Infanrix or IPV or to complete a hepatitis B vaccine (recombinant) series. Not recommended for completion of the first 3 doses of the DTaP vaccination series initiated with a DTaP vaccine from a different manufacturer. |
| **Twinrix**<br>Hepatitis A inactivated & Hepatitis B [recombinant] vaccine) | **Inj:** (Hepatitis A-Hepatitis B) 720 ELISA U-20mcg/mL | **Adults ≥18 yrs:** 3-Dose Schedule: 1mL IM in deltoid region at 0, 1, and 6 months. Alternative 4-Dose Schedule: 1 mL IM in deltoid region on Days 0, 7, and 21-30, followed by booster dose at 12 months. | |
| **HEPATITIS C TREATMENT**<br>**Biological Response Modifiers** | | | |
| **Infergen**<br>(Interferon alfacon-1) | **Inj:** 9mcg/0.3mL, 15mcg/0.5mL | **Adults ≥18 yrs:** 9mcg 3x/week (TIW) SQ for 24 wks, wait 48 hrs between doses. If No Response or Relapse: 15mcg TIW SQ as a single injection for up to 48 wks. | Hold dose temporarily in presence of severe adverse effects and reduce to 7.5mcg. |
| **Intron-A**<br>(Interferon alfa-2b, recombinant) | **Inj:** 10 MIU, 18 MIU, 50 MIU, 3 MIU/0.2mL, 5 MIU/0.2mL, 10 MIU/0.2mL, 3MIU/0.5mL, 5MIU/0.5mL | **Adults ≥18 yrs:** 3 MIU IM/SQ TIW for 18-24 months | If severe adverse reactions develop, reduce dose by 50% or temporarily stop therapy. |
| **Roferon-A**<br>(Interferon alfa-2a, recombinant) | **Inj:** 3 MIU/0.5mL, 6 MIU/0.5mL, 9 MIU/0.5mL | **Adults ≥18 yrs:** 3 MIU TIW SQ for 12 months (48-52 weeks) OR 6 MIU TIW for 12 weeks then 3 MIU for 36 wks. | D/C treatment if no response within 3 months. Retreat if tolerated and partial or complete response to therapy but relapsed. Retreatment: 3 MIU TIW OR 6 MIU TIW for 6 to 12 months. If intolerant to prescribed dose, temporarily reduce dose by 50%. If adverse events resolve, reinitiate prescribed dose. |

*(Continued)*

| BRAND NAME (GENERIC) | HOW SUPPLIED | ADULTS | COMMENTS |
|---|---|---|---|
| **Nucleoside Analog** | | | |
| **Copegus** (Ribavirin) | **Tab:** 200mg | **Adults ≥18 yrs:** Give bid in divided doses. Treat for 24-48 wks with Pegasys 180mcg. Genotypes 1 and 4: <75kg: 1000mg/day for 48 wks. ≥75kg: 1200mg/day for 48 wks. Genotypes 2 and 3: 800mg/day for 24 wks. HCV/HIV: 800mg PO QD. Treat for 48 wks with Pegasys 180mcg SQ once weekly. | **Dose Modifications:** Reduce to 600mg/day for Copegus if Hgb <10g/dL with no cardiac history, or if Hgb decreases by ≥2g/dL during a 4-week period with stable cardiac disease. D/C Copegus if Hgb <8.5g/dL with no cardiac history or if Hgb <12g/dL after 4 wks of dose reduction with stable cardiac disease. After dose modification, may restart Copegus at 600mg/day, then may increase to 800mg/day. CrCl <50mL/min: Avoid use. |
| **Rebetol** (Ribavirin) | **Cap:** 200mg; **Sol:** 40mg/mL [100mL] | **Adults ≥18 yrs:** With Intron A: ≤75kg: 400mg qam and 600mg qpm PO. >75kg: 600mg qam and 600mg qpm PO. Treat for 24-48 wks in interferon-naive patients; In relapsed patients, treat for 24 wks. With Peg-Intron: 400mg bid, qam and qpm with food. **Pediatrics ≥3 yrs:** 15mg/kg/day PO in divided doses qam and qpm. Use solution if ≤25kg or cannot swallow caps. With Intron A: 25-36kg: 200mg bid PO, qam and qpm. 37-49kg: 200mg PO qam and 400mg qpm. 50-61kg: 400mg bid PO, qam and qpm. >61kg: Dose as adult. Genotype 1: Treat for 48 wks. Genotype 2/3: Treat for 24 weeks. Reduce to 7.5mg/day (divided dose AM and PM) if Hgb <10g/dL with no cardiac history, or if Hgb decreases by ≥2g/dL during a 4 week-period with a cardiac history. (Intron A for ≥3 yrs: 3 MIU/$m^2$ 3 times weekly SQ). | **Adults:** Reduce to 600mg qd if Hgb <10g/dL with no cardiac history, or if Hgb decreases by ≥2g/dL during a 4 week-period with a cardiac history. **Adults/Peds:** D/C if Hgb <8.5g/dL with no cardiac history or if Hgb <12g/dL after 4 wks of dose reduction with a cardiac history. CrCl <50mL/min: Avoid use. |
| **Ribasphere** (Ribavirin) | **Tab:** 200mg, 400mg, 600mg; **Cap:** 200mg | **Adults ≥18 yrs:** Give bid in divided doses. Treat for 24-48 wks with Pegasys 180mcg. Genotypes 1 and 4: <75kg: 1000mg/day for 48 wks. ≥75kg: 1200mg/day for 48 wks. Genotypes 2 and 3: 800mg/day for 24 wks. HCV/HIV: 800mg PO QD. Treat for 48 wks with Pegasys 180mcg SQ once weekly. | **Dose Modifications:** Reduce to 600mg/day for Ribasphere if Hgb <10g/dL with no cardiac history, or if Hgb decreases by ≥2g/dL during a 4-week period with stable cardiac disease. D/C Ribasphere if Hgb <8.5g/dL with no cardiac history or if Hgb <12g/dL after 4 wks of dose reduction with stable cardiac disease. After dose modification, may restart Ribasphere at 600mg/day, then may increase to 800mg/day. CrCl <50mL/min: Avoid use. |

| BRAND NAME (GENERIC) | HOW SUPPLIED | ADULTS | COMMENTS |
|---|---|---|---|
| **Pegylated Virus Proliferation Inhibitor** | | | |
| **Pegasys** (Peginterferon alfa-2a) | **Inj:** Prefilled syringe: 180mcg/0.5mL; **Single Dose Vial:** 180mcg/mL | **Adults ≥18 yrs:** Monotherapy: 180mcg SQ (in abdomen or thigh) once weekly for 48 weeks. Combination Therapy With Copegus: 180mcg SQ once weekly for 24 weeks with Genotypes 2 and 3 or 48 wks with Genotypes 1 and 4. HCV/HIV: Monotherapy: 180mcg SQ in abdomen or thigh once weekly for 48 weeks. Combination Therapy with Copegus: 180mcg SQ once weekly for 48 wks, regardless of genotype. | Adjust dose based on hematological parameters and depression severity (see PI for dose modifications). |
| **PegIntron** (Peginterferon alpha-2b) | **Inj:** 50mcg/0.5mL, 80mcg/0.5mL, 120mcg/0.5mL, 150mcg/0.5mL | **Adults ≥18 yrs:** Monotherapy: 1mcg/kg/wk SQ for 1 yr administered on the same day of the week. Combination Therapy With Rebetol: 1.5mcg/kg/wk plus Rebetol 800-1400mg/day PO based on patient's body weight for 48 wks in Genotype 1, and 24 wks in Genotype 2 and 3 patients. CrCl <50mL/min: D/C therapy. Adjust dose based on hematological parameters and depression severity (see PI for dose modifications). **Pediatrics 3-17 yrs:** Combination Therapy With Rebetol: 60mcg/m$^2$/wk SQ plus Rebetol 15mg/kg/day in 2 divided doses for 48 wks in Genotype 1, and 24 weeks in Genotype 2 and 3 patients. | **Adults:** Renal Impairment: CrCl 30-50mL/min: Reduce PegIntron dose by 25%. CrCl 10-29mL/min: Reduce PegIntron dose by 50%. D/C therapy if renal function decreases, if there is not at least a 2 log$^{10}$ drop or loss of HCV-RNA at 12 wks, or whose HCV-RNA levels remain detectable after 24 wks of therapy. CrCl <50mL/min: D/C therapy. Adjust dose based on hematological parameters and depression severity (see PI for dose modifications). **Pediatrics:** Renal Impairment: CrCl 30-50mL/min: Reduce PegIntron dose by 25%. CrCl 10-29mL/min: Reduce PegIntron dose by 50%. D/C if renal function decreases, HCV-RNA dropped <2 log$^{10}$ at 12 wks, or HCV-RNA levels remain detectable after 24 wks. |

# ORAL AND SYSTEMIC ANTIBIOTICS

| DRUG | BRAND | HOW SUPPLIED | INDICATIONS |
|---|---|---|---|
| **AMINOGLYCOSIDES** | | | |
| Amikacin sulfate | Amikacin | **Inj:** 50mg/mL, 250mg/mL | Short-term treatment of serious infections caused by gram-negative bacteria such as septicemia, and respiratory tract, bone/joint, CNS (including meningitis), skin and soft tissue, and intra-abdominal infections; burns and postoperative infections; complicated and recurrent urinary tract infections (UTI); and staphylococcal disease. |
| Amikacin sulfate | | **Inj:** 50mg/mL | Concomitant therapy with a penicillin-type drug as treatment of neonatal septicemia. |
| Gentamicin sulfate | | **Inj:** 10mg/mL, 40mg/mL | Treatment of bacterial neonatal sepsis, bacterial septicemia, and serious bacterial infections of the CNS (meningitis), urinary tract, respiratory tract, GI tract (including peritonitis), skin, bone and soft tissue (including burns) caused by susceptible strains of microorganisms. |
| Streptomycin sulfate | | **Inj:** 1g/ampule | Treatment of moderate to severe infections such as mycobacterium tuberculosis (TB) and non-TB infections (eg, plague, tularemia, chancroid, brucella, donovanisis, granuloma inguinale, *H. influenzae* and *K. pneumoniae* infections, UTI, gram-negative bacillary bacteremia, endocardial infections). |
| Tobramycin | TOBI | **Sol:** 60mg/mL (300mg/ampule) | Management of cystic fibrosis patients with *P. aeruginosa*. |
| Tobramycin sulfate | | **Inj:** l0mg/mL, 40mg/mL, l.2g | Treatment of infections including serious lower respiratory tract, CNS (eg, meningitis), intra-abdominal, bone, skin and skin structure, and complicated/recurrent UTIs; and septicemia caused by susceptible strains of microorganisms. |
| **CARBAPENEMS** | | | |
| Doripenem | Doribax | **Inj:** 500mg | Treatment of infections such as complicated intra-abdominal and UTIs, including pyelonephritis, caused by susceptible microorganisms. |
| Ertapenem sodium | Invanz | **Inj:** 1g | Treatment of complicated intra-abdominal infections, SSSI (including diabetic foot infections without osteomyelitits), CAP, complicated UTI (including pyelonephritis), and acute pelvic infections (including postpartum endomyometritis, septic abortion, and post surgical gynecologic infections); also used in prophylaxis of surgical-site infection following elective colorectal surgery. |
| Meropenem | Merrem | **Inj:** 500mg, 1g | Treatment of intra-abdominal infections, bacterial meningitis (in pediatric patients >3 months), and complicated SSSI caused by susceptible strains of microorganisms. |
| **CEPHALOSPORINS, FIRST GENERATION** | | | |
| Cefadroxil monohydrate | | **Cap:** 500mg; **Sus:** 250mg/5mL [50mL, 100mL], 500mg/5mL [50mL, 75mL, 100mL]; **Tab:** 1g | Treatment of SSSI and UTI, pharyngitis, and tonsillitis. |
| Cefazolin | | **Inj:** 500mg, 1g, 10g, 20g | Treatment of respiratory tract, UTI, SSSI, biliary tract, bone and joint, and genital infections, septicemia, and endocarditis caused by susceptible strains of microorganisms. Perioperative prophylaxis for surgical procedures classified as contaminated or potentially contaminated. |
| Cephalexin | Keflex | **Cap:** 250mg, 500mg, 750mg; **Sus:** 125mg/5mL, 250mg/5mL [100mL, 200mL]; **Tab:** 250mg, 500mg | Treatment of otitis media and SSSI; bone, genitourinary tract, and respiratory tract infections. |

*(Continued)*

| DRUG | BRAND | HOW SUPPLIED | INDICATIONS |
|---|---|---|---|
| **CEPHALOSPORINS, SECOND GENERATION** | | | |
| Cefaclor | | **Cap:** 250mg, 500mg; **Sus:** 125mg/5mL [75mL, 150mL], 187mg/5mL [50mL, 100mL], 250mg/5mL [75mL, 150mL], 375mg/5mL [50mL, 100mL] | Treatment of otitis media, pharyngitis, tonsillitis, lower respiratory tract, urinary tract, and SSSI caused by susceptible strains of microorganisms. |
| Cefaclor ER | | **Tab, Extended-Release:** 375mg, 500mg | Acute bacterial exacerbation of chronic bronchitis (ABECB), secondary bacterial infections of acute bronchitis, pharyngitis, tonsillitis, and uncomplicated SSSI caused by susceptible strains of microorganisms. |
| Cefoxitin sodium | | **Inj:** 1g, 2g, 2g/50mL, 10g | Treatment of lower respiratory tract, UTI, intra-abdominal, gynecological, SSSI, and bone and joint infections, and septicemia. For surgical prophylaxis. |
| Cefprozil | Cefzil | **Sus:** 125mg/5mL, 250mg/5mL [50mL, 75mL, 100mL]; **Tab:** 250mg, 500mg | Mild to moderate pharyngitis/tonsillitis, otitis media, acute sinusitis, secondary bacterial infection of acute bronchitis, ABECB, and uncomplicated SSSI. |
| Cefuroxime | Zinacef | **Inj:** 750mg, 1.5g, 7.5g, 750mg/50mL, 1.5g/50mL | Treatment of septicemia; meningitis; gonorrhea; lower respiratory tract, UTI, SSSI, and bone and joint infections caused by susceptible strains of microorganisms. For preoperative and perioperative surgical prophylaxis. |
| Cefuroxime axetil | Ceftin | **Sus:** 125mg/5mL [100mL], 250mg/5mL [50mL, 100mL]; **Tab:** 250mg, 500mg | (Sus/Tab) Pharyngitis/tonsillitis, acute otitis media (Sus) Impetigo. (Tab) Uncomplicated SSSI and UTI, gonorrhea, early Lyme disease, acute bacterial maxillary sinusitis, acute bacterial ABECB and secondary bacterial infections of acute bronchitis. |
| **CEPHALOSPORINS, THIRD GENERATION** | | | |
| Cefdinir | Omnicef | **Cap:** 300mg; **Sus:** 125mg/5mL, 250mg/5mL [60mL, 100mL] | In adults, used to treat CAP, ABECB, acute maxillary sinusitis, pharyngitis/tonsillitis, uncomplicated SSSI; in pediatric patients, used to treat acute bacterial otitis media, pharyngitis/tonsillitis, uncomplicated SSSI. |
| Cefditoren pivoxil | Spectracef | **Tab:** 200mg, 400mg | Treatment of ABECB, pharyngitis/tonsillitis, CAP, and uncomplicated SSSI in adults and adolescents >12 yrs. |
| Cefixime | Suprax | **Sus:** 100mg/5mL [50mL, 75mL, 100mL], 200mg/5mL; **Tab:** 400mg | (Sus/Tab) Pharyngitis, tonsillitis, acute bronchitis, ABECB, uncomplicated UTIs, and cervical/urethral gonorrhea caused by susceptible strains. Otitis media should be treated with suspension. |
| Cefotaxime sodium | Claforan | **Inj:** 500mg, 1g, 2g, 10g | Treatment of lower respiratory tract, genitourinary, gynecologic, intra-abdominal, SSS, bone and joint, and CNS infections (eg, meningitis), as well as bacteremia and septicemia; administered preoperatively to reduce incidence of certain infection from surgical procedures (abdominal hysterectomy, GI and genitourinary tract surgery) that may be classified as contaminated/potentially contaminated; administered during cesarean section postoperatively and intraoperatively (after clamping the umbilical cord) to reduce certain postoperative infections. |
| Cefpodoxime proxetil | | **Sus:** 50mg/mL [50mL, 100mL], 100mg/5mL [50mL, 75mL, 100mL]; **Tab:** 100mg | Acute otitis media, pharyngitis/tonsillitis, CAP, ABECB, acute uncomplicated urethral and cervical gonorrhea, acute uncomplicated ano-rectal infections in women, uncomplicated SSSI, acute maxillary sinusitis, uncomplicated UTI. |

*(Continued)*

| DRUG | BRAND | HOW SUPPLIED | INDICATIONS |
|---|---|---|---|
| **CEPHALOSPORINS, THIRD GENERATION** *(Continued)* | | | |
| Ceftazidime | | **Inj:** 500mg, 1g, 2g, 6g | Treatment of infections such as lower respiratory tract (eg, pneumonia), skin and skin structure (SSSI), bone and joint, gynecologic, CNS (eg, meningitis), intra-abdominal, and UTI, and bacterial septicemia. For use alone in sepsis, or with other antibiotics in severe and life-threatening infections and in immunocompromised patients. |
| Ceftazidime | Fortaz | **Inj:** 500mg, 1g, 1g/50mL, 2g, 2g/50mL, 6g | Treatment of infections such as lower respiratory tract (eg, pneumonia), SSSI, bone and joint, gynecologic, CNS (eg, meningitis), intra-abdominal, and complicated and uncomplicated UTI, and bacterial septicemia. |
| Ceftibuten | Cedax | **Cap:** 400mg; **Sus:** 90mg/5mL [60mL, 90mL, 120mL] | Treatment of individuals with mild-to-moderate infections caused by susceptible strains of the designated microorganisms in ABECB, acute bacterial otitis media, pharyngitis and tonsillitis. |
| Ceftriaxone sodium | | **Inj:** 250mg, 500mg, 1g, 10g | Treatment of lower respiratory tract infections, SSSI, bone and joint infections, intra-abdominal infections, acute otitis media, uncomplicated gonorrhea, pelvic inflammatory disease, UTI, bacterial septicemia, and meningitis. For surgical prophylaxis. |
| **CEPHALOSPORINS, FOURTH GENERATION** | | | |
| Cefepime HCl | Maxipime | **Inj:** 500mg, 1g, 2g | Treatment of uncomplicated/complicated UTI, uncomplicated SSSI, and complicated intra-abdominal infections, and (mild to moderate) pneumonia. Emperic therapy for febrile neutropenia. |
| **FLUOROQUINOLONES** | | | |
| Ciprofloxacin HCl | Cipro | **Sus:** 250mg/5mL, 500mg/5mL [100mL]; **Tab:** 250mg, 500mg, 750mg | (Adults) Treatment of infections such as lower respiratory tract (LRTI), complicated intra-abdominal, SSSI, bone and joint, and UTI; acute exacerbations of chronic bronchitis, acute sinusitis, acute uncomplicated cystitis in females, chronic bacterial prostatitis, infectious diarrhea, typhoid fever, uncomplicated cervical and urethral gonorrhea; (Adults/Pediatrics): Post-exposure inhalation anthrax; (Pediatrics): Complicated UTIs and pyelonephritis. |
| Ciprofloxacin HCl | Proquin XR | **Tab, Extended-Release:** 500mg | Treatment of uncomplicated UTIs (acute cystitis) caused by *E. coli* and *K. pneumoniae.* |
| Ciprofloxacin | Cipro IV | **Inj:** 10mg/mL, 200mg/100mL, 400mg/200mL | (Adults) Treatment of SSSI, bone and joint, complicated intra-abdominal infections, LRTI, and UTI; nosocomial pneumonia, acute sinusitis, chronic bacterial prostatitis, and empirical therapy for febrile neutropenia; (Adults/Pediatrics) Post-exposure inhalation anthrax; (Pediatrics) Complicated urinary tract infections and pyelonephritis. |
| Ciprofloxacin | Cipro XR | **Tab, Extended-Release:** 500mg, 1000mg | Uncomplicated (acute cystitis) and complicated UTI, and acute uncomplicated pyelonephritis due to *E. coli.* |
| Gemifloxacin | Factive | **Tab:** 320mg | Treatment of mild to moderate CAP, including multi-drug resistant *Streptococcus pneumoniae* (MDRSP), and ABECB. |
| Levofloxacin | Levaquin | **Inj:** 5mg/mL, 25mg/mL; **Sol:** 25mg/mL; **Tab:** 250mg, 500mg, 750mg [Leva-pak, 5s] | Uncomplicated and complicated SSSI, uncomplicated and complicated UTI, acute bacterial sinusitis, ABECB, CAP, nosocomial pneumonia, chronic bacterial prostatitis (CBP), and acute pyelonephritis caused by susceptible strains of microorganisms. To reduce the incidence or progression of disease of inhalational anthrax following exposure to *Bacillus anthracis.* |

*(Continued)*

| DRUG | BRAND | HOW SUPPLIED | INDICATIONS |
|---|---|---|---|
| **FLUOROQUINOLONES** *(Continued)* | | | |
| Moxifloxacin HCl | Avelox | **Inj:** 400mg/250mL; **Tab:** 400mg | Acute bacterial sinusitis, ABECB, uncomplicated and complicated SSSI, complicated intra-abdominal infections (cIAI), and CAP (including multidrug resistant *S. pneumoniae*). |
| Norfloxacin | Noroxin | **Tab:** 400 mg | Treatment of adults with UTI (including cystitis), prostatitis, and uncomplicated cervical and urethral gonorrhea, caused by susceptible strains of microorganisms. |
| Ofloxacin | | **Tab:** 200mg, 300mg, 400mg | Treatment of complicated UTI and uncomplicated SSSI, ABECB, CAP, acute uncomplicated urethral and cervical gonorrhea, nongonococcal urethritis and cervicitis, mixed infections of the urethra and cervix, acute pelvic inflammatory disease (PID), uncomplicated cystitis, prostatitis. |
| **MACROLIDES** | | | |
| Azithromycin | Zithromax | **Inj:** 500mg; **Sus:** 100mg/5mL [15mL], 200mg/5mL [15mL, 22.5mL, 30mL], 1g/pkt [3s 10s]; **Tab:** 250mg [Z-Pak, 6 tabs], 500mg [Tri-Pak, 3 tabs], 600mg | (PO): 600mg tab & 1g packet: Treatment of nongonococcal urethritis and cervicitis due to *Chlamydia trachomatis*, as well as prophylaxis (with or without rifabutin) and treatment (in combination with ethambutol) of disseminated mycobacterium avium complex disease in advanced HIV infection; 100mg/5mL, 200mg/5mL, and 250 & 500mg tabs: (Adults) Treatment of acute bacterial exacerbations of COPD, acute bacterial sinusitis (ABS), CAP, pharyngitis/tonsillitis, uncomplicated SSSI, urethritis/cervicitis, genital ulcer disease (men); (Pediatrics): Acute otitis media, pharyngitis/tonsillitis, community acquired pneumonia; (IV) Treatment of CAP and pelvic inflammatory disease. |
| Azithromycin | Zmax | **Sus, Extended-Release:** 2g | Treatment of mild to moderate acute bacterial sinusitis in adults due to *Haemophilus influenzae*, *Moraxella catarrhalis*, or *Streptococcus pneumoniae*. Treatment of CAP in adults and pediatric patients (6 months and older) due to *Chlamydophila pneumoniae*, *Haemophilus influenzae*, *Mycoplasma pneumoniae*, or *Streptococcus pneumoniae* in patients appropriate for oral therapy. |
| Clarithromycin | Biaxin | **Sus:** 125mg/5mL, 250mg/5mL [50mL, 100mL]; **Tab:** 250mg, 500mg | (Adults) Pharyngitis/tonsillitis, acute maxillary sinusitis, ABECB, CAP, uncomplicated SSSI, disseminated mycobacterial infections, combination therapy for *H. pylori* infection with duodenal ulcers; Mycobacterium Avium Complex (MAC) prophylaxis in advanced HIV. (Pediatrics): Pharyngitis/tonsillitis, CAP, acute maxillary sinusitis, acute otitis media, uncomplicated SSSI, disseminated mycobacterial infections, MAC prophylaxis in advanced HIV. |
| Clarithromycin | Biaxin XL | **Tab, Extended-Release:** 500mg [PAC 14s, 60s, 100s] | Treatment of acute maxillary sinusitis, CAP, and ABECB. |
| Erythromycin | ERYC | **Cap, Delayed-Release:** 250mg | Mild to moderate upper and lower RTI and SSSI, listeriosis, pertussis, diphtheria, erythrasma, intestinal amebiasis, acute pelvic inflammatory disease (PID) (*N. gonorrhoeae*), primary syphilis (caused by *Treponema pallidum*) in PCN allergy, Legionnaires' disease, chlamydial infections (eg, newborn conjunctivitis, urethral, endocervical, or rectal, etc), and nongonococcal urethritis (caused by *Ureaplasma urealyticum*). Used as prophylaxis with regards to prevention of initial and recurrent attacks of rheumatic fever with PCN allergy. |

*(Continued)*

| DRUG | BRAND | HOW SUPPLIED | INDICATIONS |
|---|---|---|---|
| **MACROLIDES** *(Continued)* | | | |
| Erythromycin | Ery-Tab | **Tab, Delayed-Release:** 250mg, 333mg, 500mg | Mild to moderate upper and lower RTIs, SSSIs, listeriosis, pertussis, diphtheria, erythrasma, intestinal amebiasis, acute pelvic inflammatory disease (PID) (*N. gonorrhoeae*), primary syphilis in PCN allergy, Legionnaires' disease, chlamydial infections (eg, newborn conjunctivitis, urethral, endocervical, rectal, etc), and nongonococcal urethritis (when tetracyclines are contraindicated or not tolerated). Prophylaxis with regards to prevention of initial and recurrent attacks of rheumatic fever. |
| Erythromycin | Erythromycin | **Cap, Delayed-Release:** 250mg | Mild to moderate upper and lower RTIs, SSSIs, listeriosis, pertussis, diphtheria, erythrasma, intestinal amebiasis, acute pelvic inflammatory disease (PID) (*N. gonorrhoeae*), primary syphilis in PCN allergy, Legionnaires' disease, chlamydial infections (eg, newborn conjunctivitis, urethral, endocervical, rectal, etc), and nongonococcal urethritis (when tetracyclines are contraindicated or not tolerated). Prophylaxis with regards to prevention of initial and recurrent attacks of rheumatic fever. |
| Erythromycin | PCE | **Tab, Delayed-Release:** 333mg, 500mg | Mild to moderate upper and lower RTIs, SSSIs, listeriosis, pertussis, diphtheria, erythrasma, intestinal amebiasis, acute pelvic inflammatory disease (PID) (*N. gonorrhoeae*), primary syphilis in PCN allergy, Legionnaires' disease, chlamydial infections (eg, newborn conjunctivitis, urethral, endocervical, rectal, etc), and nongonococcal urethritis (when tetracyclines are contraindicated or not tolerated). Prophylaxis with regards to prevention of initial and recurrent attacks of rheumatic fever. |
| Erythromycin Base | | **Tab:** 250mg | Mild to moderate upper and lower RTI, SSSI, listeriosis, pertussis, diphtheria, erythrasma, intestinal amebiasis, acute pelvic inflammatory disease (PID) (*N. gonorrhoeae*), primary syphilis in PCN allergy, Legionnaires' disease, chlamydial infections (eg, newborn conjunctivitis, urethral, endocervical, rectal, etc), and nongonococcal urethritis (when tetracyclines are contraindicated or not tolerated). Prophylaxis with regards to prevention of initial and recurrent attacks of rheumatic fever. |
| Erythromycin ethylsuccinate | E.E.S. | **Sus (in liquid and granule premix form):** 200mg/5mL, 400mg/5mL (100mL, 480mL); **Tab:** 400mg | Mild to moderate upper and lower RTIs, SSSI, listeriosis, pertussis, diphtheria, erythrasma, intestinal amebiasis, acute pelvic inflammatory disease (PID) (*N. gonorrhoeae*), primary syphilis in PCN allergy, Legionnaires' disease, chlamydial infections (eg, newborn conjunctivitis, urethral, endocervical, rectal, etc), and nongonococcal urethritis (when tetracyclines are contraindicated or not tolerated). Prophylaxis with regards to prevention of initial and recurrent attacks of rheumatic fever. |
| Erythromycin ethylsuccinate | EryPed | **Sus:** 200mg/5mL, 400mg/5mL [5mL, 100mL, 200mL] | Mild to moderate upper and lower RTI, SSSI, listeriosis, pertussis, diphtheria, erythrasma, intestinal amebiasis, acute pelvic inflammatory disease (PID) (*N. gonorrhoeae*), primary syphilis in PCN allergy, Legionnaires' disease, chlamydial infections (eg, newborn conjunctivitis, urethral, endocervical, rectal, etc), and nongonococcal urethritis (when tetracyclines are contraindicated or not tolerated). Prophylaxis with regards to prevention of initial and recurrent attacks of rheumatic fever. |
| Erythromycin ethylsuccinate/ Sulfisoxazole | | **Sus:** 200/600 [100mL, 200mL] | For treatment of acute otitis media in children that is caused by susceptible strains of *Haemophilus influenzae*. |

*(Continued)*

| DRUG | BRAND | HOW SUPPLIED | INDICATIONS |
|---|---|---|---|
| **MACROLIDES** *(Continued)* | | | |
| Erythromycin stearate | Erythrocin | **Tab:** 250mg, 500mg | Mild to moderate upper and lower RTIs, SSSI, listeriosis, pertussis, diphtheria, erythrasma, intestinal amebiasis, acute pelvic inflammatory disease (PID) (*N. gonorrhoeae*), primary syphilis in PCN allergy, Legionnaires' disease, chlamydial infections (eg, newborn conjunctivitis, urethral, endocervical, rectal, etc), and nongonococcal urethritis (when tetracyclines are contraindicated or not tolerated). Prophylaxis with regards to prevention of initial and recurrent attacks of rheumatic fever. |
| **MONOBACTAM** | | | |
| Aztreonam | Azactam | **Inj:** 1g, 2g, 1g/50mL, 2g/50mL | Treatment of septicemia and lower RTIs (eg, pneumonia, bronchitis), SSSIs (eg, postoperative wounds, ulcers, burns), complicated/uncomplicated UTIs including pyelonephritis and initial/recurrent cystitis, gynecologic infections (eg, endometritis, pelvic cellulitis), and intra-abdominal (eg, peritonitis) infections caused by susceptible microorganisms. Adjunct therapy to surgery for management of infections caused by susceptible microorganisms (eg, abscesses, hollow viscus perforation infections, cutaneous infections, infections of serous surfaces). |
| Aztreonam | Cayston | **Inj:** 75mg/vial (Lyophilized) | Respiratory symptoms in cystic fibrosis patients with *Pseudomonas aeruginosa*. |
| **PENICILLINS** | | | |
| Amoxicillin | Amoxil | **Cap:** 250mg, 500mg; 125mg/5mL [80mL, 100mL, 150mL], 200mg/5mL [50mL, 75mL, 100mL], 250mg/5mL [80mL, 100mL, 150mL], 400mg/5mL [50mL, 75mL, 100mL]; **Tab:** 500mg, 875mg; **Tab, Chewable:** 200mg, 400mg **Tab, Dispersible:** 200mg, 400mg, 600mg | Infections of the ear, nose, throat, genitourinary tract, SSSI, and lower RTI due to susceptible (beta-lactamase negative) organisms, as well as gonorrhea (acute, uncomplicated). Also used in *H. pylori* eradication to reduce the risk of duodenal ulcer recurrence. |
| Amoxicillin | Moxatag | **Tab, Extended Release:** 775mg | Treatment of tonsillitis and/or pharyngitis secondary to *Streptococcus pyogenes* in adults and pediatric patients ≥12 yrs. |
| Amoxicillin-Clavulanate potassium | | **(Amoxicillin-Clavulanate) Sus:** 125-31.25mg/5mL [75mL, 100mL, 150mL] 200-28.5mg/ 5mL [50mL, 75mL, 100mL], 250-62.5mg/5mL [75mL, 100mL, 150mL], 400-57mg/ 5mL [50mL, 75mL, 100mL]; **Tab:** 250-125mg, 500-125mg, 875-125mg; **Tab, Chewable:** 125-31.25mg, 200-28.5mg, 250-62.5mg, 400-57mg | Treatment of lower RTI, SSSI, and UTI, as well as otitis media and sinusitis. |
| Amoxicillin-Clavulanate potassium | Augmentin ES-600 | **Sus:** (Amoxicillin-Clavulanate) 600mg-42.9mg/5mL [75mL, 125mL, 200mL] | Treatment of pediatric patients with recurrent or persistent acute otitis media. |

*(Continued)*

| DRUG | BRAND | HOW SUPPLIED | INDICATIONS |
|---|---|---|---|
| **PENICILLINS** *(Continued)* | | | |
| Amoxicillin-Clavulanate potassium | Augmentin XR | **Tab, Extended-Release:** (Amoxicillin-Clavulanate) 1000mg-62.5mg | Treatment of CAP or acute bacterial sinusitis due to confirmed or suspected β-lactamase producing pathogens and *S. pneumoniae* with reduced susceptibility to penicillin. |
| Ampicillin sodium | Ampicillin | **Inj:** 125mg, 250mg, 500mg, 1g, 2g, 10g | Treatment of respiratory tract, urinary tract, and GI infections, bacterial meningitis, septicemia, endocarditis. |
| Ampicillin sodium/ Sulbactam sodium | Unasyn | **Inj:** (Ampicillin-Sulbactam) 1g-0.5g, 2g-1g, 10g-5g | Treatment of SSSI, intra-abdominal, and gynecological infections caused by susceptible microorganisms. |
| Carbenicillin sodium | | **Tab:** 382mg | Treatment of acute and chronic infections of the upper and lower UTI and asymptomatic bacteriuria. |
| Dicloxacillin sodium | | **Cap:** 250mg, 500mg | Infections caused by penicillinase-producing *staphylococci*. |
| Penicillin G benzathine-Penicillin G procaine | Bicillin C-R | **Inj:** (Penicillin G Benzathine-Penicillin G Procaine) 600,000-600,000 U/2mL | Treatment of moderately severe to severe URTI and skin and soft-tissue infections (SSTI), scarlet fever and erysipelas due to *streptococci*. Treatment of moderately severe pneumonia and otitis media due to *pneumococci*. |
| Penicillin G benzathine-Penicillin G procaine | Bicillin C-R 900/300 | **Inj:** (Penicillin G Benzathine-Penicillin G Procaine) 900,000-300,000 U/2mL | Treatment of moderately severe to severe URTI and SSTI, scarlet fever and erysipelas due to *streptococci*. Treatment of moderately severe pneumonia and otitis media due to *pneumococci*. |
| Penicillin G benzathine | Bicillin L-A | **Inj:** 300,000 U/mL, 600,000 U/mL, 1,200,000 U/2mL, 2400000 U/4mL | Treatment of mild to moderate URTI due to *streptococci*, and venereal infections (eg, syphilis, yaws, bejel, pinta); prophylaxis to prevent recurrence of rheumatic fever or chorea. |
| Penicillin G benzathine | Permapen | **Inj:** 600,000 U/mL | Treatment of microorganisms susceptible to low and very prolonged serum levels in upper respiratory tract infections (*streptococci* group A, without bacteremia), syphilis, yaws, bejel, and pinta; prophylaxis for rheumatic fever and/or chorea. Follow-up prophylactic therapy for rheumatic heart disease and acute glomerulonephritis. |
| Penicillin G potassium | Pfizerpen | **Inj:** 5 MU, 20 MU | For therapy of severe infections when rapid and and high blood levels of penicillin required. Management of streptococcal, pneumococcal, staphylococcal, clostridial, fusospirochetal, listeria, gram negative bacillary, and pasteurella infections. For anthrax, actinomycosis, diphtheria, erysipeloid, meningitis (including *meningococci*), endocarditis, bacteremia, rat-bite fever, syphilis, and gonorrheal endocarditis and arthritis; with combined oral therapy, prophylaxis against endocarditis in patients with congenital heart disease, rheumatic disease, or other acquired valvular heart disease undergoing dental procedures or surgical procedures of upper respiratory tract. |
| Penicillin V potassium | Penicillin VK | **Sus:** 125mg/5mL, 250mg/5mL [100mL, 200mL]; **Tab:** 250mg, 500mg | Mild to moderately severe bacterial infections including scarlet fever, mild erysipelas, mild to moderate infections of the respiratory tract, mild to moderately severe oropharynx infections, and mild infections of skin and soft tissue. Prevention of recurrence following rheumatic fever and/or chorea. |
| Piperacillin | | **Inj:** 2g, 3g, 4g, 40g | Treatment of serious intra-abdominal, urinary tract, gynecologic, lower respiratory tract, SSSI, bone and joint, and gonococcal infections; septicemia, and perioperative surgical prophylaxis. |

*(Continued)*

| DRUG | BRAND | HOW SUPPLIED | INDICATIONS |
|---|---|---|---|
| **PENICILLINS** *(Continued)* | | | |
| Piperacillin sodium/ Tazobactam sodium | Zosyn | **Inj:** 40mg-5mg/mL, 60mg-7.5mg/mL, 2g-0.25g, 3g-0.375g, 4g-0.5g, 4g-0.5g/ 100mL, 36g-4.5g | Treatment of appendicitis, peritonitis, uncomplicated/complicated SSSIs, postpartum endometritis, pelvic inflammatory disease, moderate severity of CAP, and moderate to severe nosocomial pneumonia. |
| Ticarcillin-Clavulanate potassium | Timentin | **Inj:** (Ticarcillin-Clavulanate) 3g-100mg, 3g-200mg, 30g-1g | Treatment of lower respiratory tract, bone and joint, SSS, UTI, gynecologic, and intra-abdominal infections, as well as septicemia. |
| **TETRACYCLINES** | | | |
| Demeclocycline HCl | | **Tab:** 150mg, 300mg | Treatment of infections due to rickettsiae, respiratory tract infections due to *Mycoplasma pneumoniae*, relapsing fever due to *B. recurrentis*, agents of psittacosis, lymphomagranuloma venereum or granuloma inguinale. |
| Doxycycline | Oracea | **Cap:** 40mg | Treatment of only inflammatory lesions (papules and pustules) of rosacea in adults. |
| Doxycycline | Vibramycin | **Cap:** (Doxycycline Hyclate) 50mg, 100mg; **Syrup:** (Doxycycline Calcium) 50mg/5mL; **Sus:** (Doxycycline Mono hydrate) 25mg/5mL [60mL] | Treatment of susceptible infections including respiratory, urinary, lymphogranuloma, psittacosis, trachoma, inclusion conjunctivitis, uncomplicated urethral/endocervical/rectal infections, relapsing fever, nongonococcal urethritis, illnesses caused by rickettsiae, chancroid, plague, cholera, campylobacter fetus infections, brucellosis, bartonellosis, and granuloma inguinale. When penicillin is contraindicated, treatment of uncomplicated gonorrhea, syphilis, listeriosis, *Clostridium* species infections, actinomycosis, yaws, and Vincent's infection. Adjunct therapy for amebiasis (adjunct to amebicides) and severe acne. Prophylaxis of malaria. |
| Doxycycline hyclate | Doryx | **Tab:** 75mg, 100mg, 150mg | Treatment of susceptible infections including RTI, UTI, uncomplicated urethral/endocervical/rectal, lymphogranuloma, psittacosis, trachoma, inclusion conjunctivitis, replapsing fever due to borrelia recurrentis, nongonococcal urethritis, rickettsiae, chancroid, plague, cholera, brucellosis, bartonellosis, campylobacter fetus infections, tularemia, relapsing fever, inhalation anthrax (post exposure). When penicillin is contraindicated, treatment of syphilis, listeriosis, yaws, Vincent's infection, actinomycosis, and infections from *Clostridium* species. Adjunct therapy for amebiasis and severe acne. Prophylaxis of malaria. |
| Doxycycline hyclate | Periostat | **Tab:** 20mg | Adjunct to scaling and root planing to promote attachment level gain and reduces pocket depth in patients with adult periodontitis. |
| Doxycycline hyclate | Vibra-tabs | **Tab:** 100mg | Treatment of susceptible infections including respiratory, urinary, lymphogranuloma, psittacosis, trachoma, inclusion conjunctivitis, uncomplicated urethral/endocervical/rectal infections, relapsing fever, nongonococcal urethritis, illnesses caused by rickettsiae, chancroid, plague, cholera, campylobacter fetus infections, brucellosis, bartonellosis, and granuloma inguinale. When penicillin is contraindicated, treatment of uncomplicated gonorrhea, syphilis, listeriosis, *Clostridium* species infections, actinomycosis, yaws, and Vincent's infection. Adjunct therapy for amebiasis (adjunct to amebicides) and severe acne. Prophylaxis of malaria. |

*(Continued)*

| DRUG | BRAND | HOW SUPPLIED | INDICATIONS |
|---|---|---|---|
| **TETRACYCLINES** *(Continued)* | | | |
| Doxycycline monohydrate | Monodox | **Cap:** 50mg, 75mg, 100mg | Treatment of RTI, UTI, and SSSIs, uncomplicated urethral/endocervical/ rectal infection caused by *C. trachomatis*, illnesses due to rickettsiae, relapsing fever, nongonococcal urethritis caused by *U. Urealyticum*, lymphogranuloma venereum, psittacosis, trachoma & inclusion conjunctivitis caused by *C. trachomatis*, chancroid, plague, cholera, brucellosis, tularemia, campylobacter fetus infections, bartonellosis, and granuloma inguinale. Treatment of uncomplicated gonorrhea, syphilis, listeriosis, anthrax, *Clostridium* species infections, actinomycosis, Vincent's infection, and yaws, all when PCN is contraindicated. Adjunct therapy for amebicides (adjunct to amebicides) and severe acne. |
| Minocycline HCl | Dynacin | **Tab:** 50mg, 75mg, 100mg | Treatment of respiratory tract, urinary tract, and skin and skin structure infections, lymphogranuloma, psittacosis, trachoma, uncomplicated urethral/endocervical/rectal infection caused by Chlamydia, nongonococcal urethritis, chancroid, plague, tularemia, cholera, brucellosis, inclusion conjunctivitis, bartonellosis, campylobacter fetus infections, granuloma inguinale, relapsing fever, and illnesses due to rickettsiae. When PCN is contraindicated, treatment of uncomplicated gonorrhea, syphilis, listeriosis, anthrax, *Clostridium* species infections, yaws, Vincent's infection, actinomycosis. Adjunct therapy for amebicides (in acute intestinal amebiasis) and severe acne. |
| Minocycline HCl | Minocin | **Cap:** 50mg, 100mg | Treatment of inclusion conjunctivitis, trachoma, relapsing fever, lymphogranuloma vereneum, rickettsiae, chancroid, plague, tularemia, campylobacter fetus infections, brucellosis, bartenollosis, granuloma inguinale nongonococcal urethritis, and other infections (eg, respiratory tract, endocervical, rectal, urinary tract, skin and skin structure) caused by susceptible strains of microorganisms. Alternative treatment in certain other infections (eg, uncomplicated urethritis, yaws, listeriosis, Vincent's infection, actinomycosis, syphilis, anthrax). Adjunctive therapy in acute intestinal amebiasis and severe acne. Treatment of Mycobacterium marinum and asymptomatic carriers of *Neisseria meningitidis*. |
| Minocycline HCl | Solodyn | **Tab, Extended-Release:** 45mg, 90mg, 135mg | Treatment of inflammatory lesions of non-nodular moderate to severe acne vulgaris in patients ≥12 yrs. |
| Tetracycline HCl | Sumycin | **Sus:** 125mg/5mL; **Cap:** 250mg, 500mg | Treatment of RTI, UTI, and SSSIs, lymphogranuloma, psittacosis, trachoma, uncomplicated urethral/ endocervical/rectal infection caused by Chlamydia, nongonococcal urethritis, chancroid, plague, tularemia, cholera, brucellosis, inclusion conjunctivitis, bartonellosis, campylobacter fetus infections, granuloma inguinale, relapsing fever, and illnesses due to rickettsiae. When PCN is contraindicated, treatment of uncomplicated gonorrhea, syphilis, listeriosis, anthrax, *Clostridium* species infections, yaws, Vincent's infection, actinomycosis. Adjunct therapy for amebicides (in acute intestinal amebiasis) and severe acne. |

*(Continued)*

| DRUG | BRAND | HOW SUPPLIED | INDICATIONS |
|---|---|---|---|
| **MISCELLANEOUS** | | | |
| Clindamycin | Cleocin | **Cap:** (HCl) 75mg, 150mg, 300mg; **Inj:** (Phosphate) 150mg/mL, 300mg/50mL, 600mg/50mL, 900mg/50mL; **Pediatric Solution:** palmitate (HCl) 75mg/5mL [100mL] | Serious infections caused by anaerobes, *streptococci*, *pneumococci*, and *staphylococci*. |
| Colistimethate sodium | Coly-Mycin M | **Inj:** 150mg | Treatment of acute or chronic infections due to certain gram-negative bacilli (eg, *Pseudomonas aeruginosa*, *Enterobacter aerogenes*, *E. coli*, *Klebsiella pneumoniae*). |
| Dalfopristin-Quinupristin | Synercid | **Inj:** (Dalfopristin-Quinupristin) 350mg-150mg per 500mg vial; 420mg-180mg per 600mg vial | Treatment of serious or life-threatening infections associated with vancomycin-resistant *Enterococcus faecium* (VREF) bacteremia and complicated SSS caused by *Staphylococcus aureus* (methicillin susceptible) or *Streptococcus pyogenes*. |
| Dapsone | Dapsone | **Tab:** 25mg, 100mg | Treatment of leprosy and dermatitis herpetiformis. |
| Daptomycin | Cubicin | **Inj:** 500mg/vial | Susceptible complicated SSSI. *Staphylococcus aureus* bloodstream infections (bacteremia). |
| Fosfomycin tromethamine | Monurol | **Pow:** 3g/sachet | Uncomplicated UTI (acute cystitis) in women due to susceptible strains of *Escherichia coli* and *Enterococcus faecalis*. |
| Isoniazid-Rifampin | Rifamate | **Cap:** (Isoniazid-Rifampin) 150mg-300mg | For pulmonary TB when patient has been titrated on the individual components and it has been established that fixed dosage is therapeutically effective. Not for initial therapy or prevention of TB. |
| Isoniazid-Rifampin-Pyrazinamide | Rifater | **Tab:** (Isoniazid-Pyrazinamide-Rifampin) 50mg-300mg-120mg | For initial phase of short-course treatment of pulmonary TB. |
| Lincomycin HCl | Lincocin | **Inj:** 300mg/mL | Treatment of serious infections due to *streptococci*, *pneumococci*, and *staphylococci*. Reserve for PCN allergy or if PCN is inappropriate. |
| Linezolid | Zyvox | **Inj:** 2mg/mL [100mL, 200mL, 300mL]; **Sus:** 100mg/5mL; **Tab:** 600mg | Vancomycin-resistant *Enterococcus faecium* (VRE) infections, nosocomial pneumonia caused by *S. Aureus* (methicillin-susceptible and resistant strains) or *S. Pneumoniae* (including multidrug-resistant strains [MDRSP]), complicated SSSI including diabetic foot infections without concomitant osteomyelitis (caused by *S. Aureus* [methicillin-susceptible and resistant strains], *S. Pyogenes*, or *S. Agalactiae*), uncomplicated SSSIs caused by *S. Aureus* (methicillin-susceptible only) or *S. Pyogenes*, CAP caused by *S. Pneumoniae* (MDRSP) or *S. Aureus* (methicillin-susceptible strains only). |
| Methenamine hippurate | Hiprex | **Tab:** 1g | Prophylaxis or suppression of recurrent UTIs when long-term therapy is necessary. For use only after infection is eradicated by other appropriate antimicrobials. |
| Metronidazole | Flagyl | **Cap:** 375mg; **Tab:** 250mg, 500mg | Treatment of symptomatic and asymptomatic trichomoniasis, asymptompatic consorts, amebiasis, and anaerobic bacterial infections; in combination with IV metronidazole, treatment of intra-abdominal, SSSI, gynecologic, bone and joint, CNS (eg, meningitis), and lower RTIs, as well as endocarditis and bacterial septicemia. |
| Metronidazole HCl | Flagyl IV | **Inj:** 500mg (RTU) | Treatment of anaerobic intra-abdominal, SSSI, gynecologic, bone and joint, CNS, and lower respiratory tract infections, as well as endocarditis and bacterial septicemia. Prophylaxis preoperatively, intraoperatively, and postoperatively to reduce incidence of postoperative infection in patients undergoing elective colorectal surgery. |

*(Continued)*

| DRUG | BRAND | HOW SUPPLIED | INDICATIONS |
|---|---|---|---|
| **MISCELLANEOUS** *(Continued)* | | | |
| Nitrofurantoin | Furadantin | **Sus:** 25mg/5mL | Treatment of UTIs when due to susceptible strains of *Escherichia coli, enterococci, Staphylococcus aureus*, and certain susceptible strains of *Klebsiella* and *Enterobacter* species. |
| Nitrofurantoin macrocrystals | Macrodantin 100mg | **Cap:** 25mg, 50mg, 100mg | Treatment of UTIs when due to susceptible strains of *Escherichia coli, enterococci, Staphylococcus aureus*, and certain susceptible strains of *Klebsiella* and *Enterobacter* species. |
| Nitrofurantoin monohydrate | Macrobid | **Cap:** 100mg | Treatment of acute uncomplicated UTIs (acute cystitis). |
| Rifampin | Rifadin | **Cap:** 150mg, 300mg; **Inj:** 600mg | Treatment of all forms of TB. Treatment of asymptomatic carriers of *Neisseria meningitidis* to eliminate *meningococci* from the nasopharynx. |
| Sulfamethoxazole-Trimethoprim | | Sulfamethoxazole ([SMX]-Trimethoprim [TMP]) **Inj:** 80mg-16mg/mL; **Sus:** 200mg-40mg/5mL [100mL, 473mL]; **Tab:** 400mg-80mg; **Tab, DS:** 800mg-160mg (Generic available in tablet and DS form, as well as Suspension (in 473mL and 20ml sizes) | Treatment of UTI, PCP, and enteritis caused by Shigella. Treatment of AECB, travelers' diarrhea, and acute otitis media. |
| Telavancin | Vibativ | **Inj:** 250mg, 750mg | Treatment of adult patients with complicated SSSI caused by susceptible gram-positive microorganisms. |
| Telithromycin | Ketek | **Tab:** 300mg [20$^s$], 400mg [60$^s$, Ketek Pak, 100$^s$] | Treatment of mild to moderate community-acquired pneumonia (CAP) due to *S. pneumoniae* (including MDRSP), *H. influenzae, M. catarrhalis, C. pneumoniae*, or *M. pneumoniae* for patients >18 yrs. |
| Trimethoprim HCl | Primsol | **Sol:** 50mg/5mL | Treatment of acute otitis media in pediatrics and UTI in adults. |
| Trimethoprim-Sulfamethoxazole | Bactrim | (Sulfamethoxazole [SMX]-Trimethoprim [TMP]) **Tab:** 400mg-80mg; **Tab, DS:** 800mg-160mg | Treatment of UTI, acute otitis media, AECB, travelers' diarrhea, shigellosis, and PCP. |
| Tygecycline | Tygacil | **Inj:** 50mg/5mL, 50mg/10mL [vial] | Treatment of complicated SSSI, complicated intra-abdominal infections (cIAI), and community-acquired bacterial pneumonia (CABP) caused by susceptible strains of indicated pathogens in patients ≥18 yrs. |
| Vancomycin HCl | | **Inj:** 500mg/100mL, 1g/250mL 500mg/vial, 750mg/vial, 1g/vial, 5g/vial, 10g/vial | Treatment of severe infections caused by susceptible strains of methicillin-resistant *staphylococci*. Indicated for penicillin-allergic patients, those who cannot receive or have failed to respond to other drugs, and for vancomycin-susceptible organisms that are resistant to other antimicrobials. |
| Vancomycin HCl | Vancocin Oral | **Cap:** 125mg, 250mg | Treatment of enterocolitis caused by *Staphylococcus aureus* (including methicillin-resistant strains) and antibiotic-associated pseudomembranous colitis caused by *C. difficile*. |

# SYSTEMIC ANTIFUNGALS

| GENERIC | BRAND | INDICATION | DOSAGE FORM | DOSAGE |
|---|---|---|---|---|
| Amphotericin B | | Progressive, potentially life-threatening fungal infections: Aspergillosis, cryptococcosis, North American blastomycosis, systemic candidiasis, coccidioidomycosis, histoplasmosis, zygomycosis, sporotrichosis, and infections due to *Conidiobolus* and *Basidiobolus* species. | **Inj:** 50mg | Initial: 0.25mg/kg. Titrate: Increase by 5-10mg/day, depending on cardio-renal status, up to 0.5-0.7mg/kg/day. |
| Amphotericin B cholesteryl sulfate | Amphotec | Treatment of invasive aspergillosis in patients with renal impairment, unacceptable toxicity, or previous failure to amphotericin deoxycholate. | **Inj:** 50mg, 100mg | 3-4mg/kg/day IV at 1mg/kg/hr. |
| Amphotericin B lipid complex injection | Abelcet | Invasive fungal infections in patients who are refractory to or intolerant of conventional amphotericin B therapy. | **Inj:** 5mg/mL | Single infusion 5mg/kg. |
| Amphotericin B liposome injection | AmBisome | Treatment of patients with *Aspergillus* species, *Candida* species, and/or *Cryptococcus* species infections refractory to amphotericin B deoxycholate or in patients where renal impairment or unacceptable toxicity precludes the use of amphotericin B deoxycholate. Treatment of visceral leishmaniasis. Empirical therapy for presumed fungal infections in febrile neutropenic patients. Treatment of cryptococcal meningitis in HIV-infected patients. | **Inj:** 50mg | 3-6mg/kg/day. Empiric therapy = 3mg/kg/day IV. Systemic infections (*Aspergillus, Candida, Cryptococcus*): 3-5mg/kg/day IV. Cryptococcal Meningitis in HIV: 6mg/kg/day IV. Visceral Leishmaniasis for Immunocompetent patients: 3mg/kg/day on Days 1-5 and 3mg/kg/day on Days 14, 21. Visceral Leishmaniasis in Immunocompromised patients: 4mg/kg/day on Days 1-5 and 4mg/kg/day on Days 10, 17, 24, 31, 38. |
| Anidulafungin | Eraxis | Treatment of candidemia and other forms of *Candida* infections, esophageal candidiasis. | **Inj:** 50mg, 100mg | Candidemia: LD 200mg on Day 1, MD 100mg x 14d. Esophageal Candidiasis: LD 100mg qd x 1 day then 50mg qd x 14 days. |
| Caspofungin Acetate | Cancidas | Treatment of candidemia and the following *Candida* infections: intra-abdominal abscesses, peritonitis and pleural space infections and esophageal candidiasis, fungal infections in febrile, neutropenic patients, invasive aspergillosis in patients who are refractory to or intolerant of other therapies. | **Inj:** 50mg, 70mg | 70mg LD on Day 1 and then 50mg qd. Esophageal candidasis: 50mg qd. |
| Clotrimazole | Mycelex Troche | Oropharyngeal candidiasis. To prevent oropharyngeal candidiasis in immunocompromised conditions. | **Loz/Troche:** 10mg | 1 troche in mouth 5 times/day for 14 days. Prophylaxis: 1 troche tid. |

*(Continued)*

| GENERIC | BRAND | INDICATION | DOSAGE FORM | DOSAGE |
|---|---|---|---|---|
| Fluconazole | Diflucan | Treatment of vaginal candidiasis, oropharyngeal, and esophageal, candidiasis. The treatment of *Candida* urinary tract infections, peritonitis, and systemic *Candida* infections including candidemia, disseminated candidiasis, and pneumonia. Treatment of cryptococcal meningitis. Prophylaxis in patients undergoing BMT. | **Inj:** 200mg/100mL, 400mg/200mL; **Sus:** 350mg/35mL, 1400mg/35mL [35mL]; **Tab:** 50mg, 100mg, 150mg, 200mg | Vaginal *Candida*: 150mg po x 1 day. **Cryptococcal meningitis:** 400mg on Day 1 then 200mg qd. **Prophylaxis in patients undergoing bone marrow transplantation:** 400mg qd. All other: 200mg on Day 1, then 100mg qd. Max: 400mg/day. |
| Flucytosine | Ancobon | Treatment of septicemia, endocarditis, and urinary tract infections caused by *Candida*. Treatment of meningitis and pulmonary infection caused by *Cryptococcus*. | **Cap:** 250mg, 500mg | 50-150mg/kg/day given q6h. |
| Griseofulvin | Grifulvin V | Treatment of ringworm. | **Sus:** 125mg/5mL [120mL]; **Tab:** 500mg | 0.5-1g qd. |
| Griseofulvin | Gris-PEG | Treatment of ringworm. | **Tab (ultramicrosize):** 125mg, 250mg | 375mg as a single dose or in divided doses. |
| Itraconazole | Sporanox | Onychomycosis of the toenail and fingernail, blastomycosis and histoplasmosis. Treatment of aspergillosis if refractory to or intolerant of amphotericin B. (Sol) Treatment of oropharyngeal and esophageal candidiasis. | **Cap:** 100mg; **Inj:** 10mg/mL; **Sol:** 10mg/mL [150mL] | **(Cap)** Blastomycosis: 200mg once daily (2 capsules). Aspergillosis: 200-400mg. Max: 400mg/day. **(Inj):** 200mg bid for 4 doses, followed by 200mg once daily for up to 14 days. **(Sol):** Swish (20mL at a time) for several seconds and swallow. |
| Ketoconazole | Nizoral | Candidiasis, chronic mucocutaneous candidiasis, oral thrush, candiduria, blastomycosis, coccidioidomycosis, histoplasmosis, chromomycosis, and paracoccidioidomycosis. Treatment of patients with severe recalcitrant cutaneous dermatophyte infections not responsive to topical therapy or oral griseofulvin. Not for treatment of fungal meningitis. | **Tab:** 200mg | 200mg qd. Max: 400mg qd. |
| Micafungin sodium | Mycamine | Esophageal candidiasis and prophylaxis of *Candida* infection in HSCT patients. Treatment of candidemia, acute disseminated candidiasis, *Candida* peritonitis, and abscesses. | **Inj:** 50mg, 100mg | Treatment of Candidemia, Acute Disseminated Candidiasis, *Candida* Peritonitis and Abscesses: 100mg IV qd (usual range 10-47 days). Treatment of Esophageal Candidiasis: 150mg/day (usual range 10-30 days); Prophylaxis (HSCT): 50mg IV qd (usual range 6-51 days). |
| Posaconazole | Noxafil | Prophylaxis of invasive *Aspergillus* and *Candida*, oropharyngeal candidiasis, including oropharyngeal candidiasis refractory to itraconazole and/or fluconazole. | **Sus:** 40mg/mL [105mL] | Prophylaxis: 200mg tid. Oropharyngeal Candidiasis: 100mg bid x 1 day, 100mg qd x 13 days. Oropharyngeal Candidiasis refractory to itraconazole and/or fluconazole = 400mg bid. |

*(Continued)*

| GENERIC | BRAND | INDICATION | DOSAGE FORM | DOSAGE |
|---|---|---|---|---|
| Terbinafine HCl | Lamisil | (Tab): Onychomycosis of the toenail or fingernail. (Granules): Tinea capitis in patients ≥4 years old. | **Tab:** 250mg; **Granules:** 125mg/packet and 187.5mg/packet | **(Tab)** 250mg po qd for 6 weeks for fingernail and 12 weeks for toenail. **(Gran)** ≤25kg: 125mg/day, 25-35kg: 187.5mg/day, >35kg: 250mg/day. Take for 6 weeks. |
| Voriconazole | Vfend | Invasive aspergillosis, esophageal candidiasis, serious fungal infections caused by *Scedosporium apiospermum* and *Fusarium* spp. including *Fusarium solani*, candidemia in nonneutropenic patients. | **Inj:** 200mg; **Sus:** 40mg/mL [100mL]; **Tab:** 50mg, 200mg | 200mg po q12h. IV LD: 6mg/kg q12h for first 24h. IV MD: 3-4mg/kg q12h. |

# ANKYLOSING SPONDYLITIS AGENTS

| DRUG (BRAND) | HOW SUPPLIED | USUAL DOSE RANGE | MAX DOSE |
|---|---|---|---|
| **COX-2 INHIBITOR** | | | |
| **Celecoxib** (Celebrex) | **Cap:** 50mg, 100mg, 200mg, 400mg | 200mg qd or 100mg bid. | 400mg/day with food. |
| **MONOCLONAL ANTIBODIES/TNF-RECEPTOR BLOCKERS** | | | |
| **Adalimumab** (Humira) | **Inj:** 20mg/0.4mL, 40mg/0.8mL | 40mg SQ every other wk. | n/a |
| **Golimumab** (Simponi) | **Inj:** 50mg/0.5mL | 50mg SQ every month. | n/a |
| **Infliximab** (Remicade) | **Inj:** 100mg [20 mL] | 5mg/kg as IV infusion repeat at 2 and 6 wks then every 6 wks thereafter. | 20mg/kg. |
| **NSAIDs** | | | |
| **Diclofenac sodium** (Voltaren, Voltaren XR) | **Tab, Delayed-Release:** 75mg; (generic) 25mg, 50mg, 75mg **Extended-Release:** 100mg | 25mg qid and 25mg qhs prn. | 125mg/day. |
| **Indomethacin** (Indocin) | **Cap:** 25mg, 50mg; **Sus:** 25mg/5mL [237mL]; **Cap, Extended-Release:** (Generic) 75mg | Take with food. **Cap/Sus:** 25mg bid-tid; may increase by 25-50mg/day at wkly intervals. **ER:** 75mg qd; may increase by 75mg/day. | **Cap/Sus:** 150-200mg/day. **ER:** 150mg/day. |
| **Naproxen** (EC-Naprosyn, Naprosyn) | **Sus:** 25mg/mL; **Tab:** 250mg, 375mg, 500mg; **Tab, Delayed-Release:** (EC) 375mg, 500mg | 250mg, 375mg, or 500mg bid. | 1500mg/day. |
| **Naproxen sodium** | | | |
| (Anaprox) | **Tab:** 275mg | 275mg bid or 550mg bid. | 1500mg/day. |
| (Anaprox DS) | **Tab:** 550mg* | 275mg bid or 550mg bid. | 1500mg/day. |
| (Naprelan) | **Tab, Extended-Release:** 375mg, 500mg, 750mg | 750mg-1g qd. | 1500mg/day. |
| **Sulindac** (Clinoril) | **Tab:** 150mg, 200mg* | 150mg bid with food. | 400mg/day with food. |
| **TNF-RECEPTOR BLOCKER** | | | |
| **Etanercept** (Enbrel) | **Inj:** 25mg [vial], 50mg/mL [syringe] | 50mg SQ per wk, given as one 50-mg injection or two 25-mg injections. | 50mg/wk. |

*Scored.

# BONE MINERAL DENSITY CLASSIFICATION/TESTS

| World Health Organization (WHO) Definition of Osteoporosis | |
|---|---|
| Normal | Bone mineral density within 1 standard deviation (SD) of the young adult mean (T-score $\geq -1.0$) |
| Osteopenia (low bone mass) | Bone mineral density between 1.0 and 2.5 SD below the young adult mean ($-2.5 <$ T-score $< -1.0$) |
| Osteoporosis | Bone mineral density 2.5 SD or more below the young adult mean (T-score $\leq -2.5$) |
| Note: The definitions above should not be applied to premenopausal women, men <50 years of age, and children. | |

## Bone mineral density (BMD) tests

- BMD tests provide a measurement of T-score for bone density at hip and spine to:
  - —Establish and confirm a diagnosis of osteoporosis
  - —Predict future fracture risk
  - —Measure response to osteoporosis treatment
- BMD is measured in grams of mineral per square centimeter scanned (g/cm$^2$) and compared to the expected BMD for the patient's age and sex (Z-score) or compared with "normal adults" of the same sex (T-score).
- The difference between the patient's score and the optimal BMD is expressed in standard deviations (SD) above and below the mean. Usually 1 SD equals about 10-15% of the bone density value in g/cm$^2$.
- Negative values for T-score, such as $-1.5$, $-2$, or $-2.5$, indicate low bone mass.
- The greater the negative score, the greater the risk of fracture.

# DIETARY CALCIUM INTAKE

**Recommended Calcium Intakes***

| Age | Daily Intake (mg) |
|---|---|
| Birth-6 months | 210 |
| 6 months-1 year | 270 |
| 1-3 years | 500 |
| 4-8 years | 800 |
| 9-13 years | 1300 |
| 14-18 years | 1300 |
| 19-30 years | 1000 |
| 31-50 years | 1000 |
| 51-70 years | 1200 |
| 70 years or older | 1200 |
| **Pregnant or Lactating** | |
| 14-18 years | 1300 |
| 19-50 years | 1000 |

*Source: National Institute of Arthritis and Musculoskeletal and Skin Diseases (NIAMS); National Institutes of Health

**Estimating Daily Dietary Calcium Intake**

**Step 1:** Estimate calcium intake from calcium-rich foods.*

| Product | Servings/Day | Calcium/Serving (mg) | | Calcium (mg) |
|---|---|---|---|---|
| Milk (8 oz) | ______ | × 300 | = | ______ |
| Yogurt (8 oz) | ______ | × 400 | = | ______ |
| Cheese (1 oz, or 1 cubic inch) | ______ | × 200 | = | ______ |
| Fortified foods or juices | ______ | × 80-1000** | = | ______ |

**Step 2:** Total from above + 250 mg for nondairy sources = total dietary calcium.

* About 75-80% of the calcium consumed in American diets is from dairy products.
** Calcium content of fortified foods varies.

**Factors related to vitamin D that may affect calcium absorption:**

- National Osteoporosis Foundation recommends an intake of 800 to 1000 International Units (IU) of vitamin $D_3$ per day for adults over age 50
- Desired level for the average adult's serum 25(OH)D concentration is 30 ng/mL (75 nmol/L) or higher
- Safe upper limit for vitamin D intake for normal adult population was set at 2000 IU per day in 1997
- Patients with malabsorption (eg, celiac disease) or chronic renal insufficiency, or those who are housebound, chronically ill, or have limited sun exposure, may need vitamin D supplements

**Source:** National Institute of Arthritis and Musculoskeletal and Skin Diseases (NIAMS), National Institutes of Health, National Osteoporosis Foundation.

# Gout Agents

| DRUG (BRAND) | HOW SUPPLIED | USUAL DOSE RANGE | MAX DOSE |
|---|---|---|---|
| **ALKALINIZING AGENTS** | | | |
| **Citric Acid/ Potassium Citrate** (Cytra-K Crystals) | 1002mg-3300mg/pack [100[s]] | 1 packet qid, pc and hs. Reconstitute with at least 6 oz of cool water or juice. | |
| **Citric Acid Monohydrate/ Potassium Citrate Monohydrate/ Sodium Citrate Dihydrate** (Cytra-3) | **Syr:** (Citric Acid Monohydrate-Potassium Citrate Monohydrate-Sodium Citrate Dihydrate) 334mg-550mg-500mg/5mL | 15-30mL diluted with water, qid, pc and hs. | |
| **Citric Acid Monohydrate/ Potassium Citrate Monohydrate** (Cytra-K) | (Citric Acid Monohydrate-Potassium Citrate Monohydrate) 334mg-1100mg/5mL | 10-15mL diluted with a glassful of water, qid, pc and hs. | |
| **CORTICOSTEROIDS** | | | |
| **Hydrocortisone sodium succinate** (A-Hydrocort) | **Inj:** 100mg/2mL | **Acute Gout:** Individualized dosing. May repeat dose at intervals of 2,4, or 6 hours based on patient response. | |
| **Hydrocortisone** (Cortef) | **Tab:** 5mg, 10mg, 20mg | **Acute Gout:** Individualized dosing. | |
| **Methylprednisolone** (Medrol) | **Tab:** 4mg, 8mg, 16mg, 32mg | **Acute Gout:** Individualized dosing. | |
| **Prednisone** | **Tab:** 1mg, 2.5mg, 5mg, 10mg, 20mg, 50mg; **Sol:** 5mg/mL, 5mg/5mL | **Acute Gout:** Individualized dosing. | |
| **NSAIDs** | | | |
| **Indomethacin** (Indocin) | **Cap:** (Generic) 25mg, 50mg; **Sus:** 25mg/5mL [237mL] | **Acute Gout:** 50mg PO tid until pain is tolerable, then d/c. | |
| **Naproxen** (Naprosyn) | **Sus:** 25mg/mL; **Tab:** 250mg*, 375mg, 500mg* | **Acute Gout:** 750mg followed by 250mg q8h until attack subsides. | |
| **Naproxen Sodium** (Anaprox) | **Tab:** 275mg | **Acute Gout:** 825mg followed by 275mg q8h. | |
| (Anaprox DS) | **Tab:** 550mg* | **Acute Gout:** 825mg followed by 275mg q8h. | |
| (Naprelan) | **Tab, Controlled-Release:** 375mg, 500mg, 750mg | **Acute Gout:** 1-1.5g qd x 1 day, then 1g qd until attack subsides. | 1.5g/day. |
| **Sulindac** (Clinoril) | **Tab:** (Generic) 150mg (Clinoril, Generic) 200mg* | **Acute Gout:** 200mg bid, usually for 7 days. | 400mg/day |
| **PHENANTHRENE DERIVATIVE** | | | |
| **Colchicine** | **Tab:** 0.6mg | **Acute Gout:** 0.6-1.2mg, then 0.6mg/hr or 1.2mg q2h until pain relieved or diarrhea ensues (wait 3 days between courses). **Prophylaxis:** <1 attack/yr: 0.6mg/day given 3-4x/wk; >1 attack/year, 0.6mg qd. **Prophylaxis in Patients Undergoing Surgery:** 0.6mg tid for 3 days before and 3 days after surgery. | |
| (Colcrys) | **Tab:** 0.6mg | **Acute Gout:** 1.2mg at first sign of flare, then 0.6mg one hr later. **Prophylaxis:** 0.6mg qd-bid. | 1.8mg over 1 hr period. 1.2mg/day. |

*(Continued)*

| DRUG (BRAND) | HOW SUPPLIED | USUAL DOSE RANGE | MAX DOSE |
|---|---|---|---|
| **URICOSURIC AGENT** | | | |
| **Probenecid** | **Tab:** 500mg | **Initial:** 250mg bid x 1 wk<br>**Maint:** 500mg bid.<br>**Titrate:** May increase by 500mg every 4 wks. | 2g/day. |
| **XANTHINE OXIDASE INHIBITORS** | | | |
| **Allopurinol** (Zyloprim) | **Tab:** 100mg*, 300mg* | **Mild Gout: Usual:** 200-300mg/day.<br>**Moderately-Severe Gout: Usual:** 400-600mg/day. | 800mg/day. |
| **Febuxostat** (Uloric) | **Tab:** 40mg, 80mg | **Initial:** 40mg qd. Increase to 80mg qd if serum uric acid >6mg/dL after 2 weeks. | |
| **COMBINATION** | | | |
| **Colchicine/ Probenecid** | **Tab:** (Colchicine-Probenecid) 0.5mg-500mg | 1 tab qd x 1 wk, then 1 tab bid.<br>**Titrate:** May increase by 1 tab/day every 4 wks. | 4 tabs/day. |
| *Scored. | | | |

# OSTEOARTHRITIS AGENTS

| DRUG (BRAND) | HOW SUPPLIED | USUAL DOSE RANGE | MAX DOSE |
|---|---|---|---|
| **COX-2 INHIBITOR** | | | |
| **Celecoxib** (Celebrex) | **Cap:** 50mg, 100mg, 200mg, 400mg | 200mg qd or 100mg bid. | |
| **NSAIDs** | | | |
| **Diclofenac epolamine** (Flector) | **Patch:** 180mg [5[s]] | Apply 1 patch to most painful area bid. | 1 patch bid. |
| **Diclofenac potassium** (Cataflam) | **Tab:** 50mg | 50mg bid-tid | 150mg/day. |
| **Diclofenac sodium** (Voltaren) | **Tab, Delayed-Release:** (Generic) 25mg, 50mg, 75mg (Voltaren) 75mg | 50mg bid-tid or 75mg bid. | 150mg/day. |
| (Voltaren-XR) | **Tab, Extended-Release:** 100mg | 100mg qd. | 100mg/day. |
| (Voltaren Gel) | **Gel:** 1% [20g, 100g] | Measure onto enclosed dosing card to appropriate 2g or 4g line. Lower Extremities: Apply 4g to affected foot, knee, or ankle qid. Upper Extremities: Apply 2g to affected hand, elbow, or wrist qid. | Lower Extremities: 16g/day to any single joint. Upper Extremities: 8g/day to any single joint. 32g/day over all affected joints. |
| (Pennsaid) | 1.5% [15mL, 60mL, 150mL] | 40 drops per knee qid. | |
| **Diflunisal** | **Tab:** 500mg | 250-500mg bid. | 1500mg/day. |
| **Etodolac** | **Cap:** 200mg, 300mg; **Tab:** 400mg, 500mg | 300mg bid-tid or 400-500mg bid. | 1000mg/day. |
| (Etodolac XR) | **Tab, Delayed-Release:** 400mg, 500mg, 600mg | 400-1000mg qd. | 1000mg/day. |
| **Fenoprofen calcium** (Nalfon) | **Cap:** (Nalfon) 200mg, 400mg; **Tab:** (Generic) 600mg | 400-600mg tid-qid. | 3200mg/day. |
| **Flurbiprofen** (Ansaid) | **Tab:** 50mg, 100mg | 200-300mg/day given bid, tid or qid. | 300mg/day or 100mg/dose. |
| **Ketoprofen** | **Cap:** 50mg, 75mg; **Cap, Extended-Release:** 100mg, 150mg, 200mg | 75mg tid or 50mg qid. **ER:** 200mg qd. | 300mg/day. **ER:** 200mg/day. |
| **Ibuprofen** | **Sus:** 100mg/5mL [120mL, 473mL] | 300mg qid or 400mg, 600mg, or 800mg tid-qid. | 3200mg/day. |
| | **Tab:** 400mg, 600mg, 800mg | 400mg, 600mg, or 800mg tid-qid. | 3200mg/day. |
| (Motrin IB) | **Tab:** 200mg | 200mg q4-6h. 400mg if no response. | |
| **Indomethacin** (Indocin) | **Cap:** (Generic) 25mg, 50mg; **Cap, Extended-Release:** (Generic) 75mg; **Sus:** (Indocin) 25mg/5mL | **Initial:** 25mg bid-tid. **Titrate:** Increase by 25 or 50mg at weekly intervals until reach satisfactory response. **ER: Initial:** 75mg qd. **Titrate:** May increase to 75mg bid. | 200mg/day. **ER:** 150mg/day. |
| **Meclofenate sodium** | **Cap:** 50mg, 100mg | 200-400mg/day in 3-4 divided doses. | 400mg/day. |
| **Meloxicam** (Mobic) | **Sus:** 7.5mg/5mL; **Tab:** 7.5mg, 15mg | 7.5mg qd. | 15mg/day. |
| **Nabumetone** | **Tab:** 500mg, 750mg | 1000mg qd. | 2000mg/day. |
| **Naproxen** (Naprosyn) | **Sus:** 25mg/mL; **Tab:** 250mg, 375mg, 500mg. | 250, 375, or 500mg bid. | 1500mg/day. |
| (EC-Naprosyn) | **Tab, Delayed-Release:** 375mg, 500mg | 375 or 500mg bid. | 1500mg/day. |
| **Naproxen sodium** (Anaprox) | **Tab:** 275mg | 275mg bid. | 1500mg/day. |
| (Anaprox DS) | **Tab:** 550mg* | 550mg bid. | 1500mg/day. |
| (Naprelan) | **Tab, Extended-Release:** 375mg, 500mg, 750mg | 750mg-1g qd. | 1.5g/day. |

*(Continued)*

| DRUG (BRAND) | HOW SUPPLIED | USUAL DOSE RANGE | MAX DOSE |
|---|---|---|---|
| **NSAIDs** *(Continued)* | | | |
| **Oxaprozin** (Daypro) | **Tab:** 600mg* | 1200mg qd. | 1800mg/day or 26mg/kg/day in divided doses (whichever is lower) |
| **Piroxicam** (Feldene) | **Cap:** 10mg, 20mg | 20mg qd or 10mg bid. | 20mg/day |
| **Sulindac** (Clinoril) | **Tab:** (Generic) 150mg, (Clinoril, generic) 200mg* | 150mg bid with food. | 400mg/day with food. |
| **Tolmetin** | **Cap:** 400mg; **Tab:** 200mg*, 600mg | 200-600mg tid. | 1800mg/day. |
| **NSAID COMBINATION** | | | |
| **Diclofenac sodium/Misoprostol** (Arthrotec) | **Tab:** 50mg-0.2mg, 75mg-0.2mg | 50mg tid. Do not crush, chew or divide. | **Diclofenac:** 150mg/day; **Misoprostol:** 200mcg/dose, 800mcg/day. |
| **NON-SALICYLATE ANALGESIC** | | | |
| **Acetaminophen** (Tylenol Arthritis Pain) | **Tab, Extended-Release:** 650mg | 1300mg q8h. | 3900mg/day (6 caps/day) |
| **SALICYLATE** | | | |
| **Aspirin** (Genuine Bayer Aspirin) | **Tab:** 325mg | 1-2 tabs every 4 hrs or 3 tabs every 6 hrs. | 12 tabs/day. |
| (Extra Strength Bayer Aspirin) | **Tab:** 500mg | 1-2 tabs every 4-6 hrs. | 8 tabs/24 hrs. |
| (Ecotrin) | **Tab, Delayed-Release:** 81mg, 325mg, 500mg | Up to 3g/day in divided doses. | 3g/day. |
| **Salsalate** | **Tab:** 500mg, 750mg | 3000mg daily, given as 1500mg bid or 1000mg tid. | |
| **MISCELLANEOUS** | | | |
| **Botanical/Mineral substances** (Traumeel Inj) | **Inj:** 2.2mL amps [10s] | 1 amp qd for acute disorders, otherwise 1 amp 1-3 times per week. May administer IV, IM, SQ, or periarticularly. | NA |
| **Flavocoxid** (Limbrel) | **Cap:** 250mg, 500mg | 250-500mg q12h. | 500-1000mg/day. |
| **Hyaluronan** (Euflexxa) | **Inj:** 1% [2mL] | Inject 2mL intra-articularly into the knee weekly for 3 wks. Total 3 injections. | 3 injections. |
| (Hyalgan) | **Inj:** 2mL | 2mL by intra-articular injection once a wk. Some patients may experience benefit with 3 injections given at weekly intervals. | 5 injections. |
| (Orthovisc) | **Inj:** 30mg/2mL | 30mg intra-articularly once a wk. Total 3-4 injections. | 3-4 injections. |
| (Supartz) | **Inj:** 2.5mL | 2.5mL by intra-articular injection once a wk. Total 5 injections. Some patients may experience benefit with 3 injections given at weekly intervals. | 5 injections. |
| **Hylan G-F 20** (Synvisc) | **Inj:** 8mg/mL | Intra-articular injection once weekly (one wk apart). Total 3 injections. | 3 injections. |

*Scored

# OSTEOPOROSIS AGENTS

| DRUG (BRAND) | INDICATIONS | HOW SUPPLIED | DOSAGE |
|---|---|---|---|
| **BISPHOSPHONATES & COMBINATIONS** | | | |
| **Alendronate Sodium** (Fosamax) | Treatment and prevention of osteoporosis in postmenopausal women. Treatment to increase bone mass in men with osteoporosis. Treatment of glucocorticoid-induced osteoporosis. | Sol: 70mg [75mL]; Tab: 5mg, 10mg, 35mg, 40mg, 70mg | Osteoporosis: Treatment: 70mg once weekly or 10mg qd. Prevention: 35mg once weekly or 5mg qd. Increase bone mass in men with osteoporosis: 70mg once weekly or 10mg qd. Glucocorticoid-Induced: 5mg qd; 10mg qd for post-menopausal women not on estrogen.Take at least 30 min before the first food, beverage (other than plain water), or medication. Take tabs with 6-8 oz plain water or 2oz with oral sol. Do not lie down for at least 30 min and until after 1st food of day. |
| **Alendronate Sodium/ Cholecalciferol** (Fosamax Plus D) | Treatment of osteoporosis in postmenopausal women. Treatment to increase bone mass in men with osteoporosis. | Tab: (Alendronate Sodium-Cholecalciferol) 70mg-2800 IU, 70mg-5600 IU | Adults: 1 tab (70mg/5600 IU or 70mg/2800 IU) once weekly. Take at least 30 min before 1st food, beverage (other than plain water), or medication. Do not lie down for at least 30 min and until after 1st food of day. |
| **Ibandronate Sodium** (Boniva) | (Inj) Treatment of osteoporosis in postmenopausal women. (PO) Treatment and prevention of postmenopausal osteoporosis. | Inj: 3mg/3mL; Tab: 150mg | Inj: 3mg IV over 15-30 sec every 3 months. PO: 150mg once monthly. Swallow whole with 6-8 oz plain water. Do not lie down for 60 min after dose. Take at least 60 min before 1st food, drink (other than plain water), medication, or supplementation. |
| **Risedronate Sodium** (Actonel) | Prevention and treatment of osteoporosis in postmenopausal women, glucocorticoid-induced osteoporosis in men and women. Increase bone mass in men with osteoporosis. | Tab: 5mg, 30mg, 35mg, 150mg | Postmenopausal Osteoporosis Prevention/Treatment: 5mg qd or 35mg once weekly or 75mg on 2 consecutive days each month or 150mg once a month. Glucocorticoid-Induced Osteoporosis: 5mg qd. Increase Bone Mass in Men with Osteoporosis: 35mg once weekly. Take at least 30 min before the first food or drink of the day other than water. Swallow tab in upright position with 6-8 oz of plain water. Do not lie down for 30 min after dose. |
| **Risedronate Sodium/ Calcium Carbonate** (Actonel with Calcium) | Treatment and prevention of postmenopausal osteoporosis. | Tab: (Risedronate Sodium) 35mg; Tab: (Calcium Carbonate) 1250mg | Risedronate: 35mg once weekly (Day 1 of 7-day treatment cycle). Take at least 30 min before 1st food or drink of day other than water. Swallow tab in upright position with 6-8 oz of plain water. Do not lie down for 30 min after dose. Calcium: 1250mg qd with food on each of remaining 6 days (Days 2-7 of the 7-day treatment cycle). |
| **Zoledronic Acid** (Reclast) | Treatment and prevention of osteoporosis in post-menopausal women. Treatment to increase bone mass in men with osteoporosis. Treatment and prevention of corticoid-induced osteoporosis in men and women. | Sol: 5mg/100mL [100mL] | Osteoporosis (Men and Post-menopausal Women): 5mg IV once a year over >15 min at a constant infusion rate. Prevention of Osteoporosis (Postmenopausal Women): 5 mg IV given every 2 yrs over >15 min at a constant infusion rate. Treatment/Prevention of Glucocorticoid-Induced Osteoporosis: 5mg IV once a year over >15 min at a constant infusion rate. |

| DRUG (BRAND) | INDICATIONS | HOW SUPPLIED | DOSAGE |
|---|---|---|---|
| **HORMONE THERAPY** | | | |
| **Conjugated Estrogens** (Premarin Tabs) | Prevention of postmenopausal osteoporosis. | Tab: 0.3mg, 0.45mg, 0.625mg, 0.9mg, 1.25mg | 0.3mg qd continuous or cyclically (eg, 25 days on, 5 days off). |
| **Conjugated Estrogens/ Medroxyprogesterone Acetate** (Premphase) | Prevention of postmenopausal osteoporosis in women with intact uterus. | Tab: 0.625mg (Estrogens, Conjugated) and 0.625mg-5mg (Estrogens, Conjugated-Medroxyprogesterone) | 0.625mg tab qd on Days 1-14 and 0.625mg-5mg tab qd on Days 15-28. Re-evaluate periodically. |
| **Conjugated Estrogens/ Medroxyprogesterone Acetate** (Prempro) | Prevention of postmenopausal osteoporosis in women with intact uterus. | Tab: (Estrogens, Conjugated-Medroxyprogesterone) 0.3mg-1.5mg, 0.45mg-1.5mg, 0.625mg-2.5mg, 0.625mg-5mg | Take 1 tab qd. Re-evaluate periodically. |
| **Estradiol** (Alora) | Prevention of postmenopausal osteoporosis. | Patch: 0.025mg/ 24 hrs [8s], 0.05mg/ 24 hrs [8s, 24s], 0.075mg/24 hrs, 0.1mg/24 hrs [8s] | Apply to lower abdomen, upper quadrant of the buttocks or the hip; avoid breasts and waistline. Rotate application sites. Osteoporosis: Apply 0.025mg/day twice weekly. Titrate: May increase depending on bone mineral density and adverse events. |
| **Estradiol** (Climara) | Prevention of postmenopausal osteoporosis. | Patch: 0.025mg/day, 0.0375mg/day, 0.05mg/day, 0.06mg/day, 0.075mg/day, 0.1mg/day [4s] | Apply 1 patch weekly to lower abdomen or upper area of buttocks (avoid breasts and waistline). Rotate application sites. Minimum Effective Dose: 0.025mg/day once weekly. Re-evaluate as clinically appropriate. |
| **Estradiol** (Estrace) | Prevention of osteoporosis. | Tab: 0.5mg*, 1mg*, 2mg* *scored | Lowest effective dose has not been determined. When prescribing solely for the prevention of postmenopausal osteoporosis, therapy should be considered only for women at significant risk of osteoporosis and for whom non-estrogen medications are not considered to be appropriate. |
| **Estradiol** (Estraderm) | Prevention of postmenopausal osteoporosis. | Patch: 0.05mg/24 hrs, 0.1mg/24 hrs [8s, 24s] | Initial: 0.05mg/day. May give continuously without intact uterus. May give cyclically (3 weeks on, 1 week off) with intact uterus. Apply to clean, dry area on trunk of body. Do not apply to breast or waistline. Replace twice weekly. Rotate application site. |
| **Estradiol** (Menostar) | Prevention of postmenopausal osteoporosis. | Patch: 14mcg/day [4s] | Apply 1 patch weekly to lower abdomen (avoid breasts, waistline, and areas where sitting would dislodge the patch). Rotate application sites. |
| **Estradiol** (Vivelle, Vivelle-Dot) | Prevention of postmenopausal osteoporosis. | Patch: (Vivelle) 0.05mg/day, 0.1mg/day [8s]; (Vivelle-Dot) 0.025mg/day, 0.0375mg/day, 0.05mg/day, 0.075mg/day, 0.1mg/day [8s, 24s] | Minimum Effective Dose: 0.025mg/day twice weekly. Apply to clean, dry area of the trunk; avoid breasts and waistline. Rotate sites; allow 1 week between same site. Without intact uterus, may give continuously; with intact uterus, may give cyclically (3 weeks on, 1 week off) with a progestin. |

| DRUG (BRAND) | INDICATIONS | HOW SUPPLIED | DOSAGE |
|---|---|---|---|
| **HORMONE THERAPY** *(Continued)* | | | |
| **Estradiol/Levonorgestrel** (Climara Pro) | Prevention of postmenopausal osteoporosis. | Patch: (Estradiol-Levonorgestrel): 0.045mg-0.015mg/day [4[s]] | Apply 1 patch weekly to lower abdomen (avoid breasts and waistline). Rotate application site; allow 1 week between same site. Re-evaluate periodically (3-6 month intervals). |
| **Estradiol/Norethindrone** (Activella) | Prevention of postmenopausal osteoporosis in women with intact uterus. | Tab: (Estradiol-Norethindrone) 1mg-0.5mg, 0.5mg-0.1mg | 1 tab qd. |
| **Estradiol/Norgestimate** (Prefest) | Prevention of postmenopausal osteoporosis in women with intact uterus. | Tab: (Estradiol) 1mg and (Estradiol-Norgestimate) 1mg-0.09mg | 1 estradiol (pink color) tab for three days followed by 1 estradiol-norgestimate (white color) tab for three days. Repeat regimen continuously. |
| **Estropipate** (Ogen) | Prevention of postmenopausal osteoporosis. | Tab: 0.625mg* (0.75mg estropipate), 1.25mg* (1.5mg estropipate), 2.5mg* (3mg estropipate), *scored | 0.75mg (as estropipate) qd for 25 days of 31-day cycle. |
| **Ethinyl Estradiol/ Norethindrone** (Femhrt) | Prevention of postmenopausal osteoporosis in women with intact uterus. | Tab: (Ethinyl Estradiol-Norethindrone) 2.5mcg-0.5mg, 5mcg-1mg | 1 tab qd. Assess response by measuring bone mineral density. |
| **MISCELLANEOUS** | | | |
| **Calcitonin-Salmon** (Miacalcin) | Treatment of postmenopausal osteoporosis in females >5 yrs postmenopause. | Inj: 200 IU/mL; Nasal Spray: 200 IU/inh | (Inj) 100 IU IM/SQ every other day. If >2mL, use IM injection. (Spray) 200 IU qd intranasally. Alternate nostrils daily. Take with supplemental calcium and vitamin D for postmenopausal osteoporosis. |
| **Calcitonin-Salmon** (Fortical) | Treatment of postmenopausal osteoporosis in females >5 yrs postmenopause in conjunction with an adequate calcium and vitamin D intake. | Nasal Spray: 200 IU/inh | 200 IU qd intranasally. Alternate nostrils daily. |
| **Raloxifene** (Evista) | Treatment and prevention of osteoporosis in postmenopausal women. | Tab: 60mg | 60mg qd. |
| **Teriparatide** (Forteo) | Treatment of postmenopausal women with osteoporosis at high risk for fracture. To increase bone mass in men with primary or hypogonadal osteoporosis at high risk for fracture. Treatment of men and women with glucocorticoid-induced osteoporosis at high risk for fracture. | Inj: 250mcg/mL [2.4mL, 3mL pen] | 20mcg qd SQ into thigh or abdominal wall. Administer initially under circumstances where patient can sit or lie down if symptoms of orthostatic hypotension occur. Discard pen after 28 days. Use for >2 yrs is not recommended. |

# RHEUMATOID ARTHRITIS AGENTS

| DRUG (Brand) | HOW SUPPLIED | USUAL DOSE RANGE | MAX DOSE |
|---|---|---|---|
| **5-AMINOSALICYLIC ACID DERIVATIVE** | | | |
| **Sulfasalazine** (Azulfidine EN) | **Tab, Delayed-Release:** 500mg | 1g bid. | 3g/day. |
| **COPPER CHELATING AGENT** | | | |
| **Penicillamine** (Cuprimine, Depen) | **Cap:** (Cuprimine) 250mg; **Tab:** (Depen) 250mg* | **Initial:** 125-250mg/day **Maint:** 500-750mg/day | 1.5g/day. |
| **COX-2 INHIBITOR** | | | |
| **Celecoxib** (Celebrex) | **Cap:** 50, 100mg, 200mg, 400mg | 100-200mg bid. | |
| **DIHYDROFOLIC ACID REDUCTASE INHIBITOR** | | | |
| **Methotrexate sodium** (Trexall) | **Inj:** 25mg/mL; **Tab:** 2.5mg, 5mg, 7.5mg, 10mg, 15mg | 7.5mg once weekly. | 20mg/wk. |
| **GOLD AGENT** | | | |
| **Auranofin** (Ridaura) | **Cap:** 3mg | 6mg qd or 3mg bid. | 9mg/day. |
| **IMMUNOSUPPRESSANTS** | | | |
| **Azathioprine** (Imuran) | **Tab:** 50mg*; **Inj:** (Generic) 100mg/20mL | **Initial:** 1mg/kg/day given qd-bid. **Titrate:** Increase by 0.5mg/kg/day after 6-8 wks, then at 4 wk intervals. | 2.5mg/kg/day. |
| **Cyclosporine** (Neoral) | **Cap:** 25mg, 100mg; **Sol:** 100mg/mL [50mL] | **Initial:** 1.25mg/kg bid. **Titrate:** Increase by 0.5-0.75mg/kg/day after 8 wks, again after 12 wks. D/C if no benefit by wk 16. | 4mg/kg/day. |
| **INTERLEUKIN-1 RECEPTOR ANTAGONIST** | | | |
| **Anakinra** (Kineret) | **Inj:** 100mg/0.67mL | 100mg SQ qd. | |
| **INTERLEUKIN-6 RECEPTOR ANTAGONIST** | | | |
| **Tocilizumab** (Actemra) | **Inj:** 20mg/mL [80mg/4mL, 200mg/10mL, 400mg/20mL] | **Initial:** 4mg/kg every 4 weeks as 60 min infusion. **Titrate:** Increase to 8mg/kg based on response. | 800mg/infusion. |
| **MONOCLONAL ANTIBODIES/CD20-BLOCKER** | | | |
| **Rituximab** (Rituxan) | **Inj:** 10mg/mL | Two-1000mg IV infusions separated by 2 wks, with MTX. | 400mg/hr infusion rate |
| **MONOCLONAL ANTIBODIES/TNF-BLOCKERS** | | | |
| **Adalimumab** (Humira) | **Inj:** 20mg/0.4mL, 40mg/0.8mL [Prefilled Glass Syringe], 40mg/0.8mL [Prefilled Pen] | 40mg SQ every other wk. | 40mg every week w/o MTX. |
| **Golimumab** (Simponi) | **Inj:** 50mg/0.5mL | 50mg SQ once a month. Give with MTX. | |
| **Infliximab** (Remicade) | **Inj:** 100mg/20mL | 3mg/kg IV infusion repeat at 2 and 6 wks. **Maint:** 3mg/kg every 8 wks. | 10mg/kg or every 4 wks. |
| **NONSTEROIDAL ANTI-INFLAMMATORY DRUGS (NSAIDs)** | | | |
| **Diclofenac Potassium** (Cataflam) | **Tab:** 50mg | 50mg tid-qid. | 200mg/day. |
| **Diclofenac Sodium** (Voltaren) | **Tab, Delayed-Release:** (Generic) 25mg, 50mg, 75mg, (Voltaren) 75mg. | 50mg tid-qid or 75mg bid. | 200mg/day. |
| (Voltaren XR) | **Tab, Extended-Release:** 100mg | 100mg qd-bid. | 200mg/day. |

*(Continued)*

| DRUG (Brand) | HOW SUPPLIED | USUAL DOSE RANGE | MAX DOSE |
|---|---|---|---|
| **NONSTEROIDAL ANTI-INFLAMMATORY DRUGS (NSAIDs)** *(Continued)* | | | |
| **Diflunisal** | **Tab:** 500mg | 250-500mg bid. | 1500mg/day. |
| **Etodolac** | **Cap:** 200mg, 300mg<br>**Tab:** 400mg, 500mg | 300mg bid-tid or 400-500mg bid. | 1000mg/day. |
| (Etodolac XR) | **Tab, Extended-Release:** 400mg, 500mg, 600mg | 400-1000mg qd. | 1000mg/day. |
| **Fenoprofen Calcium** (Nalfon) | **Cap:** (Nalfon) 200mg, 400mg<br>**Tab:** (Generic) 600mg | 400-600mg tid-qid. | 3200mg/day. |
| **Flurbiprofen** (Ansaid) | **Tab:** 50mg, 100mg | 200-300mg/day given bid, tid or qid. | 300mg/day<br>100mg/dose. |
| **Ibuprofen** | **Sus:** 100mg/5mL [120mL, 473mL] | 300mg qid or 400mg, 600mg, or 800mg tid-qid. | 3200mg/day. |
| | **Tab:** 400mg, 600mg, 800mg | 400mg, 600mg, or 800mg tid-qid. | 3200mg/day. |
| (Motrin IB) | **Tab:** 200mg | 200mg q4-6h. 400mg if no response. | 1200mg/day. |
| **Indomethacin** (Indocin) | **Cap:** (Generic) 25mg, 50mg<br>**Cap, Extended-Release:** (Generic) 75mg<br>**Sus:** (Indocin) 25mg/5mL | **Initial:** 25mg bid-tid<br>**Titrate:** Increase by 25mg or 50mg at weekly intervals until reach satisfactory response.<br>**ER: Initial:** 75mg qd.<br>**Titrate:** May increase to 75mg bid. | 200mg/day<br>**ER:** 150mg/day. |
| **Ketoprofen** | **Cap:** 50mg, 75mg;<br>**Cap, Extended-Release:** 100mg, 150mg, 200mg | 75mg tid or 50mg qid.<br>**ER:** 200mg qd | 300mg/day.<br>**ER:** 200mg/day. |
| **Meclofenamate Sodium** | **Cap:** 50mg, 100mg | 200-400mg/day in 3-4 divided doses. | 400mg/day. |
| **Meloxicam** (Mobic) | **Sus:** 7.5mg/5mL; **Tab:** 7.5mg, 15mg | 7.5mg qd. | 15mg/day. |
| **Nabumetone** (Relafen) | **Tab:** 500mg, 750mg | 1000mg qd. | 2000mg/day. |
| **Naproxen** (Naprosyn) | **Sus:** 25mg/mL; **Tab:** 250mg, 375mg, 500mg | 250, 375, or 500mg bid. | 1500mg/day. |
| (EC-Naprosyn) | **Tab, Delayed-Release:** 375mg, 500 mg | 375 or 500mg bid. | 1500mg/day. |
| **Naproxen Sodium** (Anaprox) | **Tab:** 275mg | 275mg bid. | 1500mg/day. |
| (Anaprox DS) | **Tab:** 550mg* | 550mg bid. | 1500mg/day. |
| (Naprelan) | **Tab, Extended-Release:** 375mg, 500mg, 750mg | 750mg-1g qd. | 1.5g/day. |
| **Oxaprozin** (Daypro) | **Tab:** 600mg* | 1200mg qd. | 1800mg/day or 26mg/kg/day (whichever is lower) |
| **Piroxicam** (Feldene) | **Cap:** 10mg, 20mg | 20mg qd or 10mg bid. | 20mg/day. |
| **Sulindac** (Clinoril) | **Tab:** (Generic) 150mg, (Clinoril, generic) 200mg* | 150mg bid with food. | 400mg/day. |
| **Tolmetin** | **Cap:** 400mg; **Tab:** 200mg*, 600mg | 200-600mg tid. | 1800mg/day. |
| **NSAID/PROSTAGLANDIN $E_1$ ANALOGUE** | | | |
| **Diclofenac/Misoprostol** (Arthrotec) | **Tab:** (Diclofenac-Misoprostol) 50mg-0.2mg, 75mg-0.2mg | 50mg tid-qid. Do not crush, chew, or divide. | **Diclofenac:** 225mg/day<br>**Misoprostol:** 800mcg/day<br>200mcg/dose |
| **PYRIMIDINE SYNTHESIS INHIBITOR** | | | |
| **Leflunomide** (Arava) | **Tab:** 10mg, 20mg, 100mg | **Load:** 100mg qd for 3 days.<br>**Maint:** 20mg/day. | 20mg/day |

| **DRUG** (Brand) | **HOW SUPPLIED** | **USUAL DOSE RANGE** | **MAX DOSE** |
|---|---|---|---|
| **SALICYLATE** | | | |
| **Aspirin** (Genuine Bayer Aspirin) | **Tab:** 325mg | 1-2 tabs every 4 hrs or 3 tabs every 6 hrs. | 12 tabs/day. |
| (Extra Strength Bayer Aspirin) | **Tab:** 500mg | 1-2 tabs every 4-6 hrs. | 8 tabs/24 hrs. |
| (Ecotrin) | **Tab, Delayed-Release:** 81mg, 325mg, 500mg | Up to 3g/day in divided doses. | 3g/day. |
| **Salsalate** | **Tab:** 500mg, 750mg | 3000mg daily, given as 1500mg bid or 1000mg tid. | 3000mg/day. |
| **SELECTIVE COSTIMULATION MODULATOR** | | | |
| **Abatacept** (Orencia) | **Inj:** 250mg | **Initial:** <60kg: 500mg; 60-100kg: 750mg; >100kg: 1g. **Maint:** Give at 2 and 4 wks after initial infusion, then q 4 wks thereafter. | |
| **TNF-RECEPTOR BLOCKER** | | | |
| **Certolizumab pegol** (Cimzia) | **Inj:** 200mg/mL | **Initial:** 400mg SQ at weeks 2 and 4, followed by 200mg every other week. **Maint:** 400mg SQ every 4 weeks. | |
| **Etanercept** (Enbrel) | **Inj:** 25mg [vial], 50mg/mL [syringe] | 50mg SQ per wk. | 50mg/week. |
| **MISCELLANEOUS** | | | |
| **Hydroxychloroquine** (Plaquenil) | **Tab:** 200mg | **Initial:** 400-600mg qd. **Maint:** When good response is obtained (usually in 4-12 wks), 200-400mg qd with meal or milk. | |

*scored

# ADHD Agents

| BRAND (GENERIC) | HOW SUPPLIED | ADULT DOSE | PEDIATRIC DOSE |
|---|---|---|---|
| **Adderall** (Amphetamine plus dextroamphetamine) | Tab: 5mg*, 7.5mg*, 10mg*, 12.5mg*, 15mg*, 20mg*, 30mg* *scored | | **3-5 yrs:** Initial: 2.5mg qd. Titrate: May increase by 2.5mg weekly. **≥6 yrs:** 5mg qd-bid. May increase by 5mg weekly. Give 1st dose upon awakening and add'l doses q4-6h. Max (usual): 40mg/day. |
| **Adderall XR*** (Amphetamine salt combo) | Cap: 5mg, 10mg, 15mg, 20mg, 25mg, 30mg | Initial: 20mg qam. Currently Using Adderall: Switch to Adderall XR at the same total daily dose, taken once daily. Titrate at weekly intervals as needed. | **≥6 yrs:** Initial: 10mg qam. Titrate: May increase weekly by 5-10mg/day. Max: 30mg/day. **13-17 yrs:** Initial: 10mg/day. Titrate: May increase to 20mg/day after one week. Currently Using Adderall: Switch to Adderall XR at the same total daily dose, taken once daily. Titrate at weekly intervals as needed. |
| **Concerta**** (Methylphenidate HCl) | Tab, Extended-Release: 18mg, 27mg, 36mg, 54mg | Methylphenidate-Naive or Receiving Other Stimulant: Initial: 18 or 36mg qam. Titrate: Adjust dose at weekly intervals. Previous Methylphenidate Use: Initial: 18mg qam if previous dose 10-15mg/day; 36mg qam if previous dose 20-30mg/day; 54mg qam if previous dose 30-45mg/day; 72mg qam if previous dose 40-60mg/day. Initial conversion should not exceed 72mg/day. Titrate: Adjust dose at weekly intervals. Max: 72mg/day. Reduce dose or d/c if paradoxical aggravation of symptoms occur. D/C if no improvement after appropriate dosage adjustments over 1 month. | **≥6 yrs:** Methylphenidate-Naive or Receiving Other Stimulant: Initial: 18mg qam. Titrate: Adjust dose at weekly intervals. Max: **6-12 yrs:** 54mg/day; **13-17 yrs:** 18-72mg/day not to exceed 2mg/kg/day. Previous Methylphenidate Use: Initial: 18mg qam if previous dose 10-15mg/day; 36mg qam if previous dose 20-30mg/day; 54mg qam if previous dose 30-45mg/day; 72mg qam if previous dose 40-60mg/day. Initial conversion should not exceed 72mg/day. Titrate: Adjust dose at weekly intervals. Max: 72mg/day. Reduce dose or d/c if paradoxical aggravation of symptoms occur. D/C if no improvement after appropriate dosage adjustments over 1 month. |
| **Daytrana** (Methylphenidate transdermal system) | Patch: 10mg/9 hrs, 15mg/9 hrs, 20mg/9 hrs, 30mg/9 hrs [30[S]] | Individualize dose. Apply to hip area 2 hrs before effect is needed and remove 9 hrs after application. Recommended Titration Schedule: Week 1: 10mg/9 hrs. Week 2: 15mg/9 hrs. Week 3: 20mg/9 hrs. Week 4: 30mg/9 hrs. | **≥6 yrs:** Individualize dose. Apply to hip area 2 hrs before effect is needed and remove 9 hrs after application. Recommended Titration Schedule: Week 1: 10mg/9 hrs. Week 2: 15mg/9 hrs. Week 3: 20mg/9 hrs. Week 4: 30mg/9 hrs. |
| **Desoxyn** (Methamphetamine HCl) | Tab: 5mg | | **≥6 yrs:** Initial: 5mg qd-bid. Titrate: Increase weekly by 5mg/day until optimum response. Usual: 20-25mg/day; may be given in 2 divided doses. |
| **Dexedrine** (Dextroamphetamine sulfate) | Cap, Extended-Release: (Spansules) 5mg, 10mg, 15mg | | **≥6 yrs:** 5mg qd-bid. Titrate: Increase weekly by 5mg/day. Max: 40mg/day. |

*(Continued)*

| BRAND (GENERIC) | HOW SUPPLIED | ADULT DOSE | PEDIATRIC DOSE |
|---|---|---|---|
| (Dextroamphetamine sulfate) | Tab: 5mg*, 10mg* *scored | | **3-5 yrs:** Initial: 2.5mg/day. Titrate: Increase weekly by 2.5mg/day until optimum response. ≥**6 yrs:** Initial 5mg qd-bid. Titrate: Increase weekly by 5mg/day until optimum response. Give 1st dose upon awakening, and additional doses q4-6h. |
| **Focalin** (Dexmethylphenidate HCl) | Tab: 2.5mg, 5mg, 10mg | Take bid at least 4 hrs apart. Methylphenidate-Naive: Initial: 2.5mg bid. Titrate: Increase weekly by 2.5-5mg/day. Max: 20mg/day. Currently on Methylphenidate: Initial: Take ½ of methylphenidate dose. Max: 20mg/day. Reduce or d/c if paradoxical aggravation of symptoms occur. D/C if no improvement after appropriate dosage adjustments over 1 month. | ≥**6 yrs:** Take bid at least 4 hrs apart. Methylphenidate-Naive: Initial: 2.5mg bid. Titrate: Increase weekly by 2.5-5mg/day. Max: 20mg/day. Currently on Methylphenidate: Initial: Take ½ of methylphenidate dose. Max: 20mg/day. Reduce or d/c if paradoxical aggravation of symptoms occur. D/C if no improvement after appropriate dosage adjustments over 1 month. |
| **Focalin XR*** (Dexmethylphenidate HCl) | Cap, Extended-Release: 5mg, 10mg, 15mg, 20mg, 30mg | Methylphenidate-Naive: Initial: 10mg/day. Titrate: May adjust weekly by 10mg/day. Max: 40mg/day. Currently on Methylphenidate: Initial: Take ½ of methylphenidate dose. Max: 40mg/day. Currently on Focalin: May switch to same daily dose of Focalin XR. Reduce or d/c if paradoxical aggravation of symptoms occur. D/C if no improvement after appropriate dosage adjustments over 1 month. | ≥**6 yrs:** Methylphenidate-Naive: Initial: 5mg/day. Titrate: May adjust weekly by 5mg/day. Max: 30mg/day. Currently on Methylphenidate: Initial: Take ½ of methylphenidate dose. Max: 30mg/day. Currently on Focalin: May switch to same daily dose of Focalin XR. Reduce or d/c if paradoxical aggravation of symptoms occur. D/C if no improvement after appropriate dosage adjustments over 1 month. |
| **Intuniv**** (Guanfacine) | Tab, Extended-Release: 1mg, 2mg, 3mg, 4mg | | **6-17 yrs:** Initial: 1mg/day. Titrate: Adjust dose by increments of ≤1mg/week. Maint: 1-4mg/day based on clinical response and tolerability. Range: 0.05-0.08mg/kg/day. If well tolerated, doses up to 0.12mg/kg/day may provide additional benefit. Max: 4mg/day. Renal/Hepatic Impairment: Consider dose adjustment. |
| **Metadate CD*** (Methylphenidate HCl) | Cap, Extended-Release: 10mg, 20mg, 30mg, 40mg, 50mg, 60mg | Usual: 20mg qam before breakfast. Titrate: Increase weekly by 10-20mg depending on tolerability/efficacy. Max: 60mg/day. Reduce dose or d/c if paradoxical aggravation of symptoms occur. D/C if no improvement after appropriate dose adjustments over 1 month. | ≥**6 yrs:** Usual: 20mg qam before breakfast. Titrate: Increase weekly by 10-20mg depending on tolerability/efficacy. Max: 60mg/day. Reduce dose or d/c if paradoxical aggravation of symptoms occur. D/C if no improvement after appropriate dose adjustments over 1 month. |
| **Metadate ER**** (Methylphenidate HCl) | Tab, Extended-Release: 10mg, 20mg | (Immediate-Release Methylphenidate) 10-60mg/day given bid-tid 30-45 min ac. If insomnia occurs, take last dose before 6 pm.† | ≥**6 yrs:** (Immediate-Release Methylphenidate) Initial: 5mg bid before breakfast and lunch. Titrate: Increase gradually by 5-10mg weekly. Max: 60mg/day. Reduce dose or d/c if paradoxical aggravation of symptoms occur. D/C if no improvement after appropriate dose adjustment over 1 month.† |

| BRAND (GENERIC) | HOW SUPPLIED | ADULT DOSE | PEDIATRIC DOSE |
|---|---|---|---|
| **Methylin****<br>(Methylphenidate HCl) | Sol: 5mg/5mL [500mL], 10mg/5mL [500mL]; Tab: 5mg, 10mg, 20mg; Tab, Chewable: 2.5mg, 5mg, 10mg; Tab, Extended-Release: 10mg, 20mg | (Sol/Tab/Tab, Chewable) 10-60mg/day given bid-tid 30-45 min ac. If insomnia occurs, take last dose before 6 pm.† | **≥6 yrs:** (Sol/Tab/Tab, Chewable) Initial: 5mg bid before breakfast and lunch. Titrate: Increase gradually by 5-10mg weekly. Max: 60mg/day. Reduce dose or d/c if paradoxical aggravation of symptoms occur. D/C if no improvement after appropriate dose adjustment over 1 month.† |
| **Ritalin, Ritalin LA***,<br>**Ritalin SR****<br>(Methylphenidate HCl) | Cap, Extended-Release (Ritalin LA): 10mg, 20mg, 30mg, 40mg; Tab (Ritalin): 5mg, 10mg*, 20mg*; Tab, Extended-Release (Ritalin SR): 20mg **scored* | (Tab) 10-60mg/day given bid-tid 30-45 min ac. Take last dose before 6 pm if insomnia occurs. (Cap, ER) Initial: 20mg qam. Titrate: Adjust weekly by 10mg. Max: 60mg qam.† Previous Methylphenidate Use: May use as qd in place of IR dosed bid or daily dose of methylphenidate-SR. Reduce dose or d/c if paradoxical aggravation of symptoms occur. D/C if no improvement after appropriate dose adjustment over 1 month.† | **≥6 yrs:** (Tab) Initial: 5mg bid before breakfast and lunch. Titrate: Increase gradually by 5-10mg weekly. Max: 60mg/day. (Cap, ER) Initial: 20mg qam. Titrate: Adjust weekly by 10mg. Max: 60mg qam. Previous Methylphenidate Use: May use as qd in place of IR dosed bid or daily dose of methylphenidate-SR. Reduce dose or d/c if paradoxical aggravation of symptoms occur. D/C if no improvement after appropriate dose adjustment over 1 month.† |
| **Strattera**<br>(Atomoxetine HCl) | Cap: 10mg, 18mg, 25mg, 40mg, 60mg, 80mg, 100mg | Initial: 40mg/day given qam or evenly divided doses in the am and late afternoon/early evening. Titrate: Increase after minimum of 3 days to target dose of about 80mg/day. After 2-4 weeks, may increase to max of 100mg/day. Max: 100mg/day. Dose adjust in hepatic insufficiency and when used with concomitant CYP450 2D6 inhibitors. See PI for detailed dosing information. | **≥6 yrs:** ≤70kg: Initial: 0.5mg/kg/day given qam or evenly divided doses in the am and late afternoon or early evening. Titrate: Increase after minimum of 3 days to target dose of about 1.2mg/kg/day. Max: 1.4mg/kg/day or 100mg, whichever is less. >70kg: Initial: 40mg/day given qam or evenly divided doses in the am and late afternoon/early evening. Titrate: Increase after minimum of 3 days to target dose of about 80mg/day. After 2-4 weeks, may increase to max of 100mg/day. Max: 100mg/day. Dose adjust in hepatic insufficiency and when used with concomitant CYP450 2D6 inhibitors. See PI for detailed dosing information. |
| **Vyvanse**<br>(Lisdexamfetamine dimesylate) | Cap: 20mg, 30mg, 40mg, 50mg, 60mg, 70mg | Individualize dose. Usual: 30mg qam. Titrate: If needed, may increase in increments of 10mg or 20mg at weekly intervals. Max: 70mg/day. Swallow caps or dissolve contents in glass of water; do not store once dissolved. Re-evaluate periodically. | Individualize dose. **6-12 yrs:** Usual: 30mg qam. Titrate: If needed, may increase in increments of 10mg or 20mg at weekly intervals. Max: 70mg/day. Swallow caps or dissolve contents in glass of water; do not store once dissolved. Re-evaluate periodically. |

ADHD = attention-deficit/hyperactivity disorder.
*Swallow cap whole or open cap and sprinkle contents on applesauce; do not chew beads.
**Swallow whole; do not chew, crush, or divide.
†Tab, Extended-Release: May use in place of immediate-release tabs when the 8-hr dose corresponds to the titrated 8-hr immediate-release dose.

# ALZHEIMER'S DISEASE AGENTS

| DRUG (BRAND) | INDICATIONS | HOW SUPPLIED | DOSAGE | SIDE EFFECTS |
|---|---|---|---|---|
| **Donepezil HCl** (Aricept) | Treatment of dementia of the Alzheimer's type. | Tab: 5mg, 10mg; Tab, Disintegrating: 5mg, 10mg | Mild to Moderate Alzheimer's Disease: Initial: 5mg qd. Titrate: May increase to 10mg after 4-6 weeks. Severe Alzheimer's Disease: 10mg qd. Start with 5mg qd and increase to 10mg after 4-6 weeks. | Nausea, diarrhea, insomnia, vomiting, muscle cramps, fatigue, anorexia, dizziness, depression, weight decrease, infection, HTN, back pain, abnormal dreams, ecchymosis |
| **Ergoloid Mesylates** (Ergoloid mesylates) | Treatment of symptomatic decline in mental capacity of unknown etiology (eg, Alzheimer's dementia, multi-infarct dementia). | Tab: 1mg | Usual: 1mg tid. | Transient nausea, gastric disturbances |
| **Galantamine HBr** (Razadyne, Razadyne ER) | Treatment of mild to moderate dementia of the Alzheimer's type. | Sol: (Razadyne) 4mg/mL [100mL]; Tab: (Razadyne) 4mg, 8mg, 12mg. Cap, Extended-Release; (Razadyne ER) 8mg, 16mg, 24mg | (Sol, Tab) Initial: 4mg bid with am and pm meals. Titrate: Increase to 8mg bid after 4 weeks if tolerated, then increase to 12mg bid after 4 weeks if tolerated. Usual: 16-24mg/day. Max: 24mg/day. (Cap, ER) Initial: 8mg qd with am meal. Titrate: Increase to 16mg qd after 4 weeks, then increase to 24mg qd after 4 weeks if tolerated. Usual: 16-24mg/day. Max: 24mg/day. If therapy is interrupted, restart at lowest dose and increase to current dose. See PI for dose modification in moderate renal/hepatic impairment. | Nausea, vomiting, diarrhea, anorexia, weight loss, fatigue, dizziness, headache, depression, insomnia, abdominal pain, dyspepsia |
| **Memantine HCl** (Namenda) | Treatment of moderate to severe dementia of the Alzheimer's type. | Sol: 2mg/mL [360mL]; Tab: 5mg, 10mg; Titration-Pak: 5mg [28$^{S}$], 10mg [21$^{S}$] | Initial: 5mg qd. Titrate: Increase at intervals of at least one week to 5mg bid, then 5mg and 10mg as separate doses, then to 10mg bid. Severe Renal Impairment: Reduce dose. | Dizziness, confusion, headache, constipation, coughing, HTN, pain, vomiting, somnolence, hallucinations |
| **Rivastigmine tartrate** (Exelon) | Treatment of mild to moderate dementia of the Alzheimer's type. | Cap: 1.5mg, 3mg, 4.5mg, 6mg; Sol: 2mg/mL [120mL]; Patch: 4.6mg/24 hrs, 9.5 mg/24 hrs [30$^{S}$] | Initial: 1.5mg bid. Titrate: May increase by 1.5mg bid every 2 weeks. Max: 12mg/day. If not tolerating, suspend therapy for several doses and restart at same or next lower dose. If interrupted longer than several days, reinitiate with lowest daily dose and titrate as above. (Patch) Initial: Apply 4.6mg/24 hrs patch qd to clean, dry, hairless intact skin. Maint: Increase dose after 4 weeks. Max: 9.5mg/24 hrs if well tolerated. Switching from Capsules/Oral Sol: Total Oral Daily Dose <6mg: Switch to 4.6mg/24 hrs patch. Total Oral Daily Dose 6-12mg: Switch to 9.5mg/24 hrs patch. Apply 1st patch on day following last oral dose. | Nausea, vomiting, abdominal pain, dyspepsia, constipation, somnolence, anorexia, asthenia, headache, dizziness, fatigue, diarrhea, tremor, depression |

# ANTIPARKINSON'S AGENTS

| DRUG (BRAND) | INDICATIONS | HOW SUPPLIED | DOSAGE | SIDE EFFECTS |
|---|---|---|---|---|
| **Bromocriptine mesylate** (Parlodel) | Treatment of symptoms of Parkinson's disease; adjunctive treatment to levodopa. | Tab, Snap: 2.5mg*; Cap: 5mg *scored | Initial: 1.25mg bid. Titrate: If needed, increase by 2.5mg/day every 2-4 weeks. Max: 100mg/day. Take with food. See PI for detailed dosing information with levodopa. | Headache, dizziness, GI effects, orthostatic hypotension, fatigue, arrhythmia, insomnia, hallucinations, abnormal involuntary movements, depression, syncope |
| **Carbidopa** (Lodosyn) | For use with Sinemet or levodopa in treatment of symptoms of idiopathic Parkinson's disease, postencephalitic parkinsonism, and symptomatic parkinsonism. For use in patients for whom the dosage of Sinemet provides less than adequate daily dosage (usually 70mg daily) of carbidopa. | Tab: 25mg* *scored | With Sinemet or Levodopa: Determine dose by careful titration. Most patients respond to a 1:10 proportion of carbidopa: levodopa provided carbidopa dose is ≥70mg/day. Max: 200mg/day. Consider amount of carbidopa in Sinemet when calculating dose. See PI for detailed dosing information. | Dyskinesia, psychotic episodes, delusions, hallucinations, paranoid ideation, depression with or without suicidal tendencies, dementia |
| **Carbidopa/levodopa** (Sinemet, Sinemet CR) | Treatment of symptoms of idiopathic Parkinson's disease, postencephalitic parkinsonism, and symptomatic parkinsonism. | Tab: (Carbidopa-Levodopa) 10mg-100mg*, 25mg-100mg*, 25mg-250mg*; Tab, Extended Release: (Carbidopa-Levodopa) 25mg-100mg, 50mg-200mg* *scored | (Tab) 25mg-100mg tab: Initial: 1 tab tid. Titrate: Increase by 1 tab qd or every other day up to 8 tabs/day. 10mg-100mg tab: Initial: 1 tab tid-qid. Titrate: Increase by 1 tab qd or every other day up to 2 tabs qid. 70-100mg/day carbidopa required. Max: 200mg/day carbidopa. (Tab, Extended-Release) No Prior Levodopa Use: Initial: 1 50mg-200mg tab bid at intervals >6 hrs. Titrate: Increase or decrease dose or interval accordingly. Adjust dose every 3 days. Usual: 400-1600mg/day levodopa, given in 4-8 hr intervals while awake. Conversion to Extended-Release Tabs: See PI. | Dyskinesia, nausea, cardiac irregularities, hypotension, dark saliva, GI bleeding, psychotic episodes, NMS, confusion, agitation, dizziness, somnolence, dream abnormalities |
| **Carbidopa/levodopa** (Parcopa) | Treatment of symptoms of idiopathic Parkinson's disease, postencephalitic parkinsonism, and symptomatic parkinsonism. | Tab, Disintegrating: (Carbidopa-Levodopa) 10mg-100mg*, 25mg-100mg*, 25mg-250mg* *scored | 25mg-100mg tab: Initial: 1 tab tid. Titrate: Increase by 1 tab qd or qod up to 8 tabs/day. 10mg-100mg tab: Initial: 1 tab tid-qid. Titrate: Increase by 1 tab qd or qod up to 2 tabs qid. 70-100mg/day carbidopa required. Max: 200mg/day carbidopa. | Dyskinesia, choreiform, dystonic and other involuntary movements, nausea |

| DRUG (BRAND) | INDICATIONS | HOW SUPPLIED | DOSAGE | SIDE EFFECTS |
|---|---|---|---|---|
| **Carbidopa/levodopa/entacapone** (Stalevo) | Treatment of idiopathic Parkinson's disease to substitute for equivalent doses of previously administered carbidopa/levodopa and entacapone, or for those experiencing signs and symptoms of end-of-dose "wearing off" and taking up to 600mg/day levodopa without experiencing dyskinesias. | Tab: (Carbidopa/Levodopa/Entacapone): Stalevo 50: 12.5mg/50mg/200mg; Stalevo 75: 18.75mg/75mg/200 mg; Stalevo 100: 25mg/100mg/200mg; Stalevo 125: 31.25mg/125mg/200mg; Stalevo 150: 37.5mg/150mg/200mg; Stalevo 200: 50mg/200mg/200mg | Currently Taking Carbidopa/Levodopa and Entacapone: May switch directly to corresponding strength of levodopa/carbidopa/entacapone. Currently Taking Carbidopa/Levodopa, but not Entacapone: First, titrate individually with carbidopa/levodopa product and entacapone product, then transfer to corresponding dose. Max dose: 8 tabs/day except Stalevo 200. Max: 6 tabs/day. | Dyskinesia, hyperkinesia, hypokinesia, dizziness, nausea, diarrhea, abdominal pain, constipation, vomiting, urine discoloration, back pain, fatigue |
| **Diphenhydramine HCl Injection** | For parkinsonism when oral therapy is not possible or contraindicated. | Inj: 50mg/mL | Usual: 10-50mg IV at ≤25 mg/min or up to 100mg IM if needed. Max: 400mg/day. | Sedation, drowsiness, dizziness, disturbed coordination, epigastric distress, thickening of bronchial secretions |
| **Pramipexole dihydrochloride** (Mirapex) | Treatment of signs and symptoms of idiopathic Parkinson's disease. | Tab: 0.125mg, 0.25mg*, 0.5mg*, 0.75mg, 1mg*, 1.5mg* *scored | Initial: 0.125mg tid. Titrate: May increase every 5-7 days (eg, Week 2: 0.25mg tid; Week 3: 0.5mg tid; Week 4: 0.75mg tid; Week 5: 1mg tid; Week 6: 1.25mg tid; Week 7: 1.5mg tid). Maint: 0.5-1.5mg tid. Max: 1.5mg tid.† | Nausea, dizziness, somnolence, insomnia, constipation, asthenia, hallucinations, vision abnormalities, peripheral edema, arthritis, dry mouth, postural hypotension, chest pain, malaise |
| (Mirapex ER) | | (Tab, ER): 0.375mg, 0.75mg, 1.5mg, 3mg, 4.5mg | (Tab, ER) Initial: 0.375mg qd. Titrate: May increase gradually not more frequently than q 5-7 days, first to 0.75mg/day and then by 0.75mg increments based on efficacy and tolerability. Max: 4.5mg/day. Refer to PI for more detailed dosing information. | (Tab, ER) Somnolence, N/V, constipation, dizziness, fatigue, hallucinations, dry mouth, muscle spasms, peripheral edema. |
| **Rasagiline mesylate** (Azilect) | Treatment of signs and symptoms of idiopathic Parkinson's disease as initial monotherapy and adjunct therapy to levodopa. | Tab: 0.5mg, 1mg | Monotherapy: 1mg qd. Adjunctive Therapy: Initial: 0.5mg qd. Titrate: May increase to 1mg qd. Adjust dose of levodopa with concomitant use. Concomitant Ciprofloxacin or Other CYP1A2 Inhibitors/Hepatic Impairment: 0.5mg qd. | Headache, arthralgia, depression, fall, flu syndrome, dyskinesia, accidental injury, nausea, weight loss, constipation, postural hypotension, vomiting, dry mouth, rash, somnolence |
| **Rivastigmine** (Exelon) | Treatment of mild to moderate dementia associated with Parkinson's disease. | Cap: 1.5mg, 3mg, 4.5mg, 6mg; Patch: 4.6mg/24h, 9.5mg/24h; Sol: 2mg/mL (120mL) | (Cap, Sol): Initial: 1.5mg bid with meals in am and pm. Titrate: May increase at 4-week intervals to 3mg bid, then 4.5mg bid, and 6mg bid if tolerable. Usual: 1.5-6mg bid. Patch: Initial: 4.6mg/24h. Titrate: After 4 weeks, may increase to 9.5mg/24h if tolerated. Recommended: 9.5mg/24h. | Nausea, vomiting, anorexia, tremor, chest pain, dyskinesia, dyspepsia, back pain |

*(Continued)*

| DRUG (BRAND) | INDICATIONS | HOW SUPPLIED | DOSAGE | SIDE EFFECTS |
|---|---|---|---|---|
| **Ropinirole HCl** (Requip) (Requip XL) | Treatment of symptoms of idiopathic Parkinson's disease. | Tab: 0.25mg, 0.5mg, 1mg, 2mg, 3mg, 4mg, 5mg Tab, Extended-Release: 2mg, 4mg, 6mg, 8mg, 12mg | Initial: 0.25mg tid. Titrate: May increase weekly by 0.25mg tid (0.75mg/day) for 4 weeks. After Week 4, may increase weekly by 1.5mg/day up to 9mg/day, then by 3mg/day weekly to 24mg/day. Max: 24mg/day. Withdrawal: Decrease dose to bid for 4 days, then qd for 3 days. (Requip XL) Tab, Extended-Release: Initial: 2mg qd for 1-2 weeks. Swallow whole. Titrate: May increase at ≥1 week intervals by 2mg/day. Max: 24mg/day. Levodopa dose may be gradually decreased as tolerated. Switching from IR to ER: Closely match total daily IR dose with initial extended-release dose. See PI for detailed information. | Neuralgia, increased BUN, hallucinations, somnolence, vomiting, headache, sweating, asthenia, edema, fatigue, syncope, orthostatic symptoms |
| **ADJUNCT THERAPY** | | | | |
| **Amantadine HCl** | Treatment of parkinsonism and drug-induced extrapyramidal reactions. | Tab: 100mg | Parkinsonism: Initial: 100mg bid. Serious Associated Illness/ Concomitant High-Dose Antiparkinson Agent: Initial: 100mg qd. Titrate: May increase to 100mg bid. | Nausea, dizziness, insomnia, depression, anxiety, hallucinations, confusion, anorexia, dry mouth, constipation, ataxia |
| **Apomorphine HCl** (Apokyn) | Acute, intermittent treatment of hypomobility, "off" episodes (end-of-dose "wearing off" and unpredictable "on/off" episodes) associated with advanced Parkinson's disease. | Inj: 10mg/mL [3mL] | Initial: Test Dose: 2mg SC; monitor BP closely. Titrate: Increase by 1mg every few days; assess efficacy/tolerability. Max: 6mg/day. Renal Impairment: Initial: 1mg SC. | Yawning, dyskinesia, nausea, vomiting, somnolence, dizziness, rhinorrhea, edema, chest pain, increased sweating, flushing, pallor |
| **Benztropine mesylate** (Cogentin) | Adjunct in all forms of parkinsonism. Control of drug-induced extrapyramidal disorders. | Inj: 1mg/mL; Tab (generic): 0.5mg, 1mg, 2mg | Parkinsonism: Initial: 0.5-1mg PO IV/IM qhs. Titrate: May increase every 5-6 days by 0.5mg. Usual: 1-2mg PO IV/IM qhs. Max: 6mg/day. Extrapyramidal Disorders: 1-4mg PO IV/IM qd-bid. Acute Dystonic Reactions: 1-2mg IM/IV, then 1-2mg PO bid. | Tachycardia, paralytic ileus, constipation, vomiting, nausea, dry mouth, confusion, blurred vision, urinary retention, heat stroke, hyperthermia, fever |
| **Entacapone** (Comtan) | Adjunct to levodopa/carbidopa for treatment of idiopathic Parkinson's disease if experience signs of end-of-dose "wearing-off." | Tab: 200mg | 200mg with each levodopa/carbidopa dose. Max: 1600mg/day. Withdraw slowly for discontinuation. | Sweating, back pain, dyskinesia, hyperkinesia, hypokinesia, nausea, diarrhea, abdominal pain, urine discoloration |

| DRUG (BRAND) | INDICATIONS | HOW SUPPLIED | DOSAGE | SIDE EFFECTS |
|---|---|---|---|---|
| **Hyoscyamine sulfate** (Levsin, Levbid) | To reduce rigidity and tremors of Parkinson's disease. | (Levbid) Tab, Extended-Release: 0.375mg. (Levsin) Tab: 0.125mg*; Tab, Sublingual: 0.125mg*. *scored | May also chew or swallow SL tab. Levsin: (Tab and Tab, SL) 0.125-0.25mg q4h or prn. Max: 1.5mg/24 hrs. Levbid: (Tab, Extended-Release) 0.375-0.75mg q12h. Max: 1.5mg/24 hrs. Do not crush or chew. | Anticholinergic effects, drowsiness, headache, nervousness |
| **Selegiline HCl** (Eldepryl) | Adjunct to levodopa/carbidopa for management of Parkinson's disease. | Cap, Tab: 5mg | 5mg bid, at breakfast and lunch. Max: 10mg/day. May reduce levodopa/carbidopa by 10-30% after 2-3 days of therapy. May reduce further with continued therapy. | Nausea, dizziness, lightheadedness, fainting, abdominal pain, confusion, hallucinations, dry mouth |
| **Selegiline HCl** (Zelapar) | Adjunct in the management of Parkinson's disease in patients exhibiting a deteriorated response to levodopa/carbidopa therapy. | Tab, Orally Disintegrating: 1.25mg | 1.25mg qd for 6 weeks. Titrate: After 6 weeks, may increase to 2.5mg qd if desired benefit not achieved. Max: 2.5mg/day. | Nausea, dizziness, pain, headache, insomnia, rhinitis, skin disorders, dyskinesia, backache, dyspepsia, stomatitis, constipation, hallucinations, pharyngitis, rash |
| **Tolcapone** (Tasmar) | Adjunct to levodopa/carbidopa for the treatment of symptoms of idiopathic Parkinson's disease. | Tab: 100mg, 200mg | Initial: 100mg tid. Use 200mg tid only if clinical benefit is justified. May need to decrease levodopa dose. | Dyskinesia, nausea, dystonia, excessive dreaming, anorexia, muscle cramps, orthostatic complaints, diarrhea, dizziness, headache |
| **Trihexyphenidyl HCl** | Adjunct treatment for all forms of parkinsonism (postencephalitic, arteriosclerotic, and idiopathic). For control of extrapyramidal disorders caused by CNS drugs. | Sol: 2mg/5mL [473mL]; Tab: 2mg*, 5mg* *scored | Idiopathic Parkinsonism: 1mg on Day 1. Titrate: Increase by 2mg every 3-5 days. Usual: 6-10mg/day. Max: 15mg/day. Drug-Induced Parkinsonism: Initial: 1mg. If extrapyramidal manifestations not controlled in a few hrs, increase dose until achieve control. Usual: 5-15mg/day. | Dry mouth, blurred vision, dizziness, nausea, nervousness, constipation, drowsiness, urinary hesitancy/retention, tachycardia, pupil dilation, increased intraocular tension, vomiting, weakness, headache |

†For specific dosing information on different creatinine clearance values, see full Prescribing Information.

# Opioid Products

| GENERIC | BRAND | DOSAGE FORMS | ORAL EQUI-ANALGESIC DOSE | EQUI-ANALGESIC DOSE | USUAL ADULT DOSE | MAX DOSE | INDICATION | DEA SCHEDULE |
|---|---|---|---|---|---|---|---|---|
| Codeine | | **Inj:** 15mg/mL, 30mg/mL; **Tab:** 15mg, 30mg, 60mg | 200mg. | 120mg. | PO, IM, SC 15-60mg up to q4h prn. | 360mg/24 hrs. | Relief of mild to moderately severe pain. | Schedule II |
| Codeine phosphate/Acetaminophen | | **Elixir:** 12mg-120mg/5mL | | | 15mL q4h prn. | Codeine: 360mg/day. APAP: 4g/day. | Relief of mild to moderately severe pain. | Schedule V |
| | | **Tab:** 15mg-300mg | | | 15-60mg codeine/dose and 300-1000mg APAP. Doses may be repeated q4h. | | | Schedule III |
| | Tylenol #3 | **Tab:** 30mg-300mg | | | | | | Schedule III |
| | Tylenol #4 | **Tab:** 60mg-300mg | | | | | | Schedule III |
| Fentanyl | Duragesic | **Patch:** 12.5mcg/hr, 25mcg/hr, 50mcg/hr, 75mcg/hr, 100mcg/hr | | 0.1mg. | Initial: 25mcg/hr for 72 hrs. Individualize dose. | | Management of persistent, moderate to severe chronic pain that requires continuous, around-the-clock opioid administration for an extended period of time, and cannot be managed by other means such as non-steroidal analgesics, opioid combination products, or immediate-release opioids. | Schedule II |
| Fentanyl citrate | Actiq | **Loz:** 200mcg, 400mcg, 600mcg, 800mcg, 1200mcg, 1600mcg | | | 200mcg. Dispense no more than 6 units. Individually titrate. | 4 units/day. | Management of breakthrough cancer pain in patients with malignancies who are already receiving and are tolerant to opioid therapy for their underlying persistent cancer pain. | Schedule II |

*(Continued)*

| GENERIC | BRAND | DOSAGE FORMS | ORAL EQUI-ANALGESIC DOSE | EQUI-ANALGESIC DOSE | USUAL ADULT DOSE | MAX DOSE | INDICATION | DEA SCHEDULE |
|---|---|---|---|---|---|---|---|---|
| Fentanyl citrate *(continued)* | Fentora | **Tab, Buccal:** 100mcg, 200mcg, 300mcg, 400mcg, 600mcg, 800mcg | | | Initial:100mcg. Converting from Actiq doses ≥600mcg: 200mcg; proceed using multiples of this strength. Titrate: If 100mcg Initial Dose: Give two 100-mcg tabs (one on each side of mouth); may increase to four 100-mcg tabs (two on each side of the mouth). Use multiples of 200-mcg tabs for doses >400mcg. | 2 doses/episode of breakthrough pain separated by 30 min. Wait 4 hrs between episodes. Not more than 4 tabs simultaneously. | Management of breakthrough pain in patients with cancer who are already receiving and who are tolerant to opioid therapy for their underlying persistent cancer pain. | |
| | Onsolis | **Film, Buccal:** 200mcg, 400mcg, 600mcg, 800mcg, 1200mcg | | | Initial: 200mcg. Titrate: Use multiples of 200-mcg films. Increase by 200mcg per subsequent episode until effect. | Not more than four 200-mcg films simultaneously. If tolerant to 800mcg, give one 1200-mcg film. Single doses are given 2 hrs apart; use once per breakthrough pain episode. | Management of breakthrough pain in patients with cancer, ≥18 yrs who are already receiving and who are tolerant to opioid therapy for their underlying persistent cancer pain. | |
| Hydrocodone bitartrate/ Acetaminophen | | **Tab:** 5mg-325mg, 7.5mg-325mg, 5mg-500mg, 7.5mg-650mg | | | (5/325, 5/500) 1-2 tabs q4-6h. (7.5/325, 7.5/650) 1 tab q4-6h. | (5/325): 12 tabs/day. (5/500, 7.5/325): 8 tabs/day. (7.5/650): 6 tabs/day. | Relief of moderate to moderately severe pain. | Schedule III |
| | | **Cap:** 5mg-500mg | | | 1-2 caps q4-6h prn. | 8 caps/day. | | |
| | Lorcet Plus, Lorcet 10/650 | **Tab:** (Plus) 7.5mg-650mg, (10/650) 10mg-650mg | | | 1 tab q4-6h prn. | 6 tabs/day. | | |
| | Lortab Elixir Lortab | **Sol:** 7.5mg-500mg/15mL **Tab:** 2.5mg-500mg, 5mg-500mg, 7.5mg-500mg, 10mg-500mg | | | (Sol) 1 tbs q4-6h prn. (2.5/500, 5/500): 1-2 tabs q4-6h prn. (7.5/500,10/500): 1 tab q4-6h prn. | (Sol) 6 tbs/day. (2.5/500, 5/500): 8 tabs/day. (7.5/500, 10/500): 6 tabs/day. | | |
| | Maxidone | **Tab:** 10mg-750mg | | | 1 tab q4-6h prn. | 5 tabs/day. | | |

| GENERIC | BRAND | DOSAGE FORMS | ORAL EQUI-ANALGESIC DOSE | EQUI-ANALGESIC DOSE | USUAL ADULT DOSE | MAX DOSE | INDICATION | DEA SCHEDULE |
|---|---|---|---|---|---|---|---|---|
| Hydrocodone bitartrate/ Acetaminophen *(continued)* | Norco | **Tab:** 5mg-325mg, 7.5mg-325mg, 10mg-325mg | | | (5/325): 1-2 tabs q4-6h prn. (7.5/325, 10/325): 1 tab q4-6h prn. | (5/325): 8 tabs/day. (7.5/325): 6 tabs/day. (10/325): 6 tabs/day. | | |
| | Vicodin | **Tab:** 5mg-500mg | | | 1-2 tabs q4-6h prn. | 8 tabs/day. | | |
| | Vicodin ES | **Tab:** 7.5mg-750mg | | | 1 tab q4-6h prn. | 5 tabs/day. | | |
| | Vicodin HP | **Tab:** 10mg-660mg | | | 1 tab q4-6h prn. | 6 tabs/day. | | |
| | Zydone | **Tab:** 5mg-400mg, 7.5mg-400mg, 10mg-400mg | | | (5/400): 1-2 tabs q4-6h prn. (7.5/400, 10/400): 1 tab q4-6h prn. | (5/400): 8 tabs/day. (7.5/400, 10/400): 6 tabs/day. | | |
| Hydrocodone bitartrate/Ibuprofen | Vicoprofen | **Tab:** 7.5-200mg | | | 1 tab q4-6h prn. | 5 tabs/day. | Short-term (generally <10 days) management of acute pain. | Schedule III |
| Hydromorphone HCl | Dilaudid, Dilaudid-HP | **Tab:** 2mg, 4mg, 8mg; **Sol:** 1mg/mL; **Inj:** 1mg/mL, 2mg/mL, 4mg/mL; **HP:** 10mg/mL, **Pow:** 250mg | 7.5mg. | 1.5mg. | Tab: 2-4mg, PO every 4 to 6 hours. Sol: 2.5-10mL q3-6h as directed. Inj: 1-2mg SC or IM q4-6h. HP: Individualized for each patient. | | Management of pain. (HP) Relief of moderate to severe pain in opioid-tolerant patients who require larger than usual doses of opioids to provide adequate pain relief. | Schedule II |
| Meperidine HCl | Demerol | **Syr:** 50mg/5mL; **Tab:** 50mg, 100mg; **Inj:** 25mg/mL, 50mg/mL, 75mg/mL, 100mg/mL | | 60-80mg. | Tab: 50-150mg q3-4h prn. Inj: 50-150mg IM/SC q3-4h prn; 50-100mg IM/SC 30-90 min prior to anesthesia for pre-op use or at 1- to 3-hr intervals during obstetrical analgesia. | | Moderate to severe pain. Inj: also for preoperative medication, anesthesia support, and obstetrical analgesia. | Schedule II |
| Methadone HCl | Dolophine | **Tab:** 5mg, 10mg; **Inj:** 10mg/mL | 20mg. | 10mg. | 2.5mg to 10mg every 8 to 12 hrs, slowly titrated to effect. | | To treat moderate to severe pain not responsive to non-narcotic analgesics. | Schedule II |

*(Continued)*

| GENERIC | BRAND | DOSAGE FORMS | ORAL EQUI-ANALGESIC DOSE | EQUI-ANALGESIC DOSE | USUAL ADULT DOSE | MAX DOSE | INDICATION | DEA SCHEDULE |
|---|---|---|---|---|---|---|---|---|
| Morphine sulfate | Astramorph PF | **Inj:** 0.5mg/mL, 1mg/mL | 30mg. | 10mg. | IV: 2-10mg/70kg of body weight. Epidural: 2-4mg/24 hrs. IT: 0.2-1mg/24 hrs. | Epidural: 10mg q24h. | Management of pain not responsive to non-narcotic analgesics. | Schedule II |
| | Avinza | **Cap, ER:** 30mg, 60mg, 90mg, 120mg | | | 30mg q24h. | 1600mg/day. | Relief of moderate to severe pain requiring continuous opioid therapy for an extended period of time. | |
| | Depodur | **Inj:** 10mg/mL, 15mg/1.5mL | | | Epidural: 10-15mg | | Treatment of pain following major surgery. | |
| | Duramorph | **Inj:** 0.5mg/mL, 1mg/mL | | | IV: 2-10mg/70kg of body weight. Epidural: 2-4mg/24 hrs. IT: 0.2-1mg/24 hrs. | Epidural: 10mg q24h. | Management of pain not responsive to non-narcotic analgesics. | |
| | Infumorph | **Inj:** 10mg/mL (200mg), 25mg/mL (500mg) | | | 1-10mg/day | | Treatment of intractable chronic pain in microinfusion devices. | |
| | Kadian | **Cap, ER:** 10mg, 20mg, 30mg, 50mg, 60mg, 80mg, 100mg, 200mg | | | Give 50% of daily oral morphine dose q12h or give 100% oral morphine dose q24h. | Do not give more frequently than q12h. | Management of moderate to severe pain when a continuous, around-the-clock opioid analgesic is needed for an extended period of time. | |
| | MS Contin | **Tab, ER:** 15mg, 30mg, 60mg, 100mg, 200mg | | | Give 50% of pts 24-hr requirement q12h or $^{1}/_{3}$ of pts 24-hr requirement q8h. | | Relief of moderate to severe pain for patients who require repeated dosing with potent opioid analgesics over periods of more than a few days. | |
| | Oramorph SR | **Tab, ER:** 15mg, 30mg, 60mg, 100mg | | | Single dose is 1/2 of daily morphine requirement q12h. | | Relief of pain in patients who require opioid analgesics for more than a few days. | |
| Morphine sulfate/ Naltrexone HCl | Embeda | **Cap, ER:** 20mg-0.8mg, 30mg-1.2mg, 50mg-2mg, 60mg-2.4mg, 80mg-3.2mg, 100mg-4mg | | | May be administered qd or bid. The lowest dose should be used. Titrate to 1-2 tabs/day. Titrate no more frequently than qod. | | Management of moderate to severe pain when a continuous, around-the-clock opioid analgesic is needed for an extended period of time. | Schedule II |

| GENERIC | BRAND | DOSAGE FORMS | ORAL EQUI-ANALGESIC DOSE | EQUI-ANALGESIC DOSE | USUAL ADULT DOSE | MAX DOSE | INDICATION | DEA SCHEDULE |
|---|---|---|---|---|---|---|---|---|
| Oxycodone/Acetaminophen | Percocet | **Tab:** 2.5mg-325mg, 5mg-325mg, 7.5mg-325mg, 7.5mg-500mg,10mg-325mg, 10mg-650mg | | | (2.5/325): 1-2 tabs q6h. (5/325): 1 tab q6h prn. (7.5/500): 1 tab q6h prn. (10/650): 1 tab q6h prn. (7.5/325): 1 tab q6h prn. (10/325): 1 tab q6h prn. | (2.5/325): 12 tabs/day. (5/325):12 tabs/day. (7.5/500): 8 tabs/day. (10/650) 6 tabs/day. (7.5/325): 8 tabs/day. (10/325): 6 tabs/day. | Relief of moderate to moderately severe pain. | Schedule II |
| | Tylox | **Cap:** 5mg-500mg | | | 1 cap q6h prn. | APAP: 4g/day. | | |
| Oxycodone/Ibuprofen | Combunox | **Tab:** 5mg-400mg | | | 1 tab/dose. | 4 tabs/day for 7 days. | Short term (<7 days) management of acute, moderate to severe pain. | Schedule II |
| Oxycodone HCl | OxyContin | **Tab, ER:** 10mg, 15mg, 20mg, 30mg, 40mg, 60mg, 80mg | 20mg. | | 10mg q12h. Titrate: May increase the q12h dose (not the dosing frequency). May increase the total daily dose by 25-50% of the current dose. | | Management of moderate to severe pain when a continuous, around-the-clock analgesic is needed for an extended period. Only for postoperative use in patients already receiving the drug before surgery or those expected to have moderate-severe postoperative pain for an extended period of time. | Schedule II |
| | | **Cap, IR:** 5mg; **Sol:** 5mg/5mL, 20mg/mL (concentrate) | | | Cap, IR: 5mg q6h prn; Sol: 10-30mg q4h prn. | | | |
| | Roxicodone | **Sol:** 5mg/5mL; **Liq:** 20mg/mL; **Tab:** 5mg,15mg, 30mg | | | Tab: 5-15mg q4-6h prn; Sol/Liq: 5-15mg q4-6h prn. | | Relief of moderate to moderately severe pain. | |
| Oxycodone HCl/Aspirin | Percodan | **Tab:** 4.8355mg-325mg | | | 1 tab q6h prn. | 12 tabs/day or ASA 4g/day. | Relief of moderate to moderately severe pain. | Schedule II |

*(Continued)*

| GENERIC | BRAND | DOSAGE FORMS | ORAL EQUI-ANALGESIC DOSE | EQUI-ANALGESIC DOSE | USUAL ADULT DOSE | MAX DOSE | INDICATION | DEA SCHEDULE |
|---|---|---|---|---|---|---|---|---|
| Oxymorphone HCl | Opana | **Inj:** 1mg/1mL<br>**Tab:** 5mg, 10mg | 10mg. | 1mg. | Inj: SQ/IM: 1-1.5mg q4-6h, IV: 0.5mg initial.<br>Tab: 10-20mg q4-6h. | | Relief of moderate to severe acute pain. For preoperative medication, for support of anesthesia, for obstetrical analgesia, and for relief of anxiety in patients with dyspnea associated with pulmonary edema secondary to acute left ventricular dysfunction.<br>(Tab, ER) Relief of moderate to severe pain in patients requiring continuous, around-the-clock opioid treatment for extended period of time. | Schedule II |
| | Opana ER | **Tab:** 5mg, 7.5mg, 10mg, 15mg, 20mg, 30mg, 40mg | | | 5mg q12h. Titrate individually at increments of 5-10mg q12h every 3-7 days. | | | |
| Propoxyphene HCl | Darvon | **Cap:** 65mg | | | 65mg q4h prn. | 390mg/day. | Relief of mild to moderate pain. | Schedule IV |
| Propoxyphene napsylate | Darvon-N | **Tab:** 100mg | | | 100mg q4h prn. | 600mg/day. | Relief of mild to moderate pain. | Schedule IV |
| Propoxyphene napsylate/ Acetaminophen | Darvocet-N 50 | **Tab:** 50mg-325mg | | | 100mg propoxyphene napsylate/650mg APAP q4h prn. | 600mg propoxyphene napsylate/day. APAP: 4g/day. | Relief of mild to moderate pain. | Schedule IV |
| | Darvocet-N 100 | **Tab:** 100mg-650mg | | | | | | |
| | Darvocet-A 500 | **Tab:** 100mg-500mg | | | 100mg propoxyphene napsylate/500 mg APAP q4h prn. | 6 tabs q24h. | | |
| Tapentadol | Nucynta | **Tab:** 50mg, 75mg, 100mg | | | 50mg, 75mg, or 100mg q4-6 hrs depending upon pain intensity. A second dose may be given 1hr after first dose. | 700mg/day on first day of therapy; 600mg/day on sub-. sequent days of therapy. | Relief of moderate to severe acute pain in patients ≥18 yrs. | Schedule II |

Reference: "Principles of Analgesic Use in the Treatment of Acute Pain and Cancer Pain," 6th ed, Glenview, IL: The American Pain Society. 2008.

# ORAL ANTICONVULSANTS

| DRUG (BRAND) | INDICATIONS | USUAL ADULT DOSE* | THERAPEUTIC SERUM LEVELS |
|---|---|---|---|
| **BARBITURATES** | | | |
| **Mephobarbital** (Mebaral) | Grand mal and petit mal epilepsy | 400-600mg/day | NA |
| **Phenobarbital** | Generalized and partial | 60-200mg/day | 10-40mcg/mL |
| **Primidone** (Mysoline) | Tonic-clonic, psychomotor, focal | 750-2000mg/day | 5-12mcg/mL |
| **BENZODIAZEPINES** | | | |
| **Clonazepam** (Klonopin, Klonopin Wafers) | Myoclonic, akinetic, Lennox-Gastaut syndrome, absence seizures (if failed succinimides) | 1.5-20mg/day | NA |
| **Clorazepate dipotassium** (Tranxene, Tranxene-SD) | Adjunct therapy in partial seizures | 22.5-90mg/day | NA |
| **Diazepam** (Valium) | Adjunct in convulsive disorders | 4-40mg/day | NA |
| **HYDANTOIN** | | | |
| **Ethotoin** (Peganone) | Tonic-clonic, Partial (psychomotor) | 2000-3000mg/day | N/A |
| **Phenytoin** (Dilantin, Phenytek) | Tonic-clonic partial (psychomotor, temporal lobe), prevent/treat seizures during/ following neurosurgery. | 300-600mg/day | 10-20mcg/mL |
| **SUCCINIMIDES** | | | |
| **Ethosuximide** (Zarontin) | Absence | 500mg-1.5g/day | 40-100mcg/mL |
| **Methsuximide** (Celontin) | Absence | 300-1200mg/day | Toxic level: >40mcg/mL |
| **MISCELLANEOUS** | | | |
| **Carbamazepine** (Carbatrol, Tegretol) | Tonic-clonic, mixed, partial (psychomotor, temporal lobe) | 800-1200mg/day | 4-12mcg/mL |
| **Divalproex sodium** (Depakote, Depakote ER, Depakote Sprinkles) **Valproic acid** (Depakene, Stavzor) | Absence, partial | 10-60mg/kg/day | 50-100mcg/mL |
| **Felbamate**** (Felbatol) | Partial with or w/o generalization (adults), partial/ generalized with Lennox-Gastaut syndrome (pediatrics) | 1200-3600mg/day | NA |
| **Gabapentin** (Neurontin) | Partial with and without secondary generalization (>12 yrs), partial (pediatrics) | 900-1800mg/day | NA |
| **Lacosamide** (Vimpat) | Partial | 200-400mg/day | NA |
| **Lamotrigine** (Lamictal, Lamictal CD, Lamictal ODT, Lamictal XR) | Partial, generalized seizures of Lennox-Gastaut syndrome, tonic-clonic (≥2 yrs) | 100-400mg/day (Lamictal XR) 200-600mg/day | NA |
| **Levetiracetam** (Keppra, Keppra XR) | Partial, myoclonic, primary generalized tonic-clonic (Keppra XR): Partial | 1000-3000mg/day | NA |

*(Continued)*

| DRUG (BRAND) | INDICATIONS | USUAL ADULT DOSE* | THERAPEUTIC SERUM LEVELS |
|---|---|---|---|
| **MISCELLANEOUS** (*Continued*) | | | |
| **Oxcarbazepine** (Trileptal) | Partial | 600-2400mg/day | NA |
| **Pregabalin** (Lyrica) | Partial | 150-600mg/day | NA |
| **Rufinamide** (Banzel) | Lennox-Gastaut syndrome | 3200mg/day | NA |
| **Tiagabine** (Gabitril) | Partial | 32-56mg/day | NA |
| **Topiramate** (Topamax, Topamax Sprinkle) | Partial, tonic-clonic, Lennox-Gastaut syndrome (≥2 yrs) | 200-400mg/day | NA |
| **Trimethadione** (Tridione) | Refractory petit mal | 900-2400mg/day | NA |
| **Vigabatrin** (Sabril) | Refractory complex partial seizures | 3000mg | NA |
| **Zonisamide** (Zonegran) | Partial | 100-400mg/day | NA |

*Please refer to complete monograph for pediatric dosing.

**For severe epilepsy refractory to other treatment where the risk of aplastic anemia and/or liver failure is deemed acceptable. Fully advise patient and obtain written, informed consent before treatment. Closely monitor patient.

NA = Not Available.

# TRIPTANS FOR ACUTE MIGRAINE

| DRUG | BRAND | HOW SUPPLIED | INITIAL & (MAX) DOSE* | HEPATIC/RENAL DOSE ADJUSTMENT* |
|---|---|---|---|---|
| Almotriptan malate | Axert | Tab: 6.25mg, 12.5mg | 6.25-12.5mg. May repeat after 2 hours. (2 doses/24 hours) | Initial: 6.25mg. Max: 12.5mg/24 hours. |
| Eletriptan hydrobromide | Relpax | Tab: 20mg, 40mg | 20-40mg. May repeat after 2 hours. (40mg/dose or 80mg/day) | Severe Hepatic Impairment: Avoid use. |
| Frovatriptan succinate | Frova | Tab: 2.5mg | 2.5mg. May repeat after 2 hours. (7.5mg/day) | No adjustment. |
| Naratriptan hydrochloride | Amerge | Tab: 1mg, 2.5mg | 1-2.5mg. May repeat after 4 hours. (5mg/24 hours) | Severe Renal/Hepatic Impairment: Avoid use.<br>Mild-Moderate Renal/ Hepatic Impairment: Use lower dose. Max: 2.5mg/24 hours. |
| Rizatriptan benzoate | Maxalt | Tab: 5mg, 10mg | 5-10mg. May repeat after 2 hours. (30mg/24 hours) | No adjustment. |
| | Maxalt-MLT | Tab, Disintegrating: 5mg, 10mg | 5-10mg. May repeat after 2 hours. (30mg/24 hours) | No adjustment. |
| Sumatriptan | Imitrex, Sumavel DosePro | (Imitrex, Sumavel DosePro) Inj**: 6mg/ 0.5mL, (Imitrex) Inj**, stat dose system: 4mg, 6mg | (Imitrex, Sumavel DosePro) 6mg SQ. May repeat after 1 hour. (12mg/24 hours) | (Imitrex) Severe Hepatic Impairment: Avoid use. |
| | | Nasal Spray: 5mg, 20mg | 5mg, 10mg, or 20mg single dose into 1 nostril. May repeat after 2 hours. (40mg/24 hours) | Severe Hepatic Impairment: Avoid use. |
| | | Tab: 25mg, 50mg, 100mg | 25-100mg. May repeat after 2 hours. (200mg/24 hours) | Severe Hepatic Impairment: Avoid use. Hepatic Disease: Max: 50mg/single dose. |
| Zolmitriptan | Zomig | Nasal Spray: 5mg | 5mg. May repeat after 2 hours. (10mg/24 hours) | Hepatic Impairment: Use lower dose. |
| | | Tab: 2.5mg, 5mg | 2.5mg or lower. May repeat after 2 hours. (10mg/24 hours) | Hepatic Impairment: Use lower dose. |
| | Zomig-ZMT | Tab, Disintegrating: 2.5mg, 5mg | 2.5mg or lower. May repeat after 2 hours. (10mg/24 hours) | Hepatic Impairment: Use lower dose. |
| **COMBINATION DRUG** | | | | |
| Naproxen-Sumatriptan | Treximet | Tab: (Naproxen-Sumatriptan): 500mg/85mg [9s] | 1 tab; may repeat after 2 hrs. (2 tabs/24 hrs) Do not split, crush, or chew. | Advanced renal disease: Avoid use. |

***NOTE:** Dosages shown are for adults ≥18 yrs. For more detailed information, refer to the individual monograph or the drug's FDA-approved labeling.

**Also indicated for acute treatment of cluster headaches.

# HORMONE THERAPY

| DRUG | BRAND | DOSAGE (mg) |
|---|---|---|
| **INTRAMUSCULAR ESTROGEN PRODUCTS** | | |
| Estradiol valerate | Delestrogen | **(mg/mL)**<br>10mg/mL, 20mg/mL, 40mg/mL |
| Estradiol cypionate | Depo-Estradiol | 5mg/mL |
| **ORAL ESTROGEN PRODUCTS** | | |
| Conjugated equine estrogens | Premarin | 0.3, 0.45, 0.625, 0.9, 1.25 |
| | Enjuvia | 0.3, 0.45, 0.625, 0.9, 1.25 |
| **SYNTHETIC CONJUGATED ESTROGEN PRODUCTS** | | |
| Estradiol acetate | Femtrace | 0.45, 0.9, 1.8 |
| Synthetic conjugated estrogens | Cenestin | 0.3, 0.45, 0.625, 0.9, 1.25 |
| Esterified estrogens | Menest | 0.3, 0.625, 1.25, 2.5 |
| Micronized 17ß-estradiol | Estrace, Innofem | 0.5, 1, 2 |
| Estropipate (piperazine estrone sulfate) | Ortho-Est | 0.75, 1.5 |
| | (Generic) | 0.75 (0.625), 1.5 (1.25), 3 (2.5) |
| **TRANSDERMAL ESTROGEN PRODUCTS** | | |
| 17ß-estradiol matrix patch | Alora | **RELEASE RATE (mg/day)**<br>0.025, 0.05, 0.075, 0.1 |
| | Climara | 0.025, 0.0375, 0.05, 0.06, 0.075, 0.1 |
| | Vivelle, Vivelle-Dot | 0.025, 0.0375, 0.05, 0.075, 0.1 |
| 17ß-estradiol reservoir patch | Estraderm | 0.05, 0.1 |
| 17ß-estradiol | Elestrin | (0.06% gel): 1 metered pump actuation/day applied to upper arm. Adjust dosage as necessary. |
| 17ß-estradiol | Estrogel | (0.06% gel): 1 metered pump actuation/day applied to arm (from wrist to shoulder). |
| Estradiol hemihydrate | Estrasorb | (emulsion): 3.48g/day (two 1.74g pouches) applied qam to each leg from thigh to calf. Rub for 3 minutes until absorbed. |
| 17ß-estradiol | Evamist | (spray): Initial: 1 metered spray/day qam (1.53mg/spray). Usual: 1-3 sprays/day qam to adjacent, non-overlapping areas on inner forearm, start near elbow. |
| **VAGINAL ESTROGEN PRODUCTS** | | |
| **Vaginal Creams**<br>17ß-estradiol | Estrace Vaginal Cream | 2-4g/day x 1-2 wks, reduce to 1-2g/day x 1-2 wks, then 1g/day x 1-3x/wk |
| Conjugated equine estrogens | Premarin Vaginal Cream | 0.5-2g/day x 3 wks on 1 wk off |
| **Vaginal Ring**<br>17ß-estradiol | Estring | Releases 0.0075mg/day x 90 days |
| | Femring | Releases 0.05 or 0.1mg/day x 90 days |
| **Vaginal Tablet**<br>Estradiol hemihydrate | Vagifem | Intravaginal: 1 tab qd x 2 wks then 1 tab biw (started at 10mcg) |
| **PROGESTOGEN ONLY PRODUCTS** | | |
| Medroxyprogesterone acetate | Provera | 2.5, 5, 10 |
| Norethindrone acetate | Aygestin | 5 |
| Progesterone USP (in peanut oil) | Prometrium | 100, 200 |

*(Continued)*

| DRUG | BRAND | DOSAGE (mg) | | |
|---|---|---|---|---|
| **ESTROGEN + PROGESTOGEN COMBINATIONS** | | | | |
| **Oral continuous-cyclic regimen**<br>Conjugated equine estrogens (E) + Medroxyprogesterone acetate (P) | Premphase | 0.625mg (E), 5mg (P) [E alone for days 1-14, followed by E+P on days 15-28] | | |
| 17ß-estradiol (E) + Norgestimate (P) | Prefest | 1mg (E), 0.09mg (P) [E alone for days 1-3, followed by E+P on days 4-6, repeat continuously] | | |
| **Oral continuous-combined regimen**<br>Conjugated equine estrogens (E) + Medroxyprogesterone (P) | Prempro | 0.3mg (E) + 1.5mg (P) | 0.45mg + 1.5mg | 0.625mg + 2.5 or 5mg |
| Ethinyl estradiol (E) + Norethindrone acetate (P) | femhrt | 2.5mcg (E) + 0.5mg (P); 5mcg (E) + 1mg (P) | | |
| 17ß-estradiol (E) + Norethindrone acetate (P) | Activella | 1mg (E) + 0.5mg (P); 0.5mg (E) + 0.1mg (P) | | |
| **Transdermal continuous-cyclic or continuous-combined regimen**<br>17ß-estradiol (E) + Norethindrone acetate (P) | CombiPatch | 0.05mg/day (E) + 0.14 or 0.25mg/day (P) | | |
| Estradiol (E) + Levonorgestrel (P) | Climara Pro | 0.045mg/day (E) + 0.015mg/day (P) | | |
| **ESTROGEN + ANDROGEN COMBINATIONS** | | | | |
| **Oral cyclic regimen**<br>Esterified estrogens (E) + | Estratest* | 1.25 (E) + 2.5 (A) | | |
| Methyltestosterone (A) | Estratest H.S.* | 0.625 (E) + 1.25 (A) | | |

**NOTE:** This list is not inclusive of all estrogen and progestogen products available. Indications vary among the different products. For more detailed information please refer to the individual monograph listings or the drug's FDA-approved labeling. Unopposed estrogen replacement therapy (ERT) is for use in women without an intact uterus. For women with an intact uterus, progestin must be added to the estrogen (HRT) for protection against estrogen-induced endometrial cancer. As with any therapy, the lowest possible effective dosage should be used. Re-evaluate periodically.

* This product has not obtained FDA premarket approval applicable for new drugs.

# Oral Contraceptives

| DRUG | ESTROGEN | PROGESTIN | STRENGTH (ESTROGEN/PROGESTIN) |
|---|---|---|---|
| **MONOPHASIC** | | | |
| Aviane 28, Lessina 28, Sronyx 28** | Ethinyl Estradiol | Levonorgestrel | 20mcg/0.1mg |
| Brevicon, Modicon | Ethinyl Estradiol | Norethindrone | 35mcg/0.5mg |
| Demulen 1/35 | Ethinyl Estradiol | Ethynodiol Diacetate | 35mcg/1mg |
| Demulen 1/50 | Ethinyl Estradiol | Ethynodiol Diacetate | 50mcg/1mg |
| Desogen, Ortho-Cept | Ethinyl Estradiol | Desogestrel | 30mcg/0.15mg |
| Nordette-28 (Jolessa, Levlen, Levora, Portia 28**) | Ethinyl Estradiol | Levonorgestrel | 30mcg/0.15mg |
| Loestrin 21 1/20, Loestrin Fe 1/20, Loestrin 24 Fe (Junel, Microgestin**) | Ethinyl Estradiol | Norethindrone Acetate | 20mcg/1mg |
| Loestrin 21 1.5/30, Loestrin Fe 1.5/30 (Junel, Microgestin**) | Ethinyl Estradiol | Norethindrone Acetate | 30mcg/1.5mg |
| Lo/Ovral (Cryselle, Low-Ogestrel-28**) | Ethinyl Estradiol | Norgestrel | 30mcg/0.3mg |
| Lybrel* | Ethinyl Estradiol | Levonorgestrel | 20mcg/0.09mg |
| Norinyl 1/35, Ortho-Novum 1/35 | Ethinyl Estradiol | Norethindrone | 35mcg/1mg |
| Norinyl 1/50, (Necon 1/50**) | Mestranol | Norethindrone | 50mcg/1mg |
| Ortho-Cyclen (Previfem, Sprintec**) | Ethinyl Estradiol | Norgestimate | 35mcg/0.25mg |
| Ovcon 35 (Balziva**) | Ethinyl Estradiol | Norethindrone | 35mcg/0.4mg |
| Ovcon 50* | Ethinyl Estradiol | Norethindrone | 50mcg/1mg |
| Ovral (Ogestrel 28**) | Ethinyl Estradiol | Levonorgestrel | 50mcg/0.5mg |
| Seasonale (Quasense**) | Ethinyl Estradiol | Levonorgestrel | 30mcg/0.15mg |
| Yasmin (Ocella**) | Ethinyl Estradiol | Drospirenone | 30mcg/3mg |
| YAZ* | Ethinyl Estradiol | Drospirenone | 20mcg/3mg |
| **BIPHASIC** | | | |
| Mircette (Kariva**) | Ethinyl Estradiol | Desogestrel | **Phase 1:** 20mcg/0.15mg<br>**Phase 2:** 10mcg/NONE |
| Loseasonique* | Ethinyl Estradiol | Levonorgestrel | 0.1mg, 0.02mg, 0.01mg |
| Seasonique* | Ethinyl Estradiol | Levonorgestrel | 0.01mg, 30mcg/0.15mg |
| **TRIPHASIC** | | | |
| Cyclessa (Velivet**) | Ethinyl Estradiol | Desogestrel | **Phase 1:** 25mcg/0.1mg<br>**Phase 2:** 25mcg/0.125mg<br>**Phase 3:** 25mcg/0.15mg |
| Estrostep Fe (Tri-legest Fe**) | Ethinyl Estradiol | Norethindrone Acetate | **Phase 1:** 20mcg/1mg<br>**Phase 2:** 30mcg/1mg<br>**Phase 3:** 35mcg/1mg |

*(Continued)*

| DRUG | ESTROGEN | PROGESTIN | STRENGTH (ESTROGEN/PROGESTIN) |
|---|---|---|---|
| **TRIPHASIC** *(Continued)* | | | |
| Ortho-Novum 7/7/7 (Nortrel 7/7/7**) | Ethinyl Estradiol | Norethindrone | **Phase 1:** 35mcg/0.5mg<br>**Phase 2:** 35mcg/0.75mg<br>**Phase 3:** 35mcg/1mg |
| Ortho Tri-Cyclen (Tri-Previfem, Trinessa, Tri-Sprintec**) | Ethinyl Estradiol | Norgestimate | **Phase 1:** 35mcg/0.18mg<br>**Phase 2:** 35mcg/0.215mg<br>**Phase 3:** 35mcg/0.25mg |
| Ortho Tri-Cyclen Lo (Tri-Lo-Sprintec) | Ethinyl Estradiol | Norgestimate | **Phase 1:** 25mcg/0.18mg<br>**Phase 2:** 25mcg/0.215mg<br>**Phase 3:** 25mcg/0.25mg |
| Tri-Levlen, Trivora 28, Enpresse 28** | Ethinyl Estradiol | Levonorgestrel | **Phase 1:** 30mcg/0.05mg<br>**Phase 2:** 40mcg/0.075mg<br>**Phase 3:** 30mcg/0.125mg |
| Tri-Norinyl | Ethinyl Estradiol | Norethindrone | **Phase 1:** 35mcg/0.5mg<br>**Phase 2:** 35mcg/1mg<br>**Phase 3:** 35mcg/0.5mg |
| **PROGESTIN ONLY** | | | |
| Nor-Q.D. (Camila, Errin, Jolivette**) Ortho-Micronor | | Norethindrone | 0.35mg |
| Plan B (Next Choice**) | | Levonorgestrel | 0.75mg |
| Plan B One Step | | Levonorgestrel | 1.5mg |

*Currently NO generics available.
**Other branded generics.

# Breast Cancer Risk Factors

| Unmodifiable risk factors | |
|---|---|
| Gender | Women > men |
| Age | 1 out of 8 breast cancer diagnoses are among women <45 yrs, while about 2 out of 3 occur in women >55 yrs |
| Genetic | BRCA1 and BRCA2, ATM gene, CHEK2 gene, p53 tumor suppressor gene, PTEN gene mutations, CDH |
| Race | Whites > African Americans |
| Family history | Having a first-degree relative with breast cancer doubles risk; having 2 first-degree relatives increases risk about 5-fold |
| Personal history of breast cancer | Women with cancer in one breast have 3- to 4-fold increased risk of developing a new cancer in another area of the same breast or in the opposite breast |
| Abnormal breast biopsy | Nonproliferative lesions, proliferative lesions with or without atypia |
| Early menarche | Women who started menstruating at an early age (<12 yrs) |
| Age at menopause | Women who went through menopause at a late age (>55 yrs) |
| Personal history of breast abnormalities | Two breast tissue abnormalities–ductal carcinoma in situ (DCIS) and lobular carcinoma in situ (LCIS)–are associated with increased risk for developing invasive breast cancer |
| Earlier breast radiation exposure | Women who had radiation therapy to the chest area as treatment for another cancer |
| Breast density | Women with a higher proportion of dense breast tissue (eg, connective and milk duct tissue) |

**Lifestyle factors associated with increased risk of breast cancer**

- Alcohol (2 drinks/day)
- High body mass index
- Not having children or having them when >30 yrs
- Lack of physical activity
- Not breastfeeding

**Drugs associated with increased risk of breast cancer**

- Birth control pills
- DES (diethylstilbestrol)
- Postmenopausal hormone therapy or hormone replacement therapy

**Uncertain risk factors**

- Antiperspirants
- Bras
- Breast implants
- High-fat diets
- Induced abortion
- Miscarriages
- Night work
- Pollution (chemicals)
- Smoking (active or passive)

**Sources:** American Cancer Society and National Cancer Institute.

# BREAST CANCER TREATMENT OPTIONS

| DRUG (BRAND) | INDICATIONS | HOW SUPPLIED | DOSAGE |
|---|---|---|---|
| **ANDROGENS** | | | |
| **Fluoxymesterone** (Halotestin) | Palliation of androgen-responsive recurrent mammary cancer in females who are 1 to <5 yrs post-menopausal or who have a hormone-dependent tumor as shown by previous beneficial response to castration. | Tab: 2mg*, 5mg*, 10mg* *scored | 10-40mg/day in divided doses tid-qid. Continue therapy for at least 1 month for satisfactory subjective response, and for 2-3 months for objective response. |
| **Methyltestosterone** (Testred) | Secondary treatment of advancing inoperable metastatic (skeletal) breast cancer in females who are 1-5 yrs postmenopausal. | Cap: 10mg | 50-200mg/day. |
| **Testosterone** (Delatestryl) | Secondary treatment of advancing inoperable metastatic (skeletal) mammary cancer who are 1-5 years postmenopausal. | Inj: 200mg/mL | 200-400mg every 2-4 weeks. |
| **ANTIESTROGEN** | | | |
| **Faslodex** (Fulvestrant) | Treatment of hormone receptor positive metastatic breast cancer in postmenopausal women with disease progression following anti-estrogen therapy. | Inj: 50mg/mL [2.5mL, 5mL] | 250mg IM into buttock once monthly as either a single 5mL injection or two concurrent 2.5mL injections. Administer slowly. |
| **ESTROGENS** | | | |
| **Estradiol** (Estrace) | Palliative treatment of metastatic breast cancer. | Tab: 0.5mg*, 1mg*, 2mg* *scored | 10mg tid for at least 3 months. |
| **Menest** (Esterified estrogens) | Palliative therapy for metastatic breast cancer in selected men and women. | Tab: 0.3mg, 0.625mg, 1.25mg, 2.5mg | 10mg tid for at least 3 months. |
| **Premarin Tablets** (Conjugated estrogens) | Palliative treatment of breast cancer in patients with metastatic disease. | Tab: 0.3mg, 0.45mg, 0.625mg, 0.9mg, 1.25mg | 10mg tid for minimum 3 months. |
| **LHRH AGONIST** | | | |
| **Zoladex 1-Month** (Goserelin) | Palliative treatment of advanced breast cancer in pre-and perimenopausal women. | Implant: 3.6mg | Inject SQ into anterior abdominal wall below navel line. 3.6mg every 28 days. |
| **PROGESTIN** | | | |
| **Megestrol** (Megestrol) | Palliative treatment of advanced breast carcinoma (eg, recurrent, inoperable or metastatic disease). | Tab: 20mg*, 40mg* *scored Susp: 40mg/mL | 40mg qid for a minimum of 2 months. Elderly: Start at lower end of dosing range. |
| **SELECTIVE ESTROGEN RECEPTOR MODULATORS** | | | |
| **Raloxifene** (Evista) | Reduction in risk of invasive breast cancer in post-menopausal women with osteoporosis or at high risk for invasive breast cancer. | Tab: 60mg | 60mg qd. |

| DRUG (BRAND) | INDICATIONS | HOW SUPPLIED | DOSAGE |
|---|---|---|---|
| **SELECTIVE ESTROGEN RECEPTOR MODULATORS** *(continued)* | | | |
| **Tamoxifen** (Tamoxifen) | Treatment of metastatic breast cancer in women and men. Treatment of node-positive and axillary node-negative breast cancer in women following mastectomy, axillary dissection and breast irradiation. To reduce risk of invasive breast cancer in women with DCIS (Ductal carcinoma in-situ). Reduction of breast cancer incidence in high risk women. Use for up to 5 yrs. | Tab: 10mg, 20mg | 20-40mg qd. Divide dosages >20mg into AM and PM doses. Risk Reduction/DCIS: 20mg qd for 5 yrs. |
| **Toremifene** (Fareston) | Treatment of metastatic breast cancer in post-menopausal women with estrogen-receptor positive or unknown tumors. | Tab: 60mg | 60mg qd. Treat until disease progression is evident. |
| **SELECTIVE NONSTEROIDAL AROMATASE INHIBITORS (POSTMENOPAUSAL WOMEN ONLY)** | | | |
| **Anastrozole** (Arimidex) | Adjuvant treatment of post-menopausal women with hormone-receptor positive early breast cancer. First-line treatment of post-menopausal women with hormone-receptor positive or hormone-receptor unknown locally advanced or metastatic breast cancer. Treatment of advanced breast cancer in post-menopausal women with disease progression following tamoxifen therapy. Patients with ER-negative disease and patients who did not respond to previous tamoxifen therapy rarely respond. | Tab: 1mg | 1mg qd. Continue until tumor progression with advanced breast cancer. |
| **Letrozole** (Femara) | Adjuvant treatment of postmenopausal women with hormone-receptor positive early breast cancer. Extended adjuvant treatment of early breast cancer in postmenopausal women who have received 5 yrs of adjuvant tamoxifen therapy. First-line treatment of hormone-receptor positive or hormone-receptor unknown locally advanced or metastatic breast cancer in postmenopausal women. Treatment of advanced breast cancer with disease progression following antiestrogen therapy in postmenopausal women. | Tab: 2.5mg | 2.5mg qd. Continue until tumor progression is evident. Cirrhosis/ Severe Liver Dysfunction: 2.5mg every other day. |

| DRUG (BRAND) | INDICATIONS | HOW SUPPLIED | DOSAGE |
|---|---|---|---|
| **CHEMOTHERAPY AGENTS** | | | |
| **ANTHRACYCLINES** | | | |
| **Doxorubicin** | To produce regression in disseminated neoplastic conditions such as breast carcinoma. Adjuvant therapy in women with evidence of axillary lymph node involvement following resection of primary breast cancer. | Inj: (2mg/mL) 10mg, 20mg, 50mg, 200mg | Monotherapy: 60-75mg/m² IV every 21 days. Use the lower dose with inadequate bone marrow reserves due to old age, prior therapy, or neoplastic marrow infiltration. Concomitant Chemotherapy: 40-60mg/m² IV every 21-28 days. Hyperbilirubinemia: Reduce dose by 50% if 1.2-3mg/dL; reduce dose by 75% if 3.1-5mg/dL. See PI for pediatric dosing. |
| **Epirubicin** (Ellence) | Adjuvant treatment of primary breast cancer with axillary node tumor involvement following resection of primary breast cancer. | Inj: 2mg/mL [25mL, 100mL] | Initial: 100-120mg/m² IV infusion, repeat at 3-4 week cycles. May give total dose on Day 1 of each cycle or divide equally on Days 1 and 8. Bone Marrow Dysfunction: Initial: 75-90mg/m². Hepatic Dysfunction: Bilirubin 1.2-3mg/dL or AST 2-4X ULN: Give 1/2 of initial dose. Bilirubin >3mg/dL or AST 4X ULN: Give 1/4 of initial dose. Severe Renal Dysfunction: Serum Creatinine >5mg/dL: Lower dose. Give prophylactic therapy with SMZ-TMP or fluoroquinolone with 120mg/m² regimen. Consider pretreatment with antiemetics. Adjust dose after 1st treatment cycle based on hematologic and nonhematologic toxicities (see PI). |
| **ANTIMICROTUBULE AGENT** | | | |
| **Ixabepilone** (Ixempra) | In combination with capecitabine for treatment of patients with metastatic or locally advanced breast cancer resistant to treatment with an anthracycline and a taxane, or whose cancer is taxane resistant and for whom further anthracycline therapy is contraindicated. As monotherapy for treatment of metastatic or locally advanced breast cancer in patients whose tumors are resistant or refractory to anthracyclines, taxanes, and capecitabine. | Inj: 15mg, 45mg | 40mg/m² IV infusion over 3 hrs every 3 weeks. Adjust dose based on toxicities (see PI). Premedicate with H1-antagonist (eg, diphenhydramine 50mg PO) and H2-antagonist (eg, ranitidine 150-300mg PO) approximately 1hr before infusion. Also premedicate with corticosteroid (eg, dexamethasone 20mg, IV 30 min before infusion or PO 60 min before infusion) if prior hypersensitivity reaction to ixabepilone. Hepatic Impairment: Monotherapy: Mild: AST and ALT ≤2.5x ULN and Bilirubin ≤1x ULN: 40mg/m². AST or ALT ≤10x ULN and Bilirubin ≤1.5x ULN: 32mg/m². Moderate (AST and ALT ≤10x ULN and Bilirubin >1.5 to ≤3x ULN): 20-30mg/m². Strong CYP3A4 Inhibitors: Avoid or reduce dose to 20mg/m². |
| **KINASE INHIBITOR** | | | |
| **Lapatinib** (Tykerb) | Treatment of patients with advanced or metastatic breast cancer, in combination with capecitabine, whose tumors overexpress HER2 and received prior therapy including an anthracycline, a taxane, and trastuzumab. In combination with letrozole for treatment of | Tab: 250mg | Usual: 1250mg qd on Days 1-21 continuously with capecitabine 2000mg/m²/day (2 doses 12 hrs apart) on Days 1-14 in a repeating 21-day cycle. Give at least 1 hr before or after a meal (however, give capecitabine with food). ≥ Grade 2 LVEF: D/C dose. If LVEF recovers and asymptomatic after 2 weeks, restart at 1000mg/day. Hepatic Impairment (Child-Pugh |

| DRUG (BRAND) | INDICATIONS | HOW SUPPLIED | DOSAGE |
|---|---|---|---|
| **KINASE INHIBITOR** *(continued)* | | | |
| | postmenopausal women with hormone receptor positive metastatic breast cancer overexpressing HER2 receptor, for whom hormone therapy is indicated. | | Class C): Consider dose reduction to 750mg/day. Concomitant Strong CYP3A4 Inhibitors: Avoid use. Concomitant Strong CYP3A4 Inducers: Avoid use and if must coadminister titrate gradually from 1250mg/day up to 4500mg/day based on tolerability. ≥ Grade 2 NCI CTC Toxicity: D/C or interrupt dose and restart with 1250mg/day when toxicity <Grade 1. Restart at 1000mg/day if toxicity recurs. |
| **MISCELLANEOUS** | | | |
| **Capecitabine** (Xeloda) | Treatment of metastatic breast cancer in combination with docetaxel after failure of prior anthracycline-containing chemotherapy. Treatment of metastatic breast cancer in patients resistant to paclitaxel and anthracycline-containing chemotherapy or resistant to paclitaxel and for whom further anthracycline therapy is not indicated. | Tab: 150mg, 500mg | Take with water within 30 min after meals. Usual/Concomitantly w/ docetaxel: 1250mg/m² bid for 2 weeks, then 1 week off. Give as 3-week cycles. CrCl 30-50mL/min: Reduce to 75% of starting dose. Interrupt and/or reduce dose if toxicity occurs. Readjust according to adverse effects (see PI for details). |
| **Cyclophosphamide** (Cytoxan) | Treatment of breast carcinoma. | Inj (Lyophilized): 500mg, 1g, 2g; Tab: 25mg, 50mg | Malignant Diseases (Without Hematologic Deficiency): Monotherapy: Initial: 40-50mg/kg IV in divided doses over 2-5 days, or 10-15mg/kg IV given every 7-10 days, or 3-5mg/kg twice weekly. Oral Dosing: Initial/Maint: 1-5mg/kg/day PO. Adjust dose according to antitumor activity and/or leukopenia. May need to reduce dose when combined with other cytotoxic drugs. See PI for pediatric dosing. |
| **Dexrazoxane** (Zinecard) | To reduce the incidence and severity of cardiomyopathy associated with doxorubicin in women with metastatic breast cancer who received a cumulative doxorubicin dose of 300mg/m² and who will continue doxorubicin therapy. | Inj: 250mg, 500mg | IV: 10:1 ratio of dexrazoxane: doxorubicin (eg, 500mg/m² dexrazoxane: 50mg/m² doxorubicin). Hepatic Impairment: Reduce dose proportionally. Give by slow IV push or rapid IV infusion. Give doxorubicin within 30 min after start of infusion. If CrCl <40 mL/min, the recommended dosage ratio is 5:1 (dexrazoxane: doxorubicin) |
| **Fluorouracil** | Palliative management of breast carcinoma. | Inj: 50mg/mL, [10mL] | 12mg/kg IV qd for 4 days. Max: 800mg/day. If no toxicity, give 6mg/kg IV on 6th, 8th, 10th, and 12th days. Skip Days 5, 7, 9, and 11. Inadequate Nutritional State: 6mg/kg IV for 3 days. If no toxicity, give 3mg/kg IV on 5th, 7th, and 9th days. Max: 400mg/day. Skip Days 4, 6, and 8. Maint (Use Schedule 1 or Schedule 2): Schedule 1: If no toxicity, repeat 1st course every 30 days after last day of previous course. Schedule 2: When toxic signs from initial course subside, give 10-15mg/kg/week IV single dose; do not exceed 1g/week. |

| DRUG (BRAND) | INDICATIONS | HOW SUPPLIED | DOSAGE |
|---|---|---|---|
| **MISCELLANEOUS** *(continued)* | | | |
| **Methotrexate** (Methotrexate) | Adjuvant treatment of breast cancer. | Inj: 25mg/mL, Tab: 2.5mg* *scored | 40mg/m² IV on Days 1 and 8. (Refer to NCCN guidelines for regimen details.) |
| **MONOCLONAL ANTIBODY/HER2 BLOCKER** | | | |
| **Transtuzumab** (Herceptin) | Adjuvant treatment of HER2-overexpressing node-positive/negative breast cancer. 1st-line treatment of HER2-overexpressing metastatic breast cancer in combination with paclitaxel. Single agent for adjuvant treatment of HER2-overexpressing breast cancer in patients who received 1 or more chemotherapy regimens for metastatic disease. | Inj: 440mg | Adjuvant Treatment: Following Anthracycline/Concurrently With Paclitaxel for First 12 Weeks: IV infusion: Initial: 4mg/kg over 90 min. Maint: 2mg/kg/week over 30 min for total 52 doses. Following Completion of All Chemotherapy: IV Infusion: Initial: 8mg/kg. Maint: 6mg/kg every 3 weeks for total of 17 doses; give doses ≥4mg/kg over 90 min. Metastatic Breast Cancer: IV Infusion: Alone or With Paclitaxel: Initial: 4mg/kg over 90 min. Maint: 2mg/kg/week over 30 min until disease progression. |
| **NUCLEOSIDE ANALOGUE/ANTIMETABOLITE** | | | |
| **Gemcitabine** (Gemzar) | Adjunct with paclitaxel for 1st-line treatment of metastatic breast cancer after failure of prior anthracycline-containing adjuvant chemotherapy, unless anthracyclines were clinically contraindicated. | Inj: 200mg, 1g | 1250mg/m² IV on Days 1 and 8 of each 21-day cycle. Give paclitaxel 175mg/m² IV on Day 1 before gemcitabine. All IV infusions given over 30 min. Adjust dose based on hematologic toxicity. |
| **TAXANES** | | | |
| **Docetaxel** (Taxotere) | Treatment of locally advanced or metastatic breast cancer after failure of prior chemotherapy. In combination with doxorubicin and cyclophosphamide for the adjuvant treatment of operable, node-positive breast cancer. | Inj: 20mg/0.5mL, 80mg/2mL | Premedicate with oral corticosteroids. Adjust dose based on febrile neutropenia, neutrophil count, cutaneous reactions, peripheral neuropathy, neurosensory signs/symptoms, or GI toxicities (see PI). Breast Cancer: 60-100mg/m² IV over 1 hr every 3 weeks. Adjuvant Treatment Operable Node-Positive Breast CA: 75mg/m² 1 hr after doxorubicin 50mg/m² and cyclophosphamide 500mg/m² every 3 weeks for 6 courses. Administer every 3 weeks for 3 cycles. |
| **Paclitaxel** (Taxol) | Treatment of breast cancer after failure with combination chemotherapy for metastatic disease or relapse within 6 months of adjuvant chemotherapy. Adjuvant treatment of node-positive breast cancer administered sequentially to doxorubicin-containing chemotherapy. | Inj: 6mg/mL | 175mg/m² over 3 hrs every 3 weeks for 4 courses. Reduce dose of subsequent courses by 20% if neutrophils <500 cells/mm³ for ≥1 week or severe peripheral neuropathy occurs. Premedicate prior to administration with appropriate medications; see PI for additional information. |
| **Paclitaxel protein-bound particle for injectable suspension** (Abraxane) | Treatment of breast cancer after failure of combination chemotherapy for metastatic disease or relapse within 6 months of adjuvant chemotherapy. Prior therapy should have included an anthracyline unless clinically contraindicated. | Inj: 100mg | 260mg/m² IV over 30 min every 3 weeks. Severe neutropenia (neutrophil <500 cells/mm³ for week or longer) or severe sensory neuropathy (Grade 3 or 4): Hold dose until neutrophil >1500 cells/mm³ or sensory neuropathy resolves to Grade 1 or 2. Reduce subsequent courses to 220mg/m², if recurrence reduce subsequent courses to 180mg/m². |

| DRUG (BRAND) | INDICATIONS | HOW SUPPLIED | DOSAGE |
|---|---|---|---|
| **VASCULAR ENDOTHELIAL GROWTH INHIBITOR** | | | |
| **Bevacizumab** (Avastin) | Treatment of patients who have not received chemotherapy for metastatic HER2 negative breast cancer, in combination with paclitaxel. | Inj: 25mg/mL [4mL, 16mL] | 10mg/kg every 2 weeks. Give as IV infusion over 90 min, if 1st infusion is well tolerated, give 2nd infusion over 60 min and subsequent doses over 30 min. |
| **VINCA ALKALOID** | | | |
| **Vinblastine** | Palliative treatment of breast carcinoma unresponsive to appropriate endocrine surgery and hormonal therapy. | Inj: 1mg/mL [10mL] | Dose at intervals of ≤7 days. 1st Dose: 3.7mg/m². 2nd Dose: 5.5mg/m². 3rd Dose: 7.4mg/m². 4th Dose: 9.25mg/m². 5th Dose: 11.1mg/m². Max: 18.5mg/m². Do not increase dose after that dose which reduces WBC to 3000 cells/mm³. Maint: Use dose of 1 increment smaller than this dose at weekly intervals. Reduce to 50% dose if direct serum bilirubin >3mg/100mL. Only dose if WBC ≥4000 cells/mm³. |

# Chemotherapy Regimens*†

| CANCER TYPE | PREFERRED THERAPIES | ALTERNATIVE REGIMENS |
|---|---|---|
| **Bladder** | *Non-muscle invasive:* Bacillus Calmette-Guerin (BCG)<br><br>*Neoadjuvant, adjuvant, and metastatic:* Gemcitabine/cisplatin (preferred); or Methotrexate/vinblastine/doxorubicin/cisplatin (MVAC) | *Non-muscle invasive:* Mitomycin C (MMC)<br><br>*Neoadjuvant, adjuvant, and metastatic:* Carboplatin and taxane-based therapy or single-agent therapy |
| **Breast** | | |
| Risk reduction | Tamoxifen (premenopausal); tamoxifen or raloxifene (postmenopausal) | |
| Adjuvant (trastuzumab containing) | Doxorubicin/cyclophosphamide followed by paclitaxel + trastuzumab (AC → T + trastuzumab)<br>Docetaxel, carboplatin, trastuzumab (TCH) | Docetaxel + trastuzumab → fluorouracil/epirubicin/cyclophosphamide (FEC)<br>Chemotherapy followed by trastuzumab sequentially<br>Doxorubicin/cyclophosphamide (AC) → docetaxel + trastuzumab |
| Adjuvant (non-trastuzumab containing) | Docetaxel/doxorubicin/cyclophosphamide (TAC)<br>Dose-dense doxorubicin/cyclophosphamide (AC) → weekly paclitaxel<br>Docetaxel and cyclophosphamide (TC)<br>Doxorubicin/cyclophosphamide (AC) | Fluorouracil/doxorubicin/cyclophosphamide (FAC/CAF)<br>Cyclophosphamide/epirubicin/fluorouracil (FEC/CEF)<br>Cyclophosphamide/methotrexate/fluorouracil (CMF)<br>Doxorubicin/cyclophosphamide (AC) → docetaxel every 3 weeks<br>Epirubicin/cyclophosphamide (EC)<br>Doxorubicin followed by paclitaxel followed by cyclophosphamide (every 2-week regimen) with filgrastim support (A → T → C)<br>Fluorouracil/epirubicin/cyclophosphamide followed by docetaxel (FEC → T)<br>Fluorouracil/epirubicin/cyclophosphamide (FEC) followed by weekly paclitaxel |
| Neoadjuvant | Paclitaxel + trastuzumab followed by cyclophosphamide/epirubicin/fluorouracil + trastuzumab (T + trastuzumab → CEF + trastuzumab) | |
| Recurrent or metastatic | *Single agents:* Anthracyclines: Doxorubicin, epirubicin, pegylated liposomal doxorubicin. Taxanes: paclitaxel, docetaxel, albumin-bound paclitaxel. Antimetabolites: capecitabine, gemcitabine. Other microtubule inhibitors: vinorelbine.<br>*Combinations:* Cyclophosphamide/doxorubicin/fluorouracil (CAF/FAC); fluorouracil/epirubicin/cyclophosphamide (FEC); epirubicin/cyclophosphamide (EC); doxorubicin/docetaxel, doxorubicin/paclitaxel (AT); cyclophosphamide/methotrexate/fluorouracil (CMF); docetaxel/capecitabine; gemcitabine/paclitaxel (GT); bevacizumab + paclitaxel | *Other single agents:* Cyclophosphamide, mitoxantrone, cisplatin, etoposide (po), vinblastine, fluorouracil CI, ixabepilone.<br>*Other combinations:* ixabepilone + capecitabine. |
| HER2-positive metastatic disease | 1) Trastuzumab + (paclitaxel ± carboplatin) or (docetaxel) or (vinorelbine) or (capecitabine)<br>2) Lapatnib + capecitabine or trastuzumab + (other first-line agents) or (capecitabine) or (lapatnib) | |

(Continued)

| CANCER TYPE | PREFERRED THERAPIES | ALTERNATIVE REGIMENS |
|---|---|---|
| **Colorectal** | *Adjuvant Stage III:* 5-FU + oxaliplatin + leucovorin (FOLFOX)<br><br>*Metastatic: Intensive-Therapy Appropriate: Initial Therapy:* 5-FU + oxaliplatin + leucovorin (FOLFOX) + bevacizumab or CapeOX + bevacizumab or 2) FOLFOX or CapeOX + cetuximab (KRAS wild-type [WT] gene only) or 3) FOLFIRI + bevacizumab or 4) FOLFIRI + cetuximab (KARS WT gene only) or 5-FU/LV + bevacizumab or 5) FOLFOXIRI. *Refer to NCCN guidelines for therapy after first and second progression and for non–intensive-therapy appropriate patients.* Bevacizumab + 1) 5-FU + oxaliplatin + leucovorin (FOLFOX) or 2) irinotecan + leucovorin (FOLFIRI) + 5-FU or 3) oxaliplatin + capecitabine (CapeOX) or 4) 5-FU/LV | *Adjuvant Stage III:* 5-FU/LV or capecitabine |
| **Esophageal** | | |
| Definitive chemoradiation | Cisplatin + 5-FU | Cisplatin + 1) irinotecan or 2) paclitaxel or 3) docetaxel<br>Docetaxel or paclitaxel + 5-FU or capecitabine<br>Oxaliplatin + fluoropyrimidine (5-FU or capecitabine) |
| Recurrent or metastatic | Docetaxel/cisplatin/5-FU (DCF)<br>Epirubicin/cisplatin/5-FU (ECF) | Irinotecan + cisplatin or fluoropyrimidine (5-FU or capecitabine)<br>Oxaliplatin + fluoropyrimidine (5-FU or capecitabine)<br>Paclitaxel-based regimen<br>Trastuzumab |
| **Leukemia** | | |
| Acute lymphocytic leukemia (ALL) - Adults | *Induction:* Vincristine/anthracycline prednisone with or without asparaginase<br>*Refer to guidelines for CNS prophylaxis, consolidation, maintenance, and recurrent therapies.* | *Induction:* Imatinib mesylate (Ph1 positive ALL)<br>*Recurrent:* Dasatinib (imatinib-resistant BCR/ABL mutants) |
| Acute myeloid leukemia (AML) | *Induction:* (pt <60) Cytarabine + 1) daunorubicin or 2) idarubicin<br>*Induction:* (pt >60) Cytarabine + idarubicin or daunorubicin or mitoxantrone<br>*Post-induction:* (pt <60) High-dose cytarabine; or standard-dose cytarabine + idarubicin or daunorubicin<br>*Post-induction:* (pt >60) Standard-dose cytarabine + idarubicin or daunorubicin or mitoxantrone | *Induction:* (pt <60) High-dose cytarabine (HiDAC) + idarubicin or daunorubicin<br>*Induction:* (pt >60) Low-intensity subQ cytarabine or 5-azacytidine or decitabine; or intermediate-intensity clofarabine; or best supportive care (hydroxyurea) |
| Acute promyelocytic leukemia (APL) | *Induction:* Able to tolerate anthracyclines: All-trans retinoic acid (ATRA) + daunorubicin + cytarabine. Not able to tolerate anthracyclines: ATRA + arsenic trioxide<br>*Relapse:* Arsenic trioxide ± ATRA | *Relapse:* Gemtuzumab ozogamicin |
| Chronic lymphocytic leukemia (CLL) | *First-line therapy (without 17p del):* (pt ≥70) Chlorambucil + prednisone; bendamustine; cyclophosphamide, vincristine, prednisone (CVP) + rituximab; alemtuzumab; rituximab; fludarabine + rituximab (pt <70) Fludarabine, cyclophosphamide, rituximab (FCR); fludarabine, rituximab (FR); pentostatin, cyclophosphamide, rituximab (PCR); bendamustine; chlorambucil + prednisone; fludarabine; alemtuzumab. *Refer to guidelines for relapsed/refractory therapy and therapy for CLL with del (17p).* | |

*(Continued)*

| CANCER TYPE | PREFERRED THERAPIES | ALTERNATIVE REGIMENS |
|---|---|---|
| Chronic myelogenous leukemia (CML) | *Primary Treatment:* Imatinib 400mg | *Follow-up Therapy:* Dasatinib<br>Nilotinib<br>Interferon therapy |
| Hairy cell leukemia | Cladribine or pentostatin | Interferon alpha |
| **Liver** (hepatocellular carcinoma) | Sorafenib (Child-Pugh Class A [category 1] or B) | |
| **Lung** | | |
| Non-small cell | *First-line:* Chemotherapy; or bevacizumab + chemotherapy; or cisplatin/pemetrexed; or erlotinib for EGFR mutation positive.<br>*Second-line:* Docetaxel; or pemetrexed; or erlotinib<br>*Third-line:* Erlotinib | *First-line:* Cetuximab/vinorelbine/cisplatin<br>*Second-line:* Platinum doublet |
| Small cell | Cisplatin or carboplatin + etoposide | Cisplatin/irinotecan<br>Carboplatin/irinotecan<br>Cyclophosphamide/doxorubicin/vincristine |
| **Lymphoma** | | |
| Hodgkin's disease/lymphoma | Doxorubicin/bleomycin/vinblastine/dacarbazine (ABVD) | Bleomycin/etoposide/doxorubicin/cyclophosphamide/vincristine/procarbazine/prednisone (BEACOPP) |
| | Doxorubicin/vinblastine/mechlorethamine/etoposide/vincristine/bleomycin/prednisone (Stanford V) | |
| Non-Hodgkin's lymphoma | | |
| Follicular lymphoma | Rituximab (monotherapy)<br>Cyclophosphamide or chlorambucil (monotherapy)<br>Cyclophosphamide/doxorubicin/vincristine/prednisone + rituximab (R-CHOP)<br>Cyclophosphamide/vincristine/prednisone (CVP) + rituximab<br>Fludarabine/cyclophosphamide/mitoxantrone + rituximab (FCM-R)<br>Fludarabine/mitoxantrone/dexamethasone (FND) + rituximab | Bendamustine ± rituximab |
| Mantle cell lymphoma | Cyclophosphamide/doxorubicin/vincristine/prednisone + rituximab (R-CHOP) | Bendamustine + rituximab |
| | Rituximab + etoposide/prednisone/vincristine/cyclophosphamide/doxorubicin (R-EPOCH) | Bortezomib |
| | Rituximab and cyclophosphamide/vincristine/doxorubicin/dexamethasone (R-Hyper CVAD) alternating with methotrexate and cytarabine | Lenalidomide + rituximab |
| Diffuse large B-cell | Rituximab + Cyclophosphamide/doxorubicin/vincristine/prednisone (CHOP) + rituximab<br>Dose dense CHOP 14 + rituximab<br>Dose adjusted EPOCH + rituximab<br>*Refer to guidelines for therapy with poor left ventricular function.* | Dexamethasone/cisplatin/cytarabine (DHAP) ± rituximab<br>Etoposide/methylprednisone/cytarabine/cisplatin (ESHAP) ± rituximab<br>Gemcitabine/dexamethasone/cisplatin (GDP) ± rituximab<br>Ifosfamide/carboplatin/etoposide (ICE) ± rituximab<br>Mesna/ifosfamide/mitoxantrone/etoposide (MINE) ± rituximab |

*(Continued)*

| CANCER TYPE | PREFERRED THERAPIES | ALTERNATIVE REGIMENS |
|---|---|---|
| Burkitt's | *Low risk-combination:* CALGB 9251 regimen: Cyclophosphamide + prednisone → ifosfamide or cyclophosphamide; high-dose methotrexate, LV, vincristine, dexamethasone, and doxorubicin or etoposide or cytarabine; or intrathecal triple therapy (methotrexate, cytarabine, hydrocortisone).<br>Cyclophosphamide/vincristine/doxorubicin/ high-dose methotrexate ± rituximab (CODOX-M).<br>Cyclophosphamide/vincristine/doxorubicin/ dexamethasone. Dose-adjusted EPOCH: (etoposide, prednisone, vincristine, cyclophosphamide, doxorubicin) + rituximab (min 3 cycles plus one additional beyond CR) + intrathecal methotrexate.<br>(HyperCVAD) alternating with methotrexate + cytarabine + rituximab.<br>*High risk-combination:* CALGB 9521 regimen. Cyclophosphamide/vincristine/doxorubicin/ high-dose methotrexate (CODOX-M) alternating with ifosfamide/etoposide and high-dose cytarabine (IVAC) ± rituximab.<br>Cyclophosphamide/vincristine/doxorubicin/ dexamethasone. Dose-adjusted EPOCH.<br>(Hyper CVAD) alternating with methotrexate and cytarabine ± rituximab | |
| Lymphoblastic | Standard BFM (Berlin-Frankfurt-Munster) regimen<br>Augmented BFM regimen<br>CALGB ALL regimen<br>HyperCAVD regimen<br>LMB-86 regimen<br>Maintenance chemotherapy<br>*Refer to guidelines for specific information on each regimen.* | |
| Peripheral T-cell | Cyclophosphamide/doxorubicin/vincristine/ prednisone (CHOP)<br>Cyclophosphamide/vincristine/doxorubicin/ dexamethasone (Hyper CVAD) alternating with high-dose methotrexate + cytarabine | Dexamethasone/cisplatin/cytarabine (DHAP)<br>Etoposide/methylprednisolone/ cytarabine/cisplatin (ESHAP)<br>Gemcitabine/dexamethasone/ cisplatin (GDP)<br>Gemcitabine/oxaliplatin (GemOX)<br>Ifosfamide/carboplatin/etoposide (ICE)<br>Mesna/ifosfamide/mitoxantrone/ etoposide (MINE)<br>Pralatrexate<br>*Refer to guidelines for regimens in non-candidates for high-dose therapy with stem-cell rescue.* |
| **Ovarian** | *Primary Chemotherapy/Adjuvant:* Paclitaxel/ carboplatin | Docetaxel/carboplatin<br>Paclitaxel/cisplatin<br>Bevacizumab |
| Germ cell tumor | Bleomycin/etoposide/platinum (BEP) | Paclitaxel/ifosfamide/cisplatin (TIP) |
| **Pancreatic** | Locally advanced or metastatic: Gemcitabine | Gemcitabine + erlotinib or cisplatin or fluoropyrimidine<br>Capecitabine or 5-FU/LV or CapeOX |
| **Prostate** | Docetaxel/prednisone<br>Androgen deprivation therapy: Finasteride or dutasteride | Docetaxel/estramustine, docetaxel/prednisone, mitoxantrone/prednisone |

**Abbreviations:** MTX: methotrexate; 5-FU: 5-fluorouracil; LV: leucovorin.

* Selected cancers. For more detailed information, refer to the individual monograph listings or the drug's FDA-approved labeling.

† Source: National Comprehensive Cancer Network Clinical Practice (NCCN) Guidelines in Oncology, 2010.

# COLORECTAL CANCER TREATMENT OPTIONS

| DRUG (BRAND) | INDICATIONS | HOW SUPPLIED | DOSAGE |
|---|---|---|---|
| **Bevacizumab** (Avastin) | First- or second-line treatment of metastatic carcinoma of the colon or rectum, in combination with 5-fluorouracil-based chemotherapy. | Inj: 25mg/mL [4mL, 16mL] | 5mg/kg (in combination with bolus IFL) or 10 mg/kg (in combination with FOLFOX4) given once every 14 days. Give as IV infusion over 90 min; if 1st infusion is well tolerated, give 2nd infusion over 60 min and subsequent doses over 30 min. |
| **Capecitabine** (Xeloda) | First-line treatment of metastatic colorectal carcinoma when fluoropyrimidine therapy alone is preferred. Adjuvant treatment in patients with Dukes' C colon cancer who have undergone complete resection of the primary tumor when treatment with fluoropyrimidine therapy alone is preferred. | Tab: 150mg, 500mg | 1250mg/m$^2$ bid for 2 weeks followed by 1-week rest period given as 3-week cycles. Take with water within 30 min after meals. Dukes' C Colon Cancer: Give as 3-week cycles for a total of 8 cycles (24 weeks). CrCl 30-50mL/min: Reduce to 75% of starting dose. Interrupt and/or reduce dose if toxicity occurs; readjust based on toxicity grade (refer to PI for details). |
| **Cetuximab** (Erbitux) | In combination with irinotecan for the treatment of epidermal growth factor receptor (EGFR)-expressing, metastatic colorectal carcinoma in patients who are refractory to irinotecan-based chemotherapy. As monotherapy, for the treatment of EGFR-expressing, metastatic colorectal carcinoma after failure of both irinotecan- and oxaliplatin-based regimens or in patients intolerant to irinotecan-based therapy. | Inj: 2mg/mL [50mL, 100mL] | Premedication with $H_1$ antagonist (eg, diphenhydramine 50mg) IV 30-60 min prior to 1st dose is recommended. Initial: 400mg/m$^2$ IV infusion over 120 min. Maint: 250mg/m$^2$ IV infusion over 60 min once weekly. Max Infusion Rate: 10mg/min. Refer to PI for dose modifications with infusion reactions and severe acneform rash. |
| **Fluorouracil** | Palliative management of colon, rectum, breast, stomach, and pancreatic carcinomas. | Inj: 50mg/mL [10mL, 20mL] | 12mg/kg IV qd for 4 days. Max: 800mg/day. If no toxicity, give 6mg/kg IV on 6th, 8th, 10th, and 12th days. Skip Days 5, 7, 9, and 11. Inadequate Nutritional State: 6mg/kg IV for 3 days. If no toxicity, give 3mg/kg IV on 5th, 7th, and 9th days. Max: 400mg/day. Skip Days 4, 6, and 8. Maint (Use Schedule 1 or Schedule 2): Schedule 1: If no toxicity, repeat 1st course every 30 days after last day of previous course. Schedule 2: When toxic signs from initial course subside, give 10-15mg/kg/ week IV single dose; do not exceed 1g/week. |
| **Irinotecan hydrochloride** (Camptosar) | First-line therapy in combination with 5-fluorouracil (5-FU) and leucovorin (LV) for metastatic colon or rectal carcinomas, and for disease that has progressed or recurred following initial 5-FU-based therapy. | Inj: 20mg/mL [2mL, 5mL] | Refer to PI for dosage regimens and dose modifications: Combination Therapy (5-FU/LV): 125mg/m$^2$ IV over 90 min on days 1, 8, 15, 22 for 6 weeks; or 180mg/m$^2$ IV over 90 min on days 1, 15, and 29 for 6 weeks. Both regimens: Begin next cycle on Day 43. Single Therapy: 125mg/m$^2$ IV over 90 min on days 1, 8, 15, 22, followed by a 2-week rest; or 350mg/m$^2$ IV over 90 min once every 3 weeks. Premedicate with therapy. Dose modifications for reduced UGT1A1 activity, neutropenia, diarrhea, and antiemetics at least 30 min prior to other toxicities. Refer to PI. All dose modifications should be based on worst preceding toxicity. |

*(Continued)*

| DRUG (BRAND) | INDICATIONS | HOW SUPPLIED | DOSAGE |
|---|---|---|---|
| **Leucovorin calcium** | Adjunct to 5-fluorouracil (5-FU) for palliative treatment of advanced colorectal cancer. | Inj: 50mg, 100mg, 200mg, 350mg, 500mg | 200mg/m$^2$ slow IV push over 3 min followed by 5-FU 370mg/m$^2$ IV qd for 5 days, or 20mg/m$^2$ IV qd followed by 5-FU 425mg/m$^2$ IV qd for 5 days. Administer leucovorin and 5-FU separately to avoid precipitation. May repeat at 4-week intervals for 2 courses, then at 4-5 week intervals. May increase 5-FU dose by 10% if no toxicity. Reduce 5-FU dose by 20% with moderate GI/hematologic toxicity and by 30% with severe toxicity. |
| **Oxaliplatin** (Eloxatin) | In combination with infusional 5-fluorouracil (5-FU) and leucovorin (LV) for treatment of advanced metastatic carcinoma of colon or rectum and adjuvant treatment of Stage III colon cancer patients who have undergone complete resection of the primary tumor. | Inj: 50mg, 100mg | Advanced Disease: Day 1: 85mg/m$^2$ IV with LV 200mg/m$^2$; give over 120 min in separate bags using a Y-line; followed by 5-FU 400mg/m$^2$ bolus over 2-4 min, then 5-FU 600mg/m$^2$ as a 22 hr-infusion. Day 2: LV 200mg/m$^2$ over 120 min; followed by 5-FU 400mg/m$^2$ bolus over 2-4 min, then 5-FU 600mg/m$^2$ as a 22 hr-infusion. Repeat cycle every 2 weeks until disease progression or unacceptable toxicity. See PI for dose modifications for persistent grade 2 neurosensory events, grade 3 or 4 GI or grade 4 hematologic toxicity. Adjuvant Therapy: Recommended cycle every 2 weeks for 6 months (12 cycles). |
| **Panitumumab** (Vectibix) | Treatment of EGFR-expressing, metastatic colorectal carcinoma with disease progression on or following fluoropyrimidine-, oxaliplatin-, and irinotecan-containing chemotherapy regimens. | Inj: 20mg/mL [5mL, 10mL, 20mL] | 6mg/kg IV infusion over 60 min every 14 days. Infuse doses >1000mg over 90 min. Refer to PI for dose modifications with mild or severe infusion reactions and dermatologic toxicities. |

# PROSTATE CANCER TREATMENT OPTIONS

| DRUG (BRAND) | INDICATIONS | HOW SUPPLIED | DOSAGE |
|---|---|---|---|
| **BISPHOSPHONATE** | | | |
| **Zoledronic acid** (Zometa) | Treatment of documented bone metastases from solid tumors (progressive prostate cancer after treatment with one hormonal therapy), in conjunction with standard antineoplastic therapy. | **Inj:** 4mg/5mL | 4 mg as a single-dose IV infusion over ≥15 min q3-4wks with CrCl >60mL/min. Reduce with renal impairment. Coadminister calcium 500mg orally and 400 IU vitamin D daily. |
| **CHEMOTHERAPY AGENTS** | | | |
| **Docetaxel** (Taxotere) | Treatment of androgen-independent (hormone refractory) metastatic prostate cancer in combination with prednisone. | **Inj:** 20mg/0.5mL, 80mg/2mL | Premedicate with oral corticosteroids. Adjust dose based on febrile neutropenia, neutrophil count, cutaneous reactions, peripheral neuropathy, neurosensory signs/symptoms, or GI toxicities (see PI). Usual: 75mg/m$^2$ every 3 weeks over 1 hr; administer with prednisone 5mg bid continuously. |
| **Estramustine phosphate sodium** (Emcyt) | Palliative treatment of metastatic and/or progressive prostate carcinoma. | **Cap:** 140mg | Usual: 14mg/kg/day given tid-qid. Take with water at least 1 hr before or 2 hrs after meals. Treat for 30-90 days before determining possible benefits of continued therapy. |
| **Mitoxantrone** (Novantrone) | Initial treatment of patients with pain related to advanced hormone-refractory prostate cancer in combination with corticosteroids. | **Inj:** 2mg/mL | 12-14mg/m2/day IV every 21 days. |
| **ESTROGENS** | | | |
| **Conjugated estrogens tablets** (Premarin) | Palliative treatment of advanced androgen-dependent carcinoma of the prostate. | **Tab:** 0.3mg, 0.45mg, 0.625mg, 0.9mg, 1.25mg | 1.25-2.5mg tid. Effectiveness of therapy judged by phosphatase determinations and symptomatic improvement. |
| **Esterified estrogens tablets** (Menest) | Palliative therapy for advanced prostatic carcinoma. | **Tab:** 0.3mg, 0.625mg, 1.25mg, 2.5mg | 1.25-2.5mg tid. Effectiveness of therapy judged by phosphatase determinations and symptomatic improvement. |
| **Estradiol tablets** (Estrace) | Palliative treatment of advanced androgen-dependent prostate carcinoma. | **Tab:** 0.5mg*, 1mg*, 2mg* *scored | 1-2mg tid. Effectiveness of therapy judged by phosphatase determinations and symptomatic improvement. |
| **Estradiol valerate injection** (Delestrogen) | Palliative treatment of advanced androgen-dependent prostate carcinoma. | **Inj:** 10mg/mL, 20mg/mL, 40mg/mL | 30mg or more every 1 or 2 weeks. |
| **GnRH ANALOGUES** | | | |
| **Goserelin acetate implant** (Zoladex 3.6mg) | Palliative treatment of advanced prostatic carcinoma. Adjunct to and during radiotherapy, and in combination with flutamide, for management of locally confined Stage B2-C prostate cancer. | **Implant:** 3.6mg | Inject SQ into anterior abdominal wall below navel line. Advanced Prostatic Carcinoma: 3.6mg every 28 days. Stage B2-C Prostatic Carcinoma: 3.6mg starting 8 weeks before radiotherapy, then 10.8mg depot formulation 28 days after 1st injection, or 4 doses of 3.6mg at 28-day intervals (2 before and 2 during radiotherapy). |

| DRUG (BRAND) | INDICATIONS | HOW SUPPLIED | DOSAGE |
|---|---|---|---|
| **GnRH ANALOGUES** *(continued)* | | | |
| **Goserelin acetate implant** (Zoladex 10.8mg) | Palliative treatment of advanced prostate cancer. Adjunct to radiotherapy and flutamide for management of locally confined Stage B2-C prostate cancer. | **Implant:** 10.8mg | Inject SQ into anterior abdominal wall below navel line. Advanced Prostate Cancer: 10.8mg every 12 weeks. Stage B2-C Prostate Cancer: 3.6mg depot formulation 8 weeks before radiotherapy, followed by 10.8mg 28 days after 1st injection. |
| **GnRH ANTAGONIST** | | | |
| **Degarelix for injection** (Firmagon) | Treatment of advanced prostate cancer. | **Inj:** 80mg, 120mg | Initial: 240mg (as two SQ injections of 120mg) at 40mg/mL concentration. Maint: 80mg subcutaneously every 28 days at 20mg/mL concentration. |
| **LHRH AGONISTS** | | | |
| **Histrelin implant** (Vantas) | Palliative treatment of advanced prostate cancer. | **Implant:** 50mg | 50mg every 12 months. Inject SQ into inner aspect of the upper arm. Refrain from wetting the inserted arm for 24 hrs. Refrain from heavy lifting or strenuous exercise of the inserted arm for 7 days after implant insertion. Must remove after 12 months of therapy. |
| **Leuprolide acetate** (Eligard) | Palliative treatment of advanced prostate cancer. | **Inj:** 7.5mg, 22.5mg, 30mg, 45mg | 7.5mg SQ monthly, 22.5mg SQ every 3 months, 30mg SQ every 4 months, or 45mg SQ every 6 months. Rotate injection sites. |
| **Leuprolide acetate** (Lupron) | Palliative treatment of advanced prostate cancer. | **Inj:** 5mg/mL | 1mg SQ qd. Rotate injection sites. |
| **Leuprolide acetate** (Lupron Depot) | Palliative treatment of advanced prostate cancer. | **Inj:** (1-month) 7.5mg, (3-month) 22.5mg, (4-month) 30mg | 7.5mg IM as single dose monthly, 22.5mg IM single dose every 3 months, or 30mg IM single dose every 4 months. Rotate injection site. |
| **Leuprolide acetate** (Viadur) | Palliative treatment of advanced prostate cancer. | **Implant:** 65mg | Insert 1 implant SQ in upper arm every 12 months. |
| **Triptorelin pamoate injection, suspension** (Trelstar) | Palliative treatment of advanced prostate cancer. | **Inj:** (Depot) 3.75mg, (LA) 11.25mg | (Depot) 3.75mg IM every month or (LA) 11.25mg IM every 84 days. |
| **NONSTEROIDAL ANTIANDROGENS** | | | |
| **Bicalutamide** (Casodex) | Treatment of Stage D2 metastatic carcinoma of the prostate in combination with an LHRH analogue. | **Tab:** 50mg | 50mg qd at same time (morning or evening). Initiate simultaneously with an LHRH analogue. |
| **Flutamide** (flutamide) | Treatment of Stage D2 metastatic carcinoma of the prostate in combination with an LHRH analogue. | **Cap:** 125mg | 250mg q8h. Max: 750mg/day. |
| **Nilutamide** (Nilandron) | Treatment of Stage D2 metastatic prostatic cancer in combination with surgical castration. | **Tab:** 150mg | Initial: 300mg/day for 30 days beginning on the day of, or on the day after, surgical castration. Maint: 150mg qd. |

**Abbreviations:** LHRH = luteinizing hormone-releasing hormone; GnRH = gonadotropin-releasing hormone.

**Sources:**

FDA-approved product labeling.

Initial hormonal management of androgen-sensitive metastatic, recurrent, or progressive prostate cancer: 2007 update of an American Society of Clinical Oncology Practice Guideline. *J Clin Oncol.* 2007;25:1596-1605.

National Comprehensive Cancer Network Clinical Practice Guidelines in Oncology; Prostate Cancer. Version 1.2010.

# ADMINISTRATION GUIDELINES FOR EYE DROPS & OINTMENT

**Administration guidelines for eye drops:**

1. Wash hands thoroughly.
2. Tilt head back.
3. Gently pull the lower eyelid away from the eye to create a pocket.
4. Hold the bottle upside down and look up just before applying a single drop. **NOTE:** To prevent contamination, do not let the tip of the eye drop applicator touch any surface (including the eye or eyelid). When not in use, keep the container tightly closed.
5. After applying the drop, look down for several seconds (still holding the eyelid away from the eye).
6. Slowly release the eyelid and close the eyes for 1 to 2 minutes. Do not blink.
7. Gently press on the inside corner of the eye (where the eyelid meets the nose) with a finger.
8. Blot excessive solution from around the eye with a tissue.

**Administration guidelines for eye ointment:**

1. Wash hands thoroughly.
2. Tilt head back.
3. Gently grasp lower outer eyelid below lashes, and pull eyelid away from the eye.
4. Place ointment tube over eye by directly looking at it. With a sweeping motion, place ¼ to ½-inch of ointment inside the lower eyelid by gently squeezing the tube. **NOTE:** To prevent contamination, do not let the tip of the tube touch any surface (including the eye or eyelid). When not in use, keep the tube tightly closed.
5. Slowly release eyelid and close eyes for 1 to 2 minutes.
6. Blot excessive ointment from around the eye with a tissue.
7. Vision may be temporarily blurred. Until vision clears, avoid activities requiring good visual ability.

**Counseling tips:**

- If having difficulty determining whether an eye dropper has touched the eye surface, keep the dropper in a refrigerator (not in a freezer).
- If more than one drop is needed, wait at least 5 minutes before instilling the next drop to prevent flushing away or diluting the first drop.
- If both eye drop and ointment therapy are needed, instill the eye drop at least 10 minutes before the ointment.

# GLAUCOMA AGENTS

| BRAND (generic) | INGREDIENT/STRENGTH | DOSE |
|---|---|---|
| **BETA-BLOCKER, NONSELECTIVE** | | |
| Betagan (levobunolol HCl) | **Sol:** 0.25% [5mL, 10mL], 0.5% [2mL, 5mL, 10mL, 15mL] | **Adults:** (0.5%): 1-2 drops in affected eye(s) qd; bid for more severe or uncontrolled glaucoma. (0.25%): 1-2 drops in affected eye(s) bid. |
| Betimol (timolol) | **Sol:** 0.25%, 0.5% [5mL, 10mL, 15mL] | **Adults: Initial:** 1 drop in affected eye(s) 0.25% bid. May increase to max of 1 drop 0.5% bid. **Maint:** If adequate control, may try 1 drop of 0.25%-0.5% qd. |
| Carteolol (carteolol HCl) | **Sol:** 1% [5mL, 10mL, 15mL] | **Adults:** 1 drop in affected eye(s) bid. |
| Istalol (timolol maleate) | **Sol:** 0.5% [2.5mL, 5mL] | **Adults:** 1 drop in affected eye(s) qam. |
| Ocupress (carteolol HCl ) | **Sol:** 1% [10mL] | **Adults:** 1 drop in affected eye(s) bid. |
| OptiPranolol (metipranolol) | **Sol:** 0.3% [5mL, 10mL] | **Adults:** 1 drop in affected eye(s) bid. |
| Timolol GFS (timolol maleate) | **Sol, Gel-Forming:** 0.25%, 0.5% [2.5mL, 5mL] | **Adults: Initial:** 1 drop in affected eye(s) 0.25%-0.5% qd. Evaluate IOP 4 weeks after starting treatment. **Max:** 1 drop 0.5% qd. Dose other ophthalmic drugs 10 min prior to gel-forming drops. |
| Timoptic (timolol maleate) | **Sol:** (Timoptic) 0.25% [5mL, 10mL], 0.5% [5mL, 10mL] | **Adults: Initial:** 1 drop in affected eye(s) 0.25% bid. May increase to max of 1 drop 0.5% bid. **Maint:** If adequate control, may try 1 drop of 0.25%-0.5% qd. |
| Timoptic-XE (timolol maleate) | **Sol, Gel-Forming:** 0.25%, 0.5% [5mL]. | **Adults: Initial:** 1 drop in affected eye(s) 0.25%-0.5% qd. Evaluate IOP 4 weeks after starting treatment. **Max:** 1 drop 0.5% qd. Dose other ophthalmic drugs 10 min prior to gel-forming drops. |
| **BETA-BLOCKER, SELECTIVE** | | |
| Betaxolol Ophthalmic (betaxolol HCl) | **Sol:** 0.5% [5mL, 10mL, 15mL] | **Adults:** 1-2 drops in the affected eye(s) bid. |
| Betoptic S (betaxolol HCl) | **Sus:** 0.25% [2.5mL, 5mL, 10mL, 15mL] | **Adults:** 1 drop in the affected eye(s) bid. |
| **CARBONIC ANHYDRASE INHIBITORS** | | |
| Acetazolamide | **Cap, Extended-Release:** 500mg; **Inj:** 500mg; **Tab:** 125mg, 250mg | **Adults:** (Cap, ER) Glaucoma: 500mg bid. Inj: Open-Angle Glaucoma: Usual: 250mg-1g IV/PO qd in divided doses. Secondary Glaucoma/Pre-op Treatment of Closed-Angle Glaucoma: (IV/PO) 250mg q4h or 250mg bid if on short-term therapy or 500mg followed by 125mg or 250mg q4h in severe cases. |
| Azopt (brinzolamide) | **Sus:** 1% [5mL, 10mL, 15mL] | **Adults:** 1 drop in affected eye(s) tid. Space dosing of other ophthalmic drugs by 10 min. |
| Methazolamide | **Tab:** 25mg, 50mg | **Adults:** 50-100mg bid-tid. May use with miotic or osmotic agents. |
| Trusopt (dorzolamide HCl) | **Sol:** 2% [5mL, 10mL] | **Adults:** 1 drop in affected eye(s) tid. Space dosing of other ophthalmic drugs by 10 min. |

*(Continued)*

| BRAND | INGREDIENT/STRENGTH | DOSE |
|---|---|---|
| **CHOLINERGIC AGENTS** | | |
| Isopto Carbachol | **Sol:** 1.5% [15mL], 3% [15mL, 30mL] | **Adults:** 2 drops in eye up to tid. |
| Phospholine Iodide (echothiophate iodide) | **Sol:** 0.125% [5mL] | **Adults:** Early Chronic Simple Glaucoma: (0.03%): 1 drop in affected eye(s) bid, am and hs. Advanced Chronic Simple Glaucoma/Glaucoma Secondary to Cataract Surgery: **Initial:** (0.03%): 1 drop bid, am and hs. **Titrate:** May increase to higher strengths prn. |
| Pilocarpine | **Sol:** 0.5%, 1%, 2%, 3%, 4%, 6% [15mL] | **Adults:** 2 drops tid-qid or more if needed. Heavily pigmented irises may require higher strengths. |
| Pilopine HS (pilocarpine HCl) | **Gel:** 4% [4g] | **Adults:** Apply ½ inch into conjunctival sac hs. |
| **PROSTAGLANDIN ANALOGS** | | |
| Lumigan (bimatoprost) | **Sol:** 0.03% [2.5mL, 5mL, 7.5 mL] | **Adults:** 1 drop qd in affected eye(s) pm. **Max:** Once-daily dosing. Space dosing of other ophthalmic drugs by 5 min. |
| Travatan (travoprost) | **Sol:** 0.004% [2.5mL, 5mL] | **Adults:** 1 drop qd in affected eye(s) pm. **Max:** Once-daily dosing. Space dosing of other ophthalmic drugs by 5 min. |
| Travatan Z (travoprost) | **Sol:** 0.004% [2.5mL, 5mL] | **Adults:** 1 drop qd in affected eye(s) pm. **Max:** Once-daily dosing. Space dosing of other ophthalmic drugs by 5 min. |
| Xalatan (latanoprost) | **Sol:** 0.005% [2.5mL, 2.5mL x 3] | **Adults:** 1 drop qd in affected eye(s) pm. **Max:** Once-daily dosing. Space dosing of other ophthalmic drugs by 5 min. |
| **COMBINATION DRUGS** | | |
| Combigan (brimonidine tartrate-timolol maleate) | **Sol:** (brimonidine-timolol) 0.2%-0.5% [5mL, 10mL] | **Adults:** 1 drop in affected eye(s) bid approximately 12 hrs apart. Space dosing of other ophthalmic products at least 5 min apart. |
| Cosopt (dorzolamide HCl-timolol maleate) | **Sol:** (dorzolamide-timolol) 2%-0.5% [10mL] | **Adults:** 1 drop in affected eye(s) bid. Space dosing of other ophthalmic drugs by 10 min. |
| **MISCELLANEOUS** | | |
| Alphagan P (brimonidine tartrate) | **Sol:** 0.1% [5mL, 10mL, 15mL], 0.15% [5mL, 10mL, 15mL] (contains Purite) | **Adults:** 1 drop in affected eye(s) tid, approximately q8h. Space dosing of other ophthalmic products that lower IOP by 5 min. |
| Iopidine (apraclonidine HCl) | **Sol:** 0.5% [5mL, 10mL], 1% [0.1mL, 24s] | **Adults:** (0.5%): 1-2 drops in affected eye(s) tid. Space dosing of other ophthalmic drugs by 5 min. (1%): 1 drop 1 hr pre-op, then 1 drop immediately post-op. |
| Propine (dipivefrin HCl) | **Sol:** 0.1% [10mL, 15mL] | **Adults:** Usual: 1 drop in affected eye(s) q12h. |

# ANTIDEPRESSANTS

| DRUG (BRAND) | HOW SUPPLIED | DAILY DOSE Initial (I), Usual (U), Max (M) | TITRATE |
|---|---|---|---|
| **AMINOKETONE** | | | |
| **Bupropion HCl** (Wellbutrin) | **Tab:** 75mg, 100mg | **(I)**200mg **(U)**300mg **(M)**450mg | Increase by 100mg/d q3d. |
| (Wellbutrin SR) | **Tab, SR:** 100mg, 150mg, 200mg | **(I)**150mg **(U)**300mg **(M)**400mg | Increase by 150mg/d q4d. |
| (Wellbutrin XL) | **Tab, ER:** 150mg, 300mg | **(I)**150mg **(U)**300mg **(M)**450mg | Increase by 150mg/d q4d. |
| **Bupropion HBr** (Aplenzin) | **Tab, Extended-Release:** 174mg, 348mg, 522mg | **(I)**174mg **(U)**348mg **(M)**522mg | Increase by 174mg/d q4d. |
| **MONOAMINE OXIDASE INHIBITORS** | | | |
| **Phenelzine** (Nardil) | **Tab:** 15mg | **(I)**45mg **(U)**15mg qd or qod | Increase rapidly to 60-90mg/d then decrease to maintenance dose. |
| **Tranylcypromine** (Parnate) | **Tab:** 10mg | **(I,U)**30mg **(M)**60mg | Increase by 10mg/d q1-3 weeks. |
| **PHENYLETHYLAMINE** | | | |
| **Venlafaxine** (Effexor) | **Tab:** 25mg*, 37.5mg*, 50mg*, 75mg*, 100mg* | **(I)**75mg **(U)**150-225mg **(M)**375mg | Increase by 75mg/d q4d. |
| (Effexor XR) | **Cap, ER:** 37.5mg, 75mg, 150mg | **(I)**37.5-75mg **(U)**75-225mg **(M)**225mg | Increase by 75mg/d q4d. |
| **Selegeline** (Emsam) | **Patch:** 6mg/24 hrs, 9mg/24 hrs, 12mg/24 hrs | **(I)**6mg/24 hrs **(U)**6mg/24 hrs **(M)**12mg/24 hrs | Increase by 3mg/24 hrs q2wk. |
| **PHENYLPIPERAZINE** | | | |
| **Nefazodone** | **Tab:** 50mg, 100mg*, 150mg*, 200mg, 250mg | **(I)**200mg **(U)**300-600mg **(M)**600mg | Increase by 100-200mg/d in no less than 1 week. |
| **SELECTIVE SEROTONIN NOREPINEPHRINE REUPTAKE INHIBITORS** | | | |
| **Duloxetine** (Cymbalta) | **Cap:** 20mg, 30mg, 60mg | **(I,U)**40-60mg **(M)**60mg | N/A |
| **Desvenlafaxine** (Pristiq) | **Tab, Extended-Release:** 50mg, 100mg | **(I)**50mg **(M)**400mg | N/A |
| **SELECTIVE SEROTONIN REUPTAKE INHIBITORS** | | | |
| **Citalopram** (Celexa) | **Sol:** 10mg/5mL; **Tab:** 10mg, 20mg*, 40mg* | **(I)**20mg **(U)**40mg **(M)**60mg | Increase by 20mg/d qwk. |
| **Escitalopram** (Lexapro) | **Sol:** 5mg/5mL; **Tab:** 5mg, 10mg*, 20mg* | **(I)**10mg **(U)**10-20mg **(M)**20mg | Increase to 20mg/d after 1 week. |
| **Fluoxetine** (Prozac) | **Cap:** 10mg, 20mg, 40mg; **Sol:** 20mg/5mL; **Tab:** 10mg* 90mg weekly capsule | **(I)**20mg **(U)**20-80mg **(M)**80mg 90mg weekly capsule initiated 7 days after the last dose of 20mg | Consider after several weeks of therapy. |
| **Paroxetine** (Paxil) | **Sus:** 10mg/5mL; **Tab:** 10mg*, 20mg*, 30mg, 40mg | **(I)**20mg **(M)**50mg | Increase by 10mg/d qwk. |
| (Paxil CR) | **Tab, CR:** 12.5mg, 25mg, 37.5mg | **(I)**25mg **(M)**62.5mg | Increase by 12.5mg/d qwk. |
| (Pexeva) | **Tab:** 10mg, 20mg, 30mg, 40mg | **(I)**20mg **(M)**50mg | Increase by 10mg/d qwk. |
| **Sertraline** (Zoloft) | **Sol:** 20mg/mL; **Tab:** 25mg*, 50mg*, 100mg* | **(I)**50mg **(M)**200mg | Increase at 1-week intervals. |

*(Continued)*

| DRUG (BRAND) | HOW SUPPLIED | DAILY DOSE Initial (I), Usual (U), Max (M) | TITRATE |
|---|---|---|---|
| **TETRACYCLIC** | | | |
| **Maprotiline** | **Tab:** 25mg*, 50mg*, 75mg* | **(I)**OP: 25mg-75mg maintain for 2 weeks<br>IP:100mg-150mg<br>**(U)**OP: 75mg-150mg<br>IP:150mg-225mg<br>**(M)**225mg | Increase by 25mg gradually. |
| **Mirtazapine** | **Tab:** 15mg*, 30mg*, 45mg; **Tab, Disintegrating:** 15mg, 30mg, 45mg | **(I)**15mg **(M)**45mg | Increase q1-2 wk. |
| **TRIAZOLOPYRIDINE** | | | |
| **Trazodone** (Desyrel) | **Tab:** 50mg*, 100mg*, 150mg*, 300mg* | **(I)**150mg **(M)**400-600mg | Increase by 50mg/d q3-4d. |
| (Oleptro) | **Tab Extended-Release:** 150mg*, 300mg* | **(I)**150mg<br>**(U)**150-375mg<br>**(M)**375mg | Increase by 75mg/d q3d. |
| **TRICYCLICS** | | | |
| **Amitriptyline** | **Tab:** 10mg, 25mg, 50mg, 75mg, 100mg, 150mg | **(I)**OP: 50-100mg, IP: 100mg<br>**(U)**50-100mg<br>**(M)**OP: 150mg, IP: 300mg | OP: Increase by 25-50mg/d.<br>IP: Increase to 200mg/d. |
| **Amoxapine** | **Tab:** 25mg*, 50mg*, 100mg*, 150mg* | **(I)**100-150mg **(U)**200-300mg<br>**(M)**OP: 400mg IP: 600mg | Increase to 100mg bid-tid by end of first week. |
| **Clomipramine** (Anafranil) | **Cap:** 25mg, 50mg, 75mg | **(I)**25mg **(U)**100-250mg<br>**(M)**250mg | Increase to 100mg/d in 2 weeks, then increase gradually. |
| **Desipramine** (Norpramin) | **Tab:** 10mg, 25mg, 50mg, 75mg, 100mg, 150mg | **(I,U)**100-200mg **(M)**300mg | N/A |
| **Doxepin** (Sinequan) | **Cap:** 10mg, 25mg, 50mg, 75mg, 100mg, 150mg; **Sol:** 10mg/mL | **(I)**75mg **(U)**75-150mg<br>**(M)**300mg | Increase gradually. |
| **Imipramine** (Tofranil PM) | **Cap:** 75mg, 100mg, 125mg, 150mg | **(I)**OP: 75mg, IP: 100mg<br>**(U)**75-150mg **(M)**OP: 200mg, IP: 250-300mg | OP: Increase to 150mg/d.<br>IP: Increase to 200mg/d. |
| (Tofranil) | **Tab:** 10mg, 25mg, 50mg | **(I)**OP: 75mg, IP: 100mg<br>**(U)**50-150mg **(M)**OP: 200mg, IP: 250-300mg | OP: Increase to 150mg/d.<br>IP: Increase to 200mg/d. |
| **Nortriptyline** (Aventyl, Pamelor) | **Cap:** 10mg, 25mg, 50mg, 75mg; **Sol:**10mg/5mL | **(I,U)**75-100mg **(M)**150mg | N/A |
| **Protriptyline** (Vivactil) | **Tab:** 5mg, 10mg | **(I)**15mg<br>**(I,U)**15-40mg **(M)**60mg | Titrate morning dose. |
| **Trimipramine** (Surmontil) | **Cap:** 25mg, 50mg, 100mg | **(I)**OP: 75mg, IP: 100mg<br>**(U)**OP: 50-150mg, IP: 200mg<br>**(M)**OP: 200mg, IP: 250-300mg | OP: Increase to 150mg/d.<br>IP: Increase to 200mg/d. |
| **Abbreviations:** IP=Inpatient; OP=Outpatient | | *Scored. | |

# ANTIPSYCHOTIC AGENTS

| DRUG (BRAND) | HOW SUPPLIED (mg)* | INITIAL & (MAX) DOSE** | USUAL DOSE RANGE** |
|---|---|---|---|
| **ATYPICAL** | | | |
| **Aripiprazole** (Abilify) | **Tab:** 2, 5, 10, 15, 20, 30 **Sol:** 1mg/mL; **Inj:** 7.5mg/mL | 10-15mg qd (30mg/day) | 10-15mg qd |
| (Abilify Discmelt) | **Tab, Orally Disintegrating:** (Discmelt) 10, 15 | 10-15mg qd (30mg/day) | 10-15mg qd |
| **Clozapine** (Clozaril) | **Tab:** 12.5†, 25, 50†, 100, 200† | 12.5mg qd-bid (900mg/day) | 100-900mg/day given tid |
| (Fazaclo) | **Tab, Orally Disintegrating:** 12.5, 25*, 100* *scored | 12.5mg qd-bid (900mg/day) | 100-900mg/day given tid |
| **Iloperidone** (Fanapt) | **Tab:** 1mg, 2mg, 4mg, 6mg, 8mg, 10mg, 12mg | Schizophrenia: Initial: 1mg bid. Titrate: Must titrate dose slowly to avoid orthostatic hypotension. Day 2: 2mg bid. Day 3: 4mg bid. Day 4: 6mg bid. Day 5: 8mg bid. Day 6: 10mg bid. Day 7: 12mg bid. Max: 12mg bid (24mg/day) | 6-12mg bid |
| **Olanzapine** (Zyprexa, Zyprexa Zydis) | **Tab:** 2.5, 5, 7.5, 10, 15, 20 **Tab, Orally Disintegrating:** 5, 10, 15, 20 | Schizophrenia: 5-10mg qd Bipolar Mania: 10-15mg qd (20mg/day for both) | Schizophrenia: 10-15mg qd Bipolar Mania: 5-20mg qd |
| (Zyprexa IntraMuscular) | **Inj:** 10 | Agitation: 10mg IM (3 doses) | Agitation: 2.5-10mg IM |
| (Zyprexa Relprevv) | **Inj, Extended-Release:** 210, 300, 405 | Establish tolerability with oral olanzapine prior to initiating treatment. (405mg q4 weeks or 300mg q2 weeks) | 150-300mg/2 weeks or 405mg/4 weeks |
| **Paliperidone** (Invega) | **Tab, Extended-Release:** 1.5, 3, 6, 9 | 6mg qd (12mg/day) | 3-12mg/day |
| (Invega Sustenna) | **Inj, Extended-Release:** 39, 78, 117, 156, 234 | 234mg IM on treatment Day 1 and 156mg IM after 1 week. (234mg IM). | 39 mg to 234 mg IM |
| **Quetiapine fumarate** (Seroquel) | **Tab:** 25, 50, 100, 200, 300, 400 | Schizophrenia: 25mg bid Bipolar Mania: 50mg bid (800mg/day for both) | Schizophrenia: 150-750mg/day Bipolar Mania: 400-800mg/day |
| (Seroquel XR) | **Tab, Extended-Release:** 50, 150, 200, 300, 400 | Initial: 300mg/day (800mg/day) | 400-800mg/day |
| **Risperidone** (Risperdal) | **Sol:** 1mg/mL **Tab:** 0.25, 0.5, 1, 2, 3, 4 | Schizophrenia: 1mg bid (16mg/day) | Schizophrenia: 4-8mg/day Bipolar Mania: 1-6mg/day |
| (Risperdal M-Tab) | **Tab, Orally Disintegrating:** 0.5, 1, 2 (6mg/day) 3, 4 | Bipolar Mania: 2-3mg qd | |
| (Risperdal Consta) | **Inj:** 12.5, 25, 37.5, 50 | Schizophrenia: 25mg IM (50mg IM q2wk) | Schizophrenia: 25-50mg IM q2wks |
| **Ziprasidone HCl** (Geodon) | **Cap:** 20, 40, 60, 80 | Schizophrenia: 20mg bid (100mg bid) Bipolar Mania: 40mg bid | Schizophrenia: 20-80mg bid Bipolar Mania: 40-80mg bid |
| **Ziprasidone mesylate** (Geodon) for Injection) | **Inj:** 20mg/mL | 10mg IM q2h or 20mg IM q4h (40mg/day) | Switch to oral for long-term therapy |

*(Continued)*

| DRUG (BRAND) | HOW SUPPLIED (mg)* | INITIAL & (MAX) DOSE** | USUAL DOSE RANGE** |
|---|---|---|---|
| **CONVENTIONAL** | | | |
| **Chlorpromazine** | **Cap, Extended-Release:** 30, 75, 150; **Inj:** 25mg/mL; **Sup:** 25, 100; **Syrup:** 10mg/5mL; **Tab:** 10, 25,50, 100, 200 | 10-25mg PO bid-qid or 25mg IM (1000mg/day PO) | PO: 10-800mg/day<br>IM: 25-50mg IM q4-6h‡<br>Switch to PO when controlled |
| **Fluphenazine HCl** (Prolixin) | **Elixir:** 2.5mg/5mL<br>**Sol, Conc:** 5mg/mL<br>**Tab:** 1†, 2.5, 5, 10 | 2.5mg-10mg/day in divided doses (40mg/day) | 1-5mg qd |
| | **Inj:** 2.5mg/mL | 1.25mg IM q6-8h (10mg/day) | |
| **Fluphenazine decanoate** (Prolixin Decanoate) | **Inj:** 25mg/mL | 12.5-25mg IM/SQ q4-6 wks (100mg/dose) | Individualize to patient. |
| **Haloperidol** | **Sol, Conc:** 2mg/mL<br>**Tab:** 0.5, 1, 2, 5, 10, 20 | Moderate: 0.5-2mg bid-tid<br>Sev/Resist: 3-5mg bid-tid (100mg/day) | 2-20mg/day |
| **Haloperidol lactate** (Haldol) | **Inj:** 5mg/mL | 2-5mg IM q4-8h or hourly if needed (100mg/day) | Individualize to patient. |
| **Haloperidol decanoate** (Haldol Decanoate) | **Inj:** 50mg/mL, 100mg/mL | 10-20x daily oral dose up to 100mg/dose (450mg/month) | 10-15x daily oral dose |
| **Loxapine succinate** (Loxitane) | **Cap:** 5, 10, 25, 50 | 10mg bid, up to 50mg/day (250mg/day) | 60-100mg/day |
| **Molindone** (Moban) | **Tab:** 5, 10, 25, 50 | 50-75mg/day (225mg/day) | 5-25mg tid/qid |
| **Perphenazine** | **Tab:** 2, 4, 8, 16 | Non-hospitalized: 4-8mg tid<br>Hospitalized: 8-16mg bid-qid. (64mg/day) | Reduce dose as soon as possible to minimum effective dose. |
| **Prochlorperazine maleate** | **Tab:** 5, 10 | 5-10mg tid-qid | Moderate/Severe: 50-75mg/day<br>Severe: 100-150mg/day |
| **Thioridazine HCl** (Mellaril) | **Tab:** 10†, 25†, 50†, 100 | 50-100mg tid (800mg/day) | 200-800mg/day given bid-qid |
| **Thiothixene** (Navane) | **Cap:** 1, 2, 5, 10, 20<br>**Inj:** 5mg/mL | Mild: 2mg tid<br>Severe: 5mg bid (60mg/day)<br>Inj: 4mg bid-qid (30mg/day) | 20-30mg/day<br>Inj: 16-20mg/day IM<br>Switch to PO when controlled |
| **Trifluoperazine HCl** | **Tab:** 1, 2, 5, 10 | 2-5mg bid (40mg/day or higher if needed) | 15-20mg/day |

Note: This list is not inclusive of all antipsychotic agents. Indications may vary among the different products.

* Unless otherwise indicated.

** Doses shown are for adults. For pediatric dosing and additional information please refer to the individual monograph listings or the drug's FDA-approved labeling. Dosages need to be adjusted by titration to individual patient needs and may need to be reduced in the elderly, debilitated, or with renal/hepatic impairment. Periodically reassess to determine the need for maintenance treatment.

† Available only in generic forms.

‡ Severe cases may require up to 2g/day or 400mg/dose IM.

# BIPOLAR DISORDER PHARMACOTHERAPY

| DRUG | BRAND | HOW SUPPLIED | USUAL DOSE | COMMENTS |
|---|---|---|---|---|
| **MOOD STABILIZER** | | | | |
| Lithium | Various | **Cap:** 150mg, 300mg, 600mg; **Tab:** 300mg; **Tab, Extended-Release:** 300mg, 450mg; **Sol:** 8mEq/5mL | **Adults/Pediatrics:** $\geq$**12 yrs:** Acute Mania: 600mg tid or (300mg ER tab) 900mg in am and 900mg in pm or 600mg tid to achieve effective serum levels of 1-1.5mEq/L; monitor levels twice a week untilstabilized. Maintenance Therapy: 300mg tid-qid or (300mg ER tab) 600mg in am and 600mg in pm or administered on tid dosing interval up to 1200mg/d or (450mg ER tab) 450mg bid to maintain serum levels of 0.6-1.2mEq/L; monitor levels every 2 months. (Sol): 10mL (16mEq) tid. | Treatment of manic episodes of bipolar disorder and maintenance treatment of bipolar disorder. Do not crush or chew ER tab. |
| **ANTICONVULSANTS** | | | | |
| Carbamazepine | Equetro | **Cap, Extended-Release:** 100mg, 200mg, 300mg | **Adults:** Initial: 400mg/day, given in divided doses, bid. Titrate: 200mg qd. **Max:** 1600mg/day. Do not crush or chew. | Treatment of acute manic and mixed episodes associated with bipolar I disorder. |
| Divalproex sodium | Depakote ER | **Tab, Extended-Release:** 250mg, 500mg | **Adults:** Mania: Initial: 25mg/kg/day given once daily. Titrate: Increase dose rapidly to clinical effect. **Max:** 60mg/kg/day. Conversion from Depakote: Administer Depakote ER qd using a dose 8-20% higher than the total daily dose of Depakote. If cannot directly convert to Depakote ER, consider increasing to next higher Depakote total daily dose before converting to appropriate total daily Depakote ER dose. Elderly: Give lower initial dose and titrate slowly. Decrease dose or discontinue if decreased food or fluid intake or if excessive somnolence occurs. Swallow whole; do not crush or chew. | Acute manic or mixed episodes associated with bipolar disorder. |
| | Depakote | **Tab, Delayed-Release:** 125mg, 250mg, 500mg | **Adults:** Mania: 750mg daily in divided doses. Titrate: Increase dose rapidly to clinical effect. **Max:** 60mg/kg/day. Decrease dose or discontinue if decreased food or fluid intake or if excessive somnolence occurs. | Treatment of mania associated with bipolar disorder. |
| Lamotrigine | Lamictal | **Tab:** 25mg*, 100mg*, 150mg*, 200mg*; **Tab, Chewable:** (Lamictal CD) 2mg, 5mg, 25mg *scored **Tab, Disintegrating:** (Lamictal ODT) 25mg, 50mg, 100mg, 200mg | **Adults:** Bipolar Disorder: Patients not taking carbamazepine, other enzyme-inducing drugs (EIDs) or VPA: **Weeks 1 and 2:** 25mg qd. **Weeks 3 and 4:** 50mg qd. **Week 5:** 100mg qd. **Weeks 6 and 7:** 200mg qd. Patients taking VPA: **Weeks 1 and 2:** 25mg every other day. **Weeks 3 and 4:** 25mg qd. **Week 5:** 50mg qd. **Weeks 6 and 7:** 100mg qd. Patients taking carbamazepine (or other EIDs) and not taking VPA: **Weeks 1 and 2:** 50mg qd. **Weeks 3 and 4:** 100mg qd (divided doses). **Week 5:** 200mg qd (divided doses). **Week 6:** 300mg qd (divided doses). **Week 7:** Up to 400mg qd (divided doses). After discontinuation of psychotropic drugs excluding VPA, carbamazepine, or other EIDs: Maintain current dose. After discontinuation | Maintenance treatment of bipolar I disorder to delay the time to occurrence of mood episodes (depression, mania, hypomania, mixed episodes) in patients treated for mood episodes with standard therapy. |

*(Continued)*

| DRUG | BRAND | HOW SUPPLIED | USUAL DOSE | COMMENTS |
|---|---|---|---|---|
| **ANTICONVULSANTS** *(Continued)* | | | | |
| Lamotrigine *(continued)* | | | of VPA and current lamotrigine dose of 100mg qd: **Week 1:** 150mg qd. Week 2 and onward: 200mg qd. After discontinuation of carbamazepine or other EIDs and current lamotrigine dose of 400mg qd: **Week 1:** 400mg qd. **Week 2:** 300mg qd. **Week 3 and onward:** 200mg | |
| Valproic Acid | **Stavzor** | **Cap, Delayed Release:** 125mg, 250mg, 500mg | **Adults:** Mania: Initial: 750mg daily in divided doses. Titrate: Increase rapidly to produce the desired clinical effect or plasma level (50-125mcg/mL). **Max:** 60mg/kg/day. | Acute treatment of manic episodes associated with bipolar disorder. |
| **CONVENTIONAL ANTIPSYCHOTIC** | | | | |
| Chlorpromazine HCl | **Thorazine** | **Cap, Extended-Release:** 30mg, 75mg, 150mg, **Inj:** 25mg/mL; **Sup:** 25mg, 100mg; **Syrup:** 10mg/5mL; **Tab:** 10mg, 25mg, 50mg, 100mg, 200mg | **Adults:** Inpatient: Acute Schizophrenic/ Manic State: 25mg IM, then 25-50mg IM in 1 hr if needed. Titrate: Increase over several days up to 400mg q4-6h until controlled then switch to PO. Usual: 500mg/day PO. **Max:** 1000mg/day PO. Less acutely disturbed: 25mg PO tid. Titrate: Increase gradually to 400mg/day. Outpatient: 10mg PO tid-qid or 25mg PO bid-tid. More Severe: 25mg PO tid. Titrate: After 1-2 days, increase by 20-50mg twice weekly until calm. Prompt control of severe symptoms: 25mg IM, may repeat in 1 hr then 25-50mg PO tid. | Control manifestations of manic type of manic-depressive illness. |
| **ATYPICAL ANTIPSYCHOTICS** | | | | |
| Aripiprazole | **Abilify** | **Tab:** 2mg, 5mg, 10mg, 15mg, 20mg, 30mg; **Tab, Disintegrating:** 10mg, 15mg, (Discmelt) **Sol:** 1mg/mL [50mL, 150mL, 480mL]. **Inj:** 7.5mg/mL | **Adults:** (PO) Bipolar Disorder (Monotherapy or Adjunct): Initial/Target: 15mg/day. Max: 30mg/day. (Inj) Agitation: 9.75mg IM. Range: 5.25-15mg IM. Max: 30mg/day; initiate PO therapy as soon as possible. **Pediatrics:** Bipolar Disorder (Monotherapy or Adjunct) (10-17 yrs): Initial: 2mg/day. Titrate: 5mg after 2 days. May adjust dose in 5mg/day increments. Recommended: 10mg/day. Max: 30mg/day. Periodically reassess need for maintenance therapy. Oral sol can be given on mg-per-mg basis up to 25mg. Patients receiving 30mg tabs should receive 25mg of oral sol. Concomitant Strong CYP3A4 Inhibitors (eg, ketoconazole, clarithromycin): Reduce usual aripiprazole dose by 50%. Concomitant CYP2D6 Inhibitors (eg, quinidine, fluoxetine, paroxetine): Reduce usual aripiprazole dose by 50%. Concomitant CYP3A4 Inducers (eg, carbamazepine): Double aripiprazole dose. MDD: Initial: 2-5mg/day. Titrate: May adjust dose at increments up to 5mg/day at intervals ≥1 week. Usual: 2-15mg/day. Periodically reassess need for maintenance therapy. | (PO) Acute and maintenance treatment of manic and mixed episodes associated with bipolar I disorder with or without psychotic features in adults and pediatrics aged 10-17 yrs. Adjunctive therapy to either lithium or valproate for the acute treatment of manic and mixed episodes associated with bipolar I disorder with or without psychotic features in adults and pediatrics aged 10-17 yrs. (Inj) Acute treatment of agitation associated with schizophrenia or bipolar disorder, manic or mixed, in adults. Adjunctive therapy to antidepressants for acute treatment of major depressive disorder (MDD) in adults. |

*(Continued)*

| DRUG | BRAND | HOW SUPPLIED | USUAL DOSE | COMMENTS |
|---|---|---|---|---|
| **ATYPICAL ANTIPSYCHOTICS** *(Continued)* | | | | |
| Olanzapine | **Zyprexa, Zyprexa Zydis** | **Inj:** 10mg; **Tab:** 2.5mg, 5mg, 7.5mg, 10mg, 15mg, 20mg; **Tab, Disintegrating:** (Zydis) 5mg, 10mg, 15mg, 20mg | **Adults:** Bipolar I Disorder (Manic or Mixed Episodes): Initial: 10-15mg qd. Titrate: May increase/decrease dose by 5mg daily at intervals of not less than 24 hrs. Maint: 5-20mg/day. Periodically re-evaluate. **Max:** 20mg/day. With Lithium or Valproate: Initial/Usual: 10mg qd. **Max:** 20mg/day. Concomitant Use with Fluoxetine: Depressive Episodes Associated with Bipolar I Disorder/Resistant Depression: Initial: 5mg with 20mg fluoxetine qd in the evening. Titrate: Adjust dose based on efficacy and tolerability. Usual: 5-12.5mg with 20-50mg fluoxetine (depressive episodes associated with bipolar I disorder) or 5-20mg with 20-50mg fluoxetine (resistant depression). **Max:** 18mg plus fluoxetine 75mg. Hypotension Risk/Hepatic Impairment/Slow Metabolizers/Sensitivity to Olanzapine Effects: Initial: 2.5-5mg plus fluoxetine 20mg qd. Titrate: Increase cautiously. (IM) Agitation: Initial: 10mg IM. Usual: 2.5-10mg IM. Assess for orthostatic hypotension prior to subsequent dosing. **Max:** 3 doses of 10mg IM q 2-4h. Elderly: 5mg IM. Debilitated/Hypotension Risk/Sensitivity to Olanzapine Effects: 2.5mg IM. May initiate PO therapy when clinically appropriate. **Pediatrics:** Bipolar I Disorder (Manic or Mixed Episodes): Initial: 2.5-5mg qd. Target dose: 10mg/day. Titrate: Adjust by dose increments/decrements of 2.5-5mg. **Max:** 20mg/day. Periodically re-evaluate. | Acute treatment of manic or mixed episodes associated with bipolar I disorder and maintenance treatment of bipolar I disorder in adults and adolescent patients (ages 13-17 yrs). Adjunct to lithium or valproate for the treatment of manic episodes or mixed episodes associated with bipolar I disorder in adults. In combination with fluoxetine for the treatment of depressive episodes associated with bipolar I disorder and treatment-resistant depression. (Inj) Treatment of acute agitation associated with schizophrenia and bipolar I mania. |
| Olanzapine-fluoxetine | **Symbyax** | **Cap:** (Olanzapine-Fluoxetine): 3-25mg, 6-25mg, 6-50mg, 12-25mg, 12-50mg | Depressive Episodes Associated with Bipolar I Disorder/Treatment Resistant Depression: Initial: 6mg-25mg qd in evening. Range: 6-12mg (olanzapine)-25-50mg (fluoxetine). Adjust dose based on efficacy and tolerability. **Max:** 18mg-75mg/day. Re-examine the need for continued pharmacotherapy periodically. Hypotension Risk/Hepatic Impairment/Slow Metabolizers/Olanzapine-Sensitive: Initial: 3mg-25mg to 6mg-25mg qd in evening. Titrate: Increase cautiously. | Treatment of depressive episodes associated with bipolar disorder and treatment-resistant depression (MDD patients who do not respond to 2 separate trials of different antidepressants of adequate dose and duration in the current episode) in adults. |
| Quetiapine | **Seroquel** | **Tab:** 25mg, 50mg, 100mg, 200mg, 300mg, 400mg | **Adults:** Bipolar I Disorder: Manic Episodes: Monotherapy/Adjunct: Give bid. Day 1: 100mg/day, increase to 400mg/day on Day 4 in increments of up to 100mg/day and further adjust to 800mg/day by Day 6 in increments ≤200mg/day. **Max:** 800mg/day. Depressive Episodes: Give qd at hs. Day 1: 50mg/day. Day 2: 100mg/day. Day 3: 200mg/day. Day 4: 300mg/day. Maint (Bipolar I Disorder): 400-800mg/day given bid as adjunct therapy to lithium or divalproex. Hepatic Impairment: | Acute treatment of manic episodes associated with bipolar I disorder, both as monotherapy and as an adjunct therapy to lithium or divalproex in adults and pediatrics (10-17 yrs). Monotherapy for acute treatment of depressive episodes associated with bipolar disorder in adults. |

*(Continued)*

| DRUG | BRAND | HOW SUPPLIED | USUAL DOSE | COMMENTS |
|---|---|---|---|---|
| **ATYPICAL ANTIPSYCHOTICS** *(Continued)* | | | | |
| Quetiapine *(continued)* | | | Initial: 25mg/day. Titrate: May increase by 25-50mg/day to an effective dose, depending on response and tolerability. See PI for more details. **Pediatrics:** Bipolar I Disorder: Manic Episodes: 10-17 yrs: Administer bid or tid based on response and tolerability. Day 1: 50mg/day. Day 2: 100mg/day. Day 3: 200mg/day. Day 4: 300mg/day. Day 5: 400mg/day. After Day 5, adjust dose based on response and tolerability within recommended range of 400-600mg/day with increments of ≤100mg/day. Max: 600mg/day. See PI for more details. | Maintenance treatment of bipolar I disorder as adjunct therapy to lithium or divalproex. |
| Quetiapine | **Seroquel XR** | **Tab, Extended Release:** 50mg, 150mg, 200mg, 300mg, 400mg | **Adults:** Bipolar Disorder: Bipolar Mania: Monotherapy/Adjunct: Give qd in pm. Day 1: 300mg/day. Day 2: 600mg/day. Titrate: May adjust dose between 400-800mg beginning on Day 3 depending on response and tolerance. Depressive Episodes: Give qd in pm. Day 1: 50mg/day. Day 2: 100mg/day. Day 3: 200mg/day. Day 4: 300mg/day. Maint (Bipolar I Disorder): 400-800mg/day as adjunct therapy to lithium or divalproex. Periodically reassess the need for maintenance treatment and the appropriate dose. MDD, Adjunctive Therapy with Antidepressants: Initial: 50mg qd in pm. Increase dose to 150mg qd in pm on Day 3. Range: 150-300mg/day. **Max:** 300mg/day. Elderly/Hepatic Impairment: Initial: 50mg/day. See PI for more details. | Acute treatment of manic or mixed episodes associated with bipolar I disorder, both as monotherapy and as an adjunct to lithium or divalproex. Acute treatment of depressive episodes associated with bipolar disorder. Maintenance treatment of bipolar I disorder as adjunct therapy to lithium or divalproex. Adjunctive therapy to antidepressants for treatment of major depressive disorder (MDD). |
| Risperidone | **Risperdal** | **Sol:** 1mg/mL [30mL]; **Tab:** 0.25mg, 0.5mg, 1mg, 2mg, 3mg, 4mg; **Tab, Disintegrating:** (M-Tab) 0.5mg, 1mg, 2mg, 3mg, 4mg **Inj:** (Risperdal Consta) 12.5mg, 25mg, 37.5mg, 50mg | **Adults:** Bipolar Mania: Initial: 2-3mg qd. Titrate: Adjust dose at intervals no <24 hrs and in increments/decrements of 1mg/day. Range: 1-6mg/day. **Max:** 6mg/day. **Pediatrics:** 10-17 yrs: Bipolar Mania: Initial: 0.5mg qd in morning or evening. Titrate: Adjust dose, if needed, in increments of 0.5 or 1mg/day and at intervals not <24 hrs, as tolerated, to recommended dose of 2.5mg/day. **Max:** 6mg/day. Elderly/Debilitated/Hypotension/Severe Renal or Hepatic Impairment: Initial: 0.5mg bid. Titrate: Adjust dose in increments not >0.5mg bid. Increases to doses >1.5mg bid shouldoccur at intervals of ≥1 week. Periodically reassess to determine maintenance treatment. Inj: Establish PO tolerability prior to IM treatment. Usual: 25mg IM q2 weeks. Titrate: Upward dose adjustment should not be more frequent than q4 weeks. Max: 50mg IM q2 weeks. | Short-term treatment of acute manic or mixed episodes associated with bipolar I disorder as monotherapy (Adults and Adolescents 10-17 yrs) or in combination with lithium or valproate (Adults). Inj: Maintenance treatment of bipolar I disorder as monotherapy or in combination with lithium or valproate. |
| Ziprasidone | **Geodon** | **Cap:** (HCl) 20mg, 40mg, 60mg, 80mg **Inj:** 20mg/mL | **Adults:** Bipolar Mania: Initial: 40mg bid with food. Titrate: Increase to 60-80mg bid on 2nd day of treatment Maint: 40-80mg bid. Inj: 10-20mg IM. 10-mg doses may be administered q2 hrs. 20-mg doses may be administered q4 hrs. Max: 40mg/d IM. PO therapy should replace IM as soon as possible. | Treatment of acute manic or mixed episodes associated with bipolar disorder, with or without psychotic features. |

Source: FDA approved labeling.

# ADMINISTRATION GUIDELINES FOR DRY POWDER INHALERS

## Guidelines for Specific Products

### Spiriva HandiHaler Administration

1. Open the dust cap of the HandiHaler by pressing the green button. Pull the dust cap upward.
2. Open the mouthpiece by pulling it upward and away from the base.
3. Insert one Spiriva capsule in the center chamber of the HandiHaler device. Close the mouthpiece firmly until you hear a click. Leave the dust cap open.
4. Hold the HandiHaler device with the mouthpiece upward and press the green button until it is flush against the base, then release. Only press the green button once. **Note:** Do not block the air intake vents.
5. Exhale completely. **Note:** Do not exhale into the HandiHaler mouthpiece.
6. Raise the HandiHaler device to your mouth and close your lips tightly around the mouthpiece.
7. Keep your head upright and breathe in slowly and deeply until your lungs are full. You should hear or feel the Spiriva capsule vibrate.
8. Hold your breath as long as is comfortable and remove the HandiHaler from your mouth. Breathe normally again.
9. To get the full dose of Spiriva, exhale completely and inhale medication again as in steps 6-8.
10. Remove and discard empty capsule. Close mouthpiece and replace dust cap for storage.

**Counseling Tips:**

- Spiriva capsules should not be removed from the package until ready to use. Do not store the capsules in the HandiHaler device. Discard any unused capsules that are exposed to the air.
- Do not swallow Spiriva capsules.
- If you do not hear or feel the capsule vibrate, hold the HandiHaler upright and tap the device gently on a hard surface. Check to see that the mouthpiece is completely closed and continue steps.
- Clean the HandiHaler device at least once a month. Rinse with warm water and allow to air dry completely for 24 hours. **Note:** Do not use cleaning agents.
- Keep the HandiHaler device and Spiriva capsules in a dry place.

Source: Spiriva HandiHaler Prescribing Information.

## Guidelines for Specific Products

### Foradil Aerolizer Administration

1. Remove Aerolizer inhaler cover. Hold the base of Aerolizer and twist the mouthpiece in direction of arrow to open.
2. Place the Foradil capsule in capsule chamber. **Note:** Do not place capsule directly in mouthpiece.
3. Hold the mouthpiece upright and press both buttons at the same time once, then release. You should hear a click as the capsule is pierced. **Note:** If the buttons stay depressed, grasp the wings on the buttons and pull them out. Do not push the buttons a second time.
4. Exhale fully. **Note:** Do not exhale into Aerolizer mouthpiece.
5. Tilt head back slightly and keep inhaler level with blue buttons to left and right (not up and down).
6. Raise the inhaler to your mouth and close your lips tightly around the mouthpiece. Inhale quickly and deeply. **Note:** You will hear a whirring noise and experience a sweet taste.
7. Remove inhaler from the mouth. Continue to hold your breathe as long as you can then exhale.
8. Open the inhaler and check that the capsule is empty. If not, close inhaler and repeat steps 4-7.
9. Remove and discard the empty capsule. Close mouthpiece and replace cover for storage.

**Counseling Tips:**

- Never take the Aerolizer apart.
- Use Aerolizer in a level position.
- If you do not hear whirring noise, the capsule may be stuck. Open inhaler and loosen the capsule. **Note:** Do not press the buttons again.
- Do not wash Aerolizer inhaler. Keep inhaler and Foradil capsules in a dry place.
- Do not store the capsules in the Aerolizer inhaler.
- Use new Aerolizer inhaler with each refill.

Source: Foradil Aerolizer Prescribing Information, http://www.spfiles.com/piforadil.pdf.

[illegible]

## [illegible] for Specific Products

[illegible]

# ADMINISTRATION GUIDELINES FOR METERED-DOSE INHALERS

## General Guidelines

1. Remove dust cap and hold inhaler upright.
2. Shake canister well before each use.
3. Prime the inhaler before using the first time and in cases where the inhaler has not been used for extended periods of time. (Refer to product prescribing information for complete instructions.)
4. Tilt head back slightly and breathe out slowly and completely.
5. For **closed mouth** technique: Place mouthpiece in mouth and close lips tightly around (not recommended for steroid inhaler). For **open mouth** technique: Hold inhaler 1 to 2 inches from open mouth (about the width of 2 fingers).
6. Inhale slowly and deeply, and press down on the inhaler to release the medication. (The slower the breath, the greater the likelihood that the drug will reach the smaller airways.) **NOTE:** If needed, a spacer or holding chamber can be used in children or elderly patients having difficulty with coordination of technique. If using a spacer, put the mouthpiece of the spacer between teeth, and into mouth. Then, close mouth around the spacer. With the device in place, actuate the inhaler once and inhale the medication immediately after actuating the aerosol.
7. Breathe in slowly and hold breath for about 10 seconds to allow the medication to go into lungs.
8. Breathe out slowly and wait about 30 seconds to 1 minute before administering second inhalation. **NOTE:** Expect relief of symptoms within 5 to 15 minutes. Seek medical attention if symptomatic relief takes longer than 20 minutes (this should occur with short-acting medications like albuterol).
9. If using a steroid inhaler, rinse mouth with water after use. **NOTE:** Spit out the water after last puff; do not swallow.

## Counseling Tips:

- Rinse only the inhaler mouthpiece and cap with warm running water and air dry. Do not wash the canister or immerse in water.
- Keep the dust cap over the mouthpiece of the inhaler when not in use.
- Do not puncture the canister. The contents are under pressure.
- Store the canister at room temperature (15°C to 30°C), away from heat (>48.9°F) or open flames.

## Guidelines for Specific Products

### Advair Diskus Administration

1. Hold the Diskus in one hand. Then, push the thumbgrip back as far as it will go, until the mouthpiece appears and snaps into position.
2. Hold the Diskus in a level, flat position with the mouthpiece towards you.
3. Slide the lever away as far as it will go until it clicks.
4. Breathe out completely while holding the Diskus level and away from your mouth.
5. Put the mouthpiece between the lips. Breathe in quickly and deeply through the Diskus. **NOTE:** Do not breathe in through the nose.
6. Remove the Diskus from the mouth.
7. Hold breathe for about 10 seconds. Then, breathe out slowly. **NOTE:** Do not use another dose if you do not feel or taste the medicine.
8. Close the Diskus by sliding the thumbgrip back as far as it will go.
9. Rinse the mouth with water after each dose and spit out. Do not swallow.

**Counseling Tips:**

- Never breathe into the Diskus.
- Never take the Diskus apart.
- Use the Diskus in a level, flat position.
- Do not use with a spacer device.
- After each dose, rinse mouth with water and spit the water out. Do not swallow.
- Never wash the mouthpiece or any part of the Diskus.
- Keep the Diskus in a dry place, away from heat.

Source: Advair Diskus Prescribing Information, http://us.gsk.com/products/assets/us_advair.pdf.

*(Continued)*

**Pulmicort Flexhaler Administration**
Loading a dose:

1. Turn the cover and lift it off.
2. Hold the Flexhaler upright, with mouthpiece up.
3. Twist the brown grip fully in one direction as far as it will go and twist back again in the opposite direction as far as it will go until it clicks. **NOTE:** It does not matter which way you turn it first.

**Inhaling the dose:**

1. Turn your head away from the Flexhaler and breathe out completely. **NOTE:** Do not shake the inhaler after loading it.
2. Place the mouthpiece in your mouth, close your lips around the mouthpiece, and inhale deeply and forcefully.
3. Remove the Flexhaler from the mouth and breathe out. **NOTE:** Do not blow into the mouthpiece.
4. Replace the cover and twist shut when finished.
5. Rinse mouth with water after each dose. Spit out the water after last puff and do not swallow the water.

**Counseling Tips:**

- A new Flexhaler needs to be primed once before its first use. No further priming is indicated, even if it has been put aside for a long time.
- Flexhaler will deliver only one dose at a time, regardless of number of times you click the brown grip. **NOTE:** The dose indicator will continue to advance.
- Do not repeat inhalations even if you do not feel the sensation of medication when inhaling.
- Do not use with a spacer device.
- Do not chew or bite on the mouthpiece.
- Do not use Flexhaler if it has been damaged or if the mouthpiece has become detached.
- Wipe the outside of the mouthpiece once a week with a dry tissue.
- Keep the Flexhaler in a dry place, away from heat.

Source: Pulmicort Prescribing Information.

# ASTHMA & COPD MANAGEMENT

| DRUG (BRAND) | DOSAGE FORM | ADULT DOSE | CHILD DOSE |
|---|---|---|---|
| **ANTICHOLINERGICS** | | | |
| **Ipratropium** (Atrovent HFA)† | **MDI:** 0.017mg/inh [12.9g] | 2 inh qid. | |
| **Tiotropium** (Spiriva)† | **Cap, Inhalation:** 18mcg | 1 cap qd. | |
| **COMBINATION AGENTS** | | | |
| **Budesonide/Formoterol** (Symbicort) | **MDI:** (Budesonide-Formoterol) 80mcg-4.5mcg/inh, 160mcg-4.5mcg/inh [10.2g] | 2 puffs bid of 80/4.5 or 160/4.5 depending on asthma severity. **Max:** 640mcg/18mcg (2 puffs bid of 160/4.5). | **≥12 yrs:** 2 puffs bid of 80/4.5 or 160/4.5 depending on asthma severity. **Max:** 640mcg/18mcg (2 puffs bid of 160/4.5). |
| **Fluticasone/Salmeterol** (Advair Diskus)* | **DPI:** 100, 250, 500mcg/50mcg | 1 inh bid. | **4-11 yrs:** (100mcg/50mcg) 1 inh bid. |
| **Fluticasone/Salmeterol** (Advair HFA) | **MDI:** (45/21) 0.045mg-0.021mg/inh, (115/21) 0.115mg-0.021mg/inh, (230/21) 0.230mg-0.021mg/inh | **Initial:** 2 inh bid. **Max:** 2 inh of 230/21 bid. | **≥12 yrs: Initial:** 2 inh bid. **Max:** 2 inh of 230/21 bid. |
| **Ipratropium/Albuterol** (Combivent)† | **MDI:** (Albuterol-Ipratropium) 0.09mg-0.018mg/inh [14.7g] | 2 inh qid. | |
| **Ipratropium/Albuterol** (Duoneb)† | **Sol, Inhalation:** (Albuterol-Ipratropium) 3mg-0.5mg/3mL | 3mL qid via nebulizer. | |
| **CORTICOSTEROIDS** | | | |
| **Beclomethasone dipropionate HFA** (QVAR) | **MDI:** 40mcg/inh, 80mcg/inh | **Initial:** 40-160mcg bid. **Max:** 320mcg bid. | **5-11 yrs: Initial:** 40mcg bid. **Max:** 80mcg bid. |
| **Budesonide DPI** (Pulmicort Flexhaler, Pulmicort Turbuhaler) | **DPI:** 90mcg/inh, 180mcg/inh (Pulmicort Flexhaler) 200mcg/inh (Pulmicort Turbuhaler) | **Initial:** 180-360mcg bid. (Flexhaler) 200-800mcg bid. (Turbuhaler) **Max:** 720mcg bid. (Flexhaler) 400-800mcg bid. (Turbuhaler) | **≥6 yrs: Initial:** 180-360mcg bid. (Flexhaler) 200mcg bid. (Turbuhaler) **Max:** 360mcg bid. (Flexhaler) 400mcg bid. (Turbuhaler) |
| **Budesonide Neb** (Pulmicort Respules) | **Sol, Inhalation:** 0.25mg/2mL, 0.5mg/2mL, 1mg/2mL | | **12 months to 8 yrs: Initial:** 0.25mg/day-1mg/day via nebulizer. **Max:** 1mg/day. |
| **Ciclesonide** (Alvesco) | **MDI:** 80 mcg, 160mcg/inh | **Initial:** 80mcg bid-320mcg bid. **Max:** 160mcg bid-320mcg bid. | **≥12 yrs: Initial:** 80mcg bid-320mcg bid. **Max:** 160mcg bid-320mcg bid. |
| **Flunisolide** (Aerobid) | **MDI:** 250mcg/inh | **Initial:** 500mcg bid. **Max:** 1000mcg bid. | **6-15 yrs: Initial/Max:** 500mcg bid. |
| **Fluticasone propionate** (Flovent Diskus) | **DPI:** 50, 100, 250mcg/inh | **Initial:** 100mcg bid-1000mcg bid. **Max:** 500mcg bid-1000mcg bid. | **4-11 yrs: Initial:** 50mcg bid. **Max:** 100 mcg bid. |
| **Fluticasone propionate** (Flovent HFA) | **MDI:** 44, 110, 220mcg/inh | **Initial:** 88mcg bid-440mcg bid. **Max:** 440mcg bid- 880mcg bid. | **4-11 yrs: Initial/Max:** 88mcg bid. |
| **Mometasone furoate** (Asmanex Twisthaler) | **DPI:** 110mcg, 220mcg/inh | **Initial:** 220mcg qd hs-440mcg bid. **Max:** 440mcg-880mcg. | **4-11 yrs: Initial/Max:** 110mcg qd hs. |
| **Triamcinolone acetonide** (Azmacort) | **MDI:** 75mcg/inh | **Initial:** 150mcg tid-qid or 300mcg bid. **Max:** 1200mcg/day. | **6-12 yrs: Initial:** 75-150 mcg tid-qid or 150mcg-300mcg bid. **Max:** 900mcg/day. |
| **CROMOLYN** | | | |
| **Cromolyn** (Intal Inhalation Solution) | **Sol, Inhalation:** 10mg/mL | 20mg nebulized qid. | **≥2 yrs:** 20mg nebulized qid. |

*(Continued)*

| DRUG (BRAND) | DOSAGE FORM | ADULT DOSE | CHILD DOSE |
|---|---|---|---|
| **LEUKOTRIENE MODIFIERS** | | | |
| **Montelukast** (Singulair) | **Tab:** 10mg; **Tab, Chewable:** 4mg, 5mg; **Granules:** 4mg | 10mg qhs. | **6-23 mo:** 4mg granules qhs. **2-5 yrs:** 4mg qhs. **6-14 yrs:** 5mg qhs. **15 yrs:** 10mg qhs. |
| **Zafirlukast** (Accolate) | **Tab:** 10mg, 20mg | 20mg bid. | **≥12 yrs:** 20mg bid. **5-11 yrs:** 10mg bid. |
| **Zileuton** (Zyflo, Zyflo CR) | **Tab:** 600mg; **Tab, Extended-Release:** 600mg | 600mg qid, **ER:** 1200mg bid. | **≥12 yrs:** 600mg qid, **ER:** 1200mg bid |
| **LONG-ACTING $\beta_2$-AGONISTS** | | | |
| **Aformoterol** (Brovana)† | **Sol, Inhalation:** 15mcg/2mL | 15mcg bid via nebulizer. | |
| **Formoterol** (Foradil)* | **DPI:** 12mcg | 1 cap (inh) q12 hrs. | **≥5 yrs:** 1 cap (inh) q12 hrs. |
| **Formoterol** (Perforomist)† | **Sol, Inhalation:** 20mcg/2mL | 2mL q12 hrs via nebulizer. | |
| **Metaproterenol** 0.4% | **Syrup:** 10mg/5mL; **Tab:** 10mg, 20mg; **Sol, Inhalation:** 0.6%, tid-qid. | 20mg tid-qid. **(Sol)** one vial per nebulization tid-qid. | **6-9 yrs or <60 lbs:** 10mg tid-qid. **>9 yrs or >60 lbs:** 20mg **Sol (≥12 yrs):** one vial per nebulization tid-qid. |
| **Salmeterol** (Serevent)* | **DPI:** 50mcg/blister | 1 blister q12 hrs. | **≥4 yrs:** 1 blister q12 hrs. |
| **Terbutaline** | **Tab:** 2.5mg, 5mg | 2.5-5mg q6 hrs 3 times daily; **Max:** 15mg/day. | **12-15 yrs:** 2.5mg tid. **Max:** 7.5mg/day. |
| **METHYLXANTHINE** | | | |
| **Theophylline** (Elixophyllin) | **Elixir:** 80mg/15mL | **Adults & Children >45 kg** **Initial:** 300mg/day divided q6-8 hrs. After 3 days if tolerated: 400mg/day divided q6-8 hrs. After 3 more days if needed: 600mg/day divided q6-8 hrs. | **1-15 yrs (Children <45 kg): Initial:** 12-14mg/kg/day. (**Max:** 300mg/day divided q4-6 hrs.) After 3 days if tolerated: 16mg/kg/day. (**Max:** 400mg/day divided q4-6 hrs.) After 3 more days if needed: 20mg/kg/day. (**Max:** 600mg/day divided q4-6 hrs.) |
| **Theophylline** (Theo-24) | **Cap, Extended Release:** 100mg, 200mg, 300mg, 400mg | **Adults & Children >45 kg** **Initial:** 300-400mg/day q24 hrs. After 3 days if tolerated: 400-600mg/day q24 hrs. After 3 more days if needed: Doses >600mg should be titrated according to blood levels (See PI). | **12-15 yrs (Children >45 kg): Initial:** 12-14mg/kg/day. (**Max:** 300mg/day q24 hrs.) After 3 days if tolerated: 16mg/kg/day. (**Max:** 400mg/day q24 hrs.) After 3 more days if tolerated: 20mg/kg/day. (**Max:** 600mg/day q24 hrs.) |
| **Theophylline** (Theochron, Theo-Dur) | **Tab, Extended Release:** (generic) 100mg, 200mg, 300mg, 400mg, 450mg, 600mg (Theochron): 100mg, 200mg, 300mg (Theo-Dur): 200mg | **Adults & Children >45 kg** **Initial:** 300mg/day divided q12 hrs. After 3 days if tolerated: 400mg/day divided q12 hrs. After 3 more days if needed: 600mg/day divided q12 hrs. | **6-15 yrs (Children <45 kg): Initial:** 12-14mg/kg/day. (**Max:** 300mg/day divided q12 hrs.) After 3 days if tolerated: 16mg/kg/day. (**Max:** 400mg/day divided q12 hrs.) After 3 more days if needed: 20mg/kg/day. (**Max:** 600mg/day divided q12 hrs.) |

| **DRUG** (BRAND) | **DOSAGE FORM** | **ADULT DOSE** | **CHILD DOSE** |
|---|---|---|---|
| **METHYLXANTHINE** *(Continued)* | | | |
| **Theophylline** (Uniphyl) | **Tab, Extended Release:** 400mg, 600mg | **Adults & Children >45 kg Initial:** 300-400mg/day. After 3 days if tolerated: 400-600mg/day. After 3 more days if needed: Doses >600mg should be titrated according to blood levels (See PI). | **12-15 yrs (Children <45 kg): Initial:** 12-14mg/kg/day. (**Max:** 300mg/day). After 3 days if tolerated: 16mg/kg/day. (**Max:** 400mg/day). After 3 more days if needed: 20mg/kg/day. (**Max:** 600mg/day). |
| **MONOCLONAL ANTIBODY/IgE-BLOCKER** | | | |
| **Xolair** (Omalizumab) | **Inj:** 150mg/5mL | 150-375mg SQ q2 or 4 weeks. Determine dose and dosing frequency by serum total IgE level (IU/mL), measured before the start of treatment, and body weight (kg). See PI for dose determination charts. | **≥12 yrs:** 150-375mg SQ q2 or 4 weeks. Determine dose and dosing frequency by serum total IgE level (IU/mL), measured before the start of treatment, and body weight (kg). See PI for dose determination charts. |
| **SHORT-ACTING $\beta_2$-AGONISTS** | | | |
| **Albuterol** | **MDI:** 0.09mg/inh; **Sol, Inhalation:** 0.083%, 0.5%; **Syrup:** 2mg/5mL; **Tab:** 2mg*, 4mg*; **Tab, Extended-Release (Repetabs):** 4mg, 8mg *scored | 2 inh q4-6h or 1 inh q4h. **(Repetabs) Initial:** 4-8mg q12h. **Max:** 32mg/day. **(Sol)** 2.5mg tid-qid via nebulizer. **(Syrup, Tabs)** 2-4mg tid qid. **Max:** 32mg/day (8mg qid). | **(Syrup) Initial:** 2-4mg tid-qid. **Max:** 8mg (Aerosol) 2 inh q4-6h or 1 inh q4h. **(Sol)** 2.5mg tid-qid by nebulizer. **(Tabs) Initial:** 2-4mg tid-qid. |
| **Albuterol Sulfate** (ProAir HFA, Proventil HFA, Ventolin HFA) | **MDI:** 90mcg/inh | 2 inh q4-6h or 1 inh q4h. | **≥4 yrs:** 2 inh q4-6h or 1 inh q4h. |
| **Levalbuterol** (Xopenex, Xopenex HFA) | **Sol, Inhalation:** 0.31mg/3mL, 0.63mg/3mL, 1.25mg/3mL (HFA) 45mcg/inh | 0.63mg tid q6-8h via nebulizer. (HFA) 2 inh (90mcg) q4-6h or 1 inh (45mcg) q4h. | **6-11 yrs:** 0.31mg tid (max: 0.63mg tid) q6-8h **≥4 yrs:** (HFA) 2 inh (90mcg) q4-6h or 1 inh (45mcg) q4h. |
| **Pirbuterol** (Maxair) | **Autohaler:** 0.2mg/inh; **MDI:** 0.2mg/inh [14g] | 1-2 inh q4-6h. | **≥12 yrs:** 1-2 inh q4-6h. |
| **SYSTEMIC CORTICOSTEROIDS** | | | |
| **Methylprednisolone** | **Tab:** 2, 4, 8, 16, 32mg | 7.5-60mg qd in a single dose or qod prn for control. Short course "burst": 40-60 mg/day as single dose or 2 divided doses for 3-10 days. | **≤11 yrs:** 0.25-2mg/kg qd in a single dose or qod prn for control. Short course "burst": 1-2mg/kg/day. **Max:** 60mg/day or 3-10 days. |
| **Prednisolone** | **Tab:** 5mg; **Liq:** 5mg/5mL, 15mg/5mL | | |
| **Prednisone** | **Tab:** 1, 2.5, 5, 10, 20, 50mg **Liq:** 5mg/mL, 5mg/5mL | | |

MDI: metered-dose inhaler; DPI: dry powder inhaler.
†Indicated for COPD only
*Indicated for Asthma & COPD
Adopted from: The NAEPP Expert Panel Report: Guidelines for the Diagnosis and Management of Asthma–Update on Selected Topics 2007. http://www.nhlbi.nih.gov/guidelines/asthma/asthsumm.htm

# Asthma Treatment Plan

| CLASSIFICATION | LUNG FUNCTION | STEPWISE APPROACH TO THERAPY IN PATIENTS >12 YEARS OF AGE |
|---|---|---|
| **Intermittent**<br>• Symptoms $\leq$2 days a week<br>• Short-acting $\beta_2$-agonist use for symptom control $\leq$2 days a week<br>• Nighttime awakenings $\leq$2 times/month<br>• Interference with normal activity - none | • Normal $FEV_1$ b/w exacerbations<br>• $FEV_1$ $\geq$80% predicted<br>• $FEV_1$/FVC - normal | **Step 1**<br>• **Short-acting inhaled $\beta_2$-agonists as needed (2-4 puffs prn).**<br>• Severe exacerbations may occur, separated by long periods of normal lung function and no symptoms; a course of systemic corticosteroids is recommended. |
| **Mild persistent**<br>• Symptoms >2 days/week but not daily<br>• Short-acting $\beta_2$-agonist use for symptom control >2 days/wk but not daily, and not more than 1x on any day<br>• Nighttime awakenings 3-4x/month<br>• Interference with normal activity - minor limitation | • $FEV_1$ $\geq$80% predicted<br>• $FEV_1$/FVC - normal | **Step 2**<br>• **Low-dose inhaled corticosteroids.**<br>• **Short-acting inhaled $\beta_2$-agonists as needed (2-4 puffs prn).**<br>ALTERNATIVE TREATMENT:<br>• Cromolyn, leukotriene modifier, nedocromil OR theophylline |
| **Moderate persistent**<br>• Daily symptoms<br>• Short-acting $\beta_2$-agonist use for symptom control daily<br>• Nighttime awakenings >1x/wk but not nightly<br>• Interference with normal activity - some limitation | • $FEV_1$ >60% but <80% predicted<br>• $FEV_1$/FVC reduced 5% | **Step 3**<br>• **Low- to medium-dose inhaled corticosteroids**<br>AND<br>• **Long-acting inhaled $\beta_2$-agonists.**<br>• **Short-acting inhaled $\beta_2$-agonists as needed (2-4 puffs prn).**<br>ALTERNATIVE TREATMENT:<br>• Low-dose ICS + either LTRA, theophylline, OR Zileuton |
| **Severe persistent**<br>• Symptoms throughout the day<br>• Short-acting $\beta_2$-agonist use for symptom several times per day<br>• Nighttime awakenings often >7x/week<br>• Interference with normal activity - extreme limitation | • $FEV_1$ $\leq$60% predicted<br>• $FEV_1$/FVC reduced >5% | **Step 4, Step 5 or Step 6**<br>• **Medium-dose ICS + LABA OR**<br>• **High-dose ICS + LABA OR**<br>• **High-dose ICS + LABA + oral corticosteroid**<br>AND<br>• Consider Omalizumab for patients who have allergies<br>• **Short-acting inhaled $\beta_2$-agonists as needed (2-4 puffs prn).**<br>ALTERNATIVE TREATMENT:<br>• Medium-dose ICS + either LTRA, Theophylline, OR Zileuton |

**Note: Preferred treatments are in bold.**

**Key Points:**

- Stepwise approach presents general guidelines. Review treatment every 1 to 6 months; a gradual stepwise reduction in treatment may be possible. If control is not maintained, consider step up.
- The presence of one of the features of severity is sufficient to place a patient in that category. An individual should be assigned to the most severe grade in which any feature occurs (PEF is % of personal best; FEV is % predicted).
- Intensity of treatment will depend on severity of exacerbation; up to 3 treatments at 20-minute intervals or a single nebulizer treatment as needed. Course of systemic corticosteroids may be needed.
- Use of short-acting beta$_2$-agonists >2 days/week for a symptom relief generally indicates inadequate control and the need to step up treatment
- Airflow obstruction is indicated by reduced $FEV_1$ and $FEV_1$/FVC values relative to reference or predicted values.
- Abnormalities of lung function are categorized as restrictive and obstructive defects. A reduced ratio of $FEV_1$/FVC (eg, <65%) indicates obstruction to the flow of air from the lungs, whereas a reduced FVC with a normal or increased $FEV_1$/FVC ratio suggests a restrictive pattern.

**Abbreviations:** $FEV_1$: Forced expiratory volume in one second. FVC: Forced vital capacity. ICS: Inhaled corticosteroid. LABA: Long-acting inhaled beta$_2$-agonist; LTRA: Leukotriene receptor antagonist.

*Adapted from the Full Report 2007 *Guidelines for the Diagnosis and Management of Asthma.* NAEPP Expert Panel Report III.

# ERECTILE DYSFUNCTION TREATMENT

| **DRUG** (BRAND) | **HOW SUPPLIED** | **DOSING** |
|---|---|---|
| **Alprostadil** (Caverject, Caverject Impulse) | **Inj:** 5, 10, 20, 40mcg (sterile powder); **Inj:** 10, 20mcg (Impulse) | Vasculogenic, Psychogenic, or Mixed Etiology: Initiate: 2.5mcg. Increase to 5mcg within 1 hr if partial response. Max 2 doses during initial titration within 24 hrs. Increase by 5-10mcg if additional titration required ≥24 hrs apart until erection of 1 hr max duration. No Response to 2.5mcg: Initiate: 7.5mcg within 1 hr. Max 2 doses during initial titration within 24 hrs. Increase by 5-10mcg if additional titration required ≥24 hrs apart until erection. Pure Neurogenic Etiology (Spinal Cord Injury): Initiate: 1.25mcg. Increase to 2.5mcg within 1 hr. Max 2 doses during initial titration within 24 hrs. If additional titration required, give 5mcg within next 24 hrs. Thereafter, give 5mcg doses ≥24 hrs apart until erection of 1 hr max duration. Patient must stay in physician's office until complete detumescence. |
| **Alprostadil** (Edex) | **Inj:** 10, 20, 40mcg (sterile powder) | Vasculogenic, Psychogenic, or Mixed Etiology: Initiate: 2.5mcg. Increase to 5mcg, then by 5-10mcg based on response until erection of 1 hr max duration. No Response to 2.5mcg: Initiate: 7.5mcg, followed by 5-10mcg increments. Pure Neurogenic Etiology (Spinal Cord Injury): Initiate: 1.25mcg. Increase to 2.5mcg, followed by 2.5mcg dose, then increase by 5mcg increments until erection of 1 hr max duration. Patient must stay in physician's office until complete detumescence. If no response, give next higher dose within 1 hr. If response, min 24 hrs before next dose. |
| **Alprostadil** (Muse) | **Suppositories, Urethral:** 125, 250, 500, 1000mcg | Initial: 125-250mcg. Titration: Increase or decrease dose based on individual response. Max: 2 administrations within 24 hrs. |
| **Sildenafil** (Viagra) | **Tablets:** 25, 50, 100mg | Usual: 50mg prn 1 hr prior to sexual activity. Titration: Increase to 100mg qd or 25mg qd based on efficacy/tolerability. |
| **Tadalafil** (Cialis) | **Tablets:** 2.5, 5, 10, 20mg | PRN use: Initial: 10mg qd. Titration: Increase to 20mg qd or decrease to 5mg qd based on efficacy/tolerability. QD use: 2.5mg qd. Titration: Increase to 5mg qd based on efficacy/tolerability. |
| **Vardenafil** (Levitra) | **Tablets:** 2.5, 5, 10, 20mg | Usual: 10mg prior to sexual activity qd. Titration: Increase to 20mg qd or decrease to 5mg qd based on efficacy/tolerability. |

# UROLOGICAL THERAPIES

| OVERACTIVE BLADDER AGENTS | | | | |
|---|---|---|---|---|
| **DRUG** | **BRAND** | **HOW SUPPLIED** | **DOSING** | **COMMENTS** |
| Darifenacin | Enablex | **Tab, ER:** 7.5mg, 15mg | **Initial:** 7.5mg qd. **Max:** 15mg qd. | Swallow whole. Moderate Hepatic Impairment/ Concomitant Potent CYP3A4 Inhibitors: Do not exceed 7.5mg/day. Severe Hepatic Impairment: Avoid use. |
| Fesoterodine | Toviaz | **Tab, ER:** 4mg, 8mg | **Initial:** 4mg qd. **Max:** 8mg/day | Swallow whole. CrCl <30mL/min. Concomitant Potent CYP3A4 Inhibitors: Do not exceed 4mg/day. Severe Hepatic Impaiment: Avoid use. |
| Oxybutynin | Ditropan | **Syrup:** 5mg/5mL **Tab:** 5mg | **Usual:** 5mg bid-tid. **Max:** 5mg qid. | A lower starting dose of 2.5mg bid-tid is recommended for elderly patients. |
| | Ditropan XL | **Tab, ER:** 5mg, 10mg, 15mg | **Initial:** 5mg or 10mg qd. **Max:** 30mg/day. | Swallow whole. Increase dose by 5mg weekly if needed. |
| | Gelnique | **Gel:** 10% (1g/pkt) | Apply contents of 1 pkt qd to skin on abdomen, upper arms/shoulders, or thighs. | Rotate application sites. |
| | Oxytrol | **Patch:** 3.9mg/day | **Usual:** Apply 1 patch twice weekly (every 3-4 days). | Rotate application sites. |
| Solifenacin | VESIcare | **Tab:** 5mg, 10mg | **Usual:** 5mg qd. **Max:** 10mg qd. | Swallow whole. Renal (CrCl <30mL/min)/Hepatic (Child Pugh B)/Concomitant Potent CYP3A4 Inhibitors: Do not exceed 5mg/day. Hepatic (Child Pugh C): Avoid use. |
| Tolterodine | Detrol | **Tab:** 1mg, 2mg | **Initial:** 2mg bid. | Decrease dose to 1mg bid if needed. Significant Hepatic/Renal Dysfunction/Concomitant CYP3A4 Inhibitors: 1mg bid. |
| | Detrol LA | **Cap, ER:** 2mg, 4mg | **Initial:** 4mg qd. | Swallow whole. Decrease dose to 2mg qd if needed. Significant Hepatic/ Renal Dysfunction/ Concomitant CYP3A4 Inhibitors: 2mg qd. |
| Trospium | Sanctura | **Tab:** 20mg | **Usual:** 20mg bid. | Take 1 hr before meals or on empty stomach. CrCl <30mL/min: 20mg qhs. Elderly ≥75 yrs: May titrate to 20mg qd based upon tolerability. |
| | Sanctura XR | **Cap, ER:** 60mg | **Usual:** 60mg qam | Take on empty stomach, 1 hr before meal. CrCl <30mL/min: Avoid use. |
| **BENIGN PROSTATIC HYPERTROPHY AGENTS** | | | | |
| **DRUG** | **BRAND** | **HOW SUPPLIED** | **DOSING** | **COMMENTS** |
| **ALPHA-BLOCKERS** | | | | |
| Alfuzosin | Uroxatral | **Tab, ER:** 10mg | **Usual:** 10mg qd. | Take dose immediately after the same meal each day. Swallow whole. |
| Doxazosin | Cardura | **Tab:** 1mg, 2mg, 4mg, 8mg | **Initial:** 1mg qd. **Max:** 8mg/day. | Stepwise titration every 1-2 weeks if needed. |
| | Cardura XL | **Tab, ER:** 4mg, 8mg | **Initial:** 4mg qd. **Max:** 8mg qd. | Take with breakfast. Swallow whole. Titrate after 3-4 weeks if needed. |
| Silodosin | Rapaflo | **Cap:** 4mg, 8mg | **Usual:** 8mg qd. | Take with food. CrCl 30-50mL/min: 4mg qd. |
| Tamsulosin | Flomax | **Cap:** 0.4mg | **Initial:** 0.4mg qd. **Max:** 0.8mg qd. | Take dose ½ hour after the same meal each day. Titrate after 2-4 weeks if needed. Restart at initial dose if therapy is interrupted. |
| Terazosin | Hytrin | **Tab/cap:** 1mg, 2mg, 5mg, 10mg | **Initial:** 1mg qhs. **Usual:** 10mg/day. **Max:** 20mg/day. | Increase stepwise as needed. Restart at initial dose if therapy is interrupted. |
| **5-ALPHA-REDUCTASE INHIBITORS** | | | | |
| Dutasteride | Avodart | **Cap:** 0.5mg | **Usual:** 0.5mg qd. | Swallow whole. May be administered with tamsulosin. |
| Finasteride | Proscar | **Tab:** 5mg | **Usual:** 5mg qd. | May be administered with doxazosin with or without meals. |

# RECOMMENDED IMMUNIZATION SCHEDULE FOR PERSONS AGED 0-6 YEARS

| Vaccine ▼ Age ► | Birth | 1 month | 2 months | 4 months | 6 months | 12 months | 15 months | 18 months | 19–23 months | 2–3 years | 4–6 years |
|---|---|---|---|---|---|---|---|---|---|---|---|
| Hepatitis B[1] | HepB | HepB | | | HepB | | | | | | |
| Rotavirus[2] | | | RV | RV | RV[2] | | | | | | |
| Diphtheria, Tetanus, Pertussis[3] | | | DTaP | DTaP | DTaP | *see footnote*[3] | DTaP | | | | DTaP |
| *Haemophilus influenzae* type b[4] | | | Hib | Hib | Hib[4] | Hib | | | | | |
| Pneumococcal[5] | | | PCV | PCV | PCV | PCV | | | | PPSV | |
| Inactivated Poliovirus[6] | | | IPV | IPV | IPV | | | | | | IPV |
| Influenza[7] | | | | | Influenza (Yearly) | | | | | | |
| Measles, Mumps, Rubella[8] | | | | | | MMR | | | *see footnote*[8] | | MMR |
| Varicella[9] | | | | | | Varicella | | | *see footnote*[9] | | Varicella |
| Hepatitis A[10] | | | | | | HepA (2 doses) | | | | HepA Series | |
| Meningococcal[11] | | | | | | | | | | MCV | |

Range of recommended ages for all children except certain high-risk groups

Range of recommended ages for certain high-risk groups

This schedule includes recommendations in effect as of December 15, 2009. Any dose not administered at the recommended age should be administered at a subsequent visit, when indicated and feasible. The use of a combination vaccine generally is preferred over separate injections of its equivalent component vaccines. Considerations should include provider assessment, patient preference, and the potential for adverse events. Providers should consult the relevant Advisory Committee on Immunization Practices statement for detailed recommendations: **http://www.cdc.gov/vaccines/pubs/acip-list.htm**. Clinically significant adverse events that follow immunization should be reported to the Vaccine Adverse Event Reporting System (VAERS) at **http://www.vaers.hhs.gov** or by telephone, **800-822-7967**.

1. **Hepatitis B vaccine (HepB).** (Minimum age: birth)
   **At birth:**
   - Administer monovalent HepB to all newborns before hospital discharge.
   - If mother is hepatitis B surface antigen (HBsAg)-positive, administer HepB and 0.5 mL of hepatitis B immune globulin (HBIG) within 12 hours of birth.
   - If mother's HBsAg status is unknown, administer HepB within 12 hours of birth. Determine mother's HBsAg status as soon as possible and, if HBsAg positive, administer HBIG (no later than age 1 week).

   **After the birth dose:**
   - The HepB series should be completed with either monovalent HepB or a combination vaccine containing HepB. The second dose should be administered at age 1 or 2 months. Monovalent HepB vaccine should be used for doses administered before age 6 weeks. The final dose should be administered no earlier than age 24 weeks.
   - Infants born to HBsAg-positive mothers should be tested for HBsAg and antibody to HBsAg 1 to 2 months after completion of at least 3 doses of the HepB series, at age 9 through 18 months (generally at the next well-child visit).
   - Administration of 4 doses of HepB to infants is permissable when a combination vaccine containing HepB is administered after the birth dose. The fourth dose should be administered no earlier than age 24 weeks.
2. **Rotavirus vaccine (RV).** (Minimum age: 6 weeks)
   - Administer the first dose at age 6 through 14 weeks (maximum age: 14 weeks 6 days). Vaccination should not be initiated for infants aged 15 weeks 0 days or older.
   - The maximum age for the final dose in the series is 8 months 0 days.
   - If Rotarix is administered at ages 2 and 4 months, a dose at 6 months is not indicated.
3. **Diphtheria and tetanus toxoids and acellular pertussis vaccine (DTaP).** (Minimum age: 6 weeks)
   - The fourth dose may be administered as early as age 12 months, provided at least 6 months have elapsed since the third dose.
   - Administer the final dose in the series at age 4 through 6 years.
4. ***Haemophilus influenzae* type b conjugate vaccine (Hib).** (Minimum age: 6 weeks)
   - If PRP-OMP (PedvaxHIB or Comvax [HepB-Hib]) is administered at ages 2 and 4 months, a dose at age 6 months is not indicated.
   - TriHiBit (DTaP/Hib) and Hiberix (PRP-T) should not be used for doses at ages 2, 4, or 6 months for the primary series but can be used as the final dose in children aged 12 months through 4 years.
5. **Pneumococcal vaccine.** (Minimum age: 6 weeks for pneumococcal conjugate vaccine [PCV]; 2 years for pneumococcal polysaccharide vaccine [PPSV])
   - PCV is recommended for all children aged younger than 5 years. Administer 1 dose of PCV to all healthy children aged 24 through 59 months who are not completely vaccinated for their age.
   - Administer PPSV 2 or more months after last dose of PCV to children aged 2 years or older with certain underlying medical conditions, including a cochlear implant. See *MMWR* 1997;46(No. RR-8).

*(Continued)*

**6. Inactivated poliovirus vaccine (IPV)** (Minimum age: 6 weeks)

- The final dose in the series should be administered on or after the fourth birthday and at least 6 months following the previous dose.
- If 4 doses are administered prior to age 4 years a fifth dose should be administered at age 4 through 6 years. See *MMWR* 2009;58(30):829-30.

**7. Influenza vaccine (seasonal).** (Minimum age: 6 months for trivalent inactivated influenza vaccine [TIV]; 2 years for live, attenuated influenza vaccine [LAIV])

- Administer annually to children aged 6 months through 18 years.
- For healthy children aged 2 through 6 years (i.e., those who do not have underlying medical conditions that predispose them to influenza complications), either LAIV or TIV may be used, except LAIV should not be given to children aged 2 through 4 years who have had wheezing in the past 12 months.
- Children receiving TIV should receive 0.25 mL if aged 6 through 35 months or 0.5 mL if aged 3 years or older.
- Administer 2 doses (separated by at least 4 weeks) to children aged younger than 9 years who are receiving influenza vaccine for the first time or who were vaccinated for the first time during the previous influenza season but only received 1 dose.
- For recommendations for use of influenza A (H1N1) 2009 monovalent vaccine see *MMWR* 2009;58(No. RR-10).

**8. Measles, mumps, and rubella vaccine (MMR).** (Minimum age: 12 months)

- Administer the second dose routinely at age 4 through 6 years. However, the second dose may be administered before age 4, provided at least 28 days have elapsed since the first dose.

**9. Varicella vaccine.** (Minimum age: 12 months)

- Administer the second dose routinely at age 4 through 6 years. However, the second dose may be administered before age 4, provided at least 3 months have elapsed since the first dose.
- For children aged 12 months through 12 years the minimum interval between doses is 3 months. However, if the second dose was administered at least 28 days after the first dose, it can be accepted as valid.

**10. Hepatitis A vaccine (HepA).** (Minimum age: 12 months)

- Administer to all children aged 1 year (i.e., aged 12 through 23 months). Administer 2 doses at least 6 months apart.
- Children not fully vaccinated by age 2 years can be vaccinated at subsequent visits.
- HepA also is recommended for older children who live in areas where vaccination programs target older children, who are at increased risk for infection, or for whom immunity against hepatitis A is desired.

**11. Meningococcal vaccine.** (Minimum age: 2 years for meningococcal conjugate vaccine [MCV4] and for meningococcal polysaccharide vaccine [MPSV4])

- Administer MCV4 to children aged 2 through 10 years with persistent compliment component deficiency, anatomic or functional asplenia, and certain other conditions placing them at high risk.
- Administer MCV4 to children previously vaccinated with MCV4 or MPSV4 after 3 years if first dose administered at age 2 through 6 years. See *MMWR* 2009;58:1042-3.

The Recommended Immunization Schedules for Persons Aged 0–18 Years are approved by the Advisory Committee on Immunization Practices **(http://www.cdc.gov/vaccines/recs/acip)**, the American Academy of Pediatrics **(http://www.aap.org)**, and the American Academy of Family Physicians **(http://www.aafp.org)**.

# RECOMMENDED IMMUNIZATION SCHEDULE FOR PERSONS AGED 7-18 YEARS

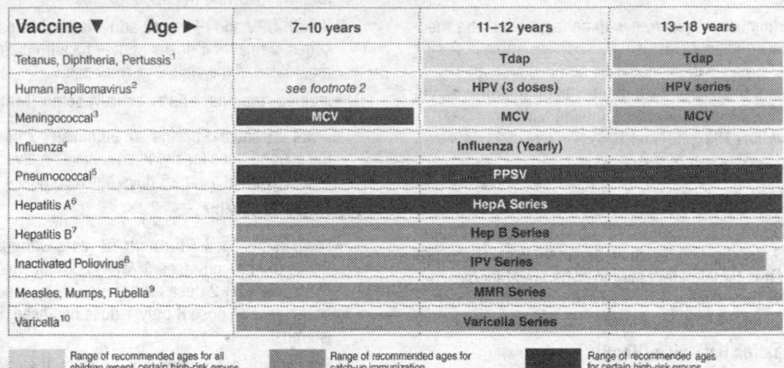

| Vaccine ▼ Age ► | 7–10 years | 11–12 years | 13–18 years |
|---|---|---|---|
| Tetanus, Diphtheria, Pertussis[1] | | Tdap | Tdap |
| Human Papillomavirus[2] | see footnote 2 | HPV (3 doses) | HPV series |
| Meningococcal[3] | MCV | MCV | MCV |
| Influenza[4] | Influenza (Yearly) | | |
| Pneumococcal[5] | PPSV | | |
| Hepatitis A[6] | HepA Series | | |
| Hepatitis B[7] | Hep B Series | | |
| Inactivated Poliovirus[8] | IPV Series | | |
| Measles, Mumps, Rubella[9] | MMR Series | | |
| Varicella[10] | Varicella Series | | |

Range of recommended ages for all children except certain high-risk groups — Range of recommended ages for catch-up immunization — Range of recommended ages for certain high-risk groups

This schedule includes recommendations in effect as of December 15, 2009. Any dose not administered at the recommended age should be administered at a subsequent visit, when indicated and feasible. The use of a combination vaccine generally is preferred over separate injections of its equivalent component vaccines. Considerations should include provider assessment, patient preference, and the potential for adverse events. Providers should consult the relevant Advisory Committee on Immunization Practices statement for detailed recommendations: **http://www.cdc.gov/vaccines/pubs/acip-list.htm**. Clinically significant adverse events that follow immunization should be reported to the Vaccine Adverse Event Reporting System (VAERS) at **http://www.vaers.hhs.gov** or by telephone, **800-822-7967**.

1. **Tetanus and diphtheria toxoids and acellular pertussis vaccine (Tdap).** (Minimum age: 10 years for Boostrix and 11 years for Adacel)
   - Administer at age 11 or 12 years for those who have completed the recommended childhood DTP/DTaP vaccination series and have not received a tetanus and diphtheria toxoid (Td) booster dose.
   - Persons aged 13 through 18 years who have not received Tdap should receive a dose.
   - A 5-year interval from the last Td dose is encouraged when Tdap is used as a booster dose; however, a shorter interval may be used if pertussis immunity is needed.
2. **Human papillomavirus vaccine (HPV).** (Minimum age: 9 years)
   - Two HPV vaccines are licensed: a quadrivalent vaccine (HPV4) for the prevention of cervical, vaginal and vulvar cancers (in females) and genital warts (in females and males), and a bivalent vaccine (HPV2) for the prevention of cervical cancers in females.
   - HPV vaccines are most effective for both males and females when given before exposure to HPV through sexual contact.
   - HPV4 or HPV2 is recommended for the prevention of cervical precancers and cancers in females.
   - HPV4 is recommended for the prevention of cervical, vaginal and vulvar precancers and cancers and genital warts in females.
   - Administer the first dose to females at age 11 or 12 years.
   - Administer the second dose 1 to 2 months after the first dose and the third dose 6 months after the first dose (at least 24 weeks after the first dose).
   - Administer the series to females at age 13 through 18 years if not previously vaccinated.
   - HPV4 may be administered in a 3-dose series to males aged 9 through 18 years to reduce their likelihood of acquiring genital warts.
3. **Meningococcal conjugate vaccine (MCV4).**
   - Administer at age 11 or 12 years, or at age 13 through 18 years if not previously vaccinated.
   - Administer to previously unvaccinated college freshmen living in a dormitory.
   - Administer MCV4 to children aged 2 through 10 years with persistent complement component deficiency, anatomic or functional asplenia, or certain other conditions placing them at high risk.
   - Administer to children previously vaccinated with MCV4 or MPSV4 who remain at increased risk after 3 years (if first dose administered at age 2 through 6 years) or after 5 years (if first dose administered at age 7 years or older). Persons whose only risk factor is living in on-campus housing are not recommended to receive an additional dose. See *MMWR* 2009;58:1042–3.
4. **Influenza vaccine (seasonal).**
   - Administer annually to children aged 6 months through 18 years.
   - For healthy nonpregnant persons aged 7 through 18 years (i.e., those who do not have underlying medical conditions that predispose them to influenza complications), either LAIV or TIV may be used.
   - Administer 2 doses (separated by at least 4 weeks) to children aged younger than 9 years who are receiving influenza vaccine for the first time or who were vaccinated for the first time during the previous influenza season but only received 1 dose.

*(Continued)*

- For recommendations for use of influenza A (H1N1) 2009 monovalent vaccine see *MMWR* 2009;58(No. RR-10).

**5. Pneumococcal polysaccharide vaccine (PPSV).**

- Administer to children with certain underlying medical conditions, including a cochlear implant. A single revaccination should be administered after 5 years to children with functional or anatomic asplenia or an immunocompromising condition. See *MMWR* 1997;46(No. RR-8).

**6. Hepatitis A vaccine (HepA).**

- Administer 2 doses at least 6 months apart.
- HepA is recommended for children aged older than 23 months who live in areas where vaccination programs target older children, who are at increased risk for infection, or for whom immunity against hepatitis A is desired.

**7. Hepatitis B vaccine (HepB).**

- Administer the 3-dose series to those not previously vaccinated.
- A 2-dose series (separated by at least 4 months) of adult formulation Recombivax HB is licensed for children aged 11 through 15 years.

**8. Inactivated poliovirus vaccine (IPV).**

- The final dose in the series should be administered on or after the fourth birthday and at least 6 months following the previous dose.
- If both OPV and IPV were administered as part of a series, a total of 4 doses should be administered, regardless of the child's current age.

**9. Measles, mumps, and rubella vaccine (MMR).**

- If not previously vaccinated, administer 2 doses or the second dose for those who have received only 1 dose, with at least 28 days between doses.

**10. Varicella vaccine.**

- For persons aged 7 through 18 years without evidence of immunity (see *MMWR* 2007;56[No. RR-4]), administer 2 doses if not previously vaccinated or the second dose if only 1 dose has been administered.
- For persons aged 7 through 12 years, the minimum interval between doses is 3 months. However, if the second dose was administered at least 28 days after the first dose, it can be accepted as valid.
- For persons aged 13 years and older, the minimum interval between doses is 28 days.

The Recommended Immunization Schedules for Persons Aged 0–18 Years are approved by the Advisory Committee on Immunization Practices **(http://www.cdc.gov/vaccines/recs/acip)**, the American Academy of Pediatrics **(http://www.aap.org)**, and the American Academy of Family Physicians **(http://www.aafp.org)**.

# CATCH-UP IMMUNIZATION SCHEDULE FOR PERSONS AGED 4 MONTHS–18 YEARS WHO START LATE OR WHO ARE MORE THAN 1 MONTH BEHIND

| PERSONS AGED 4 MONTHS THROUGH 6 YEARS | | | | | |
|---|---|---|---|---|---|
| Vaccine | Minimum Age for Dose 1 | Minimum Interval Between Doses | | | |
| | | Dose 1 to Dose 2 | Dose 2 to Dose 3 | Dose 3 to Dose 4 | Dose 4 to Dose 5 |
| Hepatitis B[1] | Birth | 4 weeks | 8 weeks (and at least 16 weeks after first dose) | | |
| Rotavirus[2] | 6 wks | 4 weeks | 4 weeks[2] | | |
| Diphtheria, Tetanus, Pertussis[3] | 6 wks | 4 weeks | 4 weeks | 6 months | 6 months[3] |
| *Haemophilus influenzae* type b[4] | 6 wks | 4 weeks if first dose administered at younger than age 12 months<br>8 weeks (as final dose) if first dose administered at age 12–14 months<br>No further doses needed if first dose administered at age 15 months or older | 4 weeks[4] if current age is younger than 12 months<br>8 weeks (as final dose)[4] if current age is 12 months or older and first dose administered at younger than age 12 months and second dose administered at younger than 15 months<br>No further doses needed if previous dose administered at age 15 months or older | 8 weeks (as final dose) This dose only necessary for children aged 12 months through 59 months who received 3 doses before age 12 months | |
| Pneumococcal[5] | 6 wks | 4 weeks if first dose administered at younger than age 12 months<br>8 weeks (as final dose for healthy children) if first dose administered at age 12 months or older or current age 24 through 59 months<br>No further doses needed for healthy children if first dose administered at age 24 months or older | 4 weeks if current age is younger than 12 months<br>8 weeks (as final dose for healthy children) if current age is 12 months or older<br>No further doses needed for healthy children if previous dose administered at age 24 months or older | 8 weeks (as final dose) This dose only necessary for children aged 12 months through 59 months who received 3 doses before age 12 months or for high-risk children who received 3 doses at any age | |
| Inactivated Poliovirus[6] | 6 wks | 4 weeks | 4 weeks | 6 months | |
| Measles, Mumps, Rubella[7] | 12 mos | 4 weeks | | | |
| Varicella[8] | 12 mos | 3 months | | | |
| Hepatitis A[9] | 12 mos | 6 months | | | |
| PERSONS AGED 7 THROUGH 18 YEARS | | | | | |
| Tetanus, Diphtheria/ Tetanus, Diphtheria, Pertussis[10] | 7 yrs[10] | 4 weeks | 4 weeks if first dose administered at younger than age 12 months<br>6 months if first dose administered at 12 months or older | 6 months if first dose administered at younger than age 12 months | |
| Human Papillomavirus[11] | 9 yrs | Routine dosing intervals are recommended[11] | | | |
| Hepatitis A[9] | 12 mos | 6 months | | | |
| Hepatitis B[1] | Birth | 4 weeks | 8 weeks (and at least 16 weeks after first dose) | | |
| Inactivated Poliovirus[6] | 6 wks | 4 weeks | 4 weeks | 6 months | |
| Measles, Mumps, Rubella[7] | 12 mos | 4 weeks | | | |
| Varicella[8] | 12 mos | 3 months if person is younger than age 13 years<br>4 weeks if person is aged 13 years or older | | | |

The table above provides catch-up schedules and minimum intervals between doses for children whose vaccinations have been delayed. A vaccine series does not need to be restarted, regardless of the time that has elapsed between doses. Use the section appropriate for the child's age.

1. **Hepatitis B vaccine (HepB).**
   - Administer the 3-dose series to those not previously vaccinated.
   - A 2-dose series (separated by at least 4 months) of adult formulation Recombivax HB is licensed for children aged 11 through 15 years.
2. **Rotavirus vaccine (RV).**
   - The maximum age for the first dose is 14 weeks 6 days. Vaccination should not be initiated for infants aged 15 weeks 0 days or older.
   - The maximum age for the final dose in the series is 8 months 0 days.
   - If Rotarix was administered for the first and second doses, a third dose is not indicated.
3. **Diphtheria and tetanus toxoids and acellular pertussis vaccine (DTaP).**
   - The fifth dose is not necessary if the fourth dose was administered at age 4 years or older.
4. ***Haemophilus influenzae* type b conjugate vaccine (Hib).**
   - Hib vaccine is not generally recommended for persons aged 5 years or older. No efficacy data are available on which to base a recommendation concerning use of Hib vaccine for older children and adults. However, studies suggest good immunogenicity in persons who have sickle cell disease, leukemia, or HIV infection, or who have had a splenectomy; administering 1 dose of Hib vaccine to these persons who have not previously received Hib vaccine is not contraindicated.
   - If the first 2 doses were PRP-OMP (PedvaxHIB or Comvax), and administered at age 11 months or younger, the third (and final) dose should be administered at age 12 through 15 months and at least 8 weeks after the second dose.
   - If the first dose was administered at age 7 through 11 months, administer the second dose at least 4 weeks later and a final dose at age 12 through 15 months.

(Continued)

**5. Pneumococcal vaccine.**

- Administer 1 dose of pneumococcal conjugate vaccine (PCV) to all healthy children aged 24 through 59 months who have not received at least 1 dose of PCV on or after age 12 months.
- For children aged 24 through 59 months with underlying medical conditions, administer 1 dose of PCV if 3 doses were received previously or administer 2 doses of PCV at least 8 weeks apart if fewer than 3 doses were received previously.
- Administer pneumococcal polysaccharide vaccine (PPSV) to children aged 2 years or older with certain underlying medical conditions, including a cochlear implant, at least 8 weeks after the last dose of PCV. See *MMWR* 1997;46(No. RR-8).

**6. Inactivated poliovirus vaccine (IPV).**

- The final dose in the series should be administered on or after the fourth birthday and at least 6 months following the previous dose.
- A fourth dose is not necessary if the third dose was administered at age 4 years or older and at least 6 months following the previous dose.
- In the first 6 months of life, minimum age and minimum intervals are only recommended if the person is at risk for imminent exposure to circulating poliovirus (i.e., travel to a polio-endemic region or during an outbreak).

**7. Measles, mumps, and rubella vaccine (MMR).**

- Administer the second dose routinely at age 4 through 6 years. However, the second dose may be administered before age 4, provided at least 28 days have elapsed since the first dose.
- If not previously vaccinated, administer 2 doses with at least 28 days between doses.

**8. Varicella vaccine.**

- Administer the second dose routinely at age 4 through 6 years. However, the second dose may be administered before age 4, provided at least 3 months have elapsed since the first dose.
- For persons aged 12 months through 12 years, the minimum interval between doses is 3 months. However, if the second dose was administered at least 28 days after the first dose, it can be accepted as valid.
- For persons aged 13 years and older, the minimum interval between doses is 28 days.

**9. Hepatitis A vaccine (HepA).**

- HepA is recommended for children aged older than 23 months who live in areas where vaccination programs target older children, who are at increased risk for infection, or for whom immunity against hepatitis A is desired.

**10. Tetanus and diphtheria toxoids vaccine (Td) and tetanus and diphtheria toxoids and acellular pertussis vaccine (Tdap).**

- Doses of DTaP are counted as part of the Td/Tdap series.
- Tdap should be substituted for a single dose of Td in the catch-up series or as a booster for children aged 10 through 18 years; use Td for other doses.

**11. Human papillomavirus vaccine (HPV).**

- Administer the series to females at age 13 through 18 years if not previously vaccinated.
- Use recommended routine dosing intervals for series catch-up (i.e., the second and third doses should be administered at 1 to 2 and 6 months after the first dose). The minimum interval between the first and second doses is 4 weeks. The minimum interval between the second and third doses is 12 weeks, and the third dose should be administered at least 24 weeks after the first dose.

Information about reporting reactions after immunization is available online at **http://www.vaers.hhs.gov** or by telephone, 800-822-7967. Suspected cases of vaccine-preventable diseases should be reported to the state or local health department. Additional information, including precautions and contraindications for immunization, is available from the National Center for Immunization and Respiratory Diseases at **http://www.cdc.gov/vaccines** or telephone, **800-CDC-INFO (800-232-4636)**.

# RECOMMENDED ADULT IMMUNIZATION SCHEDULE

## Recommended adult immunization schedule, by vaccine and age group

| VACCINE ▼ / AGE GROUP ▶ | 19–26 years | 27–49 years | 50–59 years | 60–64 years | ≥65 years |
|---|---|---|---|---|---|
| Tetanus, diphtheria, pertussis (Td/Tdap)[1,*] | Substitute 1-time dose of Tdap for Td booster; then boost with Td every 10 yrs | | | | Td booster every 10 yrs |
| Human papillomavirus (HPV)[2,*] | 3 doses (females) | | | | |
| Varicella[3,*] | 2 doses | | | | |
| Zoster[4] | | | | 1 dose | |
| Measles, mumps, rubella (MMR)[5,*] | 1 or 2 doses | | 1 dose | | |
| Influenza[6,*] | 1 dose annually | | | | |
| Pneumococcal (polysaccharide)[7,8] | 1 or 2 doses | | | | 1 dose |
| Hepatitis A[9,*] | 2 doses | | | | |
| Hepatitis B[10,*] | 3 doses | | | | |
| Meningococcal[11,*] | 1 or more doses | | | | |

*Covered by the Vaccine Injury Compensation Program.

For all persons in this category who meet the age requirements and who lack evidence of immunity (e.g., lack documentation of vaccination or have no evidence of prior infection)

Recommended if some other risk factor is present (e.g., on the basis of medical, occupational, lifestyle, or other indications)

No recommendation

Report all clinically significant postvaccination reactions to the Vaccine Adverse Event Reporting System (VAERS). Reporting forms and instructions on filing a VAERS report are available at **www.vaers.hhs.gov** or by telephone, 800-822-7967.

Information on how to file a Vaccine Injury Compensation Program claim is available at **www.hrsa.gov/vaccinecompensation** or by telephone, 800-338-2382. To file a claim for vaccine injury, contact the U.S. Court of Federal Claims, 717 Madison Place, N.W., Washington, D.C. 20005; telephone, 202-357-6400.

Additional information about the vaccines in this schedule, extent of available data, and contraindications for vaccination is also available at **www.cdc.gov/vaccines** or from the CDC-INFO Contact Center at 800-CDC-INFO (800-232-4636) in English and Spanish, 24 hours a day, 7 days a week.

Use of trade names and commercial sources is for identification only and does not imply endorsement by the U.S. Department of Health and Human Services.

## Vaccines that might be indicated for adults based on medical and other indications

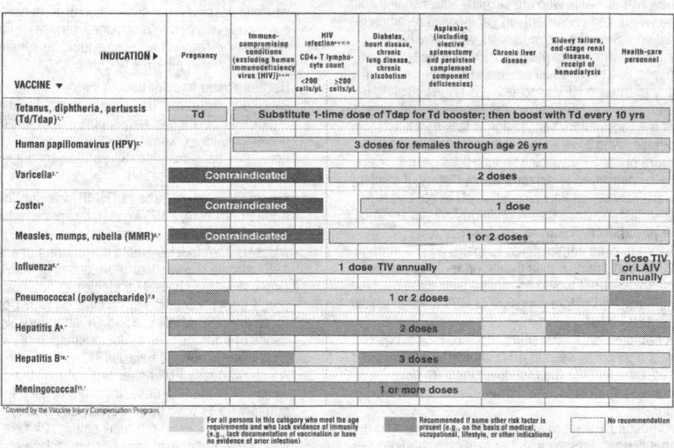

| VACCINE ▼ / INDICATION ▶ | Pregnancy | Immunocompromising conditions (excluding human immunodeficiency virus [HIV]) | HIV infection, CD4+ T lymphocyte count <200 cells/μL | HIV infection, CD4+ T lymphocyte count ≥200 cells/μL | Diabetes, heart disease, chronic lung disease, chronic alcoholism | Asplenia (including elective splenectomy and persistent complement component deficiencies) | Chronic liver disease | Kidney failure, end-stage renal disease, receipt of hemodialysis | Health-care personnel |
|---|---|---|---|---|---|---|---|---|---|
| Tetanus, diphtheria, pertussis (Td/Tdap)[1,*] | Td | Substitute 1-time dose of Tdap for Td booster; then boost with Td every 10 yrs | | | | | | | |
| Human papillomavirus (HPV)[2,*] | | 3 doses for females through age 26 yrs | | | | | | | |
| Varicella[3,*] | Contraindicated | | | 2 doses | | | | | |
| Zoster[4] | Contraindicated | | | | 1 dose | | | | |
| Measles, mumps, rubella (MMR)[5,*] | Contraindicated | | | 1 or 2 doses | | | | | |
| Influenza[6,*] | 1 dose TIV annually | | | | | | | | 1 dose TIV or LAIV annually |
| Pneumococcal (polysaccharide)[7,8] | 1 or 2 doses | | | | | | | | |
| Hepatitis A[9,*] | 2 doses | | | | | | | | |
| Hepatitis B[10,*] | 3 doses | | | | | | | | |
| Meningococcal[11,*] | 1 or more doses | | | | | | | | |

*Covered by the Vaccine Injury Compensation Program.

For all persons in this category who meet the age requirements and who lack evidence of immunity (e.g., lack documentation of vaccination or have no evidence of prior infection)

Recommended if some other risk factor is present (e.g., on the basis of medical, occupational, lifestyle, or other indications)

No recommendation

These schedules indicate the recommended age groups and medical indications for which administration of currently licensed vaccines is commonly indicated for adults ages 19 years and older, as of January 1, 2010. Licensed combination vaccines may be used whenever any components of the combination are indicated and when the vaccine's other components are not contraindicated. For detailed recommendations on all vaccines, including those used primarily for travelers or that are issued during the year, consult the manufacturers' package inserts and the complete statements from the Advisory Committee on Immunization Practices **(www.cdc.gov/vaccines/pubs/acip-list.htm)**.

*(Continued)*

1. **Tetanus, diphtheria, and acellular pertussis (Td/Tdap) vaccination.** Tdap should replace a single dose of Td for adults aged 19 through 64 years who have not received a dose of Tdap previously. Adults with uncertain or incomplete history of primary vaccination series with tetanus and diphtheria toxoid-containing vaccines should begin or complete a primary vaccination series. A primary series for adults is 3 doses of tetanus and diphtheria toxoid-containing vaccines; administer the first 2 doses at least 4 weeks apart and the third dose 6–12 months after the second; Tdap can substitute for any one of the doses of Td in the 3-dose primary series. The booster dose of tetanus and diphtheria toxoid-containing vaccine should be administered to adults who have completed a primary series and if the last vaccination was received ≥10 years previously. Tdap or Td vaccine may be used, as indicated.
   If a woman is pregnant and received the last Td vaccination ≥10 years previously, administer Td during the second or third trimester. If the woman received the last Td vaccination <10 years previously, administer Tdap during the immediate postpartum period. A dose of Tdap is recommended for postpartum women, close contacts of infants aged <12 months, and all health-care personnel with direct patient contact if they have not previously received Tdap. An interval as short as 2 years from the last Td is suggested; shorter intervals can be used. Td may be deferred during pregnancy and Tdap substituted in the immediate postpartum period, or Tdap can be administered instead of Td to a pregnant woman. Consult the ACIP statement for recommendations for giving Td as prophylaxis in wound management.
2. **Human papillomavirus (HPV) vaccination.** HPV vaccination is recommended at age 11 or 12 years with catch-up vaccination at ages 13 through 26 years.
   Ideally, vaccine should be administered before potential exposure to HPV through sexual activity; however, females who are sexually active should still be vaccinated consistent with age-based recommendations. Sexually active females who have not been infected with any of the four HPV vaccine types (types 6, 11, 16, 18 all of which HPV4 prevents) or any of the two HPV vaccine types (types 16 and 18 both of which HPV2 prevents) receive the full benefit of the vaccination. Vaccination is less beneficial for females who have already been infected with one or more of the HPV vaccine types. HPV4 or HPV2 can be administered to persons with a history of genital warts, abnormal Papanicolaou test, or positive HPV DNA test, because these conditions are not evidence of prior infection with all vaccine HPV types.
   HPV4 may be administered to males aged 9 through 26 years to reduce their likelihood of acquiring genital warts. HPV4 would be most effective when administered before exposure to HPV through sexual contact.
   A complete series for either HPV4 or HPV2 consists of 3 doses. The second dose should be administered 1–2 months after the first dose; the third dose should be administered 6 months after the first dose.
   Although HPV vaccination is not specifically recommended for persons with the medical indications described in Figure 2, "Vaccines that might be indicated for adults based on medical and other indications," it may be administered to these persons because the HPV vaccine is not a live-virus vaccine. However, the immune response and vaccine efficacy might be less for persons with the medical indications described in Figure 2 than in persons who do not have the medical indications described or who are immunocompetent. Health-care personnel are not at increased risk because of occupational exposure, and should be vaccinated consistent with age-based recommendations.
3. **Varicella vaccination.** All adults without evidence of immunity to varicella should receive 2 doses of single-antigen varicella vaccine if not previously vaccinated or the second dose if they have received only 1 dose, unless they have a medical contraindication. Special consideration should be given to those who 1) have close contact with persons at high risk for severe disease (e.g., health-care personnel and family contacts of persons with immunocompromising conditions) or 2) are at high risk for exposure or transmission (e.g., teachers; child-care employees; residents and staff members of institutional settings, including correctional institutions; college students; military personnel; adolescents and adults living in households with children; nonpregnant women of childbearing age; and international travelers).
   Evidence of immunity to varicella in adults includes any of the following: 1) documentation of 2 doses of varicella vaccine at least 4 weeks apart; 2) U.S.-born before 1980 (although for health-care personnel and pregnant women, birth before 1980 should not be considered evidence of immunity); 3) history of varicella based on diagnosis or verification of varicella by a health-care provider (for a patient reporting a history of or presenting with an atypical case, a mild case, or both, health-care providers should seek either an epidemiologic link with a typical varicella case or to a laboratory-confirmed case or evidence of laboratory confirmation, if it was performed at the time of acute disease); 4) history of herpes zoster based on diagnosis or verification of herpes zoster by a health-care provider; or 5) laboratory evidence of immunity or laboratory confirmation of disease.
   Pregnant women should be assessed for evidence of varicella immunity. Women who do not have evidence of immunity should receive the first dose of varicella vaccine upon completion or termination of pregnancy and before discharge from the health-care facility. The second dose should be administered 4–8 weeks after the first dose.
4. **Herpes zoster vaccination.** A single dose of zoster vaccine is recommended for adults aged ≥60 years regardless of whether they report a prior episode of herpes zoster. Persons with chronic medical conditions may be vaccinated unless their condition constitutes a contraindication.
5. **Measles, mumps, rubella (MMR) vaccination.** Adults born before 1957 generally are considered immune to measles and mumps.
   *Measles component:* Adults born during or after 1957 should receive 1 or more doses of MMR vaccine unless they have 1) a medical contraindication; 2) documentation of vaccination with 1 or more doses of MMR vaccine; 3) laboratory evidence of immunity; or 4) documentation of physician-diagnosed measles.
   A second dose of MMR vaccine, administered 4 weeks after the first dose, is recommended for adults who 1) have been recently exposed to measles or are in an outbreak setting; 2) have been vaccinated previously with killed measles vaccine; 3) have been vaccinated with an unknown type of measles vaccine during 1963–1967; 4) are students in postsecondary educational institutions; 5) work in a health-care facility; or 6) plan to travel internationally.
   *Mumps component:* Adults born during or after 1957 should receive 1 dose of MMR vaccine unless they have 1) a medical contraindication;



*(Continued)*

2) documentation of vaccination with 1 or more doses of MMR vaccine; 3) laboratory evidence of immunity; or 4) documentation of physician-diagnosed mumps.
A second dose of MMR vaccine, administered 4 weeks after the first dose, is recommended for adults who 1) live in a community experiencing a mumps outbreak and are in an affected age group; 2) are students in postsecondary educational institutions; 3) work in a health-care facility; or 4) plan to travel internationally.
*Rubella component:* 1 dose of MMR vaccine is recommended for women who do not have documentation of rubella vaccination, or who lack laboratory evidence of immunity. For women of childbearing age, regardless of birth year, rubella immunity should be determined and women should be counseled regarding congenital rubella syndrome. Women who do not have evidence of immunity should receive MMR vaccine upon completion or termination of pregnancy and before discharge from the health-care facility.
Health-care personnel born before 1957: For unvaccinated health-care personnel born before 1957 who lack laboratory evidence of measles, mumps, and/or rubella immunity or laboratory confirmation of disease, health-care facilities should consider vaccinating personnel with 2 doses of MMR vaccine at the appropriate interval (for measles and mumps) and 1 dose of MMR vaccine (for rubella), respectively.
During outbreaks, health-care facilities should recommend that unvaccinated health-care personnel born before 1957, who lack laboratory evidence of measles, mumps, and/or rubella immunity or laboratory confirmation of disease, receive 2 doses of MMR vaccine during an outbreak of measles or mumps, and 1 dose during an outbreak of rubella.
Complete information about evidence of immunity is available at **www.cdc.gov/vaccines/recs/provisional/default.htm**.

6. **Seasonal Influenza vaccination.** Vaccinate all persons aged ≥50 years and any younger persons who would like to decrease their risk of getting influenza. Vaccinate persons aged 19 through 49 years with any of the following indications.
*Medical:* Chronic disorders of the cardiovascular or pulmonary systems, including asthma; chronic metabolic diseases, including diabetes mellitus; renal or hepatic dysfunction, hemoglobinopathies, or immunocompromising conditions (including immunocompromising conditions caused by medications or HIV); cognitive, neurologic or neuromuscular disorders; and pregnancy during the influenza season. No data exist on the risk for severe or complicated influenza disease among persons with asplenia; however, influenza is a risk factor for secondary bacterial infections that can cause severe disease among persons with asplenia.
*Occupational:* All health-care personnel, including those employed by long-term care and assisted-living facilities, and caregivers of children aged <5 years.
*Other:* Residents of nursing homes and other long-term care and assisted-living facilities; persons likely to transmit influenza to persons at high risk (e.g., in-home household contacts and caregivers of children aged <5 years, persons aged ≥50 years, and persons of all ages with high-risk conditions).
Healthy, nonpregnant adults aged <50 years without high-risk medical conditions who are not contacts of severely immunocompromised persons in special-care units may receive either intranasally administered live, attenuated influenza vaccine (FluMist) or inactivated vaccine. Other persons should receive the inactivated vaccine.

7. **Pneumococcal polysaccharide (PPSV) vaccination.** Vaccinate all persons with the following indications.
*Medical:* Chronic lung disease (including asthma); chronic cardiovascular diseases; diabetes mellitus; chronic liver diseases, cirrhosis; chronic alcoholism; functional or anatomic asplenia (e.g., sickle cell disease or splenectomy [if elective splenectomy is planned, vaccinate at least 2 weeks before surgery]); immunocompromising conditions including chronic renal failure or nephrotic syndrome; and cochlear implants and cerebrospinal fluid leaks. Vaccinate as close to HIV diagnosis as possible.
*Other:* Residents of nursing homes or long-term care facilities and persons who smoke cigarettes. Routine use of PPSV is not recommended for American Indians/Alaska Natives or persons aged <65 years unless they have underlying medical conditions that are PPSV indications. However, public health authorities may consider recommending PPSV for American Indians/Alaska Natives and persons aged 50 through 64 years who are living in areas where the risk for invasive pneumococcal disease is increased.

8. **Revaccination with PPSV.** One-time revaccination after 5 years is recommended for persons with chronic renal failure or nephrotic syndrome; functional or anatomic asplenia (e.g., sickle cell disease or splenectomy); and for persons with immunocompromising conditions. For persons aged ≥65 years, one-time revaccination is recommended if they were vaccinated ≥5 years previously and were younger than aged <65 years at the time of primary vaccination.

9. **Hepatitis A vaccination.** Vaccinate persons with any of the following indications and any person seeking protection from hepatitis A virus (HAV) infection.
*Behavioral:* Men who have sex with men and persons who use injection drugs.
*Occupational:* Persons working with HAV–infected primates or with HAV in a research laboratory setting.
*Medical:* Persons with chronic liver disease and persons who receive clotting factor concentrates.
*Other:* Persons traveling to or working in countries that have high or intermediate endemicity of hepatitis A (a list of countries is available at **wwwn.cdc.gov/travel/contentdiseases.aspx**).
Unvaccinated persons who anticipate close personal contact (e.g., household contact or regular babysitting) with an international adoptee from a country of high or intermediate endemicity during the first 60 days after arrival of the adoptee in the United States should consider vaccination. The first dose of the 2-dose hepatitis A vaccine series should be administered as soon as adoption is planned, ideally ≥2 weeks before the arrival of the adoptee.
Single-antigen vaccine formulations should be administered in a 2-dose schedule at either 0 and 6–12 months (Havrix), or 0 and 6–18 months (Vaqta). If the combined hepatitis A and hepatitis B vaccine (Twinrix) is used, administer 3 doses at 0, 1, and 6 months; alternatively, a 4-dose schedule, administered on days 0, 7, and 21–30 followed by a booster dose at month 12 may be used.

10. **Hepatitis B vaccination.** Vaccinate persons with any of the following indications and any person seeking protection from hepatitis B virus (HBV) infection.

*(Continued)*

*Behavioral:* Sexually active persons who are not in a long-term, mutually monogamous relationship (e.g., persons with more than one sex partner during the previous 6 months); persons seeking evaluation or treatment for a sexually transmitted disease (STD); current or recent injection-drug users; and men who have sex with men.
*Occupational:* Health-care personnel and public-safety workers who are exposed to blood or other potentially infectious body fluids.
*Medical:* Persons with end-stage renal disease, including patients receiving hemodialysis; persons with HIV infection; and persons with chronic liver disease.
*Other:* Household contacts and sex partners of persons with chronic HBV infection; clients and staff members of institutions for persons with developmental disabilities; and international travelers to countries with high or intermediate prevalence of chronic HBV infection (a list of countries is available at **wwwn.cdc.gov/travel/content diseases.aspx**).
Hepatitis B vaccination is recommended for all adults in the following settings: STD treatment facilities; HIV testing and treatment facilities; facilities providing drug-abuse treatment and prevention services; health-care settings targeting services to injection-drug users or men who have sex with men; correctional facilities; end-stage renal disease programs and facilities for chronic hemodialysis patients; and institutions and nonresidential daycare facilities for persons with developmental disabilities.
Administer or complete a 3-dose series of HepB to those persons not previously vaccinated. The second dose should be administered 1 month after the first dose; the third dose should be administered at least 2 months after the second dose (and at least 4 months after the first dose). If the combined hepatitis A and hepatitis B vaccine (Twinrix) is used, administer 3 doses at 0, 1, and 6 months; alternatively, a 4-dose schedule, administered on days 0, 7, and 21–30 followed by a booster dose at month 12 may be used.
Adult patients receiving hemodialysis or with other immunocompromising conditions should receive 1 dose of 40 μg/mL (Recombivax HB) administered on a 3-dose schedule or 2 doses of 20 μg/mL (Engerix-B) administered simultaneously on a 4-dose schedule at 0, 1, 2 and 6 months.

11. **Meningococcal vaccination.** Meningococcal vaccine should be administered to persons with the following indications.
*Medical:* Adults with anatomic or functional asplenia, or persistent complement component deficiencies.
*Other:* First-year college students living in dormitories; microbiologists routinely exposed to isolates of *Neisseria meningitidis;* military recruits; and persons who travel to or live in countries in which meningococcal disease is hyperendemic or epidemic (e.g., the "meningitis belt" of sub-Saharan Africa during the dry season [December through June]), particularly if their contact with local populations will be prolonged. Vaccination is required by the government of Saudi Arabia for all travelers to Mecca during the annual Hajj.
Meningococcal conjugate vaccine (MCV4) is preferred for adults with any of the preceding indications who are aged ≤55 years; meningococcal polysaccharide vaccine (MPSV4) is preferred for adults aged ≥56 years. Revaccination with MCV4 after 5 years is recommended for adults previously vaccinated with MCV4 or MPSV4 who remain at increased risk for infection (e.g., adults with anatomic or functional asplenia). Persons whose only risk factor is living in on-campus housing are not recommended to receive an additional dose.
12. **Selected conditions for which *Haemophilus influenzae* type b (Hib) vaccine may be used.** Hib vaccine generally is not recommended for persons aged ≥5 years. No efficacy data are available on which to base a recommendation concerning use of Hib vaccine for older children and adults. However, studies suggest good immunogenicity in patients who have sickle cell disease, leukemia, or HIV infection or who have had a splenectomy. Administering 1 dose of Hib vaccine to these high-risk persons who have not previously received Hib vaccine is not contraindicated.
13. **Immunocompromising conditions.** Inactivated vaccines generally are acceptable (e.g., pneumococcal, meningococcal, influenza [inactivated influenza vaccine]) and live vaccines generally are avoided in persons with immune deficiencies or immunocompromising conditions. Information on specific conditions is available at **www.cdc.gov/vaccines/pubs/acip-list.htm**.

# ALCOHOL-FREE PRODUCTS

The following is a selection of alcohol-free products grouped by therapeutic category. This list is not comprehensive. Generic and alternate brands may exist. Always check product labeling for definitive information on specific ingredients.

| Product | Manufacturer |
|---|---|
| **Analgesics** | |
| Advil Children's Suspension | Wyeth Consumer |
| APAP Elixir | Bio-Pharm |
| Motrin Children's Suspension | McNeil Consumer |
| Motrin Infants' Suspension | McNeil Consumer |
| Silapap Infant's Drops | Silarx |
| Tylenol Children's Suspension | McNeil Consumer |
| Tylenol Extra Strength Solution | McNeil Consumer |
| Tylenol Infant's Suspension | McNeil Consumer |
| **Antiasthmatic Agent** | |
| Dy-G Liquid | Cypress |
| **Anticonvulsant** | |
| Zarontin Syrup | Pfizer |
| **Antiviral Agent** | |
| Epivir Oral Solution | GlaxoSmithKline |
| **Cough/Cold/Allergy Preparations** | |
| Accuhist PDX Drops Solution | Pediamed |
| Accuhist PDX Syrup | Pediamed |
| Alacol Solution | Ballay |
| Alacol DM Syrup | Ballay |
| Allanhist PDX Syrup | Allan |
| Andehist DM NR Syrup | Cypress |
| Andehist NR Syrup | Cypress |
| Aridex Solution | Gentex |
| Aridex-D Solution | Gentex |
| Baltussin Solution | Ballay |
| Banophen Elixir | Major |
| Benadryl Allergy Solution | Pfizer Consumer |
| Benadryl-D Allergy & Sinus Children's Solution | Johnson & Johnson Consumer |
| Bromaline Syrup | Rugby |
| Bromaline DM Elixir | Rugby |
| Bromhist PDX Solution | Cypress |
| Bromhist Pediatric Solution | Cypress |
| Bromhist-DM Pediatric Syrup | Cypress |
| Bromhist-DM Solution | Cypress |
| Bromhist-NR Solution | Cypress |
| Bromhist-PDX Syrup | Cypress |
| Bromphenex DM Solution | Breckenridge |
| Bromphenex HD Solution | Breckenridge |
| Bromplex DM Solution | Prasco |
| Bromplex HD Solution | Prasco |
| Bromtuss DM Solution | Breckenridge |
| Broncotron Liquid | Seyer Pharmatec |
| Broncotron-D Suspension | Seyer Pharmatec |
| B-Tuss Liquid | Blansett |
| Carbaphen 12 Ped Suspension | Gil |
| Carbaphen 12 Suspension | Gil |
| Carbatuss Liquid | GM |
| Carbatuss-12 Suspension | GM |
| Carbatuss-CL Solution | GM |
| Carbetaplex Solution | Breckenridge |
| Carbetaplex TS Suspension | Breckenridge |
| Carbofed DM Syrup | Hi-Tech Pharmacal |
| Cardec DM Solution | Qualitest |
| Children's Dimetapp Cold & Allergy Solution | Wyeth Consumer |
| Children's Dimetapp Long Acting Cough Plus Cold Solution | Wyeth Consumer |
| Children's Dimetapp Nighttime Flu Syrup | Wyeth Consumer |
| Children's Dimetapp DM Cold & Cough Solution | Wyeth Consumer |
| Children's Mucinex Cold Solution | Adams |
| Children's Mucinex Cough Syrup | Adams |
| Children's Mucinex Syrup | Adams |
| Chlordex GP Syrup | Cypress |
| Chlor-Mes D Solution | Cypress |
| Codal-DM Syrup | Cypress |
| Complete Allergy Elixir | Cardinal Health |
| Corfen DM Solution | Cypress |
| Coughtuss Solution | Breckenridge |
| Crantex HC Syrup | Breckenridge |
| Crantex Syrup | Breckenridge |
| Creomulsion Cough Syrup | Summit Industries |
| Creomulsion for Children Syrup | Summit Industries |
| Dacex-DM Solution | Cypress |
| Dallergy Solution | Laser |
| De-Chlor DM Solution | Cypress |
| De-Chlor DR Solution | Cypress |
| Dehistine Syrup | Cypress |
| Despec Liquid | International Ethical |
| Dex PC Syrup | Boca Pharmacal |
| Diabetic Tussin Allergy Relief Liquid | Health Care Products |
| Diabetic Tussin Cough Lozenges | Health Care Products |
| Diabetic Tussin Night Time Formula Solution | Health Care Products |
| Diabetic Tussin Solution | Health Care Products |
| Diabetic Tussin DM Solution | Health Care Products |
| Diabetic Tussin DM Maximum Strength Liquid | Health Care Products |
| Diabetic Tussin EX Liquid | Health Care Products |

| Cough/Cold/Allergy Preparations (Continued) | |
|---|---|
| Dimetapp Decongestant Pediatric Drops | Wyeth Consumer |
| Donatussin Solution | Laser |
| Donatussin DC Syrup | Laser |
| Donatussin DM Solution | Laser |
| Donatussin DM Suspension | Laser |
| Donatussin DM Syrup | Laser |
| Double-Tussin DM Liquid | Reese |
| Duratuss AC12 Suspension | Victory |
| Duratuss DM Solution | Victory |
| Duratuss DM12 Suspension | Victory |
| Dynatuss EX Syrup | Breckenridge |
| Dynatuss HC Solution | Breckenridge |
| Father John's Medicine Plus Drops | Oakhurst |
| Ganidin NR Liquid | Cypress |
| Gani-Tuss NR Liquid | Cypress |
| Gani-Tuss-DM NR Liquid | Cypress |
| Genebronco-D Liquid | PGD |
| Genecof-HC Liquid | PGD |
| Genecof-XP Liquid | PGD |
| Genecof-XP Syrup | PGD |
| Genedel Syrup | PGD |
| Genedotuss-DM Liquid | PGD |
| Genepatuss Liquid | PGD |
| Genetuss-2 Liquid | PGD |
| Genexpect-DM Liquid | PGD |
| Genexpect-PE Liquid | PGD |
| Genexpect-SF Liquid | PGD |
| Giltuss Liquid | Gil |
| Giltuss Pediatric Liquid | Gil |
| Giltuss Ped-C Solution | Gil |
| H-C Tussive Syrup | Vintage |
| Histacol DM Pediatric Syrup | Breckenridge |
| Histinex HC Syrup | Ethex |
| Histinex PV Syrup | Ethex |
| Hydramine Elixir | Teva |
| Hydro-Tussin HC Syrup | Ethex |
| Hydro-Tussin HD Liquid | Ethex |
| Hydro-Tussin XP Syrup | Ethex |
| Jaycof Expectorant Syrup | Pharmakon |
| Jaycof-HC Liquid | Pharmakon |
| Jaycof-XP Syrup | Pharmakon |
| Lodrane D Suspension | ECR |
| Lohist D Syrup | Larken |
| Lohist DM Syrup | Larken |
| Marcof Expectorant Syrup | Marnel |
| M-Clear Jr Solution | McNeil, R.A. |
| M-Clear Solution | McNeil, R.A. |
| Medi-Brom Elixir | Medicine Shoppe |
| Mintuss G Syrup | Breckenridge |
| Mintuss MR Syrup | Breckenridge |
| Mintuss MS Syrup | Breckenridge |
| Mintuss NX Solution | Breckenridge |
| Motrin Cold Children's Suspension | McNeil Consumer |
| Myhist-DM Solution | Larken |
| Myhist-PD Solution | Larken |
| Nalex DH Liquid | Blansett Pharmacal |
| Nalex-A Liquid | Blansett Pharmacal |
| Nasop Suspension | Hawthorn |
| Neotuss S/F Liquid | A.G. Marin |
| Neotuss-D Liquid | A.G. Marin |
| Norel DM Liquid | U.S.Pharmaceutical |
| Organidin NR Liquid | Meda |
| PediaCare Cough + Cold Children's Liquid | Johnson & Johnson Consumer |
| PediaCare Decongestant & Cough Liquid | Johnson & Johnson Consumer |
| PediaCare Long-Acting Cough Solution | Johnson & Johnson Consumer |
| PediaCare Multi-Symptom Cold Liquid | Johnson & Johnson Consumer |
| PediaCare Nightrest Liquid | Johnson & Johnson Consumer |
| Pediahist DM Syrup | Boca Pharmacal |
| Pedia-Relief Liquid | Major |
| Phanasin Diabetic Choice Syrup | Pharmakon |
| Phanasin Syrup | Pharmakon |
| Phanatuss Syrup | Pharmakon |
| Phanatuss DM Diabetic Choice Syrup | Pharmakon |
| Phanatuss-HC Diabetic Choice Solution | Pharmakon |
| Phena-HC Solution | GM |
| Phena-S Liquid | GM |
| Phena-S 12 Suspension | GM |
| Poly Hist DM Solution | Poly |
| Poly Hist HC Solution | Poly |
| Poly Hist PD Solution | Poly |
| Poly-Tussin Solution | Poly |
| Poly-Tussin AC | Poly |
| Poly-Tussin DHC | Poly |
| Poly-Tussin DM Syrup | Poly |
| Poly-Tussin HD Syrup | Poly |
| Poly-Tussin XP Solution | Poly |
| Pro-Clear Solution | Pro-Pharma |
| Prolex DM Liquid | Blansett Pharmacal |
| Pro-Red Solution | Pro-Pharma |
| Q-Tussin Liquid | Qualitest |
| Q-Tussin PE Liquid | Qualitest |
| Rescon-DM Liquid | Capellon |

**Cough/Cold/Allergy Preparations (Continued)**

| | |
|---|---|
| Rescon-GG Liquid | Capellon |
| Rindal HD Liquid | Breckenridge |
| Rindal HD Plus Solution | Breckenridge |
| Robitussin Chest Congestion Syrup | Wyeth Consumer |
| Robitussin Cough & Allergy Solution | Wyeth Consumer |
| Robitussin Cough & Cold CF Syrup | Wyeth Consumer |
| Robitussin Cough, Cold & Flu Nighttime Solution | Wyeth Consumer |
| Robitussin Cough & Congestion Liquid | Wyeth Consumer |
| Robitussin Cough DM Syrup | Wyeth Consumer |
| Robitussin Head & Chest Congestion PE Syrup | Wyeth Consumer |
| Robitussin Pediatric Cough & Cold CF Solution | Wyeth Consumer |
| Robitussin Pediatric Cough & Cold Long-Acting Solution | Wyeth Consumer |
| Robitussin Pediatric Night Relief Liquid | Wyeth Consumer |
| Rondec Solution | Sciele |
| Rondec DM Drops | Sciele |
| Rondec DM Solution | Sciele |
| Ru-Tuss DM Solution | Carwin |
| Scot-Tussin Diabetes CF Liquid | Scot-Tussin |
| Scot-Tussin DM Solution | Scot-Tussin |
| Scot-Tussin Expectorant Solution | Scot-Tussin |
| Scot-Tussin Original Solution | Scot-Tussin |
| Scot-Tussin Senior Solution | Scot-Tussin |
| Siladryl Allergy Solution | Silarx |
| Sildec Syrup | Silarx |
| Sildec-DM Syrup | Silarx |
| Sildec-PE Solution | Silarx |
| Sildec PE-DM Solution | Silarx |
| Siltussin DAS Liquid | Silarx |
| Siltussin DM DAS Cough Formula Syrup | Silarx |
| Siltussin SA Syrup | Silarx |
| Simply Cough Liquid | McNeil Consumer |
| Sudafed Children's Cold & Cough Solution | Johnson & Johnson |
| Sudafed Children's Solution | Johnson & Johnson |
| Sudatuss DM Syrup | PGD |
| Sudatuss-2 Liquid | PGD |
| Sudatuss-SF Liquid | PGD |
| Triant-HC Solution | Hawthorn |
| TriTuss Solution | Everett |
| Tusdec-DM Solution | Cypress |
| Tusnel Pediatric Solution | Llorens |
| Tusnel Solution | Llorens |
| Tussafed-EX Syrup | Everett |
| Tussafed-EX Pediatric Drops | Everett |
| Tussafed-HC Syrup | Everett |
| Tussafed-HCG Solution | Everett |
| Tussall Solution | Everett |
| Tussinate Syrup | Pediamed |
| Tussi-Organidin DM NR Solution | Victory |
| Tussi-Organidin DM-S NR Solution | Victory |
| Tussi-Organidin NR Solution | Victory |
| Tussi-Organidin-S NR Solution | Victory |
| Tussi-Pres Liquid | Kramer-Novis |
| Tussi-Pres Pediatric Solution | Kramer-Novis |
| Tylenol Cold Children's Suspension | McNeil Consumer |
| Tylenol Cold Infants' Drops | McNeil Consumer |
| Tylenol Cold Plus Cough Children's Suspension | McNeil Consumer |
| Tylenol Cold Plus Cough Infants' Suspension | McNeil Consumer |
| Tylenol Flu Children's Suspension | McNeil Consumer |
| Tylenol Flu Night Time Max Strength Liquid | McNeil Consumer |
| Tylenol Sinus Children's Suspension | McNeil Consumer |
| Vazol Solution | Wraser Pharm |
| Vicks 44E Pediatric Liquid | Procter & Gamble |
| Vicks 44M Pediatric Liquid | Procter & Gamble |
| Vicks Dayquil Multi-Symptom Liquid | Procter & Gamble |
| Vicks Nyquil Children's Liquid | Procter & Gamble |
| V-Tann Suspension | Breckenridge |
| Welltuss EXP Solution | Prasco |
| Z-Cof 12 DM Suspension | Zyber |
| Z-Cof 8 DM Suspension | Zyber |
| Z-Cof DM Solution | Zyber |
| Z-Cof DMX Solution | Zyber |
| Z-Cof HC Solution | Zyber |
| Z-Cof HCX Solution | Zyber |
| Z-Tuss DM Syrup | Magna |

**Ear/Nose/Throat Products**

| | |
|---|---|
| 4-Way Saline Moisturizing Mist Spray | Bristol-Myers |
| Ayr Baby Saline Spray | Ascher |
| Bucalcide Spray | Seyer Pharmatec |
| Bucalsep Solution | Gil |
| Bucalsep Spray | Gil |
| Cheracol Sore Throat Spray | Lee |
| Fresh N Free Solution | Geritrex |
| Gly-Oxide Solution | GlaxoSmithKline |

**Ear/Nose/Throat Products (Continued)**

| Product | Manufacturer |
|---|---|
| Larynex Lozenges | Dover |
| Listermint Solution | Johnson & Johnson Consumer |
| Nasal Moist Gel | Blairex |
| Orajel Baby Day & Night Gel | Del |
| Orajel Baby Nighttime Teething Pain Medicine Gel | Del |
| OraMagic Plus Powder | MPM Medical |
| OraMagicRx Powder | MPM Medical |
| Orasept Mouthwash/ Gargle Liquid | Pharmakon |
| Tanac Liquid | Del |
| Throto-Ceptic Spray | S.S.S. |
| Triaminic Sore Throat Spray | Novartis Consumer |
| Vicks Sinex Spray | P&G Company |
| Vicks Sinex 12 Hour Spray | P&G Company |
| Zilactin Baby Extra Strength Gel | Zila |

**Gastrointestinal Agents**

| Product | Manufacturer |
|---|---|
| Axid Solution | Braintree |
| Colidrops Pediatric Drops | A.G. Marin |
| Colace Solution | Purdue |
| Gas Relief Solution | Perrigo |
| Imogen Liquid | PGD |
| Kaodene NN Suspension | Pfeiffer |
| Kaopectate Advanced Formula Suspension | Pharmacia Consumer |
| Liqui-Doss Liquid | Ferndale |
| Mylicon Infants' Drops | Johnson & Johnson/ Merck |

**Topical Products**

| Product | Manufacturer |
|---|---|
| Aloe Vesta 2-N-1 Antifungal Ointment | Convatec |
| Dermatone Lips N Face Protector Ointment | Dermatone |
| Dermatone Moisturizing Sunblock Cream | Dermatone |
| Dermatone Skin Protector Cream | Dermatone |
| Fleet Pain Relief Pads | Fleet |
| Fresh & Pure Douche Solution | Unico |
| Handclens Solution | Woodward |
| Joint-Ritis Maximum Strength Ointment | Naturopathic |
| Neutrogena Acne Wash Liquid | Neutrogena |
| Neutrogena Antiseptic Solution | Neutrogena |
| Neutrogena Clear Pore Gel | Neutrogena |
| Neutrogena T/Derm Liquid | Neutrogena |
| Neutrogena Toner Solution | Neutrogena |
| Podiclens Spray | Woodward |
| Sea Breeze Foaming Face Wash Gel | Clairol |
| Sportz Bloc Cream | Med-Derm |
| Therasoft Anti-Acne Cream | SFC |
| Therasoft Skin Protectant Cream | SFC |
| Tiger Balm Arthritis Rub Lotion | Prince of Peace |

**Vitamins/Minerals/Supplements**

| Product | Manufacturer |
|---|---|
| Adaptosode For Stress Liquid | HVS |
| Adaptosode R+R For Acute Stress Liquid | HVS |
| Apetigen Elixir | Kramer-Novis |
| Biosode Liquid | HVS |
| Detoxosode Products Liquid | HVS |
| Genesupp-500 Liquid | PGD |
| Genetect Plus Liquid | PGD |
| Multi-Delyn Liquid | Silarx |
| Multi-Delyn w/Iron Liquid | Silarx |
| Nutrivit Solution | Llorens |
| Poly-Vi-Sol Drops | Mead Johnson |
| Poly-Vi-Sol w/Iron Drops | Mead Johnson |
| Protect Plus Liquid | Gil |
| Strovite Forte Syrup | Everett |
| Supervite Liquid | Seyer Pharmatec |
| Suplevit Liquid | Gil |
| Tri-Vi-Sol w/Iron Drops | Mead Johnson |
| Vitafol Syrup | Everett |

**Miscellaneous**

| Product | Manufacturer |
|---|---|
| Cytra-2 Solution | Cypress |
| Cytra-K Solution | Cypress |
| Fluorinse Solution | Oral B |
| Namenda Solution | Forest |
| Primsol Solution | FSC |

# COMMON LABORATORY TEST VALUES

Listed below are generally accepted normal values for a selection of common laboratory assays conducted on serum, plasma, and blood. Remember that norms may vary from laboratory to laboratory in accordance with the methodology and quality control measures employed by the facility. When in doubt, check with the laboratory that performed the analysis.

"SI range" refers to Système International d'Unités, a uniform system of reporting numerical values that permits interchangeability of information among nations and disciplines.

| TEST | US RANGE | SI RANGE |
|---|---|---|
| Acid phosphatase | ≤2.5 ng/mL | ≤2.5 µg/L |
| Prostatic Total | ≤5.8 U/L | <97 nkat/L |
| Alanine aminotransferase [ALT] (SGPT) | ≤48 U/L | ≤0.8 µkat/L |
| Albumin, serum | 3.5-5.5 g/dL | 35-55 g/L |
| Alkaline phosphatase | 20-125 U/L | 0.33-2.08 µkat/L |
| Ammonia [$NH_3^+$] | 10-80 µg/dL | 6-47 µmol/L |
| Amylase, serum | 60-180 U/L | 0.8-3.2 µkat/L |
| Antinuclear antibodies (ANA) | Negative at 1:40 dilution | |
| Aspartate aminotransferase (AST) (SGOT) | ≤42 U/L | <0.7 µkat/L |
| Bilirubin | | |
| Total | 0.3-1.0 mg/dL | 5.1-17 µmol/L |
| Direct | 0.1-0.3 mg/dL | 1.7-5.1 µmol/L |
| Indirect | 0.2-0.7 mg/dL | 3.4-12 µmol/L |
| Blood urea nitrogen/creatinine ratio | 10:1-20:1 | Average 15:1 |
| Calcium, plasma | 9-10.5 mg/dL | 2.2-2.6 mmol/L |
| Calcium, ionized | 4.5-5.6 mg/dL | 1.1-1.4 mmol/L |
| Chloride, serum | 95-108 mEq/L | 95-108 mmol/L |
| Cholesterol (total plasma) | | |
| Desirable level | <200 mg/dL | <5.20 mmol/L |
| Moderate risk | 200-240 mg/dL | 5.2-6.3 mmol/L |
| High risk | >240 mg/dL | >6.3 mmol/L |
| Copper | 70-140 µg/dL | 11-22 µmol/L |
| Cortisol, serum | | |
| 0800 hours | 5-25 µg/dL | 140-690 nmol/L |
| 1600 hours | 3-12 µg/dL | 80-330 nmol/L |
| Creatinine kinase (CK) | | |
| Isoenzymes | CK-MM: 97-100% of total<br>CK-MB: <3% of total<br>CK-BB: 0% of total | CK-MM: 0.97-1.00 of total<br>CK-MB: <0.03 of total<br>CK-BB: 0 of total |
| Total | Male: ≤235 U/L<br>Female: ≤190 U/L | Male: ≤3.92 µkat/L<br>Female: ≤3.17 µkat/L |
| Creatinine, serum | <1.5 mg/dL | <133 µmol/L |
| Creatinine clearance | 75-125 mL/min | 1.24-2.08 mL/sec |
| Digoxin | | |
| Therapeutic | 0.8-2.0 ng/mL | 1.0-2.6 nmol/L |
| Toxic | >2.5 ng/mL | >3.2 nmol/L |
| Erythrocyte count (RBC) | 4.15-4.90 × $10^6$/mm$^3$ | 4.15-4.90 × $10^{12}$/L |
| Erythrocyte sedimentation rate (ESR) | | |
| Male | 0-20 mm/hr | 0-20 mm/hr |
| Female | 0-30 mm/hr | 0-30 mm/hr |
| Ferritin | | |
| Male | 15-400 ng/mL | 15-400 µg/L |
| Female | 10-200 ng/mL | 10-200 µg/L |
| Folic acid | 3-16 ng/mL | 7-36 nmol/L |

| TEST | US RANGE | SI RANGE |
|---|---|---|
| Follicle-stimulating hormone (FSH) | | |
| Female | 1.4-9.6 mIU/mL | 1.4-9.6 IU/L |
| Ovulation | 2.3-21 mIU/mL | 2.3-21 IU/L |
| Postmenopausal | 34-96 mIU/mL | 34-96 IU/L |
| Male | 0.9-15 mIU/mL | 0.9-15 IU/L |
| Gamma-glutamyl transferase (GGT) | | |
| Male | ≤65 U/L | ≤1.08 μkat/L |
| Female | ≤45 U/L | ≤0.75 μkat/L |
| Gases, arterial blood | | |
| $pO_2$ | 80-100 mmHg | 11-13 kPa |
| $pCO_2$ | 35-45 mmHg | 4.7-6 kPa |
| Glucose, plasma | | |
| Fasting | 75-115 mg/dL | 4.2-6.4 mmol/L |
| Postprandial (2 h) | <140 mg/dL | <7.8 mmol/L |
| Immunoglobulins (Ig) | | |
| IgG | 800-1500 mg/dL | 8.0-15.0 g/L |
| IgA | 90-325 mg/dL | 0.9-3.2 g/L |
| IgM | 45-150 mg/dL | 0.45-1.5 g/L |
| IgD | 0-8 mg/dL | 0-0.08 g/L |
| IgE | <0.025 mg/dL | <0.00025 g/L |
| Iron, serum | 50-150 μg/dL | 9-27 μmol/L |
| Iron binding capacity | 250-370 μg/dL | 45-66 μmol/L |
| Iron saturation | 20-45% | |
| Lactic acid (plasma, venous) | 9-16 mg/dL | 1.0-1.8 mmol/L |
| Lactic dehydrogenase (LDH) | 100-190 U/L | 1.7-3.2 μkat/L |
| Lead | <20 μg/dL | 1.0 μmol/L |
| Leukocyte count (WBC) | $4.3\text{-}10.8 \times 10^3$ | $4.3\text{-}10.8 \times 10^9$/L |
| Lipase | 0-160 U/L | 0-2.66 μkat/L |
| Lipoproteins (desirable levels) | | |
| Low density (LDL) | <130 mg/dL | <3.36 mmol/L |
| High density (HDL) | >60 mg/dL | >1.55 mmol/L |
| Lithium ion (therapeutic) | 0.6-1.2 mEq/L | 0.6-1.2 mmol/L |
| Luteinizing hormone | | |
| Female | 0.8-26 mIU/mL | 0.8-26 IU/L |
| Ovulation | 25-57 mIU/mL | 25-57 IU/L |
| Postmenopausal | 40-104 mIU/mL | 40-104 IU/L |
| Male | 1.3-13 mIU/mL | 1.3-13 IU/L |
| Osmolality, plasma | 285-295 mOsm/kg | 285-295 mmol/kg |
| Phenytoin | | |
| Therapeutic | 10-20 mg/L | 40-80 μmol/L |
| Toxic | >30 mg/L | >120 μmol/L |
| Phosphorus, serum | 2.5-4.5 mg/dL | 0.8-1.45 mmol/L |
| Potassium, serum | 3.5-5 mEq/L | 3.5-5 mmol/L |
| Prolactin | 2-15 ng/mL | 2-15 μg/L |
| Prostate-specific antigen (PSA) | ≤4 ng/mL | ≤4 μg/L |
| Protein | | |
| Total | 5.5-8.0 g/dL | 55-80 g/L |
| Albumin | 3.5-5.5 g/dL | 35-55 g/L |
| Globulin | 2.0-3.5 g/dL | 20-35 g/L |
| Reticulocyte count | 0.5-2.3% of RBCs | 0.005-0.023 of RBCs |
| Rheumatoid factor | <40 IU/mL | <40 kIU/L |
| Sodium, serum | 136-145 mEq/L | 136-145 mmol/L |
| Theophylline (therapeutic) | 10-20 mg/L | 55-110 μmol/L |
| Thyroxine-binding globulin (TBG) | 16-34 mg/L | 16-34 mg/L |

| TEST | US RANGE | SI RANGE |
|---|---|---|
| Thyroid-stimulating hormone (TSH) | 0.4-5 μU/mL | 0.4-5 mU/L |
| Thyroxine ($T_4$) | | |
| Free | 0.8-1.8 ng/dL | 10-23 pmol/L |
| Total | 4.5-12.5 μg/dL | 58-161 nmol/L |
| Transferrin | 230-390 μg/dL | 2.3-3.9 mg/L |
| Triglycerides | <160 μg/dL | <1.8 mmol/L |
| Triiodothyronine ($T_3$) | 70-190 ng/dL | 1.1-2.9 nmol/L |
| $T_3$ uptake | 25-35% | 0.25-0.35 (proportion of 1.0) |
| Urea nitrogen, blood (BUN) | 7-30 mg/dL | 2.5-10.7 mmol/L |
| Uric acid | | |
| Male | 4.0-8.5 mg/dL | 238-506 μmol/L |
| Female | 2.5-7.5 mg/dL | 149-446 μmol/L |
| Vitamin $B_{12}$ | 200-600 pg/mL | 148-443 pmol/L |

**SOURCES:**

Beers MH, Porter RS, Jones TV, et al. *Merck Manual of Diagnosis and Therapy,* ed 18. Whitehouse Station, NJ: Merck Research Laboratories; 2006.

Cahill M. *Illustrated Guide to Diagnostic Tests,* ed 2. Springhouse, PA: Springhouse Corporation; 1998.

Fauci AS, Braunwald E, Kasper DL, et al. *Harrison's Principles of Internal Medicine,* ed 17. New York, NY: McGraw Hill; 2008.

Goldman L, Ausiello D. *Cecil Medicine,* ed 23. Philadelphia, PA: Saunders Elsevier; 2008.

Sacher RA, McPherson RA, Campos JM. *Wildmann's Clinical Interpretation of Laboratory Tests.* Philadelphia, PA: FA Davis Company; 2000.

# Cytochrome P450 Enzymes: Substrates, Inducers, and Inhibitors

| SUBSTRATES | INDUCERS | INHIBITORS |
|---|---|---|
| **CYP1A2** | | |
| Acetaminophen | Broccoli | Amiodarone HCl |
| Aminophylline | Brussels Sprouts | Anastrozole |
| Amiodarone HCl | Carbamazepine | Cimetidine |
| Amitriptyline HCl | Charbroiled Food | Ciprofloxacin |
| Amoxapine | Citalopram Hydrobromide | Clarithromycin |
| Anagrelide HCl | Diltiazem HCl | Desogestrel |
| Caffeine | Erythromycin | Esomeprazole Sodium |
| Chlordiazepoxide | Escitalopram Oxalate | Ethinyl Estradiol |
| Cimetidine HCl | Esomeprazole Sodium | Fluvoxamine |
| Ciprofloxacin | Fluvoxamine | Gatifloxacin |
| Clomipramine HCl | Hypericum | Gemifloxacin Mesylate |
| Clopidogrel Bisulfate | Insulin | Grapefruit |
| Clozapine | Lansoprazole | Isoniazid |
| Cyclobenzaprine | Nafcillin Sodium | Ketoconazole |
| Desipramine HCl | Nicotine | Levofloxacin |
| Diazepam | Omeprazole | Levonorgestrel |
| Diltiazem HCl | Phenobarbital | Mestranol |
| Doxepin HCl | Phenytoin | Methoxsalen |
| Erythromycin | Primidone | Mexiletine HCl |
| Estradiol | Rifampicin | Moxifloxacin HCl |
| Flutamide | Rifampin | Nalidixic Acid |
| Fluticasone Propionate | Ritonavir | Norethindrone |
| Fluvoxamine Maleate | Tobacco | Norfloxacin |
| Haloperidol | | Norgestrel |
| Imipramine HCl | | Ofloxacin |
| Levobupivacaine HCl | | Omeprazole |
| Maprotiline HCl | | Paroxetine |
| Methadone HCl | | Ranitidine HCl |
| Mexiletine HCl | | Ritonavir |
| Mirtazapine | | Sildenafil Citrate |
| Moxifloxacin HCl | | Tacrine HCl |
| Nafcillin Sodium | | Ticlopidine HCl |
| Naproxen | | Trovafloxacin Mesylate |
| Nicotine | | Vardenafil HCl |
| Norethindrone Acetate | | Zileuton |
| Norfloxacin | | |
| Nortriptyline HCl | | |
| Ofloxacin | | |
| Olanzapine | | |
| Ondansetron | | |
| Phenobarbital | | |
| Phenytoin | | |
| Propafenone HCl | | |
| Propranolol HCl | | |
| Protriptyline HCl | | |
| Riluzole | | |
| Ritonavir | | |
| Ropinirole HCl | | |
| Ropivacaine HCl | | |
| Tacrine HCl | | |

*(Continued)*

| SUBSTRATES | INDUCERS | INHIBITORS |
|---|---|---|
| **CYP1A2** *(Continued)* | | |
| Tamoxifen Citrate | | |
| Theobromine | | |
| Theophylline | | |
| Tizanidine | | |
| Trimethaphan Camsylate | | |
| Trimipramine Maleate | | |
| Trovafloxacin Mesylate | | |
| Verapamil HCl | | |
| Warfarin Sodium | | |
| Zileuton | | |
| Zolmitriptan | | |
| **CYP2C18** | | |
| Naproxen | | Cimetidine |
| Omeprazole | | |
| Piroxicam | | |
| Propranolol HCl | | |
| Tretinoin | | |
| Warfarin Sodium | | |
| **CYP2C19** | | |
| Amitriptyline HCl | Carbamazepine | Cimetidine |
| Amoxapine | Norethindrone | Citalopram Hydrobromide |
| Carisoprodol | Phenobarbital | Delavirdine Mesylate |
| Cilostazol | Phenytoin | Desogestrel |
| Citalopram Hydrobromide | Prednisone | Efavirenz |
| Clomipramine HCl | Rifampin | Ethinyl Estradiol |
| Cyclophosphamide | | Ethynodiol Diacetate |
| Desipramine HCl | | Felbamate |
| Dextromethorphan | | Fluoxetine |
| Diazepam | | Fluvastatin Sodium |
| Divalproex Sodium | | Fluvoxamine |
| Doxepin HCl | | Indomethacin |
| Esomeprazole Magnesium | | Isoniazid |
| Ethosuximide | | Ketoconazole |
| Ethotoin | | Lansoprazole |
| Felbamate | | Letrozole |
| Formoterol Fumarate | | Levonorgestrel |
| Fosphenytoin | | Mestranol |
| Gabapentin | | Modafinil |
| Imipramine HCl | | Norethindrone |
| Indomethacin | | Norethynodrel |
| Lamotrigine | | Norgestimate |
| Lansoprazole | | Norgestrel |
| Levetiracetam | | Omeprazole |
| Maprotiline HCl | | Oxcarbazepine |
| Mephenytoin | | Paroxetine HCl |
| Mephobarbital | | Ritonavir |
| Meprobamate | | Sertraline HCl |
| Methsuximide | | Sildenafil Citrate |
| Midazolam HCl | | Sulfaphenazole |
| Nelfinavir Mesylate | | Telmisartan |
| Nilutamide | | Ticlopidine HCl |

*(Continued)*

| SUBSTRATES | INDUCERS | INHIBITORS |
|---|---|---|
| **CYP2C19** *(Continued)* | | |
| Nortriptyline HCl | | Tolbutamide |
| Omeprazole | | Topiramate |
| Oxcarbazepine | | Vardenafil HCl |
| Pantoprazole Sodium | | Voriconazole |
| Pentamidine Isethionate | | |
| Phenacemide | | |
| Phenobarbital | | |
| Phenytoin | | |
| Primidone | | |
| Progesterone | | |
| Proguanil HCl | | |
| Propranolol HCl | | |
| Protriptyline HCl | | |
| Rabeprazole Sodium | | |
| Sertraline HCl | | |
| Teniposide | | |
| Thioridazine | | |
| Tiagabine HCl | | |
| Tolbutamide | | |
| Topiramate | | |
| Trimethadione | | |
| Trimipramine Maleate | | |
| Valproate Sodium | | |
| Valproic Acid | | |
| Voriconazole | | |
| Warfarin Sodium | | |
| Zonisamide | | |
| **CYP2C8** | | |
| Amiodarone HCl | Carbamazepine | Anastrozole |
| Amitriptyline HCl | Phenobarbital | Cimetidine |
| Amoxapine | Primidone | Gemfibrozil |
| Benzphetamine HCl | Rifabutin | Nicardipine |
| Carbamazepine | Rifampin | Omeprazole |
| Clomipramine HCl | | Sulfaphenazole |
| Desipramine HCl | | Sulfinpyrazone |
| Diazepam | | Trimethoprim |
| Diclofenac Sodium | | |
| Docetaxel | | |
| Doxepin HCl | | |
| Fluvastatin Sodium | | |
| Imipramine HCl | | |
| Isotretinoin | | |
| Maprotiline HCl | | |
| Mephobarbital | | |
| Nortriptyline HCl | | |
| Omeprazole | | |
| Paclitaxel | | |
| Phenytoin | | |
| Pioglitazone HCl | | |
| Protriptyline HCl | | |
| Repaglinide | | |
| Rosiglitazone Maleate | | |

*(Continued)*

| SUBSTRATES | INDUCERS | INHIBITORS |
|---|---|---|
| **CYP2C8** *(Continued)* | | |
| Rosiglitazone/Metformin | | |
| Tolbutamide | | |
| Tretinoin | | |
| Trimipramine Maleate | | |
| Verapamil HCl | | |
| Vitamin A | | |
| Warfarin Sodium | | |
| **CYP2C9** | | |
| Acarbose | Aprepitant | Amiodarone HCl |
| Amitriptyline HCl | Carbamazepine | Anastrozole |
| Candesartan Cilexetil | Dexamethasone | Bendroflumethiazide |
| Carbamazepine | Phenobarbital | Chloramphenicol |
| Carvedilol | Phenytoin | Chlorothiazide |
| Celecoxib | Primidone | Chlorpropamide |
| Chlorpropamide | Rifampin | Cimetidine |
| Clomipramine HCl | Rifapentine | Clopidogrel Bisulfate |
| Desogestrel | Secobarbital Sodium | Clotrimazole |
| Dextromethorphan | | Diclofenac Epolamine |
| Diazepam | | Disulfiram |
| Diclofenac Potassium | | Efavirenz |
| Dronabinol | | Fenofibrate |
| Eprosartan Mesylate | | Fluconazole |
| Etodolac | | Fluorouracil |
| Fenoprofen Calcium | | Fluoxetine HCl |
| Fluoxetine HCl | | Flurbiprofen |
| Flurbiprofen | | Fluvastatin Sodium |
| Fluvastatin Sodium | | Fluvoxamine Maleate |
| Glimepiride | | Gemfibrozil |
| Glipizide | | Glipizide |
| Ibuprofen | | Glyburide |
| Imipramine HCl | | Hydrochlorothiazide |
| Indomethacin | | Hydroflumethiazide |
| Irbesartan | | Imatinib Mesylate |
| Ketoprofen | | Isoniazid |
| Ketorolac Tromethamine | | Itraconazole |
| Lansoprazole | | Ketoconazole |
| Losartan Potassium | | Ketoprofen |
| Meclofenamate Sodium | | Leflunomide |
| Mefenamic Acid | | Lovastatin |
| Meloxicam | | Methyclothiazide |
| Metformin HCl | | Metronidazole |
| Miglitol | | Miconazole |
| Mirtazapine | | Modafinil |
| Montelukast Sodium | | Nifedipine |
| Nabumetone | | Omeprazole |
| Naproxen | | Oxiconazole Nitrate |
| Nateglinide | | Paroxetine HCl |
| Nifedipine | | Phenylbutazone |
| Omeprazole | | Polythiazide |
| Oxaprozin | | Ritonavir |
| Phenylbutazone | | Sertraline HCl |
| Phenytoin | | Sildenafil Citrate |

*(Continued)*

| SUBSTRATES | INDUCERS | INHIBITORS |
|---|---|---|
| **CYP2C9** *(Continued)* | | |
| Pioglitazone HCl | | Sulfacytine |
| Piroxicam | | Sulfamethizole |
| Repaglinide | | Sulfamethoxazole |
| Rofecoxib | | Sulfasalazine |
| Rosiglitazone Maleate | | Sulfinpyrazone |
| Sildenafil Citrate | | Sulfisoxazole Acetyl |
| Sulfamethoxazole | | Terconazole |
| Sulindac | | Ticlopidine HCl |
| Suprofen | | Tolazamide |
| Tamoxifen Citrate | | Tolbutamide |
| Telmisartan | | Vardenafil HCl |
| Tolazamide | | Voriconazole |
| Tolbutamide | | Zafirlukast |
| Tolmetin Sodium | | |
| Torsemide | | |
| Valsartan | | |
| Vardenafil HCl | | |
| Verapamil HCl | | |
| Voriconazole | | |
| Warfarin Sodium | | |
| Zafirlukast | | |
| Zileuton | | |
| **CYP2D6** | | |
| Amitriptyline HCl | Carbamazepine | Amiodarone HCl |
| Amphetamine Aspartate | Ethanol | Amitriptyline HCl |
| Atomoxetine HCl | Hypericum | Amoxapine |
| Bisoprolol Fumarate | Phenobarbital | Bupropion HCl |
| Captopril | Phenytoin | Celecoxib |
| Carvedilol | Primidone | Chloroquine |
| Cevimeline HCl | Rifampin | Chlorpheniramine |
| Chlorpromazine | Ritonavir | Cimetidine |
| Chlorpropamide | | Citalopram Hydrobromide |
| Clomipramine HCl | | Clomipramine HCl |
| Clozapine | | Cocaine HCl |
| Codeine Phosphate | | Desipramine HCl |
| Cyclobenzaprine HCl | | Diphenhydramine |
| Desipramine HCl | | Doxepin HCl |
| Dexfenfluramine HCl | | Escitalopram Oxalate |
| Dextromethorphan Hydrobromide | | Fluoxetine |
| Dolasetron Mesylate | | Fluphenazine Decanoate |
| Donepezil HCl | | Fluvoxamine Maleate |
| Doxepin HCl | | Haloperidol |
| Fentanyl | | Hydroxychloroquine Sulfate |
| Flecainide Acetate | | Imatinib Mesylate |
| Fluoxetine | | Imipramine HCl |
| Fluphenazine Decanoate | | Maprotiline HCl |
| Fluvoxamine Maleate | | Methadone HCl |
| Formoterol Fumarate | | Nortriptyline HCl |
| Galantamine Hydrobromide | | Paroxetine HCl |
| Haloperidol | | Perphenazine |
| Hydrocodone Bitartrate | | Propafenone HCl |
| Imipramine HCl | | Propoxyphene HCl |

*(Continued)*

| SUBSTRATES | INDUCERS | INHIBITORS |
|---|---|---|
| **CYP2D6** *(Continued)* | | |
| Labetalol HCl | | Protriptyline HCl |
| Lidocaine | | Quinacrine HCl |
| Maprotiline HCl | | Quinidine |
| Meperidine HCl | | Ranitidine Bismuth Citrate |
| Methadone HCl | | Ritonavir |
| Methamphetamine HCl | | Sertraline HCl |
| Metoprolol Succinate | | Sildenafil Citrate |
| Mexiletine HCl | | Terbinafine HCl |
| Mirtazapine | | Thioridazine HCl |
| Morphine Sulfate | | Trimipramine Maleate |
| Nelfinavir Mesylate | | Vardenafil HCl |
| Nortriptyline HCl | | |
| Olanzapine | | |
| Omeprazole | | |
| Ondansetron | | |
| Oxycodone HCl | | |
| Paclitaxel | | |
| Paroxetine HCl | | |
| Pindolol | | |
| Propafenone HCl | | |
| Propoxyphene HCl | | |
| Propranolol HCl | | |
| Quetiapine Fumarate | | |
| Quinidine Gluconate | | |
| Risperidone | | |
| Ritonavir | | |
| Tamoxifen Citrate | | |
| Teniposide | | |
| Testosterone | | |
| Thioridazine | | |
| Timolol Maleate | | |
| Tolterodine Tartrate | | |
| Tramadol HCl | | |
| Trazodone HCl | | |
| Triazolam | | |
| Trimipramine Maleate | | |
| Venlafaxine HCl | | |
| Vinblastine Sulfate | | |
| Zonisamide | | |
| **CYP3A4** | | |
| | | **Potent inhibitors** |
| Alfentanil HCl | Allium sativum | Amprenavir |
| Alprazolam | Aminoglutethimide | Atazanavir |
| Amiodarone HCl | Aprepitant | Clarithromycin |
| Amitriptyline HCl | Betamethasone | Delaviridine |
| Amlodipine Besylate | Bosentan | Delavirine |
| Aprepitant | Carbamazepine | Fosamprenavir Calcium |
| Astemizole | Ciprofloxacin | Indinavir Sulfate |
| Atorvastatin Calcium | Cisplatin | Itraconazole |
| Belladonna Ergotamine | Cortisone Acetate | Ketoconazole |
| Buspirone HCl | Dexamethasone | Lopinavir |
| Busulfan | Doxorubicin HCl | Nefazodone HCl |

*(Continued)*

| SUBSTRATES | INDUCERS | INHIBITORS |
|---|---|---|
| **CYP3A4** *(Continued)* | | |
| | | **Potent inhibitors, cont.** |
| Carbamazepine | Efavirenz | Nelfinavir Mesylate |
| Chlorpheniramine | Ethosuximide | Ritonavir |
| Cisapride | Felbamate | Saquinavir |
| Clarithromycin | Fludrocortisone Acetate | Telithromycin |
| Cyclosporine | Fosphenytoin Sodium | Voriconazole |
| Desogestrel | Garlic Extract | |
| Diazepam | Hydrocortisone | **Inhibitors (potency not specified)** |
| Dihydroergotamine Mesylate | Hypericum | Acetazolamide |
| Diltiazem HCl | Mephenytoin | Amiodarone HCl |
| Disopyramide | Methsuximide | Amprenavir |
| Disulfiram | Methylprednisolone | Anastrozole |
| Doxorubicin HCl | Modafinil | Aprepitant |
| Dronabinol | Nafcillin Sodium | Atazanavir |
| Ergotamine Tartrate | Nevirapine | Cimetidine |
| Erythromycin | Oxcarbazepine | Ciprofloxacin |
| Estradiol | Phenobarbital | Clarithromycin |
| Ethinyl Estradiol | Phenytoin | Clotrimazole |
| Ethosuximide | Prednisolone | Conivaptan HCl |
| Ethynodiol Diacetate | Prednisone | Cyclosporine |
| Etoposide | Primidone | Dalfopristin |
| Felodipine | Rifabutin | Danazol |
| Fentanyl | Rifampicin | Darunavir |
| Haloperidol | Rifampin | Dasatinib Monohydrate |
| Indinavir Sulfate | Rifapentine | Delavirdine Mesylate |
| Isradipine | Sulfinpyrazone | Delaviridine |
| Itraconazole | Theophyllinate | Delavirine |
| Ixabepilone | Theophylline | Desloratadine |
| Ketoconazole | Triamcinolone | Diltiazem HCl |
| Levonorgestrel | | Efavirenz |
| Lidocaine | | Erythromycin |
| Lovastatin | | Esomeprazole Magnesium |
| Mestranol | | Fluconazole |
| Methadone HCl | | Fluoxetine |
| Midazolam HCl | | Fluvoxamine Maleate |
| Nefazodone HCl | | Fosamprenavir Calcium |
| Nelfinavir Mesylate | | Grapefruit |
| Nicardipine HCl | | Imatinib Mesylate |
| Nifedipine | | Indinavir Sulfate |
| Nimodipine | | Isoniazid |
| Nisoldipine | | Itraconazole |
| Nitrendipine | | Ketoconazole |
| Norethindrone | | Lapatinib |
| Norgestrel | | Lopinavir |
| Ondansetron | | Loratadine |
| Paclitaxel | | Metronidazole |
| Pimozide | | Miconazole |
| Polyestradiol Phosphate | | Mifepristone |
| Quinidine Gluconate | | Nefazodone HCl |
| Rifabutin | | Nelfinavir Mesylate |
| Ritonavir | | Nevirapine |
| Saquinavir | | Niacin |

*(Continued)*

| SUBSTRATES | INDUCERS | INHIBITORS |
|---|---|---|
| **CYP3A4** *(Continued)* | | |
| Sertraline HCl | | **Inhibitors** |
| Sildenafil Citrate | | **(potency not specified, cont.)** |
| Simvastatin | | Niacinamide |
| Sirolimus | | Nicotinamide |
| Tacrolimus | | Nifedipine |
| Tadalafil | | Norfloxacin |
| Tamoxifen Citrate | | Omeprazole |
| Tiagabine HCl | | Paroxetine HCl |
| Tolterodine Tartrate | | Posaconazole |
| Trazodone HCl | | Propoxyphene HCl |
| Triazolam | | Quinidine |
| Vardenafil HCl | | Quinine |
| Verapamil HCl | | Quinupristin |
| Vinblastine Sulfate | | Ranitidine HCl |
| Vincristine Sulfate | | Ritonavir |
| Warfarin Sodium | | Saquinavir |
| | | Sertraline HCl |
| | | Sildenafil Citrate |
| | | Telithromycin |
| | | Troglitazone |
| | | Valproate Sodium |
| | | Vardenafil HCl |
| | | Verapamil HCl |
| | | Voriconazole |
| | | Zafirlukast |
| | | Zileuton |
| **CYP3A** | | |
| Alfentanil HCl | Allium sativum | Amiodarone HCl |
| Alprazolam | Aprepitant | Amprenavir |
| Aminophylline | Carbamazepine | Aprepitant |
| Amitriptyline HCl | Dexamethasone | Cimetidine |
| Amlodipine Besylate | Efavirenz | Ciprofloxacin |
| Aprepitant | Ethosuximide | Clarithromycin |
| Astemizole | Modafinil | Cyclosporine |
| Atorvastatin Calcium | Nevirapine | Delavirdine Mesylate |
| Buspirone HCl | Phenobarbital | Diltiazem HCl |
| Busulfan | Phenytoin | Efavirenz |
| Carbamazepine | Rifabutin | Erythromycin |
| Chlorpheniramine | Rifampicin | Fluconazole |
| Cisapride | Rifampin | Fluoxetine |
| Clarithromycin | Rifapentine | Fluvoxamine Maleate |
| Cyclosporine | | Grapefruit |
| Desogestrel | | Indinavir Sulfate |
| Dexamethasone | | Isoniazid |
| Diazepam | | Itraconazole |
| Dihydroergotamine Mesylate | | Ketoconazole |
| Diltiazem HCl | | Lopinavir |
| Disopyramide Phosphate | | Metronidazole |
| Doxorubicin HCl | | Miconazole |
| Dronabinol | | Nefazodone HCl |
| Dyphylline | | Nelfinavir Mesylate |
| Ergotamine Tartrate | | Nifedipine |

*(Continued)*

| SUBSTRATES | INDUCERS | INHIBITORS |
|---|---|---|
| **CYP3A** *(Continued)* | | |
| Erythromycin | | Norfloxacin |
| Estrogen | | Paroxetine HCl |
| Ethinyl Estradiol | | Quinine |
| Ethosuximide | | Ritonavir |
| Ethynodiol Diacetate | | Saquinavir |
| Etoposide | | Sertraline HCl |
| Felodipine | | Venlafaxine HCl |
| Fentanyl | | Verapamil HCl |
| Glyburide | | Voriconazole |
| Haloperidol | | Zafirlukast |
| Imipramine HCl | | Zileuton |
| Indinavir Sulfate | | |
| Isradipine | | |
| Itraconazole | | |
| Ketoconazole | | |
| Levonorgestrel | | |
| Lidocaine | | |
| Lovastatin | | |
| Mestranol | | |
| Methadone HCl | | |
| Midazolam HCl | | |
| Nefazodone HCl | | |
| Nelfinavir Mesylate | | |
| Nicardipine | | |
| Nifedipine | | |
| Nimodipine | | |
| Nisoldipine | | |
| Norethindrone | | |
| Norgestrel | | |
| Ondansetron HCl | | |
| Paclitaxel | | |
| Pimozide | | |
| Quinidine Gluconate | | |
| Quinine | | |
| Rifabutin | | |
| Ritonavir | | |
| Saquinavir | | |
| Sertraline HCl | | |
| Sildenafil Citrate | | |
| Simvastatin | | |
| Sirolimus | | |
| Tacrolimus | | |
| Tamoxifen Citrate | | |
| Testosterone | | |
| Theophylline | | |
| Tiagabine HCl | | |
| Tolterodine Tartrate | | |
| Trazodone HCl | | |
| Triazolam | | |
| Venlafaxine HCl | | |
| Verapamil HCl | | |
| Vinblastine Sulfate | | |
| Vincristine Sulfate | | |
| Warfarin Sodium | | |

Note: This list is not comprehensive. For more information, refer to the specific product's full Prescribing Information.

# DRUGS EXCRETED IN BREAST MILK

The following list is not comprehensive; generic forms and alternate brands of some products may be available. When recommending drugs to pregnant or nursing patients, always check product labeling for specific precautions.

Accolate
Accuretic
Aciphex
Actiq
Activella
Actonel
Actonel with Calcium
ActoPlus Met
Adalat
Adderall
Advicor
Aggrenox
Aldactazide
Aldactone
Alesse
Alfenta
Allegra-D
Aloprim
Altace
Ambien
Amerge
Anafranil
Anaprox
Androderm
Aplenzin
Apresoline
Aralen
Arthrotec
Asacol
Ativan
Augmentin
Avalide
Avandamet
Axid
Azactam
Azasan
Azathioprine
Azulfidine
Bactrim
Baraclude
Benadryl
Bentyl
Betapace
Bexxar
Bicillin
Boniva
Brethine
Brevicon
Brontex
Byetta
Caduet
Cafergot
Calan
Campral
Capoten
Capozide
Captopril
Carbatrol
Cardizem
Cataflam
Catapres
Ceclor
Cefotan
Ceftin
Celebrex
Celexa
Cerebyx
Ceredase
Cipro
Ciprodex
Claforan
Clarinex
Claritin
Claritin-D
Cleocin
Climara
Clozaril
Codeine
Combigan
CombiPatch
Combivir
Combunox
Compazine
Cordarone
Corgard
Cortisporin
Corzide
Cosopt
Coumadin
Covera-HS
Cozaar
Crestor
Crinone
Cyclessa
Cymbalta
Cytomel
Cytotec
Dapsone
Daraprim
Darvon
Darvon-N
Deconsal II
Demerol
Demulen
Depacon
Depakene
Depakote
DepoDur
Depo-Provera
Desogen
Desoxyn
Desyrel
Dexedrine
DextroStat
D.H.E. 45
Diabinese
Diastat
Diflucan
Digitek
Dilacor
Dilantin
Dilaudid
Diovan
Diprivan
Diuril
Dolobid
Dolophine
Doral
Doryx
Droxia
Duraclon
Duragesic
Duramorph
Duratuss
Duricef
Dyazide
Dyrenium
E.E.S.
EC-Naprosyn
Ecotrin
Effexor
Elavil
EMLA
Enduron
Epzicom
Equetro
ERYC
EryPed
Ery-Tab
Erythrocin
Erythromycin
Esgic-plus
Eskalith
Estrogel
Estrostep
Evista
Factive
FazaClo
Felbatol
Feldene
femhrt
Fiorinal
Flagyl
Floxin
Foradil
Fortamet
Fortaz
Fosamax
Furosemide
Gabitril
Galzin
Garamycin
Glucophage
Glucovance
Glumetza
Glyset
Halcion
Haldol
Helidac
Hycamtin
Hydrocortone
Ifex
Imitrex
Imuran
Inderal
Indocin
INFeD
Inspra
Invanz
Invega
Isoptin
Janumet
Kadian
Kaletra
Keflex
Keppra
Kerlone
Ketek
Klonopin
Kronofed-A
Lamictal
Lamisil
Lamprene
Lanoxicaps
Lanoxin
Lariam
Lescol
Letairis
Levbid
Levitra
Levlen
Levlite
Levora
Levothroid
Levoxyl
Levsin
Levsinex
Lexapro
Lexiva
Lialda
Lindane
Lioresal
Lithium
Lithobid
Lo/Ovral
Loestrin
Lomotil
Lopressor
Lortab
Lotensin
Lotrel
Luminal
Luvox
Lyrica
Macrobid
Macrodantin
Marinol
Maxipime
Maxzide
Menostar
Metaglip
Methergine
Methotrexate
MetroCream/Gel/Lotion

*(Continued)*

Micronor
Microzide
Migranal
Minocin
Mirapex
Mircette
M-M-R II
Mobic
Modicon
Monodox
Monopril
Morphine
MS Contin
Myambutol
Mycamine
Mysoline
Namenda
Naprelan
Naprosyn
Nascobal
Necon
Nembutal
Neoral
Neurontin
Niaspan
Nicotrol
Niravam
Nizoral
Norco
Nor-QD
Nordette
Norinyl
Noritate
Normodyne
Norpace
Norpramin
Novantrone
Nubain
Nucofed
Nydrazid
Oramorph
Ortho-Cept
Ortho-Cyclen
Ortho-Novum
Ortho Tri-Cyclen
Orudis
Ovcon
Oxistat
OxyContin
OxyIR
Pacerone
Pamelor
Pancrease
Paxil
PCE
Pediapred
Pediazole
Pediotic
Pentasa
Pepcid
Periostat
Persantine
Pfizerpen
Phenergan
Phenobarbital
Phenytek
Phrenilin
Plan B
Ponstel
Prandimet
Pravachol
Premphase
Prempro
Prevacid
Prevacid NapraPAC
PREVPAC
Prinzide
Pristiq
Prograf
Prometrium
Pronestyl
Propofol
Prosed/DS
Protonix
Provera
Prozac
Pseudoephedrine
Pulmicort
Pyrazinamide
Quinidex
Quinine
Reglan
Relpax
Renese
Requip
Reserpine
Restoril
Retrovir
Rifadin
Rifamate
Rifater
Risperdal
Rocaltrol
Rocephin
Roxanol
Rozerem
Sanctura
Sanctura XR
Sandimmune
Sarafem
Seconal
Sectral
Semprex-D
Septra
Seroquel
Seroquel XR
Soma
Sonata
Soriatane
Spiriva
Sprycel
Stadol
Stavzor
Streptomycin
Stromectol
Symbyax
Synthroid
Tagamet
Tambocor
Tapazole
Tarka
Tasigna
Tavist
Tazicef
Tegretol
Tenoretic
Tenormin
Thalitone
Theo-24
Theo-Dur
Thorazine
Tiazac
Timoptic
Tindamax
Tobi
Tofranil
Toprol-XL
Toradol
Trandate
Tranxene
Trental
Tricor
Triglide
Trileptal
Tri-Levlen
Tri-Norinyl
Triostat
Triphasil
Trisenox
Trivora
Trizivir
Truvada
Tygacil
Tylenol
Tylenol with Codeine
Ultane
Ultram
Unasyn
Uniphyl
Uniretic
Unithroid
Valium
Valtrex
Vancocin
Vantin
Vaseretic
Vasotec
Ventavis
Verelan
Vermox
Vibramycin
Vibra-Tabs
Vicodin
Vigamox
Viramune
Voltaren
Vytorin
Vyvanse
Wellbutrin
Xanax
Xolair
Zantac
Zarontin
Zaroxolyn
Zegerid
Zemplar
Zestoretic
Zetia
Ziac
Zinacef
Zithromax
Zoloft
Zomig
Zonalon
Zonegran
Zosyn
Zovia
Zovirax
Zyban
Zydone
Zyloprim
Zyprexa
Zyrtec

# Drugs That May Cause Photosensitivity

The drugs in this table are known to cause photosensitivity in some individuals. Effects can range from itching, scaling, rash, and swelling to skin cancer, premature skin aging, skin and eye burns, cataracts, reduced immunity, blood vessel damage, and allergic reactions. The list is not all-inclusive, and shows only representative brands of each generic. When in doubt, always check specific product labeling. Individuals should be advised to wear protective clothing and to apply sunscreens while taking the medications listed below.

| GENERIC | BRAND |
|---|---|
| Acamprosate calcium | Campral |
| Acetazolamide | Diamox |
| Acitretin | Soriatane |
| Acyclovir | Zovirax |
| Alendronate | Fosamax |
| Alendronate/cholecalciferol | Fosamax Plus D |
| Almotriptan malate | Axert |
| Amiloride HCl/HCTZ | |
| Aminolevulinic acid HCl | Levulan Kerastick |
| Amiodarone HCl | Cordarone, Pacerone |
| Amitriptyline HCl | |
| Amitryptyline HCl/ chlordiazepoxide | Limbitrol, Limbitrol DS |
| Amitryptyline HCl/ perphenazine | |
| Amlodipine/HCTZ/ valsartan | Exforge HCT |
| Amphetamine aspartate/ amphetamine sulfate/ dextroamphetamine saccharate/ dextroamphetamine sulfate | Adderall XR |
| Anagrelide HCl | Agrylin |
| Atenolol/chlorthalidone | Tenoretic |
| Atorvastatin | Lipitor |
| Atorvastatin/Amlodipine | Caduet |
| Atovaquone/proguanil HCl | Malarone |
| Azithromycin | Zithromax, Zmax |
| Benazepril HCl | Lotensin |
| Benazepril HCl/HCTZ | Lotensin HCT |
| Bendoflumethizaide/nadolol | Corzide |
| Benzoyl proxide/erythromycin | Benzamycin Pak |
| Bexarotene | Targretin |
| Bismuth subcitrate potassium/metronidazole/ tetracycline HCl | Pylera |
| Bismuth subsalicylate/ metronidazole/ tetracycline HCl | Helidac Therapy |
| Brompheniramine maleate/ carbetapentane citrate/ phenylephrine HCl | Vazotan Tannate |
| Brompheniramine maleate/ dextromethorphan HBr/ phenylephrine HCl | Alacol DM |
| Brompheniramine maleate/ phenylephrine HCl | Vazobid Tannate |
| Bupropion HBr | Aplenzin |
| Bupropion HCl | Budeprion SR, Budeprion XL, Buproban, Wellbutrin SR, Zyban |
| Candesartan Cilexetil/HCTZ | Atacand HCT |
| Capecitabine | Xeloda |
| Captopril | Capoten |
| Captopril/HCTZ | Capozide |
| Carbamazepine | Carbatrol, Epitol, Equetro, Tegretol, Tegretol-XR |
| Carbinoxamine maleate | Palgic |
| Carvedilol | Coreg |
| Carvedilol phosphate | Coreg CR |
| Celecoxib | Celebrex |
| Cetirizine HCl/ pseudoephedrine HCl | Zyrtec-D 12 Hour |
| Cevimeline HCl | Evoxac |
| Chloroquine Phosphate | Aralen |
| Chlorothiazide | Diuril |
| Chlorpheniramine maleate/ dextromethorphan HBr/ pseudoephedrine HCl | Atuss DS |
| Chlorpheniramine maleate/ pseudoephedrine HCl | Sudal-12 |
| Chlorpheniramine tannate/ dextromethorphan tannate/ pseudoephedrine tannate | Dicel DM |
| Chlorpromazine HCl | |
| Chlorpropamide | Diabinese |
| Chlorthalidone | Thalitone |
| Chlorthalidone/clonidine HCl | Clorpres |
| Cidofovir | Vistide |
| Ciprofloxacin HCl | Cipro, Cipro XR, Proquin XR |
| Citalopram HBr | Celexa |
| Clemastine Fumarate | |
| Clindamycin phosphate | Clindagel |
| Clomipramine HCl | Anafranil |
| Clozapine | Clozaril, FazaClo |
| Codeine phosphate/ phenylephrine HCl/ promethazine HCl | Promethazine VC with Codeine |
| Codeine phosphate/ promethazine HCl | Promethazine with Codeine |
| Cyclobenzaprine HCl | Flexeril |
| Cyproheptadine HCl | |
| Dacarbazine | DTIC-Dome |
| Demeclocycline HCl | Declomycin |
| Desipramine HCl | Norpramin |
| Dextromethorphan HBR/ Promethazine HCl | Dextromethorphan HBR/ Promethazine HCl |
| Diclofenac potassium | Cataflam, Zipsor |
| Diclofenac sodium | |
| Diclofenac sodium/ misoprostol | Arthrotec |
| Diflunisal | |
| Diltiazem HCl | Cardizem LA, Tiazac |
| Diphenhydramine HCl | Benadryl |
| Divalproex sodium | Depakote, Depakote ER |
| Doxepin HCl | Sinequan |
| Doxorubicin HCl | |
| Doxycycline | Oracea |
| Doxycycline hyclate | Doryx, Periostat |
| Duloxetine HCl | Cymbalta Delayed-Release |
| Enalapril maleate | |
| Enalapril maleate/felodipine | |
| Enalapril maleate/HCTZ | |
| Enalaprilat | Enalaprilat |
| Epirubicin HCl | Ellence |

*(Continued)*

| GENERIC | BRAND |
|---|---|
| Eprosartan mesylate/HCTZ | Teveten HCT |
| Erythromycin ethylsuccinate/ sulfisoxazole acetyl | |
| Escitalopram oxalate | Lexapro |
| Esomeprazole magnesium | Nexium |
| Esomeprazole sodium | Nexium I.V. |
| Estazolam | |
| Estradiol | Elestrin |
| Estradiol cypionate | Depo- Estradiol |
| Ethinyl Estradiol/ Norelgestromin | Ortho Evra |
| Ethionamide | Trecator |
| Etodolac, Etodolac ER | |
| Ezetimibe/simvastatin | Vytorin |
| Feboxostat | Uloric |
| Felbamate | Felbatol |
| Fenofibrate | Antara, Lipofen, Lofibra, Tricor, Triglide |
| Floxuridine | Sterile FUDR for Intra-Arterial Infusion |
| Flucytosine | Ancobon |
| Fluorouracil | Efudex |
| Fluoxetine HCl | Prozac, Sarafem |
| Fluoxetine/Olanzapine | Symbyax |
| Fluphenazine HCl | |
| Flurbiprofen | Ansaid |
| Flutamide | Eulexin |
| Fluvoxamine maleate | |
| Fosinopril sodium | Monopril |
| Fosinopril sodium/HCTZ | |
| Fosphenytoin | Cerebyx |
| Furosemide | Lasix |
| Gabapentin | Neurontin |
| Gemfibrozil | Lopid |
| Gemifloxacin mesylate | Factive |
| Gentamicin sulfate | |
| Glatiramer acetate | Copaxone |
| Glimepiride/pioglitazone HCl | Duetact |
| Glimeperide | Amaryl |
| Glimeperide/ rosiglitazone maleate | Avandaryl |
| Glipizide | Glucotrol |
| Glyburide | DiaBeta, Glynase PresTab, Micronase |
| Griseofulvin | Grifulvin V |
| Haloperidol decanoate | Haldol Decanoate |
| Haloperidol lactate | Haldol |
| Hexachlorophene | pHisoHex Detergent Cleanser |
| HCTZ | |
| HCTZ/aliskiren hemifumarate | Tekturna HCT |
| HCTZ/bisoprolol fumarate | Ziac |
| HCTZ/irbesartan | Avalide |
| HCTZ/lisinopril | Prinzide, Zestoretic |
| HCTZ/losartan potassium | Hyzaar |
| HCTZ/methyldopa | |
| HCTZ/metoprolol tartrate | Lopressor HCT |
| HCTZ/moexipril HCl | Uniretic |
| HCTZ/propranolol HCl | Inderide |
| HCTZ/quinapril HCl | Accuretic |
| HCTZ/spironolactone | Aldactazide |
| HCTZ/telmisartan | Micardis HCT |
| HCTZ/triamterene | Dyazide, Maxzide |
| HCTZ/valsartan | Diovan HCT |
| Hydroxychloroquine sulfate | Plaquenil |
| Ibuprofen | Motrin |
| Imatinib mesylate | Gleevec |
| Imipramine HCl | Tofranil |
| Imipramine pamoate | Tofranil-PM |
| Indapamide | Indapamide |
| Interferon alfa-2b | Intron A |
| Interferon alfa-n3 | Alferon-N |
| Interferon beta-1a | Avonex |
| Inferferon beta-1b | Betaseron |
| Isocarboxazid | Marplan |
| Isoniazid/ pyrazinamide/rifampin | Rifater |
| Isotretinoin | Accutane, Amnesteem, Claravis, Sotret |
| Itraconazole | Sporanox |
| Ketoprofen | Ketoprofen |
| Ketorolac tromethamine | Toradol |
| Lamotrigine | Lamictal, Lamictal XR |
| Lansoprazole/naproxen | Prevacid NapraPAC 500 |
| Leuprolide acetate | Lupron, Lupron Depot |
| Levofloxacin | Levaquin |
| Lisinopril | Prinivil, Zestril |
| Losartan potassium | Cozaar |
| Lovastatin | Altoprev, Mevacor |
| Maprotiline HCl, USP | |
| Mefenamic acid | Ponstel |
| Mesalamine | Pentasa |
| Methotrexate | |
| Methyclothiazide | |
| Methyl aminolevulinate HCl | Metvixia |
| Metolazone | Zaroxolyn |
| Metoprolol succinate | Toprol-XL |
| Metoprolol tartrate | Lopressor |
| Minocycline HCl | Dynacin, Minocin, Solodyn |
| Mirtazapine | Remeron, RemeronSolTab |
| Moexipril HCl | Univasc |
| Moxifloxacin HCl | Avelox |
| Nabilone | Cesamet |
| Nabumetone | |
| Naproxen | EC-Naprosyn, Naprosyn |
| Naproxen sodium | Anaprox, Anaprox DS, Naprelan |
| Naratriptan HCl | Amerge |
| Nefazodone HCl | Nefazodone HCl |
| Nifedipine | Adalat CC, Nifediac CC, Nifedical XL, Procardia, Procardia XL |
| Nilotinib HCl monohydrate | Tasigna |
| Nisoldipine | Sular |
| Norfloxacin | Noroxin |
| Nortriptyline HCl | Pamelor |
| Ofloxacin | Floxin |
| Olanzapine | Zyprexa, Zyprexa ZYDIS |
| Olsalazine sodium | Dipentum |
| Omeprazole magnesium | Prilosec |
| Omeprazole/ sodium bicarbonate | Zegerid |
| Oxaprozin | Daypro, Daypro Alta |

| GENERIC | BRAND |
|---|---|
| Oxcarbazepine | Trileptal |
| Paclitaxel | Abraxane |
| Panitumumab | Vectibix |
| Pantoprazole sodium | Protonix |
| Paroxetine HCl | Paxil, Paxil CR |
| Paroxetine mesylate | Pexeva |
| Pentosan polysulfate sodium | Elmiron |
| Perphenazine | Perphenazine |
| Phenylephrine HCl/ promethazine HCl | Promethazine VC |
| Pilocarpine HCl | Salagen |
| Pimozide | Orap |
| Poly-L-lactic acid | Sculptra |
| Porfimer sodium | Photofrin |
| Pramipexole DiHCl | Mirapex |
| Pravastatin sodium | Pravachol |
| Pregabalin | Lyrica |
| Prochlorperazine | Compro Suppositories |
| Promethazine HCl | Phenadoz, Phenergan, Promethegan |
| Protriptyline HCl | Vivactil |
| Pyrazinamide | |
| Quetiapine fumarate | Seroquel |
| Quinapril HCl | Accupril |
| Quinidine gluconate | |
| Quinidine sulfate | |
| Quinine sulfate | Qualaquin |
| Ramipril | Altace |
| Rasagiline mesylate | Azilect |
| Riluzole | Rilutek |
| Ritonavir | Norvir |
| Rizatriptan benzoate | Maxalt, Maxalt-MLT |
| Ropinirole HCl | Requip |
| Saquinavir mesylate | Invirase |
| Selegiline | Emsam Transdermal System |
| Selegiline HCl | Eldepryl |
| Sertraline HCl | Zoloft |
| Sibutramine HCl | Meridia |
| Sildenafil citrate | Viagra |
| Simvastatin | Zocor |
| Sotalol HCl | Betapace, Betapace AF, Sorine |
| Sulfamethoxazole/ trimethoprim | Bactrim, Bactrim DS, Septra, Septra DS, Sulfatrim |
| Sulfasalazine | Azulfidine, Azulfidine EN-tabs |
| Sulindac | Clinoril |
| Sumatriptan | Imitrex Nasal Spray |
| Sumatriptan succinate | Imitrex |
| Tacrolimus | Prograf, Protopic |
| Tetracycline HCl | Sumycin |
| Thalidomide | Thalomid |
| Thioridazine HCl | Thioridazine HCl |
| Thiothixene | Navane |
| Tiagabine HCl | Gabitril |
| Tigecycline | Tygacil |
| Tipranavir | Aptivus Oral Solution |
| Tolazamide | |
| Tolbutamide | |
| Topiramate | Topamax |
| Tretinoin | Avita, Retin-A |
| Triamcinolone acetonide | Azmacort Inhalation Aerosol |
| Triamterene | Dyrenium |
| Trifluoperazine HCl | Trifluoperazine HCl |
| Trimipramine maleate | Surmontil |
| Valacyclovir HCl | Valtrex Caplets |
| Valproate sodium | Depacon |
| Valproic acid | Depakene, Stavzor |
| Vardenafil HCl | Levitra |
| Varenicline | Chantix |
| Venlafaxine HCl | Effexor, Effexor XR |
| Verteporfin | Visudyne |
| Vibramycin calcium | Vibramycin Calcium |
| Vibramycin hyclate | Vibra-Tabs |
| Vibramycin monohydrate | Vibramycin Monohydrate |
| Voriconazole | VFEND |
| Zaleplon | Sonata |
| Ziprasidone HCl | Geodon |
| Zolmitriptan | Zomig, Zomig-ZMT |
| Zolpidem tartrate | Ambien, Ambien CR, Edluar, Zolpimist |

# DRUGS THAT MAY CAUSE QT PROLONGATION

| BRAND NAME | GENERIC NAME |
|---|---|
| Abilify | Aripiprazole |
| AcipHex | Rabeprazole sodium |
| Advair | Fluticasone propionate/ salmeterol xinafoate |
| Advair HFA | Fluticasone propionate/ salmeterol xinafoate |
| Aloxi Injection | Palonosetron HCl |
| Amerge | Naratriptan HCl |
| Amitriptyline | Amitriptyline |
| Anzemet | Dolasetron mesylate |
| Apokyn | Apomorphine HCl |
| Avelox | Moxifloxacin HCl |
| Betapace | Sotalol HCl |
| Betapace AF | Sotalol HCl |
| Biaxin | Clarithromycin |
| Brovana | Arformoterol tartrate |
| Celexa | Citalopram HBr |
| Cipro | Ciprofloxacin |
| Cipro XR | Ciprofloxacin |
| Cordarone | Amiodarone HCl |
| Corvert | Ibutilide fumarate |
| Detrol LA | Tolterodine tartrate |
| Dolophine | Methadone HCl |
| Doxepin | Doxepin |
| E.E.S. | Erythromycin ethylsuccinate |
| Effexor XR | Venlafaxine HCl |
| Eraxis | Anidulafungin |
| ERYC | Erythromycin |
| EryPed | Erythromycin ethylsuccinate |
| Erythrocin stearate | Erythromycin stearate |
| Erythromycin Base Filmtab | Erythromycin |
| Erythromycin Delayed-Release | Erythromycin |
| Exelon Patch | Rivastigmine |
| Factive | Gemifloxacin mesylate |
| Fleet Enema/Enema Extra/ Enema for Children | Monobasic sodium phosphate/dibasic sodium phosphate |
| Foradil | Formoterol |
| Geodon | Ziprasidone HCl |
| Haldol | Haloperidol |
| Halfan* | Halofantrine HCl |
| Imitrex Injection | Sumatriptan succinate |
| Inapsine | Droperidol |
| Invega | Paliperidone |
| Ketek | Telithromycin |
| Levaquin | Levofloxacin |
| Levitra | Vardenafil HCl |
| Lexapro | Escitalopram oxalate |
| Maxaquin | Lomefloxacin HCl |
| Methadose | Methadone HCl |
| Namenda | Memantine HCl |
| Nizoral | Ketoconazole |
| Noroxin | Norfloxacin |
| Norpace | Disopyramide phosphate |
| Norpramin | Desipramine |
| Noxafil | Posaconazole |
| Orap | Pimozide |
| OsmoPrep | Sodium phosphate monobasic monohydrate/ sodium phosphate dibasic anhydrous |
| Pacerone | Amiodarone HCl |
| PCE | Erythromycin particles |
| Perforomist | Formoterol fumarate |
| Plenaxis* | Abarelix |
| Pletal | Cilostazol |
| PREVPAC | Lansoprazole/amoxicillin/ clarithromycin |
| Procainamide | Procainamide |
| Prograf | Tacrolimus |
| Prozac | Fluoxetine |
| Quinidine gluconate | Quinidine gluconate |
| Quinidine sulfate | Quinidine sulfate |
| Ranexa | Ranolazine |
| Raxar* | Grepafloxacin |
| Razadyne | Galantamine HBr |
| Risperdal Consta | Risperidone |
| Rythmol SR | Propafenone HCl |
| Serentil* | Mesoridazine besylate |
| Serevent | Salmeterol |
| Seroquel | Quetiapine fumarate |
| Sporanox | Itraconazole |
| Sprycel | Dasatinib |
| Strattera | Atomoxetine HCl |
| Sutent | Sunitinib malate |
| Symbicort | Budesonide/formoterol fumarate dihydrate |
| Symbyax | Olanzapine/fluoxetine HCl |
| Tambocor | Flecainide acetate |
| Tasigna | Nilotinib |
| Tequin* | Gatifloxacin |
| Thioridazine HCl | Thioridazine HCl |
| Tikosyn | Dofetilide |
| Tofranil, Tofranil-PM | Imipramine |
| Trisenox Injection | Arsenic trioxide |
| Tykerb | Lapatinib |
| Uroxatral | Alfuzosin HCl |
| Vascor* | Bepridil HCl |
| VFEND | Voriconazole |
| Viracept | Nelfinavir mesylate |
| Visicol | Sodium phosphate |
| Zagam* | Sparfloxacin |
| Zanaflex | Tizanidine |
| Zmax | Azithromycin |
| Zofran | Ondansetron HCl |
| Zolinza | Vorinostat |
| Zoloft | Sertraline HCl |
| Zomig | Zolmitriptan |
| Zomig-ZMT | Zolmitriptan |

* Drug no longer available in the U.S.

NOTE: This list does not include all of the drugs that may cause QT disturbance. For more information, please refer to the specific product's full Prescribing Information.

# DRUGS THAT MAY CAUSE STEVENS-JOHNSON SYNDROME AND TOXIC EPIDERMAL NECROLYSIS (TEN)

| BRAND NAME | GENERIC NAME |
|---|---|
| ACAM2000 | Smallpox vaccine, live |
| AcipHex | Rabeprazole sodium |
| Adderall XR | Dextroamphetamine sulfate/dextroamphetamine saccharate/amphetamine sulfate/amphetamine aspartate |
| Advicor | Niacin/lovastatin |
| Agenerase | Amprenavir |
| Aggrenox | Aspirin/dipyridamole |
| Albenza | Albendazole |
| Aldoril | Methyldopa/ hydrochlorothiazide |
| Aloprim | Allopurinol sodium |
| Altace | Ramipril |
| Amoxil | Amoxicillin |
| Anaprox | Naproxen |
| Ancobon | Flucytosine |
| Ansaid | Flurbiprofen |
| Arava | Leflunomide |
| Arimidex | Anastrozole |
| Arthrotec | Diclofenac sodium/ misoprostol |
| Atacand HCT | Candesartan cilexetil/ hydrochlorothiazide |
| Atripla | Efavirenz/emtricitabine/ tenofovir disoproxil fumarate |
| Attenuvax | Measles virus vaccine, live |
| Augmentin | Amoxicillin/clavulanate potassium |
| Avalide | Irbesartan/ hydrochlorothiazide |
| Avandamet | Rosiglitazone maleate/ metformin HCl |
| Avandia | Rosiglitazone maleate |
| Avelox | Moxifloxacin HCl |
| Azulfidine | Sulfasalazine |
| Bactrim | Sulfamethoxazole/ trimethoprim |
| Betagan | Levobunolol HCl |
| Betoptic S | Betaxolol HCl |
| Biaxin | Clarithromycin |
| Bleph-10 | Sulfacetamide sodium |
| Blephamide | Sulfacetamide sodium/ prednisolone acetate |
| Caduet | Amlodipine besylate/ atorvastatin calcium |
| Capoten | Captopril |
| Carbatrol | Carbamazepine |
| Cataflam | Diclofenac potassium |
| Ceftin | Cefuroxime axetil |
| Celebrex | Celecoxib |
| Cialis | Tadalafil |
| Cimzia | Certolizumab pegol |
| Cipro | Ciprofloxacin |
| Cleocin vaginal ovules | Clindamycin phosphate vaginal suppositories |
| Clinoril | Sulindac |
| Clorpres | Clonidine HCl/chlorthalidone |
| Clozaril | Clozapine |
| Combivir | Lamivudine/zidovudine |
| Combunox | Oxycodone HCl/ibuprofen |
| Comvax | *Haemophilus* b conjugate (meningococcal protein conjugate)/ hepatitis B (recombinant) vaccine |

| BRAND NAME | GENERIC NAME |
|---|---|
| Covera-HS | Verapamil HCl |
| Crixivan | Indinavir sulfate |
| Cymbalta | Duloxetine HCl |
| Daraprim | Pyrimethamine |
| Daypro | Oxaprozin |
| Depakote ER | Divalproex sodium |
| Diamox | Acetazolamide |
| Didronel | Etidronate disodium |
| Dilantin | Phenytoin sodium |
| Diovan HCT | Valsartan/ hydrochlorothiazide |
| Diuril | Chlorothiazide |
| Dolobid | Diflunisal |
| Donnatal Extentabs | Phenobarbital |
| Duac Topical Gel | Clindamycin, 1%/benzoyl peroxide, 5% |
| Dynacin | Minocycline HCl |
| EC-Naprosyn | Naproxen |
| E.E.S. | Erythromycin ethylsuccinate |
| Effexor XR | Venlafaxine HCl |
| Emend | Aprepitant |
| Engerix-B Vaccine | Hepatitis B vaccine (recombinant) |
| Epzicom | Abacavir sulfate/lamivudine |
| Equetro | Carbamazepine |
| EryPed | Erythromycin ethylsuccinate |
| Ethyol | Amifostine |
| Etodolac | Etodolac |
| Exelon | Rivastigmine tartrate |
| Fansidar | Sulfadoxine/pyrimethamine |
| Feldene | Piroxicam |
| Flebogamma 5% | Immune globulin intravenous (human) |
| Flector | Diclofenac epolamine topical patch |
| Fluarix | Influenza virus vaccine |
| Fortaz | Ceftazidime for injection |
| Fosamax | Alendronate sodium |
| Fosamax Plus D | Alendronate sodium/ cholecalciferol |
| Furadantin | Nitrofurantoin |
| Gammagard | Immune globulin intravenous (human) |
| Gamunex | Immune globulin intravenous (human), 10% caprylate/ chromatography purified |
| Gantrisin | Acetyl sulfisoxazole |
| Gleevec | Imatinib mesylate |
| Hyzaar | Losartan potassium/ hydrochlorothiazide |
| Inderal LA | Propranolol HCl |
| Intelence | Etravirine |
| Intron A | Interferon alfa-2b |
| Lozol | Indapamide |
| Indocin | Indomethacin |
| Lamictal | Lamotrigine |
| Lamisil | Terbinafine HCl |
| Lariam | Mefloquine HCl |
| Lescol | Fluvastatin sodium |
| Leukeran | Chlorambucil |
| Leustatin | Cladribine |
| Levaquin | Levofloxacin |
| Lexapro | Escitalopram oxalate |
| Lexiva | Fosamprenavir calcium |
| Lipitor | Atorvastatin calcium |
| Lyrica | Pregabalin |

## Drugs That May Cause Stevens-Johnson Syndrome and TEN

| BRAND NAME | GENERIC NAME |
|---|---|
| Malarone | Atovaquone/proguanil HCl |
| Maxalt | Rizatriptan benzoate |
| Mefoxin | Cefoxitin injection |
| Merrem | Meropenem for injection |
| Meruvax II | Rubella virus vaccine, live |
| Mevacor | Lovastatin |
| Micardis HCT | Telmisartan/ hydrochlorothiazide |
| Minocin | Minocycline HCl |
| Mintezol | Thiabendazole |
| M-M-R II | Measles, mumps, and rubella virus vaccine, live |
| Mobic | Meloxicam |
| Moduretic | Amiloride HCl/ hydrochlorothiazide |
| Motrin | Ibuprofen |
| Mumpsvax | Mumps virus vaccine, live |
| Nalfon | Fenoprofen calcium |
| Namenda | Memantine HCl |
| Naprelan | Naproxen sodium |
| Naprosyn | Naproxen |
| Neurontin | Gabapentin |
| Nexium | Esomeprazole magnesium |
| Niravam | Alprazolam orally disintegrating |
| Noroxin | Norfloxacin |
| Norvir | Ritonavir |
| Nuvigil | Armodafinil |
| Nystatin Oral | Nystatin |
| Omnicef | Cefdinir |
| Orthoclone OKT3 Sterile Solution | Muromonab-CD3 |
| Ovace | Sodium sulfacetamide |
| Paxil | Paroxetine HCl |
| PCE | Erythromycin particles in tablets |
| PegIntron | Peginterferon alfa-2b |
| Pepcid | Famotidine |
| Phenytek | Phenytoin sodium |
| Plavix | Clopidogrel bisulfate |
| Pletal | Cilostazol |
| Ponstel | Mefenamic acid |
| Prevacid NapraPAC | Lansoprazole/naproxen |
| PREVPAC | Lansoprazole/ amoxicillin/clarithromycin |
| Prezista | Darunavir |
| Primaxin I.M./I.V. | Imipenem/cilastatin |
| Prinivil | Lisinopril |
| Prinzide | Lisinopril/ hydrochlorothiazide |
| Prograf | Tacrolimus |
| Proleukin | Aldesleukin |
| ProQuad | Measles, mumps, rubella and varicella virus vaccine, live |
| Protonix | Pantoprazole sodium |
| Provigil | Modafinil |
| Prozac | Fluoxetine |
| Raniclor | Cefaclor |
| Recombivax HB | Hepatitis B vaccine (recombinant) |
| Relafen | Nabumetone |
| Remicade for IV Injection | Infliximab |
| Rescriptor | Delavirdine mesylate |
| Retrovir | Zidovudine |
| Reyataz | Atazanavir sulfate |
| Rituxan | Rituximab |
| Rosula NS | Sodium sulfacetamide |
| Septra | Trimethoprim/ sulfamethoxazole |
| Seroquel | Quetiapine fumarate |
| Solodyn | Minocycline HCl |
| Stromectol | Ivermectin |
| Suprax | Cefixime for oral suspension |
| Sustiva | Efavirenz |
| Tamiflu | Oseltamivir phosphate |
| Tarka | Trandolapril/verapamil HCl |
| Taxotere | Docetaxel |
| Tegretol | Carbamazepine |
| Teveten HCT | Eprosartan mesylate/ hydrochlorothiazide |
| Thalomid | Thalidomide |
| Tiazac | Diltiazem HCl |
| Ticlid | Ticlopidine HCl |
| Timentin | Ticarcillin disodium/ clavulanate potassium |
| Timolide | Timolol maleate/ hydrochlorothiazide |
| Tindamax | Tinidazole |
| Topamax | Topiramate |
| Tricor | Fenofibrate |
| Trileptal | Oxcarbazepine |
| Trizivir | Abacavir sulfate/ lamivudine/zidovudine |
| Trusopt | Dorzolamide HCl |
| Twinrix | Hepatitis A inactivated/ hepatitis B (recombinant) vaccine |
| Vancocin | Vancomycin HCl |
| Varivax | Varicella virus vaccine, live |
| VFEND | Voriconazole |
| Viramune | Nevirapine |
| Voltaren | Diclofenac sodium |
| VoSpire ER | Albuterol sulfate |
| Vytorin | Ezetimibe/simvastatin |
| Vyvanse | Lisdexamfetamine dimesylate |
| Wellbutrin | Bupropion HCl |
| Zegerid | Omeprazole/sodium bicarbonate |
| Ziagen | Abacavir sulfate |
| Zinacef | Cefuroxime for injection |
| Zmax | Azithromycin extended release for oral suspension |
| Zocor | Simvastatin |
| Zoloft | Sertraline HCl |
| Zonegran | Zonisamide |
| Zosyn | Piperacillin/tazobactam |
| Zovirax | Acyclovir |
| Zyban | Bupropion HCl |
| Zyvox | Linezolid |

Note: This list is not comprehensive. For more information, refer to the specific product's full Prescribing Information.

# DRUGS THAT SHOULD NOT BE CRUSHED

Listed below are various slow-release as well as enteric-coated products that should not be crushed or chewed. Slow-release (sr) represents products that are controlled-release, extended-release, long-acting, or timed-release. Enteric-coated (ec) represents products that are delayed-release.

In general, capsules containing slow-release or enteric-coated particles may be opened and their contents administered on a spoonful of soft food. Instruct patients not to chew the particles, though. (Patients should, in fact, be discouraged from chewing any medication unless it is specifically formulated for that purpose.)

This list should not be considered all-inclusive. Generic and alternate brands of some products may exist. Tablets intended for sublingual or buccal administration (not included in this list) should also be administered only as intended, in an intact form.

| DRUG | MANUFACTURER | FORM |
|---|---|---|
| AcipHex | Eisai | ec |
| Adalat CC | Schering Plough | sr |
| Adderall XR | Shire U.S. | sr |
| Advicor | KOS | sr |
| Aerohist | Aero | sr |
| Aerohist Plus | Aero | sr |
| Afeditab CR | Watson | sr |
| Aggrenox | Boehringer Ingelheim | sr |
| Ala-Hist | Poly | sr |
| Ala-Hist D | Poly | sr |
| Aleve Cold & Sinus | Bayer Healthcare | sr |
| Aleve Sinus & Headache | Bayer Healthcare | sr |
| Allegra-D 12 Hour | sanofi-aventis | sr |
| Allegra-D 24 Hour | sanofi-aventis | sr |
| Allerx | Cornerstone | sr |
| Allerx-D | Cornerstone | sr |
| Allfen | MCR American | sr |
| Allfen-DM | MCR American | sr |
| Alophen | Numark | ec |
| Altoprev | First Horizon | sr |
| Ambien CR | sanofi-aventis | sr |
| Ambifed-G | MCR American | sr |
| Ambifed-G DM | MCR American | sr |
| Amdry-C | Prasco | sr |
| Amdry-D | Prasco | sr |
| Amibid LA | Actavis | sr |
| Amrix | ECR | sr |
| Anextuss | Cypress | sr |
| Aplenzin | Biovail | sr |
| Apriso | Salix | sr |
| Arthrotec | Pfizer | ec |
| Asacol | Procter & Gamble | ec |
| Ascriptin Enteric | Novartis Consumer | ec |
| Atrohist Pediatric | Celltech | sr |
| Augmentin XR | GlaxoSmithKline | sr |
| Avinza | King | sr |
| Azulfidine Entabs | Pfizer | ec |
| Bayer Aspirin Regimen | Bayer Healthcare | ec |
| Biaxin XL | Abbott | sr |
| Bidex-A | SJ | sr |
| Bidhist | Cypress | sr |
| Bisac-Evac | G & W | ec |
| Biscolax | Global Source | ec |
| Blanex-A | Blansett | sr |
| Bontril Slow-Release | Valeant | sr |
| Bromfed | Victory | sr |
| Bromfed-PD | Victory | sr |
| Bromfenex | Ethex | sr |
| Bromfenex PD | Quality Care | sr |
| Bromfenex PE | Quality Care | sr |
| Bromfenex PE Pediatric | Ethex | sr |
| Budeprion SR | Teva | sr |
| Budeprion XL | Teva | sr |
| Buproban | Teva | sr |
| Calan SR | Pfizer | sr |
| Campral | Forest | ec |
| Carbatrol | Shire U.S. | sr |
| Cardene SR | Roche | sr |
| Cardizem CD | Biovail | sr |
| Cardizem LA | KOS | sr |
| Cardura XL | Pfizer | sr |
| Cartia XT | Watson | sr |
| Cemill 500 | Miller | sr |
| Cemill 1000 | Miller | sr |
| Certuss-D | Capellon | sr |
| Chlorex-A | Cypress | sr |
| Chlor-Phen | Truxton | sr |
| Chlor-Trimeton Allergy | Schering Plough | sr |
| Chlor-Trimeton Allergy Decongestant | Schering Plough | sr |
| Cipro XR | Schering Plough | sr |
| Clarinex-D 24 Hour | Schering Plough | sr |
| Claritin-D | Schering | sr |
| Claritin-D 12 Hour | Schering | sr |
| Claritin-D 24 Hour | Schering | sr |
| Coldamine | Breckenridge | sr |
| Concerta | McNeil Pediatrics | sr |
| Contac 12-Hour | GlaxoSmithKline | sr |
| Correctol | Schering Plough | ec |
| Coreg CR | GlaxoSmithKline | sr |
| Covera-HS | Pfizer | sr |
| CPM 8/PE 20/MSC 1.25 | Cypress | sr |
| CPM-12 | Brighton | sr |
| Creon 5 | Solvay | ec |
| Creon 10 | Solvay | ec |
| Creon 20 | Solvay | ec |
| Cymbalta | Eli Lilly | ec |
| Dairycare | Plainview | ec |

**Enteric-coated = ec** **Slow-released = sr**

| DRUG | MANUFACTURER | FORM |
|---|---|---|
| Dallergy | Laser | sr |
| Dallergy-Jr | Laser | sr |
| Deconamine SR | Kenwood Therapeutics | sr |
| Deconsal II | Cornerstone | sr |
| Deconex | Poly | sr |
| Deconex DM | Poly | sr |
| Depakote | Abbott | ec |
| Depakote ER | Abbott | sr |
| Depakote Sprinkles | Abbott | ec |
| Despec SR | International Ethical | sr |
| Detrol LA | Pfizer | sr |
| Dexedrine Spansules | GlaxoSmithKline | sr |
| D-Feda II | Dexo | sr |
| D-Hist D | Midlothian | sr |
| Diabetes Trio | Mason Vitamins | sr |
| Diamox Sequels | Duramed | sr |
| Dilacor XR | Watson | sr |
| Dilantin | Pfizer | sr |
| Dilantin Kapseals | Pfizer | sr |
| Dilatrate-SR | UCB | sr |
| Diltia XT | Andrx | sr |
| Dilt-CD | Apotex | sr |
| Disophrol Chronotab | Schering Plough | sr |
| Ditropan XL | Ortho-McNeil | sr |
| Donnatal Extentabs | PBM | sr |
| Doryx | Warner Chilcott | ec |
| D-Phen 1000 | Midlothian | sr |
| Drihist SR | Prasco | sr |
| Drysec | A.G. Marin | sr |
| D-Tab | Palm | sr |
| Dulcolax | Boehringer Ingelheim | ec |
| Duomax | Capellon | sr |
| Durahist | Kowa | sr |
| Durahist D | Kowa | sr |
| Durahist PE | Kowa | sr |
| Duratuss | Physicians Total Care | sr |
| Duratuss DA | Victory | sr |
| Dynacirc CR | GlaxoSmithKline | sr |
| Dynahist-ER Pediatric | Breckenridge | sr |
| Dynex LA | Athlon | sr |
| Dynex VR | Athlon | sr |
| Dytan-CS | Hawthorn | sr |
| Easprin | Rosedale | ec |
| EC Naprosyn | Roche | ec |
| Ecotrin | GlaxoSmithKline | ec |
| Ecotrin Adult Low Strength | GlaxoSmithKline | ec |
| Ecotrin Maximum Strength | GlaxoSmithKline | ec |
| Ecpirin | Prime Marketing | ec |
| Ed A-Hist | Edwards | sr |
| Effexor-XR | Wyeth | sr |
| Embeda | Alpharma | sr |
| Enablex | Novartis | sr |
| Entercote | Global Source | ec |
| Entex LA | Andrx | sr |
| Entex PSE | Andrx | sr |
| Entocort EC | Prometheus | ec |
| Equetro | Shire U.S. | sr |
| ERYC | Warner Chilcott | sr |
| Ery-Tab | Abbott | ec |
| Eskalith-CR | GlaxoSmithKline | sr |
| Extendryl G | Auriga | sr |
| Extendryl Jr | Auriga | sr |
| Extendryl SR | Auriga | sr |
| Extress-30 | Key | sr |
| Exetuss-DM | Larken | sr |
| Extress-60 | Key | sr |
| Feen-A-Mint | Schering Plough | ec |
| Femilax | G & W | ec |
| Fero-Folic-500 | Abbott | sr |
| Fero-Grad-500 | Abbott | sr |
| Ferro-Sequels | Inverness Medical | sr |
| Ferrous Fumarate DS | Vita-Rx | sr |
| Fetrin | Lunsco | sr |
| Flagyl ER | Pharmacia | sr |
| Fleet Bisacodyl | Fleet, C.B. | ec |
| Focalin XR | Novartis | sr |
| Folitab 500 | Rising | sr |
| Fortamet | First Horizon | sr |
| Fumatinic | Laser | sr |
| Genacote | Teva | ec |
| GFN 600/ Phenylephrine 20 | Cypress | sr |
| GFN 600/PSE 60/DM 30 | Cypress | sr |
| GFN 1200/DM 60 | Cypress | sr |
| GFN 1200/ Phenylephrine 40 | Cypress | sr |
| Gilphex TR | Gil | sr |
| Giltuss TR | Gil | sr |
| Glucophage XR | Bristol-Myers Squibb | sr |
| Glucotrol XL | Pfizer | sr |
| Glumetza | Depomed | sr |
| Guaifenex DM | Ethex | sr |
| Guaifenex GP | Ethex | sr |
| Guaifenex PSE 60 | Ethex | sr |
| Guaifenex PSE 80 | Ethex | sr |
| Guaifenex PSE 85 | Ethex | sr |
| Guaifenex PSE 120 | Ethex | sr |
| Halfprin | Kramer | ec |
| Hemax | Pronova | sr |
| Histacol LA | Breckenridge | sr |
| Humavent LA | Dexo | sr |
| Humibid | Adams | sr |
| Humibid DM | Cornerstone | sr |
| Humibid LA | Cornerstone | sr |
| Iberet-500 | Abbott | sr |
| Iberet-Folic-500 | Abbott | sr |
| Icar-C Plus SR | Hawthorn | sr |
| Imdur | AstraZeneca | sr |
| Inderal LA | Wyeth | sr |
| Indocin SR | Forte Pharma | sr |

| DRUG | MANUFACTURER | FORM |
|---|---|---|
| Innopran XL | GlaxoSmithKline | sr |
| Intuniv | Shire | sr |
| Invega | Janssen | sr |
| Isochron | Forest | sr |
| Isopro | Rugby | sr |
| Isoptin SR | Ranbaxy | sr |
| Kadian | Alpharma | sr |
| Kapidex | Takeda | sr |
| Kaon-Cl 10 | Savage | sr |
| Keppra XR | UCB | sr |
| Klor-Con 8 | Upsher-Smith | sr |
| Klor-Con 10 | Upsher-Smith | sr |
| Klor-Con M10 | Upsher-Smith | sr |
| Klor-Con M15 | Upsher-Smith | sr |
| Klor-Con M20 | Upsher-Smith | sr |
| K-Tab | Abbott | sr |
| K-Tan | Prasco | sr |
| Lamictal XR | GlaxoSmithKline | sr |
| Lescol XL | Novartis | sr |
| Levall G | Auriga | sr |
| Levbid | Alaven | sr |
| Levsinex | Alaven | sr |
| Lialda | Shire | ec |
| Lipram 4500 | Global | ec |
| Lipram-PN10 | Global | ec |
| Lipram-PN16 | Global | ec |
| Lipram-PN20 | Global | ec |
| Liquibid-D | Capellon | sr |
| Liquibid-D 1200 | Capellon | sr |
| Liquibid-PD | Capellon | sr |
| Lithobid | JDS Pharmaceuticals | sr |
| Lodrane-12 Hour | ECR | sr |
| Lodrane-12D | ECR | sr |
| Lodrane 24 | ECR | sr |
| Lodrane 24D | ECR | sr |
| Lohist-12 | Larken | sr |
| Lohist-12D | Larken | sr |
| Luvox CR | Jazz Pharmaceuticals | sr |
| Mag Delay | Major | ec |
| Mag64 | Rising | ec |
| Mag-SR Plus Calcium | Cypress | sr |
| Mag-Tab SR | Niche | sr |
| Maxifed | MCR American | sr |
| Maxifed DM | MCR American | sr |
| Maxifed DMX | MCR American | sr |
| Maxifed-G | MCR American | sr |
| Maxiphen DM | MCR American | sr |
| Medent DM | SJ | sr |
| Medent PE | SJ | sr |
| Mega-C | Merit | sr |
| Menopause Trio | Mason Vitamins | sr |
| Mestinon Timespan | Valeant | sr |
| Metadate CD | UCB | sr |
| Metadate ER | UCB | sr |
| Methylin ER | Mallinckrodt | sr |
| Micro-K | Ther-Rx | sr |
| Micro-K 10 | Ther-Rx | sr |
| Mild-C | Carlson, J.R. | sr |
| Montephen | Monte Sano | sr |
| Moxatag | Middlebrook | sr |
| MS Contin | Purdue | sr |
| Mucinex | Adams | sr |
| Mucinex D | Adams | sr |
| Mucinex DM | Adams | sr |
| Multiret Folic-500 | Actavis | sr |
| Mydocs | Centurion | sr |
| Myfortic | Novartis | ec |
| Nalex-A | Blansett | sr |
| Naprelan | Victory | sr |
| Nasatab LA | ECR | sr |
| New Ami-Tex LA | Actavis | sr |
| Nexium | AstraZeneca | ec |
| Niaspan | Abbott | sr |
| Nicomide | Sirius | sr |
| Nifediac CC | Teva | sr |
| Nifedical XL | Teva | sr |
| Nitro-Time | Time-Cap | sr |
| Nohist | Larken | sr |
| Nohist-Plus | Larken | sr |
| Nohist-Plus Jr | Larken | sr |
| Norel SR | U.S. Pharmaceutical | sr |
| Norpace CR | Pfizer | sr |
| Obstetrix EC | Seyer Pharmatec | ec |
| Omnihist LA | Dexo | sr |
| Opana ER | Endo | sr |
| Oramorph SR | Xanodyne | sr |
| Oracea | Collagenex | sr |
| Oxycontin | Purdue | sr |
| Palcaps 10 | Breckenridge | ec |
| Palcaps 20 | Breckenridge | ec |
| Pancrease MT 10 | McNeil Consumer | ec |
| Pancrease MT 16 | McNeil Consumer | ec |
| Pancrease MT 20 | McNeil Consumer | ec |
| Pancrecarb MS-4 | Digestive Care | ec |
| Pancrecarb MS-8 | Digestive Care | ec |
| Pancrecarb MS-16 | Digestive Care | ec |
| Pangestyme CN-10 | Ethex | ec |
| Pangestyme CN-20 | Ethex | ec |
| Pangestyme EC | Ethex | ec |
| Pangestyme MT16 | Ethex | ec |
| Pangestyme UL12 | Ethex | ec |
| Pangestyme UL18 | Ethex | ec |
| Pangestyme UL20 | Ethex | ec |
| Panocaps | Breckenridge | ec |
| Panocaps MT 16 | Breckenridge | ec |
| Panocaps MT 20 | Breckenridge | ec |
| Para-Time SR | Time-Cap | sr |
| Paser | Jacobus | sr |
| Pavacot | Truxton | sr |
| Paxil CR | GlaxoSmithKline | sr |

| DRUG | MANUFACTURER | FORM |
|---|---|---|
| PCE Dispertab | Abbott | sr |
| PCM LA | Cypress | sr |
| Pendex | Cypress | sr |
| Pentasa | Shire U.S. | sr |
| Pentoxil | Upsher-Smith | sr |
| Phenabid | Gil | sr |
| Phenabid DM | Gil | sr |
| Phenavent D | Ethex | sr |
| Phendiet-105 | Truxton | sr |
| Phenytek | Mylan Bertek | sr |
| Phlemex-PE | Cypress | sr |
| Plendil | AstraZeneca | sr |
| Poly Hist Forte | Poly | sr |
| Poly-Vent | Poly | sr |
| Poly-Vent Jr | Poly | sr |
| Prehist D | Marnel | sr |
| Prevacid | Tap | ec |
| Prilosec | AstraZeneca | ec |
| Prilosec OTC | Procter & Gamble | sr |
| Pristiq | Wyeth | sr |
| Procardia XL | Pfizer | sr |
| Prolex PD | Blansett | sr |
| Prolex-D | Blansett | sr |
| Pronestyl-SR | Bristol-Myers Squibb | sr |
| Proquin XR | Depomed | sr |
| Protid | Lunsco | sr |
| Protonix | Wyeth | ec |
| Prozac Weekly | Eli Lilly | ec |
| Pseudocot-C | Truxton | sr |
| Pseudocot-G | Truxton | sr |
| Pseudovent DM | Ethex | sr |
| Ralix | Cypress | sr |
| Ranexa | CV Therapeutics | sr |
| Razadyne ER | Ortho-McNeil | sr |
| Reliable Gentle Laxative | Ivax | ec |
| Requip XL | GlaxoSmithKline | sr |
| Rescon-Jr | Capellon | sr |
| Rescon-MX | Capellon | sr |
| Respa-AR | Respa | sr |
| Respa-BR | Respa | sr |
| Respahist-II | Respa | sr |
| Respaire-60 SR | Laser | sr |
| Respaire-120 SR | Laser | sr |
| Rhinacon A | Breckenridge | sr |
| Risperdal Consta | Janssen | sr |
| Ritalin LA | Novartis | sr |
| Ritalin-SR | Novartis | sr |
| Rodex Forte | Legere | sr |
| Ru-Tuss | Carwin | sr |
| Rythmol SR | GlaxoSmithKline | sr |
| Ryzolt | Purdue | sr |
| SAM-e | Pharmavite | ec |
| Sanctura XR | Allergan | sr |
| Scopohist-PE | Larken | sr |
| Seroquel XR | AstraZeneca | sr |
| Simcor | Abbott | sr |
| Sinemet CR | Bristol-Myers Squibb | sr |
| Sinutuss DM | Dexo | sr |
| Sinuvent PE | Dexo | sr |
| Slo-Niacin | Upsher-Smith | sr |
| Slow Fe | Novartis Consumer | sr |
| Slow Fe With Folic Acid | Novartis Consumer | sr |
| Slow-Mag | Purdue | ec |
| Solodyn | Medicis | sr |
| St. Joseph Pain Reliever | McNeil Consumer | ec |
| Stahist | Magna | sr |
| Stavzor | Noven | sr |
| Sudafed 12 Hour | Johnson & Johnson | sr |
| Sudafed 24 Hour | Johnson & Johnson | sr |
| Sudahist | Larken | sr |
| Sudatrate | Larken | sr |
| Sudex Tab | Atley | sr |
| Sular | Sciele | sr |
| Sulfazine EC | Qualitest | ec |
| Symax Duotab | Capellon | sr |
| Symax-SR | Capellon | sr |
| Tarka | Abbott | sr |
| Taztia XT | Andrx | sr |
| Tegretol-XR | Novartis | sr |
| Theo-24 | UCB | sr |
| Theochron | Forest | sr |
| Theo-Time | Major | sr |
| Tiazac | Forest | sr |
| Toprol XL | AstraZeneca | sr |
| Totalday | National Vitamin | sr |
| Touro Allergy | Dartmouth | sr |
| Touro CC | Dartmouth | sr |
| Touro CC-LD | Dartmouth | sr |
| Touro DM | Dartmouth | sr |
| Touro HC | Dartmouth | sr |
| Touro LA | Dartmouth | sr |
| Touro LA-LD | Dartmouth | sr |
| Toviaz | Pfizer | sr |
| Tranxene-SD | Ovation | sr |
| Trental | sanofi-aventis | sr |
| Treximet | GlaxoSmithKline | ec |
| Trilipix | Abbott | ec |
| Trituss-ER | Everett | sr |
| Tussafed-LA | Everett | sr |
| Tussall-ER | Everett | sr |
| Tussi-Bid | Capellon | sr |
| Tussicaps | Mallinckrodt | sr |
| Tusso-DM | Everett | sr |
| Tusso-HC | Everett | sr |
| Tylenol Arthritis | McNeil Consumer | sr |
| Ultrabrom | Dexo | sr |
| Ultrabrom PD | Dexo | sr |
| Ultracaps MT 20 | Breckenridge | ec |
| Ultram ER | Ortho-McNeil | sr |
| Ultrase | Axcan Scandipharm | ec |

| DRUG | MANUFACTURER | FORM |
|---|---|---|
| Ultrase MT12 | Axcan Scandipharm | ec |
| Ultrase MT18 | Axcan Scandipharm | ec |
| Ultrase MT20 | Axcan Scandipharm | ec |
| Uniphyl | Purdue | sr |
| Urocit-K 5 | Mission | sr |
| Urocit-K 10 | Mission | sr |
| Uroxatral | sanofi-aventis | sr |
| Utira | Hawthorn | sr |
| Veracolate | Numark | ec |
| Verelan | UCB | sr |
| Verelan PM | UCB | sr |
| Videx EC | Bristol-Myers Squibb | ec |
| Vivitrol | Cephalon | sr |
| Voltaren | Novartis | ec |
| Voltaren-XR | Novartis | sr |
| Vospire | Dava | sr |
| Vospire ER | Dava | sr |
| Votrient | GlaxoSmithKline | ec |
| We Mist LA | WE Pharmaceuticals | sr |
| We Mist II LA | WE Pharmaceuticals | sr |
| Wellbid-D | Prasco | sr |
| Wellbid-D 1200 | Prasco | sr |
| Wellbutrin SR | GlaxoSmithKline | sr |
| Wellbutrin XL | GlaxoSmithKline | sr |
| Wobenzym N | Marlyn | ec |
| Woman's Wellbeing Menopause Relief | Consumer Choice | sr |
| Xanax XR | Pfizer | sr |
| Xedec II | Cypress | sr |
| Xpect-AT | Hawthorn | sr |
| Xpect-HC | Hawthorn | sr |
| Xpect PE | Hawthorn | sr |
| Zmax | Pfizer | sr |
| Zorprin | Par | sr |
| Zotex-12D | Vertical | sr |
| Zyban | GlaxoSmithKline | sr |
| Zyflo CR | Critical Therapeutics | sr |
| Zyrtec-D | McNeil Consumer | sr |

# LACTOSE- AND GALACTOSE-FREE DRUGS

The following is a selection of lactose- and galactose-free products. The list is not comprehensive. Generic and alternate brands may exist. Always check product labeling for definitive information on specific ingredients.

| TRADE NAME (OTC) | FORM |
|---|---|
| Advil | Tablets, Caplets, Gel Caplets, Liquigels |
| Advil PM | Liquigels |
| Advil Cold and Sinus | Caplets |
| Aleve | Caplets, Gelcaps, Tablets, Gel Tablets |
| Aleve Smooth Gels | Gel Tablets |
| Align | Capsules |
| Alka-Mints | Tablets |
| Alka-Seltzer | Effervescent Tablets |
| Alka-Seltzer Plus Cold | Effervescent Tablets |
| Ascriptin | Tablets |
| Axid AR | Tablets |
| Benadryl | Liquid, Tablets |
| Benadryl Allergy & Cold | Caplets |
| Caltrate 600 PLUS | Tablets |
| Claritin-D 24 | Tablets |
| Claritin-D Reditabs | Tablets |
| Colace | Capsules |
| Dramamine Chewable | Tablets |
| Elecare | Powder |
| Enfamil Poly-Vi-Sol | Drops |
| Enfamil Poly-Vi-Sol with Iron | Drops |
| Enfamil Tri-Vi-Sol | Drops |
| Enfamil Tri-Vi-Sol with Iron | Drops |
| Ensure | Liquid, Powder, Pudding |
| Ensure Fiber | Liquid |
| Ensure High Calcium | Liquid |
| Ensure High Protein | Liquid |
| Ensure Plus | Liquid |
| Excedrin Extra-Strength | Caplets |
| Ex-Lax Maximum Strength | Tablets |
| Ex-Lax Regular Strength | Tablets |
| Ex-Lax Regular Strength Chocolate | Chewable |
| Fergon Iron | Tablets |
| Gaviscon Regular Strength | Tablets |
| Imodium A-D | Liquid, Tablets |
| Imodium A-D EZ Chews | Tablets |
| Imodium Multi Symptom Relief Chewable | Tablets, Caplets |
| Jevity | Liquid |
| Kaopectate Cherry | Liquid |
| Kaopectate Peppermint | Liquid |
| Kaopectate Peppermint Extra Strength | Liquid |
| Kaopectate Stool Softener | Softgel |
| Kaopectate Vanilla | Liquid |
| Konsyl | Powder |
| Lactaid | Tablets |
| Lactaid Fast Act | Caplets, Chewables |
| MCT Oil | Oil |
| Medi-Lyte | Tablets |
| Metamucil | Powder, Wafers |
| Metamucil Heart and Digestive Health | Capsules |
| Metamucil Strong Bones | Capsules |
| Motrin Children's | Suspension |
| Motrin Children's Cold | Suspension |
| Motrin IB | Tablets |
| Motrin Infant's | Drops |
| Motrin Junior Strength | Caplets, Tablets |
| Mylanta Children's | Tablets |
| Mylanta Gas | Tablets |
| Mylanta Gas Maximum Strength | Softgels |
| Mylanta Maximum Strength | Liquid |
| Mylanta Regular Strength | Liquid |
| Mylanta Supreme | Liquid |
| Mylanta Ultimate Strength | Liquid, Tablets |
| Mylicon Infants' | Drops |
| Nepro | Liquid |
| Ocuvite Vitamin and Mineral Supplement | Tablets |
| One-A-Day Cholesterol Plus | Tablets |
| One-A-Day Energy | Tablets |
| One-A-Day Essential | Tablets |
| One-A-Day Maximum | Tablets |
| One-A-Day Men's | Tablets |
| One-A-Day Men's Health Formula | Tablets |
| One-A-Day Men's 50+ Advantage | Tablets |
| One-A-Day Weightsmart Advanced | Tablets |
| One-A-Day Women's | Tablets |
| One-A-Day Women's 50+ Advantage | Tablets |
| One-A-Day Women's Active Mind & Body | Tablets |
| One-A-Day Women's Prenatal | Tablets |
| Pepto-Bismol | Suspension, Tablets |
| Pepto-Bismol Max. Strength | Suspension |
| Percy Medicine | Liquid |
| Polycose | Liquid, Powder |
| Portagen | Powder |
| Prilosec OTC | Tablets |
| Promote | Liquid |
| Promote with Fiber | Liquid |
| Pulmocare | Liquid |
| RCF | Liquid |
| Simply Sleep | Caplets |
| St. Joseph Adult Low Strength Aspirin | Tablets |
| Sucrets Maximum Strength | Lozenges |
| Sudafed | Tablets |
| Sudafed Children's | Liquid |
| Sudafed OM Sinus Congestion Spray | Liquid |
| Sudafed PE Cold and Cough | Caplets |
| Sudafed PE Maximum Strength Sinus & Allergy | Tablets |
| Sudafed PE Nighttime Cold | Caplets |
| Sudafed PE Non-Drying Sinus | Caplets |
| Sudafed PE Severe Cold Formula | Caplets |
| Sudafed PE Sinus Headache | Caplets |
| Sudafed Sinus | Tablets |
| Titralac | Tablets |
| Titralac Plus | Tablets |
| Tums | Tablets |
| Tums E-X 750 | Tablets |
| Tums E-X Sugar Free | Tablets |
| Tums Kids | Tablets |
| Tums Quik Pak | Powder |
| Tums Smoothies | Tablets |
| Tums Ultra 1000 | Tablets |
| Tylenol | Drops, Liquid, Tablets |
| Tylenol Children's Plus Cold | Liquid |
| Tylenol Children's Plus Cold & Allergy | Liquid |
| Tylenol Children's Plus Cough & Runny Nose | Liquid |
| Tylenol Children's Plus Cough & Sore Throat | Liquid |
| Tylenol Children's Plus Flu | Liquid |
| Tylenol Children's Plus Multi-Symptom Cold | Liquid |
| Tylenol Meltaways Jr. | Tablets |
| Unisom SleepTabs | Gels, Melts, Tablets |
| Zantac 75 | Tablets |
| Zantac 150 Cool Mint | Tablets |
| Zantac Maximum Strength 150 | Tablets |

| TRADE NAME (Rx) | FORM |
|---|---|
| Actigall | Capsules |
| Advicor | Tablets |
| Aldactazide | Tablets |
| Aldactone | Tablets |
| Allegra Oral | Suspension |
| Allegra | Solution, Tablets |
| Allegra-D 12 Hr, 24 Hr | Tablets |
| Allernase | Liquid |
| Altace | Capsules |
| Amicar | Solution, Tablets |
| Amnesteem | Capsules |
| Antivert | Tablets |
| Aplenzin | Tablets |
| Apriso | Capsule |
| Aromasin | Tablets |
| Augmentin Chewable | Tablets |
| Augmentin ES 600 | Powder |
| Augmentin XR | Tablets |
| Augmentin | Suspension, Tablets |
| Axid | Capsules, Solution |
| Bactrim | Tablets |
| Biaxin Granules | Suspension |
| Calan SR | Tablets |
| Cambia | Solution |
| Carafate | Suspension, Tablets |
| Cardene | Capsules |
| Cardizem CD | Capsules |
| Ceftin | Suspension, Tablets |
| Cefzil | Suspension, Tablets |
| Cipro XR | Tablets |
| Cipro | Suspension, Tablets |
| Citranatal RX | Tablets |
| Clinoril | Tablets |

| Drug | Form |
|---|---|
| Coartim | Tablets |
| Combivir | Tablets |
| Comtan | Tablets |
| Covera-HS | Tablets |
| Creon | Capsules |
| Cytotec | Tablets |
| Daypro | Tablets |
| Demerol | Tablets |
| Depakene | Capsules |
| Depakote Sprinkle | Capsules |
| Depakote | Tablets |
| Detrol LA | Tablets |
| Detrol | Tablets |
| DiaBeta | Tablets |
| Diabinese | Tablets |
| Diovan HCT | Tablets |
| Diovan | Tablets |
| E.E.S. | Suspension, Tablets |
| Edluar | Tablets |
| Embeda | Capsules |
| Entereg | Capsules |
| Epivir | Tablets, Solution |
| Epivir-HBV | Tablets |
| Ery-Tab | Tablets |
| Esgic-Plus | Capsules, Tablets |
| Exelon | Capsules |
| Exforge HCT | Tablets |
| Fibricor (fenofibric acid) | Tablets |
| Fioricet with Codeine | Capsules |
| Fioricet | Tablets |
| Flomax | Capsules |
| Gleevec | Tablets |
| Glucotrol XL | Tablets |
| Glucovance | Tablets |
| Glyset | Tablets |
| GoLYTELY | Powder |
| Granisol | Liquid |
| Grifulvin V | Suspension, Tablets |
| Inderal LA | Capsules |
| Isoptin SR | Tablets |
| Kaletra | Solution, Tablets |
| Kapidex | Capsules |
| Keppra | Solution, Tablets |
| K-Lor | Powder |
| K-Phos Neutral | Tablets |
| K-Phos Original Formula | Tablets |
| K-Tab | Tablets |
| Lamisil | Tablets |
| Lescol XL | Tablets |
| Lescol | Capsules |
| Levaquin | Solution, Tablets |
| Levothroid | Tablets |
| Levoxyl | Tablets |
| Lexapro | Suspension, Tablets |
| Librium | Capsules |
| Lomotil | Solution, Tablets |
| Lopid | Tablets |
| Lysteda | Tablets |
| Malarone Pediatric | Tablets |
| Malarone | Tablets |
| Maxzide | Tablets |
| Methylin ER | Tablets |
| Micardis | Tablets |
| Micro-K | Capsules |
| Micronase | Tablets |
| Minipress | Capsules |
| Minocin | Capsules |
| Moxatag | Tablets |
| Niaspan | Tablets |
| Niferex-150 | Capsules, Elixir |
| Niferex-150-Forte | Capsules |
| Norpramin | Tablets |
| Norvasc | Tablets |
| Omnicef | Capsules, Suspension |
| Onsolis | Buccal film |
| Pamelor | Capsules, Suspension |
| Pamine Forte | Tablets |
| Pancrease MT | Capsules |
| Patanase | Liquid |
| Paxil | Suspension, Tablets |
| Pepcid | Suspension, Tablets |
| Percocet | Tablets |
| Percodan | Tablets |
| Plaquenil | Tablets |
| Pletal | Tablets |
| PrandiMet | tablets |
| Prandin | Tablets |
| Precare | Tablets |
| Precose | Tablets |
| Prevacid | Capsules, Suspension |
| Prinivil | Tablets |
| Pristiq | Tablets |
| ProAmatine | Tablets |
| Procardia XL | Tablets |
| Procardia | Capsules |
| Promacta | Tablets |
| Prometrium | Capsules |
| Protonix | Suspension, Tablets |
| Prozac | Capsules, Solution |
| Qualaquin | Tablets |
| Questran Light | Powder |
| Questran | Powder |
| Rapaflo | Capsules |
| Remeron SolTab | Tablets |
| Rifadin | Capsules |
| Robaxin | Tablets |
| Ryzolt | Tablets |
| Sabril | Solution, Tablets |
| Saphris | Tablets |
| Sarafem | Pulvules, Tablets |
| Savella | Tablets |
| Sectral | Capsules |
| Sinemet CR | Tablets |
| Sinemet | Tablets |
| Soma | Tablets |
| Stalevo | Tablets |
| Stavzor | Capsules |
| Sucraid | Solution |
| Symmetrel | Syrup, Tablets |
| Tamiflu | Capsules, Suspension |
| Tegretol/Tegretol-XR | Suspension, Tablets |
| Tenoretic | Tablets |
| Tenormin | Tablets |
| Tessalon | Capsules |
| Tiazac | Capsules |
| Ticlid | Tablets |
| Tikosyn | Capsules |
| Tofranil-PM | Capsules |
| Toprol-XL | Tablets |
| Treanda | Powder |
| Trental | Tablets |
| Treximet | Tablets |
| Trileptal | Suspension, Tablets |
| Trilipix | Capsules |
| Trizivir | Tablets |
| Twynsta | Tablets |
| Tyvaso | Liquid |
| Ultrase MT | Capsules |
| Ultrase | Capsules |
| Uniphyl | Tablets |
| Urex | Tablets |
| Valcyte | Tablets |
| Valtrex | Caplets |
| Valturna | Tablets |
| Vibramycin Hyclate | Capsules, Suspension |
| Vicodin ES | Tablets |
| Vicodin HP | Tablets |
| Vicodin | Tablets |
| Vicoprofen | Tablets |
| Videx EC | Capsules, Delayed Release |
| Vimpat | Capsules |
| Visicol | Tablets |
| Vistaril | Capsules, Suspension |
| Votrient | Tablets |
| Welchol | Tablets |
| Wellbutrin SR | Tablets |
| Wellbutrin XL | Tablets |
| Wellbutrin | Tablets |
| Xenical | Capsules |
| Zantac | Efferdose Tablets, Syrup, Tablets |
| Zarontin | Capsules, Solution |
| Zebeta | Tablets |
| Zenpep | Capsules |
| Zestril | Tablets |
| Ziac | Tablets |
| Ziagen | Solution, Tablets |
| Zipsor | Capsules |
| Zofran | Solution, Tablets (disintegrating) |
| Zoloft | Oral Concentrate, Tablets |
| Zolpimist | Solution |
| Zonegran | Capsules |
| Zyban | Tablets |
| Zyvox | Suspension, Tablets |

# Poison Antidote Chart

**WARNING:** While every effort has been made to ensure the accuracy of this chart, it is not intended to serve as the sole source of information on antidotes. Guidelines may need to be adjusted based on factors such as anticipated usage in the hospital's local area, the nearest alternate sources of antidotes, and distance to tertiary care institutions. Contact your nearest regional poison control center (1-800-222-1222) for treatment information regarding any exposure, including indications for use of antidote therapy. Directions in this chart assume that all basic life support and decontamination measures have been initiated as needed.

| ANTIDOTE | POISON/DRUG/TOXIN | SUGGESTED MINIMUM STOCK QUANTITY | COMMENTS |
|---|---|---|---|
| N-Acetylcysteine (Acetadote®, Mucomyst®) | Acetaminophen<br>Carbon tetrachloride<br>Other hepatotoxins | Oral product: 600 mL in 10 mL or 30 mL vials of 20% solution<br>IV product: One carton of four 30 mL vials of 20% solution | Acetaminophen is the most common drug involved in intentional and unintentional poisonings. 600 mL (120 g) of the oral product provides enough antidote to treat an adult for an entire 3-day course of therapy, or enough to treat three adults for 24 h. Several vials may be stocked in the ED to provide a loading dose and the remaining vials in the pharmacy for the q 4 h maintenance doses. The IV product dose of 120 mL (24 g) will treat one adult patient for an entire 20-hour IV protocol. |
| Amyl nitrite, sodium nitrite, and sodium thiosulfate (Cyanide antidote kit) | Acetonitrile<br>Acrylonitrile<br>Bromates (thiosulfate only)<br>Chlorates (thiosulfate only)<br>Cyanide (e.g., HCN, KCN and NaCN)<br>Cyanogen chloride<br>Cyanogenic glycoside natural sources (e.g., apricot pits and peach pits)<br>Hydrogen sulfide (nitrites only)<br>Laetrile<br>Mustard agents (thiosulfate only)<br>Nitroprusside (thiosulfate only)<br>Smoke inhalation (combustion of synthetic materials) | One to two kits<br>Each kit contains:<br>Twelve 0.3 mL amyl nitrite ampules<br>Two vials 3% sodium nitrite, 10 mL each<br>Two vials 25% sodium thiosulfate, 50 mL each | Stock one kit in the ED. Consider also stocking one kit in the pharmacy.<br>Note: This kit has a short shelf life of 24 months. Note: Stocking this kit may be unnecessary if an adequate supply of hydroxocobalamin is available. |
| Antivenin, *Crotalidae* Polyvalent (equine origin) | Pit viper envenomation (e.g., rattlesnakes, cottonmouths, copperheads, and timber rattlers) | None | As of March 31, 2007, this product is no longer available from the manufacturer. See Antivenin, *Crotalidae* Polyvalent Immune Fab–Ovine in this chart. |

*(Continued)*

This chart is adapted from material furnished by the Illinois Poison Center, a program of the Metropolitan Chicago Healthcare Council (MCHC).

| ANTIDOTE | POISON/DRUG/TOXIN | SUGGESTED MINIMUM STOCK QUANTITY | COMMENTS |
|---|---|---|---|
| Antivenin, *Crotalidae* Polyvalent Immune Fab–Ovine (CroFab®) | Pit viper envenomation (e.g., rattlesnakes, cottonmouths, copperheads, and timber rattlers) | Four to six vials | Advised in geographic areas with endemic populations of copperhead, water moccasin, eastern massasauga, or timber rattlesnake. In low-risk areas, know nearest alternate source of antivenin. This product may have a lower risk of hypersensitivity reaction than previously marketed equine product. Average dose in premarketing trials was 12 vials, but more may be needed. Stock in pharmacy. Store in refrigerator. Equine unavailable after March 31, 2007. |
| Antivenin, *Latrodectus mactans* (Black widow spider) | Black widow spider envenomation | Zero to one vial | Serious *Latrodectus* envenomations are rare. This product is only used for severe envenomations. Antivenin must be given in a critical care setting since it is an equine-derived product. Know the nearest source of antidote. Note: Product must be refrigerated at all times. |
| Atropine sulfate | $Alpha_2$ agonists (e.g., clonidine, guanabenz, and guanfacine)<br>Alzheimer's drugs (e.g., donepezil, galantamine, rivastigmine, tacrine)<br>Antimyesthenic agents (e.g., pyridostigmine)<br>Bradyarrhythmia-producing agents (e.g., beta blockers, calcium channel blockers, and digitalis glycosides)<br>Cholinergic agonists (e.g., bethanechol)<br>Muscarine-containing mushrooms (e.g., Clitocybe and Inocybe)<br>Nerve agents (e.g., sarin, soman, tabun, and VX)<br>Organophosphate and carbamate insecticides | Total 100 mg to 150 mg<br>Available in various formulations:<br>0.4 mg/mL (1 mL, 0.4 mg ampules)<br>0.4 mg/mL (20 mL, 8 mg vials)<br>0.1 mg/mL (10 mL, 1 mg ampules)<br>Atropine sulfate military-style auto-injectors: (Atropen®) 2mg/0.7 mL, 1 mg/0.7 mL, 0.5 mg/0.7 mL, 0.25 mg/0.3 mL<br>Atropine sulfate 2.1 mg/0.7 mL with pralidoxime chloride 600 mg/2 mL (DuoDote®) | The product should be immediately available in the ED. Some may also be stored in the pharmacy or other hospital sites, but should be easily mobilized if a severely poisoned patient needs treatment. Note: Product is necessary for adequate preparedness for a weapon of mass destruction (WMD) incident; the suggested amount may not be sufficient for mass-casualty events. Auto-injectors are available from Bound Tree Medical, Inc. Drug stocked in chempack container is intended only for use in mass-casualty events. |
| Calcium disodium EDTA (Versenate®) | Lead<br>Zinc salts (e.g., zinc chloride) | One 5 mL ampule (200 mg/mL) | Stock in pharmacy. One vial provides one day of therapy for a child. More may be needed in lead-endemic areas. Important note: Edetate disodium (Endrate®) is not the same as calcium disodium EDTA, and is used primarily as an IV chelator for emergent treatment of hypercalcemia, etc. |
| Calcium chloride and Calcium gluconate | Beta blockers<br>Calcium channel blockers<br>Fluoride salts (e.g., NaF)<br>Hydrofluoric acid (HF)<br>Hyperkalemia (not digoxin-induced)<br>Hypermagnesemia | 10% calcium chloride: fifteen 10-mL vials<br>10% calcium gluconate: five 10-mL vials | Stock in ED. More may be stocked in pharmacy. Many ampules of calcium chloride may be necessary in life-threatening calcium channel blocker or hydrofluoric acid poisoning. |

*(Continued)*

| ANTIDOTE | POISON/DRUG/TOXIN | SUGGESTED MINIMUM STOCK QUANTITY | COMMENTS |
|---|---|---|---|
| Deferoxamine mesylate (Desferal®) | Iron | Twelve 500-mg vials | Stock in pharmacy. Note: Per package insert, the maximum daily dose is 6 g (12 vials). However, this dose may be exceeded in serious poisonings. |
| Digoxin immune Fab (Digibind®, DigiFab®) | Cardiac glycoside-containing plants (e.g., foxglove and oleander)<br>Digitoxin<br>Digoxin | Ten vials | Stock in ED or pharmacy. This amount (ten vials) may be given to a digoxin-poisoned patient in whom the digoxin level is unknown. This amount would effectively neutralize a steady-state digoxin level of 14.2 ng/mL in a 70-kg patient. More may be necessary in severe intoxications. Know nearest source of additional supply. |
| Dimercaprol (BAL in oil) | Arsenic<br>Copper<br>Gold<br>Lead<br>Lewisite<br>Mercury | Two 3mL-ampules (100 mg/mL) | Stock in pharmacy. This amount provides two doses of 3 to 5 mg/kg/dose given q 4 h to treat one seriously poisoned adult or provides enough to treat a 15-kg child for 24 h. |
| Ethanol | Ethylene glycol<br>Methanol | 10% alcohol in $D_5W$ was discontinued in 2004; 5% alcohol in $D_5W$ was discontinued in 2007. However, 10% alcohol can be prepared from dehydrated alcohol and $D_5W$. 180 mL of 100% ethanol or equivalents. Consult regional poison control center. | Stock in pharmacy. This amount provides enough to treat two adults with a loading dose followed by a maintenance infusion for 4 hours each. More alcohol or fomepizole will be needed during dialysis or prolonged treatment. 95% or 40% alcohol diluted in juice may be given po if IV alcohol is unavailable. Note: Ethanol is unnecessary if fomepizole is stocked. See also fomepizole in this chart. |
| Flumazenil (Romazicon®) | Benzodiazepines<br>Zaleplon<br>Zolpidem | Total 1 mg: two 5 mL vials (0.1 mg/mL) | Suggested minimum is for ED stocking. Due to risk of seizures, use with extreme caution, if at all, in poisoned patients. More may be stocked in the pharmacy for use in reversal of conscious sedation. |
| Folic acid and Folinic acid (Leucovorin) | Formaldehyde/Formic Acid<br>Methanol<br>Methotrexate, trimetrexate<br>Pyrimethamine<br>Trimethoprim | Folic acid: three 50-mg vials<br>Folinic acid: one 50-mg vial | Stock in pharmacy. For methanol-poisoned patients with an acidosis, give 50 mg folinic acid initially, then 50 mg of folic acid q 4 h for six doses. |
| Fomepizole (Antizol®) | Ethylene glycol<br>Methanol | Two 1.5-g vials<br>Note: Available in a kit of four 1.5-g vials | Stock in pharmacy. Know where nearest alternate supply is located. One vial will provide at least one initial adult dose. Hospitals with critical care and hemodialysis capabilities should consider stocking one kit of four vials (enough to treat one patient for up to several days). Note: Product has a 2-year shelf life; however, the manufacturer offers a credit for unused, expired product. Ethanol is unnecessary if adequate supply of fomepizole is stocked. |

*(Continued)*

| ANTIDOTE | POISON/DRUG/TOXIN | SUGGESTED MINIMUM STOCK QUANTITY | COMMENTS |
|---|---|---|---|
| Glucagon | Beta blockers<br>Calcium channel blockers<br>Hypoglycemia<br>Hypoglycemic agents | Fifty 1-mg vials | Stock 20 mg in ED and remainder in pharmacy. The total amount (50 mg) provides approximately 5 to 10 hours of high-dose therapy in life-threatening beta blocker or calcium channel blocker poisoning. A protocol using high doses of insulin/dextrose also may be considered. Consult regional poison center for guidelines. |
| Hydroxocobalamin (Cyanokit®) | Acetonitrile<br>Acrylonitrile<br>Cyanide (e.g., HCN, KCN and NaCN)<br>Cyanogen chloride<br>Cyanogenic glycoside natural sources (e.g., apricot pits and peach pits)<br>Laetrile<br>Nitroprusside<br>Smoke inhalation (combustion of synthetic materials) | Two to four kits<br>Each kit contains two 2.5 g vials<br>Note: Diluent is not included in the kit. | Seriously poisoned cyanide patients may require 5-10 g (one or two kits). Stock two kits in ED. Consider also stocking two kits in the pharmacy. The product has a shelf-life of 30 months post-manufacture. Due to its favorable safety profile, this product may be used in a pre-hospital setting. |
| Hyperbaric oxygen (HBO) | Carbon monoxide<br>Carbon tetrachloride<br>Cyanide<br>Hydrogen sulfide<br>Methemoglobinemia | Post the location and phone number of nearest HBO chamber in the ED. | Consult IPC to determine if HBO treatment is indicated. |
| Methylene blue | Methemoglobin-inducing agents including:<br>Aniline dyes<br>Dapsone<br>Dinitrophenol<br>Local anesthetics (e.g., benzocaine)<br>Metoclopramide<br>Monomethylhydrazine-containing mushrooms (e.g., Gyromitra)<br>Naphthalene<br>Nitrates and nitrites<br>Nitrobenzene<br>Phenazopyridine | Three 10-mL ampules (10 mg/mL) | Stock in pharmacy. This amount provides three doses of 1 to 2 mg/kg (0.1 to 0.2 mL/kg) for an adult patient. |
| Nalmefene (Revex®) and Naloxone (Narcan®) | ACE inhibitors<br>Alpha$_2$ agonists (e.g., clonidine, guanabenz, and guanfacine)<br>Coma of unknown cause<br>Imidazoline decongestants (e.g., oxymetazoline and tetrahydrozoline)<br>Loperamide<br>Opioids (e.g., codeine, dextromethorphan, diphenoxylate, fentanyl, heroin, meperidine, morphine, and propoxyphene) | Nalmefene: none required<br>Naloxone: total 40 mg, any combination of 0.4 mg, 1 mg, and 2 mg ampules | Stock 20 mg naloxone in the ED and 20 mg elsewhere in the institution. Note: Nalmefene has a longer duration of action but it offers no therapeutic advantage over a naloxone infusion. |
| D-Penicillamine (Cuprimine®) | Arsenic<br>Copper<br>Lead<br>Mercury | None required as an antidote.<br>Available in bottles of 100 capsules (125 mg or 250 mg/capsule) | D-Penicillamine is no longer considered the drug of choice for heavy-metal poisonings. It may be stocked in the pharmacy for other indications such as Wilson's disease or rheumatoid arthritis. |

*(Continued)*

| ANTIDOTE | POISON/DRUG/TOXIN | SUGGESTED MINIMUM STOCK QUANTITY | COMMENTS |
|---|---|---|---|
| Physostigmine salicylate (Antilirium®) | Anticholinergic alkaloid-containing plants (e.g., deadly nightshade and jimson weed)<br>Antihistamines<br>Atropine and other anticholinergic agents<br>Intrathecal baclofen | Two 2-mL ampules (1 mg/mL) | Stock in ED or pharmacy. Usual adult dose is 1 to 2 mg slow IV push. Note: Duration of effect is 30 to 60 min. |
| Phytonadione (Vitamin $K_1$) (AquaMEPHYTON®, Mephyton®) | Indandione derivatives<br>Long-acting anticoagulant rodenticides (e.g., brodifacoum and bromadiolone)<br>Warfarin | Two 0.5-mL ampules (2 mg/mL) and ten 1-mL ampules (10 mg/mL)<br>5-mg tablets available in packages of 10, 14, 20, 30, and 100 | Stock in pharmacy. |
| Pralidoxime chloride (2-PAM) (Protopam®) | Antimyesthenic agents (e.g., pyridostigmine)<br>Nerve agents (e.g., sarin, soman, tabun, and VX)<br>Organophosphate insecticides<br>Tacrine | Six 1-g vials<br>Pralidoxime chloride military-style auto-injectors: 600 mg/2 mL | Stock in ED or pharmacy. Note: Serious intoxications may require 500 mg/h (12 g/day). Product is necessary for adequate preparedness for a weapon of mass destruction (WMD) incident; the suggested amount may not be sufficient for mass-casualty events. Auto-injectors are available from Bound Tree Medical, Inc. Drug stocked in chempack container is intended only for use in mass-casualty events. |
| Protamine sulfate | Enoxaparin<br>Heparin | Variable, consider recommendation of hospital P&T Committee<br>Available as 5-mL ampules (10 mg/mL) and 25-mL vials (250 mg/25 mL) | Stock in pharmacy. |
| Pyridoxine hydrochloride (Vitamin $B_6$) | Acrylamide<br>Ethylene glycol<br>Hydrazine<br>Isoniazid (INH)<br>Monomethylhydrazine-containing mushrooms (e.g., Gyromitra) | 100 1-mL vials (100 mg/mL vials) | Stock in ED or pharmacy. Usual dose is 1 g pyridoxine HCl for each gram of INH ingested. If amount ingested is unknown, give 5 g of pyridoxine. Repeat dose if seizures are uncontrolled. Know nearest source of additional supply. For ethylene glycol, a dose of 100 mg/day enhances the clearance of toxic metabolite. |
| Sodium bicarbonate | Chlorine gas<br>Hyperkalemia<br>Serum alkalinization: Agents producing a quinidine-like effect as noted by widened QRS complex on EKG (e.g., amantadine, carbamazepine, chloroquine, cocaine, diphenhydramine, flecainide, propafenone, propoxyphene, tricyclic antidepressants, quinidine, and related agents)<br>Urine alkalinization: Weakly acidic agents (e.g., chlorophenoxy herbicides, chlorpropamide, phenobarbital, and salicylates) | Twenty 50-mEq vials | Stock 10 vials in the ED and 10 vials elsewhere in the hospital. |
| Succimer (Chemet®) | Arsenic<br>Lead<br>Lewisite<br>Mercury | One bottle of 100 capsules (100 mg/capsule) | Stock in pharmacy. FDA-approved only for pediatric lead poisoning; however, it has shown efficacy for other heavy-metal poisonings. |

# SUGAR-FREE PRODUCTS

The following is a selection of products by therapeutic category that contain no sugar. When recommending these products to diabetic patients, keep in mind that many may contain sorbitol, alcohol, or other sources of carbohydrates. This list is not all-inclusive and generics and alternate brands may be available. Check product labeling for a current listing of inactive ingredients.

**Analgesics**

| Product | Manufacturer |
|---|---|
| Addaprin Tablets | Dover |
| Aminofen Tablets | Dover |
| Aminofen Max Tablets | Dover |
| Aspirtab Tablets | Dover |
| Back Pain-Off Tablets ‡ | Medique |
| Buffasal Tablets | Dover |
| Dyspel Tablets | Dover |
| I-Prin Tablets ‡ | Medique |
| Medi-Seltzer Effervescent Tablets | Medique |
| Methadose Sugar Free Oral Concentrate | Mallinckrodt |
| Ms.-Aid Tablets ‡ | Medique |
| Children's Silapap Liquid | Silarx |

**Antacids/Antiflatulants**

| Product | Manufacturer |
|---|---|
| Alcalak Chewable Tablets*† ‡ § | Medique |
| Dimacid Chewable Tablets | Otis Clapp & Son |
| Diotame Chewable Tablets*† ‡ § | Medique |
| Neutralin Tablets | Dover |
| Pepto-Bismol Caplets † ‡ | Procter & Gamble |
| Tums E-X Sugar Free Tablets* § | GlaxoSmithKline Consumer |

**Anti-asthmatic/Respiratory Agents**

| Product | Manufacturer |
|---|---|
| Jay-Phyl Syrup | JayMac |

**Antidiarrheals**

| Product | Manufacturer |
|---|---|
| Diarrest Tablets | Dover |
| Imogen Liquid | Pharm Generic |

**Blood Modifiers/Iron Preparations**

| Product | Manufacturer |
|---|---|
| I.L.X. B-12 Elixir | Kenwood |
| Nephro-Fer Tablets ‡ | Rugby |

**Corticosteroid**

| Product | Manufacturer |
|---|---|
| Pediapred Solution* § | UCB |

**Cough/Cold/Allergy Preparations**

| Product | Manufacturer |
|---|---|
| Alacol DM Syrup | Ballay |
| Alacol Solution | Ballay |
| Anaplex DMX Syrup | ECR |
| Andehist DM NR Syrup | Cypress |
| Andehist NR Syrup | Cypress |
| Aquatab C Tablets | Deston |
| Aridex Solution | Gentex |
| Baltussin Solution | Ballay |
| Children's Benadryl-D Allergy & Sinus Liquid*† § | Johnson & Johnson |
| Bromhist-DM Solution | Cypress |
| Bromhist Pediatric Solution | Cypress |
| Bromphenex DM Solution*† § | Breckenridge |
| Bromplex DM Solution*† § | Prasco |
| Broncotron Liquid | Seyer Pharmatec |
| Broncotron-D Suspension | Seyer Pharmatec |
| B-Tuss Liquid | Blansett |
| Carbaphen 12 Ped Suspension | Gil |
| Carbaphen 12 Suspension | Gil |
| Carbatuss-12 Suspension | GM |
| Carbatuss-CL Solution | GM |
| Carbetaplex Liquid* § | Breckenridge |
| Carbofed DM Liquid | Hi-Tech |
| Carbofed DM Syrup | Hi-Tech |
| Cardec DM Syrup | Qualitest |
| Cardec Solution | Qualitest |
| Cetafen Cough & Cold Tablets ‡ | Hart Health and Safety |
| Cetafen Cold Tablets ‡ | Hart Health and Safety |
| Cheratussin DAC Liquid | Qualitest |
| Chlordex GP Syrup | Cypress |
| Codal-DM Syrup | Cypress |
| Coldcough PD Syrup* § | Breckenridge |
| Coldcough Syrup* § | Breckenridge |
| Coldonyl Tablets | Dover |
| Corfen DM Solution | Cypress |
| Crantex Syrup | Breckenridge |
| Dacex-DM Solution | Cypress |
| Dallergy Drops*† § | Laser |
| De-Chlor DM Solution | Cypress |
| De-Chlor DR Solution | Cypress |

* Contains sorbitol.
† May contain other sugar alcohols (eg, glycerol, isomalt, maltitol, mannitol, xylitol).
‡ May contain other sources of carbohydrates (eg, cellulose, lactose, maltodextrin, polydextrose, starch).
§ May contain natural or artificial flavors.

| Product | Manufacturer |
|---|---|
| De-Chlor HD Solution | Cypress |
| Despec Liquid | International Ethical |
| Despec-SF Liquid | International Ethical |
| Diabetic Tussin | Health Care Products |
| Diabetic Tussin Allergy Relief Tablets | Health Care Products |
| Diabetic Tussin Cold & Flu Gelcaplets † | Health Care Products |
| Diabetic Tussin DM Liquid § | Health Care Products |
| Diabetic Tussin EX Liquid § | Health Care Products |
| Diabetic Tussin Solution§ | Health Care Products |
| Diphen Capsules ‡ | Medique |
| Donatussin Drops*† § | Laser |
| Double Tussin DM Liquid | Reese |
| Duratuss DM Elixir*† ‡ § | Victory |
| Dytan-CS Tablets | Hawthorn |
| Emagrin Forte Tablets | Otis Clapp & Son |
| Emagrin Tablets | Otis Clapp & Son |
| Endacof-PD Solution † § | Larken Laboratories |
| Ganidin NR Liquid | Cypress |
| Gani-Tuss NR Liquid | Cypress |
| Gani-Tuss-DM NR Liquid | Cypress |
| Genebronco-D Liquid | Pharm Generic |
| Genecof-HC Liquid | Pharm Generic |
| Genecof-XP Liquid | Pharm Generic |
| Genedel Syrup | Pharm Generic |
| Genedotuss-DM Liquid | Pharm Generic |
| Genelan Liquid | Pharm Generic |
| Genetuss-2 Liquid | Pharm Generic |
| Genexpect DM Liquid | Pharm Generic |
| Genexpect SF Liquid | Pharm Generic |
| Gilphex TR Tablets | Gil |
| Giltuss Liquid§ | Gil |
| Giltuss Ped-C Solution§ | Gil |
| Giltuss Pediatric Liquid§ | Gil |
| Giltuss TR Tablets | Gil |
| Guiadex DM Liquid*† § | Breckenridge |
| Halotussin AC Liquid | Axiom |
| Halotussin DAC Solution | Axiom |
| Lodrane D Suspension | ECR |
| Lohist-PD Solution*† § | Larken |
| Marcof Expectorant Syrup | Marnel |
| Metanx Tablets‡ | Pamlab |
| Nalex DH Liquid | Blansett |
| Nalex A Liquid | Blansett |
| Neo DM Drops*† § | Laser |
| Neo DM Syrup*† § | Laser |
| Neotuss-D Liquid † § | A.G. Marin |
| Neotuss S/F Liquid † § | A.G. Marin |
| Niferex Elixir* ‡ § | Ther-Rx |
| Norel DM Liquid*† § | U.S. Pharmaceutical |
| Nycoff Tablets | Dover |
| Organidin NR Liquid † § | Meda |
| Organidin NR Tablets ‡ | Meda |
| Phanasin Syrup | Pharmakon |
| Phanasin Diabetic Choice Syrup | Pharmakon |
| Phanatuss Syrup | Pharmakon |
| Phanatuss DM Diabetic Choice Syrup | Pharmakon |
| Phanatuss-HC Diabetic Choice Solution | Pharmakon |
| Phena-HC Solution | GM |
| Phenabid Tablets | Gil |
| Phenabid DM Tablets | Gil |
| Phena-S 12 Suspension | GM |
| Phena-S Liquid | GM |
| Poly Hist DM | Poly |
| Poly Hist PD Solution | Poly |
| Prolex DM Liquid | Blansett |
| Quintex Syrup | Qualitest |
| Rescon-DM Liquid* § | Capellon |
| Rondec DM*† | Sciele |
| Ru-Tuss DM Syrup*† § | Carwin |
| Safetussin Liquid | Kramer |
| Scot-Tussin Diabetes CF Liquid | Scot-Tussin |
| Scot-Tussin DM Cough Chasers Lozenge | Scot-Tussin |
| Scot-Tussin DM Maximum Strength | Scot-Tussin |
| Scot-Tussin Diabetes CF | Scot-Tussin |
| Scot-Tussin Expectorant Solution | Scot-Tussin |
| Scot-Tussin Senior Solution | Scot-Tussin |
| Siladryl Allergy Solution* § | Silarx |
| Sildec Syrup*† § | Silarx |

* Contains sorbitol.
† May contain other sugar alcohols (eg, glycerol, isomalt, maltitol, mannitol, xylitol).
‡ May contain other sources of carbohydrates (eg, cellulose, lactose, maltodextrin, polydextrose, starch).
§ May contain natural or artificial flavors.

| | |
|---|---|
| Sildec DM Syrup*† § | Silarx |
| Sildec PE-DM Syrup*† § | Silarx |
| Sildec-PE Syrup*† § | Silarx |
| Siltussin DAS Liquid*† § | Silarx |
| Siltussin DM DAS Cough Formula Syrup*† § | Silarx |
| Siltussin SA Liquid*† § | Silarx |
| Statuss Green Liquid* § | Magna |
| Children's Sudafed PE Cough & Cold Liquid*† § | Pfizer |
| Children's Sudafed Nasal Decongestant Liquid*† § | Pfizer |
| Sudanyl Tablets | Dover |
| Sudatuss-SF Liquid | Pharm Generic Developers |
| Supress DX Pediatric Drops † § | Kramer-Novis |
| Suttar-SF Syrup | Gil |
| Tanacof XR Suspension*† ‡ § | Larken |
| Tusdec-DM Solution*† § | Cypress |
| Tusnel Solution | Llorens |
| Tussall Solution* § | Everett |
| Tussi-Pres Liquid † § | Kramer-Novis |
| Vazol Solution | Wraser |
| Z-Tuss DM Syrup † § | Magna |
| Ztuss Expectorant Solution* § | Magna |
| **Fluoride Preparations** | |
| Fluor-A-Day Tablets*† § | Pharmascience |
| Fluor-A-Day Liquid | Pharmascience |
| Lozi-Flur Lozenge* § | Dreir |
| Sensodyne with Fluoride Cool Gel*† ‡ § | GlaxoSmithKline Consumer |
| Sensodyne Tartar Control with Whitening † ‡ § | GlaxoSmithKline Consumer |
| Sensodyne w/Fluoride Toothpaste Original Flavor*† ‡ § | GlaxoSmithKline Consumer |
| **Laxatives** | |
| Benefiber Powder | Novartis |
| Citrucel Powder ‡ § | GlaxoSmithKline Consumer |
| Colace Liquid 1% Solution | Purdue Products |
| Fiber Choice Tablets* ‡ § | GlaxoSmithKline Consumer |
| Fibro-XL Capsules | Key |
| Genfiber Powder | Teva |
| Konsyl Easy Mix Formula Powder ‡ | Konsyl |
| Konsyl Orange Powder ‡ § | Konsyl |
| Konsyl Powder ‡ | Konsyl |
| Metamucil Smooth Texture Powder ‡ | Procter & Gamble |
| Reguloid Powder Regular Flavor ‡ | Rugby |
| Reguloid Powder Orange Flavor ‡ § | Rugby |
| **Mouth/Throat Preparations** | |
| Cepacol Dual Relief Sore Throat Spray † § | Combe |
| Cepacol Maximum Strength Spray*† § | Combe |
| Cepacol Sore Throat + Coating Relief Lozenge † § | Combe |
| Cepacol Sore Throat Lozenges † § | Combe |
| Cheracol Sore Throat Spray † | Lee |
| Chloraseptic Spray*† § | Prestige |
| Diabetic Tussin Cough Drops † § | Health Care Product |
| Fisherman's Friend Sugar Free Mint Lozenges* | Mentholatum |
| Fresh N Free Liquid | Geritrex |
| Larynex Lozenges | Dover |
| Listerine Pocketpaks Film ‡ § | Johnson & Johnson |
| Luden's Sugar Free & Wild Cherry Throat Drops † § | Johnson & Johnson |
| Medikoff Sugar Free Drops † | Medique |
| N'ice Lozenges* § | Heritage/Insight |
| Oragesic Solution* § | Parnell |
| Oragel Dry Mouth Moisturizing Gel*† ‡ § | Del |
| Orajel Dry Mouth Moisturizing Spray † ‡ § | Del |
| Sepasoothe Lozenges* ‡ § | Medique |
| Thorets Maximum Strength Lozenges | Otis Clapp & Son |
| Triaminic Sore Throat Spray*† § | Novartis |
| **Vitamins/Minerals/Supplements** | |
| Action Tabs Made for Men ‡ | Action Labs |
| Adaptoside R+R For Stress Liquid | HVS |
| Adaptoside R+R For Acute Stress Liquid | HVS |
| Alamag Tablets*† ‡ § | Medique |
| Alcalak Tablets*† ‡ | Medique |

| Product | Manufacturer |
|---|---|
| Apetigen Elixir*† | Kramer-Novis |
| Apptrim Capsules | Physician Therapeutics |
| Apptrim-D Capsules | Physician Therapeutics |
| Bevitamel Tablets | Westlake |
| Biosode Liquid | HVS |
| Biotect Plus Caplet | Gil |
| Bugs Bunny Complete | Bayer |
| C&M Caps-375 Capsules | Key |
| Cal-Cee Tablets | Key |
| Calcet Plus Tablets | Mission Pharmacal |
| Calcimin-300 Tablets | Key |
| Cal-Mint Chewable Tablets*† ‡ | Freeda Vitamins |
| Cerefolin NAC Tablets | Pamlab |
| Chromacaps ‡ | Key |
| Delta D3 Tablets ‡ | Freeda Vitamins |
| Detoxosode Liquids | HVS |
| Dexfol Tablets ‡ | Rising |
| DHEA Capsules | ADH Health Products |
| Diatx ZN Tablets ‡ | Pamlab |
| Dimacid Tablets | Otis Clapp & Son |
| Diucaps Capsules | Legere |
| DL-Phen-500 Capsules | Key |
| Enterex Diabetic Liquid ‡ | Victus |
| Evening Primose Oil Capsules † | National Vitamin |
| Ex-L Tablets Tablets ‡ | Key |
| Extress Tablets | Key |
| Eyetamins Tablets ‡ | Rexall Consumer |
| Fem-Cal Citrate Tablets ‡ | Freeda Vitamins |
| Fem-Cal Tablets ‡ | Freeda Vitamins |
| Fem-Cal Plus Tablets | Freeda Vitamins |
| Ferrocite Plus Tablets ‡ | Breckenridge |
| Folacin-800 Tablets ‡ | Key |
| Folbee Plus Tablets ‡ | Breckenridge |
| Folbee Tablets ‡ | Breckenridge |
| Folplex 2.2 Tablets ‡ | Breckenridge |
| Foltx Tablets ‡ | Pamlab |
| Gabadone Capsules | Physician Therapeutics |
| Gram-O-Leci Tablets*† ‡ | Freeda Vitamins |
| Herbal Slim Complex Capsules | ADH Health Products |
| Hypertensa Capsules ‡ | Physician Therapeutics |
| Lynae Calcium/Vitamin C Chewable Tablets | Boscogen |
| Lynae Chondroitin/ Glucosamine Capsules | Boscogen |
| Lynae Ginse-Cool Chewable Tablets | Boscogen |
| Mag-Ox 400 Tablets | Blaine |
| Mag-SR Tablets ‡ | Cypress |
| Mag-SR Plus Calcium Tablets ‡ | Cypress |
| Magimin Tablets ‡ | Key |
| Maginex Tablets ‡ | Logan |
| Magnacaps Capsules ‡ | Key |
| Mangimin Tablets ‡ | Key |
| Medi-Lyte Tablets ‡ | Medique |
| Metanx Tablets ‡ | Pamlab |
| Multi-Delyn with Iron Liquid † | Silarx |
| Natelle C Tablets | Azur |
| Natelle Tablets | Azur |
| Nephro-Fer Tablets ‡ | Rugby |
| New Life Hair Tablets ‡ | Rexall Consumer |
| Niferex Elixir* ‡ § | Ther-Rx |
| Nutrisure OTC Tablets | Westlake |
| Nutrivit Solution*† § | Llorens |
| Ob Complete Tablets | Vertical |
| O-Cal Fa Tablets ‡ | Pharmics |
| Os-Cal 500 + D Tablets ‡ | GlaxoSmithKline Consumer |
| Powervites Tablets ‡ | Green Turtle Bay Vitamin |
| Prostaplex Herbal Complex Capsules | ADH Health Products |
| Protect Plus Liquid | Gil |
| Protect Plus Liquid NR Softgels | Gil |
| Pulmona Capsules | Physician Therapeutics |
| Quintabs-M Tablets ‡ | Freeda Vitamins |
| Replace Capsules ‡ | Key |
| Replace w/o Iron Capsules ‡ | Key |

* Contains sorbitol.

† May contain other sugar alcohols (eg, glycerol, isomalt, maltitol, mannitol, xylitol).

‡ May contain other sources of carbohydrates (eg, cellulose, lactose, maltodextrin, polydextrose, starch).

§ May contain natural or artificial flavors.

| | |
|---|---|
| Resource Arginaid Powder ‡ | Novartis Nutrition |
| Ribo-100 T.D. Capsules | Key |
| Samolinic Softgels † | Key |
| Sea Omega 30 Softgels † | Rugby |
| Sea Omega 50 Softgels † | Rugby |
| Sentra AM Capsules | Physician Therapeutics |
| Sentra PM Capsules | Physician Therapeutics |
| Soy Care for Menopause Capsules | Inverness Medical |
| Span C Tablets ‡ | Freeda Vitamins |
| Strovite Forte Syrup | Everett |
| Sunnie Tablets | Green Turtle Bay Vitamin |
| Sunvite Tablets † ‡ | Rexall Naturalist |
| Super Dec B100 Tablets ‡ | Freeda Vitamins |
| Super Quints B-50 Tablets ‡ | Freeda Vitamins |
| Supervite Liquid | Seyer Pharmatec |
| Suplevit Liquid | Gil |
| Theramine Capsules | Physician Therapeutics |
| Triamin Tablets | Key |
| Triamino Tablets* ‡ | Freeda Vitamins |
| Ultramino Powder | Freeda Vitamins |
| Uro-Mag Capsules ‡ | Blaine |
| Vitafol Tablets † ‡ | Everett |
| Vitamin C/Rose Hips Tablets | ADH Health Products |
| Vitrim Jr Chewable Tablets † ‡ § | Mason Vitamins |
| Xtramins Tablets | Key |
| Yohimbe Power Max 1500 for Women Tablets ‡ | Action Labs |
| Ze Plus Softgel | Everett |

**Miscellaneous**

| | |
|---|---|
| Acidoll Capsules | Key |
| Alka-Gest Tablets | Key |
| Bicitra Solution † § | Ortho-McNeil |
| Cafergot Tablets ‡ | Sandoz |
| Cytra-2 Solution* § | Cypress |
| Cytra-K Solution* § | Cypress |
| Cytra-K Crystals | Cypress |
| Melatin Tablets ‡ | Mason Vitamins |
| Namenda Solution*† § | Forest |
| Polycitra-K Crystals | Ortho-McNeil |
| Prosed/DS Tablets ‡ | Ferring |
| Questran Light Powder ‡ § | Par |
| Soltamox Solution*† ‡ | Cytogen |

# SULFITE-CONTAINING PRODUCTS

The following is a selection of products that contain sulfites, a common allergic trigger. Please remember, however, that the list is not comprehensive. Always check product labeling for definitive information on specific ingredients.

| PRODUCT | GENERIC NAME |
|---|---|
| Alphaquin HP | Hydroquinone |
| Amikacin Sulfate Injection | Amikacin sulfate |
| Amikin Injectable | Amikacin sulfate |
| Apokyn | Apomorphine hydrochloride |
| Aramine Injection | Metaraminol |
| Betagan Liquifilm | Levobunolol |
| Betagan Ophthalmic Solution, USP | Levobunolol hydrochloride |
| Campral (residual traces) | Acamprosate calcium |
| Corlopam Injection | Fenoldopam mesylate |
| Cortisporin Otic Solution | Hydrocortisone/neomycin sulfate/polymyxin B |
| Dilaudid Ampules, Dilaudid Tablets, Dilaudid Non-Sterile Powder | Hydromorphone |
| Dilaudid-HP Injection, Dilaudid-HP Lyophilized Powder 250 mg | Hydromorphone |
| Dilaudid Oral Liquid; Dilaudid Tablets - 2 mg, 4 mg, 8 mg | Hydromorphone |
| Dobutamine Injection | Dobutamine Injection |
| Dopamine HCl Injection | Dopamine HCl |
| Eldopaque Forte 4% | Hydroquinone |
| Eldoquin Forte 4% | Hydroquinone |
| EpiPen Auto-Injector | Epinephrine |
| EpiPen Jr. Auto-Injector | Epinephrine |
| EpiQuin Micro | Hydroquinone |
| Gentamicin Sulfate Injection | Gentamicin sulfate |
| Innohep Injection | Tinzaparin sodium |
| Ketoconazole Cream | Ketoconazole |
| Klaron Lotion 10% | Sodium sulfacetamide |
| Levophed Injection | Norepinephrine |
| Lustra | Hydroquinone |
| Lustra-AF | Hydroquinone |
| Marcaine Hydrochloride/ Epinephrine 1:200,000 | Bupivacaine/epinephrine bitartrate |
| Melpaque HP | Hydroquinone |
| Melquin HP | Hydroquinone |
| Morphine Sulfate Injection | Morphine sulfate |
| Nizoral A-D | Ketoconazole |
| Norflex Injection | Orphenadrine |
| Novocain Hydrochloride for Spinal Anesthesia | Procaine |
| Nubain Ampules/Multiple-Dose Vials | Nalbuphine |
| Nuquin HP | Hydroquinone |
| Orphenadrine Citrate Injection | Orphenadrine citrate |
| Perphenazine Tablets | Perphenazine |
| Phenergan Injection | Promethazine hydrochloride |
| Pred Forte Ophthalmic Solution | Prednisolone acetate |
| Pred Mild Ophthalmic Solution | Prednisolone acetate |
| Propofol Injectable Emulsion | Propofol |
| Rowasa Enema | Mesalamine |
| Sensorcaine with Epinephrine Injection | Bupivacaine/epinephrine bitartrate |
| Sensorcaine-MPF with Epinephrine Injection | Bupivacaine/epinephrine bitartrate |
| SMZ-TMP Concentrate | Trimethoprim/sulfamethoxazole |
| Solaquin Forte 4% Cream; 4% Gel | Hydroquinone |
| Soma Compound with Codeine | Carisoprodol/aspirin/ codeine |
| Streptomycin Sulfate Injection | Streptomycin sulfate |
| Sulfamylon Cream | Mafenide acetate |
| Sumycin Suspension | Tetracycline hydrochloride |
| Talacen | Pentazocine hydrochloride/ acetaminophen |
| Tobramycin Sulfate Injection | Tobramycin sulfate |
| Torecan Injection | Triethylperazine maleate |
| Tri-Luma | Fluocinolone acetonide/ hydroquinone/tretinoin |
| Twinject Injection | Epinephrine |
| Tylenol with Codeine Tablets | Acetaminophen/codeine |
| Tylox Capsules | Acetaminophen/oxycodone |
| Vibramycin Syrup | Doxycycline calcium |
| Xibrom Ophthalmic | Bromfenac |
| Xylocaine with Epinephrine Injection | Lidocaine/epinephrine |

# USE-IN-PREGNANCY RATINGS

The U.S. Food and Drug Administration's Use-in-Pregnancy rating system weighs the degree to which available information has ruled out risk to the fetus against the drug's potential benefit to the patient. Below is a listing of drugs (by generic name) for which ratings are available.

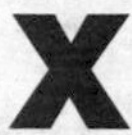

**Contraindicated in pregnancy**

*Studies in animals or humans, or investigational or postmarketing reports, have demonstrated fetal risk, which clearly outweighs any possible benefit to the patient.*

Acetohydroxamic Acid
Acitretin
Ambrisentan
Amlodipine Besylate/
Atorvastatin Calcium
Atorvastatin Calcium
Bexarotene
Bicalutamide
Bosentan
Cetrorelix Acetate
Clomiphene Citrate
Degarelix Acteate
Desogestrel/Ethinyl Estradiol
Diclofenac Sodium/Misoprostol
Dihydroergotamine Mesylate
Dronedarone
Dutasteride
Estazolam
Estradiol
Estradiol Acetate
Estradiol Valerate
Estradiol/Levonorgestrel
Estradiol/Norethindrone Acetate
Estrogens, Conjugated
Estrogens, Conjugated, Synthetic A
Estrogens, Conjugated/
Medroxyprogesterone Acetate
Estrogens, Esterified
Estrogens, Esterified/
Methyltestosterone
Estropipate
Ethinyl Estradiol/Drospirenone
Ethinyl Estradiol/Ethynodiol Diacetate
Ethinyl Estradiol/Etonogestrel
Ethinyl Estradiol/Ferrous
Fumarate/Norethindrone Acetate
Ethinyl Estradiol/Levonorgestrel
Ethinyl Estradiol/
Norelgestromin
Ethinyl Estradiol/
Norethindrone Acetate
Ethinyl Estradiol/Norgestimate
Ethinyl Estradiol/Norgestrel
Ezetimibe/Simvastatin
Finasteride
Fluorouracil
Flurazepam Hydrochloride
Fluvastatin Sodium
Follitropin Alfa
Follitropin Beta
Ganirelix Acetate
Goserelin Acetate
Histrelin Acetate
Iodine I 131 Tositumomab/
Tositumomab
Isotretinoin
Leflunomide
Leuprolide Acetate
Levonorgestrel
Lovastatin
Lovastatin/Niacin
Medroxyprogesterone Acetate
Megestrol Acetate
Mequinol/Tretinoin
Mestranol/Norethindrone
Methotrexate Sodium
Methyltestosterone
Miglustat
Misoprostol
Nafarelin Acetate
Niacin/Simvastatin
Norethindrone
Norethindrone Acetate
Oxandrolone
Oxymetholone
Pitavastatin Calcium
Pravastatin Sodium
Raloxifene Hydrochloride
Ribavirin
Rosuvastatin Calcium
Simvastatin
Tazarotene
Testosterone
Testosterone Enanthate
Thalidomide
Tositumomab
Triptorelin Pamoate
Warfarin Sodium

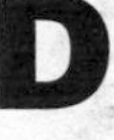

**Positive evidence of risk**

*Investigational or postmarketing data show risk to the fetus. Nevertheless, potential benefits may outweigh the potential risk.*

Aliskiren*
Aliskiren/Hydrochlorothiazide
Aliskiren/Valsartan
Alitretinoin
Alprazolam
Altretamine
Amiodarone Hydrochloride
Amlodipine Besylate/
Benazepril Hydrochloride
Amlodipine Besylate/
Olmesartan Medoxomil*
Amlodipine Besylate/Valsartan
Amlodipine Besykate/
Valsartan/HCTZ
Amlodipine/Telmisartan
Anastrozole
Arsenic Trioxide
Aspirin/Dipyridamole
Atenolol
Azacitidine
Azathioprine
Azathioprine Sodium
Benazepril Hydrochloride
Benazepril Hydrochloride/
Hydrochlorothiazide
Bendamustine Hydrochloride
Bortezomib
Busulfan
Candesartan Cilexetil*
Candesartan Cilexetil/
Hydrochlorothiazide*
Capecitabine
Captopril*
Carbamazepine
Carboplatin
Carmustine (BiCNU)
Chlorambucil
Cladribine
Clofarabine
Clonazepam
Cytarabine Liposome
Dactinomycin
Dasatinib
Daunorubicin Citrate Liposome
Daunorubicin Hydrochloride
Demeclocycline Hydrochloride
Dexrazoxane
Diazepam
Divalproex Sodium
Docetaxel
Doxorubicin Hydrochloride
Doxorubicin Hydrochloride Liposome
Doxycycline
Doxycycline Calcium
Doxycycline Hyclate
Doxycycline Monohydrate
Efavirenz
Enalapril Maleate*
Enalapril Maleate/
Hydrochlorothiazide*

* Category C or D depending on the trimester the drug is given.

Epirubicin Hydrochloride
Eprosartan Mesylate
Erlotinib
Everolimus
Exemestane
Floxuridine
Fludarabine Phosphate
Flutamide
Fosinopril Sodium*
Fosinopril Sodium/
  Hydrochlorothiazide*
Fosphenytoin Sodium
Fulvestrant
Gemcitabine Hydrochloride
Gemtuzumab Ozogamicin
Goserelin Acetate
Idarubicin Hydrochloride
Ifosfamide
Imatinib Mesylate
Irbesartan*
Irbesartan/Hydrochlorothiazide*
Irinotecan Hydrochloride
Ixabepilone
Letrozole
Lisinopril*
Lisinopril/Hydrochlorothiazide*
Lithium Carbonate
Losartan Potassium*
Losartan Potassium/
  Hydrochlorothiazide*
Mechlorethamine Hydrochloride
Melphalan Hydrochloride
Mephobarbital
Mercaptopurine
Methimazole
Midazolam Hydrochloride
Minocycline Hydrochloride
Mitoxantrone Hydrochloride
Moexipril Hydrochloride*
Moexipril Hydrochloride/
  Hydrochlorothiazide
Mycophenolate Mofetil
Mycophenolic Acid
Nelarabine
Neomycin Sulfate/
  Polymyxin B Sulfate
Nicotine
Nilotinib
Nilotinib Hydrochloride Monohydrate
Olmesartan Medoxomil
Oxaliplatin
Pamidronate Disodium
Paroxetine Hydrochloride
Paroxetine Mesylate
Pazopanib HCl
Pemetrexed
Penicillamine
Pentobarbital Sodium
Pentostatin
Perindopril Erbumine
Phenytoin
Procarbazine Hydrochloride
Quinapril Hydrochloride*
Quinapril Hydrochloride/
  Hydrochlorothiazide*
Ramipril*
Romidepsin
Sorafenib
Streptomycin Sulfate
Sunitinib
Tamoxifen Citrate
Telmisartan*
Telmisartan/
  Hydrochlorothiazide*
Temozolomide
Temsirolimus
Thioguanine
Tigecycline
Tobramycin
Topotecan Hydrochloride
Toremifene Citrate
Trandolapril*
Trandolapril/Verapamil
  Hydrochloride*
Tretinoin
Valproate Sodium
Valproic Acid
Valsartan
Valsartan/Hydrochlorothiazide
Vinorelbine Tartrate
Voriconazole
Zoledronic Acid

**Risk cannot be ruled out**

*Human studies are lacking, and animal studies are either positive for risk or are lacking as well. However, potential benefits may outweigh the potential risk.*

Abacavir Sulfate
Abacavir Sulfate/Lamivudine
Abacavir Sulfate/
  Lamivudine/Zidovudine
Abciximab
Acamprosate Calcium
Acetaminophen
Acetaminophen/
  Butalbital/Caffeine
Acetaminophen/Caffeine/
  Chlorpheniramine Maleate/
  Hydrocodone Bitartrate/
  Phenylephrine Hydrochloride
Acetazolamide
Acetazolamide Sodium
Acyclovir
Adapalene
Adefovir Dipivoxil
Adenosine
Albendazole
Albumin (Human)
Albuterol Sulfate
Albuterol Sulfate/
  Ipratropium Bromide
Alclometasone Dipropionate
Aldesleukin
Alemtuzumab
Alendronate Sodium
Alendronate Sodium/
  Cholecalciferol
Aliskiren*
Allopurinol Sodium
Almotriptan Malate
Alpha1-Proteinase Inhibitor (Human)
Alprostadil
Alteplase
Amantadine Hydrochloride
Amifostine
Aminocaproic Acid
Aminohippurate Sodium
Aminolevulinic Acid Hydrochloride
Amlodipine Besylate
Amlodipine Besylate/
  Olmesartan Medoxomil*
Amoxicillin/Clarithromycin/
  Lansoprazole
Amphetamine Aspartate/
  Amphetamine Sulfate/
  Dextroamphetamine Saccharate/
  Dextroamphetamine Sulfate
Anagrelide Hydrochloride
Anthralin
Antihemophilic Factor (Human)
Antihemophilic Factor (Recombinant)
Anti-Inhibitor Coagulant Complex
Anti-Thymocyte Globulin
Apomorphine Hydrochloride
Aripiprazole
Armodafinil
Arnica Montana/Herbals,
  Multiple/Sulfur
Artemther/Lumefantrine
Asenapine Maleate
Asparaginase
Atomoxetine Hydrochloride
Atovaquone
Atovaquone/Proguanil Hydrochloride
Atropine Sulfate/Hyoscyamine
  Sulfate/Scopolamine
  Hydrobromide
Azelastine Hydrochloride
Bacitracin Zinc/Neomycin
  Sulfate/Polymyxin B Sulfate
Baclofen
BCG, Live (Intravesical)
Becaplermin
Beclomethasone Dipropionate
Beclomethasone Dipropionate
  Monohydrate
Bendroflumethiazide
Benzocaine
Benzonatate
Benzoyl Peroxide
Benzoyl Peroxide/Clindamycin

Benzoyl Peroxide/Erythromycin
Bepotastine Besilate
Besifloxacin HCl
Betamethasone Dipropionate
Betamethasone Dipropionate/Clotrimazole
Betamethasone Valerate
Betaxolol Hydrochloride
Bethanechol Chloride
Bevacizumab
Bimatoprost
Bisacodyl/Polyethylene Glycol/Potassium Chloride/Sodium Bicarbonate/Sodium Chloride
Bisoprolol Fumarate
Bisoprolol Fumarate/Hydrochlorothiazide
Black Widow Spider Antivenin (Equine)
Botulinum Toxin Type A
Botulinum Toxin Type B
Brimonidine Tartrate/Timolol Maleate
Brinzolamide
Brompheniramine Maleate/Dextromethorphan Hydrobromide/Phenylephrine Hydrochloride
Budesonide
Bupivacaine Hydrochloride
Bupivacaine Hydrochloride/Epinephrine Bitartrate
Buprenorphine Hydrochloride
Buprenorphine Hydrochloride/Naloxone Hydrochloride
Bupropion Hydrobromide
Bupropion Hydrochloride
Butalbital/Acetaminophen
Butenafine Hydrochloride
Butoconazole Nitrate
Butorphanol Tartrate
Caffeine Citrate
Calcipotriene
Calcitonin-Salmon
Calcitriol
Calcium Acetate
Canakinumab
Candesartan Cilexetil*
Candesartan Cilexetil/Hydrochlorothiazide*
Capreomycin Sulfate
Captopril*
Carbetapentane Tannate/Chlorpheniramine Tannate
Carbidopa/Entacapone/Levodopa
Carbidopa/Levodopa
Carbinoxamine Maleate/Dextromethorphan Hydrobromide/Pseudoephedrine Hydrochloride
Carteolol Hydrochloride
Carvedilol
Caspofungin Acetate
Celecoxib
Cetirizine Hydrochloride
Cetuximab
Cevimeline Hydrochloride
Chloramphenicol
Chloroprocaine Hydrochloride
Chlorothiazide
Chlorothiazide Sodium
Chlorpheniramine Maleate/Pseudoephedrine Hydrochloride
Chlorpheniramine Polistirex/Hydrocodone Polistirex
Chlorpheniramine Tannate/Phenylephrine Tannate
Chlorpropamide
Chlorthalidone/Clonidine Hydrochloride
Choline Magnesium Trisalicylate
Ciclesonide
Cidofovir
Cilostazol
Cinacalcet Hydrochloride
Ciprofloxacin Hydrochloride
Ciprofloxacin Hydrochloride/Hydrocortisone
Ciprofloxacin/Dexamethasone
Citalopram Hydrobromide
Clarithromycin
Clobetasol Propionate
Clonidine
Clonidine Hydrochloride
Codeine Phosphate/Acetaminophen
Colistimethate Sodium
Colistin Sulfate/Hydrocortisone Acetate/Neomycin Sulfate/Thonzonium Bromide
Corticorelin Ovine Triflutate
Cyanocobalamin
Cycloserine
Cyclosporine
Cytomegalovirus Immune Globulin
Dacarbazine
Daclizumab
Dantrolene Sodium
Dapsone
Darbepoetin Alfa
Darifenacin
Deferoxamine Mesylate
Delavirdine Mesylate
Denileukin Diftitox
Desloratadine
Desloratadine/Pseudoephedrine Sulfate
Desoximetasone
Desvenlafaxine
Dexamethasone
Dexamethasone Sodium Phosphate
Dexmethylphenidate Hydrochloride
Dexrazoxane
Dextroamphetamine Sulfate
Diazoxide
Diclofenac Epolamine
Diclofenac Potassium
Diclofenac Sodium
Diflorasone Diacetate
Diflunisal
Digoxin
Digoxin Immune Fab (Ovine)
Diltiazem Hydrochloride
Dimethyl Sulfoxide
Dinoprostone
Diphtheria & Tetanus Toxoids and Acellular Pertussis Vaccine Adsorbed
Diphtheria & Tetanus Toxoids and Acellular Pertussis Vaccine Adsorbed/Hepatitis B Vaccine, Recombinant/Poliovirus Vaccine Inactivated
Dofetilide
Donepezil Hydrochloride
Dorzolamide Hydrochloride
Dorzolamide Hydrochloride/Timolol Maleate
Doxazosin Mesylate
Dronabinol
Drotrecogin Alfa (Activated)
Duloxetine Hydrochloride
Echothiophate Iodide
Econazole Nitrate
Eflornithine Hydrochloride
Eletriptan Hydrobromide
Enalapril Maleate*
Enalapril Maleate/Hydrochlorothiazide*
Entacapone
Entecavir
Epinastine Hydrochloride
Epinephrine
Epoetin Alfa
Eprosartan Mesylate
Erythromycin Ethylsuccinate/Sulfisoxazole Acetyl
Escitalopram Oxalate
Eszopiclone
Ethionamide
Ethotoin
Etidronate Disodium
Exenatide
Ezetimibe
Factor IX Complex
Febuxostat
Felodipine
Fenofibrate
Fentanyl
Fentanyl Citrate
Fentanyl Hydrochloride
Ferumoxytol
Fexofenadine Hydrochloride
Fexofenadine Hydrochloride/Pseudoephedrine Hydrochloride
Filgrastim
Flecainide Acetate
Fluconazole

* Category C or D depending on the trimester the drug is given.

Flucytosine
Fludrocortisone Acetate
Flumazenil
Flunisolide
Fluocinolone Acetonide
Fluocinolone Acetonide/
Hydroquinone/Tretinoin
Fluocinonide
Fluorometholone
Fluorometholone/
Sulfacetamide Sodium
Fluoxetine Hydrochloride
Fluoxetine Hydrochloride/
Olanzapine
Flurandrenolide
Flurbiprofen Sodium
Fluticasone Furoate
Fluticasone Propionate
Fluticasone Propionate HFA
Fluticasone Propionate/
Salmeterol Xinafoate
Fluvoxamine Maleate
Formoterol Fumarate
Fosamprenavir Calcium
Foscarnet Sodium*
Fosinopril Sodium*
Fosinopril Sodium/
Hydrochlorothiazide*
Frovatriptan Succinate
Furosemide
Gabapentin
Gallium Nitrate
Ganciclovir
Ganciclovir Sodium
Gemfibrozil
Gemifloxacin Mesylate
Gentamicin Sulfate
Gentamicin Sulfate/
Prednisolone Acetate
Glimepiride
Glimepiride/Rosiglitazone Maleate
Glipizide
Glipizide/Metformin Hydrochloride
Globulin, Immune (Human)
Globulin, Immune (Human)/
Rho (D) Immune Globulin
(Human)
Glyburide
Gramicidin/Neomycin Sulfate/
Polymyxin B Sulfate
Guaifenesin/Hydrocodone
Bitartrate
Haemophilus B
Conjugate Vaccine
Haemophilus B Conjugate
Vaccine/Hepatitis B Vaccine,
Recombinant
Halobetasol Propionate
Haloperidol Decanoate
Hemin
Heparin Sodium
Hepatitis A Vaccine, Inactivated
Hepatitis A Vaccine,
Inactivated/Hepatitis B Vaccine,
Recombinant
Hepatitis B
Immune Globulin (Human)
Hepatitis B Vaccine, Recombinant
Homatropine Methylbromide/
Hydrocodone Bitartrate
Homeopathic Formulations
Hyaluronidase Recombinant Human
Hydralazine Hydrochloride/
Isosorbide Dinitrate
Hydrochlorothiazide
Hydrocodone Bitartrate
Hydrocodone Bitartrate/
Acetaminophen
Hydrocodone Bitartrate/
Ibuprofen
Hydrocortisone
Hydrocortisone Acetate
Hydrocortisone Acetate/
Neomycin Sulfate/
Polymyxin B Sulfate
Hydrocortisone Butyrate
Hydrocortisone Probutate
Hydrocortisone/Neomycin
Sulfate/Polymyxin B Sulfate
Hydromorphone Hydrochloride
Hydroquinone
Hyoscyamine Sulfate
Ibandronate Sodium
Ibutilide Fumarate
Iloperidone
Iloprost
Imiglucerase
Imipenem/Cilastatin
Imiquimod
Immune Globulin
Intravenous (Human)
Indinavir Sulfate
Indocyanine Green
Influenza Virus Vaccine
Insulin Aspart Protamine,
Human/Insulin Aspart, Human
Insulin Glargine
Insulin Glulisine
Interferon Alfa-2B, Recombinant
Interferon Alfacon-1
Interferon Alfa-N3
(Human Leukocyte Derived)
Interferon Beta-1A
Interferon Beta-1B
Interferon Gamma-1B
Iodoquinol/Hydrocortisone
Irbesartan*
Irbesartan/Hydrochlorothiazide*
Iron Dextran
Isoniazid/Pyrazinamide/
Rifampin
Isosorbide Mononitrate
Isradipine
Itraconazole
Ivermectin
Ketoconazole
Ketorolac Tromethamine
Ketotifen Fumarate
Labetalol Hydrochloride
Lamivudine
Lamivudine/Zidovudine
Lamotrigine
Lanreotide Acetate
Lanthanum Carbonate
Latanoprost
Levalbuterol Hydrochloride
Levalbuterol Tartrate
Levamisole Hydrochloride
Levetiracetam
Levobunolol Hydrochloride
Levofloxacin
Linezolid
Lisdexamfetamine
Lisinopril*
Lisinopril/Hydrochlorothiazide*
Lopinavir/Ritonavir
Losartan Potassium*
Losartan Potassium/
Hydrochlorothiazide*
Loteprednol Etabonate
Lubiprostone
Mafenide Acetate
Magnesium Salicylate Tetrahydrate
Measles Virus Vaccine, Live
Measles, Mumps & Rubella Virus
Vaccine, Live
Mebendazole
Mecasermin [rDNA Origin]
Mefenamic Acid
Mefloquine Hydrochloride
Meloxicam
Meningoccal Polysaccharide
Diphtheria Toxoid Conjugate
Vaccine
Meningococcal Polysaccharide
Vaccine
Meperidine Hydrochloride
Mepivacaine Hydrochloride
Metaproterenol Sulfate
Metaraminol Bitartrate
Metformin Hydrochloride/
Pioglitazone Hydrochloride
Metformin Hydrochloride/
Repaglinide
Metformin Hydrochloride/
Rosiglitazone Maleate
Methamphetamine Hydrochloride
Methazolamide
Methenamine Mandelate/
Sodium Acid Phosphate
Methocarbamol
Methoxsalen
Methoxy Polyethylene Glycol/
Epoetin Beta
Methscopolamine Nitrate/
Pseudoephedrine Hydrochloride

Methyldopa/Hydrochlorothiazide
Methylphenidate Hydrochloride
Metipranolol
Metoprolol Succinate
Metoprolol Tartrate
Metoprolol Tartrate/
Hydrochlorothiazide
Metyrosine
Mexiletine Hydrochloride
Micafungin Sodium
Midodrine Hydrochloride
Milnacipran HCl
Modafinil
Moexipril Hydrochloride*
Moexipril Hydrochloride/
Hydrochlorothiazide*
Mometasone Furoate
Mometasone Furoate Monohydrate
Morphine Sulfate
Morphine Sulfate, Liposomal
Morphine sulfate/Naltrexone HCl
Moxifloxacin Hydrochloride
Mumps Virus Vaccine, Live
Muromonab-CD3
Nabumetone
Nadolol
Nadolol/Bendroflumethiazide
Naloxone Hydrochloride/
Pentazocine Hydrochloride
Naltrexone Hydrochloride
Naphazoline Hydrochloride
Naproxen Sodium
Naratriptan Hydrochloride
Natamycin
Nateglinide
Nebivolol
Nefazodone Hydrochloride
Neomycin Sulfate/Polymyxin B
Sulfate/Prednisolone Acetate
Nesiritide
Nevirapine
Niacin
Nicardipine Hydrochloride
Nifedipine
Nilutamide
Nimodipine
Nisoldipine
Nitroglycerin
Norfloxacin
Ofatumumab
Ofloxacin
Olanzapine
Olmesartan Medoxomil/
Hydrochlorothiazide
Olopatadine Hydrochloride
Olsalazine Sodium
Omega-3-Acid Ethyl Esters
Omeprazole
Oprelvekin
Orphenadrine Citrate
Oseltamivir Phosphate
Oxcarbazepine

Oxycodone Hydrochloride/
Acetaminophen
Oxycodone Hydrochloride/
Ibuprofen
Oxymorphone Hydrochloride
Palifermin
Paliperidone
Palivizumab
Pancrelipase
Paricalcitol
Peg-3350/Potassium Chloride/
Sodium Bicarbonate/
Sodium Chloride
Pegademase Bovine
Pegaspargase
Pegfilgrastim
Peginterferon Alfa-2A
Peginterferon Alfa-2B
Pemirolast Potassium
Pentazocine Hydrochloride/
Acetaminophen
Pentoxifylline
Phenoxybenzamine Hydrochloride
Phentermine Hydrochloride
Pilocarpine Hydrochloride
Pimecrolimus
Pimozide
Pioglitazone Hydrochloride
Pirbuterol Acetate
Piroxicam
Plasma Fractions, Human/
Rabies Immune Globulin (Human)
Plasma Protein Fraction (Human)
Pneumococcal Vaccine, Diphtheria
Conjugate
Pneumococcal Vaccine, Polyvalent
Podofilox
Polyethylene Glycol
Polyethylene Glycol/
Potassium Chloride/Sodium
Bicarbonate/Sodium Chloride
Polyethylene Glycol/Potassium
Chloride/Sodium
Bicarbonate/Sodium
Chloride/Sodium Sulfate
Polymyxin B Sulfate/
Trimethoprim Sulfate
Porfimer Sodium
Potassium Acid Phosphate
Potassium Chloride
Potassium Citrate
Pralidoxime Chloride
Pramipexole Dihydrochloride
Pramlintide Acetate
Pramoxine Hydrochloride/
Hydrocortisone Acetate
Prazosin Hydrochloride
Prednisolone Acetate
Prednisolone Acetate/
Sulfacetamide Sodium
Prednisolone Sodium
Phosphate

Pregabalin
Promethazine Hydrochloride
Propafenone Hydrochloride
Proparacaine Hydrochloride
Propranolol Hydrochloride
Pseudoephedrine Hydrochloride
Pyrimethamine
Quetiapine Fumarate
Quinapril Hydrochloride*
Quinidine Sulfate
Rabies Vaccine
Raltegravir Potassium
Ramelteon
Ramipril*
Ranolazine
Rasburicase
Remifentanil Hydrochloride
Repaglinide
Reteplase
Rho (D) Immune Globulin (Human)
Rifampin
Rifapentine
Rifaximin
Riluzole
Rimantadine Hydrochloride
Risedronate Sodium
Risedronate Sodium/
Calcium Carbonate
Risperidone
Rituximab
Rizatriptan Benzoate
Rocuronium Bromide
Romiplostim
Ropinirole Hydrochloride
Rosiglitazone Maleate
Rubella Virus Vaccine, Live
Sacrosidase
Salmeterol Xinafoate
Sapropterin Dihydrochloride
Sargramostim
Scopolamine
Selegiline Hydrochloride
Selenium Sulfide
Sertaconazole Nitrate
Sertraline Hydrochloride
Sevelamer Carbonate
Sevelamer Hydrochloride
Sibutramine Hydrochloride
Monohydrate
Sirolimus
Sodium Benzoate/
Sodium Phenylacelate
Sodium Phenylbutyrate
Sodium Polysterene Sulfonate
Sodium Sulfacetamide/Sulfur
Solifenacin Succinate
Somatropin
Somatropin (rDNA Origin)
Stavudine
Streptokinase
Succimer
Sulfacetamide Sodium

* Category C or D depending on the trimester the drug is given.

Sulfamethoxazole/Trimethoprim
Sulfanilamide
Sumatriptan
Sumatriptan Succinate
Tacrine Hydrochloride
Tacrolimus
Tapendalol HCl
Televancin HCl
Telithromycin
Telmisartan*
Telmisartan/
Hydrochlorothiazide*
Tenecteplase
Terazosin Hydrochloride
Teriparatide
Tetanus & Diphtheria Toxoids
Adsorbed
Tetanus Immune Globulin (Human)
Theophylline
Theophylline Anhydrous
Thiabendazole
Thrombin
Thyrotropin Alfa
Tiagabine Hydrochloride
Tiludronate Disodium
Timolol Maleate
Tinidazole
Tiotropium Bromide
Tipranavir
Tizanidine Hydrochloride
Tobramycin/Dexamethasone
Tobramycin/Loteprednol Etabonate
Tolcapone
Tolterodine Tartrate
Tolvaptan
Topiramate
Tramadol Hydrochloride
Tramadol Hydrochloride/
Acetaminophen
Trandolapril*
Trandolapril/Verapamil
Hydrochloride*
Travoprost
Tretinoin
Triamcinolone Acetonide
Triamterene
Triamterene/Hydrochlorothiazide
Trientine Hydrochloride
Triethanolamine Polypeptide Oleate-
Condensate
Trifluridine
Trimethoprim Hydrochloride
Trimipramine Maleate
Tropicamide/
Hydroxyamphetamine
Hydrobromide
Trospium Chloride
Tuberculin Purified Protein Derivative,
Diluted
Typhoid Vaccine Live
Oral Ty21a
Urea
Valganciclovir Hydrochloride
Varenicline Tartrate
Varicella Virus Vaccine, Live
Venlafaxine Hydrochloride
Verapamil Hydrochloride
Verteporfin
Vigabatrin
Vitamin K1
Yellow Fever Vaccine
Zaleplon
Zanamivir
Zidovudine
Ziprasidone Mesylate
Zolmitriptan
Zolpidem Tartrate
Zonisamide

# B

**No evidence of risk in humans**

*Either animal findings show risk while human findings do not, or, if no adequate human studies have been done, animal findings are negative.*

Acarbose
Acrivastine
Acyclovir
Acyclovir Sodium
Adalimumab
Agalsidase Beta
Alefacept
Alfuzosin Hydrochloride
Alosetron Hydrochloride
Alvimopan
Amiloride Hydrochloride
Amiloride Hydrochloride/
Hydrochlorothiazide
Amoxicillin
Amoxicillin/Clavulanate Potassium
Amphotericin B
Amphotericin B Lipid Complex
Amphotericin B, Liposomal
Amphotericin B/Cholesteryl Sulfate
Complex
Ampicillin Sodium/
Sulbactam Sodium
Anakinra
Antithrombin III
Aprepitant
Aprotinin
Argatroban
Arginine Hydrochloride
Atazanavir Sulfate
Azelaic Acid
Azithromycin
Azithromycin Dihydrate
Aztreonam
Balsalazide Disodium
Basiliximab
Bivalirudin
Brimonidine Tartrate
Bromocriptine Besylate
Budesonide
Cabergoline
Cefaclor
Cefazolin Sodium
Cefdinir
Cefditoren Pivoxil
Cefepime Hydrochloride
Cefixime
Cefotetan Disodium
Cefoxitin Sodium
Cefpodoxime Proxetil
Cefprozil
Ceftazidime Sodium
Ceftibuten Dihydrate
Ceftriaxone Sodium
Cefuroxime
Cefuroxime Axetil
Cephalexin
Cetirizine Hydrochloride
Certolizumab Pegol
Ciclopirox
Ciclopirox Olamine
Cimetidine Hydrochloride
Cisatracurium Besylate
Clindamycin Hydrochloride/
Clindamycin Phosphate
Clindamycin Palmitate Hydrochloride
Clindamycin Phosphate
Clopidogrel Bisulfate
Clotrimazole
Clozapine
Colesevelam Hydrochloride
Cromolyn Sodium
Cyclobenzaprine Hydrochloride
Cyproheptadine Hydrochloride
Dalfopristin/Quinupristin
Dalteparin Sodium
Dapiprazole Hydrochloride
Daptomycin
Desflurane
Desmopressin Acetate
Dexlansoprazole
Dicyclomine Hydrochloride
Didanosine
Diphenhydramine Hydrochloride
Dipivefrin Hydrochloride
Dipyridamole
Dolasetron Mesylate
Doripenem
Dornase Alfa
Doxapram Hydrochloride
Doxepin Hydrochloride
Doxercalciferol
Edetate Calcium Disodium
Emtricitabine
Emtricitabine/Tenofovir Disoproxil
Fumarate
Enfuvirtide
Enoxaparin Sodium
Eplerenone
Epoprostenol Sodium

Ertapenem
Erythromycin
Erythromycin Ethylsuccinate
Erythromycin Stearate
Esomeprazole Magnesium
Esomeprazole Sodium
Etanercept
Ethacrynate Sodium
Ethacrynic Acid
Etravirine
Famciclovir
Famotidine
Fenoldopam Mesylate
Fondaparinux Sodium
Galantamine Hydrobromide
Glatiramer Acetate
Glucagon
Glyburide/Metformin Hydrochloride
Guanfacine HCl
Granisetron Hydrochloride
Hydrochlorothiazide
Ibuprofen
Indapamide
Infliximab
Insulin Aspart
Insulin Lispro Protamine, Human/Insulin Lispro, Human
Insulin Lispro, Recombinant
Ipratropium Bromide
Iron Sucrose
Isosorbide Mononitrate
Lactulose
Lansoprazole
Lansoprazole/Naproxen
Laronidase
Lepirudin
Levocarnitine
Levocetirizine Dihydrochloride
Lidocaine Hydrochloride
Lidocaine/Prilocaine
Lindane
Loperamide Hydrochloride
Loratadine
Malathion
Maraviroc
Meclizine Hydrochloride
Memantine Hydrochloride
Meropenem
Mesalamine
Metformin Hydrochloride
Metformin Hydrochloride/Sitagliptin
Methohexital Sodium
Methyldopa
Methylnaltrexone Bromide
Metolazone
Metronidazole
Miglitol
Montelukast Sodium
Mupirocin
Mupirocin Calcium
Naftifine Hydrochloride
Nalbuphine Hydrochloride
Naloxone Hydrochloride
Naproxen Sodium
Nedocromil Sodium
Nelfinavir Mesylate
Nitazoxanide
Nitrofurantoin Macrocrystals
Nitrofurantoin Macrocrystals/Nitrofurantoin Monohydrate
Nizatidine
Octreotide Acetate
Omalizumab
Ondansetron Hydrochloride
Orlistat
Oxiconazole Nitrate
Oxybutynin
Oxybutynin Chloride
Oxycodone Hydrochloride
Palonosetron Hydrochloride
Pancrelipase
Pantoprazole Sodium
Pegvisomant
Penciclovir
Penicillin G Benzathine
Penicillin G Benzathine/Penicillin G Procaine
Penicillin G Potassium
Pentosan Polysulfate Sodium
Permethrin
Piperacillin Sodium
Piperacillin Sodium/Tazobactam Sodium
Prasugrel HCl
Praziquantel
Progesterone
Propofol
Pseudoephedrine Hydrochloride
Psyllium Preparations
Rabeprazole Sodium
Ranitidine Hydrochloride
Retapamulin
Rifabutin
Ritonavir
Rivastigmine Tartrate
Ropivacaine Hydrochloride
Saquinavir Mesylate
Saxagliptin
Sevoflurane
Sildenafil Citrate
Silver Sulfadiazine
Sitagliptin Phosphate
Sodium Ferric Gluconate
Somatropin
Sotalol Hydrochloride
Sucralfate
Sulfasalazine
Tadalafil
Tamsulosin Hydrochloride
Tenofovir Disoproxil Fumarate
Teprostinil
Terbinafine Hydrochloride
Ticarcillin Disodium/Clavulanate Potassium
Ticlopidine Hydrochloride
Tirofiban Hydrochloride
Torsemide
Tranexamic Acid
Trastuzumab
Treprostinil Sodium
Urokinase
Ursodiol
Ustekinumab
Valacyclovir Hydrochloride
Vancomycin Hydrochloride
Vardenafil Hydrochloride
Zafirlukast

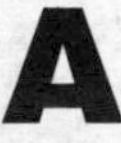


**Controlled studies show no risk**

*Adequate, well-controlled studies in pregnant women have failed to demonstrate risk to the fetus.*

Liothyronine Sodium
Liotrix
Nystatin

* Category C or D depending on the trimester the drug is given.

# VITAMIN COMPARISON TABLE

For easy comparison, the grid below lists the contents of an assortment of widely available vitamin/mineral supplements. It includes entries for all vitamins and minerals—except sodium—assigned a Recommended Dietary Allowance (Daily Value) by the U.S. Food and Drug Administration.

The grid is divided into two parts: the first covers general multivitamin/mineral supplements for adults; the second focuses on supplements sold especially for children.

Many of the brands in the grid include other ingredients that have nutritional importance but lack an official Recommended Dietary Allowance from the government. The presence of additional ingredients is noted in the last column of the grid.

The amounts listed are drawn from the manufacturer's package labeling, primarily as published in the *PDR® for Nutritional Supplements, 2nd Edition.* For easy comparison, the figures have been converted as necessary from the unit of measure used by the manufacturer to the measurement most frequently employed in the industry. **Amounts listed are those found in the total daily dose.** Check package labeling for other usage information provided by the manufacturer.

To conserve space, units of measure are not shown in the grid; see the following key for the measurement used for a particular ingredient.

| Ingredient | Measure |
|---|---|
| Vitamin A (retinol, beta-carotene) | International Units |
| Vitamin B1 (thiamin) | Milligrams |
| Vitamin B2 (riboflavin) | Milligrams |
| Vitamin B3 (niacin) | Milligrams |
| Vitamin B5 (pantothenic acid) | Milligrams |
| Vitamin B6 (pyridoxine) | Milligrams |
| Vitamin B9 (folic acid) | Micrograms |
| Vitamin B12 (cobalamin) | Micrograms |
| Vitamin C (ascorbic acid) | Milligrams |
| Vitamin D | International Units |
| Vitamin E | International Units |
| Biotin | Micrograms |
| Calcium | Milligrams |
| Copper | Milligrams |
| Iodine | Micrograms |
| Iron | Milligrams |
| Magnesium | Milligrams |
| Phosphorus | Milligrams |
| Potassium | Milligrams |
| Zinc | Milligrams |

| BRAND | A | B1 | B2 | B3 | B5 | B6 | B9 | B12 | C | D | E | BIOTIN | CALCIUM | COPPER | IODINE | IRON | MAGNESIUM | PHOSPHORUS | POTASSIUM | ZINC | OTHER |
|---|---|---|---|---|---|---|---|---|---|---|---|---|---|---|---|---|---|---|---|---|---|
| **ADULTS** | | | | | | | | | | | | | | | | | | | | | |
| **ACES (Carlson)** | 5,000 | — | — | — | — | — | — | — | 500 | — | 200 | — | — | — | — | — | — | — | — | — | y |
| **Adult Chewable Multivitamin (Puritan's Pride)** | 5,000 | 15 | 15 | — | 20 | 15 | 400 | 15 | 150 | 400 | 100 | 20 | 10 | 0.05 | 100 | 5 | 0.145 | — | — | 0.325 | y |
| **Advanced Prenatal** *per 3 tabs* | 2,700 | 3 | 3.4 | — | 10 | 3 | 800 | 12 | 120 | 400 | 45 | 300 | 125 | 2 | 75 | 30 | 125 | — | 25 | 25 | y |
| **Centamin Liquid** *per 15 ml* | 1,300 | 1.5 | 1.7 | 20 | 10 | 2 | — | 6 | 60 | 400 | 30 | 300 | — | — | 150 | 9 | — | — | — | 3 | |
| **Centrum** | 3,500 | 1.5 | 1.7 | 20 | 10 | 2 | 400 | 6 | 60 | 400 | 30 | 30 | 200 | 0.5 | 150 | 18 | 50 | 20 | 80 | 11 | y |
| **Centrum Cardio** | 1,750 | 0.75 | 0.85 | 10 | 5 | 2.5 | 200 | 100 | 30 | 200 | 15 | 15 | 54 | 0.35 | 75 | 3 | 20 | 40 | 32 | 3.75 | y |
| **Centrum Chewable** | 3,500 | 1.5 | 1.7 | 20 | 10 | 2 | 400 | 6 | 60 | 400 | 30 | 45 | 108 | 2 | 150 | 18 | 40 | 50 | — | 15 | y |
| **Centrum Performance** | 3,500 | 4.5 | 5.1 | 40 | 12 | 6 | 400 | 18 | 120 | 400 | 60 | 50 | 100 | 0.9 | 150 | 18 | 40 | 48 | 80 | 11 | y |
| **Centrum Silver** | 2,500 | 1.5 | 1.7 | 20 | 10 | 3 | 400 | 25 | 60 | 500 | 50 | 30 | 220 | 0.5 | 150 | — | 50 | 20 | 80 | 11 | y |
| **Daily Multi (Sundown)** | 2,500 | 1.5 | 1.7 | 20 | 10 | 2 | 400 | 6 | 60 | 400 | 30 | 30 | 155 | 2 | 150 | 18 | 100 | 105 | 80 | 15 | y |
| **Duet by Stuartnatal** | 3,000 | 1.8 | 4 | 20 | — | 25 | 1,000 | 12 | 120 | 400 | 30 | — | 200 | 2 | — | 29 | 25 | — | — | 25 | y |

(Continued)

| BRAND | A | B1 | B2 | B3 | B5 | B6 | B9 | B12 | C | D | E | BIOTIN | CALCIUM | COPPER | IODINE | IRON | MAGNESIUM | PHOSPHORUS | POTASSIUM | ZINC | OTHER |
|---|---|---|---|---|---|---|---|---|---|---|---|---|---|---|---|---|---|---|---|---|---|
| **Duet Chewable by Stuartnatal** | 3,000 | 1.8 | 4 | — | — | 25 | — | 12 | 120 | 400 | 30 | — | 100 | 2 | — | 29 | 25 | — | — | 25 | y |
| **Folgard Rx 2.2** | — | — | — | — | — | 25 | 2,200 | 1,000 | — | — | — | — | — | — | — | — | — | — | — | — | |
| **Formula 100 (Puritan's Pride)** | 10,000 | 100 | 100 | 100 | 100 | 100 | 400 | 100 | 250 | 400 | 150 | 100 | 100 | 0.5 | 150 | 18 | 50 | — | 10 | 15 | y |
| **Geritol Complete** | 6,100 | 1.5 | 1.7 | 20 | 13 | 2 | 380 | 6.7 | 57 | 400 | 30 | 44 | 148 | 1.8 | 120 | 16 | 86 | 118 | 36 | 13.5 | y |
| **Goldline Prenatal S** | 4,000 | 1.84 | 1.7 | — | — | 2.6 | 800 | 4 | 100 | 400 | 11 | — | 200 | — | — | 27 | — | — | — | 25 | y |
| **Green Source** *per 3 tabs* | 5,000 | 25 | 25 | 25 | 30 | 25 | 400 | 250 | 500 | 800 | 100 | 300 | 237 | 0.5 | 150 | 15 | 125 | — | 50 | 15 | y |
| **Hair, Skin & Nails Formula (Nature's Bounty)** *per 3 tabs* | 5,000 | 5 | 5 | 25 | 15 | 5 | 200 | 8 | 120 | 100 | 15 | 3,000 | 707 | — | 112.5 | 3 | 100 | 150 | — | 7.5 | y |
| **Hep-Forte** | 1,200 | 1 | 1 | 10 | 2 | 0.5 | 60 | 1 | 10 | — | 10 | 3.3 | — | — | — | — | — | — | — | 2 | y |
| **Mega Vita Gel Iron Free** *per 2 softgels* | 10,000 | 50 | 50 | 50 | 50 | 50 | 400 | 50 | 300 | 400 | 300 | 50 | 200 | 2 | 150 | — | 50 | 50 | 30 | 15 | y |
| **Mini-Multi (Carlson Laboratories)** | 5,000 | 1.5 | 1.7 | 20 | 10 | 2 | 400 | 6 | 120 | 400 | 60 | 30 | 20 | 2 | 75 | — | 40 | — | — | 15 | |

| | | | | | | | | | | | | | | | | | | | | | |
|---|---|---|---|---|---|---|---|---|---|---|---|---|---|---|---|---|---|---|---|---|---|
| Mini-Prenatal (Freeda Vitamins) | 2,000 | 2 | 3 | 20 | 10 | 3 | 800 | 10 | 100 | 400 | 15 | 100 | 200 | 2 | — | 27 | 60 | — | — | 15 | |
| Multi-Day Plus Minerals (Nature's Bounty) | 5,000 | 1.5 | 1.7 | 20 | 10 | 2 | 400 | 6 | 60 | 400 | 30 | 30 | 162 | 2 | 150 | 18 | 100 | 109 | 80 | 15 | |
| Myadec | 5,000 | 1.7 | 2 | 20 | 10 | 3 | 400 | 6 | 60 | 400 | 30 | 30 | 162 | 2 | 150 | 18 | 100 | 125 | 40 | 15 | y |
| Ocuvite | 1,000 | — | — | — | — | — | — | — | 200 | — | 60 | — | — | 2 | — | — | — | — | — | 40 | |
| One A Day Active | 5,000 | 4.5 | 5.1 | 40 | 10 | 6 | 400 | 18 | 120 | 400 | 60 | 40 | 110 | 2 | 150 | 9 | 40 | 48 | 200 | 15 | y |
| One A Day Men's 50+ Advantage | 2,500 | 4.5 | 3.4 | 20 | 15 | 6 | 400 | 25 | 120 | 400 | 33 | 30 | 120 | 2 | 150 | — | 100 | — | 40 | 22.5 | y |
| One A Day Men's | 3,500 | 1.2 | 1.7 | 16 | 5 | 3 | 400 | 18 | 90 | 400 | 45 | 30 | 210 | 2 | — | — | 120 | — | 100 | 15 | y |
| One A Day Women's | 2,500 | 1.5 | 1.7 | 10 | 5 | 2 | 400 | 6 | 60 | 800 | 30 | 30 | 450 | 2 | — | 18 | 50 | — | — | 15 | y |
| One A Day Women's 50+ Advantage | 2,500 | 4.5 | 3.4 | 20 | 15 | 6 | 400 | 25 | 60 | 800 | 33 | 30 | 405 | 2 | 150 | — | 50 | — | — | 22.5 | y |
| One A Day Women's Prenatal | 4,000 | 1.7 | 2 | 20 | 10 | 2.5 | 800 | 8 | 60 | 400 | 30 | 300 | 300 | 2 | 150 | 28 | 50 | — | — | 15 | y |
| Optisource Chewable | 1,875 | 0.375 | 0.425 | 5 | 2.5 | 0.5 | 200 | 125 | 15 | 100 | 125 | 75 | 250 | 0.5 | 37.5 | 7.5 | 100 | 50 | — | 7.5 | y |
| PreCare Chewable | — | — | 2 | — | — | 2 | 1,000 | — | 50 | 6mcg | 3.5 | — | 250 | 2 | — | 40 | 50 | — | — | 15 | y |
| PreCare Conceive | — | 3 | 3.4 | 20 | — | 50 | 1,000 | 12 | 60 | — | 30 | — | 200 | 2 | — | 30 | 100 | — | — | 15 | y |

*(Continued)*

| BRAND | A | B1 | B2 | B3 | B5 | B6 | B9 | B12 | C | D | E | BIOTIN | CALCIUM | COPPER | IODINE | IRON | MAGNESIUM | PHOSPHORUS | POTASSIUM | ZINC | OTHER |
|---|---|---|---|---|---|---|---|---|---|---|---|---|---|---|---|---|---|---|---|---|---|
| **PremesisRx Tablets** | — | — | — | — | — | 75 | 1,000 | 12 | — | — | — | — | 200 | — | — | — | — | — | — | — | |
| **Prenatal Vitamins (Nature's Bounty)** | 4,000 | 1.8 | 1.7 | 20 | — | 2.6 | 800 | 8 | 120 | 400 | 30 | — | 200 | — | — | 28 | — | — | — | 25 | |
| **Prenatal Vitamin (Puritan's Pride)** | 4,000 | 1.84 | 1.7 | 18 | — | 2.6 | 800 | 4 | 100 | 400 | 11 | — | 200 | — | — | 27 | — | — | — | 25 | |
| **Puritan's Pride Complete One** | 10,000 | 25 | 25 | 50 | 50 | 50 | 400 | 50 | 250 | 400 | 30 | 50 | 54 | 2 | 150 | 10 | 100 | 23 | 1 | 15 | y |
| **Strovite Advance** | 3,000 | 20 | 5 | 25 | 15 | 25 | 1,000 | 50 | 300 | 400 | 100 | 100 | — | 1.5 | — | — | 50 | — | — | 25 | y |
| **Stuart Prenatal** | 4,000 | 1.8 | 1.7 | 20 | — | 2.6 | 800 | 8 | 120 | 400 | 30 | — | 200 | — | — | 28 | — | — | — | 25 | |
| **Viactiv Chews** | 2,500 | 1.5 | 1.7 | 15 | 10 | 2 | 400 | 6 | 60 | 400 | 33 | 30 | 200 | — | — | — | — | — | — | — | |
| **CHILDREN** | | | | | | | | | | | | | | | | | | | | | |
| **Carlson for Kids Chewable** | 5,000 | 1.5 | 1.7 | 5 | 10 | 2 | 400 | 6 | 120 | 400 | 60 | 150 | 50 | 1 | 75 | 9 | 25 | 22 | 2.5 | 7.5 | y |
| **Centrum Kids** | 3,500 | 1.5 | 1.7 | 20 | 10 | 2 | 400 | 6 | 60 | 400 | 30 | 45 | 108 | 2 | 150 | 18 | 40 | 50 | — | 15 | y |
| **Flintstones** | 3,000 | 1.5 | 1.7 | 15 | 10 | 2 | 400 | 6 | 60 | 400 | 30 | 40 | 100 | 2 | 150 | 18 | 20 | 100 | — | 12 | y |
| **GNC Kid's Chewable** *per 2 tabs* | 5,000 | 5 | 5 | 20 | 15 | 5 | 400 | 10 | 90 | 400 | 30 | 100 | 30 | 0.2 | 100 | 12 | 15 | 15 | — | 3 | y |

| | | | | | | | | | | | | | | | | | | | | | |
|---|---|---|---|---|---|---|---|---|---|---|---|---|---|---|---|---|---|---|---|---|---|
| **One A Day Kids Bugs Bunny** | 3,000 | 1.5 | 1.7 | 15 | 10 | 2 | 400 | 6 | 60 | 400 | 30 | 40 | 100 | 2 | 150 | 18 | 20 | 100 | — | 12 | y |
| **One A Day Kids Scooby-Doo Complete** | 3,000 | 1.5 | 1.7 | 15 | 10 | 2 | 400 | 6 | 60 | 400 | 30 | 40 | 100 | 2 | 150 | 18 | 20 | 100 | — | 12 | y |
| **One A Day Kids Scooby-Doo Plus Calcium** | 2,500 | 1.05 | 1.2 | 13.5 | — | 1.05 | 300 | 4.5 | 60 | 400 | 15 | — | 200 | — | — | — | — | — | — | — | y |

*USP units.

# BRAND/GENERIC INDEX

Organized alphabetically, this index includes the brand and generic names of each drug in the Product Information section. Brand-name drug entries are capitalized; generic names are not. If more than one brand name is associated with a generic, each brand can be found under the generic entry.

## A

## E

## I

## J



## K



## L

## N

## O

## T

# THERAPEUTIC CLASS INDEX

Organized alphabetically, this index includes the therapeutic class of each drug in the Product Information section. Therapeutic class headings are based on information provided in the drug monographs. The drug entries listed under each bold therapeutic class are organized alphabetically by brand name or monograph title (shown in capitalized letters), followed by the generic name in parentheses.

## A

## C

## F



## G

## K

## N

## S

## U



## V

## W



## X

# VISUAL IDENTIFICATION GUIDE*

## ACIPHEX

RX (rabeprazole sodium)
**EISAI**

20 mg

Delayed-Release Tablets

## ACTONEL

RX (risedronate sodium)
**PROCTER & GAMBLE**

5 mg 30 mg

35 mg 150 mg

## ACTOS

RX (pioglitazone HCl)
**TAKEDA**

15 mg 30 mg 45 mg

## ACTOPLUS MET

RX (pioglitazone HCl/metformin HCl)
**TAKEDA**

15 mg/500 mg 15 mg/850 mg

## ADVICOR

RX (niacin/lovastatin)
**ABBOTT**

500 mg/20 mg

750 mg/20 mg

1000 mg/20 mg

1000 mg/40 mg

Extended-Release Tablets

## ALLEGRA

RX (fexofenadine HCl)
**sanofi-aventis**

30 mg 60 mg

180 mg

## ALLEGRA-D 12 HOUR

RX (fexofenadine HCl/pseudoephedrine HCl)
**sanofi-aventis**

60 mg/120 mg

Extended-Release Tablets

## ALLEGRA-D 24 HOUR

RX (fexofenadine HCl/pseudoephedrine HCl)
**sanofi-aventis**

180 mg/240 mg

Extended-Release Tablets

## AMBIEN

C-IV (zolpidem tartrate)
**sanofi-aventis**

5 mg 10 mg

## ARICEPT

RX (donepezil HCl)
**EISAI**

5 mg 10 mg

## ARICEPT ODT

RX (donepezil HCl)
**EISAI**

5 mg 10 mg

Orally Disintegrating Tablets

*Other dosage forms and strengths may be available

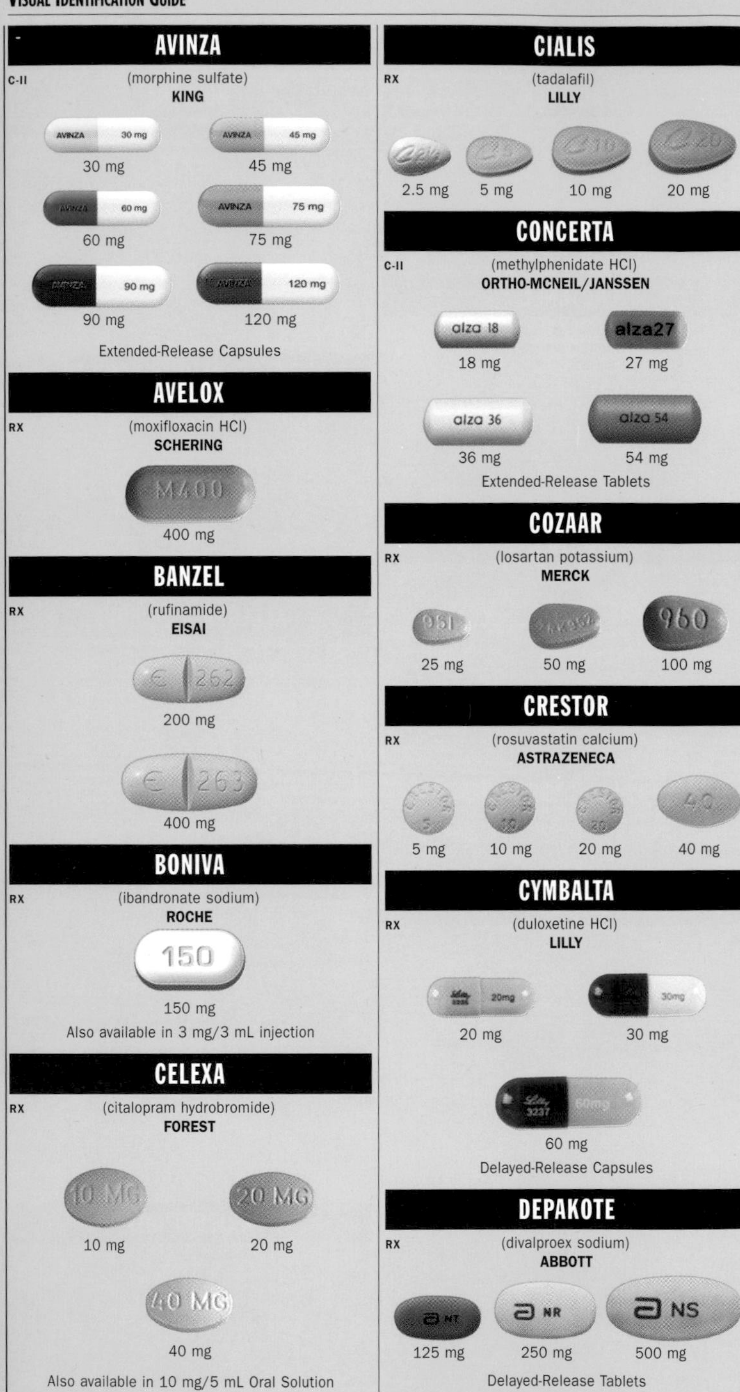
AVINZA
C-II
(morphine sulfate)
KING
30 mg
45 mg
60 mg
75 mg
90 mg
120 mg
Extended-Release Capsules
AVELOX
RX
(moxifloxacin HCl)
SCHERING
400 mg
BANZEL
RX
(rufinamide)
EISAI
200 mg
400 mg
BONIVA
RX
(ibandronate sodium)
ROCHE
150 mg
Also available in 3 mg/3 mL injection
CELEXA
RX
(citalopram hydrobromide)
FOREST
10 mg
20 mg
40 mg
Also available in 10 mg/5 mL Oral Solution
CIALIS
RX
(tadalafil)
LILLY
2.5 mg
5 mg
10 mg
20 mg
CONCERTA
C-II
(methylphenidate HCl)
ORTHO-MCNEIL/JANSSEN
18 mg
27 mg
36 mg
54 mg
Extended-Release Tablets
COZAAR
RX
(losartan potassium)
MERCK
25 mg
50 mg
100 mg
CRESTOR
RX
(rosuvastatin calcium)
ASTRAZENECA
5 mg
10 mg
20 mg
40 mg
CYMBALTA
RX
(duloxetine HCl)
LILLY
20 mg
30 mg
60 mg
Delayed-Release Capsules
DEPAKOTE
RX
(divalproex sodium)
ABBOTT
125 mg
250 mg
500 mg
Delayed-Release Tablets

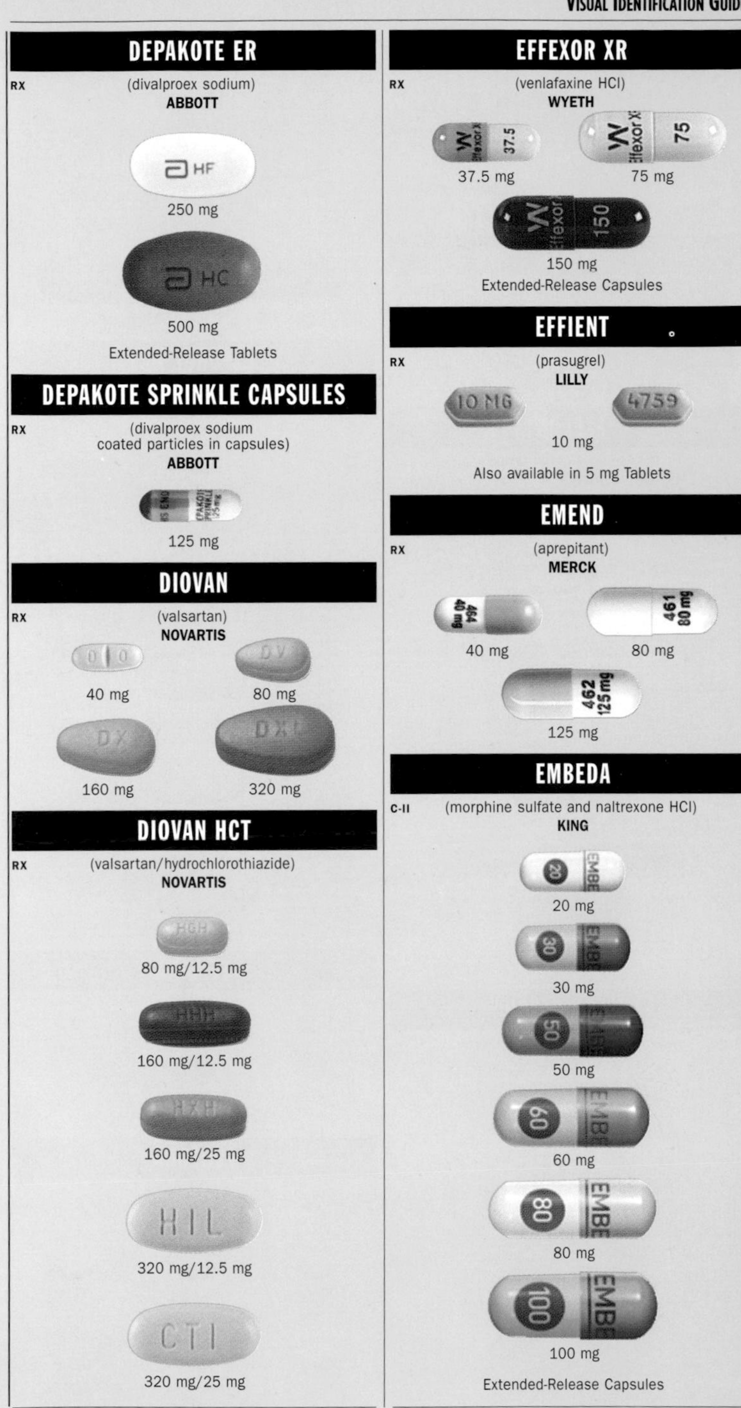

## DEPAKOTE ER

RX

(divalproex sodium)
**ABBOTT**

250 mg

500 mg

Extended-Release Tablets

## DEPAKOTE SPRINKLE CAPSULES

RX

(divalproex sodium coated particles in capsules)
**ABBOTT**

125 mg

## DIOVAN

RX

(valsartan)
**NOVARTIS**

40 mg

80 mg

160 mg

320 mg

## DIOVAN HCT

RX

(valsartan/hydrochlorothiazide)
**NOVARTIS**

80 mg/12.5 mg

160 mg/12.5 mg

160 mg/25 mg

320 mg/12.5 mg

320 mg/25 mg

## EFFEXOR XR

RX

(venlafaxine HCl)
**WYETH**

37.5 mg

75 mg

150 mg

Extended-Release Capsules

## EFFIENT

RX

(prasugrel)
**LILLY**

10 mg

Also available in 5 mg Tablets

## EMEND

RX

(aprepitant)
**MERCK**

40 mg

80 mg

125 mg

## EMBEDA

C-II

(morphine sulfate and naltrexone HCl)
**KING**

20 mg

30 mg

50 mg

60 mg

80 mg

100 mg

Extended-Release Capsules

## ENABLEX

RX

(darifenacin)

**NOVARTIS**

7.5 mg | 15 mg

Extended-Release Tablets

## EVISTA

RX

(raloxifene HCl)

**LILLY**

60 mg

## EXELON

RX

(rivastigmine tartrate)

**NOVARTIS**

1.5 mg

3 mg

4.5 mg

6 mg

Also available in 2 mg/mL Oral Solution

## EXELON PATCH

RX

(rivastigmine transdermal system)

**NOVARTIS**

4.6 mg/24 hours

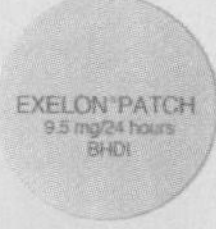


9.5 mg/24 hours

## EXFORGE

RX

(amlodipine/valsartan)

**NOVARTIS**

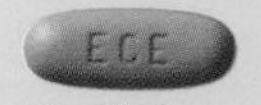


5 mg/160 mg

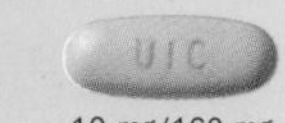


10 mg/160 mg

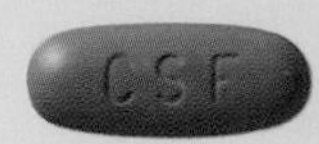


5 mg/320 mg

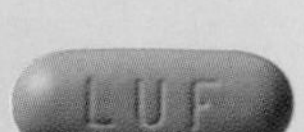


10 mg/320 mg

## EXFORGE HCT

RX

(amlodipine/valsartan/hydrochlorothiazide)

**NOVARTIS**

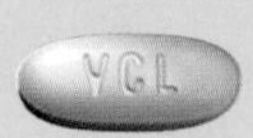


5/160/12.5 mg

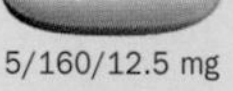

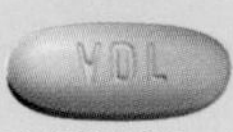


10/160/12.5 mg

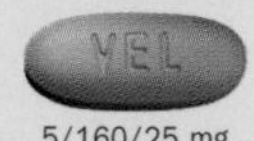


5/160/25 mg

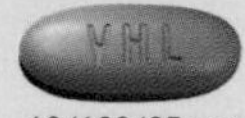


10/160/25 mg

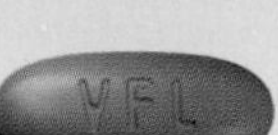


10/320/25 mg

## FEMARA

RX

(letrozole)

**NOVARTIS**

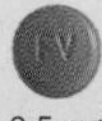


2.5 mg

## FENTORA

C-II

(fentanyl buccal tablet)

**CEPHALON**

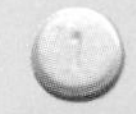

100 mcg

200 mcg

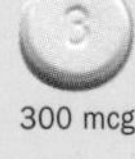


300 mcg

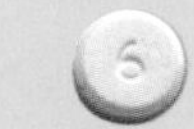

400 mcg | 600 mcg | 800 mcg

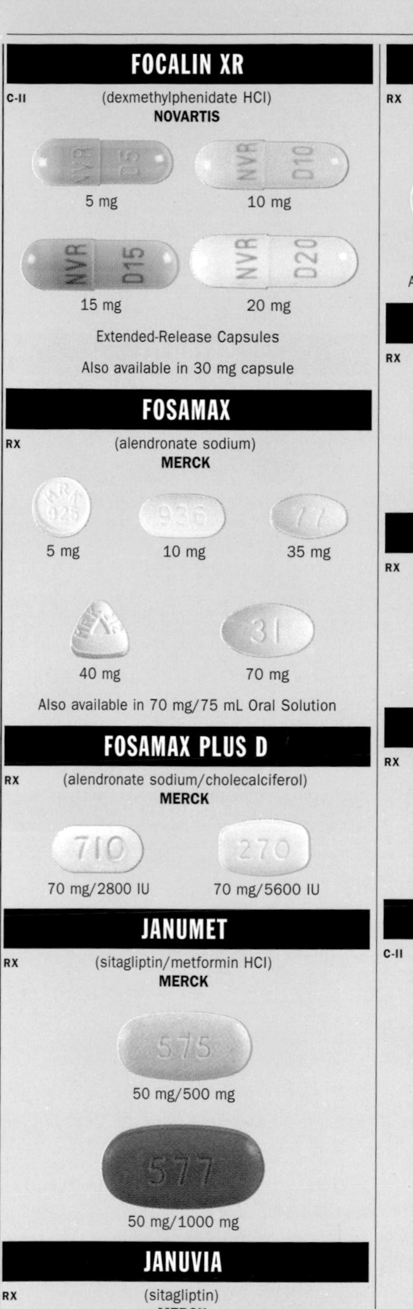

## FOCALIN XR

C-II (dexmethylphenidate HCl)
**NOVARTIS**

5 mg | 10 mg

15 mg | 20 mg

Extended-Release Capsules

Also available in 30 mg capsule

## FOSAMAX

RX (alendronate sodium)
**MERCK**

5 mg | 10 mg | 35 mg

40 mg | 70 mg

Also available in 70 mg/75 mL Oral Solution

## FOSAMAX PLUS D

RX (alendronate sodium/cholecalciferol)
**MERCK**

70 mg/2800 IU | 70 mg/5600 IU

## JANUMET

RX (sitagliptin/metformin HCl)
**MERCK**

50 mg/500 mg

50 mg/1000 mg

## JANUVIA

RX (sitagliptin)
**MERCK**

25 mg | 50 mg | 100 mg

## KALETRA

RX (lopinavir/ritonavir tablets)
**ABBOTT**

100 mg/25 mg | 200 mg/50 mg

Also available in 80 mg-20 mg/mL Oral Solution

## LEXAPRO

RX (escitalopram oxalate)
**FOREST**

5 mg | 10 mg | 20 mg

Also available in 5 mg/5 mL Oral Solution

## NAMENDA

RX (memantine HCl)
**FOREST**

5 mg | 10 mg

Also available in 2 mg/mL Oral Solution

## NEXIUM

RX (esomeprazole magnesium)
**ASTRAZENECA**

20 mg | 40 mg

Delayed-Release Capsules

## OPANA ER

C-II (oxymorphone HCl)
**ENDO**

5 mg | 7.5 mg

10 mg | 15 mg

20 mg | 30 mg

40 mg

Extended-Release Tablets

## ORTHO TRI-CYCLEN LO

RX (norgestimate/ethinyl estradiol)
**ORTHO-MCNEIL**

## PERCOCET

C-II (oxycodone HCl/acetaminophen)
**ENDO**

2.5 mg/325 mg

5 mg/325 mg

7.5 mg/325 mg

7.5 mg/500 mg

10 mg/325 mg

10 mg/650 mg

## PLAVIX

RX (clopidogrel bisulfate)
**BRISTOL-MYERS SQUIBB/ sanofi-aventis**

75 mg

300 mg

## PROTONIX

RX (pantoprazole sodium)
**WYETH**

20 mg

40 mg

Also available in 40 mg/packet for Delayed-Release Oral Suspension

## ROZEREM

RX (ramelteon)
**TAKEDA**

8 mg

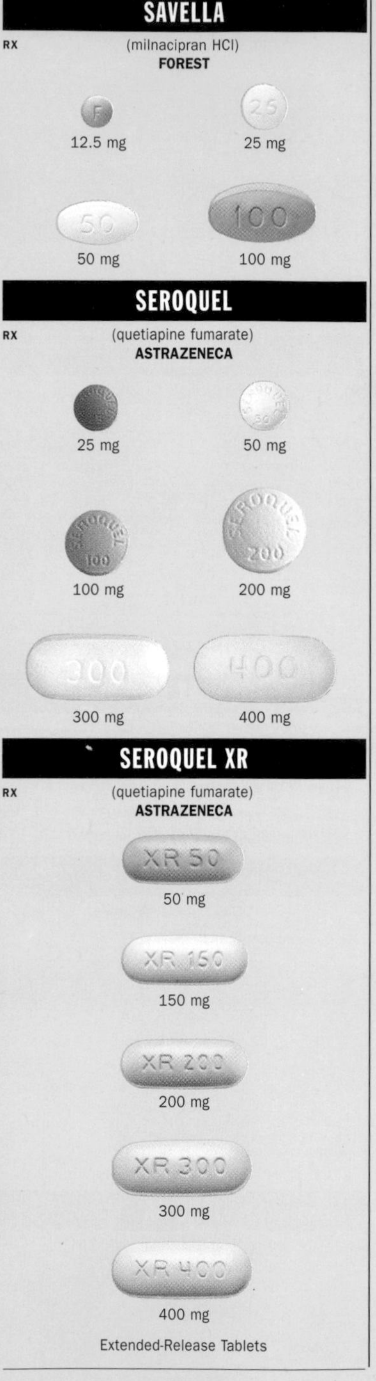

## SAVELLA

RX (milnacipran HCl)
**FOREST**

12.5 mg

25 mg

50 mg

100 mg

## SEROQUEL

RX (quetiapine fumarate)
**ASTRAZENECA**

25 mg

50 mg

100 mg

200 mg

300 mg

400 mg

## SEROQUEL XR

RX (quetiapine fumarate)
**ASTRAZENECA**

50 mg

150 mg

200 mg

300 mg

400 mg

Extended-Release Tablets

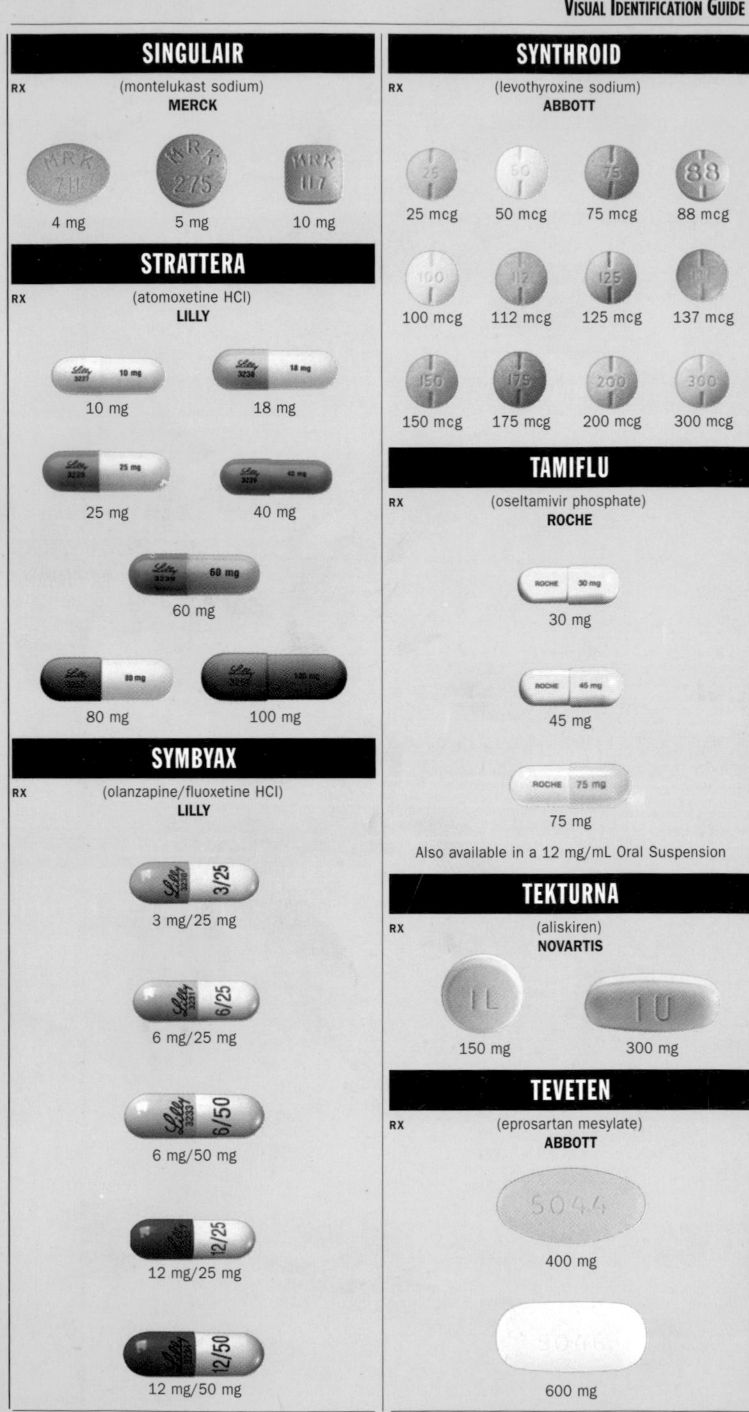


## SINGULAIR

RX

(montelukast sodium)

**MERCK**

4 mg 5 mg 10 mg

## STRATTERA

RX

(atomoxetine HCl)

**LILLY**

10 mg 18 mg

25 mg 40 mg

60 mg

80 mg 100 mg

## SYMBYAX

RX

(olanzapine/fluoxetine HCl)

**LILLY**

3 mg/25 mg

6 mg/25 mg

6 mg/50 mg

12 mg/25 mg

12 mg/50 mg

## SYNTHROID

RX

(levothyroxine sodium)

**ABBOTT**

25 mcg 50 mcg 75 mcg 88 mcg

100 mcg 112 mcg 125 mcg 137 mcg

150 mcg 175 mcg 200 mcg 300 mcg

## TAMIFLU

RX

(oseltamivir phosphate)

**ROCHE**

30 mg

45 mg

75 mg

Also available in a 12 mg/mL Oral Suspension

## TEKTURNA

RX

(aliskiren)

**NOVARTIS**

150 mg 300 mg

## TEVETEN

RX

(eprosartan mesylate)

**ABBOTT**

400 mg

600 mg

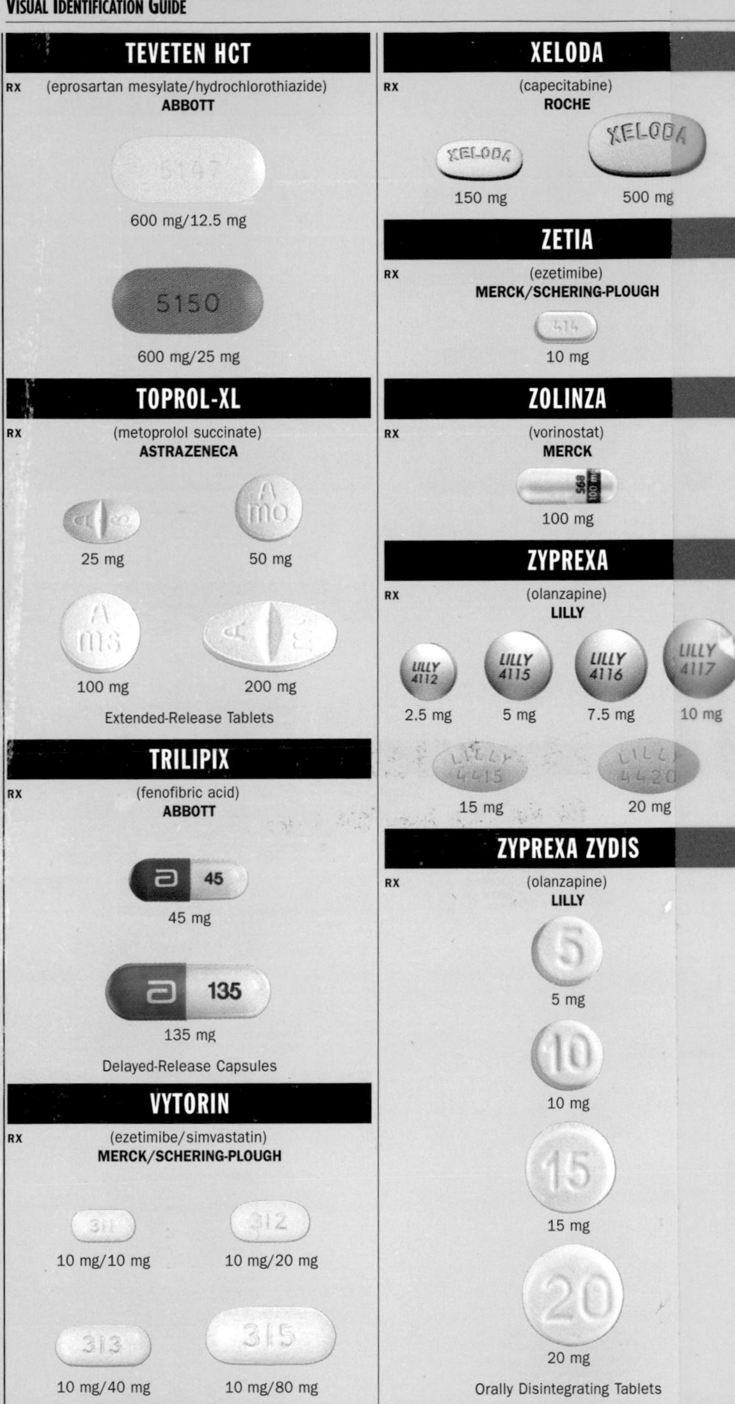

## TEVETEN HCT

RX (eprosartan mesylate/hydrochlorothiazide)
**ABBOTT**

600 mg/12.5 mg

600 mg/25 mg

## TOPROL-XL

RX (metoprolol succinate)
**ASTRAZENECA**

25 mg | 50 mg

100 mg | 200 mg

Extended-Release Tablets

## TRILIPIX

RX (fenofibric acid)
**ABBOTT**

45 mg

135 mg

Delayed-Release Capsules

## VYTORIN

RX (ezetimibe/simvastatin)
**MERCK/SCHERING-PLOUGH**

10 mg/10 mg | 10 mg/20 mg

10 mg/40 mg | 10 mg/80 mg

## XELODA

RX (capecitabine)
**ROCHE**

150 mg | 500 mg

## ZETIA

RX (ezetimibe)
**MERCK/SCHERING-PLOUGH**

10 mg

## ZOLINZA

RX (vorinostat)
**MERCK**

100 mg

## ZYPREXA

RX (olanzapine)
**LILLY**

2.5 mg | 5 mg | 7.5 mg | 10 mg

15 mg | 20 mg

## ZYPREXA ZYDIS

RX (olanzapine)
**LILLY**

5 mg

10 mg

15 mg

20 mg

Orally Disintegrating Tablets